REPLACEMENT OF RENAL FUNCTION BY DIALYSIS

Fourth edition

DRUKKER, PARSONS and MAHER

REPLACEMENT OF RENAL FUNCTION BY DIALYSIS

Fourth edition

Edited by

C. JACOBS

C. M. KJELLSTRAND

K. M. KOCH

J. F. WINCHESTER (editor-in-chief)

Springer-Science+Business Media, B.V.

Library of Congress Cataloging in Publication Data

Replacement of renal function by dialysis / edited by Claude Jacobs
... [et al.]. -- 4th ed.
    p.   cm.
    Includes bibliographical references and index.

    1. Hemodialysis.   I. Jacaobs, Claude.
    [DNLM: 1. Hemodialdsis.   WJ 378 R425 1995]
    RC901.7.H45R46 1995
    617.4'61059--dc20
    DNLM/DLC
    for Library of Congress   95-31081

ISBN 978-94-017-4178-1   ISBN 978-0-585-36947-1 (eBook)
DOI 10.1007/978-0-585-36947-1

Printed on acid-free paper

Cover illustration:
The illustration on the cover is meant to visualize a blood contacting biomaterial by an artistic concept of molecular modelling.
The colours indicate the hydrophilicity of the functional groups ranging from deep blue (hydrophilic) to reddish (hydrophobic).
It shows a Hemophan® hemodialysis membrane, with its hydrophobic DEAE substituents evolving
from the hydrophilic cellulose backbone.
Copyright by C. Hahn and M. Diamantoglou, Akzo Nobel Central Research

FOREWORD TO THE FOURTH EDITION

BELDING H. SCRIBNER

Within these pages the reader will find detailed descriptions of dialysis techniques and equipment whose excellence is to this old timer almost unbelievable. The question that has bothered me more and more these past few years is whether or not we nephrologists are making the best use of all this largess. On the basis of disappointing survival data, especially in the United States, the answer is 'No.' Of course there are outstanding exceptions and I will discuss some of these below.

Why have survival results, especially among patients on dialysis in the United States, been so disappointingly poor? Some of the answers will be found in the pages of this long overdue 4th edition. However, 2 factors seem to stand out above all others The first cause of shortened survival is gross underdialysis of large numbers of patients. Gotch was among the first to identify this serious problem in a classic paper in which he studied visitors to his unit in San Francisco (1). Since then this fact of widespread underdialysis has been repeatedly documented.

I believe that underdialysis is caused mainly by the widespread misuse of the technique of high efficiency *shortened time* hemodialysis. This misuse results from the fact that it is very easy to shorten dialysis time because everybody is in favor of it – especially the patients and the 'bottom liners.' In sharp contrast it is extremely difficult to increase hemodialysis efficiency, unless special equipment is used and special precautions are taken. Most hemodialysis units simply do not have the equipment and/or the know-how to increase dialysis efficiency. In this connection it is important to remember that whenever a dialysis technique is pushed toward the upper limit of performance, as it must be in high efficiency dialysis, the chances of error and malfunction increase exponentially. Therefore those readers who do get involved with high efficiency/shortened time dialysis should study very carefully the chapters in this volume that deal with this subject.

Even when properly carried out, I believe that high efficiency/shortened time dialysis has very limited application. It should be used only on the minority of patients who can maintain normal blood pressure despite the marked reduction in dialysis time. Two to three hours of dialysis simply does not allow sufficient time to remove the salt water accumulated since the last dialysis. This fact brings me to a brief discussion of the second major factor responsible for the low survival among hemodialysis patients, namely failure to control blood pressure.

Despite the fact that the classic paper by Haire and Sherrard on the adverse effect of hypertension (and smoking) on survival of patients on dialysis was published back in 1978 (2), surprisingly few papers and presentations at meetings have dealt with this all important subject. Important exceptions are the publications of Charra and his colleagues from Tassin in France (3, 4). Indeed their 1992 paper (4) sets the gold standard for survival on dialysis. Because they were using a very long low efficiency dialysis technique, they were able to deliver a very large dose of dialysis and provide a large protein intake to the 445 patients in their series thereby eliminating these two important factors that could adversely affect survival. That made it possible to pinpoint excellent control of blood pressure as the major factor that accounted for their outstanding survival data. Readers of this volume should pay particular attention to the chapters that deal with control of blood pressure both during the years before starting dialysis as well as control while on dialysis and after transplantation if survival figures among patients on renal replacement therapy are to improve significantly in the future.

As this is being written in the spring of 1994, studies are in progress on Charra's patients to try and determine whether or not the long 8 hour dialysis also lowers blood pressure by removing a uremic toxin that increases blood pressure, as suggested in a recent publication by Ritz (5). If Ritz's postulate is correct, this toxin must behave during dialysis like a middle molecule, whose removal, unlike urea, is mainly a function of time on dialysis (6). For a more general discussion of this topic of uremic toxins, see Chapter 1 by Vanholder.

Of emerging importance is the observation that nutritional parameters may also affect survival. Several analytic studies in hemodialysis (7), and in CAPD (8) and confirmed by the US Renal Data System (9), show that a serum albumin lower than normal increases the relative risk of death on dialysis. This deserves further study, and attention to detail in nutritional management of dialysis patients.

The experience we have had over the years with some of our original patients sheds additional light on matters under discussion here. Patient #2 in our series, who began dialysis on March 20, 1960, survived 28 years and died suddenly of an acute myocardial infarction while playing golf at Palm Springs, California in the winter of 1989. This death probably was due to the accelerated atherosclerosis (10) that he may have developed during his early years on dialysis when we did not understand the importance of blood pressure control. Patient #5, who began dialysis in the summer of 1960, currently is in his 34th year of hemodialysis and as such is the longest survivor in the world. He has had a very successful career in academia as a Professor of Physics. In January of 1963 we accepted for temporary treatment a young medical student from Guy's Hospital in London. Now 30 years later this patient is a world renowned dermatologist on the faculty of the University of London. His health is good, having received a cadaveric transplant, which was performed by Mr Peter Morris at Oxford in 1991. This patient has provided a fascinating account of what it was like to be a chronic hemodialysis patient during the early years (11). Even though they are anecdotal, these early successful outcomes stand in sharp contrast to what is being reported today in terms of survival and quality of life among dialysis patients. These outcomes are all the more remarkable when one takes into account the fact that by today's standards, all 3 of these early patients received very poor care during their first decade on renal replacement therapy because we simply did not know what constituted good dialysis care.

Finally, a word about quality of life among dialysis patients. The recent literature reports that quality of life on dialysis is good in only a minority of patients. These poor results are encountered despite the fact that the improvement in anemia with erythropoietin promised a considerable improvement in quality of life. The reasons for the disappointing quality of life are multifactorial. There is no question that the modern dialysis patient not only is older, but has more intercurrent conditions (diabetes, cardiac disease, drug addiction, aids, etc) and complications of those conditions (blindness, amputations, etc) than his/her early dialysis predecessor. The disabilities entailed by aging or non-renal complications cannot be overcome by dialysis itself, and demand much from the practicing nephrologist. Such patients present a medical challenge to the modern dialysis practitioner, and consequently place more demands on the medical community for adequate training. It is my observation that there may be a serious deficiency in the training that we nephrologists have received over the years. During fellowships, most nephrologists learn about dialysis by taking care of patients with acute potentially reversible renal failure and with rare exceptions get very little exposure to the day to day care of chronic dialysis patients. Recently there are indications that this neglected area of training may be corrected. If and when this task is undertaken, I believe it is important to keep in mind the often overlooked fact that patients with chronic renal failure suffer from a *chronic disease*. This fact in turn means that nephrologists must be taught the same skills used in the care of chronic illness that are taught routinely to fellows in rehabilitation medicine and rheumatology. Perhaps if that is done, then the quality of life of dialysis patients will improve and thereby indicate that the best use is being made of the marvelous knowledge and technology presented in this volume.

References

1. Gotch FA, Yarian S, Keen M: A kinetic survey of US hemodialysis prescriptions. *Am J Kidney Dis* 5: 511, 1990
2. Haire HM, Sherrard DJ, Scarpadane O, Curtis FK, Brunzell JD: Smoking, hypertension and mortality in a maintenance dialysis population. *Cardiovasc Med* 3: 1163, 1978
3. Charra B, Calemard E, Laurent G: Control of hypertension and prolonged survival on maintenance hemodialysis. *Nephron* 33: 96, 1983
4. Charra B, Calemard E, Ruffet M, Chazot C, Terrat JC, Vanel T, Laurent G: Survival as an index of adequacy of dialysis. *Kidney Int* 41: 286, 1992
5. Ritz E: Hypertension and cardiac death in dialysis patients – should target blood pressure be lowered? *Semin Dial* 6: 227, 1993
6. Babb AL, Farrell P, Uvelli D, Scribner BH: Hemodialyzer evaluation by examination of solute molecular spectra. *Trans Am Soc Artif Intern Organs* 18: 98, 1972
7. Lowrie EG, Lew NL: Death risk in hemodialysis patients: The predictive value of commonly measured variables and an evaluation of death rate differences between facilities. *Am J Kidney Dis* 15: 458, 1990
8. Teehan BT, Schleifer C, Brown J, *et al*: Urea kinetic analysis and in CAPD. A five year longitudinal study. *Adv Peritoneal Dial* 6: 181, 1990
9. US Renal Data System, USRDS 1992 Annual Data Report, The National Institutes of Health, National Institute of Diabetes and Digestive and Kidney Diseases, Bethesda, MD, August 1992.
10. Lindner A, Charra B, Sherrard DJ, Scribner BH: Accelerated atherosclerosis in prolonged maintenance hemodialysis. *N Engl J Med* 290: 697, 1974
11. Eady RAJ: A patient's experience of over one thousand haemodialyses. *Proc Eur Dial Transplant Assoc* 8: 50, 1971

INTRODUCTION AND TRIBUTE TO DRUKKER, PARSONS AND MAHER

CLAUDE JACOBS, CARL M. KJELLSTRAND, KARL M. KOCH and JAMES F. WINCHESTER

The years 1978, 1983, and 1989 were the publication dates for the three previous editions of this book, the first two editions having all three editors in place, while the last was edited by Jack Maher alone. This book has been a global resource and considered as the prime textbook for information on dialysis for many years. As Maher wrote in his introduction in 1989, they were all 'first generation nephrologists', and in our opinion at the leading edge of clinical and research nephrology of the times. Sadly, we cannot call on them for advice, as all have passed away. However, we have gleaned knowledge from them in the past in person, and by their written word. We have also been aided in having the same publisher, Boudewijn Commandeur, for this edition as in all previous. He has served as a lynchpin for the project. Therefore, during the construction of this book we have as much as possible tried to keep the same flavor, of first outlining the principles of a subject, and then its clinical application.

First, we asked is there a need for this book? Despite our cumulative nephrology experience of at least a century, we were unanimous in our affirmative answer. There, of course, are other books related to dialysis available, but what made the previous editions unique, were the careful eye to detail, in theory and in application, the introduction of topics never previously discussed in a single text (e.g. in this text, dialysis in developing countries), and finally the comprehensive nature of all previous editions, and hopefully this edition as well. We strived to make this book a repository of information, as a reference text, as well as a practical clinical tool. We want this book to become familiar to seasoned nephrologists, nephrology trainees, dialysis nurses and technicians, and perhaps to students as well – it is our wish to see this book used – even torn and tattered. We have, therefore, gathered together, those whom we consider leaders in this subject, be it theoretical, or be it practical.

In acute renal failure, we have become more cognizant of the fact that multi-organ involvement is associated with a poor outcome. This has led to continuous therapies, such as arterio-venous and veno-venous hemodialysis and hemofiltration, to automated machines to accomplish these tasks, to the use of biocompatible membranes, to citrate anticoagulation, and to intensive nutritional support. All of these subjects are covered in detail. Similarly, the infrastructure necessary to perform acute or chronic hemodialysis and peritoneal dialysis is covered – namely, water preparation, dialysate composition, bacterial contamination, and machine design. Today's dialysis machines are largely automated and have built in safety controls, blood pressure monitors, continuous anticoagulation, programmable sodium delivery, in-line solute measurement. The fledgling nephrologist might easily by-pass the theory and the nuances of dialysis understanding. We hope that this text will be used to overcome and give understanding of the complexities of modern dialysis apparatus, whose starting point was the simple physical process discovered by Thomas Graham in 1861, that solutes travel down a concentration gradient.

We have tried to address the current problems in dialysis practice today. Over half a million patients receive dialysis world-wide. There appears to be no shortage of patients, nor trends towards a global decrease in patients reaching end-stage renal disease from the most common diseases, such as diabetes, hypertension, glomerulonephritis, or inherited renal disorders. Despite demonstrations that control of hypertension, and control of diabetes may slow the progress of, or prevent, end-stage kidney disease, and the identification of genetic abnormalities, any effect on prevalence of patients requiring dialysis has yet to filter down to the nephrology community at large. We must not forget that, while life span has increased in the modern world this brings with it reduction in renal function, and intercurrent conditions which make the application of dialysis that much more difficult (mostly related to vascular disease), as well as diabetes and severe hypertension. For these reasons we have added sections specifically to address these issues. How do we as specialists assess the effect of dialysis? After all it is a substitute only for the solute excretory component of renal function. Yes, we can now replace the renal hormones erythropoietin and 1,25 dihydroxycholecalciferol, but what of the other hormonal derangements, the lipid disorders, the impaired immunological function, etc. Most importantly, perhaps, how do we know if we are prescribing enough, or if the patient is receiving enough, dialysis – these issues are at the forefront of investigation and clinical application. Each of these topics and more are dealt with in detail.

Continuous ambulatory peritoneal dialysis is now the preferred home dialysis therapy throughout the world, and we have concentrated on discussion of its application, its amplification by machine delivered peritoneal fluid, its limitations and its complications. Like the problems facing the hemodialysis patient with angioaccess, also described in this book, the peritoneal dialysis patient also faces problems with access to the peritoneal cavity. These topics are addressed in a special section. Because of renewed interest in home hemodialysis, we have added a section to cover that topic.

How does the patient feel about dialysis? Can he/she work? Can he/she play? Is dialysis long-term survival or outcome the same all over the world? When should we let our patients tell us that it is time to stop, and let them die? These issues are real ones, and we may have been remiss in the past by not addressing them in detail. For that reason we have added sections on quality of life, and a new section on outcome analysis, lacking in the previous editions.

What other 'new' problems face the dialysis patient, and perhaps dialysis staff in the late 1990s. We are all familiar with the hepatitis B outbreaks and deaths of the 1970s, and the often observed bacteremia in hemodialysis patients. But what of the diseases of the 1990s – human immunodeficiency virus, hepatitis C, and tuberculosis. Each has unique characteristics, management problems, complications and affects to a great extent staffing and organization of dialysis units. Currently, the Centers for Disease Control, in Atlanta, Georgia, does not recommend isolation of patients with HIV nor hepatitis C, yet for the latter the debate may not be definitively closed.

Tuberculosis has its own 1990s uniqueness, drug resistance and association with recent immigration or HIV. All these topics can be found in this text.

We have also striven to make sure that all the topics covered are correct in detail, but we wish the reader to make judgements as to validity of concept, a prescription, a formula, a diagram, and to use such judgement to adjust therapy in clinical application. Due to the ever changing nature of medicine, and technology, differences of opinion are to be found in this book, and the publisher and editors assume no responsibility for these differences of opinion, rather publishing them as written to improve the academic impact of our text.

Finally, what have we left and what have we taken away. We felt that the previous chapter on the history of dialysis as written by Drukker could not be bettered, and in deference to him we omitted it. We have changed many of the authors in this text, not for changes sake, but to bring in new and younger, and perhaps the fourth or fifth generation nephrologists. This is a changing field, steeped in tradition, and to honor that tradition it was our decision to retain the name of the text as Drukker, Parsons and Maher, our first generation nephrology colleagues and friends. In keeping with the changing nature of investigation, to molecular biology, we have replaced the familiar cover diagram of middle molecule peak 7c, with a schematic of molecular modeling of a well known cellulosic dialysis membrane.

Claude Jacobs, Paris
Carl M. Kjellstrand, Edmonton
Karl M. Koch, Hannover
James F. Winchester, Washington

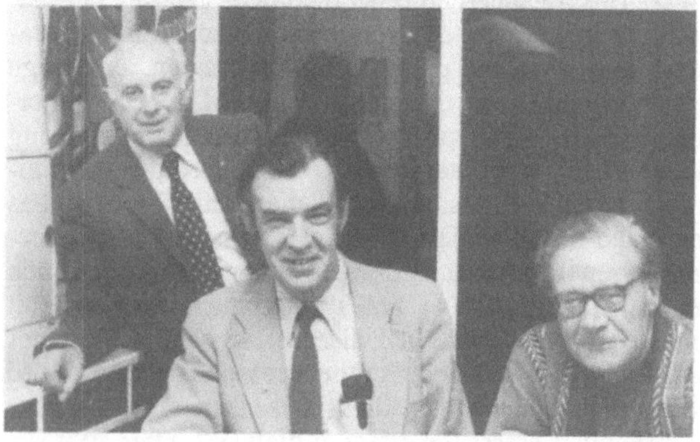

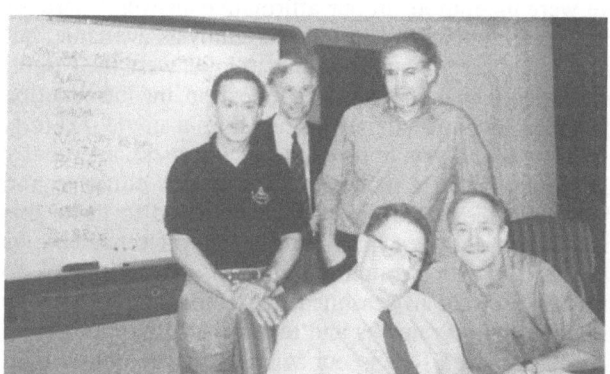

Figure 1. William Drukker, Jack Maher, Frank Parsons.

Figure 2. Jim Winchester, Boudewijn Commandeur (Publisher), Karl Koch, Claude Jacobs, Carl Kjellstrand.

CONTRIBUTING AUTHORS

T. Agishi, M.D.
Kidney Center
Tokyo Women's Medical College
Department of Surgery
8-1 Kawada-Cho, Shinjuku-ku
Tokyo 162, Japan
Chapter 58C

J. Ahlmén, M.D., Ph.D.
Department of Nephrology
Central Hospital
S-541 85 Skövde, Sweden
Chapter 62B

Alfred C. Alfrey, M.D.
Veterans Affairs Medical Center
1055 Clermont Street
Denver, CO 80220, USA
Chapter 51

G.S. Arbus, M.D.
Department of Nephrology
Hospital for Sick Children
555 University Avenue
Toronto, ON, Canada M5G 1X8
Chapter 58F

R.S. Barsoum, M.D.
The Cairo Kidney Center
P.O. Box 91
Bab-el-Louk
Cairo 11513, Egypt
Chapter 60

Robert H. Barth, M.D.
Hemodialysis Unit
VA Medical Center
800 Poly Place
Brooklyn, NY 11209, USA
Chapter 16

William M. Bennett, M.D., Ph.D.
Division of Nephrology and Hypertension
Oregon Health Sciences University
3181 SW Sam Jackson Park Road
L 455 Portland, OR 97201, USA
Chapter 29

Christopher Blagg, M.D.
Northwest Kidney Centers
700 Broadway
Seattle, WA 98122, USA
Chapter 56

Peter Blake, M.D.
University of Western Ontario
Victoria Hospital Corp.
P.O. Box 5375, 375 South Street
London, Ontario N6A 4G5, Canada
Chapter 24

Marcel Broyer, M.D.
Department of Pediatric Nephrology
Hospital for Sick Children
Paris, France
Chapter 31

C.E. Butler, M.D.
Brigham & Women's Hospital
Department of Surgery
Boston, MA 02115, USA
Chapter 10

Bernard J.M. Canaud, M.D.
Division of Nephrology
Lapeyronie University Hospital
F-34295 Montpellier, France
Chapter 8

Cyril Chantler, M.D.
Evelina Children's Department
Guy's and St. Thomas' Hospital
Guy's Hospital
London, England
Chapter 31

D.N. Churchill, M.D.
Division of Nephrology
McMaster University
Hamilton, Ontario, Canada L8N 4A6
Chapter 23

Allan J. Collins, M.D.
Regional Kidney Disease Program
914 S. 8th Street
Minneapolis, MN 55404, USA
Chapters 46, 61

C.K. Colton, Ph.D.
Department of Chemical Engineering
Massachusetts Inst. of Technology
25 Amnes St., Room 66-452
Cambridge, MA 02139, USA
Chapter 3

P.F. Copleston, M.D.
Canadian Organ Replacement Register
Canadian Institute for Health Information
Box 3900
Don Mills, Ontario, Canada M3C 2T9
Chapter 58F

Ronald Cranford, M.D.
Hennepin County Medical Centre
701 Park Ave S
Minneapolis Minnesota 55415, USA
Chapter 63

John Daugirdas, M.D., Ph.D.
University of Illinois at Chicago
Department of Research (151)
Westside VA Medical Center
820 South Damen Avenue
Chicago, Illinois 60612, USA
Chapter 24

Alex M. Davison, M.D., Ph.D.
Department of Renal Medicine
St. James's University Hospital
Beckett Street
Leeds LS9 7TF, England
Chapter 54

R. De Smet, M.D.
Nephrology Department
University Hospital
De Pintelaan 185
B-9000 Ghent, Belgium
Chapter 1

Wilfried A. De Backer, M.D.
Department of Pulmonary Medicine
University Hospital Antwerp
Wilrijkstraat 10
B-2650 Edegem-Antwerpen, Belgium
Chapter 41

Marc E. De Broe, M.D., Ph.D.
Department of Nephrology-Hypertension
University Hospital Antwerp
Wilrijkstraat 10
B-2650 Edegem-Antwerpen, Belgium
Chapter 41

Françoise Degos, M.D.
Service d'Hépato-Gastro-Entérologie 2
Hôpital Beaujon
100 Boulevard du Gen. Leclerc
92110 Clichy, France
Chapter 47B

Barbara G. Delano, M.D.
Department of Medicine
State University of New York
Health Science Center Brooklyn
450 Clarkson Ave, Box 52
Brooklyn, NY 11203, USA
Chapter 55A

B. Descamps-Latscha, M.D., Ph.D.
INSERM U.25
GH Necker-Enfants Malades
161 rue de Sèvres
75015 Paris, France
Chapter 45

Marie Desmeules, M.D.
Laboratory Centre for Disease Control
LCDC Building, Rm22-c
Tunney's Pasture
Ottawa, ON, Canada K1A 0L2
Chapter 58F

J.A. Diaz-Buxo, M.D.
Metrolina Nephrology Associates P.A.
928 Baxter Street
Charlotte, NC 28204-2879, USA
Chapter 21

A.P.S. Disney, M.D.
The Queen Elizabeth Hospital
28 Woodville Road
Woodville South
Adelaide, South Australia 5011
Chapter 58E

Raymond Donckerwolcke, M.D.
Department of Nephrology
Alberta Children's Hospital
1820 Richmond Road SW
Calgary, Alberta
Canada T2T 5C7
Chapter 31

Jochen H.H. Ehrich M.D.
Charité University Hospital
Humboldt University
Berlin, Germany
Chapter 33

Joseph W. Eschbach, M.D.
Department of Medicine
University of Washington
515 Minor Ave.
Seattle, WA 98104, USA
Chapter 43

Aldo Fabris, M.D.
Department of Nephrology
St. Bortolo Hospital
Via Rodolfi
I-36100 Vicenza, Italy
Chapters 9, 40

S.A. Fenton, M.D.
Toronto Hospital-General Division
200 Elizabeth Street, EN13-232
Toronto, Ontario, Canada M5G 2C4
Chapter 58F

Mariano Feriani, M.D.
Department of Nephrology
St. Bortolo Hospital
Via Rodolfi
I-36100 Vicenza, Italy
Chapters 9, 20, 40

M.J. Flanigan, M.D.
Department of Internal Medicine, W336-16
University of Iowa Hospitals and Clinics
200 Hawkins Drive
Iowa City, IA 52246, USA
Chapter 49

R.N. Foley, M.D.
Division of Nephrology
The Health Sciences Center
Memorial University
St. Johns, Newfoundland, Canada A1B 3V6
Chapter 38

Denis Fouque, M.D.
Department of Nephrology
Hôpital Edouard Herriot
University Claude Bernard
69437 Lyon Cédex 03, France
Chapter 52

Ulrich Frei, M.D.
Virchow-Klinikum of Humboldt-University
Medical Clinic and Policlinic
Department of Internal Medicine and Nephrology
Augustenburger Platz 1
13353 Berlin, Germany
Chapter 34

Eli A. Friedman, M.D.
SUNY Health Science Center
450 Clarkson Ave, Box 52
Brooklyn, NY 11203, USA
Chapters 17, 35

Daniel H. Froment, M.D.
Service de Néphrologie
Hôpital Notre Dame
Université du Montréal
Montréal, Québec, Canada
Chapter 58F

Ram Gokal, M.D.
Manchester Royal Infirmary
Department of Renal Medicine
Oxford Road
Manchester M13 9WL, England
Chapter 25

Thomas A. Golper, M.D.
University of Arkansas
College of Medicine, Mail Slot 501
Department of Internal Med./Div. of Nephrology
4301 West Markham Street
Little Rock, AR 72205, USA
Chapter 29

Frank A. Gotch, M.D.
University of California
45 Castro Street # 227
San Francisco, CA 94114, USA
Chapter 2

E. Grapsa, M.D.
Division of Nephrology
Toronto Hospital – Western Division
399 Bathurst Street
Toronto, Ontario, Canada M5T 2S8
Chapter 32

A. Grassmann, Ph.D.
AKZO Nobel Faser AG
Business Unit Membrana
Öhder Strasse 28
D-42289 Wuppertal, Germany
Chapter 28

A.P. Guérin, M.D.
Nephrology and Hemodialysis Department
Center Hospitalier Manhès
8 Grande Rue
91700 Fleury Mérogis, France
Chapter 37

Rolf W. Günther, M.D.
Department of Diagnostic Radiology
University of Technology
Pauwelsstrasse
D-52057 Aachen, Germany
Chapter 11

Hans Gurland, M.D.
Nephrology Division
Medical Department I
Klinikum Grosshadern
Marchioninistrasse 15
D-8000 Munich 70, Germany
Chapter 18

Raymond M. Hakim, M.D., Ph.D.
Renal Division
S-3307 MCN, VUMC
1161 21st Avenue S. and Garland
Nashville, TN 37232-2372, USA
Chapter 6

J.D. Harnett, M.D.
Division of Nephrology
The Health Sciences Center
Memorial University
St. Johns, Newfoundland, Canada A1B 3V6
Chapter 38

Philip J. Held, Ph.D.
Department of Health Services Management and Policy
University of Michigan
Ann Arbor, MI 48103, USA
Chapter 58B

Lee W. Henderson, M.D.
Baxter Healthcare Corp.
1620 Waukegan Rd
McGaw Park, IL 60085-6730, USA
Chapter 4

J. Himmelfarb, M.D.
Maine Nephrology Associates P.A.
1600 B Congress Street
Portland, ME 04102, USA
Chapter 6

Nicholas A. Hoenich, Ph.D.
Department of Medicine, Medical School
University of Newcastle upon Tyne
Newcastle-upon-Tyne NE2 4HH, England
Chapter 7

C. Hsu, M.D., Ph.D.
Nephrology Division
Department of Medicine
University of Michigan Medical School
Ann Arbor, MI 48103, USA
Chapter 1

Todd Ing, M.D.
Loyola University, Chicago
Stritch School of Medicine
Maywood, IL 60153, USA
Chapter 26

I. Ishikawa, M.D.
Department of Internal Medicine
Kanazawa Medical University
1-1 Daigaku, Uchinada-Machi
Kahoku-gun, Ishikawa-ken, 920-02 Japan
Chapter 58C

Katsumi Ito, M.D.
Department of Surgery
Kidney Center
Tokyo Women's Medical College
8-1 Kawada-Cho-Shinjuku-Ku
Tokyo 162, Japan
Chapter 58F

Claude Jacobs, M.D.
Service de Néphrologie
Hôpital de La Pitié
83, Blvd. de l'Hôpital
75013 Paris, France
Chapter 57

John J. Jeffery, M.D.
Section of Nephrology
Health Sciences Center
820 Sherbrook Street
Room GE-441
Winnipeg, MB, Canada
Chapter 58F

Paul Jungers, M.D.
Department of Nephrology
GH Necker-Enfants Malades
161 rue de Sèvres
75015 Paris, France
Chapters 45, 47B

A.A. Kaplan, M.D.
University of CT Health Center
Division of Nephrology, MC 1405
Farmington, CT 06030, USA
Chapter 15

B.L. Kasiske, M.D.
Hennepin County Medical Center
Div. of Nephrology
701 Park Ave. S.
Minneapolis, MN 55415, USA
Chapter 36

Michael Kaye, M.D.
Montreal General Hospital
2650 Cedar Ave
Montreal Quebec H3G 1A4, Canada
Chapter 63

William F. Keane, M.D.
University of Minnesota
Division of Nephrology
Department of Medicine
Hennepin County Medical Center
701 Park Avenue
Minneapolis, MN 55415, USA
Chapter 46

Carl M. Kjellstrand, M.D., Ph.D.
Department of Medicine
2E3-31 W. McKenzie
University of Alberta Hospital
Edmonton, Alberta, Canada T6G 2B7
Chapters 26, 30, 58F, 63

Saul Klahr, M.D.
Department of Medicine
The Jewish Hospital of St. Louis
216 South Kingshighway
St. Louis, Missouri 63110, USA
Chapter 59

Karl M. Koch, M.D.
Department of Nephrology
Medizinische Hochschule Hannover
Postfach 610180
D-3000 Hannover 61, Germany
Chapters 27, 53

Joe D. Kopple, M.D.
Harbor-UCLA Medical Center
1000 W. Carson Street
Torrance, CA 90509, USA
Chapter 52

S. Koshikawa, M.D.
Department of Internal Medicine
Showa University Fujigaoka Hospital
1-30 Fujigaoka, Midori-ku
Yokohama-Shi, 227 Japan
Chapter 58C

Raymond T. Krediet, M.D., Ph.D.
Renal Unit, F4-215
Academic Medical Center
Meibergdreef 9
1105 AZ Amsterdam, The Netherlands
Chapter 5

Giuseppe La Greca, M.D.
Department of Nephrology
St. Bortolo Hospital
Via Rodolfi
I-36100 Vicenza, Italy
Chapters 20, 40

J.M. Lazarus, M.D.
Brigham and Women's Hospital
Nephrology Department
75 Francis Street
Boston, MA 02215, USA
Chapter 42

H. Lemke, M.D.
AKZO Nobel
D-63785 Obernburg, Germany
Chapter 28

N.W. Levin, M.D.
Division of Nephrology
Beth Israel Medical Center
1st Avenue at 16th Street
New York, NY 10003, USA
Chapter 13

V.S. Lim, M.D.
Department of Internal Medicine
W336-16
University of Iowa Hospitals and Clinics
200 Hawkins Drive
Iowa City, IA 52246, USA
Chapter 49

Robert MacGregor Lindsay, M.D.
University of Western Ontario
375 South Street
London, Ontario N6A 4G5, Canada
Chapter 44

Robert R. Lins, M.D., Ph.D.
Department of Nephrology
A.Z. Stuivenberg
Lange Beeldekensstraat 267
B-2060 Antwerpen, Belgium
Chapter 41

Francisco Llach, M.D.
Beth Israel Medical Center
201 Lyons Avenue
Newark, NJ 07112, USA
Chapter 48

Gérard London, M.D., Ph.D.
Nephrology and Hemodialysis Department
Center Hospitalier Manhès
8 Grande Rue
91700 Fleury Mérogis, France
Chapter 37

G. Lonnemann, M.D.
Department of Nephrology
Medizinische Hochschule Hannover
Postfach 610180
D-3000 Hannover 61, Germany
Chapter 27

Michael J. Lysaght, Ph.D.
Division of Biology and Medicine
Brown University
Providence, RI, USA
Chapters 3, 18

Netar P. Mallick, M.D.
Manchester Royal Infirmary
Department of Renal Medicine
Oxford Road
Manchester M13 9WL, England
Chapters 58A, 58D

D.A. Mandelbrot, M.D.
250 Longwood Ave.
Seeley Mudd Bldg, Rm 504
Boston, MA 02115, USA
Chapter 42

S. Marchais, M.D.
Nephrology and Hemodialysis Department
Center Hospitalier Manhès
8 Grande Rue
91700 Fleury Mérogis, France
Chapter 37

M.A. Marx, Ph.D.
Asst. Professor of Pharmacy Practice
College of Pharmacy
University of Arkansas for Med. Sciences
Little Rock, AR 72205, USA
Chapter 29

Anne Marie V. Miles, M.D.
SUNY-Health Science Center at Brooklyn
450 Clarkson Avenue-Box 52
Brooklyn, NY 11203, USA
Chapters 17, 35

Charles M. Mion, M.D.
Division of Nephrology
Lapeyronie University Hospital
F-34259 Montpellier Cédex, France
Chapters 8, 22

Salim K. Mujais, M.D.
Northwestern University School of Medicine
Section of Nephrology
Chicago, IL 60153, USA
Chapter 26

Iraj Nadjafi, M.D.
Nephrology-Dialysis-Transplant Unit
Dr Shariaty Hospital
University of Tehran
Kargar Avenue
Tehran, Iran
Chapter 61

H. Nihei, M.D.
Kidney Center
Tokyo Women's Medical College
Department of Surgery
8-1 Kawada-Cho, Shinjuku-ku
Tokyo 162, Japan
Chapter 58C

M. Nowicki, M.D.
Department Nephrology
Silesian School of Medicine
Katowice, Poland
Chapter 39

Dimitrios G. Oreopoulos, M.D.
Division of Nephrology
Toronto Hospital – Western Division
399 Bathurst Street
Toronto, Ontario, Canada M5T 2S8
Chapter 32

K. Ota, M.D.
Kidney Center
Tokyo Women's Medical College
Department of Surgery
8-1 Kawada-Cho, Shinjuku-ku
Tokyo 162, Japan
Chapter 58C

Patrick S. Parfrey , M.D., Ph.D.
Division of Nephrology
The Health Sciences Center
Memorial University
St. Johns, Newfoundland, Canada A1B 3V6
Chapter 38

Beth Piraino, M.D., Ph.D.
Medical Center
F1159 Presbyterian University Hospital
200 Lothrop Street
Pittsburgh, PA 15213, USA
Chapter 19

Hans D. Polaschegg, Ph.D.
Grünswiesenweg 9
D-61440 Oberursel, Germany
Chapter 13

Frederick K. Port, M.D.
University of Michigan
Kidney Epidemiology and Cost Center
315 W. Huron St., Suite 240
Ann Arbor, MI 48103. USA
Chapter 58B

Eduard A. Quellhorst, M.D.
Nephrology Center Niedersachsen
Vogelsang 105
D-34346 Hannover-Münden, Germany
Chapter 14

V.E. Quijada, M.D.
Department of Nephrology
Georgetown University Medical Center
3800 Reservoir Road
Washington, DC 20007, USA
Chapter 44

T.K. Sreepada Rao, M.D.
SUNY Health Science Center at Brooklyn
450 Clarkson Ave., Box 52
Brooklyn, NY 11203-2098, USA
Chapter 47A

Giuseppe Remuzzi, M.D.
Division of Nephrology and Dialysis
Ospedali Riuniti di Bergamo
I-24100 Bergamo, Italy
Chapter 12

Ann Rinehart, M.D.
Hennepin County Medical Center
Department of Medicine/Div. of Neprohology
701 Park Avenue
Minneapolis, MN 55415, USA
Chapter 46

Severin Ringoir, M.D., Ph.D.
Nephrology Department
University Hospital
De Pintelaan 185
B-9000 Ghent, Belgium
Chapter 1

E. Ritz, M.D., Ph.D.
Ruperto Carola University
Department of Internal Medicine
Bergheimerstr. 58
D-69115 Heidelberg, Germany
Chapter 39

Gianfranco Rizzoni, M.D.
Division of Nephrology and Dialysis
Department of Pediatric Research and Teaching
Ospedale Bambino Jesu
Rome, Italy
Chapter 31

Claudio Ronco, M.D.
Department of Nephrology
St. Bortolo Hospital
Via Rodolfi
I-36100 Vicenza, Italy
Chapters 7, 9, 20, 40

G. Said, M.D.
Service de Neurologie
Center Hospitalier Universitaire
Bicêtre
78, Ave. de Général Leclerc
94275 Le Kremlin
Bicêtre Cédex, France
Chapter 50

Walter Samtleben, M.D.
Nephrology Division
Medical Department I. Klinikum Grosshadern
University of Munich
München, Germany
Chapter 18

John A. Sargent, Ph.D.
5901 Christie Avenue
Suite 201
Emeryville, CA 94608, USA
Chapter 2

J. Schaeffer, M.D.
Division of Nephrology – 6840
Hannover Medical School
D-30623 Hannover, Germany
Chapter 53

A. Schieppati, M.D.
Mario Negri Inst. for Pharmacol. Res.
Clinical Res.Cntr. for Rare Diseases 'Aldo e Cele Dacco'
Villa Camozzi
I-24020 Ranica, Italy
Chapter 12

Belding H. Scribner, M.D.
Division of Nephrology
University of Washington
Mailstop Rm 11
Seattle, WA 98195, USA
Foreword

Neville H. Selwood, Ph.D.
UK Transplant Service
Southmead Hospital
Bristol, England
Chapter 57

Stanley Shaldon, M.D.
86, Rue de Grezac
F-34100 Montpellier, France
Chapter 28

A. Shinoda, M.D.
Department of Internal Medicine
Kanazawa Medical University
1-1 Daigaku, Uchinada-Machi
Kahoku-gun, Ishikawa-ken, 920-02 Japan
Chapter 58C

C. Shuler, M.D.
Division of Nephrology and Hypertension
Oregon Health Sciences University
3181 SW Sam Jackson Park Road
L 455
Portland, OR 97201, USA
Chapter 29

Heinz-Günther Sieberth, M.D.
Department Internal Medicine II
University of Technology
Pauwelsstrasse
D-52057 Aachen, Germany
Chapter 11

Kim Solez, M.D.
Department of Laboratory Medicine
5B4.02 W. MacKenzie Center
University of Alberta Hospitals
Edmonton, Alberta, Canada T6G 2R7
Chapter 61

B.P. Teehan, M.D.
Lankenau Medical Center # 135
100 Lancaster Avenue
Wynnewood, PA 19096, USA
Chapter 30

S. Teraoka, M.D., Ph.D.
Kidney Center
Tokyo Women's Medical College
8-1 Kawada-Cho, Shinjuku-ku
162 Tokyo, Japan
Chapter 58C

Nicholas L. Tilney, M.D.
Division of Transplant Surgery
Brigham and Women's Hospital
75 Francis Street
Boston, MA 02115, USA
Chapter 10B

H. Toma, M.D.
Kidney Center
Tokyo Women's Medical College
Department of Surgery
8-1 Kawada-Cho, Shinjuku-ku
Tokyo 162, Japan
Chapter 58C

Sato Tsuyoshi, M.D.
Tokai University School of Medicine
Department of Transplantation I, Boseidai, Isehara-shi
Kanagawa-ken, 269-11 Japan
Chapter 58F

M.N. Turenne, M.D.
Department of Medicine and Epidemiology
University of Michigan
Ann Arbor, MI 48103, USA
Chapter 58B

R. Uldall, M.D. (deceased)
Wellesley Hospital
Room 372
160 Wellesley Str., Bruce Wing 3-372
Toronto, Ontario M4Y 1J3, Canada
Chapter 10A

Raymond Vanholder, M.D., Ph.D.
Nephrology Department
University Hospital
De Pintelaan 185
B-9000 Ghent, Belgium
Chapter 1

Claude Verger, M.D.
Hôpital René Dubos
Unité de Dialyse
Avenue de l'Ile de France
F-95301 Pontoise, France
Chapter 55B

Jorg Vienken, M.D.
Fresenius AG
Medical Department
Borkenberg 14
D-61440 Oberursel, Germany
Chapter 28

G. Vigano, M.D.
Mario Negri Inst. for Pharmacol. Res.
Clinical Res.Cntr. for Rare Diseases 'Aldo e Cele Daccò'
Villa Camozzi
I-24020 Ranica, Italy
Chapter 12

P. Vogeleere
Nephrology Department
University Hospital
De Pintelaan 185
B-9000 Ghent, Belgium
Chapter 1

Dierk Vorwerk, M.D.
Department of Diagnostic Radiology
University of Technology
Pauwelsstrasse
D-52057 Aachen, Germany
Chapter 11

A. Wiecek, M.D.
Department of Nephrology
Silesian School of Medicine
Francuska 20
40-027 Katowice, Poland
Chapter 39

P.G. Wilson, M.D.
Department of Psychiatry
Cornell University Medical Center
525 68th Street
New York, NY 10021, USA
Chapter 62A

James F. Winchester, M.D.
Department of Nephrology
Georgetown University Medical Center
3800 Reservoir Road
Washington, DC 20007, USA
Chapters 18, 44

Antony J. Wing, M.D.
Department of Renal Medicine
St. George's Hospital
Blackshaw Road, Tooting
London SW17 0QT, England
Chapter 33

C. Woffindin, M.D.
Renal Unit
Royal Victoria Infirmary
Queen Victoria Road
Newcastle upon Tyne, NE1 4LP, England
Chapter 7

Ali-Reze Atef Zafarmand, M.D.
Nephrology-Dialysis-Transplant Unit
Dr Shariaty Hospital
University of Tehran
Kargar Avenue
Tehran, Iran
Chapter 61

TABLE OF CONTENTS

SECTION I
Pathophysiology of the uremic syndrome.
Principles and biophysics of dialysis

SECTION II
Technology of dialysis and associated methods

SECTION III
Quantification and prescription of dialysis

SECTION IV
Complications of dialysis

SECTION V
Pharmacological considerations

SECTION VI
Special clinical situations

SECTION VII
Organ system and metabolic complications in chronic dialysis

SECTION VIII
Organization and results of chronic dialysis

THE URAEMIC SYNDROME

R. VANHOLDER, R. DE SMET, P. VOGELEERE, C. HSU and S. RINGOIR

INTRODUCTION

The uraemic syndrome is characterized by a deterioration of biochemical and physiologic functions, in parallel with the progression of renal failure, and results in important but variable symptomatology. Although well known for more than 160 years (1), our knowledge about the responsible factors remains inconsistent and incomplete. The quest for 'the' uraemic toxin has been overemphasized, not taking into account the uraemic syndrome as the result of a cumulative retention of innumerable compounds. The extrapolation of *in vitro* data to the clinical situation has sometimes resulted in incorrect hypotheses, whereas trivial factors with a potential bias on the results have not been taken into account.

The uraemic syndrome results from the retention of compounds, that are cleared by the healthy kidneys; the intake of precursors, mainly via nutrition, also plays a role. This concept is underscored by the success of dialysis in end-stage renal failure and the symptomatic improvement following decreases in dietary protein intake. The uraemic syndrome is however not only the result of retention of compounds but also of deranged hormonal and enzymatic homeostasis.

Several secondary factors contribute to the uraemic syndrome, such as the speed of progression of renal failure and fluctuations in toxin concentration. In analogy to pharmaca, peak levels may be more important than through levels, possibly one of the reasons why patients on continuous ambulatory dialysis (CAPD) display a satisfactory clinical condition, in spite of higher concentrations of uraemic solutes, compared to patients on chronic intermittent haemodialysis.

In this chapter, the current science about the uraemic syndrome, its clinical and biochemical characteristics, and the factors playing a role in its development will be reviewed.

CLINICAL CHARACTERISTICS

The uraemic syndrome is characterized by a quantitative and qualitative overall deterioration of performance (Table 1). The clinical characteristics are aspecific, mimicking the picture of exogenous poisoning, e.g. by drug overdosage. The most pronounced changes are found in the cardio-vascular, neurologic, haematologic and immunologic status, the basic patho-physiologic mechanisms being related to the derangement of several functional systems (Table 2).

Cardio-vascular system

Cardio-vascular anomalies occur almost invariably in the progression of renal failure (2), their epiphenomena being multiple: hypertension, congestive heart failure, valvular stenosis or insufficiency, accelerated atheromatosis and uraemic pericarditis (3). Survival with and without symptomatic heart disease is however hardly different (4).

With the advent of adequate dialysis strategies, the incidence of *pericarditis* became rare, except in those cases waiting too long to start dialysis and/or in patients with major access problems. If not treated by efficient dialysis, pericarditis may result in cardiac tamponnade.

Cardiac *hypertrophy* and *dilated cardiomyopathy* are current findings in end-stage renal failure (5). Myocardial dysfunction is related to an increase in myocardial calcium content especially in patients undergoing chronic dialysis (6). Increased cytosolic Ca^{++} is related to peripheral vascular resistance and hence hypertension (7).

In view of a potential ouabain-like effect in uraemic serum of Na^+, K^+-ATPase, it could be expected that uraemia induces a positive inotropic effect; this hypothesis has been confirmed, at least in acute renal failure, in older studies (8, 9), but seems in conflict with the clinical findings of frequent cardiac decompensation.

Experimental studies are compatible with a *diminished responsiveness of the cardiac alpha- and beta-receptors* (10). This may be related to uraemic polyneuropathy of

Table 1. The uraemic syndrome – clinical alterations

1) *Nervous system*

– Stupor, coma	– Polyneuritis
– Sleep disorders	– Convulsions
– Fatigue	– Dementia
– Asterixis	– Motor weakness
– Malaise	– Concentration disturbances
– Insomnia	– Drowsiness
– Erratic memory	– Headache
– Slurred speech	– Irritability
– Reduced sociability	– Restless legs
– Flapping tremor	– Cramps
– Tics	– Meningismus
– Disturbance brain stem evoked potentials	

2) *Gastro-intestinal system:*

– Hiccup	– Stomatitis
– Parotitis	– Pancreatitis
– Gastritis	– Gastro-intestinal ulcers
– Anorexia	– Nausea, vomiting

3) *Haematological system:*

– Anaemia	– Bleeding
– Red cell fragility	

4) *Immunologic system:*

– Susceptibility to infection	– Cancer
– Burn-out of immune disorders (e.g. SLE)	

5) *Cardiovascular system:*

– Pericarditis	– Hypertension
– Atheromatosis	– Cardiomyopathy
– Edema	– Hypotension
– Decreased diastolic compliance	

6) *Pulmonary system:*

– Pleuritis	— Pulmonary edema
– Uraemic lung	

7) *Skin:*

– Pruritus	– Melanosis
– Retarded wound healing	– Nail atrophy

8) *Endocrinology:*

– Glucose intolerance	– Growth retardation
– Hyperlipidaemia	– Hypogonadism
– Hyperparathyroidism	– Impotence, diminished libido

9) *Bone disease:*

– Osteodystrophy	– Amyloidosis (β_2-microglobulin)
– Hyperparathyroidism	– Defective calcitriol metabolism

10) *Miscellaneous:*

– Thirst	– Uraemic foetor
– Weight loss	– Hypothermia

Table 2. The uraemic syndrome – pathophysiology

1) *Haematologic disturbances:*
– Inappropriate erythropoietin production
– Fragility of red blood cells
– Erythrocyte membrane fluidity
– Iron transport
– Erythropoiesis
– Erythrocyte osmotic fragility
– Modulatory function IGF-1

2) *Immunologic system:*
– T-cell growth and activation
– T-cell subset identification
– B7/CD28 pathway
– 3 H-thymidine uptake of lymphocytes
– Bone marrow thymidine incorporation
– Lymphocyte immune response, with and without stimulation
– E-rosette forming capacity
– Cytokine production
– B cell activation and immunoregulation
– Interleukin-2 production
– Phagocytic response: – locomotion, chemotaxis and phagocytosis
                         – granulocyte and macrophage differentiation
                         – adherence
                         – chemiluminescence
                         – uptake of radiolabelled particles
                         – skin window test
                         – phagocytic glucose metabolism
– Immunoglobulin levels

3) *Coagulation:*
– Platelet cyclo-oxygenase activity
– Platelet aggregation
– Platelet adherence
– Platelet glycolysis
– Exposure of fibrinogen receptors
– Increased von Willebrand factor activity
– Increased bleeding time

4) *Metabolic processes or enzymatic activities:*
– Gluconeogenesis
– Sodium-potassium ATP-ase activity
– Lactate dehydrogenase activity
– Mitochondrial storage of calcium
– Mitochondrial activity
– Alkaline phosphatase activity
– Insulin degradation
– Glutathione peroxidase activity
– Cellular calcium pumps
– Methylation of phenols
– Production and clearance of 1,25 diOH-vit D

Table 2. (continued)

5) *Heart cell function:*
– Beating rate of heart cells
– Heart cell contractility
– Heart cell survival
– Cardiovascular reflexes
– Effect of adenylate cyclase stimulation
– Beta-adrenoceptor density and affinity
– Diminished responsiveness to alpha- and beta-receptors
– Decrease in diastolic compliance
– Increased volume of interstitial cells
– Vasoconstrictor response to postural changes

6) *Endocrine function:*
– Glucose utilization
– Insulin receptors
– Decreased number of glucose transport sites
– Impaired insulin release
– Suppressed TSH-release
– Suppressed pituitary responsiveness
– Reproduction abnormalities
– Response to growth and reproductive hormones
– Production and clearance of calcitriol

7) *Drug protein binding:*
– Decrease for acidic drugs
– Increase for alkaline drugs

8) *Nerve function:*
– Isolated sural nerve conductivity
– Microtubule formation
– Polymerization of tubulin
– Brain synaptosome neurotransmitter production

9) *Overall:*
– DNA repair ability
– Recovery of RNA synthesis after UV irradiation
– Cell membrane organic acid transport

the autonomic nervous system, and occurs in spite of elevated circulating catecholamine levels. Vasoconstrictive response during postural stress is lacking (11). Moreover, the binding properties to vascular and myocardial adrenergic receptors may be altered (12).

Apart from changes in systolic cardiac contractility, a *decrease in diastolic compliance* plays a major pathophysiologic role (13), related to myocardial interstitial fibrosis, resulting in a decreased cardiac compliance (14). This defect is probably not related to previous hypertension. The basic mechanism is associated with an activation of interstitial cells and increased volume of interstitial cell nuclei and cytoplasm, whereby uraemia increases myocardial interstitial ground substance.

Neurologic system

Uraemic encephalopathy, and peripheral neuropathy, may develop alone or in combination (15). The spectrum of central neuropathy is variable and ranges from minor obtundation to coma (16). *Sleep disorders*, mainly sleep-apnea syndrome based on obstructive events, are among the major actual problems (17). Brain stem evoked potentials are disturbed (18). Dialysis prevents major *encephalopathy*, so that this complication is observed only exceptionally, in patients not seeking medical help until late in their course, or when dialysis is abandoned because of grave disease, e.g. incurable cancer.

Peripheral polyneuropathy has also become exceptional today, although less pronounced forms still persist, even in patients apparently treated by adequate dialysis. The formation of microtubules by polymerization of tubulin is an essential process for the functional activity of nervous axon cells, and was shown to be depressed by a chromatographic fraction of uraemic plasma (19).

Haematology

Until the development and therapeutic application of genetically engineered recombinant erythropoietin (20), uraemic anaemia was one of the major factors responsible for the malaise and bad condition in renal failure.

This anaemia with hypoproliferative marrow is mainly due to inappropriate erythropoietin production by the failing kidneys, defective body iron stores, vitamin deficiency and haemolysis. Contributing factors are changes in erythrocyte fragility, membrane fluidity, iron transport and osmotic resistance, in part related to hyperparathyroidism (21).

The causative role of inhibitors of erythropoiesis remains a matter of debate (22). Two proven inhibitors of *in vitro* haematopoiesis are the polyamines spermine and spermidine (23). Segal et al. however suggested that their inhibitory effect was aspecific (24). Kushner et al., in contrast, demonstrated that polyamines inhibited erythroid colony formation in a dose dependent manner (25). Insulin-like growth factor I (IGF-I) may be a modulator of erythropoiesis and an enhancer of erythropoietin effect in uraemia: according to Urena et al. a highly significant correlation was found between IGF-I and haematocrit values (26).

Coagulation

Disturbances of coagulation are related to a varied spectrum of possibilities, from bleeding tendency to hypercoagulability. Other, non-toxic factors (e.g. related to the bioincompatibility of dialysis membranes and/or to intradialytic anticoagulation) are involved.

Uraemic *bleeding tendency* has a multifactorial origin: platelet related alterations (adherence, aggregation) (27, 28), together with uraemic anaemia, hyperparathy-roidism, disturbances in prostaglandin production from arachidonic acid and inefficient thromboxane generation. Until recently, no specific 'toxin' could be designed that interferes with coagulation. Recent data, however, incriminate nitric oxide (NO) as an important inductor of defective coagulation in uraemia (29).

Currently, the circulating number of *thrombocytes* is not altered. There is more concern about functional changes: retention by glass beads (30), aggregation response to adenosine disphosphate and collagen, exposure of fibrinogen receptors (31), cyclo-oxygenase activity (32) and glycolysis (33) are all disturbed.

In spite of a general tendency to bleeding, isolated defects point to *hypercoagulability*: elevated amplitudes at thromboelastography (34) and increased von Willebrand factor activity (35).

Immune status

Susceptibility to infection, including tuberculosis, increased incidence of cancer, burn-out of immunologic disorders, inadequate production of antibodies, e.g. against hepatitis B vaccination, are all current clinical problems of uraemia that point to immune deficiency.

Here also the problem is not entirely toxic: other factors may be involved, such as contact of the vascular bed with the external world via access systems, bioincompatibility of artificial organs, Vitamin D deficiency or resistance, and/or the presence of anatomical lesions prone to infection (e.g. polycystic kidney disease, ureteral reflux, heart valve damage etc) (36).

Uraemic immune depression is registered at different levels: inefficacy of muco-cutaneous barriers, granulocyte abnormalities (locomotion, phagocytosis), changes in immunoglobulin levels and synthesis, reticulo-endothelial function, and cell-mediated immunity (36, 37). Currently, the circulating number of white blood cells is not altered. There is more concern about functional changes.

A central position in the host-defense against bacterial infection is occupied by neutrophils and monocytes (Figure 1) (38). Although the number of circulating phagocytes is not affected, granulocytic and macrophagic differentiation may be altered (39). Specific *phagocytic functions*, such as microparticle ingestion and killing of bacteria have extensively been studied, with contradictory results, the majority of the results however pointing to depression (36, 37). A cross-sectional study by the authors, evaluating the metabolic response of phagocytes to stimuli by estimating glucose metabolization indicates that there is a depression of phagocytic metabolism once serum creatinine is higher than 6 mg/100 mL (Table 3) which corresponds to a creatinine clearance of ±15 mL/min (40). The start of haemodialysis induces a further depression in polymorphonuclear functional response, but this is possibly related to bioincompatibility rather than to uraemic toxic effects (40, 41). Surprisingly, polymorph functional capacity in response

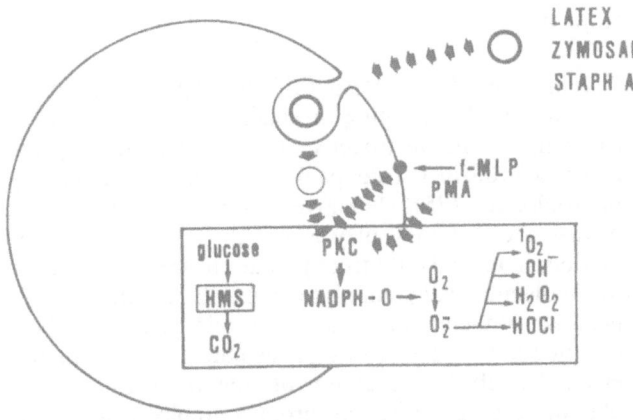

Figure 1. Metabolic processes involved with phagocytic cell function. Abbreviations are: f-MLP, formyl-methionine-leucine-phenylalanine; PMA, phorbol myristic acid; PKC, protein kinase C; NADPH-O, NAD(P)H-oxidase; HMS: hexose monophosphate shunt. Various stimuli are illustrated: particles (latex, zymosan, Staphylococcus Aureus) and soluble stimuli (f-MLP, PMA). Only the particles stimulate metabolic function following ingestion (phagocytosis). The two remaining stimuli challenge function, either via a membrane receptor (f-MLP) or via direct activation of PKC (PMA). The subsequent process consists of the production of oxygen free radicals by NAD(P)H-oxidase. The necessary energy is delivered by the HMS. (Reproduced with permission from Vanholder et al., *Kidney Int* 42: S91, 1992).

to phagocytosis tends to improve when patients stay on dialysis for prolonged periods (Table 3) (42).

The responsible factors for the depression of phagocytic function in uraemia are far from being identified. Apart from the abovementioned factors such as deficient barriers and dialysis incompatibility, possible candidates are a lack of circulating opsonins (e.g. fibronectin) (43), iron overload (44), uraemic anaemia (45) and overconcentration of circulating suppressants (endomorphins, phenols, indoles, parathyroid hormone, high and middle molecular weight compounds) (36). Hörl and his coworkers recently identified two peptidic structures with marked inhibitory effect on various immune functions (46, 47); the second compound showed structural resemblance to part of the β_2-microglobulin molecule (47).

Cellular immunity primarily involves T-lymphocytes and the lymphokines they produce. There is an interrelation with granulocytes and macrophages as effector cells of this system. Suppression of cell-mediated immunity in uraemia involves intrinsically normal cells in a primarily suppressive milieu. There is a substantial number of cellular dysfunctions (48): T-cell growth factor activity, T-cell subset identification, metabolic responsiveness, lymphatic immune response and/or proliferation, and E-rosette forming capacity. Raskova et al. demonstrated that B-cell activation and immunoregulation, as well as helper T-cell functions, were quantitatively deficient (49).

Table 3. Polymorphonuclear metabolic response in different stages of renal failure[a]

	Latex	Zymosan
Non-dialyzed patients		
Screa (mg/100 mL)		
< 1.3 (controls)	154 ± 7	339 ± 15
1.3–1.9	140 ± 11	339 ± 23
2.0–2.9	124 ± 13	318 ± 26
3.0–3.9	131 ± 14	340 ± 33
4.0–5.9	134 ± 7	360 ± 15
6.0–7.9	$102 \pm 7^*$	$268 \pm 21^*$
≥ 8.0	$70 \pm 8^{**}$	$183 \pm 19^{**}$
Haemodialyzed patients		
Dialytic age		
< 2 years	$46 \pm 4_{**}$	$72 \pm 7^{**}$
> 2 years	$70 \pm 5^{**}$	$180 \pm 8^{**}$

[a]Data expressed as Desintegrations per Minute (DPM) per 10^3 polymorphonuclear cells (PMNLs), as an index of $^{14}CO_2$-production from radiolabelled glucose (in response to standard quantities of latex and zymosan as stimulants (means $\pm$ SEM). Non-dialyzed patients are divided according to renal function, as indicated by Screa, haemodialyzed patients are divided according to dialytic age.
$^*p < 0.05$.
$^{**}p < 0.01$ vs controls with normal renal function. Screa: serum creatinine.

A defective interleukin-2 production (50) and the retention of guanidino-compounds (51) have been recognized as potential causative factors. Lymphocyte response to stimulation is disturbed in cultured cells from dialysed patients (52). Correction was possible after addition of interleukin-2 (IL-2) but not of interleukin-1 (IL-1). T-cell adhesion to extracellular matrix proteins was shown to be depressed in the presence of uraemic sera (53). Impaired proliferation of peripheral blood leukocytes and T-cell activation defect was recently attributed to an accessory cell defect in the B7/CD28 pathway (54). *In vitro* restoration of this B7/CD28 pathway reconstituted leukocytic cellular functions.

Endocrinology

The endocrine dysfunction of uraemia affects carbohydrate metabolism, and thyroid, growth and reproductive hormones, resulting in a progressive catabolic status (55).

Carbohydrate metabolism

Changes in carbohydrate metabolism consist of alterations of glucose metabolism, pancreatic glucose-induced insulin secretion, metabolism and target organ sensitivity of insulin (56), resulting in abnormal glucose tolerance (57). These changes are apparently not related to a decrease of insulin receptor binding or receptor kinase activity (58), but possibly to a decrease of glucose transport sites (59, 60). Surprisingly, 1,25-dihydroxycholecalciferol corrects glucose intolerance in haemodialysis patients (61).

Mac Galeb et al. characterized and partially purified a factor from uraemic serum inducing insulin resistance, but an exact identification was not obtained, unless for the peptidic nature of the substance (62). Dzúrik et al. first suggested hippuric acid (63) and later also pseudouridine (64) as potential inhibitors of glucose tolerance.

The uraemic status impairs insuline release. According to Fadda et al., this abnormality is reversed by parathyroidectomy (65).

Glucagon levels are elevated, due to defective metabolization by the kidneys (66).

Thyroid hormone

Levels of T3 and T4 may be low normal or depressed, the pituitary responsiveness being abnormal, in spite of an euthyroid appearance (67). Thyroid stimulating hormone (TSH) release is suppressed, possibly by a dopamine-dependent mechanism (68).

Growth hormones

Basal levels of growth hormone are elevated in uraemia, in proportion with renal failure. Nevertheless, growth retardation is one of the onerous facets in uraemic children. Contributing factors are malnutrition, acidosis, renal osteodystrophy, and inadequate gonadotropic hormone secretion. The administration of excess doses of recombinant human growth hormone corrects the growth disturbances of paediatric uraemics (69), and improves protein utilization in stable haemodialysed adults (70). Acute induction in the liver of insulin-like growth factor-1 (IGF-1) mRNA is reduced in uraemic rats (71).

Reproductive hormones

Advanced renal failure results in reproductive abnormalities in both males and females, related to hormonal disturbances. In uraemic women, FSH, progesteron and estradiol tend to approximate and LH tends to be higher than the levels seen in the follicular phase of the menstrual cycle in normal women (72). The normal cyclical peaks that occur immediately before ovulation do not occur.

Uraemic men may be infertile and/or impotent, which is associated with an increased LH and a decreased testosteron. Spermatogenesis is compromised, related to increased FSH levels. Prolactin levels may be elevated, inducing galactorrhea and amenorrhea in women and gyneco masty impotence and gyneco masty in men (73).

Growth retardation is one of the epiphenomena of reduced gonadotropin pulsatility during pubertal maturation (74).

Bone disease

Uraemic bone disease is a multifactorial problem, depending upon such diverging mechanisms as hyperparathyroidism, aluminum toxicity, vitamin D deficiency and resistance, intrinsic osteopenia, and accumulation of β_2-microglobulin (75). Defective production of insulin-like growth factor-1 may play a role in deficient bone formation, independently from parathormone levels (76). A low molecular weight inhibitor of cartilage sulfation, with negative influence on bone cell proliferation, has been detected in the plasma of dialysis patients (77). Andress et al. described an inhibitor of osteoblast mitogenesis, obtained after gel filtration chromatography, with a molecular weight range between 750 and 900 Daltons, inhibiting osteoblast mitogenesis (78). Hsu and coworkers found evidence that uraemic retention solutes reduced renal 24-hydroxylase activity due to a decrease in genomic synthesis (79).

Pruritis

Pruritis is a disturbing epiphenomenon of uraemia, with unclear patho-physiologic mechanisms. Several different factors have been incriminated: increased levels of serum vitamin A, hyperparathyroidism, high skin contents of divalent cations, mast cell proliferation with increased release of histamine, and/or abnormal pattern of cutaneous innervation with prolific sprouting of neuron-specific enolase immunoreactive nerve fibers on skin biopsy (80). Responsible toxins, if any, have not been incriminated, apart from parathormone.

Progression of renal disease

Motojima et al. found compelling evidence that one or more ultrafiltrable uraemic retention solutes were involved in the advancement of glomerulosclerosis (81).

End-stage renal failure

Renal failure may progress relentlessly, until the terminal stage is reached, when it becomes necessary to pursue solute elimination by haemodialysis, peritoneal dialysis, or transplantation. Renal replacement is currently started when creatinine clearance reaches a level of 5 mL/min, or even earlier, in diabetics and hypertensives. Some authors advocate the start of dialysis at an earlier stage (Ccrea 10–15 mL/min) (82), and this approach has been claimed to improve outcome after transplantation.

The authors currently enroll patients for transplantation from a creatinine clearance of 15 mL/min on, without start of dialysis, allowing some of them to be transplanted without need to dialyse.

If no renal replacement therapy is started, the patient may remain in acceptable condition for an unpredictable period. Sudden deterioration may occur, due to increased catabolism, infection, fluid overload, hypertension, etc. Dialysis is currently started when the patient is still in good condition. Major complications are prevented by not waiting until the patient is gravely ill. In the rare patient that waits too long before seeking medical help, terminal intoxication is characterized by progressive alterations of the central nervous state, ending with convulsions, coma and death. Additional problems are an enhanced bleeding tendency (ecchymoses, haematoma, gastro-intestinal bleeding), dermatologic alterations (uraemic frost), peripheral and pulmonary edema, hypertension, hyperventilation (due to acidosis), pericarditis and gastro-intestinal problems such as anorexia and vomiting.

On the other hand, the availability of erythropoietin for treatment of uraemic anaemia may mask one of the primary signs of intoxication, by the way increasing the need for objective markers of dialysis adequacy, such as urea kinetic calculations.

Differential diagnosis

Renal patients may develop symptoms mimicking the uraemic state because of alternative reasons: their primary disease, as well as the concomitant presence of hepatic or cerebro-vascular disease, diabetes mellitus, disturbances of electrolyte and water homeostasis, drug intoxication etc. Also, acute renal failure may develop on top of baseline chronic renal failure.

If incorrectly understood, renal replacement therapy will be started without necessity.

Interfering factors due to renal replacement therapy

Renal replacement therapy, in spite of its beneficial effect on uraemic retention, may cause a number of side-effects or trade-off effects mimicking uraemic toxicity.

Dialysis with dialyzers containing complement and leukocyte activating membranes may affect the immunologic, metabolic, and haematologic status, irrespective of general toxicity (40, 83). The insertion of central vein catheters for acute haemodialysis as well as the use of peritoneal dialysis catheters may enhance the risk of infection (84, 85). Both fresh and spent peritoneal dialysis fluid affect leukocyte functional capacity (86–88), but in spent dialysate part of the functional depression may be the consequence of the presence of toxic solutes in the fluid (88).

Arterio-venous fistulae may cause cardiac decompensation. The use of immunosuppressive agents after renal transplantation and in immune disorders enhances the risk of infection and cancer. All these factors may cause problems that at first glance could be related to uraemia.

BIOCHEMICAL ALTERATIONS

Enzymatic processes

A host of enzymatic and metabolic functions are depressed, as reviewed (89, 90): gluconeogenesis, lactate dehydrogenase, mitochondrial storage of calcium, mitochondrial oxygen consumption, alkaline phosphatase isoenzyme activity, insulin degradation etc.

New data have been accumulated over the recent years that added to this knowledge.

Na^+, K^+ *pump* suppression (91–93) results in an increased cellular sodium content, arterial hypertension, and plasmatic digitalis- or ouabain-like activity (94). The mechanism for defective cation transport is multifactorial and tissue-specific (95). In parallel, sodium-dependent amino acid transport is also decreased, pointing to the general influence of this defect on cellular metabolism.

The activity of *glutathione peroxidase* and erythrocyte reduced glutathione contents are decreased in chronic renal failure (96, 97), oxidized glutathione levels being higher (97).

Extra- and intracellular *serine depletion* in the presence of high plasma glycine, even in non-malnourished uraemic patients, reflects a defect in the metabolism of glycine to serine, related to a lack of renal tissue (98).

Due to a host of enzymatic and functional disturbances, resting *cellular and cytosolic Ca++-contents* are enhanced, resulting in the impairment of various metabolic processes, e.g. pancreatic glucose-dependent insulin secretion (99). Increased intracellular or cytosolic Ca^{++} has been related to increased peripheral vascular resistance and hence hypertension (100), as well as to a blunted phagocytic response (101). According to Gafter et al., uraemic high RBC calcium can at least in part be attributed to deficient extrusion after deactivation of Ca^{++}-ATPase (102). Convincing data collected by Lindner et al. demonstrated the presence of a circulating inhibitor of the RBC membrane calcium pump in uraemic plasma ultrafiltrate (103). The responsible factor was partially identified and characterized by a low molecular weight, and by being dialysable and heat stable.

Further studies, based on ^{31}P-magnetic resonance spectroscopy evidenced *mitochondrial dysfunction* in uraemia due either to limitation of oxygen supply, reduced mitochondrial content, or an intrinsic mitochondrial defect (104). Correction of this defect after erythropoietin administration suggests that anaemia contributes to these metabolic anomalies. At maximum workload, major depletion of phosphocreatine and ATP with a fall in intracellular pH were demonstrated, equally pointing to a defect of oxidative metabolism, compensated for by an increase in anaerobic glycolysis (105).

Metabolization through *methylation of phenols* by phenyl-O-methyltransferase is blunted in red blood cell membranes of patients on maintenance haemodialysis

(106), which may add to the toxic accumulation of phenols.

Tubular anion transport has been shown to be depressed by plasma extracts from haemodialysed patients, probably due to competition with anionic uraemic solutes (107). Sera from spontaneously hypertensive rats (SHR) also contain a factor(s) inhibiting renal organic anion transport. Hypertension and organic anion transport were significantly correlated, suggesting an extension of the patho-physiologic impact of these findings to hypertension (108).

Both *production and metabolic clearance of calcitriol* were demonstrated to be disturbed in acute as well as chronic renal failure (109–111). Parathyroidectomy had no effect on this process. In further studies, it was demonstrated that uraemic ultrafiltrate contained factors inhibiting both production and metabolization of calcitriol (112). Some of these factors showed an elution pattern on HPLC, conform with purines, such as uric acid, or xanthine, and administration of purines induced similar alterations as uraemic ultrafiltrate (113). Infusion of uraemic ultrafiltrate to normal rats further reduced the intestinal calcitriol receptor concentration as well as the receptor interaction with DNA *in vitro*, hence pointing to a reduction of the biological action of calcitriol in renal failure (114).

Depressed DNA repair ability and effete recovery of RNA synthesis after damage, e.g. after UV irradiation, may contribute to the enhanced susceptibility for cancer (115).

From these data it becomes clear that a host of biological processes are depressed or altered in uraemia, and that the causative factors are variable and remain to a large part unidentified.

Drug protein binding

Drug plasma protein binding in renal failure has been the subject of several reviews (116, 117). Two binding defects are possible: one group of mostly *acidic drugs* shows a decreased binding, which means an increase of the free, active fractions; since for most drugs, total (bound plus unbound) concentrations are monitored, lower than normal total concentrations should be pursued in this situation; at 'normal' levels toxic side effects should be expected. Current examples are theophyllin, phenytoin, methotrexate, diazepam, digoxin, salicylate (Table 4) (118–120). *Basic drugs*, e.g. propanolol, cimetidine, clonidine, imipramine, show an increased protein binding (Table 4). This causes a decrease of available free concentration, diminishing the therapeutic effect. For these drugs higher total concentrations should be pursued.

Attempts to identify the ligands responsible for decreased protein binding have been scant. Several studies suggest that hippuric acid would be one of the main contributing compounds (Figure 2) (119–122), but its relative importance remains undefined. Other potential

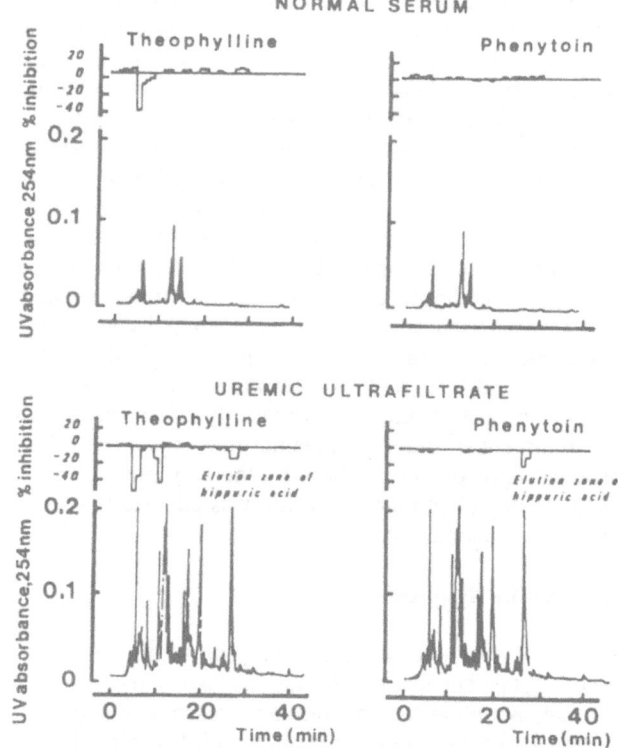

Figure 2. High performance liquid chromatogram of ultrafiltrate of normal (upper panel) and uraemic serum (lower panel) with corresponding UV absorbance (below) and percent protein binding inhibition of the different fractions (above) for theophylline (left) and phenytoin (right). For normal serum ultrafiltrate, theophylline protein binding is inhibited in one elution zone, whereas phenytoin binding is not influenced. For ultrafiltrate of uraemic serum, theophylline protein binding is inhibited in 3 different elution zones. Phenytoin binding is inhibited in only one elution zone. The asterisk indicates the elution zone of hippuric acid. (Reproduced with permission from Vanholder et al., *Kidney Int* 33: 996, 1988).

competitors are indoxyl sulfate (121), derivates of furanpropanoic acid (123, 124) and other furancarboxylic acids (125), β-(m-hydroxyphenyl)-hydracrylate and p-hydroxyphenylacetate (122).

One of the problems with research for protein binding inhibitors is that this research has been focussed on uraemic ultrafiltrate, that by definition only contains an incomplete fraction of protein bound compounds. Studies on deproteinized sera, offered a much larger yield of protein binding inhibitors (Figure 3) (126).

In addition to the myriad of compounds that are potential competitors for drug protein binding, structural changes of albumin, e.g. due to carbamylation, may also induce changes in binding capacity (127).

The rise in binding site number for basic drugs is related to a rise in alpha$_1$-acid glycoprotein concentration (128), due to its decreased removal by the kidneys.

Table 4. Percentage drug protein binding according to renal function

	Serum creatinine (mg/100 mL)			Haemodialyzed patients
	< 1.3	1.3 to 6.0	> 6.0	
Acidic drugs				
Theophylline	63.6 ± 1.9	57.4 ± 4.7[a]	48.8 ± 8.7[b]	43.5 ± 9.5[b]
Phenytoin	91.6 ± 0.7	85.1 ± 1.4[b]	81.7 ± 2.7[b]	75.6 ± 6.2[b]
Methotrexate	42.8 ± 1.6	42.5 ± 5.9	36.2 ± 9.1[a]	27.7 ± 7.7[b]
Diazepam	98.3 ± 1.0	98.0 ± 0.3	97.1 ± 1.1[a]	96.6 ± 1.1[b]
Prazosin	94.0 ± 0.5	91.8 ± 0.5[b]	89.9 ± 0.6[b]	92.4 ± 3.1
Alkaline drugs				
Imipramine	96.2 ± 0.8	97.4 ± 0.5[a]	96.7 ± 0.6	96.2 ± 1.3
Propanolol	90.2 ± 2.0	94.1 ± 1.3[a]	94.1 ± 1.8	93.6 ± 1.2[b]
Cimetidine	8.9 ± 2.2	15.9 ± 2.7[b]	15.5 ± 3.7[b]	14.4 ± 3.0[b]
Clonidine	44.4 ± 7.1	52.1 ± 4.4[a]	52.4 ± 6.7	56.2 ± 6.8[b]

[a] $p < 0.05$.
[b] $p < 0.01$ vs control (serum creatinine < 1.3 mg/100 mL). Expressed as mean ± SD.

The altering relations between bound and unbound drug fractions emphasize the importance of monitoring free rather than total drug concentrations in uraemic patients.

It should be stressed that changes in drug protein binding are not the only by-effects of uraemia related to pharmacology. Decreased renal clearance and/or metabolization, and changes in distribution volume may also enhance drug toxicity. Increments in active concentration may be compensated by alternative pathways of metabolization, e.g. hepatic or intestinal. In addition, accumulation of active drug metabolites may add to the toxicity of the accumulation of the genuine drug *per se*, as is the case for theophylline (129).

Protein binding is not only related to efficacy and toxicity of drugs. In addition, uraemic solute protein binding also may alter toxicity, as conceivably only free, nonbound compounds may exert toxicity. Many potential toxins are protein bound (e.g. indoxyl sulfate, the hippuric and propionic acids, phenols and indoles (Table 5). Peritoneal dialysate may be a much richer source of protein bound compounds than haemodialysate (130), removal of entire albumin-ligand complex being demonstrated as the only rewarding attitude to eliminate substantial amounts of protein bound compounds (130, 131).

URAEMIC SOLUTE RETENTION

General classification of uraemic solutes

The progression of renal failure is characterized by a gradual retention and increase in serum concentration of a large number of organic compounds. Some are metabolites of protein, although a substantial group may be of non-proteinacious origin. Not only small molecules are retained. As concentration increases, partial metabolization and elimination by other than renal pathways becomes more prominent. Some of the retained compounds have been proven to be toxic. Toxicity is not an overall process whereby one or a few toxins affect many different metabolic processes at a time. As of today, the current knowledge points to the fact that each metabolic function may be altered by different retention solutes. Other substances are not toxic but can be used as markers of retention.

Under normal conditions, molecules with a molecular weight up to ± 58,000 Daltons are cleared by the glomerular filter. All these substances are supposed to be retained in uraemia; an additional role should be attributed to changes in tubular secretion and reabsorption.

Uraemic retention products are arbitrarily subdivided in several groups, according to their molecular weight, going from molecules with a low molecular weight (MW) up to 300 Daltons, e.g. urea (MW: 60), creatinine (MW: 113), via substances with a middle molecular weight (300 to 12,000 Daltons), e.g. parathormone (MW: 9,424), beta 2-microglobulin (MW: 11,818), up to those with a high molecular weight (> 12,000 Daltons) e.g. larger molecules like myoglobulins.

The exact nature of the so-called middle molecules should be questioned. Schoots et al. stated that chromatographic middle molecular fractions contained a considerable amount of low molecular weight compounds (132). Uraemic solutes may behave chromatographically and during dialysis like middle molecules, in spite of a low molecular weight, due to electrostatic charges, molecular configuration and protein binding, in spite of a lower

Table 5. Biochemical characteristics of uraemic retention solutes. (Reproduced with permission from Vanholder et al., *Sem Nephrol* 14: 205, 1994. Ref. (134))

Name	Hydrophobic	Protein-bound	Multicompartment	Toxic
Classical 'small' molecules:				
Urea	−	−	−	−
Creatinine	−	−	−	−
Pseudouridine	−	−	−	−
Myo-inositol	−	−	?	±
Purines	−	−	−	+
Organic phosphates	−	−	+	+
Oxalate	−	−	−	±
Ascorbic acid (conj)	−	−	−	−
Dimethylarginine	−	−	−	+
Classical 'middle' molecules:				
Peptides	−	−	+	+
Parathormone	−	−	+	+
β_2-microglobulin	−	−	+	+
'Small' molecules with 'middle' molecular behaviour,				
New definition 'middle' molecules:				
Methylguanidine	−	−	+	+
Guanidinosuccinic acid	−	−	+	+
Indoxyl sulfate	+	+	+	+
Hippuric acid	±	+	+	+
O-OH hippuric acid	±	+	+	±
P-OH hippuric acid	±	+	+	−
Phenylacetylglutamine	±	−	+	−
Polyamines	+	+	+	+
Phenols & indoles	+	+	+	+
Trace metals	−	∓	?	?
CMPF	+	+	+	+
Chloramines (org)	∓	∓	∓	+

Those molecules scoring + for hydrophobicity, protein binding and/or multicompartmental distribution behave like larger molecules and can be considered as small molecules with middle molecular behavior. Many solutes not conforming with either one or two definitions of middle molecules are not toxic. Data on hydrophobicity/hydrophilicity are in general obtained from HPLC-analysis of behavior in formiate/methanol gradient.
Conj: conjugated, org: organic, CMPF: 3-carboxy-4-methyl-5-propyl-2-furanpropionic acid.

molecular weight. Substances like hippurate, are small molecules, that behave like middle molecules due to high protein binding. Consequently, the definition of middle molecules is too rough and aspecific, to accept them as a homogenous group of well defined uraemic toxins (133, 134).

Separation and identification methods

The concentration of most known low molecular weight organic substances, can be determined chemically. The study of uraemia becomes more complex, when the reten-

tion pattern of unidentified compounds is evaluated. Historically, this research has been concentrated on middle molecules, most separation methods having been chosen in function of this aim.

Gel chromatography

Different types of gel have been used, most frequently Sephadex G-15 (135–137). Although some separation is obtained, the resolution is often insufficient, so that other separation strategies are to be associated.

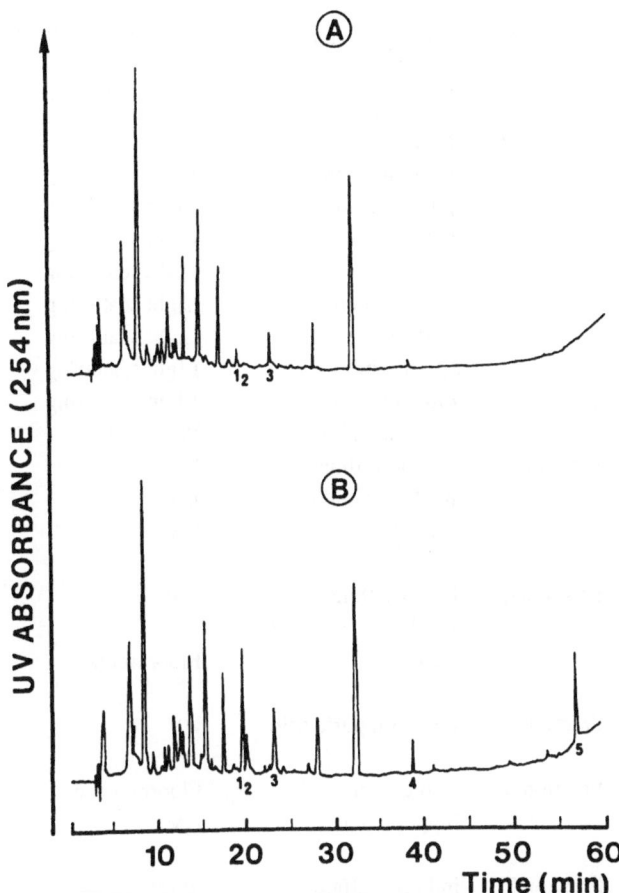

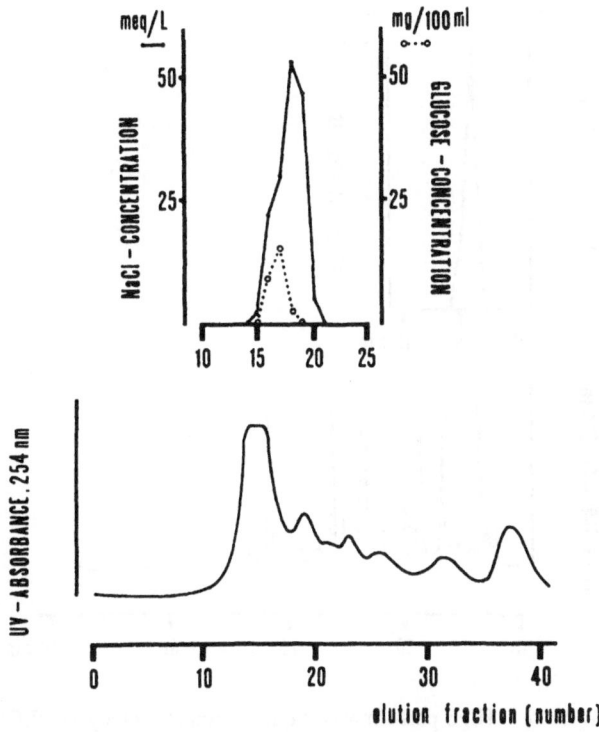

Figure 3. C$_{18}$ reversed-phase HPLC of the same serum sample, once submitted to ultrafiltration (A), and once to deproteinization by heat denaturation (B). Peak height is related to concentration. Peak height is increasing after deproteinization (B) for a number of compounds, especially at the right hand side of the chromatogram: this suggests substantial protein binding of these solutes. At the extreme right hand side, a number of peaks appear in (B) that were totally absent in (A), pointing to their ± 100% protein binding. 1: indoxyl sulfate; 2: tryptophan; 3: hippuric acid; 4: indole-3-acetic acid; 5: 3-carboxy-4-methyl-5-propyl-2-furanpropionic acid (CMPF); IS: internal standard.

Gel chromatography in combination with other separation strategies

In many studies, gel filtration was used as first line separation, followed by a second technique to allow a more accurate definition of the substances under study (multicomponent analysis): gel chromatography in conjunction with amino acid analysis, isotachophoresis, ion exchange chromatography on DEAE A-25 Sephadex, high pressure liquid chromatography, ultraviolet spectroscopy, or 1H-13C nuclear magnetic resonance (132, 135, 136, 138–140).

Only a limited number of groups have by this method separated an earlier unidentified single middle molecular

Figure 4. Gel chromatography (Sephadex G15) of uraemic serum with registration of UV absorbance at 254 nm (below), together with sodium chloride (full lines) and glucose concentrations (broken lines) in the corresponding fractions. Only those fractions containing a significant amount of sodium chloride and glucose are illustrated. Each elution fraction was collected over 20 minutes. More than 5 fractions, corresponding to a zone of major UV absorption, contain sodium chloride and glucose. These compounds may interfere with biochemical tests, performed with lyophilizates of the corresponding fractions. (Reproduced with permission from Vanholder and Ringoir, *Oxford Textbook of Clinical Nephrology*, 1992, p 1236).

component of relative purity from uraemic serum (139–146).

Disadvantages of gel chromatography

Gel chromatography may give rise to elution patterns that induce interpretation problems. Artifacts in plasma middle molecule determination might be induced by some drugs (147). It is known that salicylic acid modifies the chromatographic pattern of the middle molecule fractions in normal subjects and uraemic patients (148, 149). Resolution is not very good and peaks still contain numerous compounds. Even if a fraction causes inhibition of a biochemical function, it is virtually impossible to come to an identification of the responsible compound, in view of the complex composition of the fractions.

Gel chromatography should also be used with care when combined with biochemical tests, as the latter might be suppressed by excess NaCl and glucose, present in sev-

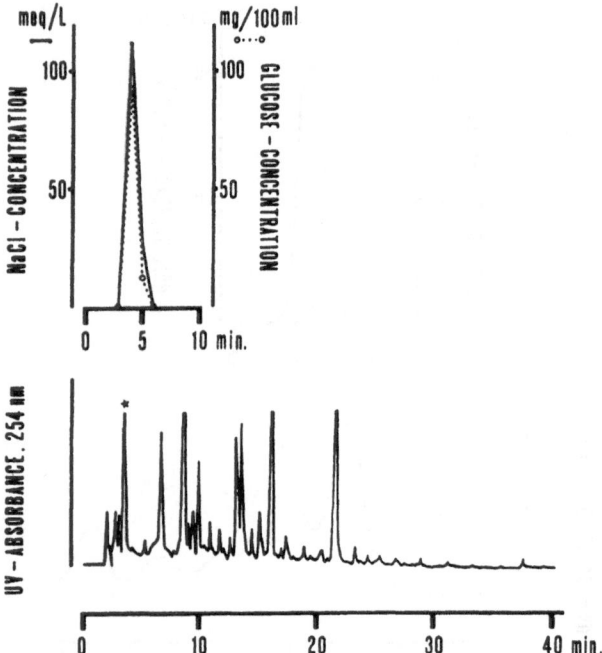

Figure 5. High performance liquid chromatography (HPLC) (reverse phase C_{18}-5 μm) on uraemic serum (below), together with sodium chloride (full lines) and glucose concentration (broken lines) in the corresponding fractions (above). Only two fractions contain NaCl and glucose. In only one of them concentration is elevated. These two fractions contain only one important uraemic solute: creatinine (asterisk). (Reproduced with permission from Vanholder and Ringoir, *Oxford Textbook of Clinical Nephrology*, 1992, p 1236).

eral fractions (Figure 4). NaCl and glucose will be restricted to a narrow elution zone with other separation strategies, such as HPLC (Figure 5). Middle molecular mass regions may contain substantial quantities of substances of low molecular weight molecules, carbohydrates, organic acids, amino acids, and ultraviolet absorbing solutes (132).

High performance liquid chromatography (HPLC)

The HPLC-technique combines several advantages in the search for uraemic retention solutes. Known and unknown solutes are analyzed simultaneously with sufficient resolution, without need for chemical modification. The method is non-destructive; adequate collection of fractions facilitates further characterization of solutes with respect to biochemical activity. Exact quantification is possible by the estimation of peak height or area. HPLC allows a clear cut separation of close to 30 different components, that are visualized by UV-absorbance or by fluorescence emission (Table 6). Molecular mass in the eluted fractions can be defined by combination with light scattering analysis. Electrolytes and glucose are eluted in only 1 or 2 fractions (Figure 5). The HPLC-technique enables

Table 6. Major uraemic retention solutes identifiable on HLPC[a]

Fraction	Compound	Detection method
Fraction 2	creatinine	UV
	guanidinoacetic acid	UV
	guanidinosuccinic acid	Light scattering
	arginine	Light scattering
	urea	Light scattering
	β-endorphin	Light scattering
	spermine	Light scattering
	spermidine	Light scattering
	dimethylamine	Light scattering
	inorganic phosphates	Photometry
Fraction 3	pseudouridine	UV
	methylguanidine	UV
	uric acid	UV
Fraction 4	hypoxanthine	UV
	xanthine	UV
	tyrosine	Fluorescence
Fraction 5	p-OH hippuric acid	UV
Fraction 6	tryptophan	Fluorescence
	hippuric acid	UV
Fraction 7	indoxyl sulfate	Fluorescence
Fraction 8	o-OH hippuric acid	UV
Fraction 9	phenol	Fluorescence
	benzylalcohol	UV
Fraction 11	indole-3-acetic acid	Fluorescence
Fraction 21	p-cresol	Fluorescence
	o-cresol	Fluorescence
Fraction 15	CMPF	UV

[a]HPLC C_{18}, 10 μm, preparative set-up, gradient from 100% 50 mmol/L formiate buffer, pH 4.0 to 100% methanol in 60 min. Fractions are collected over 4 min each.
UV: ultraviolet absorption (254 nm). Fluorescence: extinction 280 nm (emission 340 nm). CMPF: 3-carboxy-4-methyl-5-propyl-2-furanpropionic acid.

to recognize subtle differences in intradialytic extraction ratios between different dialysis strategies (Figure 6) (150–152), that could not be recognized earlier with gel chromatography (153). HPLC can also be used for the fractionation of uraemic samples in the study of biochem-

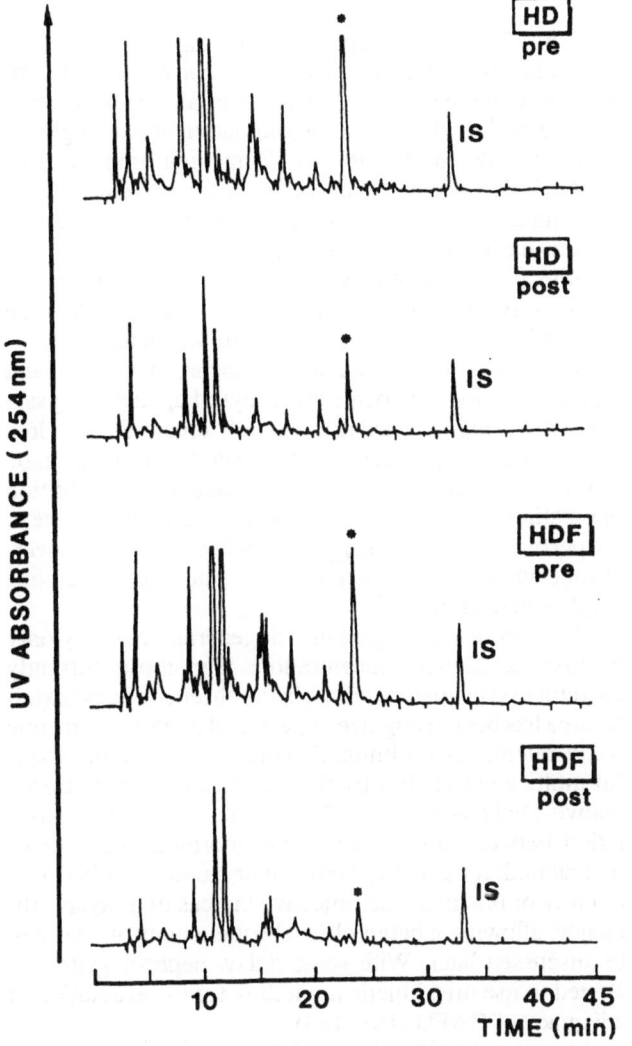

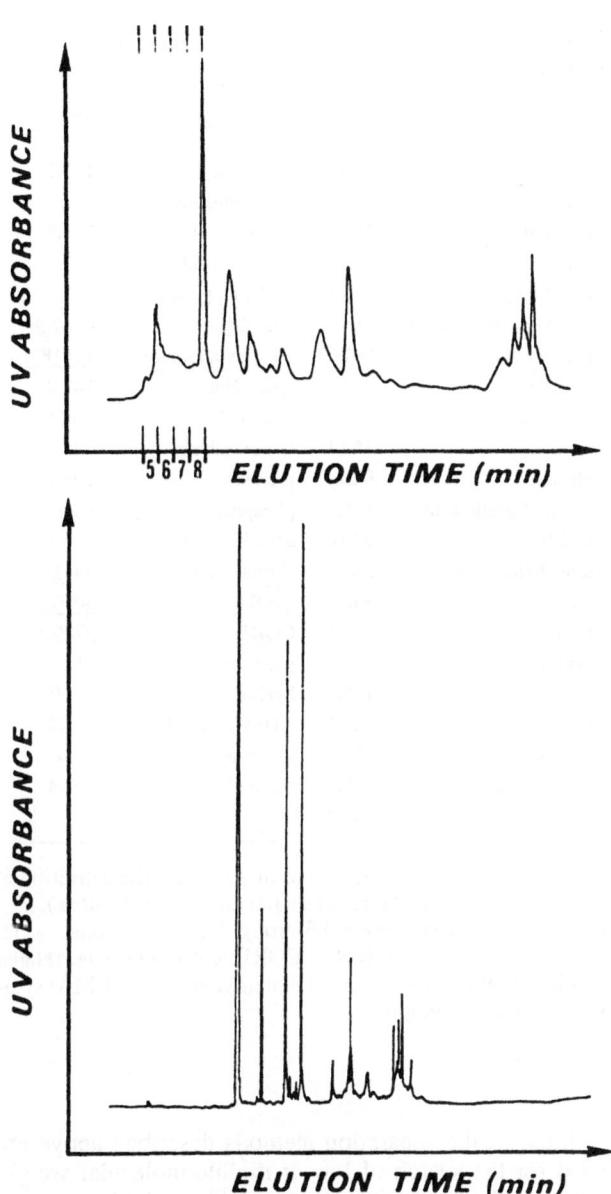

Figure 6. Analytical C_{18} reversed phase HPLC-profile with UV-absorbance peak detection of blood samples drawn before (pre) and after treatment (post) for haemodialysis (HD) (above) and haemodiafiltration (HDF) (below). Peak height is in proportion with solute concentration. Solute removal is more pronounced for HDF, especially on the right hand side of the chromatogram. *: hippuric acid; IS: internal standard.

Figure 7. UV absorbing peak pattern after reversed phase C_{18}-5 μm HPLC of uraemic ultrafiltrate on a formiate/methanol gradient (above). Subfraction 8 (*) seemingly contains only one major peak. Rechromatography of this subfraction 8 on an aminopropyl column with acetonitrile and phosphate buffer as an eluent however reveals the presence of a whole cluster of peaks.

ical dysfunction (112, 119, 120, 126). One can play with the composition of packings and eluates in order to pursue the separation of solutes with different characteristics. A classical set-up is the use of analytical or preparative C_{18}-reversed phase HPLC, with a gradient from 100% formiate to 100% methanol, in order to separate hydrophilic from hydrophobic compounds. Small fractions, obtained by the latter methodology, can then be submitted to separation by other set-ups, e.g. aminopropyl-columns with acetonitrile gradient (Figure 7). Our experience learns that narrow elution fractions, obtained with one separation method, still contain a large number of compounds (Figure 7), and

that one single peak may conceal several compounds, that can only be detected by other identification methods. It is also our experience that one single separation technique in the search for uraemic compounds is not enough in most cases. Identification becomes even more difficult when one is on the outlook for low concentration, high activity compounds.

Table 7. Some major uraemic retention solutes and their molecular weight (Daltons)

Compound	MW	Compound	MW
urea	60.1	creatinine	113.1
pseudouridine	244.2	methylguanidine	73.1
guanidinosuccinic acid	175.1	indoxyl sulfate	251.3
myo-inositol	180.2	hippuric acid	179.2
o-OH hippuric acid	195.1	p-OH hippuric acid	195.
phenylacetylglutamine	264.0	endothelin	4282.9
parathormone	9424.7	β₂-microglobulin	11818.0
spermine	202.3	spermidine	145.2
putrescine	88.1	uric acid	168.1
xanthine	152.1	hypoxanthine	136.1
phenol	94.1	p-cresol	108.1
indole-3-acetic acid	175.2	phosphate	96.0
CMPF	240.0	ascorbic acid	176.1
dimethylarginine	202.0	β-endorphin	3465.0
arginine	74.2	ANF	3080.5
benzylalcohol	108.1	CGRP	3789.3
cytidine	234.2	guanidinoacetic acid	117.1
homocysteine	135.2	hyaluronic acid	> 10⁶
melanine	126.1	ADMA/SDMA	202.3
nitric oxide	30.0	oxalic acid	90.0
trichloromethane	119.4	tryptophan	202.4
tyrosine	181.2		

The underlined compounds conform with the strict definition of middle molecules (MW between 300 and 12,000 Daltons). CMPF: 3-carboxy-4-methyl-5-propyl-2-furanpropionic acid, ANF: atrial natriuretic factor, CGRP: calcitonin gene related peptide, ADMA: asymmetrical dimethylarginine, SDMA: symmetrical dimethylarginine.

Most of the separation methods described above are used for the search of low or middle molecular weight compounds. Specific chromatographic methods are available for the search of compounds with higher molecular weight: e.g. HPLC on TSK columns.

Major uraemic retention products

Several substances retained in uraemia influence one or more biological activities, mostly in concentrations that correspond to those found in uraemia. Other compounds have no directly proven toxicity, but may be useful markers of uraemic retention. A review of the most currently known uraemic retention solutes with their molecular weight is given in Table 7 (133, 134). It should be acknowledged that such trivial and anorganic compounds as water, potassium and sodium may as well exert toxicity, and even mortality, if they are not sufficiently removed in renal failure. In what follows, however, emphasis will be on organic retention compounds.

Urea

Urea has been held responsible for the overconcentration of haemoglobin A1C that is currently found in non-diabetic uraemics (154). Fluckiger et al. suggested that this was mainly due to the carbamylation of haemoglobin by isocyanate formed *in vivo* from high ambient urea levels (155). A correlation between time averaged urea concentrations and carbamylated haemoglobin concentrations has been described (156).

Other proteins probably undergo structural changes in a similar way, this being a potential mechanism of abnormal metabolism and/or altered protein binding in uraemia.

Toxic symptoms such as headache, vomiting and fatigue, develop if patients are dialysed against dialysate containing high concentrations of urea (157). Urea decreases the output response of isolated guinea pig hearts (158). This effect is even accentuated by the addition of creatinine, guanidinosuccinate and methylguanidine to the perfusion medium, suggesting that a mixture of several substances may cause more toxic side effects than one single solute alone.

However, it is accepted that in general, urea may only be toxic at higher concentrations than those currently encountered in uraemia. Even in the absence of any toxicity, urea has been recognized as a useful marker of uraemic solute retention and elimination in dialysed patients. Careful multicenter studies by the American National Cooperative Dialysis study (NCDS) revealed a direct correlation between urea kinetics and morbidity of patients on haemodialysis (159, 160). Their studies resulted in a number of practical and objective indices of dialysis efficiency, allowing a better clinical patient control, that will be discussed later. With some delay, nephrologists also started to use urea kinetic modelling for the evaluation of adequacy of CAPD (161–163).

As urea not only reflects solute retention and removal, but also protein break-down, and hence intake, high blood urea nitrogen before dialysis not necessarily reflects inadequate dialysis, but possibly high protein intake, and hence good metabolic status. High pre-dialysis urea may therefore be related to a better survival and a better quality of life than a low value. Low urea reduction ratios during dialysis, are on the contrary associated with increased odds ratios for death (160).

Creatinine

Creatinine, a product of muscle break-down, is progressively retained during uraemia. The rise in serum creatinine during renal failure is not linearly related to the decrease in glomerular filtration (GFR), that may decrease by 50% or more without marked changes in serum creatinine. Changes become more prominent in the lower range of filtration. Creatinine clearances are often used as a more accurate parameter of GFR, however, associated with an overestimation of true GFR, due to tubular secretion of creatinine. This would be no problem if this tubular secretion showed some parallellism with the evolution of

GFR, but unfortunately such a correlation is totally lacking.

There are virtually no convincing arguments in favor of a toxic effect of creatinine, although it may be a precursor of the toxic compound methylguanidine (164).

As serum creatinine is not only the resultant of uraemic retention but also of muscular break-down, a high serum creatinine may be at the same time a marker of muscular mass, and hence metabolic well-being. Low morbidity and mortality has in haemodialysed patients been demonstrated to be directly and positively correlated with high creatinine concentration, hence, the higher serum creatinine, the better patient outcome (165).

Pseudouridine

Pseudouridine is accumulated in uraemia in parallel to creatinine (166). Until recently, no convincing evidence could be found for the toxicity of this solute, but in a recent paper, Dzúrik et al. demonstrated inhibition of glucose utilization in isolated rat soleus muscle at the level of Ca^{++}-modulation in the insulin regulatory cascade (64). Other pyrimidine derivatives, such as orotic acid, orotidine, uridine and thymine are also accumulated in uraemia, the concentration of orotic acid and orotidine being further enhanced after allopurinol administration (167).

Methylguanidine and other guanidines

Methylguanidine, when injected to healthy dogs, causes a picture of heavy intoxication, characterized by anorexia, vomiting, diarrhea, gastric ulceration and polyneuritis (168, 169). *In vitro* brain Na^+, K^+-ATPase of uraemic rats (170) and heart cell contractility of guinea pigs (158) are inhibited. Generally, guanidines are believed to be only toxic in concentrations that are higher than those found in uraemic patients. Guanidinosuccinic acid and methylguanidine are however present in uraemic serum at levels that are currently toxic *in vitro* (171). Guanidinosuccinic acid has been shown to interfere with activation of ADP-induced platelet factor 3 (172) at concentrations currently found in haemodialysed uraemics (173, 174). Guanidines may also be related to uraemic polyneuropathy and have experimentally been shown to be epileptogenic (168, 175). A mixture of guanidino-compounds was shown to suppress the natural killer cell response to interleukin-2 (51). Guanidinosuccinic acid suppresses the production rate of calcitriol (111).

Methylguanidine distributes over several body pools. In spite of a molecular weight of only 73 Daltons, its intradialytic behavior is comparable to that of larger molecules (176). Similar kinetics are seen with guanidinosuccinic acid and other guanidines.

Indoxyl sulfate

Indoxyl sulfate, an indole derivative, is found at high concentrations in uraemic serum, however to a large extent bound to protein. Indoxyl sulfate has been associated with decreases in drug protein binding (121), and to defects of cellular organic acid transport (177).

Reduction of serum indoxyl sulfate concentration, by intra-intestinal absorption of the precursor indole, reduced uraemic itching (178). Indoxyl sulfate is not removed effectively during haemodialysis, due to its high protein binding (179). Removal by CAPD is more effective (180).

Due to its substantial protein binding (about 100% in normals, and 90% in uraemics), it has an intradialytic behavior that is not typical of other small, water soluble compounds such as creatinine. For example, the percentage removal for creatinine during one haemodialysis session was reported to be approximately 50%, compared to about 0 to 20% for indoxyl sulfate (152, 180). Under certain conditions, even a rise in indoxyl sulfate concentration has been observed during dialysis. This may be related to the competitive release of indoxyl sulfate from protein binding sites by heparin-induced increases in free fatty acid concentration and/or by the competition for protein binding sites with other uraemic retention solutes.

Myo-inositol

A decrease of sciatic nerve conduction velocity was found in rats given myo-inositol (181), pointing to a possible role in peripheral neuropathy. In uraemic nervous tissue (cauda equina nerve) an increased concentration of myo-inositol has been found (182). Myo-inositol also inhibited proliferation of Schwann cells, as estimated from their [^{3}H]-thymidine uptake, again pointing to neurotoxicity (183).

Apart from these reports, there are not many arguments in the recent literature in favor of the toxicity of this compound.

Hippuric acid

Hippuric acid interferes with several biochemical functions. Already in 1975, Boumendil-Podevin et al. demonstrated that hippuric acid inhibits para-amino-hippurate and uric acid transport at the cortical tubular level (177), suggesting that hippuric acid might interfere with the transport of a variety of organic acids. Especially the renal tubules, the chorioid plexus of the brain, the ciliary body of the eye, the thyroid, the liver and erythrocytes might be sensitive to this influence (184).

It was also demonstrated by Porter et al. that hippuric acid causes net fluid secretion in proximal straight tubules isolated from rabbit kidneys (185). Indirect data reported by MacNamara et al. (121), and by Gulyassy et al. (122), and more direct studies from the authors on ultrafiltrate collected in dialysed patients (119), demonstrated an interference of hippuric acid with the protein binding of drugs, such as phenytoin and theophylline. Finally, according to Dzúrik et al., hippurate interferes with glucose tolerance (63).

In parallel to indoxyl sulfate, hippuric acid (MW: 179D) behaves like a larger molecule, due to its protein binding; protein binding even tends to increase during dialysis (186).

Hippuric acid belongs to a large group of related compounds; its intradialytic behaviour might be representative for large groups of uraemic substances in a more accurate way than some current markers of uraemia, like urea or creatinine (152), were it not that no information is available about the concentration that should be pursued.

Ortho-hydroxyhippuric acid

Ortho-hydroxyhippuric acid is a substance with structural relationship to hippurate. It can be considered as a middle molecule (187, 188) in spite of its molecular weight, due to its protein binding. Ortho-hydroxyhippuric acid interferes with defective binding of acid drugs to serum albumin (189). The glycine conjugate is excreted at an increased rate in the urine of patients with enhanced catabolism (190). Possible precursors are compounds in the tyrosine-dopa-catecholamine pathway, but also salicylate; as salicylate abuse was current in uraemics at the moment of the detection of ortho-hydroxyhippuric acid, this finding casts some doubts on its endogenous toxicity.

Para-hydroxyhippuric acid

Another compound with structural relationship to hippurate is para-hydroxyhippuric acid. Up to now, no real biochemical effects have been attributed to this compound. One of the major non-identified compounds eluting on HPLC of uraemic serum (peak 6) was identified as para-hydroxyhippuric acid (191), and its possible role as a marker has been pointed out (193).

Phenylacetylglutamine

Phenylacetylglutamine, a metabolite of phenylalanine, is found in increased concentrations in uraemic plasma and ultrafiltrate (194), but to our knowledge no toxicity was demonstrated. Removal pattern and inter- and intradialytic kinetics are more conform with hippuric acid than with urea and creatinine (195).

Peptides

Peptides constitute a heterogenous group. Unless their structure is exactly known, isolation and identification remains complex and labor intensive. Several peptides have been shown to be retained in uraemia (196). Peptides may also influence biochemical functions.

Abiko et al., were able to isolate a peptide from the haemodialysate of a uraemic patient with immunodeficiency, that inhibited lymphocyte stimulation (197). The same polypeptide was also shown to interfere with rosette forming capacity, proliferation of T-cells and induction of suppressor cells (198). Conflicting results on the retention of endorphins have been reported (199, 200). If uraemic retention of endorphins occurs, they might interfere with neurologic and immunologic functions.

Concentration changes of vasoactive peptides may play a role in the regulation of blood pressure in uraemic patients. Endothelin has been isolated in 1988 (201), and is especially retained in patients with hypertension (202). Calcitonin gene-related peptide (CGRP) is a potent vasodilator (203). The concentration of atrial natriuretic factor (ANF-atriopeptide), may be elevated in uraemia, especially in fluid overload, e.g. before the start of haemodialysis (204, 205). Although this factor might be protective against pulmonary edema by inducing peripheral vasodilatation, it may also cause third spacing, which is a non-desired by-effect. The effect of haemodialysis on vasoactive peptide concentration has recently been evaluated (206): whereas endothelin decreased only with high flux dialyzers and CGRP only with polyacrilonitrile, atriopeptide decreased with all types of dialyzers, irrespective of their pore size, due to decrease of volume overload.

Break-down products of larger protein moieties like parathormone, are a potential source for the production of various peptides (207). Two polypeptides, extracted from ultrafiltrate from haemodialysed patients, one of which showing structural homology with a part of the β_2-microglobulin moiety, were shown by Hörl and coworkers to have immune-suppressive properties (208, 209).

Most peptides have multicompartment kinetics during haemodialysis.

Parathormone

Parathormone (PTH), a middle molecule with a molecular weight of $\pm$ 9,000 Daltons is now recognized as a uraemic toxin, mainly due to the efforts of Massry and his coworkers. It is oversecreted during uraemia as a result of an abortive effort of the organism to correct for hypocalcaemia and hyperphosphataemia. Hyperparathyroidism can be prevented or attenuated by the timely correction of these disturbances. Recent data suggest that elevation of serum phosphate affects PTH levels only in half of haemodialysis patients, the non-responders possibly being characterized by aluminum accumulation (210).

Hyperparathyroidism will result in:
1. increase in intracellular calcium;
2. a change in membrane permeability, integrity and phospholipid turnover;
3. a stimulation of cyclic AMP production;
4. soft tissue calcification, related to a raised calcium-phosphorus product;
5. protein catabolism (211).

PTH is related to glucose intolerance probably by suppressing insulin secretion which would be a normal response to the insulin resistant state (211). Remuzzi et al. documented an inhibition of human platelet function (212). PTH induces cardiomyopathy (213) due to a disturbance of fatty acid metabolism. Skeletal muscle fatty acid oxidation is similarly affected (214). Pancreatic glucose-induced insulin release is disturbed as a result of a rise of resting levels of cytosolic Ca^{++} of islet cells (99). Potassium-induced insulin release is disturbed (215). Further inhibitory effects are related to erythropoiesis (216), heart cell contractility (217), red cell osmotic resistance (21), synaptosome function (218, 219), T-cell function (220), B-cell proliferation (221) and fatty acid oxidation (222).

Although PTH manifests itself as a virtually ubiquitous uraemic toxin, affecting a myriad of biological functions, it certainly is only a part of the explanation of the complex defects occurring during uraemia.

The molecular weight of PTH fully conforms with that of the classical middle molecules. Its concentration is the result of a number of compensatory mechanisms ('trade off'), increasing production in response to hypovitaminosis D, hypocalcaemia and hyperphosphataemia. Although PTH removal by dialysis has a rather weak influence on concentration (223), serum PTH can be an indirect parameter of long-term adequacy of dialysis, since its production is related to long-term phosphate accumulation.

Beta 2-microglobulin (β_2-M)

β_2-Microglobulin (MW $\pm$ 11,000 D) also conforms with the most strict, classical definition of middle molecules. β_2M, a break-down product of the major histocompatibility antigen, is accumulated in renal failure (224) and distributes as an unbound monomer in two body water compartments: plasma and interstitial fluid (225).

It is not clear whether some feedback mechanism exists for the generation of β_2-M. The amyloidosis, frequently registered after prolonged dialysis, is caused by a local deposition of β_2-M (226, 227). β_2-M amyloidosis only presents after a prolonged period of exposure. It is not entirely clear, whether this disorder is related to accumulation as such: a chronic inflammatory state due to membrane or dialysate contact in haemodialysis may equally play a role.

The evolution of β_2-M concentration during dialysis is different with different types of dialyzers (228). Haemodialysis with dialyzers with low biocompatibility towards complement and leukocytes and a small pore size, like cuprophane, are characterized by a rise in β_2-M concentration, due to haemoconcentration, without removal (229). Considering dialyzers with identical pore size where leukocyte activation is minimized, the latter biocompatibility related fact does not influence intradialytic β_2-M concentration in a significant way. These data suggest that at least intradialytic concentration is rather related to the interplay of removal and haemoconcentration than to extra production due to bioincompatibility. Removal only occurs during dialysis with high flux dialyzers (230), but even those eliminate only a minor fraction of the total body β_2-M pool per dialysis.

Patients treated solely by open polyacrylonitrile (AN69) membranes have less signs of bone amyloidosis than those treated by cellulosic membranes (231). It is not clear whether these results are best attributed to better elimination or, rather, to lower generation in the context of better biocompatibility.

Thus, the exact patho-physiology of β_2-M amyloidosis remains undefined. Intradialytic elimination and enhanced production in relation to neutrophil break-down after membrane contact may be of less importance. Overall concentration, mainly influenced by residual renal function, and the chronic inflammatory state related to some types of dialysis and to contact with contaminated dialysate, are probably more important contributing factors. Nevertheless, β_2-M amyloidosis develops in patients treated by peritoneal dialysis (232), and in patients treated during a substantial period of time with dialyzers containing membranes with a low complement and leukocyte activating capacity (233).

Polyamines

Spermine is a polycationic polyamine, which inhibits erythropoiesis (23). Other polyamines like spermidine, putrescine and cadaverine, also found in increased concentration in renal failure, inhibit erythroid colony formation in a dose dependent manner (25). Polyamines have a high affinity for body proteins and cells. They play a role in anorexia, vomiting, ataxia, seizures, hypothermia and immune deficiency (234). Possible adverse effects at the cellular level are:

1. changes in cAMP messenger activity;
2. inhibition of receptor recycling by plasma membrane sequestration;
3. disturbed regulation of cellular calcium entry and/or distribution;
4. inhibition of protein kinase;
5. disturbances of protein synthesis;
6. depression of cellular response to activating stimuli (234).

Purines

Uric acid is related to gout. In spite of high serum concentrations in uraemia, gout is rarely observed, except in association with lead toxicity. Several other purine analogues are also retained in uraemia: xanthine and hypoxanthine have been implicated as modulators of neurotransmission and may be related to poor appetite and weight loss (235). Recently, the purines were demonstrated to be involved in disturbances of both calcitriol production and metabolization, with the emphasis on production (113). Administration of allopurinol to chronic renal failure patients resulted in a rise of plasma calcitriol levels, in association to a fall in plasma uric acid (236).

In young children with chronic renal failure, cytidine is found in cerebrospinal fluid in concentrations that are at least ten times higher than normal, and that are also higher than the corresponding concentrations in blood (237). This finding has been related to delayed cognitive development, albeit on indirect arguments.

Phenols and indoles

Substantial retention of phenols and indoles in uraemia has been recognized since long (238–241). Our knowledge in this area became more fundamental by the availability of HPLC-techniques, allowing the separation, identification and evaluation of their concentration.

Phenolic acids were shown to suppress several enzyme systems related to cerebral metabolism, especially respiration and anaerobic glycolysis (242). Rabiner and Molinas attributed a role to phenol and phenolic acids in the thrombocytopathy and the defective platelet aggregation of uraemia (243). P-cresol was shown to inhibit cerebral oxygen uptake, as well as oxygen uptake in liver slices (244). Phenol depressed various functional parameters of vital enzymatic activity in polymorphonuclear leukocytes (245). A depressive effect of phenol was demonstrated on the 3':5'-cyclic monophosphate response of the neostriatum to dopamine (246). This effect was abolished after conjugation of phenol to phenylglucoronide. These findings may be relevant to hepatic and uraemic coma. The authors could recently demonstrate an inhibitory effect of p-cresol and phenol on respiratory burst response to phagocytosis (247). Metabolic effects may also be related to their activity as free radical scavengers (248), causing inadequate bacterial killing.

Phenols and cresols are lipophilic compounds, with a low molecular weight in the range of 90–110 Daltons. Due to their chemical characteristics, they are protein bound and show a multicompartmental distribution.

Indoles, especially indole-3-acetic acid, are plant growth hormones (249), but, on the other hand, indole derivatives, e.g. indole-3-carbinol, are known as tumor growth inhibitors (250, 251). The relevance for human pathology is as yet unknown.

Trace elements

Trace elements may accumulate in uraemia. Sources are dialysate, food intake, drugs or prosthetic materials. Accumulation is then enhanced by insufficient renal elimination.

The most current example is aluminum; excess accumulation is due to presence in the dialysate, and excessive intake of aluminiumhydroxide as a phosphate binder. It results in mental changes (aluminum encephalopathy), and the cation aluminum competes with calcium in the bone matrix, resulting in osteomalacia.

Other elements, like copper, iron, cadmium, mercury and molybdene may also be accumulated (252, 253). In recent studies, retention of arsenicum was evidenced in a substantial segment of the uraemic population (253, 254). For some trace elements a decreased concentration is observed: zinc, bromine, selenium, rubidium and cesium have been reported (253, 255–258).

Organic phosphates

A high level of organic phosphates may be related to itching. Accumulation stimulates parathyroid activity, resulting in hyperparathyroidism. Until recently, hyperphosphataemia was currently corrected by the administration of aluminum containing phosphate binders, that in turn exerted toxicity.

Phosphorus concentration is the result of protein intake and catabolism as well as other dietary phosphate sources. Intradialytic kinetics are not straightforward and are not comparable to those of urea, creatinine or uric acid (259). Dialytic phosphate removal is followed by a marked rebound (260), suggesting multicompartmental behavior and does not correlate with urea elimination. As a marker, its behavior is too specific, and not representative of other compounds.

Urofuranic acids

The compound of this group that attracted most attention is 3-carboxy-4-methyl-5-propyl-2-furanpropionic acid (CMPF), originally described by Mabuchi and Nakahashi as 'Factor P' (123). This factor was later identified by Takeda et al. (261). Its main effect is a strong inhibition of drug protein binding. Due to its own important protein binding (98–100% both in healthy subjects and uraemics), it is not removed by haemodialysis but well by haemoperfusion and CAPD (180, 262). Mabuchi and Nakahashi demonstrated a suppressive effect on hepatic glutathione S-transferases (263), whereas Niwa et al. also showed dose dependent inhibition of ADP-stimulated oxidation of NADH-linked substrate in isolated mitochondria, even in the presence of appropriate concentrations of serum albumin (264).

Pesticides

Pesticides, probably entering the blood stream from dialysate, may accumulate in uraemia (265) and are possibly related to toxic side effects, such as polyneuropathy.

Carcinogenic heterocyclic amines

A remarkable discovery is the registration of an increased accumulation of several imidazole derivatives in uraemia (Glu-P-1 and Glu-P-2), known to have a carcinogenic effect (266). This would suggest a decreased elimination of these amines in uraemia, and indicates that uraemic patients are continuously exposed to the carcinogenic properties of these substances. They may contribute to the depressed DNA repair ability registered in peripheral lymfocytes of chronic renal failure patients (115), although this defect was missing in dialysed uraemic patients.

Hyaluronic acid

Hyaluronic acid is elevated above the normal range in 90% of patients with chronic renal failure (267). Concentrations do not correlate with serum creatinine, but show a significant correlation with serum β_2-microglobulin. High values are especially found in patients with deteriorating clinical condition. The molecule presents mainly in two forms, one with molecular weight > 1 million Daltons, a second depolymerized form having a molecular weight of 25 kD. Data regarding potential toxicity are to our knowledge not available.

Glomerulopressin

Circulating levels of glomerulopressin, a small molecular weight (< 500 D) hepatic hormone, which increases glomerular capillary pressure and enhances glomerular filtration rate (268), are elevated in chronic renal failure (269). Removal by dialysis is 75% that of urea. Production may be stimulated by increased dietary protein ingestion (270), so that this hormone might at least in part be related to the progressive deterioration of renal function in relation to high protein intake.

These data may somehow be connected with the finding that uraemic toxin(s) induce(s) the progressive loss of intact nephrons in rats with chronic renal failure (81). A compound with renotropic activity was recently extracted and partially purified from plasma of uninephrectomized subjects (271).

Oxalate

Increased plasma oxalate, causing the deposition of calcium oxalate in various tissues, is correlated with time on dialysis, and occurs in spite of increased removal by haemodialysis, compared to normal kidney function (272).

Conjugates of ascorbic acid

Gallice et al. detected after multistep gel-chromatic separation associated to nuclear magnetic resonance (NMR) spectroscopy, various conjugates of ascorbic acid in a middle molecular fraction (273). One of these was identified as ascorbic acid$_2$-sulfate. The question arises how the metabolism is triggered to conjugate an essentially water soluble compound. No toxicity was demonstrated up to now.

Trihalomethanes

Trihalomethanes, entering in dialysate as they may be present in tap water and as they are not entirely eliminated by water treatment systems, are found in increased concentration in blood of haemodialysed patients (274). They are potentially carcinogenic and neurotoxic.

Dimethylarginine

Asymmetrical dimethylarginine (N^G,N^G-dimethylarginine, ADMA) is an endogenous structure analogue of L-arginine, the latter compound being a precursor of nitric oxide (NO)-synthesis. NO-synthesis is blocked by excess ADMA accumulation in the blood, which is the case in chronic renal failure (275). Since NO has been held responsible for systemic peripheral vasodilation, NO-blockade in uraemia may contribute to the development of hypertension.

Nitric oxide

Nitric oxide (NO) per se may exert its own toxicity. The compound is a potent vasodilator which also inhibits platelet adhesion and may be responsible for dialysis hypotension. Prolonged bleeding time in uraemic rats normalizes by the administration of the NO-synthesis inhibitor N-monomethyl-L-arginine (L-NMMA) (276), pointing to the possible role of excessive NO synthesis in uraemic bleeding. In a recent study, Noris et al. demonstrated that uraemic platelets generated more NO than control platelets, and that uraemic plasma induced NO synthesis (29). These data are seemingly in contradiction with those reported by Vallance et al. (275), who emphasize on the patho-physiologic role of endogenous NO-inhibitors (see above). However, *in vivo* concentrations in uraemia of these NO-inhibitors apparently do not reach active concentration (29). Nitric oxide and its congeners may also contribute to neurotoxicity (277).

Methylamines

Di- and trimethylamines are retained in uraemia, and intracellular concentration is even higher than concentration in plasma (278). Apart from a study by Maxfield et al. (279), demonstrating *in vitro* inhibition of fibroblast cellular function, data on toxicity is lacking.

Complement factor D

Complement factor D is accumulated in uraemia, essentially due to a diminution of its renal elimination (280, 281). This is one of the factors potentially responsible for the hyperactivability of the complement system in chronic renal disease.

Melatonin and 6-sulfatoxymelatonin

The pineal hormone melatonin may play a role in the regulation of the hypothalamic-pituitary axis, target gland function, sleep pattern, mood changes, cellular immunity, antibody response, skin pigmentation, all of which are altered in end-stage renal disease. Vaziri et al. however found no differences in early morning serum melatonin and its metabolite 6-sulfatoxymelatonin between healthy subjects and dialysed uraemics (282). In addition, haemodialysis had no effect on the concentration of these compounds. The fluctuating concentration pattern, normally occurring in healthy subjects, was however, missing in dialysed uraemics (282).

Organic chloramines

Organic chloramines are created by the chemical binding of hypochlorite, produced as a free radical after leukocyte activation with retained organic compounds (283). They have a longer life-span than genuine hypochlorite. In as far as binding occurs with liposoluble compounds, e.g. spermine or spermidine (284), removal by haemodialysis will be hampered, whereas the capacity to penetrate cellular membranes and to cause toxic metabolic effects will be enhanced.

Homocysteine

Hyperhomocysteinemia has been reported to occur in renal failure and to increase in inverse relation to the evolution of renal function (285). Hyperhomocysteinemia has also been shown to be a risk factor for premature arterial occlusion, which is a frequent complication of chronic renal failure (286).

Middle molecules and middle molecule-like substances

Middle molecules are hypothetical uraemic toxins with a molecular weight roughly between 300 and 12,000 Daltons (287), but when strictly adhering to the definition proposed in the seventies, it may be extremely difficult to name more than a few uraemic retention solutes that conform with this definition (Tables 5 and 7). It should be stressed that most of the basic data emanating from the 'middle molecule' or the 'square meter hour hypothesis' were based on *in vitro* data and on the kinetics of a non-uraemic marker with a molecular weight within the middle molecular range: vitamin B_{12} (MW: 1353 D).

The major problem was thus the lack of well defined representative solutes of middle molecular range that could serve as a marker. With improved analytical techniques, it became evident that presumed middle molecular fractions are in fact heterogenous mixtures containing many lower molecular weight compounds (132). The reason why those molecules behave like middle molecules during haemodialysis and on chromatography, may be that molecular weight is only one factor influencing solute behavior in uraemia. Factors which play an additional role include: electrostatic charge, hydrophilicity/phobicity, steric configuration, protein binding, multicompartmental behavior, and resistance of cell membranes towards gradient dependent solute transfer. Each of these factors may slow intradialytic solute movement, either from the plasma to the dialysate compartment or from the intracellular compartment to the plasma. As a result, a removal pattern may be found that is comparable to that of larger molecules; *thus the definition of middle molecules may be extended to much smaller molecules with protein binding and/or multicompartmental distribution.* In spite of the fact that we do not have an exact name for the molecules that are present in the middle molecular fractions, there are a number of biochemical

arguments that support their toxicity. Failure of the early peritoneal dialysis patients to develop neuropathy, in spite of their higher blood urea concentrations, suggested that the peritoneum is more permeable to larger molecules than haemodialysis membranes (136). In at least 10 studies in haemodialysed patients, reduction of urea elimination, coupled to an unchanged or enhanced 'middle molecule' removal, caused no deterioration of clinical condition (288). Most studies were however uncontrolled, involved small patient groups, and occurred over short periods.

Up to now, dialysis efficacy is most currently evaluated by kinetic behavior of urea, a small, water soluble compound, with an intradialytic evolution far away from that of 'middle molecules', whatsoever their definition. This is the result of the large multicenter effort from the American National Cooperative Dialysis Study (NCDS) (159). The above-mentioned facts underscore the need for a large multicenter study, where, in parallel to the NCDS, the impact on morbidity and mortality is evaluated with a better differentiation between small versus large molecule removal. It should be recalled that in the NCDS, length of dialysis, which is related to middle molecule removal, had a significant effect on morbidity within the high TAC_{urea} groups. On this basis, it has been recommended choosing a membrane with good clearance rates for high as well as low molecular weight solutes.

In several recent uraemic toxicity studies, it was observed that lipophilic and/or protein bound compounds interfere with manifold biochemical functions (133), a finding that supports the hypothesis that the uraemic syndrome is the result of more than the accumulation of small, non-protein bound, water-soluble compounds (such as urea).

Hörl et al. recently identified a high molecular weight compound with various immune inhibiting properties (209). More recently, this group also isolated from uraemic ultrafiltrate a structure homologue of β_2-microglobulin, with depressive effect on several aspects of immune response (208). Andress et al. described an inhibitor of osteoblast mitogenesis, with a molecular weight in the range between 750 and 900 Daltons, that inhibited osteoblast mitogenesis (78). If we use the broader definition of middle molecules which includes not only large solutes, but also small solutes with middle molecular behavior, a substantial number of known uraemic toxins will qualify as middle molecules (133, 134): methylguanidine and other guanidines, indoxyl sulfate, hippuric acid, peptides, parathormone, β_2-microglobulin, phenols, cresols, 3-carboxy-4-methyl-5-propyl-2-furanpropionic acid (CMPF), spermine and other polyamines (Table 5).

The concept of overall retention

Numerous identified and unidentified substances are retained in uraemia. All of them are potential toxins. In

Table 8. Factors influencing solute concentration in dialysed patients

Solute related factors
  Compartmental distribution
  Intracellular concentration
    Resistance of cell membrane
  Protein binding
  Electrostatic charge
  Steric configuration
  Molecular weight

Patient related factors
  Distribution volume and body weight
  Intake and generation
    Solute
    Metabolic precursors
  Residual renal function
  Access quality
  Absorption from intestine
  Haematocrit
  Blood viscosity

Dialysis related factors
  Dialysis time
  Interdialytic intervals
  Blood flow
    Mean blood flow
    Blood flow pattern
    Shear in dialyzer
  Dialysate flow
  Dialysate distribution
  Dialyzer surface
  Dialyzer volume
  Dialyzer membrane resistance
  Dialyzer pore size
  Dialyzer hydrophilicity/hydrophobicity
  Adsorption
    On the membrane
    On other constituents of the circuit
  Ultrafiltration rate
  Intradialytic changes in efficacy
  Changes with direct effect on solute related factors
    Blood pH
    Heparinization
    Free fatty acid concentration

view of the enormous amount of potential retention products, it is clear that our knowledge about toxic actions is incomplete.

The uraemic syndrome is the consequence of the cumulative retention of several different solutes with different action modes (89). Even if single functions are considered, a complex interwoven system is playing a role. Single compounds as such may be non-toxic. The uraemic syndrome is thus to be defined as the resultant of overall retention of solutes. Therefore, if treatment modalities like dialysis are considered, an optimum overall solute elimination should be pursued. Differences in overall retention and removal may occur in absence of differences in retention or removal of current marker compounds.

FACTORS INFLUENCING PLASMA CONCENTRATION OF URAEMIC SOLUTES

Multiple factors influence the concentration of uraemic solutes (Table 8) (288). A current example is urea: its concentration depends mainly on protein intake, general metabolic status, residual renal function, and dialysis performance; protein binding is virtually nil and urea is essentially distributed over the body water.

Most other substances are subjected to more complex rules, due to a multicompartmental distribution, effects of protein binding and production sources other than nutrition. The concentration of hippuric acid e.g. is influenced by the intake of foods and beverages containing sodium benzoate as a preservative, the break-down of phenylalanine or phenyl containing fatty acids with an odd number of carbon atoms, environmental contact with xylenes and/or toluenes, production by the intestinal flora, and endogenous production (192). Renal elimination is controlled both by the glomerular filtration and tubular processing. In dialysed patients, further production may result from the metabolization of benzyl alcohol used as a preservative in heparin solutions (186).

β_2-microglobulin is related to the expression of the HLA antigen on cells, and appears in the blood as a result of cellular break-down and shedding. A possible additional source of circulating β_2-microglobulin would be the cellular break-down of leukocytes after their activation during haemodialysis with non-biocompatible membranes; however there is no clear relationship between intradialytic neutropenia and β_2-microglobulin concentration (229). These levels rather seem to be influenced by the ultrafiltered volume, the dialyzer pore size, and by adsorption on the dialyzer membrane (289).

Uraemic solute elimination via the urine remains of physiologic importance, even once dialysis has been started. Assuming a GFR of 5 mL/min, the kidneys still clear ± 50 L per week, to be compared with a clearance of 100 to 150 L per week through artificial kidneys, if the relation between total dialyzer clearance and distribution volume (Kt/V) is taken as 1. At that moment, residual renal function still contributes substantially to overall clearance; when GFR falls to 1 mL/min, the weekly contribution of renal clearance drops to 10 L; once the stage

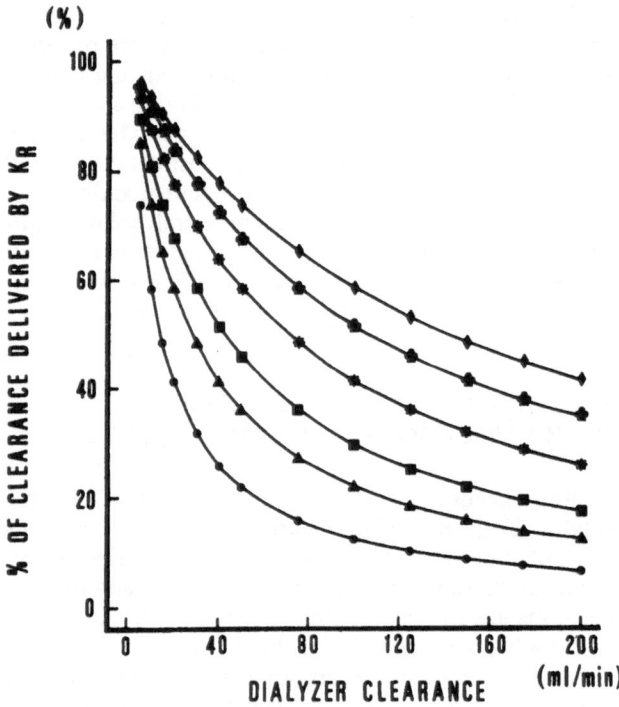

Figure 8. Percentage of total clearance delivered by residual renal clearance (K_R) in function of dialyzer clearance, for 3 ∗ 4 hours haemodialysis per week. Symbols are: (◆) K_R 10 mL/min; (♣) K_R 7.5 mL/min; (■) K_R 5 mL/min; (▲) K_R 2 mL/min; (●) K_R 1 mL/min. The contribution of K_R is related inversely to dialyzer clearance and is especially important for the lower dialyzer clearances. (Reproduced with permission from Vanholder and Ringoir, *Kidney Int* 42: 540, 1992.)

of anuria is reached, this contribution of course drops to zero (Figure 8).

DEFICIENCIES

The uraemic syndrome is not only defined by solute accumulation but also by deficiencies. Current examples of inadequate renal production are erythropietin and vitamine D deficiencies. Inadequate production by organs other than the kidney, plays a role in the inefficient secretion of several hormones. Deficient blood levels of trace elements have been observed. Current examples are bromine and zinc (258). Zinc deficiency has been related to immune deficiency, gonadal dysfunction and neurosensory changes (255).

Fibronectin, an opsonin enhancing phagocytic ingestion, has been demonstrated to be deficient in uraemia (43) although the causative factors are not clearly defined. This may play a role in the immunologic disturbances currently observed in uraemia, although other influencing factors are probably more important (36).

MARKERS OF URAEMIC RETENTION

Markers in non-dialysed patients

Serum concentrations of urea and creatinine are influenced by factors that are not related to renal function, like dietary protein intake, muscle mass, certain drugs affecting tubular secretion etc, so that their serum concentrations as such give an inaccurate estimation of glomerular filtration rate. Therefore, the determination of clearances is preferred.

Urea clearance being unreliable due to important tubular reabsorption, e.g. in volume depletion, creatinine clearance has become a standard procedure in the follow-up of renal function. Tubular secretion of creatinine currently results in an overestimation of glomerular filtration (290). Virtually all endogenous uraemic solutes show tubular secretion and/or reabsorption. Therefore, exogenous substances administered via injection or infusion (e.g. inulin, EDTA), are to be preferred for an exact estimation of glomerular filtration. Those give however no indication about tubular secretion. Therefore, the tubular secretion of creatinine is probably not a complete disadvantage for its use as a marker. In addition, decisions to start dialysis have always been based on experience with creatinine clearance: the use of true GFR estimates may incite to start dialysis earlier than when using creatinine clearance. Currently, the critical clearance before starting renal replacement therapy is accepted to be 5 mL/min, except for hypertensive or diabetic patients, although some authors propagate an earlier start (82).

Markers in dialysed patients

After the start of dialysis, the picture becomes even more complex. *In vitro* study of dialyzer clearances has been performed with creatinine, urea, inulin, vitamine B12 and EDTA as markers, the latter three substances being no genuine uraemic solutes, but substitutes for middle molecules, having the same hypothetical molecular weight.

Urea kinetic modelling

A reliable index of *in vivo* dialysis efficacy has been lacking, until the development of urea kinetic modelling in the context of the American National Cooperative Dialysis Study (NCDS), allowing a dynamic evaluation of the removal and production of urea. Urea kinetics allow the calculation of three critical parameters:
1. TAC_{urea}, the time averaged concentration of urea over a one week period;
2. PCR (protein catabolic rate), an index of dietary protein intake in equilibrated patients;
3. Kt/V, total clearance over distribution volume (291).

The expected normal values together with some figures obtained in the author's dialysis population and in the National Cooperative Dialysis Study are illustrated in Table 9. The NCDS showed definitely that urea kinet-

Table 9. Urea kinetic data obtained in the national dialysis cooperative study, in groups I and III (groups with low morbidity) and in the author's unit

	Group I	Group II	Own series	
			1989	1993
TAC$_{urea}$				
(mg/100 mL)	51 ± 1	54 ± 1	54 ± 1	–
PCR				
(g/kgBW 24 h)	0.8 to 1.4	0.8 to 1.4	1.0 ± 0.3	1.0 ± 0.2
Kt/V	> 0.9	> 0.9	1.1 ± 0.2	1.3 ± 0.3
Dialysis duration				
(min)	269 ± 3	199 ± 3	236 ± 13	232 ± 12
Dialyzer surface				
(m^2)	> 1.3	1.3	1.3 ± 2.8	> 1.3

Means ± SD. Abbreviations: TAC – time averaged concentration; PCR – protein catabolic rate; BW – body weight; Kt – total clearance; V – distribution volume; note the rise in Kt/V over time in the authors' series.

ic results that were divergent from these normal values, were related to a higher patient morbidity (159).

Dialyzer clearances should be obtained during the session where pre- and post-dialysis urea measurements are also obtained (292). These are the basic elements for an iterative calculation of *urea distribution volume* (V) and *generation rate* (G).

Once G is known, this can be transformed in *protein catabolic rate* (PCR) according to Borah et al. (293). In equilibrated patients PCR is considered as a parameter of protein intake. PCR is unreliable as an index of protein intake in overt catabolic or anabolic states (294), arousing some questions about its validity as an ubiquitous index of protein intake.

There is much debate whether computerized iteration should be used or not. Non-iteration presumes a fixed relation of V to body weight (e.g. 58%); this is however not necessarily the case in uraemia, so that this approach might give incorrect results.

In the iterative model, dialyzer clearance should be estimated directly, and corrected for recirculation. Sometimes, *in vitro* clearances procured by the manufacturer are used, currently resulting in an overestimation of the true clearance, and subsequently, of V, G and PCR.

A reliable and not too complex method in our hands has been the calculation of clearances based on pre- and post-dialysis urea concentrations and distribution volumes according to Watson et al. (295).

Another method is the one using dialysate and urea collection over a given period (direct quantification method) (296). This method is simple as a concept but has some practical drawbacks in view of the large volumes that are to be collected.

In our hands, each of the methods gave comparable results (297). The current calculations of urea kinetics are based on a single pool model, although urea follows two pool kinetics, especially during short high efficiency dialysis. A correction for this multicompartmental behaviour should be introduced in the calculations. A rebound phenomenon at the end of dialysis is obvious, especially after short dialysis, due to ongoing shifts from the tissue stores to the blood. Although for current dialysis a Kt/V of 1 to 1.2 should be pursued for urea, therefore, during short dialysis, the aim should be 20–30% higher. The concept of an ideal Kt/V, with a threshold value, above which morbidity reaches a plateau, has been challenged. Keshaviah and Collins, reconsidering the NCDS database, claim that morbidity linearly declines as Kt/V increases, and that there is no optimum Kt/V (298). In analogy, Shen and Hsu found a hospitalization rate to be inversely proportional to Kt/V (299). It is clear that threshold values for calculation of Kt/V have been increased progressively over time.

A drawback of urea kinetics is that the basic experience was gained with cellulosic dialyzers with a small pore size, that are incompatible versus the leukocyte-complement system (40, 300) and possibly have a catabolic effect (301). Other dialyzers with a larger pore size and a better compatibility may be characterized by a better overall solute elimination in spite of similar urea kinetics. Those may require a lower delivery of urea clearance and/or PCR than cuprophane (302). There is an urgent need for prospective studies analyzing this issue.

Incomplete delivery of dialysis prescription (303) induces, when not recognized, flaws in kinetic calculations. Errors in registration of dialysis time due to connection, disconnection, turning down the blood flow and interruptions, manufacturer clearances that overestimate true clearance, dialysis devices that overestimate true blood flow, and lack of correction of recirculation, all will result in a misconception of dialysis dose, and hence of G and V (304–306).

It should also not be forgotten that urea kinetics are nothing more than an index of dialysis efficiency. They give no estimation of clinical condition. A clinical deterioration, even in the presence of perfect urea kinetics, should rather suggest an error in the kinetic modelling than an error in the interpretation of the clinical status. Moreover, calculations should be performed carefully, and according to appropriate methods. On the other hand, kinetic modelling may be of help demonstrating changes in dialysis adequacy, in the absence of overt clinical signs of underdialysis, e.g. in the case of erythropoietin administration, whereby anaemia is eliminated as one of the cardinal signs of patient non-wellbeing.

In a recent paper, care has been advocated with the use of commercial packages for the determination of urea kinetics, as substantial differences in the results were registered (307).

Alternatives

Finally, one should dissect the validity of urea as a marker for the removal and generation of other uraemic toxins. This may be the case for other, small and water soluble compounds, such as uric acid, pseudouridine and creatinine, but most of these have no or only weak proven toxicity. Among the compounds with proven toxicity, there are many substances with different hydrophilicity and higher molecular weight, compared to urea (Table 5) (133, 134). On the other hand, its generation can only be representative for the compounds that result solely and purely from protein break-down. Again many toxins do not conform with this rule. Hence, one may question the validity of urea as an ubiquitous marker. There is an urgent need for alternative markers, being representative for the larger/hydrophobic/protein-bound/multicompartmentally distributed molecules. Among those, the most valuable candidates today are hippuric acid and β_2-M, although we miss for both data about their concentration being related to clinical outcome (288). It may be necessary to evaluate a group of known and unknown compounds together, whereby HPLC of uraemic sera may turn out to be a valuable tool.

CONCLUSIONS

The uraemic syndrome is related to a complex set of biochemical and patho-physiological disturbances, resulting in a state of generalized malaise and dysfunction. It is related to the retention of a host of compounds, due to altered glomerular filtration and other factors of renal dysfunction. Although solute accumulation is one of the major patho-physiologic events, deficiencies may play a role as well. A host of substances are accumulated in renal failure, and many of them exert a negative effect on physiological and biochemical functions, subsequently being identified as uraemic toxins. The uraemic syndrome appears to be the result of the overall accumulation of multiple interfering factors, rather than of one single substance. The concept of overall retention, and of overall elimination during dialysis, thus appears to be important. Current markers of uraemia, such as urea and creatinine, may be less relevant in this context.

Solute clearance eventually reaches a plateau as dialyzer blood flow and/or dialysate flow are increased; this plateau is reached much sooner for molecules with a higher molecular weight. As a result, clearance of middle molecules *stricto sensu* is relatively blood and dialysate flow independent. Removal of middle molecules as originally defined, can be enhanced mainly by increasing dialysis time, dialyzer surface area, ultrafiltration rate and/or dialyzer pore size.

For solutes that behave like larger molecules due to their protein binding, multicompartmental distribution and/or lipophilicity, removal will be less affected by the use of high flux dialyzers and/or dialyzers with a larger pore size. To improve clearances of these 'new definition' middle molecules, it may be necessary to develop renal replacement systems with different characteristics, e.g. specific adsorption systems and/or procedures that allow a slower exchange of solutes. Adsorption of protein bound compounds may make the difference, although some lipophilic compounds may not be protein bound and necessitate alternative extraction and adsorption procedures. The question arises however whether this increase in efficacy will be sufficient to induce a perceptible difference in toxic phenomena.

Removal and generation can hardly be predicted by urea, a small water soluble compound generated from protein, whereas most of these other toxins are hydrophobic and/or not generated from protein break-down. To improve clearances of 'new definition' middle molecules, it may be necessary to develop renal replacement strategies with newly conceived characteristics, e.g. specific adsorption systems and/or procedures that allow a slower exchange of solutes.

It is clear that CAPD is better in the elimination of protein bound solutes, not only because of a more gradual exchange than with conventional haemodialysis, but also because some protein is lost in the dialysate. The solute exchange for the other newer, continuous dialysis strategies, such as continuous arteriovenous haemofiltration (CAVH) and haemodialysis (CAVHD), is also more gradual than with intermittent haemodialysis, so that removal of middle molecules or middle molecule-like compounds may be improved. Earlier work on charcoal adsorption, eventually largely abandoned, was perhaps not such a bad idea, especially for the removal of organic acids, among which there are probably numerous compounds with toxic characteristics. More specific adsorptive systems may be needed, however. As an alternative, adsorption of toxins or of their precursors may be pursued at the intestinal level. Using an adsorbent of indoles, Niwa et al. (178) could decrease indoxyl sulfate concentration, by the way reducing also the intensity of uraemic itching. Another alternative to be considered is dialysis against recycled albumin-containing dialysate solution, allowing a better diffusion of protein bound toxic compounds (308, 309), although cost of dialysate may become an important drawback here. It should nevertheless be considered that some of the known morbidity associated with dialysis may relate to the unphysiologic concentration of anions (acetate$^-$, D,L-lactate$^-$) and hence toxicity of dialysis fluids (309).

Finally, another alternative could be the use of protein permeable membranes, removing larger molecules as well as protein bound substances (310). The question that arises here is however whether the amount of removal will be sufficient to reduce uraemic toxicity.

Whether the cost of such procedures will outweigh the benefit remains a matter of debate. One should also consider the risk of introducing various compounds with potential toxicity, such as aluminum, by adding albumin to the dialysate, or by using adsorbents.

Another question is related to the follow-up of the retention and of the dialytic removal of these potentially toxic, mainly organic acid compounds. In this context, HPLC has become a valuable tool, since it allows the evaluation of concentration of several hydrophilic/hydrophobic compounds at a time (Table 6). Perhaps hippuric acid may become useful as a marker for the behavior of various organic acid compounds (152, 311), in view of its easy detection, and its relatively high free concentrations.

The role of peroral sorbents as an aid in decreasing toxin concentration should be further corroborated. Niwa et al. demonstrated significant concentration changes for the solutes indoxyl sulfate (178) and p-cresol (312) after the administration of an oral sorbent (AST-120).

What we really need is a more specific removal of uraemic toxins. However, for this to come to pass, we will need to know more about both the basic metabolic disturbances that take place in uraemia and about the toxic compounds responsible for the disturbances.

We are convinced that our views on how to enhance dialysis efficacy need to be changed. Increasing pore size, alone or in combination with adaptations in dialyzer geometry, is certainly not the only solution, and may not be a solution at all.

In the last decade, in spite of the introduction of various new strategies of dialysis, toxin removal was hardly improved (152). To pursue newer and efficient modes of elimination of uraemic toxins, some creativity will be needed.

REFERENCES

1. Prevost JL, Dumas JA: Examen du sang et de son action dans les divers phénomènes de la vie. *Ann Chimie et Physiol* 23: 90, 1821
2. Lazarus JM, Lowrie EG, Hampers CL, Merrill P: Cardiovascular disease in uremic patients on hemodialysis. *Kidney Int* 7: S167, 1975
3. Wray TM, Stone WJ: Uremic pericarditis: a prospective echocardiographic and clinical study. *Clin Nephrol* 6: 295, 1976
4. Parfrey PS, Harnett JD, Barre PE: The natural history of myocardial disease in dialysis patients. *J Am Soc Nephrol* 2: 2, 1991
5. Parfrey PS, Harnett JD, Griffiths SM, Gault MH, Barré PE: Congestive heart failure in dialysis patients. *Arch Intern Med* 148: 1519, 1988.
6. Rostand SG, Sanders C, Kirk KA, Rutsky EA, Fraser RG: Myocardial calcification and cardiac dysfunction in chronic renal failure. *Am J Med* 85: 651, 1988
7. Lindner A, Kenny M, Meacham A: Effects of a circulating factor in patients with essential hypertension on intracellular free calcium in normal platelets. *N Engl J Med* 316: 509, 1987
8. Mason MF, Resnik H, Minot AS, Rainey J, Pitcher C, Harrison TR: Mechanism of experimental uremia. *Arch Intern Med* 60: 312, 1937
9. Raab W: Cardiotoxic substance in the blood and heart muscle in uremia. *J Lab Clin Med* 29: 715, 1944
10. Rambausek M, Mann JFE, Mall G, Kreusser W, Ritz E: Cardiac findings in experimental uremia. *Contr Nephrol* 52: 125, 1986
11. Kong CH, Thompson FD: Hemodynamic responses to head-up tilt in uremic patients. *Clin Nephrol* 33: 283, 1990
12. Meggs LG, Ben-Ari J, Gammon D, Choudhury M, Goodman AI: Effect of chronic uremia on the cardiovascular alpha receptor. *Life Sciences* 39: 169, 1986
13. Mall G, Rambausek M, Neumeister A, Kollmar S, Vetterlein F, Ritz E: Myocardial interstitial fibrosis in experimental uremia – implications for cardiac compliance. *Kidney Int* 33: 804, 1988
14. Kramer W, Wizemann V, Kinder M, Thormann J: Urämische Herzkrankheit: Inzidenz und Klinische Wertigkeit nicht-invasiver kardialer Befunde bei dialysepflichtiger Niereninsuffizienz. *Med Welt* 36: 1228, 1985
15. Fraser CL, Arieff AI: Nervous system complications in uremia. *Ann Inter Med* 109: 143, 1988
16. Vanholder RC: Neuropsychiatric alterations in uraemia. in *Oxford Textbook of Clinical Nephrology*, edited by Cameron S, Davison AM, Grünfeld JP, Kerr DS, Ritz E, Oxford University Press, Oxford, 1992, p 1396
17. Kimmel PL, Miller G, Mendelson WB: Sleep apnea syndrome in chronic renal disease. *Am J Med* 86: 308, 1989
18. Shvili Y, Gafter U, Zohar Y, Talmi YP, Levi J: Brainstem auditory evoked responses in rats with experimental renal failure. *Clin Science* 76: 415, 1989
19. Braguer D, Gallice P, Yatzidis H, Berland Y, Crevat A: Restoration by biotin of the *in vitro* microtubule formation inhibited by uremic toxins. *Nephron* 57: 192, 1991
20. Eschbach JW, Kelly MR, Haley NR, Abels RI, Adamson JW: Treatment of the anemia of progressive renal failure with recombinant human erythropoietin. *N Engl J Med* 321: 158, 1989
21. Bogin E, Massry SG, Levi J, Djaldetti M, Bristol G, Smith J: Effect of parathyroid hormone on osmotic fragility of human erythrocytes. *J Clin Invest* 69: 1017, 1982
22. Pavlovic-Kentera V, Clemons GK, Djukanovic L, Biljanovic-Paunovic L: Erythropoietin and anemia in chronic renal failure. *Exp Hematol* 15: 785, 1987
23. Radtke HW, Rege AB, La Marche MB, Bartos D, Bartos F, Campbell RA, Fischer JW: Identification of spermine as an inhibitor of erythropoiesis in patients with chronic renal failure. *J Clin Invest* 67: 1623, 1981
24. Segal GM, Stueve T, Adamson JW: Spermine and spermidine are non-specific inhibitors of *in vitro* hematopoiesis. *Kidney Int* 31: 72, 1987
25. Kushner D, Beckman B, Nguyen L, Chen S, Della Santina C, Husserl F, Rice J, Fisher JW: Polyamines in the anemia of end-stage renal disease. *Kidney Int* 39: 725, 1991
26. Ureña P, Bonnardeaux A, Eckardt KU, Kurtz A, Drüeke TB: Insulin-like growth factor I: a modulator of erythropoiesis in uraemic patients? *Nephrol Dial Transplant* 7: 40, 1992
27. Larsson SO: On coagulation and fibrinolysis in renal failure. *Scand J Haematol* 15 (Suppl): 1, 1971

28. Remuzzi G: Bleeding in renal failure. *Lancet* 1: 1205, 1988
29. Noris M, Benigni A, Boccardo P, Aiello S, Gaspari F, Todeschini M, Figliuzzi M, Remuzzi G: Enhanced nitric oxide synthesis in uremia: implications for platelet dysfunction and dialysis hypotension. *Kidney Int* 44: 445, 1993
30. Remuzzi G, Livio M, Marchiaro G, Mecca G, de Gaetano MG: Bleeding in renal failure: altered platelet function in chronic uraemia only partially corrected by haemodialysis. *Nephron* 22: 347, 1978
31. Di Minno G, Cerbone A, Usberti M, Cianciaruso B, Cortese A, Farace MJ, Martinez J, Murphy S: Platelet dysfunction in uremia. II. Correction by arachidonic acid of the impaired exposure of fibrinogen receptors by adenosine diphosphate or collagen. *J Lab Clin Med* 108: 246, 1986
32. Remuzzi G, Benigni A, Dodesini P, Schieppati A, Livio M, De Gaetano G, Day JS, Smith WL, Pinca E, Patrignani P, Patrono C: Reduced platelet thromboxane formation in uremia. Evidence for a functional cyclo-oxygenase defect. *J Clin Invest* 71: 762, 1983
33. Tison P, Cernacek P, Silvanova E, Dzúrik R: Uremic 'toxins' and blood platelet carbohydrate metabolism. *Nephron* 28: 192, 1981
34. Holloway DS, Vagher JP, Caprini JA, Simon NM, Mockros LF: Thrombelastography of blood from subjects with chronic renal failure. *Thromb Res* 45: 817, 1987
35. Warren RP, Hultin MB, Coller BS: Increased factor VIII/von Willebrand factor antigen and von Willebrand factor activity in renal failure. *Am J Med* 66: 226, 1979
36. Vanholder R, Ringoir S: Infectious morbidity and defects of phagocytic function in end-stage renal disease: a review. *J Am Soc Nephrol* 3: 1541, 1993
37. Goldblum SE, Reed WP: Host defenses and immunologic alterations associated with chronic hemodialysis. *Ann Int Med* 93: 597, 1980
38. Lewis SL, Van Epps DE: Neutrophil and monocyte alterations in chronic dialysis patients. *Am J Kidney Dis* 9: 381, 1987
39. Ponassi A, Morra L, Gurreri G, Moccia F, Giusti M, Caristo G, Sacchetti C: Alterations of granulopoiesis in chronic uremic patients treated with intermittent hemodialysis. *Acta Haematol* 77: 220, 1987
40. Vanholder R, Ringoir S, Dhondt A, Hakim R: Phagocytosis in uremic and hemodialysis patients: a prospective and cross sectional study. *Kidney Int* 39: 320, 1991
41. Vanholder R, Ringoir S: Polymorphonuclear cell function and infection in dialysis. *Kidney Int* 38: S91, 1992
42. Vanholder R, Van Biesen W, Ringoir S: Contributing factors to the inhibition of phagocytosis in hemodialyzed patients. *Kidney Int* 44: 208, 1993
43. Schena FP, Pertosa G: Fibronectin and the kidney. *Nephron* 48: 177, 1988
44. Flament J, Goldman M, Waterlot Y, Dupont E, Wybran J, Vanherweghem JL: Impairment of phagocyte oxidative metabolism in hemodialyzed patients with iron overload. *Clin Nephrol* 25: 227, 1986
45. Veys N, Vanholder R, Ringoir S: Correction of deficient phagocytosis during erythropoietin treatment in maintenance hemodialysis patients. *Am J Kidney Dis* 19: 358, 1992

46. Hörl WH, Haag-Weber M, Georgopoulos A, Block LH: Physicochemical characterization of a polypeptide present in uremic serum that inhibits the biological activity of polymorphonuclear cells. *Proc Natl Acad Sci USA* 87: 6353, 1990
47. Haag-Weber M, Mai B, Hörl WH: Isolation of a granulocyte inhibitory protein in uremia: homology to beta$_2$-microglobulin. *Nephrol Dial Transplant* 9: 382, 1994
48. Keane WF, Maddy MF: Host defense and infectious complications in maintenance hemodialysis patients. in *Replacement of Renal Function by Dialysis*, edited by Maher JF, Kluwer Academic Publishers, Dordrecht, 1989, p 865
49. Raskova J, Ghobrial I, Czerwinski DK, Shea SM, Eisinger RP, Raska K: B-cell activation and immunoregulation in end-stage renal disease patients receiving hemodialysis. *Arch Int Med* 147: 89, 1987
50. Langhoff E, Ladefoged J, Odum N: Effect of interleukin-2 and methylprednisolone on *in vitro* transformation of uremic lymphocytes. *Int Arch Allergy Applied Immunol* 81: 5, 1986
51. Asaka M, Iida H, Izumino K, Sasayama S: Depressed natural killer cell activity in uremia. *Nephron* 49: 291, 1988
52. Ladefoged J, Langhoff E: Accessory cell functions in mononuclear cell cultures from uremic patients. *Kidney Int* 37: 126, 1990
53. Hershkovitz R, Rathaus M, Mekori YA, Lider O, Bernheim J: Uraemic serum inhibits peripheral blood mononuclear cell and purified T-cell adhesion to extracellular matrix glycoproteins. *Nephrol Dial Transplant* 8: 951, 1993 (Abstract)
54. Girndt M, Köhler H, Schiedhelm-Weick E, Meyer zum Büschenfelde KH, Fleischer B: T cell activation defect in hemodialysis patients: evidence for a role of the B7/CD28 pathway. *Kidney Int* 44: 359, 1993
55. Baliga R, George VT, Ray PE, Holliday MA: Effects of reduced renal function and dietary protein on muscle protein synthesis. *Kidney Int* 39: 831, 1991
56. Mak RHK, DeFronzo RA: Glucose and insulin metabolism in uremia. *Nephron* 61: 377, 1992
57. De Fronzo RA, Andres R, Edgar P, Walker WG: Carbohydrate metabolism in uremia: a review. *Medicine (Baltimore)* 52: 469, 1973
58. Cecchin F, Ittoop O, Sinha MK, Caro JF: Insulin resistance in uremia: insulin receptor kinase activity in liver and muscle from chronic uremic rats. *Am J Physiol* 254: E394, 1988
59. Schmitz O, Arnfred J, Orskov L, Hother Nielsen O, Orskov H, Posborg V: Influence of hyperglycemia on glucose uptake and hepatic glucose production in nondialyzed uremic patients. *Clin Nephrol* 30: 27, 1988
60. Jacobs DB, Hayes GR, Truglia JA, Lockwood DH: Alterations of glucose transporter systems in insulin-resistant uremic rats. *Am J Physiol* 257: E193, 1989
61. Mak RHK: Intravenous 1,25 dihydrocholecalciferol corrects glucose intolerance in hemodialysis patients. *Kidney Int* 41: 1049, 1992
62. MacCaleb ML, Izzo MS, Lockwood DH: Characterization and partial purification of a factor from uremic human serum that induces insulin resistance. *J Clin Invest* 75: 391, 1985

63. Dzúrik R, Spustová V, Gerykova M: Pathogenesis and consequences of the alteration of glucose metabolism in renal insufficiency. in *Uremic Toxins*, edited by Ringoir S, Vanholder R, Massry SG, Plenum Press, New York, 1987, p 105

64. Dzúrik R. Spustová V, Lajdová I: Inhibition of glucose utilization in isolated rat soleus muscle by pseudouridine: implications for renal failure. *Nephron* 65: 108, 1993

65. Fadda GZ, Akmal M, Premdas FH, Lipson LG, Massry SG: Insulin release from pancreatic islets: effects of CRF and excess PTH. *Kidney Int* 33: 1066, 1988

66. Katz AI, Emmanouel DS: Metabolism of polypeptide hormones by the normal kidney and in uremia. *Nephron* 22: 69, 1978

67. Kalk WJ, Morley JE, Gold CH, Meyers A: Thyroid function tests in patients on regular hemodialysis. *Nephron* 25: 173, 1980

68. Elias AN, Vaziri ND, Pandian MR, Iyer K, Ansari MA: Dopamine and TSH secretion in uremic male rats. *Hormone Res* 27: 102, 1987

69. Lippe B, Fine RN, Koch VH, Sherman BM: Accelerated growth following treatment of children with chronic renal failure with recombinant human growth hormone (Somatrem): a preliminary report. *Acta Paed Scand* 343 (Suppl): 127, 1988

70. Ziegler TR, Lazarus JM, Young LS, Hakim R, Wilmore DW: Effects of recombinant human growth hormone in adults receiving maintenance hemodialysis. *J Am Soc Nephrol* 2: 1130, 1993

71. Chan W, Valerie KC, Chan JCM: Expression of insulin-like growth factor-1 in uremic rats: growth hormone resistance and nutritional intake. *Kidney Int* 43: 790, 1993

72. Bommer J: Sexual dysfunction in chronic renal failure. in *Oxford Textbook of Clinical Nephrology*, edited by Cameron S, Davison AM, Grunfeld JP, Kerr D, Ritz E, Oxford University Press, Oxford, 1992, p 1329

73. Biasioli S, Mazzali A, Foroni R, D'Andrea G, Feriani M, Chiaramonte S, Cesaro A, Micieli G: Chronobiological variations of prolactin (PRL) in chronic renal failure. *Clin Nephrol* 30: 86, 1988

74. Schaefer F, Stanhope R, Scheil H, Schönberg D, Preece MA, Schärer K: Pulsatile gonadotropin secretion in pubertal children with chronic renal failure. *Acta Endocrin* 120: 14, 1989

75. Ritz E, Matthias S, Seidel A, Reichel H, Szabo A, Hörl WH: Disturbed calcium metabolism in renal failure – pathogenesis and therapeutic strategies. *Kidney Int* 42: S37, 1992

76. Andress DL, Pandian MR, Endres DB, Kopp JB: Plasma insulin-like growth factors and bone formation in uremic hyperparathyroidism. *Kidney Int* 36: 471, 1989

77. Phillips LS, Fusco AC, Unterman TG, Del Greco F: Somatomedin inhibitor in uremia. *J Clin Endocrinol Metab* 59: 764, 1984

78. Andress DL, Howard GA, Birnbaum RS: Identification of a low molecular weight inhibitor of osteobast mitogenesis in uremic plasma. *Kidney Int* 39: 942, 1991

79. Hsu CH, Patel SR, Young EW: Mechanism of decreased calcitriol degradation in renal failure. *Am J Physiol* 262: F192, 1992

80. Ponticelli C, Bencini PL: Uremic pruritus: a review. *Nephron* 60: 1, 1992

81. Motojima M, Nishijima F, Ikoma M, Kawamura T, Yoshioka T, Fogo AB, Sakai T, Ichikawa I: Role for uremic toxins in the progressive loss of intact nephrons in chronic renal failure. *Kidney Int* 40: 461, 1991

82. Bonomini V, Feletti C, Stefoni S, Vangelista A: Early dialysis and renal transplantation. *Nephron* 44: 267, 1986

83. Vanholder R, Dell'Aquila R, Jacobs V, Dhondt A, Veys N, Waterloos MA, Van Landschoot N, Van Biesen W, Ringoir S: Depressed phagocytosis in hemodialyzed patients: *in vivo* and *in vitro* mechanisms. *Nephron* 63: 409, 1993

84. Vanholder R, Hoenich N, Ringoir S: Morbidity and mortality of central venous catheter hemodialysis: a review of 10 year's experience. *Nephron* 47: 274, 1987

85. Piraino B, Bernardini J, Sorkin M: Catheter infections as a factor in the transfer of continuous ambulatory peritoneal dialysis. *Am J Kidney Dis* 13: 365, 1989

86. Duwe AK, Vas SI, Weatherhead JW: Effects of the composition of peritoneal dialysis fluid on chemiluminescence, phagocytosis, and bactericidal activity in vitro. *Infect Immun* 33: 130, 1981

87. Jörres A, Topley N, Steenweg L, Müller C, Köttgen E, Gahl GM: Inhibition of cytokine synthesis by peritoneal dialysate persists throughout the CAPD cycle. *Am J Nephrol* 12: 80, 1992

88. Vanholder R, Lameire N, Waterloos MA, Van Landschoot N, De Smet R, Vogeleere P, Ringoir S: Depression of PMNL-response to phagocytic challenge in the presence of CAPD-effluent. *J Am Soc Nephrol* 4: 419, 1993 (Abstract)

89. Ringoir S, Schoots A, Vanholder R: Uremic toxins. *Kidney Int* 33: S4, 1988

90. Vanholder RC, Ringoir SMG: The uraemic syndrome. in *Oxford Textbook of Clinical Nephrology*, edited by Cameron S, Davison AM, Grunfeld JP, Kerr D, Ritz E, Oxford University Press, Oxford, 1992, p 1236

91. Boero R, Guarena C, Berto IM, Deabate MC, Rosati C, Quarello F, Piccoli G: Erythrocyte Na, K pump activity and arterial hypertension in uremic dialyzed patients. *Kidney Int* 34: 691, 1988

92. Gallice P, Monti JP, Baz M, Murisasco A, Crevat A: ^{23}Na Nuclear magnetic resonance study of Na$^+$, K$^+$ pump inhibition by a fraction from uremic toxins. *Clin Chem* 34: 2044, 1988

93. Aparicio M, Vincendeau P, Combe C, Caix J, Gin H, de Precigout V, Bezian JH, Bouchet JL, Potaux L: Improvement of leucocytic Na$^+$K$^+$ pump activity in uremic patients on low protein diet. *Kidney Int* 40: 238, 1991

94. Deray G, Pernollet MG, Devynck MA, Zingraff J, Touam A, Rosenfeld J, Meyer P: Plasma digitalis-like activity in essential hypertension or end-stage renal disease. *Hypertension* 8: 632, 1986

95. Druml W, Kelly A, May RC, Mitch WE: Abnormal cation transport in uremia. Mechanisms in adipocytes and skeletal muscle from uremic rats. *J Clin Invest* 81: 1197, 1988

96. Seth RK, Saini AS, Aggarwal SK: Glutathione peroxidase activity and reduced glutathione content in erythrocytes of patients with chronic renal failure. *Scand J Haematol* 35: 201, 1985

97. Costagliola C, Romano L, Sorice P, Di Benedetto A: Anemia and chronic renal failure: the possible role of the oxidative state of glutathione. *Nephron* 52: 11, 1989

98. Bergström J, Alvestrand A, Fürst P: Plasma and muscle free amino acids in maintenance hemodialysis patients without protein malnutrition. *Kidney Int* 38: 108, 1990

99. Fadda GZ, Hajjar SM, Perna AF, Zhou XJ, Lipson LG, Massry SG: On the mechanism of impaired insulin secretion in chronic renal failure. *J Clin Invest* 87: 255, 1991

100. Raine AEG, Bedford L, Simpson AWM, Ashley CC, Brown R, Woodhead JS, Ledingham JGG: Hyperparathyroidism, platelet intracellular free calcium and hypertension in chronic renal failure. *Kidney Int* 43: 700, 1993

101. Alexiewicz JM, Smogorzewski M, Fadda GZ, Massry SG: Impaired phagocytosis in dialysis patients: studies on mechanisms. *Am J Nephrol* 11: 102, 1991

102. Gafter U, Malachi T, Barak H, Levi J: Red blood cell calcium level in chronic renal failure: effect of continuous ambulatory peritoneal dialysis. *J Lab Clin Med* 116: 386, 1990

103. Lindner A, Gagne ER, Zingraff J, Jungers P, Drüeke T, Hannaert P, Garay R: A circulating inhibitor of the RBC membrane calcium pump in chronic renal failure. *Kidney Int* 42: 1328, 1992

104. Thompson CH, Kemp GJ, Taylor DJ, Ledingham JGG, Radda GK, Rajagopalan B: Effect of chronic uraemia on skeletal muscle metabolism in man. *Nephrol Dial Transplant* 8: 218, 1993

105. Durozard D, Pimmel P, Baretto S, Caillette A, Labeeuw M, Baverel G, Zech P: ^{31}P NMR spectroscopy investigation of muscle metabolism in hemodialysis patients. *Kidney Int* 43: 885, 1993

106. Pazmiño P, Rogoff F, Weinshilboum R: Inhibition of human erythrocyte phenol-O-methyltransferase in uremia. *Clin Pharmacol Ther* 26: 464, 1979

107. Depner TA: Suppression of tubular anion transport by an inhibitor of serum protein binding in uremia. *Kidney Int* 20: 511, 1981

108. Gharib N, Gao CY, Areas JL, El Zein M, Preuss HG: Correlation of renal organic anion and cation transport with blood pressure in SHR. *Clin Nephrol* 36: 87, 1991

109. Hsu CH, Patel SR, Young EW, Simpson RU: Production and degradation of calcitriol in renal failure rats. *Am J Physiol* 253: F1015, 1987

110. Hsu CH, Patel SR, Young EW, Simpson RU: Production and metabolic clearance of calcitriol in acute renal failure. *Kidney Int* 33: 530, 1988

111. Hsu CH, Patel S: Factors influencing calcitriol metabolism in renal failure. *Kidney Int* 37: 44, 1990

112. Hsu CH, Vanholder R, Patel S, De Smet RR, Sandra P, Ringoir SMG: Subfractions in uremic plasma ultrafiltrate inhibit calcitriol metabolism. *Kidney Int* 40: 868, 1991

113. Hsu CH, Patel SR, Young EW, Vanholder R: Effects of purine derivatives on calcitriol metabolism in rats. *Am J Physiol* 260: F596, 1991

114. Hsu CH, Patel SR, Vanholder R: Mechanism of decreased intestinal calcitriol receptor concentration in renal failure. *Am J Physiol* 264: F662, 1993

115. Malachi T, Zevin D, Gafter U, Chagnac A, Slor H, Levi J: DNA repair and recovery of RNA synthesis in uremic patients. *Kidney Int* 44: 385, 1993

116. Piafsky KM: Disease-induced changes in the plasma binding of basic drugs. *Clin Pharmacokin* 5: 246, 1980

117. Lindup WE, Bishop KA, Collier R: Drug binding defect of uraemic plasma: contribution of endogenous binding inhibitors. in *Protein Binding and Drug Transport*, edited by Tillement JP, Lindenlaub E, Schattauer Verlag, Stuttgart, 1986, p 397

118. Roman S, Gulyassy PF, Depner TA: Inhibition of salicylate binding to normal plasma by extracts of uremic fluids. *Am J Kidney Dis* 4: 153, 1984

119. Vanholder R, Van Landschoot N, De Smet R, Schoots A, Ringoir S: Drug protein binding in chronic renal failure: evaluation of nine drugs. *Kidney Int* 33: 996, 1988

120. Vanholder R, De Smet R, Ringoir S: Factors influencing drug protein binding in patients with end stage renal failure. *Eur J Clin Pharmacol* 44: S17, 1993

121. MacNamara PJ, Lalka D, Gibaldi M: Endogenous accumulation products and serum protein binding in uremia. *J Lab Clin Med* 98: 730, 1981

122. Gulyassy PF, Bottini AT, Stanfel LA, Jarrad EA, Depner TA: Isolation and chemical identification of inhibitors of plasma ligand binding. *Kidney Int* 30: 391, 1986

123. Mabuchi H, Nakahashi H: Profiling of endogenous ligand solutes that bind to serum proteins in sera of patients with uremia. *Nephron* 43: 110, 1986

124. Mabuchi H, Nakahashi H: Isolation and characterization of an endogenous drug-binding inhibitor present in uremic serum. *Nephron* 44: 277, 1986

125. Niwa T, Takeda N, Maeda K, Shibata M, Tatematsu A: Accumulation of furancarboxylic acids in uremic serum as inhibitors of drug binding. *Clin Chim Acta* 173: 127, 1988

126. Vanholder R, Hoefliger N, De Smet R, Ringoir S: Extraction of protein bound ligands from azotemic sera: comparison of 12 deproteinization methods. *Kidney Int* 41: 1707, 1992

127. Dengler TJ, Robertz-Vaupel GM, Dengler HJ: Albumin binding in uraemia: quantitative assessment of inhibition by endogenous ligands and carbamylation of albumin. *Eur J Clin Pharmacol* 43: 491, 1992

128. Paxton JW: Alpha 1-acid glycoprotein and binding of basic drugs. *Meth Findings Exp Clin Pharmacol* 5: 635, 1983

129. Nicot G, Charmes JP, Lachatre G, Sautereau D, Valette JP, Eichler B, Leroux-Robert C: Theophylline toxicity risks and chronic renal failure. *Int J Clin Pharmacol* 27: 398, 1989

130. Gulyassy P: Can dialysis remove protein-bound toxins that accumulate due to renal secretory failure? *ASAIO J* 40: 92, 1994

131. Gulyassy PF, Depner TA, Shearer GC: Peritoneal versus serum protein binding in CAPD patients. *Abstracts Am Soc Artif Organs Meeting*, New Orleans, May, 1993, p 91

132. Schoots AC, Mikkers FEP, Claessens HA, De Smet R, Van Landschoot N, Ringoir S: Characterization of uremic 'middle molecular' fractions by gas chromatography, mass spectrometry, isotachophoresis and liquid chromatography. *Clin Chem* 28: 45, 1982

133. Vanholder R: Middle molecules as uremic toxins: still a viable hypothesis? *Sem Dial* 7: 65, 1994

134. Vanholder R, De Smet R, Hsu C, Vogeleere P, Ringoir S: Uremic toxicity: the middle molecule hypothesis revisited. *Sem Nephrol* 14: 205, 1994

135. Fürst P, Bergström J, Gordon A, Johnson E, Zimmerman L: Separation of peptides of 'middle' molecular weight from biological fluids of patients with uremia. *Kidney Int* 7: S272, 1975

136. Fürst P, Zimmerman L, Bergström J: Determination of endogenous middle molecules in normal and uremic body fluids. *Clin Nephrol* 5: 178, 1976

137. De Smet R, Van Landschoot N, Van Der Stiggel G, Ringoir S: Isotachophoresis pattern of LDH inhibiting fractions obtained from uremic ultrafiltrate by gel chromatography. *Int J Artif Org* 6: 67, 1983

138. Bultitude FW, Newham SJ: Identification of some abnormal metabolites in plasma from uremic subjects. *Clin Chem* 21: 1329, 1975

139. Zimmerman L, Fürst P, Bergström J, Jornvall H: A new glycine containing compound with a blocked amino group from uremic body fluids. *Clin Nephrol* 14: 109, 1980

140. Gallice P, Monti JP, Crevat A, Durand C, Murisasco A: A compound from uremic plasma and from normal urine isolated by liquid chromatography and identified by nuclear magnetic resonance. *Clin Chem* 31: 30, 1985

141. Cueille G, Man NK, Farges JP, Funck-Brentano JL: Characterization of sub-peak b4.2 middle molecule. *Artif Organs* 4: 28, 1980

142. Abiko T, Kumikawa M, Ishizaki M, Takahashi H, Sekino H: Identification of a tripeptide in ECUM fluid of an uremic patient. *Biophys Bioch Res Com* 83: 357, 1978

143. Abiko T, Kumikawa M, Higuchi H, Sekino H: Identification and synthesis of a heptapeptide in uremic fluid. *Biophys Bioch Res Com* 84: 184, 1978

144. Weisshaar G, Brunner H, Friebolin H, Baumann W, Mann H, Opferkuch HJ, Sieberth HG: Isolation of sialylcompounds from hemofiltrate of chronic uremic patients and identification by nuclear magnetic resonance. *Adv Exp Med Biol* 223: 219, 1987

145. Klein A, Sarnecka-Keller M, Hanicki Z: Middle sized ninhydrin positive molecules in uremic patients treated by repeated haemodialysis. II. Chief peptide constituents of the fraction. *Clin Chim Acta* 90: 7, 1978

146. Gallice P: Toxines urémiques: leur rôle dans l'inhibition de la pompe sodium chez les patients insuffisants rénaux chroniques traités par hémodialyse. Thèse de doctorat d'état, Marseille, 1993

147. Chapman GV, Ward RA, Farrell PC: Separation and quantification of the middle molecules in uremia. *Kidney Int* 17: 82, 1980

148. Faguer P, Man NK, Cueille G, Funck-Brentano JL: Drug interaction in middle molecule analysis, with special reference to acetylsalicyclic acid. *Artif Organs* 8: 226, 1984

149. Asaba H, Zimmerman L, Bergström J: On drug artifacts in middle molecule analysis. *Nephron* 39: 73, 1985

150. Schoots AC, Homan HR, Gladdines MM, Cramers C, De Smet R, Ringoir S: Screening of UV-absorbing solutes in uremic serum by reversed phase HPLC-change of blood levels in different therapies. *Clin Chim Acta* 146: 37, 1985

151. Vanholder R, Krause A, De Smet R, Ringoir S: *In vivo* solute extraction by a new polysulfone membrane with low ultrafiltration capacity. *Trans Am Soc Artif Intern Organs* 34: 598, 1988

152. Vanholder RC, De Smet RV, Ringoir SM: Assessment of urea and other uremic markers for quantification of dialysis adequacy. *Clin Chem* 38: 1429, 1992

153. Ringoir S, De Smet R, Becaus I: Serum middle molecules in different dialysis strategies. in *Aktuelle Probleme der Dialyseverfahren und der Niereninsuffizienz*, edited by von Dittrich P, Kopp K, Verlag Bindernagel, Friedburg, 1977, p 128

154. Haley RJ, Ward DM: Nonenzymatically glucosylated serum proteins in patients with end-stage renal disease. *Am J Kidney Dis* 8: 115, 1986

155. Flückiger R, Harmon W, Meier W, Loo S, Gabbay KH: Hemoglobin carbamylation in uremia. *N Engl J Med* 304: 823, 1981

156. Kwan JTC, Carr EC, Neal AD, Burdon J, Raftery MJ, Marsh FP, Barron JL, Bending MR: Carbamylated haemoglobin, urea kinetic modelling and adequacy of dialysis in haemodialysis patients. *Nephrol Dial Transplant* 6: 38, 1991

157. Johnson WJ, Hagge WW, Wagoner RD, Dinapoli RP, Rosevaer JW: Effects of urea loading in patients with far-advanced renal failure. *Mayo Clin Proc* 47: 21, 1972

158. Scheuer J, Stezoski SW: The effects of uremic compounds on cardiac function and metabolism. *J Mol Cell Cardiol* 5: 287, 1973

159. Lowrie EG, Laird NM, Parker TF, Sargent JA: Effect of the hemodialysis prescription on patient morbidity. *N Engl J Med* 305: 1176, 1980

160. Owen WF, Lew NL, Liu Y, Lowrie EG, Lazarus JM: The urea reduction ratio and serum albumin concentration as predictors of mortality in patients undergoing hemodialysis. *N Engl J Med* 329: 1001, 1993

161. Lameire NH, Vanholder R, Veyt D, Lambert MC, Ringoir S: A longitudinal, five year survey of urea kinetic parameters in CAPD patients. *Kidney Int* 42: 426, 1992

162. Lysaght MJ, Pollock CA, Hallet MD, Ibesl LS, Farrell PC: The relevance of urea kinetic modeling to CAPD. *Trans Am Soc Artif Intern Organs* 35: 784, 1989

163. Blake PG, Sombolos K, Abraham G, Weissgarten J, Pemberton R, Chu GL, Oreopoulos DG: Lack of correlation between urea kinetic indices and clinical outcomes in CAPD patients. *Kidney Int* 39: 700, 1991

164. Yokozawa T, Fujitsuka N, Oura H: Studies on the precursor of methylguanidine in rats with renal failure. *Nephron* 58: 90, 1991

165. Lowrie EG, Lew NL: Death risk in hemodialysis patients: the predictive value of commonly measured variables and an evaluation of death rate differences between facilities. *Am J Kidney Dis* 15: 458, 1990

166. Dzúrik R, Lajdová I, Spustová V, Opatrny K: Pseudouridine excretion in healthy subjects and its accumulation in renal failure. *Nephron* 61: 64, 1992

167. Daniewska-Michalska D, Motyl T, Gellert R, Kukulska W, Podgurniak M, Opechowska-Pacocha E, Ostrowski K: Efficiency of hemodialysis of pyrimidine compounds in patients with chronic renal failure. *Nephron* 64: 193, 1993

168. Giovannetti S, Balestri PL, Barsotti G: Methylguanidine in uremia. *Arch Intern Med* 131: 709, 1973

169. Giovannetti S, Barsotti G: Uremic intoxication. *Nephron* 14: 123, 1975

170. Minkoff L, Gaertner G, Darab M, Mercier D, Levin ML: Inhibition of brain sodium-potassium ATP-ase in uremic rats. *J Lab Clin Med* 80: 71, 1972

171. De Deyn PP, Marescau B, Swartz RD, Hogaerth R, Possemiers I, Lowenthal A: Serum guanidino compound levels and clearances in uremic patients treated with continuous ambulatory peritoneal dialysis. *Nephron* 54: 307, 1990

172. Horowitz H, Cohen B, Martinez P, Papayoanou M: Defective ADP-induced platelet factor 3 activation in uremia. *Blood* 30: 331, 1977

173. De Deyn P, Marescau B, Lornoy W, Becaus I, Lowenthal A: Guanidino compounds in uraemic dialysed patients. *Clin Chim Acta* 157: 143, 1986

174. De Deyn P, Marescau B, Lornoy W, Becaus I, Van Leuven I, Van Gorp L, Lowenthal A: Serum guanidino compound levels and the influence of a single hemodialysis in uremic patients undergoing maintenance hemodialysis. *Nephron* 45: 291, 1987

175. D'Hooge R, Pei YQ, Manil J, De Deyn PP: The uremic guanidino compound guanidinosuccinic acid induces behavioral convulsions and concomitant epileptiform electrocorticographic discharges in mice. *Brain Res* 598: 326, 1992

176. Giovannetti S, Barsotti G: Dialysis of methylguanidine. *Kidney Int* 6: 177, 1974

177. Boumendil-Podevin EF, Podevin RA, Richet G: Uricosuric agents in uremic sera. Identification of indoxyl sulfate and hippuric acid. *J Clin Invest* 55: 1142, 1975

178. Niwa T, Emoto Y, Maeda K, Uehara Y, Yamada N, Shibata M: Oral sorbent suppresses accumulation of albumin-bound indoxyl sulphate in serum of haemodialysis patients. *Nephrol Dial Transplant* 6: 105, 1991

179. Niwa T, Takeda N, Tatematsu A, Maeda K: Accumulation of indoxyl sulfate, an inhibitor of drug-binding, in uremic serum as demonstrated by internal-surface reversed-phase liquid chromatography. *Clin Chem* 34: 2264, 1988

180. Niwa T, Yazawa T, Kodama T, Uehara Y, Maeda K, Yamada K: Efficient removal of albumin-bound furancarboxylic acid, an inhibitor of erythropoiesis, by continuous ambulatory peritoneal dialysis. *Nephron* 56: 241, 1990

181. Clements RS, De Jesus PV, Winegrad AT: Raised plasma myoinositol levels in uraemia experimental neuropathy. *Lancet* 1: 1137, 1973

182. Niwa T, Asada H, Maeda K, Yamada K, Ohki T, Saito A: Profiling of organic acids and polyols in nerves of uraemic and non-uraemic patients. *J Chromatogr* 377: 15, 1986

183. Niwa T, Sobue G, Maeda K, Mitsuma T: Myoinositol inhibits proliferation of cultured Schwann cells: evidence for neurotoxicity of myoinositol. *Nephrol Dial Transplant* 4: 662, 1989

184. Cathcart-Rake W, Porter R, Whittier F, Stein P, Carey M, Grantham J: Effect of diet on serum accumulation and renal excretion of aryl acids and secretory activity in normal and uremic man. *Am J Clin Nutr* 28: 1110, 1975

185. Porter RD, Cathcart-Rake WF, Suk Han Wan, Whittier FC, Grantham JJ: Secretory activity and aryl acid content of serum, urine and cerebrospinal fluid in normal and uremic man. *J Lab Clin Med* 85: 723, 1975

186. Farrell PC, Gotch FA, Peters JH, Berridge BJ, Lam M: Binding of hippurate in normal plasma and in uremic plasma pre- and post-dialysis. *Nephron* 20: 40, 1978

187. Asaba H: Accumulation and excretion of middle molecules. *Clin Nephrol* 1991: 116, 1983

188. Zimmerman L, Bergström J, Jörnvall H: A method for separation of middle molecules by high performance liquid chromatography: application in studies of glucuronyl-o-hydroxyhippurate in normal and uremic subjects. *Clin Nephrol* 25: 94, 1986

189. Lichtenwalner DM, Byungse S, Lichtenwalner MR: Isolation and chemical characterization of 2-hydroxybenzoylglycine as a drug binding inhibitor in uremia. *J Clin Invest* 71: 1289, 1983

190. Altschule MD, Hegedus ZL: Orthohydroxyhippuric (salicyluric) acid – its physiologic and clinical significance. *Clin Pharmacol Ther* 15: 111, 1974

191. Schoots A, Dijkstra JB, Ringoir SMG, Vanholder R, Cramers CA: Are the classical markers sufficient to describe uremic solute accumulation in dialyzed patients? Hippurates reconsidered. *Clin Chem* 34: 1022, 1988

192. Vanholder R, Schoots A, Cramers C, De Smet R, Van Landschoot N, Wizemann V, Botella J, Ringoir S: Hippuric acid as a marker. in *Uremic Toxins*, edited by Ringoir S, Vanholder R, Massry SG, Plenum Press, New York, 1987, p 59

193. Flöge J, Granolleras C, Shaldon S, Koch KM: Dialysis-associated amyloidosis and beta-2-microglobulin. *Contrib Nephrol* 61: 27, 1988

194. Zimmerman L, Egestad B, Jörnvall H, Bergström J: Identification and determination of phenylacetylglutamine, a major nitrogenous metabolite in plasma of uremic patients. *Clin Nephrol* 32: 124, 1989

195. Zimmerman L, Jörnvall H, Bergström J: Phenylacetylglutamine and hippuric acid in uremic and healthy subjects. *Nephron* 55: 265, 1990

196. Röhr U, Spiteller G, Tripier D: Isolierung und Strukturaufklärung der mittelmolekularen Fraktion aus urämischem Hämofiltrate. *J Liebig's Ann Chem* 96: 881, 1988

197. Abiko T, Onodera T, Sekino HA: A peptide isolated from the hemodialysate of a uremic patient with immunodeficiency inhibits lymphocyte stimulation. *J Appl Biochem* 3: 562, 1981

198. Niese D, Gilsdorf K, Hiester E, Dressen P, Michels S, Dengler HJ: Immunomodulating properties of the uremic pentapeptide H-Asp-Leu-Trp-Glu-Lys-OH *in vitro*. *Klin Wochenschrift* 64: 642, 1986

199. Aronin N, Krieger DT: Plasma immunoreactive beta-endorphin is elevated in uraemia. *Clin Endocrinol* 18: 459, 1983

200. Elias AN, Vaziri ND, Maksy M: Plasma beta-endorphin and beta-lipotropin in patients with end-stage renal disease – effects of hemodialysis. *Nephron* 43: 173, 1986

201. Yanagisawa M, Kurihara H, Kimura S, Tomobe Y, Kobayashi M, Mitsui Y, Yazaki Y, Goto K, Masaki T: A novel potent vasoconstrictor peptide produced by vascular endothelial cells. *Nature* 332: 411, 1988

202. Shichiri M, Hirata Y, Ando K, Emori T, Ohta K, Kimoto S, Ogura M, Inoue A, Marumo F: Plasma endothelin levels in hypertension and chronic renal failure. *Hypertension* 15: 493, 1990

203. Brain SD, Williams TJ, Tippins JR, Morris HR, MacIntyre I: Calcitonin gene-related peptide is a potent vasodilator. *Nature* 313: 54, 1985

204. Kojima S, Inoue I, Hirata Y, Kimura G, Saito F, Kawano Y, Satani M, Ito K, Omae T: Plasma concentrations of immunoreactive-atrial natriuretic polypeptide in patients on hemodialysis. *Nephron* 46: 45, 1987

205. Rascher W, Tulassay T, Lang RE: Atrial natriuretic peptide in plasma of volume-overloaded children with chronic renal failure. *Lancet* 2: 303, 1985

206. Niwa T, Fujishiro T, Uema K, Tsuzuki T, Tominaga Y, Emoto Y, Miyazaki T, Maeda K: Effect of hemodialysis on plasma levels of vasoactive peptides: endothelin, calcitonin-gene related peptide and human atrial natriuretic peptide. *Nephron* 64: 552, 1993

207. Bazilinski N, Dunea G: Peptidic uremic retention products. *Int J Artif Organs* 14: 619, 1991

208. Hörl WH, Haag-Weber M, Georgopoulos A, Block LH: Physicochemical characterization of a polypeptide present in uremic serum that inhibits the biological activity of polymorphonuclear cells. *Proc Natl Acad Sci USA* 87: 6353, 1990

209. Haag-Weber M, Mai B, Hörl W: Impaired cellular host defence in peritoneal dialysis by two granulocyte inhibitory proteins. *Nephrol Dial Transplant* 9: 1769, 1994

210. Fine A, Cox D, Fontaine B: Elevation of serum phosphate affects parathyroid hormone levels in only 50% of hemodialysis patients, which is unrelated to changes in serum calcium. *J Am Soc Nephrol* 3: 1947, 1993

211. Massry SG: Parathyroid hormone: a uremic toxin. in *Uremic Toxins*, edited by Ringoir S, Vanholder R, Massry SG, Plenum Press, New York, 1987, p 1

212. Remuzzi G, Dodesini P, Livio M, Mecca G, Benigni A, Schieppati A, Poletti E, de Gaetano G: Parathyroid hormone inhibits human platelet function. *Lancet* 2: 1321, 1981

213. Smogorzewski M, Perna AF, Borum PR, Massry SG: Fatty acid oxidation in the myocardium: effects of parathyroid hormone and CRF. *Kidney Int* 34: 797, 1988

214. Perna AF, Smogorzewski M, Massry SG. Verapamil reverses PTH- or CRF-induced abnormal fatty acids oxidation in muscle. *Kidney Int* 34: 774, 1988

215. Fadda GZ, Thanakitcharu P, Comunale R, Lipson LG, Massry SG: Impaired potassium-induced insulin secretion in chronic renal failure. *Kidney Int* 40: 413, 1991

216. Meytes D, Bogin E, Ma A, Dukex PP, Massry SG: Effect of parathyroid hormone on erythropoiesis. *J Clin Invest* 67: 1263, 1981

217. Bogin E, Massry SG, Harary I: Effect of parathyroid hormone on rat heart cells. *J Clin Invest* 67: 1215, 1981

218. Smogorzewski M, Campese VM, Massry S: Abnormal norepinephrine uptake and release in brain synaptosomes in chronic renal failure. *Kidney Int* 36: 458, 1989

219. Ni Z, Smogorzewski M, Massry SG: Derangements in acetylcholine metabolism in brain synaptosomes in chronic renal failure. *Kidney Int* 44: 630, 1993

220. Shasha SM, Kristal B, Barzilai M, Makov UE, Shkolnik T: *In vitro* effect of PTH on normal T cell functions. *Nephron* 50: 212, 1988

221. Alexiewicz JM, Klinger M, Pitts TO, Gacoing Z, Linker-Israeli M, Massry SG: Parathyroid hormone inhibits B cell proliferation: implications in chronic renal failure. *J Am Soc Nephrol* 1: 236, 1990

222. Perna AF, Smogorzewski M, Massry SG: Effects of verapamil on the abnormalities in fatty acid oxidation of myocardium. *Kidney Int* 36: 453, 1989

223. D'Amour P, Jobin J, Hamel L, L'Ecuyer N: iPTH values during hemodialysis: role of ionized Ca, dialysis membranes and iPTH assays. *Kidney Int* 38: 308, 1990

224. Vincent C, Revillard JP, Galland M, Traeger J: Serum beta-2-microglobulin in hemodialyzed patients. *Nephron* 21: 260, 1978

225. Sargent JA, Gotch FA: Principles and biophysics of dialysis. in *Replacement of Renal Function by Dialysis*, edited by Maher JF, Kluwer Academic, Dordrecht, 1989, p 87

226. Shirahama T, Skinner M, Cohen AS, Gejyo F, Arakawa M, Suzuki M, Hirasawa Y: Histochemical and immunohistochemical characterization of amyloid associated with chronic hemodialysis as beta-2-microglobulin. *J Lab Invest* 53: 705, 1985

227. Gejyo F, Odani S, Yamada T, Honma N, Saito H, Suzuki Y, Nakagawa Y, Kobayashi H, Maruyama Y, Hirasawa Y, Suzuki M, Arakawa M: Beta-2-microglobulin: a new form of amyloid protein associated with chronic hemodialysis. *Kidney Int* 30: 385, 1986

228. Hauglustaine D, Waer M, Michielsen P, Goebels J, Vandeputte M: Haemodialysis membranes, serum beta-2-microglobulin, and dialysis amyloidosis. *Lancet* 1: 1211, 1986 (Letter)

229. Vanholder RC, Ringoir SM: Intradialytic body weight changes and dialyzer pore size as main contributing factors to the evolution of beta-2-microglobulin in dialysis. *Blood Purif* 8: 32, 1990

230. Petersen J, Moore RM, Kaczmarek RG, Singh B, Yeh I, Hamburger S, Kankam M: The effects of reprocessing cuprophane and polysulfone dialyzers on β_2-microglobulin removal from hemodialysis patients. *Am J Kidney Dis* 17: 174, 1991

231. van Ypersele de Strihou C, Jadoul M, Malghem J, Maldague B, Jamart J: Effect of dialysis membrane and patient's age on signs of dialysis-related amyloidosis. *Kidney Int* 39: 1012, 1991

232. Gagnon RF, Somerville P, Thomson DM: Circulating form of beta-2-microglobulin in dialysis patients. *Am J Nephrol* 8: 379, 1988

233. Renaud H, Fournier A, Morinière Ph, Westeel PF, El Esper N, Belbrik S, Marie A, Cohen-Solal HE, Sebert JL: Erosive osteoarthropathy associated with β_2-microglobulin amyloidosis in a uremic patient treated exclusively by long-term hemofiltration with biocompatible membranes. *Nephrol Dial Transplant* 3: 820, 1988

234. Campbell RA: Polyamines and uremia. in *Uremic Toxins*, edited by Ringoir S, Vanholder R, Massry SG, Plenum Press, New York, 1987, p 47

235. Simmonds HA, Cameron JS, Morris GS, Fairbanks LD, Davies PM: Purine metabolites in uraemia. in *Uremic Toxins*, edited by Ringoir S, Vanholder R, Massry SG, Plenum Press, New York, 1987, p 73

236. Hsu CH, Patel S, Vanholder R: Effect of uric acid on plasma levels of calcitriol in renal failure. *J Am Soc Nephrol* 4: 1035, 1993.

237. Gerrits GPMJ, Monnens LAH, De Abreu RA, Schröder CH, Trijbels JMF, Gabreëls, FJM: Disturbances of cerebral purine and pyrimidine metabolism in young children with chronic renal failure. *Nephron* 58: 310, 1991

238. Ludwig GD, Senesky D, Bluemle LW, Elkinton JR: Indoles in uremia: identification by countercurrent distribution and paper chromatography. *Am J Clin Nutr* 21: 436, 1968

239. Wengle B, Hellström K: Volatile phenols in serum of uraemic patients. *Clin Science* 43: 493, 1972

240. Wardle EN, Wilkinson K: Free phenols in chronic renal failure. *Clin Nephrol* 6: 361, 1976

241. Niwa T, Maeda K, Ohki T, Saito A, Kobayashi K: A gas chromatographic-mass spectrometric analysis for phenols in uremic serum. *Clin Chim Acta* 110: 51, 1981

242. Hicks JM, Young DS, Wootton IDP: The effect of uraemic blood constituents on certain cerebral enzymes. *Clin Chim Acta* 9: 228, 1964

243. Rabiner SF, Molinas F: The role of phenol and phenolic acids on the thrombocytopathy and defective platelet aggregation of patients with renal failure. *Am J Med* 49: 346, 1970

244. Lascelles PT, Taylor WH: The effect upon tissue respiration *in vitro* of metabolites which accumulate in uraemic coma. *Clin Science* 31: 403, 1966

245. Wardle EN, Williams R: Polymorph leukocyte function in uraemia and jaundice. *Acta Haemat* 64: 157, 1980

246. Turner GA, Wardle EN: Effect of unconjugated and conjugated phenol and uraemia on the synthesis of adenosine 3′:5′ cyclic monophosphate in rat brain homogenates. *Clin Science Mol Med* 55: 271, 1978

247. Vanholder R, De Smet R, Waterloos MA, Van Landschoot N, Ringoir S: Characterization of p-cresol and phenol as uremic toxins inhibiting polymorphonuclear (PMNL) respiratory burst response to phagocytosis. *J Am Soc Nephrol* 4: 786, 1993 (Abstract)

248. Wardle EN: Chemiluminescence and superoxide anions generated by phagocytes in uraemia. *Nephron* 40: 37D, 1985 (Letter)

249. Bartling D, Seedorf M, Mithofer A, Weiler EW: Cloning and expression of an Arabidopsis nitrilase which can convert indole-3-acetonitrile to the plant hormone, indole-3-acetic acid. *Eur J Biochem* 205: 417, 1992

250. Efimov S, Shevehenko V, Shchukin I, Preobrazhenskaya M: The influence of 1′-methyl- and 1′-ethylascorbigen on metabolism of arachidonic acid in murine spleen cells. *Biochem Biophys Res Commun* 190: 895, 1993

251. Suto A, Bradlow HL, Wong GY, Osborne MP, Telang NT: Persistent estrogen responsiveness of res oncogene-transformed mouse mammary epithelial cells. *Steroids* 57: 262, 1992

252. Wallaeys B, Cornelis R, Mees L, Lameire N: Trace elements in serum, packed cells and dialysate in CAPD patients. *Kidney Int* 30: 599, 1986

253. Van Renterghem D, Cornelis R, Vanholder R: Behaviour of 12 trace elements in serum of uremic patients on hemodiafiltration. *J Trace Elem Electrolytes Health Dis* 6: 169, 1992

254. De Kimpe J, Cornelis R, Mees L, Van Lierde S, Vanholder R: More than tenfold increase of arsenic in serum and packed cells of chronic hemodialysis patients. *Am J Nephrol* 13: 429, 1993

255. Mahajan SK: Zinc metabolism in uremia. *Int J Artif Organs* 11: 223, 1988

256. Cornelis R, Ringoir S, Lameire N, Mees L, Hoste J: Blood bromine in uremic patients. *Min Electrol Metab* 2: 186, 1979

257. Cornelis R, Mees L, Ringoir S, Hoste J: Serum and red blood cell Zn, Se, Cs and Rb in dialysis patients. *Min Electrol Metab* 2: 88, 1979

258. Van Renterghem D, Cornelis R, Mees L, Vanholder R: The effect of adding Br and Zn supplements to the dialysate on the concentrations of Br and Zn in the blood of hemodialyzed patients. *J Trace Elem Electrolytes Health Dis* 6: 105, 1992

259. Sugisaki H, Onohara M, Kunimoto T: Dynamic behavior of plasma phosphate in chronic dialysis patients. *Trans Am Soc Artif Intern Organs* 28: 302, 1982

260. Haas T, Hillion D, Dongradi G: Phosphate kinetics in dialysis patients. *Nephrol Dial Transplant* 6 (Suppl 2): 108, 1991

261. Takeda N, Niwa T, Tatematsu A, Suzuki M: Identification and quantification of a protein-bound ligand in uremic serum. *Clin Chem* 33: 682, 1987

262. Mabuchi H, Nakahashi H: A major endogenous ligand substance involved in renal failure. *Nephron* 49: 277, 1988

263. Mabuchi H, Nakahashi H: Inhibition of hepatic glutathione S-transferases by a major endogenous ligand substance present in uremic serum. *Nephron* 49: 281, 1988

264. Niwa T, Aiuchi T, Nakaya K, Emoto Y, Miyazaki T, Maeda K: Inhibition of mitochondrial respiration by furancarboxylic acid accumulated in uremic serum in its albumin-bound and non-dialyzable form. *Clin Nephrol* 39: 92, 1993

265. Rutten GA, Schoots AC, Vanholder R, De Smet R, Ringoir S, Cramers CA: Hexachlorobenzene and 1,1-di(4-chlorophenyl)-2,2-dichloroethene in serum of uremic patients and healthy persons: determination by capillary gas chromatography and electron capture detection. *Nephron* 48: 217, 1988

266. Manabe S, Yanagisawa H, Ishikawa S, Kitagawa Y, Kanai Y, Wada O: Accumulation of 2-amino-6-methyldipyrido(1,2-a:3,′2-′-d)imidazole and 2-aminodipyrido(1,2-a:3′,-2′-d)imidazole, carcinogenic glutamic acid pyrolysis products, in plasma of patients with uremia. *Cancer Res* 47: 6150, 1987

267. Turney JH, Davison AM, Forbes MA, Cooper EH: Hyaluronic acid in end-stage renal failure treated by haemodialysis: clinical correlates and implications. *Nephrol Dial Transplant* 6: 566, 1991

268. del Castillo E, Fuenzalida R, Uranga J: Increased glomerular filtration rate and glomerulopressin activity in diabetic dogs. *Horm Metab Res* 9: 46, 1975

269. Zhou XJ, Vaziri ND, Kaupke CJ: Effects of chronic renal failure and hemodialysis on plasma glomerulopressin. *Int J Artif Organs* 16: 180, 1993

270. Alvestrand A, Bergström J: Glomerular hyperfiltration and protein ingestion, during glucagon infusion, and in insulin-dependent diabetes is induced by a liver hormone: deficiency production of this hormone in hepatic failure causes hepatorenal syndrome. *Lancet* 1: 195, 1984

271. Garcia-Ocaña A, Ortega J, González-García Y, García-Cantón C, Esbrit P: Partial purification of a renotropic activity from plasma of uninephrectomized human subjects. *Nephron* 64: 547, 1993

272. Costello JF, Sadovnic MJ, Cottington EM: Plasma oxalate levels rise in hemodialysis patients despite increased oxalate removal. *J Am Soc Nephrol* 1: 1289, 1991

273. Gallice PM, Monti JP, Braguer DL, Baz M, Elsen RE, Berland YF, Crevat AD: Ascorbic acid derivatives in two different fractions of uremic toxins. *Int J Artif Organs* 14: 754, 1991

274. Cailleux A, Subra JF, Riberi P, Allain P: Uptake of trihalomethanes by patients during hemodialysis. *Clin Chim Acta* 181: 75, 1989

275. Vallance P, Leone A, Calver A, Collier J, Moncada S: Accumulation of an endogenous inhibitor of nitric oxide synthesis in chronic renal failure. *Lancet* 339: 572, 1992

276. Remuzzi G, Perico N, Zoja C, Corna D, Macconi D, Viganò GL: Role of endothelium-derived nitric oxide in the bleeding tendency of uremia. *J Clin Invest* 86: 1768, 1990

277. Lipton SA, Choi YB, Pan ZH, Lei SZ, Chen HSV, Sucher NJ, Loscalzo J, Singel DJ, Stamler JS: A redox-based mechanism for the neuroprotective and neurodestructive effects of nitric oxide and related nitroso-compounds. *Nature* 364: 626, 1993

278. Ihle BU, Cox RW, Dunn SR, Simenhoff ML: Determination of body burden of uremic toxins. *Clin Nephrol* 22: 82, 1984

279. Maxfield FR, Willingham MC, Davies PJ, Pastan I: Amines inhibit the clustering of α-macroglobulin and EGF on the fibroblast cell surface. *Nature* 277: 661, 1979

280. Pascual M: Le facteur D du complément: toxine urémique? *Néphrologie* 12: 215, 1991

281. Pascual M, Schifferli JA: Adsorption of complement factor D by polyacrylonitrile dialysis membranes. *Kidney Int* 43: 903, 1992

282. Vaziri ND, Oveisi F, Wierzbiezki M, Shaw V, Sporty LD: Serum melatonin and 6-sulfatoxymelatonin in end-stage renal disease: effect of hemodialysis. *Artif Organs* 17: 764, 1993

283. Witko V, Nguyen AT, Descamps-Latscha B: Microtiter plate assay for phagocyte-derived taurine-catecholamines. *J Clin Lab Anal* 6: 47, 1993

284. Thomas EL, Grisham MB, Jefferson MM: Myeloperoxidase-dependent effect of amines on functions of isolated neutrophils. *J Clin Invest* 72: 441, 1983

285. Chauveau P, Chadefaux B, Coude M, Aupetit J, Hannedouche T, Kamoun P, Jungers P: Hyperhomocysteinemia, a risk factor for atherosclerosis in chronic uremic patients. *Kidney Int* 43: S72, 1993

286. Clarke R, Daly L, Robinson K, Naughten E, Cahalane S, Fowler B, Graham I: Hyperhomocysteinemia: an independent risk factor for vascular disease. *N Engl J Med* 324: 1149, 1991

287. Schoots A, Mikkers F, Cramers C, De Smet R, Ringoir S: Uremic toxins and the elusive middle molecules. *Nephron* 38: 1, 1984

288. Vanholder R, Ringoir S: Adequacy of dialysis: a critical analysis. Editorial review. *Kidney Int* 42: 540, 1992

289. Goldman M, Lagmiche M, Dhaene M, Amraoui Z, Thayse C, Vanherweghem JL: Adsorption of β_2-microglobulin on dialysis membranes: comparison of different dialyzers and effects of reuse procedures. *Int J Artif Organs* 12: 373, 1989

290. Shemesh O, Golbetz H, Kriss JP, Myers BD: Limitations of creatinine as a filtration marker in glomerulopathic patients. *Kidney Int* 28: 830, 1985

291. Sargent JA, Gotch FA: Mathematic modeling of dialysis therapy. *Kidney Int* 18: S2, 1980

292. Vanholder R, Hoenich N, Ringoir S: Adequacy studies of fistula single-needle dialysis. *Am J Kidney Dis* 10: 417, 1987

293. Borah MF, Schoenfeld PY, Gotch FA, Sargent JA, Wolfson M, Humphreys MH: Nitrogen balance during intermittent dialysis therapy of uremia. *Kidney Int* 14: 491, 1978

294. Buur T, Timpka T, Lundberg M: Urea kinetics and clinical evaluation of the haemodialysis patient. *Nephrol Dial Transplant* 5: 347, 1990

295. Watson PE, Watson ID, Batt RD: Total body water volumes for adult males and females estimated from simple anthropometric measurements. *Am J Clin Nutr* 33: 27, 1980

296. Malchesky PS, Ellis P, Nosse G, Magnusson M, Lankhorst B, Nakamoto S: Direct quantification of dialysis. *Dial Transplant* 11: 42, 1982

297. Vanholder R, Van Trimpont P, Ringoir S: Urea kinetic modelling: comparison of three methods. *J Med Engin Technol* 13: 87, 1989

298. Keshaviah P, Collins A: A re-appraisal of the National Cooperative Dialysis Study (NCDS). *Kidney Int* 33: 227 1988 (Abstract)

299. Shen FH, Hsu KT: Lower mortality and morbidity associated with higher Kt/V in hemodialysis patients. *J Am Soc Nephrol* 1: 377, 1990 (Abstract)

300. Hakim RM, Fearon DT, Lazarus JM: Biocompatibility of dialysis membranes: effects of chronic complement activation. *Kidney Int* 26: 194, 1984

301. Gutierrez A, Alvestrand A, Wahren J, Bergström J: Effect of *in vivo* contact between blood and dialysis membranes on protein catabolism in humans. *Kidney Int* 38: 487, 1990

302. Lindsay RM, Spanner E: A hypothesis: the protein catabolic rate is dependent upon the type and amount of treatment in dialyzed uremic patients. *Am J Kidney Dis* 13: 382, 1989

303. Sargent JA: Shortfalls in the delivery of dialysis. *Am J Kidney Dis* 15: 500, 1990

304. Ellis PW, Malchesky PS, Magnusson MO, Goormastic M, Nakamoto S: Comparison of two methods of kinetic modeling. *Trans Am Soc Artif Intern Organs* 30: 60, 1984

305. Ilstrup K, Hanson G, Shapiro W, Keshaviah P: Examining the foundations of urea kinetics. *Trans Am Soc Artif Intern Organs* 31: 164, 1985

306. Aebischer P, Schorderet D, Juillerat A, Wauters JP, Fellay G: Comparison of urea kinetics and direct dialysis quantification in hemodialysis patients. *Trans Am Soc Artif Intern Organs* 31: 164, 1985

307. Hoenich NA, Keir MJ, Hildreth K, Woffindin C, Goodall R, Vanholder R, Ward MK: Urea kinetic modeling: comparing the options. *Artif Organs* 17: 813, 1993

308. Stange J, Ramlow W, Mitzner S, Schmidt R, Klinkmann H: Dialysis against a recycled albumin solution enables the removal of albumin-bound toxins. *Artif Organs* 17: 809, 1993

309. Veech RL: The untoward effects of the anions of dialysis fluids. *Kidney Int* 34: 587, 1988

310. Chiu WY, Yamada K, Saito A, Ogawa H, Takagi T, Chung TG: Comparison of serum protein removal in haemodialysis therapy by partly protein-permeable haemodialysers. *J Chromatogr* 428: 25, 1988

311. Vanholder R, De Smet R, Schoots A, Ringoir S: Correlation of a colorimetric and a HPLC method for the determination of serum hippuric acid concentrations in uremia. *Nephron* 49: 164, 1988

312. Niwa T, Ise M, Miyazaki T, Maeda K: Suppressive effect of an oral sorbent on the accumulation of p-cresol in the serum of experimental uremic rats. *Nephron* 65: 82, 1993

PRINCIPLES AND BIOPHYSICS OF DIALYSIS

JOHN A. SARGENT and FRANK A. GOTCH

INTRODUCTION

Intermittent dialysis therapy is used in chronic uremia to re-establish body water solute concentrations that cannot be achieved by the natural organ. In this sense, the dialyzer becomes an artificial kidney and it is through the transport of substances by this device that chemical and biophysical control consistent with continued survival is achieved. This chapter is organized as shown in Figure 1 and consists of two basic lines of development:

1. Consideration of the dialyzer and its operating principles.
2. Application of mass balance principles to various solute systems and the effect of dialyzer use on solute control during intermittent dialysis therapy.

Biophysical treatment of hemodialysis requires quantitative description of the interacting variables involved in this therapy; such a description, to be unambiguous, must use mathematical relationships. Certain fundamental relationships, because of their central role, have been developed in detail, such as clearance measurements and single pool solute kinetics. For solution techniques of equations and relationships that are mainly descriptive, such as double pool kinetics of larger molecules, the reader is either referred to the Appendix or to specific texts on applied mathematics. The Appendix discusses independent and dependent variables, as well as the quantitative use of relational (linear) analysis. In most cases symbols are defined in the text. For reader convenience, however, a list of symbols used appears under Nomenclature at the end of the chapter.

The dialyzer will be considered initially, starting with a brief discussion of the fundamentals of diffusion embodied in Fick's law. The practical application of these concepts to dialyzer development or clinical use, however, requires the definition of several coefficients that can aid in either the design of dialyzers or their use in the clinic; these two aspects will be discussed in turn. The mechanistic view of transport is intended to describe what influences dialyzer properties; the discussion of the operational aspects of a dialyzer, which concerns itself with the development of relationships for dialysance and clearance, will be of value in the second part of the chapter when mass balance is considered with respect to the patient-dialyzer system.

The section which considers the mass balance of intermittent dialysis therapy begins with the fundamentals of conservation of matter and from them develops kinetic and steady state relationships that govern concentration control in dialyzed patients; these concepts are then applied to several solute systems.

FUNDAMENTALS OF MASS TRANSPORT

To remove a substance from the blood with a dialyzer, the species must move out of the blood across a membrane and into the dialysate by diffusion which is governed by Fick's Law:

$$J = -DA\frac{dc}{dx} = -DA\frac{\Delta c}{\Delta x}.$$ [1]

This expression states that the flux, J, of a material over a short distance, dx, is proportional to its concentration difference, dc, over this distance and the area of the diffusion front, A. The phenomenological constant of proportionality resulting in equality of the above statements is the diffusivity, D, which has units of cm^2/sec and will be a unique property of the solute-solvent at a specific temperature. Finally, the sign convention is adopted that diffusion will be in the positive direction; material moves from the region of higher to that of lower activity so that concentration will be decreasing ($dc/dx < 0$) in the direction of flux; mathematically, therefore, the right hand side of the equation must carry a negative sign.

Equation [1] is the fundamental relationship for unidimensional diffusive movement of material and is the mass transfer analog to Fourier's Law which governs heat conduction. For practical use in the study of the operation of dialyzers, however, it is necessary to put Equation [1] in less general form so that the mechanisms of transport of specific devices can be evaluated. This mechanistic approach is generally taken by engineers who desire to improve the operating characteristics and efficiency of a dialyzer. It can also be helpful to physicians in understanding the anticipated effects of different operational conditions on dialyzer performance. Typical changes in operational conditions would be dialyzer clotting, variable ultrafiltration, and non-standard flow rates. This approach also can give increased insight into what to expect from changes in the components of a dialyzer such as the use of a different dialysis membrane.

MECHANISMS OF TRANSPORT

If the value of Δx in Equation [1] is relatively constant in any one dialyzer design, the major variables that determine flux for the dialyzer will be concentration difference and area, D being a constant at any particular temperature for a specific chemical species. This being the case, Equation [1] can be written as:

$$J = -K_oA\Delta C.$$ [2a]

Here ΔC is an appropriately defined concentration difference. In Equation [2a] a new proportionality constant, the overall mass transfer coefficient, K_o, has appeared and is defined as:

$$K_o = \frac{J/A}{-\Delta C} = \frac{\text{unit flux}}{\text{driving force}}.$$ [2b]

K_o has units of cm/min and is independent of ΔC in the concentration range experienced in dialysis. Comparison

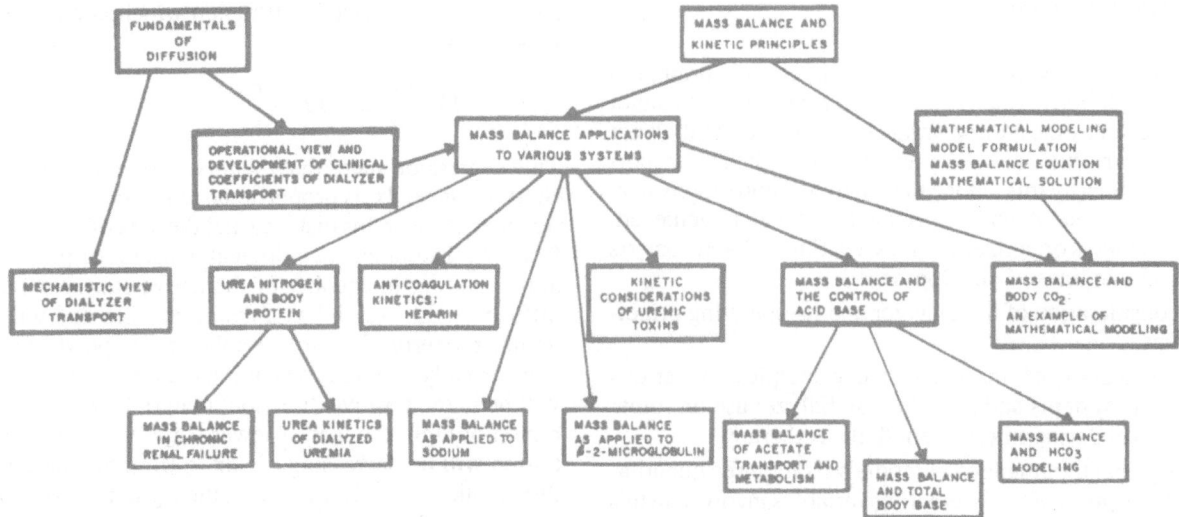

Figure 1. Diagrammatic outline of chapter organization.

of Equations [1] and [2a] shows that K_o is proportional to the diffusivity of the solute being transferred and inversely proportional to the diffusion distances characteristic of the dialyzer; this transport coefficient can be calculated from basic transport values if blood and dialysate flow rates are known as will be shown below (1–3). If Equation [2a] is further rewritten, the flux per unit area can be described as:

$$\text{unit flux} = \frac{J}{A} = \frac{-\Delta C}{1/K_o} = \frac{-\Delta C}{R_o}. \qquad [2c]$$

If $1/K_o$ is viewed as a resistance to transport (R_o), Equation [2c] can be written as:

$$\frac{\text{Mass transfer}}{\text{per unit area}} = \frac{\text{Driving force}}{\text{Resistance to transport}}. \qquad [3]$$

Equation [3] is a quantitative statement of a fundamental physical principle which applies throughout the physical sciences. It states that there will be a flux of material proportional to the driving force and that that flux will be opposed by (or is inversely proportional to) certain resistances. This is the same form as Ohm's law of electric current flow, it is the same law that is applied to conductive heat flow, and it is in the same form as the relationship that is used to calculate peripheral resistance in circulation physiology (4).

Specifically, Equation [3] shows that mass transfer is the result of the driving force relative to the resistance to transfer and is useful in that it demonstrates that flux per unit area can be improved only by increasing the driving force or decreasing the resistance. The overall resistance is an index of the difficulty in getting from the center of the blood stream to the center of the dialysate stream and

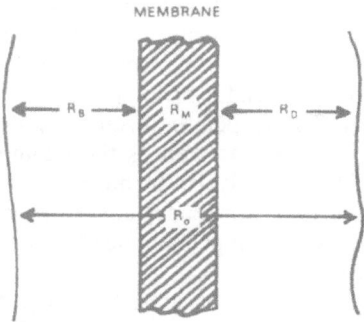

Figure 2. Schematic representation of resistances to transport in a dialyzer.

is the sum of all the resistances of which it is composed (see Figure 2):

$$R_o = R_B + R_M + R_D \qquad [4]$$

where R_B = blood side resistance; R_M = membrane resistance; R_D = dialysate side resistance.

In this way, the diffusion path is divided into three segments representing the three fundamental elements of a dialyzer.

K_o was defined above as proportional to $D/\Delta x$ so that R_o, being proportional to $1/K_o$, is proportional to $\Delta x/D$. In the three segments described above, R will be:

$$R_B = \frac{\Delta x_B}{D_B}$$

$$R_M = \frac{\Delta x_M}{k D_M} = \frac{\Delta x_M}{D_M^*}$$

$$R_D = \frac{\Delta x_D}{D_D}$$

where k is the solute distribution coefficient between the membrane material and the solution.

For any particular solute, the diffusivity in blood (D_B) and dialysate (D_D) of a given composition will be constant. Moreover, it should have the same value irrespective of the dialyzer being a solution constant at operational temperatures. As a consequence, the R_B and R_D in a specific dialyzer will be governed by the Δx_B and Δx_D terms; these terms are the effective diffusion distances from the main stream to and from the membrane. To the extent that blood flows are swift and fluid channels are small, the value of Δx for both blood and dialysate will be small as will the values for R_B and R_D. The membrane resistance R_M still depends on Δx_M (the thickness of the membrane) but in addition, will be sensitive to the effective diffusivity in the membrane (D_M^*) which can vary considerably as a result of its chemical composition. In this context, a thin (small Δx_M) permeable (large D_M^*) membrane would have a small value for R_M. It should be noted, however, that the resistances are additive so that while a dialyzer with a highly permeable membrane will have low values for R_M, R_o may be high due to large values for R_B and R_D. Dialyzer efficiency can be best increased, therefore, by reducing the value of the largest resistance in Equation [4]. The relative values for the above resistances in four dialyzer-membrane combinations which were in common use in the early days of dialysis serves to illustrate the importance of the various resistances (see Table 1). The improvement in dialyzer design that occurred in the 1970s was spurred by the desire to reduce the overall resistance shown in Table 1.

It becomes evident from Table 1 that for urea, the predominant resistances to transport in the prototype parallel plate, Kiil dialyzer, were R_B and R_D, (i.e., in the fluid streams), whereas in the hollow fiber devices with narrow fluid paths, the major resistance is in the membrane. The overall resistance, however, is lower in the latter explaining why, in general, hollow fiber dialyzers have better urea transport. For large molecules all of these dialyzers, except the one with the non-cellulosic membrane, have over two thirds of the resistance in the membrane.

The overall resistance, R_o (or overall mass transfer coefficient, K_o), can be readily calculated from the diffusive dialysance, D, and knowledge of blood and dialysate flow rates, (see below for discussion of diffusive dialysance). Conversely, if R_o or K_o is known the expected diffusive dialysance under specific clinical conditions of flow can be calculated (see below).

CONCENTRATION DIFFERENCE, THE DRIVING FORCE

Equation [2a] states that with a specific dialyzer (K_oA a constant) the removal of solute will depend directly on the concentration difference, ΔC. It is important to develop

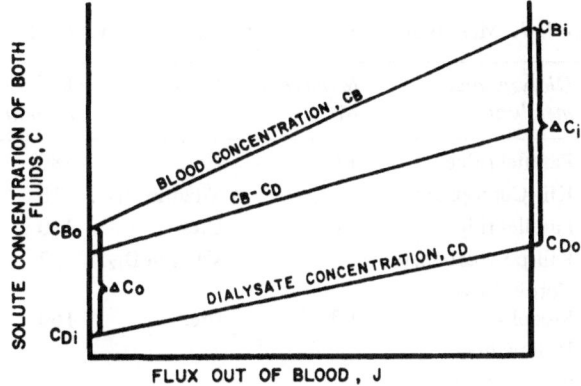

Figure 3. Graphical representation of blood and dialysate concentration as a function of flux between the two fluid streams.

this variable further so that it can be used in computations to follow.

Logarithmic mean concentration difference

There will be a linear change in concentrations of the blood and dialysis solution as solute transfers from one to the other (shown diagrammatically in Figure 3). This figure is for counter-current flows and shows solute levels in the blood decreasing from its entry into the dialyzer at the right while concentrations in the dialysis fluid increase from its entry into the dialyzer at the left. The concentration difference at any point in the dialyzer is represented by the difference between these two lines (see the intermediate line) and it is this concentration that will determine the local flux (see Equation [2a]). A similar figure can be constructed for co-current flow and the analytical results to be developed below will apply equally to this case. In Figure 3 the slope of the concentration difference line will be:

$$\text{slope} = \frac{d(\Delta C)}{dJ} = \frac{\Delta C_i - \Delta C_o}{J} \qquad [5]$$

If Equation [2a] is differentiated and evaluated for the very small transport area, dA, then substituted into Equation [5] for dJ:

$$\frac{d(\Delta C)}{-K_o dA \Delta C} = \frac{\Delta C_i - \Delta C_o}{J} \; .$$

Rearrangement yields:

$$\frac{d(\Delta C)}{\Delta C} = \frac{-K_o(\Delta C_i - \Delta C_o)\, dA}{J} \; .$$

Integration and solving the resulting expression for flux yields:

$$J = K_o A \left[\frac{\Delta C_i - \Delta C_o}{\text{Ln}(\Delta C_i / \Delta C_o)} \right] . \qquad [6]$$

Table 1. Mass transfer resistances for various dialyzer-solute combinations

Dialyzer and membrane	Membrane M²	Solute	$K_B{}^a$ ml/min	$R_B{}^b$ ml/min	R_M min/cm	$R_D{}^b$ min/cm	R_o min/cm	$\dfrac{R_B + R_D}{R_o}$	$\dfrac{R_M}{R_o}$	Ref
Parallel ridge	1.0	Urea	80	24	19	16	59	0.68	0.32	(5)
Kiil-Cuprophane		Vitamin B₁₂	18	101	362	45	508	0.29	0.71	(5)
Parallel ridge	1.0	Urea	110	24	14	16	54	0.74	0.26	(6)
Kiil-polycarbonate		Vitamin B₁₂	37	101	90	45	236	0.62	0.38	(6)
Cordis-Dow Model 4	1.3	Urea	160	4	21	7	32	0.34	0.66	(7)
Hollow fiber regenerated cellulose		Vitamin B₁₂	23	17	–	20	519	0.07	0.93	(7)
Cordis-Dow Model 5	2.5	Urea	185	5	21	9	35	0.40	0.60	(7)
Hollow fiber regenerated cellulose		Vitamin B₁₂	40	21	–	25	536	0.09	0.91	(7)

[a] Clearances based on Q_B = 200 ml/min, Q_D 500 ml/min and 37°C vitamin B₁₂ *in vitro*.
[b] The value of R_B and R_D have been established from (R Urea, hollow fiber kidney/R urea Kill) (R vitamin B₁₂, Kiil) = R vitamin B₁₂, hollow fiber kidney.

The expression in parentheses in Equation [6] is the logarithmic mean concentration difference which can be expanded as:

$$\Delta C \text{ (Log-mean)} = \frac{(C_{Bi} - C_{Do}) - (C_{Bo} - C_{Di})}{\text{Ln}[(C_{Bi} - C_{Bo}) / (C_{Bo} - C_{Di})]} \cdot [7]$$

The log-mean concentration difference as represented in Equation [7] is an operationally exact statement of the integrated concentration driving force in a dialyzer being operated in either counter-current or co-current mode. Equation [7], however, contains both inlet and outlet blood and dialysate concentrations which in the clinical operation of a dialyzer are tedious to obtain.

It is considerably more convenient to define a surrogate concentration driving force, $(C_{Bi} - C_{Di})$ in the clinical setting. This concentration difference can be shown to be directly proportional to the log-mean concentration difference and is clinically more convenient than Equation [7] because it uses undialyzed blood and inlet dialysis fluid as reference levels to evaluate and calculate dialyzer performance. This measurement of concentration difference also adapts well to system modeling because it is possible to determine fluxes from patient's systemic concentrations alone.

OPERATIONAL CHARACTERISTICS OF THE DIALYZER

During dialysis treatment the dialyzer is the point at which mass transfer takes place either from the patient (e.g., potassium and protein catabolites) or to the patient (e.g.,

calcium or acetate). There is also a transfer of water from the patient to the dialysate for volume control. The two mechanisms of transport are different and are effected by virtue of dissimilar driving forces: concentration differences for the various chemical constituents and a pressure difference in the case of water. To describe the operational characteristics of a dialyzer for clinical use, it is desirable to define operational coefficients which are the analog of K_o in Equation [2b], and which result in a linear proportionality relating flux and driving force. The two coefficients for dialyzer water and solute flux are the ultrafiltration coefficient (K_{UF}) and dialysance (D); clearance (K) is a special case of dialysance as will be discussed below.

Ultrafiltration coefficient

Ultrafiltration Coefficient [K_{UF} (ml/min/mmHg)] =

$$= \frac{\text{water flux}}{\text{transmembrane pressure}} = \frac{Q_F}{P_B - P_D} \cdot [8]$$

The water flux is referred to as the ultrafiltration rate (Q_F ml/min) and the driving force is the difference in mean pressures from the blood side (P_B) to the dialysate side (P_D).

Mass transport and solute flux

Consideration of flow rates

A dialyzer is operated by manipulation of blood and dialysate flow rates. It is, therefore, appropriate to define the basis for these flows.

Because dialysate and ultrafiltrate are homogeneous aqueous fluids, their flow rates are unambiguous and represent those flows which would be calculated if a timed, volumetric collection were done. Blood, in contrast, is a heterogeneous fluid which contains proteins and cellular elements. Its bulk flow rate will always exceed its water flow rate; indeed at times it non-cellular water flow rate (or plasma water) is a more relevant flow, as in the case of inulin transport; the non-cellular flow adjusted for cellular water participation is more appropriate when considering materials such as bicarbonate which readily enters cells but is in much lower cellular concentration due to Donnan effects (8–10). Bulk blood flow (Q_B), however, is routinely measured clinically and throughout the evolution of the dialysis field this quantity has been used.

In the development of the expressions to follow, Q_B will be used as the flow rate of the portion of the blood appropriate to the solute being discussed. Consequently, the quantity, $Q_B C_B$, will represent the mass of material in the flowing stream and Q_B will take its units from C_B (e.g., if C_B for bicarbonate is in mEq/l of blood water adjusted for red cell water and Donnan effects then Q_B will be in units of l/min of effective blood water flow). It should be recognized, however, that much dialysis literature and product information (such as dialyzer performance data) use the clinically measurable values of Q_B so that if other flow rates are desired they must be computed from the bulk flow and blood constants.

Protein binding

Many substances bind to plasma and body proteins (11). The relevant solute concentration with regard to dialyzer transport will be the free concentration in plasma water. However, the bound material will be in equilibrium with bound solutes to the extent of the particular solute system's solute protein binding coefficient (11). The practical effect of solute-protein binding will be that solute analyses of plasma will yield the sum of the bound and free concentrations and will overstate the concentration driving force present. Secondly, as free solute is removed there will be unbinding of solute with the effect of supporting the free concentrations. Consequently, depending on the kinetics of binding/unbinding – the free concentration in inlet blood, relative to dialysate concentrations, will understate the concentration driving force present during the transit of a dialyzer by the plasma.

Dialysance and clearance

Consider the dialyzer under single pass conditions as shown in Figure 4. Once flows have stabilized after the start of dialysis, the system will be nominally at steady state under which condition the mass balance will be:

$$Q_{Bi} C_{Bi} + Q_{Di} C_{Di} = (Q_{Bi} - Q_F) C_{Bo} + (Q_{Di} + Q_F) C_{Do}.$$

Rearrangement of this expression yields:

$$Q_{Bi} (C_{Bi} - C_{Bo}) + Q_F C_{Bo} = Q_{Di} (C_{Do} - C_{Di}) + Q_F C_{Do}. \quad [9]$$

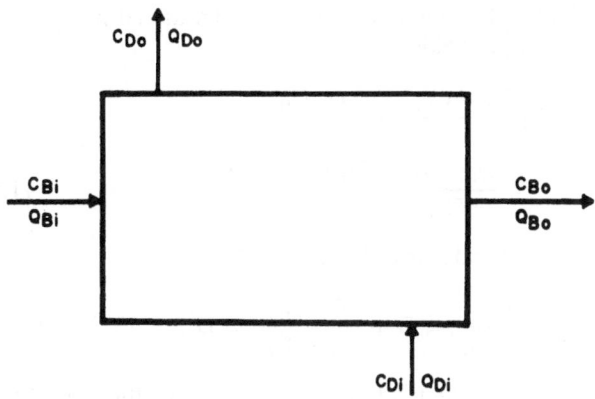

Figure 4. Schematic representation of flows and concentrations for a dialyzer operated with counter-current flows.

The first term on each side of Equation [9] can be viewed as the diffusive component of flux whereas the second term shows the deviation from the purely diffusive case when there is a convective contribution. Both sides of the Equation are expressions of solute flux during the transit of the dialyzer. The left hand side represents the solute leaving the blood; the right hand side is the solute appearing in the dialysate.

We now define a term called diffusive dialysance (D) (12), which will be a constant for a dialyzer at any specific blood and dialysis fluid flow rate.[1]

$$D = \frac{\text{Change in solute content of incoming blood}}{\text{Concentration driving force}}.$$

Dialysance is the magnitude of flux to be expected per unit of concentration driving force. The next step in the mathematical development is to divide Equation [9] by the concentration driving force from the blood to the dialysate. Using the inlet concentrations as discussed above the generalized inlet concentration driving force will be: $C_{Bi} - C_{Di}$. The term α, is a 'Donnan factor' defined as the ratio of ionic concentrations in dialysate and blood at equilibrium and is relevant to diffusive transport of ions.

$$\alpha = \frac{\text{Equilibrium ion concentration in dialysate}}{\text{Equilibrium ion concentration in plasma water}}$$

$$D = \frac{Q_{Bi}(C_{Bi} - C_{Bo})}{\alpha C_{Bi} - C_{Di}} = \frac{Q_{Di}(C_{Do} - C_{Di})}{\alpha C_{Bi} - C_{Di}}. \quad [10]$$

When non-charged solutes are being considered, $\alpha = 1$ and Equation [10] becomes:

$$D = \frac{Q_{Bi}(C_{Bi} - C_{Bo})}{C_{Bi} - C_{Di}} = \frac{Q_{Di}(C_{Do} - C_{Di})}{C_{Bi} - C_{Di}}. \quad [11]$$

---

[1] It should be noted that this is the special case of dialysance (which will appear later) and that in this unique case, ultrafiltration, Q_F, is zero.

Dividing Equation [9] by the concentration driving force, $C_{Bi} - C_{Di}$, yields:

$$\frac{Q_{Bi}(C_{Bi} - C_{Bo})}{C_{Bi} - C_{Di}} + \frac{Q_F C_{Bo}}{C_{Bi} - C_{Di}}$$
$$= \frac{Q_{Di}(C_{Do} - C_{Di})}{C_{Bi} - C_{Di}} + \frac{Q_F C_{Do}}{C_{Bi} - C_{Di}} . \qquad [12]$$

The left hand side of Equation [12] becomes:

$$\frac{J}{C_{Bi} - C_{Di}} = D + \frac{Q_F C_{Bo}}{C_{Bi} - C_{Di}} = D', \qquad [13a]$$

where D' is the total dialysance (12). The flux out of the blood compartment is then:

$$J = D(C_{Bi} - C_{Di}) + Q_F C_{Bo}. \qquad [13b]$$

If $Q_F \ll Q_B$, Equation [11] can be considered to represent the approximate relationship of blood inlet and outlet concentrations. In such a case, which is generally true during hemodialysis, Equation [11] can be solved for C_{Bo}. If this rearrangement is substituted into the above expression:

$$J = D(C_{Bi} - C_{Di}) + Q_F \left[C_{Bi} - \frac{D}{Q_{Bi}} (C_{Bi} - C_{Di}) \right].$$

And expanding and rearranging:

$$J = \left[D \left(1 - \frac{Q_F}{Q_{Bi}} \right) + Q_F \right] C_{Bi}$$
$$- D \left(1 - \frac{Q_F}{Q_{Bi}} \right) C_{Di}. \qquad [14]$$

Equation [14] when solved for D yields:

$$D = \frac{(J/C_{Bi} - C_{Di}) - (Q_F C_{Bi}/C_{Bi} - C_{Di})}{1 - Q_F/Q_{Bi}} . \qquad [15]$$

The flux in Equation [15] can either be measured by the amount of solute lost from the blood or the amount appearing in the dialysate. Equation [9] indicates that by using the left hand side as the value for J, an expression for dialysance based on the blood side results, D_B. Analogous steps and using the right hand side of Equation [9] will result in D_D.

An important special case of these expressions is when $C_{Di} = 0$ which is the case with most single pass dialyzers and metabolic wastes. In this case, Equation [11] becomes the definition of diffusive clearance K, which is the analog of the physiological concept (13):

$$K = \frac{Q_{Bi}(C_{Bi} - C_{Bo})}{C_{Bi}} \qquad [16]$$

and Equation [13a] and [15] become:

$$\frac{J}{C_{Bi}} = K + Q_F \frac{C_{Bo}}{C_{Bi}} = K' \qquad [17a]$$

$$K = \frac{(J/C_{Bi}) - Q_F}{1 - (Q_F/Q_{Bi})} . \qquad [17b]$$

Rearrangement of this expression, or alternatively, simplification of Equation [14] when $C_{Di} = 0$ yields:

$$J = [K(1 - Q_F/Q_{Bi}) + Q_F]C_{Bi} = K'C_{Bi}. \qquad [18]$$

Here K' is the total clearance and is defined as the total flux divided by the inlet blood concentration. Equations [13] and [17a] mathematically combine diffusive and convective components of transport into a single first order term D' or $K'.^2$

Because these linear coefficients relate flux to the concentration driving force, they are very useful in the kinetic description of dialysis. It should be pointed out, however, that these terms are no longer constant for a given set of blood and dialysis fluid flow rates because of their dependence on the ultrafiltration rate, Q_F.

The appearance of a diffusive and a convective term in Equations [14] and [18] should not be taken as identifying the mechanism of convective transport but as a description of the net contribution that ultrafiltration will make to flux and corresponding dialysance and clearance. It is seen in Equations [14] and [18] that clearance and dialysance will increase with ultrafiltration to the extent of the actual concentration present in the outflow blood.

That these equations mathematically (as opposed to physically) describe net transport is illustrated by considering Equation [13a] for a cation such as K^+. In such a case, the cation will be retained as plasma is ultrafiltered due to Donnan effects and $C_{Bo} > C_{Bi}$. In fact it is possible to conceive of cases where the increased dialysance above the diffusive value, due to Q_F, may be greater than the ultrafiltration flux itself as a result of the second term of Equation [13a] $- C_{Bo}/(\alpha C_{Bi} - C_{Di}) > 1$.

Potassium presents an illustrative case. If D(potassium) $= 0.100$ l/min, $C_{Bi} = 4$ mmol/l, $C_{Di} = 2$ mmol/l and $\alpha = 0.95$ (Gotch FA, Falkenhagen D, Sargent JA: Unpublished data), C_{Bo} will be approximately 3 mmol/l, and $C_{Bo}/(\alpha C_{Bi} - C_{Di}) = 1.67$, and there would be an increase of more than 3 ml/min in dialysance for each 2 ml/min of ultrafiltration.

Measurement of dialysance and clearance
In the context of Equation [12] dialysance and clearance values should be identified as flux measured from blood or dialysis fluid and the selection of the location for sampling would appear to be based on the convenience of sampling and the analytical sensitivity of the assays used. While this is true *in vitro*, *in vivo* measurements are complicated by the complexity of blood. The unstated assumption of Figure 4 and Equation [12] is that the blood flow rate, Q_B, is that of a homogeneous fluid at concentration C_B. *In vivo* conditions are at variance with this assumption: 1) Blood

---

[2] These expressions are those generally used in defining clearance and dialysance and also appear in Chapters 6 and 13.

is heterogeneous because of suspended red cells which will result in transmural solute disequilibrium for large materials and rapid transits through the dialyzer, 2) Blood is composed of certain non-aqueous constituents so that water flow (the distribution space for dissolved unbound solutes) equals the product of blood flow and the aqueous fraction.

In light of these difficulties, using dialysate values allows direct measurement of fluxes without the complexities described above. It is prudent, however, to obtain both blood and dialysate side values as a check on methods and analysis. In general, dialysance and clearance measurements used throughout this chapter, will be specified in terms of the dialysate side (K_D).

It should be noted that there are preferred methods of measuring the values in Equation [9]. Operationally Q_{Do} and C_{Do} can be determined from a timed aliquot of outflow dialysate; historically the preferred method of determining Q_B has been from bubble time measurement (14). The bubble time method has always been clinically tedious and this is particularly true with the advent of more rapid blood flow. An alternate method is to time blood pump revolutions (Sargent JA: Unpublished data). The sequence of blood and dialysate samples should be C_{Bo} and C_{Do} then C_{Bi} and C_{Di} so that sampling does not upset flow patterns. Q_F is determined from the product of ultrafiltration coefficient (K_{UF}) and the blood-dialysate pressure drop ($P_B - P_D$) a rearrangement of Equation [8].

$$Q_F = K_{UF}(P_B - P_D). \qquad [19]$$

Effective blood water flow for various solutes

Blood water is the solvent for most materials, diffusively transported by the dialyzer. In general, blood water can be considered to be divided into extracellular or plasma water and intercellular or red cell water. If the hematocrit (HCT), plasma, and red cell water fractions (F_P, F_R) are known the portion of blood water flow of each can be estimated.

$$\text{Plasma water flow rate} = Q_B \left(1 - \frac{HCT}{100}\right) F_P$$

$$\text{Red cell water flow rate} = Q_B \frac{HCT}{100} F_R$$

and total blood water flow rate will be:

$$Q_{BW} = Q_B \left[F_P - \frac{HCT}{100} (F_P - F_R)\right]. \qquad [20]$$

Some substances resist somewhat transport out of the red blood cell and the contribution of the red blood cell to overall mass transfer can be modified by a coefficient γ which represents the fraction of red blood cell water that participates in the transfer during a transit of the dialyzer. That is, if during a transit of the dialyzer the plasma concentration is dropped to half its inlet value while the red blood cell concentration is reduced by only 25% γ would be 0.5. For a material for which the red blood cell membrane is essentially transparent, γ will be 1.0. For charged particles the Donnan ratio (R_D) must also be added to Equation [20], where:

$$R_D = \frac{\text{anion concentration in red cells}}{\text{anion concentration in plasma water}}$$

$$= \frac{1}{\alpha} \text{ (red cell to plasma).}$$

Substituting these factors into Equation [20] the general expression for effective blood flow rate (Q_E) is:

$$Q_E = Q_B \left[F_P - \frac{HCT}{100} (F_P - F_R \gamma R_D)\right]. \qquad [21]$$

Effective blood flow rate for bicarbonate

The bicarbonate ion is a charged particle for which the red cell membrane is very permeable (8), and $\gamma = 1.0$.

Because of its charge, bicarbonate concentration in red cell water will be lower than in plasma water (i.e., $R_D < 1.0$). For bicarbonate Equation [21] becomes:

$$Q_E = Q_B \left(F_P - \frac{HCT}{100} (F_P - F_R R_D)\right). \qquad [22]$$

For values of: $F_P = 0.94$, $F_R = 0.72$, and $R_D = 0.69$, Equation [22] reduces to (10):

$$Q_E = Q_B \, 0.94 - 0.443 \frac{HCT}{100}. \qquad [23]$$

The effective flow, Q_E, can then be used in place of Q_B in the foregoing expressions and those to be developed relating D, Q_D and Q_B to K_oA.

The effect of increasing hematocrit on transport

With the anticipated introduction of recombinant human erythropoietin (15, 16) the long sought ability to correct the anemia seen in most dialysis patients may become a reality. However considering Equation [21] this advance would be expected to be accompanied by a reduction in effective blood flow and lower dialyzer performance at the same blood flows. The effect of doubling hematocrit on Q_E for three hypothetical substances is shown in Table 2 as calculated using Equation [21]. The first substance represents a small solute evenly distributed in blood water (urea would be an example). For this substance effective blood flow would decrease slightly and a 5% increase in blood flow rate would be required to compensate. The effect has been merely to add more protein (in the form of red blood cells) to the blood. The second case is a substance such as potassium that either does not distribute in red cell water or is large enough, (or metabolically retained in the red cell), that it does not appreciably move

Table 2. Effective blood flow at different hematocrits for various substances (see Equation [21]). Calculations assume blood flow of 250 ml/min, $F_P = 0.94$, and $F_R = 0.72$

HCT	γ	R_D	Q_E	Q_B to keep Q_E const	% increase Q_B
20	1	1	224	–	
40	1	1	213	263	5%
20	0	1	188	–	
40	0	1	141	333	33%
20	1	0.69	213	–	
40	1	0.69	191	279	12%

The values in Table 2 show the increases in blood flow rate required to keep solute fluxes constant for substances with a range of plasma – red cell distribution characteristics. It is also clear that different substances will require different adjustments so that compensation for flux rate changes for all materials will not be possible by increases in blood flow alone.

out of red cells during transit through the dialyzer. In this case the effective blood flow rate equals the plasma water flow rate and will be reduced accordingly. An increase of 33% in blood water flow rate will be required in this case to keep effective blood flow (plasma flow) rate constant. The final case is for a charged material which is easily transported out of red cells (e.g., bicarbonate). In this case the Donnan effect keeps its concentration low in cells relative to plasma and as HCT increases, the effective blood flow decreases by about 10%. An increase in blood flow of 12% would be required to keep the effective blood flow constant in this case. The effect of intermediate cases (i.e., $0 < \gamma < 1$) can be estimated from Table 2 or can be calculated using Equation [21].

Reduced fluxes can also be compensated for by changes in dialysis fluid composition. To keep flux rates of a substance constant the right side of Equation [14] must be constant when the individual variables change. With increased hematocrit the dialysate concentrations C_{Di} will have to change (from C_{D1} to C_{D2}) to account for reduction in Q_E (from Q_{E1} to Q_{E2}) which will also cause D to decrease (from D_1 to D_2 – see below).

If the left side of Equation [14] remains the same, equating the right side at different hematocrits, the dialysate concentration required to keep flux of a substance constant will be:

$$C_{D2} = \frac{D_1 C_{D1} \left(1 - \frac{Q_F}{Q_{E1}}\right) - C_B \left[D_1 \left(1 - \frac{Q_F}{Q_{E1}}\right) - D_2 \left(1 - \frac{Q_F}{Q_{E2}}\right)\right]}{D_2 \left(1 - \frac{Q_F}{Q_{E2}}\right)}. \quad [24]$$

Consider the case of bicarbonate with hematocrit increasing from 20 to 40% with $C_{D1} = 35$ mEq/l at average plasma levels of 25 mEq/l. Effective blood flows (Q_{E1} and Q_{E2}) can be read from Table 2 as 0.213 and 0.191 l/min respectively. As will be discussed below, D_2 will be lower than D_1 because of the reduced effective blood flow (10). If $D_1 =$

0.150 l/min, $D_2 = 0.142$ l/min at $Q_f = 0.01$ l/min, Equation [24] indicates that C_{D2} will have to be 35.62 mEq/l to keep bicarbonate flux constant.

Similar manipulation of Equation [14] can determine what new plasma levels would result if dialysis fluid concentrations are not (or cannot) be changed (Figures 5 and 6).

For the majority of patients required dialysis fluid potassium levels can be computed with the help of Equation [24]. There could be a problem, however, with patients who are poorly compliant with respect to dietary K^+ restriction and have normal or high plasma K^+ level with low HCT controlled by use of zero potassium dialysis solution. Consider a patient with short dialysis (Dialysis time – td – 2 h), plasma K^+ of 5.0 mEq/l with HCT = 20. Figure 5 shows that K^+ removal in 2 h with $C_D K = 0$ is approximately 148 mEq and that if HCT increased to 40 the CpK would have to rise to 6.0 to remove the same amount of potassium. In this case serious pre-dialysis hyperkalemia could result.

The effect of decreasing inorganic phosphate (iP) dialysance (DiP) on phosphate removal is complicated because of the double pool nature of phosphate. Moreover, the bulk of phosphate removal is through the gut and mediated by binders. However, estimates of the effect of decreased phosphorus dialysance due to increased HCT can be made by a double pool analysis shown in the Appendix. The results of this analysis for a short (td = 2 h) treatment are shown in Figure 6.

The rise in pre-dialysis phosphorus levels required to maintain zero iP balance as dialysance drops with constant gut removal was computed and is shown in Figure 6a as a function of HCT. It is apparent that as HCT increases from 20 to 40% the rise in pre-treatment phosphorus would be less than 0.5 mg/dl, a modest increase.

The increase in iP binder mediated gut removal required to maintain pre-dialysis levels constant at 5 mg/dl with decreasing DiP was also computed with results shown in Figure 6b. A 3% increase in iP binders would be required as HCT increases from 20 to 40%.

It can be concluded from the above that efficiency of dialyzer removal of the major low molecular solutes analyzed will not be seriously compromised by normalization of HCT with erythropoietin therapy. It would appear that normal HCTs will not jeopardize the current interest in the use of high flux dialyzers with short treatment times in the range of 2 h.

The interrelationship of operational constants, D, Q_B and Q_D and the overall mass transfer coefficient-membrane area product

It is useful to determine the relationship between the operational clinical constant, diffusive dialysance, and the overall mass transfer coefficient. Equation 6 shows that for a given dialyzer K_o will be a constant and flux will be determined solely by the magnitude of blood and dialysate concentrations; the value of K_o will not change as flows

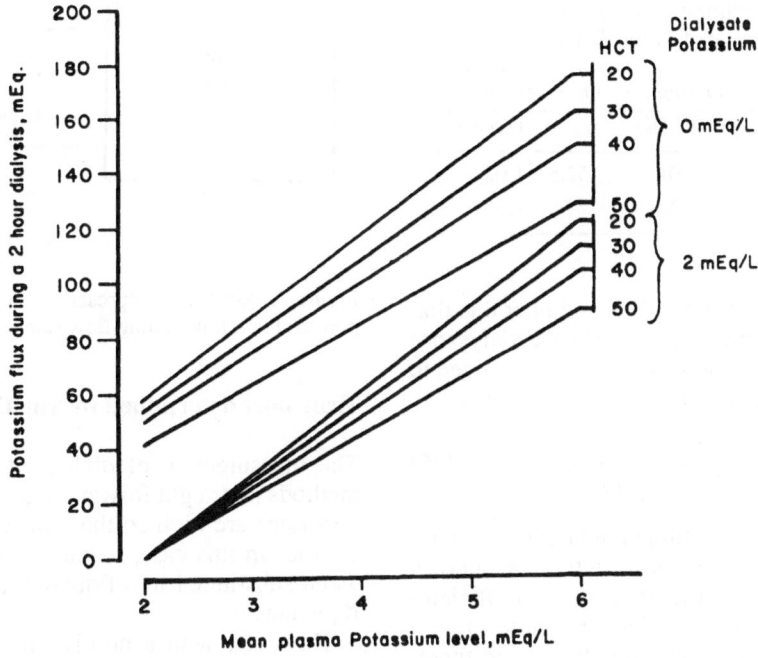

Figure 5. The effect of hematocrit on potassium transport during dialysis.

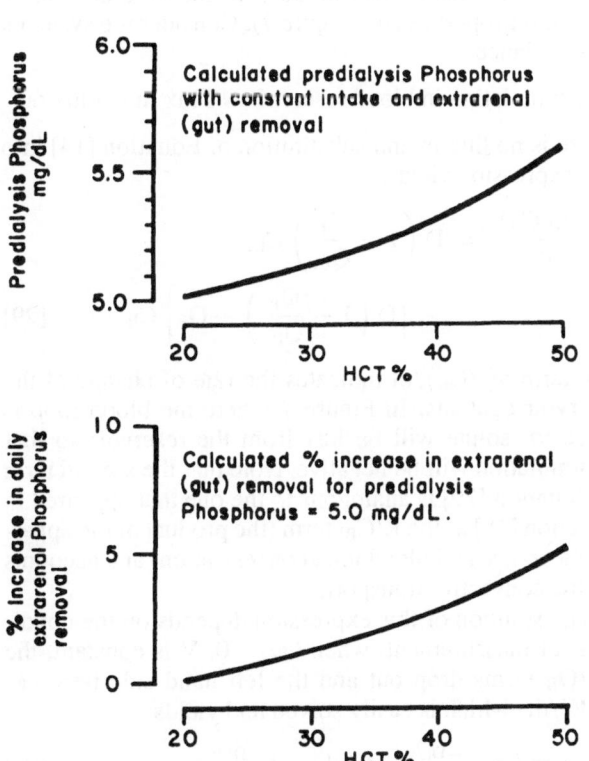

Figure 6. Expected phosphorus levels and extrarenal removal requirements with increasing hematocrit.

or concentrations change. Inspection of Equations [10] and [11] shows that this is not true for diffusive dialysance and that the value of this constant depends directly on the flow rate. Hence, under any particular flow conditions there should be a relationship between D and K_o, (or K_oA) which would be useful in determining the value of the dialyzer constant K_o from a set of clinical chemistries. Conversely, it should be possible to determine what clinical performance a dialyzer should have when blood or dialysate flow rates change or when dialyzer membrane is compromised such as in the case of clotting.

It is possible to relate K_oA and D by equating solute flux in a dialyzer using Equation [14] (when $Q_F = 0$), the definition of D (see Equation [11], and Equations [6] and [7]. Such a combination and rearrangement yields:

$$D\,(C_{Bi} - C_{Di}) = K_oA\,\frac{(C_{Bi} - C_{Do}) - (C_{Bo} - C_{Di})}{\text{Log}(C_{Bi} - C_{Do}/C_{Bo} - C_{Di})}\,.$$

Manipulation of Equation [11] yields the inlet and outlet concentration differences:

$$C_{Bi} - C_{Do} = (C_{Bi} - C_{Di})(1 - D/Q_D)$$

and

$$C_{Bo} - C_{Di} = (C_{Bi} - C_{Di})(1D/Q_B).$$

Substitution of these concentration terms into the equation above and rearrangement yields:

$$K_oA = \frac{Q_B}{1 - Q_B/Q_D}\,\text{Log}\,\frac{1 - D/Q_D}{1 - D/Q_B}\,. \qquad [25]$$

Table 3. The effect of ultrafiltration on solute clearance for materials easily and poorly cleared by the dialyzer

Solute	K_d	$Q_F = 5\ ml/min$		$Q_F = 10\ ml/min$	
	$Q_F = 0$	K_d'	K_d'/K_d	K_d'	K_d'/K_d
Urea	150	151.25	1.01	152.5	1.02
Solute 'X'	20	24.5	1.23	29.0	1.45

This is the expression describing K_oA and how this dialyzer constant can be computed from diffusive dialysance and clinical flows. This relationship can be rearranged to yield dialysance as a function of K_oA and flow rates:

$$D = \frac{e + (K_oA\,(1 - Q_B/Q_D)/Q_B) - 1}{\frac{e + (K_oA(1 - Q_B/Q_D)/Q_B)}{Q_B} - (1/(Q_D))} \qquad [26]$$

Equation [25] is extremely useful in predicting the dialysance (or clearance) of a particular solute under known flow conditions if the overall mass transfer coefficient-membrane area product (K_oA) is known. Quite often a family of dialyzers will have the same design and therefore similar transport resistances. In such cases, the clinical performance of other dialyzers of same type can be accurately estimated merely by scaling the value of K_oA by the differing membrane areas in the various devices.

Equations [25] and [26] are for counter current flow. Similar expressions can be developed for co-current flow for K_oA:

$$K_oA = \frac{Q_B}{1 + Q_B/Q_D} \, \text{Log} \frac{Q_B}{Q_B - D(1 + Q_B/Q_D)} . \qquad [27]$$

and upon rearrangement for D:

$$D = Q_B \frac{1 - e - (K_oA(1 + Q_B/Q_D)/Q_B)}{1 + Q_B/Q_D} . \qquad [28]$$

Effective clearance of larger solutes with ultrafiltration

It is generally recognized that convective transport (ultrafiltration) augments solute transport (17, 18). Equation [18] indicates that with smaller solutes and high clearance values (K), the effective clearance (K') will not be greatly influenced by ultrafiltration. This is not the case, however, with larger substances where K may be of the same order of magnitude as Q_F. The effect of ultrafiltration on mass transport of solutes of different size can be illustrated using urea and a hypothetical, large molecular weight, substance which is poorly removed by diffusive transport (see Table 3). The data in Table 3 confirm that ultrafiltration plays an extremely limited role in the case of a highly cleared solute as urea (adding only 2% at high rates of ultrafiltration) but can be a major means of transport of material with limited diffusive transport potentially augmenting clearance by as much as 45%.

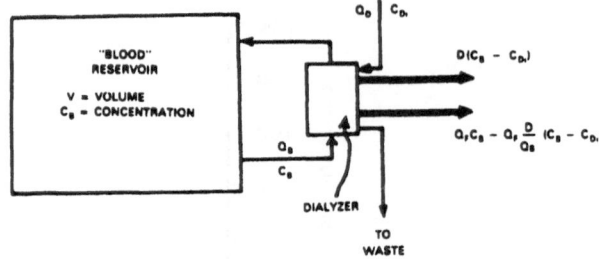

Figure 7. Schematic representation of recycle circuit for transport evaluation including flow rates and removal rates.

Transport determined by kinetic methods

The measurement of dialyzer transport by single pass methods is straight forward and accurate as long as transport rates are high so that concentration differences are sizable. In this case, values for Q_{Do}, C_{Do}, Q_F, and C_{Bi} when substituted into Equation [17b] will yield reliable K_d values.

However, with a poorly diffusing solute where C_{Do} values may be small as will the drop in blood values, a closed loop method will yield more accurate results. With this procedure either the blood circuit or the dialysate circuit is recycled through a reservoir, and the rate of solute accumulation can be used to measure accurately transport properties (see Figure 7). Consider the system's mass balance:

Accumulation in blood reservoir = Flux in − Flux out.

There is no flux in and substitution of Equation [14] into this expression yields:

$$\frac{d(VC_B)}{dt} = D\left(1 - \frac{Q_F}{Q_{Bi}}\right)C_{Di}$$
$$- \left[D\left(1 - \frac{Q_F}{Q_{Bi}}\right) + Q_F\right]C_B. \qquad [29]$$

The term $d(VC_B)/dt$ indicates the rate of change of the reservoir contents. In Figure 7 where the blood loop is recycled, solute will be lost from the reservoir so that accumulation will be negative. Note that the second term of Equation [29] is analogous to the one that appeared in Equation [18] as the $K'C_{Bi}$ term (the product of the apparent clearance and blood inlet concentration) and accounts for the convective transport.

The solution of this expression depends on the conditions of measurement; when $Q_F = 0$, V is constant, the Q_F/Q_B terms drop out and the left hand side becomes $V(dC/dt)$ which is easily solved and yields:

$$C_B = C_{Bo}\, e^{-Dt/v} + C_{Di}(1 - e^{-Dt/v}). \qquad [30a]$$

Rearranging and solving for D:

$$D = \frac{v}{t}\, \text{Log} \frac{C_{Bo} - C_{Di}}{C_{Bt} - C_{Di}} . \qquad [30b]$$

Table 4. Commonly used solute markers for transport studies

Solute	Molecular weight	Ref
NaCl	58	(2)
Urea	60	(2)
Creatinine	113	(2)
Uric acid	168	(2)
Dextrose	180	(2)
Sucrose	342	(2)
Raffinose	594	(2)
Bromsulfophthalein (BSP)	838	(19)
Cyclohepta-amylose or β Schardinger or Cyclodextrin	1,152	(2, 21)
Vitamin B_{12}	1,355	(2, 19)
Bacitracin	1,411	(2, 19)
Insulin	5,200	(2, 19)
Cytochrome C	13,400	(2, 19)

Note that if the reservoir of Figure 7 is placed on the dialysate side, an equivalent expression to Equation [29] results which when solved yields analogous solutions where the 'B' and 'D' sub-scripts are reversed. If Q_F is not zero, Equation [29] must be solved and yields a more complicated expression which is the analog to Equation [30a]. (This case is solved in the Appendix.)

Using the closed loop method for clearance determination, one of the streams is recycled through a reservoir and the reservoir concentration is sampled at two times, t minutes apart. The first concentration becomes C_{Bo} (or C_{Do}), the second C_{Bt} (or C_{Dt}). The dialysance can then be calculated from Equation [30b]. Another method using this recycle technique and Equation [30b] is to take serial reservoir samples and to plot the logarithm term as a function of time. The slope of the resulting straight line will then be D/V from which the value of D can be obtained, V being known.

This technique is most suitable for materials that are poorly transported by the dialyzer so that the reservoir concentration does not change rapidly. The model shown in Figure 7 assumes that all of the material in the system is in the reservoir which is well mixed. In actuality, a significant fraction of the recycle loop can be outside (i.e., the dialyzer volume and tubing) so that this assumption is not strictly true. If D is small and V is large, however, this non-ideality becomes negligible.

The use of marker solutes

It is common practice to describe a dialyzer or membrane by the transport properties of a series of marker substances such as those listed in Table 4 (19–23). These materials

when used in controlled *in vitro* studies yield transport as a function of molecular weight relationships that characterize the particular dialyzer. The difficulty with such characterizations is that *in vivo* performance cannot be predicted accurately from *in vitro* transport data because of the presence of proteins and the probability of their interaction with the membrane, the possibility of Donnan effects, and other phenomena unique to physiologic solutions. An added complication is that less than half of the listed materials (predominantly those of lower molecular weight) can be used *in vivo* so that the relationship between *in vitro* and *in vivo* values cannot be obtained easily. Finally, results of transport studies with higher molecular mass substances should be used circumspectly; membrane permeability depends on factors other than molecular mass such as molecular conformation (2, 19, 20) so that a substance of 1355 Daltons (the mass of vitamin B_{12}), for example, may have transport properties far different *in vivo* from those observed for vitamin B_{12} *in vitro*.

MASS BALANCE PRINCIPLES APPLIED TO INTERMITTENT DIALYSIS: SOLUTE KINETIC MODELING

Uremia results from the body's loss of control over its internal chemistry through the diminished capacity of the chemical regulating organ, the kidney. The fundamental assumption of dialysis treatment is that some uremic abnormalities depend on the concentration of ingested or metabolically produced toxic materials which are normally excreted by the natural kidney. The ability to keep the uremic patient alive by hemodialysis and peritoneal dialysis emphasizes that if some degree of chemical control can be restored, however imperfect, the results of uremia (particularly the predictable and imminent mortality) can be, in part, reversed. It is clear, therefore, that the passive transport of water, solutes and electrolytes which is the sole capability of dialysis, is sufficient to control the chemical imbalances which result from kidney failure.

In dialysis treatment a large number of materials, many of unknown composition (24–36) and toxicity are being removed, at unequal rates. To 'control' dialysis treatment, therefore, one might hope to select a key compound which would provide an index of treatment. To date there is no such compound although there have been numerous attempts to define one in order to develop an index of adequate treatment (5, 37, 38). In reality although control of toxic substances may be the goal of dialysis treatment, levels of a limited number of solutes, balance of fluid and electrolytes, and control of acid-base constitute the basis of current treatment adequacy on a day-to-day basis. It is with regard to the measurement and control of such substances that the concept of mass balance and solute kinetics can provide powerful tools and insights to guide treatment.

Dialysis was first mathematically modeled over three decades ago (12) with similar analysis continuing until the present time (22, 37–49). Clinical dialysis, however, has not kept pace with these advances in the quantitative understanding and ability to describe and monitor treatment. The reasons for this vary. Not all physicians consider the task of clinical management of the dialysis patient as a completely quantifiable one, a view that is at least partially justified because of the multifactorial nature of most medical problems. In addition, much of the information required by some models is unavailable to the practising physician in the time span required for his treatment decisions. These restrictions notwithstanding, the ability to describe quantitatively biochemical and physiologic processes, and the abnormalities that exist in uremic patients make the process of modeling an important one for greater understanding of the disease state and better management of subsequent therapy.

Mathematical modeling of dialysis therapy represents the structured application of the principles of conservation of matter to the patient undergoing dialysis. There are many advantages to this structured approach:

1. It can describe a specific biochemical system and thereby monitor or investigate various physiologic processes, such as net rates of protein catabolism (50–52).
2. It enables one to prescribe the appropriate dialysis treatment to achieve a desired therapeutic goal, or to investigate the predictable results of altered treatment (42, 43, 53, 54).
3. It increases understanding of the controlling physiologic biochemical mechanisms from the type of model required to describe the kinetics of a particular substance (10, 47, 55).
4. It allows determination of the controlling factors in any solute system through evaluation of the order of magnitude of various routes of input and output in a quantitatively defined system (10).
5. It allows discrimination of the causes of clinical observations and problems such as hypertension caused by sodium flux or hypoxia during acetate dialysis (10, 47).

Mathematical modeling can be viewed as 'quantified intuition' in that it mathematically relates events that are known to take place. Two aspects of mathematical modeling that should be stressed are:

1. An individual who has a thorough basic understanding of the physiologic system being modeled is best able to construct and benefit from the model (i.e., the physician who deals with specific clinical problems).
2. Putting the qualitative relationship in a mathematical context increases its value and the usefulness of information by vastly extending its range of application and the value of analyzed data (see discussion of mathematical elements in the appendix).

The basic steps of modeling are shown in Figure 8 and consist of: formulating the system description (step one)

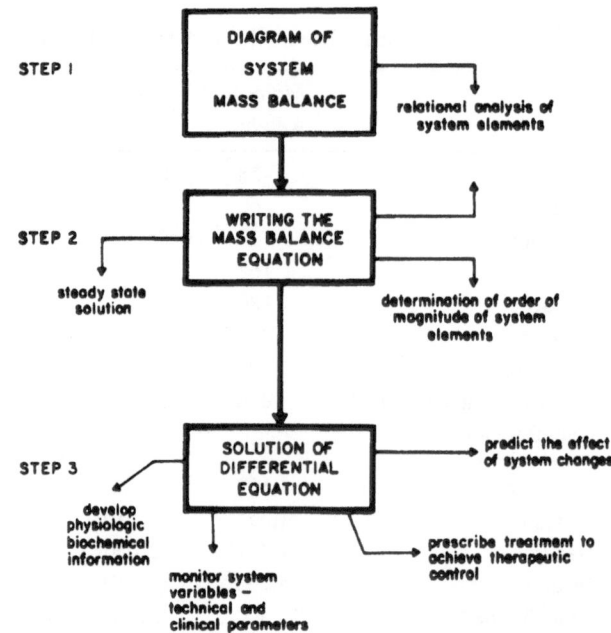

Figure 8.   Diagram illustrating the steps in formulating and representing a mathematical model. Figure includes indications of uses of each stage of formulation.

which usually involves a diagrammatic representation of the system; writing the mass balance equation (step two) using the diagram; and solving the mass balance equation (step three). It should be noted that only step three requires any degree of advanced mathematical skills.

MASS BALANCE CONSIDERATIONS AS APPLIED TO QUANTIFICATION OF INTERMITTENT DIALYSIS TREATMENT

The concept of conservation of matter or mass balance appears to be obvious; it is in the application of this law to a physical system, however, that it becomes an increasingly complex but an extremely powerful analytical and conceptual tool.

The Law of Conservation of Mass can be restated in the word equation:

$$\begin{matrix} \text{Accumulation} \\ \text{(increase in} \\ \text{system content)} \end{matrix} = \begin{matrix} \text{input} \\ \text{to} \\ \text{system} \end{matrix} - \begin{matrix} \text{output} \\ \text{from} \\ \text{system} \end{matrix} \qquad [31]$$

Equation [31] forms the basis for a substantial portion of this chapter in that most relationships to follow are either applications or solutions of it.

Formulation of a model: elements of the mass balance diagram

While the application of mass balance principles to a specific system would appear not to pose any great problem, in practice it is the most difficult aspect of modeling. The difficulty lies in the need to understand fully and isolate quantitatively the specific system being modeled. It should be stressed that once the model is formulated the mathematical description of the system is predetermined, so that a deliberate attempt to represent the system accurately and quantitatively will assure the validity of subsequent steps. It is helpful if the model is formulated by use of a structured diagram. Such a diagram consists of boxes for the system and arrows for inputs and outputs.

In the following systems the model is shown as a box with arrows going into and out of it; these figures exemplify the two formal elements of this approach. The box describes the system content (generally in units of mass), such as the product of volume and concentration. Inputs add to the system content, and outputs decrease it. The manner (if any) that the inputs or outputs relate to the system content or concentration is indicated with respect to the appropriate arrows. In the case of a single box (the vast amount of figures shown in this chapter), the system is 'single pool' or one well mixed compartment.

The system content is the total mass present at any instant. It can be contained in any physical space, such as the vascular space, the red blood cell, or the amount of dialysate recirculating through a dialyzer. The system content is the product of the compartment volume and the concentration in that space. Alternatively it can be the total system mass (irrespective of its distribution space) or simply the effect of the total mass such as in the case of heparin (56).

The quantitative description of system inputs and outputs must be consistent with the description of system content. In general, there are two common types of input/outputs: those that depend on the amount of material present in the system (first-order processes) and those that are constant (zero-order processes). The clearance of a dialyzer (K_D) is a first-order process, because material is removed as a product of K_D and concentration (see Equation [18]). In contrast, an effectively saturated metabolic process (such as acetate metabolism in most dialyzed patients) (55) is a constant output, or zero-order process.

The process of model formulation is best illustrated with an example.

Carbon dioxide transport in dialyzed patients

The transport of CO_2 in dialysis patients attracted considerable attention during the 1970s (57–61) and represents a good illustration of modeling techniques. The first step is to define what is meant by the CO_2 system. One must decide what forms of CO_2 are to be included, (eg, should bicarbonate be considered part of the system?) so that all

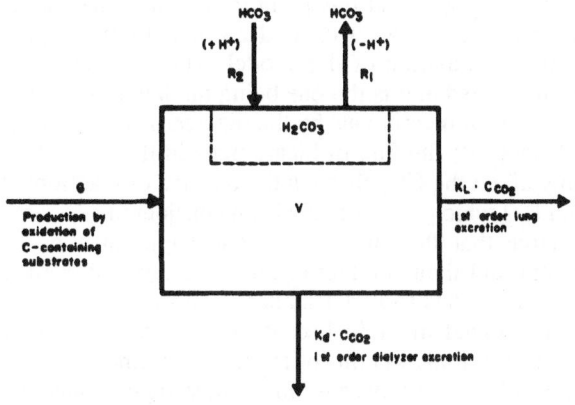

Figure 9. Model describing the CO_2 in the dialysed patient. (Reprinted from *Kidney International*, with permission.)

elements of the model are consistent. For this analysis we will let the CO_2 system be the total dissolved CO_2 gas in body water and let it also include the hydrated form of CO_2 (carbonic acid), but not bicarbonate. We can then draw a box such as Figure 9, that will represent the total body content of CO_2 gas at any time shown as the product of body water and CO_2 concentration (10).

Once the system is identified it is necessary to define how CO_2 is added to, and leaves the system. There are two major means of CO_2 production. The first is the oxidative metabolism of carbon containing substrates which is the ultimate origin of all body CO_2. The other is the neutralization of acid (H^+) by body bicarbonate (see reaction R-2).

$$CO_2 + H_2O \underset{\longleftarrow}{\overset{\longrightarrow}{}} H_2CO_3 \underset{\longleftarrow}{\overset{\longrightarrow}{}} H^+ + HCO_3 \quad \begin{matrix} \text{[R-1]} \\ \text{[R-2]} \end{matrix}$$

Carbon dioxide readily reacts with water to form carbonic acid, which will dissociate to yield H^+ and bicarbonate by reaction R-1. This system of reactions is reversible and moves to the left by reaction R-2, which represents the neutralization of acid (H^+) by bicarbonate to form H_2CO_3 and generation of CO_2. In fact, both of these reactions continue and to the extent that they are unbalanced there is net generation or consumption of CO_2.

There are two major means by which CO_2 is removed from the body water in the non-dialyzed patient. It is apparent that if reaction R-1 predominates CO_2 is removed from the system. The other route of removal is by exhalation in the lungs which will be a first order process and which will depend on the CO_2 concentration (C_{CO_2}) of the system with the lungs representing a first order excretion route which can be viewed as a lung clearance, K_L. The amount of CO_2 removed by the lungs, therefore, is $K_L C_{CO_2}$. In the patient not on dialysis this completely defines the system. In the dialyzed patient, however, the dialyzer will also have a CO_2 clearance (K_D) and flux by this route is $K_D C_{CO_2}$.

It is important, at this point to re-emphasize the need for an unambiguous, structured, and quantitative approach to the formulation of this model. The CO_2 system has been isolated and is the one being modeled. As such the transport of bicarbonate by the dialyzer is not relevant to the analysis; the flux of bicarbonate in the dialyzer will only affect the CO_2 through the balance of reactions R-1 and R-2 which have already been considered.

Note that the units of K_D and C_{CO_2} must be consistent and their product equal the dialyzer flux of dissolved gaseous CO_2. Clearances will most conveniently be expressed in l/min because CO_2 concentrations are most commonly in units of grams or millimoles per liter. This is important, because many investigators have been under the impression that the dialyzer totally 'clears' incoming blood of CO_2 having CO_2 clearances equaling or exceeding blood flow (10, 60, 61). The CO_2 content of incoming blood, however, when expressed in appropriate units is very low (about 1.1 mmol/l) so that the CO_2 removed by the dialyzer is very small (10, 47). Analysis of the system (which will be completed below) will show that a much more significant route of CO_2 removal during dialysis is reaction R-1 which is promoted by bicarbonate loss and body re-alkalinization using acetate during treatment.

This completes the formulation of the CO_2 model. The CO_2 system itself is carbon dioxide, present as dissolved gas and its hydrated form (carbonic acid). CO_2 is generated by metabolic processes and the production of carbonic acid when acids are neutralized by combining with bicarbonate. It is removed by the reversal of this reaction (dissociation of H_2CO_3) and the first order removal, (CO_2 clearance) represented by the lungs (K_L) and the dialyzer (K_D).

Writing the mass balance equation

Once the system has been formulated the mass balance equation is written. This is basically a mechanical step of substituting terms into Equation [31].

The accumulation, or change in system content, will be the rate of change of the system content with time (first derivative with respect to time of the system content: d(content)/dt). It should be noted that although this term gives the intimidating appearance of 'higher mathematics' it is merely a quantitative symbol of the time dependent change of system content (i.e., accumulation). The only aspect that will change from one system to another is the representation of 'content'. In the current example, total dissolved CO_2 'content' will be the product of total body water and CO_2 concentration (not PCO_2):

$$CO_2 \text{ Content} = V\, C_{CO_2}$$

$$\text{Change in system content} = \frac{d(V_{CO_2})}{dt}.$$

The input and output are taken directly from the system diagram (Figure 9) and will be the algebraic sum of all

Table 5. Typical values in a 70 kg patient undergoing acetate dialysis

Interdialytic	Intradialytic	Ref
V = 40 l	40 l	–
C = 1.05 mmol/l		
(P_{CO_2} = 35 mmHg)	1.05 mmol/l	(10)
G = 11 mmol/min	11 mmol/min	(60, 61)
R_1 = –	2.3 mmol/min	–
R_2 = –	0	(10)
K_L = 10.5 l/min	8.1 l/min	(10, 60)
K_D = 0	0.20 l/min	(10)
dC = –	0.3 mmol	–
	(10 mmHg)	
d(VC)/dt = –	0.05 mm/min	–
$K_L C_{CO_2}$ = 11 mmol	8.5 mmol	–
$K_D C_{CO_2}$ = 0	0.21 mmol	–
R_2 = –	2.29 mmol	–

the arrows in the diagram. The zero-order terms will be constants and the first order terms will be the product of first order constants (clearances) and the system concentration. Substitution of all of these terms in Equation [31] yields:

$$\frac{d(V_{CO_2})}{dt} = G + R_2 - R_1 - K_L C_{CO_2} - K_D C_{CO_2}. \quad [32]$$

Equation [32] is the mass balance equation for body CO_2 and, as has been stated, is a strictly mechanical reduction of the elements of the formulation, shown in Figure 9, to a mathematical form.

Use of the mass balance equation

One may be inclined to solve the above expression immediately to obtain the body CO_2 content as a function of time. For this substance this is not a very productive approach. The most useful mathematical relationship in this case, and a valuable one generally, is the mass balance equation itself.

It is instructive to consider all the terms in the specific equation to determine their relative magnitude and relation to one another. Common values for the terms listed are shown in Table 5.

Consider first the accumulation term on the left hand side of Equation [32]. Computation of body CO_2 content using the values in Table 5 (i.e., V = 40 l; C_{CO_2} = 1.05 mmol/l show body CO_2 content is about 42 mmol. This is an interesting value from two standpoints. First, it should be appreciated that the entire body content of CO_2 represents only 4 min of body CO_2 production. Stated differently, there is very little 'CO_2 storage' in the body. The physiological impact of this, as is widely appreciated, is that ventilation can have a pronounced second to second effect on CO_2 levels which is extremely important in pH control through respiratory compensation in response to an acid/base insult. The second point is that a P_{CO_2} change of 10 mmHg over a 4 h dialysis represents an average rate of change in body CO_2 content of: $d(V_{CO_2})/dt = (40)(10)(0.03)/240 = 0.05$ mmol/min or less than 0.5% of the rate of body production. It becomes clear that the change in body CO_2 content represents a small difference between two very large numbers (the rate of production at the rate of removal) and that in fact the body is effectively in steady state with respect to CO_2 content. Intuitively it would be difficult to conclude otherwise.

The system being at steady state, all the terms on the right hand side of Equation [32] must add to zero. Between dialyses Equation [32] reduces to: $G = K_L C_{CO_2}$ the generated CO_2, is exhaled. During dialysis the situation is more complicated. The generation of CO_2 would be expected to remain relatively constant. which from the standpoint of energetics is reasonable. During acetate dialysis reaction R-1 will predominate and R2 will equal zero. Bicarbonate loss in itself will not affect this model. Usually, however, the HCO_3 lost in the dialyzer is almost quantitatively replaced by reaction R-1. If plasma bicarbonate levels are 18 mEq/l approximately 2.3 mEq/min will be lost and replaced by reaction R-1.

Examination of the three routes of removal indicates that the effect of dialyzer CO_2 transport is vanishingly small (2%, see Table 5) and can be neglected with respect to its effect on P_{CO_2}. This fact has not been widely appreciated (60, 61).

At steady state rearrangement of Equation [32] yields:

$$G - R1 - K_D C_{CO_2} = K_L C_{CO_2}.$$

Solving for K_L

$$K_L = G/C_{CO_2} - R1/C_{CO_2} - K_D. \qquad [33]$$

The 'normal' steady state relationship (in the non-dialyzed patient) of G, K_L, K_{Ln}, and C_{CO_2} is:

$$K_{Ln} = G/C_{CO_2}. \qquad [34]$$

If Equation [33] is divided by Equation [34] the relative value of K_L will be

$$\frac{K_L}{K_{Ln}} = 1 - \frac{R1}{G} - \frac{K_D}{K_{Ln}}. \qquad [35]$$

Substituting values into this expression from Table 5 lung clearance would be expected to drop to 77% of its normal value.

Adjustments of CO_2 levels to control pH is part of respiratory feed back in the normal individual (8, 62) although this may be complicated by hypoxia particularly at low P_{CO_2} values. During dialysis P_{CO_2} remains relatively stable (59) and Equation [35] indicates that this must reflect

a reduction in K_L (which is directly related to respiratory rate) to approximately three quarters of non-dialysis values in order to adjust for extrapulmonary CO_2 excretion. It is important, therefore, that the reduced ventilation predicted by Equation [35] be explained when the observed dialysis hypoxia is analyzed (58–61).

Solution of the mass balance equation

Most kinetic models (and all those to be considered) are in the form of a first order linear differential equation for which solutions and solution techniques by classical methods of applied mathematics are well known (63, 64). The solutions describe the system concentration (or system content) as function of time. Essentially the expression can then be used to predict the effect of treatment changes on a particular solute being modeled and to monitor various system parameters. This aspect of modeling has been most extensively developed for urea as described below. In the case of the CO_2 model the system is essentially at steady state (as discussed above). Consequently, a third step will not be taken for this system.

These are the key steps of modeling. It is good to emphasize again that the actual mathematical steps of writing the mass balance equation and solving it (steps two and three in Figure 8) are mechanical operations which totally depend upon the model formulation (step one). Consequently the entire validity of the solutions depends on the correct and rigorous formulation of the model itself.

MASS BALANCE AS APPLIED TO VARIOUS SOLUTE SYSTEMS

Urea nitrogen mass balance

Urea is of interest because it is the major product of protein catabolism so it can be used as an index of the patient's catabolic status and, by extension, nutritional state. Furthermore, development of the uremic syndrome depends to a large extent on protein catabolism (65–69) for which urea[3] generation provides a quantitative measure (see Equation [A-16] in the Appendix).

Although urea is not considered highly toxic, its presence in high blood concentrations may accompany increased morbidity in dialysis patients (70–73). It has been demonstrated in a large well controlled cooperative study that elevation of BUN in the presence of adequate protein intake is associated with increased rates of hospitalization (74–78). In addition, some nitrogenous compounds that are commonly found in the dialysis patient may be stoichiometrically related to the rate of protein

---

[3] Because it is the nitrogen component of urea that is derived from protein, urea nitrogen is the expression used in quantitative considerations herein, but the solute itself is referred to as urea.

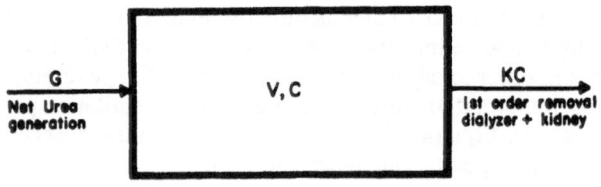

Figure 10.   Model of urea nitrogen in the dialyzed patient. (Reprinted from *Kidney International* with permission.)

catabolism and, consequently, to the rate of urea production.

Urea distribution and metabolism can be described quantitatively as shown in Figure 10. This figure considers urea nitrogen to be distributed in a single pool (physically approximating total body water) (79) with one route of net entry (or net generation) and one route of removal by first order processes.

Urea will enter the pool of body water as amino acids are oxidized (80, 81). As such its minute rate of net generation (absolute synthesis – absolute degradation) will not, in fact, be constant. The urea content of the body, however, is a thermodynamic property (its value being path independent) and will increase in a quasi-linear manner between dialyses. As a result, the assumption that net urea generation is zero-order (constant) is considered to have practical validity.

Routes of removal are considered to be entirely first order (i.e., proportional to concentration) and accounted for solely by the residual kidney and the dialyzer. Urea diffuses into the gut where its nitrogen is converted into ammonia which is reabsorbed by the portal circulation (82, 83). Because this path is internal to the model no net gut contribution to urea removal from total body water is considered.

The analysis of this model then proceeds by writing the mass balance relationship:

$$\text{Accumulation} = \text{Input} - \text{Output}$$
$$\frac{d(VC)}{dt} = G - (K_R + K_D)C. \qquad [36]$$

Further expansion of Equation [36] yields:

$$V\frac{dC}{dt} + C\frac{dV}{dt} = G - (K_R + K_D)C. \qquad [37]$$

Consideration of steady state: chronic renal failure

Before considering the solution of Equation [37] it is appropriate to contemplate the mass balance equation itself with respect to the special, but more usual case of steady state when dC/dt and dV/dt are both negligible. These two quantities will always have some value, but when dialysis is not required there will be no net accumulation of body urea or water and these terms can be neglected. With respect to body solutes steady state is

commonly called 'homeostasis' and in this physiological situation the left hand side of Equation [37] is zero (steady state with respect to body protein is usually called zero nitrogen or protein balance). Considering Equation [37] steady state for urea nitrogen can be represented as:

$$G = K_R C. \qquad [38a]$$

There are two other forms of this expression

$$K_R = G/C \qquad [38b]$$

and

$$C = G/K_R. \qquad [38c]$$

Figure 11 interrelates the three parameters shown in Equations [38]. The figure shows BUN as a function of time at two different levels of protein intake as renal function (urea clearance) declines. The K_R as a linear function of time is shown in a secondary K-time plot in the same figure (lower left). This figure makes use of net rate of urea nitrogen production resulting from a known quantity of protein catabolism. As is discussed further in the Appendix this accurately relates the net amount of urea that will be generated for net protein catabolic rates (PCR) from 20 to 350 g/day in uremic and normal individuals (51, 81, 84, 85). The two forms of this relationship are (with G expressed in mg/min):

$$G = \frac{PCR - 0.294V}{9.35} \qquad [39a]$$

which when rearranged yields

$$PCR = 9.35G + 0.294V. \qquad [39b]$$

Figure 11 represents a progression of steady states as renal function declines. In this figure there is no change in generation. As 70 g of protein is ingested and a like amount catabolized a net quantity of 6.23 mg/min of urea nitrogen or 13.4 mg/min of urea, (i.e., 233 μmol/min) is produced, both in the uremic patient with 10 ml/min of renal function, and in a normal individual. This same amount is excreted in both cases. The difference between the two is that because the flux is equal to the product of K_R and C (Equation [38a]) the BUN must be far higher in the uremic patient which is obviously the case.

There will be some BUN level above which every physician will consider dialysis appropriate. For this discussion 1 mg/dl (214 mg/dl of urea or 35.7 mmol/l) has been chosen as this value, to illustrate the use of steady state expressions shown in Equations [38].

When K_R drops to 6 ml/min, BUN will be slightly above 100 mg/dl (35.7 mmol/l of urea) (see Equation [38c]). At this point the clinical decision may be to start dialysis. As seen from the figure, however, a reduction in protein intake to 50 g/day would decrease the BUN to below 70 mg/dl (25 mmol/l) and delay dialysis for an extended period. This has been the historic approach of the

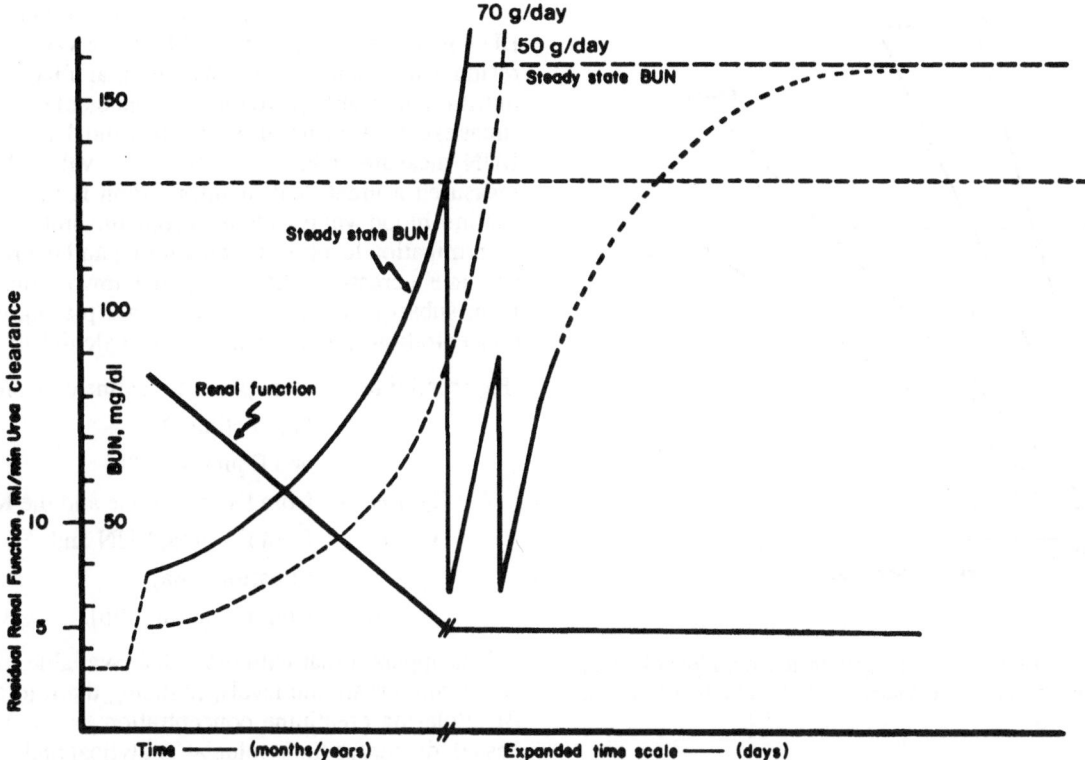

Figure 11. Blood urea nitrogen in a patient with chronic renal failure with decreasing renal function (see superimposed plot in bottom left of figure). Relationship is shown for two levels of protein intake (and net catabolism) up to the point where dialysis is instituted.

management of uremia (65, 86, 87). This, in fact, is the spontaneous physiologic result of uremia and anorectic feed back. With an intake of 50 g/day (G = 4.09 mg/min) the BUN will reach 100 mg/dl (35.7 mmol/l) when K_R is approximately 4 ml/min (see Equation [38c]). Once again the intake may be reduced.

At some point, however, dialysis will be initiated to allow a tolerable intake with acceptable BUN. It is important to realize, however, that a steady state concentration still exists, a mathematical value that may never really be attained. For an intake of 70 g/day with a K_R of 2 ml/min steady state BUN it would be 312 mg/dl (111.4 mmol/l) for example. The patient undergoes dialysis to keep BUN below this level. But at the end of a dialysis, BUN starts to increase towards this level and only the next dialysis interrupts it. The build up of BUN to a steady state value post-dialysis is curvilinear because as BUN increases the remnant kidney removes more material and blunts the rate of rise (see right hand side of Equation [38a] and Figure 11). It is also important to recognize that as long as there is some kidney function there is mathematically a steady state BUN, which will change as K_R does. In some cases K_R will improve slightly; in such cases a re-evaluation of intake and treatment is appropriate (88).

Establishing a level of K_R

In Figure 11 the level of renal function is the major parameter to which all others must adjust. In steady state its value is shown by Equation [38b] which can be expanded to yield:

$$K_R = \frac{G}{C} = \frac{\text{Excretion rate}}{C} = \frac{V_{ur} C_{ur}}{T_{ur}} \frac{1}{C_B}. \qquad [40]$$

This expression is a general form of the classical formula for clearance: $K_R = UV/P$, where U = urine concentration (C_{ur}), V = the volume of a 24 h urine collection divided by 1440 min/day (V_{ur}/T_{ur}) and P = plasma solute level (C_B). Equation [40] recognizes that collection intervals may differ from an exact 24 h.

The right hand side of Equation [40] is general for all solutes and does not rely on the presence of steady state. In this case C_B will be the average blood value during the urine collection (see Appendix for the mathematical determination of this quantity during dialysis). What is required is a urine collection of known volume, V_{ur}, and analysis of the solute concentration in that urine volume, C_{ur}, (urea nitrogen, creatinine, etc) the duration of the collection, T_{ur}, and the average prevailing blood level of that solute C_B. In the case described above (see Figure 11), typical values for a 1500 ml 24 h collection with

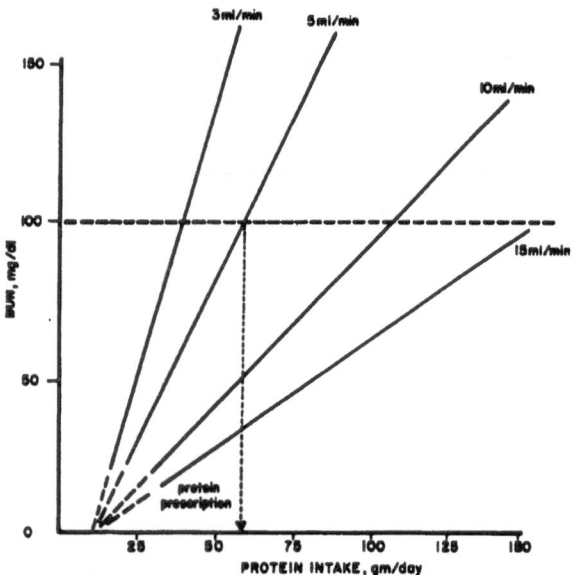

Figure 12. Blood urea nitrogen in the nutritionally stable adult chronic renal failure patient in relation to intake (and net catabolism).

urine urea nitrogen (C_{ur}) 600 mg/dl (214 mmol/l) and creatinine 92 mg/dl (8.1 mmol/l) respectively would yield excretory rates (and generation for the steady state) of 9 g/day (6.25 mg/min) for urea nitrogen and 1380 mg/day (0.96 mg/min) for creatinine. For BUN and creatinine levels of 104 mg/dl (37.1 mmol/l) and 8 mg/dl (708 μmol/l) respectively, clearances will be K_R urea = 6 ml/min; K_R creatinine = 12 ml/min.

This information is useful in several ways. The net rate of urea generation obtained from this urine collection can be used in Equation [39b] to compute net protein catabolism. Such data are useful in many disease states (not just uremia) to assess protein nutritional status and are readily available from urine collections analyzed for urea nitrogen. The rate of creatinine generation is useful as a nutritional parameter (89). Creatinine generation rate is also a convenient check on the accuracy of the urine collection; its value is relatively stable because it is produced at a reasonably constant rate from muscle tissue. Consequently, variability of this parameter suggests inaccuracy in urine collection (either V_{ur}, or T_{ur}) or analysis (C_{ur}).

The ratio of K_R urea to K_R creatinine is also a useful parameter because in chronic renal failure the ratio of these two clearances tends to remain relatively constant and can be used to estimate K_R urea from K_R creatinine values (90, 91). Once K_R urea is known, it is possible to use Equations [38a] both to determine the level of protein intake required to keep BUN below a desired value, and the actual protein intake when a patient presents with an elevated BUN (90).

This approach is shown graphically in Figure 12 where BUN is plotted as a function of PCR for various levels of residual urea clearance. It illustrates that if K_R is known in nutritionally stable (zero nitrogen balance) patients. PCR (intake) can be accurately prescribed and determined from BUN measurements. Once clearance values have been measured a great deal of information is available from routine blood values alone. From the initial clearance determination levels of G (creatinine) and the ratio of K_R urea to K_R creatinine (K_R ratio) are known. Consequently, from subsequent values of BUN and plasma creatinine concentrations the following can be calculated:

K_R creatinine — from plasma creatine concentration, G (creatinine) and Equation [38b]

K_R urea — from K_R creatinine and the K_R ratio

G urea — from K_R urea, BUN and Equation [38a]

PCR — from Equation [39b].

It is apparent that with these data available from BUN and serum creatinine levels, reducing them to a ratio of BUN/plasma creatinine concentration as has been suggested, decreases their value as analytical and nutritional parameters (92).

The technique of evaluating net protein catabolic rate using K_R ratio and G (creatinine) is useful in non-dialyzed patients and has been successfully applied to acute ill patients (91). In unpublished studies of 84 post-transplant patients, burn trauma patients, geriatric patients and normal subjects the average deviation of estimated PCR relative to those computed from 24 h urine collections was less than 10%. The value of this technique is that it permits the monitoring of catabolism in the patient who is undergoing nutritional support as well as the monitoring of renal status and nutrition in the patient with chronic renal failure.

Equation [38c] shows the general determinants of BUN and creatinine levels in the undialyzed (not necessarily uremic) patient. The solute levels relate directly to net rates of generation and inversely to clearances. The widespread use of the reciprocal of plasma creatinine concentration as an index of renal function (93) and the tendency to view elevated BUNs as indicators of renal failure should be examined in the context of Equation [38c]. Plasma creatinine levels reflect renal function only when creatinine generation is constant. When wasting occurs simultaneously with decreasing renal function, creatinine concentration may remain relatively stable because G creatinine and K_r creatinine are decreasing at the same rate. Similarly, elevated BUN reflects the net rate of generation relative to clearance. Consequently, a high BUN may reflect a high rate of catabolism or intake (84) or reduced renal function or both. Appropriate clinical and nutritional management require that the determinants of mass balance as represented by Equation [38c] be evaluated individually.

Urea nitrogen kinetics in the dialyzed patient

At the point in Figure 11 when dialysis is instituted, solute concentration will oscillate at a point below steady state and the object of dialysis is to keep it within a tolerable range. Equation [37] must, therefore, be considered in its entirety.

When there is no significant change in the system volume the second term on the left of Equation [37] can be dropped $(dV/dT = 0)$ and:

$$V\frac{dC}{dt} = G - (K_R + K_D)C \qquad [41a]$$

$$\frac{dC}{dt} = \frac{G}{V} - \frac{K_R + K_D}{V} C. \qquad [41b]$$

It should be pointed out that in the steady state analysis concentration was insensitive to the system volume because there was no solute accumulation. Once dialysis is needed, however, body water serves as a container that stores solutes between treatments. Equation [41b] describes this, and shows that V will significantly influence the rate of concentration increase, dC/dt, and by extension the corresponding treatment required.

The more general case, however, in the uremic patient is for V to change due to fluid retention between treatments and ultrafiltration during dialysis. In this case V as a function of time is represented as:

$$V = V_0 + \beta t \qquad [42a]$$

and

$$\frac{dC}{dt} = \beta, \qquad [42b]$$

where β is the rate of weight gain. Combining Equations [37, 42a] and [42b] and letting $K = K_R + K_D$, yields:

$$\frac{dC}{G - (K + \beta)C} = \frac{dt}{V_0 + \beta} . \qquad [43]$$

Solution of Equations [41a] and [43] by classical techniques (63, 64) yields analogous expression for concentration as a function of time:

$$C = C_0 e^{-Kt/V} + \frac{G}{K}[1 - e^{-Kt/V}] \qquad [44a]$$

$$C = C_0 \left(\frac{V_0 + \beta t}{V_0}\right)^{-K+\beta/\beta}$$

$$+ \frac{G}{K + \beta}\left[1 - \left(\frac{V_0 + \beta t}{V_0}\right)^{-K+\beta/\beta}\right]. \qquad [44b]$$

Manipulations of Equation [44a] for the guidance of dialysis therapy have been discussed elsewhere (42). Analogous rearrangements of Equation [44b] provide for the same monitoring and guidance of treatment in the more general case in renal failure where volumes are changing due to expanding and contracting quantities of body water during different intervals of the therapy.

Equations [44] are used to predict the BUN concentration that will result from a specific set of therapy (t, K, and schedule) and patient (V_0, G, and β) parameters.

Although Equation [44b] is the more general solution of Equation [37] examination of Equation [44a] can give some insight into the nature of these expressions. Reference to Equation [38c] shows that the coefficient of the second term on the right side of Equation [44a] is the steady state concentration if dialysis was performed indefinitely. Equation [44a] can then be written as:

$$C = C_0 - e^{-Kt/V} + Css[1 - e^{-Kt/V}]. \qquad [45]$$

The term, $e^{-Kt/V}$ is one that describes the rate of concentration decay in a first order system of volume V where material is being cleared at a rate K. It represents the reciprocal of $e^{+Kt/V}$ and, therefore, becomes small, approaching zero, as t becomes large. The second term is that for a system approaching steady state with constant input and first order removal. Consequently, Equation [45] represents the combination of 1st order removal of material originally present in the system (1st term) plus the build up of additional material (2nd term).

By definition, any number, including e, raised to the power 0 will equal 1, so that when t = 0, Equation [45] reduces to the trivial expression $C_B = C_{Bo}$ which is the case by definition at t = 0. Conversely, as t becomes large C_B approaches Css.

If the patient is dialyzed for an infinite period of time, the exponential terms will approach zero, as mentioned above. The rate at which this happens will depend on the relative values of $(K_R + K_D)$ and V. If the numerator of the exponent $(K_R + K_D)$ is large compared to V, then the exponent will disappear rapidly; if the converse is true, it will remain a significant factor for long intervals. When the exponential is no longer significant, Equation [45] reduces to the steady state (i.e., when the concentration has ceased to change) and the rate of material entering equals the rate of material leaving and there is no accumulation. Rarely is the patient actually dialyzed to steady state although it is important to note that even if long dialyses are used, the lowest possible concentration is that described by the ratio G/K (which is the analogue of Equation [38c]).

A similar analysis of Equation [44b] will not lead to the same relationships. This is because the analysis that led to Equation [44b] is based on volume changing at a constant rate over time, and at large values of t the inescapable and impossible result is that during very long treatments V could become negative; (i.e., $-Q_F t$ would be larger than V_0, β being Q_F during dialysis – see Equation [42a].

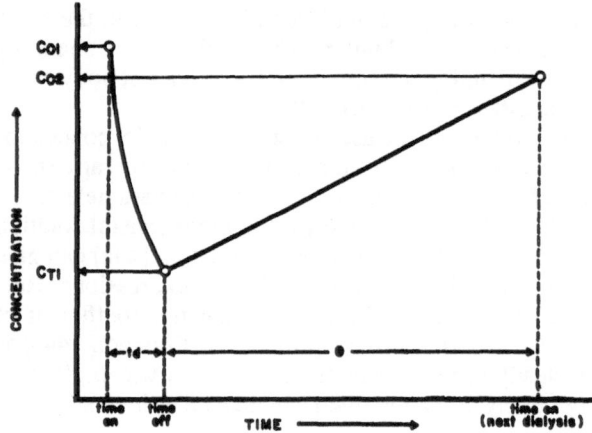

Figure 13. Blood urea nitrogen in the dialyzed patient during one dialysis cycle.

Use of mass balance equation solution

Equation [44b] is used in two ways: to establish patient parameters (V and G) from clinical data (42, 94) and to predict the effect of therapy changes and prescribe dialysis treatment to achieve clinical goals (42, 43, 58, 94–96).

It is clear from Equation [44b] that desired BUN concentration can be achieved by manipulation of K_D and T_D (the two direct therapy parameters). Dialysis frequency is also a treatment parameter which will determine the interval over which BUN is allowed to increase between treatments (96). The use of Equation [44b] for predictive and prescriptive computations, however, presupposes knowledge of the patient parameters V and G. Initially values for these parameters must be developed from clinical data for the specific patient for whom the model is to be used. If the patient's level of renal function is known, examination of Equation [44b] shows that with BUN concentrations at the start and end of an interval as well as weight changes and treatment variables the only remaining undefined parameters in these expressions are patient volume, V_0, and urea nitrogen generation rate, G. Taking each of these constants separately, if one of them were known the other could be calculated directly from a single interval. It follows that both can be computed if the treatment parameters and BUN concentrations are known over two intervals, such as a dialysis and an inter-dialytic period (see Figure 13). The computations to obtain V and G as well as the predictive use of these solutions have been discussed elsewhere (42, 43, 47, 94).

Attempts to simplify urea kinetic modeling

There have been several investigators who have attempted to substitute 'simplified' arithmetic methods as a substitute for urea kinetic modeling. These methods have concentrated solely on estimating KT/V from the dialytic

drop in BUN (112–115). The formula presented by Daugirdas is an example:

$$\frac{KT}{V} = \ln\left(\frac{Ct}{Co} - 0.03 - \frac{uf}{w}\right), \qquad [46]$$

where uf/w is total liters of fluid removed divided by body weight. In practice this expression has provided a remarkably good estimation of sp(KT/V). The empirical relationship between the urea reduction ratio (UUR) and sp(KT/V) suggested by Lowrie *et al.* (116) is considerably less precise and inspection of the relationship between these two parameters (115) shows that the 95% confidence limits are approximately ±40% of the mean value – an excessive degree of variation for clinical use.

The limits of these approaches, and using Daugirdas as an example, is that although they may reliably approximate sp(KT/V), they provide no estimates of the other key parameter that is available from urea kinetic modeling, PCR. This parameter, which allows monitoring of protein intake in important in analyzing the quality of care delivered and quantitative analysis of treatment changes that are needed to correct the level of care prescribed. For example, if the observed sp(KT/V) is either too high or too low relative to that desired, treatment modification must be done by trial and error. That is, changes in dialyzer types, blood and/or dialysate flow rates, treatment times, etc, must be guessed with no method of prospectively analyzing the effect of such changes on the actual delivery of therapy. In contrast, when formal urea kinetic modeling is used, the individual or combined effects of dialyzers, flows, and treatment times can quickly be evaluated from the model solutions and the best clinical choice can be selected.

Deviation of urea from single pool behavior

It is important to appreciate the nature of the assumption of a single well mixed compartment, ie, a single pool model. The body has virtually an infinite number of physical compartments. Modeling attempts simplification by viewing the body as a system that acts as a single unit (single pool) or as a few discrete volumes which interconnect (multipool). For a multipool model there is mass transport between the compartments and to the extent that some of these compartments behave similarly they can be lumped as a modeled volume. Consequently, it is common to consider intracellular water as a discrete space when, in fact, it is composed of a large number of individual cells; other 'compartments' are treated similarly. Single pool modeling assumes that the body acts as a single well mixed container and relies not only on the high permeability of cells to the material being modeled, but also on the transport of the material throughout the body (i.e., the mixing) by rapidly flowing blood through a totally perfused body. Consequently, a patient in shock would tend to deviate from these assumptions, not because of

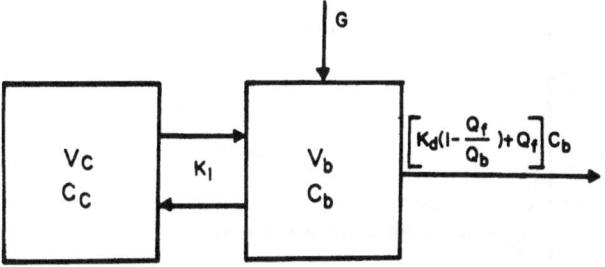

Figure 14. Two pool model for urea nitrogen in the dialyzed patient.

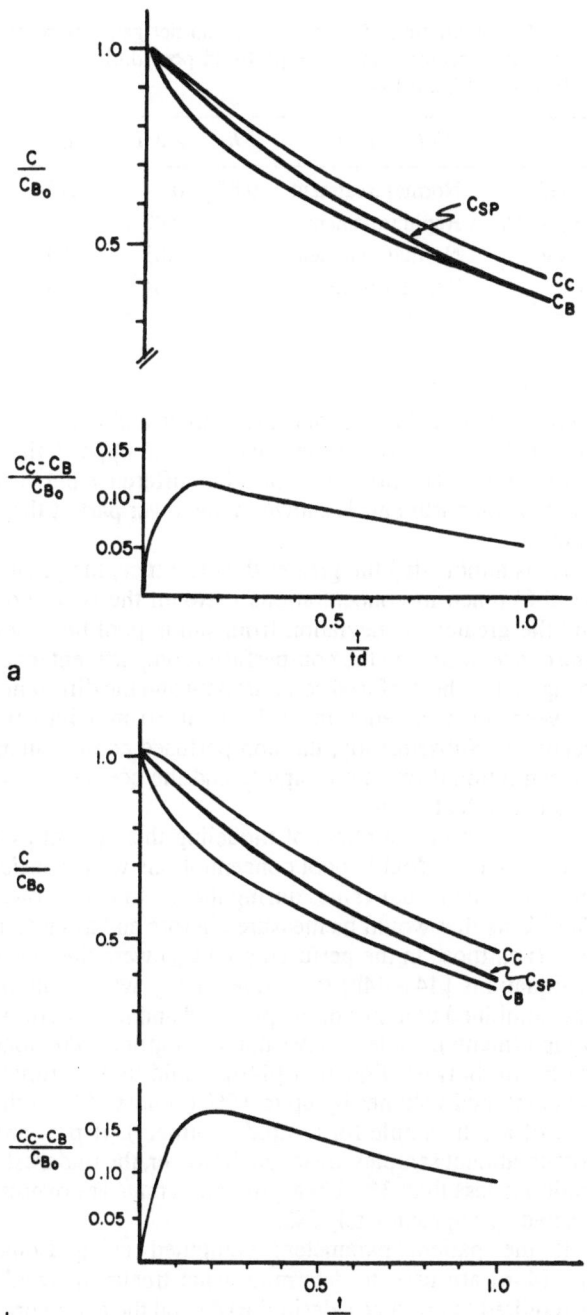

Figure 15. Urea levels (C) during dialysis computed from Two Pool Model for different dialysis times and dialyzer clearances: (A) 4 h with $K_d = 175$ ml/min; (B) 2.5 h with $K_d = 280$ ml/min.

any lack of permeability of cells, but because there is an upset in the normally well mixed nature of the system.

The simplifying assumption of a single pool for urea during dialysis has general validity as long as the movement of urea into and out of cells (a non-perfused compartment) from an extracellular 'compartment' is more rapid than movement of material out of this extracellular space (as happens during dialysis). When the urea transport constants from non-perfused to perfused spaces are of the same order as that of dialysis, urea will exhibit behavior that increasingly deviates from that of single pool kinetics.

With the trend toward increased dialyzer efficiency and 'rapid dialysis (97, 98) an examination of the validity of single pool modeling of urea and other materials is important. The double pool model for urea in the dialyzed patient is shown in Figure 14. This model shows urea generation into a perfused compartment which is often considered as extracellular space (V_B, C_B). This site of urea production is considered reasonable because urea is produced in the liver and enters body water from the portal circulation. The perfused compartment is shown to communicate with the non-perfused compartment (V_C, C_C) along a concentration gradient with an intercompartmental transfer coefficient, K_1. It is important to repeat that this constant K_1 will be a combination of cell permeability and the rates of tissue perfusion. The term K_1 which combines these effects has been evaluated in dialysis patients by several investigators and has been determined to have a value of 760–1000 ml/min (39, 45, 99). Urea clearance with highly efficient dialyzers and rapid blood and dialysis fluid flow rates now approaches 1/4 to 1/3 of theses values of K_1.

To determine the effect of normal and elevated urea clearances on the use of the single pool urea model discussed, concentrations in the two compartments during treatment were computed with a 'normal' dialysis (4 h with dialyzer urea clearance of 175 ml/min) and a 'rapid' dialysis (2.5 h with dialyzer urea clearance of 280 ml/min). The mass balance equations for this system and their solution appear in the Appendix. The hypothetical patient used for these computations was a 72 kg male undergoing dialysis, eating 1.0 g protein/kg-day, with compartment

volumes of 141 (perfused, V_B) and 281 (non-perfused, V_C).

The urea concentrations for both compartments are shown in Figures 15A and 15B for the first dialysis of the week (assuming thrice weekly treatment). The total body urea concentration that would be expected if the

Table 6. Calculation of urea volume and net generation rates from urea concentration in the perfused pool during different dialysis (see Figure 14)

	Dialysis time	1 h	2/3 T_D	T_D
V_{SP}/	Normal treatment	0.85	0.94	0.99
$V_B + V_C$	Rapid treatment	0.77	0.90	0.97
G_{SP}/	Normal treatment	1.01	1.03	1.04
G	Rapid treatment	1.01	1.04	1.06

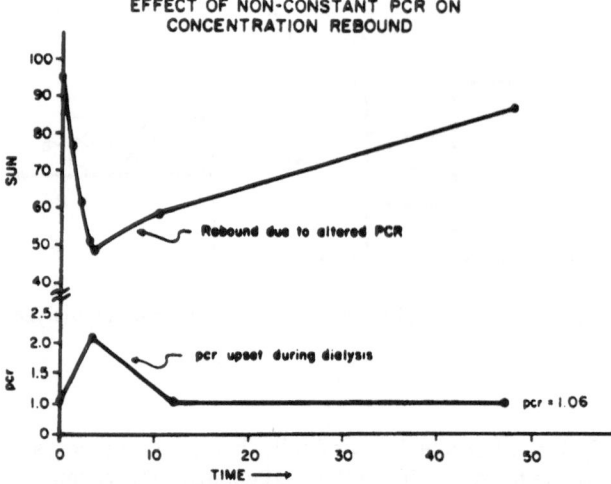

Figure 16. Illustration of the BUN (SUN) during and after dialysis in the case of non-constant net protein catabolism showing an apparent urea rebound due to increased net urea generation during and immediately after dialysis. (Reprinted from *Uremia: Pathobiology of Patients Treated for 10 Years or More,* edited by Giordano C, Friedman EA, Milan, Wichtig Editore, 1981, with permission.)

body acted as a single pool is also shown and is intermediate between the two other curves in the upper half of those figures. The urea concentration difference between the two compartments is shown in the lower part of these figures.

As is anticipated the greater the clearance, the greater the difference in concentrations between the two pools and the greater the deviation from single pool behavior. The concentration in the non-perfused compartment tends to lag that in the perfused compartment and the difference between the two tends to peak about 30 min into the treatment. Subsequently, the non-perfused compartment concentration drops more rapidly and the concentration, C_c tends to 'catch up'.

To determine the effect of modeling this system as a single pool the double pool concentrations were considered to be the actual values during the treatments shown. The BUNs that would be measured before and after dialysis, (i.e., those in the perfused pool C_B) were then used in Equations [44a–44b] to estimate body water volume (the combined volumes of the perfused and non-perfused compartments). Table 6 shows that if sampling were done 'early' in dialysis, Equation [44b] would underestimate the combined volumes by up to 15% (almost 25% in the case of a 1 h sample for a rapid treatment). If pre- and post-treatment samples are taken, however, the underestimation is less than 3%. Urea generation rates are overestimated by approximately 5%.

If the patient parameters computed using Equation [44b] are used to determine what treatment would be required to produce a desired BUN and the actual urea level achieved in the perfused compartment is calculated using these treatment factors and the double pool model the actual BUNs exceed those expected by 2 to 4%.

Multicompartmental models, while more mathematically elegant, present at least two difficulties: first, more physiological/anatomical parameters are needed for a complete modeling definition of the patient and second, the model may be deceptive because of the need to define the internal metabolic mechanisms in greater detail. In most multicompartment model (45) the magnitude of many patient parameters are taken to be those published (44, 99) so that actual values are not calculated. This approach predetermines certain parameters. Thus,

the model does not actually describe the specific patient and no truly individual treatment can be achieved. The assumption of parameter values, however, is required in complex models because actual calculation of patient values would require a large amount of clinical data such as interdialytic as well as pre-post solute levels. This approach makes modeling for clinical treatment inordinately complex. In contrast, a single pool model requires only pre-post concentrations for parameter calculations (42). It is this simplicity that makes a single pool model so attractive and clinically usable for the individualization of treatment (43, 53, 94).

Postulation of a multicompartmental model presumes knowledge of internal metabolic events in some detail and in this regard may be misleading. For example, the two pool model describes the well known rebound effect of solutes following dialysis (39) while the single pool does not. In so doing it attributes the rebound to concentration differences at the end of treatment between the two pools. There is ample evidence, however, to indicate that much of the urea rebound is due to change in rates of protein catabolism following treatment (50, 100–103). Figure 16 shows the type of rebound curve that would result from a doubling of net protein catabolic rates post-dialysis, returning to pre-dialysis levels in 8 to 10 h. Thus, although a two pool model can describe a rebound curve, it may mask some of the actual determinants of these solute levels ascribing them to concentration differences in compartments rather than a perturbation of metabolic rates. In contrast the simpler model may be more clinically significant because it is less tightly defined. It allows

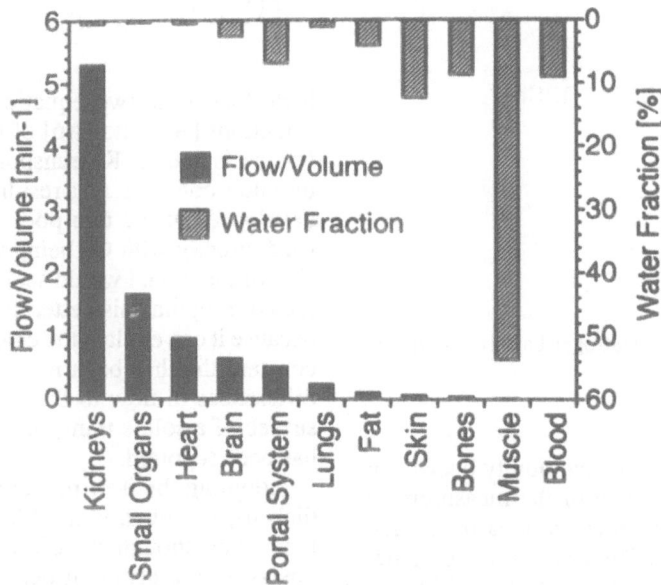

Figure 17. Blood flow at water content at different body space. Data for Schneditz (reprinted for (109A)).

more flexible interpretation of data which can result in greater physiological or nutritional insights because of its generality (41, 51, 90, 104).

The effect of cardiopulmonary recirculation on the delivery of treatment

As has been described, the single pool model assumes one well mixed pool (i.e., that all blood is at the same well mixed concentration). In fact, there will be differing concentrations in different parts of the body as dialyzer clearance increases. The concept of cardiopulmonary recirculation stems from the observation that when dialyzer urea clearance is high and a peripheral access is used, the mixed arterial blood will be at a lower urea concentration than the venous return from the tissues. This is because the dialyzed blood returning to the circulation from the dialyzer is at a much lower concentration than the blood return from the tissues, where it has picked up more urea. As these two streams mix the resulting urea concentration will be at a lower concentration which will on the next circuit be the dialyzer inlet concentration. This phenomenon has always existed, but it was not until high blood flow and high clearance dialysis that it had much affect on the delivery of dialysis. With aggressive therapy the model deviates from what is shown in Figure 10 because the concentration of the mixed pool shown in the figure is not what is entering the dialyzer.

To correct for the difference between the actual venous urea concentration and the concentration of blood entering the dialyzer the dialyzer clearance term should be modified using a constant coefficient to correct for the lower blood urea levels that will be present at the dialyzer inlet.

$$\text{Fsum} = \frac{\text{CO} - \text{Qac})}{(\text{CO} - \text{Qac} + \text{K}_d)} , \qquad [46]$$

where Fsum is the correction factor for the BUN being lower in the access than in the venous blood; CO is cardiac output; Qac is the access flow. Using Equation [46] the mass balance equation becomes:

$$\frac{\text{d(VCv)}}{\text{dt}} = \text{G} - \text{K}_d(\text{Fsum})\text{Cv}, \qquad [47]$$

where Cv is the venous return concentration and the measure of systemic BUN.

It is clear from Equation [46] that as K_d gets large, Fsum decreases. It is also apparent that when K_d was small relative to CO, which was the case before rapid dialysis that Fsum was very close to unity so that cardiopulmonary recirculation could be ignored in modeling. Note that the term '(Fsum)Cv' in Equation [47] is the K_dC term used in the previous modeling discussions but is now corrected to reflect the lower dialyzer inlet levels of urea and consequent lower transport that will result.

The perfusion model as the cause of two pool effects

It has been common to view the multipool effects of dialysis as is shown in Figure 14. This figure, as has been discussed, assumes that there are two discrete volumes between which urea is transported down a concentration gradient. Each pool in this model is considered well mixed and the transport resistance between pools is defined to be an intercompartmental transport coefficient. This model

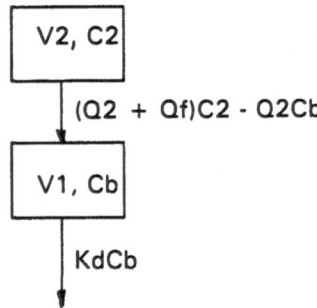

Figure 18. Two pool model for urea nitrogen based on perfusion of body space.

has had appeal in the nephrology community because it has the form consistent with much of the measurement of anatomical spaces that was an active area of investigation in the 1950s and 1960s. There are, however, other possible explanations for the two pool behavior of the dialyzer/patient system during dialysis. One can also suspect that a different model may be better, because it is common to find that the value of patient constants calculated from the concentration model are not easily reproduced (39, 45, 104). It is in this context that a perfusion explanation of two pool behavior should be viewed.

Figure 17 shows both the blood flow volume to different organ systems as well as the water faction contained by each of these systems. It is clear that there is a large discrepancy between the contained water and the flow to each of these organs. Of particular note is the contained water versus the flow rate to muscle.

The urea content of the body will be distributed consistent with the water content. Consequently, muscle will contain most of the body urea. However, the flow to muscle is quite small so that the ability to move urea from the muscle to the blood and to remove it from the body by dialysis will be limited by the flow to and from the muscle mass. Intuitively, one can appreciate that at the end of a dialysis there may be a rebound of urea from the delay in moving urea from muscle to the blood and not from any lack of cell membranes permeability for urea.

Consider the model shown in Figure 18 which is the analogue to that shown in Figure 14 but defines the perfusion relationships.

In this model the perfused compartment is assumed to be well mixed and supplying blood at this well mixed concentration to the poorly-perfused compartment. The transport between these compartments is strictly a mass balance – blood arrives at a mass content of Q_2C_b and picks up ultrafiltrate to increase the flow volume to $Q_2 + Q_f$; the increased flow is at equilibrium with this pool and leaves at a concentration of C_2.

The mass balance expressions for this model are:

$$\frac{d(V_2C_2)}{dt} = C_2C_b - (Q_2 + Q_f)C_2 \qquad [48a]$$

$$\frac{d(V_1, C_b)}{dt} = G - K_dC_b + (Q_2 + Q_F)C_2 - Q_2C_b. [48b]$$

Note that these two equations are of the same form as Equations [A5] and [A6] of the Appendix. The only difference is that the K_1 transport constant has been replaced by a flow constant. As a result the equations that have been developed for the two pool concentration model can be used directly with Q_2 being substituted for K_1. This version of the model would seem to describe the behavior of urea during dialysis better than the concentration version because it can explain the changing nature of the transport constant that has been noted by several investigators by differences in flow to the poorly-perfused. That is, it is suspect if a solute transport constant varies widely as K_1 has been reported.

Adopting the flow model as the most realistic one for dialysis, however, is troublesome because it is apparent that, even though it describes the urea concentrations observed in dialysis, it depends on the perfusion of the tissues, Q_2. Clearly, this parameter depends on factors that are hard to control during treatment.

Estimating the mixed end dialysis urea concentration to adapt the single pool model to the two pool case

It is logical to deal with the two pool model in a manner that is totally analogous to the single pool case. That is, one would be expected to use concentration excursions that result from treatment to define the values of the model parameters and then use those parameters to analyze treatment and urea generation as well as prescribe the dialysis treatment that meets adequacy criteria. This classical approach analyzes the concentration-time relationship during and after dialysis to develop patient specific values for the modeling constants, V_b, V_c, K_1, and G. Inspection of Equation [A11] shows that the BUN is described by two exponentials. The time course of BUN both during dialysis and post-dialysis are analyzed logarithmically to yield values for the two exponents, alpha and beta. This commonly requires that the details of the rebound be examined and that the patient stay up to an hour after treatment for blood values to be drawn. One can equally analyze the intradialytic concentration to generate model parameters.

The advantage of using the end dialysis values is that the rebound, which is the most obvious departure from single pool behavior most manifests itself once dialysis is over. In addition, the analysis of this part of the dialysis cycle is somewhat easier. The disadvantage of using the rebound to characterize two pool behavior is that patients have to remain at the dialysis facility for an additional hour after treatment.

There was considerable value in being able to define model parameters in the single pool case. The calculated value of the urea distribution volume gave an indication of the validity of the data used for the calculation (i.e., a value that exceeded body weight indicated that there was an error in input data and probably a short fall in the magnitude of treatment delivered (105); the urea generation rate yielded net protein catabolic rate which in the stable dialysis patient equals the dietary protein intake. This latter parameter is currently taking on considerable significance because of the recent observations that mortality in dialysis is related very strongly to low albumin levels as well as other nutritional parameters (106).

In contrast to the single pool model, the factors that define the double pool model (V_b, V_c, and K_1) do not have great significance in characterizing the patient, and in fact, if the model is a perfusion one they may not have significance in and of themselves; that is their main use may be to provide predictive computations. Consequently, from the standpoint of clinical utility it may be a reasonable approach to determine what the rebound concentration is for a particular dialysis and use this value as the end dialysis concentration in the single pool calculations. What such an assumption means is that the total body concentration at the start of dialysis will be reasonably close to the blood urea levels and that the end dialysis concentration, which can be measured an hour after dialysis is over, can be used to compute KT/V as well as G.

This simplified approach can be supported by considering that the drop in systemic urea is the dialysis effect desired. Ever since the field started to use KT/V to define the magnitude of treatment and establish values that are desirable for adequate dialytic care it was the effective dropping of urea that was used as the indicator of treatment delivery. That is, if the BUN is reduced from 100 to 35 mg/dl it does not matter that it was done in 2 or 4 h (i.e., the KT in KT/V remained the same). On this basis the single pool model can be used; the only frustration is that if rapid dialysis is used it is difficult to measure the end dialysis concentration without compelling the patient to remain in the dialysis unit for an inconvenient period after treatment.

The other kinetic parameter of interest is G, the net rate of urea generation, from which the net protein catabolic rate, PCR, can be calculated. Net urea production is easily calculated from the single pool model if an accurate value of total system, end dialysis urea concentration can be determined. Once again if one can measure the post-rebound urea concentration this value can be used in single pool calculations to obtain an accurate value of G and PCR. A desirable approach is to estimate the degree of rebound that will occur by measuring intradialytic parameters that will permit such an estimation. With such an estimate the single pool model can be used without the concern introduced by double pool effects.

Smye has developed a technique to estimate an equilibrated end dialysis concentration using intradialytic urea levels. One is referred to his analysis of the details of this estimation technique (107). By measuring urea levels 70 minutes into dialysis (the time at which the larger exponent in Equations [11, 12] has become small), the end

dialysis concentration, corrected for rebound, C_∞, can be estimated:

$$C_{T\infty} = C_{02} \exp(-LT),$$

where L is:

$$L = \left[\frac{1}{(T - t)}\right] \ln\left(\frac{C_t}{C_T}\right).$$

This technique is then used to adjust the measured end dialysis value of C_T so that accurate estimates of delivered KT/V and G can be calculated. The computation process computes the equilibrated KT/V (e(KT/V), the effective treatment that resulted in the measured drop in systemic BUN.

$$e\left(\frac{KT}{V}\right) = sp\left(\frac{KT}{V}\right) - RT', \qquad [49]$$

where sp(KT/V) is the KT/V calculated from the end dialysis BUN, rather than the post-rebound value, C_∞, and RT' is the fractional rebound defined as C_∞/C_t. This value can be rearranged to yield:

$$sp\left(\frac{KT}{V}\right) = e\left(\frac{KT}{V}\right) + RT' \qquad [50]$$

where RT' can be computed by the Smye analysis (107) as:

$$RT' = 0.44\left(\frac{K_d}{K_1}\right) + 0.14\left(\frac{K_d}{K_1}\right)^2. \qquad [51]$$

The computation process is:
1. Measure C_0, C_{70}, and C_t for three dialyses.
2. From these values compute $C_{t\infty}$ and use $C_{t\infty}$ to compute e(KT/V) from Equation [49] and the value of RT' computed as RT' = $C_{t\infty}/C_t$; also compute the average value of RT' for these three treatments (RT'bar).
3. The average value of RT' permits the computation of K_1, which can be used to estimate RT' when therapy changes, as: 0.5

$$K_1 = \frac{K_d}{[5(0.1936 + 0.4RT'bar) - 2.2]}.$$

4. If changes in K_d are anticipated, an estimated value for RT' can be computed from Equation [51].
5. With this parameter estimated the required sp(KT/V) can be computed from Equation [50].

It is clear that the estimating of therapy changes will be an iterative process. For example:
− Current e(KT/V) is too low.
− Increase K_d to adjust for a desired level of e(KT/V) and compute the new estimate of RT' from Equation [51].
− Compute sp(KT/V) to be used in individualize the treatment to the target e(KT/V) from Equation [50].

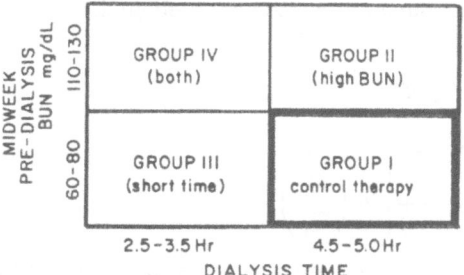

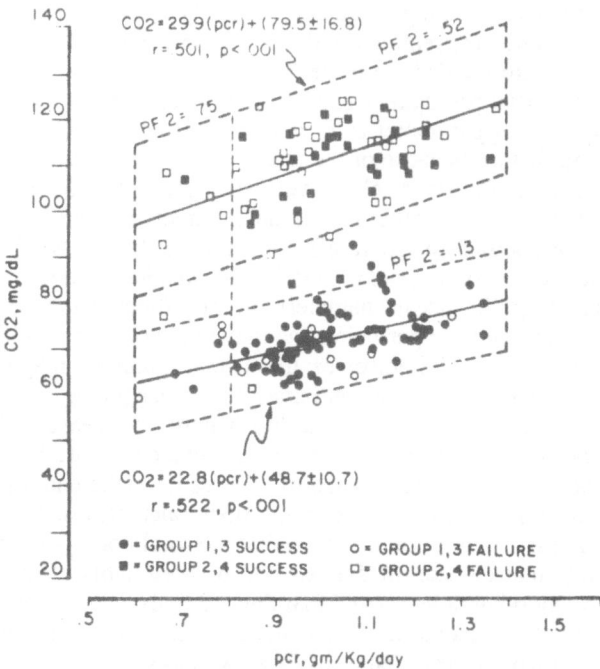

Figure 19. The design of the National Cooperative Dialysis Study.

- Using the single pool kinetic model, select the desired options to individualize the treatment.
- If this individualization results in a change in K_d recompute RT' and sp(KT/V) and adjust the individualization process.

Figure 20. The locus of all patients in the National Cooperative Dialysis Study mapped by average mid-week pre-dialysis BUN (CO_2 mg/dl) and PCR (g/kg/day). Symbols are: O, group 1, 3 success; P, group 1, 3 failure; [ ], group 2, 4 success; [ ], group 2, 4 failure. (Reprinted from *Kidney International*, with permission.)

The National Cooperative Dialysis Study (NCDS): The clinical application of urea kinetics and operational relationships

The NCDS was conducted in the United States between 1976 and 1981. It was designed as shown in Figure 19 (76) and represents a unique example of quantitatively prescribed solute levels using a mathematical model and implementation of the dialyzer operating constants as described in this chapter to achieve them (49, 95).

There were four groups of patients in the experimental phase of the NCDS representing the combinations of the two independent variables of mid week pre-dialysis BUN and dialysis time (see Figure 19). The study was designed to hold BUN at nominal values of 70 mg/dl (25 mmol/l) and 120 mg/dl (42.9 mmol/l) mid week during dialyses of 4.5 to 5.0 h (long) and 2.5 to 3.5 h (short dialysis). All patients were initially treated in the control phase with 'long' dialysis times and 'low' BUN treatment. After successful completion of 3 months of control therapy they were randomly assigned to the four groups shown in Figure 19.

Because dialysis time was reasonably fixed for the protocol (see Figure 19) dialyzer clearance was the main treatment parameter that was adjusted. The dialyzer clearance required to maintain each patient initially in the control group and eventually in the specific experimental group was determined from Equation [44b] (and mathematical rearrangements thereof) (94). With knowledge of residual kidney urea clearance present the value of 'K' in Equation [44b] was used to determine the dialyzer clearance required for a specific patient (i.e., for specific values of V_0, G, and β). Equations [26] and [28] were then used to determine what blood and dialysate flows (Q_B and Q_D)

were needed to produce this urea clearance for the dialyzer in use (K_oA). Clearances that were possible to achieve in the NCDS protocol using dialyzers and clinical blood and dialysate flows in use at that time ranged from approximately 90 ml/min with all dialyzers to a maximum of approximately 200 to 250 ml/min (the former value was for the smaller dialyzers used; the latter was for dialyzers with nominal 2.5 m^2 membrane area) (94).

A graphical representation of the NCDS results is shown in Figure 20 (78) as a map relating average mid week pre-dialysis BUN (CO_2: C – BUN; 0 – pre-dialysis at T – 0; 2 – second dialysis) to protein catabolic rate PCR – g/kg/day. Protein catabolic rate for patients in nutritional steady state (such as those in the NCDS) will be equivalent to protein intake (108).

The two regions that are blocked off by parallelograms signify the BUN regions explored in the study with the upper region representing the patients with high BUNs (groups 2 and 4 of Figure 19) and the lower region representing those patients with low BUNs (groups 1 and 3 in Figure 19). Figure 20 shows that by using the operational relationships developed in this chapter (i.e., Equations [25–28] which relate K_oA, Q_B and Q_D, to desired K_D) and the urea kinetics model, a carefully controlled multicenter, clinical study protocol, such as that described in Figure 19, can be successfully implemented.

Extension of NCDS results to clinical therapy

The results of the NCDS and the use of KT/V as indicator of therapy adequacy have resulted in:
- wide use of this therapy index,
- attempts to reduce treatment times by increasing dialyzer performance (K) in order to reduce the length of treatment (T, by keeping KT constant),
- trying to establish the value of KT/V necessary for dialysis adequacy from other databases,
- attempting to 'simplify' the calculation with estimation formulae which in most cases are less accurate than the kinetic model that they strive to duplicate and do not provide PCR estimates.

Attempts to reduce treatment time

After the results of the NCDS were analyzed and reported (78) clinicians introduced protocols that increased dialyzer clearance (K) by combinations of dialyzer size and blood and dialysate flow rates in order to reduce dialysis time. The goal was to use increased clearance to enable shorter times for the benefit of the patient and the efficient use of dialysis staff. These rapid treatments took at least two forms:
- increase in small molecular weight transport (High Efficiency Dialysis),
- increase in both small and larger molecular weight transport (High Flux).

The former was a strict extrapolation of the NCDS results in that if the overall transport of small molecular weight substances could be kept constant adequate dialysis could be achieved in a shorter time. The second, High Flux dialysis, used open membranes which could clear larger substances, such as beta-2-microglobulin which is thought to cause considerable morbidity for long term ESRD patients.

The goal of a universal radically shorter treatment (i.e., treatment times in the range of two hours) has not been universally achieved. In addition to technical difficulties that have frustrated this goal, analyses of treatment results from national data (reference Held, USRDS) as well as observations of others have suggested that more treatment is required. These results are complex. The studies used to support longer treatments are either retrospective, in which case it is not possible to verify the actual level of treatment delivered, or conducted in such a way that there was sufficient variation in delivered treatment (i.e., high variable KT/V) that a cause effect argument is difficult to support.

Attempts to redefine adequacy from other retrospective analyses and other studies

Subsequent to the NCDS several investigators attempted to evaluate mortality and morbidity from institutionally maintained databases by retrospectively evaluating KT/V using ordered treatment (109) or from prospective studies (110). For retrospective analyses to yield valid results the

actual treatment provided must be identical to the intended, which other studies have put in doubt (105). These retrospective studies have yielded recommended treatment levels of KT/V of 1.2 to 1.4 as adequate. There are several problems with these analyses. First the quantification of the delivery of the expected treatment is suspect. In contrast to the NCDS, the actual treatment delivery was not determined at frequent intervals, if at all by actual measurement of urea levels that resulted from treatment.

Secondly, the level of KT/V reported as 'adequate' is the average of all values from the data analysis. The individual values of KT/V in these studies, however, varied widely. This is possibly because of the tendency in the field to provide the same amount of treatment to all patients (i.e., KT is relatively constant) which would result in a wide range of KT/V in these studies. It was found in the analysis of the NCDS that there is a threshold level of KT/V which produced greater morbidity and once treatment level exceeded this level the morbidity was steady and low (78). With a wide range of KT/V there would have to be a high average value of this parameter for the patients being treated in the lower range to receive adequate therapy. This explanation also fits with prospective studies where a wide range of KT/V produced high average values that seemed to indicate adequacy. In these studies, however many patients' KT/V were below 1.0, the threshold value of the NCDS, and it with a fairly standard treatment required that this standard be raised, elevating the entire range of therapy to get the lowest above 1.0.

Analyses of clinical experience have shown that a sizable number of dialyses are not conducted as prescribed and recorded in the patient's record and are in fact under delivered (105). This analysis showed that on the average KT/V delivered was approximately 10 to 20% lower than the intended level and that many values were substantially lower. The reasons for the short falls were various and included undelivered blood flow, dialyzers not performing to manufacturer's specifications (111), shortened dialysis time, recirculation, and other factors that lowered the performance of the dialyzer. If this experience can be applied to the KT/V reported in the retrospective analyses the actual delivered KT/V would be expected to be closer to 1.0 which is consistent with NCDS result (78).

Recent reports of mortality and KT/V which concluded that values of 1.2–1.4 are needed for adequate care, exhibit the same flaws in that the range of KT/V delivered covered a wide range with a significant number of values below 1.0. One is forced to conclude that there was not uniform distribution of deaths over all of the KT/V values, but that they were concentrated at the lower ones and that the average KT/V that the authors say are necessary for adequate therapy are a combination of high values for which there is very low mortality and low values where mortality is high.

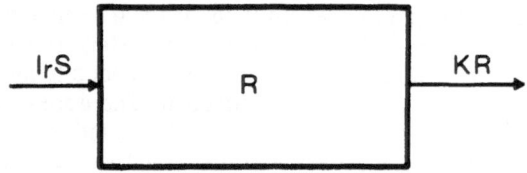

Figure 21. Model of heparin.

Modeling the anticoagulation activity of heparin

Heparin is the usual anticoagulant for hemodialysis. The need to model this material stems from the fact, which has generally been ignored in the pharmacology literature that biological sensitivity and elimination of heparin varies widely (56). In formulating this model, a slightly different approach is followed. The characteristic of interest with heparin is its anticoagulant effect, measured as the clotting time prolongation (56) rather than concentration. Consequently, it is this response to heparin that is the appropriate parameter to model. In this analysis, therefore, the anticoagulation response (R) or clotting time prolongation relative to baseline levels resulting from systemic heparinization, will be considered a direct measure of the system content (see Figure 21).

Input to the system, after initial heparin loading is a zero order infusion rate, I_r, quantified as units/hour. A coefficient is required to convert the infusion rate to increased clotting time response, so input is I_rS. This coefficient, S (clotting time prolongation per unit), is the 'sensitivity' of the clotting system to added heparin. This response is found to be linear and insensitive to dose level for therapeutic quantities of this drug (56). Output or deactivation of anticoagulation in response to heparin is first order(117–119) and described as the product of the response and an elimination constant, K. This completes the model formulation.

Mass balance is then written:

$$\frac{dR}{dt} = I_rS - K_R. \qquad [52a]$$

At steady state the right side of Equation [53a] will equal zero and the steady state infusion rate necessary for the required response will be:

$$I_r = \frac{K_R}{S}. \qquad [52b]$$

Solution of Equation [53a] yields:

$$R_t = R_oe^{-Kt} + (1 - e^{-Kt}). \qquad [53]$$

Both S and K are individual patient constants and must be determined for each individual. The sensitivity, S, is evaluated by measurement of the change in clotting response to a step change in heparin as represented by bolus dose:

$$S = \frac{R - R_o}{Dose}. \qquad [54]$$

It is apparent from Equation [54] that the elimination or deactivation constant, K, can be calculated from the decrease clotting response with time once heparin infusion has stopped from,

$$K = -\frac{1}{T} Ln \frac{R_T}{R_o}.$$

The technique of having to discontinue heparin administration in order to determine a value for K, however, is inconvenient because it may require a patient to remain after the dialysis is discontinued or be at risk of unacceptable clotting levels during treatment. Recognizing this, a method was developed to calculate the heparin elimination constant from serial clotting times for a dialysis patient receiving a constant heparin infusion. Examination of Equation [55] shows that K appears both in the I_rS/K term as well as the exponent, and as such this expression cannot be directly solved for K although there will be a unique value for this metabolic constant for any specific value of R_T, R_o, I_r, and S. A specific rearrangement of Equation [55] which avoids the use of logarithms, common in analogous urea kinetic solution (42) is shown in Equation [56].

$$K = \frac{I_rS(1 - e^{Kt})}{R_I - R_Te^{Kt}}. \qquad [55]$$

Equation [56] is used when the infusion rate, I_r, is known and the sensitivity, S, has been calculated for clotting time response values after the start of dialysis as shown in Figure 22. Both R_i and R_t are measured by standard techniques (although some form of the whole blood partial thromboplastin time is preferred because of its speed and reproducibility). The computation requires that Equation [56] be 'primed' with a 'starting' value of K. This value is then used to compute the right hand side of Equation [56], which will yield a 'closer' value for K (the left hand side of the equation). This new K value is then used to recompute another value of K until this system of calculations converges to a unique value.

The red cell mass

The red cell mass represents the volume of red cells in the blood at any time. It is generally viewed that it is the change of total red cell mass rather than its concentration (hematocrit, HCT) that governs generation of new cells through the synthesis of endogenous erythropoietin. Red cell mass is not directly measurable because it represents the product of red cell concentration and blood volume. In dialysis this is particularly troublesome because blood volume can change as water is added to the patient (between treatments) or is removed (during treatments). This fact is of practical concern because it is important to know if HCT changes are due to hydration changes, which will change blood volume, and may be a result of the body's blood pressure control mechanisms, or due to actual changes in the red cell mass.

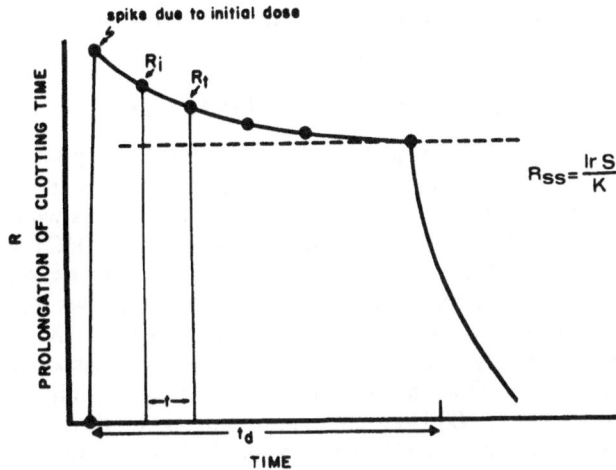

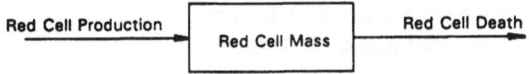

Figure 23. Model for red cell mass.

Figure 22. Clotting time prolongation in a dialysis patient with systemic heparinization consisting of a loading dose and a constant infusion thereafter.

The red cell mass will depend on the rate of red cell production and death as well as the red cell life span (tau days). The change in true red cell mass will be the difference between the rate of red cell production and the rate of red cell death. Clearly, red cell life span (tau) also has a direct impact on red cell mass. That is, at the same rate of production and death, if survival time increases the red cell mass will increase. If production of red cells increases – the mechanism of EPO therapy – red cell mass will increase because for tau days the death rate will remain at the pre-EPO level. Once the EPO generated cells achieve their life span (i.e., they are in the system for tau days) the death rate will increase and equal the increased production rate. The transient increase in red cell mass will remain as long as the production rate is maintained, and the red cell life span does not change. It is clear, particularly with EPO therapy, that when production rates are changed there will be a transient in red cell mass (increasing if production is increased; decreased if production is decreased) which will be followed tau days later by a corresponding change in death rate. Although there may be changes in red cell life span, the main impact of the availability of exogenous EPO has been the ability of clinicians to manipulate the production rates of red cells. However, the nature of the transient before newly produced cells die presents a challenge in the control of red cell mass that presents difficulties of the control of anemia in dialysis patients.

As was alluded to above, under stable production and death rates the life span of the red cell will also have a profound impact on the red cell mass. That is for a given production/death rate a halving of the life span for the red cell population will halve the red cell mass. This is particularly important in uremic patients because of the documented shortening of life span associated with this disease. A useful way to look at the interacting effect of

these two patient variables is by use of the 'zero order' or 'populations' model.

Modeling of erythropoietic therapy

An organized way to understand changes in HCT is important in prescribing and monitoring EPO therapy. An accurate and useful model of this therapy is that referred to as the population model, where individuals (red cells) are produced live a fixed life span after which they die. This model is referred to as a 'population' model because its behavior is similar to the aggregate number or population of a living species under stable or changing production (birth) and death rates with a constant average life span. It can be appreciated that certain events can influence production or birth rates but changing these events and hence the production rate will not change the presence of those individuals whose life span is not yet complete.

Using EPO to correct anemia in ESRD patients, one can only manipulate the production rate of red cells. In this case the immediate and linear increase in HCT when EPO therapy is initiated will reflect the additive population of the various cohorts of red cell age. In this case one has control only of the rate of red cell production with the death rate dependent on the cells that are currently at the end of their life. In systems, such as the use of medications, where elimination is first order – increased levels result in increased metabolism – one has far greater control over concentration, the analogue of HCT, than in the case with the red cell mass. Initial attempts at prescription schemes treated EPO, and its measurable outcome – HCT, as analogous to drug therapy (i.e., a loading dose followed by a maintenance dose) (15).

Using these borrowed pharmacological dosing protocols has caused difficulties in controlling HCT levels in dialysis. Individual experiences vary but commonly include seemingly unpredictable swings in HCT that are not the result of nor are they responsive to the day to day levels of EPO administration. The conclusion drawn from these observations is that the dynamics of HCT in the dialysis patient receiving EPO can be better understood if one recognizes that the drug analogue does not apply to this medication and uses a model that incorporates the unique nature of red cell production, death, and life span.

Formulation of the model

The model of red cell mass itself is quite simple. The system is the red cell mass. The input is zero order (a constant at any one time) and represents the red cell production rate, which will depend on EPO stimulation of the bone marrow and the availability of the needed substrates (eg, iron, amino acids, etc). Removal of red cells from the system occurs upon their death and is also zero order. In addition, it should be recognized that the death rate will be close to the reverse of the production rate when the current cohort of dying red cells was produced. That is, if the production rate of red cells that will live 120 days is 20 ml/day, the death rate 120 days hence will also be 20 ml/day, and if there is a rapid and sustained increase in red cell production (as a result of EPO) HCT will increase until the first cohort of these cells live out their life span at which time the HCT will stabilize at a new, higher, level (increased production equaling increased death).

An example of the change in HCT with constant EPO therapy is shown in Figure 24a. HCT rises relative to baseline values as a result of increased production until the life span of the new red cells is reached. At this point the HCT stabilizes at a new level where the new production rate is exactly countered by the new and elevated death rate. It can be observed in Figure 24a that the length of time between the start of the increase in HCT and its leveling is a reasonable measure of the red cell life span (tau) which is known to be less than normal in uremic individuals; in this figure tau is approximately 45 days. Using this model consider several clinical scenarios:

a) Stopping EPO before tau is reached – The 'Loading' Dose Method: If EPO were to be stopped before tau is reached in Figure 24a the HCT would stabilize at the level where this change in therapy occurred because the newly produced red cells will remain as a younger cohort (i.e., not the ones that are reaching the end of their life). When the first EPO cohort finally attains its life span they will die at an accelerated rate (relative to the baseline, pre-EPO cohorts). Once the HCT starts to drop, re-initiating EPO therapy at the original level will not increase HCT but will stabilize it at the current level. This is because the new production rate will equal the death rate until the cohorts of the original EPO group have all died.

b) Manipulating EPO dose to adjust to changing HCT: Continuing to adjust EPO to control the HCT discussed in a), after EPO has been terminated prior to t – tau, leads to seemingly counter intuitive results. For example, if EPO is restarted when HCT has decreased, but is not yet at baseline levels, the HCT will level. If EPO is increased further HCT will go up, but the patient will appear less sensitive to EPO's effects. In fact, the apparent insensitivity results from a large increase in red cell production that barely exceeds the elevated death rate of cells produced from the first EPO regimen. Once the first group of EPO produced red cells finally dies the increased production rate, now not countered by a high death rate will result in a dramatic rate of HCT rise. The concerned clinician may once again terminate the EPO to halt this rapid rise in HCT and see it level at a high value once again. This difficulty in day to day management of HCT using EPO has baffled many concerned physicians

trying to provide the benefits of this new medication to their patients.

Example of intuitive guidance of EPO therapy

Ironically the frustration with HCT control is highest for those who are trying the hardest to impose day-to-day control of HCT by frequent changes in EPO doses which can result in seemingly random excursions of HCT in response to EPO administration. An example of these difficulties is shown in Figure 24. This example shows HCT over nearly 18 months for a patient receiving EPO who has been actively monitored. The figure shows a reasonably linear slope from the point that EPO therapy was initiated at a level of 100 U/kg until approximately 80 days later. At this point the HCT was 35% and EPO was reduced to 50 U/kg in order to control the rate of HCT increase. It can be conjectured that the point of dose change was close to the red cell life span and consequently HCT would have been expected to level at this point if the original dose had been continued, as was the case in Figure 23. Nevertheless, at the point of EPO dose reduction the HCT started to drop at a rate of approximately half of the rate of HCT build up (this can be explained by the new production rate, over baseline, being half the death rate of the initial EPO generated cohort that were dying). This view is supported by the re-starting of the original dose (at day 140) causing HCT to level (when the new red cell production rate equaled the death rate from the initial 100 U/kg dose).

Somewhere around day 180–200 a complicating factor emerges, once all of the originally produced red cells (from the first 100 U/kg dose) have died and the EPO has been increased to 150 U/kg; this increase in EPO has no apparent effect on HCT. At this point intravenous iron is given with the result that HCT increases from 30 to 45% over the next 3–4 weeks – at a rate roughly 1.5 times the original slope for the 100 U/kg dose. At these high HCTs, EPO is stopped and the HCT gradually decreases over the next 150 days. Even though EPO is re-started at 75 U/kg it is not until more iron is given that HCT starts to rise once more. Several points can be drawn from the data in Figure 24b:

– The population model describes the HCT excursions resulting from erythropoietic therapy.
– Intuitive monitoring and rapid changes in EPO doses for patients, as shown in Figure 24b, is frustrating and seldom will result in stable HCT long term.
– Although outside of the model parameters, monitoring and active management of iron therapy is an essential part of EPO therapy and a confounding element of this treatment.

Using the model to guide EPO therapy

The guiding of EPO therapy is both simple and complex. Both the simplicity and complexity are illustrated in Figures 24a and 24b. The model helps to simplify the delivery of EPO because of the understanding of how HCT will

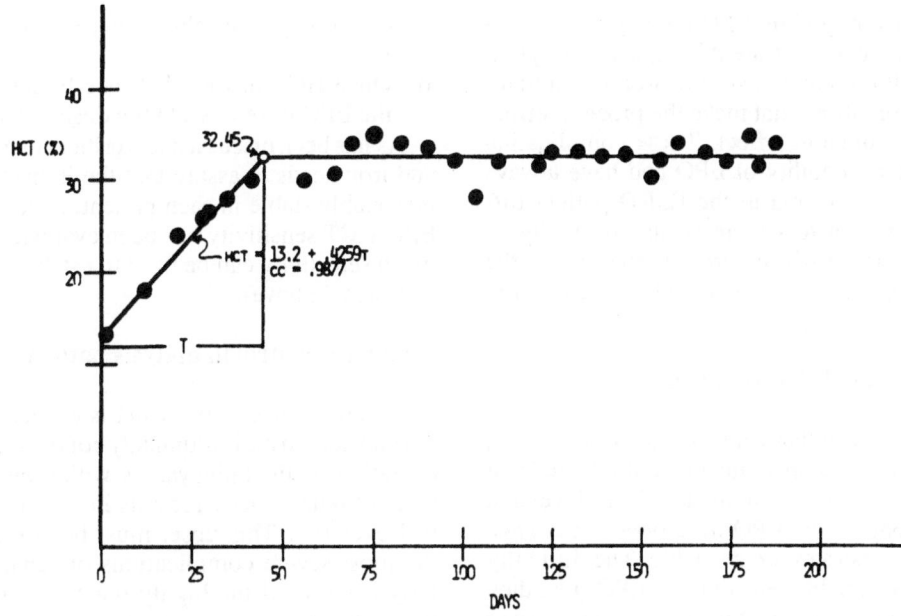

Figure 24a. Normal course of hematocrit rise with constant EPO therapy.

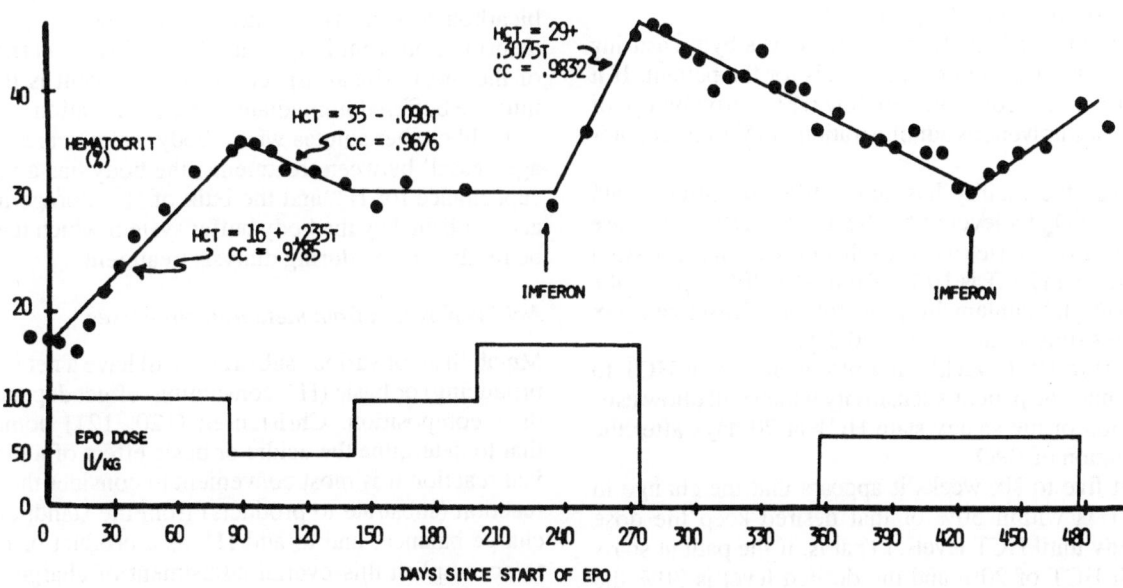

Figure 24b. An example of hematocrit excursions for intuitive use of EPO without guidance of a model. This figure also illustrates the model for the monitoring of iron status when EPO is used.

react to EPO stimulation. The basic practical lesson to be drawn from these data is to avoid trying to react to each excursion in HCT that results from use of this medication. The model does give the practitioner confidence that a steady linear HCT increase will eventually level once tau days have passed since the initiation of EPO therapy.

There are clearly limits, however, regarding the desired maximum for HCT based on possible high HCT clinical effects, and unfortunately in the United States, the misguided reimbursement policies of the Medicare program that question payment over HCT of 36%.

The complexities of guiding EPO therapy involve the multiple factors that can frustrate the impact of EPO on stimulating red cell production, such as iron and inflammatory diseases, conditions that make the process refractory to the EPO stimulating effect. These complicating factors predate the availability of EPO and have always made management of anemia in the ESRD patient difficult. Some of these factors increase this difficulty as HCT rises because there will be greater iron loss as the patient loses blood, because of the blood's increased red cell content.

Suggested approach to EPO treatment

From Figure 24a it is clear that with a steady dose of EPO, the HCT will increase in a linear manner until the red cell life span is attained. At this point the HCT will level and stay constant as long as the EPO dose does not change and the necessary substrates are available. The difficulty is that patients have variable sensitivity to EPO (i.e., they will produce differing amounts of red cells in response to a 'standard' dose of EPO) and the red cell survival time (tau) will also vary. The suggested approach is to start all patients assuming that they have average EPO parameters, measure the actual values of these patient constants under constant EPO dosing, and correct the dose once a steady state has been achieved. Specifically:

1. Assure that adequate iron status exists by measuring iron saturation and ferritin levels for the patient. If it appears that iron stores are low replete iron by use of oral or intravenous administration of IV iron preparations.
2. Unless the facility has actual EPO sensitivity data start EPO at a level of 5 U/kg per % desired increase in HCT on a thrice weekly schedule (i.e., if the desired increase in HCT is 10% – from 20 to 30% – prescribe 50 U/kg). Maintain this protocol for at least five to six weeks (this assumes tau = 70 days).
3. Measure HCT weekly and plot increases in HCT to estimate the patient's sensitivity which will allow estimation of the steady state HCT at 70 days after the initiation of EPO.
4. If at five to six weeks it appears that the change in HCT is within 50% of that desired keep the dose steady until HCT levels. (That is, if the patient starts with HCT of 20% and the desired level is 30% the change is 10%. If at five to six weeks projection of changed HCT in ten weeks – 70 days – is between 5% and 15%, maintain the EPO dose until it levels.)
5. If at five to six weeks the EPO sensitivity is outside of this range the EPO dose should be altered based on the relationship:

$$\text{EPOdoseB} = \left(\frac{\text{dHCTdesired}}{\text{dHCTobserved}} \right) \text{EPOdoseA}; \quad [56]$$

where dHCT is the change in HCT that has resulted from EPOdoseA. Only one correction should be made

– and only if absolutely necessary – before the HCT levels.
6. Once HCT has leveled, use Equation [57] to adjust the EPO dose to yield the desired long term HCT.

As has been discussed it is critical to monitor blood loss and iron needs to assure that the impact of EPO remains reasonably stable in each patient. Note that once average EPO/HCT sensitivity has been evaluated a more accurate mean sensitivity can be used to establish initial treatment (see step 2 above).

Acid base control in dialysis patients

The maintenance of body pH is a fundamental aspect of normal homeostasis ultimately controlled through net acid excretion by the kidneys. As with other solutes, impairment of renal function results in loss of homeostatic control over H^+. This upset must be considered as one of the most severe complications of renal failure, particularly because of the highly reactive nature of acids and bases and the narrow range of pH consistent with life (approximately 6.8 to 7.8 in man). The entire metabolic structure of the body relies on the maintenance of optimal pH; the clinical signs of lowered pH in acidosis are well known: hyperventilation due to respiratory compensation, K^+ elevation due to cellular neutralization of H^+, low bicarbonate from H^+ neutralization, and eventual bone deterioration from long term H^+ buffering. Perhaps one of the most critical aspects of this problem is that acid must be buffered immediately upon generation.

Unlike other solutes where body water acts as a 'storage vessel' between treatments, the body has a very low capacitance for H^+ and the bulk of H^+ storage must be accomplished by the body buffer system which then must be re-alkalinized during dialysis treatment.

Acid generation from metabolic processes

Metabolism of various substrates will have a net acid (H^+ producing) or basic (H^+ consuming) effect depending on their composition. Christensen (120, 121) pointed out that to determine the acidic or basic effect of a biochemical reaction it is most convenient to consider the overall reaction (substrate to products) from the standpoint of a charge balance, and to add H^+ as a product or reactant to accomplish this overall adjustment of charge. In this manner acid producing reactions yield products that are more negative than their reactants and generate H^+. Conversely, reactions whose products have a more positive electrical charge than the reactants, have consumed H^+ and have a basic effect. Consideration of NH_4Cl, which is a typical material to produce experimental acidosis, illustrates Christensen's point.

$$NH_4Cl(+CO_2) \rightarrow urea + H_2O + Cl^-. \quad [R\text{-}3]$$

The complete catabolism of ammonium chloride will yield urea and water from the oxidation of nitrogen and will strand Cl^- in body water. The net effect is the same as adding equivalent amounts of HCl. To balance the reactions with respect to charge H^+ must be added to the right hand side of the reaction

$$2NH_4Cl(+CO_2) = urea + H_2O + 2(Cl^- + H^+). \quad [R\text{-}4]$$

Metabolism of an organic anion will have the reverse effect as can be illustrated with the acetate anion whose products are neutral CO_2 and water:

$$\text{Organic anion} + H^+ = H_2O + CO_2 \quad [R\text{-}5a]$$

$$acetate + (H^+) = 2H_2O + 2CO_2. \quad [R\text{-}5b]$$

Writing this expression in traditional biochemical form tends to confuse this point.

$$
\begin{array}{ll}
\text{ATP} & \text{AMP} + \text{PP} \\
\text{Acetate} & \text{Acetyl-S-CoA} + H_2O . \\
\text{HSCoA} &
\end{array} \quad [R\text{-}6]
$$

Chemical balance shows, however, that as written there is one more hydrogen in the products than in the reactants.

Reactions R-5 and R-6 illustrate that the popular concept that acetate produces bicarbonate is figurative at best (60, 61), the alkalinizing effect of acetate being through its consumption of H^+ as it is metabolized. Bicarbonate is produced by the unique reaction of carbonic acid dissociation (see reaction R-1 above). The only connection between these two reactions is that one consumes hydrogen ion (acetate metabolism) whereas the other produces it (dissociation of carbonic acid).

This method of considering metabolic reactions would then predict that ingested citric acid, formic acid (even nitric acid) would have no net effect on body acid base status because these compounds are electrically neutral on ingestion and will produce only neutral products. Although pH will decrease transiently, metabolism of the anion (base equivalent) will eventually reverse the response.

Net acid generation as related to protein catabolism and intake

Catabolism of protein should have a predictable acidic effect. This is because of the two sulfur containing amino acids – cystine and methionine – which when metabolized will abandon their sulfur as a negatively charged sulfate ion.

$$
\begin{array}{l}
\text{H}\quad\text{H H H} \\
\text{H-C-S-C-C-C-COO}^- \rightarrow H_2O + CO_2 + \text{Urea} + SO_4^= + (2H^+) \\
\text{H}\quad\text{H H N} \\
\qquad\qquad / | \backslash \\
\qquad\qquad \text{H H H} \\
\text{(methionine)}
\end{array}
$$

$$[R\text{-}7]$$

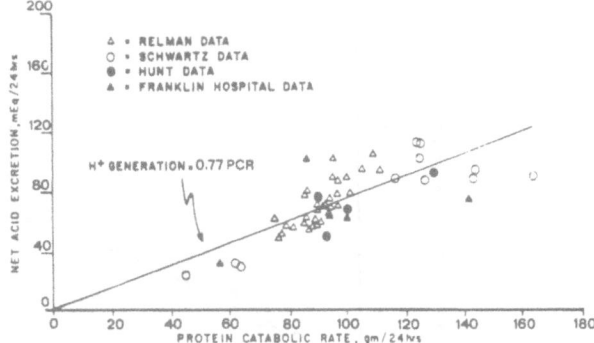

Figure 25. Hydrogen ion (acid) generation as a function of net rates of protein catabolism.

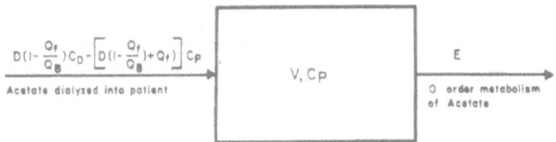

Figure 26. Model of acetate transport and metabolism in dialyzed patients.

In addition to its direct acidic effect, protein is a good index of general intake of various substances (49, 122). Analysis of metabolically and clinically controlled studies where both H^+ and nitrogen balances were done (Figure 25) shows that net rates of protein catabolism can be used to obtain good estimates of the net quantity of acid being produced (0.77 mEq/g of protein catabolized) (123–127).

Acetate metabolism

Appreciation of the alkalinizing effect of acetate metabolism, shown in reaction R-5, led Mion and coworkers in 1965 to substitute this anion for the more commonly used bicarbonate (128). This opened the way for the development of single concentrate dialysis proportioning system (129). The disadvantages of using bicarbonate in dialysate solutions are its poor solubility, its instability, and the requirement of high concentrations of dissolved CO_2, to keep pH in the range where magnesium and calcium will remain soluble (130). The advantages of acetate are its high solubility and perceived rapid rate of metabolism (131, 132).

Model formulation of acetate metabolism presents a major problem. Once again a single pool is sought (see Figure 26). Input to the system is uncomplicated being diffusive transport from dialysate to blood in the dialyzer as described in Equation [14]. The output from the system presents some difficulty, however. A typical acetate concentration profile during and immediately after dialysis is shown in Figure 27 and is the one that is commonly found in dialysis patient (55, 133). Examination of this figure

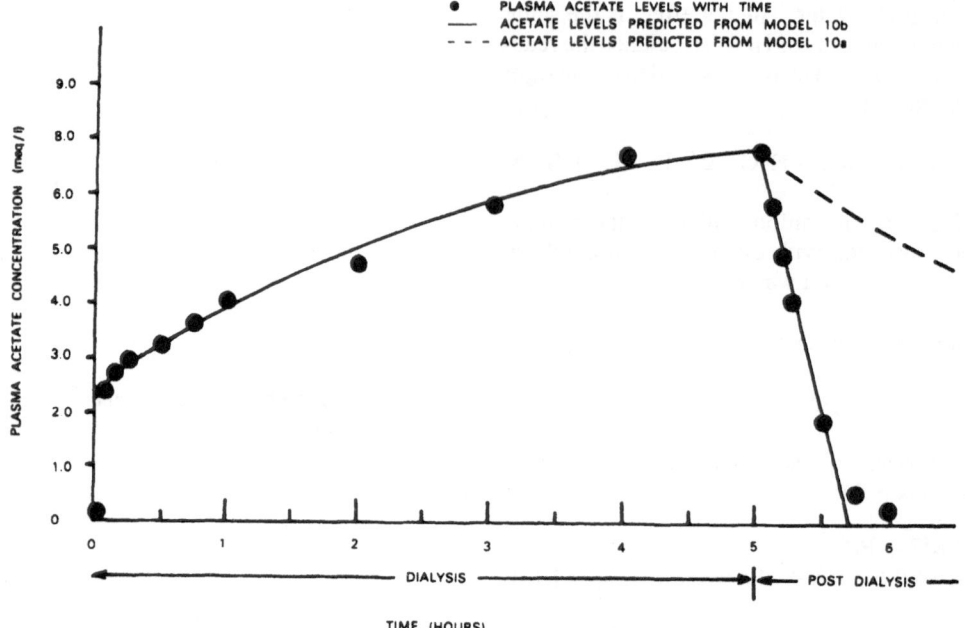

Figure 27. Acetate concentration with time in a typical dialysis patient during and shortly after a 5-hour treatment.

reveals an asymmetry between the concentration build-up, which may take as long as 2 to 3 h during dialysis and the rapid reduction of acetate to low plasma levels in less than an hour after dialysis. These kinetics are not consistent with a first order metabolic process.

Many metabolic systems show non-linear behavior as described by Michaelis–Menten type kinetics and shown in Figure 28. The type of system shown indicates first order metabolism at low substrate levels (eg, a doubling of metabolic rate for a doubling of substrate); as substrate builds up, however, there is less of an increase in metabolic rate approaching saturation levels. If acetate metabolism were in the shaded region of the figure its conversion to acetyl C_oA shown in reaction R-6 would show very little sensitivity to changing acetate levels and would be effectively constant (or zero order). When this output is used, the model in Figure 26 results. This yields the mass balance expression:

$$\frac{d(VC_P)}{dt} = D\left(1 - \frac{Q_F}{Q_B}\right)C_D$$
$$- \left[D\left(1 - \frac{Q_F}{Q_B}\right) + Q_F\right]C_P - E. \quad [58a]$$

If ultrafiltration can be neglected (i.e., Q_F and dV/dt approach zero) then Equation [58a] becomes:

$$V\frac{d(C_P)}{dt} = D(C_{Di} - C_P) - E. \quad [58b]$$

Using the assumption of constant ultrafiltration (see Equations [42a] and [42b] and solving for acetate concentration

during dialysis yields:

$$C_P = C_{Po}\left(\frac{V_0 - Q_Ft}{V_0}\right)^{D(1/Q_F - 1/Q_B)}$$
$$+ \left[D\left(1 - \frac{Q_F}{Q_B}\right) - E\right]$$
$$\times \left[1 - \left(\frac{V_0 - Q_Ft}{V_0}\right)^{D(1/Q_F - 1/Q_B)}\right]. \quad [59a]$$

And when extracellular volume can be considered constant (dV/dt and Q_F are negligible see Equation [49b]) an analogous expression results:

$$C_P = C_{Po}e^{-Dt/V} + \frac{DC_{Di} - E}{D}\left(1 - e^{-Dt/V}\right) \quad [59b]$$

and after dialysis in both cases:

$$C_P = C_{Pt} - \frac{E}{V}t. \quad [60]$$

From Figure 27 it is clear that acetate metabolism slows when acetate concentration is below 2 mEq/l post-dialysis. Reference to Figure 28 would indicate that below these acetate levels the metabolic reaction is below the shaded region and in the linear range (the reaction is now first order).

It is seen that Equation [59b] is of the same form as Equation [45] and that $(DC_{Di} - E)/D$ will be the steady state plasma level (C_{Pss}) at large values of t (i.e., when

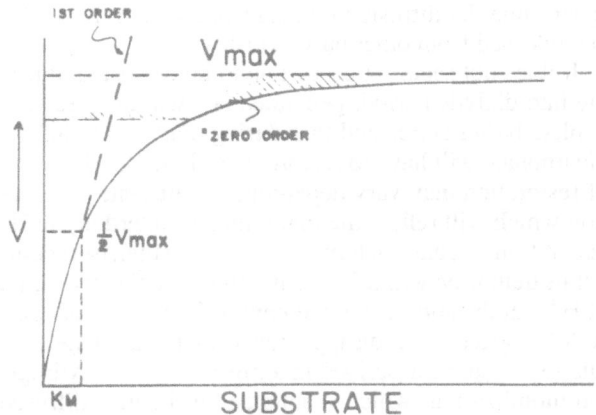

Figure 28. Velocity of metabolic reaction (V mEq/min) as a function of substrate levels (mEq/l) which would result from Michaelis-Menten kinetics.

Table 7. Acetate concentration in a patient dialyzed with 39 mmol/l in the dialysis fluid for 5 h. D acetate = 0.120 l/min

Time: t-relative to the start of dialysis, 0-relative to its end (min)	Plasma concentration (mmol/l)	E (from Equation [54])	E (from Equation [53])
0	0	–	–
60	4.0	3.63	–
120	4.7	3.87	–
180	5.8	3.74	–
240	6.7	3.66	–
300	6.8	3.73	–
		3.73	3.74

$e^{-Dt/V}$ is very small). It is clear that if steady state concentrations are known or can be approximated and D is known then the value of E can be estimated from

$$E = D(C_{Di} - C_{Pss}) \qquad [61]$$

rearrangement of Equation [59] allows another computation of E:

$$E = D\left(C_{Di} - \frac{C_P - C_{Po}e^{-Dt/V}}{1 - e^{-Dt/V}}\right), \qquad [62]$$

where V is assumed to be extracellular water and is taken as 1/3 of total body water (or V urea from the urea kinetic calculations). Values of E computed by both methods for the data shown in Figure 27 are shown in Table 7 and agree very closely.

Body base

Because of the critical nature of acid base control it is important to describe quantitatively the elements of H^+ and buffer base in the patient.

Table 8. Magnitude of elements in H^+ balances over one dialysis cycle

Hydrogen generation (from dietary sources)	100–200 mEq
Bicarbonate loss during acetate dialysis	500 mEq
Acetate uptake	600–800 mEq
Organic acid production	0–200 mEq
Organic anion loss (net H^+ production)	0-0100 mEq
Body H^+ content	0.0017 mEq

Ironically, from a strict mass balance sense, the modeled species (H^+) can be ignored because it is present in negligible quantities. In fact, H^+ balance is so treated, and the difference between H^+ production and elimination is taken as equal to the degree of buffer depletion (i.e., R-8 goes to completion and $d(H^+)/dt = 0$). In the discussion to follow, the model is of the body content of basic equivalents. and their increase or decrease in content can be considered as the negative of H^+ balance. In this context body buffer (i.e., adding basic equivalents) is 'negative H^+ balance', and acidification of body buffer (i.e., removing basic equivalents) is a 'positive H^+ balance'.

Acid-base kinetics are conceptually complex because of the labile nature of the solute, H^+, for which mass balance equations must be written. In addition, although several hundred milliequivalents of H^+ may be generated and removed during a complete dialysis cycle, the free concentration in body water remains vanishingly small (0.000030 – 0.000045 mEq/l) because of instantaneous reactions between H^+ and the large buffer pool in the body.

$$H^+ + buffer^- = bufferH. \qquad [R-8]$$

This can be more fully appreciated by reference to Table 8 which shows the various elements of H^+ balance in a 70 kg dialysis patient ingesting from 0.8 to 1.6 g protein/kg/day dialyzed with acetate dialysate using a 1.3 m² regenerated cellulose dialyzer.

Body base model formulation requires an in depth consideration of all elements that affect acid base status and consequently becomes quite complex. Step 1 of Figure 8 indicates that it is first necessary to define the system. However, consideration of the bicarbonate system is appropriate before the body base system is defined.

Bicarbonate modeling

Bicarbonate is traditionally and superficially treated pharmacokinetically as distributed in a single pool volume (generally estimated to be 40% body weigh) (124, 125, 134). If a general model of bicarbonate is formulated for dialysis with dialytic uptake of HCO_3^- and its removal by H^+ generation (gH^+) Figure 29a results. If a fixed dis-

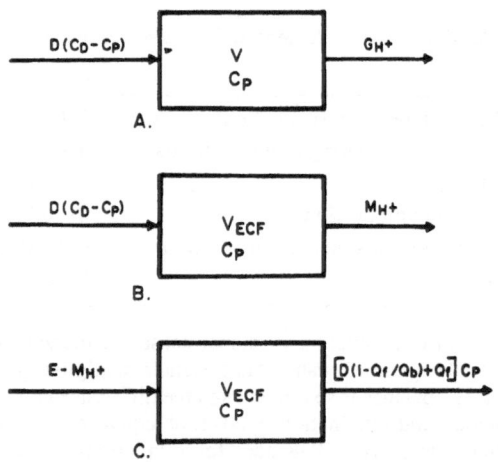

Figure 29. Models of the bicarbonate system during bicarbonate dialysis showing two versions of the model: (a) using apparent bicarbonate space, (b) using a fixed volume approximating extracellular volume and a mobilization constant, and (c) during acetate dialysis.

tribution volume is assumed the mass balance equation becomes:

$$V\frac{dC_P}{dt} = D(C_{Di} - C_{Pi}) - gH^+.$$ [63a]

Solution of this expression yields:

$$C_P = C_{Po}e^{-Dt/V} + \left(C_{Di} - \frac{gH^+}{D}\right)(1 - e^{-Dt/V}).$$ [63b]

Rearrangement of Equation [63b] yields an expression for V:

$$V = Dt \, \text{Log} \frac{C_{Po} - (C_{Di} - gH^+/D)}{C_{Pt} - (C_{Di} - gH^+/D)}.$$ [63c]

From the change in plasma concentration under known dialysis conditions of D and C_{Di} during bicarbonate dialysis, V can be calculated (where gH^+/D is considered negligible).

Values calculated using this equation occasionally show large and variable bicarbonate volumes (135). Similar variation of bicarbonate space depending on the level of acidosis has been reported (136).

Re-evaluation of the model shows that the fault may lie with the use of traditional pharmacokinetic techniques as embodied in Figure 29a and Equation [63c]. Such methods are normally applied to a specific solute which occupies a unique physical volume. This may be modified in the case of protein binding because an additional storage capacity for the substance is present and V is correspondingly larger (i.e., 'distribution volume' for a bound substance will be larger than its physical distribution space). Bicarbonate, however, because of its interrelation with H^+ and through it the other buffer systems, represents a highly labile material which may disappear from extracellular

space either by diffusion into cells or by neutralization of H^+ released from other buffers (134).

It does not seem unreasonable to consider that during the interdialytic period, generated H^+ will progressively deplete buffer stores and that during dialysis the infused bicarbonate will have to restore these buffers. The extent of restoration may vary depending on the state of depletion which will reflect the magnitude of interdialytic H^+ generation. A constant term like g_{H^+} must then be retained but its definition will differ as it will not be the generation of H^+ but the apparent movement of HCO_3^- out of extracellular space. The disappearance of bicarbonate from this space can be described in terms of m_{H^+} or 'hydrogen ion mobilization' which is intended to include diffusive movement of HCO_3^- out of the extracellular volume. The V term in the equation then becomes a constant whose value is known or can be determined. Rearrangement of the mass balance equation for the model shown in Figure 29b yields:

$$V_{ecf}\frac{dC_P}{dt} = D(C_D - C_P) - m_H.$$ [64a]

$$m_{H^+} = D\left[(C_D - C_{Po}) - \frac{(C_{Bi} - C_{Bo})}{1 - e^{-Dt/V}}\right].$$ [64b]

Note in this expression C_{Po} represents bicarbonate concentration at the start of dialysis. Equation [64b] shows that m_{H^+} is the difference of two terms, the initial rate of diffusive flux into extracellular space, and a term that contains the amount of rise of bicarbonate in that space. The second term accounts for the fact that HCO_3^- content of extracellular space is increasing. Examination of this expression shows what intuition would suggest, that the greater the rise in bicarbonate ($C_{Bt} > C_{Bo}$) during a treatment the smaller the alkalinization of other buffers will be. The lack of equivalence of this increased content with the flux from the dialyzer is accounted for by basic equivalents that have moved into other anatomical areas. Consequently, using typical intradialytic values for C_D, C_{Po}, C_{Pt}, V, D, and t, the extent of titration of buffers can be calculated. Thus if $C_D = 35$ mEq/l, $C_{Po} = 20$ mEq/l, $C_{Pt} = 23$ mEq/l over a 1 h period and V = 131, D = 0.100 l/min, the bicarbonate is disappearing (mH^+) at a rate of 0.69 mmol/min during this interval. The average flux into the patient $D(C_D - C_B)$ would be approximately 0.1 (35 − 21.5) or 1.35 mmol/min of which 49% would contribute to a rise in extracellular bicarbonate concentration. These illustrative data demonstrate an analytical technique that can estimate the H^+ balance during the process of acid-based correction with dialysis treatment. The adoption of model b in Figure 29 should increase understanding of what is actually occurring in the body, whereas a 'distribution space' for bicarbonate tends to blur the fact that the kinetics of this substance are interrelated both to the movement of H^+ and the status of body buffers.

Expected bicarbonate levels during acetate dialysis

The model shown in Figure 29c depicts bicarbonate mass balance during acetate dialysis. This model is the reverse of models 25a and 25b, which described bicarbonate dialysis. In this case bicarbonate is being dialyzed out of extracellular space; this model also incorporates volume changes during treatment. There will be some addition of HCO_3^- to the system resulting from the alkalinizing effect of acetate metabolism and the consumption of H^+, some of which will come from reaction R-1. The rate of HCO_3^- production is shown as the rate of alkalinization by metabolic conversion of acetate to acetyl-co-a (E) modified to account for the fact that only part of the H^+ consumed by this reaction will come from H_2CO_3 (see R-1). This modification is indicated as the acetate conversion rate less the hydrogen ion mobilization term ($E - mH^+$). Because of the relatively small contribution of gH^+ and the difficulty of separating it from the mH^+ term it is included in this term for the purposes of this model.

The mass balance equation becomes:

$$\frac{d(V_{ecf}C_P)}{dt} = V_{ecf}\frac{dC_P}{dt} + C_P\frac{dV_{ecf}}{dt}$$
$$= (E - mH^+) - \left[D\left(1 - \frac{Q_F}{Q_B}\right) + Q_F\right]C_P. \quad [65a]$$

If most of the intradialytic volume change comes from changes in extracellular water volume, Equations [42a] and [42b] can be used to define the change in this space. With this substitution solution of Equation [65a] yields:

$$C_P = C_{Po}\left(\frac{V_0 - Q_Ft}{V_0}\right)^{D(I/Q_F - I/Q_B)}$$
$$+ \frac{E - m_{H+}}{D(1 - Q_F/Q_B)}$$
$$\times \left[1 - \left(\frac{V_0 - Q_Ft}{V_0}\right)^{D(I/Q_F - I/Q_B)}\right]. \quad [65b]$$

Equations [59a] and [59b] can be used to calculate the expected end dialysis plasma acetate and bicarbonate levels that would result with increasing dialyzer flux rates of these materials. The following patient and dialyzer parameters were used to examine these relationships: urea volume 361; V_{ecf}(end) = 121; V_{ecf}(start) = 14.51; E = 3.8 mEq/min; C_PHCO_3(start) = 20 mEq/l; with treatment delivered during a dialysis designed to provide total urea clearance equal to urea volume (i.e., KT/V urea = 1.0) but conducted over differing intervals. Under these conditions dialyzer clearances will increase as dialysis time is shortened. Bicarbonate and acetate dialysance values were taken to be 83 and 70% of the required urea clearance respectively; C_D(acetate) = 37 mEq/l; mH^+ (the alkalinization required to restore body base equivalents depleted between treatments) is 123 mEq divided by the

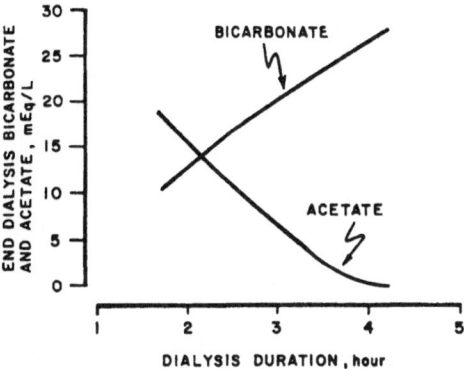

Figure 30. End dialysis bicarbonate and acetate levels during different length treatments where normalized treatment (KT/V) remains the same.

length of dialysis in minutes. Dialysis times were varied from 4 to 2 h.

The end dialysis bicarbonate and acetate levels expected to result from these treatment conditions are shown in Figure 30. It can be seen that acetate levels are near zero at the end of a 4 h treatment but steadily increase as treatment becomes more rapid reaching a level of 15 mEq/l at the end of a 2 h treatment. This curve reflects acetate flux increasing beyond the acetate metabolic rate with more rapid dialysis.

Bicarbonate levels at the end of treatment decrease as dialysis becomes more rapid due to increasing net dialyzer bicarbonate loss which exceeds the rate of alkalinization from acetate metabolism and its contribution to the H_2CO_3 neutralization reaction (see R-1). At the end of a 2 h dialysis, the blood acetate level is 15 mEq/l and higher than blood bicarbonate which is 13 mEq/l. The analysis indicates that acute metabolic acidosis and striking acetatemia would result if high flux 2 h dialysis was performed using dialysis fluid buffered with acetate. It cannot be concluded that net correction of acidosis would be inadequate since the large extracellular acetate inventory will be rapidly metabolized over 30 to 45 min after dialysis and will result in rapid bicarbonate generation. The magnitude of post-dialysis acetate metabolism can be estimated from the patient parameters used for this analysis. The acetate inventory in V_{ecf} can be calculated from this volume and end dialysis acetate concentrations = 12(15) = 180 mEq. Thus 180 mEq H^+ will be consumed and result in some combination of cell buffer alkalinization and bicarbonate production. Since in this analysis it was assumed that m_{H+} during dialysis resulted in full alkalinization of cell buffers during dialysis (which is not likely to be strictly correct), the rise in bicarbonate post-dialysis could be estimated as 180/12 = 15.0 mEq/l and the plasma bicarbonate 30 to 40 min after dialysis would be 13 + 15 = 28 mEq/l. In fact, it would be expected that a similar percentage of the alkalinizing potential of the conversion of acetate to acetyl-co-A would go to alkalinize

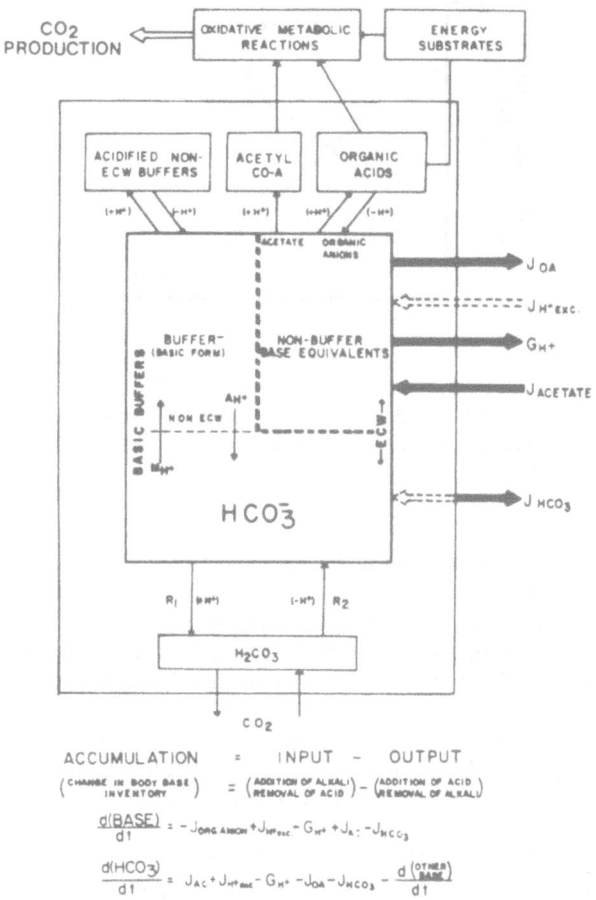

ACCUMULATION = INPUT − OUTPUT

$$\begin{pmatrix}\text{CHANGE IN BODY BASE}\\ \text{INVENTORY}\end{pmatrix} = \begin{pmatrix}\text{ADDITION OF ALKALI}\\ \text{REMOVAL OF ACID}\end{pmatrix} - \begin{pmatrix}\text{ADDITION OF ACID}\\ \text{REMOVAL OF ALKALI}\end{pmatrix}$$

$$\frac{d(BASE)}{dt} = -J_{ORG.ANION} + J_{H^+Exc} - G_{H^+} + J_A - J_{HCO_3}$$

$$\frac{d(HCO_3)}{dt} = J_{AC} + J_{H^+Exc} - G_{H^+} - J_{OA} - J_{HCO_3} - \frac{d\begin{pmatrix}\text{OTHER}\\ \text{BASE}\end{pmatrix}}{dt}$$

Figure 31. Model of body base equivalents.

other buffers and a smaller rise in ultimate plasma HCO_3^- would be expected.

The curves in Figure 29b demonstrate that acetate will not be a suitable dialysate buffer for correction of metabolic acidosis as dialysis times are shortened and as dialyzer flux rates increase. The point at which it is necessary to change from acetate to bicarbonate for an individual patient will clearly depend on his parameters as shown in Equations [59a] and [65b] (particularly the value of E). In any event, as bicarbonate flux rates progressively exceed acetate metabolic rates progressive acetatemia and metabolic acidosis will be induced during dialysis followed by very rapid post-dialysis alkalinization from acetate metabolism.

The body base model

The model shown in Figure 29b represents only the bicarbonate portion of the overall base content of the body. Figure 31 shows its incorporation into the overall model of body base equivalents. It is included as the bottom half of the inner box which is the bicarbonate portion of buffer base equivalents, that are capable of interact-

ing with other body buffers. The inner box represents the body base equivalents and is separated into three sections. Base equivalents in extracellular water are illustrated as including the HCO_3^-, just discussed, as well as the non-buffer materials in extracellular water (top right) such as lactate, acetate, and other organic anions (see R-5). The top left section of this box represents the non-extracellular buffers in basic form. The size of the space belies its extent which is actually greater than half of the total buffer base capacity of the body (134). Communication between these three compartments is indicated. As was discussed, addition of HCO_3^- to the extracellular pool will not quantitatively increase the extracellular bicarbonate content because there will be 'mobilization' of bicarbonate (or transfer of base equivalents) to other buffer systems. Similarly, when the buffers are acidified the buffer load will distribute among bicarbonate and other buffer systems as shown by the H^+ accumulation term A_{H^+} which indicates that as the extracellular compartment sustains an acid load, base equivalents will move into that compartment to restore partially the bicarbonate level (i.e., non-extracellular buffers will neutralize some of the added H^+). In Figure 31 the outer box encloses the system but also contains internal sources capable of producing buffer base if alkalinized, such as carbonic acid, organic acids, and acidified non-extracellular buffers.

Consider the example of lactic acid production by anaerobic metabolism:

$$\text{glucose} = \text{lactate-} + (H^+). \qquad \text{[R-9]}$$

Glucose (an energy substrate – upper right) has produced lactic acid (an organic acid). Both lactate and H^+ are added to the internal box of the figure. H^+, however, will combine with a buffer base, HCO_3^- for example, and produce H_2CO_3, which may in turn be exhaled in its anhydrous form CO_2. These reactions, however, will have no effect on the total base content because the decrease in HCO_3^- has been matched by the addition of lactate, a base equivalent (i.e., a substance capable of removing H^+ from the system when it is metabolized see R-5a).

It should be emphasized that carbon dioxide interaction with the body base system will have no net effect on the base content, for it is a neutral substance, although it can profoundly effect the system pH through its relation with the carbonic acid-bicarbonate system. The net excretion or retention of carbon dioxide, however, will not effect the body base content.

With reference to Figure 31 only the bold arrows represent net inputs and outputs for the system. All other arrows represent the transfer of neutral materials which have no net effect on the overall acid base status.

Consider first the inputs of the system: The ways that the body buffer system content can increase. A total of three inputs are considered. Renal excretion of acids (j_{H^+} Exc) will effect a net increase because net removal of hydrogen ion will cause a net movement of base equivalents from one of the internal buffer systems (eg, alkalinization of non-extracellular buffers or dissociation of H_2CO_3 by reaction R-1). Body base can be increased directly by flux of acetate into the patient (direct addition of base equivalents).

Alternatively, bicarbonate (if used in the dialysis fluid) can be a pathway to increase base content of the system. Note that once in the system, the acetate to acetyl-CoA conversion will be coupled to one of the other internal systems alkalinizing a non-extracellular buffer or net dissociation of H_2CO_3. In this light it is apparent that non-stoichiometric appearance of bicarbonate during acetate metabolism (60, 61) should, in fact, be predicted because of the variety of substances capable of providing the hydrogen ion consumed in the acetate metabolic reaction.

Routes of output or ways in which base equivalents will be removed from the system will be: by removal of organic anions which are themselves base equivalents (eg, lactate); by acid generation g_{H+}, or by bicarbonate loss during acetate dialysis. These outputs (and inputs) are totally general. If the diet is low in protein and high in alkaline, material (sodium citrate for example) g_{H+} will be negative and there will be a net base increase. Also if bicarbonate is given by mouth or some other unbalanced organic anion, such as monosodium glutamate is ingested, this contribution can be dealt with by incorporating the flux of these substances in J_{HCO_3} or J_{OA} terms and appropriate adjustment of algebraic sign.

Referring to the section 'Formulation of a model' and Figure 8 it will be apparent that the model in Figure 31 has not been completely specified. The normal step would be to relate the inputs and outputs to the system content. In this case 'body base' consists of a collection of substances which may interrelate in a manner that cannot be defined on the basis of current research. These difficulties of specifying this model further will be discussed below.

Writing the mass balance equation yields

$$\frac{d(\text{Base})}{dt} = -J_{OA} + J_{H+}\text{Exc} - g_{H+} + J_{AC} - J_{HCO_3^-}. \quad [66a]$$

This expression is totally general and not restricted to dialysis or even uremia. Consider the stable individual not on dialysis (i.e., $J_{AC} = 0$), presumably in steady state $(d(\text{base})/dt = 0)$

$$J_{H+}\text{Exc} = g_{H+} + J_{OA} + J_{HCO_3^-}. \quad [66b]$$

This indicates that H^+ excretion will balance H^+ generation plus the loss of organic anions and bicarbonate. Acid base upsets can also be described by Figure 31 and Equations [66a] and [66b]. Consider, for example, ketoacidosis in diabetes mellitus. When fat is a major energy substrate, there is generation and neutralization of organic acids represented by their dissociation into the buffer pool. The immediate effect will be neutralization of H^+ by some other buffer, which the organic anion will replace

as a body base equivalent, the body base content staying constant. The elevated levels of organic anions, however, will result in urinary excretion of these materials (J_{OA}). If $J_{H+}\text{Exc}$ can increase to accommodate the buffer loss (see Equation [66b]), there will be no net acidification of the system. If not, base content will be reduced (see Equation [66a]).

If body base is separated into bicarbonate and other buffers, Equation [66a] can be rewritten and solved for the HCO_3^- terms:

$$\frac{d(HCO_3^-)}{dt} + H_{HCO_3^-} = J_{AC} - g_{H+} - J_{OA}$$
$$- \frac{d(\text{other base})}{dt} + J_{H+}\text{Exc}. \quad [67]$$

Equation [67] indicates that HCO_3^- removal from the system plus the increase in HCO_3^- content will equal the combination of the five terms on the right side. It should, once again, be noted that for acetate flux and metabolism to be equal to HCO_3^- mass balance, as has been anticipated by some (60, 61), the algebraic sum of the last four terms must be zero, an improbable result during such a metabolically disruptive event as dialysis. Consequently, the non-equivalence of acetate uptake and bicarbonate appearance described by others (60, 61) should not be surprising.

Control of acid base: solution of the model

The goal of acid base control during dialysis treatment is to minimize the depletion of body buffers between dialyses and the non-extracellular buffers (bone) long term, and to restore adequately the basic buffer forms during treatment.

As alluded to above there is very little therapeutic control of interdialytic base depletion. That primarily results from acid forming foods in the diet and appears in the forgoing relationships as g_{H+}. In addition, intake of fluid, which will not have an overall effect on body buffers, causes movement of base equivalents into the extracellular compartment to supply buffer to this space as it expands (dilutional acidosis) (136). Hence, while Figure 31 represents a useful model it cannot yet be adequately formulated.

The system content as represented by the internal box in Figure 31 cannot be accurately specified. More information about the composition and interrelation of buffers as implied by the terms aH^+ and mH^+ is required. Because HCO_3^- is the measurable component of body buffer and the one to which output and input relate knowledge of how HCO_3^- and other buffers interact is required. Also of interest is the location of the acetate alkalinization step and whether it has its effect directly on extracellular buffers or through non-extracellular buffers. The dashed lines shown in Figure 31 may have certain resistances associated with them so that the addition of HCO_3^- to the extracellular fluid may have a different effect than equivalent alkalinization using acetate and indications of this possibility have been observed. The alkalinizing effect of acetate may also depend on transport of a co-ion, eg, sodium, and therefore complete specification of the model will rely on another solute system which is changing during dialysis. For these reasons the model as described in Figure 31 must be considered as partially specified, for which the mass balance equation (Equations [66a–67]) are an accurate representation, but for which insufficient information is available for complete formulation for the purposes of guiding treatment.

The effect of fluid retention and removal

A few comments are appropriate with respect to the marginal ability to correct acid base during dialysis. The acidification of the system between treatments was discussed primarily with respect to protein and acid generation. In addition, as fluid is consumed and retained in body water some dilutional acidosis occurs (i.e., base equivalents move into extracellular fluid acidifying cell buffers in the process, to sustain extracellular buffer levels). Although this will not change total body base equivalents, intracellular buffers will be depleted. The need to remove the retained fluid during dialysis, however, markedly blunts the ability to alkalinize the patient. Equation [14] shows that with Q_F of zero and 15 ml/min under the same bicarbonate conditions discussed above (see bicarbonate model) flux would be 1.35 mEq/min versus 0.91 mEq/min or a 31% drop when (Q_F = 15 ml/min (900 ml/h).

Creatinine

Creatinine is traditionally grouped with urea as a major uremic catabolite, the concentration of which should be controlled (137–139). That plasma creatinine concentration provides valuable nutritional information through its relationship to body muscle mass is well established (89). In this regard, it can be more accurate to view creatinine, or at least its production rate, as an outcome measure of dialysis therapy rather than control variable.

Plasma creatinine concentration is widely used in the pre-dialysis patient as a rough inverse correlate to kidney function (93), although there is evidence that creatine production drops in chronic uremia disproportionally to the decrease in lean body mass (140–142). Nevertheless, the relative constancy of creatinine production from the spontaneous and non-enzymatic dehydration of creatine phosphate has made it useful as an endogenous marker in progressive renal failure. Through its utility as a marker of renal function it has become associated with other catabolites and has assumed an importance that is unwarranted for its role as a metabolic product. It does not represent the end product of major metabolic pathway, although it is associated with the energy pathway in muscle tissue through its connection with the creatine–phosphocreatine system. It can be shown that creatinine follows single pool kinetics (138) although not as closely as urea (139).

Sodium

There continues to be significant intradialytic morbidity associated with regular dialysis therapy. This morbidity comprises multiple symptoms including headache, nausea and vomiting, fatigue, hypotension and severe muscle cramps. The most frequent and objective symptoms are hypotension and muscle cramps which require medical intervention and occur in 15 to 40% of treatments in different centers.

Several studies have shown that increasing the dialysis fluid concentration of Na (C_{DNa}) reduces morbidity during dialysis (143–145). This therapeutic maneuver has been effective but can cause excessive body Na content and volume overload. Consequently a model would seem highly desirable for quantitative assessment of interdialytic Na and volume loading and intradialytic Na and volume removal.

Hemofiltration has been widely reported to reduce morbidity compared to hemodialysis (146–157). In view of the strong dependence of treatment morbidity during dialysis on dialysate sodium concentration an evaluation of comparative hemofiltration morbidity should include assessment of Na flux in the compared therapies.

Measurement of sodium concentration and activity

Until recently blood and dialysate inlet Na concentrations (C_B, C_D) have been routinely measured by the flame photometer (F) in clinical practice. The Na diffusion gradient or driving force for diffusive Na flux (J) across the dialyzer however, is a function of the Na activity in the blood and dialysate streams which is correctly measured with an ion selective electrode (ISE). The flame photometer correctly measures Na concentration of the two streams but does not provide a correct measure of the Na activity; the ion selective electrode does.

The reason for these differences is that the electrode measures the ionized Na concentration in the aqueous phase of each stream but does not include Na ionically complexed with anions, particularly protein (158), bicarbonate (159) and acetate. The flame method measures total Na content per unit volume irrespective of ionization state and sample water fraction. These differences between measurement methods indicate that the Na diffusion gradient across the dialyzer should be measured by ion selective electrode and Na flux should be measured by flame photometry.

These relationships have been verified in *in vitro* and *in vito* studies (159). These studies also showed that the osmotic distribution of Na in the blood stream is equal to the total water content of red cells plus plasma since Na mass balance between the blood and dialysate streams was achieved when Q_B was defined by the aqueous phase flow rate. Thus Q_e for sodium equals the total blood water flow rate.

Table 9. The relationship of ion selective electrode and flame photometer determination of sodium concentration in blood and dialysate samples

Fluid	Relationship	References	Equation
Blood plasma	$C_PE/C_PF = 1.01$	(139–141)	[68a]
Dialysate	$C_DE/C_DF = 0.99e^{-0.00063Ca}$	(139)	[68b]

Solution of the dialysate equation in Table 9 for typical dialysate acetate or bicarbonate concentration of 40 mEq/l shows that $C_DE/C_DF = 0.965$.

Relationships between measurement methods for blood and dialysate

The flame and electrode measurements of Na agree fairly closely in blood under usual conditions (160–162). In dialysate they differ substantially with electrode values typically being lower than flame values due to the high concentrations of acetate or bicarbonate. A predictable relationship has been reported between electrode and flame methods for both blood and dialysate in the presence of acetate or bicarbonate anions (Ca), as shown in Table 9.

The impact of measurement methods on clinical practice

There are important clinical consequences of the relationships in Table 9. In order to achieve a zero Na diffusive gradient across the dialyzer the Na activity in blood and dialysate must be equal and from the above considerations it follows that $1.01C_PF = 0.965C_DF$ or $C_DF = 1.05C_PF$. Thus if $C_PF = 140$, for a zero diffusion gradient C_DF must be 147 mEq/l or about 7 mEq/l higher than blood Na.

These relationships have resulted in some controversy in recent years between dialysate manufacturers and consumers. Many clinical laboratories now use electrode measurements because of its technical simplicity compared to flame measurements. Consequently, dialysate concentrate which is prepared to provide a Na content (determined correctly by F) of 140 mEq/l with standard 35:1 dilution will show Na concentration measured by electrode of only 135 mEq/l. When the consumer finds a dialysate electrode Na value of 135 mEq/l he is likely to conclude the concentrate is 4% low while the manufacturers data shows the actual Na content is 140 mEq/l. Both measurements are correct but confusion results because the parameters being measured (concentration or activity) are not widely understood by most clinicians.

Equivalency of Na flux in hemodialysis and hemodiafiltration studies

The relationships between flame and electrode measurement of Na shown in Table 9 also have significant implications with respect to comparative Na flux in hemodialysis (J_{HD}) and post-dilution hemofiltration (J_{HF}). Sodium flux into the patient during hemodialysis is described by a version of Equation [14].

$$J_{HD} = D(1 - Q_F/Q_E)C_D - [D(1 - Q_F/Q_E) + Q_F]C_P, \quad [68]$$

where D is Na dialysance, Q_F is ultrafiltration rate, Q_E is blood water flow rate, C_D is inlet dialysate Na concentration, and C_P is inlet plasma Na concentration. The values for C_D and C_P represent the Na activity so when C_D and C_P are measured by flame photometer, the effective concentrations are:

$$
\begin{aligned}
J_{HD} = {} & D(1 - Q_F/Q_E)(0.965C_DF) \\
& - [D(1 - Q_F/Q_E) + Q_F](1.01C_PF). \quad [69]
\end{aligned}
$$

In the case of post-dilution hemofiltration Na flux can be described by:

$$J_{HF} = (Q_{HF} - Q_F)C_S - Q_{HF}(C_F), \quad [70]$$

where J_{HF} is Na flux into the patient, Q_{HF} is an analogue of D and represents the total hemofiltration rate, Q_F is net fluid removal rate, $(Q_{HF} - Q_F)$ is substitution fluid infusion rate, C_S is substitution fluid Na concentration, C_F is hemofiltrate Na concentration.

When C_S and C_F are measured by flame photometer, the effective Na concentrations will be:

$$J_{HF} = (Q_{HF} - Q_F)C_SF - Q_{HF}(0.985C_PF). \quad [71]$$

There is no correction for C_SF because it is infused directly into the blood stream. The coefficient 0.985 is applied to the term C_PF based on several reports indicating the mean ratio $C_FF/C_PF = 0.985$ (163–165).

The C_DF value relative to C_SF required for $J_{HD} = J_{HF}$ can be calculated by combining Equations [69b] and [71] and solving for C_DF as follows:

$$
\begin{aligned}
C_DF = {} & \frac{1}{0.965D(1 - Q_F/Q_E)} \\
& \times [Q_{HF}(C_SF - 0.985C_PF) - Q_F(C_SF - 1.10C_PF)] \\
& + [D(1 - Q_F/Q_E)1.01C_PF]. \quad [72]
\end{aligned}
$$

Equation [72] can be evaluated for the following set of typical treatment parameters: $D = Q_HF = 0.160$ l/min; $Q_F = 0.010$ l/min; $Q_E = 0.200$ l/min; $C_PF = C_SF = 140$ mEq/l.

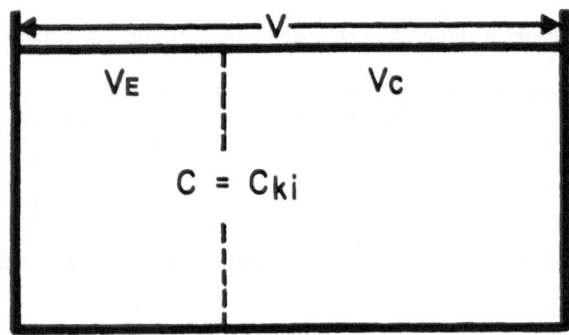

Figure 32. Two compartment distribution of osmotically active sodium and potassium in body water.

Solution of Equation [72] for these data results in $C_DF = 149$ mEq/l when $C_SF = 140$ mEq/l and $J_{HD} = J_HF$.

There has been considerable controversy regarding the ratio of C_FF/C_PF (14, 166, 167). If it is assumed that this ratio is 1.00 (i.e., the first two terms in the numerator of Equation [72] are neglected), solution of the above data shows $C_DF = 147$ when $C_SF = 140$ mEq/l and $J_{HD} = J_{HF}$.

This analysis of the effective Na concentrations in hemodialysis and hemofiltration indicates that dialysate Na concentrations must be 7 to 9 mEq/l higher than substitution fluid Na concentration for equal Na flux with both therapies. Dialysate Na concentration is known to influence strongly treatment morbidity which in hemofiltration has been reported to be lower than for hemodialysis when $C_DF = C_SF$. Consideration of the effective Na concentrations with these two therapies indicates that reduced morbidity with hemofiltration may be due to lower Na removal in hemofiltration when $C_DF = C_SF$.

The difference between these two treatments under the same initial dialysis conditions can be illustrated further by computing the difference in sodium flux resulting from both therapies. Substituting the initial parameters used in the above computation into Equations [69] and [70] assuming that $C_DF = J_{HF}$ 140 mEq/l and computing the flux difference yields J_{HD}, $_{HF}$, and $J_{HD} - J_{HF}$ of -2.37 mEq/min – 1.06, = -1.31 mEq/min. The instantaneous effect of this difference on the vascular compartment would be to move 1.31/140 = 0.0094 l/min (9.4 ml/min) out of the extracellular compartment which would have the same effect early in dialysis of nearly doubling the ultrafiltration rate (i.e., 10 ml/min ultrafiltration plus 9.4 ml/min osmotically drawn into cells).

Sodium distribution volume

It has long been known that osmotic equilibrium exists throughout body water (168). Although there are multiple small anatomical subdivisions of total body water (V) (169), with respect to osmotic equilibrium it can be described as a two compartment system comprised of extracellular and intracellular water (V_E and V_C) as diagrammed in Figure 32. Osmotic equilibrium exists between compartments because of the high hydraulic permeability of cell membranes; any change in the osmotically active solute content of V_C or V_E selectively results in net water flux until the concentration of solute in both compartments is again equal.

Owing to the passive nature of water flux between V_E and V_C due only to the osmotic driving force, it follows that the volume of each compartment will be determined by the relative contents of osmotically active solute in each compartment and the total amount of water distributed between the compartments. Although there are multiple solutes present in body water, the bulk of osmolality in V_E is contributed by sodium salts and in V_C it is contributed by potassium salts. The asymmetric distribution of Na and K is achieved by active transport mechanisms in cell membranes resulting in high transcellular concentration gradients for Na and K. It has been shown by isotope dilution studies that plasma Na (C_{Na}) over a wide concentration range linearly depends on the rapidly exchangeable body sodium and potassium content (Na_{Ex}, K_{Ex}) and total body water, V.

The relationship found was (170):

$$C_{Na} = \frac{Na_{Ex} + K_{Ex}}{V} . \tag{73}$$

The rapidly exchangeable quantities, $Na_{Ex} + K_{Ex}$, were postulated to be measures of the osmotically active Na and K salts in V_E and V_C respectively. The relationship in Equation [73] provided confirmation of this postulate and demonstrated that the effective osmotic driving force controlling body water distribution between V_E and V_C was determined by Na and K salts in the two compartments respectively. The sum of Na_{Ex} and K_{Ex} can be considered equal to the total osmotically active cation (C^+) in body water and Equation [73] can then be written.

$$C_{Na} = \frac{C^+}{V} . \tag{74}$$

Equation [74] is a powerful physiologic statement showing that C^+ can readily be calculated from the product $C_{Na}V$. Serial change in C^+ can be computed from serial changes in C_{Na} if V is either constant or undergoes a quantified change, ΔV. This can be illustrated as follows: Consider initial composition to be represented by C_{Na_1}, V_1, and C_I^+ assume that C_{Na_2} is measured after a known ΔV and unknown change in C^+ due to changes in body water content of Na and K, ΔNa and ΔK.

The serial composition relationships will be:

$$C_{Na_1} = \frac{C_I^+}{V_1} \tag{75a}$$

$$C_{Na_2} = \frac{C_I^+ + \Delta Na + \Delta K}{V_1 + \Delta V} . \tag{75b}$$

The change in C^+, which is by definition $\Delta Na + \Delta K$, can be determined by subtraction of Equation [75a] from [75b] and rearrangement:

$$(\Delta Na + \Delta K) = (C_{Na_2} - C_{Na_1})V_1 + (C_{Na_2})(\Delta V). \quad [75c]$$

Assuming all quantities on the right hand side of Equation [75c] can be measured, the relationships in Equation [75c] provide a simple method to calculate ΔC^+ or $\Delta Na + \Delta K$.

The clinical material used to establish the relationships in Equation [73] was comprised of a spectrum of patients with chronic illness with C_{Na} ranging from hyponatremic to modest hypernatremic levels (170). In the hyponatremia of chronic illness, depletion of cellular K^+ often was the major compositional change present causing H_2O to move out of cells diluting Na^+ in extracellular fluid.

In the dialysis patient there are regular small oscillations in body water K^+ content with interdialytic loading of excess K^+ followed after 2 or 3 days by dialytic removal of the excess. Thus the body K^+ content, in the absence of an associated severe K^+ depleting chronic illness, oscillates between mild excess and normal.

Because of normal K^+ sequestration in cells, potassium loads should result in small changes in plasma K^+ levels (167, 171, 172). Studies in dialysis patients, however, indicate that K^+ loading and removal can be accurately estimated by considering changes in potassium levels to extend over total body water. That is, a 3 mEq/l reduction in K^+ in a patient with 40 l of total body water will reflect 120 mEq of potassium removal. The reasons behind this apparent contradiction of asymmetric potassium distribution are not clear. It may relate to the small changes in potassium which makes this approximation usable. Thus, ΔK is negligible and Equation [75b] can be rewritten as:

$$\Delta Na = C_{Na_2}(V_1 + \Delta V)(C_{Na_1})(V_1). \quad [76]$$

It is apparent from Equation [76] that although anatomically Na is confined to V_E, its osmotic distribution is V, and a single pool equal to total body water can be used to model sodium in steady state. It should be emphasized that the magnitude of change in the Na^+ content of body water can be computed from Equation [76] only if there are no unusual asymmetrically distributed solutes which are loaded or removed from body water during the dialysis cycle. Consequently, if solutes such as dextrose or mannitol are present Equation [76] should not be used to calculate the change in body Na content. Both of these materials can accumulate in V_E. Consequently, in the diabetic patient with substantial changes in blood sugar during dialysis or in the mannitol treated patient, Equation [76] would be invalid due to unaccounted for changes in osmotically active solute in V_E resulting in net transcompartmental water flux independent of ΔNa.

A third solute which can have a significant impact on these relationships is urea. At steady state there is concentration equilibrium between V_E and V_C for urea and thus

urea will not influence water distribution between these components. During dialysis a urea concentration gradient develops between the two compartments (i.e., cellular urea concentration will be higher than extracellular concentration – see Figure 15) which will transiently pull water into cells. This urea disequilibrium then introduces another osmotic effect in addition to that of Na and as in the case of mannitol and dextrose Equation [76] should be used with caution.

Calculation of ΔNa and ΔV over the dialysis treatment cycle

A flow diagram of body compositional relationships over the dialysis treatment cycle is shown in Figure 33. In order to calculate values for interdialytic dietary Na loading and subsequent intradialytic sodium removal from serial values of C_{Na} it is necessary to determine V and ΔV. Total body water is coextensive with the urea distribution volume (79) so that the variable volume urea kinetic model described earlier can be used to determine end-dialysis volume (V_t). Over short 2 to 3 day interdialytic intervals, change in body weight is traditionally used as a measure of change in V (volume loading, V_L). Similarly, change in body weight from pre- to post-dialysis is used to measure the volume of fluid removal, V_R.

The magnitude of sodium removal is equal to $C_{02}^+ - C_{t1}^+$ (see Figure 33) and described by:

$$\text{sodium loading} = C_{02}(V_{t1} + V_L) - (C_{t1}(V_{t1}). \quad [77]$$

The magnitude of sodium removal is equal to $C_{02}^+ - C_{t2}^+$ and described by:

$$\begin{aligned} \text{sodium removal} \\ = C_{02}(V_{t1} + V_L) - C_{t2}(V_{t1} + V_L - V_R). \quad [78] \end{aligned}$$

Sodium balance $\Delta(C_{Na}V)$ over the treatment cycle by definition equals sodium loading less sodium removal and can be determined by subtracting Equation [78] from [77] resulting in:

$$\Delta C_{Na}V = (C_{t2} - C_{t1})V_{t1} + C_{t2}(V_L - V_R). \quad [79]$$

Equations [77] to [79] provide a simple method to quantify Na loading, removal and balance over the treatment cycle from several measured values of C_{Na} and use of urea kinetics to determine V, and changes in weight to determine V_L and V_R.

The usual therapeutic goal for each treatment cycle is to achieve zero Na and V balance; that is, to remove during dialysis exactly the quantity of dietary sodium and water loaded since the previous dialysis. Inspection of Equation [79] shows that to achieve this, the end dialysis sodium concentration must always be returned to the same value ($C_{t2} = C_{t1}$) and the net fluid removed during dialysis must equal the interdialytic weight gain ($V_L = V_R$). The first term on the right side of Equation [79] can be viewed as being controlled by the diffusive Na concentration gradient between blood and dialysate: the second

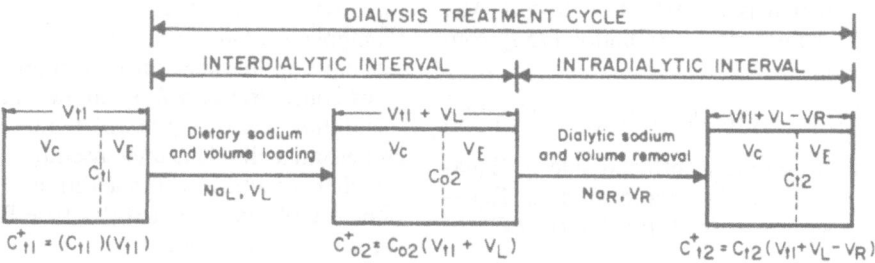

Figure 33. Flow diagram of interdialytic Na⁺ and volume loading and intradialytic Na and volume removal.

term can be viewed as being controlled by the magnitude of ultrafiltration. Current state of the art dialysis therapy provides reasonable assurance that $V_R = V_L$ by matching the ultrafiltration to the interdialytic weight gain but does not assure that $C_{t2} = C_{t1}$ since there is no attempt to individualize the diffusive Na gradient for each treatment. This would require measurement of C_{02} and use of a model to individualize dialysis fluid Na⁺ concentration as will be discussed.

The relative impact on Na⁺ balance resulting from mismatch of diffusive gradient and ultrafiltration can he shown by consideration of Equation [79]. Assume average values of $V_t = 38.01$ and $C_{t2} = 140$ mmol/l. For a 1.0 mmol/l difference between C_{t2} and C_{t1} there will be a 38 mmol change in Na balance, and for each 0.11 mismatch between V_L and V_R there will be a difference of 14 mmol. It is apparent that both diffusion and ultrafiltration must be individualized for each treatment if no change in Na balance is to result.

Modeling extracellular water and osmotic interactions

The preceding discussion provides the theoretical basis for a single pool Na distribution model as well as methods to compute change in Na and water balance over the interdialytic and intradialytic intervals. Sodium and volume loading between dialyses will depend entirely on dietary Na and water intake and can be quite variable. In order to achieve zero Na balance over each dialysis cycle reliably, it is necessary to target a constant end-dialysis Na concentration irrespective of pre-dialysis concentration as shown by Equation [79]. Sodium concentration, however, depends on the amount of Na present as well as the volume of extracellular water which will change during dialysis depending on ultrafiltration and on osmotic factors.

In addition, extracellular water is the system of interest because its content will directly influence hypotension and intradialytic patient morbidity. Extracellular water will be influenced, however, by two major factors: The ultrafiltration rate across the dialyzer induced by a blood-dialysate pressure difference (the analogue of convective transport of a solute); and the osmotic movement of water due to

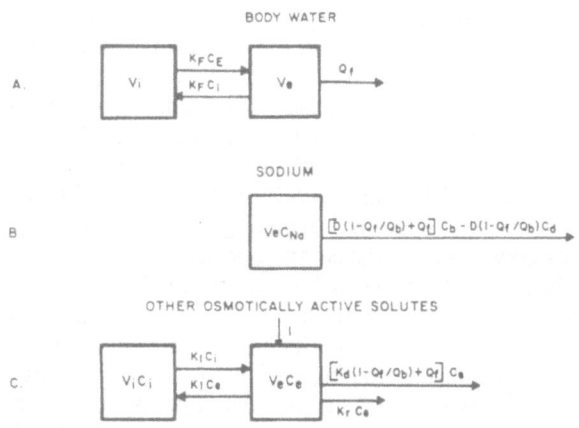

Figure 34. Model for body water and osmotically active solutes during dialysis.

changes in osmotically active solutes (the analogue of diffusive transport of a solute). The model for this system, therefore, involves other systems in a similar manner as did the body base model.

There are three interacting systems that will influence extracellular water content and these systems are shown in Figure 34. They are: 1. The body water system (Figure 34a), 2. The sodium system (Figure 34b); and 3. The system designated as that for 'other osmotically active solutes' (Figure 34c). This latter system is general and will be seen to be the same as Figure 14 for urea if 'I' is equated to urea generation rate (G) and if Q_F is set to zero. This model, however, can also be used to describe such osmotic agents as mannitol with 'I' as an infusion rate and with K_1 approaching zero (effectively confining mannitol to extracellular water).

Each of these models will be considered in turn. Although extracellular water is the system of interest it is actually part of total body water as described in Figure 34a. This system is considered as consisting of two compartments – intracellular and extracellular water. Movement of water out of the extracellular space occurs by ultrafiltration (Q_F) across the dialyzer and depends on the hydraulic permeability of the dialyzer (its ultrafiltration coefficient) and the mean transmembrane pressure (see

Equation [19]). For purposes of this model the ultrafiltration rate is considered constant which is generally the case during dialysis. Movement of water between intra- and extracellular compartments depends on the relative concentration of osmotically active solutes in these compartments (CI and CE). Higher concentrations in extracellular water (CE) cause movement of water into this compartment. Conversely, higher concentrations in intracellular water (CI) cause water to move from the extracellular space into cells. In general, therefore, it is desirable for (CE – CI) to be positive or zero so that there will be refilling of the extracellular volume or at least no volume change. If (CE – CI) is negative, water will move out of the extracellular space both across the dialyzer and into cells in which case hypotension and some degree of vascular collapse is likely.

Osmotically active solutes (CI and CE above) will consist of electrolytes (predominantly sodium as discussed above) and non-electrolytes (such as urea). The model for sodium is shown in Figure 34b. It is a single pool model and its content will be influenced, during dialysis, by diffusive and convective transport as described in Equation [14].

Figure 34c describes other osmotically active solutes (non-electrolytes) examples of which are urea and exogenous materials. A specific case of this model for urea was presented in Figure 14. In this system the intracellular pool is basically passive with the only route of solute entry being diffusion from the extracellular space. Material enters the extracellular space either through generation (urea: I – G) or by constant infusion (in the case of exogenous solutes). The second route by which material is added to the extracellular space is by diffusion from the intracellular space down a concentration gradient controlled by an intercompartmental transfer coefficient of K_L. Material is removed from this compartment by dialysis (see Equation [14] or continuing renal clearance (K_R) of this material or both.

Considering each of these systems separately, the mass balance equations will be:

Body water system (Figure 34a):

$$\frac{d(V_i)}{dt} = K_F(CI - CE) \tag{80a}$$

$$\frac{d(V_e)}{dt} = -Q_F - K_F(CI - CE). \tag{80b}$$

Sodium system (Figure 34b):

$$\frac{d(V_e C_{Na})}{dt} = -\left[D\left(1 - \frac{Q_F}{Q_B}\right) + Q_F\right]C_{Na}$$
$$+ D\left(1 - \frac{Q_F}{Q_B}\right)C_d. \tag{81}$$

Other osmotically active solutes (Figure 34c):

$$\frac{d(V_i C_i)}{dt} = -K_1(C_i - C_e) \tag{82a}$$

$$\frac{d(V_e C_e)}{dt} = K_1(C_i - C_e) + I$$
$$- \left[K_D\left(1 - \frac{Q_F}{Q_B}\right) + Q_F\right]C_e - K_R C_e. \tag{82b}$$

A model similar to the one shown in Figures 34 has been used to obtain *in vivo* measurements of the whole-body cell ultrafiltration (K_F) and urea mass transfer (K_1) coefficients (99). In these studies the Q_F and $C_D Na$ were manipulated to remove either 1.01 of Na free water or 130 mEq Na without water removal over 30 min of dialysis (99). Frequent measurements of blood Na and urea during the 30 min of dialysis and a following 30 min period of equilibration were used to calculate K_F and K_1 values from numerical solution of the mass balance expressions (Equations [80] to [82]).

These studies yielded mean values of K_1 of 760 ml/min which agrees with other reported values (22, 39). Contrary to common intuition, that water transport into and out of cells is 'rapid', values of K_F were 0.2 ml/min/mmHg (i.e., the entire body cell diffusion area is less permeable to water than most dialyzers). The transcapillary ultrafiltration coefficient is considerably higher and of the order of 5 ml/min/mmHg (173).

It is clear from Figure 34 that extracellular volume with potential impact on intradialytic morbidity requires a complex and a multisystem model. In contrast, however, to the body base system, most of the interrelationships between the water, sodium, and urea systems can be quantitatively defined. What is also clear is that intradialytic hypotension is far more complicated than has perhaps been appreciated and depends on more factors than strictly ultrafiltration rates for its control.

Clinical applications of the extracellular water model

A major goal of each dialysis is removal of dietary Na$^+$ and water that has accumulated since the previous treatment with minimal risk of intradialytic morbidity such as symptomatic hypotension and muscle cramps. At present, there are not clear guidelines for optimizing Na$^+$ and H$_2$O removal. A number of empirically developed dialysate Na$^+$ profiles have been reported to reduce morbidity associated with ultrafiltration (174) but a consensus has not been reached regarding their value. It would seem probable that clinical optimization of ultrafiltration will require quantification of the relationships between several different systems including various body fluid compartments and definition of circulatory hemodynamics. Unfortunately such information is not yet available.

Decreasing intradialytic morbidity can be viewed as a problem of selecting the best means of removing the interdialytic Na$^+$ and water load during dialysis. The means of accomplishing this removal remains ultrafiltration and the selecting of an appropriate dialysis solution Na$^+$ concentration. However, with the current designs of dialysis fluid delivery equipment it is increasingly possible to have both of these parameters change during the course of dialysis. This evolution in dialytic control makes it possible to investigate if variable, or even individualized, prescriptions for Na^+ and water removal may provide more optimal treatment.

Current understanding of water 'kinetics' as described above provides the basis for considering possible optimization of Na^+ and water removal. For balance over the treatment cycle the interdialytic Na^+ load should be removed during the subsequent treatment. The ultrafiltration rate, Q_F may be variable but the integrated product of ultrafiltration rate and dialysis time over the course of a treatment should equal the patient's interdialytic weight gain. Examination of Figure 34b and Equation [81] indicates that the dialysis fluid Na+ concentration required to produce a specific rate of change in the extracellular Na^+ is:

$$C_d = \frac{d(V_eC_{Na})/dt + [D(1 + Q_F/Q_B) + Q_F]C_{Na}}{D(1 + Q_F/Q_B)} . \quad [83]$$

It may be useful to select the desired value for $d(V_eC_{Na})/dt$ (either constant or variable) during the course of a treatment. An illustration of possible methods of removing accumulated Na^+ is shown in Figure 35. In each case the pre- and post-dialysis extracellular Na^+ content are the same, but the rate of change is different. The top line indicates the major decrease in Na+ content is toward the end of the treatment. This might be the case if there were concern that large urea flux combined with Na^+ removal would contract extracellular volume (V_e) too rapidly and Na^+ removal would be delayed until much of the urea load had been removed (see Figure 15 above). The lower line is the opposite case where there is accelerated removal of sodium early in dialysis. This case is more of a logical contrast to the previous case and may have limited clinical use because of the rapid decrease in extracellular volume that would be intuitively expected if this option were used. The intermediate (straight) line indicates a constant decrease in extracellular Na^+ during the treatment.

It should be noted that the term $d(V_eC_{Na})/dt$ indicates the slope of the line in Figure 35. For the straight line, where the slope is constant, this term will be constant and negative. For the upper line this term will change with time and will be increasingly negative during the treatment; for the bottom line this term will also be a function of time and will be increasingly positive (i.e., will be less negative) throughout the dialysis.

It should also be stressed that the relationships shown in Figure 35 do not directly show what is happening to either Na^+ concentration (C_{Na}) or extracellular volume (V_e) but their product. Consequently, the upper line could be produced by a rapid initial decrease in extracellular volume and a rise in sodium concentration as well as a relatively constant or increasing extracellular volume and more rapidly decreasing Na^+ concentrations. Consequently, a prescription of the Na^+ removal rate may also require some control of the rate of change of either extracellular

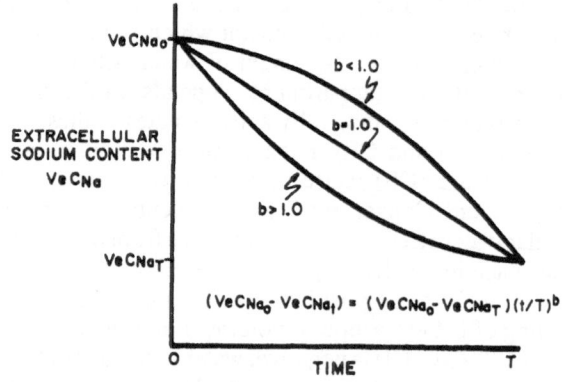

Figure 35. Possible means of decreasing extracellular sodium content during dialysis.

volume or Na^+ concentrations. In fact further investigation may indicate that either of these rates may be the parameter that should be controlled during dialysis rather than their product recognizing that

$$\frac{d(V_eC_{Na})}{dt} = V_e\left(\frac{dC_{Na}}{dt}\right) + C_{Na}\left(\frac{dV_e}{dt}\right).$$

Nonetheless, a prescriptive expression for curves such as those shown in Figure 35 can be expressed as:

$$\begin{bmatrix} \text{Total change} \\ \text{in sodium content} \\ \text{at any time} \end{bmatrix}$$

$$= \begin{bmatrix} \text{Total change in sodium} \\ \text{content during the} \\ \text{course of the treatment} \end{bmatrix} \left(\frac{t}{T}\right)^b$$

$$V_eC_{Na_o} - V_eC_{Na_t} = (V_eC_{Na_o} - V_eC_{Na_T})\left(\frac{t}{T}\right)^b$$

and

$$V_eC_{Na_t} = V_eC_{Na_o} - (V_eC_{Na_o} - V_eC_{Na_T})\left(\frac{t}{T}\right)^b .[84a]$$

Differentiation of Equation [84a] yields:

$$\frac{d(V_eC_{Na})}{dt} = -b(V_eC_{Na_o} - V_eC_{Na_T})\left(\frac{t}{T}\right)^{b-1} . \quad [84b]$$

Equation [84b] can be used to develop values for $d(V_eC_{Na})/dt$ in Equation [83] at specific times during the treatment. It is apparent that Equation [83] now defines the dialysate Na^+ concentration as a function of both C_{Na} and time and should be solved using general methods for nonlinear systems. These methods require that the terms in Equation [83], for example, be determined over very short intervals of time to produce new system values for recomputation. For example, in Equation [83] if intervals of a minute were chosen the value of $[D(1+Q_F/Q_B)+Q_F]C_{Na}$ would be computed using the initial value of C_{Na}. The value of $(d/V_eC_{Na})/dt$ would be computed from Equation [84b] at mid-interval (i.e., $t = 0.5$ min) and C_{DNa} could be computed for the first minute of dialysis. The value of V_e would then be computed from the multisystem model described above. This value would then be used in either Equations [81] and [82] to determine C_{Na} after one minute. This value would then be used to compute C_{dNa} during the second minute, etc.

It should be apparent from examination of Equations [80] to [82] that a substantial number of physiologic parameters must be estimated and historic data must be assumed to represent current patient values for implementation of the extracellular water model described above. These requirements may limit the clinical accuracy of the model and a clinical data base will be required to evaluate its precision in actual use.

Use of the extracellular water–sodium model to counter the intradialytic urea gradient

It should also be possible to use the above model to determine a dialysate Na_a^+ profile to counter balance the transcellular osmotic urea gradient $(C_iU - C_eU)$ with an osmotic cation gradient $(C_e - C_i)$ and thus prevent any water movement into cells during dialysis. This application may be particularly useful in dialysis of patients with acute renal failure or during the initial dialyses of patients with chronic renal failure and high BUNs.

The goal of this therapeutic maneuver is to determine the dialysate Na^+ profile, as defined by $d(V_eC_{Na})/dt$, to exactly counter the urea gradient in order to solve Equation [83] for the dialysate Na^+ concentration throughout the treatment.

The desired extracellular sodium profile will be:

$$\frac{dC_e}{dt} = \frac{dC_{Na}}{dt} = \frac{d(C_iU - C_eU)}{dt}$$
$$= \frac{dC_iU}{dt} - \frac{dC_eU}{dt}. \qquad [85]$$

The rate of change in extracellular Na^+ shown in Equation [83] can be described as:

$$\frac{d(V_eC_e)}{dt} = V_e\frac{dC_e}{dt} + C_e\frac{dV_e}{dt}.$$

If intracellular volume is to remain constant, ultrafiltration will be exclusively from the extracellular fluid (i.e., $V_e = V_{eo} - Q_Ft$) and:

$$\frac{d(V_eC_e)}{dt} = (V_{eo} - Q_Ft)\frac{dC_e}{dt} - C_eQ_F. \qquad [86]$$

Combining Equations [85] and [86]:

$$\frac{d(V_eC_{Na})}{dt}$$
$$= (V_{eo} - Q_Ft)\left(\frac{dC_iU}{dt} - \frac{dC_eU}{dt}\right) - C_{Na}Q_F. \quad [87a]$$

Because of the constraints of the treatment (i.e., holding intracellular volume constant) $d(C_iU)/dt$ and $d(C_eU)/dt$ can be determined by use of Equations [82a] and [82b]:

$$\frac{dC_iU}{dt} = -\frac{K_1}{V_i}(C_iU - C_eU) \qquad [87b]$$

and

$$\frac{dC_eU}{dt} = \frac{1}{V_{eo} - Q_Ft}[K_1(C_iU - C_eU)$$
$$+ G - K_D(1 - Q_F/Q_B)C_eU - K_RC_eU]. \qquad [87c]$$

Equation [87a] is used with Equation [83] as Equation [84b] was above over short intervals to compute the desired dialysis solution Na^+ concentration during dialysis. In this case the value of $d(V_eC_{Na})/dt$ is computed from Equation [87a] using Equations [87b] and [87c] to compute values for dC_iU/dt and dC_eU/dt. These expressions use values of C_eU and C_iU which are calculated from Equations [82a] and [82b] (adapted for urea).

The use of osmotically active solutes to counter urea disequilibrium

Another approach to balancing the urea gradient and associated water movement in acute or high BUN dialysis is to use an exogenous osmotically active solute such as mannitol. If the intracellular volume can be kept constant (as in the previous case) this case is computationally somewhat easier because Equation [82b] (adapted for mannitol, ie, $K_1 = 0$) can be solved in the same manner as the single pool variable volume urea model. If this is done, and the impact of renal excretion of mannitol during dialysis is considered negligible (i.e., $K_R = 0$) the expression for mannitol concentration at any time will be:

$$C_M = C_{Mo}\left(\frac{V_{eo} - Q_Ft}{V_{eo}}\right)^{K(1/Q_F-1/Q_B)}$$
$$+ \frac{I}{K(1 - Q_F/Q_B)}$$
$$\times \left[1 - \left(\frac{V_{eo} - Q_Ft}{V_{eo}}\right)^{K(1/Q_F-1/Q_B)}\right]. \qquad [88]$$

Equation [88] can then be rearranged to yield the infusion rate necessary to keep the mannitol at the desired concentration which in this case will be the difference between urea concentrations in the two modeled compartments $(C_iU - C_eU)$.

For intracellular volume to be constant Na^+ must be controlled to assure that there is no intercompartmental water movement due to unbalanced cation concentrations. If Na^+ is not controlled, the assumptions of $dV_i/dt = 0$ and $V_e = V_{eo} - Q_Ft$ may not be valid and mannitol concentration will not be an analytical function of time as shown in Equation [88]. If the volumes V_i and V_e are not controlled this system must be solved in the manner as the previous two cases – by step-wise calculations using small increments of time to determine the mannitol infusion rate with time.

If the assumptions of constant intracellular volume and ultrafiltration from the extracellular compartment alone are valid then this system of Equations may be solved analytically. That is, the concentrations in the extracellular and intercellular compartments (presuming that these coincide with the perfused and non-perfused compartments described above for urea) are distinct functions of time. Consequently, it is possible to describe the infusion rate of mannitol to counter this urea disequilibrium as an analytical function, ie, iterative methods should not be needed.

It should be noted that consistent with the discussion of modeling compartments above, it is important to appreciate that the models shown in Figure 34 may not be the same physiological spaces. That is, the 'non-perfused' urea compartment may not be coincident with the intracellular compartment. To the extent that this is the case the methods described to control urea induced water movement may be inexact. For example, the mean whole body K, of 760 ml/min may represent some combination of cell membrane resistance to urea transport and non-ideality of cell perfusion. In this case a therapeutically induced increase in osmotically active materials (i.e., Na^+ or mannitol) extracellularly could result in local regions of cell dehydration transiently.

The transcellular urea gradient and total osmolar drop in BUN have been discussed above and indicate that greater problems with urea induced water movement should be encountered at high urea removal rates. Reports to date have generally indicated less intradialytic morbidity with high flux dialysis times in the range of 2 h (175). However, these short treatment times have generally been accompanied by conversion from acetate to bicarbonate dialysis, the use of volumetric ultrafiltration control systems and more biocompatible membranes all of which very likely contributed heavily to decreased morbidity. There is still significant morbidity in the range of 10% with optimized high flux dialysis which could in part be due to the increased transcellular urea gradient.

Intradialytic morbidity studies using mannitol infusions have been designed to evaluate symptoms with infusion rates high enough to counterbalance the total osmolar drop in BUN during dialysis (176–178). These designs will result in infused mannitol doses that are four or five times those required to prevent cell swelling, and should cause cell dehydration, expansion of extracellular volume and high plasma mannitol levels at the end of dialysis. If the purpose of mannitol is to prevent osmotically driven cell swelling due to the transcellular urea gradient, much smaller infusions during the first half hour of dialysis adequate to counterbalance the transcellular urea osmotic gradient should be administered.

The computations described above to counter urea gradients with extracellular sodium were performed to cal-

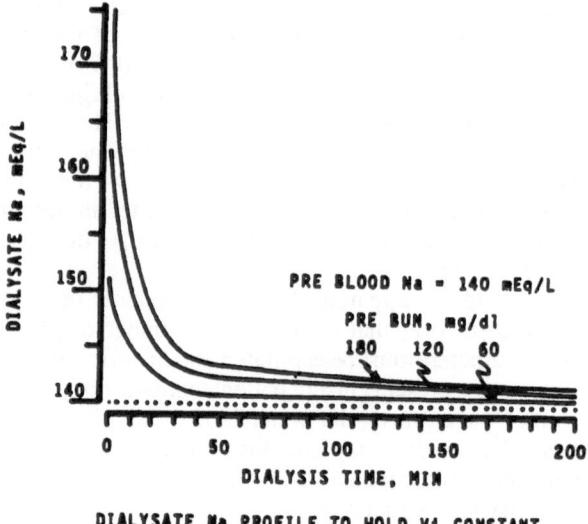

Figure 36.   Dialysate sodium concentration required during dialysis to counteract urea gradient.

culate the C_{DNa} profile which would be required to hold V_i constant with results shown in Figure 36. Average physiologic parameters were used and the rate of dialysis was such that t = 220 min for KT/V urea = 1.0. It can be seen that the initial C_{DNa} would have to be 10 to 35 mEq/l greater than CeNa. The profiles for high flux dialysis would be very similar since although the initial transcellular urea osmotic gradient is higher, the dialysance of Na^+ is much higher so the dialysate to blood Na^+ gradient would not he appreciably different.

The multisystems model for extracellular water shown in Figure 34, as with the body base model, is very flexible. It can be used to guide the ultrafiltration aspect of normal dialysis when deliberate removal of both water and Na is required, particularly in the presence of a possible urea gradient which can 'pull' water into cells. It can be used to guide a wider range of 'non-routine' treatments when efficient removal of water, electrolytes, and solutes are required, such as described as above. At this time the extent of application of this model has not been extensively evaluated. Nevertheless it has the potential for greatly enhanced control of dialysis treatment with the goal of reducing intradialytic patient morbidity.

The single pool interdialytic and double pool intradialytic models of Na^+, urea and water flux can be used to write dialysis prescriptions which will achieve targeted changes in Na^+ balance and intracellular and extracellular compartment volume during dialysis. At present there is not an adequate clinical data base to assess the utility of this model in reducing intradialytic morbidity in routine chronic dialysis.

We have had preliminary experience using the double pool Na^+ model to prescribe either a dialysate Na profile or a mannitol infusion to hold V_i constant during the initial dialyses in four patients with acute renal failure and pre-dialysis BUN ranging from 110 to 200 mg/dl. In each instance a full treatment was provided in the first dialysis of these patients resulting in a 60 to 70% drop in BUN over 3 to 4 h. The modeled therapy was highly successful in these patients who did not manifest dialysis disequilibrium.

Beta₂ microglobulin

Over the past several years evidence has accumulated linking beta₂ microglobulin (β_2m) to long term complications in dialysis patients (179, 180). The toxicity of β_2m results from its possible polymerization reactions which produce amyloid material (179–182) which preferentially deposits in synovia and bone (179) (where it may result in tumoral masses and pathological fractures) but also in skin (183) and many viscera (184).

The function of β_2m is not known. It is structurally associated with the general class of globulins involved with the immune system. However, little is known about this substance such as the regulation of its production and what may affect it; if it is a degradation product of some other process; or if it is a primary material produced to fill some, yet unknown, physiologic role.

Blood levels of β_2m are 20 to 50 times normal in dialysis patients. This has led to speculation that the rate of amyloid formation in these patients is in some way β_2m concentration dependent and that lowering blood levels through enhanced removal by dialysis might reduce amyloid formation.

It is reasonably well established that β_2m distributes as an unbound monomer (185) in two body water compartments, plasma (V_P) and interstitial fluid (V_{is}) (186, 187) as depicted in Figure 37a. As in other double pool models there will be concentration dependent transfer between compartments as described by a first order intercompartmental transfer coefficient (K_1).

Figure 34a shows generation of β_2m into V_{is} and removal from V_P primarily by renal clearance in normal subjects. It is not known if production of β_2m in a specific individual is constant or whether there is some degree of feedback control over its production or product inhibition. Other aspects of β_2m production will be discussed below.

The model indicates that removal (in the absence of dialysis) will be by renal clearance and metabolic routes (K_m and Γ). Monomeric β_2m is readily filtered at the glomerulus and reabsorbed into the proximal tubule where it is quantitatively catabolized (188). Thus plasma clearance is proportional to glomerular filtration rate (GFR).

The relationship between β_2m clearance and inulin clearance (K_1) has been studied by Vincent *et al.* (186) at low levels of renal function (inulin clearances from 0 to 10 ml/min). From these studies the clearance of β_2m appears to follow the relationship: $K_{\beta_2 m} = 0.6 K_i + 1.9$.

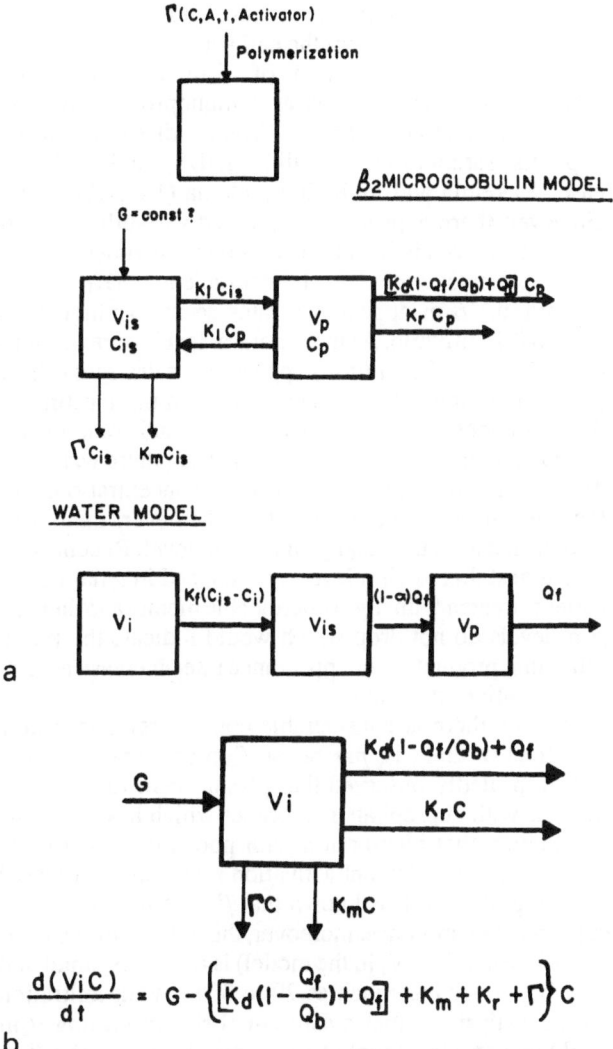

Figure 37. Model for beta-2 microglobulin and body water: (A) considering beta-2 microglobulin as distributed in two pools; (B) treating beta-2 microglobulin as distributed in a single pool.

This relationship would seem to indicate that renal clearance of β_2m is approximately 60% of GFR.

The above clearance relationship also indicates that there is some degree of β_2m catabolism or a metabolic clearance (K_m) which is approximately 2 ml/min. This term is shown in Figure 37a as β_2m removal from interstitial water at the rate of $K_m C$. The model also indicates the possibility of β_2m serving as a substrate for biochemical reactions such as the postulated polymerization to amyloid at a rate ΓC_{is}. If this reaction exists, its rate of reaction (expressed as a clearance, Γ) may be variable and may depend on other factors not shown in this strictly concentration model.

The turnover of β_2m on lymphocyte cell membranes has been studied in tissue culture and found to be quite variable with $T_{1/2}$ ranging from 1.5 to 11.7 h (189). A large portion of the turnover in these studies appears to be via shedding of β_2m from the cell surface.

Whole body production of β_2m is substantially increased in such diseases as lymphoproliferative diseases, rheumatoid arthritis, Crohn's disease, chronic hepatitis, sarcoidoses, vasculitis, AIDS, Hodgkin's disease, leukemia and multiple myeloma (185, 190, 191). However, there appears to be marked variability in β_2m appearance even in the absence of these disorders.

In patients with renal insufficiency ($K_{R\beta_2m}$ < 40 ml/min) β_2m appearance rates seem to range from 0.04 to 0.25 mg/min. At more normal levels of renal function ($K_{R\beta_2m}$ > 70 ml/min) appearance rates range from 0.12 to 0.25 mg/min. It is apparent from these estimates that β_2m appearance is highly variable and some degree of product inhibition may be present (i.e., there was some decrease in β_2m appearance at high concentrations and low clearances). This observation, however, cannot be established at a statistically significant level. Recent studies suggest that as β_2m levels are reduced in renal failure patients treated with highly permeable membrane therapy, β_2m levels do not drop which would indicate the possibility that production or appearance rates increase as β_2m concentrations decrease.

Finally, there is considerable controversy concerning the effect of dialysis, *per se*, on β_2m appearance. It has been repeatedly observed that plasma β_2m rises during dialysis with cuprophan membranes which has led to the speculation that membranes with poor biocompatibility resulting in complement activation may cause increased shedding of β_2m. It is known that β_2m is not cleared by cuprophan membranes, moreover, the volume of distribution for β_2m ($V_P + V_i$ in the model) is relatively small and may be reduced as much as 20 to 30% by ultrafiltration during dialysis so that a substantial rise in plasma β_2m could be expected simply from concentration of the β_2m present.

Bergstrom and co-workers (192) have reported that plasma β_2m is unchanged after cuprophan dialysis when the level is corrected for ultrafiltration. Shaldon *et al.* (193) reported that there is no change in plasma β_2m with sham dialysis but a substantial rise occurs with isovolemic dialysis with cuprophan. This has been interpreted to reflect increased cell shedding of β_2m due to cell swelling, resulting from the fall in osmolality because of urea removal. The effect of osmolality has been studied by Mahiout *et al.* (194) who correlated the change in plasma β_2m with change in plasma osmolality during dialysis with dialysate Na^+ of 140 and 155 mEq/l. However, it is very likely that this correlation is due entirely to large changes in extracellular fluid volume related to dialysate Na^+.

The model shown in Figure 37a ignores the role of biocompatability in β_2m appearance (if present) and shows β_2m addition to the interstitial compartment only. If blood-membrane interactions are important, an appearance term should also be associated with the plasma compartment.

The model shows dialytic removal of β_2m as described in Equation [14]. Cellulose and cellulose acetate membranes that have historically been used in chronic hemodialysis are virtually impermeable to β_2m. In this case Kd is zero, and this term drops out of the model. More recently, dialysis membranes of materials such as polysulfone and polyacrylonitrile have been developed that have increased permeability to materials in this size range.

The mass balance equation for the models shown are:

Beta-2 microglobulin model:

$$\frac{d(V_{is}C_{is})}{dt} = G - K_1(C_{is} - C_P) - K_M C_{is} - \Gamma C_{is} \quad [89a]$$

$$\frac{d(V_P C_P)}{dt} = K_1(C_{is} - C_P)$$
$$- \left[K_D \left(1 - \frac{Q_F}{Q_B} \right) + Q_F \right] C_P - K_R C_P. \quad [89b]$$

Water model:

$$\frac{dV_i}{dt} = -K_F(C_{is} - C_i) \quad [89c]$$

$$\frac{dV_{is}}{dt} = K_F(C_{is} - C_i) - (1 - a)Q_F \quad [89d]$$

$$\frac{dV_P}{dt} = (1 - a)Q_F - Q_F = -aQ_F. \quad [89e]$$

It should be apparent that some of the terms in the above relationships are unknown such as Γ. In addition, some may be variable and depend on factors other than concentration or time such as G and Γ. As such it will be difficult to solve these relationships in an unequivocal manner.

Consider initially the situation of steady state with traditional dialyzers. In this case β_2m dialyzer clearance can be considered negligible and $K_D = 0$. In the absence of kidney function Equation [89b] shows that β_2m content will remain reasonably stable in the plasma compartment with the concentration increasing as V_P decreases (due to ultrafiltration) and content will change somewhat if plasma volume changes cause differences in C_P and C_{is}. In fact, the plasma concentration will basically reflect what is occurring in the interstitial compartment.

If the system is truly in steady state (i.e., content of both compartments is not changing) then it is clear that β_2m appearance will be off-set by removal: $G = K_m C_{is} - \Gamma C_{is}$. If, as expected ΓC_{is} is very small with respect to $K_m C_{is}$ it can be neglected and: $C_{is} = G/K_m$. It is apparent from this steady state expression that with K_m being small and G varying considerably (0.04 to 0.24 mg/min) a wide range of C_{is} can be expected. The above relationship would predict C_P values ranging from 20 to 120 mg/l which, in fact, are seen in clinical reports. This wide range in C_P, however, may not be entirely due to variation in β_2m appearance since small variations in K_m would also result in wide dispersion of C_P steady state values.

Until recently, conventional dialyzers were virtually impermeable to substances of the size of β_2m (both diffusively and connectively). With newer membranes such as polyacrylonitrile and polysulfone it is now possible to achieve clearance for β_2m in the range of 40 to 90 ml/min and by using such devices it should be possible to lower concentrations of this material.

The impact of using dialyzers that are highly permeable to β_2m can be investigated using the model shown in Figure 37a and Equations [89a–89e]. For calculation purposes, the postulated conversion of β_2m to amyloid (ΓC_{is}) can be ignored because such a pathway (while important if present) is small from a mass flow standpoint. Consequently, this term can be dropped from Equation [89a]. Even with this simplification, solution of the equations shown should be used with caution. Much of the information shown in Figure 38a is based on estimates (V_P, V_{is}, K_1, K_m, a, etc). In addition, G may be variable and increase with β_2m removal.

Preliminary, unpublished studies suggest that despite high flux dialysis pre-dialysis β_2m concentrations are not reduced. The conclusion generally drawn from these observations is that as β_2m is removed with more permeable dialyzer membranes its appearance rate increases so that the original pre-dialyzer levels are restored. However, it must be pointed out that β_2m mass balance measurement has not been attempted in these studies and would be required to establish this conclusion. For example, the β_2m concentrations (both before and after dialysis) depend strongly on extracellular volume which may vary up to 30% and, if not accounted for, could result in considerable scatter in pre-dialysis concentrations. Further, the magnitude of removal has generally not been documented carefully. The large molecular mass of β_2m (12 kilodaltons) places this solute in the region where membrane permeability is decreasing rapidly as a function of molecular size. The variability in a commercial membrane permeability to β_2m *in vivo* has not been carefully studied nor has the effect of various cleaning agents on membrane β_2m permeability been studied. Consequently, the level of *in vivo* β_2m clearance provided may have been poorly controlled.

The solution of Equations [89a–89e] is complex, generally requiring a computer and iterative solution. An alternative approach is to simplify the model shown in Figure 37a (see Figure 37b) to a single pool model. As long as the dialyzer clearances remain at values approximately 0.5 K_1 or less the single pool model will reasonably estimate β_2m concentrations to be expected using dialytic and filtration therapy. Calculation using V_P/V_{is} of 3/121 and K_D of 90 ml/min (the highest clearance now available) indicate that calculated post-treatment concentrations are underestimated by approximately 20%. When clearance is 40 ml/min calculated post-treatment β_2m levels are underestimated by 5%.

The use of the models shown in Figure 37 (a and b) will be along the lines of other models such as the urea model: that is, to determine what β_2m concentrations will result from a given level of therapy; to estimate β_2m production rates; or to evaluate how much treatment (clearance and time) is needed for a specific patient to control β_2m levels.

At this time it is not known what adequate treatment is regarding β_2m. It should be remembered that its toxicity is inferred from the presence of identical material in excised amyloid for and the assumption that production of amyloid is caused by the higher than normal levels of β_2m present in dialysis patients. Although this is a reasonable hypothesis, the mechanism by which β_2m may result in amyloid production is not clear. Concentrations of β_2m are high shortly after the initiation of chronic hemodialysis (195) while amyloid formation, is either delayed almost a decade despite virtually constant β_2m concentrations or this length of time may be required to recognize its formation. There is some indirect evidence suggesting that aluminum may augment the rate of amyloid appearance since there is a correlation between excess body burden of aluminum and the clinical appearance of amyloid (179, 182, 191). Another mystery is why there is a predilection for amyloid deposition in synovia and bone and not other anatomical regions.

Kinetic consideration of uremic toxins

The concept of a uremic toxin is an old one. It is normal to consider that as other regulated substances accumulate in the absence of excretory capacity, so do certain substances that are systemic toxins. This concept is in part supported by the unresponsiveness of some lesions to the regulation of the commonly measured materials by dialysis. Toxic substances have been generally presumed to be certain peptides which are normally excreted. This presumption has been supported by detection of various substances in normal urine (196) which are found in uremic plasma but are absent in uremic urine (29, 31). Peptide production can be pictured by the hypothetical scheme shown in Figure 38.

In this scheme are shown a protein and substance γ; the protein is initially cleaved to A and B, and these two peptide fragments subsequently break down into various intermediate peptides until the final products G, H, I, and L result which are normally excreted in the urine. Substance γ is some other material that undergoes various metabolic steps which result in Z; Z may or may not be excreted by the kidney. It is only reasonable to presume in this scheme that the impaired removal of these hypothetical catabolic products will cause disruptions, perhaps toxic in nature. There has been the feeling that one or more of such substances are toxins and that their accumulation results in various uremic lesions (18, 33, 37, 38, 197).

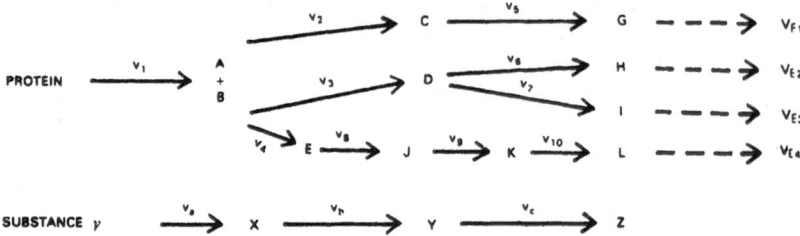

Figure 38. Hypothetical metabolic scheme involving catabolism of a protein and the biochemical pathways for some other substance γ.

This concept was pursued in the early 1970s by attempting to accelerate 'toxin' removal using different dialysis protocols (5, 198, 199), and more permeable dialysis membranes: in addition, certain quantifications and indices of therapy, partially based on these materials, were proposed (5, 37, 38). The rationale behind these studies was that the materials to be removed vary in size so that during dialysis they would be removed at different rates, the smaller ones being removed more rapidly than the larger ones (i.e., during dialysis the rates of elimination, V_{e1}, V_{e2}, V_{e3}, and V_{e4}, which might be similar in the natural organ, are different and depend on the size of the individual solute and the dialyzer characteristics). Consequently, the larger materials or 'middle molecules' (32, 197) would accumulate to a greater extent than the smaller catabolites and if toxic, would aggravate a given uremic lesion, the neurological system being one of the target areas (200).

In this regard, it has been suggested that the peritoneum is a far more permeable membrane than those used in hemodialyzers and that removal of 'middle molecules' is more efficient with peritoneal dialysis (5). Observation of patients undergoing this therapy supports this hypothesis by the less frequent occurrence of neuropath (201) a lesion thought to result from middle molecule accumulation (5, 21). More recent analysis of peritoneal dialysis questions this contention (202). Other analyses of patients undergoing peritoneal dialysis, however, suggests that there may be a lower rate of some catabolic reactions (protein catabolism and urea generation) than in hemodialysis patients (17), this would lower correspondingly the level of several of the hypothetical catabolic materials discussed above but because this is caused by lower overall catabolic rates some level of undernutrition should be expected in such cases.

Nevertheless the presence of several catabolic materials G, H, I and L in high concentrations and the possible toxicity of one or more of these substances is certainly valid. The analysis becomes immediately more complex, however, due to the size of the materials involved and the heterogeneity of the body. Kinetic analysis of such solute systems requires multicompartmental models in order that the levels of these unknown catabolites which will result from different types of dialysis therapy can be estimated

and the effects of different dialyzers and protocols can be evaluated.

The steps of model formulation are similar to those discussed above with the exception that it is now necessary to abandon the simplicity of a single well mixed system. Two basic models are shown in Figure 39 (a and b), the difference between the two being the site of solute generation. Figure 39a indicates that material is generated into the perfused pool which would be the case if the solute in question were produced in the liver so that it had to traverse the extracellular system to reach cells. Figure 39b represents the case where the material is produced in cells. In either case there is a resistance to movement between the two compartments. The transport constant in this case is the intercompartmental transport coefficient (K_1) which has units of flow. Note that the model shown in Figure 39a was used to model urea and is the same as that in Figures 14 and 34c.

These models have been discussed at length by others (22, 45) but it is instructive to consider briefly the basic differences between them. In 'case A' the peripheral pool acts as a capacitance, and the perfused compartment will go through large swings, the concentration being low immediately post-dialysis and building up to levels higher than the peripheral compartment as the interdialytic period progresses. There will be solute movement alternately out of and into the peripheral pool during the dialysis cycle.

In contrast, 'case B' shows that the peripheral pool connects the site of generation and the site of excretion. As such the peripheral pool concentration will be elevated, because it is only through a high concentration difference that material can be transported into the perfused pool. Ironically, in 'case B' the uremic levels are closer to normal (relatively) because the same transport situation exists in health, ie, large concentration gradients being required for transport out of cells. This may be seen more clearly if steady state mass balance is examined in the two pools of model 35b:

$$G = K_1(C_{C_{Ss}} - C_{B_{Ss}}) \qquad [90a]$$

$$K_1(C_{C_{Ss}} - C_{B_{Ss}}) = K_R C_{B_{Ss}}. \qquad [90b]$$

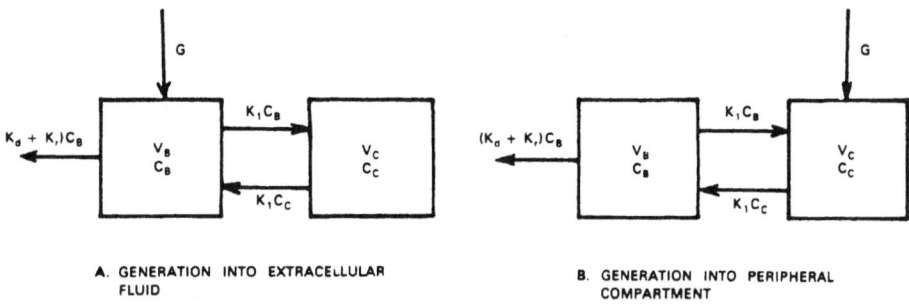

Figure 39. Two versions of a two compartment model for large molecular weight substances. Model a shows generation of material into the perfused (extracellular) compartment; model b shows generation into the peripherial (cellular) compartment.

Solution of these equations for the steady state concentration in pool C yields:

$$C_{S_{Ss}} = \frac{G}{K_R} 1 + \frac{K_R}{K_1}. \qquad [91]$$

Equation [91] shows that for peripheral generation the concentration will approach G/K_R when K_1 becomes large but will be higher with decreasing values of K_1 (eg, for $K_1 = 5$ ml/min and K_R (normal) of 125 ml/min, the K_R/K_1 term results in normal steady state concentrations in the peripheral pool 26 times G/K_R). Thus, a minimal toxic effect of decreased transport out of extracellular space with model 35b would be expected if the effecter site was situated in pool C because of the high normal levels in this pool.

In models such as Figures 39a and 39b mass balance expressions are written for each pool and the resulting differential equations are then solved simultaneously. Solutions for each of these cases are shown in the Appendix.

The case with metabolic interactions

The foregoing discussion of middle molecules in a multicompartmental setting is entirely hypothetical; such analyses point up the difficulties to be encountered when 'toxic' substances are not measured and their site of action is not known. In addition, the complexity of the kinetic system requiring knowledge of production rates and rates of transport between compartments coupled with the paucity of knowledge of these fundamental parameters makes this area of research a very demanding one.

Attempts to date to demonstrate a cause and effect relationship with respect to lowering levels of middle molecular weight toxins have been somewhat ambiguous (33, 203). There have been reports of improved blood pressure control (204) and decreased neuropathy (205) with similar high permeability protocols.

The two pool analysis of uremic toxins views the metabolic network shown in Figure 38 as a series of independent reactions that will depend on the removal rate alone for their level in the body. Reconsidering this fig-

ure shows that while this approach may be attractive, it is probably overly simplistic.

Consider the path for the protein to fragment B and the three pathways resulting in end products H, I, and L. If the clearances of L, H, and I are restricted, these substances will build up uniformly. However, if L is removed more rapidly than H and I, as would be the case during dialysis with urea (L) and large molecules, then the levels of H and I would be much higher relative to normal than the level of L would be; this interrelationship of catabolites has been the basis of the preceding discussion.

It is instructive, however, to consider the case where the paths are not independent. Let reaction V_4 be much faster than V_3 so that comparatively small amounts of H and I are formed with respect to L. At steady state, ie, with the natural kidney still functioning, V_4, V_8, V_9, V_{10} and V_{e4} will all be equal because none of the intermediates E, J, or K are accumulating. This will also be true of the chain of reactions resulting in H and I, ie, $V_3 = V_6 + V_7 = V_{e2} + V_{e3}$. In this system, the complete blockage of pathways V_6 and V_7 will not significantly increase production of E because the predominant reaction is already in this direction. Reduction of V_{e4}, however, would cause reaction V_{10}, V_9 and V_8 to slow which would increase B and the rates of reactions V_3, V_6, and V_7. If L is a common catabolite, such as urea, then its elevation in the steady state case would cause corresponding elevation of the levels of K, J, E, and B. Urea's immediate precursor, arginine, has, in fact, been shown to be higher than normal in uremic patients (206). In addition, if pathway V_3 existed, higher levels of D, H, and I would be expected. In fact, H and I would increase more than L even if they were cleared at the same rate because V_3 has been increased with respect to V_4. In the dialysis patient where V_{e2} and V_{e3} would possibly be less than V_{e4}, levels of H and I would be that much higher.

Up to this point, we have considered the ultimate products of these hypothetical biochemical reactions to be the potentially toxic materials. It is quite possible that intermediate substances C, D, E, J, or K might be metabolically active materials. As such, the elevated concentrations existing when the described pathways are blocked

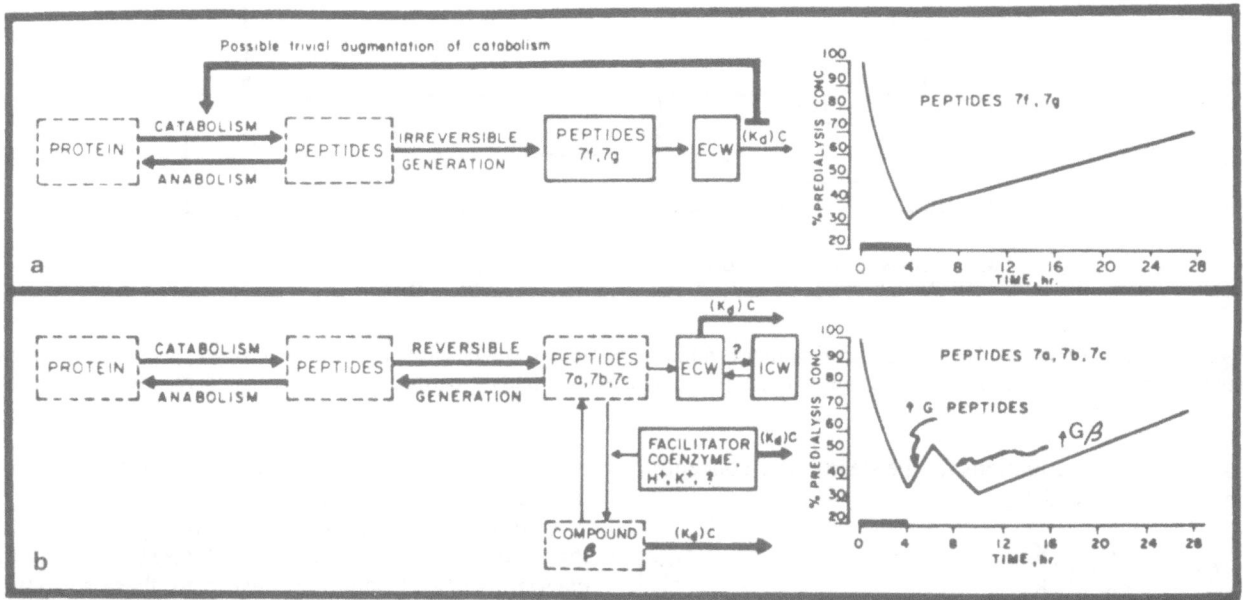

Figure 40.   Concentration/time behavior or two types of peptides reported by Asaba *et al.* (36) showing possible explanations for the kinetics of these materials. Reprinted by permission from 'Middle Molecules in Uremia and Other Diseases' (Supplement to Volume 4, *Artificial Organs*). Copyright ©1981 by the International Society for Artificial Organs.

might reach toxic levels, or one of these materials (D, for example) might inhibit reaction Vb in another metabolic pathway. This in turn might result in either toxic levels of X in the metabolic reaction series in which D does not itself participate, or the creation of some lesion because of the abnormally low levels of substance Z.

The above discussion has viewed the series of reactions with regard to what may occur at different steady state levels. In the dialysis patient, however, the levels of G, H, I and L will be continually changing, which will cause the levels of intermediates to change with lags appropriate to the kinetics of the individual reactions. This would then cause a system of metabolic perturbations to exist in the dialysis patient and would be a new syndrome not found in non-dialyzed patients and the perturbations themselves might cause toxic effects that would not be the result of any specific compound.

That the above discussion describes some catabolites is indicated by the kinetic behavior of various 'middle molecular' weight compounds (36) (see Figure 40). Two 'typical' curves shown in this figure demonstrate markedly different behavior. Figure 40a shows classical double pool behavior (39) for compounds 7f and 7g of Asaba *et al.* (36). The modest concentration rebound and short transient times indicate that there is only slight multipool behavior. The short rebound transient also indicates that K_1 values are probably large relative to the dialyzer clearance so that re-equilibration takes place rapidly. The behavior shown by these materials is not much different than that of urea, creatinine, or uric acid (39, 137, 138).

Figure 40b shows a totally different and confusing concentration pattern, particularly post-dialysis. It is clear from this curve, (which is a composite of peptides 7a, 7b, and 7c of Asaba and coworkers (36)), that both models shown in Figure 39 are inadequate. What is most disturbing about these compounds is the rapid rise post-treatment followed by a drop even below post-dialysis levels. The model in Figure 40b should be viewed as a specific but hypothetical example of the general diagram shown in Figure 38 and constructed to represent a possible explanation of the concentration behavior of the peptide shown.

Consider that these peptides are metabolic intermediates and are ultimately catabolized to compound beta. Both the peptides and beta are dialyzable and will accumulate in the uremic patient after dialysis. Further, the metabolic reaction of the peptide to beta requires a facilitator, co-enzyme, or cofactor (be it an electrolyte, optimal pH, etc). Consider what, under these specific conditions, would happen as a result of dialysis. During dialysis all of these materials – the peptide, the facilitator, and beta – decrease in concentration. Immediately at the end of treatment there is a marked increase in peptide levels both because of re-equilibration between intracellular and extracellular water and the increased production of this material from the precursor peptide. In addition, because the facilitator has been dialyzed to low concentrations, the degradation of 7a, b and c to beta is temporarily blocked. The combination of increased production of these peptides into a 'dead-ended' system will result in a rapid rise in their concentration post-dialysis.

The facilitator is gradually repleted post-dialysis to the point where the catabolism of the peptide to beta can proceed and there is a rapid decrease of peptide levels as beta (which was also removed during treatment) increases. Once this reaction scheme is back to 'normal' the concentration of the peptides gradually rises as levels of beta increase, dependent on the reaction constant for the peptide/beta reaction. Note also, that the final slope of peptide build-up is more gradual than that immediately post-dialysis because the same amount of peptide generation is both accumulating and supplying substrate for the 'beta' reaction.

This reaction scheme, while entirely hypothetical, is a possible explanation of curves such as the one shown in Figure 40b. Moreover, what this figure shows is not a traditional 'toxin' but a very labile compound which appears and is degraded by multiple pathways, and which depends on the level of reactants and products for its kinetic behavior, and which may require cofactors and certain optimum biochemical conditions for normal reactions to take place. In short, it is a typical biochemical compound in a uremic setting. Curves such as that in Figure 40b serve to remind us that uremia, particularly dialyzed uremia, where homeostasis no longer exists, is a very disruptive metabolic state. And it is very likely that there is a high degree of 'toxicity' associated with such metabolic chaos.

APPENDIX

Dialyzer transport measurements: the case with ultrafiltration

The use of recycle methods of dialyzer transport measurement were described above for the case where there is no ultrafiltration. When ultrafiltration is present ($Q_F \neq 0$) a solution different from Equations [30] results. Reconsider Equation [29] with the left hand side expanded:

$$V\frac{dC_B}{dt} + C_B\frac{dV}{dt} = D\left(1 - \frac{Q_F}{Q_B}\right)C_{Di}$$
$$- \left[D\left(1 - \frac{Q_F}{Q_B}\right) + Q_F\right]C_B. \quad [A1]$$

The size of the 'blood' reservoir volume as a function of time will be:

$$V = V_0 - Q_F t$$

and

$$\frac{dV}{dt} = -Q_F.$$

Substitution of these relationships into Equation [A1] rearrangement and solution yield:

$$C_{Bt} = C_{Di} + (C_{Bo} - C_{Di})$$
$$\times [(V_0 - Q_F t)/V_0]^{D(1/Q_F - 1/Q_B)}. \quad [A2]$$

Solving for D:

$$D = \frac{Q_F}{1 - Q_F/Q_B} \frac{\log(C_{Bt} - C_{Di})/(C_{Bo} - C_{Di})}{\log(V_0 - Q_F t)/(V_0)}. \quad [A3]$$

Appropriate reservoir sampling for equation variables will yield dialysance values (see text).

Average blood concentration during urine collection

Figure A1 shows that when concentration build up between dialyses is considered linear, it follows from the principle of similarities (207) that:

$$\frac{C_o - C_t}{\theta_t} = \frac{C_{01} - C_t}{\theta_1} = \frac{C_{02} - C_t}{\theta_2}.$$

The value of starting and ending collection concentration (C_{01} and C_{02}) will be:

$$C_{01} = C_t + (C_o - C_t)\frac{\theta_1}{\theta_2}$$

and

$$C_{02} = C_t + (C_o - C_t)\frac{\theta_2}{\theta_1}.$$

The average collection concentration will be the average of C_{01} and C_{02} or:

$$\bar{C}_B = C_t + \frac{(C_o - C_t)(\theta_1 + \theta_2)}{2\theta_1}. \quad [A4]$$

Two pool analysis of 'middle molecule' kinetics

The model in Figure 39 assumes distribution in two well mixed spaces: Compartment B, a perfused space and Compartment C, a non-perfused space. Between these two compartments there is transport by first order mechanism K_1. Two variations of the model are considered: (A) with generation into the perfused space and (B) with generation into the non-perfused space.

The removal of 'middle molecules' from the system is by first order elimination from compartment B by the dialyzer and natural organ if present. Note for simplicity both models assume constant pool volumes, ie,

$$\frac{dV_C}{d_c} = \frac{dV_B}{dc} = 0.$$

As has been discussed, this assumption is not entirely valid in dialysis where fluid volume increases between dialysis and where a major treatment consideration is its decrease during a treatment session. As was considered during the analysis of extracellular volume, the manner of changes in both C_B and C_C will depend on ultrafiltration rates and transport of osmotically active solutes.

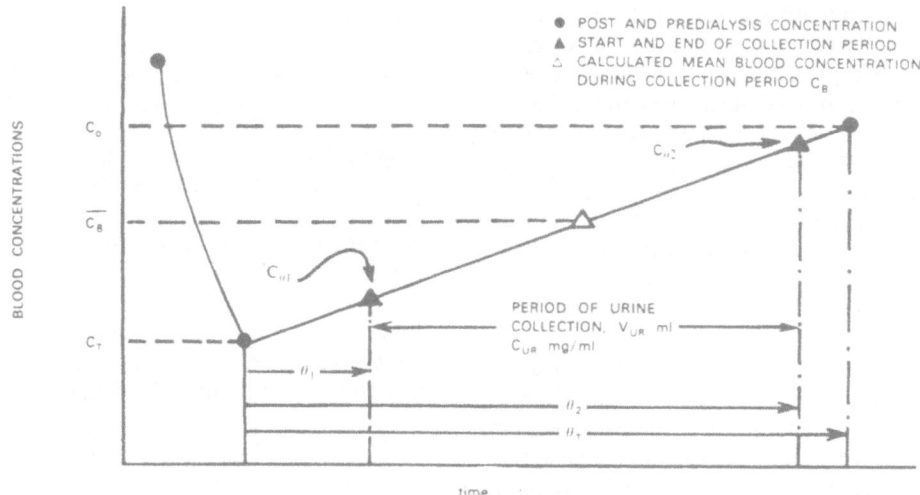

Figure A1. Blood concentration and time values post-dialysis required to calculate residual kidney clearance in the dialyzed patient.

However, it is felt that for general consideration of middle molecules assuming constant volumes will permit more useful mathematical expressions while not compromising the analysis significantly.

Model A represents the case where the solute is generated into the perfused space, for example if such substances were synthesized in the liver during protein catabolism. The defining equations for this model during all phases of dialysis are:

$$V_B \frac{dC_B}{dt} = G - K_1(C_B - C_C) - (K_R + K_D)C_B \quad [A5]$$

(compartment B)

$$V_C \frac{dC_C}{dt} = K_1(C_B - C_C) \quad [A6]$$

(compartment C).

The method of solution employed has been to put both Equations [A5] and [A6] into Laplace transform space and alternately solve them simultaneously for the transformed concentration in each space. These expressions are then easily inverted by standard techniques to yield (63, 64):

$$C_B = \left[\frac{C_{Co}K_1}{V_B} + \frac{C_{Bo}K_1}{V_C} + \frac{G}{V_B} \right.$$
$$\left. - \frac{GK_1}{V_B V_C} \frac{1}{\beta} - C_{Bo}\beta \right] \frac{e^{-\beta t}}{\alpha - \beta}$$
$$- \left[\frac{C_{Co}K_1}{V_B} + \frac{C_{Bo}K_1}{V_C} + \frac{G}{V_B} \right.$$
$$\left. - \frac{GK_1}{V_B V_C} \frac{1}{\alpha} - C_{Bo}\alpha \right] \frac{e^{-\alpha t}}{\alpha - \beta}$$
$$+ \frac{GK_1}{V_B V_C \alpha \beta} \quad [A7]$$

$$C_C = \left[\frac{C_{Bo}K_1}{V_C} + \frac{C_{Co}(K_1 + K_R + K_D)}{V_B} \right.$$
$$\left. - \frac{GK_1}{V_B V_C} \frac{1}{\beta} - C_{Co}\beta \right] \frac{e^{-\beta t}}{\alpha - \beta}$$
$$- \left[\frac{C_{Bo}K_1}{V_C} + \frac{C_{Co}(K_1 + K_R + K_D)}{V_B} \right.$$
$$\left. - \frac{GK_1}{V_B V_C} \frac{1}{\alpha} - C_{Co}\alpha \right] \frac{e^{-\alpha t}}{\alpha - \beta}$$
$$+ \frac{GK_1}{V_B V_C \alpha \beta} , \quad [A8]$$

where α and β are defined by:

$$\alpha \text{ and } \beta = \frac{1}{2} \left[\frac{K_1}{V_C} + \frac{K_1 + K_R + K_D}{V_B} \right.$$
$$\left. \pm \left[\frac{K_1}{V_C} + \left(\frac{K_1 + K_R + K_D}{V_B} \right)^2 - 4 \frac{K_1(K_R + K_D)}{V_B V_C} \right]^{1/2} \right.$$

Off dialysis these equations still hold except in the case of the anephric patient; this special case can be approximated by letting K_R approach zero (i.e., by letting K_R have a very small value). C_{Bo} and C_o will be the initial values for the particular interval being considered; pre-dialysis for the dialytic period, end-dialysis values for the period between treatments. Model B represents the case where the solute is generated into the peripheral space in a manner similar to creatinine. The defining equations for this model during all phases of dialysis are:

$$V_B \frac{dC_B}{dt} = -K_1(C_B - C_C) - (K_R + K_D)C_B \quad [A9]$$

$$V_C \frac{dC_C}{dt} = G + K_1(C_B - C_C). \qquad [A10]$$

The same solution method described above was used to solve Equations [A9] and [A10] and results in:

$$
\begin{aligned}
C_B = &\left[\frac{C_{Co}K_1}{V_B} + \frac{C_{Bo}K_1}{V_C}\right. \\
&\left. - \frac{GK_1}{V_B V_C}\frac{1}{\beta} - C_{Bo}\beta\right]\frac{e^{-\beta t}}{\alpha - \beta} \\
&- \left[\frac{C_{Co}K_1}{V_B} + \frac{C_{Bo}K_1}{V_C}\right. \\
&\left. - \frac{GK_1}{V_B V_C}\frac{1}{\alpha} - C_{Bo}\alpha\right]\frac{e^{-\alpha t}}{\alpha - \beta} \\
&+ \frac{GK_1}{V_B V_C \alpha\beta} \qquad [A11]
\end{aligned}
$$

$$
\begin{aligned}
C_C = &\left[\frac{C_{Bo}K_1}{V_C} + \frac{C_{Co}(K_1 + K_R + K_D)}{V_B} + \frac{G}{V_B}\right. \\
&\left. - \frac{G(K_1 + K_R + K_D)}{V_C V_B}\frac{1}{\beta} - C_{Co}\beta\right]\frac{e^{\beta t}}{\alpha - \beta} \\
&- \left[\frac{C_{Bo}K_1}{V_C} + \frac{C_{Co}(K_1 + K_R + K_D)}{V_B} + \frac{G}{V_B}\right. \\
&\left. - \frac{G(K_1 + K_R + K_D)}{V_C V_B}\frac{1}{\alpha} - C_{Co}\alpha\right]\frac{e^{-\alpha t}}{\alpha - \beta} \\
&+ \frac{G(K_1 + K_R + K_D)}{V_B V_C \alpha\beta}. \qquad [A12]
\end{aligned}
$$

The value of α and β will be the same for the two models. Inspection of Equations [A11] and [A12] shows that a steady state (i.e., $e^{-\alpha t}$ and $e^{-\beta t}$ equal zero) the concentration is represented by the constant term which is different for two compartments B and C. In the non-dialysis case, C_B will be less than C_C because the residual clearance, K_R, appears in the numerator of the constant term for Equation [A12] but not in the corresponding one in Equation [A11]. What is indicated is that in the normal patient where K_R may exceed 100 ml/min, there will be a profound intercompartmental concentration difference in the case of model B which was discussed previously.

Inorganic phosphorus balance in dialysis patients

A two pool model for analysis of inorganic phosphorus balance during dialysis is shown in Figure A2. Input is via dietary phosphorus intake, in the gut into the extracellular pool (V_e). There is phosphorus distribution into the intracellular pool (V_i) but this pool remains passive much as model A discussed above. Transfer between compartments is described by the intracompartmental transfer

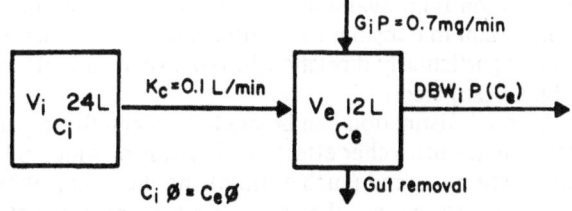

Figure A2. Model for phosphorus mass balance in dialyzed patients.

Table A1. Typical parameters for phosphorus model

V_i:	24 l
V_e:	12 l
K_C:	0.100 l/min
$G_I P$:	100 mg/day
$C_{Oi}P$:	5.0 mg/dl
$K_P A_i P$:	0.62 l/min
Q_B:	0.40 l/min
Q_D:	0.80 l/min
Q_F:	0.021 l/min
H_{ct}:	20 to 40%
gamma:	0

coefficient (K_C). Removal of phosphorus is by dialysis $D_{BWi}P$ (C_e) and gut removal using phosphorus binders.

Mass balance equations for the system shown in Figure A2 are:

$$\frac{d(V_i C_i)}{dt} = -K_C(C_i - C_c) \qquad [A13a]$$

$$
\begin{aligned}
\frac{d(V_e C_e)}{dt} = &-K_C(C_i - C_e) + G_i P \\
&- D_{BWi}P(C_e) - \text{gut}. \qquad [A13b]
\end{aligned}
$$

Solution of these relationships are analogous to those shown in Equations [A7] and [A8]. Using this model and the following system parameters phosphorus removal during 2 h, thrice weekly dialysis was computed (see Table A1).

Removal through the gut using phosphorus binders was computed as the difference in intake and removal during dialysis. The results of this dialysis have been discussed and are shown in Figure 6.

Mathematical concepts and relational analysis

Independent and dependent variables and linear regressions

Medical science and clinical practice are characterized by, among other things, the vast amounts of data and information both available and obtained for patients. It is important to consider such clinical data in a structured manner particularly if relationships between variables are to be investigated.

A broad distinction can be made between those parameters that cause other effects, or in terms of which other effects are measured (such as time) and the effects themselves. Those that are the cause or reference parameters are generally referred to as *independent variables* and their effects or results are *dependent variables*. Thus, as will be discussed below, when protein is catabolized, urea is generated. The protein being catabolized will cause the urea to be generated (not the other way around) so that the amount of protein being catabolized is considered to be the independent variable. The amount of urea produced is considered to be the dependent variable.

This independent/dependent variable relationship in many biological systems is linked. For example, protein catabolism will also produce acid (H^+), another dependent variable; the production of acid, however, will lower plasma bicarbonate concentration which will neutralize the generated acid and in this context H^+ generation will be an independent variable and HCO_3 will be a dependent variable. Bicarbonate will be an independent variable in the buffer reactions which will cause respiratory changes (as quantitatively described by the Henderson–Hasselbalch Equation). These examples of related physiological variables illustrate that the examination of clinical data can be much more meaningful when the concept of independent and dependent variables is kept in mind.

This is clearly the case when relationships and correlations between variables are investigated using linear analysis. Analysis for linear correlations is an attempt to obtain a direct relationship between two variables. Most commonly when such a relationship is found, the analysis is considered complete when in fact it has only begun.

This is the starting point for in depth analysis because a non-trivial relationship between variables allows a fundamental property of that variable system to be described in an unequivocal mathematical form of a straight line. In addition, analysis of composite data will often reveal a fundamental relationship that is more accurate than any of the points that make it up. An example of this is the determination of bicarbonate dialysance values from the slope of a plot of flux as a function of concentration driving force $J = f(C_{Bi} - C_{Di})$ rather than by direct computation using Equation [10] (10).

The relationship that results from a linear regression analysis is:

$$Y = aX + b. \tag{A14}$$

The presence of an expression, in this exact form, on a linear regression plot, ie, the use of y rather than the actual variables being related, however, belies a reluctance to take the next step. In addition, it should be noted that this general mathematical form indicates that the dependent variable should be plotted on the vertical axis (ordinate)

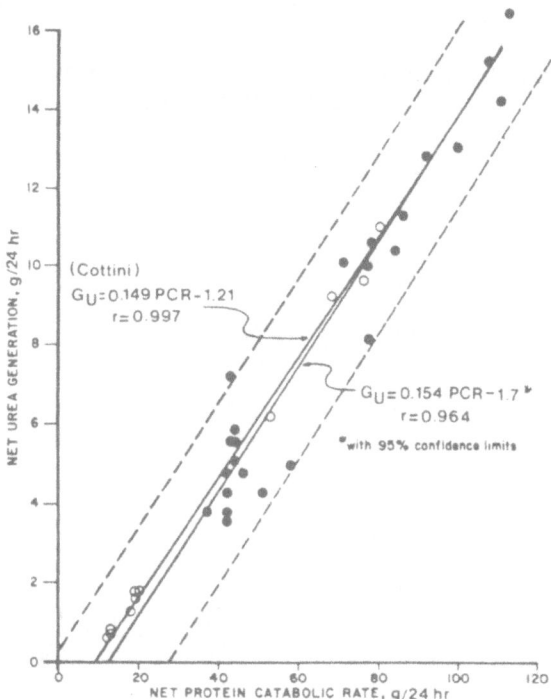

Figure A3. Relationship between net protein catabolic rate and net urea nitrogen generation in uremic subjects. Data shown are those from two populations: Cottini (197) and Borah (50). Reprinted by permission, *Dialysis & Transplantation* 10: 314, 1981.

as a function of the independent variable on the horizontal axis (abscissa) so that Equation [A13] shows what can be expected to happen to Y (a dependent variable) when X (an independent variable) changes.

Consider, for example, the data of Borah and colleagues (50, 51, 208) relating net urea generation rate and net rates of protein catabolism (see Figure A3) the dependent variable will be the net urea generation because it is caused by protein catabolism and oxidation of amino acids; the net rate of protein catabolism will be the independent variable. The linear regression is shown in Figure A3 and results in the relationship:

$$G = 0.154 PCR - 1.7 (not\ Y = (0.154X - 1.7). \tag{A15a}$$

This relationship can now be used in various ways. First, it can be used to estimate what the rate of urea generation will be at various levels of intake, eg, 400 g/day protein intake such as the patient of Richards and Brown (94). Second, it is important to consider the equation constants, specifically the coefficient of PCR and the intercept.

The slope indicates that for each 10 g of protein catabolized, 1.54 g of urea nitrogen will be generated. This is 96% of the nitrogen content of protein and indicates that there may be some other non-urea catabolites that will be produced in a linear manner when protein is catabolized.

A slight dependence of creatinine generation on protein generation has been found (209) and there may be other trace catabolites whose net production increases as the net amount of protein catabolism does.

The intercept (-1.7) should also be considered. There are two intercepts that should be evaluated (when G = 0 and when PCR = 0). When PCR = 0, ie, when there is no net catabolism, extrapolation of the relationship would indicate that there will be negative generation (or that urea will be consumed). Physically what this would mean is that urea would be consumed to produce the other nitrogen base materials that are produced and excreted at a fixed rate (see below). It appears that this conclusion is more a result of the mathematics than actual physiology, and would not be expected to occur under normal circumstances: the relationship will become discontinuous at some point before G = 0. In this context it is important to emphasize that one should be cautious in extrapolating relationships into domains outside the range of the data used. Extrapolation into ranges where discontinuity would be expected (very low levels of protein catabolism in the present case) should be attempted with caution. Evaluation of the PCR intercept (where G = 0) gives other information:

$$0 = 0.154PCR - 1.7$$
$$PCR = 1.7/0.154 = 11.014. \qquad [A15b]$$

The PCR intercept indicates that in the patients Borah and coworkers (50) studied there is an obligatory rate of catabolism (i.e., not linearly related to PCR) of 11 g/day. This obligatory catabolic rate includes creatinine production and nitrogen excretion in stool. If, as is likely, this rate of obligatory nitrogen loss is a function of body size then the Borah relationship can be generalized by adjusting this intercept value relative to body size by keeping the same slope, ie, the same linear relation of G to PCR. In this case when the intercept is scaled by the volume of total body water (in Borah's patients 37.6 liters) the relationship when solved for the PCR becomes

$$PCR = 6.49G + 0.294V \qquad [A16a]$$

or if G is in mg/min:

$$PCR = 9.35G + 0.294V. \qquad [A16b]$$

Graphically, this adaptation to body size shifts the G/PCR line to the left (for smaller individuals) and to the right (for larger ones) with the slope remaining the same. Such a modification has been shown to be valid for estimation of PCR in pediatric patients (81, 209). Similarly, if obligatory or fixed losses are known to be different, ie, as they would be in peritoneal dialysis, a similar shift in the relation of Figure A3 would be appropriate. Data from Blumenkrantz *et al.* (85) from CAPD patients shows such a shift, although the analysis did not follow the lines described above.

This example, while fundamental to the urea nitrogen discussion in this chapter, is meant to illustrate the logical progression and extensive use that can be made of linear relational analysis.

It is critical to add that if there is a linear relationship between variables, an extended evaluation of the elements of that relationship is important. If such analysis (examination of slopes and intercepts) does not result in useful information) then it is likely that the key, or fundamental, variables are not being related.

Therapeutic extension of clinical information through mathematical reduction or data

Nutritional management of acute dialysis

Linear reduction of data reduces clinical information to quantitative form, increasing its therapeutic use as has been discussed above. It can also extend these collective data to broader areas of therapy and treatment decision. The relation of net rates of catabolism as a function of energy and protein intake in the acute dialysis patient provides a pertinent example (51, 210, 211).

Often in the acute dialysis patient undergoing total parenteral nutrition a relation will exist between the rate of energy input to the patient and the net rate of protein catabolism (see Figure A4) (51, 251). Such relationships have been found by many investigators (213–217) and clinical observations are commonly made of negative nitrogen balance in patients with large energy demands that are not met, eg, protein-calorie malnutrition.

This clinical 'understanding' of the interaction of net protein catabolism and energy intake, however, can be further extended and made into a powerful therapeutic tool if it is reduced to quantitative form. The relationship shown in Figure A4 is a PCR-energy relationship for an acute dialysis patient receiving total parenteral nutrition (energy in the form of 70% dextrose). In this figure, energy is the independent variable because, as is shown, the change in the energy level is the factor influencing the net rate of protein catabolism. It should be noted that the metabolic interrelationships in the acute dialysis patient are clearly complex, but in terms of Figure A4 it is the change in energy that is shown to influence the PCR. For this particular patient during this specific illness the relation was:

$$PCR = 59 - 0.007 \, Kcal. \qquad [A17]$$

Equation [A17] indicates that for each 1000 Kcal (4,200 KJ) of additional dextrose energy given the PCR will be reduced by 7 g/day. When no exogenous dextrose is given the PCR will be 59 g/day. It should be stressed that Figure A4 is specific for the patient-illness for which it was determined. A different patient will have a different relation; moreover, the effect of dextrose input would be expected to be different for the same patient during another illness.

This expression which reduces the multiple PCR/energy observations to a mathematical relation can then be used

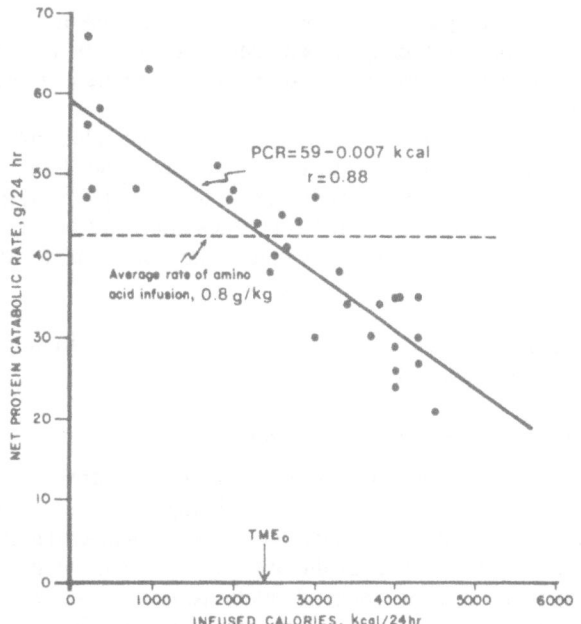

Figure A4. Net protein catabolic rate as a function of glucose calorie infusion in a 73 year old male with acute renal failure. PCR = 59 − 0.007 Kcal. Reprinted by permission, *Dialysis & Transplantation* 10(4): 314, 1981.

to determine the probable effect of giving more or less energy in the form of dextrose, much the way that the G/PCR relation (see Figure A3) was used to determine the effect of increased catabolism on BUN or to determine the PCR from computed G values. The analysis, however. should not stop here.

In addition to the problems of catabolite accumulation in acute dialysis patients, there is the problem of volume control. As more protein and dextrose are administered there is an obligatory addition of water. This added volume load using an energy 'stock solution' with C_e Kcal/ml 'energy concentration' and an amino acid stock solution of C_{aa} mg amino acids/ml, however, can be accurately estimated and can be shown to be:

$$V = \frac{PPI}{(1000 - E/C_e)C_{aa}} + V_a. \qquad [A18]$$

In this expression PPI is the 'effective parenteral protein intake' and V is the additional volume required to supply the desired electrolytes to the intravenous solution. For 70% dextrose monohydrate C_e will be 2.38 Kcal/ml; C_{aa} will be 0.085 g amino acids/ml for standard amino acid solutions.

The amount of protein administered for a specific energy input, E, and volume of solution, V, will be:

$$PPI = (1000 - E/C_e)C_{aa}(V - V_a). \qquad [A19]$$

For the degree of nitrogen balance PPI − PCR = dP/dt. Equations [A17] (in general form) and [A19] can be

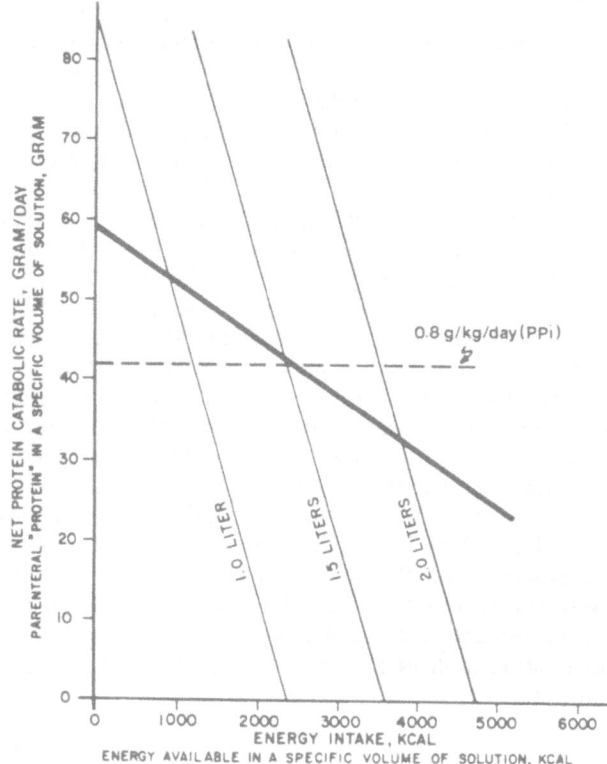

Figure A5. The energy-catabolism-volume relationships in the acute renal failure patient. Isovolumic lines for total volumes of 1, 1.5, and 2 liters are shown superimposed on the PCR/Energy relation of Figure A-3. The figure shows the nutritient constraints of parenteral fluid mixing as well as the therapeutic constraints of treating such a patient. Reprinted by permission, *Dialysis & Transplantation* 10(4): 314, 1981.

combined (see graphical representation Figure A5) to yield:

$$dP/dt = (1000 - E/C_e)C_{aa}(V - V_a) - (PCR_0 - bE). [A20]$$

In Equation [A20] PCR_0 is the PCR when no energy is given (the PCR intercept) and b is the slope of the PCR/E relation (see Figure A4). Equation [A20] presents the treatment/nutritional problem in unequivocal form. The three clinical factors that have to be considered, and how they interrelate, are shown:

1. dP/dt: The degree of protein balance (positive, negative, or zero)
2. E: The amount of energy to be administered.
3. V_f: The amount of fluid to be administered.

The choice of independent variable now rests with the physician. Volume may be controlling and dP/dt and E will then have to adjust to the need for control of fluid. Or the status of protein balance (dP/dt) may be the primary clinical consideration.

The effect of amino acid administration

It is common when a patient is found to be protein depleted or in negative nitrogen balance, to supply intravenous amino acids. The methods of prescribing amino acid administration and the degree of evaluation of this therapy has been found to be somewhat arbitrary (91).

Administration of amino acids will increase protein catabolism because on an intuitive basis it is highly unlikely that additional protein (irrespective of its 'quality') will be quantitatively anabolized. Consequently, it would be useful to evaluate PCR as a function of PPI. If this were done and the slope of this analysis proved equal to 1.0, one could conclude that the administration of amino acids was having little effect on the catabolic state of the patient. If, however, the slope was less than 1.0, this would indicate an anabolic effect and the magnitude of that effect could be determined.

It should be noted that energy and protein will have counteracting effects on PCR (energy lowers it, protein increases it). Consequently, the common practice of modifying nutritional support by increasing or decreasing the quantity of solutions (containing both energy and amino acids) administered, may show no effect on PCR (91).

Summary

The essential point to be drawn from the foregoing development is that there is information contained in clinical data that remains untapped, even when such information is analyzed by elegant statistical techniques. The need is generally not for more data or more sophisticated analysis: it is for a more structured analysis of the information available to provide greater understanding.

The initial step, as in the process of modeling, is a conceptual one: which variables are controlling (the independent variables), and which ones respond (the dependent variables). The independent-dependent variable statistical analysis will yield certain direct (or linear) relationships. The question must be asked: Do they make sense? An important means to answer this question is by examination of the slope and intercept values of the specific linear relationship. If these show physically or physiologically impossible situations there is reason to re-examine the original data. If these basic parameters seem devoid of any physical meaning it is likely that a different presentation of the data will yield more important information.

Finally, once a linear relation has been discovered and found to be relevant it represents a precise analytical and clinical tool. The tool should be examined, 'fashioned', and used to predict clinical behavior and estimate the magnitude of metabolic events. Such a tool, which represents the quantitative distillation of physiological properties and behavior in man, provides a unique means to use clinical information and an opportunity to greatly expand the domain of clinical investigation and medical understanding.

NOMENCLATURE

A Area: cm^2; dA: differential area

α Donnan factor; fraction of ultrafiltration from plasma volume

aH^+ Addition of H^+ to extracellular water from intracellular water; this term is the reverse of mH^+; mEq/min

b Exponent of expression for control of extracellular sodium content during dialysis

C Concentration; mg/ml, mEq/l; C_{aa}: amino acid concentration in stock solution for parenteral nutrition; C_B: blood concentration; C_C: concentration in pool C in a two pool model; $\boxed{}$: concentration of gaseous CO_2; C_D: dialysate concentration; C_e: energy concentration of glucose stock solution for parenteral nutrition; C_F: concentration in hemofiltrate; C_O: initial concentration – pre-dialysis; C_t: end-dialysis concentration; C_{UR}: urine concentration: C_{SS}, $\boxed{}$, $\boxed{}$: steady state concentration; C_{01}, C_{02}, C_0 for two sequential dialyses; C_{Bi}, C_{Di}: inlet concentrations; C_{Na}: sodium concentration; C_P: plasma concentrations – C_{Po}, C_{PT}, and $\boxed{}$ C_{Pss} represent initial, end dialysis, and steady state values; C_{PR}: concentration of proteins in plasma $\bar{C}_B$: mean concentration: ΔC: concentration difference in flux expressions dc/dx: change of concentration with distance indicates a concentration gradient $\Delta c / \Delta x$: gradient over the fixed distance Δx: C(Log-mean): concentration driving force in a dialyzer; dC/dt: time rate of change in concentration C_+ total osmotically active caption, $Na_{ex} + K_{ex}$; mEq

D Diffusive dialysance; ml/min, l/min, D': apparent dialysance initial, end dialysis, and steady state values; C_{PR}: concentration of proteins in plasma

d ( )/dt Rate of change of ( ) with respect to time

D $\boxed{}$ Diffusivity, cm^2/sec: **Db**: diffusivity in blood; **Dd**: diffusivity in dialysate; **Dm**: diffusivity in the membrane; **Dm***: effective diffusivity in the membrane:

E Zero order enzymatic conversion rate of acetate to acetyl-C_oA: mEq/min; glucose energy infused as part of parenteral nutrition: Kcal

F Fraction; F_F: filtration fraction in hemofiltration; F_P: water fraction in plasma; F_R: water fraction of the red cell

G Generation rate: mg/min, mM/min, mEq/min; in the case of urea G: the net rate of urea nitrogen generation from net protein catabolism; g_{H+}: rate of hydrogen ion production

Γ Rate of beta-2 microglobulin removal from interstitial water to form amyloid, expressed as a clearance, ml/min

HCT hematocrit, per cent

Ir Infusion rate of heparin: units/h

J Flux; mass/time, mg/min, mEq/min; J_{ac}: flux of acetate into a patient: J_{H+Exc}: flux of H^+ out of patient by renal excretion; J_{HCO_3}: flux of bicarbonate out of patient; J_{OA}: flux of organic anions

K   Diffusive clearance or transport constant; K_o: overall mass transfer coefficient, cm/min; K: clearance, ml/min, l/min; K_B: clearance based on blood side flux; K_D: clearance based on dialysate side flux; K_L: lung clearance (of CO_2); K_{Ln}: normal lung clearance: K_R: Residual renal clearance; K': apparent clearance; K_1: intercompartmental transport coefficient in a two pool model; K_{UF}: ultrafiltration coefficient, ml/min/mmHg

k   Solute distribution coefficient

K_{ex} Total exchangeable potassium: mEq

mH^+ Mobilization of H^+ out of extracellular water into other buffers: mEq/min

Na_{ex} Total exchangeable sodium: mEq

P   Pressure: mmHg; P_b: blood side pressure; P_d: dialysate side pressure; P: average pressure

P   Tissue protein content of the body: g; dP/dt: rate of change of tissue protein content with time–protein balance

PCR   Net rate of protein catabolism: g/day; PCR: net rate of protein catabolism relative to normal body weight

PPI   Parenteral protein intake; g/day

Q   Flow rate; ml/min, l/min: Q_B: blood flow; Q_D: dialysate flow; Q_E: effective blood water flow rate: Q_F ultrafiltrate flow; Q_F: ultrafiltration rate; Q_{Bi}, Q_{Di}: inlet flow rates to the dialyzer; Q_S: rate of addition of substitution fluid in hemofiltration

R   Mass transfer resistance, min/cm; R_B: mass transfer resistance in blood phase; R_D: mass transfer resistance in dialysate phase; R_m: mass transfer resistance in the membrane; R_o: overall mass transfer resistance

R   Response of body clotting mechanism to a heparin load; prolongation of clotting time: sec; R_i: R at the start of an interval; R_o: initial value of R – baseline value; R_t: R at the end of an interval

S   Sensitivity of an individual to heparin: response/unit; see clotting prolongation/unit of heparin

T(t)   Time: minutes; t_d: duration of dialysis; T_{ur}: length of a urine collection

V   Volume: ml, l; volume of distribution of specific species; volume of parenteral solutions given to a patient; V_a: volume of electrolytes added to parenteral solutions; V_B: volume of compartment b in a two pool model; V_C: volume of compartment c in a two compartment model; V_{ecf}: volume of extracellular fluid; V_f: amount of fluid to be administered to the patient receiving total parenteral nutrition; V_L: interdialytic volume loading; V_R: intradialytic volume removal; V_0: initial volume; V_{ur}: volume of a urine collection; dV/dt: time rate of change in volume

X(x)   Distance, cm; dx: differential distance; Δx: diffusion distance; ΔB: thickness of blood film; Δx_D: thickness of dialysate film; Δx_M: membrane thickness

α, β Exponent in two pool analysis, min^{-1}

β Rate of weight gain: g/min, kg/day

θ Interdialytic interval; min

REFERENCES

1. Michaels AS: Operating parameters and performance criteria for hemodialyzers and other membrane-separation devices. *Trans Am Soc Artif Intern Organs* 12: 387, 1966

2. Gotch FA, Autian J, Colton CK, Ginn HE, Lipps BJ, Lowrie EG: *The Evaluation of Hemodialyzers*, DHEW Publication No (NIH) 72–103, 1971–1972

3. Klein E, Autian J, Bower ID, Buffaloe G, Centella L, Colton CK, Darby TD, Farrell PC, Holland FF, Kennedy RS, Lipps B Jr, Mason R, Nolph KD, Villarroel F, Wathen RL: *Evaluation of Hemodialyzers and Dialysis Membranes.* DHEW Publication No (NIH) 77–1294, 1977

4. Guyton AC: *Textbook of Medical Physiology*, 6th Edition, Philadelphia, WB Saunders, 1981, p 208

5. Babb AL, Popovich RP, Christopher TG, Scribner BH: The genesis of the square meter-hour hypothesis. *Trans Am Soc Artif Intern Organs* 17: 81, 1971

6. Klein E: Membranes and materials evaluation. in *Proc 7th Annu Contractors's Conf Artif Kidney-Chronic Uremia Program NIAMDD*, edited by Krueger KK, DHEW Publ No (NIH), Vol 85, 1974, 75–248

7. Gotch FA, Sargent JA, Keen ML, Seid MA, Foster R: Comparative treatment time with Kiil, Gambro and Cordis-Dow Kidneys. *Proc Clin Dial Transplant Forum* 3: 217, 1973

8. Comroe JH: *Physiology of Respiration*, 2nd Edition, Chicago, Year Book Medical Publishers, 1975, p 60

9. Pitts RF: *Physiology of the Kidney and Body Fluids*, 2nd Edition, Chicago, Year Book Medical Publishers, 1968, p 29

10. Sargent JA, Gotch FA: Bicarbonate and carbon dioxide transport during dialysis therapy. *ASAIO J* 2: 61, 1979

11. Farrell PC, Grib NL, Fry DL, Popovich RP, Broviac JW, Babb AL: A comparison of *in vitro* and *in vivo* solutes-protein binding interactions in normal and uremic subjects. *Trans Am Soc Artif Intern organs* 18: 268, 1972

12. Wolf AV, Remp DG, Killey JE, Currie GD: Artificial kidney function: kinetics of hemodialysis. *J Clin Invest* 30: 1062, 1951

13. Smith HW: *The Kidney: Structure and Function in Health and Disease*, New York, Oxford University Press, 1951, p 39

14. Gotch FA: Hemodialysis: Technique and kinetic considerations. in *The Kidney*, edited by Brenner BM, Rector FC Jr, Philadelphia, WB Saunders Company, 1976, p 1673

15. Eschbach JW, Egrie JC, Downing MR, Browne JK, Adamson JW: Correction of the anemia of end-stage renal disease with recombinant human erythropoietin: results of a combined phase I and phase II clinical trial. *N Eng J Med* 316: 73, 1987

16. Erslev A: Erythropoietin coming of age. *N Eng J Med* 316: 1987

17. Nolph KD, Nothum RJ, Maher JF: Effects of ultrafiltration on dialysance in commercially available coils. *Kidney Int* 2: 293, 1972

18. Nolph KD, Nothum RJ, Maher JF: Ultrafiltration: A mechanism for removal of intermediate molecular weight substances in coil dialyzers. *Kidney Int* 6: 55, 1974

19. Farrell PC, Babb AL: Estimation of the permeability of cellulosic membranes from solute dimensions and diffusivities. *J Biomed Mater Res* 7: 25, 1973

20. Bottomley S, Parsons FM, Broughton PMG: The dialysis of non-electrolytes through regenerated cellulose (Cuprophane). I. The effect of molecular size. *J Appl Polym Sci* 16: 2115, 1972

21. Babb AL, Farrell PC, Uvelli DA, Scribner BH: Hemodialyzer evaluation by examination of solute molecular spectra. *Trans Am Soc Artif Intern Organs* 18: 98, 1972

22. Popovich RP, Hlavinka DO, Bomar JB, Monerief JW, Dechard IF: The consequences of physiological resistances on metabolic removal from the patient-artificial kidney system. *Trans Am Soc Artif Intern Organs* 21: 108, 1975

23. French D: The Schardinger dextrins. *Adv Carbohydrate Chem* 12: 189,1957

24. Schreiner GE: The search for the uremic toxin(s). *Kidney Int* 7 (Suppl 3): S270, 1975

25. Horowitz HI: Uremic toxins and platelet function. *Arch Intern Med* 127: 823, 1970

26. Cohen BD: Guanidinosuccinic acid in uremia. *Arch Intern Med* 126: 846, 1970

27. Giovannetti S, Biagini M, Cioni L: Evidence that methyl guanidine is retained in chronic renal failure. *Experientia* 24: 341, 1968

28. Schmidt EG, McElvian NS, Bowen JJ: Plasma amino acids and the ether soluble phenols in uremia. *Am J Clin Path* 20: 253, 1950

29. Gordon A, Bergstrom J, Furst P, Zimmerman L: Separation and characterization of uremic metabolites in biologic fluids. A screening approach to the definition of uremic toxins. *Kidney Int* 7 (Suppl 3): S45, 1975

30. Giovanetti S, Barsotti G: Dialysis of methylguanidine. *Kidney Int* 6: 177, 1974

31. Furst P, Bergstrom J, Gordon A, Johnsson E, Zimmerman L: Separation of peptides of 'middle' molecular weight from biological fluids of patients with uremia. *Kidney Int* 7 (Suppl 3): S272, 1975

32. Funck-Brentano J, Man NK, Sausse A. Zingraff J, Boudet J, Becker A, Cueiile GF: Characterization of a 1100–1300 MW uremic neurotoxin. *Trans Am Soc Artif Intern Organs* 22: 163, 1976

33. Bergstrom J, Furst P, Zimmerman L: Uremic middle molecules exist and are biologically active. *Clin Nephrol* 11: 229, 1979

34. Bergstrom J, Furst P: Uremic toxins. *Kidney Int* 12 (Suppl 8): S9, 1978

35. Asaba H, Bergstrom J, Furst P, Oules R, Zimmerman L: Accumulation and excretion of middle molecules. *Proc Eur Dial Transplant Assoc* 13: 481, 1976

36. Asaba H, Furst P, Oules R, Ward M, Yahiel V, Zimmerman L, Bergstrom J: The effect of hemodialysis on endogenous middle molecules in uremic patients. *Clin Nephrol* 11: 257, 1979

37. Babb AL, Strand MJ, Uvelli DA, Milutinovic J, Scribner BH: Quantitative description of dialysis treatment: a dialysis index. *Kidney Int* 7 (Suppl 2): S23, 1975

38. Babb AL, Strand MJ, Uvelli DA, Scribner BH: The dialysis index: a practical guide to dialysis treatment. *Dial Transplant* 6: 9, 1977

39. Bell RL, Curtis FK, Babb AL: Analog simulation of the patient-artificial kidney system. *Trans Am Soc Artif Intern Organs* 11: 183, 1965

40. King PH, Baker WR, Ginn HE, Frost AB: Computer optimization of hemodialysis. *Trans Am Soc Artif Intern Organs* 14: 389, 1968

41. Dedrick RL: Pharmacodynamic considerations for chronic hemodialysis. *Kidney Int* 7 (Suppl 2): S7, 1975

42. Sargent JA, Gotch FA: The analysis of concentration dependence of uremic lesions in clinical studies. *Kidney Int* 7 (Suppl 2): S35, 1975

43. Gotch FA, Sargent JA, Keen ML, Lee M: Individualized quantified dialysis therapy of uremia. *Proc Clin Dial Transplant Forum* 4: 27, 1974

44. Gotch FA, Farrell PC, Sargent JA: Theoretical considerations of molecular transport in dialysis and sorbent therapy for uremia. *J Dial* 1: 105, 1976

45. Frost TH, Kerr DNS: Kinetics of hemodialysis: A theoretical study of the removal of solutes in chronic renal failure compared to normal health. *Kidney Int* 12: 41, 1977

46. Sargent JA: Kinetic modeling in the guidance of dialysis therapy. *Dial Transplant* 8: 1101, 1979

47. Sargent JA, Gotch FA: Mathematical modeling of dialysis therapy. *Kidney Int* 18 (Suppl 10): S2, 1980

48. Sargent JA: Which mathematical model to guide clinical dialysis? in *Uremia-Pathobiology of Patients Treated for Ten Years or More*, edited by Giordano C, Friedman EA, Milan, Wichtig Editore, 1980, p 209, Milano

49. Sargent JA, Lowrie EG: Which mathematical model to study uremic toxicity? *Clin Nephrol* 17: 303, 1982

50. Borah MF, Schoenfeld PY, Gotch FA, Sargent JA, Wolfson M, Humphreys MH: Nitrogen balance during intermittent dialysis therapy of uremia. *Kidney Int* 14: 491, 1978

51. Sargent JA, Gotch FA, Borah M, Piercy L, Spinozzi N, Schoenfeld P, Humphreys M: Urea kinetics: a guide to nutritional management of renal failure. *Am J Clin Nutr* 31: 1696, 1978

52. Cogan MG, Sargent JA, Yarbrough SG, Vincenti F, Amend WJ: Prevention of prednisone-induced negative nitrogen balance. *Ann Intern Med* 95: 158, 1981

53. Gotch FA, Sargent JA, Keen ML, Lam M, Prowitt M, Grady M: Clinical results of intermittent dialysis therapy (IDT) guided by ongoing kinetic analysis or urea metabolism. *Trans Am Soc Artif Intern Organs* 22: 175, 1976

54. Sargent JA: Urea kinetics: A quantitative guide to nutrition and treatment in renal disease. *Dial Transplant* 10: 275, 1981

55. Sargent JA: The role of acetate in acid base corrections during hemodialysis treatment, Doctoral dissertation, University of California, Berkeley, 1976

56. Gotch FA, Keen ML: Precise control of minimal heparinization for high bleeding risk hemodialysis. *Trans Am Soc Artif Intern Organs* 23: 168, 1977

57. Sherlock JE, Yoon Y, Ledwith JW, Letteri JM: Respiratory gas exchange during hemodialysis. *Proc Clin Dial Transplant Forum* 2: 171, 1972

58. Sherlock JE, Ledwith JW, Letteri JM: Hypoventilation and hypoxemia during hemodialysis: reflex response to removal of CO_2 across the dialyzer. *Trans Am Soc Artif Intern Organs* 23: 406, 1977

59. Aurigemma NM, Feldman NT, Gottlieb M, Ingram RH, Lazarus JM, Lowrie EG: Arterial oxygenation during hemodialysis. *N Engl J Med* 297: 871, 1977

60. Tolchin N, Rogers JL, Hayashi J, Lewis EJ: Metabolic consequences of high mass-transfer hemodialysis. *Kidney Int* 11: 366, 1977

61. Tolchin N, Roberts JL, Lewis EJ: Respiratory gas exchange by high efficiency hemodialysis. *Nephron* 21: 137, 1978

62. Guyton AC: *Textbook of Medical Physiology*, 6th Edition, Philadelphia, WB Saunders, 1981, p 518

63. Kreyszig E: *Advanced Engineering Mathematics*, New York, John Wiley and Sons, 1972, p 24, 147

64. Sokolnikoff IS, Redheffer RM: *Mathematics of Physics and Modern Engineering*, New York, McGraw Hill, 1958, p 23, 756

65. Giovanetti S, Maggiore Q: A low nitrogen diet with proteins of high biological value for severe chronic uremia. *Lancet* 1: 1000, 1964

66. Shaw AB, Bazzard FJ, Booth EM, Nilwarangkur S, Berlyne GM: The treatment of chronic renal failure by modified Giovannetti diet. *Q J Med* 34: 237, 1965

67. Kerr DNR, Robson A, Elliott RW, Ashcroft R: Diet in chronic renal failure. *Proc Roy Soc Med* 60: 115, 1967

68. Franklin SS, Gordon A, Kleeman CR, Maxwell MH: Use of a balanced low-protein diet in chronic renal failure. *JAMA* 202: 477, 1967

69. Kopple JD, Sorensen MK, Coburn JW, Gordon A, Rubini ME: Controlled comparison of 20 g and 40 g protein diets in the treatment of chronic uremia. *Am J Clin Nutr* 21: 553, 1968

70. Hewlett AW, Gilbert QO, Wickett AD: The toxic effects of urea on normal individuals. *Arch Intern Med* 18: 636, 1916

71. Grollman EF, Grollman A: Toxicity of urea and its role in the pathogenesis of uremia. *J Clin Invest* 38: 749, 1959

72. Cohen BD, Handelsman DG, Narayan Pai B: Toxicity arising from the urea cycle. *Kidney Int* 7 (Suppl 3): S285, 1975

73. Johnson WJ, Hagge WW, Wagoner RD, Dinapoli RP, Rosevear JW: Toxicity arising from urea. *Kidney Int* 7 (Suppl 3): S288, 1975

74. Lowrie EG, Laird NM, Parker TF, Sargent JA: Effect of the Hemodialysis prescription on patient morbidity: report from the national cooperative dialysis study. *N Engl J Med* 305: 1176, 1981

75. Luke RG: Uremia and the BUN. *N Engl J Med* 305: 1213, 1981

76. Lowrie EG, Laird NM, Henry RP: Protocol for the national cooperative dialysis study. *Kidney Int* 23 (Suppl 13): S11, 1983

77. Laird NM, Berry CS, Lowrie EG: Modeling success or failure of dialysis therapy: the national cooperative dialysis study. *Kidney Int* 23 (Suppl 13): S101, 1983

78. Gotch FA, Sargent JA: A Mechanistic analysis of the national cooperative dialysis study (NCDS). *Kidney Int* 28: 526, 1985

79. Steffenson KA: Some determinations of the total body water in man by means of intravenous injections of urea. *Acta Physiol Scand* 13: 282, 1947

80. Lehnnger AL: *Biochemistry*, New York, Worth Publishers, 1970, p 433

81. Sargent JA, Gotch FA: Is urea generation adaptive? *Controv Nephrol* 1: 451, 1979

82. Walser M, Bodenlos LJ: Urea metabolism in man. *J Clin Invest* 38: 1617, 1959

83. Wolpert E, Phillips SF, Summerskill WHJ: Transport or urea and ammonia production in the human colon. *Lancet* 2: 1387, 1971

84. Richards P, Brown CL: Urea metabolism in an azotemic woman with normal renal function. *Lancet* 2: 207, 1975

85. Blumenkrantz MJ, Kopple JD, Moran JK, Grodstein GP, Coburn JW: Nitrogen and urea metabolism during continuous ambulatory peritoneal dialysis. *Kidney Int* 20: 78, 1981

86. Berlyne GM, Shaw AB, Nilwaramgkur S: Dietary treatment of chronic renal failure. Experience with a modified Giovanetti diet. *Nephron* 2: 129, 1965

87. Walser M: The conservative management of the uremic patient. in *The Kidney*, edited by Brenner BM, Rector FC, Philadelphia, WB Saunders Co, 1976, p 1613

88. Bennett N: Urea kinetics: A dietitian's clinical tool in the nutritional management of patients with end stage renal disease. *Dial Transplant* 10: 332, 1981

89. Forbes G, Bruining GJ: Urinary creatinine excretion and lean body mass. *Am J Clin Nutr* 29: 1359, 1976

90. Sargent JA, Gotch FA: Mass balance: A quantitative guide to clinical nutritional therapy I: the predialysis renal disease patient. *J Am Dietetic Assoc* 75, 547, 1979

91. Sargent JA: Assessing the utility and improving the effectiveness of nutritional support. *Nutr Clin Prac* 1: 29, 1986

92. Kopple JD, Coburn JW: Evaluation of chronic uremia. Importance of serum urea nitrogen, serum creatinine, and their ratio. *JAMA* 227: 41, 1974

93. Rutherford WE, Blondin J, Miller JP, Greenwalt AS, Vavra JD: Chronic progressive renal disease: rate of change of serum creatinine concentration. *Kidney Int* 11: 62, 1977

94. Sargent JA: Control of dialysis by a single-pool urea model; the national cooperative dialysis study. *Kidney Int* 23 (Suppl 13): S2, 1983

95. Cestero RVM, Thunberg B, Jain VK, Fain VK: Diagnostic value of modeled therapy: nutritional status and technical problems of treatment. *Dial Transplant* 10: 302, 1981

96. Acchiardo SR, Moore LW: Urea kinetics: the possibility of selectively reduced treatment frequency. *Dial Transplant* 10: 295, 1981

97. Collins A, Kesaviah P, Berkseth R, Ilstrup K, McMichael C, Ebben J: Short efficient hemodialysis with reduced symptoms. *Kidney Int* 27: 158, 1985

98. Keshaviah P, Collins A: Rapid high-efficiency bicarbonate hemodialysis. *Trans Am Soc Artif Intern Organs* 32: 17, 1986

99. Heineken FG, Evans MC, Keen ML, Gotch FA: Intercompartmental fluid shifts in hemodialysis patients. *Biotechnol Progr* 3:2, 1987

100. Shackman R, Chisholm GD, Holden AJ, Pigott RW: Urea distribution in the body after haemodialysis. *Br Med J* 2: 355, 1962

101. Wathen R, Keshaviah P, Hommeyer R, Cadwell K, Comty C: Role of dialysate glucose in preventing gluconeogenesis during hemodialysis. *Trans Am Soc Artif Intern Organs* 23: 393, 1977

102. Wathen RL, Keshaviah P, Hommeyer P, Cadwell K, Comty CM: The metabolic effects of hemodialysis with and without glucose in the dialysate. *Am J Clin Nutr* 31: 1870, 1978

103. Farrell PC, Hone PW: Dialysis induced catabolism. *Am J Clin Nutr* 33: 1417, 1980

104. Wineman RJ, Sargent JA, Piercy L: Nutritional implications of renal disease, II. The dietitian's key role in studies of dialysis therapy. *J Am Diet Assoc* 70: 483, 1977

105. Sargent J: Shortfalls in the delivery of dialysis. *Am J Kidney Dis* 15: 500, 1990

106. Lowrie EG, Lew NL: Death risk in hemodialysis patients: the predictive value of commonly measured variables and an evaluation of death rate differences between facilities. *Am J Kidney Dis* 15: 458–482, 1990

107. Smye SW, Evans JHC, Wills E, Brocklebank JT: Paediatric haemodialysis: estimation of treatment efficiency in the presence of urea rebound. *Clin Phys Physiol Meas* 13(1): 51–62, 1992

108. Sargent JA, Gotch FA, Henry RA, Bennett N: Mass balance: a quantitative guide to clinical nutritional therapy. *J Am Diet Assoc* 75: 551, 1979

109. Collins AJ, Ma JZ, Umen A, Keshaviah P: Urea index and other predictors of hemodialysis patient survival. *Am J Kid Dis* 23(5): 272–282, 1994 23: 272, 1994

109a. Schneditz D, Van Stone JC, and Davgirdas JT: A regional blood circulation alternative to in-series two compartment urea kinetic modeling. *Am Soc Artif Int Organs* 39(3): M573–M577

110. Hakim RA, Breyer J, Nuhad I, Schulman G: Effects of dose of dialysis on morbidity and mortality. *Am J Kid Dis* 23(5): 661–669, 1994

111. Delmez JA, Weerts CA, Hasamear PD *et al.*: Severe dialyzer dysfunction undetectable by standard reprocessing validation tests. *Kidney Int* 36: 478, 1989

112. Basile C, Casino F, Lopez T: Percent reduction in blood urea concentration during dialysis estimates Kt/V in a simple and accurate way. *Am J Kid Disease* 15: 40, 1990

113. Jindal K, Manuel A, Goldstein M: Percent reduction in blood urea concentration during hemodialysis (PRU). *Trans Am Soc Artif Intern Organs* 33: 286, 1987

114. Daugirdas J: Rapid methods of estimating Kt/V: three formulas compared. *ASAIO Trans* 36: M362, 1990

115. Lowrie E, Lew N: The urea reduction ratio (URR): A simple method for evaluating hemodialysis treatment. *Cont Dial Nephrol* Feb: 11, 1991

116. Lowrie EG, Laird NM, Parker TF, Sargent JA: Effect of the hemodialysis prescription on patient morbidity. Report from the National Cooperative Dialysis Study. *N Engl J Med* 305: 1176–1181, 1981

117. Olsson P, Lagergen H, Er S: The elimination from plasma of intravenous heparin. *Acta Med Scand* 173: 619, 1963

118. Eiber HB, Danishefsky I, Borelli JJ: Studies with radioactive heparin in humans. *Angiology* 2: 40, 1960

119. Estes JW: The kinetics of heparin. *Ann N Y Acad Sci* 179: 187, 1971

120. Christensen HN: General concepts of neutrality regulation. *Am J Surg* 103: 286, 1962

121. Christensen HN: *Diagnostic Biochemistry: Quantitative Distribution of Body Constituents and Their Physiological Interpretation*, New York, Oxford University Press, 1959, p 122

122. Isaksson B: Urinary nitrogen output as a validity test in dietary surveys. *Am J Clin Nutr* 33: 4, 1980

123. Gotch FA, Sargent, JA: Measurement of H$^+$ balance during acetate and bicarbonate dialysis therapy. *Kidney Int* 16: 887, 1979

124. Relman AS, Schwartz WB: The effects of DOCA on electrolyte balance in normal man and its relation to sodium chloride intake. *Yale J Biol Med* 24: 540, 1952

125. Schwartz WB, Jenson RL, Relman AS: The disposition of acid administered to sodium-depleted subjects: the renal response and the role of the whole body buffers. *J Clin Invest* 33: 687, 1954

126. Schwartz WB, Orning KJ, Porter R: The internal distribution of hydrogen ions with varying degrees of metabolic acidosis. *J Clin Invest* 36: 373, 1957

127. Hunt JH: The influence of dietary sulfur on the urinary output of acid in man. *Clin Sci* 5: 119, 1956

128. Mion CM, Hegstrom RM, Boen ST, Scribner BH: Substitution of sodium acetate for sodium bicarbonate in the bath fluid for hemodialysis. *Trans Am Soc Artif Intern Organs* 10: 110, 1964

129. Grimsrud L, Cole JJ, Lehman GA, Babb AL, Scribner BH: A central system for the continuous preparation and distribution of hemodialysis fluid. *Trans Am Soc Artif Intern Organs* 10: 107, 1964

130. Sargent JA, Gotch FA, Lam MA, Prowitt M, Keen ML: Technical aspects of on line proportioning of bicarbonate dialysate. *Proc Clin Dial Transplant Forum* 7: 109, 1977

131. Krebs HA: The biochemical lesions in ketosis. *Arch Intern Med* 107: 119, 1961

132. Lundquist F: Production and utilization of free acetate in man. *Nature* 193: 579, 1962

133. Kaiser BA, Potter DE, Bryant RE, Vreman HJ, Weiner MW: Acid-base changes and acetate metabolism during routine and high-efficiency hemodialysis in children. *Kidney Int* 19: 70, 1981

134. Swan RC, Pitts RF: Neutralization of infused acid by nephrectomized dogs. *J Clin Invest* 34: 205, 1955

135. Gotch FA, Borah MF, Keen ML, Lam MA, Provitt M, Sargent JA: The solute kinetics of intermittent dialysis therapy. *Third Annual Report of Artificial Kidney Chronic Uremia Program NIAMDD* 1977, p 48

136. Garella S, Dana CL, Chazan JA: Severity of metabolic acidosis as a determinant of bicarbonate requirements. *N Engl J Med* 289: 121, 1973

137. Dombec DH, Klein E, Wendt RP: Evaluation of two pool model for predicting serum creatinine levels during intra and interdialytic periods. *Trans Am Soc Artif Intern Organs* 21: 117, 1975

138. Sanfelippo ML, Hall DA, Walker WE, Swenson RS: Quantitative evaluation of hemodialysis therapy using a simple mathematical model and a programmable pocket calculator. *Trans Am Soc Artif Intern Organs* 21: 125, 1975

139. Katz MA, Hull AR: Transcellular creatinine disequilibrium and its significance in hemodialysis. *Nephron* 12: 171, 1974

140. Jones JD, Burnett PC: Implication of creatinine and gut flora in the uremic syndrome: Induction of 'creatinine' in colon contents of the rat by dietary creatinine. *Clin Chem* 18: 280, 1972

141. Jones JD, Burnett PC: Creatinine metabolism in humans with decreased renal function: creatinine deficit. *Clin Chem* 20: 1204, 1974

142. Mitch WE, Walser M: A proposed mechanism for reduced creatinine excretion in severe chronic renal failure. *Nephron* 21: 248, 1978

143. Wehle B, Asaba H, Castenfors J, Furst P, Grahn A, Gunnarson B, Shaldon S, Berstrom J: The influence of dialysis fluid composition on the blood pressure response during dialysis. *Clin Nephrol* 10: 62, 1978

144. Ogden DA: A double crossover comparison of high and low sodium dialysis. *Proc Clin Dial Transplant Forum* 8: 157, 1978

145. Van Stone JC, Cook J: Decreased postdialysis fatigue with increased dialysate sodium concentration. *Proc Clin Dial Transplant Forum* 8: 152, 1978

146. Quellhorst D, Reiger J, Doht B, Beckman H, Jacob I, Kraft B, Mietzsch G, Scheler F: Treatment of chronic uraemia by an ultrafiltration kidney-first clinical experience. *Proc Eur Dial Transplant Assoc* 13: 314, 1976

147. Maekawa M, Kishimoto T, Ohyama T, Tanaka H: Present status of hemofiltration and hemodiafiltration in Japan. *Artif Organs* 4: 85, 1980

148. Kakagwa S: Multifactorial evaluation of hemofiltration therapy in comparison with conventional hemodialysis. *Artif Organs* 4: 94, 1980

149. Streicher E, Schneider H: Clinical experience in hemofiltration. *Int J Artif organs* 3: 221, 1980

150. Schneider H, Streicher D, Hachmann H, Chmiel H, von Mylius U: Clinical experience with haemofiltration. *Proc Eur Dial Transplant Assoc* 14: 136, 1977

151. Baldamus CA, Knobloch M, Schoeppe W, Koch KM: Hemodialysis/hemofiltration. A report of a controlled cross-over study. *Int J Artif Organs* 3: 211, 1980

152. Shaldon S, Beau MC, Claret G, Deschodt G, Oules R, Ramperez P, Mion H, Mion C: Haemofiltration with sorbent regeneration of ultrafiltrate: first clinical experience in end stage renal disease. *Proc Eur Dial Transplant Assoc* 15: 220, 1978

153. Shaldon, Deschodt G, Beau MC, Claret G, Mion H, Mion C: Vascular stability during high flux haemofiltration (HF). *Proc Eur Dial Transplant Assoc* 16: 695, 1979

154. Shaldon S, Beau MC, Deschodt G, Ramperez P, Mion C: Vascular stability during hemofiltration. *Trans Am Soc Artif Intern Organs* 26: 391, 1980

155. Baldamus CA, Ernst W, Fassbinder W, Koch KM: Differing haemodynamic stability due to differing sympathetic response: comparison of ultrafiltration, haemodialysis and haemofiltration. *Proc Eur Dial Transplant Assoc* 17: 205, 1980

156. Shaldon S, Beau MC, Deschodt G, Flavier JL, Gullberg CA, Ramperez P, Mion C: Two years clinical experience with short hour high efficiency haemofiltration (HF). *Abstracts Clin Dial Transplant Forum*, 1980, p 52,

157. Quellhorst E, Schuenemann B, Hildebrand U, Falda Z: Response of the vascular system to different modification of haemofiltration and haemodialysis. *Proc Eur Dial Transplant Assoc* 17: 197, 1980

158. Ladenson JH: Direct potentiometric analysis of sodium and potassium in human plasma: evidence for electrolyte interaction with a non protein, protein-associated substance (S). *J Lab Clin Med* 90: 654, 1977

159. Shyr C, Young CC: Effect of sample protein concentration on results of analysis for sodium and potassium in serum. *Clin Chem* 26: 1517, 1980

160. Coleman RL: Differences in electrolyte results as measured by direct potentiometry (ISE) and flame photometry. *Bulletin from Nova Biomedical*, Newton, MA

161. Gotch FA, Evans MC, Keen ML: Measurement of the effective dialyzer Na diffusion gradient *in vitro* and *in vivo*. *Trans Am Soc Artif Inters Organs* 31: 354, 1985

162. Flannery JM: Differences in electrolyte results as measured by direct potentiometry (ion selective electrode) and flame photometry. *Bulletin from Nova Biomedical*, Newton, MA

163. Bijster P, Vader HL, Vink CLJ: An evaluation of the Corning 902 direct potentiometric sodium/potassium analyzer. *J Automatic Chem* 4: 125, 1982

164. Aluer A, Belledonne M, Saciaggi A, Glabman S, Bosch J: Sodium fluxes during hemodialysis. *Trans Am Soc Artif Intern Organs* 29: 684, 1983

165. Nolph KD, Stoltz ML, Carter CB, Fox M, Maher JF: Factors affecting the composition of ultrafiltrate from hemodialysis coils. *Trans Am Soc Artif Intern Organs* 16: 495, 1970

166. Shinaberger JH, Brautbar N, Miller JH, Gardner PN: Successful application of sequential hemofiltration followed by diffusion dialysis with standard dialysis equipment. *Trans Am Soc Artif Intern Organs* 24: 677, 1978

167. Flear CTG, Bhattacharya SS, Sung CM: Solute and water exchanges between cells and extracellular fluids in health and disturbances after trauma. *J Pen J Parenter Entera/Nutr* 4: 98, 1980

168. Maffly RH: The body fluids: Volume, composition, and physical chemistry. in *The Kidney* edited by Brenner BM, Rector FC, Philadelphia, WB Saunders Co, 1976, p 65

169. Edelman IS, Leibman J: Anatomy of body water and electrolytes. *Am J Med* 27: 256, 1959

170. Edelman IS, Leibman J, O'Meara MP, Birkenfeld LW: Interrelations between serum sodium concentration, serum osmolarity and total exchangeable sodium, total exchangeable potassium and total body water. *J Clin Invest* 37: 1236, 1958

171. Feig PU, Shook A, Sterns RH: Effect of potassium removal during hemodialysis on the plasma potassium concentration. *Nephron* 27: 25–30, 1981

172. Feig PU, Pring M, Guzzo J, Singer I: Disposition of intravenous potassium in anuric man: a kinetic analysis. *Kidney Int* 15: 651–660, 1979

173. Landis EM, Pappenheimer JR: Exchange of substances through the capillary walls. in *Handbook of Physiology*, Section II, Circulation, Volume 22, Washington DC, Am Physiol Soc, 1963, p 961

174. Maeda K, Saito A, Kawaguchi S: Hemodiafiltration with sodium concentration-controlled dialysate *Artif Organs* 4: 121, 1980

175. Keen M, Evans M, Gotch FA: Comparison of morbidity in high flux dialysis (HFD) and conventional dialysis (CD). *Kidney Int* 31: 235, 1987

176. Acchiardo S, Burk L, Bannister D: High-flux (HF) hemodialysis (HD). *Kidney Int* 31: 226, 1987

177. Kjellstrand CM, Rosa AA, Shideman JR: Hypotension during hemodialysis: osmolality fall is an important pathogenetic factor. *ASAIO J* 3: 11, 1980

178. Heinrich EL, Woodard TD, Blackley JD, Gomez-Sanchez C, Pettinger W, Cronin RE: Role of osmolality in blood pressure stability after dialysis and ultrafiltration. *Kidney Int* 18: 480, 1980

179. DiRaimondo C, Stone W: B_2M amyoidosis. *Int J Artif Organs* 10: 281, 1987

180. Sethi D, Gower P: Synocial fluid B₂-M levels in dialysis arthropathy. *N Engl J Med* 315: 1419, 1986

181. Gejyo F, Odani S, Yamada R, Honma N, Saito H, Suzuki Y, Nakagawa Y, Kobayashi H, Maruyama Y, Hirasawa Y, Suzuki M, Arakawa M: B₂-microglobulin: a new form of amyloid protein associated with chronic hemodialysis. *Kidney Int* 30: 385, 1986

182. Gorevic P, Munoz P, Casey T: Polymerization of intact B₂/microglobulin in tissue cases amuloidosis in patients on chronic hemodialysis. *Proc Natl Acad Sci USA* 83: 7908, 1986

183. Kachel H, Altmeyer P, Baldamus C, Koch K: Deposition of amyloid-like substance as a possible complication of regular dialysis treatment. *Contrib Nephrol* 36: 127, 1983

184. Ogawa H, Saito A, Hirabayashi N, Hara K: Amyloid deposition in systemic organs in long-term hemodialysis patients. *Clin Nephrol* 28: 199, 1987

185. Messmer RP: B₂-microglobulin: an old molecule assumes a new look. *J Lab Clin Med* 104: 141, 1984

186. Vincent C, Pozet N, Revillard J: Plasma B₂-microglobulin turnover in renal insufficiency. *Acta Clin Belg* 35 (Suppl 10): 1, 1980

187. Karlsson F, Groth T, Sege K, Wibell L, Peterson P: Turnover in humans of B₂-microgolulin: The constant chain of HLA-antigens. *Euro J Clin Invest* 10: 293, 1980

188. Schardijn G, Statius Van Eps L: B₂-microglobulin: Its significance in the evaluation of renal function. *Kidney Int* 32: 635, 1987

189. Cresswell P, Springer T, Strominger JL, Turner MU, Grey HM, Kubo RT: Immunological identity of the small subunit of HLA antigens and B₂-microglobulin and its turnover on the cell membrane. *Proc Nat Acid Sci USA* 71: 2123, 1974

190. Statius Van Eps L, Schardijn G: B₂-microglobulin and the renal tubule. in *Non-Invasive Diagnosis of Kidney Disease*, edited by Lubec G, Basel, Karger, 1983, p 103

191. Bhalla R, Safai B, Mertelsmann R, Schwartz MK: Abnormally high concentrations of B₂-M in acquired immunodeficiency syndrome (AIDS) patients. *Clin Chem* 29: 1560, 1983

192. Bergstrom J, Wehle B: No change in corrected B₂-M concentration after cuprophane hemodialysis. *Lancet* 1: 628, 1987

193. Shaldon S, Koch KM, Dinarello CA, Colton CK, Knudsen PJ, Floege J, Granolleras C: B₂-microglobulin and haemodialysis. *Lancet* 1: 925, 1987

194. Mahiout A, Ludat K, Schultze G: Alteration of blood osmolality induces a shift of B₂-M plasma levels in patients undergoing hemodialysis. *Nephrol Dial Transplant* 2: 448, 1987

195. Geiyo F, Homma N, Suziki Y, Arakawa M: Serum levels of Beta-2-microglobulin as a new form of amyloid protein in patients undergoing long-term hemodialysis. *N Engl J Med* 314: 585, 1986

196. Burzynski SR: Biologically active peptides in human urine: I. Isolation of a group of medium size peptides. *Physiol Chem Physics* 5: 437, 1973

197. Scribner BH, Babb AL: Evidence for toxins of middle molecular weight. *Kidney Int* 7 (Suppl 3): S349, 1975

198. Shinaberger JH, Miller JH, Rosenblatt MG, Gardner PW, Carpenter GW, Martin FE: Clinical studies of 'low flow' dialysis with membranes highly permeable to middle weight molecules. *Trans Am Soc Artif Intern Organs* 18: 82, 1972

199. Rattazzi T, Wathen R, Comty C, Raij L, Leonard A, Shapiro F: The comparison of low flow (Qd200) to regular flow (Qd500) dialysis. *Trans Am Soc Artif Intern Organs* 20: 402, 1974

200. Ginn HE, Teschan PE, Walker PJ, Bourne JR, Macalyne F, Ward JW, McLain LW, Johnson HB, Hamel B: Neurotoxicity in uremia. *Kidney Int* 7 (Suppl 3): S357, 1975

201. Tenckhoff H, Curtis FK: Experience with maintenance peritoneal dialysis in the home. *Trans Am Soc Artif Intern Organs* 16: 90, 1970

202. Gotch FA: A quantitative evaluation of small and middle molecule toxicity in therapy of uremia. *Dial Transplant* 9: 183, 1980

203. Gotch FA, Sargent JA, Modelling of middle molecules in clinical studies. Symposium on present status and future orientation of middle molecules in uremia and other diseases. *Artif Organs* 4: 133, 1980

204. Henderson LW, Stone RA, Ford CA, Lysagth MJ: Blood pressure control with hemodiafiltration. *Proc 10th Annu Contractors: Conf Artif Kidney* – Chronic Uremia Program NIAMDD, DHEW Publication No (NIH) 77–1442, 1977, p 110

205. Funck-Brentano JL, Man NK, Sausse A, Cueille G, Zingraff J, Drueke T, Jungers P, Billon JP: Neuropathy and 'middle' molecule toxins. *Kidney Int* 7 (Suppl 3): S352, 1975

206. Gulyassy PRF, Peters JH, Lin SC, Ryan PM: Hemodialysis and plasma amino acid composition in chronic renal failure. *Am J Clin Nutr* 21: 565, 1968

207. Bartsch HJ: *Handbook of Mathematical Formulas*, Translated by Liebscher H, New York, Academic Press, 1974, p 139

208. Cottini ERP, Gallina DK, Dominguez JE: Urea excretion in adult humans with varying degrees of kidney malfunction fed milk, egg or an amino acid mixture: assessment of nitrogen balance. *J Nutr* 103: 11, 1973

209. Bleiler RE, Schedl HP: Creatinine excretion: variability in relationship to diet and body size. *J Lab Clin Med* 59: 945, 1962

210. Harmon WE, Spinozzi N, Meyer A, Grupe WE: Use of protein catabolic rate to monitor pediatric hemodialysis. *Dial Transplant* 10: 324, 1981

211. Sargent JA, Gotch FA: Nutrition and treatment of the acutely ill patient using urea kinetics. *Dial Transplant* 10: 314, 1981

212. Sargent JA: Urea mass balance: Nutrition and treatment of the acutely ill patient. *Nutr Support Services* 2: 2, 1982

213. Cuthbertson DP: The metabolic response to injury and its nutritional implications: retrospect and prospect. *J Parenter Enteral Nutr* 3: 1078, 1979

214. Long JM, Wilmore DW, Mason AD: Effect of carbohydrate and fat intake on nitrogen excretion during total intravenous feeding. *Ann Surg* 185: 417, 1977

215. Clowes GHA Jr, O'Donnell TF Jr, Blackburn GL *et al.*: Energy metabolism and proteolysis in traumatized and septic man. *Surg Clin North Am* 56: 1169, 1976

216. Clowes GHA Jr, O'Donnell TF Jr, Ryan NT: Energy metabolism in sepsis: treatment based on different patterns in shock and high output stage. *Ann Surg* 179: 684, 1974

217.   Wolfe BM, Culebras JM, Sim AJW, Ball MR, Moore FD: Substrate interaction in intravenous feeding: comparative effects of carbohydrate and fat on amino acid utilization in fasting man. *Ann Surg* 186: 518, 1977

MEMBRANES FOR HEMODIALYSIS

CLARK K. COLTON and MICHAEL J. LYSAGHT

INTRODUCTION

Not only have the number and type of hemodialyis membranes proliferated over the past decade, but expectations of what a membrane should, and should not, do have altered to the extent that researchers and clinicians alike now find it difficult to understand the patient consequences of hemodialyzer membrane selection. The associated literature is extensive, e.g. Medline® contains over 1500 citations to hemodialysis membranes, but several comprehensive technical reviews are available (1–11). This chapter begins with a brief introduction and history. Then it describes and classifies currently available membranes and summarizes our current understanding of how a membrane's physical properties and chemical structure determine its transport characteristics and biocompatibility.

Membranes may be described as thin barriers capable of providing selective transport between adjacent phases. In the case of hemodialysis, transport is selective because smaller species permeate the membrane at a higher velocity than do larger species. This is partially due to steric factors and also as a consequence of the intrinsically higher Stefan–Boltzman velocity of smaller molecules. Two modes of transport are important in hemodialysis: *diffusion* and *convection*. Diffusion has its roots in the Latin word *diffundere*, a term of art in the dyestuff industry, meaning 'to spread out in all directions'. More rigorously, diffusion refers to molecular movement of solutes from a region of greater concentration to a region of lesser concentration at a rate that is proportional to the gradient in concentration. The diffusion rate of solutes in a common environment varies inversely with the square root of molecular weight; thus inulin with a molecular weight of ~ 5200 Daltons will diffuse a little under 10 times more slowly than urea with a molecular weight of 60 Daltons. The driving force for a diffusive process cannot be augmented externally and dissipates as a separation moves toward completion. Diffusion is effective at moving small molecules across short distances; it is less efficient in unit operations of larger scale. Convection is a broad term and refers to the bulk movement of fluid in response to a hydraulic or osmotic force. It derives from the participle of the Latin verb *convehere*, 'to carry together'. Convection is not intrinsically discriminating but relies upon some form of selective media, such as a membrane, to realize a separation between solvent or solute or between two solutes. The rate of convection can be augmented by changing conditions of pressure or flow and convection can be an efficient method of large-scale mass transfer. In early hemodialysis formats, most solute removal occurred by diffusion, and convection was responsible only for fluid removal. Formal treatments of the process assumed that the two modes were independent and additive and often simply ignored solute removal by convection. With the introduction of newer membranes and with interest in removal of larger species, such as β_2 microglobulin, convective transport has become increasingly more significant. In the increasingly-popular so-called high-flux formats, treatment of diffusion and convection as simultaneous independent processes is questionable and possibly misleading.

EARLY MEMBRANES

In Kolff and Berk's original dialyzer (12), the membrane was nothing more than commercially available sausage casing. Prepared from regenerated cellulose in the form of continuous seamless tubes, this material had long been adapted for laboratory dialysis because it was thin, strong, and reasonably permeable. Thalhimer had earlier recognized its utility for artificial kidney applications and used it in place of the fragile colloidin membranes hand-cast from cellulose nitrate by Abel et al. (13) and other earlier investigators. During the 1940s hemodialyzer designs multiplied, but regenerated cellulose, variously called Visking, Cellophan, or Bemberg Pt, was the only widely employed material (14); alternatives began to be investigated seriously in the 1960s and introduced clinically in

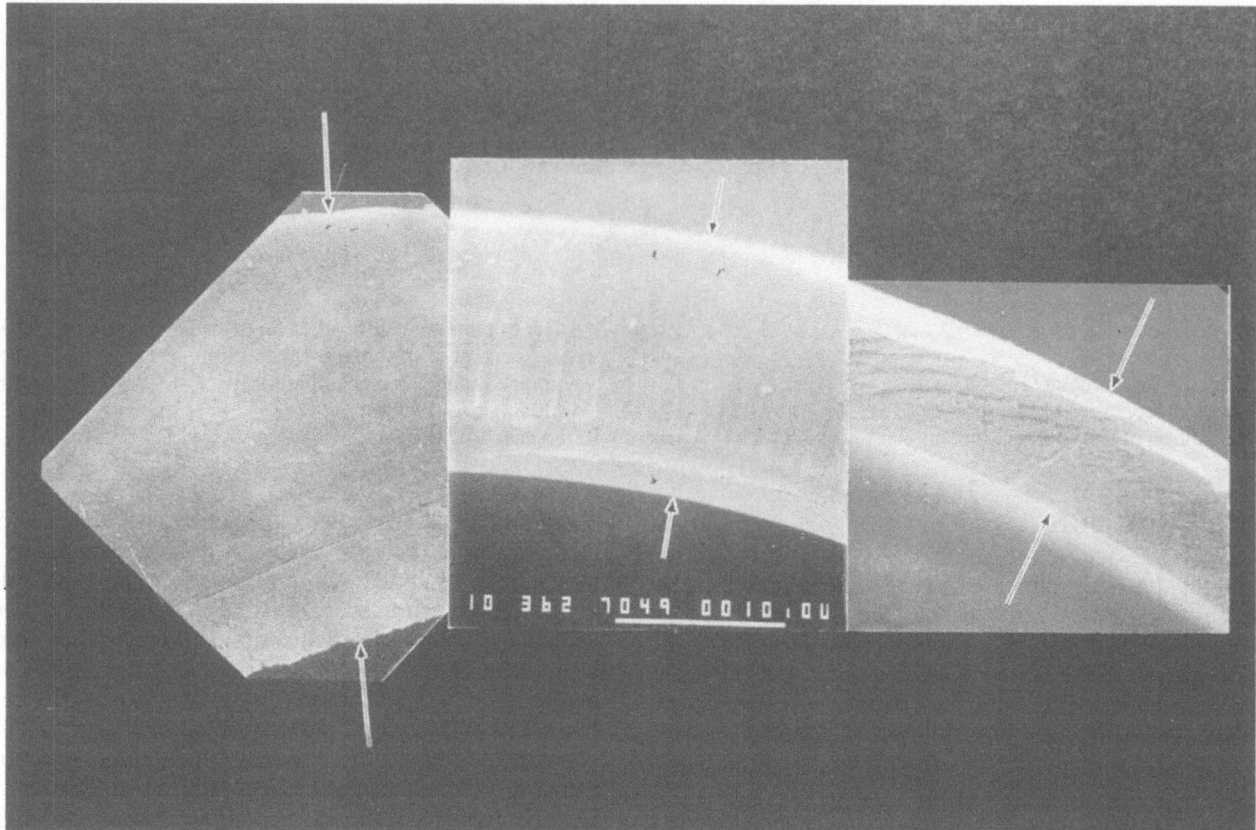

Figure 1. Trend towards a decrease in the dry wall thickness of cellulosic hollow fibers. The three SEM panels all taken at the same nominal magnification demonstrate the decreasing thickness of hollow fiber cellulosic membranes from 16 microns (late 1970s) to 12 microns (mid-1980s) to 8 microns late 1980s). The reduction in wet thickness is comparable and the thinnest membrane offers only half the resistance to transport of its thicker counterpart. This permits a reduction in overall membrane surface area with no loss in performance and leads to the design and utilization of more cost-effective hemodialyzers.

the 1970s. From the late 1940s to early 1960s several ingenious designs were advanced to replace Kolff's rotating drum. Few had any moving parts and most were suitable for pressure-driven ultrafiltration. The two designs which were initially most popular after the introduction of chronic hemodialysis were the Kiil flat plate and the Kolff twin coil. Disposable flat plate designs soon followed. Hollow fiber hemodialyzers were introduced around 1970. The principle motivation behind the design of these devices was the reduction in slow-moving or quasi-stagnant layers adjacent to the membranes. Such 'boundary layer' effects were particularly prominent in the blood pathway of coil designs and added significantly to the transport resistance of early devices. The improved hydrodynamic characteristics of later designs resulted in considerably improved device performance at no increase in membrane surface area. Both flat plate and hollow fiber designs effectively minimized perimembrane boundary layers. Hollow fiber designs ultimately proved to be the most popular format because the membrane served as its own support and thus eliminated the costly struts needed to provide flow chan-

nels in disposable parallel plate designs. There have been no basic advances in the hemodialyzer device geometry over the past 25 years.

In addition to being deployed in more efficient geometric formats, membranes have become progressively thinner. This is illustrated in Figure 1 for cellulosic hollow fibers, whose dry wall thickness has decreased since the mid-1970s from 16 microns to its current level of 8 microns ... or from 8 to 4% of the fiber diameter. Cellulosic membranes swell and increase in thickness when contacted with fluid. Nevertheless, a 50% reduction in width is a significant accomplishment with major transport implications. For any homogeneous membrane material, permeability is inversely proportional to thickness while selectivity is independent of thickness. Thus an 8 micron membrane offers half the transport resistance of a 16 micron membrane. Full sized hemodialyzers prepared from thinner fibers require less membrane surface area to achieve the same transport as otherwise identical hemodialyzers with thicker membranes. Because of boundary layers and nonlinearity of scaling, a twofold

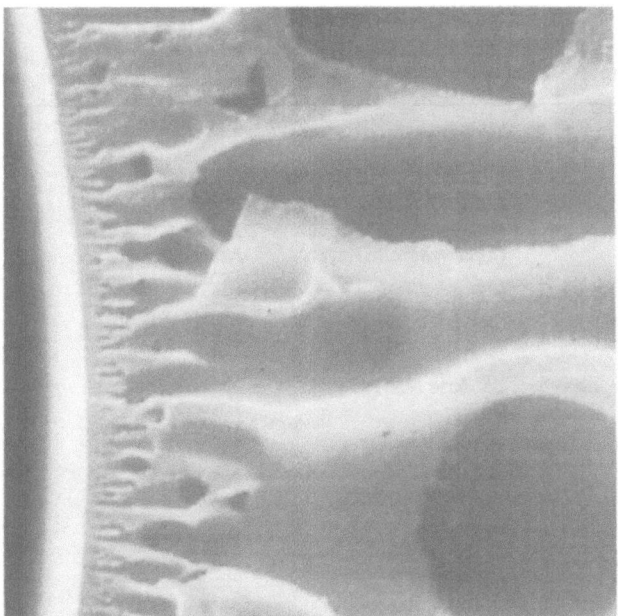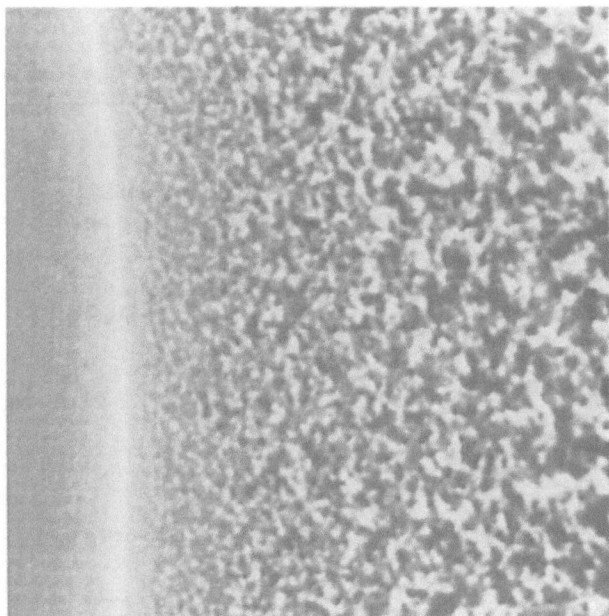

Figure 2. SEM of synthetic membranes, which were introduced in the 1980s and now account for about 35% or more of overall dialysis utilization. On the left is the classic macroreticular anisotropic structure introduced by Amicon for hemofiltration; on the right the more foam-like structure later developed by Fresenius. The foam-like structure offers greater strength at equivalent levels of transport.

increase in membrane transport rate does not permit a twofold decrease in device size, but the resultant reduction in area, bulk, and cost is nonetheless important. This is apparent from a comparison of contemporary hemodialyzers with those first introduced in the 1970s.

Original hemodialysis membranes were primarily homogeneous cellulosic films. Starting in the mid-1980s dialysis membranes became available in a wide variety of synthetic materials, morphologies, and microgeometries (Figure 2). Formulators were able to vary and tailor transport properties over a much wider range than had been possible with earlier cellulosic fibers. The clinical community has rapidly moved toward more open membranes, with their higher clearance of larger solutes, and has been willing to tolerate the obligatory backfiltration of dialysate into blood which inevitably accompanies such loose membranes. The utilization of synthetic membrane is now around 35% and is increasing yearly.

CHEMISTRY AND STRUCTURE

Hemodialysis membranes vary in chemical compositional structure, transport properties and biocompatibility. Hemodialysis membranes are fabricated from three classes of materials: regenerated cellulose, modified cellulose, and synthetics (9). The chemical composition of commercially available dialysis membranes is shown in Table 1. Regenerated cellulose is most comonly prepared by the cuproammonium process and is macroscopically homogenous. These extremely hydrophilic structures sorb water, bind it tightly and form a hydrogel. Solute diffusion occurs through highly water-swollen amorphous regions in which the cellulose polymer chains are in constant random motion and would actually dissolve if they were not tied down by the presence of crystalline regions. Their principle advantage is low unit cost, complemented by the strength of the highly crystalline cellulose, which allows polymer films to be made very thin. These membranes provide effective small-solute transport in relatively small exchange devices. The drawbacks of regenerated cellulose are their limited capacity to transport middle molecules and the presence of labile nucleophilic groups which trigger complement activation and transient leukopenia during the first hour of exposure to blood. The advantages appear to outweigh the disadvantages, since 40–50% of all hemodialyzers are still prepared from cellulosics, the most common of which is supplied by Akzo under the trade name Cuprophan (see book cover).

A variety of other hydrophilic polymers account for 20–30% of total hemodialyzer production, including derivatized cellulose, such as cellulose acetate, diacetate, triacetate, and synthetic materials such as polycarbonate (PC), ethylenevinylalcohol (EVAL), and polyacrylonitrile-sodium methallyl sulfonate copolymer (PAN-SO_3), all of which can be fabricated into homogenous films.

Table 1. Membranes used for the treatment of end-stage renal failure

CELLULOSE AND ITS DERIVATIVES

Polymer	Chemical Structure	Common Name or Abbreviation	Manufacturer
Regenerated Cellulose		Cuprophan Cuprammonium Rayon Saponified Cellulose Ester	Akzo Asahi Medical Terumo Teijin Althin Medical
Cellulose Diacetate	R= –C–CH₃	Cellulose Acetate CA	Althin Medical Toyobo Teijin
Cellulose Triacetate	Replace all hydroxyl groups	CTA	Toyobo
Derivatized Cellulose	< 1% hydroxyl groups replaced	Hemophan	Akzo

SYNTHETIC POLYMERS

Polyethylene/Vinyl Alcohol	–CH₂–CH₂–····–CH₂–CH(OH)–	EVAL	Kawasumi
Polymethyl Methacrylate	–CH₂–C(CO-OCH₃)(CH₃)–	PMMA	Toray
Polyacrylonitrile/ Methyl Acrylate	–CH₂–CH(CO-OCH₃)–····–CH₂–CH(C≡N)–	PAN	Asahi Medical
Polyacriyonitrile/ Sodium Methallyl Sulfonate	–CH₂–CH(C≡N)–····–CH₂–C(CH₃)(CH₂SO₃Na)–	AN-69	Gambro/ Hospal
Polysulfone Admixed with polyvinylpyrrolidone		PS	Akzo Fresenius Kawasumi Kurary Toray
Polyamide (Trogamide) [Polytrimethylhexamethyl-eneterephthalamide] Admixed with polyvinylpyrrolidone		Polyflux	Gambro
Polycarabonate/Polyether		Gambrane	Gambro

At the opposite end of the spectrum are membranes prepared from synthetic engineered thermoplastics, such as polysulfones, polyamides and polyacrylonitrilepolyvinylchloride copolymers. These hydrophobic materials, which account for 30–40% of the hemodialyzer market, form asymmetric and anisotropic membranes with solid structures and open void spaces (unlike the highly mobile polymeric structure of regenerated cellulose). These membranes are characterized by a skin on one surface, typically a fraction of a micron thick, which contains very fine pores and constitutes the discriminating barrier determining the hydraulic permeability and solute retention properties of the membrane. The bulk of the membrane is composed of a spongy region, with interstices that cover a wide size range and with a structure ranging from open to closed cell foam. The primary purpose of the spongy region is to provide mechanical strength; the diffusive permeability of the membrane is usually determined by the properties of this matrix. As the convective and diffusive transport properties of these membranes are, to a large extent, associated independently with the properties of the skin and spongy matrix, respectively, it is possible to vary independently the convective and diffusive transport properties with these asymmetric structures. There is often a second skin on the other surface, usually much more open than the primary barrier. These materials are usually less activating to the complement cascade than are cellulosic membranes. The materials are also less restrictive to the transport of middle and large molecules. Drawbacks are increased cost and such high hydraulic permeability as to require special control mechanisms to avoid excess fluid loss and to raise concerns over the biologic quality of dialysate fluid because of the possibility of backfiltration carrying pyrogenic substances to the bloodstream.

The discovery of asymmetric membrane structures launched the modern era of membrane technology by motivating research on new membrane separation processes. Asymmetric membranes proved useful in ultrafiltration, and a variety of hydrophobic materials have been used including polysulfone (PS), polyacrylonitrile (PAN), and its derivatives, its copolymer with polyvinylchloride (PVC), polyamide (PA), and polymethylmethacrylate (PMMA). PMMA does not form an obvious skin surface and should perhaps be placed in a class of its own.

TRANSPORT PROPERTIES OF MEMBRANES

Definition of transport coefficients

A membrane is a thin film across which mass is transferred in response to a chemical potential driving force. For artificial kidneys the driving forces of interest arise from differences in solute concentration and pressure across the membrane.

When transport across the membrane is predominantly diffusive as a result of a concentration driving force, the process is called *dialysis*. When transport is primarily convective as a result of bulk flow across the membrane induced by a pressure driving force, the process is called *ultrafiltration* if the membrane passes small solutes but rejects macromolecules.

We first consider steady-state liquid phase membrane transport resulting from a concentration difference between the upstream (1) and downstream (2) sides of the membrane. We assume that Fick's first law, defined in terms of an appropriate membrane diffusion coefficient D_m, is valid locally within the membrane. The integrated form is given by

$$N = D_m \frac{(C_{1m} - C_{2m})}{L} . \qquad [1]$$

This relationship is defined in terms of the concentration within the membrane, C_m, whereas it is normally only the concentration in solutions, C_s, that is measurable experimentally. The ratio between the concentration in the membrane and the concentration in the adjacent solution at equilibrium is called the equilibrium partition coefficient and is defined by

$$K_p = \left(\frac{C_m}{C_s} \right)_{eq} . \qquad [2]$$

Equations [1] and [2] can be combined to give a flux expression in terms of the concentration difference between the solutions on either side of the membrane:

$$N = D_m K_p \frac{(C_{1s} - C_{2s})}{L} = P_m (C_{1s} - C_{2s}). \qquad [3]$$

The membrane diffusive permeability, P_m, plays a role analogous to that of a mass transfer coefficient. It is defined by

$$P_m = \frac{D_m K_p}{L} = \frac{D_{eff}}{L} \qquad [4]$$

which except for the inclusion of K_p in D_{eff} is analogous to the definition of a mass transfer coefficient for diffusion across a stagnant film. In analogy with the behavior of mass transfer coefficients the reciprocal of the membrane permeability is the membrane mass transfer resistance

$$R_m = \frac{1}{P_m} . \qquad [5]$$

When pressure and concentration driving forms are present simultaneously, both convective and diffusive transport occur at the same time. This more complicated situation is conveniently described by using the irreversible thermodynamic description of membrane transport:

$$J_v = L_p (\Delta P - \sigma \Delta \pi) \qquad [6]$$

$$J_s = \bar{C}_s(1 - \sigma)J_v + \omega\Delta\pi, \qquad [7]$$

where J_v is the net volume flux (equivalent to the superficial velocity across the membrane), and J_s is the solute flux (equivalent to N). L_p, σ and ω are the hydraulic permeability, Staverman reflection coefficient, and diffusive permeability coefficient, respectively. $\bar{C}_s$ is the mean solute concentration in the membrane, and ΔP and $\Delta\pi$ are the hydrostatic and osmotic pressure differences between the solutions on either side of the membrane. L_p is equivalent to the symbol K_{UF} which is often used in describing the hydraulic permeability properties of a hemodialyzer.

The derivation of Equation [6] uses the Van't Hoff equation for dilute solutions, which relates osmotic pressure to concentration by

$$\pi = RTC_s. \qquad [8]$$

When $\Delta C_s = 0$, only bulk flow occurs, according to

$$J_v = L_p\Delta P. \qquad [9]$$

When ΔC_s is also finite, the driving force for volume transport is reduced by the effective osmotic pressure difference, $\sigma\Delta\pi$. The quantity σ, which varies from 0 to 1, is a measure of how easily the solute can get through the membrane during convective transport. If the solute is unhindered, then $\sigma = 0$, whereas $\sigma = 1$ applies to a solute that cannot pass through the membrane.

For the case of zero or negligible volume flow,

$$J_s = \omega RT\Delta C_s. \qquad [10]$$

Comparison of Equations [3] and [10] shows that

$$P_m = \omega RT. \qquad [11]$$

Equations [6] and [7] provide a useful framework for recognizing that three parameters are required for a complete description of membrane transport. However, the simple additivity of diffusive and convective transport, as represented in Equation [7], is valid only for small driving forces. When this resection does not hold, as is the case for most practical situations, a more complicated, nonlinear relationship applies that is valid for any combination of driving forces (16).

Effect of membrane properties on device performance

The rate of mass transfer M of a specific species from blood to dialyzer in a hemodialyzer may be expressed by (17)

$$M = k_oA\Delta C, \qquad [12]$$

where k_o is the average overall mass transfer coefficient of the dialyzer, A is the membrane area for transport, and ΔC is an average concentration difference between blood and dialyzate, usually taken to be the log-mean concentration

driving force appropriate to the contacting geometry of the hemodialyzer (usually countercurrent flow). For each of the three phases in a hemodialyzer, one may associate a mass transfer coefficient and its reciprocal, a mass transfer resistance, the sum of which is the overall mass transfer resistance, R_o given by

$$R_o = R_b + R_m + R_d \qquad [13]$$

or, equivalently

$$\frac{1}{k_o} = \frac{1}{k_b} + \frac{1}{P_m} + \frac{1}{k_d}, \qquad [14]$$

where subscripts b, m, and d refer to blood, membrane and dialyzate phases, respectively.

As a consequence of there being three mass transfer resistances in series, the mass transfer performance of a hemodialyzer is determined not solely by the membrane permeation properties but also by the properties of the concentration boundary layers in the blood and in dialysate. The relative contribution of each of the individual phases to the overall mass transfer resistance has been examined in detail in only one study for the case of a hollow fiber dialyzer commercialized in the mid-1970s (17). The results, shown in Figure 3, are representative of currently available hollow fiber dialyzers except that current membranes are more permeable than those available in the 1970s. In any event, the resistances of blood, membrane, and dialysate are roughly comparable in magnitude for a low molecular weight solute such as urea. As molecular weight increases, the membrane resistance becomes more important, and it is clearly the dominant resistance for middle and higher molecular weight solutes over 1000 Daltons in molecular weight.

Measurement of membrane transport properties

Membrane permeability P_m is most easily measured with membranes in the form of flat sheets (18, 19). Typically, the membrane is placed between two cylindrical chambers filled with solution in the equivalent of a diaphragm diffusion cell, often called a batch dialyzer. Solute is placed in one chamber and its permeation into the other chamber is followed with time, from which the overall mass transfer coefficient is calculated. This value must be corrected for the presence of mass transfer boundary layer resistances on each side of the membrane, which themselves must be estimated from separate experimental measurements. Hollow fiber membranes, used in almost all commercial hemodialyzers today, are more difficult to characterize (17). The lumen (blood side) mass transfer resistance can be estimated from theoretical analysis previously carried out. However, there is no way to predict the dialysate resistance because it is very sensitive to the details of fiber packing. The dialysate resistance can be estimated from experiments in which the overall mass transfer coefficient is measured as dialysate flow rate is varied over a wide range and the data then extrapolated to infinite

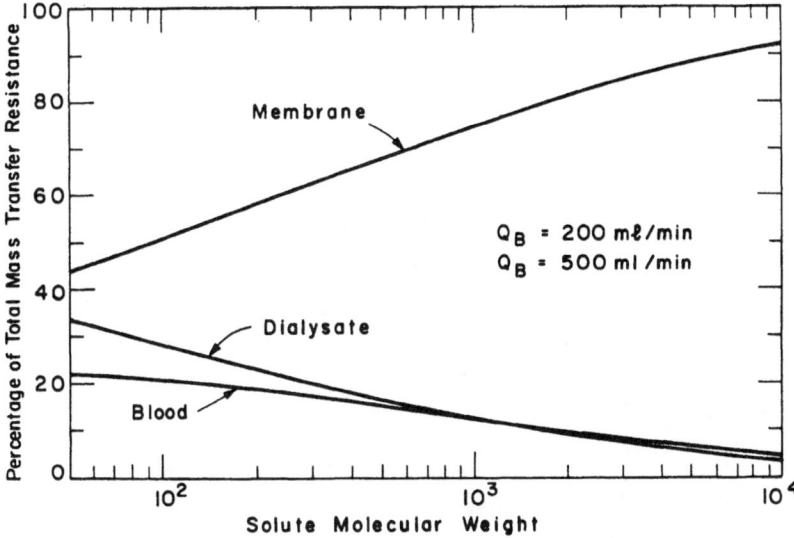

Figure 3. Fraction of total mass transfer resistance in a hollow fiber dialyzer accounted for by the individual phases. Adapted from Colton and Lowrie, 1981 (17).

dialysate flow rate using a procedure called a 'Wilson Plot'. Because accurate, repetitive measurements must be made, this analysis has been carried out in very few studies.

The hydraulic permeability is easily measured with membranes in any configuration by imposing a known hydrostatic pressure difference across the membrane and measuring the volumetric flow rate.

MEMBRANE-INDUCED BIOINCOMPATI-BILITY

Biocompatibility is a state, perhaps unattainable, in which all possible pathways to bioincompatibility are absent or inactive. These pathways become active when the extracorporeal system interacts with the bloodstream. The need for eliminating sources of bioincompatibility is considerable in processes used for end stage renal disease (ESRD) because (1) the process is employed chronically and frequently, and (2) the blood is exposed to both materials of construction, especially the large membrane surfaces, and to exogenous agents contained in the dialysate (or replacement fluid) that can permeate across the membrane. In this section we consider the sources of bioincompatibility associated with the membrane (20). There is a variety of initiating events that can manifest themselves as bioincompatibility pathways (21). There are significant interactions between them that further magnify the complexity of their interpretation.

Figure 4 illustrates some of these interactions in terms of surface-induced bioincompatibility. The surface is viewed as being composed of (1) covalently bound proteins derived from the complement system, and (2) a layer of physically adsorbed proteins derived from all of the plasma proteins. These protein-coated surfaces are shown interacting with the coagulation and complement systems as well as with platelets and immune cells. (Other protein systems that also interact but are not shown include the kinin and fibrinolytic systems.)

Virtually all surfaces foreign to blood activate complement to some degree via the alternative pathway, leaving on the surface covalently bound C3b which is eventually converted to iC3b or to C3 and C5 convertases (22) that serve to amplify the complement cascade. The latter tvo enzymes catalyze the cleavage of C3 and C5, respectively, to produce the cationic polypeptides C3a and C5a. The extent of complement activation and anaphylatoxin appearance in blood depends upon the number and reactivity of surface nucleophiles, especially hydroxyl groups, the degree of facilitation or inhibition of convertase activity, and binding of the fragments to negatively charged surfaces. Surfaces lacking nucleophiles, such as some hydrophobic membranes, are not completely free of complement activation because any plasma glycoproteins that denature on the surface would provide the requisite hydroxyls for C3b deposition.

Platelets and immune cells can also be adherent to certain proteins on the surface. For example, phagocytic cells, as well as red cells, B cells, and some T cells, have CR1 receptors that bind to C3b; phagocytes with CR3 receptors bind to iC3b. Complement fragment generation causes a C5a-induced increase in expression of adhesion receptors by phagocytes, leading to pulmonary leukosequestration. The anaphylatoxins mediate other functions of phagocytic cells (22, 23) and also activate other cells, including eosinophils, basophils, and mast cells (24). However, it appears that C5a does not directly mediate

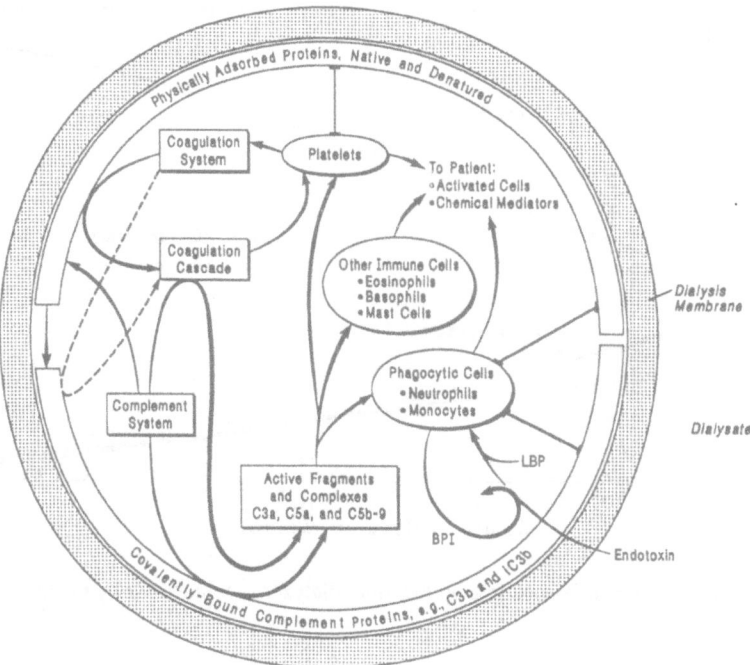

Figure 4. Interactions of membrane-induced bioincompatibility pathways. (Colton et al., 1994) (20).

significant neutrophil degranulation and that complement-independent mechanisms are responsible for the degranulation observed to occur in hemodialysis (22, 23). Shear rates at values found in ESRD therapies can cause lysosomal enzyme release from neutrophils (17). It is not known if there are other complement-independent mechanisms that cause degranulabon.

When blood contacts a foreign surface there is very rapid adsorption of plasma proteins at the interface (26). These proteins are physically adsorbed by noncovalent forces. Each adsorbed protein may retain its native configuration, undergo a conformational change, or be denatured. The composition and state of the proteins and their relationship to the nature of the material are not well understood. In general the composition of adsorbed proteins changes with time. Initially it is dominated by the most prevalent proteins in plasma: albumin, fibrinogen and IgG. With time these are replaced by trace proteins such as high-molecular-weight kininogen and Hageman factor (factor XII) (27, 28), which participate in initiating the coagulation cascade through contact activation as well as activating the platelet adhesion/aggregation reaction (21). The general reactions occurring in these processes have been worked out (29), but the precise steps involved with activation in whole blood are not as well known as that of complement activation. Heparin is used in extracorporeal circulation to prevent clotting. Because it acts late in the coagulation cascade, heparin does not block protein adsorption nor activation of coagulation. Even in the presence of heparin, some localized clot formation

often occurs, usually in regions of flow separation where reduced mass transport rates allow build-up of activated clotting factors (17).

Both coagulation and complement systems are composed of serine proteinases. As pointed out by Johnson (22), certain proteinases in one cascade have the capacity to act on proteins in the others and *vice versa*. For example, C3 convertase can cleave prothrombin to thrombin and factor XIIa, thrombin, and plasmin can cleave C3 and C5. This latter capability provides another mechanism for generation of active complement fragments with materials lacking surface nucleophiles.

The representation of cells in Figure 4 indudes cells in the bloodstream as well as cells adherent to materials of the extracorporeal circuit. Cells rarely, perhaps never, adhere directly to a foreign material but rather to intervening proteins. Platelets adhere to physically adsorbed proteins. Phagocytes can bind to covalently bound complement components via complement receptors and to physically adsorbed proteins via receptors to other molecules (30). Various plasma proteins such as fibrinogen and fibronectin adsorb to surfaces and can modulate phagocyte adhesion and activation. Lipopolysaccharide (LPS)-induced IL-1 secretion by monocytes cultured on, and adherent to, various polymeric surfaces is increased substantially when the surfaces are first contacted with plasma proteins. The secretion rate varies over a wide range, depending on the nature of the polylner and the adsorbed protein (31). Bound complement C3 derivatives together with fibronectin are necessary for maximizing monocyte adhesion. Monocytes adhere to hydroxylated polystyrene surfaces in the presence of C3-depleted human serum. These observations sugest that adhesion of monocytes to membrane surfaces is not necessarily limited to complement-activating materials. Our knowledge about the state of plasma proteins physically adsorbed to well-defined surfaces is relatively primitive. To further complicate interpretation, reused dialyzers probably present to the bloodstream an interface comprised of totally denatured plasma proteins (32). Beyond providing sites for complement activation, the manner in which such an interface interacts with circulating blood cells is unknown.

Endotoxin which permeates across the membrane (25) is shown interacting only with phagocytes in Figure 2 for clarity. In fact, endotoxin and other dialysate contaminants of microbial origin interact with virtually everything represented in Figure 4 and more. Endotoxin stimulates the coagulation, complement (classical and alternate pathways), kinin, and fibrinolytic systems. Following stimulation by endotoxin, platelets aggregate and degranulate, granulocytes become more adherent, degranulate, and increase their bactericidal activity, monocytes secrete cytokines, platelet activating factor, and arachidonic acid metabolites, and endothelial cells increase their adhesiveness for circulating leukocytes (33–36).

The net effect of all of these interactions is to return in the venous blood line going to the patient a multitude of activated cells and chemical mediators which may act on other cellular and humoral effector systems, locally or systemically. With our current knowledge it is not possible to predict the consequences of this periodic shower of hiologically active species. For example, intercellular communication between immune cells is very complex and exhibits several important characteristics, including redundancy, synergy, and cooperation (37). Furthermore, the effect of any single agent may depend on the totality of the signals presented. Lastly, the activated cells and chemical mediators induced by ESRD therapy are superimposed on abnormalities attributable to uremia, for example the various defects in both humoral and cellular immune responses recognized in non-dialyzed uremics (38).

CONCLUDING PERSPECTIVES

One measure of the dialysis membrane is how effectively it contributes to the basic hemodialyzer mission of mass exchange. The combination of improved format and geometry, particularly thin-walled hollow fibers, and the large-pore structure of the hydrophobic materials has lead to significant increases in solute transport rates. This is illustrated in Figure 5, a plot of estimated clearance *vs* permeant molecular weight for Kiil (1966), twin coil (1966), early hollow fiber (1976) and contemporary hollow fiber (1992) hemodialyzers. Small molecule clearances have

IMPROVEMENT IN DIALYZER PERFORMANCE

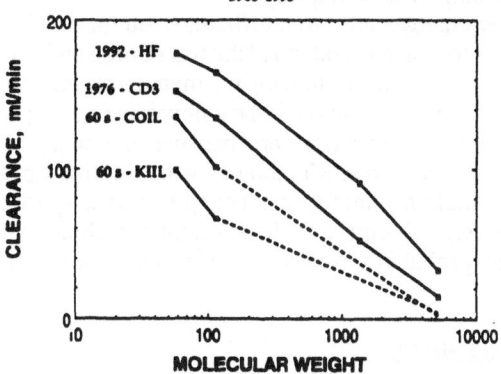

Figure 5. Increased transport efficiency in hemodialyzers since 1963. Lines (bottom to top) show estimated clearance *vs* molecular weight of Kiil dialyzers (~1966), coils from the same period, for early hollow fiber dialyzers (mid-1970s), and for contemporary hollow fibers. Dotted lines are estimates. Redrawn from reference (39) with permission.

doubled at equivalent blood flow rates (200 ml/min), and this is probably an underestimate of actually-realized improvements since blood flow rates are now more typically 300 ml/min. Large solute clearances have increased by an order of magnitude although accurate estimates of this parameter for early-stage hemodialyzers are not available. Overall, improvements in membranes have lead to a quadrupling of device efficiency and an even greater increase in the rate of middle molecule clearance.

What then of the future? One factor which may drive change is the growing concern over the environmental impact of even life-saving medical technologies. Membranes are vulnerable to environmental concerns. Their manufacture involves large quantities of water and caustic or toxic solvents. Moreover, a single hemodialysis session generates considerable biohazards which must be incinerated. This produces gaseous pollutants from polymers containing chlorine (e.g., PVC), sulfur (polysulfone), or nitrogen (e.g., polyacrylonitrile, polyamide). Reuse, while limiting source pollution, creates large quantities of aqueous wastes containing toxins or potentially toxic effluents which are rarely treated before being discharged. None of these considerations are appropriate in the early stages of development of a heroic life-saving technique. But they could become important in a therapy which is routinely applied 70 million times per year. The manufacture of membranes by low polluting processes or of hemodialyzers from environmentally friendly materials would have enormous appeal to the green movement. Development of a fluid cycler containing a permanent nondisposable dialyzing element made from ceramic or metallic membranes, which could be thermally depyrogenated and autoclaved *in situ* between uses, is within current technological reach and has the potential for destablizing the *status quo*.

Other changes are more difficult to endorse. The hollow fiber format has withstood the test of time and become firmly entrenched in the industry manufacturing culture. Devices incorporating secondary flow have never proven productive in hemodialyzers because boundary layers are already very low. Membranes with reactive surfaces, either containing anticoagulant or sorbents for a particular species (e.g., β_2-micro globulin) remain technically feasible but probably too expensive for routine use (39).

REFERENCES

1. Lonsdale HK: The growth of membrane techology. *J Membr Sci* 10: 81, 1982
2. Pusch W, Walch A: Synthetic membranes – preparation, structure, and applications. *Angew Chem* 21: 685, 1982
3. Ward RA, Feldhoff PW, Klein E: Membrane materials for therapeutic applications. in *Materials Science of Synthetic Membranes*, edited by Lloyd DR, ACS Symp Series. Washington, American Chemical Society, 1985 No 269, p 100
4. Goehl H, Konstantin P: Membranes and filters for hemofiltration. in *Hemofiltration*, edited by Henderson LW, Quellhorst EA, Baldamus CA, Lysaght M, Berlin, Springer, 1986, p 1211
5. Colton CK: Technical foundations of renal prosthesis. in: *Uremia Therapy - Perspectives for the Next Quarter Century*, edited by Gurland HJ, Berlin, Springer, 1987, p 187
6. von Sengbusch G, Lemke HD, Vienken J: Evolution of membrane technology; possibilities and consequences. in *Uremia Therapy – Perspectives for the Next Quarter Century*, edited by Gurland HJ, Berlin, Springer, 1987, p 187
7. Lysaght MJ: Hemodialysis membranes in transition. in *Nephrology and Dialysis Update*, edited by D'Amico G, Colasanti G, Contrib Nephrol, Vol 61, Basel, Karger, 1988, p 1
8. Strathmann H, Goehl H: Membranes for blood purification – state of the art and new developments. in *Terminal Renal Failure: Therapeutic Problems, Possibilities, and Potentials*, edited by Klinkmann H, Smeby LC, Contrib Nephrol, Vol 78, Basel, Karger, 1990, p 119
9. Lysaght MJ, Baurmeister U: *Dialysis*. Kirk Othmer Encyclopedia of Chemical Technology, ed 4. 1993, Vol 8, p 59
10. Vienken J: Biocompatibility: what role does the haemodialysis membrane play? *Biocompatibility Monograph EDTNA/ERCA* 1993, 7
11. Radovich JM: Composition of polymer membranes for therapies of end stage renal disease. in *Dialysis Membranes: Structure and Predictions*, edited by Bonomini V, Berland Y, Contrib Nephrol, Vol 113, Basel, Karger, 1995, p 11
12. Kolff WJ, Berk HT: De kunstmatige nier, een dialysator met groot oppervlak. *Ned Tijdschr Geneeskd* 87: 1684, 1943
13. Abel JJ, Rowntree LG, Turner BB: On the removal of diffusable substances from the circulation of living animals by dialysis. *J Pharmacol Exp Ther* 5: 275, 1914
14. Thalhimer W: Experimental exchange transfusions for reducing azotemia. Use of artificial kidney for this purpose. *Proc Soc Exp Biol Med* 641, 1937
15. Colton CK: A review of the development and performance of hemodialyzers. Special report of the AKCUP-NIAMD, 1967. Fed Clearinghouse Accession No PB 183-281
16. Ofsthun NJ, Colton CK, Lysaght MJ: Determinants of fluid and solute removal rates during hemofiltration. in *Hemofiltration*, edited by Henderson LW, Quellhorst EA, Baldamus CA, Lysaght MJ, New York, Springer-Verlag, 1986, p 17
17. Colton CK, Lowrie EG: Hemodialysis: physical principles and technical considerations. in *The Kidney*, 2nd ed, edited by Brenner BM, Rector FC, Vol II, Philadelphia, WB Saunders, 1981, p 2425
18. Colton CK, Smith KA, Merrill EW, Farrell PC: Permeability studies with cellulosic membranes. *J Biomed Materials Research* 5: 459, 1971
19. Klein E, Buffaloe G, Colton CK et al.: Evaluation of hemodialyzers and dialysis membranes. Nat Inst of Arthritis, Metabolism, and Digestive Diseases, NIH (1977). DHEW Publication No (NIH) 77-1294. Also, *Artificial Organs* 1: 21, 1977
20. Colton CK, Ward RA, Shaldon S: Scientific basis for assessment of biocompatibility in extracorporeal blood treatment. *Nephrol Dial Transplant* 9 (Suppl 2): 11, 1994
21. Lane DA, Bowry SK: Scientific basis for selection of measures of thrombogeneticity. *Nephrol Dial Transplant* 9 (Suppl 2): 18, 1994
22. Johnson R: Complement activation during extracorporeal therapy: biochemistry, cell biology and clinical relevance. *Nephrol Dial Transplant* 9 (Suppl 2): 36, 1994
23. Ward RA: The use phagocytic cell function as an index of biocompatibility. *Nephrol Dial Transplant* 9 (Suppl 2): 9, 46
24. Goetze O: The role of basophilic leukocytes and mast cells. *Nephrol Dial Transplant* 9 (Suppl 2): 57, 1994
25. Colton CK: Analysis of membrane processes for blood purification. *Blood Purif* 5: 202, 1987
26. Baier RE, Dutton RC: Initial events in interaction of blood with foreign surfaces. *J Biomed Mater Res* 3: 191, 1969
27. Vroman L: The life of an artificial device in contact with blood: initial events and their effect on its final state. *Bull NY Acad Med* 64: 352, 1988
28. Brash JL, Scott CF, ten Hove P, Wojciechowski P, Colman RW: Mechanism of transient adsorption of fibrinogen from plasma to solid surfaces: role of the contact and fibrinolytic systems. *Blood* 71: 932, 1988
29. Saltzman EW, Merrill EW: Interaction of blood with artificial surfaces. in *Hemostatis and Thrombosis*, 2nd ed., edited by Colman RW, Hirsh J, Maider VJ, Salzmon EW, New York, Lippincott, 1987, p 1335
30. Patarroyo M, Prieto J, Beatty PG, Clark EA, Gatimberg CG: Adhesion-mediating molecules of human monocytes. *Cell Immunol* 113: 278, 1988
31. Anderson JM, Bonfield TL, Ziats NP: Protein adsorption and cellular adhesion and activation on biomedical polymers. *Int J Artif Organs* 13: 375, 1990
32. Shaldon S: Dialyzer reuse: a practice that should be abandoned. *Semin Dial* 6: 11, 1993
33. Morrison DC, Ulevitch RJ: The effects of bacterial endotoxins on host mediation systems. *Am J Pathol* 93: 525, 1978

3: Membranes for Hemodialysis

34. Kreger VE, Craben DE, McCabe WR: Gram-negative bacteremia. IV. Reevaluation of clinical features and treatment in 612 patients. *Am J Med* 68: 344, 1980

35. Duma RJ: Gram-negative bacillary infections: pathogenic and pathophysiologic correlates. *Am J Med* 78: 154, 1985

36. Morrison DC, Ulevitch RJ: Endotoxins and disease mechanisms. *Ann Rev Med* 38: 417, 1987

37. Nany CA, Green SJ, Leiby DL et al.: Intercellular communication: macrophages and cytokines. in *Molecular Aspects of Immune Response and Infectious Diseases*, edited by Kiyoni H, Jinllo E, Desimone C, New York, Raven Press, 1990, p 47

38. Tetta C, Camussi G, Mariano F, Triolo G, Vercellone A: Immunomodulation and biomaterials. *Biomat Art Cells & Immob Biotech* 21: 253, 1993

39. Lysaght MJ: Evolution of hemodialysis membranes. in *Dialysis Membranes: Structure and Predictions*, edited by Bonomini V, Berland Y, Contrib Nephrol, Vol 113, Basel, Karger, 1995, p 1

BIOPHYSICS OF ULTRAFILTRATION AND HEMOFILTRATION

LEE W. HENDERSON

INTRODUCTION

Removal of excess body water is an important function of both the artificial kidney and peritoneal dialysis. More recently, solute removal in conjunction with ultrafiltration has been exploited as an alternative to diffusion as a means for cleaning uremic blood. This chapter deals with the practical and theoretical aspects of ultrafiltration and convective mass transfer across the artificial kidney and peritoneal mass transfer barriers.

THEORETICAL BACKGROUND

Hemodialysis

When a concentration gradient exists across a semipermeable membrane, both solute and water tend with time to move in a direction to discharge that gradient. For a single-component system, solute and water move in opposite directions across the membrane to achieve equilibrium. The gradient may be expressed in terms emphasizing the solute (e.g. number of milligrams per deciliter of solute on side A, minus that number on side B) or in terms emphasizing the water (e.g. number of milliosmoles on side A, minus that number on side B). Osmolality indicates the number of solute particles per kilogram of water. Alternatively, osmolality may be conceptualized as the number of water molecules per kilogram of solution, i.e. the 'concentration of water'. While the concentration of water is not commonly spoken about by physical chemists, it may be helpful conceptually to understand the intimate events in the small domain of the water filled channels in dialysis membranes.

There are two ways that a concentration gradient for water may be achieved: osmotically and hydrostatically. For artificial kidney membranes both osmotic and hydrostatic (hydraulic) force may be used to cause ultrafiltration, i.e. the separation of plasma water from macromolecular constituents such as protein and cellular elements. For reasons that will become apparent hydrostatic force is the more effective.

An equation that relates ultrafiltration rate to these forces is frequently written

$$J_f = Q_f/A = L_p(\Delta P + \Delta\pi). \qquad [1]$$

Ultrafiltration rate per unit area of membrane = (permeability of membrane to water) × (hydrostatic force + osmotic force) where J_f = the volume flux rate per unit membrane area across the membrane for water (ml/min/cm^2);[1] L_p = the hydraulic permeability of the membrane for water, i.e. the volumetric flow rate of water per unit area of membrane per unit pressure gradient (ml/min/cm^2/mmHg); Q_f = flow rate of ultrafiltrate (ml/min); A = area of the membrane (cm^2); ΔP = the hydraulic pressure gradient from blood path to dialysis fluid path (mmHg); $\Delta\pi$ = the osmotic pressure gradient from blood path to dialysis fluid path (mmHg); $\Delta\pi$ is frequently expressed as mOsm/l and may be converted to mmHg using 1.0 mOsm ≈ 19 mmHg.

The hydrostatic and osmotic forces are summed in this equation, since with hemodialysis there is a deliberate,

---

[1] Because ml = cm^3 the unit expression can be reduced to that of a velocity, i.e. cm/min.

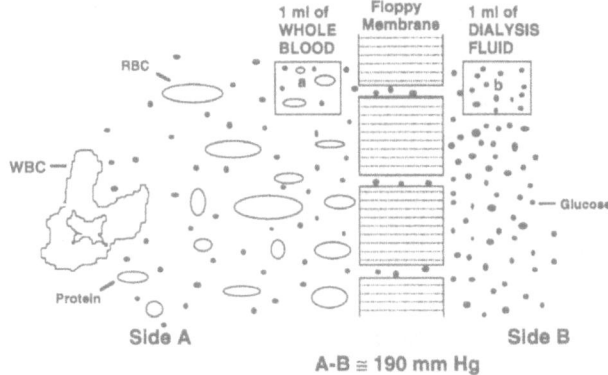

Figure 1. Diagram of a semipermeable membrane dividing whole blood (side A) and dialysis fluid (side B). Glucose (anhydrous) is present on side B at 280 mg/dl (15.6 mmol/l). The pores in the membrane are too small to allow passage of cell elements and protein. An osmolar gradient from A to B of approximately 190 mmHg is shown diagrammatically in 1 ml control volumes, a and b, where the amount of water per milliliter of solution is greater in a than in b (see text for further discussion). .

usually hydrostatic, gradient favoring water movement from blood to dialysate. When isotonic dialysis fluid is used, the osmotic pressure provided by the plasma proteins favors water movement from the dialysis solution to the blood and the contribution of $\Delta\pi$ to J_f is negative. The two forces, $\Delta\pi$ and ΔP, may be examined conceptually for an artificial kidney membrane with the aid of Figures 1 and 2. Consider Figure 1 showing two perfectly mixed solutions (blood and dialysis fluid) separated by a membrane that contains homogeneously distributed water filled pores (drawn in cross section as right circular cylinders). Further, the membrane is perfectly semipermeable with respect to blood proteins and formed elements. That is, no cells or protein traverse the pores which have a diameter that is too small to accommodate these comparatively large molecules and even larger blood cells. Figure 1 shows the events at the pore when an osmotically active solute such as glucose (as anhydrous d-glucose, mass – 180 Daltons) is present in high concentration (280 mg/dl – 15.6 mmol/l) on the dialysis fluid side of the membrane (side B). As noted, the 'concentration' of water is inversely related to the concentration of solute. That is, for a given volume of solution the greater number of dissolved solute particles (molecules, ions) the fewer number of water molecules can be present. The osmolality of the plasma in the present example is 300 mOsm/l. Figure 1 depicts the instant after these two solutions appear on each side of the membrane. Further, there is no difference in hydrostatic pressure across the membrane (consider the membrane 'floppy', such that no hydrostatic pressure gradient can be sustained). At this instant, there is a concentration gradient for water across the pores from A to B. The magnitude of this pressure gradient is 10 mOsm/l or 190 mmHg (1.0 mOsm/l – 19 mmHg). Water moves

very swiftly to discharge such concentration gradients. Water rarely, if ever, moves primarily by single molecule diffusion,[2] but rather by 'bulk' or 'plug' flow in which movement of 'blocks' of water occur much as you would consider the movement of pure water in a pipe when an inlet to outlet pressure gradient is applied. It is apparent that in subsequent instants this rather straightforward conceptualization becomes much more complicated. To cite some of the events, glucose is small enough to move by diffusion down its concentration gradient from B to A reducing the osmotic driving force; further, the water arriving on side B reduces the glucose concentration adjacent to the membrane lengthening the diffusion path over which the concentration gradients apply and slowing their discharge. Further, protein, a macromolecular structure present in solution on the blood side (A), cannot cross the membrane and will exert an osmotic effect (oncotic pressure) favoring water reabsorption from side B, the dialysate. Finally, ionic charges on the solute particles and the requirement for electroneutrality across the membrane will modulate the movement of electrolytes in response to their concentration gradient.

Before moving to a somewhat more rigorous description, it is helpful to consider a comparable conceptualization for the circumstance in which an hydraulic (hydrostatic) pressure gradient exists. Figure 2 depicts a rigid membrane with blood on side A and dialysis fluid on side B. As in the previous example, the composition of electrolytes in plasma water and dialysis fluid are identical as are the measured osmolalities. For this example there is no difference in glucose concentration. The plunger on side A exerts 190 mmHg of hydrostatic pressure. A single pore in the membrane is depicted in the lower part of Figure 2. The higher hydrostatic pressure on side A is a measure of the greater number of bombardments per second of solute and solvent particles on a given surface area of the container, one surface of which is our semipermeable membrane. An 'average' water molecule just outside the pore in the membrane is shown for each side. The average magnitude and direction of water molecule movement is given by the vector arrows. In the bulk phase of solution outside the pore such motion is random and is schematically shown in Figure 2 as four arrows of equal length reflecting the sums of all intermediate vectors for each quadrant. The greater number of bombardments at the pore entrance on side A, as opposed to that on side B, results in a net movement of water from A to B through the pore. It should be noted that solute particles that are small enough not to be hindered by the pore, (the pore diameter being substantially larger than the hydrated radius of the solute), will move with the water. This is because the frictional forces between water and the solute particle substantially exceed those between the solute particle and the walls of the pore. This convectiive movement of solutes along with water through

---

[2] Tritiated water in a beaker can distribute by single molecule diffusion.

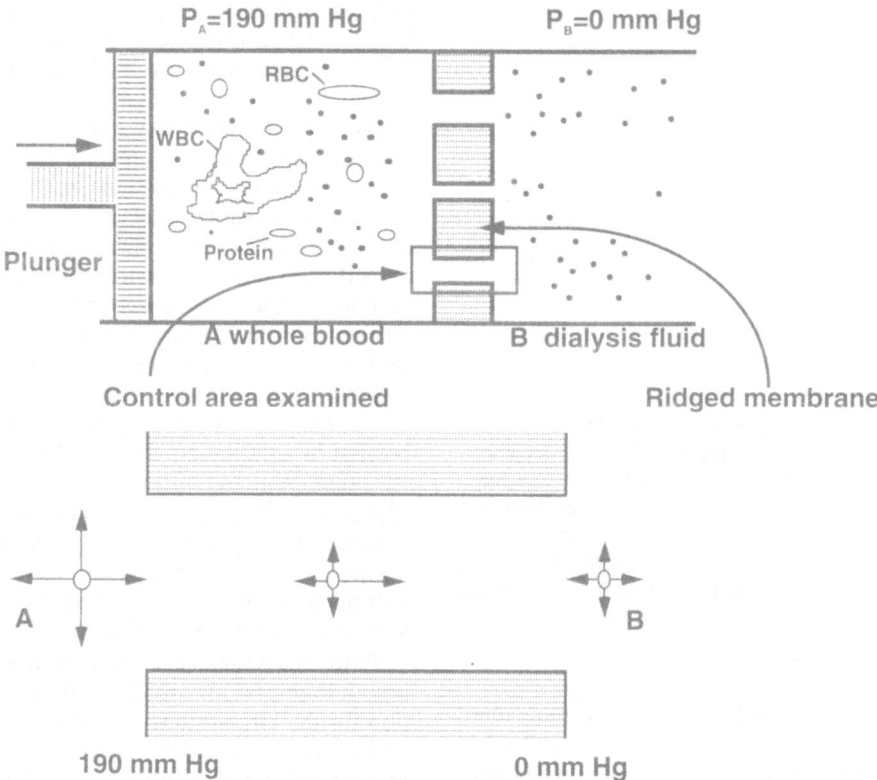

Figure 2. Diagram of a rigid membrane dividing whole blood (side A) and iso-osmolar dialysis fluid (side B). A piston on side A provides 190 mmHg pressure on the whole blood. A single pore in the membrane is depicted below. An average water molecule just outside each end of the pore is depicted as an open circle (○). Vectors for the random motion of these molecules are given. The length of the vector depicts the number of water molecules moving in the direction indicated. An imbalance in the vectors within the pore is such that more water molecules are moving into the pore from side A than from side B with resultant net flow from A to B down the length of the pore. For simplicity, the pore is depicted to be free of solute. See text for interaction between hydrostatic and osmotic fluid movement.

a membrane in response to a pressure gradient (osmotic or hydrostatic) is termed 'solvent drag'. If the membrane does not hinder solute transport and the solute passes unrestrained across the membrane, then the terms 'bulk', 'plug' or 'Poiseuillien' flow describe the event. Of course, in the present example protein and cellular elements are blocked from crossing the membranes by pore size restriction resulting in a change in the solute concentration of plasma water as the ultrafiltrate is formed.

Osmotic and hydrostatic forces, while commonly considered to give the same result in terms of water movement, differ in an important respect. In order for a solute to exert sustained osmotic force it is necessary for the solute particle to be of such a size that there is resistance to its movement through the channels in the membrane. The hydrated radius of the solute then must approach the mean radius of the pores in the membrane. For a small solute such as glucose, only membranes containing pores with radii near in size to that of glucose participate in the osmotically driven generation of ultrafiltrate. Treating these channels as a parallel array of right circular cylinders

or pores has proven useful in simplifying the arithmetic commonly employed to describe them but must not be considered an accurate description of the actual physical circumstance. In a membrane with heterogeneously dispersed pore sizes it will mean that pores with radii substantially larger than the diameter of the glucose molecule do not participate in the osmotically driven flow of water. Quite the contrary would be true for an hydrostatic driving force as water flow through a pore is directly proportional to the fourth power of the radius (r) of that pore, i.e. r^4. As such, large pores dominate in conducting hydrostatic ultrafiltration.

Let us return now to equation 1, and a more formal description of the above events. In general, the hydraulic pressure gradient of equation 1 (ΔP) may be taken as the average blood path pressure (P_B) minus the dialysate path pressure (P_D). These values are routinely measured in most artificial kidney machines. The osmotic pressure gradient is somewhat more complicated to compute. Van 't Hoff's Law of Osmotic Pressure adequately describes the osmotic pressure difference between two adjacent solutions (eg blood and dialysis fluid) at their interface and in the absence of a membrane:

$$\Delta\pi = \left[\sum_{j=1}^{m} C_j^B - \sum_{j=1}^{n} C_j^D \right] \qquad [2]$$

where B and D identify blood and dialysis fluid and $\sum_{j=1}^{m} C_j^B$ = the sum $(1 + 2 + 3 \ldots m)$ of the concentrations[3] of all solute particles in blood (B); $\sum_{j=1}^{n} C_j^D$ = the sum of the concentrations of all solute particles in dialysis fluid (D); T = the temperature in degrees Kelvin; R = the gas constant = 0.0623 when units of (liter × mmHG/mmol × degree) are used.

However, we wish to compute the $\Delta\pi$ across a semipermeable membrane. An ideal semipermeable membrane permits permeation of one species, e.g. water, with no resistance while blocking entry to all other species, e.g. protein. Conventional cellulosic dialysis membranes may be considered to be ideally semipermeable for water and protein. In the dialysis setting, however, there are a host of other osmotically active solutes, most of which diffuse across the membrane. To assess the contribution a given solute makes to the overall transmembrane osmotic pressure gradient, it is necessary to know how readily it permeates the membrane compared to water in response to an applied hydraulic pressure gradient. This may be expressed as

$$C_f = \frac{N}{Q_f} = C_s(1 - \varepsilon), \qquad [3]$$

where N = the net flux rate of solute movement across the membrane (moles/min); Q_f = the net flux rate of water movement across the membrane (ml/min); C_f = the solute concentration in the ultrafiltrate (moles/ml); C_s = the concentration of the solute in the solution to be ultrafiltered (moles/ml; ε = a property of the membrane/solute system termed the 'rejection coefficient' and is a measure of the degree to which the membrane restrains movement of the solute under a given set of experimental conditions. This restraint may either be physical, electrostatic, or both, depending on whether pore size and/or charge on the membrane impact on the solute particle size and/or charge. If the membrane pore is much larger than both the water molecule and the solute particle, both will traverse the membrane without hindrance, and the ultrafiltrate's concentration (C_f)

$$C_f = \frac{N}{Q_f} \qquad [4]$$

---

[3] Partially or completely dissociated electrolytes contribute more solute particles to the solution than their molar concentration would identify. For example, NaCl at concentrations used in dialysis fluid, dissociates almost completely into its constituent ions, providing nearly double the number of osmotically active particles that would be expected from the molality and Avogadro's number.

is unchanged from the retentate, i.e. the concentration of the solution does not change as it crosses the membrane. In this instance

$$C_f = C_s$$

and by equations (3) and (4)

$$\varepsilon = 0 = \text{rejection coefficient}.$$

For protein, which is completely rejected by the membrane, however,

$$\varepsilon = 1.$$

The rejection coefficient, therefore, will have values that range from zero to 1, depending on the degree of stearic or electrostatic hindrance presented by the membrane to the hydrated solute particle. At times, it is more convenient to refer to the sieving coefficient (S) of a membrane for a given solute:

$$\varepsilon = 1 - S \qquad [5]$$

$$S = \frac{C_f}{C_s}. \qquad [6]$$

The Van 't Hoff equation applied across the membrane may be written using Staverman's reflection coefficient (σ), which may be considered the measure of a membrane's 'semipermeability' for a given solute. The reflection coefficient is closely related to, but different from the rejection coefficient (ε)[4]

$$\Delta\pi = RT\sigma_j \left[\sum_{j=1}^{m} C_j^B - \sum_{j=1}^{n} C_j^D \right] \qquad [7]$$

or, converting concentration terms for each side of the membrane into osmolar gradients we have the more useful

$$\Delta\pi = \sum_{j=1}^{n} (\Delta\pi_j \sigma_j) \qquad [8]$$

$$= (\Delta\pi_1 \sigma_1) + (\Delta\pi_2 \sigma_2) + \ldots \text{etc.} \qquad [9]$$

---

[4] ε is readily measured during clinical or bench experiments with ultrafiltration. It may be considered a phenomenologic parameter that will be reflective of such things as the rate of flow (velocity) of the solution through the membrane, the mixing present at the membrane surface as well as the pore structure of the membrane. σ on the other hand must be computed from ε values taking into account these phenomenologic parameters. As such, σ is an intrinsic property of the membrane/solute pair and remains a constant number over a wide range of operating conditions. S, ε and σ are dimensionless (i.e. do not have a unit of measure). The relationship between ε and σ is analogous to the relationship between dialyzer solute clearance, which depends on experimental conditions, and mass transfer resistance (R_m), an intrinsic property of the membrane/solute pair.

Equation 1 may now be written more precisely as

$$Q_f = AL_p(\Delta P + \sum_{j=1}^{n} \Delta\pi_j\sigma_j). \qquad [10]$$

Under carefully controlled conditions the concentration of the ultrafiltrate C_f not only depends on σ, but, as has been shown by Spiegler and Kadem (1) and expressed in equation 11, varies with the volume flow rate J_f (ml/min/cm^2) of ultrafiltrate.

$$C_f = \frac{J_s}{J_f} = (1 - \varepsilon)C_s, \qquad [11]$$

where J_s is the solute flux rate (mol/min/cm^2). ε then may be related to σ using the Spiegler equation (2):

$$\varepsilon = \sigma\frac{\varepsilon^\beta - 1}{\varepsilon^\beta - \sigma}, \qquad [12]$$

where $\beta = J_f(l - \sigma)/P_m$ and P_m = the diffusive permeability of the membrane for the solute considered (cm/min).

When J_f is very large, compared to P_m, convection dominates and ε approaches σ.

When J_f is very small, compared to P_m, diffusion dominates and ε approaches $J_f\sigma/P_m$.[5]

These relationships of ε and σ point out that the difference between σ, the intrinsic property of the membrane/solute pair, and ε the phenomenologic coefficient, may be considered as the contribution made by diffusive transport toward the observed net movement of the solute. Diffusion of solute across the filtering membrane will lessen the amount of measured rejection, thus requiring that ε will always be less than σ.

The ultrafiltration rate in the human glomerulus and capillary beds, such as that in the splanchnic circulation, interestingly, are dominated by oncotic pressure. The importance of oncotic pressure lies not in its magnitude, which is small in absolute terms (1 to 1.5 mOsm/l or 19 to 28 mmHg), but rather because it is asymmetrically present (interstitium to lumen) and is nearly equal to the hydraulic pressure gradient (lumen to interstitium) across the capillary wall. As such, it plays a major role in modulating the flow rate of water across the membrane. By contrast, in the artificial kidney, under usual operating conditions (where length averaged transmembrane pressure ranges from 20 to 250 mmHg), hydraulic pressure (ΔP) almost invariably exceeds oncotic pressure and oncotic pressure is commonly neglected in calculating the membrane ultrafiltration rate. Unlike protein, small solutes present in dialysis fluid or in uremic plasma (e.g. glucose and urea) contribute substantially to the osmolality of the solution (25 to 100 mOsm/l or 475 to 1900 mmHg), but cause less

---

[5] In the engineering literature this dimensionless ratio is referred to as the Peclet number.

water flux across the membrane than would larger solutes of similar osmolality because their reflection coefficient across cellophane are significantly less than unity. The peritoneal membrane turns out to be surprisingly 'tight' ($S = 0.4 \pm 0.04$) for glucose, and this coupled with the use of high concentrations of glucose in the dialysis fluid (4.25%) make it the major driving force for fluid flow in peritoneal dialysis.

Peritoneal dialysis

A detailed description of the peritoneum appears in Chapter 5. Concepts of the peritoneal mass transfer resistance have recently become more complex with both the invoking of models that comprise capillaries uniformly distributed within supporting interstitium, the so called distributed model (3, 4), and the postulating of two functional barriers to transport configured in series (5) to better explain the performance of this 'membrane'. In addition, the role of the lymphatics in both water and solute transport must now be taken into account (6–8). To begin with, our analysis considers the peritoneal membrane as the domain that separates the bulk phase of plasma water from that of well-mixed dialysis fluid. Such a description then comprises both the anatomical structures such as the vascular endothelium and mesothelium, and in addition, all of their attendant unstirred layers. Unlike hemodialysis, ultrafiltration across the peritoneal membrane is accomplished almost exclusively by osmotic force.

The peritoneal membrane is not perfectly semipermeable (i.e. is somewhat leaky) for the solutes to be considered, making rigorous quantitation of the driving force for ultrafiltration more complicated. Glucose moves across the peritoneal membrane by diffusion at a rate consonant with its rather small size (180 Daltons). Protein molecules such as albumin (69,000 Daltons) traverse the peritoneal membrane to a small extent.

As noted for the artificial kidney, the peritoneal membrane is not ideally semipermeable for a host of solutes and the correction factor (σ) for each solute concentration gradient ($\Delta\pi$) must be applied to adjust that gradient for the degree of the membrane's 'semipermeability' for that solute. Analogous to equation 10 for artificial membranes these concepts are mathematically described as follows:

$$Q_f = AL_p(\Delta\pi_1\sigma_1 \text{ and } \Delta\pi_2\sigma_2 + \dots \text{ etc.}, \qquad [13]$$

where: $\Delta\pi_1\sigma_1$ represents the osmotic driving gradient for sodium $\Delta\pi_2 s_2$ that for potassium, etc, until each solute present on each side of the membrane is represented. This equation was previously written for the artificial kidney (equation 10) with a term to express the hydrostatic driving force resulting from the hydrostatic pressure gradient from blood to bath (ΔP). Because the peritoneal space under normal circumstances is free of significant quantities of fluid, we may reasonably assume that the flow which results from hydrostatic and oncotic forces at play across the capillary membrane from arteriolar to venular end (Starling flow) is in balance with lymphatic run off. To effect net accumulation of ultrafiltrate in the peritoneal space, these forces must be unbalanced by the osmotic force contributed by the dialysis fluid. The only hydrostatic force contributed by a 2 liter exchange added to the peritoneal space results from the elastic recoil of the abdominal wall (12–14 cm H_2O or 0.9–1.0 mmHg) or the hydrostatic head of pressure generated by the 'column' of water above the dependent portion of the peritoneal membrane, or both (8). As such, it would be expected to be small and to favor net uptake across the peritoneal membrane from 'bath to blood'. To be precise, this force must be added to equation 13 as a component of ΔP. Lastly, in considering this simplification of dropping out ΔP there is the unlikely possibility that hypertonic dialysis fluid by some mechanism may alter the afferent/efferent resistances of the peritoneal capillary bed in such a manner as to enhance the hydrostatic pressure gradient thereby causing increased ultrafiltration. Solutes that were equal or nearly equal in concentration on both sides of the membrane would, of course, contribute little or no driving force for ultrafiltration. Solutes such as glucose, urea and protein, which by therapeutic intent or biological circumstance will have significant concentration gradients across the membrane, may contribute significant osmotic driving force.

To understand just how much (or even relatively how much) force for ultrafiltration across the peritoneal membrane would be contributed by a given solute (for example, when glucose is contrasted with protein or urea) requires further exploration of the term σ and an appreciation that the larger the molecular weight of a solute, the less likely it is to be present in biologic solutions at a concentration that contributes much to the total osmolality. Albumin, for example, has a reasonable high σ. That is to say, albumin moves through the membrane with difficulty. It is commonly present in the plasma at a concentration of 3.5 g/dl. Taking a low average molecular mass (for ease of calculation and remembrance) of 60,000 and assuming $\sigma = 1$, the osmolar contribution of albumin to resisting movement of plasma water into the peritoneal space is only

$$\frac{35 \text{ g/kg } H_2O}{60000} = 0.006 \text{ Osm/kg } H_2O$$

$$= 0.6 \text{ mOsm/kg } H_2O = 11 \text{ mmHg}$$

On the other hand, glucose (dextrose monohydrate), at a concentration of 1.5 or 4.25 g/dl in the dialysis fluid[6] and 100 mg/dl in plasma, would contribute a maximum potential osmolar driving gradient for ultrafiltration of either

---

[6] Dextrose (d-glucose) is added to dialysis solution to provide an osmotic gradient for ultrafiltration. Expressed as d-glucose · H_2O (dextrose monohydrate, 198 Daltons), the concentrations are 1.5 g/dl or 4.25 g/dl, whereas the concentrations of dextrose anhydrous are 1.36 and 3.86 g/dl.

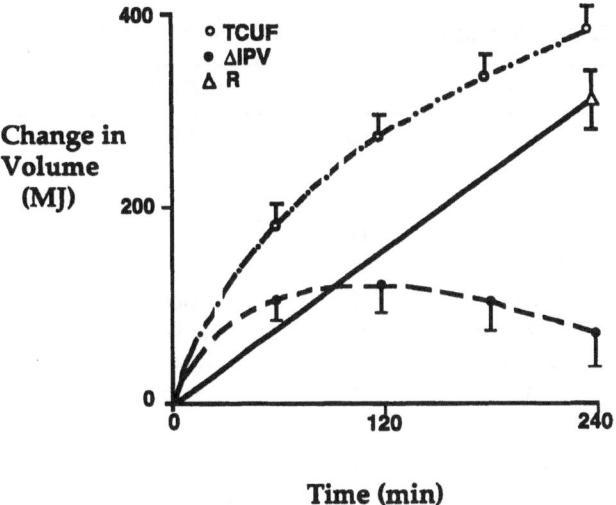

Figure 3. The respective contributions to overall peritoneal volume over time (ΔIPV) during an hypertonic exchange from transcapillary ultrafiltration (TCUF) and reabsorption of fluid into the lymphatic channels and interstitial space (R).

70 mOsm (1330 mmHg) or 209 mOsm (3987 mmHg). This maximum is never manifested, however, because σ for dextrose across the peritoneal membrane is less than unity. Furthermore, with time, the concentration gradient deteriorates. The two components that discharge this gradient are diffusion of dextrose into the plasma and convection of water countercurrent to the flow of dextrose. Clinically, the net movement of water is obtained as the difference between inflow and outflow volumes. As such, it represents an average value. Fluid reabsorption into lymph channels and the interstitial spaces from the cavity (not commonly measured) modulates this net movement of water (6–8).

Figure 3, taken from Krediet et al. (9) shows the respective contributions of transcapillary ultrafiltration, net reabsorption (lymphatic uptake plus backfiltration into the interstitial space) to overall peritoneal volume over time in 9 study subjects, measured using indicator dilution technique with dextran 70 as described by Pust et al. (10, 11).

Note that reabsorption of ultrafiltrate from the peritoneal cavity may reduce net ultrafiltration by as much as 50%. At present, there is rather limited information about σ for the peritoneal membrane and the various solutes that are present in the peritoneal dialysis system (i.e. soluble constituents of uremic plasma water and dialysis fluid) (5, 12, 13–21). As with hemodialysis, what is usually measured clinically is the sieving coefficient (equation 6) or rejection coefficient (ε) as described in equations 5 and 6. Table 1 lists these values for several relevant solutes. To gain insight into the relationship between the rejection coefficient and Staverman's reflection coefficient for the peritoneal membrane where direct measurements are

Table 1. Sieving and reflection coefficients measured for the adult human peritoneal membrane[a]

Solute	Daltons	Hydrated radius (Å)	S ± SEM	1 − σ (range)	Ref.
Urea	60	2.7	0.81 ± 0.03		18
			0.63 ± 0.06[c]		21
				0.82 (0.9–0.73)	12
Creatinine	113	–	0.57 ± 0.09[c]	0.67 (0.83–0.51)	21
Uric acid	168	–	–	0.63 (0.83–0.54)	12
Chloride	35	3.86	0.78 ± 0.2	–	19
Potassium	37	3.96	0.36 ± 0.2	–	20
Dextrose	180	4.4	0.40 ± 0.04[c]	0.62 (0.82–0.57)	21
Sodium	23	5.12	0.54 ± 0.2	–	19
			0.56 ± 0.04[c]		
Inulin	5,200	12.0	0.83 ± 0.04	0.63 (0.91–0.30)	18
			0.41 ± 0.08[c]		
Albumin	69,000	35.5	< 0.02	–	a

[a] See text for explanation.
[b] S = sieving coefficient (± one standard error of the mean).
[c] Sieving coefficient values for these studies were obtained using 4.25% dextrose monohydrate containing solutions, a 30 min dwell and 20 min drain time. The other values reported are for 7% soution, a 30 min dwell and 30 min drain time.

difficult to make, consider the following empirical formulation. With reference to equations 11 and 12:

— When J_f is large, ε approaches σ as a limit.
— When J_f is small, ε approaches $J_f\sigma/P_m$, the Peclet number, as a limit.

A reasoned estimate for the functional area (vs anatomic area) of the peritoneal membrane, participating in the transport process, is 0.5 m² (22). The maximum net ultrafiltration rate measured at the onset of a 4.25% exchange when the glucose gradient is greatest, ranges from 12 to 16 ml/min (23). Adding substantial fluid reabsorption (see Figure 3) might raise the 'true' maximum ultrafiltration rate to 20 ml/min. 'True' in this instance refers to the ultrafiltration rate of fluid into the peritoneal space not the net amount (usually measured as drained volume) after fluid reabsorption has occurred. For the estimated membrane functional area of 0.5 m², J_f computes to 8×10^{-3} ml/min/cm², a value that would be considered 'small' in the context of equations 11 and 12, and ε approaches the Peclet number as a limit. Consider hemodialysis where a 1.0 m² hollow fiber Cuprophan® dialyzer is typically expected to remove 5 liters of excess total body water over a 4 h treatment period: $J_f \approx 2 \times 10^{-3}$ ml/min/cm². This value for Cuprophan® is of the same order of magnitude as that for peritoneal ultrafiltration and is also considered 'small'. Hence, for a given solute moving convectively across the peritoneum it is expected that $\varepsilon \approx J_f\sigma/P_m$. This relationship has been used by us and others to compute σ values from the experimental parameters of filtration flow rate (J_f) and measured rejection coefficient (ε) (12, 15).

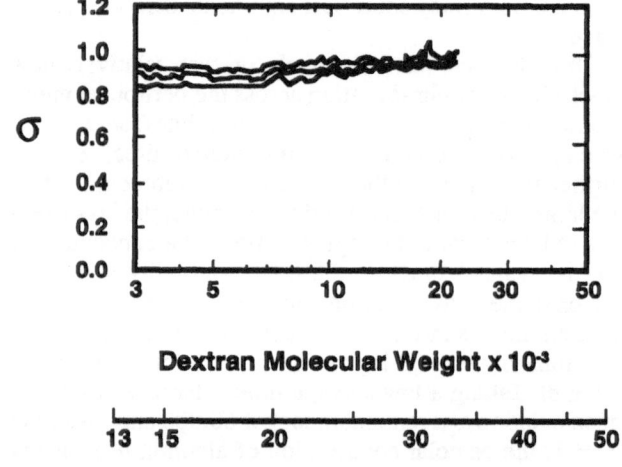

Dextran Molecular Weight x 10⁻³

Dextran Stokes Radius (Å)

Figure 4. The values for the reflection coefficient (σ) of neutral dextran for the periotneal membrane of the rabbit are plotted as a function of molecular weight and Stokes radius. The mean value is shown with bracketing curves at ±1 SEM. For reference, inulin (5,200 Daltons) has a Stokes radius of approximately 13 Å and albumin (69,000 Daltons) of 35 Å.

Figure 4 plots σ vs molecular weight in a rabbit model using neutral dextran studied in a size dispersion that corresponds in molecular size range from inulin (13 Å, 5.2 kiloDaltons [kd]) to albumin (35 Å, 69 kd). Of note are

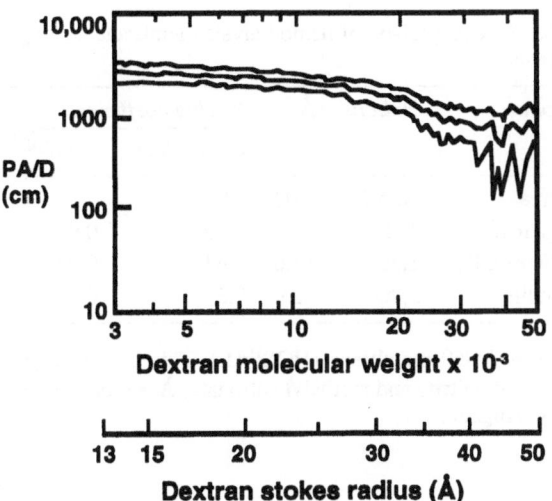

Figure 5. The overall mass transfer coefficient, or permeability-area product (PA), value for neutral dextran for the peritoneal membrane of the rabbit divided by its diffusion coefficient (D) in isotonic saline, is plotted as a function of molecular weight and Stokes radius. The mean value is shown with bracketing curves at ± 1 SEM.

the uniformly high values that are relatively independent of molecular size. This pattern points out that the peritoneal membrane of the rabbit is remarkably 'tight' when studied by ultrafiltration (5). This same surprising conclusion may be reached for human peritoneal membrane by examining Table 1, which shows that even solutes as small as urea and creatinine are held back by this membrane which is considered to be quite open when tested using diffusion-based methods. Figure 5 is a plot of the same polydispersed neutral dextran in the rabbit, but this time the experiment was conducted in order to compute the diffusive mass transference coefficient, or permeability-area product (PA). PA for each sized dextran molecule has been divided by its diffusion coefficient in water (D) in order to factor out the resistance imposed by the water present in the diffusion path traversed by a dextran molecule on its way from plasma water to dialysate. PA/D compares the rate of diffusive transport across the peritoneal membrane to that across a simple film of water of comparable thickness. The point of interest is that PA/D is independent of molecular size between 13 and 30 Å. This indicates that there is little if any size dependence of transport through these barriers. When tested by diffusion in the rabbit model, the peritoneal membrane behaves as if it were very open in its pore structure.

MODELS OF PERITONEAL TRANSPORT

There have been several efforts to reconcile this paradox of a membrane which behaves as an open membrane to diffusion and as a tight membrane to convection. One theory postulates that two pore sizes participate in such a way that when glucose is used to induce ultrafiltration, only the small (tight) pores are brought to bear. Nolph et al. (24) have laid out this theory including considerable anatomical support for the presence of two pore sizes in the peritoneal membrane. Rippe et al. (13, 14) have mathematically formulated a multiple pore model to try to fit their experimental data more closely. Conceptually, for diffusion using a dual pore model, while both small and large pores are postulated to participate, the large pores predominate making the membrane appear open to diffusion. When hypertonic solutions induce osmotically, driven convective transport, only the small pores are presumed to participate, as glucose can only exert an osmotic driving force on a pore for which it exhibits a σ of greater than zero. The large pore is postulated to exhibit a radius that is significantly larger than that of glucose for which $\sigma = 0$. In an effort to test these theoretical models, experiments were performed in the rabbit model employing intraperitoneal vacuum as the driving force for ultrafiltration. The results are at odds with an heteroporosity model of the peritoneal membrane (25, 26). With vacuum driven ultrafiltration, convective transport of water and solute should primarily occur through the large pores and, hence, σ values should be lower than for osmotically driven ultrafiltration. Hydrostatically driven transport does not show the more open pattern of transport that would be expected if heteroporosity was the full explanation. More recent work by Chen et al. (27), in which the natural hydrostatic ultrafiltration of Starling's forces across the peritoneal capillary wall has been examined and contrasted with glucose driven osmotic flux, is at odds with a heteroporous model as well. The results of these experiments do not support heteroporosity alone as an explanation for the behavior of the peritoneal transport barrier. This is not to say that mathematical models using the assumptions of a heteroporous transport barrier cannot be made to fit the experimental observations. It only raises a warning flag that should limit our acceptance of the anatomic reality of these variously sized pores.

A second effort at reconciliation of the paradox may be found in rabbit work which postulates the functional equivalent of two mass transfer resistances, coupled in series, that separate the capillary lumen from the peritoneal cavity. The anatomical candidates for these two resistances and their special characteristics are as follows. The proximal membrane would be the capillary endothelium which anatomically has been shown to be but a few microns thick (28). Its transport characteristics for diffusion would be dominated by its very thinness, recognizing that membrane permeability is proportional to the diffusivity of the solute in the membrane and inversely proportional to the thickness of the membrane (length of the diffusion path within the membrane) i.e.

$$P_m \propto \frac{D_{eff}}{L} \quad \text{or}$$

$$P_m = K_p \frac{D_{eff}}{L} \qquad\qquad [14]$$

where P_m = the permeability of the membrane for a given solute; D_{eff} = the diffusivity of the given solute within the membrane L = the length of the diffusion path (thickness of the membrane); and K_p = the partition coefficient of the solute between the bulk dialysate and the membrane.

The thinness of the capillary endothelium then would make it highly permeable. The other property of the endothelium must be that it predominantly contains pores that are 'tight'. This would serve as the dominant restraining barrier during osmotic convective transport making the peritoneal membrane appear tight when studied using convective transport.

The second or distal barrier would be the interstitium and its overlying mesothelial membrane. This barrier would have two important properties, an openness to both convective and diffusive transport and a substantial thickness (50 to 100 microns). Anatomically, this thickness has been shown to be correct (28). Diffusive transport then would display the familiar size dependence commonly reported and imposed simply by the length of the diffusion path that it adds between blood and dialysate. Little or no additional resistance would be imposed by the membrane itself, a feature compatible with the flat PA/D curve shown in Figure 5.

Should this model be anatomically correct, there are theoretical reasons (29) as to why such a dual barrier to transport should result in asymmetric functional characteristics, i.e. rectification. For convective transport from blood to dialysate the peritoneal 'membrane' should appear 'tighter' than convective transport from dialysate to blood (5). Tests of the rectifying properties of this membrane, however, were negative (30) in one experimental model. Re-examination of this animal model, in light of recent modeling studies on the rectifying properties of synthetic membranes (74, 84), calls this study design into question on grounds that the rate of ultrafiltration per unit area of membrane is likely too slow to result in rectification (unpublished observations – Zydney, Leypoldt, Henderson). More work on this problem is needed to identify which interpretation is correct.

Recent work by Flessner et al. (4) and Dedrick et al. (3) using a rat model of peritoneal dialysis puts forward a distributed model of peritoneal transport. The underlying concept of the distributed model is that for analytical purposes the capillary is 'smeared' evenly throughout the tissue considered, in this instance the peritoneal membrane. The permeability area product employed here applies to the capillary wall rather than the overall peritoneal membrane. This model shows a remarkably good degree of 'fit' with diffusive experimental data both presented by Flessner et al. and Dedrick et al. and taken from the literature (3). This model is not intended to be anatomically correct but rather to be mathematically reflective of experimental data when certain known physiological parameters are used. As of this writing there are still many uncertain-

Table 2. Comparison of hemodialysis membrane sieving coefficients

Solute	Daltons	Å	Sieving coefficients	
			Cuprophane	AN69®
Urea	60 5.1	1.00	1.00	
Sucrose	342	9.2	0.79	0.98
Vitamin B$_{12}$	1,355	14.6	0.63	0.94
Inulin	5,200	22.9	0.31	0.78

PAN = AN69 membrane (HOSPAL). This is a copolymer of polyacrylonitrile and methalyl sulfonate; Å = molecular diameter in Angstra.

ties about these models as pointed out by Leypoldt (26). This model has been extended to examine diffusive bidirectional convective transport (31). Difficulty with this model arises when the interstitial tissue and not the capillary wall is the dominant diffusive solute transport barrier. In this instance the predictions from a distributed model look like those of the dual membrane barrier model and, if anatomically valid, should display rectifying properties. As noted above, studies to confirm this property in rabbits were negative (30), raising the same concerns as noted above for the dual membrane model. Suffice it to say that several models offer a satisfactory fit of clinically derived data (4, 5, 14–16).

SIEVING COEFFICIENT MEASUREMENT

Hemodialysis

The clinical benefit is small from measuring sieving coefficients for hemodialysis membranes such as Cuprophan® which have comparatively low hydraulic permeability (approximately ten or more times less) when contrasted with hemofiltration membranes. At maximum, 5 l of excess total body water would be removed per treatment. As such, the maximum amount of urea, creatinine and other small uremic solutes to be removed would be that contained in 5 l of uremic plasma water. Furthermore, measurements by Green et al. (32) show small but significant rejection of solutes as small as sucrose (MW = 342 Daltons) by Cuprophan® (Table 2).

If the traditional concern is accepted that solutes of 500 Daltons or less, rather than 'middle molecules' are important for removal in uremia, then hemodialysis treatment may be considered to be dominated by the diffusive rather than the convective component of mass transfer. Transport of such small solutes by convection may be considered as quantitatively insignificant when contrasted with diffusive transport obviating the need to know about the membrane sieving properties for them.

Table 3. Inulin sieving coefficients for hemofiltration membranes at common clinical operating parameters

Membrane	Inulin sieving coefficient	
	Saline	Whole blood
Polysulfone-XP-50 (Amicon)	0.97 ± 0.04	0.28 ± 0.08
PAN*-15 (Asahi)	0.94 ± 0.09	0.13 ± 0.05
PAN*-AN69® (Hospal)	0.84 ± 0.01	0.78 ± 0.05

*Polyacrylonitrile.

Electrolyte transport, however, is an important exception. Sodium, for example, commonly appears in dialysis fluid in a concentration nearly equivalent to that in plasma water. As such, the diffusive transport is markedly reduced making the relative contribution of convective loss dominate the net balance of sodium per treatment. For example, if 3.0 l of plasma water at a sodium concentration of 140 mmol/l are removed during a 4.0 h treatment, then the 420 mmol of sodium lost by ultrafiltration far exceeds that lost down the modest 2 mmol/l concentration gradient (for total equilibration with bath sodium the value is 240 mmol) established when the bath sodium concentration is 138 mmol/l. Sorbent cartridge dialysis with dialysis fluid sodium concentrations that start well below and rise to supernormal levels during treatment relies in no small measure on convective sodium removal to restore sodium balance in the sodium and volume overloaded patient (33). Calcium concentrations in the dialysis fluid (6 ± 1 mg/dl, or 1.5 mmol/l) also exceed somewhat those in normal plasma water (5 mg/dl or 1.25 mmol/l). The protein bound calcium of course is not available for convective loss due to nearly complete restraint of protein by the membrane. Net negative calcium balance during therapy may result if 3.0 l of plasma water are removed, each containing 5.0 mg/dl (1.25 mmol/l) of unbound calcium. The 150 mg (3.75 mmol) of calcium removed will offset, in part, that moving into the plasma down the modest 1 to 2 mg/dl (0.25 to 0.5 mmol/l) bath to blood concentration gradient. In the case of potassium, convective loss augments the diffusive loss down the usual blood to bath gradient chosen for that ion.

It should be noted that ionic charge can affect electrolyte distribution across a dialysis membrane. There have been relatively few experiments with artificial kidney membranes to examine this phenomenon (34). The experimental design of these studies does not permit a clear judgment as to whether the influence of a charge bearing protein, such as albumin present on the blood side of the membrane, exerts a Gibbs–Donnan like charge effect during isolated ultrafiltration through the membrane, or whether sufficient diffusive interchange between the 'blood' and the ultrafiltered droplet hanging on the membrane (no dialysate was circulated) resulted in the observed deviations from unity in the sieving coefficient.

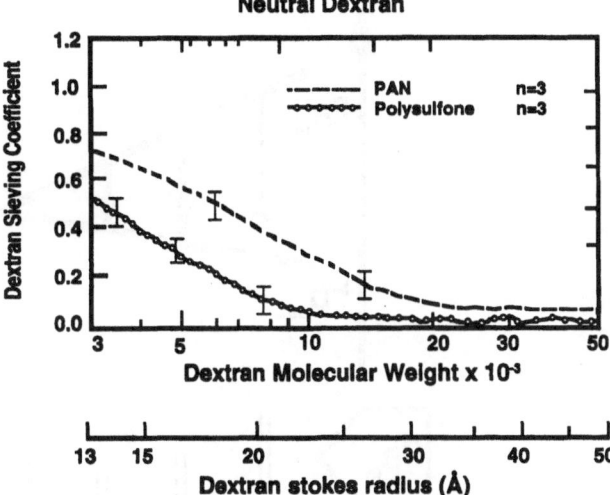

Figure 6. Sieving coefficients for polydispersed neutral dextran are plotted vs molecular weight and Stokes radius for two hollow fiber membranes used for hemofiltration. The polyacrylonitrile membrane from Hospal (Biospal 3000) is contrasted with the polysulfone membrane from Fresenius (F-60). Means values with error bar (± 1 SEM) are shown.

In this system, the cation and anion concentration distribution are quantitatively very similar to that expected at diffusion equilibrium as described by Donnan (35). As a practical matter when the 'plasma' concentrations of cations are corrected for both the displaced volume effect of protein ('Protocrit') and for Gibbs–Donnan distribution, the concentrations in the plasma water are virtually the same as those in the ultrafiltrate (34, 36).

Convective transport is also significant in the removal of 'middle molecules.' The plasma clearance for inulin (5,200 Daltons), a test 'middle molecule', across 1 m^2 of Cuprophan® is 4 ml/min by diffusion (22). For a 3.0 l fluid removal over a 4.0 hour hemodialysis treatment, the convective clearance would be of the order of 12 ml/min if the membrane did not restrain the passage of the solute. Cuprophan® is a relatively 'tight' membrane and the sieving coefficient for inulin is 0.3 (Table 2), which reduces the purely convective clearance to 4 ml/min (32). Cuprophan® is likely to be typical of the other low flux dialysis membranes such as cellulose acetate or cellophane for which there are few studies of sieving properties.

High flux dialysis membranes used for hemodialysis such as the polyacrylonitrile membrane from Hospal (3000S) or polysulfone membrane from Fresenius (F-60) or cellulose triacetate from Baxter (CT-190G) have a far higher hydraulic permeability than Cuprophan® as well as a more open pore structure. They require special fluid cycling equipment in order to use them for hemodialysis. They may also be used for both hemofiltration and hemodiafiltration. Sieving coefficients for two of these

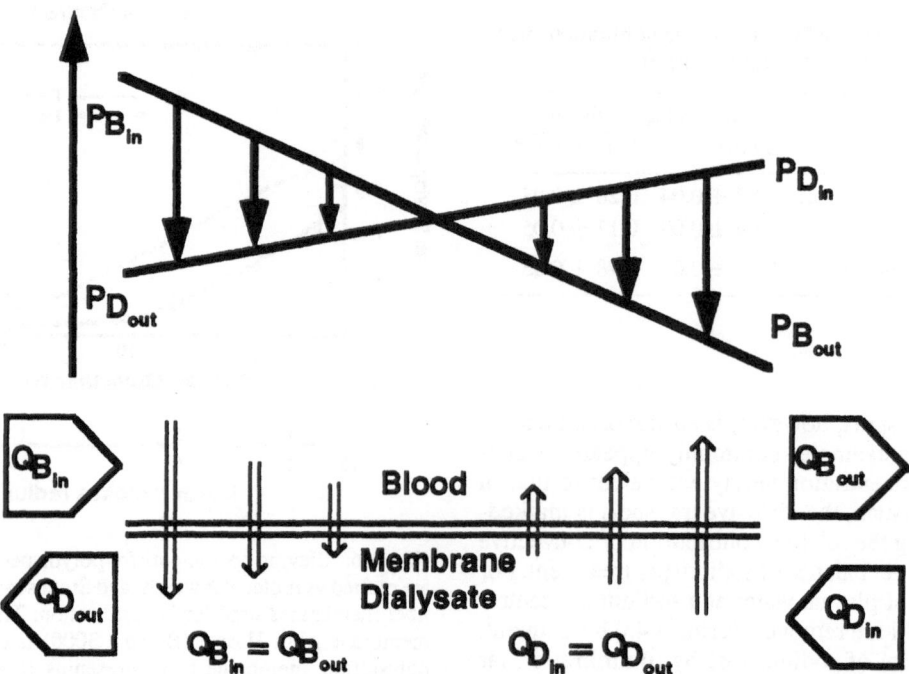

Figure 7. The pair of lines in the upper half of the figure represent the pressure on the dialysis fluid (P_D) and blood side (P_B) of the membrane. The heavy solid arrows are vectors indicating the magnitude (length) of the driving pressure along the length of the flow paths from inflow (in) to outflow (out). In the lower half of the figure the vertical open arrows represent the direction and magnitude of flow of ultrafiltrate over the length of the flow paths. It is clear that ultrafiltered plasma water leaves the blood path and is swept to drain with the spent dialysate. Similarly, fresh dialysis fluid is ultrafiltered into the blood at the blood outflow end of the membrane. These conditions exist when membranes with high hydraulic permeability are operated at zero net ultrafiltration (23).

membranes are shown in Figure 6. Convective transport of middle molecules can readily be accomplished with these more open membranes (37, 38), even under circumstances where these membranes are presumably being used for pure hemodialysis, i.e. high flux dialysis. During high flux dialysis, because of the membrane's high hydraulic permeability, the fluid cyclers must control the amount of ultrafiltration during treatment to prevent rapid fluid loss. This requirement, coupled with the pressure drop in the blood path from inflow to outflow end, sets up an internal convection loop in which ultrafiltration occurs from blood to dialysate at the inflow end of the membrane and from dialysate to blood at the outflow (Figure 7) (39). Schmidt has explored these events in a quantitative manner for a polysulfone hollow fiber membrane (39). Schmidt, in a manner analogous to Starling's capillary flow *in vivo* (40), and Leypoldt (41) contrasted backfiltration rates in both the polysulphone and Cuprophan® membranes, with respective hydraulic permeabilities of 40 and 6 ml/h/mmHg. Schmidt concludes that convective transport accounts for some 25% of the net clearance of inulin sized molecules in this 'inadvertent' hemodiafiltration mode. With reference to Figure 8 Soltys et al. (42) note that one may calculate an estimate of the magnitude of backfiltration as a function of net ultrafiltration (NF) using the simple expression

$$\mathrm{BF} = F_c \times \left[\frac{(1 - (\mathrm{NF}/F_c))}{2} \right]^2, \qquad [15]$$

where F_c = the critical or obligatory filtration rate for the dialyzer under operating conditions where the transmembrane pressure at the blood outlet end of the dialyzer is zero. Filtration occurs from blood to dialysate along the length of the dialyzer in this instance. Having determined F_c the calculation of BF at any net filtration rate may now be performed. Errors exist in the literature with regard to the way backfiltration is calculated (see, for example, Lonneman et al. (38)).

Peritoneal dialysis

For peritoneal dialysis, certain experiments to measure the sieving coefficient (S) have involved infusing hypertonic peritoneal dialysis fluid that contains the relevant solute in a concentration equal to that in plasma water (18, 27). The average concentration of this solute in ultrafiltrate $\bar{C}_f$ = mmol/ml may be computed from the concentrations of the solute measured on inflowing and outflowing dialysis fluid. The number of millimoles of solute transported by convection into the peritoneal space is computed as the difference in concentrations divided by the time of the exchange to obtain an average rate of solute removal

($\bar{Q}_s$ = mmol/min). Similarly, the volume of dialysis fluid removed in excess of that infused provides the volume of ultrafiltrate which is also divided by the exchange time ($\bar{Q}$ = ml/min) as

$$\bar{C}_f = \frac{J_s(\text{mmol/min} \cdot \text{membrane area})}{J_f(\text{ml/min} \cdot \text{membrane area})}\text{[7]} \qquad [16]$$

$$\bar{C}_f = \frac{\bar{Q}_s}{\bar{Q}_f} \cdot \qquad [17]$$

The concentration of the solute in the plasma water available from a peripheral vessel (artery or vein) is then measured and is presumed to represent the concentration of that solute on the 'blood side' of the peritoneal membrane. Peripheral blood water is usually estimated by sampling plasma concentration (C_p) and applying a correction factor to convert the measured value to plasma water concentration (C_w).

$$\frac{\bar{C}_f}{C_w} = S = 1 - \varepsilon \qquad [18]$$

$$C_w = \frac{C_p}{1 - \varphi}, \qquad [19]$$

where φ, the volume fraction of hydrated protein, is taken as 0.0107 times the concentration of total plasma proteins (7.4 g/dl) in normal plasma (43).

In criticism of this method, the potential impact of transport from the peritoneal cavity via lymphatic flow and into the interstitial space is not addressed. In addition, loss of volume from the peritoneal cavity to the vascular space via reabsorption will mean, first, that the true volume of ultrafiltrate generated will be underestimated (i.e. a low $\bar{Q}_f$). Secondly, the solute flux via the ultrafiltrate will appear to be less due to loss via reabsorption, reducing mass of solute in the dialysate (low $\bar{Q}_s$). It is apparent from equation 17 that the error induced by ignoring reabsorption may to some degree be self-canceling. This suggests that the values for S reported in Table 1 using this 'diffusion blocked' methodology may well be quite reasonable values. At present the reported studies (43) are in conflict about the best means for quantitating reabsorptive flow rates from the cavity.

More recent experiments (5, 12) employ mathematical relationships found in equation 12 to compute the values of s rather than the diffusion blocked methodology previously employed to determine sieving coefficients. To perform these calculations and derive σ accurately, it is a prerequisite to measure accurately peritoneal fluid volume and its changes with time. This method is subject

to significant errors as well (45). The reasonable agreement noted between the values reported in Table 1 using these different methods lends confidence to their validity. Methods for measuring peritoneal volume will be addressed in a subsequent section on solute transport by ultrafiltration.

The observed sieving coefficients for the electrolytes that are below unity (Table 1), should make the clinician expect hypernatremia and hyperchloridemia when substantial fluid removal occurs. As with hemodialysis, potassium[8] is removed by diffusion in addition to convection (unlike sodium and chloride) and offers few problems. Treatment of these iatrogenic concentration increments may be accomplished either by offering sodium chloride-free water in amounts calculated to offset the sodium chloride-free water lost as ultrafiltrate, or by alternating hypotonic or isotonic fluid with hypertonic exchanges, to permit diffusion equilibrium or water reabsorption to readjust these high values toward normal. At times plasma glucose levels rise considerably above the usual values of 300 to 500 mg/dl (16.7 to 27.8 mmol/l) when dialysis fluid containing 4.25% dextrose monohydrate is used, resulting in an osmolar shift of water out of cells. This would artifactually ameliorate the hypernatremia induced by serial hypertonic exchanges. With the return to isotonic exchanges or discontinuance of the dialysis, hyperglycemia would abate and water would move intracellularly revealing the true degree of hypernatremia. At present there is no information on sieving coefficients for other electrolytes.

CLINICAL APPLICATION OF ULTRAFILTRATION

Reabsorption of peritoneal fluid

Work from the Missouri group has focused attention on this important subject from a quantitative point of view (6, 7, 46). With reference to equation 10, filtration across a semipermeable membrane may logically be divided according to the forces that drive fluid movement (i.e. hydrostatic (ΔP) and osmotic ($\Delta \pi \sigma$) reabsorp-

---

[7] It is assumed that the area of the membrane for movement of the solute is the same as that for movement of water and hence, may be cancelled out of the ratio, a point that needs experimental verification.

---

[8] It is noteworthy that dialysis fluid left to equilibrate in the peritoneal space approaches a limit for potassium concentration equivalent to that in plasma water. This underscores the lack of contribution of intracellular potassium concentration to this equilibration. Active transport mechanisms, of course, sustain the intracellular concentration making the cell membranes functionally 'unavailable' for potassium diffusion to achieve equilibration. As the mass transfer-area coefficient for potassium (P_kA) is the same order of magnitude as that of the extracellular cation sodium ($P_{Na}A$), i.e. $P_{Na}A \cong P_kA$, and the charge and atomic size of these two cations is similar, it would suggest that the diffusional area for equilibration for these two cations is comparable as well, i.e., considerably smaller than the simple anatomic area covered by mesothelium.

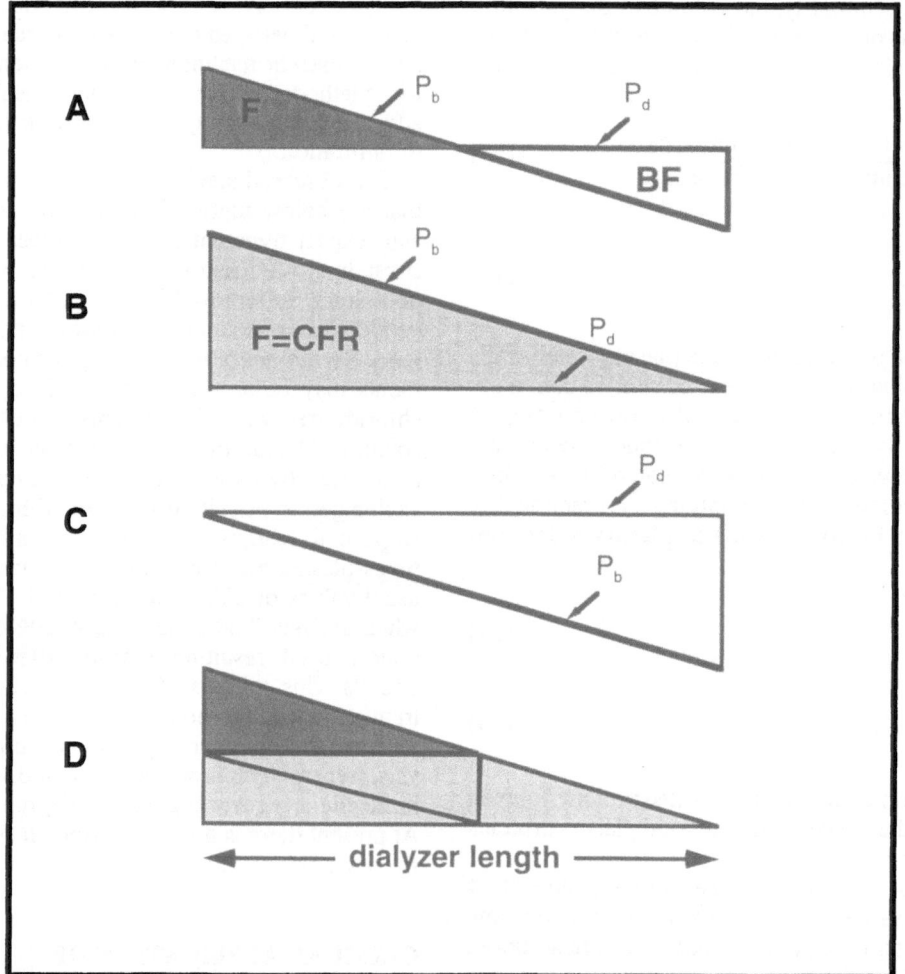

Figure 8. Approximate filtration pattern in a high flux dialyzer at (A), zero net ultrafiltration; at (B), the (positive) critical filtration rate (CFR), i.e., the lowest ultrafiltration rate which results in no backfiltration; at (C), i.e., the smallest negative ultrafiltration which results in no positive filtration. The convection at (D), zero net ultrafiltration has been shown to be equal to one-fourth of the CFR (42). P_D = pressure in the dialysate path. P = pressure in the blood path. P_D = pressure in the dialysate path. P_B = pressure in the blood path.

tion). Osmotic forces that drive fluid reabsorption from the peritoneal cavity derive from both oncotically important large solutes, predominantly albumin (for reasons discussed previously) and smaller solutes such as glucose, urea and electrolytes. With reference to Figure 9, water movement at the beginning of an exchange is driven by the osmolar gradient presented by the high concentration of glucose in the fresh dialysate. With time, this small molecule concentration gradient first deteriorates and eventually equilibrates with plasma water. The osmolar gradient, as noted above, is a composite of contributions from each of the solutes on both sides of the peritoneal transport barrier. Glucose dominates simply because of its presence in such high concentration. Diffusion equilibrium across the barrier is not ever achieved as a result of asymmetrical presence of albumin on the 'blood side'. As the

glucose gradient deteriorates, the oncotic force of albumin supersedes the glucose osmotic force and reabsorption of peritoneal fluid occurs. Left unperturbed, the peritoneal space would return to 'dry' state in a matter of hours-to-days. The shape of the curves in Figure 9 is only in part explained by this interplay of forces.

It is apparent from Figure 3 that fluid departs the cavity even during net osmotic movement of fluid into the cavity. There appear to be two components to this departure. First, is lymphatic drainage predominantly through subdiaphramatic lacunae, with reabsorbed fluid and its contents, returned to the vascular space. Second, is movement of fluid and its contents into the interstitial space surrounding the cavity and separated from it by the mesothelial cell barrier (i.e. the 'peritoneal membrane'). The forces that result in this movement have yet to be clearly described.

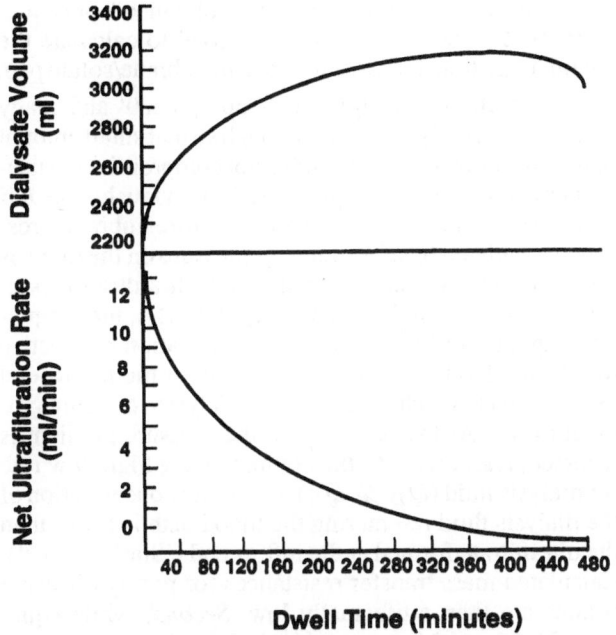

Figure 9a. Diagram of changes in d-glucose concentration and osmolality (a) and volume and ultrafiltration rate.

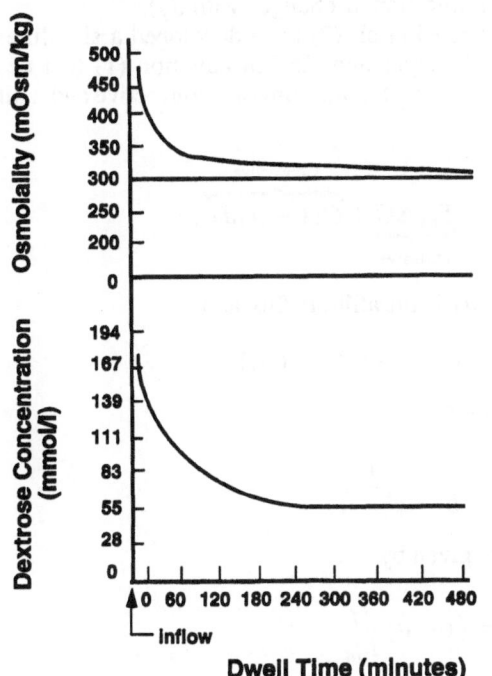

Figure 9b. Plotted against dwell time in man for a 2 liter exchange containing 4.25% dextrose monohydrate.

The characteristics of both paths of movement are those of convection (bulk flow). Both classical lymph flow and

this interstitial 'migration' are not size discriminatory in nature and appear to be uninfluenced by osmotic gradients (47). In a rabbit model, increased hydrostatic pressure within the cavity of 5–10 mmHg (68–137 cm H$_2$O) reduces this effluent flow (48) for reasons that at present remain speculative, e.g. possibly lymph channels and/or interstitial spaces are physically collapsed by this pressure. On the other hand, a more usual intra-abdominal pressure in man (15 cm H$_2$O) results in increased fluid reabsorption on the order of 70 ml/2hours/cm H$_2$O for a 3 l fill volume (8).

A recent symposium on lymphatic and non-lymphatic fluid loss from the peritoneal cavity provides reports from all major workers in this area and bears reading for those who wish to find experimental detail and informed speculation (44). More investigation is clearly needed in this complex area as fluid reabsorption may fall in the 10–50% range of the net amount of fluid removed from the peritoneal cavity in response to hypertonic dialysate and, as such, has real clinical significance with regard to net fluid balance.

Alternative osmotic agents

Recent use of the glucose polymer (maltodextrin) for clinical trials clinically has interesting implications (49). The selection of an average molecular weight for this polymer of $\cong$ 16–17 Kd means that, on average, this polymer overall will have a much higher reflection coefficient than glucose. This translates into the use of lower concentrations of solute to accomplish the clinical goal of fluid balance. There appear to be three potential clinical advantages with this compound: a) a more 'physiologic' osmolality for the fresh dialysate; b) possibly a slightly lower calorie load than might otherwise be possible when monomolecular glucose is used, and c) the possibility to use a somewhat larger initial fill volume, e.g. 2.2 l since there is no need to accommodate the overshoot volume in the abdomen that occurs with, for example, 3.86% glucose containing solution.

This polymer is branch chained and the two bonds between glucose molecules are α1–4 (90%) and α1–6 (at the branch point). The point of uncertainty about this agent is the effect of the long term presence in the uremic plasma of the polymer and its fragments. The polymer is slowly degraded in the uremic patient. Two years of study in a small, carefully followed, functionally anephric population has shown no evidence of depositional problems in the cornea or liver on routine slit lamp and liver function study; this, in spite of carrying significant concentrations of the large molecular weight component of the polymer in the plasma water. I expect that this will be the first in a series of polymeric molecules that will be used to achieve a more prolonged ultrafiltration profile for patients with high permeability transport characteristics maintained on peritoneal dialysis.

SOLUTE TRANSPORT BY ULTRAFILTRATION DURING DIALYSIS

Hemodialysis

While the concept of solute rejection by the membrane is important, in order to understand why $\Delta\pi\sigma$ contributes comparatively little to the transmembrane pressure when fluid is removed from a patient during dialysis, it is vital to the understanding of convective mass transfer. From equation 3 it is apparent that the membrane property (ε) dictates the respective velocities of solute (N) and solvent (Q_f) movement across the membrane. While transport by diffusion always requires a concentration gradient and is always size-dependent (i.e. small solutes are transported faster than large ones), convective mass transfer is not necessarily dependent on solute size, and solute transport does not require a concentration gradient. The respective contributions of convection and diffusion in conventional dialyzers has long been ignored, largely because of the comparatively low hydraulic permeability of Cuprophan®. The advent of more water permeable ('high flux') membranes, however, has directed interest to this area. At present there is comparatively little information on sieving coefficients for uremic solutes across cellulosic dialysis membranes. Current fluid cycling equipment, however, permits the use of high hydraulic permeability membranes for hemodialysis making a quantitative understanding of convective transport important. In Table 2 the sieving properties of Cuprophan® are compared with those of the most open of the currently available dialysis membranes.

An expression for combined diffusive and convective clearance (and dialysance) may be derived from equations for clearance (and dialysance) and from consideration of mass balance across a dialyzer in which ultrafiltration is occurring:

$$Q_{Bi}C_{Bi} = Q_{Bo}C_{Bo} + Q_fC_f \qquad [20]$$

$$\text{Clearance} = \frac{Q_{Bo}(C_{Bi} - C_{Bo})}{C_{Bi}} + Q_f \qquad [21]$$

$$= \frac{Q_{Di}(C_{Do} - C_{Di})}{C_{Bi}} + \frac{Q_fC_{Do}}{C_{Bi}} \qquad [22]$$

$$\text{Dialysance} = \frac{Q_{Bo}(C_{Bi} - C_{Bo}) + Q_FC_{Do}}{C_{Bi} - C_{Di}} \qquad [23]$$

$$= \frac{Q_{Di}(C_{Do} - C_{Di}) + Q_FC_{Do}}{C_{Bi} - C_{Di}}. \qquad [24]$$

These equations provide a clinically satisfactory means for describing mass transfer when both solute transport processes are ongoing. Two points of importance should be noted. *First*, equations relating dialysance and membrane mass transfer resistances are not valid in the presence of ultrafiltration. Hence, values obtained from equations 21, 23 and 24 should not be used to calculate the overall mass transfer resistance of a membrane/solute pair. The hydraulic permeability of Cuprophan® and many other clinical dialyzers is low enough so that small amount of ultrafiltration that occurs does not compromise the useful application of these equations. As previously noted, if high flux membranes are used and transmembrane pressure is regulated by adjustment of pressure on the dialysis fluid side of the membrane to block net ultrafiltration (see, for example, Schmidt (39) or Leypoldt (41)), these equations again will be in error. In this situation convective flux from blood to dialysate will occur at the inflow end of the blood path where a blood-to-dialysate pressure gradient exists. At the outflow end the pressure gradient is reversed, and, owing to the comparatively high flow rate for dialysis fluid ($Q_D \gg Q_B$), the solute concentration of the dialysis fluid re-entering the blood path is lower than the ultrafiltrate formed at the inflow end ('Starling flow'). Calculated mass transfer resistances for poorly diffusing solutes are then artifactually low. *Second*, while equations 21, 23 and 24 are useful in deriving expected chemical benefits from treatment, they offer little insight into the interaction between convection and diffusion when both are operating in a given dialyzer (as noted in the section on ultrafiltration, σ changes with J_f).

Villarroel et al. (2) have developed a simplified form of the Spiegler and Kadem equation (1) that describes solute transport as the sum of a convective and a diffusive term:

$$J_s = \underbrace{P_m\Delta C}_{\text{Diffusive}} + \overbrace{C(1 - \sigma)J_f}^{\text{Convective}}, \qquad [25]$$

where J_f is ultrafiltrate flux and

$$C = C_B - Z(C_B - C_D) \qquad [26]$$

and (the factor)

$$Z = \frac{1}{b} - \frac{1}{\varepsilon^b - 1}. \qquad [27]$$

Beta is given by

$$\beta = (1 - \sigma)\frac{J_f}{P_m} \qquad [28]$$

If $0 < \beta < 3$ then $\frac{1}{3} < Z < \frac{1}{2}$ \qquad [29]

If $\beta > 3$ then $Z = \frac{1}{\beta}$ and $J_s = C_b(1 - \sigma)J_f$ \qquad [30]

These relationships point out that as *in vitro*, ultrafiltration rate, increases, the relative contribution to net solute transport made by diffusion becomes negligible, an observation already made by Nolph and associates (50, 51). The

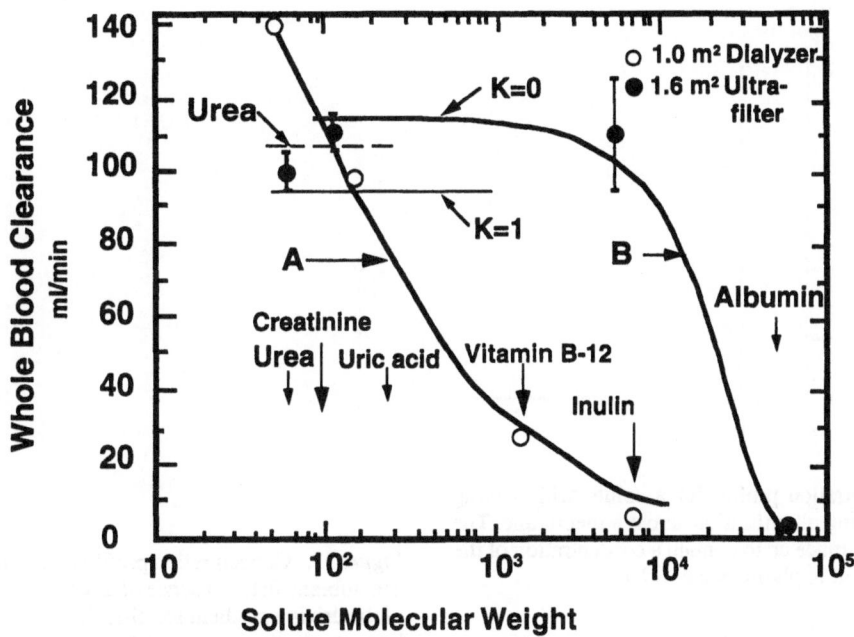

Figure 10. Whole blood clearance is plotted against the log of solute molecular weight. Curve A shows the solute clearance pattern for a 1.0 m² dialyzer operated with no ultrafiltration where solute transport is by diffusion. Curve B shows such a pattern for a 1.6 m² ultrafilter where solute transport is by convection. Normal human kidneys display a clearance pattern very similar to curve B. Small solutes (< 200 molecular weight) are better cleared by diffusion. *K* ranges from 0 to 1 and describes the distribution of solute between plasma and the red blood cell (see text on hemofiltration for further discussion of *K*).

studies of Villarroel et al. (2) demonstrated that for dialysis membranes tested *in vitro*, equation 25 shows a reasonable degree of agreement (within 5%) with the results obtained with the more rigorous and complex Spiegler equation. As can be predicted, the impact of convective mass transport is most impressive on solutes that diffuse poorly through the membrane. Figure 10 plots clearance by diffusion (curve A) and clearance by convection (curve B) against log molecular weight (52, 53). It is apparent that for 'conventional' uremic solutes (less than 200 Daltons) curve A shows a higher clearance than curve B. Figure 10 shows two extreme cases for comparison. Clearance is plotted vs molecular weight for diffusion using a Cuprophan® membrane (curve A). This contrasts with curve B where clearance by pure convection is plotted. As we move toward use of more hydraulically permeable membranes where the interplay between convection and diffusion may not be externally apparent in terms of net water movement, we will see an improvement in the transport of larger molecules that is more reflective of curve B. Hemodiafiltration will be commented upon in a subsequent section.

Peritoneal dialysis

The ability of solutes to move across the peritoneal membrane in the absence of a driving concentration gradient was demonstrated in 1966 for urea (54). Important to the understanding of the mechanisms for movement of solutes into the dialysis fluid is the role that the peritoneal membrane plays in restraining or modulating such movement. The concept of membrane sieving or rejection as explored above, is central to an understanding of how solute movement occurs. Solute mass transfer and its quantitation has been dealt with in some detail elsewhere. Therefore, these comments are restricted to convective mass transfer across the peritoneal barrier and the impact that this may have on simultaneously occurring diffusive mass transfer. The usual calculation of peritoneal clearance using the conventional relationship

$$\text{Clearance} = \frac{\text{average mass removed per minute in the dialysis}}{\text{plasma concentration}}$$

will provide an average rate of plasma clearance that will not distinguish the comparative contributions of convection and diffusion, but which is perfectly satisfactory for clinical judgments relating to the rate at which plasma is cleared of solute. Table 1 offers sieving coefficient values for urea, inulin, glucose, sodium, potassium and chloride. At present, data in humans on larger biologically relevant solute is scant. Figure 4 shows sieving coefficients for neutral polydispersed dextrans over the range of sizes from inulin (5,200 Daltons) to protein sized molecules in a rabbit model.

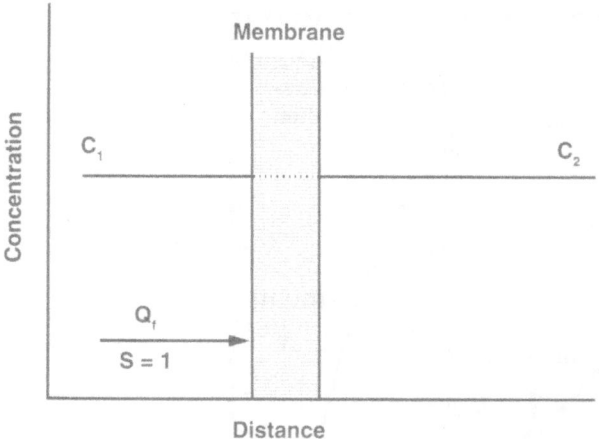

Figure 11. Concentration profile for a solute with sieving coefficient $S = 1$ during ultrafiltration across a membrane. The dialysis fluid has been made up to contain a concentration of the solute (C_2) equal to that in plasma water (C_1).

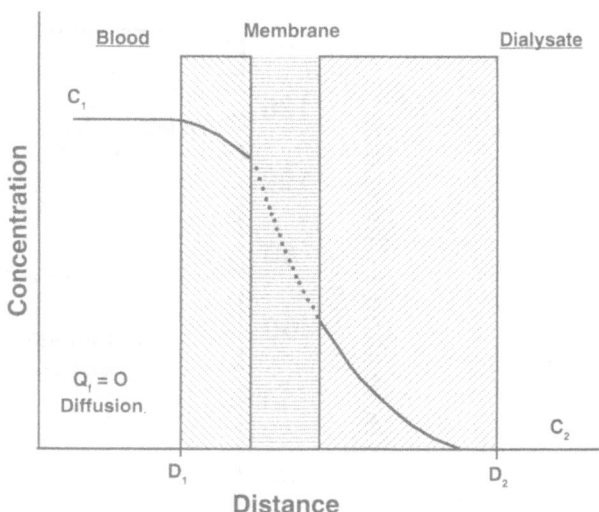

Figure 12. Concentration profile for a solute that diffuses across a membrane in the absence of any ultrafiltration. The 'steepness' of the driving gradient for diffusion is depicted by the difference in concentrations between the bulk phase of the plasma water (C_1) and that of the dialysis fluid (C_2) acting over the distance D_1 to D_2, i.e. $(C_1 - C_2)/(D_1 - D_2)$.

Consider an uncharged solute of small weight for which $S \cong 1$. Let us assume for the moment that urea fulfills these criteria. Figure 11 depicts this concentration profile across a membrane separating blood and dialysis fluid. The concentration for urea has been adjusted to be equal in plasma water and dialysis fluid. The concentration profile is drawn for the conditions existing a few moments after the onset of ultrafiltration and is linear. That is, there is no change in the concentration of the ultrafiltered plasma water as it crosses the membrane and its attendant 'unstirred' layers. In this circumstance, the average convective clearance of urea will be the product of the sieving coefficient and the ultrafiltration rate.

$$S_u = \frac{\bar{C}_{Fu}}{\bar{C}_{Wu}} \qquad [31]$$

$$S_u \bar{Q}_r = \frac{\bar{C}_{Fu}}{\bar{C}_{Wu}} \bar{Q}_f$$

$$= \text{Average clearance of urea from}$$
$$\text{plasma water by convection} \qquad [32]$$

Average convective clearance of urea ($\bar{C}_{fu}$) =

$$\frac{\text{Mass removed by ultrafiltration exchange/time}}{\text{Plasma water concentration}} .$$

$\bar{Q}_f$ would usually be obtained as the volume difference (inflow volume − outflow volume) divided by the exchange time. It is apparent that the average convective clearance for a solute with $S = 1$ is equal to the ultrafiltration rate.

For peritoneal dialysis the measurement of the ultrafiltration rate as usually performed clinically provides

an average value, since the glucose-generated osmotic gradient deteriorates exponentially with time. The convective clearance described then is also an average value for the plasma cleared over the time interval of the exchange rather than an instantaneous value as obtained with hemodialysis. As previously noted, there is a significant absorption of fluid across the peritoneal transport barrier, both by lymphatic uptake and transport into the interstitial space surrounding the peritoneal cavity. Studies show that the fluid reabsorbed carries with it a full complement of solute up to and including molecules as large as Dextran 70, commonly used as a 'dye dilution marker' for studying volume changes with time (11). This bulk flow out of the peritoneal space then does not result in a change in concentration of solute present in the dialysate and, hence, does not introduce any error into the calculation of $\bar{C}_{fu}$.

In the usual clinical situation, where one may wish to quantify the convective clearance for a solute such as urea, it is important to remember that there is no urea present initially in the dialysis fluid. Diffusion and convection then occur simultaneously during the exchange. At present a rigorous calculation of the respective contributions of diffusion and convection must await determination of 'backfiltration' of fluid from the peritoneal cavity. A conceptual understanding of this interaction for both peritoneal and hemodialysis is, however, useful.

Conceptualizing the impact of convection on diffusion during dialysis

While there are theoretical treatments for the comparative contributions of diffusion and convection to overall clearance rate for the peritoneal (55, 56) and hemodialysis membranes (2, 57), there are only a few *in vivo* experiments to substantiate the respective contributions of these forces to net mass transfer (5, 14, 15, 54, 56). Reasoning from this work and from analogy with synthetic membranes *in vitro*, a qualitative appreciation of the interaction between these two modes of solute transport may be developed. Figure 12 differs from Figure 11 in that there is no ultrafiltration occurring, and there is no urea in the dialysis fluid. Figure 12 depicts the concentration profile when diffusion alone occurs. The fall in concentration from bulk phase plasma to the surface of the membrane represents the 'blood side' unstirred layer that is partially depleted of solute by diffusion across the membrane into the dialysis fluid. Similarly, the 'dialysate side' unstirred layer is depicted as a continuing reduction in concentration with distance in the dialysis fluid before achieving the dialysate bulk phase concentration (which at the start will be zero). With peritoneal dialysis there is comparatively little mixing of unstirred layers of dialysate when compared with hemodialysis. In a conceptually amusing experiment, Levitt et al. (58) mounted rats on a conventional laboratory shaker and determined the change in permeability area product (PA) for urea, creatinine and glucose for stationary animals and at various shaker speeds. Values increased with increasing shaker speed and plateaued for shaken rats at a value for all three solutes that was four times higher than that measured in stationary animals. These experiments are the *in vivo* analog of experiments conducted with cellulosic membrane in a stirred cell (59) where the revolutions per minute (RPM) of the stirring rotor on either side of a suspended membrane were plotted against the overall mass transfer resistance (R_e) of the membrane for a test solute. By linearizing such a plot (60) (expressing RPM as a 0.5 power) one may then extrapolate to an infinite stirrer speed (or plateau in the shaking rat experiment) and arrive at the intrinsic resistance of the membrane without any attendant 'unstirred layers' of fluid that contribute to the overall mass transfer resistance to diffusion. One must conclude, if the rat is a reasonable model for the human, that the unstirred layer of dialysate is a significant component of the resistance to transport for peritoneal dialysis.

Imposing a transmembrane driving force for ultrafiltration on the conditions shown in Figure 12 results in the changes shown in Figure 13. The reduction to zero (or toward zero for a more diffusively permeable solute) of the blood side fluid film will enhance diffusion by shortening the length of the path over which the gradient for diffusion is acting (D_1 to D_2) between bulk phase blood and bulk phase dialysate. In addition, the drop in concentration within the membrane has been obliterated, further

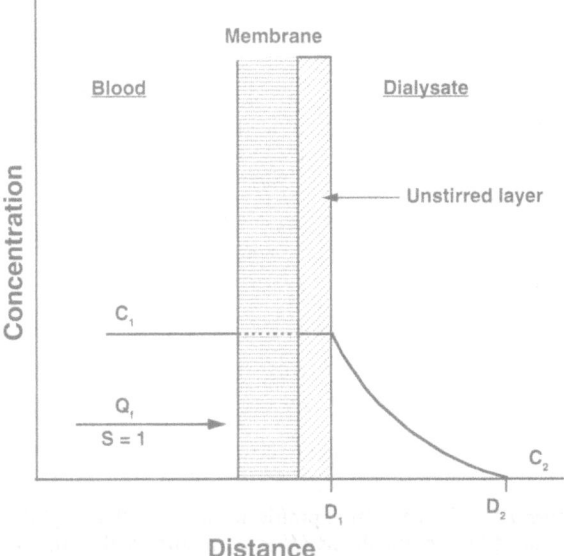

Figure 13. Concentration profile for a solute with $S = 1$ moments after ultrafiltration has begun. Note the steeper driving gradient for diffusion created by the obliteration of the unstirred layer on the blood side, i.e. D_1 to D_2 for diffusion (Figure 11) is larger than that depicted here.

shortening the path over which the concentration gradient occurs. Finally, the dialysate side stagnant film shifts away from the membrane. In the event that mechanical mixing may be somewhat better some distance from the membrane, there will be some enhancement of diffusion. Alternatively, if mechanical mixing is less good the diffusion path may be lengthened and diffusive transport reduced (51). This circumstance arises only from adding an osmotic gradient to drive ultrafiltration and assumes no changes in the membrane to alter its permeability characteristics.

Figure 14 shows the effect of ultrafiltration for a larger uncharged solute for which there is significant membrane restraint ($1 - \sigma \cong S < 1$). The solute is convected to the membrane surface where the concentration builds up ('concentration polarization' or 'solute polarization') (61). The concentration within the membrane falls with distance and the dialysate side film is displaced in a manner analogous to the situation in Figure 13. Again, the overall effect is to steepen the concentration gradient between blood and dialysate, enhancing the diffusive component of transport. Precise quantitation of this enhancement for the solutes routinely dealt with in uremic plasma is not possible presently for the peritoneal membrane, and may not be in view of data that indicate that exposure to hypertonic solutions not only increases membrane permeability, but membrane area (increase in number of capillary loops perfused?) as well (18).

Finally, in considering the impact of convection on diffusion it should be apparent that solute size is impor-

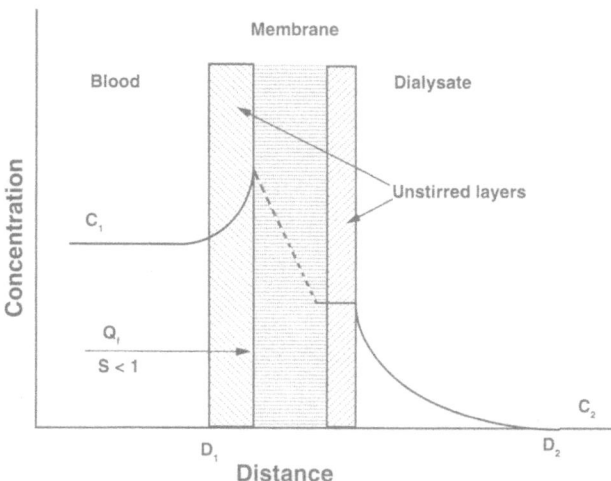

Figure 14. Concentration profile for a solute that is partially restrained by the membrane ($S < 1$) moments after the onset of ultrafiltration. The concentration gradient is made steeper by the buildup of solute on the membrane and acts over a shorter distance than was the case for simple diffusion (as in Figure 11).

tant. For larger solutes with poor diffusive permeability in the membrane (referred to now without its attendant fluid films), if the sieving coefficient for that solute is high enough, convective mass transport can contribute the major portion of the total mass transported. As a corollary, the fraction of overall mass transfer resistance to diffusion contributed by unstirred fluid films becomes less important as the solute considered becomes larger as the membrane then dominates the serial resistance to transport (62).

Albumin, the smallest of the traditional plasma proteins and plasma protein in general, merit special comment with respect to peritoneal dialysis. The presence of protein on first catheter placement (i.e. the 'ascites' present) and its subsequent decline over the next few exchanges to a steady state level is evidence that under usual circumstances there is a slow loss of protein from the plasma across the capillary and into the peritoneal space, from whence it is returned to the vascular space via the lymphatics. Albumin is the predominant protein transported in this manner. Table 1 lists a sieving coefficient (S) for albumin of < 0.02. Glomerular restraint of albumin in animals is somewhat more complete with $S \approx 0.003$ (63). The sieving coefficient given in Table 1 for the peritoneal membrane is not rigorously arrived at, as there are no experiments reported so far that determine this value. Rather, it is derived from data for protein (measured by trichloracetic acid precipitation) loss in a series of isotonic exchanges (1.3 ± 0.1 g, $n = 13$) taken after washout and subtracted from losses for exchanges using hypertonic solution (1.7 ± 2 g) to which no protein had been added to block diffusion. The ultrafiltrate concentration of 0.06 g/dl divided by a normal plasma albumin

of 3.5 g/dl equals 0.02. This figure is purely an estimate as diffusive loss is not blocked, and it is assumed that only albumin is convected when, in point of fact, small amounts of other proteins are also present. Further, the presence of protein in spent peritoneal dialysate is frequently cited as evidence that the peritoneal membrane is 'very permeable' when contrasted with hemodialysis or hemofiltration membranes. It should be noted, however, that for convective transport more than 98% of the protein is held back by this 'very permeable' membrane, even under the stress of hypertonic solutions.

Recent interesting work by Leypoldt and Blindauer (64) in which selected proteins were added to the peritoneal dialysate (Ringers lactate) of rabbits surprisingly showed a reduction in the loss of these proteins. This finding indicates that diffusion plays a major role in protein transport which is contrary to the conventional wisdom which specifies that protein transport occurs by convection. This work would suggest that the above computed S for albumin of < 0.02 is high and may well be closer to the 0.003 as noted for the glomerulus. Examination of Figure 4 also supports the 'tightness' of this membrane in the rabbit when tested with convective transport. For perspective, Cuprophan® PT-150 has a transmittance (T_r) value ($T_r \approx S$) for egg albumin (44,000 Daltons, 46.6 Å) of 0.002 and the more permeable HOSPAL AN 69 (polyacrylonitrile) dialysis membrane has a value of 0.04 (32).

The massive dilution of protein by dialysis fluid would, of course, 'trap' protein lost from the capillary that without this dilution would, under steady state circumstances, be either returned to the vascular space via previously described reabsorptive forces or, less likely, be convected back across the venular end of the capillary bed. As noted above, these forces accomplish solute transport by a mechanism that is independent of solute size, i.e., bulk flow of peritoneal fluid through open channels rather than by diffusion. The quantitative importance of this transport path is now under study. Work in rats and rabbits place its quantitative importance at 10 to 50% of the net water transaction taking place during an hypertonic exchange (44).

An important consideration in studies of peritoneal ultrafiltration is the method used to measure the volume of peritoneal dialysate and how it changes with time during the exchange. The rigor with which this is done will determine the rigor of mass transport parameters such as the reflection coefficient (σ) for convection and the permeability area product (PA) or dialysance parameter for diffusion. The latter may be computed from either isotonic or hypertonic exchanges. Its accuracy when computed from hypertonic exchanges depends on accurate volume measurements. Studies of this problem by indicator dilution methodology show that lymphatic uptake of the marker solute (e.g. radiolabeled albumin, Evans Blue albumin complex, red blood cells) is significant and dilution of the marker solute by ultrafiltered water results in a systematic error that overestimates the volume due to loss through the lymphatics (10, 11). Accurate volumes could be obtained by using both the traditional method of placing an index solute in the infused dialysate at the beginning of the exchange and following its concentration serially with time, as well as employing a second index solute applied at intervals for an 'instantaneous' indicator dilution measure of volume. The latter technique requires repeated additions of index solute for instantaneous assessment and gave values comparable to those obtained by simply draining the abdomen and measuring the volume with a graduated cylinder. On formulating a model of fluid transport that included 'lymphatic'[9] run-off, it was possible to determine from mathematical first principles that for the most rigorous assessment of mass transport parameters, it was necessary to use both volume measurements, i.e. that from the common way of using the index solute with its systematic error and the instantaneous value (11). Further, if only one of these volume methods is to be used the best (and quite reasonable) values for computed mass transfer parameters are given by the common method. Comparison of actual data obtained in a rabbit model confirmed this mathematical prediction (11); that is, values for PA and σ computed in the most rigorous manner using both methods were compared with values computed using the volume measurement or the other indicator dilution methods alone. Happily, this work validates many fine studies using the volume measurement method conducted without knowledge of the systematic error it introduces. One may speculate that the common method provides the most accurate figure to compute PA and σ because this volume with its systematic error is somehow more truly reflective of the area of membrane involved in transport.

HEMOFILTRATION

Hemofiltration in pure form is not widely practiced today although it has received sufficient study to permit reasonably accurate characterization. Hemodiafiltration in various forms, which utilizes dialysis fluid and diffusive

---

[9] Methods for measuring lymphatic flow rate from the cavity entail quantitating the departure of a large index solute, e.g. radiolabeled or dye labeled albumin. Work by Flessner et al. in the rat (65) and Rippe et al. (66) in CAPD patients show that there is a significant departure of such index solutes from the peritoneal cavity and that at 3 to 4 h these solutes remain sequestered in the interstitial tissues. That is, they have not entered the vascular space as would be expected had they departed the peritoneal cavity via the lymphatics. As much as 50% of radiolabeled fibrinogen departing the peritoneal cavity of the rat does not return to the vascular space during the 4 h study. Our model does not assume loss of the index solute from the cavity via a lymphatic path but rather assumes the general case of its departure by any non size discriminatory pathway. Hence, the use of the term 'lymphatic' in quotes. The quantitative impact of true lymphatic drainage of the peritoneal cavity will await further clarification of this problem.

Predilution / Post Dilution

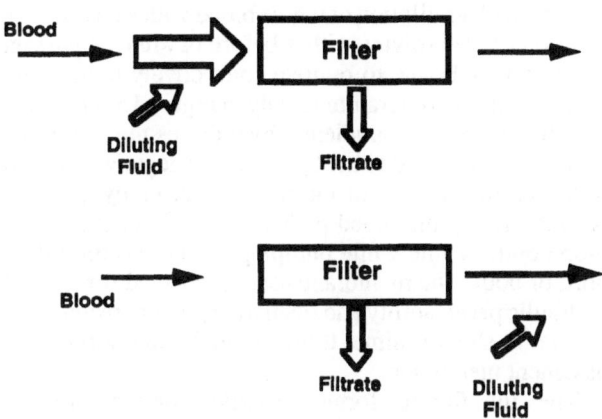

Figure 15. Diagram of hemofiltration showing two modes of replacing ultrafiltrate to the blood path.

transport in addition to that provided by convection, is now quite rationally and commonly used. Hemodiafiltration is now practiced with a wide variety of techniques, and rigorous characterization of their performance is not available. The treatment options range from simple use of membranes with high hydraulic permeability (hemofilters) paired with conventional dialysate cycling equipment and run in the same manner as routine hemodialysis. In this technique fluid balance is maintained with removal of only excess total body water in amounts adjusted only to correct for pretreatment overhydration. At the other extreme, there is the system employing a special dialysate cycler with two full sized hemofiltration membranes. The first is run at maximum filtration velocities; the second run in maximum reverse (reabsorption) filtration velocity while simultaneously putting 1000 ml/min of dialysate through the system to utilize the diffusive transport characteristics of these two membranes. These hemodiafiltration systems do not lend themselves to a generic discussion/description. What follows is a generic description of hemofiltration with specific comments on derivative techniques.

Theoretical aspects

Solute removal by hemodialysis as a diffusion-based process is size discriminatory, i.e. small molecules such as the conventionally recognized uremic solutes, (urea (60 Daltons), creatinine (113), uric (168)) diffuse rapidly in water and through water-filled 'pores' in membranes and are removed, with commonly available dialysis equipment at clearances that are similar to those for intact human kidneys. It should be remembered, however, that the continuously functioning human kidney provides a net weekly clearance that dramatically exceeds even the most efficient artificial kidney applied for 12 to 15 h per week. On the other hand, large solutes that diffuse poorly are cleared slowly by hemodialysis. The process of hemofiltration involves dilution of whole blood with a physiologic solution of electrolytes, either before or after its passage across a membrane, to remove convectively undesirable solutes is shown diagrammatically in Figure 15. The transmembrane pressure gradient which drives the ultrafiltration is accomplished either by creating a negative pressure in the casing outside of the membrane, or by positively pressurizing the blood path by partially clamping the blood outflow line while pumping blood into the inflow port, or both. The membrane used is selected for its high hydraulic permeability and open transport characteristics. The latter should mimic those of the human glomerular basement membrane.

The ultrafiltrate formed should contain little or no macrosolutes (protein) and no cellular elements. Microsolutes, e.g. electrolytes, urea, creatinine, uric acid, glucose, phosphate and sulfate should be present in the ultrafiltrate in the same concentration as in plasma water. Intermediate molecular weight solutes (500 up to 30,000 Daltons), identified (but not fully characterized) as present in abnormal concentrations in uremic plasma, will be removed convectively along with the microsolutes. Depending on the size of the membrane pores and the solute particles, a certain percentage of these intermediate molecular weight solutes will be retained. Figure 10 shows the clearance pattern for a polysulphone ultrafilter. It is apparent that, like the human kidney, inulin with a molecular weight of 5,200, is cleared at the same rate (approximately 100 ml/min) as creatinine (113 Daltons) at the operating conditions of this experimental 1.6 m² device.

It is obvious that replacement of water, desirable electrolytes and glucose, simulating 'tubular reabsorption,' are required to maintain a satisfactory blood volume and composition. With reference to Figure 15, diluting fluid may be introduced into the blood path, either upstream of (predilution) or downstream from (postdilution) the ultrafilter.

At present, there are at least four membrane types with high enough hydraulic permeability for hemofiltration. Most are noncellulosic, i.e. polysulfone, polyacrylonitrile and polyamide. One formulation of cellulose (cellulose triacetate) has proven satisfactory. The solute transport characteristics of two of these formulations are compared in Figure 6.

Factors affecting ultrafiltration flow rate

Solute mass transfer rate across the membrane in hemofiltration is governed by the rate of ultrafiltration and the sieving coefficient of the membrane. Equation 1 gives the general form of the relationship of forces governing the ultrafiltrate flux (J_f) across membranes with relatively low hydraulic permeability. A more useful equation for membranes having a high hydraulic permeability and used

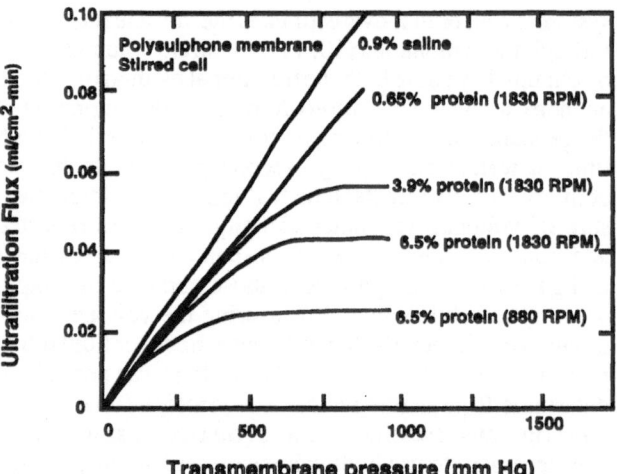

Figure 16. Ultrafiltration flux rate in a stirred cell with sheet ultrafiltration membrane is plotted against transmembrane pressure. The influence of changes in protein concentration can be seen. For saline (0% protein) the response is linear. Increasing protein concentration in the bulk solution decreases the plateau value for the flux rate of water. Increasing stirrer speed reduces the thickness of the polarized layer of protein on the membrane and increases the flux rate for water at any given protein concentration. (RPM = stirrer speed, revolutions per minute, see text).

to ultrafilter protein containing solutions, such as plasma or blood, is needed and will be developed. Figure 16 shows the results of an experiment in which a sheet of high flux membrane is placed in a stirred cell and transmembrane pressure is induced. Saline flux is linearly related to transmembrane pressure. When protein is present, however, the flux rate varies linearly at low transmembrane pressures, but eventually reaches a plateau, at which time pressure increments do not increase flux rate. An increase in protein concentration of the solution being filtered results in a lower plateau of water flux, while increasing stirrer speed elevates this level. Experiments such as these have permitted a reasonable empirical description of the events at the membrane level (52, 53, 61, 67–68). Figure 17 is a diagrammatic representation of such events.

During the ultrafiltration of blood, protein containing solution moves to the membrane surface, where water and the microsolutes continue to move unimpeded across the discriminating surface. Protein, however, is sieved out and remains behind (concentration polarization). The thickness of this polarized protein layer is determined by the amount of protein delivered to the surface (protein concentration in the bulk phase of plasma times the flow rate for water through the membrane) and the amount diffusing back from the surface (back flux). Factors that influence the back flux are the concentration gradient between the bulk phase of the solution and the polarized layer of protein at the membrane and the shear forces that 'stir' the protein layer. In the stirred cell with sheet membrane,

Concentration Polarization

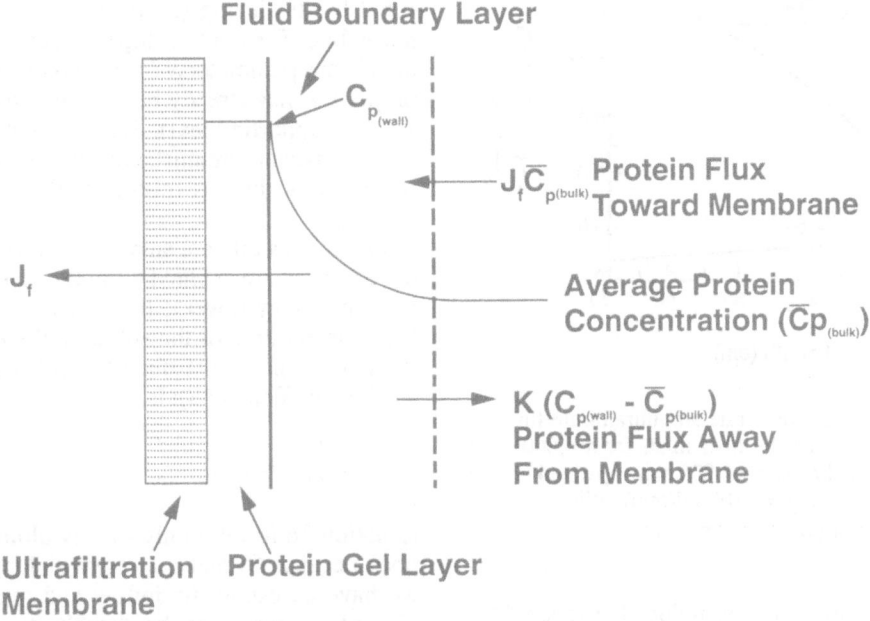

Figure 17. Diagram of the events at the membrane during ultrafiltration of a protein containing solution. Protein is moved to the membrane surface (polarized) in conjunction with the water traversing the membrane. It is moved away from the membrane by diffusion and shear forces generated by flow over the membrane. Thickness of the protein layer at steady state represents the net balance of these two processes. The concentration profile for protein is shown.

used to generate the data for Figure 16, increasing stirrer speed decreases the thickness of the polarized protein layer and increases the water flux rate. In a hollow fiber unit, increasing flow rate down the fiber reduces the thickness of this layer. Previous work (52, 53) with hollow fiber ultrafilters using plasma permitted several useful correlations relating variables of protein concentration in the bulk phase of plasma (C_p), the slope of the velocity profile for whole blood at the fiber wall (that is, the shear rate (γ_w)), and the fiber length from the inlet (X):

$$J_f = 3.40 \times 10^{-5} \left[\frac{\gamma_w}{X} \right]^{1/3} \ln \frac{28.7}{C_p} . \qquad [33]$$

This semiempirical relationship for the ultrafiltration of plasma in a hollow fiber unit states that J_f, the water flux rate averaged across the entire membrane, falls with increasing plasma protein concentration; that the faster the end-to-end flow rate down the fiber the higher the flux, but the longer the fiber length, the lower the flux rate. The impact of introducing red blood cells, i.e., ultrafiltering whole blood as studied by Okazaki and Yoshida (67) changes these relationships as red cells augment the diffusion of protein away from the membrane, i.e., act as a stirring force. As such, there is an increasing influence on γ_w as hematocrit rises, i.e. the exponent on γ_w rises

from 0.3 to 0.8 as hematocrit was changed from 0.0 to 44%. While more work needs to be done in refining these relationships into a truly predictive equation, this semiempirical relationship remains useful to help conceptualize the interaction of the forces that govern water flux rate across the membrane.

Vilker et al. (69, 70), using an optical method to determine the concentration profile of the polarized protein layer at the solution membrane interface, studied a variety of single proteins in water. These studies showed that the oncotic pressure of polarized albumin is of sufficient magnitude to largely offset the hydrostatic pressure driving ultrafiltration, i.e., that the ultrafiltration flow rate in response to a transmembrane pressure gradient (ΔP) applied to plasma or whole blood is determined by the rise in oncotic pressure ($\Delta \pi$), i.e.

$$J_f = \frac{\Delta P - \Delta \pi}{R_m + R_p} , \qquad [34]$$

where R_m is the resistance of the membrane and R_p is the resistance of the polarized protein layer to water flow. Larger plasma proteins such as globulins do not contribute much to ($\Delta \pi$) because of their size and concentration but add a small amount to R_p. It is widely appreciated that polysulfone membrane adsorbs protein to its surface

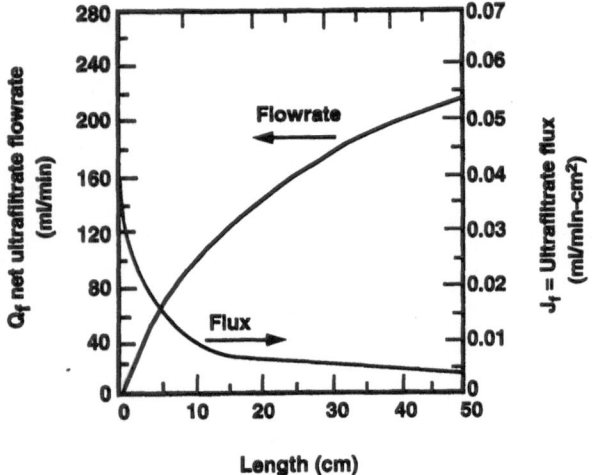

Figure 18. Net ultrafiltrate flow rate and ultrafiltrate flux are plotted against distance from the fiber inlet, for a 4,000 fiber unit with fiber internal diameter of 200 mm operated in the predilution mode ($Q_B = Q_f = 200$ ml/min). With a 20 cm length, a 1.0 m² total transport area is present.

and its hydraulic permeability is reduced 'irreversibly' on exposure to plasma protein; solute sieving is reduced as well. Original transport may be restored by chemical removal of this adsorbed protein but not by simple flushing/back flushing maneuvers (71–73). Polyacrylonitrile membrane similarly adsorbs protein, but shows a much less reduction in hydraulic permeability and solute sieving. Cuprophan® does not show these changes on blood exposure. Recent studies by Langsdorf and Zydney (74) compare transport properties for polyacrylonitrile and Cuprophan® membranes before and after exposure to blood. They find that they can rigorously describe the changes seen with polyachrilonitrile membrane mathematically using a two-layer membrane model. This model could account for both the decrease in sieving coefficients and the fall in diffusive permeability of the membrane.

Another useful expression (68) relates net ultrafiltration flow rate (Q_f) to the membrane area of the device (A), the diameter of the fiber (d) and the blood flow rate entering the device:

$$Q_f \propto (A/d)^{2/3}(Q_{Bi})^{1/3}. \qquad [35]$$

This points out that Q_f is independent of fiber length as long as (A/d) is held constant. It might be assumed incorrectly that for a given total membrane area, J_f could be increased by shortening the length of the fibers and increasing their numbers, holding total surface area constant. However, this is not true; if a given blood flow is directed into a greater number of fibers the shear rate in each fiber will fall and J_f will decrease as a result. Figure 18 depicts the differences in net flow of ultrafiltrate (Q_f) and ultrafiltrate flux (J_f) and their dependence on fiber length, i.e., (A/d) increasing.

Factors affecting solute transport

The other factor governing clearance of a solute is, of course, the degree of openness of the membrane as measured by its sieving (S) or reflection (σ) coefficient for that solute. The relationship between the phenomenologic membrane parameter S (or ε) and the intrinsic membrane property σ has already been explored (see equations 11, 12 and supporting text). What is important to note here are the special circumstances that pertain to hemofiltration and how they are relevant to the relationship between S and σ.

For solutes that are small in comparison with the pore diameter and are not held back, the concentration does not change as they traverse the pores in the membrane, i.e., the concentration of the solute in the ultrafiltrate (C_f) is the same as in the plasma water (C_w), and their ratio, the sieving coefficient (S), is 1.0:

$$S = \frac{C_f}{C_w} = 1. \qquad [36]$$

Equation 36 is valid only locally along the length of the fiber, because C_f and C_w vary with length. Operationally, we have access to the inflow and outflow blood of the ultrafilter as well as to the ultrafiltrate. S can be measured using the average of inflow and outflow plasma water concentration as an approximation of C_w for solutes with $S < 1$, i.e.

$$S = \frac{2C}{C_{wi} + C_{wo}}. \qquad [37]$$

This approximation has been shown to be reasonably accurate (better than 1%) for flow conditions reported with hollow fiber hemofiltration (52, 53). In this instance ($S = 1$), there will be no concentration gradient for the solute across the membrane to drive diffusion; as such, there is no contribution by diffusion to S, and S and σ may be considered operationally equivalent. These operating conditions, of course, do not occur with hemodialysis where $S \neq \sigma$. For solutes of such a size that $S < 1$ for the membrane, there is potentially a very different situation. The build up of protein ($S = 0$) at the membrane surface referred to as concentration polarization has been discussed above. An analogous circumstance applies to a partially sieved solute (e.g. $S = 0.5$). One may envision a concentration profile that is qualitatively the same as that shown for protein in Figure 17, or as depicted for the peritoneal membrane in Figure 14. At steady state (i.e. after a minute or two of operation), there will be a significant concentration gradient for diffusive transport from blood to ultrafiltrate. That is, the concentration of the solute in the polarized layer will be higher than that in the plasma water being ultrafiltered and, by virtue of membrane restraint, the concentration in the ultrafiltrate will be lower than that in the plasma water. With reference to Figures 14 and 17, the barrier to diffusion between the polarized solute layer and the ultrafiltrate stream is reduced to only the thickness of the separating synthetic membrane. The unstirred layers of fluid on both sides of the membrane, so important to the overall mass transfer resistance for diffusive transport, are swept away by the filtrate stream. Our expectation then is for values of S (or ε) to depart significantly ($S > \sigma$) from values of σ, by virtue of solute added to the filtrate stream by diffusion.

Hemofiltration is usually conducted with a transmembrane pressure gradient that falls on the plateau region of the plot of ultrafiltration flux rate and transmembrane pressure (see Figure 16). For clinical hemofiltration membranes this would be approximately 200 mmHg or above. As such, the filtrate flux rate (J_f) is at its maximum for the membrane, flow and concentration conditions present. With reference to equations 11 and 12, J_f is considered large and the relative contribution of diffusion to solute transport is small, i.e. ε approaches σ.

A second point to consider is that both logic and theory would predict that if a solute with $S < 1$ is polarized to the wall of an ultrafiltering membrane, this higher concentration will, in point of fact, perturb measured sieving coefficients such that they will be higher than would occur in the absence of such a concentration build up at the membrane, i.e., the solution being ultrafiltered by the membrane carries a solute concentration that is higher than we are aware of by measuring concentrations in the well-mixed domain remote from the membrane on the 'blood side'. These influences on S push in opposite directions as filtrate flux rate (J_f) is increased. The diffusive component of transport drops away and S falls, approaching σ whereas solute brought to and held at the membrane surface by the filtrate stream should make S rise above σ. One would expect, as J_f increased, to see a nadir reached for S that would be close to but still greater than σ, and that with further increase in J_f the measured S would rise in response to polarization of the test solute.

In a pragmatic check of these theoretical circumstances in the range of clinically relevant operating parameters, we conducted experiments with hemofiltration membranes that were being operated in the plateau region (75). Our test solute was polydispersed neutral dextran of sizes that ranged between full rejection by the membrane and nearly uninhibited passage. Two widely differing 'blood flows' (of plasma *in vitro*) were used (100 and 700 ml/min). Our aim at the higher flow rate was to sweep away the polarized layer of dextrans at the membrane surface and, hence, establish the true sieving coefficient. We were unable to show any difference in S for test solutes of any size at the two flow rates. In a second set of experiments in which 'blood flow rate' was held constant, and the filtration rate per unit area of membrane (J_f) was increased, the dextran S fell in a manner consonant with the dependence of S on J_f previously described. We were unable to show a rise in S as J_f increased to its maximum for the membrane used, suggesting that within practical operating limits of the hemofiltration membranes used, diffusive augmentation of S above σ is more important than the enhancement of

S caused by increased solute deposition at the membrane surface. The relationship may be rigorously stated as:

$$S = \frac{1 - \sigma}{1 - \sigma}\left[-J_v \frac{(1 - \sigma)}{P_m}\right] \qquad [38]$$

(Note the lack of a term implicating concentration polarization of the test solute.)

As noted for biological filtration membranes the charge of the solute molecule may contribute to its degree of sieving for certain membranes. Recent work (76, 77) points out that anionic dextran sulfate is preferentially rejected by the negatively charged polyacrylonitrile membrane (Biospal 3000S) but moves identically with neutral dextran of the same size across the uncharged polysulfone membrane (Fresenius F-60). Whether this is purely the effect of charge-charge interaction or whether membrane composition plays a role remains to be clarified. More work in this area of solute charge and transport is clearly needed to develop a full understanding of the intimate mechanisms involved in what clearly is a complex interaction[10]

Previous comment indicates that solute sieving for some membranes is reduced by the presence of protein. An 'irreversible' (to saline rinsing) fouling of these membranes lowers sieving coefficients for solutes of all sizes (73). Work by Langsdorf and Zydney using a hemodialysis membrane (AN69® polyacrylonitrile) has shown that this protein fouling layer (as distinct from the polarized layer of protein that develops as protein is convected to the surface of the membrane) may be satisfactorily modeled as a second filtration membrane in series with the first (83). This two-layer membrane model accurately describes the changes in sieving coefficients and diffusive permeabilities that are observed on blood contact. This two membrane model also describes the observed asymmetric convective transport properties (i.e. rectification) of this blood exposed (dual) membrane.

Solute concentration in plasma water (C_w) is related to the measured concentration of that solute (in the absence of protein binding) by:

$$\frac{C_p}{C_w} = 1 - \varphi, \qquad [39]$$

---

[10] Recent work on glomerular basement membrane (GBM) transport properties for dextran sulfate (a negatively charged polymer) casts strong doubt on the classical understanding of this subject taken from the work of Chang et al. (78, 79) and reviewed by Deen et al. (80). Studies by Tay and Comper (81, 82) indicate that this biological membrane takes up dextran sulfate by a metabolically driven, receptor mediated, mechanism probably lodged at the endothelial cell level. These receptors release desulfated dextran sulfate which then is transported through the GBM and gives the appearance at urinalysis of restrained transport of the charged, but not the uncharged, dextran. Synthetic membrane experiments then will provide a clearer understanding of the impact of solute charge on membrane transport.

where φ (the volume fraction of plasma proteins – the 'protocrit') may be calculated as the product of 0.0107 and the total concentration of plasma proteins in g/dl (43). Whole blood concentration (C_B) is related to plasma concentration as

$$\frac{C_B}{C_P} = 1 - H + HK, \qquad [40]$$

where H is the hematocrit, expressed as a decimal, and K is the distribution coefficient between red cells and plasma. For a solute entirely excluded from the red cell, such as inulin, $K = 0$, whereas if there is no difference in concentration across the red cell membrane then $K = 1$. The high hemoglobin concentration precludes K ever reaching 1.0 for passively distributed solutes. Typical K values (52, 53) for some solutes are

Inulin = 0.00
Urea = 0.86
Creatinine = 0.73.

Clearance

We may now express solute clearance in terms of flow rates and the sieving coefficient for that solute. By definition, clearance is the mass of solute removed divided by the concentration of that solute in the whole blood or plasma. The mass removed in the ultrafiltrate ($C_f Q_f$) is easily determined.

$$\text{Plasma clearance} = \frac{C_f Q_f}{C_w} = Q_f S. \qquad [41]$$

For certain solutes where the assay employed gives a significant reading (blank value) when no solute is present, e.g. for inulin, a particular form of the clearance equation may be useful if balanced operation pertains (ie the flow rates for diluting fluid and ultrafiltrate are equal).

$$\text{Whole blood clearance} = Q_B \frac{C_{pi} - C_{po}}{C_{pi}}. \qquad [42]$$

Note that it is not necessary to know K and H as they cancel out of the fraction. In predilution mode, C_{pi} should be sampled before dilution. In postdilution mode C_{po} should be sampled after dilution.

Measurements of solute concentration and flow on the blood side of the membrane make it possible to compute a mass balance for a particular solute:

$$C_{bi} Q_i - C_{Bo} Q_{bo} = Q_f C_f. \qquad [43]$$

The principle of the mass balance is that the mass lost from blood should appear in the ultrafiltrate. This calculation has also been used to assess adsorption of solute by the membrane since one reason for a mass balance not to 'close' is that mass is lost from the fluids examined. However, this is a relatively insensitive index in that the mass remaining is measured, rather than that adsorbed,

and the latter quantity is likely to fall within the error of measurement of the former.

Figure 19 illustrates the impact of sieving coefficient on whole blood clearance rate for solutes with K values that range 0 to 1, and compares predilution and postdilution modes of operation for a fixed set of flow conditions (52, 53, 68). It should be noted that for a given clearance rate, the amount of replacement fluid required in the postdilution mode is roughly half that required for operation in the predilution mode. Further, for a given sieving coefficient, and at these flow rates, clearance is higher in the predilution mode. Figure 20 shows the impact of the hematocrit on whole blood clearance for solutes with the range of K from 0 to 1 at the same flow conditions as in Figure 19. The apparent advantage of the linear increase in postdilution whole blood clearance is offset by the increased filtration flow rate in predilution mode due to the lower protein concentration of the diluted blood entering the device (52, 53, 68). The sieving coefficient was held at 1.0. Finally, Figure 21 shows the impact of ultrafiltration flow rate on whole blood clearance. It should be noted that for the postdilution mode there is a limit placed on the ultrafiltration flow rate by the concentration of plasma protein and red cells. The filtration fraction (glomerular filtration rate/renal plasma flow rate) achieved by the human glomerulus is 0.20 ± 0.05. Higher values occur in congestive heart failure or other abnormal circumstances. What filtration fraction is permissible in ultrafiltration from the standpoint of protein denaturation, red cell damage and plugging of the ultrafilter from overly viscous 'blood' is only now coming under study. Jenkins et al. (84, 85) have developed a mathematical model that predicts an 'operational instability' beginning at a post filter hematocrit of 50. Limited clinical tests support the model's conclusions. For hemofiltration in which a blood pump is employed this operational instability swiftly moves the system without any further manipulation to rupture of the blood path at its weakest point. For systems in which no pump is employed, e.g., continuous arteriovenous hemofiltration, there is simply stagnation of flow and clotting of the blood path. The curves for post dilution are plotted up to a filtration fraction of 0.5 in Figure 21.

For clearance calculations with hemofiltration, it is important to identify the volume of distribution of the solute in whole blood so that the appropriate expression for clearance can be used. Clearance is commonly expressed for either plasma or whole blood depending on the solute concentration. If a solute is distributed exclusively in the plasma water then:

$$C_{Bi} < C_{pi} < C_{wi} \text{ and } C_{Bo} < C_{po} < C_{wo}. \qquad [44]$$

Continuity requires that

$$Q_{Bi}(C_{Bi} - C_{Bo}) = Q_{pi}(C_{pi} - C_{po})$$
$$= Q_{wi}(C_{wi} - C_{wo}) \qquad [45]$$

and it follows that clearance from whole blood > clearance from plasma > clearance from plasma water.

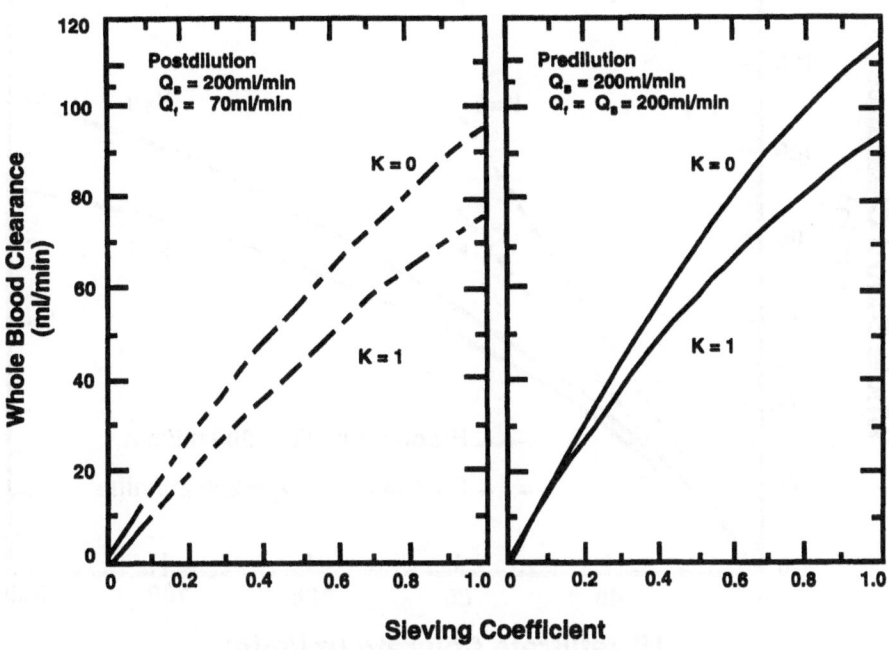

Figure 19. Whole blood clearance is plotted against sieving coefficient with pre- and postdilution for the range of K from 0 to 1 for 200 ml/min blood flow. Predilution results in a higher clearance.

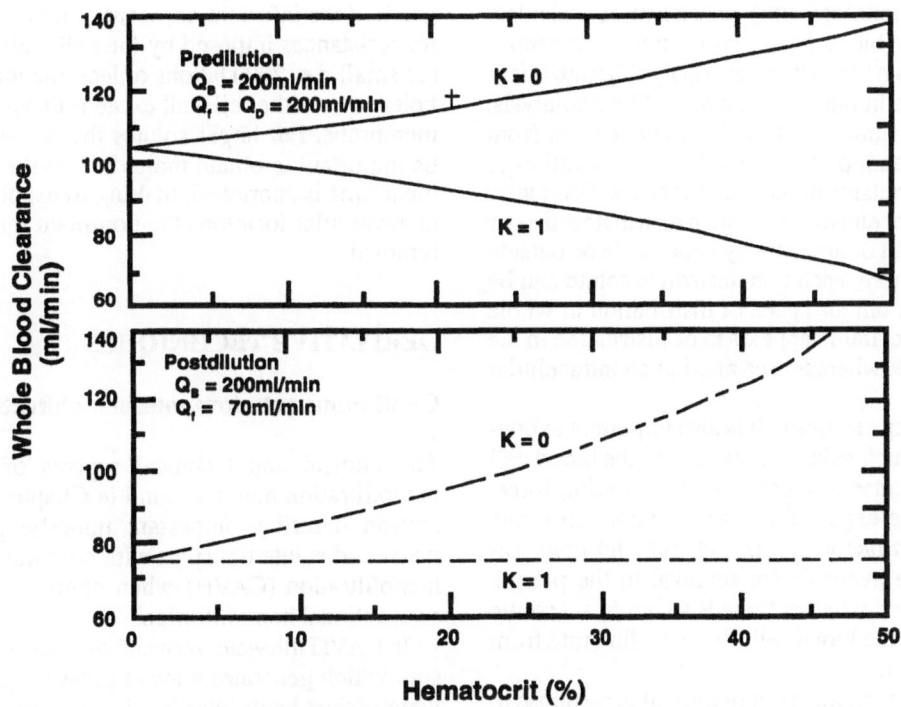

Figure 20. Effect of hematocrit on whole blood clearance by hemofiltration for the range of solute distributions ($K = 0$ to 1) in predilution and postdilution mode. For an intracellular solute in ready equilibrium with plasma water ($K = 1$) there is no change in clearance with hematocrit in the postdilution mode.

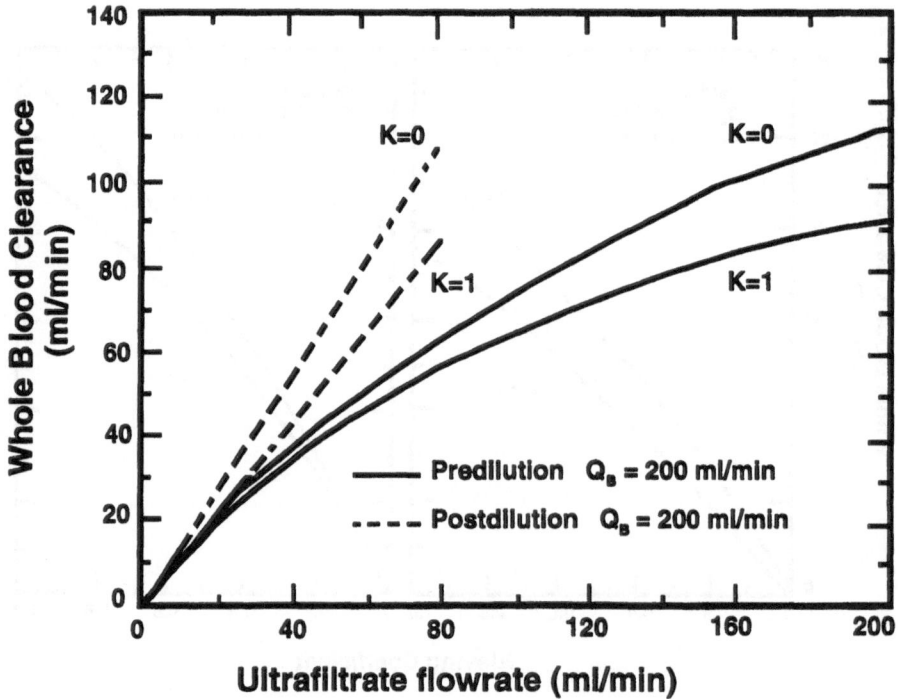

Figure 21. The effect of ultrafiltration flow rate on whole blood clearance, plotted for predilution and postdilution mode. The postdilution mode curves are terminated at a filtration fraction of 0.5 (see text).

It is not (methodologically) consistent to calculate clearance of whole blood from plasma solute concentrations (C_p) and whole blood flow rate (Q_B) although this is a common practice in the clinical world of hemodialysis. That calculation assumes that blood is homogeneous from a concentration standpoint, i.e. that the concentration of solutes inside and outside the cell are the same. This clearly does not apply for electrolytes which distribute either by Donnan equilibrium or are actively kept inside or outside the cells. Furthermore, each nonelectrolyte solute can be expected to have a unique space of distribution in whole blood. For example, inulin appears to be distributed in the plasma water alone, whereas urea also has an intracellular distribution.

When calculating clearance, it is also important to consider the rate at which solutes move across the blood cell membrane in response to a concentration driving force. Each solute can be expected to have a unique flux rate depending on such factors as size, charge and lipid solubility. The solute available for removal in the plasma water will depend on whether there is a significant solute distribution within the blood cell and on its flux rate from cell to plasma water.

Studies on urea movement out of the cell in response to the concentration gradient established by 50% dilution of whole blood in predilution mode hemofiltration indicate swift equilibration between red cell and plasma water (86). This, likely, will not be the case for other larger solutes or those bearing a charge. Frost et al. (87) summarized

much of the information, scant as it is, on the mass transfer resistances imposed by the cell wall. For solutes that are small, i.e. 200 Daltons or less, the mass transfer coefficient across the cell wall exceeds that across the dialyzer membrane. For larger solutes the reverse is true. It will be important to obtain more data on this subject as treatment time is shortened, making transport of solutes from extravascular locations the dominant resistance to solute removal.

DERIVATIVE TECHNIQUES

Continuous arteriovenous hemofiltration

The clinical and technical aspects of this variant of hemofiltration may be found in Chapter 15. The present section describes important underlying differences in water and solute transport with continuous arteriovenous hemofiltration (CAVH) when contrasted with those for conventional hemofiltration.

In CAVH the water movement stems from arterial pressure which generates a lower pressure gradient than that which drives hemofiltration, i.e., transmembrane pressure is commonly less than 100 mmHg in CAVH. This means that the filter is operated well below the plateau region noted in Figure 16, where filtration rate is plotted against transmembrane pressure; i.e. concentration polarization

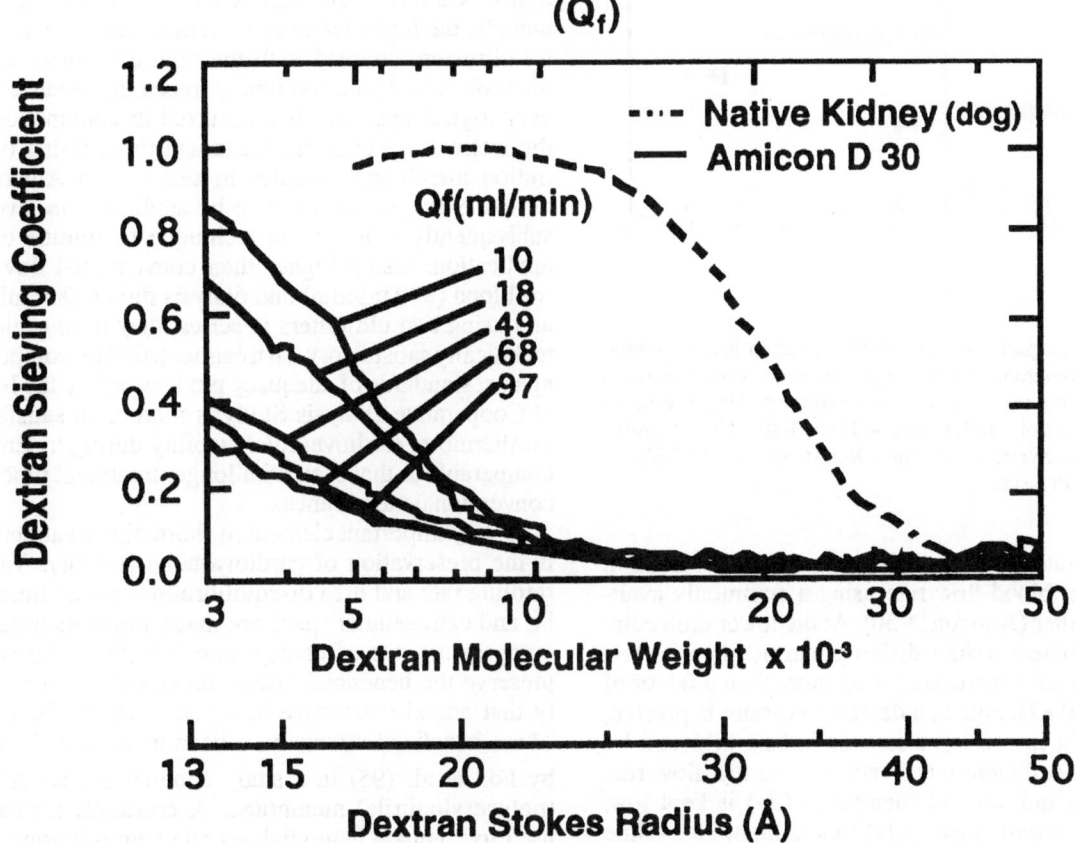

Sieving profile for a 0.5m² membrane at various ultrafiltration flow rates (Q_f)

Figure 22. The sieving profile for an Amicon D-30 CAVH filter is compared with that for dog glomerular membrane over the range of dextran sizes from 13 to 50 Å. At increasing ultrafiltration rate the D-30 membrane shows a fall in sieving coefficient. Clearance ($Q_f \times S$) however rises as ultrafiltration rate increases.

of protein does not limit the water flux rate (J_f). This has important implications for filter design as it means that membrane hydraulic permeability (after exposure to blood) is the most important determinant of the filtration flow rate during clinical operation of CAVH filters (88). This is contrary to transport with routine hemofiltration where the polarized protein layer, not the membrane hydraulic permeability, governs J_f. Return of the control of this important governing parameter for clearance to the hands of the design engineer has not as yet been translated into membranes with hydraulic permeability exceeding that of devices routinely used for hemofiltration. Hydraulic permeability for these latter membranes has not been systematically optimized at driving pressures relevant to CAVH. However, the previously discussed reduction of solute and solvent transport as a result of blood exposure modeled as a dual layer membrane (for

AN69® (polyacrylonitrile)) will apply to this membrane used for CAVH. Polysulfone membrane also has been shown to adsorb protein and show reduced transport properties (89). It is likely that high flux cellulose triacetate membrane will behave like Cuprophan® (also cellulosic in composition) which does not adsorb much protein. It seems likely that a new set of filters designed to operate at 150 mmHg or less will be forthcoming. In addition to preventing flux deterioration by protein adsorption, they will also permit better clearance at lower pressures than are currently available from hemofiltration membranes scaled down in size for use in CAVH.

As is predictable from prior considerations (equations 5, 11, 12) when a CAVH filter is operated at these low flows there is a significant diffusive component to the clearance, i.e. S is larger than σ. Figure 22 plots the dependence of neutral dextran sieving coefficients on ultrafil-

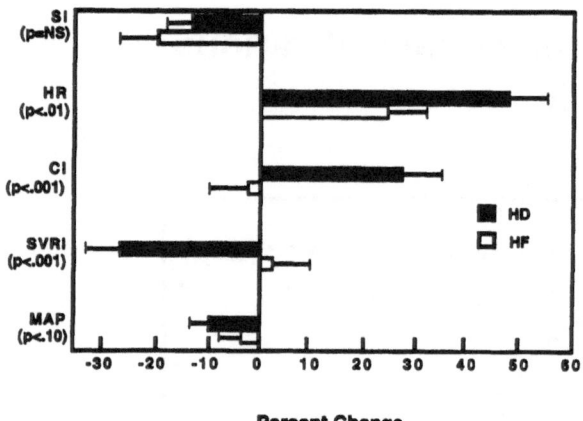

Figure 23.   Comparison of percent changes in hemodynamic indices at end-treatment relative to pre-treatment values between HD and HF using polyacrylonitrile membrane. Data are mean ± SEM. SI = Stroke Index; HR = Heart Rate; CI = Cardiac Index; SVRI = Systemic Vascular Resistance Index; MAP = Mean Arterial Pressure.

tration flow rate (75), over the range 10 to 97 ml/min for a constant blood flow rate using a commonly available CAVH filter (Amicon D-30). At the lower molecular weight end, there is a sharp difference in sieving with low ultrafiltration rates increasing S by more than a factor of two (0.39 to 0.82). Again, a design constraint is present, indicating that increasing clearance is best achieved by providing: a) sufficient membrane area so that flow rate of filtrate per unit area of membrane (J_f) is kept low, b) an overall filtration rate (Q_f) that is high, Net solute transport rate then will have the convective transport component augmented by diffusion.

The principle identified in the above paragraph is logically applied to further enhance the transport efficiency of CAVH membranes by providing a concentration gradient, even for solutes that pass the membrane with a sieving coefficient of unity. This is readily achieved by circulating dialysis fluid through the casing of the filter at a slow (10 to 15 ml/min) rate, i.e. continuous arteriovenous hemodiafiltration (CAVHD) (90). Recalling that the principle barrier for difusive transport is the length of the diffusion path, optimum design of a CAVHD membrane would require that, in addition to being permeable to convective solute transport, they also be thin. This thinness would provide a short diffusion path from blood to 'dialysate' and thus high diffusive permeability. Because of the differences in mechanical strength, most asymmetric membranes used for hemofiltration are thick and spongy (40 to 60 microns) as opposed to cellulose and cellulose derivatives (10 to 15 microns or less when wet). Again, deliberate exploitation by industry of this potential advantage is expected.

It is apparent that optimizing membranes for CAVH and CAVHD is a different matter than for HF.

Hemodiafiltration

The combination of hemodialysis and hemofiltration was first exploited by Leber et al. (91), with the deliberate aim of capturing the best features of both techniques, namely, the high clearance of conventional small solutes by diffusion, coupled with the high clearances of middle molecules by convection. A recent resurgence in this very logical approach has occurred in conjunction with the interest in shortening treatment time. Using two filtration membrane modules in series. von Albertini et al. (92–94) have shown it to be applicable *in vivo*, and subsequently reduced the technique to routine clinical application. Using higher than conventional flow rates for blood (500 ml/min) and dialysis fluid (1000 ml/min), and using two ultrafilters in series, they have achieved a technically satisfactory 2 h treatment, that by computation against standards of adequacy put forward by the National Cooperative Dialysis Study is more than satisfactory. Furthermore, cardiovascular stability during treatment is comparable to that seen with longer treatment times with conventional membranes.

A very important element in shortening treatment time is the preservation of cardiovascular stability. Vascular refilling rate and urea disequilibrium between intracellular and extracellular space are made worse materially by compressing 4 h of change into 2 h (94). The need to preserve the beneficial effects on cardiovascular stability that attend convective transport then will be crucial. These beneficial effects have been underscored recently by Fox et al. (95) in a study conducted with AN69® (polyacrylonitrile) membrane. A crossover format was used to compare hemodialysis and hemofiltration in the same patient in order to identify potential mechanisms for their disparate hemodynamic responses. With reference to Figure 23, it is apparent that systemic vascular resistance drops profoundly with hemodialysis and does not change with hemofiltration. This disparity is not readily explained by presently understood mechanisms of response to these two blood cleansing techniques. A role for an as yet unidentified vasodilatory substance, generated during dialysate exposure or convectively removed (as contrasted with adsorptively removed) during hemofiltration, remain intriguing possibilities.

ACKNOWLEDGEMENTS

I should like to thank my friend and administrative assistant, Ms. Marlene Ziemniak, for her help with the preparation of this manuscript and in particular for her meticulous attention to the details of format and for preparation of the figures. In addition, I am indebted to my colleagues, Norma Ofsthun, PhD and Gretchen Kunas, MS for their careful proofreading of the final manuscript.

REFERENCES

1. Spiegler KS, Kadem O: Thermodynamics of hyperfiltration (reverse osmosis): Criteria for efficient membranes. *Desalination* 1: 311, 1966
2. Villarroel F, Klein E, Holland F: Solute flux in hemodialysis and hemofiltration membranes. *ASAIO J* 23: 225, 1977
3. Dedrick RL, Flessner MF, Collins JM, Schultz JS: Commentary: is the peritoneum a membrane? *ASAIO J* 5: 1, 1982
4. Flessner MF, Dedrick RL, Schultz JS: A distributed model of peritoneal-plasma transport: theoretical considerations. *Am J Physiol* 246: R597, 1984
5. Leypoldt JK, Parker HR, Frigon RP, Henderson LW: Molecular size dependence of peritoneal transport. *J Lab Clin Med* 110: 207, 1987
6. Nolph KD, Mactier R, Khanna R: Twardowski ZJ, Moore H, McGary T: The kinetics of ultrafiltration during peritoneal dialysis: the role of the lymphatics. *Kidney Int* 32: 219, 1987
7. Mactier RA, Khanna R, Twardowski Z, Moore H, Nolph KD: Contribution of lymphatic absorption to loss of ultrafiltration and solute clearances in continuous ambulatory peritoneal dialysis. *J Clin Invest* 80: 1311, 1987
8. Durand P, Chanliau J, Gamberoni J, Hestin D, Kessler M: Intraperitoneal hydrostatic pressure and ultrafiltration volume in CAPD. *Adv Perit Dial* 9: 233, 1993
9. Krediet RT, Imholz ALT, Struijk DG, Koomen GCM, Arisz L: Effects of tracer, volume, osmolality and infection on fluid kinetics during CAPD. *Blood Purif* 10: 173, 1992
10. Pust AH, Leypoldt JK, Frigon RP, Henderson LW: Peritoneal dialysate volume measured by indicator dilution measurements. *Kidney Int* 33: 64, 1988
11. Leypoldt JK, Pust AH, Frigon RP, Henderson LW: Dialysate volume measurements required for determining peritoneal solute transport. *Kidney Int* 34: 254, 1988
12. Pyle WK, Moncrief JW, Popovich RP: Peritoneal transport evaluation in CAPD. in *CAPD Update; Continuous Ambulatory Peritoneal Dialysis*, edited by Moncrief JW, Popovich RP, New York, Masson Publ USA Inc, 1981
13. Rippe B, Stelin G, Haraldsson B: Computer simulations of peritoneal fluid transport in CAPD. *Kidney Int* 40: 315, 1991
14. Rippe B, Haraldsson B: Transport of macromolecules across microvascular walls: the two-pore theory. *Physiol Rev* 74: 163, 1994
15. Waniewski J, Verynski A, Heimburger O, Lindholm B: A comparative analysis of mass transport in peritoneal dialysis. *ASAIO J* 37: 65, 1991
16. Vonesh EF, Rippe B: Net fluid absorption under membrane transport models of peritoneal dialysis. *Blood Purif* 10: 209, 1992
17. Daniels FH, Leonard EF, Cortell S: Glucose and glycerol compared as osmotic agents for peritoneal dialysis. *Kidney Int* 25: 20, 1984
18. Henderson LW, Nolph KD: Altered permeability of the peritoneal membrane after using hypertonic peritoneal fluid. *J Clin Invest* 48: 922, 1969
19. Nolph KD, Hano JE, Teschan PE: Peritoneal sodium transport during hypertonic peritoneal dialysis. *Ann Intern Med* 70: 931, 1969
20. Brown ST, Ahearn DJ, Nolph KD: Potassium removal with peritoneal dialysis. *Kidney Int* 4: 67, 1973

21. Rubin J, Klein E, Bower JD: Investigation of the net sieving coefficient of the peritoneal membrane during peritoneal dialysis. *ASAIO J* 5: 9, 1982
22. Henderson LW: The problem of peritoneal membrane area and permeability. *Kidney Int* 3: 409, 1973
23. Rubin J, Nolph KD, Popovich RP, Moncrief JW, Prowant B: Drainage volume during continuous ambulatory peritoneal dialysis. *ASAIO J* 2: 54, 1979
24. Nolph KD, Miller FN, Pyle WK, Popovich RP, Sorkin Ml: An hypothesis to explain the ultrafiltration characteristics of peritoneal dialysis. *Kidney Int* 20: 543, 1981
25. Bell JL, Leypoldt JK, Frigon RP, Henderson LW: Hydraulically-induced convective solute transport across the rabbit peritoneum. *Kidney Int* 38: 19, 1990
26. Leypoldt JK: Evaluation of peritoneal membrane pore models. *Blood Purif* 10: 227, 1992
27. Chen TW, Khanna R, Moore H, Twardowski ZJ, Nolph KD: Sieving and reflection coefficients for sodium salts and glucose during peritoneal dialysis in rats. *J Am Soc Nephrol* 2: 1092, 1991
28. Nolph KD, Twardowski ZJ: The peritoneal dialysis system. in *Peritoneal Dialysis*, 2nd ed, edited by Nolph KD, The Hague, Martinus Nijhoff Publishers, 1985, p 23
29. Patlak CS, Goldstein DA, Hoffman JF: The flow of solute and solvent across a two-membrane system. *J Theor Biol* 5: 426, 1963
30. Leypoldt JK, Chiu AS, Frigon RP, Henderson LW: Dialysate to blood transport of macromolecules during peritoneal dialysis. *Am J Physiol* 275: H1851, 1989
31. Leypldt JK, Henderson LW: The effect of convection on bidirectional peritoneal transport: predictions from a distributed model. *Ann Biomed Enginr* 20: 463, 1992
32. Green DM, Antwiler GD, Moncrief JW, Decherd JF, Popovich RP: Measurement of the transmittance coefficient spectrum of Cuprophan and RP 69 membranes: Applications to middle molecule removal via ultrafiltration. *ASAIO J* 22: 627, 1976
33. Henderson LW: Redy® or not. *ASAIO J* 2: 49, 1979
34. Nolph KD, Stoltz ML, Carter CB, Fox M, Maher JF: Factors affecting the composition of ultrafiltrate from hemodialysis coils. *ASAIO J* 16: 495, 1970
35. Donnan FG: Theory of membrane equilibria. *Chem Reviews* 1: 73, 1924–1925
36. Ramenofsky JA, Prestidge H, Ford C, Sanfelippo ML, Henderson LW: Novel applications for hemofiltration membranes. *ASAIO J* 27: 613, 1981
37. Floege J, Granolleras C, Deschodt G, Heck M, Baudin G, Branger B, Tournier O, Reinhard B, Eisenbach GM, Smeby LC, Koch KM, Shaldon S: High flux synthetic versus cellulosic membranes for beta-2-microglobulin removal during hemodialysis, hemodiafiltration and hemofiltration. *Nephrol Dial Transplant* 4: 653, 1989
38. Lonnemann G, Behme T, Lenzner B, Floege J, Schulze M, Colton CK, Koch KM, Shaldon S: Permeability of dialyzer membranes to TNFα-inducing substances derived from water bacteria. *Kidney Int* 42: 61, 1992
39. Schmidt M, Baldamus CA, Schoeppe W: Back filtration in hemodialyzers with highly permeable membranes. *Blood Purif* 2: 108, 1984
40. Starling EH, Tubby AH: On absorption from and secretion into the serous cavities. *J Physiol* 16: 140, 1894

41. Leypoldt JK, Schmidt B, Gurland HJ: Measurement of backfiltration rates during hemodialysis with high permeability membranes *Blood Purif* 9: 74, 1991

42. Soltys PJ, Ofsthun NJ, Leypoldt JK: Critical analysis of formulas for estimating backfiltration in hemodialysis. *Blood Purif* 10: 326, 1992

43. Colton CK, Smith KA, Merrill EW, Friedman S: Diffusion of urea in flowing blood. *Am Inst Chem Enginr* 117: 800, 1971

44. Ofsthun NJ, Schockley TR (Eds): Lymphatic and non-lymphatic fluid loss from the peritoneal cavity. *Blood Purif* 10: 109, 1992

45. Leypoldt JK, Blindauer KM: Peritoneal solvent drag reflection coefficients are within the physiological range. *Blood Purif.* In press

46. Mactier RA, Khanna R, Twardowski Z, Nolph KD: Role of the peritoneal cavity lymphatic absorption in peritoneal dialysis. *Kidney Int* 32: 165, 1987

47. Zink J, Greenway CV: Control of ascites absorption in anesthetized cats: affects of intraperitoneal pressure, protein and furosemide diuresis. *Gasteroenterol* 73: 1119, 1977

48. Okamoto SN, Fox SD, Leypoldt JK, Henderson LW: Abdominal compression reduces fluid absorption during peritoneal dialysis in the rabbit. *Kidney Int* 35 (Abstract): 274, 1989

49. Mistry CD, Mallick NP, Gokal R: Ultrafiltration with an isosmotic solution during long peritoneal dialysis exchange. *Lancet* 178, 1987

50. Nolph KD, Fox M, Maher JF: Factors affecting the ultrafiltration rate from standard dialysis coils. *ASAIO J* 16: 487, 1970

51. Husted FC, Nolph KD, Vitale FC, Maher JF: Detrimental effects of ultrafiltration on diffusion in coils. *J Lab Clin Med* 87: 435, 1976

52. Colton CK, Henderson LW, Ford CA, Lysaght MJ: Kinetics of hemodiafiltration I. *In vitro* transport characteristics of a hollow fiber blood ultrafilter. *J Lab Clin Med* 85: 355, 1975

53. Henderson LW, Colton CK, Ford C: Kinetics of hemodiafiltration. II. Clinical characterization of a new blood cleansing modality. *J Lab Clin Med* 85: 372, 1975

54. Henderson LW: Peritoneal ultrafiltration dialysis: enhanced urea transfer using hypertonic peritoneal dialysis fluid. *J Clin Invest* 45: 950, 1966

55. Babb AL, Johansen PJ, Strand MJ, Tenckhoff H, Scribner BH: Bidirectional permeability of the human peritoneum to middle molecules. *Proc Eur Dial Transplant Assoc* 10: 247, 1973

56. Randerson DH, Farrell PC: Mass transfer properties of the human peritoneum. *ASAIO J* 3: 140, 1980

57. Andreoli TE, Schafer JA, Troutman SL: Coupling of solute and solvent flows in porous lipid bilayer membranes. *J Gen Physiol* 57: 479, 1971

58. Levitt MD, Kneip JM, Overdahl MC: Influence of shaking on peritoneal transfer in rats. *Kidney Int* 35: 1145, 1989

59. Leonard E, Bluemle LW Jr: The permeability concept as applied to dialysis. *Trans Am Soc Artif Intern Organs* 6: 33, 1960

60. Wilson EE: A rational design for heat transfer apparatus *Trans Am Soc Mech Enginr* 37: 47, 1916

61. Blatt WF, Dravid A, Michaels AS, Nelson L: Solute polarization and cake formation in membrane ultrafiltration: causes, consequences and control techniques. in *Membrane Science and Technology*, edited by Flinn JE, New York, Plenum Corporation, 1970

62. Colton CK: Permeability and transport studies in batch and flow dialyzers with application to hemodialysis. PhD Thesis Massachusetts Institute of Technology, Cambridge, MA, 1969

63. Renkin EM, Gilmore JP: Glomerular filtration. in *Handbook of Physiology*, edited by Orloff J, Berliner RW, Am Physiological Society, Washington, DC, 1973

64. Leypoldt JK, Blindauer KM: Convection does not govern plasma to dialysate transport of protein. *Kidney Int* 42: 1412, 1992

65. Flessner MF, Parker RJ, Sieber SM: Peritoneal lymphatic uptake of fibrinogen and erythrocytes in the rat. *Am J Physiol* 244: H89, 1983

66. Rippe B, Stelin G, Ahlem J: Lymph flow from the peritoneal cavity in CAPD patients. in *Frontiers in Peritoneal Dialysis*, edited by Maher JF, Winchester JF, New York, Field, Rich and Assoc, 1986

67. Okazaki M, Yoshida F: Ultrafiltration of blood: effect of hematocrit on ultrafiltration rate. *Ann Biomed Enginr* 4: 138–150, 1976

68. Lysaght MJ, Ford CA, Colton CK, Stone RA, Henderson LW: Mass transfer in clinical blood ultrafiltration devices – a review. in *Technical Aspects of Renal Dialysis*, edited by Frost TH, Tunbridge Wells, Pitman Medical Publ Co, 1978

69. Vilker VL, Colton CK, Smith KA: Concentration polarization in protein ultrafiltration. *Am Inst Chem Enginr* 47: 632, 1981

70. Vilker VL, Colton CK, Smith KA, Green DL: The osmotic pressure of concentrated protein and lipoprotein solutions and its significance to ultrafiltration. *J Memb Sci* 20: 63, 1984

71. Leypoldt JK, Frigon RP, Alford MF, Uyeji SN, Henderson LW: The effects of plasma protein on sieving properties of hemofilters. in *Progress in Artificial Organs – 1983*, edited by Atsumi KA, Maekawa M, Ota K, Cleveland, ISAO (presentation) 1984, p 580

72. Leypoldt JK, Frigon RP, Henderson LW: Dextran sieving coefficients of hemofiltration membranes. *Trans Am Soc Artif Intern Organs* 29: 678, 1983

73. Frigon RP, Leypoldt JK, Alford MF, Uyeji SN, Henderson LW: Hemofilter solute sieving is not governed by dynamic polarized protein. *Trans Am Soc Artif Intern Organs* 30: 486, 1984

74. Langsdorf LJ, Zydney AL: Diffusive and convective solute transport through hemodialysis membranes: a hydrodynamic analysis. *J Biomed Materials Res.* In press

75. Henderson LW, Leypoldt JK, Frigon RP: The impact of membrane area on solute clearance in continuous arteriovenous hemofiltration. in *Proc Int Symp on Continuous Arteriovenous Hemofiltration*, edited by La Greca G, Fabris A, Ronco C, Milan, Wichtig Editore, 1986, p 37

76. Leypoldt JK, Frigon RP, Henderson LW: Macromolecular charge effects hemofilter solute sieving. *Trans Am Soc Artif Intern Organs* 32: 384, 1986

77. Leypoldt JK, Frigon RP, Okamoto S, Henderson LW: Macrosolute charge independent of sign decreases sieving coefficient. Abstract 5th Annual Mtg Int Soc Blood Purification. *Blood Purif* 5: 268, 1988

78. Chang RLS, Ueki IF, Troy JL, Deen WM, Robertson CR, Brenner BM: Permselectivity of the glomerular capillary wall to macromolecules. II. Experimental studies in rats using neutral dextran. *Biophyics J* 15: 887, 1975

79. Chang RLS, Deen WM, Robertson CR, Brenner BM: Perselectivity of the glomerular capillary wall. III. Restricted transport of polyanions. *Kidney Int* 8: 212, 1975

80. Deen WM, Satvat B, Jamieson JM: Theoretical model for glomerular filtration of charged solutes. *Am J Physiol* 241: F126, 1980

81. Tay M, Comper WD, Singh AK: Charge selectivity in kidney ultrafiltration is associated with glomerular uptake of transport probes. *Am J Physiol* 260: F549, 1991

82. Comper WD, Tay M, Wells X, Dawes J: Desulphation of dextran sulphate during kidney ultrafiltration. *Biochem J* 297: 31, 1994

83. Langsdorf LJ, Zydney AL: Effect of blood contact on the transport properties of the hemodialysis membranes: a two-layer membrane model. *Blood Purif*. In press

84. Jenkins RD, Funk JE, Chen B, Golper T: A mathematical model for flow, pressure and ultrafiltration rate in extracorporeal filtration of blood. *Blood Purif* 10: 282, 1992

85. Jenkins RD, Funk JE, Chen B, Golper T: Operational instability in extracorporeal filtration of blood. *Blood Purif* 10: 292, 1992

86. Cheung AK, Alford MF, Wilson MM, Leypoldt JK, Henderson LW: Urea movement across erythrocyte membrane during artificial kidney treatment. *Kidney Int* 23: 866, 1983

87. Frost TH, Kerr DNS: Kinetics of hemodialysis: A theoretical study of the removal of solutes in chronic renal failure compared to normal health. *Kidney Int* 12: 41, 1977

88. Lysaght MJ, Schmidt B, Gurland HJ: Filtration rates and pressure driving forces in AV filtration. *Blood Purif* 1: 178, 1983

89. Röckel A, Hertel J, Fiegel P, Abdelhamid S, Panitz N, Walb D: Permeability in secondary membrane formation of a high-flux polysulphone hemofilter. *Kidney Int* 30: 429, 1986

90. Schneider NS, Geronemus RP: Continuous arteriovenous hemodialysis. *Kidney Int* 33 (Suppl 24): S159, 1988

91. Leber HW, Wizemann V, Goubeaud G, Rawer P, Schutterle G: Simultaneous hemofiltration/hemodialysis: an effective alternative to hemofiltration and conventional hemodialysis in the treatment of uremic patients. *Clin Nephrol* 9: 115, 1978

92. von Albertini B, Miller JH, Gardner PW, Shinaberger JH: High flux hemodiafiltration: Under six hours per week treatment. *Trans Am Soc Artif Intern Organs* 30: 227, 1984

93. Miller JH, von Albertini B, Gardner BW, Shinaberger JH: Technical aspects of high flux hemodiafiltration for adequate short [under two hours] treatment. *Trans Am Soc Artif Intern Organs* 30: 377, 1984

94. von Albertini B, Garcia-Valdecasa J, Barlee V, Lew SQ, Bosch JP: Solute rebound in highly efficient: Impact on quantification of therapy. *J Am Soc Nephrol* (Abstract) 4: 393, 1993

95. Fox SD, Henderson LW: Cardiovascular response during hemodialysis and hemofiltration: Thermal membrane and catecholamine influences. *Blood Purif* 11: 224, 1993

PERITONEAL ANATOMY AND PHYSIOLOGY DURING PERITONEAL DIALYSIS

RAYMOND T. KREDIET

ANATOMY

The peritoneum is the largest serous membrane in the body. It is a sac that covers the inner side of the abdominal wall, forms the mesentery to which loops of bowel are suspended, and reflects over the contained viscera (Figure 1). In the male the sac is closed, in the female the free end of the uterine tubes open into the peritoneal cavity. The part that lines the abdominal wall is named the parietal peritoneum, the part that covers the viscera constitutes the visceral peritoneum. Loosely arranged extraperitoneal connective tissue is present between the parietal peritoneum and the abdominal wall. The visceral peritoneum on the other hand is firmly united to the viscera which it covers. The parietal and visceral layers are in actual contact, but the virtual space between them is named the peritoneal cavity. It consists of a main portion, named the greater sac (*cavum peritonei*) and a diverticulum from this, termed the lesser sac (*omental bursa*), situated behind the stomach and adjoining structures. Both sacs are connected by the epiploic foramen. The peritoneal cavity is lined with a layer of flattened mesothelium and lubricated by a small quantity of serous fluid. This allows movement of the viscera with a minimum of friction (1). During peritoneal dialysis the peritoneal cavity is filled with dialysis fluid.

Anatomic studies on the surface area of the peritoneum are scarce. Wegener mentioned a surface area of 1.72 m^2 in one adult woman, but no information was given on the method of measurement (2). Putiloff reported a similar value of 2.07 m^2 in one adult male (3). Much lower values of about 1 m^2 in adults have been found in two

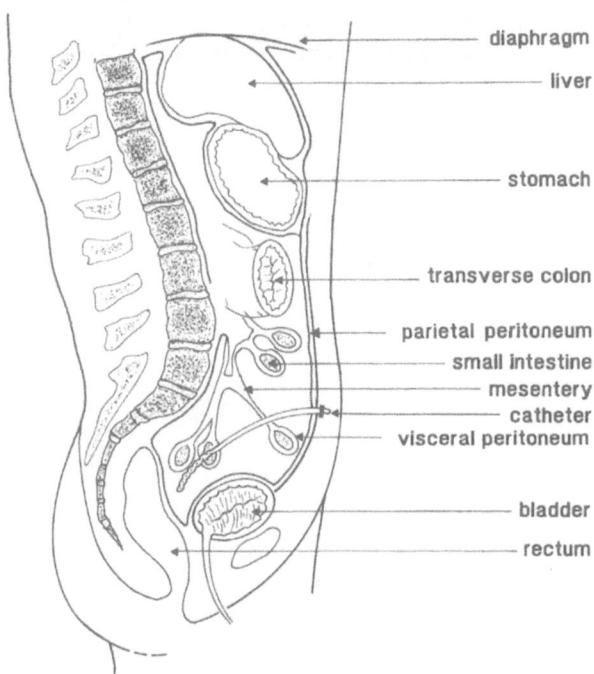

Figure 1. A sagittal section through the peritoneal cavity. A peritoneal catheter is in place.

more recent studies (4, 5). About 60% of the peritoneum consists of visceral peritoneum (10% of this covers the liver), 30% of mesenterium and omentum, and 10% is parietal peritoneum. The latter 38% of which covers the diaphragm (4). The ratio between peritoneal surface area and body weight in adults is about half that found in a newborn infant (4). The contribution of the various parts of the peritoneum to solute transport during peritoneal dialysis may be different. Evisceration was found to lead to a marked reduction in the transport of creatinine in rabbits (6), but not in rats (7, 8). Effective peritoneal dialysis has been described in a neonate with extensive resection of the small intestine (9). It has recently been suggested that especially the peritoneum covering the liver may be important in solute transport during peritoneal dialysis, because of the close relationship with the liver sinusoids (10). The diaphragmatic part of the peritoneum is especially involved in the absorption of solutes and fluid from the peritoneal cavity into the lymphatic system (11).

The parietal peritoneum derives its arterial supply from the arteries perfusing the abdominal and pelvic walls, its veins and lymphatics join the systemic veins in the neighbouring parts of the body wall. They eventually drain into the caval vein and the thoracic duct. The visceral peritoneum derives its arterial supply from the arteries supplying the appropriate viscera, its veins join the visceral vessels (1). The visceral veins drain into the portal vein. The visceral lymphatics drain into parietal lymph nodes and from there to the thoracic duct. The lymphatic drainage of the peritoneal cavity is mainly by subdiaphragmatic gaps in the mesothelium, so called stomata. These occur only at the sites of lymphatic lacunae. The lymph is collected in the peritoneal diaphragmatic plexus, that communicates with the pleural diaphragmatic plexus. From there, the lymph is transported in collecting ducts associated with the internal mammary blood vessels to the anterior mediastinal lymph nodes. These structures mainly drain into the right lymphatic duct. In addition, some of the lymphatic drainage from the peritoneal cavity passes into the thoracic duct (11).

HISTOLOGY AND CELL BIOLOGY

The peritoneal cavity is lined with mesothelial cells. They originate from the embryonic mesodermal layer, as do endothelial cells. This probably occurs by differentiation from subserosal multipotent cells, the mesenchymal stemcells. These cells have characteristics of myofibroblasts, such as the expression of vimentin, but also epithelial markers like cytokeratin. Vimentin disappears during the differentiation to mesothelial cells (12–14). The mesothelium consists of a flat layer of polygonal cells forming a mosaic structure. The cells lie on a thin basement membrane and overlap each other like roof tiles (15–18). They are covered with microvilli and often have a cilium. Besides tight junctions between the cells, communicating and macular junctions have also been found, making them resemble the endothelium found in the venules (19). The width of the intercellular channels in rabbits averaged 423 Å in one study (17). The nuclei are ovoid or ellipsoid and contain nucleoli. The cytosol contains

many organelles such as a rough endoplasmatic reticulum, a prominent Golgi apparatus and sometimes lamellar bodies (20). The latter are composed of phospholipids and probably store phosphatidylcholine, the main constituent of the lubricant in the peritoneal cavity (21). Mesothelial cells of uremic non-dialyzed patients are normal on light microscopy (16, 23), but contain cytoplasmic inclusions when examined by transmission electron microscopy. They consist of densely osmophilic filaments within the cisterna of the rough endoplasmatic reticulum (23), and may be involved in the pathogenesis of uremic serositis (24).

The mesothelium during peritoneal dialysis has some special features: the cells have a more cubic form and the number of cells per unit of surface area is higher. This leads to an increase of the total length of the intercellular junctions. These junctions can be wider than normal. The cells have been described as reactive; the number of microvilli is decreased. Sometimes degeneration of mesothelial cells is present. Scanning electron microscopy often shows blisters and blebs on the cell surface. Hyperplasia of the rough endoplasmatic reticulum, the Golgi apparatus and the lamellar bodies is found (16, 17, 25–27). A comparison between normal mesothelial cells and those during peritoneal dialysis is shown in Figure 2.

Mesothelial cells are capable of synthesizing and excreting various substances. The presence of lamellar bodies in mesothelial cells and the demonstration of surface active material containing phosphatidylcholine in peritoneal effluent of CAPD patients (28) are in favour of its synthesis by the mesothelium. This is probably by a process of exocytosis of the lamellar bodies from the apical part of mesothelial cells, similar to surfactant production of type II pneumocytes (29, 30). The role of phosphatidylcholine in serous cavities is probably to decrease friction between the various organs that they contain (31). The effect on the decrease of surface tension is only present at the fluid air interface. The phosphatidylcholine concentration in peritoneal effluent may therefore be regarded as an indicator of the functional status of the mesothelium. Peritoneal effluent of CAPD patients also contains proteoglycans (32, 33), mainly chondroitin/dermatan sulphate, but also hyaluronan. It is likely that hyaluronan can be synthesised by mesothelial cells, because it is present in high concentrations in exudates of patients with malignant mesotheliomas (34). Gel permeation chromatography of hyaluronan present in effluent of CAPD patients, showed that the elution profile was similar to that of cultured peritoneal mesothelial cells (35). Cancer antigen (CA) 125 is a 220 kD glycoprotein that is present in ascites of patients, also with non-malignant conditions (36). It has been shown recently that this protein can also be detected in the effluent of CAPD patients, and in supernatants of cultured mesothelial cells (37). Evidence was obtained that it can probably be regarded as a marker of the total mesothelial cell mass.

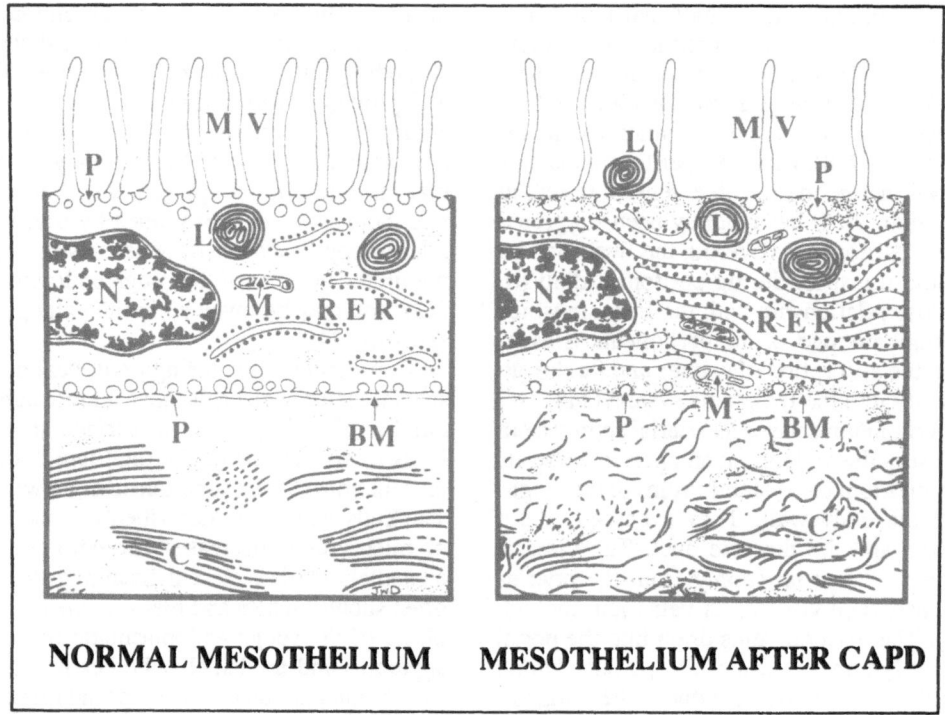

Figure 2. Diagrammatic representation of the ultrastructure of the mesothelium and subjacent serosal stroma in normal individuals and CAPD patients as determined by electron-microscopic examination of peritoneal biopsies. The most striking differences are found in the decrease in numbers of mesothelial microvilli (MV) and micropinocytotic vesicles (P), and the hyperplasia of the RER in biopsies from CAPD patients as opposed to the findings in normal controls. There are also differences in the submesothelium in CAPD patients where variations in texture of ground substance and disposition of collagen fibres (C) may be observed. L = lamellar bodies; M = mitochondria; N = nucleus; BM = basement membrane. Published with permission from reference (27) and of Karger AG.

Cultured mesothelial cells are capable of synthesizing prostaglandins, especially PGE_2 and prostacyclin (38–41). They also release IL-1 after stimulation with endotoxin and TNFα (42), as well as IL-6 (43) and IL-8 (44). Also, spent peritoneal dialysate stimulated these cells to secrete IL-6 in one study (45). These cytokines are present in effluents of CAPD patients. TNFα probably diffuses from the circulation to the dialysate in stable CAPD patients, but is locally produced in the acute phase of peritonitis (46). IL-6 can be detected in dialysate of non-infected CAPD patients (47, 48), and increases markedly during peritonitis (47, 49). This cytokine is probably locally produced, just as IL-8 (50, 51). Mesothelial cell cultures are also capable of synthesizing fibrinolytic factors (52). Stimulation with TNFα leads to a decrease of the tissue plasminogen activator concentration and to an increase in the plasminogen activator inhibitor type 1 concentration in the supernatant, and so to decreased fibrinolysis (53). Chronic intraperitoneal administration of dialysate in rats caused an increase in the peritoneal fibrinolytic activity (54), which could be an explanation for the low incidence of peritoneal adhesions in stable CAPD patients. Tissue plasminogen activator and plasminogen activator inhibitor type 1 can also be detected in peritoneal effluent.

Their concentrations were higher than could be expected on the basis of their molecular weights (55). All these studies show that the mesothelium during CAPD is not just a covering cell layer, but that it consists of metabolic active cells that are able to secrete a large number of substances. Some of these activities are probably provoked by the dialysis procedure.

Besides the mesothelial cell layer, the peritoneal microvessels that are embedded in interstitial tissue are involved in the transport of solutes and fluid during peritoneal dialysis. The interstitial tissue is composed of oriented bundles of collagen fibres and reticuloform elastic laminae in a relatively acellular ground substance (17, 27). Fibroblasts and occasional mast cells and macrophages are normally present (17, 23). The number of blood vessels is rather low. Capillary lymphatics and larger lymphatic lacunae were found more frequently than blood vessels in the mesentery of rabbits, suggesting a role in the absorption of solutes from the peritoneal cavity (17). In CAPD patients the superficial collagen bundles show increasing irregularity of distribution and disposition, associated with diffuse or patchy expansion of the ground substance (27). In addition, fibrosis has been found (22).

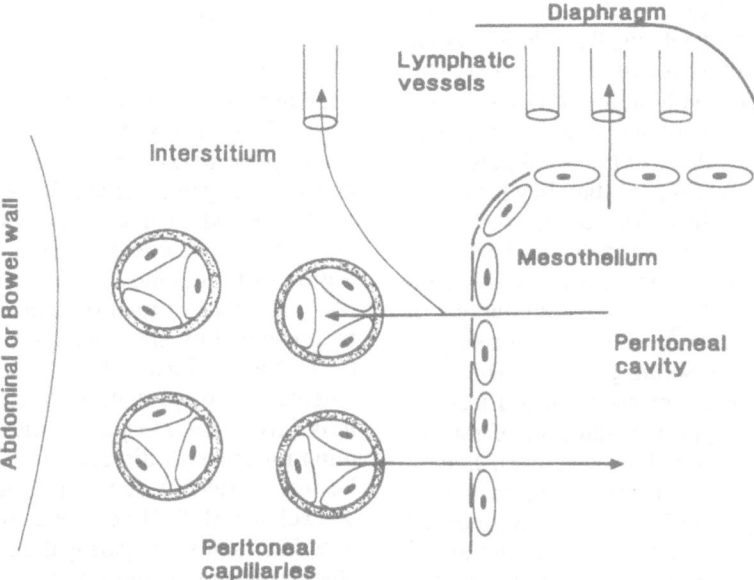

Figure 3. A schematic representation of the peritoneal membrane. Diffusion and transcapillary ultrafiltration occur in two directions. Lymphatic absorption from the peritoneal cavity is partly directly into the subdiaphragmatic lymphatics and partly into the lymphatics that drain the interstitium. Published with permission from reference (121) and of Multimed Inc.

The interstitial matrix is largely composed of mucopolysaccharides such as hyaluronan and chondroitin sulphate (56). It is often regarded as a two-phase system of a colloid rich gel phase, interspersed with a free fluid phase (57–60). Procollagen peptides and hyaluronan are present in peritoneal effluents of CAPD patients (32, 33, 61). Cultured peritoneal fibroblasts are capable of secretion of IL-6 after stimulation with IL-1β and TNFα (62). It implies that the functional state of the peritoneal interstitium may be reflected in the concentration of these locally produced substances in the effluent.

The endothelium of the peritoneal capillaries is mainly of the continuous type, but a small fraction of the peritoneal microvasculature has fenestrated endothelial cells, covered with diaphragms (63). The capillaries have a continuous basement membrane (17). During CAPD reduplications of this membrane are sometimes found (23, 64, 65). These alterations resemble the vascular changes present in patients with diabetes mellitus.

The effects of uncomplicated peritoneal dialysis on the morphology of the peritoneum can be summarized as follows: reactive changes are present in the mesothelium. The cells can show signs of degeneration, but also of high metabolic activity. The collagen in the interstitial tissue is irregular and reduplication of the capillary basement membrane occurs.

PHYSIOLOGY OF SOLUTE TRANSPORT DURING PERITONEAL DIALYSIS

Pathways and barriers

Solutes passing from the blood in the peritoneal capillaries to the dialysate filled peritoneal cavity have to pass at least three structures that can offer resistance: the capillary wall, the interstitial tissue and the mesothelial cell layer (Figure 3). Stagnant fluid layers have also been proposed as sites of resistance (66), but more recent data on solute diffusivity in the interstitial tissues have made this less likely (67). The mesothelium is also probably not a very important restriction barrier to the transport of solutes. Studies on the diffusion properties of an isolated avascular part of mesentery, thus representing transport in a diffusion chamber across two layers of mesothelium divided by interstitial tissue, have shown that the diffusion of particles with a molecular weight up to 500,000 Daltons was similar to the expected values on the basis of their molecular weights (68, 69). A pore radius of 0.68 μm could be calculated (68). The barrier function of the interstitium to the transport of solutes and fluid during peritoneal dialysis is not elucidated. It appeared non-size selective in the studies using an isolated mesentery. In contrast, the study by Fox and Wayland (70) using *in vivo* microscopy of the rat mesentery, pointed to an important role of the interstitial matrix in the restriction of the diffusion of macromolecules.

The capillary wall is probably the most important restriction barrier. Solute transport occurs size-selectively and is generally considered to take place through a system of pores (71). This physiologically defined system can be described by the two-pore theory (72, 73). This model proposes small pores with radii of 40 to 50 Å that are involved in the transport of low molecular weight solutes. The anatomic equivalents of the small pores may be the interendothelial clefts (74, 75), but they have never been identified with certainty. Also transport through plasmalemmal vesicle forming channels has been suggested (76). In addition, the model proposes a small number of large pores, less than 0.1% of the total number of pores. Their radii exceed 150 Å, allowing the transport of macromolecules, such as serum proteins. The morphological equivalent has not been established. Electron-microscopic studies also suggested transport of macromolecules through plasmalemmal vesicles (77). Such a transport route would however require active metabolic processes and hence energy. Cooling experiments reduced the transcapillary passage of albumin only to the extent that cooling reduced passive transcapillary filtration, but not to the extent that would be expected due to decreased cell metabolism (78). The large venular interendothelial gaps that can be provoked by the administration of histamine are an attractive alternative for representing the large pores (79). Such gaps could also be induced by other locally produced vasodilating substances. This would imply that the large pore radius is not a constant value, but that it could be subject to variations. In other words: the capillary wall is a heteroporous membrane that can be described by the combination of a set of small pores with uniform radii and an additional small set of large pores with different radii. The radius calculated for the large pores is in fact the mean value of the various radii. This concept is similar to that employed for the glomerular filter barrier (80).

Recently this two pore theory has been extended by assuming very small transcellular pores (< 5 Å) that are only involved in the transport of water and exclude solute transport because of their size (81, 82). This assumption was based on computer simulation studies. However, at the same time a 28 kD protein was discovered, present in the plasma membrane of red blood cells and Xenopus oocytes, that appeared to be involved in channel-mediated water transport (83). This protein, CHIP 28 or aquaporin was subsequently found to be the water channel in the proximal tubular cells of the kidney (84). Furthermore, it could be detected in capillary endothelia of the continuous type (85). This implies that aquaporin CHIP could be the ultrasmall pore involved in the osmotic induced water transport during peritoneal dialysis. The hypothesis that ultrasmall pores are involved in water transport during peritoneal dialysis, is attractive, because it can explain why glucose and other low molecular weight osmotic agents are effective, and also why apparent sieving of small solutes is present during convection (86).

Electric charge

Using ruthenium red, fixed negative electric charges have been demonstrated in peritoneal microvessels of rats not exposed to peritoneal dialysis (87). They were especially found on the basal lamina of the capillary endothelial cells and also along interstitial collagen fibres. It is however, not established whether, and how, they influence solute transport during peritoneal dialysis. Intraperitoneal administration of protamine sulphate to rabbits led to increased concentrations of total protein in the effluent, that could be prevented by simultaneous administration of heparin (88). This was interpreted as an effect of neutralization of anionic sites by protamine. Such an effect would particularly favour the transport of the negatively charged albumin molecules. A direct toxic effect on mesothelial cells leading to release of tissue proteins however could not be excluded (89). No evidence for charge selectivity was found in a study comparing the transport of the negatively charged serum albumin with a dextran fraction of a similar diffusion radius in CAPD patients (90). An apposite finding was reported in a study in rabbits that compared the transport of intravenously administered neutral- and charged dextrans (90). Especially the positively charged dextrans were hindered in their transperitoneal transport. This could be explained by the assumption that the colloid rich phase of the peritoneal interstitium behaves as a cation exchange column, facilitating the transport of negatively charged solutes through the tissue and retarding that of cationic macromolecules. Such effects are likely to disappear during steady state conditions, as present for serum proteins during CAPD. In that situation the concentrations of serum proteins in the interstitium are probably in equilibrium with their plasma concentrations. Therefore comparisons were done between the transport of proteins with (near) identical sizes, but different charges. IgG subclasses range in isoelectric points (p I) between less than 6 to 8.7. Their clearances in CAPD patients however were not different (92). Also comparisons between the peritoneal clearances of albumin and transferrin, β_2-microglobulin and lysozyme gave no indication for a charge selective barrier (93). Only the clearances of LDH subclasses suggested charge selectivity (44). Observations during peritonitis showed that an alternative explanation is more likely. Fixed negative charges disappear during peritonitis (45). However, during peritonitis in CAPD patients signs of increased charge selectivity for LDH were found (93). This could be explained by release of LDH by the cells present in the peritoneal effluent.

Taken together, most evidence points to an absence of charge selectivity of the peritoneum in the transport of macromolecules. This may be explained by the lower density of fixed negative charges in the peritoneum compared to the glomerular basement membrane.

Transport models

Because of the very complex structure of the various barriers to the peritoneal transport of solutes and fluid, the so-called distributed models are probably the most complete ones to describe peritoneal exchange (67, 96–98). They are however very complicated and based on a large number of assumptions. A much simpler approach is to consider the peritoneal tissues involved in the exchange of solutes and fluids, as a single membrane that separates two well-mixed pools: the blood compartment and the peritoneal cavity compartment. In this membrane concept the peritoneal dialysis system is compared with an artificial membrane having cylindrical, fluid filled pores, similar to the situation for transcapillary transport.

Every membrane can be characterized by its surface area and its intrinsic permeability. Henderson made a comparison between the transport characteristics of urea and inulin during peritoneal dialysis, and those during haemodialysis using cuprophane and cellulose-acetate membranes of a defined surface area (99). It could be concluded that the effective surface area of the peritoneal membrane, i.e., the part that actually participates in solute transport, had to be considerably less than the 1 m^2 found in anatomic studies. This can be explained by the observation that under basal circumstances only about one-quarter of the peritoneal capillaries is perfused (100). The instillation of dialysate, on the contrary, leads to an increase in the blood flow to splanchnic organs (101). The total splanchnic blood volume may even be more important than the flow for the determination of the effective peritoneal surface area (102). Also, studies on the effects of intraperitoneally administered nitroprusside (100, 103) have made it likely that the effective peritoneal surface area is mainly dependent on the number of perfused peritoneal capillaries, and thus on the number of pores available for transport. This implies that the effective surface area is not a static property of the peritoneum, but that it can vary depending on internal and external factors.

Peritoneal blood flow

The number of perfused peritoneal capillaries is dependent on peritoneal blood flow and blood volume (102). Based on the anatomic situation, splanchnic blood flow is probably much more important than the flow in the abdominal wall. Splanchnic blood flow averages 1200 ml/min in normal adults (104). Its distribution over the various splanchnic organs is markedly influenced by the instillation of dialysate. Experiments in rats using microspheres showed marked increases in the blood flow to the mesentery, omentum, intestinal serosa and parietal peritoneum (101). There was no effect on total splanchnic blood flow. Using the peritoneal clearance of hydrogen gas in rabbits (105) a value of 4.2 ml/min/kg body weight was found. Similar values could be calculated during peritoneal dialysis in rats with the microsphere

technique (101). Using the peritoneal clearance of carbon dioxide in rats an average value of 4.9 ml/min/kg was found after the instillation of an isotonic solution and of 8.1 ml/min/kg with a hypertonic dialysis fluid (106).

Lower values per kg body weight are probably present in peritoneal dialysis patients. The peritoneal blood flow has been assumed to average 60 to 100 ml/min (107). Studies in a limited number of intermittent peritoneal dialysis patients using the peritoneal mass transfer area coefficient of carbon dioxide, yielded values ranging between 68 and 82 ml/min (108), or of about 150 ml/min (109). A much lower value of 25 ml/min has been calculated in one study (110, 111). This was based on the relationship between the hydrostatic pressure and the plasma protein concentration obtained with a hollow-fiber hemofilter, and extrapolated to the situation in peritoneal dialysis. It can be concluded that most evidence suggests that peritoneal blood flow probably averages 100 ml/min, and that it is markedly influenced by the tonicity of the dialysate.

The regulation of splanchnic blood flow is complex. Intrinsic and extrinsic control mechanisms ar involved (112). The intrinsic regulation consists of a pressure-flow autoregulation, while also the venous pressure and the ingestion of meals have effects (113). The intrinsic regulation is mediated by myogenic factors, metabolic factors and locally produced substances such as vasoactive peptides and autocoids like prostaglandins (112). Extrinsic control mechanisms are predominantly mediated by the sympathetic noradrenergic nerves and by circulating vasoactive substances, such as catecholamines, vasopressin and angiotensin II (112). Alpha-adrenergic stimulation causes intestinal vasoconstriction, stimulation of β_2-receptors leads to dilatation. Intra-arterial infusion of nor-epinephrine causes intestinal vasoconstriction and a decrease in capillary density (112). A similar effect is present for epinephrine in high doses, but β_2-receptor mediated vasodilation prevails after the administration of a low dose. Vasopressin and angiotensin II cause generalized vasoconstriction with a disproportionate reduction in mesenteric blood flow (114). Vasopressin also causes a decrease in the density of perfused capillaries (112). Angiotensin II is probably mainly involved in the control of mesenteric blood flow during volume depletion (115). The administration of glucagon leads to splanchnic dilatation (116), but its role in the regulation of splanchnic blood flow is not established (112). The extrinsic control mechanisms of splanchnic blood flow regulation are mainly involved in the decrease that is present during shock and exercise (117).

Mechanisms of solute transport

Diffusion and convection are the mechanisms involved in the transport of solutes during peritoneal dialysis. Diffusion through a membrane takes place when a concentration gradient is present. According to Fick's first law of diffusion, the rate of transfer of a solute is determined by the diffusive permeability of the peritoneum to that solute (the ratio between the free diffusion coefficient of that solute and the diffusion distance), the surface area available for its transport, and the concentration gradient:

$$J_s = \frac{D_f}{\Delta x} \cdot A\Delta C \qquad [1]$$

in which J_s is the rate of solute transfer, D is the free diffusion coefficient, Δx is the diffusion distance, A is the surface area and ΔC is the concentration gradient. $D \cdot A/\Delta x$ is called the permeability surface area product or the mass transfer area coefficient (MTAC). During peritoneal dialysis ΔC is the concentration difference between the plasma concentration of a solute (P) and its dialysate concentration (D):

$$J_s = MTAC(B - D). \qquad [2]$$

Convective transport or solute drag occurs in conjunction with the transport of water, and thus during ultrafiltration. It is determined by the water flux (J_v), the mean solute concentration (C) in the membrane and the solute reflection coefficient (σ):

$$J_s = J_v \bar{C}(1 - \sigma). \qquad [3]$$

For reasons of simplicity C is often approached as:

$$\bar{C} = (P + D)/2. \qquad [4]$$

Staverman's reflection coefficient σ is the fraction of the maximal osmotic pressure a solute can exert across a semipermeable membrane. It equals 1.0 for an ideal semipermeable membrane and 0 when the membrane offers no resistance to the transport of a solute. With an isoporous membrane $\sigma = 1 - S$, in which S is the sieving coefficient. S is the ratio between the concentration of a solute in the filtrate divided by its concentration in plasma when no diffusion occurs. The peritoneum is not an isoporous membrane. This is the explanation that sieving coefficients of low molecular weight solutes during peritoneal dialysis are between 0.8 (118) and 0.6 (119) for urea, between 0.6 (119) and 0.7 (6) for creatinine and 0.7 for glucose (86). However, the reflection coefficient of glucose was estimated to be 0.02 in cats (120) and 0.05 in CAPD patients (121) using intraperitoneally administered solutions with various osmolalities. A value of 0.03 was found in a more recent study in CAPD patients (122). A value of 0.02 was calculated using a distributed model of peritoneal transport (123). It is likely that the marked differences between the reflection coefficients and one minus the sieving coefficients are caused by the heteroporosity of the peritoneum, especially by the presence of transcellular water channels and restricting properties of the interstitium.

Parameters of solute transport

The time-course of the dialysate/plasma (D/P) concentration ratio for various low molecular weight solutes and macromolecules is shown in Figure 4. A hyperbolic relationship is present for low molecular weight solutes, due to saturation of the dialysate during the dwell. In contrast, the relationship is about linear for macromolecules. This implies that peritoneal clearances of low molecular weight solutes are highest during the initial phase of the dwell and gradually decrease during the subsequent hours. Once equilibrium has been reached, the clearance is only dependent on the dialysate flow rate, i.e. the drained dialysate volume divided by the dwell time. Therefore, given that peritoneal clearances of low molecular weight solutes during long dwells as employed in CAPD, only provide information on the net mass transfer of the solute removed from the body, they cannot be used to assess the permeability characteristics of the peritoneal membrane.

The peritoneal equilibration test (PET) as developed by Twardowski et al. (124), is the most simple approach to estimate the transport properties of the peritoneal membrane. It gives the D/P ratio of urea and creatinine in a standardized way, using 2.5% dialysate glucose during a 4 h dwell. Also the ratio between the dialysate glucose concentration at the end of the dwell and that before inflow (D/D_o) is calculated. In addition, the drained volume after 4 h, and the residual volume can be assessed. The PET is attractive because of its simplicity, but it also has its limitations, especially when used for the assessment of membrane characteristics. It should be realized that D/P creatinine using 2.5% dialysate glucose is not only dependent on diffusion, but also partly on convective transport. Similarly D/D_o glucose is determined mainly by diffusion, but also by uptake of glucose into the lymphatic system. The drained volume can be used to calculate net ultrafiltration, but this is in fact the difference between transcapillary ultrafiltration and lymphatic absorption. The residual volume in the PET is calculated from the dilution of various low molecular weight solutes or combinations of them. These values overestimate the actual residual volume caused by diffusion. The best method for the determination of the residual volume is by the dilution of intraperitoneally administered high molecular weight solutes such as inulin or dextran 70 (125). When this is not available, albumin corrected for diffusion is the best approximation.

It has been claimed that D/P ratios have a high reproducibility in individual patients. This has been found within a period of three months (126), but changes may occur on the long term (126, 127). Good correlations have been reported between D/P ratios and MTAC values (128, 129), but the largest deviations are found in patients with very low and very high MTAC values (Figure 5). This suggests that D/P ratios may be rather insensitive to detect subtle changes in the permeability of the peritoneal membrane. PET D/P ratios have been used to extrapolate the total removal of urea and creatinine per 24 h in order to estimate the adequacy of peritoneal dialysis. It has now been shown that this can introduce considerable

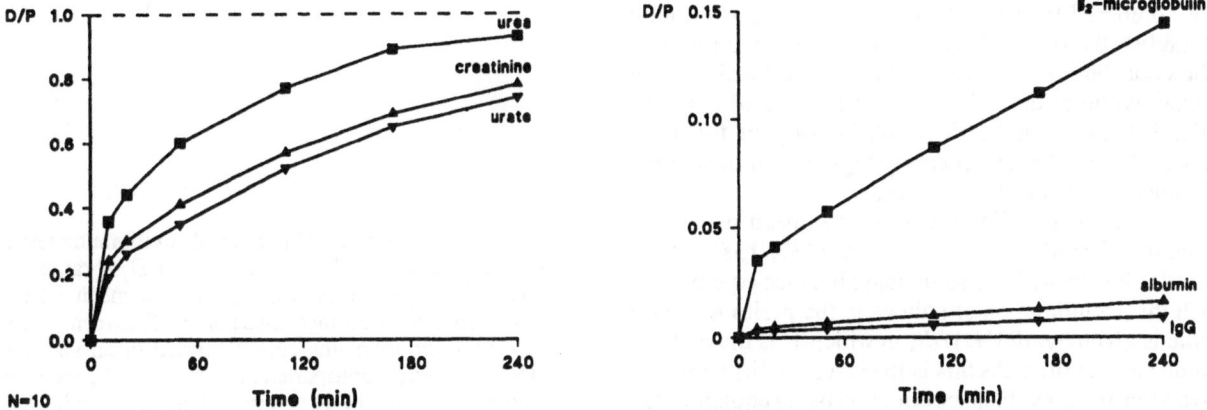

Figure 4. The time course of dialysate/plasma (D/P) ratios of urea (MW 60 Daltons), creatinine (MW 113 Daltons), urate (MW 168 Daltons), β_2-microglobulin (MW 11,800 Daltons), albumin (MW 69,000 Daltons) and IgG (MW 150,000 Daltons). Mean values of 10 stable CAPD patients are given. Reprinted with permission of the Boerhaave Committee for postgraduate medical education of the faculty of medicine, Leiden University, The Netherlands.

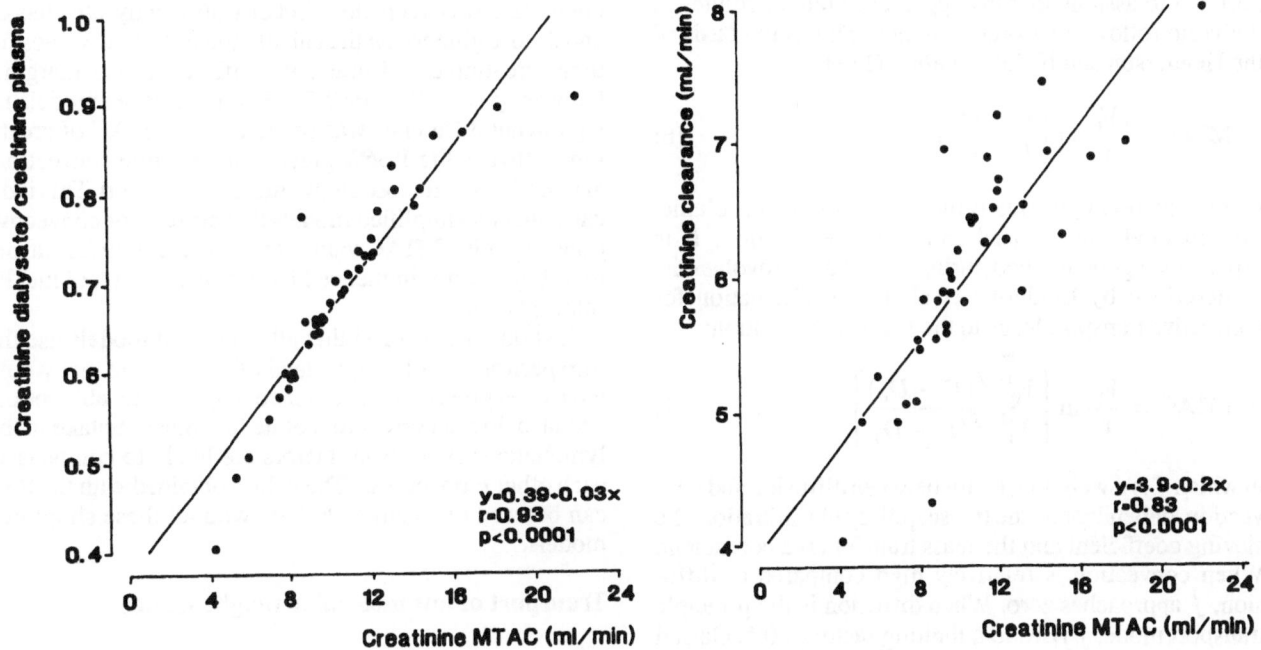

Figure 5. Relationship between creatinine D/P versus creatinine MTAC (left panel) and creatinine clearance versus creatinine MTAC (right panel) from the study of Struijk et al. (128). With permission from the author and from Kluwer Academic Publishers.

errors (130). For estimating solute removal 24 h dialysate collections should be used.

The calculation of the mass transfer area coefficient, i.e., the theoretical maximal clearance by diffusion at time zero, before solute transport has started, is the preferred way to characterize peritoneal permeability. The calculation requires complicated models that cannot be solved analytically, but depends on numerical solutions requiring the use of a computer. Such models are for instance the

Pyle–Popovich (131) and the Randersson model (132). A more simple approach to estimate the MTAC is the assessment of peritoneal clearances during short dwell times. This can easily be done by multiplying the D/P ratio after e.g. 1 h with the drained volume, divided by the dwell time. This was the conventional technique during intermittent peritoneal dialysis, and has also been employed in CAPD patients (123). It may seem attractive, but the method has a number of disadvantages. First, the contribution of the time of inflow and drainage is relatively large compared to the dialysis time, making it difficult to establish the precise dwell time. The second problem is the contribution of convective transport, leading to an overestimation of the MTAC. Another cause of overestimation is the finding that the MTAC during the first hour of a CAPD dwell is significantly higher than during the subsequent hours (129, 134–136).

A number of simplified methods has been developed to calculate MTAC values in patients (137, 138). These methods all start with the same mass balance equation, in which the accumulation of solutes in the peritoneal fluid in time is given by: $d(VD)/dt$, in which V is the dialysis volume and t is time. As this is the result of diffusion and convection, the mass balance equation using equations (2) to (4) is:

$$\frac{d}{dt}(VD) = \text{MTAC}(P-D)+0.5J_v(P+D)(1-\sigma).[5]$$

The most simple approach to solve this differential equation is to neglect the contribution of convective transport and to assume that the appearance rate of solutes in dialysate follows first order kinetics. This is the basis of the Henderson and Nolph equation (118).

$$\text{MTAC} = \frac{V_t}{t}\ln\left[\frac{P-D_o}{P-D_t}\right].\qquad[6]$$

In this equation V_t is usually the drained dialysate volume. This method can be used as a rough estimation. It is especially a good method during a period of isovolaemia, as described by Lindholm et al. (139). Correction for convective transport leads to the following equation:

$$\text{MTAC} = \frac{V_t}{t}\ln\left[\frac{V_0^{1-f}(P-D_o)}{V_t^{1-f}(P-D)}\right]\qquad[7]$$

in which f is a weighing factor between diffusion and convection, dependent on the transcapillary ultrafiltration, the sieving coefficient and the mass transfer area coefficient. When convection is relatively high compared to diffusion, f approaches zero. When diffusion is the principle transport mode, f rises to a limiting factor of 0.5. Garred et al. (140) developed a simple model based on multiple dialysate samplings, and assuming $f = 0$ and $S = 1$:

$$\text{MTAC} = \frac{V}{t}\ln\left[\frac{V_o(P-D_o)}{V_t(P-D_t)}\right].\qquad[8]$$

This model could also be used taking samples only before instillation and after drainage, and taking the drained volume for V (141). Waniewski et al. (142) pointed out that f values of 0.33 for a large degree of convective transport and of 0.5 for negligible convection are more justified (142). In addition plasma concentrations of small solutes should be corrected for aqueous solute concentrations, either by a correction factor of 1.05 or using the

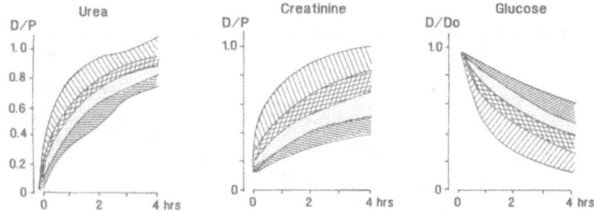

Figure 6. The results of 103 peritoneal equilibration test using 2.5% glucose dialysate. The upper zones of D/P ratios of urea and creatinine represent high transporters (> mean + SD), the adjacent zones high average transporters (between mean and mean + SD), the following zone (between mean and mean – SD) the low average transporters, and the lowest zone (< mean – SD) represents the low transporters. The same symbols, but in a mirrow view indicate the same transport categories for D/Do glucose. Redrawn from reference (124), with permission from the author and of Pergamon Press).

total protein concentration in plasma (143). However, in a comparison between the effect of 1.36% dialysate glucose and 3.86% glucose on the calculation of MTAC values for urea, creatinine and urate, the difference was marginal between $f = 0$, 0.33 or 0.5 (136). In all three models no significant difference was found for the MTAC of creatinine between the 1.36% glucose study (little convection) and the 3.86% glucose study (more convection). This indicates that all simplified models that correct for convective transport, give MTAC values that represent diffusion and that they are not influenced by convection in a clinically relevant degree.

It should be realized that all simplified models use the intraperitoneal volume, instead of the volume that would have been present in the absence of lymphatic absorption, and also do not correct for solute loss due to uptake in the lymphatic system. Both factors are likely to compensate each other more or less. The values obtained with the PET can be used to calculate MTAC with all these simplified models.

Transport of low molecular weight solutes

Diffusion is quantitatively the most important transport mechanism for low molecular weight solutes, such as urea, creatinine, and uric acid. This is especially the case when the osmolality of the dialysate is low. Figure 6 shows the D/P ratios of urea and creatinine during 2.5% dialysate glucose in the population of 86 patients studied by Twardowski et al. (124). The mean values of the MTAC's of urea, creatinine and uric acid as obtained in a cross sectional study using 1.36% dialysate glucose in 64 adult patients (144) are given in Table 1. It appeared that some relationship was present between MTAC creatinine and body surface area, but the variation was rather large (Figure 7). This could indicate some relationship between peritoneal surface area and body surface area.

Table 1. Results of standard permeability analysis in 64 CAPD patients treated for more than 3 months. Mean values, standard deviations and ranges are given. Data partly presented in reference (144)

Parameters	Mean ± SD	Range
Time on CAPD (yrs)	2.4 ± 2.2	0.4–10.3
MTAC urea (ml/min)	18.6 ± 3.9	10.2–30.3
MTAC creatinine (ml/min)	11.0 ± 3.2	6.1–19.2
MTAC urate (ml/min)	9.8 ± 3.6	4.9–20.1
Cl β_2-microglobulin (μl/min)	949 ± 395	399–2070
Cl albumin (μl/min)	101 ± 45	10–250
Cl IgG (μl/min)	53 ± 28	12–150
Cl α_2-macroglobulin (μl/min)	19 ± 14	1–70
Restriction coefficient	2.37 ± 0.40	1.62–3.80
Glucose absorption (%)	60 ± 10	37–87
Transcapillary UF rate (ml/min)	1.33 ± 0.80	0.10–6.16
Effective lymphatic absorption rate (ml/min)	1.28 ± 0.70	0.34–4.35
Net UF rate (ml/min)	0.05 ± 0.62	−1.37–2.41
Residual volume (ml)	245 ± 143	62–824

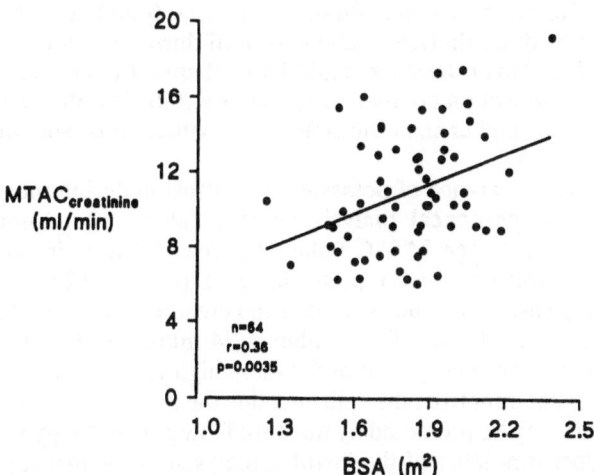

Figure 7. Relationship between MTAC creatinine and body surface area in 64 adult CAPD patients who underwent their first standard peritoneal permeability analysis. Based on reference (144).

The coefficients of intra-individual variation for the MTAC of low molecular weight solutes were originally reported to range between 15 and 20% (141). A more recent study in a larger number of patients with better standardization yielded values ranging between 2 and 11%, mean 7% (145). Most of this variability can be ascribed to biological variation and not to variations in the assays (145). This emphasizes the need to characterize the permeability characteristics of the peritoneal membrane in a functional way.

A functional characterization is possible by relating transport by diffusion of various solutes to their molecular weights. When a particle is an ideal sphere, the relationship between its radius (r) and molecular weight (MW) is given by:

$$\text{MW} = \frac{4}{3}\, \Pi r^3. \qquad [9]$$

The relationship between the free diffusion coefficient (D_f) of a solute and its radius is given in the Einstein–Stokes equation:

$$D_f = \frac{RT}{6\Pi \eta r N} \qquad [10]$$

in which R is Bolzmann's gas constant, T is the absolute temperature, η is the viscosity of the solvent and N is Avagadro's number. This implies that in the case of an ideal sphere, the free diffusion coefficient of a solute is related to the cubic root of its molecular weight:

$$D_f = a\text{MW}^{-0.33} \qquad [11]$$

in which a is a constant.

It is evident from the above that relationships between solute transport and molecular weight should be expressed as power functions:

$$y = ax^b \qquad [12]$$

or

$$\ln y = b \ln x + \ln a. \qquad [13]$$

This implies that the power (b) is the slope of the correlation line that is obtained when x and y are plotted on a double logarithmic scale. Most solutes are not ideal spheres. When the free diffusion coefficients in water of urea, glucose and inulin were plotted against their molecular weights on a double logarithmic scale, the slope of the correlation line was −0.46 (146, 147). This implies that values up to −0.46 are consistent with free diffusion across the peritoneal membrane. In that case only the surface area determines the maximal transport capacity. Values exceeding −0.46 imply restricted diffusion. This means that the membrane itself (the pore size or the interstitium) offers an additional barrier to the transport of solutes. For the clearances of low molecular weight solutes up to β_2-microglobulin (MW 11,800 Daltons)

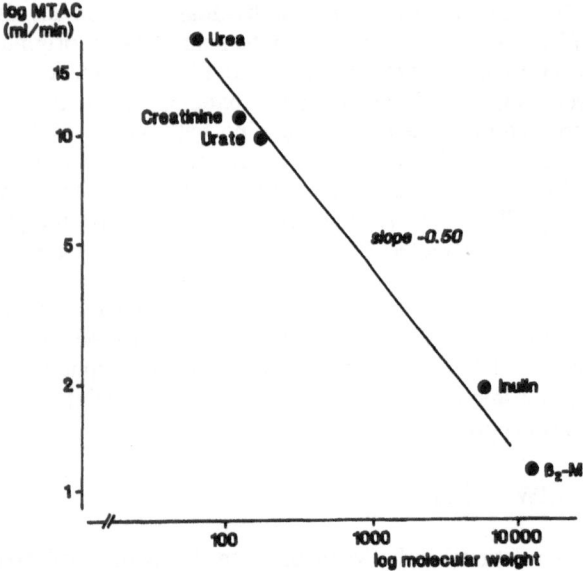

Figure 8. The power relationship between the mass transfer area coefficients of urea, creatinine, urate, and the clearances of inulin and β_2-microglobulin (β_2-m) on a double logarithmic scale. Mean values taken from references (90) and (136). The slope of 0.5 indicates a process of mainly free diffusion. See text for explanation.

a value of -0.44 was found during intermittent peritoneal dialysis (148). During CAPD we found a value of -0.50 (Figure 8). These data give no indication for a size-selective restriction barrier for low molecular weight solutes during peritoneal dialysis, but are more in favour of a transport process, similar to free diffusion in water. This implies that the functional or effective peritoneal surface area is the only membrane characteristic that influences the MTAC of a low molecular weight solute. Consequently, the MTAC of such a solute, for example creatinine, can be used as a functional measurement of the effective peritoneal surface area. Changes in the MTAC of creatinine in individual patients reflect changes in their effective peritoneal surface area.

Transport of electrolytes

The dialysate concentration of sodium decreases during the initial phase of a dialysis dwell using hypertonic solutions, followed by a gradual rise (86, 143, 149–151). The minimum value is usually reached after 1 h. It is likely that this apparent sieving of sodium is caused by transcellular water transport through ultrasmall pores or, alternatively, temporal binding of Na^+ in the interstitial tissue. This implies that during short dwells using hypertonic dialysate much more water than sodium is removed from the extracellular volume. This can lead to hypernatraemia (152). The gradual rise during the subsequent hours is probably caused by diffusion of sodium from the circulation.

The MTAC of sodium is difficult to calculate due to the small differences in dialysate and plasma concentrations. Using 3.86% dialysate glucose an average value of 4 ml/min has been reported during a period of isovolaemia (143, 151). Using dialysate with a sodium concentration of 102 mmol/l a value of 8 ml/min was found (122). Corrections for Gibbs-Donnan equilibrium were applied in these calculations. The MTAC of chloride was 9 ml/min (122). Both for Na^+ (MW 23 D) and Cl^- (MW 35.5 D) the MTAC values were considerably below those of urea (MW 60 D), creatinine (MW 113 D) and urate (MW 168 D). As a consequence these electrolytes are transported at a lower rate than expected on the basis of their molecular weight. Also the molecular radii of anhydrated sodium (0.98 Å) and chloride (1.81 Å) are smaller than those estimated during peritoneal dialysis, based on computer simulations (2.3 Å for sodium and chloride) (82). It is conceivable that interactions of these ions with H_2O molecules leading to a water shell, may cause transport characteristics that suggest a higher molecular weight. In the study of Imholz et al. the calculated radius of sodium during peritoneal dialysis was 2.68 Å and that of chloride 2.42 Å (122). The lower MTAC of sodium than that of chloride is in accordance with the lower permeability coefficient of sodium compared to that of chloride, present for transport across synthetic lipid bilayer membranes *in vitro* (154).

The finding that sodium diffuses as a larger molecule during peritoneal dialysis has focussed attention to the potential use of ultralow sodium dialysis solutions to improve net ultrafiltration, especially as Nakayama et al. reported favourable results of such a solution in a small number of overhydrated CAPD patients (155, 156). In a study comparing dialysate with a normal sodium concentration with a dialysate containing sodium 102 mmol/l, that was made isosmotic by addition of more glucose, a slightly better net ultrafiltration was found with the low sodium dialysate: about 100 ml during a 6 h dwell (122). This difference could be explained by the calculated reflection coefficient of glucose (0.0326), that was slightly higher than the reflection coefficient of sodium (0.0297).

The clearance of potassium by diffusion during intermittent peritoneal dialysis averages about 17 ml/min (157). Average MTAC values between 12 ml/min and 16 ml/min have been reported in CAPD patients (122, 143, 151), in-between those of urea and creatinine. During the first hour of a dwell the value is 24 ml/min (122). The most probable explanation for these high values is release of potassium from the cells that line the peritoneal cavity. This may be promoted by the initial low pH and/or by the hyperosmolality of the instilled dialysate. It is also supported by the finding of sieving coefficients of potassium exceeding 1.0 (142, 158). It can be concluded that charged electrolytes are transported at lower rates than expected on the basis of their molecular weights, irrespective of the charge being positive or negative. For potassium release from intracellular sources during the initial phase of a dialysis dwell is likely to occur.

Transport of macromolecules

Macromolecules, such as serum proteins, are transported from the circulation to the peritoneal cavity at a much lower rate than low molecular weight solutes. Therefore, their dialysate consentrations are low and do not reach equilibrium with serum (Figure 4). Consequently their clearances can be used as an approximation of MTAC's. Normal values for the clearances of β_2-microglobulin (MW 11,800 D), albumin (MW 69,000 D), IgG (MW 150,000 D) and α_2-macroglobulin (MW 820,000 D) are given in Table 1. The transport of macromolecules is size-selective, both for proteins and uncharged dextran molecules (90, 159). Similar to low molecular weight solutes, the relationship between clearances and molecular weights can be described as a power relationship (159, 160). The slope of the regression line between molecular weights and clearances is however much steeper (−0.69) than that between molecular weights and free diffusion coefficients (−0.36) (159). This indicates that the transperitoneal transport of macromolecules is hindered by a restriction barrier within the peritoneal membrane. Unlike the transport of low molecular weight solutes, that is dependent only on the effective surface area of the peritoneum, the transport of macromolecules is determined both by surface area and intrinsic permeability.

It is still controversial whether the main transport mechanism of macromolecules during peritoneal dialysis is by convection (161, 162) or by restricted diffusion (79, 90, 163, 164). *In vitro* studies using endothelial monolayers on polycarbonate filters suggest that macromolecular transport in this system is caused by both diffusion and convection (165). Restricted diffusion was especially present with highly confluent monolayers on filters with pores of about 400 Å, a situation probably similar to that in peritoneal dialysis. Convection requires fluid transport. This can occur by hydrostatic forces and by osmotic forces. An effect of osmotically induced convection has only been demonstrated for the low molecular weight protein β_2-microglobulin, but not for larger proteins such as albumin, transferrin, IgG and α_2-macroglobulin, which are transported through the large pores (136). A mathematical approach has been used in an attempt to demonstrate that proteins larger than 50 Å reach the peritoneal cavity exclusively by hydrostatic convection through the large pore system (81). However, this can only occur when the pressure in the peritoneal blood vessels exceeds that in the interstitial tissue. The intraperitoneal pressure during CAPD averages 8 mm Hg during recumbency (166). This value is lower than that in the arterioles, but similar to that in the venules. It implies that the localization of the large pores determines whether hydrostatic convection across them is likely to occur. Increasing the intraperitoneal pressure by 10 mm Hg with the application of external

compression decreases the clearances of proteins (166). This effect is most pronounced for proteins with the highest molecular weights, suggesting an effect on the size of the pores. The measured data could be explained by convection through large pores with a radius of about 180 Å, but also by diffusion through large pores with an average radius of 1000 Å. The large venular interendothelial gaps with radii from 500–5000 Å, which can be found after the application of vasoactive substances, such as histamine (79), suggest that the latter value is not unrealistic.

It can be concluded that the peritoneal transport of albumin and larger proteins presumably occurs through the large pore system, and is size-selectively restricted. The mechanism involved may be restricted diffusion, or hydrostatic induced convection, or a combination of both. The localization and size of the large pore system determine which mechanism prevails.

Individual characterization of surface area and intrinsic permeability

Power relationships are present between the MTAC of solutes and their molecular weights. The slope of the regression line between these two parameters indicates whether the diffusion is restricted by intrinsic barriers within the membrane, or not. This can be done by making comparisons with the slopes obtained with the free diffusion coefficients in water, as explained in the sections on the transport of low molecular weight solutes and that on the transport of macromolecules.

The molecular weight of a solute is not the only determinant of its diffusion velocity. The density and the shape of a molecule can also have an effect. This is evident for non protein macromolecules, such as dextrans. Based on the equation: radius = 3.05 MW$^{-0.47}$ (167), as derived from the data of Granath and Kvist (168), it can be calculated that the dextran fraction with a diffusion radius identical to that of β_2-microglobulin (MW 11,800 D) has a molecular weight of only 4600 D. For α_2-macroglobulin (MW 820,000 D) the molecular weight of the corresponding dextran fraction is 176,000 D (169). Since diffusion is the most important mechanism for the transport of low molecular weight solutes, and restricted diffusion may be the most important mechanism for the transport of macromolecules, the establishment of power relationships between the MTAC of solutes and their free diffusion coefficients in water, is a more rational approach than the use of the molecular weights. A power relationship was found for peritoneal clearances (C) of proteins and their free diffusion coefficients in water (Dw) (170), according to the equation:

$$C = aDw^{rc} \qquad [14]$$

in which the slope (rc) was called the peritoneal restriction coefficient. The restriction coefficient represents the intrinsic permeability of the peritoneal membrane: high values mean a low permeability. The application of the

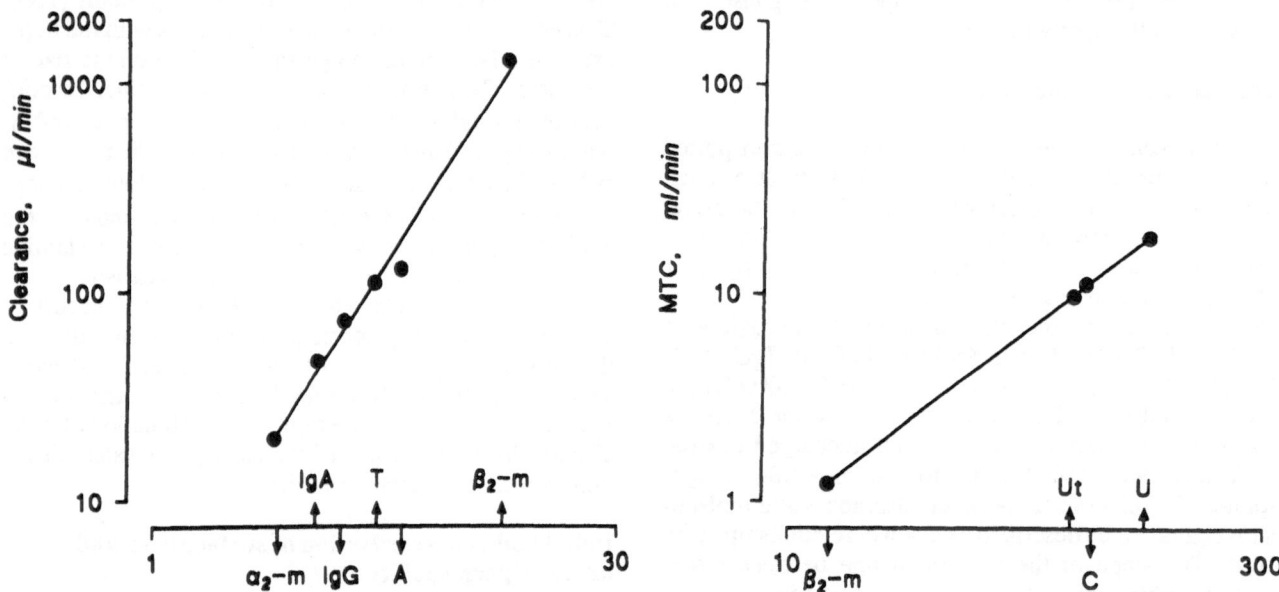

Figure 9. The power relationship between the mass transfer area coefficients (n = 10) of urea (U), creatinine (C), urate (Ut) and β_2-microglobulin (β_2-m) and their free diffusion coefficient in water ($D_{20,w}$) (right panel), and the power relationship between the protein clearances (n = 9) of β_2-microglobulin (β_2-m), albumin (A), transferrin (T), IgG, IgA and α_2-macroglobulin (α_2m), and their free diffusion coefficient in water (left panel) on a double logarithmic scale. The slope of the regression line represents the restriction coefficient. A restriction coefficient of 1.0 means that a linear relationship is present between clearances of solutes and their free diffusion coefficients in water. For the low molecular weight solutes a slope of 1.24 ± 0.03 and for the proteins a slope of 2.37 ± 0.04 were found. Published with permission of reference (136) and of Blackwell Scientific Publications.

Table 2. The relationship between membrane characteristics and parameters of solute transport

	Effective surface area	Intrinsic permeability
MTAC creatinine		
C β_2-microglobulin	+	−
C macromolecules	+	+
Restriction coefficient	−	+

restriction coefficient in individual patients was validated both for proteins (171) and for dextran fractions (172).

A restriction coefficient that equals 1.0 means a linear relationship between MTAC's and free diffusion coefficients, and no hindrance by the restriction barrier. In this situation differences in free diffusion coefficients of solutes are the only determinants of their clearances, and so the effective peritoneal surface area is the only membrane characteristic that determines solute transport. In a study in 10 CAPD patients a mean value of the restriction coefficient of 1.24 was found for low molecular weight solutes and of 2.37 for serum proteins (Figure 9) (136). This is consistent with a mainly free diffusion process for low molecular weight solutes and restricted transport

for macromolecules. In Table 2 a summary is given of the relationship between the parameters of solute transport and the permeability characteristics of the peritoneal membrane. The effective surface area can be characterized by the MTAC of creatinine, or, when this is not possible because of long dwell times, and consequently equilibrium of small solute concentrations, by the clearance of β_2-microglobulin. The intrinsic permeability can be characterized by the calculation of the restriction coefficient. The effective surface area can be considered as a reflection of the number of pores, whereas the restriction coefficient mainly represents the size of the large pores.

Regulation of surface area and permeability

The effective peritoneal surface area is determined by the area of the membrane that is in direct contact with the dialysate and by the number of perfused peritoneal capillaries. The dialysate is evenly distributed throughout the peritoneal cavity in the supine position, but it accumulates mainly in the subumbilical region in the upright position (173). This may be the explanation for lower solute clearances and MTAC's that have been found when upright than during recumbency (173–175). Also, an increase in intraperitoneal pressure decreases MTAC's of solutes (166). Both the effective surface area and the intrinsic permeability show marked day-to-day variabili-

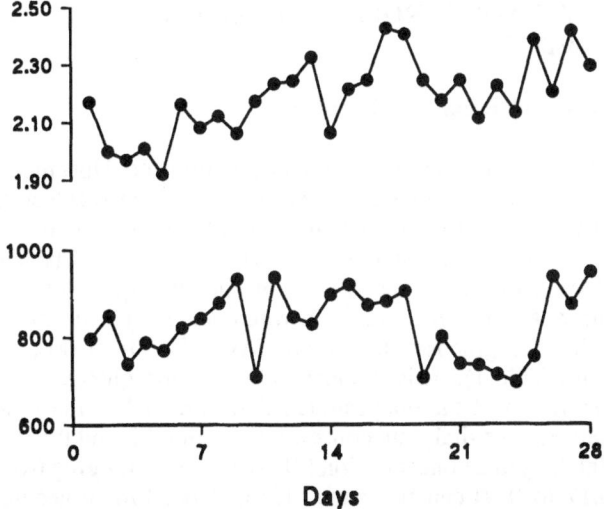

Figure 10. Day-to-day variations of the restriction coefficient representing the intrinsic peritoneal permeability (upper panel) and the clearance of β_2-microglobulin (μl/min), characterizing the effective peritoneal surface area (lower panel). Based on data from reference (169) and reprinted with permission of the Boerhaave Committee for postgraduate medical education of the faculty of medicine, Leiden University, The Netherlands.

ty. These variations do not run parallel (Figure 10) (170). The splanchnic blood flow is likely to be involved in the regulation of the permeability characteristics of the peritoneum. Possible effects of splanchnic blood flow have been studied in situations in which changes are likely to occur, in studies focussed on substances known to influence splanchnic blood flow, and experiments in which these substances are administered. Changes in splanchnic blood flow occur during shock, exercise and after a meal. An effect of hypotension on the peritoneal clearance of urea has been found in dogs with haemorrhagic shock (176). However, a decrease in mean arterial pressure to 38% of the initial value caused a decrease in urea clearance to 74% of it. After restoration of the blood pressure to 58% of the initial value, the urea clearance exceeded the control value by 28%. Physical exercise by CAPD patients has been reported to have no effect on D/P ratios of low molecular weight solutes in one study (173), but a decrease in the clearances of albumin and IgG was found in another (92). The ingestion of a meal produced a marginal increase only in the clearances of these proteins.

Plasma levels of catecholamines, vasopressin, ANP, aldosterone and plasma renin activity are elevated in CAPD patients (177–180). This does not necessarily imply increased sympathetic activity, but could also be the result of decreased clearance (178). Dialysate concentrations of catecholamines have been measured in one study (177). The D/P ratio for epinephrine was 0.69 and 1.17 for norepinephrine, suggesting local production in the peritoneal cavity. Prostaglandins and cytokines are also likely to be produced locally in the peritoneal cavity. This

has been shown both for vasodilating and vasoconstricting eicosanoids. The vasodilating prostaglandins were present in the highest concentrations (181–183). Drained peritoneal effluent also contains the cytokines, TNFα (46, 184), interleukin-1 (IL-1) (185, 186), IL-6 (47, 48) and IL-8 (50, 51). The presence of TNFα in the dialysate of uninfected CAPD patients is probably caused by diffusion from the circulation (46, 184), while the other cytokines mentioned above are produced locally within the peritoneal cavity. A relationship has been reported between very high dialysate IL-6 levels in stable CAPD patients and a low peritoneal restriction coefficient, representing high intrinsic permeability to macromolecules (48).

Possible effects of solutes generally considered to be involved in the regulation of the permeability characteristics of the peritoneum, have been analyzed by studying transport kinetics during peritoneal dialysis, after their intraperitoneal or intravenous administration. These factors include the dialysate itself, hormones such as catecholamines, gastrointestinal hormones and vasopressin, and also histamine, nitroprusside and prostaglandins. The administration of hypertonic and acid dialysate in the rat causes arteriolar vasodilation in the cremaster muscle preceded by initial vasoconstriction (187, 188), and also vasodilation of cecal arterioles (189). This effect was more pronounced for acetate buffered, than for lactate buffered, dialysate, and also more pronounced for 1.5% glucose than for 0.5% glucose containing dialysate. This may explain why the instillation of commercial dialysate leads to a redistribution of splanchnic blood flow (101), and the finding that the MTAC values are highest during the beginning of a dwell, when the osmolality is maximal and the pH is minimal (129, 134–136). Increasing the glucose concentration from 1.36% to 3.86% has no effect on the indices of the effective peritoneal surface area (136); a decrease in these indices has been reported using glycerol based dialysate (190). The effects of aminoacid containing dialysate are not equivocal. One percent aminoacid dialysis fluid only marginally influenced the equilibration of urea and creatinine (191). The MTAC values of low molecular weight solutes were increased during the use of a 2.67% amino acid solution, but statistical significance was not always reached (158, 192). One percent commercially available dialysis solution caused an increase in the protein loss in the effluent of 20%, which occurred directly after the start of treatment, and which appeared reversible after discontinuation (193). Another 2.6% aminoacid solution had a similar effect (194). Glucose polymer containing dialysate increases the clearance of β_2-microglobulin, probably by increased convective transport, but has no effect on other permeability characteristics (195–197).

Intravenous administration of norepinephrine in rabbits leads to a decrease in effective surface area as judged from the clearances of urea and creatinine (198). In contrast, intravenous glucagon increases the clearances of these solutes (199, 200). As glucagon, a peptide with a molecular weight of 3484 D, was not effective after intraperitoneal administration, these findings support a direct effect on the peritoneal vasculature. The effects of glucagon have also been confirmed in dogs (201). Vasopressin administered either intraperitoneally (202) or intravenously (203) leads to a fall in solute kinetics consistent with a decreased effective peritoneal surface area. Topical application of histamine causes arteriolar vasodilation with leakage of proteins, both in skeletal muscles and in the mesenteric vasculature (79, 204). This would suggest an action on the effective surface area and on the intrinsic permeability. Intraperitoneal administration of histamine in rats caused a 10 to 20% increase in the clearance of urea (205). This effect was not confirmed in rabbits, but a marked increase was reported for the protein loss in the dialysate (206). The histamine-induced protein loss could be blocked by H_1 and H_2 receptor antagonists. These antagonists were not effective when given alone, or during desoxycholate induced chemical peritonitis. Intraperitoneal administration of the nitric oxide donor nitroprusside during intermittent peritoneal dialysis, leads to an increase in the clearances of urea and creatinine (100, 103, 207). Other vasodilators like hydralazine, phentolamine, isoprenaline and diazoxide had no such effects (103). The effect of nitroprusside on the clearance of inulin and on protein loss in the effluent was even more pronounced than its effect on the clearance of urea and creatinine (100, 103). This suggests that vasodilation without activation of the nitric oxide system has no effect on peritoneal permeability.

The possible role of vasodilating and vasoconstricting prostaglandins on the effective peritoneal surface area has been studied by intravenous and intraperitoneal administration in rabbits (208–210). In general, the effects were more pronounced after intraperitoneal administration. Arachidonic acid and the vasodilating prostaglandins led to an increase in the effective peritoneal surface area, while the vasoconstricting $PGF_{2\alpha}$ decreased the clearances of urea and creatinine. The oral administration of the cyclo-oxygenase inhibitor indomethacin had no effect in these animals. Intraperitoneally administered mefenamic acid marginally reduced the clearance of creatinine, but not that of urea. The intraperitoneal administration of indomethacin in CAPD patients during peritonitis has been reported to lead to a reduction in peritoneal protein loss in one study (183), but the effect was less pronounced in another (211).

It can be concluded that many factors, that are involved possibly in the regulation of the effective peritoneal surface area and the intrinsic permeability have been identified, but their relative importance and interactions in the day to day variability of these parameters during peritoneal dialysis still remain unclarified.

TRANSPORT FROM THE PERITONEAL CAVITY

Low molecular weight solutes

The clearance of intraperitoneally administered low molecular weight solutes from the dialysate is size-selective (147, 212), at least up to the size of inulin. This mainly suggests a diffusive process. The absorption of lactate (MW 90 D) averages 82% of the instilled quantity during a 4 h dwell (data from reference 147). The mean value for glucose absorption (MW 180 D) is 60% in 4 h (Table 1). This is independent on the glucose concentration of the dialysate (213). Expressed as the ratio between the dialysate concentration after 4 h and the initial dialysate concentration (D/Do), values ranging from 0.12 to 0.60 can be found (124). Other low molecular weight solutes that can be used as osmotic agents, such as glycerol and aminoacids, are also absorbed according to their molecular weights. The absorption of glycerol (MW 92 D) averages 84% after a 6 h dwell (190), and that of aminoacids (average MW 145 D) 73 to 90% (191, 214). The absorption of these solutes mainly occurs in the portal circulation (215).

The disappearance rates or clearances of intraperitoneally administered solutes always exceed the values found after intravenous administration with an average value of 1 to 2 ml/min. This was found for sucrose, vitamin B_{12} (216) and inulin (217, 218), as well as for the clearances of the non-protein bound antibiotics fosfomycin (219) and cefamandole (220). A similar difference was found when intraperitoneally administered 5-flucytosine (MW 129 D) was compared to the transport of creatinine (MW 113 D) from the circulation to the dialysate (212), and also between intraperitoneally administered haemoglobin (MW 68,000 D) and albumin (MW 69,000 D) transported to the peritoneal cavity (221). Assuming that the peritoneal restriction barrier is uniform in its hindrance to diffusion, i.e., there is bidirectional equivalency for diffusive mass transfer, then a molecular weight-independent, convective transport from the peritoneal cavity of 1 to 2 ml/min should be present for intraperitoneally administered solutes. Although such a bidirectional equivalency to diffusion has not been proven, it is supported by the fact that the absolute difference between the two transport routes is always of the same order of magnitude, irrespective of the size of the solutes. However, the relative difference ranges, from 16% for low molecular weight solutes, to more than 1000% for albumin. When diffusion would not occur equally in both directions, but would always be systematically higher for intraperitoneally administered solutes, a constant relative difference would have been expected. The presence of a convective, size independent transport of 1 to 2 ml/min out of the peritoneal cavity may be caused by uptake into the lymphatic system. This was supported by Leypoldt et al. who compared the bidirectional transport of creatinine in rabbits using a kinetic model that included lymphatic absorption. In this situation no difference between the two routes was found (222).

The contribution of convection to diffusive transport is relatively small for low molecular weight solutes, but becomes increasingly more important the higher the molecular weight of a solute. The convection/diffusion ratio is about 0.1 for glucose, 1.0 for inulin (217), but 10 for intraperitoneally administered autologous haemoglobin (221), making the disappearance rate of macromolecules relatively independent of molecular size.

Macromolecules

Intraperitoneally administered particles, such as blood cells and bacteria, are taken up into the diaphragmatic lymphatics (reviewed in reference (11)). Accordingly, a proportion of intraperitoneally administered macromolecules during peritoneal dialysis, disappears from the peritoneal cavity. Gjessing used dextran 70 as a dialysis solution in peritoneal dialysis patients treated with 30 minute dwells. The recovery of dextran 70 in the dialysate averaged 92% after the dwell (223). Recoveries of intraperitoneally administered macromolecules of 70–90% after 4 to 7 h dwells in patients have been reported for radio-iodine tagged serum albumin (150, 224–228), for unlabelled human albumin (229), for dextran 70 10 g/l (230) and 1 g/l (231), and for autologous haemoglobin (218, 227). In only one study a recovery of autologous haemoglobin in excess of 95% has been reported (232). A high recovery of one batch of unlabelled human albumin was found in another study (233). This was shown to be caused by a high transport of endogenous albumin, because this particular batch contained a high concentration of prekallikrein activator that caused an inflammatory reaction.

The disappearance rate of intraperitoneally administered macromolecules is independent of molecular size, both in animals (234–236) and in CAPD patients (237). A proportion is taken up directly into the subdiaphragmatic lymphatic plexus, as has been shown in experiments using India ink (238). Also, transmesothelial uptake, especially in the anterior abdominal wall has been shown in rats using radio-labelled fibrinogen (239) and albumin (240). Uptake of radio-labelled albumin in peritoneal tissues is also likely to be present in peritoneal dialysis patients (224). In mice this phenomenon is transient (241), probably by subsequent uptake into the lymphatics that drain the interstitium.

FLUID TRANSPORT

Transcapillary ultrafiltration

Fluid transport during peritoneal dialysis consists of water transport from the peritoneal capillaries into the peritoneal cavity by transcapillary ultrafiltration and by fluid loss out of the peritoneal cavity. The latter consists of transcapillary backfiltration and by fluid uptake into the lymphatic system. As a consequence, the changes in the *in situ* intraperitoneal volume are determined by the magnitude of the transcapillary ultrafiltration and lymphatic absorption. The water removal from the body at the end of a dwell period, defined as net ultrafiltration, is therefore the difference between the cumulative transcapillary ultrafiltration and fluid uptake into the lymphatic system.

The transport of water across the capillary wall occurs through the small pore system and probably through ultrasmall transcellular water channels (see section on Pathways and barriers). The small pores are mainly involved in transport by hydrostatic and colloid osmotic forces, transport through the ultrasmall pores is dependent on the osmotic gradient across the endothelial cells. It has been assumed that, during CAPD, 40% of the filtered fluid volume passes through transcellular water channels (81). According to Starling's law, the transcapillary ultrafiltration rate in peritoneal dialysis is determined by the ultrafiltration coefficient of the peritoneal membrane and the driving forces between the peritoneal capillaries and the abdominal cavity. These forces are exerted by hydrostatic, crystalloid osmotic and colloid osmotic pressure gradients. The ultrafiltration coefficient of the peritoneum is the product of the hydraulic permeability and the effective surface area. Little is known about determinants of the hydraulic permeability. It is most likely dependent on the combination of intracapillary pressure, and the number and size of the pores. The state of the interstitial tissue, possibly containing sites of fibrosis, may also be one of the determinants. In computer simulations of peritoneal transport values of 0.04 and 0.08 ml/min/mm Hg have been calculated for the ultrafiltration coefficient (242).

The hydrostatic pressure in the peritoneal capillaries is assumed to be 17 mm Hg (243). The intraperitoneal pressure during CAPD has been reported to average 2 mm Hg (244) and 8 mm Hg (166) in the supine position, depending on the choice of reference point. It exceeds 20 mm Hg while walking (244), and is dependent on the instilled dialysate volume (245). This implies that the hydrostatic pressure gradient is determined mainly by the intraperitoneal pressure. The colloid osmotic pressure in the peritoneal capillaries probably averages 26 mm Hg (243). The contribution of the dialysate to the colloid osmotic pressure gradient can be neglected because of its low protein content. Using dialysate without an osmotic agent in CAPD patients we found an average transcapillary backfiltration rate of 0.4 ml/min after the establishment of osmotic equilibrium. The crystalloid pressure gradient is mainly determined by glucose. The effectiveness of this osmotic agent depends on the resistance the membrane exerts on its transport. This is expressed as the osmotic reflection coefficient (see section on Mechanisms of solute transport). It can range from 1 (no passage, ideal

Table 3. A summary of the pressure gradients across the peritoneal membrane during peritoneal dialysis. See text for further explanation

	Pressure in peritoneal capillaries	Pressure in dialysate filled peritoneal cavity	Pressure gradient
Hydrostatic pressure (mm Hg)	17	8 recumbent	9
		20 walking	−3
Colloid osmotic pressure (mm Hg)	26	0.1	26
Osmolality (mosmol/kg)	305	347 (glucose 1.36%)	
		486 (glucose 3.86%)	
Maximal crystalloid osmotic pressure gradient (mm Hg)			23 (glucose 1.36%)
			104 (glucose 3.86%)

semipermeable membrane) to 0 (passage not hindered, no osmotic effect). In case of a reflection coefficient of 1, every mosmol exerts an osmotic pressure of 19.3 mm Hg according to van 't Hoff's law. The reflection coefficient for glucose during CAPD is probably between 0.02 and 0.05 (120–123), so very low. It must be appreciated however, that these are mean values. The reflection coefficient for glucose across the ultrasmall pores will be 1.0, and will approach zero across the large pores.

The hyperosmolality of commercial dialysis fluid when compared to uremic plasma is about 45 mosmol/kg H_2O for the lowest glucose concentration (1.36%) and 180 mosmol/kg H_2O for the highest glucose concentration (3.86%). The osmotic pressure exerted by these solutions across the peritoneal membrane can therefore be estimated as 45×0.03 (reflection coefficient) $\times 19.3 =$ 23 mm Hg (lowest glucose concentration), and similarly 104 mm Hg (highest glucose concentration). The various pressure gradients are summarized in Table 3. The values for the crystalloid osmotic pressure gradients are the maximum values, as present during the initial phase of a dialysis dwell. They will decrease in time due to absorption of glucose from the dialysate. These figures imply that dialysate with a low glucose concentration will only induce a small amount of transcapillary ultrafiltration. The maximal transcapillary ultrafiltration rate during the initial phase of a dwell is 12 to 16 ml/min using 3.86% glucose dialysate (151, 246, 247). The average transcapillary ultrafiltration rate during a 4 h dwell was reported as 1.2 ml/min with 1.39% glucose and 3.4 ml/min with 3.86% glucose dialysate (136). The value of 1.3 ml/min as given in Table 1 is in close agreement with this. Using the values given in Table 3 and assuming an intraperitoneal pressure of 8 mm Hg, a reflection coefficient for glucose of 0.03, and a maximal transcapillary ultrafiltration rate of 15 ml/min using glucose 3.86% dialysate, it can be calculated that the ultrafiltration coefficient of the peritoneal membrane during CAPD averages 0.17 ml/min/mm Hg. This value is about two times higher than that used in computer simulations (82).

Lymphatic absorption

Direct measurement of the lymphatic flow from the peritoneal cavity is impossible in humans. Therefore, indirect methods have been used. They include the disappearance rate (clearance) of intraperitoneally administered macromolecules from the peritoneal cavity, and their appearance rate in the circulation. Using the disappearance rate it is assumed that the administered macromolecule is removed from the peritoneal cavity by absorption into the lymphatic system. Human albumin (229), radio-iodated serum albumin (RISA) (150, 151), autologous haemoglobin (221, 248) and dextran 70 (230) have all been used. This approach is justified, because the disappearance rate of these solutes is constant in time (231, 249) and independent of molecular size (237) (see also the section on Transport from the peritoneal cavity). Using these tracers average values of 1.0 to 1.5 ml/min have been found in CAPD patients (150, 151, 221, 228–230). The validity of this method has been questioned, because the appearance rate of intraperitoneally administered RISA in the circulation is only about 20% of the disappearance rate (224, 225). But, half this difference can be explained by the fact that only 40 to 50% of the total albumin mass is intravascular (250). Local accumulation of i.p. RISA has been found in the anterior abdominal wall of rats (240), most likely caused by transmesothelial transport. It is probable that macromolecules in the peritoneal interstitial tissue will eventually be taken up into the lymphatic system, as has been made plausible in mice (241). This is supported by the observation that saturation of the peritoneal interstitium in CAPD patients by continuous administration of dextran 70 did not alter the appearance rate of this macromolecule (231).

Direct measurement of lymphatic flow from the peritoneal cavity has been done by the group of Johnston, both in anaesthetized and conscious sheep (251–254). In these animals the right lymphatic duct could not be cannulated. Anesthesia appeared to have a pronounced effect on the flow in the cannulated lymphatics, probably because of reduced movements of the diaphragm. The mean lymph flow in conscious sheep ranged from 1 to 1.5 ml/hr/kg body weight, depending on estimations for flow in the right lymphatic duct. Comparisons of these measured flow rates with disappearance – and appearance rates of RISA in sheep are difficult, because the disappearance rate of RISA was very high and the RISA appearance rate was 60% of the disappearance rate, so a much smaller difference than in human CAPD patients. Also, the amount of RISA intraperitoneally administered, recovered in the blood and in the drained lymphatic vessels was always equal to the amount lost from the peritoneal cavity during a 6 h dwell. This is not supportive of marked accumulation of RISA in the anterior abdominal wall. The flow from the caudal mediastinal lymph node can be raised 200% in the awake sheep model by intraperitoneal administration of fluid (255). In analogy, the disappearance rate of intraperitoneally administered autologous haemoglobin is higher in CAPD patients after the administration of a 3 liter dialysate volume than with a volume of 2 liters (147). Also, increasing the intraperitoneal pressure in rats that underwent peritoneal dialysis increased the RISA disappearance rate (256). It had however no effect on its appearance rate in the systemic circulation. Combining this observation with those in awake sheep and CAPD patients, strongly suggests that the disappearance rate of macromolecules is a better way of assessing lymphatic absorption in CAPD patients than the appearance rate.

It has been suggested that fluid transport associated with the disappearance of macromolecules should not be called lymphatic flow nor lymphatic absorption, but simply fluid loss (257). This is a simplification, because reabsorption of fluid into the capillaries by the colloid osmotic pressure gradient is not associated with the transport of macromolecules, as has been shown in studies using normal saline (224), or hypotonic dialysate without an osmotic agent (218). The amount of saline absorbed during a 7 h dwell was 24% in the former study, but the amount of RISA that had disappeared was only 17%. In the latter study the dialysate concentration of intraperitoneally administered dextran 70 increased 10% during a 4 h dwell, most likely because of transcapillary backfiltration of water, caused by the colloid osmotic pressure gradient. This underlines that fluid loss from the peritoneal cavity is coupled mainly to the disappearance of macromolecules (lymphatic absorption), but is also partly uncoupled (backfiltration by colloid osmosis). Based on these data it can be concluded that the disappearance rate of intraperitoneally administered macromolecules cannot be used alone as a measurement of lymph flow through the subdiaphragmatic lymphatics, but also cannot be used as an over-all indicator of fluid loss from the peritoneal cavity, irrespective of the mechanism involved. It is plausible that the disappearance rate can be used as a functional approach for the calculation of the effective lymphatic absorption from the peritoneal cavity during CAPD. It implies that all pathways of lymphatic drainage from the peritoneal cavity, both subdiaphragmatic and interstitial,

are included in the definition of the effective lymphatic absorption rate. The term 'effective' is analogous to the effective renal plasma flow, where clearance is used to estimate flow.

The combined effects of transcapillary ultrafiltration and effective lymphatic absorption on the time course of net ultrafiltration are shown in Figure 11. Intraperitoneal pressure is likely to be one of the determinants of the effective lymphatic absorption. Intraperitoneal administration of saline in rats causes an increase in the number of patent subdiaphragmatic stomata, that was not present when the intraperitoneal pressure was kept constant (258). Also, a relationship has been found between intraperitoneal pressure in CAPD patients and the disappearance rate of intraperitoneally administered dextran 70 (259). Increasing the intraperitoneal pressure 10 mm Hg by external compression, leads to a marked increase in the effective lymphatic absorption rate (166), and consequently a lower net ultrafiltration. Net ultrafiltration is also somewhat (16%) lower in the upright position compared to recumbency (175), caused by the combination of a small increase in the dextran disappearance rate and a slight decrease in the transcapillary ultrafiltration rate. The effects of higher intraperitoneal pressure in the upright position are probably counter-balanced by the effect of gravity leading to a decreased contact between the dialysate and the subdiaphragmatic lymphatics. The coefficients of intra-individual variation of the parameters of fluid transport average 17% (145). Net ultrafiltration is inversely related to the MTAC of creatinine and to the effective lymphatic absorption rate (Figure 12).

Failure of net ultrafiltration

The magnitude of the drained volume that is required for the definition of net ultrafiltration failure is rather arbitrary, especially because it is very much dependent on the length of the dwell time and the glucose concentration used. In the longitudinal study of Struijk et al. (260), performed in 61 patients with a maximal follow-up of two years, in whom 211 peritoneal permeability tests were done using 1.36% glucose dialysate during a 4 h dwell, negative net ultrafiltration was found in 30% of the examinations. The frequency distribution was similar in the first and the second year. In the cross-sectional study shown in Table 1 negative net ultrafiltration was present in 45% of the patients. This figure may be too high, since some of the patients were investigated because of clinical problems. The prevalence of net ultrafiltration failure in other studies has been reported to range between 1.3 and 100% (150, 261–267). It was especially frequent in patients on long-term treatment and in those using dialysate with acetate as buffer. The definition of loss of ultrafiltration was based on a clinical picture of overhydration despite frequent use of 3.86% glucose dialysis solutions in most of the studies.

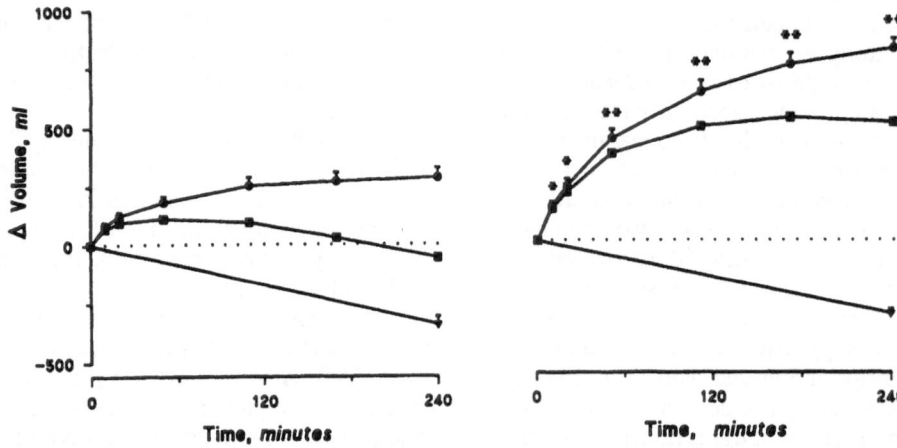

Figure 11.   For 10 patients the time course of transcapillary ultrafiltration (dots), lymphatic absorption (triangles) (calculated indirectly as the dextran disappearance rate from the peritoneal cavity) and the resulting chances in intraperitoneal volume (squares) with 1.36% glucose (left panel) and 3.86% glucose (right panel) are given as mean values $\pm$ SEM. $*p < 0.01$, $**p < 0.001$ when compared to 1.36% glucose. Published with permission from reference (136) and of Blackwell Scientific Publications.

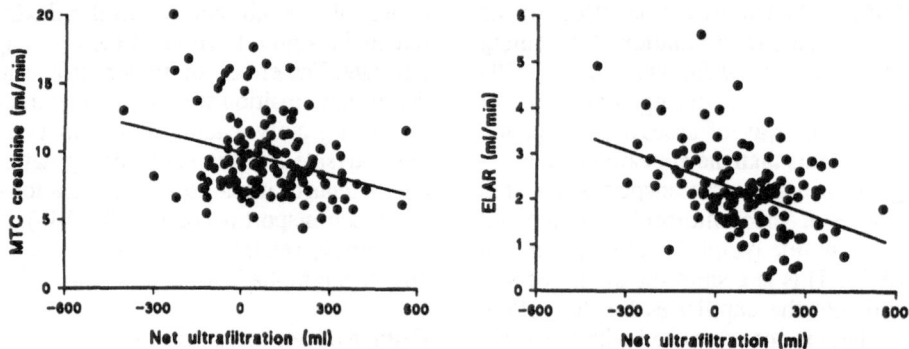

Figure 12.   The relationship between net ultrafiltration and the mass transfer area coefficient of creatinine (left panel, $r = 0.30$, $p < 0.001$), and the effective lymphatic absorption rate (ELAR, right panel, $r = 0.43$, $p < 0.001$). Data from reference (121).

Verger et al. have distinguished two types of net ultra-filtration failure (268): type 1 is associated with intact or high solute transport rates, while solute transport is impaired in type 2. Type 1 ultrafiltration failure occurs more frequently than type 2. Mechanisms for type 1 net ultrafiltration failure include a large volume of distribution of dialysate, e.g. with leaks from the peritoneal cavity to the pleural cavity, but also a large residual volume leading to instantaneous dilution of the administered glucose. Most important however is the presence of a large effective peritoneal surface area leading to rapid disappearance of glucose (150, 263, 265). Type 2 ultrafiltration failure, caused by a small effective peritoneal surface area is probably rare. It has been described in some patients with sclerosing peritonitis (269). Others with this condition tend to have indices of a large effective peritoneal surface area. A transition from high to low transport rates has been described (270). A high effective lymphatic absorption rate is another cause of net ultrafiltration failure. Remark-

ably little is known about the frequency of its occurrence. One case history has been reported from the United States (271). In a study from Sweden, performed in nine CAPD patients with permanent net ultrafiltration failure, indices of a large effective surface area were found in seven, and of a high effective lymphatic absorption rate in two (150). The most likely explanation that this cause of net ultrafiltration failure has been described rarely, is the fact that macromolecules have to be administered intraperitoneally to determine it appropriately, and this technique has not been employed in many instances.

Twenty-nine of the patients shown in Table 1 had negative net ultrafiltration. This was associated with the following transport characteristics, or their combination: a MTAC creatinine exceeding 12 ml/min was present in 34%, a MTAC creatinine less than 7 ml/min in 24%, an effective lymphatic absorption rate exceeding 2 ml/min in 21%, and a residual volume of more than 400 ml in 7%. However, the cause of ultrafiltration failure remained unexplained in 31% of these patients. This raises the question whether impairment of transcellular water transport can contribute to net ultrafiltration failure. One of the ways to approach this problem is to study the dialysate sodium concentration during a hypertonic dialysis exchange. The minimum dialysate sodium concentration is reached after 60 to 90 minutes (149–151). Impairment of transcellular water transport can be expected to abolish the decrease in dialysate sodium concentration. One patient on long-term CAPD with loss of ultrafiltration, associated with no decrease in dialysate sodium has been described (272). This was also found in four other patients with loss of net ultrafiltration, whose indices for effective peritoneal surface area and lymphatic absorption rates were within the normal range (273). These data are too preliminary to guess what the contribution of impaired transcellular water transport is in the genesis of ultrafiltration failure, and also the causes are unknown. Possible mechanisms could include non-enzymatic glycosylation of the aquaporin CHIP protein, caused by the high glucose concentrations in the dialysate. Such an explanation is supported by the diabetes-like alterations in the basement membranes of peritoneal capillaries that have been described in patients treated with CAPD (23, 64, 65).

Treatment of net ultrafiltration failure often consists of decreasing the dialysate dwell time, increasing the number of exchanges and avoiding the long night dwell. Therapeutic options based on the underlying mechanism are more interesting, but partly experimental. Patients with net ultrafiltration impairment caused by a large effective surface area have, theoretically, a large area available for transcapillary ultrafiltration, but the effect is counteracted by the rapid absorption of the osmotic agent. A high molecular weight osmotic agent, that is mainly removed from the peritoneal cavity by uptake into the lymphatic system, could therefore be beneficial by inducing marked ultrafiltration in this condition. Icodextrin, a glucose polymer, is an osmotic agent with a molecular weight of about 16,000 D (274). Preliminary results suggest that it may be very effective in these patients (196, 197, 275), and the mechanism of inducing transcapillary ultrafiltration appears to be a process of colloid osmosis, which will be effective mainly across the small pores. It is speculative that it can also be used for patients with impairment of the transcellular route.

Intraperitoneal administration of phosphatidylcholine leads to improvement in net ultrafiltration (276–280). This pharmacological effect is caused probably by decreased lymphatic absorption from the peritoneal cavity due to constriction of the subdiaphragmatic stomata (281, 282). It is controversial whether orally administered phosphatidylcholine increases net ultrafiltration. This was suggested in some studies (277, 283), but could not be confirmed in others (284, 285). The reason for this difference is not clear. Amphotericin B has been reported to increase net ultrafiltration after intraperitoneal administration in rabbits (286, 287), without affecting solute transport. This suggests increased hydraulic permeability of the peritoneum. Evidence has been obtained *in vitro* that this effect could have been caused by interactions of amphotericin B with cell membrane-bound cholesterol, resulting in the formation of pores, with radii in the range of 7 to 10.5 Å, enhancing transcellular water transport (288). The effect of amphotericin B on water transport is counterbalanced by a chemical peritonitis, caused by its solvent desoxycholate (289). Recently, the enhancing effect of amphotericin B on net ultrafiltration has been described in three CAPD patients (290). Amphotericin B increased transcapillary ultrafiltration, but had no influence on solute transport, nor on effective lymphatic absorption. In situations with impaired net ultrafiltration caused by a small effective peritoneal surface area, the intraperitoneal administration of nitroprusside may lead to increase ultrafiltration. This drug has been used only in intermittent peritoneal dialysis (100, 103, 207). Other vasodilating agents used in the treatment of hypertension are not effective (103). The results of treatment with calcium-channel blocking agents are controversial (291, 292).

It can be concluded that, currently, no drugs are available to improve net ultrafiltration after oral administration. The use of high molecular weight osmotic agents, such as icodextrin, is likely to be beneficial in a proportion of patients with net ultrafiltration failure, depending on the cause.

PERITONITIS

Infectious peritonitis

Peritonitis is accompanied more or less by extensive loss of the mesothelial cell layer (25, 293, 294). Four stages of inflammation have been distinguished (27): (1) fibrin exudation and cuboidal transformation of mesothelial cells; (2) mesothelial exfoliation, fibrin insudation of serosa; (3) fibrin resorption and remesothelialization and; (4) remodelling of submesothelium and/or fibrosis. Healing of the mesothelium was found ten days after discontinuation of peritoneal dialysis (293). Inflammation causes hyperaemia, and, therefore changes in the permeability characteristics of the peritoneal membrane are likely to occur. 'Membrane failure', as judged from deteriorating biochemical control has been reported in four of 35 IPD patients with peritonitis (295). In contrast, increased clearances of creatinine and urea during peritonitis have been found in four IPD patients who were studied both in the absence of, and in the presence of, peritonitis (296). As the effluent volume was similar, increased permeability caused by inflammation was the most likely explanation.

The most striking clinical finding in CAPD patients with peritonitis is impaired net ultrafiltration, leading to weight gain and other signs of fluid overload (297).

This phenomenon is associated with increased transport of low molecular weight solutes and increased absorption of glucose (146, 298–302). These phenomena point to an increased effective peritoneal surface area, leading to rapid disappearance of the osmotic gradient, and thus to a reduced net ultrafiltration. In this situation a high molecular weight osmotic agent should be able to induce more transcapillary ultrafiltration. This was recently confirmed by the use of icodextrin, which led to increased, instead of decreased, net ultrafiltration during peritonitis (303). Using autologous hemoglobin as a volume marker, it was shown that the maximal intraperitoneal volume during peritonitis is reached at about 1 h after instillation of the dialysis fluid, compared to 2.5 h after recovery (146). This may explain why a decrease in net ultrafiltration has not been observed during peritonitis in IPD patients. In addition, a high effective lymphatic absorption rate from the peritoneal cavity may also contribute to the decreased net ultrafiltration during peritoneal inflammation (304).

Protein loss in the dialysis effluent is also markedly increased during peritonitis (146, 159, 296, 300, 305, 306). In IPD the losses can be as high as 48 grams per dialysis and often remain elevated for several weeks (305). These proteins could be produced locally, or originate from the circulation (307). Serum proteins are quantitatively the most important in peritoneal effluent. The increment in their clearances of more than 100% during peritonitis, favours increased transport (146, 159), due both to the increased effective surface area and increased peritoneal permeability to macromolecules (159). In a longitudinal study in CAPD patients with peritonitis, Zemel et al. showed an increase in the effective peritoneal surface area and a decrease in the restriction coefficient during the acute phase of the inflammation (49). Both parameters returned to normal during follow-up. Possible causes of the increase in surface area and permeability include endotoxin and complement activation (308), as well as prostaglandins (181–183), IL-6 (47, 49) and TNFα (49). It was shown that the increased effective peritoneal surface area was associated with changes in IL-6 and TNFα, while the decreased restriction coefficient was associated mainly with changes in PGE$_2$ and to a lesser extent with changes in IL-6 (49). All alterations in peritoneal transport of fluids, solutes and macromolecules, as well as the dialysate levels of the various cytokines and eicosanoids are reversible after resolution of peritonitis (49, 146, 302).

Sclerosing encapsulating peritonitis

Sclerosing encapsulating peritonitis is a life threatening complication of chronic peritoneal dialysis (309, 310). Its precise etiology is still unclarified. Contributing factors to its development include the length of time undergoing peritoneal dialysis, recurrent peritonitis (311), acetate as a dialysate buffer (309), the use of bacterial filters (185, 312), the use of antiseptic agents such as chlorhex-idine (313–315) and treatment with β-blocking drugs (316). Spontaneous sclerosing encapsulation of bowel in patients not on peritoneal dialysis has been reported (317). The principal finding is a thickened leathery, fibro-connective sheath of marbled appearance that envelopes the small intestine. The bulk of the encapsulating sheath lies anteriorly, and parietal involvement may be present. Histopathology reveals dense fibrous tissue with a chronic inflammatory infiltrate. Fibrin depositions are also found (318).

Loss of net ultrafiltration is the most prominent sign of changed peritoneal transport in patients with this complication (269, 309, 319–324). Reduced clearance of urea and creatinine has been described in two IPD patients who developed this condition (325). One CAPD patient has been described who, initially, had loss of net ultrafiltration associated with increased glucose absorption, that was followed by a normal glucose absorption at a stage where sclerosing peritonitis was present (320). In another study serial measurements of peritoneal transport kinetics were reported in four CAPD patients, who developed sclerosing peritonitis (269); loss of net ultrafiltration was associated with an increase in glucose absorption and an increase in transperitoneal solute transport in three of them. In the other patient a decrease in all these parameters was found. These data suggest that sclerosing peritonitis can either be associated with a small, or with a large effective peritoneal surface area. Local production of interleukin-1 has been hypothesized as a pathogenetic mechanism (185, 312). As in later years the IL-1 bio assay also appeared to measure IL-6, and because IL-6 is continuously released in the peritoneal cavity, it may well be that IL-6 is also involved in the development of sclerosing peritonitis. The secretion of this cytokine in the peritoneal cavity could lead to an increased production of collagen by peritoneal fibroblasts, but also to release of prostacyclin by the vascular endothelium. It is conceivable that the vasodilating properties of this eicosanoid augment the peritoneal permeability characteristics by increasing the number of perfused capillaries. In addition, the formation of connective tissue could lead to an increase in the number of blood vessels in the poorly vascularized parts of the peritoneum. It is possible that the differences in solute transport in patients with sclerosing peritonitis can be explained by interindividual variations in the susceptibility to either formation of collagen, or the effect of prostacyclin and neovascularization. The former would lead to low, and the latter to high, transport rates.

LONG DURATION PERITONEAL DIALYSIS

Peritoneal dialysis leads to activation, and sometimes degeneration of mesothelial cells (see section on Histology and cell biology). This leads to an increased turn-over of the mesothelium. Histologic abnormalities can develop when remesothelization is impaired. In this situation the peritoneum is lined by acellular hyalinized collagen, the so-called cellular dessert (24, 318). It is often accompanied by diabetiform vascular changes in the submesothelial tissue. Development into the so-called tanned peritoneum can occur. In this condition the outer portion of the peritoneum has been replaced by an acellular rind of hyalinized collagen, but its thickness is normal. The cause of the light brown coloration of the peritoneum in this condition is unknown, but it is possible that products of oxidative degradation of glucose, such as 3-acetylacrylic acid contribute to it (318). Data from the peritoneal biopsy registry suggest that the tanned peritoneum is most commonly encountered in patients who have been on CAPD for many years (24, 318). It can probably proceed to mural fibrosis and sclerosing encapsulating peritonitis, but the factors that are directly involved in such a development are unknown.

The effect of time on the efficiency of intermittent peritoneal dialysis has been studied by Finkelstein et al. in eight patients during a follow-up of 10 months (326). A decrease was found for the clearances of urea, creatinine and glucose in all patients. It is unclear whether this was due to decreased drainage volumes or to decreased dialysate/plasma ratios. All other studies on solute transport during long-duration peritoneal dialysis have been done in CAPD patients. The first study in 12 CAPD patients showed no significant differences for 1 h clearances of low molecular weight solutes, except for an increased inulin clearance during the first 6 months on CAPD (327).

In the last decade at least 9 cross sectional studies (265, 328–335) on the effect of the duration of CAPD on peritoneal solute transport parameters, and 16 longitudinal studies (260, 265, 267, 329, 333, 336–346) have been published. The effect of time on loss of net ultrafiltration has been analyzed in 17. Large differences were present between the studies in the duration of follow-up, the methods used to measure solute transport and the solutes analyzed. The studies that report clearances of low molecular weight solutes are difficult to interpret, since the drained volume can contribute significantly to the result. This may be the explanation for the contrasting finding of reduced creatinine clearance in combination with increased glucose absorption in the study of Nikolakakis et al. (330). In three studies only patients were included who were treated with CAPD for at least 3 years (345), 4 years (341), and 5 years (346). They therefore represent an interesting, but selected population.

It is evident from the published studies that MTAC values or D/P ratios are not reduced during CAPD. This implies that the capability of the peritoneum to remove uremic toxins remains intact. In general, most studies report loss of net ultrafiltration in some long-term CAPD patients. In 14 of the 25 studies no effect of time on the transport of low molecular weight solutes was found (265, 329, 331–336, 338, 339, 341, 342, 344, 346), in the other 11 an increase was reported indicating a large effective

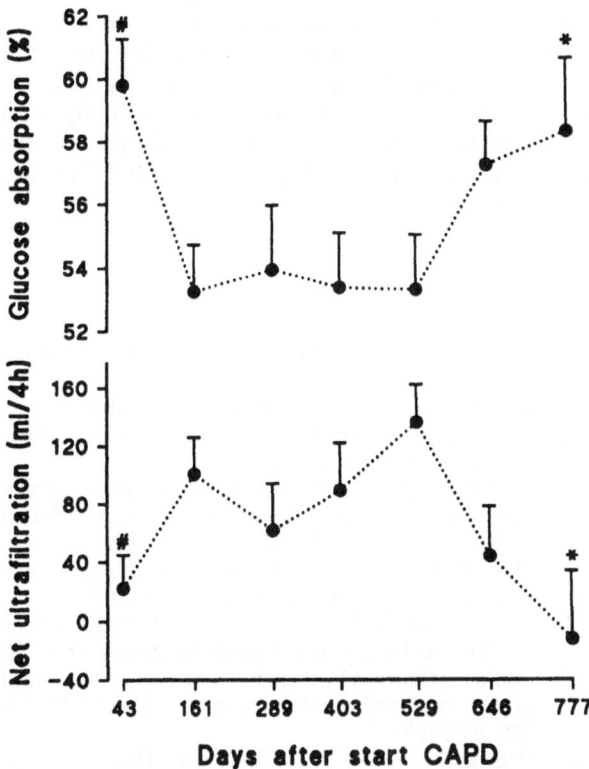

Figure 13. Glucose absorption (mean ± SEM, %) and net ultrafiltration (ml/4h/1.73m^2), measured every four months in 61 CAPD patients for a period of two years. The median days at each interval are given. The symbol # indicates a significant difference between day 43 and 161, whereas * symbolizes a significant trend from day 161 to 777. Published with permission from reference (260) and of Blackwell Scientific Publications.

peritoneal surface area (260, 265, 267, 328–330, 333, 337, 340, 343, 345). This discrepancy may be explained by the fact that solute transport parameters, when measured shortly after the initiation of CAPD are higher and net ultrafiltration is lower than after 4 months (Figure 13), suggesting that baseline values are not reached within three months on CAPD (260).

The clearances of serum proteins were in general not increased, despite the development of a large effective peritoneal surface area, and it would suggest a decrease in the intrinsic permeability of the peritoneum. This was supported by the finding of a higher restriction coefficient in patients treated with CAPD for more than 4 years, when compared to matched controls who were studied within the first three months of CAPD (328). It may, however, be a late effect, because the restriction coefficient showed no changes during the first 2 years (260).

It can be concluded that long-duration CAPD does not lead to functional deterioration of the peritoneal membrane, as far as solute transport is concerned. The modest alterations found in some studies suggest an increase in the effective peritoneal surface area. This is one of the

168   *Raymond T. Krediet*

causes for the loss of net ultrafiltration that can occur in some patients treated for several years. The large effective surface area does not lead to increased protein loss in the effluent, because the intrinsic permeability of the membrane to macromolecules tends to decrease. Up to now precise morphological functional relationships have not been elucidated.

REFERENCES

1. Davies DV, Davies F: *Gray's Anatomy*, 33rd ed, London, Longmans, 1964, p 1421
2. Wegener G: Chirurgische Bemerkungen über die peritoneale Hole, mit besondere Berucksichtigung der Ovariotomie. *Arch Klin Chir* 20: 51, 1877
3. Putiloff PV: Materials for the study of the laws of growth of the human body in relation to the surface area: the trial on Russian subjects of planigraphic anatomy as a mean of exact anthropometry. Presented at the Siberian branch of the Russian Geographic Society, Omsk, 1886
4. Esperanca MJ, Collins DL: Peritoneal dialysis efficiency in relation to body weight. *J Paediatric Surg* 1: 162, 1966
5. Rubin JL, Clawson M, Planch A, Jones Q: Measurements of peritoneal surface area in man and rat. *Am J Med Sci* 245: 453, 1988
6. Bell JL, Leypoldt JK, Frigon RP, Henderson LW: Hydraulically-induced convective solute transport across the rabbit peritoneum. *Kidney Int* 38: 19, 1990
7. Rubin J, Jones Q, Planch A, Stanek K: Systems of membranes involved in peritoneal dialysis. *J Lab Clin Med* 110: 448, 1987
8. Fox SD, Leypoldt JK, Henderson LW: Visceral peritoneum is not essential for solute transport during peritoneal dialysis. *Kidney Int* 40: 612, 1991
9. Alon U, Bar-Maor JA, Bar-Joseph G: Effective peritoneal dialysis in an infant with extensive resection of the small intestine. *Am J Nephrol* 8: 65, 1988
10. Flessner MF, Dedrick RL: Importance of the liver in peritoneal dialysis (PD). *J Am Soc Nephrol* 4 (Abstract): 404, 1993
11. Khanna R, Mactier R, Twardowski ZJ, Nolph KD: Peritoneal cavity lymphatics. *Perit Dial Bull* 6: 113, 1986
12. Raftery AT: Regeneration of parietal and visceral peritoneum: an electron microscopical study. *J Anat* 115: 375, 1973
13. Bolen JW, Hammer SP, McNutt MA: Serosal tissue: reactive tissue as a model for understanding mesotheliomas. *Ultrastruct Pathol* 11: 251, 1987
14. Dobbie JW: New concepts in molecular biology and ultrastructural pathology of the peritoneum: their significance for peritoneal dialysis. *Am J Kidney Dis* 15: 97, 1990
15. Odor L: Observations of the rat mesothelium with the electron and phase microscopes. *Am J Anat* 95: 433, 1954
16. Dobbie JW, Zaki M, Wilson L: Ultrastructural studies on the peritoneum with special reference to chronic ambulatory peritoneal dialysis. *Scott Med J* 26: 213, 1981
17. Gotloib L, Digenis GE, Rabinovich S, Medline A, Oreopoulos DG: Ultrastructure of normal rabbit mesentery. *Nephron* 34: 248, 1983
18. Lloyd JK, Hauch WN, Dobbie JW: Comparative ultrastructural studies on animal peritoneal mesothelium. *Adv Perit Dial* 4: 27, 1988
19. Simionescu M, Simionescu N: Organization of cell junctions in the peritoneal mesothelium. *J Cell Biol* 74: 98, 1977
20. Dobbie JW: Morpho-functional correlations in human mesothelium. in *Peritoneal Dialysis*, edited by La Greca G, Ronco C, Feriani M, Chiaramonte S, Conz P, Milano, Wichtig Editore, 1991, p 33
21. Dobbie JW: Ultrastructural similarities between mesothelial and type II pneumocytes and their relevance to phospholipid surfactant production by the peritoneum. *Adv Perit Dial* 4: 32, 1988
22. Pollock CA, Ibels LS, Eckstein RP, Graham JC, Caterson RJ, Makony JF, Sheil AGR: Peritoneal morphology on maintenance dialysis. *Am J Nephrol* 9: 198, 1989
23. Dobbie JW, Lloyd JK, Gall CA: Categorization of ultrastructural changes in peritoneal mesothelium, stroma and blood vessels in uremia and CAPD patients. *Adv Perit Dial* 6: 3, 1990
24. Dobbie JW, Anderson JD, Hind C: Long-term effects of peritoneal dialysis on peritoneal morphology. *Perit Dial Int* 14 (Suppl 3): S16, 1994
25. Di Paolo N, Sacchi G, De Mia M, Gaggiotti E, Capotondo L, Rossi P, Bernini M, Pucci AM, Ibba L, Sabatelli P, Alessandrini C: Morphology of the peritoneal membrane during continuous ambulatory peritoneal dialysis. *Nephron* 44: 204, 1986
26. Gotloib L, Schostack A, Bar-Sella P, Cohen R: Continuous mesothelial injury and regeneration during long term peritoneal dialysis. *Perit Dial Bull* 7: 148, 1987
27. Dobbie JW: Morphology of the peritoneum in CAPD. *Blood Purif* 7: 74, 1989
28. Grahame GR, Torchia MG, Dankewich KA, Ferguson IA: Surface-active material in peritoneal effluent of CAPD patients. *Perit Dial Bull* 5: 109, 1985
29. Dobbie JW, Pavlina T, Lloyd JK, Johnston RC: Phosphatidylcholine synthesis by peritoneal mesothelium: its implications for peritoneal dialysis. *Am J Kidney Dis* 12: 31, 1988
30. Dobbie JW, Lloyd JK: Mesothelium secretes lamellar bodies in a similar manner to type II pneumocyte secretion of surfactant. *Perit Dial Int* 9: 215, 1989
31. Williams JD, Beavis JM: Phosphatidylcholine and peritoneal dialysis. *Contrib Nephrol* 85: 142, 1990
32. Strapans I, Piel CF, Felts JM: Analysis of selected plasma constituents in continuous ambulatory peritoneal dialysis effluent. *Am J Kidney Dis* 6: 490, 1986
33. Davies M, Stylianou E, Young S, Thomas GJ, Coles GA, Williams JD: Proteoglycans of CAPD-dialysate fluid and mesothelium. *Contrib Nephrol* 85: 134, 1990
34. Roboz J, Greaves J, Silides D, Chahinian AP, Hollund JF: Hyaluronic acid content of effusions as a diagnostic aid for malignant mesothelioma. *Cancer Res* 45: 1850, 1985
35. Davies M, Young S, Coles GA: The possible significance of hyaluronan in the peritoneal cavity of CAPD patients. *J Am Soc Nephrol* 3: 408, 1992
36. Molina R, Fitella X, Bruix J, Mengual P, Bosch J, Calvet X, Jo J, Ballesta AM: Cancer antigen 125 in serum and ascitic fluid of patients with liver diseases. *Clin Chem* 37: 1379, 1991

37. Koomen GCM, Betjes MGH, Zemel D, Krediet RT, Hoek FJ: Cancer antigen 125 is locally produced in the peritoneal cavity during continuous ambulatory peritoneal dialysis. *Perit Dial Int* 14: 132, 1994

38. Hermon AG, Claeys M, Moncada S, Vane JR: Biosynthesis of prostacyclin (PGI$_2$) and 12L-hydroxy-5, 8, 10, 14-eicosatraenoic acid (HETE) by pericardium, pleura, peritoneum, and aorta of the rabbit. *Prostaglandins* 18: 434, 1979

39. Stylianou E, Mackenzie R, Davies M, Coles GA, Williams JD: The interaction of organism, phagocyte and mesothelial cell. *Contr Nephrol* 85: 30, 1990

40. Stylianou E, Jenner LA, Davies M, Coles GA, Williams JD: Isolation, culture and characterization of human peritoneal mesothelial cells. *Kidney Int* 37: 1563, 1990

41. Topley N, Mackenzie R, Jörres A, Coles GA, Davies M, Williams JD: Cytokine networks in continuous ambulatory peritoneal dialysis: interactions of resident cells during inflammation in the peritoneal cavity. *Perit Dial Int* 13 (Suppl 2): S282, 1993

42. Rappoport J, Douvdevani A, Conforti A, Zlotnik M, Chaimovitz C: Peritoneal mesothelial cells synthesize IL-1. *J Am Soc Nephrol* 3: 416, 1992

43. Topley N, Jörres A, Luttmann W, Peterson M, Lang M, Thierausch K, Müller C, Coles G, Davies M, Williams J: Human peritoneal mesothelial cells synthesize IL-6: induction by IL-1β and TNFα. *Kidney Int* 43: 226, 1993

44. Topley N, Brown Z, Jörres A, Westwick J, Coles G, Davies M, Williams J: Human peritoneal mesothelial cells synthesize IL-8: synergistic induction by interleukin-1β and tumor necrosis factor α. *Am J Pathol* 142: 1876, 1993

45. Topley N, Witowski J, Jörres A, Mackenzie R, Coles GA, Williams JD: Synthesis of IL-6 by human peritoneal mesothelial cells: superinduction by spent dialysate and PMϕ derived cytokines. *J Am Soc Nephrol* 4: 419, 1993

46. Zemel D, Imholz ALT, de Waart DR, Dinkla C, Struijk DG, Krediet RT: The appearance of tumor necrosis factor α and soluble TNF receptors I and II in peritoneal effluent during stable and infectious CAPD. *Kidney Int* 46: 1422, 1994

47. Goldman M, Vandenabeele P, Moulart J, Amraoui Z, Abramovicz D, Nortier J, Vanherweghem JL, Fiers W: Intraperitoneal secretion of interleukin-6 during continuous ambulatory peritoneal dialysis. *Nephron* 56: 277, 1990

48. Zemel D, ten Berge RJM, Struijk DG, Bloemena E, Koomen GCM, Krediet RT: Interleukin-6 in CAPD patients without peritonitis; relationship to the intrinsic permeability of the peritoneal membrane. *Clin Nephrol* 37: 97, 1992

49. Zemel D, Koomen GCM, Hart AAM, ten Berge RJM, Struijk DG, Krediet RT: Relationship of TNFα, interleukin-6, and prostaglandins to peritoneal permeability for macromolecules during longitudinal follow-up of peritonitis in continuous ambulatory peritoneal dialysis. *J Lab Clin Med* 122: 686, 1993

50. Lin CY, Lin CC, Huang TP: Serial changes of interleukin-6 and interleukin-8 levels in drain dialysate of uremic patients with continuous ambulatory peritoneal dialysis during peritonitis. *Nephron* 63: 404, 1993

51. Zemel D, Krediet RT, Koomen GCM, Kortekaas WMR, Geertzen HGM, ten Berge RJM: Interleukin-8 during peritonitis in patients treated with CAPD; an in-vivo model of acute inflammation. *Nephrol Dial Transplant* 9: 169, 1994

52. Whitaker D, Papadimitrou JM, Wolters M: The mesothelium: its fibrinolytic properties. *J Pathol* 136: 291, 1982

53. Hinsbergh van VWM, Kooistra T, Scheffer MA, Bockel van JH, Muyen van GNP: Characterization and fibrinolytic properties of human omental tissue mesothelial cells. Comparison with endothelial cells. *Blood* 75: 1450, 1990

54. Slater ND, Lope GH, Raftery AT: Peritoneal plasminogen activator activity after chronic exposure to dialysis fluid. *Perit Dial Int* 12: 262, 1992

55. Gries E, Kopp J, Thomal U, Kuhlmann H: Regulation of intraperitoneal and intravascular coagulation and fibrinolysis related antigen in peritoneal dialysis. *Thromb Haemostas* 63: 356, 1990

56. Laurent TC: II. The ultrastructure and physical-chemical properties of interstitial connective tissue. *Pfluegers Arch* (Suppl) 336: S21, 1972

57. Gerch I, Catchpole HR: The nature of ground substances of connective tissue. *Perspect Biol Med* 3: 282, 1960

58. Watson PD, Grodins FS: An analysis of the effects of the interstitial matrix on plasma-lymph transport. *Microvasc Res* 16: 19, 1978

59. Laurent TC: Interaction between proteins and glycosaminoglycans. *Fed Proc* 36: 24, 1977

60. Aukland K, Reed RD: Interstitial-lymphatic mechanisms in the control of extracellular fluid volume. *Physiol Rev* 73: 1, 1993

61. Joffe P, Jensen CT: Type I and III procollagens in CAPD: markers of peritoneal fibrosis. *Adv Perit Dial* 7: 158, 1991

62. Jörres A, Ladat K, Lang J, Sander K, Gahl GM, Williams JD, Topley N: Human peritoneal fibroblasts synthesize IL-6 in response to IL-1β and TNFα. *Nephrol Dial Transplant* 9: 1023, 1993

63. Gotloib L, Shustak A, Bar-Sella P, Eiali V: Fenestrated capillaries in human parietal and rabbit diaphragmatic peritoneum. *Nephron* 41: 200, 1985

64. Gotloib L, Bar-Sella P, Shostak A: Reduplicated basal lamina of small venules and mesothelium of human parietal peritoneum. *Perit Dial Bull* 5: 212, 1985

65. Di Paolo N, Sacchi G: Peritoneal vascular charges in continuous ambulatory peritoneal dialysis (CAPD): an *in vivo* model for the study of diabetic microangiopathy. *Perit Dial Int* 9: 41, 1989

66. Nolph KD, Miller F, Rubin J, Popovich R: New directions in peritoneal dialysis concepts and applications. *Kidney Int* 18 (Suppl 10): S111, 1980

67. Flessner MF: Peritoneal transport physiology: insights from basic research. *J Am Soc Nephrol* 2: 122, 1991

68. Nagel W, Kuschinsky W: Study of the permeability of the isolated dog mesentery. *Eur J Clin Invest* 1: 149, 1970

69. Rasio EA: Metabolic control of permeability in isolated mesentery. *Am J Physiol* 226: 962, 1974

70. Fox JR, Wayland H: Interstitial diffusion of macromolecules in the rat mesentery. *Microvasc Res* 18: 255, 1979

71. Grotte G: Passage of dextran molecules across the blood-lymph barrier. *Acta Chir Scand* 211 (Suppl): 1, 1956

72. Rippe B, Haraldsson B: Transport of macromolecules across microvascular walls: the two-pore theory. *Physiol Rev* 74: 163, 1994

73. Renkin EM: Relation of capillary morphology to transport of fluid and large molecules: a review. *Acta Physiol Scand* 463 (Suppl): 81, 1979

74. Karnovsky MJ: The ultrastructural basis of capillary permeability studied with peroxidase as a tracer. *J Cell Biol* 35: 213, 1967

75. Rippe B, Haraldsson B: How are macromolecules transported across the capillary wall? *News Physiol Sci* 2: 135, 1987

76. Simionescu N, Simionescu M, Palade GE: Permeability of muscle capillaries to exogenous myoglobin. *J Cell Biol* 57: 424, 1973

77. Simionescu N, Simionescu M, Palade GE: Permeability of muscle capillaries to small heme-peptides. *J Cell Biol* 64: 586, 1975

78. Rippe B, Kamiya A, Folkow B: Transcapillary passage of albumin; effects of tissue cooling and of increases in filtration and plasma colloid osmotic pressure. *Acta Physiol Scand* 105: 171, 1979

79. Fox J, Galey F, Wayland H: Action of histamine on the mesenteric microvasculature. *Microvasc Res* 19: 108, 1980

80. Deen WM, Bridges CR, Brenner BM, Myers BD: Heteroporous model of glomerular size selectivity: application to normal and nephrotic humans. *Am J Physiol* 249: F374, 1985

81. Rippe B, Stelin G: Simulations of peritoneal solute transport during CAPD. Application of two-pore formalism. *Kidney Int* 35: 1234, 1989

82. Rippe B, Stelin G, Haraldsson B: Computer simulations of peritoneal fluid transport in CAPD. *Kidney Int* 40: 315, 1991

83. Preston GM, Carroll TP, Guggino WB, Agre P. Appearance of water channels in Xenopus oocytes expressing red cell CHIP 28 protein. *Science*, Washington DC 256: 385, 1992

84. Dempster JA, van Hoek AN; van Os CH: The quest for water channels. *News Physiol Sci* 7: 172, 1992

85. Agre P, Preston GM, Smith BL, Jung JS, Raina S, Moon C, Guggino WB, Nielsen S: Aquaporin CHIP: the archetypal molecular water channel. *Am J Physiol* 265: F463, 1993

86. Chen TW, Khanna R, Moore H, Twardowski ZJ, Nolph KD: Sieving and reflection coefficients for sodium salts and glucose during peritoneal dialysis. *J Am Soc Nephrol* 2: 1092, 1991

87. Gotloib L, Bar-Sella P, Jaichenko J, Shustack A: Ruthenium-red-stained polyanionic fixed charges in peritoneal microvessels. *Nephron* 47: 22, 1987

88. Galdi P, Shostak A, Jaichenko J, Fudin R, Gotloib L: Protamine sulfate induces enhanced peritoneal permeability to proteins. *Nephron* 57: 45, 1991

89. Alavi N, Lianos E, Andres G, Bentzel CJ: Effect of protamine on the permeability and structure of rat peritoneum. *Kidney Int* 21: 44, 1982

90. Krediet RT, Koomen GCM, Koopman MG, Hoek FJ, Struijk DG, Boeschoten EW, Arisz L: The peritoneal transport of serum proteins and neutral dextran in CAPD patients. *Kidney Int* 35: 1064, 1989

91. Leypoldt JK, Henderson LW: Molecular charge influences transperitoneal macromolecule transport. *Kidney Int* 43: 837, 1993

92. Krediet RT, Struijk DG, Koomen GCM, Zemel D, Boeschoten EW, Hoek FJ, Arisz L: Peritoneal transport of macromolecules in patients on CAPD. *Contrib Nephrol* 89: 161, 1991

93. Buis B, Koomen GCM, Imholz ALT, Struijk DG, Arisz L, Krediet RT: Is the transperitoneal transport of macromolecules charge dependent? *Perit Dial Int* 14 (Suppl 1): S33, 1994

94. Haraldsson B: The peritoneal membrane acts as a negatively charged barrier restricting anionic proteins. *J Am Soc Nephrol* 4: 407, 1993

95. Gotloib L, Shustuk A, Jaichenko J: Loss of mesothelial electronegative fixed charges during murine septic peritonitis. *Nephron* 51: 77, 1989

96. Flessner MF, Dedrick RL, Schultz JS: A distributed model of peritoneal plasma transport: theoretical considerations. *Am J Physiol* 246: R597, 1984

97. Flessner MF, Fenstermacher JK, Dedrick RL, Blasberg RG: A distributed model of peritoneal plasma transport: tissue concentration gradients. *Am J Physiol* 248: F425, 1985

98. Seasmes EL, Moncrief JW, Popovich RP: A distributed model of fluid and mass transfer in peritoneal dialysis. *Am J Physiol* 258: 958, 1990

99. Henderson LW: The problem of peritoneal membrane area and permeability. *Kidney Int* 3: 409, 1973

100. Nolph KD, Ghods A, Brown P, Miller F, Harris P, Pyle K, Popovich R: Effects of nitroprusside on peritoneal mass transfer coefficients and microvascular physiology. *Trans Am Soc Artif Intern Organs* 23: 210, 1977

101. Granger DN, Ulrich M, Perry MA, Kvietys PR: Peritoneal dialysis solutions and feline splanchnic blood flow. *Clin Exp Pharmacol Physiol* 11: 473, 1984

102. Pietrzak I, Hirszel P, Shostak A, Welch PG, Lee RE, Maher JF: Splanchnic volume, not flow rate, determines peritoneal permeability. *Trans Am Soc Artif Intern Organs* 35: 583, 1989

103. Nolph KD, Ghods AJ, van Stone J, Brown PA: The effects of intraperitoneal vasodilators on peritoneal clearances. *Trans Am Soc Artif Intern Organs* 22: 586, 1976

104. Bradley SE: Variations in hepatic flow in man during health and disease. *N Engl J Med* 240: 456, 1949

105. Aune S: Transperitoneal exchange. Peritoneal blood flow estimated by hydrogen gas clearance. *Scand J Gastroent* 5: 99, 1970

106. Grzegorzewska AE, Moore HL, Nolph KD, Chen TW: Ultrafiltration and effective peritoneal blood flow during peritoneal dialysis in the rat. *Kidney Int* 39: 608, 1991

107. Maher JF: Transport kinetics in peritoneal dialysis. *Perit Dial Bull* (Suppl): S4, 1983

108. Nolph KD, Popovich RP, Ghods AJ, Twardowski ZJ: Determinants of low clearances of small solutes during peritoneal dialysis. *Kidney Int* 13: 117, 1978

109. Grzegorzewska AE, Antoniewicz K: An indirect estimation of effective peritoneal capillary blood flow in peritoneally dialyzed uremic patients. *Perit Dial Int* 13 (Suppl 2): S39, 1993

110. Ronco C, Brendolan A, Braglantini L, Chiaramonte S, Feriani M, Fabris A, La Greca G: Studies on ultrafiltration in peritoneal dialysis: influence of plasma proteins and capillary blood flow. *Perit Dial Bull* 6: 93, 1986

111. Ronco G, Feriani M, Chiaramonte S, Brendolan A, Bragantini L, Conz P, Dell'Aquilla R, Milan M, La Greca G:

Pathophysiology of ultrafiltration in peritoneal dialysis. *Perit Dial Int* 10: 119, 1990

112. Crissinger KD, Granger DN. Gastrointestinal blood flow. in *Textbook of Gastroenterology*, edited by Yamada T, Philadelphia, Lippincott, 1991, p 447

113. Brandt JL, Castleman L, Ruskin HD, Greenwald J, Kelly JJ Jr, Jones A: The effect of oral protein and glucose feeding on splanchnic blood flow and oxygen utilization in normal and cirrhotic subjects. *J Clin Invest* 34: 1017, 1955

114. Rocha E, Silva M, Rosenberg M: The release of vasopressin in response to haemorrhage and its role in the mechanism of blood pressure regulation. *J Physiol, London* 202: 535, 1969

115. Suvannapara A, Levens NR: Local control of mesenteric blood flow by the renin-angiotensin system. *Am J Physiol* 225: G267, 1988

116. Rayford PL, Miller TA, Thompson J: Secretin, cholecystokinin and newer gastrointestinal hormones. *N Engl J Med* 244: 1093, 1976

117. Wade OL, Combes B, Childs AW, Wheeles HO, Cournand A, Bradley SE: The effect of exercise on the splanchnic blood flow and splanchnic blood volume in normal man. *Clin Sci* 15: 457, 1956

118. Henderson LW, Nolph KD: Altered permeability of the peritoneal membrane after using hypertonic peritoneal dialysis fluid. *J Clin Invest* 48: 992, 1969

119. Rubin J, Klein E, Bower JD: Investigation of the net sieving coefficient of the peritoneal membrane during peritoneal dialysis. *ASAIO J* 5: 9, 1982

120. Rippe B, Perry MA, Granger DN. Permselectivity of the peritoneal membrane. *Microvasc Res* 29: 89, 1985

121. Krediet RT, Imholz ALT, Struijk DG, Koomen GCM, Arisz L: Ultrafiltration failure in continuous ambulatory peritoneal dialysis. *Perit Dial Int* 13 (Suppl 2): S59, 1993

122. Imholz ALT, Koomen GCM, Struijk DG, Arisz L, Krediet RT: Fluid and solute transport in CAPD patients using ultralow sodium dialysate. *Kidney Int* 46: 333, 1994

123. Leypoldt JK: Interpreting peritoneal osmotic reflection coefficients using a distributed model of peritoneal transport. *Adv Perit Dial* 9: 3, 1993

124. Twardowski ZJ, Nolph KD, Khanna R, Prowant BF, Ryan CP, Moore HL, Nielsen MP: Peritoneal equilibration test. *Perit Dial Bull* 7: 138, 1987

125. Imholz ALT, Koomen GCM, Struijk DG, Arisz L, Krediet RT: Residual volume measurements in CAPD patients with exogenous and endogenous solutes. *Adv Perit Dial* 8: 33, 1992

126. Davies SJ, Brown B, Bryan J, Russel GI: Clinical evaluation of the peritoneal equilibration test: a population-based study. *Nephrol Dial Transplant* 8: 64, 1993

127. Nolph KD: Clinical implications of membrane transport characteristics on the adequacy of fluid and solute removal. *Perit Dial Int* 14 (Suppl 3): S78, 1994

128. Struijk DG, Krediet RT, Koomen GCM, Boeschoten EW, Arisz L: Measurement of peritoneal transport for low molecular weight solutes; which test should be used? *Nephrol Dial Transplant* 5: 721, 1990

129. Heimbürger O, Waniewski J, Werynski A, Park MS, Lindholm B: Dialysate to plasma solute concentration (D/P) versus peritoneal transport parameters in CAPD. *Nephrol Dial Transplant* 9: 47, 1994

130. Burkart JM, Jordan JR, Rocco MV: Assessment of dialysis dose by measured clearance versus extrapolated data. *Perit Dial Int* 13: 184, 1993

131. Pyle WK: Mass transfer in peritoneal dialysis. Thesis. University of Texas at Austin, University Microfilms International, Ann Arbor, Michigan, 1982

132. Randersson DH, Farrell P: Mass transfer properties of the human peritoneum. *ASAIO J* 3: 140, 1980

133. Rubin J, Nolph KD, Arfania D, Brown P, Prowant B: Follow-up of peritoneal clearances in patients undergoing continuous ambulatory peritoneal dialysis. *Kidney Int* 16: 619, 1979

134. Kagan A, Bar-Khayim Y, Shafer Z, Fainara M: Kinetics of peritoneal protein loss during CAPD: I. Different characteristics for low and high molecular weight proteins. *Kidney Int* 37: 971, 1990

135. Rippe B, Stelin G, Haraldsson B: Understanding the kinetics of peritoneal transport. in *Nephrology*, edited by Hatano M, Tokyo, Springer, 1991, p 1563

136. Imholz ALT, Koomen GCM, Struijk DG, Arisz L, Krediet RT: The effect of dialysate osmolarity on the transport of low molecular weight solutes and proteins during CAPD. *Kidney Int* 43: 1339, 1993

137. Lysaght MJ, Farrell PC: Membrane phenomena and mass transfer kinetics in peritoneal dialysis. *J Membr Sci* 44: 5, 1984

138. Waniewski J, Werynski A, Heimbürger O, Lindholm B: A comparative analysis of mass transport models in peritoneal dialysis. *Trans Am Soc Artif Intern Organs* 37: 65, 1991

139. Lindholm B, Werynski A, Bergström J: Kinetics of peritoneal dialysis with glycerol and glucose as osmotic agents. *Trans Am Soc Artif Intern Organs* 33: 19, 1987

140. Garred LJ, Canaud B, Farrell PC: A simple kinetic model for assessing peritoneal mass transfer in chronic ambulatory peritoneal dialysis. *ASAIO J* 6: 131, 1983

141. Krediet RT, Boeschoten EW, Zuyderhoudt FMJ, Strackee J, Arisz L: Simple assessment of the efficacy of peritoneal transport in continuous ambulatory peritoneal dialysis patients. *Blood Purif* 4: 194, 1986

142. Waniewski J, Werynski A, Heimbürger O, Lindholm B: Simple models for description of small solute transport in peritoneal dialysis. *Blood Purif* 9: 129, 1991

143. Waniewski J, Heimbürger O, Werynski A, Lindholm B: Aqueous solute concentrations and evaluation of mass transport coefficients in peritoneal dialysis. *Nephrol Dial Transplant* 7: 50, 1992

144. Krediet RT, Imholz ALT, de Waart DR, Langedijk MJ, Schouten M, Pannekeet MM, Struijk DG: Clinical experience with the standard peritoneal permeability analysis (SPA). *Nephrol Dial Transplant* 9: 1022, 1994

145. Imholz ALT: Peritoneal fluid and solute transport in CAPD patients. Thesis, University of Amsterdam: 44, 1994

146. Krediet RT, Zuyderhoudt FMJ, Boeschoten EW, Arisz L: Alterations in the peritoneal transport of water and solutes during peritonitis in continuous ambulatory peritoneal dialysis patients. *Eur J Clin Invest* 17: 43, 1987

147. Krediet RT, Boeschoten EW, Struijk DG, Arisz L: Differences in the peritoneal transport of water, solutes and proteins between dialysis with two- and with three-litre exchanges. *Nephrol Dial Transplant* 2: 198, 1988

148. Lasrich M, Maher JM, Hirszel P, Maher JF: Correlation of peritoneal transport rates with molecular weight: a method for predicting clearances. *ASAIO J* 2: 107, 1979

149. Nolph KD, Twardowski ZJ, Popovich RP, Rubin J: Equilibration of peritoneal dialysis solutions during long-dwell exchanges. *J Lab Clin Med* 93: 246, 1979

150. Heimbürger O, Waniewski J, Werynski A, Tranaeus A, Lindholm B: Peritoneal transport in CAPD patients with permanent loss of ultrafiltration capacity. *Kidney Int* 38: 495, 1990

151. Heimbürger O, Waniewski J, Werynski A, Lindholm B: A quantitative description of solute and fluid transport during peritoneal dialysis. *Kidney Int* 41: 1320, 1992

152. Nolph KD, Hano JE, Teschan PE: Peritoneal sodium transport during hypertonic peritoneal dialysis. *Ann Intern Med* 70: 931, 1989

153. Weast RC, Selby SM, Hodgman CD: *Handbook of Chemistry and Physics*, 64th ed, Ohio, Rubber, 1965, p F-117

154. Stryer L: *Biochemistry*, 2nd ed, Freeman, San Francisco 1981, p 205

155. Nakayama N, Yokoyama K, Kubo H, Watanabe S, Kawaguchi Y, Sakai O: Effects of ultralow Na concentration dialysate (ULNaD) for overhydrated patients undergoing CAPD. *Perit Dial Int* 12 (Suppl 1): S143, 1992

156. Nakayama N, Kawaguchi Y, Kubo H, Miura Y, Sakai O: Clinical effect of low Na concentration dialysate (120 mEq/l) for CAPD patients. *Perit Dial Int* 13 (Suppl 1): S76, 1993

157. Brown ST, Ahearn J, Nolph KD: Potassium removal with peritoneal dialysis. *Kidney Int* 4: 67, 1973

158. Waniewski J, Werynski A, Heimbürger O, Park MS, Lindholm B: Effect of alternative osmotic agents on peritoneal transport. *Blood Purif* 11: 248, 1993

159. Krediet RT, Zuyderhoudt FMJ, Boeschoten EW, Arisz L: Peritoneal permeability to proteins in diabetic and non-diabetic continuous ambulatory peritoneal dialysis patients. *Nephron* 42: 133, 1986

160. Bonomini V, Zucchelli P, Mioli V: Selective and unselective protein loss in peritoneal dialysis. *Proc Eur Dial Transplant Assoc* 4: 146, 1967

161. Taylor AE, Granger DN: Exchange of macromolecules across the microcirculation. in *Handbook of Physiology. Sec 2. The Cardiovascular System*, edited by Renkin EM, Michell CC, American Physiological Society, 1984, p 465

162. Rippe B, Haraldsson B: Fluid and protein fluxes across small and large pores in the microvasculature. Applications of two-pore equations. *Acta Physiol Scand* 131: 411, 1987

163. Nolph KD, Miller FN, Pyle WK, Popovich RP, Sorkin MI: An hypothesis to explain the ultrafiltration characteristics of peritoneal dialysis. *Kidney Int* 20: 543, 1981

164. Leypoldt JK, Blindauer KM: Convection does not govern plasma to dialysate transport of protein. *Kidney Int* 42: 1412, 1992

165. Schaeffer RC jr, Bitrick MS, Holberg WC III, Katz MA: Macromolecular transport across endothelial monolayers. *Int J Microcirc Clin Exp* 11: 181, 1992

166. Imholz ALT, Koomen GCM, Struijk DG, Arisz L, Krediet RT: Effect of an increased intraperitoneal pressure on fluid and solute transport during CAPD. *Kidney Int* 44: 1078, 1993

167. Leypoldt JK, Frigon RP, De Vore KW, Henderson LW: A rapid renal clearance methodology for dextran. *Kidney Int* 31: 855, 1987

168. Granath KA, Kvist BE: Molecular weight distribution analysis by gel chromatography on sephadex. *J Chromatogr* 28: 69, 1967

169. Krediet RT, Struijk DG, Zemel D, Koomen GCM, Arisz L: The transport of macromolecules across the human peritoneum during CAPD. in *Peritoneal Dialysis*, edited by La Greca G, Ronco C, Feriani M, Chiaramonte S, Conz P, Milano, Wichtig Editore, 1991, p 61

170. Zemel D, Krediet RT, Koomen GCM, Struijk DG, Arisz L: Day-to-day variability of protein transport used as a method for analyzing peritoneal permeability in CAPD. *Perit Dial Int* 11: 217, 1991

171. Krediet RT, Zemel D, Struijk DG, Koomen GCM, Arisz L: Individual characterization of the peritoneal restriction barrier to the transport of serum proteins. in *Current Concepts in Peritoneal Dialysis*, edited by Ota K, Maher JF, Winchester JF et al., Amsterdam, Excerpta Medica 1992, p 49

172. Krediet RT, Zemel D, Struijk DG, Koomen GCM, Arisz L: Individual characterization of the peritoneal restriction barrier to macromolecules. *Adv Perit Dial* 7: 15, 1991

173. Zonosi S, Winchester JF, Kloberdanz N, Preuss H, Fox S, Cocker C, Sanders K, Barnard W, Fox L: Upright position and exercise lower peritoneal transport rates. *Kidney Int* 23: 165, 1983

174. Caratola G, Zoccali C, Crucitti S, Pastorino D, Siclari F, Cuzzucri A, Maggiore Q: Effect of posture on peritoneal clearance in CAPD patients. *Perit Dial Int* 8: 58, 1988

175. Imholz ALT, Koomen GCM, Struijk DG, Arisz L, Krediet RT: Fluid and solute transport during CAPD in upright and recumbent position. *Nephrol Dial Transplant* 9: 1021, 1994

176. Erbe RW, Greene JA Jr, Weller JM: Peritoneal dialysis during hemorrhagic shock. *J Appl Physiol* 22: 131, 1967

177. Selgas R, Munoz IM, Conesa J, Madero R, Gancedo PG, Carmona AR, Martinez ME, Huarte E, Fontan MP, Sicilia L: Endogenous sympathetic activity in CAPD patients: its relationship to peritoneal diffusion capacity. *Perit Dial Bull* 6: 205, 1986

178. Ratge D, Augustin R, Wisser H: Plasma catecholamines and α- and β-adrenoceptors in circulating blood cells in patients on continuous ambulatory peritoneal dialysis. *Clin Nephrol* 28: 15, 1987

179. Zabetakis PM, Kumar DN, Gleim GW, Gavdenswartz MH, Agrawal M, Robinson AG, Michelis MF: Increased levels of plasma renin, aldosterone, catecholamines and vasopressin in chronic ambulatory peritoneal dialysis (CAPD) patients. *Clin Nephrol* 28: 147, 1987

180. Plum J, Ziyail M, Kemmer FW, Passlick-Deetjen J, Grabensee B: Intraindividual comparison of ANP, cGMP and plasma catecholamines between HD and CAPD. *Adv Perit Dial* 6: 211, 1990

181. Steinhauer HB, Günter B, Schollmeyer P: Stimulation of peritoneal synthesis of vasoactive prostaglandins during peritonitis in patients on continuous ambulatory peritoneal dialysis. *Eur J Clin Invest* 15: 1, 1985

182. Steinhauer HB, Günter B, Schollmeyer P: Enhanced peritoneal generation of vasoactive prostaglandins during peritonitis in patients undergoing CAPD. in *Frontiers in*

Peritoneal Dialysis, edited by Maher JF, Winchester JF, New York, Field, Rich 1986, p 604

183. Steinhauer HB, Schollmeyer P: Prostaglandin-mediated loss of proteins during peritonitis in continuous ambulatory peritoneal dialysis. *Kidney Int* 29: 584, 1986

184. Hain H, Jörres A, Gahl M, Pastelnik A, Müller C, Köttgen E: Peritoneal permeability for proteins in uninfected CAPD patients: a kinetic study. in *Current Concepts in Peritoneal Dialysis*, edited by Oka K, Winchester JF, Hirszel P et al., Amsterdam, Excerpta Medica, 1992, p 59

185. Shaldon S, Koch KM, Quelhorst E, Dinarello CA: Hazards of CAPD: interleukin-1 production. in *Frontiers in Peritoneal Dialysis*, edited by Maher JF, Winchester JF, New York, Field, Rich 1986, p 630

186. Shaldon S, Dinarello CA, Wyler DJ: Induction of interleukin-1 during CAPD. *Contrib Nephrol* 57: 207, 1987

187. Miller FN: Effects of peritoneal dialysis on rat microcirculation and peritoneal clearances in man. *Dial Transplant* 7: 818, 1978

188. Miller FN, Nolph KD, Joshua IG, Wiegman DL, Harris PD, Anderson DB: Hyperosmolality, acetate, and lactate: dilatory factors during peritoneal dialysis. *Kidney Int* 20: 347, 1981

189. Miller FN, Nolph KD, Joshua IG: The osmolality component of peritoneal dialysis solutions. in *Continuous Ambulatory Peritoneal Dialysis*, edited by Legrain M, Amsterdam, Excerpta Medica 1980, p 12

190. Heaton A, Ward MK, Johnston DG, Nicholson DV, Alberti KGMM, Kerr DNS: Short-term studies on the use of glycerol as an osmotic agent in continuous ambulatory peritoneal dialysis (CAPD). *Clin Sci* 67: 121, 1984

191. Goodship THJ, Lloyd S, McKenzie PW, Earnshaw M, Smeaton I, Bartlett K, Ward MK, Wilkinson R: Short-term studies on the use of aminoacids as an osmotic agent in continuous ambulatory peritoneal dialysis. *Clin Sci* 73: 471, 1987

192. Lindholm B, Werynski A, Bergström J: Peritoneal dialysis with aminoacid solutions: fluid and solute transport kinetics. *Artif Organs* 12: 2, 1988

193. Young GA, Dibble JB, Taylor AE, Kendall S, Brownjohn AM: A longitudinal study on the effects of amino-acid-based CAPD fluid on aminoacid retention and protein losses. *Nephrol Dial Transplant* 4: 900, 1989

194. Steinhauer HB, Lubrick-Birkner I, Klutte R, Baumann G, Schollmeyer P: Effect of aminoacid based dialysis solution on peritoneal permeability and prostanoid generation in patients undergoing continuous ambulatory peritoneal dialysis. *Am J Nephrol* 12: 61, 1992

195. Mistry CD, O'Donoghue DN, Nelson S, Gokal R, Ballardi FW: Kinetic and clinical studies of β_2-microglobulin in continuous ambulatory peritoneal dialysis: influence of renal and enhanced peritoneal clearances using glucose polymer. *Nephrol Dial Transplant* 5: 513, 1990

196. Imholz ALT, Brown CB, Koomen GCM, Arisz L, KKrediet RT: The effects of glucose polymers on water removal and protein clearances during CAPD. *Adv Perit Dial* 9: 25, 1993

197. Krediet RT, Brown CB, Imholz ALT, Koomen GCM: Protein clearance and icodextrin. *Perit Dial Int* 14 (Suppl 2): S39, 1994

198. Hirzel P, Lasrich M, Maher JF: Augmentation of peritoneal mass transport by dopamine. *J Lab Clin Med* 94: 747, 1974

199. Hirszel P, Maher JF, Le Grow W: Increased peritoneal mass transport with glucagon acting at the vascular surface. *Trans Am Soc Artif Intern Organs* 24: 136, 1978

200. Maher JF, Hirszel P, Lasrich M: Effects of gastrointestinal hormones on transport by peritoneal dialysis. *Kidney Int* 16: 130, 1979

201. Felt J, Richard C, McCaffrey C, Levy M: Peritoneal clearance of creatinine and inulin during dialysis in dogs: effect of splanchnic vasodilators. *Kidney Int* 16: 459, 1979

202. Hare HG, Valtin H, Gosselin RE: Effect of drugs on peritoneal dialysis in the dog. *J Pharmacol Exp Ther* 145: 122, 1964

203. Henderson LW, Kintzel JE: Influence of antidiuretic hormone on peritoneal membrane area and permeability. *J Clin Invest* 40: 2437, 1971

204. Miller FN, Joshua IG, Andersson GL: Quantitation of vasodilator-induced macromolecular leakage by *in vivo* fluorescent microscopy. *Microvasc Res* 24: 56, 1982

205. Brown EA, Kliger AS, Goffinet J, Finkelstein FO: Effect of hypertonic dialysate and vasodilators on peritoneal dialysis clearances in the rat. *Kidney Int* 13: 271, 1978

206. Shostak A, Chakrabarti E, Hirszel P, Maher JF: Effects of histamine and its receptor antagonists on peritoneal permeability. *Kidney Int* 34: 786, 1988

207. Nolph KD, Ghods AJ, Brown PA, Twardowski ZJ: Effects of intraperitoneal nitroprusside on peritoneal clearances in man with variation of dose, frequency of administration and dwell times. *Nephron* 24: 114, 1979

208. Maher JF, Hirszel P, Lasrich M: Modulation of peritoneal transport rates by prostaglandins. *Adv Prostaglandin Thromboxane Res* 7: 965, 1980

209. Hirszel P, Lasrich M, Maher JF: Arachidonic acid increases peritoneal clearances. *Trans Am Soc Artif Intern Organs* 27: 61, 1981

210. Maher JF, Hirszel P, Lasrich M: Prostaglandin effects on peritoneal transport. in *Adv Perit Dial*, edited by Gahl GM, Kessel M, Nolph KD, Amsterdam, Excerpta Medica, 1981, p 64

211. Zemel D, Koomen GCM, Struijk DG, ten Berge RJM, van Acker BAC, Krediet RT: Inflammatory mediators and peritoneal permeability (P Perm) in CAPD patients given cyclooxygenase inhibition (Cyl) during peritonitis. *Perit Dial Int* 14 (Suppl 1): S31, 1994

212. Krediet RT, Boeschoten EW, Struijk DG, Arisz L: Pharmacokinetics of intraperitoneally administered 5-fluorocytosine in continuous ambulatory peritoneal dialysis. *Nephrol Dial Transplant* 2: 453, 1987

213. Krediet RT, Boeschoten EW, Zuyderhoudt FMJ, Arisz L: The relationship between glucose absorption and body fluid loss by ultrafiltration during continuous ambulatory peritoneal dialysis. *Clin Nephrol* 27: 51, 1987

214. Williams PF, Marliss EB, Andersson GH, Oren A, Stein AN, Khanna R, Pettit J, Brandes L, Rodella H, Mupas L, Dombros N, Oreopoulos DG: Amino-acid absorption following intraperitoneal administration in CAPD patients. *Perit Dial Bull* 2: 124, 1982

215. Lukas G, Brindle SD, Greengard P: The route of absorption of intraperitoneally administered compounds. *J Pharm Exp Ther* 178: 562, 1971

216. Babb AL, Johansen PJ, Strand MJ, Tenckhoff H, Scribner BH: Bi-directional permeability of the human peritoneum to middle molecules. *Proc Eur Dial Transplant Assoc* 10: 247, 1973

217. Struijk DG, Krediet RT, Koomen GCM, Boeschoten EW, Reijden HJ van der, Arisz L: Indirect measurement of lymphatic absorption with inulin in continuous ambulatory peritoneal dialysis (CAPD) patients. *Perit Dial Int* 10: 141, 1990

218. Struijk DG, Imholz ALT, Krediet RT, Koomen GCM, Arisz L: The use of the disappearance rate for the measurement of lymphatic absorption during CAPD. *Blood Purif* 10: 182, 1992

219. Bouchet JL, Albin H, Quentin C, De Barbeyrac B, Vinçon G, Martin-Dupont Ph, Potaux L, Aparicio M: Pharmacokinetics of intravenous and intraperitoneal fosfomycin in continuous ambulatory peritoneal dialysis. *Clin Nephrol* 29: 35, 1988

220. Janicke DM, Morse GD, Apicella MA, Jusko WJ, Walshe JJ: Pharmacokinetic modelling of bidirectional transfer during peritoneal dialysis. *Clin Pharmacol Ther* 40: 209, 1986

221. Krediet RT, Struijk DG, Boeschoten EW, Hoek FJ, Arisz L: Measurement of intraperitoneal fluid kinetics in CAPD patients by means of autologous hemoglobin. *Neth J Med* 33: 281, 1988

222. Leypoldt JK, Pust AH, Frigon RP, Henderson LW: Dialysate volume measurements are required for determining peritoneal solute transport. *Kidney Int* 34: 254, 1988

223. Gjessing J: The use of dextran as a dialyzing fluid in peritoneal dialysis. *Acta Med Scand* 185: 237, 1969

224. Daugirdas JT, Ing TS, Ghandi VC, Hano JE, Chen WT, Yuan L: Kinetics of peritoneal fluid absorption in patients with chronic renal failure. *J Lab Clin Med* 95: 351, 1980

225. Rippe B, Stelin G, Ahlmen J: Lymph flow from the peritoneal cavity in CAPD patients. in *Frontiers in Peritoneal Dialysis*, edited by Maher JF, Winchester JF, New York, Field, Rich, 1986, p 24

226. Spencer PC, Farrell PC: Solute and water transfer kinetics in CAPD. in *Continuous Ambulatory Peritoneal Dialysis*, edited by Gokal R, Edinburgh, Churchill Livingstone 1986, p 38

227. De Paepe M, Belpaire F, Schelstraete K, Lameire N: Comparisons of different volume markers in peritoneal dialysis. *J Lab Clin Med* 111: 421, 1988

228. Lindholm B, Heimbürger O, Waniewski J, Werynski A, Bergström J: Peritoneal ultrafiltration and fluid reabsorption during peritoneal dialysis. *Nephrol Dial Transplant* 4: 805, 1989

229. Mactier RA, Khanna R, Twardowski ZJ, Moore H, Nolph KD: Contribution of lymphatic absorption to loss of ultrafiltration and solute clearances in continuous ambulatory peritoneal dialysis. *J Clin Invest* 80: 1311, 1987

230. Krediet RT, Struijk DG, Koomen GCM, Arisz L: Peritoneal fluid kinetics during CAPD measured with intraperitoneal dextran 70. *Trans Am Soc Artif Intern Organs* 37: 662, 1991

231. Struijk DG, Koomen GCM, Krediet RT, Arisz L: Indirect measurement of lymphatic absorption in CAPD patients is not influenced by trapping. *Kidney Int* 41: 1668, 1992

232. Brouard R, Tozer TN, Baumelou A, Gambertoglio JG: Transfer of autologous haemoglobin from the peritoneal cavity during peritoneal dialysis. *Nephrol Dial Transplant* 7: 57, 1992

233. Struijk DG, Bakker JC, Krediet RT, Koomen GCM, Stekkinger P, Arisz L: Effect of intraperitoneal administration of two different batches of albumin solutions on peritoneal solute transport in CAPD patients. *Nephrol Dial Transplant* 6: 198, 1991

234. Flessner MF, Dedrick RL, Schultz JS: Exchange of macromolecules between peritoneal cavity and plasma. *Am J Physiol* 248: H15, 1985

235. Hirszel P, Shea-Donohue F, Chakrabarti E, Montcalm E, Maher JF: The role of the capillary wall in restricting diffusion of macromolecules. *Nephron* 44: 58, 1988

236. Cheek TR, Twardowski ZJ, Moore HL, Nolph KD: Absorption of inulin and high-molecular weight gelatin isocyanate solutions from peritoneal cavity in rats. in *Ambulatory Peritoneal Dialysis*, edited by Avram MM, Giordano C, New York, Plenum, 1990, p 149

237. Krediet RT, Struijk DG, Koomen GCM, Hoek FJ, Arisz L: The disappearance of macromolecules from the peritoneal cavity during continuous ambulatory peritoneal dialysis (CAPD) is not dependent on molecular size. *Perit Dial Int* 10: 147, 1990

238. Mactier RA, Khanna R, Twardowski ZJ, Moore H, Nolph KD: Influence of phosphatidylcholine on lymphatic absorption during peritoneal dialysis in the rat. *Perit Dial Int* 8: 179, 1988

239. Flessner MF, Parker RJ, Sieber SM: Peritoneal lymphatic uptake of fibrinogen and erythrocytes in the rat. *Am J Physiol* 244: H89, 1983

240. Flessner MF, Fenstermacher JD, Blasberg RG, Dedrick RL: Peritoneal absorption of macromolecules studied by quantitative autoradiography. *Am J Physiol* 248: H26, 1985

241. Nagy JA: Lymphatic and nonlymphatic pathways of peritoneal absorption in mice: physiology versus pathology. *Blood Purif* 10: 148, 1992

242. Stelin G, Rippe B: A phenomenological interpretation of the variation in dialysate volume with dwell time on CAPD. *Kidney Int* 38: 465, 1990

243. Rose BD: *Clinical Physiology of Acid-base and Electrolyte Disorders*, 2nd ed, New York, McGraw-Hill, 1984, p 33

244. Twardowski ZJ, Khanna R, Nolph KD, Scalamogna A, Metzler MH, Schneider TW, Prowant BF, Ryan LP: Intraabdominal pressures during natural activities in patients treated with continuous ambulatory peritoneal dialysis. *Nephron* 44: 129, 1986

245. Twardowski ZJ, Prowant BF, Nolph KD, Martinez AJ, Lampton LM: High volume, low frequency continuous ambulatory peritoneal dialysis. *Kidney Int* 23: 64, 1983

246. Rubin J, Nolph KD, Popovich RP, Moncrieff JW, Prowant B: Drainage volumes during continuous ambulatory peritoneal dialysis. *ASAIO J* 2: 54, 1979

247. Canaud B, Liendo-Liendo C, Claret C, Mion H, Mion C: Etude 'in situ' de la cinetique de l'ultrafiltration en cours de dialyse péritonéale avec périodes de diffusion prolongée. *Nephrologie* 1: 126, 1980

248. Krediet RT, Imholz ALT, Struijk DG, Koomen GCM, Arisz L: Effects of tracer, volume, osmolarity and infection on fluid kinetics during CAPD. *Blood Purif* 10: 173, 1992

249. Nolph KD, Mactier RA, Khanna R, Twardowski ZJ, Moore H, McCary T: The kinetics of ultrafiltration during peritoneal dialysis: the role of lymphatics. *Kidney Int* 32: 219, 1987

250. Kaysen GA, Schoenfeld PY: Albumin homeostasis in patients undergoing continuous ambulatory peritoneal dialysis. *Kidney Int* 25: 107, 1984

251. Abernathy HJ, Clin W, Hay JB, Rodela H, Oreopoulos D, Johnston MG: Lymphatic removal of dialysate from the peritoneal cavity of anesthetized sheep. *Kidney Int* 40: 174, 1991

252. Johnston MG: Studies on lymphatic drainage of the peritoneal cavity in sheep. *Blood Purif* 10: 122, 1992

253. Tran LP, Rodella H, Abernathy NJ, Yuan Z-Y, Hay JB, Oreopoulos D, Johnston MG: Lymphatic drainage of hypertonic solution from the peritoneal cavity of anesthetized and conscious sheep. *J Appl Physiol* 74: 859, 1993

254. Tran LP, Rodella H, Hay JB, Oreopoulos DG, Johnston MG: Quantitation of lymphatic drainage of the peritoneal cavity in sheep: comparison of direct cannulation techniques with indirect methods to estimate lymph flow. *Perit Dial Int* 13: 270, 1993

255. Drake RE, Gabel JC: Diaphragmatic lymph vessel drainage of the peritoneal cavity. *Blood Purif* 10: 132, 1992

256. Rippe B, El Rashied Z: Peritoneal fluid and albumin kinetics in the rat; effects of increases in intraperitoneal hydrostatic pressure. *Perit Dial Int* 13 (Suppl 1): S74, 1993

257. Shockley TR, Ofsthun NJ: Pathways for fluid loss from the peritoneal cavity. *Blood Purif* 10: 115, 1992

258. Tsilibary EC, Wissig SL: Lymphatic absorption from the peritoneal cavity: regulation of patency of mesothelial stomata. *Microvasc Res* 25: 22, 1983

259. Abensur H, Romao JE Jr, Brando de Almeida Prado E, Kakahaski E, Sabbaga E, Marcoudes M: Influence of the hydrostatic intraperitoneal pressure and the cardiac function on the lymphatic absorption rate of the peritoneal cavity in CAPD. *Adv Perit Dial* 9: 41, 1993

260. Struijk DG, Krediet RT, Koomen GCM, Boeschoten EW, Hoek FJ, Arisz L: A prospective study of peritoneal transport in CAPD patients. *Kidney Int* 45: 1739, 1994

261. Verger C, Brunshvig O, Le Carpentier Y, Lavergne A, Vantelon J: Structural and ultrastructural peritoneal membrane changes and permeability alterations during continuous ambulatory peritoneal dialysis. *Proc Eur Dial Transplant Assoc* 18: 199, 1981

262. Slingeneyer A, Canaud B, Mion C: Permanent loss of ultrafiltration capacity of the peritoneum in long-term peritoneal dialysis: an epidemiological study. *Nephron* 33: 133, 1983

263. Wideröe TE, Smeby LC, Mjåland S, Dahl K, Berg KJ, Aas TW: Long-term changes in transperitoneal water transport during continuous ambulatory peritoneal dialysis. *Nephron* 38: 238, 1984

264. Faller B, Marichal JF: Loss of ultrafiltration in continuous ambulatory peritoneal dialysis: a role for acetate. *Perit Dial Bull* 4: 10, 1984

265. Krediet RT, Boeschoten EW, Zuyderhoudt FMJ, Arisz L: Peritoneal transport characteristics of water, low-molecular weight solutes and proteins during long-term continuous ambulatory peritoneal dialysis. *Perit Dial Bull* 6: 61, 1986

266. Gokal R, Jakubowski C, King J, Hunt L, Bogle S, Baillod R, Marsh F, Ogg C, Oliver D, Ward M, Wilkinson R: Outcome in patients on continuous ambulatory peritoneal dialysis and hemodialysis; 4-year analysis of a prospective multicentre study. *Lancet* 2: 1105, 1987

267. Pollock CA, Ibels LS, Caterson RJ, Mahoney JF, Waugh DA, Cocksedge B: Continuous ambulatory peritoneal dialysis. Eight years of experience at a single center. *Medicine* 68: 293, 1989

268. Verger C, Larpent L, Celicout B. Clinical significance of ultrafiltration failure on CAPD. in *Peritoneal Dialysis*, edited by La Greca G, Chiaramonte S, Fabris A, Feriani M, Ronco C, Milano, Wichtig Editore, 1986, p 91

269. Krediet RT, Struijk DG, Boeschoten EW, Koomen GCM, Stouthard JML, Hoek FJ, Arisz L: The time course of peritoneal transport kinetics in continuous ambulatory peritoneal dialysis patients who develop sclerosing peritonitis. *Am J Kidney Dis* 13: 299, 1989

270. Verger C, Celicout B: Peritoneal permeability and encapsulating peritonitis. *Lancet* 1: 986, 1985

271. Mactier RA, Khanna R, Twardowski ZJ, Nolph KD: Ultrafiltration failure in continuous ambulatory peritoneal dialysis due to excessive peritoneal cavity lymphatic absorption. *Am J Kidney Dis* 10: 461, 1987

272. Dobbie JW, Krediet RT: Twardowski ZJ, Nichols WK: A 39 year old man with loss of ultrafiltration. *Perit Dial Int* 14: 384, 1994

273. Monquil MCJ, Imholz ALT, Struijk DG, Krediet RT: Does impaired transcellular water transport contribute to net ultrafiltration failure during CAPD? *Perit Dial Int* 15: 42, 1995

274. Mistry CD, Mallick NP, Gokal R: Ultrafiltration with an isosmotic solution during long peritoneal dialysis exchanges. *Lancet* 2: 178, 1987

275. Stein A, Peers E, Hattersley J, Harris K, Feehally J, Walls J: MIDAS Study Group. Clinical experience with icodextrin in continuous ambulatory peritoneal dialysis patients. *Perit Dial Int* 14 (Suppl 2): S51, 1994

276. Di Paolo N, Buoncristiani U, Capotondo L, Gaggiotti E, de Mia M, Rossi P, Sansoni E, Bernini M: Phosphatidylcholine and peritoneal transport during peritoneal dialysis. *Nephron* 44: 365, 1986

277. Di Paolo H, Capotondo L, Ciccoli L, Gaggiotti E, Rossi P, Sansoni E: Phosphatidylcholine: a physiological modulator of the peritoneal membrane. in *Ambulatory Peritoneal Dialysis*, edited by Avram MM, Giordano CG, New York, Plenum, 1990, p 44

278. Dombros N, Balaskas E, Savidis N, Tourkantonis A, Sombolis K. Phosphatidylcholine increases ultrafiltration in continuous ambulatory peritoneal dialysis. in *Ambulatory Peritoneal Dialysis*, edited by Avram MM, Giordano GC, New York, Plenum, 1990, p 44

279. Querques M, Procaccini DA, Pappani A, Strippoli P, Passione A: Influence of phosphatidylcholine on ultrafiltration and solute transfer in CAPD patients. *Trans Am Soc Artif Intern Organs* 30: M581, 1990

280. Krack G, Viglino C, Cavalli PL, Gandolfo CF, Magliano G, Cantaluppi A, Peluso F: Intraperitoneal administration of phosphatidylcholine improves ultrafiltration in continuous ambulatory peritoneal dialysis patients. *Perit Dial Int* 12: 354, 1992

281. Mactier RA, Khanna R, Twardowski ZJ, Moore H, Nolph KD: Influence of phosphatidylcholine on lymphat-

ic absorption during peritoneal dialysis in the rat. *Perit Dial Int* 8: 179, 1988

282. Struijk DG, van der Reijden HJ, Krediet RT, Koomen GCM, Arisz L: Effect of phosphatidylcholine on peritoneal transport and lymphatic absorption in a CAPD patient with sclerosing peritonitis. *Nephron* 51: 577, 1989

283. Chan H, Abraham G, Oreopoulos DG: Oral lecithin improves ultrafiltration in patients on peritoneal dialysis. *Perit Dial Int* 9: 203, 1989

284. De Vecchi A, Calstelnovo C, Guerra L, Scalamogna A: Phosphatidylcholine administration in continuous ambulatory peritoneal dialysis (CAPD) patients with reduced ultrafiltration. *Perit Dial Int* 9: 207, 1989

285. Chan PCK, Tam SCF, Robinson JD, Yu L, Ip MSM, Chan CY, Chen IKP: Effect of phosphatidylcholine on ultrafiltration in patients on continuous ambulatory peritoneal dialysis. *Nephron* 59: 100, 1991

286. Maher JF, Hirszel P, Bennett RR, Chakrabarti E: Amphotericin selectively increases peritoneal ultrafiltration. *Am J Kidney Dis* 4: 285, 1984

287. Maher JF, Hirszel P, Bennett RR, Chakrabarti E: Augmentation of peritoneal hydraulic permeability by amphotericin B: locus of action. *Perit Dial Bull* 4: 229, 1984

288. Andreoli TE, Dennis VW, Weigl AM: The effect of amphotericin B on the water and nonelectrolyte permeability of thin lipid membranes. *J Gen Physiol* 53: 133, 1969

289. Maher JF, Hirszel P, Chakrabarti E, Bennett RR: Contrasting effects of amphotericin B and the solvent desoxycholate on peritoneal transport. *Nephron* 43: 38, 1986

290. Imholz ALT, Koomen GCM, Struijk DG, Arisz L, Krediet RT: The effect of amphotericin B on fluid kinetics and solute transport in CAPD. *Adv Perit Dial* 9: 12, 1993

291. Lamperi S, Carozzi S, Nasini MG: Calcium antagonists improve ultrafiltration in patients on continuous ambulatory peritoneal dialysis (CAPD). *Trans Am Soc Artif Intern Organs* 33: 657, 1987

292. Favazza A, Montanaro D, Mesa P, Antonucci F, Gropuzzo M, Mion G: Peritoneal clearances in hypertensive CAPD patients after oral administration of clonidine, enalapril and nifedipine. *Perit Dial Int* 12: 287, 1992

293. Gotloib L, Shostack A, Bar-Sella P, Cohen R: Continuous mesothelial injury and regeneration during long term peritoneal dialysis. *Perit Dial Bull* 7: 148, 1987

294. Suassuna J, Neves F, Glancey G, Cameron JS, Ogg C, Hartley B: Mesothelial and endothelial cell markers of activation in the peritoneal membrane of continuous ambulatory peritoneal dialysis patients. *Nephrol Dial Transplant* 5: 271, 1990

295. Heale WF, Letch KA, Dawborn JK, Evans SM: Long term complications of peritonitis. in *Peritoneal Dialysis*, edited by Atkins RC, Thomson NM, Farrell PC, Edinburgh, Churchill Livingstone, 1981, p 284

296. Rubin J, McFarland S, Hellems EW, Bower JD: Peritoneal dialysis during peritonitis. *Kidney Int* 19: 460, 1981

297. Prowant BF, Nolph KD. Clinical criteria for diagnosis of peritonitis. in *Peritoneal Dialysis*, edited by Atkins RC, Thomson NM, Farrell PC, Edinburgh, Churchill Livingstone, 1981, p 257

298. Smeby LC, Wideröe TE, Jörstad S: Individual differences in water transport during peritonitis. *ASAIO J* 4: 17, 1981

299. Raja RM, Kramer MS, Rosenbaum JL, Bolisay C, Krug M: Contrasting changes in solute transport and ultrafiltration with peritonitis in CAPD patients. *Trans Am Soc Artif Intern Organs* 27: 68, 1981

300. Rubin J, Ray R, Barnes T, Bower J: Peritoneal abnormalities during infectious episodes of continuous ambulatory peritoneal dialysis. *Nephron* 29: 124, 1981

301. Smeby LC, Wideröe TE, Svartås TM, Jörstad S: Changes in water removal due to peritonitis during continuous ambulatory peritoneal dialysis. in *Adv Perit Dial*, edited by Gahl GM, Kessel M, Nolph KD, Amsterdam, Excerpta Medica, 1981, p 287

302. Raja RM, Kramer MS, Barber K: Solute transport and ultrafiltration during peritonitis in CAPD patients *ASAIO J* 7: 8, 1984

303. Gokal R, Mistry CD, Peers EM et al.: Peritonitis occurrence in a multicentre study of icodextrin and glucose in CAPD. *Perit Dial Int* 15: 226, 1995

304. Krediet RT, Arisz L: Fluid and solute transport across the peritoneum during continuous ambulatory peritoneal dialysis (CAPD). *Perit Dial Int* 9: 15, 1989

305. Blumenkrantz MJ, Gahl GM, Kopple JD, Kamdar AV, Jones MR, Kessel M, Coburn JW: Protein losses during peritoneal dialysis. *Kidney Int* 19: 593, 1981

306. Katirtzoglou A, Oreopoulos DG, Husdan H, Leung M, Ogilvie R, Dombros N: Reappraisal of protein losses in patients undergoing continuous ambulatory peritoneal dialysis. *Nephron* 26: 230, 1980

307. Dulaney JT, Hatch JR FE: Peritoneal dialysis and loss of proteins: a review. *Kidney Int* 26: 253, 1984

308. Miller FN, Hammerschmidt DE, Anderson GL, Moore JN: Protein loss induced by complement activation during peritoneal dialysis. *Kidney Int* 25: 480, 1984

309. Slingeneyer A, Mion C, Mourad G, Canaud B, Faller B, Béraud JJ: Progressive sclerosing peritonitis: a late and severe complication of maintenance peritoneal dialysis. *Trans Am Soc Artif Intern Organs* 29: 633, 1983

310. Ing TS, Daugirdas JT, Ghandi VD: Peritoneal sclerosis in peritoneal dialysis patients. *Am J Nephrol* 4: 173, 1984

311. Novello AC, Port FK: Sclerosing encapsulating peritonitis. *Int J Artif Organs* 9: 393, 1986

312. Shaldon S, Koch KM, Quellhorst E, Dinarello CA. Pathogenesis of sclerosing peritonitis in CAPD. *Trans Am Soc Artif Intern Organs* 30: 193, 1984

313. Junor BJR, Briggs JD, Forwell MA, Dobbie JW, Henderson I: Sclerosing peritonitis; the contribution of chlorhexidine in alcohol. *Perit Dial Bull* 5: 101, 1985

314. Oulès R, Challah S, Brunnes FP: Case-control study to determine the cause of sclerosing peritoneal disease. *Nephrol Dial Transplant* 3: 66, 1988

315. Mackow RC, Aray WP, Winchester JF et al.: Sclerosing encapsulating peritonitis in rats induced by long-term intraperitoneal administration of antiseptics. *J Lab Clin Med* 112: 363, 1988

316. Grebfberg N, Nilsson P, Andréen T: Sclerosing obstructive peritonitis, beta-blockers and continuous ambulatory peritoneal dialysis. *Lancet* 2: 733, 1983

317. Narayama R, Bhargava BV, Kabra SA, Saugal BC: Idispathic Sclerosing encapsulating peritonitis. *Lancet* 2: 127, 1989

318. Dobbie JW: Pathogenesis of peritoneal fibrosing syndromes (sclerosing peritonitis) in peritoneal dialysis. *Perit Dial Int* 12: 14, 1992

319. Rottembourg J, Gahl GM, Poignet JL, Mertani E, Strippoli P, Langlois P, Tranbaloc P, Legrain M: Severe abdominal complications in patients undergoing continuous ambulatory peritoneal dialysis. *Proc Eur Dial Transplant Assoc* 20: 236, 1983

320. Verger C, Celicout B: Peritoneal permeability and encapsulating peritonitis. *Lancet* 1: 986, 1985

321. Manos J, Postlethwaite RJ, Mallick NP, Gokal R: Sclerosing encapsulating peritonitis and other complications of CAPD peritonitis. in *Frontiers in Peritoneal Dialysis*, edited by Maher JF, Winchester JF, New York, Field, Rich, 1986, p 634

322. McWhinnie DL, Bradley JA, Bramwell SP, Hamilton DNH, Macpherson SG, Cram LP, Moore IAR, Forwell MA, Smith WGJ, Briggs JD, Junor BJR: Sclerosing peritonitis – a further complication of CAPD. in *Frontiers in Peritoneal Dialysis*, edited by Maher JF, Winchester JF, New York, Field, Rich, 1986, p 638

323. Rottembourg J, Issad B, Langlois P, de Groc F, Legrain M. Sclerosing encapsulating peritonitis during CAPD. Evaluation of the potential risk factors. in *Frontiers in Peritoneal Dialysis*, edited by Maher JF, Winchester JF, New York, Field, Rich, 1986, p 643

324. Tanaka Y, Shirai D: Clinical aspects of sclerosing peritonitis. in *Current Concepts in Peritoneal Dialysis*, edited by Ota K, Maher JF, Winchester JF et al., Amsterdam, Excerpta Medica, 1992, p 112

325. Gandhi VC, Ing TS, Daugirdas JT, Hagen C, Blumenkrantz MJ, Jablokow VR: Failure of peritoneal dialysis due to peritoneal sclerosis. *Int J Artif Organs* 6: 97, 1983

326. Finkelstein FO, Kliger AS, Bastl C, Yap P: Sequential clearance and dialysance measurements in chronic peritoneal dialysis patients. *Nephron* 18: 342, 1977

327. Rubin J, Arfania D, Nolph KD, Prowant B, Fruto L, Brown P, Moore H: Peritoneal clearances after 6–12 months on continuous ambulatory peritoneal dialysis. *Trans Am Soc Artif Intern Organs* 25: 104, 1979

328. Struijk DG, Krediet RT, Koomen GCM, Hoek FJ, Boeschoten EW, van der Reijden HJ, Arisz L: Functional characteristics of the peritoneal membrane in long-term continuous ambulatory peritoneal dialysis. *Nephron* 59: 213, 1991

329. Selgas R, Rodrigues-Carmona A, Martinez ME, Perez-Fontan M, Salinas M, Escuin F, Rinon C, Martinez-Ara J, Sanchez-Sicilia L: Peritoneal mass transfer in patients on long-term CAPD. *Perit Dial Bull* 4: 153, 1984

330. Nikolakakis N, Rodger RSC, Goodship THJ, Fletcher K, Ashcroft R, Wilkinson R, Ward MK: The assessment of peritoneal function using a single hypertonic exchange. *Perit Dial Bull* 5: 186, 1985

331. Hallet MD, Kush RD, Lysaght MJ, Farrel PC: The stability and kinetics of peritoneal mass transfer. in *Peritoneal Dialysis*, edited by Noph KD, Dordrecht, Kluwer Academic Publishers, 1989, p 380

332. Park MS, Lee J, Lee MS, Baick SH, Hwang SD, Lee HB: Peritoneal solute clearances after four years of continuous ambulatory peritoneal dialysis (CAPD). *Perit Dial Int* 9: 75, 1989

333. Passlick-Deetjen J, Chlebowski H, Koch M, Ziegelmayer C, Grabensee B: Evaluation of long-term changes in peritoneal membrane function. in *Peritoneal Dialysis*, edited by La Graeca G, Ronco C, Feriani M, Chiaramonte S, Cour P, Milano, Wichtig, 1991, p 109

334. Coronel F, Tornero F, Mucia M, Sánchez A, De Oleo P, Naranjo P, Barrientos A: Peritoneal clearances, protein losses and ultrafiltration in diabetic patients after four years on CAPD. *Adv Perit Dial* 7: 35, 1991

335. Lee HB, Park MS, Chung SH, So IN, Han DC, Lee SK, Hwang SD, Moon C: Peritoneal membrane performance after 5 years on CAPD. in *Current Concepts in Peritoneal Dialysis*, edited by Ota K, Maher JF, Winchester JF et al., Amsterdam, Excerpta Medica, 1992, p 84

336. Spencer PC, Farrell PC: Solute and water transfer kinetics in CAPD. in *Continuous Ambulatory Peritoneal Dialysis*, edited by Gokal R, Edinburgh, Churchill Livingstone, 1986, p 38

337. Rubin J, Nolph KD, Arfania D, Brown P, Prowant B: Follow-up of peritoneal clearances in patients undergoing continuous ambulatory peritoneal dialysis. *Kidney Int* 16: 619, 1979

338. Farrell PC, Randerson JH: Membrane permeability changes in long-term CAPD. *Trans Am Soc Artif Intern Organs* 26: 197, 1980

339. Randerson DH, Farrell PC: Long-term peritoneal clearance in CAPD. in *Peritoneal Dialysis*, edited by Atkins RC, Thomson NM, Farrell PC, Edinburgh, Churchill Livingstone, 1981, p 21

340. Selgas R, Rodrigues-Carmona A, Martinez ME, Conesa J, Perez-Fontan M, Huarte E, Ortega O, Sanchez-Sicilia L: Follow-up of peritoneal mass transfer properties in long-term CAPD patients. in *Frontiers in Peritoneal Dialysis*, edited by Maher JF, Winchester JF, New York, Field, Rich, 1986, p 53

341. Selgas R, Muños J, Cigarran S, Ramos P, L-Revuelta K, Escuin F, Miguel JL: Peritoneal functional parameters after five years on continuous ambulatory peritoneal dialysis (CAPD): The effect of late peritonitis. *Perit Dial Int* 9: 329, 1989

342. Blake PG, Abraham G, Sombolos K, Izatt S, Weissgarten J, Ayiomamitis A, Oreopoulos DG: Changes in peritoneal membrane transport rates in patients on long term CAPD. *Adv Perit Dial* 5: 3, 1989

343. Kush RD, Hallett MD, Ota K, Yamushita A, Kumano K, Watenabe N, Sakai T, Hidai H, Farrell PC: Long-term continuous ambulatory peritoneal dialysis; mass transfer and nutritional and metabolic stability. *Blood Purif* 8: 1, 1990

344. Bordoni E, Lombardo V, Bibiano L, Carletti P, Francialli E, Gaffi G, Perilli A, Mioli V: Peritoneal clearances, ultrafiltration and diuresis in long-term continuous ambulatory peritoneal dialysis. in *Ambulatory Peritoneal Dialysis*, edited by Avram MM, Giordano C, New York, Plenum, 1990, p 87

345. Chan PCK, Chan CY, Wu PG, Cheng IKP, Chan MK: Long-term peritoneal clearances in patients on continuous ambulatory peritoneal dialysis. *Int J Artif Organs* 13: 707, 1990

346. Lameire NH, Vanholder R, Veyt D, Lambert M-C, Ringoir S: A longitudinal, five year survey of urea kinetic parameters in CAPD patients. *Kidney Int* 42: 426, 1992

BIOCOMPATIBILITY – PRINCIPLES

RAYMOND M. HAKIM and JONATHAN HIMMELFARB

INTRODUCTION

The contact of blood with biomaterials used in hemodialysis, elicits an organized inflammatory response that involves the activation of the body's defense against 'nonself'. These reactions include not only the enzymatic cleavage of proteins, such as the complement, contact and coagulation pathways, but in addition, cellular events that are part of the inflammatory response. Activation of these cellular pathways can result indirectly from the products of activation of these protein pathways or from the direct interaction of these cells with foreign surfaces. In this chapter, several of these inflammatory responses which are relevant to the hemodialysis procedure will be outlined. The clinical relevance of these reactions are detailed elsewhere in this volume.

PROTEIN PATHWAYS

The complement system

The complement system is an important component of the host's defense against non-self and plays a pivotal role in the mediation of immunological tissue injury.

The complement system consists of at least 20 plasma proteins that are normally present in inactive form (zymogens). Similar to the coagulation pathway, the complement proteins can be divided into two pathways; the first is the so-called 'classical' pathway, and the other is the 'alternative' pathway (Figure 1). These two pathways are distinguished by the entities that are involved in their initial activation but they share a common 'terminal' pathway that is independent of the initial pathway of activation. Also, similar to the coagulation pathway, the activation

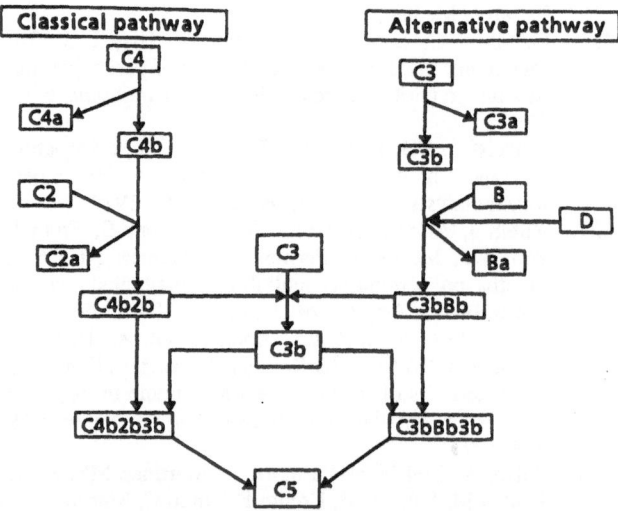

Figure 1. Analogous action of the classical and alternative complement activation pathways. Both pathways generate a C3 convertase: C4b2b (classical pathway) and C3bBb (alternative pathway). In the classical sequence, C1 activated by complexed antibody splits C4 and C2 with the loss of the small fragments C4a and C2a: the major components form C4b2b. In the alternative route, pre-existing C3b binds Factor B, which is split releasing a small fragment, Ba. The major fragment, Bb, remains bound to form C3bBb. This converts more C3, so continuing the feedback cycle. Activator surfaces, on microorganisms for example, facilitate the combination of Factor B and C3b, and promote alternative pathway activation. The C3 convertases of both pathways may bind further C3b to yield the enzymes which activate the next component of the complement system, C5: classical pathway C5 convertase, Crb2b3b, and alternative pathway C5 convertase C3bBb3b (IC – immune complexes).

of either pathway involves a cascade of sequential activation of different proteins and its propagation is governed by regulatory proteins, which are intrinsic components of the complement system and are either inhibitory or amplifying (1, 2). The specific components of the complement system are normally inactive in plasma, although a continuous low grade, short-lived, and labile activation of C3 in the fluid phase reportedly occurs (3). The complement proteins also have the ability to transfer themselves from solution to the surface of biological particles and to function as solid phase enzymes.

Although the interaction of the complement system with biomaterials involves almost exclusively the activation of the alternative pathway, it is useful to review the general scheme of activation common to both pathways. An initial event catalyzes the formation and stabilization of target-bound C3 convertase (i.e., the enzyme that activates C3), which is made up of different components in the classical and alternate pathways; in turn, C3 convertase catalyzes the formation of the target-bound C5 convertase, which is also made up of different components, depending on the pathway of activation. This latter enzyme then sets in motion the self-assembly of the membrane attack complex C5b-9 (4). Because of the central role that C3 activation plays in the propagation of the complement pathway (both classical and alternate), a number of control mechanisms are available for the inactivation of the C3 convertase, limiting their propagation or deposition on 'self' surfaces. Among these, decay accelerating Factor (DAF) and the receptor for iC3b) inhibit the association of Factor B and C3b and act as a co-factor for the catabolism of C3b and C4b by Factor I (5).

Alternative pathway

Stimuli for the alternative pathway of complement activation include 'foreign' surfaces such as plant, fungal and bacterial polysaccharides and lipopolysaccharides on the outer wall of bacteria. The initial event of the alternative pathway is the activation of C3 and formation of C3a and C3b. There is evidence that this process occurs spontaneously from the low grade proteolysis of C3 (3). Activation of the alternative pathway proceeds following the covalent attachment of C3b to the foreign surface. Such attachment favors assembly of Factor B with C3b (see Figure 2). If attachment of C3b to an activating surface does not occur quickly, it is inactivated as discussed below.

The propagation of the alternative pathway is critically dependent on Factor B, a zymogen, which, when acted upon by Factor D, dissociates into Ba and Bb fragments (2, 5). Once activated, the Bb fragments combine with C3b to form C3bBb, a C3 convertase. Clustering of multiple C3b around the C3 convertase $(C3b)_n$ Bb results in the formation of C5 convertase and permits further propagation of the common pathway. Inhibitory regulatory proteins control the further propagation of this pathway at an early stage. This inhibitory control is provided by

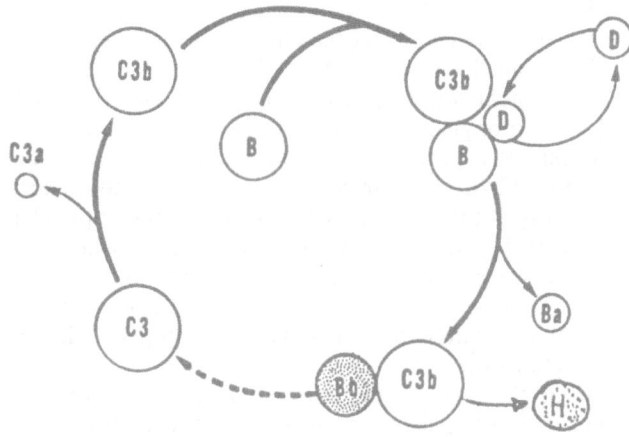

Figure 2. The sequence of reactions in alternative pathway complement activation. Initiation is a continuous process which begins with spontaneous hydrolysis of the thioster in native C3. $C3(H_2O)$ forms a fluid phase C3 convertase and cleaves C3. The resulting metastable C3b attaches randomly on host and nonhost particles. Only on activators of the pathway does C3b escape inactivation by Factors H and I. C3b is amplified on these particles. C5 convertases are formed, and the cytolytic pathway is activated (163).

Factor H. The attachment of Factor H to C3b prevents further interaction of Factor B with C3b and may even displace the activated Factor B (Bb) from its attachment to C3b. Factor H is not consumed in this process. Thus, the newly formed C3bBb can be inactivated by the competitive binding of Factor H to C3b, leading to its further degradation to iC3b (and subsequently to C3c and C3d) by Factor I. Thus, Factor H and Factor I control and limit propagation of the alternative pathway of complement (5).

Membrane attack pathway

Lysis of cells as a result of the activation of the complement system depends on the propagation of the membrane attack pathway (MAC) or terminal pathway (4, 6). This pathway is made up of complement proteins C5 to C9. These five precursor proteins form a loose complex, but upon cleavage of C5 (by C5 convertase) into C5a (which remains in the fluid phase) and C5b, this assembly becomes a stable complex. This complex can bind to cell surfaces and cause cell lysis, either by forming a transmembrane protein channel or by reorganization of the cellular lipid layer with formation of a transmembrane lipid channel. Both mechanisms of cell lysis result in equilibration of the ionic gradient across the cell membrane and cell damage with consequent cell death (7–9). In the absence of biological membranes, this complex may bind to other lipoproteins such as S protein and thereby becomes soluble. Binding to these plasma proteins therefore serves to inhibit bystander lysis.

In addition to its ability to cause cell lysis, the MAC has the potential to induce the release of prostanoids, such as PGE_2 and thromboxane A_2, and to trigger the synthesis of other mediators of inflammation such as interleukin-1 (IL-1) and oxygen radicals by cells such as monocytes, Kupffer cells, granulocytes, and platelets (10–12). The effect of MAC on platelets is of particular importance. Assembly of the MAC has been shown to trigger platelet activation by allowing calcium in flux and activation of protein kinases, and activation of its prothrombinase activity (13). These events are not accompanied by aggregation, and thus these activated platelets may persist in the circulation (14).

As is the case for the other components of complement activation, there are several control proteins that limit the extent of complement-mediated lysis and the propagation of the common pathway. During the initial stepwise formation of MAC, the assembly of C5b, C6 and C7 is unstable unless it binds to a biological surface within a short time. C8 binding protein or homologous restriction factor has recently been identified. Although this protein is known to be anchored to the cell membrane by a phosphatidylinositolglycan tail, little else is known at this time about its mechanism of action (8). Finally, the attachment of these nascent complexes to circulating lipoproteins, such as S-protein, also serve to inhibit propagation (9).

Activation of complement by biomaterials

During the past decade, interest in determining the complement activating potential of biomaterials has increased considerably. This interest stems from several factors. First is the development of precise and relatively rapid radioimmunoassays for the determination of specific products of complement activation, such as the measurements of the anaphylatoxins (C3a, C4a, C5a), which are known to possess important biological properties. Second is the increasing awareness that complement activation represents an inflammatory response of the host toward the biomaterials and is therefore an important parameter of biocompatibility. Finally, there is increasing evidence that the extent of complement activation has important short-term and long-term clinical sequelae (15–22).

Much research has been devoted to the determination of surface structures, moieties or general principles that govern the activation of the alternative pathway by biomaterials (19, 23). Although there are important exceptions, it is generally agreed that hydroxyl-nucleophiles contribute importantly to the complement activating potential of a biomaterial.

Another factor that discriminates between activating and non-activating surfaces is the relative capacity of the surface to bind Factor H: a surface that promotes preferential binding of Factor H and does not favor the binding of Factor B is a material that does not trigger extensive complement activation. Binding of Factor H leads to inactivation of C3b and termination of the propagation of the complement cascade (19). As shown in Figure 3, there is a strict correlation of the ability of a surface to bind Factor H and the generation of the terminal membrane attack complex.

Relatively minor modification (only a few percent of the hydroxyl groups) markedly influences Factor H binding and complement activation. Thus, covalent modification of a few hydroxyl groups by DEAE or acetate on the surface of cellulosic molecules transforms the surface from a high complement activating 'cuprophane' to a moderate complement activating 'Hemophane' or cellulose acetate membrane respectively (24).

Net activation by biomaterials may also depend on other distinct characteristics of the membrane. For example, the Polyacrylonitrile (PAN) membrane has a surface that vigorously activates the alternative pathway of complement, but because it also has the ability to absorb significant quantities of those activated complement products, the patient dialyzed with such membranes is not exposed to these products or experience the consequences of such a vigorous activation (25, 26).

Host factors in complement activation

Discussion of the complement activation by biomaterials should also include host (i.e., patient) factors that impact on the extent of complement activation. As mentioned earlier, Factor D plays a pivotal role in the propagation of the alternative pathway of complement via its modulation of Factor B. Factor D, a molecule of approximately 24 KD, is excreted by glomerular filtration as well as renal catabolism. Because of this, Factor D accumulates in patients with chronic renal failure and end-stage renal disease, and the levels of Factor Ba and baseline levels of C3a is therefore elevated in such patients (27). It is also likely that this elevated level of Factor D participates in the high complement activation by low-flux membranes, and the attenuation of complement activation by high-flux membranes that allow the clearance of Factor D (24, 27).

Similarly, different levels of Factor D may explain inter-individual variations in the extent of complement activation in different patients exposed to the same surface or to the same individual exposed to a new high-flux membrane acutely or chronically (24). Finally, although complement activation by biomaterials occurs predominantly via the alternative complement pathway, its activation may well be modulated by the presence of 'natural' antibodies against complex carbohydrates, which can be detected by their interaction with Dextran or in patients with reaginic antibodies against the commonly used sterilant ethylane oxide (28).

Relevance of measurement of C3a and C5a

The biological properties of C3a and C5a (and to a lesser extent C4a) share several common features (29). C3a has the ability to release histamine from mast cells and basophils, induce contraction of smooth muscle cells, and

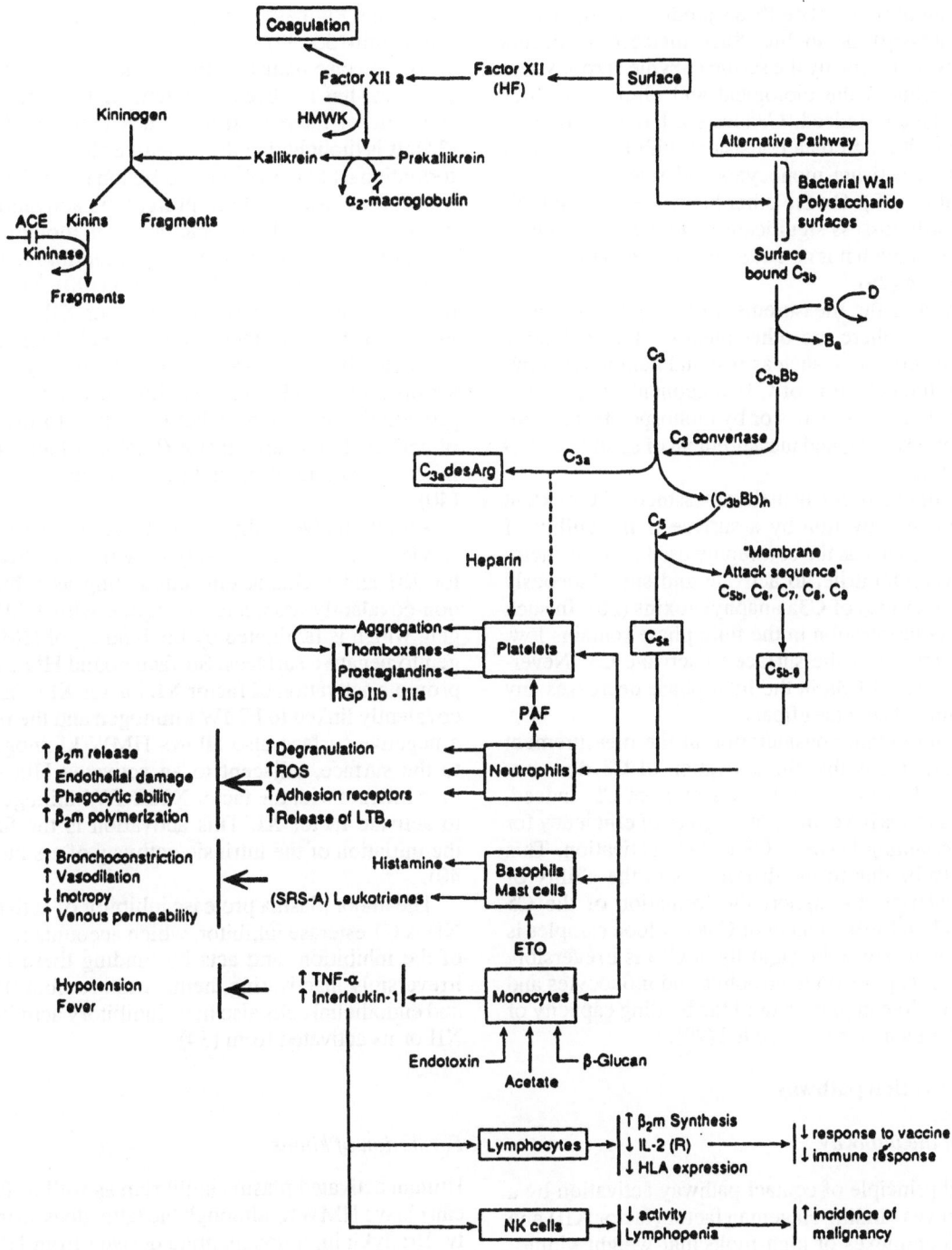

Figure 3. Schematic outline of the interactions of the coagulation, fibrinolytic, kallikrein-kinin and complement systems.

increase capillary permeability. C5a, in addition to its spasmogenic activity on vascular beds, has potent chemotactic ability for polymononuclear cells and is an activator of monocytes and other leukocytes. For example, it induces polymorphonuclear cells to release oxidative products and lysosomal enzymes. These collective bio-

logical properties of the complement fragments have led to their designation as anaphylatoxins, since their infusions in animals results in an anaphylactic response.

It should be recalled, however, that these properties require a C-terminal arginine for full physiological activity and are, therefore, exhibited fully in non-plasma samples that cannot metabolize these products to their des-Arginine (desArg) metabolite. Such metabolism occurs very quickly in plasma by the serum enzyme carboxypeptidase and reduces the biological and clinical potency of these products. Indeed, C3adesArg has little biological activity, although data consistent with the ability of C3adesArg to activate monocytes and release IL-1 has been described (30). On the other hand, the desArg moiety of C5a still possess significant biological and clinical potency even though it is considerably less than the parent (C5a) molecule (29).

In addition to the measurement of anaphylatoxins in the fluid phase, there are other methods for evaluating complement activation, such as residual hemolytic activity (CH50), the detection of C3 components on surfaces by radiolabelled C3 moieties or by monospecific or monoclonal antibody (31), and measurement of soluble C5b-9 complexes (32).

A more difficult problem in the assessment of the extent of complement activation by a surface is the ability of some surfaces, such as the commonly used dialysis membrane, polyacrylonitrile, to activate and simultaneously bind large quantities of C3a anaphylatoxins (26). In such cases, C3a concentration in the fluid phase remains low, despite the ability of the surface to activate C3. Nevertheless, the lack of C3a in the fluid phase decreases any potential clinical adverse effects.

Another important consideration in the measurement of anaphylatoxins is that the activation of C3 does not invariably lead to an equimolar activation of C5. Indeed, different materials have different degrees of efficiency for enzymatic coupling between C3 and C5 activation. This is thought to be due to the differences in the ability of different materials to support the formation of the C5 convertase (17). Measurement of C5a in blood samples is also problematic since the majority of C5a is irreversibly bound to its receptors on neutrophils and monocytes and it is not found free in plasma until the binding capacity of these cellular elements is exceeded (29).

Contact activation pathway

Initiation of the pathway

The general principle of contact pathway activation by a surface involves binding Hageman factor (factor XII) and circulating complexes of high-molecular-weight kininogen (HMWK) with prekallikrein. Activation of Hageman factor into Hfa and prekallikrein into kallikrein continues at the surface, subject to regulation by the plasma inhibitors, C1 inactivator, α2 macroglobulin and antithrombin III. Once activated, kallikrein is potent in liberating bradykinin from HMWK (33, 34). The activation of the contact pathway has been implicated in the development of anaphylactoid reactions during dialysis with some membranes that have a negative charge on their surface, particularly in patients who are taking angiotensin converting enzyme inhibitors, which also

inhibit the kininase enzyme and thus the degradation of bradykinin (35–39).

The precise nature of the surfaces that initiate contact activation has not been well defined, but a common characteristic of these surfaces is a negative surface charge (34). It is thought that this negative charge induces a conformational change of surface-bound factor XII, such that it becomes susceptible to proteolytic activation (autoactivation). Surface-bound factor XII is thought to be several orders of magnitude more susceptible to proteolytic activation than factor XII in solution (40). The conformational change of surface-bound factor XII also promotes interaction between factor XII and prekallikrein, which is facilitated by surface-bound HMW kininogen. The interaction of factor XII with prekallikrein results in reciprocal proteolytic activation of both, leading to the formation of activated Hageman factor (Hfa) and kallikrein, which is several orders of magnitude faster than autoactivation (40).

An alternative pathway of Hageman factor activation is via a reciprocal proteolytic activation between factor XII and prekallikrein, circulating as a bimolecular, non-covalently associated complex with HMW kininogen, which is facilitated by the binding of HMW kininogen to negative surfaces. Surface bound Hfa can, in turn, promote activation of factor XI. Factor XI is usually non-covalently linked to HMW kininogen and the presence of a negative surface also allows HMW kininogen to bind to the surface, adjacent to an activated Hfa which can then interact with the factor XI/HMW kininogen complex to activate factor XI. This activation is the first step in the initiation of the intrinsic pathway of coagulation (34, 40).

The major plasma protease inhibitor of activated factor XII is C1 esterase inhibitor, which accounts for over 90% of the inhibition, and acts by binding these factors and irreversibly inactivating them. Antithrombin III, heparin, and endothelial cells also have inhibitory activity of factor XII or its activated form (34).

Formation of kinins

Human activated plasma kallikrein as well as factor XIIa can cleave HMWK, although the latter does so more slowly. Bradykinin, a nonapeptide derived from HMWK has profound vascular affects. It stimulates endothelial cells to induce prostacyclin PGI_2 (a vasodilator) as well as superoxide formation and nitric oxide, the endothelium derived relaxing factor. Finally, bradykinin also induces the release of cytokines, via the BK receptors on endothelial cells (41).

The major plasma inactivator of bradykinin is the kininase II enzyme, which has been shown to be identical to the angiotensin converting enzyme. Nevertheless, although the biological half-life of kinins is on the order of seconds, they are very potent vasodilators (41).

Importance of contact pathway activation in dialysis

Recent studies have reported an increased incidence of anaphylactic-type reactions during dialysis (35–38). In contrast to earlier reports, which affected primarily patients dialyzed with cuprophane (CUP) membranes, these more recent reports appear to implicate the combined use of angiotensin-converting enzyme (ACE) inhibitors and predominantly the polyacrylonitrile (PAN) membrane. A recent report that surveyed dialysis centers reporting anaphylactic reactions showed that of 72 patients on a combination of ACE inhibitors and the PAN membrane, 41 developed anaphylactic reactions, whereas none of the 71 patients taking ACE inhibitors but dialyzed with other membranes, and only 2 of 519 patients (0.4%) dialyzed with PAN membrane but no on ACE inhibitors, developed anaphylactic reactions (35–39). A more recent report has documented a number of anaphylactoid reactions involving polysulfone dialyzers reused with peracetic acid/hydrogen peroxide-based solution (Renalin®). Again, this report found an eight-fold higher risk of these reactions in patients using ACE inhibitors (42). However, the relative contribution of the membrane, the reuse procedure, or the reuse agent in this report is not well defined.

Because of the well-known ability of ACE inhibitors to inhibit the kininase II enzyme, the hypothesis to explain these anaphylactic reactions is that the contact of blood with specific membranes during dialysis leads to rapid generation and, in patients taking ACE inhibitors, results in persistently high levels of bradykinin after the initiation of dialysis (36).

Another report lends support to this hypothesis. Thus, Lemke and Fink have shown that the generation of bradykinin in *in vitro* experiments where blood is in contact with PAN dialysis membranes is significantly higher in the presence of ACE inhibitors in a dose-dependent manner. Neither endotoxin nor C5a resulted in histamine release when blood was in contact with the PAN membrane (39).

It is difficult to explain with this hypothesis the episodic nature of the anaphylactic reactions. It is possible that this is related to the timing of the intake of these ACE inhibitors in relationship to the start of the dialysis session. If ACE inhibitors are ingested close to the start of the dialysis session, their blood level and presumably their ability to block the kininase system will be highest at the time of the initial contact between the blood and the dialysis membrane. However, such data are not available from published reports. Because the effects of bradykinin can also be mediated locally, differences in the tissue and circulating bioactivity of the kininase enzyme level may also lead to differences in individual susceptibility (36).

In summary, contact pathway activation also occurs during dialysis, and is particularly vigorous with some specific dialysis membranes that are known to have negative surface charges on their surface. In the presence of ACE inhibitors, such activation can prolong the half-life of bradykinin and lead to anaphylactic reactions.

Activation of the clotting cascade

Extracorporeal thrombogenesis remains a major problem when blood interacts with artificial surfaces. Thrombus formation depends not only on the nature and the composition of the surface of the biomaterials, but also on the flow condition of blood. For example, turbulent flow enhances and laminar flow decreases the possibility of thrombosis (43).

Numerous studies have documented the complex sequential and simultaneous deposition of various plasma proteins on artificial surfaces. In the early stages, thrombin adsorption may be a critical initial step, since it appears to be adsorbed in an enzymatically active form, and can become a site for platelet adhesion and further thrombin deposition, thus resulting in a nidus for thrombus formation (44).

Although the use of heparin can effectively blunt the activation of thrombin and the formation of fibrin, heparin at doses commonly used in clinical practice does not blunt platelet adherence to surfaces (45). In fact, heparin has been shown to stimulate platelet aggregation and the platelet release reaction in the presence of subthreshold concentrations of aggregating agents (46). Further, it is possible that the release of platelet factor 4 from adherent platelets can lead to the neutralization of the anticoagulating properties of heparin (47).

Nevertheless, because of the general effectiveness of heparin in blunting thrombus formation, modifications of surfaces of biomaterials that contact blood has been primarily directed at bonding heparin to the surface, by covalent or ionic bonding (48). Such a procedure, if successful, would be applicable to most biomaterial surfaces, and would obviate the need for extensive modification of the chemical or surface structure of these surfaces.

In summary, the complexities of extracorporeal thrombogenesis has made it difficult to elucidate the simultaneous and sequential steps that are involved in the interaction of biomaterials with the clotting cascade, and at present, no effective method other than the use of heparin intravenously, has been found to be clinically effective in blunting this interaction.

CHANGES IN CELLULAR FUNCTION

Leukocytes

Leukopenia

In addition to the marked changes in plasma proteins that occur with the extracorporeal circulation of blood, changes have also been noted in leukocyte number, activation and function. Numerous studies have shown a correlation between the transient development of leukopenia during hemodialysis and activation of the alternative pathway of complement (21, 25, 49).

Studies in dogs and rabbits have also demonstrated that dialysis-induced leukopenia was associated with pulmonary neutrophil sequestration (51, 52). Infusion of cellophane-incubated plasma also caused engorgement of pulmonary vessels with leukocytes. Initial studies using Sephadex chromatography have demonstrated that a plasma factor(s) with a molecular weight between 7,000 and 20,000 daltons was responsible for the development of leukopenia and pulmonary leukostasis, with the suggestion that these factors might be C3a and C5a anaphylatoxins (52). Subsequently, studies using radioimmunoassay techniques have confirmed the causative role of complement activation in the development of leukopenia (20, 21).

Rebound leukocytosis

In addition to the development of leukopenia during dialysis with cellulose-containing membranes, the characteristic rapid reversal of leukopenia has also been intensively studied. Within 30–60 minutes of hemodialysis initiation, leukocyte counts have returned to predialysis levels. By the end of the dialysis procedure, a rebound leukocytosis, usually to 140% of initial values has usually occurred.

Many investigators have assumed that the reversal of hemodialysis induced leukopenia occurs by return of sequestrated leukocytes to the circulation. However, several recent studies, measuring either intracellular enzyme concentrations (granulocyte elastase or lactoferrin) (53) or cell surface proteins (L-selectin) (54, 55) suggest that, in addition to the return of the neutrophils from the lung capillaries, the reversal of leukopenia also occurs by recruitment of leukocytes from the marginated pool or bone marrow stores.

Mechanisms of leukopenia and rebound leukocytosis

One of the earliest events in the inflammatory response is the adhesion of activated granulocytes to the endothelium and to other granulocytes. Adherent neutrophils then migrate through the capillary wall to reach their site of action. The control of granulocyte adherence plays a major role in the development of inflammation. CD11b/CD18 (MAC1) has been found to be essential for binding of granulocytes to iC3b, homotypic adhesion, stimulated adhesion to human endothelial cells, and phagocytosis of opsonized particles in neutrophils (56).

Complement activation results in a dramatic upregulation of granulocyte cell surface MAC1 (CD11b/CD18) (54, 55, 57) and the peak increase of granulocyte surface CD11b/CD18 expression coincides with the peak of plasma C5adesArg levels. Subsequent studies have confirmed that the hemodialysis-induced increases in granulocyte MAC1 (CD11b/CD18) expression appears to play a causative role in the development of granulocytopenia (57).

While the importance of increased granulocyte MAC-1 expression in causing granulocytopenia has been demonstrated, granulocyte cell surface MAC-1 levels remain elevated throughout much of the course of dialysis, despite the early reversal of granulocytopenia beginning after the initiation of dialysis. Thus, while increased cell surface MAC1 expression may result in the development of dialysis granulocytopenia, it is not sufficient to maintain a granulocytopenic state, and other mechanisms must be involved in the reversal of granulocytopenia.

Early investigation using granulocyte aggregation assays, proposed that the reversal of hemodialysis granulocytopenia and pulmonary leukostasis was due to selective downregulation of granulocyte responsiveness to C5a (58), or to internalization of C5a receptors on granulocytes (59). Other investigators, also employing granulocyte aggregometry, recently postulated that the transience of granulocytopenia during hemodialysis is caused by the decline of plasma C5a levels below a critical threshold needed to induce granulocyte aggregation (60). Support for the view that the reversal of dialysis-induced granulocytopenia is not due to downregulation of granulocyte responsiveness to C5a comes from recent reports demonstrating that granulocytopenia can recur if complement-activating membranes are changed during the procedure (61, 62). Finally, other studies measuring granulocyte cell surface C5a receptor density have not demonstrated a downregulation of C5a receptors during hemodialysis with cuprophane membranes (see below) (63, 64).

In addition to the integrin family of cell adhesion molecules, the primary structures of three glycoproteins defining a novel class of adhesion receptors, termed selectins, have recently been determined (65, 66). All members of the selectin family (P-selectin, L-selectin and E-selectin) appear to be involved in the adhesion of circulating blood cells to the endothelium. Recently, shedding or downregulation of L-selectin from human granulocytes *in vitro* upon activation with chemotactic factors has been demonstrated (67) and a role for L-selectin shedding in regulating cell adhesion and transendothelial cell migration has been proposed. Other studies have identified L-selectin as playing a crucial role in leukocyte rolling and in some of the earliest steps in transendothelial cell migration (68).

Two groups have recently demonstrated that hemodialysis with complement-activating membranes causes a decrease or shedding of granulocyte L-selectin expression along with increased granulocyte MAC1 expression (54, 55). The downregulation or shedding of L-selectin was prevented by the multiple reuse of cellulosic dialysis membranes, which attenuates complement activation (54). Furthermore, granulocytes harvested during hemodialysis with first-use cellulosic dialysis membranes lost the ability to bind to endothelial cell monolayers, a phenomenon that was not seen with non-complement activating dialysis membranes (54).

In summary, during the early (first five minutes) stages of first-use cellulosic hemodialysis, complement activation leads to rapid upregulation by incorporation of CD11b/CD18 receptors on granulocyte cell surfaces and increased adhesiveness both to other granulocytes and to endothelium, resulting in granulocytopenia. In the absence of endothelial derived signals and transendothelial migration, activated granulocytes shed their L-Selectin receptors and detach from the endothelium, leading to the reversal of granulocytopenia. Recruitment of new granulocytes into the circulation also helps reverse the granulocytopenia. A recent report demonstrates that hemodialysis with cuprophane membranes also leads to decreased expression of granulocyte CD43, a major sialoglycoprotein involved in homotypic leukocyte adhesion (55). Decreased granulocyte CD43 expression may play a synergistic role in the reversal of hemodialysis-associated granulocytopenia.

Changes in leukocyte function

In addition to the cyclical changes in granulocyte function, several studies have documented substantial changes in the function of these granulocytes when exposed to membranes that activate complement. Although recent studies, using soluble complement receptor type 1 show that several indices of granulocyte activation have a complement dependent and a complement independent mechanisms that participate in their activation during *in vitro* circulation, the predominant mechanism in the clinical setting is complement mediated (69, 70).

Depression in chemotactic responsiveness to several chemotactic stimuli after *in vivo* exposure to complement activating dialysis membranes, as well as decrements in additional production of reactive oxygen species (via the respiratory burst) of granulocytes harvested during dialysis with cellulosic membranes have been documented in response to heat fixed staphylococcus aureus organisms (71).

Impairment of the phagocytic process following exposure to complement activating membranes have also been recently documented (72). On the other hand, granulocyte enzyme release such as lactoferrin elastase and cathapsin G_1 (neutrol proteases) appears to be a process that involves an equivalent stimulation by complement and non-complement (?mechanical trauma) processes (70). Therefore, the correlation of granulocyte enzymes release with the complement activating properties of the membrane is less well established.

In summary, most of the observed changes in granulocyte function during the hemodialysis procedure are at least temporally associated with complement activation. Virtually all studies to date have shown a relationship between the extent of complement activation induced by various types of dialyzers and the extent of the development of leukopenia. Furthermore, the time of maximal complement activation coincides with the maximal development of leukopenia. Similarly, changes in granulocyte cell adhesion molecules and complement receptors induced by the dialysis procedure have been clear-

ly associated with complement activation. Upregulation of MAC1 (CD11b-CD18) occurs only with new cuprophane dialysis membranes, which activate the complement cascade vigorously (57) and the downregulation of L-selectin (LAM-1) induced by cuprophane hemodialysis membranes is also prevented by their reuse and attenuation of the activation of complement cascade (54). Changes in granulocyte cell surface CR1 (complement receptor 1, a receptor for C3b) have also been demonstrated to be specific for complement activating dialysis membranes (67). Functional changes in granulocytes induced by extracorporeal dialysis have generally also been shown to be confined largely to the use of dialysis membranes which activate complement.

Nevertheless, other pathways by which dialysis membranes could cause alterations in granulocyte function have not be sufficiently explored. The contact activation pathway, a surface-mediated blood activation pathway, can participate in inflammatory injury (73). The activated contact proteins kallikrein and factor XIIa induce neutrophil aggregation and release of human neutrophil elastase (74, 75). Inhibition of the contact activation pathway with aprotinin has been demonstrated to decrease granulocyte elastase release during simulated cardiopulmonary bypass but has not been studied during hemodialysis (76). Further work will be needed to clarify the relative roles of complement activation, contact activation, and other pathways of granulocyte activation during hemodialysis.

REFERENCES

1. Schreiber RD, Muller-Eberhard HJ: Complement and renal disease. in *Immunologic Mechanisms of Renal Disease, Vol 3*, edited by Wilson CB, Brenner BM, Stein JH, New York, Churchill Livingstone, 1979, p 67
2. Muller-Eberhard HJ: Molecular organization and function of the complement system. *Ann Rev Biochem* 57: 321, 1988
3. Pangburn MK, Schreiber RD, Muller-Eberhard HJ: Formation of the initial C3 convertase of the alternative complement pathway: acquisition of C3b-like activities by spontaneous hydrolysis of the putative thioester in native C3. *J Exp Med* 154: 856, 1981
4. Esser AF: The membrane attack pathway of complement. *Year Immunol* 6: 229, 1989
5. Pangburn MK: Initiation and activation of the alternative pathway of complement. in *Cytolytic Lymphocytes and Complement Effectors of the Immune System*, edited by Podack ER, Boca Raton, CRC Press, 1988, p 41
6. Podack ER: Assembly and structure of the membrane attack (MAC) of complement. in *Cytolytic Lymphocytes and Complement Effectors of the Immune System*, edited by Podack ER, Boca Raton, CRC Press, 1988, p 173
7. Dalmasso AP, Benson BA: Pore size of lesions induced by complement on red cell membranes and its relation to C5b-8, C5b-9 and Poly C9. in *Cytolytic Lymphocytes and Complement Effectors of the Immune System*, edited by Podack ER, Boca Raton, CRC Press, 1988, p 207

8. Young JD-E, Cohn ZA, Podack ER: Pore size and functional properties of defined MAC and poly C9 complexes: reconstitution into model lipid membranes. in *Cytolytic Lymphocytes and Complement Effectors of the Immune System*, edited by Podack ER, Boca Raton, CRC Press, 1988, p 221

9. Shin ML, Carney DF: Mechanisms of the cellular defense response of nucleated cells to membrane attack by complement. in *Cytolytic Lymphocytes and Complement Effectors of the Immune System*, edited by Podack ER, Boca Raton, CRC Press, 1988, p 229

10. Seeger W, Suttorp N, Hellwig A, Bhakdi S: Noncytolytic terminal complement complexes may serve as calcium gates to elicit leukotriene B4 generation in human polymorphonuclear leukocytes. *J Immunol* 137: 1286, 1986

11. Hansch GM, Seitz M, Martinotti G, Betz M, Rauterberg EW, Gemsa D: Macrophages release arachidonic acid, prostaglandin E2, and thromboxane in response to late complement components. *J Immunol* 133: 2145, 1984

12. Salama A, Mueller-Eckhardt C, Boschek B, Bhakdi S: Haemolytic 'efficiency' of C5b-9 complexes in drug-induced immune haemolysis: role of cellular C5b–9 distribution. *Br J Haematol* 65: 217, 1987

13. Weidmer T, Esmon CT, Sims PJ: On the mechanisms by which complement proteins C5b–9 increase platelet prothrombinase activity. *J Biol Chem* 261: 14587, 1986

14. Rinder CS, Bohnert J, Rinder HM, Mitchell J, Ault K, Hillman R: Platelet activation and aggregation during cardiopulmonary bypass. *Anesthesiology* 75: 388, 1991

15. Chenoweth DE: Complement activation in extracorporeal circuits. *Ann NY Acad Sci* 516: 306, 1987

16. Chenoweth DE: The properties of human C5a anaphylatoxin. The significance of C5a formation during hemodialysis. *Contrib Nephrol* 59: 51, 1987

17. Chenoweth DE: Complement activation produced by biomaterials. *Trans Am Soc Artif Intern Organs* 32: 226, 1986

18. Chenoweth DE: Complement activation produced by biomaterials. *Artif Organs* 12: 502, 1991

19. Janatova J, Cheung AK, Parker CJ: Biomedical polymers differ in their capacity to activate complement. *Complement Inflamm* 8: 61, 1991

20. Cheung AK: Biocompatibility of hemodialysis membranes. *J Am Soc Nephrol* 1: 150, 1990

21. Hakim RM, Fearon DT, Lazarus JM: Biocompatibility of dialysis membranes: effects of chronic complement activation. *Kidney Int* 26: 94, 1984

22. Chenoweth DE, Cooper SW, Hugli TE, Stewart RW, Blackstone EH, Kirklin JW: Complement activation during cardiopulmonary bypass. Evidence for generation of C3a and C5a anaphylatoxins. *N Engl J Med* 304: 497, 1981

23. Meri S, Pangburn MK: Discrimination between activators and nonactivators of the alternative pathway of complement: regulation via a sialic acid/polyanion binding site on factor H. *Proc Natl Acad Sci USA* 87: 3982, 1990

24. Deppisch R, Ritz E, Hansch GM, Schols M, Rauterberg EW: Bioincompatibility – Perspectives in 1993. *Kidney Int* 54; 44: S77, 1994

25. Cheung AK, Parker CJ, Wilcox L, Janatova J: Activation of the alternative pathway of complement by hemodialysis membranes. *Kidney Int* 36: 257, 1989

26. Cheung AK, Chenoweth DE, Otsuka D, Henderson LW: Compartmental distribution of complement activation products in artificial kidneys. *Kidney Int* 30: 74, 1986

27. Oppermann M, Kurts C, Zierz R, Quentin E, Weber MH, Gotze O: Elevated plasma levels of the immunosuppressive complement fragment Ba in renal failure. *Kidney Int* 40: 939, 1991

28. Maillet F, Kazatchkine MD: Specific antibiotics enhance alternative complement pathway activation by cuprophan. *Nephrol Dial Transplant* 6: 193, 1991

29. Hugli TE: Biochemistry and biology of anaphylatoxins. *Comp* 3: 111, 1986

30. Haeffner-Cavaillon N, Cavailon JM, Laude M, Kazatchkine MD: C3a (C3adesArg) induces production and release of interleukin-1 by cultured human monocytes. *J Immunol* 139: 794, 1987

31. Cheung AK, Parker CJ, Janatova J: Analysis of the complement C3 fragments associated with hemodialysis membranes. *Kidney Int* 35: 576, 1989

32. Deppisch R, Schmitt V, Bommer J, Hansch G, Ritz E, Rauterberg EW: Fluid phase generation of terminal complement complex as a novel index of biocompatibility. *Kidney Int* 37: 696, 1990

33. Salzman EW: Interaction of blood with artificial surfaces. in *Hemostasis and Thrombosis*, edited by Colman RW, Hirsh J, Marder VJ, Salzman EW, New York, Lippincott, 1987, p 1335

34. Schmeier AH: Contact activation. in *Thrombosis and Hemorrhage*, edited by Loscalzo J, Schafer AI, Boston, Blackwell Scientific Publications, 1994, p 87

35. Parnes EL, Shapiro WB: Anaphylactoid reactions in hemodialysis patients treated with the AN69 dialyzer. *Kidney Int* 40: 1148, 1991

36. Schulman G, Hakim R, Arias R, Silverberg M, Kaplan AP, Arbeit L: Bradykinin generation by dialysis membranes: possible role in anaphylactic reaction. *J Amer Soc Neph* 3: 1563, 1993

37. Tielemans C, Madhoun P, Lenaers M, Schandene L, Goldman M, Vanderweghem JL: Anaphylactoid reactions during hemodialysis on AN69 membranes in patients receiving ACE inhibitors. *Kidney Int* 38: 982, 1990

38. Verresen L, Waer M, Vanrenterghem Y, Michielsen P: Angiotensin-converting-enzyme inhibitors and anaphylactoid reactions to high-flux membrane dialysis. *Lancet* 336: 1360, 1990

39. Lemke HD, Fink E: Accumulation of bradykinin formed at the AN69 or polyacrylonitrile 17DX membrane is due tot he presence of an angiotensin-converting enzyme inhibitor *in-vitro* (Abstract). *Blood Purif* 10: 92, 1992

40. Williams DF: Blood physiology and biochemistry: hemostasis and thrombosis. in *Blood Compatibility, Vol 1*, edited by Williams DF, Boca Raton, CRC Press, 1987, p 5

41. Carretero O: Vasoactive mediators: kinins and kallikreins. in *Manual of Vascular Mediators*, edited by Ward P, New York, Hospital Practice, 1993

42. Pegues DA, Beck-Sague CM, Woollen SW et al.: Anaphylactoid reactions associated with reuse of hollow-fiber hemodialyzers and ACE inhibitors. *Kidney Int* 42: 1232, 1992

43. Mohammad SF: Extracorporeal thrombogenesis: mechanisms and prevention. in *Replacement of Renal Function by Dialysis, Vol 3*, edited by Maher JF, Boston, Kluwer Academic Publishers, 1989, p 229

44. Chuang HYK, Mohammad SF, Sharma NC, Mason RG: Interaction of human a-thrombin with artificial surfaces

and reactivity of adsorbed a-thrombin. *J Biomed Mater Res* 14: 467, 1980

45. Lindon J, Rosenberg R, Merrill E, Salzman E: Interaction of human platelets with heparinized agarose gel. *J Lab Clin Med* 91: 47, 1978

46. Mohammad SF, Anderson WH, Smith JB, Chuang HYK, Mason RG: Effects of heparin on platelet aggregation, release reaction and thromboxane A2 production. *Am J Pathol* 104: 132, 1981

47. Kaplan KL, Owen J: Plasma levels of beta-thromboglobulin and platelet factor 4 as indices of platelet activation *in vivo*. *Blood* 57: 199, 1981

48. Cheung AK, Parker CJ, Janatova J, Brynda E: Modulation of complement activation on hemodialysis membranes by immobilized heparin. *J Am Soc Nephrol* 8: 1328, 1992

49. Kaplow L, Goffinet J: Profound neutropenia during the early phase of hemodialysis. *JAMA* 203: 133, 1968

50. Toren M, Goffinet JA, Kaplow LS: Pulmonary bed sequestration of neutrophils during hemodialysis. *Blood* 36: 337, 1970

51. Craddock PR, Fehr J, Brigham KL, Kronenberg RS, Jacob HS: Complement and leukocyte-mediated pulmonary dysfunction in hemodialysis. *N Eng J Med* 296: 769, 1977

52. Craddock PR, Fehr J, Dalmasso AP, Brigham K, Jacob HS: Hemodialysis leukopenia: pulmonary vascular leukostasis resulting from complement activation by dialyzer cellophane membranes. *J Clin Invest* 59: 879, 1977

53. Schaefer RM, Herfs N, Ormanns W, Horl WH, Heidland A: Change of elastase and cathepsin G content in polymorphonuclear leukocytes during hemodialysis. *Clin Nephrol* 29: 307, 1988

54. Himmelfarb J, Zaoui P, Hakim RM, Holbrook D: Modulation of granulocyte LAM1 and MAC1 during dialysis – a prospective, randomized controlled trial. *Kidney Int* 41: 388, 1992

55. Alvarez PR, Campanero MR, Pariaso V, Landazuri MO, Sanchez-Madrid F: Differentially regulated cell surface expression of leukocyte adhesion receptors on neutrophils. *Kidney Int* 40: 899, 1991

56. Arnaout MA: Structure and function of the leukocyte adhesion molecules CD11/CD18. *Blood* 75: 1037, 1990

57. Arnaout MA, Hakim RM, Todd RF, Dana N, Colten HR: Increased expression of an adhesion-promoting surface glycoprotein in the granulocytopenia of hemodialysis. *N Engl J Med* 312: 457, 1985

58. Skubitz KM, Craddock PR: Reversal of hemodialysis granulocytopenia and pulmonary leukostasis: a clinical manifestation of selective down-regulation of granulocyte responses to C5a desArg. *J Clin Invest* 67: 1383, 1981

59. Craddock PR, Hammerschmidt DE: Complement-mediated granulocyte activation and down-regulation during hemodialysis. *ASAIO J* 7: 50, 1984

60. Gardinalli M, Hugli TE, Ward DM, Agostoni A: PMN C5a-receptor-down-regulation is not involved in recovery from C5a-induced neutropenia. *ASAIO J* 10: 482, 1987

61. Brubaker LH, Nolph KD: Mechanism of recovery from neutropenia induced by hemodialysis. *Blood* 38: 623, 1971

62. Smith EKM, Jobbins K: Observation on neutropenia associated with hemodialysis. *Br Med J* 4: 70, 1969

63. Lewis SL, Van Epps DE, Chenoweth DE: Leukocyte C5a receptor modulation during hemodialysis. *Kidney Int* 31: 112, 1987

64. Himmelfarb J, Gerard NP, Hakim RM: Intradialytic modulation of granulocyte C5a receptors. *J Am Soc Nephrol* 2: 920, 1991

65. Butcher EC: Cellular and molecular mechanisms that direct leukocyte traffic. *Am J Path* 136: 3, 1990

66. Springer TA: Adhesion receptors of the immune system. *Nature* 346: 425, 1990

67. Kishimoto TK, Jutila MA, Berg EL, Butcher EC: Neutrophil MAC-1 and MEL-14 adhesion proteins inversely regulated by chemotactic factors. *Science* 245: 1238, 1989

68. Lawrence MB, Springer TA: Leukocytes roll on a selectin at physiologic flow rates: distinction from and prerequisite for adhesion through integrins. *Cell* 65: 859, 1991

69. Cheung AK, Hohnholt M, Gilson J: Adherence of neutrophils to hemodialysis membranes: Role of complement receptors. *Kidney Int* 40: 1123, 1991

70. Cheung AK, Parker CJ, Hohnholt M: Soluble complement receptor type 1 inhibits complement activation induced by hemodialysis membranes *in vitro*. *Kidney Int* 46: 1680, 1994

71. Himmelfarb J, Lazarus JM, Hakim RM: Reactive oxygen species production by monocytes and polymorphonuclear leukocytes during dialysis. *Am J Kidney Dis* 17: 271, 1991

72. Vanholder R, Ringoir S, Dhondt A, Hakim R: Phagocytosis in uremic and hemodialysis patients: a prospective and cross sectional study. *Kidney Int* 39: 320, 1991

73. Schamier AH, Silverberg M, Kaplan AP, Colman RW: Contact activation and its abnormalities. in *Hemostasis and Thrombosis, Vol 2*, edited by Colman RW, Hirsh J, Marder VJ, Salzman WE, Philadelphia, JB Lippincott Co, 1987

74. Wachtfogel TY, Kuchich U, James HL, Scott CF, Schapira M, Zimmerman M, Cohen AB, Colman RW: Human plasma kallikrein releases neutrophil elastase during blood coagulation. *J Clin Invest* 72: 1672, 1983

75. Wachtfogel YT, Pixley RA, Kucich U, Abrams W, Weinbaum G, Schapira M, Colman RW: Purified plasma factor XIIa aggregates human neutrophils and causes degranulation. *Blood* 67: 1731, 1986

76. Van Oeverin W, Jansen NJG, Bidstrup BP, Royston D, Westaby S, Neuhof H, Wildevuur CRH: Effects of aprotinin on hemostatic mechanisms during cardiopulmonary bypass. *Ann Thorac Surg* 44: 640, 1987

HAEMODIALYSERS AND ASSOCIATED DEVICES

NICHOLAS A. HOENICH, CELIA WOFFINDIN and CLAUDIO RONCO

INTRODUCTION

The principle of haemodialysis is simple. Blood and dialysis fluid are circulated on opposite sides of a semipermeable membrane which permits the passage of metabolites elevated as a consequence of renal failure but restricts the transfer of blood proteins and formed elements. The device containing the semi-permeable membrane is the haemodialyser. Removal of water occurs by control of the hydrostatic pressure gradient across the membrane and may be supplemented by increasing the dialysis fluid osmolality by the addition of glucose.

Haemodialysis has been synonymous with the treatment of chronic renal failure since its inception and remains the most widely used mode of treatment. The past decade has, however, seen the evolution and clinical application of various extracorporeal treatment modalities, not only for the treatment of chronic renal failure

Table 1. Characteristics of an ideal haemodialyser or associated device

High clearance of small and middle weight uremic toxins
Negligible loss of vital solutes (eg. amino acids, low molecular weight proteins)
Adequate ultrafiltration range
Minimal backfiltration at low ultrafiltration rates
Low-blood compartment volume
Non-toxic and non-thrombogenic materials of construction
Good washback characteristics
High reliability
Low cost
Potentially reusable without adverse effects

Table 2. Membranes available for use in haemodialysers and associated devices for the treatment of renal failure

Membrane material		Common name
Cellulose	Regenerated Cellulose	Cuprophan
		Cellophane
		Bioflux
	Cuprammonium rayon	
Modified cellulose		
		Hemophan®
	Cellulose diacetate	Dicea™
	Cellulose hydrate	
	Cellulose acetate	
	Cellulose triacetate	
	Saponified Cellulose Ester	SCE
	Cellulose 2–5 diacetate	Diaphan®
Synthetic		
	Polyacrylonitrile	AN69, SPAN, PAN
	Polysulfone	PS, Biosulfane®
	Polyethylvinylalcohol	EVAL
	Polymethylmethacrylate	PMMA
	Polycarbonate	Gambrane®
	Polyamide	

but also for the treatment of acute renal failure. Each of these new treatment modalities retain reliance on a device containing a semi-permeable membrane.

The rationale for the development and use of these modes of treatment are discussed elsewhere in this book. This chapter will focus on the devices used to deliver the therapy, their physical properties, functional performance and reactions mediated by their use.

THE IDEAL HAEMODIALYSER

The requirements of an ideal dialyser are summarised in Table 1. Many of these requirements are inter-related; for example, low blood compartment volume not only enhances solute clearance but also minimises the volume required to rinse the dialyser at the termination of treatment, while others are mutually exclusive, e.g., low cost and high reliability. Some demands are unmet since the membranes used are non-selective, high middle or large molecular weight solute removal is inevitably associated with loss of proteins and amino acids (1, 2). Each device, therefore, represents the manufacturer's solution to meet these ideal requirements.

MEMBRANES USED IN HAEMODIALYSERS AND ASSOCIATED DEVICES

Many of the characteristics of an ideal dialyser are governed by the membrane used. The ideal membrane must have a high permeability for a range of molecular weights but, at the same time, loss of vital solutes must be negligible. The membrane's ultrafiltration (or convective transport properties) must be controllable and reproducible. Membranes incorporated in haemodialysers and associated devices represent the largest contact area with blood and they must be biocompatible. Their physical and mechanical properties must be such as to ensure negli-

gible leak rate during production and use, and they should be able to be sterilised by a variety of processes without alteration in their diffusive or convective transport properties and their biocompatibility.

Membranes in clinical use may be classed into either cellulose based or synthetic categories (Table 2).

Cellulose based membranes

The first chemical extraction of cellulose from wood was made in 1885 by Charles Cross and Edward Bevan working in the Jodrell laboratory of the Royal Botanic Garden, Kew. The first clinical use of cellulose based membranes (celloidin) may be traced back to 1914 (3). Cellulose based membranes may be produced by a variety of processes which govern the membranes physicochemical properties, their hydraulic and solute permeabilities and their biocompatibility. The chemical structure of cellulose may be modified through substitution of the hydroxyl (OH) groups. Such substitution may be by the use of tertiary amino groups such as di-ethyl-amino-ethyl (DEAE) to produce Hemophan or with acetate groups to produce cellulose acetate, cellulose diacetate or cellulose triacetate. Currently, over 30 different variants of cellulose based membranes in either flat sheet or more commonly hollow fibre format are available for clinical use, and they are used in over 80% of the extracorporeal circulatory procedures that are performed world-wide (4).

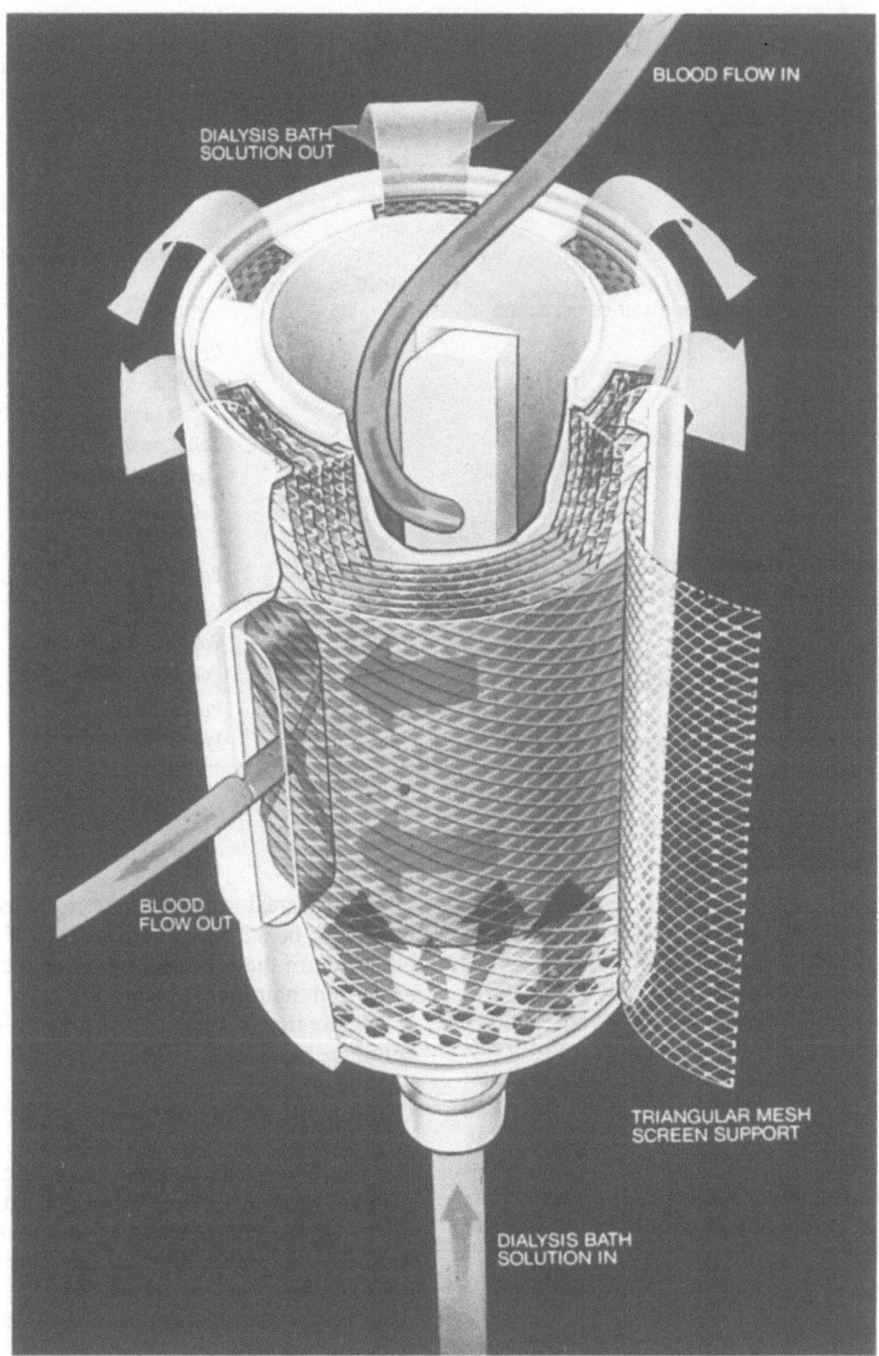

Figure 1. Coil haemodialyser.

Synthetic membranes

Synthetic membranes were used in between 10–12% of the haemodialysis treatments undertaken in 1992 (4). Such membranes are co-polymers and their introduction into clinical practice may be traced to the middle molecule hypothesis (5) which stressed the importance of middle molecular weight solutes in the development of some of the manifestations of uraemia such as peripheral neuropathy, coupled with the poor removal of these compounds by the then used haemodialysis membranes. This led to the search for membranes with improved middle molecular weight removal, the first of which was polyacrylonitrile (AN 69, Rhone Poulenc), introduced clinically in 1972 (6) and used by 4% of European patients by 1984 (7).

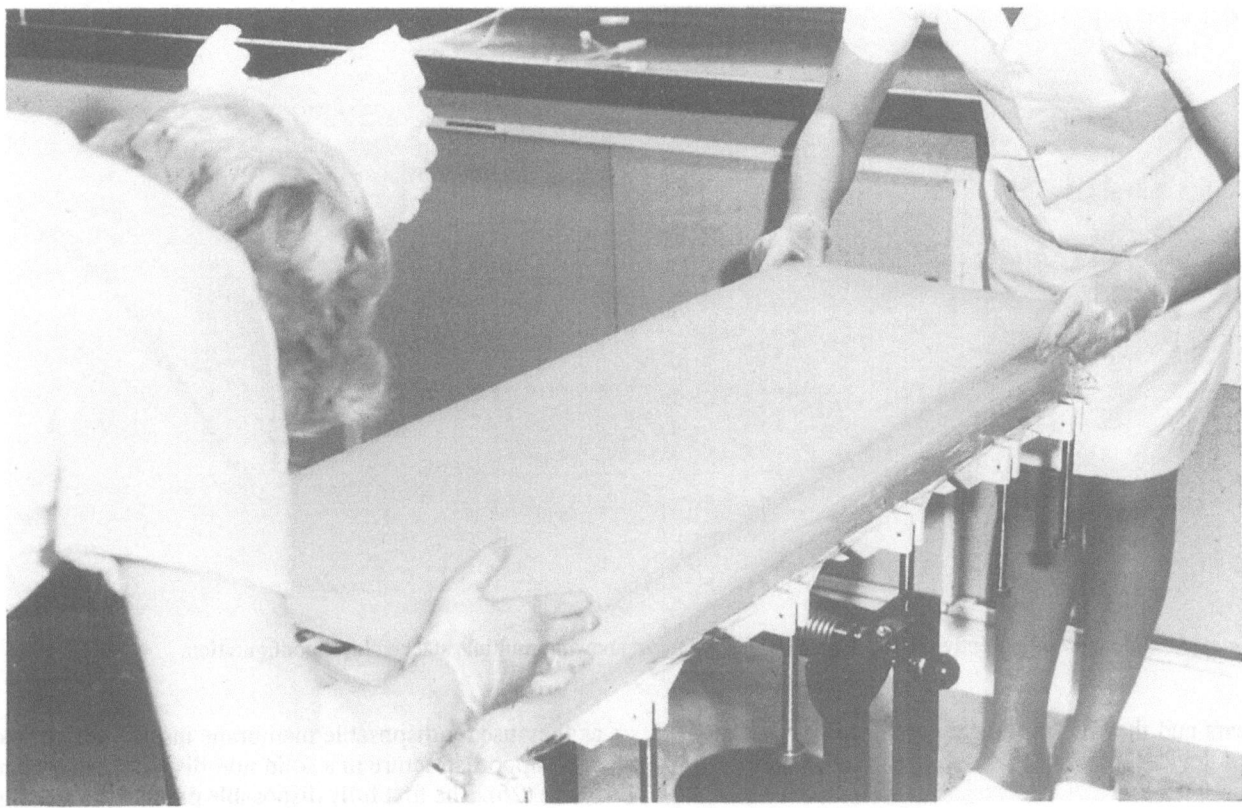

Figure 2. A rebuildable parallel plate haemodialyser. The illustration shows the support plate being laid onto the membrane.

Although synthetic membranes offered enhanced solute removal compared with their cellulose based counterparts, recently produced cellulose based membranes are not only comparable in respect of solute removal, but also in their biocompatibility profile (8). The cost of synthetic membranes is higher than for other membranes and this price difference is partly responsible for their low clinical utilisation.

CONTEMPORARY HAEMODIALYSERS AND ASSOCIATED DEVICES

Extracorporeal techniques for the treatment of renal failure owe their origins to the pioneering work of Abel, Rowntree and Turner (3) who used a fore-runner of todays hollow fibre in their experiments. The first use of the technique on humans was by Kolff and Berk (9) who used a rotating drum kidney in their treatment. These were subsequently sent to other centres in the world and sowed the seeds of haemodialysis treatment. These early developments have been reviewed elsewhere (10–12).

Today three basic haemodialyser designs are available – coil, flat plate and hollow fibre. They are available not only in a range of sizes suitable for the treatment of children, to the delivery of rapid high efficiency therapy, and in parallel with the development of membranes, they can incorporate either cellulose based or synthetic membranes.

Coil designs

The coil haemodialyser was the first single use haemodialyser produced. The original design manufactured by Travenol Laboratories utilised a tubular membrane supported by a fibre glass mesh. The membrane and support were stitched together and wrapped around a central core. The commercially produced device owed its origins to a design originally described by Kolff and Watschinger (13).

Early designs of this type of dialyser had a high blood compartment volume, necessitating priming with blood prior to use, an unpredictable solute removal due to the uneven flow of dialysate in the device and a high basal ultrafiltration rate, resulting from the high pressure drop across the blood pathway. The fibre glass mesh was subsequently replaced by a truncated pyramid support developed by Hoeltzenbein (14) and the device encased in a solid outer casing (Figure 1). Such dialysers required a recirculating dialysate supply to permit use although some were produced for use with conventional single pass dialysate systems. Their use has declined over the past few

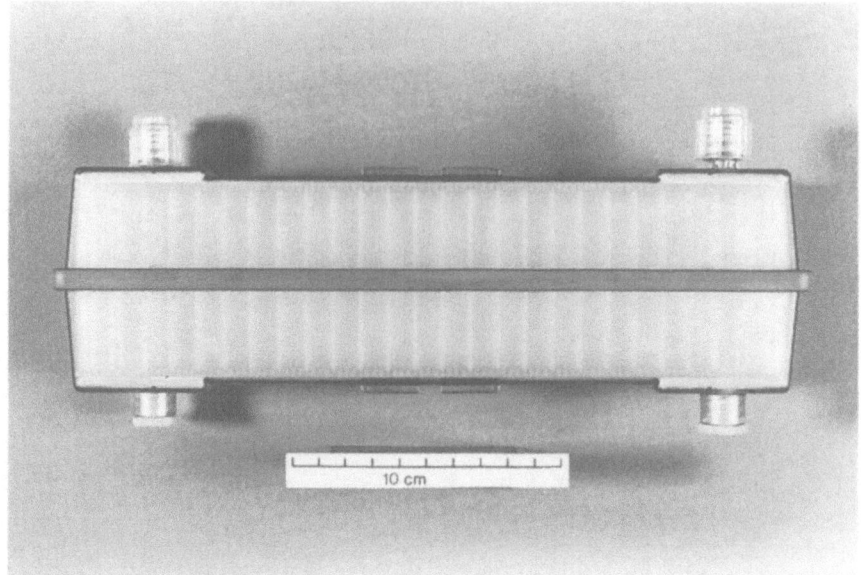

Figure 3. Side view of currently produced parallel plate dialyser showing multiple stacked layer configuration.

years and they are no longer considered as *'state of the art'* devices.

Parallel plate designs

Early parallel plate designs owe their origin to the Skeggs-Leonard dialyser (15) which used sheets of membrane sandwiched between grooved rubber plates supported by a metal backing plate on either side of each plate-membrane-plate layer. This design was followed by that of Kiil (16) which retained the twin blood layer concept and was extensively used in the early 1960's. By the 1970's it was largely replaced by multipoint variants (17, 18) which offered a substantial improvement in solute removal due to the reduction of the contact area between membrane and support and improved mixing of the dialysis fluid during its passage through the device.

While such devices offered high solute removal, they could be used without a blood pump due to their low flow resistance. They needed to be built either weekly or prior to each dialysis. Such dialysers were bulky (Figure 2) which made their handling difficult. They were sterilised with formaldehyde which was difficult to eliminate prior to use (19–21), resulted in the formation of anti-N antibodies (19, 22–24) and was implicated as a cause of haemolysis (25). Repeated staff exposure to formaldehyde led to respiratory and dermatological problems (25). With the availability of pre-sterilised single use parallel plate designs, the use of multiple use parallel plate devices declined.

Early variants of single use disposable parallel flow designs were a compromise between today's designs and the previously discussed multiple use devices in as much

as they used a disposable membrane insert with an integral support structure in a solid non-disposable clamping frame (26). The first fully disposable parallel plate design was the Alwall dialyser (27), the fore-runner of the Lundia series produced by Gambro (Lund, Sweden) (28). These designs were smaller than their multiple use counterparts with the reduction in size being achieved by the use of multiple, stacked layer configuration (Figure 3).

Early variants of multiple layer devices were prone to uneven flow distribution through the multiple layers, resulting in a variable performance (29), their efficiency was further compromised by inadequately degassed dialysis fluid produced by the then used single patient proportionating systems (30).

Currently produced devices have been further reduced in size (Figure 4). This reduction being achieved by the use of thinner membrane support plates than those used in earlier devices.

Hollow fibre designs

The predecessor of current hollow fibre designs was that described by Stewart et al. (31) based upon hollow fibres manufactured by the Dow Chemical Company for desalination. Stewart's design criteria for the device were low blood compartment volume and low resistance to blood flow – features which characterise current designs.

Early commercially produced hollow fibre devices consisted of a bundle of fibres encased in a perspex tubular housing. The bundle was bonded at the two ends and a screw cap manifold was used (Figure 5). Blood entered and left the device via the manifolds which were designed to optimise both blood velocity and pressure drops at all

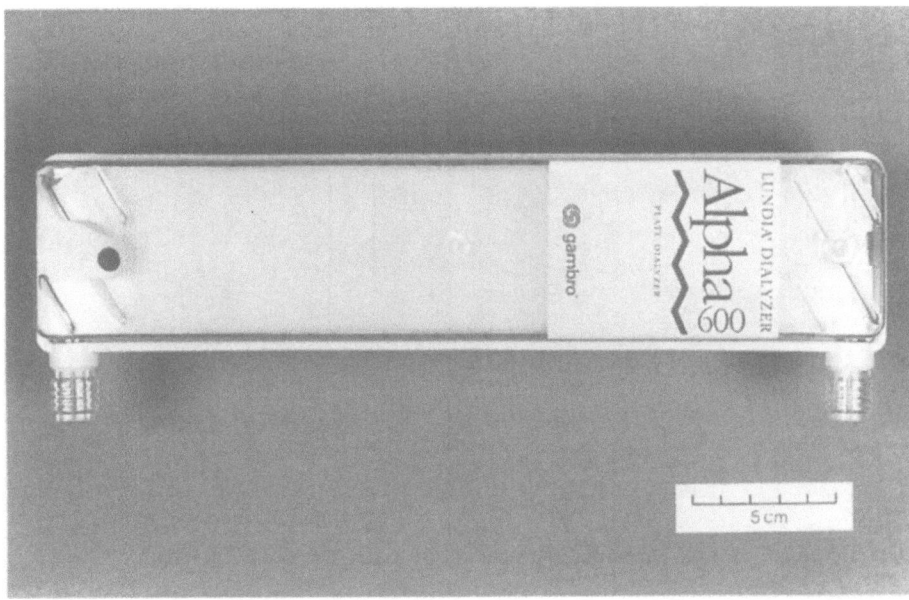

Figure 4. Miniature multiple layer parallel flow haemodialyser utilising moulded herringbone patterned membrane support plates.

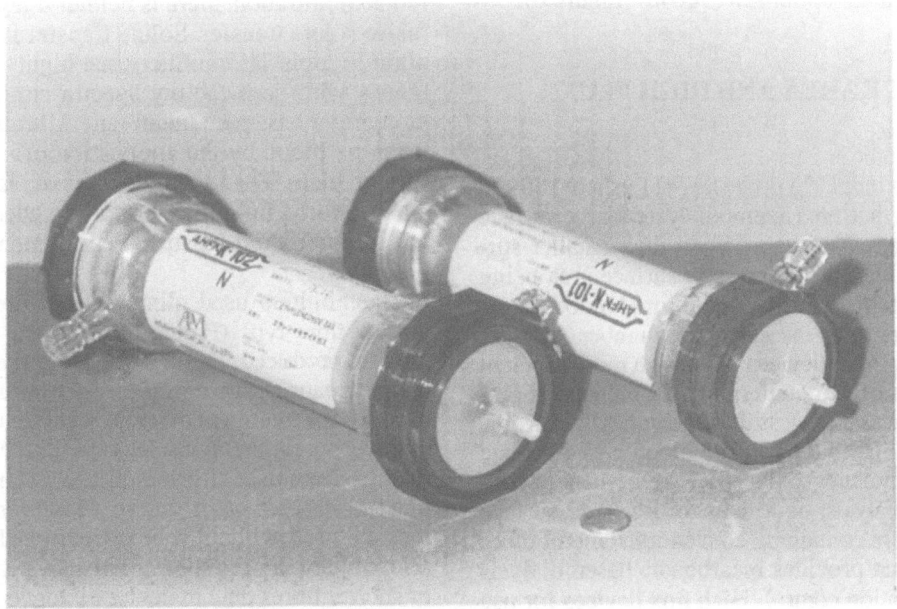

Figure 5. Early production version of hollow fibre haemodialyser utilising screw endcaps.

points in the manifold thereby ensuring an even distribution of the blood in the fibre bundle. Problems with such designs included excessive thrombus formation in the manifolds and clotted fibres due to irregular flow distribution in the fibre bundle (32, 33). Early designs also experienced problems with an uneven dialysate flow through the fibre bundle. To eliminate this problem, a number of alternate design solutions were introduced including the arrangement of the fibres in a rectangular block (34),

or the use of multiple bundles (35). Other methods of improving dialysate flow distribution included the use of a central core around which the fibres were wound in a spiral manner or the use of wound knitted hollow fibre mats. Blood flow distribution was improved by the introduction of tangential flow (36) or by redesigned manifolds (37).

Due to technical problems (38) and high manufacturing costs, these alternatives to a single bundle have largely dis-

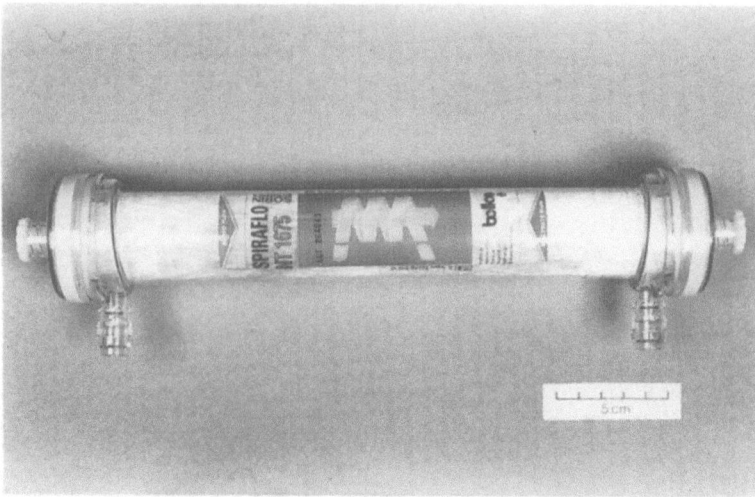

Figure 6. Currently produced hollow fibre haemodialyser with optimised fibre spacing and length.

appeared from clinical use and todays dialysers retain the classical format in which the fibre spacing within the bundle and fibre length are optimised (38–40) (Figure 6).

LARGE SURFACE AREA AND HIGH FLUX DEVICES

The *'square meter hour'* hypothesis (41) ushered in the era of the large surface area haemodialyser. Large surface area haemodialysers were based upon their smaller surface counterparts with the increase in surface area being achieved by the incorporation of additional blood layers for flat plate designs or by increasing the number or length of fibres for hollow fibre devices. Although more efficient than their smaller surface counterparts, the increase in performance offered was often less than theoretically possible due to poor flow distribution in the blood and dialysate pathways. High efficiency dialysis, a development of conventional haemodialysis, continues to use large surface area haemodialysers containing conventional membranes with equipment that provides bicarbonate based dialysis fluid and ultrafiltration control. High flux devices for use in haemodialysis were developed to provide high diffusive and convective transport of middle and large molecules. Their use is not confined to haemodialysis and they are also used in haemodiafiltration, acetate free biofiltration or paired filtration. In contrast to conventional haemodialysis, such modes of treatment offer enhanced removal of middle weight molecular solutes such as β_2 microglobulin. However, the necessity for relatively high blood flow rates and the complexity of the equipment with which they are used has, to date, prevented their wide spread routine use.

HAEMOFILTERS

In haemofiltration, there is neither dialysate flow nor diffusive solute transfer. Solute transfer is by convection or ultrafiltration. Haemofilters use highly permeable membranes with permeability spectra similar to that of the glomerular basement membrane. Ultrafiltrate is extracted from the blood by the application of a hydrostatic pressure gradient. The fluid thus removed is then replaced by a substitution fluid in a proportion adequate to maintain the patient's fluid balance; replacement may be pre- or post-filter.

Haemofilters used clinically are predominantly of a hollow fibre type (Figure 7) although flat plate designs are also produced. The use of haemofilters is not confined to the treatment of chronic renal failure, they are also used for the treatment of acute renal failure by continuous extracorporeal therapies. The membranes used are identical to those used in haemofilters intended for the treatment of chronic renal failure. However, as such devices may be used without a blood pump, they must possess a low hydraulic resistance which is achieved by the use of shorter fibres than in devices intended for pump driven haemofiltration (Figure 8). Characteristics of haemofilters used in the treatment of acute renal failure are summarised in Table 3.

PLASMA SEPARATORS

Plasma separation from whole blood by membrane containing devices is a well established technique used for plasma collection from donors and in the treatment of various autoimmune diseases (42). The technique also permits the extracorporeal manipulation of the plasma globulins and other macromolecules in the specific humoral immune

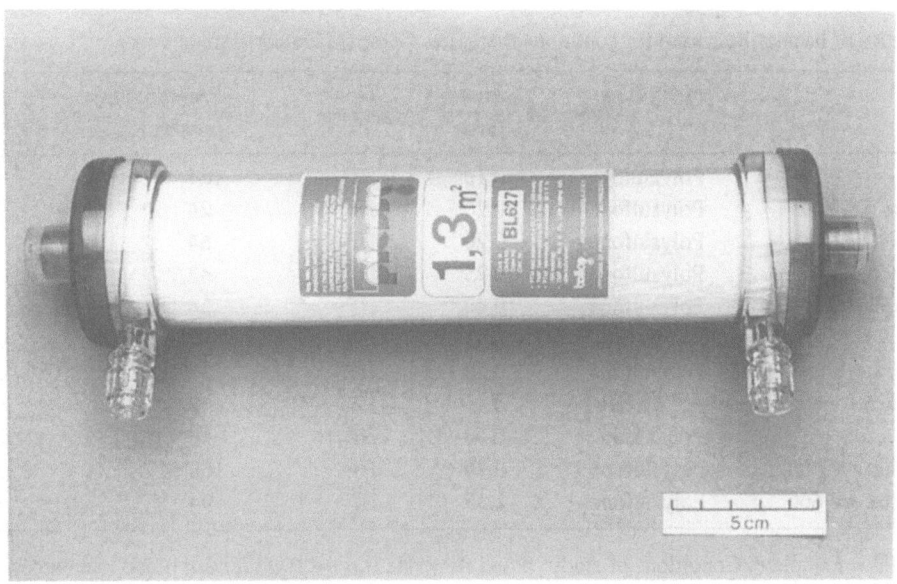

Figure 7. Hollow fibre haemodialyser utilising high permeability polysulfone membranes suitable for use for haemodialysis and haemodiafiltration.

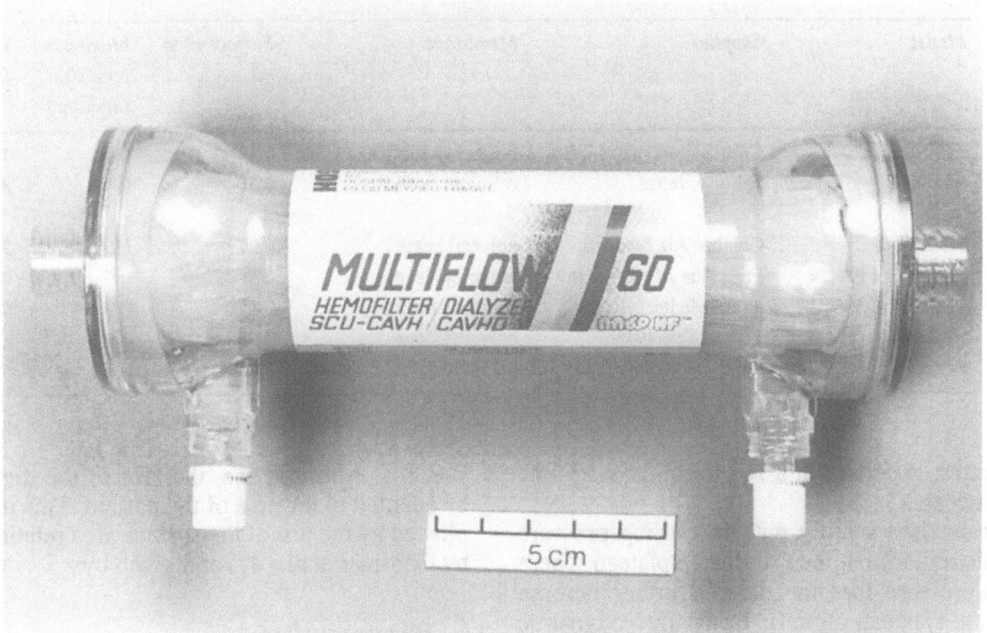

Figure 8. Hollow fibre device for use in continous renal replacement therapies. Note the relationship between fibre length and casing diameter compared to devices used for haemodialysis.

response. Early devices used sheet membranes; and were subject to problems in the maintenance of a blood film thickness compatible with a high shear rate across the membrane, a prerequisite for the maintenance of flux across the membrane (43). Current clinical devices are predominantly of a hollow fibre configuration (Table 4), although the Cobe Laboratories TPE system, as well as an experimental high efficiency system utilising oscillating vortex mixing (44) retain a parallel plate configuration.

The membranes used in plasma separators generally have pore sizes ranging from 0.2–0.65 microns in size, which permit the separation of solutes of several million Daltons molecular weight from cellular elements. The

Table 3. Characteristics of haemofilters used for continous therapies. Comparative performance data

Filter	Membrane	Area (m^2)	Design	Pressure drop (mmHg)	Filtration rate (mmHg)*
Gambro FH22	Polyamide	0.16	HF	164	1.5
Amicon Diafilter 10	Polysulfone	0.20	HF	24	10.5
Bellco BL634	Polysulfone	0.20	HF	64	7.5
Renaflo HF 250	Polysulfone	0.25	HF	42	12.6
Amicon Diafilter 20	Polysulfone	0.40	HF	34	16
Hospal AN 69S	AN 69 S	0.43	FP	72	5.5
Renaflo HF 500	Polysulfone	0.50	HF	36	22.5
Hospal Multiflow 60	AN 69 HF	0.55	HF	52	9.7
Gambro FH66	Polyamide	0.60	HF	58	13
Fresenius Ultraflux AV 400	Polysulfone	0.70	HF	168	34.3
Fresenius Ultraflux AV 600	Polysulfone	1.35	HF	94	37.5

HF = Hollow fibre; FP = Flat plate; Conditions of study: blood flow rate (Q_b) = 100 ml/min; blood haematocrit 42 ± 3.5%; blood total protein content 53.8 ± 2.0 g/l.
*Collection reservoir 50 cm below centre of filter.

Table 4. Characteristics of plasma separators in clinical use

Type	Model	Supplier	Membrane	Surface area m^2	Maximum pore size (microns)	Priming volume (ml inner/outer)
Parallel plate	TPE	Cobe Laboratories, USA	polyvinylchloride	0.13	0.6	18/NA
	PS 4000	Terumo, Japan	cellulose acetate	0.50	0.45	80/120
Hollow fibre	PC 1000	Gambro Ab, Sweden	polycarbonate	0.27	N/A	24/NA
	Plasmaflux P2	Fresenius AG, Germany	polypropylene	0.5	0.5	48/290
	Plasmaflo AP-06-M	Asahi Medical, Japan	cellulose diacetate	0.65	0.2	95/NA
	Hemaplex BT 900	Dideco Spa, Italy	polypropylene	0.20	0.5	18/NA
	PlasmaxPS-05	Toray Industries, Japan	polymethylmethacrylate	0.50	0.5	59/102

plasma flow rates, generated at a 100 ml/min blood flow rate, range between 25–35%.

Filtration rate rises sharply with increasing pressure (hydrodynamic region) but then reaches a plateau where an increase in pressure does not lead to a further increase in filtration rate (plateau region). In the hydrodynamic region, the filtrate is haemolysis free, but haemolysis will be observed at higher pressures in the plateau region. Such behaviour may be explained by mathematical models of cellular concentration polarisation (45, 46).

PAEDIATRIC DESIGNS

Many of the smaller surface area hollow fibre haemodialysers are suitable for paediatric use. A number of manufacturers also produce devices suitable for the treatment of small children or neonates. When selecting a haemodial-yser for paediatric use, the size of the dialyser needs to be adapted to the size of the patient. This may be accomplished by the use of the surface area relationship derived by Gardiner et al. (47) and given by:

$$\frac{\text{Dialyser surface}}{\text{Patient surface}} = 0.75.$$

Other parameters that require adaptation are extracorporeal circuit volume, clearance and ultrafiltration rate and blood flow rate.

For children the volume of the extracorporeal circuit should be below 10% of the child's blood volume. Larger volumes may lead to hypotension during treatment and fluid overload at the termination of treatment.

Dialysis induced disequilibrium may be avoided by maintaining urea clearance below 4 ml/min/kg. This is generally achieved by appropriate selection of blood flow

Table 5. Number of different types of haemodialyser and associated devices used clinically in Europe during the period 1982–1992

Year	Non-disposable flat plate	Disposable flat plate	Coil	Hollow fibre	Haemo-filter	Total
1982	10	81	34	141	23	289
1983	10	86	28	158	29	311
1984	10	87	28	197	30	352
1985	10	92	28	258	34	422
1986	2	70	19	260	37	388
1987	2	86	21	352	42	503
1988	2	73	8	338	34	455
1989	2	50	4	364	37	457
1990	2	37	3	351	35	425
1991	2	36	2	368	49	457
1992	2	39	2	372	50	465

Table 6. Demography of European haemodialyser use during the period 1982–1992 (% of patients using each category)

Year	Non-disposable flat plate	Disposable flat plate	Coil	Hollow filter	Haemo-fibre
1982	1.3	37.1	7.0	52.6	2.1
1983	0.8	31.2	5.3	60.6	22.1
1984	0.5	27.2	4.0	66.3	2.0
1985	0.4	25.4	2.7	69.4	2.0
1986	0.4	22.9	1.5	73.6	1.6
1987	0.3	21.2	0.7	76.2	1.6
1988	0.3	19	0.2	79.1	1.4
1989	0.2	16.3	0.1	81.5	1.9
1990	0.2	14.2	0.1	83.7	1.8
1991	< 0.1	10.6	< 0.1	86.9	2.5
1992	0	6.4	0	93.6	N/A

Values shown based on responses to EDTA-ERA patient questionaire which asked for the most commonly used dialyser in a given year. N/A: Not available.

Table 7. Demography of haemodialyser use in the United Kingdom during the period 1982–1992 (% of patients using each category)

Year	Non-disposable flat plate	Disposable flat plate	Coil	Hollow filter	Haemo-fibre
1982	9.7	41.4	6.8	41.9	0.2
1983	6.4	42.6	2.5	48.3	0.1
1984	2.0	41.7	4.1	52.1	0.1
1985	1.3	31.3	1.7	65.7	0.2
1986	0.7	27.6	1.7	69.8	0.2
1987	0.4	23.8	1.7	72.6	0.1
1988	0.1	23.7	1.9	76	0.1
1989	0.1	19.5	0.1	80.2	0.2
1990	0	19.6	0	80.1	0.3
1991	0	12.4	0	84.8	2.8
1992	N/A	N/A	N/A	N/A	N/A

Values shown based on responses to EDTA-ERA patient questionaire which asked for the most commonly used dialyser in a given year. N/A: Not available.

rate. The general guideline for paediatric blood flow rates are based upon the patient's weight, namely:

$$Q_B = 2.5 \times \text{Body weight (kg)} + 100.$$

For children weighing less than 10 kg the flow rate should not exceed 75 ml/min, while for children weighing more than 40 kg, adult blood flow rates may be used. It is advisable to keep ultrafiltration rates during dialysis less than 5% of body weight to avoid side effects. The high calorie, protein and fluid intake requirement of children necessitates more dialysis in relation to body weight than adults and in view of this, paediatric dialysis schedules should be more frequent than for adults. This is often impractical necessitating the use of longer treatments which may increase the incidence of dialysis related complications.

CLASSIFICATION AND DEMOGRAPHY OF HAEMODIALYSERS IN USE

Haemodialysers in current clinical use either parallel plate or hollow fibre devices, both of which may be used for the newer modalities of treatment, as well as for the continuous therapies.

Other types of device such as coil and multiple use or rebuildable parallel plate devices are no longer in widespread clinical use. A wide range of designs in each of the above categories are available (Table 5). The percentage of patients using the principal categories of dialyser in Europe has been monitored by the European Dialysis and Transplant Association, European Renal Association (EDTA-ERA) and is shown in Table 6. Individual countries may vary in their use of devices and the data for the United Kingdom over the period 1981–1992 is shown for comparison in Table 7.

DEVICE PERFORMANCE

As shown in Table 5 the choice of devices for the treatment of renal failure has continued to grow. In reviewing device performance we have not set out to provide the reader with a catalogue of device performance but have drawn on our studies performed on behalf of the Medical Devices Agency (MDA) of the Department of Health in the United Kingdom (details of which are available on request to potential purchasers of haemodialysers, as well as manufacturers) and have selected the devices whose physical

Table 8. Physical characteristics of standard haemodialysers

Type	Name	Manufacturer	Surface area (m²)	Membrane characteristics	
				Type	Thickness (micron)
Flat plate	Lundia Alpha 400	Gambro Ab, Sweden	0.7	Cuprophan	8.0
	Lundia Alpha 600	Gambro Ab, Sweden	1.0	Cuprophan	8.0
Hollow fibre	CentrySystem 100HG	Cobe Laboratories, USA	0.2	Hemophan	6.5
	CentrySystem 200	Cobe Laboratories, USA	0.7	Cuprophan	11.0
	F4	Fresenius AG, Germany	0.7	Low Flux Polysulfone	40.0
	FB 70U	Nissho Corp, Japan	0.7	Cellulose triacetate	15.0
	HT80	Baxter Healthcare, USA	0.8	Hemophan	8.0
	Focus 90	NMC, Ireland	0.9	Cuprophan	8.0
	CentrySystem 400HG	Cobe Laboratories, USA	0.9	Hemophan	6.5
	Alwall GFE 12	Gambro GmbH, Germany	1.2	Cuprophan	8.0
	Disscap 160E	Hospal, France	1.2	Cuprophan	9.5
	CA 130	Baxter Healthcare, USA	1.3	Cellulose acetate	15.0
	F6	Fresenius AG, Germany	1.3	Low flux Polysulfone	40.0
	BL 643LF	Bellco Spa, Italy	1.4	Low flux Polysulfone	40.0
	EDG 1.5/32	Althin, USA	1.5	EVAL	32.0
	Clirans SE 15	Terumo Corp, Japan	1.5	Cuprammonium rayon	26.0

Table 9. Characteristics of large surface area and high flux devices

Type	Name	Manufacturer	Surface area (m²)	Membrane characteristics	
				Type	Thickness (micron)
Flat plate	Crystal 2800	Hospal, France	1.04	AN69XS Polyacrylonitrile	19.0
	Crystal 3400	Hospal, France	1.25	AN69XS Polyacrylonitrile	19.0
Hollow fibre	F40	Fresenius AG, Germany	0.7	Polysulfone FPS 600	40.
	F60	Fresenius AG, Germany	1.25	Polysulfone FPS 600	40.0
	BL 627 Rapido	Bellco Spa, Italy	1.3	Polysulfone	40.0
	Focus 160H	NMC, Ireland	1.6	Hemophan	8.0
	Altraflux	Althin, USA	1.7	Meltspun Cellulose Diacetate	30.0
	F8	Fresenius AG, Germany	1.8	Low flux Polysulfone	40.0

characteristics are summarised in Tables 8–9 for comparison of device performance, their measurement and influencing factors. Our own data has been supplemented with that provided by manufacturers in their product literature where appropriate, such data is shown in italics where it is included. This should allow clinicians to make rational choices, permit their own studies and allow reasons for differences between devices to be analysed.

Blood flow

Blood flow through haemodialysers and associated devices is an important factor in determining device performance and behaviour. Accurate knowledge of the blood flow rate is critical in obtaining optimum device performance.

In vitro measurement of flow through haemodialysers and associated devices may be accomplished by a timed collection at the outflow of the device. The measured flow rate must be corrected for ultrafiltration prevailing at the time of measurement. *In vivo* measurement or measurement in the laboratory using a closed circuit is more difficult. A commonly used technique is the use of calibrated blood pumps, the calibration being performed either at the beginning or the end of the study. Such a calibration assumes that the flow generated is a product of the rotational speed of the pump and the volume contained in the pump insert, and forms the basis of the flow rate dis-

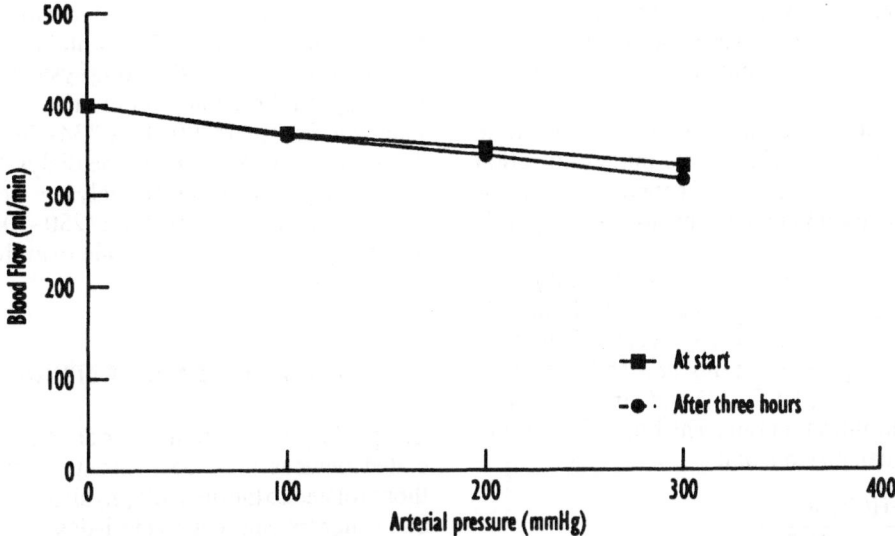

Figure 9. The effect of inlet pressure and alteration of pump insert dimensions on delivered blood flow rate. Adapted from Collins (254).

play in proportionating systems. While this is acceptable for routine clinical use, the flow delivered may be lower than indicated due to a high arterial (pump inlet) pressure causing deformation and incomplete filling of the pump insert, resulting in an under delivery of set flow rate. Figure 9 shows the magnitude of decrease in the delivered blood flow rate during dialysis with increasing inlet negative pressure. Maintenance of the flow rate over a three hour period further reduces the flow rate due to loss of compliance in the pump segment.

The bubble transit technique is an accurate, inexpensive method of blood flow determination, routinely used in connection with our haemodialyser studies. We use a 200 cm race track, giving an accuracy of ± 3% over the clinical range of blood flows. At high blood flows, a longer race track (350 cm) is used to minimise errors. A single air bubble is injected (0.5 ml) and its passage timed in triplicate using a stop watch capable of measuring 0.01 second. Blood flow rate is calculated from a relationship established using bank blood whose haematocrit is of a comparable range to that experienced clinically. Such calibrations are performed for each batch of race tracks used. The race tracks are kept horizontal during use to minimise errors introduced by the lower density of air compared with blood and its length measured at the commencement of dialysis to minimise stretching when the blood is flowing through the extracorporeal circuit. To prevent the ingress of the injected air into the dialyser during the course of measurements, a bubble chamber is inserted into the extracorporeal circuit pre-dialyser. Since the internal diameter of the tubing used for the race track is 5 mm, the additional burden for the patient in respect of the extracorporeal volume is small.

Blood flow profile in extracorporeal circuit when using double pump mechanical system of single needle dialysis (pressure-pressure operation)

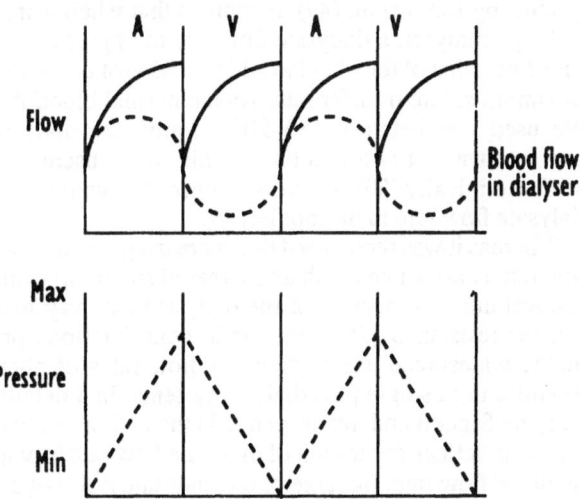

Figure 10. Blood flow during double pump single needle haemodialysis.

A modification of this technique is used in single needle dialysis which generates a cyclic blood flow pattern through the extracorporeal circuit consisting of high transient flow rates during the aspiration (arterial) and return (venous) phases of the cycle. In such systems, a 500 cm rack track is used and this race track is placed between the dialyser venous outlet and the venous compliance chamber as in this portion of the extracorporeal circuit. The flow rate is independent of the cyclic variations induced by the blood pump since they are damped out by the dialyser (Figure 10).

This technique of measurement of blood flow time involves repeated insertion of a needle into an injection site and because of the risk of aerosol generation the technique should not be used in patients positive for hepatitis or HIV.

For the measurement of blood flow in continuous haemofiltration (CAVH), the use of bubble transit times is impractical and a method described by Bosch (48) may be used. This method requires sampling pre- and post-filter for haematocrit (HCT_{inlet}, HCT_{outlet}) and simultaneously establishing the ultrafiltration rate. The blood flow at the filter inlet may be calculated from:

$$Q_{Bin} = \frac{Q_F HCT_{outlet}}{HCT_{outlet} - HCT_{inlet}}$$

while the plasma flow at the inlet is calculated from:

$$Q_{Pin} = Q_{Bin} - \frac{Q_{Bin} HCT_{inlet}}{100}.$$

Dialysate flow

In a review of engineering aspects of artificial kidney systems by Babb et al. (49), recounted that when using a Kiil type dialyser, a dialysate flow rate of approximately three times that of the blood would give 95% of theoretical maximum solute transfer rate. As the normal blood flow rate used was between 150–200 ml/min, the dialysate flow rate was set at 500 ml/min. This was subsequently verified clinically (50) and is the origin of this widely used dialysate flow rate in haemodialysis.

Whereas it was recognised that increasing the dialysate flow rate is associated with an increased small molecular removal due to reduction of the dialysate pathway mass transfer resistance (R_D), economic considerations precluded widespread use of dialysate flow rates of above 500 ml/min in single pass dialysis systems. In a detailed study by Sigdell and Tersteegen (51) the authors showed that the practical upper limit of dialysate flow rate is twice the blood flow rate. Increase of the dialysate flow beyond this upper limit would result in only a minimal improvement in solute removal.

The interest in high efficiency and high flux treatments has reawakened the interest in using non-standard dialysate flow rates, since in these treatment modalities the blood flow rate is in excess of 300 ml/min, such treatments are generally undertaken at a dialysate flow rate of 800 ml/min. Many of today's proportionating systems offer the option of performing treatment at three fixed dialysate flow rates, viz: 300, 500 and 800 ml/min.

Traditionally, measurement of dialysate flow has been undertaken at the drain from the proportionating system. This poses a number of problems. The volume flowing

to drain may not have all passed through the dialyser, it may be phased, and it also contains the ultrafiltrate. As the majority of proportionating systems no longer display the dialysate flow rate, in our studies we use an electromagnetic flow meter (Tosflow 334 – Toshiba Corporation, Tokyo, Japan) connected to the dialysate lines at the inlet to the dialyser to measure dialysate flow rate. This flow meter has a range of 15–60 l/h (250–1000 ml/min) and its accuracy is ±0.4% of full scale over the operating range 0–50% range.

PERFORMANCE PARAMETERS

The performance parameters of haemodialysers and associated devices have been grouped into two categories; those related to the device's physical properties, and solute and water transport characteristics.

PERFORMANCE PARAMETERS RELATED TO PHYSICAL PROPERTIES OF THE DEVICE

Blood compartment volume

The volume contained in the device is of importance not only from the clinical viewpoint, but also from the engineering viewpoint. The clinician views the haemodialyser as part of the circulatory system and the volume contained in the device is a major constituent of the extracorporeal circuit volume. In engineering terms, it is an important factor in determining the efficiency of solute transport.

Haemodialysers may be considered as comprising either a series of parallel layers or as a bundle of tubes permitting the definition of the contained volume in terms of the blood pathway geometry. Thus, for a device consisting of parallel layers the blood compartment volume may be expressed as (see Nomenclature for explanation):

$$LW h_b N$$

while for those consisting of a series of tubes or hollow fibres, as:

$$\frac{\pi d^2 LN}{4}.$$

Both of these relationships depend upon the device's geometric surface area which for parallel plate devices is given by:

$$A = 2LWN$$

and for hollow fibre containing devices by:

$$A = \pi NdL.$$

Historically the blood compartment volume of the dialyser was important. Early devices required blood priming,

Table 10. Blood compartment volume of standard haemodialysers

	Blood compartment volume (ml)
Lundia Alpha 400	70*
Lundia Alpha 600	83*
CentrySystem 100HG	19
CentrySystem 200	40
F4	41
FB 70U	49
HT80	58
Focus 90	53
CentrySystem 400HG	53
Alwall GFE 12	70
Disscap 160E	81
CA 130	77
F6	80
BL 643LF	85
EDG 1.5/32	110
Clirans SE 15	99

*At a transmembrane pressure of 50 mm Hg

Table 11. Blood compartment volume of large surface area and high flux devices

	Blood compartment volume (ml)
Crystal 2800	110*
Crystal 3400	120*
F40	42
F60	83
BL 627	86
Focus 160H	97
Altraflux	101
F8	100

*At a transmembrane pressure of 50 mmHg.

however, since the 1960's there has been a gradual reduction in this parameter and today the volume contained in many devices is less than that contained in the blood lines (Tables 10–11).

Dialysate compartment volume

This parameter is generally not shown in product literature and may be determined experimentally. When undertaking such measurements it should be borne in mind that the membranes in the device are permeable and consequently, for the most accurate determination a non-perfusable

Table 12. Surface areas measured using fibre dimensions for hollow fibre haemodialysers

Dialyser	Inner dry surface area (m^2)	Inner wet surface area (m^2)	Average wet surface area (m^2)
Bellco BL 611HB	0.96	1.15	1.2
Bellco BL 613H	1.14	1.32	1.43
Gambro GF80H	0.7	0.9	0.94
Gambro GF 120H	1.0	1.2	1.26
Sorin NT 1108	1.1	1.31	1.38
Sorin NT 1808	1.52	1.81	1.9

fluid should be used. The value of this parameter is of limited clinical interest, but it is used in determination of residence times in the dialysate pathway when analyzing device fluid dynamic behaviour.

Device surface area

The surface area available for mass and fluid transfer is one of the fundamental parameters of the device. Considerable variation in the measurement of surface areas of haemodialysers and associated devices exist. The device's effective surface area differs from the geometric or planar surface area. In parallel plate devices the latter is generally expressed as the area bounded by the sealing gasket. The effective surface area is the planar surface area corrected for the loss of area due to contact with the membrane support. This contact area is, however, not constant and is influenced by the fluid dynamic conditions within the device as well as the applied pressure.

In hollow fibre devices the length of the fibres determines the surface area. However, the surface area is also influenced by the swelling of the membrane following wetting. Measurements by Sigdell (39) indicate that for Cuprophan membranes there is a 13.5% swelling upon fibre wetting and a 100% increase in the wall thickness for a fibre of 200 micron internal diameter. These dimensional changes may differ in synthetic membranes. A change in length of the fibres may also occur and consequently, we can consider different fibre diameters – namely, inner dry diameter (d_{id}), inner wet diameter (d_{iw}), the average inner dry diameter (d_{ia}), the average inner wet diameter (d_{iw}) from which the inner dry surface, the inner wet surface and the average wet surface may be determined. Table 12 demonstrates the differences in surface areas based on the above fibre dimensions.

With the increased utilisation of hollow fibre devices, mention must be made of a number of other parameters.

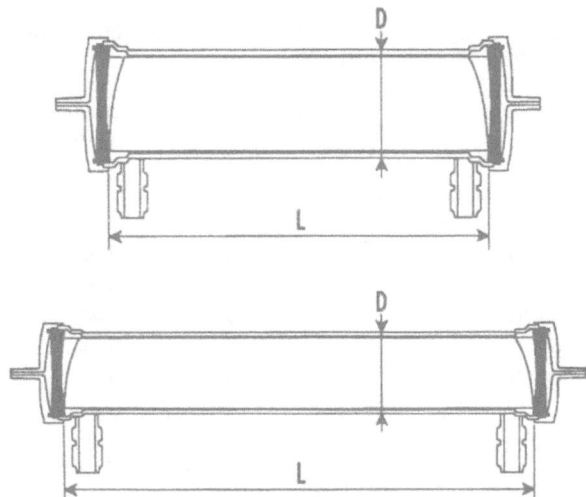

Figure 11. Fibre length and casing diameter ratios for conventional haemodialysers and devices used for continous renal replacement therapy.

Internal diameter of outer casing

The knowledge of the dimensions of the internal diameter of the casing containing the fibres is useful since it permits the ability to determine some characteristic design parameters, notably the fibre length/casing internal diameter ratio which provides an index of distribution within the device. Figure 11 shows that this ratio increases as the optimal flow configuration is achieved, particularly for haemodialysers. For haemofilters and haemodiafilters, this parameter is important in the minimisation of stagnation and improving flow distribution.

In general, due to manufacturing processes employed to produce the casing, there may be some variation in this parameter along the length of the casing.

The coefficient of filling

This parameter is defined as the ratio occupied by the fibres and the internal cross section of the casing, it provides a measure of the proportion of space occupied by the fibres relative to the available area contained within the casing. This parameter is primarily of interest to the engineer since it provides an indication of how well the fibres are placed within the casing. This is important since it provides information whether flow maldistribution in the dialysate pathway or excessive pressure drops are likely during clinical use. This parameter may be determined either wet or dry.

Fibre density

Fibre packing density of hollow fibre devices is primarily of interest to the engineer, and may be optimised by

Table 13. Influence of haematocrit on blood pathway pressure drop in a hollow fibre haemodialyser. Adapted from Ofstun et al. (112)

Blood flow (ml/min)	Haematocrit		
	25	30	35
200	1.0	1.063	1.23
300	1.0	1.071	1.26
400	1.0	1.075	1.26

Pressure changes relative to 25% haematocrit; number of fibers 8000; fiber length 230 mm; fibre internal diameter 200 micron.

configuring spacing between the fibres. In an optimum arrangement, the fibres form a hexagonal array so that the centres of any three adjacent fibres form an equilateral triangle. The optimisation process to achieve such spacing has been described by Sigdell (39).

A practical measure of the fibre density can be obtained by consideration of the ratio between the number of fibres in the centre of the device and the cross-sectional area of the casing. This ratio is generally expressed as the number of fibres per square mm of cross sectional surface area.

FLUID DYNAMIC CHARACTERISTICS

Blood pathway flow resistance

Haemodialysers may be considered as a series of parallel blood compartments. In hollow fibre devices, the geometry of the blood compartments is circular while in parallel plate devices, it is rectangular.

The pressure drop in hollow fibre devices may be calculated from consideration of the Hagen–Poiseuille formula:

$$\Delta P_B = \frac{128 \mu L}{\pi d_i^4 N} Q_B$$

while for parallel plate devices with a large width to height ratio, the flow resistance is given by:

$$\Delta P_B = \frac{12 \mu L}{W h^3 N} Q_B$$

Caution must be exercised in using the appropriate units in the above relationships since they express the pressure drop in dynes/cm^2. To convert the pressure drops to the more commonly used, the equations must be multiplied by 7.5×10^{-4} (mmHg/dyne/cm^2).

These relationships indicate that the pressure drops are directly proportional to the flow rate and are dependent upon both viscosity and pathway geometry. The relationships also assume that the blood pathway is impermeable.

The Hagen–Poiseuille's equation presumes that viscosity of the fluid flowing within the geometry is constant and the fluid is Newtonian. At sufficiently high shear rates blood fulfils the latter, blood viscosity, however, varies with haematocrit and protein concentration. To calculate pressure drops in the device, blood viscosity must be related to these parameters. This may be achieved by consideration of the empiric relationships of Charm and Kurland (52). Blood rheology in CAVH has been studied by Pallone and Petersen (53) who extended the work of Charm and Kurland to consider the viscosity of plasma to total protein concentration.

The blood flow resistance of devices may be measured *in vitro* using blood or an aqueous solution whose viscosity is similar to blood e.g., sucrose or glycerol/water mixture (54, 55) or *in vivo*.

Table 13 shows the expected pressure drops in a hollow fibre over the clinical range of blood flow rates and haematocrits. In general, actual pressure drops exceed those predicted from theory, due to differences in fluid dynamic conditions within the device during use, influencing the viscosity as well as the presence of small clots in the manifold region.

Dialysate pathway flow resistance

The equations governing dialysate pathway resistance and flow rate are comparable to those derived for the blood pathway. In the case of hollow fibre devices the flow resistance will be governed not only by the pathway dimensions, but also by the fibre packing density.

For an ordered hexagonal array of parallel equi-spaced fibres, the dialysate side pressure drop has been derived by Sigdell (36) and is given by:

$$\Delta P_D = \frac{8\mu L t^4}{\pi N r_e^4 F(t)} Q_D$$

where t is a parameter relating to the fibre packing density in the bundle and is given by:

$$t = r e \sqrt{\frac{\pi N}{\text{Fibre bundle area}}}$$

and

$$F(t) = (t^2 - \log_e t) - 3 - t^4.$$

Dialysate pathway resistance, in practice, ranges between 20–40 mmHg, depending upon the design, and is a function of the dialysate flow as well as the flow distribution. In some clinically used designs the dialysate pathway may be modified to permit a uniform flow through the fibre bundle. This distribution, while avoiding the presence of preferential streaming in the fibre bundle, may cause an increase in the compartment resistance.

In parallel plate dialysers the resistance in the dialysate pathway is related to the positive pressure applied to the blood pathway due to the latter's compliance.

Flow distribution

Essentially, all devices may be considered as a series of parallel flow paths which are rectangular in the case of parallel plate devices, and circular for hollow fibre devices. Ideally, in the absence of flow maldistribution, the flow in each of the pathways will be the same and generate an identical pressure drop. However, the pressure drop in parallel plates varies inversely with the cube of the spacing, while for hollow fibres, the flow resistance varies inversely with the fourth power of the hollow fibre diameter; consequently, a 10% variation in fibre diameter will produce a 46% variation in the flow through the fibres. Maldistribution in devices may arise from either dimensional variations or variations attributable to the design of the device. The magnitude of such non-ideal flow may be assessed by a stimulus response technique using either non-diffusible dyes or radioactive tracers (56, 57).

Two important parameters are derived from stimulus response studies. First, the location of the distribution (mean residence time), and the spread (or the variance) of the distribution.

The residence time in the blood compartment may be obtained by consideration of:

$$\bar{t}_B = \frac{\text{Priming volume}}{\text{Blood flow}} .$$

This parameter depends upon the device geometry and may influence solute transport processes. A high residence time may reduce concentration gradients and lead to a lower efficiency. It will also influence filtration rate, a factor that becomes important in continuous therapies where at high residual times, filtration pressure equilibrium leading to clotting, may occur.

For the dialysate pathway the residence time is given by:

$$\bar{t}_D = \frac{\text{Priming volume}}{\text{Dialysate flow}} .$$

As for the blood compartment, a high or long residence time reduces the diffusion gradients and compromises diffusion. In haemodiafiltration, the long residence may further reduce solute transport due to the presence of ultrafiltrate on the dialysate side of the device.

Details of the underlying mathematical theory are given by Levenspiel (58).

Characterisation of flow distribution in haemodialysers and associated devices

Characterisation of the flow through the blood compartment of the device may be by the injection of contrast medium into the arterial or inlet line to the device and undertaking sequential imaging as shown in Figure 12. In

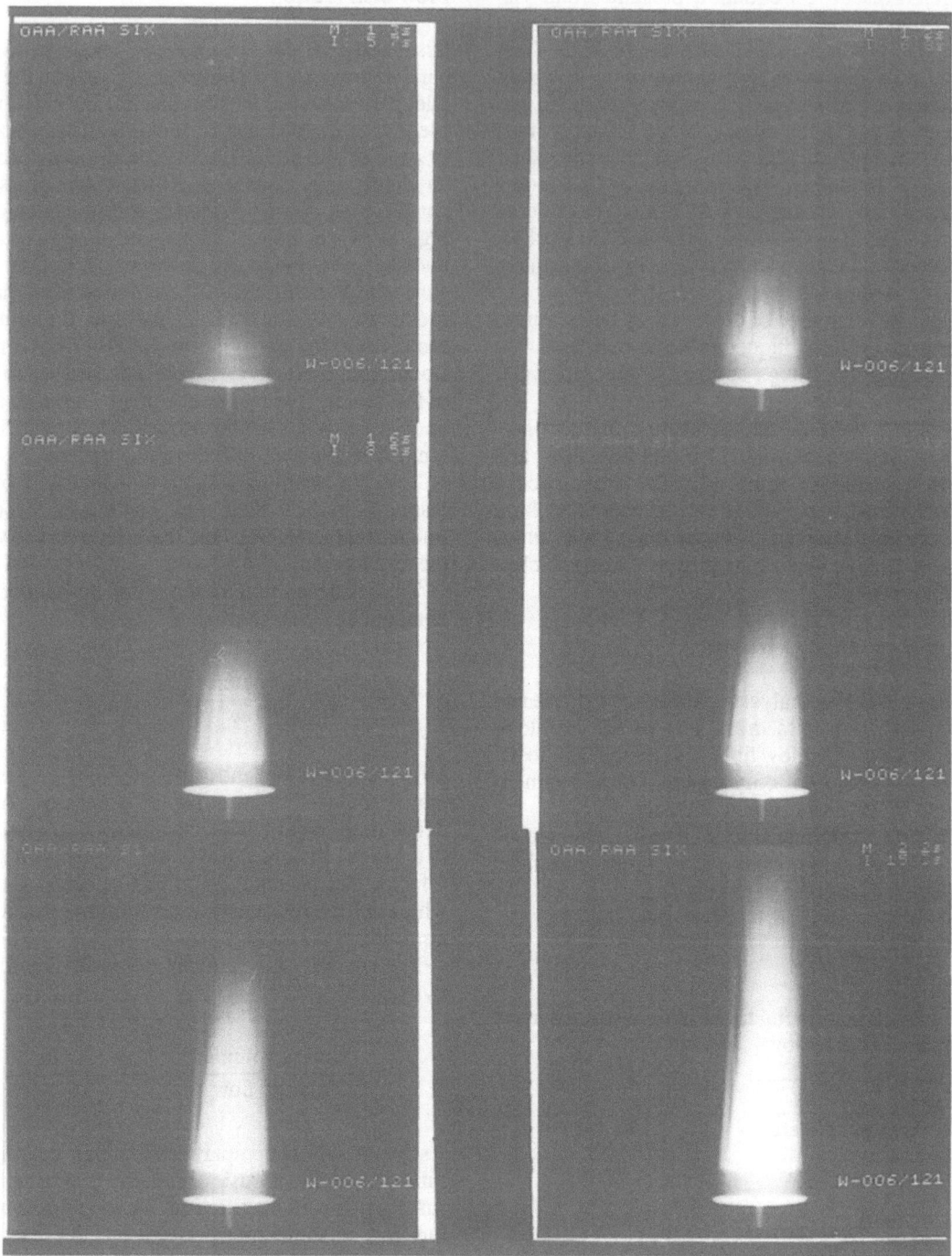

Figure 12. Flow distribution in hollow fibre device characterised by contrast medium injected at the device inlet. An area of non-perfusion may be seen in the last photograph of the series.

such studies the average flow velocity per fibre may be calculated from the relationship:

$$V = \frac{4Q_B}{\pi d_{\text{fw}}^2 N} .$$

This parameter may be used to determine the effect of blood flow on the boundary layers at the blood membrane interface.

Table 14. Fluid blood loss observed during clinical use of standard haemodialysers

	Fluid blood retained (ml)		Saline rinse	Rinse volume/
	Mean	Range	(ml)	Circuit volume
Lundia Alpha 400	2.0	0.8–3.0	500	1.41
Lundia Alpha 600	5.1	3.4–7.4	600	1.56
CentrySystem 100HG	N/A	N/A	N/A	N/A
CentrySystem 200	1.7	0.4–3.9	600	1.84
F4	3.5	0.4–8.7	500	2.04
FB 70U	N/A	N/A	N/A	N/A
HT80	4.6	0.6–12.2	500	2.15
Focus 90	1.5	0.6–2.9	600	1.77
CentrySystem 400HG	3.2	0.7–5.0	500	1.88
Alwall GFE 12	2.1	0.2–5.8	500	1.64
Disscap 160E	4.2	1.5–7.8	500	1.66
CA 130	3.9	1.1–6.5	500	1.50
F6	2.0	0.5–3.1	500	1.62
BL 643LF	4.9	0.8–13.5	500	2.14
EDG 1.5/32	9.0	3.8–17.5	500	1.47
Clirans SE 15	5.7	0.7–8.6	500	1.38

N/A: Not available.

Table 15. Fluid blood loss observed during clinical use of large surface area and high flux devices

	Fluid blood retained (ml)		Saline rinse	Rinse volume/
	Mean	Range	(ml)	Circuit volume
Crystal 2800	2.3	1.0–4.3	600	1.46
Crystal 3400	1.5	0.6–2.4	600	1.56
F40	1.8	0.7–4.9	500	1.78
F60	2.0	0.8–3.1	500	1.55
BL 627	6.7	1.6–13.6	500	1.56
Focus 160H	10.3	0.4–25.1	500	1.49
Altraflux	< 1.0			
F8	5.6	4.1–7.2	500	1.4

Blood loss

After the completion of treatment, the contents of the extracorporeal circuit are rinsed with saline to return as much of the blood contained in the circuit to the patient. This process may be broken down into discrete elements, each of which are discussed below.

The reinfusion process

During reinfusion of saline to the extracorporeal circuit, the concentration of blood decreases. The rate of decrease will be governed by a number of factors: the volume of the extracorporeal circuit relative to the rinse volume, the rate of rinsing, the presence of clots in the dialyser or the extracorporeal circuit. Currently practiced short dialysis schedules with high efficiency low volume devices require the optimisation of the rinseback process to maximise blood return and minimise blood retained. The percentage blood retained may be plotted against the washback volume (expressed in units of circuit volume). The construction of such a curve is, however, subject to scatter introduced by the thrombus generating potential of the patient, the presence of clots in the extracorporeal circuit, and variations in haematocrit and viscosity. Theoretical and experimental studies on the purging of extracorporeal circuits has been described elsewhere (59–61).

Blood retained in the haemodialyser

All currently used devices are sufficiently thrombogenic to require the administration of an anticoagulant-heparin. Despite this thrombus generation in the extracorporeal circuit occurs. This may be a consequence of the inactivation of heparin (62), the binding of heparin to the material surface (63) and the presence of heparin binding or neutralising proteins in the plasma (64) and the blood air interface (65), technique of rinsing and the degree of anticoagulation achieved during the procedure.

An additional factor may be the loss of heparin through the membrane during treatment. This effect probably occurs to a limited extent only when unfractionated heparin (molecular weight range 4–35 kD) is used, but is likely to be more pronounced when low molecular weight heparin (molecular weight 4–10 kD) is used, particularly in combination with high flux membranes.

Thrombus formation is also influenced by the surface properties of the material in contact with the blood (66–68) as well as local fluid dynamic conditions.

A reduction in the amount of thrombus formation is of critical importance, particularly in devices intended for continuous therapies and has led to the development of antithrombotic surfaces (69).

The blood retained at the termination of treatment has two distinct components. First, the fluid blood component which is related to the volume used to rinse the extracorporeal circuit, the technique of rinsing and the device design. The second component is the irretrievable clotted residue. Measurement of these two components differ. Fluid residue retained in the extracorporeal circuit may be estimated using haemoglobinometry, where the haemoglobin content of the patient's blood (taken immediately prior to the termination of treatment) is compared to that contained in the extracorporeal circuit after the usual rinse back volume had been used.

In our own studies of this parameter we recirculate the contents of the extracorporeal circuit under minimal ultrafiltration conditions for a period of ten minutes to ensure thorough mixing, through one litre of ammoniated water (0.04% NH_3). The optical density of the patient's blood and a sample of the ammoniated water is measured spectrophotometrically at 540 nm and the blood retained calculated from the formula:

$$\text{RBV} = \frac{U}{200S} [1000 + X],$$

where U = haemoglobin concentration of recirculated fluid; S = haemoglobin concentration of a sample of arterial blood taken immediately prior to the commencement of the reinfusion process which has been diluted 1:200 with 0.04% NH_3; X = Extracorporeal circuit volume.

The circuit volume is determined separately. To establish the volume retained in the dialyser alone the blood is returned in the normal manner but the blood lines are disconnected and replaced by clean blood tubing prior to recirculation.

Table 16. Scoring system for the assessment of clotted residue in haemodialysers and associated devices

Clotted fibres Rating	Number of clotted fibres observed
1	1–10
2	11–50
3	51–100
4	101–500
5	> 500

Clots in device header Rating	Number of clots observed
1	1–3 small clots
2	Large circular clots
3	Several large clots
4	Header completely clotted

Fluid blood retained in haemodialysers studied at our centre is shown in Tables 14–15. These results show a scatter but the overall loss from this source is small when compared with losses due to biochemical sampling. Variation in the dialyser or the extracorporeal circuit volume has only a small effect on the final result unless the volumes are large.

The most appropriate method of quantifying clotted residue is by the use of radioisotopically labelled red cells. As the technique involves the administration of radioisotopes to the patient, it is not widely used. It may also be assessed visually, by the use of a scoring system (Table 16). This method is subjective, and can be associated with errors, particularly in the case of clotted fibres since the method only estimates the number of visible fibres rather than the total number of fibres (70).

SOLUTE TRANSPORT

In a haemodialyser a semi-permeable membrane replaces the renal glomeruli and tubules. Blood passes on one side of the membrane while dialysis fluid made up of a buffered electrolyte solution passes on the other. Across the membrane, diffusive and convective mass transfer occurs. The clinician views the haemodialyser as part of the circulatory system whose function is to remove metabolites elevated as a consequence of renal insufficiency, while an engineer views the haemodialyser as a mass exchanger and his primary interest is in the understanding and improvement of the device efficiency. For the most effective understanding of solute transport in haemodialysers and associated devices, an inter-disciplinary approach is necessary.

Mechanism of solute transport

In order to understand why haemodialysers vary in efficiency, it is helpful to visualise three distinct elements of the diffusion of a molecule from the blood to the dialysate stream. The molecule must first diffuse through the blood layer to the membrane boundary, cross the membrane, enter the dialysate layer and then move away from the point of entry. The overall rate of mass transport may be represented by a differential equation in which the rate of mass transfer (K_T) is defined in terms of the membrane area and the concentration driving force such that the net flux (dN) is:

$$dN = K_T(C_B - C_D)dA$$

which when integrated is:

$$N = K_T A \Delta C.$$

ΔC represents the log mean concentration driving force for solute mass transfer. This parameter is dependent upon the directions of the blood and dialysis fluid flow to one another, which for the commonly used contra-parallel flow configuration is given by:

$$\Delta C = \frac{(C_{Bi} - C_{Do}) - (C_{Bo} - C_{Di})}{\log e \left[\dfrac{C_{Bi} - C_{Do}}{C_{Bo} - C_{Di}}\right]}.$$

Rearrangement results in:

$$K_o = \frac{N}{A\Delta C},$$

where K_o is the overall transport coefficient which defines the fundamental physical property of the device. This parameter is constant provided that no channelling or maldistribution in the blood and dialysate pathways is present, nor changes in surface area of the device occur over the operational range of blood and dialysate flow rates.

The reciprocal of K_o may be considered as the average overall mass transfer resistance (R_T) which is the sum of the individual average mass transfer resistances in the blood (R_B), dialysate (R_D) and the membrane (R_M) elements.

The measurement of blood side mass transfer coefficient or resistance is not possible in practice but may be estimated by theoretical analysis assuming fully developed steady laminar flow through the blood compartment of the device in the case of flat plate devices (71). For hollow fibre devices Sigdell (72) has derived relationships for both R_B and R_D assuming a regular hexagonal array of hollow fibres.

The value of R_T may be influenced by dialyser design (73), increased dialysate flow rate (74), or alteration of the membrane permeability. However, the relative importance of these will vary according to molecular weight since for low molecular weight solutes, the principal barriers to diffusion lie in the boundary layers adjacent to the membrane, while for large molecules, the barrier is in the membrane itself.

Clearance and dialysance

Analogous to the clearance concept of the human kidney, the solute transport characteristics of a haemodialyser may also be expressed in terms of clearance. Clearance in this context focuses on the removal of solute from the patient by the device and it may be defined as the amount of solute removed from the blood per unit of time, divided by incoming blood concentration and thus represents the volumetric rate of removal by the device. By consideration of the mass balance across the dialyser, the clearance may be expressed in terms of concentration gradients and flow rates such that:

$$\begin{bmatrix} \text{Solute transferred} \\ \text{from blood to dialysate} \end{bmatrix} = \begin{bmatrix} \text{Solute mass} \\ \text{entering device} \end{bmatrix} - \begin{bmatrix} \text{Solute mass} \\ \text{leaving device} \end{bmatrix}.$$

In the presence of ultrafiltration

$$Q_{Bi} - Q_{Bo} = Q_F.$$

Since the definition of clearance is the mass removal rate divided by the incoming concentration, thus:

$$K_B = Q_{Bi}\frac{(C_{Bi} - C_{Bo})}{C_{Bi}} + Q_F\frac{C_{Bo}}{C_{Bi}}.$$

Since the solutes removed are in the dialysate (assuming negligible adsorption on the membrane), an equivalent relationship for the dialysate side is given by:

$$K_D = Q_{Di}\frac{(C_{Di} - C_{Do})}{C_{Bi}} + Q_F\frac{C_{Do}}{C_{Bi}}.$$

The first terms of these equations may be viewed as the diffusive components of solute transport, while the second represents the convective component. In the case of negligible ultrafiltration or negligible convective mass transport, the relationships reduce to:

$$K_B = Q_B\frac{(C_{Bi} - C_{Bo})}{C_{Bi}}$$

and

$$K_D = Q_D\frac{(C_{Di} - C_{Do})}{C_{Bi}}.$$

Dialysance is used by engineers in the comparison of overall solute removal by different blood dialysate flow configurations and is defined as the amount of solute removed from the blood per unit of time divided by the concentration difference between incoming blood and dialysis fluid.

In a manner similar to that shown above, general relationships for the blood and dialysate sides of the dialyser are given by:

$$D_B = Q_{Bi} \frac{(C_{Bi} - C_{Bo})}{(C_{Bi} - C_{Di})} + Q_F \frac{C_{Bo}}{(C_{Bi} - C_{Di})}$$

and

$$D_D = Q_{Di} \frac{(C_{Do} - C_{Di})}{(C_{Bi} - C_{Di})} + Q_F \frac{C_{Do}}{(C_{Bi} - C_{Di})}$$

may be derived. The equivalent simplified versions (i.e., in the absence of ultrafiltration) are given by:

$$D_B = Q_B \frac{(C_{Bi} - C_{Bo})}{C_{Bi} - C_{Di}}$$

and

$$D_D = Q_D \frac{(C_{Di} - C_{Do})}{C_{Bi} - C_{Di}} \; .$$

The relative importance of dialysance has diminished over the past decade as the clinical use of haemodialysers and associated devices rely on single pass rather than recirculating dialysate supply systems. In such systems C_{Di} is zero and the two relationships are equivalent. It is, however, important to bear in mind that in the case of devices whose construction is such that a single pass system can not be used, e.g., coil dialysers, clearance and dialysance are only equivalent in the initial minutes of the treatment and thereafter the dialysance is higher than the clearance since the relationship between the parameters is governed by the formula:

$$K_B = \frac{C_{Bi} - C_{Di}}{C_{Bi}} D_B.$$

The recirculating dialysate systems have largely been replaced by recirculating single pass systems (RSP). In such systems a small volume (5–10 litres) is recirculated through the dialyser at a rate similar to that used by pure recirculating systems but simultaneously the recirculation dialysate flows to waste and is replaced by fresh dialysis fluid. To maintain a hydrostatic balance in the system, the rate of addition is equal to the rate of discharge to waste (0.5–1.0 litres/minute). The relationship between clearance and dialysance for such systems assuming a well mixed dialysate is given by:

$$K_B = \frac{D_B}{1 + \dfrac{D_B}{Q_D}}$$

and permits the comparison of coil dialysers with the more commonly used parallel plate or hollow fibre designs.

Clearance, therefore, may be considered as the operational parameter of clinical interest that focuses upon the removal of solute from the blood and ultimately from the patient and can, therefore, be used to predict concentration changes in the body.

Unfortunately, the dialysance parameter has often been misinterpreted in clinical dialysis as it was thought to be equivalent to clearance. This is only true in the case of single pass dialysis fluid flow and the use of dialysance should be confined to such situations that require comparisons of different dialysate flow configurations.

While these relationships hold for aqueous solutions, *in vivo* measurements are complicated by the heterogeneous nature of blood and consequently caution must be exercised in extrapolating 'in vitro' solute removal data obtained using aqueous homogenous solutions to the clinical setting as the diffusive transfer of solutes may be slower due to the presence of plasma proteins and the movement of solute from the formed elements into the plasma and plasma water. Despite these potential limitations, the measurement of whole blood clearance provides a useful method of comparing the solute removal characteristics of devices from different manufacturers.

The relationships discussed above refer to the clearance in the haemodialyser itself, not the removal of metabolite from the patient. To understand metabolite removal from the patient during therapy, the concept of effective clearance needs to be introduced, since this represents the true volumetric rate at which the patient's systemic blood is being cleared of the solute.

Effective clearance may, therefore, be considered as a refinement of clearance. This refinement is required to correct for the partial recirculation of blood that may occur in the dialyser. Such recirculation may originate from patient access problems or the access device. By consideration of the mass balance, Gotch (75) has derived a modification given by:

$$K_R = \frac{(1 - R')}{1 - R' \left(1 - \dfrac{K_B}{Q_B}\right)} K_B.$$

By rearrangement of this relationship the percentage reduction in clearance at a specific recirculation rate may be established. The influence of recirculation on solute removal is shown schematically for two solutes with differing clearance characteristics (Figure 13).

Haematocrit and plasma water and solute protein binding also influence solute clearance and their role is important not only in conventional haemodialysis, but also in the newer modalities of treatment such as the continuous therapies and haemofiltration, since in these modes of treatment the principal route of solute removal is by convection.

The impact of haematocrit on dialyser solute removal has been discussed by Morcos and Nissenson (76) who derived a correction factor (Q_E) to replace Q_B in the conventional formula such that:

$$Q_E = Q_B \left[F_P - \frac{HCT}{100} (F_P - F_R k' \gamma) \right],$$

Influence of recirculation on small and middle molecular clearance

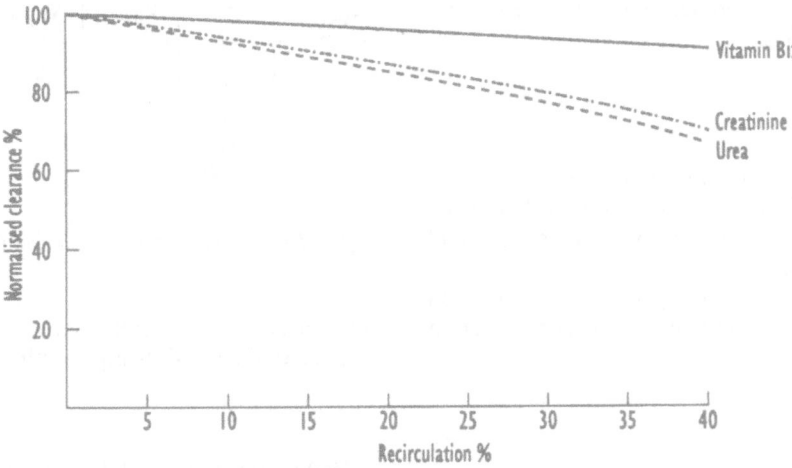

Figure 13. Effect of recirculation on solute removal during haemodialysis.

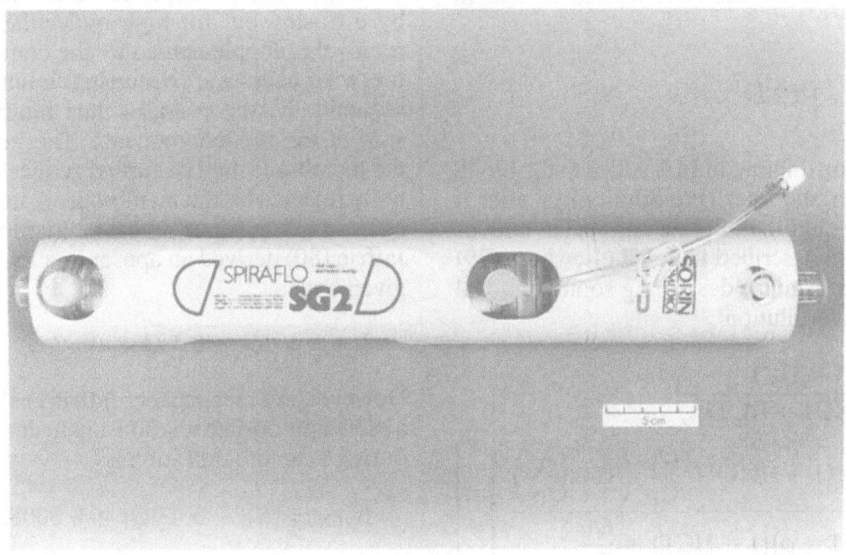

Figure 14. Combined haemodialyser and haemofilter used in paired filtration dialysis (PFD).

where F_P – Plasma water fraction; F_R – Red cell water fraction; k' – Equilibrium distribution coefficient; γ – Fraction of red blood cell water that participates in solute transfer during a transit of blood through the dialyser.

It may be seen that the effective clearance is reduced as haematocrit increases. The effect, however, is modulated by the values for k' and γ so that for solutes that do not move out rapidly from the red cells during a transit through the dialyser. The effective blood flow rate would be close to the plasma flow rate and, consequently, their removal would be diminished as haematocrit increases. For solutes such as urea, the impact would be reduced

since the equilibrium distribution coefficient approaches unity (77).

In the case of continuous therapies as well as haemofiltration, solute is cleared from the blood by the removal of plasma water. Greater attention must be paid to the precise distribution of solute. To permit equivalent calculations to those used in haemodialysis it is necessary to introduce the concept of sieving coefficient, a ratio of the solute concentration in the ultrafiltrate to the concentration of bulk plasma water, such that:

$$S = \frac{C_F}{C_W}$$

for $S = 1$ when the solute passes freely across the membrane, while for $S = 0$ the solute is completely rejected and does not cross the membrane. In practice the sieving coefficient is calculated as:

$$S = \frac{2C_F}{C_{Wi} + C_{Wo}}.$$

For retentive membranes this approximation of sieving coefficient does not hold and a more rigorous characterisation involving the relationship derived by Spiegler and Kadem (78) is required.

In the absence of protein binding solute concentration in the plasma water is related to the plasma concentration by:

$$\frac{CP}{C_W} = 1 - \phi,$$

where ϕ is the volume fraction of hydrated proteins and is $0.0107\ C_P$ (79).

The concentration in the blood is related to that in plasma by:

$$\frac{CP}{C_W} = 1 - HCT + HCTk'.$$

During haemofiltration diluting fluid is added to the blood either before it enters the filter (pre-dilution) or after it leaves the filter (post-dilution). Solute removal in both of these models has been described in detail elsewhere (79) and only the derived formulae describing solute removal are given below for pre-dilution:

$$K_B = Q_B \left(\frac{1 - HCT}{1 - HCT + HCTk'} \right)$$
$$\times \left[1 - \left\{ \frac{(1 - \phi)(1 - HCT) + \frac{Q_B}{Q_D}\left(1 - \frac{Q_F}{Q_D}\right)}{(1 - \phi)(1 - HCT) + \frac{Q_D}{Q_B}} \right\}^S \right]$$

for post-dilution the formula is:

$$K_B = Q_B \left(\frac{1 - HCT}{1 - HCT + HCTk'} \right)$$
$$\times \left[1 - \left\{ \frac{(1 - \phi)(1 - HCT) + \frac{Q_B}{Q_D}}{(1 - \phi)(1 - HCT)} \right\}^S \right].$$

In the case of solute removal for post-dilution e.g., during CVVH or CAVH the whole blood clearance is equivalent to the plasma clearance such that:

$$K_B = \frac{Q_F C_F}{C_{Bi}}.$$

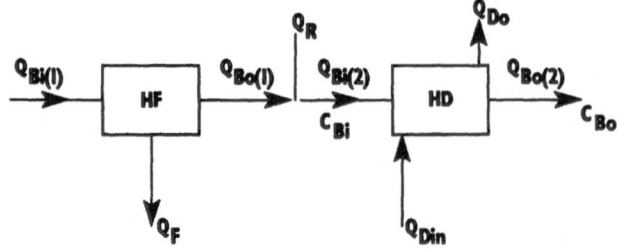

Figure 15. Paired filtration dialysis flow configuration.

If the effects of exclusion volume of hydrated proteins are neglected, the relationship simplifies to:

$$K_B = Q_F S$$

Haemodiafiltration (HDF) is a technique for the treatment of chronic renal failure which combines conventional haemodialysis with significant (40–80 ml/min) ultrafiltration. The principal route of removal for solutes is by diffusion but for high molecular weight solutes the removal is supplemented by the convective transport. As the two processes are occurring simultaneously rather than sequentially, the overall solute removal is less than the sum of the two components. The mass transport across the membrane may be further reduced if the solute is partially rejected by the membrane. A mathematical analysis of the mass transport in haemodiafiltration by Gupta and Jaffrin (80) derived an approximation of the mass transfer given by:

$$K_{HDF} = K_B + 0.5\ Q_F.$$

However, in a recent paper Jaffrin et al. (81) suggested that a more appropriate relationship to describe solute removal during haemodiafiltration is:

$$K_{HDF} = K_B + 0.43\ Q_F + 0.00083\ Q_F^2$$

which for $Q_F < 70$ ml/min approximates to

$$K_{HDF} = K_B + 0.43\ Q_F.$$

In order to circumvent the problems of simultaneous diffusive and convective mass transport in the device, Ghezzi et al. (82) have described a two chamber system of dialysis known as paired filtration haemodialysis which combines a haemodialyser and haemofilter (Figure 14).

In paired filtration dialysis the haemofilter is located before the dialyser and provides the convective mass transport element of the system while the haemodialyser provides the diffusive element. As the transmembrane pressure in the dialyser is maintained as close as possible to zero and to avoid excessive increases in blood viscosity for the blood entering the dialyser, an infusion of 0.9% NaCl is infused between the two elements of the system

(Figure 15). The total clearance for small molecules in this situation is given by:

$$K_{\text{PFD}} = Q_F + Q_{\text{Bi2}} \left[\frac{(C_{\text{Bi}} - C_{\text{Bo}})}{C_{\text{Bi}}} \right] \left[\left(\frac{Q_{\text{Bi1}} - Q_F}{Q_{\text{Bi2}}} \right) \right]$$

assuming $Q_F = 0$ at the dialyser and $S = 1$ at the haemofilter.

A similar relationship may be derived if the haemodialyser is located before the haemofilter:

$$K_{\text{TOTAL}} = A + \frac{C_F}{C_{\text{Bo}}} \left[1 - \frac{A}{Q_{\text{Bi}}} \right] Q_F$$

where

$$A = Q_{\text{Bi}} \left(1 - \frac{C_{\text{Bo}}}{C_{\text{Bi}}} \right).$$

A variation in the technique of haemodiafiltration is continuous arteriovenous haemodiafiltration which is a combination of continuous arteriovenous haemodiafiltration with slow continuous dialysis. A mathematical model of continuous arteriovenous haemodiafiltration whereby the diffusive mass transfer coefficient for a solute may be derived from flow rates and solute concentrations has been described by Vincent et al. (83).

Interdisciplinary approach

An interdisciplinary approach involves the combination of the descriptive term for clearance and the overall mass transfer coefficient (R_T). Table 17 gives the relationship of these terms for the three commonly used flow configurations. These relationships were first derived by Leonard and Bluemle (84) and Michaels (85) and are based upon equations for heat transfer, rigorous derivations of which may be found in textbooks dealing with the subject.

In the absence of significant ultrafiltration, the relationships may be used not only to analyse the mass transfer phenomena occurring within dialysers, but also to provide a predictive indication of the expected performance under specific conditions. In making use of the formula for predictive purposes, the underlying assumption is that R_T does not change.

SOLUTE TRANSPORT CHARACTERISTICS OF HAEMODIALYSERS AND ASSOCIATED DEVICES

Solute transport characteristics of haemodialysers and associated devices are related to the blood flow through the device at a given dialysis fluid flow rate (Figure 16). The shape of this relationship governed by constraints imposed by the blood flow (flow limited mass transfer) and the overall mass transfer coefficient (membrane limited mass transfer). A similar relationship exists for solute transport as a function of dialysis fluid flow rate at a given blood flow rate and forms the basis of high efficiency treatments.

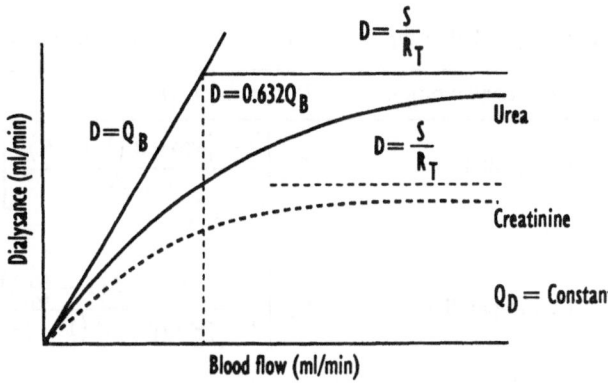

Figure 16. The relationship between blood flow and solute removal. This relationship is applicable to any device.

Since the relationship between blood flow and clearance is the same for all designs and solutes, this allows comparison between different designs to be made. To permit such comparisons to be made, a method used in our studies is the plot of $(1 - (C_{\text{Bo}}/C_{\text{Bi}}))$ against Q_B using a method of least squares fit procedure via the equation

$$\frac{1}{K_B} = a + \frac{b}{Q_B}$$

which satisfies the conditions that the clearance is zero when the blood flow rate is zero and it approaches an asymptotic rate as the blood flow rate increases. An alternate, but mathematically questionable method is the fitting of a polynomial (normally a cubic) curve to the experimental data with the use of higher blood flow rates. In clinical practice we have recently reviewed our method of establishing the blood flow clearance relationship and currently use an equation of the form

$$C_{\text{Bout}} = C_{\text{Bin}} \frac{\frac{1}{Q_{\text{Bin}}} - \frac{1}{Q_D}}{\frac{T}{Q_{\text{Bin}}} - \frac{1}{Q_D}}$$

and

$$T = \exp\left(\frac{S}{R_T} \left(\frac{1}{Q_D} - \frac{1}{Q_{\text{Bin}}} \right) \right).$$

The parameters in this relationship, with the exception of R_T, are measurable quantities. The necessary curve fitting may be achieved by a variety of software packages. Initially, it was assumed that R_T was constant; however, it became apparent that this assumption was incorrect and it was necessary to assume that the overall mass transfer resistance (R_T) varies with blood flow (Q_{Bin}) in accordance with a relationship given by

$$R_T = \alpha + \frac{\beta}{Q_{\text{Bin}}}$$

Table 17. Relationship between dialysance and overall mass transfer resistance for commonly used flow configurations

Flow configuration	Dialysance (D)	Total mass transfer resistance (R_T)
Co-parallel	$Q_B \left[\dfrac{1 - \left[\exp -J\left(1 + \frac{Q_B}{Q_D}\right)\right]}{1 + \frac{Q_B}{Q_D}} \right]$	$\dfrac{S(Q_B + Q_D)}{Q_B Q_D \ln\left[\frac{1}{1 - \frac{D}{Q_B} - \frac{D}{Q_D}}\right]}$
Contra-parallel	$Q_B \left[\dfrac{1 - \left[\exp -J\left(1 - \frac{Q_B}{Q_D}\right)\right]}{1 - \frac{Q_B}{Q_D} \exp\left[-J\left(1 - \frac{Q_B}{Q_D}\right)\right]} \right]$	$\dfrac{S(Q_B - Q_D)}{Q_B Q_D \ln\left[\frac{1 - \frac{D}{Q_B}}{1 - \frac{D}{Q_D}}\right]}$
Cross-flow*	$\dfrac{Q_B}{2} \left\{ \left[\dfrac{1 - \left[\exp -J\left(1 + \frac{Q_B}{Q_D}\right)\right]}{1 + \frac{Q_B}{Q_D}} \right] + \left[\dfrac{1 - \left[\exp -J\left(1 - \frac{Q_B}{Q_D}\right)\right]}{1 - \frac{Q_B}{Q_D} \exp\left[-J\left(1 - \frac{Q_B}{Q_D}\right)\right]} \right] \right\}$	$\dfrac{S}{2Q_B Q_D}\left[\dfrac{(Q_B + Q_D)}{\ln\left[\frac{1}{1 - \frac{D}{Q_B} - \frac{D}{Q_D}}\right]} + \dfrac{(Q_B - Q_D)}{\ln\left[\frac{1 - \frac{D}{Q_B}}{1 - \frac{D}{Q_D}}\right]} \right]$

where $J = \dfrac{S}{R_T Q_B}$

*Approximation only. For exact solution refer to Kays and London: *Compact Heat Exchangers*, 2nd ed, New York, McGraw-Hill, 1964.

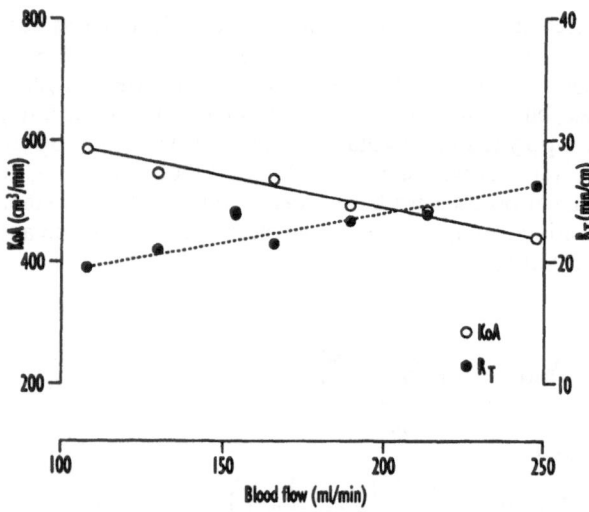

Figure 17. Relationship betweeen overall mass transfer resistance R_T and mass transfer coefficient area product (koA) and blood flow rate for a hollow fibre haemodialyser.

such that the overall mass transfer resistance decreases as the blood flow rate increases, but never has a value less than α.

These methods provide accurate prediction of the clearance at specific flow rates based upon measurements over a range of flow rates. An alternate approach to use R_T or its derivative KoA to predict the clearance at a specific set of operating conditions based on measurements. This process assumes that the value of R_T remains constant at all blood and dialysate flow rates. Figure 17 shows such a relationship and indicates that this assumption may not be the case.

In describing device performance it is common practice to characterise the device's solute removal by commonly used small molecular weight solutes such as urea (60), creatinine (113) and phosphate (134) while middle molecular clearance is represented by vitamin B_{12} (135). Tables 18–19 summarise the mean *in vivo* clearance data of haemodialysers and associated devices based on our studies on patients whose mean haematocrit was 27% at a blood flow rate of 200 ml/min. Equivalent *in vitro* results, as well as those for vitamin B_{12} are shown in Tables 20–21.

Long term haemodialysis therapy is associated with elevated β_2 microglobulin levels and the development of amyloidosis (86) due to inadequate clearance of β_2 microglobulin, although evidence is emerging that the synthesis and release of β_2 microglobulin may also be influenced by the interaction of peripheral blood cells with the membrane (87, 88).

This issue is complicated by the fact that some membranes are highly permeable and are able to clear small or medium size molecules which may counterbalance any production (89) while in others the route of removal is not via transfer across the membrane, but by adsorption

Table 18.   In vitro clearance characteristics of standard haemodialysers

	Clearance (ml/min)			
	Urea	Creatinine	Phosphate	Vitamin B_{12}
Lundia Alpha 400	149	120	103	32.2
Lundia Alpha 600	171	145	131	42.9
CentrySystem 100HG*	73	56	50	14.9
CentrySystem 200	145	114	94	24.3
F4	143	115	76	24.3
FB 70U	168	149	143	82.0
HT80	157	131	120	33.5
Focus 90	159	132	114	28.6
CentrySystem 400HG	161	137	127	39.1
Alwall GFE 12	169	143	127	36.3
Disscap 160E	176	153	139	45.7
CA 130	169	144	120	60.4
F6	170	150	117	40.2
BL 643LF	164	145	116	52.8
EDG 1.5/32	137	110	87	33.1
Clirans SE 15	171	154	148	84.9

*Clearance data at a blood flowrate of 100 ml/min.

Table 19.   In vitro clearance characteristics of high flux haemodialysers and haemofilters

	Clearance (ml/min)			
	Urea	Creatinine	Phosphate	Vitamin B_{12}
Crystal 2800	155	134	120	78
Crystal 3400	158	135	123	81
F40	149	128	125	81.3
F60	169	156	154	106.1
BL 627	161	145	143	87
Focus 160H	184	170	164	73.9
Altraflux	159	142	134	79.9
F8	176	164	139	76.8

Table 20.   In vivo clearance characteristics of standard haemodialysers

	Clearance (ml/min)		
	Urea	Creatinine	Phosphate
Lundia Alpha 400	152	119	124
Lundia Alpha 600	170	136	145
CentrySystem 100HG	N/A	N/A	N/A
CentrySystem 200	144	104	97
F4	143	115	58
FB 70U	N/A	N/A	N/A
HT80	156	128	125
Focus 90	164	125	115
CentrySystem 400HG	169	143	137
Alwall GFE 12	167	143	132
Disscap 160E	170	139	121
CA 130	167	134	123
F6	172	136	106
BL 643LF	169	145	112
EDG 1.5/32	152	123	95
Clirans SE 15	179	148	148

N/A: Not available.

Table 21. In vivo clearance characteristics of high flux and large surface area haemodialysers

	Clearance (ml/min)		
	Urea	Creatinine	Phosphate
Crystal 2800	152	121	127
Crystal 3400	159	128	143
F40	154	130	128
F60	179	159	154
BL 627	159	135	141
Focus 160H	184	146	159
Altraflux	166	134	136
F8	181	163	126

FACTORS INFLUENCING SOLUTE TRANSPORT

Operating conditions

The relationship between blood flow and solute clearance is shown in Figure 16. The relationship is similar for solute clearance and dialysate flow rate. Studies by Sigdell and Tersteegen (99) showed that the practical upper limit of dialysate flow is $Q_D = 2Q_B$, beyond which the gain in solute removal is minimal and any improvement must be balanced by the extra cost. Consequently the use of high dialysate flow rates to enhance solute removal should be

to the membrane (90, 91). In view of this the kinetics of β_2 microglobulin has received study not only during haemodialysis (92–94), but also other modes of therapy (95, 96). Beta 2 microglobulin removal by membranes now forms part of the characterisation of new membranes used in haemodialysers and associated devices (8, 97, 98).

confined to blood flow rates in excess of 300 ml/min. The impact of ultrafiltration or convective mass transport on solute removal has received extensive study (80, 100–103). However, no universal agreement exists in between a theoretically correct and practically useful method of predicting the effect of ultrafiltration on solute clearance.

Blood composition

Following the availability of recombinant human erythropoietin (r-HuEPO) as a treatment for anaemia associated with chronic renal failure, the effect of haematocrit on dialyser solute clearance has been studied by a number of investigators. The findings of these studies which have been reviewed elsewhere (104) and show reduced solute clearances following the rise in haematocrit, a finding that has also been observed following blood transfusion (105). Since blood is a non-homogenous medium, disequilibrium between plasma and red cells may also be present and further influence *in vivo* solute removal (106) particularly in rapid high efficiency therapies.

Membrane properties

The overall performance of blood purification devices is determined by the mass transport properties of the membrane which are related to membrane structure. Mathematical relationships describing solute flux across membranes have been derived in the literature (107) and show that:

a) In haemodialysis and haemofiltration, the transmembrane transport rate is proportional to the porosity of the membrane and the sieving coefficient and is inversely proportional to the membrane thickness.

b) In haemofiltration the transmembrane transport rate is effected by the radius of the pores in the membrane and fluid viscosity and is independent of the molecular weight provided the sieving coefficient approaches unity. Other membrane related factors which influence solute transport include the structure and surface charge which not only influences the removal of negatively charged solutes such as phosphate (108–110) but is also implicated in adhesion of cellular elements on the membrane (J. Vienken, pers. comm.).

WATER TRANSPORT CHARACTERISTICS

During haemodialysis, haemodiafiltration and haemofiltration, plasma water is removed. The fluid removal has two components – the first due to the hydrostatic pressure gradient exerted as the blood flows through the device ($Q_{F(h)}$), the other is due to the osmotic transmembrane pressure gradient ($Q_{F(osm)}$) such that:

$$Q_F = Q_{F(h)} + Q_{F(osm)}.$$

During haemodialysis, the overall contribution from the latter component is dependent upon the composition of the dialysis fluid. A special case of the osmotic pressure gradient is the pressure exerted by the proteins in plasma, since the proteins used in renal replacement therapy are considered to be impermeable to proteins.

The colloid-osmotic or oncotic pressure may be estimated from consideration of the serum globulin and albumin concentrations. At normal plasma protein concentrations this pressure is about 25 mmHg.

The transmembrane pressure in the device is given by:

$$TMP = \frac{P_{Bin} + P_{Bout}}{2} + \frac{P_{Din} + P_{Dout}}{2} - P_{osm}.$$

The relative importance of this correction is small when the hydrostatic pressure gradient dominates the fluid removal.

The water transport characteristics of haemodialysers and associated devices may be expressed in terms of the device's surface area, membrane hydraulic permeability and the hydrostatic pressure gradient such that:

$$Q_F = [L_h A]TMP.$$

This relationship may be most easily studied *in vitro* where in contrast to the clinical situation, monitoring of the pressures may be practical. Extrapolation of *in vitro* data, if established using aqueous solutions is difficult, since the pressure drop in the blood pathway may be influenced by thrombus formation during clinical use, fouling of the membrane by proteins and blood components as well as the variable relationship between haematocrit and viscosity.

In practice, a linear relationship exists between the mean transmembrane pressure applied and the ultrafiltration rate, although deviations from linearity may occur due to membrane fouling by proteins or blood components, while in parallel plate devices, draping of the membrane over the support structure may contribute to such deviation. In haemofiltration the filtrate flux is less dependent upon the hydrostatic pressure and is governed by the haemodynamic conditions in the device. Theoretical relationships that describe the ultrafiltration flux for both flat sheet and hollow fibre devices in terms of geometric dimensions, mean flow rate through the device, and wall shear rate have been described elsewhere (111).

Tables 22–23 summarise the *in vitro* and, where available, the *in vivo* ultrafiltration coefficients. During clinical use, the amount of protein which adsorbs onto the membrane and the oncotic pressure may vary and, as a result of these factors, *in vivo* ultrafiltration coefficients determined directly may be some 20–25% lower than those measured *in vitro* by the use of bovine blood diluted by saline (112).

The clinical use of haemodialysers utilising high permeability membranes represents a special situation. Since

Table 22. Ultrafiltration characteristics of standard haemodialysers

	Ultrafiltration coefficient (ml/h/mmHg)	
	In vitro	*In vivo*
Lundia Alpha 400	4.4	3.0
Lundia Alpha 600	5.3	5.0
CentrySystem 100HG	2.1	1.8
CentrySystem 200	2.6	2.4
F4	3.0	3.0
FB 70U	83.6	N/A
HT80	4.5	4.2
Focus 90	3.8	4.3
CentrySystem 400HG	6.8	5.5
Alwall GFE 12	5.0	5.9
Disscap 160E	6.9	N/A
CA 130	9.7	N/A
F6	7.5	N/A
BL 643LF	8.0	7.9
EDG 1.5/32	9.8	5.2
Clirans SE 15	21.5	9.0

N/A: Not available.

Table 23. Ultrafiltration characteristics of large surface area and high flux devices

	Ultrafiltration coefficient (ml/h/mmHg)	
	In vitro	*In vivo*
Crystal 2800	45.6	
Crystal 3400	75.0	
F40	20[a]	
F60	40[a]	
BL 627	63[b]	
Focus 160H	11.0	8.5[c]
Altraflux	64.0	18.0[c]
F8	10.6	8.1[c]

[a]Manufacturers data *ex vivo*.
[b]Manufacturers data *in vitro*.
[c]Manufacturers data expected *in vivo*.

such membranes are used in conjunction with proportionating systems incorporating ultrafiltration control, whereby the pressure generated in the blood pathway is offset by the pressure in the dialysate pathway to minimise fluid removal. In such situations, water flux may occur in two directions – first from the blood to the dialysate, i.e., ultrafiltration and second, from the dialysate to the blood, termed back filtration. Although it has been suggested that this is principally a feature of high flux membranes, the phenomenon of back filtration still occurs with high efficiency dialysers, albeit at a lesser degree (113, 114).

Back filtration during haemodialysis varies with axial position and depends upon the pressure profiles in the blood and dialysate pathways. At any location within the device, the opposing pressure forces in the blood and dialysate compartments govern the direction of filtration. Several approaches have been proposed to model back filtration and, therefore, predict the amount of dialysate infused into the blood during treatment; these have been analysed and compared by Soltys et al. (115).

The clinical significance of back filtration is yet to be determined. However, concern has been expressed that in the presence of reverse ultrafiltration contaminants from the dialysate such as pyrogens can enter the patient's blood stream, cause fever and stimulate the release of biologically active cytokines (116–121). These concerns are not without justification inasmuch as contamination of the dialysate either from the water used or from the concentrate is well recognised (122–124).

FACTORS INFLUENCING WATER TRANSPORT

Water transport in haemodialysers and associated devices are dependent upon a range of factors, some of which are interlinked and related to the characteristics of the membrane, operating conditions, device geometry, blood composition and temperature.

Membrane characteristics

Membranes used in haemodialysers and associated devices are batch produced and subject to interbatch variation. Manufacturers' product sheets for Cuprophan membranes indicate that the variation in ultrafiltration is of the order of ± 8–10% depending upon the membrane type. Between batches of the same membrane, ultrafiltration may also be influenced by storage conditions, particularly temperature and humidity (125), and it is important to follow manufacturer's instructions in storing haemodialysers. Membrane structure and thus hydraulic permeability may also be influenced by the method of sterilisation (126).

In parallel plate devices, changes in membrane permeability may result from the stretching of the membrane over the support structure, although in practice, such an increase may be negated by concomitant loss of surface area (127).

Blood composition

The influence of plasma protein concentration on ultrafiltration rate for conventional haemodialysers is small. However, for haemofiltration and haemodiafiltration the protein concentration in the plasma water, haematocrit and blood viscosity affect the rate of ultrafiltration. At low blood flow rates, the ratio between ultrafiltration rate and plasma flow may exceed 30%, and under such circumstances the plasma protein concentration rises. The oncotic pressure thus generated will act against the filtration. Proteins may also be deposited on the membrane during use and form a secondary or concentration-polarisation layer which will influence the membrane permeability. This effect may be minimised by the use of high flow rates through the blood pathway which induces a high shear rate at the membrane-blood interface and minimise deposition.

Haematocrit influences filtration rates in both conventional and continuous therapies since haemoconcentration occurs as blood passes through the device which in turn influences the filtration rate (128).

The effect of high haematocrit on ultrafiltration rates in haemodialysis has been studied by Ofsthun et al. (112), who showed that increases in haematocrit can lead to axial variation of transmembrane pressure which, if ignored, result in inaccurate fluid removal during treatment. The effect of increased haematocrit on the rate of back filtration has been investigated by Robertson and Curtin (129) who showed that the rate of back filtration is increased from 10.1 ml/min at a haematocrit of 20% to 15.7 ml/min when the haematocrit rises to 33%.

Fluid dynamic conditions

The dependence of ultrafiltration on the fluid dynamic conditions within haemodialysers and associated devices is complex and for this reason it has not been studied. Its role is particularly important in haemofilters where the filtration flux is dependent upon the shear rate or the velocity gradient at the blood membrane interface. It may also be important in the context of patients receiving erythropoietin therapy.

Temperature

During haemodialysis, temperature differences between the blood and dialysate pathway may be present and this, in turn, may influence fluid flux.

PLASMA FILTRATION

In contrast to haemodialysis and related therapies where only plasma water is removed during treatment, in plasma filtration, or plasma separation, the plasma proteins pass through the membrane but the cellular elements of blood are retained. This separation is a function of the membrane properties, the characteristics of the blood (i.e., its constituents) and the flow dynamics. A number of theories describing plasma separation have been reviewed elsewhere (130). Where the rate of filtration is dependent upon the applied pressure, in contrast to haemodialysis, a plateau is reached at which increase in pressure does not result in an increase in filtration rate due to flux limiting phenomena. A new process called dynamic filtration to enhance plasma filtration by the use of a pulsation generator has recently been described (131). Haemolysis or the damage of red cells due to their deformation as they are forced through the pores of the membrane is another limiting factor of plasma separation.

STERILISATION

Early haemodialysers were sterilised by the use of formaldehyde. Today, haemodialysers and associated devices may be sterilised either by ethylene oxide (ETO), ionising radiation (γ rays), heat, or by the use of aqueous disfectant solutions (aldehydes, peracetic acid, hypochlorite, hydrogen peroxide).

ETO sterilisation is the method of choice for the sterilisation of many medical disposables, since most materials are unaffected by the sterilisation process. Furthermore, because of the highly diffusive nature of ETO, the devices may be sterilised ready packed for shipment. A disadvantage of the diffusive nature of ETO, is its adsorption into polymers that are used in haemodialysers (132). IgE antibodies against ETO have been suspected as a causative factor in the acute hypersensitivity reactions observed at the onset of haemodialysis (133); while residual ETO in sterilised plastic tubing, has been also reported as a cause of haemolysis in heart lung bypass (134). Two other important factors associated with ethylene oxide sterilisation of devices are penetration and aeration. To permit the former and facilitate the latter, the packaging of the device must contain materials that allow ETO diffusion. Such material should also be impermeable to microbes to maintain sterilising during storage. Although extensively used, occupational exposure to ETO represents a potential health hazard and stringent occupational exposure limits are imposed (135). This, coupled with environmental concerns, is likely to limit future use of this method of device sterilisation.

Sterilising of haemodialysers and associated devices by ionising radiation is increasingly being employed as an alternative to ETO sterilisation (Figure 18). In Europe in 1986, it was used in 2% of produced dialysers, while by 1992, its use has grown to 8.4%. Its use in Japan is much higher. The sterilisation is accomplished by the use of γ rays generated from ^{60}Cobalt. The product is placed in close proximity to the source until the required dose level has been obtained. Dosimetric methods are used to control the radiation process and the general irradiation level is 2.5 Megarads (or 2.5 KGy). More recently, there has been much interest in reducing the sterilisation dose to 2.0 Megarads provided that the product bioburden is low since lower radiation exposure limits membrane degradation (136, 137). The radiation resistance of

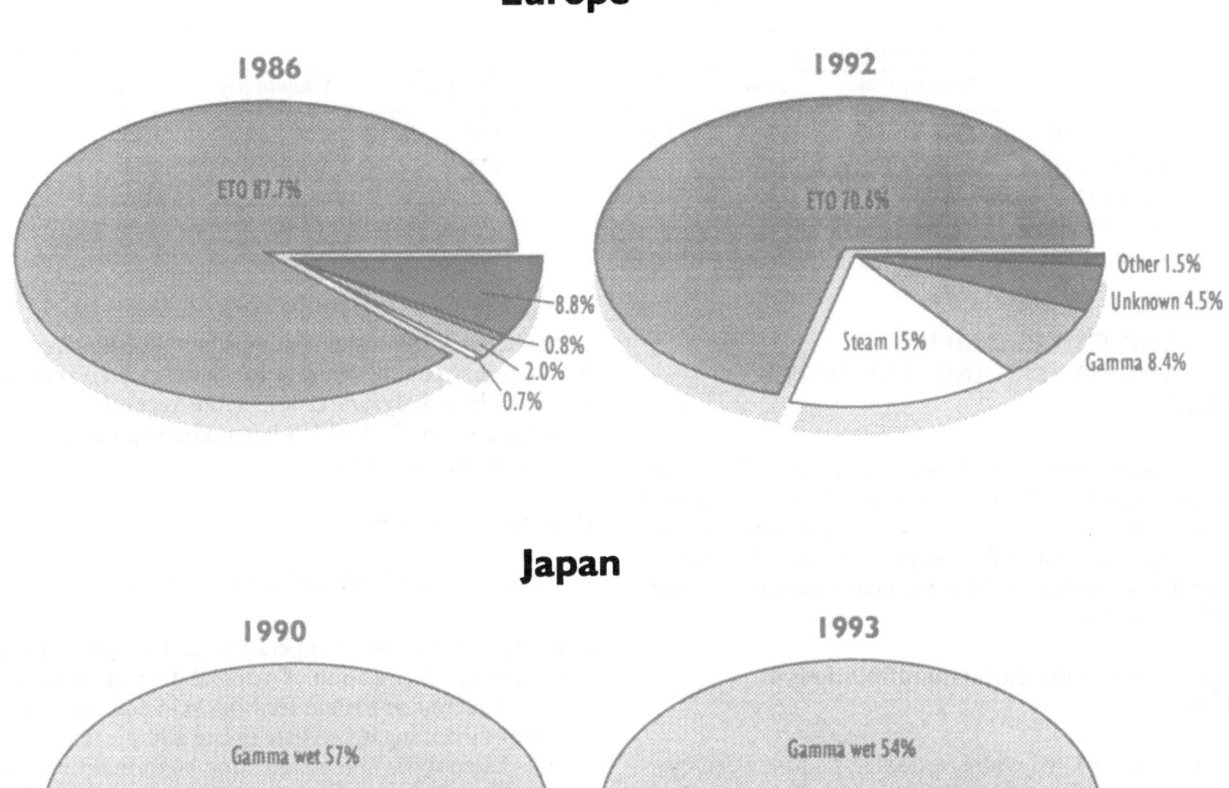

Figure 18. Methods used to sterilise haemodialysers and associated devices in Europe and Japan. Data courtesy of Dr J Vienken IMMA, Akzo-Nobel.

commonly used materials varies (138), discoloration may occur following irradiation while aromatic polyurethane compounds may release carcinogenic methylene dianiline (MDA) following irradiation (139, 140).

Steam sterilisation of medical devices is widely used and pre-vacuum high temperature steam sterilisers are the most practical method of sterilising a wide range of products. Destruction of bacteria by this method is dependent upon the time exposed and the temperature of exposure. A typical procedure for haemodialysers would involve heating the device for 20 minutes at a temperature of 121°C followed by venting, cooling and drying phases. With this technique there is absence of chemical residues following sterilisation. As with gamma irradiation careful selection of materials must be made since membrane degradation can occur but may be minimised by its pre-treatment with glycerin-water mixture. In contrast with ethylene oxide

and gamma sterilisation procedures, steam sterilisation cannot be undertaken in the shipping case.

Sterilisation with aqueous solutions is usually performed during reuse of haemodialysers. The procedure is simple, but membrane performance or integrity may change following exposure to the sterilising agent (141, 142), the presence of air bubbles on the material surface may reduce the effectiveness of sterilisation. The effect of sterilisation on haemodialyser functional performance is shown in Table 24. This data indicates that, whereas ETO and gamma irradiation yield comparable performance with steam sterilisation, the performance is lower due to the structural changes induced in the membrane by the sterilisation process. These findings are consistent with those of Takesawa et al. (143).

Table 24. Influence of sterilisation procedure on haemodialyser performance

Dialyser	Clearance (ml/min)					Ultrafiltration (ml/h/mmHg)
	Sterilisation	Urea	Creatinine	Phosphate	Vitamin B$_{12}$	
Althin AFB 12 08	Steam	156	135	119	42.1	6.8
Althin AFE 12 08	ETO	167	145	132	46.6	6.1
Althin AFG 12 08	γ ray	169	147	132	46.8	6.8

Results shown at zero ultrafiltration for a blood flow rate of 200 ml/min.

REACTIONS MEDIATED BY HAEMODIALYSERS AND ASSOCIATED DEVICES

Extracorporeal circulatory procedures involve the repeated exposure of blood to components of the extracorporeal circuit, namely the haemodialyser or associated device, the tubing comprising the circuit and possible residues remaining in the system from the manufacturing and sterilisation processes.

Classification and clinical manifestations of reactions

Reactions associated with haemodialysis have been classified by Daugirdas and Ing (144) as either Type A or Type B reactions. In Type A reactions such as those described by Nicholls and Platts (145) the onset of the symptoms is usually immediate or within the first few minutes of dialysis, but on occasion, the reactions may be delayed up to 20 minutes following the start of treatment. Such reactions varied in their severity but were typical of anaphylaxis. The second type of reaction (Type B) were generally milder and were not associated with anaphylactic or allergic type of symptoms. The onset of these symptoms were often later (20–40 minutes) after the commencement of treatment and usually abated after the first hour (144).

Incidence of hypersensitivity reactions during haemodialysis

When non-disposable, reusable parallel plate haemodialysers were used, febrile reactions during treatment were frequently seen. Although it was suggested that such reactions were due to endogenous factors such as infection rather than exogenous factors, their cause was never satisfactorily explained and it is possible that as well as some of the causes discussed below, the manual assembly and soaking of the membranes in saline and chemical sterilisation all contributed. The epidemiology of reactions during haemodialysis have been the subject of recent studies in the United States, which have shown that the greatest incidence of reactions was noted in patients dialysing with hollow fibre devices compared with parallel plate devices, with the incidence of observed reactions in the former group being 3.3/thousand patients/annum compared with 0.3/thousand patients/annum for patients dialysing with parallel plate dialysers (146). More recently, reactions were reported in 31% of US haemodialysis centres when using new dialysers (147).

Responsible factors

Ethylene oxide and its breakdown products

Ethylene oxide is a low temperature sterilising agent widely used in the sterilisation of medical devices. It has long been considered an irritant for both skin and mucosa and capable of inducing immediate or late allergic reactions as well as haemolysis and coagulation abnormalities (148). It was first suggested that it may be a mediator of Type A reactions as early as 1975 (149). Ethylene oxide (ETO) when conjugated to human serum albumin (HSA) to form ETO-HSA acts as an allergen. A strong association of anaphylactoid reactions in the presence of IgE against ETO-HSA is well documented (150, 151) and is established by the use of a radioallergosorbent assay (RAST). The finding that reactions were much rarer with plate dialysers focused attention on its cause; it was found that the potting compound used in hollow fibre devices acted as a reservoir for ethylene oxide which was inadequately removed during preparation prior to use (152, 153).

Leachables

Patients undergoing regular extracorporeal circulatory procedures are particularly prone to the problem of leachables from the extracorporeal circuit as they are repeatedly exposed to the same material over a long time. Such leachables include the plasticiser from the blood tubing (154) and have led to the search for alternatives to the commonly used di–2-ethylhexyl-phthalate (DEHP) (155, 156) and the development of co-extruded tubings (157). Leachables originating from the haemodialyser include isopropylmyristrate, methanol, and freon, used in the production of hollow fibres while potting compounds made from polyurethane generate isocyanates (158, 159). Other unidentified materials have been implicated as the cause of iritis and scleritis in haemodialysis patients (160). Haemodialysers also contain particulate matter (161, 162) but no reactions have been specifically attributed to such particles.

Blood membrane interactions

During contact of blood with the membrane contained in the haemodialyser, several physiological pathways as well as cellular mechanisms are activated. The details of the activation is outside the scope of this chapter. Instead, discussion is confined to the role of the haemodialyser or associated device in these reactions.

Activation of the coagulation system

Activation of the coagulation system occurs as soon as the blood comes into contact with a foreign surface. If the process is not controlled by the administration of an anti-coagulant, thrombus formation occurs with subsequent clotting. The first event in this process is protein adsorption onto the surface with simultaneous platelet activation. The interaction of platelets with the surface depends not only upon the surface, but also the local haemodynamic and rheological forces (163) and, consequently, plate and capillary dialysers would be expected to affect platelets differently. However, experimental studies by Taylor et al. (164) failed to demonstrate such differences. The role of the membrane in mediating both protein adsorption and platelet activation has been studied by a number of investigators (165–167) and the observed differences may be influenced by not only membrane structure but also membrane permeability and surface characteristics (168).

Activation of the contact pathway

The body's defence mechanisms in plasma consist of a series of interlinked biochemical pathways which include the fibrinolytic and kinin systems. Blood contact with the surface involves the binding of Hageman factor (Factor XII) and circulating complexes of high molecular weight kininogen with pre-kallikrein. The activation of Hageman factor and pre-kallikrein results in the formation of kallikrein at the surface. This pathway of activation is influenced by the membrane charge (169). Following discoveries made by Ferreira (170) and Erdos (171). A series of bradykinin potentiating compounds (angiotensin converting enzyme inhibitors, ACEIs) have been developed and now constitute a group of drugs used in the treatment of hypertension and congestive heart failure. Such drugs not only block the angiotensin converting enzyme, but also the kininase enzyme (172) and thus in the presence of ACE inhibitors bradykinin is not degraded leading to elevated levels in the circulation resulting in adverse biological sequelae. Several reports in the literature have appeared describing such reactions particularly when using AN69 membranes (173–175), and LDL apheresis (176) which utilises negatively charged dextran surface particles. Following these clinical observations, the ability of negatively charged membranes to generate bradykinin has been demonstrated in laboratory studies (177) which did not find generation in either Cuprophan or the recently developed SPAN membrane (Akzo-Nobel).

Activation of the immune system

Complement is the principal mediator of the acute inflammatory response. Biomaterial surfaces in contact with blood activate the complement system. Interest in the activation of complement during haemodialysis stems from the work of Craddock et al. (178) which implicated this process as the cause of granulocytopenia during haemodialysis. Although activation of the complement system can occur via two distinct pathways, the classical or alternate pathway, it is the alternate pathway that is primarily involved in the activation following blood contact with biomaterials. Activation is initiated by the deposition of C3b on the membrane surface which with Factor B forms C3 and C5 convertases. These enzymes are able to cleave the anaphylatoxins C3a and C5a from C3 and C5 respectively by an auto-catalytic process. In plasma the C-terminal arginine is removed and C3a des Arg and C5a des Arg are formed. It is the measurement of these fractions that is undertaken when haemodialysis induced complement activation is quantified. The cleavage of C5 by C5 convertase results not only in the production of C5a but also in C5b which initiates a macromolecular complex of proteins, the membrane attack complex (MAC) which is composed of C5b, C6, C7, C8 and C9 and is alternatively known as C5b-9 complex.

Haemodialysis membranes differ in their ability to induce not only C3 and C5 activation (8, 179–183) but also in their capacity to form C5bb-9 (184, 185).

The ability of cellulose based membranes to activate complement is probably related to the structure of cellulose since modification of this structure alters the magnitude of complement activation. However, there does not seem to be a straightforward relationship between the number of OH groups replaced in the basic structure or by the type of replacement (179) and it is more probable that the differences are a consequence of the ability of the membranes to bind regulatory proteins (Factor B, a promoter of activation, Factor H an inhibitor of activation) (186). Adsorption of the complement fractions on the membrane also contributes to the observed differences (187). The long term sequelae associated with repeated complement activation are at present unclear and require further investigation. Hakim et al. (188) described excessive generation of C3a des Arg in patients suffering from hypersensitivity reactions and suggested that not only the enhanced generation but also the diminished degradation of the components were contributory factors in these reactions. A subsequent study by Lemke et al. (133), however, failed to demonstrate differences in the patterns of complement activation in patients with and without hypersensitivity reactions.

Cellular changes and activation

Platelets

Platelets play an important role in the evolution of thrombus formation following blood membrane contact in a haemodialyser. Associated with the adherence of platelets is platelet activation leading to the release of platelet factor 4 (PF4) and β thromboglobulin. The activation of platelets during haemodialysis may be assessed by monitoring such changes (189). However, the interpretation of changes is difficult due to their dependence on heparin administered during treatment.

Leucocytes

Leucocytes may be classified as polymorphonuclear granulocytes (neutrophils, eosinophils, basophils), monocytes and lymphocytes. In the early stages of haemodialysis a drop in the number of leucocytes occurs reaching a nadir at 15 minutes, and is reversed by the first hour of treatment, a phenomenon first described by Kaplow and Goffinet (190). The magnitude of the changes is membrane dependent, and the fall in leucocyte count is due to sequestration in the lung vasculature resulting from changes in cell surface antigen expression following complement activation (191–193). The transient leucopenia during haemodialysis has been used extensively to characterise different membranes. However, the associated events rather than the leucopenia itself, are likely to be more important in the long term. It has been postulated that the repeated contact of activated neutrophils and the pulmonary endothelium may be implicated in the development of haemodialysis related amyloidosis (194), as well as being partly responsible for the hypoxia observed during haemodialysis (195, 196).

Contact with haemodialysis membranes results in the release of proteinases (197, 198) which have been used to characterise membrane induced cell activation. Granulocyte activation and release reactions are, however, influenced by heparin which is able to reduce elastase release, superoxide production and adhesion of stimulated granulocytes to endothelial cells (199) while the dialyser configuration may also influence granulocyte activation (200). Eosinophilia is known to occur during haemodialysis (201). Its incidence and cause has been reviewed by Vanherweghem et al. (202) and showed that in 971 patients treated with various strategies it was found at least once in 35.4% of the patients and that the incidence increased with duration on dialysis. Eosinophilia was higher in patients treated with hollow fibre dialysers compared with parallel plate devices suggesting a role for ETO. More recently, Hertel et al. (203) demonstrated a link between eosinophilia and cytokine production. Between 2–8% of the total leucocytes are monocytes. There is increasing evidence that monocytes are stimulated to produce Interleukin 1 (IL-1) (204–206). The mechanisms involved in this stimulation are:

a) bacterial contamination of the dialysate and the back transfer into the blood across the dialyser membrane
b) direct contact between monocytes and the membrane contained in the haemodialyser
c) the action of the complement components activated by the membrane on the monocytes

More recently, attention (in respect of this dialysis related phenomenon) has focused upon the measurements of IL-1 receptor antagonist (IL-1Ra), a molecule structurally related to IL-1 which is present in much larger quantities than IL-1 making its measurement much easier (207). Although the membranes themselves have been implicated in the production of IL-1, production resulting from stimulation by particles originating from dialysis tubing has also been described (208).

Red cells

During extracorporeal circulatory procedures damage to red cells can occur which, in extreme cases, may lead to haemolysis. The cause of such damage may be a result of fluid mechanical factors such as pump malocclusion, kinked blood lines (209), abnormalities of the dialysate (210) or the presence of chemicals in the dialysate circuit originating from reuse or sterilisation (211, 212). Other causes reported have included undetected excessive ultrafiltration (213) and arterial negative pressure (214) during treatment. Red blood cells act as a major site for deposition of C5b-9, the membrane attack complex leading to lysis and sublethal or lethal damage. The potential clinical relevance of this aspect of membrane biocompatibility has not been studied to date.

Pyrogens and bacteria

Infection remains a common complication of haemodialysis and associated treatments. Although a large number of these are the consequence of vascular access infections (215). The use of bicarbonate dialysate, facilitating the growth of pathogenic organisms in the dialysate pathway, may also increase the risk of infection in patients receiving regular dialysis therapy (147) particularly in view of the fact that membranes used in renal replacement therapy, while impermeable to bacteria, may permit the passage of bacterial fragments (121, 216–217). This has focused attention on the microbiological quality of water and concentrate used in haemodialysis and related therapies (218, 219) and methods of minimising such contamination (220–223).

When non-disposable dialysers were used pyrogen reactions were frequently encountered. Early disposable dialysers also contained significant levels of leachable bacterial endotoxin (224). Gordon et al. (225) studied the epidemiology of febrile reactions in patients receiving haemodialysis and observed an incidence of 0.7 pyrogenic reactions per 1000 treatments when using heavily contaminated dialysate. Both studies agreed that the bacterial contamination of the dialysate was the principal factor involved and suggested that to avoid the risk of pyrogenic reactions, compliance with dialysate water standards should be supplemented by filtration of the dialysate prior to its entering the dialyser (226). Recent studies concerning the incidence of pyrogen reactions in other modes of renal replacement therapy are unavailable, but Schaeffer et al. (227) studied the occurrence of fever during haemodialysis compared with haemofiltration and demonstrated an occurrence of 4.84% compared with 0.81%.

SPECIAL APPLICATIONS OF HAEMODIALYSERS AND ASSOCIATED DEVICES

Haemodialysers and associated devices may be considered as single mass exchanges or devices used for filtration. As such, they have been used in a number of non-renal applications. Such applications include ascites filtration and reinfusion (228–232), combined treatment of refractory ascites and renal insufficiency (233, 234), artificial liver support (235, 236) and respiratory support (237, 238). Haemodialysis has also been used for the treatment of accidental hypothermia (239). Its use in other non-uremic situations has been reviewed by Splendiani (240).

CHOOSING A HAEMODIALYSER OR ASSOCIATED DEVICE

The choice of device for delivery of therapy is a complex decision, involving not only the functional performance of the device, the device's biocompatibility profile but also the philosophy of treatment and available equipment. With the wide range of devices and performances, the clinician is often faced with a considerable dilemma in aiming at the most appropriate choice.

To help in the choice and to enable a number of parameters to be compared, a graphical representation enabling several devices to be compared on multiple criteria is useful (241). Radar graphs or star charts, part of spreadsheet programmes for personal computers or standalone graphics packages facilitate such comparisons since lines radiating from the centre represent each category, with values shown by the distance from the centre. An example of such representation is shown in Figure 19.

FUTURE TRENDS

Prior to discussing future trends, it is useful to reflect upon the advances and developments of the last decade in respect of haemodialysers and associated devices. Early design efforts were concerned with the improvement of solute transport. The influence of design variables on clinical performance are shown in Table 25. Of these surface area, blood and dialysate pathway geometry and minimisation of boundary layers have all been improved and have led to an overall improvement in device performance. Improvements in manufacturing technology have resulted in the production of highly reliable devices so that blood leaks during clinical use are rare and can usually be traced to a faulty preparation procedure or incorrect storage and handling. The options for further improvement of existing devices has, however, become limited. Enhanced molecular clearance and ultrafiltration may be achieved by using pulsable flow (242) or by the use of extraluminal flow (ELF), a concept described by Catapano et al. (243) in which the conventionally used fibre bundle is replaced by layered knitted membrane mats wrapped around a central solid core in which the blood flows through the membrane mesh generating secondary flow patterns. This concept is particularly appropriate in haemofiltration and plasma separation where the blood side resistance is the limiting factor in mass transfer across the membrane.

Depending on the membrane material and the production processes involved, it is possible to construct different membrane structures. The membrane permeability as well as its biocompatibility will be dependent upon such structural aspects. However, such membranes are likely to be non-specific in their removal of metabolites and future developments will include some specificity possibly in the form of sites for specific adsorption. Until the availability of such membranes, existing devices may be combined with adsorbent columns which would enhance the removal of molecules such as β_2 microglobulin (244) and phosphate.

At present, clinically used devices use a single type of membrane. The concept of devices containing blended membranes to enhance performance has been described by Tanaka (245) but has not seen widespread application.

Considerable differences in patient survival between countries exist (246). The cause of this difference is a matter of some debate. However, in connection with the long term complications arising from regular dialysis therapy, interest has inevitably focused upon biocompatibility. It is true that the numerous studies that have been undertaken in this area have increased our knowledge and understanding of the phenomena involved. Their correlation with clinical outcome remains largely unsubstantiated. However, recent studies suggest that the clinical outcome and patient morbidity may be influenced by membrane biocompatibility (247–249).

Coagulation of blood following contact with a foreign surface has long been recognised as a problem. In haemodialysis, heparin is used as an anticoagulant. This form of anticoagulation may give rise to complications (250) or be unsuitable for patients at risk from haemorrhage. Since the efficacy of continuous therapies depends

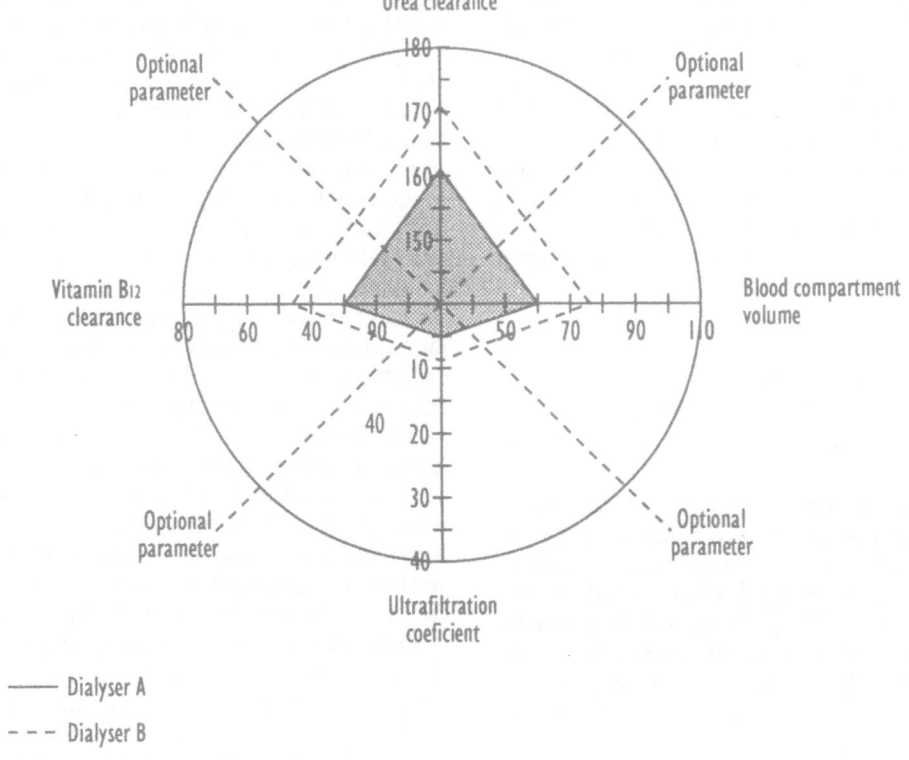

Figure 19. Comparison of haemodialyser performance using multiple criteria.

Table 25. Device design variables and their influence on performance

		Clearance		Ultrafiltration	Flow resistance	Blood contained	Blood loss
		Small molecules	Large molecules				
Device	Surface area	↑	↑	↑	↑	↑	↑
	Blood pathway geometry	↑	↑	↑	↑	↑	↑
	Dialysate pathway geometry	↑	↔	↑		↔	↔
Membrane	Permeability	↔	↑	↑	↔	↔	↔
	Thrombogenecity	↑	↑	↑	↑		↑

↔: No effect.
↑: Positive influence.

in a large part on the continuous maintenance of adequate solute and water removal rates at a constant level over a long period, the use of coatings such as Duraflo II (Baxter Healthcare Corporation) is likely to lead to the attainment of this important requirement without use of additional heparinisation and additionally will permit safe use of continous modalities of treatment in patients for whom systemic anticoagulation is contraindicated (251–253).

Pressures to contain health care costs will inevitably hinder major developments, lead to product rationalisation and company mergers. Many of the materials used in existing devices will need to be reconsidered not only in respect of their biocompatibility but also to permit change from the current ethylene oxide to gamma or other methods of sterilisation due to environmental pressure which will also influence the disposal of haemodialysers and associated devices.

NOMENCLATURE

A	Area
C	Concentration
D	Dialysance
HCT	Haematocrit
K	Clearance
L	Length
Lh	Permeability
N	Integer
P	Pressure
Q	Flow
R	Mass transfer resistance
R'	Recirculation
S	Surface area, sieving coefficient
W	Width
π	Universal constant
d	Diameter
h	Blood film thickness
k'	Equilibrium solute partition coefficient
μ	Viscosity
ϕ	Volume fraction of hydrated proteins

Subscripts

B, b	Blood
D	Dialysate
F	Filtrate
HDF	Haemodiafiltration
M	Membrane
P	Plasma
PFD	Paired filtration dialysis
T	Total
W	Water
i, in, inlet	Inlet
o, out, outlet	Outlet
h	Hydraulic
osm	Osmotic

REFERENCES

1. Davies SP, Reaveley DA, Brown EA, Kox WJ: Amino-acid clearances and daily losses in patients with acute-renal-failure treated by continuous arteriovenous hemodialysis. *Critical Care Med* 19: 1510, 1991
2. Brunner H, Schafer U, Mann H, Stiller S, Sieberth HG: Molecular-weight distribution in ultrafiltrates of different filters used for continuous arteriovenous hemofiltration. *Chromatographia* 22: 399, 1986
3. Abel JJ, Rowntree LG, Turner BB: On removal of diffusible substances from circulating blood of living animals by dialysis. *J Pharmacol Exp* 5: 275, 1913–1914
4. Vienken J: Dialysis with cellulosic membranes 1992. Analysis of recent clinical and statistical data. *Eur Dial Transplant Nurse Assoc-Eur Renal Care Assoc J* 18: 13, 1992
5. Babb AL, Farrell PC, Uvelli DA, Scribner BH: Haemodialyzer evaluation by examination of solute molecular spectra. *Trans Am Soc Artif Intern Organs* 18: 98, 1972
6. Man NK, Granger A, Rondon-Nucete M, Zingraff J, Jungers P, Sausse A et al.: One year follow up of short dialysis with a membrane highly permeable to middle molecules. *Proc Eur Dial Transplant Assoc* 10: 236, 1973
7. Drukker W: Haemodialysis: A historical review. in *Replacement of Renal Function by Dialysis*, 3rd ed, edited by Maher JF, Dordrecht, Boston, Lancaster, Kluwer Academic Publishers, 1989, p 21
8. Hoenich NA, Woffindin C. Matthews JNS, Goldfinch ME, Turnbull J: Clinical comparison of high-flux cellulose acetate and synthetic membranes. *Nephrol Dial Transplant* 9: 60, 1994
9. Kolff WJ, Berk HThJ: The artificial kidney – a dialyser with a great area. *Acta Med Scand* 117: 121, 1944
10. McBride PT: *Genesis of the Artificial Kidney*, 2nd ed, Baxter Healthcare Corporation, 1987
11. Colton CK: *A Review of the Development and Performance of Hemodialyzers. Artificial Kidney – Chronic Uremia Program*, National Institute of Arthritis and Metabolic Diseases, US Dept of Health Education and Welfare, Washington, 1967
12. Colton CK: Technical foundations of renal prostheses. in *Uremia Therapy*, edited by Gurland HJ, Berlin, Springer Verlag, 1987, p 187
13. Kolff WJ, Watschinger B. Further development of a coil kidney: disposable artificial kidney. *J Lab Clin Med* 47: 969, 1956
14. Hoeltzenbein J: Efficient and inexpensive, no-prime, no-blood-loss haemodialysis system. *Proc Eur Dial Transplant Assoc* 5: 316, 1968
15. Skeggs LT, Leonards JR: Studies on artificial kidney: preliminary results with new type of continuous dialyzer. *Science* 108: 212, 1948
16. Kiil F: Development of a parallel-flow artificial kidney in plastics. *Acta Chir Scand* (Suppl) 253: 142, 1960
17. von Hartitzsch B, Hoenich NA: Meltec Multipoint Haemodialyser. *Br Med J* 1: 237, 1972
18. Edson H, Keen M, Gotch F: Comparative solute transport and therapeutic effectiveness of multiple point support and standard Kiil hemodialyzers. *Trans Am Soc Artif Intern Organs* 18: 113, 1972
19. Lewis KJ, Dewar PJ, Ward MK, Kerr DNS: Formation of anti-N-like antibodies in dialysis patients: Effect of different methods of dialyzer rinsing to remove formaldehyde. *Clin Nephrol* 15: 39, 1981
20. Hakim RM, Friedrich RA, Lowrie EG, Mantilla JM, Lee C: Formaldehyde kinetics and bacteriology in dialyzers. *Kidney Int* 28: 936, 1985
21. Woffindin C, Hoenich NA: Some aspects of residual formaldehyde testing when reusing haemodialysers. *Int J Artif Organs* 8: 313, 1985
22. Howell ED, Perkins HA: Anti-N-like antibodies in the sera of patients undergoing chronic hemodialysis. *Vox Sang* 23: 291, 1972
23. Fassbinder W, Seidl S, Koch KM: The role of formaldehyde in the formation of haemodialysis-associated anti-N-like antibodies. *Vox Sang* 35: 41, 1978
24. Orringer EP, Mattern WD: Formaldehyde-induced hemolysis during chronic hemodialysis. *N Engl J Med* 294: 1416, 1976

25. Fielder RJ, Sorrie GS, Bishop CM, Van Den Heuvel M, Fletcher AP: *Formaldehyde, Toxicity Review*, Her Majesty's Stationery Office, London, 1985
26. Hoenich NA, von Hartitzsch B, Samson PJ, Erickson J, Reed B, Kerr DNS: The Dasco SP 400 disposable dialyser. *Proc Eur Dial Transplant Assoc* 9: 592, 1972
27. Alwall N: A new disposable artificial kidney: Experimental and clinical experience. *Proc Eur Dial Transplant Assoc* 5: 18, 1968
28. von Hartitzsch B, Hoenich NA, Erickson J, Jolly D, Samson P, Reed BR et al.: The Gambro Lundia – a new disposable multilayer dialyser. *Proc Eur Dial Transplant Assoc* 9: 601, 1972
29. Hoenich NA, Conceicao S, White T, Ward MK, Kerr DNS: Large surface area dialysers – a question of performance. *Proc Eur Soc Artif Organs* 3: 185, 1976
30. von Hartitzsch B, Hoenich NA, Johnson J, Brewis RAL, Kerr DNS: The problem of de-aeration – cause, consequence, cure. *Proc Eur Dial Transplant Assoc* 9: 605, 1972
31. Stewart RD, Baretta ED, Cerny JC, Mahon HI: An artificial kidney made from capillary fibres. *Inv Urology* 3: 614, 1966
32. Lindsay RM, Burton JA, Edward N, Dargie HJ, Prentice CRM, Kennedy AC: Dialyser blood loss. *Clin Nephrol* 1: 29, 1973
33. Agishi T, Ota K, Nose Y: Is hollow fibre occlusion due to maldistribution of blood? *Proc Eur Dial Transplant Assoc* 12: 519, 1975
34. Nakagawa S, Koshikawa S, Ishida Y, Uematsu M, Ishibashi K: Development of a flat type hollow fibre dialyser (NF-01). Achievement of better performance than cylinder type with same membrane area. in *Technical Aspects of Renal Dialysis*, edited by Frost TH, Tunbridge Wells, Pitman Medical, 1977, p 29
35. Lee KH, Taylor JA: Multi-chambered dialyzers and their efficiencies. *Artif Organs* 3: 137, 1979
36. Sigdell JE: A Mathematical Theory for the Capillary Artificial Kidney, Stuttgart, Hippokrates Verlag, 1974
37. Ronco C, Mantovani F: *Criteri generali per la valutazione tecnica e clinica dei dializzatori e delle membrane per emodialisi*, Trattato Italiano di Dialisi, Milan, Wichtig Editore, 1992
38. Sigdell JE: New hollow fibre dialyzers. *Artif Organs* 9: 69, 1985
39. Sigdell JE: Operating characteristics of hollow-fiber dialyzers. in *Clinical Dialysis*, 2nd ed, edited by Nissenson AR, Fine RN, Gentile DE, Connecticut, Appleton Lange, 1990, p 97
40. Sakai K: Technical determination of optimal dimensions of hollow fibre membranes for clinical dialysis. *Nephrol Dial Transplant* 4 (Suppl): 73, 1989
41. Babb AL, Popovich RP, Christopher TG, Scribner BH: The genesis of the square meter-hour hypothesis. *Trans Am Soc Artif Intern Organs* 17: 81, 1971
42. Kambic HE, Nose Y: Plasmapheresis: Historical perspective, therapeutic applications, and new frontiers. *Artif Organs* 17: 850, 1993
43. Malchesky PS, Wojcicki J, Horinchi T, Lee JM, Nose Y: Membrane Separation Processes for Macromolecule Removal. in *Plasmapheresis*, edited by Nose Y, Malchesky P, Smith JW, Cleveland, Int Soc Artif Organs Press, 1983, p 51
44. Bellhouse BJ, Lewis RWH: A high efficiency membrane separator for donor plasmapheresis. *Trans Am Soc Artif Intern Organs* 34: 747, 1988
45. Zydney AL, Colton CK: Continuous flow membrane plasmapheresis: Theoretical models for flux and hemolysis prediction. *Trans Am Soc Artif Intern Organs* 28: 408, 1982
46. Malbrancq JM, Jaffrin MY, Bouveret E, Angleraud R, Vantard G: Factors governing plasma filtration rate in plasmapheresis by plane microporous membranes. *Proc Eur Soc Artif Organs* 11: 46, 1982
47. Gardiner AOP, Sawyer AN, Donckerwolcke RA, Haycock GB, Murphy A, Ogg CS et al.: Assessment of dialysis requirement for children on regular hemodialysis. *Dial Transplant* 11: 754, 1982
48. Bosch JP: Continuous Arteriovenous Hemofiltration. in *Hemofiltration*, edited by Henderson LW, Quellhorst EA, Baldamus CA, Lysaght MJ, Berlin, Heidelberg, Springer-Verlag, 1986, p 234
49. Babb AL, Grimsrud L, Bell RL, Layno SB: Engineering aspects of artificial kidney systems. in *Chemical Engineering in Medicine and Biology*, edited by Hershey D, New York, Plenum Press, 1967, p 289
50. Fry D, Hoover PL: Single pass dialysate flow for the Seattle pumpless hemodialysis system. *Trans Am Soc Artif Intern Organs* 10: 98, 1964
51. Sigdell JE, Tersteegen B: Clearance for a dialyzer under varying operating conditions. *Artif Organs* 10: 219, 1986
52. Charm S, Kurland G: Viscometry of human blood for shear rates 0–100,000 sec^{-1}. *Nature* 206: 617, 1965
53. Pallone TH, Petersen J: Continuous arteriovenous hemofiltration: an *in vitro* simulation and mathematical model. *Kidney Int* 33: 685, 1988
54. Pallone TL, Petersen J: A mathematical model of continuous arteriovenous hemofiltration predicts performance. *Trans Am Soc Artif Intern Organs* 33: 304, 1987
55. Sheely ML: Glycerol viscosity tables. *Industrial and Engineering Chemistry* 24: 1060, 1932
56. Takesawa S, Terasawa M, Sakagami M, Kobayashi T, Hidai H, Sakai K: Nondestructive evaluation by X-ray computed tomography of dialysate flow patterns in capillary dialyzers. *Trans Am Soc Artif Intern Organs* 34: 794, 1988
57. Gunnarsson B: Single photon emission tomographic studies of a capillary dialyzer. *ASAIO J* 4: 103, 1981
58. Levenspiel O: *Chemical Reaction Engineering*, 2nd ed, New York, John Wiley, 1972
59. Tello R, March R, Lowrie EG: A model of the reinfusion process at termination of hemodialysis. *Dial Transplant* 12: 444, 1983
60. Saleh TAM: *Investigation into the Washout Characteristics of Flat Plate Rectangular Channels with Supply Systems and Their Application to Haemodialysers*, University of Newcastle upon Tyne, 1978
61. Clayton CB, Hoenich NA, Keir MJ: The measurement of dialyser washout characteristics. in *Technical Aspects of Renal Dialysis*, edited by Frost TH, Tunbridge Wells, Pitman Medical, 1977, p 65
62. Pijl AJ, Solen KA, Mohammad SF, Monson R, Yu LS, van Griensven J et al.: Loss of anticoagulant effect of heparin during circulation of human blood *in vitro*. *Artif Organs* 14: 125, 1990

63. Holland FF, Gidden HE, Mason RG, Klein E: Thrombogenecity of heparin bound DEAE cellulose hemodialysis membranes. *ASAIO J* 1: 24, 1978

64. Lane DA: Heparin binding and neutralising proteins. *Heparin: Chemical and Biological Properties, Clinical Applications*, edited by Lane DA, Lindahl U, London, Edward Arnold, 1989, p 363

65. Kitamoto Y, Fukui H, Matsushita K, Sato T, Soejima H, Noguchi Y et al.: Supression of thrombin formation during hemodialysis with triglyceride. *ASAIO J* 39: M581, 1993

66. Lins LE, Boberg U, Jacobson SH, Kjellstrand C, Ljunberg B, Skroder, R: The influence of dialyzer geometry on blood coagulation and biocompatibility. *Clin Nephrol* 40: 281, 1993

67. Verbeelen D, Jochmans K, Herman AG, van der Niepen P, Sennesael J, de Waele M: Evaluation of platelets and haemostasis during hemodialysis with six different membranes. *Nephron* 59: 567, 1991

68. Leitienne Ph, Trzeciak MC, Adeleine P, Ville D, Dechavanne M, Traeger J et al.: Comparison of hemostasis with two high flux hemocompatible dialysis membranes. *Int J Artif Organs* 14: 227, 1991

69. Arakawa M, Aoike I, Sizuki Y, Gejyo F, Terada R, Sugaya H et al.: Antithrombogenecity of polyacrylonitrile-polyethyleneoxide hollow fiber membrane developed for designing an antithrombogenic continuous ultrafiltration system. *Artif Organs* 16: 146, 1992

70. Bowry SK: Dialyser redness: its measurement and meaning. *Eur Dial Transplant Assoc-Eur Renal Care Assoc J* 18: 43, 1992

71. Colton CK: Analysis of membrane processes for blood purification. *Blood Purif* 5: 202, 1987

72. Sigdell JE: Calculation of combined diffusive and convective mass transfer. *Int J Artif Organs* 5: 361, 1982

73. Hoenich NA, Frost TH: Influence of design and operating variables on conventional haemodialysis. in *Renal Dialysis*, edited by Whelpton D, London, Sector Publishing, 1974, p 85

74. Babb AL, Maurer CJ, Fry DL, Popovich RP, McKee RE: The determination of membrane permeabilities and solute diffusivities with applications to hemodialysis. *Chemical Engineering Symposium Series* 64: 59, 1968

75. Gotch FA: Models to predict recirculation and its effect on treatment time in single-needle dialysis. in *First International Symposium on Single-Needle Dialysis*, edited by Ringoir S, Vanholder R, Ivanovich P, Cleveland, Int Soc Artif Organs Press, 1984, p 47

76. Morcos AWB, Nissenson AR: Erythropoietin and high-efficiency dialysis. in *Contemporary Issues in Nephrology 27 – Hemodialysis High-Efficiency Treatments*, edited by Bosch JP, New York, Churchill Livingstone, 1993, p 151

77. Shinaberger JH, Miller JH, Gardner PW: Erythropoietin alert: risks of high hematocrit hemodialysis. *Trans Am Soc Artif Intern Organs* 34: 179, 1988

78. Spiegler KS, Kedem O: Thermodynamics of hyperfiltration (reverse osmosis): Criteria for efficient membranes. *Desalination* 1: 311, 1966

79. Lysaght MJ, Ford CA, Colton CK, Stone RA, Henderson LW: Mass transfer in clinical blood ultrafiltration devices – a review. in *Technical Aspects of Renal Dialysis*, edited

by Frost TH, Tunbridge Wells, Pitman Medical, 1978, p 81

80. Gupta BB, Jaffrin MY: *In vitro* study of the combined convection-diffusion mass transfer in hemodialysers. *Int J Artif Organs* 7: 263, 1984

81. Jaffrin MY, Ding L, Laurent JM: Simultaneous convective and diffusive mass transfers in a hemodialyser. *Trans ASME Journal of Biomechanical Engineering* 112: 212, 1990

82. Ghezzi PM, Sanz-Moreno C, Gervasio R, Nigrelli S, Botella J: Technical requirements for rapid high-efficiency therapy in uremic patients. Paired filtration-dialysis (PFD) with a two-chamber technique. *Trans Am Soc Artif Intern Organs* 33: 546, 1987

83. Vincent HH, van Ittersun FJ, Akcahuseyin E, Vos MC, van Duyl WA, Schalekamp MADH: Solute transport in continuous arteriovenous hemodiafiltration. A new mathematical model applied to clinical data. *Blood Purif* 8: 159, 1990

84. Leonard EF, Bluemle LW Jr: Factors influencing the permeability in extracorporeal hemodialysis. *Trans Am Soc Artif Intern Organs* 4: 4, 1958

85. Michaels AS: Operating parameters and performance criteria for hemodialyzers and other membrane separation devices. *Trans Am Soc Artif Intern Organs* 12: 387, 1966

86. Campistol JM, Skinner M: β_2-microglobulin amyloidosis: an overview. *Semin Dial* 6: 117, 1993

87. Zaoui PH, Stone WJ, Hakim RM: Effects of dialysis membranes on β_2 microglobulin production and cellular expression. *Kidney Int* 38: 962, 1990

88. Jahn B, Betz M, Deppisch R, Janssen O, Hansch GM, Ritz E: Stimulation of β_2 microglobulin synthesis in lymphocytes after exposure to Cuprophan dialyzer membranes. *Kidney Int* 40: 285, 1991

89. Zingraff J, Druecke T: Can the nephrologist prevent dialysis related amyloidosis? *Am J Kidney Dis* 18: 1, 1991

90. David S, Canino F, Ferrari ME, Cambi V: The role of adsorption in β_2 microglobulin removal. *Nephrol Dial Transplant* (Suppl 2): 64, 1991

91. Klinke B, Rockel A, Abdelhamid S, Fiegel P, Walb D: Transmembranous transport and adsorption of β_2 microglobulin during hemodilyais using polysulfone, polyacrylonitrile, polymethyl methacrylate and cuprammonium rayon membranes. *Int J Artif Organs* 12: 697, 1989

92. Lian JD, Cheng CH, Chang YL, Hsiong CH, Lee CJ: Clinical experience and model analysis on β_2-microglobulin kinetics in high-flux hemodialysis. *Artif Organs* 17: 758, 1993

93. Di Raimondo CR, Pollack VE: β_2 microglobulin kinetics in maintenance haemodialysis. A comparison of conventional and high flux dialyzers and the effects of dialyser reuse. *Am J Kidney Dis* 13: 390, 1989

94. Skroeder NR, Jacobson SH, Holmquist B, Kjellstrand P, Kjellstrand CM: β_2 microglobulin generation and removal in long slow and short fast hemodiaylsis. *Am J Kidney Dis* 21: 519, 1993

95. Floege J, Wilks M, Shaldon S, Koch KM, Smeby LC: β_2 microglobulin kinetics during haemofiltration. *Nephrol Dial Transplant* 3: 784, 1988

96. Kaiser JP, Hagemann J, von Herrath D, Schaefer K: Different handling of β_2-microglobulin during hemodialysis and hemofiltration. *Nephron* 48: 132, 1988

97. Floege J, Granolleras C, Deschodt G, Heck M, Baudin G, Branger B et al.: High flux synthetic versus cellulosic membranes for β_2 microglobulin removal during hemodialysis, hemodiafiltration and hemofiltration. *Nephrol Dial Transplant* 4: 653, 1989

98. Ward RA, Schaefer RM, Falkenhagen D, Joshua MS, Heidland A, Klinkmann H et al.: Biocompatibility of a new high-permeability modified cellulose membrane for haemodialysis. *Nephrol Dial Transplant* 8: 47, 1993

99. Sigdell JE, Tersteegen B: Clearance of a dialyser under varying operating conditions. *Artif Organs* 10: 219, 1986

100. Tyagi VP, Abbas M: An exact analysis for solute transport, due to simultaneous dialysis and ultrafiltration in a hollow-fibre artificial kidney. *Bull Math Biol* 49: 697, 1987

101. Waniewski J, Lucjanek P, Werynski A: Alternative descriptions of combined diffusive and convective mass transport in hemodialyzer. *Artif Organs* 17: 3, 1993

102. Hootkins R, Bourgeois B: The effect of ultrafiltration on dialysance. Mathematical theory and experimental verification. *Trans Am Soc Artif Intern Organs* 37: M375, 1991

103. Waniewski J, Werynski A, Abrenholz P, Lucjanek P, Judycki W, Esther G: Theoretical basis and experimental verification of the impact of ultrafiltration on dialyser clearance. *Artif Organs* 15: 70, 1991

104. Morcos AWB, Nissenson AR: Erythropoietin and high efficiency dialysis. in *Hemodialysis – High Efficiency Treatments*, edited by Bosch JP, Stein JH, New York, Churchill Livingstone, 1993, p 151

105. Collins A, Keshaviah P, Berkseth R, Opsahl J, Abraham P: Impact of erythropoietin (EPO) therapy (RX) on rapid high efficiency hemodialysis (RHED). (Abstract). *Kidney Int* 35: 243, 1989

106. Descombes E, Perriard F, Fellay G: Diffusion kinetics of urea, creatinine and uric acid in blood during hemodialysis. Clinical Implications. *Clin Nephrol* 40: 286, 1993

107. Strathmann H, Gohl H: Membranes for blood purification. State of the art and new developments. in *Terminal Renal Failure, Therapeutic Problems, Possibilities and Potentials. Contributions to Nephrology*, edited by Klinkmann H, Smeby LC, Basel, Karger, 1990, p 119

108. Suzuki Y, Kanamori T, Sakai K: Zeta potential of hollow fiber dialysis membranes and its effects on hydrogen phosphate ion permeability. *ASAIO J* 39: M301, 1993

109. Okada M, Watanabe T, Imamura K, Tsurumi T, Suma Y, Sakai K: Ionic strength affects diffusive permeability to an inorganic phosphate ion of negatively charged dialysis membranes. *Trans Am Soc Artif Intern Organs* 36: M324, 1990

110. Higa M, Kira A, Tanioka A, Miyasaka K: New hemodialysis method using positively charged membrane dialyzer and/or polycation dialysate. *Ind Eng Chem Res* 32: 917, 1993

111. Gohl H, Konstantin P: Membranes and filters for hemofiltration. in *Hemofiltration*, edited by Henderson LW, Quellhorst EA, Baldamus CA, Lysaght MJ, Berlin, Springer-Verlag, 1986, p 42

112. Ofsthun NJ, Jensen JC, Kay M: Effect of high haematocrit and high blood flow rates on transmembrane pressure and ultrafiltration rate in hemodialysis. *Blood Purif* 9: 169, 1991

113. Petersen J, Hyver SW, Cajias J: Backfiltration during dialysis. A critical assessment. *Semin Dial* 5: 13, 1992

114. Ronco C: Back filtration in clinical dialysis: nature of the phenomenon, mechanisms and possible solutions. *Int J Artif Organs* 13: 11, 1990

115. Soltys PJ, Ofsthun N, Leypoldt JK: Critical analysis of formulas for estimating back filtration in hemodialysis. *Blood Purif* 10: 326, 1992

116. Ronco C: Back filtration. A controversial issue in modern dialysis. *Int J Artif Organs* 11: 69, 1988

117. Baurmeister U, Vienken J, Daum V: High flux dialysis membranes: Endotoxin transfer by back filtration can be a problem. *Nephrol Dial Transplant* 4 (Suppl): 89, 1989

118. Laude Sharp M, Caroff M, Simard L, Pusineri C, Kazatchkine MD, Haeffner Cavailion N: Induction of IL-1 during hemodialysis. Transmembrane passage of intact endotoxins (LPS). *Kidney Int* 38: 1089, 1990

119. Kumano K, Vokota S, Nanbu M, Sakai T: Do cytokine inducing substances penetrate through dialysis membranes and simulate monocytes. *Kidney Int* 43 (Suppl 41): S205, 1993

120. Evans RC, Holmes CJ: *In vitro* study of the transfer of cytokine inducing substances across selected high flux hemodialysis membranes. *Blood Purif* 9: 92, 1991

121. Urena P, Herbelin A, Zingraff J, Lair M, Khoa Man N, Deschamps Latscha B et al.: Permeability of cellulose and nono-cellulosic membranes to endotoxin subunits and cytokine production during *in vitro* haemodialysis. *Nephrol Dial Transplant* 7: 16, 1992

122. Harding GB, Klein E, Pass T, Wright R, Million C: Endotoxin and bacterial contamination of dialysis center water and dialysate; a cross sectional survey. *Int J Artif Organs* 13: 39, 1990

123. Oliver JC, Bland LA, Oettinger CW, Arduino MJ, Garrard M, Pegues DA et al.: Bacteria and endotoxin removal from bicarbonate dialysis fluids for use in conventional, high efficiency, and high-flux hemodialysis. *Artif Organs* 16: 141, 1992

124. Gordon SM, Oettinger CW, Bland LA et al.: Permeability of cellulosic and non cellulosic membranes to endotoxin subunits and cytokine production during *in vitro* haemodialysis. *Nephrol Dial Transplant* 7: 16, 1992

125. Sato H, Kidaka T: Effect of moisture on and kinetic features of the ultrafiltration rate of dialysis membranes. *Artif Organs* 5: 286, 1981

126. Takesawa S, Ohmi S, Konno Y, Sekiguchi M, Shitaokoshi S, Takahashi T et al.: Varying methods of sterilisation and their effects on the structure and permeability of dialysis membranes. *Nephrol Dial Transplant* 1: 254, 1987

127. Potter LJ, Frost TH: The effect of strain and pretensions on the permeability of cellulose membranes and on the performance of flat bed dialysers. in *Technical Aspects of Renal Dialysis*, edited by Frost TH, Tunbridge Wells, Pitman Press, 1977, p 112

128. Okazaki M, Yoshida F: Ultrafiltration of blood: effect of hematocrit on ultrafiltration rate. *Ann Biomed Eng* 4: 138, 1976

129. Robertson BC, Curtin C: Effects of EPO therapy on backfiltration of dialysate in high flux dialysis. *Trans Am Soc Artif Intern Organs* 36: M447, 1990

130. Gupta BB, Jaffrin MY, Ding LH: Modelling of plasma separation through microporous membranes. *Int J Artif Organs* 12: 51, 1989

131. Ding L, Laurent JM, Jaffrin MY: Dynamic filtration of blood: a new concept for enhancing plasma filtration. *Int J Artif Organs* 14: 365, 1991

132. Henne W, Dietrich W, Pelger M, von Sengbusch G: Residual ethylene oxide in hollow fiber dialyzers. *Artif Organs* 8: 306, 1984

133. Lemke H-D, Heidland A, Schaefer RM: Hypersensitivity reactions during haemodialysis: role of complement fragments and ethylene oxide antibodies. *Nephrol Dial Transplant* 5: 264, 1990

134. Szycher M: Sterilization of medical devices. in *Blood Compatible Materials and Devices*, edited by Sharma CP, Szycher M, Lancaster, Technomic Publishing Co, 1990, p 87

135. Dorman-Smith V: Considerations when using ethylene oxide for the sterilization of medical devices. *Med Dev Technol* 42, 1991

136. Klimentov AS, Martynenko AI, Fiodorov AL, Ershov BG: Influence of γ-radiation on the molecular-mass distribution of cellulose. *Radiochem Radioanal Let* 48: 137, 1981

137. Takesawa S, Satoh S, Hidai H, Sekiguchi M, Sakai K: Degradation by gamma irradiation of regenerated cellulose membranes for clinical dialysis. *Trans Am Soc Artif Intern Organs* 33: 584, 1987

138. Landfield H: Sterilization of medical devices based on polymer selection and stabilization techniques. in *Biocompatible Polymers, Metals, and Composites*, edited by Szycher M, PA, Technomic Publ Inc, 1983, p 975

139. Shintani H, Nakamura A: Analysis of a carcinogen, 4,4'-methylenedianiline, from thermosetting polyurethane during sterilization. *J Anal Toxicol* 13: 354, 1989

140. Shintani H, Nakamura A: Analysis of the carcinogen 4,4'-methylenedianiline (MDA) in gamma-ray and in autoclave-sterilised polyurethane. *Fresenius Zeitschrift für Analytische Chemie* 333: 637, 1989

141. Hoenich NA, Goodship THJ, Ward MK, Ringoir S: Technical aspects of reuse in Europe. in *Guide to Reprocessing of Hemodialyzers*, edited by Deane N, Wineman RJ, Bemis JA, Boston, Martinus Nijhoff Publishers, 1986, p 107

142. Bland LA, Favero MS, Oxborrow GS, Aguero SM, Searcy BP, Danielson JW: Effect of chemical germicides on the integrity of hemodialyzer membranes. *Trans Am Soc Artif Intern Organs* 34: 172, 1988

143. Takesawa S, Ohmi S, Konno Y, Sekiguchi M, Shitaokoshi S, Takahashi T et al.: Varying methods of sterilisation and their effects on the structure and permeability of dialysis membranes. *Nephrol Dial Transplant* 1: 254, 1987

144. Daugirdas JT, Ing TS: First-use reactions during hemodialysis: A definition of subtypes. *Kidney Int* 33 (Suppl 24): S37, 1988

145. Nicholls AJ, Platts MM: Anaphylactoid reactions due to haemodialysis, haemofiltration or membrane plasma separation. *Br Med J* 285: 1607, 1982

146. Villaroel F, Clarkowski AA: A survey of hypersensitivity reactions in hemodialysis. *Artif Organs* 9: 231, 1985

147. Alter MJ, Favero MS, Moyer LA, Bland LA. National surveillance of dialysis-associated diseases in the United States, 1989. *Trans Am Soc Artif Intern Organs* 37: 97, 1991

148. Alomar A, Camarasa JMG, Noguera J, Aspinolea F: Ethylene-oxide dermatitis. *Contact Derm* 7: 205, 1981

149. Poothullil J, Shimizu A, Day RP, Dolovich J: Anaphylaxis from the product(s) of ethylene oxide gas. *Ann Intern Med* 82: 58, 1975

150. Grammer LC, Patterson R: IgE against ethylene oxide altered human serum albumin (ETO-HSA) as an etological agent in allergic reactions of hemodialysis patients. *Artif Organs* 11: 97, 1987

151. Dolovich J, Marshall CP, Smith EKM, Shimizu A, Pearson FC, Sugona MA et al.: Allergy to ethylene oxide in chronic hemodialysis patients. *Artif Organs* 8: 334, 1984

152. Ing TS, Daugirdas JT: Extractable ethylene oxide from cuprammonium cellulose plate dialyzers: Importance of potting compound. *Trans Am Soc Artif Intern Organs* 32: 108, 1986

153. Ansorge W, Pelger M, Dietrich M, Baurmeister U: Ethylene oxide in dialyser rinsing fluid: effect of rinsing technique, dialyser storage time and potting compound. *Artif Organs* 11: 118, 1987

154. Neergaard J, Nielsen B, Faurby V, Christensen DH, Nielsen OF: On the exudation of plasticizers from PVC haemodialysis tubings. *Nephron* 14: 263, 1975

155. Flaminio LM, de Angelis L, Ferazza M, Mannovich M, Galli G, Galli CL: Leachability of a new plasticiser tri(2-ethyl-hexyl) trimellitate from haemodialysis tubing. *Int J Artif Organs* 11: 435, 1988

156. Blass CR, Jones C, Courtney JM: Biomaterials for blood tubing: the application of plasticised poly (vinyl chloride). *Int J Artif Organs* 15: 200, 1992

157. Hoenich NA, Thompson J, Varini E, McCabe EJ, Appleton D: Particle spallation and plasticizer (DEHP) release from extracorporeal circuit tubing materials. *Int J Artif Organs* 13: 55, 1990

158. Chanard J, Lavaud S, Lavaud F, Toupance O, Kochman S: IgE antibodies to isocyanates in hemodialyzed patients. *Trans Am Soc Artif Intern Organs* 33: 551, 1987

159. Grammer LC, Harris KE, Shaughnessy MA, Dolovich J, Patterson R, Evans S: Antibodies to toluene di isocyanate in patients with and without dialysis anaphylaxis. *Artif Organs* 15: 2, 1991

160. Oba T, Tsuji K, Nakamura A, Shintani H, Mizumachi S, Kickuchi H et al.: Migration of acetylated hemi cellulose from capillary hemodialyser to blood causing scleritis and/or iritis. *Artif Organs* 8: 429, 1984

161. Hoenich NA, Thompson J, McCabe J, Appleton DR: Particle release from haemodialysers. *Int J Artif Organs* 13: 803, 1990

162. Inagaki H, Hamazaki T, Kuroda H, Yano S: Foreign particles contaminating hemodialyzers and methods of removing them by rinsing. *Nephron* 46: 343, 1987

163. Remuzzi A, Boccardo P, Benigni A: *In vitro* platelet adhesion to dialysis membranes. *Nephrol Dial Transplant* 6 (Suppl 2): 36, 1991

164. Taylor J, McLaren M, Mactier R, Henderson I, Stewart W, Belch J: Effect of dialyser geometry during hemodialysis with cuprophane membranes. *Kidney Int* 42: 442, 1992

165. Kuwahara T, Markert M, Wauters JP: Proteins adsorbed on hemodialysis membranes modulate neutrophil function. *Artif Organs* 13: 427, 1989

166. Panichi V, Biachi AM, Parrini M, Casarosa L, Cirami C, Grazi G et al.: Biocompatibility evaluation of five dialysis membranes: protein layer and anaphylatoxin generation. *Int J Artif Organs* 12: 579, 1989

167. Verbeelen D, Jochmans K, Herman AG, van der Niepen P, Sennesael J, deWaele M: Evaluation of platelets and hemostasis during hemodialysis with six different membranes. *Nephron* 59: 567, 1991

168. Lim F, Cooper SL: The effect of surface hydrophilicity on biomaterial-leukocyte interactions. *Trans Am Soc Artif Intern Organs* 37: M146, 1991

169. Matsuda T: Biological responses at non physiological interfaces and molecular design of biocompatible surfaces. *Nephrol Dial Transplant* 4 (Suppl 4): 60, 1989

170. Ferreira SH: A bradykinin-potentiating factor (BPF) present in the venom of *Bothrops jararaca*. *Br J Pharmacol* 24: 163, 1965

171. Erdos EG: Angiotensin-1 converting enzyme and the changes in our concepts through the years. *Hypertension* 16: 363, 1990

172. Zusman RM: Renin- and non-renin-mediated antihypertensive actions of converting enzyme inhibitors. *Kidney Int* 25: 969, 1984

173. Tielemanns C, Madhoun P, Lenaers M, Schandene L, Goldman M, Vanherwegem J: Anaphylactoid reactions during hemodialysis on AN69 membranes in patients receiving ACE inhibitors. *Kidney Int* 38: 982, 1990

174. Verresen L, Waer M, Vanrentergheim Y, Michielsen P: Angiotensin converting enzyme inhibitors and anaphylactoid reactions to high flux membranes. *Lancet* 336: 1360, 1990

175. Parnes E, Shapiro W: Anaphylactoid reactions in hemodialysis patients treated with AN69 dialysers. *Kidney Int* 40: 1148, 1991

176. Olbricht C, Schaumann D, Fischer D: Anaphylactoid reactions, LDL apheresis with dextran sulphate and ACE inhibitors. *Lancet* 340: 908, 1992

177. Lemke H, Fink E: Generation of bradykinin in human plasma using AN69 and PAN17DX membranes in the presence of ACE inhibitor *in vitro*. *Nephrol Dial Transplant* 7: 728, 1992

178. Craddock P, Fehr J, Dalmasso A, Brigham K, Jacog H: Hemodialysis leukopenia: pulmonary vascular leukostasis resulting from complement activation by dialyser cellophane membranes. *J Clin Invest* 59: 879, 1977

179. Woffindin C, Hoenich NA, Matthews JNS: Cellulose based haemodialysis membranes: Biocompatibility and functional performance compared. *Nephrol Dial Transplant* 7: 340, 1992

180. Amadori A, Candi P, Sasdelli M, Massai G, Favilla S, Passaleva A et al.: Hemodialysis leukopenia and complement function with different dialyzers. *Kidney Int* 24: 775, 1983

181. Bergesio F, Monzani G, Manescalchi F, Boccabianca I, Passaleva A, Frizzi V: Leukocytes, eosinophils and complement function during hemodialysis with polysulphone and polymethylmethacrylate membranes: Comparison with Cuprophan and polyacrylonitrile. *Blood Purif* 6: 16, 1988

182. Moll S, de Moerloose P, Reber G, Schifferli J, Leski M: Comparison of two hemodialysis membranes, polyacrylonitrile and cellulose acetate on complement and coagulation systems. *Int J Artif Organs* 13: 273, 1990

183. Bingel M, Arndt W, Schulze M, Floege J, Shaldon S, Koch KM et al.: Comparative study of C5a plasma levels with different hemodialysis membranes using an enzyme-linked immunosorbent assay. *Nephron* 51: 320, 1989

184. Schaefer RM, Rauterberg EW, Deppisch R, Vienken J: Assembly of terminal SC5b-9 complement complexes: a new index of blood-membrane interaction. *Miner Electrolyte Metab* 16: 73, 1990

185. Deppisch R, Schmitt V, Bommer J, Hansch G, Ritz E, Rauterberg E: Fluid phase generation of terminal complement complex as a novel index of biocompatibility. *Kidney Int* 37: 696, 1990

186. Cheung A: Biocompatibility of hemodialysis membranes. *J Am Soc Nephrol* 1: 150, 1990

187. Kandus A, Ponikvar R, Drinovec J, Kladnik S, Ivanovich P: Anaphylatoxins C3a and C5a adsorption on polyacrylonitrile membrane of hollow fibre and plate dialyser: an *in vivo* study. *Int J Artif Organs* 13: 176, 1990

188. Hakim RM, Breillatt HJ, Lazarus JM, Port FK: Complement activation and hypersensitivity reactions to dialysis membranes. *N Engl J Med* 311: 878, 1984

189. Sultan Y, London GM, Goldfarb B, Toulon P, Marchais SJ: Activation of platelets, coagulation and fibrinolysis in patients on long-term haemodialysis: influence of Cuprophan and Polyacrylonitrile membranes. *Nephrol Dial Transpl* 5: 362, 1990

190. Kaplow LS, Goffinet JA: Profound neutropenia during early phase of hemodialysis. *JAMA* 203: 133, 1968

191. Arnaout MA, Hakim RM, Todd RF, Dana N, Colten HR: Increased expression of adhesion promoting surface glycoprotein in the granulocytopenia of hemodialysis. *N Engl J Med* 312: 457, 1985

192. Himmelfarb J, Zaoui P, Hakim R: Modulation of granulocyte LAM-1 and MAC-1 during dialysis. A prospective randomised controlled trial. *Kidney Int* 41: 388, 1992

193. Kolb G, Fischer W, Schoenemann H, Bathke K, Hoffken H, Muller T et al.: Effect of Cuprophan, hemophan and polysulfone membranes on the oxidative metabolism, degranulation reaction, enzyme release and pulmonary sequestration of granulocytes. in *Improvements in Dialysis Therapy*, Contributions to Nephrology, Vol 74, edited by Baldamus CA, Mion C, Shaldon S, Basel, Karger, 1989, p 10

194. Hakim RM: Clinical implications of hemodialysis membrane biocomptibility. *Kidney Int* 44: 484, 1993

195. Francos GC, Besarab A, Burke JF Jr, Peters J, Tahamont MV, Gee MH et al.: Dialysis induced hypoxemia: Membrane dependent and membrane independent causes. *Am J Kidney Dis* 5: 191, 1985

196. Kishimoto T, Tanaka H, Maekawa M, Ivanovich P, Levin N, Bergstrom J et al.: Dialysis-induced hypoxaemia. *Nephrol Dial Transplant* 8 (Suppl 2): 25, 1993

197. Horl WH, Riegel W, Schollmeyer P, Rautenberg W, Neumann S: Different complement and granulocyte activation in patients dialyzed with PMMA dialysers. *Clin Nephrol* 25: 304, 1986

198. Hoerl W, Schafer R, Heidland A: Effect of different dialysers on proteinases and proteinase inhibitors during hemodialysis. *Am J Nephrol* 5: 320, 1985

199. Bazzoni G, Nunez AB, Mascellani G, Bianchini P, Dejana E, del Maschio A: Effect of heparin, dermatan sulfate and related oligo derivatives on human polymorphonuclear leukocyte functions. *J Lab Clin Med* 121: 268, 1993

200. Schaefer RM, Heidland A, Horl WH. Effect of dialyser geometry on granulocyte and complement activation. *Am J Nephrol* 7: 121, 1987

201. Friedberg M, Joffe P, Nielsen B, Nielsen LP: Eosinophilia in hemodialysis patients. *Artif Organs* 11: 90, 1987
202. Vanherweghem J-L, Goldman M, Tielemans C: Eosinophilia in chronic dialysis. *Semin Dial* 3: 171, 1990
203. Hertel J, Kimmel PL, Phillips TM, Bosch JP: Eosinophilia and cellular cytokine responsiveness in hemodialysis patients. *J Am Soc Nephrol* 3: 1244, 1992
204. Haeffner Cavallion N, Jahns G, Poignet J-L Kazatchkine MD: Induction of Interleukin 1 during hemodialysis. *Kidney Int* 43 (Suppl 39): S139, 1993
205. Kimmel PL, Phillips TM, Phillips E, Bosch JP: Effect of renal replacement therapy on cellular cytokine production in patients with renal disease. *Kidney Int* 38: 129, 1990
206. Schaefer RM, Paczek L, Heidland A: Cytokine production by monocytes during haemodialysis. *Nephrol Dial Transplant* 6 (Suppl 2): 14, 1991
207. Pereira BJG, King AJ, Poutsiaka DD, Strom JA, Dinarello CA: Comparison of first use and reuse of Cuprophan membranes on Interleukin 1 receptor antagonist and Interleukin 1β production by blood mononuclear cells. *Am J Kidney Dis* 22: 288, 1993
208. Bommer J, Weinreich T, Lovett DH, Bouillon R, Ritz E, Gemsa D: Particles from dialysis tubing stimulate Interleukin 1 secretion by macrophages. *Nephrol Dial Transplant* 5: 208, 1990
209. Gault MH, Duffett S, Purchase L, Murphy J: Hemodialysis intravascular hemolysis and kinked blood lines. *Nephron* 62: 267, 1992
210. Said R, Quintanilla A, Levin N, Ivanovich P: Acute hemolysis due to profound hypo-osmolality. *J Dial* 1: 447, 1977
211. Pun KK, Yeung CK, Chan TK: Acute intravascular hemolysis due to accidental formalin intoxication during hemodialysis. *Clin Nephrol* 21: 188, 1984
212. Gordon SM, Bland CA, Alexander SR, Newman HF, Arduino MJ, Jarvis WR: Hemolysis associated with hydrogen peroxide at a pediatric dialysis center. *Am J Nephrol* 10: 123, 1990
213. Hudson S, Taylor JE, Stewart WK: Undetect excessive ultrafiltration and serious haemolysis during maintenance haemodialysis. *Nephrol Dial Transplant* 8: 477, 1993
214. Francos GC, Burke JF Jr, Besarab A, Martinez J, Kirkwood RG, Hummel LA: An unsuspected cause of acute hemolysis during hemodialysis. *Trans Am Soc Artif Intern Organs* 29: 140, 1983
215. Kessler M, Hoen B, Mayeux D, Hestin D, Fontenaille C: Bacteremia in patients on chronic hemodiaylsis – a multicenter prospective survey. *Nephron* 64: 95, 1993
216. Komuro T, Nakazawa R: Detection of low molecular size lipopolysaccharide contaminated in dialysates used for hemodialysis therapy with polyacrylonitride gel electrophoresis in the presence of sodium deoycholate. *Int J Artif Organs* 16: 245, 1993
217. Smollich BP, Falkenhagen D, Schneidewind J, Mitzner S, Klinkmann H: Importance of endotoxins in high flux diaylsis. *Nephrol Dial Transplant* 6 (Suppl 3): 83, 1991
218. Harding GB, Klein E, Pass T, Wright R, Million C: Endotoxin and bacterial contamination of dialysis center and dialysate: a cross sectional survey. *Int J Artif Organs* 13: 39, 1990
219. Klein E, Pass T, Harding GB, Wright R, Million C: Microbial and endotoxin contamination in water and dialysate in the central United States. *Artif Organs* 14: 85, 1990
220. Oliver JC, Bland LA, Oettinger CW, Arduino MJ, Garrard M, Pegues DA et al.: Bacteria and endotoxin removal from bicarbonate dialysis fluids for use in conventional high-efficiency and high-flux hemodialysis. *Artif Organs* 16: 141, 1992
221. Gault MH, Duffett AL, Murphy JF, Purchase LH: In search of sterile, endotoxin-free dialysate. *ASAIO J* 38: M431, 1992
222. Di Felice A, Cappelli G, Facchini F, Tetta C, Cornia F, Aimo G et al.: Ultrafiltration and endotoxin removal from dialysis fluids. *Kidney Int* 43 (Suppl 41): S201, 1993
223. Cappelli G, Tetta C, Cornia F, Defelice A, Facchini F, Neri R et al.: Removal of limulus reactivity and cytokine-inducing capacity from bicarbonate dialysis fluids by ultrafiltration. *Nephrol Dial Transplant* 8: 1133, 1993
224. Petersen NJ, Carson LA, Favero MS: Bacterial endotoxin in new and reused hemodialyzers: a potential cause of endotoxemia. *Trans Am Soc Artif Intern Organs* 27: 155, 1981
225. Gordon SM, Oettinger CW, Bland LA, Oliver JC, Arduino MJ, Aguero SM et al.: Pyrogenic reactions in patients receiving conventional high-efficiency, or high-flux hemodialysis treatments with bicarbonate dialysate containing high concentrations of bacteria and endotoxin. *J Am Soc Nephrol* 2: 1436, 1992
226. Pegues DA, Oettinger CW, Bland LA, Oliver JC, Arduino MJ, Aguero SM et al.: A prospective study of pyrogenic reactions in hemodialysis patients using bicarbonate dialysis fluids filtered to remove bacteria and endotoxin. *J Am Soc Nephrol* 3: 1002, 1993
227. Schaefer K, von Herrath D, Hufler M, Pauls A: The occurrence of fever during hemodialysis and hemofiltration. A comparative study. *Int J Artif Organs* 9: 247, 1986
228. Hariprasad MK, Paul PK, Eisinger RB, Gary NE, Timins JE, Miller JW: Extracorporeal dialysis of ascites. *Arch Intern Med* 141: 1550, 1981
229. Hwang ER, Sherman RA, Mehta S, Walker JA, Goodling KA, Hariprasad MK et al.: Dialytic ascitic ultrafiltration in refractory ascites. *Am J Gastroenterol* 77: 652, 1982
230. Assadi FK, Gordon D, Kecskes SA, John E: Treatment of refractory ascites by ultrafiltration – reinfusion of ascitic fluid peritoneally. *J Paediatrics* 106: 943, 1985
231. Landini S, Coli U, Fracasso A, Morachiello P, Righetto F, Scanferia F et al.: Spontaneous ascites filtration and reinfusion (SAFR) in cirrhotic patients. *Int J Artif Organs* 8: 277, 1985
232. Lai KN, Leung JWC, Loke J, Panesar NS, Swaminathan R, Vallance-Owen J: Ultrafiltration by hemofilter – a new therapeutic measure in intractable ascites. *Int J Artif Organs* 10: 109, 1987
233. Adler AJ, Feldman J, Friedman EA, Berlyne GM: Use of extracorporeal ascites dialysis in combined hepatic and renal-failure. *Nephron* 30: 31, 1982
234. Lai KN, Leung JWC, Vallance-Owen J: Dialytic ultrafiltration by hemofilter in treatment of patients with refractory ascites and renal insufficiency. *Am J Gastroenterol* 82: 665, 1987
235. Yoshiba M, Sekiyama K, Iwamura Y, Sugata F: Development of a reliable artificial liver support (ALS). Plasma exchange in combination with hemodiafiltration using high performance membranes. *Dig Dis Sci* 38: 469, 1993
236. Rozga J, Williams F, Ro M-S, Neuzil DF, Giorgio TD, Backfisch G et al.: Development of a bioartificial liver:

Properties and function of a hollow-fiber module inoculated with liver cells. *Hepatology* 17: 258, 1993

237. Gille JP, Lautier A, Tousseul B: ECCO2R in respiratory support – artificial lung or kidney – experimental study. *Ann de Chir* 46: 71, 1992

238. Nolte SH, Jonitz WJ, Grau J, Roth H, Assenbaum ER: Hemodialysis for extracorporeal bicarbonate/CO_2 removal (ECBicCO2R) and apneic oxygenation for respiratory failure in the newborn. *Trans Am Soc Artif Intern Organs* 35: 30, 1989

239. Hernandez E, Praga M, Alcazar JM, Morales JM, Montejo JC, Jimenez MJ et al.: Hemodialysis for treatment of accidental hypothermia. *Nephron* 63: 214, 1993

240. Splendiani G, Giammaria U, Daniele M, Tancredi M: Dialysis in nonuremia. in *Biotechnology in Renal Replacement Therapy*, Contributions to Nephrology, Vol 70, edited by Bonomini V, Scolari MP, Stefoni S, Basel, Karger, 1989, p 277

241. Tufte ER: *The Visual Display of Quantitative Information*, Godalming, Graphics Press, 1983

242. Runge TM, Briceno JC, Scheller ME, Moritz CE, Sloan L, Bohls FO et al.: Hemodialysis: evidence of enhanced molecular clearance and ultrafiltration volume by using pulsatile flow. *Int J Artif Organs* 16: 645, 1993

243. Catapano G, Wodetzki A, Baurmeister U: Blood flow outside regularly spaced hollow fibres: the future concept of membrane devices. *Int J Artif Organs* 15: 327, 1992

244. Nakazawa R, Azuma N, Suzuki M, Nakatani M, Nankou T, Furuyoshi S et al.: A new treatment for dialysis-related amyloidosis with β_2-microglobulin adsorbent column. *Int J Artif Organs* 16: 823, 1993

245. Tanaka H: Quality of membrane: High flux membrane and its future. in *Evolution of Dialysis Adequacy*, Contributions to Nephrology, Vol 103, edited by Bonomini V, Basel, Karger, 1993, p 112

246. Shaldon S, Koch KM: Survival and adequacy in long term hemodialysis. *Nephron* 59: 353, 1991

247. Bergamo Collaborative Dialysis Study Group: Acute intradialytic well being. Results of a clinical trial comparing polysulfone with Cuprophan. *Kidney Int* 40: 714, 1991

248. Chandran PKG, Liggett R, Kirkpatrick B: Patient survival on PAN/AN69 membrane hemodialysis. A ten year analysis. *J Am Soc Nephrol* 4: 1199, 1993

249. Hakim RM, Wingard RL, Lawrence P, Parker RA, Schulman G: Use of biocompatible membranes improves outcome and recovery from acute renal failure. *J Am Soc Nephrol* 3: 367 (Abstract), 1992

250. Hall AV, Clark WF, Parbtani A: Heparin-induced thrombocytopenia in renal failure. *Clin Nephrol* 38: 86, 1992

251. Tong S-D, Hsu L-C: Non-thrombogenic hemofiltration system for acute renal failure treatment. *ASAIO J* 38: M702, 1992

252. Arakawa M, Suzuki Y, Nagao M, Aoike I, Koda Y, Terada R et al.: Development of a new antithrombogenic continuous ultrafiltration system (ACUS) and its clinical evaluation. *Nephrol Dial Transplant* 6 (Suppl): S249, 1991

253. Arakawa M, Aoike I, Sizuki Y, Geyo F, Terada R, Sugaya H et al.: Antithrombogenecity of polyacrylonitrile-polyethyleneoxide hollow fiber membrane developed for designing an antithromogenic continuous ultrafiltration system. *Artif Organs* 16: 146, 1992

254. Collins AJ: High-efficiency treatments using conventional equipment. in *Hemodialysis High-Efficiency Treatments*, Contemporary Issues in Nephrology, Vol 27, edited by Bosch JP, New York, Churchill Livingstone, 1993, p 91

WATER TREATMENT FOR CONTEMPORARY HEMODIALYSIS

BERNARD J.M. CANAUD and CHARLES M. MION

RATIONALE FOR WATER TREATMENT IN HEMODIALYSIS

Maintenance hemodialysis is an accepted life support system ensuring long term survival of half a million end stage renal failure patients worldwide. Hemodialysis patients are regularly exposed to 300–400 liters of hemodialysis fluids per week during dialysis. The quality of water used to dilute the concentrated dialysate fluid is important because of the nature of the contact between dialysate and the patient's blood. The end stage renal failure patient is the last link of a complex chain leading to the hemodialysis process, where patient's blood is exposed to dialysate. One can look at the hemodialysis system as the end point of an hydraulic circuit where city water is changed in water for HD through municipal water supply, water treatment system, distribution system and delivering dialysate through the artificial kidney (Figure 1).

From the early days of dialysis it is known that water used for hemodialysis must be purified in order to prevent clinical side effects due to contamination of water (1–4). Water for dialysis must be considered as a pharmaceutical product exposed to patient's blood system requiring a specific and more stringent purification approach (5–7). Drinking regulation standards for water are based on a weekly exposure of 14 liters with a selective gut barrier. Hemodialysis patients are exposed to 300–400 liters per week through a non-selective artificial dialyzer membrane. Furthermore, dialysis patients having non urinary excretion capacity are exposed to higher risk of toxic substances accumulation particularly for those who are bound to protein and/or tissue. Contemporary dialysis has introduced new risks directly related to the quality and purity of water used in dialysis (8–11). Hemodialysis using highly permeable membrane and ultrafiltration controller is responsible for backfiltration and/or backdiffusion from dialysate (12–17). On the one hand, such an unapparent convective transport phenomenon is capable of transferring toxic and/or pyrogenic substances from dialysate to blood resulting in febrile reaction (18–21). On the other hand, dialysate contaminants may contribute to the activation of various protein systems, enzymes and cells circulating in the blood compartment (22, 23). In-line production of substitution fluid used in some dialysis modalities (e.g., in-line hemofiltration, HF or hemodiafiltration, HDF) infuse a large fraction of dialysate fluid directly into the patient's blood stream enhancing risks for direct toxicity and/or pyrogenicity (24, 25). Dialyzer reconditioning using water from the dialysis unit is associated with hazards of introducing pyrogenic material and/or bacteria within the lumen of the dialyzer fibers (26–35). Water treatment system therefore must provide the dialysis facility and the hemodialysis machine with a pure water which has been cleared from all contaminants (36–38).

Water purity requirements have changed over the past three decades. Hemodialysis has been used routinely as maintenance therapy in end stage renal disease patients for thirty years. Schematically, water purity has considerably improved according to a three stage periods.

The first decade (1960–1970) was a pioneering period. The objectives were essentially the development of dialysis program in order to ensure survival of end stage renal failure patients. Water treatment system used during this

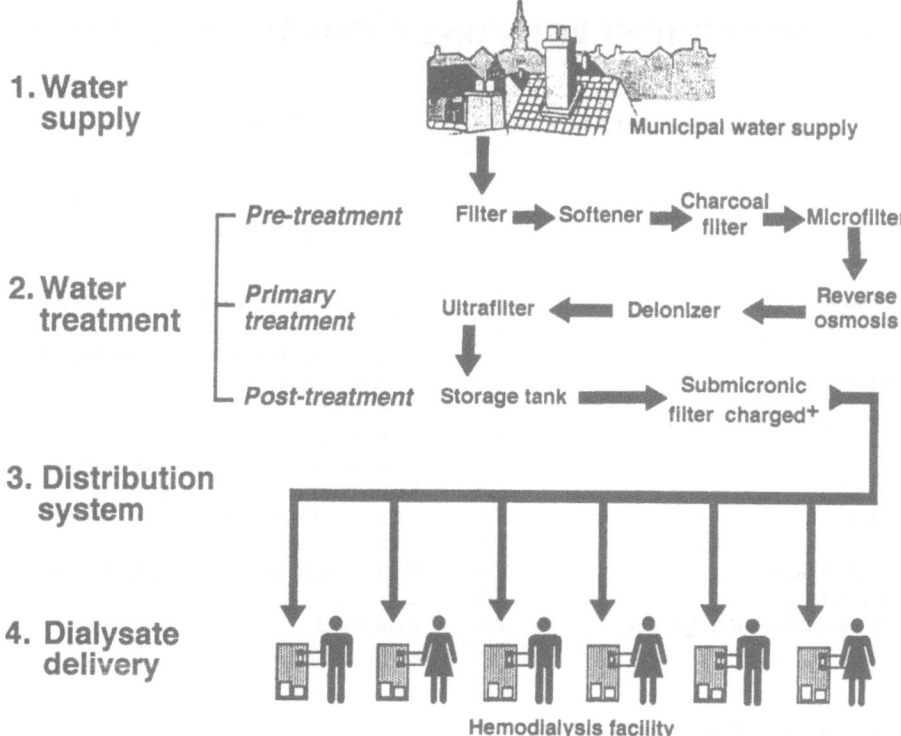

Figure 1. Schematic representation of the different steps of the water purification system, starting from the municipal water supply and ending at the dialysate delivery system.

period was basically designed to remove colloid particulates, calcium, magnesium, chlorine and toxic substances in order to prevent mainly 'hard water syndrome' and also to prevent pyrogenic reactions. Indeed, from the early Seattle experience, it was shown that the bacteriologic contamination of the dialysis fluid was a potential risk for the hemodialysis patient (39).

The second decade (1970–1980) revealed the hazards of various substances added to city water to control turbidity (aluminium sulfate) or bacteriologic contamination (chlorine, chloramine). Aluminium intoxication revealed by the epidemic occurrence of 'dialysis dementia' was particularly stressed (40–44). Water treatment system improvement consisted in generalizing the use of reverse osmosis system and/or the deionizers (mixed beds) to prevent the risk of aluminium intoxication, and activated charcoal to remove chlorine and chloramine from city water (45–49).

The third decade (1980–1990) was characterized by the introduction of major changes in hemodialysis technology. Bicarbonate dialysis, highly permeable membranes, ultrafiltration controllers were soon identified as new hazards requiring a higher degree of water purity with reduced bacteriologic and endotoxin contamination (8). In this context, water became a component of the complex problem hemodialysis hemocompatibility. The Interleukin-1

hypothesis was the starting point of a new research area in water and dialysate purity leading to the use of ultrapure water and dialysate in hemodialysis (22).

In this chapter, the various water purification options available to the dialysis practionner will be described. Details will be provided concerning the nature of water treatment systems, the physical principles involved, and the monitoring approach necessary to optimize water treatment production for hemodialysis. The quality standards required to satisfy contemporary dialysis needs and to ensure patient's safety on a long term basis will also be discussed.

WATER CONTAMINANTS

There are three major groups of water contaminants: particulates, dissolved substances and microorganisms which are presented in Figure 2.

Depending on the source, water will contain varying amounts of particulates. These particulates are responsible for water turbidity: they include minerals (clay, sand, iron) or colloids (silica soluble or polymerised).

Dissolved substances are inorganics or organics, microorganisms and pyrogens.

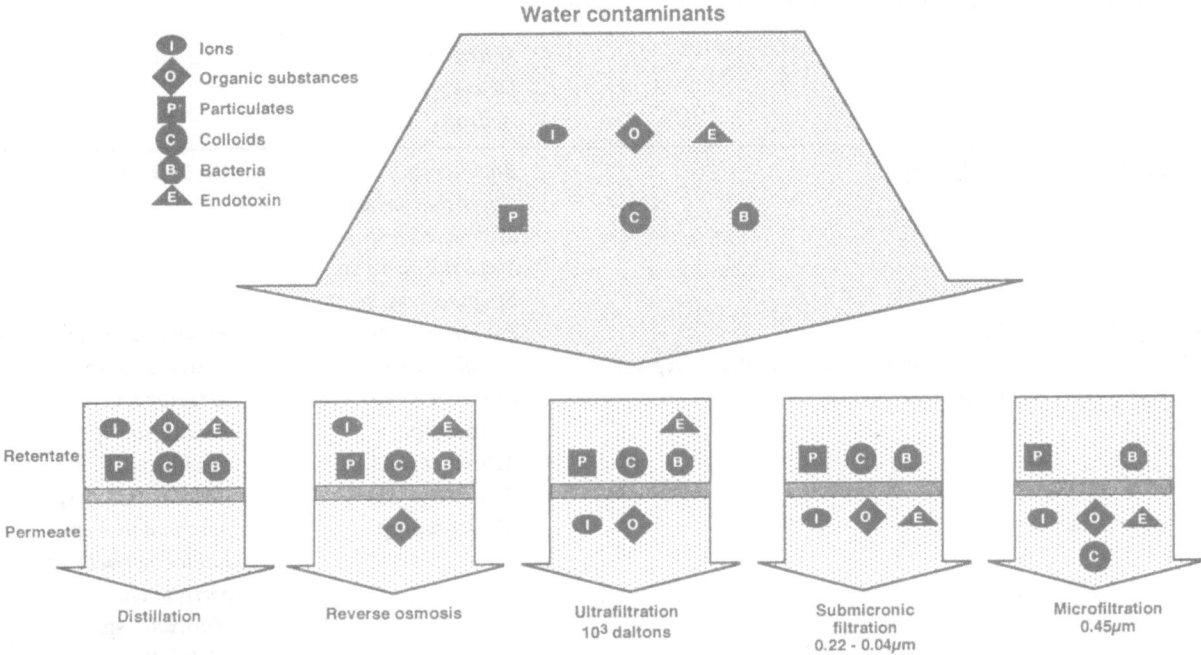

Figure 2. Water contaminants. Efficacy of several water purification devices currently used in water treatment system.

Table 1. Contaminants of water and their toxic effects as documented in hemodialysis patients

Contaminants	Toxic effects
Aluminium	Dialysis encephalopathy, bone disease, microcytic anemia
Calcium-Magnesium	Hard water syndrome: nausea, vomiting, muscular weakness, headache, hypertension, malaise
Chloramines	Hemolysis, anemia, methemoglobinemia
Copper	Nausea, chills, headache, severe hemolysis, hepatitis
Fluoride	Bone disease: osteomalacia
Nitrate	Methemoglobinemia, cyanosis, hypotension, nausea
Sodium	Hypertension, pulmonary oedema, confusion, headache, thirst, tachycardia, seizures, coma
Sulfate	Nausea, vomiting, metabolic acidosis
Zinc	Anemia, nausea, vomiting, fever
Microbial	Chills, fever, nausea, septicemia
Pyrogen	Pyrogenic reaction, hypotension, cyanosis, shock

The main inorganic species are represented by ions, salts, Ca, Fe, Zn. Among the organic substances, the main common species are by-product from natural substances (tannin, lignine) or from agricultural (pesticide, insecticide, fertilizer) or industrial (oil, mining, municipal dumps) processes. Contaminants of water which have documented toxicity in hemodialysis have been listed in Table 1.

Microorganisms are mainly represented by bacteria, although fungi, viruses, protozoan are occasionally encountered. Bacteria contamination with living organisms lead also to release of degradation products (endotoxin, peptidoglycanes) (50, 51). The main microorganisms observed in city and/or dialysis water are listed in Table 2.

Water treatment options should take into account the degree of contamination of the incoming water and requirements for purity grade of the final water product. Furthermore, it must be emphasized that municipal water supplies may have seasonal variations (52). Chemical substances, such as aluminum, chlorine, chloramine, fluoride, that are added by municipal authorities to clear or to make water safe for drinking make unsafe the water for hemodialysis (53–74). In addition, the distribution piping system may itself contribute to water contamination: toxic material such as copper, brass, zinc and lead may leach into the water supply during distribution or prolonged stagnation; poorly designed hydraulic systems will facilitate bacterial growth.

Table 2. Waterborne bacteria usually identified in water treatment system

Bacteria	Tap water	Softeners Deionizers Activated charcoal	Dialysate
Gram positive	*Bacillus* sp.	*Bacillus* sp. *Corynebacterium* sp. *Micrococcus* sp. *Staphylococcus* sp. *Streptococcus* sp.	*Bacillus* sp.
Gram negative	*Pseudomonas* sp. (*P. aeruginosa, P. maltophilia, P. cepacia*) *Flavobacterium* sp.	*Eschericia coli* *Pseudomonas* sp. *Flavobacter* sp. *Serratia* sp. *Achromobacter* sp. *Aerobacter* sp. *Alcaligenes* sp.	*Pseudomonas* sp. *Flavobacter* sp. *Acinetobacter* sp. *Alcaligenes* sp. *Erwinia* sp. *Achromobacter* sp. *Aeromononas* sp. *Xanthomononas* sp. *Serratia* sp. *Moraxella* sp. *Klebsiella* sp. *Enterobacter cloacae*
Anaerobic	*Mycobacteria* *M. chelonei* *M. xenopi* *M. gordonae* *M. scrofulaceum*	*Clostridium* sp. *Mycobacter* sp.	*M. chelonei* *M. chelonei*-like

WATER TREATMENT DEVICES

Activated carbon filters

Activated carbon filter is usually used as pre-treatment for removing dissolved organic contaminants and chlorine, chloramines from water supply (75–78).

Granular activated carbon is embedded in cartridge. Carbon filter may be utilized both as an adsorptive device and a pre-treatment clearing media filter. However, it has to be mentioned that activated carbon is not an efficient media filter since the equally sized carbon particles tend to occlude at the top of the media causing rapid increases in delta pressure drop in turbid water situations. Carbon filter should be used for first stage oxident removal and not as media filter.

Activated carbon has a microporous structure offering a very large surface area to weight ratio that facilitates surface adsorption of chlorine, chloramine utilized to sanitize water distribution system and organic removal (Figure 3).

The adsorption capacity and the rate of removal varies with the carbon used. The activated charcoal efficiency is function of various parameters: volume of charcoal,

particle sizing, source, nature and degree of activation of charcoal. Overall efficacy of charcoal filter, is depending upon cartridge geometry, incoming water flow and content of chlorine and chloramines. Regarding the proper configuration of carbon filter the most critical factor is the water contact time with the charcoal bed. The choice of a carbon filter must be appropriately sized according to water contamination degree and volume to be treated. Periodic backwashing of carbon filter will permit cleansing of accumulated organic substances while restoring adsorptive capacity by unpacking media and preventing channeling occurrence.

When adsorptive capacity is exceeded and activated carbon exhausted, 'spill-over' of chlorine, chloramines and dissolved organics may occur in the effluent water. Permanent monitoring of the concentration of chlorine in the effluent is therefore a convenient and easy method for monitoring the efficacy of activated carbon. Carbon filter may not be regenerated effectively and must be used as a disposable cartridge or repackable with fresh granular activated charcoal. Periodic replacement of carbon filter cartridge is therefore necessary to maintain optimal functioning of the device.

Table 3. Advantages and drawbacks of the different water treatment modules

Activated carbon

Advantages
- Remove adequately organic contaminants chloride, chloramine
- Large adsorptive capacity
- Low cost

Drawbacks
- Release abrasive particles (fines)
- Limitation in adsorptive capacity (spill-over)
- Facilitate bacterial proliferation
- Difficult to sanitize

Distillation

Advantages
- Remove all type of contaminants
- Indefinite reusability
- Prevent using chemical agent
- Spare environment from polution

Drawbacks
- High consumption of energy
- Non effective on volatile contaminants
- Require strict attention

Softeners

Advantages
- Reduce effectively 'water hardness'
- Regenerable at ease
- Low cost

Drawbacks
- Non effective for removing particles, organic components, or other ions
- Salt release is a function of hardness of water degree
- Facilitate growth of bacteria
- Difficult to sanitize
- Aging of softener and exhaustion of resins is associated with
- Risk of 'hard water syndrome'

Mixed bed of deionization

Advantages
- Eliminate ions
- Regenerable without limitations
- Low cost in use

Drawbacks
- Non effective in organic components, nor micro-oganisms
- Potentiate bacterial growth
- Release of particles
- Exhaustion of resins

Continuous Electric Deionizer

Advantages
- Eliminate adequately ions
- Permanent regeneration
- Low cost of maintenance
- Not source for bacterial growth

Drawbacks
- Non effective for organic components, particles and micro-organisms
- Sensitivity of membranes
- Aging and loss of efficacy with time

Microfiltration

Advantages
- Eliminate all micro-organisms, particles according to permeability of the membrane
- Limited maintenance

Drawbacks
- No regeneration
- Non effective for dissolved mineral, pyrogens, nor colloids
- Saturation and release risks
- Bacterial growth and contamination risk

Reverse osmosis

Advantages
- Remove most ions dissolved
- Eliminate lipolysaccharides and part of incoming bacterial

Drawbacks
- Require a pre-treatment system
- Consumption of large quantity of water
- Wearing of the RO membrane

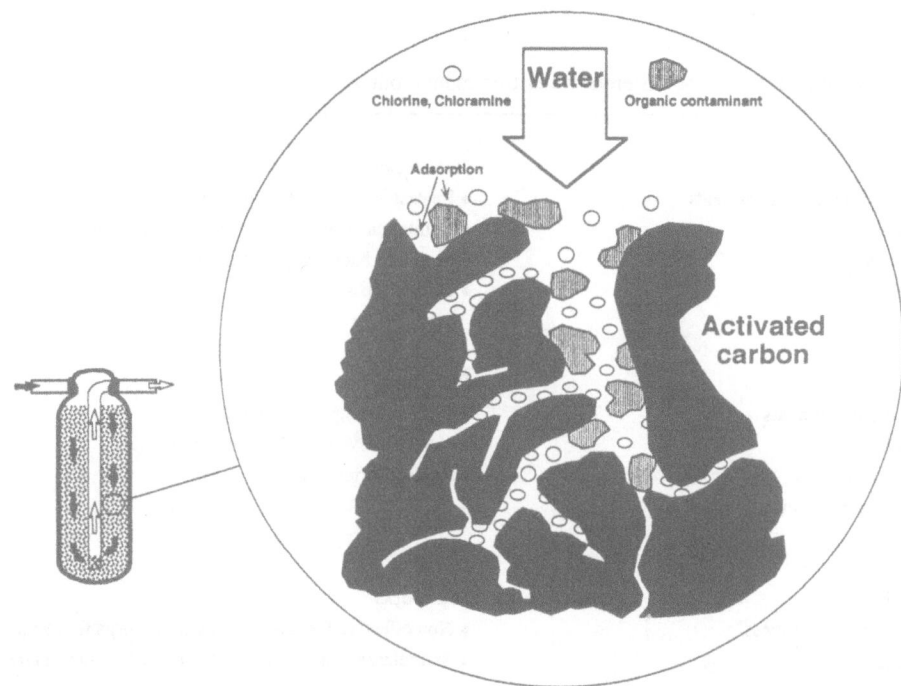

Figure 3. Activated carbon module (left part) and its mode of action in water purification (right and enlarged part).

Carbon filter, because of its granular structure, tends to release abrasive particles called fines. Microfilters are therefore placed in series with carbon filter to prevent downstream plugging and deleterious effects of fines on reverse osmosis membrane.

Microporous structure of activated carbon and organic substances accumulation represent a perfect media favoring microbial contamination. Furthermore, removal of chlorine by activated carbon facilitates bacterial growth. Carbon filter contributes largely to increase levels of bacteria and endotoxins in treated water. Periodic sanitization of carbon filter is therefore necessary to prevent reaching critical levels of bacteria proliferation (10^6 to 10^7 CFU/ml) with major risk of downstream seeding. Flushing carbon filter with high concentration chlorine may be used to reduce level of bacterial contamination without altering activated carbon functionality. Advantages and drawbacks of activated carbon filtration are summarized in Table 3.

Distillation

Distillation is the oldest approach and the reference method used for water purification by the pharmaceutical industry (9). Two stage distillation remains the European Pharmacopoeia standard method to produce water for injection (WFI).

Distillation is based on change of water state with large consumption of energy: liquid water is converted to the

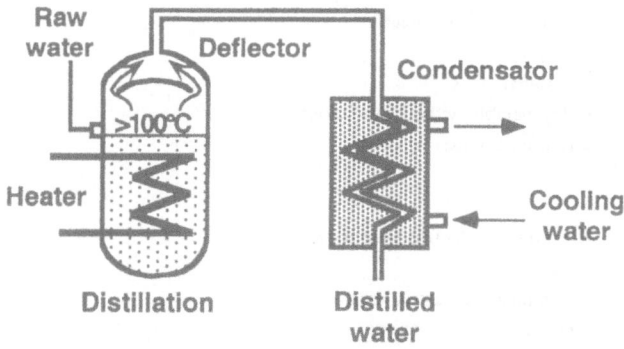

Figure 4. Water distillation system used in an industrial or pharmaceutical setting.

vapor phase with a subsequent condensation of the vapor to water by cooling (Figure 4).

Distillation is effective in removing non volatile organic and inorganic substances, particulate, colloids substances, microorganisms and pyrogens. On the opposite it is not effective for volatile substances which may be found in distillate.

Although distillation is an effective modality, it is not commonly used in water treatment for hemodialysis. Two main reasons for that: first, it requires an expensive chain of production (tubing system, stainless steel storage tanks) which is prone to recontamination; second, it consumes large amount of energy both for heating and cooling water;

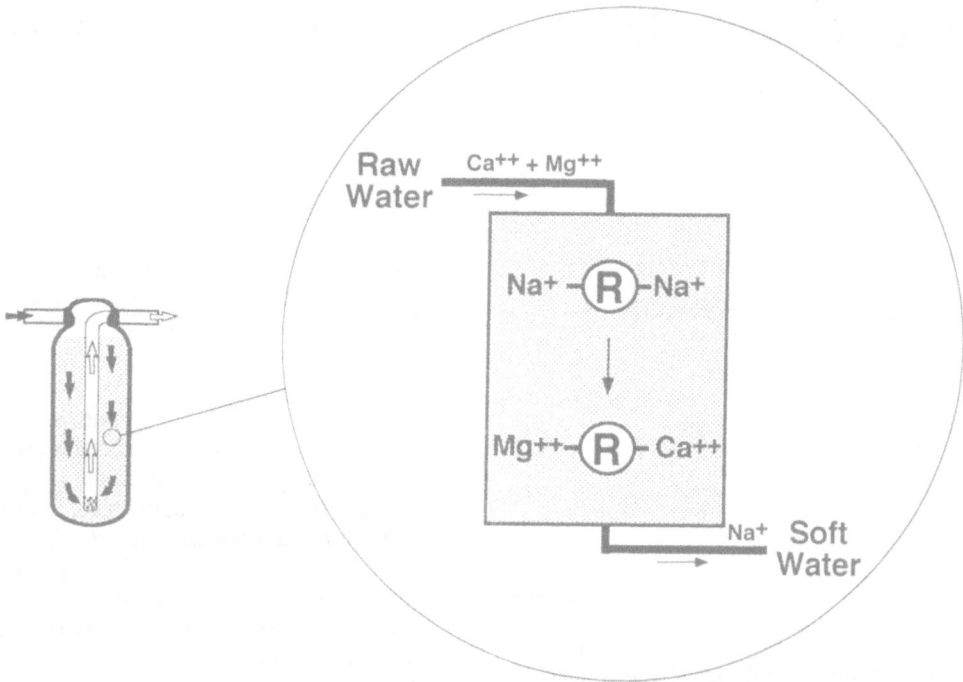

Figure 5. Water softener module (left part) and its mode of action in water purification (right and enlarged part).

although recent technological improvement have substantially reduced these expenses. Advantages and drawbacks of distillation are summarized in Table 3.

Softening

Water softening is necessary to reduce total hardness of incoming municipal supply water (< 1 ppm). It consists in removing calcium and magnesium from water by ionic exchange with cation fixed on resin beads (9). Water softeners are used commonly in the pre-treatment stage of water to reduce divalent ion charge and to protect membrane of equipment downstream from build up and scaling. It is essential to prevent 'hard water syndrome'.

Water softeners are ion exchangers (Figure 5). The resin of the module is a cationic form that exchanges two Na^+ ions for Ca^{++} and Mg^{++} as well as other cation ions (iron, manganese).

Volume of resins (15–75 l) determines roughly the volume of softened water available for consumption (1–4 m^3). Effectiveness of softeners is a function of total hardness of incoming water, flow production and/or consumption ratio, functional quality of resins used and frequency of regeneration cycles. When all Na^+ ions have been exchanged the resin is exhausted and has to be regenerated to prevent hard water syndrome. Regeneration cycles are programmed to start automatically out of dialysis running hours. Softeners must be equipped with a by-pass, shunting the water flow during the regeneration

process. Regular softener regeneration is accomplished on site with brine sodium chloride solution by reverting the ion exchange process. Na^+ ions are then reinstated on the resin by exchange with divalent ions fixed. Regeneration of exhausted resins may be done industrially outside from site.

Softener performances optimization have been achieved by using monodispersed resin beads: the homogeneity of such resin particles improves the softener ion exchange capacity resulting in a reduced volume of resin required for water softening.

Calcium release from exhausted resin may lead to 'hard water syndrome'. This must be prevented by continuous or daily hardness monitoring (Testomat®) and by frequent automated regeneration cycles ensuring a safety reserve in softening capacity of the resin.

Softener resin, favoring water stagnation, is prone to bacterial growth with seeding downstream. Frequent regeneration cycles with back washing will reduce bacterial proliferation as well as the accumulation of particulates in resin bed. Continuous chlorine infusion upstream is effective in preventing bacterial proliferation within resin beads. Periodic sanitization performed either by flushing the softener with a highly concentrated sodium hypochlorite solution or the peracetic acid may be helpful to reduce the level of bacterial contamination without altering resin functionality. Advantages and drawbacks of softening are summarized in Table 3.

Conventional Filtration

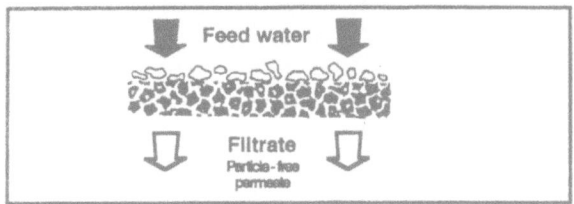

Cross-Flow Filtration

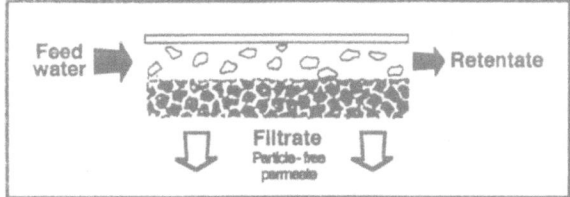

Figure 6. Water filtration principles: conventional filtration (perpendicular) favoring built-up and accumulation of contaminants at the membrane surface; cross-flow (tangential) preventing accumulation of contaminants at the membrane surface.

Microfilter
Microporous filter
Ultrafilter
Molecular filter

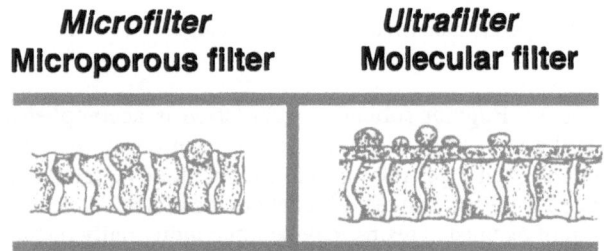

Figure 7. Illustration of the retentive capacity of microfilter compared to ultrafilter.

Filtration

Sediment filtration, as the name states, is a membrane filter process, used to remove particulate of large size from the water supply (79–84). It prevents plugging and fouling of water treatment equipment downstream. Filtration is accomplished by particulate size exclusion while water percolates through porous medium with nominal porosity less than that particulate one (Figure 6). According to size particulate removed there are three stages of filtration: pre-filtration, micro-filtration and sub-micronic filtration:

— Pre-filtration is a crude process designed to clarify raw supply water. It eliminates the large size particulate (5–500 μm) from incoming water preventing fouling of equipment downstream;
— Micro-filtration is a more refined process, removing smaller size particulate (1–5 μm diameter) (Figure 7);
— Sub-micronic filtration is used to exclude lower size water particulate and bacteria. Membranes with pore

Depth filter   Screen filter

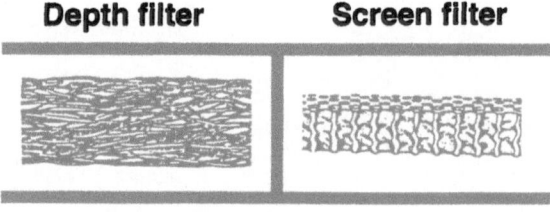

Figure 8. Microfilter types: depth filters are made of an arrangement of packed fibers knot-works in bundle; Screen filter are made of porous inert and homogenous matrix.

size in the range of 0.45 μm down to 0.1 μm are commercially available with surface areas large enough to reduce hydraulic resistance to a minimum and in various fittings (i.e., cartridges, flat disks). Microbial filtration is defined as absolute with 0.22 μm pore size membranes. It has been shown, however, that some bacterial species of minute size can cross 0.22 μm pores, and will be removed only with 0.1 μm pore size membranes.

Except for the removal of microorganisms, filtration never reach the efficacy of reverse osmosis (RO) or ultrafiltration (UF) that work at molecular size filtration.

Filters commercially available are of two main types: depth filter (packed fibers); surface or screen filter (porous matrix) (Figure 8):

— Depth filters are made of an arrangement of closely packed fibers knot-works in a bundle determining a variable thickness. Particulates are excluded by hazard retention (inertial impacting to media) or by adsorption into fibers.
— Screen filters are made of porous, inert and homogeneous matrix sieving incoming particulates. Retention on matrix surface is then absolute for particulates larger than medium pore diameter.

Stability of filtering media is most helpful from a clinician point of view to ensure the safety of filtering process. Filters are then best classified either in stable or unstable media according to pressure flow regimen changes.

— Unstable media structure are characterized by a porosity size that increases with filtration pressure forbidding nominal retention rating. Such a condition facilitates the release of medium and permeation of particulates above the nominal porosity of filter. This is mainly observed with depth and fiber filters.
— Stable media means that the pore size determined during the manufacturing process remains stable whatever pressure regimen flow is used. Such filters ensure an absolute retentive capacity for particulates larger than the pore size. This is obtained mainly with screen filters.

The choice of a filter depends on its planned use:

— In-depth or unstable filters used for prefiltration remove in an inexpensive way 90–98% of suspended particulates and prevent fouling and build up in equipment downstream.

- Screen filters (surface filters) on the contrary are used for post-treatment to exclude small size contaminants (resin fragments, particulate of activated charcoal, colloidal substances ...)

Combining filters of different retentive capacity in series permits to optimize and to improve the overall effectiveness of the filtering system: serial association with down rating filtering capacity is designed to enhance final purity of water: parallel association of filters is designed to increase the production capacity while maintaining the loss of pressure charge at a low level.

Functional performances of a filter are usually defined according to their retentive capacity rating. However two major points must be underlined. First, from a terminology standpoint it is important to differentiate absolute and nominal retentive rating. Absolute retentive rating represents the diameter of the largest particulates that cannot pass through a filter in fixed conditions. Nominal retentive rating is determined by the manufacturing process and corresponds to the media pore size that is supposed to exclude incoming particulates with a larger diameter. Second, from an effective efficacy standpoint, a filtration process is defined as a reduction percentage of incoming contaminants. Therefore, the efficacy of a filtering system will also depend upon the purity of the feeding water.

Charge-modified filter is a new and promising approach enlarging filter properties by adding a removal capacity for pyrogens. Based on the positive zeta potential of their membrane surface, such filters are able to remove negatively charged lipopolysaccharide from deionized, reverse-osmosis treated, and distilled water (85–86).

Filter fouling may be monitored by differential pressure changes occurring from pre- to post-filter in fixed functional conditions. Periodic filter changes are therefore necessary to prevent reduction of filtering capacity.

Bacterial growth is a major problem with filters. This is due to colloid and organic substances accumulation and to water stagnation, both conditions favoring bacterial proliferation.

Filters are usually not regenerable meaning that with time progressive build up of particulate matter is occurring within the membrane. When filter membrane is saturated, retention capacity may be exceeded and particulates break-through may occur. Retentive capacity is then overflowed. Filter must be replaced periodically to ensure optimal functioning and to prevent unexpected release of particulates from saturated membrane. Advantages and drawbacks of filtration are summarized in Table 3.

Ultrafiltration

Ultrafiltration (UF) is a membrane filtration process based mainly on a molecular sieving exclusion (Figure 7). It has a molecular cut off higher than reverse osmosis but lower than submicronic filtration. Ultrafilter splits incoming water in two streams: on one side permeating the membrane is the ultrafiltrate cleared of contaminants; on the other side excluding from the membrane is the retentate a concentrate of rejected particulates (Figure 6). UF is effective in removing microorganisms, pyrogens, colloids and particulates (submicronic) with a molecular size higher than cut off point of the membrane (88–95).

Ultrafilters are made from highly permeable membrane usually synthetic (polyamide, polysulfone ...) arranged and packed in a plate or hollow fiber unit.

The performances of an ultrafilter depend on the characteristics of the membrane, including hydraulic permeability, sieving molecular cut off, surface electric charges and surface area. Performances are also influenced by flow rate regimen, purity of incoming water and transmembrane pressure. Membrane adsorption, due to the chemical reactivity and zeta potential of the synthetic membranes, may also contribute significantly in removing charged particles of inflowing water. Such property extending functional capacity of ultrafilter to reactive species have been clearly demonstrated for lipopolysaccharides (87–95).

The nature of the membrane is a critical factor determining efficacy and resistance of UF to water contaminants and corrosive action of chemical disinfectant. As a membrane filtration process, ultrafiltration reduces contaminant titer of inlet water, meaning that effectiveness of UF is also a function of purity of incoming water. Optimal functioning of UF requires permanent tangential filtration flux and/or intermittent flushing preventing plugging and build up at the membrane surface. Association of ultrafilters in series enhances the overall efficacy of the UF system by reducing hazards of permeating contaminants. Programmed changes of ultrafilters is also a safe and necessary way to prevent unexpected passage of contaminants in case of ultrafilter saturation.

Ultrafilters are particularly useful and highly effective in removing pyrogens at a reasonable cost. Ultrafilter may also be used to protect RO membranes or to ensure final ultrapurity of water produced. Ultrafilters are usually placed in water posttreatment. Regeneration of industrial ultrafilter may be performed on site by chemical cleaning and back flushing. Advantages and disadvantages of UF are summarized in Table 3.

Reverse osmosis (RO)

Reverse osmosis is a membrane filtration process based on molecular sieving ($\approx$ 300 Daltons) and ionic exclusion with 90–99% rejection (9) (Figure 9). RO is the more cost competitive effective method to purify water from dissolved organic and inorganic particulates including bacteria and endotoxins (96–101).

Osmosis occurs when two solutions of different ionic concentrations are separated by a semi permeable membrane. Osmosis describes the phenomenon of solvent flowing from the less concentrated to the more concentrated side. The driving force responsible for this movement

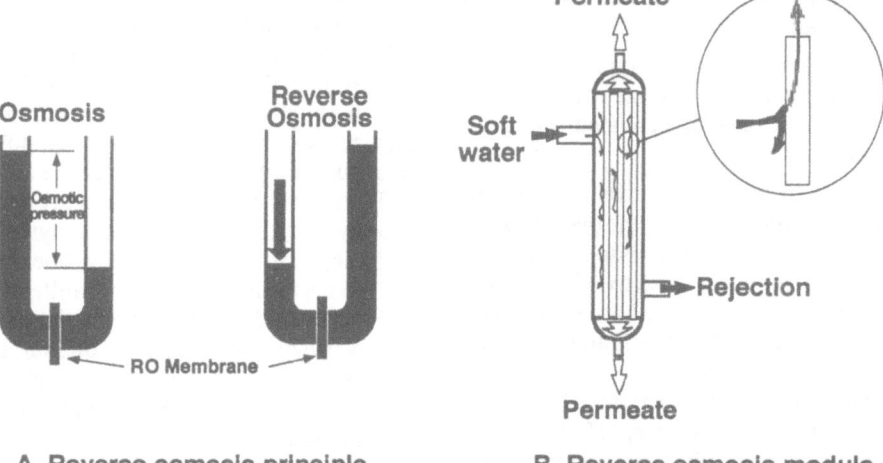

Figure 9. Reverse osmosis (RO). A. Physic principle of reverse osmosis. B. Reverse osmosis module and its mode of action (enlarged part). RO splits incoming soft water in two fluxes, permeate (purified water) and retentate (rejected and concentrated water).

being known as the osmotic pressure as shown on Figure 9 (left panel). If the hydraulic pressure applied on the concentrated side is higher than the osmotic pressure, then the solvent flow is reverse and move from the more concentrated to the less concentrated side. The process is then called reverse osmosis. The RO acts as a selective sieving filter rejecting solute above the membrane cut off. RO separates incoming water flow in two fluxes: RO water (permeate) on one side; rejected water (concentrate) contains 90–99% of water contaminants as shown on Figure 9 (right panel).

RO membranes include two major types: cellulosic (cellulose acetate) and synthetic (polyamide, polysulfone). Thin composite membranes, recently developed for clinical use, seem more promising as they ally high performance and strong resistance. RO membranes are fitted in modules with various geometrical configuration: plate membrane frame, spiral wound and hollow fibers.

RO performances depend upon different factors: membrane and module characteristics (structure, surface area, nature), inflowing water temperature, pH, water contaminant concentration and production/rejection ratio. Optimal performances and life span of RO are function both of the pretreatment system efficacy and of the RO membrane maintenance (flushing, cleaning, disinfecting) (101).

Resistance of the RO membranes to the destructive action of chemical species (pH, chlorine, chloramine), disinfectant (peracetic acid, formaldehyde ...) or bacteria is directly related to the nature of the membrane: cellulose acetate is highly sensitive to the bacteria destructive action; synthetic membranes are more sensitive to the corrosive action of chemical species; thin composite membranes appears conversely highly resistant to all agents.

The performance of the RO system is monitored by continuous measurement of resistivity of both product water and of rejected water. A production/rejection ratio of 0.85–0.95 is obtained with an efficient RO system while a value below 0.80 indicates the need to change the membrane module. RO water quality can deteriorate with time because of fouling and/or scaling of membrane. Such problems depend mainly on the purity of the inflowing pretreated water. Periodic flushing of membrane is then required for scrubbing concentrated particles at the membrane surface and then to restore optimal functioning of RO.

The RO process is effective in decontaminating water, if membrane integrity is preserved: RO removes bacteria (provided the bacterial load of affluent water is limited and the tightness of the frame is adequate), viruses and lipopolysaccharides (LPS) (47, 48). It must be emphasized however that its efficiency is highly dependent of nature of the RO membrane and its interaction with the chemical and/or bacteria species of water.

Overall efficacy of RO may be overwhelmed in case of incoming water of high ionic strength. A deionizer may be added downstream of the RO system to 'polish' water: this approach introduces a major risk of microbiological contamination of the purified RO water by the resins of the deionizer. Advantages and drawbacks of reverse osmosis are summarized in Table 3.

Deionization

Water deionization consists in removing dissolved inorganic ions using their electrical and charged properties. It is based on a ion-exchange process. According to the nature of the media used for exchange, deionizers may be classified in two types: solid phase deionizer (mixed bed)

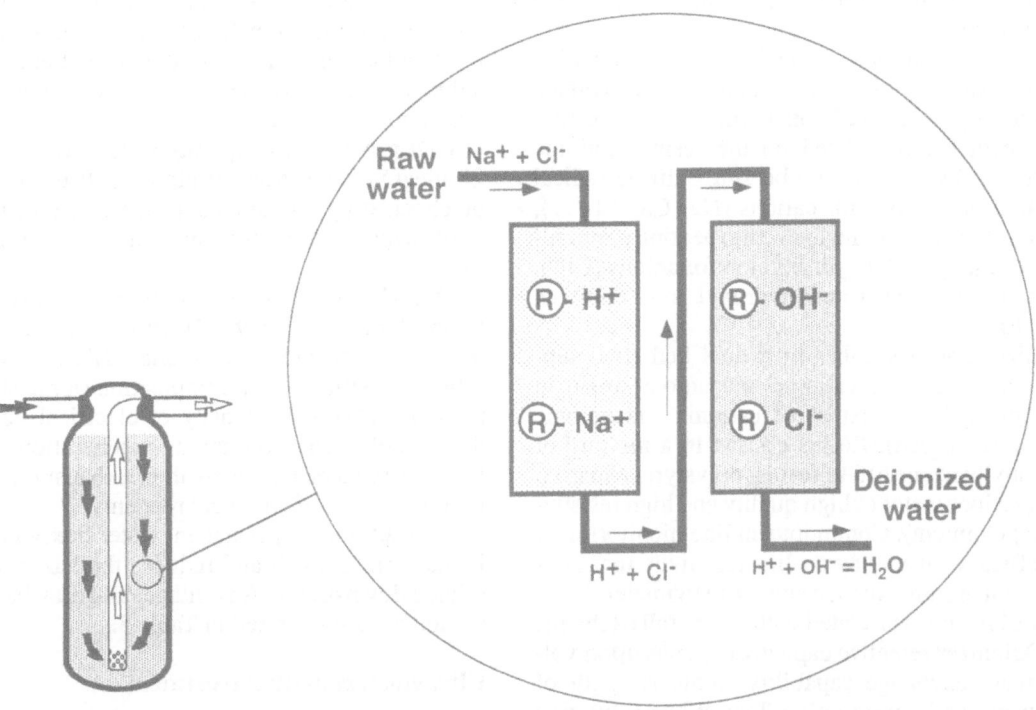

Figure 10. Mixed bed deionizer module (left part) and its mode of action (right and enlarged part) as a ion resin exchanger (cationic and anionic resins).

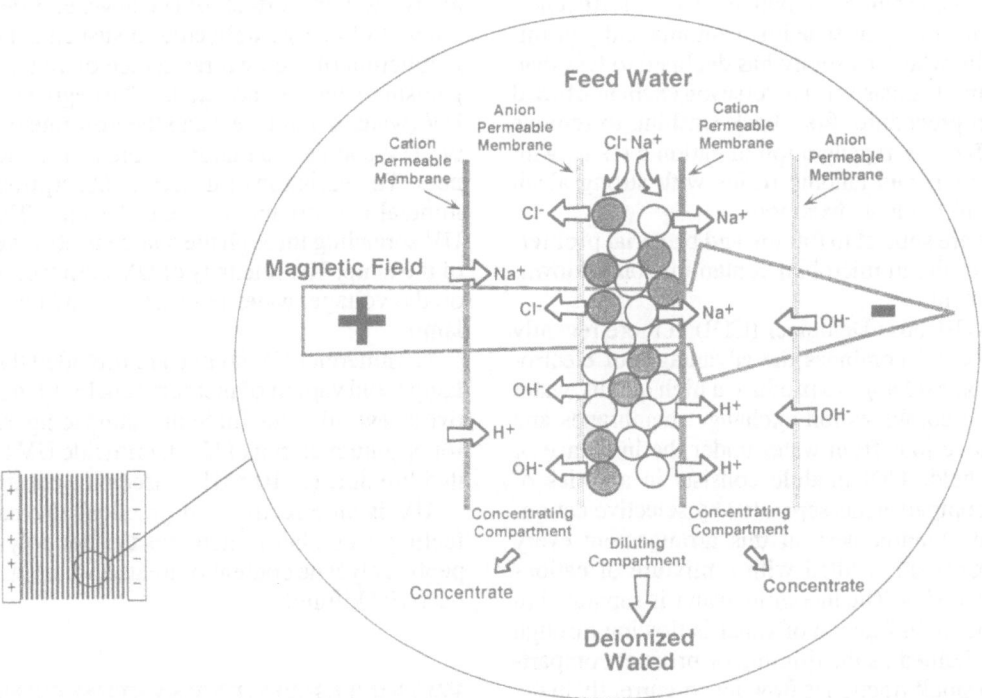

Figure 11. Continuous Electric Deionizer (CDI) module combines electrodialysis (magnetic field, arrow) and ion exchange (resin and membrane) to produce high quality water.

(Figure 10); Continuous Electric Deionizer (Figure 11) (CDI) (102–104).

Deionizer in solid phase consists in a percolation of water in resin of cationic and anionic types (mixed bed) (Figure 10). Dissolved ion particles of water are exchanged with the ions fixed on the resins, cationic resins (styrene, divinylbenzene) bearing sulfuric radical exchange hydrogens ions for cations (Na, Ca, Al ...), anionic resins (styrene, divinylbenzene) bearing ammonium radical exchanges OH hydroxyl ion for anions (Cl^-). The exchanged hydrogen and hydroxyl ions combine together to form water.

A deionizer consists either in a dual bed (two separate beds one each, for cationic and anionic resin in series) or mixed bed (mixture of cationic and anionic resins in the same bed). Resins consist in a mixture of styrene/divinylbenzene bed to form a polystyrene matrix. Deionizer produce water of high quality and high resistivity (> 1 megOhm/cm). Continuous in line monitoring of deionizer efficacy insured by on-line resistivity measurement with temperature compensated resistivimeter.

Efficacy of resin is correlated with its overall exchange capacity. Deionizer retentive capacity depends upon volume and resin exchange capability, ionic strength of inflowing water and consumption flow. When saturation of exchange sites is reached, the resin is exhausted. Regeneration is then necessary to prevent release of fixed cations (Ca^{++}, Mg^{++}) and anions (NO_3, SO_4 ...). Effluent water may also become acidic because of the imbalance between cations and anions exchange capacities. Regeneration of deionizer may be scheduled automatically or initiated manually when resistivity has declined to less than 1 megOhm/cm. It consists in a reverse ion exchange based on a two step procedure: first, back washing to remove particulates; second, regeneration of cationic resins with strong acid (HCl) and anionic resins with strong alcali (NaOH, bleach) to eluate fixed ions.

Deionizers are subject to fouling and bacterial proliferation which results in microbial contamination of downstream equipment.

Continuous Electric Deionizer (CDI), a more recently developed process, combines the advantages of electrodialysis and ion exchange to produce a high quality water (Figure 11). It combines ion exchange membranes and resins to remove ions from water under the influence of an electrical field. CDI module consists in a series of thin parallel compartments separated by selective cationic and anionic membranes; in this arrangement every second compartment is filled with a mixture of cationic and anionic resins. The incoming water is separated in two fluxes: the main fraction of water is flowing through mixed resins defined as the diluting or product compartment, while a small fraction is flowing co-currently in the adjacent compartments designed as concentrate compartments. Electrical field force ions to migrate from product compartment to dilute pathway according to polarity of field and selectivity of membranes as shown in Figure 11.

The resin facilitates ion transfer by providing a low resistance path for the transfer of ions. In addition as the water product become very pure, the current applied in excess splits water into hydrogen and hydroxyl ions regenerating continuously the resin.

CDI provides high quality water with resistivity up to 20 megOhm/cm. Monitoring of CDI performances may be checked by continuous measurement of resistivity on outflowing water with temperature compensated conductimeter.

Overall efficacy depends upon geometrical and functional characteristics of CDI (surface area exchange, number of compartment, membranes, dilute/concentrate flow ratio), incoming water composition (ionic strength, temperature, pH) and intensity of electrical field acting on the module. The continuous regeneration of the resins by electrodialysis prevents their exhaustion and does not require the use of chemical reagents.

In addition, the permanent water flux within CDI limits bacterial growth and reduces the hazards of pyrogen release downstream. Advantages and drawbacks of deionization are summarized in Table 3.

Ultraviolet radiation treatment

Ultraviolet (UV) radiation is a ionization process that is able to destroy all types of waterborne bacteria whatever their state, vegetative or sporulated. Microorganisms withstand considerably more to UV in water than in dry air. Bactericidal effects of UV in water is depending on the amount of energy delivered to suspended organisms and is function of the own resistance of waterborne microorganism to the UV radiations. The degree of penetration of UV (water depth layer) and the flow rate of water through the UV source are major factors of germicidal effectiveness. The variation of degree of absorption is function of mineral and organic content of water. The reduction of UV spreading through the source is observed with scaling of the lamp. The intensity of UV output of a lamp depends on the voltage, water temperature and burning hours of a lamp.

Commercial UV source are provided through mercury lamp (cold vapour of mercury) enclosed in a quartz protective sleeve allowing for higher lamp temperatures required for optimum output of UV. Germicide UV lamps have limited life time (5–10000 h) based on a continuous flow.

UV is an effective and practical alternative for disinfecting water, but it increases the lipopolysaccharide and peptidoglycane content of treated water due to process of bacterial killing.

WATER TREATMENT SYSTEM CONCEPT

None of the individual water treatment devices described above offers the possibility of producing high purity water on a long term basis. The association of several water

Table 4. Purified water according to European and US Pharmacopeia. Highly purified water (ultrapure water) according to semiconductor industry needs

Constituent	Purified water (European &) US pharmacopoeia)	Ultrapure water 5 MΩ cm
pH	5.0–7.0	5.0–7.0
Chloride, mg/l	≤ 0.50	≤ 0.06
Sulfate, mg/l	≤ 0.10	≤ 0.08
Ammonia, mg/l	≤ 0.10	≤ 0.03
Calcium, mg/l	≤ 1.00	≤ 0.04
Carbon dioxide, mg/l	≤ 5.00	≤ 0.20
Heavy metals, mg/l	≤ 0.10	≤ 0.01
Total solids, mg/l	≤ 10.0	≤ 0.50
Total bacteria count, CFU/ml	≤ 100	≤ 10.0
Pyrogen Endotoxin, UE/ml	?	≤ 0.25

treatment options is required to achieve a regular and constant production of high grade quality water. A water treatment system in all cases will be a chain associating several units assembled either in series or in parallel, each one having a specific function. The major contribution of water engineering should be to optimize the performance of each component to enhance the quality of final product (105–108). The assemblage of various components to make a water treatment chain results frequently in an antagonism between the chemical and microbiologic criteria of ultrapure water. For example, the improvement of ion removal by adding resins to a RO system enhances bacterial proliferation with a deleterious effect on microbiological purity.

Water treatment is a complex process that starts from water mains and ends at patient bed-side in the dialysate production. Final purity of water distributed to the hemodialysis machine will therefore integrate all imperfections in the water treatment chain.

Water treatment systems for hemodialysis include usually four sections assembled in series, which include: (1) water pre-treatment; (2) water purification system; (3) water storage (reserve) and distribution system (piping, net delivery system); (4) dialysate preparation and delivery system (dialysis machine) (Figure 1). Most dialysis machines are also a final filtration device (submicronic filter and/or ultrafilter) to ensure the microbial purity of the water feeding dialysis machine and/or the dialysate delivered to the patient's dialyzer.

The complexity of such water treatment chain explain easily the difficulties in maintaining high quality grade standards for water. It is also important to remind that the final quality of the delivered water will be negatively influenced by the worst quality segment of the water chain.

Water pre-treatment and purification systems

Chemical purification is the first stage of the water treatment system. It is one of the most important since conditioning the final purity grade of the water distributed. Water purification consists in three steps which includes: (1) pre-treatment consisting in filters, softener, carbon filter, microfilters; (2) primary treatment consisting in a reverse osmosis (one or two RO) and deionizer for 'polishing' water; (3) post-treatment consisting in ultrafiltration and submicronic filtration with or without storage tank. Various grades of water may be achieved depending directly upon complexity and cost of water purification options used. According to our present knowledge, pharmaceutical quality grade water appears as a new and generalized standard for contemporary hemodialysis. Of these waters two types are suitable for hemodialysis as presented in Table 4: (1) purified water; (2) highly purified water (ultrapure water). The chemical specifications for hemodialysis water are similar to those of water for injection. Absence of bacteria and endotoxin and a resistivity superior to 5 megOhm/cm are the main characteristic of the latter.

a. Purified water may be obtained from a relatively simple water purification system made of a pretreatment (softener) and reverse osmosis (RO) module assembled in series. Such water treatment system should represent now, the basic and common denominator for all conventional hemodialysis system.

According to the quality of the municipal water supply different options of filtration may be proposed. Basically, such water treatment purification system consists of a pretreatment followed by a deionization by RO with straight and direct distribution system. Microfiltration may be occasionally associated as a final quality insurance. A flow diagram of such water purification treatment showing the different components is given in Figure 12.

The pretreatment consists in series of filters for large particulate removal, a cation exchange softener, an activated charcoal cartridge and a filtration down to 1.0–0.45 μm. Permanent sanitization of resins may achieved by continuous chlorine injection in tap water.

b. Highly purified water (ultrapure water). Chemical and microbiological (bacteria viable organisms and endotoxins) limits are most stringent in this case. Quality standards are those required for water for injection with the only difference that conditions of production and instantaneous consumption preclude any microbiological control to be performed (Table 4).

Highly purified water may be produced using different treatment options. Schematically, three different types of water treatment chains are presented that seem to offer the best quality insurance consisting in:

1. The first type presented in Figure 13, consists in a pretreatment system followed by two stage deioniza-

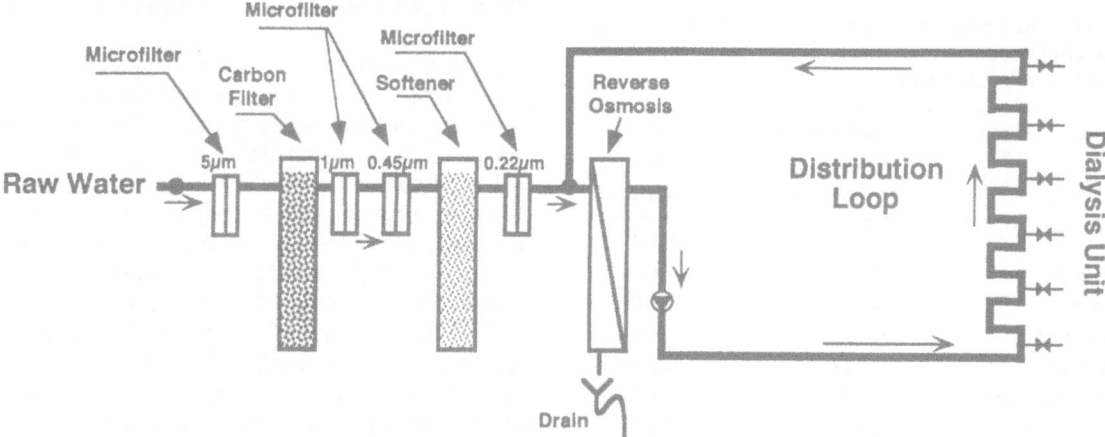

Figure 12. Basic water treatment chain for hemodialysis consists in a pre-treatment (microfiltration, activated carbon, softener) completed by a RO module and a direct production of treated water to the dialysis unit through a recirculating loop.

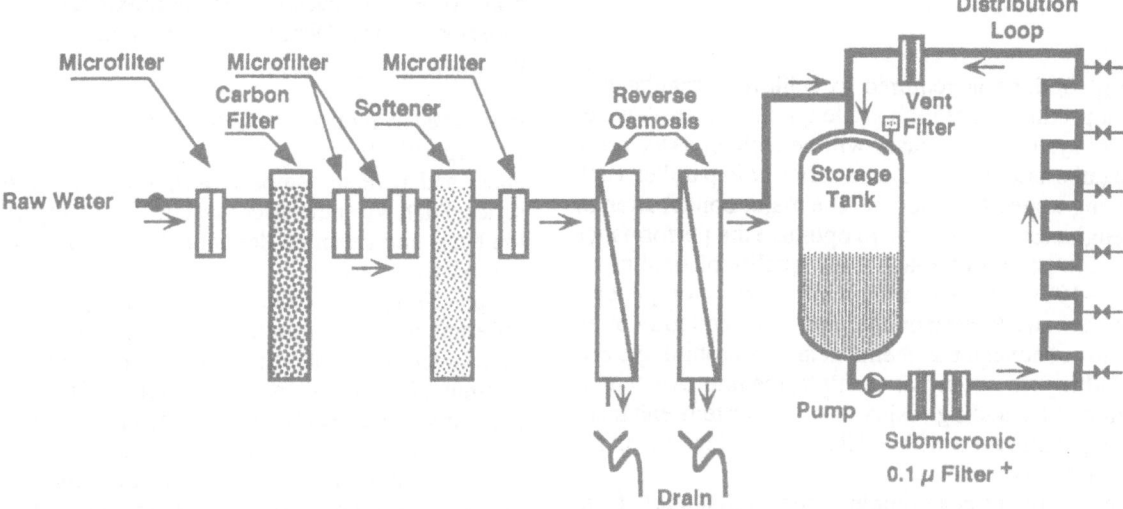

Figure 13. Water treatment chain designed to produce highly purified water. It consists in a pre-treatment followed by a two stages RO treatment. Storage tank is used in this case to prevent any imbalance due to peak flow consomption. Microbiologic purity of water is insured by a permanent recirculation through two serial positively charged submicronic (0.1 μm) filter.

tion by RO completed by a final filtration using a 0.1 μm pore size filter membrane. The treated water is distributed to the dialysis machines through a recirculation loop. The pretreatment uses a series of filters for large particulate removal (5–1 μm), a dual softener and activated carbon filter followed by a filtration down to 0.45 μm. The water treatment consists in two RO units placed in series. An intermediary storage tank may be useful to prevent any RO dysfunction by fluid imbalancing. Rejection flow is discarded on the first RO module while it is recirculated and mixed with softened water on the second RO module. RO modules use cellulose acetate or composite membrane.

2. The second type of chain shown in Figure 14, consists in a pretreatment system followed by primary deionization by RO, completed by polishing deionization by CDI and a final ultrafiltration or microfiltration (0.22 or 0.1 μm positively charged). Pretreatment is the same as previously described. RO unit uses synthetic or composite membrane. RO is operated at 50–60% rejection to reduce the rate of fouling. The CDI unit is a single stage, 30 parallel plate cell designed to produce a nominal product flow of 20 l/min. CDI is operated at 80–85% recovery. The ultrafilter unit is made of a spiral synthetic membrane or a hollow fiber used at a low rejection rate and/or with periodi-

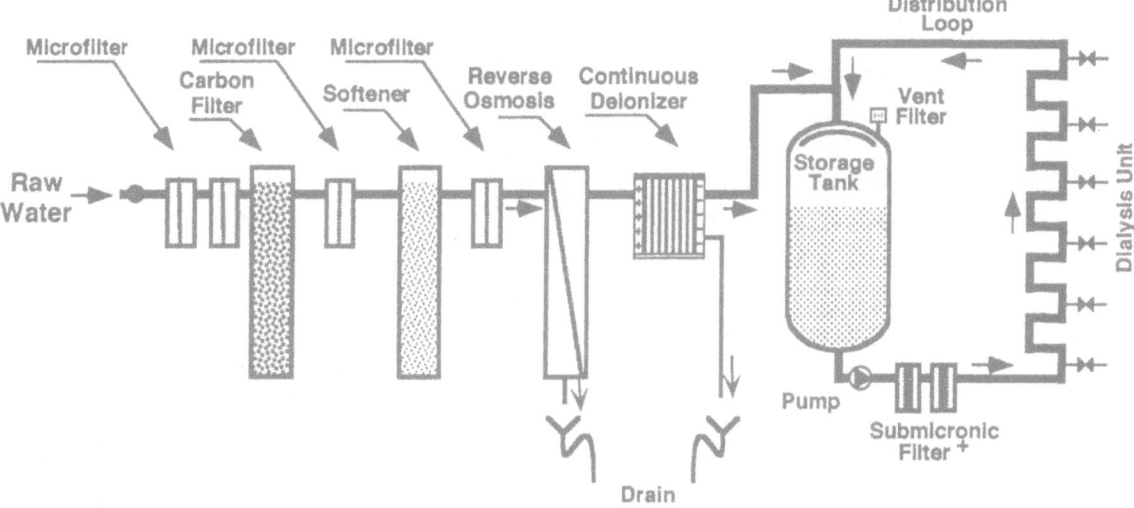

Figure 14. Water treatment chain designed to produce highly purified water. It consists in a pre-treatment completed by RO treatment then polished by Continuous Electric Deionizing (CDI). Storage tank is used in this case to prevent any imbalance due to peak flow consumption. Microbiologic purity of water is insured by a permanent recirculation through serial positively charged submicronic (0.1 μm) filter.

cal flushing of the membrane. The RO, CDI and UF should be sanitized at regular intervals at least monthly and preferably weekly. Chemical disinfection may be performed, according to the manufacturer recommendations, using appropriate concentrations of formaldehyde or peracetic acid or chlorine. Simplification of sanitization has been made possible through the use of a single and common chemical agent both for RO, CDI and ultrafilters.

3. The third type of chain shown in Figure 15 consists in a pretreatment system followed by a primary deionization (mixed bed) then enhancing microbiological quality by final filtration (ultrafiltration or preferably microfiltration); RO can be used for that purpose, but the rejection flow should be recirculated and mixed with the afferent water feeding the deionizer. Deionizer consists in a mixed anionic cationic resin exchange unit. RO unit uses a synthetic or a composite membrane. Ultrafiltration unit or submicronic filtration insure the final purity of water produced to the dialysis unit by eliminating endotoxins and bacteria.

Water storage

A water tank is not always required in a water distribution circuit: whenever possible, it is preferable to avoid it, as water stagnation in a reservoir favors bacterial growth. A tank can be avoided when the production capacity of the water treatment system exceeds at all times the consumption needs of the dialysis units (Figure 12). A reservoir will be necessary when water consumption in the dialysis unit varies during the day with peak consumption

flow exceeding the instantaneous production capacity of the water treatment system; it is also requisite to keep a water safety reserve in a large dialysis unit or to prevent flow and hydrostatic pressure imbalances between the various components of the water treatment system. In practice, water storage can be dispensed with in small dialysis units (e.g., self dialysis or limited care facilities) or in home hemodialysis, while it becomes mandatory in large dialysis facilities. When water storage is required, a reservoir should be designed specifically and integrated into the water distribution system (Figures 13–15). Closed stainless steel storage tank offers the best choice for this purpose. Vessel design is important to prevent water stagnation. The interior of the reservoir is concave at both ends. The internal surface is polished to discourage bacterial adhesion. Water arrives at the upper entry point of the reservoir, impinges into a concave baffle which directs the water stream along the inner surface of the vessel, thus assuring permanent lavage of the wall. Water is continually pumped into the circuit from the bottom of the reservoir either forward in the distribution loop for dialysis use or backward in the water treatment system when dialysis unit is not running.

Reservoir is maintained under pressure of water supply circuit when placed before RO. Event of the reservoir are protected from bacterial contamination by microfilters (0.1 μm). Level probes (max and min) are also necessary to check filling state and action automatically filling/emptying cycles.

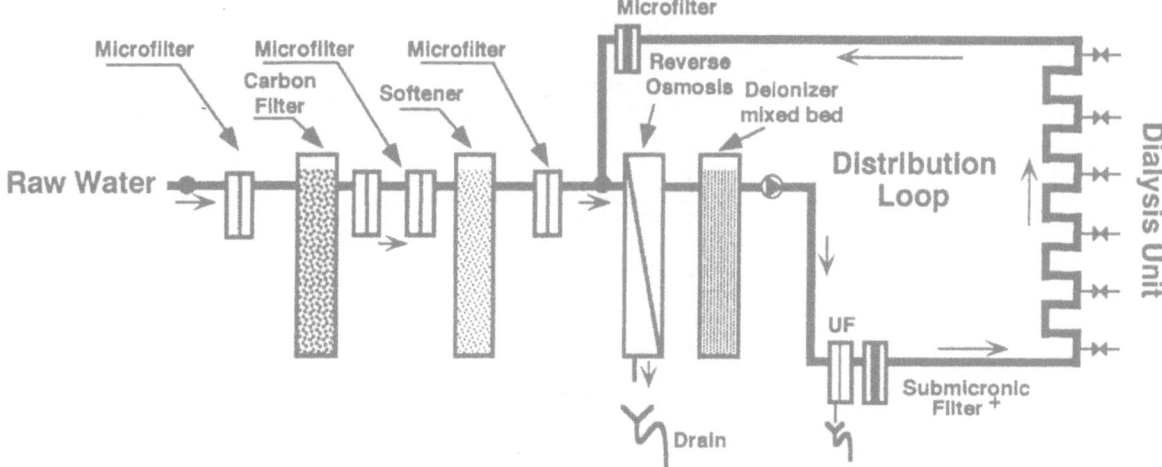

Figure 15. Water treatment chain to produce highly purified water. It consists in a pre-treatment completed by RO treatment then polished by mixed bed deionizing. Treated water is directly flowed to the dialysis unit without storage then recirculated. Microbiologic purity of water is insured by a permanent recirculation through serial submicronic (0.1 μm) filter and/or ultrafilter.

Water and dialysate distribution system

The hydraulic circuit starts from the water mains, supplying the dialysis unit and leads into the dialysate compartment of the dialyzer. It forms a complex path that comprises three major segments:

— The first segment includes the pretreatment and treatment water systems. As indicated above, it is the most complex part of the hydrostatic circuit and it will not be discussed further here.

— The second segment, that should be linear, may include a reservoir and ends into the various ports of utilisation in the dialysis center; it includes the tubes connecting the hemodialysis machines to the main piping.

— The third segment consists of as many hydraulic circuits as they are HD machines. The complexity of the hydraulic pathway inside the machines creates numerous niches facilitating bacterial adhesion and proliferation. To prevent bacterial contamination of dialysis water and of dialysate, the hydraulic circuit should be carefully designed by the manufacturer.

The design of the hydraulic installation is a critical point that will have a major impact on the degree of bacterial contamination of water and thus of dialysate. Since the extra cost in this area is modest the greatest effort should be made to obtain the best plumbing configuration. Without entering into details of such technical points, four principal criteria that must be adhered to should be underscored.

First, hydraulic circuit requires a design that insures linear circulation of the water. Elimination of any by-pass creating stagnation zones. If valves are required on the water distribution piping, they should be placed on lateral

arms whose length does not exceed the diameter of the principal circuit.

Second, to prevent bacterial adhesion to the inner surface of the piping, high water velocity and shear rate should be obtained by selecting a pipe with the smallest inner diameter compatible with the required flow. The material chosen should have a smooth and polished inner surface and joints that disrupt piping continuity should be avoided. Stainless steel, that can be welded without crack formation at the inner surface, thus preventing the formation of bacterial niches, is the ideal material. Its high cost, however, has been an impediment to its routine use. High grade PVC is more commonly used, because of its lower cost: high bacterial quality can be obtained provided the piping installation is carefully designed and regularly disinfected.

Third, continuous water circulation is a basic necessity to prevent water stagnation and bacterial growth. If possible, storage reservoir should be avoided. If this impossible, reservoir with a recirculating loop including a filtration system must be operated 24 h a day.

Fourth, dead space and lateral arms (manyfolds) must be avoided or reduced to a minimum. Tubing connecting the distribution loop to the dialysis machine should be as short as possible as shown in Figure 16.

Final filtration

When a storage tank is used, water flow in the recirculation loop is provided by dual centrifugal pumps which maintain the hydrostatic pressure at the level required for proper functioning of the various systems fed with ultrapure water. A cold sterilisation system, made of an ultrafilter or preferably a submicronic filters with positive zeta potential at the filter membrane surface (0.1 μm

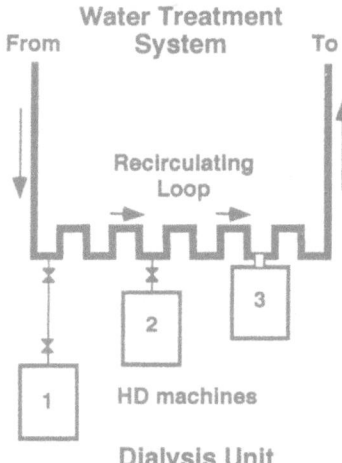

Figure 16. Tubing connecting the water distribution loop to the dialysis machine must be as short as possible to reduce dead space and water stagnation. This is illustrated by the 3 mode of connection: 1. Conventional tubing. 2. Short tubing connecting system. 3. Total suppression of tubing dead space with a specific connecting device.

pore size, Posidyne®, Pall, NY, USA) is placed after the pumps, at the inlet of the recirculation loop. This system should eliminate all the bacteria that may have grown in the water stagnant into the reservoir. The recirculation loop returns to the reservoir, the water not utilized in the dialysis center. Optimal functioning of such a distribution closed loop system is based on four major rules: first, permanent water flux and bacterial absolute filtration to lower bacterial growth in the reservoir and to eliminate bacteria and endotoxins from the water running into the loop; second, high flow rate to impede the bacterial colonization of the pipes; third, careful cleaning and disinfection of the hydraulic circuit at regular intervals to prevent biofilm formation and bacterial contamination; fourth, prevention of back contamination through lateral arms by regular disinfection and physical disconnection of the HD machines when they are not in use.

WATER TREATMENT SYSTEM MAINTENANCE AND HYGIENE OF DIALYSIS

As discussed previously, both proper design of the hydraulic circuit and adequate hygienic measures are the two key conditions to obtain high quality water for dialysis. The careful maintenance of a water treatment system is essential to insure the continuous production and distribution of ultrapure water. Thus maintenance relies on three complementary measures: disinfection; filters and/or resins changes; biofilm destruction.

Disinfection

Disinfection is necessary to reduce the degree of bacterial contamination in a water treatment system production (109–112). It must be adapted to the segment of the water treatment chain considered and to the level of contamination (Figure 17).

Bacteria lodging inside in depth filters, softeners resins and activated charcoal are very difficult to remove. All these material, easily penetrated by water-borne bacteria, offer excellent niches facilitating bacterial growth. To reduce microbial multiplication in this critical sector of the water treatment chain, several measures are required: (1) permanent addition of bleach to raw water to enhance free chlorine level to reach 0.3 mg/l within filters and softener resins; (2) pulse disinfection of activated charcoal by high bleach flushing once a week; (3) suppression of activated charcoal if possible and free chlorine neutralization by downstream infusion of thiosulfate.

Periodic disinfection of RO, CDI and ultrafilters may be achieved by using a chemical disinfectant. The choice of disinfectant must be done in accordance with material specifications and manufacturer recommendations to prevent any damaging effect. Periodicity, concentration and time exposure to the agent are dependent upon the nature of the disinfected material, the degree of contamination and the kinetics of recontamination.

Filter and resin changes

Filters, softeners, activated charcoal and deionizers represent an ideal support for microbial growth. On the one hand, porosity of these material facilitate adhesion and penetration by circulating water-borne bacteria. On the other hand, presence of organic substances enhance bacteria growth by providing nutrient media. When bacteria have colonized such material they are very difficult to dislodge by a back-washing or to kill by disinfectants and/or chemical germicides. Moreover, heavily contaminated filters overpassing their retentive capacity are subject to release with risk of downstream contamination of equipment. Disinfection permits to reduce bacterial contamination of a water treatment system in a limited and/or an acceptable range. However disinfection alone cannot insure sterility for a prolonged period of time when filters or resins are contaminated. Therefore, periodical changes of filters and resins, combined with frequent disinfection cycles, is the only way to optimize microbiological results and to insure on the long term the production of ultrapure water (113).

Biofilm synthesis and destruction

Bacterial adhesion to inert surface material occurs inevitably in all water distribution piping network (114). Such adhesion is facilitated by reduced water flow and low shear rates at the water-tubing interface by areas of

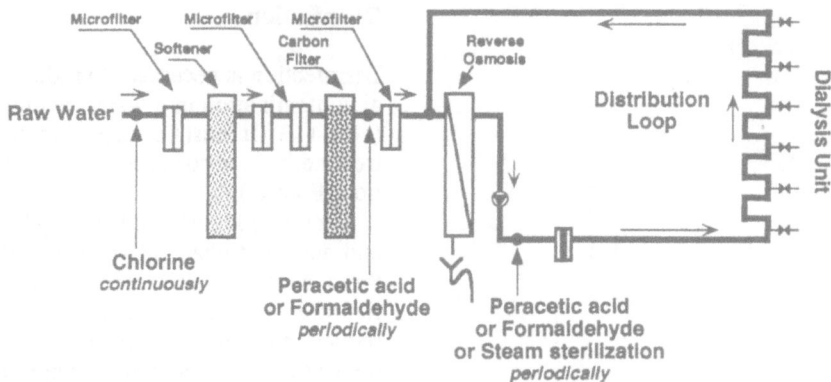

Figure 17. Dinsinfection procedures. 1. Permanent chlorine infusion in the pre-treatment part prevents bacterial growth. Chlorine is then removed by the activated carbon. 2. Periodic disinfection may be realized with biocide (formaldehyde, peracetic acid, hypochlorite) with appropriate concentration and optimal periodicity. 3. Daily seam disinfection may be performed in the stainless steel recirculating loop.

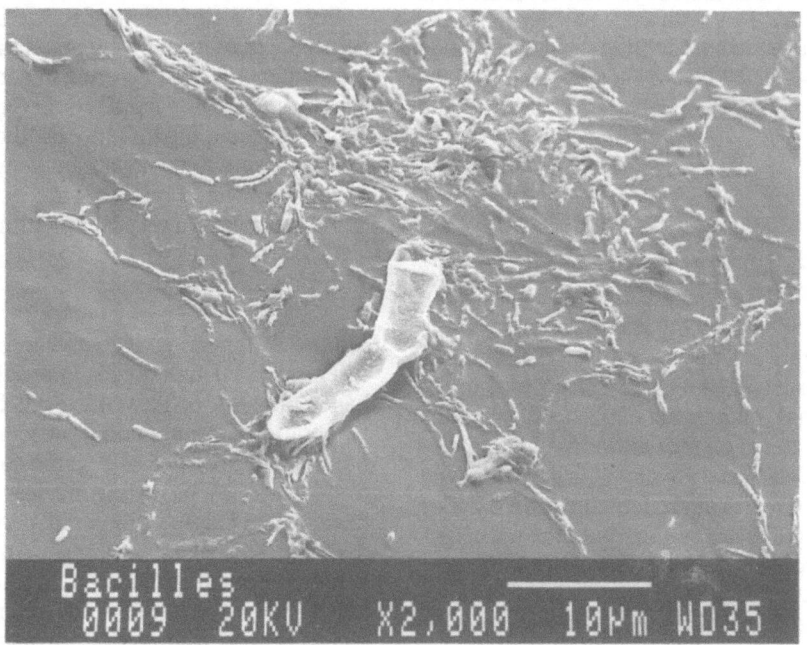

Figure 18. Biofilm, as it can be observed in the PVC water piping feeding a dialysis machine not regularly disinfected (courtesy of Rémy Nicolle, Biocides Department, SEPPIC, Paris-France).

water and/or by defect and cracks at the inner surface of the pipe walls (storage tank, valves). However, water borne bacteria may stick to surfaces even at high water fluxes. Moreover fixed bacteria facilitate the adhesion of other circulating microorganisms leading to a progressive bacterial build-up. Interaction of bacteria is initially reversible, but it becomes eventually irreversible. In nutrient poor environment such as ultrapure water most bacteria grow attached to surfaces mainly because of their hydrophobicity. Initially, sessile bacteria adhere randomly to tubing surfaces by means of their glycocalyx. Then, the

production of the exopolysaccharide and the reproduction of bacteria leads to the production of a continuous biofilm at the inner part of the colonized surface (Figure 18). Biofilm provides a protection from natural or synthetically produced antimicrobial agents (biocides). It facilitates bacterial proliferation in which in turn metabolic products stimulate the growth of the other organisms. An aggregate of microorganisms leads to molecular or proton exchanges which in turn is associated with microbial corrosion. The corrosion process can be initiated by formation of proton concentration gradients inside and around the bacteria,

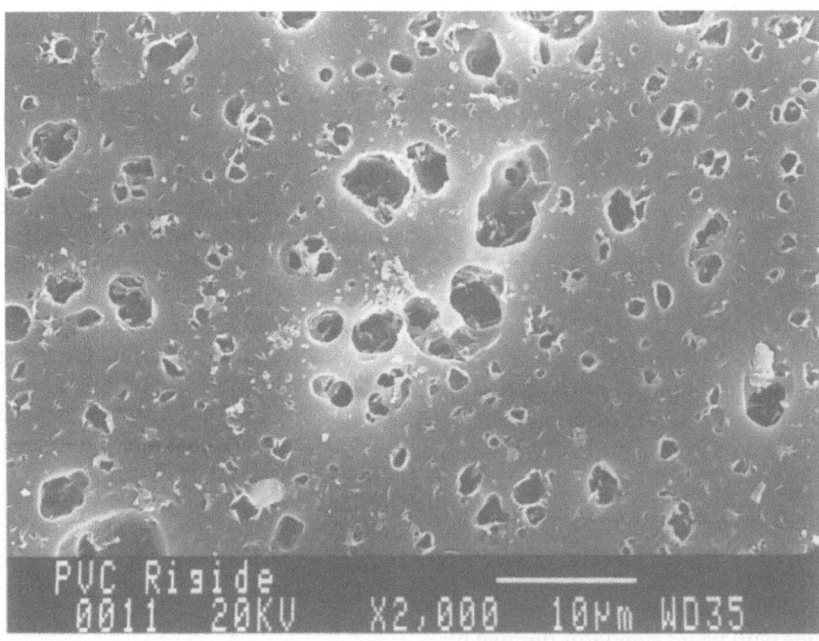

Figure 19. Biofilm striping effect of a peracetic acid solution (Dialox®, CFPO, Paris-France). PVC tubing appears clean and germ-free. Only silicium deposits can be observed at the tubing surface (courtesy of Rémy Nicolle, Biocides Department, SEPPIC, Paris-France).

which generate electrochemical forces within the biofilm. High grade stainless steel is the only material resistant to this corrosion phenomenon.

Most plastics contains synthetic polymers which are resistant to microbial degradation with the exception for low molecular weight polyethylene and polyesters. Plastics may also contains plasticizers, pigments, stabilizers, lubricants that may serve as nutrients for bacteria and fungi. Even though the plastic is not degraded, its resistance may be altered. Bacterial growth may cause plastic pipes to become brittle and crack. Fungi may grow inside plastic material and on their surface modifying their aspect.

Prevention and destruction of biofilm is therefore an essential aim in the hygiene of the water distribution systems. Few detergent agents can induce the hydrolysis of the exopolysaccharide shield. Bleach, sodium hydroxide and peroxyacetic acid preparation which demonstrate detergent properties, should be periodically employed to strip the biofilm away from the inner surface of the pipe wall and disinfect adequately the water distribution pipes (Figure 19).

WATER TREATMENT QUALITY CONTROL

Chemical purity

The methods used for monitoring the effectiveness of each water treatment options have been discussed in paragraphs above. Basic requirements for an adequate control of the chemical purity of the water produced are summarized in this section (115).

The effectiveness of the softener may be monitored either periodically (daily or weekly) by measuring the hardness of the effluent water using suitable titration kits (resolution of less < 1 mg/l) or permanently by a sensitive automated probe (Testomat®) equipped with appropriate alarms which will inform the nursing personnel of the dialysis center if the hard water is not adequately softened.

The filters (sediment filters, ultrafilter) capability must be monitored to prevent plugging and sloughing risks. It is therefore important to monitor the pressure drop across the filters by suitable pressure gauges; the filters will be discarded and replaced when the pressure gradient across the filter reaches the safety limits specified by the manufacturer.

Chlorine removal by activated charcoal is important to prevent RO membrane damage. The effectiveness of activated charcoal must be monitored by measuring chlorine concentration in the effluent. This control can be performed periodically with appropriate dosage kits or permanently monitored by an appropriate probe under automated control.

The effectiveness of a desionizer (conventional mixed bed or CDI) and of a RO system can be monitored permanently by measuring the resistivity of the effluent water produced using an adequate resistivimeter. With RO the

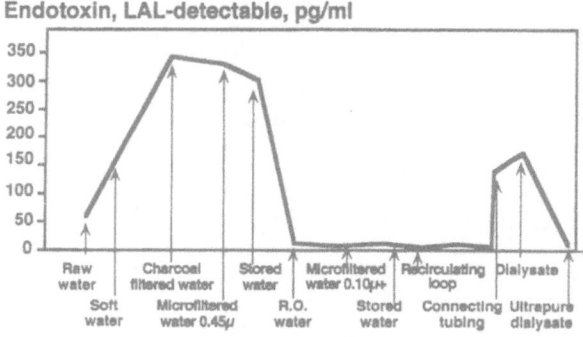

Endotoxin, LAL-detectable, pg/ml

Figure 20. Endotoxin concentration profile of a water treatment chain from raw water to dialysate delivery system.

rejection/production ratio permits to adjust the quality of treated water according to ionic strength of affluent water.

For monitoring the quality of the final water produced and to ensure compliance with water standards defined by pharmacopoeia, water contaminant concentrations have to be determined at the end point of water treatment production and at the inlet of the distribution system. Analytical methods complying with pharmacopoeia recommendations should be used to control the chemical purity of water.

Microbiological purity

To guarantee the reliable and reproducible production of an ultrapure water, it is important to organize a surveillance protocol documenting the degree of water contamination along the water chain (116–118). Water sampling devices should be placed in judiciously chosen sites to permit easy and efficient microbiologic surveillance of the water treatment chain, reservoir and water delivery system. Samples of water should be cultured regularly once or twice a week to verify that the installation is operating properly and that adequate disinfection is being implemented.

The most practical method for conducting the bacteriologic surveillance of a water treatment production and distribution system is to culture 0.45 μm membranes following filtration of adequate volume of the water to be tested (from few milliliters up to one liter) according to the expected degree of contamination. A convenient membrane support (Swinnex, Millipore, Bedford, MA, USA) will simplify this operation (119–121). Following sample filtration the membrane is placed on a culture medium favoring the growth of water born bacteria; in spite of the recommendations of culturing on trypticase-soya media by various pharmacopoeia, the R2A poor nutrient medium will offer a more sensitive method to detect the presence of these bacteria and to quantify the degree of water contamination and to evaluate the risk of pyrogenic reactions (122–129).

Bacteriologic surveillance should concentrate on the critical areas of the installation: after resins and activated charcoal cartridges, at the entrance and at the outlet of the cold sterilization system of the recirculating loop. Monitoring should be more frequent when an installation is put out of service in order to detect abnormalities in the hydraulic circuit (126–139). The experience and data gained provide to the user a bacteriologic and lipopolysaccharide contamination profile of the water treatment system and can be used to establish the points and frequency of subsequent monitoring (Figure 20). Endotoxin level in the water should be evaluated using the LAL test (134, 135). Under usual conditions of use this test has a detection limit of 0.1 EU/ml, but a sensitive automated assay using a chromogenic method lowers the detection threshold down to 0.005 EU/ml.

WATER STANDARDS FOR CONTEMPORARY DIALYSIS

Various grades of water may be used for hemodialysis. From the early days of dialysis, it is known that softened water was necessary to prevent the occurrence of the 'hard water syndrome'. Later on it was shown that purified water using reverse osmosis or deionizer was a basic requirement to prevent aluminium intoxication. Eventually, according to our present knowledge and conditions of contemporary dialysis, it became clear that highly purified water was required (140–149). Water used for hemodialysis must be close to pharmaceutical grade (i.e., water for injection) which is achievable with the modern technology of water treatment (143–144). Of these waters, two are of primary interest for hemodialysis, purified water and ultrapure water. In Table 4 a summary of the water quality standards is presented permitting to differentiate both type of water. The term 'ultrapure water' has been coined mainly to satisfy the needs of the semiconductor industry. In this definition, a strong emphasis is given to a higher chemical purity expressed in terms of a water resistivity equal or superior to 5 megOhms/cm. This definition includes also stringent requirements concerning the degree of bacterial contamination, with less than 100 CFU/liter and undetectable levels of lipopolysaccharides. For dialysis purposes, RO treated water with a resistivity in the range of 0.1–0.3 megOhm/cm is quite satisfactory; in this context, the term ultrapure water refers mainly to a very low level of bacterial and endotoxin contamination(i.e., $\leq$ 100 CFU/liter; undetectable levels of endotoxin with a sensitive assay). This microbiologic purity is required particularly when high flux dialysis methods (with high convection rates) are utilized or when reuse of dialyzers is performed.

CONCLUSIONS

Contemporary dialysis has created new needs for the water purification system. Treated water utilized in hemodialysis machine must satisfy more stringent constraints of purity both for chemical and microbiological.

Pharmaceutical grade or highly purified water, so called ultra-pure water, has become a new standard for the dialysis of the 90s. Several reasons support this need. Limitations of conventional dialysis as a long term treatment modality (> 10 years) has become largely evident over the last decade. A growing number of patients are suffering from the bone and joint long term dialysis syndrome induced by β2-microglobulin amyloidosis.

Hemoincompatibility of the hemodialysis system has been regularly raised as a potential causal factor. Release of pro-inflammatory mediators from protein and cell system activation occuring through the blood-membrane interaction is enhanced by water contaminant and/or by-products. Role of bacteria fragments such as lipopolysacharides or muramyl-dipeptides appears particularly important in this context. Highly purified water, used to produce ultra-pure dialysate, must be considered as a major component of the hemodialysis hemocompatibility complex.

Technical conditions of contemporary dialysis enhance the risk and the hazards of using contaminated dialysate. Bicarbonate buffer largely used in dialysis units facilitate bacterial growth with a subsequent production of endotoxin in dialysate. Highly permeable membrane increasingly used for their solute removal performances tend to facilitate penetration of endotoxin fragments into the blood stream. Ultrafiltration controller used for highly permeable dialyzers enhance the backfiltration and/or the backdiffusion phenomenon that may potentiate the microbiological hazards of contaminated dialysate.

Newly developed methods increasing the convective part in the dialysis efficacy, based on the on-line production of substitution fluid such as hemofiltration (HF) or hemodiafiltration (HDF), are more widely applied. High microbiologic water purity is an essential pre-requisite to insure the safety of these alternative methods to standard hemodialysis.

Reconditioning dialyzer process using treated water require also ultra-pure water. The use of such a high purity water is mandatory to prevent the introduction of pyrogenic substances within the blood compartment of the dialyzer.

The routine use of ultrapure water in the dialysis center is one of the major attainments of the 90s. Progress in water treatment technology and improved understanding of water borne ecology permits the safe and easy production of pharmaceutical grade water (i.e., water for injection according to pharmacopeia specifications). Using a bacteria free water, cleared from lipopolysaccharides, is the simplest approach to minimize the patient-hemodialysis interactions (i.e., blood monocytes activation and cytokines production). Time will tell wether this purified environment provided by ultrapure dialysate delays (or prevents) the occurrence of late dialysis complications such as β2M-amyloidosis. Ultrapure water was developed mainly to satisfy the stringent specification of the semiconductor industry. Due to increased awareness of the biological hazards of extra-corporeal circulation and blood transmembrane contact with a polluted dialysis fluid is a strong stimulus to provide hemodialysis patient with a sterile endotoxin free dialysate (140).

REFERENCES

1. Man NK, Funck-Brentano JL: Dialyzers and water treatment. in *Therapy of Renal Diseases and Related Disorders*, edited by Suki WN, Massry SG, Boston, Martinus Nijhoff Publishers, 1984, p 545
2. Easterling RE: Mechanical aspects of dialysis including dialysate delivery systems and water for dialysate. in *Clinical Dialysis*, edited by Nissenson AR, Fine RN, Gentile DE, Philadelphia, Hanley & Belfus, Inc, 1984, p 53
3. Luehmann DA: Water purification for hemodialysis. *Med Instrum* 20: 74, 1986
4. Comty CM, Shapiro FL: Pretreatment and preparation of city water for hemodialysis. in *Replacement of Renal Function by Dialysis*, edited by Drukker W, Parsons FM, Maher JF, Martinus Nijhoff Publishers, 1986, p 155
5. Laskey DA, Schell D: Addressing new water treatment standards and technologies. *Contemp Dial Nephrol* 10: 35, 1989
6. Vallot D: Purified water fror hemodialysis: present needs (Part 1) (in French). *Techniques Hospitalières* 529: 65, 1989
7. Vallot D: Purified water fror hemodialysis: present needs (Part 2) (in French). *Techniques Hospitalières* 529: 45, 1989
8. Man NK, Ciancioni CH, Guyomard S, Blais D, Delons S, Funck-Brentano JL: Risks and hazards of contaminated dialysate associated with high flux membranes. in *Prevention in Nephrology*, edited by Buccianti G, Masson, Italia, 1987, p 227
9. Keshaviah P, Luehmann D: The importance of water treatment in haemodialysis and haemofiltration. *Proc Eur Dial Transplant Assoc Eur Renal Assoc* 21: 111, 1984
10. Meeks JN: Water refining considerations for high flux dialysis (Part 1). *Contemp Dial Nephrol* 10: 27, 1989
11. Meeks JN: Water refining considerations for high flux dialysis (Part 2). *Contemp Dial Nephrol* 10: 38, 1989
12. Baurmeister U, Travers M, Vienken J, Harding G, Millon C, Klein E, Pass T, Wright R: Dialysate contamination and back filtration may limit the use of high-flux dialysis membranes. *Trans Am Soc Artif Intern Organs* 35: 519, 1989
13. Leypoldt JK, Schmidt B, Gurland HJ: Measurement of backfiltration rates during hemodialysis with highly permeable membranes. *Blood Purif* 9: 74, 1991
14. Leypoldt JK, Schmidt B, Gurland HJ: Net ultrafiltration may not eliminate backfiltration during hemodialysis

with highly permeable membranes. *Artif Organs* 15: 164, 1991

15. Vanholder R, Van Haecke E, Ringoir S: Endotoxin transfer through dialysis membranes: small-versus large-pore membranes. *Nephrol Dial Transplant* 7: 333, 1992
16. Petersen J, Hyver SW, Cajias J: Backfiltration during dialysis: a critical assessment. *Semin Dial* 5: 13, 1992
17. Klinkmann H, Ebbighausen H, Uhlenbusch I, Vienken J: High-flux dialysis, dialysate quality and backtransport. in *Contrib Nephrol*, Vol 103, Basel, Karger, 1993, p 89
18. Favero MS, Petersen NJ, Carson LA, Bond WW, Hindman SH: Gram-negative water bacteria in hemodialysis systems. *J Am Soc Microbiol* (HLS) 12: 321, 1975
19. Petersen NJ, Boyer KM, Carson LA, Favero MS: Pyrogenic reactions from inadequate disinfection of a dialysis fluid distribution system. *Dial Transplant* 7: 52, 1978
20. Watzke H, Mayer G, Schwartz HP, Stanek G, Rotter M, Hirschl AM, Graf H: Bacterial contamination of dialysate in dialysis-associated endotoxaemia. *J Hosp Infect* 13: 109, 1989
21. Goetz A, Yu VL, Hanchett JE, Rihs JD: Pseudomonas Stutzeri bacteriemia associated with hemodialysis. *Arch Intern Med* 143: 1909, 1983
22. Dinarello CA, Krueger JM: Induction of interleukin 1 by synthetic and naturally occuring muramyl peptides. *Fed Proc* 45: 2545, 1986
23. Bingel M, Lonnemann G, Shaldon S, Koch KM, Dinarello CA: Human Interleukin-1 production during hemodialysis. *Nephron* 43: 161, 1986
24. Mion CM, Canaud B: 'On-site' preparation of sterile apyrogenic electrolyte solutions for hemofiltration and hemodiafiltration. in *Short Dialysis*, edited by Cambi V, Boston, Martinus Nijhoff Publishers, 1987, p 261
25. Canaud B, Flavier JL, Argiles A, Stec F, Nguyen QV, Bouloux Ch, Garred LJ, Mion C: Hemodiafiltration with on-line production of substituion fluid: long-term safety and quantitative assessment of efficacy. *Contrib Nephrol* 108: 12, 1994
26. Petersen NJ, Carson LA, Favero MS: Bacterial endotoxin in new and reused hemodialyzers: a potential cause of endotoxinemia. *Trans Am Soc Artif Intern Organs* 28: 155, 1981
27. Bolan G, Reingold AL, Carson LA, Silcox VS, Woodley CL, Hayes PS, Hightower AW, McFarland L, Brown JW, Petersen NJ, Favero MS, Good RC, Broome CV: Infections with Mycobacterium Chelonei in patients receiving dialysis and using processed hemodialyzers. *J Infect Dis* 152: 1013, 1985
28. Lowry PW, Beck-Sague CM, Bland LA, Aguero SM, Arduino MJ, Minuth AN, Murray RA, Swenson JM, Jarvis WR: Mycobacterium chelonae infection among patients receiving high-flux dialysis in a hemodialysis clinic in California. *J Infect Dis* 161: 85, 1990
29. Alter MJ, Favero MS, Miller JK, Moyer LA, Bland LA: National surveillance of dialysis-associated diseases in the United States, 1987. *Trans Am Soc Artif Intern Organs* 35: 820, 1989
30. Vanholder R, Vanhaecke E, Ringoir S: Waterborne Pseudomonas septicemia. *Trans Am Soc Artif Intern Organs* 36: M215, 1990
31. Alter MJ, Favero MS, Moyer LA, Bland LA: National surveillance of dialysis-associated diseases in the United States. *Trans Am Soc Artif Intern Organs* 37: 97, 1991

32. Held PJ, Levin NW, Bovbjerg RR, Pauly MV, Diamond LH: Mortality and duration of hemodialysis treatment. *JAMA* 265: 871, 1991
33. Gordon SM, Oettinger CW, Bland LA, Oliver JC, Arduino MJ, Aguero SM, McAllister SK, Favero MS, Jarvis WR: Pyrogenic reactions in patients receiving conventional, high-efficiency, or high-flux hemodialysis treatments with bicarbonate dialysate containing high concentrations of bacteria and endotoxin. *J Am Soc Nephrol* 2: 1436, 1992
34. Tokars JI, Alter MJ, Favero MS, Moyer LA, Bland LA: National surveillance of hemodialysis associated diseases in the United States. *ASAIO J* 39: 71, 1993
35. Bland L, Alter M, Favero M, Carson L, Cusick L: Hemodialyzer reuse: practices in the united states and implication for infection control. *Trans Am Soc Artif Intern Organs* 31: 556, 1985
36. Canaud B, Peyronnet P, Armynot AM, Nguyen QV, Attisso M, Mion C: Ultrapure water: A need for future dialysis. *Proc Eur Dial Transplant Assoc-Eur Renal Assoc* 23 (Abstract): 113, 1986
37. McNulty J: The proper sizing of ultrapure water delivery systems. *Contemp Dial Nephrol* 12: 30, 1991
38. McNulty J: Improving your water-treatment system? Here is how to get the latest technology and cut costs. *Contemp Dial Nephrol* 13: 18, 1992
39. Curtis JR, Wing AJ, Coleman JC: Bacillus cereus bacteraemia: a complication of intermittent haemodialysis. *Lancet* 1: 136, 1967
40. Alfrey AC, Mishell JM, Burks J, Contiguglia SR, Rudolph H, Lewin E, Holmes JH: Syndrome of dyspraxia and multifocal seizures associated with chronic hemodialysis. *Trans Am Soc Artif Intern Organs* 18: 257, 1972
41. Ward MK, Pierides AM, Fawcett P, Shaw DA, Perry RH, Tomlinson BE, Kerr DNS: Dialysis encephalopathy syndrome. *Proc Eur Dial Transplant Assoc* 13: 348, 1976
42. Flendring JA, Kruis H, Das HA: Aluminium intoxication: the cause of dialysis dementia? *Proc Eur Dial Transplant Assoc* 13: 355, 1976
43. Alfrey AC, Legendre GR, Kaehny WD: Dialysis encephalopathy syndrome. *N Eng J Med* 294: 184, 1976
44. Salvadeo A, Minoia C, Segagni S, Villa G: Trace metal changes in dialysis fluid and blood of patients on hemodialysis. *Int J Artif Organs* 2: 17, 1979
45. Platts MM, Owen G, Smith S: Water purification and the incidence of fractures in patients receiving home haemodialysis supervised by a single centre: evidence for 'safe' upper limit of aluminium in water. *Br Med J* 288: 969, 1984
46. Abreo K, Brown ST, Sella ML: Correction of microcytosis following elimination of an occult source of aluminium contamination of dialysate. *Am J Kidney Dis* 13: 465, 1989
47. Kabei N, Kolff WJ, Foux A: Evaluation of hollow-fiber osmosis permeator for use in peritoneal dialysis. *Dial Transplant* 6: 59, 1977
48. Wathen RL, Burcham CW: Reverse osmosis technology: its applications in water treatment for hemodialysis. *Contemp Dial Nephrol* 13: 28, 1992
49. Petrie JJB, Fleming R, McKinnon P, Winney RJ, Cowie J: The use of ion exchange to remove aluminium from water used in hemodialysis. *Am J Kidney Dis* 4: 69, 1984

50. Bernick JJ, Port FK, Favero MS: *In vivo* studies of dialysis-related endotoxemia and bacteremia. *Nephron* 27: 307, 1981

51. Du Moulin GC, Coleman EC, Hedley-Whyte J: Bacterial colonization and endotoxin content of a new renal dialysis water system composed of acrylonitrile butadiene styrene. *Appl Environ Microbiol* 53: 1322, 1987

52. Clements MC: Why validate? *Contemp Dial Nephrol* 12: 37, 1991

53. Arduino MJ, Bland LA, Favero MS: Adverse patient reactions due to chemical contamination of hemodialysis fluids. *Dial Transplant* 18: 655, 1989

54. Kroneld R, Reunanen M: Volatile halocarbons in haemodialysis therapy. *Bull Environ Contam Toxicol* 35: 583, 1985

55. Villforth JC, FDA Issues Safety Alert: Chloramine contamination of hemodialysis water supplies (Letter). *Am J Kidney Dis* 11: 447, 1988

56. Carson LA, Bland LA, Cusick LB, Favero MS, Bolan GA, Reingold AL, Good RC: Prevalence of nontuberculous Mycobacteria in water supplies of hemodialysis centers. *Appl Environ Microbiol* 54: 3122, 1988

57. Becker FF, Janowsky U, Overath H, Stetter D: Removability of pesticides during the production of dialysis water (Part 1). *Biomed Tech* 34: 139, 1989

58. Becker FF, Janowsky U, Overath H, Stetter D: Removability of pesticides during the production of dialysis water (Part 2). *Biomed Tech* 34: 215, 1989

59. Hopfer SM, Fay WP, Sunderman FW: Serum nickel concentrations in hemodialysis patients with environmental exposure. *Ann Clin Lab Sci* 19: 161, 1989

60. Davenport A, Roberts NB: Accumulation of aluminium in patients with acute renal failure. *Nephron* 52: 253, 1989

61. Piccoli A, Andriani M, Mattiello G, Nordio M, Modena F, Dalla Rosa C: Serum aluminium level in the veneto chronic haemodialysis population: cross-sectional study on 1026 patients. *Nephron* 51: 482, 1989

62. Chazan JA, Abuelo JG, Blonsky SL: Plasma aluminum levels (unstimulated and stimulated): clinical and biochemical findings in 185 patients undergoing chronic hemodialysis for 4 to 95 months. *Am J Kidney Dis* 13: 284, 1989

63. Brem AS, Di Mario C, Levy DL: Perceived aluminum-related disease in a dialysis population. A report from the End-Stage Renal Disease Network 28. *Arch Intern Med* 149: 2541, 1989

64. Tsukamoto Y, Saka S, Kumano K, Iwanami S, Ishida O, Marumo F: Abnormal accumulation of vanadium in patients on chronic hemodialysis. *Nephron* 56: 368, 1990

65. Gordon SM, Drachman J, Bland LA, Reid MH, Favero M, Jarvis WR: Epidemic hypotension in a dialysis center caused by sodium azide. *Kidney Int* 37: 110, 1990

66. Gordon SM, Bland LA, Alexander SR, Newman HF, Arduino MJ, Jarvis WR: Hemolysis associated with hydrogen peroxide at a pediatric dialysis center. *Am J Nephrol* 10: 123, 1990

67. Bello VA, Gitelman HJ: High fluoride exposure in hemodialysis patients. *Am J Kidney Dis* 15: 320, 1990

68. Smith RP, Willhite CC: Chlorine dioxide and hemodialysis. *Regul Toxicol Pharmac* 11: 42, 1990

69. Tipple MA, Shusterman N, Bland LA, McCarthy MA, Favero MS, Arduino MJ, Reid MH, Jarvis WR: Illness in hemodialysis patients after exposure to chloramine contaminated dialysate. *Trans Am Soc Artif Intern Organs* 37: 588, 1991

70. Montagnac R, Schillinger F, Roquebert MF, Croix JC, Eloy C: Contamination par des champignons d'un circuit de traitement d'eau en autodialyse. *Néphrologie* 7: 27, 1991

71. Petersen MD, Thomas SB: The new EPA lead and copper rule. *Contemp Dial Nephrol* 12: 26, 1991

72. Gitelman HJ, Alderman FR, Perry SJ: Silicon accumulation in dialysis patients. *Am J Kidney Dis* 19: 140, 1992

73. FDA Issues Safety Alert: Dialysis patients in Chicago die from fluoride poisoning. *Contemp Dial Nephrol* 14: 10, 1993

74. Steinbergs CZ: Removal of by-products of chlorine and chlorine dioxide at a hemodialysis center. *Res Technol (Journal AWWA)*: 94, 1986

75. Weiss LG, Danielson BG, Fellstrom B, Wikstrom B: Aluminum removal with hemodialysis, hemofiltration and charcoal hemoperfusion in uremic patients after desferrioxamine infusion. A comparison of efficiency. *Nephron* 54: 179, 1990

76. Jourdan JL, Maingourd C, Meguin C, Nivet H, Martin C, Moulier MC: Possible aluminium release from activated charcoal filters used in home hemodialysis. *Néphrologie* 4: 153, 1986

77. Petersen NJ, Carson LA, Favero MS, Marshall JH, Aguero SM: Removal of bacteria and bacterial endotoxin from dialysis fluids by sorbents. *ASAIO J* 3: 6, 1979

78. Muirhead N, Mitton R: Use of bone char as an adsorbent in preparation of water for dialysis. *ASAIO J* 38: M334, 1992

79. Perlmuter BA: Principles of Filtration. Pall Well Technology Corporation – Technical Notes, 1982

80. Sweadner KJ, Forte M, Nelsen LL: Filtration removal of endotoxin (pyrogens) in solution in different states of aggregation. *Appl Envir Microbiol* 34: 382, 1977

81. Howard G, Duberstein R: A case of penetration of 0.2 μm rated membrane filters by bacteria. *J Parenter Drug Assoc* 34: 95, 1980

82. Hou K, Gerba CP, Goyal SM, Zerda KS: Capture of latex beads, bacteria, endotoxins, and viruses by charge-modified filters. *Appl Environ Microbiol* 40: 892, 1980

83. Gerba CP, Hou KC, Babineau RA, Fiore JV: Pyrogen control by depth filtration. *Pharm Technol* 5: 32, 1980

84. Pall DB, Kirnbauer EA, Allen BT: Particulate retention by bacteria retentive membrane filters. *Colloids and Surfaces* 1: 235, 1980

85. Carazzone M, Arecco D, Fava M, Sancin: A new type of positively charged filter: preliminary test results. *J Parenter Sci Technol* 39: 69, 1985

86. Gerba CP, Hou KC, Babineau RA: Pyrogen control by charge-modified filters. *Pharm Enginr* 6: 32, 1981

87. Cradock JC, Guder LA, Francis DL, Morgan SL: Reduction of pyrogens: applications of molecular filtration. *J Pharm Pharmac* 30: 198, 1978

88. Abramson D, Butler LD, Chrai S: Depyrogenation of a parenteral solution by ultrafiltration. *J Parenter Sci Technol* 35: 3, 1981

89. Nelsen LL: Removal of pyrogens from parenteral solutions by ultrafiltration. *Pharm Technol* 8: 30, 1978

90. Rechen HC: The role of ultrafiltration in the production of pyrogen-free purified water. *Pharm Manu* 10: 29, 1984

91. Klinkmann H, Falkenhagen D, Smollich BP: Investigation of the permeability of highly permeable polysulfone membranes for pyrogen. *Contrib Nephrol* 46: 174, 1985

92. Kumano K, Yokota S, Nanbu M, Sakai T: Methods of minimizing endotoxin level in dialysate. *Dial Transplant* 22: 147, 1993

93. Di Felice A, Cappelli G, Facchini F, Tetta C, Cornia F, Aimo G, Lusvarghi E: Ultrafiltration and endotoxin removal from dialysis fluids. *Kidney Int* 43: 201, 1991

94. Cappelli G, Tetta C, Cornia F, Di Felice A, Facchini F, Neri R, Lucchi L, Lusvarghi E: Removal of limulus reactivity and cytokine-inducing capacity from bicarbonate dialysis fluids by ultrafiltration. *Nephrol Dial Transplant* 8: 1133, 1993

95. Kumano K, Yokota S, Nanbu M, Sakai T: Do cytokine-inducing substances penetrate through dialysis membranes and stimulate monocytes? *Kidney Int* 41 (Suppl): S205, 1993

96. White D, Layman R: Reverse osmosis element design evolution and its effects. *Contemp Dial Nephrol* 12: 20, 1991

97. Williamson J: Getting comfortable with your reverse osmosis machine. *Contemp Dial Nephrol* 13: 52, 1992

98. Layman-Amato R: How to maintain your reverse osmosis system. *Contemp Dial Nephrol* 13: 54, 1992

99. Healey RJ: Reverse osmosis and distribution. *Contemp Dial Nephrol* 13: 24, 1992

100. Chapman WF, Williamson JL: Recordkeeping for reverse osmosis performance analysis. *Contemp Dial Nephrol* 14: 24, 1993

101. Schwarzbeck A, Wagner L, Squarr HU, Straugh M: Clotting in dialyzers due to low pH dialysis fluid. *Clin Nephrol* 7: 125, 1977

102. Ganzi GC, Egozy Y, Giuffrida AJ, Jha AD: High purity water by electrodeionization: performance of Ionpure® continuous deionization system. *Ultrapure Water* 4: 3, 1987

103. Ganzi GC: Electrodeionization for high purity water production. AIChE Symposium Series. in *New Membrane Materials and Processes for Separation*, edited by Sirkar KK, Lloyd DR, New York, AIChE, 1988, p 73

104. Parise PL, Parekh BS, Waddington G: The use of Ionpure® continuous deionization for the production of pharmaceutical and semiconductor grades of water. *Ultrapure Water Expo '90*, 1990, p 63

105. Hudson MV: What role do dialysis professionals play in the design and operation of water-treatment systems? *Contemp Dial Nephrol* 13: 26, 1992

106. Schultze N, Morelle C, Egly JC: Les traitements de l'eau destinée au laboratoire. *Biofutur* 55: 117, 1992

107. Cartwright PS: Hemodialysis water treatment: a consultant's perspective. *Dial Transplant* 21: 130, 1992

108. Healey RJ, Nicol CW: Economical operation of a dialysis water purification system. *Contemp Dial Nephrol* 12: 16, 1991

109. Grabow WOK, Gauss-Müller V, Prozesky OW, Deinhardt F: Inactivation of hepatitis A virus and indicator organisms in water by free chlorine residuals. *Appl Environ Microbiol* 46: 619, 1983

110. Klein E: Effects of disinfectants in renal dialysis patients. *Environmental Health Perspectives* 69: 45, 1986

111. Besarab A, DeLuca T, Picarello D, Jungkind D: Formaldehyde, sodium hypochlorite and metabisulphite are equally effective as sterilants for central delivery systems. *ASAIO J* (Abstract) 39: 82, 1993

112. Matsushima H, Sakurai N: A selected ion monitoring assay for chlorhexidine in medical waste water. *Biomed Mass Spectrometry* 11: 203, 1984

113. Mayr HU, Stec F, Canaud B, Mion CM, Shaldon S: Microbiological aspects of the batch preparation of replacement fluid for hemofiltration. *Blood Purif* 2: 158, 1985

114. Sifontes JR, Block S: Preservation of metals from microbial corrosion. in *Disinfection, Sterilization and Preservation*, edited by Block SS, Philadelphia, London, Lea & Febiger, 1991, p 948

115. Meeks JN: Water quality monitoring and the AAMI hemodialysis standards. *Contemp Dial Nephrol* 10: 41, 1989

116. Bernick JJ, Port FK, Favero MS, Brown DG: Bacterial and endotoxin permeability of hemodialysis membranes. *Kidney Int* 16: 491, 1979

117. Vos T, Roodvoets AP, Staal J: Bacterial proliferation in dialysis fluid. *Clin Nephrol* 2: 235, 1974

118. Dawids SG, Vejlsgaard R: Bacterial and clinical evaluation of different dialysate delivery systems. *Acta Med Scand* 199: 151, 1976

119. Sladek KJ, Suslavitch RV, Sohn BI, Dawson FW: Optimum membrane structures for growth of coliform and fecal coliform organisms. *Appl Environ Microbiol* 30: 685, 1975

120. Tobin RS, Dutka BJ: Comparison of the surface structure, metal binding, and fecal coliform recoveries of nine membrane filters. *Appl Environ Microbiol* 34: 69, 1977

121. Logan KB, Rees GE, Seeley ND, Primrose SB: Rapid concentration of bacteriophages from large volumes of fresh water: evaluation of positively charged, microporous filters. *J Virol Methods* 1: 87, 1980

122. Harding GB, Pass T, Million C, Wright R, DeJarnette J, Klein E: Bacterial contamination of hemodialysis center water and dialysate: are current assays adequate? *Artif Organs* 13: 155, 1989

123. Clements MC: Investigation of microbial contamination of hemodialysis water systems. *Contemp Dial Nephrol* 37, 1989

124. Ward RA, Luehmann DA, Klein E: Are current standards for the microbiological purity of hemodialysis adequate? *Semin Dial* 2: 69, 1989

125. Tominaga H, Tanaka S, Tominaga N: Endotoxin level of sterile injection solutions and substitution fluid for hemofiltration in Japan and Australia. *Nephron* 42: 128, 1986

126. Harding GB, Klein E, Pass T, Million C: Endotoxin and bacterial contamination of dialysis center water and dialysate; a cross sectional survey. *Int J Artif Organs* 13: 39, 1990

127. Klein E, Pass T, Harding GB, Wright R, Million C: Microbial and endotoxin contamination in water and dialysate in the Central United States. *Artif Organs* 14: 85, 1990

128. Gaynes R, Friedman C, McLaren C, Swartz R: Hemodialysis-associated febrile episodes: surveillance before and after major alteration in the water treatment system. *Int J Artif Organs* 13: 482, 1990

129. Wathen RL: High-flux dialysis and pyrogenic reactions. *Semin Dial* 3: 193, 1990

130. Umeda M, Niwa M, Yamagami S, Kishimoto T, Maekawa M, Sawada Y: Novel endotoxin materials, polymyxin-sepharose and polyethylene membrane for removal of endotoxin from dialysis systems. *Biomater Artif Cells Artif Organs* 18: 491, 1990

131. Canaud B, Imbert E, Kaaki M, Assounga A, Nguyen QV, Stec F, Garred LJ, Bostroem M, Mion C: Clinical and microbiological evaluation of a post-dilutional hemofiltration system with in-line production of substitution fluid. *Blood Purif* 8: 160, 1990

132. Arduino MJ, Bland LA, Aguero SM, Carson L, Ridgeway M, Favero M: Comparison of microbiologic assay methods for hemodialysis fluids. *J Clin Microbiol* 29: 592, 1991

133. Arduino MJ, Bland LA, Aguero SM, Favero MS: Effects of incubation time and temperature on microbiologic sampling procedures for hemodialysis fluids. *J Clin Microbiol* 29: 1462, 1991

134. Murray J: The merits of LAL testing: *Contemp Dial Nephrol* 12: 32, 1991

135. Gould MJ, Novitsky TJ: Endotoxin as a measure of water quality for hemodialysis. *Contemp Dial Nephrol* 13: 48, 1992

136. Harding GB, Pass T, Wright R: Bacteriology of hemodialysis fluids: are current methodologies meaningful? *Artif Organs* 16: 448, 1992

137. Pollak VE, Kant S, Pesce A, Cathey M: Continuous quality improvement in chronic disease: early detection of a mini-cluster of pyrogenic reactions during hemodialysis and effect of on-line monitoring. *Dial Transpl* 21: 330, 1992

138. Harding GB, Sharp W: Possible risks to dialysis patients by 48-hour 37°C bacterial culturing of fluids. *Blood Purif* (Abstract) 10: 78, 1992

139. Layman-Amato R: Taking the 'bugs' out of bacterial monitoring. *Contemp Dial Nephrol* 14: 29, 1993

140. Mion CM, Canaud B, Garred LJ, Stec F, Nguyen QV: Sterile and pyrogen-free bicarbonate dialysate: a necessity for hemodialysis today. *Adv Nephrol* 19: 275, 1990

141. Bambauer R, Meyer S, Jung H, Goehl H, Nystrand R: Sterile versus non-sterile dialysis fluid in chronic hemodialysis treatment. *Trans Am Soc Artif Intern Organs* 3: M317, 1990

142. Bambauer R, Schmidt R, Falkenhagen D, Walther J, Jung WK: Sterile and endotoxin free dialysis fluid for hemodialysis. *Biomater Artif Cells Immob Biotech* 19: 71, 1991

143. Baz M, Durand C, Ragon A, Jaber K, Andrieu D, Merzouk T, Purgus R, Olmer M, Reynier JP, Berland Y: Using ultrapure water in hemodialysis delays carpal tunnel syndrome. *Int J Artif Organs* 14: 681, 1991

144. Gunderson RW, Concannon MF: Five years of experience with a pure water system designed for hemodialysis. *Contemp Dial Nephrol* 12: 40, 1991

145. Bambauer R, Schauer M, Vienken J: Contamination of dialysis water and dialysate. A survey of 30 centers. *Blood Purif* (Abstract) 9: 32, 1991

146. Oliver JC, Bland LA, Oettinger CW, Arduino MJ, Garrard M, Pegues DA, McAllister S, Moone T, Aguero S, Favero MS: Bacteria and endotoxin removal from bicarbonate dialysis fluids for use in conventional, high efficiency, and high-flux hemodialysis. *Artif Organs* 16: 141, 1992

147. Gault MH, Duffett AL, Murphy JF, Purchase LH: In search of sterile, endotoxin-free dialysate. *ASAIO J* 431, 1992

148. Henderson L, Ward RA, Mion CA, Canaud B, Bosch JP, Charytan C, Spinowitz BS, Gupta BK, Maindel N, Bland LA, Favero MS, Arduino MJ: Should hemodialysis fluid be sterile? *Semin Dial* 6: 26, 1993

149. Berland Y, Brunet P, Ragon A, Frenkian G, Crevat A: *Dialysate Biocompatibility: Evaluation and Expectations*, Contrib Nephrol, Vol 103, Basel, Karger, 1993, p 76

HEMODIALYSIS FLUID COMPOSITION

CLAUDIO RONCO, ALDO FABRIS and MARIANO FERIANI

INTRODUCTION

In a general sense, the hemodialysis fluid should be considered as a temporary 'extension' of the patient's extracellular fluid (1).

When blood comes in contact with dialysate a bidirectional diffusion process takes place and solutes tend to reach similar concentrations in both sides of dialysis membrane. Thus highly concentrated blood uremic toxins tend to diffuse across the membrane into the toxin free dialysate. On the contrary, higher concentrations of ionized calcium and buffers in dialysate permit to achieve a backtransport into the blood, with consequent correction of hypocalcemia and uremic acidosis.

The concentration gradients are maintained along the length of the dialyzer thanks to the countercurrent flow configuration, and act as a driving force for solute transport. Convection is also bidirectionally present, and solute transport by filtration and backfiltration must be considered for the final mass balance calculation.

Therefore, the composition of dialysis fluid is crucial in achieving the wanted blood purification and body fluid and electrolyte homeostasis. Finally, not only the chemical composition of the fluid is important, but also its physical and microbiological characteristics. These aspects will be discussed in detail in the following section.

HISTORICAL NOTICES

The first time the now familiar term '*dialysis*' was used in the literature was in 1854 (2). Thomas Graam used it to describe the movement of various solutes through a membrane into a less concentrated solution. From that moment, the characteristics of the 'dialyzing solution' appeared to be of great importance.

From these studies, John J. Abel started with Rowntree and Turner, his experiments on 'vividiffusion' in animals at Johns Hopkins University in Baltimore (3). The device developed was surprisingly similar to the modern hollow fiber dialyzers and the blood was circulated in numerous collodion tubes surrounded by a cylindrical jacket. When the device was in use, dialysis solution was introduced into the jacket, passed around the tubes and than it was removed. The authors selectively introduced, into the solution, substances they did not want to remove from the blood during the diffusion process. Their basic solution contained 0.9% sodium chloride and variable potassium. Lately, all researchers involved in dialysis development, focused their attention on dialysis fluid composition as a crucial point of the procedure (4–6).

In the 40s, Willelm Kolff (7) studied the variation of toxins concentration in a pool of blood separated from a isotonic solution by a cellulose acetate membrane. From these studies, Kolff started his experiments leading to the development of the rotating drum kidney (8). A batch of dialysate was prepared in advance and placed in the wooden slat where the drum was rotating. To adjust the pH of the solution, Kollf bubbled carbon dioxide or oxigen through the fluid. He also tried to control dialysate temperature to obtain maximum molecular movement and patient confort. Furthermore, sugar was added to the dialysis solution in order to increase its osmotic power and remove fluid from the blood. Kollf now feels that high blood sugars resulting from this use of glucose in the dialysate, probably prevented the disequilibrium syndrome (9).

Negative pressure on the dialyzing solution was firstly applied by Alwall in 1949 by placing a pump on the dialysate effluent line at the bottom of the hermetically sealed vertical drum used as artificial kidney (10). A modified version of the Alwall kidney, the Westinghouse unit, was also including a system for circulation and stirring of the dialysate bath.

In 1948 the Kollf-Brigham kidney was used at the P.B. Brigham hospital in Boston and a dialysate batch of 100 liters was standardized for a dialysis session; the problem of high pH of the solution and consequent precipitation of calcium salts in the presence of bicarbonate was approached by bubbling CO_2 in the dialysis fluid and lowering the calcium content in the solution. Calcium supplementation had to be given intravenously (11).

When early coil-type dialyzers became available, a fixed volume of dialysis fluid was prepared to perform dialysis treatment (Travenol-Kollf Tank) and the dialyzer was completely immesed in this fixed volume of fluid. However, to increase solute removal, the dialysate bath had to be substituted every two hours (12). Dialysate pH was adjusted to 7.4 with lactic acid and bubbled CO_2. Calcium chloride was finally added.

As the pioniering phase of dialysis ended and renal replacement therapy entered a new era, a central delivery system for dialysate was utilized, serving up to 30 dialysis stations. In such condition, a standardization of dialysate composition was achieved permitting the preparation of large quantities of ready-to-use dialysis fluid (13, 14). A typical composition of the dialysis fluid used for 30 patients symultaneously was Na = 140, K = 1.5, Ca = 1.87, Mg = 0.5 mmol/l. The content of dextrose, previously high to permit osmotic ultrafiltration, was progressively reduced and even eliminated in some cases.

Scribner at that time proposed the use of 27 mmol/l of bicarbonate as a buffer in dialysate. This was creating problems of calcium precipitation and easy bacterial contamination (15). For this reason, in 1964, Mion et al. (16) introduced the use of acetate as alkaline equivalent in the dialysis fluid. Acetate containing solutions were easily prepared, chemically stable and microbiologically safe (16).

The central preparation and delivery of dialysate was certainly offering some advantages in terms of standardization and constant quality of the fluid. On the other hand this was precluding any type of personalization of the treatment at least as far as dialysate was concerned. Individualized prescribing of dialysate concentration became possible after 1976 when dialysis machines equipped with bedside proportioning systems for dialysate started to be available on the market (17). The new era of a freshly prepared dialysis fluid from treated water and concentrated salts, took over quickly and new criteria of personalization of treatment characterized the subsequent evolution of dialysis therapy (18). Since that time, in fact, purity, electrolyte concentration and buffer content of dialysate, represented a main field of interest in dialysis research and clinical routine of treatment (19, 20).

Table 1. Ranges of solute concentration in the final dialysate

	Acetate dialysis	Bicarbonate dialysis
Sodium [Na^+] (mmol/l)	132–145	137–144
Potassium [K^+] (mmol/l)	0–3	0–3
Calcium [CA^{++}] (mmol/l)	1.5–2.0	1.25–2.0
Magnesium [Mg^{++}] (mmol/l)	0.75	0.25–0.75
Chloride [Cl^-] (mmol/l)	99–110	98–112
Acetate [CH_3COO^-] (mmol/l)	31–45	2.5–10
Bicarbonate [HCO_3^-] (mmol/l)	–	27–35
Glucose [$C_6H_{12}O_6$] (mmol/l)	0–5.5	0–5.5

Note: In the present table most commonly used ranges for standard acetate and bicarbonate solutions are reported. Special solutions designed for experimental purposes or special clinical requirements are not included and may therefore present different components or concentrations.

DIALYSATE COMPOSITION

The composition of dialysis fluid is today prescribed for each single patient in an attempt to individualize the dialysis therapy and to meet personal needs and requirements. Dialysis fluid has become a real 'drug' and, as a consequence, a pharmacological preparation is needed to meet criteria of quality and standards. This has been made possible by the modern dialysis machines that, not only permit an accurate proportioning of treated water and concentrated salts, but also guarantee a continuous monitoring on the accuracy of the final composition and a constant maintenance of the desired values.

Several formulas are today commercially available. The typical ranges for various components of the final dialysate are reported in Table 1. Each dialysate type is generally offered as a standard for one center according to clinical requirements and doctors convinciments. In other cases, a single center may use more than one dialysate type to better meet the patients individual needs.

In the following sections we will try to analyze why various dialysis fluid concentrations are needed in the dialysis routine.

Sodium

Since Sodium is the major determinant of volume and tonicity of extracellular fluids, and since it easily crosses dialytic membranes, sodium dialysate concentration plays an important role in determining cardiovascular stability of the patients undergoing extracorporeal treatments. Therefore, it is very important do define the kinetics of this electrolyte to achieve a correct dialytic balance.

Plasma is an acqueous solution containing substances both of low molecular weight such as cristalloids, and high molecular weight such as proteins.

Considering an average protein concentration of 70 g/l, the volume occupied by plasma water in a liter of plasma will be 930 cc. Thus, since plasma water occupies a volume lower than 1000 cc, its sodium concentration will be always greater than that measured in total plasma.

To obtain plasma water sodium concentration [Na]$_{pw}$, plasma concentration [Na]$_p$ must be corrected for the volume occupied by proteins, utilizing several formulas (21, 22), being the lipid concentration negligible in normal conditions (23).

Not all the sodium present in plasma water however, is able to cross dialysis membranes. Indeed, sodium concentration in the ultrafiltrate [NA]$_{uf}$ is lower than that in plasma water (24–26). In fact, due to Donnan's effect (27), cations, and particularly sodium, must be kept in the blood to balance the negative charges of plasma proteins not able to cross dialysis membranes. Therefore, the ultrafiltrate is hyponatric to plasma water (28) and thus, the electroneutrality on both sides of the membrane is maintained. To evaluate the active sodium, i.e., the sodium available for diffusion, [Na]$_{pw}$ must be corrected for the Donnan factor (23, 29).

It is worthy to mention that active [Na]$_{pw}$ can be directly measured by potentiometry (30) or indirectly calculated if the [Na]p concentration is measured by flame photometry (31). Nevertheless, both calculated and directly measured [Na]$_{pw}$ have to be corrected for the Donnan factor to obtain the concentration of sodium available for diffusion (29).

In the seventies, in order to correct arterial hypertension, dialysate sodium concentration [Na]$_d$ was maintained below plasma sodium concentration to favour diffusive sodium losses. By using a hyponatric dialysate with [Na]$_d$ of 130 mmol/l, patients had nor thirst nor great interdialytic weight gain (32–34). On the other hand, in some patients, the negative sodium balance could stimulate renin secretion with maintenance of high blood pressure levels (35). Negative sodium balance obtained with hyponatric dialysate, led to a reduction of natremia and plasma osmolality with fluid shifts from extracellular into the intracellular space (36). Then, dialytic dehydration was mainly obtained at the expenses of the extracellular volume, while the intracellular space was overhydrated. The osmolar changes, with consequent fluid shifts generated during these unphysiological treatments were responsible for the high incidence of dialysis disequilibrium, cramps and hypotension (37, 38).

In the following years, with the coming of short dialysis and with the improvement of the dialytic technology, leading to the development of more permeable membranes, the use of hyponatric baths were not longer acceptable, and higher [Na]$_d$ were utilized with increased well-being and clinical tolerance.

Wilkinson et al., increasing [Na]$_d$ from 130 to 136 mmol/l, noted a marked reduction of muscle cramps (39).

Stewart et al. compared the results obtained in some patients treated with [Na]$_d$ of 132.5 mmol/l with those obtained in the same patients with [Na]$_d$ of 145 mmol/l (40). With higher [Na]$_d$, the patients felt better and complained of less cephalea, nausea and vomiting. Furthermore, hypertension was better controlled when patients were treated with higher dialysate sodium concentration, when appropriate dry body weight was achieved.

Similar clinical results have been reached by Redaelli et al. (28). The authors increased dialysate sodium concentration from 135 to 142 mmol/l. This concentration was kept constant for 18 months and then it was adjusted to the [Na]$_{pw}$ of each patient. Such concentration was defined 'adequate', because it prevented any fall in plasma osmolality secondary to diffusive plasma sodium losses (28).

Locatelli et al. dialyzed for a long time their patients with [Na]$_d$ of 142 mmol/l, similar to their [Na]$_{pw}$ corrected for the Donnan factor (41). They defined such concentration 'physiological'. In this condition, sodium diffusion was avoided, and the amount removed was obtained together with water only by convection (41). With the further increase of dialysate sodium concentration to 148 mmol/l (similar to the patient [Na]$_{pw}$ and called 'pharmacologically high'), cardiovascular stability improved and blood pressure did not show significant increase (41).

The use of [Na]$_d$ higher than [Na]$_{pw}$, has been suggested because the Na/Water ratio in the ultrafiltrate is higher than the Na/Water ratio in the fluid introduced in the interdialytic period (42). In these circumstances, if isonatric dialysate would be utilized, sodium losses with ultrafiltration would exceed the amount of sodium introduced, with possible cardiovascular instability. Therefore, convective sodium losses in excess to sodium introduced must be counterbalanced by a diffusive gain employing a dialysate sodium concentration higher than 'physiological' (42).

Funk-Brentano et al. considered as adequate, a [Na]$_d$ which maintains a normal [Na]$_p$ at the end of dialysis treatment (43). Since daily sodium and water intake is usually 100 mmol and 1 liter respectively, adequate [Na]$_d$ should be that permitting a Na/Water mass removal ratio of 100. This, results in [Na]$_d$ of 145 mmol/l (43).

From these and other studies (43–46), that underline the importance of an adequate [Na]$_d$, some considerations can be drawn.

Dialytic treatment is aimed at removing the quantity of salt and water accumulated during the interdialytic period. This removal is carried out by diffusion and convection (28, 47). Diffusion is more important during hyponatric dialysis which, however, is considered unphysiological (41).

Its negative sodium balance, triggers remarkable extracellular dehydration and intracellular overhydration with several acute side effects (41, 48).

When $[Na]_d$ approaches $[Na]_{pw}$, diffusion becomes less important and evenctually ceases. In this setting, water and salt mass transport occurs only by convection (28, 41, 49) and ultrafiltration and backfiltration fluxes must be carefully evaluated (50). In fact, in this condition ultrafiltrate is hyponatric because of Donnan effect, while sodium concentration in backultrafiltrate is similar to that of dialysate (50). If an hyponatric ultrafiltrate is produced in absence of diffusive sodium losses and backfiltration, a compensation is achieved by varying the UF volume (28, 47).

The constant osmolality obtained with dialysate containing more physiological sodium concentrations prevents important extracellular dehydration and intracellular overhydration accounting for a less incidence of muscular cramps, nausea and vomiting.

Furthermore, by preventing hypovolemia and collapse, a more complete correction of overall hyperhydration and a better control of hypertension can be obtained. In this setting, a dry body weight lower than that obtained during hyponatric dialysis, can be reached thanks to a better correction of cellular hyperhydration (28, 47). Nevertheless, high $[Na]_d$ increases thirst and may provoke important interdialytic weight gains, with circulatory overload, hypertension and possible pulmonary oedema (51, 52). Some Authors suggest that this augmented sense of thirst may be transient if $[Na]_d$ is increased gradually (53).

Others, proposed dialysis with variable $[Na]_d$, i.e., high sodium in the first part of the treatment to avoid osmolar changes secondary to urea losses and lower sodium at the end of the session to avoid hypernatremia (54, 55).

In conclusion, since sodium plays an important role in cardiovascular hemodynamics, it is necessary to reach an exact dialytic sodium balance to avoid adverse effects. Factors involved in this balance that must be evaluated are sodium intake, interdialytic weight gain, duration of dialysis and total body water (42).

Recently, computer-based sodium models have been introduced. These models allow computation of sodium concentration in the dialysate necessary to modulate sodium transfer in order to match individual needs and reach a target $[Na]_p$ at the end of treatment.

The clinical application of these models has improved cardiovascular stability and reduced side effects linked to inadequate sodium and water removals during hemodialysis.

Petitclerc et al. introduced a biofeedback module (BM) designed for optimization of dialysate conductivity during dialysis. The authors used conductivity measurements instead of sodium measurements and defined the effective conductivity of the patient as the conductivity of dialysate at equilibrium with plasma water (56).

At the beginning of dialysis BM requires input of several data such as duration of the session, pre-dialysis weight, desired weight loss and expected effective conductivity at the end of the session.

In several patients, with different predialytic sodium concentrations, ranging from ≤ 130 mmol/l to ≥ 140 mmol/l, BM automatically adjusted dialysate conductivity to the predialytic $[Na]_p$ in order to obtain at the end of the session an effective conductivity of the patient of 14.2 mS/cm. This value was arbitrarily chosen because the authors demonstrated that it led to a post-dialytic $[Na]_p$ in the physiological range (56).

The introduction of highly efficient short dialysis techniques in the clinical routine has spurred new interest on this subject. Since short treatment time often require ultrafiltration rates higher than those programmed in standard hemodialysis, maximal care is placed in maintaining a good clinical tolerance and in avoiding symptomatic hypotension. In these treatments a minimal sodium concentration in dialysate of 140 mmol/l has been suggested and satisfatory clinical results have been achieved with this approach (57). The search of enhanced dialysis efficiency and improved clinical tolerance has also spurred new interest in alternative dialysis techniques (58).

Hemodiafiltration (HDF) is a dialytic technique introduced in 1978 by Leber et al., in which the use of highly permeable membrane allows the symultaneous application of hemodialysis and hemofiltration (59). Therefore, in this technique, dialysate and substitution fluids must be combined to achieve the final electrolyte and acid-base balance.

Diffusion takes place due to chemical concentration gradients while convective transport of solutes is achieved because of high filtration rates. Since ultrafiltration exceeds the amount of fluid required to achieve the dry body weight, replacement solution must be infused in adequate amount. The dialysate and replacement solutions used in hemodiafiltration by different authors are reported in Table 2 (59–62).

In spite of many papers dealing with this topic, very few kinetic studies were described. In mixed diffusion-convection transport, the final balance of sodium is a complex result of diffusion fluxes, convective removal and reinfusion with substitution fluid. In these conditions, the risk of side effects due to water and sodium imbalances is even greater. In fact, not only dialysate sodium is important, but also sodium content in the substitution fluid is critical to influence sodium balance and thus final $[Na]_{pw}$.

Pedrini et al. developed a computer model which predicts changes in $[Na]_{pw}$ and solute transfer during HDF, using different dialysate and substitution fluid sodium concentrations (63). The model demonstrated that there is a close correlation between changes of $[Na]_{pw}$ and sodium gradient between plasma water and dialysate, sodium concentration in the substitution fluid and ultrafiltration.

Table 2. Composition of dialysate and substitution fluid in hemodiafiltration

| | Author, Reference # | | | |
	Leber (59)	Cambi (60)	Von Albertini (61)	Wizemann (62)
Dialysate (mmol/l)				
Sodium	138	130	140	143
Potassium	2.0	2.0	2.0	2.0
Calcium	1.8	2.0	2.3	1.8
Magnesium	0.5	0.8	0.4	1.0
Chloride	112.5	112.5	108.2	115.0
Bicarbonate	–	–	35.0	–
Acetate	32.0	25.0	4.0	35.0
Glucose	16.7	5.5	5.6	11.1
Substitution fluid (mmol/l)				
Sodium	135	275	Back	140
Potassium	2.0	–	Filtered	2.0
Calcium	1.9	–	Dialysate	2.1
Magnesium	1.0	–		0.8
Chloride	102.7	150		112.0
Bicarbonate	–	125		–
Lactate	40	–		35.8
Glucose	30.5	–		8.3

During HDF performed with infusion of 49 to 66 ml/min of a solution containing 140 to 145 mmol/l of sodium, the mean gradient to avoid sodium changes was 9.5 mmol/l. This gradient was greater than that observed in the hemodialysis sessions performed during the same study. Such gradient for diffusion, permitted to counterbalance the sodium retention caused by substitution fluid infusion and the production of an hyponatric ultrafiltrate (Donnan effect was enhanced by the high ultrafiltration rates) (63).

Potassium

Hyperkalaemia is a dangerous complication frequently occurring in acute and chronic renal failure (64). Potassium tends to accumulate during the interdialytic interval. To achieve an adequate removal, dialysate K concentration ($[K]_d$) is generally maintained between 1.5 and 2 mmol/l. Such concentration is generally adequate to generate a diffusion gradient throughout the entire duration of the dialysis session.

However, to achieve an exact potassium balance, the dietary intake, the type of dialysis, the duration and frequency of treatment, the metabolic status and intercurrent illness in the patient must be taken into account.

Furthermore, intracellular potassium, which is the real marker of body potassium content, is strongly affected by

acid-base balance. It is well known that metabolic acidosis causes the exit of potassium from the cells, with consequent reduction of the intracellular content; therefore, the buffer concentration in dialysis fluid as well as the level of correction of metabolic acidosis, are important determinants of potassium balance during hemodialysis. In these circumstances, the polarization of the cell is affected and the intra/extra cellular concentration ratio $[K]_i/[K]_e$ represents one of the factors governing cardiac rythm and contractility and, as a consequence, the cardiovascular tolerance to hemodialysis.

In acute renal failure, where several other variables may interfere with potassium balance, $[K]_d$ should be more flexible and complete personalization of the dialysis fluid composition is required.

Lower dialysate concentrations are generally required during the oliguric phase of acute renal failure.

In traumatized patients with internal bleeding or wide hematomas, potassium release from red blood cells may produce a severe condition of hyperkalaemia. In these cases a dialysate containing low or no potassium is required to maintain adequate blood levels, even though a possible potassium depletion may occur in the long run.

On the contrary, when daily dialysis is performed, in patients with poor potassium intake or in presence of potassium losses through vomiting or diarrhoea, a dialysis fluid containing 4 mmol/l of K may be strongly advised to prevent dangerous hypokalaemia (19).

In patients undergoing chronic dialysis on free diet, daily potassium intake generally varies between 60 and 80 mmol. In this case, a thrice weekly hemodialysis seems to produce an acceptable potassium balance when dialysate contains 1.5 to 2.0 mmol/l of K (19).

In high-efficiency hemodialysis, Dalal et al. (65), utilized three different solutions containing lactate, acetate or bicarbonate as a buffer. Dialysate K content was 2.0 or 3.0 mmol/l. In their study the Authors did not note any difference in dialysate recovery of potassium and in post-dialitic kaliaemia with the three different solutions. Because pre-dialytic Kalaemia was about 4.8 mmol/l, one could speculate that dilysate K content would have not been adequate, if pre-dialytic potassium values were more elevated than those reported in this study.

Obviously, also in chronic uremic patients, dialysis fluid must be settled to clinical needs, especially when intercourrent illness modify body potassium content.

Dialysis patients on inotropic therapy with digoxin or with poor dietary potassium intake, may experience dangerous arrhytmias when potassium removal is excessive or too rapid. For these patients, higher K dialysate concentrations are suggested instead of those routinely utilized.

The above reported observations, stress the importance of an accurate evaluation of the 'adequate' dialysate concentration of potassium for each single patient.

This concept has been further outlined by Redaelli and coworkers (66). These authors hypothesized that rapid removal of potassium during dialysis, secondary to inadequate content in the dialysis fluid, might limit the correction of metabolic acidosis. The cellular hyperpolarization caused by a rapid fall in serum potassium, might in fact interfere with the extraction of H^+ from the cells and the cellular uptake of HCO_3. In this case, a rapid decrese of dialytic transmembrane gradient of HCO_3 is likely to occur. The acid-base status would than be characterized by an extracellular alkalosis with persistent intracellular acidosis. The same cellular hyperpolarization could produce an increased entry of calcium into the cells with various possible consequences. Theoretically, hemodialysis-mediated modifications of potassium metabolism, could interfere on calcium and phosphate metabolism and on acid-base regulation, leading in the long run, to accelerated atherosclerosis and enhanced risk of osteodistrophy (66).

Recently, Redaelli et al. have experimentally studied a computerized unit, able to modulate the concentration of potassium in the dialysate such to maintain during dialysis a constant gradient for diffusion (67). This 'biofeedback' approach will certainly be part of future studies designed to reduce dialysis unphysiology, devoted to decrease clinical complications related to sudden $[K]_i/[K]_e$ alterations, and oriented to permit a better maintenance of body fluid and electrolyte homeostasis.

Calcium

The content of calcium in the dialysate is extremely important to maintain calcium homeostasis, and to avoid adverse effects due to altered calcium levels in the patient (68).

Calcium concentration in dialysis fluids generally range between 1.5 and 2 mmol/l.

Occasionally, calcium levels of 3.6 mmol/l (14.4 mg/dl) have been reported after failure of the systems for water treatment. In such circumstances an acute syndrome was described including nausea, vomiting, hypertension, sweating, progressive lethargy and weakness.

This cohort of symptoms was described as 'hard water syndrome' (69, 70) and, although uncommon, it must be considered as a potential risk for the patient.

The advent of softeners, deionizers and reverse osmosis water treatments, and the continuous monitoring of treated water resistivity, has permitted to avoid such incovenient and the syndrome is practically disappeared at the present time.

Calcium content in treated water is today irrelevant and the final concentration in the dialysate is only depending on pure water mixing with calcium containing liquid concentrates.

Since in most patients a positive calcium balance is required to maintain adequate calcium homeostasis, a sufficient concentration gradient between dialysate calcium and ionized calcium in the blood must be established thoughout the dialysis session.

Typical uremic patients have a constant level of hypocalcemia unless hyperparathyroidism has reached

its final phase with unpredictable calcium levels in the blood.

The diffusable fraction of calcium in uremic patients has been reported to be higher than in normal subjects (68). Values ranging between 57.6 and 64.3% of total plasma calcium have been reported. This is the amount of Calcium available for the dialytic exchanges that corresponds to an average concentration of 1.6 mmol/l (6.5 mg/dl) in case of total plasma calcium concentrations near normal. Considering a condition of mild hypocalcemia, an average concentration of calcium in the dialysate of 1.5 mmol/l is generally able to provide a net calcium balance during dialysis near zero or slightly positive (68). On the other hand, a calcium concentration in dialysate of 1.62 mmol/l has been shown to provide net calcium balances of 650 mg/session either positive or negative (71).

Other studies demonstrated a negative calcium balance and consequent calcium losses from the skeleton when 1.5 mmol/l of calcium containing dialysate was used (72). The increase to 1.75 mmol/l of the calcium concentration in dialysate, prevented the fall in the metacarpal bone index, while a further increase to 2.0 mmol/l determined an increase in total body calcium in dialyzed patients with osteomalacia (73).

As in the case of other ions, the dialytic mass transport of calcium is affected by the concentration gradient between dialysate and blood, by the performance of the dialyzer and by the rate of ultrafiltration. Significant amounts of ultrafiltration may in fact determine a remarkable calcium loss via convective transport. In some cases these losses may even exceed the amount of calcium gained by backdiffusion (68, 74).

Based on these observations, a suitable concentration of calcium in dialysate has been established between 1.25 and 1.75 mmol/l (71, 74). The calcium concentration should however be adjusted to each single patient according to the conditions of the mineral metabolism, the levels of PTH and calcemia, and the possible assumption of calcium containing phosphate binders in order to avoid dangerous hypercalcemia and soft tissue calcifications (75–78).

In the case of hemodiafiltration, the concentration of calcium in the dialysate must be adapted to the patient requirement and to the wanted corrections in the body pool (79). It is evident that calcium content in the replacement solutions may strongly affect final calcium balance, and a correct evaluation of all these components must be carried out to obtain the right final mass balance (80, 81).

In convective treatments such as hemofiltration or hemodiafiltration, lactate based replacement solutions are also containing calcium. When bicarbonate is used as a buffer in the replacement solution, calcium cannot be added at the same time and calcium free substitution fluids are generally employed. In these cases, calcium content in the dialysate has been increased to overcome its convective losses. Recently however, replacement solutions containing calcium and bicarbonate simultaneously have been made available thanks to a new design of the containers. The acid solution containing calcium and the basic solution with bicarbonate are mixed just before use, and sufficient stability of the solution is therefore obtained. The container is divided into two compartments (bags) generally separated by a partition wall with a breakable valve that allow for the mixing of the solutions before use.

For several years, a constant tendency to increase dialysate calcium concentration was observed in standard hemodialysis (75). This was done in an attempt to correct patient's hyperparathyroidism and uremic osteodistrophy. However, even slight increases up to 1.75–2.0 mmol/l have shown to present some risks of postdialytic hypercalcemia, alterations of the vascular tone and cardiac contractility, hypertension and cardiac arrhythmias (82, 83). On the other hand, the effect of transient postdialytic hypercalcemia and high dialysate calcium on the suppression of parathyroid function is not totally clear. In this condition, an adequate administration of 1,25 (OH)2 cholecalciferol may result in a greater benefit for the patient with a more constant effect in normalizing calcium levels (84–91).

In patients treated with oral supplementations of calcium, calcium containing phosphate binders and vitamin D analogues, the concentration of calcium in the dialysate has been recently reduced to 1.05–1.35 mmol/l with satisfactory results in terms of ionized calcium levels and control of the osteodistrophy (92). On the other hand, other Authors have shown that a reduction of dialysate calcium concentrations at these levels and in general under 1.5 mmol/l may definitely worsen the secondary hyperparathyroidism (93, 94).

In conclusion, the concentration of calcium in the dialysate cannot be standardized for all patients. An average concentration between 1.25 and 1.75 mmol/l is sufficient in most patients to avoid a negative calcium balance during dialysis. Special adjustments must be done when hemodiafiltration techniques are used, when high ultrafiltration rates are scheduled during treatment and finally when oral calcium supplementations, calcium containing phosphate binders and vitamin D analogues are administered to the patients. In these circumstances, the intestinal absorption and the dialytic mass transfer may vary significantly and an adequate concentration of calcium in the dialysate must be accurately chosen.

Magnesium

The importance of magnesium content in dialysate has been poorly studied in clinical dialysis and its role is still under evaluation (95).

Magnesium is a prevalently intracellular ion, largely present in the bone tissue. Therefore, magnesium plasma levels (ranging 0.6–1.0 mmol/l) only partially reflect significant changes in the total body pool. Furthermore, magnesium is partially binded to proteins and only 70% is diffusible across dialysis membranes (95, 96).

Although Magnesium intake is reduced in uremic patients undergoing low protein diet, Magnesium levels in blood may be slightly increased because of impaired elimination in the urine (96). The gastrointestinal absorption is one of the main factors influencing plasma levels and may vary significantly in uremic patients. Thus, plasma levels may be finally decreased, increased or even normal.

Therefore, magnesium concentration in the dialysate may strongly affect the overall balance of the ion in dialysis patients (97–104). Most commercial dialysis solution have a magnesium concentration ranging between 0.25 and 0.75 mmol/l. It must be observed however, that magnesium based drugs may be frequently administered to dialysis patients (IV Infusion, chelating agents, irrigations, laxatives) making the final balance of the ion rather complex.

Nevertheless, the average magnesium concentration in dialysate has been adjusted in order to achieve a slight increase in plasma levels. This effect has been considered responsible for a partial inhibition on PTH secretion. This however has been found to be the case, only in the case of acute hypermagnesemia, while chronic increases seem to have a limited effect (96–99).

Inversely, recent studies have proposed that a severe hypo-magnesemia may reduce the clinical signs of uremic osteoporosis and osteomalacia (104–108). Based on these findings, a lower concentration of magnesium in dialysate has been suggested (0.2–0.35 mmol/l). In these study predialysis plasma levels were nearly normal, while post-dialysis values were slightly reduced. The tissue content was however unchanged.

In order to avoid aluminum containing phosphate binders, other agents containing magnesium hydroxide or magnesium carbonate have been recently utilized. In patients undergoing this kind of treatment, the use of low magnesium concentrations in dialysate is strongly recommended. In some cases, the use of magnesium free dialysate has also been proposed to avoid significant hypermagnesemia (101, 102).

In conclusion, the dialytic balance of magnesium depends on several factors including concentration gradients (plasma levels of diffusible Mg versus Dialysate Mg concentration), the amount of ultrafiltration (causing a magnesium convective removal) and the dialyzer performance at given blood and dialysate flow rates (109–116).

In bicarbonate hemodiafiltration, the replacement solution is generally magnesium free to avoid precipitation of calcium and magnesium salts. In such circumstance, an adequate adjustment of dialysate concentration is recommended. Lactate replacement solution may or may not contain magnesium and the level in dialysate should be therefore adjusted according to patient's clinical requirements and contingent situations.

Buffers

Correction of metabolic acidosis in the uremic patient represents one of the foundamental aims of dialysis. Hemodialysis therapy cannot remove large quantities of free hydrogen ion (H^+) because of its low concentration in the blood. As hydrogen ions are produced, they are rapidly buffered by plasma bicarbonate and other body buffers thus remaining at very low concentration in plasma water (116).

Therefore, in hemodialysis, the process of H^+ removal from the blood is mainly achieved by the flux of alkaline equivalents from dialysate into the blood, with replacement of the buffers previously utilized in the chemical process of buffering.

The amount of buffer to be administered in order to achieve an adequate correction of metabolic acidosis with dialysis, should at least equal the overall acid production in the patient during the interdialytic interval. In clinical dialysis, base transfer across dialysis membrane, is achieved by using acetate or bicarbonate containing dialysate. The chemical gradient between dialysate and blood acts as a driving force for diffusion of the buffer contained in the dialysate.

Kolff in 1943 (118), and later Scribner (119), used a dialysis solution with 27 mmol/L of bicarbonate as a buffer. Bicarbonate containing dialysate was prepared in large containers before the dialysis session. When calcium and magnesium were added to the fluid, bicarbonate was rapidly reacting, the solution was becoming unstable with precipitation of calcium and magnesium carbonate crystals.

For this reason, and for the easy microbiological contamination of bicarbonate fluid, Mion et al. (16) introduced in 1964 the use of acetate as alkaline equivalent in the dialysis fluid. The solution was chemically stable and microbiologic contamination was avoided.

Rapidly, acetate solutions became widely applied in the clinical routine of dialysis being used world wide for more than 20 years. The low cost, the equimolar conversion to bicarbonate in the body and the bacteriostatic effect in the solution, made acetate a first choice substrate for the correction of acid-base derangements in hemodialysis. Acetate solutions rendered hemodialysis more simple thus stimulating the proliferation of renal replacement therapy.

In the early 1980s, new dialytic strategies, based on large dialyzers and highly permeable membranes, that permitted to increase efficiency and to shorten dialysis treatment time, uncovered technical and clinical limitations imposed by acetate. Hence, the use of bicarbonate in clinical dialysis was reintroduced, supported this time by new procedures of dialysate preparation, mixing and delivery. The improved clinical tolerance and the more physiologic correction of uremic acidosis, together with the advances in technology of the new proportioning systems for dialysate preparation, led to the wide application

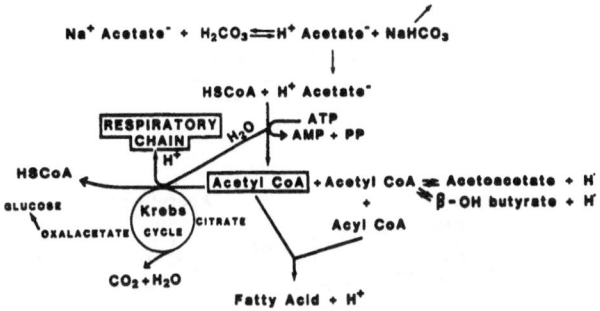

Figure 1. Mechanism of bicarbonate generation from acetate and metabolic pathways of acetate.

of bicarbonate dialysis in the clinical routine and to the almost complete substitution of acetate dialysis.

Buffer Chemistry

Sodium salts of organic acids (OA) can generate alkaline equivalents according to the formula:

$$NaOA + H_2CO_3 \rightarrow HOA + NaHCO_3$$

This process takes place only when the anion is completely metabolized to a neutral compound or decarboxylated to CO_2 and H_2O. Despite several potential substrates have been proposed in the past as alkaline equivalents in humans, e.g., succinate, fumarate and ketoglutarate (120, 121), evident side effects discouraged their use and only acetate was utilized in clinical dialysis.

Acetate

Sodium acetate, originally proposed by Mudge (122), has a molecular weight of 136 Daltons. It is almost completely dissociated in the body fluids because of its low pK (4.7). Acetate is mostly metabolized in peripheral tissues (123), although in the past, the liver was considered the main site of metabolism (124).

Acetate thiokinase activates the reaction between acetate and CoA to form Acetyl CoA, and one hydrogen ion is captured in this process.

Acetyl CoA may enter different metabolic pathways such as decarboxylation in the Krebs cycle, condensation to keton bodies or transformation into fatty acids and glucose via gluconeogenesis (Figure 1).

The buffering effect takes place only when the hydrogen ion is transferred to the respiratory chain and Acetyl CoA is decarboxylated. When alternative pathways are entered or the decarboxylation process is incomplete, the buffering effect is delayed until the intermediate products are completely decarboxylated.

Several attempts have been made to quantify the amount of acetate infused during dialysis that is immediately oxydized in the Krebs cycle. Tolchin et al. (125), by measuring the rate of conversion into bicarbonate, found approximate values of 93% while Davidson et al. (126)

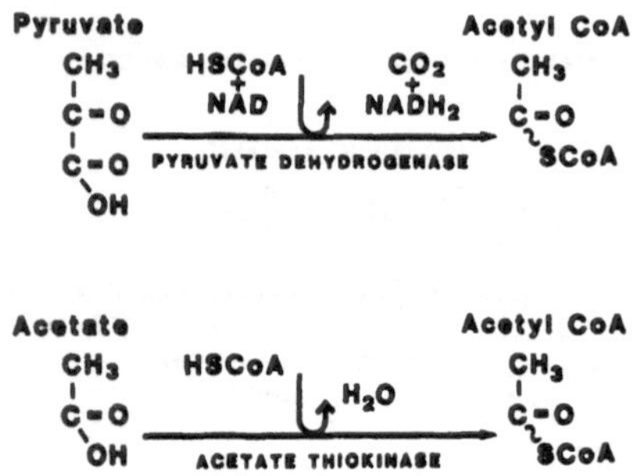

Figure 2. Mechanisms of Acetyl CoA generation from pyruvate and acetate.

and Morin et al. (127) have shown values of 70% using ^{14}C acetate. More recently Skutches et al. (128), using a sophysticated radioisotopic method, demonstrated that only 54% of the infused acetate is immediately oxidized during dialysis while 46% enters alternative pathways. This low rate of oxidation might be explained by the fact that acetate is not a usual major metabolic fuel and differences may arise in the way the Krebs cycle handles acetate as compared to pyruvate (Figure 2). In pyruvate metabolism only 3-carbon moieties are concerned when oxalacetate is transformed into citrate (Krebs cycle), compared to 2-carbon moieties for acetate (129). The significance of this difference remains to be established.

During dialysis, acetate is the main source of Acetyl CoA representing about 65% of the energy requirement (128). As a consequence the β-oxydation of long chain fatty acids is spared and triglicerydes synthesis is favoured (130). This fact may explain the potential lipogenetic action of acetate.

When glucose free dialysate is used, a remarkable increase of free fatty acids, keton bodies and gluconeogenesis precursors can be noted (131). Concurrently, serum insulin levels fall suggesting a possible role of this hormon in acetate metabolism. High levels of acetoacetate and β-hydroxybutirate can also be found in highly efficient dialysis treatments, probably depending on the large acetate load (132). These metabolites commonly dissociate in body fluids, and release hydrogen ions, so their previous buffering effect vanishes. However, when not lost in the dialysate, they can still operate as buffers being reconverted to Acetyl CoA. Acetate metabolism depends on an intact oxydative phosphorilation system; since Krebs cycle activity is regulated by the ATP/ADP ratio, when ATP concentration increases acetate metabolism is slowed down (133).

Lundquist (123) estimated in 5 mmol/min, the maximal rate of acetate metabolism in normal subjects. Such a rate seems to be lower in, dialysis patients (3–4 mmol/min) because of a possible impairment of the Krebs cycle activity. Yamakawa et al. (133) have found that malate and citrate increase during acetate dialysis and isoci-

trate becomes detectable in the blood when acetate levels exceed 7 mmol/L.

The complete decarboxylation of 1 mol of acetate, leads to the production of 2 mol of CO_2 and consumes 2 mol of O_2.

Since 1 mol of CO_2 is consumed in the acetate → acetic acid reaction, the final CO_2/O_2 ratio is 1/2 (134).

$$CO_2[\text{consumed}] + H_2O + CH_3COONa$$
$$\leftrightarrow NaHCO_3 + CH_3COOH$$

$$CH_3COOH + 2O_2[\text{consumed}]$$
$$= 2CO_2[\text{produced}] + 2H_2O$$

Therefore, if the buffer would be the main source of energy, the RQ should be reduced; however, several factors may interfere with this metabolic pathway, and the final value of this ratio may be variously affected.

Bicarbonate
Bicarbonate is the physiologic buffer in the body fluids. It has a molecular weight of 61 Daltons and a pK of 6.305 at 37°C. Bicarbonate is part of a complex system including carbonic acid, carbonate and carbon dioxyde:

$$CO_2 + H_2O \leftrightarrow HCO_3^- \leftrightarrow H^+ + HCO_3^-$$
$$\leftrightarrow 2H^+ + CO_3^=$$

When acid is added or dissolved CO2 leaves the system, the reaction quickly shifts to the left, while the reaction to the right is slow in the absence of carbonic anhydrase (135, 136). However, since this enzyme is almost ubiquitous (137), the carbonic acid concentration in body fluids is proportional to the dissolved CO2 concentration. At the temperature and ionic strenght of the body fluids, the equilibrium

$$H_2O + CO_2 \leftrightarrow H_2CO_3$$

is greatly towards CO_2 formation with a H_2CO_3/CO_2 ratio of 1/340. The concentration of dissolved CO_2 is proportional, according to Henry's law, to the partial pressure of CO_2 gas or:

$$dCO_2 = \alpha \, pCO_2$$

where α is the CO_2 solubility coefficient which in the blood is 0.0301 mmol/l/mmHg.

The first dissociation of carbonic acid

$$H_2CO_3 \leftrightarrow H^+ + HCO_3^-$$

occurs instantaneously and equilibrium is reached when pH becomes equal to the pK of carbonic acid. The true pK of carbonic acid is 3.8. However carbonic acid appears to be a much weaker hydrogen ion donor than this dissociation constant would imply, and the first dissociation, called 'first apparent dissociation', has a pK of 6.10 in the blood.

The second dissociation of carbonic acid

$$HCO_3^- \leftrightarrow H^+ + CO_3^=$$

has a pK of 9.8 and therefore it has not practical relevance in body fluids except for the buffering activity in bone. This however, is important in dialysis solutions containing bicarbonate which may reach a pH of 8.4. Under this condition bicarbonate and carbonate may exist according to the following equilibrium:

$$Na^+ + HCO_3^- \leftrightarrow Na^+ + CO_3^= + H^+$$

Since in the dialysate, divalent anions such as Ca and Mg are also present, the following equilibrium will be achieved:

$$NaHCO_3 + CaCl_2 \leftrightarrow CaCO_3 + NaCl + HCl$$

When pH of the solution is higher than 7, $CaCO_3$ will begin to precipitate thus reducing the bicarbonate concentration. An high CO_2 content may avoid this precipitation shifting to the left the following reaction:

$$Ca[HCO_3]_2 \leftrightarrow CaCO_3 + H_2O + CO_2$$

forming a soluble salt of calcium.

Since CO_2 is volatile, the CO_2 content of the solution tends to be reduced over a prolonged period of time facilitating $CaCO_2$ formation. This problem can be solved by the separation of Ca and bicarbonate in two containers and mixing them just before the filter. Meanwhile by the formula:

$$NaHCO_3 + CH_3COOH \leftrightarrow CH_3COONa + H_2O + CO_2$$

small amounts of acetic acid in solution containing calcium, permit to achieve an high CO_2 content in the final mixed dialysate.

During the 80s the availability of new highly automated dialysis machines with proportional pumps enabled to separate the concentrated solutions with bicarbonate and calcium into two containers thus solving the practical problems related to the above mentioned chemical reactions.

Several reports about contamination with viable bacteria of liquid bicarbonate concentrate have been published in the late 80s (138–140). Recently a cartridge with bicarbonate powder has been introduced as an alternative to the liquid bicarbonate concentrate (141).

The bicarbonate powder is packed in a sealed container, which can be stored dry for many years without either bacterial growth or chemical decomposition. The cartridge is attached to the dialysis machine, where the powder is automatically and continuously dissolved into a concentrate solution which is proportioned by the machine (142). The final dialysis fluid is prepared just before the use.

Buffer concentration in dialysis fluids

A variety of factors, i.e., blood and dialysate flows, type and surface area of dialyzer, dialysate buffer concentration, and ultrafiltration rate, may affect base balance and therefore the correction of acidosis in dialysis patients. Currently, the concentration of buffer in the dialysate appears to be somewhat arbitrarily chosen and acetate or bicarbonate are added to dialysate at fixed concentration for every patient (143). This can explain the large variability of the acid base results amongs different studies (144), since a single buffer concentration may not be adequate for all patients.

In acetate dialysis, acetate concentration in dialysate usually ranges from 35 to 40 mmol/l. Several studies, using different blood flows (200–300 ml/min), various dialyzer surface areas (1.3–2.5 m²) and different acetate dialysate concentrations (34–41 mmol/l), have reported an acetate influx ranging from 3.8 to 5.1 mmol/min (117, 125, 132). The concurrent loss of bicarbonate in the dialysate mainly depends on blood bicarbonate concentration, being about 2.5 mmol/min with a blood bicarbonate level of 20 mmol/l (145). Since the acetate metabolic rate in dialyzed patients cannot exceed 3–4 mmol/min (125, 146), it is evident that a maximal net buffer gain of about 0.5–1.5 mmol/min can be achieved in acetate dialysis. Hence, in a 4 hour dialysis session, a total amount of 120–360 mmols of buffer can be gained by the patients. This amount may be lower than the metabolic acid production during the interdialytic period. From a clinical point of view these kinetic observations are confirmed by the low pre-dialysis blood bicarbonate levels (16–20 mmol/l) that are usually seen in patients treated with an acetate dialysate (147–150).

On the other hand, acetate transport across the dialysis membrane can be increased by using a more efficient dialysis technique or an higher acetate concentration in the dialytic bath. However if acetate influx exceeds the metabolic capacity, depending on large acetate loads or reduced metabolism, the normal oxidative pathways becomes overloaded. This may lead to a progressive increase of the plasma acetate levels that are associated with severe symptoms during and after dialysis (125, 151).

In the meantime, since bicarbonate losses into dialysate are depending on CO_2 dialysance, they dramatically increase when high dialytic clearances are achieved during treatment. In acetate dialysis, CO_2 and urea clearances display a parallel behaviour. The higher is urea clearance, the higher will be the amount of bicarbonate lost in the dialysate. Therefore, when urea clearance exceeds 180 ml/min, the possibility of correction of uremic acidosis by acetate dialysis is definitely reduced because of an insufficient net base gain.

In bicarbonate dialysis, the bicarbonate concentration in dialysate usually ranges from 30 to 35 mmol/min. However a certain amount of acetate is added to dialysate in order to maintain the chemical stability of the solution. This amount of acetate contributes, even in a little extent, to base balance.

During bicarbonate dialysis, the dialysate/plasma concentration gradient permits to avoid bicarbonate losses and determines the quantity of bicarbonate that will be transferred into the blood (145).

When diffusion is the main form of solute transport, bicarbonate concentration in the dialysis fluid can be maintained at levels slightly higher than those of the desired plasma concentration.

However, when high ultrafiltration rates are utilized and large ultrafiltrate volumes are produced, higher bicarbonate dialysate levels are needed to compensate for the convective loss of bicarbonate (145).

Gotch et al. (117) have studied a weekly base balance in 8 patients undergoing bicarbonate dialysis with 1.3–1.8 m^2 dialyzers, blood flow of 200 ml/min, dialysate flow of 400 ml/min, and 36 mmol/l of bicarbonate in the dialysate. Bicarbonate mass transfer was 618 mmol/week (206 mmol/session). The net final base gain was +175 mmol/week. In case of body buffer depletion this positive balance may contribute to restore the acid-base equilibrium and to replenish the body buffer stores.

Controlled studies of patients treated with bicarbonate dialysis for more than 12 weeks demonstrated the high risk of postdialytic alkalosis with plasma bicarbonate levels exceeding 30 mmol/l and blood pH higher than 7.55. This acute alkalosis may cause nausea, vomiting and letargy and such chronic effects as calcium deposition in soft tissues. On the basis of these observations Ward et al. (147) suggested progressive reduction of dialysate bicarbonate concentration over time. On the other hand, studies carried out with dialysis solutions containing 31 mmol/l of bicarbonate and 5 mmol/l of acetate, have shown insufficient correction of metabolic acidosis and no significant differences from the results achieved with acetate dialysis (152).

Chloride

Chloride concentration in most dialysis fluids varies from 98 to 112 mmol/l.

Since sodium potassium calcium and magnesium are usually present in the concentrates as chloride salts, the concentration of chloride in the dialysate is determined by the electrochemical relationship wherein total anion charges must equal total cation charges. Sodium salts of buffers are used to achieve the final concentration of sodium and buffer in the fluid and thus the concentration of chloride can be derived from the formula

$$[Cl^-] = [Na^+] + [K^+] + [Ca^{++}]$$
$$+ [Mg^{++}] - [Acetate + Bicarbonate]$$

As pointed out by Stewart (19), in this situation, the equivalent concentration must be equal and not the molar concentration. It is also evident that the amount of buffer and the total chloride concentration are inversely correlated since no other anions are present in the solution.

Dextrose

At the beginning of the dialytic era, dextrose was utilized in the dialysis solution to generate an osmotic pressure leading to fluid withdrawal from the blood. Concentrations in the range of 5 g/l were often utilized in the early dialysis treatment (8). While this approach is still valid in peritoneal dialysis, the evolution of hemodialysis machines has permitted the modulation of the transmembrane pressure to achieve ultrafiltration, and the presence of dextrose in the dialysis solution has become ininfluent from this point of view.

The importance of glucose in the dialysate has however been claimed also for its capacity of inducing hyperglycemia during treatment and thus to avoid the possible disequilibrium syndrome secondary to rapid removal of urea from the blood. A 2.7 g/l glucose containing dialysate appeared adequate to reduce of about 50% the fall in osmolality during hemodialysis (153). This advantage was shown to be even greater in infants and children where the postdialytic rebound in urea concentration is compensated by a rapid glucose metabolization.

Contemporary dialysis fluids can be dextrose-free, isoglycemic or they may contain glucose at a concentration slightly higher than that of blood glucose (0–200 mg/dl) (19, 131, 154).

Glucose losses of 30 ± 9 grams/session have been reported using a dextrose-free dialysate, while a positive balance of 15.8 ± 12 g/session has been noted in patients treated with a dialysate glucose concentration of 2 g/dl (155).

Despite these differences, significant adverse reactions or symptoms were not clearly reported and contraddictory results have been presented in the literature (154–158). Recent studies suggest that patients on hemodialysis may have hypercholesterolemia and hypertriglyceridemia irrespective of the dextrose concentration in the dialysate (157). Higher insulin and growth hormon levels reported in hemodialysis patients were reported in association with higher dextrose concentration in the dialysate, although they seemed not to influence the patient's lipid status. In some cases, the presence of dextrose in the dialysate, has been related to the capacity of avoiding hypotension, neurological disorders and changes in serum osmolality (153). The real clinical impact, however, is still unclear. Certainly the presence of dextrose may avoid the occurrence of hypoglycemic symptoms in those patients who are displaying such acute events during dextrose-free hemodialysis. The real nutritional impact of dextrose containing dialysis fluids is controversial (153–158). It should be noted however that in acute patients and in children, hemodialysis may lead to a dramatic amelioration of the peripheral utilization of glucose and consequently, in such conditions, it is absolutely important to maintain glucose levels within physiologic levels. This can easily be achieved with a 1 g/l dextrose containing dialysate in a regular dialysis treatment.

The presence of dextrose in the dialysate has also been correlated with a better buffer balance during dialysis. In absence of glucose, in fact, the krebs cycle may be slowed down and intermediate products may accumulate increasing their levels in the blood. As a consequence, an increased loss of organic anions potentially acting as buffers is observed and the buffering power of the blood is slightly impaired (131, 159).

Finally, dextrose-free solutions appear to be less easily contaminated by bacteria and seem to present less bacterial growth once some contamination has occurred (155).

DIALYSATE QUALITY

The problem of dialysate quality has been underestimated over the past several years (160). New interest in this field has been spurred by the wide use of highly permeable membranes in clinical practice, and by the increased number of pyrogenic reaction and side effects reported in the literature (161–163). In addition, an increased number of possible contaminants have been found, both in tap water and in the dialysate, thanks to new and more sophisticated analytic methods. Therefore, water treatment for hemodialysis must efficiently remove all different types of contaminants in order to make extremely pure and refined water available at the individual dialysis bed station.

The same level of care must be given to the final preparation of dialysate. Dialysate quality must be checked and defined in terms of chemical, physical and microbiologic characteristics. The choice of concentrates and the disinfection of the dialysis machine as well as the microbiologic control of the final dialysate, are crucial points in the achievement of a 'pure' dialysate (164).

Different water treatment modalities will not be deeply discussed in this section, since they are completely described in another chapter of this book. We should only mention that, in case of malfunction or inaccurate maintenance, they may become themselves a dangerous surce of dialysate contamination (164).

Treated water is one of the main components of final dialysate, and its quality is definitely affected by the initial degree of purity and the correct function of treatment modalities (165). Several factors contribute to the increasing contamination of tap water. Increased water consumption, large urban areas, high population density, industrial waste products and use of fertilizers in agriculture, account for the most common sources of contamination. Mineral, vegetal and organic compounds may contribute to a significant degree of physical, chemical and microbiologic pollution. Different substances can be removed with various modalities applied in series. Particles such as beach sand, coal dust or vegetable particulates can be removed by sediment or media filters. Organic contaminants such as chloramine can be removed by absorbing carbon filters. Inorganic chemical contaminants such as

Table 3. Various contaminants and water treatment systems

Substance	Sediment filters	Carbon filters	Softeners	Deionizers	Reverse osmosis
Aluminum				X	X
Arsenic				X	X
Barium				X	X
Cadmium				X	X
Calcium			X	X	X
Chloram.		X			
Chlorine		X			
Chromium				X	X
Copper				X	X
Fluoride				X	X
Lead				X	X
Magnesium			X	X	X
Mercury				X	X
Nitrate				X	X
Potassium				X	X
Selenium				X	X
Silver				X	X
Sodium				X	X
Sulphate				X	X
Zinc				X	X
Viruses		X		X	X
Organic C.		X		X	X
Endotoxins		X		X	X
Particles	X	X		X	X
Bacteria	X	X		X	X

X = effective.

aluminum, fluoride, sodium, calcium, magnesium, iron, copper and manganese originating from industrial waste or substances in the ground can be effectively removed by softeners, deionizers and reverse osmosis equipment. Various contaminants and the relative removal capacity of different equipment are schematically outlined in Table 3. All systems can be used in series to obtain the wanted standard of water purity (166–171). The standards for dialysis water recommended by the American Association for the Advancement of Medical Instrumentation (AAMI) and the Canadian Science Association (CSA) are outlined in Table 4. In the absence of specific rules, the European Community also follows these standards as a model including a maximal content of chlorinated derivatives (30 ppb).

The presence of trace elements in the dialysate has been considered a potential risk for patients undergoing chronic hemodialysis (19). In particular, Aluminum has received increasing attention due to the occurrence of dialysis related encephalopathy and aluminum induced osteomalacia. While in the original description of Aluminum intoxication (172, 173) the source of the contaminant was inadequately treated tap water, today this trace element

Table 4. Proposed water standards for hemodialysis maximal allowable level (mg/l) or (ppm)

Substance	Chem. symbol	AAMI	CSA
Sodium	Na	70	70
Potassium	K	8	8
Calcium	Ca	10	10
Magnesium	Mg	4	4
Fluoride	F	0.2	0.2
Chloride	Cl	0.5	0.5
Chloramines	NH_2Cl, $NHCl_2$, NCl_3	0.1	0.1
Nitrate	NO_3	2	2
Sulphate	SO_4	100	100
Copper	Cu	0.1	0.1
Barium	Ba	0.1	0.1
Zinc	Zn	0.1	0.1
Arsenic	As	0.05	0.05
Chromium	Cr	0.05	0.05
Lead	Pb	0.05	0.05
Silver	Ag	0.05	0.05
Cadmium	Cd	0.01	0.01
Selenium	Se	0.01	0.01
Aluminium	Al	0.01	0.01
Mercury	Hg	0.002	0.0002
Colony Count	CFU	< 200/ml	< 200 ml

can be found in dialysate because of its presence in the powder used for concentrates. The EEC imposes today a limit < 30 μg/l for dialysis fluid and water (1 μmol/l) in order to prevent toxic effects. We should be aware however, that even small concentrations of trace elements may lead to long term accumulation, because hemodialysis patients are exposed to an enormous amount of dialysis fluid (more than 300 liters/week) compared to the amount of water intake per os. For this reason a great care must be placed in monitoring serum levels of such contaminants. A similar consideration should be made for fluorinated compounds, even though their accumulation in hemodialysis patients and their clinical effects are still anecdotal and conjectural (174, 175).

As previously noted, all systems for water treatment can become potential sources of contamination because of bacterial infestation, system failure or exhaustion. In these circumstances, despite the remarkable quality of treated water, chemical and microbiologic contaminants can be found in significant amount in the final dialysate (176).

Therefore, several clinical symptoms may be related to malfunction of the various systems and the clinical tolerance to the treatment may be strongly influenced.

When adequately functioning, the above mentioned procedures render the treated water almost 100% free

of contaminants, as demonstrated by a resistivity higher than 1 megaohm/cm. Analysis of final dialysate, however, demonstrate a significant presence of trace elements and bacterial contamination. Trace elements are contained in the salts used for preparation of the concentrates. Despite innovative procedures, such as complexation with macromolecules (e.g., transferrin), significant improvement in dialysate quality from this point of view cannot be anticipated at present. Dialysate contamination may depend on several other factors acting after the water treatment system: storage tanks, piping and dialysis machines can be sites of bacterial contamination (177–181). Water stagnation, inadequate piping layout and inaccurate disinfection may lead to a highly contaminated dialysate. Contamination may also depend on quality and age of the concentrate. While acid concentrates preclude bacterial growth because of their pH and osmolality, liquid bicarbonate concentrate may easily be colonized by bacteria Several authors have reported the presence of bacterial contamination and bacterial degradation products in commercial containers of liquid bicarbonate concentrate (176–178). Such contaminants deriving from gram negative bacteria can be found in various concentrations in the final dialysate and include the intact lipopolysaccharide (100,000 Daltons) as well as LAL-positive fragments with molecular weights ranging between 1,000 and 20,000 Daltons. Enzymatic degradation of gram positive bacteria may also release peptidoglycans such as muramyldipeptides, LAL-negative, able to cause monocyte activation and Interleukin-1 production. Minimal doses of these substances (1–2 ng/Kg) may produce pyrogenic reactions in humans (180, 181). Therefore, the series of pyrogenic reactions described in the literature, has been correlated with the observation of endotoxin contentrations in the dialysate ranging between 0.1 and 200 ng/ml (177, 179, 182–184). The question whether endotoxins are able to cross dialysis membranes is still matter of controversy. Adsorption and trapping of endotoxins in the membrane structure, might lead to their possible contact with pseudopods of human monocytes. Under such conditions, the release of cytokines from monocytes can be observed even in the absence of detectable endotoxin levels in the blood. Nevertheless, several reports have shown that various fragments may cross dialysis membranes both by backfiltration and backdiffusion (185, 186). While the last mechanism is frequently observed in cellulosic thinner membranes, the first one is more frequent in highly porous synthetic membranes. Synthetic membranes however, have demonstrated a remarkable capacity of retention of endotoxins and endotoxin fragments because of their adsorbitive capacity. These feature has been utilized to reduce endotoxin content in dialysate by placing large ultrafilters in the dialysate line just before the dialyzer. These filters, whose characteristics are reported in Table 5, have been demonstrated to be effective in reducing dialysate contamination and in achieving a sort of 'ultrapure dialysate'. Most companies presently supply

Table 5. Filters for the treatment of dialysate

	Company				
	Amicon	*Bellco*	*Fresenius*	*Gambro*	*Hospal*
Product name	Diaclean	Multiclean	Diasafe	UH 7000	Diaclear
Membrane type	Polysulf. 75 μ	Polysulf. 75 μ	Polysulf. 30 μ	Polyamide hydrophil	Polyamide hydrophil
Surf. area (m^2)	2.4	2.4	1.8	1.4	1.4
Pr. drop (Qd = 500)	40 mmHg	40 mmHg	135 mmHg	75 mmHg	75 mmHg
Bacterial retention	100%	100%	100%	100%	100%
Endotoxin red. factor	5	5	7.5	4	4

Native endotoxin reduction factor is calculated from the ratio (log endotoxin units in challenge suspension/log endotoxin units in the filtrate). Experimental conditions: log bacterial challenge = 7; log endotoxin challenge = 4.

a built-in system for ultrafiltration of dialysate, consisting on a large ultrafilter equipped with a synthetic membrane and a special circuit to guarantee complete sterilization and periodical wash-out of the membrane. Such systems permit to maintain high quality and purity of dialysate during treatment.

Despite dialysate treatment is not a standard procedure yet, we would like to stress its importance in view of the following consideration: all water treatment systems may be hidden sources of contamination when disinfection procedures are inadequate. Even in the case of properly operating water treatment, several possible contamination sites may be present in the circuit such as the piping system, liquid bicarbonate concentrate, the dialysis machine itself. Therefore, not only is stringent disinfection of the whole system required, but final dialysate treatment, just before the dialyzer is also recommended.

Recently, pyrogen free, sterile concentrates have been produced by the industry. They are supplied in bags sealed and directly connected to the proportioning system line of the machine without open contact with the air. This approach, although costly, may cartainly contribute to an improved quality of the final dialysate delivered to the patient.

PHYSICAL CHARACTERISTICS OF THE DIALYSIS FLUID

Dialysis fluids are exposed to physical factors such as pressure and temperature. In such conditions it may become important to exert a certain control on the final composition, temperature and partial pressure of gases (19, 20).

Temperature control

Dialysate temperature must be accurately regulated and maintained within specific ranges to achieve patient confort and neutral thermic balance during the hemodialysis session.

Dialysate temperature is therefore generally maintained between 36.5 and 38°C at the inlet of the dialyzer. To achieve such result, heat exchangers are provided in the dialysis machines together with a temperature monitor. Higher temperature of dialysate may result in fever, hyperventilation, tachycardia, nausea, vomiting hypotension and patient discomfort. In some cases where a temperature monitor failure occurred, severe hemolysis has been reported (187–189). Lower temperature may result in sense of cold, chills, and hypothermia with shivering in the patient.

Maggiore et al. however, have recently proposed that a lower temperature of the dialysis solution may permit an improved vascular stability in hypotension prone patients (189). This has been confirmed by other Authors that have tried a similar approach (190). In other cases however, the studies had to be interrupted because of frequent discomfort and chills and possible hypoxemia (191). Nevertheless, an increased vascular tone and increased levels of norepinephrin are the rule utilizing cold dialysate, and this may lead to an improved tolerance to fluid withdrawal during hemodialysis (192).

Acchiardo et al. have proposed that dialysate temperature may modulate the activity of endothelial cells. In uremic patients, reduced lipoprotein lipase activity might be secondary to an autonomic nervous system mediated vasoconstriction. Increased dialysate temperature (hyperthermic dialysis) might expose endothelial cells to the effects of heparin and increased lipoprotein lipase activity. This could have an impact on progression of atherosclerosis in dialyzed patients (193).

Recently, temperature control monitors have been experimentally placed both on the dialysate inlet and in the outlet line to perform thermal balance and recirculation studies in dialyzed patients (194, 195).

This represents one of the several approaches to achieve on-line signals from the patient to be evenctually used in a complex system of automatic biofeedback.

Deaeration

The solubility of gases in water depends on the temperature and the partial pressure of each gas at the gas/water interface. Therefore when dialysate is heated, the appearance of air bubbles is likely to occur. Furthermore, when ultrafiltration control systems determine a negative pressure on the dialysate compartment to increase ultrafiltration, a further air bubling is likely to occur. Air bubbles represent a possible loss of efficiency, since they effectively reduce the surface available for dialytic exchanges. In fact, when air is present on one side of the dialysis membrane, the diffusion process ceases and a reduction in solute transfer immediately occur. In some cases, this microbubble formation may also occur in the blood compartment when high blood flows and small size needles are utilized. A possible transfer of of gas across the dialysis membrane has also been postulated with a consequent increase in air trapping and blood foaming in the venous drip chanber of the blood circuit (196–198).

One of the problems created by the air bubble formation in the dialysate compartment is the need for a deaeration device in the dialysis machine. These devices generally utilize ventilation valves, sudden changes in temperature (pasteuriation-like process) or negative pressure chambers. Despite all these procedures, air bubbles are still present in the final dialysate and the better dialyzer performance is obtained with a blood/dialysate countercurrent flow with the dialysate inlet at the bottom and the outlet at the top of the dialyzer.

USE OF DIALYSATE AS A REPLACEMENT SOLUTION

In recent years, the use of highly permeable membranes has introduced a series of problems related to the kinetics of water transport in highly efficient hemodialysis treatments (186, 199). In particular, high flux membranes can be used both in hemodiafiltration and in high flux dialysis modes (200). While the former technique, requires a replacement solution to balance the large amount of ultrafiltrate produced, the latter, does not require any replacement solution since the amount of ultrafiltration produced in the proximal portion of the dialyzer is balanced by a significant amount of backfiltration taking place in the distal part of the dialyzer (200). In this condition, backfiltration fluxes of 30–50 ml/min have been described (199). Therefore, the composition of the dialysis fluid must be carefully considered and adequately adjusted in order to achieve the desired solute balance. In some cases, an on-line production of replacement solution from fresh incoming dialysate has been proposed. Such treatments defined on-line hemofiltration or on-line hemodiafiltration, maintain high filtration rates in the dialyzer, while the fluid balance is achieved by reinfusion of on-line filtered fresh dialysate (201). In this case, the buffer and electrolyte balances may be variously affected and adequate adjustments must be done to avoid any possible complication. Furthermore, in some countries, these procedures cannot be performed, since adequate quality control of on-line produced fluid cannot be ensured.

FROM PERSONALIZATION TO BIOFEEDBACK

The modern machines for hemodialysis permit a complete manipulation of the dialysate composition, temperature, flows and pressure. This ensures that, according to patient needs and medical prescription, a refined personalization of the dialysis treatment can be scheduled. This approach has led to an improvement of the correction of metabolic acidosis, of electrolyte imbalances and derived clinical symptoms. On the other hand, the accurate evaluation and monitoring of the dialysis session has shown that the patient entering the session, may vary his clinical condition during treatment and may definitely change his requirements throughout each single session. For this reason, new dialysis monitors are equipped with a computerized program able to perform operational changes along the lenth of the session, in response to adequate inputs. In this way, sodium, potassium and bicarbonate concentrations in the dialysate can be profiled for the entire duration of the treatment and the dialysis machine may operate the programmed changes during the session. These profiles of dialysate concentration have been studied in an attempt to optimize buffer and electrolyte fluxes during treatment, thus avoiding transient but dangerous imbalances. Bicarbonate concentration is therefore profiled in an attempt to avoid acute postdialytic alkalemia while potassium concentration is programmed such to maintain a constant gradient between plasma water and dialysate. Sodium profiling has been proposed to mitigate osmolal changes and to reduce hypotension episodes due to fluid withdrawal from the patient.

All these profiles, however, must be designed in advance, according to previous clinical observations and the clinical history of the patient. Therefore, they somehow represent a static view of the patient and they do not correspond to the real changes occurring to the patient in that specific dialysis session. To overcome this aspect, a new generation of biosensors are today under evaluation in order to achieve an on-line monitoring of the biochemical changes occurring to the patients undergoing hemodialysis. Ion selective electrodes, refratometric cells or immobilized enzymes are used to monitor on line the composition of the effluent dialysate. Assuming that the composition of the spent dialysate is strictly correlated to the changes occurring to the patient, an adaptive response in terms of changes in dialysate composition, ultrafiltration rate and blood flow, may be operated as an active biofeedback. For the moment this has only been studied with an open loop requiring the autorization of the operator before performing any change. However, this may be the future way to improve dialysis efficiency and tolerance in response to the actual requirements and patient needs. Chemical and physical signals can be recorded from the patient and they may become a trigger signal for an efferent branch of the loop operating changes in the dialysis regimen and dialysis fluid composition.

The composition of spent dialysate may definitely offer some instantaneous information on the efficiency of the dialysis session. The on-line measurement of urea concentration has permitted to evaluate dialysis adequacy in a series of patients (202). For this purpose, an on-line urea monitor (Biostat1000®, Baxter, USA) was utilized. A pH sensitive electrode was able to detect the variation in cation concentration following the instantaneous metabolization of urea into ammonia by urease. In this way, Kt/V, PCR and solute removal could be timely measured and when predicted final values were different from those expected on the basis of the efficiency prescription, treatment parameters vere modified.

This is a typical example of the possible utilization of spent dialysate and it appears evident that dialysate composition is also important after the passage through the dialyzer.

CONCLUSIONS

The composition of dialysis fluid represents today one of the most critical aspects in the personalized treatment of end stage renal disease. Dialysis fluid must be considered a drug and therefore it must be prescribed both in quantity and quality adequate to fulfill the patient clinical requirement. A continuous surveillance on the quality and standards of the delivered dialysis fluid ensure an optimal performance of the dialysis treatment and a complete personalization of the therapy. The on-line monitoring of the spent dialysate composition and the possible use of the dialysis fluid as a source of information for a biofeedback loop with consequent modification of the dialysis operational parameters, might be of great importance in further developments of the dialysis therapy in the coming future.

REFERENCES

1. Smith HW: From Fish to Philosopher, Boston, Little Brown & Co, 1966

2. Graham T: The Bakerian Lecture – on osmotic force. *Philos Trans R Soc Lond* 144: 177, 1854

3. Abel JJ, Rowntree LG, Turner BB: The removal of diffusible substances from the circulating blood of living animals by dialysis. *J Pharmacol Exp Ther* 5: 275, 1914

4. Alwall N: On the artificial kidney. I. Apparatus for dialysis of the blood *in vivo*. *Acta Med Scand* 128: 317, 1947

5. Aoyama S, Kolff W: Treatment of renal failure with the disposable artificial kidney. Results in fiftytwo patients. *Am J Med* 23: 565, 1957

6. Coleman BK, Merrill JP: The artificial kidney. *Am J Nurs* 52: 327, 1952

7. Haas G: Die Methoden der Blutauswaschung. *Abderhalden's Handb Biol Arbeitsmethoden* 8: 7-17, 1935

8. Kolff WJ, Berk HT: The artificial kidney: A dialyzer with a great area. *Acta Med Scand* 117: 121, 1944

9. McBride PT: *The Genesis of the Artificial Kidney*, Travenol Laboratories Inc, 1979

10. Alwall N: On the artificial kidney. XI Some supplementary constructional details of the dialyzer intended for rabbit and homo. *Acta Med Scand* 133 (Suppl 229): 20, 1949

11. Teschan P: Personal communication, Chicago, 1982

12. Wolf AV, Remp DG, Kiley JE, Currie GD: Artificial kidney function: kinetics of hemodialysis. *J Clin Invest* 30: 1062, 1951

13. Grimsrud L, Cole JJ, Lehman GA, Babb AL, Scribner BH: A central system for the continuous preparation and distribution of hemodialysis fluid. *Trans Am Soc Artif Intern Organs* 10: 107, 1964

14. Scribner BH, Babb AL: Chronic hemodialysis in Seattle 1960–1966, Part II. *Dial Tranplant* 11: 324, 1982

15. Sherris JC, Cole JJ, Scribner BH: Bacteriology of continuous flow hemodialysis. *Trans Am Soc Artif Intern Organs* 7: 37, 1961

16. Mion CM, Hegstrom RM, Boen ST, Scribner BH: Substitution of sodium acetate for bicarbonate in the bath fluid for hemodialysis. *Trans Am Soc Artif Intern Organs* 10: 110, 1964

17. Drukker W. Haemodialysis: a historical review. in *Replacement of Renal Function by Dialysis, 3rd Ed*, edited by Maher JF, Dordrecht, Kluwer Academic Publisherss 1989, p 20

18. Merrill JP, Schupak E, Cameron E, Hampers CL: Hemodialysis in the home. *JAMA* 190: 466, 1964

19. Stewart SK: The composition of dialysis fluid. in *Replacement of Renal Function by Dialysis, 3rd Ed*, edited by Maher JF, Dordrecht, Kluwer Academic Publishers, 1989, p 199

20. Ronco C, Brendolan A, Crepaldi C: Water and dialysate treatment for hemodialysis. in *Hemodialysis: High Efficiency Treatments*, edited by Bosch JP, New York, Churchill Livingstone, 1993, p 41

21. Waugh WH: Utility of expressing serum sodium per unit of water in assessing hyponatremia. *Metabolism* 18: 706, 1969

22. Gotch FA, Lam MA, Prowitt M, Keen M: Preliminary clinical results with sodium-volume modeling of hemodialysis therapy. *Proc Dial Transplant Forum* 10: 12, 1980

23. Locatelli F, Ponti R, Pedrini L, Di Filippo S: Sodium and dialysis: a deeper insight. *Int J Artif Organs* 12: 71, 1989

24. Nolph KD, Stotz ML, Carter CB et al.: Factors affecting the composition of ultrafiltrate from hemodialysis coils. *Trans Am Soc Artif Intern Organs* 16: 495, 1970

25. Gotch FA, Sargent JA: Hemofiltration: an unnecessarily complex method to achieve hypotonic sodium removal and controlled ultrafiltration. *Blood Purif* 1: 9, 1983

26. Locatelli F, Ponti R, Pedrini L et al.: Sodium kinetics across dialysis membranes. *Nephron* 38: 174, 1984

27. Donnan FG: The theory of membrane equilibria. *Chem Rev* 1: 73, 1924

28. Redaelli B, Sforzini S, Bonoldi G et al.: Hemodialysis with 'adequate' sodium concentration in dialysate. *Int J Artif Organs* 2: 133, 1979

29. Bosch J, Ponti R, Glabman S, Lauer A: Sodium fluxes during hemodialysis. *Nephron* 45: 860, 1987

30. Worth HGJ: A comparison of the measurement of sodium and potassium by flame photometry and ion-selective electrode. *Ann Clin Biochem* 22: 343, 1985

31. Lauer A, Belledonne M, Saccaggi A et al.: Sodium fluxes during hemodialysis. *Trans Am Soc Artif Intern Organs* 29: 684, 1983

32. Comty C, Rottka H, Shaldon S: Blood pressure control in patients with end-stage renal failure treated by intermittent hemodialysis. *Proc Eur Dial Tranplant Assoc* 1: 209, 1964

33. Drukker W, Jungerius NA, Alberts C: Report on regular dialysis treatment in Europe. *Proc Eur Dial Tranplant Assoc* 4: 3, 1967

34. Boquin E, Parnell S, Grondin G et al.: Cross-over study of the effect of different dialysate sodium concentrations in large surface area short-term dialysis. *Proc Clin Dial Tranplant Forum* 7: 48, 1977

35. Weidman P, Maxwell MH, Lupu AN et al.: Plasma renin activity and blood pressure in terminal renal failure. *N Engl J Med* 285: 757, 1971

36. Van Stone JC, Bauer J, Carey J: The effect of dialysate sodium concentration on body fluid distribution during hemodialysis. *Trans Am Soc Artif Intern Organs* 26: 383, 1980

37. Bosl R, Shideman JR, Meyer RM et al.: Effects and complications of high efficiency dialysis. *Nephron* 15: 151, 1975

38. Levine J, Falk B, Henriquez M et al.: Effects of varying dialysate sodium using large surface area dialyzers. *Trans Am Soc Artif Intern Organs* 24: 139, 1978

39. Wilkinson R, Barber SG, Robson V: Cramps, Thirst and hypertension in hemodialysis patients – the influence of dialysate sodium concentration. *Clin Nephrol* 7: 101, 1977

40. Stewart WK, Fleming LV, Manuel MA: Benefits obtained by the use of high sodium dialysate during maintenance hemodialysis. *Proc Eur Dial Tranplant Assoc* 9: 111, 1972

41. Locatelli F, Pedrini L, Ponti R et al.: Physiological and pharmacological dialysate sodium concentrations. *Int J Artif Organs* 5: 17, 1982

42. Locatelli F, Di Filippo S, Ponti R et al.: Changes in dialysate composition related to new dialysis techniques. *Contrib Nephrol* 77: 106, 1990

43. Funck-Brentano JL, Man NK: Optimization of Na content in dialysis fluid. *Nephron* 36: 197, 1984

44. Port FK, Johnson WJ, Klass DW: Prevention of dialysis disequilibrium syndrome by use of high sodium concentration in the dialysate. *Kidney Int* 3: 327, 1973

45. Ogden DA: A double blind cross-over comparison of high and low sodium dialysis. *Proc Clin Dial Transplant Forum* 8: 157, 1978

46. Van Stone JC, Cook J: Decreased post-dialysis fatigue with increased dialysate sodium concentration. *Proc Clin Dial Transplant Forum* 8: 152, 1978

47. Locatelli F, Pedrini L, Ponti R et al.: Long-term hemodialysis treatment with sodium removal by convection. *Proc Eur Dial Tranplant Assoc* 18: 146, 1981

48. Kjellstrand CM, Evans RL, Petersen RJ et al.: The 'unphysiology' of dialysis: a major cause of side effects? *Kidney Int* 2: 5, 1975

49. Locatelli F, Costanzo R, Di Filippo S: High sodium dialysate (letter). *Int J Artif Organs* 2: 171, 1979

50. Ronco C: Backfiltration: a controversial issue in clinical dialysis. *Int J Artif Organs* 2: 69, 1988

51. Robson R, Oren A, Ravid M: Dialysate sodium concentration, hypertension and pulmonary oedema in hemodialysis patients. *Dial Transplant* 7: 678, 1978

52. Sellars L, Robson B, Wilkinson R: Sodium retention and hypertension with short dialysis. *Br Med J* 1: 520, 1979

53. Locatelli F, Costanzo R, Di Filippo S et al.: Controlled sequential ultrafiltration-dialysis, iso-osmotic dialysis, iso-natric dialysis: pathophysiological and clinical evaluations. *Dial Transplant* 8: 622, 1979

54. Daugirdas JT, Al-Kudsir R, Ing TS, Norusis MJ: A double blind evaluation of sodium gradient hemodialysis. *Am J Nephrol* 5: 163, 1985

55. Dumler F, Grondin G, Levin NW: Sequential high/low sodium hemodialysis: an alternative to ultrafiltration. *Trans Am Soc Artif Intern Organs* 25: 351, 1979

56. Petitclerc T, Hamani A, Jacobs C: Optimization of sodium balance during hemodialysis by routine implementation of kinetic modeling. *Blood Purif* 10: 309, 1992

57. Keshaviah P, Luehmann D, Ilstrup K, Collins A: Technical requirements for rapid high efficiency therapies. *Artif Organs* 10: 189, 1986

58. Ronco C, Brendolan A, Bragantini L et al.: Technical and clinical evaluation of four different shor dialysis techniques. *Contrib Nephrol* 61: 46, 1988

59. Leber HW, Wizemann V, Goubeaud G: Simultaneous hemofiltration/hemodialysis: an effective alternative to hemofiltration and conventional hemodialysis in the treatment of uremic patients. *Clin Nephrol* 9: 115, 1978

60. Cambi V, Buzzio C, Arisi L et al.: Vascular stability and middle-molecule removal in hypertonic hemodiafiltration. *Artif Organs* 5: 59, 1981

61. von Albertini B, Miller JH, Gardner PV, Shinaberger JH: High flux hemodiafiltration: under six hours/week treatment. *Trans Am Soc Artif Intern Organs* 30: 227, 1984

62. Wizemann V, Kramer W, Knopp G et al.: Ultrashort hemodiafiltration: efficiency and hemodinamic tolerance. *Clin Nephrol* 19: 24, 1983

63. Pedrini LA, Ponti R, Faranna P et al.: sodium modeling in hemodiafiltration. *Kidney Int* 40: 525, 1991

64. Tannen RL: *Disorders of Potassium Balance. The Kidney*, Philadelphia, WB Saunders, 1991, p 805

65. Dalal S, Yu AW, Goupta DK et al.: L-lactate high-efficiency hemodialysis: Hemodynamics, blood gas

changes, potassium-phosphorus and symptons. *Kidney Int* 38: 896, 1990

66. Redaelli B, Sforzini S, Bonoldi L: Potassium removal as a factor limiting the correction of acidosis during hemodialysis. *Proc Eur Dial Tranplant Assoc* 19: 366, 1982
67. Redaelli B: Unpublished data. Personal communication
68. Wing AJ: Optimum calcium concentration of dialysis fluid for maintenance haemodialysis. *Br Med J* 4: 145, 1968
69. Freeman RM, Lawton RL: The hard-water syndrome. *Med Instrum* 8: 201, 1974
70. Drukker W: The hard water syndrome: a potential hazard during regular dialysis treatment. *Proc Eur Dial Transplant Assoc* 5: 284, 1968
71. Carney SL, Gillies AHG: Effect of an optimum dialysis fluid calcium concentration on calcium mass transfer during maintenance hemodialysis. *Clin Nephrol* 24: 28, 1985
72. Bone JM, Davison AM, Robson JS: Role of dialysate calcium concentration in osteoporosis in patients on haemodialysis. *Lancet* 1: 1047, 1972
73. Denney JD, Sherrard DJ, Nelp WB et al.: Total body calcium and long-term calcium balance in chronic renal disease. *J Lab Clin Med* 82: 226, 1973
74. Goldsmith RS, Furszyfer J, Johnson WJ, Beeler GW Jr, Taylor WF: Calcium flux during hemodialysis. *Nephron* 20: 132, 1978
75. Ritz E: Azotemic osteodystrophy – indications for intervention. *Prog Biochem Pharmacol* 17: 251, 1980
76. Johnson WJ: Persistent severe hypercalcemia during maintenance hemodialysis. *Ann Intern Med* 93: 272, 1980
77. Zawada ET Jr, Bennett EP, Stinson JB, Ramirez G: Serum calcium in blood pressure regulation during hemodialysis. *Arch Intern Med* 141: 657, 1981
78. Kuzela DC, Huffer WE, Conger JD, Winter SD, Hammond WS: Soft tissue calcification in chronic dialysis patients. *Am J Pathol* 86: 403, 1977
79. Malberti F, Surian M, Marchini M, Minetti L: Bilancio del calcio e variazioni intradialitiche della calcemia in emodiafiltrazione a camere separate (PFD) in relazione al contenuto di calcio nel dialisato e nel reinfusato. Effetto sulla funzione paratiroidea di 6 mesi di trattamento. *Giorn It Nefrol* 6: 249, 1989
80. Memoli B, Gazzotti RM, Dello Russo A, Libetta C, Andreucci VE: Bicarbonate and calcium kinetics in post-dilutional hemodiafiltration. *Nephron* 58: 1974, 1991
81. Malberti F, Surian M: Ionized calcium changes and parathyroid hormone secretion in hemodiafiltration in relation to substitution fluid calcium content. *Nephrol Dial Transplant* 6: 104, 1991
82. Zawada ET, Simmons J, Sica D: The importance of divalent ions to blood pressure regulation during hemodialysis. *Int J Artif Organs* 7: 245, 1984
83. Henrich WL, Hunt JM, Nixon JV: Increased ionized calcium and left ventricular contractility during hemodialysis. *N Engl J Med* 310: 19, 1984
84. Haddy FJ, Scott JB, Emerson TE, Overbeck HW, Daugherty RM: Effect of generalized changes in plasma electrolyte concentration and osmolarity on blood pressure in the anesthetized dog. *Circ Res* 24 (Suppl I): 59, 1969
85. Blachley JD, Blankenhip DM, Menter A, ParKer TF, Knochel JP: Uremie pruritus: skin divalent ion content and response to ultraviolet phototheraopy. *Am J Kidney Dis* 5: 237, 1985

86. Winney RJ, Bone JM, Anderson TJ, Robson JS: Treatment of renal osteodystrophy with 1 alpha-hydroxycholecalciferol (1 alpha-OH-D) in conjunction with a high dialysate calcium. *Calcif Tissue Res* 22 (Suppl): 94, 1977
87. Goldsmith RS, Furszyfer J, Johnson WJ, Fournier AE, Sizemore GW, Arnaud CD: Etiology of hyperparathyroidism and bone disease during chronic hemodialysis III. Evaluation of parathyroid suppressibility. *J Clin Invest* 52: 173, 1973
88. Drueke T, Bordier Pj, Man NK, Jungers P, Marie P: Effects of high dialysate calcium concentration on bone remodelling serum biochemistry, and parathyroiid hormone in patients with renal osteodystrophy. *Kidney Int* 11: 267, 1977
89. Bouillon R, Verberckmoes R, de Moor P: Influence of dialysate calcium concentration and vitamin D on serum parathyroid hormone during repetitive dialysis. *Kidney Int* 7: 422, 1975
90. Cundy T, Kanis Ja, Earnshaw M, Woods CG: Comparative effects of alphacalcidol and parathyroidectomy with vitamin D in hyperparathyroid renal bone disease. *Q J Med* 60: 659, 1986
91. Kwan JTC, Almond MK, Beer JC, Nooan K, Evans SJW, Cunningham J: Pulse oral calcitriol in uraemic patients: rapid modification of parathyroid response to calcium. *Nephrol Dial Transplant* 36: 829, 1992
92. Sawyer N, Noonan K, Altmann P, Marsh F, Cunningham J: High dose calcium carbonate with stepwise reduction in dialysate calcium concentration: effective phosphate control and aluminum avoidance in hemodialysis patients. Nephrol *Dial Tranplant* 4: 105, 1989
93. Malberti F, Surian M, Montoli A et al.: Effect of dialysate calcium concentration changes on plasma calcium and PTH in dialysis patients treated with calcium carbonate as a phosphate binder. in *Current Therapy in Nephrology*, edited by Andreucci VE, Dal Canton A, Boston, Kluwer Academic Publishers, 1989, p 401
94. Malberti F, Montoli A, Surian M: Long term effect of low calcium dialysate on parathyroid activity in dialysis patients treated with calcium carbonate as a phosphate binder. *Nephrol Dial Transplant* 4: 165, 1989
95. Massry SG: The clinical pathophysiology of magnesium. *Contrib Nephrol* 14: 64, 1978
96. Schmidt P, Kotzaurek R, Zazgornik J, Hysek H: Magnesium metabolism in patients on regular dialysis treatment. *Clin Sci* 41: 131, 1971
97. Brautbar N, Kleeman CR: Disordered divalent ion metabolism in kidney disease: comments on pathogenesis and treatment. *Adv Nephrol* 8: 179, 1979
98. Gonella M: Plasma and tissue levels of magnesium in chronically hemodialyzed patients: effects of dialysate magnesium levels. *Nephron* 34: 141, 1983
99. Heidland A, Wetzels E: Discussion: magnesium metabolism. *Contrib Nephrol* 38: 203, 1984
100. Brunner FP, Thiel G: The use of magnesium-containing phosphate binders in patiens with end-stage renal disease on maintenance haemodialysis (letter). *Nephron* 32: 266, 1982
101. Brewer J, Monitz C, Baldwin D, Parsons V: The effect of zero magnesium dialysate and magnesium supplements on ionized calcium concentration in patients on regular dialysis treatment. *Nephrol Dial Transplant* 2: 347, 1987

102. O'Donovan R, Monitz C, Baldwin D et al.: Control of hyper-phosphatemia by oral magnesium carbonate on zero magnesium dialysate without aluminum binders. *Eur Dial Transplant Nurse Assoc Eur Renal Care Assoc* 22: 1229, 1985

103. Drueke T: Does Mg excess play a role in renal osteodystrophy. *Contrib Nephrol* 38: 195, 1984

104. Massry SG: Magnesium homeostasis in patients with renal failure. *Contrib Nephron* 38: 175, 1984

105. Mandelbaum JM, Heistand ML, Schardin KE: Six months' experience with PD-2 solution. *Dial Transplant* 12: 259, 1983

106. Johnny KV, Lawrence Jr, O'Halloran MW, Weilby ML: Effect of haemodialysis on erythrocyte and plasma potassium, magnesium sodium and calcium. *Nephron* 8: 81, 1971

107. Stewart WK, Fleming LW: The effect of dialysate magnesium on plasma and erythrocyte magnesium and potassium concentration during maintenance haemodialysis. *Nephron* 10: 22, 1973

108. Fleming LW, Lenmman JAR, Stewart WK: Effect of magnesium om nerve conduction velocity during regular dialysis treatment. *J Neurol Neurosurg Psychiatry* 35: 342, 1972

109. Graf H, Kovarik J, Stummvoll HK, Wolf A: Disappearance of uraemic pruritus after lowering dialysate magnesium concentration. *Br Med J* 2: 1478, 1979

110. Burnell JM, Teubner E: Effects of decreasing dialysate magnesium in patients with chronic renal failure. *Proc Clin Dial Transplant Forum* 5: 191, 1976

111. Catto GRD, Reid IW, MacLeod M: The effect of low magnesium dialysate on plasma, ultrafiltrable erytrocyte and bone magnesium concentrationa from patients on maintmenace haemodialysis. *Nephron* 13: 372, 1974

112. Alfrey AC, Miller NL: Bone magnesium pools in uraemia. *J Clin Invest* 52: 3019, 1973

113. Posner AS, Betts F, Blumenthal NC: Role of ATP and Mg in the stabilization of biological and synthetic amorphous calcium phosphates. *Calcif Tissue Res* 22 (Suppl): 208, 1977

114. Meema HE, Oreopoulos DG, Rapoport A: Serum magnesium level and arterial calcification in end-stage renal disease. *Kidney Int* 32: 388, 1987

115. Terasaki M, Rubin H: Evidence that intracellular magnesium is present in cells at a regulatory concentration for protein synthesis. *Proc Nat Acad Sci USA* 82: 7324, 1985

116. Kenny MA, Casillas E, Ahmad S: Magnesium, calcium and PTH relationships in dialysis patients after magnesium repletion. *Nephron* 46: 199, 1987

117. Gotch FA, Sargent JA, Keen ML: Hydrogen ion balance in dialysis therapy. *Artif Organs* 6: 388, 1982

118. Kolff WJ: Le rein artificiel: un dialyseur à grande surface. *Presse Medicale* 52: 103, 1944

119. Scribner BH, Caner JEZ, Buri R: The technique of continuous hemodialysis. *Trans Am Soc Artif Intern Organs* 6: 88, 1960

120. Kirkendol PL, Devia CJ, Bower JD, Holbert RD: A comparison of the cardiovascular effects of sodium acetate, sodium bicarbonate and other potential sources of fixed base in hemodialysate solutions. *Trans Am Soc Artif Intern Organs* 23: 399, 1977

121. Wathen RL, Ward RA, Harding GB, Meyer LC: Acid-base and metabolic responses to anion infusion in the anesthetized dog. *Kidney Int* 21: 592, 1982

122. Mudge GH, Manning JA, Gilman A: Sodium acetate as a source of fixed base. *Proc Soc Exp Biol Med* 71: 136, 1949

123. Lundquist F: Production and utilization of free acetate in man. *Nature* 193: 579, 1962

124. Harper PV, Neal WB, Hlavacek GR: Acetate utilization in dog. *Metabolism* 2: 62, 1953

125. Tolchin N, Roberts JL, Hayashi J, Lewis EJ: Metabolic consequences of high mass-transfer hemodialysis. *Kidney Int* 11: 366, 1977

126. Davidson WD, Morin RJ, Srikantaiah M, Basset L: The role of acetate in dialysate for hemodialysis. in *11th Annual Contractor's Conf Artif Kidney Program Natl Institute Arthritis, Metabol Digest Dis*, Washington D.C., Department of Health, Education, and Welfare, 1978, p 75

127. Morin RJ, Guo LSS, Rorke SJ, Davidson WD: Lipid metabolism in non-uremic dogs during and after hemodialysis with acetate. *J Dial* 2: 113, 1978

128. Skutches CL, Singler MH, Teehan BP, Cooper JH, Reichard GA: Contribution of dialysate acetate to energy metabolism: Metabolic implications. *Kidney Int* 23: 57, 1983

129. Wathen RL, Ward RA: Disturbances in fluid, electrolyte, and acid base in the dialysis patient. in *Textbook of Nephrology, Vol 2, 1st Ed*, edited by Massry SG, Glassok RJ, Baltimore, Williams & Wilkins 1983, p 798

130. Karlsson N, Fellenius E, Kiessling KH: Influence of acetate on the metabolism of palmitate in the perfused hindquarter of the rat. *Acta Physiol Scand* 99: 156, 1977

131. Wathen RL, Keshaviah P, Hommeyer P, Cadwell K, Comty CM: The metabolic effects of hemodialysis with and without glucose in the dialysate. *Am J Clin Nutr* 31: 1870, 1978

132. Vreman HJ, Assomull VM, Kaiser BA, Blaschke TF, Weiner MW: Acetate metabolism and acid-base homeostasis during hemodialysis: Influence of dialyzer efficiency and rate of acetate metabolism. *Kidney Int* 18 (Suppl 10): S62, 1980

133. Yamakawa M, Yamamoto T, Kishimoto T et al.: Serum levels of acetate and TCA cycle intermediates during hemodialysis in relation to symptoms. *Nephron* 32: 155, 1982

134. Oh MS, Uribarri J, Del Monte ML, Friedman EA, Carroll HJ: Consumption of CO2 in metabolism of acetate as an explanation for hypoventilation and hypoxemia during hemodialysis. *Proc Clin Dial Transplant Forum* 9: 226, 1979

135. Gibbson BH, Edsall JT: Rate of hydration of carbon dioxide and dehydration at 25°C. *J Biol Chem* 238: 3501, 1963

136. Gray BA: The rate of approach to equilibrium in uncatalyzed CO₂ hydration reactions: The teoretical effect of buffering capacity. *Respir Physiol* 11: 223, 1971

137. Maren TH: Carbonic anhydrase: chemistry, physiology and inhibition. *Physiol Rev* 47: 595, 1967

138. Blandt LA, Ridgeway MR, Aguero SM, Carson LA, Favero MS: Potential bacteriologic and endotoxin hazard associated with liquid bicarbonate concentrate. *Trans Am Soc Artif Intern Organs* 33: 542, 1987

139. Ebben JP, Hirsch DN, Luehmann DA, Collins AJ, Keshaviah PR. Microbiological contamination of liquid bicarbonate concentrate for hemodialysis. *Trans Am Soc Artif Intern Organs* 33: 269, 1987

140. Mion C, Canaud B, Francesqui MP et al.: Bicarbonate concentrate: A hidden source of microbial contamination of dialysis fluid. *Blood Purif* 5 (Abstract): 299, 1987

141. Delin K, Attman PO, Dahlberg M, Aurell M: A clinical test of a new device for on-line preparation of dialysis fluid from bicarbonate powder: The Gambro BiCart. *Dial Transplant* 17: 468, 1988

142. Ledebo I: *Acetate vs Bicarbonate in Everyday Dialysis*, Gambro AB Lund, Sweden, 1990, p 128

143. Feriani M, Bragantini L, Milan M, Ronco C, La Greca G: Optimization of base balance in diffusive-convective treatments. in *Issues in Nephron Science*, edited by D'Amico G, Colasanti G, Milan, Wichtig Editore, 1991, p 12

144. Zucchelli P, Santoro A: Correction of acid-base balance by dialysis. *Kidney Int* 43 (Suppl 41): S179, 1993

145. Sargent JA, Gotch FA: Bicarbonate and carbon dioxide transport during hemodialysis. *asaio J* 2: 61, 1979

146. Kveim M, Nesbakken R: Utilization of exogenous acetate during hemodialysis. *Trans Am Soc Artif Intern Organs* 21: 138, 1975

147. Ward RA, Wathen RL, Williams TE: Effects of long-term bicarbonate hemodialysis [BHD] on acid-base status. *Trans Am Soc Artif Intern Organs* 28: 295, 1982

148. Metha BR, Fischer D, Ahmad M, Dubose TD Jr: Effects of acetate and bicarbonate hemodialysis on cardiac function in chronic dialysis patients. *Kidney Int* 24: 782, 1983

149. Hakim RM, Pontzer MA, Tilton D, Lazarus JM, Gottlieb MN: Effects of acetate and bicarbonate dialysis in stable chronic dialysis patients. *Kidney Int* 28: 535, 1985

150. Henrich WL, Woodard TD, Meyer BD, Chappell TR, Rubin LJ: High sodium bicarbonate and acetate hemodialysis: Double-blind crossover comparison of hemodynamic and ventilatory effects. *Kidney Int* 24: 240, 1983

151. Graefe U, Milutinovich J, Follette WC, Vizzo JE, Babb AL, Scribner BH: Less dialysis-induced morbidity and vascular instability with bicarbonate dialysate. *Ann Int Med* 88: 332, 1978

152. La Greca G, Feriani M, Bragantini L, Petrosino L, Santoro A, Altieri P: Effects of acetate and bicarbonate dialysate on vascular stability: a prospective multicentric study. *Int J Artif Organs* 10: 15, 1987

153. Ramirez G, Bercaw BL, Butcher DE, Mathis HL, Brueggemeyer C, Newton JL: The role of glucose in hemodialysis: the effects of glucose free dialysate. *Am J Kidney Dis* 7: 413, 1986

154. Wathen R, Keshaviah P, Hommeyer P, Caldwell K, Comty C. Role of dialysate glucose in preventing gluconeogenesis during hemodialysis. *Trans Am Soc Artif Intern Organs* 23: 393, 1977

155. Ward RA, Wathen R, Williams TE, Harding GB: Hemodialysate composition and intradialytic metabolic, acid-base and potassium changes. *Kidney Int* 32: 129, 1987

156. Ward RA, Shirlow MJ, Hayes JM, Chapman GV, Farrell PC: Protein catabolism during hemodialysis. *Am J Clin Nutr* 32: 2443, 1979

157. Ramirez G, Butcher DE, Morrison AD: Glucose concentration in the dialysate and lipid abnormalities in chronic hemodialysis patients. *Int J Artif Organs* 10: 31, 1987

158. Swamy AP, Cestero RVM, Campbell RG, Freeman RB: Long term effect of dialysate glucose on the lipid levels of maintenance hemodialysis patients. *Trans Am Soc Artif Intern Organs* 22: 54, 1976

159. La Greca G, Fabris A, Feriani M, Chiaramonte S, Ronco C: Acid base homeostasis in clinical dialysis. in *Replacement of Renal Function by Dialysis*, 3rd ed, edited by Maher JF, Dordrecht, Kluwer Academic Publishers, 1989, p 808

160. Bommer J, Ritz E: Water quality: a neglected problem in hemodialysis. *Nephron* 46: 1, 1987

161. Keshaviah P, Luehmann D, Ilstrup K, Collins A: Technical requirements for rapid high efficiency therapies. *Artif Organs* 3: 189, 1987

162. Raij L, Shapiro FL, Michael F: Endotoxemia in febrile reactions during hemodialysis. *Kidney Int* 4: 57, 1973

163. Graf H, Watzke H, Stanek H.P, Schwarz I, Mayer G: Bacterial contamination of dialysate in dialysis-associated endotoxemia. *Blood Purif* 5: 284, 1987

164. Keshaviah PR. Pretreatment and preparation of city water for hemodialysis. in *Replacement of Renal Function by Dialysis*, 3rd ed, edited by Maher JF, Dordrecht, Kluwer Academic Publishers, 1989, p 188

165. Canaud B, Peyronnet P, Annynot AM, Nguyen QV, Attisso M, Mion C: Ultrapure water: a need for future dialysis. *Eur Dial Transplant Assoc* (Abstract): A: 115, 1986

166. Keshaviah P, Luehman F, Shapiro F, Compty C: Investigation of the risks and hazards associated with hemodialysis system. (Technical Report Contract 223-78-5046) Silver Spring MD, US Dep. of Health and Human Service, Food and Drug Administration, Bureau of Medical Devices, 1980

167. Kjellestrand CM, Eaton JW, Yawata Y et al.: Hemolysis in dialysed patients caused by chloramines. *Nephron* 13: 427, 1974

168. Manzler AD, Schreiner AW: Copper induced acute hemolytic anemia. *Ann Intern Med* 73: 409, 1970

169. Webster JD, Parker TF, Alfrey AC et al.: Acute nickel intoxication by dialysis. *Ann Intern Med* 92: 631, 1980

170. Gallery EDM, Blomfield J, Dixon SR: Acute zinc toxicity in hemodialysis. *Br Med J* 4: 331, 1972

171. Scanziani R.: La qualità delle acque nel trattamento dialitico. *Dialisi Oggi* 25: 37, 1989

172. Ward MK, Feets TG, Ellis HA et al.: Osteomalacic dialysis osteodistrophy: evidence for a water born aetiological agent, probably aaluminum. *Lancet* 1: 84, 1978

173. Alfrey AC, Le Gendre GR, Kaehny WD: The dialysis encephalopathy syndrome. Possible aluminum intoxication. *N Engl J Med* 294: 184, 1976

174. Johnson WJ, Taves DR: Exposure to excessive fluoride during hemodialysis. *Kidney Int* 5: 451, 1974

175. McIvor M, Baltazar RF, Beltram J et al.: Hyperkalemia and cardiac arrest from fluoride exposure during hemodialysis. *Am J Cardiol* 51: 901, 1983

176. Kjellstrand CM: Toxicity of material and medications used in dialysis. *Trans Am Soc Artif Intern Organs* 24: 764, 1978

177. Mion C, Canaud B, Francesqui MP et al.: Bicarbonate (HCO₃) Concentrate (CONC). A hidden source of micro-

276   *Claudio Ronco, Aldo Fabris and Mariano Feriani*

bial contamination of dialysis fluid. *Blood Purif* 5: 299, 1987

178. Ebben JP, Hirsch DN, Luehmann DA, Collins AJ, Keshaviah PR: Microbiological contamination of Liquid Bicarbonate Concentrate (LBC) for hemodialysis (HD). *Trans Am Soc Artif Intern Organs* 33: 269, 1987

179. Man NK, Ciancioni C, Guyomard S, Blais D, Delous S, Funk Brentano JL: Risks and hazards of contaminated dialysate associated with high flux membrane. *Prev Nephrol* 227, 1987

180. Port FK, VanDeKerkhove KM, Kunkel SL, Kluger MH: The role of dialysate in the stimulation of interleukin-1 production during clinical hemodialysis. *Am J Kidney Dis* 10: 118, 1987

181. Dinarello CA, Kreuger JM: Induction of interleukin-1 by synthetic and naturally occuris muramyl peptides. *Fed Proc* 45: 2534, 1986

182. Ronco C: Backfiltration in clinical dialysis: nature of the phenomenon and possible solutions. *Int J Artif Organs* 13: 11, 1990

183. Petersen NJ, Boyer KM, Carson LA, Favero MS: Pyrogenic reactions from inadequate disinfection of a dialysis fluid distribution system. *Dial Transplant* 7: 56, 1978

184. Port FK, Bernick JJ: Pyrogen and endotoxin reactions during hemodialysis. *Contrib Nephrol* 36: 100, 1983

185. Bernick JJ, Port FK, Favero MS, Brown DG: Bacterial and endotoxin permeability of hemodialysis membranes. *Kidney Int* 16: 491, 1979

186. Colton CK: Analysis of membrane processes for blood purification. *Blood Purif* 5: 202, 1987

187. Berkes SL, Kahn SI, Chazan JA, Garella S: Prolonged hemolysis from overheated dialysate. *Ann Intern Med* 83: 363, 1975

188. Fortner RW, Nowakowski A, Carter CB, King LH, Knepshield GH: Death due overheated dialysate during dialysis. *Ann Intern Med* 73: 443, 1970

189. Maggiore Q, Pizzarelli F, Sisca S, Catalano C, Delfino D: Vascular stability and heat in dialysis patients. *Contrib Nephrol* 41: 398, 1984

190. Lindholm T, Thysell H, Yamamoto Y, Forresberg B, Gullberg CA: Temperature and vascular stability in hemodial-ysis. *Nephron* 39: 130, 1985

191. Marcen R, Quereda C, Lamas S et al.: Hypoxemia and dialysate temperature. *Nephron* 45: 74, 1987

192. Van Kuijk W, Luik A, van Hooff J, de Leeuw P, Leunissen K: Are both the vascular and sympathetic response improved by lowering the dialysate temperature? *Am Soc Nephrol* 4 (Abstract): 393, 1993

193. Acchiardo SR, Kang E, Burk L, Smith SJ, Cardoso S: Effect of hyperthermic dialysis upon autonomic nervous system and plasma lypoprotein lipase activity in patients with ESRD. *Am Soc Nephrol* 4 (Abstract): 329, 1993

194. Kaufman AM, Steil H, Morris AT, Polaschegg HD, Levin NW: Clinical application of on-line effective dialyzer clearance measurement. *Am Soc Nephrol* 4 (Abstract): 358, 1993

195. Hootkins R, Husni L: Comparison of current access recirculation methods vis-à-vis the thermodilution technique. *Am Soc Nephrol* 4 (Abstract): 355, 1993

196. Von Hartitzsch B, Hoenich NA, Johnson J, Brewis RAL, Kerr DNS: The problem of de-aeration: cause, consequence, cure. Proc *Eur Dial Transplant Assoc* 9: 605, 1972

197. Drukker W, van de Werff B, Meinsma K: De-aeration of dialysis fluid. *Dial Transplant* 33: 3, 1974

198. Ronco C, Feriani M, Chiaramonte S et al.: Impact of high blood flows on vascular stability in hemodialysis. *Nephrol Dial Transplant* (Suppl 1): 109, 1990

199. Ronco C, Brendolan A, Feriani M et al.: A new scintigraphic method to characterize ultrafiltration in hollow fiber dialyzers. *Kidney Int* 41: 1383, 1992

200. Ronco C: Hemofiltration and hemodiafiltration. in *Hemodialysis: High Efficiency Treatments*, edited by Bosch JP, New York, Churchill Livingstone, 1993, p 119

201. Canaud B, Nguyen QV, Kaaki M, Stec F, Mion C: Bicarbonate hemodiafiltration with in line production of substitution fluid: short dialysis of high efficiency in uncompliant patients and the elderly. *Blood Purif* 6: 348, 1988

202. Ronco C, Brendolan A, Crepaldi C, La Greca G: Accuracy of nutritional assessment and dialysis delivery by on-line urea monitoring. *Am Soc Nephrol* 4 (Abstract): 378, 1993

HEMODIALYSIS ACCESS
PART A – TEMPORARY

ROBERT ULDALL

INTRODUCTION

Since hemodialysis was first practiced clinically as a substitute for absent renal function, access to the circulation has always been a demanding and, at times, frustrating exercise. In the beginning hemodialysis was only performed for relatively short periods for acute reversible renal failure in young people with good blood vessels. Almost any method of access was adequate for this purpose. Shaldon's semi-stiff tapered catheter with a single cylindrical lumen inserted over a guide-wire by the Seldinger technique into the femoral vein provided one blood flow pathway for removal or return of blood (1). A second conduit could be provided by means of a second catheter in the same or a different vein and these catheters could be left in place for two or three treatments. Evidence for the crucial importance and desirability of this technique is apparent in the fact that it remains widely practiced today when no safe alternative can be found. Because of its superficial position, just medial to the femoral artery in the groin, the femoral vein is easy to cannulate, even by inexperienced operators. The relatively low incidence of serious or fatal complications from femoral cannulation compared to those from cannulating the subclavian and jugular veins, in which there may be injury to the heart and lungs, explains why femoral cannulation has and probably always will remain widely used.

The development by Quinton, Dillard and Scribner of the silastic-teflon shunt allowed dialysis to be performed repeatedly from the same access site, not only for 2–3 weeks for an episode of acute reversible renal failure, but also for several months or years in patients with end-stage renal failure, thus opening up the possibility for long-term maintenance dialysis (2). Although the silastic-teflon shunt, now largely of historical interest, has been rightly replaced by arteriovenous fistulae and grafts for long-term dialysis (3, 4), their use can still be justified for episodes of acute reversible renal failure (even though they destroy a pair of peripheral blood vessels) as long as it can be confidently predicted that long-term dialysis will not be required. Shunts can be placed in the leg in order to preserve vessels at the wrist for fistula formation (5), but for obvious reasons this operation can only be done twice (providing two separate periods of temporary vascular access). Occasionally a patient with a silastic-teflon shunt placed at the wrist, for what is presumed to be reversible acute renal failure, may turn out to have end-stage renal damage, and hence may require long-term hemodialysis. In such a case it may be possible to convert the shunt into an arteriovenous fistula and so preserve the precious forearm vessels (6).

Moreover there are now easier and less damaging ways to provide vascular access for two or three weeks and this explains why most centres have not used silastic-teflon shunts for many years. Some might still wish to justify their use for the performance of continuous arteriovenous hemofiltration (CAVH) for complicated oliguric acute renal failure (7) as an alternative to femoral arterial and venous catheters (8). Femoral artery cannulation is sometimes difficult in arteriopathic individuals, and is also not without risk, but most centres are moving to pump-assisted methods of slow continuous blood purification which only require venous access (9). Thus the days of silastic-teflon shunts are numbered, if not over, and their surgical insertion is a dying art. Numerous texts are available for those who wish to continue to use them. They will not therefore be discussed further except to acknowledge their rightful place in medical history as a brilliant innovation in the evolution of access for both temporary and long-term dialysis.

Cannulation of the subclavian vein for repeated hemodialysis, first reported by Erben et al. (10) and popularized by Uldall et al. (11) and DeCubber et al. (12), owes its wide acceptance to the ease of the technique for doctors and nurses and the great convenience for patients who can remain mobile and go home. The global love affair with subclavian cannulation soon became tempered by reports of fatal traumatic complications (13–16), and later on by the realization, especially since the advent of double-lumen catheters, that subclavian cannulation, even in skilled hands, is associated with an unacceptably high incidence of subclavian vein damage in the form of thrombosis and stenosis which, by interfering with the proximal venous drainage of the upper limb, leads to intolerable swelling of the arm in the presence of an ipsilateral arteriovenous fistula (17–23). By contrast, jugular vein cannulation for temporary vascular access, does not damage the proximal venous drainage of the arm (24). The main message of this chapter is that although subclavian vein cannulation for hemodialysis may still be justified, like the silastic-teflon shunt, for predictably reversible acute renal failure, it cannot any longer be justified in patients with end-stage renal failure, any or all of whom may at some stage require a prolonged period of hemodialysis and hence need intact proximal venous drainage on the side of an arteriovenous fistula or graft. Good and reliable technology is now available for repeated short-term or long-term cannulation of the jugular veins for hemodialysis. The method is so inherently safe that traumatic complications can be largely avoided and, because the subclavian veins will never be cannulated, they will not become thrombosed or stenosed.

Temporary vascular access now depends almost exclusively on central venous cannulation of the femoral, subclavian and jugular veins. Although subclavian cannulation is still the most widely practiced I believe that very soon it will properly be restricted to patients with acute reversible renal failure. Each of these methods will be discussed; and on the principle that first and above all we should do no harm, emphasis will be on the avoidance of complications (25).

Temporary vascular access for extracorporeal blood purification is needed for three main indications:

— Acute reversible renal failure.
— The management of severe poisoning
— End-stage renal failure.

ACUTE REVERSIBLE RENAL FAILURE

In many patients with acute renal failure one can predict fairly confidently that dialysis will only be required for

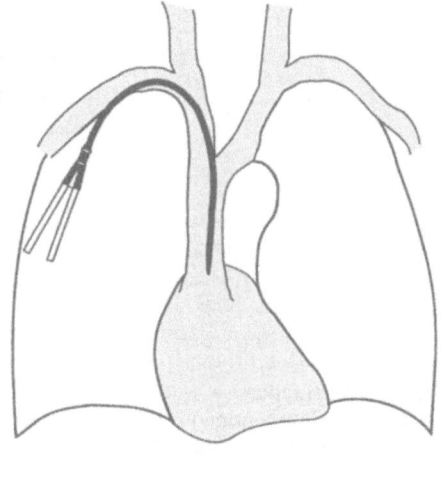

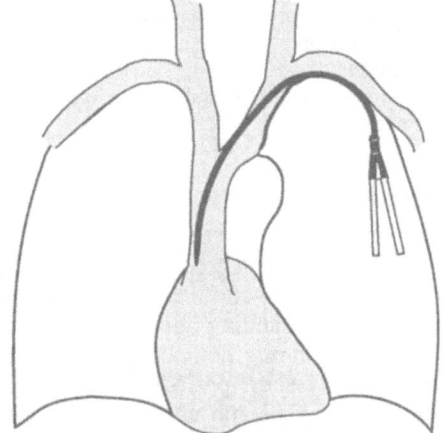

Figure 1.   (a) The correct position for a subclavian catheter introduced from the right side. (b) The correct position for a subclavian catheter introduced from the left side. In many patients this catheter would have to be 24 cm in length from the tip to the hub.

about 2 weeks. Once recovery of renal function occurs it is no more likely to be needed again in the future than it would be in any other previously healthy person.

If the patient is not fluid-overloaded and can lie flat without discomfort, insertion of a subclavian catheter which can be left in place throughout the period of treatment is easy and convenient (Figure 1). When no longer needed, the catheter is simply pulled out by the nurse and gentle pressure applied for a few minutes (26). If, on the other hand, the patient is in pulmonary edema and cannot lie flat, or has some other reason for respiratory distress, subclavian cannulation should not be attempted (25). An accidental pneumothorax, always a possibility even in skilled hands, is too great a risk. Femoral cannulation should be used to provide access for the first one or two treatments until the patient is stable enough for a subclavian catheter (Figure 2) One should never attempt

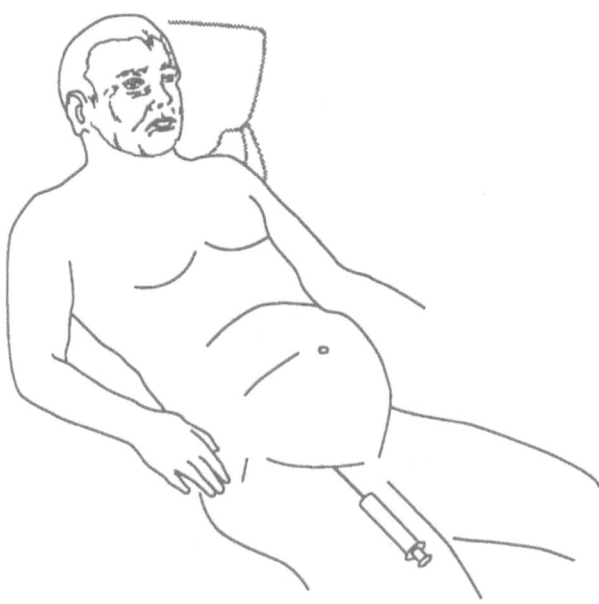

Figure 2. For a patient in pulmonary edema femoral cannulation can be performed safely with the patient with his back-rest elevated.

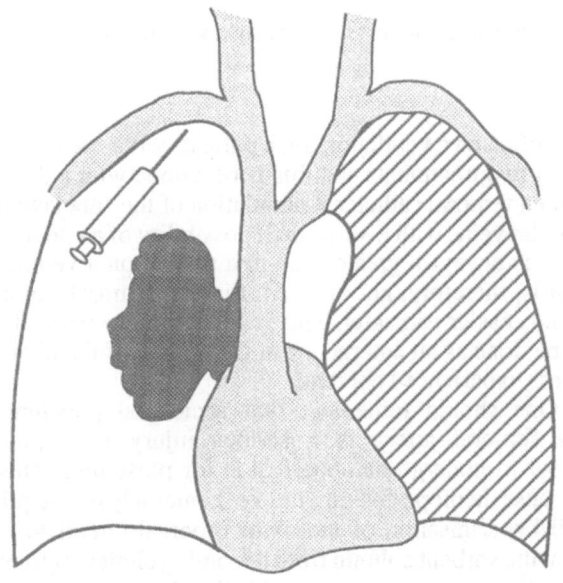

Figure 3. Subclavian cannulation on the right in the presence of a non-functioning lung on the left. A complete pneumothorax may result in death of the patient.

subclavian cannulation on the side of the only healthy lung (even in the absence of dyspnoea). A large pneumothorax on this side may result in death of the patient (27, 28) (Figure 3). The catheter should always be inserted on the opposite side.

VASCULAR ACCESS FOR SLOW CONTINUOUS BLOOD PURIFICATION

In those centres which still practice CAVH, rather than pump-assisted methods of veno-venous blood purification, the silastic-teflon shunt has largely been replaced by wide bore catheters in the femoral artery and vein (Figure 4). A silastic-teflon shunt is still a good method in young patients with good peripheral blood vessels. It is likely to last for the duration of the treatment and is less dangerous than a femoral artery catheter. The two best positions for a shunt are the radial artery and cephalic vein at the wrist and the posterior tibial artery and long saphenous vein at the ankle (Figure 5). One has to be wary of using the posterior tibial artery in elderly patients with peripheral arterial disease. This may lead to ischemia of the foot which may necessitate reconstituting the posterior tibial artery, a difficult exercise in a vessel which has been ligated.

Cannulation of the femoral vessels is quicker and easier but here the danger is to the femoral artery. All the following complications should be anticipated and prevented:

1. Exsanguination caused by the femoral catheter slipping out accidentally. Some method should be used to anchor the catheter so that this cannot happen. Suturing the catheter wings to the skin is fairly effective.
2. Infection at the arterial puncture site leading to mycotic aneurysm formation. At least one young man has had to have an amputation at the top of the thigh when an infected iatrogenic aneurysm could not be repaired (personal communication).
3. Difficulty in controlling the bleeding when the arterial catheter is removed. Remember that the longer the catheter is left in, the more organised will be the track through the arterial wall and the longer it will take to stop the bleeding. Probably no patient should be left with a catheter in the same artery for more than about 5 days. It is also important to remove both the arterial and venous catheters as soon as hemodialysis or hemofiltration is no longer needed. To leave the catheters in place after treatment is over and systemic heparinisation has been discontinued is to invite the risk of arterial or venous thrombosis (29).

It is worth remembering that vascular access problems are significantly more frequent with CAVH than with veno-venous methods which do not depend on arterial cannulation (30). There is now some evidence from controlled trials that pump-assisted systems produce better survival results (31).

DIALYSIS AND HEMOPERFUSION IN THE MANAGEMENT OF SEVERE POISONING

Most of the patients requiring extracorporeal therapy for poison removal will be lying flat in an intensive care unit

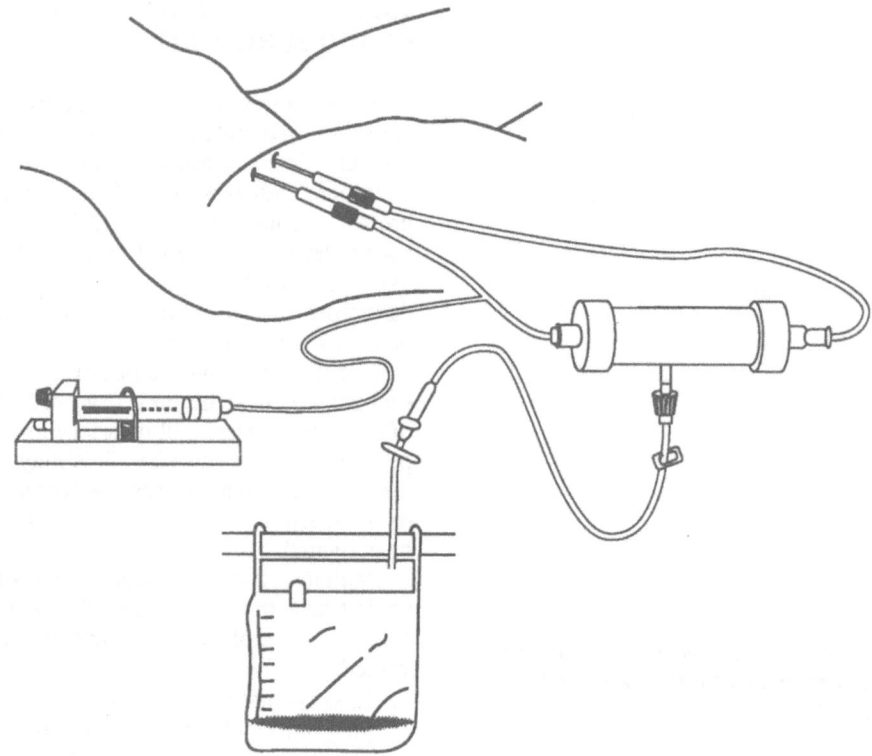

Figure 4. The method, first described by Kramer, using wide bore catheters in the femoral artery and vein to perfuse a high-flux filter for the performance of arteriovenous hemofiltration.

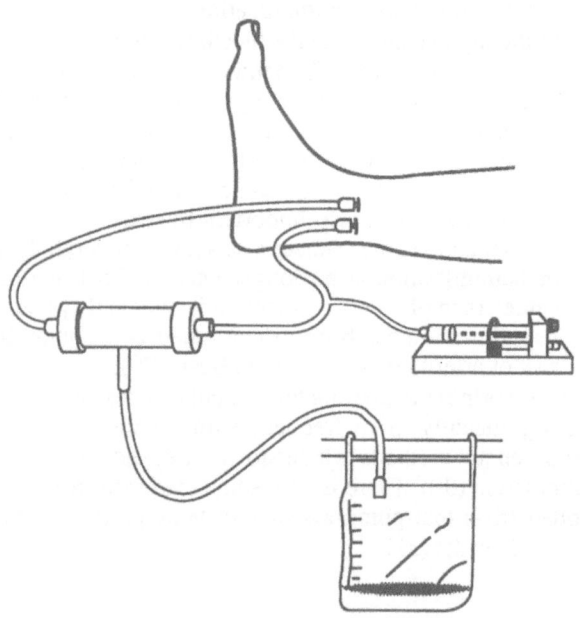

Figure 5. The method, popularised by Paganini et al. (6) for performing arteriovenous hemofiltration by means of a silastic-teflon shunt in the leg.

and often on a ventilator. Such patients will need one or at most two treatments and this is best done with a double-lumen femoral catheter. Cannulation of the subclavian or jugular veins with even a small possibility of a pneumothorax is always a greater risk in a patient on a ventilator, and is, therefore, not justified. Finally, femoral cannulation is easier and safer. This is an advantage when it has to be done as an emergency in the middle of the night by a less experienced operator.

One should remember that accidental puncture of the femoral artery is a serious injury in a patient about to undergo hemoperfusion for poisoning. This is because hemoperfusion, unlike hemodialysis, requires full heparinisation of the extracorporeal circuit to prevent the sorbent column from becoming clotted. Systemic heparin may cause serious bleeding in a patient with a recent femoral artery puncture.

TEMPORARY ACCESS IN PATIENTS WITH END-STAGE RENAL FAILURE

If everything went according to plan, all patients with ed-stage renal failure would have an arteriovenous fistula, using the radial artery and cephalic vein at the wrist, created well in advance of need (Figure 6). This remains

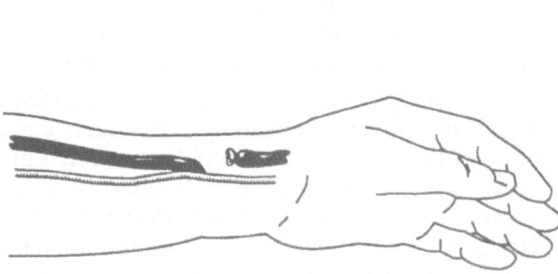

Figure 6. A good radial-cephalic fistula at the wrist, created well in advance of need, may be the only vascular access the patient will ever need.

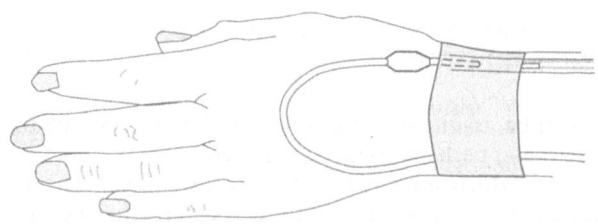

Figure 7. An intravenous infusion in the dorsal forearm vein may irreparably damage the vein, making it unfit for creation of an arteriovenous fistula.

the gold standard, more durable than any other form of vascular access, and in some fortunate patients it may be the only access they will ever need. Reality in most renal centres is sadly different, and vascular access problems remain the commonest reason for admission to hospital for most patients with end-stage renal failure (32). Although preservation of forearm vessels will be discussed in the sections on permanent vascular access, it is so important that it should be emphasised again here. Temporary vascular access in end-stage renal failure patients would never be necessary if they all had a functioning fistula. By far the most important and potentially preventable cause of failure to create a good fistula is the unnecessary destruction of dorsal forearm veins by inappropriately placed intravenous infusions (Figure 7). No renal failure patient who may ever need long-term hemodialysis should have an I-V infusion placed in a vein which might be used for creation of an A-V fistula. A plastic cannula placed in one of these veins even for a few hours may cause irreparable damage and render the vein unusable.

To some extent patients themselves should take responsibility for preserving their own veins. A bracelet on the non-dominant wrist reminding would-be intruders that the dorsal forearm vein is off limits is a strategy which seems worth pursuing (Figure 8). Ironically the growth of CAPD programs has made the situation worse, since, frequent-

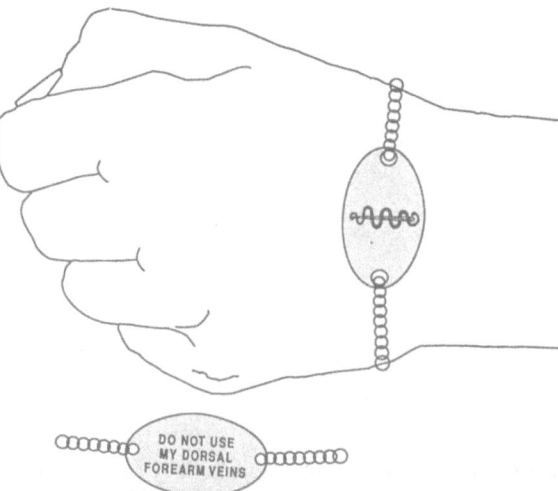

Figure 8. The patient is wearing a bracelet on the wrist of the non-dominant arm. The inside of the bracelet bears the message 'DO NOT USE MY DORSAL FOREARM VEINS'.

ly, these patients go straight to peritoneal dialysis without having a fistula made for future hemodialysis. If hemodialysis finally becomes necessary, all the forearm veins may have been destroyed during a series of hospital admissions. Attempts to give all CAPD patients a prophlylactic A-V fistula have met with only limited success and in at least one comparative study this practice was found to be of questionable value (33). Ultimately the answer may be to make the proscription of I-V infusions in dorsal forearm veins of all patients as basic and well known amongst all nurses in training as the correct position for an intramuscular injection in the buttock. In other words, the dorsal forearm veins will not be used for I-V infusion in anybody, except perhaps for those receiving terminal care in whom we know that dialysis will never be used. However, the acceptance of this principle would require a widespread agreement among all doctors and nurses, and realistically it is unlikely to happen in the near future. In the meantime, the placing of an I-V infusion in the dorsal forearm vein of a renal patient should be regarded as absolutely contraindicated. It is clear that the nephrology community is facing an educational challenge which has yet to be tackled with real determination.

FEMORAL VEIN CANNULATION

Femoral catheter insertion is the method of choice for most emergencies:

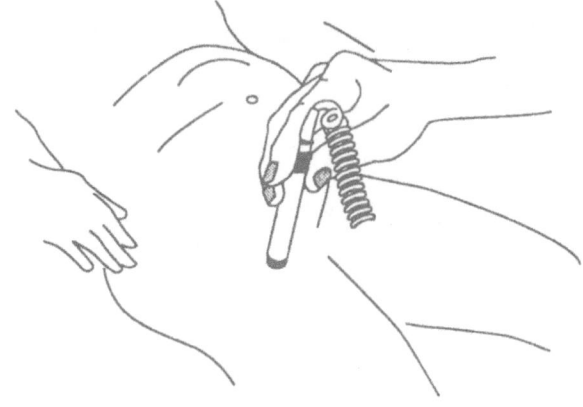

Figure 9. A hand-held audible doppler may assist in locating the position of the femoral artery when this is difficult to palpate.

1. It should be used in all patients with pulmonary edema who cannot lie flat, even if only for one or two treatments until the fluid overload is corrected.
2. It should be used in any patient in respiratory distress in whom an accidental pneumothorax, though unlikely, would be a serious event.
3. It should be used for all cases of dialysis or hemoperfusion for poisoning in which only one, or at most two, treatments will be required.

Special points of technique which may be helpful are:

1. In obese patients with a pendulous abdomen the abdominal adipose tissue which would otherwise fall down and cover the groin can be held up out of the way by means of adhesive strapping during the procedure.
2. Femoral vein catheters should always be at least 20 cm in length from the hub to the tip. Fifteen centimetre catheters tend not to reach as far as the inferior vena cava. They provide inferior flow rates with a high percentage of blood recirculation (34). Probably 24 cm catheters would be ideal for most femoral insertions.
3. In patients in whom it is difficult to palpate the artery one can often locate it accurately with a small hand-held portable doppler (Figure 9).
4. The commonest mistake of inexperienced operators is to make the venous puncture too close to the artery and puncture the artery by mistake. It is better to start too far medial and gradually come more laterally until one finds the vein.
5. It is a good idea to use a fine gauge needle (gauge 21) to locate the vein first before using the Seldinger needle to introduce the guide wire.

6. If one inadvertently punctures the femoral artery with the Seldinger needle it is wise to avoid the use of heparin for at least 24 hours – hence the difficulties ensuing from a femoral artery puncture in a patient who needs hemoperfusion (and hence full systemic heparin therapy) for management of severe poisoning.
7. The commonest undiagnosed complication of femoral vein cannulation for hemodialysis is a traumatic arteriovenous fistula (35). It should be suspected in any patient with persistent discomfort in the groin. There is usually a loud bruit audible with the stethoscope. The diagnosis can be confirmed by ultrasound; and when found this injury should always be repaired. If left untreated it will cause or aggravate an existing high output cardiac failure (36). If not suspected and routinely looked for, it may be missed.

SUBCLAVIAN CANNULATION FOR HEMODIALYSIS

It can be assumed that this approach will continue to be used, and perhaps rightly so, for episodes of acute renal failure which are predicted to be reversible. The need for an A-V. fistula in the future is assumed to be highly unlikely. First some points of technique.

Prevention of infection

The traditional povidone-iodine for skin preparation should now be replaced by chlorhexidine because the latter seems to be more reliable (37).

When cannulating the subclavian vein, should one make a subcutaneous tunnel? In the author's view the small amount of extra work in doing so is justified, because: (a) a subcutaneous tunnel allows the catheter to be stabilised more easily on the anterior chest wall; (b) in the event of the catheter slipping out accidentally there will be less danger of serious bleeding or accidental air embolus because the subcutaneous tunnel will collapse and close; and (c) a subcutaneous tunnel should reduce the incidence of catheter-related infection. Controlled trials of subcutaneous tunnels in other clinical settings would support this (38), though a controlled trial of tunnelling versus no tunnelling by Dahlberg et al. (39) showed no reduction in infection by tunnelling for hemodialysis access catheters. Certainly the very low incidence of infections in jugular catheters with long subcutaneous tunnels suggests that tunnels have value in preventing infection.

The next point relates to the matter of which type of dressing to use to seal the exit site. We have always used the double transparent dressing technique (11) and have reported a blood stream infection rate of one for every 50 subclavian cannulation episodes (22).

On the other hand Levin et al. (40) in a controlled trial of double transparent dressings versus dry gauze dressings and povidine-iodine ointment at the exit site, showed a clear superiority of the latter technique in their centre. Double transparent adhesive dressings have certainly been very successful with very low infection rates in silastic jugular catheters. They have the additional advantage of stabilising the catheter without the need for skin sutures to hold it in place; and also the ability to see the exit site at all times. Usually the dressings do not need to be changed more than once a week. Smith and Nephew (Hull, UK) have a new porous dressing called IV 3000 which allows evaporation of water vapor through the skin, especially useful in patients who sweat profusely. This dressing seems to cause less skin irritation than either Tegaderm (3M, Minneapolis, USA) or OP-SITE (Smith and Nephew, Hull, UK) and in initial studies by Maki the infection rates were comparable to those achieved with dry gauze (41).

Finally, the matter of silver impregnation of the catheter or the cuff of the catheter at the exit site to discourage infection continues to be a tantalising idea whose full potential has probably yet to be realised (42).

Avoidance of trauma

If one is going to continue to use subclavian cannulation for patients with acute reversible renal failure, one has an obligation to make it safe (25) The following is a set of rules and guidelines formulated to make subclavian cannulation as safe as possible and thereby avoid tragedy:

1. Subclavian cannulation should only be performed by skilled operators or carefully supervised trainees. For the most part these will be nephrologists and interventional radiologists and their trainees.
2. Straight guide wires should never be used, because, occasionally, they may perforate the heart and cause cardiac tamponade (43).
3. A chest X-ray should always be taken after a subclavian cannulation to assess the position of the catheter. Whether the catheter is introduced from the left or the right, the tip should be low in the superior vena cava (SVC) so that the catheter is lying parallel with the vein wall (Figure 1).

The most serious mistakes with a right sided insertion are:

a) Perforation of the left wall of the SVC so that the catheter tip enters the pericardial cavity (13, 14) This will lead rapidly to fatal pericardial tamponade when dialysis is started (Figure 10).
b) Perforation of the wall of the right atrium when a full-sized catheter is used in a small individual (16). This would not normally happen immediately, but only after hours or days when the catheter tip drills its way through the atrial wall which is constantly contracting against it (Figure 11). This injury is almost invariably fatal no matter how quickly one tries to get the patient to the operating room, though in the case reported by Hansbrough et al. (44) the patient's life was saved by opening the chest and evacuating pericardial blood at

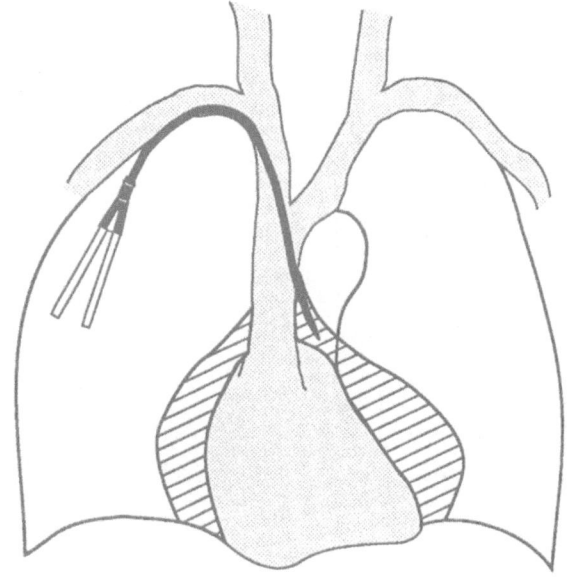

Figure 10. If a subclavian catheter inserted from the right side perforates the wall of the superior vena cava and enters the pericardial cavity, the patient will be in mortal danger from pericardial tamponade when dialysis is started. Immediate cessation of dialysis may save the patient's life.

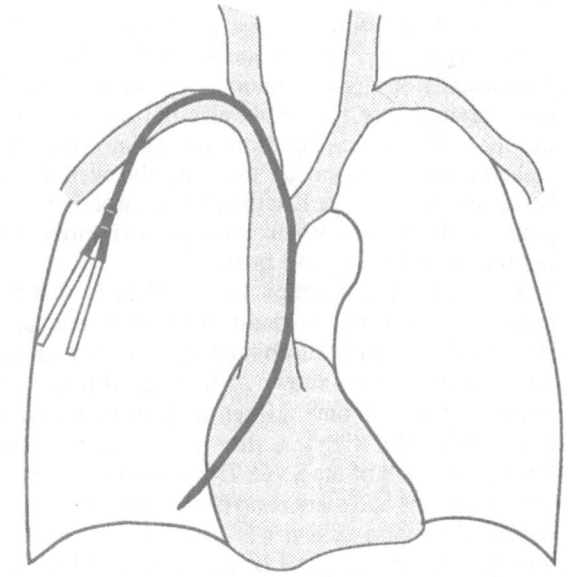

Figure 11. A full-sized subclavian catheter inserted from the right side in a small patient may perforate the wall of the right atrium. This injury is nearly always fatal.

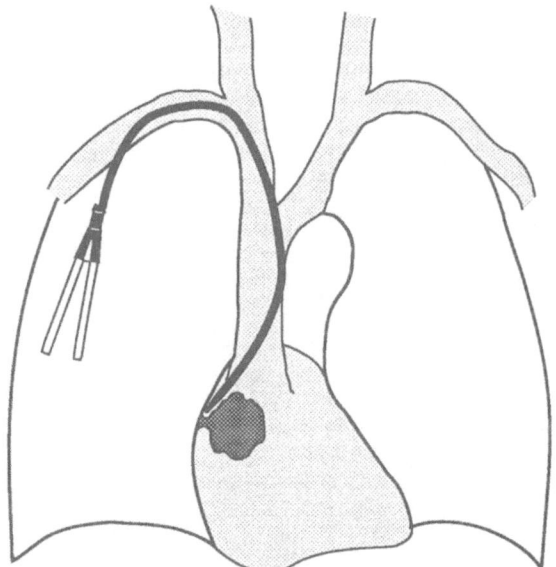

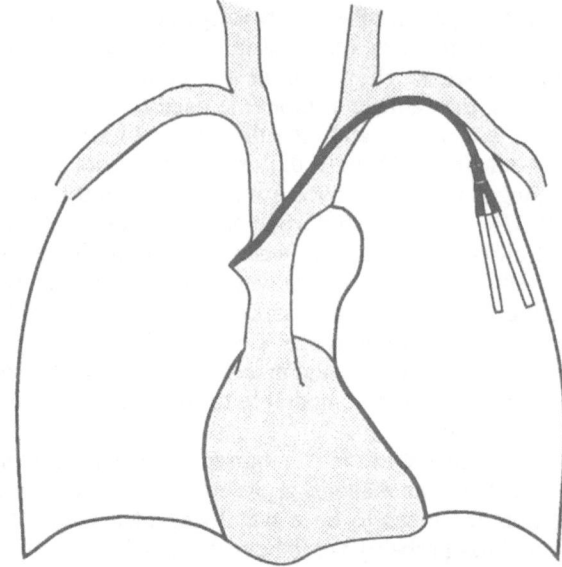

Figure 12. If a right sided catheter ends up with the tip in contact with the upper part of the wall of the right atrium it may slowly cause the development of a pedunculated ball thrombus. This may kill the patient by obstructing the passage of blood through the tricuspid valve.

Figure 13. A subclavian catheter inserted from the left side is 'tenting' the right wall of the superior vena cava. The danger is that after one or more dialyses it will perforate the wall.

the bedside. Prevention lies in making sure that the catheter is never allowed to protrude into the cavity of the right atrium. Shorter catheters must be used for smaller patients.

c) A catheter tip sitting against the right wall of the upper atrium can cause an atrial ball thrombus (45). This usually occurs over many weeks or months. On echocardiography it looks like an atrial myxoma (Figure 12). If it is arising from the point where the catheter tip is seen to be touching the wall it can be assumed to be a pedunculated ball thrombus. The patient will require open heart surgery to remove it. If not removed it may prove fatal.

d) With a left-sided insertion the problem is that the catheter tends to point towards the wall of the superior vena cava and the pointed tip may stretch the wall, an appearance known as 'tenting' (Figure 13). After a period of time, which may include one or more uneventful dialyses, the catheter tip may pop through the wall of the SVC. This event causes minimal symptoms and there is no danger until dialysis is started. As soon as dialysis is started blood is drawn through the arterial ports of the catheter which are usually still intravascular and discharged out through the distal 'venous' ports of the catheter which may be lying outside the wall of the vena cava. Blood will either enter the parenchyma of the lung (Figure 14), causing very alarming and profuse bright red hemoptysis or may track down the mediastinum into the right

hemithorax (46) (Figure 15). Paradoxically the first of these injuries is less dangerous because it immediately alerts the nurse and physician to the nature of the problem. Dialysis will be discontinued and an X-ray will immediately show what has happened.

Bleeding into the thorax is much more dangerous because hypotension and chest pain may be attributed to other reasons. In one such case the dialysis was not stopped until shock was far advanced and the patient did not recover though successfully resuscitated after a cardiac arrest (Personal communication).

The lessons from all of these cases are as follows:

1. Always take a chest X-ray after a catheter insertion to be sure that the catheter is in a safe position.
2. If the catheter is pointing at, and 'tenting', the wall of the superior vena cava, it should be replaced by a longer catheter which lies parallel with the wall.
3. Catheters should never be allowed to protrude into the cavity of the right atrium. If they are seen to do so they should immediately be replaced by a shorter one.
4. In any patient on dialysis with a semi-stiff, tapered catheter, whether it is the first or a subsequent treatment, the catheter should be suspected if chest pain, breathlessness or hypotension occur soon after the start of dialysis. The dialysis should be stopped, the physician should be called at once, and a chest X-ray should be taken to check the position of the catheter.

In a case of pericardial tamponade the patient's life may be saved by drawing back on the venous limb of the catheter with a syringe (47). If this fails to remove blood

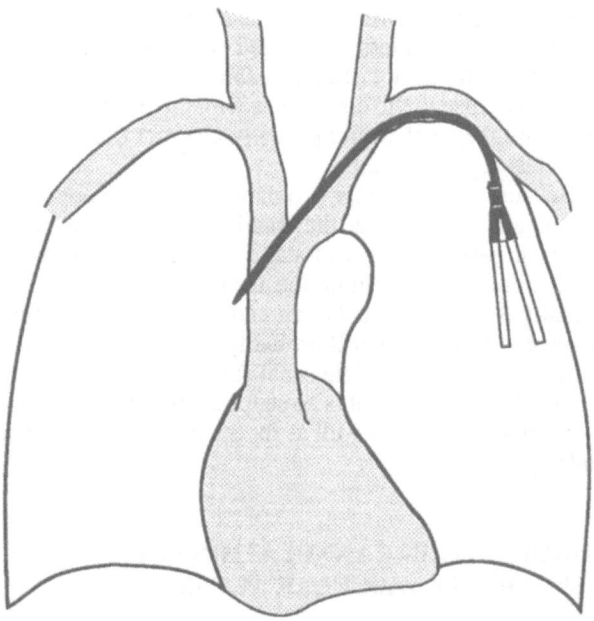

Figure 14. A subclavian catheter introduced from the left side has perforated the wall of the superior vena cava so that the tip is lying in the parenchyma of the lung. There may be no symptoms until the start of dialysis when the patient will experience profuse bright red hemoptysis.

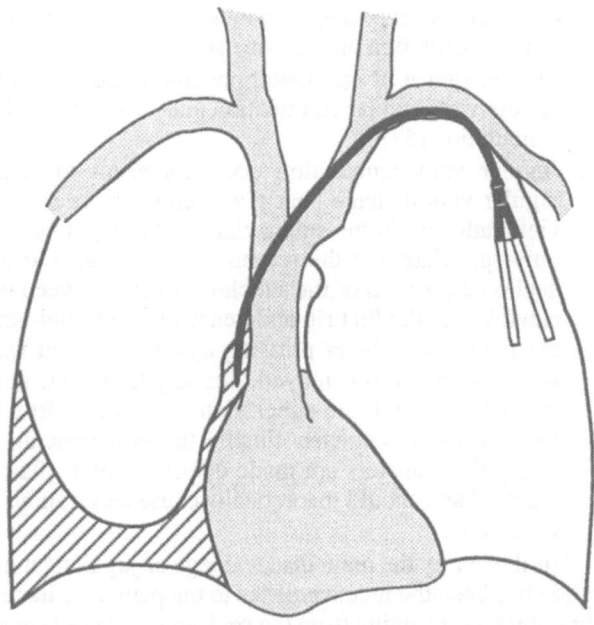

Figure 15. A left-sided subclavian catheter has perforated the SVC. Blood is tracking down into the right hemithorax. Continuation of dialysis may result in death.

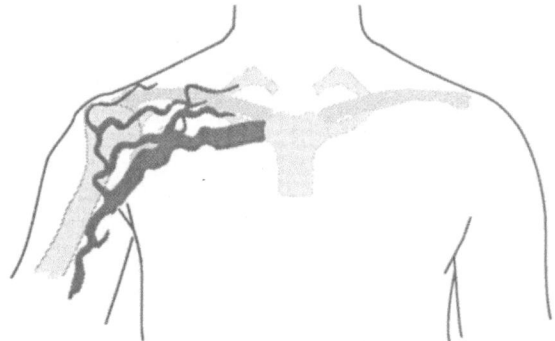

Figure 16. If a subclavian vein thrombosis is not detected early it will become permanent and essentially untreatable. Tell-tale collateral veins will be seen coursing over the shoulder.

from the pericardial cavity a pericardiocentesis should be done by needle aspiration (48). A hemothorax will require a chest tube drain and blood transfusion.

Diagnosis and management of subclavian vein thrombosis and stenosis

The incidence of subclavian vein damage is almost certainly related to the size and duration of insertion of the subclavian catheter. Single lumen catheters (of smaller diameter) probably cause less damage (49). Single-lumen subclavian catheters used with single-needle, double pump systems have been used successfully in Europe for many years. Vanholder has reported an incidence of subclavian vein thrombosis of 0.5% (50). However, since double-lumen subclavian catheters were developed (51), of which Mahurkar's design with the double-D configuration has become the almost universal choice (52), the incidence of subclavian vein damage has been found to be very significant. Although single-lumen catheters are still popular in Europe, where single-needle technology is well developed, it seems unlikely that they will ever replace double-lumen catheters in the United States.

Longer duration of insertion seems to increase the likelihood of venous stenosis (20). Therefore the duration of insertion should be kept as short as possible.

Complete subclavian vein thrombosis occurred in 6% of the series of Brady et al. (22) and in 19% of that reported by Vanherweghem (18). When stenosis has been investigated prospectively by venography the incidence has been remarkably consistent at about 40–50% (20, 23, 24, 53). In fact subclavian vein thrombosis and stenosis is clearly the second commonest cause (after destruction of forearm veins by I-V infusions) of failure to create an arteriovenous fistula. Thrombosis frequently is a clinically silent event because the collateral venous drainage of the upper limb is so generous. There may be no edema. Frequently the diagnosis only becomes apparent after a delay of several weeks when collateral veins develop

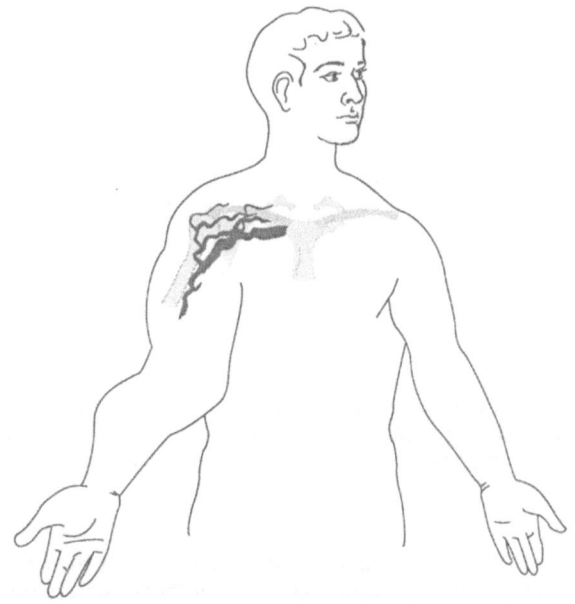

Figure 17. When an A-V fistula is created on the same side as a subclavian vein thrombosis or stenosis, the patient will develop massive congestive edema of the arm. Usually the only treatment is to ligate or dismantle the fistula.

over the shoulder. By this time the thrombus is organised and not treatable by heparin or thrombolysis (Figure 16). Alternatively the subclavian vein thrombosis only comes to light after a fistula has been constructed in the ipsilateral arm and the arm swells up to twice its normal size (Figure 17). The only way to deal with this is to ligate or dismantle the fistula. Although surgical by-pass of the obstruction has been described, most vascular surgeons are reluctant to attempt it (54).

Early diagnosis depends on a high index of suspicion, and frequent and early use of ultrasound to ascertain patency of the subclavian vein (22). This should be followed by a venogram in positive cases. Diagnosis within 2–3 days of the event allows recanalisation with systemic heparin therapy. A delay of 2–3 weeks will necessitate the use of local thrombolytic infusion administered through a fine catheter advanced until the tip is buried in the clot (22). With serial venograms it will be seen that the clot is receding and the infusion catheter can be advanced until complete lysis of the clot occurs. This may take up to 36 hours. Dissolution of the thrombus in a patient who is already bleeding from some other site such as the gastro-intestinal tract is a real challenge. We have been successful at least once in this situation with the use of Ancrod. The subclavian vein thrombosis was cleared without provoking any new bleeding. In order not to miss the diagnosis of subclavian vein thrombosis there is a strong argument to be made for routine doppler ultrasound studies in all patients whose subclavian catheters have just been removed.

Unfortunately stenosis, once it occurs, is usually permanent (22, 55). This is because even after angioplasty it always recurs unless the dilated vein is kept open by a stent (56). This is not often possible because the stenosis is usually close to the confluence with the internal jugular vein, and the stent would partially obstruct the mouth of the internal jugular vein.

Because of all of these problems we have in our centre completely discontinued the practice of subclavian cannulation in patients with end-stage renal failure. However, until jugular vein cannulation technology becomes universally available, subclavian cannulation will continue to be practiced and it will probably remain the method of choice in acute reversible renal failure for some time to come. This is because it is so seductively easy and convenient for the patient as well as for the medical and nursing staff.

JUGULAR VEIN CANNULATION FOR TEMPORARY VASCULAR ACCESS

A number of authorities have for some time advocated jugular vein cannulation for temporary vascular access for hemodialysis (24). The obvious advantages seem to be:

1. Avoidance of damage to the subclavian veins. If we never cannulate the subclavian veins in any patient with end-stage renal failure we will presumably cause no more iatrogenic subclavian vein thrombosis and stenosis. This will allow the proximal venous drainage of the upper limb to remain intact for A-V fistula and graft construction on the same side.
2. The incidence of accidental pneumothorax seems to be less with jugular cannulation than with subclavian cannulation (57).
3. Jugular vein cannulation does not seem to cause jugular vein damage nearly as frequently as subclavian catheters in the subclavian veins (53). One can only speculate that the reason may be related to the anchored position of the subclavian vein between the clavicle and the first rib and hence more intimal trauma from the catheter pressing against the vein wall whenever the arm is moved. The jugular vein is generally larger than the subclavian vein and is free to move with the catheter. Finally the new generation of jugular catheters are made of soft flexible silastic material and should theoretically cause less trauma to vein walls.

Until recently the main disadvantage of jugular cannulation has been the inconvenience to the patient of having the catheter protruding from the neck and anchored somewhere next to the ear.

The Quinton PermCath is designed to curve through 180° over the top of the clavicle and exit through a subcutaneous tunnel on the anterior chest wall (58). It was designed to be inserted surgically, and if it has to be

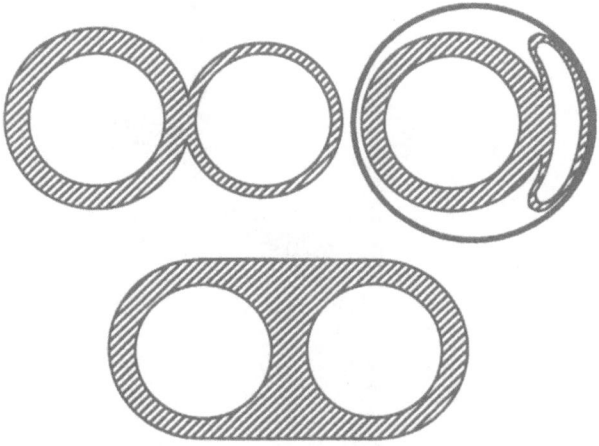

Figure 18. The silastic jugular catheter from Cook Critical Care is compressible during insertion: (a) to allow it to be passed through a relatively small peel-away sheath. (b) The upper part of the catheter has a smooth exterior where it goes through the vein wall.

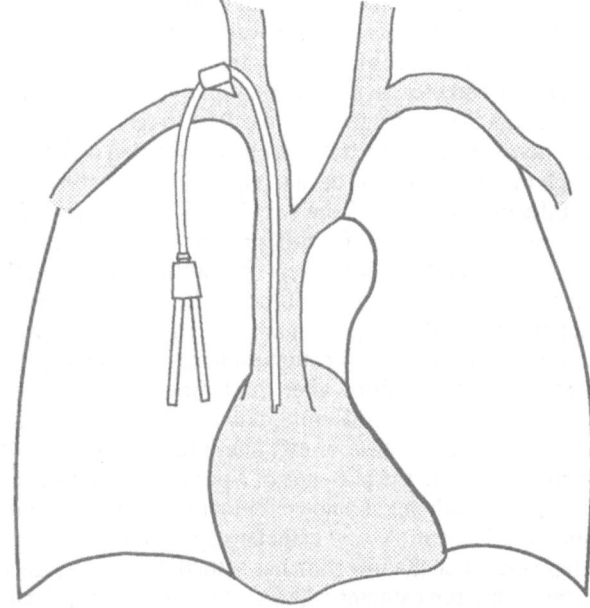

Figure 19. The optimal position for a silastic jugular catheter with a soft blunt end (parallel cylindrical lumens) is one in which the tip is just inside the entrance to the right atrium.

removed it would be very hard to insert it surgically a second time in the same vein (59). It has proved extremely successful for long-term access in patients with refractory access problems but because of the difficulty of repeated surgical insertion it is not really suitable for temporary vascular access. Although it can be inserted percutaneously through a French gauge 18 peel-away sheath, it takes a lot of courage to place such a large dilator and sheath in the jugular vein (60). Furthermore, the procedure tends to be associated with bleeding.

Canaud has developed a technique for inserting two separate single lumen silastic catheters percutaneously side-by-side in the jugular vein, one for withdrawal and the other for return of blood (61). This method has been successful both for temporary as well as long-term access, but there is the disadvantage of two separate catheters and two separate percutaneous insertions.

More recently Uldall, in collaboration with Cook Critical Care, has developed a double-lumen silastic catheter with parallel cylindrical lumens which, being compressible during insertion, can be passed percutaneously through a French gauge 13 peel-away sheath (62). The distal section of the catheter has a thick-walled lumen lying beside a thin-walled lumen. The thin-walled lumen can be compressed against the thick-walled lumen to allow the catheter to be passed through the relatively small sheath (Figure 18). Once it is in the vein the catheter regains its former shape. Although the thick-walled lumen was designed for negative pressure removal of blood and the thin-walled lumen for positive pressure return of blood, in practice the lumens can be reversed and blood is removed from the patient through whichever lumen provides the best blood flow. A flow of 400 ml/min should be obtainable at every dialysis if the catheter is placed in a good position and provided that there is no

thrombus clinging to the catheter to act as a non-return valve when dialysis is started. The method for catheter insertion has been described in detail (62), as has the method for changing the catheter over a guide wire to eradicate blood-stream infection in the presence of a clean exit site (63). A few selected comments about the technique are worth making here.

None of the components of the method is any more technically difficult than with subclavian cannulation. There are more steps involved and the method is more time-consuming, taking 35–45 minutes as compared to 20 minutes for a straightforward subclavian cannulation. The method is specially suited to the skills of an interventional radiologist who has the advantage of fluoroscopy for those cases in which blind guide wire manipulation cannot be done. The majority at our institution have been done in a procedure room without the benefit of fluoroscopy. Initial ultrasound localisation of the vein significantly increases the chance of first attempt cannulation (64). When inserting the catheter blindly from the left side it may occasionally end up in the right innominate vein instead of dropping down into the superior vena cava. When this is observed on the chest X-ray the easiest way to correct the malposition is by pulling it down by means of a hooked catheter passed up percutaneously through the femoral vein (65).

The catheter functions best when the tip is just inside rather than above the entrance to the right atrium (Figure 19). It is quite safe to position the tip in the middle of the right atrium as long as it is not touching the tricuspid valve. The tip is so soft and blunt that it could not conceivably perforate any vein wall. The catheter is available in different sizes in 2 cm increments from 24–32 cm. A 26 cm catheter is most commonly used on the right side and a 30 cm catheter on the left, to take account of the increased distance travelled by a left sided catheter to reach the superior vena cava (a right-sided structure).

Infection rates have been very low. Blood stream infection rates at the time of writing are one every 30 patient months and exit site infections (pus at the exit site in the absence of fever or positive blood culture) are one every 12 patient months (66). Both are treated with appropriate antibiotics followed by catheter-changing over a guide wire (63). This is done after the temperature has come down in a case of septicemia, and after the exit site has become clean in a case of exit site infection. When septicemia occurs in the presence of a purulent exudate at the exit site the catheter should be removed as quickly as possible and left out. A new catheter can be inserted on the other side when the infection has settled down. Any delay in removing the catheter when septicemia is complicated by a purulent exit site is an unacceptable risk for septic shock, especially if the organism is Staphylococcus aureus. The new Cook catheter can be inserted repeatedly in the same vein for separate periods of temporary hemodialysis. The incidence of jugular vein thrombosis attributable to this catheter has been shown to be 2% of all veins cannulated, even with repeated cannulation of the same vein for short or long duration (67).

Thrombus obstruction of the catheter is caused by fibrin and blood clot clinging to the outside of the catheter and this can be dealt with very effectively by administration of a bolus dose of urokinase (250,000 units) intravenously (68). This can be repeated after 3 hours if necessary. Two doses are not usually necessary and even less frequently one may need 3 doses. Recurrent clotting, involving expensive administration of urokinase can usually be prevented by low-dose anticoagulation with warfarin (65). At the Wellesley Hospital in the last 16 months there have been no bleeding complications from this therapy although previously we did encounter some hemorrhagic complications including a fatal subdural hematoma in a patient on warfarin where the diagnosis was missed. Freedom from hemorrhagic complications depends on excluding bleeding sources, at least weekly monitoring of the International Normalised Ratio (INR) by taking blood from the catheter itself before dialysis (69), and a conservative approach involving maintenance of the INR below 3.0 (70).

When clotting appears to be occurring at every dialysis one should suspect the presence of a superior vena cava stenosis (71)· (Figure 20). This may even be the cause of failure to introduce a catheter in the first place. It can be dilated by angioplasty but will recur if a stent is not used to keep the vena cava wide open. At present there is still some difficulty in availability of large diameter stents. Almost certainly all the cases of superior vena cava

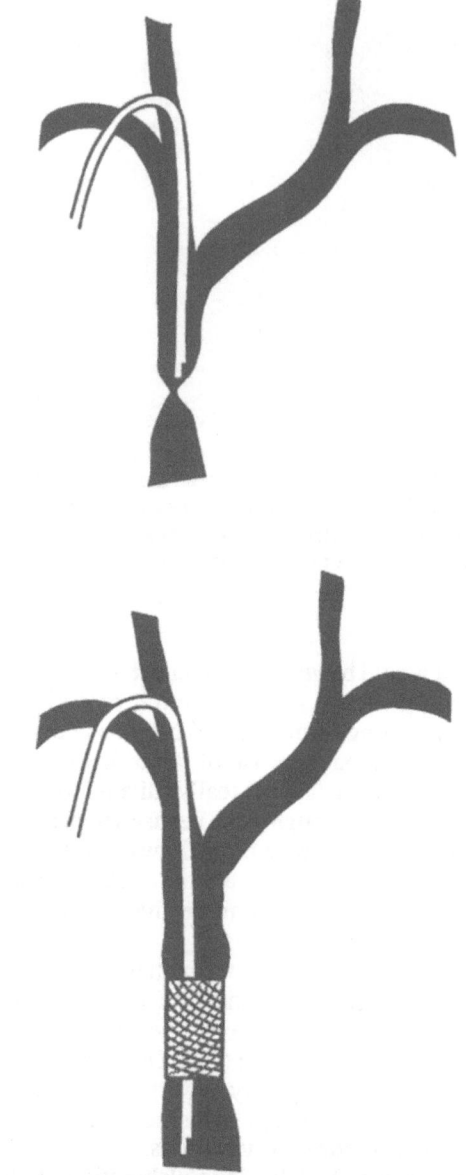

Figure 20. Multiple cannulations of the subclavian veins may traumatise the wall of the superior vena cava and cause severe SVC stenosis. (a) One should suspect this if urokinase is needed frequently to establish good blood flow. (b) Angioplasty followed by placement of a superior vena cava stent may allow the catheter to be passed freely into the upper part of the right atrium.

stenosis we have seen have been caused by the presence of multiple previous semi-stiff tapered subclavian catheters. One hopes that this condition will become rare when this type of catheter is no longer used in patients with end-stage renal failure.

POTENTIAL DANGERS FROM ALL TYPES OF CENTRAL VENOUS CATHETERS

The potential for strokes from paradoxical cerebral emboli from central venous catheters

In one patient with a long-term silastic jugular catheter (PermCath), we observed a series of strokes in which the cerebral infarctions were clearly seen in a series of computerized axial tomography (CAT) scans of the brain. After her third stroke, a particularly devastating hemiplegia with total aphasia, dialysis was withdrawn and the patient was allowed to die. Autopsy revealed blood clot clinging to the catheter tip in the superior vena cava and a widely patent foramen ovale. Paradoxical embolisation was revealed as the cause of her strokes. Following this episode we carried out transesophageal echocardiograms in 26 patients with silastic jugular catheters to look for other clinically silent communications between the right and left side of the heart and we found none. This experience demonstrated that a patent foramen ovale is a serious risk in any hemodialysis patient with a central venous catheter. If an unexpected stroke occurs in such a patient a search should be made for a patent foramen ovale. If a communication is found one may wish to avoid central venous catheters completely or keep the patient permanently on warfarin. It seems highly likely that small fragments of blood clot are becoming intermittently detached from central venous catheters in most hemodialysis patients who have them, and that they are accommodated without damage by the body's own fibrinolytic processes. One is tempted to suggest that an important function of the lungs in a hemodialysis patient is to trap blood clots which would otherwise pass to the brain. Interestingly, it has been shown that the prevalence of patent foramen ovale declines progressively with age, but with increasing age the openings become larger (72).

Danger of bleeding caused by the heparin lock

All medical and nursing staff should know that, in the intervals between dialysis, central vein catheters have their dead-space partially or wholly filled with heparin to prevent clotting. Over filling of this space will cause systemic heparinisation and this could be dangerous if the patient is about to undergo surgery. If an intravenous infusion is attached the heparin should be removed first or it will be flushed straight into the circulation with the potential danger of bleeding.

Accidental disconnection

All central vein catheters should be closed off with Luer-lock caps and also clamped with removable clamps on the clamping limbs. If a cap slips off and there is no clamp in place the patient may exsanguinate during sleep without ever waking up. Intravenous infusions should have Luer-locks and should be taped. Snug fit infusion sets can slip out with tragic consequences. Finally the new 'Interlink' system of connection (Becton Dickinson & Co, Franklin Lakes, NJ) is safe for an I-V infusion but not safe during dialysis because the venous blood line may slip out of the catheter and allow bleeding from the venous blood tubing. The narrow aperture at the distal end of the Interlink may prevent a sufficient drop in venous pressure to activate the venous pressure alarm. We recently observed an example of just this accident. The patient's life was saved by the sharp eyes and quick response of the nurse. Prior to this episode with the Interlink we had not observed an accidental disconnection in the last 7 years.

Use of hemodialysis catheters for intravenous infusions in the intervals between dialysis

Apart from the danger of accidental disconnection of intravenous infusion sets from central venous catheters (and the necessity for Luer-lock connections), the question whether to use hemodialysis catheters at all for intravenous infusions remains controversial. The argument has been made that any additional invasion of the integrity of the hemodialysis catheter for the purpose of infusion will increase the likelihood of blood stream infection. Therefore they should never be used for this purpose, except in the case of a life-threatening problem (e.g., hyperkalemia). A separate central venous line should be inserted on the other side for example for the delivery of total parenteral nutrition (TPN). The trouble with this strategy is that if a fever appears in association with a positive blood culture one has no way of knowing which of the catheters is responsible. All central venous lines have to be removed and there may be no clean site left for the new insertion. This might be an attractive indication for the use of the rapid technique (supposedly within one hour) for diagnosis of central venous catheter sepsis described by Rushforth and colleagues (73) because theoretically it should identify which catheter is to blame. In our view it is preferable to keep the number of central venous lines down to a minimum. If the patient already has a hemodialysis catheter this should be used for the TPN but with careful attention to aseptic technique. In this case there may be a strong argument for using the Interlink system, which theoretically should reduce the chance of contamination. If the Interlink were to come away from the sealed cap, the only complication would be leakage of the intravenous infusion. In this context it is worth remembering that, when using TPN containing high concentrations of glucose, the likelihood of superior vena cava thrombosis is much greater if the catheter tip is lying in the superior vena cava, much less if it is lying in the right atrium (74), an additional reason if one be needed for trying to place the tips of soft silastic catheters inside the right atrium. It does not, however, justify placing the tips of semi-stiff tapered catheters inside the right atrium, for all the reasons quoted above.

Failure of central vein catheters to activate pressure alarms in the event of cardiac arrest

This danger was brought to our attention when a patient being dialysed through a subclavian catheter pulled his sheet over his head to go to sleep. When his nurse went to check his vital signs 30 minutes later she found him dead. Attempts at cardiac resuscitation not surprisingly failed since the patient may have died anything up to 29 minutes before. He was last seen alive 30 minutes previously. This brought home to us that cardiac arrest does not generate alarms in the extracorporeal circuit when a central vein catheter is being used as long as blood in the central reservoir of the vena cava remains fluid. The same cardiac arrest in a patient being dialysed with a fistula would immediately cause an arterial negative pressure alarm because of cessation of blood flow through the fistula. This highlighted the rule that patients on dialysis with central vein catheters must be visible at all times or have a cardiac or pulse monitor attached.

SUMMARY AND CONCLUSIONS

Temporary access to the circulation for hemodialysis has evolved and improved ever since the first two most important innovations, namely Shaldon's femoral catheter and Scribner's silastic-teflon shunt, were described. Subclavian cannulation became popular largely because of the ease and convenience of the technique. However, I have tried to show that for patients with end-stage renal failure, subclavian cannulation is no longer justified because of the high incidence of damage to the subclavian veins from subclavian vein thrombosis and stenosis, which interfere with the proximal venous drainage of the arm and hence with the creation of arteriovenous fistulas and grafts. I have also emphasised the dangers of semi-stiff pointed catheters which may cause serious and sometimes fatal perforating injuries.

Fortunately we now have available soft, flexible catheters with blunt tips which are incapable of causing perforating injuries. More importantly these new catheters are suitable for temporary cannulation of the jugular veins. Their adoption should bring to a halt the terrible toll of subclavian vein damage and also greatly reduce the incidence of traumatic complications. If the initial observations of the low incidence of damage to jugular veins from these devices continues to hold true, then we may find that we have the best of both worlds. We may have a central venous cannulation technique with a remarkably low incidence of serious complications which is convenient and acceptable to patients, and which can be used repeatedly at different times in the same vein. The new techniques of central venous cannulation have huge advantages to

patients as well as to doctors and nursing staff but we have an obligation to make them very safe. It looks as though, for the next few years at least, femoral catheters will continue to be used in unstable patients with pulmonary edema or other causes for respiratory distress. Jugular cannulation with the new generation of percutaneously inserted, soft, flexible silastic catheters with blunt tips will become the mainstay of temporary vascular access. Another obvious advantage is that they are also suitable for long-term use; so there is no hurry to remove them in the event that hemodialysis has to be continued because of difficulty in constructing an A-V fistula. Whether these catheters will be inserted and changed mainly by nephrologists, interventional radiologists, or vascular access surgeons will be a matter for each center to decide. A high success rate and low incidence of complications will depend on developing good collaboration and high standards of practice at all levels.

REFERENCES

1. Shaldon S, Chiandussi L, Higgs SB: Hemodialysis by percutaneous catheterisation of the femoral artery and vein with regional heparinisation. *Lancet* 2: 857, 1961
2. Quinton WE, Dillard DH, Scribner BH: Cannulation of blood vessels for prolonged hemodialysis. *Trans Am Soc Artif Intern Organs* 6: 104, 1960
3. Brescia MJ, Cimino JE, Appel K, Hurwich K: Chronic hemodialysis using venipuncture and surgically created arteriovenous fistula. *N Eng J Med* 275: 1089, 1966
4. Sabanayagam P, Schwartz AB, Soricelli PR, Lyons P, Chinitz JA: A comparative study of 402 bovine heterografts and 225 reinforced expanded PTFE grafts as AVF in the ESRD patient. *Trans Am Soc Artif Intern Organs* 26: 88, 1980
5. Bell PRF, Calman KC: Vascular access in dialysis. in *Replacement of Renal function by Dialysis*, 1st ed, edited by Drukker W, Parsons F, Maher JF, The Hague, Martinus Nijhoff Medical Division, 1978, p 182
6. Simonian SJ, Stuart FP, Hill JL, Mahajan SK: Conversion of a Scribner shunt to an arteriovenous fistula for chronic dialysis. *Surgery* 82: 448, 1977
7. Paganini EP, Nakamoto S: Continuous slow ultrafiltration in oliguric acute renal failure. *Trans Am Soc Artif Intern Organs* 26: 201, 1980
8. Kramer P, Boehler J, Kehr A, Gröne HJ, Schrader J, Matthaei D, Scheler F: Intensive care potential of continuous arteriovenous hemofiltration. *Trans Am Soc Artif Intern Organs* 28: 28, 1982
9. Tam P, Huraib SO, Mahan B, LeBlanc D, Lunski C, Holtzer C, Doyle CA, Vas SI, Uldall PR: Slow continuous hemodialysis for the management of complicated oliguric acute renal failure in an intensive care unit. *Clin Nephrol* 23: 79, 1988
10. Erben J, Kvasnicka J, Bastecky J et al.: Experience with routine use of subclavian cannulation in hemodialysis. *Proc Eur Dial Transplant Assoc* 6: 59, 1969
11. Uldall PR, Dyck RF, Woods F, Merchant N, Martin GS, Cardella CJ, Sutton D, deVeber G: A subclavian cannu-

la for temporary vascular access for hemodialysis and plasmaphoresis. *Dial Transplant* 8: 963, 1979

12. DeCubber A, DeWolf C, Lameire N: Single-needle hemodialysis with the double headpump via the subclavian vein. *Dial Transplant* 7: 1261, 1978

13. Fine A, Churchill D, Gault H: Fatality due to subclavian dialysis catheter. *Nephron* 29: 99, 1981

14. Merrill RH, Raab SO: Dialysis catheter-induced pericardial tamponade. *Arch Intern Med* 142: 1751, 1982

15. Barton BR, Hermann G, Weil R: Cardiothoracic emergencies associated with subclavian hemodialysis catheters. *JAMA* 250: 2660, 1983

16. Tapson JS, Uldall PR: Fatal hemothorax caused by a subclavian hemodialysis catheter. *Arch Intern Med* 144: 1685, 1984

17. El Nachef MW, Rashad E, Ricanati ES: Occlusion of the subclavian vein: a complication of indwelling subclavian venous catheters for hemodialysis. *Clin Nephrol* 24: 42, 1985

18. Vanherwegem JL, Yassine T, Goldman M et al.: Subclavian vein thrombosis: a frequent complication of subclavian vein cannulation for hemodialysis. *Clin Nephrol* 26: 235, 1986

19. Glaze RC, McDougall ML, Weigmann TB: Thrombotic arm edema as a complication of subclavian vein catheterisation and arteriovenous fistula formation for hemodialysis. *Am J Kidney Dis* 7: 439, 1986

20. Barrett N, Spencer S, McIvor J, Brown EA: Subclavian stenosis: a major complication of subclavian dialysis catheters. *Nephrol Dial Transplant* 3: 423, 1988

21. Clark DD, Albina JE, Chezan JA: Subclavian vein stenosis and thrombosis: a potential serious complication in chronic hemodialysis patients. *Am J Kidney Dis* 15: 256, 1990

22. Brady HR, Fitzcharles B, Goldberg H, Huraib S, Simons M, Uldall PR: Diagnosis and management of subclavian vein thrombosis occurring in association with subclavian cannulation for hemodialysis. *Blood Purif* 7: 210, 1987

23. Spinowitz BS, Galler M, Golden RA et al.: Subclavian vein stenosis as a complication of subclavian catheterisation for hemodialysis. *Arch Int Med* 147: 305, 1987

24. Cimochowski GE, Worley E, Rutherford WE, Sartain J, Blondin J, Harter H: Superiority of the internal jugular over the subclavian access for temporary dialysis. *Nephron* 54: 154, 1990

25. Tapson JS, Uldall PR: Avoiding deaths from subclavian cannulation for hemodialysis. *Int J Artif Organs* 6: 227, 1983

26. Uldall PR: Subclavian cannulation for hemodialysis: the present state of the art. *Artif Organs* 6: 73, 1982

27. Ward ME, Lee PF: Pneumothorax and contralateral hydrothorax following subclavian vein catheterisation. *Br J Anaesth* 45: 227, 1973

28. Holt S, Kirkham N, Myerscough E: Haemothorax after subclavian vein cannulation. *Thorax* 32: 101, 1977

29. Gröne HJ, Kramer P: Puncture and long-term cannulation of the femoral artery and vein in adults. in *Arteriovenous Hemofiltration. A Kidney Replacement Therapy for the Intensive Care Unit*, edited by Kramer P, Berlin, Springer-Verlag, 1985

30. Bellomo R, Parkin G, Love J, Boyce N: A prospective comparative study of continuous arteriovenous hemodiafiltration and continuous venovenous hemodiafiltration in critically ill patients. *Am J Kidney Dis* 21: 400, 1993

31. Storck M, Hartl WH, Zimmerer E, Inthorn D: Comparison of pump-driven and spontaneous continuous hemofiltration in post-operative acute renal failure. *Lancet* 337: 452, 1991

32. Lazarus JM: Complications in haemodialysis: An overview. *Kidney Int* 18: 783, 1980

33. Farrington K, Brown AL, Mathias MT, Karim MS, Cattell WR, Baker LRI: Simultaneous creation of peritoneal and vascular access in patients commencing continuous ambulatory peritoneal dialysis. *Nephron* 59: 323, 1991

34. Kelber J, Delmez JA, Windus DW: Factors affecting delivery of high efficiency dialysis using temporary vascular access. *Am J Kidney Dis* 22: 243, 1993

35. Fuller TJ, Mahoney JJ, Juncos LI et al: Arteriovenous fistula after femoral vein catheterisation. *JAMA* 236: 2943, 1976

36. Ahearn DJ, Maher JF: Heart failure as a complication of haemodialysis arteriovenous fistula. *Ann Intern Med* 77: 201, 1972

37. Maki DG, Ringer M, Alvarado CJ: Prospective randomised trial of povidone-iodine, alcohol and chlorhexidine for prevention of infection associated with central venous and arterial catheters. *Lancet* 338: 339, 1991

38. Keohane PP, Jones BJM, Attril H et al.: Effect of catheter tunnelling and a nutrition nurse on catheter sepsis during parenteral nutrition. A controlled trial. *Lancet* 2: 1388, 1983

39. Dahlberg PJ, Yutuc WR, Newcomer KL: Subclavian hemodialysis catheter infections. *Am J Kidney Dis* 7: 421, 1986

40. Levin A, Mason AJ, Jindal KK, Fong IW, Goldstein MB: Prevention of hemodialysis subclavian vein catheter infections by topical povidone-iodine. *Kidney Int* 40: 934, 1991

41. Maki DG, Wheeler S, Stolz SM: Study of a novel highly permeable polyurethane dressing for IV catheters. Presented at the Hospital Infection Society International Meeting, London, 1990

42. Maki DG, Cobb L, Garman JK et al.: An attachable silver-impregnated cuff for prevention of infection with central venous catheters: a prospective randomized multi-center trial. *Am J Med* 85: 307, 1988

43. Blake PG, Uldall PR: Cardiac perforation by a guide wire during subclavian catheter insertion. *Int J Artif Organs* 2: 111, 1989

44. Hansbrough JFG, Narrod JA, Stiegman V: Cardiac perforation and tamponade from a malpositioned subclavian dialysis catheter. *Nephron* 32: 363, 1982

45. Wijeyesinghe ECR, Pei Y, Fenton S, Uldall PR: Right atrial ball thrombus as a complication of subclavian catheter insertion for hemodialysis. *Int J Artif Organs* 10: 102, 1987

46. Mattox KL, Fisher RG: Persistent hemothorax secondary to malposition of a subclavian venous catheter. *J Trauma* 17: 387, 1977

47. Karnauchow PN: Cardiac tamponade from central vein catheterisation. *Can Med Assoc J* 135: 1145, 1986

48. Gebert E: Non-operative treatment of cardiac tamponade. *Crit Care Med* 14: 519, 1986

49. Vanholder R, Hoenich N, Ringoir S: Morbidity and mortality of central venous catheter hemodialysis: a review of 10 years experience. *Nephron* 47: 274, 1987

50. Vanholder R, Lameire N, Verbanck J, van Rattinghe R, Kunnen M, Ringoir S: Complications of subclavian

catheter hemodialysis: a 5 year prospective study in 257 consecutive patients. *Int J Artif Organs* 5: 297, 1982

51. Uldall PR, Woods F, Merchant N, Crichton E, Carter H: A double-lumen subclavian cannula (DLSC) for temporary hemodialysis access. *Trans Am Soc Artif Intern Organs* 26: 93, 1980

52. Tapson JS, Hoenich NA, Wilkinson R: Dual lumen subclavian catheters for haemodialysis. *Int J Artif Organs* 8: 195, 1985

53. Schillinger F, Schillinger D, Montagnac R, Milcent T: Post catheterisation vein stenosis in haemodialysis: comparative angiographic study of 50 subclavian and 50 internal jugular accesses. *Nephrol Dial Transplant* 6: 722, 1991

54. Currier CB Jr, Widder S, Ali A, Kunsisto E, Sidawy A: Surgical management of subclavian and axillary vein thrombosis in patients with a functioning arteriovenous fistula. *Surgery* 100: 25, 1986

55. Glanz S, Gordon DH, Lipkowitz GS, Brett KMH, Hong J, Sclafani SJS: Axillary and subclavian vein stenosis: percutaneous angioplasty. *Radiology* 168: 371, 1988

56. Uchida BT, Putnam JS, Rosch J: Modifications of Gianturco expandable wire stents. *Am J Radiol* 150: 1185, 1988

57. Campistol JM, Almiral J, Rello J, Revert L: Jugular vein cannulation for hemodialysis access. *Nephron* 50: 391, 1988

58. Shusterman NH, Kloss K, Mullen JL: Successful use of double-lumen silicone rubber catheters for permanent hemodialysis access. *Kidney Int* 35: 887, 1989

59. Blake PG, Huraib S, Wu G, Uldall PR: The use of dual-lumen jugular venous catheters as definitive long-term access for hemodialysis. *Int J Artif Organs* 13: 26, 1990

60. McDowell DE, Pillai L, Goldstein RM: A simplified technique for percutaneous insertion of permanent vascular access catheters in patients requiring chronic hemodialysis. *J Vasc Surg* 7: 574, 1988

61. Canaud B, Saumier F, Beraud JJ, Joyeux H, Mion C: La cannulation jugulaire interne avec deux cathéters silastic. Une nouvelle méthode d'acces vasculaire pour hemodialyse. *Néphrologie* 7: 57, 1986

62. Uldall PR DeBruyne M, Besley M, McMillan J, Simons M, Francoeur R: A new vascular access catheter for hemodialysis. *Am J Kidney Dis* 21: 270, 1993

63. Carlisle EJF, Blake PG, McCarthy F, Vas S, Uldall PR: Septicemia in long-term jugular hemodialysis catheters; eradicating infection by changing the catheter over a guidewire. *Int J Artif Organs* 14: 150, 1991

64. Denys BG, Uretsky BF, Reddy PS, Ruffner RJ, Sandhu JS, Breishlatt WM: An ultrasound method for safe and rapid central venous access. *N Eng J Med* 324: 566, 1991

65. Hawkins IF, Page RM: Redirection of malpositioned central venous catheters. *Am J Radiol* 140: 393, 1983

66. Mustata S, Less P, Uldall PR: Further experience with a percutaneously inserted double-lumen silastic catheter for end-stage renal failure patients with refractory vascular access problems. *Am Soc Artif Intern Organs*, San Francisco, 1994

67. Agraharkar M, Mendelssohn D, Zevallos G, Uldall PR: Does percutaneous jugular vein cannulation for hemodialysis access cause jugular vein damage? *Am Soc Artif Organs*, San Francisco, 1994

68. Uldall PR, Besley ME, Thomas A, Salter S, Nuezca LA, Vas M: Maintaining the patency of double-lumen silastic jugular catheters for haemodialysis. *Int J Artif Organs* 16: 37, 1993

69. Besley ME, Thomas A, Salter S, Sang YY, Vas M, Uldall PR: Control of oral anticoagulation in patients using long-term internal jugular catheters for haemodialysis access. *Int J Artif Organs* 15: 277, 1992

70. Landefeld CS, Beyth RJ: Anticoagulant-related bleeding: clinical epidemiology, prediction and prevention. *Am J Med* 95: 315, 1993

71. Khanna S, Sniderman K, Simons M, Besley ME, Uldall PR: Superior vena cava stenosis associated with hemodialysis catheters. *Am J Kidney Dis* 21: 278, 1993

72. Hagen PT, Scholz DG, Edwards WD: Incidence and size of patent foramen ovale during the first 10 decades of life: an autopsy study of 965 normal hearts. *Mayo Clinic Proc* 59: 17, 1984

73. Rushforth JA, Hoy CM, Kite P, Puntis JWL: Rapid diagnosis of central venous catheter sepsis. *Lancet* 342: 402, 1993

74. Pithie A, Soutar JS, Pennington CR: Catheter tip position in central vein thrombosis. *J Parenteral Enteral Nutr* 12: 613, 1988

10

HEMODIALYSIS ACCESS
PART B – PERMANENT

CHARLES E. BUTLER and NICHOLAS L. TILNEY

INTRODUCTION

The introduction of extracorporeal dialysis of blood by Kolff et al. (1) in 1943 provided a means whereby patients with end stage renal failure could be sustained for prolonged periods by intermittent filtering of uremic toxins from the blood. Temporary access to the circulation by catheterization of distal arteries and veins using glass or metal cannulae was performed originally, with the used portions of the vessels ligated following each dialysis treatment. Chronic dialysis was not feasible until the introduction of the external arteriovenous shunt by Quinton, Dillard and Scribner in 1960 (2) and the endogenous fistula by Brescia, Cimino and colleagues in 1966 (3), approaches that afforded routine intermittent access to the circulation without sacrifice of the vessels after each treatment. The increased availability of synthetic vascular prostheses, especially expanded polytetrafluoroethylene (PTFE), has allowed a greater procedural choice, particularly in chronic dialysis patients whose peripheral venous sites have been exhausted or whose native veins are inadequate for the creation of an endogenous fistula. In recent years, the frequency of placement of external shunts has diminished coincident with the greater popularity of permanent subcutaneous vascular grafts for long-term use or vascular catheters for acute use inserted either percutaneously or surgically. In this chapter we will review general techniques of placement, care, complications, revision and repair of chronic vascular access for dialysis as well as expectations for their long term patency.

GENERAL PRINCIPLES OF CHRONIC DIALYSIS ACCESS

Arteriovenous fistulae are fashioned either of endogenous vein or prosthetic material. They are optimally placed just deep to the dermis to prevent erosion through the skin, while still permitting convenient puncture. Provided that a cephalic vein of adequate size is easily visible, the endogenous (Cimino) fistula at the wrist or antecubital space is preferred as a first procedure because of its long-term patency and low incidence of infection. In addition, the rate of complications requiring operative intervention is significantly lower than that of prosthetic grafts, with thrombosis secondary to localized areas of stenosis accounting for most of the failures (4). Attempts to create such fistulae are impractical in patients whose cephalic veins are sclerosed or thrombosed, are buried deeply in subcutaneous fat or are fragile as in many postmenopausal women. They are also often unsuccessful in diabetic patients because of inadequate arterial inflow, particularly at the wrist. Preoperative planning includes adequate hydration, prevention of hypotension and vasoconstriction, and perioperative antibiotics, particularly when prosthetic materials are used. Repeated venipuncture or placement of indwelling intravenous catheters in the arm to be used for access is anathema.

In selecting a fistula site (5, 6), the upper extremity is preferred because the incidence of infection is significantly lower and development of arterial steal syndrome less likely than in the leg. These considerations are especially important in patients at risk for atherosclerosis and ischemia, such as the elderly or those with diabetes. Similarly, the saphenous vein should be spared when possible for future peripheral or coronary arterial reconstruction. This vein is also not a particularly satisfactory conduit for

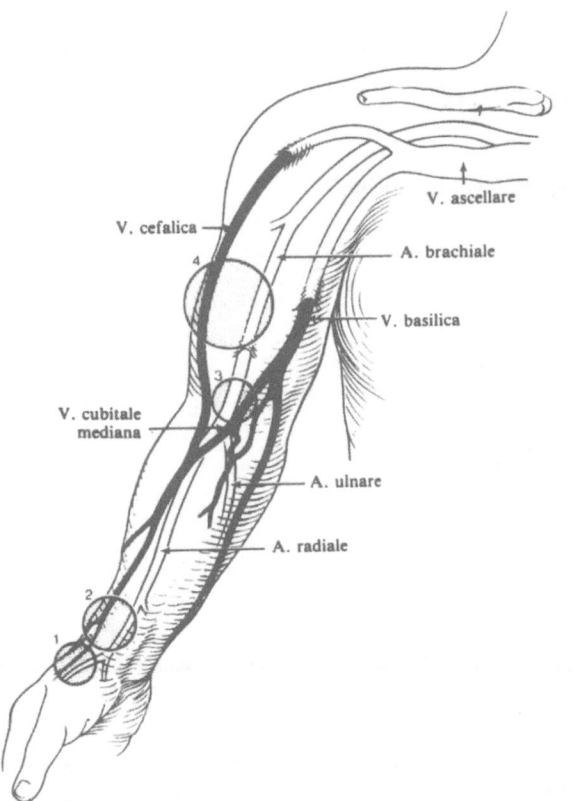

Figure 1. The most widely used sites for the creation of arteriovenous fistula. (Reprinted with permission of WB Saunders Co.)

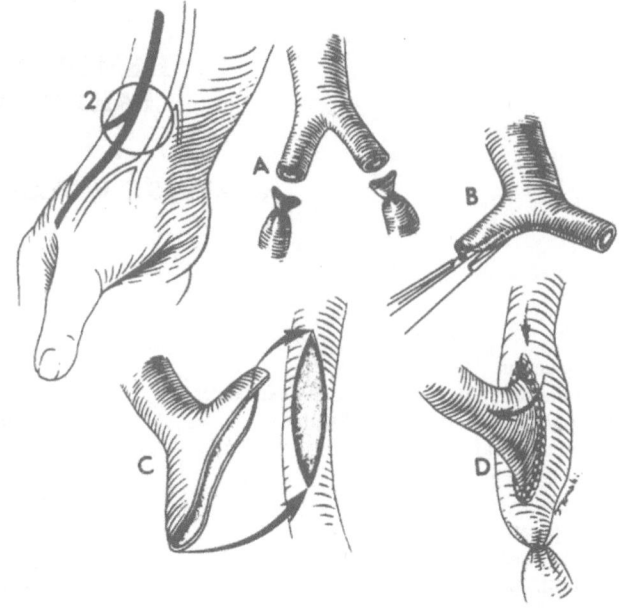

Figure 2. Cimino fistulae are made most commonly at the wrist (Area 2). A. The cephalic vein is isolated at its bifurcation and the distal branches ligated. B. The bifurcation is opened. C. The widened area is trimmed to create a patch graft. D. An end-to-side anastomosis is performed using fine suture. The distal radial artery can be ligated if desired. (Reprinted with permission of WB Saunders Co.)

access as it tends to develop stenoses and aneurysms. The most distal available site in the upper extremity should be used to keep maximal vessel length for future revision or placement of new grafts. Finally, the non-dominant arm is preferable to keep the dominant arm free during dialysis.

ENDOGENOUS ARTERIOVENOUS FISTULAE

For permanent initial access, use of the patient's own vein is desirable despite a relatively high initial failure rate. The radial artery and cephalic vein at the wrist are preferred for the initial site of a Cimino fistula, although other upper extremity locations can be used (Figure 1). Although the side-to-side anastomosis was first described for wrist fistulae, an end-vein to side-artery anastomosis with preservation of the distal radial artery should be performed, as it results in a reduced incidence of arterial steal and distal venous hypertension (7–9). Furthermore, patency rates for the two approaches were reported to be equal in one study of 71 patients, 79.2% and 78.6% at nine months for side-to-side and end-to-side, respectively (9). The majority of failures occur soon after placement; once

a Cimino fistula is established, it usually functions well for extended periods. A radiocephalic fistula may also be created more distally at the anatomic snuffbox if desired, although the advantages of this approach are not clear.

Performed under local anesthesia as an outpatient procedure, the wrist Cimino fistula is constructed by exposing the radial artery and distal cephalic vein via a transverse incision (Figure 2). After distal ligation, the vein is divided and a small catheter passed proximally to irrigate, dilate and ensure patency. The end-to-side anastomosis is then performed with continuous 6–0 monofilament suture. If possible, the confluence of two major venous tributaries are used as an onlay patch after each distal branch has been ligated and divided a few millimeters from their junction. The vein proximal to the anastomosis should be isolated from surrounding tissue for 2 to 3 cm to allow maximal dilation for arterial flow. On completion of the anastomosis and release of the occlusive vessel loops, a thrill should be palpable over the proximal vein. Absence of a thrill and a bounding pulse suggest venous outflow obstruction which will usually result in fistula failure.

Proximal forearm or upper arm endogenous arteriovenous fistulae may be created in individuals with inadequate wrist vessels but obvious proximal cephalic or antecubital veins, or in those with a previous failed distal Cimino fistula which has produced proximal venous dilatation. The cephalic vein can be mobilized, divided and anasto-

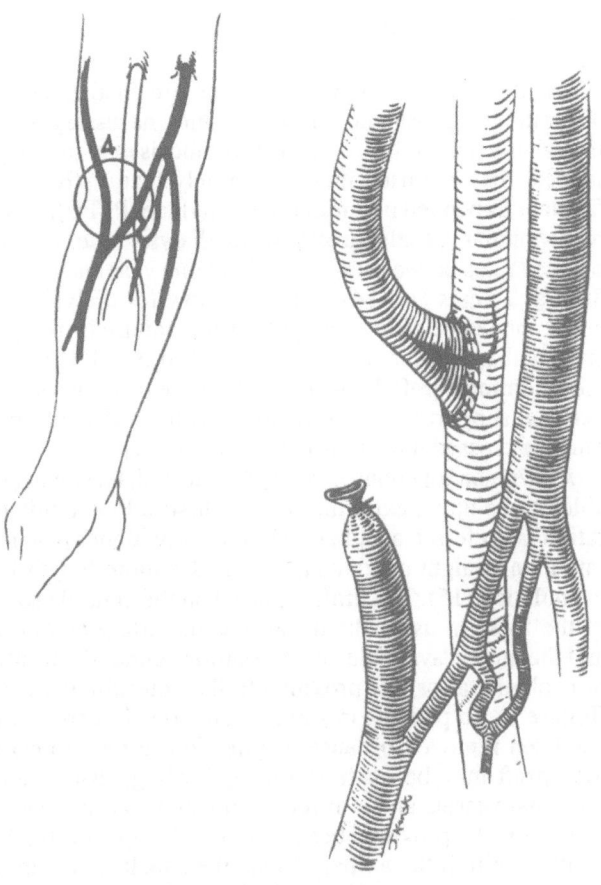

Figure 3. The cephalic vein can be anastomosed to the brachial artery to create an upper arm Cimino fistula (Area 4). (Reprinted with permission of WB Saunders Co.)

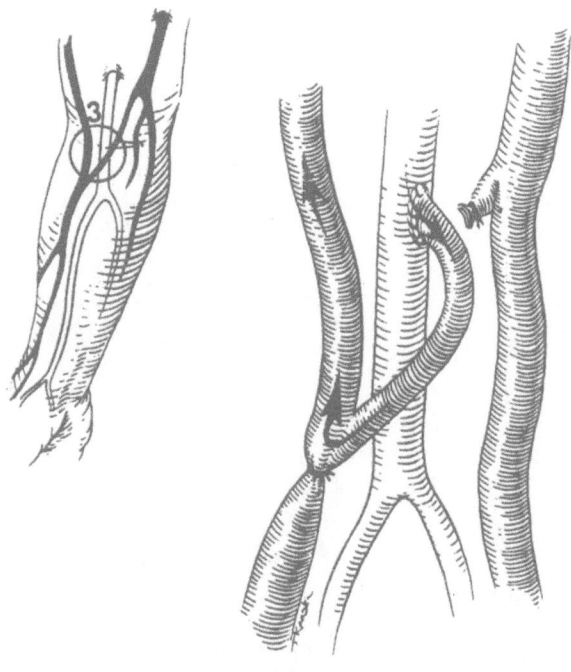

Figure 4. The median cubital vein can be anastomosed to the brachial artery to create an upper arm Cimino fistula (Area 3). (Reprinted with permission of WB Saunders Co.)

mosed, end-to-side, more proximally to the radial artery in the distal third of the forearm. Anastomoses in this area are more difficult as the artery lies deeply beneath the flexor muscles. Use of the cephalic vein in the upper arm, if large, joined to the brachial artery immediately above the antecubital crease often provides an excellent fistula (Figure 3). If buried deeply in subcutaneous fat, it can be exteriorized to lie more superficially by blunt dissection along its course. Alternatively, the median cubital vein can be isolated from its junction with the basilic system above the elbow and anastomosed end-to-side to the proximal brachial artery (Figure 4). This provides arterial flow into the cephalic system, retrograde through the median cubital vein; the cephalic vein should be ligated distal to its junction with the median cubital vein to reduce venous hypertension.

If large and easily visible veins are not available in the upper extremity, an endogenous fistula may be created by lateral transposition of the basilic vein. Although not commonly performed, the transposed brachiobasilic fistula may provide a satisfactory alternative to a prosthetic graft (10). Through a medial longitudinal incision, a length of

basilic vein is mobilized from the axillary vein to an area immediately beyond the antecubital fossa and transected distally. The vein is then tunneled anterolaterally through the subcutaneous tissue to a separate transverse incision just proximal to the antecubital crease and anastomosed to the brachial artery in an end-to-side fashion. In most cases, failure of this fistula does not prevent the future construction of a prosthetic graft if satisfactory venous outflow is still available. Alternatively, an anastomosis can be created between brachial artery and brachial vein and the vein left *in situ* until it matures. The dilated and thickened vein can then be transposed after several weeks in a second operation; to accomplish this, the vein must be divided at or near the original anastomosis, its length isolated, positioned appropriately, then re-anastomosed.

When the venous anatomy of the arm precludes creation of an endogenous fistula, a saphenous vein segment may occasionally be used as an autograft through a looped or curved tunnel between an adequate upper extremity artery and vein (4, 8, 11). This technique may be useful in those individuals who seem to be allergic to PTFE or who react adversely to the material with sterile inflammation. Although the incidence of infection in such grafts is less than with prosthetic ones, the long term occurrence of diffuse stenosis is higher (12). More commonly, the saphenous vein may be used *in situ* as a loop fistula in the thigh (Figure 5). It is isolated through a series of longitudinal incisions from the groin to the knee. Branches are carefully ligated. The saphenofemoral junction is

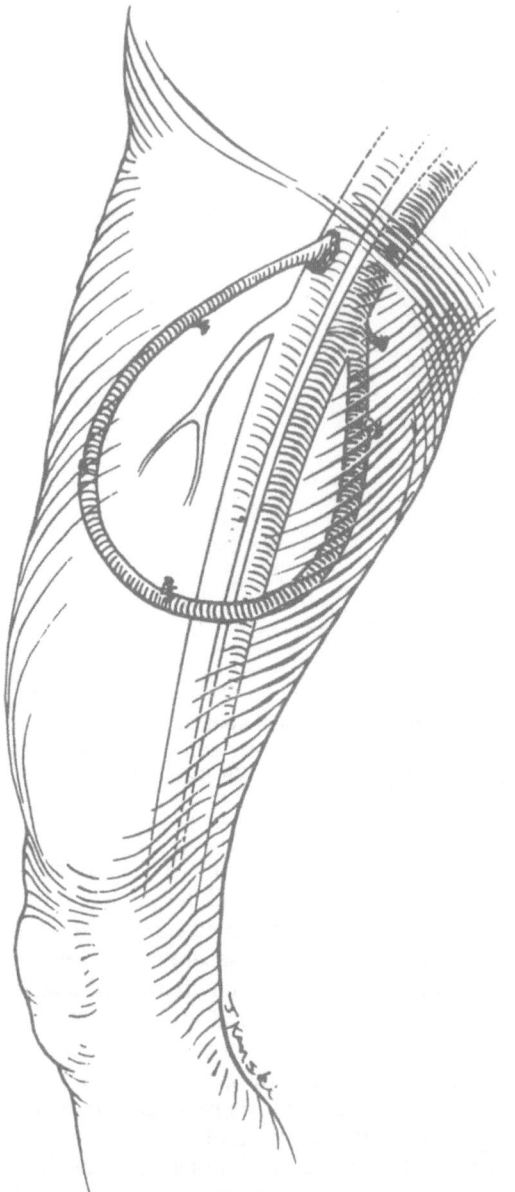

Figure 5.   An autogenous saphenous vein loop fistula can be created in the groin when upper arm sites have been exhausted. The saphenous vein is isolated carefully from just below the knee to the saphenofemoral junction and all branches are carefully ligated. The vein is then positioned in the superficial tunnel and its distal end anastomosed to the femoral artery. (Reprinted with permission of WB Saunders Co.)

kept intact and the vein passed in a U-shaped tunnel to the common femoral artery where it is anastomosed end-to-side. Although used as a last resort, this technique is effective in some difficult long-term patients with limited remaining potential access sites. Because of its propensity to develop stenoses and aneurysms along its length, it is not an optimal solution.

PROSTHETIC GRAFTS

When the patient's superficial veins are inadequate or unavailable, prosthetic grafts become necessary even though the rate of infection and thrombosis may increase; indeed, they are used more commonly than native vein fistulae. Expanded polytetrafluoroethylene (PTFE), is the most popular vascular prosthesis for dialysis access; it has patency rates between 58 and 95% at one year and 36 and 86% at 2 years (12–14). Adequate flow for dialysis and a low incidence of high output cardiac failure or peripheral steal syndrome are achieved with 6 mm PTFE, the most common graft diameter used. Those bearing a spiral external support are occasionally beneficial if joint lines must be crossed, but are usually unnecessary.

As with endogenous fistulae, the most distal site available on the upper extremity is used first; a loop configuration is preferred as it has a significantly higher patency rate than straight conduits and provides more length for cannulation (15). The graft is placed on the ventral aspect of the forearm using the distal brachial artery as inflow and the largest available vein as outflow, either the basilic or cephalic, at or just proximal to the antecubital crease (Figure 6). In patients in whom a previous forearm graft has been removed because of infection, a new forearm loop graft may be made following healing, using more proximal vessels and a different subcutaneous course. If necessary, the proximal basilic vein in the upper arm, the axillary vein in the axillary fossa, the subclavian vein in the infraclavicular position or the internal jugular vein just above the clavicle may be used (Figure 7). In the upper arm, the graft should be positioned on the lateral aspect of the biceps, as it is not only difficult to cannulate for dialysis on the medial aspect but also uncomfortable for the patient to hold the arm in external rotation during the treatment.

Techniques in placement of access prostheses are the same as those used in standard peripheral vascular surgery. After isolating the appropriate vessels at a chosen site, the graft is tunneled subcutaneously in a loop configuration using a curved tunneler (16); some surgeons prefer a straight forearm graft between the radial artery at the wrist and a vein at the antecubital space. Such tunnelers should be the same diameter as the graft to prevent seroma and hematoma formation. Kinking or twisting of the graft must be avoided; many grafts now have longitudinal stripes to help prevent this. Adequate venous outflow is confirmed by irrigating the proximal vein with heparinized saline via a catheter introduced through the longitudinal venotomy created for the venous anastomosis. After the vessels are occluded with loops, the graft is beveled obliquely and anastomosed end-to-side to the vessel using continuous 5-0 or 6-0 monofilament suture. Upon completion of the first anastomosis, heparinized saline is placed in the vessel, the graft clamped and the second anastomosis constructed. Systemic heparinization is rarely necessary. As with the Cimino fistula, it is helpful

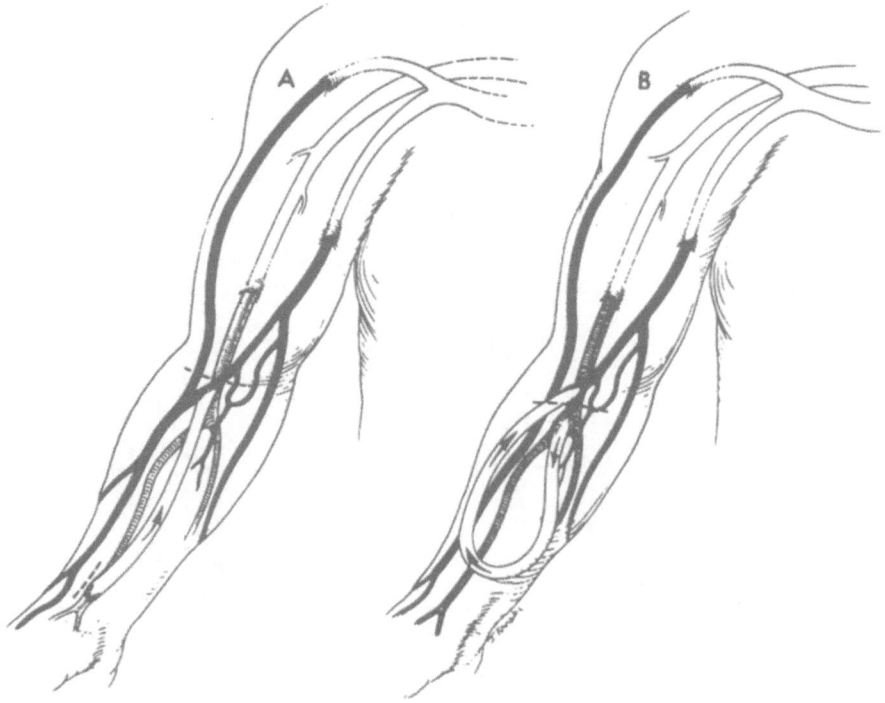

Figure 6. PTFE is commonly used for dialysis access in the forearm. A. A straight graft can be run between the distal radial artery and a convenient venous channel at the antecubital space. B. A forearm loop prosthesis is placed in a U configuration between the brachial artery and a convenient venous channel at the antecubital space. The loop configuration provides more length for cannulation and a higher patency rate than the straight graft. (Reprinted with permission of WB Saunders Co.)

to isolate a short segment of vein proximal to the anastomosis to allow dilatation with arterial flow. A venous thrill should be palpable after this maneuver. By temporarily occluding the graft with direct finger pressure the proximal graft pulse should increase; when the finger is subsequently released, the pulse should diminish. A bounding pulse in the absence of a thrill suggests venous obstruction. As with Cimino fistulae, such a finding at the end of an otherwise satisfactory procedure cannot always be explained or corrected.

As a last resort in difficult or long term patients with multiple previous access failures, vessels of the lower extremity may be used . Prosthetic grafts may be positioned between the distal superficial femoral or popliteal artery and the proximal saphenous or femoral vein. Alternatively, a femoro-femoral loop can be constructed over the anterior medial aspect of the upper thigh between the common or proximal superficial femoral artery and saphenous or femoral vein (17). Some have advocated axillary-axillary or brachial-internal jugular grafts in such patients, although grafts running across the neck or sternum are disfiguring and cannula placement and stabilization unpleasant (18). Grafts in the lower extremity should be avoided in patients with diabetes or peripheral vascular compromise.

ALTERNATIVE GRAFT MATERIAL

Although no graft material has been thoroughly satisfactory for dialysis access, biological materials in particular have not lived up to their potential. The one year patency rates of bovine grafts, prepared from cow carotid artery treated with aldehyde and alcohol, range from 33 to 95% in several series; however, at 2 years, patency rates fall to 6 to 24% (12, 19–22). Stenoses at the venous anastomosis are common and the rate of infection high. Most problematic, if they become infected, they rapidly degenerate, leaving only a blood-filled subcutaneous tunnel lined with sludge. Similarly, while human umbilical vein grafts have been available since 1974, little enthusiasm has been shown for their use (23, 24).

PREOPERATIVE CARE

The site for access placement should be chosen to offer the greatest long-term function, preservation of potential future locations and convenience to the patient. A distal site in the non-dominant arm is optimal, if available. Venipunctures and intravenous catheters must be avoided in the chosen extremity. If a Cimino fistula is planned, the cephalic vein should be evaluated by applying a tourni-

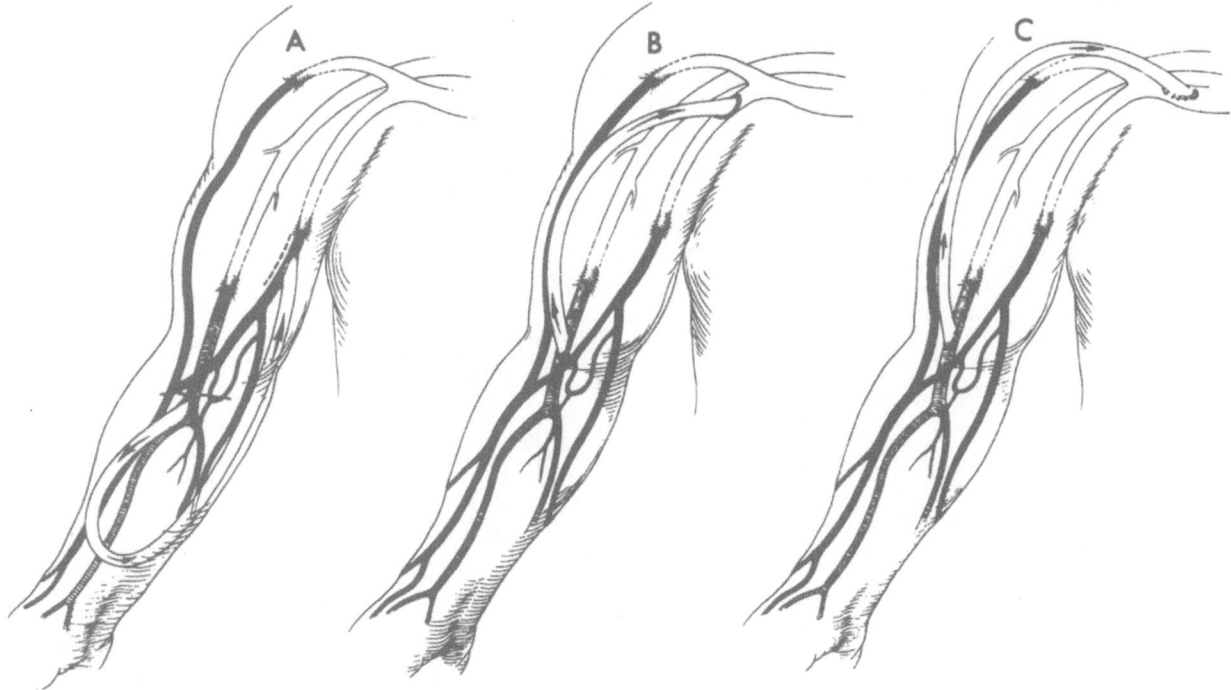

Figure 7.   A. When distal veins have all been used, the venous limb of the prosthesis can be anastomosed more proximally to the basilic vein. B. A new prosthetic graft may be placed between the brachial artery and the proximal brachial vein in the axilla. C. The venous end can also be anastomosed to either the subclavian vein in the infraclavicular position (pictured) or the internal jugular vein just above the clavicle (not pictured). (Reprinted with permission of WB Saunders Co.)

quet to the upper arm and observing its location and size. Both ulnar and radial arterial flow should be confirmed with an Allen test. The incidence of clinically unsuspected but significant subclavian stenosis has been reported to be 40% in patients who have had a prior indwelling subclavian vein dialysis catheter (25). As this can lead to reduced access outflow with venous hypertension and thrombosis, a preoperative venogram may be helpful if access surgery is planned for an extremity of such an individual. Preoperative venography is not indicated for the asymptomatic patient with a prior internal jugular dialysis catheter as the incidence of significant, clinically unsuspected subclavian stenosis using this approach is low (26). Construction of a permanent fistula several weeks prior to the initiation of dialysis will avoid the need for temporary access as incisions will heal and the graft will become incorporated into the surrounding tissues. If the patient is currently undergoing dialysis treatments, surgery should be coordinated with the dialysis schedule, paying careful attention to the preoperative volume status and serum potassium levels. There should be no evidence of either local or systemic infection, especially if prosthetic material is to be used. A temporary dialysis catheter; such as a Quinton–Hickman inserted into the contralateral jugular vein, may be placed at the time of permanent access surgery to allow convenient dialysis until the new fistula can be used.

POSTOPERATIVE CARE

Cimino fistulae are often created as outpatient procedures in an ambulatory surgery setting. They should not be used for several weeks to allow the fistula to dilate and the vein wall to thicken. Intermittent tourniquet application proximal to the fistula is carried out to facilitate this maturation process.

Some PTFE grafts tend to extrude beads of serum into the perigraft space which can cause significant arm edema and discomfort immediately after their placement. The extremity should be continuously elevated for 24 to 48 hours postoperatively to reduce pain and swelling. Care should be taken to prevent systemic hypotension and external compression of the graft site which can cause early thrombosis. The graft should not be used for dialysis for at least 3 weeks to allow the surrounding tissues to heal firmly around the graft, preventing perigraft hematoma.

PATENCY RATES

In a review of 324 arteriovenous conduits constructed over a 4 year period at the Brigham and Women's Hospital, satisfactory rates of function were demonstrated for both Cimino fistulae and PTFE grafts by life table analysis (14). The results confirmed those obtained previously by others (4, 13, 15, 27) and suggested that the cumulative patency rates for PTFE in particular exceed most other grafts, particularly those of biological origin (12, 28, 29). In the Brigham series, the cumulative patency of 163 PTFE grafts was 83% at one year and 70% at 2 years. In contrast, 64% of 154 Cimino fistulae were patent at one year and 50% at 2 years; the lower survival of the native vein fistulae resulted from early failures, usually in the first postoperative month. Although in most cases such failure was secondary to the use of veins of marginal quality, as noted at operation, it was elected to proceed in the hope that the use of a synthetic graft could be avoided. There was no difference in patency of Cimino fistulae created at the wrist and in the antecubital fossa. Importantly, when the earlier failures were not considered, PTFE grafts and endogenous fistulae had equivalent survival over a 4 year period. Once established, however, Cimino fistulae develop fewer complications than PTFE grafts and usually function for more prolonged periods.

COMPLICATIONS

Thrombosis and stenosis

Thrombosis is the most common cause of fistula failure and may occur early or late after placement. Early thrombosis (within the first few months) is less common and usually the result of technical error or inadequate vascular inflow or outflow. In the Brigham series, 50% of PTFE grafts required thrombectomy or revision to maintain their function; recurrent thrombosis represented 56% of the total (14). Although thrombosis may be induced by external pressure on the fistula, dehydration, hypotension, hypovolemia (usually associated with dialysis), or a hypercoaguable state often occurring after surgery, outflow stenosis is at fault in the majority of instances. This usually occurs in the vein, at or near the venous anastomosis, secondary to neointimal fibrous hyperplasia from the arterial flow. Diffuse areas of stenosis may also develop within the fistula, presumably due to accumulation of organized laminar clot and scarring at frequently used puncture sites. Some individuals develop a progressively occlusive dense neointima, tightly adherent to the graft lumen. This is usually impossible to remove and often necessitates placement of a new PTFE graft. Atherosclerotic changes have been described in this neointima (30).

Although usually performed soon after thrombosis to keep within the dialysis schedule, successful thrombectomies of PTFE fistulae can be accomplished as long as 2 weeks later, as the clot seems to organize exceedingly slowly. As initial treatment, thrombectomy under local or regional anesthesia is performed. The fistula is opened surgically through a small transverse incision placed near the

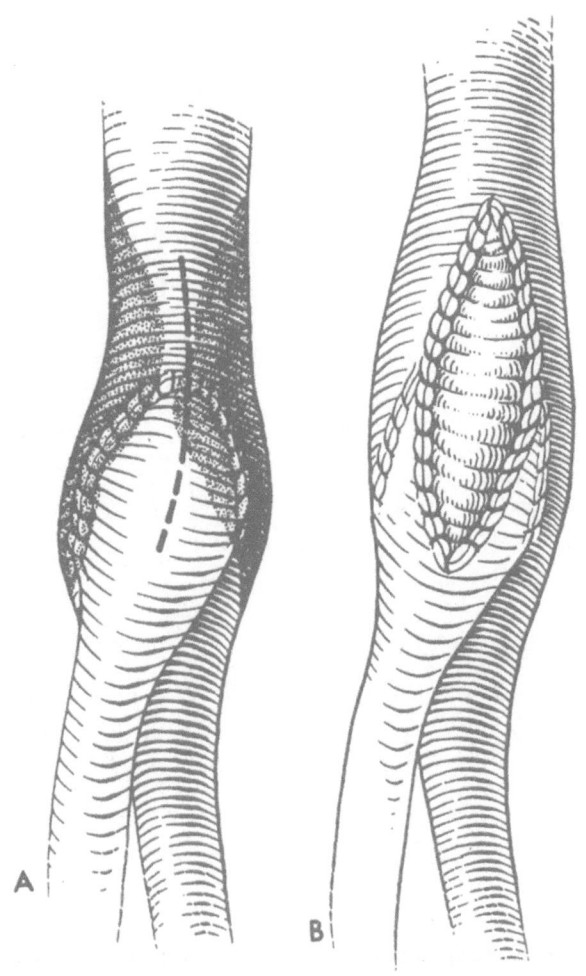

Figure 8. A stenosis at or near the graft venous anastomosis can be patched using a native vein patch or prosthetic material. (Reprinted with permission of WB Saunders Co.)

anastomosis of Cimino fistulae or adjacent to the venous anastomosis in synthetic grafts. Clot is removed using an appropriate Fogarty balloon-tipped catheter. If fistula thrombosis is due to mechanical obstruction, discovered at the time of thrombectomy, surgical revision or repair should be performed either then or conveniently thereafter.

A short stenotic segment found within a Cimino fistula can be repaired locally using a vein patch (Figure 8). When the stenosis occurs at the anastomotic site, however, a new fistula should be created by using the already dilated vein and a more proximal arterial site, or reconstituted by using a short PTFE jump graft between a new arterial site and the vein. Rarely, a Cimino fistula will clot secondary to external pressure. These can be reopened using a fine Fogarty catheter; and must be undertaken relatively promptly as thrombus seems to adhere rapidly to vascular

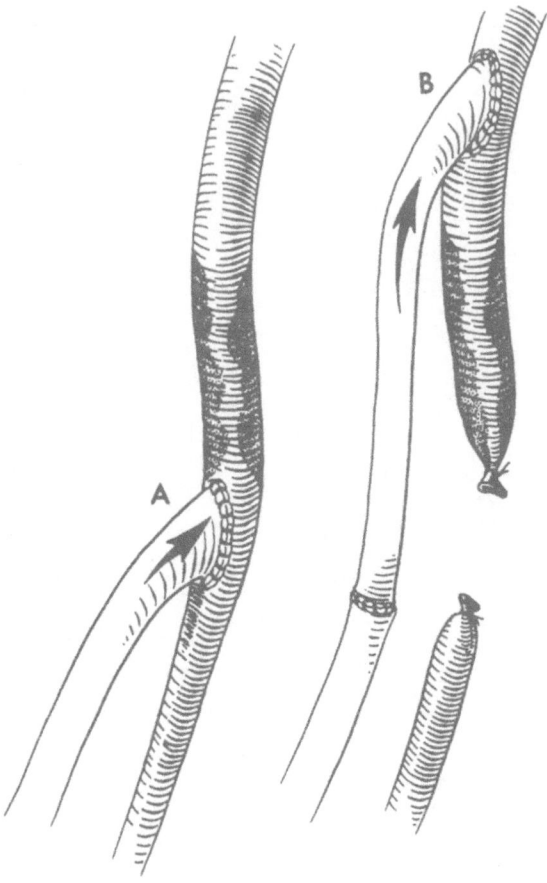

Figure 9. Lengthy stenoses proximal to the graft venous anastomosis can be bypassed using a jump graft anastomosed to an uninvolved proximal segment of vein. (Reprinted with permission of WB Saunders Co.)

endothelium. If thrombophlebitis develops, thrombectomy is useless as the inflamed vein will reclot.

Correction of stenosis may result in prolonged PTFE graft survival equivalent to that of unrevised grafts (14). It is noteworthy that for such devices, a significantly higher cumulative patency was noted if an outflow stenosis was bypassed as compared either to simple thrombectomy or the use of a patch (14); a jump graft of prosthetic material may easily be run between the original prosthesis to a more proximal uninvolved portion of the vein (Figure 9). In addition, a focal intragraft stenosis can be isolated and bypassed with an interposed segment of PTFE using an end-to-end anastomosis on each side.

A recent approach to thrombosis involves clot lysis with thrombolytic agents administered directly into the thrombus through percutaneous catheters. Following clot dissolution (usually after several hours) a fistulogram is performed which may demonstrate a stenosis as the cause which may be amenable to immediate angioplasty. Alternatively, and usually more effectively, the anatomic infor-

mation gained from a fistulogram will allow appropriate surgical revision. Although angioplastied stenoses often recur within a relatively short time; the maneuver may allow corrective surgery to be scheduled at a more convenient later time.

Aneurysm and pseudoaneurysm

Aneurysmal complications of arteriovenous fistulae may be an additional cause for thrombosis. True aneurysms of Cimino fistulae occur primarily at the anastomotic site and along areas of the vein where the wall is weakened by multiple venipunctures. Most remain asymptomatic, although occasionally the overlying skin may become attenuated and ulcerate or the aneurysm can become thrombosed or infected. If symptomatic, cosmetically unacceptable, or bothersome after successful transplantation, the aneurysm can be excised after proximal and distal ligation. If desired, a new access can then be constructed elsewhere. Thrombosis can occur from stagnation of blood and progressive layering of laminar clot both in sacular aneurysms and in large fusiform aneurysms involving much of the venous limb. Although it is sometimes possible to remove such a clot with a Fogarty catheter or by expressing the thrombus from the aneurysm by direct pressure via a venotomy, one often has to open into the sac to remove the clot. Most Cimino fistulae with thrombosed aneurysms should be revised if possible or established elsewhere, as thrombosis tends to recur.

Pseudoaneurysms in PTFE grafts may result from unsealed needle puncture sites anywhere along their course, particularly in areas which are repeatedly cannulated. Like true aneurysms, they may become thrombosed, locally symptomatic, cosmetically undesirable or infected. Overall, pseudoaneurysm formation in PTFE accounts for only 2% of malfunctions (14); treatment is by local excision, closure, or restoration of continuity with an interposition graft if necessary. True aneurysms of PTFE grafts occasionally occur and are usually caused by repeated cannulations at the same site along the graft. Their management is identical to that of pseudoaneurysms.

Ischemia

Ischemic symptoms of the hand or forearm distal to a well functioning fistula occur relatively infrequently, most often in diabetic patients, and may be difficult to resolve. Both arterial insufficiency and venous hypertension may contribute to the low flow state. Insufficient arterial inflow to the hand may result in a vascular steal phenomenon whereby blood to the already compromised distal vessels is shunted directly to the proximal fistula or where blood flows retrograde from the palmar arches through the radial artery into the fistula. For example, when thumb blood pressure was used as an index of perfusion, occlusion of the radial artery distal to a Cimino fistula resulted in a significant increase in pressure in 88% of patients studied, only a small proportion of whom had ischemic symptoms (31). In one series (32), 42% of patients with side-to-side radiocephalic fistulae and 16% of those with end-to-side fistulae had intermittent hand claudication with exercise. A cool, bluish, and painful hand with rest pain is often relieved by placing the hand in a dependent position. Rarely, a fixed and functionless hand may result, and occasionally overt necrosis of the fingertips may occur.

As the majority of ischemic symptoms improve within several weeks following fistula placement, a period of temporization is essential. Occasionally, symptoms are severe enough to demand surgical recourse; in the case of PTFE grafts, this entails narrowing the diameter by banding it, use of a tapered graft or by replacing the arterial limb of the existing graft with a smaller diameter step graft, maneuvers which are only occasionally effective. Reduced fistula flow, at least theoretically, drives more arterial blood distally into the hand. In the case of the end-to-side Cimino fistula, ischemic symptoms may be alleviated by ligating the radial artery just distal to the fistula. This reduces retrograde radial blood flow and improves perfusion to the hand and requires a patent ulnar artery. Promising results have been reported using a revascularization technique for the treatment of both prosthetic and endogenous angioaccess-induced ischemia; this involves ligation the artery just distal to the fistula followed by an arterial bypass from a point proximal to the origin of the fistula to a point distal to the ligature (33).

The situation may be different when a patient presents with venous hypertension. A proximal venous occlusion or stenosis of a major vein may sometimes be demonstrated by angiography with major collateralization around it and often with significant retrograde venous flow into the distal venous system. This condition may occur secondary to axillary vein thrombosis of any cause or following an indwelling subclavian vein catheter. Such occlusions may rarely be improved with angioplasty or surgical bypass; however, if extensive or very proximal, a new access should be created at another site so as to stop arterial fistula flow into the site of stenosis.

Congestive heart failure

High output cardiac failure may be associated with arteriovenous fistulae in a few patients with pre-existing cardiac disease, including congestive heart failure of any cause, prolonged hypertension, or coronary artery disease (34). Excessive flow through the fistula, usually between 20 to 50% of the cardiac output, with a concomitant increase in venous return, may cause a deleterious rise in cardiac preload. Occasionally, venous fistulae may hypertrophy enormously, carrying very large amounts of blood flow (Figure 10). By reducing fistula flow with simple ligation, banding, or interposition of a tapered synthetic segment, cardiac performance may be increased, although such manipulations are usually not particularly effective. A large fistulae may need to be ligated or removed, and a

new fistula created. Peritoneal dialysis may be an alternative in such fragile individuals.

Infection

A common cause of prosthetic access failure is infection; for example, at Brigham and Women's Hospital, graft sepsis accounted for 19% of PTFE graft complications (14). The incidence of sepsis appears to correlate with the completeness of the neointimal lining and time following graft insertion (12, 35, 36). In contrast, infection of Cimino fistulae is rare, usually localized to a needle site and often treated effectively by antibiotics and local care. In descending order of frequency; Staphylococcus aureus, Staphylococcus epidermidis, other gram positive cocci, and a variety of gram negative organisms are causative agents. Bacteria may be inoculated during graft puncture for dialysis; the presence of a peri-graft hematoma, aneurysm with associated thrombus, operative thrombectomy or reconstructive procedures increases the risk (37, 38). Therefore, strict aseptic technique during dialysis and perioperative antibiotics at operation are mandatory (4, 36). In inner city populations, direct injection of illicit street drugs into the access is a surprisingly common source of infection. HIV is becoming an increasing problem in the dialysis population, especially among patients with a history of drug abuse or multiple blood transfusions. The immunosuppression inherent in this disease inhibits host defenses against and masks the signs and symptoms of infection.

Prosthetic graft infection has a variable presentation. Although pain, tenderness, swelling, erythema or fluid collections around the superficially placed graft are easily identified, the process can also be extremely subtle, with few obvious manifestations. Occasionally, the interior of the graft may be colonized without overt inflammation in the febrile patient with positive blood cultures. Once all other possibilities for sepsis have been ruled out, the graft should be removed.

With a severe abscess or septicemia secondary to an infected Cimino fistula or aneurysm, the infected vein must be excised and the subcutaneous tunnel drained (35). In 50% of infected PTFE prostheses, it is possible to bypass a localized septic area with a jump graft, close the new incisions, then excise and drain the involved portion (14). If the infection is generalized and purulent material tracks along the length of the prosthesis, or if an anastomosis is involved, the entire graft should be removed and the tunnel packed open (14, 36, 39). Although resection of the venous and arterial anastomoses has been recommended in the face of extensive tunnel infection (36), subsequent repair of the involved artery to ensure patency can be problematic, particularly if the edges of the arteriotomy are friable or if the patient is a diabetic. Isolation of the artery in an inflamed or infected site may be difficult. To obviate this problem, a 2 to 3 mm oversewn cuff of PTFE may be safely left at the arterial anastomosis if

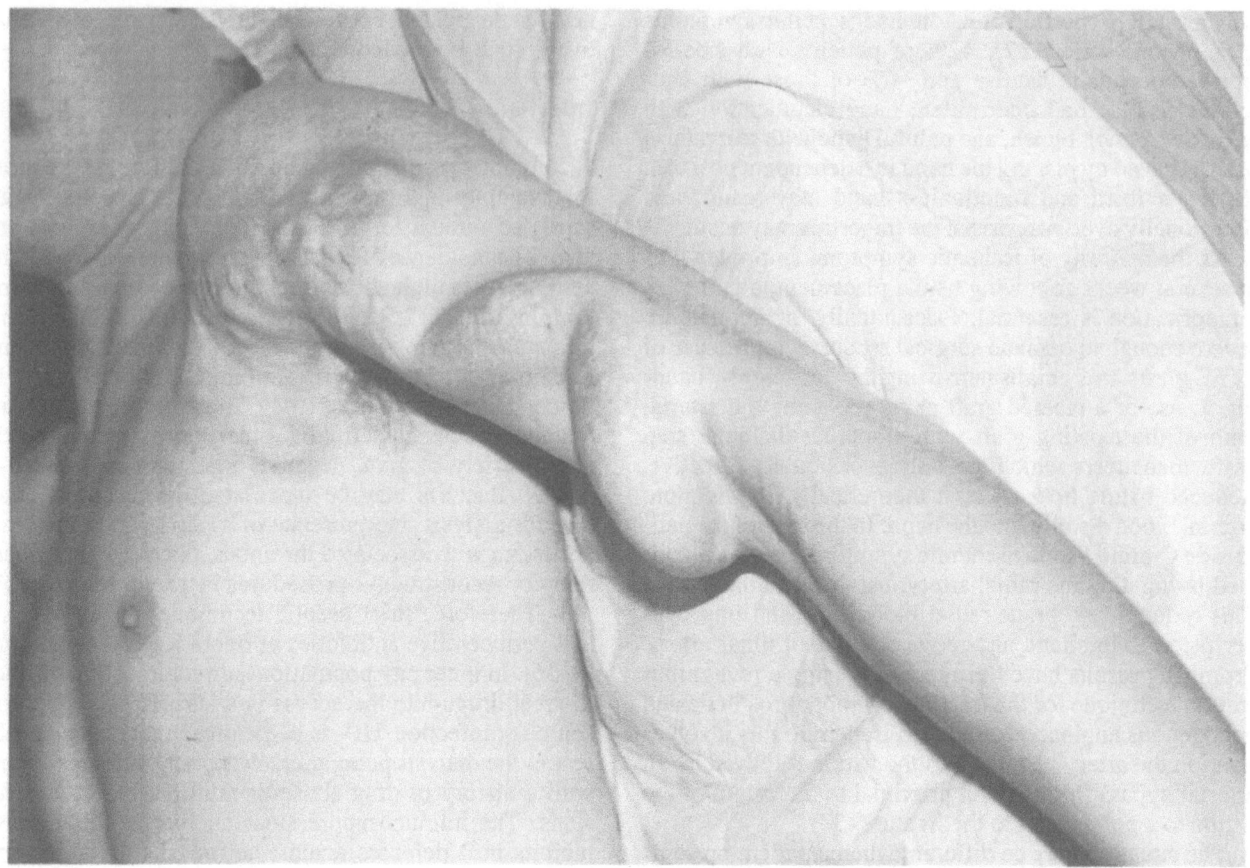

Figure 10. Cimino fistulae occasionally become enormous because of dilatation or aneurysms. These can cause superficial skin erosion, congestive heart failure or cosmetic dissatisfaction. This patient required excision of the dilated cephalic vein because of incipient congestive heart failure.

the remainder of the graft, including the venous anastomosis, is excised and the entire tunnel tract debrided and irrigated with antibiotics. This method is recommended if progressive, severe infection stops short of the arterial anastomotic site (39). The skin incision over the vessels is usually closed primarily, the remainder allowed to heal by secondary intention. Another graft may be placed later in the healed extremity, using more proximal vessels.

The type and location of the access influences rates of infection and treatment. As noted, the incidence of infection in biological grafts (bovine carotid artery, human umbilical vein) is higher than in native vessels; once infected, such grafts dissolve (40). Furthermore, the incidence of bacteremic episodes in individuals with prosthetic grafts is twice that of endogenous fistulae and three times higher for patients with fistulae placed in the groin regardless of the material used (41). Infections in the femoral triangle are especially difficult to control. In one large series, 27 out of 161 patients (17%) with groin fistulae developed infection (42). Overall mortality and amputation rate of those patients developing groin sepsis was reported to be 18 and 22%, respectively. Bacteremia from

a septic focus may also produce serious complications, including septic pulmonary emboli, myocardial abscess, endocarditis, empyema, meningitis, osteomyelitis, or infection of joint prostheses. However, in the aforementioned study, most patients with an infected groin access were treated appropriately for 4 to 6 weeks beginning within 48 h of discovery; 71% of these became afebrile within 3 days (40). Nine cases of endocarditis, usually of the aortic valve (2.7% of those on chronic hemodialysis), were reported in another study; the diagnosis was difficult, although the development of murmurs, central nervous system abnormalities of varying degrees of seriousness, and occasional peripheral emboli were described (43).

Diabetes

The patient with diabetes mellitus and end-stage kidney failure often poses difficult problems for the surgeon. Anastomosis may be challenging as arteries of the upper extremity are often small with diffuse arteriosclerosis, fragility of the wall, and calcification of the media. Arterial inflow may be unsatisfactory. The groin should not be used as an access site in these individuals because of their increased propensity for infection and because diffuse peripheral vascular involvement of the lower extremities is almost invariable and the potential threat of steal ominous. Access infections in this population are potential hazards regardless of the type of prosthesis used (44). As noted, necrosis and painful ulceration of the finger tips have been described in diabetic patients bearing upper extremity fistulae, presumably secondary to vascular steal in conjunction with compromised microcirculation (45) and inability of the distal arterial tree to dilate. Rarely in such individuals, the entire hand is compromised with a Volkman's contracture, or may develop gangrene and be lost.

Another difficulty that occasionally occurs in this patient population is their inability to heal small skin incisions made over graft thrombectomy sites. Often, many days after the procedure, the graft itself or the suture line may be seen at the bottom of a small non-healing area in the skin. This site inevitably becomes infected, a jump graft can be run around the area and the exposed portion removed.

CONCLUSION

Despite a significant early failure rate, a Cimino fistula should be considered first when hemodialysis access becomes necessary as it may provide many years of successful function with infrequent complication. A PTFE graft offers an excellent alternative when native vessels are inadequate or unavailable. It allows a versatility of location and can usually function for prolonged periods, with repair or revision as necessary.

REFERENCES

1. Graham WB: Historical aspects of hemodialysis. *Transplant Proc* 9: xlix, 1977
2. Quinton WE, Dillard DH, Scribner BH: Cannulation of blood vessels for prolonged hemodialysis. *Trans Am Soc Artif Intern Organs* 6: 104, 1960
3. Brescia MJ, Cimino JE, Appel K, Hurwich BJ: Chronic hemodialysis using venipuncture and a surgically created arteriovenous fistula. *N Engl J Med* 275: 1089, 1966
4. Jenkins AM, Buist TAS, Glover SD: Medium-term follow-up of forty autogenous vein and forty polytetrafluorethylene (Gortex) grafts for vascular access. *Surgery* 88: 667, 1980
5. Whittemore AD: Vascular access for hemodialysis, in *Surgical Care of the Patient with Renal Failure*, edited by Tilney NL, Lazarus JM, Philadelphia, WB Saunders Co, 1982, p 49
6. Tilney NL, Whittemore AD: Dialysis access in difficult patients, in *Vascular Surgery*, edited by Bell PRF, Tilney NL, London, Butterworths, 1984, p 175
7. Bossell JA, Abbott JA, Lim RC: A radial steal syndrome with arteriovenous fistula for hemodialysis. *Ann Intern Med* 75: 387, 1971
8. May J, Tiller D, Johnson J, Stewart J, Sheil AG: Saphenous vein arteriovenous fistula in regular dialysis treatment. *N Engl J Med* 280: 770, 1969
9. Wedgwood KR, Wiggins PA, Guillou PJ: A prospective study of end-to-side vs side-to-side arteriovenous fistulas for haemodialysis. *Br J Surg* 71: 540, 1984
10. Rivers SP, Scher LA, Sheehan E, Lynn R, Veith FJ: Basilic vein transposition: an underused autologous alternative to prosthetic dialasis angioaccess. *J Vasc Surg* 18: 391, 1993
11. Gerardet RE, Hackett RE, Goodwin NJ, Friedman EA: Thirteen months' experience with the saphenous vein graft arteriovenous fistula for maintenance hemodialysis. *Trans Am Soc Artif Intern Organs* 16: 285, 1970
12. Morgan AP, Dammin GJ, Lazarus JM: Failure modes in secondary vascular access for hemodialysis. *ASAIO J* 1: 44, 1978
13. Hammill FS, Johnson GG, Collins GM: A critical appraisal of the changing approaches to vascular access for chronic dialysis. *Proc Eur Dial Transplant Assoc* 9: 325, 1980
14. Palder SB, Kirkman RL, Whittemore AD, Hakim RM, Lazarus JM, Tilney NL: Vascular access for hemodialysis. *Ann Surg* 202: 235, 1985
15. Munda R, First MR, Alexander JW, Linneman CC Jr, Fidler JP, Kittur D: Polytetrafluoroethylene graft survival in hemodialysis. *JAMA* 249: 219, 1983
16. Salvatierra O Jr, Feduska NJ: Construction of the optimal tunnel for interposition arteriovenous hemodialysis fistulas. *Surgery* 94: 508, 1983
17. Mandel SR, McDougal EG: Popliteal artery to saphenous vein vascular access for hemodialysis. *Surg Gynecol Obstet* 160: 358, 1985
18. Haimov M: Vascular access for hemodialysis – new modifications for the difficult patient. *Surgery* 92: 109, 1982
19. Rosenthal JJ, Spigelman A, Gaspar MR, Mavius HJ: Problems with bovine heterografts for hemodialysis. *Am J Surg* 130: 182, 1975
20. Johnson JM, Kenoyer MR, Johnson KE, Potter DJ, Nickas GM, Williams T: The modified bovine heterograft in vascular access for chronic hemodialysis. *Ann Surg* 183: 62, 1976
21. Hurt AV, Batello-Cruz M, Skipper BJ, Teaf SR, Sterling WA Jr: Bovine carotid artery heterograft versus polytetrafluoroethylene grafts. *Am J Surg* 146: 844, 1983
22. Naimov M, Jacobson NJ: Experience with modified bovine arterial heterograft in peripheral reconstruction and vascular access for hemodialysis. *Ann Surg* 180: 291, 1974
23. Mindich BP, Silverman MJ, Elguezabel A, Levowitz BS: Umbilical cord vein fistula for vascular access in hemodialysis. *Trans Am Soc Artif Intern Organs* 21: 273, 1975
24. Dardik H, Ibrahim IK, Dardik I: Arteriovenous fistulas constructed with modified human umbilical cord vein graft. *Arch Surg* 111: 60, 1976
25. Surratt RS, Picus D, Hicks ME, Darcy MD, Kleinhoffer M, Jendrisak M: The importance of preoperative evaluation of the subclavian vein in dialysis access planning. *Am J Roentgenol* 156: 623, 1991
26. Cimochowski GE, Worley E, Rutherford WE, Sartain J, Blondin J, Harter H: Superiority of the internal jugular over the subclavian access for temporary dialysis. *Nephron* 54: 154, 1990

27. Etheredge EE, Haid SD, Maeser MN, Sicard GA, Anderson CB: Salvage operations for malfunctioning polytetrafluoroethylene hemodialysis access grafts. *Surgery* 94: 464, 1983

28. Tellis VA, Kohlberg WI, Bhat DJ, Driscoll B, Veith FJ: Expanded polytetrafluoroethylene graft fistula for chronic hemodialysis. *Ann Surg* 189: 101, 1979

29. Sabanayagam P, Soricelli R, Schwartz A: Experience with 225 expanded PTFE arteriovenous fistulae for chronic maintenance hemodialysis. Presented at the Annual Meeting of the European Society for Artificial Organs, Geneva, Switzerland, Sept 29–Oct 1, 1979

30. Selman SH, Rhodes RS, Anderson JM, DePalma RG, Clowes AW: Atheromatous changes in expanded polytetrafluorethylene grafts. *Surgery* 87: 630, 1980

31. Duncan H, Ferguson L, Faris I: Incidence of the radial steal syndrome in patients with Brescia fistula for hemodialysis: its clinical significance. *J Vasc Surg* 4: 144, 1986

32. Kinnaert P, Strugven J, Mathieu J, Vereerstraeten P, Toussaint C, Van Geertruyden J: Intermittent claudication of the hand after creation of an arteriovenous fistula in the forearm. *Am J Surg* 139: 838, 1980

33. Schanzer H, Sklandany M, Haimov M: Treatment of angioaccess-induced ischemia by revascularization. *Vasc Surg* 16: 861, 1992

34. Anderson CB, Codd JR, Graff RA, Groce MA, Harter HR, Newton WT: Cardiac failure and upper extremity arteriovenous dialysis fistulas. Case reports and a review of the literature. *Arch Intern Med* 136: 292, 1976

35. Nsouli KA, Lazarus JM, Schoenbaum SC, Gottlieb MN, Lowrie EG, Shocair M: Bacteremic infection in hemodialysis. *Arch Intern Med* 139: 1255, 1979

36. Bhat DJ, Tellis VA, Kohlberg WI, Driscoll B, Veith FJ: Management of sepsis involving expanded polytetrafluoroethylene grafts for hemodialysis access. *Surgery* 187: 445, 1980

37. Malone JM, Moore WS, Campagna G, Bean B: Bacteremic infectability of vascular grafts: the influence of pseudointimal integrity and duration of graft function. *Surgery* 78: 211, 1975

38. Roon AJ, Malone JM, Moore WS, Bean B, Campagna G: Bacteremic infectability: a function of vascular graft material and design. *J Surg Res* 22: 489, 1977

39. Gifford RM: Management of tunnel infections of dialysis polytetrafluoroethylene grafts. *J Vasc Surg* 2: 854, 1985

40. Dobkin JF, Miller MH, Steigbigel NA: Septicemia in patients on chronic hemodialysis. *Ann Intern Med* 88: 28, 1978

41. O'Brien TF: Infection in dialysis and transplant patients. in *Surgical Care of the Patient with Renal Failure*, edited by Tilney NL, Lazarus JM, Philadelphia, WB Saunders Co, 1982, p 67

42. Morgan AP, Knight DC, Tilney NL, Lazarus JM: Femoral triangle sepsis in dialysis patients. *Ann Surg* 191: 460, 1980

43. Leonard A, Raij L, Shapiro FL: Bacterial endocarditis in regularly dialyzed patients. *Kidney Int* 4: 407, 1973

44. Morgan AP, Lazarus JM: Vascular access for dialysis. *Am J Surg* 129: 432, 1975

45. Najarian JS, Sutherland DER, Simmons RL, Howard RJ, Kjelistrand CM, Mauer SM, Kennedy W, Ramsay R, Barbosa J, Goetz FC: Kidney transplantation for the uremic diabetic patient. *Surg Gynecol Obstet* 144: 682, 1977

MALFUNCTIONING HEMODIALYSIS ACCESS: DIAGNOSIS AND PERCUTANEOUS TREATMENT

DIERK VORWERK, ROLF W. GÜNTHER and HEINZ-GÜNTHER SIEBERTH

Malfunction of hemodialysis access is a frequent problem in hemodialysis patients and requires an adequate diagnostic and therapeutic approach thus making percutaneous interventions a technique of growing importance for interventional radiologists.

An increasing number of patients are joining chronic dialysis programs which are no longer restricted to a highly selected subgroup of younger patients. About 150 to 200 individuals (1) – according to modern statistics more than 300 – per million are involved in Western countries (1). Despite of refinement of dialysis techniques, prognosis of shunt function, however, is still limited. There are approximately no more than 15% of shunts permanently well functioning (2). Even primary patency of noncomplicated hemodialysis fistulae is low. Keller et al. found a 1-year primary patency of 65% for Brescia–Cimino AV fistulae and 50% for graft shunts (3). For Brescia–Cimino shunts, primary patency after 2 years and 4 years was 60 and 45% respectively; for graft shunts it was even lower with 43 and 10% (3). In case shunt repair was included, overall patency of shunts improved slightly. Keller reported 70% (1-year overall patency), about 60% after 2 years and 40–60% after 3 years of follow-up. A significantly better overall patency for Brescia–Cimino fistulae was found after 4 years with 55 vs 29% (graft shunts). Similar overall patencies were reported by other groups such as Palder's (3, 4). Generally, early failure during the maturation period is more common in native shunts while implant shunts mostly have a good early patency but are burdened with a higher rate of late failure due to thrombosis. Thrombosis is the most important reason for shunt failure (5, 6); repair of pseudoaneurysm, infection or steal syndromes are comparably less frequent. Shunt stenosis has been found to be an important co-factor for shunt thrombosis if intervention as a prophylaxis against complete occlusion has been therefore advocated (7).

DIAGNOSIS

Clinical symptoms of malfunction

Several simple clinical symptoms are helpful in order to detect shunt malfunction even in an early stage. Most simple, auscultation of the typical bruit tests sufficiency of shunt flow and can be easily performed on shunts being suspicious for failure or as a test following percutaneous or surgical revision. Absence and discontinuity of the bruit may indicate a stenotic area (8). Although being most important to detect major function problems, it remains a relatively nonspecific test for detection of minor lesions that may also be treated to prevent shunt thrombosis (7).

Palpation of the shunt is a most useful test to get more information on shunt morphology, vessel run and shunt pulsation. It helps to identify stenotic areas which are characterised by a retracted venous wall or poststenotic venous dilatation. Palpation mostly gives a suitable information on thrombus formation and its extension within the vein. If a tourniquet is additionally applied at the upper arm, draining veins can be palpated for collateral pathways and areas can be identified which are suitable for retrograde puncture in case a percutaneous intervention is planned – even if the shunt flow is minimal or absent. Palpation of the shunt should be, therefore, regularly performed not only by the dialysis staff but also by the interventionalist prior to any intervention in order to plan the procedure.

Table 1. Diagnostic techniques

Function	Morphology
Venous pressure	Ultrasound
Doppler ultrasound	Colour-coded duplex sonography
Recirculation fraction	Shuntogram
	Transbrachial fine-needle arteriography
	(Transfemoral angiography)

Several indicators for shunt failure become available during dialysis itself. Collapse by suction during dialysis or needle blockage on the arterial side indicates inflow problems that may be located in the feeding artery at any level, at the anastomotic site or in any distal venous shunt segment close to the anastomosis. Palpation of the radial and brachial artery pulse in combination with Doppler analysis may help to localize the site of inflow obstruction because location of the obstruction site is difficult to assess by clinical means only.

Increase of venous pressure during dialysis serves as an important parameter indicating venous outflow obstruction, which may.be located in the proximal shunt veins or more centrally. Although monitoring of venous counter pressure is easy to perform during hemodialysis, generally relevant data indicating access malfunction are difficult to obtain and strictly requires a standardized procedure of measurement in order to deliver comparable data. Venous counter pressure highly depends on individual data in each patient such as dialysis flow, needle size and position. Thus, in the literature inconsistent data are given that may indicate shunt outflow problems. Schwab and co-workers considered a pressure greater than 150 mm Hg (blood flow 200 ml/min via a 16 G needle) as a threshold indicating venous obstruction (7). However, use of rapid blood flow exceeding 400 ml/min compromises diagnostic sensitivity of elevated venous pressure (9, 10). Far better, marked increase of venous pressure over a period of time in an individual patient undergoing dialysis under comparable circumstances should be strongly suspicious for shunt malfunction thus requiring further diagnostic evaluation by angiography or colour duplex.

Recirculation as a main consequence of shunt malfunction may be also used as a diagnostic parameter. Problem of recirculation depends on the blood flow used for hemodialysis and becomes more evident with high-flow hemodialysis. Windus and co-workers found that urea-based measurement of recirculation exceeding 0.15 was associated with a venous shunt obstruction in 82% and was found to be an excellent indicator for shunt malfunction in high-flow hemodialysis (11). The finding, however, is nonspecific for the location of shunt malfunction.

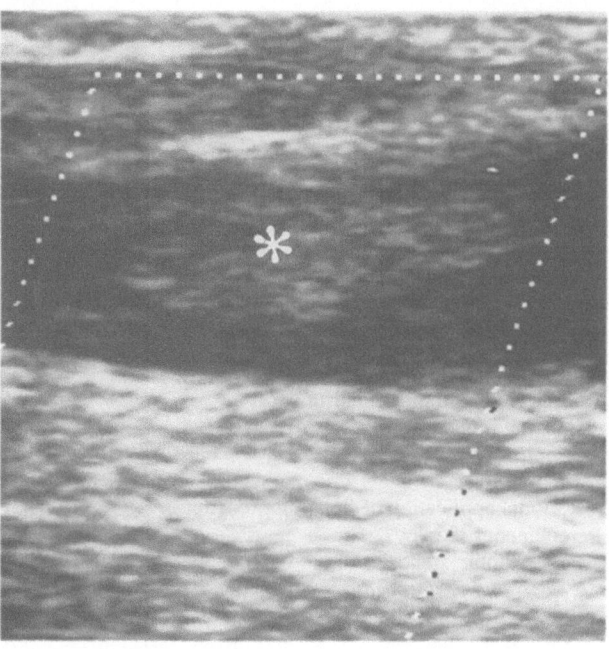

Figure 1. Real-time ultrasound showing thrombus (∗) within a shunt vein.

Imaging procedures

Adequate imaging of hemodialysis fistulae is a prerequisite for shunt intervention. Clinical investigation, doppler and duplex ultrasound and – more recently – color-coded duplex sonography offer important information on the underlying problem (Table 1). They are, however, of limited importance for planning and on-line monitoring of the intervention.

Sonography

Real-time ultrasound is an excellent tool to investigate hemodialysis fistulae both dynamically and morphologically. B-mode sonography is able to depict narrowing of the venous outflow tract or thrombus formation that can be mostly identified by its slightly increased echogenicity (Figure 1). Recent thrombus, however, may be markedly hypoechoic and missed by B-mode sonography alone. Duplex sonography allows additional evaluation of shunt flow by measuring flow velocity and flow volume (11). Introduction of color-coded duplex sonography facilitates sonographic evaluation of hemodialysis shunts by rapid identification of shunt vessels and flow direction. Real-time flow observation allows easy identification of vessel morphology and topography. Flow measurement can be sampled in selected shunt areas. Use of different ultrasound probes varying from 7.5 to 3.0 MHz allows evaluation of all parts from the anastomosis to the upper arm but is of limited accuracy for the central venous portion (12). Combination of narrowing and increase of turbulent flow allows identification of significantly stenosed segments, absence of flow identifies thrombosis. Therefore, color-duplex represents an important noninvasive imaging modality and should be applied – if easily accessible – to shunts being suspicious for failure.

There are, however, several drawbacks limiting the importance of color-duplex for practical routine. Morphological evaluation remains incomplete or confusing when complex morphology is present that includes branching vessel run or extensive collateralization. Only small segments are documented simultaneously and presentation to a third party is difficult requiring (cost-) extensive hardcopy documentation with considerable lack of anatomic orientation (13). Shunt interventions guided by sonography alone have been infrequently reported and may render several practical problems.

Several authors favor duplex sonography as a valuable tool for quantitative analysis of shunt flow in order to evaluate maturity of a newly created fistula or to depict flow obstruction (12, 14, 15). It has, however, to be stressed that quantitative measurements are problematic (10). Firstly, there is no general consensus on the area where flow quantification should be obtained. Some authors use the draining vein although multiple pathways may be present. The anastomotic area is problematic for measuring, since mostly turbulent flow is found there and straight segments are rare (15). Therefore, some authors recommend measurement of the radial artery as a single feeder vessel for the forearm vessels (15) and tissue supply has been assumed to be no more than 10% of whole blood volume (15). Correlation between shunt flow and doppler shunt flow, however, has been found to be rather inaccurate and inconsistent along the shunt varying from one segment to another. Oates and co-workers found that shunt flow may be overestimated by 200 to 600 ml/min (15). Variables that influenced accuracy of measurement were due to doppler angle and measurement of vessel area, filters, beam nonuniformity and doppler system velocity (15). Furthermore shunt flow depends on the age, site and type of the arteriovenous communication thus making it difficult to define general data on doppler shunt flow limits that should request for invasive diagnosis or intervention.

Angiography

Angiography is an accurate but invasive method for diagnosis of shunt problems and for monitoring of therapy. Application of digital subtraction angiography is most important in order to keep the whole amount of contrast low and to achieve maximum information of both the fistula and the draining venous system (16). Access to the vascular system depends on the type of shunt investigated.

In Brescia–Cimino fistulae, we prefer an arterial access for shuntography. The brachial artery is punctured by a 22 G sheathed needle under local anesthesia at the elbow where it usually runs beneath the aponeurosis.

Shuntogram is performed by hand-injection of dilute contrast medium (1 : 2 to 1 : 3) so a total of 20 ml of contrast is mostly sufficient to complete a diagnostic study. We did not encounter any event of a serious complication with this technique over a period of 7 years. Brachial arterial approach has been previously described by Glanz and co-workers using an 18 G sheath needle without reporting complications in a series of 125 shuntograms (17). Other than Zijlstra (18) we recommend brachial access in all cases accessible. Therefore, transfemoral angiography has only exceptional indications and should be limited to selected cases in which a proximal arterial problem is assumed that cannot be diagnosed by a brachial approach. Due to the general morbidity of the vascular system in chronic hemodialysis patients, transfemoral angiography is considered more risky and more difficult. Furthermore, transfemoral approach cannot be easily performed on an outpatient basis.

Direct puncture of the shunt is applied in upper arm native shunts and Goretex implant shunts. For diagnostic studies, we also use a 22 G sheath needle in order to minimize traumatization. Retrograde imaging of the arterial anastomosis is readily obtained by compression of the venous outflow while contrast injection (19).

Both arterial and venous techniques can be applied on outpatients. Shuntograms should always be completed by imaging of the draining upper-arm and central veins in order to exclude additional lesions.

Rational application of imaging procedures

A rational approach to imaging procedures depends on individual circumstances in each patient and facilities in each center.

If a therapeutic intervention seems inevitable or highly probable from clinical information, and percutaneous intervention is the regular approach, angiography should be performed primarily without being preceded by color-duplex since most information of ultrasound will be equally delivered by angiographic data.

If surgery represents the regular approach and the surgeon relies on clinical and sonographic data, angiography may be dropped prior to intervention. If the surgeon, however, requests for angiography prior to intervention, angiography should be done first instead of sonography in order to save time and costs.

It has, however, to be stressed that color-duplex sonography and angiography may be adjunctive rather than competitive under numerous circumstances. If a moderate stenosis is found angiographically, ultrasound may help to judge on its hemodynamic relevance. Furthermore, ultrasound may serve as a noninvasive follow-up instrument after percutaneous intervention for noninvasive monitoring of the acute and interval course. In case of complete shunt occlusion, ultrasound is superior to angiography to determine the extension of the thrombosed segment (14).

Table 2. Type of complication and treatment

	Percutaneous	Surgery
Stenosis		
Arterial stenosis	PTA	New shunt, Neoanastomosis
Anastomotic stenosis	PTA	Neoanastomosis
Venous stenosis	PTA	Patch, neoanastomosis, Jump graft
Central stenosis	PTA + *Stent*	(Bypass)
Thrombosis		
– small thrombus mass	PTA	Thrombectomy, Neoanastomosis
– large thrombus mass	Pharmacological, hydrodynamic or mechanical thrombolysis	Thrombectomy
Chronic venous occlusion		
Peripheral veins	PTA (+ Stent)	Jump graft, neoanastomosis, new shunt
Central veins	PTA + *Stent*	Shunt ligation, (bypass)
Infection	–	Explantation
Aneurysm	(Stent)	Excision
Steal syndrome	–	Shunt banding, ligation

PERCUTANEOUS THERAPY

Percutaneous techniques and predominantly balloon angioplasty has been recommended to be applicable only to a small subset of shunt problems such as short segment stenosis (19). New developments and growing experience on that field, however, have enlarged indications to a greater extent as an alternative to surgical revision (Table 2). Choice of various methods, however, depends on a number of different factors. These include type of shunt (native or goretex implant shunt), type of obstruction (stenosis or occlusion), diameter and location of the lesion. Several percutaneous techniques have been applied to failing shunts that include balloon dilatation (PTA) as the most important technique, atherectomy, stenting, thrombolysis and mechanical thrombectomy. Furthermore, a combination of percutaneous intervention and surgical revision techniques offers various alternatives.

PTA of shunt stenosis

Shunt stenosis is a frequent problem in hemodialysis shunts. Several factors contribute to their development such as high flow, recurrent puncture traumatization, insufficient variation of puncture site, residual venous valves and previous damage to veins used for shunt operation. Stenosis of the distal feeding artery, at the anastomosis of native shunts or stenoses of the venous anastomosis which is frequent in graft shunts (21) are often due to technical problems of underlying surgery. Stenoses may both occur in the punctured section or in draining veins not used for shunt puncture (18). They lead to decreased shunt flow, elevated venous counter-pressure (7), increase of recirculation (22) or arm-swelling in case of central obstruction. Furthermore, they increase the risk of shunt thrombosis (7). Revision of stenotic lesions in time has been shown to be effective in avoiding recurrent shunt thrombosis thus improving the overall patency (7).

It remains, sometimes, difficult to decide on the hemodynamic relevance of stenotic lesions found in hemodialysis fistulae in order to decide on intervention or to determine the endpoint of a procedure. Sullivan and co-workers performed pressure monitoring along forearm implant shunts and found different types of pressure loss along the shunt depending on the location of obstruction (22, 23). Moreover, they found a significant pressure increase once the stenosis exceeds 40% (22, 23). In combination with a low peripheral resistance that is present in arteriovenous shunts, stenosis seems to become hemodynamically relevant even with a moderate degree of stenosis (22, 23).

First choice for percutaneous treatment of stenosis is balloon dilatation. Recent developments in interventional radiology such as small balloon shafts of 5 F and supergliding guidewires are beneficial for the intervention. Access for intervention is regularly established by ante- or retrograde venous puncture depending on the location of the lesion. In order to limit the risk of malpuncture, we prefer a double puncture technique starting with a 22 G sheath needle. After introduction of an 0.018 in guidewire, the needle is coaxially exchanged for a 16 G sheath needle. After insertion of the larger sheath, a 0.035 in guidewire can be safely introduced. In contrast, graft fistulae can be primarily punctured by a 16 or 18 G sheath needle. We prefer to pass the stenosis by combining 5 F catheters and supergliding guidewires. In our institution, puncture of the shunt is performed by the interventional radiologist for intervention. Some authors, however, recommend shunt puncture to be performed by experienced staff members of the dialysis department (18).

There is a great variation in the type of stenotic lesions found in hemodialysis fistulae. Besides simple concentric stenoses that are easy to dilate, highly rigid concentric stenoses are more frequently found than in arteries that do not well respond to balloon dilatation (Figure 2). They may be particularly associated with stenotic venous valves

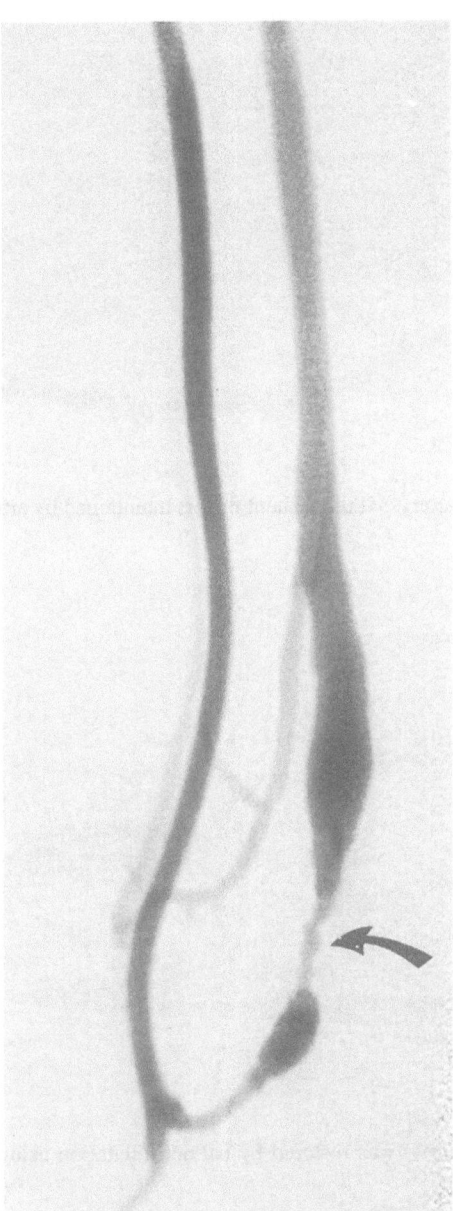

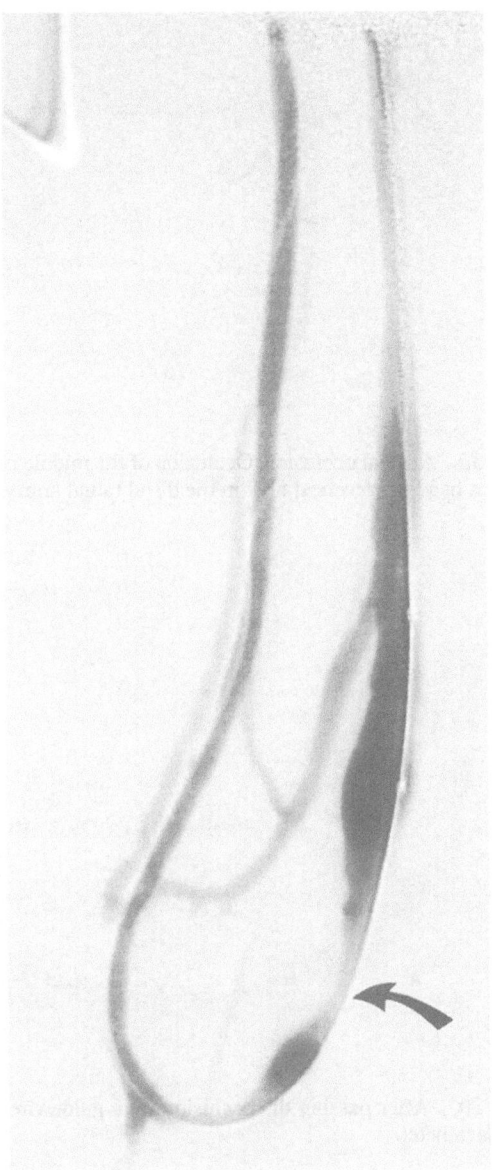

Figure 2a. Resistant venous stenosis. Concentric but somewhat irregular stenosis of the distal shunt vein close to the anastomosis (arrow).

Figure 2b. After balloon dilatation, vein is enlarged but a major residual stenosis is still present (arrow).

(24). Most authors therefore recommend prolonged dilatation time and/or high-pressure balloons (10–15 atm) for those lesions (18). Zijlstra experienced an optimal dilatation time of 20 minutes or even additional 10 minutes after complete distension of the balloon opening. In order to avoid adjacent thrombosis due to shunt blockage, Zijlstra described a balloon catheter that allows shunt circulation via the catheter during dilatation (18). It has to be mentioned, however, that considerable pain is frequently experienced with dilatation of rigid stenosis which sometimes

requires analgesia or may compromise feasibility of prolonged dilatation. Local application of anesthetics around the stenosis may be performed but subcutaneous edema may compress the shunt vein. Regional plexus anesthesia would be another choice but has been used rarely in our experience because of its potential complications.

For shunt dilatation, normally no special instrumentation is necessary. We prefer 5 F low profile balloon catheters without access sheath whenever possible. Larger punctures should be avoided in order to minimize dam-

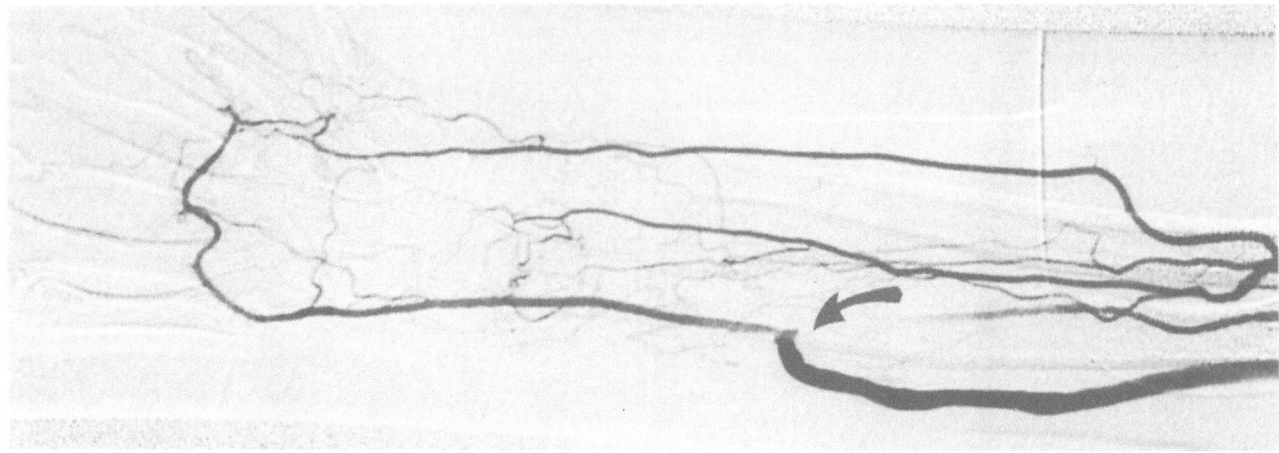

Figure 3a.   Arterial occlusion. Occlusion of the middle portion of the radial artery. Minimal shunt flow is maintained by arterial steal from the hand via reversed flow in the distal radial artery.

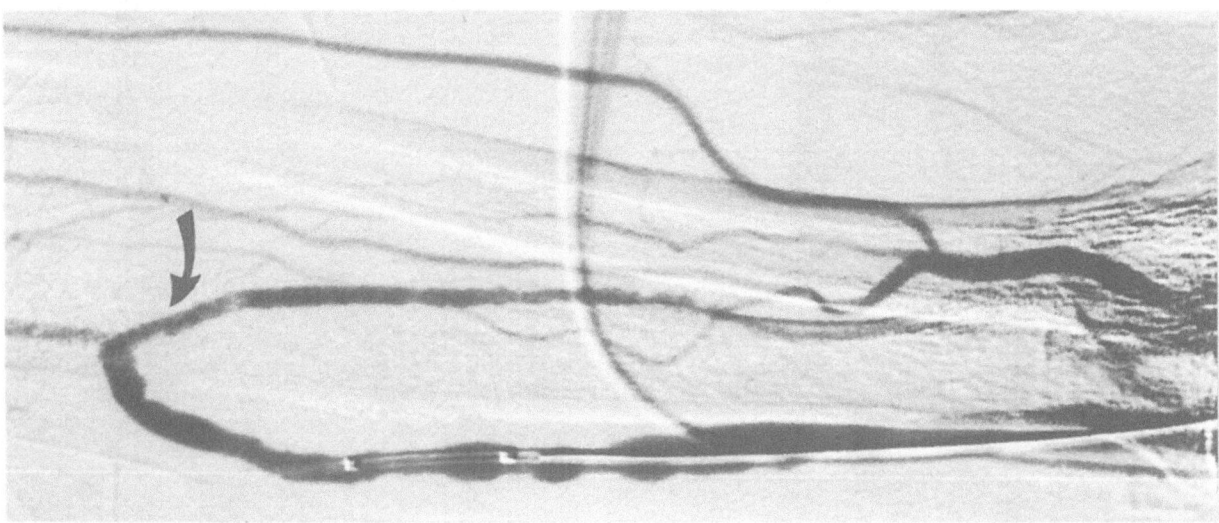

Figure 3b.   After passing the occlusion by a guidewire arterial patency (arrow) was restored by balloon dilatation using a 4 mm balloon catheter.

age to the shunt veins, but 7 or 9 F sheath accesses even in forearm shunts may be used without major problems of bleeding ceasure or severe hematomas. If dilatation of the puncture site is performed stepwise, concerns on hemostasis problems do not seem relevant.

Another type of stenosis is the recoil type that nicely opens during balloon dilatation but collapses right after deflation. Balloon dilatation alone is mostly insufficient to keep these lesions open. These lesions are more often found in larger veins at the upper arm and central veins. In this location, shunt flow frequently leads to venous enlargement and elongation that may result in a kinked stenosis. These lesions also respond well to balloon dilatation, but after deflation, minor success is maintained.

Location of the stenosis varies considerably and depends on the type of shunt. An arterial stenosis is some-

times found in lower arm arteries and frequently leads to incurable shunt insufficiency (Figure 3). They may undergo transvenous balloon dilatation if circumscribed. For this purpose, recently developed balloon catheters of 3–4 mm with supergliding coating and excellent tractability are useful to overcome the arteriovenous anastomosis and to enter the distal arterial segment. Sometimes, severe atherosclerosis of hemodialysis patients may lead to obstruction in otherwise unusual locations such as the axillary or brachial artery (Figure 4). Approach to those lesions depends on the individual situation and may be achieved by a transfemoral, transbrachial or retrograde transvenous access.

In Brescia–Cimino fistulas, shunt stenoses mostly occur in the puncture area or may be found close to the arteriovenous anastomosis. In Goretex shunts, stenosis

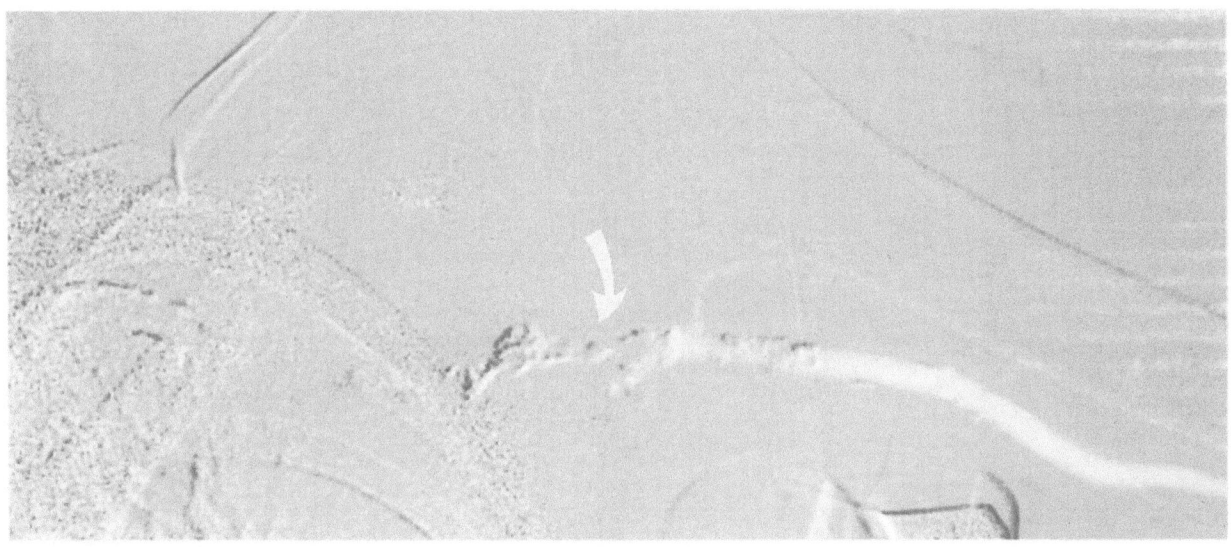

Figure 4.   Occlusion of brachial artery due to calcified atherosclerotic plaques (arrow) that was demonstrated by retrograde carbondioxide angiography.

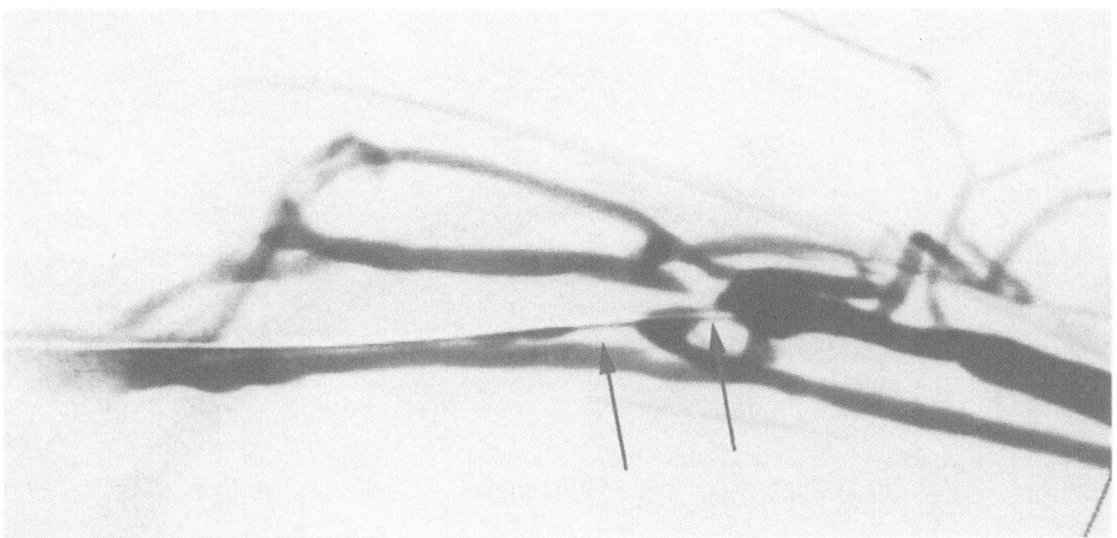

Figure 5a.   Double stenosis of proximal brachial vein draining an implant shunt (double arrow).

due to neointima may occur inside the loop but is more frequently found in the venous section closely proximal to the loop-venous anastomosis. Upper arm (Figure 5) or central vein stenosis occur with no respect to the shunt type used, but have been described to be due to prior placement of large bore temporary subclavian Sheldon catheters (25).

A true venous stenosis may be mimicked by venous spasm that occurs sometimes in an area recently punctured. Furthermore compression of the vein due to surrounding hematoma may lead to misdiagnosis of stenosis but may be excluded by palpation or ultrasound.

Post- and periprocedural care

Periprocedural heparinization is mandatory and does not affect puncture closure within a reasonable time. We administer 5000 IU of heparin intravenously at the beginning of the procedure. Normally, the patient is transferred to the dialysis unit right after the procedure. Both in Brescia–Cimino fistulas and Goretex shunts, the shunt is used for dialysis right after the intervention. Heparinization is maintained during dialysis but is normally not extended afterwards. Full heparinization for additional 24 h is only performed in selected cases after percutaneous shunt revision for stenosis. Chronic medication by

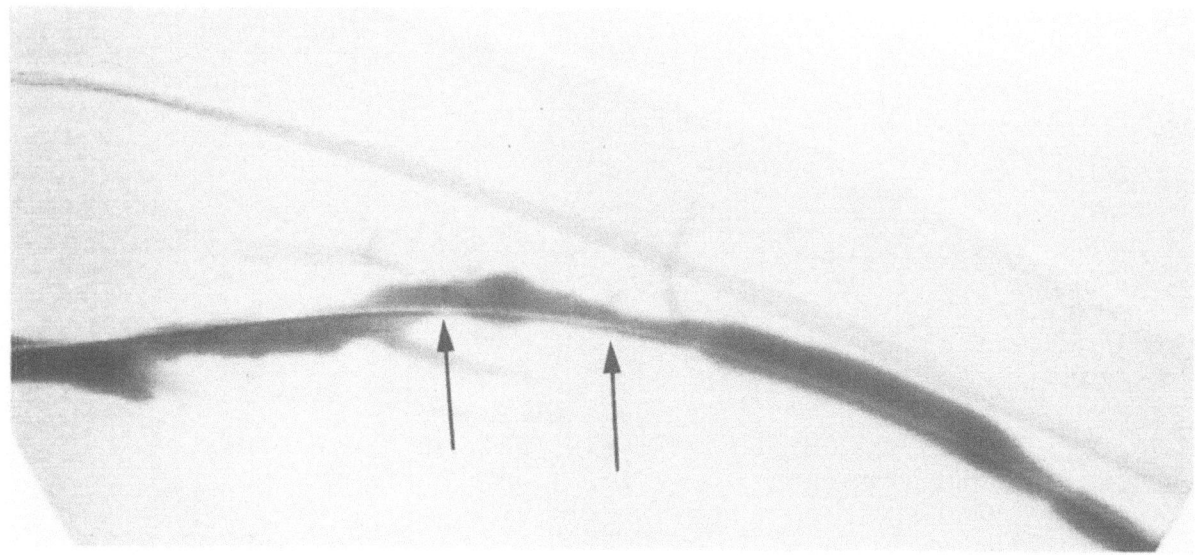

Figure 5b. After balloon dilatation no major residual stenosis is present (double arrow).

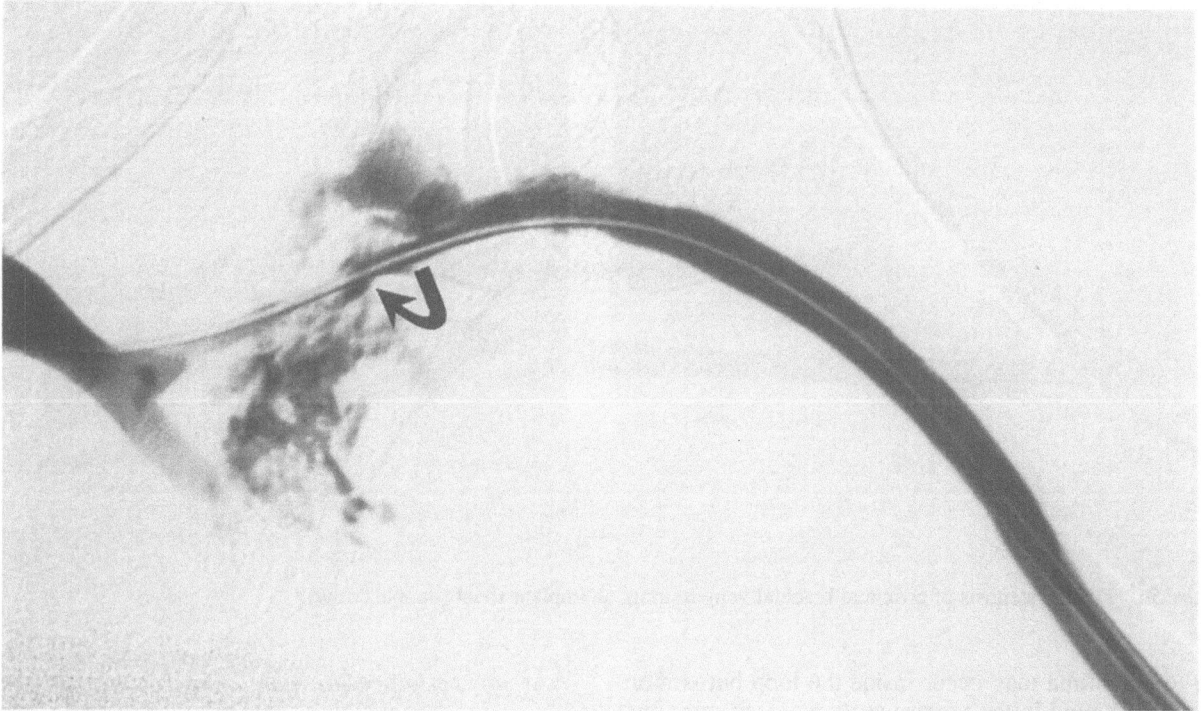

Figure 6. Rupture of the cephalic vein close to the axillary junction after balloon dilatation. Major extravasation of contrast (arrow) but minor and self-limiting hematoma.

acetyl salicylic acid may help to prevent shunt thrombosis.

Complications

Balloon dilatation of shunts is a relatively safe procedure. Most authors only report on small complication rates (17, 18, 28). Main complication is venous rupture, that occurs in up to 2% (24). Although it may be combined by an impressing extravasation of contrast medium, clinical sequelae are mostly minor if occurring in larger veins. Circumscribed rupture of the shunt vein (Figure 6) and concominant venous hematoma may, however, lead to venous compression and subsequent shunt occlusion (24). Thus,

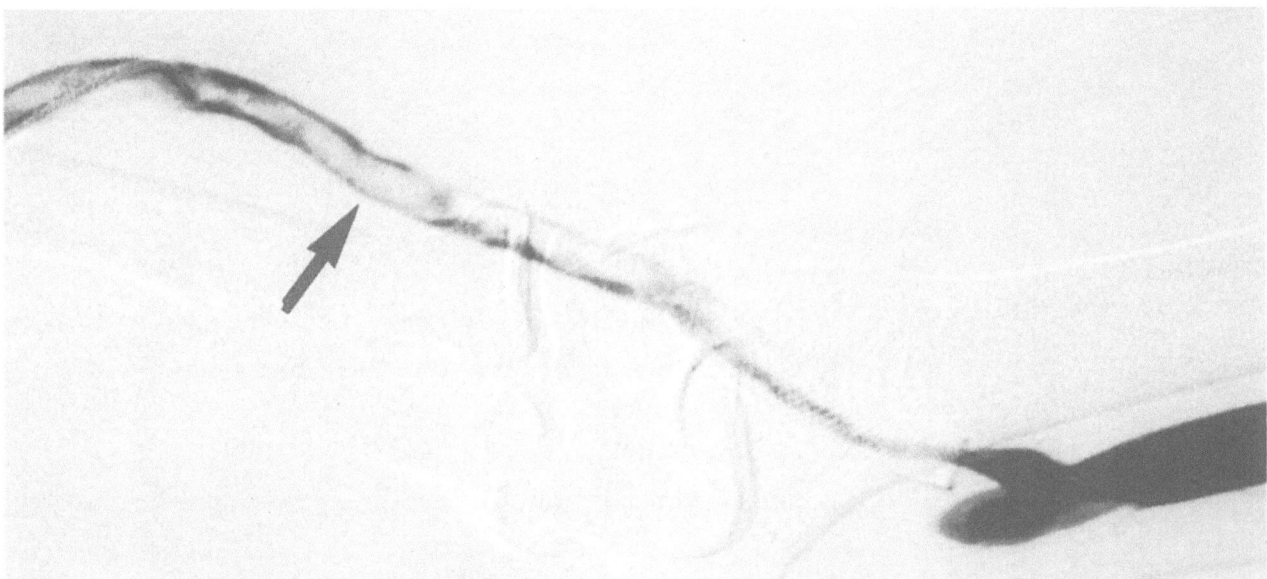

Figure 7. Thrombosis of Goretex implant shunt with fresh clot within the graft (arrow).

overdistension should be avoided. Aneurysm formation as a late sequelae of dilatation has been described by Gmelin and Karnel (28). Venous dissection is infrequently found after PTA. Arterial damage is rarely due to percutaneous shunt intervention if atraumatic wires and catheter material are used. Balloon rupture may occur because of high pressure applied but is mostly without consequences (18). Shunt infection is another possible complication after percutaneous shunt intervention although no specific rates have been reported. Its potential risk, however, requires utmost sterility available in an angiography unit.

Efficacy of balloon dilatation

Numerous publications were made on PTA of hemodialysis shunts. In larger series involving more than a hundred of interventions (17, 24, 27, 28), a similar high technical success ranging from 82 to 94% (17, 24, 27, 28) was reported. Only few and less severe complications occurred ranging from 2 to 6% (24, 27) and included venous rupture with hematoma, formation of pseudoaneurysms and eventually subsequent shunt occlusion.

Gmelin and Karnel reported on a reduced technical success for treatment of shunt occlusions (27). They reported on 80 cases with occluded venous segments that represented a mixed group of recent and older obstructions. In 25 cases they used thrombolysis as an adjunct to PTA with a technical success of 14 of 25 cases (56%), in the remaining 55 instances they exclusively applied PTA being successful in 36/55 cases (65%).

Follow-up patency showed a high rate of reobstruction and failure in all series reported. Gmelin and Karnel found a 6-month, 1-year and 2-year patency of 75, 62 and 34% (28) for stenoses and 73, 54 and 14% for occlu-

sions respectively. Glanz and co-workers (17) reported an patency on 57% (6 months), 45% (1 year) and 24% (2 years). Both groups did not use life-table analysis for evaluation of their data which was done by Beathard (24). He reported on a cumulative patency of 61% after 6 months, 38% after 1 year and 22% after 2 years. Although these results may look disappointing, PTA in failing hemodialysis fistulas is able to improve overall patency of failing shunts. Bohndorf and co-workers (28) were able to achieve an overall patency for both failing PTFE shunts and Brescia–Cimino fistulas, that corresponded well to the one and two-year overall patency of a general shunt population after primary shunt surgery (3, 4). This was in contrast to the poor primary patency for this negatively biased subgroup of failing hemodialysis fistulae (28) which was considerably lower compared to the general shunt population (3). Therefore, a 'normalized' overall function rate can be expected even for complicated shunts after percutaneous revision.

Differences in long-term success between surgical versus percutaneous revision are marginal. Although early reports on PTA (29, 30) advocated surgery to be superior to PTA, Dapunt and co-workers (31) did not find a significant advantage of surgery over PTA. Overall patencies achieved by surgical revision only (3, 4) do not outnumber overall patency after PTA (2).

Repeat PTA does not compromise patency rates. Beathard found similar results with no relation to the first, second or third PTA performed (24). Although in previous papers long-segment stenoses (> 6 cm in length) were considered not to respond well to PTA (32, 33) Beathard did not find a significant difference for that subgroup of lesions nor for midgraft stenoses in Goretex shunts which were also advocated to be not amenable to balloon

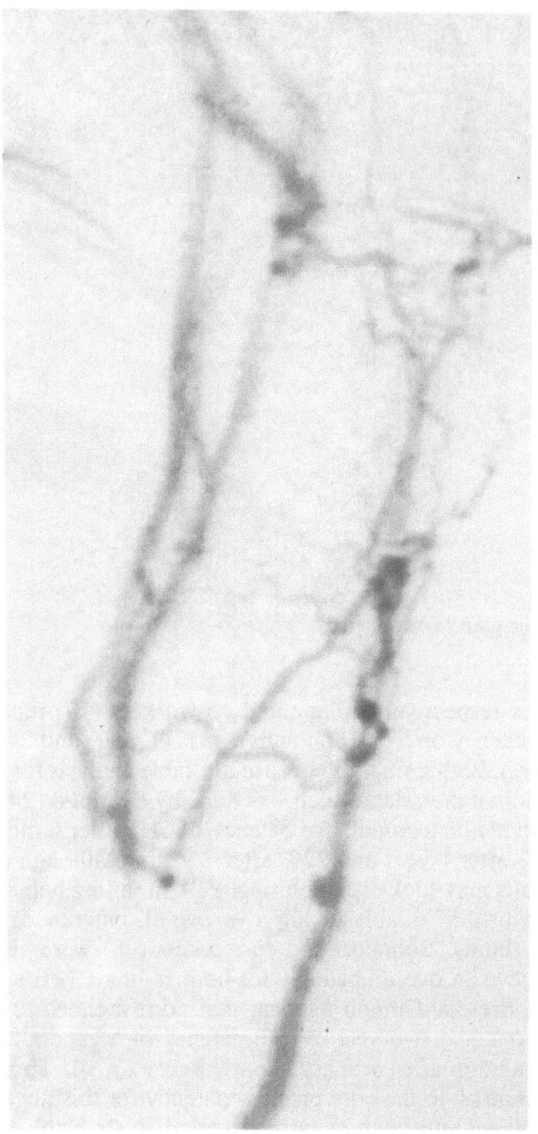

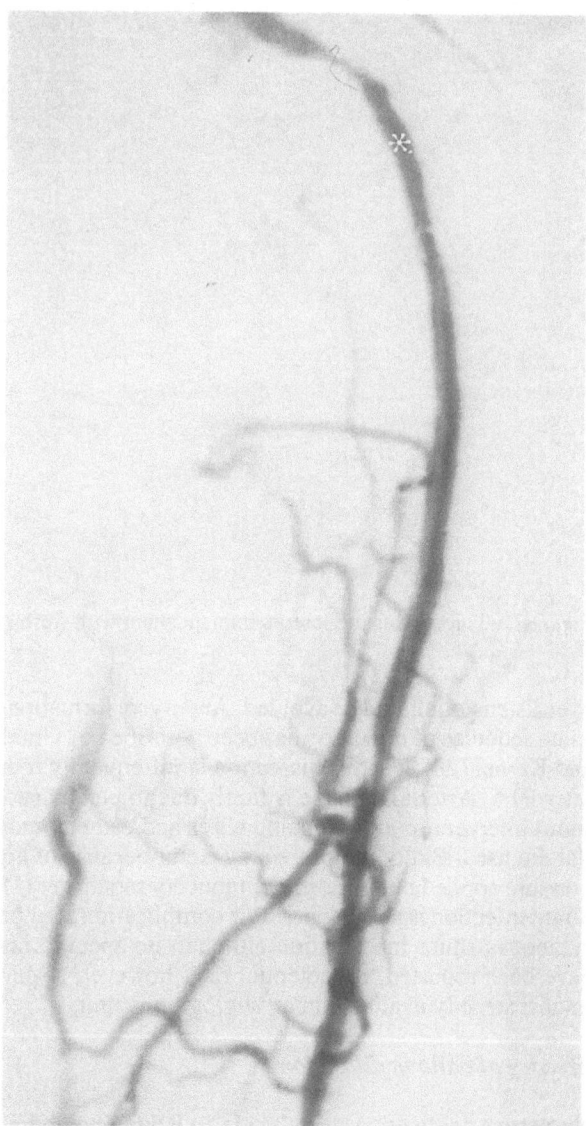

Figure 8a. Chronic venous stenosis. Occlusion of the left cephalic vein (open arrow) and shunt flow via collateral veins to the basilic vein (small arrows).

Figure 8b. Combining balloon dilatation and stent placement, cephalic vein was recanalized up to its outflow to the axillary vein (⋆).

dilatation (24). There is only a subgroup of central venous obstruction which showed an early tendency of recurrence in the early postprocedural follow-up (24, 32, 33).

Alternative techniques

As an alternative to balloon dilatation, percutaneous atherectomy has been described for treatment of shunt stenosis (34). Follow-up results, however, are not yet better compared to PTA. Specific indications for atherectomy are removal of neointimal hyperplasia from grafts or stents within shunt vessels. This is a reasonable approach to smaller vessels up to 7 mm of diameter but atherecto-

my is of limited use in large diameter vessels and stent restenosis in central veins is therefore, preferably treated by balloon dilatation.

As a specific approach to resistant shunt stenosis, Zwaan and co-workers used pulse dye laser therapy which was described to be highly successful in cases when PTA failed (35). Wider clinical application, however, is limited by lacking feasibility of appropriate laser technology in most institutions.

Shunt thrombosis

Shunt thrombosis is a more severe complication in failing hemodialysis shunts. Underlying causes are manifold: clotting abnormalities, thrombocytosis, disturbed fluid balance as well as hypotension may lead in combination with an additional shunt stenosis to shunt occlusion that has been considered in the past as a relative contraindication to percutaneous intervention. There are, however, different types of shunt thrombosis that differently respond to percutaneous intervention. To this respect, digital palpation of the occluded shunt is important to classify the type of thrombosis prior to intervention.

Recent shunt thrombosis in Brescia-Cimino fistulas may be due to a very short-segment plug-like thrombus selectively obstructing the arteriovenous anastomosis. The draining shunt veins are very soft at palpation. If digital manipulation fails, this type of obstruction is an ideal candidate for PTA, since the small thrombus can be macerated by balloon inflation alone and flow can be restored immediately. Treatment, however, should be started soon to avoid propagated thrombus formation. Short segment thrombosis of the draining vein may also undergo percutaneous treatment by combining local lysis therapy and balloon dilatation.

Palpation easily depicts cases where shunt thrombosis is due to an underlying severe stenosis and subsequent thrombus formation. If this happens close to the arteriovenous anastomosis, the amount of thrombus is mostly small and balloon dilatation alone may be sufficient for recanalization.

Long-segment thrombosis of Brescia-Cimino fistulas and complete thrombosis of Goretex implant shunts, however, are more problematic for percutaneous intervention. Local thrombolysis therapy with several modifications have been described as a suitable approach. More recently, various types of percutaneous mechanical thrombectomy have been proposed but have not yet been fully established. Since long-segment Brescia–Cimino fistulas thrombosis may require neoanastomosis, Goretex shunts are most frequently declotted using Fogarty balloons after surgical cut-down (37). Combination with balloon dilatation and thrombus cracking for older thrombus formation has been recommended and combined surgical-radiological intervention is a suitable approach to that problem in order to image the shunt morphology after thrombectomy and to treat underlying stenosis by PTA (36, 37).

Thrombolysis

Percutaneous thrombolysis of thrombosed hemodialysis grafts (Figure 7) may be performed with different application techniques of the lytic agent. Early reports used systemic (38) or infusion techniques (39) via the feeding artery. The latter technique, however, was tested insufficient with a high number of bleeding complications. Transcutaneous injection of lytic agents into the thrombus using ultrasonic guidance may be performed as an alternative approach. Direct transcatheter infusion of lytic agents into the thrombosed graft in combination with mechanical maceration of the thrombus by balloon dilatation was described by several authors to obtain improved results (26, 40, 41). Davis and co-workers described a technique which utilizes two catheters inserted in a criss-cross manner into the thrombosed segment (26). Urokinase (2000 IU/min) was directly infused into the thrombus up to a total of 400000 IU after mechanical lacing of the thrombus by the infusion catheters. They were able to restore flow in 37 of 41 patients (90%) within a mean time of 86 ± 57 min. Major complications did not occur. Poulain and co-workers reported less successful results with a similar technique that also included mechanical aspiration thrombectomy in case of residual thrombus formation (40). They reported a success in 38 of 64 events (59%). Recanalization period was 7 ± 3 hours and thrombolysis had to be combined with balloon angioplasty and thromboaspiration in 80%. Both groups reported no (26) or only minor bleeding (40) complications. Both of them described a case of embolization to distal forearm arteries (26, 40). Poulain and co-workers stated that with increasing experience a primary success my be achievable in about 80%. Valji and co-workers modified thrombolysis therapy by introducing a spray-lysis technique where highly-concentrated urokinase is forcefully injected through a specially designed catheter with multiple small side holes thus spraying the lytic agent into the thrombus mass (41). They applied 150000 IU of urokinase within 15–20 min with two pulses per minute and continued with one pulse per minute (mean total 300000 IU) until shunt flow was restored. Using this technique, they were able to reduce moderately the total amount of urokinase but to shorten the treatment period to 46 ± 21 min. Gmelin and co-workers replaced Urokinase by rTPA as lytic agents (27). It is important to mention that 114 of 117 cases of Valji and all cases of Davis were implant grafts (26, 41). Therefore, suitability of shunt lysis for native shunts is still questionable. Poulain reported a success rate of 75% for this shunt type which, however, represented only a quarter the shunts treated (40). Thrombolysis combined with PTA may be helpful in recent central venous occlusion (42).

Time delay and potential complications, however, compromise a wider acceptance of thrombolysis in shunt declotting. Furthermore, sophisticated techniques such as spray-lysis therapy require considerable experience to gain excellent results. Surgical thrombectomy using Fogarty balloons, in contrast, is a safe, easy and quick procedure. Therefore, potential risks may limit importance of thrombolysis as an alternative to surgery.

To avoid major drawbacks of lysis therapy, different mechanical instruments were tested for mechanical thrombectomy in single cases (43–46). These instruments mainly combined suction and mechanical fragmentation by rotating or oscillating probes for thrombus removal and

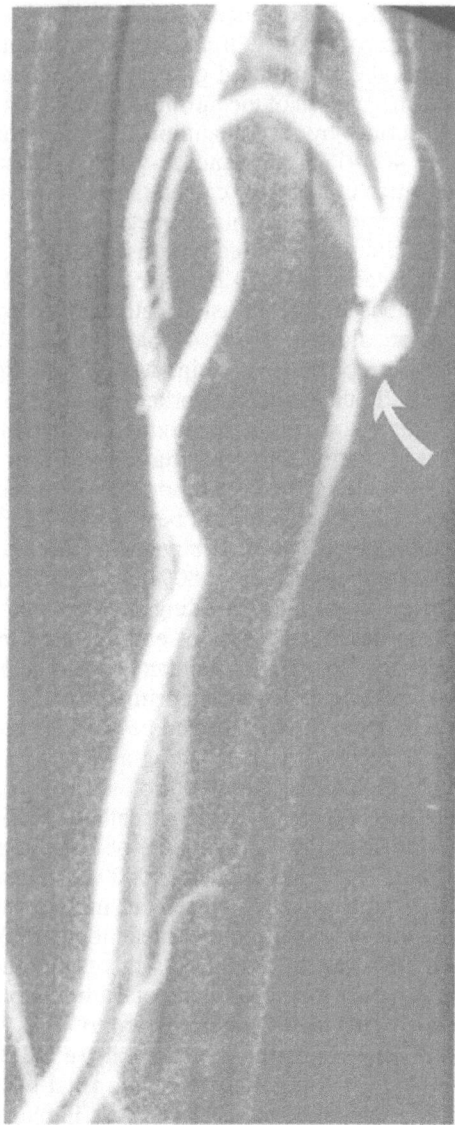

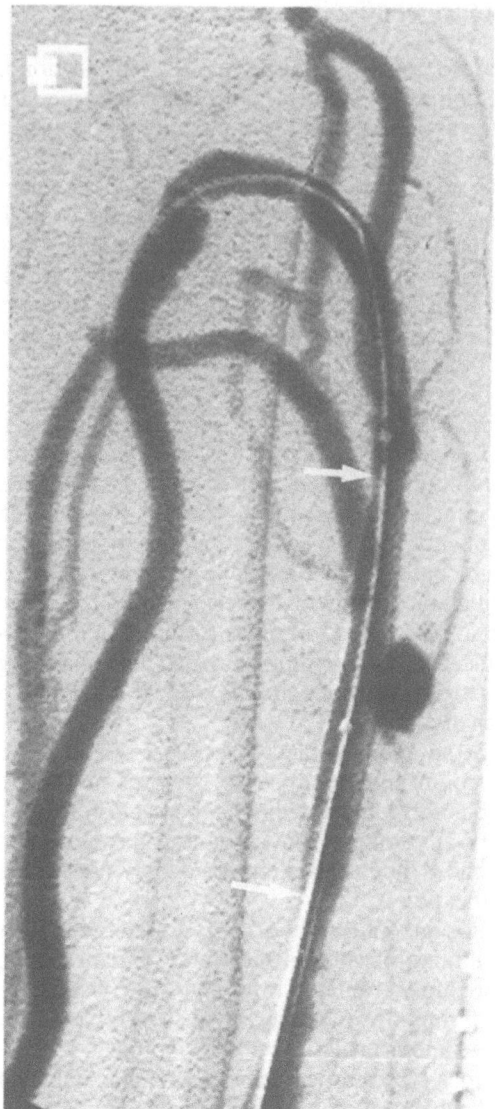

Figure 9a. Peripheral stent. False aneurysm (curved arrow) combined with severe stenosis (arrow) of the draining distal shunt vein of a BC forearm shunt.

Figure 9b. Stent (arrows) was placed to treat the stenosis thus facilitating resection of aneurysm.

were used with success in graft shunts but turned out to be less effective in native veins which collapsed when suction was applied (43). Schmitz-Rode described a stent basket for mechanical thrombectomy (44, 45). Hydrodynamic thrombectomy using specially designed catheters utilizing the Venturi effect (46) has been tested more recently and showed promising results to be effective for nonsurgical thrombectomy avoiding application of lytic agents (47).

Chronic venous occlusion

In some cases, older segmental venous occlusion may be present but was missed for earlier diagnosis because venous outflow has been preserved via collateral veins (Figure 8). Clinical signs in those patients often include elevated venous counter-pressure and prolonged bleeding time after dialysis. The occluded venous segment is mainly free from nonorganized thrombotic material and the vein itself is atrophic. In those cases, percutaneous recanalization may be tried but technical success has been reported to be moderate (27). In our experience, combination of a straight guidewire and a multipurpose catheter is most helpful to overcome the obstructed segment that is followed by balloon dilatation. Successful passage of the complete obstruction is, however, mandatory before balloon dilatation should be performed. The failure rate is relatively high, but complications are also rare and shunt

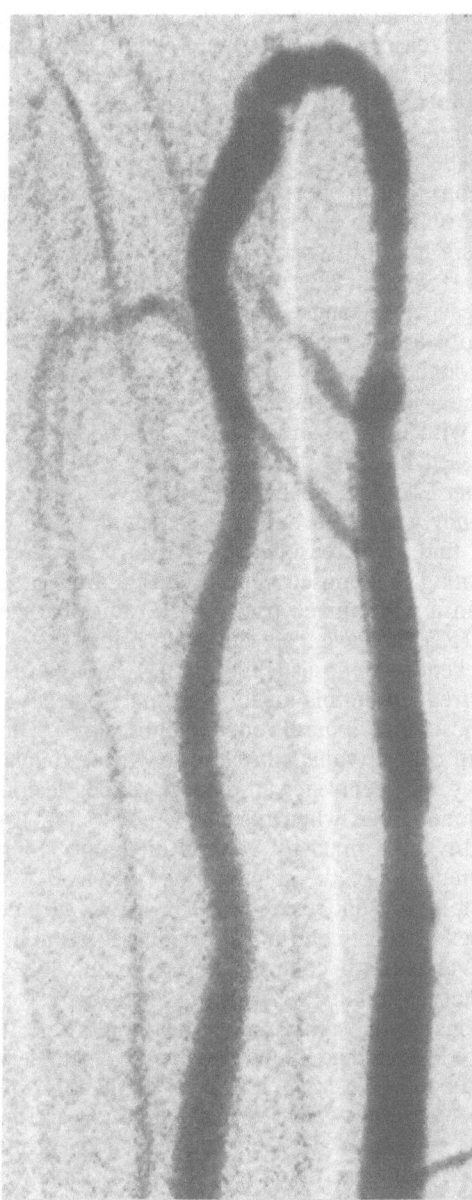

Figure 9c.   After resection of aneurysm, patency is fully restored; puncture site is limited to the nonstented venous segment.

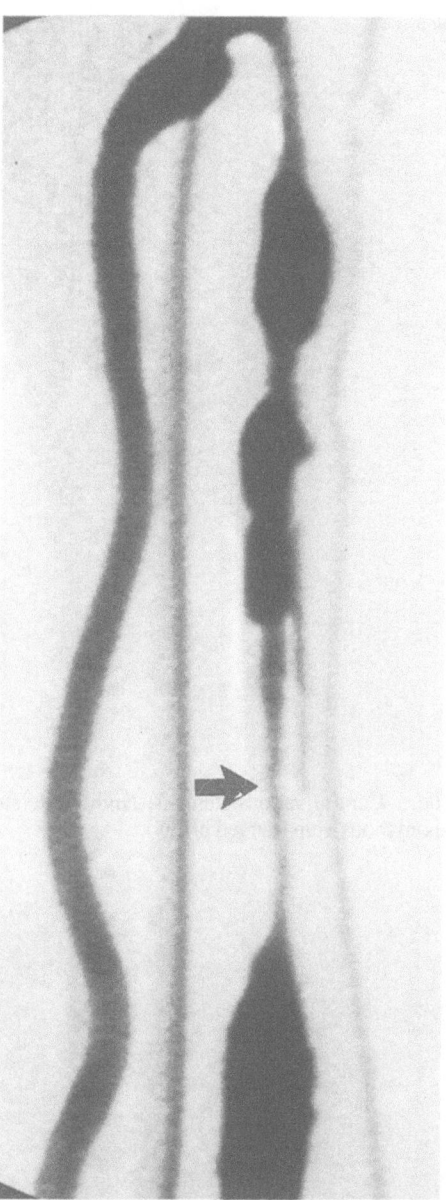

Figure 9d.   After 6 months, severe restenosis within the stent and adjacent venous segment (arrows) is present that was treated by balloon dilatation.

patency in general is not endangered as long as collateral flow is preserved. In some cases, additional application of stents are required to keep the newly created venous outflow tract open (48).

Endoprostheses (Stents)

Several types of metallic endoprostheses has been used in the venous system and particularly for shunt stenoses and occlusions (49–54).

Table 3. Indications for stent placement

Primary	Secondary
Central venous obstruction	Kinked stenosis
Dissection	Collapsing stenosis
Circumscribed perforation	Resistant stenosis
	Chronic venous occlusion

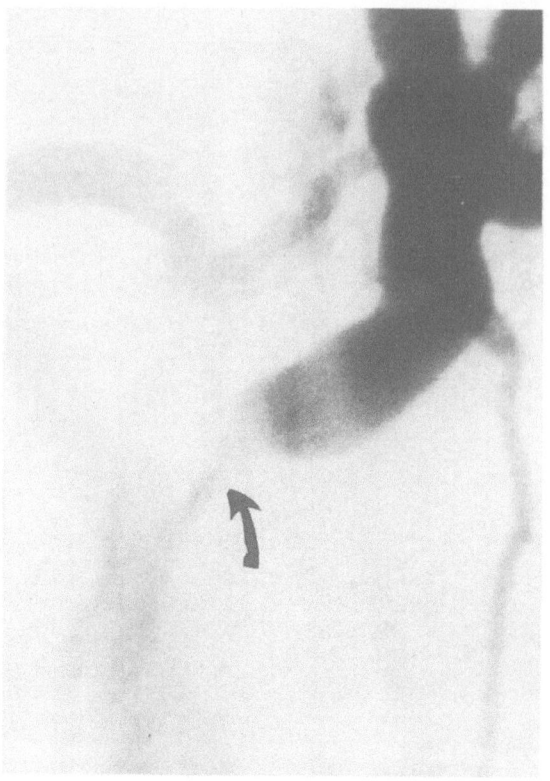

Figure 10a. Central venous stenosis. High-grade stenosis of the left anonymous vein (curved arrow).

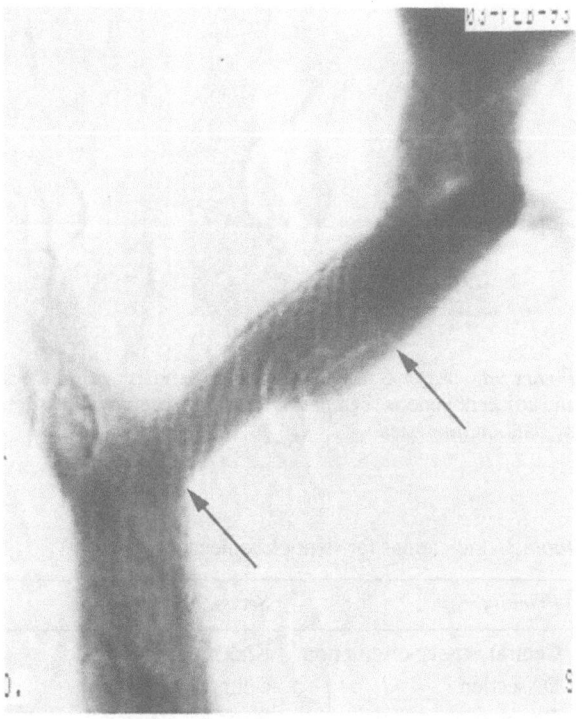

Figure 10b. After placement of a 12 mm large self-expanding stent patency of the vein is restored.

The main indication for stents in shunts is related to technical reasons (Figure 9) and should be mainly considered if PTA failed or complicated (Table 3). Stents are helpful particularly in kinked and collapsing stenoses, for sealing of dissections or circumscribed perforations and can be utilized to establish patency of chronic venous occlusions. Results post PTA of highly resistant stenoses can be improved by stent implantation. Furthermore, stents are helpful to remodel venous outflow in special situations. In contrast, stents should not be placed in puncture areas, since long-term effects of recurrent traumatization of stented areas are not yet evaluated.

Although never proven, stents have been advocated as a potential tool to prevent restenosis. In our own experience with more than 50 cases, it has to be, however, stressed, that the rate of restenosis is very similar to that after PTA, so no benefit on the long-term primary patency was achieved (53). Beathard and co-workers did not find an increased patency using Gianturco stents for stenting of stenosed venous anastomoses of Goretex grafts in a randomized trial (54). From our own experience (53), however, we advocate primary stenting of central venous stenoses (Figure 10). Although restenosis is also frequent in this location, primary patency is similar to those of peripheral venous stenoses (53). Therefore, stents in central veins can slow down the much higher tendency for recurrence in central venous lesions after PTA alone. Even when restenosis occurs, revision can be readily performed by balloon dilatation (Figure 11) or atherectomy of the stented area; the latter we prefer for peripheral stent restenosis. Thus, overall patency is increased both for central and peripheral stents in shunts but is even better in central lesions reaching 90% 2 years after intervention in our own experience (53).

In conclusion, stent application should be limited to selective lesions that are technically not treatable by PTA alone. In those lesions, however, application of stents can clear an otherwise desperate situation and helps to preserve the shunt. Except central venous obstruction, improved long-term patency is not likely to achieve, but an adequate overall patency can be accomplished by percutaneous reintervention.

Contraindications for percutaneous treatment

There are a few contraindications to percutaneous treatment. Immature shunts are no candidates for balloon dilatation or other percutaneous techniques. Particularly, fresh anastomotic strictures are no indication for PTA in order to avoid rupture of the anastomosis. Insufficient venous outflow due to small draining veins is not likely to be corrected by percutaneous intervention and should undergo PTA only in case of a circumscribed lesion or in the presence of concominant central venous obstruction.

Long-segment or multifocal arterial disease are not ideal for PTA since the chance of restenosis is high. A circum-

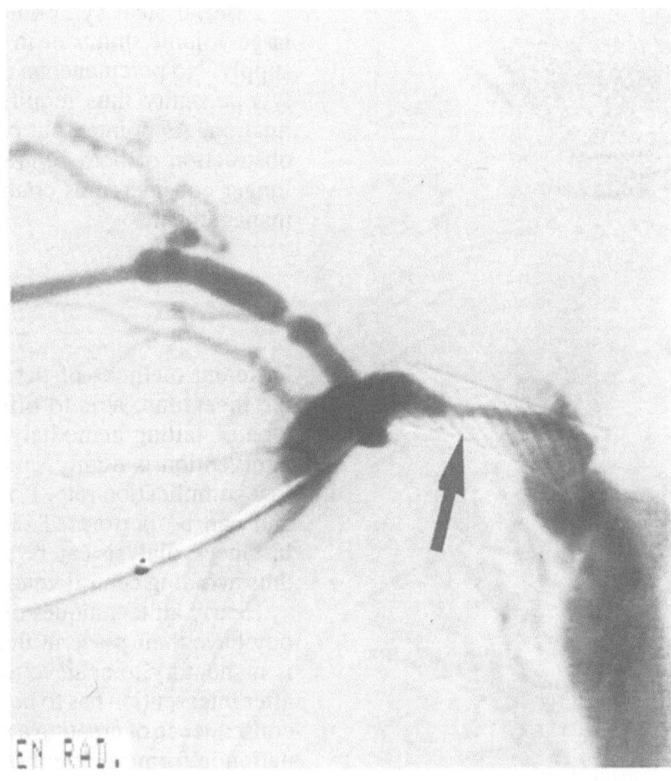

Figure 11a. Recurrent central stenosis. Restenosis within right subclavian vein after stent placement due to neointimal hyperplasia.

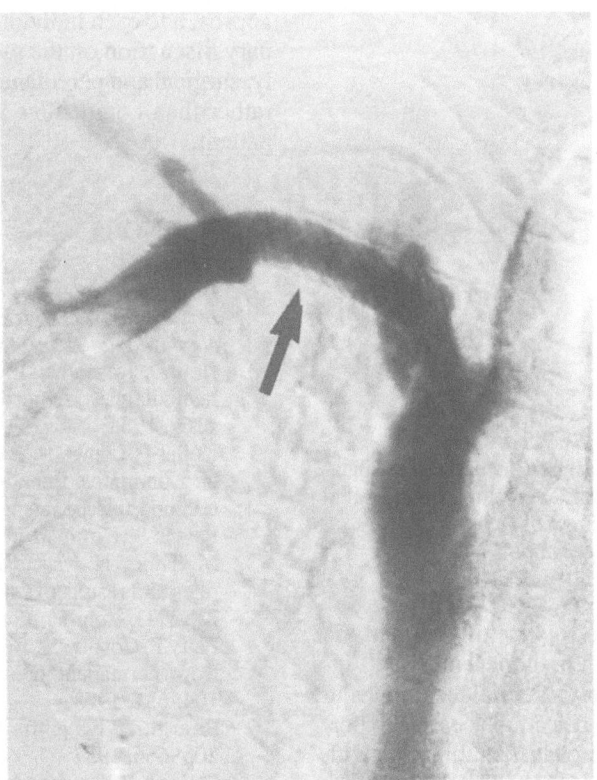

Figure 11b. Restenosis has been sufficiently treated by balloon dilatation.

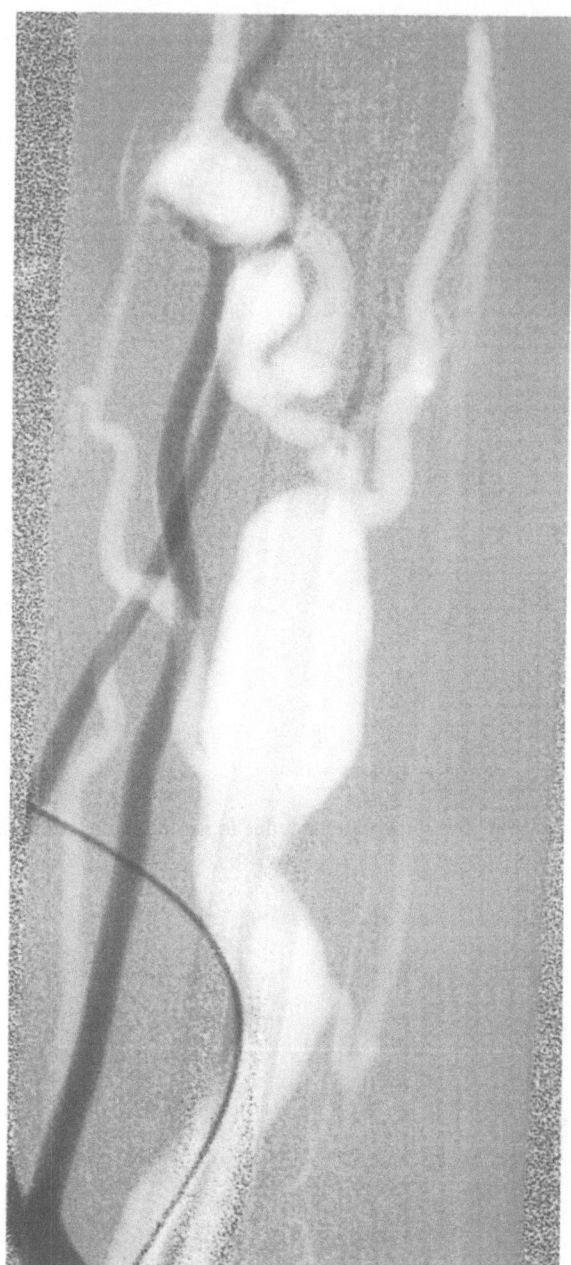

Figure 12. Transbrachial DSA of shunt. Aneurysmatic dilatation of shunt vein (white vessel). Black vessel represents radial artery; small arrows indicate flow direction.

scribed arterial stenosis may be successfully treated via a transvenous approach. Arterial pseudoaneurysms (Figure 12) have been treated by interventional techniques in selected cases (55), but surgical resection is easier to perform and a more reasonable approach. Combination with stenting may be helpful in selected cases (Figure 9). Shunt infection, of course, remains a domain for conservative and surgical treatment (56).

Arterial steal syndrome may occur after creation of large volume shunts or in case of impaired distal arterial supply. No percutaneous approach exists to this relatively rare entity thus requiring surgical banding or shunt ligation. As pointed out previously, also chronic venous obstruction of both central and peripheral veins can no longer considered as contraindications for percutaneous management.

SUMMARY

Different methods of percutaneous management are, in the meantime, able to offer an approach to nearly each type of failing hemodialysis fistulae. Technically, shunt intervention is highly successful and accompanied by a low complication rate. It is quick, relatively inexpensive and can be performed on an outpatient basis. In most instances, dialysis can be performed via the shunt treated thus avoiding central venous cannulation.

Nearly all techniques of modern interventional radiology have their place in that strategy and skilled training is mandatory to achieve excellent results. Reobstruction after intervention has to be, however, accepted as a natural consequence of creating a nonphysiological high-flow situation in formerly low-flow vessels to gain access to circulation. Timely reintervention is therefore part of shunt maintenance and protection.

It has, however, to be stressed, that the adequate approach to each individual case requires an interdisciplinary discussion on the most suitable approach. Frequently, surgical and percutaneous methods are then adjunctive rather than competitive in the best management for the patient.

REFERENCES

1. Burger H, Kootstra G, de Charro F, Lepers P: A survey of vascular access for haemodialysis in the Netherlands. *Nephrol Dial Transplant* 6: 5, 1991
2. Bell D, Rosenthal J: Arteriovenous graft life in chronic hemodialysis. A need for prolongation. *Arch Surg* 123: 1169, 1988
3. Keller F, Loewe H, Bauknecht K, Schwarz A, Offermann G: Kumulative Funktionsraten von orthotopen Dialysefisteln und Interponaten. *Dtsch Med Wschr* 113: 332, 1988
4. Palder S, Kirkman R, Whittemore A, Hakim R, Lazarus M, Tilney N: Vascular access for hemodialysis. Patency rates and results of revision. *Am Surg* 202: 235, 1985
5. Zibari G, Rohr M, Landreneau M, Bridges R, DeVault G, Petty F, Costley K, Brown S, McDonald J: Complications from permanent hemodialysis vascular access. *Surgery* 104: 681, 1988
6. Raju S: PTFE grafts for hemodialysis access. *Ann Surg* 206: 666, 1987
7. Schwab S, Raymond J, Saeed M, Newman G, Dennis P, Bollinger R: Prevention of hemodialysis fistula thrombo-

sis. Early detection of venous stenoses. *Kidney Int* 36: 707, 1989

8. Thomsen M, Stenport G: Evaluation of clinical examination preceding surgical treatment of av fistula problems. *Acta Chir Scand* 151: 133, 1985

9. Windus D: Permanent vascular access: a nephrologist's view. *Am J Kidney Dis* 21: 457, 1993

10. Windus D, Audrain J, Vanderson R, Jendrisak M, Picus D, Delmez J: Optimization of high-efficiency hemodialysis by detection and correction of fistula dysfunction. *Kidney Int* 38: 337, 1990

11. Kathrein H: Duplexsonographie von Dialyseshunts. Nichtinvasive Beurteilung der arteriovenösen Fistel bei Dialysepatienten. *Fortschr Med* 111: 313, 1993

12. Vorwerk D, Günther RW, Bohndorf K, Asgarzadeh A, Borchers K: Farbkodierte Duplexsonographie (Angiodynographie) in der Beurteilung arteriovenöser Shunts. *Fortschr Roentgenstr* 148: 265, 1988

13. Nonnast-Daniel B, Martin R, Lindert O, Mügge A, Schaefer J, vd Lieth H, Söchtig E, Galanski M, Koch KM, Daniel W: Colour doppler ultrasound assessment of arteriovenous haemodialysis fistulas. *Lancet* 339: 143, 1992

14. Forsberg L, Tylen T, Olin T, Lindstedt E: Quantitative flow estimations of arteriovenous fistulas with doppler and dye dilution techniques. *Acta Radiol Diagn* 21: 465, 1980

15. Oates C, Williams E, McHugh M: The use of a diasonics DRF 400 duplex ultrasound scanner to measure volume flow in arterio-venous fistulae in patients undergoing haemodialysis: an analysis of measurement uncertainties. *Ultrasound Med Biol* 16: 571, 1990

16. Picus D, van Breda A, Katzen B, Steinberg D: Use of digital subtraction angiography for evaluation of vascular access for hemodialysis. *Cardiovasc Intervent Radiol* 10: 210, 1987

17. Glanz S, Gordon D, Butt K, Hong J, Lipkowitz G: The role of percutaneous angioplasty in the management of chronic hemodialysis fistulas. *Ann Surg* 206: 777, 1987

18. Zijlstra J: Percutaneous transluminal angioplasty in vascular access for hemodialysis. Proefschrift ter verkrijging van de graad van doctor aan de Rijksuniversiteit te Utrecht. Utrecht, 19897

19. Staple T: Retrograde venography of subcutaneous arteriovenous fistulas created surgically for hemodialysis. *Radiology* 106: 223, 1973

20. Shu M, Hwang N: Haemodynamics of angioaccess venous anastomoses. *J Biomed Eng* 13: 103, 1991

21. Nardi L, Bosch J: Recirculation: review, techniques for measurement and ability to predict hemoaccess stenosis before and after angioplasty. *Blood Purif* 6: 85, 1988

22. Sullivan K, Besarab A, Dorell S, Moritz M: The relationship between dialysis graft pressure and stenosis. *Invest Radiol* 27: 352, 1992

23. Sullivan K, Besarab A, Bonn J, Shapiro M, Gardiner G, Moritz M: Hemodynamics of failing dialysis grafts. *Radiology* 186: 867, 1993

24. Beathard G: Percutaneous transvenous angioplasty in the treatment of vascular access stenosis. *Kidney Int* 42: 1390, 1992

25. Surratt R, Picus D, Hicks M, Darcy M, Kleinhoffer M, Jendrisak M: The importance of preoperative evaluation of the subclavian vein in dialysis access planning. *Am J Roentgenol* 156: 623, 1991

26. Davis G, Dowd C, Bookstein J, Maroney T, Lang E, Halasz N: Thrombosed dialysis grafts. Efficacy of intrathrombic deposition of concentrated urokinase, clot maceration and angioplasty. *Am J Roentgenol* 149: 177, 1987

27. Gmelin E, Karnel F: Radiologische Rekanalisation von Venen, Gefäßprothesen und Arterien bei insuffizienten Dialysefisteln. *Fortschr Roentgenstr* 153: 432, 1990

28. Bohndorf K, Gladziwa U, Kistler D, Kretschmer K, Vorwerk D, Sieberth H, Günther RW: Rekanalisation von stenosierten oder verschlossenen Hämodialyseshunts. *Fortschr Roentgenstr* 158: 525, 1993

29. Brooks J, Sigley R, May K, Mack R: Transluminal angioplasty versus surgical repair for stenosis of hemodialysis grafts. A randomized study. *Am J Surg* 153: 530, 1987

30. Tortolani E, Tan A, Butchart S: Percutaneous transluminal angioplasty. An ineffective approach to failing vascular access. *Arch Surg* 119: 221, 1984

31. Dapunt O, Feuerstein M, Rendl K, Prenner K: Transluminal angioplasty versus conventional operation in the treatment of haemodialysis fistula stenosis: results from a 5-year study. *Br J Surg* 74: 1004, 1987

32. Glanz S, Gordon D, Lipkowitz G, Butt K, Hong J, Sclafani S: Axillary and subclavian vein stenosis: percutaneous angioplasty. *Radiology* 168: 371, 1988

33. Schwab S, Quarles L, Middleton J, Cohan R, Saaed M, Dennis V: Hemodialysis-associated subclavian vein stenosis. *Kidney Int* 33: 1156, 1988

34. Gray R, Dolmatch B, Buick M: Directional atherectomy treatment for hemodialysis access: early results. *J Vasc Intervent Radiol* 3: 497, 1992

35. Zwaan M, Weiss H, Gmelin E, Rinast E, Scheu M: Lasergestützte Ballonangioplastie insuffizienter Hämodialysefisteln. *Fortschr Roentgenstr* 159: 456, 1993

36. Kistler D, Bohndorf K, Günther RW: Kombiniert chirurgisch-radiologisches Vorgehen beim Verschluß eines Hämodialyseshunts. *Chirurg* 61: 84, 1990

37. Smith T, Hunter D, Darcy M, Castaneda-Zuniga W, Amplatz K: Thrombosed synthetic hemodialysis access fistulas: the success of combined thrombectomy and angioplasty (Technical note). *Am J Roentgenol* 147: 161, 1986

38. Brittinger W, Twittenhoff W: *Anschlußverfahren an die künstliche Niere. Technische und klinische Aspekte*, Bindernagel, Friedberg, 1975, p 68

39. Young A, Hunter D, Castaneda-Zuniga W, So S, Mercado S, Cardella J, Amplatz K: Thrombosed synthetic hemodialysis access fistulas: failure of fibrinolytic therapy. *Radiology* 154: 639, 1985

40. Poulain F, Raynaud A, Bourquelot P, Knight C, Rovani X, Gaux J: Local thrombolysis and thromboaspiration in the treatment of acutely thrombosed arteriovenous hemodialysis fistulas. *Cardiovasc Intervent Radiol* 14: 98, 1991

41. Valji K, Bookstein J, Roberts A, Davis G: Pharmacomechanical thrombolysis and angioplasty in the management of clotted hemodialysis grafts: early and late clinical results. *Radiology* 178: 243, 1991

42. Newman G, Saeed M, Himmelstein S, Cohan R, Schwab S: Total central vein obstruction: resolution with angioplasty and fibrinolysis. *Kidney Int* 39: 761, 1991

43. Guenther RW, Vorwerk D: Aspiration catheter for percutaneous thrombectomy: clinical results. *Radiology* 175: 271, 1990

44. Schmitz-Rode T, Bohndorf K, Guenther RW: Rekanalisation thrombosierter Hämodialyseshunts mit Oszillations-

Aspiration und Maschenkorb. *Fortschr Roentgenstr* 158: 49, 1993

45. Schmitz-Rode T, Bohndorf K, Guenther RW: New 'Mesh basket' for percutaneous removal of wall-adherent thrombi in dialysis shunts. *Cardiovasc Intervent Radial* 16: 7, 1993

46. Reekers J, Kromhout J, van der Waal K: Catheter for percutaneous thrombectomy: first clinical results. *Radiology* 188: 871, 1993

47. Vorwerk D, Guenther RW, Sohn M, Schuermann K, Hoogeveen Y: Percutaneous mechanical thrombectomy of hemodialysis shunts with use of the hydrolyser system (Abstract). SCVIR Meeting, San Diego 1994. *JVIR* 5: 37, 1994

48. Vorwerk D, Guenther RW, Bohndorf K, Kistler D: Self-expanding stents in peripheral and central veins used for arteriovenous shunts: five years of experience (abstract). *Radiology* 189(P): 174, 1993

49. Günther R, Vorwerk D, Bohndorf K, Klose K, Kistler D, Mann H, Sieberth H, El-Din A: Venous stenosis in dialysis shunts: treatment with self-expanding metallic stents. *Radiology* 170: 401, 1989

50. Quinn S, Schuman E, Hall L, Gross G, Uchida B, Standage B, Rosch J, Ivancev K: Venous stenoses in patients who undergo hemodialysis: treatment with self-expandable endovascular stents. *Radiology* 183: 499, 1992

51. Bosnjakovic P, Ivkovic T, Ilic M, Aracki S: Strecker stent in stenotic hemodialysis Brescia–Cimino arteriovenous fistulas. *Cardiovasc Intervent Radiol* 15: 217, 1992

52. Landwehr P, Lackner K, Gotz R: Dilatation and balloon-expandable stents for the treatment of central venous stenosis in dialysis patients. *Fortschr Roentgenstr* 153: 239, 1990

53. Vorwerk D, Günther RW, Bohndorf K, Kistler D, Gladziwa U, Sieberth HG: Follow-up results after stent placement in failing arteriovenous shunts: a three-year experiment. *Cardovasc Intervent Radiol* 14: 285, 1991

54. Beathard GA: The use of the Gianturco intravascular stent in stenotic hemodialysis fistulas. *ASAIO Trans* 37: M234, 1991

55. Selby J, Pruett T, Westervelt F, Tegtmeyer C, Poole L: Treatment of hemodialysis fistula pseudoaneurysms with detachable balloons: technique and preliminary results. *J Vasc Intervent Radiol* 3: 505, 1992

56. Gaylord G, Taber T: Long-term hemodialysis access salvage: problems and challenges for nephrologists and interventional radiologists. *J Vasc Intervent Radiol* 4: 103, 1993

THROMBOGENESIS AND ANTICOAGULATION IN PATIENTS UNDERGOING CHRONIC HEMODIALYSIS

GIANLUIGI VIGANÒ, ARRIGO SCHIEPPATI and GIUSEPPE REMUZZI

INTRODUCTION

A tendency toward thrombosis (particularly of the arterovenous shunt) is a frequent complication of uremic patients on hemodialysis. It is well known that uremia is associated with complex coagulation abnormalities (1–4) which include both bleeding diathesis (for a review see chapter by Winchester JF) and hypercoagulability. Table 1 shows the factors involved in the latter disturbance. The results of the global coagulation screening tests in uremic patients are generally normal. Most consistent findings are an increased level of fibrinogen (5) and decreased protein C anticoagulant activity with normal amidolytic activity and antigen (6, 7). Recently, it has been documented that the reduced protein C anticoagulant activity is due to the presence of a soluble plasma inhibitor that interferes specifically with the anticoagulant activity of activated protein C (8). Given the role of fibrinogen and protein C in coagulation homeostasis, it is not surprising that these abnormalities contribute to the increased risk of thrombosis episodes in these patients. *In vivo* studies have also demonstrated enhanced platelet activity in this population (9–11). However, conflicting data have been reported concerning *in vitro* platelet aggregation which was normal (12, 13), reduced (14, 15), or increased (16) according to different patient population and experimental conditions of the various studies.

The presence of lupus anticoagulant and anticardiolipin antibody (autoantibodies directed against negatively charged phospholipids) have also been described in uremic patients (17, 18) with a high prevalence both in conservatively treated (22%) and hemodialyzed (30%) patients. It has also been suggested that the presence of lupus anticoagulant and anticardiolipin antibody in these patients may represent a possible index of poor biocompatibility of dialyzer membranes (17, 18). Indeed, Garcia-

Table 1. Factors involved in the increased thrombotic risk of patients undergoing chronic hemodialysis

– Enhanced level of fibrinogen
– Reduced level of protein C anticoagulant activity
– Prevalence of lupus anticoagulant and anticardiolipin antibody
– Blood-artificial surface interaction
– Treatment with recombinant human erythropoietin

Martin and coworkers (17) found that patients dialysed with cuphropane membranes showed a greater incidence of anticardiolipin antibody compared to patients in whom more biocompatible membranes were used. Moreover, a possible link between the inhibitory effect of this activity and the system of protein C has been suggested (19).

The exposure of blood to an artificial surface also leads to a number of reactions of the hemostatic cascade. Indeed, immediately following the exposure of most artificial surfaces to blood, various plasma proteins begin to be adsorbed (20). The interaction between plasma proteins with artificial surfaces can initiate the activators of the intrinsic and extrinsic blood coagulation pathways. The consequent series of events culminate ultimately in the formation of a white mural thrombus mainly composed of fibrin, platelets, leukocytes, and erythrocytes (21). Numerous factors influence formation of the mural thrombi including the chemical and physical nature of the artificial surface itself, rheologic factors, stasis or vortical flow (21). Similarly, alterations in the reactivity of platelets and leukocytes brought about by their contact with artificial surfaces or by shear stress-induced changes enable these activated cells to enhance their contribution toward the thrombotic process. Therefore, the interaction

Table 2. Causes of fistula thrombosis in hemodialysis patients

- Venous or arterial stenosis
- Excessive postdialysis fistula compression
- Technical errors during fistula construction
- Hypotension
- Hypovolemia
- Fistula compression during sleeping position
- Hypercoagulable state

between blood and artificial surfaces represents an important mechanism of thrombogenesis and may itself explain the increased incidence of arteriovenous shunt thrombosis in hemodialysis patients.

The effect of artificial surfaces in activating blood coagulation and promoting thrombus formation have made necessary the use of anticoagulants in patients undergoing hemodialysis. Heparin is the most commonly used anticoagulant, both as a soluble anticoagulant and to coat artificial surfaces in efforts to improve their blood compatibility. Heparin can be indeed covalently bonded to a surface with resultant decrease in formation of thrombi. Antiplatelet agents such as aspirin, dypiridamole, sulphinpyrazone and prostacyclin have also been employed to reduce the activation of coagulation induced by artificial surfaces, however they are not routinely used as anticoagulants in hemodialyis.

VASCULAR ACCESS THROMBOSIS

A frequent cause of hospitalization in patients undergoing chronic hemodialysis is replacement, repair, removal or treatment of infection of an arteriovenous shunt or fistula (22). Approximately, 0.5–0.8 episodes of fistula thrombosis occur per patient year on dialysis (22). Table 2 reports the most common causes of fistula thrombosis. Usually, about 75% of all access thromboses are associated with stenotic lesions in the venous system (23). In the absence of an anatomic lesion the thrombosis may result from the application of excessive fistula compression to achieve hemostasis after dialysis and occasionally hypotension, decreased cardiac output, or hypovolemia also cause vascular access thrombosis (24, 25). It has been also documented that factors unrelated to fistula blood flow can contribute: anticardiolipin antibodies and the hypercoagulable states are associated with recurrent graft thrombosis (26). Alterations in the levels of protein C and S and antithrombin III (27, 28) have uncertain clinical significance.

The rate of access trombosis is also influenced by the access type. Indeed, it has been documented that synthetic grafts have a higher incidence of clotting than endogenous fistulae (29–31) mainly due to thrombogenicity of the graft material, turbulence of access blood flow, or progressive deterioration caused by repeated cannulation.

During the last decade, the cloning of the gene coding for erythropoietin and the production of the recombinant human erythropoietin have provided clinicians with a powerful tool for correcting the anemia of chronic renal failure. Erythropoietin treatment reverses the anemia of uremic patients eliminating their dependency upon transfusion (32–37). The treatment was also associated with a significant shortening of the bleeding time: a study (34) in 20 dialysis patients with a prolonged bleeding time (more than 15 minutes) randomly allocated to receive erythropoietin or no specific treatment, showed that an erythropoietin dose of 150 to 300 U/kg/week increased the hematocrit to a range of 27–32% and normalized bleeding times in all patients. The increase in the hematocrit value with erythropoietin raised concern that hemodialyis patients may suffer more frequent thrombotic events, including clotting of dialyzers and vascular access. Recently, Taylor et al. (38) studied the effect of erythopoietin therapy on blood coagulation and fibrinolysis in hemodialyzed patients. They showed that erythropoietin was associated with significant increase in the endothelial product Factor VIII von Willebrand factor antigen and fibrinogen to levels comparable to those observed in the untreated patients. Whole blood platelet aggregation also increased following erythropoietin treatment. Changes were also noted in thrombin-antithrombin III complex, prostacyclin stimulating factor and protein C (38). Macdougall et al. (39) studied the incidence of fistula thromboses in patients receiving erythropoietin therapy by measuring fistula blood flow, blood viscosity and a variety of tests of coagulation in 10 patients undergoing chronic hemodialysis and treated with erythropoietin. They showed that fistula blood flow was not altered during a 1-year of observation despite an increase in whole blood viscosity. Bleeding time improved in all the patients. No significant changes were found in prothrombin time, kaolin cephalin clotting time, antithrombin III or platelet aggregability to ADP after erythropoietin therapy. However, protein C and protein S levels significantly decreased over the first 4 months of therapy. By 8 to 12 months, these levels returned to pretreatment values. The Authors suggested that these alterations may predispose to thromboses of the fistula for hemodialysis (39). These findings were also confirmed in another study (40) showing that a higher incidence of graft thrombosis was detected between 2 and 5 months after the start of erythropoietin therapy.

However, a recent prospective placebo-controlled study investigating the relationship between hemorrheological changes caused by erythropoietin treatment and alterations in fistula function and heparin requirements in home hemodialyzed patients documented that erythropoietin induced a rise in high shear rate blood viscosity, but tests of fistula function and heparin requirements were similar both in patients receiving erythropoietin and in those receving placebo (41). Similar results were obtained by Standage et al. (42) who examined 64 hemodialyzed patients utilizing polytetrafluoroethylene grafts and treated with erythropoietin. The patients served as their own historical controls. There were 1.19 thrombectomies and 0.222 mechanical problems per 1,000 patient-days before erythropoietin use and 0.656 and 0.222 respectively after erythropoietin. There were no statistically significant differences between patients receiving low, medium or high erythropoietin dosages, suggesting that erythropoietin therapy was not associated with an increased incidence of graft thrombosis.

TREATMENT OF VASCULAR ACCESS THROMBOSIS AND ANTITHROMBOTIC PROPHYLAXIS

The surgical thrombectomy has long been established as the procedure of choice for the treatment of shunt thrombosis. A Fogarty-type catheter is usually employed (22). The procedure can be delayed for 24–48 hours, but the best result is obtained if the procedure is performed before the thrombus becomes organized.

The management of acute graft thrombosis also includes therapy with thrombolytic agents but the results are disappointing. Indeed, graft patency can be reestablished in fewer than 60% of cases (43–48), whereas serious bleeding complications and embolization of clot fragmentation also occur (45, 48), although the adjustments in thrombolytic dosing may improve the results. Using catheters with multiple side ports to minimize thrombolytic dispersion, the crossed catheter (49) and pulsed spray (50) techniques combine mechanical clot disruption with urokinase infusion. A 90% incidence of success was described in early reports within 1 hour from injection or infusion (43). Brunner and coworkers (49) have treated 11 out of 14 consecutive hemodialysis access occlusions with a dose of 1–1.25 million IU of urokinase delivered at a rate of 20,000 IU/min infused via the crossed-catheter technique. Such therapy restored patency within 1 hour without any significant complication. However, no study exists on the efficacy and a cost analysis is not available to compare these techniques with surgical thrombectomy.

Recently, it has been documented that a systemic streptokinase infusion was successful in 53% of hospitalized patients with internal shunt thrombosis without serious complication (51) and the authors suggested that systemic streptokinase treatment for acute shunt declotting followed by radiological evaluation of the vessels can be a reasonable alternative to urgent surgical declotting.

The use of the thrombolytic agent tissue plasminogen activator (t-PA) to declot arteriovenous accesses of hemodialyzed patients has also been described (52). t-PA was infused directly into the vascular access at a 10 mg dose, at 2 hour intervals, to a maximum of 30 mg. In 10 out of 15 patients t-PA completely restored graft patency, 3 patients reclotted within 24 hours and one had post-dialysis bleeding 5 days later after dialysis requiring compression of the vascular access, which resulted in reclotting.

Since platelet activation has been proposed to play a role in the development of neointimal hyperplasia as an important factor associated with vascular access thrombosis, several studies have been carried out to assess the efficacy of antiplatelet drugs in the prolongation of patency of vascular grafts. Although in some trials a significant protection against shunt thrombosis was obtained with aspirin, sulfinpyrazone and ticlopidine (53–56), the results cannot be considered conclusive because most studies lack randomized or double-blind design, have a very short follow-up period (a few weeks or months) or enrolled patients with external shunts. In 1979 Harter and coworkers reported in a randomized double-blind trial that aspirin (160 mg/day) helped prevent shunt thrombosis in chronic renal failure (57). The aim of the study was to determine the efficacy of aspirin versus placebo in prevention of shunt-thrombosis in 44 patients undergoing chronic hemodialysis. It was found that thrombi occurred in 18 of 25 (75%) of patients receiving placebo and 6 of 19 (32%) of those given aspirin ($p < 0.01$). Thus the incidence of thrombosis was reduced from 0.46 thrombi per patient/month in the placebo to 0.16 thrombi per patient month in the aspirin group ($p < 0.005$). However, the use of aspirin in uremic patients needs extreme caution. Indeed, two studies (58, 59) showed that low dose aspirin significantly prolonged bleeding time – the best hallmark of clinical bleeding in uremia (60) – in hemodialyzed patients. In the majority of patients bleeding time after aspirin was extremely prolonged (> 15 minutes) (58, 59). It has been also reported that a 56-year old hemodialyzed woman had a severe gastrointestinal bleeding following therapy with 50 mg/day of aspirin given to prevent thrombosis of an arteriovenous graft. Her hemoglobin fell to 3.1 g/dl, the hematocrit was 9% and bleeding time greater than 30 minutes (61). A gastroscopy documented a diffuse bleeding of the gastric mucosa with several superficial erosions, a picture typical for acute NSAID-induced gastritis. Therefore, even at very low dose, aspirin may be dangerous in uremic patients.

Recently, a meta-analysis of 9 studies (including 418 patients) indicated that antiplatelet treatment (with different drug regimens) obtained a reduction of 70% of the graft occlusions (62). However, these results suffer from several limitations, including the fact that the majority of the studies were carried out more than a decade ago, when the dialytic procedures and the incidence of thrombotic episodes were different. Thus, further studies are needed to address the exact role of antiplatelet treatment in preventing the clotting of vascular access for hemodialysis, avoiding bias in selecting subcategories of patients, considering a longer duration and using a randomized controlled design.

The results of a recent prospective, double-blind, placebo-controlled study has suggested a potential role for dipyridamole in preventing graft thrombosis in patients with a new arteriousvenous expanded polytetrafluoroethylene (ePTFE) graft (63). Two patients groups were studied: group I (with a new ePTFE graft) and group II (with thrombectomy and/or revision of a previously placed ePTFE graft). The aim of the study was to examine if dipyridamole and/or aspirin treatment could decrease the rate of thrombi of ePTFE graft in hemodialysis patients. Patients were randomly assigned to one of four drug regimens; dipyridamole 75 mg three times a day (tid) with aspirin placebo once a day (qd); dipyridamole placebo tid with aspirin 325 mg qd; dipyridamole 75 mg tid with aspirin 325 mg qd; or dipyridamole placebo tid with aspirin placebo qd. The results showed that patients on dipyridamole alone had a graft patency rate of 79% at the end of the observation period (1 year) in comparison with those treated with dipyridamole and aspirin combined who had a 75% rate. The authors concluded that dipyridamole was beneficial in patients with a new ePTFE grafts and that aspirin did not improve the risk of thrombosis in ePTFE grafts. Neither dipyridamole nor aspirin had any beneficial effect in patients with prior thrombosis of ePTFE grafts.

THE ANTICOAGULATION FOR HEMODIALYSIS

Heparin

Heparin is the anticoagulant most widely used to prevent clotting in the extracorporeal blood circuit in hemodialyzed patients. It is a highly anionic charged sulphated glycosaminoglicane extracted from bovine and porcine lung or intestine. Heparin accelerates the formation of a molecular complex between antithrombin III (AT III), a constituent of normal plasma, and coagulation factors of the intrinsic coagulation system. AT III, together with heparin, inhibits the activated clotting factors IX, X, XI, XII and thrombin. There is also evidence for a second heparin cofactor (HC II) active against thrombin (64), but it seems to be more specific for dermatan sulphate than for heparin itself.

Heparin preparations are a heterogenous mixture of molecules (2,000 to 40,000 molecular weight, averaging around 15,000 to 18,000) and the anticoagulant activity is related to its molecular size: by decreasing the molecular weight there is an increase in factor Xa inhibition and a reduction in thrombin inhibition. Low molecular weight heparin has a higher affinity for AT III and strongly inhibits factor Xa and XIIa, but only weakly inhibits thrombin and factor IX and XI. The size of heparin molecule also influences its interaction with platelets, and the interaction of platelets with dialyzer membranes (65, 66). Heparin is usually administered either by an infu-

sion pump or by bolus. A bolus dose of heparin, usually 50 U/kg of lean body weight is given followed by a constant infusion of 500 to 1,000 U of heparin per hour. The infusion is stopped 30 to 60 minutes before the end of the dialysis session.

A precise control of heparin anticoagulation is necessary. This used to be achieved by whole blood clotting time (WBCT). With the systemic used of heparin, WBCT is usually between 15 to 20 minutes. This method is however time-consuming and rapid adjustments in heparin dose cannot be made. Determination of the standard partial thromboplastin time as a control needs a coagulation laboratory available and is time-consuming. Therefore, adequate tests for bedside monitoring of anticoagulation during hemodialyis are the whole blood activated clotting time (WBACT) and the whole blood activated partial thromboplastin time. The WBACT is similar to WBCT but differs in that an activator, such as kaolin, is added to accelerate clotting. A normal WBACT is between 90 to 140 seconds, and allows close monitoring of clotting. For systemic anticoagulation the WBACT is kept 1.5 time greater than baseline. The whole blood activated partial thromboplastin time is based on the same principle except that the activator contains a platelet lipid surrogate as well as surface contact activators (normal range between 50 and 80 seconds). During hemodialysis the optimal WBACT is between 200 and 240 seconds and the whole blood activated partial thromboplastin time is between 120 and 160 seconds.

Side effects of a long-term treatment with heparin

The standard heparinization procedure includes administration of an initial bolus of heparin prior to the connection of the patient to the extracorporeal circuit and continuous infusion of heparin during hemodialysis.

Several undesiderable side effects may result from the long term therapy with heparin in hemodialysis patients, including the risk of bleeding complications and the possibility of chronic occult blood loss (67), thus leading to a further deterioration of the anemia in these patients. Heparin is also known to adversely affect both the coagulation and immune system as well as the plasma lipoproteins (68–70). In particular it has been described that heparin can induce an immuno-mediated thrombocytopenia (71). Some investigators have reported an increased amount of IgG on the surface of platelets from affected individuals, and others have isolated IgG fractions from patient serum that activate platelets in the presence of heparin (68, 69, 72–74). Adelmann et al. (71) have also demonstrated that intact IgG is necessary suggesting a role for the platelet Fc receptor.

Osteoporosis has been suggested as a further complication to long-term treatment with heparin. The development of osteoporosis may be related to the dosage of heparin rather than to the duration of therapy, but there is no conclusive evidence from controlled clinical trials

(75). Whether hemodialyzed patients may have a further aggravation of their abnormal bone metabolism by the continued exposure to treatment with heparin remains to be established. The mechanism by which heparin could induce osteoporosis is unknown but available data suggest that there could be a combination of decreased synthesis and increased resorption of bone (75, 76). Recently, it has been suggested by technetium-labeled heparin kinetics, that the accumulation of heparin in bone tissue due to impaired renal excretion could play a role in mineral metabolism resulting in osteopenia in hemodialysis patients (77).

Low molecular weight heparins (LMWH)

LMWH have been obtained by the depolymerization of the various chains of unfractioned heparin by chemical or enzymatic reactions which results in a molecule of an average molecular weight of approximately 5,000 Daltons. Due to the difference in production in procedures, available LMWHs have different characteristics and are structurally heterogenous (78–80). Specific biological properties of LMWH include a greater inhibition of factor Xa than thrombin activity and less interaction with platelets (78–80).

The influence of LMWH and unfractioned standard heparin on blood clotting and other routine laboratory parameters was investigated by Schrader and coworkers in a long-term cross-over study in hemodialysis patients (81). It has been shown that safe and effective dialysis can be performed using LMWH for anticoagulation. In a previous study (70) the same group of investigators comparing the efficacy of LMWH and unfractioned heparin in hemodialysis/hemofiltration found no overt bleeding complications in either groups, but the patients treated with LMWH required significantly fewer erythrocyte concentrates as compared to an 'unfractioned heparin group'. They suggest that LMWH may offer potential advantages in terms of less blood transfusion requirement and less derangement of certain metabolic parameters, such as triglycerides and plasma lipase activity (81). Nurmohamed et al. (82) in a randomized 6 month open follow-up study in 70 patients undergoing hemodialysis reported no major bleeding complication or adverse experiences during a total of 2,000 dialytic procedures with LMWH. Clot formation in the extracorporeal circuit was comparable between patients receiving LMWH or standard heparin and no accumulation of LMWH-anticoagulant activity was noted.

Regional heparinization and citrate anticoagulation

Regional heparinization procedure consists in a constant infusion of heparin into the inlet line of the dialyzer and a constant infusion of protamine sulfate into the outlet line before the blood returns to the patient (83–85). Howev-

Table 3. Characteristics of patients eligible for citrate anticoagulation or heparin-free dialysis

- Active bleeding
- Recent surgery (cardiovascular, ophtalmic, renal transplant, brain surgery)
- Pericarditis
- Intracranial hemorrhages
- Thrombocytopenia due to heparin sensitivity

er, it is difficult to determine the proper infusion rate of heparin to achieve extracorporeal but not systemic anticoagulation. An 'heparin rebound' phenomenon may occur after regional heparinization from 2 to 4 hours after cessation of dialysis for up to 10 hours. This rebound is caused by a heparin-protamine complex being broken down in the reticulo-endothelial system and heparin reentering the circulation (86, 87). This technique is rarely employed at present.

The citrate anticoagulation is mainly adopted for patients at high risk of bleeding who are actively bleeding. Table 3 shows the characteristics of selected patients in whom citrate anticoagulation is recommended. Blood is anticoagulated by chelating calcium with sodium citrate and by using a zero-calcium dialysate bath. At the same time, calcium chloride is given to the patient through the venous limb distal to the dialyzer. The risk of clotting with this method is low. Regional citrate anticoagulation has been successfully used in the treatment of both acute (88–90) and chronic (91–93) renal failure. Recently, it was shown (94) in a controlled comparison between citrate and low-dose heparin in patients at increased risk of bleeding, that the incidence of dialysis associated bleeding was significantly more frequent in those patients receiving low-dose heparin (50%) than in those given citrate anticoagulation (18%). One of the advantages of citrate anticoagulation is that systemic anticoagulation can be avoided. Disadvantages include the need for additional equipment, increased ultrafiltration and potential risk of hypercalcemia, hypocalcemia, hypernatremia, and metabolic alkalosis caused by citrate intoxication (95). The citrate infusion rate is adapted according to WBACT (measured in the arterial line, downstream from citrate infusion, and aimed at 100% prolongation).

Prostacyclin

Prostacyclin, an arachidonic acid metabolite, was first used by Turney et al. (96, 97) to reduce heparin requirement in patients at increased risk of bleeding. Further studies have documented the efficacy of this method both in acute (98–100) and chronic (98, 99, 101) hemodialysis. Prostacyclin induces a complete inhibition of platelet aggregation and does not cause bleeding when given at a mean dose of 5 ng/kg/min. Side effects of prostacy-

328   *Gianluigi Viganò, Arrigo Schieppati and Giuseppe Remuzzi*

clin therapy include headache, lightheadness and facial flushing at lower doses and hypotension at higher doses (98, 99, 102). With the lower doses (4–8 ng/kg/min) it has been possible to perform dialysis despite vasodilation (98, 103). A recent prospective trial has documented a significant decrease in bleeding complications using prostacyclin as compared to low-dose heparin in a high risk group of hemodialyzed patients (98). It was also documented that prostacyclin prevented the drop in platelet count due to extracorporeal aggregation (104) and the rise in plasma free-fatty acid concentrations (101) found in hemodialyzed patients using heparin as anticoagulant. The advantages of prostacyclin include the fact that hemodialysis can be performed without systemic anticoagulation, and that the bleeding risk is reduced (98). Disadvantages include the cost of the agent, hypotension secondary to vasodilation, tachycardia, headache, nausea, chest and abdominal pain, requiring close hemodynamic monitoring and physician attendance.

Hemodialysis without anticoagulation

In patients with active bleeding or at increased risk of bleeding or when heparin is contraindicated, heparin-free hemodialysis can be successfully performed (105–107). This technique involves pretreatment of both the blood lines and the dialyzer with a heparin-containing solution. Usually 2,000–5,000 U of heparin are added to a liter of saline and the solution is flushed across the dialyzer and blood lines. After initiation of dialysis, periodic saline rinses with 300 ml every 15 minutes are needed. One-to-one nursing is usually required for this technique to be successful. In patients with subclavian or femoral catheters or with blood flow lower than 300 ml/min, heparin-free hemodialysis is not recommended. Sanders and coworkers (106) in reviewing their retrospective experience documented the successfulness of the technique in mantaining solute clearances and avoiding the need for anticoagulation. In a prospective clinical trial performed in intensive care unit patients with acute renal failure the success of this technique was documented in more than 92% of the treatments without need to resort to anticoagulants (108). A temporary venous catheter was used in the majority of patients. Due to clotting in the extracorporeal circuit, about 7% of patients required conversion to other techniques of dialyses. Raja et al. (109) described 20 such heparin-free dialysis with a cellulate hollow fiber artificial kidney in 14 stable chronic hemodialysis patients. No severe episodes of clotting occurred. Caruana et al. (110) proposed heparin-free dialysis with rapid blood flow and without saline flushes as the first strategy to be used in dialysis patients at increased risk of bleeding. The obvious advantage of this technique is that no anticoagulants of any type are required. Specific disadvantages include the close monitoring of the venous and the arterial pressure alarms and careful monitoring for early signs of clotting in the extracorporeal circuit. Additionally, high blood flows

(250–300 ml/min) are required and transfusion should not be performed via the hemodialysis circuit because of the danger of hemoconcentration.

Dermatan sulphate

Recently, the infusion of dermatan sulphate has been proposed as anticoagulant agent in alternative to heparin during hemodialysis (111, 112). Dermatan sulphate is a naturally occurring glycosaminoglycan found in the connective tissues. It contains less sulphate glycosaminoglycan than heparin and in animal models it was found that dermatan sulphate caused less bleeding than heparin (113). This lower hemorrhagic property may be attributable to its reduced effect on platelet function. The dose-finding studies performed so far have shown that dermatan sulphate allowed a successful completion of the dialysis procedure at doses ranging from 6 to 10 mg/kg, depending on the type of the dialyzer and dialysis duration (112, 113). Usually dermatan sulphate is given as a single pre-dialysis bolus (4–5 mg/kg) followed by a constant infusion ranging between 0.65 mg/kg/h to 1 mg/kg/h. However, clinical experience is limited and future studies must address the clinical efficacy of dermatan sulphate in hemodialysis patients.

CONCLUSION

In conclusion, several methods to prevent extracorporeal circulation clotting during the hemodialysis procedure have been employed. Heparin is the mainstay of anticoagulant therapy and different heparin regimens are used according to patient's risk of development of complications due to the anticoagulation. Periodically evaluations for risks of bleeding and assessment of the appropriate anticoagulation regimen are needed.

In patients with active bleeding or with a recent history of hemorrhagic episodes hemodialysis procedure can be performed without any anticoagulation or with regional anticoagulation (citrate anticoagulation). These patients require close monitoring and in some cases close physician attendance.

Future directions should address alternative methods to heparin anticoagulation for hemodialysis which may also avoid possible complication associated with long-term heparin treatment such as osteoporosis, trombocytopenia and lipid abnormalities.

ACKNOWLEDGEMENT

The authors are grateful to Doctor Guido Finazzi for fruitful cooperation.

REFERENCES

1. Remuzzi G: Bleeding in renal failure. *Lancet* 1: 1205, 1988
2. Llach F: Hypercoagulability, renal vein thrombosis, and other thrombotic complications of nephrotic syndrome. *Kidney Int* 28: 429, 1985
3. Hocking WG: Hematologic abnormalities in patients with renal disease. *Hematol Oncol Clin North Am* 1: 229, 1987
4. Viganò G, Remuzzi G: Disorders of hemostasis in dialysis patients. in *The Principles and Practice of Dialysis*, edited by Henrich WL, Baltimore, Williams & Wilkins, 1994, p 287
5. Koppensteiner R, Stockenhuber F, Derfler K et al.: Fibrinogen in kidney disease. in *Fibrinogen: A New Cardiovascular Risk Factor*, edited by Ernest E, Koening W, Lowe GDO, Meade TW, Wien, Blackwell-MZV, 1992, p 301
6. Sorensen PJ, Knudsen F, Nielsen AH et al.: Protein C assay in uremia. *Thromb Res* 301, 1989
7. Sorensen PJ, Nielsen AH, Knudsen E, Dyerberg J: Defective protein C in uremia. *Blood Purif* 5: 29, 1987
8. Faioni EM, Franchi F, Krachmalnicoff A et al.: Low levels of the anticoagulant activity of Protein C in patients with chronic renal insufficiency: an inhibitor of Protein C is present in uremic plasma. *Thromb Haemostas* 66: 420, 1991
9. Viener A, Aviram M, Better OS, Brook JG: Enhanced *in vitro* platelet aggregation in hemodialysis patients. *Nephron* 43: 139, 1986
10. Lindsay RM, Prentice CRM, Davidson JF et al.: Haemostatic changes during dialysis associated with thrombus formation on dialysis membranes. *Br Med J* 4: 454, 1972
11. George CPR, Slichter SJ, Quadracci LJ et al.: A kinetic evaluation of hemostasis in renal disease. *N Engl J Med* 293: 1111, 1974
12. Smith MC, Dunn MJ: Impaired platelet thromboxane production in renal failure. *Nephron* 29: 133, 1981
13. Jorgenson KA, Ingeborg S: Platelets and platelet function in patients with chronic uremia on maintenance hemodialysis. *Nephron* 23: 233, 1979
14. Nenci GG, Berrettini M, Agnelli G et al.: Effects of peritonela dialysis, hemodialysis and kidney transplantation on blood platelet function. *Nephron* 23: 287, 1979
15. Lindsay RM, Moorthy AV, Koens F, Linton AL: Platelet function in dialyzed and non-dialyzed patients with chronic renal failure. *Clin Nephrol* 4: 52, 1975
16. Bemis J, Rigney J, Sosin A, Deane N: Enhanced platelet aggregation in chronic renal failure patients receiving hemodialysis treatment. *Trans Am Soc Artif Intern Organs* 23: 48, 1977
17. Garcia-Martin F, De Arriba G, Carrascosa T et al.: Anticardiolipin antibodies and lupus anticoagulant in end-stage renal disease. *Nephrol Dial Transplant* 6: 543, 1991
18. Quereda C, Pardo A, Lamas S et al.: Lupus-like *in vitro* anticoagulant activity in end-stage renal disease. *Nephron* 49: 39, 1988
19. Freyssinet JM, Ravanat C, Grunebaum L et al.: Antiphospholipid autoantibodies in thrombosis: cause and/or consequence of the disruption of the protein C-dependent hemostatic balance. in *Phospholipid-binding Antibodies*, edited by Harris EN, Exner T, Hughes GRV, Asherson TA, Boca Raton, CRC Press, 1991, p 255
20. Forbes CD, Prentice CRM: Thrombus formation and artificial surfaces. *Br Med Bull* 34: 201, 1978
21. Lindsay RM, Mason RG, Kim SW, Andrade JD, Hakim RM: Blood surface interactions – report of ASAIO panel conference. *Trans Am Soc Artif Intern Organs* 26: 603, 1980
22. Fan P, Schwab SJ: Hemodialysis vascular access. in *The Principles and Practice of Dialysis*, edited by Henrich WL, Williams & Wilkins, Baltimore, 1994, p 22
23. Galbraith S, Fan P, Collins D, Schawb S: Hemodialysis fistula thrombosis: a prospective evaluation of anatomic vs nonanatomic causes. *J Am Soc Nephrol* 3: 365, 1992
24. Feldman HI, Held PJ, Stoiber E et al.: Dialysis vascular access morbidity in the USA. *J Am Soc Nephrol* 1: 356, 1991
25. Del Greco F, Soper WS, Krumlovsky FA et al.: Thrombosis of vascular access for hemodialysis. in *Haemostasis and the Kidney*, edited by Remuzzi G, Rossi EC, Butterworths, London, 1989, p 303
26. Kirschbaum B, Mullinax F, Curry N, Mallory J: Association between anticardiolipin antibody and frequent clotting problems in hemodialysis patients. *J Am Soc Nephrol* 2: 232, 1991
27. Alegre A, Vicente V, Gonzales R, Alberca I: Effect of hemodialysis on Protein C. *Nephron* 46: 386, 1987
28. Lai KN, Yin JA, Yuen PMP, Li PKT: Effect of hemodialysis on protein C, protein S, and antithrombin III levels. *Am J Kidney Dis* 17: 38, 1991
29. Palder SB, Kirkman RL, Wittermore AD, Hakim RM, Lazarus JM, Tilney NL: Vascular access for hemodialysis. *Ann Surg* 202: 235, 1985
30. Zibari GB, Rohr MS, Landreneau MD et al.: Complications from permanent hemodialysis vascular access. *Surgery* 104: 681, 1988
31. Raju S: PTFE grafts for hemodialysis access. *Ann Surg* 206: 666, 1987
32. Winearls CG, Pippard MJ, Dowing MR et al.: Effect of human erythropoietin derived from recombinant DNA on the anaemia of patients maintained by chronic haemodialysis. *Lancet* 2: 1175, 1986
33. Ad Hoc Committee for the National Kidney Foundation: Statement on the clinical use of recombinant erythropoietin in anemia of end-stage renal disease. *Am J Kidney Dis* 14: 163, 1989
34. Viganò G, Benigni A, Mendogni D, Mingardi G, Mecca G, Remuzzi G: Recombinant human erythropoietin to correct uremic bleeding. *Am J Kidney Dis* 18: 44, 1991
35. Eschbach JW: Erythropoietin 1991 – an overview. *Am J Kidney Dis* 18 (Suppl 1): 3, 1991
36. Eschbach JW, Adamson JW: Guidelines for recombinant human erythropoietin therapy. *Am J Kidney Dis* 14 (Suppl 1): 2, 1989
37. Eschbach JW, Adamson JW: Recombinant human erythropoietin: implication for nephrology. *Am J Kidney Dis* 11: 203, 1988
38. Taylor JE, Belch JJ, McLaren M, Henderson IS, Stewart WK: Effect of erythropoietin therapy and withdrawal on blood coagulation and fibrynolysis in hemodialysis patients. *Kidney Int* 44: 182, 1993
39. MacDougall IC, Davies ME, Hallett I, Cichlin DL, Hutton RD, Coles GA, Williams JD: Coagulation studies and fistula blood flow during erythropoietin therapy in

haemodialysis patients. *Nephrol Dial Transplant* 6: 862, 1991

40. Muirhead N, Laupacis A, Wong C: Erythropoietin for anaemia in haemodialysis patients: results of a maintenance study. *Nephrol Dial Transplant* 7: 811, 1992

41. Shand BI, Buttimore AL, Hurrell MA et al.: Hemorheology and fistula function in home hemodialysis patients following erythropoietin treatment: a placebo-controlled study. *Nephron* 64: 53, 1993

42. Standage BA, Schuman ES, Ackerman D, Gross GF, Rangsdale JW: Does the use of erythropoietin in hemodialysis patients increase dialysis graft thrombosis rates? *Am J Surg* 165: 650, 1993

43. Zeit RM, Cope C: Failed hemodialysis shunts. *Radiology* 154: 353, 1985

44. Young AT, Hunter DW, Castaneda-Zuniga WP et al.: Thrombosed synthetic hemodialysis access fistulas: failure of thrombolytic therapy. *Radiology* 154: 639, 1985

45. Mangiarotti G, Canavese C, Thea A et al.: Urokinase treatment for arteriovenous fistulae declotting in dialyzed patients. *Nephron* 36: 60, 1984

46. Schilling JJ, Eiser AR, Slifkin RF, Withney JT, Neff MS: The role of thrombolysis in hemodialysis access occlusion. *Am J Kidney Dis* 10: 92, 1987

47. Rodkin RS, Bookstein JJ, Heeney DJ, Davis GB: Streptokinase and transluminal angioplasty in the treatment of acutelythrombosed hemodialysis access fistulas. *Radiology* 149: 425, 1983

48. Tordoir JHM, Herman JMMPH, Kwan TS, Diderich PM: Long-term follow-up of the polytetrafluoroethylene (PFTE) prosthesis as an arteriovenous fistula for haemodialysis. *Eur J Vasc Surg* 2: 3, 1987

49. Brunner MC, Matalon TA, Patel SK, McDonald V, Jensik SC: Ultrarapid urokinase in hemodialysis access occlusion. *J Vasc Intervent Radiol* 2: 503, 1991

50. Valji K, Bookstein JJ, Roberts AC, Davis GB: Pharmacomechanical thrombolysis and angioplasty in the management of clotted hemodialysis grafts: early and late clinical results. *Radiology* 178: 243, 1991

51. Matuszkiewicz-Rowinska J, Billip T, Omecka Z, Rowinski W, Sicinski A: Systemic streptokinase infusion for declotting of hemodialysis arteriovenous fistulas. *Nephron* 66: 67, 1994

52. Ahmed A, Shapiro WB, Porush JG: The use of tissue plasminogen activator to declot arteriovenous accesses in hemodialysis patients. *Am J Kidney Dis* 21: 38, 1993

53. Sreedhara R, Himmelfarb J, Lazarus JM, Hakim RM: Antiplatelet therapy in expanded polytetrafluoroethylene (ePTFE) graft thrombosis: results of a randomized double-blind study. *J Am Soc Nephrol* 4: 388 (Abstract 9P), 1993

54. Michie DD, Wombolt DG: Use of sulfilnpyrazone to prevent thrombus formation in arteriovenous fistulas and bovine grafts of patients on chronic hemodialysis. *Ther Res* 22: 196, 1977

55. Kobayashi K, Maeda K, Koshikawa S et al.: Antithrombotic therapy with ticlopidine in chronic renal failure patients on maintenance hemodialysis – a multicenter collaborative double blind study. *Thromb Res* 20: 255, 1980

56. Domoto DT, Bauman JE, Joist JH: Combined aspirin sulfynpirazone in the prevention of recurrent hemodialysis vascular access thrombosis. *Thromb Res* 82: 737, 1991

57. Harter HR, Burch JW, Majerus PW et al.: Prevention of thrombosis in patients on hemodialysis by low dose aspirin. *N Engl J Med* 301: 577, 1979

58. Livio M, Benigni A, Viganò G, Mecca G, Remuzzi G: Moderate doses of aspirin and risk of bleeding in renal failure. *Lancet* 1: 414, 1986

59. Gaspari F, Viganò G, Orisio S, Bonati M, Livio M, Remuzzi G: Aspirin prolongs bleeding time in uremia by a mechanism distinct from platelet cyclooxygenase inhibition. *J Clin Invest* 79: 1788, 1987

60. Steiner RW, Coggins C, Carvalho ACA: Bleeding time in uremia. *Am J Hematol* 7: 107, 1979

61. Viganò G, Remuzzi G: Low-dose aspirin and bleeding in uremia. *Am J Hematol* 42: 235, 1993

62. Antiplatelet Trialists' Collaboration: Collaborative overview of randomized trials of antipylatelet therapy. II: Maintenance of vascular graft of arterial patency by antiplatelet therapy. *Br Med J* 308: 159, 1994

63. Sreedhara R, Himmelfarb J, Lazarus JM, Hakim RM: Antiplatelet therapy in graft thrombosis: results of a prospective, randomized double-blind study. *Kidney Int* 45: 1477, 1994

64. Tollefaen DM, Majerus DW, Blank MK: Heparin cofactor II. *J Biol Chem* 257: 2162, 1982

65. Salzman EW, Rosenberg RD, Smith MH, Lindon JN, Favreau L: Effect of heparin and fractions on platelet aggregation. *J Clin Invest* 65: 64, 1980

66. Hirsh J, Ofosu F, Buchanan M: The rationale behind the development of low molecular weight heparin derivatives. *Semin Thromb Haemostas* 11, 13, 1985

67. Koch KM, Bechstein PB, Fassbinder W, Kaltwasser P, Schoeppe W: Occult blood loss and iron balance in chronic renal failure. *Proc Eur Dial Transplant Assoc* 12: 681, 1975

68. Larsson SO: On coagulation and fibrinolysis in uraemic patients on maintenance hemodialysis. *Acta Med Scand* 189: 453, 1971

69. Wessel-Aas T, Blomhoff JP, Wirum E, Nilson T: Hemodialysis and cell toxicity *in vitro* related to plasma triglycerides, post-heparin lipolytic activity and free fatty acids. *Acta Med Scand* 216: 75, 1984

70. Schrader J, Stibbe W, Armstrong VW et al.: Comparison of low molecular weight heparin to standard heparin in hemodialysis/hemofiltration. *Kidney Int* 33: 890, 1988

71. Adelman B, Sobel M, Fuhimura Y, Ruggero ZM, Zimmerman TS: Heparin-associated trombocytopenia: observations on the mechanism of platelet aggregation. *J Lab Clin Med* 113: 204, 1989

72. Chong BH, Grace CS, Rozenberg MC: Heparin-induced trombocytopenia: effect of heparin platelet antibody on platelets. *Br J Haematol* 49: 531, 1981

73. Chong BH, Pitney WR, Castaldi PA: Heparin-induced thrombocytopenia: association of thrombotic complications with heparin-dependent IgG antibody that induces thromboxane synthesis in platelet aggregation. *Lancet* 2: 1246, 1982

74. Stead RB, Schafer AI, Rosenberg RD et al.: Heterogeneity of heparin lots associated with thrombocytopenia and thromboembolism. *Am J Med* 77: 185, 1984

75. Matzsch T, Bergqvist D, Hedner U, Nilsson B, Ostergaard P: Heparin-induced osteoporosis in rats. *Thromb Haemost* 56: 293, 1986

76. Ringe JD, Becker K: Osteoporoseentwicklung bei Heparinlangzeit Therapie. *Med Mo Pharm* 8: 80, 1955

77. Majdalani G, Chomat J, Kanchko A, Yanai M, Man NK: Kinetics of technetium-labeled heparin in hemodialyzed patients. *Kidney Int* 41 (Suppl): 5131, 1993

78. Salzman EW: Low molecular weight heparin. Is small beautiful? *N Engl J Med* 315: 957, 1986

79. Thomas DR, Barrowwcliffe TW, Curtis AD. Low molecular weight heparin: a better drug? *Haemostasis* 16: 87, 1986

80. Ireland H, Lane DA, Curtis JR: Objective assessment of heparin requirements for hemodialysis in humans. *J Lab Clin Med* 103: 643, 1984

81. Schrader J, Stibbe W, Kandt M, Warneke G, Armstrong V, Muller HJ, Scxheler F: Low molecular weight heparin versus standard heparin. A long term study in hemodialysis and hemofiltration patients. *Trans Am Soc Artif Intern Organs* 36: 28, 1990

82. Nurmohamed MT, Ten Cate J, Stevens P, Hoeh JA, Lins RL, Ten Cate JW: Long term efficacy and safety of a low molecular weight heparin in chronic hemodialysis patients. A comparison with standard heparin. *Trans Am Soc Artif Intern Organs* 37: M459, 1991

83. Lindholm DD, Murray JS: A simplified method of regional heparinization during hemodialysis according to a predetermined dosage formula. *Trans Am Soc Artif Intern Organs* 10: 92, 1964

84. Spencer P, Cozzi E, Easterling RE, Penner JA: Regional heparinization with hollow fiber artificial kidney. *Proc AANNT* 4: 69, 1977

85. Gordon LA, Somon ER, Rukes JM, Richards V, Perkins HA: Studies in regional heparinization. *N AE J Med* 255: 1063, 1956

86. Blaufox MD, Hampers CL, Merril JP: Heparinization for hemodialysis. *Trans Am Soc Artif Intern Organs* 12: 207, 1966

87. Hampers CL, Blaufox MD, Merrill JP: Anticoagulation rebound after hemodialysis. *N Engl J Med* 275: 776, 1966

88. Pinnick E, Wiegmanson TE, Diederick DA: Regional citrate anticoagulation for hemodialysis in the patient at high risk for bleeding. *N Engl J Med* 308: 258, 1983

89. Lohr JW, Slusher S, Diederich D: Safety of regional citrate hemodialysis in acute renal failure. *Am J Kidney Dis* 13: 104, 1989

90. Collart F, Tielemans C, Wens R, Drawta M: Local experience of regional anticoagulation with sodium citrate for hemodialysis in patients at risk of bleeding. *Proc Eur Dial Transplant Assoc-Eur Renal Assoc* 22: 325, 1985

91. Morita Y, Johnson RW, Dorn RE, Hall DS: Regional anticoagulation during hemodialysis using citrate. *Am J Med Sci* 242: 32, 1961

92. Von Brecht JH, Flanigan MJ, Freeman RM et al.: Regional anticoagulation. Hemodialysis with hypertonic trisodium citrate. *Am J Kidney Dis* 8: 196, 1986

93. MacDougall M, Seaton R, Diederich D, Wiegmann T: Effects of both composition and dialyzer membrane on leukocytes and oxygenation during hemodialysis with citrate anticoagulation. *Kidney Int* 25: 188, 1984

94. Flanigan MJ, Von Brecht J, Freeman RM, Lim VS: Reducing the hemorrhagic complications of dialysis. A controlled comparison of low dose heparin and citrate anticoagulation. *Am J Kidney Dis* 9: 147, 1987

95. Kelleher SP, Schulman G: Severe metabolic alkalosis complicating regional citrate hemodialysis. *Am J Kidney Dis* 9: 235, 1987

96. Turney JH, Fewell MR, Williams LC, Parsons V, Weston MJ: Platelet protection and heparin sparing with protsacyclin during regular dialysis therapy. *Lancet* 2: 219, 1980

97. Turney JH, Woods HF, Weston MJ: The use of prostacyclin in extracorporeal circuits. in *Hemostasis, Prostaglandins and Renal Disease*, edited by Remuzzi G, Mecca G, de Gaetano G, New York, Raven Press, 1980, p 353

98. Swartz RD, Flamenbaum W, Dubrow A, Hall JC, Crow JW, Cato A: Epoprostenol during high risk hemodialyis – preventing further bleeding complications. *J Clin Pharmacol* 28: 818, 1988

99. Zussman RM, Rubin RH, Cato AE, Cocchetto DM, Crow JW, Tolkoff-Rubin N: Hemodialysis using prostacyclin instead of heparin as the sole antithrombotic agent. *N Engl J Med* 304: 934, 1981

100. Hory B, Saint-Hiller Y, Perol JC: Prostacyclin as the sole anti-thrombotic agent for acute renal failure hemodialysis. *Nephron* 33: 71, 1983

101. Davies SJ, Hobson SM, Young GA, Turney JH: Acute changes in plasma free fatty acid concentratioon during hemodialysis comparing heparin with epoprostenol as anticoagulant. *Proc Eur Dial Transplant Assoc-Eur Renal Assoc* 22: 321, 1985

102. Smith MC, Danviriyasup K, Crow JW, Cato AE, Park GD, Hassid A, Dunn MJ: Prostacyclin substitution for heparin in long-term hemodialysis. *Am J Med* 73: 669, 1982

103. Dubrow A, Flamenbaum W, Mittman N, Hall J, Zinn T: Safety and efficacy of epoprostenol (PGI2) versus heparin in hemodialysis. *Trans Am Soc Artif Intern Organs* 30: 52, 1984

104. Addonizio VP, Fisher CA, Bowen JC, Palatianos GC, Colman RW, Edmunds LH: Prostacyclin in lieu of anticoagulation with heparin for extracorporeal circulation. *Trans Am Soc Artif Intern Organs* 27: 304, 1981

105. Glaser P, Guesde R, Rouby JJ, Eurin B: Hemodialysis without heparin is possible. *Lancet* 2: 579, 1980

106. Sanders PW, Taylor H, Curtis JJ: Hemodialysis without anticoagulation. *Am J Kidney Dis* 5: 32, 1985

107. Casati S, Moia, Graziani G et al.: Hemodialysis without anticoagulants: efficiency and hemostatic aspects. *Clin Nephrol* 21: 102, 1984

108. Schwab SJ, Omorato JJ, Sharar LR, Dennis PA: Hemodialysis without anticoagulation. One year prospective trial in hospitalized patients at risk of bleeding. *Am J Med* 83: 405, 1987

109. Raja RM, Kramer M, Rosenbaum JL et al.: Haemodialysis without heparin infusion using CORDIS DOW 3500 hollow filter. *Proc Dial Transplant Forum* 10: 39, 1980

110. Caruana RJ, Raja RM, Bush JV, Kramer MS, Goldsmith SJ: Heparin free dialysis: comparative data and results in high risk patients. *Kidney Int* 31: 1351, 1987

111. Ryan KE, Lane DA, Flynn A et al.: antithrombotic properties of dermatan sulphate (MF 701) in haemodialyis for chronic renal failure. *Thromb Haemost* 68: 563, 1992

112. Nurmohamed MT, Roggekamp M, Buller HR, Erkamp R, Stevens P, Ten Cate JW: A randomized cross-over study of dermatan sulphate and combination with heparin as

anticoagulant in chronic haemodialysis patients. *Thromb Haemost* 65 (Abstract): 925, 1991

113. Fernandez F, Van Ryn J, Ofosu FA, Hirsh J, Buchanan MR: The haemorrhagic and antithrombotic effects of dermatan sulphate. *Br J Haematol* 64: 309, 1986

HEMODIALYSIS MACHINES AND MONITORS

HANS-DIETRICH POLASCHEGG and NATHAN W. LEVIN

INTRODUCTION

The last decade has seen not only an enormous growth in the number of hemodialysis patients but also a concomitant growth in the number of hemodialysis machines produced every year by fewer companies than 10 years ago. Because the risk of accidents increases with the number of different machines in the field, standard organizations and government authorities worldwide have issued standards and laws that regulate the design of hemodialysis machines. Both effects have slowed the development of new concepts and the effective use of modern technology in hemodialysis machines. The extracorporeal circuit has remained unchanged for more than twenty years. Bicarbonate dialysis with single patient machines and volumetric ultrafiltration control which were developed in the late 70s took more than 10 years to be generally accepted. Cost pressure has been an effective driving force for the introduction of new technology. High-efficiency dialysis was introduced in order to reduce treatment time. Underdialysis of many patients was the result because in many cases the shortening of the treatment time was not sufficiently compensated for by the increased efficacy of the dialysis process. This triggered the development of devices that allow monitoring of dialysis efficacy. It became apparent that intradialytic symptomatic episodes, blood access problems and long-term complications contribute significantly to the overall cost of hemodialysis. This has already triggered the development of innovative monitors for the feed-back loop control of the hemodialysis process. It is hypothesized that these monitors will allow more physiological control of hemodialysis and thus reduce the number of intradialytic symptoms. While the introduction of these monitors in addition to existing monitoring devices will temporarily increase the cost of hemodialysis equipment this new technology is potentially cost saving. The new monitors for feedback control using physiological parameters can replace the existing more costly mechanical controls of hemodialysis parameters (1). This chapter describes current technology of hemodialysis machines as well as recent developments for dialysis quantification and feed-back control of dialysis parameters that may become standard features by the year 2000.

GENERAL SAFETY DESIGN

Safety standards

Because of the paramount importance of safety, national and international authorities and committees have developed regulations and standards. Standards describe the established technology, the state of the art. They are voluntary but can be referenced by authorities. Internationally IEC, the International Electrical Commission (2), issues standards for medical electrical equipment, and those relevant for dialysis (3). ISO, the International Standard Organization (4) publishes standards for disposables, such as dialyzers and blood lines (5, 6). The European counterparts are CENELEC (7) and CEN (8) respectively. The European standards mostly adapt the international ones. These standards are translated into the various European languages to become national standards. In the US a comprehensive standard on hemodialysis equipment is published by AAMI (9, 10).

Safety and reliability

A technical device is safe when any malfunction can be excluded. Because every manmade device wears out and develops defects, it is impossible to manufacture an ultimately reliable device. In practice any safety design has to take defects into account. One example for safe design is the use of additional protective systems that switch the device into a safe mode in case of malfunction of the control or operating system.

Fail safe design

Dialysis machines are fail-safe! This term is used to describe systems with at least two safe modes of operation, normal operation being the first one. In case of a hazard the machine is automatically switched into the second mode (usually the operation is halted). The definition given by Grimsrud et al (11) is still applicable: "In the event of an excursion of the variables outside their control limits, or a breakdown of the monitoring or control equipment itself, the system will automatically return to a safe configuration. The term 'safe configuration' means that condition in which the patient is isolated and thereby protected from the malfunction and its effects."

Safety under single-fault condition

A hazard might be caused by a single defect of a device (e.g., loss of control function of the blood pump so that the pump runs at maximum speed) or by two or multiple defects, independent of each other. The development and production cost of any device increases non-linearly with the number of defects a device can safely tolerate. Safety is a relative measure depending on risk and risk acceptance. For medical devices the risk caused by two defects within one treatment period is generally accepted. As can be shown it is less than the risk of a normal life accident: In a typical dialysis machine production of dialysis fluid is performed by a mixing system that is monitored by an independent conductivity monitor. Quality and repair statistics show that the likelihood for any of the two systems to fail is less than 10^{-4}/h. For both systems to fail the likelihood is therefore less than 10^{-8}/h, which is less than the natural likelihood of death. This rare event is accepted by the dialysis industry and national and international standards. Fortunately a double fault does not necessarily

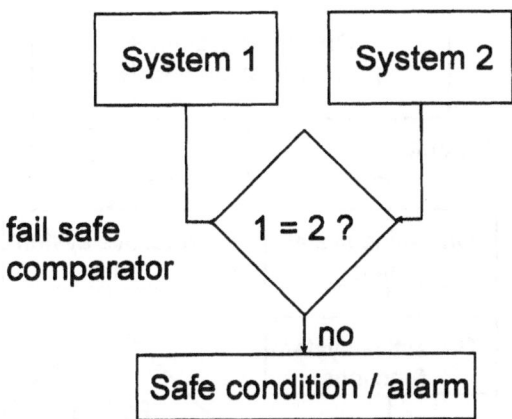

Figure 1. Design principles for safety under single-fault condition: Redundancy of protective systems.

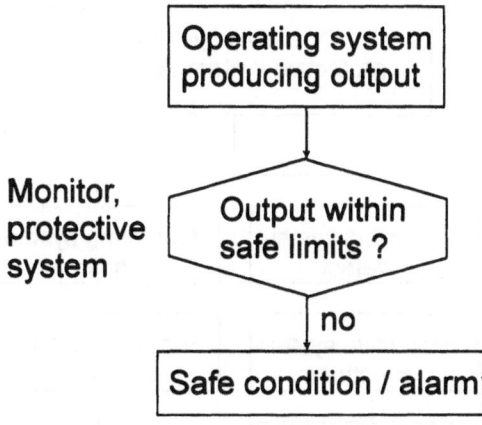

Figure 2. Design principles for safety under single-fault condition: Operating system and protective system (monitor).

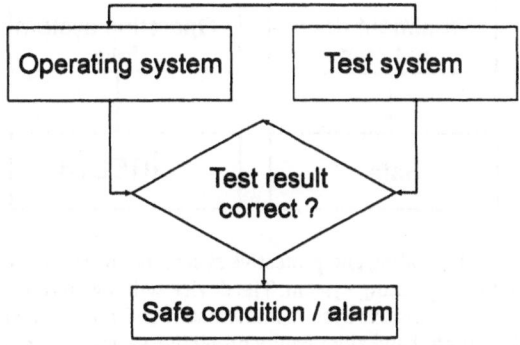

Figure 3. Design principles for safety under single-fault condition: Periodic test of the operating system by a test system.

lead to a severe accident. In most cases the user is able to react before the patient is harmed.

Design principles for safety under single-fault condition

Fault exclusion: For some components, especially mechanical ones, faults can be excluded because they are highly unlikely. To use fault exclusion for safety design, long lasting experience with the specific kind of component must exist and the component must not be used at its maximum rating. An example for such a component is the spring in a spring loaded clamp. In some cases only specific faults can be excluded. An example is the relay with mechanically coupled contacts. It can be excluded that the contacts are in different positions, opposite or it can be assumed that all contacts are either open or closed.

Inherent fail safe design: In some cases it is possible to design a component or device such that in case of a malfunction it automatically returns to a safe position. One example is the spring loaded clamp often used to shut the extracorporeal circuit. This clamp is so designed that mechanical faults can be excluded. In case of an electrical fault the clamp will automatically be closed by the spring.

Redundancy (Figure 1): If the safety of the patient or user depends only on a protective system (monitoring device), a malfunction of this device causes a hazard to the patient. In this case a second device can be added and the output of the two devices be compared by a fail safe comparator. In case the two outputs are different the fail safe comparator will switch the device into a safe position. This design is often used for air detectors.

Protective system in addition to an operating system (Figure 2): If the safety of the patient or user depends on the correct function of an operating system an additional protective system can be used to achieve safety under a single-fault condition. An example for the operating

system is dialysate mixing with the conductivity monitor serving as protective system.

Periodic test of the operating system (Figure 3): This is a cost effective means applied when an additional protective system that monitors the output of the operating system would be too expensive or too difficult to design. In this case the operating system is periodically checked for correct function by an automatic test system. An example for this design is the automatic pressure holding test for volumetric ultrafiltration control devices. In this design the test system serves as a protective system.

Test of protective systems prior to use: The above mentioned limitation to single-faults is justified only, when the likelihood for double faults is small. This is only the case when a first fault becomes or is made obvious to the user within a limited period of time. Because not every fault occurring during dialysis will become immediately obvious to the user the protective systems periodically have to be tested. Generally it is required to test the system prior to each dialysis. If field records prove that the likelihood of a fault is sufficiently low the time between tests can be increased. Most machines produced in the 1980s do

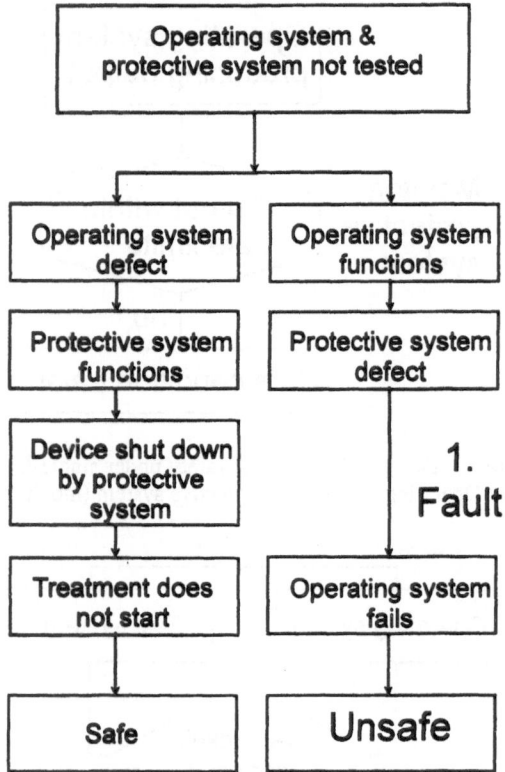

Figure 4. Operating and protective system not tested. Left hand side: Faulty operating system. The device will not start working because the protective system immediately switches it into a safe position. Right hand side: Faulty protective system, not obvious to the user. The device will start working. A first fault of the operating system will cause an immediate hazard to the patient.

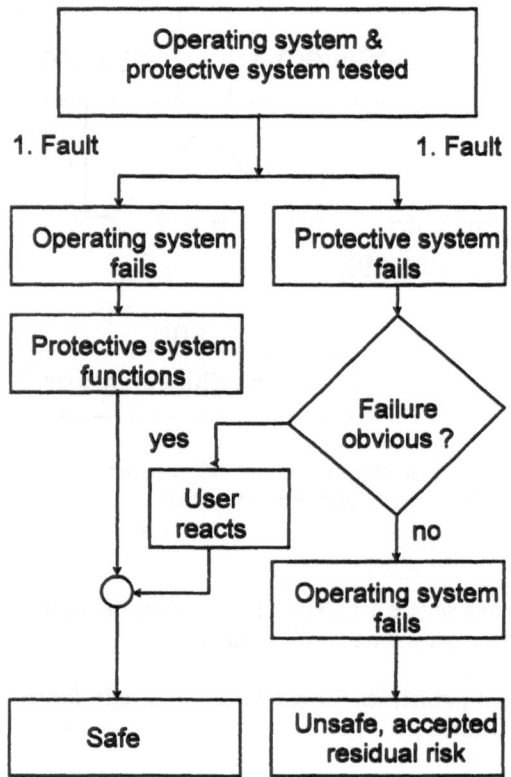

Figure 5. Operating and protective system tested prior to use. Left hand side: First fault on operating system. In this case the protective system will switch the device into a safe position. Right hand side: First fault on protective system. No immediate hazard to the patient because the operating system still functions normally. The fault might become obvious to the user and the user will react. If it does not become obvious and a second fault occurs that leads to a malfunction of the operating system then the patient is in danger. This risk is low and generally accepted when the system is tested prior to each use.

not test automatically the protective systems. Failure to do this manually is the cause of most accidents reported. The flow of events in case of systems tested properly or not tested is sketched in Figures 4 and 5.

User error: Even within the limits mentioned above safety can only be achieved by proper operation of the device. The most common user error is the inappropriate use of the override function of a protective system and the unjustified readjustment of alarm limits after an alarm. Modern electronic technology allows the design of dialysis machines without manual alarm settings and override buttons.

THE EXTRACORPOREAL CIRCUIT

Dialysis requires that blood is transported through the dialyzer. The driving force for this flow is a pressure difference between inlet and outlet. Historically, Kolff (12) used gravity as a driving force by lifting a burette with blood collected from the patient to the ceiling of the room. Later, arterio-venous pressure differences were utilized to propel blood through the extracorporeal circuit.

This technique is still in use in intensive care for CAVH (continuous arterio-venous hemofiltration) and CAVHD (continuous arterio-venous hemodialysis). It was reintroduced in 1977 (13) because it is not dependent on technical devices. An extracorporeal circuit, even if operated only by the arterio-venous pressure difference, might pose a hazard in case of a fault. A possible fault is disconnection of the line with a large blood loss to the environment. Deaths have been reported caused by such disconnections (14). Nevertheless this procedure is accepted as safe by regulatory authorities and the medical community. This is a good example of risk acceptance being higher when no technology is involved.

Hemodialysis machines today work almost exclusively with pump driven extracorporeal circuits comprising peristaltic pumps. Either cannulas or catheters are used as blood access. Figure 6 shows the principal components of the extracorporeal circuit. The part between the arterial cannula and the dialyzer is called the arterial blood line,

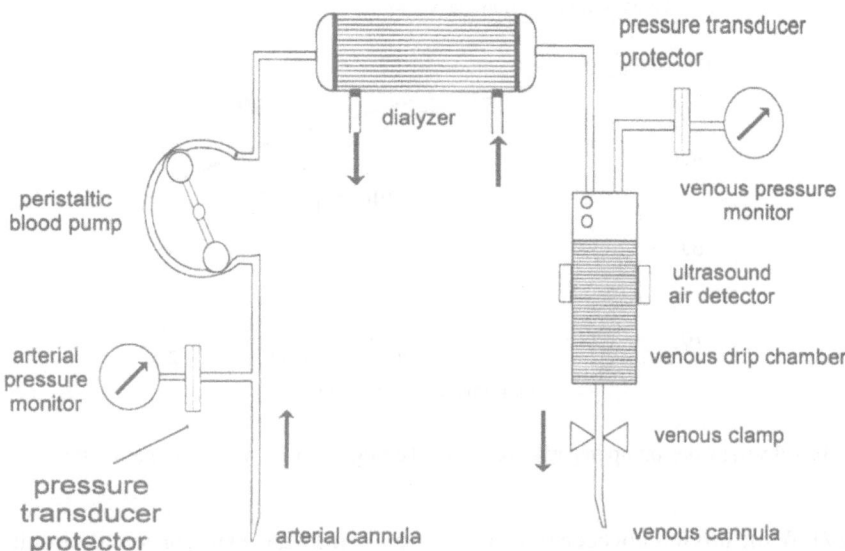

Figure 6. Main components of the extracorporeal circuit. The blood circuit might additionally have an arterial drip chamber positioned either upstream or downstream of the blood pump and one or more injection or sampling ports.

the part between the dialyzer and the venous cannula the venous blood line.

Pumps

Practically all pumps used today are of the rotary peristaltic type with two spring loaded rollers. The rationale for two rollers is a compromise between the ability to load simply and physical damage to blood. With other parameters kept constant blood damage is proportional to the number of rollers. On the other hand the pump bed must cover at least an angle of $360°/n$ with n being the number of rollers. For two rollers the result is $> 180°$ which allows entrance and exit on the same side. The stroke per revolution is calculated by equation [1]:

$$V_s = D * \pi * a,$$ [1]

with D [cm] being the diameter of the pump bed at the tubing axis, and a [cm^2] the cross section of the tube V_s, measured in [ml]. For an ideal tube of circular cross section a is calculated by equation [2]:

$$a = \frac{d^2 * \pi}{4}.$$ [2]

For typical dimensions ($D = 9$, and $d = 0.8$ [cm]), $V_S = 14$ ml per revolution. Note that the stroke per revolution is independent of the number of rollers employed.

The flow speed is the product of the stroke volume and rotary speed (equation [3]):

$$Q_b = V_s * r.$$ [3]

Most dialysis machines calculate blood pump rate from this equation for a pre-set tubing diameter. Some machines

allow input of tubing diameter for blood flow calculation.

The tubing collapses under negative pressure. This reduces the cross section and thus the pumping speed. It leads to a reduction of blood flow versus the value calculated by equation [3] of typically 13% with PVC and 20% with silicon tubing at a negative pressure of -200 mmHg (Figure 7). At least one commercial dialysis machine comprises software that takes this into account (15).

Making the tubing softer leads to earlier collapse of the tubing under negative pressure. This can be used to limit the negative pressure the pump is capable of creating physically, but the shear stress resulting from the narrow slit formed by the collapsed tubing might lead to hemolysis.

The pump speed is independent of the positive pressure created downstream of the pump, up to a certain limit defined by the force of the springs employed to occlude the tubing and by the tubing rigidity. Older pumps were capable of producing pressures of more than 6 bar which was sufficient to rupture most lines. More recent ones utilize springs that limit the maximum pressure the pump might produce to 2 bar with PVC tubing at 37°C. Above this pressure the pump is no longer fully occluding. Whether or not this leads to hemolysis is still unknown.

Self-loading pumps: Many pumps require manual loading of the pump tubing: The pump has to be stopped, a door opened and the tubing put in with one hand while the other one manually operates the rotor. Inventors successfully simplified this procedure by developing self loading pumps as described (16). Particle spallation: Particles released from silicon blood pump tubing have been

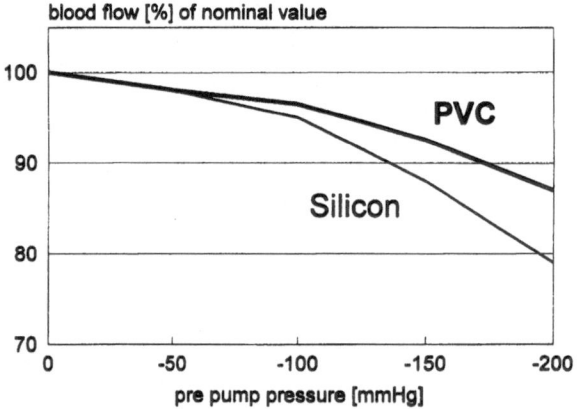

Figure 7. Reduction of blood versus pre-pump negative pressure. Tubing 8 mm id, wall thickness 2 mm.

detected in patients (17). While this has not been related to any patient morbidity it has caused concern and initiated research in this field. It was found that the problem is not limited to silicone, since particles are also released from PVC blood pump tubing although their detection in tissue is much more difficult. Reducing the occlusive force of the rollers has been found effective in reducing spallation (18).

Bubble traps

Blood lines traditionally include a venous and more recently also an arterial bubble trap. Usually the venous bubble trap holds a particle filter within it. These bubble traps were introduced during the development of the extracorporeal circuit and are by no means required if state of the art monitoring is applied. In fact these bubble traps and filters promote clotting.

Historical development: The first extracorporeal circuits were pumpless and blood flow was measured by the bubble transit time method: An air bubble was injected into the line and its transit time for a given length of tubing was determined (19). This bubble had to be removed before entering into the patient. A 'bubble catcher' or 'bubble trap' was therefore placed into the line. Later this bubble trap was found to be a convenient place to add a pressure line that permitted measurement of the pressure in the extracorporeal circuit in order to gain some control of ultrafiltration. Another purpose was the estimate of blood flow from the number of drops into the chamber. The venous bubble trap is therefore also called 'drip chamber'. The arterial bubble trap was introduced because it was found that air from the pre-pump arterial pressure sensor line entered the dialyzer when blood flow was increased and pre-pump pressure decreased (became more negative).

It is well known that air interfaces, as well as stagnant areas, introduced by bubble traps cause clotting. When heparin-free dialysis is performed the basic rules are to fill bubble traps completely to avoid air-blood interfaces

and rinse the extracorporeal circuit frequently, to clear stagnant areas of blood. The filter usually found in the venous bubble trap has a mesh size of 120–200 μm. Its intended use is to trap particles and emboli emerging from the dialyzer or the blood pump. Capillary dialyzers that account for more than 80% of all used dialyzers do not allow the passage of particles larger than 200 μm. The filter in the bubble trap only catches particles in the diameter range of 120 to 200 μm. If such particles still come out of modern dialyzers they are caught during the priming procedure instead of washed away during priming. The filters are another site for clot formation. If clots are found in these filters close inspection reveals that they are downstream of the mesh. No problems have been reported by clinicians not using filters in bubble traps. While no purpose seems to exist for the use of filters in conjunction with capillary dialyzers the situation might be different for parallel plate dialyzers. Filters might give some protection if large clots formed inside the dialyzer are released.

Priming of the extracorporeal circuit

The extracorporeal circuit has to be primed with an isotonic fluid, usually a sodium chloride solution with a concentration of 155 mmol/l. The purpose is to rinse the circuit, remove remaining particles and sterilants and also to remove air from the circuit. The precise priming procedure depends on the dialyzer and dialysis machine used. An important part of the procedure not described in instruction manuals is the priming of the arterial pressure line. This part is primed under positive pressure. Later during dialysis if negative pressure is created, air in the pressure line expands and enters the blood line. The arterial bubble trap was introduced to collect this air. Air released from the line can be avoided if at one point during the priming procedure the blood tubing upstream of the pressure line is clamped and a negative pressure equal to the greatest occurring during operation is created.

In order to fill the blood and the dialysate side of the dialyzer, as well as purge all air from both circuits the dialyzer is first rinsed on one side from bottom to top then turned and filled from the other side. Several procedures have been developed or proposed that allow keeping the dialyzer in place: Reversal of blood side flow was used in the Seratron machine (Seratronics, Walnut Creek, CA, USA), reversal of dialysate flow by valves or pumps (20, 21), evacuation of the circuit (22) and filling by backfiltration (23, 24). When the extracorporeal circuit is completely filled with fluid, it is flushed of sterilants and particles. Isotonic fluid is then recirculated until the circuit is eventually connected to the patient. In general the arterial end is connected to the extracorporeal circuit first and blood enters the system, while the filling solution is discarded. Many dialysis machines include optical sensors downstream of the venous drip chamber to indicate when blood arrives at this point during the priming procedure. The blood pump stops automatically to allow connection of the venous side. The optical sensor also indicates the end of the flush back procedure at the end of dialysis. This optical sensor was introduced with the A2008C machine (Fresenius AG, Oberursel, Germany) and later improved (25).

Devices and procedures to prevent clotting in the extracorporeal circuit

The bubble traps, injection ports and pressure measuring lines of the extracorporeal circuits common today are areas of stagnant flow and air-blood interfaces that promote clotting. This clotting is either prevented by the application of drugs, mostly heparin or by periodic flushing of the circuit with saline. Both procedures can be performed manually but mechanical devices such as pumps or controllers are common.

Heparin pumps: Mostly syringe pumps are used for heparin injection into the extracorporeal circuit. Standard heparin contains 5000 IU/ml. An infusion rate of 600–3000 IU/h is required to maintain anticoagulation during dialysis (26). A syringe size of 5 ml and pump rates of 0.1 to 1 ml/h would be appropriate. Most dialysis machines have pumps adapted for larger syringes. In this case heparin has to be diluted to allow precise anticoagulation. Traditionally, the point of infusion is between the blood pump and the dialyzer to avoid the risk of air-infusion. With air-detectors obligatory today, heparin could as well be infused pre-pump. In this case the pump could be replaced by a simple controller (27). Heparin can be infused on the venous side as well because the purpose of this infusion is the replacement of heparin lost by metabolism.

Regional anticoagulation: For regional anticoagulation either heparin or citrate is used as an anticoagulating agent and infused in front of the dialyzer. Protamine sulfate and calcium chloride, respectively, are used to reverse anticoagulation downstream of the dialyzer. The infusion rate for heparin is approximately 0.3 IU/ml (28). This converts into an infusion rate of 2 ml/h at a blood

flow of 500 ml/min. Syringe pumps using 10 to 20 ml syringes would be appropriate for this treatment. Larger volumes are required for anticoagulation with sodium citrate where isoosmotic trisodium citrate is infused at a rate of 2.5–7.5% of blood flow. This has to be combined with increased ultrafiltration to compensate for the infused volume, calcium free dialysate and $CaCl_2$ (5% solution) infusion at a rate of 0.5 ml/min (29). If hyperosmolar trisodium citrate is used standard syringe pumps can be used.

Anticoagulation-free dialysis: An extracorporeal blood circuit can be operated without anticoagulation if it is flushed with saline solution at intervals of 15–30 minutes. Approximately 200 ml of saline are used for each flush which accumulates to 2–3 liters of saline that additionally have to be ultrafiltered. In general the procedure is performed manually. Automatic devices have been described in the patent and general literature. Donatelli (30) described a system comprised of two clamps that are alternatively closed and opened. The first one is on the blood line, the second one on an infusion line that branches from the pre-pump arterial line. These clamps are switched by an automatic timer. A system that uses on-line prepared substitution fluid for the flushing procedure is described (31). No adjustment of the ultrafiltration rate is necessary in this system.

Safety monitors of the extracorporeal circuit

The use of a pump able to create negative and positive pressure introduces additional hazards. Safety standards (IEC, AAMI) list these hazards as blood loss to the environment, blood loss by clotting and air embolism. Additional hazards, not addressed by standards include: Damage of vessel walls by elevated sucking pressure and hemolysis caused by high shear stress in kinked or otherwise obstructed blood lines.

Pressure monitors

The venous pressure monitor is a limited protective system against blood loss to the environment. Blood might leak through open clamps on infusion lines that branch from the blood tubing or through faulty connections in the blood line. Because blood flow per minute accounts for 5–10% of the patient's total blood volume, a leak has to be detected immediately. Venous pressure monitors are generally accepted as a protective system against blood loss to the environment. They are sensitive to pressure changes caused by reduced flow through the blood access needle that accounts for the larger part of the flow resistance. The sensitivity is limited to major leaks. The monitor is not capable of detecting blood loss when the needle slips from a forearm-fistula because pressure in this kind of blood access is close to environmental pressure. Fistula pressure is about 10 mmHg, venous pressure at a blood flow of 400 ml/min might be 210 mmHg depending on the cannula type used. The 210 mmHg pressure in this example is the sum of the fistula pressure (10 mmHg) and the pressure drop caused by the flowing blood and the flow resistance. An alarm limit might be set at 190 mmHg close to the operating pressure. In order to trigger the alarm the pressure has to drop by 20 mmHg. If the needle slips from the fistula the pressure will drop only by 10 mmHg, not triggering the alarm. Any other blood leak must exceed 20/200 = 10% of the blood flow to reduce the pressure by 20 mmHg. Thus a blood loss of up to 40 ml/min might go undetected.

Pressure is sensed through a completely or partially air filled tube that connects the venous bubble trap with a luer lock connector connected to the sensor. To avoid cross contamination in case blood enters this line and wets the machine-side connection, pressure transducer protectors are inserted into this line. Most common are hydrophobic membranes but impermeable flexible membranes have been used as well. When hydrophobic membranes become accidentally wetted pressure changes are no longer transmitted to the sensor and the monitor becomes inoperative. This situation is normally not detected automatically by the monitor. Sensing pressure pulses that are produced by the blood pump have recently been described as a means to detect such faults (32).

Better alternatives to pressure monitoring generally are not yet available. A cassette type device developed for a dialysis machine for intensive care use, uses a conductivity sensor that senses small amounts of fluid leaking inside the cassette (33). The tube leading from the cassette to the cannula is uninterrupted by injection ports or other components. Pressure pulses produced by blood pumps might be used to detect misplaced or slipped needles. This technology was developed for infusion pumps and could be applied to monitor extracorporeal circuits.

Another purpose of the venous pressure monitor is to detect obstructions downstream of the sensor which might otherwise lead to line ruptures. It must be pointed out that obstructions upstream of the sensor, i.e., between the blood pump and the venous bubble trap, are not detected. Such obstructions can cause line ruptures or hemolysis even if only partial (34).

To avoid a common user error, safety standards demand that upper and lower alarm limits only simultaneously can be adjusted. This makes it impossible to set alarm limits to the ends of the scale which would render the monitor useless. More recent microprocessor controlled machines set the alarm limits automatically and do not allow hazardous interference by the operator.

The future might bring better use of existing microprocessor and signal processing technology that allow for more reliable detection of blood leaks to the environment, while on the other hand nuisance alarms, which are so common today, will be avoided.

The arterial pressure monitor is not required by safety standards and is often positioned pre-pump, i.e., between the arterial cannula and blood pump. Traditionally, with pressure controlled ultrafiltration, it was positioned post-pump to allow for more precise ultrafiltration control. The pre-pump arterial pressure monitor allows for calculation of net blood flow and detection of obstructions in the pre-pump blood access or blood line. While low arterial pressure (high negative pressure) is not hazardous by itself, it indicates high shear rates and probably turbulence at the cannula or catheter entrance that might cause hemolysis (35). Negative pressures down to −200 mmHg are common and no adverse effects have been related to this.

Air detector

Air infusion is the most dangerous hazard in dialysis because the infusion of 50 ml or even less, may be lethal if immediate and corrective action is not taken to rescue the patient. Air can enter the circuit in case of a leak on the negative pressure side. This is the only way larger amounts of air can enter the system. Blood will not degas and release air at pressures above −500 mmHg and air can only enter from the dialysate side through the dialyzer membrane by diffusion. This will lead to oversaturation and air release only if the dialysate pressure is above the blood pressure; this is prevented by the transmembrane pressure monitor. Air accumulating in the bubble trap is either air left in the circuit after priming or entering through a leak on the negative pressure side.

Safety standards require a fail-safe air detector on the venous side. In addition the signal paths that close the venous clamp and stop the blood pump have to be redundant. If air enters through a leak in the arterial line foam is likely to be created. This foam is as dangerous as larger air boluses and also has to be detected.

Various physical principles can be used to detect air. Because the initial models used capacitive and optical detectors were unable to detect foam, these principles have been abandoned. This does not mean, however, that these principles cannot be applied to detect foam. Today ultrasonic sensors are used that are placed either on the bubble trap or on the line below it. When air is detected the venous clamp placed below the air detector is closed and the blood pump is stopped. If the air detector is placed on the line, pressure has to be released from the bubble trap before the clamp is opened to remove the air and suck blood back into the bubble trap. Otherwise, air in the bubble trap will expand and might reach the patient. The sensitivity of air detectors can be tested by lowering the level or injecting air bubbles. Ultrasound contrast agents that create foam can be used to detect the sensitivity for foam (36). To avoid air infusion through the arterial line reverse operation of the blood pump must not be possible during dialysis.

SINGLE-NEEDLE DIALYSIS

Single-needle dialysis is more than 20 years old but has not gained wide acceptance as the preferred method for

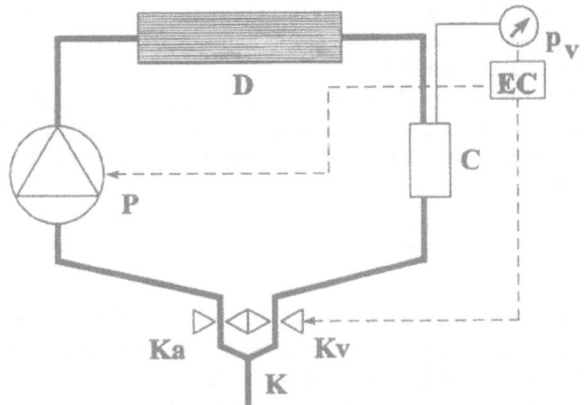

Figure 8. K: Single lumen cannula, K_a: arterial clamp, K_v: venous clamp, P: blood pump, D: dialyzer, C: compliance vessel, p_v: venous pressure monitor, EC: electronic control.

hemodialysis outside a few centers in Belgium and the UK. Elsewhere in Europe it is mostly applied when a failing fistula no longer allows the use of two needles or when a catheter has to be used. In the US it has been almost completely replaced by conventional dialysis with double lumen catheters. For a review of technical systems see Hoenich et al (37).

Principle and mean blood flow

The two principles developed 20 years ago are still popular: The pump/clamp system and the double-pump system. The pump clamp system as described by Kopp (38) is shown in Figure 8. The extracorporeal circuit consists of the single cannula with connected Y-piece. From the Y-piece the arterial line leads to the dialyzer. Before or after the dialyzer a compliance vessel is inserted into the line (the venous drip chamber can serve as compliance vessel but the storage capacity is low). From the dialyzer the venous line leads back to the Y-piece. The lines can be occluded alternately by the clamps K_a and K_v. The blood pump runs either continuously or is operated simultaneously with K_a.

During the arterial pumping cycle K_a is open, K_v closed and blood is pumped to the dialyzer and stored in the compliance vessel. After some time (usually a few seconds) K_a is closed and K_v opened and the blood returns through the venous line, the Y-piece and the cannula to the patient. The first part of the cycle is called arterial cycle with arterial cycle time T_a, the second part venous cycle (venous cycle time T_v). The total cycle time is T. Blood flow is Q_a, which is normally constant during the arterial cycle and Q_v during the venous cycle. Q_v decreases with time if a bubble trap or air filled chamber is used as compliance vessel.

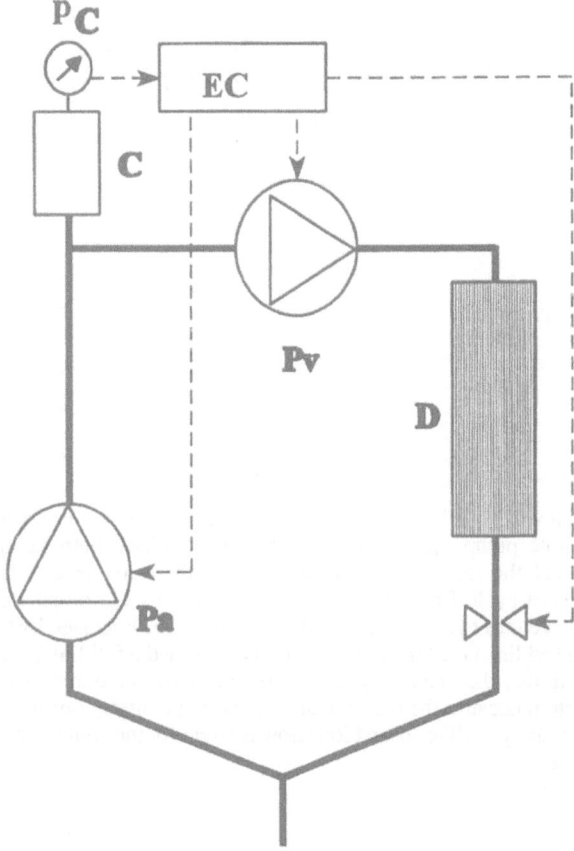

Figure 9. P_a: arterial blood pump, P_v: venous blood pump, p_C: compliance vessel pressure.

Double pump system

This system first described in (39) is shown in Figure 9. In this system the two pumps are operated alternately. The venous clamp is switched either simultaneously with the venous pump or remains open. Initially the arterial pump runs until the compliance vessel C is full which is sensed by a pressure or volume sensor. At this point the arterial pump is stopped and the venous pump activated by the electronic control unit. Blood is pumped through the dialyzer to the fistula. When the level in C reaches a lower limit the venous pump is stopped and the arterial pump activated again, and so on.

Calculation of net flow

The flow characteristic for both systems is illustrated by Figure 10.

With Q_a, the arterial blood flow, and Q_v, the venous blood flow known and constant we derive the mean blood flow Q_m:

$$Q_m = \frac{Q_a * Q_v}{Q_a + Q_v}. \qquad [4]$$

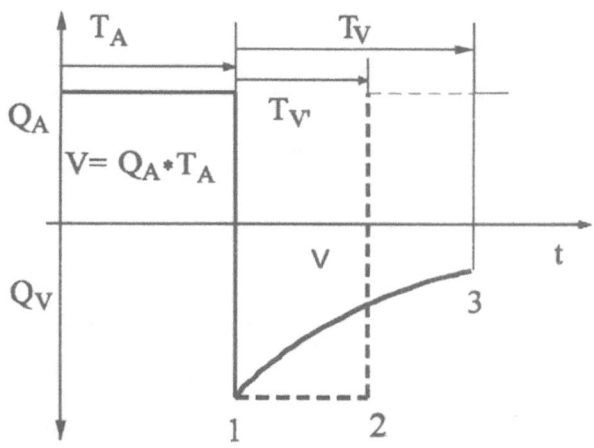

Figure 10. Flow characteristics of the pump-clamp and the double pump system. During the arterial phase both pumps propel the same amount of blood with the same speed. The arterial cycle for both systems is indicated by the broad line. The venous cycle of the double pump system is indicated by the dashed line (1, 2) the pump/clamp system by the full line (1, 3). Note that the venous cycle time is longer for the pump/clamp system because the pressure and flow is not constant during the venous cycle. The mean blood flow is larger for the double pump system.

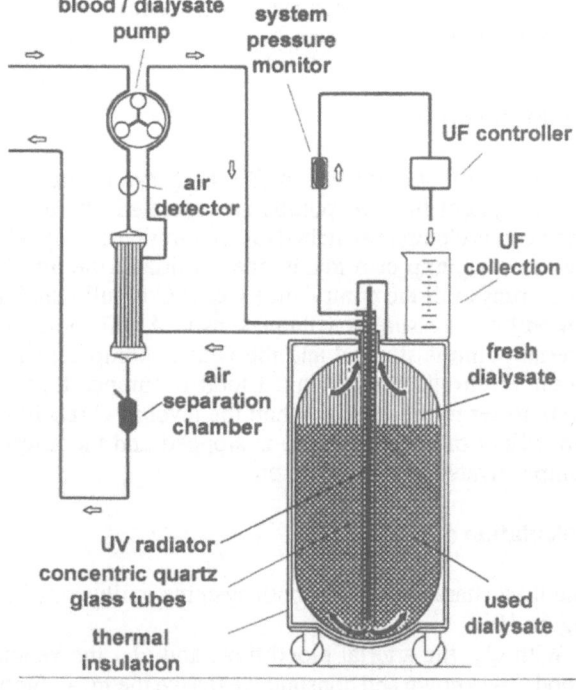

Figure 11. The Tersteegen dialysis machine.

Q_a and Q_v are constant if a standard S-N device with two blood pumps is used. If Q_a and Q_v is equal then Q_m is half of Q_a (and Q_v).

For the pump-clamp system the venous blood flow is not constant. The mean blood flow can be calculated from the constant arterial blood flow, the arterial and the total cycle time.

$$Q_m = \frac{Q_a * T_a}{T} . \qquad [5]$$

Some devices directly display mean blood flow. This is useful especially when the flow is not constant during either the arterial or the venous cycle.

Consideration of ultrafiltration leads to:

$$Q_m = \frac{Q_a * (Q_v + \text{UFR})}{Q_a + Q_v} \qquad [6]$$

for double pump systems.

Features influencing efficacy

The efficacy of the system depends on the mean blood flow and recirculation. The latter is mainly caused by the compliance of the tubing system. The cumulated length of the tubing system between the cannula and the arterial and venous clamp or pump respectively is approximately 2 to 3 meters. This part of the system is exposed to positive venous pressure during the venous cycle and to negative arterial pressure during the arterial cycle. During the venous cycle some already cleansed blood is forced into the arterial branch of the tubing. At the beginning of the arterial cycle this blood and some additional blood which is sucked from the venous branch is recirculated. The arterial pressure line contributes approximately 50% to the recirculation volume of 3–10 ml. This is related to the stroke volume, which is usually 30–50 ml. The recirculation can therefore reduce the efficacy by 6 to 30%. The volume of blood in the cannula or catheter is recirculated also, but this volume is less than 1 ml if special single needle cannulas are used and can be neglected.

Safety aspects

In principle, the potential hazards for a single needle system are the same as for conventional double needle extracorporeal circuits: blood loss to the environment (due to a rupture or disconnection of the blood line) and air embolism. The specific features of the single needle system offers one additional pathway for air entry: assume that a small leak occurs in the venous line downstream of the air detector. During the arterial cycle air might enter the line which is pumped into the patient during the venous cycle. It is therefore recommended not to integrate injection ports downstream of the air detector. Many single needle systems utilize the venous pressure sensor to sense the filling status of the compliance vessel. In these systems the venous pressure can no longer serve as a conventional protective system for blood loss to the environment. Most single needle systems therefore control the cycle time. If the cycle time exceeds a certain limit, the blood pumps are stopped and the venous clamp closed. The reaction time of this protective system can be 10–20 seconds which means that blood losses of 100–200 ml might occur in case of a rupture. Such systems are also more prone to line ruptures. In case of a small leak at the venous pressure transducer protector the venous pressure sensor might become inoperative. The system will then not be switched from arterial to venous cycle at the appropriate upper pressure level. The pressure will rise and eventually destroy the line if an additional monitoring system does not stop the pump.

Blood access

Single-needle mode is recommended for acute dialysis where blood access is made through a central venous catheter. Often double lumen catheters are used when a single needle system is not available. It should be pointed out, that the flow resistance of single lumen catheters is only one quarter of each channel of a double lumen catheter as long as the outer diameter is kept constant. This means that a single lumen catheter operated in single-needle mode allows twice the mean blood flow as compared to a double lumen catheter.

THE DIALYSATE CIRCUIT

Early in the history of dialysis dialysate was produced in large tanks from water and various salts and recirculated through the dialyzer. Two major problems were inherent in this system. First, efficacy was reduced because spent and fresh dialysate were mixed in the tank which reduced the concentration driving force, and, second bacteria proliferated rapidly in the dialysate mixture. In order to reduce bacterial growth the dialysate tank was cooled and blood rewarmed downstream of the dialyzer (40). This reduced urea clearance further by approximately 25% because diffusion is temperature dependent.

A modern batch type dialysis machine

In 1994 a device was presented to the market that comprises the simplicity of the original tank systems but overcomes the deficiencies mentioned above by an ingenious use of basic physical principles and rules of hygiene (41). A thermally insulated glass tank ($V = 75$ l) is filled with the total amount of dialysate mixed mostly from dry ingredients and pre-heated ultrapure water. This process is completely automated. The dialysate composition can be freely individualized according to a physician's prescription and is intended to include desirable additives. Fresh dialysate is taken from the top and is returned at the bottom of the vessel. Due to differences in terms of

temperature, solute loading and other factors the used dialysate layers below the fresh dialysate with a sharp interface. As a result of a hygienic design (geometry, materials, connections, handling, integrated UV radiator, etc) the system in practice operates with sterile dialysate. The automated cleaning/disinfection procedure has been proven to be highly effective for bacteria as well as for viruses. In a closed system such as this, completely filled with fluid and having no compliance, true volumetric UF control is simply achieved by controlling the outflow from the dialysate tank, which is kept permanently under positive pressure; this also prevents degassing of the dialysate. Blood and dialysate flow is driven by a double-sided roller pump with the flow ratio $Q_b : Q_d = 1 : 1$. Because a dialysate heater (typically operated at line voltage) is not necessary, the system is supplied by 25 V either from a transformer system or from a chargeable integrated battery pack lasting for at least 8 h of treatment independent of any electrical supply. Due to its design this machine is safe without most of the protective systems used in conventional dialysis machines. It has passed the approval procedure according to IEC601-1 and IEC601-2-16 and has been used prior to market introduction for more than 150,000 treatments.

Continuous production of dialysate

Historically the problems with the original tank systems were overcome by the development of continuous mixing devices for dialysate either as central dialysate delivery or as single patient machines.

Most machines produce dialysate continuously by mixing liquid or solid concentrates with water. In general these devices also heat and degas water or dialysate. While central dialysate delivery systems are still in use in a few centers in Europe, in the US and more often in Japan, single-patient machines are predominant today. Some single patient machines combine elements used for dialysate mixing with elements for ultrafiltration control, reducing the number of components (42). Because faults in the system can cause hazards to the patient the machines also utilize appropriate safety monitors.

Heating water or dialysate

The basic reason dialysate has to be heated to a physiological temperature of 35–37°C is the thermal energy loss the patient would otherwise suffer. There is no damage to blood at lower temperatures, as is well known from heart-lung machine experience. Furthermore, blood was successfully dialyzed at 4°C in the early days of dialysis. The dialyzer is an almost ideal heat exchanger. The thermal energy loss through the dialyzer is approximately 0.063 W/(°C * ml/min) or 375 W at a blood flow of 400 ml/min and 15°C temperature difference. Other influences of temperature on dialysis are the reduction of clearance (43) due to reduced diffusivity, the reduction of clotting

(44) and complement activation (45). The amount of energy necessary to heat dialysate depends on the temperature of the incoming water and dialysate flow and can exceed 2 kW at a dialysate flow of 1000 ml/min and a water input temperature of 5°C. Heat exchangers are therefore an integral part of almost all dialysis machines. Whether central heating of water is cost saving depends on the local cost for electrical and thermal energy. In countries close to the equator where water temperatures are high, a heat exchanger is not cost effective because the energy savings are negligible.

Accuracy of dialysate temperature: the AAMI standard specifies ± 1.5°C at the position of the dialyzer. This poses no problem for state of the art dialysis machines. The effective dialysate temperature might vary by 1°C during dialysis. Because the point of control is upstream the dialyzer and dialysate will cool on the way to the dialyzer, depending on dialysate flow and environmental temperature. If a heat sterilization program precedes the dialysis session, dialysate temperature might increase relative to the controlled value because the interior of the dialysis machine might still be above 37°C. For a more detailed discussion of the influence of dialysate temperature on cardiovascular stability during hemodialysis see Thermal energy balancing later in this chapter.

In general, feedback loops are used to control water or dialysate temperature: a control sensor measures the temperature of the heated fluid downstream of the heater. The measured temperature is compared with the set temperature. The heater is switched on whenever the measured temperature is lower and switched off whenever the measured temperature is higher than the set temperature. Microprocessor technology now also allows use of feed-forward control processes (46): With this technique the incoming water temperature is measured. From dialysate flow and the difference between the set temperature, and the water inlet temperature the required heating power is calculated and the heater appropriately controlled.

Independent safety monitors are required that prevent dialysis against overheated dialysate. The temperature limits set by safety standards are 41°C (IEC) and 42°C (AAMI). Hemolysis and even death was reported from overheated dialysate at temperatures above 45°C. No serious accidents involving overheated dialysate were published recently but an FDA (Food and Drug Administration) report, covering the period from 1985–1989 listed two incidents (47). In general the temperature safety sensor is positioned downstream of the heating and proportioning system as part of the conductivity monitor. Whenever the dialysate temperature exceeds the preadjusted upper limit, flow to the dialyzer is stopped.

Degassing water

The solubility of air in water depends on temperature. If water, already saturated with air, is heated it becomes oversaturated. If no nucleation cores are available water

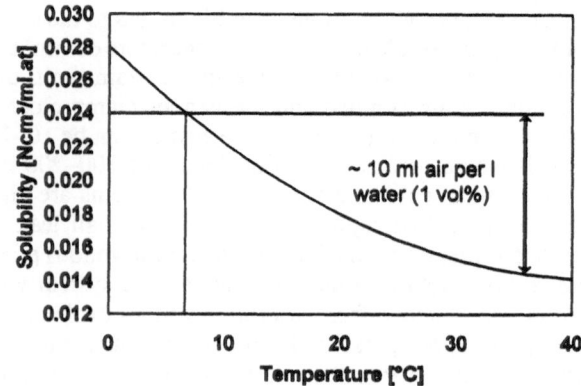

Figure 12.   Solubility of air in water. Data from Landolt-Börnstein.

will remain oversaturated for a long period (48). If already oversaturated fluid comes into contact with nucleation cores, rapid degassing will occur. This is the case with the dialyzer membrane. Air saturated water at 5°C contains approximately 25 Nml of air per l of water (49) (Figure 12). Nml is the volume of gas measured in ml at atmospheric pressure. At 35°C the solubility is only 15 Nml/l. At a dialysate flow of 500 ml/min 5 ml of air will be released per min. The contribution of air from concentrate is negligible. Concentrate contributes only 3–5% of total dialysate flow. In addition the solubility of air in concentrated salt solutions is very low.

When single-pass dialysis at 37°C dialysate temperature was first tested it was recognized that gas bubbles formed in the venous line downstream of the dialyzer (50). It was suspected that this was caused by gas-transfer from the dialysate to the blood side and subsequently dialysate degassing was introduced (51). Gas transfer that leads to oversaturation of blood is only likely with highly oversaturated dialysate, high dialysate flow and low blood flow.

Another motivation for the degassing of water is to avoid the accumulation of air on the dialysate side of the hemodialyzer which might reduce the effective surface area. Whether this is the case depends on the dialyzer geometry and position. Kolobow (52) was able to show even an increase of efficiency when air bubbles were injected into the dialysate stream. He interpreted this as an effect of turbulence created by the air bubbles. A further reason for degassing is the sensitivity of volumetric fluid balancing devices to air.

There are two methods for degassing incoming water. Either water is heated close to the boiling point or the pressure is decreased to approximately 150–200 mmHg absolute (−550 to −600 mmHg relative). In both cases the partial pressure of air in water becomes higher than the pressure of exposure and if nucleation cores are provided, air will be released. Either large surfaces or vortices can serve as nucleation cores. In both cases the air has to be released to the environment. Degassing by heat, once

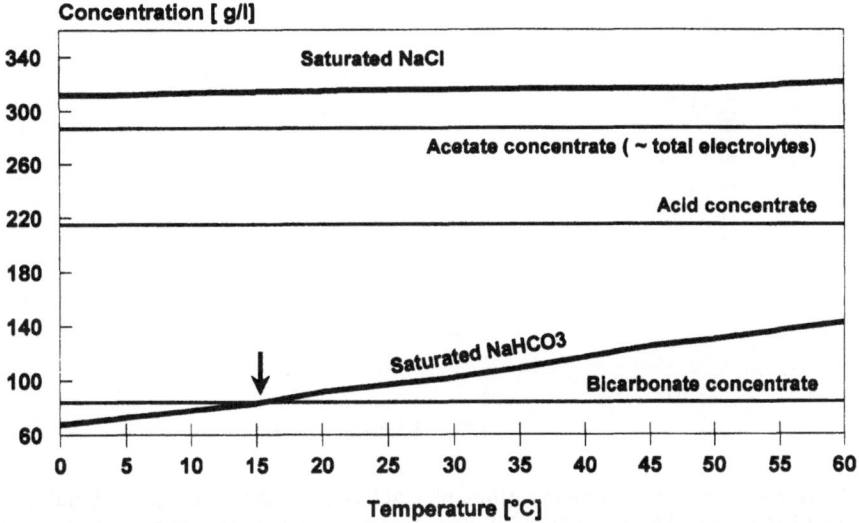

Figure 13. Saturation of sodium chloride and sodium bicarbonate in water versus temperature.

popular, requires an additional heat exchanger to cool the water after passage and is therefore less cost effective, therefore modern machines solely rely now on negative pressure degassing of either water or dialysate.

Malfunction of the degassing system causes no immediate hazard to the patient. In most cases air will accumulate in the dialyzer and the error will be detected. No protective system against dialysate oversaturation with air is required by safety standards.

Proportioning dialysate and monitoring dialysate composition

In tank systems dialysate is mixed either from salts and water or liquid concentrates and water. The first system for continuous proportioning was designed in Seattle (53) as a central dialysate supply system to overcome the deficiencies of previously used tank systems. The volumetric proportioning system consisted of two positive displacement pumps with a fixed volume ratio of 1:35 driven by a single motor. Dialysate flow was set to 500 ml/min as a result of studies that showed that dialysance increased only very little above this flow for the Kiil dialyzer used at this time (54). The original design was for a three stream mixing system for bicarbonate dialysis, but this was abandoned when acetate was found to be an effective replacement for bicarbonate in dialysate (55). This basic design principle is still in use.

The other method widely used today is feed-back controlled proportioning based on dialysate conductivity. This was probably first described in a patent (56). The latest development is the on-site production of dialysate from solid concentrate and water.

Bicarbonate (HCO_3^-) containing dialysate has to be produced from at least two concentrates. One contains

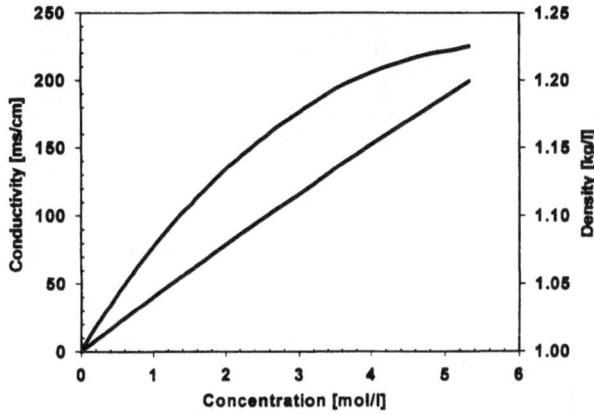

Figure 14. Conductivity and density at 20°C of NaCl in water. Data from CRC Handbook of Chemistry and Physics, 67th Ed.

sodium bicarbonate the second one calcium and magnesium salts. The other constituents can be put in either concentrate. Most commonly is the use of a 1-molar sodium bicarbonate concentrate and a so called 'acid-concentrate' that contains sodium-, potassium-, calcium- and magnesium chloride as well as some acetic acid to adjust dialysate pH to approximately 7.3. The strength of concentrate is limited by saturation. Acid and acetate concentrate contains mostly sodium chloride. The saturation limit of sodium chloride is more than 5-molar (Figure 13) allowing for a 35-fold concentration for acetate concentrate and up to 45-fold for acid concentrate. Acid concentrates are available 1:34 (35-fold), 1:35.83 and 1:44. Sodium bicarbonate saturation is temperature dependent. The saturation temperature of the widely used 1-molar solution is approximately 15°C.

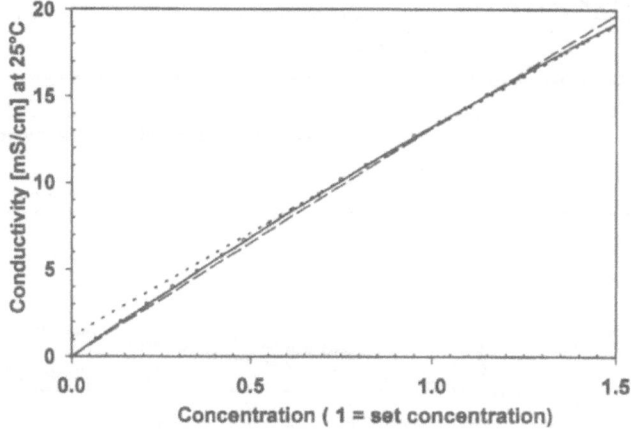

Figure 15. Conductivity versus concentration for HD04 (Fresenius AG, Bad Homburg, Germany). Solid line: Cubic approximation to measured data: Cond $= 14.16 * c - 1.133 * c^2 + 0.11 * c^3$. Dashed line: Straight line through origin and set value: Cond $= 13.141 * c$. Dotted line: Tangent at set point: Cond $= 13.141 + (c - 1) * 12$.

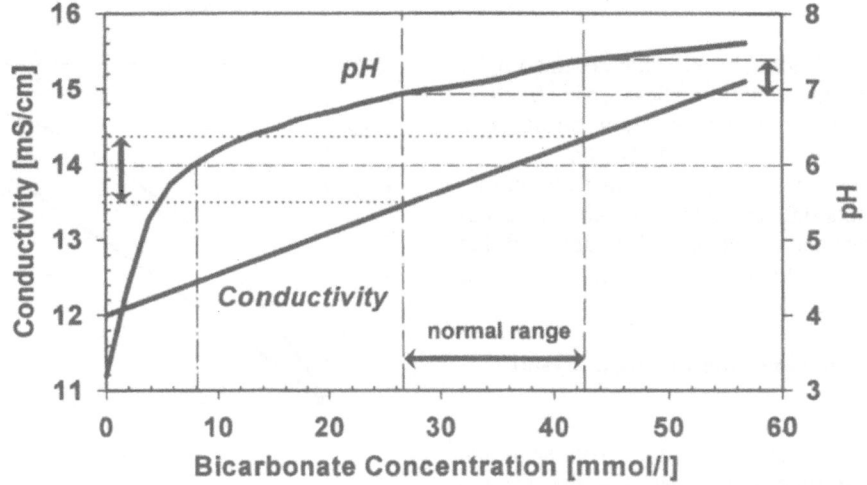

Figure 16. Conductivity and pH versus bicarbonate concentration in dialysate. Below the alarm trigger level of pH $= 6$ bicarbonate concentration is below 10 mmol/l.

Safety monitoring is required for dialysate composition because any malfunction of the mixing system may result in hypo- or hyperosmolar or buffer-free or buffer-rich dialysate which is potentially harmful to the patient. Various physical parameters can be used as a measure of dialysate concentration. Conductivity of an ionic fluid is non-linearly dependent on concentration while density follows a more linear function (Figure 14). Both parameters vary with temperature. In order to use conductivity as a measure of concentration it has to be measured at a standardized temperature (25°C) or the measured conductivity has to be normalized for this temperature. The temperature coefficient is 0.021/°C and linear over the range of 20–40°C. Figure 14 shows conductivity and density of NaCl versus concentration at 20°C. By tradition conductivity is used for safety monitoring while density

measurement is used for checking concentrates. With new technologies available density monitoring might become more cost effective especially when combined with ultrasound level monitoring.

The conductivity of acetate dialysate versus concentration around the set point is shown in Figure 15. This function can be used also for bicarbonate dialysate, as long as the total concentration is varied. The slope of the tangent is only 91% of the slope of the straight line between origin and set point (12/13.141 $=$ 0.91). The practical importance of this finding is, that for any variation dc/c of the concentration about the set point the relative change of conductivity $dcond/cond$ will only be 91% of the concentration change. In other words: if the concentration is increased by 10%, conductivity will only increase by 9%. Figure 16 shows conductivity and pH for dialysate with a constant amount of acid concentrate in solution and variable bicarbonate concentration. From this figure it becomes obvious that conductivity is a more sensitive parameter for monitoring bicarbonate concentration than pH. Only for differentiating between no buffer and some buffer in dialysate, pH would be more sensitive.

Volumetric proportioning of liquid concentrates and water

Volumetric proportioning follows either equation [7] or equation [8]:

$$V_{\text{Dialysate}} = V_{\text{Water}} + V_{\text{Conc.1}} + V_{\text{Conc.2}} \qquad [7]$$

$$V_{\text{Water}} = V_{\text{Dialysate}} - V_{\text{Conc.1}} - V_{\text{Conc.2}}. \qquad [8]$$

In the first case metered amounts of concentrates are added to a metered amount of water resulting in a total amount of dialysate that is the sum of the three volumes. In the second case concentrates are diluted by water until a pre-determined amount of dialysate is produced. The amount of water necessary is the difference between the preset amount of dialysate and the amount of concentrates. These two principles are shown in Figures 17a and b. Various pump designs can be used: Piston, membrane and bellow pumps with rotating or linear mechanical drive as well as pneumatic and hydraulic pumps. Modern dialysis machines comprise pumps with adjustable stroke volumes allowing variable dialysate concentration within safe limits.

Accuracy: The typical volumetric accuracy is 1%. Accuracy of dialysate composition also depends on concentrate tolerance. Adding 2% tolerance for the sodium concentration of concentrates, dialysate concentration tolerance is 3% or approximately ± 5 mmol/l for sodium.

Monitoring: Temperature compensated conductivity measurement is commonly used for safety monitoring. Upper and lower alarm limits are set at ± 5% of the expected conductivity. If conductivity is below or above this window, dialysate flow is bypassed from the dialyzer. For this purpose dialysis machines comprise at least one dialyzer valve leading from the dialysate source to the dialyzer and one bypass valve leading from the dialysate source to drain. Dialysate conductivity monitoring guarantees safety in case of single faults in the mixing system but not for any case of mixup of concentrates (57). If bicarbonate and acid concentrate are mixed up and the proportioning pumps are adjusted to rather uncommon albeit possible settings the conductivity of the final dialysate can still be in the range of scale of the safety monitor. Either mechanical coding of concentrate containers or the automatic setting of conductivity limits based on theoretical conductivity for a specific dialysate composition can prevent harm to the patient from this user error. More severe is a mixup of a 1:44 acid concentrate with acetate concentrate. Because 1:44 concentrates are used with a specific brand of dialysis machine, only accidents for this

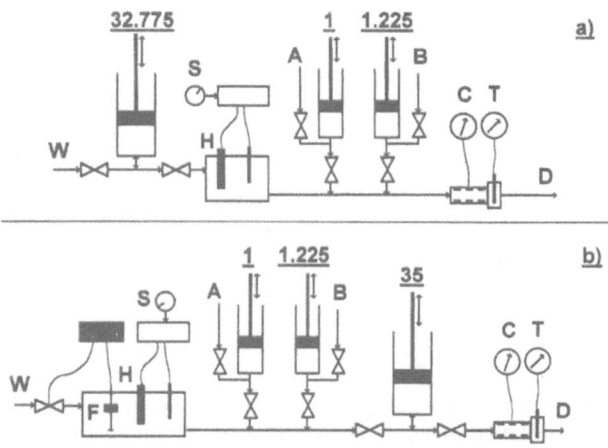

Figure 17. Volumetric mixing with a) water metering, b) dialysate metering. A: 'acid' concentrate. B: bicarbonate concentrate. C: conductivity monitor. D: dialysate outlet. F: float, water level sensor. H: heater. S: dialysate temperature set point. Underlined numerals: Volumes (arbitrary units).

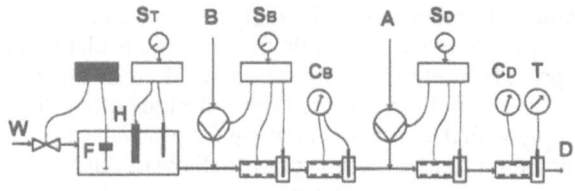

Figure 18. Conductivity controlled proportioning system. S_B (S_D): set bicarbonate (total) conductivity. Two redundant albeit non-diverse conductivity monitors serve as protective system: C_B for the bicarbonate and C_D for total concentration.

brand were reported, although other machines potentially are prone to the same user error. Measurement of concentrate conductivity can provide safety also in this case of concentrate mixup (58).

Closed-loop control proportioning systems

In this type of proportioning system a physical parameter proportional to dialysate concentration is measured downstream of the mixing point. The result is compared with a set-value and the difference is used to control the concentrate flow in order to reduce the difference to a minimum. It is inherent for this kind of control system, that the difference cannot be permanently zero. Electrical conductivity is the only parameter used for this purpose today. In most cases, redundant conductivity monitors are used as protective system against single faults in the mixing part of the device (Figure 18). Some machines monitor concentrate volume (59), others include conductivity monitors of an alternative kind, e.g., contactless sensors (60) to overcome the inherent safety problems of redundant non-diverse sensors. The use of non-diverse sensors for control and monitoring poses the inherent risk that the

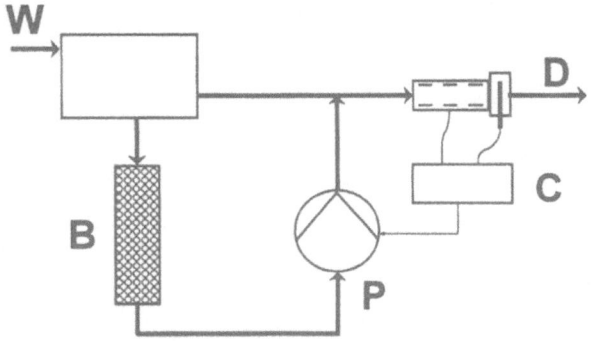

Figure 19. Continuous production of bicarbonate concentrate by percolation of water through powder. B: bicarbonate cartridge. C: control system for dialysate mixing. D: dialysate. P: concentrate pump. W: water inlet.

sensitivity of both sensors can be adversely changed by the same process. Such an alteration could result in higher or lower dialysate concentration without indication by the monitor. In other words the dialysate concentration can be hyper- or hypotonic while the machine is alarm-free. To provide safety for such cases, some dialysis machines have additional pH sensors. These designs often do not comply with the basic requirement for protective systems demanding functional tests prior to dialysis. Also, a malfunction of the pH sensor does not necessarily become obvious to the user during operation. These 'pseudo' safety monitors therefore do not provide safety under single fault condition. The cause of events that led to dialysis against hypertonic dialysate is described in Williams et al (61): high pH in bicarbonate concentrate resulting in a moderate increase in dialysate pH led to precipitation of calcium carbonate that reduced the sensitivity of both the control and the monitoring conductivity sensor. Bicarbonate dialysate is generally oversaturated with calcium carbonate that tends to precipitate spontaneously at pH above 7.4. Because only a moderate increase in pH might trigger precipitation this cannot be detected by a pH monitor. Malfunction of the pH sensor was reported by Sethi et al (62). As currently used, the pH sensor is an unreliable monitor unable to guarantee safety as required by accepted safety standards.

On-site production of concentrate

Liquid concentrate can be produced from dry concentrate and water, either continuously or prior to dialysis by integrated systems or added to single patient dialysis machines. A system for continuous production of a saturated bicarbonate concentrate that is subsequently diluted with water to produce dialysate was invented by Jönsson and co-workers (63). Water percolates through a cartridge filled with bicarbonate powder. The liquid exiting this cartridge at the bottom is a saturated bicarbonate solution (see Figure 19). This liquid is fed by a concentrate pump

that is part of a control loop to the water stream to produce dialysate. The feedback control is required because the concentration of the saturated bicarbonate concentrate varies with temperature. If the water used for concentrate production is not sufficiently degassed, air is released in the cartridge because the solubility of air in a concentrated salt solution is low. In addition bicarbonate is in equilibrium with CO_2 at a pressure of a few tenths of an atmosphere depending on the quality of the powder. The patent by Jönsson describes various ways to remove this air. Further improvements comprising a recirculation loop for the concentrate are described in two further patents (64, 65). Alternative technical solutions using the same principle utilize bags instead of cartridges (66) and feed-forward control of the mixing pump (67). The percolation principle can be applied for other salts but not for salt-mixtures as otherwise used for the batch-wise production of acid-concentrates.

Ultrafiltration control systems

Pressure controlled systems

The single patient machines that replaced the tank machines historically used pressure control to achieve ultrafiltration (equation [9]).

$$\text{UFR} = \text{TMP} * \text{UFK}. \tag{9}$$

UFK is the ultrafiltration coefficient assumed to be constant. TMP, the transmembrane pressure is adjusted. The ultrafiltration rate UFR is the result. Whenever UFK changes, the ultrafiltration rate will change as well. Because the ultrafiltration coefficient depends on various parameters, e.g., hematocrit and might also change intradialytically the resulting ultrafiltration rate is likely to deviate from the intended one. This was a nuisance but not dangerous as long as conventional, low-flux dialyzers (UFK < 10 ml/h * mmHg) were used. The transmembrane pressure is calculated from four pressures: p_{Bi} (blood in, post-pump arterial), p_{Bo} (blood out, venous), p_{Di} (dialysate in) and p_{Do} (dialysate out) by equation [10]:

$$\text{TMP} = \frac{p_{Bi} - p_{Bo}}{2} - \frac{p_{Di} - p_{Do}}{2}. \tag{10}$$

Equation [10] must be used literally. In dialysis, pressures are measured relative to atmospheric pressure. Dialysate pressure can become negative. In this case the second term on the right hand side becomes positive when multiplied with the minus sign. The hydraulic principle is shown in Figure 20. Some systems use three or two pressure measurements only for the calculation of TMP. The error introduced by this simplification is usually small if compared with the tolerance of the ultrafiltration coefficient. Later, systems were designed that measured the actual ultrafiltration coefficient periodically during dialysis and subsequently adjusted the transmembrane pressure automatically. These principle is no longer used for modern

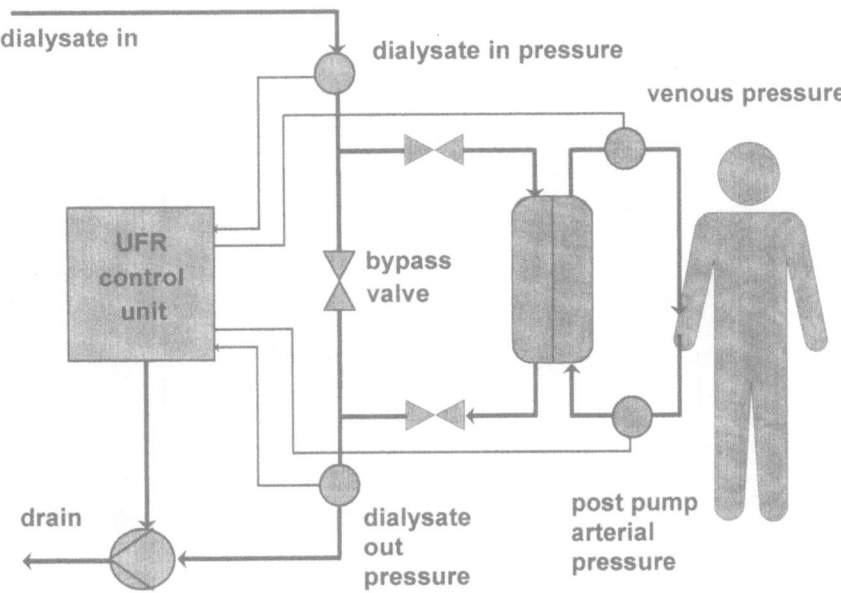

Figure 20. Transmembrane-pressure (TMP) controlled ultrafiltration. TMP is calculated from up- and downstream pressures on both sides of the dialyzer.

dialysis machines. For a review of these and other ultrafiltration control methods see Polaschegg (68).

Direct control of ultrafiltration

When high-flux dialyzers became available the demand for a more direct method to control ultrafiltration increased. Initially batch type machines as the one shown in Figure 1 were used for volumetric control of ultrafiltration. The device used by Kiil (69) measured the increase of fluid in the tank as the result of spontaneous ultrafiltration caused by the pressure on the blood side of the dialyzer. Bower and Magee (70) were the first to apply the principle of a closed dialysate system for ultrafiltration control. In their rarely quoted paper they describe a Seattle-type tank closed air tight by a lid. From this tank fluid was drawn to a suction bottle connected to a vacuum source. The negative pressure could be adjusted to deliver the required amount of ultrafiltration. The next step was the replacement of the suction bottle by a positive displacement pump that allowed pre-adjustment of the ultrafiltration rate (71).

Ultrafiltration control based on differential flow measurement

This method relies on accurate flowmeters in the dialysate path as input to a feedback loop that controls the dialysate effluent pump as shown in Figure 21. An additional ultrafiltration pump in parallel to the dialysate-out flowmeter is used by some devices. This allows the use of low-cost flowmeters that are operated at equal flow. Three types of flowmeters are commonly used: The electromagnet-

ic (72) and the turbine-flowmeter (73) are sensitive to volume flow while, the Coriolis force flowmeter (74) is sensitive to mass only. Volumetric flowmeters are sensitive to air. Most systems therefore comprise a secondary degassing chamber between the dialyzer outlet and the spent dialysate flowmeter. The flowmeters can be calibrated intradialytically whenever the dialysate system is switched into bypass mode.

Volumetric ultrafiltration

This method relies on balancing chambers to create a temporarily closed system as originally described by Bower and Magee but without recirculation of dialysate. These balancing chamber systems are also called 'flow equalizers' because they equalize the flow of fresh and spent dialysate. The principle is shown in Figure 22. A balancing chamber is separated into a 'fresh dialysate' and a 'spent dialysate' compartment by a membrane to avoid mixing of fresh and spent dialysate. The membrane is not essential for fluid balancing. Some systems use long, thin, rigid tubes as balancing chambers without any membrane. In membraneless balancing tubes, mixing of fresh and spent dialysate is very much reduced but cross contamination cannot be avoided. Operation: the balancing chamber is first filled with fresh dialysate. Simultaneously spent dialysate is forced to drain. Next it is separated from the dialysate source and drain by closing valves 1 and 3. Dialysate circulates from the 'fresh dialysate' side of the balancing chamber through the dialyzer to the 'spent dialysate' side of the balancing chamber. Because the volume of the system does not change, no net fluid transport takes place through the dialyzer membrane. With an addi-

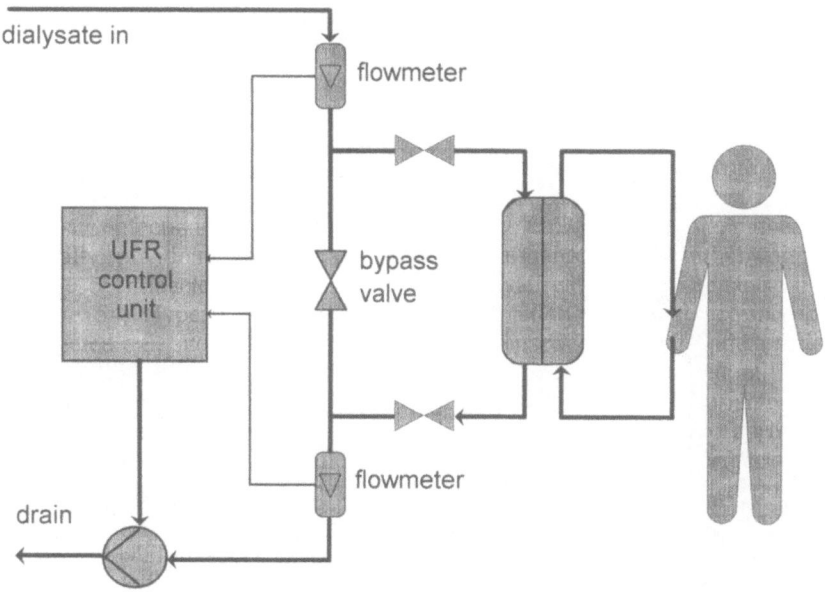

Figure 21. Ultrafiltration control by difference-flow measurement. The system can be tested prior to dialysis and intradialytically in bypass mode.

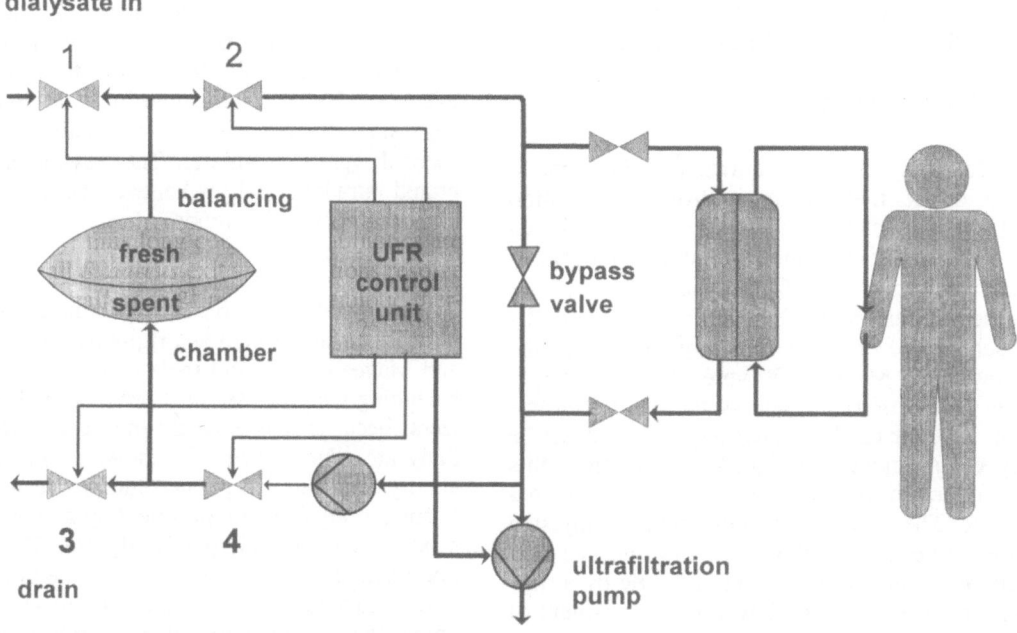

Figure 22. Ultrafiltration control with balancing chambers.

tional ultrafiltration pump fluid can be removed from the dialysate circuit. Because the only connection to the environment is through the dialyzer membrane and the patient this fluid is sucked from the patient. In other words: the action of the ultrafiltration pump reduces the pressure in the dialysate system creating a pressure gradient between blood and dialysate side. This causes ultrafiltration that commences until the pressure between blood and dialysate is again equalized. At this point precisely the same amount is ultrafiltered as previously withdrawn by the ultrafiltration pump. To achieve a more uniform dialysate flow two balancing chambers are operated sequentially. Fluid circulates through one while the other one is filled.

Schultheis (75) presumably was the first one to describe this principle. His design differs from the one used today by separate chambers for fresh and spent dialysate. Beelen (76) described a system that is functionally equivalent to the system in Figure 21, but uses pistons rather than balancing chambers. Pinkerton (77) described a piston operated balancing system in which the volume of fresh dialysate could be reduced by an idler rod that allowed adjustment of a predetermined volume difference for ultrafiltration control. The first balancing chamber used in hemodialysis and almost identical in design to the current models, is described in a patent by Kozlov, Khaitlin and Lisitsina from Russia in 1972 (78). Many different designs have been developed since.

The method of withdrawing fluid from the dialysate circuit and the size of the balancing chamber are major design differences. The system described by Schael (42) has an ultrafiltration pump positioned downstream of the dialyzer where the dialysate pressure might be positive or negative. Because it is technically difficult to make a precise pump that works under varying input pressure conditions, designs that position the ultrafiltration pump hydraulically at a point of constant positive pressure are more common. This could be either on the fresh or on the spent dialysate side.

The size of the balancing chamber is crucial for the influence of operational characteristics on efficacy. As is shown for single-needle dialysis (79) and (80) for the dialysate side, pulsatile flow is as equally efficient as continuous flow if the volume of the pulses is smaller than the filling volume of the dialyzer. This is the case for the balancing chambers of dialysis machines produced by Fresenius AG, Bad Homburg, Germany. Small volume balancing chambers therefore allow an overlap for the closure of all valves of the balancing chamber system that increases the fault tolerance. In addition it allows operation with only one balancing chamber, thus reducing the cost of the system. As for systems working with volume-flow meters degassing of spent dialysate occurs in most dialysis machines with volume controlled ultrafiltration.

Safety of ultrafiltration control systems under single-fault condition

Older, pressure controlled hemodialysis machine comprised no safety means for single faults in the dialysate pressure control system; because the ultrafiltration coefficient of the dialyzer was low at this time and the accuracy of control poor anyway this was not regarded as hazardous. This changed when systems that allow direct control of ultrafiltration became available.

$$TMP = \frac{UFK}{UFR} \qquad [11]$$

Because ultrafiltration is controlled precisely, any large deviation is regarded as potentially hazardous. None of the safety standards, however, specifies the tolerable ultrafiltration error. Generally inverse ultrafiltration resulting in unintended weight gain of the patient is regarded as hazardous. As long as the ultrafiltration coefficient of the dialyzers used was moderate, transmembrane pressure could serve as a diverse – redundant protective system against severe ultrafiltration errors under single fault condition. The transmembrane pressure builds up as a result of ultrafiltration. Assuming that the ultrafiltration coefficient (UFK) of the dialyzer remains constant during dialysis TMP alarm limits are set around the actual TMP when it stabilizes at the beginning of dialysis as reputed by Grimsrud et al (11). Appropriately, the lower TMP alarm limit is set at zero to avoid net back-filtration and weight gain and the upper alarm limit is set close to the start value. The TMP that settles within the first minutes should be checked for plausibility because there is a small chance that a fault occurred between the pre-dialysis test of the dialysis machine (see paragraph on general safety) and settling of TMP.

With increased use of high-flux dialyzers with an UFK of 40 ml/mmHg $*$ h and larger, TMP monitoring is no longer sufficient to prevent large ultrafiltration errors caused by single faults in the ultrafiltration control system (81). As shown in Figure 23 TMP changes only by 12.5 mmHg for an ultrafiltration error of 0.5 l/h. The resolution of most TMP monitors is 20 mmHg or coarser. A high resolution of better than 5 mmHg is possible but would cause frequent nuisance alarms because of short time pressure fluctuations caused by patient movements and the variation of the ultrafiltration coefficient throughout dialysis. Appropriate safety can be achieved by TMP monitoring in combination with periodic test of the ultrafiltration control system (82) (see also: Design principles for safety . . .: Periodic test of the operating system).

Blood leak detectors

A blood loss to the dialysate is defined as a loss of erythrocytes. This is possible in the case of a leak in the membrane or the potting material of a dialyzer, large enough to allow passage of erythrocytes. This requires pores or cracks larger than a few micrometers in diameter or width. The normal pore size of a dialyzer membrane is much smaller. Any defects between the normal diameter of a membrane pore and the size that allows the passage of erythrocytes does not cause blood loss according to this definition, but can cause plasma loss. Blood loss also requires that the transmembrane pressure at the position of the membrane leak is positive (the pressure gradient is from blood to dialysate). Blood leaks can be severe and therefore hazardous for the patient. In batch type machines spent dialysate is recirculated and blood leaks can be detected visually. This is not possible in single pass machines. The prototypes designed for unattended overnight dial-

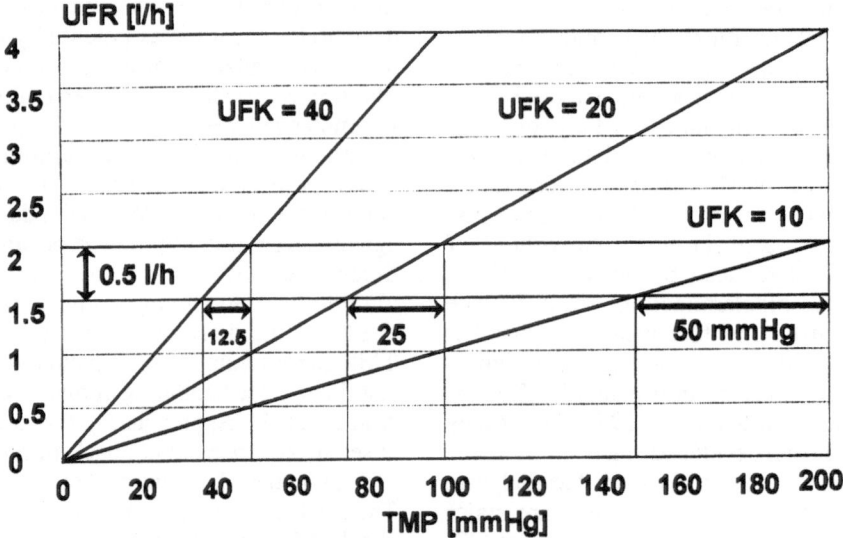

Figure 23. TMP change for an ultrafiltration error of 0.5 l/h.

ysis were equipped with blood leak detectors (50). The single wavelength blood leak detectors were sensitive to gas bubbles and non-specific turbidity of spent dialysate or contamination of the optical pathway. Dual wavelength blood leak detectors were developed (83, 84) that have a hemoglobin sensitive channel, and a background turbidity channel the latter usually working in the infrared range. The blood leak detector described by Eschbach et al (50) was able to detect 0.1 ml of blood in 1 l of dialysate. Today's safety standards require a detection sensitivity of 0.35–0.5 ml/min of blood loss to the dialysate. With 500 ml/min dialysate flow these two specifications are equivalent.

Membrane leaks that do not cause a blood leak

In high-flux dialyzers transmembrane pressure is not uniformly positive throughout the flow path. Because of counter current operation and differential pressure drops, transmembrane pressure reverses at some point between the ends of the dialyzer. In low-flux dialyzers (dialyzers with KUF < 10 ml/h * mmHg) this can be avoided by an appropriately high ultrafiltration rate. In high-flux dialyzers normally this is not possible. A leak in a region of negative transmembrane pressure might not be detectable but might allow transfer of bacteria from contaminated dialysate to blood. Such membrane leaks could influence patient outcome. Taking into account that a large number of patients die from infections and that membrane leaks in re-used dialyzers are not rare, the risk of backflow of contaminated dialysate through membrane leaks should not be neglected. Currently the only protective system against such events is sterile filtration of dialysate.

Disinfection or sterilization of the dialysate fluid path

Problems caused by bacterial contamination of dialysate became obvious early in the history of hemodialysis and persist today. The source of bacterial contamination of dialysate in single-pass, single-patient machines is usually the water and sometimes the bicarbonate concentrate. Because dialysate is an excellent growth medium, bacteria rapidly proliferate in this environment. Bacteria can enter blood through membrane leaks under certain circumstances (see paragraph on sterile filtration of dialysate). A secondary product of bacterial growth are endotoxins. Some active parts of these endotoxins e.g., Lipid A have molecular weights of less than 2000 Daltons and readily can pass the pores of a dialyzer membrane if they are not adsorbed by the membrane material. Large endotoxin concentrations cause acute symptoms summarized, manifest as pyrogenic reactions, but even low concentrations reportedly produce intradialytical symptoms such as hypotensive episodes (85), and are also suspected to have long term adverse effects. For an overview on the importance of sterile dialysate see Mion et al (86). The relationship between equipment design, disinfection procedure, bacterial contamination and pyrogenic reactions is described in an exemplary paper by Petersen et al (87). While the system investigated in the latter was a central dialysate supply system, all findings are pertinent to single patient machines: the pyrogenic reactions were traced back to contamination of distribution pipes that never were disinfected due to a combination of design and operational errors. While dialysis machines have only partial influence on the quality of dialysate they should at least guarantee that bacterial proliferation is minimized.

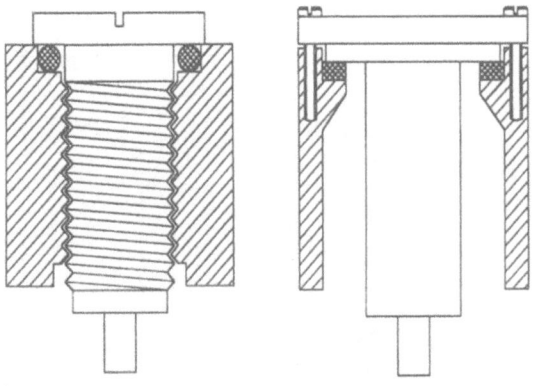

Figure 24. Left hand side: The fluid in the narrow gaps of the screw between the open fluid path and the O-ring seal is stagnant. Disinfectant can only enter by diffusion which might take many days. Right hand side: No stagnant areas between the open fluid path and the sealing quad-ring.

That the design of the dialysate fluid path was crucial, was recognized by the early pioneers (88). Until recently many components used in dialysis machines were not specially developed for applications sensitive to bacterial growth. A typical example is shown in Figure 24.

After dialysis or at the end of a dialysis day the dialysate fluid path is rinsed with water and afterwards subjected to a chemical or heat disinfection procedure. Because bicarbonate dialysis leads to precipitation of more or less calcium carbonate in the dialysis fluid path, a rinse procedure with an acid (either acetic acid (vinegar) or citric acid) is added. Some acidic disinfectants are able to remove carbonates and make an additional acid rinse redundant. The disinfection procedure should guarantee that no bacterial growth can take place between the end of the procedure and the beginning of the next treatment.

Chemical disinfection

Dialysis machines with a volumetric dialysate proportioning system, frequently use this system to produce a disinfecting solution from a concentrated solution and water. Other machines provide separate inlets for the disinfection concentrate. The disinfectant is added after the machine is rinsed of dialysate and is preferably allowed to dwell until the machine is prepared for the next dialysis session. This allows for sufficient exposure time to the disinfectant and avoids recontamination in the dialysis free interval by contaminated water. The water connecting tube and the water inlet components are not disinfected by this procedure.

Special designs guarantee safety of the patient and reduce the risk of dialyzing with a disinfectant solution or with dialysate contaminated with disinfectant residues. Disinfectant concentrates are connected only during the disinfection procedure. Connection is to special inlets that are often mechanically coded or equipped with sensors.

Disinfection is initiated through a special program that can be started only when the dialysate lines are in a special interlock which guarantees that they are not connected to a dialyzer. Whenever the disinfectant concentrate is connected to the machine and/or the disinfection program is started the operation of the blood pump is automatically interrupted. In general two or more machine faults have to accumulate for dialysis with a disinfectant to be possible. This makes up for the difficulty of automatically testing some of the safety functions. Because most disinfectants have a low specific electrical conductivity, dialysis with a pure disinfectant solution is not possible as long as the conductivity monitor is functioning. This is, however, not the case with sodium hypochlorite (bleach), which can be proportioned to produce a solution with conductivity within the lower range of dialysis conductivity monitors. Operational procedures must therefore guarantee that bleach cannot be mixed up with dialysate concentrate. To avoid dialysis with residues of disinfectant, dialysis machine interlocks in the machine or machine program only allow dialysis after completion of a rinse program.

Handling of disinfectant concentrates is not without risk. Some substances are chemically aggressive, e.g., bleach and peracetic acid, while others are potentially carcinogenic, e.g., formaldehyde. A system has been described that allows the permanent connection of the disinfectant container to the dialysis machine (89). The mixing point for the disinfectant concentrate is downstream of the dialyzer to increase the number of independent faults to 4 faults necessary to accidentally dialyze with a disinfectant solution. The dialysis machine designed according to this system is rinsed with reverse osmosis water after initiation of the disinfection program. After a 5–10 minute rinse the outlet and inlet of the machine is connected through a recirculation loop normally closed by a valve. At this time disinfectant concentrate is metered to the system and the resulting disinfectant solution is recirculated through the dialysate pathway at an elevated temperature up to 85°C. By this means the solution is continuously in motion, the amount of disinfectant required is low, while its activity is increased due to the higher temperature. Another system has been described that uses a special refillable cartridge with liquid disinfectant concentrate in combination with a valve manifold to create a recirculation loop (90, 91). The recirculation loop includes the water pipe connecting the water loop with the dialysis machine and the dialysis machine drain line enabling the cleaning and disinfection of parts that are frequently not disinfected at all.

Heat sanitation/disinfection/sterilization

Hot water at 85°C was used successfully to reduce the bacterial contamination of the Seattle central dialysate delivery system. This method is still used by many commercial machines today. The method poses much less risk for patient and staff as compared to chemical disinfection.

Heat will also reach dead space parts within the dialysate loop. It is effective if the complete fluid distribution system of a dialysis unit (the water treatment system downstream of the reverse-osmosis membrane and the water distribution loop included) is rinsed simultaneously with hot water as in the Seattle system. If the disinfection procedure is limited to the dialysis machine the machine is recontaminated continuously by in-flowing water. A hot-disinfection program is effective then only immediately before dialysis. To overcome this problem, recirculation loops have been introduced (92). In such systems the dialysis machine remains separated and sterile after the end of the heat-disinfection program. The drain line, however, is not disinfected which might pose a problem for direct dialysis quantification where total dialysate is collected and analyzed. The system described in (91) avoids this problem. A valve manifold includes the fresh water and spent dialysate line in the recirculation loop.

HEMOFILTRATION AND HEMODIAFILTRATION

Solute removal in hemofiltration is by convection rather than diffusion. Ultrafiltrate is replaced by a substitution fluid of a composition similar to dialysate. Proponents of this method emphasize the similarity to the natural kidney and the more effective removal of larger molecules. On the other hand removal of low molecular substances is reduced as compared to hemodialysis because at best 45% of blood can be ultrafiltered in post-dilution hemofiltration. Hemodiafiltration combines hemodialysis and hemofiltration and combines the advantages of both methods. A review of the history of hemofiltration is presented by Henderson (93), one of the inventors of this method. Today maintenance hemofiltration is used only in a small number of patients because of the high cost of commercial replacement fluid and the high blood flow required to perform the treatment in reasonable time. Hemofiltration with or without fluid replacement is a preferred treatment modality for acute renal failure.

Hemofiltration machines

Hemofiltration machines for chronic treatment comprise the same extracorporeal pumping and monitoring systems as hemodialysis machines. The dialysate circuit is replaced by a fluid balancing and warming system.

Substitution fluid is added to blood upstream to the filter and filtrate is produced as the result of the increased pressure in the blood circuit. This method is called pre-dilution hemofiltration. To be clinically effective more than 70 l of substitution fluid is required. Because of the high cost of commercial substitution fluid this method never became widely accepted. More common is the post-dilution method (Figure 25) because less substitution fluid

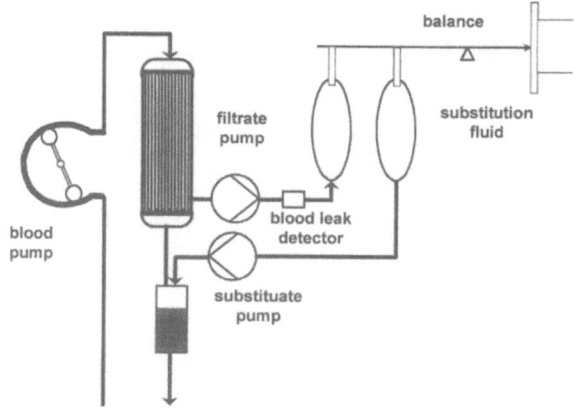

Figure 25. Principle of post-dilution hemofiltration. The fluid removed by ultrafiltration is replaced by an equal amount of substitution fluid.

is required. Originally only 20 l were exchanged but this was increased later to 30 l or more.

Various systems have been proposed for fluid balancing: The system originally designed by Henderson and co-workers (94) used a double roller pump to balance blood. Alternative ways of fluid balancing in the extracorporeal circuit were proposed but never gained practical importance. Gravimetric fluid balancing as shown in Figure 25 (95) is the most common method. Ultrafiltrate is withdrawn by the ultrafiltrate pump into a bag or container that hangs or stands on a balance platform. Substitution fluid from a bag hanging or laying on the same platform is pumped by another pump to the venous drip chamber. Net fluid removal is achieved either by an additional ultrafiltration pump or by a programming unit that controls the substitution pump to deliver less fluid than removed by the filtration pump (96). No information regarding filtration rate can be gained from the balance or the control unit but has to be derived from the pump speeds. Some devices therefore have two separate balances for filtrate and substitute (95). This allows calculation of the exchange rate from weight increase or decrease of the filtrate and substitute balance respectively. One inherent problem of gravimetric fluid balancing is the total amount of substitution fluid that has to be placed on the balance at the beginning of dialysis. With 30 l required for an effective treatment, this poses a practical problem. At the end of treatment the same amount of filtrate has to be discarded manually. Safety designs of gravimetric balancing systems have been described in patents. A typical hazard in a balancing system as described in Figure 1 is the dislocation of the ultrafiltration or substitution line. When ultrafiltrate or substitution fluid is spilled, fluid removed from the patient is not replaced. Either a dynamic approach with non continuous filtrate or substitute flow or alternatively filtrate and substitute pump monitoring can be used to detect gross balancing errors.

Volumetric fluid balancing systems have been proposed (97) but had not been developed by industry until recently (98). In this volumetric system a disposable balancing chamber similar to those used in volummetrically controlled hemodialysis machines is used for fluid balancing.

Heating of substitution fluid is necessary to avoid unacceptable negative thermal energy balance. Electrical heaters are used to indirectly heat fluid either in the tubing or a bag. Temperature control quality of indirect heating is poor and the temperature of substitution fluid is usually lower than blood temperature. This causes a moderately negative thermal energy balance and stabilization or moderate reduction of the patient's body temperature. This technical deficiency led to Maggiore et al (99) pioneering work on the influence of dialysate or substitution fluid temperature on blood pressure stability. The device described in Beden et al (98) uses a directly heated stainless steel tube which allows more precise control of substitution fluid temperature.

Blood leak detectors are required as in hemodialysis monitors. Because blood is not diluted by dialysate, the sensitivity can be reduced. To avoid infusion of air into the drip chamber most machines also have an air detector in the substitution fluid line.

Hemodiafiltration machines

Hemodiafiltration, a combination of hemodialysis and hemofiltration can be performed by combining an extracorporeal circuit with a hemofilter and a hemodialyzer with a hemofiltration and a hemodialysis machine (100). Hemodialysis machines with volumetrically controlled ultrafiltration can be adapted easily for hemodiafiltration which is more cost-effective. The most common approach is the removal of spent or fresh dialysate by a separate hemofiltration pump. This fluid is exchanged by an equal amount of substitution fluid by a balance controlled pump. Net fluid removal from the patient is achieved as in dialysis mode. Technically even simpler, but potentially more hazardous is the removal of all ultrafiltrate by the ultrafiltration pump of the hemodialysis machine and partial replacement by a separate volumetric infusion pump (101). This is especially the case when bicarbonate is exclusively supplied by the substitution pump and the dialysate is buffer-free.

Fluid exchange capacity of most commercial hemodiafiltration modules is limited to 10 l. The clinical usefulness of low exchange volumes is questionable. Canaud and coworkers reported only moderate improvements with fluid exchange of 15–20 l per session (102). Higher reimbursement rates for hemodiafiltration, even with low exchange volumes, in Germany (103) and probably other European countries might be the motivation for the ongoing use of low volume hemodiafiltration. The volumetric fluid balancing system described in Beden et al (98) allows unlimited uninterrupted volume exchange. It has been successfully integrated as a module into a hemodialysis machine.

ON-LINE PRODUCTION OF STERILE DIALYSATE AND SUBSTITUTION FLUID

Sterile filters as protective system against bacterial contamination of blood under single fault condition

As mentioned earlier, backfiltration of dialysis fluid into blood within the dialyzer is unavoidable in high-flux dialysis. As long as the dialyzer membrane is leak free no bacteria can pass from dialysate to blood. A leak in the membrane or potting material of a high-flux dialyzer can be at a position of positive or negative transmembrane pressure (TMP varies within the dialyzer, the TMP displayed by dialysis machine monitors is the mean TMP). Membrane leaks in a membrane area of positive TMP are detected as blood leaks and presumably will not cause bacterial contamination of blood (104). If the membrane leak is in an area of negative TMP, backfiltration of potentially bacteria contaminated dialysate will not be detected and might lead to bacterial contamination of blood (Figure 26). The occurrence of membrane leaks is low with modern dialyzers and the risk small. When dialyzers are re-used, blood leaks and hence membrane leaks are more frequent and the risk of blood contamination is no longer negligible. This risk is explicitly addressed in the IEC-standard for safety of hemodialysis equipment (3). It can either be avoided by the use of sterile dialysate in a sterilized dialysate circuit (as in CAVHD) or by sterile filtration of dialysate. The sterile filter in the dialysate fluid path serves as a protective device. As for other protective devices, means must be provided to test membrane integrity prior to treatment. A system that complies with this requirement is shown in Figure 27. The dialysate filter can be submitted to a pressure holding test: The filter is vented through the venting valve with the bypass valve closed and the ultrafiltration pump is started. After all fluid is removed from the raw dialysate side, the pressure on the filtrate side will decrease because air cannot penetrate the hydrophilic membrane in absence of a leak (diffusion can be neglected for this step). The ultrafiltration pump is stopped when the pressure reaches approximately −400 mmHg. The pressure increases slowly in absence of a membrane leak due to diffusion of air through the water filled pores. A single broken fiber will prevent build-up of negative pressure at filtration rates of 4 l/h. Smaller leaks will be detected by an increase of pressure after the ultrafiltration pump is stopped. Leaks with a few μm diameter might not be detectable, but the filtration rate through leaks of this size is small and the likelihood of bacteria transfer is low, if bacteria do not accumulate because the filter is periodically flushed. This is the case in the system of Figure 27 but not when filters are operated

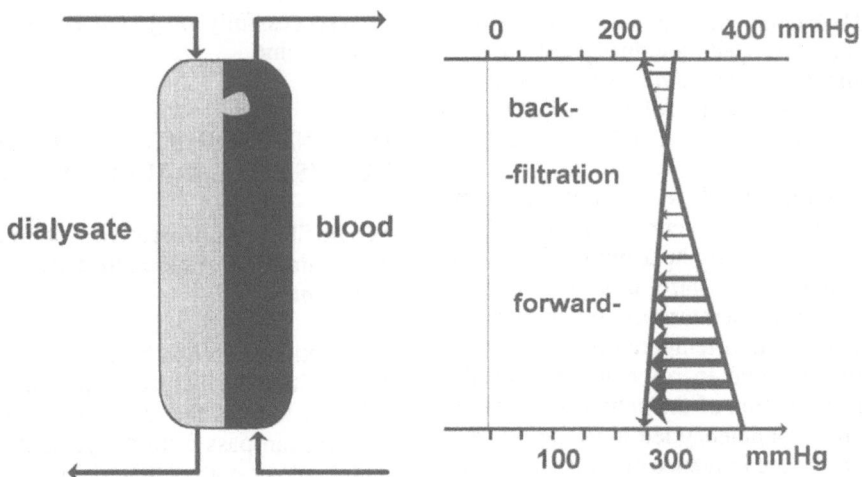

Figure 26. Right hand side: Blood and dialysate side pressure (schematic). At the blood entrance blood pressure is higher than dialysate pressure (positive TMP) resulting in forward filtration. At the other end, TMP is negative and dialysate is back-filtered into blood. Left hand side: Dialysate enters the blood side through a leak.

in dead-end mode. Challenging tests of this system have confirmed bacteria free dialysate downstream of the filter (105, 106). Tests in clinics have demonstrated rejection rates of > 10^6 (107).

It must be pointed out that a dialysate filter does not make regular disinfection of the system superfluous. The dialysate path might become contaminated when the dialyzer is connected or disconnected. In addition retrograde contamination is possible during no-flow periods.

The production of low endotoxin dialysate

The term 'low endotoxin' was chosen because 'endotoxin free' would not be correct. Absence of endotoxins is a matter of test sensitivity rather than clinical relevance. General discussion of this subject can be found (108). The contribution of backfiltration to endotoxin transfer from blood to dialysate is small as compared to backdiffusion (109, 110). The active fractions of endotoxins as Lipid A have a molecular weight of 2000 Daltons or less and are retained by adsorption rather than filtration. Retention of endotoxins is therefore membrane-material specific. Even modification of a basic material might change the retention capacity (111). The acceptable limit of endotoxin concentration in dialysate is controversial. Oettinger and coworkers (112) in a prospective study came to the conclusion that endotoxin contamination commonly found in dialysate is not clinically relevant. Quellhorst and Schünemann (113) were able to show a reduction of beta-2-microglobulin pre-dialysis plasma concentration with the use of sterile as compared to moderately contaminated dialysate and Cuprophane dialyzers. With Polysulphone dialyzers the production rate of beta-2-M was significantly increased with non-sterile as compared to sterile dialysate. Because of the comparably high clearance for beta-2-M this was

not reflected by the plasma concentration with polysulphone membranes.

The highest endotoxin concentration in dialysate reported by Oettinger (112) was 10 ng/ml. Frinak and co-workers (105) were unable to produce more than 30–300 ng/ml of endotoxin concentration in dialysate in mimicked dialysis. Lonnemann (114) used 500 ng/ml, Laude-Sharp (115) and co-workers 800 ng/ml, Fischbach and co-workers 5000 ng/ml and Urena and co-workers up to 25000 ng/ml for laboratory challenge tests. Endotoxin of different bacterial origin was used. The controversial results on endotoxin transfer through synthetic membranes can be interpreted easily as the result of different experimental settings. Endotoxins are retained by adsorption which is a surface interaction depending on temperature and pH. It is also cross-sensitive to other substances which might reduce or enhance the adsorption capacity. In addition it is load dependent. Taking the results of Oettinger (112) and Frinak (105) into account it can be assumed that it is possible to reduce endotoxin concentration in dialysate to a level below clinical relevance in a typical dialysis environment. A material that works satisfactorily as a dialysate filter might not necessarily be safe as a dialyzer regarding endotoxin transfer because uremic substances might compete with adsorption sites or otherwise enhance the endotoxin permeability.

Hemodiafiltration and hemofiltration with on-line produced substitution fluid

The concept of fluid replacement through a sterile filter was conceived by Bluemle, who presented his idea in the discussion following the paper by Henderson et al (94). He proposed a filter consisting of two sheets of membrane with blood flowing between the sheets as in a parallel

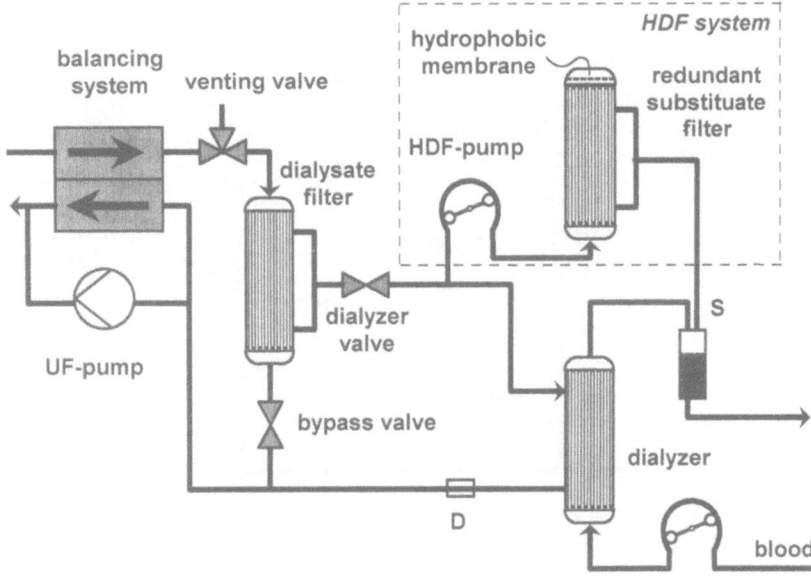

Figure 27. Flow diagram of hemodialysis machine with volumetric fluid balancing, dialysate filter for sterile filtration of dialysate and on-line HDF module. For disinfection the substitution line S is connected to connector D on the spent dialysate line.

plate dialyzer, and ultrafiltration through one membrane and substitution through the other.

A description of on-line filtration of substitution fluid through two capillary ultrafilters in series and direct infusion into blood was published in 1978 (116). A commercial dialysate delivery machine was used to prepare substitution fluid for pre-dilution hemofiltration. The filters were disinfected together with the dialysis machine. Prior to each treatment the fluid between the two filters was checked for absence of endotoxins.

Both principles mentioned above are used for hemodiafiltration (HDF) today. Bluemle's idea is applied in backfiltration-HDF and push-pull HDF. The second principle, infusion of the substitution fluid into the extracorporeal circuit pre- or post-hemofilter is used in modern commercial hemodialysis machines that can be modified for HF or HDF. Backfiltration was proposed by Sausse (117) to increase large molecular clearance. He patented a dialyzer with increased flow resistance on both the dialysate side and the blood side to allow forward-filtration in the first part of the dialyzer and backfiltration in the second part. Fluid control was provided by a closed system. This principle was further developed and clinically applied by Shinzato et al (118) and later by Miller and von Albertini et al (119) who used two high-flux dialyzers in series with some flow resistance control in the dialysate path between the filter. No modification of HD machines comprising volumetric UF control and a dialysate filter is required for this procedure. The hemofiltration flux can be measured with the help of a flowmeter in the dialysate line between the two dialyzers. Hemofiltration rate is equal to the dif-

ference between fresh dialysate flow and mid dialysate flow measured by the flow meter. The pressure drop is a function of blood and dialysate flow and can be varied on the dialysate side by the clamp. The principle is shown in Figure 28.

In push-pull HDF (120) filtration of up to 300 ml is followed by backfiltration of the same amount of fluid through the same membrane. HD machines that comprise a closed dialysate system can easily be adapted for push-pull by adding a piston-like pump. It is claimed that this system avoids build up of a protein layer on the membrane that reduces the ultrafiltration coefficient. This was reported for low blood flows of 200 ml/min. Whether this is still significant at higher shear rates has to be evaluated.

Safety under single fault condition in this system is provided by a dialysate filter, integrity tested prior to treatment. The dialyzers are either single use ones and tested by the manufacturer or reused ones that were tested by the reuse machine.

Hemodiafiltration with direct infusion of the on-line prepared substitution fluid into the extracorporeal circuit requires at least two filters in series to provide safety under single fault condition. The filters either have to be tested prior to dialysis by the machine or separately or must be single-use filters. Figure 27 shows the flow diagram of a commercial machine that tests both filters prior to use: Fresh dialysate is filtered and than pumped by the HDF-pump through a redundant substitute filter. This filter can be operated in dead end mode because it is not contaminated with bacteria or endotoxin as long as the dialysate filter is intact. Both filters have to be replaced if a leak

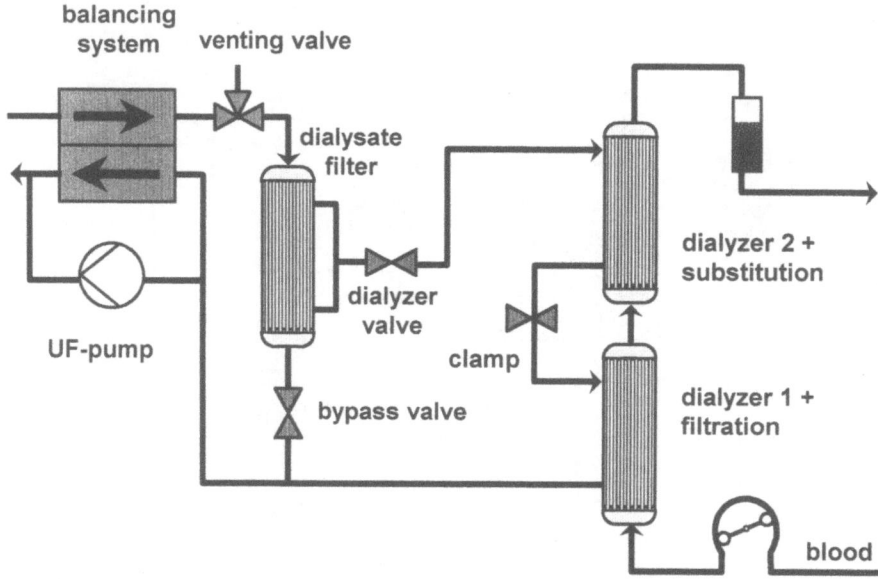

Figure 28. Backfiltration-HDF. Filtration takes place in dialyzer 1, substitution in dialyzer 2, Filtration rates can be increased by increasing flow resistance in the dialysate path with a clamp between dialyzers.

is detected in the dialysate filter. For disinfection and the simultaneous test of both filters the substitute line S is connected with the spent dialysate line at D. The dialysate lines are in a fluid interlock that connects the fresh and the spent dialysate line during disinfection. The bypass valve is closed and the venting valve opened. Operation of the UF-pump removes all fluid from the raw dialysate side of the dialysate filter and the input side of the substitute filter. The latter is vented through a hydrophobic membrane at the top of the filter. The pressure holding test is then performed as described above for the dialysate filter. Short, disposable connecting lines are used to connect the substitute line with the venous drip chamber for the next treatment. Reused dialyzers can be tested simultaneously if required. In this case dialyzer and blood lines are set up as for dialysis. The substitute line is connected to the spent dialysate line. For the pressure holding test the dialyzer membrane must be wet (which is usually the case with reused dialyzers). The blood side of the dialyzer is vented through the pressure transducer protector of the venous pressure monitor. The pressure holding test can be performed as described but will take longer. A slightly different approach is used in another commercial device (121). The substitute filter is used for a single treatment only and need not be tested on-site prior to dialysis.

HDF systems with separate preparation of substitution fluid as described can be used for pre- and post-dilution hemodiafiltration or hemofiltration. With additional flow control devices pre-, post- and mid-dilution techniques can be combined. Mid dilution is a technique where two dialyzers or filters are used in series and substitution is between both filters. The first one is operated in post-, the second one in pre-dilution mode. Hemofiltration

has no advantages as compared to hemodiafiltration. If for research purposes the contribution of hemofiltration and hemodialysis must be varied dialysate flow and filtrate flow can both be adjusted. For pure hemofiltration dialysate can be bypassed (122).

Filtered dialysate can be used to prime the extracorporeal circuit or replace saline for the treatment of hypotensive episodes. On-line HDF allows anticoagulation-free dialysis with automatic, periodic flush of the extracorporeal circuit (123, 124): Filtered fluid is collected in a bag connected to the extracorporeal system upstream of the blood pump (on the negative pressure side) through a line normally closed by an electrically operated clamp. This clamp is opened periodically and the bag is emptied into the extracorporeal circuit. The substitution pump rate is adjusted to match typical flushing volumes of 200 ml and time intervals of 20 min.

MODELLED VARIATION OF TREATMENT PARAMETERS

Treatment parameters such as dialysate (sodium) concentration, ultrafiltration rate, blood and dialysate flow are varied intradialytically in an attempt to increase or maintain efficacy and/or reduce intradialytic symptoms. The objective is to keep the overall treatment goal (e.g., ultrafiltration volume, electrolyte balance, sodium removal) unchanged. The variation either follows a kinetic model or, more often, 'clinical judgement'. With microprocessor technology not only available but the most cost effective means to control dialysis machines, variation of parameters has become a favored marketing tool. In this paragraph the term 'variation' is used for the variation of treatment parameters while 'modeling' is used for kinetic models.

Electrolyte variation

Among other parameters, dialysate sodium, potassium and calcium are known to influence intradialytic blood pressure and symptoms. Most 'sodium variation devices' change total dialysate concentration rather than sodium alone but some devices vary these parameters individually.

For variation of total dialysate concentration the mixing ratio of volumetric proportioning machines is changed according to the programmed profile. Alternatively the conductivity goal is varied for conductivity controlled proportioning devices. In the latter case the slope of the conductivity versus concentration function has to be taken into account. As mentioned earlier this slope is approximately 0.91 which means that a 10% increase in conductivity leads to an 11% increase of concentration.

Variation of individual concentrates is performed by volumetric proportioning of individual electrolyte concentrates to the basic dialysate. Saito and co-workers (125) described a device where proportioning of dialysis concentrate and 10% NaCl is performed with the same pump. Water, acetate concentrate and 10% saline is connected through individual valves to the inlet of a constant flow pump. The proportioning ratio is adjusted by the opening time of the valves. Murisasco and co-workers (126) added sodium and potassium concentrate by computer controlled individual pumps to dialysate centrally produced. A module allowing individual profiling of Na, K, and bicarbonate by addition of $NaCl$, $NaHCO_3$ and KCl to dialysate was designed by one of the authors (127). This device also allows simultaneous profiling of ultrafiltration. Pumps and ultrafiltration are controlled by a computer that also allows calculation of intra-extracellular water shifts, plasma sodium concentration and sodium balance by a single pool sodium model. Profiles can be programmed individually and the projected outcome calculated by the model before treatment. Several applications have been reported for this device (128–130).

Another application for sodium profiles was proposed as 'cell wash' dialysis. In this modality bi-directional intra-extracellular fluid shifts are produced by large intermittent variations of dialysate sodium. The objective is to increase intra-extracellular solute transfer by convection (a kind of osmotically driven push-pull filtration) (131).

Clinically these profiles might have a beneficial effect. It can be hypothesized, however, that this could have been achieved by a more careful adjustment of basic parameters. Because all profiles are based on sodium added to a baseline concentration the sodium balance, with such profiles is more positive and is known to reduce symptoms. The usefulness of the single pool sodium model for the

prediction of fluid shifts and plasma sodium is questionable because post-dialysis electrolyte rebound has been demonstrated (26, 132).

Safety aspects: Safety design for profiling controllers requires redundant storage of profiles. One possibility is the storage of preprogrammed concentration profiles in a memory area of the microprocessor control unit reserved for the proportioning system and a corresponding conductivity profile in an independent area for the adjustment of the conductivity alarm limits. Individual programming of profiles by the user requires sophisticated input routines to guarantee correct storage of the information in the two separate memory areas. Systems that add concentrates are safer inherently because dialysate concentration cannot decrease below the basic concentration, which excludes the risk of hemolysis by hypoosmolar dialysate. The risk of hypernatremia or hyperkalemia can be limited by restricting the pump speeds of the concentration pumps.

Variation of ultrafiltration rate

Intradialytic symptoms, especially hypotension, are closely related to ultrafiltration. Removal of fluid from the vascular system is only partially compensated by refilling from the interstitium. This results in a decrease of blood volume that eventually might lead to symptoms. The refilling rate decreases as the patient approaches dry weight. Attempts have been made to either match ultrafiltration rate and refilling capacity or enhance refilling capacity by special ultrafiltration profiles. Decreasing rate profiles (133) or intermittent ultrafiltration (134) combined with sodium profiles have been used for this purpose.

In dialysis machines having ultrafiltration pumps independent of dialysate pumps, profiling is performed by variation of the ultrafiltration pump speed. Safety against a fault in the programming unit can be provided by an independent ultrafiltration volume limiter that stops the ultrafiltration pump when the pre-programmed volume is ultrafiltered. Safety design in machines with flow difference programming is more complicated because the volume integrator cannot stop ultrafiltration in case of a controller error. A possible solution is the separation of the dialyzer by two valves up- and downstream in the dialysate path in case of an error. In this case dialysis has to be terminated because dialysate flow is stopped. For both variants the commonly used transmembrane pressure control offers only marginal safety against excessive fluid loss because the ultrafiltration coefficient is individually different and not a true constant in relation to ultrafiltration rate. Safety can be achieved by periodic tests of the ultrafiltration control system whenever the ultrafiltration rate is changed as described above.

Variation of blood and dialysate flow

The objective of programmed intradialytic variation of clearance is linearization of solute removal. Under normal conditions solute removal at the beginning of dialysis is rapid, causing intra-extracellular osmotic differences. A model to calculate the appropriate blood flow versus time function based on single pool urea kinetics was published by Lewis and Frost (135). There is no indication that this approach is clinically significant. Model calculations show that intra-extracellular osmotic differences caused by urea become insignificant after 30 minutes of dialysis. The same goal can be achieved by variation of dialysate flow. For safety reasons the latter is preferable because pressure monitors in the extracorporeal circuit need not be changed.

TOWARDS MORE PHYSIOLOGICAL DIALYSIS: FEEDBACK-CONTROL

Maintenance dialysis is still accompanied by many unpleasant side effects and is costly for providers. Modelled variation of treatment parameters has been tried with little success. The underlying cause is that patient specific momentary parameters usually are unknown. Attempts were made during the last two decades to develop monitors that could be used for feedback control of dialysis machine parameters such as dialysate concentration, and temperature, as well as ultrafiltration rate and volume. The authors who have contributed to this development in the scientific and industrial field have introduced the term 'physiological dialysis' for this approach. The principle is illustrated in Figure 29.

BLOOD VOLUME CONTROL

Blood volume changes have an important influence on intra-dialytic blood pressure. In 1970 Kim et al (136) measured blood volume by means of radioactive labeled erythrocytes. Since then much work has been devoted to the development of monitoring methods applicable to routine dialysis.

Principle of blood volume measurement

Blood volume and blood volume changes usually are measured with the help of an indicator injected into blood. From the amount of indicator injected and the concentration of the diluted indicator the diluting factor and the blood volume can be calculated. For the measurement of blood volume changes, erythrocytes or total blood protein (plasma protein + erythrocyte protein) can be used as internal indicator.

The method to calculate blood volume changes from hematocrit changes is illustrated in Figure 30. With hematocrit HCT0 measured at time 0 and HCT1 at time 1 blood volume changes can be calculated as follows:

$$VE = HCT0 * BV0 = HCT1 * BV1 \qquad [12]$$

$$\frac{BV1}{BV0} = \frac{HCT0}{HCT1} \qquad [13]$$

$$dBV = \frac{BV0 - BV1}{BV0} = 1 - \frac{HCT0}{HCT1}. \qquad [14]$$

If blood volume changes are known it is only a small step to create a feed back device in order to control ultrafiltration and limit blood volume reduction.

Methodology of continuous blood water concentration monitoring

Various physical methods can be used for continuous hematocrit or total blood protein monitoring: electrical conductivity, optical density, blood viscosity and physical density (Figure 31).

Blood volume measurement by electrical conductivity

Electrical conductivity was developed as a method for hematocrit measurement at the end of the 19th century. It was known already at this time that electrical conductivity of whole blood is a function of serum conductivity, number of corpuscles in blood (hematocrit, hct) and temperature (137–139). Gram (140) published experimental and calculated data which displays the relationship between the quotient of blood and serum conductivity and cell volume (hct). During dialysis total plasma protein (tpr), plasma lipid content and hct concentration changes because water is ultrafiltered. Plasma water conductivity changes as well due to electrolyte transfer to and from dialysate. To separate these two effects and correct whole blood conductivity for plasma water conductivity changes three methods can be applied: Stiller and coworkers (141) used a setup which consists first of a conductivity and temperature sensor for whole blood, a small plasma filter and second a conductivity and temperature sensor for plasma conductivity. With this and similar devices Stiller et al (142, 143) and other authors were able to demonstrate the effect of ultrafiltration and saline infusion on blood volume. Maeda et al (144) reported a similar system. Thomasset (145) proposed a system which is based on whole blood conductivity measurement at high and low frequencies. The conductivity at high frequency reflects the plasma conductivity while whole blood conductivity is measured at low frequencies. This frequency dependence of whole blood conductivity was known earlier (146). The same principle is used by Ishihara et al (147). A method to calculate plasma conductivity changes from electrolyte differences continuously measured in dialysate up- and downstream of the dialyzer was patented by Polaschegg (148).

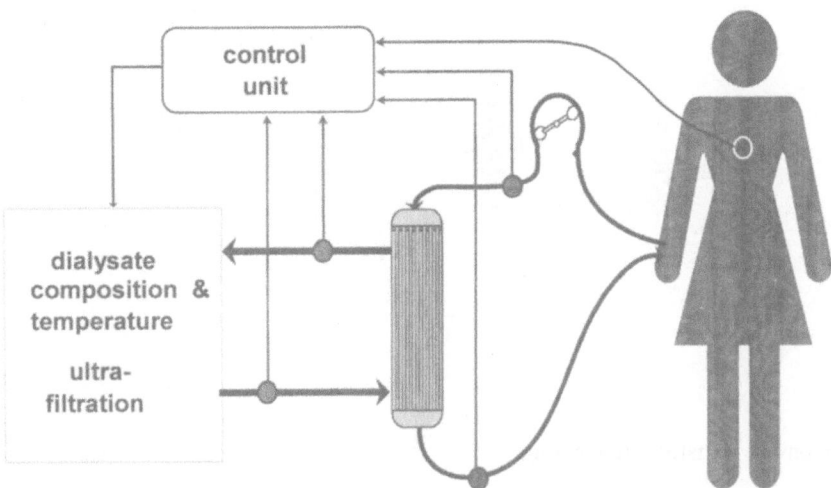

Figure 29. 'Physiological dialysis'. Physiological parameters measured in dialysate, in the extracorporeal system and/or on the patient are used for feedback control of dialysis parameters.

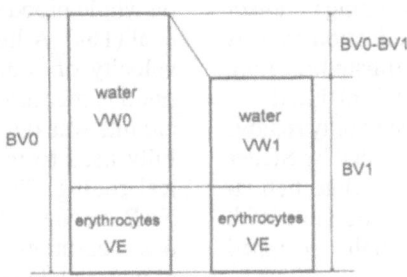

Figure 30. Reduction of water space becomes apparent as an increase of hematocrit or blood density. This can be used to calculate relative blood volume change.

Conductivity measurement usually requires electrodes. With special blood tubing forming a closed electrical circuit for blood, contact-less conductivity sensors can be used (149). Whole blood conductivity is not only sensitive to changes of blood volume but also reflects changes of erythrocyte volume caused by osmotic shifts. This effect was used to measure erythrocyte volume changes by de Vries et al (150). Recently a commercial device without any compensation for these effects was presented on the market and described (151).

Blood volume measurement by optical density

Optical absorption is the standard method to measure hemoglobin concentration in the clinical laboratory. Hemoglobin content in the vascular space remains constant during dialysis. Optical measurement of hemoglobin concentration changes can therefore be used to record intradialytic blood volume changes. In whole blood hemoglobin is contained in erythrocytes. The application of optical methods for hemoglobin concentration in the extracorporeal circuit is hampered by the strong non-

linearity of the optical density at higher hemoglobin levels (152) and the dependence of the absorption coefficient on oxygen saturation.

The non-linearity of the optical transmission function versus hematocrit is caused by multiple scattering effects. At low hematocrit, photons are scattered only one time by an erythrocyte and then absorbed somewhere on the wall of the measuring system. With increasing numbers of erythrocytes the likelihood increases that the photon is scattered again. Scattering problems were avoided by Schallenberg et al (153) by continuous hemolysis of a small amount of whole blood sampled from the extracorporeal circuit. Hypotonic ammonia solution (pH = 10) was used to create 99% oxidized hemoglobin.

With whole blood the oxygen saturation problem can be overcome by measuring at or close to the isobestic point (about 805 nm). At the isobestic point light absorption is independent of oxygen saturation of hemoglobin. This method was used successfully to record blood volume changes by Wilkinson et al (154). The same approach is used by Mancini et al (155). The latter paper reports linear dependence of optical absorption for a hemoglobin

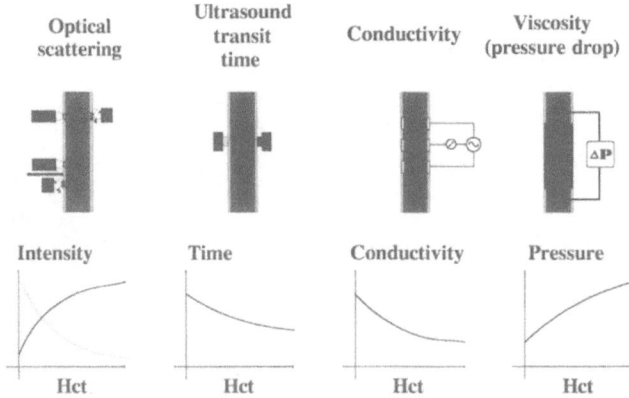

Figure 31. Methods for on-line hematocrit monitoring.

content of 70 to 100 g/l. In order to compensate for scattering effects a device patented by Adamo (156) uses a reflecting coating around the optical sensor.

De Vries et al (157) describe a device working in reflection rather than transmission mode. The reflection angle is about 130° and the penetration depth is estimated at 2 mm. Linearity and independence of blood flow is claimed.

While all these devices are able to measure only relative changes of hematocrit a novel device described by Steuer et al (158) allows the measurement of absolute hematocrit as well as oxygen saturation. This is possible with a multi wavelength technique and a specially designed cuvette.

Blood volume measurement by viscosity

It is well known that blood viscosity changes with hematocrit. Greenwood et al (159) demonstrated *in vitro* that this effect can be used to measure blood volume changes. The device consists of a capillary and pressure sensors. Polaschegg (160) proposed a system that calculates blood volume and fistula pressure changes, from pre-pump arterial and post-pump venous pressure in the extracorporeal circuit. No clinical application of this method is known to the authors. A practical device also would require blood temperature measurement, because viscosity of whole blood depends on temperature.

Blood volume measurement by density

Density of whole blood is slightly different from water. The difference is caused mainly by the total protein content of plasma and erythrocytes. Because erythrocyte proteins dominate, the total amount of proteins in whole blood during dialysis can be assumed as constant and therefore used to measure blood volume changes.

Blood density was used successfully to record blood volume changes by means of a mechanical oscillator technique (161, 162). Because of the rather complicated mechanical system which requires special preparation

and sterilization of the measuring system this method never found wide acceptance. The velocity of sound depends on the density of the medium. This effect was confirmed on whole blood by Bradley and Sacerio (163) and Bakke et al (164). A linear relationship between hematocrit and velocity of sound was found. A device allowing continuous measurement of blood density in extracorporeal circuits was developed by Roob et al (165) and successfully used to measure blood volume changes in a clinical setting. This principle was independently patented by Polaschegg (166). This method requires simultaneous measurement of blood temperature because density of material depends on temperature.

Technical comparison of blood volume sensors

All methods described with the exception of the optical ones require blood temperature measurement. The optical and conductivity methods are sensitive to osmolarity changes caused by electrolytes because these changes alter the volume of the erythrocytes. This has to be compensated by a multi wavelength and/or multiple sensor technology. Figure 32 shows the result of simultaneous blood volume measurement with 3 devices.

MONITORING AND CONTROL OF BLOOD TEMPERATURE AND THERMAL ENERGY BALANCE

The pioneering work of Maggiore et al (167) on blood pressure stability in hemodialysis versus hemofiltration described the important clinical finding, that decreases in the number of hypotensive episodes were related to dialysate or substitution fluid temperature and not to the method of treatment. These findings were supported by others but it became apparent that reduction of dialysate temperature to 34 or 35°C caused shivering and discomfort in many patients.

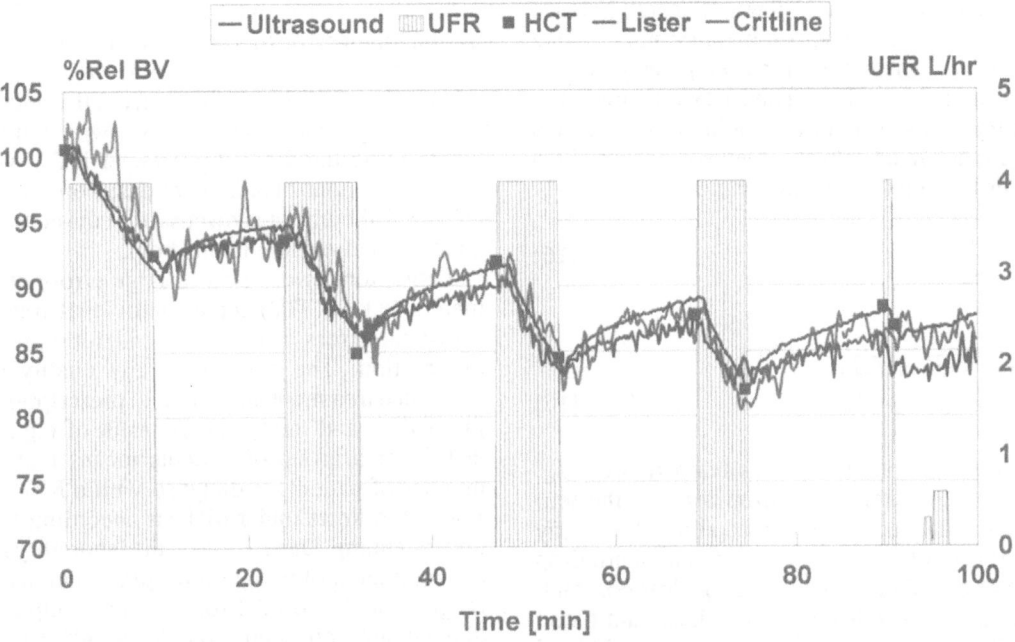

Figure 32. Blood volume changes measured continuously with two optical devices (Lister: experimental device (154), Critline: CRIT-LINE® instrument, In-Line diagnostics Corporation, Riverdale, Utah) one ultrasound device (Blood Water Monitor, Fresenius AG, Bad Homburg, Germany) and calculated from hematocrit (HCT). Blood volume drops during ultrafiltration and increases in pauses.

Intradialytic body temperature change is governed by thermal energy balance and heat capacity of the human body. The contribution of vasoconstriction and the extracorporeal circuit can be estimated: Resting energy expenditure of a 70 kg male adult person is 116 Watt (168). This energy is normally dissipated to the environment by evaporation (22%), conduction (18%) and radiation (60%). Thermal regulation tries to keep the body temperature close to an individual set temperature by changing the radiant heat loss through vasoconstriction and vasodilation. Temperature sensors are positioned in the skin and deep body tissue. If the body is no longer able to keep the central temperature within a narrow range around the set value the temperature regulation center in the hypothalamus initiates sweating (positive deviation) or shivering (negative deviation). The core temperature at which sweating starts depends not only on the set temperature but also on skin temperature as shown by Benzinger (169).

The extracorporeal circuit influences intradialytic thermal energy balance. The dialyzer is a perfect heat exchanger. Blood leaves the dialyzer in thermal equilibrium with dialysate. The energy balance in the dialyzer is a function of the difference between arterial blood temperature and dialysate temperature, blood flow Q_b, specific heat c and density ϱ of blood:

$$dE = (T_a - T_d) * Q_b * c * \varrho. \qquad [15]$$

Specific heat c of whole blood is 3.64 J/g and density $\varrho = 1.052$ g/ml at 37°C. The energy balance for a temperature difference of 1°C at 400 ml/min blood flow is 25 W. Another contribution comes from energy loss in the venous blood line. For blood flows > 100 ml/min the temperature drop becomes small as compared to the blood-environment temperature difference. In this case the energy loss is independent of blood flow and depends on blood-environment temperature difference and length and type of tubing only. For 20°C environmental temperature, and standard PVC blood tubing (inner diameter 4.5 mm) of 2.8 m length, the energy loss is approximately 10 W.

Body temperature changes during dialysis depend on the difference between pre-dialysis core temperature and dialysate temperature. Pre-dialysis body temperature varies about 1.5°C between patients (mean values) and up to 2°C from treatment to treatment (170). Considering all effects, the intradialytic energy flux can vary between ± 80 W. The pre-post temperature difference of a 70 kg patient can vary between ± 2.8°C in 2.5 h under these assumptions. This is normally not the case because the body will react with sweating or shivering which was not taken into account. This estimate however shows the importance of the extracorporeal circuit for thermal energy balance.

Recently a blood temperature monitor (BTM, Fresenius AG, Bad Homburg, Germany) became available that allows continuous monitoring of thermal energy balance and feedback control of body temperature (171). This non-invasive device measures blood temperature in the arterial and venous blood line. The surface temperature of the blood line is measured by a platinum sensor. This sensor is positioned in an actively shielded housing (172) that minimizes heat loss to the environment.

$$\Delta T = 62 * \frac{L}{Q} \qquad [16]$$

$$T_a(\text{fistula}) = T_a + \Delta T,$$
$$T_v(\text{fistula}) = TV - \Delta T. \qquad [17]$$

The measured arterial and venous temperatures (T_a, T_v) are corrected for temperature drop between the sensor heads and the fistula. As mentioned above the energy loss is independent of blood flow. The temperature drop can therefore be calculated from the energy loss constant, length of tubing between fistula, sensor head and blood flow [16]. ΔT is measured as °C, L as meters and blood flow Q as ml/min. This corrected temperatures represent the temperatures at the point of entry into the fistula [17].

From the difference between these temperatures, blood flow and heat capacity of blood, thermal energy balance is calculated as already mentioned above. In absence of recirculation, arterial blood represents core temperature. In order to monitor body temperature the device is capable of measuring recirculation (see paragraph Recirculation measurement later in this chapter) and correct for this effect. As a monitor this device displays energy balance and body temperature, as a control device it allows control of thermal energy balance or body temperature. For safety reasons the module cannot increase dialysate temperature above the set value.

With the BTM it was possible to measure the patient related thermal effects (173). In the energy balancing mode a body temperature increase of 0.5°C was recorded at zero thermal energy balance in the extracorporeal circuit while in the body temperature control mode 100 kJ had to be removed during a 2.5 h dialysis session in order to maintain body temperature. An example that demonstrates stabilization of blood pressure by thermal feedback control in a patient who otherwise experiences blood pressure reduction during dialysis is shown in Figures 33 and 34.

CONTINUOUS MONITORING OF BLOOD OR DIALYSATE BIOCHEMICAL PARAMETERS

Kinetic models were developed for a better understanding of pathophysiology of end stage renal disease treated by hemodialysis and for quality control of prescription and performance. This models allow the calculation of

mass balances from intradialytic and interdialytic concentration changes of biochemical substances such as urea, creatinine, beta-2-microglobulin, sodium, potassium and others. Conclusions are drawn from this models based on clinical experience. The best known examples are urea kinetics and the derived parameter KT/V which is used as a quality control parameter based on findings from the NCDS. This subject is discussed in the chapter of Sargent and Gotch elsewhere in this book.

Laboratory errors lead to large errors of model parameters (e.g., KT/V) for an individual treatment, while statistical errors will be reduced for large numbers of observation. The purpose of any quality control is to guarantee treatment according to prescription for any single patient and treatment. A result of e.g., KT/V = 1.2 ± 0.3 for a group of patients means that a substantial number of patients is dialyzed with a KT/V of less than 1 which reflects under-dialysis according to our current understanding. Depending on the laboratory method used, the coefficient of variation for plasma urea concentration ranges from 1.3 to 9.3% for reference samples close to pre-dialysis urea concentrations to 2–14% for post-dialysis values. This converts into KT/V tolerances of ± 0.07 for the best and more than ± 0.3 for the lowest laboratories (95% confidence interval).

Dialysate sodium concentration influences cardiovascular stability during dialysis. Precise control of the plasma–dialysate sodium gradient is therefore essential. The laboratory error for plasma or serum sodium is approximately 1.8 mmol/l (standard deviation) (174). This means that more than 30% of samples show a deviation from the reference value larger than 1.8 mmol/l. If dialysate concentration is adjusted without laboratory control the concentrate tolerance (± 2%) (175) and the tolerance of the proportioning system has to be taken into account. The latter can be estimated to be ± 2% as well. Assuming that both tolerances follow a normal distribution and that 2% corresponds to σ (standard deviation) the likelihood of more than 2 mmol/l deviation from the set value of dialysate sodium concentration is again more than 30%. The tolerance for the concentration driving force is therefore ± 3.8 mmol/l (one standard deviation). This tolerance exceeds the difference between low and high sodium concentration used in some of the controlled studies on dialysate sodium. Another source of error comes from the influence of plasma proteins on the thermodynamic equilibrium between ions (Gibbs–Donnan-effect) but also from the analysis technique used. As pointed out in (176) ion-selective electrodes and flame photometry measure different properties and give different results. Altogether, the modeling approach is of little help for the individual dialysis session.

Continuous intradialytic measurement of biochemical parameters follows the goal of increasing accuracy by reducing the statistical error and obtaining better information about the time course allowing more precise calculation of important dynamic model parameters. Information

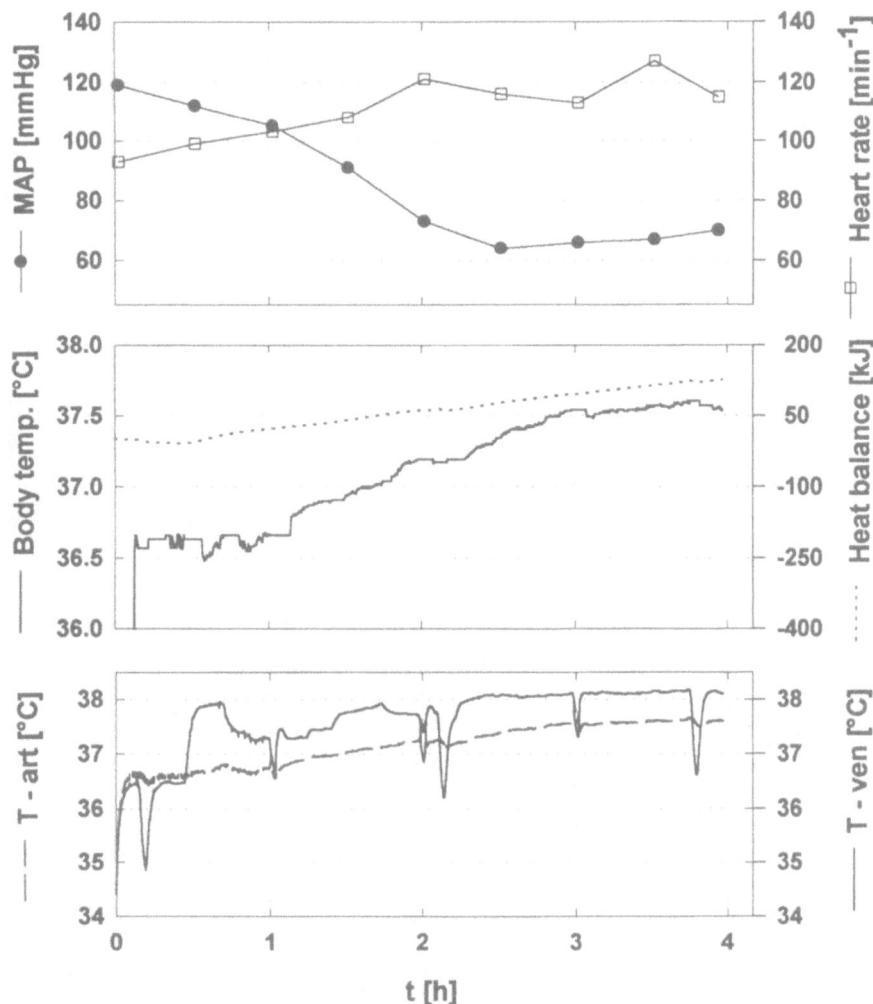

Figure 33. Dialysis with constant dialysate temperature: Venous temperature is higher than arterial temperature. Energy balance is positive and body temperature increases. Heart rate increases and blood pressure decreases (Krämer M, Christmann-Braun H, Rode C, unpublished data).

is instantaneous and available results within treatment, allow corrective measures. Correction can be achieved manually (e.g., by increasing treatment time) or automatically by feedback control.

Continuous urea measurement

Most analytical techniques employ the enzyme urease to convert urea to ammonium. The end product of this reaction is either measured directly by an ion selective electrode or indirectly. Under near neutral pH the reaction may be expressed as follows:

$$CO(NH_2) + 3H_2O \Rightarrow 2NH_4^- + HCO_3^- + OH^-. \quad [18]$$

The ammonium ion can be measured directly by ion sensitive electrodes (177). The reaction also changes pH and conductivity of the solution. Both parameters can

be used to measure urea indirectly, but only the conductivity method has found application. Buffers are added to samples because the reaction described above is pH dependent (178). The conventional laboratory method employs additional reagents to allow quantification by optical adsorption in the UV range at 340 nm. These laboratory tests are available from SIGMA, St Louis, Missouri, USA and other reagent suppliers. Urease is either applied in liquid form or is immobilized on membranes or beads. An alternative to enzymatic methods would be optical spectroscopy in the far infrared range at wavenumber 1617 cm^{-1} (179).

For continuous measurement of plasma water concentration either a sampling filter or a sampling dialyzer is used. Kabei et al (180) describe a sampling filter and ion sensitive electrodes for continuous measurement of urea and electrolytes. Thavarungkul et al (181) equilibrated

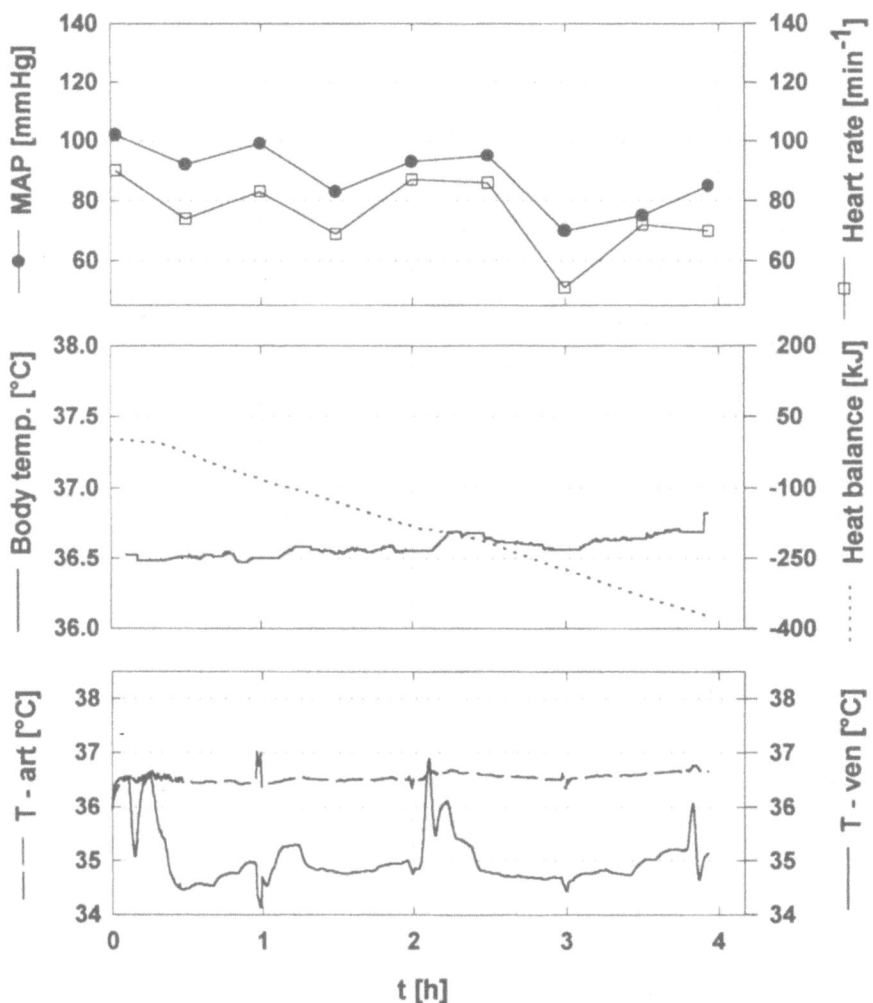

Figure 34. Feedback control of body temperature. Venous temperature is lower than arterial temperature. Heat balance is negative and body temperature remains constant as does heart rate and blood pressure (Krämer M, Christmann-Braun H, Rode C, unpublished data).

blood with dialysate in a sampling dialyzer. The dialysate was either pumped through a column with immobilized urease to a conductivity sensor or bypassed to measure conductivity differences caused by the conversion of urea to ammonium ions. An integrated sensor that comprises a membrane with immobilized urease and a conductivity sensor is described by Jacobs et al (182).

An alternative to the measurement of plasma water concentrations is measurement in dialysate. This was described by Klein and Montalvo (183) who mixed aliquots of spent dialysate with a buffer concentrate and pumped the mixture through a column containing immobilized urease. An ammonium sensitive electrode served as sensor. In modern devices the ammonium sensitive electrode is covered with a disposable membrane containing immobilized urease. The lifespan of such a membrane at room temperature is a few days. Bacteria will prolifer-

ate in this environment and might have an adverse effect on accuracy. A filter that prevents contamination of the sensor device by bacteria and particulates is advisable. Sensor sensitivity depends on many parameters, is variable, as known for enzymatic processes, and ion sensitive electrodes. Devices for clinical use therefore comprise means for automatic two point calibration of the sensor. The Nonactin-PVC sensor normally used in urea measurement assemblies is also sensitive to potassium. This cross sensitivity has to be taken into account. A commercial device, the BioStat 1000® from Baxter Healthcare Corp, McGaw Park, Illinois, USA combines all the mentioned features with a sampling device and a proprietary modeling program that calculates relevant treatment results. Marketing for this product has triggered renewed interest in continuous urea measurement and also alternative developments. Clinical results demonstrate good agreement with direct dialysis quantification (DDQ) for urea removed but a 5% overestimation of KT/V (184).

A novel method originally developed for glucose measurement is microdialysis of interstitial fluid (185): A single dialysis fiber of 30 mm length is placed under the subcutaneous tissue. Microbore tubing is glued to both ends and dialysate is slowly pumped through the interior of the fiber. The effluent from the other end is collected and analyzed.

Continuous measurement of creatinine

Creatinine is another accepted, albeit less frequently used, marker for dialysis kinetic modeling. KT/V for creatinine can be calculated from intradialytic decrease of creatinine in blood over time and can be translated into KT/V for urea. Creatinine can also be measured by enzymatic methods. Of practical interest is optical absorption in the UV range because it does not require special equipment or techniques, but can be performed with standard laboratory photometers. This method was employed by Gal and Grof (186) who were able to demonstrate an exponential fall in UV absorption intradialytically in spent dialysate at 210 nm. Absorption in this range is not only by creatinine but also by other uremic substances at lesser concentration. Progress in the technology of solid state electronics with integrated optics might allow the development of low cost spectrometers that can be integrated into the dialysate path and can be employed as blood leak detectors but also for quantification of creatinine, bilirubin and other substances.

Continuous measurement of electrolytes

Sampling filters or dialyzers are usually employed to measure not only urea but also electrolytes intradialytically (180, 187). Murisasco et al (188)described a feed-back system with such a sampling device. Direct measurement of whole blood sampled from the extracorporeal circuit of heart-lung machines has been described (189, 190). The commercial device used was the GEM–6 from Diamond Sensor Systems now marketed by Mallinckrodt, Ann Arbor, Michigan, USA. This device measures Na, K, Ca, Hct, pO_2, pCO_2 and pH. The disposable cartridges are rather expensive which is a serious obstacle for the application of such devices in dialysis. A more cost effective approach developed by industry is the IONOFLOW® (Fresenius AG, Bad Homburg, Germany) (191): Dialysate is sampled continuously by a double channel sampling pump at comparably high speed up- and downstream of the dialyzer to reduce delay time. Samples are taken automatically from the lines downstream the sampling pump and fed into an electrolyte analyzer (IONOMETER, Fresenius AG, Bad Homburg, Germany). Electrolyte balances were measured that agreed closely with results from electrolyte models based on pre-dialysis and post-equilibrium blood samples (132).

Indirect electrolyte measurement and electrolyte balancing

When optimal dialysate sodium concentration was investigated in the seventies, Gotch and coworkers (192) applied the variable volume single pool sodium model to this problem and showed that total body sodium increases slightly during high Na treatment probably compensating for potassium loss, as pointed out in the discussion. They proposed control of the patient's individual post dialysis plasma electrolyte composition to minimize intra- and inter-dialytic symptoms. Individual treatment based on kinetic models requires precise knowledge of pre-dialysis plasma electrolyte concentration and equally precise control of dialysate electrolytes.

There are three ways for individualized and/or quantitative sodium therapy: Sodium prescription based on sodium modeling, feedback control of dialysate concentration by on-line measurement of plasma sodium and sodium balancing.

Sodium modeling: Individualized therapy with the goal of achieving a pre-determined post-dialysis plasma sodium concentration requires knowledge of pre-dialysis plasma sodium, extra- and intracellular volume, total plasma protein and dialyzer clearance to start with. With the help of sodium model programs the required dialysate sodium or sodium profile can be calculated. As mentioned above analytical errors and dialysate tolerances render this approach useless. For this reason researchers began to look for better alternatives in the late 70s and developed or proposed various methods to measure plasma sodium concentration directly or indirectly and control dialysate sodium through a feedback loop.

On-line measurement and feedback control: One alternative to the modeled prescription of dialysate sodium concentration is on-line measurement of plasma sodium and feedback control of dialysate concentration as proposed in (192). It compensates for dialysate concentration tolerances but does not take intra-extracellular fluid transfer resistance (193) (two-pool effects) into account, and is also prone to measurement errors related to sodium measurement in plasma or whole blood. No device that allows continuous measurement in whole blood as proposed in (192) has so far being described for hemodialysis because of problems related to sensor technology (187). Man et al (194) described a system that allows equilibration of dialysate with blood by means of a temporary recirculation loop. Initially the plasma Na concentration and the Na concentration of the equilibrated dialysate is measured. During dialysis the concentration of the equilibrated dialysate is measured periodically and from this data plasma Na concentration is calculated. The system was further modified by adding a conductivity sensor to the recirculation loop (195). Plasma water conductivity is calculated that correlates with plasma sodium. With this data a manual feedback loop, programmed to achieve the prescribed end dialysis plasma Na concentration, is used to adjust dialysate sodium concentration (196).

Electrolyte balancing: Another alternative is electrolyte or sodium balancing as described by Polaschegg and Husar (197): Dialysate electrolyte concentration is measured up- and downstream of the dialyzer. The difference of the concentrations multiplied by the dialysate flow rate is equal to the transfer rate of electrolytes to or from blood. The method also allows calculation of the equilibrium plasma sodium concentration. The transfer rate integrated over dialysis time is equal to the total electrolyte balance for the dialysis session. Either single, multiple or total electrolytes can be measured by appropriate sensors. Because total electrolytes rather than sodium changes are relevant for osmotic shifts, conductivity sensors can be employed. Dialysate conductivity and dialysate flow can be measured much more accurately as compared to blood side biochemical parameters. Dialysate conductivity or concentration measurement is also more cost effective. Feedback control based on electrolyte balancing allows removal of a prescribed amount of electrolytes. A balancing goal of zero keeps plasma sodium or electrolyte concentration constant. If a specific reduction of plasma sodium is intended the necessary sodium balance can be calculated from total body water and intended plasma sodium change. The algorithm to calculate plasma concentration from dialysate concentrations up- and downstream of the dialyzer has been described (198). Later patents describe similar approaches (199, 200).

MONITORS FOR DIALYSIS QUANTIFICATION

Models for dialysis quantification are described elsewhere in the book. A simplified version is presented here as introduction to monitors used for dialysis quantification. Quantification includes measurement of solute quantity removed during dialysis and intradialytic reduction of solid concentration. For simplicity it is assumed that the solute is urea, no solutes are generated intradialytically and the only pathway for removal is dialysis.

For practical purposes multi-compartment models have been simplified to two-pool or one-pool compartment models. The latter became popular following the NCDS study. Newer approaches are therefore translated back into the one-pool model. A rebound factor allows correction for solute rebound usually seen during the first hour after dialysis ends. Alternatively a modeled one-pool clearance can be calculated to describe the solute concentration reduction from start to equilibration after end of dialysis. This is illustrated in Figure 35. It shows intra- and extracellular urea concentration versus time as described by the two-pool model and the modeled one-pool extracellular concentration.

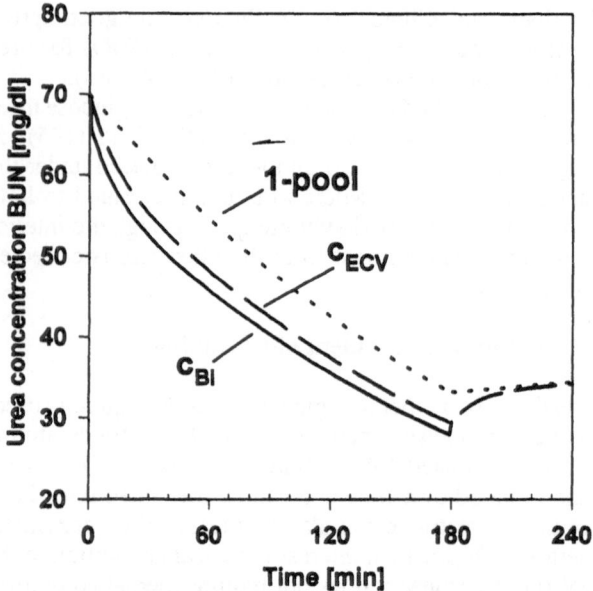

Figure 35. 2-pool urea kinetics without ultrafiltration. Dashed line: extracellular concentration c_{ECV}. Solid line: plasma concentration c_{Bl}. The difference between extracellular and plasma concentration is caused by recirculation. Dotted line: single pool simulation (1-pool) based on post-dialysis equilibrium concentration corrected for urea generation rate.

Monitors for urea quantification must take this effect into account. This is the case with the BioStat 1000® device mentioned in the previous paragraph. It measures dialysate urea concentration and calculates 'patient clearance' with the help of a built-in two-pool model. Integration of dialysate urea concentration multiplied by dialysate flow over time gives total urea removed. A first estimate of KT/V is available after 90 minutes which is too late to correct dialysis settings or change dialyzers. Operational cost of this device might limit its use to monthly checks of patient clearance and urea removal. Quality control, however, must guarantee that every single treatment is according to prescription and that immediately deficiencies are corrected. On line measurement of electrolyte dialysance which is equivalent to effective urea clearance is a cost effective method that can be used for this purpose.

On-line automatic intradialytic clearance measurement using conductivity

Electrolyte clearance is proportional to urea clearance. The proportionality factor is equal to one within errors of measurement. Electrolyte clearance can therefore replace urea clearance as quality control parameter. Albers and Smith (201) demonstrated that like urea clearance 'conductivity' clearance is blood- and dialysate-flow dependent. Electrolyte concentration is indirectly measured by conductivity. The conductivity versus concentration function is non-linear but can be approximated by a cubic function with sufficient accuracy. Aqueous clearance of a dialyzer can be measured *in vitro* with deionized water replacing blood. Dialysance = Clearance can be calculated from dialysate in and out concentrations according to equation [19].

$$D = Q_D \frac{C_{Di} - C_{Do}}{C_{Di}} . \qquad [19]$$

If conductivity is used, concentration can be calculated with equation [20]. C is the normalized concentration (concentration divided by the nominal concentration) and σ the normalized conductivity (conductivity divided by the conductivity at nominal concentration).

$$C = 0.912 * \sigma + 0.087 * \sigma^2. \qquad [20]$$

This non-linearity was neglected by Boag and Vlchek (202). Resnick (203) consequently found a deviation of 7% between blood side and dialysate clearance with this method that is the error introduced by the use of conductivity instead of concentration. Equation [19] can only be applied for in vitro tests with $C_{Bi} = 0$. *In vivo*, equation [21] is to be used:

$$D = Q_D * \frac{C_{Di} - C_{Do}}{C_{Di} - \alpha * C_{Bi}}. \qquad [21]$$

If only dialysate side parameters (Q_D, C_{Di}, C_{Do}) are known, equation [21] contains two unknowns: Dialysance D and $\alpha * C_{Bi}$, the blood water electrolyte concentration multiplied by the Donnan-coefficient. With two unknowns, two equations are necessary to solve this problem. This is done by using two different dialysate input concentrations (equations [22] and [23]).

$$D = Q_D * \frac{C_{Di}(1) - C_{Do}(1)}{C_{Di}(1) - \alpha * C_{Bi}} \qquad [22]$$

$$D = Q_D * \frac{C_{Di}(2) - C_{Do}(2)}{C_{Di}(2) - \alpha * C_{Bi}} . \qquad [23]$$

Calculation of $\alpha * C_{Bi}$ from one equation and substitution into the other allows calculation of dialysance D (204) (equation [24]).

$$D = Q_D * \frac{[C_{Di}(2) - C_{Do}(2)] - [C_{Di}(1) - C_{Do}(1)]}{C_{Di}(2) - C_{Di}(1)} . \qquad [24]$$

For easier interpretation of equation [24] let us assume that electrolyte balance is zero before the measurement starts ($C_{Di}(1) = C_{Do}(1)$). Equation [24] is reduced to equation [25]:

$$D = Q_D * \frac{C_{Di}(2) - C_{Do}(2)}{C_{Di}(2) - C_{Di}(1)} . \qquad [25]$$

An increase of dialysate-in concentration C_{Di} is followed by an increase of dialysate-out concentration C_{Do}.

For an 'ideal' dialyzer the additional electrolytes completely are transferred to the blood side hence C_{Do} remains unchanged and with the assumption made above $C_{Do}(2) = C_{Do}(1) = C_{Di}(1)$ the fraction becomes 1 and dialysance D equals dialysate flow Q_D. If no electrolytes are transferred $C_{Do}(2)$ follows $C_{Di}(2)$ and the numerator becomes zero as well as dialysance D.

Hardware setup (Figure 36): Because dialysis machines already have a conductivity sensor upstream of the dialyzer, only one additional conductivity sensor downstream is required. Automatic measurements can be performed intradialytically by increasing dialysate concentration by 10% for approximately two minutes. It was shown by Polaschegg (204) that the dialysance calculated by equation [24] is effective dialysance which is dialysance reduced by recirculation (205).

Figure 37 shows the time course of conductivity during automatic clearance measurement which takes less than 10 minutes and can be repeated several times during dialysis. Accuracy is mostly limited by accuracy of dialysate flow measurement. Influence of resolving power and noise of conductivity sensors is negligible. Baseline shifts can be neglected as long as steep electrolyte gradients (profiles) are avoided during dialysis. *In vivo* comparison of results from this measuring principle with 'the gold standard' blood side clearance method is hampered by the large error of the 'gold standard' combining blood side input and output plasma urea measurement, evaluation of blood flow and total recirculation (= access recirculation and cardiopulmonary recirculation) and calculation of blood water flow. *In vivo* tests so far demonstrate agreement of automatically and conventionally measured mean values of effective clearance (206).

Partial dialysate collection

DDQ (direct dialysis quantification), a standard method of dialysis quantification measures directly total amount of solute removed during dialysis (207): Spent dialysate is collected and total amount of solute removed calculated from concentration and volume. This approach is not limited to urea but easily can be expanded to other solutes. The result can be used for various purposes. The distribution volume can be calculated from pre-dialysis and post-rebound plasma water concentration and total solute removed.

With TSR being total solute removed and V the distribution volume the mass balance equation can be written as

$$C_{pre} * V - C_{post} * V = TSR \qquad [26]$$

and we get

$$V = \frac{TSR}{C_{pre} - C_{post}} . \qquad [27]$$

From pre-dialysis plasma water concentration, total solute removed, and dialysate time, a single-pool simulated clearance can be calculated.

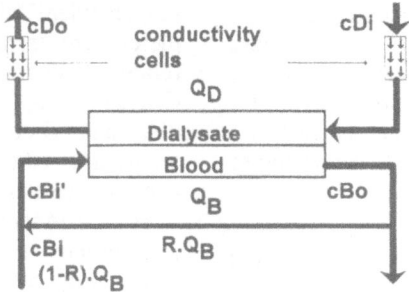

Figure 36. Setup for automatic clearance measurement and electrolyte balancing. Conductivity cells are placed up- and downstream of the dialyzer in the dialysate flow path. Dialysate side mass balance $Q_D * (c_{Di} - c_{Do})$ reflects the influence of recirculation.

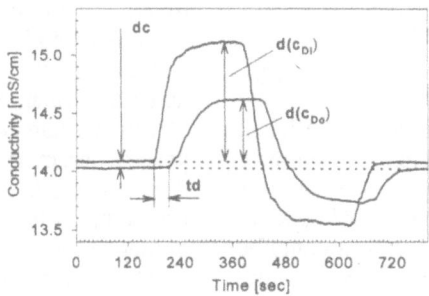

Figure 37. Automatic clearance measurement. Dialysate-in concentration is automatically increased by $d(c_{Di})$. Dialysate out-concentration increases with delay time $td(d(c_{Do}))$. The positive electrolyte bolus is compensated by the following negative one. dc, the baseline difference reflects the diffusive electrolyte gradient which, integrated over dialysis time is the electrolyte balance. From td and Q_D (dialysate flow) the filling volume of the dialyzer can be calculated which can be used for automatic identification of dialyzer size. Data from Harald Peter/Fresenius USA.

Keshaviah and Star (208) proposed the solute removal index SRI as a measure for dialysis quantity with

$$SRI = \frac{TSR}{C_{pre}} . \qquad [28]$$

DDQ requires the collection of approximately 100–150 l of dialysate. Spent dialysate is carefully stirred before a sample is taken for analysis and volume is measured. Bacterial contamination must be avoided because bacteria consume urea (209). In spite of its simplicity DDQ never has found routine application.

Partial dialysate collection offers the same information without the inconvenience of handling large waste volumes. Several methods have been described in the literature. With all methods sampling time need not be matched precisely with dialysis time. If sampling commences after dialysis the dialysate will be diluted but proportionally the volume will increase.

Partial dialysate collection with constant volume pumps (210, 211)

A volumetric pump pumps a small portion of waste dialysate to a receptacle. The rate of the sampling pump is proportional to the dialysate flow rate.

$$TSR = c * \left(V_s * \frac{Q_D}{sr} + UF \right) . \qquad [29]$$

Total dialysate volume can be calculated from partial dialysate volume collected and the ratio of dialysate flow to sampling rate. Ultrafiltration volume has to be added to total volume calculated. With Q_D being the dialysate flow, sr the sampling rate, V_s the sampled volume, UF the ultrafiltration volume and c the concentration of the solute of interest, total solute removed can be calculated by equation [29]. Accuracy is limited by the stability of dialysate flow and the sampling pump. If the sampling pump works non-continuously additional errors might be introduced by alarms that switch the machine into bypass or stop blood flow. If a sample is taken at this time it might not be representative of the period between two sampling points.

Partial dialysate collection with a flow divider

A device patented by Stiller (212) consists of many parallel capillaries. One of these capillaries is used for sampling while the others carry the rest of the spent dialysate stream. This device samples continuously and is free of the above mentioned technical limitations. However, such devices are prone to other specific problems. Capillaries can be blocked by small particles and flow distribution might change with dialysate flow. Ing and co-workers simply placed a cannula in the spent dialysate tube to collect aliquots of dialysate (213). No reproducibility can be expected for this simple approach.

Volumetric partial dialysate collection

Dialysis machines with volumetric ultrafiltration control comprising balancing chambers offer a cost effective and reliable way for dialysate sampling: At equidistant intervals a balancing chamber of spent dialysate is bypassed to the sampling receptacle. If the samples are taken at mid-time of the predefined sampling interval only three samples are sufficient to produce results accurate within $\pm 3\%$ provided solute removal can be described by a single pool model. With 30 or more samples the error will always be less than 1% if the solute concentration follows any monotone falling function between begin and end of sampling time, which is the case during dialysis. With a balancing chamber volume of 30 ml sampling volume approximately is one liter. Because the sampling interval is large this method is prone to errors from periods of reduced solute removal during alarms that cause stop of blood flow or bypass of dialysate. Samples must not be taken during this interval. Time delays between alarm and actual arrival of fluid at the sampling point as well as fluid mixing has to be taken into account. In a practical setting 'time out' for sampling starts four balancing chamber cycles after beginning of an alarm and ends 40 balancing chamber cycles after switch back to normal operation. The subsequent sample might be delayed but this error is negligible. Total dialysate volume is calculated automatically by the dialysis machine from balancing chamber volume and number of balancing chamber cycles. Counting starts nine balancing chamber cycles after blood is sensed by the venous optical detector of the machine. Alarm periods are excluded. Total solute removed is calculated according to equation [30] with V_D being total dialysate spent as displayed by the dialysis machine.

$$\text{TSR} = c * (V_D + \text{UF}). \qquad [30]$$

Common problems

A few problems are common to total and partial dialysate collection. Bacteria stemming from contaminated water or concentrate proliferate rapidly in spent dialysate. Urea is converted into other nitrogen containing substances. Because most analytical devices today measure urea directly rather than total nitrogen bacterial contamination might lead to an incorrect measure of concentration and consequent incorrect modeling results. Filtering fresh dialysate through a dialysate filter significantly will reduce the risk of contamination. It is also advisable to analyze samples immediately after dialysis, or if not possible to keep the sample refrigerated until analysis. Failure to mix sampled dialysate before analysis is another common error. Analytical errors from high dilution occur: If dialysate flow exceeds clearance by a factor of five or more, the concentrations of urea or other solutes in the dialysate sample might be too low for reliable analysis. The relative accuracy of urea measurement decreases with decreasing concentration.

BLOOD ACCESS ASSESSMENT MONITORS

Blood access has always been the weakest link in the dialysis chain. This has become even more obvious with decreased treatment times and the attempt to increase dialysis efficacy. Early detection of recirculation and access failure is crucial for the prevention of underdialysis.

Recirculation of blood in the extracorporeal circuit reduces the efficacy of dialysis because cleansed blood is mixed with blood from the patient and the concentration driving force is reduced (Figure 36). The reduction of clearance (205) is described by equation [31].

$$K_{\text{eff}} = \frac{1 - R}{1 - R * \left(1 - \frac{K}{Q_{\text{Bi}}}\right)} * K. \qquad [31]$$

K_{eff} is the effective clearance, K the dialyzer clearance, Q_{Bi} the blood flow through the dialyzer and R the fraction of the total blood flow through the dialyzer that is recirculated. No recirculation $R = 0$ leads to $K_{\text{eff}} = K$ and total recirculation $R = 1$ to $K_{\text{eff}} = 0$ as can be expected. With fistulas or grafts, recirculation is the consequence of extracorporeal blood flow exceeding access flow. When extracorporeal blood flow exceeds access flow, clearance will not increase further, but will in fact decrease (214). In single-needle dialysis recirculation in the extracorporeal circuit is unavoidable because the volume of the access device is always recirculated. In addition compliance of the extracorporeal circuit adds to recirculation. Another contribution is cardiopulmonary recirculation (215), occurring as a consequence of the arterio-venous fistula or graft. Cleansed blood returning from the blood access is mixed in the cardiopulmonary system with blood equilibrated with the tissue and returns to the access without further equilibration. Catheter access to a central vein is always free of cardiopulmonary recirculation but double lumen catheters are not free of access recirculation, especially when used in a flow reverse mode because of clotting problems (216).

$$R = \frac{C'_{\text{Bi}} - C_{\text{Bi}}}{C'_{\text{Bi}} - C_{\text{Bo}}}, \qquad [32]$$

with C_{Bi} being the solute (urea) concentration on the arterial side of the dialyzer, C_{Bo} the concentration on the venous side and C'_{Bi} the unaffected reference sample, recirculation can be calculated from equation [32]. If urea or another physiological solute is used, C'_{Bi} is the systemic reference sample taken where or when no recirculation is present. The so called 'three sample method' with a reference sample taken from the collateral arm was state of the art until the beginning of the 90s when it became apparent that this method produces artifacts (217, 218). Today the reference sample is taken from the arterial blood line within 20 seconds – 2 minutes (access *vs* access + cardiopulmonary recirculation) after blood flow is reduced to 50 ml/min. If a non-physiological tracer substance is injected on the venous side C'_{Bi} is zero and recirculation simply is C_{Bi}/C_{Bo}. Using urea for recirculation measurement is neither simple nor accurate. Three accurately timed samples have to be taken and analyzed. The result is not immediately available and the analytical error converts into an error of 8–12% recirculation. The need for a more reproducible and simpler method that gives immediate results was seen by some researchers already at the beginning of the eighties (219). Since then various recirculation monitors and methods for fistula assessment have been developed. All have in common that a blood parameter (temperature, conductivity, hematocrit, density) is temporarily changed on the venous side and the variation of the same parameter on the arterial side within 10 to 120 seconds afterwards is used as an indicator for recirculation. The thermal, conductivity or density bolus on the venous side can be caused by an injection or by the variation of a dialysate parameter (temperature, conductivity). Variation of a dialysate parameter is advantageous because blood flow parameters are not changed and an additional contamination risk is avoided. For the calculation of effective clearance the combined effect of access and cardiopulmonary recirculation has to be taken into account. A time resolving power of 10 sec or better is necessary to separate both effects (215).

Recirculation measurement with temperature sensors

If blood temperature on the venous side is reduced either by injection of cold saline or by the reduction of dialysate temperature the temperature bolus travels down the venous line and, if blood is recirculated, can be detected on the arterial side. This method was pioneered by Aldridge, Greenwood (219, 220) and coworkers. More recently a commercial device, the blood temperature monitor (BTM, Fresenius AG, Bad Homburg, Germany (221)) has been adapted automatically to measure recirculation. Initiated by the user the BTM automatically commands the dialysis machine to reduce dialysate temperature by approximately 3°C (Figure 38). This temperature decrease is transmitted by the dialyzer to the venous side of the extracorporeal circuit. Recirculation

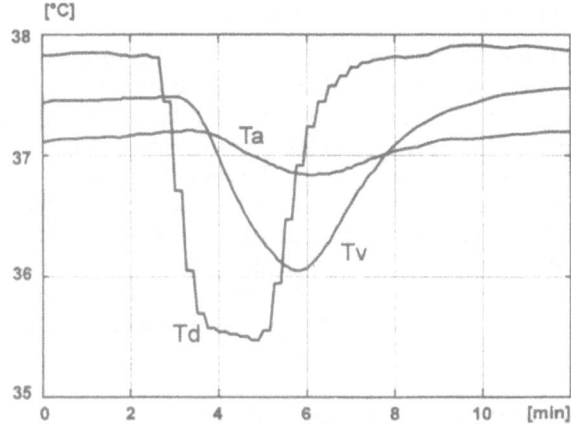

Figure 38. From Reference (215), with permission. T_d dialysate cold temperature bolus automatically generated. T_v temperature bolus as measured by the venous temperature sensor. T_a recirculated temperature bolus. Recirculation (22%) is calculated from the bolus amplitudes.

becomes apparent by a small transient arterial temperature decrease. Temperature sensors are non-invasive with a time constant of approximately 1 to 2 minutes. Total recirculation which is the sum of access and cardiopulmonary recirculation is therefore measured integrally. Accuracy is ± 3%, a factor of 2 to 3 better as the standard urea technique.

Recirculation measurement with optical sensors

This method too was pioneered by Aldridge and Greenwood (222) in England and was combined with arterial and venous pressure measurement in a device called 'Fistula Assessment Monitor'. This device used optical transmission. The optical sensors are housed in an assembly which simply clips onto the blood tubing. Typically 10 ml of normal saline are injected into the venous drip chamber within a few seconds. This reduces the hematocrit of the venous blood which is detected as an increase in light transmission through the blood line. The appearance of an arterial signal is used for the quantification of recirculation. The wavelength used is close to the isobestic point (810 nm), the wavelength at which light absorption is independent of oxygen saturation. Seven years later this method was reinvented in the US (223).

Recirculation measurement by ultrasound density

Ultrasound speed is proportional to the density of the medium. This method is sensitive to the total concentration of proteins (the sum of plasma proteins and red cell protein) and solutes in blood. This density is reduced when a bolus of saline is injected into the venous drip chamber. This method was used to demonstrate the time delay between access and cardiopulmonary recirculation

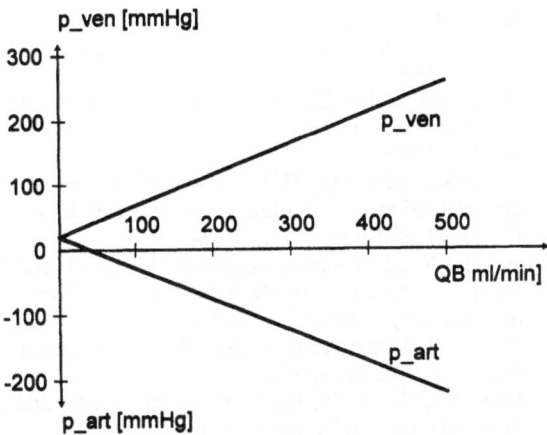

Figure 39. Pressure versus blood flow characteristic for a fistula without stenosis (schematic). At zero blood flow the pressure is the fistula pressure ± the pressure caused by the height difference between fistula and sensors. With the same cannulas on arterial and venous side the slope of arterial and venous pressure versus flow has the same magnitude but opposite sign.

(215). Access recirculation becomes apparent 10 sec after injection of a saline bolus while cardiopulmonary recirculation is detected after 1 to 2 minutes. The principle is used in a commercial device in combination with ultrasound blood flow measurement (Transonic Systems Inc, Ithaca, NY, USA).

Recirculation measurement by conductivity

This method applies conductivity sensors in the arterial and venous blood lines. A bolus of hypertonic saline is injected into the drip chamber and the subsequent increase of whole blood conductivity on the venous and on the arterial side is used for the quantitative evaluation of recirculation. Contactless conductivity sensors are used by a commercial device (COBE Renal Care, Inc, Lakewood, CO, USA) (224). For this method, special blood lines are required. A bolus-injection method combined with paired-filtration dialysis (PFD) was described by Canaud and co-workers (225). In PFD ultrafiltrate is collected separately from dialysate. The conductivity change in ultrafiltrate caused by a bolus injected on the venous side was normalized by the variation caused by an arterial bolus to calculate recirculation. In principal, bolus injection can be replaced by automatically increasing dialysate sodium for a short period. This method, however, has not yet been described in the literature.

Access assessment by pressure measurement

Again Aldridge and Greenwood (219, 220) were the pioneers who developed a method for fistula assessment based on the evaluation of the arterial and venous pressure as a function of flow in the extracorporeal circuit. Because the resolving power of standard monitors used for pressure measurement in dialysis is not sufficient for this purpose they developed a special monitoring device that allowed the precise recording of pressure changes while blood flow was increased by manual adjustment of the blood pump. The principle of this measurement is shown in Figure 39. More pragmatically Schwab and coworkers (226) recognized that venous pressure was a good predictor of access stenosis. Whenever venous pressure during dialysis exceeded 150 mmHg a fistulogram was performed and stenosis found in more than 80%. This method worked because blood flow and hematocrit was uniform at the time of this investigation but failed later when a wider range of blood flows was used. Combining the ideas of Aldridge, Greenwood and coworkers and Schwab and coworkers, Polaschegg (227) described a method to calculate fistula pressure and blood volume changes from pressure drop. Any deviation of the pressure flow characteristic from symmetry would translate into a change of fistula pressure. The pressure increase(decrease) at the beginning of dialysis when the blood flow is increased could be used to test for a stenosis.

REFERENCES

1. Kaufman AM, Polaschegg HD: What technological advances will significantly alter the future care of dialysis patients? *Semin Dial* 7: 321, 1994
2. IEC – International Electrotechnical Commission: 3 rue de Varembé, Ch–1211, Geneva 20
3. IEC 601-2-16: Medical electrical equipment, Part 2, Particular requirements for safety of haemodialysis equipment
4. ISO – International Standard Organisation, Case postale 56, Ch–1211 Geneva 20
5. ISO 8637: Haemodialysers, haemofilters and haemoconcentrators
6. ISO 8638: Extracorporeal blood circuit for haemodialysers, haemofilters and haemoconcentrators
7. CENELEC – European Committee for Electrotechnical Standardization: Central Secretariat, rue des Stassart 35, B–1050 Brussels
8. CEN – European Committee for Standardization: rue de Stassart 36, B–1050 Brussels
9. AAMI 3330: Washington Boulevard, Suite 400, Arlington, VA 22201–4598, USA
10. ANSI/AAMI RD5-1992: American National Standard, Hemodialysis Systems
11. Grimsrud L, Cole JJ, Eschbach JW, Babb AL, Scribner BH: Safety aspects of hemodialysis. *Trans Am Soc Artif Intern Organs* 13: 1, 1967
12. Kolff WJ: The beginning of the artificial kidney. *Artif Organs* 17: 293, 1993
13. Kramer P, Wigger W, Rieger J, Matthaei D, Scheler F: Artero-venous hemofiltration: a new simple method for treatment of overhydrated patients resistant to diuretics. *Klin Wschr* 55: 1121, 1977
14. Eisenhauer Th: Development and actual performance of continuous arteriovenous hemofiltration (CAVH). in

Continuos Arteriovenous Hemofiltration (CAVH), edited by Sieberth HG, Mann H, Basel, Karger, 1985

15. Polaschegg HD (inventors), Fresenius AG (assignee): Vorrichtung zur Bestimmung des behandelten Blutvolumens bei der Hämodialyse. EP patent 0513421. 11/19/92

16. Finsterwald PM, Eilers GJ (inventors), Cobe Laboratories Inc (assignee): Peristaltic pumps. GB patent 2190145. 11/11/87

17. Leong ASY, Disney AP, Gove DW: Spallation and migration of silicone from blood-pump tubing in patients on hemodialysis. *N Engl J Med* 306: 135, 1982

18. Bommer J: Silikonablagerungen in den Organen von Dialysepatienten – Derzeitiger Stand der Untersuchungen. *Nieren- u. Hochdruckkrankheiten* 12: 250, 1983

19. Scribner BH, Caner JEZ, Buri R, Quinton W: The Technique of continuous hemodialysis. *Trans Am Soc Artif Intern Organs* 6: 88, 1960

20. Schnell WJ (inventors), Baxter Travenol Laboratories Inc (assignee): Flow reversal in a dialyzer. US patent 4324662. 4/13/82

21. Polaschegg HD (inventors), Fresenius AG (assignee): Hämodialysevorrichtung mit Entlüftungseinrichtung. EP patent 0366950. 12/16/92

22. Polaschegg HD (inventors), Fresenius AG (assignee): Verfahren zum Füllen eines Blutschlauchsystems einer Hämodialysevorrichtung mit einer physiologischen Kochsalzlösung. EP patent 0161686. 2/13/91

23. Polaschegg HD (inventors), Fresenius AG (assignee): Dialysegerät. DE patent 3442744. 7/28/88

24. Eigendorf HG (inventors), Medical Support GmbH (assignee): Verfahren und Anordnung zum Spülen und Befüllen des extrakorporalen Blutkreislaufs von Dialysemaschinen. DE patent 4208274. 10/21/93

25. Paolini F, Rossi A (inventors), Hospal AG (assignee): Equipment for detecting the presence of a tube and/or the presence of blood within it. EPA patent 0467805. 1/22/92

26. Ward RA, Farrell PC: Precise antikoagulation for routine hemodialysis using nomograms. *Trans Am Soc Artif Intern Organs* 24: 439, 1978

27. Polaschegg HD (inventors), Fresenius AG (assignee): Apparatus for infusion of medicaments into an extracorporeal blood circuit. GB patent 2225954. 6/17/92

28. Lindholm DD, Murray JS: A simplified method of regional heparinization during hemodialysis according to a predetermined dosage formula. *Trans Am Soc Artif Intern Organs* 10: 92, 1964

29. Lohr JW, Schwab SJ: Minimizing hemorrhagic complications in dialysis patients. *Am Soc Nephrol* 2: 961, 1991

30. Donatelli D (inventors), Donatelli D (assignee): Device for the automatic actuation of haemodialysis without anticoagulants. EP patent 0235591. 9/9/87

31. Wamsiedler R, Polaschegg HD, Tattersall JE: Heparin-free dialysis with an on-line hemodiafiltration system. *Artif Organs* 17: 948, 1993

32. Polaschegg HD, Christmann-Braun H: A fail-safe protective system against blood loss to the environment for extracorporeal circuits. *Proc 14th Ann Int Conf IEEE-EMBS* 14: 1302, 1992

33. Polaschegg HD (inventors), Fresenius AG (assignee): Apparatus for removing water from blood. US patent 4713171. 12/15/87

34. Gault MH, Duffet S, Purchase L, Murphy J: Hemodialysis intravascular hemolysis and kinked blood lines. *Nephron* 62: 267, 1992

35. Dhaene M, Gulbis B, Lietaer N, Gammar N: Red blood cell destruction in single-needle dialysis. *Clin Nephrol* 31: 327, 1989

36. Wojke R, Polaschegg HD: Ein einfaches Testverfahren zur Detektion von Mikroblasen im extrakorporalen Blutkreislauf. *Biomed Tech* 38: 34, 1993

37. Hoenich NA, Downing N, Pearson S: Review of mechanical systems for single-needle hemodialysis. in *First International Symposium on Single-Needle Dialysis*, edited by Ringoir S, Vanholder R, Ivanovich P, Cleveland, ISAO Press, No. 305, 1984, p 22

38. Kopp KF, Gutch CF, Kolff WJ: Single needle dialysis. *Trans Am Soc Artif Intern Organs* 18: 75, 1972

39. van Waeleghem JP, Boone L, Ringoir S: New technique on the one needle system during haemodialysis. *Proc Eur Dial Transplant Assoc* 1: 10, 1973

40. Scribner BH, Canez JEZ, Buri R, Quinton W: The technique of continuous hemodialysis. *Trans Am Soc Artif Intern Organs* 6: 88, 1960

41. Tersteegen B, van Endert G (inventors), Tersteegen (assignee): Haemodialysegeraet und Arbeitsverfahren zur Ultrafiltrationssteuerung mit diesem Geraet. DE patent 3115665. 11/4/82

42. Schael W (inventors), Fresenius AG (assignee): Hemodialysis apparatus. US patent 4267040. 5/12/81

43. Freeman N, Connally Th (Eds): *Proceedings, Conference on Hemodialysis, NIH, November 9–10, 1964*, Public Health Service Publication No 1349, 1964, p 128

44. Weiss C, Jelkmann W: Funktionen des Blutes: Blutungstillung und Blutgerinnung. in *Physiologie des Menschen*, 24th Ed (English title: *Human Physiology*), edited by Schmidt RF, Thews G, Berlin, Springer-Verlag, 1994, p 439

45. Maggiore Q, Enia G, Catalano C, Mundo A: Dialysate temperature and complement activation. *Contrib Nephrol* 59: 72, 1987

46. Shouldice David Robert (inventors), Cobe Laboratories Inc (assignee): Heater control for liquid flowing through a chamber. US patent 4769151. 9/6/88

47. Mackison F, Warren J: Hemodialysis Systems Conformance Assessment Report, edited by Center for Devices and Radiological Health, FDA, 1990, p 1

48. Harvey EN, Barnes DK, McElroy WD, Whiteley AH, Pease DC, Cooper KW: Bubble formation in animals. *J Cell Compar Physiol* 24: 1, 1944

49. Kruis A, May A: Lösungsgleichgewichte von Gasen in Flüssigkeiten. in *Landolt-Börnstein: Eigenschaften der Materie in ihren Aggregatzuständen, 2. Teil*, edited by Schäfer K, Lax E, Berlin, Springer-Verlag, 1962

50. Eschbach Jr JW, Wilson Jr WE, Peoples RW, Wakefield AW, Babb AL, Scribner BH: Unattended overnight home hemodialysis. *Trans Am Soc Artif Intern Organs* 12: 346, 1966

51. Grimsrud L, Lorentzen O, Cappelen C: A truly portable, fully automatic, fluid preparation and control unit for hemodialysis. *Trans Am Soc Artif Intern Organs* 14: 160, 1968

52. Kolobow N, Thomas Connally (Eds): *Proceedings, Conference on Hemodialysis, NIH, November 9–10, 1964*, Public Health Service Publication No 1349, 1964, p 87

53. Grimsrud L, Cole JL, Lehman GA, Babb AL, Scribner BH: A central system for the continuous preparation and distribution of hemodialysis fluid. *Trans Am Soc Artif Intern Organs* 10: 107, 1964

54. Grimsrud L, Babb AL: Optimization of dialyzer design for the hemodialysis system. *Trans Am Soc Artif Intern Organs* 10: 101, 1964

55. Mion CM, Hegstrom RM, Boen ST, Scribner BH: Substitution of sodium acetate for sodium bicarbonate in the bath fluid for hemodialysis. *Trans Am Soc Artif Intern Organs* 10: 110, 1964

56. Serfass EJ, Troutner VH (inventors), Milton Roy Comp (assignee): Portable dialysate supply system. US patent 3508656. 4/28/70

57. Breitenfelder W: Technische Aspekte der Bikarbonat-Haemodialyse, Teil 2. *Medizintechnik* 106: 121, 1986

58. Polaschegg HD (inventors), Fresenius AG (assignee): Apparatus for hemodialysis. US patent 4895657. 1/23/90

59. Gambro AB, Lund, Sweden: AK100 leaflet HCE–7416

60. Ogawa FT (inventors), Cobe Laboratories Inc (assignee): Remote conductivity sensor having transformer coupling in fluid flow path. US patent 4740755. 4/26/88

61. Williams DJ, Jugurnauth J, Harding K, Woolfson RG, Mansell MA: Acute hypernatraemia during bicarbonate-buffered haemodialysis. *Nephrol Dial Transplant* 9: 1170, 1994

62. Sethi D, Curtis JRT, Topham DL, Gower PE: Acute metabolic alkalosis during haemodialysis. *Nephron* 51: 119, 1989

63. Jönsson ULP, Carlsson PAV, Jönsson D, Jönsson SA, Knutsson SL, Tryggvason R (inventors), Gambro AB (assignee): A system for preparing a fluid intented for a medical procedure by mixing at least one concentrate in powder form with water and a cartridge intended to be used in said system. EPB patent 0278100. 7/15/92

64. Jönsson Lennart, Knutsson Stefan Lars (inventors), Gambro AB (assignee): System for preparation of a fluid intended for medical use. EPA patent 0443324. 8/28/91

65. Chevallet J, Gauckler J, inventors: Hospal Industrie (assignee): Preparation d'une solution à usage medical par dissolution concentres pulverulents avec recirculation d'une. FR patent 2647349. 11/30/90

66. Polaschegg HD, Pieper W, Weber D, inventors: Fresenius AG (assignee): Beutel zur Aufnahme von Konzentrat. EP patent 0575970. 12/29/93

67. Polaschegg HD, Walter C (inventors), Fresenius AG (assignee): Einrichtung zur Herstellung einer medizinischen Flüssigkeit. EP patent 0548537. 6/30/93

68. Polaschegg HD: History and methods of ultrafiltration monitoring. in *Proc 9th Annual Symp on Renal Technology*, Warwick July 15–17. Assoc of Renal Technicians, edited by Kilvington M, Lawrence A, 1984

69. Kiil F, Amundsen B: Haemodialysis and controlled ultrafiltration. *Lancet* 340, 1961

70. Bower JD, Magee JH: The use of the Seattle hemodialysis system in renal homotransplantation. *Trans Am Soc Artif Intern Organs* 10: 251, 1964

71. Granger A, Sausse A (inventors), Rhône-Poulenc Ind (assignee): Artificial kidney and a method of ultrafiltering a liquid. US patent 3939069. 2/17/76

72. Gray OJ, Sanderson ML, Mallick NP: Automatically controlled ultrafiltration during haemodialysis using the Kiil haemodialyser. *Proc Eur Dial Transplant Assoc* 7: 474, 1970

73. Aid JD, Cameron NF, Hartranft TP (inventors), Baxter International Inc (assignee): Improved flow measurement system. EP patent 0298587. 1/11/89

74. Multimat System: Company brochure. Bellco advertising office 09/92–3000SHE000

75. Schultheis R: Gerät zur volumetrischen Bestimmung der abgezogenen Flüssigkeitsmenge bei der Haemodialysebehandlung. *Biomed Tech* 20: 81, 1975

76. Beelen R (inventors), Beelen R (assignee): Distributor voor de dialysatomloop in een kunstnier. BE patent 831895. 11/17/75

77. Pinkerton HE (inventors), Pinkerton HE (assignee): Proportioning fluids. US patent 4037616. 7/26/77

78. Kozlov JG, Khaitlin AE, Lisitsina K (inventors), Kozlov GK, Khaitlin AE, Lisitsina K (assignee): Device for preparation of a dialyzing solution. US patent 3804107. 4/16/74

79. Polaschegg HD, Wojke R: Constant blood flow during single-needle dialysis is unnecessary. *Int J Artif Organs* 16: 505, 1993

80. Polaschegg HD (inventors), Fresenius AG (assignee): Hämodialysegerät mit einer Bilanzkammer. EPA patent 0615760. 9/21/94

81. FDA-M.D.R. Report dated 1/16/91. Publication date: 9101. 00162549 MDR-219086 Subfile: MDR Product(s): 11-218 Hemodialysis units

82. Polaschegg HD (inventors), Fresenius AG (assignee): Verfahren zur Feststellung der Funktionsfähigkeit einer Teileinrichtung eines Hämodialysegerätes und Vorrichtung zur Durchführung dieses Verfahrens. EP patient 0604753. 7/6/94

83. DePalma JR, Pecker EA, Gordon A, Maxwell MH: A new compact automatic home hemodialysis system. *Trans Am Soc Artif Intern Organs* 14: 152, 1968

84. Shintani Motoaki, Wada Yoshikazu, Nakamachi Hideo (inventors), Takeda Chemical Ind (assignee): Blutleckdetektor und damit ausgeruesteter Blutdialysator. DE patient 2631686. 1/20/77

85. Dawids SG, Vejlsgaard R: Bacteriological and clinical evaluation of different dialysate delivery system. *Acta Medica Scandinavia* 199: 151, 1976

86. Mion CM, Canaud B, Garred LJ, Stec F, Nguyen QV: Sterile and pyrogen-free bicarbonate dialysate: a necessity for hemodialysis today. *Adv Nephrol* 19: 275, 1990

87. Petersen NJ, Boyer KM, Carson LA, Favero MS: Pyrogenic reactions from inadequate disinfection of a dialysis fluid distribution system. *Dial Transplant* 7: 52, 1978

88. Cole JJ, Fritzen JR, Vizzo JE, van Paaschen WH, Grimsrud L: One year's experience with a central dialysate supply system in a hospital. *Trans Am Soc Artif Intern Organs* 11: 22, 1965

89. Polaschegg HD (inventors), Fresenius AG (assignee): Hämodialysevorrichtung. DE patent 3447989. 7/16/87

90. NN, inventors: ASM Anlagen und Systeme für Medizintechnik GmbH (assignee): Vorrichtung zum Zuführen zweier Flüssigkeiten. DE patent 3913008. 8/22/91

91. NN (inventors), ASM Anlagen und Systeme für Medizintechnik GmbH (assignee): Desinfektionsverfahren eines Dialysierflüssigkeitskreislaufs, Gerät zur Durchführung derartiger Desinfektionsverfahren, Wasserversorgungs-

einrichtung für Dialysegerät und Dosiereinrichtung. DE patent 3941103. 12/17/92

92. Cappelen Chr, Grimsrud L (inventors), Cappelen Chr Jr (assignee): Method for the sterilization of a system for preparation of a liquid mixture. US patent 3738382. 6/12/73

93. Henderson LW: The beginning of hemofiltration. *Contrib Nephrol* 32: 1, 1982

94. Henderson LW, Besarab A, Michaels A, Bluemle LW: Blood purification by ultrafiltration and fluid replacement (diafiltration). *Trans Am Soc Artif Intern Organs* 13: 216, 1967

95. Kramer P, Wigger W, Matthaei D, Langescheid C, Rieger J, Fuchs C, Rumpf KW, Scheler F: Clinical experience with continuously monitored fluid balance in automatic hemofiltration. *Artif Organs* 2: 147, 1978

96. NN (inventors), Fresenius AG (assignee): Vorrichtung zur Steuerung des Flüssigkeits-Ausgleichs eines Patienten bei der Hämodiafiltration. DE patent 2629717. 5/6/82

97. Streicher E (inventors), Streicher E (assignee): Vorrichtung zur volumengleichen Ersetzung einer ersten Fluessigkeit durch eine zweite Fluessigkeit, insbes. zur HDF. DE patent 2755882. 2/18/82

98. Beden J, Flaig HJ, Polaschegg HD, Steinbach B: Volumetric Fluid Balancing for Hemo- and Plasmafiltration, in *Proc 2nd European Conf on Engineering and Medicine*, edited by Faust UR, Stuttgart, April 25–29, Amsterdam, Elsevier Science Publishers, 1993, p 149

99. Maggiore Q, Pizzarelli F, Zoccali C, Sisca S, Nicolo F, Parlongo S: Effect of extracorporeal blood cooling on dialytic arterial hypotension. *Proc Eur Dial Transplant Assoc* 28: 597, 1981

100. Marangoni R, Savino R, Colombo R, Civadi F: Short time treatment with high-efficiency paired filtration dialysis for chronic renal failure. *Artif Organs* 16: 547, 1992

101. Zucchelli P, Santoro A, Ferrari G, Spongano M: Acetate-free biofiltration: hemodiafiltration with base-free dialysate. *Blood Purif* 8: 14, 1990

102. Canaud B, Kerr P, Argilés A, Flavier JL, Stec F, Mion C: Is hemodiafiltration the dialysis modality of choice for the next decade? *Kidney Int* 43: S296, 1993

103. Klauber J, Reichelt H: Probleme und Perspektiven der Dialyseversorgung in den westlichen Bundesländern. WIdO-Materialien, Band 34, WIdO(Wissenschaftliches Institut der Ortskrankenkassen), 1992

104. Tierno PM, Aboody R: Risk of bacterial infection resulting from a blood leak during hemodialysis. *Nephron* 6: 110, 1969

105. Frinak S, Polaschegg HD, Levin NW, Pohlod DJ, Dumler F, Saravolatz LD: Filtration of dialysate using an on-line dialysate filter. *Int J Artif Organs* 14: 691, 1991

106. Brunet P, Ragon A, Gulian C, Mege JL, Clement JC, Tehhani E, Capo C, Berland Y: On-line production of infusion fluid for hemodiafiltration (Hdf) from contaminated dialysate. *J Am Soc Nephrol* 5: 410, 1994

107. Pegues DA, Oettinger CW, Bland LA, Favero MS: A prospective study of pyrogenic reactions in hemodialysis patients using bicarbonate dialysis fluids filtered to remove bacteria and endotoxin. *J Am Soc Nephrol* 3: 1002, 1992

108. Mion CM, Canaud B, Garred LJ, Stec F, Nguyen QV: Sterile and pyrogen-free bicarbonate dialysate: a necessity for hemodialysis today. *Adv Nephrol* 19: 275, 1990

109. Hosoya N, Sakai K: Backdiffusion rather than backfiltration enhances endotoxin transport through highly permeable dialysis membranes. *Trans Am Soc Artif Intern Organs* 36: M311, 1990

110. Takesawa S, Saito H, Hidai H, Suzuki M, Sakai K: Measurement of back clearance. *Trans Am Soc Artif Intern Organs* 36: M441, 1990

111. Bommer J, Becker KP, Urbaschek R: Endotoxin permeability of highflux polysulfon membranes. *J Am Soc Nephrol* 5: 408, 1994

112. Oettinger CW, Arduino MJ, Oliver JC, Bland LA: The clinical relevance of dialysate sterility. *Semin Dial* 7: 263, 1994

113. Quellhorst E, Schünemann B: Beta-2-amyloidosis and haemofiltration. in *Dialysis Amyloidosis*, edited by Gejyo F, Brancaccio D, Bardin T, Milan, Wichtig Editor, 1989

114. Lonnemann G: Dialysate bacteriological quality and the permeability of dialyzer membranes to pyrogens. *Kidney Int* 43: S195, 1993

115. Laude-Sharp M, Caroff M, Simard L, Pusinieri C, Kazatchkine MD, Haeffner-Cavaillon N: Induction of IL-1 during hemodialysis: transmembrane passage of intact endotoxins (LPS). *Kidney Int* 38: 1098, 1990

116. Henderson JW, Sanfelippo ML, Beans E: 'On line' preparation of sterile pyrogen-free electrolyte solution. *Trans Am Soc Artif Intern Organs* 24: 465, 1978

117. Sausse A (inventors), Rhône-Poulenc Ind (assignee): Artificial kidney. US patent 4024059. 5/17/77

118. Shinzato T, Sezaki R, Usuda M, Maeda K, Ohbayashi S, Toyoto T: Infusion-free hemodiafiltration: simultaneous hemofiltration and dialysis with no need for infusion fluid. *Artif Organs* 6: 453, 1982

119. Miller JH, von Albertini B, Gardner PW, Shinaberger JH: Technical aspects of high-flux hemodiafiltration for adequate short (under 2 hours) treatment. *Trans Am Soc Artif Intern Organs* 30: 378, 1984

120. Usuda M, Shinzato T, Sezaki R, Kawanishis A, Maeda K, Kawaguchi S, Shibata M, Toyoda T, Asakura Y, Ohbayashi S: New simultaneous HF and HD with no infusion fluid. *Trans Am Soc Artif Intern Organs* 28: 24, 1982

121. Sternby J: A decade of experience with on-line hemofiltration/hemodiafiltration. in *Effective Hemodiafiltration: New Methods*, edited by Maeda K, Shinzato T, Basel, Karger, 1994, p 1

122. Canaud B, N'guyen QV, Lagarde C, Stec F, Polaschegg HD, Mion C: Clinical evaluation of a multipurpose dialysis system adequate for hemodialysis or for postdilution hemofiltration/hemodiafiltration with on-line preparation of substitution fluid from dialysate. *Contrib Nephrol* 46: 184, 1985

123. Polaschegg HD (inventors), Fresenius AG (assignee): Vorrichtung zur Hämodialyse ohne Antikoagulation. DE patent 4240681. 9/8/94

124. Wamsiedler R, Polaschegg HD, Tattersall JE: Heparin-free dialysis with an on-lne hemodiafiltration system. *Artif Organs* 17: 948, 1993

125. Saito A, Koyama M, Sakurai K, Ohta K, Maeda K, Haraguchi S: A new dialysate delivery system to control osmotic pressure and ultrafiltration rate: description and clinical evaluation, in *Proc Third Metting ISAO*, edited by Funck-Brentano JL, Klinkmann H, Man NK, Paris, 1981, p 696

126. Murisasco A, Boobes Y, Elsen R, El Mehdi M, Baz M, Durand C, Crevat A, Monti JP, Fondarai J: Control of K⁺ homeostasis in ESRD patients treated with chronic hemodialysis. in *Progress in Artificial Organs – 1985*, edited by Nosé Y, Kjellstarnd C, Ivanovich P, Cleveland, ISAO Press No 205, 1986, 1985, p 197–203

127. Fresenius AG, Oberursel, Germany: Brochure 'Computer Modelling System 08, CMS08'

128. Deuber HJ, Schulz W, Rebstöck W: Improved stability of circulation during computer modelling dialysis. *Kidney Int* 32: 433, 1987

129. Stefoni S, Coli L, Zaca F, Bombardini T, Puddu G, Feliciangeli G, Cianciolo G, Facchini MG: Modulated dialysis: a new strategy for the treatment of intradialytic intolerance. *Nephrol Dial Transplant* (Suppl): 154, 1990

130. Ebel H, Saure B, Laage Ch, Dittmar A, Keuchel M, Stellwaag M, Lange H: Influence of computer-modulated profile haemodialysis on cardiac arrhythmias. *Nephrol Dial Transplant* (Suppl): 165, 1990

131. Maeda K, Kawaguchi S, Kobayashi S, Niwa T, Kobayashi K, Saito A, Iyoda S, Ohta K: Cell-wash dialysis (CWD). *Trans Am Soc Artif Intern Organs* 26: 213, 1980

132. Gotch F, Evans M, Metzner K, Westphal D, Polaschegg H: An on-line monitor of dialyzer Na and K flux in hemodialysis. *Trans Am Soc Artif Intern Organs* 36: M359, 1990

133. Stefoni S, Coli L, Zacà F, Bombardini T, Feliciangeli, Stagni B, Puddu G, Cianciolo G, Puddu P, Bonomini V: The CMS 08 modulated dialysis. *Contrib Nephrol* 74: 221, 1989

134. Perschel WT, Röckel A, Klinke B, Reinhardt B, Behnken LJ, Abdelhamid S, Fiegel P, Walb D: Variation of ultrafiltration and dialysate sodium. *Contrib Nephrol* 74: 176, 1989

135. Lewis AED, Frost TH: Programmed clearance dialysis to minimize osmotic disequilibrium: A technique for microprocessor-controlled dialysis machines. *Artif Organs* 5: 364, 1981

136. Kim KE, Neff M, Cohen B, Somerstein M, Chinitz J, Onesti G, Swartz C: Blood volume changes and hypotension during hemodialysis. *Trans Am Soc Artif Intern Organs* 16: 508, 1970

137. Bugarsky S, Tangl F: Physikalisch-chemische Untersuchungen über die molecularen Concentrationsverhältnisse des Blutserums. *Arch Ges Physiol* 72: 531, 1898

138. Stewart GN: The relative volume or weight of corpuscles and plasma in blood. *J Physiol* 24: 356, 1899

139. Oker-Blom M: Thierische Säfte und Gewebe in physikalisch-chemischer Beziehung. *Arch Ges Physiol* 79: 111, 1900

140. Gram HC: Cell volume and electrical conductivity of blood. *J Biol Chem* 59: 33, 1924

141. Stiller S, Mann H: Automatische Kontrolle des Blutvolumens bei extrakorporaler Dialyse und Filtration. *Biomed Tech* 25 (Ergaenzungsband): 286, 1980

142. Stiller S, Mann H, Byrne T: Continuous monitoring of blood volume during hemodialysis. *Proc Eur Soc Artif Organs* 7: 167, 1980

143. Bonnie E, Lee WG, Stiller S, Mann H: Influence of fluid overload on vascular refilling rate in hemodialysis: continuous measurements with the conductivity method. in *Progress in Artificial Organs – 1985*, edited by Nosé Y, Kjellstrand C, Ivanovich P, Cleveland, ISAO Press, 1986, p 135

144. Maeda K, Shinzato T, Yoshida F, Tsuruta Y, Usuda M, Yamada K, Ishihara T, Inagaki F, Igarashi I, Kitano T: Newly developed circulating blood volume-monitoring system and its clinical application for measuring changes in blood volume during hemofiltration. *Artif Organs* 10: 452, 1986

145. Thomasset AL (inventors), Thomasset AL (assignee): Appareillage pour le controle des séances d'hémodialyse. EP patent 0029793. 8/24/83

146. Schaefer H: Hochfrequenzleitfähigkeit des Blutes bei Ultrakurzwellen von 3–6 m Wellenlänge. *Klin Wochenschr* 2: 102, 1933

147. Ishihara T, Igarashi I, Kitano T, Shinzato T, Maeda K: Continuous hematocrit monitoring method in an extracorporeal circulation system and its application for automatic control of blood volume during artificial kidney treatment. *Artif Organs* 17: 708, 1993

148. Polaschegg HD (inventors), Fresenius AG (assignee): Vorrichtung zur Bestimmung der Veränderung des intravasalen Blutvolumens während der Hämodialyse. EP patent 0272414. 10/23/91

149. Ogawa FT: Remote conductivity sensor having transformer coupling in fluid flow path. US Patent 4740755, 04/26/88

150. de Vries PMJM, Kouw PM, Meijer JH, Oe LP, Schneider H, Donker AJM: Changes in blood parameters during hemodialysis as determined by conductivity measurements. *Trans Am Soc Artif Intern Organs* 34: 623, 1988

151. Baudin S, Jussiaux P (inventors), Laboratoire Eugedia (assignee): Procédé et appareil de surveillance du déroulement de l'hémodialyse. EPA patent 0551043. 7/14/93

152. Anderson NM: Light-absorbing and scattering properties of non-haemolysed blood. *Phys Med Biol* 12: 173, 1967

153. Schallenberg U, Stiller S, Mann H: A new method of continuous haemoglobinometric measurement of blood volume during haemodialysis. *Life Support Systems* 5: 293, 1987

154. Wilkinson JS, Fleming SJ, Greenwood RN, Catell WR, Aldridge C: Continuous measurement of blood hydration during ultrafiltration using optical methods. *Med Biol Enginr Comput* 25: 317, 1987

155. Mancini E, Santoro A, Spongano M, Paolinifer H. Hochfrequ F, Rossi M, Zucchelli P: Continuous on-line optical absorbance recording of blood volume changes during hemodialysis. *Artif Organs* 17: 691, 1993

156. Caleffi Adamo (inventors), Hospal AG (assignee): Optical detector for equipment for measuring a substance in a liquid. EPA patent 0467804. 1/22/92

157. de Vries JPPM, Olthof CG, Visser V, Kouw PM, van Es A, Donker AJM, de Vries PMJM: Continuous measurement of blood volume during hemodialysis by an optical method. *ASAIO J* 38: M181, 1992

158. Steuer RR, Harris DH, Conis JM: A new optical technique for monitoring hematocrit and circulating blood volume: its application in renal dialysis. *Dial Transplant* 22: 260, 1993

159. Greenwood RN, Aldridge C, Catell WR: Serial blood water estimations and in-line blood viscometry: the continuous measurement of blood volume during dialysis procedures. *Clin Sci* 66: 575, 1984

160. Polaschegg HD (inventors), Fresenius AG (assignee): Vorrichtung zur Ultrafiltrationskontrolle und Ultrafiltrationsregelung bei Blutreinigungsverfahren. DE patent 4024434. 6/11/92

161. Kenner T, Hinghofer-Szalkay H, Leopold H, Pogglitsch H: The relation between the density of blood and the arterial pressure in animal experiments and in patients during hemodialysis. *Z Kardiol* 66: 399, 1977

162. Holzer H, Pogglitsch H, Hinghofer-Szalkay H, Kenner T, Leopold H, Passath A: Die kontinuierliche Messung der Blutdichte waehrend der Haemodialyse. *Wien klin Wochenschr* 91: 762, 1979

163. Bradley EL, Sacerio J: The velocity of ultrasound in human blood under varying physiologic parameters. *J Surg Res* 12: 290, 1972

164. Bakke T, Gytre T, Haagensen A, Giezendanner L: Ultrasonic measurement of sound velocity in whole blood. A comparison between an ultrasonic method and the conventional packed-cell-vlume test for hematocrit determination. *Scand J Clin Lab Invest* 35: 473, 1975

165. Roob JM, Schneditz D, Haas GM, Horina JH, Pogglitsch H: Kontinuierliche Messung von Blutvolumenaenderungen waehrend der Haemodialyse mit einer Ultraschallmethode. *Wien klin Wochenschr* 102: 131, 1990

166. Polaschegg HD: Vorrichtung zum Messen der Änderung des intravasalen Blutvolumens während der Blutfiltration in einer Blutreinigungseinrichtung. Deutsche Patentschrift 3827553

167. Maggiore Q, Pizzarelli F, Zoccali C, Sisca S, Nicolo F, Parlongo S: Effect of extracorporeal blood cooling on dialytic arterial hypotension. *Proc Eur Dial Transplant Assoc* 28: 597, 1981

168. Guyton AC: Energetics and metabolic rate. in *Textbook of Medical Physiology*, Eight Ed, WB Saunders Company, 1991, p 789

169. Benzinger TH: Heat regulation: Homeostasis of central temperature in man. *Physiol Rev* 49: 671, 1969

170. Tattersall J, Lister Hospital Stevenage UK: Personal communication, 1993

171. Polaschegg HD: Verfahren und Vorrichtung zum Entziehen von Waerme aus Blut im extrakorporalen Kreislauf. European Patent 0265795, priority date 30.10.1986

172. Kraemer M, Steil H, Polaschegg HD: Optimization of a sensor head for blood temperature measurement during hemodialysis. in *Proc 14th Ann Int Conf IEEE-EMBS*, Paris, 1992, p 1610

173. Kraemer M, Polaschegg HD: Control of blood temperature and thermal energy balance during hemodialysis. in *Proc 14th Ann Int Conf IEEE-EMBS*, Paris, 1992, p 2299

174. College of American Pathologists Quality Assurance Services: Group Summary, New York IX Regional Chemistry Q/C Program, October 1991

175. American National Standard ANSI/AAMI RD5-1992: Association for the Advancement of Medical Instrumentation, Arlington, VA, USA, 1993

176. Sargent JA, Gotch FA: Principles and Biophysics of Dialysis. in *Replacement of Renal Function by Dialysis*, 3rd Ed, edited by Maher JF, Dordrecht, Kluwer Academic Publishers, 1989, p 118

177. Garred LJ, Amour NRS, McCready WG, Canaud BC: Urea kinetic modeling with a prototype urea sensor in the spent dialysate stream. *ASAIO J* 39: M337, 1993

178. Hanss M, Rey A: Application de la conductimétrie à l'étude de réactions enzymatique. *Biochim Biophys Acta* 227: 630, 1971

179. Zeller H, Novak P, Landgraf R: Blood glucose measurement by infrared spectroscopy. *Int J Artif Organs* 12: 129, 1989

180. Kabei N, Machiyama E, Yamada A, Kikuchi M, Sakurai Y: Blood chemical continuous monitoring system for hemodialysis. *Trans Am Soc Artif Intern Organs* 24: 468, 1978

181. Thavarungkul P, Hakanson H, Holst O, Mattiasson B: Continuous monitoring of urea in blood during dialysis. *Biosens Bioelectron* 6: 101, 1991

182. Jacobs P, Suls J, Sansen W, Hombrouckx R: A disposable urea sensor for continuous monitoring of hemodialysis efficiency. *ASAIO J* 39: M353, 1993

183. Klein E, Montalvo JG: Continuous monitoring of urea and inorganic phosphate during hemodialysis: II. Clinical trials. *Int J Artif Organs* 1: 175, 1978

184. Bosticardo GM, Avalle U, Giacchino F, Molino A, Alloatti S: Accuracy of an on-line urea monitor compared with urea kinetic model and direct dialysis quantification. *ASAIO J* 40: M426, 1994

185. Metry GS, Attman PO, Lönnroth P, Beshara SN, Aurell M: Urea kinetics during hemodialysis measured by microdialysis – a novel technique. *Kidney Int* 44: 622, 1993

186. Gal G, Grof J: Continuous UV photometric monitoring of the efficiency of hemodialysis. *Int J Artif Organs* 3: 338, 1980

187. Kuhlmann U, Gräf R, Schindler J, Lange H: Continuous ionography (CIG) in haemodialysis by ion-selective carrier membrane electrodes (ISCME) with solid cement contact for flow-through measurement. *Int J Artif Organs* 15: 209, 1992

188. Murisasco A, Leblond G, Elsen R, Stroumza P, Durand C, Jeannigros E, Crevat A, Reynier JP: Equilibration of body water distribution and Na^+ balance during hemodialysis (HD) with an ion specific electrode feedback system and integrated computer. *Trans Am Soc Artif Intern Organs* 30: 254, 1984

189. Bashein G, Greydanus WK, Kenny MA: Evaluation of a blood gas and chemistry monitor for use during surgery. *Anesthesiology* 70: 123, 1989

190. Parault B: Technique for improved patient care: initial experience with the GEM-6. *J Extra-corporeal Technol* 20: 47, 1988

191. Polaschegg HD (inventors), Fresenius AG (assignee): Apparatus for the drawing off of untreated and treated dialyzing liquid and/or blood from a dialysis device. US patent 4662208. 5/5/87

192. Gotch FA, Lam MA, Prowitt M, Keen M: Preliminary clinical results with sodium-volume modeling of hemodialysis therapy. *Proc Dial Transplant Forum* 10: 12, 1980

193. Heineken, FG, Evans, MC, Keen, ML, Gotch FA: Intercompartmental fluid shifts in hemodialysis patients. *Biotechnol Prog* 3: 69, 1987

194. Man NK, Petitclerc T, Tien NQ, Jehenne G, Funck-Brentano JL: Clinical validation of a predictive modeling equation for sodium. *Artif Organs* 9: 150, 1985

195. Petitclerc T, Man NK, Goureau Y, Guilleaume J, Funck-Brentano JL: Optimization of sodium dialysate con-

centration by plasma water conductivity monitoring.in *Progress in Artificial Organs – 1985*, edited by Nosé Y, Kjellstrand C, Ivanovich P, Cleveland, ISAO Press, 1986, p 234

196. Petitclerc T, Hamani A, Jacobs C: Optimization of sodium balance during hemodialysis by routine implementation of kinetic modeling. *Blood Purif* 10: 309, 1992

197. Polaschegg HD, Husar D (inventors), Fresenius AG (assignee): Dialysis apparatus with regulated mixing of the dialysis solution. US patent 4508622. 4/2/85

198. Polaschegg HD (inventors), Fresenius AG (assignee): Vorrichtung zum Bestimmen des intravasalen Blutvolumens während der Hämodialyse. DE patent 3640089. 12/22/88

199. Sternby JP (inventors), Gambro AB (assignee): Dialysis system. EPA patent 0547025. 6/16/93

200. Chevallet J (inventors), Hospal Industrie (assignee): Method for determining a patients blood sodium level and artificial kidney for the application thereof. US patent 4923613. 5/8/90

201. Albers, JR, Smith, JM: A conductivity technique for rapid measurement of *in vitro* dialyzer performance. *Trans Am Soc Artif Intern Organs* 11: 161, 1965

202. Boag J, Vlchek D: Clearance testing of dialyzers using conductivity. *Contemp Dial Nephrol* 11, 1987

203. Resnick D: QA testing of hemodialyzers in a clinical setting. *Dial Transplant* 19: 136, 1990

204. Polaschegg HD: Automatic, noninvasive intradialytic clearance measurement. *Int J Artif Organs* 16: 185, 1993

205. Gotch FA: Models to predict recirculation and its effect on treatment time in single-needle dialysis. in *First International Symposium on Single-Needle Dialysis*, edited by Ringoir S, Vanholder R, Ivanovich P, Cleveland, ISAO Press, No 305, 1984, p 47

206. Steil H, Kaufman AM, Morris AT, Levin NW, Polaschegg HD: *In vivo* verification of an automatic noninvasive system for real time Kt evaluation. *ASAIO J* 39: M348, 1993

207. Malchesky PS, Ellis P, Nosse C, Magnusson M, Lankhorst B, Nakamoto S: Direct quantification of dialysis. *Dial Transplant* 11: 42, 1982

208. Keshaviah P, Star R: A new approach to dialysis quantification: an adequacy index based on solute removal. *Semin Dial* 7: 85, 1994

209. Kidd EE: Bacterial contamination of dialysing fluid of artificial kidney. *Br Med J* 1: 880, 1964

210. Aviram A, Peters JH, Gulyassy PF. Dialysance of amino acids and related substances. *Nephron* 8: 440, 1971

211. Garred LJ, Rittau M, McReady W, Canaud B: Urea kinetic modeling by partial dialysate collection. *Int J Artif Organs* 12: 96, 1989

212. Stiller S, Schaefer U (inventors), Stiller S (assignee): Passiver Dialysatfluss-Teiler. DE patent 3312909. 10/18/84

213. Ing TS, Yu AW, Khalaf MN, Tiwari P, Rafiq M, Khan AA, Nawab ZM: Collection of hemodialysate aliquot whose

composition reflects that of total dialysate. *Am Soc Artif Intern Organs Abs* 85, 1994

214. Krämer M, Polaschegg HD: Automated measurement of recirculation. *Proc Eur Dial Transplant Assoc-Eur Renal Care Assoc* 19: 6, 1993

215. Schneditz D, Polaschegg HD, Lewin NW, Cu GA, Morris AT, Krämer M, Daugirdas JT, Kaufman AM: Cardiopulmonary recirculation in dialysis. An underrecognized phenomenon. *ASAIO J* 38: M194, 1992

216. Sohi PS, Laurin L, Lowery M, Twolan C, Posen GA: Hemodialysis (HD) catheter malfunction: impact on recirculation rate (RR) and dialysis efficiency, *J Am Soc Nephrol* 4: 387, 1993

217. Depner TA, Rizwan S, Cheer AY, Wagner JM, Eder LA: High venous urea concentration in the opposite arm. A consequence of hemodialysis-induced compartment disequilibrium. *Trans Am Soc Artif Intern Organs* 37: M141, 1991

218. Aldridge C, Tattersall J, Tomlinson C, Greenwood R: Haemodialysis recirculation detected by the three sample method is an artefact. *Proc Eur Dial Transplant Assoc-Eur Renal Care Assoc* 19: 2, 1993

219. Aldridge C, Greenwood RN, Cattell WR, Barrett RV: The assessment of arteriovenous fistulae created for haemodialysis from pressure and thermal dilution measurements. *J Med Eng Technol* 8: 118, 1984

220. Greenwood RN, Aldridge C, Goldstein L, Baker LRI: Assessment of arteriovenous fistulae from pressure and recirculation studies. Clinical experience in 186 fistulae. *Clin Nephrol* 23: 189, 1985

221. Polaschegg HD (inventors), Fresenius AG (assignee): Vorrichtung zur Behandlung von Blut im extrakorporalen Kreislauf. EP patent 0265795. 6/5/91

222. Aldrige C, Greenwood RN, Frampton CF, Wilkinson JS: Instrument design for the bedside assessment of arteriovenous fistulae in hemodialysis patients. *Proc Eur Dial Transplant Assoc-Eur Renal Care Assoc* 14: 255, 1985

223. Hester RL, Ashcraft D, Curry E, Bower J: Non-invasive determination of recirculation in the patient on dalysis. *ASAIO J* 38: M190, 1992

224. Buffaloe GW, Brugger JM, Ogawa FT (inventors), Cobe Laboratories Inc (assignee): Differential conductivity recirculation monitor. EPA patent 0590810. 4/6/94

225. Canaud B, Tetta C, Bosc JY, Berti M, Mazzocchi C, Mion C: Routine on-line evaluation of access recirculation (R) without blood sampling. *J Am Soc Nephrol* 5: 411, 1994

226. Schwab SJ, Raymond JR, Saeed M, Newman GE, Dennis PA, Bollinger RR: Prevention of hemodialysis fistula thrombosis. Early detection of venous stenoses. *Kidney Int* 36: 707, 1989

227. Polaschegg HD (inventors), Fresenius AG (assignee): Vorrichtung zur Ultrafiltrationskontrolle und Ultrafiltrationsregelung bei Blutreinigungsverfahren. DE patent 4024434. 6/11/92

ULTRAFILTRATION/HEMOFILTRATION PRACTICE

EDUARD A. QUELLHORST

HISTORICAL OVERVIEW

The first device to perform ultrafiltration in vivo was described by Brull in France (1) and Geiger (2) in Jerusalem using collodium membranes. They observed an undiminished concentration of chlorides, dextrose and non-protein nitrogen in the filtrate whereas phosphorus and calcium were partially retained. The first ultrafiltration with the aim to prolong the life of uremic animals was achieved by Malinow and Korzon in 1947 (3). Using cellophane tubes a filtrate flow of 15–20 ml/min could be obtained at a trans-membrane pressure of 500 mm Hg. Since they substituted the blood filtrate of test animals by injecting Ringer–Krebs-solution and since they made use of the arteriovenous pressure difference as the driving force for the filtration these investigators performed the first 'spontaneous arteriovenous hemofiltration'. A dialyzer-filter design with membrane support systems enabling a rapid fluid removal by ultrafiltration was described by Alwall in 1963 (4), but his first aim was to remove water and not to treat uremia.

During the 1950s reports appeared by Leonards (Cleveland Clinic) together with Skeggs and Kahn (5) or Kolff (6) demonstrating the possibility of fluid removal in dogs and humans by ultrafiltration.

The modern era of hemofiltration began not earlier than 1967 when L. Bluemle and L. Henderson (7) published their experience with highly permeable 'polyelectrolyte' membranes enabling blood purification by fluid and solute removal, preventing the individual from being dehydrated by fluid substitution. Whereas Bluemle and Henderson favoured the substitution of the filtrate before the filter ('pre-dilution') another group developing hemofiltration independently in Germany (8) preferred 'post-dilution', e.g. the infusion of substitution fluid behind the filter thereby reducing the amount of the substitution fluid to about fifty percent. In 1976, Bergström et al (9) published experiments by which they demonstrated a remarkable stability of the cardiovascular system to isolated ultra-

Table 1. Comparison of a typical hemofilter and a pair of human kidneys (13)

	Conventional Hemofilter	Human Kidney
Membrane area (m^2)	0.5–1.5	1.5
Number of fibers/capillaries	4,000–12,000	5×10^6
Transmembrane pressure difference (mm Hg)	200–500	50
Maximum blood flow rate	200–400	1.200
Filtration fraction	0.35–0.50	0.2

filtration, an observation, which could be extended to hemofiltration by Quellhorst et al (10). In 1979 Henderson first described sterile fluid generation (11).

In 1977 'spontaneous' or 'continuous' hemofiltration was described by Kramer (12), a method enabling continuous filtration making use of the arteriovenous pressure difference.

Fluid and solute removal during hemofiltration

In hemofiltration solutes are removed by a convective transport imitating the filtration process in the glomerulus of natural kidneys. Within the limits of the pore size all solutes pass the filter with the same velocity and to the same amount depending on the solute concentration of the retentate and the trans-membrane pressure difference. Water and vital solutes are replenished in hemofiltration either before (pre-dilution) or after (post-dilution) the ultrafiltration step.

In Table 1 a comparison a typical hemofiltration device and a pair of human kidneys is given concerning various filtration parameters. It has to be stressed that a hemofilter with approximately the same membrane area as the natural kidneys is restricted to a lower blood flow and requires a

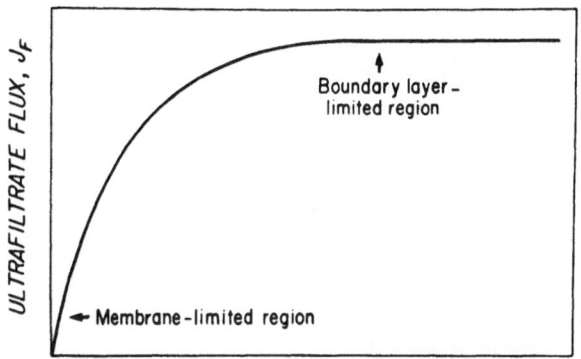

Figure 1. Relation between trans-membrane pressure difference and ultrafiltration flux in hemofiltration (13).

greater blood pressure difference to achieve a filtrate flux comparable to that of a pair of human kidneys.

THEORETICAL CONSIDERATIONS

In ultrafiltration, the volumetric flow rate of ultrafiltrate is denoted by Q_F. The ultrafiltrate flux, J_F is the volumetric flow rate per unit membrane surface area **A** (13). Thus

$$J_F = \frac{Q_F}{A}$$

being equivalent to the superficial velocity of ultrafiltrate across the membrane. The mass removal rate M of a given solute is defined by

$$M = Q_F c_F,$$

where c_F is the solute concentration in the ultrafiltrate being equivalent to the solute concentration in the bulk plasma water c_{wb}, by the observed sieving coefficient S_O

$$S_O = \frac{c_F}{c_{wb}}.$$

If there is no restriction for the solute by the membrane $S_O = 1$, if the solute is completely retained $S_O = 0$. The solute flux, thus, can be defined as by

$$J_s = \frac{M}{A} = J_F c_{wb} S_O.$$

It has to be noted that the reflection coefficient (R_O) is inversely correlated to the sieving coefficient: $R_O = 1 - S_O$.

ULTRAFILTRATION FLOW

In hemofiltration the ultrafiltration flow rate is determined by the following parameters: membrane hydraulic permeability, trans-membrane pressure difference, blood flow rate, device geometry and dimensions as well as blood protein concentration. Moreover protein composition, hematocrit and temperature influence the filtrate flux.

Figure 1 shows a typical plot of ultrafiltrate flux vs membrane pressure. At low trans-membrane pressures the flux shows a linear relation to the trans-membrane pressure difference. In this 'membrane limited' region trans-membrane pressure difference and membrane hydraulic permeability completely determine the flux. At high applied pressures the filtration flux is independent of the trans-membrane pressure difference and the membrane permeability. In this 'boundary layer-limited' region the ultrafiltration rate is determined by blood flow rate, device geometry and protein concentration. Thus, the flux can be increased by increasing the blood flow rate, decreasing the channel diameter and decreasing the protein concentration.

Especially in post-dilution hemofiltration in which all solutes are eliminated by removing the plasma water the compartmentalization between plasma water, proteins and the red blood cells has to be considered. Here, the whole blood clearance C is of more importance than the plasma clearance for the characterization of its effectiveness. It can be defined as the removal rate of a solute divided by its initial concentration in whole blood, c_B.

$$C = \frac{M}{c_B}.$$

Here, the solute removal rate (M) in a hemofilter is equal to the ultrafiltration rate Q_F, times the solute concentration in the plasma filtrate, c_F.

Pre-dilution hemofiltration makes more substances previously bound or sequestered to red cells available for the filtration process than post-dilution does.

Figure 2 (14) shows the relations between the sieving coefficient and whole blood clearances with respect to the distribution of solutes in red blood cells and plasma water ($K = 1$: solute equally distributed between red blood cells and plasma water, $K = 0$: solute cannot permeate through the red cell membrane). Two facts can be derived from Figure 2: a) the higher the sieving coefficient the more the whole blood clearance is influenced by the solute distribution and b) solutes for which most membranes have a sieving coefficient of nearly 1 (like urea or creatinine) are removed more effectively by pre-dilution than by post-dilution hemofiltration.

Membranes and devices

Whereas Alwall (4) used cellophane tubings for his first ultrafiltration experiments the development of new polymers at the end of the 60s was the main presupposition for the construction of hemofilters. In contrast to hemodialysis, in which thin membranes are necessary to enhance the diffusion process, the porosity of the membrane and not

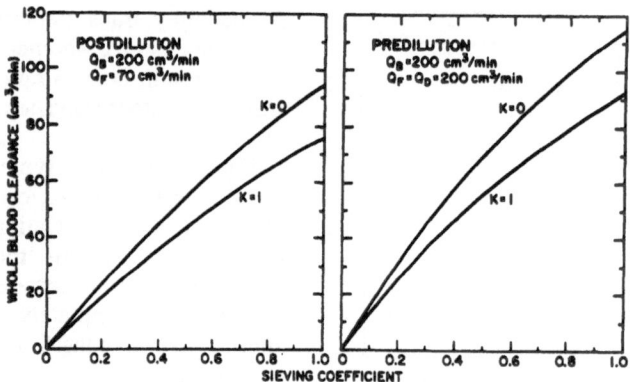

Figure 2. Relation between sieving coefficient and whole blood clearance. $K = 0$ and $K = 1$: Distribution pattern between red blood cells and plasma (14).

the wall thickness is of importance for the hemofiltration process.

A membrane has to fulfill the following properties in order to be used for hemofiltration: Good blood compatibility, high plasma water flux and total retention of albumin. Ideally hemofiltration membranes are 'asymmetric' hollow fiber membranes, consisting of a 'support' layer and a 'filtering' layer where the former is responsible for the mechanical stability of the membrane and the latter for its permeability. Thus, polyamide, polycarbonate, polysulfone, cellulose acetate, polyacrylonitrile and polymethyl methacrylate have been used for the production of hemofiltration membranes. With the exception of polyacrylonitrile (flat sheet) all membranes are mounted as capillary hemofilters.

Quite different from a hemodialysis system the functionally most genuine part of the hemofiltration apparatus is the balancing system providing the substitution of the ultrafiltrate (minus the fluid volume desired to be removed) gravimetrically or volumetrically. Since an imbalance of ultrafiltration and substitution could rapidly lead to a life-threatening volume depletion the ultrafiltration rate must be continuously monitored with the aim of a suitable fluid replacement. Substitution fluids have to be sterile and free of pyrogens and, thus, are very expensive. High costs of the substitution fluid were one important reason for the preference of post-dilution over pre-dilution hemofiltration where considerably smaller amounts of fluid are necessary, taking into account a minor effectiveness concerning the elimination of substances with a smaller molecular weight. With the construction of hemofiltration systems (11) allowing the production of ultra-clean substitution fluids using processed tap water and concentrates cost arguments have lost their importance. It may be speculated that these systems will favour the spread of pre-dilution hemofiltration in the near future. Figure 3 presents a volumetric balancing system, allowing pre- or post-dilution hemofiltration under conditions of an ultra-pure substitution fluid produced using processed water

and concentrate. These devices are now commercially available.

SUBSTITUTION FLUID

During the course of one hemofiltration (post-dilution technique) at least 30–40 l of extracellular fluid, removed by ultrafiltration, have to be replaced by a fluid with a composition as close as possible to the composition of normal extracellular fluid. In contrast to hemodialysis the electrolyte balance in hemofiltration depends primarily on the composition and volume of the replacement fluid. For example: a negative fluid balance of about 2 l induces a negative sodium balance of somewhat less than 300 mmol per treatment. The close correlation between fluid and electrolyte balance in hemofiltration was initially demonstrated by Fuchs et al (15) who showed that the calcium and fluid balance in an individual patient was equilibrated when the calcium concentration in the diluting fluid was 1.9 mmol/l (7.6 mg/dl) and fluid removal was 3.9 kg per treatment. Fluid loss exceeding this amount caused a negative calcium balance while less ultrafiltration resulted in a positive calcium balance. Such a correlation also applies to other electrolytes and has to be considered when large fluid volumes must be removed by hemofiltration. In spite of the fact, that a considerable amount of various substances (e.g. amino acids) is lost by hemofiltration, there is no need to add amino acids or dextrose to the substitution fluid. Some investigators, however, have contrary views and recommend the addition of dextrose to stabilize the extracellular osmotic pressure.

Whereas the effectiveness of hemodialysis concerning the elimination of molecules is mainly time-dependent, the effect of hemofiltration depends on the volume of fluid filtered. There is a consensus of opinion that the fluid volume exchanged during each treatment with the post-dilution technique should exceed 30 l per treatment. Baldamus et al (16) have proposed a formula to predict

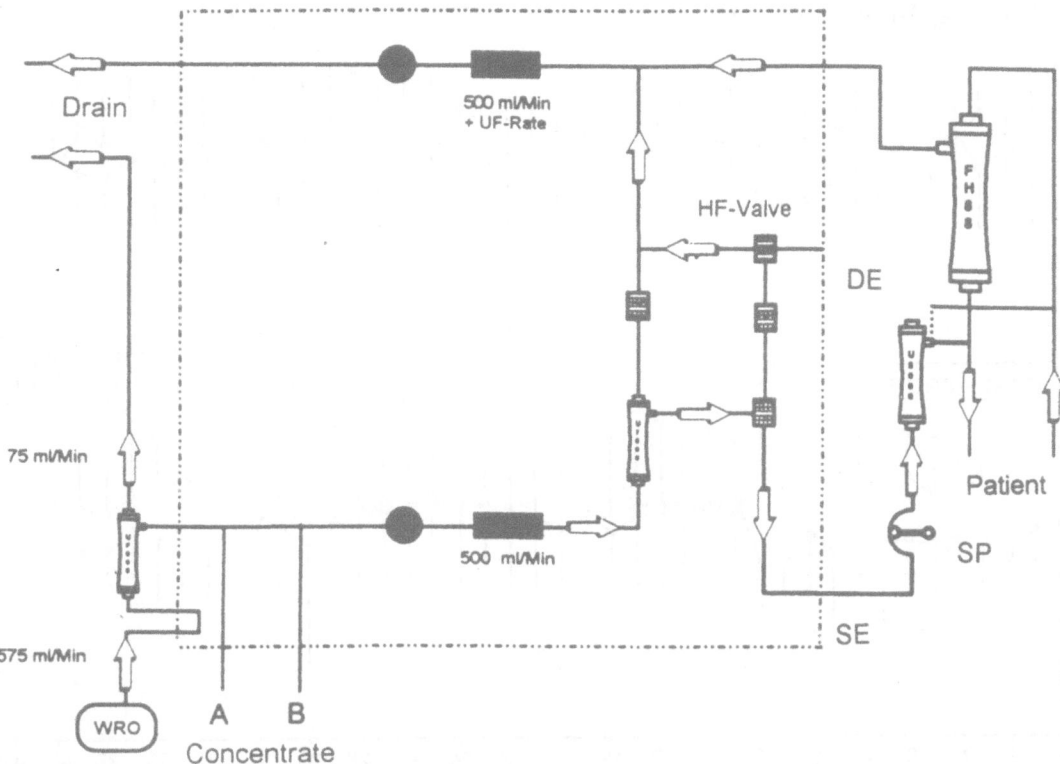

Figure 3. Flow diagram of a typical hemofiltration system allowing the 'on-line' production of substitution fluid (WRO = reverse osmosis system; DE = dialysis fluid exit, SE = substitution fluid exit, SP = substitution pump).

the efficiency of the removal of low molecular weight substances, e.g. for urea:

$$V\tfrac{1}{2} = 0.47 \times \text{BW} - 3.03,$$

where $V\tfrac{1}{2}$ is the volume of fluid necessary to reduce serum levels to 50% and BW = body weight. No prescription exists as yet for the operation of hemofiltration in the pre-dilution mode. The system currently available allows the production of 99 l of substitution fluid per treatment or 27 l per hour.

Clinical experience with hemofiltration

Indications

Long-term hemofiltration treatment of patients with terminal chronic renal failure started in 1974. With increasing experience the new method became increasingly popular. Some patients now have been on regular hemofiltration treatment for more that 20 years. Since the early 1980s the proportion of patients on regular hemofiltration or hemodiafiltration treatment has leveled off to less than 10% of the total population on artificial kidney treatment registered in the EDTA statistics. Two reasons may be responsible for this situation: a) hemofiltration in comparison to hemodialysis is very expensive because of higher

costs for filters and substitutions fluid, and b) the experience made in hemofiltration has induced an improvement of hemodialysis making use of a controlled ultrafiltration process and bicarbonate as buffers in dialysis fluids.

In addition an increasing number of patients with acute renal failure have been treated by hemofiltration. Other applications reported in the literature are glycoside and diuretic resistant cardiac failure with pulmonary edema, exogenous intoxications and hepatic coma (17).

Influence on the cardiovascular system

Under similar conditions of fluid removal, total peripheral resistance remains unchanged or increases slightly during hemofiltration but decreases during hemodialysis (18–20). Thus, the cardiovascular system reacts in a more physiologic way to fluid removal by hemofiltration than to combined ultrafiltration and hemodialysis. It could be also demonstrated that serum catecholamine levels remained stable during hemofiltration but decreased considerably during hemodialysis (18–20).

A more pronounced stability of the vascular system in hemofiltration than in hemodialysis treatment could be confirmed by the results obtained from a comparative study of two groups each of 30 patients. Both groups were alternately treated with hemofiltration and hemodialysis

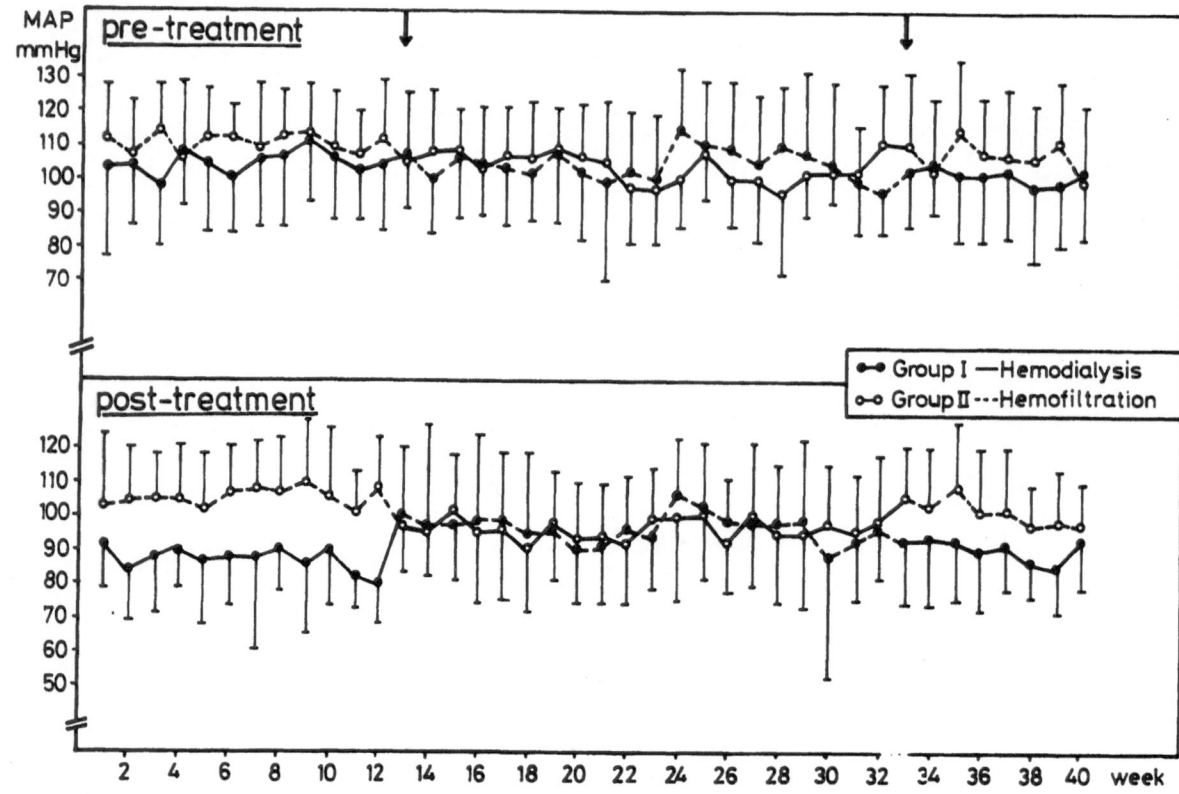

Figure 4. Pre- and post-treatment mean arterial blood pressure (MAP) in two groups of 30 patients each. The mean fluid removal per treatment was kept constant in both groups ($\bar{x} \pm$ SD).

for periods of three months, according to an A–B–A or B–A–B sequence (A = hemodialysis, B = hemofiltration). Mean pre-treatment arterial blood pressure readings did not differ in the two groups. Post-treatment blood pressures were however significantly higher during hemofiltration treatment (Figure 4). The number of hypotensive episodes with collapse reactions during and after treatment with hemofiltration was only one tenth of the number of collapse reactions observed with hemodialysis.

In spite of removal of more body fluid with hemofiltration the extracellular volume is obviously reduced to a lesser degree by hemofiltration than by hemodialysis (21), which may be explained by a more substantial fluid shift to the extracellular space (Figure 5). Evidence for this 'refilling phenomenon' was presented for ultrafiltration by Rouby et al (22) and was confirmed by observations from Sausse and co-workers (23) who calculated the extracellular volume on the basis of the sodium free water clearance. Hypertensive patients in the hemodialysis population can be divided into two groups: In one (large) group hypertension is predominantly volume dependent. In this group blood pressure can be lowered by fluid removal. In a small group of patients (about 5–10% of the dialysis population) hypertension is volume independent and cannot be corrected by ultrafiltration. In the former group plasma renin activity is usually normal or only slightly elevated. The latter group usually shows very high plasma renin levels and blood pressure can be dramatically reduced by the administration of ACE-blockers. Both groups of hypertensive patients may profit from hemofiltration: Volume dependent hypertension can be favourably influenced by this method which, in contrast to hemodialysis, allows a linear fluid removal without collapse reactions. Because of the minimal number of hypotensive episodes saline infusion are usually unnecessary, which facilitates correction of hypertension. But also volume-independent, dialysis and antihypertensive drug resistant hypertension may react favourably during hemofiltration treatment. In one study (24) blood pressure could be normalized in 13 patients who were transferred from hemodialysis to hemofiltration because of dialysis resistant severe hypertension. Ten patients had a very high renin activity at the start of hemofiltration treatment which could be normalized in all patients except one, during an 8 month course of treatment. Similar results were obtained by Henderson et al (25), but another group of investigators (16) observed no differences between hemofiltration and hemodialysis in the control of hypertension. It has to be emphasized, however, that blood pressure values in these patients at the start of treatment were considerably lower than in the patients of the other two studies.

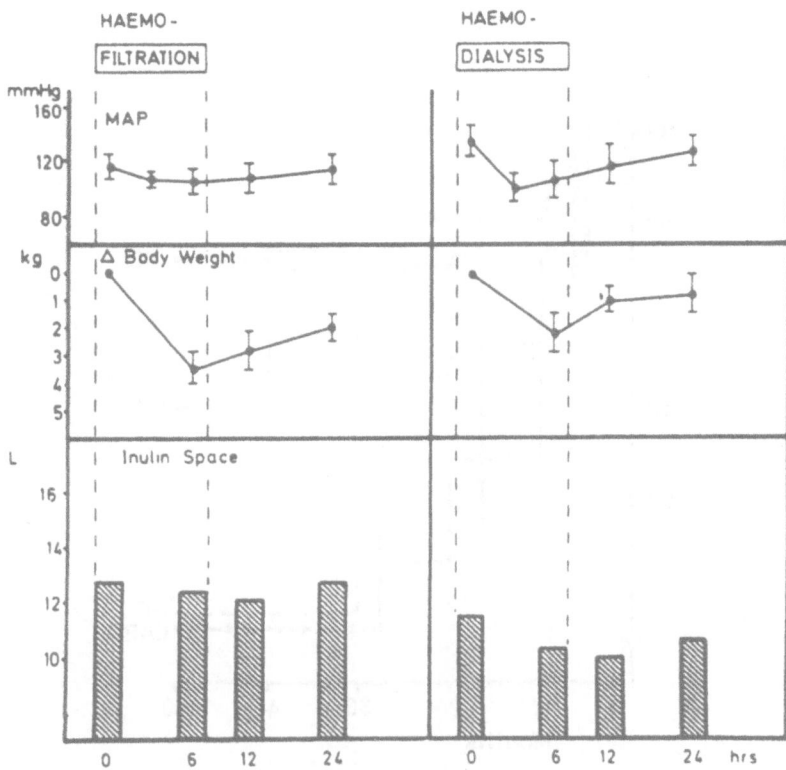

Figure 5.   Changes of insulin space, body weight and mean arterial pressure (MAP) in 4 patients undergoing post-dilution hemofiltration and, after restitution of their initial body weight, hemodialysis treatment.

Hemofiltration in diabetic nephropathy

Thanks to technical improvement and to the introduction of new methods of treatment, the results of long-term artificial kidney treatment in patients with diabetic nephropathy have been improved during the last two decades. However, compared to patients with renal insufficiency of non-diabetic origin they are still poor, mainly because of non-renal complications (e.g. cardiac infarction, gangrene).

In one study (26) morbidity and mortality rates were investigated in 394 patients with renal insufficiency because of type I diabetic nephropathy, depending on the method of treatment. In these patients the results of hemofiltration were compared to those of intermittent hemodialysis, intermittent peritoneal dialysis (IPD) and continuous ambulatory peritoneal dialysis (CAPD).

Approximately 90% of the patients with a nephropathy due to diabetes mellitus suffered from hypertension or needed antihypertensive drug treatment upon initiation of renal replacement therapy (Figure 6), but progress was different according to the type of treatment. In patients with type I diabetes, hemofiltration and CAPD yielded substantially more favourable results than hemodialysis and, particularly, IPD. While only about 35% of the hemodialysis and CAPD groups were suffering from hypertension or required antihypertensive drug therapy after 5 years of treatment, this applied to 62% of the hemodialysis patients and nearly 76% of the IPD-patients.

As shown in Figure 7 proliferative diabetic retinopathy existed in 12–25% of the patients at the initiation of renal replacement therapy. Its incidence increased in all treatment groups over a 5-year period, whereby the hemodialysis group displayed the least favourable results: in this group, 63% of the patients were suffering from a proliferative retinopathy by the end of the treatment period. The results in the other treatment groups were significantly more favourable, CAPD and hemofiltration showing the least progression. The difference in the development of proliferative retinopathy between hemofiltration and hemodialysis may serve as a strong argument against heparin being particularly responsible for retinal changes, as this anticoagulant is used in both procedures. The influence of hypertension suggests itself much more readily, particularly since the procedures with less favourable influence on blood pressure (IPD and hemodialysis) also display the most rapid progression of diabetic retinopathy. An unfavourable effect on the progression of this serious complication is to be expected not only from hypertension, but also from fluctuations in blood pressure, which occur much more frequently under hemodialysis and IPD than under the two other procedures.

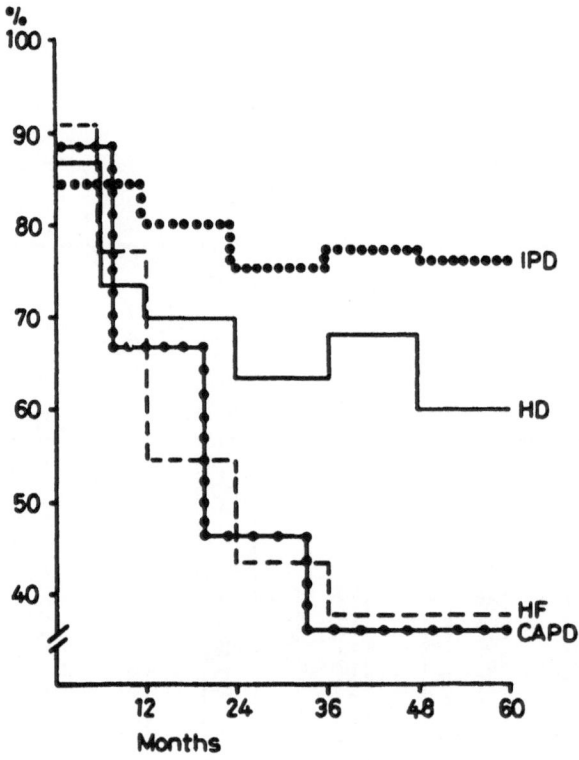

Figure 6. Percentage of patients with hypertension or needing antihypertensive drug therapy in relation to the method of treatment.

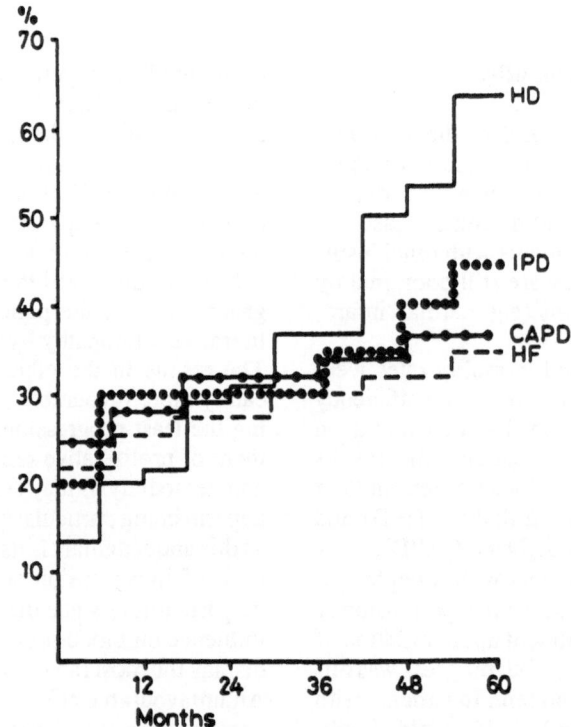

Figure 7. Behaviour of proliferative retinopathy in patients with diabetic nephropathy in relation to the different methods of treatment.

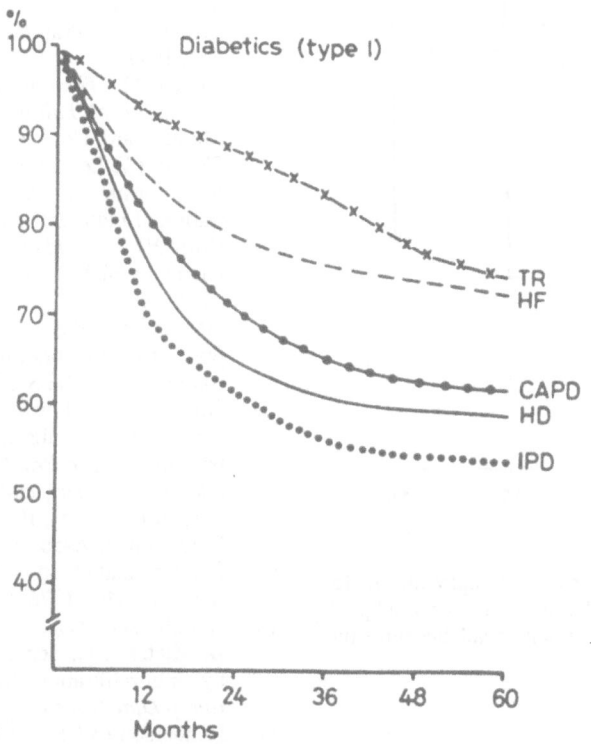

Figure 8. Survival rates of patients with diabetic nephropathy (type I diabetes mellitus) in relation to the method of treatment.

Mortality rates showed different tendencies in patients with diabetic nephropathy in relation to the method of treatment: As can be demonstrated in Figure 8, from the third year of treatment onwards there is a significantly more favourable course in patients who received a kidney transplant and those under hemofiltration than in patients on CAPD, hemodialysis and IPD. After 5 years, the survival rate of hemofiltration patients and patients who received a transplant is around 76–78% but only between 58 and 69% in patients of the other treatment groups. As expected, the results in all treatment groups are significantly less favourable in diabetics than in non-diabetics of approximately the same age.

HEMOFILTRATION AND AMYLOIDOSIS

Amyloidosis is one of the most severe complications of long term dialysis treatment provoking arthralgia amongst other clinical symptoms (e.g., the carpal tunnel syndrome and myalgia). Since only few patients have been exclusively treated by hemofiltration for longer periods of time and since signs and symptoms of 'dialysis amyloidosis' are generally observed not earlier than after the 6th to 8th year of artificial kidney treatment statistically relevant answers cannot be given to the question whether long term hemofiltration has any benefits concerning the

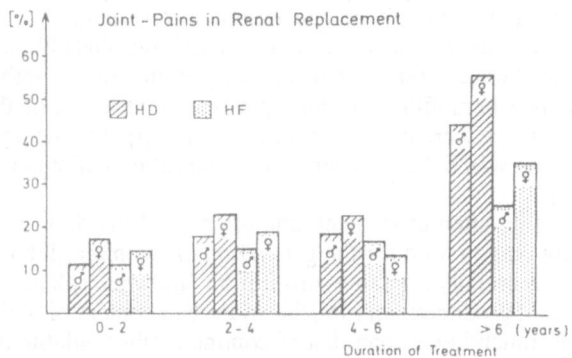

Figure 9. Influence of the time of treatment on the development of arthralgia (HD = hemodialysis, HF = hemofiltration).

development of this complication. In one study (27) 260 hemodialysis and 155 hemofiltration patients who had been on their specific treatment for at least 3 years were asked whether they suffered from joint pains and, if so, to describe the intensity and distribution pattern. As Figure 9 shows the percentage of patients with arthralgia increased substantially after the 6th year of treatment, in hemofiltration, however, to a lesser degree than in hemodialysis patients of both sexes.

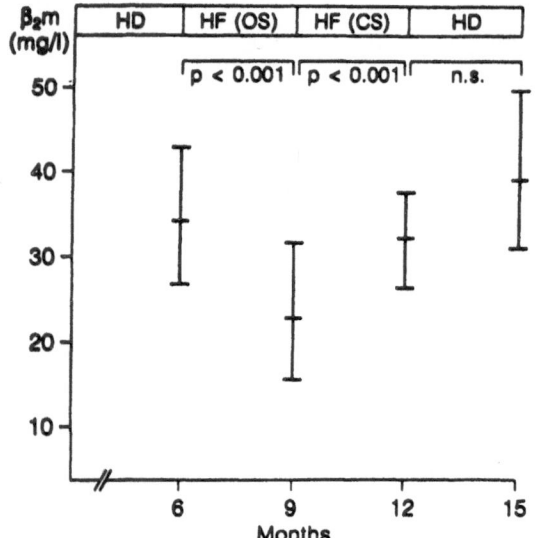

Figure 10.   Mean serum levels of Beta-2-microglobulin in 15 patients after different treatment modalities (OS = 'on-line' produced substitution fluid, CS = commercially available substitution fluid).

The discovery of β_2-microglobulin as the main constituent of dialysis-associated amyloidosis has not only cast light on the pathophysiology of this complication but also raises hopes for its prevention or treatment.

In earlier publications, it had been shown that although hemofiltration removes β_2-microglobulin more effectively than hemofiltration, high pre-treatment levels of this substance were measured (28) and the carpal tunnel syndrome was detected even in hemofiltration patients (29, 30).

In an attempt to determine the role of the dialysis or substitution fluid for the generation of β_2-microglobulin, commercially available substitution fluid was replaced by a fluid produced 'online', the endotoxin content of which was much lower than that of commercially available fluids (30). Within an observation period of 3 months, serum levels of β_2-microglobulin declined significantly and rose again substantially after transferring the patients from 'online' hemofiltration to conventional treatment (Figure 10). It may, thus, be speculated, that higher endotoxin levels in conventional substitution fluid may be one factor responsible for a continuous inflammation resulting in β_2-microglobulin formation and amyloid deposition.

REFERENCES

1.   Brull L: Réalisation de l'ultrafiltration *in vivo. Biol C R* 99: 105, 1928
2.   Geiger A: A method of ultra-filtration *in vivo. J Physiol* 71: 111, 1931
3.   Malinow MR, Korzon W: An experimental method for obtaining an ultrafiltrate of the blood. *J Lab Clin Med* 32: 461, 1947
4.   Alwall N: *Therapeutic and Diagnostic Problems in Severe Renal Failure.* Scandinavian University Books, Münksgaard, Copenhagen, 1963
5.   Skeggs LT, Leonards JR, Kahn JR: Removal of the fluid from normal and edematous dogs by continuous ultrafiltration of blood *Lab Invest* 1: 488, 1952
6.   Kolff WJ, Leonards JR: Reduction of otherwise intractable edema by dialysis or filtration. *Cleveland Clin Quarterly* 21: 61, 1954
7.   Henderson L, Besarab A, Michaels A, Bluemle LW: Blood purification by ultrafiltration and fluid replacement (diafiltration). *Trans Am Soc Artif Int Organs* 16: 216, 1967
8.   Quellhorst E, Plashues E: Ultrafiltration: Elimination harnpflichtiger Substanzen mit Hilfe neuartiger Membranen. in *Aktuelle Probleme der Dialyseverfahren und der Niereninsuffizienz*, edited by Ditrich P, Skrabal F, Friedberg, Bindernagel, 1971, p 216
9.   Bergström J, Asaba H, Fürst P, Oules R: Dialysis, ultrafiltration and blood pressure. *Proc Europ Dial Transplant Assoc* 13: 293, 1976
10.   Quellhorst E, Rieger J, Doht B, Beckmann H, Jacob I, Kraft B, Mietzsch G, Scheler F: Treatment of chronic uremia by an ultrafiltration kidney: first clinical experience. *Proc Europ Dial Transplant Assoc* 13: 314, 1976
11.   Henderson LW, Beans E: Successful production of sterile pyrogen-free electrolyte solution by ultrafiltration. *Kidney Int* 14: 522, 1978
12.   Kramer P, Wigger W, Rieger J, Matthaei D, Scheler F: Arteriovenous haemofiltration: a new simple method for treatment of overhydrated patients resistant to diuretics. *Klin. Wochenschr* 55: 1121, 1977
13.   Ofsthun NJ, Colton CK, Lysaght M: Determinants of fluid and solute removal rates during hemofiltration. in *Hemofiltration*, edited by Henderson LW, Quellhorst EA, Baldamus CA, Lysaght RJ, Berlin, Springer Verlag, 1986, p 17
14.   Lysaght MJ, Ford CA, Colton CK, Stone RA, Henderson LW: Mass transfer in clinical blood ultrafiltration devices - a review. in *Technical Aspects of Renal Dialysis*, edited by Frost TH, Tunbridge Wells, Pitman Medical Publishing Co Ltd, 1978, p 81
15.   Fuchs C, Doht B, Dorn D, McIntosh C, Müller D, Scheler F: Parathyroid hormone, calcium and phosphate balance in hemofiltrations. *J Dialysis* 1: 631, 1977
16.   Baldamus CA, Schoeppe W, Koch KM: Comparison of haemodialysis (HD) and post dilution haemofiltration (HF) in an unselected dialysis population. *Proc Europ Dial Transplant Assoc* 15: 228, 1978
17.   Denis J, Opolon P, Delorme ML, Granger A, Darnis F: Long-term extra-corporal assistance by continuous haemofiltration during fulminant hepatic failure. *Gastroenterol Clin Biol* 3: 337, 1979
18.   Hampl H, Paeprer H, Unger V, Kessel MW: Hemodynamics during hemodialysis, sequential ultrafiltration and hemofiltration. *J Dialysis* 3: 51, 1979
19.   Shaldon S, Deschodt G, Bean MC, Claret G, Mion H, Mion C: Vascular stability during high flux haemofiltration (HF). *Proc Europ Dial Transplant Assoc* 16: 695, 1979
20.   Baldamus CA, Fassbinder W, Ernst W, Koch KM: Differing haemodynamic stability due to differing sympathetic

response: comparison of ultrafiltration, hemodialysis and hemofiltration. *Proc Europ Dial Transpl Assoc* 17: 205, 1980

21. Schuenemann B, Borghardt J, Falda Z, Jacob I, Kramer P, Kraft B, Quellhorst E: Reactions of blood pressure and body spaces to hemofiltration treatment. *Trans Am Soc Artif Int Organs* 24: 687, 1978

22. Rouby JJ, Rottembourg J, Durande JP, Basset JY, Legrain M: Importance of the refilling rate in the genesis of hypovolaemic hypotension during regular dialysis and controlled sequential ultrafiltration-haemodialysis. *Proc Europ Dial Transplant Assoc* 15: 239, 1972

23. Sausse A, Man NK, Di Gulio S, Zingraff J, Drueke T, Jungers P, Funck-Brentano JL: Evidence for Na-free water clearance during haemodialysis. *Proc Europ Soc Artif Organs* 5: 186, 1978

24. Quellhorst E, Schuenemann B, Doht B: Treatment of severe hypertension in chronic renal failure by haemofiltration. *Proc Europ Dial Transplant Assoc* 14: 129, 1977

25. Henderson LW, Ford CA, Lysaght MJ, Grosman RA, Silverstein ME: Preliminary observation on blood pressure response with maintenance diafiltration. *Kidney Int* 7 (Suppl 3): S-413, 1975

26. Quellhorst E: Treatment of end-stage renal insufficiency in diabetic nephropathy by hemofiltration. in *Diabetes and the Kidney*, edited by Heidland A, Koch KM, Heidbreder E, Contrib to Nephrol 73, Basel, Karger, 1989, p 170

27. Quellhorst E, Schuenemann B: Beta-2 amyloidosis and hemofiltration. in *Dialysis Amyloidosis*, edited by Gejyo F, Brancaccio D, Bardin T, Milan, Wichtig Editore, 1989, p 123

28. Blumberg A, Bürgi W: Behaviour of β_2-microglobulin in patient with chronic renal failure undergoing hemodialysis, hemodiafiltration and continuous ambulatory peritoneal dialysis (CAPD). *Clinical Nephrol* 27: 245, 1987

29. Argiles A, Mourad G, Berta P, Polito C, Canaud B, Robinot-Levy M, Mion C: Dialysis-associated amyloidosis in a patient on long-term post-dilutional hemofiltration. *Nephron* 46: 96, 1987

30. Quellhorst E, Hildebrand U, Solf A: Long-term morbidity: hemofiltration versus hemodialysis. in: *Dialysis Membranes: Structure and Predictions*, Contrib Nephrol 113, Basel, Karger 1995, p 110

CONTINUOUS ARTERIOVENOUS HEMOFILTRATION AND RELATED THERAPIES

ANDRE A. KAPLAN

HISTORY/BACKGROUND/DEVELOPMENT

By the late seventies, machine driven hemofiltration had been investigated as a treatment for chronic uremia (1–4). With the operational characteristics and advantages of convective based solute removal well described, the availability of low resistance hemofilters allowed for the development of filtration techniques which could be powered by the patient's arterial blood pressure. In 1977, Kramer et al. first proposed arteriovenous hemofiltration as a method of emergency fluid removal in patients resistant to diuretics (5). In 1979, Neff and colleagues used the technique for outpatient control of uremia (6). In 1980, Paganini and Nakamoto employed spontaneous filtration to maintain fluid balance in patients with acute renal failure (7) and Shaldon et al. described its use as an adjunct to chronic hemodialysis (8). Finally, in a follow up to their original work, Kramer et al. demonstrated that continuous arteriovenous hemofiltration could be used to supplant conventional dialytic techniques in the intensive care unit (9, 10).

Continuous arteriovenous hemofiltration has several potential advantages over intermittent dialytic techniques. The most obvious is that ultrafiltration is self limited since overly aggressive fluid removal results in a lowered blood pressure and a decline in the production of filtrate. A second advantage is that it is continuous, allowing for a constant readjustment of fluid and electrolyte balance and the administration of large amounts of parenteral nutrition without the risk of interdialytic volume overload. Third, is its convective mode of solute transport, known to increase middle molecule clearance when compared to diffusion based dialytic techniques (11–13). Finally, the circuit did not require expensive mechanical equipment nor the continual attendance of specially trained hemodialysis personnel. When compared to peritoneal dialysis, CAVH was not problematic in patients with abdominal surgery and offered isovolumetric fluid removal without the risk of peritonitis.

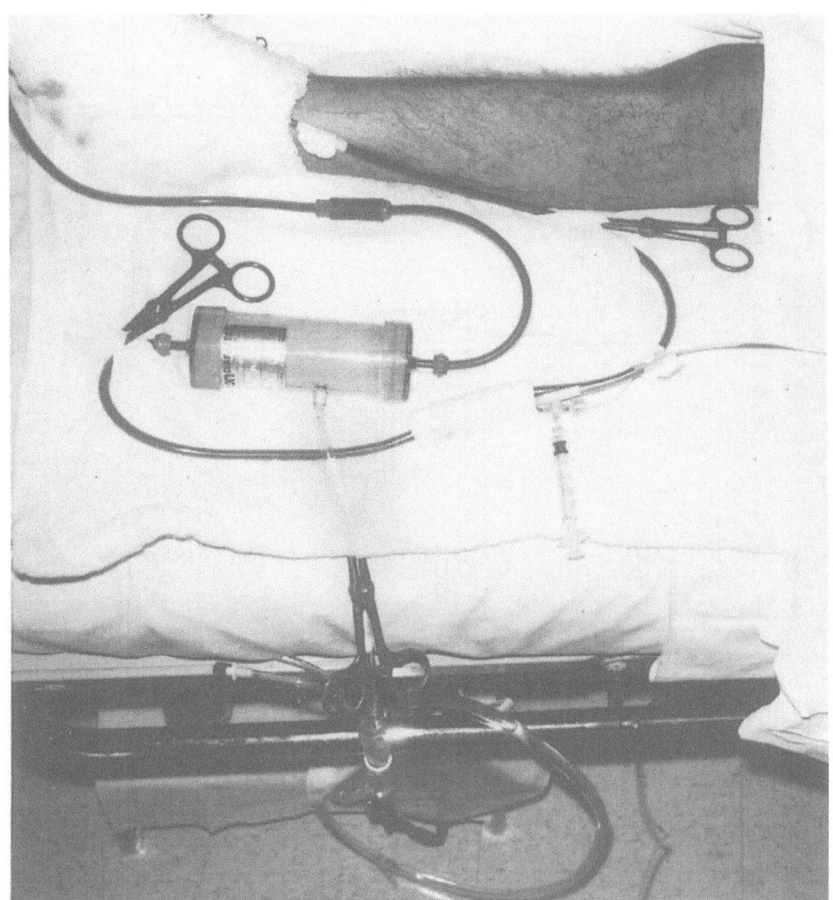

Figure 1. Continuous arteriovenous hemofiltration using a Quinton–Scribner shunt. The arterial limb of the shunt is attached with shortend dialysis tubing to the hemofilter. The filtered blood is returned to the patient via the venous limb. The resultant filtrate is collected in a standard urine bag. The arterial line is punctured at the injection port and connected to a continuous heparin infusion. Replacement fluid can be infused together with the heparin (predilution) or into the venous limb (postdilution). Reproduced with permission from Kaplan et al. (14).

OPERATIONAL CHARACTERISTICS OF THE ARTERIO-VENOUS CIRCUIT

The standard CAVH circuit is depicted in Figures 1 and 2a (14). Arterial access allows blood to flow through tubing to a low resistance hemofilter and back to a venous access. Filtrate, which is relatively protein-free (Table 1), is produced at a rate of several hundred ml/h and is collected into a bag connected to the ultrafiltrate port of the filter. In the postdilution mode, the replacement fluid is infused into the venous tubing. Continuous anticoagulation is administered through a prefilter tubing connection.

In an arterially driven circuit, blood flow (Qb) will be directly proportional to the mean arterial pressure (Figure 3a) and will be inversely related to the resistances presented by each of the circuit's components. In turn, the filtrate production rate (Qf) will be directly proportional to the blood flow (Figure 3c). Plasma is the part of blood which is available for filtration and its flow rate entering the filter is the plasma flow (Qp). The percentage of plasma which is filtered is the filtration fraction (FF).

The blood flow (Qb) can be calculated by simultaneous measurement of the hematocrit in the arterial (inlet) and venous (outlet) tubing and a timed collection of the filtrate (Qf) using the following formula (15):

$$Qb(\text{ml/min}) = \frac{(Qf(\text{ml/min}) \times Hct_{\text{outlet}})}{(Hct_{\text{outlet}} - Hct_{\text{inlet}})}$$

Alternatively, if the volume of the tubing circuit and filter are known, a reasonable estimate of the blood flow can be obtained during the initial hookup or after flushing procedures by determining the time it takes for blood to displace the priming solution from the arterial to the venous end of the circuit using the formula:

$$Qb(\text{ml/min}) = \frac{\text{circuit volume (ml)}}{\text{displacement time (minutes)}}$$

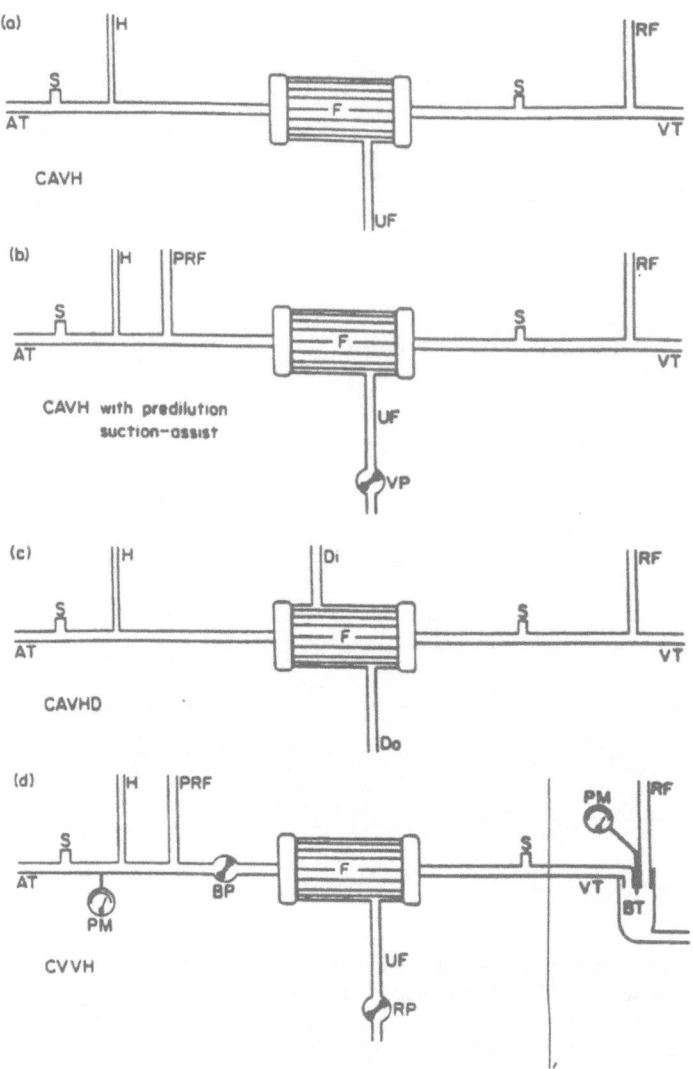

Figure 2. Circuit diagrams. (a) CAVH = continuous arteriovenous hemofiltration, (b) Suction-assisted CAVH with the predilution mode for replacement fluid administration. (c) CAVHD = continuous arteriovenous hemodialysis, (dialysate flow may be more efficient flowing countercurrent to blood flow). (d) CVVH = continuous venovenous hemofiltration. AT = arterial tubing, S = sampling port, H = heparin line, F = filter, UF = ultrafiltration fluid, RF = replacement fluid, VT = venous tubing, PRF = predilution replacement fluid, VP = vacuum pump, Di = dialysate inflow, Do = dialysate outflow, PM = pressure monitor, BP = blood pump, RP = roller pump, BT = bubble trap.

Thus, if the priming volume of the tubing and filter is 50 ml and the displacement time is 30 seconds, then Qb = 50 ml/0.5 min = 100 ml/min.

The plasma flow (Qp) can be calculated as:

$$Qp(\text{ml/min}) = Qb(\text{ml/min}) \times (1 - Hct)$$

and the filtration fraction (FF) can be calculated by one of several formulae (16, 17):

$$FF = Qf/Qp,$$
$$FF = [1 - (Hct_{\text{inlet}}/Hct_{\text{outlet}})]/1 - Hct_{\text{inlet}} \quad \text{or}$$
$$FF = 1 - (c_{\text{inlet}}/c_{\text{outlet}})$$

where c_{inlet} and c_{outlet} represent the protein concentrations in the prefilter (arterial) tubing and the postfilter (venous) tubing.

The filtration fraction will increase proportionately with the resistances provided by the filter and the venous end of the circuit. The filtration fraction will also increase directly with the transmembrane pressure (TMP), which can be defined as:

TMP = hydrostatic pressure (HP) − colloid oncotic pressure (COP)

where the hydrostatic pressure equals the average of the pre and postfilter pressures *and* the negative pressure in the

Table 1. Relation of ultrafiltrate to plasma with continuous arteriovenous hemofiltration. Reproduced with permission from Kaplan et al. (14)

	Ultrafiltrate (UF)	Plasma (P)	UF/P Ratio
Sodium, meq/l	135.3 ± 11.2	136.2 ± 10.37	0.993 ± 0.023
Potassium, meq/l	4.05 ± 0.71	4.11 ± 0.66	0.985 ± 0.055
Chloride, meq/l	103.7 ± 9.55	99.3 ± 10.8	1.046 ± 0.037
Carbon dioxide, meq/l	22.13 ± 5.08	19.78 ± 4.69	1.124 ± 0.085
Blood urea nitrogen, mg/dl	82.9 ± 38.4	79.1 ± 36.1	1.048 ± 0.024
Serum creatinine, mg/dl	6.63 ± 4.00	6.5 ± 3.86	1.020 ± 0.074
Uric acid, mg/dl	7.54 ± 3.33	7.35 ± 3.00	1.016 ± 0.081
Phosphorus, mg/dl	4.15 ± 1.29	3.94 ± 1.13	1.044 ± 0.078
Glucose, mg/dl	173 ± 84.5	164.5 ± 76.6	1.043 ± 0.055
Total proteins, g/dl	0.13 ± 0.13	6.21 ± 0.32	0.021 ± 0.021
Albumin, g/dl	0.02 ± 0.04	2.65 ± 0.46	0.008 ± 0.016
Calcium, mg/dl	5.12 ± 0.42	8.08 ± 0.61	0.637 ± 0.071
Total bilirubin, mg/dl	0.44 ± 0.55	12.1 ± 9.52	0.030 ± 0.029
Direct bilirubin, mg/dl	0.26 ± 0.31	7.35 ± 5.89	0.030 ± 0.019
Creatine phosphokinase IU	66.5 ± 88.3	80.9 ± 88.2	0.676 ± 0.215

All values are expressed as means ± SD, $n = 10$ samples.

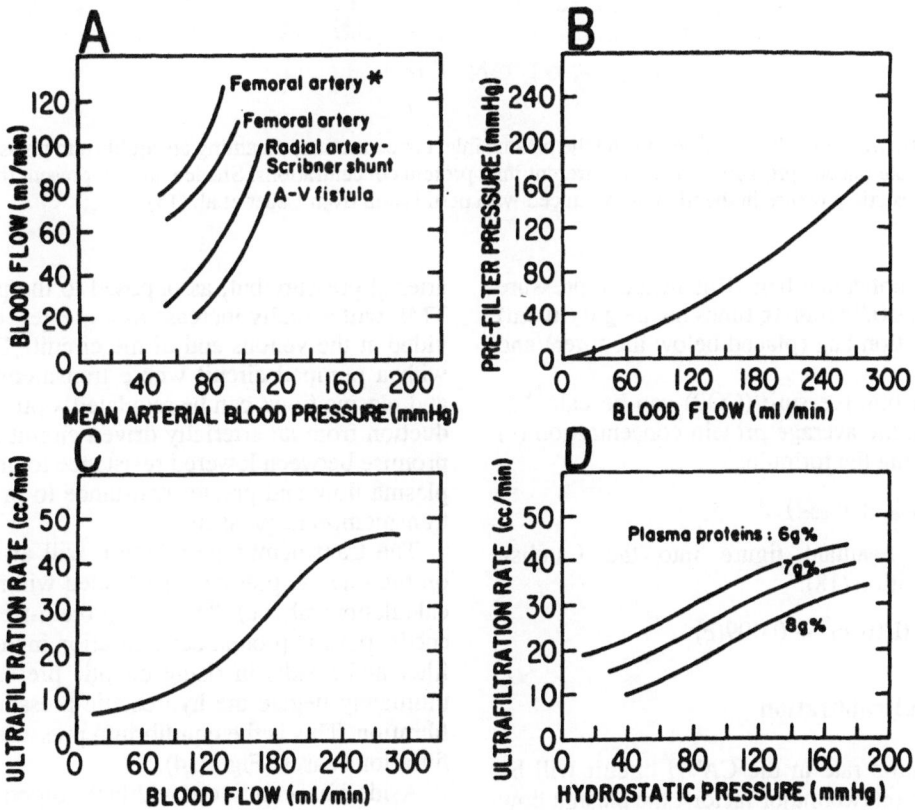

Figure 3. A: Effect of the mean arterial pressure on blood flow rate with different vascular access. Femoral artery cannulation with 14 gauge (∗) or 16 gauge catheter, radial artery cannulation with Quinton Scribner shunt or lower arm cannulation of an arteriovenous (A-V) fistula. B: Effect of pump-assisted blood flow rate on prefilter pressure. C: Effect of blood flow rate on ultrafiltration rate. (blood flow above 90 ml/min were obtained with a blood pump). D: Effect of hydrostatic pressure on ultrafiltration rate. Hydrostatic pressures above 80 mm Hg were obtained with a blood pump. Reproduced with permission from Lauer et al. (15).

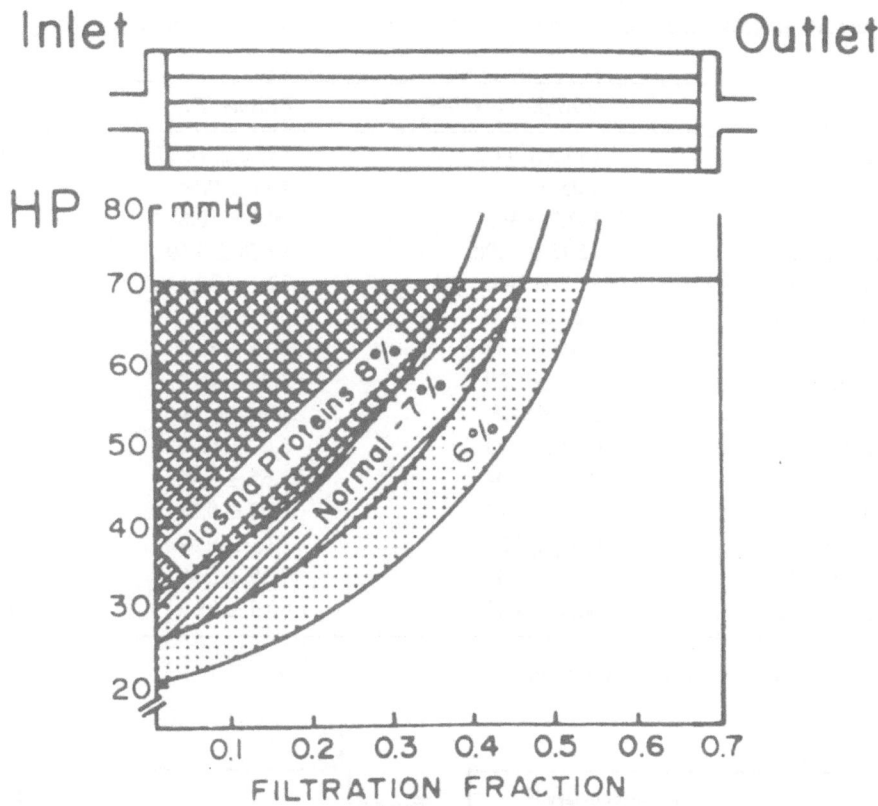

Figure 4. Relation between the filtration fraction and the plasma inlet concentration, assuming an equlibrium pressure of 77 mm Hg. The curved lines denote oncotic pressure values for different inlet protein concentrations. Shaded areas represent the transmembrane pressure. HP = hydrostatic pressure in the filter. Reproduced with permission from Lauer et al. (15).

filtrate tubing and collecting bag. This negative pressure can be calculated as 0.74 mmHg times the height (in cm) between the collection bag (placed below the filter) and the filter.

The colloid oncotic pressure (COP) can be calculated by determining the average protein concentration (c) within the filter using the formula:

$$c(\text{gm/dl}) = (c_{\text{inlet}} + c_{\text{outlet}})/2$$

and placing the resultant figure into the Landis–Pappenheimer equation (18):

$$COP = 2.1c + 0.16(c)^2 + 0.009(c)^3.$$

Determinants of ultrafiltration

The net ultrafiltration rate in the CAVH circuit will be directly dependent on two major factors, the plasma flow and the net transmembrane pressure. As discussed above, the plasma flow is directly related to the mean arterial pressure and is inversely related to the sum of the resistances provided by the circuit's components. The transmembrane pressure is also directly related to the mean arterial pressure but, as opposed to the plasma flow, the TMP will actually increase as a greater resistance is provided at the venous end of the circuit. Thus, in contrast with a pumped circuit where transmembrane pressures and plasma flows can be regulated, optimum filtrate production from an arterially driven circuit must be a compromise between lowered resistance to promote a greater plasma flow and greater resistance to provide increased transmembrane pressure.

The transmembrane pressure will also be dependent on the oncotic pressures generated within the filter (see calculations above). Thus, as protein-free filtration proceeds, plasma protein concentration increases within the filter and results in rising oncotic pressures which will ultimately negate the hydrostatic pressures which favor filtration. This is the equilibrium pressure at which point filtration ceases (Figure 4).

Aside from conditions within the blood compartment of the circuit, the transmembrane pressure is directly related to the negative pressure generated within the filtrate compartment. This negative pressure, which usually favors filtration, is a direct function of the vertical distance between the filter and the collection bag and is often in the range of 30 mmHg (40 cm × 0.74 mmHg). Although lowering the collection bag to its lowest point may provide the highest TMP, this maneuver may not always yield the highest filtration rates. In a recent study, Jenkins et al. have demonstrated that under conditions of minimal blood pressure and decreased blood flows, increases in TMP can cause a decline in plasma flow and a decrease in ultrafiltration rates (19).

If ultrafiltration declines in a previously well functioning circuit, the most common cause will be a decline in blood pressure or clotting of one or more of the circuit's components (hemoaccess, filter or tubing). An inadvertent change in the vertical distance between the filter and the collection bag can also cause a dramatic reduction in filtration rate. Kinking of the tubing or access catheters is another potential problem.

If ultrafiltration rates are insufficient at the initiation of the circuit and mean arterial pressure seems adequate (> 70 mmHg), the problem may lie in an inappropriate choice of one of the components. Possible causes include an arterial access whose internal diameter is too small or a filter which provides an inadequate amount of resistance. Once again, tubing kinks and the position of the collection bag should be checked.

Management of the circuit and maintenance of its patency is subject to a variety of procedural choices such as how often to rinse the system with saline and how often to change the filters, tubing and hemoaccess. These issues will often depend on the clinical setting and the type of system components being employed. Several procedural manuals provide useful guidelines, and often can be obtained from the filter manufacturers (20, 21). A manual endorsed by the American Association of Critical Care Nurses and the American Nephrology Nurses' Association has recently been published (22).

SYSTEM COMPONENTS

Hemoaccess

Since resistance is inversely related to the 4th power of the internal radius and changes in direct proportion with the length of the component (23), the ideal vascular access will have the largest internal diameter and shortest length. As such, a well designed hemoaccess with a large internal diameter will offer only minor resistance to flow, while smaller, more conventional hemoaccess needles will yield a much greater resistance (Figure 3a). In general, using large bore hemoaccess, the greatest resistance will be offered by the filter followed by the arterial and venous tubing (Figure 5). A small bore access will actually present a greater resistance to flow than the filter. Thus, the choice of access is critical for optimum performance in a blood pressure driven circuit (24, 25).

Although less than ideal because of the relatively small internal diameter, Quinton-Scribner shunts can often provide sufficient blood flow and can be placed in the low-

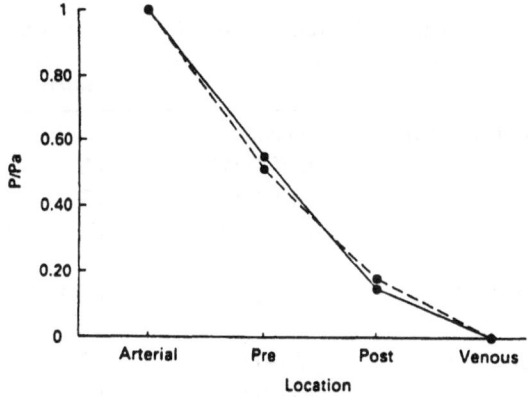

Figure 5. Hydrostatic pressures within the CAVH circuit. Pressures measured (P) are graphed as a fraction of the original arterial pressure (Pa) and are obtained at the arterial access, just prior to the filter (pre), immediately after the filter (post) and at the venous access. P/Pa = measured pressure as a fraction of original arterial pressure. Reproduced with permission from Pallone et al. (23).

er leg, thus avoiding cannulation of large arterial vessels (26). Similarly, Buselmeier shunts placed in a forearm have been successfully employed (27). Standard single lumen hemodialysis catheters can also provide useful flow, but are often limited by the small internal diameter of their tapered ends. Kramer and colleagues have described a substantial experience using a large-bore (0.3 cm inner diameter) femoral catheter with minimal taper and no side holes (10). The catheter is percutaneously placed using an inner plastic 'trocar' with a tapered tip. In view of its large inner diameter, this type of catheter presents the least resistance and provides the best blood flow to the filter.

Arterial access in neonates and pediatric patients present particularly difficult problems (28, 29) (see below). Pumped continuous therapies, such as continuous veno-venous hemofiltration or hemodialysis (CVVH, CVVHD) can be operated with any venous access capable of providing 100 to 300 ml/min of blood flow.

Filters

The ideal filters for CAVH are those which provide high water permeability with low resistance and a minimal tendency to clot. Most of these are of a hollow fiber configuration manufactured from synthetic membranes. Filters which are available commercially and suitable for an arterially driven circuit are listed in Table 2 (19, 30–40). Filters with greater surface area will usually provide higher filtration rates but, due to increased resistance, may be operational only marginally under conditions of low blood pressure and may have a greater tendency to clot. As opposed to CAVH, CAVHD is strongly dependent on diffusion and less dependent on water permeability and

Table 2. Commercially available filters for the continuous therapies. Modified from Lysaght et al. (30)

Manufacturer	Model	Material	Area	Comments (references)
Amicon Corp	Minifilter	PS	0.005	neonates (31)
	Diafilter 10	PS	0.2	low resistance (32)
	Diafilter 20	PS	0.25	(33)
	Diafilter 30	PS	0.6	high resistance, high UFR (33)
Asahi Medical	Ultrafilter CS	PAN	0.5	(19)
Fresenius AG	AV-400	PS	0.7	(34)
	AV-600	PS	1.35	high resistance, CVVH
Gambro AB	FH-22	PA	0.16	(35)
	FH-55	PA	0.6	(36)
	FH-66	PA	0.6	(37)
Hospal Ltd	Biospal 1200 S	PAN	0.5	plate configuration often used for CAVHD (38)
Minntech	Renaflo 0.25	PS	0.3	(39)
	Renaflo 0.5	PS	0.5	high resistance, pumped systems
Toray Indust Inc	Hemofeel-CH	PAN-PEO	0.25	heparin binding for decreased thrombogenesis (40)

PS = polysulphone, PAN = polyacrylonitrile, PA = polyamide, PEO = polyethyleneoxide.

thus may be more efficiently performed with a plate dialyzer, such as the Hospal unit (41).

Of increasing popularity is the use of the pumped continuous therapies, CVVH or CVVHD (see below). These pumped systems are no longer dependent on the potentially marginal pressures and flows inherent in arterially driven circuits and can thus be successfully operated with a wider variety of filters, such as those used for standard pump-driven hemodialysis (42).

Biocompatibility

All membrane filters currently available for arterio-venous circuits are made of material considered to be relatively biocompatible when compared to cuprophane. This increased biocompatibility produces more modest treatment related leukopenia, and less marked increase in complement derived anaphylatoxins (43, 44).

Tubing

Early arteriovenous hemofiltration relied on standard dialysis tubing, shortened to minimize loss of arterial pressure. Currently, specialized tubing segments are provided as a combined set with a given hemofilter. These tubing segments are offered in a variety of configurations and should be evaluated for several features. Essential components are luer lock connectors for the hemoaccess and the hemofilter thus avoiding accidental tubing disconnections. Useful sampling ports on the arterial tubing will allow for evaluation of the patient's arterial blood, prior to and after the infusion of anticoagulant (Figures 2 and 6). Sampling ports on the venous tubing will allow for evaluation of postfilter hematocrit, coagulation status and chemistries. Separate infusion lines are often provided for the anticoagulant, but may also be available for prefilter or postfilter administration of replacement fluid.

Since resistance increases linearly with the length of the component, shortening the blood tubing provides a relatively painless way to decrease system resistance and particularly short tubing segments have been proposed by Paganini (45).

REPLACEMENT FLUID

Replacement fluid for the hemofiltration based systems are designed to normalize and maintain the patient's electrolyte and acid-base status. With continuous replacement fluid administration equalling 10 to 20 liters per day, the patient's serum will begin to mimic the formula infused. A simplified set of fluids which will allow for a near normal electrolyte balance can be attained by alternating two different solutions: 1 liter of normal saline to which is

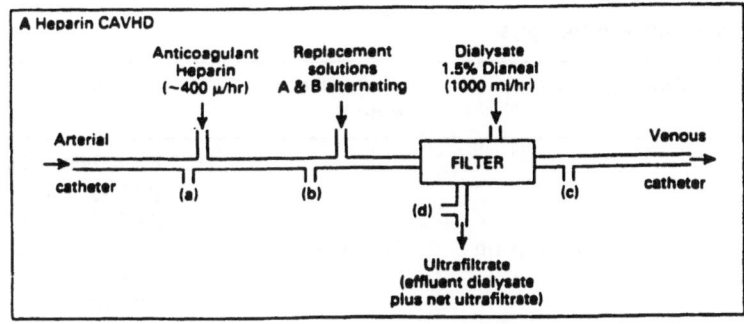

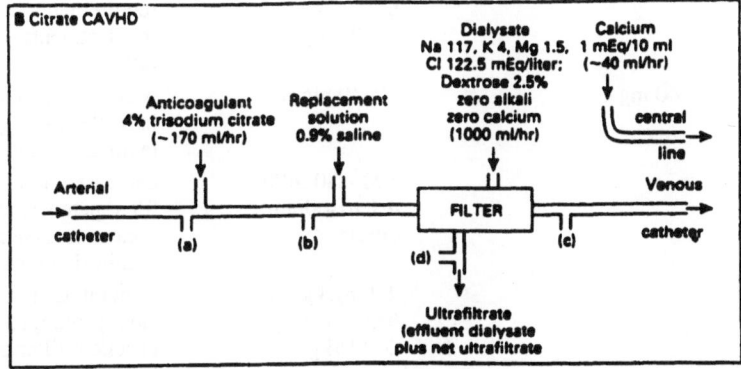

Figure 6. Comparison of circuit diagrams for heparin CAVHD (A) and citrate CAVHD (B). Sampling ports are marked (a) peripheral, (b) prefilter, (c) postfilter and (d) ultrafiltrate. Reproduced with permission from Mehta et al. (67).

added two 10 ml ampules of calcium gluconate and 1 liter of 1/2 normal saline to which is added 50 mEq of sodium bicarbonate (Table 3) (14). If hyperkalemia is not present, 3–4 mEq/l of potassium can be added to each liter to maintain normokalemia. If parenteral nutrition is employed and filtration rates are high, magnesium and phosphorus must be monitored and replaced accordingly. Ringer's lactate offers a readily available solution which has been widely used but hepatic conversion of lactate to bicarbonate may be hampered under conditions of severe hemodynamic compromise or liver failure. Olbricht et al. have reported that, compared to lactate, bicarbonate may also be advantageous by decreasing net negative nitrogen balance (46).

Dialysate

Technical modifications of the CAVH circuit which employ diffusion (CAVHD, CVVHD, see below) will require dialysate to provide buffer replacement and appropriate electrolyte balance. Standard peritoneal dialysis solution can be used and is most often employed at a rate of 1 liter per hour (38). The addition of 3 to 4 mEq (3 to 4 mEq/L) of potassium may be necessary to avoid hypokalemia. It should be kept in mind that the dextrose-rich peritoneal dialysate will result in a substantial amount of glucose transfer into the patient. These calories should

Table 3. Bedside preparation of replacement fluid used in continuous arteriovenous hemofiltration. Reproduced with permission from Kaplan et al. (14)

	Solution 1	Solution 2	Combined concentration
Sodium	154	127	140.5
Chloride	154	77	115.5
Calcium	8	–	4
Bicarbonate	–	50	25
Gluconate	8	–	4

Solution 1 is composed of 1 liter of normal saline and 2 ampules of (10%) calcium gluconate. Solution 2 is composed of 1 liter of 1/2 normal saline and 50 mEq of sodium bicarbonate. There may be small differences in the combined concentrations of both solutions due to dilution with additives (bicarbonate, calcium, etc).

be accounted for when calculating net energy requirements for hyperalimentation (see below, CAVHD) (47). In some cases of metabolic acidosis, lactate and acetate solutions may be inadequate and bicarbonate based dialysis fluid may be preferred (48).

Table 4. Anticoagulation for the continuous therapies

Method	Loading dose	Maintenance dose	Comments (see text)
Saline flush			least hemorrhagic risk, short filter patency, most successful with low platelets, short tubing and predilution
Heparin	1000–2000 U heparin	5–10 U/kg/h	standard technique, easy reversibility with protamine, risk of thrombocytopenia
Regional heparinization	1000–2000 U heparin	5–20 U/kg/h, protamine at 10–20 mg/h	reduced risk of bleeding, variable requirements for protamine, frequent readjustments of heparin/protamine ratio
LMW heparin	40 mg	10–40 mg/h	decreased risk of bleeding, prolonged half-life, incomplete reversal with protamine, specialized monitoring
Regional citrate		100–180 ml/h, 4% trisodium citrate	decreased risk of bleeding, excellent filter patency, requires diffusive component to system (CAVHD), extensive monitoring required
Prostacyclin		4–8 ng/kg/min heparin at 2–4 U/kg	difficult to monitor, risk of hypotension, prolonged action, no reversibility, excellent filter patency, often used with heparin
Nafomostate mesilate		0.1 mg/kg/h	excellent potential, limited experience

ANTICOAGULATION

In general, CAVH and its related therapies require continuous anticoagulation in order to maintain a reasonable duration of filter patency. Unfortunately, during the early application of these techniques, hemorrhagic complications were common (14, 49, 50). Considering the extreme variability in system operation (blood flows, intrafilter pressures, etc) and its highly variable kinetics, it is not surprising that the continuous administration of heparin would produce dosing difficulties previously unencountered during its use for standard hemodialysis. In response there has been a substantial effort to identify better tolerated means of maintaining filter patency. At present there is a considerable choice of anticoagulant strategies which have been applied to the continuous therapies (Table 4) (51, 52). An ideal anticoagulant regimen will provide at least 1 to 2 days of adequate filter patency, minimal systemic effect, easy monitoring, a means of rapid reversibility and minimal secondary effects. The currently available choices will be addressed below.

Heparin

Kramer et al. demonstrated that the continuous administration of 10 IU/kg/h of heparin was capable of providing adequate anticoagulation within the filter while avoiding systemic anticoagulation in the patient (53, 54). Further, it was suggested that maintaining a constant heparin dose would provide for increased anticoagulant concentrations during periods of decreased blood flow when filter clotting was more common. Kaplan et al. employing the same dosing schedule in high risk patients, reported hemorrhagic complications in 6 of 15 patients and performed protamine neutralization studies suggesting that, even at this low dose, prolonged administration could result in substantial systemic heparinization (14). Olbricht et al. adjusted the heparin infusion in order to achieve a 50% prolongation in whole blood PTT and observed a 20% bleeding rate (49). Subsequently, several dosing schedules have been proposed which usually involve a heparin rinse of the filter prior to use (5000 to 10,000 IU of heparin in 2 l of saline) and an hourly dose ranging from 250 to 1000 IU/h. Lauer et al. have proposed a dosing schedule directly related to the circuit's blood flow, a technique which may be best suited to pumped systems where blood flow can be maintained at a relatively constant rate (15).

Repetitive monitoring of prefilter and systemic anticoagulation is essential, especially when one considers the highly variable half life of heparin (45 minutes to 4.5 hours) (55) and the prolongation of half lives as the total dose administered is increased (56). Prefilter partial thromboplastin times (PTT) should be 1.5 times normal or, alternatively, activated clotting times (ACT) should be between 200 and 250 seconds. Concomitant monitoring of the patient's prothrombin time (PT) can provide evidence for a non-heparin induced endogenous coagulopathy. Golper has suggested that diluting the heparin solution will ensure a more constant delivery (57), while Shurek and Biela propose a more uniform heparin delivery using a three-way stop cock as a 'Venturi' mixing chamber (58).

Advantages to heparin include its rapid neutralization by protamine, disadvantages include highly variable kinetics and heparin induced thrombocytopenia.

Regional heparinization with protamine neutralization

The postfilter neutralization of heparin with protamine was originally proposed by Maher et al. as a means of limiting systemic anticoagulation during hemodialysis (59). The technique had lost favor due to the phenomena of heparin rebound (60, 61) and the reported risk of anaphylactoid reactions (62). Kaplan and Petrillo reconsidered its use for CAVH, noting that the slow, continuous infusion of heparin and protamine would preclude heparin rebound and would limit the risk of protamine-induced anaphylactic reactions, reported with rapid infusions of high doses. Using an initial dosing regimen of 1000 units per hour of heparin and a postfilter infusion of 10 mg/hour of protamine, the technique was capable of providing substantial anticoagulation in the filtered blood (mean PTT of 130 seconds) with minimum effect on the patient's systemic anticoagulation (63). Monitoring was performed 3 times daily with PT and PTT determinations obtained concurrently from the postheparin and postprotamine tubing and from the patient's systemic circulation (preheparin portion of the arterial tubing). Postprotamine neutralization of the heparin was limited in order to avoid venous catheter clotting. Prolonged utilization of the technique demonstrated a wide variability in protamine neutralization requirements, ranging from 0.6 to 2 mg of protamine for 100 units of heparin. In a small series of 10 high risk patients, only one developed a hemorrhagic complication. Average duration of filter patency was 41 hours.

Regional heparinization offers reasonable filter patency with decreased hemorrhagic risk. Disadavantages are the requirements for frequent monitoring and dosing modifications.

Low molecular weight heparin

Low molecular weight (LMW) fractions of heparin (4000 to 7000 Daltons) are more active in inhibiting Factor Xa and less active in inhibiting the clotting cascade as is determined by PTT. These qualities provide a basis for considering LMW heparin as an anticoagulant with increased antithrombotic effects and a decreased risk of hemorrhagic tendencies. To date, experience with the continuous therapies has been limited (54, 64). Monitoring is by measuring anti-FXa activity, a test which may not be readily available. PTT determinations are inconclusive.

Potential advantages to LMW heparin are a decrease in hemorrhagic risk. Disadvantages include a prolonged half-life (> 10 h), incomplete neutralization with protamine and limited availability of the monitoring technique.

Citrate

Citrate anticoagulation has been found to be a reasonable alternative to heparin for conventional hemodialysis, where the citrate-calcium complex can be rapidly removed by diffusion (65, 66). Modifying this technique to the rather modest diffusive capabilities of an arterio-venous circuit, Mehta et al. have employed prefilter infusion of trisodium citrate (3 to 7% of blood flow rate) neutralized by postfilter infusion of calcium chloride (67). In order to avoid citrate induced alkalosis and hypernatremia, the dialysate must be hyponatric (117 mEq/L) and devoid of alkali (Figure 6). In a comparison study of heparin *vs* citrate for CAVHD, these investigators found citrate to ensure a greater urea clearance and a more prolonged filter life (63 h *vs* 44 h). Serious bleeding developed in 30% of heparinized patients and in none of the citrate treated patients. Citrate induced alkalosis was found in 26% of patients, most commonly in those with hepatic insufficiency. Recommended monitoring involves repetitive determinations of ionized calcium and acid base status. Because of the need to remove at least some of the citrate-calcium complex, this technique seems to require a diffusive component and is most suited for CAVHD or CVVHD.

Advantages include excellent filter ptency with no systemic anticoagulation. Disadvantages include increased complexity in monitoring and risks of metabolic alkalosis and hypocalcemic induced arrhythmias.

Prostacyclin

Prostacyclin (PGI$_2$) inhibits platelet aggregation and adhesion and appears to provide substantial protection against filter clotting. It has been successfully used during standard hemodialysis and has been considered safer than heparin because of its relatively short half life (2 minutes) (68, 69). Unfortunately, its antiplatelet activity is still present 2 hours after cessation of therapy with no known means for rapid reversal. Furthermore, dosage monitoring requires platelet aggregation studies. The major secondary effect is systemic hypotension, which appears to be directly dose related. Considering the above drawbacks, it is not surprising that most of the published experience for the continuous therapies involves some combination of low dose prostacyclin, presumably to limit its hypotensive effects, and some other form of anticoagulation. Zobel et al. treated six pediatric patients with a combination of low dose heparin (2.5 to 5 IU/kg/h) and prostacyclin (4 to 8 ng/kg/min), demonstrating prolonged filter patency without bleeding or hypotension (70). Similar combinations have been reported for CAVHD (71) and CVVH (72). Using a dose of 5 to 9 ng/min/kg, Pataca et al. have used prostacyclin as a sole anticoagulant for CAVHD (73). When compared to heparin, they found no particular advantage to prostacyclin but speculated that it might provide a therapeutic advantage in patients with respiratory failure. Ponikvar et al. infused 4 ng/kg/min of prostacyclin as the sole anticoagulant for CVVH (74). At this low dose they reported no hemodynamic compromise but there was also a 30% reduction in duration of filter patency when compared to heparin.

Prostacyclin can provide excellent filter patency. Disadvantages include inconvenient monitoring, risk of hypotension and prolonged antiplatelet effect with no means for rapid reversal.

Nafamostat mesilate

Nafamostat mesilate is a serine protease inhibitor which can inhibit thrombin, factor Xa and factor XIIa. Ohtake et al. have described its use in CAVH and CAVHD using a dose of 0.1 mg/kg/h to achieve an ACT (activated clotting time) of 150 seconds (75, 76). A comparison study with heparin and low-molecular weight heparin (LMWH) demonstrated a 67% incidence of bleeding with heparin, a 29% incidence with LMWH and a 5% incidence with nafamostat mesilate. Duration of filter patency was not reported. Half life is reported to be between 5 and 8 minutes. Further study is warranted but has been hindered due to limited availability.

Non-anticoagulated techniques

Considering the common occurrence of endogenous coagulopathies, several authors have attempted to maintain reasonable filter patency without anticoagulation. Using the predilution mode for fluid replacement (see below), Kaplan et al. found adequate filter patency could be maintained without anticoagulation if the platelet counts were less than 100,000 mm^3 (14). In contrast, preexisting elevations in the partial thromboplastin time (PTT), without thrombocytopenia, did not protect against filter clotting. Smith et al. were successful in providing no-heparin SCUF and CAVH in patients with either thrombocytopenia or elevations in the prothrombin time (PT) (77). Paganini has speculated that these results may have been possible due to shortened tubing and has demonstrated similar success in patients having undergone open heart surgery (78). In a recent preliminary report involving CVVH, Martin et al. found thrombocytopenia to be the only parameter predicting success without using an anticoagulant (79).

Antithrombotic circuits

A recent development has been the production of a particularly antithrombotic circuit which combines a poly- acrylonitrile (PAN)-polyethyleneoxide (PEO) membrane with ionically bound heparin-coated catheters, tubing and modular headers. In unheparinized dogs, the system has provided continuous system patency for a mean 458 hours (40). In 15 patients, these circuits remained patent for a mean 26 hours, with a range of 5 to 216 hours (80).

TECHNICAL MODIFICATIONS

Slow continuous ultrafiltration (SCUF)

In 1980, Paganini and Nakamoto employed blood pressure driven filtration as a means of providing continuous, isosmotic fluid removal for aid in the management of oliguric patients (8). Using shortened dialysis tubing, an Amicon 20 Diafilter was placed in series with a Quinton–Scribner shunt producing a mean 220 ml/h of filtrate. Although intermittent hemodialysis was still required for solute removal, the authors were able to maintain stable blood pressure despite removal of approximately 3000 ml of fluid. Further observations with this technique demonstrated its utility as a means of maintaining fluid balance in patients intolerant of aggressive fluid removal and in those with cardiodynamic instability such as seen during aortic balloon pumping or during open heart surgery (78, 81–85).

Suction-assisted CAVH

In an attempt to increase the filtration rates of the CAVH system without resorting to a blood pump, Kaplan et al. increased the transmembrane pressure by producing a pumped negative pressure on the filtrate outflow port (86). Using vacuum outlets in the ICU designed for nasogastric or endotracheal aspiration, 200 mmHg of negative pressure was added to the filtrate port. This approach virtually doubled filtration rates but at a cost of significantly increasing net filtration fractions and creating a risk of aggressively high hemoconcentration. Although this difficulty can be easily overcome with the predilution mode of fluid replacement (see below), other disadvantages to this system include the loss of the 'self-limited' fluid removal which was an inherent feature of the blood pressure driven system. Thus, applications of suction-assist required increased blood pressure surveillence. Nonetheless, several authors have found this technique to provide a simple means for enhancing filtration rates under conditions of insufficient blood flows and inadequate solute removal (14, 87, 88). A useful extension of this technique consists of placing a constant infusion pump on the filtrate line in order to provide the negative pressure while at the same time controlling the rate of filtrate removal. Using several combinations of this procedure, Golper et al. demonstrated that transmembrane pressures never exceeded 150 mmHg, despite pump settings as high as 900 ml/h (89).

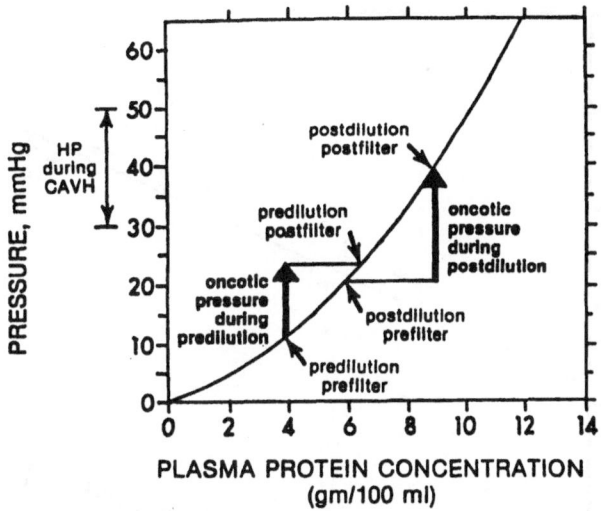

Figure 7. Range of oncotic pressures seen during CAVH. The conditions generated by the postdilution mode are contrasted with the conditions generated by the predilution mode. These oncotic pressures can be compared to the hydrostatic pressures (HP) within the filter. During the postdilution mode, the oncotic pressures generated by increasing protein concentrations can attain values capable of negating the hydrostatic pressure which favors filtration. Predilution reduces oncotic pressures allowing for continued net filtration. Reproduced with permission from Kaplan (93).

Predilution

The infusion of replacement fluid into the prefilter tubing segment of the circuit had been proposed by Henderson for use with machine driven hemofiltration (90). *In-vitro* (91) and *in-vivo* (92) evaluation of the predilution technique demonstrated that the prefilter dilution of urea plasma promoted the transfer of intraerythrocytic urea into the plasma compartment where it would be available for removal in the filtrate. Considering filtrate limiting increases in oncotic pressure and hemoconcentration resulting from the use of suction-assisted CAVH (see above), Kaplan applied the predilution mode to offset these difficulties. In an *in vivo* crossover study of CAVH without suction assist, the predilution mode increased net filtrate outputs by 22% and, despite an approximate 15% dilution of the filtrate with predilution fluid, there was a net 18% increase in urea clearance (93). The potential benefits in avoiding filtration equilibrium (see above, Figure 4) are depicted graphically in Figure 7. Although some authors have been unable to document an increased efficiency with the predilution mode, the amount of predilution fluid administered was limited (36). Studies combining the predilution mode with suction-assisted CAVH (Figure 2b) demonstrated a markedly enhanced efficiency with filtrate outputs averaging 1300 ml/h and net urea clearances of more than 18 ml/min (94–96). The potential advantages of the predilution mode include enhanced urea clearance and the possibility of increasing filter patency by the prefilter dilution of hematocrit, clotting factors and platelets. Disadvantages include the increased cost of replacement fluid

and the dilution of the filtrate chemistries when compared to the plasma levels.

Continuous arterio-venous hemodialysis/hemodiafiltration (CAVHD)

In 1984, Geronemus and Schneider proposed a modification to the CAVH circuit which added a diffusive component in order to enhance urea clearance (97). The circuit is essentially the same as that for CAVH with the addition of a constant infusion of dialysate into the filtrate compartment of the filter (Figure 2c). At the relatively slow blood flow rates encountered with an arterio-venous circuit, complete equilibrium of urea and creatinine is achieved (98) and clearance rates increase linearly with dialysis fluid flow rates up to 33.3 ml/min (2 l/h) (47). Further increases in dialysate flow do not allow for complete equilibrium but clearances can still be enhanced and dialysate flows up to 4 l/h can yield urea clearances of 49 ml/min (47). In most clinical situations, however, dialysate flow rate is set at 1 l/h yielding an approximate 17 ml/min of urea clearance by diffusion. Further operational characteristics were elucidated by Sigler and Teehan who demonstrated that the additional diffusive clearance was completely independent from the amount of net filtration (Figure 8) (38). A preliminary report suggested that a flat plate dialyzer may be best for this modality (41) but successful treatments are clearly obtainable with the hollow fiber configuration. The major advantage to this system is the enhanced solute clearance and there is a substantial amount of published experience demonstrating its utility in the treatment of the critically ill patient (71, 99–

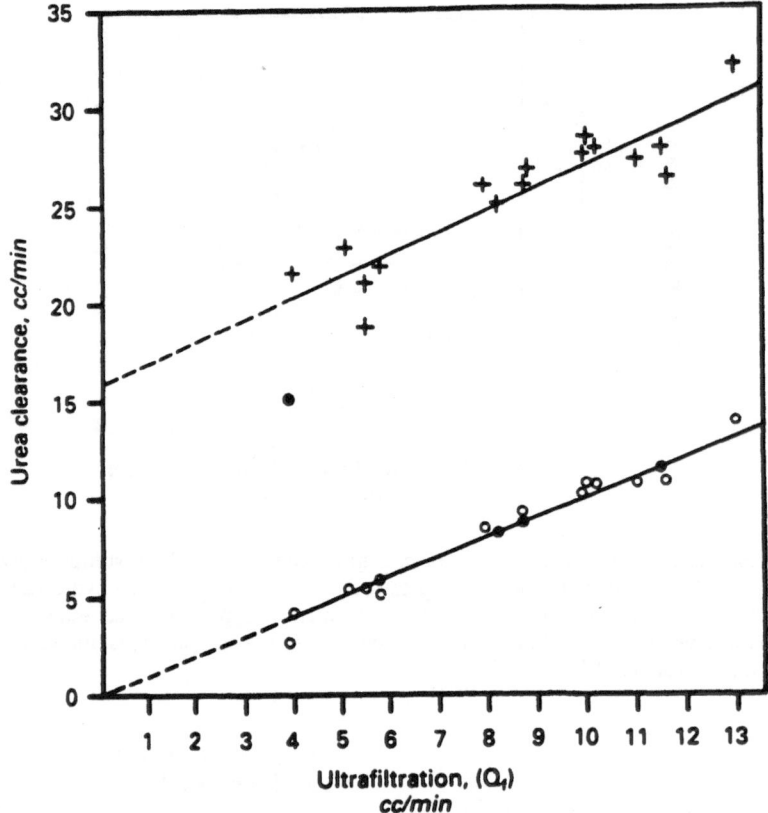

Figure 8. Whole blood urea clearance versus ultrafiltration rate. Each total clearance (+) has its corresponding convective component (o) plotted directly under it on the lower line. The distance between the two lines represents clearance by diffussion. Dialysate was infused at a rate of 1 l/h (16.6 ml/min). Reproduced with permission from Sigler et al. (38).

104). The substantially enhanced clearance capabilities has also allowed the technique to be applied to certain intoxications (105, 106).

An interesting issue is the amount and nature of back-filtration which can occur with this technique. Bonnardeaux et al. noted that about 60% of the dialysate's glucose can be absorbed through a poylacrylonitrile (PAN) hollow fiber membrane (47). At the common flow rate of 1 l/h, a standard 1.5% dextrose containing dialysis fluid produced a net glucose transfer averaging 120 mg/min (175 gm/day) while a 4.25% solution would yield 415 mg/min (600 gm/day). It is obvious that these amounts of carbohydrate infusions must be accounted for when considering the patient's nutritional and insulin requirements. Although Golper and Leone confirmed the backfiltration of glucose and inulin in an *in-vitro* model employing a PAN membrane, they found no backfiltration of either inulin nor glucose through a polysulphone membrane (107). A possible explanation is that the asymmetric polysulphone was not as conducive to diffusion from the filtrate compartment into the blood compartment. Although an increasing number of membranes have been found to allow sufficient blood to dialysate diffusion

(108), the amount and size limitations of backfiltration remains unclear.

Continuous veno-venous hemofiltration (CVVH)

In an attempt to eliminate the need for arterial access and provide more predictable filtrate outputs, several investigators have initiated the use of continuous veno-venous hemofiltration (109–115). The circuit requires a blood pump and an air detector and is often equipped with arterial and venous pressure monitors (Figure 2d). This technique has the clear advantage of avoiding the potential complications of arterial access and is capable of providing an almost limitless amount of convection-based clearance. The relatively rapid blood flow rates, commonly above 150 ml/min, allow for decreased filter clotting and limit the dosage requirement for anticoagulants. In a comparison study of conventional CAVH and CVVH, Storck et al. found that the pumped system was associated with an increased net filtration (16 l/day *vs* 7 l/day) and an improved overall survival (29% *vs* 13%) (114). Although the authors employed none of the available techniques for increasing solute clearance with arterially driven circuits (CAVHD, predilution and suction-assist, see above), the results did demonstrate that daily filtration rates under 7.5 liters were less likely to be associated with survival than rates of 15 liters or more. In another study, comparing CAVH and CAVHD to pump driven CVVH. Macias et al. reported decreased hemorrhagic and vascular complications (115).

In the United States there has been resistance from the ICU nursing staff to take on the added responsibility of a pump driven circuit. This difficulty can be overcome by allowing shared responsibility for the circuit's maintenance, with dialysis personnel priming the circuit and providing advice on troubleshooting the system (115).

Continuous veno-venous hemodialysis/hemodiafiltration (CVVHD)

The addition of a diffusive component to the CVVH system allows for the maximum clearance capabilities of any of the continuous therapies. The basic circuit resembles that of CVVH (Figure 2d) but allows a variable amount of dialysate to flow past the filtrate compartment of the filter. The machines utilized are similar to those employed for CVVH (see below) but several more innovative circuits have been proposed (117–119). In a prospective study of 53 patients, Bellomo et al. compared CAVHD with CVVHD and found no significant difference in urea clearance (33 l/day *vs* 37 l/day) nor in survival (43% *vs* 52%) (120). There was, however, a substantial difference in the number of vascular access complications (10 *vs* 2).

Pumped systems for the continuous therapies

Although the pumped continuous therapies were originally performed with standard dialysis monitors and roller pumps (Renal Systems, Redy 2000, Drake Willock, etc) (Figure 9) there are currently two commercially available machines specifically designed for these treatments. The Hospal BSM-22 and the Baxter BM-11. The Hospal unit strongly resembles the Gambro AK-10 and has an additional roller pump which can be used for the infusion of dialysate or replacement fluid or to control the ultrafiltration rate (116). The Baxter BM-11 resembles an ICU infusion pump and may therefore elicit a less negative response from uninitiated ICU staff. A comparison of these two machines found them to be comparable in blood flows (up to 300 ml/min) and maximum filtration rates (121).

CLINCIAL MANAGEMENT

Nitrogen balance and treatment prescription

Studies regarding the prophylactic prescription of dialytic therapy suggest that maintaining blood urea nitrogen (BUN) at or below 100 to 120 mg/dl improves survival in acute renal failure (122–125). Supporting this concept

of 'adequate' urea clearance, a recent study comparing pumped (CVVH) and non-pumped (CAVH) treatments demonstrated statistically improved survival as urea clearance increased from less than 7.5 to more than 15 liters per day, regardless of the technique employed (114). Given the above considerations, it is often useful to calculate the urea nitrogen appearance (UNA) and determine the amount of urea clearance required to maintain the BUN at or below 100 mg/dl. Under conditions of neutral nitrogen balance, the UNA depends on protein ingestion and can be calculated as follows:

$$UNA = protein\ (g/day)/6.25 - NUN$$

assuming every 6.25 g of protein contains 1 g of nitrogen and that the daily production of non-urea nitrogen (NUN) is 31 mg/kg/day of lean body mass (126). The minimum amount of urea clearance required to remove a given amount of UNA can be calculated using the formula:

$$Urea\ clearance\ (l/day) = [UNA\ (mg/day)]/[BUN\ (mg/l)]$$

Using the above formulae, a 70 kg patient receiving 1 g/kg/d protein will ingest 11 g of nitrogen (70 g/6.25). Approximately 2 g will form nitrogenous wastes other than urea (NUN = 70 kg × 31 mg/kg/day), while the remaining 9 g will form urea. For a continuous therapy, assuming a stable BUN of 100 mg/dl, this amount of urea nitrogen will be removed wth a urea clearance of 9 liters per day (127). Kramer has created a nomogram which assumes neutral nitrogen balance and predicts the resultant BUN with a given amount of amino acid infusion (Figure 10). A clinical example of the dependence of BUN on protein nitrogen intake is depicted in Figure 11.

The above calculations will work reasonably well when the patient exhibits neutral nitrogen balance. Under conditions of negative nitrogen balance, when the patient is catabolising endogenous protein, UNA can greatly exceed the amount calculated from ingested protein. Under these conditions, UNA can be determined using the formula:

$$UNA = [(BUN_2 - BUN_1)] \times TBW + UN$$

where BUN_1 and BUN_2 are determined at the initiation and termination of a 24 hour urine collection; TBW equals total body water in liters, estimated as 60% of lean body mass plus the amount of extra edema fluid; and UUN is the urea nitrogen found in the 24 hour urine collection. If a continuous therapy is already in progress, the total amount of urea removed within the same 24 hour period is added to the UUN.

Nutrition

The impressive fluid removal capabilities of the continuous therapies allow for a voluminous nutritional support without the fluid balance oscillations inherent with intermittent techniques. Thus it is not surprising that attempts

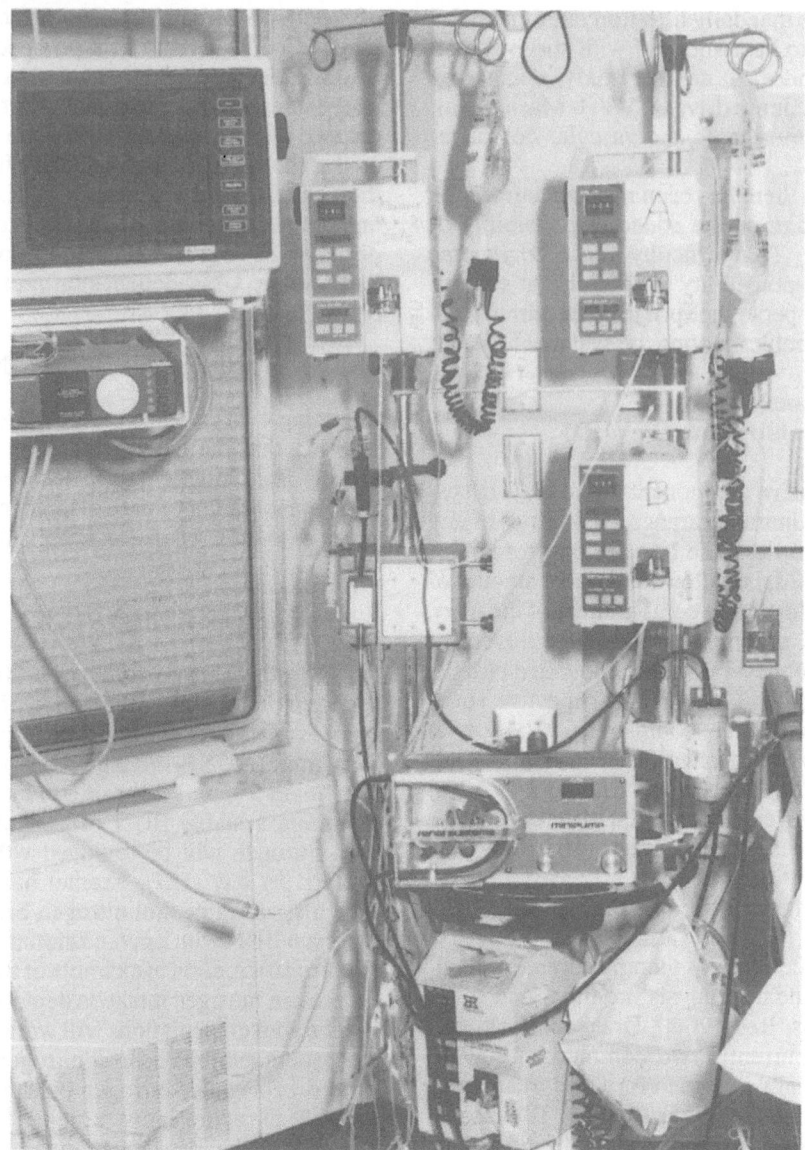

Figure 9. Continuous veno-venous hemofiltration: The entire CVVH apparatus is contained on a single support stand. The circuit consists of arterial venous blood tubing (Travenol 5M 4033, Baxter Travenol, Deerfield, IL) and a hemofilter (Amicon D-20, Amicon Division of WR Grace & Co, Danvers, MA). Blood flow throught the circuit is generated by a roller blood pump (RS-7800, Minntech, Minneapolis, MN). Ultrafiltrate production is regulated by an infusion pump (attached to the lower portion of the support stand). The replacement fluids, delivered by the infusion pumps labeled A and B and heparin are administered via a prepump infusion port. A bubble/foam detector with blood line clamp (RS-3220A, Minntech) is attached to the venous drip chamber and blood line. The pressure within the circuit is measured by a standard hemodynamic pressure transducer and the in-unit monitor (upper left corner). Photo kindly provided by Drs WR Clark and WL Macias.

to compare the continuous therapies to standard hemodialysis often involve an assessment of each modality's ability to allow for sufficient nutritional support (128–130). Originally, using the standard CAVH circuit, nitrogen waste removal was often insufficient in the hypercatabolic patient. Currently, the available technical modifications provide an almost limitless capability (in terms of urea

clearance) and compare very favorably to the most aggressive intermittent prescriptions (Table 5) (131–132).

Aside from providing the volume removal to allow for the 2 to 3 liters of hyperalimentation which may be required, several continuous techniques can provide significant caloric infusion as a result of the replacement fluid or dialysis fluid employed (47) (see above, CAVHD). In contrast, one must also be aware of amino acid and glucose

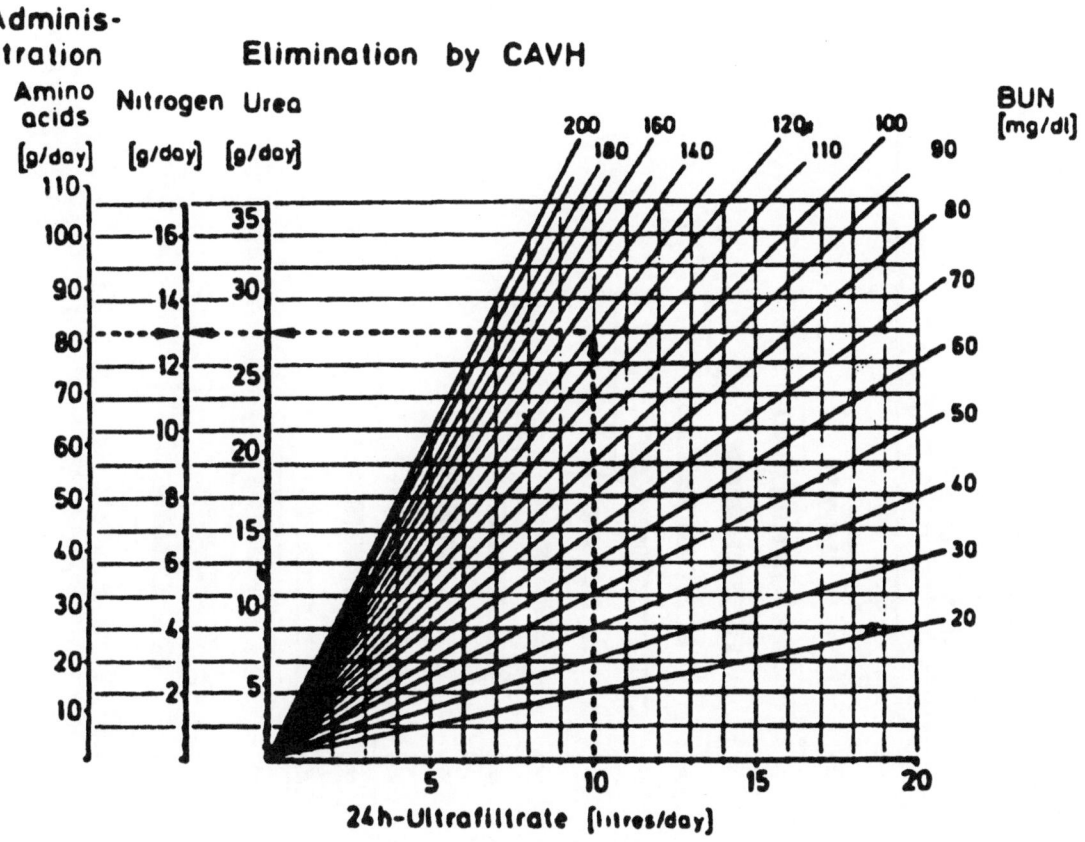

Figure 10. resultant urea nitrogen level in mg/dl as a function of the 24 hour filtrate production in liters per day and the total amino acid administration in grams per day. The normogram assumes neutral nitrogen balance. To convert from mg/dl BUN to millimoles per liter urea, divide by 2.8. Reproduced with permission from Kramer et al. (133).

Table 5. Time averaged urea clearance for renal replacement therapies

Technique	Prescription	Urea clearance		
		ml/min	l/d	l/wk
Hemodialysis[a]	3 × 4 hr/wk	14.3	21	144
	7 × 4 hr/wk	33.3	48	336
Peritoneal dialysis	2 l/h	16.7	24	168
CAVH	14 l/h	6.9	10	70
CAVH (enhanced)[b]	24 l/h	9.7	14	98
CAVHD[c]	1–2 l/h[d]	19–35	27–51	189–357
CVVH	1–2 l/h	17–33	24–48	168–336
CVVHD[c]	1–2 l/h[d]	19–35	27–51	189–357

[a] Assumes urea clearance of 200 ml/min.
[b] With vacuum suction on filtrate port and predilution infusion.
[c] Assumes 3 l/d net filtrate.
[d] Infused dialysate.

losses which are directly related to the net solute clearance provided by a given therapy and which can amount to substantial negative values if not accounted for and replaced (81, 133–135). For example, during the infusion of hyperalimentation, Paganini et al. measured an approximate 4 g amino acid loss with SCUF therapy providing a modest 4 liters per day of filtrate (81), while Sigler et al. demonstrated a loss of 15 g/d during CAVHD delivering a net clearance of 30 liters per day (134). Finally the net protein loss should be considered, which has been measured to be 77 mg/dl of filtrate (14) and which might amount to 18 g/d in a hemofiltration circuit operating at 1 liter per hour. Of note is that protein losses have not been measured in the continuous therapies involving a diffusive component (CAVHD and CVVHD).

Drug clearances

Although there are increasing data regarding drug kinetics during CAVH (105, 136–143), this has not been measured for most medications. Therefore the clinician should consider the factors which govern removal and potential dosage adjustments of drugs. Four major factors which must be considered: molecular weight; the degree of protein binding; the drug's volume of distribution and the

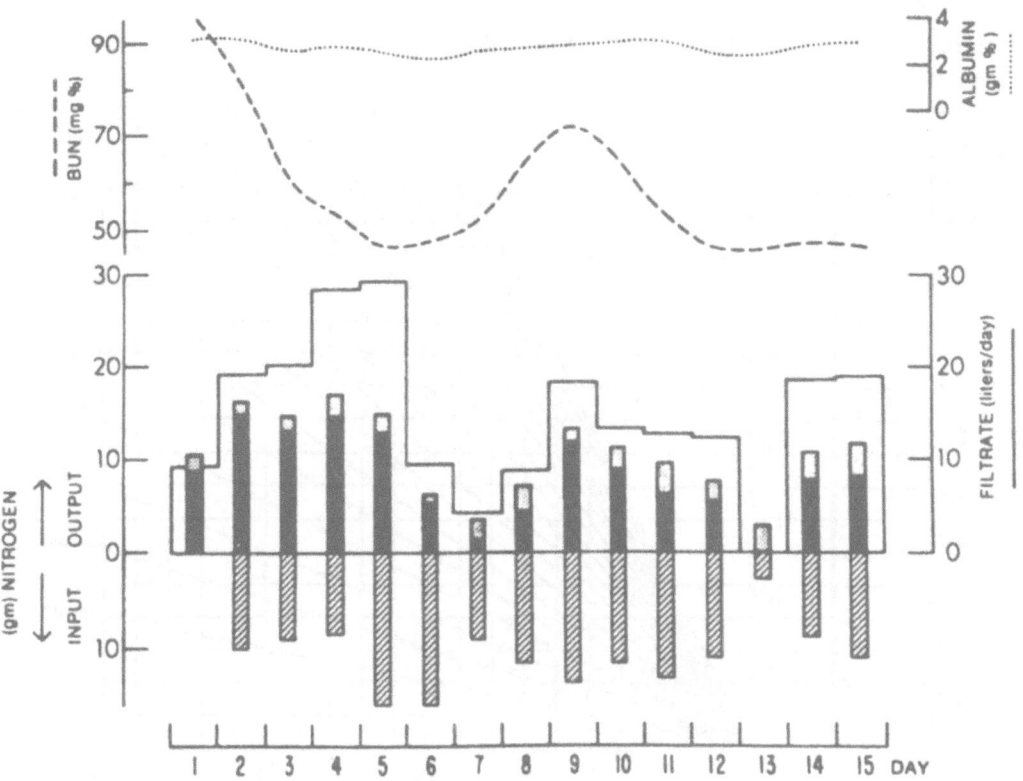

Figure 11. Urea nitrogen balance in a 35 year old man with postsurgical acute renal failure, cirrhosis and septic shock. Parenteral nutrition is represented below the abscissa as vertical bars and is given as grams of nitrogen (10 g of nitrogen = 65 g of amino acids). Urea nitrogen removal is represented by vertical bars above the abscissa. The black area represents urea removal through filtration; the speckeled area represents urea removal through residual renal function. Filtration rate is represented by the wide clear bars above the abscissa. Replacement fluid rate is not shown but was approximately equal to the filtrate output. Note that the blood urea nitrogen (BUN) level declined steadily over the first few days as urea nitrogen removal exceeded nitrogen input (dashed line). The BUN level then rose slightly when filtration rates dropped and urea removal failed to match nitrogen input. Despite daily infusions of between 60 and 100 g of amino acids, BUN levels remained between 50 to 70 mg/dl until return of adequate renal function. To convert from mg/dl BUN to millimoles per liter urea, divide by 2.8. Reproduced with permission from Kaplan et al. (14).

drug's endogenous clearance. Aside from these factors, which will be discussed below, the clinician must consider the efficiency of the system being employed. If a drug is removable by a continuous filtration technique, the net clearance provided must be ascertained. Clearly, the amount of drug removed by 10 liters of filtrate from a CAVH circuit will not equal that which is removed by 50 liters of filtrate provided by CVVH. The multiple factors which must be considered and the great interpatient variability in drug metabolism renders periodically obtained blood levels to be invaluable when dealing with medications of narrow therapeutic index.

Molecular weight

Although small increments in molecular weight might have a great effect in limiting the diffusibility of a drug by standard dialytic technique, the convective mode of transport inherent in the CAVH procedure will allow unimpeded flow of solutes up to a limit of 5 to 10,000 Daltons. Thus, molecular weight is unlikely to have a substantial effect in limiting removability during hemofiltration based procedures. An exception might be the use of genetically engineered proteins (i.e., erythropoietin, cytokine receptor antagonists) whose molecular weights approach values which may exceed several thousand Daltons. It should be kept in mind that some drugs, like vancomycin (1400 Daltons) which are classically considered to be 'non-dialyzable' because of their size may be easily removed by filtration. Similarly, the relatively slow blood flows of the CAVHD circuit may allow for the sieving of larger molecular weight solutes than would normally be removed during standard machine driven dialysis.

Degree of protein binding

Most drug binding proteins (albumin, specific binding proteins, etc) are larger than the 10,000 Dalton limit of

Table 6. Drug sieving coefficients

Drug	Sieving coefficient[a] UF/P
Amikacin	0.88
Amphotericin	0.40
Ampicillin	0.69
Cefoperazone	0.27 (140)
Cefotaxime	0.51
Cefoxitin	0.64 (139)
Ceftazidime	0.70 (140)
Ceftriaxone	0.71
Cefuroxime	0.86 (140)
Ceftizoxime	0.63 (140)
Cephapirin	1.48 (137)
Ceftriaxone	0.73 (140)
Clindamycin	0.98
Digoxin	0.96
Erythromycin	0.37
Gentamicin	0.81
Imipenem	0.80 (142)
Metronidazole	0.86
Moxalactam	0.44 (140)
Nafcillin	0.54
Oxacillin	0.02
Phenytoin	0.45
Procainamide	0.86
Procainamide (*n*-acetyl)	0.92
Ranitidine	0.74 (139)
Streptomycin	0.30
Theophyline	0.85
Thiocyanate	1.07 (137)
Tobramycin	0.78
Valproic acid	0.18 (138)
Vancomycin	0.76

[a] Sieving coefficient defined as concentration in the ultrafiltrate (UF) divided by the concentration in the plasma (*P*). Values may vary with different membranes (138).
All values are from Golper et al. (136), except where noted in parentheses.

most hemofilters and the percentage of a drug which is protein bound is not available for removal. Golper et al., as well as others have published lists of drug 'sieving coefficients' (136–140) which are defined as the percentage of the drug's plasma level which can be found in the filtrate (Table 6). For the most part (ignoring membrane adsorption), the percentage of the plasma drug concentration which passes through a hemofilter *is* the non-protein bound fraction. Thus, if the specific sieving coefficient for a given drug has not been published, it can be reasonably estimated by ascertaining its percentage protein binding.

Factors which may affect protein binding include serum albumin, free fatty acids, bilirubin and uremia, which can either enhance or decrease protein binding. It should be noted that a high sieving coefficient (approaching one) is not, in itself, sufficient to suggest clinically significant drug removal, since the volume of distribution and the drug's endogenous clearance may be an overiding limiting factor (see below).

Using the sieving coefficients, the net amount of drug removed by a given filtration treatment can be calculated by multiplying the drug's plasma level by its sieving coefficient and multiplying the resulting value by the net amount of ultrafiltration.

Volume of distribution

Drugs with low water solubility, high lipid affinity or membrane receptor interaction may be highly concentrated within cells or on cell membranes. These drugs will have large 'apparent' volumes of distribution, well in excess of total body water (0.6 l/kg). Assuming first order kinetics, removal of 50% of a drug's accumulation (i.e., its half-life) will require a drug clearance of approximately 0.7 times its volume of distribution (136). A case in point is digoxin, which has a rather modest degree of protein binding and thus a high sieving coefficient of 0.9. Despite this, its net removal by CAVH is minimal, since its apparent volume of distribution is 5 l/kg, or approximately 350 liters in a 70 kg patient. Thus it would take approximately 245 liters (350 × 0.7) of exogenous clearance in order to lower its level by 50%; its endogenous hepatic metabolism far exceeds its meager removal by any blood purification technique.

Endogenous clearance

Drugs which undergo rapid extrarenal clearance (hepatic metabolism, enzymatic degradation, etc) are unlikely to be greatly affected by renal replacement therapies. This is the case of several of the continuously administered vasoactive catecholamines (dopamine, norepinephrine and epinephrine) which were found not to be substantially affected by either CAVHD or CVVHD, despite a substantal clearance of approximately 45 ml/min (141). An interesting complicating factor is that the non-renal clearance of some drugs may be different in acute renal failure when compared to their published values obtained in chronic renal failure, e.g., imipenem (142).

Simplified method of drug dosing

Since most drugs are eliminated by glomerular filtration rate (GFR) and since the filters used are similar in sieving to the functioning glomerulus, a reasonable starting point is to determine the normal recommendations for dosing in renal failure (143, 144) and consider the day's total filtrate as equivalent to the GFR and adjust accord-

Table 7. Complications

Technique related
Anticoagulation associated hemorrhage
Improper fluid balance: hypotension/fluid overload
Hyponatremia
Hyperglycemia
Hyperlactemia
Hypothermia
Circuit related
Tubing disconnect
Improper fluid administration
Filter rupture and blood leak
Air embolism
Access related
Hemorrhage
Thrombosis
Pulmonary embolus
Infection: sepsis/cellulitis
Arterial occlusion
Distal ischemia

ingly (145). For the diffusion based treatments, such as CAVHD, the situation is somewhat more complicated and requires determination of ongoing solute clearance.

COMPLICATIONS

Complications seen with the continuous therapies can be subdivided into three major catogories; technique related, circuit related and access related (Table 7). Of those related directly to the technique, *anticoagulation associated hemorrhage* is clearly the most onerous and most often reported (14, 49, 50, 82). It should be noted that the patients treated with these techniques are often the most likely to develop endogenous coagulopathies which may not be easily distinguishable from those induced by the treatment's anticoagulation. Several methods have been employed in order to minimize the risk of hemorrhage and these alternative methodologies should be considered when treating the high-risk patient (see above, anticoagulation). The particular risks of each type of anticoagulant should also be considered, such as heparin induced thrombocytopenia, prostacyclin induced hypotension or citrate induced alkalosis or hypocalcemia.

It is obvious that hypotension can result if large filtrate outputs are not matched with sufficient replacement fluid, particularly with the pump driven systems or when employing suction-assist on an arterially driven circuit. Similarly, fluid overload and pulmonary congestion can occur if replacement fluids exceed output. Less obvious, but not surprising considering the large amounts of fluids exchanged per day (10 to 25 liters), is that *improper fluid balance* can occur as a result of inaccurate monitoring, or as a result of minor, but repeated inaccuracies, in the measurement in the collection apparatus. Thus an apparently minor 5 to 10% error in the accuracy of the output measurement can easily translate into a 1 to 2 liter error in daily balance. When using automated measuring devices, it is advisable to validate hourly outputs by some manual means (weighing of a standard container). In order to minimize this problem, weight balancing devices which match the rate of replacement fluid administration to that of the ultrafiltration rate have been developed (58, 147). In any event, there is never any substitute for appropriate and repeated clinical evaluation of the patient's fluid status.

Hyponatremia has been reported as a result of combining hyponatric dialysate (132 mEq/L) and a sodium restricted parenteral nutrition (34). Similarly, large volumes or dextrose containing replacement fluid or dialysate may lead to *hyperglycemia* requiring supplemental insulin. *Hyperlactemia or metabolic acidosis* may result if the patient cannot metabolize large amounts of lactate or acetate (48, 148).

When large volumes are exchanged rapidly (1 to 2 liters per hour) there is a risk of systemic *hypothermia*, and gentle warming of the solutions is advisable.

As with the application of any renal replacement therapy, continued removal without adequate supplementation may result in *hypokalemia, hypocalcemia, hypophosphatemia* or *hypomagnesemia*, especially when the patient is maintained with parenteral nutrition. With some elements, the replacement solution can be formulated to contain sufficient quantities to assure proper levels such as with potassium or calcium (see above: replacement solutions). With other elements, daily replacement in the parenteral nutrition will be adequate, such as with phosphorus, magnesium or water soluble vitamins.

During the early application of CAVH, makeshift tubing connections allowed for the accidental *disconnection* from hemoaccess or filter. Currently all the commercially available devices and filter sets are made with luer lock type connections to avoid this possibility. Despite the relatively low transmembrane pressures inherent in the CAVH circuit, early experience reported a small but definite incidence of filter blood leaks (14, 82, 87) even without the use of suction-assist. This problem seems to have been successfully addressed by the manufacturer.

Air embolism has not been reported as a complication of CAVH or its related therapies. Nonetheless, the risk should be considered especially when employing one of the myriad of innovative circuits employing a blood pump. As with any pumped system, a bubble detector is an absolute requirement.

Percutaneous cannulation of the femoral vessels presents the possibility of local or retroperitoneal hemorrhage, arteriovenous fistula and nerve damage. Prolonged vessel cannulation can lead to thrombosis, cellulitis, sepsis and embolisation including pulmonary embolus. Arterial cannulation presents the added possibility of ischemia and necrosis of sites distal to the access. In a review of their experience with cannulations of up to 50 days, Kramer et al. found that the use of specially shortened catheters and a regimented administration of heparin was helpful in reducing the incidence of arterial or femoral thrombosis (133). Quinton–Scribner shunts provide their own list of difficulties, including repeated clotting, infection and distal ischemia. Although the list of access complications is impressive, reports of severe complications have been limited. In a series of 300 femoral cannulations, Grone and Kramer reported only 2 serious complications (149). In contrast, less serious complications occur more frequently. Bellomo et al. reported an incidence of 10 access related complications in 28 patients receiving arterio-venous cannulation for CAVHD *vs* only 2 complications with 25 patients given double lumen venous cannulation for CVVHD (120).

Finally, the ease and rapidity by which CAVH can provide fluid removal may result in *inadequate diagnostic measures* for determining the cause of the renal failure, such as might occur by ignoring renal obstruction (150).

SPECIAL INDICATIONS

Neonates/pediatrics

Although peritoneal dialysis remains the mainstay of renal replacement therapy in the neonate, abdominal surgeries, abdominal wall malformations and peritoneal infections may render this technique difficult or impossible. Ronco and associates have clearly demonstrated the usefulness of CAVH as an alternative therapy which can provide continuous fluid and electrolyte management with filtration rates as low as 40 ml per hour (31, 151–153). Filtration was provided by an ultrasmall minifilter (Amicon Minifilter $0.015\,m^2$, Table 2) which can operate with minimal blood flows. Arterial access can be obtained from the umbilical, femoral or brachial arteries using 18 to 20 gauge cannulas which are shortened to the minimum length necessary. Jugular or umbilical veins were used for venous access. Zobel et al. have successfully applied the technique to a neonate weighing only 1.3 kg using a 20 gauge cannula in the brachial artery and a 4 French cannula in the internal jugular, obtaining 14 ml/h of ultrafiltrate (28). In the same report, these authors described their successful experience with vascular access and filters of varying dimensions. Aside from the Amicon Minifilter, other filters employed were the Gambro U2000 ($0.1\,m^2$), the Amicon D-10 ($0.2\,m^2$) and the Amicon D-20 ($0.25\,m^2$). Choice of access is critical and is clearly limited by the vessels available Jenkins et al. have demonstrated a 39% vari-

ability in the internal diameter of commercially available catheters of minimal size (less than 2.0 mm, 5 French), yielding variations in blood flow of up to 370% (29). As previously described in adults (see above), predilution and suction-assist has been found to be useful for increasing filtration rates without significant negative effects (35, 154). In contrast, despite the use of suction-assist with the Amicon Minifilter, Leone et al. were not able to obtain useful outputs and substituted a standard Amicon D-20 in infants as small as 5.4 kg (155). In a direct comparison of the minifilter and the larger filter, in a circuit which was limited to a 27 ml volume, filtration rates increased from 4.5 ml/h to 40 ml per hour. Other technical modifications include CAVHD which tripled the small solute clearance provided by CAVH and was successful in treating hyperkalemia in a 3.5 kg neonate (156) and CVVHD which was associated with decreased heparin requirements (157).

Multiple organ failure and cytokine removal

The convective based solute transport of the CAVH treatment fueled speculation that this type of therapy might be advantageous in removing middle-molecular weight toxins which were felt to induce the instability and organ failure of the critically ill. In 1984, Coraim et al. studied patients having undergone cardiac surgery and demonstrated the existence of a 1000 Dalton myocardial depressant factor (MDF) which could inhibit *in-vitro* preparations of guinea pig papillary muscle (158). Chromatographic and pharmacologic studies confirmed the existence of this factor in the filtrate during treatment with CAVH and concurrent assessment demonstrated an improvement in cardiac function. There was, however, no data regarding the serum levels of this substance and the clinical improvement in cardiac function may have been related to a normalization in Starling forces (159). A follow up study did demonstrate a 50% decline in serum levels of MDF one hour after initiation of CAVH (160). It is unlikely, however, that this change could be achieved by one hour of filtration and this rapid decrease in serum levels is more suggestive of either filter-membrane adsorption or a decline in production.

Tumor necrosis factor (TNF) is a cytokine often implicated in the initiation of the inflammatory response and has a molecular weight of 17,000 Daltons. Bellomo et al. studied twelve septic patients and were able to demonstrate that continuous hemodiafiltration could provide a mean 27 liters per day of TNF clearance, but changes in serum levels were minimal (161). Subsequently Cottrell and Mehta presented preliminary data suggesting that the AN69 polyacrylonitrile membrane was capable of TNF adsorption (162). Once again, however, their *in-vitro* system demonstrated little change in 'serum' levels.

Using a variety of animal models, several other investigators have attempted to demonstrate the possible adavantages of the continuous therapies in the removal of inflammatory mediators (163, 164) and the subject has recently undergone extensive review (165). Of these, the most convincing data is provided by Grootendorst and colleagues demonstrating that 6 liters per hour of zero-balance filtration could remove a myocardial depressant factor from pigs in septic shock (166–168). It remains to be seen whether this amount of convective solute transfer can be practically provided to the human patient.

Regardless of whether the continuous therapies can provide clinically relevant removal of inflammatory mediators, the advantages in clinical management offered by these techniques have spurred their use in the treatment of multiple organ failure (10, 14, 27, 34, 43, 49, 71–73, 103, 111–115, 128, 129, 169–171). Although overall results are encouraging, there remains considerable controversy as to whether these treatments offer a significant advantage in mortality when compared to conventional dialytic modalities (see below).

Non-renal uses

Congestive heart failure

The well tolerated fluid removal capabilities of the continuous therapies have prompted their use in the management of patients with congestive heart failure resistant to conventional therapy. In 1984, Misler and Nidus utilized a pumped hemofiltration circuit to provide longterm management of a patient with congestive heart failure by the once weekly removal of 4 liters of fluid (172). Subsequently, utilizing the CAVH circuit, anecdotal and preliminary reports documented the salutary hemodynamic effects of slow continuous fluid removal (173–176). In 1988, Lauer et al. presented a more formal study, demonstrating improvement in cardiac index and a decrease in peripheral resistance as a result of CAVH induced fluid removal (177). More recently, Biasioli et al., using a CVVH circuit, performed fluid removal sessions on a bi-weekly or monthly schedule, suggesting that this approach could be used as a 'bridge' to cardiac transplantation (178).

Hepatic coma

In a successful attempt to treat fulminant hepatic failure, Davenport et al. demonstrated that machine driven hemofiltration increased intracranial pressure while CAVH did not (179). This finding supports previous attempts to employ hemofiltration techniques for the management of hepatic failure (180). It should be noted, however, that hemofiltration alone is unlikely to remove all the toxins associated with hepatic failure and better results have been obtained when hemofiltration is added to plasma exchange (181).

Intoxications

The slow, continuous solute removal provided by the continuous therapies has been found to be useful in the treatment of intoxications by drugs with large volumes of distribution and a tendency to 'rebound' when removed by more rapid, intermittent techniques. Domoto et al. studied the removal of N-acetyl procainamide and found that CAVH and CAVHD were more efficient than hemodialysis (105). Bellomo et al. reported that lithium toxicity could be successfully treated with CAVHD (106). Other intoxications may also possess the unique qualities which make a continuous therapy the technique of choice for their management (182).

Lactic acidosis

The ability of the continuous therapies to allow for the massive infusion of bicarbonate without the risk of hypernatremia or fluid overload has allowed these techniques to be used for the management of lactic acidosis. Raimondi et al. employed CAVH with a bicarbonate based replacement fluid and were able to infuse over 2000 mEq of bicarbonate to a cirrhotic patient in shock, while simultaeoulsy decreasing serum sodium concentration (183). Although the patient ultimately succumbed to refractory shock, the technical abilties of the therapy were defined. Using CAVHD in seven pediatric patients, Jenkins et al. found that switching from lactate or acetate to bicarbonate based dialysate fluid was more likely to control acidosis, increase bicarbonate levels and decrease anion gaps, without an increase in pCO_2 (48). Finally, Kirschbaum et al. took the novel approach of using citrate anticoagulation and its associated alkalosis as a means of treating lactic acidosis in patients with a high risk of bleeding (184).

Electrolyte abnormalities, hypercalcemia and respiratory acidosis

Considering the enormous solute removal capabilities of some of the more efficient continuous therapies (Table 5), it is clear that even the most troublesome electrolyte abnormalities can be successfully treated if the proper techniques are chosen. CAVHD for example, given a 2 l/h dialysate, can yield 50 l/day of solute clearance and its continuous application offers advantage over intermittent hemodialysis. Thus, standard CAVH has been used temporarily to treat medically resistant hypercalcemia and would have been even more successful if a more efficient modification of the CAVH procedure had been employed (185). Similarly, high volume CAVH, with predilution and suction-assist, was successful in infusing sufficient bicarbonate to control respiratory acidosis in a case of fatal ARDS (94). Although some of these attempted therapies seem futile, they serve to define the capabilities of the treatment and may ultimately allow for their successful application in the future, as was the case in the early attempt to treat lactic acidosis (see above).

Treatment of hyperthermia and total body cooling

The externalisation of the arterio-venous circuit has allowed Kramer to treat hyperthermia by placing the tubing in ice water (186). Cooling of the replacement solutions can also aid in lowering systemic temperature.

CONTINUOUS THERAPIES VS CONVENTIONAL DIALYTIC TECHNIQUES

Several studies have attempted to compare the survival of patients treated with the continuous therapies and those treated with conventional dialytic techniques. In the earliest of these, Bartlett et al. randomized 56 patients with multiple organ failure and found an improved survival in patients treated with CAVH compared to those treated with intermittent hemodialysis (28% *vs* 12%); statistically the difference was not significant (128). Nonetheless, there was significantly increased survival in patients receiving adequate nutritional support, a situation which was more likely in the patients treated with CAVH. Subsequently, Bellomo et al. retrospectively reviewed the outcome of 167 patients treated with either conventional dialytic techniques (hemodialysis or peritoneal dialysis) or with acute continuous hemodiafiltration (CAVHD or CVVHD) (129). Although overall survival was greater in those receiving continuous hemodiafiltration (41% *vs* 30%) the difference did not attain statistical significance. There was, however, a statistically significant decreased mortality in a subgroup of patients with 2 to 4 failing organs and in those with intermediate APACHE II scores (187). As with Bartlett's study, these authors also documented that the continuous therapies allowed for a more substantial nutritional support. Most recently Kruczynski et al. reviewed their experience with 12 patients treated with 'high volume' CAVH (using predilution and an infusion pump control of ultrafiltration) and 23 patients receiving conventional intermittent hemodialysis (188). Mortality was 25% in the CAVH group and 82% in the hemodialysis group ($p < 0.05$), but despite equal APACHE II scores, the CAVH group was significantly younger (45 years *vs* 61 years). Once again, the authors remarked on the improved nutrition received by those patients on CAVH.

Despite some intriguing results, these studies cannot be considered as conclusive. The difficulties in designing such a study include the geographical variability in survival rates, the need for large numbers of patients and the differing expertise of the treating units (189). Add to this the imperfect means available to stratify disease severity (APACHE II, number of failed organs, etc) (131, 190, 191) and it would seem that such a definitive study will never be completed. It is perhaps more useful to consider the advantages that the continuous therapies offer in terms of a smooth, well tolerated means of fluid removal, the ability to provide substantial nutritional support and the continuous maintenance of acid-base and electrolyte homeostasis.

ACKNOWLEDGEMENT

Aside from the numerous authors cited in the text, the author would like to acknowledge the efforts of Dr Juan Bosch, who inspired many to pursue investigations of the CAVH treatment and Dennis Battersby, of the Amicon Corporation, who was instrumental in promoting CAVH in the United States.

REFERENCES

1. Henderson LW, Silverstein ME, Ford CA, Lysaght MJ: Clinical response to maintenance hemodiafiltration. *Kidney Int* 10 (Suppl): S58, 1975
2. Quellhorst E, Rieger J, Doht B, Beckmann H, Jacob I, Kraft B, Mietzsch G, Scheller F: Treatment of chronic uraemia by an ultrafiltration kidney-first clinical experience. *Proc Eur Dial Transplant Assoc* 13: 314, 1976
3. Schneider H, Streicher E, Hachmann H, Chmeil H, von Mylius U: Clinical experience with haemofiltration. *Proc Eur Dial Transplant Assoc* 14: 136, 1977
4. Bosch JP, von Albertini B, Geronemus R, Glabman S, Kahn T: Comparison of hemofiltration and ultrafiltration plus hemodialysis to conventional hemodialysis. in *Annual Progress Report, March 1979, Artificial Kidney Program of the National Institute of Arthritis, Metabolism and Digestive Diseases*, Bethesda, Maryland, National Institute of Arthritis, Metabolic and Digestive Diseases, Publication No (NIH) NO1-AM-7-2228, 1979
5. Kramer P, Wigger W, Rieger J, Matthaei D, Scheler F: Arteriovenous haemofiltration: a new and simple method for the treatment of over-hydrated patients resistant to diuretics. *Klin Wochenschr* 55: 1121, 1977
6. Neff MS, Sadjadi S, Slifkin R: A wearable artificial glomerulus. *Trans Am Soc Artif Intern Organs* 25: 71, 1979
7. Paganini EP, Nakamoto S: Continuous slow ultrafiltration in oliguric acute renal failure. *Trans Am Soc Artif Intern Organs* 26: 201, 1980
8. Shaldon S, Beau MC, Deschodt G, Lysaght MJ, Ramperez P, Mion C: Continuous ambulatory hemofiltration. *Trans Am Soc Artif Intern Organs* 26: 210, 1980
9. Kramer P, Seegers A, De Vivie R, Matthaei D, Trautmann M, Scheler F: Therapeutic potential of hemofiltration. *Clin Nephrol* 11: 145, 1979
10. Kramer P, Kaufhold G, Grone HJ, Wigger W, Rieger J, Matthaei D, Stokke T, Burchardi H, Scheler F: Management of anuric intensive-care patients with arterio-venous hemofiltration. *Int J Artif Organs* 3: 225, 1980
11. Colton CK, Henderson LW, Ford CA, Lysaght MJ: Kinetics of hemodiafiltration: I. *In vitro* transport characteristics of a hollow fiber blood ultrafilter. *J Lab Clin Med* 85: 355, 1975
12. Henderson LW, Colton CK, Ford CA: Kinetics of hemodiafiltration: II. Clinical characterization of a new blood cleansing modality. *J Lab Clin Med* 85: 372, 1975
13. Nolph KD: Short dialysis, middle molecules and uremia. *Ann Intern Med* 86: 93, 1977
14. Kaplan AA, Longnecker RE, Folkert VW: Continuous arteriovenous hemofiltration: a report of six month's experience. *Ann Intern Med* 100: 358, 1984
15. Lauer A, Saccaggi A, Ronco C, Belledonne M, Glabman S, Bosch JP: Continuous arteriovenous hemofiltration in the critically ill patient. *Ann Intern Med* 99: 455, 1983

16. Deen WM, Troy JL, Robertson CR, Brenner BM: Dynamics of glomerular ultrafiltration in the rat: IV. Determination of the ultrafiltration coefficient. *J Clin Invest* 52: 1500, 1973

17. Bosch JP, Geronemus R, Glabman S, Lysaght M, Kahn T, von Albertini B: High flux hemofiltration. *Artif Organs* 2: 339, 1978

18. Landis EM, Pappenheimer JR: Exchange of substances through the capillary wall; in *Handbook of Physiology. Circulation, Vol 2*, Washington, Am Physiol Soc, 1963, p 962

19. Jenkins R, Chen B, Funk JE: Maximum ultrafiltration rate in continuous arteriovenous hemofiltration does not occur at the lowest level of the ultrafiltrate collection chamber. *Am Soc Artif Intern Organs* 39: M618, 1993

20. Kaplan AA: *Procedure Manual: Continuous Arterio-Venous Hemofiltration*, Clinical Protocol from the John Dempsey Hospital, University of Connecticut Health Center, Farmington, CT

21. Mault JR, Dirkes SM, Swartz RD, Bartlett RH: *Continuous Hemofiltration: A Reference Guide for SCUF, CAVH and CAVHD*, University of Michigan Medical Center, Ann Arbor, Michigan

22. Price CA: Standards of clinical practice for continuous renal replacement rherapy (excerpt). in *Standards of Clinical Practice for Nephrology Nursing*, 3rd Ed, edited by Burrows-Hudson S, Pitman, NJ, American Nephrology Nurses' Association, 1993, available from the ANNA National Office, East Holly Avenue, Box 56, Pitman, NJ 08071

23. Pallone TL, Hyver S, Petersen J: The simulation of continuous arteriovenous hemodialysis with a mathematical model. *Kidney Int* 35: 125, 1989

24. Olbricht CJ, Schurek HJ, Stolte H, Koch KM: The influence of vascular access modes on the efficiency of CAVH. in *Continuous Arteriovenous Hemofiltration*, edited by Sieberth HG, Mann H, Basel, Karger, 1985, p 14

25. Jenkins R, Funk J, Chen B, Thacker: Effects of access catheter dimensions on bloodflow in continuous arteriovenous hemofiltration. in *Continuous Hemofiltration*, Contributions to Nephrology, Vol 93, edited by Sieberth H-G, Mann H, Stummvoll HK, Basel, Karger, 1991, p 171

26. Quinton W, Dillard D, Scribner BH: Cannulation of blood vessels for prolonged hemodialysis. *Trans Am Soc Artif Intern Organs* 6: 104, 1960

27. Weiss L, Danielson BG, Wikstrom B, Hedstrand U, Wahlberg J: Continuous arteriovenous hemofiltration in the treatment of 100 critically ill patients with acute renal failure: report on clinical outcome an nutritional aspects. *Clin Nephrol* 31: 184, 1989

28. Zobel G, Trop M, Beitzke A, Ring E: Vascular access for continuous arteriovenous hemofiltration in infants and young children. *Artif Organs* 12: 16, 1988

29. Jenkins RD, Kuhn RJ, Funk JE: Clinical implications of catheter variability on neonatal continuous arteiovenous hemofiltration. *Trans Am Soc Artif Intern Organs* 34: 108, 1988

30. Lysaght MJ, Boggs DR, Ritger P, Howard DD, Jensen JJ: Membranes and transport phenomena in CAVH and CAVHD. in *CAVH: International Symposium on Continuous Arterio-Venous Hemofiltration*, edited by La Greca G, Fabris A, Ronco C, Milan, Wichtig Editore, 1986, p 77

31. Ronco C, Brendolan A, Bragantini L, Chiaramonte S, Fabris A. Feriani M, Frigiola A, La Greca G: Treatment of acute renal failure in newborns by continuous arteriovenous hemofiltration. *Trans Am Soc Artif Intern Organs* 31: 634, 1985

32. Ronco C, Bosch JP, Lew S, Fecondini L, Fabris A, Feriani M, Chiaramonte S, Brendolan A, Bragantini L, La Greca G: Technical and clinical evaluation of a new hemofilter for CAVH: theoretical concepts and practical application of a different blood flow geometry. in *CAVH: International Symposium on Continuous Arterio-Venous Hemofiltration*, edited by La Greca G, Fabris A, Ronco C, Milan, Wichtig Editore, 1986, p 55

33. Ronco C, Brendolan A, Borin D, Bragantini L, Fabris A, Feriani M, Chiaramonte S, La Greca G: Permeability characteristics of polysulfonic membranes in CAVH. in *Continuous Arteriovenous Hemofiltration*, edited by Sieberth HG, Mann H, Basel, Karger, 1985, p 59

34. Voerman HJ, Strack van Schijndel RJM, Thijs LG: Continuous arterial-venous hemodiafiltration in critically ill patients. *Crit Care Med* 18: 911, 1990

35. Zobel G, Ring E, Trop M, Grubbauer HM: Suction-supported continuous arteriovenous hemofiltration in children. *Blood Purif* 6: 37, 1988

36. Lennander O, Mulec H: CAVH by negative suction-what is the optimal pressure? in *CAVH: International Symposium on Continuous Arterio-Venous Hemofiltration*, edited by La Greca G, Fabris A, Ronco C, Milan, Wichtig Editore, 1986, p 87

37. Ronco C, Brendolan A, Bragantini L, Fabris A, Feriani M, Chiaramonte S, Milan M, Dell'Aquila R, La Greca G: Technical and clinical evaluation of a new polyamide hollow fiber hemofilter for CAVH. *Int J Artif Organs* 11: 33, 1988

38. Sigler MH, Teehan BP, Van Valkenburgh D: Solute transport in continuous hemodialysis: a new treatment for acute renal failure. *Kidney Int* 32: 562, 1987

39. Kaplan AA, Golper TA: Sieving characteristics of a new polysulfone hemofilter for use with continuous arteriovenous hemofiltration. *Int J Artif Organs* 10: 357, 1987

40. Arakawa M, Nagao M, Gejyo F, Terada R, Kobayashi T, Kunitomo T: Development of a new antithrombogenic continuous ultrafiltration system. *Artif Organs* 15: 171, 1991

41. Yohay DA, Schwab SJ, Quarles LD: Parallel plates are more effective than hollow fiber dialyzers in continuous arteriovenous hemodialysis. (Abstract) *Am Soc Nephrol* 1: 382, 1990

42. Golper TA, Price J: Continuous veno-venous hemofiltration for acute renal failure in the ICU: technical considerations. *ASAIO J* 1994. In press

43. Kramer P, Bohler J, Kehr A, Grone HJ, Schrader J, Matthaei D, Scheler F: Intensive care potential of continuous arteriovenous hemofiltration. *Trans Am Soc Artif Intern Organs* 28: 28, 1982

44. Kaplan AA, Toueg S, Kennedy TL: Complement kinetics during continuous arteriovenous hemofiltration: studies with a new polysulfone hemofilter. *Blood Purif* 6: 27, 1988

45. Paganini E: Continuous replacement modalities in acute renal dysfunction. in *Acute Continuous Renal Replacement Therapy*, edited by Paganini E, Boston, Martinus Nijhoff Publishers, 1986, p 7

46. Olbricht CJ, Schurch HJ, Huxman-Nageli D: Effect of lactate and bicarbonate-buffered substitution solutions on urea generation in continuous arteriovenous hemofiltration. (Abstract) *Blood Purif* 9: 48, 1981

47. Bonnardeaux A, Pichette V, Ouimet D, Geadah D, Habel F, Cardinal J: Solute clearances with high dialysate flow rates and glucose absorption from the dialysate in continuous arteriovenous hemodialysis. *Am J Kidney Dis* 19: 31, 1992

48. Jenkins RD, Jackson E, Kuhn R, Funk J: Benefit of bicarbonate dialysis during CAVHD. *Trans Am Soc Artif Intern Organs* 36: M465, 1990

49. Olbricht C, Mueller C, Schurek HJ: Treatment of acute renal failure in patients with multiple organ failure by continuous spontaneous hemofiltration. *Trans Am Soc Artif Intern Organs* 28: 33, 1982

50. Kohen JA, Whitley KY, Kjellstrand CM: Continuous arteriovenous hemofiltration: a comparison with hemodialysis in acute renal failure. *Trans Am Soc Artif Intern Organs* 31: 169, 1985

51. Mehta RL, Dobos GJ, Ward DM: Anticoagulation in continuous renal replacement procedures. *Semin Dial* 5: 61, 1992

52. Spinowitz B: Anticoagulation in continuous arteriovenous hemofiltration. in *Proceedings of the Third International Symposium on Acute Continuous Renal Replacement Therapy*, Fort Lauderdale, Florida, 1987, p 106

53. Kramer P, Schrader J, Bohnsack W, Grieben G, Grone HJ, Scheler F: Continuous arteriovenous haemofiltration: a new kidney replacement therapy. *Proc Eur Dial Transplant Assoc* 18: 743, 1981

54. Shrader J, Scheler F: Coagulation disorders in acute renal failure and anticoagulation during CAVH with standard heparin and with low molecular weight heparin, in *Continuous Arteriovenous Hemofiltration*, edited by Sieberth HG, Mann H, Basel, Karger, 1985, p 25

55. Bull BS, Korpman RA, Huse WM, Brigs BD: Heparin therapy during extracorporeal circulation. I. Problems inherent in existing heparin protocols. *J Thorac Cardiovasc Surg* 69: 674, 1975

56. Bjornssson TD, Wolfram KM, Kitchell BB: Heparin kinetics determined by three assay methods. *Clin Pharmacol Ther* 31: 104, 1982

57. Golper TA, Ronco C, Kaplan AA: Continuous arteriovenous hemofiltration: improvements, modifications and future directions. *Semin Dial* 1: 50, 1988

58. Schurek HJ, Biela D: Continuous arteriovenous hemofiltration: improvement in the handling of fluid balance and hepariniazation. *Blood Purif* 1: 189, 1983

59. Maher JF, Lapierre L, Schreiner GE, Geiger M, Westervelt FB Jr: Regional heparinization for hemodialysis. *N Engl J Med* 268: 451, 1963

60. Ellison N, Beatty P, Blake DR, Wurzel HA, MacVaugh H: Heparin rebound. *J Thorac Cardiovasc Surg* 67: 723, 1974

61. Hampers CL, Blaufox MD, Merill JP: Anticoagulation rebound after hemodialysis. *N Engl J Med* 275: 776, 1966

62. Milne B, Rodgers K, Cervenko F, Salerno T: Hemodynamic effects of intra-aortic administration versus intravenous administration of protamine for reversal of heparin in man. *Can Anaesth Soc J* 30: 347, 1983

63. Kaplan AA, Petrillo R: Regional heparinization for continuous arterio-venous hemofiltration (CAVH). *Trans Am Soc Artif Intern Organs* 33: 312, 1987

64. Hory B, Cachoux A, Toulemonde F: Continuous arteriovenous hemofiltration with low-molecular weight heparin. (Letter) *Nephron* 41: 125, 1985

65. Pinnick RV, Wiegmann TB, Diedrich DA: Regional citrate anticoagulation for hemodialysis in the patient at high risk for bleeding. *N Engl J Med* 308: 258, 1983

66. Von Brecht JH, Flanigan MJ, Freeman RM, Lim VS: Regional anticoagulation: hemodialysis with hypertonic trisodium citrate. *Am J Kidney Dis* 8: 196, 1986

67. Mehta RL, McDonald BR, Aguilar MM, Ward DM: Regional citrate anticoagulation for continuous arteriovenous hemodialysis in critically ill patients. *Kidney Int* 38: 976, 1990

68. Zusman RM, Rubin RH, Cato AE, Cocchetto BS, Crow JW, Tolkoff-Rubin N: Hemodialysis using prostacyclin instead of heparin as the sole antithrombotic agent. *N Engl J Med* 304: 934, 1981

69. Smith MC, Danviriyasup K, Crow JW, Cato AE, Park GD, Hassid A, Dunn MJ: Prostacyclin substitution for heparin in long-term hemodialysis. *Am J Med* 73: 669, 1982

70. Zobel G, Trop M, Muntean W, Ring E, Gleispach H: Anticoagulation for continuous arteriovenous hemofiltration in children. *Blood Purif* 6: 90, 1988

71. Stevens PE, Riley B, Davies SP, Gower PE, Brown EA, Kox CW: Continuous arteriovenous hemodialysis in critically ill patients. *Lancet* ii: 150, 1988

72. Weeden J, Smithies M, Sheppard M, Bullen K, Tinker J, Bihari D: Continuous high volume venous-venous haemofiltration in acute renal failure. *Int Care Med* 15: 358, 1989

73. Pataca MI, Ramesh BR, Parmer A, Rifkin I, Ware RJ, Parsons V: Continuous arteriovenous haemodialysis in severe combined renal and respiratory failure. *Blood Purif* 10: 262, 1992

74. Ponikvar R, Kandus A, Buturovic J, Kveder R: Use of prostacyclin as the only anticoagulant during continuous venovenous hemofiltration. in *Continuous Hemofiltration*, Contributions in Nephrology, Vol 93, edited by Sieberth HG, Mann H, Stummvoll HK, Basel, Karger, 1992, p 218

75. Ohtake Y, Hirasawa H, Sugai T, Oda S, Shiga H, Matsuda K, Kitamura N, Odaka M, Tabata Y: A study on anticoagulants in continuous hemofiltration. *Jpn J Artif Organs* 19: 744, 1990

76. Ohtake Y, Hirasawa H, Sugai T, Oda S, Shiga H, Matsuda K: Nafamostat mesilate as anticoagulant in continuous hemofiltration and continuous hemodiafiltration. in *Continuous Hemofiltration*, Contributions to Nephrology, Vol 93, edited by Sieberth HG, Mann H, Stummvol H, Basel, Karger, 1991, p 215

77. Smith D, Paganini EP, Suhoza K, Eisele G, Swann S, Nakamoto S: Non-heparin continuous renal replacement therapy is possible. in *Progress in Artificial Organs*, edited by Nose Y, Kjellstrand C, Ivanovich P, Cleveand, ISAO Press, 1986, p 226

78. Paganini EP: Continuous renal replacement therapy in open heart or artificial heart patients with acute renal failure. in *CAVH: Proceedings of the International Symposium on Continuous Arterio-Venous Hemofiltration*, edit-

414   *Andre A. Kaplan*

ed by La Greca G, Fabris A, Ronco C, Milan, Wichtig Editore, 1986, p 199

79. Martin PY, Suter P, Chevrolet JC, Favre H: Anticoagulation in patients treated by continuous veno-venous hemofiltration (CVVH): a retrospective study. (Abstract) *J Am Soc Nephrol* 4: 367, 1993

80. Arakawa M, Suzuki Y, Nagao M, Aoike I, Koda Y, Terada R, Kunitomo T: Development of a new antithrombogenic continuous ultrafiltration system (ACUS) and its clinical evaluatation. *Nephrol Dial Transplant* 2 (Suppl): 49, 1991

81. Paganini EP, Flaque J, Whitman G, Nakamoto S: Amino acid balance in patients with oliguric acute renal failure undergoing slow continuous ultrafiltration (SCUF). *Trans Am Soc Artif Intern Organs* 28: 615, 1982

82. Paganini EP, O'Hara P, Nakamoto S: Slow continuous ultrafiltration in hemodialysis resistant oliguric acute renal failure patients. *Trans Am Soc Artif Intern Organs* 30: 173, 1984

83. Desio FJ, Paganini EP: Evaluation of slow continuous ultrafiltration in oliguric patients on intraaortic balloon pumps. (Abstract) *Blood Purif* 2: 5, 1984

84. Paganini EP: Continuous replacement modalities in acute renal dysfunction. in *Acute Continuous Renal Replacement Therapy*, edited by Paganini EP, Boston, Martinus Nijhoff Publishers, 1986, p 7

85. Paganini EP: Slow continuous ultrafiltration (SCUF), in *Proceedings of the Third International Symposium on Acute Continuous Renal Replacement Therapy*, Fort Lauderdale, Florida, 1987, p 37

86. Kaplan AA, Longnecker R, Folkert VW: Suction-assisted continuous arteriovenous hemofiltration. *Trans Am Soc Artif Intern Organs* 24: 408, 1983

87. Domoto DT: Two years clinical experience with continuous arteriovenous hemofiltration in acute renal failure. *Trans Am Soc Artif Intern Organs* 31: 581, 1985

88. Zobel G, Ring E, Trop M, Grubbauer HM: Suction-supported continuous arteriovenous hemofiltration in children. *Blood Purif* 6: 37, 1988

89. Golper TA, Kaplan AA, Narasimhan N, Leone M: Transmembrane pressures generated by filtrate line suction maneuvers and predilution fluid replacement during *in vitro* continuous arteriovenous hemofiltration. *Int J Artif Organs* 10: 41, 1987

90. Henderson LW: Pre *vs* post dilution hemofiltration. *Clin Nephrol* 11: 120, 1979

91. Cheung AK, Alford MF, Wilson MW, Leypoldt JK, Henderson LW: Urea movement across erythrocyte membrane during artificial kidney treatment. *Kidney Int* 23: 866, 1983

92. Geronemus R, von Albertini B, Glabman S, Lysaght M, Kahn T, Bosch JP: Enhanced small molecular clearances in hemofiltration. *Proc Clin Dial Transplant Forum* 8: 147, 1978

93. Kaplan AA: Predilution *vs* postdilution for continuous arteriovenous hemofiltration. *Trans Am Soc Artif Intern Organs* 31: 28, 1985

94. Kaplan AA: Clinical trials with predilution and vacuum suction: enhancing the efficiency of the CAVH treatment. *Trans Am Soc Artif Intern Organs* 32: 49, 1986

95. Kaplan AA: Enhanced efficiency during CAVH: Clinical trials with predilution and suction. in *CAVH: Proceedings of the International Symposium on Continuous Arterio-Venous Hemofiltration*, edited by La Greca G, Fabris A, Ronco C, Milan, Wichtig Editore, 1986, p 49

96. Kaplan AA: The predilution mode for continuous arteriovenous hemofiltration. in *Acute Continuous Renal Replacement Therapy*, edited by Paganini EP, Boston, Martinus Nijhoff Publishers, 1986, p 143

97. Geronemus R, Schneider N: Continuous arteriovenous haemodialysis: a new modality for the treatment of acute renal failure. *Trans Am Soc Artif Intern Organs* 30: 610, 1984

98. Pallone TL, Hyver S, Petersen J: Blood-dialysate equilibrium during continuous arteriovenous hemodialysis. *Trans Am Soc Artif Intern Organs* 34: 512, 1988

99. Ronco C, Bragantini L, Brendolan A, Dell'Awuila R, Fabris A, Chiaramonte S, Feriani M, Laquaniti L, La Greca G: Arteriovenous hemodiafiltration (AVHDF) combined with continuous arteriovenous hemofiltration (CAVH). *Trans Am Soc Artif Intern Organs* 31: 349, 1985

100. Ing TS, Daugirdas H, Bregman H, Leehey DJ: Continuous arteriovenous hemodialysis. (Editorial) *Int J Artif Organs* 8: 117, 1985

101. Daugirdas JT, Bregman H, Rahman MA, Ramanujam LS, Nawab ZM, Leehey DJ, Ing TS: Ultrafiltration control during continuous arteriovenous hemodialysis using paired volumetric dialysate pumps. (letter) *Int J Artif Organs* 9: 273, 1986

102. van Geelen JA, Vincent HH, Schalekamp MADH: Continuous arteriovenous haemofiltration and haemodiafiltration in acute renal failure. *Nephrol Dial Transplant* 2: 181, 1988

103. Gibney RTN, Stollery DE, Lefebvre RE, Sharun CJ, Chan P: Continuous arteriovenous hemodialysis: an alternative therapy for acute renal failure associated with critical illness. *Can Med Assoc J* 139: 861, 1988

104. Pattison ME, Lee SM, Ogden DA: Continuous arteriovenous hemodiafiltration: an aggressive approach to the management of acute renal failure. *Am J Kidney Dis* 11: 43, 1988

105. Domoto DT, Brown WW, Bruggensmith P: Removal of toxic levels of N-acetylprocainamide with continuous arteriovenous hemofiltration or continuous arteriovenous hemodiafiltration. *Ann Intern Med* 106: 550, 1987

106. Bellomo R, Kearly Y, Parkin G, Love J, Boyce N: Treatment of life threatening lithium toxicity with continuous arteriovenous hemodiafiltration. *Crit Care Med* 19: 836, 1991

107. Golper TA, Leone M: Backtransport of dialysate solutes during *in vitro* continuous arteriovenous hemodialysis. *Blood Purif* 7: 223, 1989

108. Morabito S, Gamberini M, Marzoli G, Marinelli R, Palumbo R, Cinotti GA, Chiavarelli R, Cassese M, Marino B: Efficiency of different hollow-fiber hemofilters in continuous arteriovenous hemodiafiltration (CAVHD). (Abstract) *Am Soc Nephrol* 4: 370, 1993

109. Canaud B, Beraud JJ, Mion C: Pump assisted continuous veno-venous hemofiltration (PA-CVVH): a more flexible mode of acute uremia treatment in severely ill patients. in *CAVH: Proceedings of the International Symposium on Continuous Arterio-Venous Hemofiltration*, edited by La Greca G, Fabris A, Ronco C, Milan, Wichtig Editore, 1986, p 185

110. Bouchet JL, Bourdenx JPh, Montoriol J, Martin-Dupont Ph: Continuous veno-venous hemofiltration (CVVH):

technical and clincial experience. in *CAVH: Proceedings of the International Symposium on Continuous Arterio-Venous Hemofiltration*, edited by La Greca G, Fabris A, Ronco C, Milan, Wichtig Editore, 1986, p 319

111. Canaud B, Garred LJ, Christol JP, Aubas S, Beraud JJ, Mion C: Pump assisted continuous venovenous hemofiltration for treating acute uremia. *Kidney Int* 33: S154, 1988

112. Morgan JM, Morgan C, Evans TW: Clinical experience of pumped arteriovenous haemofiltration in the management of patients in oliguric renal failure following cardiothoracic surgery. *Int J Cardiol* 21: 259, 1988

113. Wendon J, Smithies M, Sheppard M, Bullen K, Tinker J, Bihari D: Continuous high volume venous-venous haemofiltration in acute renal failure. *Int Care Med* 15: 358, 1989

114. Storck M, Hartl WH, Zimmerer E, Inthorn D: Comparison of pump-driven and spontaneous haemofiltration in postoperative acute renal failure. *Lancet* i: 452, 1991

115. Macia WL, Mueller BA, Scarim SK, Robinson M, Rudy DW: Continuous venovenous hemofiltration: an alternative to continuous arteriovenous hemofiltration and hemodiafiltration in acute renal failure. *Am J Kidney Dis* 18: 451, 1991

116. Golper TA, Price J: Continuous veno-venous hemofiltration for acute renal failure in the ICU: technical considerations. *Trans Am Soc Artif Intern Organs*, 1994. In press

117. Kudoh Y, Iimura O: Slow continuous hemodialysis – new therapy for acute renal failure in critically ill patients – Part 1. Theoretical consideration and new technique. *Jpn Cir J* 52: 1171, 1988

118. Kudoh Y, Shiiki M, Sasa Y, Hotta D, Nozawa A, Iimura O: Slow continuous hemodialysis – new therapy for acute renal failure in critically ill patients – Part 2. Animal experiments and clinical implication. *Jpn Cir J* 52: 1183, 1988

119. Tam PYW, Huraib S, Mahan B, LeBlanc D, Lunski CA, Holtzer C, Doyle CE, Vas SI, Uldall PR: Slow continuous hemodialysis for the management of complicated acute renal failure. *Clin Nephrol* 30: 79, 1988

120. Bellomo R, Parkin G, Love J, Boyce N: A prospective comparative study of continuous arteriovenous hemodiafiltration and continuous venovenous hemodiafiltration in critically ill patients. *Am J Kidney Dis* 21: 400, 1993

121. Hertel J, Lew SQ, Barlee V, Bosch JP: Continuous veno-venous hemofiltration (CVVH) – the end of continuous arterio-venous hemofiltration/hemodialysis (CAVH/CAVHD). (Abstract) *Am Soc Nephrol* 3: 368, 1992

122. Teschan PE, Baxter CR, O'Brien TF, Freyhof JN, Hall WH: Prophylactic hemodialysis in the treatment of acute renal failure. *Am J Med* 53: 992, 1960

123. Kleinknecht D, Jungers P, Chanard J, Barbanel C, Ganeval DD: Uremic and non-uremic complications in acute renal failure. *Kidney Int* 1: 190, 1972

124. Conger JD: A controlled evaluation of prophylactic dialysis in post-traumatic acute renal failure. *J Trauma* 15: 1056, 1975

125. Gillium DM, Dixon BS, Yanover MJ, Kelleher SP, Shapiro MD, Benedetti RG, Dillingham MA, Paller MS, Goldberg JP, Tomford RC, Gordon JA, Conger JD: The role of intensive dialyis in acute renal failure. *Clin Nephrol* 25: 249, 1986

126. Maroni BJ, Steinman TI, Mitch WE: A method for estimating nitrogen intake of patients with chronic renal failure. *Kidney Int* 27: 58, 1985

127. Kaplan AA: Renal replacement therapy for acute renal failure. in *Current Therapy in Nephrology and Hypertension*, edited by Glassock RJ, Toronto, C Decker, 1992, p 264

128. Bartlett RH, Mault JR, Dechert RE, Palmer J, Swartz RD, Port FK: Continuous arteriovenous hemofiltration: improved survival in surgical acute renal failure? *Ann Surg* 100: 400, 1986

129. Bellomo R, Mansfield D, Rumble S, Shapiro J, Parkin G, Boyce N: Conventional dialysis versus acute continuous hemodiafiltration. *ASAIO J* 38: M654, 1992

130. Clark WR, Murphy MH, Alaka KJ, Mueller BA, Pastan SO, Marcias WL: Urea kinetics during continuous hemofiltration. *ASAIO J* 38: M664, 1992

131. Kaplan AA: Extracorporeal blood purification in the treatment of acute renal failure with multiorgan involvement. *Blood Purif* 1996. In press

132. Clark WR, Mueller BA, Alaka KJ, Macias WL: A comparison of metabolic control by continuous and intermittent therapies in acute renal failure. *Am Soc Nephrol* 4: 1413, 1994

133. Kramer P, Bohler J, Kehr A, Grone HJ, Schrader J, Matthaei D, Scheler F: Intensive care potential of continuous arteriovenous hemofiltration. *Trans Am Soc Artif Intern Organs* 28: 28, 1982

134. Sigler MH, Samuel S, Teehan BP: Amino acid removal during continuous arterio-venous hemodialysis (CAVHD) in acute renal failure patients receiving total parenteral nutrition (Abstract). *Blood Purif* 6: 357, 1988

135. Chima SC, Meyer L, Hummell C, Bosworth C, Heyka R, Paganini EP, Werynski A: Protein catabolic rate in patients with acute renal failure on continuous arteriovenous hemofiltration and total parenteral nutrition. *Am Soc Nephrol* 3: 1516, 1993

136. Golper TA, Wedel SK, Kaplan AA, Saad AM, Donta S, Paganini EP: Drug removal during continuous arteriovenous hemofiltration: theory and clincial observations. *Int J Artif Organs* 8: 307, 1975

137. Golper TA Pulliam J, Bennett WM: Removal of therapeutic drugs by continuous arteriovenous hemofiltration. *Arch Intern Med* 145: 1651, 1985

138. Kronfol NO, Lau AH, Colon-Rivera J, Libertin C: Effect of CAVH membrane types on drug-sieving coefficients and clearances. *Trans Am Soc Artif Intern Organs* 2: 85, 1986

139. Reyad S, Barajas M, Swartz RD, Hyneck ML, Moustafa M: Drug removal during continous arteriovenous hemofiltration. *Contemp Dial Nephrol* (May): 30, 1989

140. Lau AH, Pyle K, Kronfol NO, Libertin CR: Removal of cephalosporins by continuous arteriovenous ultrafiltration (CAVU) and hemofiltration (CAVH). *Int J Artif Organs* 12: 379, 1989

141. Bellomo R, McGrath B, Boyce N: *In vivo* catecholamine extraction during continuous hemodiafiltration in inotrope-dependent patients. *Trans Am Soc Artif Intern Organs* 37: M324, 1991

142. Mueller BA, Scarim SK, Macias WL: Comparison of imipenem pharmacokinetics in patients with acute or chronic renal failure treated with continuous hemofiltration. *Am J Kidney Dis* 21: 172, 1993

143. Bennet WM, Aronoff GR, Golper TA, Morrison G, Singer I, Brater DC: *Drug Prescribing in Renal Failure*, 2nd Ed, Philadelphia, Am Coll Phys, 1991

144. Bennet WM, Aronoff GR, Morrison G, Golper TA, Pulliam J, Wolfson M, Singer I: Drug dosing in renal failure: dosing guidelines for adults. *Am J Kidney Dis* 3: 155, 1983

145. Kaplan AA, Longnecker RE, Folkert VW: Continuous hemofiltration. (Letter) *Ann Intern Med* 101: 145, 1984

146. Roberts M, Winney RJ: Errors in fluid balance with pump control of continuous hemodialysis. *Int J Artif Organs* 15: 99, 1992

147. Schunemann B, Kramer P: Simple techniques for accurate fluid balancing during continuous arteriovenous hemofiltration. in *Arteriovenous Hemofiltration: A Kidney Replacement Therapy for the Intensive Care Unit*, edited by Kramer P, Berlin, Springer-Verlag, 1985, p 91

148. Reynolds HN: Complications related to the use of continuous arterio-venous hemofiltration with dialysis. (Abstract) *Crit Care Med* 18: S191, 1990

149. Grone HJ, Kramer P: Puncture and long-term cannulation of the femoral artery and vein in adults. in *Arteriovenous Hemofiltration: A Kidney Replacement Therapy for the Intensive Care Unit*, edited by Kramer P, Berlin, Springer-Verlag. 1985, p 35

150. Kramer P: Limitations and pitfalls of continuous arteriovenous hemofiltration. in *Arteriovenous Hemofiltration: A Kidney Replacement Therapy for the Intensive Care Unit*, edited by Kramer P, Berlin, Springer-Verlag, 1985, p 206

151. Ronco C, Brendolan A, Bragantini L, Chiaramonte S, Feriani M, Fabris A, Dell'Aquila, La Greca G: Treatment of acute renal failure in the newborn by continuous arteriovenous hemofiltration. *Kidney Int* 29: 908, 1986

152. Ronco C, Brendolan A, Bragantini S, Chiaramonte S, Fabris A, Feriani M, Menicanti L, Frigiola A, La Greca G: Treatment of acute renal failure in the newborn by continuous arterio-venous hemofiltration. in *CAVH: Proceedings of the International Symposium on Continuous Arterio-Venous Hemofiltration*, edited by La Greca G, Fabris A, Ronco C, Milan, Wichtig Editore, 1986, p 263

153. Ronco C: Continuous arteriovenous hemofiltration in infants. in *Acute Continuous Renal Replacement Therapy*, edited by Paganini EP, Boston, Martinus Nijhoff Publishers, 1986, p 201

154. Zobel G, Trop M, Ring E, Grubbauer HM: Nine months experience with CAVH in a pediatric intensive care unit. in *CAVH: Proceedings of the International Symposium on Continuous Arterio-Venous Hemofiltration*, edited by La Greca G, Fabris A, Ronco C, Milan, Wichtig Editore, 1986, p 155

155. Leone MR, Jenkins RD, Golper TA, Alexander SR: Early experience with continuous arteriovenous hemofiltration in critically ill pediatric patients. *Crit Care Med* 14: 1058, 1986

156. Jenkins RD, Jackson EC: Treatment of acute renal failure and hyperkalemia in a newborn using continuous arterio-venous hemodiafiltration (CAVHD). (Abstract) *Kidney Int* 33: 226, 1988

157. Bunchman TE, Kershaw DB, Maxvoid NJ: CVVH(D) versus CAVH(D) in infants and children: a single center experience. (Abstract) *Am Soc Nephrol* 4: 336, 1993

158. Coraim F, Fasol R, Stellwag F, Wolner E: Continuous arteriovenous hemofiltration after cardiac surgery. in *Continuous Arteriovenous Hemofiltration*, Contributions to Nephrology, Vol 93, edited by Sieberth HG, Mann H, Basel, Karger, 1985, p 116

159. Coraim F, Wolner E: Management of cardiac surgery patients with continuous arteriovenous hemofiltration. in *Continuous Arteriovenous Hemofiltration*, Contributions to Nephrology, Vol 93, edited by Sieberth HG, Mann H, Basel, Karger, 1985, p 103

160. Coraim FJ, Coraim HP, Ebermann R, Stellwag FM: Acute respiratory failure after cardiac surgery: clinical experience with the application of continuous arteriovenous hemofiltration. *Crit Care Med* 14: 714, 1986

161. Bellomo R, Tippiong P, Boyce N: Tumor necrosis factor clearances during veno-venous hemodiafiltration in the critically ill. *Trans Am Soc Artif Intern Organs* 37: M322, 1991

162. Cottrell AC, Mehta RL: Cytokine kinetics in septic ARF patients on continuous veno-veno hemodialysis. (Abstract) *Am Soc Nephrol* 3: 279, 1992

163. Gomez A, Wang R, Unruh H, Light RB, Bose D, Chau T, Correa E, Mink S: Hemofiltration reverses left ventricular dysfunction during sepsis in dogs. *Anesthesiology* 73: 671, 1990

164. Stein B, Pfenninger E, Grunert A, Schmitz JE, Deller A, Kocher F: The consequences of continuous hemofiltration on lung mechanics and extravascular lung water in a porcine endotoxic shock model. *Int Care Med* 17: 293, 1991

165. Grootendorst AF, van Bommel EFH: The role of hemofiltration in the critically-ill intensive care unit patient: present and future. *Blood Purif* 11: 209, 1993

166. Grootendorst AF, van Bommel EFH, van der Hoven B, van Leengoed LAMG, van Osta ALM: High volume hemofiltration improves hemodynamics of endotoxin-induced shock in the pig. *J Crit Care* 7: 67, 1992

167. Grootendorst AF, Bommel EFH van, Hoven B van der, Leengoed LAMG van, Osta ALM van: High volume hemofiltration improves right ventricular function of endotoxin-induced shock in thepig. *Int Care Med* 18: 235, 1992

168. van Bommel EFH, Grootendorst AF, van Leengoed LAMG: Influence of high-volume hemofiltration on hemodynamics in porcine endotoxic shock (Abstract). *Blood Purif* 10: 88, 1992

169. Ossenkoppelle GJ, van der Meulen J, Bronsveld W, Thijs LG: Continuous arteriovenous hemofiltration as an adjunctive therapy for septic shock. *Crit Care Med* 13: 102, 1985

170. DiCarlo JV, Dudley TE, Sherbotie JR, Kaplan BS, Costarino AT: Continuous arteriovenous hemofiltration/dialysis improves pulmonary gas exchange in children with multiple organ system failure. *Crit Care Med* 18: 822, 1990

171. Barzilay E, Kessler D, Berlot G, Gullo A, Geber D, Zeev IB: Use of extracorporeal supportive techniques as additional treatment for septic induced multiple organ failure patients. *Crit Care Med* 17: 634, 1989

172. Misler S, Nidus BD: Long-term ultrafiltration as a treatment of refractory congestive heart failure. *NY State J Med* 518, 1984

173. Inoue T, Morooka S, Hayashi T, Takayanagi K, Yoshihiko S, Yamamanaka T, Yamaguchi H, Fujimura H, Shimizu M, Kakoi H, Satoh T, Takabatake Y: Effectiveness of continuous arterio-venous hemofiltration (CAVH) for patients with refractory heart failure. (Abstract) *Jpn Cir J* 52: 772, 1988

174. Kaplan AA: Enhanced efficiency during CAVH: clinical trials with predilution and vacuum suction. in *CAVH: Proceedings of the International Symposium on Continuous Arterio-Venous Hemofiltration*, edited by La Greca G, Fabris A, Ronco C, Milan, Wichtig Editore, 1986, p 87

175. Bergerone S, Tognarelli G, Pacitti A, Segoloni G, Pozzi R, Dalmasso M, DiLeo M: Ultrafiltration in the treatment of refractory congestive heart failure. in *CAVH: Proceedings of the International Symposium on Continuous Arterio-Venous Hemofiltration*, La Greca G, Fabris A, Ronco C, Milan, Wichtig Editore, 1986, p 247

176. DiLeo M, Pacitti A, Bergerone S, Pozzi R, Tognarelli G, Segoloni G, Vercellone A, Brusca A: Ulatrafiltration in the treatment of refractory congestive heart failure. *Clin Cardiol* 11: 449, 1988

177. Lauer A, Alvis R, Avram M: Hemodynamic consequences of continuous arterio-venous hemofiltrationl. *Am J Kidney Dis* 12: 110, 1988

178. Biasoli S, Barbaresi F, Barbiero M, Petrosino L, Cavallini L, Zambello A, Cavalcanti G, Foroni R, Bonofiglio C: Intermittent venovenous hemofiltration as a chronic treatment for refractory and intractable heart failure. *ASAIO J* 38: M658, 1992

179. Davenport A, Will EJ, Losowsky MS, Swindells S: Continuous arteriovenous haemofiltration in patients with hepatic encephalopathy and renal failure. *Lancet* ii: 295, 1987

180. Hughes RD, Williams R: Use of sorbent columns and haemofiltration in fulminant hepatic failure. *Blood Purif* 11: 163, 1993

181. Yoshiba M, Sekiyama K, Inoue K: Development of reliable artificial liver support – plasma exchange in combination with hemodiafiltration using high performance membranes. (Abstract) Proceedings of the Fifth International Congress of the World Apheresis Association, 1994, March 9–12, Houston, p 68

182. Golper TA, Bennett WM: Drug removal by continuous arteriovenous hemofiltation – a review of the evidence in poisoned patients. *Med Toxicol Adverse Drug Exp* 3: 341, 1988

183. Raimondi F, Bianchi T, Emmi V, Braschi A, Iotti G, Bobbio Pallavicini F, Tosi P, Fischetti M, Galli F, Villa S: Use of continuous arterio-venous hemofiltration in lactic acidosis. in *CAVH: Proceedings of the International Symposium on Continuous Arterio-Venous Hemofiltration*, edited La Greca G, Fabris A, Ronco C, Milan, Wichtig Editore, 1986, p 135

184. Kirschbaum B, Galishoff M, Reines HD: Lactic acidosis treated with continuous hemodiafiltration and regional citrate anticoagalation. *Crit Care Med* 20: 349, 1992

185. Schou H, Knudsen F: Continuous arteriovenous hemofiltration – a new treatment in hypercalcemic crisis. *Blood Purif* 6: 227, 1988

186. Kramer P, Biege G: Intensive care potentials of continuous arteriovenous hemofiltration. in *Arteriovenous Hemofiltration: A Kidney Replacement Therapy for the Intensive Care Unit*, edited by Kramer P, Berlin, Springer-Verlag, 1985, p 196

187. Knaus WA, Draper EA, Wagner DP, Zimmerman JE: APACHE II: a severity of disease classification system. *Crit Care Med* 13: 818, 1985

188. Kruczynski K, Irvine-Bird K, Toffelmire EB, Morton AR: A comparison of continuous arteriovenous hemofiltration and intermittent hemodialysis in acute renal failure patients in the intensive care unit. *ASAIO J* 39: M778, 1993

189. Bellomo R, Boyce N: Does continuous hemodiafiltration improve survival in acute renal failure. *Semin Dial* 6: 16, 1993

190. Cerra FB, Negro F, Abrams J: Apache II score does not predict multiple organ failure or mortality in postoperative surgical patients. *Arch Surg* 125: 519, 1990

191. Le Gall JR, Lemeshow S: Do we need a new severity score? *Crit Care Med* 19: 857, 1991

PROS AND CONS OF SHORT, HIGH EFFICIENCY, AND HIGH FLUX DIALYSIS

ROBERT H. BARTH

INTRODUCTION

One of the characteristic features of the brief three-decade history of chronic maintenance hemodialysis has been the progressive decline of the duration of individual treatment sessions. Since the 1960s, when seven to ten hour treatment times were the standard (1, 2), progress in dialysis technique has largely been measured by the degree to which session length could be shortened – to 4 to 5 hours during the 1970s, and to 3 hours or even less during the 1980s (3, 4). From the earliest attempts at reducing treatment time, it was clear that compensatory increases in dialyzer surface area (5), or solute clearance (1, 6), would be necessary to maintain patient well-being, and so the shortening of time has been inextricably linked with the development of techniques to increase dialyzer efficiency.

During the last ten years, however, skeptical voices increasingly have been heard, suggesting that perhaps a point of diminishing returns has been reached in the relentless drive to shorten dialysis. Short treatment times have been implicated in both problems of increased morbidity (7, 8) and increased mortality (7, 9, 10) of dialysis populations, especially in the United States, where since the startling mortality figures for end stage renal disease patients first became known in 1989 (11), suspicion – and evidence – has accumulated that the widespread shortening of dialysis sessions which took place throughout the 1980s was at least partially responsible (12, 13). Nevertheless, short sessions remain popular, and the questions

need asking yet again: what is the evidence linking too short dialysis with higher mortality, and how short *is* too short?

Finally, the link between high-efficiency/high-flux dialysis and short treatment times bears closer examination. These therapies may have a number of advantages over 'conventional' hemodialysis beyond the potential for reduced treatment duration – in fact, the continuous reduction of treatment times may actually negate some of those advantages. This chapter will examine the nature, benefits, and drawbacks of hemodialysis with highly permeable membranes, and its role in the present therapeutic environment, as well as reviewing the history and clinical implications of extremely short treatment times.

THE SHORTENING OF DIALYSIS

The 1970s: Establishment of the four-hour treatment

Three factors have been essential to the development of short dialysis times: incentives, technical feasibility, and a means of medical/scientific rationalization and justification. The incentives have been consistent since the earliest era of dialysis: economics, as short dialysis means decreased labor costs per treatment; and patient wellbeing, since the disruption of life attendant on spending 24 or more hours per week undergoing hemodialysis is obvious (1, 14, 15). This correspondence of the interests of

Table 1. Short dialysis: representative clinical studies

First author	Date	Patients	Dialyzer(s)[a]	Mode[b]	t (h)	K_{urea} (ml/min)	V_{urea} (l)	Kt/V[c]	Followup (mo)
Rosenzweig (17)	1971	3	3 Ce	HD	2.0–3.0	185		0.58–0.86	1–3
Orrell (24)	1973	30	Ce	HD	5.0	144		1.08	$\leq$ 28
Man (25)	1973	5	PAN	HFH	3.5–5.0	90		0.49–0.70	12
Mirahmadi (16)	1973	14	2 Ce	HD	4.0	140	43[d]	0.79	3–13
Cambi (26)	1975	101	Ce	HD	3.5–4.0	120–130		0.68–078	$\leq$ 24
Shaldon (21)	1976	12	2 Ce	HD	4.5	140		0.94	12–18
Ben Ari (22)	1976	13	2 Ce	HD	3.0	163		0.73	2
Manji (23)	1976	11	Ce	HD	4.0–4.5	150	30[d]	1.28	12
Shaldon (27)	1981	2	2 PA	HF	2.0	263	45[d]	0.70	18
Chanard (28)	1982	70	PAN	HFH	3.1	143		0.71	6–52
Wizemann (29)	1983	6	PAN PMMA	HDF	1.8	230	37[d]	0.65	6
Cioni (30)	1984	16	PAN	HDF	2.2	305	32	1.24	5
von Albertini (31)	1984	4	2 CA	HDF	1.9	407	47[d]	0.99	0.5
Rotellar (32)	1985	25	2 Ce	HD	2.0	436	36[d]	1.44	12
Keshaviah (33)	1986	112	CA	HD	2.9	265	36[d]	1.25	10
Rubin (34)	1987	12	PAN	HFH	3.0	190		0.89	18
Dumler (35)	1992	56	PS	HFH	2.5	285	41.5	1.03	6–30

[a]CA = cellulose acetate; Ce = cellulose; PA = polyamide; PMMA = polymethylmethacrylate; PS = polysulfone; PAN = polyacrylonitrile.
[b]HD = hemodialysis; HDF = hemodiafiltration; HF = hemofiltration; HFH = high-flux hemodialysis.
[c]Best estimate of prescribed Kt/V; V estimated at 38.5 l if not provided.
[d]Calculated as 0.55 × body weight.

patient and dialysis center still powers the drive to shorten hemodialysis even in the present decade (16).

During the 1970s, when session length first began to shrink significantly, intellectual and mathematical support came from two directions. 'Middle molecule' theorists proposed a framework within which time and membrane surface area had equal weight in the determination of dialysis adequacy (5). Reducing one could be accomplished by increasing the other, thereby maintaining total large-molecular weight solute removal, and a number of early clinical trials of short dialysis were characterized by the use of increased membrane surface area, with either large or multiple dialyzers (15, 17–23) (Table 1).

Another approach was taken at the Hôpital Necker in Paris, where a small surface area dialyzer with a new membrane which was more highly permeable to middle molecules – Rhone-Poulenc sulfonated polyacrylonitrile, or PAN-SO₃ – was used to shorten session time from ten to five hours (25). The patients did not deteriorate clinically, despite a 56% increase in predialysis BUN, a result ascribed to the efficient middle molecule removal effected by the RP PAN-SO₃ membrane. The barrier to wider use of this technique was the extremely high water permeability of PAN-SO₃, which had an ultrafiltration coefficient of 22 to 27 ml · hr^{-1} · mmHg^{-1} · m^{-2}, some 10 times that of cuprophan, and thus required specially construct-

ed equipment for safe ultrafiltration (25, 36). At the same time, other investigators placed the emphasis on dialyzer clearance of small molecular weight substances. In a kinetic analysis published in 1973, Gotch et al. concluded that the reduction of dialysis time with more efficient dialyzers was limited not by the clearance of solutes in the 'middle molecule' range, such as vitamin B_{12}, but by the clearance of urea, whose generation rate they considered to be a quantitative index of protein catabolism (6). The Kiil 1.0 m^2 non-disposable parallel-plate cuprophan dialyzer which was used in the majority of dialyses during the 1960s had a urea clearance of up to about 95 ml/min in its various versions at the standard 200 ml/min blood flow rate (37, 38), and using the Kiil, treatment times ranged from 20–36 hours per week. By the early 1970s, however, dialyzer technology had advanced considerably, and new, disposable parallel plate, coil, and hollow fiber devices easily achieved urea clearances from 120 to 180 ml/min (6, 24, 36, 37), allowing reduction of time by up to one-half while maintaining urea removal equal to that of the Kiil. Cambi and his group shortened the time of all the patients in their dialysis center to 10.5–12 hours per week, reasoning that middle molecules were unimportant, that higher blood urea concentrations were well tolerated (39, 40) and that longer dialysis "cause[s] a depletion of vital substances" (41). Their treatment protocol included blood flow rates of 350 ml/min or higher, and use of newer coil and plate dialyzers, resulting in significant increases in urea clearance over the Kiil; in 1975 they reported three years of successful treatment (26).

The controversy over the importance of small vs. middle molecules to uremic toxicity and dialysis adequacy was not settled during the 1970s, but both philosophies converged with respect to shortening of dialysis time. By the end of the decade the hollow-fiber and parallel plate cellulose dialyzers with urea clearances greater than 150 ml/min which had been considered 'high-efficiency' five years earlier, were in common use, and four to five hour treatment times had become standard in both Europe and the USA.

The National Cooperative Dialysis Study and the ascendancy of urea

The most important single investigation in the development of hemodialysis prescription began patient recruitment in June, 1978. The National Cooperative Dialysis Study (NCDS), sponsored by the National Institute of Arthritis, Diabetes, Digestive and Kidney Diseases and carried out at nine dialysis centers across the United States, was intended to develop "techniques by which dialysis could be prescribed on an individualized and quantitative basis and by which it would provide the minimum exposure that would keep patients free from dialysis-responsive complications" (42). The principal hypothesis to be tested was that measurement of blood urea was the best indicator of dialysis adequacy, and the model chosen to control therapy was urea kinetics, as formulated by Sargent and Gotch (43) and Sargent (44).

The results of the NCDS were reported in 1983, and confirmed the role of urea concentration as a predictor of morbidity, although the "precise quantitative nature of the relationship" was not clear (45). Low protein intake, as measured by normalized protein catabolic rate (PCR), was also related to poor outcome, as was short dialysis time, albeit with a somewhat weaker statistical association (46), but in a summary of recommendations for dialysis prescription based on the NCDS findings, the investigators warned against attempting to equate "a particular [time-averaged concentration of urea]-PCR combination or $Kd \times Td/V$ with an exact probability of morbidity for a particular patient" (45). Nonetheless, the establishment of urea measurement as the principal valid method of monitoring dialysis therapy had been accomplished, and the groundwork laid for development and diffusion of the mathematical tools which would profoundly influence dialysis prescription in the late 1980s and lead to widespread adoption of even shorter dialysis times.

It remained for Gotch and Sargent to provide the tool itself: Kt/V – the total 'dialysis dose' (= Kt, the product of dialyzer urea clearance and treatment time) normalized to V, the urea distribution volume. This dimensionless number, which approximates the fractional urea clearance of total body water, was central to their reanalysis of the NCDS data published in 1985 (47). The authors took issue with the NCDS investigators' "conceptual implication ... that the optimal therapy prescription would be comprised of high protein intake and intensive dialysis," finding instead that outcome was a discontinuous function of Kt/V with no further improvement at levels of that variable higher than 0.9. Thus, they concluded that "a fully adequate dialysis prescription is provided with PCR = 1.0 and Kt/V = 1.0 and that prescribing higher levels of these nutritional and dialysis parameters are of no apparent clinical value" (47).

The conceptual implication of this conclusion with respect to dialysis time was clear: sufficient total dose was established (Kt/V = 1.0), and dialysis time, t, could be shortened as desired as long as a compensatory increase in dialyzer urea clearance, K, kept Kt/V constant. This strategy was adopted by the Regional Kidney Disease Program (RKDP) in Minneapolis, Minnesota, which chose to utilize newly available high-clearance cellulose acetate dialyzers to achieve the high clearances necessary to shorten time to three hours or less. The technical feasibility of extremely short dialysis times, even less than three hours, had been established by several groups using large dialyzers in series to achieve urea clearances over 400 ml/min (31, 32). Calling the RKDP approach 'rapid high-efficiency hemodialysis,' Keshaviah and Collins, in a series of descriptive publications (4, 33, 48–56), did much to popularize both the terminology and the concept of extremely short dialysis with cellulose membranes. Largely due to their usage, 'high-efficiency' has come to be used as a description of a particular hemodialysis modality; that is, high-urea clearance dialysis using cellulosic dialyzers with ultrafiltration coefficients in the range of 10 to 20 – a description derived from the characteristics of the Baxter CA-170 and CA-210 dialyzers used by the RKDP.

By the mid-eighties a number of manufacturers were producing dialyzers capable of delivering treatments which could be characterized as 'high-efficiency' by the standard of the day – that is, dialyzers with K_OA for urea higher than about 500 ml/min – but barriers existed to their widespread use. Their increased solute clearance was associated with a concomitant increase in water permeability, leading to the necessity for volumetric ultrafiltration-control devices (57). The problem of acetate intolerance during high-clearance dialysis which had been discovered and described a few years earlier (58–60) was exacerbated by the use of these even more permeable dialyzers (48, 61, 62), necessitating the use of bicarbonate as the dialysate buffer (49). Both volumetric ultrafiltration and bicarbonate buffer capability required new, more expensive delivery systems, and the dialyzers themselves were considerably more costly than the conventional cellulosic devices used in the overwhelming majority of dialysis units.

Table 2. Dialysis time in two large studies in the United States

	Patients	Weekly dialysis time		
		< 9 hr	*9–10.5 hr**	*> 10.5 hr*
National Medical Care (21)	19746	40%	18%	42%
USRDS 1986–1987 incident cohort (22)	3757	17%	52%	31%

*USRDS data are for 9–11 hr.

The response of dialyzer manufacturers was to market high-clearance dialyzers as a tool to shorten time (63), offsetting the higher cost of the devices by increasing the potential daily census of the dialysis unit, thus lowering labor costs per treatment. In the United States, with an economic environment characterized by a fixed government reimbursement per dialysis which has not increased since 1973 (64, 65), this approach found a receptive audience. Held and colleagues (66), studying the relationships between funding and treatment duration, found that the degree of reduction of time practiced in dialysis units after the reduction in Medicare reimbursement of 1983 was related to the extent of decreased funding in each unit, and that the shortest treatments were received by patients in for-profit units. The combination of marketing and economic pressure with the intellectual justification provided by urea modeling, and the easily applied reciprocal manipulation of K and t led to ferocious shortening of treatments in the US (16, 66, 67). The extent of this shortening is suggested by Table 2, which shows the results of two studies of dialysis prescription in large populations – the 237 units of the National Medical Care proprietary dialysis chain (68), and the presumably representative sample of 3,823 patients starting hemodialysis in 1986–1987 evaluated by the United States Renal Data System (USRDS) (69). As can be seen, about 60% of the patients receive 3.5 hours or less per treatment. In fact, the median weekly treatment time for the USRDS patients was 9.0 hours, indicating that fully one-half were treated for 3 hours or less (69). That these figures are representative of US practice is confirmed by the findings of the St Louis Nephrology Study Group (70), which examined hemodialysis delivery for 617 patients in 16 outpatient units in metropolitan St. Louis and found a mean treatment length of 3.2 ± 0.4 hours. Infatuation with short time appears primarily to be a United States phenomenon; USRDS data for European dialysis prescriptions shows a mean weekly treatment time of 12.1 hours and a median of 11.3 hours (69), while information showing mean treatment lengths of well over 4 hours is available from Australia (71) and Japan (72, 73).

Urea modeling and short dialysis have developed together in the US, and many of the regional regulatory agencies that oversee dialysis there have begun if not to require, at least to recommend that treatment be monitored by urea kinetics. In Europe acceptance of urea kinetic modeling has been less enthusiastic. In Germany, for example, less than 10% of dialysis centers used kinetic modeling in 1990 to prescribe and monitor therapy (74). Median treatment duration was longer – over 11 hours per week – and dialysis mortality considerably lower than in the US. The cause-and-effect relationships among these facts are not straightforward, but even in the US an association has been described between use of kinetic modeling and short treatment times (10). Precise mathematical quantification of dialysis dose, while in theory a goal greatly to be desired, has in practice been problematic (16, 74, 75), and will be reexamined in a later section with regard to adequacy of short dialysis.

Convective therapies: Middle molecules redux

Since the earliest period of chronic dialysis, there has been a parallel current of development of renal replacement therapy based on the use of synthetic, non-cellulosic membranes with increased permeability to larger molecular weight solutes and to water. Henderson and colleagues set this current in motion in 1967 with the conceptualization of 'diafiltration' (76), the removal of solutes from blood by pure convective transfer; that is, by ultrafiltration and 'solvent drag' without diffusion down a chemical gradient into dialysate. Clinical use of the technique was described by Quellhorst et al. in 1972 (77), using the same Rhone-Poulenc RP-6 dialyzer and sulfonated PAN membrane utilized by Man and his colleagues in their trial of shortened dialysis (25). Renamed 'hemofiltration' at a Swiss conference in 1977, this approach to therapy was limited in its adoption by complexity, high cost, and infectious complications (78), and its use in shortened therapy was impeded by its rather poor clearance of small molecules. Interest in the technique remained high, however, because of the impressive hemodynamic stability of patients treated with hemofiltration in comparison to those treated with acetate hemodialysis (79). One solution to the problem of limited small molecular weight clearance was the development of membranes which could increase ultrafiltration, or transmembrane fluid flux, to extremely high rates, from 120 ml/min to over 200 ml/min (79–82). Since small molecules like urea, with a sieving coefficient of unity, will be cleared at a rate equal to the ultrafiltration rate, this 'high flux' hemofiltration resulted in clearances in an acceptable range and allowed considerably shorter treatment times (79, 81, 82).

The method remained complex and expensive, requiring extremely large volumes of sterile replacement solution, but another approach was developing to exploit the high large-molecular weight permeability of the new PAN-SO$_3$, polyamide, polymethylmethacrylate, and polysulfone membranes – simultaneous hemodialysis and hemofiltration, or hemodiafiltration (83). This strategy utilized a synthetic membrane in a conventional dialysis configuration for diffusive clearance of small solutes, while using volumetric ultrafiltration control to achieve a constant, moderately high rate of ultrafiltration and resultant convective clearance of both large and small molecules (84).

Several groups used hemodiafiltration techniques either with high-performance membranes (30), or a high surface-area double-dialyzer configuration (31) to reduce treatment time to as little as six hours per week.

Hemodiafiltration retained the necessity for the administration of large volumes of sterile substitution fluid – 18 to 27 l per treatment (30) – and thus was not a practical alternative to hemodialysis. The superior hemodynamic stability with convective therapies became less of an advantage, as hemodialysis with bicarbonate dialysate and volumetric ultrafiltration control became increasingly available. The additional removal of large solutes achieved by convection had great theoretical appeal, especially to those who maintained belief in the importance of middle molecule toxicity. With ultrafiltration control, however, the membranes used in hemofiltration and hemodiafiltration could be utilized for more conventional diffusive hemodialysis, and their greater permeability resulted in markedly increased clearance of larger molecules even without the contribution of convective transfer. Inspection of Table 3 reveals the high-molecular weight clearance characteristics of the 'high-flux' membranes AN-69 (the renamed PAN-SO$_3$), PMMA, cellulose triacetate, and polysulfone. These membranes and the modified cellulose acetate marketed as a high-flux device achieve significantly higher diffusive clearances of the 1350 Dalton vitamin B$_{12}$ than do conventional membranes, at similar levels of urea removal, and only the high-flux membranes clear the 11 800 Dalton polypeptide β-2-microglobulin. Permeability of dialysis membranes to high-molecular weight solutes is related to high water permeability; among the membranes in Table 3, vitamin B$_{12}$ clearance is highly correlated with ultrafiltration coefficient ($r = 0.855$, $p < 0.001$).

Use of these synthetic membranes for diffusive hemodialysis – so-called high-flux dialysis – became a successful and fairly widely adopted strategy for reduction of session length to three hours or less (28, 34, 35, 93). By the late 1980s, high-flux was widely (and inaccurately) perceived to be synonymous with short time (94–96) again abetted by vigorous dialyzer marketing (97). There may be real advantages of high-flux dialysis other than potential time-shortening, however, which reside in the beneficial effects of improved biocompatibility and enhanced middle and large molecule clearance (62), benefits which are still not conclusively established, but which will be discussed later in this chapter.

The prevalence of high-flux treatment in the present dialysis environment is difficult to determine. The best information is probably available for the United States, where the Centers for Disease Control, in annual surveys of dialysis-associated diseases, collect data by mailed questionnaire on the use of high-efficiency and high-flux dialyzers (defined as K_{UF} 10–19 and ≥ 20 ml $\cdot$ hr^{-1} $\cdot$ mmHg^{-1}, respectively) (98) (Table 4). The number of patients so treated has increased each year since 1987, by this count having reached an estimated 17% of the total dialysis population receiving high-flux, and 12% high-efficiency dialysis by 1991.

SHORT DIALYSIS: LIMITING FACTORS

To a large extent, the effect of dialysis session length cannot be separated from that of the total dialysis dose – a function of both time and clearance – and from the additional effect of patient body size, and without doubt some of the drawbacks of short dialysis are due to inadequate dose. Nevertheless, there are a number of problems which have been closely associated with shortening of therapy – problems related to increased small molecule clearance, such as disequilibrium and acetate toxicity, and those which result more directly from the time decrease itself, such as difficulty in controlling volume overload and hypertension, and the failure to provide adequate solute removal.

Disequilibrium

The dialysis disequilibrium syndrome (DDS) is a clinical complex characterized by nausea, vomiting, headache, somnolence, lethargy, restlessness, irritability, hypertension, cardiac arrhythmias, and occasionally seizures, occurring during or shortly after hemodialysis (99–103). First reported by Kennedy et al. in 1962 (99), it is said to occur most commonly in patients with rapid and marked intradialytic falls in urea, especially when predialysis urea levels are particularly high, and during the first few hemodialysis treatments. Although several mechanisms have been proposed, no firm consensus exists regarding the cause of DDS symptoms. Most of the putative mechanisms involve an increase in intracranial pressure brought about either by a rapid fall in plasma urea with a slower change in CNS levels ('reverse urea effect') (99–101, 104), by systemic to CNS acid-base disequilibrium with (105) or without (106) the effect of CNS 'idiogenic osmoles', or by fall in plasma osmolality secondary to dialysis-induced hyponatremia (107).

Table 3. Solute clearances and ultrafiltration cofeficients of contemporary dialysis membranes (85–92)

Membrane[a]	Dialyzer	Surface area (m^2)	Clearance (ml/min)[b]			K_{UF}[c]
			Urea	B_{12}	β-2-m	
Saponified cellulose ester	Althin 135 SCE	1.5	177	43	0	3.1
Cuprophan	Baxter CF-15	1.1	173	46	0	4.2
Cellulose acetate	Althin Altra Nova 140	1.4	161	55	0	5.7
'Low-flux' polysulfone	Fresenius F6	1.3	183	56	0	5.5
'Low-flux' PMMA	Toray B2-1.5H	1.2	193	72	0	7.5
Cellulose acetate (HE)	Baxter CA 210	2.1	192	77	0	12.0
Modified cellulose acetate	CD (Althin) DuoFlux	1.4	171	88	11	15.0
Sulfonated PAN (AN69)	Hospal Filtral 16	1.6	181	91	36	38.0
PMMA	Toray B1-2.1U	2.1	192	119	[d]	17.0
Cellulose triacetate	Baxter CT-190	1.9	192	137	39	36.0
Polysulfone	Fresenius F80	1.9	196	144	54	60.0

[a]PMMA = polymethylmethacrylate; PAN = polyacrylonitrile; HE = 'high-efficiency'.
[b]All clearances measured *in vitro* at 200 ml/min test-solution flow and 500 ml/min dialysate flow.
[c]Ultrafiltration coefficient, ml · hr^{-1} · mmHg^{-1}.
[d]PMMA β-2-microglobulin removal is equal to that of polysulfone, but entirely by adsorption (89).

Table 4. Prevalence of high-flux and high-efficiency hemodialysis in the United States, 1987–1991 (98)

Year	Total centers	Total patients	High-flux[a]		High-efficiency[b]	
			Centers (%)	Patients (%)	Centers (%)	Patients (%)
1987	1,486	97,225	224 (15)	5,057 (5)	–	–
1988	1,586	107,804	284 (18)	8,351 (8)	–	–
1989	1,726	122,734	387 (22)	12,658 (12)	396 (23)	9,598 (8)
1990	1,882	140,608	478 (25)	17,363 (12)	528 (28)	14,587 (10)
1991	2,046	155,877	624 (30)	26,379 (17)	642 (31)	19,456 (12)

[a]High-flux defined as dialyzer ultrafiltration coefficient $\geq$ 20 ml/hr/mmHg.
[b]High-efficiency defined as dialyzer ultrafiltration coefficient 10–19 ml/hr/mmHg. Data on high-efficiency dialysis not collected prior to 1989.

Whatever the mechanism, disequilibrium is associated with rapid changes in serum chemistry, and is thus a feared consequence of high-efficiency therapies, especially in children (20, 108). Nonetheless, disequilibrium-type symptoms are quite rare in current patient populations undergoing short rapid therapies (109–111). Evaluation of EEG pattern and of computed tomography indicators of cerebral hydration and ventricular size (112), and measurement of intraocular pressure (113) – a correlate of intracranial pressure – have shown no changes during high-flux dialysis. The presumably exaggerated 'unphysiology' (114) of short high-clearance therapy does not appear to be associated with increased intradialytic or interdialytic symptoms, perhaps because of improvements in dialytic technique, including volumetric ultrafiltration and use of dialysate with higher sodium concentration (115) and with bicarbonate as the buffer anion.

Acetate 'intolerance'

During the mid-1970s, with rising small molecule permeability of dialysis membranes, development of extremely high intradialytic serum acetate levels was noted in some patients, and the suggestion was made that symptoms including hypotension, nausea, and vomiting were attributable at least in part to a toxic effect of the acetate anion (116). The degree of postdialysis hyperacetatemia was soon shown to be related to urea clearance, with large surface-area dialyzers and 'high-efficiency' treatments clearly related to higher levels of acetate (58, 60, 116–118). While some early studies correlated the degree of rise in serum acetate with occurrence of symptoms (116, 119), this has generally not been confirmed, and a quantitative relationship between acetate levels and incidence of symptoms has been difficult to demonstrate (120–122).

Studies comparing treatments with acetate and bicarbonate containing dialysates have consistently demonstrated a higher incidence of episodes of nausea and vomiting with acetate, but the role of dialysate acetate in hypotension has been less clear (48, 49, 61, 123–125), with only a few reports of statistically significant differences between acetate and bicarbonate in unselected patient groups (35, 128). It may be that a hypotensive response to acetate is related to a patient-specific 'acetate sensitivity', occurring in some 10 to 20% of dialysis patients (126–131).

The serum acetate levels required to show an effect in sensitive patients appear to be about 2 to 5 mmol/L – fully within the range achieved in relatively low-urea clearance dialysis. Few studies have been reported comparing the incidence of intradialytic symptoms in standard *vs* high-urea clearance acetate dialysis, and those that are available show differences in postdialysis serum acetate and bicarbonate levels, but little or no difference in incidence of symptoms (20, 48, 49, 60, 62). Nonetheless, a definition of 'high-efficiency' hemodialysis has been proposed based on a urea clearance-to-body weight ratio of 3.0 ml $\cdot min^{-1} \cdot kg^{-1}$, said to be a dialysis efficiency above which acetate-induced symptoms would become intolerable, and bicarbonate dialysate would be required (55, 56). This is, however, based on extrapolation of data from dialysis of ten infants weighing 3–14 kg, who demonstrated more nausea and vomiting but not hypotension at clearance ratios greater than 3.3 ml $\cdot min^{-1} \cdot kg^{-1}$ (132), and has not been borne out in adults. The hemodynamic effects of acetate are ameliorated by use of volumetric ultrafiltration and by a dialysate sodium concentration of 140 mEq/L or greater (121, 125, 133, 134) and several reports exist of groups of patients dialyzed with high-flux techniques and high-sodium, acetate-containing dialysate, with low rates of intradialytic symptoms (34, 135).

The incidence of symptoms in high and low clearance acetate dialysis is compared with that in bicarbonate high flux dialysis in Table 5, where it can be seen that, while the differences between dialyses with high and low acetate transfer are not striking, all methods of acetate dialysis lead to more nausea and vomiting, and more intradialytic saline administration, than bicarbonate dialysis. In short treatment strategies, which require rapid removal of volume, use of bicarbonate dialysate can only improve patient tolerance, and is certainly to be preferred. In any case, the acetate-bicarbonate 'controversy' is becoming less and less heated, as dialysis units increasingly replace outmoded delivery systems with bicarbonate-capable equipment, and as the cost differential between acetate and bicarbonate dialysate has become smaller. Data from the American Centers for Disease Control indicate that in 1986 only 22% of surveyed US dialysis centers used bicarbonate dialysate, while by 1991 that number had risen to 91% (98), virtually rendering the controversy moot.

Blood flow rate and vascular access

Short treatment times require extremely high dialyzer clearance of small molecular weight solutes, and even with the more permeable high flux membranes, the achievement of elevated clearances of urea, creatinine, potassium, and phosphate requires maneuvers which maximize diffusive transport, such as the use of large surface area dialyzers. One such maneuver, which is universally available and easily performed, is the augmentation of blood and dialysate flow rates. Increasing dialysate flow results in the use of larger quantities of concentrate per dialysis, and thus increases costs, but blood flow is free, and recent experience has made it clear that use of flow rates of 400 ml/min or more is a safe and effective means of raising small molecule clearance (136, 137). The advantage gained from blood flow increases is limited by the overall mass transfer coefficient ($K_O A$) for urea of the dialyzer (Figure 1), but almost all dialyzers in use today have $K_O A$ values for urea between 400 and 900 ml/min, and in this range significant clearance increases continue up to blood flows of at least 600 ml/min (138). Flow rates in fistulas and grafts have been measured using ultrasound techniques, and mean values range from 700 to over 1000 ml/min (139–145). There is also evidence that blood flow through polytetrafluoroethylene grafts markedly increases during dialysis, so that even an access with a lower 'resting' flow can support intradialytic extracorporeal flow rates over 400 ml/min (146).

There is still concern in many dialysis units that very high blood flow rates may increase intradialytic symptoms, or lead to 'steal' phenomena by diverting blood from the systemic circulation, but there is no evidence that this is true, either from clinical experience (34, 136), or in several studies of left ventricular function in patients dialyzed with blood flow rates up to 450 ml/min (145, 147, 148). The increased shear force generated by the high flow might be expected to cause access stenosis and a higher incidence of thrombotic complications, but the limited published information available would indicate that this is not the case (149). Intradialytic thrombosis of the dialyzer and lines may actually be reduced at high blood flows, an effect which can be important in heparin-free dialysis (150, 151).

Use of blood flow rates of 400 to 600 ml/min does require larger, 15 gauge dialysis needles, and usually leads to venous pressures in excess of 200 mmHg, a potential problem when non-volumetric ultrafiltration systems are used (152). Highly negative pre-pump pressures are also generated, which lead to partial collapse of the intra-pump segment of the blood line and consequent inaccuracy of blood flow settings. When using a flow rate of 400 ml/min the negative arterial pressure is in the range of −200 to −250 mmHg (153), and the rate indicated by the machine may overestimate actual flow by 10 to 15% (154, 155). At 600 ml/min indicated flow the error may reach 30% (153–155). This error can be extremely important, as it

Table 5. Incidence of intradialytic symptoms according to dialysate buffer and dialyzer efficiency

	I Standard acetate[a]	II High-flux acetate[b] K/Wt < 3	III High-flux acetate[b] K/Wt > 3	IV High-flux bicarbonate[b]
Patients	12	4	4	8
Treatments	191	28	32	46
K_{urea}, ml/min	192 ± 6^g	220 ± 9	239 ± 9	233 ± 11
K/Wt, ml/min/kg	2.8	2.4 ± 0.1^g	3.5 ± 0.1^g	2.9 ± 0.1
Kt/V	$1.28 \pm 0.06^{c,d,g}$	$0.84 \pm 0.03^{d,g}$	1.08 ± 0.05	1.02 ± 0.03
Wt loss, % body weight	3.0 ± 0.2^e	3.3 ± 0.3	3.7 ± 1.0	3.5 ± 0.2
Post-HD acetate (mmol/l)		$2.9 \pm 0.2^{e,g}$	5.0 ± 0.3^g	0.6 ± 0.1
Saline administered (ml)		239 ± 65^g	234 ± 53^g	82 ± 23
Incidence (%) of				
BP < 90	17	11	22	15
Nausea	16^f	14	22^f	4
Vomiting	8	3	19^g	0

[a] Standard acetate dialysis: cuprophan dialyzers, mean time 253 min, dialysate Na 140 mEq/l (49).
[b] High-flux dialysis: 1.7 m^2 AN69 dialyzers, time 180 min, dialysate Na 142–145 mEq/l (62).
[c] $P < 0.01$ vs group II.
[d] $P < 0.05$ vs group III.
[e] $P < 0.01$ vs group III.
[f] $P < 0.05$ vs bicarbonate (group IV).
[g] $P < 0.01$ vs group IV.
None of the differences in symptom incidence among acetate groups is statistically significant.

Table 6. Blood flow rate (BFR), recirculation (Recirc), and urea clearance (K_U) (151)

BFR (ml/min)	Non-stenotic accesses (N = 10)		Stenotic accesses (N = 5)	
	Recirc (%)	K_U (ml/min)	Recirc (%)	K_U (ml/min)
200	8.1 ± 1.3	146 ± 9	16.7 ± 3.6	139 ± 8
400	11.1 ± 2.0	210 ± 11	25.9 ± 3.5	182 ± 8
600	13.4 ± 1.8	263 ± 19	27.9 ± 3.4	205 ± 42

Means $\pm$ SEM. Clearances corrected for recirculation, hematocrit, ultrafiltration, and BFR inaccuracy.

may lead to systematic overestimation of delivered urea clearance.

An important concern when using high blood flows is the associated increase in access recirculation (153, 156). Even taking increased recirculation into account, urea clearance is significantly elevated by raising blood flow rates, but in a patient with a stenotic access the recirculation may reach quite high values at higher blood flows, and so may seriously compromise treatment adequacy (Table 6).

Hypertension

Eighty to ninety percent of patients beginning hemodialysis are hypertensive (157, 158). Hypertension in the dialysis population, like that in any population, has a complex pathogenesis, but in the large majority of patients the major pathogenetic factor appears to be extracellular volume expansion, with control of blood pressure frequently achievable by adequate ultrafiltration and maintenance of 'dry weight' (157–163). During a single dialysis, an ultrafiltrate volume equal to or greater than the plasma volume must often be removed, and thus the efficacy of ultrafiltration is limited by the rate of plasma refilling from the extravascular compartment (164). When dialysis time is shortened, the rate of ultrafiltration must be correspondingly increased, and may surpass the plasma refilling rate, precipitating hypotensive episodes and incomplete control of extravascular volume. Thus poor control of hypertension is a potential problem with shortened dialysis sessions.

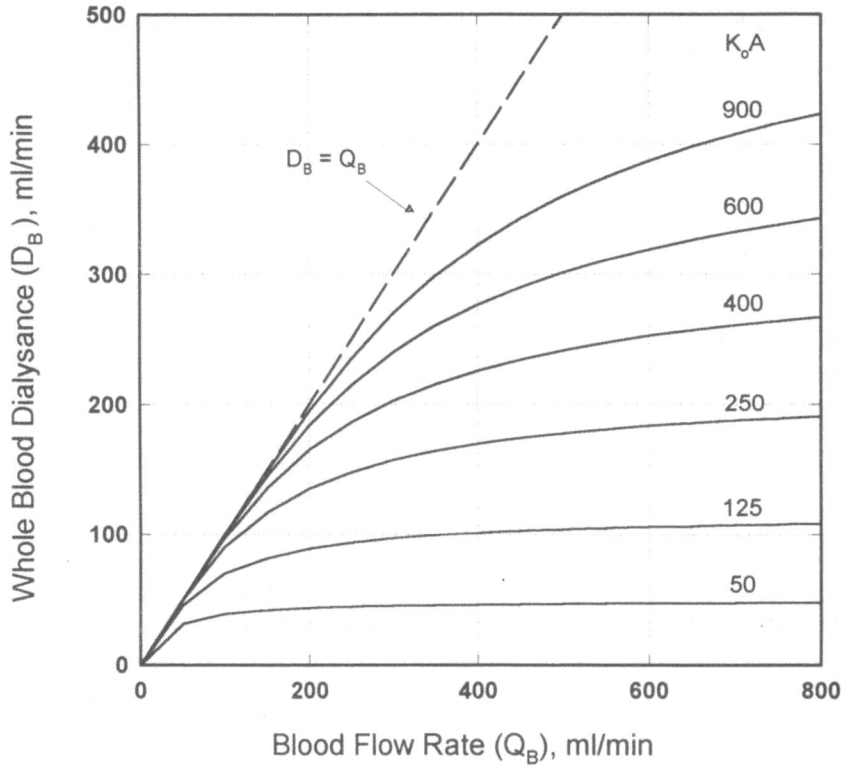

Figure 1. Dependence of dialysance on blood flow rate, plotted for different values of $K_O A$. For a solute with concentration = 0 in afferent dialysate, such as urea, dialysance is equal to clearance.

This in fact appears to be the case. Although several authors have reported long-term results of short dialysis schedules with no increase in hypertension (28, 35, 165), the majority of reported experience has been less optimistic. In an early comparison of short and long dialysis, one of the principal differences in outcome was the higher likelihood in the short dialysis group (30% *vs* 6%) of failure to control blood pressure (166). In the initial report of short treatment by Keshaviah et al. (48), the incidence of predialysis hypertension was 9% in the standard treatment group and 17 and 24% in the groups treated with rapid bicarbonate and rapid acetate dialysis. Antihypertensive medication was needed in 54% of patients treated by Raja et al. with short schedules (167) and 65% of those reported by Greenwood (168). Wizemann and Kramer (8), after eight years of application of short dialysis treatment, abandoned the approach because of poor cardiovascular tolerance, concluding that "in the vast majority of patients, short renal replacement therapy, associated with rapid fluid removal, should be avoided due to cardiac findings" – specifically, left ventricular hypertrophy or coronary artery disease. When, over four years, the mean treatment time in their program was raised from approximately 2.6 to 4 hr, there was a marked fall in hospitalization rate, and the percentage of patients requiring antihypertensive medications dropped from 73 to 20%.

A standard for comparison is available in the reports from the Centre de Rein Artificiel in Tassin, France, where as of 1994 the standard dialysis prescription remains 24 square-meter hours per week using 1 m² Kiil cuprophan dialyzers (169); session lengths, that is, of approximately eight hours. Using this regimen, satisfactory blood pressure control and discontinuation of all antihypertensive medications was achieved within six months of starting dialysis in all but 7 of 445 patients (170). The remarkable patient survival of this population – 55% at ten years, higher than any other reported figure – is ascribed, at least in part, to the striking control of extracorporeal volume and hypertension enabled by long, slow ultrafiltration (170–173). If hypertension is in fact poorly controlled in the majority of dialysis patients (162, 163), the overall trend to shorter dialysis duration may be an important contributory factor, especially in the US, where mean treatment times appear to be in the range of 3 to 3.2 hours per session. This may in part be due to increasing use of high-sodium dialysate (8, 157), but is more likely related to the difficulty in achieving adequate ultrafiltration without cramps or hypotension in 3.5 hours or less.

(In)adequacy

It has long been known and accepted that shortening of dialysis time requires increasing the rate of solute removal. With the 1980s and the use of urea kinetic modeling, the basis of measurement has become small solute clearance, particularly that of urea, and the standard for shortening dialysis sessions has been maintenance of a constant value of Kt/V. Two problems arise – the questionable applicability of the model in extremely short, high clearance dialysis, and uncertainty about the minimum safe value of Kt/V.

The mathematical model used in the NCDS, and which underlies virtually all methods of calculation of Kt/V, assumes the distribution of urea in a single compartment, roughly equal to total body water, with input from metabolic generation, output to dialytic removal with or without residual renal function, and instantaneous equilibration of concentration changes throughout the distribution space. Since urea (as well as most other solutes) is in fact distributed in at least two physical compartments – intra- and extracellular – with a barrier to diffusion between them, the single compartment model can only approximate the actual behavior of urea during and between hemodialysis treatments. This approximation is the more accurate the greater is the difference between the rate constants for dialytic elimination of the solute and for diffusion across the intercompartmental barrier. That is, if urea is removed slowly from the extracellular compartment by dialysis, but moves relatively quickly across cell membranes, its behavior will simulate distribution in a single compartment, with changes in concentration distributed throughout body water in an apparently rapid and homogeneous manner. The shorter and more efficient the dialysis, the more 'two-compartment' the behavior (174–176).

Multicompartmental mathematical models for hemodialysis can be and have been constructed (176–181) which more accurately describe the changes in intradialytic urea concentration, especially during a short dialysis. Figure 2 illustrates the differences between the concentration changes and total urea removal predicted by the most widely used single- (43) and two-compartment (176, 181) models. Compared to the multicompartment model, single-compartment kinetics overestimates urea removal for a given change in blood concentration, and this overestimate increases as duration is shortened, from 5% in the hypothetical 5-hour dialysis shown, to 12% in the shorter 2.5-hour session. Furthermore, two-compartment behavior is more marked for large, less diffusible molecules, so that the relationship of urea removal to larger molecular weight solute removal changes as hemodialysis is shortened and made more efficient. As a result, a given change in urea implies one level of middle-molecule removal in a 5-hour dialysis, and another, lower level in a shorter treatment. A Kt/V value of 1.2, therefore, does not have the

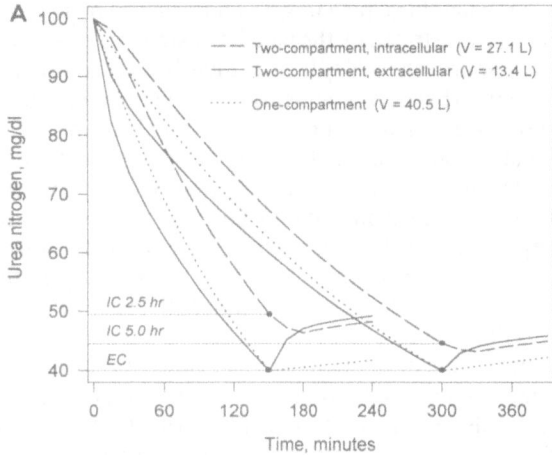

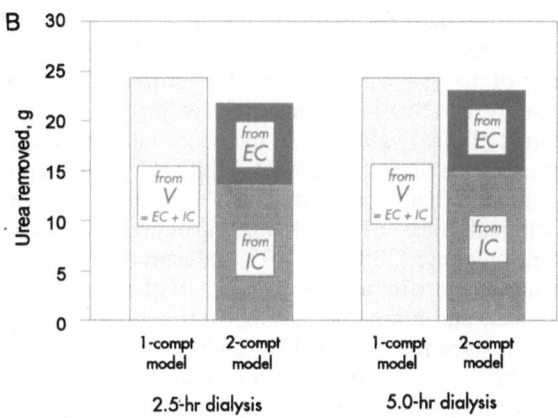

Figure 2. Prediction of urea removal by one-compartment and two-compartment fixed-volume models of urea kinetics, for two hemodialyses with identical change in blood urea concentration but different duration (2.5 vs 5.0 hr). For each dialysis, body weight = 70 kg, g = 10 mg/min, V_U = 40.6 l, intercompartmental transport coefficient for urea = 700 ml/min, urea reduction = 60%. A: Changes in urea nitrogen concentration during and after dialysis, showing end-dialysis concentration in the intracellular (IC 2.5 hr and IC 5.0 hr) and extracellular (EC) compartments. The single-compartment model assumes homogeneous distribution in a single intra- and extracellular compartment. B: Total urea removal predicted by each model for 2.5 and 5.0-hr dialyses. Single compartment model overestimates urea removal by 5% for a 5.0-hr dialysis and by 12% for a 2.5-hr dialysis.

same significance in a long, slow dialysis as it does in a rapid, high-clearance treatment (174, 175, 182–184).

The systematic underestimate of dialysis dose by single-compartment methods in short high-efficiency treatments has led some authors to recommend two-compartment modeling (182), but use of these more complex approaches are hampered by the difficulty of determining the necessary physiological parameters – in particular, intercompartmental rate constants – for individual patients (185). Others have suggested simply increasing the target values of Kt/V and urea reduction ratio (183,

184), but what those new target values should be is not at all clear, as illustrated by the fact that, using this somewhat arbitrary approach, a Kt/V of 1.2 has been recommended for high-efficiency treatments (183), while others have suggested 1.2 as a minimum value for Kt/V in any dialysis, including conventional low-clearance methods (186). A multicenter cooperative study currently being planned by the US National Institute of Diabetes, Digestive and Kidney Diseases (187) may shed some light on this question, but what is currently clear is that, especially in the US, short treatment times are common, but such levels of dialysis dose are not.

Central to the evaluation of the adequacy of short treatment methods is a definition of adequacy, and this is still an incompletely answered question. The NCDS established urea as a valid surrogate marker for uremic toxins, and ushered in the era of kinetic modeling, but did not define a standard for optimal dialysis. The statement by Gotch and Sargent in 1985 that a Kt/V of 1.0 represented a dose of dialysis which achieved the minimum possible morbidity, and that increasing dialysis further was "of no apparent clinical value" (47), has since been challenged even using the data of the NCDS itself (188). Both a reexamination of that data and of Gotch's analysis (188, 189), and clinical studies of the relationship of urea removal and patient outcome (170, 189–195) indicate that morbidity and mortality are improved by dialysis with a Kt/V of 1.2 or greater, and it may be reasonable to believe that optimal dialysis requires a Kt/V as high as 1.4 or more (189, 196). Table 7 shows the effect of higher levels of Kt/V on mortality, with USRDS data shown for comparison. While these studies largely lack simultaneous controls, the data are nonetheless striking, and strongly suggest a positive effect from increasing Kt/V well beyond even 1.2. It is probably fair to say that there is consensus in the US today that 1.2 is the minimum adequate value of Kt/V (186).

Accepting this value as a definition of adequate dialysis, one may proceed to ask what is the minimum treatment duration for delivery of this dialysis dose. The answer depends, of course, on dialyzer urea clearance and the body weight of the patient. Figure 3 presents the relationships between K, t and V (expressed as body weight, estimated as $V/0.55$) in graphic form for a dialysis which will provide $Kt/V = 1.2$. Inspection of the graph reveals that for a 3-hour dialysis, a 70 kg patient would require a dialyzer urea clearance of 276 ml/min, and for a 2.5-hour dialysis, 336 ml/min would be necessary. It is now important to know whether these are realistic clearances, obtainable with currently available equipment. Table 8 shows dialyzer clearances obtained by measurement of the urea in the entire volume of spent dialysate, an accurate measure of effective clearance. The values in the table have been corrected upward to compensate for the effect of access recirculation, measured in all cases, which was $11.4 \pm 7.9\%$ (mean $\pm$ SD). No measured clearance was higher than 300 ml/min. The larger surface-area high-

efficiency dialyzers, like the F-60, F-80 and CA210 were able to achieve 240–260 ml/min, but it is unlikely that much higher values can be reached with a single dialyzer. Thus it would seem that with the best available dialyzer, the highest blood and dialysate flows, and a well-functioning access, a patient weighing 70 kg or less *might* achieve a Kt/V of 1.2 in 3 hours. In 2.5 hours it is not possible with currently available equipment. In the US, however – where 3-hour treatment times are common – patients are apparently not being dialyzed with the largest dialyzers and the highest blood flows. A representative cohort of 3823 patients beginning hemodialysis in 1986–1987 have been studied by the United States Renal Data System, and found to be dialyzed with a median time of 9.0 hours, using dialyzers with a mean clearance of 181 ml/min and mean surface area of 0.9 m^2 at a mean blood flow rate of 248 ml/min, with high-flux dialyzers used for 3.3% of patients (69, 198). Prescribed clearances, moreover, are often based on manufacturer-supplied data, which, because they are derived from so-called *in vitro* measurements using aqueous solutions of urea, because they are frequently extrapolated from measurements made at low dialysate and blood flow rates, and because they take no account of clearance losses from intradialytic blood clotting, recirculation, and the like, almost always grossly overestimate dialyzer performance (Table 8) (199, 200). When prescriptions are formulated on the basis of these inflated clearance values, dangerously inadequate treatments may result (201). Adding to the shortfall in delivered clearance are the effects of erythropoietin-stimulated hematocrits (202, 203), access recirculation (148), and the various forms of temporal corner-cutting that often occur in a busy dialysis unit (196). All in all, it is not surprising that, to paraphrase LeFebvre et al. (204), patients do not get what the physician *thinks* he or she prescribes.

While the situation in the US does appear to be changing – the latest data from the Centers for Disease Control indicating a rise in the use of high-flux dialyzers to 17% by 1991 (98) – the great majority of American patients continue to be dialyzed with conventional cellulose dialyzers. The second part of Table 8 shows conventional dialyzer clearances at blood flows of 330–350 ml/min. The most efficient among them approaches, but does not reach, 200 ml/min; the overall mean clearance value is 176 ml/min, not much different from the mean prescribed clearance of 181 ml/min for the USRDS patients. With a dialyzer urea clearance of 190 ml/min, only a patient weighing less than 52 kg can be dialyzed in three hours with a Kt/V of 1.2 or more. A 70 kg patient cannot receive adequate dialysis in less than four hours, and a patient weighing 90 kg needs five hours. Some leeway is afforded by residual renal function, and it is probably for that reason that patients do as well as they do on short dialysis, since 1 or 2 ml/min of native glomerular filtration is the equivalent of 20–40 ml/min extra dialyzer clearance, considering only urea. As their residual renal function dis-

Table 7. Kt/V and patient survival on hemodialysis

Unit	N	Kt/V	Survival			
			1 year	*2 years*	*5 years*	*10 years*
USRDS 1993 (197)	121987	0.8?	77%	60%	28%	13%
Taiwan # 1 (190)	505	1.5		78%		
Taiwan # 2 (193)	256	1.85	95%	86%	73%	
Tassin, FR (47)	445	1.7			87%	75%
Vanderbilt* (194)	92	0.82	77%			
	114	0.96	82%			
	128	1.01	84%			
	130	1.18	91%			
Dallas* (195)	809	1.18	77%			
	869	1.21	80%			
	884	1.39	83%			
	764	1.46	83%			

*Vanderbilt and Dallas data are for consecutive years.

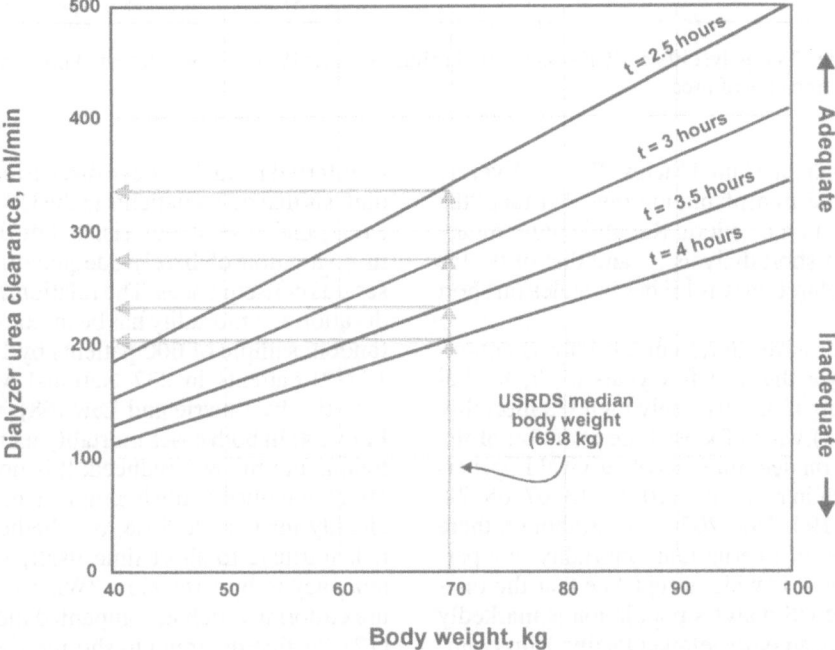

Figure 3. Dialyzer urea clearance required to provide Kt/V = 1.2 at various treatment lengths. Any clearance above the time line for a given body weight will provide $Kt/v \geq 1.2$. Thus, for a patient weighing 69.8 kg, a clearance of 202 ml/min for 4 hours or 336 ml/min for 2.5 hours will provide Kt/V = 1.2. A blood flow rate of 400 ml/min and access recirculation of 10% are assumed.

appears, however, trouble may ensue for many patients on short dialysis regimens.

Mortality

The most troubling aspect of extreme shortening of dialysis sessions is the suspicion that the survival of dialysis patients may be compromised. The NCDS results suggested an increased morbidity associated with short time, but did not address mortality (46). The earliest epidemiological evidence that shortening of dialysis might be related to deterioration of patient outcome came from the European Dialysis and Transplant Association, which had long been more effective at data collection than any

430   *Robert H. Barth*

Table 8. Dialyzer urea clearances in clinical use, by total dialysate collection and from manufacturers' data (200)

Dialyzer	Manufacturer	Membrane*	N	Blood flow (ml/min)	K by DQU (ml/min)	K from manufacturer (ml/min)
High-flux/high-efficiency:						
CA-210	Baxter	CA	7	500	253	322
Duoflux	Cordis-Dow	CA	7	486	183	252
F-60	Fresenius	PS	5	443	256	290
F-80M	Fresenius	PS	5	390	239	281
Filtral 12	Hospal	PAN-SO$_3$	23	544	196	244
Filtral 16	Hospal	PAN-SO$_3$	27	538	230	281
Total high-flux/high-efficiency:			74	517	220	273
Conventional:						
CA-90	Baxter	CA	7	311	163	210
CD-4000	Cordis-Dow	CA	5	350	148	187
135sce	Cordis-Dow	SCE	10	338	198	229
155sce	Cordis-Dow	SCE	3	350	177	234
F-5	Fresenius	PS	6	338	177	231
Total conventional:			31	335	176	219

*CA = cellulose acetate; PS = polysulfone; SCE = saponified cellulose ester; PAN-SO$_3$ = sulfonated polyacrylonitrile; DQU = dialysate quantification of urea.

similar organization in the United States. The 1981 yearly report on dialysis and transplantation revealed that "the proportion of deaths in the Federal Republic of Germany was twice as high in short dialysis ... and that of deaths due to myocardial infarction was higher in males on short dialysis" (9).

Concern over excessive shortening of dialysis continued to be voiced over the next few years (3, 7, 8), but it was the publication of the strikingly high US mortality statistics in 1989 (11) which focused the attention of the dialysis community on determinants of survival in general, and session length in particular (10, 12, 13, 67, 68, 72, 73, 170, 186, 187, 194, 195, 205–214). Although there have been criticisms of international mortality comparisons (215, 216), there is wide acceptance that the one-year mortality in the US dialysis population is markedly higher than in European or developed Pacific Rim countries, and that the mortality has not fallen significantly over the past decade (11–13, 67, 69, 186, 187, 197, 206, 213, 217). Potential explanations for the high US mortality include case mix differences ultimately deriving from the high US acceptance rate to chronic dialysis (216), but comparisons between dialysis prescriptions in the US and other countries (71, 72, 198, 217), and data like the survival figures in Table 8 have led most observers to believe that the problem is, at least in part, one of inadequate dialysis in the US (12, 13, 67, 68, 70, 186, 194, 195, 206, 208, 212, 213, 218, 219).

While session length is only one part of the dialysis prescription and not the sole determinant of dose, it can

be inferred from the above discussion of adequacy in short dialysis that many patients in the US appear to be receiving a marginal dose of dialysis, and further shortening of time in a situation of barely adequate treatment may lead to serious consequences. The relationship between treatment duration and mortality has been examined for a nationwide random sample of 600 patients by Held et al. (10) and in 12,099 patients in 237 National Medical Care dialysis facilities by Lowrie and Lew (68), with results shown in Figure 4. In both cases mortality increased significantly as treatment time was reduced. It is not certain whether this effect of reduced time is simply a matter of reduction in an already inadequate dose, or whether there is a mortality risk intrinsic to short time itself, such as the increased tendency to hypertension. "What is certain," commented the editorial which accompanied the report by Held et al. (12), "is that the trend to shorter dialysis times has led to underdialysis and adverse clinical outcomes."

Short dialysis and adequacy: A summary

With respect to short dialysis and adequacy, particularly in the United States, several conclusions may be drawn:

1. *Acceptable dialysis can be delivered in three hours or less, but only under optimal conditions*, such as low body weight, very high dialyzer urea clearance, and low access recirculation. Practically speaking, such conditions rarely obtain in the US.

2. *With most of the dialyzers in use in the United States, adequate dialysis cannot be delivered in three hours.*

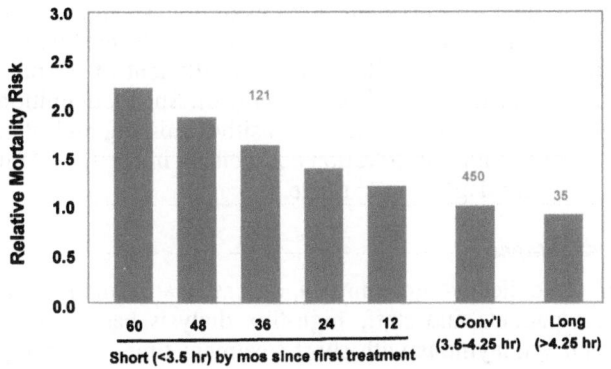

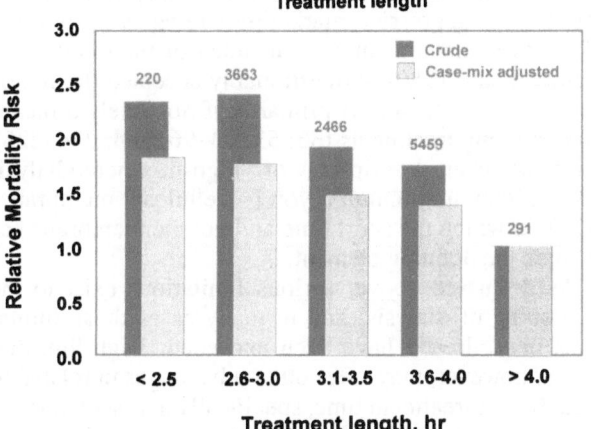

Figure 4. Relative mortality risk *vs* dialysis treatment length. A. 600 patients studied by Held et al. show higher mortality risk with treatment times less than 3.5 hours, and increasing risk with more months of exposure (10); B. National Medical Care patients show increasing mortality risk with each decrement of treatment time from greater than 4.0 to less than 2.5 hours (68). Numbers above bars are patients at risk.

Most conventional dialyzers are incapable of adequately dialyzing a 70 kg patient in less than four hours, and many high-flux/high-efficiency dialyzers cannot do it in three hours, especially in the setting of less than maximal blood flow and/or high access recirculation.

3. *Most of the dialysis delivered in the United States is inadequate. Available data indicate that most dialyses do not achieve a Kt/V of 1.0, let alone the more ambitious value of 1.2. Prescriptions are frequently founded on erroneously high dialyzer clearances supplied by manufacturers.*

4. *Short (3 hour or less) dialysis should only be used for small patients or for those who have significant residual renal function.*

HIGH-CLEARANCE HEMODIALYSIS STRATEGIES: DEFINITIONS AND ADVANTAGES

High-efficiency hemodialysis

Definition

Applied to hemodialysis, 'high-efficiency' has been and remains a relative term, referring principally to the ability of a cellulose dialyzer to clear small molecular weight solutes. Two decades ago, a hollow fiber dialyzer capable of a urea clearance of 150 ml/min was considered a high-efficiency device, while today the term is reserved for dialyzers with a $K_O A$ for urea higher than about 450 ml/min, achieving treatments with urea clearance greater than about 200 ml/min. Notwithstanding the attempts of some authors to define a precise threshold of urea clearance (220), clearance per weight (55) or clearance per distribution volume (56) above which the term would apply, there is really no strong scientific basis for such definitions. Perhaps a more practical definition is that used by the Centers for Disease Control (98); that is, use of a dialyzer with ultrafiltration coefficient between 10 and 19 ml $\cdot$ hr^{-1} $\cdot$ mmHg^{-1}. This classifies dialyzers by the necessity or not of a volumetric ultrafiltration system for their use, allows relatively objective data collection on high clearance treatments, and in the present state of the dialyzer market includes mostly cellulose devices which achieve urea clearances in the range most would consider high efficiency, excluding the synthetic high flux dialyzers with higher water permeability. The concept is imperfect, however, as is demonstrated by the existence of dialyzers which are undeniably high-flux, but fall into the CDC high-efficiency category, such as the 2.1 m^2 polymethylmethacrylate Toray B1-2.1U, which has an ultrafiltration coefficient of 17 ml $\cdot$ hr^{-1} $\cdot$ mmHg^{-1}.

ADVANTAGES

Definitions of adequate dialysis have moved toward higher and higher values of Kt/V, as survival figures like those of Table 7 have accumulated. The relatively conservative National Institutes of Health consensus development conference on morbidity and mortality of dialysis in 1993 concluded that a Kt/V of 'at least 1.2' was necessary for adequate hemodialysis (186), and in the chapter on hemodialysis adequacy in a major 1994 dialysis text, Parker states that "delivery of dialysis in a range less than 1.5 is suboptimal" (196). If dialysis doses like these are to be given in session times that are at all acceptable to providers and patients, extremely high urea clearances are necessary, as shown in Figure 3, and high-efficiency dialyzers are needed to attain them. There needs to be a paradigm shift in the dialysis community, away from defining the goal of dialysis treatment as achieving the minimal possible treatment time and toward the provision of optimal solute clearance in whatever time necessary. High-efficiency dialyzers can be tools to accomplish either of these goals; if the evolution of dialysis has followed the course of shorter rather than optimal treatments, it is perhaps largely for economic reasons. A rational reimbursement policy is needed which will allow what is now considered somewhat exotic, high-efficiency therapy to become the conventional dialysis therapy of the nineties.

High-flux hemodialysis

Definition

A good deal of confusion surrounds the term 'high flux', the 'flux' being variously conceived as blood flow, solute flux or ultrafiltration. As discussed in the section on convective therapies, 'high flux' historically refers to membrane water permeability, and was first used in connection with sulfonated polyacrylonitrile (PAN-SO_3 or AN69). Other highly permeable ('open') synthetic dialysis membranes followed, first used for hemofiltration and later for combined diffusive-convective – high-flux – hemodialysis. These membranes – polyacrylonitrile (PAN), polyamide, polymethylmethacrylate (PMMA), polysulfone, and cellulose triacetate – share certain physicochemical properties (221): they are highly permeable both to water and higher molecular weight solutes; their surfaces are hydrophobic (although often with hydrophilic microdomains) and strongly adsorptive of proteins; and they are relatively inert in biological environments, that is, 'biocompatible' (222, 223). The recent development of cellulose triacetate – a cellulose membrane which has been modified to the point of behaving more like the hydrophobic synthetics – and 'low-flux' PMMA and polysulfone with the surface characteristics but not the permeability of the high flux membranes, has blurred the distinction between cellulose and noncellulose, making classification on the basis of membrane material alone problematic.

Dialyzers constructed of these membranes are generally large enough and permeable enough to urea to achieve urea clearances well in excess of 200 ml/min when used at high blood and dialysate flows. Thus, as pointed out by Collins (56), high-flux dialyzers are also high-efficiency dialyzers, although their performance differs in important respects from treatment, even high-efficiency treatment, with cuprophan, cellulose acetate, and hemophan. The most widely accepted definition, then, for high-flux dialysis, and one which makes clinical sense, is dialysis using a hydrophobic membrane with high K_OA for urea and high ultrafiltration coefficient – at least 10 ml · hr^{-1} · $mmHg^{-1}$ · m^{-2} (35, 53, 55, 56, 62, 80, 184, 221, 224). The length of the session is secondary: high-flux dialysis is not a synonym for short dialysis.

The Centers for Disease Control, apparently aiming at a simple, easily reproducible definition suitable for use in their questionnaire surveys of dialysis units, have characterized high-flux dialysis as that performed with a dialyzer having an ultrafiltration coefficient of 20 ml · hr^{-1} · $mmHg^{-1}$ · m^{-2} or greater (98). Such a definition is relatively specific, but not sensitive, missing high-flux dialyzers with ultrafiltration coefficients in the 15–20 ml · hr^{-1} · $mmHg^{-1}$ · m^{-2} range.

Advantages

In the collective imagination, at least that of many dialysis patients and staff, high-flux dialysis has virtually been synonymous with short treatment time, especially durations less than three hours. This conception has been fostered by aggressive marketing strategies on the part of dialyzer manufacturers, but much of the dialysis literature of the 1980s unquestionably accepted the notion that high-flux therapy is primarily if not solely a means of shortening treatments (35, 53, 93–96, 184, 224–226). There are even descriptions of "high-flux hemodialysis with . . . cuprammonium rayon [= cellulose] membrane" (227), in which the short time and not the membrane has become the defining element.

As discussed above, serious limitations exist to the shortening of dialysis, and in many cases those limitations may already have been exceeded. High-flux dialyzers, however, may offer other advantages unrelated to reduction of treatment time, specifically a lesser tendency to interact with circulating cells and proteins, and a greater ability to remove large molecular weight solutes.

Metabolic effects: Biocompatibility

There are clear differences in the tendency of various membranes to interact with humoral or cellular elements and to influence metabolic processes. Contact of blood with the dialysis membrane leads to activation of complement (222, 223, 228–236); granulocytopenia (223, 228–233, 236–241); activation, degranulation and/or release of oxygen free radicals from granulocytes, with their subsequent diminished function (223, 242–260); changes in lymphocyte function (261–268); and activation of platelets and the coagulation cascade (269–283). In virtually every investigation of these effects in which comparisons have been made, cellulose membranes have been markedly more 'bioincompatible' – that is, reactive – than high-flux membranes like PMMA, AN69, and polysulfone.

Other areas of membrane reactivity have been reported, but both their nature and the degree of differences among membranes are somewhat more controversial. Intradialytic symptoms, hypotension, fever, and catabolism have been ascribed to the induction of circulating mononuclear cells to release proinflammatory cytokines like interleukin-1 (IL-1), interleukin-6 (IL-6), and tumor necrosis factor (TNF), either by membrane contact, by the effects of the products of complement activation, by exposure to dialysate contaminated by endotoxin, or by some combination of these factors (268, 284,

285). This 'interleukin hypothesis', first articulated by Henderson et al. in 1983 (286), has been both supported (287–304) and challenged (305–313) by the results of investigations of plasma and intracellular cytokine levels in hemodialysis patients. The reason for the failure of some reports to detect an intradialytic membrane-related stimulatory effect may be related to the delayed nature of the response, which appears to proceed via increased transcription of cytokine mRNA, with synthesis and release perhaps requiring a second 'message' such as endotoxin exposure (268, 285). Membrane-specificity of the effect has been difficult to establish, with some reporting a particular propensity of cuprophan over synthetic membranes to induce cytokines (289, 291, 292, 294, 299, 302–304), while others have not (295–298). This may be due to the mixed nature of the required stimulus, and the opposite tendencies of cuprophan and high-flux membranes – the former more active in direct and complement-mediated stimulation of monocytes, but possibly having less tendency to allow passage of dialysate contaminants which might provide the additional message needed for augmented cytokine release.

The reported acute catabolic effect of hemodialysis (314, 315) has also been attributed to bioincompatibility of the dialysis membrane. Hypothesizing that IL-1 and TNF induction may lead to increased lysozymal catabolism of muscle protein, Gutierrez and colleagues found that amino acid release from leg muscle was increased by sham dialysis with cuprophan, but not with biocompatible membranes (316–318). This finding was not confirmed, however, by Lim et al. (319), who used an infusion of radiolabelled leucine to investigate protein turnover during dialysis with cuprophan membrane and found no evidence of intradialytic protein degradation. Hemodialysis was a net catabolic event, but only because protein synthesis was reduced and amino acids were lost in the dialysate. Proteolytic enzymes released by the degranulation of neutrophils during dialysis might also contribute to intradialytic catabolism (320).

Another proposed manifestation of bioincompatibility has been the reported tendency of cellulose membranes to stimulate the generation of soluble β-2-microglobulin, based on the observation that serum levels increase during cellulose hemodialysis, while they fall during dialysis with high-flux membranes (321–325). The apparent intradialytic increase has persisted in some cases when levels were corrected for changes in extracellular volume (321, 325), but most investigators have found no change in concentration during cellulose dialysis when such corrections were made (89, 326–334). Mononuclear cells *in vitro* have demonstrated an increased synthesis of β-2-microglobulin in response to staphylococcal exotoxin, lipopolysaccharide, TNF, IL-1, and osmotic stimuli (335, 336), but with few exceptions (337–339) have shown no response to exposure to cuprophan membrane (329, 340–343). Finally, several groups have studied the whole-body kinetics of ^{131}I-labelled β-2-microglobulin in

dialysis patients and have found slight increases in synthesis rate over non-uremic controls, but no differences between patients dialyzed with cellulosic and high-flux membranes (344, 345). The weight of evidence would seem to indicate that membrane bioincompatibility does not affect β-2-microglobulin synthesis rates or serum levels (346).

The clinical implications of bioincompatibility are not always clear. With respect to short-term effects, the influence of membrane type on intradialytic symptoms has been investigated in three quite rigorously designed and controlled studies using volumetric ultrafiltration in all dialyses (347–349). No difference between cellulose and high-flux dialysis was found in incidence of hypotension, nausea, vomiting, cramps, headache or pruritus. An international study of the subjective effects of dialysis with seven different cellulose and synthetic membrane dialyzers found, on the contrary, a relationship between bioincompatibility and intradialytic symptoms reported by patients (350). The study was, however, unblinded, did not control for ultrafiltration method nor dialysate sodium, used acetate dialysate, and contained "wide differences in dialysis duration and blood flow between centers." It is likely that much of the differences in symptoms could be accounted for by these differences in technique, such as the effects of volumetric ultrafiltration. All in all, there is little evidence for an intradialytic effect of membrane biocompatibility on patient symptoms.

While repeated complement activation seems undesirable, long-term consequences have not been unequivocally identified. Studies in animals (351) and patients (352) suggest that C3a, C5a and thromboxane may mediate pulmonary hypertension during cellulose dialysis. Rats with ischemic acute renal failure have delayed recovery when exposed to cuprophan or to the complement-activating agent zymosan (353), a finding with important implications for the dialytic therapy of patients, and preliminary data have shown lower mortality and more rapid recovery of acute renal failure in patients dialyzed with biocompatible membranes in comparison to those dialyzed with cellulosic dialyzers (354). Anaphylactoid reactions, which occasionally occur during dialysis and may be quite severe, have been ascribed to complement activation (355), although the evidence for this is not compelling. Repeated degranulation of granulocytes, loss of phagocyte activity, and functional impairment of lymphocytes may contribute to the immunological deficits in uremia that lead to increased incidences of infections with pyogenic bacteria and tuberculosis (356). In fact, the few available outcome studies comparing conventional and high-flux hemodialysis have suggested a reduced infection risk in patients treated with biocompatible membranes. Hornberger and associates (357) found that the unadjusted monthly hospital admission rate for infection in a group of patients on cellulosic dialysis was more than twice that of a similar group on high-flux dialysis. Similarly, Levin et al. (358), comparing 438 patients treated with cellulosic dialyzers to 548 receiving high-flux treatment, reported a markedly reduced risk of death from all causes, but particularly of death from infection, in patients in the high-flux group.

Clearance of middle- and high-molecular weight solutes

As shown in Table 3, the high-flux synthetic membranes have markedly greater permeability than cellulose for higher molecular weight solutes, particularly in the range of 1000 to 12000 Daltons. When compared to conventional cellulose dialyzers, high-flux devices achieve approximately 3 times the clearance of vitamin B^{12} (1355 Daltons) (85) and 12 times that of inulin ($\sim$ 5200 Daltons) (359), while β-2-microglobulin (11800 Daltons) is cleared by synthetic high-flux membranes at about 30 to 50 ml/min (Table 3), but not at all by cuprophan. This high permeability has important implications for the therapeutic use of high-flux dialyzers.

Since molecules as large as β-2-microglobulin are removed, there has been some concern that clinically significant protein loss might occur through high-flux membranes, as pointed out by Berlyne and co-workers in 1978 (360), but this does not seem to be the case. Sieving coefficients for albumin are quite low (0.001–0.003), predicting a loss of 40 to 120 mg/L of ultrafiltrate (361, 362). Serum concentrations of small molecular weight proteins measured before and after 6 months of high-flux dialysis or hemofiltration change toward normal values (361, 363), and there is evidence that the nutritional status of patients dialyzed with polyacrylonitrile membrane is better than that of patients on cellulose dialysis (364). Significant protein loss may occur, however, with polysulfone dialyzers which are reused and sterilized with hypochlorite bleach and formaldehyde. Graeber and colleagues have reported increasing dialysate protein with increasing number of uses, ranging from approximately 1.3 mg/dl on the first use, to as much as 20 mg/dl or 18 g per treatment by the 24th reuse (365).

While the relative role of middle molecular weight substances in uremic toxicity remains controversial (366), there are some specific solutes whose effects are known, and which are more effectively cleared by high flux dialysis. Among these, β-2-microglobulin is probably the best studied, and has the clearest pathogenetic role in a uremic complication – there is little doubt that long-term exposure to high circulating levels of this small protein leads to increased morbidity in dialysis patients. The identification, in 1985, of a new form of amyloid containing β-2-microglobulin in a patient with carpal tunnel syndrome (367) was soon followed by a proliferation of reports of destructive spondyloarthropathy, intraosseous cysts and periarthritis, all associated with β-2-microglobulin-containing amyloid deposits (368, 369). Prevalence of the condition increases greatly in patients maintained on dialysis for more than a decade, and some form of β-2-microglobulin-associated arthropathy seems an almost inevitable concomitant of cuprophan dialysis lasting more than fifteen years (369–374). With the exception of renal transplantation, which normalizes rapidly serum levels of β-2-microglobulin and relieves symptoms (375–377), but has not yet been reported to bring about regression of skeletal lesions (376, 378), therapy has been ineffective. Hope for prevention springs from several reports, albeit retrospective, which indicate that symptomatic dialysis arthropathy is less prevalent in patients dialyzed with high-flux membranes, especially AN69 (371, 373, 374, 379–381). The clinical advantage of AN69 over other high-flux membranes is probably illusory since only AN69 has been in regular use long enough to demonstrate an advantage in this disease which arises in the second decade of dialysis treatment. This protective effect of high-flux dialysis is most likely due to increased removal of β-2-microglobulin by adsorption and/or filtration (89, 329–332, 334, 382–389), with long-term lowering of serum levels (329, 390). Improved biocompatibility is probably not a factor, since, as discussed above, the increase in serum β-2-microglobulin level after cellulose dialysis seems to be an artifact of hemoconcentration.

Daily synthesis of β-2-microglobulin in hemodialysis patients ranges from about 4 to 8 mg/kg (345), while high-flux dialytic removal rarely exceeds 200 mg per 4-hour treatment (89, 391), making accumulation of the protein and high serum levels inevitable, even with high-flux dialysis. In fact, use of high-flux membranes does not reverse established lesions of dialysis-related amyloidosis and does not completely prevent its development (375, 392). We have observed a patient dialyzed exclusively with AN69 for five years who during that time developed new bone cysts which led to pathological fracture of the femoral neck, and which on histological examination proved to be filled with amyloid. Nevertheless, serum β-2-microglobulin levels do fall markedly during high-flux dialysis and remain 30 to 40% lower than with cellulosic dialysis over the long term. In the absence of more effective therapy, such as selective adsorption columns for removal of β-2-microglobulin (393), high-flux dialysis is the best alternative currently available for the prevention of arthropathy in the dialysis patient in the second decade of treatment.

In both diabetics and non-diabetics with end-stage renal disease, an increased concentration of proteins altered by non-enzymatic condensation with glucose is found in the serum (394). Especially in diabetics, these advanced glycosylation end-products (AGEs) have been implicated in the pathogenesis of atherosclerosis and proliferative-fibrotic complications of diabetes and of the aging process (395–397). β-2-microglobulin modified by AGEs has been identified in samples of dialysis-related amyloid (398) and may be central to the inflammatory reaction induced by the amyloid deposits (399). AGE serum levels are affected little by conventional cellulose hemodialysis, but dialysis with high-flux AN69 and polysulfone membranes produces a 48–61% intradialytic fall in AGE levels

(394). The clinical significance of AGE removal by high-flux dialysis has not been investigated, but if early reports of improved survival with high-flux treatment (357, 400) are confirmed, reduction of AGE levels and consequent improvement in cardiovascular morbidity could be a contributory mechanism, particularly in diabetics.

Hypertriglyceridemia occurs commonly in patients with end-stage renal disease (401–405). Several groups have reported an intradialytic fall in plasma triglycerides with high-flux, but not with cellulose membranes (406–409), and longer-term studies have confirmed the effect, demonstrating lower triglyceride levels in patients undergoing chronic high-flux dialysis (411, 412). Lipase inhibitory activity of uremic plasma has been described by several investigators (402, 403, 412–416), and post-dialytic increases in both free fatty acid levels (408) and lipase activity (409) imply that the mechanism of triglyceride reduction by high-flux dialysis may be removal of a middle-molecular weight inhibitor of lipoprotein lipase.

Several reports of improvement (417–420) or stabilization (421) of peripheral neuropathy with high-flux dialysis have suggested that more efficient removal of unidentified higher molecular weight uremic neurotoxins was responsible for the reported advantage over cuprophan (422). Other, controlled studies have found little or no difference in the response of neuropathy to different membranes (423, 424). In general, the favorable reports have been either descriptions of a few cases or have not been controlled for small molecular weight solute removal, but the evidence is not conclusive one way or the other, and a case can be made for changing to high-flux dialysis with high Kt/V for patients with progressive peripheral neuropathy who are being dialyzed with cuprophan.

A number of other metabolites reportedly are cleared more effectively by high-flux membranes, including oxalate (425, 426); parathyroid hormone and its C- and N-terminal fragments (427–431); myoglobin (432); and porphyrins, in porphyria cutanea tarda (433). Hörl and co-workers (430) have isolated several small proteins in uremic serum which are inhibitory of granulocyte function (granulocyte inhibiting protein, GIP, molecular weight 28000 Daltons; and degranulation inhibiting protein, DIP, MW 14000 Daltons). Both are removed by high-flux dialysis, and not by cellulose (430). Finally, the permeability of high-flux AN69 membrane has been exploited with some success in the therapy of liver disease, for removal of bile acids and relief of pruritus in primary biliary cirrhosis (434) and in the therapy of fulminant hepatic failure to remove presumed middle molecular weight toxin(s) and improve encephalopathy (435–441).

Besides being more highly permeable to larger solutes, the hydrophobic high-flux membranes interact with plasma proteins and adsorb substantial quantities on their surface (442–444). Adsorbed proteins include fibrinogen, IgG, and albumin, and the effect contributes significantly to the total clearance of a number of compounds. Several investigators have found that the 60 to 65% of β-2-microglobulin removed by dialysis with AN69, 17 to 37% with polysulfone, and virtually 100% with PMMA, is adsorbed on the membrane (385–387, 430). Adsorbed protein appears to enhance membrane biocompatibility (444), and the adsorption of IL-1 (445), complement factor D (446), and C3a and C5a (447–449), which may further reduce the effect of cell-membrane interactions and complement activation in high-flux dialysis. Adsorption is not always desirable, as therapeutic agents like erythropoietin (450) and vancomycin (451) may also be removed from the plasma in this manner.

Drug removal

The increased permeability of high-flux membranes has important effects on the levels of drugs administered to dialysis patients, but data for specific medications are sorely lacking (452). The two best-understood examples are vancomycin, an antibiotic with a molecular weight of 1486 Daltons, and deferoxamine, a 657 Dalton compound used for the chelation of trivalent cations, particularly iron and aluminum. Vancomycin is so poorly cleared by cellulose membranes that dialysis has been reported to have no effect on serum levels of the drug, and since the half-life of vancomycin in anuria is three to seven days, the recommended dosing regimen for dialysis patients has been 500 to 1000 mg every five to eight days (453, 454). A number of investigators, however, have reported significant removal of vancomycin with high-flux dialysis using AN69 or polysulfone membranes (451, 455–458), resulting in sub-therapeutic levels for much of the week-long inter-dose period. Others have pointed out that the wide tissue distribution and slow intercompartmental transfer of vancomycin results in a large post-dialysis rebound rise in serum concentration, and have suggested that supplemental post-dialysis dosing is unnecessary (462–464). This conclusion was based on the detection of serum levels between 4 and 10 μg/ml at the end of one week following a single vancomycin dose, acceptable trough levels for the two to four times daily dosing schedules used in patients with normal renal function. For therapeutic effectiveness against staphylococci, however, a mean level of about 15 μg/ml is required (461, 465, 466). Since vancomycin has minimal 'post-antibiotic effect' against staphylococci (467, 468) if the level falls below 10 for days, as may be the case with weekly dosing during high-flux dialysis, there is a serious likelihood of therapeutic failure in any but superficial infections. In patients receiving high-flux treatment who require vancomycin therapy, we administer a 20 mg/kg loading dose followed by 500 mg doses after every subsequent dialysis. This regimen results in one-hour peak levels between 25 and 40 μg/ml and steady-state pre-dialysis serum levels of 10–20 μg/ml for periods of up to at least three weeks (459–461).

Deferoxamine is used to mobilize tissue and protein-bound aluminum for removal by dialysis. Use of polysulfone dialyzers (but not polyacrylonitrile (469, 470)) results in a two- to fourfold increase, over cellulose, in clearance of the deferoxamine-aluminum complex (471–474), and may represent an important improvement in the therapy of the aluminum encephalopathy and bone disease associated with dialysis. A similar 1.5 to threefold advantage over cellulose, has been reported for the clearance of radiocontrast agents by AN69 (475), and for the clearance of N-acetylprocainamide by polysulfone in a case of procainamide intoxication (476).

Much investigative work is needed on the pharmacokinetics of drug therapy in high-flux hemodialysis – many of the assumptions about non-dialyzable drugs in conventional cellulose dialysis come into question when highly permeable membranes are utilized. At present, the best course is to monitor pre-dialysis serum levels whenever possible, and to avoid parenteral administration until completion of the dialysis procedure of drugs intended to exert an effect during the interdialytic interval.

Drawbacks

The high permeability of high-flux membranes has caused wide concern about the potential for transport of contaminants from dialysate to blood (476–484). The nature of the pressure relationships in a countercurrent, volumetric ultrafiltration system is such that at the blood outlet/dialysate inlet end of the dialyzer, pressure on the blood side is at its lowest, and on the dialysate side its highest. There thus exists a hydrostatic pressure gradient from dialysate to blood (Figure 5). The gradient increases if blood flow rate is increased (486), since this raises the mean pressure on the blood side, and hence on the dialysate side, and exaggerates the differences at the ends of the dialyzer. The phenomenon is known as 'backfiltration', and the relevant pressures and fluid fluxes have been measured and described by a number of investigators (485–496). In a dialyzer with a very high ultrafiltration coefficient, the local fluid movement into blood may be substantial; Leypoldt et al. (493) measured backfiltration rates of 7–9 ml/min over two-thirds the length of a Fresenius F60 polysulfone dialyzer at the relatively low blood flow of 340 ml/min.

If dialysate is entering blood along much of the dialyzer length at 500 ml/min or more, and the dialyzer membrane has significant permeability to solutes with molecular weights up to 10–15,000, there is a serious possibility that products of bacterial contamination may be transported by convection into the circulation. The minimal pyrogenic dose of *E. coli* endotoxin (in the rabbit) is only 1–4 ng/kg body weight, and concentrations as low as 50 pg/ml can induce cytokine production by monocytes *in vitro* (497, 498). Sampling of incident water and dialysate in dialysis centers in the USA. (480, 481, 499), France (478), and Germany (496) has revealed frequent bacterial contamination, with dialysate often containing endotoxin concentrations higher than 1 ng/ml, so that transfer across high-flux membranes poses a potential threat. Bicarbonate dialysate is particularly vulnerable to bacterial contamination, especially when prepared in the dialysis center (478, 500). Further concern derives from *in vitro* studies which demonstrate the ability of contaminated dialysate to induce cytokine production across dialysis membranes (477, 501–504), and from detection of endotoxin or its antibody in the serum of patients dialyzed with high-flux membranes (479, 483).

Many of the *in vitro* studies which have demonstrated permeability of high-flux membranes to endotoxin or cytokine-inducing substances have used extremely high concentrations of endotoxin in the dialysate, however, and some have shown the same or greater permeability of cellulose membranes to these substances, casting some doubt on backfiltration as the mechanism (503–505), while others have been unable to demonstrate penetration of endotoxin through high-flux membranes at all (506–510). Evans and Holmes (511) found passage of cytokine-inducing activity at high dialysate endotoxin concentrations, but not at concentrations which more realistically approximated severe clinical contamination. The US Centers for Disease Control (98) has collected retrospective information, via questionnaires, about pyrogenic reactions in dialysis units, and found that the relative risk of reactions in units using high-flux dialyzers in at least some patients was 1.4 times that of units using conventional dialyzers ($p = 0.007$). All of the excess risk was in units which practiced reuse, which may particularly increase infection risk in high-flux dialyzers (512). Two prospective studies have investigated treatments with contaminated dialysate. In the first, Powell et al. (513) found no increase in circulating IL-1β or TNF-α during 5 conventional and 5 high-flux treatments with dialysate contaminated by extremely high concentrations of bacteria ($18,440 \pm 530$ CFU/ml) and endotoxin (976 ± 205 pg/ml). Gordon et al. (514) prospectively studied 26,877 conventional, high-efficiency, and high-flux treatments in three dialysis centers for 12 months. Mean dialysate bacterial and endotoxin concentrations were 19,000 CFU/ml and 380 pg/ml, respectively, but there were only 19 pyrogenic reactions (0.7/1000 treatments), with no difference in rates among treatment modalities. In summary, strong reason exists for concern about endotoxin transfer by backfiltration in high-flux dialysis, but *in vivo* evidence of its occurrence and clinical significance has not unequivocally been demonstrated. Maintenance of the AAMI standards for bacterial concentration in incident water and dialysate (200 CFU/ml and 2000 CFU/ml, respectively) should be sufficient precaution in the light of present knowledge (484, 515).

There have been a number of reports in the recent literature of hypersensitivity-like reactions, some extremely severe, even fatal, associated with the use of AN69 dialyzers (516–528). The reactions bear a resemblance to the so-called 'first-use' reaction often ascribed to ethylene oxide sensitivity (529), usually occur during the first few minutes of the dialysis treatment, and are more common, and perhaps more severe, in patients treated with

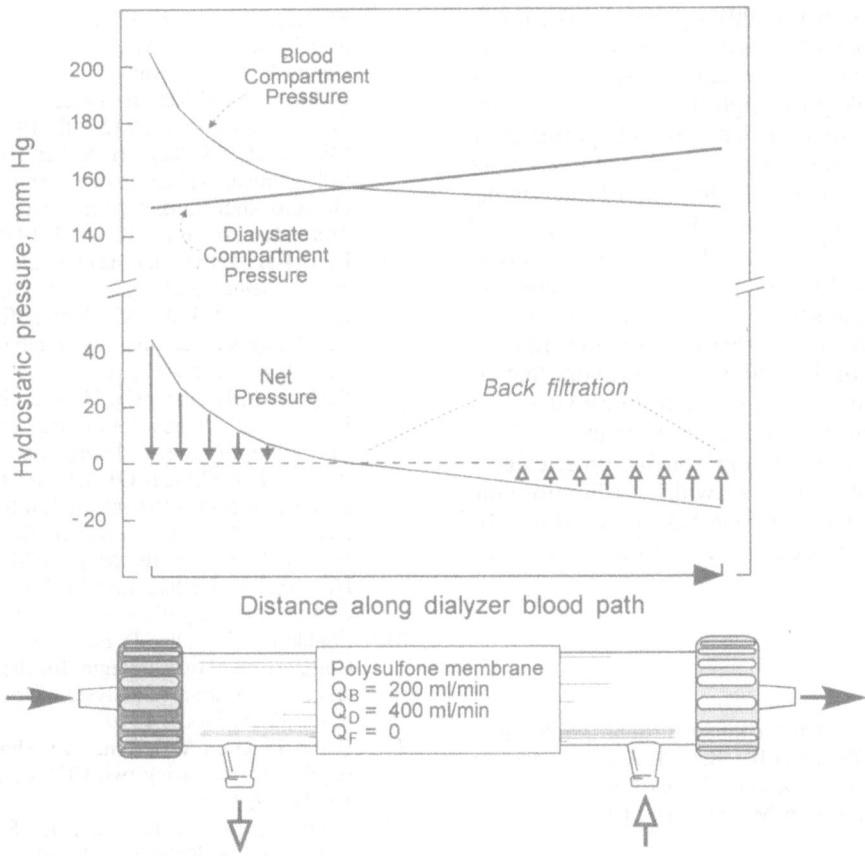

Figure 5. Backfiltration. With no net ultrafiltration, blood-side hydrostatic pressure exceeds that on the dialysate side over about the first 40% of the blood path, and there is movement of ultrafiltrate out of blood. Over the last 60% of the blood path, the pressure relationships reverse and an equivalent amount of fluid moves from dialysate to blood. Filled arrows = blood compartment; open arrows = dialysate compartment. Data from (485).

angiotensin-converting-enzyme inhibitors. In some cases further reactions were abolished by a change in the priming procedure aimed at prevention of backfiltration (482), implying that transfer of bacterial products from dialysate to blood may have been the cause, but there is no direct evidence for this, and in many instances patients have been changed to another high-flux dialyzer and the ACE-inhibitors continued, with no further reactions. The rarity of reports of similar reactions with other high-flux membranes, and the association with ACE-inhibitor therapy, may indicate that some propensity of AN69 to activate bradykinin is involved. Both *in vitro* (530) and *in vivo* (531) evidence of rapid, vigorous generation of bradykinin after blood exposure to AN69 membrane now exists; similar bradykinin generation was not stimulated by polysulfone or by cuprophan membranes. The question remains why these anaphylactoid reactions were rarely observed during almost twenty years of clinical use of AN69 prior to 1990, but sufficient evidence has accumulated to indicate that the reactions are membrane-specific,

and that the use of ACE-inhibitors in patients undergoing dialysis with AN69 membrane is contraindicated.

If backfiltration is largely a theoretical problem, there is a far more important obstacle to the expanded availability of high-flux dialysis therapy, and that is cost. In general, the price of AN69, polysulfone, and cellulose triacetate dialyzers is approximately three to four times that of cellulose devices, which in the US private market virtually precludes their use without reprocessing. The prevalence of high-flux dialysis nonetheless appears to be increasing (Table 4), and by 1990 was offered in 25% of dialysis units surveyed by the Centers for Disease Control (98).

AFTERWORD: THE ROLE OF HIGH-FLUX AND HIGH-EFFICIENCY DIALYSIS

The difference between high-efficiency and conventional hemodialysis is a quantitative one, and given the importance of small-molecular weight clearance in current concepts of dialysis adequacy, highly significant. The provision of high-efficiency clearance to as many patients as possible within the available economic framework is in fact a highly desirable goal. High-flux dialyzers – which for the most part are high-efficiency as well – differ from conventional devices in qualitative ways, the importance of which is less well established than that of small molecule clearance, but which nonetheless seem to promise improved therapy with less morbidity and, perhaps, lower mortality. Improved biocompatibility and removal of large-molecular weight solutes are both clear advantages, and the trade-offs are few: higher cost and the (largely) potential problem of backfiltration. One may hope that the direction of dialysis development will be toward the ability to deliver very high small molecule clearance – perhaps a Kt/V of 1.5 or more – in a reasonable time, using a biocompatible, high-flux dialyzer, with backfiltration controlled by asymmetrical membrane water permeability, by changes in dialyzer geometry, or by on-line sterilization of dialysate.

REFERENCES

1. Bower JD, Berman LB, Remmers R, Babb AL, Scribner BH, Gotch FA, DePalma JR, Siegel L: What is adequate dialysis? *Proc Dial Transplant Forum* 1: 61–72, 1971
2. Gotch FA: Progress in hemodialysis. *Clin Nephrol* 9: 144–155, 1978
3. Cambi V, Arisi L, David S, Bono F, Gardini G: 2-h dialysis: A realistic goal? *Contrib Nephrol* 44: 40–48, 1985
4. Collins AJ, Keshaviah PR: Are there limitations to shortening dialysis treatment? *Trans Am Soc Artif Intern Organs* 34: 1–5, 1988
5. Babb AL, Popovich RP, Christopher TG, Scribner BH: The genesis of the square meter-hour hypothesis. *Trans Am Soc Artif Intern Organs* 17: 81–91, 1971
6. Gotch FA, Sargent JA, Keen ML, Seid M, Foster R: Comparative treatment time with Kiil, Gambro, and Cordis-Dow kidneys. *Proc Dial Transplant Forum* 3: 217–228, 1973
7. Kjellstrand CM: Short dialysis increases morbidity and mortality. *Contrib Nephrol* 44: 65–77, 1985
8. Wizemann V, Kramer W: Short-term dialysis – long-term complications: Ten years experience with short-duration renal replacement therapy. *Blood Purif* 5: 193–201, 1987
9. Kramer P, Broyer M, Brunner FP, Brynger H, Donckerwolcke RA, Jacobs C, Selwood NH, Wing AJ: Combined report on regular dialysis and transplantation in Europe, XII, 1981. *Proc Eur Dial Transplant Assoc* 19: 4–59, 1983
10. Held PJ, Levin NW, Bovbjerg RR, Pauly MV, Diamond LH: Mortality and duration of hemodialysis treatment. *JAMA* 265: 871–875, 1991
11. Hull AR, Parker TF: Introduction and summary: Proceedings from the morbidity, mortality and prescription of dialysis symposium, Dallas TX, September 15 to 17, 1989. *Am J Kidney Dis* 15: 375–383, 1990
12. Berger EE, Lowrie EG: Mortality and the length of dialysis. *JAMA* 265: 909–910, 1991
13. Shaldon S, Koch KM: Survival and adequacy in long-term hemodialysis. *Nephron* 59: 353–357, 1991
14. Cambi V, Arisi L, Buzio C, Rossi E, Savazzi G, Migone L: Intensive utilisation of a dialysis unit. *Proc Eur Dial Transplant Assoc* 10: 342–348, 1973
15. Miramahdi KS, Kay JH, Miller JH, Gorman JT, Rosen SM: Clinical evaluation of patients dialysed with double Gambro 4hours, three times per week. *Proc Eur Dial Transplant Assoc* 11: 121–127, 1975
16. Barth RH. Dialysis by the numbers: The false promise of Kt/V. *Semin Dial* 2: 207–212, 1989
17. Rosenzweig J, Babb AL, Vizzo JE, Scribner BH, Ginn HE: Large surface area hemodialysis. *Proc Dial Transplant Forum* 1: 56–60, 1971
18. Sargent JA, Teisinger CL, Holmes GW, Evans MC, Gotch FA: Clinical studies with highly efficient 2 M2 hollow fiber kidney. *Proc Dial Transplant Forum* 1: 44–47, 1971
19. Raja RM, Kollmann GJ, Kramer MS, Rosenbaum JL: Solute transport with triple hollow fiber kidney in parallel and series. *Proc Dial Transplant Forum* 3: 229–233, 1973
20. Bosl R, Shideman JR, Meyer RM, Buselmeier TJ, von Hartitzsch B, Kjellstrand CM: Effects and complications of high efficiency dialysis. *Nephron* 15: 151–160, 1975
21. Shaldon S, Florence P, Fontanier P, Polito C, Mion C: Comparison of two strategies for short dialysis using 1 m² and 2 m² surface area dialysers. *Proc Eur Dial Transplant Assoc* 12: 596–605, 1976
22. Ben Ari J, Oren A, Berlyne GM: Short duration-high area regular dialysis using two UF 2 coils in series. *Nephron* 16: 74–79, 1976
23. Manji T, Maeda K, Ohta K, Saito A, Amano A, Kawaguchi S, Kobayashi K: Short time dialysis. *Proc Eur Dial Transplant Assoc* 12: 589–595, 1976
24. Orrell FL, Barbour BH, Bischel M, Austin E: Clinical response to shorter dialyses with a high performance dialyser. *Proc Eur Dial Transplant Assoc* 10: 476–478, 1973
25. Man NK, Granger A, Rondon-Nucete M, Zingraff J, Jungers P, Sausse A, Funck-Brentano JL: One year follow-up of short dialysis with a membrane highly permeable to middle molecules. *Proc Eur Dial Transplant Assoc* 10: 236–246, 1973
26. Cambi V, Savazzi G, Arisi L, Bignardi L, Bruschi G, Rossi E, Migone L: Short dialysis schedules (SDS) – finally ready to become routine? *Proc Eur Dial Transplant Assoc* 11: 112–120, 1975
27. Shaldon S, Beau MC, Deschodt G, Mion C. Mixed hemofiltration (MHF): 18 months treatment with ultrashort treatment time. *Trans Am Soc Artif Intern Organs* 27: 610–612, 1981
28. Chanard J, Brunois JP, Melin JP, Lavaud S, Toupance O: Long-term results of dialysis therapy with a highly permeable membrane. *Artif Organs* 6: 261–266, 1982
29. Wizemann V, Kramer W, Knopp G, Rawer P, Mueller K, Schütterle G: Ultrashort hemodiafiltration: Efficiency and hemodynamic tolerance. *Clin Nephrol* 19: 24–30, 1983
30. Cioni L, Palmarini N, Pilone N, Rindi P: Hemodiafiltration: Better efficiency with respect to hemodialysis and hemofiltration. *Blood Purif* 2: 30–35, 1984
31. von Albertini B, Miller JH, Gardner PW, Shinaberger JH: High-flux hemodiafiltration: Under six hours/week treatment. *Trans Am Soc Artif Intern Organs* 30: 227–231, 1984

32. Rotellar E, Martinez E, Samsó JM, Barrios J, Simó R, Mulero JF, Perez D, Bandrés S, Piñol J: Why dialyze more than 6 hours a week? *Trans Am Soc Artif Intern Organs* 31: 538–545, 1985

33. Keshaviah P, Collins A: Rapid high-efficiency bicarbonate hemodialysis. *Trans Am Soc Artif Intern Organs* 32: 17–23, 1986

34. Rubin JE, Berlyne GM: Long-term follow-up of patients on short-time dialysis. *Trans Am Soc Artif Intern Organs* 33: 540–541, 1987

35. Dumler F, Stalla K, Mohini R, Zasuwa G, Levin NW: Clinical experience with short-time hemodialysis. *Am J Kidney Dis* 19: 49–56, 1992

36. Hilderson J, Ringoir S, van Waeleghem JP, van Egmond J, van Haelst JP, Schelstraete K: Short dialysis with a polyacrylonitrilmembrane (RP) without the use of a closed recirculating dialyzate delivery system. *Clin Nephrol* 4: 18–22, 1975

37. von Hartitzsch B, Hoenich NA, Samson P, Erickson J, Ashcroft RA, Kerr DNS: A clinical evaluation of the new dialyzers. *Kidney Int* 3: 35–45, 1973

38. Hoenich NA, Frost TH, Kerr DNS: Dialysers. in *Replacement of Renal Function by Dialysis*, edited by Drukker W, Parsons FM, Maher JF, The Hague, Martinus Nijhoff, 1979, pp 80–124

39. Cambi V, Dall'Aglio P, Savazzi G, Arisi L, Rossi E, Migone L: Clinical assessment of haemodialysis patients with reduced small molecules removal. *Proc Eur Dial Transplant Assoc* 9: 67–73, 1972

40. Cambi V: Limits of dialysis technology. in *Proceedings of the Sixth International Congress of Nephrology; 1975*, edited by Giovanetti S et al., Florence, Basel, Karger, 1976, pp 624–628

41. Quadracci LJ, Cambi V, Christopher TG, Harker LA, Striker GE: Assay of serum abnormalities in uremic and dialysis patients: Evidence for depletion of vital substances in hemodialysis. *Trans Am Soc Artif Intern Organs* 17: 96–103, 1971

42. Lowrie EG: History and organization of the National Cooperative Dialyis Study. *Kidney Int* 23 (Suppl 13): S1–S7, 1983

43. Sargent JA, Gotch FA: The analysis of concentration dependence of uremic lesions in clinical studies. *Kidney Int* 7 (Suppl 2): S35–S43, 1975

44. Sargent JA: Control of dialysis by a single-pool urea model: The National Cooperative Dialysis Study. *Kidney Int* 23 (Suppl 13): S19–S25, 1983

45. Lowrie EG, Teehan BP: Principles of prescribing dialysis therapy: Implementing recommendations from the National Cooperative Dialysis Study. *Kidney Int* 23 (Suppl 13): S113, 1983

46. Harter HR: Review of significant findings from the National Cooperative Dialysis Study and recommendations. *Kidney Int* 23 (Suppl 13): S107, 1983

47. Gotch FA, Sargent JA: A mechanistic analysis of the National Cooperative Dialysis Study (NCDS). *Kidney Int* 28: 526, 1985

48. Keshaviah P, Berkseth R, Ilstrup K, McMichael C, Collins A: Reduced treatment time: Hemodialysis (HD) *versus* hemofiltration (HF). *Trans Am Soc Artif Intern Organs* 31: 176, 1985

49. Collins A, Ilstrup K, Hanson G, Berkseth R, Keshaviah P: Rapid high-efficiency hemodialysis. *Artif Organs* 10: 185, 1986

50. Keshaviah P, Luehmann D, Ilstrup K, Collins A: Technical requirements for rapid high-efficiency therapies. *Artif Organs* 10: 189, 1986

51. Ilstrup K, Collins A, Berkseth R, Keshaviah P: Therapy prescription for rapid high efficiency hemodialysis. (Abstract) *Kidney Int* 29: 215, 1986

52. Keshaviah P, Collins A, Hansen G, Ilstrup K: Rapid high efficiency bicarbonate hemodialysis. (Abstract) *Kidney Int* 31: 235, 1987

53. Keshaviah P, Collins A: High efficiency hemodialysis. *Contrib Nephrol* 69: 109, 1989

54. Collins A., Kjellstrand CM: Shortening of the hemodialysis procedure and mortality in 'healthy' dialysis patients. *Trans Am Soc Artif Intern Organs* 35: M145, 1990

55. Collins AJ, Keshaviah P: High efficiency therapies for clinical dialysis. in *Clinical Dialysis*, 2nd Ed, edited by Nissenson AR, Fine RN, Gentile DE, Norwalk, Appleton & Lange, 1990, p 687

56. Collins AJ: High-flux, high-efficiency procedures. in *Principles and Practice of Dialysis*, edited by Henrich WL, Baltimore, Williams & Wilkins, 1994, p 76

57. Buffaloe GW: Ultrafiltration control. in *Hemodialysis: High-Efficiency Treatments*, edited by Bosch JP, Stein JH, New York, Churchill Livingstone, 1993, p 79

58. Tolchin N, Roberts J, Hayashi J, Lewis EJ: Metabolic consequences of high mass-transfer hemodialysis. *Kidney Int* 11: 366, 1977

59. Tolchin N: Acetate metabolism and high-efficiency hemodialysis. *Int J Artif Organs* 2: 1, 1979

60. Kaiser BA, Potter DE, Bryant RE, Vreman HJ, Weiner MW: Acid-base changes and acetate metabolism during routine and high-efficiency hemodialysis in children. *Kidney Int* 19: 70, 1981

61. Dalal SP, Ajam M, Gupta DK, Gupta R, Nawab Z, Manahan FJ, Ing TS, Daugirdas JT: L-lactate for high-efficiency hemodialysis: Feasibility studies and a randomized comparison with acetate and bicarbonate. *Int J Artif Organs* 12: 611, 1989

62. Barth RH: High-flux hemodialysis: Overcoming the tyranny of time. *Contrib Nephrol* 102: 73, 1993

63. Travenol Laboratories: Travenol Systems to Reduce Treatment Time. Deerfield, Travenol Laboratories, Inc, 1986

64. Hull AR: Impact of reimbursement regulations on patient management. *Am J Kidney Dis* 20 (Suppl 1): 8, 1992

65. Kaserman DL: Reimbursement rates and quality of care in the dialysis industry: a policy discussion. *Issues Law Med* 8: 81, 1992

66. Held PJ, García J, Pauly MV, Cahn MA: Price of dialysis, unit staffing, and length of dialysis treatments. *Am J Kidney Dis* 15: 441, 1990

67. Barth RH: Short hemodialysis: Big trouble in a small package. in *Death on Hemodialysis: Preventable or Inevitable?*, edited by Friedman EA, Dordrecht, Kluwer Academic Publishers, 1994, p 143

68. Lowrie EG, Lew NL: Death risk in hemodialysis patients: the predictive value of commonly measured variables and an evaluation of death rate differences between facilities. *Am J Kidney Dis* 15: 458, 1990

69. US Renal Data System: USRDS 1992 Annual Data Report. Bethesda, MD: The National Institutes of Health, National Institute of Diabetes and Digestive and Kidney Diseases, 1992

70. Delmez JA, Windus DW: The St. Louis Nephrology Study Group. Hemodialysis prescription and delivery in a metropolitan community. *Kidney Int* 41: 1023, 1992

71. Disney APS: Prescription and practice of dialysis in Australia, 1988. *Am J Kidney Dis* 15: 494, 1990

72. Iseki K, Kawazoe N, Osawa A, Fukiyama K: Survival analysis of dialysis patients in Okinawa, Japan (1971–1990). *Kidney Int* 43: 404, 1993

73. Marumo F, Maeda K, Koshikawa S: ESRD registry statistics on dialysis mortality in Japan. in *Death on Hemodialysis: Preventable or Inevitable?*, edited by Friedman EA, Dordrecht, Kluwer Academic Publishers, 1994, p 45

74. Gurland HJ, Mujais SK: Treacherous fantasy: The unfulfilled promise of *Kt/V*. in *Death on Hemodialysis: Preventable or Inevitable?*, edited by Friedman EA, Dordrecht, Kluwer Academic Publishers, 1994, p 35

75. Barth RH: A model's just a model: Formal urea kinetic modeling is not a necessity. *Semin Dial* 6: 156, 1993

76. Henderson L, Besarab A, Michaels A, Bluemle LW Jr: Blood purification by ultrafiltration and fluid replacement (diafiltration). *Trans Am Soc Artif Intern Organs* 13: 216, 1967

77. Quellhorst E, Fernandez E, Scheler F: Treatment of uraemia using an ultrafiltration-filtration system. *Proc Eur Dial Transplant Assoc* 9: 584, 1972

78. Koch K-M, Baldamus CA, Frei U, Ernst W: Hemofiltration, future aspects in relation to other treatment modalities of uremia. *Contrib Nephrol* 32: 165, 1982

79. Shaldon S, Deschodt G, Beau MC, Claret G, Mion H, Mion C: Vascular stability during high flux haemofiltration (HF). *Proc Eur Dial Transplant Assoc* 16: 695, 1979

80. Bosch JP, Geronemus R, Glabman S, Lysaght M, Kahn T, von Albertini B: High flux hemofiltration. *Artif Organs* 2: 339, 1978

81. Mion C, Beau MC, Deschodt G, Gullberg CA, Ramperez P, Shaldon S: Reduction of treatment time with high flux postdilutional hemofiltration (HF). *Proc Dial Transplant Forum* 9: 63, 1979

82. Shaldon S, Beau MC, Deschodt G, Mion C: Mixed hemofiltration (MHF): 18 months experience with ultrashort treatment time. *Trans Am Soc Artif Intern Organs* 27: 610, 1981

83. Kunitomo T, Lowrie EG, Kumazawa S, O'Brien M, Lazarus JM, Gottlieb MN, Merrill JP: Controlled ultrafiltration (UF) with hemodialysis (HD): Analysis of coupling between convective and diffusive mass transfer in a new HD-UF system. *Trans Am Soc Artif Intern Organs* 23: 234, 1977

84. Kirkwood RG, Kunitomo T, Lowrie EG: High rates of controlled ultrafiltration combined with optimal diffusion: recent advances in hemodialysis technique. *Nephron* 22: 175, 1978

85. Sigdell JE: Hollow-fiber dialyzers on the market. *Artif Organs* 12: 345, 1988

86. Naitoh A, Tatsuguchi T, Okada M, Ohmura T, Sakai K: Removal of beta-2-microglobulin by diffusion alone is feasible using highly permeable dialysis membranes. *Trans Am Soc Artif Intern Organs* 34: 630, 1988

87. Jindal KK, Mcdougall J, Woods B, Nowakowski L, Goldstein MB: A study of the basic principles determining the performance of several high-flux dialyzers. *Am J Kidney Dis* 14: 507, 1989

88. Piazolo P, Brech W, Niedermayer W, Albrecht J, Hennemann H, Witter E: Clinical multicenter study of Hemoflow F6 in comparison with different standard dialyzers. *Contrib Nephrol* 74: 22, 1989

89. Klinke B, Röckel A, Perschel W, Abdelhamid S, Fiegel P, Walb D: Beta-2-microglobulin handling in dialysis. *Contrib Nephrol* 74: 139, 1989

90. Chauveau P, Poignet J-L, Kuno T, Bonete R, Kerembrun A, Naret C, Delons S, Man NK, Rist E: Phosphate removal rate: A comparative study of five high-flux dialysers. *Nephrol Dial Transplant* 2 (Suppl 2): 114, 1991

91. Baxter Healthcare Corporation: Hemodialysis Product Guide, McGaw Park, Baxter Healthcare, 1992

92. Althin Medical Inc: Product Information, Miami Lakes, Althin Medical, 1993

93. Various authors: Special issue: High flux dialysis. *Contemp Dial Nephrol* 10: 24, 1989

94. DePalma JR: High flux – high fashion? *Contemp Dial Nephrol* 8: 32, 1987

95. McClellan S, Cordova S, Chado D, Martin G, Mishell J: High flux dialysis: Results of a one-year clinical study on a large patient population. *Contemp Dial Nephrol* 10: 24, 39, 1989

96. Pollock P, Lehman JM: Administering a high flux dialysis program. *Contemp Dial Nephrol* 10: 34, 42, 1989

97. Seirup J: Industrial insight: Does patient mental status clinically improve on high flux dialysis? *Contemp Dial Nephrol* 10: 37, 1989

98. Tokars JI, Alter MJ, Favero MS, Moyer LA, Bland LA: National surveillance of dialysis associated diseases in the United States, 1991. *ASAIO J* 39: 966, 1993

99. Kennedy AC, Linton AL, Eaton JC: Urea levels in cerebrospinal fluid after haemodialysis. *Lancet* 1: 410, 1962

100. Kennedy AC, Linton AL, Renfrew S, Luke RG, Dinwoodie A: The pathogenesis and prevention of cerebral dysfunction during dialysis. *Lancet* 1: 790, 1964

101. Peterson HDC, Swanson AG: Acute encephalopathy occurring during hemodialysis: the reverse urea effect. *Arch Intern Med* 113: 877, 1964

102. Wakim KG: The pathophysiology of the dialysis disequilibrium syndrome. *Mayo Clin Proc* 44: 406, 1969

103. Mahoney CA, Arieff AI: Uremic encephalopathies: clinical, biochemical, and experimental features. *Am J Kidney Dis* 2: 324, 1982

104. Silver SM, DeSimone JA, Smith DA, Sterns RH: Dialysis dysequilibrium syndrome (DDS) in the rat: Role of the 'reverse urea effect'. *Kidney Int* 42: 161, 1992

105. Arieff AI, Lazarowitz VC, Guisado R: Experimental dialysis disequilibrium syndrome: prevention with glycerol. *Kidney Int* 14: 270, 1978

106. Klinkman H: The dysequilibrium syndrome in experimental hemodialysis. *Trans Am Soc Artif Intern Organs* 16: 523, 1970

107. Wakim KG: Predominance of hyponatremia over hypoosmolality in simulation of the dialysis disequilibrium syndrome. *Mayo Clin Proc* 44: 433, 1969

108. Kjellstrand CM, Mauer SM, Buselmeier TJ, Shideman JR, Meyer RM, von Hartitzsch B, Simmons RL, Michael A, Vernier RL, Najarian JS: Haemodialysis of premature

and newborn babies. *Proc Eur Dial Transplant Assoc* 10: 349, 1973

109. Bergamo Collaborative Dialysis Study Group: Acute intradialytic well-being: results of a clinical trial comparing polysulfone with cuprophan. *Kidney Int* 40: 714, 1991

110. Churchill DN, Bird DR, TAylor DW, Beecroft ML, Gorman J, Wallace JE: Effect of high-flux hemodialysis on quality of life and neuropsychological function in chronic hemodialysis patients. *Am J Nephrol* 12: 412, 1992

111. Collins DM, Lambert MB, Tannenbaum JS, Oliverio M, Schwab SJ: Tolerance of hemodialysis: a randomized prospective trial of high-flux *versus* conventional high-efficiency hemodialysis. *Am Soc Nephrol* 4: 148, 1993

112. Basile C, Miller JDR, Koles ZJ, Grace M, Ulan RA: The effects of dialysis on brain water and EEG in stable chronic uremia. *Am J Kidney Dis* 9: 462, 1987

113. Austin JN, Klein M, Mishell J, Contiguglia SR, Levy J, Chan L, Shapiro JI: Intraocular pressures during high-flux hemodialysis. *Renal Failure* 12: 109, 1990

114. Kjellstrand CM, Evans RL, Petersen RJ, Shideman JR, von Hartitzsch B, Buselmeier TJ: The 'unphysiology' of dialysis: a major cause of dialysis side effects? *Kidney Int* 7 (Suppl 2): S30, 1975

115. Port FK, Johnson WJ, Klass DW: Prevention of dialysis disequilibrium syndrome by use of high sodium concentration in the dialysate. *Kidney Int* 3: 327, 1973

116. Novello A, Kelsch RC, Easterling RE: Acetate intolerance during hemodialysis. *Clin Nephrol* 5: 29, 1976

117. Port FK, Easterling RE: Evaluation of acetate tolerance during highly efficient hemodialysis. *Proc Clin Dial Transplant Forum* 5: 128, 1975

118. Viljoen M, Gold CH: Danger of haemodialysis using acetate dialysate in combination with a large surface area dialyser. *S Afr Med J* 56: 170, 1979

119. Cannella G, Maiorca R: Acetate appearance curve in normotensive and hypotension-prone hemodialysis patients. *Nephron* 32: 269, 1982

120. Mansell MA, Nunan TO, Laker MF, Boon NA, Wing AJ: Incidence and significance of rising blood acetate levels during hemodialysis. *Clin Nephrol* 12: 22, 1979

121. Wehle B, Asaba H, Castenfors J, Fürst P, Grahn A, Gunnarsson B, Shaldon S, Bertström J: The influence of dialysis fluid composition on the blood pressure response during dialysis. *Clin Nephrol* 10: 62, 1978

122. Pagel MD, Ahmad S, Vizzo JE, Scribner BH: Acetate and bicarbonate fluctuations and acetate intolerance during dialysis. *Kidney Int* 21: 513, 1982

123. Vanholder R, Piron M, Ringoir S: Absence of a beneficial haemodynamic effect of bicarbonate versus acetate haemodialysis. *Proc Eur Dial Transplant Assoc-Eur Ren Assoc* 21: 195, 1985

124. Anderson LE, Nixon JV, Henrich WL: Effects of acetate and bicarbonate dialysate on left ventricular performance. *Am J Kidney Dis* 10: 350, 1987

125. Otte KE, Lillevang ST, Rasmussen AG, Christensen HK, Pedersen FB: Acetate or bicarbonate for haemodialysis: a randomised, double-blind controlled trial. *Nephrol Dial Transplant* 5: 931, 1990

126. Vreman HJ, Assomull VM, Kaiser BA, Blaschke TR, Weiner MW: Acetate metabolism and acid-base homeostasis during hemodialysis: influence of dialyzer efficiency and rate of acetate metabolism. *Kidney Int* 18 (Suppl 10): S62, 1980

127. Weiner MW: Acetate metabolism during hemodialysis. *Artif Organs* 6: 370, 1982

128. Hakim RM, Pontzer MA, Tilton D, Lazarus JM, Gottlieb MN: Effects of acetate and bicarbonate dialysate in stable chronic dialysis patients. *Kidney Int* 28: 535, 1985

129. Vinay P, Prud'Homme M, Vinet B, Cournoyer G, Degoulet P, Leville M, Gougoux A, St-Louis G, Lapierre L, Piette Y: Acetate metabolism and bicarbonate generation during hemodialysis: 10 years of observation. *Kidney Int* 31: 1194, 1987

130. Diamond SM, Henrich WL: Acetate dialysate versus bicarbonate dialysate: a continuing controversy. *Am J Kidney Dis* 9: 3, 1987

131. Bloembergen WE, Port FK: The acetate versus bicarbonate dialysate controversy. *Int J Artif Organs* 15: 692, 1992

132. Kjellstrand C-M, Shideman JR, Santiago EA, Mauer M, Simmons RL, Buselmeier TJ: Technical advances in hemodialysis of very small pediatric patients. *Proc Dial Transplant Forum* 1: 124, 1971

133. Keshaviah PR: The role of acetate in the etiology of symptomatic hypotension. *Artif Organs* 6: 378, 1982

134. Bijaphala S, Bell AJ, Bennett CA, Evans SM, Dawborn JK: Comparison of high and low sodium bicarbonate and acetate dialysis in stable chronic hemodialysis patients. *Clin Nephrol* 23: 179, 1985

135. Civati G, Guastoni C, Teatini U, Perego A, Perrino ML, Benazzi E, Minetti L: High-flux acetate haemodialysis: A single-center experience. *Nephrol Dial Transplant* 2 (Suppl 2): 75, 1991

136. Barth RH, Rubin JE, Berlyne GM: Very high blood flow rate is safe and effective in hemodialysis. (Abstract) *Am Soc Artif Intern Organs* 17: 58, 1988

137. Ronco C, Feriani M, La Greca G: Hemodynamic response to high blood flows and ultrafiltration modelling during short dialysis. (Abstract) *Kidney Int* 37: 317, 1990

138. Barth RH: Dialysis. in *Encyclopedia of Applied Physics, Vol 4*, edited by Trigg GL, New York, VCH, 1992, p 533

139. Bouthier JD, Levenson JA, Simon AC, Bariety JM, Bourquelot PE, Safar ME: A noninvasive determination of fistula blood flow in dialysis patients. *Artif Organs* 7: 404, 1983

140. Ilstrup K, Collins A, Hanson G, Keshaviah P: Repeatable access blood flow (ABF) measurement. *Trans Am Soc Artif Intern Organs* 30: 338, 1984

141. Rodriguez Moran M, Rodriguez Rodriguez JM, Ramos Boyero M, Almazan Enriquez A, Ingelmo Morin A: Flow of dialysis fistulas: noninvasive study performed with standard Doppler equipment. *Nephron* 40: 63, 1985

142. Rittgers SE, Garcia-Valdez C, McCormick JT, Posner MP: Noninvasive blood flow measurement in expanded polytetrafluoroethylene grafts for hemodialysis access. *J Vasc Surg* 3: 635, 1986

143. Kubota K, Kawauchi A, Nakajima M, Ohta H, Koike T, Ishi J: Arteriovenous shunt flow measurement by ultrasonic duplex system. *Trans Am Soc Artif Intern Organs* 33: 144, 1987

144. Krpan D, Demarin V, Prot F, Milutinovic S, Molnar V, Milutinovic E: Measurement of blood flow through AV-fistulae by means of Doppler sonography in regularly haemodialysed patients. *Int J Artif Organs* 14: 78, 1991

442   *Robert H. Barth*

145. Ronco C, Brendolan A, Bragantini L, Chiaramonte S, Fabris A, Feriani M, Dell'Aquila R, Milan M, Scabardi M, Pinna V, LaGreca G: Technical and clinical evaluation of diferent short, highly efficient dialysis strategies. *Contrib Nephrol* 61: 46, 1988

146. Pontari MA, McMillen MA: The straight radial-antecubital PTFE angio-access graft in an era of high-flux dialysis. *Am J Surg* 161: 450, 1991

147. Calzavara P, Galardi N, Vianello A, Da Porto A, Gatti PL, Bertolone G, Salandin V: Modification of blood flow during haemodialysis and effect on cardiac function. *Int J Artif Organs* 13: 323, 1990

148. Alfurayh O, Galal O, Sobh M, Fawzy M, Taher S, Qunibi W, Almeshari K, Philipp T: The effect of extracorporeal high blood flow rate on left ventricular function during hemodialysis – an echocardiographic study. *Clin Cardiol* 16: 791, 1993

149. Collins DM, Lambert MB, Middleton JP, Proctor RK, Davidson CJ, Newman GE, Schwab SJ: Fistula dysfunction: Effect on rapid hemodialysis. *Kidney Int* 41: 1292, 1992

150. Barth RH, Sodden S, Berlyne GM: Heparin-free hemodialysis with a polyacrylonitrile membrane. *Trans Am Soc Artif Intern Organs* 35: 597, 1989

151. Dewanjee MK, Kapadvanjwala M, Mao WW, Jy W, Ahn Y, Ruzius K, Ghafouripour AK, Serafini AN, Sfakianakis GN: A higher blood flow window of reduced thrombogenicity and acceptable fragmentation in a hollow fiber hemodialyzer. *ASAIO J* 39: M363, 1993

152. Daugirdas JT: Chronic hemodialysis prescription: a urea kinetic approach. in *Handbook of Dialysis*, 2nd Ed, edited by Daugirdas JT, Ing TS, Boston, Little, Brown and Company, 1994, p 92

153. Daniels ID, Berlyne GM, Barth RH: Blood flow rate and access recirculation in hemodialysis. *Int J Artif Organs* 15: 470, 1992

154. Depner TA, Rizwan S, Stasi TA: Pressure effects on roller pump blood flow during hemodialysis. *Trans Am Soc Artif Intern Organs* 31: M456, 1990

155. Schmidt DF, Schniepp BJ, Kurtz SB, McCarthy JT: Inaccurate blood flow rate during rapid hemodialysis. *Am J Kidney Dis* 17: 34, 1991

156. Sherman RA, Levy SS: Rate-related recirculation: the effect of altering blood flow on dialyzer recirculation. *Am J Kidney Dis* 17: 170, 1991

157. Klooker P, Bommer J, Ritz E: Treatment of hypertension in dialysis patients. *Blood Purif* 3: 15, 1985

158. Heyka RJ, Paganini EP: Blood pressure control in chronic dialysis patients. in *Replacement of Renal Function by Dialysis*, 3rd Ed, edited by Maher JF, Dordrecht, Kluwer Academic Publishers, 1989, p 772

159. Vertes V, Cangiano JL, Berman LB, Gould A: Hypertension in end-stage renal disease. *N Engl J Med* 280: 978, 1969

160. Diamond SM, Henrich WL: Hypertension in dialysis patients. *Int J Artif Organs* 9: 213, 1986

161. Zucchelli P, Santoro A, Zuccala A: Genesis and control of hypertension in hemodialysis patients. *Semin Nephrol* 8: 163, 1988

162. Cheigh JS, Milite C, Sullivan JF, Rubin AL, Stenzel KH: Hypertension is not adequately controlled in hemodialysis patients. *Am J Kidney Dis* 19: 453, 1992

163. Mailloux LU, Bellucci AG, Napolitano B, Mossey RT: The contribution of hypertension to dialysis patient outcomes: a point of view. *ASAIO J* 40: 130, 1994

164. Daugirdas JT: Dialysis hypotension: a hemodynamic analysis. *Kidney Int* 39: 233, 1991

165. Alloatti S, Torazza MC, Gaiter AM, Nebiolo PE, Gabella P: L'emodialisi ad alta efficienza: Revisione della letteratura e prime esperienze cliniche. *Minerva Urol Nefrol* 42: 1, 1990

166. Alvarez-Ude F, Ward M, Elliott RW, Uldall PR, Wilkinson R, Appleton DR, Kerr DNS, Petrella E, Gentile M, Romagnoni M, Orlandini G, Luciani L, Ferrandes C, D'Amico G: A comparison of short and long haemodialysis. *Proc Eur Dial Transplant Assoc* 12: 606, 1976

167. Raja R, Kramer M, Goldstein S, Caruana R, Lerner A: Short hemodialysis – 10-year follow-up. *Trans Am Soc Artif Intern Organs* 32: 374, 1986

168. Greenwood RN: High-flux short-duration haemodialysis; a new approach. in *Advanced Renal Medicine*, edited by Raine AEG, Oxford, Oxford University Press, 1992, p 405

169. Charra B: Personal communication, 1994

170. Charra B, Calemard E, Ruffet M, Chazot C, Terrat J-C, Vanel T, Laurent G: Survival as an index of adequacy of dialysis. *Kidney Int* 41: 1286, 1992

171. Scribner BH: Adequate control of blood pressure in patients on chronic hemodialysis. *Kidney Int* 41: 1286, 1992

172. Charra B: Does empirical long slow dialysis result in better survival? If so, how and why? *ASAIO J* 39: 819, 1993

173. Scribner BH: Blood pressure control: the neglected factor that affects survival of dialysis patients. in *Death on Hemodialysis: Preventable or Inevitable?*, edited by Friedman EA, Dordrecht, Kluwer Academic Publishers, 1994, p 195

174. Fabris A, La Greca G, Chiaramonte S, Feriani M, Brendolan A, Bragantini L, Milan M, Pellanda MV, Crepaldi C, Ronco C: Total solute extraction *versus* clearance in the evaluation of standard and short hemodialysis. *Trans Am Soc Artif Intern Organs* 34: 627, 1988

175. Alloatti S, Bosticardo G, Torazza M, Gaiter AM, Nebiolo PE: Transcellular disequilibrium and intradialytic catabolism reduce the reliability of urea kinetic formulas. *Trans Am Soc Artif Intern Organs* 35: 328, 1989

176. Depner TA: *Prescribing Hemodialysis: A Guide to Urea Modeling*, Boston, Kluwer Academic Publishers, 1991, p 91

177. Popovich RP, Havinka DJ, Bomar JB, Moncrief JW, Decherd JF: The consequences of physiological resistances on metabolite removal from the patient-artificial kidney system. *Trans Am Soc Artif Intern Organs* 21: 108, 1975

178. Dombeck DH, Klein E, Wendt RP: Evaluation of two pool model for predicting serum creatinine levels during intra- and inter-dialytic periods. *Trans Am Soc Artif Intern Organs* 21: 117, 1975

179. Schindhelm K, Farrel PC: Patient-hemodialyzer interactions. *Trans Am Soc Artif Intern Organs* 24: 357, 1978

180. Wellhöner HH: Predicative calculation of the efficiency of hemodialysis or hemoperfusion for the removal of drugs from the body. *Arch Toxicol* 56: 182, 1985

181. Sargent JA, Gotch FA: Principles and biophysics of dialysis. in *Replacement of Renal Function by Dialysis*, edited by Drukker W, Parsons FM, Maher JF, The Hague, Martinus Nijhoff, 1979, p 38

182. Lopot F: Is urea kinetic modeling an appropriate tool for guiding ultrashort high-flux dialysis therapy? *Nephrol Dial Transplant* 3: 86, 1991

183. Bosch JP: Prescribing high-efficiency treatments. in *Hemodialysis: High-Efficiency Treatments*, edited by Bosch JP, Stein JH, New York, Churchill Livingstone, 1993, p 135

184. von Albertini B, Bosch JP: Short hemodialysis. *Am J Nephrol* 11: 169, 1991

185. Sargent JA, Lowrie EG: Which mathematical model to study uremic toxicity?: National Cooperative Dialysis Study. *Clin Nephrol* 17: 303, 1982

186. National Institutes of Health Consensus Development Conference Statement: Morbidity and mortality of dialysis. Bethesda: National Institute of Diabetes and Digestive and Kidney Diseases, 1993

187. Kusek JW, Agodoa LY, Jones CA: Morbidity and mortality among hemodialysis patients: a plan for action. *Semin Dial* 6: 81, 1993

188. Keshaviah P, Collins A: A re-appraisal of the national cooperative dialysis study. (Abstract) *Kidney Int* 33: 227, 1988

189. Hakim RM, Depner TA, Parker TF: Adequacy of hemodialysis. *Am J Kidney Dis* 20: 107, 1992

190. Shen F-H, Hsu K-T: Lower mortality and morbidity associated with higher Kt/V in hemodialysis patients. *Am Soc Nephrol* 1: 377, 1990

191. Collins A, Liao M, Umen A, Hanson G, Keshaviah P: High-efficiency bicarbonate hemodialysis has a lower risk of death than standard acetate dialysis. *Am Soc Nephrol* 2: 318, 1991

192. Collins A, Liao M, Umen A, Hanson G, Keshaviah P: Diabetic hemodialysis patients treated with a high Kt/V have a lower risk of death than standard Kt/V. *Am Soc Nephrol* 2: 318, 1991

193. Shen F-H, Cheng K-R: High clearance hemodialysis is associated with low mortality and morbidity: 5 years experience. (Abstract). *Am Soc Nephrol* 4: 385, 1993 (Data updated to November, 1993 by personal communication from Cheng, K-R)

194. Hakim RM, Breyer J, Ismail N, Schulman G: Effects of dose of dialysis on morbidity and mortality. *Am J Kidney Dis* 23: 661, 1994

195. Parker TF III, Husni L, Huang W, Lew N, Lowrie EG, Dallas Nephrology Associates: Survival of hemodialysis patients in the United States is improved with a greater quantity of dialysis. *Am J Kidney Dis* 23: 670, 1994

196. Parker T: Hemodialysis adequacy. in *Principles and Practice of Dialysis*, edited by Henrich WL, Baltimore, Williams & Wilkins, 1994, p 63

197. US Renal Data System: USRDS 1993 Annual Data Report, Bethesda, MD, The National Institutes of Health, National Institute of Diabetes and Digestive and Kidney Diseases, 1993

198. Held PJ, Blagg CR, Liska DW, Port FK, Hakim R, Levin N: The dose of hemodialysis according to dialysis prescription in Europe and the United States. *Kidney Int* 42 (Suppl 38): S16, 1992

199. Saha LK, Van Stone JC: Differences between KT/V measured during dialysis and KT/V predicted from manufacturer clearance data. *Int J Artif Organs* 15: 465, 1992

200. Barth RH: Urea modeling and Kt/V: a critical appraisal. *Kidney Int* 43 (Suppl 41): S252, 1993

201. Galen M: Reasonably short hemodialysis time can be achieved without high-efficiency dialyzers and without ultrafiltration-controlled delivery systems. *Trans Am Soc Artif Intern Organs* 35: 255, 1989

202. Acchiardo SR, Quinn BP, Burk LB, Moore LM: Are high flux dialysis and erythropoietin treatment on a collision course? *Trans Am Soc Artif Intern Organs* 35: 308, 1989

203. Lim VS, Flanigan MJ, Fangman J: Effect of hematocrit on solute removal during high efficiency hemodialysis. *Kidney Int* 37: 1557, 1990

204. LeFebvre JM, Spanner E, Heidenheim AP, Lindsay RM: Kt/V: Patients do not get what the physician prescribes. *Trans Am Soc Artif Intern Organs* 37: M132, 1991

205. Port FK, Wolfe RA, Levin NW, Guire KE, Ferguson CW: Income and survival in chronic dialysis patients. *Trans Am Soc Artif Intern Organs* 36: M154, 1990

206. Acchiardo SR, Moore LW, Burk L: Morbidity and mortality in hemodialysis patients. *Trans Am Soc Artif Intern Organs* 36: M148, 1990

207. McClellan WM, Flanders WD, Gutman RA: Variable mortality rates among dialysis treatment centers. *Ann Intern Med* 117: 332, 1992

208. Acchiardo SR, Hatten KW, Ruvinsky MI, Dyson B, Fuller J, Moore LW: Inadequate dialysis increases gross mortality rate. *ASAIO J* 38: M282, 1992

209. Nicolucci A, Cubasso D, Labbrozzi D, Mari E, Impicciatore P, Procaccini DA, Forcella M, Stella I, Querques M, Pappani A, Passione A, Strippoli P: Effect of coexistent diseases on survival of patients undergoing dialysis. *ASAIO J* 38: M291, 1992

210. Khan IH, Catto GR, Edward N, Fleming LW, Henderson IS, MacLeod AM: Influence of coexisting disease on survival on renal-replacement therapy. *Lancet* 341: 415, 1993

211. Goldwasser P, Mittman N, Antignani A, Burrell D, Michel MA, Collier J, Avram MM: Predictors of mortality in hemodialysis patients. *Am Soc Nephrol* 3: 1613, 1993

212. Owen WF Jr, Lew NL, Liu Y, Lowrie EG, Lazarus JM: The urea reduction ratio and serum albumin concentration as predictors of mortality in patients undergoing hemodialysis. *N Engl J Med* 329: 1001, 1993

213. Charra B, Port FK, Berger EE, Lowrie EG, Parfrey PS, Foley RN, Posen GA, Collins AJ: How can the mortality rate of chronic dialysis patients be reduced? *Semin Dial* 6: 91, 1993

214. Friedman EA (Ed): *Death on Hemodialysis: Preventable or Inevitable?*, Dordrecht, Kluwer Academic Publishers, 1994

215. Friedman EA: Death on hemodialysis: Preventable or inevitable? in *Death on Hemodialysis: Preventable or Inevitable?*, edited by Friedman EA, Dordrecht, Kluwer Academic Publishers, 1994, p 1

216. Kjellstrand CM: International comparisons of dialysis survival are meaningless to evaluate differences in dialysis procedures. in *Death on Hemodialysis: Preventable or Inevitable?*, edited by Friedman EA, Dordrecht, Kluwer Academic Publishers, 1994, p 55

217. Held PJ, Akiba T, Stearns NS, Marumo F, Turenne MN, Maeda K, Port FK: Survival of middle-aged dialysis patients in Japan and the US, 1988–89. in *Death on Hemodialysis: Preventable or Inevitable?*, edited by Friedman EA, Dordrecht, Kluwer Academic Publishers, 1994, p 13

218. Lundin AP: Many deaths in hemodialysis patients are preventable. in *Death on Hemodialysis: Preventable or Inevitable?*, edited by Friedman EA, Dordrecht, Kluwer Academic Publishers, 1994, p 199

219. Lowrie EG, Huang WH, Lew NL, Liu Y: The relative contribution of measured variables to death risk among hemodialysis patients. in *Death on Hemodialysis: Preventable or Inevitable?*, edited by Friedman EA, Dordrecht, Kluwer Academic Publishers, 1994, p 121

220. Bosch JP: The evolution of high-efficiency treatments from conventional hemodialysis. in *Hemodialysis: High-Efficiency Treatments*, edited by Bosch JP, Stein JH, New York, Churchill Livingstone, 1993, p 1

221. Lysaght MJ: Hemodialysis membranes in transition. *Contrib Nephrol* 61: 1, 1988

222. Deppisch R, Ritz E, Hänsch GM, Schöls M, Rauterberg E-W: Bioincompatibility – Perspectives in 1993. *Kidney Int* 45 (Suppl 44): S77, 1994

223. Hakim RM: Choice of the hemodialysis membrane. in *Principles and Practice of Dialysis*, edited by Henrich WL, Baltimore, Williams & Wilkins, 1994, p 1

224. Shinaberger JH, Miller JH, Gardner PW: Short treatment. in *Replacement of Renal Function by Dialysis*, 3rd Ed, edited by Maher JF, Dordrecht, Kluwer, 1989, p 360

225. Francisco LL: High efficiency dialysis. *The Kidney* 21: 7, 1988

226. Riley HJ: The social work implications of high flux dialysis. *Contemp Dial Nephrol* 11: 26, 1990

227. Ronco C, Fabris A, Brendolan A, Feriani M, Chiaramonte S, Milan M, Dell'Aquila R, Biasioli S, Pisani E, La Greca G: High-flux haemodialysis with 1.5 m² modified cuprammonium rayon membrane: technical and clinical evaluation. *Nephrol Dial Transplant* 3: 440, 1988

228. Craddock PR, Fehr J, Delmasso AP, Brigham KL, Jacob HS: Hemodialysis leukopenia: pulmonary vascular leukostasis resulting from complement activation by dialyzer cellophane membranes. *J Clin Invest* 59: 878, 1977

229. Jacob AI, Gavellas G, Zarco R, Perez G, Bourgoignie JJ: Leukopenia, hypoxia and complement function with different hemodialysis membranes. *Kidney Int* 18: 505, 1980

230. Chenoweth DE, Cheung AK, Henderson LW: Anaphylatoxin formation during hemodialysis: Effects of different dialyzer membranes. *Kidney Int* 24: 764, 1983

231. Amadori A, Candi P, Sasdelli M, Massai G, Favilla S, Passaleva A, Ricci M: Hemodialysis leukopenia and complement function with different dialyzers. *Kidney Int* 24: 775, 1983

232. Hakim RM, Fearon DT, Lazarus JM, Perzanowski CS: Biocompatibility of dialysis membranes: Effects of chronic complement activation. *Kidney Int* 26: 194, 1984

233. Wegmüller E, Montandon A, Nydegger U, Descoeudres C: Biocompatibility of different hemopdialysis membranes. Activation of complement and leukopenia. *Int J Artif Organs* 9: 85, 1986

234. Vienken J, Baurmeister U: Complement activation by dialyzer membranes – *in vitro* assessment. *Artif Organs* 10: 344, 1986

235. Pertosa G, Tarantino EA, Gesualdo L, Montinaro V, Schena FP: C5b-9 generation and cytokine production in hemodialyzed patients. *Kidney Int* 43 (Suppl 41): S221, 1993

236. Himmelfarb J, Gerard NP, Hakim RM: Intradialytic modulation of granulocyte C5a receptors. *Am Soc Nephrol* 2: 920, 1991

237. Kaplow LS, Goffinet JA: Profound neutropenia during the early phase of hemodialysis. *JAMA* 203: 1135, 1968

238. Hoenich NA, Woffindin C, Qureshi M, Kerr DNS: Membrane-induced leukopenia. *Contrib Nephrol* 36: 1, 1983

239. Camussi G, Pacitti A, Tetta C, Bellone G, Mangiarotti G, Canavese C, Segoloni G, Vercellone A: Mechanisms of neutropenia in hemodialysis (HD). *Trans Am Soc Artif Intern Organs* 30: 364, 1984

240. Thylen P, Lundahl J, Fernvik E, Hed J, Svenson SB, Jacobson SH: Mobilization of an intracellular glycoprotein (Mac-1) on monocytes and granulocytes during hemodialysis. *Am J Nephrol* 12: 393, 1992

241. Lundahl J, Hed J, Jacobson SH: Dialysis granulocytopenia is preceded by an increased surface expression of the adhesion-promoting glucoprotein Mac-1. *Nephron* 61: 163, 1992

242. Nguyen AT, Lethias C, Zingraff J, Herbelin A, Naret C, Descamps-Latscha B: Hemodialysis membrane-induced activation of phagocyte oxidative metabolism detected *in vivo* and *in vitro* within microamounts of whole blood. *Kidney Int* 28: 158, 1985

243. Cappelli G, Lucchi L, Bonucchi D, Cenci AM, Montagnani G, De Palma M, Lusvarghi E: Polymorphonuclear oxygen free radical production and complement activation induced by dialysis membranes as assayed in an experimental model. *Blood Purif* 7: 293, 1989

244. Kolb G, Fischer W, Schoenemann H, Bathke K, Hoffken H, Muller T, Lange H, Joseph K, Havemann K: Effect of cuprophan, hemophan and polysulfone membranes on the oxidative metabolism, degranulation reaction, enzyme release and pulmonary sequestration of granulocytes. *Contrib Nephrol* 74: 10, 1989

245. Jacobs AA Jr, Ward RA, Wellhausen SR, McLeish KR: Polymorphonuclear leukocyte function during hemodialysis: relationship to complement activation. *Nephron* 52: 119, 1989

246. Himmelfarb J, Lazarus JM, Hakim R: Reactive oxygen species production by monocytes and polymorphonuclear leukocytes during dialysis. *Am J Kidney Dis* 17: 271, 1991

247. Kolb G, Nolting C, Eckle I, Müller T, Lange H, Havemann K: The role of membrane contact in hemodialysis-induced granulocyte activation. *Nephron* 57: 64, 1991

248. Luciak M, Trznadel K: Free oxygen species metabolism during haemodialysis with different membranes. *Nephrol Dial Transplant* 6 (Suppl 3): 66, 1991

249. Schaefer RM, Heidland A, Hörl WH: Release of leukocyte elastase during hemodialysis: Effect of different dialysis membranes. *Contrib Nephrol* 46: 109, 1985

250. Coratelli P, Rizzi R, Schena A, Pavone V, Specchia G, Liso V: Neutrophil function during hemodialysis: Effects of three different membranes. in *Immune and Metabolic Aspects of Therapeutic Blood Purification Systems*, edit-

ed by Smeby LC, Jørstad S, Widerøe T-E, Basel, Karger, 1986, p 137

251. Hörl WH, Riegel W, Schollmeyer P: Plasma levels of main granulocyte components in patients dialyzed with polycarbonate and cuprophan membranes. *Nephron* 45: 272, 1987

252. Schaefer RM, Herfs N, Ormanns W, Hörl WH, Heidland A: Change of elastase and cathepsin G content in polymorphonuclear leukocytes during hemodialysis. *Clin Nephrol* 29: 307, 1988

253. Hörl WH, Feinstein EI, Wanner C, Frischmuth N, Gösele A, Massry SG: Plasma levels of main granulocyte components during hemodialysis: comparison of new and reused dialyzers. *Am J Nephrol* 10: 53, 1990

254. Vanholder R, Ringoir S, Dhondt A, Hakim R: Phagocytosis in uremic and hemodialysis patients: a prospective and cross sectional study. *Kidney Int* 39: 320, 1991

255. Vanholder R, Ringoir S: Polymorphonuclear function and infection in dialysis. *Kidney Int* 42 (Suppl 38): S91, 1992

256. Himmelfarb J, Zaoui P, Hakim R: Modulation of granulocyte LAM-1 and MAC-1 during dialysis – a prospective, randomized controlled trial. *Kidney Int* 41: 388, 1992

257. Wehle B, Bergström J, Kishimoto T, Lantz B, Levin N, Klinkmann H: β2-Microglobulin and granulocyte elastase. *Nephrol Dial Transplant* 8 (Suppl): 220, 1993

258. Tielemans CL, Delville JP, Husson CP, Madhoun P, Lambrechts AM, Goldman M, Vanherweghem JL: Adhesion molecules and leukocyte common antigen on monocytes and granulocytes during hemodialysis. *Clin Nephrol* 39: 158, 1993

259. Cheung AK, Parker CJ, Hohnholt M: β2 integrins are required for neutrophil degranulation induced by hemodialysis membranes. *Kidney Int* 43: 649, 1993

260. Himmelfarb J, Ault KA, Holbrook D, Leeber DA, Hakim RM: Intradialytic granulocyte reactive oxygen species production: a prospective, crossover trial. *Am Soc Nephrol* 4: 178, 1993

261. Zaoui P, Green W, Hakim R: Hemodialysis with cuprophane membrane modulates interleukin-2 receptor expression. *Kidney Int* 39: 1020, 1991

262. Kay NE, Raij L: Differential effect of hemodialysis membranes on human lymphocyte natural killer function. *Artif Organs* 11: 165, 1987

263. Stefoni S, Nanni Costa A, Colì L, Bonomini M, Buscaroli A, Raimondi C, Stagni B, Cianciolo G, Bonomini V: Lymphocyte DNA synthesis and surface antigen expression in chronic dialysis: comparative effects of cuprophan and polysulfone membranes. *Contrib Nephrol* 74: 66, 1989

264. DeGiannis D, Czarnecki M, Donati D, Homer L, Eisinger RP, Raska K, Raskova J: Normal T lymphocyte function in patients with end-stage renal disease hemodialyzed with 'high-flux' polysulfone membranes. *Am J Nephrol* 10: 276, 1990

265. Donati D, Degiannis D, Combates N, Raskova J, Raska K Jr: Effects of hemodialysis on activation of lymphocytes: analysis by an *in vitro* dialysis model. *Am Soc Nephrol* 2: 1490, 1992

266. Zaoui P, Hakim RM: Natural killer-cell function in hemodialysis patients: effect of the dialysis membrane. *Kidney Int* 43: 1298, 1993

267. Stefoni S, Feliciangeli G, Nanni Costa A, Coli L, Cianciolo G, De Sanctis LB, Buscaroli A, Iannelli S, Mosconi G, Bonomini V: Approach to dialysis biocompatibility: evaluation through *in vivo* investigation of lymphocyte biology. A technical note. *Contrib Nephrol* 103: 65, 1993

268. Descamps-Latscha B, Herbelin A: Long-term dialysis and cellular immunity: a critical survey. *Kidney Int* 43 (Suppl 41): S135, 1993

269. Green D, Santhanam S, Krumlovsky FA, del Greco F: Elevated beta-thromboglobulin in patients with chronic renal failure: effect of hemodialysis. *J Lab Clin Med* 95: 679, 1980

270. Adler AJ, Berlyne GM: Beta thromboglobulin and platelet factor-4 levels during hemodialysis with polyacrylonitrile. *ASAIO J* 4: 100, 1981

271. Vicks SL, Gross ML, Schmitt GWz: Massive hemorrhage due to hemodialysis-associated thrombocytopenia. *Am J Nephrol* 3: 30, 1983

272. Docci D, Turci F, Del Vecchio C, Bilancioni R, Cenciotti L, Pretolani E: Hemodialysis-associated platelet loss: Study of the relative contribution of dialyzer membrane composition and geometry. *Int J Artif Organs* 7: 337, 1984

273. Hakim RM, Schafer AI: Hemodialysis-associated platelet activation and thrombocytopenia. *Am J Med* 78: 575, 1985

274. Martín-Malo A, Velasco F, Castillo D, Pérez R, Andrés P, Torres A, Aljama P: Factors affecting the plasma beta-thromboglobulin levels during hemodialysis. in *Immune and Metabolic Aspects of Therapeutic Blood Purification Systems*, edited by Smeby LC, Jørstad S, Widerøe T-E, Basel, Karger, 1986, p 18

275. Simon P, Ang KS, Cam G: Enhanced platelet aggregation and membrane biocompatibility: possible influence on thrombosis and embolism in hemodialysis patients. *Nephron* 45: 172, 1987

276. Amato M, Salvadori M, Bergesio F, Messeri A, Filimberti E, Morfini M: Aspects of biocompatibility of two different dialysis membranes: cuprophane and polysulfone. *Int J Artif Organs* 11: 175, 1988

277. Barth RH, Sodden S, Berlyne GM: Heparin-free hemodialysis with a polyacrylonitrile membrane. *Trans Am Soc Artif Intern Organs* 35: 597, 1989

278. Leitienne P, Trzeciak MC, Adeleine P, Ville D, Dechavanne M, Traeger J, Zech P: Comparison of hemostasis with two high-flux hemocompatible dialysis membranes. *Int J Artif Organs* 14: 227, 1991

279. Gawaz MP, Ward RA: Effects of hemodialysis on platelet-derived thrombospondin. *Kidney Int* 40: 257, 1991

280. Verbeelen D, Jochmans K, Herman AG, Van der Niepen P, Sennesael J, De Waele M: Evaluation of platelets and hemostatis during hemodialysis with six different membranes. *Nephron* 59: 567–572, 1991

281. Seyfert UT Helmling E, Hauck W, Skroch D, Albert W: Comparison of blood biocompatibility during haemodialysis with cuprophane and polyacrylonitrile membranes. *Nephrol Dial Transplant* 6: 428, 1991

282. Remuzzi A, Boccardo P, Benigni A: *In vitro* platelet adhesion to dialysis membranes. *Nephrol Dial Transplant* 6 (Suppl 2): 36, 1991

283. Reber G, Stoermann C, de Moerloose P, Ruedin P, Leski M: Hemostatic disturbances induced by two hollow-fiber hemodialysis membranes. *Int J Artif Organs* 15: 269, 1992

284. Cheung AK: Biocompatibility of hemodialysis membranes. *Am Soc Nephrol* 1: 150, 1990

285. Dinarello CA: Cyttokines: Agents provocateurs in hemodialysis? *Kidney Int* 41: 683, 1992

286. Henderson LW, Koch KM, Dinarello CA, Shaldon S: Hemodialysis hypotension: the interleukin hypothesis. *Blood Purif* 1: 3, 1983

287. Haeffner-Cavaillon N, Cavaillon JM, Ciancioni C, Bacle F, Delons S, Kazatchkine MD: *In vivo* induction of interleukin-1 during hemodialysis. *Kidney Int* 35: 1212, 1989

288. Schindler R, Lonnemann G, Shaldon S, Koch KM, Dinarello CA: Transcription, not synthesis, of interleukin-1 and tumor necrosis factor by complement. *Kidney Int* 37: 85, 1990

289. Blumenstein M, Ziegler-Heitbrock HW, Schiller B, Schmidt B, Ward RA, Gurland HJ: Differential activation of monocytes in haemodialysis patients exposed to different types of membranes. *Scand J Immunol* 31: 183, 1990

290. Tetta C, Camussi G, Turello E, Salomone M, Aimo G, Priolo G, Segoloni G, Vercellone A: Production of cytokines in hemodialyis. *Blood Purif* 8: 337, 1990

291. Ghysen J, De Plaen JF, van Ypersele de Strihou C: The effect of membrane characteristics on tumour necrosis factor kinetics during haemodialysis. *Nephrol Dial Transplant* 5: 270, 1990

292. Chollet-Martin S, Stamatakis G, Bailly S, Mery JP, Gougerot-Pocidalo MA: Induction of tumour necrosis factor-alpha during haemodialysis: influence of the membrane type. *Clin Exp Immunol* 83: 329, 1991

293. Pertosa G, Marfella C, Tarantino EA, Di Cillo M, Manno C, Russo R, Schena FP: Involvement of peripheral blood monocytes in haemodialysis: *in vivo* induction of tumour necrosis factor alpha, interleukin 6 and beta 2-microglobulin. *Nephrol Dial Transplant* 6 (Suppl 2): 18, 1991

294. Mege JL, Olmer M, Purgus R, Bertocchio P, Farnarier C, Kaplanski S, Capo C, Bongrand P: Haemodialysis membranes modulate chronically the production of TNF alpha, IL1 beta and IL6. *Nephrol Dial Transplant* 6: 868, 1991

295. Honkanen E, Gronhagen-Riska C, Teppo AM, Maury CP, Meri S: Acute-phase proteins during hemodialysis: correlations with serum interleukin-1 beta levels and different dialysis membranes. *Nephron* 57: 283, 1991

296. Donati D, Degiannis D, Homer L, Raska K Jr, Raskova J: Production and kinetics of interleukin-1 in hemodialysis. *In vivo* and *in vitro* study. *Am J Nephrol* 11: 451, 1991

297. Donati D, Degiannis D, Combates N, Raskova J, Raska K Jr: Evidence of mononuclear cell activation by hemodialysis. *Trans Am Soc Artif Intern Organs* 37: M386, 1991

298. Donati D, Degiannis D, Homer L, Raska K, Raskova J: Interleukin-1 kinetics in hemodialysis. *Trans Am Soc Artif Intern Organs* 37: M391, 1991

299. Memoli B, Libetta C, Rampino T, Dal Canton A, Conte G, Scala G, Ruocco MR, Andreucci VE: Hemodialysis related induction of interleukin-6 production by peripheral blood mononuclear cells. *Kidney Int* 42: 320, 1992

300. Nakahama H, Tanaka Y, Shirai D, Miyazaki M, Imai N, Yokokawa T, Okada M, Kubori S: Plasma interleukin-6 levels in continuous ambulatory peritoneal dialysis and hemodialysis patients. *Nephron* 61: 132, 1992

301. Hertel J, Kimmel PL, Phillips TM, Bosch JP: Eosinophilia and cellular cytokine responsiveness in hemodialysis patients. *Am Soc Nephrol* 3: 1244, 1992

302. Patarca R, Perez G, Gonzalez A, Garcia-Morales RO, Gamble R, Klimas N, Fletcher MA: Comprehensive evaluation of acute immunological changes induced by cuprophane and polysulfone membranes in a patient on chronic hemodialysis. *Am J Nephrol* 12: 274, 1992

303. Docci D, Bilancioni R, Pistocchi E, Baldrati L, Capponcini C, Delvecchio C, Feletti C: Evolution of serum prealbumin following hemodialysis: Effect of different dialysis membranes. *Nephron* 62: 145, 1992

304. Schindler R, Linnenweber S, Schulze M, Oppermann M, Dinarello CA, Shaldon S, Koch KM: Gene expression of interleukin-1 beta during hemodialysis. *Kidney Int* 43: 712, 1993

305. Vaziri ND, Kaupke CJ, Yousefi S, Gonzales E, Cesario TC: Cytokine levels during hemodialysis. *Trans Am Soc Artif Intern Organs* 37: M389, 1991

306. Powell AC, Bland LE, Oettinger CW, McAllister SK, Oliver JC, Arduino MJ, Favero MS: Lack of plasma interleukin-1 beta or tumor necrosis factor-alpha elevation during unfavorable hemodialysis conditions. *Am Soc Nephrol* 2: 1007, 1991

307. Paczek L, Schaefer RM, Heidland A: Dialysis membranes decrease immunoglobulin and interleukin-6 production by peripheral blood mononuclear cells *in vitro*. *Nephrol Dial Transplant* 6 (Suppl 3): 41, 1991

308. Schaefer RM, Paczek L, Heidland A: Cytokine production by monocytes during haemodialysis. *Nephrol Dial Transplant* 6 (Suppl 2): 14, 1991

309. Bandiani G, Camaiora E, Farina D, Nicolini MA, Perotta U, Tagliazucchi A: Long-term influence of dialysis treatment on beta 2-microglobulin, interleukin-2 R and tumour necrosis factor. *Nephrol Dial Transplant* 6 (Suppl 2): 61, 1991

310. Herbelin A, Ureña P, Nguyen AT, Zingraff J, Descamps-Latscha B: Influence of first and long-term dialysis on uraemia-associated increased basal production of interleukin-1 and tumour necrosis factor alpha by circulating monocytes. *Nephrol Dial Transplant* 6: 349, 1991

311. Powell AC, Bland LA, Oettinger CW, McAllister SK, Oliver JC, Arduino MJ, Favero MS: Enhanced release of TNF-alpha, but not IL-1 beta, from uremic blood after endotoxin stimulation. *Lymphokine Cytokine Res* 10: 343, 1991

312. Herbelin A, Urena P, Nguyen AT, Zingraff J, Descamps-Latscha B: Elevated circulating levels of interleukin-6 in patients with chronic renal failure. *Kidney Int* 39: 954, 1991

313. Putz D, Barna U, Luger A, Mayer G, Woloszczuk W, Graf H: Biocompatibility of high-flux membranes. *Int J Artif Organs* 15: 456, 1992

314. Borah MF, Schoenfeld PY, Gotch FA, Sargent JA, Wolfson M, Humphreys MH: Nitrogen balance during intermittent dialysis therapy of uremia. *Kidney Int* 14: 491, 1978

315. Bergström J, Alvestrand A, Gutierrez A: Acute and chronic metabolic effects of hemodialysis. in *Immune and Metabolic Aspects of Therapeutic Blood Purification Systems*, edited by Smeby LC, Jørstad S, Widerøe T-E, Basel, Karger, 1986, p 254

316. Gutierrez A, Alvestrand A, Wahren J, Bergström J: Effect of *in vivo* contact between blood and dialysis membranes on protein catabolism in humans. *Kidney Int* 38: 487, 1990

317. Gutierrez A, Bergström J, Alvestrand A: Protein catabolism in sham-hemodialysis: the effect of different membranes. *Clin Nephrol* 38: 20, 1992

318. Gutierrez A, Alvestrand A, Bergström J: Membrane selection and muscle protein catabolism. *Kidney Int* 42 (Suppl 38): S86, 1992

319. Lim VS, Bier DM, Flanigan MJ, Sum-Ping ST: The effect of hemodialysis on protein metabolism: a leucine kinetic study. *J Clin Invest* 91: 2429, 1993

320. Hörl WH, Heidland A: Evidence for the participation of granulocyte proteinases on intradialytic catabolism. *Clin Nephrol* 21: 314, 1984

321. Vincent C, Revillard JP, Galland M, Traeger J: Serum β_2-microglobulin in hemodialyzed patients. *Nephron* 21: 260, 1978

322. Hauglustaine D, Waes M, Michielsen P, Goebels J, Vandeputte M: Haemodialysis membranes, serum β_2-microglobulin, and dialysis amyloidosis. *Lancet* 1: 1211, 1986

323. Bommer J, Seelig P, Seelig R, Geerlings W, Bommer G, Ritz E: Determinations of plasma beta–2-microglobulin concentrations: Possible relation to membrane biocompatibility. *Nephrol Dial Transplant* 2: 22, 1987

324. DeBroe ME, Nouwen J, Waeleghem: On the mechanism and site of production of β_2 microglobulin during haemodialysis. *Nephrol Dial Transplant* 2: 124, 1987

325. Bandiani G, Camaiora E, Farina D, Nicolini MA, Perotta U, Tagliazucchi A: Long-term influence of dialysis treatment on beta 2-microglobulin, interleukin-2 R and tumour necrosis factor. *Nephrol Dial Transplant* 6 (Suppl 2): 61, 1991

326. Bergström J, Wehle B: No change in corrected beta 2-microglobulin concentration after cuprophane haemodialysis. *Lancet* 1: 628, 1987

327. Shaldon S, Koch KM, Dinarello CA, Colton CK, Knudsen PJ, Floege J, Granolleras C: β_2-microglobulin and haemodialysis. *Lancet* 1: 925, 1987

328. Honig R, Marsen T, Schad S, Barth C, Pollok M, Baldamus CA: Correlation of beta-2-microglobulin concentration changes to changes of distribution volume. *Int J Artif Organs* 11: 459, 1988

329. Zingraff J, Beyne P, Ureña P, Uzan M, Man NK, Descamps-Latscha B, Drueke T: Influence of haemodialysis membranes on beta 2-microglobulin kinetics: *in vivo* and *in vitro* studies. *Nephrol Dial Transplant* 3: 284, 1988

330. Martin-Malo A, Mallol J, Castillo D, Barrio V, Burdiel LG, Perez R, Aljama P: Factors affecting beta 2-microglobulin plasma concentration during hemodialysis. *Int J Artif Organs* 12: 509, 1989

331. DiRaimondo CR, Pollak VE: Beta 2-microglobulin kinetics in maintenance hemodialysis: a comparison of conventional and high-flux dialyzers and the effects of dialyzer reuse. *Am J Kidney Dis* 13: 390, 1989

332. Sulkova S, Votruba T, Lapcik O, Valek A: Beta 2-microglobulin serum levels during dialysis: effect of cuprophan and serum osmolality changes. *Int J Artif Organs* 13: 22, 1990

333. Skroeder NR, Jacobson SH, Holmquist B, Kjellstrand P, Kjellstrand CM: Beta 2-microglobulin generation and removal in long slow and short fast hemodialysis. *Am J Kidney Dis* 21: 519, 1993

334. Wehle B, Bergström J, Kishimoto T, Lantz B, Levin N, Klinkmann H: β_2-microglobulin and granulocyte elastase. *Nephrol Dial Transplant* 8 (Suppl 2): 20, 1993

335. Knudsen PJ, Ng A-K, Liu Z: Beta-2-microglobulin synthesis is increased during activation of human monocytes. *Blood Purif* 6: 178, 1988

336. Knudsen PJ, Leon J, Ng AK, Shaldon S, Floege J, Koch KM: Hemodialysis-related induction of beta-2-microglobulin and interleukin-1 synthesis and release by mononuclear phagocytes. *Nephron* 53: 188, 1989

337. Jahn B, Betz M, Deppisch R, Janssen O, Hansch GM, Ritz E: Stimulation of beta 2-microglobulin synthesis in lymphocytes after exposure to Cuprophan dialyzer membranes. *Kidney Int* 40: 285, 1991

338. Schoels M, Jahn B, Hug F, Deppisch R, Ritz E, Hansch GM: Stimulation of mononuclear cells by contact with cuprophan membranes: further increase of beta 2-microglobulin synthesis by activated late complement components. *Am J Kidney Dis* 21: 394, 1993

339. Zaoui PM, Stone WJ, Hakim RM: Effects of dialysis membranes on beta$_2$-microglobulin production and cellular expression. *Kidney Int* 38: 962, 1990

340. Stein G, Schauer S, Suss J, Muller A, Huller M, Schaefer K, Falkenhagen D, Linss W: Influence of membranes on generation of beta 2 M and release of leukocyte lysosomal enzymes. *Int J Artif Organs* 13: 359, 1990

341. Campistol JM, Molina R, Bernard DB, Rodriguez R, Mirapeix E, Munoz-Gomez JM, Revert L: Synthesis of beta 2-microglobulin in lymphocyte culture: role of hemodialysis, dialysis membranes, dialysis-amyloidosis, and lymphokines. *Am J Kidney Dis* 22: 691, 1993

342. Schaefer RM, Paczek L, Heidland A: Suppression of beta 2-microglobulin release from lymphocytes by dialysis membranes. *Nephrol Dial Transplant* 6 (Suppl 3): 53, 1991

343. Bonucchi D, Lucchi L, Leonardi M, Cenci AM, Lusvarghi E: Cellulosic membranes and leukocytes are not effective for *in vitro* generation of beta 2-microglobulin. *Nephrol Dial Transplant* 3: 708, 1988

344. Floege J, Bartsch A, Schulze M, Shaldon S, Koch KM, Smeby LC: Turnover of ^{131}I-β_2-microglobulin in hemodialyzed patients. *J Lab Clin Med* 118: 153, 1991

345. Chanard J, Vincent C, Caudwell V, Lavaud S, Toupance O, Wong T, Revillard J-P: Beta 2-microglobulin metabolism in uremic patients who are undergoing dialysis. *Kidney Int* 43 (Suppl 41): S83, 1993

346. Floege J, Schäffer J, Koch KM, Shaldon S: Dialysis related amyloidosis: a disease of chronic retention and inflammation? *Kidney Int* 42 (Suppl 38): S78, 1992

347. Quereda C, Orofino L, Marcen R, Sabater J, Matesanz R, Ortuño J: Influence of dialysate and membrane biocompatibility on hemodynamic stability in hemodialysis. *Int J Artif Organs* 11: 259, 1988

348. Bergamo Collaborative Dialysis Study Group: Acute intradialytic well-being: results of a clinical trial comparing polysulfone with cuprophan. *Kidney Int* 40: 714, 1991

349. Collins DM, Lambert MB, Tannenbaum JS, Oliverio M, Schwab SJ: Tolerance of hemodialysis: A randomized prospective trial of high-flux *versus* conventional high-efficiency hemodialysis. *Am Soc Nephrol* 4: 148, 1993

350. Levin NW, Zasuwa G: Relationship between dialyser type and signs and symptoms. *Nephrol Dial Transplant* 8 (Suppl 2): 30, 1993

351. Cheung AK, LeWinter M, Chenoweth DE, Lew W, Henderson LW: Cardiopulmonary effects of cuprophan-activated plasma in the swine. Role of complement activation products. *Kidney Int* 29: 799, 1986

352. Schohn DC, Jahn HA, Eber M, Hauptman G: Biocompatibility and hemodynamic studies during polycarbonate versus cuprophan membrane dialysis. *Blood Purif* 4: 102, 1986

353. Schulman G, Fogo A, Gung A, Badr K, Hakim R: Complement activation retards resolution of acute ischemic renal failure in the rat. *Kidney Int* 40: 1069, 1991

354. Hakim RM, Wingard RL, Lawrence P, Parker RA, Schulman G: Use of biocompatible membranes improves outcome and recovery from acute renal failure. (Abstract) *Am Soc Nephrol* 3: 367, 1992

355. Hakim RM, Breillatt J, Lazarus M, Port FK: Complement activation and hypersensitivity reactions to dialysis membranes. *N Engl J Med* 311: 878, 1984

356. Lundin AP, Adler AJ, Berlyne GM, Friedman EA: Tuberculosis in patients undergoing maintenance hemodialysis. *Am J Med* 67: 597, 1979

357. Hornberger JC, Chernew M, Petersen J, Garber AM: A multivariate analysis of mortality and hospital admissions with high-flux dialysis. *Am Soc Nephrol* 3: 1227, 1992

358. Levin NW, Zasuwa G, Dumler F: Effect of membrane type on causes of death in hemodialysis patients. (Abstract) *Am Soc Nephrol* 2: 335, 1991

359. Streicher E, Schneider H: The next generation of dialysis membranes – barriers or pathways? *Contrib Nephrol* 44: 127, 1985

360. Rubin JE, Adler AJ, Friedman EA, Berlyne GM: Reduced protein loss during hemofiltration using cuprophan membranes. *Artif Organs* 2: 131, 1978

361. Röckel A, Abdelhamid S, Fiegel P, Walb D: Elimination of low molecular weight proteins with high flux membranes. *Contrib Nephrol* 46: 69, 1985

362. Röckel A, Hertel J, Fiegel P, Abdelhamid S, Panitz N, Walb D: Permeability and secondary membrane formation of a high flux polysulfone hemofilter. *Kidney Int* 30: 429, 1986

363. Wizemann V, Birk HW, Techert F: Effects of a modified hemodiafiltration method on low-molecular-weight protein composition in plasma. *Blood Purif* 8: 45, 1990

364. Lindsay RM, Spanner E, Heidenheim P, Kortas C, Blake PG: PCR, Kt/V and membrane. *Kidney Int* 43 (Suppl 1): S268, 1993

365. Graeber CW, Halley SE, Lapkin RA, Graeber CA, Kaplan AA: Protein losses with reused dialyzers. (Abstract) *Am Soc Nephrol* 4: 349, 1993

366. May RC, Kelly RA, Mitch WE: Pathophysiology of uremia. in *The Kidney*, 4th Ed, edited by Brenner BM, Rector FC Jr, Philadelphia, Harcourt, Brace, Jovanovich, 1991, p 1997

367. Gejyo F, Yamada T, Odani S, Nakagawa Y, Arakawa M, Kunitomo T, Kataoka H, Suzuki M, Hirasawa Y, Shirahama T, Cohen AS, Schmidt K: A new form of amyloid protein associated with chronic hemodialysis was identified as beta 2-microglobulin. *Biochem Biophys Res Comm* 129: 701, 1985

368. Ullian ME, Hammond WS, Alfrey AC, Schultz A, Molitoris BA: Beta-2-microglobulin-associated amyloidosis in chronic hemodialysis patients with carpal tunnel syndrome. *Medicine* 68: 107, 1989

369. Sethi D, Naunton Morgan TC, Brown EA, Cary NRB, Erhardt CC, Pazianas M, Maini RN, Woodrow DF, Gower PE: Dialysis arthropathy: A clinical, biochemical, radiological and histological study of 36 patients. *Q J Med* 282: 1061, 1990

370. Schwarz A, Keller F, Seyfert S, Poll W, Molzahn M, Distler A: Carpal tunnel syndrome: a major complication in long-term hemodialysis patients. *Clin Nephrol* 22: 133, 1984

371. van Ypersele de Strihou C, Honhon B, Vandenbroucke JM, Huaux JP, Noël H, Maldague B: Dialysis amyloidosis. *Adv Nephrol* 17: 401, 1988

372. Charra B, Calemard E, Laurent G: Chronic renal failure treatment duration and mode: Their relevance to the late dialysis periarticular syndrome. *Blood Purif* 6: 117, 1988

373. Sargent MA, Fleming SJ, Chattopadhyay C, Ackrill P, Sambrook P: Bone cysts and haemodialysis-related amyloidosis. *Clin Radiol* 40: 277, 1989

374. Chanard J, Bindi P, Lavaud S, Toupance O, Maheut H, Lacour F: Carpal tunnel syndrome and type of dialysis membrane. *Br Med J* 298: 867, 1989

375. Acchiardo S, Kraus AP Jr, Jennings BR: Beta 2-microglobulin levels in patients with renal insufficiency. *Am J Kidney Dis* 13: 70, 1989

376. Jadoul M, Malghem J, Pirson Y, Maldague B, van Ypersele de Strihou C: Effect of renal transplantation on the radiological signs of dialysis amyloid osteoarthropathy. *Clin Nephrol* 32: 194, 1989

377. Hermann E, Mayet WJ, Wandel E, Scherer G, Schadmand S, Klose KJ, Poralla T, Meyer zum Buschenfelde KH, Kohler H: Rheumatologic and radiologic symptoms of dialysis-associated beta 2-microglobulin amyloidosis: long-retrospective study of 175 chronic hemodialysis patients. *Z Rheumatol* 50: 160, 1991

378. Sethi D, Brown EA, Cary NRB, Woodrow DF, Gower PE: Persistence of dialysis amyloid after renal transplantation. A case report. *Am J Nephrol* 9: 173, 1989

379. van Ypersele de Strihou C, Jadoul M, Malghem J, Maldague B, Jamart J, The Working Party on Dialysis Amyloidosis: Effect of dialysis membrane and patient's age on signs of dialysis-related amyloidosis. *Kidney Int* 39: 1012, 1991

380. Miura Y, Ishiyama T, Inomata A, Takeda T, Senma S, Okuyama K, Suzuki Y: Radiolucent bone cysts and the type of dialysis membrane used in patients undergoing long-term hemodialysis. *Nephron* 60: 268, 1992

381. Aoyagi R, Miura Y, Ishiyama T, Maruyama Y, Hasegawa H: Influence of dialysis membranes on the development of dialysis associated osteoarthropathy. *Kidney Int* 43 (Suppl 41): S111, 1993

382. Drücke T, Ureña P, Man NK, Zingraff J: Membrane transfer, membrane adsorption and possible membrane-induced generation of beta-2-microglobulin. *Contrib Nephrol* 74: 113, 1989

383. Goldman M, Nortier J, Dhaene M, Amraoui Z, Vanherweghem J-L: Fate of beta-2-microglobulin during dialysis on polysulfone and AN 69 membranes. *Contrib Nephrol* 74: 127, 1989

384. Floege J, Granolleras C, Deschodt G, Heck M, Baudin G, Branger B, Tournier O, Reinhard B, Eisenbach GM, Smeby LC et al.: High-flux synthetic versus cellulosic membranes for beta 2-microglobulin removal during hemodialysis, hemodiafiltration and hemofiltration. *Nephrol Dial Transplant* 4: 653, 1989

385. Klinke B, Rockel A, Abdelhamid S, Fiegel P, Walb D: Transmembranous transport and adsorption of beta-2-microglobulin during hemodialysis using polysulfone, polyacrylonitrile, polymethylmethacrylate and cuprammonium rayon membranes. *Int J Artif Organs* 12: 697, 1989

386. Goldman M, Lagmiche M, Dhaene M, Amraoui Z, Thayse C, Vanherweghem JL: Adsorption of beta 2-microglobulin on dialysis membranes: comparison of different dialyzers and effects of reuse procedures. *Int J Artif Organs* 12: 373, 1989

387. David S, Canino F, Ferrari ME, Cambi V: The role of adsorption in beta 2-microglobulin removal. *Nephrol Dial Transplant* 6 (Suppl 2): 64, 1991

388. Mineshima M, Hoshino T, Era K, Kitano Y, Suzuki T, Sanaka T, Teraoka S, Agishi T, Ota K: Difference in beta 2-microglobulin removal between cellulosic and synthetic polymer membrane dialyzers. *Trans Am Soc Artif Intern Organs* 36: M643, 1990

389. Floege J, Smeby L: Dialysis-related amyloidosis and high-flux membranes. *Contrib Nephrol* 96: 124, 1992

390. Simon P, Cavarle YY, Ang KS, Cam G, Catheline M: Long-term variations of serum beta$_2$-microglobulin levels in hemodialysed uremics according to permeability and biocompatibility of dialysis membranes. *Blood Purif* 6: 111, 1988

391. Kaiser JP, Hagemann J, von Herrath D, Schaefer K: Different handling of beta$_2$-microglobulin during hemodialysis and hemofiltration. *Nephron* 48: 132, 1988

392. Kessler M, Netter P, Maheut H, Wolf C, Prenat E, Cao Huu T, Gaucher A, The Cooperative Group on Dialysis-associated Arthropathy: Highly permeable and biocompatible membranes and prevalence of dialysis-associated arthropathy. *Lancet* 337: 1092, 1991

393. Geyjo F, Arakawa M: Dialysis amyloidosis: Current disease concepts and new perspectives for its treatment. *Contrib Nephrol* 78: 47, 1990

394. Makita Z, Bucala R, Rayfield EJ, Friedman E, Kaufman AM, Korbet SM, Barth RH, Winston JA, Fuh H, Vlassara H: Efficiency of removal of circulating advanced glycosylation end-products and mode of tretment in patients with ESRD. (Abstract) *Am Soc Nephrol* 3: 335, 1992

395. Vlassara H, Fuh H, Makita Z, Krungkrai S, Cerami A, Bucala R: Exogenous advanced glycosylation end products induce complex vascular dysfunction in normal animals: a model for diabetic and aging complications. *Proc Natl Acad Sci USA* 89: 12043, 1992

396. Nakamura Y, Horii Y, Nishino T, Shiiki H, Sakaguchi Y, Kagoshima T, Dohi K, Makita Z, Vlassara H, Bucala R: Immunohistochemical localization of advanced glycosylation end products in coronary atheroma and cardiac tissue in diabetes mellitus. *Am J Pathol* 143: 1649, 1993

397. Vlassara H, Bucala R, Striker L: Pathogenic effects of advanced glycosylation: biochemical, biologic, and clinical implications for diabetes and aging. *Lab Invest* 70: 138, 1994

398. Miyata T, Oda O, Inagi R, Iida Y, Araki N, Yamada N, Horiuchi S, Taniguchi N, Maeda K, Kinoshita T: β2-microglobulin modified with advanced glycation end products is a major component of hemodialysis-associated amyloidosis. *J Clin Invest* 92: 1243, 1993

399. Miyata T, Inagi R, Iida Y, Sato M, Yamada N, Oda O, Maeda K, Seo H: Involvement of beta 2-microglobulin modified with advanced glycation end products in the pathogenesis of hemodialysis-associated amyloidosis. Induction of human monocyte chemotaxis and macrophage secretion of tumor necrosis factor-alpha and interleukin-1. *J Clin Invest* 93: 521, 1994

400. Levin NW, Dumler F, Zasuwa G, Stalla K: Mortality comparison between conventional and high flux dialysis. *Am Soc Nephrol* 2: 365, 1991

401. McCosh EJ, Solangi K, Rivers JM, Goodman A: Hypertriglyceridemia in patients with chronic renal insufficiency. *Am J Clin Nutr* 28: 1036, 1975

402. Murase T, Cattran DC, Rubenstein B, Steiner G: Inhibition of lipoprotein lipase by uremic plasma, a possible cause of hypertriglyceridemia. *Metabolism* 24: 1279, 1975

403. Savdie E, Gibson JC, Crawford GA, Simons LA, Mahony JF: Impaired plasma triglyceride clearance as a feature of both uremic and posttransplant triglyceridemia. *Kidney Int* 18: 774, 1980

404. Weintraub M, Burstein A, Rassin T, Liron M, Ringel Y, Cabili S, Blum M, Peer G, Iaina A: Severe defect in clearing postprandial chylomicron remnants in dialysis patients. *Kidney Int* 42: 1247, 1992

405. Cressman MD, Hoogwerf BJ, Schreiber MJ, Cosentino FA: Lipid abnormalities and end-stage renal disease: implications for atherosclerotic cardiovascular disease? *Miner Electrolyte Metab* 19: 180, 1993

406. Barth RH, Zara AC, Berlyne GM: Reduction of serum triglycerides by heparin and high-flux hemodialysis membrane. (Abstract) *Kidney Int* 37: 288, 1990

407. Kusano E, Sakiri Y, Miyata S, Ebata S, Tetsuka T, Asano Y: Effect of polyacrylonitrile hemodialysis on lipid metabolism in the patients undergoing maintenance hemodialysis. (Abstract) *Am Soc Nephrol* 2: 334, 1991

408. Marangoni R, Civardi F, Savino R, Colombo R, Marangoni F, Mosconi C, Galli C: Plasma lipids and fatty acid levels in chronically uremic patients undergoing blood purification with different methods. *Artif Organs* 16: 625, 1992

409. Seres DS, Strain GW, Hashim SA, Goldberg IJ, Levin NW: Improvement of plasma lipoprotein profiles during high-flux dialysis. *Am Soc Nephrol* 3: 1409, 1993

410. Josephson MA, Fellner SK, Dasgupta A: Improved lipid profiles in patients undergoing high-flux hemodialysis. *Am J Kidney Dis* 20: 361, 1992

411. Blankestijn PJ, Vos PF, Rabelink AJ, van Rijn H, Jansen H, Koomans HA: High flux dialysis membranes improve lipid profiles in dialysis patients. (Abstract) *Am Soc Nephrol* 4: 334, 1993

412. Ibels SL, Reardon MF, Nestel PJ: Plasma post-heparin lipolytic activity and triglyceride clearance in uremic and hemodialysis patients and renal allograft recipients. *J Lab Clin Med* 87: 648, 1976

413. Mordasini R, Frey F, Flury W, Klose G, Greten H: Selective deficiency of hepatic triglyceride lipase in uremic patients. *N Engl J Med* 297: 1362, 1977

414. Crawford GA, Mahony JF, Stewart JH: Impaired lipoprotein lipase activation by uraemic and post-transplant sera. *Clin Sci* 60: 73, 1981

415. Chan MK, Persaud J, Varghese Z, Moorhead JF: Pathogenic roles of post-heparin lipases in lipid abnormalities in hemodialysis patients. *Kidney Int* 25: 812, 1984

416. Yukawa S, Tone Y, Sonobe M, Maeda T, Mimura K, Mune M, Fujiwara S, Tsujimoto K, Maeshima E, Saika Y et al.: Study on the inhibitory effect of uremic plasma on lipoprotein lipase. *Nippon Jinzo Gakkai Shi* 34: 979, 1992

417. Violante F, Lorenzi S, Fusello M: Uremic neuropathy: clinical and neurophysiological investigation of dialysis patients using different chemical membranes. *Eur Neurol* 24: 398, 1985

418. Manohar NL, Gorfien PC, Namba T, Louis BM, Lipner HI: Rapid improvement of uremic neuropathy on short high-efficiency hemodialysis with special reference to middle molecules. *Trans Am Soc Artif Intern Organs* 33: 274, 1987

419. Djukanović LJD, Mimi'c-Oka JI, Potić JB: The effects of hemodialysis with different membranes on middle molecules and uremic neuropathy. *Int J Artif Organs* 12: 11, 1989

420. Tattersall JE, Cramp M, Shannon M, Farrington K, Greenwood RN: Rapid high-flux dialysis can cure uraemic peripheral neuropathy. *Nephrol Dial Transplant* 7: 539, 1992

421. Malberti F, Surian M, Farina M, Vitelli E, Mandolfo S, Guri L, De Petri GC, Castellani A: Effect of hemodialysis and hemodiafiltration on uremic neuropathy. *Blood Purif* 9: 285, 1991

422. Man NK, Cueille G, Zingraff J, Boudet J, Sausse A, Funck-Brentano JL: Uremic neurotoxin in the middle molecular weight range. *Artif Organs* 4: 116, 1980

423. Di Paolo B, Di Marco T, Cappelli P, Albertazzi A: Polymethylmethacrylate in chronic hemodialysis. Is it of benefit in patients with uremic neuropathy? *Trans Am Soc Artif Intern Organs* 33: 293, 1987

424. Robles NR, Murga L, Galvan S, Esparrago JF, Sánchez-Casado E: Hemodialysis with cuprophane or polysulfone: effects on uremic polyneuropathy. *Am J Kidney Dis* 21: 282, 1993

425. Chimienti S, Mele G, Perrone F, Muscogiuri P, Cristofano C: Oxalate depuration during biofiltration with AN69 and in conventional hemodialysis in chronic renal failure patients. *Int J Artif Organs* 9 (Suppl 3): 73, 1986

426. Dell'Aquila R, Feriani M, Mascalzoni E, Bragantini L, Ronco C, La Greca G: Oxalate removal by differing dialysis techniques. *ASAIO J* 38: 797, 1992

427. Gueris J, Fournier A, Sebert JL, De Fremont JF, Ferriere C, Covoet B, Quichaud J: Comparative effects of dialysis with cuprophan *versus* polyacrylonitrile membranes on plasma immunoreactive parathyroid hormone levels in patients on chronic hemodialysis. *Calcif Tissue Res* 22 (Suppl): 434, 1977

428. Wizemann V, Velcovsky HG, Bley H, Brüning S, Schütterle G: Removal of hormones by hemofiltration and hemodialysis with a highly permeable polysulfone membrane. *Contrib Nephrol* 46: 61, 1985

429. D'Amour P, Jobin J, Hamel L, L'Ecuyer N: iPTH values during hemodialysis: role of ionized Ca, dialysis membranes and iPTH assays. *Kidney Int* 38: 308, 1990

430. Hörl WH: Removal of high-molecular-weight toxins. *Contrib Nephrol* 96: 138, 1992

431. De Francisco ALM, Amado JA, Prieto M, Alcalde G, Sanz de Castro S, Ruiz JC, Morales P, Arias M: Dialysis membranes and PTH changes during hemodialysis in patients with secondary hyperparathyroidism. *Nephron* 66: 442, 1994

432. Stefanović V, Bogićević M, Mitić M: Myoglobin elimination in end stage kidney disease patients on renal replacement therapy. *Int J Artif Organs* 16: 659, 1993

433. Carson RW, Dunnigan EJ, DuBose TD Jr, Goeger DE, Anderson KE: Removal of plasma porphyrins with high-flux hemodialysis in porphyria cutanea tarda associated with end-stage renal disease. *Am Soc Nephrol* 2: 1445, 1992

434. Hoek FJ, Grijm R, Sanders GTB, Tytgat GNJ, Wilmink JM: Removal of bile acids from the blood by hemodialysis with a polyaacrylonitril membrane: Treatment of pruritus of cholestatic disease. *Digestion* 23: 135, 1982

435. Opolon P, Rapin JR, Huguet C, Granger A, Delorme ML, Boschat M, Sausse A: Hepatic failure coma (HFC) treated by polyacrylonitrile membrane (PAN) hemodialysis (HD). *Trans Am Soc Artif Intern Organs* 22: 701, 1976

436. Silk DB, Trewby PN, Chase RA, Mellon PJ, Hanid MA, Davies M, Langley PG, Wheeler PG, Williams R: Treatment of fulminant hepatic failure by polyacrylonitrile-membrane haemodialysis. *Lancet* 2: 1, 1977

437. Denis J, Opolon P, Nusinovici V, Granger A, Darnis F: Treatment of encephalopathy during fulminant hepatic failure by haemodialysis with high permeability membrane. *Gut* 19: 787, 1978

438. Strand V, Mayor G, Ristow G, Greenbaum D, Mayle J, Rosenbaum R: Concomitant renal and hepatic failure treated by polyacrylonitrile membrane hemodialysis. *Int J Artif Organs* 4: 136, 1981

439. Gardere JJ, Castaing Y, Gbikpi-Benissan G: Hemodialysis with a high permeability membrane in the treatment of encephalopathy of fulminant hepatitis. *Ann Fr Anesth Reanim* 6: 423, 1987

440. Splendiani G, Tancredi M, Daniele M, Giammaria U: Treatment of acute liver failure with hemodetoxification techniques. *Int J Artif Organs* 13: 370, 1990

441. Yoshiba M, Sekiyama K, Iwamura Y, Sugata F: Development of reliable artificial liver support (ALS)-plasma exchange in combination with hemodiafiltration using high-performance membranes. *Dig Dis Sci* 38: 469, 1993

442. Barozzi C, Cairo G, Fumero R, Scuri S, Tanzi MC, Tieghi G: Protein-membrane interactions during hemodialysis; in *Immune and Metabolic Aspects of Therapeutic Blood Purification Systems*, edited by Smeby LC, Jørstad S, Widerøe T-E, Basel, Karger, 1986, p 1

443. Andrade JD, Hlady V: Plasma protein adsorption: the big twelve. *Ann NY Acad Sci* 516: 158, 1987

444. Kuwahara T, Markert M, Wauters JP: Proteins adsorbed on hemodialysis membranes modulate neutrophil activation. *Artif Organs* 13: 427, 1989

445. Lonnemann G, Koch KM, Shaldon S, Dinarello CA: Studies on the ability of hemodialysis membranes to induce, bind, and clear human interleukin-1. *J Lab Clin Med* 112: 76, 1988

446. Pascual M, Schifferli JA: Adsorption of complement factor D by polyacrylonitrile dialysis membranes. *Kidney Int* 43: 903, 1993

447. Cheung AK, Chenoweth DE, Otsuka D, Henderson LW: Compartmental distribution of complement activation products in artificial kidneys. *Kidney Int* 30: 74, 1986

448. Röckel A, Hertel J, Perschel WT, Walb D, Fiegel P, Panitz N, Abdelhamid S: Polyacrylonitrile complement activation attenuated by simultaneous ultrafiltration and adsorption. *Nephrol Dial Transplant* 2: 251, 1987

449. Cheung AK, Parker CJ, Wilcox LA, Janatova J: Activation of complement by hemodialysis membranes: Polyacrylonitrile binds more C3a than cuprophan. *Kidney Int* 37: 1055, 1990

450. Cheung AK, Hohnholt M, Leypoldt JK, DeSpain M: Hemodialysis membrane biocompatibility: The case of erythropoietin. *Blood Purif* 9: 153, 1991

451. Quale JM, O'Halloran JJ, Devincenzo N, Barth RH: Removal of vancomycin by high-flux hemodialysis membranes. *Antimicrob Agents Chemother* 36: 1424, 1992

452. Golper TA, Vincent HH, Gleason JR, Vos MC: Drug removal during high-efficiency and high-flux hemodialysis. in *Hemodialysis: High-Efficiency Treatments*, edited by Bosch JP, Stein JH, New York, Churchill Livingstone, 1993, p 175

453. Barcenas CG, Fuller TJ, Elms J, Cohen R, White MG: Staphylococcal sepsis in patients on chronic hemodialysis regimens: Intravenous treatment with vancomycin given once weekly. *Arch Intern Med* 136: 1131, 1976

454. Cunha BA, Quintiliani R, Deglin JM, Izard MW, Nightingale CH: Pharmacokinetics of vancomycin in anuria. *Rev Infect Dis* 3 (Suppl): S269, 1981

455. Barth RH, DeVincenzo N, Zara AC, Berlyne GM: Vancomycin pharmacokinetics in high-flux hemodialysis. (Abstract) *Am Soc Nephrol* 1: 348, 1990

456. Lanese DM, Alfrey PS, Molitoris BA: Markedly increased clearance of vancomycin during hemodialysis using polysulfone dialyzers. *Kidney Int* 35: 1409, 1989

457. Torras J, Cao C, Rivas MC, Cano M, Fernandez E, Montoliu J: Pharmacokinetics of vancomycin in patients undergoing hemodialysis with polyacrylonitrile. *Clin Nephrol* 36: 35, 1991

458. DeSoi CA, Sahm DF, Umans JG: Vancomycin elimination during high-flux hemodialysis: kinetic model and comparison of four membranes. *Am J Kidney Dis* 20: 354, 1992

459. Barth RH, DeVincenzo N, Berlyne GM: Revised vancomycin dosing schedule for high-flux hemodialysis. (Abstract) *Am Soc Nephrol* 2: 314, 1991

460. Mac-Kay MV, Sanchez Burson J, Martinez-Lanao J, Dominguez-Gil A: Drug dosage in end-stage renal disease (ESRD) patients undergoing haemodialysis. A predictive study based on a microcomputer program. *Clin Pharmacokinet* 25: 243, 1993

461. Keller F, Hörstensmeyer C, Looby M, Borner K, Pommer W, Erdmann K, Giehl M: Vancomycin dosing in haemodialysis patients and bayesian estimate of individual pharmacokinetic parameters. *Int J Artif Organs* 17: 19, 1994

462. Böhler J, Reetze-Bonorden P, Keller E, Schollmeyer P: Comment on 'Pharmacokinetics of vancomycin' by Torras et al.. *Clin Nephrol* 37: 268, 1992

463. Bohler J, Reetze-Bonorden P, Keller E, Kramer A, Schollmeyer PJ: Rebound of plasma vancomycin levels after haemodialysis with highly permeable membranes. *Eur J Clin Pharmacol* 42: 635, 1992

464. Pollard TA, Lampasona V, Akkerman S, Tom K, Hooks MA, Mullins RE, Maroni BJ: Vancomycin redistribution: dosing recommendations following high-flux hemodialysis. *Kidney Int* 45: 232, 1994

465. Moellering RC Jr, Krogstad DJ, Greenblatt DJ: Vancomycin therapy in patients with impaired renal function: a nomogram for dosage. *Ann Intern Med* 94: 343, 1981

466. Barth RH: Staphylococcal bacteremia. *Semin Dial* 6: 374, 1993

467. Ingerman MJ, Santoro J. Vancomycin: A new old agent. *Infect Dis Clin North Am* 3: 641, 1989

468. Spivey JM: The postantibiotic effect. *Clin Pharmacol* 11: 865, 1992

469. Hercz G, Norris KC, Miller JH, Shinaberger JH, Coburn JW: Aluminum removal by hemodialysis: Critical comparison of dialyzer membranes. (Abstract) *Kidney Int* 29: 215, 1986

470. Muirhead N, Hollomby DJ, Leung FY, Mitton R, Henderson AR, Keown PA, Stiller CR: Removal of aluminum during hemodialysis: effect of different dialyzer membranes. *Am J Kidney Dis* 8: 51, 1986

471. Molitoris BA, Alfrey AC, Alfrey PS, Miller NL: Rapid removal of DFO-chelated aluminum during hemodialysis using polysulfone dialyzers. *Kidney Int* 34: 98, 1988

472. Day JP, Hewitt CD, Ackrill P, Hill K: Clearance of aluminium desferrioxamine by haemodialysis using a polysulfone high flux membrane. *Contrib Nephrol* 74: 101, 1989

473. Aarseth HP, Ganss R: Removal of chelated aluminum during haemodialysis using polysulphone high-flux dialysers. *Nephrol Dial Transplant* 5: 942, 1990

474. Gouge SF, Moore J Jr, Atkins F, Hirszel P: Radiocontrast removal by dialysis membranes. *Blood Purif* 9: 182, 1991

475. Kar PM, Kellner K, Ing TS, Leehey DJ: Combined high-efficiency hemodialysis and charcoal hemoperfusion in severe N-acetylprocainamide intoxication. *Am J Kidney Dis* 20: 403, 1992

476. Bommer J, Ritz E: Water quality-A neglected problem in hemodialysis. *Nephron* 46: 1, 1987

477. Port FK, VanDeKerkhove KM, Kunkel SL, Kluger MJ: The role of dialysate in the stimulation of interleukin-1 production during clinical hemodialysis. *Am J Kidney Dis* 10: 118, 1987

478. Man NK, Ciancioni C, Faivre JM, Diab N, London G, Maret J, Wambergue FP: Dialysis-associated adverse reactions with high-flux membranes and microbial contamination of liquid bicarbonate concentrate. *Contrib Nephrol* 62: 24, 1988

479. Yamagami S, Adachi T, Sugimura T, Kishimoto T, Maekawa M, Niwa M, Shaldon S: Detection of bacteria in dialysate and its antibody in long-term hemodialysis patients. *Trans Am Soc Artif Intern Organs* 35: 331, 1989

480. Baurmeister U, Travers M, Vienken J, Harding G, Million C, Klein E, Pass T, Wright R: Dialysate contamination and back filtration may limit the use of high-flux dialysis membranes. *Trans Am Soc Artif Intern Organs* 35: 519, 1989

481. Harding GB, Klein E, Pass T, Wright R, Million C: Endotoxin and bacterial contamination of dialysis center water and dialysate; a cross sectional survey. *Int J Artif Organs* 13: 39, 1990

482. Bigazzi R, Atti M, Baldari G: High-permeable membranes and hypersensitivity-like reactions: role of dialysis fluid contamination. *Blood Purif* 8: 190, 1990

483. Mege JL, Sanguedolce MV, Purgus R, Moulin B, Bongrand P, Capo C, Olmer M: Chronic and intradialytic effects of high-flux hemodialysis on tumor necrosis factor-α production: relationship to endotoxins. *Am J Kidney Dis* 20: 482, 1992

484. Henderson L, Ward RA, Mion CM, Canaud B, Bosch JP, Charyton C, Spinowitz BS, Gupta BK, Meindel N, Bland La, Favero MS, Arduino MJ: Should hemodialysis fluid be sterile? *Semin Dial* 6: 26, 1993

485. Streicher E, Schneider H: The development of a polysulfone membrane. A new perspective in dialysis? *Contrib Nephrol* 46: 1, 1985

486. Mohammed D, Barth RH: The effect of blood flow rate on backfiltration in high flux hemodialysis. (Abstract) *Am Soc Nephrol* 4: 370, 1993

487. Schmidt M, Baldamus CA, Schoeppe W: Backfiltration in hemodialyzers with highly permeable membranes: an *in vitro* and *in vivo* investigation. *Blood Purif* 2: 108, 1984

488. Bosch T, Schmidt B, Samtleben W, Gurland HJ: Effect of protein adsorption on diffusive and convective transport through polysulfone membranes. *Contrib Nephrol* 46: 14, 1985

489. Stiller S, Mann H, Brunner H: Backfiltration in hemodialysis with highly permeable membranes. *Contrib Nephrol* 46: 23, 1985

490. Ronco C: Backfiltration: A controversial issue in modern dialysis. *Int J Artif Organs* 11: 69, 1988

491. Ronco C: Backfiltration in clinical dialysis: nature of the phenomenon, mechanisms and possible solutions. *Int J Artif Organs* 13: 11, 1990

492. Robertson BC, Curtin C: Effects of EPO therapy on backfiltration of dialysate in high flux dialysis. *Trans Am Soc Artif Intern Organs* 36: M447, 1990

493. Leypoldt JK, Schmidt B, Gurland HJ: Measurement of backfiltration rates during hemodialysis with highly permeable membranes. *Blood Purif* 9: 74, 1991

494. Leypoldt JK, Schmidt B, Gurland HJ: Net ultrafiltration may not eliminate backfiltration during hemodialysis with highly permeable membranes. *Artif Organs* 15: 164, 1991

495. Hyver SW, Petersen J, Cajias J: An *in vivo* analysis of reverse ultrafiltration during high-flux and high-efficiency dialysis. *Am J Kidney Dis* 12: 439, 1992

496. Klinkmann H, Ebbighausen H, Uhlenbusch I, Vienken J: High-flux dialysis, dialysate quality and backtransport. *Contrib Nephrol* 103: 89, 1993

497. Duff GW, Atkins E: The detection of endotoxin by *in vitro* production of endogenous pyrogen: comparison with limulus amebocyte lysate gelation. *J Immunol Methods* 52: 323, 1982

498. Ogawa Y, Murai T, Kanoh S: Characterization of the pyrogenicity of two different lipopolysaccharides and their lipid A-bovine serum albumin complexes. *J Pharmacobiodyn* 9: 722, 1986

499. Klein E, Pass T, Harding GB, Wright R, Million C: Microbial and endotoxin comtamination in water and dialysate in the central United States. *Artif Organs* 14: 85, 1990

500. Bland LA, Ridgeway MR, Aguero SM, Carson LA, Favero MS: Potential bacteriologic and endotoxin hazards associated with liquid bicarbonate concentrate. *Trans Am Soc Artif Intern Organs* 33: 542, 1987

501. Herbelin A, Ureña P, Man NK, Drüeke T, Descamps-Latscha B: *In vitro* studies of endotoxin transfer across cellulosic and noncellulosic dialysis membranes: II. Interleukin-1 production. *Contrib Nephrol* 74: 79, 1989

502. Laude-Sharp M, Caroff M, Simard L, Pusineri C, Kazatchkine MD, Haeffner-Cavaillon N: Induction of IL-1 during hemodialysis: transmembrane passage of intact endotoxin (LPS). *Kidney Int* 38: 1089, 1990

503. Ureña P, Herbelin A, Zingraff J, Lair M, Man NK, Descamps-Latscha B, Drüeke T: Permeability of cellulose and non-cellulosic membranes to endotoxin subunits and cytokine production during *in-vitro* haemodialysis. *Nephrol Dial Transplant* 7: 16, 1992

504. Lonnemann G, Behme TC, Lenzner B, Floege J, Schulze M, Colton CK, Koch KM, Shaldon S: Permeability of dialyzer membranes to TNFα-inducing substances derived from water bacteria. *Kidney Int* 42: 61, 1992

505. Watzke H, Mayer G, Schwarz HP, Stanek G, Rotter M, Hirschl AM, Graf H: Bacterial contamination of dialysate in dialysis-associated endotoxaemia. *J Hosp Infect* 13: 109, 1989

506. Bommer J, Becker KP, Urbaschek R, Ritz E, Urbaschek B: No evidence for endotoxin transfer across high flux polysulfone membranes. *Clin Nephrol* 6: 278, 1987

507. Ureña P, Herbelin A, Basile C, Zingraff J, Man NK, Drüeke T: *In vitro* studies of endotoxin transfer across cellulosic and noncellulosic dialysis membranes: I. Radiolabeled endotoxin. *Contrib Nephrol* 74: 71, 1989

508. Vanholder R, Van Haecke E, Veys N, Ringoir S: Endotoxin transfer through dialysis membranes: small- *versus* large-pore membranes. *Nephrol Dial Transplant* 7: 333, 1992

509. Klinkmann H, Falkenhagen D: Importance of endotoxins in high-flux dialysis. *Nephrol Dial Transplant* 7: 884, 1992

510. Kumano K, Yokota S, Nanbu M, Sakai T: Do cytokine-inducing substances penetrate through dialysis membranes and stimulate monocytes? *Kidney Int* 43 (Suppl 41): S205, 1993

511. Evans RC, Holmes CJ: *In vitro* study of the transfer of cytokine-inducing substances across selected high-flux hemodialysis membranes. *Blood Purif* 9: 92, 1991

512. Lowry PW, Beck-Sague CM, Bland LA, Aguero SM, Arduino MJ, Minuth AN, Murray RA, Swenson JM, Jarvis WR: *Mycobacterium chelonae* infection among patients receiving high-flux dialysis in a hemodialysis clinic in California. *J Infect Dis* 161: 85, 1990

513. Powell AC, Bland LA, Oettinger CW, McAllister SK, Oliver JC, Arduino MJ, Favero MS: Lack of plasma interleukin-1β or tumor necrosis factor-α elevation during unfavorable hemodialysis conditions. *Am Soc Nephrol* 2: 1007, 1991

514. Gordon SM, Oettinger CW, Bland LA, Oliver JC, Arduino MJ, Aguero SM, Mcallister SK, Favero MS, Jarvis WR: Pyrogenic reactions in patients receiving conventional, high-efficiency, or high-flux hemodialysis treatments with bicarbonate dialysate containing high concentrations of bacteria and endotoxin. *Am Soc Nephrol* 2: 1436, 1992

515. Petersen J, Hyver SW, Cajias J: Backfiltration during dialysis – a critical assessment. *Semin Dial* 5: 13, 1992
516. Tielemans C, Madhoun P, Lenaers M, Schandene L, Goldman M, Vanherweghem JL: Anaphylactoid reactions during hemodialysis on AN69 membranes in patients receiving ACE inhibitors. *Kidney Int* 38: 982, 1990
517. Verresen L, Waer M, Vanrenterghem Y, Michielsen P: Angiotensin-converting-enzyme inhibitors and anaphylactoid reactions to high-flux membrane dialysis. *Lancet* 336: 1360, 1990
518. Jadoul M, Struyven J, Stracher A, van Ypersele de Strihou C: Angiotension-converting-enzyme inhibitors and anaphylactoid reactions to high-flux membrane dialysis. *Lancet* 337: 112, 1991
519. van Es A, Henny FC, Lobatto S: Angiotension-converting-enzyme inhibitors and anaphylactoid reactions to high-flux membrane dialysis. *Lancet* 337: 112, 1991
520. Alvarez-Lara MA, Martin-Malo A, Espinosa M, Castillo D, Aljama P: ACE inhibitors and anaphylactoid reactions to high-flux membrane dialysis. *Lancet* 337: 370, 1991
521. Tielemans C, Vanherweghem JL, Blumberg A, Cuvelier R, De Fremont JF, Dehout F, Dupont P, Richard C, Stolear JC, Wens R: ACE inhibitors and anaphylactoid reactions to high-flux membrane dialysis. *Lancet* 337: 370, 1991
522. Petrie JJ, Campbell Y, Hawley CM, Hogan PG: Anaphylactoid reactions in patients on hemodiafiltration with

AN69 membranes whilst receiving ACE inhibitors. *Clin Nephrol* 36: 264, 1991
523. Parnes EL, Shapiro WB: Anaphylactoid reactions in hemodialysis patients treated with the AN69 dialyzer. *Kidney Int* 40: 1148, 1991
524. Lacour F, Maheut H: AN 69 membrane and conversion enzyme inhibitors: prevention of anaphylactic shock by alkaline rinsing? *Nephrologie* 13: 135, 1992
525. Rousaud Baron F, Garcia JM, Camps EM, Cubells TD, Comamala MR: ACE inhibitors and anaphylactoid reactions to high-flux membrane dialysis (AN69): clinical aspects. *Nephron* 60: 487, 1992
526. Caravaca F, Pizarro JL, Garcia MC, Cubero JJ, Arrobas M, Esparrago JF, Sanchez-Casado E: More about anaphylactoid reactions in patients dialyzed with AN69 filter and on angiotensin converting enzyme inhibitors treatment. *Nephron* 60: 372, 1992
527. Perez-Garcia R, Galan A, Garcia Vinuesa M, Anaya F, Valderrabano F: Anaphylactoid reactions during hemodialysis on AN69 membranes: role of ACE inhibitors and back-filtration. *Nephron* 61: 123, 1992
528. Brunet P, Jaber K, Berland Y, Baz M: Anaphylactoid reactions during hemodialysis and hemofiltration: role of associating AN69 membrane and angiotensin I-converting enzyme inhibitors. *Am J Kidney Dis* 19: 444, 1992
529. Daugirdas JT, Ing TS: First-use reactions during hemodialysis: A definition of subtypes. *Kidney Int* 33 (Suppl 24): S37, 1988

DIALYZER REUSE – TECHNIQUES AND CONTROVERSY

A.M. MILES and E.A. FRIEDMAN

INTRODUCTION

Hemodialyzer reuse refers to the processing of a used dialyzer cartridge with or without connecting tubing, for repeated hemodialysis in the same patient. Dialyzer reuse was first described in 1964 by Shaldon (1), who refrigerated coil dialyzers containing the patient's heparinized blood until the next dialysis. Reuse of dialyzers then underwent a series of refinements and became progressively widespread, initially for reasons of convenience in home hemodialysis programs to reduce the need for rebuilding of Kiil dialyzers, and later for cost containment and improved dialyzer biocompatibility. Dialyzer reuse today is largely limited to hollow fiber capillary dialyzers because of their near universal use, and because of difficulty in assessing the efficacy of reprocessing in parallel plate dialyzers. Automated reprocessing machines were introduced in 1980–1981 and contributed to the increasing trend to reuse dialyzers. In an effort to contain the burgeoning cost of health care in the United States, in 1983, the Federal Government discontinued the previous Medicare system of reimbursing 80% of the actual cost of each dialysis session and instituted a composite rate of reimbursement for each hemodialysis treatment, i.e.: a limited, fixed amount was paid for each dialysis. Following imposition of composite reimbursement for dialysis, further expansion of reuse programs in the United States was noted, so that while 16% of American patients on hemodialysis in 1976 used reprocessed dialyzers; in 1991, this figure had increased to 71% (2).

Dialyzer manufacturers however, still label their products for single use only, and though the Food and Drug Administration has requested the performance of clinical studies which would allow relabelling of dialyzers for multiple use (3), it seems unlikely that these studies would be performed by the manufacturers who stand to bear no gain from further expansion of reuse programs. Absence of strict quality control requirements for sterility and function of reused dialyzers, sporadic outbreaks of endotoxemia and septicemia, the possible contribution of reuse to chronic underdialysis in the USA (4), and recent reports of significant elevation of relative mortality risk in patients treated with reused dialyzers processed with particular disinfectants (5), are other problems in the field of dialyzer reuse. Chronic underdialysis and high mortality in the United States dialysis population is thought by

Table 1. Reuse of hemodialyzers by location, ownership and size (1991, United States). From Ref (2)

Type of facility	Total centers	Number (%) reusing
Location		
Hospital	711	298 (42)
Non-hospital	1334	1154 (87)
Ownership		
Profit	1144	992 (87)
Non-profit	720	404 (56)
Government	182	57 (31)
Size		
1–40 patients	620	378 (61)
41–80 patients	687	488 (71)
> 80 patients	739	587 (79)

many to comprise an 'American tragedy', in which shortened dialysis treatments (less than 3.5 hours) and multiple dialyzer reuse are the preeminent villains. Patients receiving shortened dialysis treatments are more likely to be in a dialysis center that has also begun dialyzer reuse within the previous 2 years (6). Some have gone so far as to suggest abandonment of dialyzer reprocessing (7).

Despite drawbacks, dialyzer reuse has helped cost containment in chronic hemodialysis facilities, allowed use of more expensive high flux dialyzers in many centers, reduced the incidence of first use reactions, and has ostensibly provided safe and effective hemodialysis for thousands of American dialysis patients. In addition, in many developing countries, dialyzer reuse has allowed more widespread availability of scarce and expensive dialysis treatments. This chapter will discuss the epidemiology and current techniques of reuse while assessing advantages, disadvantages and complications of dialyzer reuse.

EPIDEMIOLOGY OF REUSE

Health Care Financing Administration (HCFA) questionnaire surveys of the Medicare funded hemodialysis population in the United States revealed that the most dramatic rise in reuse prevalence occurred between 1976 and 1983: 18% (135) of dialysis centers reused dialyzers in 1976 while 52% (579) of centers practiced reuse in 1983 (Figure 1). The percentage of dialysis centers reusing dialyzers continues to increase, and in 1992, 72% (1569) of American dialysis centers treating 78% (133,348) of the hemodialysis population used reprocessed dialyzers (2) (Figures 1 and 2). The number of reuses ranged from 2 to 50 (mean = 14), and the maximum number of times

a reprocessed dialyzer was ever reused ranged from 3 to 181 (mean = 32). Reuse of dialyzer caps was reported from 62% of dialysis centers, of bloodlines from 13% of centers, and of transducer filters from 1% of centers (2). Though reuse of these disposable dialysis components was not associated with increased risks of pyrogenic reactions, septicemia or hepatitis B virus infection, reuse of transducer filters is not recommended because of the risk of cross-contamination of dialyzers by refluxed blood. In the United States, reuse is practiced mainly in large, non-hospital based, for profit facilities (2) (Table 1). In an earlier HCFA survey done in 1989 (8), 56% of dialysis centers used automated reprocessing only, 36% used manual reprocessing only, and 7% of centers used a combination of manual and automated reuse systems.

Outside of the United States, dialyzer reuse is not as widespread. In Australia in 1990, for example, only 27% of dialysis units (35% of the hemodialysis population) used reprocessed dialyzers (9). Ten percent of all European hemodialysis patients were treated with reused dialyzers in 1989 (10), but percentages have ranged from 0.1% in the Netherlands, 35.4% in the United Kingdom to 75.9% in Poland (11). Dialyzer reuse is not practiced in Japan where it is proscribed by law.

RELATIVE CONTRAINDICATIONS TO DIALYZER REUSE

Reprocessing of dialyzers should not be done in patients with an active systemic infection, in particular acute hepatitis. Because of high levels of viremia and consequent high risk of infectivity, patients with chronic hepatitis B virus (HBV) infection should not have their dialyzers reprocessed. The risk of HBV infection in patients and staff at centers reprocessing dialyzers, however, has not been reported to be increased compared to centers practicing single use dialysis (12). According to current Centers for Disease Control (CDC) recommendations, dialyzer reuse may be practiced in patients with human immunodeficiency virus (HIV) infection, as long as universal precautions are maintained. It would seem prudent however, to reprocess dialyzers from HIV-infected patients in a separate area or on a dedicated automated device, but this is not currently mandated. In hemodialysis patients with hepatitis C virus (HCV) infection, reuse practices though currently unrestricted, may be abridged as the severity and high infectivity of HCV in dialysis units becomes more fully appreciated.

REPROCESSING A USED DIALYZER

The major steps in dialyzer reprocessing are outlined in Table 2. Details of the reuse process vary from center to center. Factors which may determine the details of a reprocessing device or method are listed in Table 3. Guide-

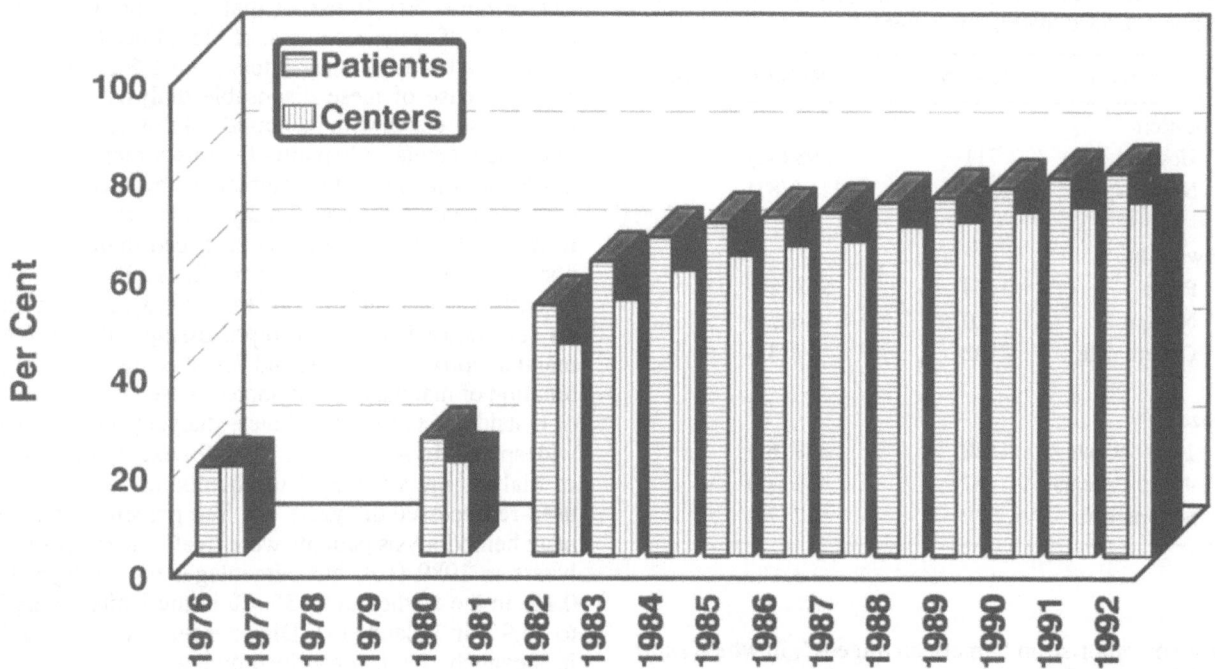

Figure 1. Increasing prevalence of reuse in American hemodialysis units (percentage of dialysis patients and dialysis centers employing reused dialyzers). Data from Ref (2).

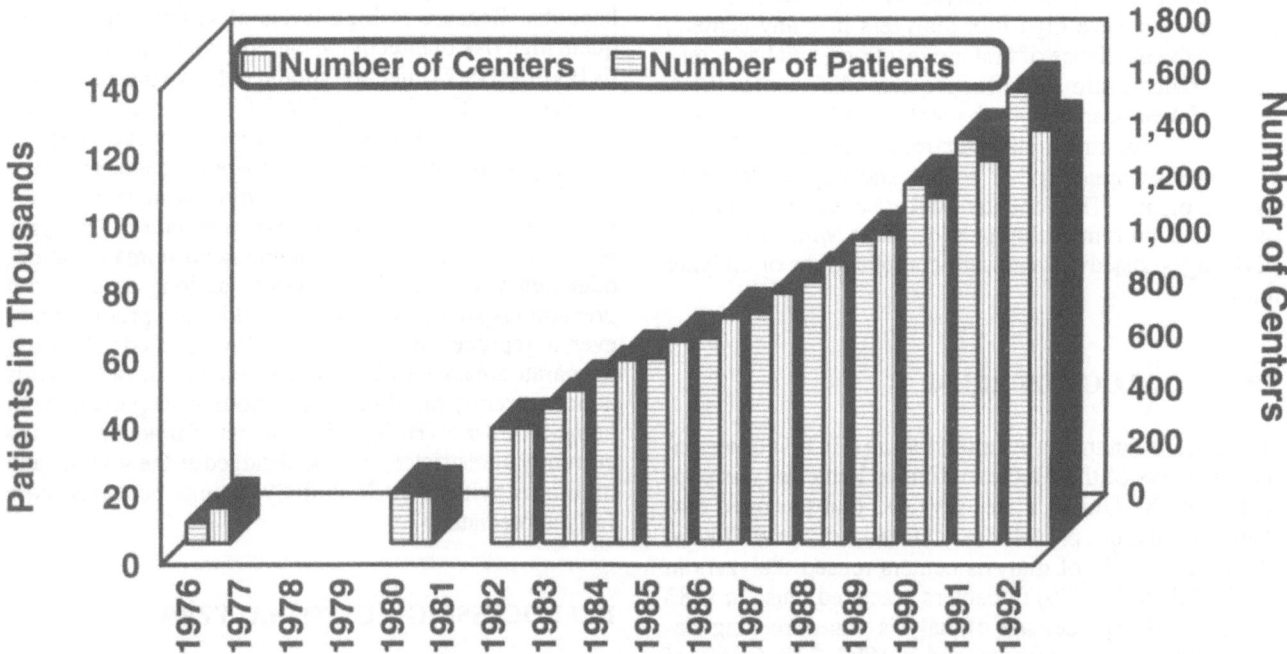

rigure 2. Increasing prevalence of reuse in American hemodialysis units (number of patients and dialysis centers employing reused dialyzers). Data from Ref (2).

REPROCESSING TECHNIQUE

Following termination of dialysis conducted with optimal heparinization in order to minimize dialyzer fiber clotting, the dialyzer is rinsed with 200–300 ml of heparinized normal saline, ensuring that air does not enter the dialyzer and later prevent complete filling of the dialyzer with disinfectant. In some centers practising manual reuse, further dialyzer pre-rinsing at the dialysis station is performed: reverse osmosis (RO)-treated water with or without added heparin is run through the dialyzer blood compartment for 8–10 minutes, or until the effluent is clear. The dialysate outflow line may be periodically clamped during pre-rinsing in order to generate positive pressure from dialysate to blood compartment, thereby loosening blood products adhering to the fibers.

The dialyzer is visually inspected for clotted fibers (if more than 10–15 fibers are clotted the dialyzer is discarded) (Figure 3), for the presence of large clots about the headers, for cracks and for potting compound damage. Multiply processed dialyzers may acquire a yellowish or brownish discoloration which is aesthetically displeasing, and also lead to the dialyzer being discarded. The dialyzer is then labelled and transported to the reprocessing area, where processing of the used dialyzer is begun, ideally, within 10 minutes. Some centers however refrigerate the dialyzer at 4°C until it is convenient to begin reprocessing (18). Once started, the reprocessing sequence should proceed to completion without interruption. A suitable label must include the patient's name, number of previous uses, date of last reprocessing, and original and residual total cell volume (TCV). Label markings should resist reprocessing damage and should not obscure pertinent information printed on the dialyzer surface. The reuse area should be: a) separate from the dialysis area, b) well ventilated (a hood with an exhaust fan is ideal), and c) free of frequent traffic of staff or patients since it is a potentially blood-contaminated area.

Dialyzers may be reprocessed manually or by using an automated device. Manual reuse may be preferred in smaller dialysis centers or for home dialysis patients. Manual reprocessing of dialyzers is more labor intensive, requires strict adherence to detail, results in variable quality control, and may result in less reuse cycles for an individual dialyzer when compared with automated reprocessing. Details of typical manual and automated dialyzer reprocessing will now be discussed.

MANUAL REPROCESSING

Rinsing

A variety of rinsing sequences may be used. Variables include the type of fluid used (RO-processed water, deionized water, saline, tap water (ideally filtered through a 5 micron filter)), rinse times, pressures, temperatures; the

---

Table 2. Steps in dialyzer reprocessing

- Termination of hemodialysis
- Pre-rinsing
- Visual inspection
- Labelling and transport to reprocessing area
- Rinsing
- Cleaning (optional)
- Performance testing
- Disinfection
- Storage
- Preparing for next dialysis
  - Inspection and patient identification
  - Verify presence of concentrated disinfectant
  - Priming and rinsing of dialyzer
  - Testing for residual disinfectant

Table 3. Factors determining details of the reuse process

Physical space and financial considerations
Personnel and supervisory requirements
Manual versus automated considerations
Processed water requirements
Type of dialyzer membrane
Interaction of patient schedules
Maintenance requirements
Environmental interactions

---

lines relating to dialyzer reprocessing have been set by the Association for the Advancement of Medical Instrumentation (AAMI) in 1986 (13) (and updated in 1993 (14). Information on reuse techniques may also be found in publications from the National Kidney Foundation (15), and the National Nephrology Foundation (16). In 1987, HCFA adopted the AAMI Recommended Practice for Reuse of Hemodialyzers as Federal guidelines for dialyzer reprocessing. Facilities failing to comply with these regulations risk losing Medicare eligibility and funding. There is no maximum number of times a dialyzer may be reused, though some centers set a maximum limit based on the frequency of failure of performance testing after a certain number of reuses. The number of times a dialyzer is reprocessed is guided by its gross appearance and by performance testing. Consequent to the raised mean hematocrit of hemodialysis patients receiving erythropoietin therapy, the number of times a dialyzer may be reused may decline after institution of erythropoietin therapy despite increases in heparin dosage (17).

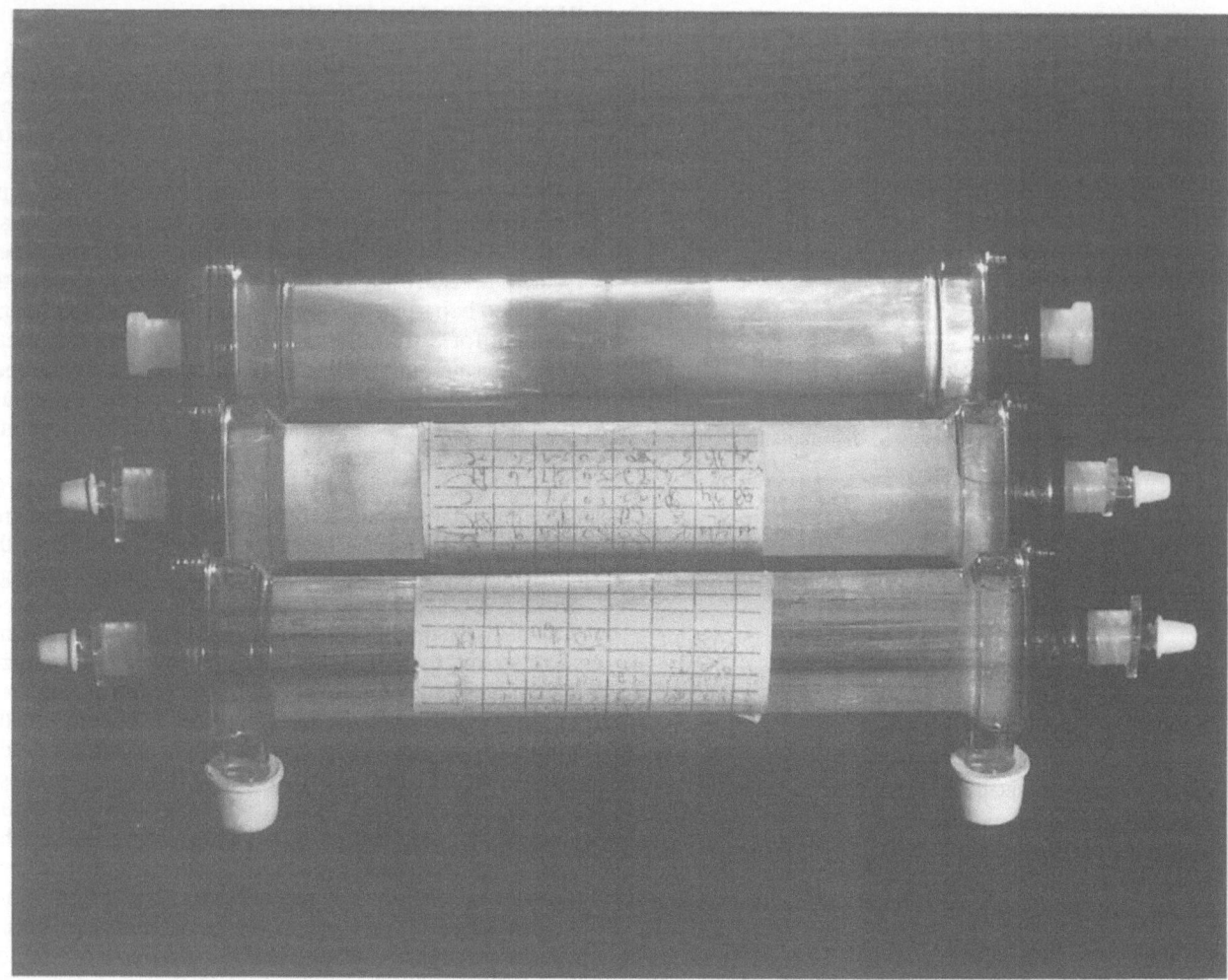

Figure 3. Visual infection of reused dialyzers. Top: new dialyzer, middle: dialyzer reused 25 times and still in use, bottom: reprocessed dialyzer rejected after 12 reuses because of multiple fiber clotting (courtesy of Edmund G. Lowrie MD).

use of pulsatile or continuous, uni- or bidirectional water flow; and the use of a reverse ultrafiltration step. All water coming into contact with dialyzer blood or dialysate compartments must be of good quality i.e.: fulfilling requirements of the Association for the Advancement of Medical Instrumentation (AAMI) of bacterial colony counts < 200 per ml and bacterial lipopolysaccharide concentration of < 1 ng/ml (5 endotoxin units(EU)/ml) as measured by the Limulus amebocyte lysate (LAL) assay (14).

The manual rinse sequence used by the National Nephrology Foundation (19) is described. The dialyzer is placed on a rack with the arterial side down. First, the blood compartment is rinsed (arterial to venous direction) at 15–20 psi (or at 3–4 l/min) with processed water. Next, 4 cycles of reverse ultrafiltration alternating with flushing with water are performed over the next hour: the dialysate side is filled with water free of air bubbles and the dialysate outflow line is clamped for 15 minutes. Then, the dialysate flow is released and the blood compartment is rinsed for

2 minutes with water at 20 psi. During this 2 minute period, the blood compartment outflow line is clamped briefly three times. The entire cycle is then repeated. The direction of fill of the dialysate compartment is changed with each cycle.

Cleaning

A cleaning step with sodium hypochlorite (bleach), hydrogen peroxide or Renalin® is optional, and is unnecessary if a prolonged rinsing sequence as described above is used. A cleaning step may be added if the dialyzer has a significant number of clotted fibers as sodium hypochlorite has been found to significantly increase the fiber bundle volume of used dialyzers by dissolving proteinaceous deposits. Hydrogen peroxide decolorizes clotted fibers but does not remove protein residues, and has fallen out of use because of difficulty in ridding the dialyzer of bubbles and debris. The blood compartment is filled with 1% sodium hypochlorite or 3% hydrogen peroxide for 30–60 seconds. Cleaning-induced damage may occur particularly with cellulosic membranes if high concentrations of bleach are used for prolonged times. Concentrations of bleach in excess of 1% with exposure times over 1 minute strips protein residues from the surface of cellulosic membranes (20), thereby restoring bioincompatibility (21, 22). Concentrations of bleach above 2%, with exposure times over 10 minutes, destroys the dialyzer membrane itself, producing increases in the ultrafiltration rate and enhancing the risk of blood leaks or membrane rupture. Use of bleach in the reprocessing of polysulfone dialyzers may alter the effective pore size of the membrane and produce loss of blood proteins in dialysate fluid (23).

Performance testing

Total cell volume (TCV)

Decreased solute transport in reprocessed dialyzers is due to occlusion of fibers by clotted blood and to protein deposition on the membrane resulting in thickening of the dialysis membrane, occlusion of membrane pores, and decreased membrane permeability to solute. Fiber occlusion is detected by measuring the TCV: the volume of aqueous liquid needed to fully prime the blood compartment of a hollow fiber dialyzer. TCV includes fiber bundle volume (FBV) and dialyzer header volume; the terms TCV and FBV are often used interchangeably however. TCV assesses the number of unclotted, functional fibers in the dialyzer and is an indirect test of clearance and solute transfer capacity of a reprocessed dialyzer. Because it is easy to quantify, TCV is the most commonly used test of dialyzer function in reuse programs. To measure TCV, an air or nitrogen rinse of the blood compartment is performed using a squeezable bulb, and the amount of liquid displaced is measured. If possible, each dialyzer should have its TCV measured before its first use in order to have a baseline for comparison after each reprocessing sequence. A decrease in TCV of 20% corresponds to a loss of urea or creatinine clearance of about 4–11% (24–26). It is thought that relatively minor reductions in urea clearance of reprocessed dialyzers despite reduced TCV is possible as long as total dialyzer blood flow remains constant, because blood flow through remaining non-occluded fibers must increase (27, 28). Small molecular weight substance clearance has been shown to remain unchanged for up to 30 dialyzer reuses (29, 30). Clearances of larger molecular weight (middle molecules) such as vitamin B_{12} (24), and inulin (31), also correlate closely with TCV and are well preserved in multiply reused dialyzers.

If the TCV falls to less than 20% of its original value, the dialyzer is discarded. The blood compartment volume of a parallel plate dialyzer changes with transmembrane pressure and hence its TCV cannot be reliably measured.

Blood path integrity testing

Pressure-leak testing

A transmembrane pressure gradient is generated across the membrane and any fall in pressure on the blood or dialysate side with time (by plotting a pressure decay curve) is noted. It is essential to perform pressure testing if a cleaning step is included in dialyzer reprocessing. The pressure gradient may be produced by running pressurized air or nitrogen (at a pressure 20% above the maximal operating pressure) into the blood side of the dialyzer or by subjecting the dialysate compartment to a negative pressure of 250 mmHg over 30 seconds. A pressure change of < 0.83 mmHg/sec indicates preserved membrane integrity. For high flux membranes, a pressure change of < 1.25 mmHg/sec is allowed. The test detects weakness in dialyzer fibers as well as in dialyzer end caps, potting compound and O-rings.

Clearance studies

In vitro urea, sodium chloride and B_{12} clearances may be determined for reused dialyzers. These measurements afford a more accurate means of assessing dialyzer clearance than TCV. Protein and lipid components in blood, the level of the hematocrit, and incomplete red cell to serum equilibration of some substances during a single passage through the dialyzer blood compartment may reduce dialyzer clearance *in vivo*. *In vitro* clearances (which are measured using aqueous media) will therefore overestimate actual *in vivo* clearance. Clearance studies are not routinely performed on all dialyzers, but on a sampling basis, once monthly. A simple method of *in vitro* clearance measurement is described. A normal saline solution containing urea (100 mg/dl), and cyanocobalamin (1000 cpm/ml) is run through the blood compartment at 200 ml/min while dialysate is circulated through the dialysate compartment at 500 ml/min with a negative pressure of zero. The system is an open-loop one in which the solutions perfusing the dialyzer are discharged to drain after a single pass. Samples from the arterial and venous lines are collected simultaneously 30 minutes later and the dialyzer clearances calculated as:

$$\frac{(\text{Inflow concentration–Outflow concentration})}{\text{Inflow concentration}} \times \text{Blood flow}$$

A 10% loss of clearance in a reprocessed dialyzer is regarded as acceptable.

Severe reduction in the clearances of certain batches of cuprophane dialyzers subjected to automated reuse at one center (32) was associated with no significant fall in the TCV. The problem was recognized during routine 2 monthly urea kinetic studies, and was found to be due to a manufacturing defect in the dialyzer fibers which resulted in non-uniform flow (channeling) of the dialysate along one side of the dialyzer. Hence, the importance of doing periodic random checks of the clearances of reused dialyzers.

In vitro ultrafiltration coefficient (Kuf) or ultrafiltration rate (Qf)

These methods of assessing dialyzer function are more often used with automated devices. The *in vitro* ultrafiltration coefficient (or its inverse, hydraulic resistance) assesses the permeability of the dialyzer membrane to water and is also an indirect measure of large molecule clearance via solute drag. It may be measured by determining the number of milliliters of water per minute (Q_f) passing through the membrane at a given pressure and temperature. Changes in the K_{uf} reflect changes in membrane surface area (reflecting the number of occluded fibers) and membrane resistance (reflecting protein coating of the membrane). The *in vitro* K_{uf} falls much less rapidly than the TCV because thrombosed fibers may still have high *in vitro* hydraulic permeability. This method may therefore overestimate the *in vivo* clearance of reused dialyzers, and close attention must be paid to expected and actual weight losses in the patient. Both entities may be calculated using the formula: $Q_f = K_{uf} \times SA \times TMP$, where SA = membrane surface area and TMP = transmembrane pressure. Dialyzers are discarded when Q_f falls below < 75% of the initial value.

Disinfection and storage

Sterilization refers to destruction of all microorganisms (bacteria, fungi and viruses), as well as bacterial endospores, such that the chance of survival of a viable microorganism is less than 1 in 10^6. Reused dialyzers are not sterilized, but are treated with chemical germicides or heat to achieve high level disinfection, i.e.: inactivation of all microorganisms except bacterial spores. High level disinfection with adequate concentration and exposure time to disinfectant may also achieve sterility or may reduce the population of bacterial spores to safe levels. Inadequate disinfection may be due to use of an inappropriate disinfectant agent, an inadequate concentration of disinfectant, contamination of the water used to dilute the disinfectant, or to too short an exposure time to the disinfectant. Water used to prepare disinfectant solutions should have a bacterial colony count of < 200 per ml and/or a bacterial lipopolysaccharide concentration of < 1 ng/ml (14), as bacterial or endotoxin contamination of water used to dilute disinfectant solutions is one of the commoner means by which reuse-related sepsis and pyrogenic reactions may occur.

Disinfectants which have been used in dialyzer reprocessing include formaldehyde, glutaraldehyde-based formulations (Cidex, Sporicidin, Nephrex), peracetic acid solutions (Renalin®), and active chlorine compounds (Warexin, Amuchina, Ren-New-D). Only formaldehyde, glutaraldehyde and peracetic acid are currently used (Table 4). Formaldehyde use has declined by over 50% from 1983 to 1991 while peracetic acid use has increased 10 fold over the same time period (2). Compounds containing active chlorine have fallen out of use

Table 4. Chemical germicides for reprocessing hemodialyzers (1983–1991). From Ref (2)

Type and concentration	Percentage of centers				
	1983 n=579	1985 n=764	1987 n=948	1989 n=1172	1991 n=1453
Formaldehyde					
Total	94	80	62	47	42
<4.0%	57	43	42	58	66
≥ 4.0%	28	47	51	37	32
Unknown	15	10	7	5	2
Renalin®	5	17	34	46	50
Glutaraldehyde	< 1	3	43	7	9

Table 5. Minimum exposure times and temperatures with commonly used disinfectants

Disinfectant	Concentration	Temperature	Minimum storage time
Formaldehyde	4%	20°C	24 hours
Renalin®	1%	20°C	11 hours
Glutaraldehyde	0.75%	20°C	1 hour

because of damage to cellulosic and polysulfone dialyzer membranes resulting in blood leaks and outbreaks of pyrogenic reactions and septicemia (33). Sporicidin and Warexin are associated with a high incidence of microbiologic failure in cellulose acetate membranes (34).

Disinfectant is run into the blood and dialysate compartments of the dialyzer. At least 4 volumes of disinfectant are passed through the dialyzer in order to ensure that disinfectant is not diluted by water remaining in the dialyzer and that the concentration of disinfectant is at least 90% of the prescribed concentration. The blood ports of the dialyzer are disinfected and then capped with new or disinfected caps. Caps for dialysate ports of reused dialyzers constitute an insignificant source of possible bacterial contamination and may be washed with soap and water instead of being disinfected (2). Blood products on the outside of the dialyzer cartridge should be removed by wiping clean or immersing briefly in a dilute bleach solution. The dialyzer label is checked for intactness and the dialyzer stored in a container on a shelf reserved for that purpose. Recommended minimum storage times with the 3 commonly used disinfectants are shown in Table 5.

Formaldehyde

Diluting 1 part concentrated formaldehyde with 9 parts water produces 4% (V/V), or 3.7% (W/W) formaldehyde (or formalin). Four percent formaldehyde is now

Table 6. Disadvantages of formaldehyde

Occupational irritant
Association with contact dermatitis and asthma
Induction of anti-N antibodies
Defective red cell metabolism with ATP depletion and hemolysis
Difficult to totally remove from dialyzers
Rebound phenomenon
Reaction with sodium hypochlorite

---

used instead of the 2% solution because non-tuberculous mycobacteria (e.g., *M. chelonae, M. kansasai*) commonly found in tap water and reverse-osmosis processed water are not inactivated by the lower dilution and outbreaks of septicemias due to these organisms were reported in Louisiana (35) and California (36). Brilliant Blue (FDC dye #1) may be added to formaldehyde batch solution to serve as visual confirmation of its presence. One percent formaldehyde has similar efficacy to the 4% solution when dialyzers are incubated at 40°C for 24 hours (37). Formaldehyde levels in reused dialyzers being prepared for their next use should be < 5 parts per million (ppm) (5 mg/l) after rinsing.

Disadvantages of formaldehyde (Table 6)

At air levels above 0.13 ppm, formaldehyde is an occupational irritant, and the threshold limit for acute exposure (short term exposure limit) is 3 ppm. Long term levels of formaldehyde levels in air should be < 0.75 ppm as a time weighted average (38). Prolonged exposure to formaldehyde has been associated with asthma (39) and contact dermatitis. Inhalation exposure of 15 ppm formaldehyde, 6 hours per day, 5 days per week, for 16 months, has produced nasopharyngeal carcinomas in rats (40), but carcinogenicity of formaldehyde has not been documented in humans.

Formaldehyde reacts with amino groups of proteins adherent to the blood compartment membrane surface of reused dialyzers, as well as to the polyurethane potting compound in dialyzer headers (41), and therefore does not rinse easily from dialyzers (particularly those with cellulosic membranes). Since complete removal of formaldehyde from reused dialyzers is not possible even when dialysis rather than saline rinsing is used (29, 42), concern has arisen about cumulative intravenous exposure to formaldehyde. Formaldehyde concentration in serum as a product of normal body metabolism is reported to be 2.6 ± 0.14 mg/l (43). It is metabolized to carbon dioxide and water or excreted by the lungs. Serum formaldehyde level is calculated to increase by only 0.3 mg/l after use of a reprocessed dialyzer in which the concentration of formaldehyde was 3–5 mg/l (3–5 ppm) (15). Hence, with dialyzer concentrations of formaldehyde of < 5 ppm, lev-els of residual formaldehyde in reused dialyzers are low. In addition, long term oral methenamine for the treatment of urinary tract infections releases more formaldehyde to the patient than does a reprocessed dialyzer and has not been associated with toxicity; and chronic toxicity from small, repeated intravenous infusions of formaldehyde has not been reported in human or animal studies. Dogs given intravenous formaldehyde (200 mg per kg body weight) daily for 21 days developed no gross toxicity (44).

Chronic intravenous exposure to small residual amounts of formaldehyde in reused dialyzers has, thus far, been proven to result in only one form of toxicity: the induction of anti-N antibodies. These are antibodies to the N antigen of the red cell surface MN antigen system. Red cell N antigens are altered by formaldehyde in a dose-dependent manner. The altered red cell N antigen induces formation of a cold agglutinin which is associated with early renal allograft rejection (45), shortening of red cell life span and difficulty in crossmatching blood. Induction of anti-N antibodies does not occur below a residual formaldehyde level of 10 ppm (1 μg/ml or 10 mg/l) (46). Formaldehyde may also contribute to hemolysis by causing red cell ATP depletion and defective red cell metabolism (47).

Formaldehyde levels in rinsed dialyzers which have been allowed to stand may rebound: increase by as much as 6 mg/l as formaldehyde diffuses from the potting compound of the dialyzer into the contained fluid. Formaldehyde and sodium hypochlorite react to form noxious fumes with resultant degradation of both compounds. Bleach should therefore be rinsed from the dialyzer before starting formaldehyde disinfection. Despite these problems, formaldehyde remains the most commonly used disinfectant because it is cheap and efficacious.

Peracetic acid

Renalin® is the most commonly used peracetic acid derivative for dialyzer reprocessing. Composed of a mixture of 2% peracetic acid, acetic acid and hydrogen peroxide, Renalin® may be used both as a disinfectant and as a cleaning agent. The agent has a less offensive smell than formaldehyde and poses little hazard to skin and eyes. Clotted dialyzer fibers are decolorized after use of Renalin® (hydrogen peroxide reacts with heme residues), an effect that is aesthetically more pleasing to patients, but which may not necessarily indicate removal of blood protein residues. Peracetic acid is reported to be as effective a disinfectant as formaldehyde (48), but may be associated with greater reductions in dialyzer K_{uf}, (both *in vivo* and *in vitro*) when compared to formaldehyde reprocessing (49, 50). After 5 reuses, automated reprocessing of cuprophane dialyzers with peracetic acid resulted in greater reductions in K_{uf} of dialyzers when compared to automated reprocessing with 3.7% formaldehyde including a cleaning step with 3% hydrogen peroxide (21.4% vs 5%) (49). Direct comparisons of clearance studies in peracetic acid-processed dialyzers and formaldehyde-processed dialyzers were not made in this study. Renalin® is unstable at dilutions of 1 in 4.7 and fresh solutions need to be prepared weekly. It is degraded to hydrogen peroxide and may cause pressure buildup in stored dialyzers. Peracetic acid reacts with bleach to form hydrochloric acid vapor, hence the two agents should never be mixed. Environmental exposure limits for peracetic acid have not been developed, for acetic acid is 10 ppm and for hydrogen peroxide is 1 ppm time weighted average (38).

Glutaraldehyde

Glutaraldehyde (0.8%) is as effective as 4% formaldehyde in its anti-microbial effect, but less glutaraldehyde is found in environmental air and less remains in the dialyzer after pre-dialysis rinsing (51). Glutaraldehyde however, leads to lower reuse rates than formaldehyde, and a cleaning phase with dilute sodium hypochlorite is recommended in order to increase the reuse rate. The OSHA environmental exposure limit for glutaraldehyde is 0.2 ppm.

Preparing for the next dialysis

Label verification

As a safety imperative, the dialyzer label must be checked by at least 2 staff members and if possible the patient, ensuring that the patient receives his own dialyzer.

Verification of presence of disinfectant

The light blue color of formaldehyde previously colored with Brilliant Blue verifies presence of formaldehyde, alternatively, Clinitest (Miles Labs, Elkhart, Indiana, USA) tablet testing of the liquid in the dialyzer will confirm the presence of concentrated formaldehyde. A colorimetric Renalin® indicator strip marketed by Renal Systems turns dark blue on exposure to concentrated Renalin®. At least one dialyzer per patient shift should be sampled and subjected to a test for presence of concentrated disinfectant.

Priming and rinsing

Disinfectant is drained from the dialyzer, dialysate lines are attached and dialysate flow begun at 500 ml/min at 37°C, while the blood compartment remains closed. A saline line is attached to an arterial line which is primed to remove air and then attached to the arterial port of the dialyzer blood compartment which is then flushed with 500 cc of normal saline. Next, a venous line is attached to the venous port of the dialyzer and primed with saline. Arterial and venous lines are joined together and saline is recirculated through the blood compartment for 15 minutes with slow normal saline infusion (1–2 l in total) and 500 mmHg negative pressure, as heated dialysate fluid continues to flow in the dialysate chamber. The dialyzer

is rotated at intervals during the flushing to release any air trapped within the dialyzer, which can retard removal of the disinfectant. An automated dialyzer rinsing device, the Seratronics DPS 4 is available from Fresenius (Walnut Creek, California).

Testing for residual disinfectant

Formaldehyde

Residual formaldehyde level in the dialyzer must be below 5 ppm (5 mg/l). Clinitest (Miles Labs, Elkhart, Indiana, USA) detects concentrations of formaldehyde above 25 mg/l, and is therefore not sensitive to low concentrations of formaldehyde. Schiff's test is a semi-quantitative visual colorimetric test that develops a purple color in the presence of equal parts of reagent and formaldehyde. A test is positive in 10 minutes at concentrations of formaldehyde > 5–10 ppm. A commercially available modified Schiff's reagent Formasure (Di-Chem, Minneapolis, Minnesota) can detect concentrations of formaldehyde as low as 3 ppm. The Hantzsch reaction is a highly sensitive assay for detecting as little as 1 μg/ml of formaldehyde. This test, however, is complicated and time consuming and therefore not suitable for routine use.

Peracetic acid

Residual levels of peracetic acid should be < 1 ppm (1 mg/l). Renal Systems (Minneapolis, Minnesota) manufactures a separate colorimetric test strip to detect residual Renalin®.

Glutaraldehyde

Residual glutaraldehyde may be tested for with a kit from Surgikos utilizing 2,4 dinitrophenol. The dialyzer solution turns turbid after 1 minute at concentrations of glutaraldehyde > 1–3 ppm.

HEAT STERILIZATION

Subjection of dialyzers to temperatures of 105°C for 20 hours effects sterilization of polysulfone dialyzers (52). Other dialyzer membranes have not been reported to be heat resistant. Advantages of heat sterilization include absence of chemical residues after sterilization and lack of staff exposure to chemicals. Pyrogenic reactions and sepsis were not reported in 180 patients receiving 9000 hemodialysis treatments using heat sterilized dialyzers reprocessed a mean of 7.4 times and limited to a maximum of 11 uses (52). *In vitro* and *in vivo* clearance studies revealed no significant decline in sodium chloride clearance after 7–8 uses. Dialyzer ultrafiltration coefficient increased from 22 ± 1 ml/min/mmHg to 158 ± 69 after 7–8 uses. This increase in ultrafiltration coefficient may be due to associated use of sodium hypochlorite for dialyzer cleaning. Addition of 1.5% citric acid to the processed water used to fill dialyzers undergoing heat sterilization

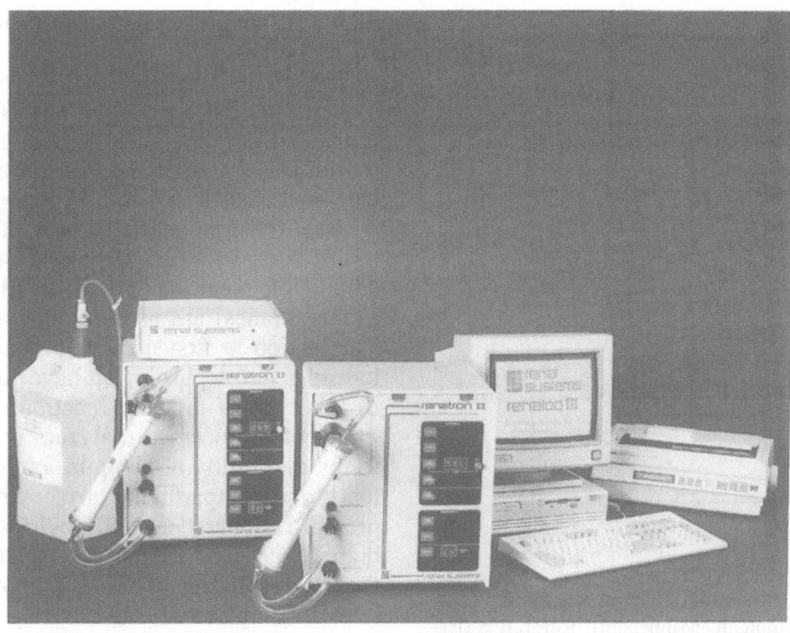

Figure 4. The Renatron single station dialyzer reprocessor (courtesy of Renal Systems, Minntech, Minnesota).

allows use of lower temperatures and lessens the risk of dialyzer damage, and is currently being evaluated. Heat sterilization is not in widespread use at present.

AUTOMATED DIALYZER REPROCESSING

Automated reprocessing devices may be single station (processing single dialyzers at a time) or multistation (processing multiple dialyzers simultaneously). Automation increases the reliability and reproducibility of the reuse process and can include features of label printing, record keeping, computerized analysis of records and results, and may reduce labor costs. A similar sequence of processing steps is employed in an automated device as with manual reprocessing. Reverse ultrafiltration, a cleaning step and a pressure leak test are always included however, and performance tests may include measuring K_{uf}, as well as TCV.

Three automated reprocessing machines are currently on market and some features of these devices are shown in Table 7 (53). A photograph and schematized drawing of a commonly used single station device, the Renatron RS-8300 (Renal Systems, Minneapolis, Minnesota, USA) are shown in Figures 4 and 5. A standard dialyzer reprocessing cycle in the Renatron includes mechanical cleaning of obstructed fibers by reverse ultrafiltration, high velocity flushing, and chemical cleaning with Renalin®. TCV and

pressure testing is performed by the machine and blood and dialysate compartments of the dialyzer filled with Renalin®. The ECHO dialyzer reprocessor (Mesa Laboratories Inc, Wheat Ridge, Colorado) is the other available single station device and employs a similar reprocessing sequence. One model of the ECHO is designed for use with peracetic acid and another for use with formaldehyde or glutaraldehyde. The Seratronics DSR 4 (Figure 6) is a multistation dialyzer reprocesser manufactured by Fresenius (Walnut Creek, California, USA). It utilizes a bidirectional rinse of the blood compartment with water heated to 40–44°C at flow rates varying between 420 ml/min to 2 l/min. A cleaning agent (usually 0.5–1% bleach) is then introduced into the blood and dialysate sides of the dialyzer and a vacuum induced on the blood side such that reverse ultrafiltration with dislodgement of membrane-coating particles on the blood side is achieved. Dialyzer K_{uf} is then measured as 400 mmHg pressure is applied on the blood side. TCV is measured by evacuating the contents of the blood side into a volume chamber using an air pump. A pressure decay curve is obtained by applying 575–675 mmHg pressure to the blood side and then opening the dialysate side to air: a pressure fall of < 60 mmHg in 60 secs is acceptable. If these 3 tests are passed, the dialyzer is filled with the disinfectant of choice and labels printed.

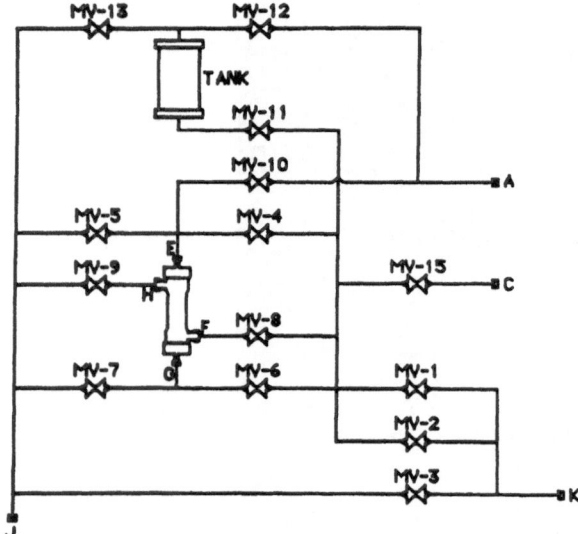

Figure 5. Renatron hydraulic tank/manifold schematic (courtesy of Renal Systems, Minntech, Minnesota). Reference designations: A: Vent header line; C: 21% Renalin line; E: Arterial header line; F: Dialysate inlet line; G: Venous header line; H: Dialysate outlet line; J: Drain header line and jet pump; K: Water inlet port; MV-1 to MV-15: Solenoid operated valves.

Table 7. Features of some automated dialyzer reprocessing devices (adapted from Ref (53))

Device Features	Mesa Center ECHO	Renatron	Seratronics DSR 4
Stations	1	1	4
Water pressure	40 psi	20 psi	25–80 psi
Flow rate (l/min)	1.5	1.75	1.8
Cleaning agent	Variable	Renalin®	NaOCl
Tests			
Pressure leak	+	+	+
TCV	+(Visual)	+	+
K_{uf}	–	–	+
Sterilant	HCHO	Renalin®	HCHO[a]
Cycle time (mins)	8–90	7.5	28/4 dialyzers
Data analysis	–	–	+

NaOCl = sodium hypochlorite, HCHO= formaldehyde.
[a] or glutaraldehyde

ADVANTAGES OF DIALYZER REUSE (TABLE 8)

Improved biocompatibility and reduction in first use reactions

Type A first use reactions due mainly to an anaphylactic reaction to ethylene oxide gas used to sterilize some dialyzers, are greatly reduced when reprocessed dialyzers are employed.

The milder type B first use reactions are manifested by chest and back pain, cramps, fever, nausea and vomiting; and are thought to be associated, at least in part, to complement activation by protruding hydroxyl radicles on unsubstituted cellulosic membranes (e.g., cuprophane). These reactions are also reduced in patients using reprocessed cellulosic dialyzers (54–57). When more biocompatible membranes (e.g., cellulose acetate or synthetic membranes) are used for dialysis, there may not be a reduction in first use symptoms with reuse (55, 58), indeed, some nephrologists have questioned the existence of this type of first use reaction. Improved biocompatibility of reprocessed dialyzers is thought to be related to the deposition of albumin, complement and fibrin on the blood compartment surfaces of the dialyzer. These protein residues coat hydroxyl ions of cellulosic membranes (59), and effectively isolate the membrane surface from subsequent blood-membrane interactions. This retards complement activation by hydroxyl moieties on reprocessed cellulosic membranes, and reduces sequelae of leukopenia due to pulmonary sequestration of leukocytes (60, 61), with resultant hypoxemia and reduction in peak expiratory flow rate (62). Activation of the kinin system, thromboxane production, histamine release and the production of various cytokines (63) may also contribute to the manifestations of dialyzer bioincompatibility.

A recent report links the use of angiotensin converting enzyme inhibitors to the development of anaphylactoid reactions in patients at a center practicing automated reuse of polysulfone, cellulose acetate and cuprophane dialyzers (64). The incidence of anaphylactoid reactions was slightly but not significantly higher with polysulfone dialyzers. Negatively charged residues on the synthetic dialyzer membrane may activate Factor 12 and lead to bradykinin generation which is potentiated in patients on ACE inhibition, as degradation of bradykinin is dependent on ACE.

Reprocessing does not decrease the ability of highly permeable membranes to adsorb or filter β_2 microglobulin (65): reuse of polysulfone dialyzers up to 24 times results in decreased pre-dialysis levels of β_2 microglobulin and increases the removal of β_2 microglobulin compared to first use values (66). Dialyzer reuse should therefore not increase the risk of dialysis-associated amyloidosis.

Decreased treatment cost

In 1980, the national savings from the practice of dialyzer reuse was estimated at $150 million (67). With 5 manual reuses, a conservative estimate of savings has been set at $3250/year per patient (68). Because it is less labor intensive, automated reuse results in further savings despite the cost of leasing or buying an automated device. Such savings have contributed to the widespread adoption of dialyzer reuse primarily by non-hospital based, for-profit

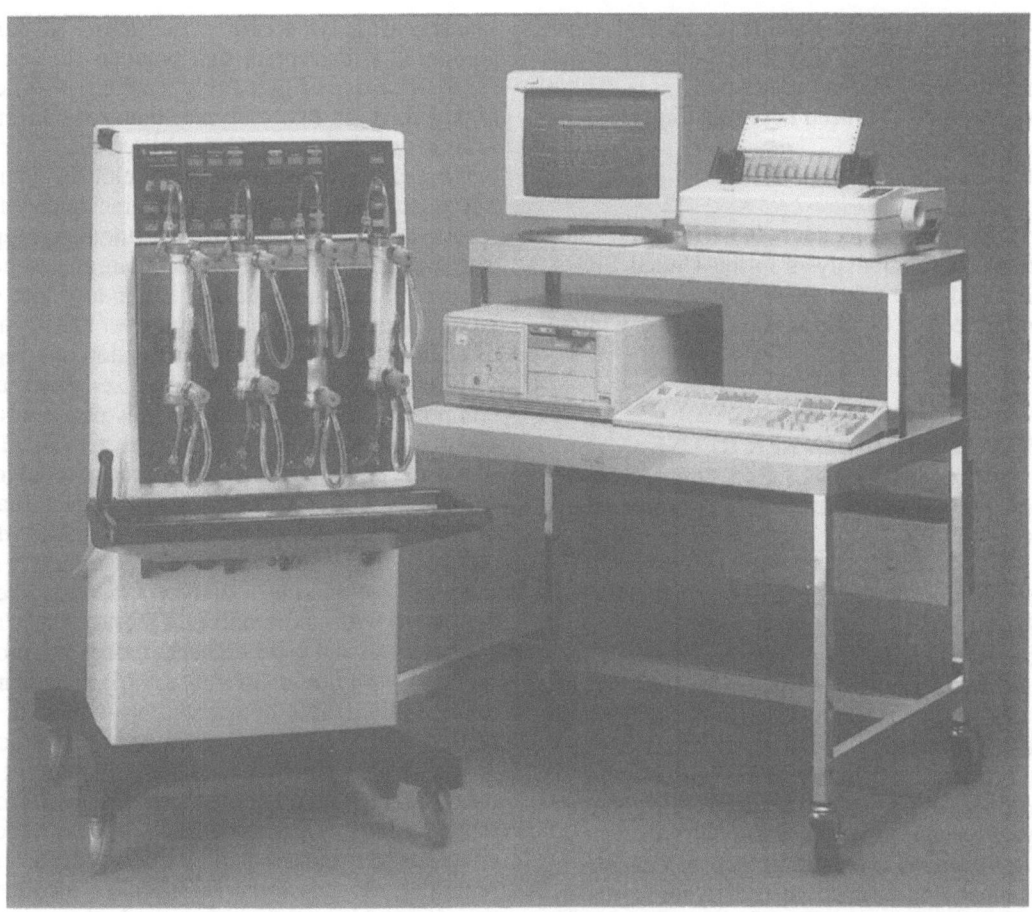

Figure 6. The Seratronics DRS4 multistation dialyzer reprocessor (courtesy of Fresenius, Walnut Creek, California).

Table 8. Advantages and disadvantages of dialyzer reuse

Advantages	Disadvantages
Reduction of first use reactions	Environmental and possible intravenous exposure to disinfectants
Improved biocompatibility	Anti-N antibodies with formaldehyde
Decreased treatment cost	Risk of pyrogenic reactions and septicemia
Allows use of more expensive (high flux) dialyzers	Decreased dialyzer efficacy with time
Reduced exposure to plasticizers and LAL-reactive material in new dialyzers	?Increased mortality with certain disinfectants

dialysis centers, and has raised ethical concerns regarding the goal of financial gain by private dialysis centers versus the best possible treatment for the patient. In some centers however, use of more expensive high flux dialyzers would not be possible if dialyzer reprocessing were not employed. In developing countries, savings related to reuse of dialyzers may facilitate wider availability of scarce dialysis treatments.

Reduced exposure to plasticizers and Limulus Amebocyte Lysate (LAL)-reactive material in new dialyzers

New dialyzers may contain particulate fibers of up to 1 mm length, plasticizers leached from PVC used in the manufacture of the dialyzer casing, as well as LAL-reactive material (69, 70). No adverse clinical reactions have been attributed to intravascular delivery of particulates in dialysis patients, but plasticizers have been associated with cutaneous necrotizing vasculitis and hepatitis (69). Contained LAL-reactive material may contribute to dialysis associated neutropenia (71), but is not pyrogenic. These contaminants are greatly reduced in reused dialyzers.

Reduced environmental bioburden

Dialyzer cartridges are non-biodegradable, and with some 170,000 patients on hemodialysis in the United States, each receiving 3 dialyses per week, almost 27 million dialyzers would need to be disposed of per year without reuse.

DISADVANTAGES OF DIALYZER REUSE

Environmental and possible intravenous exposure to disinfectants

Atmospheric exposure limits for disinfectants are regulated by OSHA (38); exposure may result in effects as described above. Inadvertent high dose intravenous exposure to formaldehyde results in burning at the site of access cannulation (72), dyspnea and hypotension, and hemolysis. Should acute formaldehyde intoxication be suspected in a patient undergoing hemodialysis, the blood pump should immediately be stopped, the venous line clamped, and the dialyzer contents tested for formaldehyde. Chronic low dose intravenous exposure to formaldehyde is of no known clinical significance when dialyzer levels are kept < 5 ppm. Close adherence to institutional reuse policies and procedures, and periodic quality control checks will prevent serious exposure of staff and patients to the disinfectants in use.

Anti-N antibodies

The association of formaldehyde use for dialyzer disinfection and the development of anti-N antibodies is discussed above.

Risk of pyrogenic reactions and septicemia

A pyrogenic reaction on dialysis is defined as a temperature elevation $\geq$ 37.8°C in an initially afebrile patient, whether asymptomatic or associated with symptoms of chills, rigors, myalgia, nausea, vomiting or hypotension; and unassociated with bacteremia. Contamination of the dialyzer with endotoxin is the key pathogenic mechanism for pyrogenic reactions in dialyzer reuse programs. Endotoxins may remain in processed water after the bacteria which produced them have been killed by disinfection. Intravascular exposure to 1 ng/kg body weight of endotoxin will produce a pyrogenic reaction, and the reaction may occur up to 90 minutes after exposure to pyrogen. Pyrogenic reactions occurring in clusters are more frequently reported in centers that reprocess dialyzers (par-

ticularly if dialyzers are reused above 40 times), when compared with centers that practice single use dialysis (2, 8). The risk of pyrogenic reactions with reuse is also higher for high flux dialyzers than for conventional cellulosic membranes, and for bicarbonate versus acetate dialysis (2, 8). If performed meticulously, manual reuse is not associated with an increased incidence of pyrogenic reactions when compared with automated reprocessing. The most common source of contamination has been the use of endotoxin-containing water to dilute concentrated disinfectant solution, or improper mixing and dilution of disinfectant. During storage, endotoxin migrates from disinfectant and adsorbs to dialyzer fibers and potting compound. Adsorbed endotoxin is not removed by predialysis aqueous rinsing of the dialyzer (70). The passage of plasma or whole blood is required to remove endotoxin from dialyzer fibers (73). At some centers, dialysis water or dialysate is passed through polysulfone dialyzers to reduce bacterial and endotoxin contamination (74). Water used to rinse and clean dialyzers may also become contaminated with endotoxin in a storage tank, and though the LAL test indicates endotoxin does not cross conventional or high flux membranes (75), fragments of endotoxins still capable of stimulating monocyte production of IL-1 and TNF can cross dialyzer membranes (74). If AAMI-quality water (i.e., water containing < 1 ng/ml or 5 endotoxin units/ml of endotoxin) is used throughout the reprocessing process, the risk of pyrogenic reactions related to dialyzer reuse is significantly reduced, and concerns regarding the possibility of pyrogen-mediated stimulation of cytokine production contributing to cachexia and hypoalbuminemia in chronic hemodialysis patients (7), are lessened.

While septicemia is reported in similar frequency in centers practicing single use and multiple use of dialyzers, sporadic, localized outbreaks of bacteremia may occur in centers reprocessing dialyzers. Gram negative bacteria (including Pseudomonas, Acinetobacter, Serratia, Alcaligenes, Flavobacterium, Xanthomonas and Moraxella) grow rapidly to levels of 10^3–10^6/ml in water prepared by reverse osmosis, deionization and carbon filtration. Adequate disinfection of water treatment systems and the water and dialysate delivery systems is therefore important. Proper dilution of disinfectant solution is also crucial: an outbreak of Pseudomonas septicemia in a Belgian center practicing automated reuse was traced to inadequate mixing of sterilant with tap water in the automated device (76). Though small amounts of microorganisms may survive in the removable header caps and O-rings of high flux dialyzers following reprocessing with 4% formalin or 4% Renalin®, contamination of the blood compartment is insignificant (77).

Highly resistant strains of non-tuberculous mycobacteria may also survive and grow in processed water, and are commonly found in domestic water supplies. These mycobacteria have been associated with outbreaks of septicemia and death in some reuse centers (35, 36). They are inactivated by 4% but not 2% formaldehyde.

Decreased dialyzer efficacy

If adequate performance testing is not routine, mass transfer characteristics of the dialyzer membrane as well as its ultrafiltration capacity may decrease with time and go undetected. The ultrafiltration capacity of some reprocessed dialyzers may increase with each reuse, particularly if a cleaning step is used, but UFR more usually undergoes reduction with continuing reprocessing. Changes in the ultrafiltration rate (UFR) of reused dialyzers are not well predicted by changes in TCV. Fluid removal must therefore be closely monitored when pressure controlled dialysis machines are used with reprocessed dialyzers. Volumetric dialysis machines which directly adjust ultrafiltrate volume obviate the need to follow changes in the UFR of reused dialyzers closely.

Many studies indicate good correlation between TCV of reused dialyzers and their clearance, and have documented preserved dialyzer clearance for large and small molecules after multiple reuses (25–31). Some studies in the early 1970s reported significant decreases in dialyzer clearance with reuse (78, 79), but dialyzer reprocessing at that time was not as effective as it is now. Dialyzers with extensive visible clotting today are not reused beyond a third reprocessing, if at all. Other studies have documented declining dialyzer clearances for small molecules of between 4–6% and for middle molecules of some 8% (49). Reduction in mean KT/v from 1.10 to 1.05 in dialyzers reprocessed 4 times and 14 times respectively has been reported in a study of 325 patients from 23 centers practicing formaldehyde reuse (80). Reduction in dialyzer clearance with reuse is therefore clearly possible, and no doubt common to lesser or greater degrees depending on the amount of dialyzer fiber clotting and efficacy of the reprocessing technique. It is therefore imperative to monitor clearances of reused dialyzers. TCV, though easy to perform and quite reliable in reflecting falls in dialyzer clearance, is an indirect measure of clearance, and not totally fail-safe (32). Periodic *in vitro* or *in vivo* clearance studies on reused dialyzers must be done. Clinical assessment of patients as well as urea kinetic modelling should also be integral parts of a reuse program.

Possible increase in mortality associated with dialyzer reuse

The possible role of multiple dialyzer reuse in chronic underdialysis and high mortality on dialysis in the United States requires investigation. Previous studies indicate equivalent or better survival in hemodialysis patients using reprocessed dialyzers. For example, the European Dialysis and Transplant Association, in 1978 (81), reported similar 1 year mortality in patients reusing dialyzers (93.2%) and those practicing single use dialysis (91.2%). Similarly, over 6–12 year periods, 259 patients in Cincinnati and 1059 Detroit patients who used reprocessed dialyzers had unadjusted case fatality rates of 70% and 96% respectively when compared to the regional renal disease networks in Ohio and Michigan (82). A study of the Medicare-funded ESRD population reported in 1987 (83) found the relative risk of death in a 5 year cohort of hemodialysis patients in reuse programs to be 0.88 compared to 1.00 in patients whose dialysis centers never practiced reuse.

In October 1992, the results of a USRDS case-mix study were made public by the FDA (5, 84). This study retrospectively examined mortality rates in 3163 ESRD patients treated with high-flux or conventional hemodialysis in 291 free-standing and hospital-based hemodialysis units who had started dialysis during 1986 and 1987. Patients were followed for 2 years, stratified for age, race, gender and disease and results were adjusted for patient comorbidity. A 33% increased mortality risk was found in patients undergoing manual reuse with peracetic acid; there was no increase in mortality risk in patients using dialyzers reprocessed automatedly with peracetic acid; or with dialyzers reprocessed with glutaraldehyde or formaldehyde. A second study from the USRDS funded by HCFA (85) combined Medicare patient demographic and survival data with dialyzer reuse data from the CDC's annual survey of dialysis-related diseases. Records of some 54,000 patients on hemodialysis in 674 free-standing units undergoing conventional dialysis were analyzed. Because of the large sample size, results were not adjusted for comorbidity. A 17% higher mortality was seen in patients treated in units which reused dialyzers with glutaraldehyde, compared to patients in units which did not practice dialyzer reuse ($p = 0.01$). An increased mortality risk of 13% was also seen in patients treated with peracetic acid-reprocessed dialyzers ($p < 0.001$). There was no significant increase in mortality risk in patients treated with formaldehyde-processed dialyzers. These studies have been the subject of great controversy and litigation (86). A direct cause and effect relationship between increased mortality and the use of particular disinfectant agents remains to be established. Long-term, controlled, prospective studies of morbidity and mortality in patients in hospital-based and free-standing units, on conventional and high flux dialysis, using dialyzers reprocessed with various disinfectants are needed, and such studies, under the aegis of the NIH are currently in progress.

QUALITY CONTROL AND QUALITY ASSURANCE IN REUSE PROGRAMS

Meticulous performance, scrupulous monitoring, recording, and periodic review and testing of all aspects of dialyzer reuse are essential to minimize adverse clinical events, to track breaks in procedure which may have resulted in an adverse event, and to protect staff and patients from hazardous environmental exposure to materials employed in reuse. Use of an automated device does not lessen or eliminate the need for strict quality control. In addition to the AAMI guidelines, the 1991 Food and Drug Administration publication on Quality Assurance Guidelines for Hemodialysis Devices (87), provides guidelines which may be individualized by dialysis facilities. Both institution and practitioner bear responsibility for safety and effectiveness of reused dialyzers, as manufacturer labels guarantee sterility and function of dialyzers for single use only. Components of good quality control in dialyzer reuse programs include:

Master file. A file containing reuse policies, specifications, materials, methods, requirements of water quality, pressure, flow rate, and temperature, as well as samples of forms and labels should be maintained with ready access to all members of the hemodialysis team.

Quality assurance log. Documented, periodic audits of the reuse program including equipment, technique, results of microbiologic testing must be performed regularly by personnel not directly involved in reprocessing dialyzers.

Reuse log. This is a record of each reused dialyzer from its entry into a facility to its disposal. The date of each reprocessing, name of the person performing the procedure and results of performance tests, residual disinfectant levels, and reasons for ultimately discarding the dialyzer must be recorded.

Water chemical analysis. A complete analysis of inorganic and organic chemicals in dialysis water should be done at least once yearly. Levels should comply with AAMI recommendations (14).

Water quality record. All water used in reprocessing should meet AAMI recommendations (14). Water used to prepare disinfectant should not contain waterborne particles larger than 5 μ. Water used to prepare disinfectant and to rinse and clean dialyzers should be cultured for bacteria and tested for endotoxin weekly, or at least monthly. Samples collected should include water from the hose or pipe used to dilute disinfectant, from the hose used to rinse dialyzers manually or at the entrance to an automated reuse machine; at various points along the water treatment system; at the entrance to a central water proportioning system; at the entrance and exit of water to the dialysis machine; and as close to the point where dialysate is formulated from dialysis water and concentrate. Samples should be sent to the microbiology lab within 30 minutes or stored at 5°C and assayed within 24 hours. 0.1–0.5 cc of a water sample should be placed directly on tryptic soy agar, spread evenly and incubated at 35–37°C for 2 days, and bacterial colonies counted with a magnifying glass. A calibrated loop should not be used to deliver dialysis water samples onto culture media as it delivers only 1 μl of liquid and hence has a sensitivity of only 1000 CFU/ml, far greater than the AAMI recommended maximum level of 200 CFU/ml. Dialysis water micro-

biologic results which consistently record 0 CFU/ml are probably not being properly cultured. Results of bacterial cultures should be charted so that trend analyses can be easily made.

Dialyzer bacterial studies. After disinfection, many centers do random bacterial culture of the contents of the dialyzer blood compartment in order to document efficacy of the disinfection process. Culture of 3–5% of reused dialyzers may be done weekly.

Environmental testing. Vapors from chemicals used in reuse should be kept below the environmental exposure limits of the Occupational Safety and Health Administration (38). Atmospheric testing for levels of appropriate chemicals should be done once monthly in the reuse area and clinical dialysis area.

Personnel health monitoring. Results of medical examinations of workers to monitor exposure to potentially toxic substances should be periodically obtained and documented.

Complaint log and incident report log. All complaints by patients or staff about failure or possible adverse reactions related to reused dialyzers should be documented, as should be results of relevant investigations into the complaint and any corrective action.

Individual patient monitoring. The importance of monitoring patients' clinical and laboratory profiles while in a program practicing dialyzer reuse cannot be overstressed. Weight removal, heparinization and frequency of dialyzer clotting, occurrence of adverse symptoms, and following parameters reflecting adequacy of dialysis such as the urea reduction ratio, formal urea kinetic modelling and serum albumin should result in detailed review of the reuse system (as well as other relevant parameters such as dialyzer type, presence of access recirculation and the presence of intercurrent illness) if abnormalities are detected.

Equipment maintenance and incoming materials log. Preventive maintenance checks on all equipment or machines used in reprocessing, and a record of the incoming date of all new supplies should be kept. Disinfection of the water system, including booster pumps and water storage tanks should be done periodically and the level of residual germicide used reduced to safe levels.

Training record. Successful completion of the facilities training course by each staff member in a reuse program should be documented. Use of protective eyewear and clothing, and the handling of chemical spills are stressed.

Informed consent. Federal law requires that patients be fully informed of the reuse process but does not require signed informed consent. Many dialysis centers however utilize a consent form detailing the possible benefits and complications of dialyzer reuse and may also include a disclaimer. The rights of the patient to refuse or withdraw from a program of dialyzer reuse are explained, and patients should not feel coerced into participating in a program of dialyzer reuse. Legal responsibility regarding liability for morbidity or mortality of patients in reuse programs rests with the institution or practitioner unless a disclaimer has been signed.

CONCLUSIONS

Reuse of hollow fiber dialyzers is common in American hemodialysis centers. Financial considerations have been a major contributor to the widespread acceptance of dialyzer reuse. While single use of preprocessed, biocompatible, high flux membranes is ideal, in order to help contain the rapidly expanding cost of ESRD treatment in the USA, it is likely that reuse of hemodialyzers will remain a feature of American hemodialysis. If properly reprocessed, reused dialyzer can provide safe and efficacious dialysis. Compliance with good technique, quality control and quality assurance measures vary widely between facilities. Some aspects of the reuse process require standardization (e.g., testing of the mass transfer characteristics of reused dialyzers, manual rinse protocols); and the possible contribution of reuse to increased mortality and underdialysis in the chronic hemodialysis population requires large scale, randomized, prospective investigation. Only then will the medical and ethical controversies surrounding the widespread practice of dialyzer reuse be settled. Meanwhile, strict adherence to reuse techniques of proven efficacy, and to quality control and assurance programs can continue to provide safe and effective dialysis for many hemodialysis patients.

REFERENCES

1. Shaldon S, Silva H, Rosen M: Technique of refrigerated coil preservation hemodialysis with femoral vein catheterization. *Br Med J* 2: 411, 1964
2. Tokars JI, Alter MJ, Favero MS, Moyer LS, Moyer LA, Bland LA: National surveillance of dialysis-associated diseases in the United States, 1991. *Am Soc Artif Int Org J* 39: 966, 1993
3. Lore G: Industry leaders respond to FDA proposed guidelines on dialyzer reuse labelling. *Contemp Dial Nephrol* 15: 14, 1994
4. Shaldon S: Unanswered questions pertaining to dialysis adequacy in 1992. *Kidney Int* 43 (Suppl 41): 274, 1993
5. US Department of Health and Human Services: *Food and Drug Administration.* Talk paper T92-46. October 13, 1992
6. Held PJ, Levin NW, Bovbjerg RR, Pauly MV, Diamond LH: Mortality and duration of hemodialysis treatment. *J Am Med Ass* 265: 871, 1991
7. Shaldon S: Dialyzer reuse: a practice that should be abandoned. *Sem Dial* 6: 11, 1993
8. Alter MJ, Favero MS, Moyer LS, Bland LA: National surveillance of dialysis-associated diseases in the United States, 1989. *Trans Am Soc Artif Int Organs* 37: 97, 1991
9. Thirteenth report of the Australia and New Zealand Dialysis and Transplant Registry (ANZDATA): *Reuse of Hemodialyzers,* 1990, p 111
10. Fassbinder W, Brunner FP, Brynger H, Ehrich JHH et al.: Combined report on regular dialysis and transplantation in Europe, XX, 1989. *Nephrol Dial Transplant* 6 (Suppl 1): 5, 1991
11. Challah S, Wing AJ, Brunner FP, Brynger HOA, Oules R, Selwood NH: Use and reuse of dialyzers in Europe. in *Guide to Reprocessing of Hemodialyzers,* edited by Deane W, Wineman RJ, Bemis JA, Massachusetts, Martinus Nijhoff, 1986, p 99
12. Favero MS, Deane N, Leger RT, Sosin AE: Effect of multiple use of dialyzers on hepatitis B incidence in patients and staff. *J Am Med Ass* 245: 166, 1981
13. Association for the Advancement of Medical Instrumentation: *Recommended Practice for Reuse of Hemodialyzers,* Arlington, VA, 1986
14. AAMI: *Recommended Practice for Reuse of Hemodialyzers,* Arlington, VA, Association for the Advancement of Medical Instrumentation, 1993
15. NKF revised standards for reuse of hemodialyzers: *Am J Kid Dis* 3:466, 1984
16. Deane M, Bemis JA: *Multiple Use of Hemodialyzers,* New York, Manhattan Kidney Center, National Nephrology Foundation, 1982, p 64
17. Veys N, Vanholder R, DeCuyper K, Ringoir S: Influence of erythropoietin on dialyzer reuse, heparin need and urea kinetics in maintenance hemodialysis patients. *Am J Kid Dis* 23: 52, 1994
18. Billiouw JM, Vanholder R, Piron M, Veirman R, Ringoir S: Automated reuse of capillary hemodialyzers. *Int J Artif Organs* 8: 83, 1985
19. Deane M, Beamis J: *Multiple Use of Hemodialyzers.* Final report to the National Institutes of Arthritis, Diabetes and Digestive and Kidney Disease. Contract NO1-AM-9-2214, 1981, p 53
20. Stein G, Lines W, Volksch G et al.: Changes of the capillary surface in reused dialyzers – electron microscopic investigations. *Int J Artif Organs* 2: 27, 1979
21. Gagnon RF, Kaye M: Hemodialysis neutropenia and dialyzer reuse: role of the cleaning agent. *Uremia Invest* 8: 17, 1984
22. Kuwahara T, Markert M, Wauters JP: Biocompatibility aspects of dialyzer reprocessing: a comparison of 3 reuse methods and 3 membranes. *Clin Nephrol* 32: 139, 1989
23. Graeber CW, Halley SE, Lapkin RA, Graeber CA, Kaplan AA: Protein losses with reused dialyzers (abstract). *J Am Soc Nephrol* 4: 349, 1993
24. Gotch FA: Quality control tests for validation of dialyzer performance. in *Hemodialyzer Reuse; Issues and Solutions.* AAMI Technology Assessment Report 10-85, Arlington, VA, Association for the Advancement of Medical Instrumentations, 1985, p 37
25. Farrell P, Eschbach J, Vizzo J, Babb L: Hemodialyzer reuse: estimation of area loss from clearance data. *Kidney Int* 5: 466, 1974
26. Gotch F: Mass transport in reused dialyzers. *Proc Clin Dial Transplant Forum* 10: 81, 1980
27. Garred LJ, Canaud B, Flavier JL et al.: Effect of reuse on dialyzer efficacy. *Artif Organs* 14: 80, 1990
28. Schmidt R, Zasuwa G, Schell D, Dumler F: Proper dialyzer reprocessing does not impair urea mass transfer. *J Am Soc Nephrol* 2: 349, 1991
29. Gagnon RF, Kaye M: Dialyzer performance over prolonged reuse. *Clin Nephrol* 24: 21, 1985

30. Kaye M, Gagnon R, Mulhearn B, Spergel D: Prolonged dialyzer reuse. *Trans Am Soc Artif Int Organs* 30: 491, 1984

31. Deane N, Bemis J: *Multiple Use of Hemodialyzers*. Final report to the National Institute of Arthritis, Diabetes and Digestive and Kidney Disease, Contract NO1-AM-9-2214, 1981, p 53

32. Delmez JA, Weerts CA, Hasamear PD, Windus DW: Severe dialyzer dysfunction undetectable by standard reprocessing validation tests. *Kidney Int* 36: 478, 1989

33. Centers for Disease Control: Bacteremia associated with reuse of hollow fiber dialyzers. *MMWR* 35: 417, 1986

34. Bland LA, Favero MS, Oxborrow GS et al.: Effect of chemical germicides on the integrity of hemodialyzer membranes. *Trans Am Soc Artif Int Organs* 34: 172, 1988

35. Bolan GA, Reingold AL, Carson LA et al.: Infections with Mycobacterium chelonei in patients receiving dialysis and using processed hemodialyzers. *J Infect Dis* 152: 1013, 1985

36. Lowry PW, Beck-Sague CM, Bland LA et al.: Mycobacterium chelonae infection among patients receiving high flux dialysis in a hemodialysis clinic in California. *J Infect Dis* 161: 85, 1990

37. Hakim RM, Friedrich RA, Lowrie EG: Formaldehyde kinetics and bacteriology in dialyzers. *Kidney Int* 28: 936, 1985

38. Occupational Safety and Health Administration Code of Federal Regulations (Chapter 29, Part 1910.20) Federal Register, May 27, 1992

39. Hendrick DJ, Lane DJ: Formalin asthma in hospital staff. *Br Med J* 1: 607, 1975

40. Formaldehyde: evidence of carcinogenicity. NIOSH Current Intelligence Bulletin 34, DHEW (NIOSH) Publication no 81-111, 1981

41. Gotch F, Keene M: Formaldehyde kinetics in reused dialyzers. *Trans Am Soc Artif Int Organs* 29: 396, 1983

42. Gotch FA: Dialyzer transport properties and germicide elution. in *Proceedings, Seminar on Reuse of Hemodialyzers and Automated and Manual Methods*, New York: National Nephrology Foundation, 1984

43. Heck H: Formaldehyde (CH_2O) concentrations in the blood of humans and Fischer-344 rats exposed to CH_2O under controlled conditions. *J Am Ind Hyg Ass* 46: 1, 1985

44. Formaldehyde: evidence of carcinogenicity: NIOSH Current Intelligence Bulletin 34, DHEW (NIOSH) Publication no 81-111, 1981

45. Belzer FO, Kountz SL, Perkins HA: Red cell cold autoagglutinins as a cause of failure of renal allotransplantation. *Transplantation* 11: 422, 1971

46. White W, Miller G, Kaehny WD: Formaldehyde in the pathogenesis of hemodialysis-related anti-N antibodies. *Transfusion* 17: 443, 1977

47. Orringer EP, Mattern WD: Formaldehyde-induced hemolysis during chronic hemolysis. *N Engl J Med* 294: 1416, 1976

48. Kline LB, Hull RD: The virucidal properties of peracetic acid. *Am J Clin Pathol* 33: 30, 1960

49. Berkseth R, Luehman D, McMichael C, Keshavian P, Kjellstrand C: Peracetic acid for reuse of hemodialyzers. Clinical studies. *Trans Am Soc Artif Int Organs* 30: 270, 1984

50. Fleming SJ, Foreman K, Schanley K, Mihrshahi A, Siskind V: Dialyzer reprocessing with Renalin. *Am J Nephrol* 11: 27, 1991

51. Husni L, Kale E, Climer C, Bostwick B, Parker TF: Evaluation of a new disinfectant for dialyzer reuse. *Am J Kid Dis* 14: 110, 1989

52. Kaufman AM, Frinak S, Godmere RO, Levin NW: Clinical experience with heat sterilization for reprocessing dialyzers. *Am Soc Artif Int Organs J* 38: M338, 1992

53. Wineman RJ: Automated reprocessing. in *Guide to Reprocessing of Hemodialyzers*, edited by Deane N, Wineman RJ, Bemis JA, Massachusetts, Martinus Nijhoff, 1986, p 163

54. Bok DV, Pascual L, Herberger C, Sawyer R, Levin NW: Effect of multiple use of dialyzers on intradialytic symptoms. *Proc Clin Dial Transpl Proc* 92, 1980

55. Robson MD, Charoenpanich R, Kant KS et al.: Effect of first and subsequent use of hemodialyzers on patient well being. *Am J Nephrol* 6: 101, 1986

56. Kant KS, Pollak VE, Cathey M et al.: Multiple use of dialyzers: safety and efficacy. *Kidney Int* 19: 728, 1981

57. Dumler F, Zasuwa G, Levin NW: Effect of dialyzer reprocessing on complement activation and hemodialyzer-related symptoms. *Artif Organs* 11: 128, 1987

58. Cheung AK: A prospective study on intradialytic symptoms associated with reuse of hemodialyzers. *Am J Nephrol* 11: 397, 1991

59. Hakim RM, Breillat J, Lazarus JM, Port FK: Complement activation and hypersensitivity reactions to dialysis membranes. *N Engl J Med* 311: 878, 1984

60. Hakim RM, Lowrie EG: Effect of dialyzer reuse on leukopenia and the total hemolytic system. *Trans Am Soc Artif Int Organs* 26: 159, 1980

61. Craddock PR, Fehr J, Dalmasso AP, Brigham KL, Jacob HS: Hemodialysis leukopenia; pulmonary leukostasis resulting from complement activation by dialyzer cellophane membranes. *J Clin Invest* 59: 879, 1977

62. Davenport A, Williams AJ: The effect of dialyzer reuse on peak expiratory flow rate. *Res Med* 84: 17, 1990

63. Zaoui P, Green W, Hakim RM: Hemodialysis with cuprophane membrane modulates interleukin 2 receptor expression. *Kidney Int* 39: 1020, 1991

64. Pegues DA, Beck-Sague CM, Woollen SW et al.: Anaphylactoid reactions associated with reuse of hollow-fiber hemodialyzers and ACE inhibitors. *Kidney Int* 42: 1232, 1992

65. Di Raimondo CR, Pollak VE: Beta-2-microglobulin kinetics in maintenance hemodialysis: a comparison of conventional and high flux dialyzers and the effects of dialyzer reuse. *Am J Kid Dis* 13: 390, 1989

66. Diaz RJ, Washburn S, Cauble L, Siskind MS, Van Wyck D: The effect of dialyzer reprocessing on performance and β_2-microglobulin removal using polysulfone membranes. *Am J Kid Dis* 21: 405, 1993

67. Easterling RE: *Invited Commentary*. National Workshop on Reuse of Consumables in Hemodialysis. Kidney Disease Coalition. Washington, DC, 1982, p 257

68. Hoffstein PA: *Reuse of Consumables in Hemodialysis*. National Workshop on Reuse of Consumables in Hemodialysis. Kidney Disease Coalition. Washington, DC, 1982, p 228

69. Ogden DA: Clinical responses to new and reprocessed hemodialyzers. in *Guide to Reprocessing of Hemodialyz-*

ers, edited by Deane W, Wineman RJ, Bemis JA, Massachusetts, Martinus Nijhoff, 1986, p 87

70. Petersen NJ, Carson JA, Favero MS: Bacterial endotoxin in new and reused hemodialyzers: a potential cause of endotoxemia. *Trans Am Soc Artif Int Organs* 27: 155, 1981

71. Pizzaconi VB, Dorson WJ, Breillat J et al.: Factors affecting complement activation and neutropenia during dialysis using cuprophane membranes. *Am Soc Artif Int Organs J* 7: 64, 1984

72. Ogden DA, Myers LE, Eskelson CD, Zeigler EJ: Iatrogenic administration of formaldehyde to hemodialysis patients. *Proc Dial Transplant Forum* 3: 141, 1973

73. Lufft V, Schindler R, Lonneman G, Shaldon S, Koch KM: Adsorption of exogenous pyrogen (EP) onto new and reused high flux dialyzers (abstract). *Nephrol Dial Transplant* 7: 729, 1992

74. Oliver JC, Bland LA, Oettinger CW et al.: Bacteria and endotoxin removal from bicarbonate dialysate fluids for use in conventional, high-efficiency and high flux hemodialysis. *Artif Organs* 16: 141, 1992

75. Lonnemann G, Bingel M, Floege J, Koch KM, Shaldon S, Dinarello CA: Detection of endotoxin-like interleukin-1 inducing activity during *in vitro* dialysis. *Kidney Int* 33: 29, 1988

76. Vanholder R, Vanhaecke E, Ringoir S: Waterborne Pseudomonas septicemia. *Am Soc Artif Int Org Trans* 36: 215, 1990

77. Bland LA, Arduino MJ, Aguero SM, Favero MS: Recovery of bacteria from reprocessed high flux dialyzers after bacterial contamination of the header spaces and O-rings. *Trans Am Soc Artif Int Organs* 35: 314, 1989

78. Nolph KD, Ahearn DJ, Esterly JA, Maher JF: Irreversible, morphological and functional changes in hollow fiber kidneys with a single dialysis. *Trans Am Soc Artif Int Organs* 20: 604, 1974

79. Lazarus JM, Friedlich RA, Merrill JP: Hollow fiber kidney reuse. *Dial Transplant* 2: 14, 1973

80. Sherman RA, Cody RP, Rogers ME, Solanchick JC: The effect of dialyzer reuse on dialysis delivery. *Am J Kid Dis.* In press

81. Jacobs C, Brunner FP, Chantler C et al.: Combined reports on regular dialysis and transplantation in Europe. *VII. Proc Eur Dial Transplant Assoc* 14: 3, 1977

82. Pollak V, Kant K, Parnell S et al.: Repeated use of dialyzers is safe: long term observations on morbidity and mortality in patients with end stage renal disease. *Nephron* 42: 217, 1986

83. Held PJ, Pauly MV, Diamond L: Survival analysis of patients undergoing dialysis. *J Am Med Assoc* 257: 645, 1987

84. Luehmann DA, Cosentino LC: Safety of dialyzer reuse with Renalin: the untold story. *Dial Transplant* 23: 248, 1994

85. Held PJ, Wolfe RA, Gaylin DS et al.: Analysis of the association of dialyzer reuse practices and patient outcomes. *Am J Kid Dis* 23: 692, 1994

86. Kjellstrand CJ: The search for scientific truth versus corporate interests (editorial). *Sem Dial* 6: 281, 1993

87. US Department of Health and Human Services: *Food and Drug Administration*. Quality Assurance Guidelines for Hemodialysis Devices, 1991

EXTRACORPOREAL BLOOD PURIFICATION TECHNIQUES: PLASMAPHERESIS AND HEMOPERFUSION

HANS GURLAND, WALTER SAMTLEBEN, MICHAEL J. LYSAGHT and JAMES F. WINCHESTER

INTRODUCTION

This chapter will focus on techniques other than dialysis for removal of chemical toxins (endogenous or exogenous), immune toxins, or other naturally occurring biochemical substances considered to produce disease. Plasmapheresis is the process of removal of plasma (by mechanical, immunoprecipitation, cryoprecipitation, or filtration techniques) which contains the substance in question. Hemoperfusion is the passage of blood over sorbent agents for removal of harmful products.

PLASMA EXCHANGE

Introduction

The therapeutic rationale of plasma exchange is removal from the circulation of high molecular weight species which are instrumental in the pathogenesis of a wide variety of disorders. Examples of well characterized and clinical relevant pathogens include:

1. uremic toxins (molecular weight range 60 up to 5,000 or more Daltons) in renal failure;
2. circulating toxins in drug intoxications as well as exogenous and endogenous poisonings;

3. autoantibodies of the IgG or IgM class (molecular weight 150,000 and 970,000 Daltons respectively) with subsequent binding to antigens in autoimmune disorders (e.g., Goodpasture's syndrome, myasthenia gravis, immune thrombocytopenia);

4. circulating immune complexes (molecular weight about 500,000 up to 3,000,000 Daltons) which cause tissue lesions by deposition;

5. excessive low density lipoprotein concentrations (molecular weight about 2,400,000 Daltons) in type II hyperlipidemia; and

6. paraproteins (intact immunoglobulins as well as free light or heavy chains) with subsequent disturbances, e.g., renal paraprotein deposition, hyperviscosity, polyneuropathy, cutaneous vasculitis and cryoglobulinemia.

Ideally, a blood purification system should remove only the pathogenic molecule and not other substances. It should also have a high removal capacity and its clinical application should be free of side effects. These three criteria have been realized for only a few systems applicable in some distinct clinical entities with well characterized pathogens (e.g., LDL removal systems). This chapter summarizes the technology and clinical application of extracorporeal macro-molecular separation processes.

Methods for unselective plasma exchange

Separation techniques

The simplest way to harvest an adequate volume of plasma from whole blood is to collect a bag of anticoagulated blood, centrifuge it and express off the plasma supernatant (1). Plasma containing the target pathogens may be discarded in which case the cells are resuspended in a saline or protein solution and returned to the patient. When repeated several times this batch process provides effective reduction in the plasma concentration of intravascular toxins (2).

In the late 1960s continuous closed centrifugal apheresis equipment was developed, originally with the aim of collecting blood cells for bone marrow transplant recipients (3) and these could also be used for separating plasma from whole blood. Originally such equipment was quite bulky. Newly developed centrifuges for therapeutic plasmapheresis have become more compact and require smaller extracorporeal priming volumes and a few are capable of performing apheresis with a single venous access. These techniques are utilized almost exclusively in blood banking and hematology.

Clinical on-line plasma separation employing membranes became available in 1978 (4). Highly permeable membranes were originally developed to recover a cell free filtrate of ascitic fluid for reinfusion in patients with advanced liver disease. Although not ideally suited for plasmapheresis (5), early studies with these membranes motivated the development of a wide variety of clinical

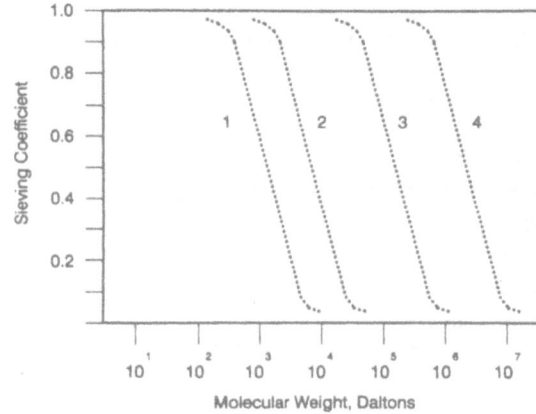

Figure 1. Schematic illustration of permeability properties (sieving coefficients) of membranes used for various extracorporeal blood purification. Curves represent: 1 – standard hemodialysis membrane; 2 – hemofiltration membrane; 3 – cascade filtration membrane; 4 – plasma separation membrane. Molecular weights (in Daltons) of referece marker molecules: urea, 60; creatinine, 113; Vitamin B 12, 1,355; β2-microglobulin, 11,800; albumin, 66,000; IgG, 150,000; IgM, 970,000; β-lipoprotein, 2,400,000.

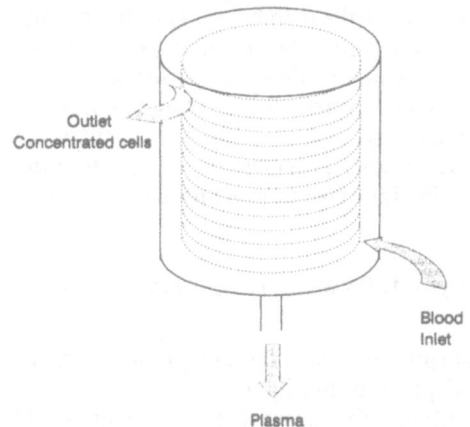

Figure 2. Schematic drawing of the plasma separation device used in the Autopheresis^R monitor. Anticoagulated blood is fed into a small slit between the housing and the rotating cylinder (3,600 rpm). The rotating cylinder consists of a highly permeable membrane. The cell free plasma is harvested at the bottom of the rotating cylinder while the cell concentrate leaves the device at the left top.

membrane filters fabricated from several different polymers (6). These filters exhibit a wide range of permeabilities (Figure 1) without significant retention of high molecular weight proteins. Furthermore, the design of membrane filters has been improved so that devices with smaller surface areas permit plasma exchanges at low blood flow rates eliminating the need for central venous access (7). A further development in the field of plasmapheresis, available since the mid 1980s, employs the com-

Table 1. Polymers used for membrane plasma separation filters

Cellulose-diacetate
Polyethylene
Polymethylmethacrylate
Polymer alloy (cellulose-diacetate based)
Polypropylene
Polysulfone
Polyvinyl alcohol
Polyvinyl chloride

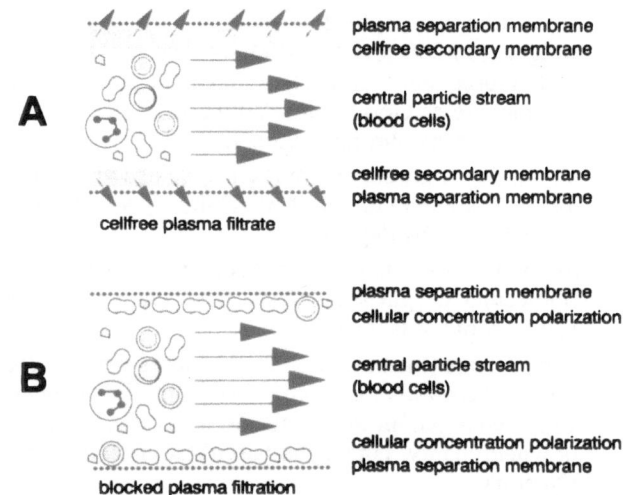

Figure 3. Illustration of the fluid-mechanic phenomena occurring when blood flows through a hollow fiber. Under ideal operating conditions (A), the cells flow centrally and a cell free secondary layer will form near to the inner membrane surface as shown in the upper panel. At a high TMP (B & region III, Figure 4), cells impinge on the membrane surface(cellular concentration polarization), block the filtration of plasma through the membrane (B), and hemolyze.

bination of centrifugal and membrane-based plasma separation (Figure 2). The shear forces are achieved by a rotating cylinder, the surface of which is 60 cm^2 (8, 9).

Membrane materials and device configuration

Polymers used for hollow fiber and flat sheet plasma separation membranes are summarized in Table 1. The diameter of all hollow fiber membranes is between 270 and 370 m with a wall thickness of 50–150 m. The nominal pore size is 0.5 m which prevents transport of normal platelets through the membrane. The effective fiber length chosen by the different manufacturers is between 13.5 and 26 cm. One flat sheet device for plasma separation, together with a cycler, became commercially available in 1980. It employs polyvinyl chloride as membrane material. Several other polymers have been used *in vitro* for characterization of the transmembrane transport of solutes (10).

Factors governing mass transport in membrane plasma separation

The transport of plasma through plasma separation membranes depends primarily on:
1. membrane filter design (flat sheet or hollow fiber, pore size, fiber diameter in hollow fiber filters or channel heights in flat sheet devices, membrane surface area);
2. blood composition (hematocrit, blood and plasma viscosity, platelet count, plasma protein composition); and
3. operating conditions (blood flow, transmembrane pressure, filtrate flux, shear rate, filtration fraction).

Membrane filter design

When the blood passes through a highly permeable hollow fiber filter, red cells and platelets together with the plasma move towards the wall and accumulate to form a secondary membrane which limits the filtration efficiency. Blood flow tangential to the membrane surface removes these blood cells from the wall by augmented particle diffusion (10), as shown in Figure 3. Under certain conditions, cells remain near to the filtering wall. This dynamic process is called cellular concentration polarization and

may, in extreme situations, completely block further plasma filtration through the membrane if the cells cannot be moved from the wall. Cellular concentration polarization is enhanced by a high filtration fraction, a high transmembrane pressure, and a low shear rate. At hematocrits usually found in the plasmapheresis population (20 to 40%), hollow fiber filters can be operated at a filtration fraction not exceeding 0.3 (10). This means that a plasma flux of 30 volume % of the blood input is filtered through the membrane. Hematocrit increases proportionally and to prevent fiber plugging, outlet hematocrit must be kept below 70% by decreasing the filtration fraction (10).

Flat sheet devices offer the advantage of allowing a far higher filtration fraction than hollow fibers. This is especially true when an automated fluid cycler (e.g., Cobe TPE) is used. This equipment automatically adjusts the channel height and the filtration rate to give an optimal shear rate and transmembrane pressure for a given blood flow. The maximum filtration fraction which can be achieved in flat sheet devices approaches 0.6 (10) allowing high yield plasma separations even at low blood flow rates when peripheral veins serve as vascular access. Surface areas of commercial membrane plasma separators for therapeutic purposes are in the range of 0.12 to 0.6 m^2 in hollow fiber devices and 0.13 m^2 for flat sheets (6).

Under appropriate operating conditions all currently available membrane plasma separation modules exhibit nearly ideal protein permeability properties without significant protein retention (6). Protein permeability can be best described by the sieving coefficient which is calculated according to the following equation:

$$SC = \frac{2Cf}{Cin + Cout} \qquad [1]$$

where SC – dimensionless sieving coefficient, Cin – protein inlet concentration, Cout – protein outlet concentration and Cf – protein concentration in the filtrate.

For adequate characterization of a plasma separation module it is necessary to determine sieving coefficients for a spectrum of proteins which cover a wide molecular weight range. This should at least include the following globularly shaped proteins (molecular weight): albumin (66,000), IgG (150,000), IgM (970,000), and β-lipoprotein (2,400,000). A sieving coefficient of 1.0 would represent the same protein concentration in the filtrate as in the blood fed into the filter. At a sieving coefficient of 0 the protein under investigation cannot be detected in the plasma filtrate. Sieving coefficients of at least 0.95 for all plasma proteins are standard for virtually all currently available membrane plasma separators (6).

Blood composition

The plasma filtration flux is independent of hematocrit in the range of 0 to 60% (10). Platelet count may decrease the filtration rate byhigh concentrations. Similarly, high molecular weight plasma constituents when present in extremely high plasma concentrations can also limit filtration efficiency. This is true for IgM (IgM paraproteinemia, Waldenström's disease) and for β-lipoprotein (hyperlipoproteinemia). Those cryoglobulins (mostly of type I – monoclonal) which are solubilized only a few degrees below physiologic temperatures might precipitate within the membrane immediately after blood withdrawal. This phenomenon can be prevented by warming the entire extracorporeal circuit including the filtering device to 37 to 38°C.

Operating conditions

Early on it was noted that membrane plasmapheresis can be performed safely only at a narrow window of operating conditions (10), which is determined primarily by the transmembrane pressure (TMP), the shear rate and the filtrate flux per unit filtering area (Figure 4). For a hollow fiber device the wall shear rate, is directly proportional to the blood flow rate and inversely correlated to the number of fibers and to the third power of the fiber radius. It is calculated according to the following equation (11):

$$gw = \frac{4 \times QB}{n \times p \times R3} \qquad [2]$$

where gw – wall shear rate (sec-1), QB – blood flow (ml/sec), n – number of fibers and R – internal fiber radius (cm). Consequently, for a given device geometry the shear rate is determined only by the blood flow rate.

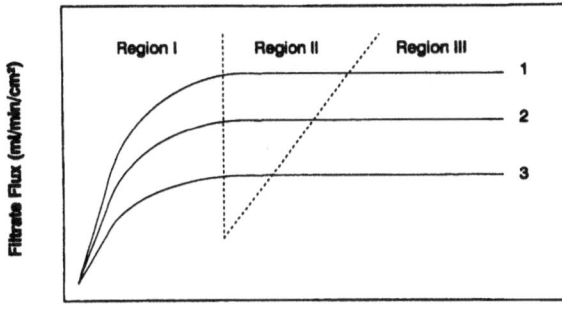

Figure 4. Schematic showing filtration behaviour in membrane plasmapheresis in the form of a plot of local filtration rate *vs* transmembrane pressure. Curve 1, 2, and 3 repesent high, median and low rates of blood velocity. In region I the membrane is the primary resistance to trasnport. Region II is a transition region. Region III represents fully developed concentration polarization. Filtration in region III is accompanied by hemolysis.

The mean TMP represents the pressure difference between the blood and the filtrate compartment:

$$TMP = \frac{1}{2} (Pin + Pout) - Pfiltr \qquad [3]$$

where Pin – pressure at the filter blood inlet, Pout – pressure at the filter blood outlet and Pfiltr – pressure at the filtrate side.

At very low TMPs, there is a nearly linear increase of the filtrate flux (per unit surface area) with increasing TMP (Figure 4, Region I). At intermediate TMPs, the plasma filtration reaches a plateau (Region II) with a filtrate flux independent of the TMP. If the TMP is further increased, this does not influence the filtrate flux positively but induces hemolysis resulting in free hemoglobin in the plasma filtrate (Region III). Region III represents unstable operating conditions with flux decay, worsening of the protein permeability of the filter and hemolysis as already mentioned (6, 7).

Sterilization of membrane plasma separators

In general, sterilization procedures for membrane plasmaseparators are adapted from those used for hemodialyzers. Only a few are still sterilized with ethylene oxide gas and at least one anaphylactoid reaction during a clinical plasma exchange treatment has been attributed to residual ethylene oxide as has been well documented with hollow fiber dialyzers (12). Gamma radiation and steam autoclavation are clearly preferrable.

Reuse

Because membrane plasma separators were expensive when first introduced commercially, same patient reuse has been investigated by several groups (13, 14). When reuse is performed properly, a filter can be reused a few

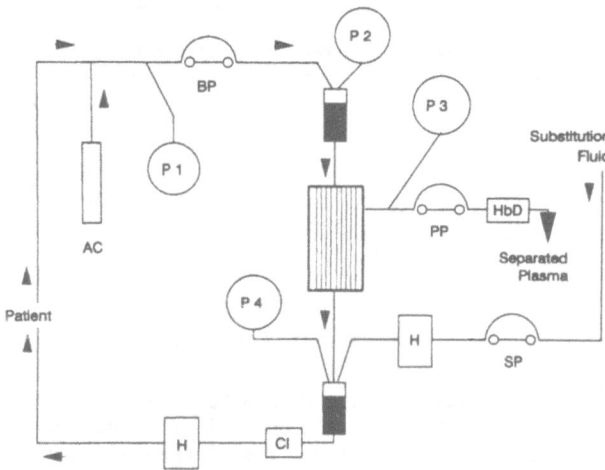

Figure 5. Schematic illustration of a membrane plasma separation circuit. For details see text.

times without significant loss in flux or protein permeability (14). Because of associated labor costs, physician liability, and decreasing disposable costs, reuse never became widespread in clinical plasmapheresis.

Hardware

Equipment for membrane plasmapheresis is available from several companies. Safety standards for this extracorporeal treatment are similar to those for hemodialysis. There are, however, some differences in safety requirements inherent in the membrane plasma separation process. Figure 5 illustrates a fully equipped membrane plasmapheresis flow diagram. An ideal system should include (labels in brackets relate to Figure 5):

1. negative pressure monitor in the blood drawing line (P1);
2. blood pump (BP) which can be operated at low blood flow rates (minimum 40, maximum 200 ml/min);
3. continuous infusion of the anticoagulant (heparin or citrate) with the option of different anticoagulant to blood application ratios (AC);
4. filter inlet and outlet pressure monitors (P2, P4);
5. air bubble detector and clamp (C1) in the venous return line;
6. pressure gauge in the plasma filtrate line (P3);
7. controlled plasma filtration via a pump in the plasma line (PP);
8. hemoglobin detector in the plasma filtrate line (HbD);
9. substitution pump (SP) adjustable to different substitution ratios in relation to the separated plasma; and
10. low volume warmers (H) in the replacement and venous return lines.

The optional equipment should display the transmembrane pressure. Adequate alarms should be included for all essential parameters (e.g., inadequate blood withdrawal, TMP, air).

Comparison of different plasma exchange procedures

A few publications compare the efficiency of centrifugal and membrane based plasmapheresis techniques (15–18). All these studies suggest that the effcacy is comparable when both methods are applied under optimal conditions. However, when a high citrate to blood ratio is used in centrifugation, the dilutional effect will reduce efficiency in comparison with membrane plasma separation where heparin anticoagulant is typically employed (18). Moreover, platelet loss is significantly greater with the centrifugation (15).

Technical aspects of membrane plasma exchange

Vascular access

For most membrane plasma separation devices a stable blood flow of 50 to 80 ml/min is sufficient. Consequently, peripheral veins these can be used for access in most cases.. Large surface area hollow fiber plasma separators (0.5 to 0.6 m^2) could be operated at blood flow rates up to 300 ml/min or more, yielding a plasma flow of up to 100 ml/min. Asside effects of plasma exchange procedures appear relate to the rate of the infused proteinaceous substitution fluid, filtration rates of less than 0 to 50 ml/min are preferred. In patients with potentially irreversible renal disease with the risk of complete loss of kidney function (e.g., all forms of rapidly progressive glomerulonephritis) a large bore central venous catheter is preferred. This access method preserves peripheral veins for fistula placement should renal replacement therapy be required later.

Anticoagulation

For anticoagulation in a routine membrane plasma exchange a bolus of heparin (2,000 to 5,000 IU) is combined with continuous heparin (300 to 1,200 IU/h) or citate infusion (ACD-A 1 ml per 15 to 30 ml of blood). In patients at a high risk for bleeding (e.g., pulmonary hemorrhage in Goodpasture's syndrome), the actual dose of the anticoagulant should be reduced to avoid bleeding complications. In those cases the anticoagulant regimen should be monitored during treatment by an appropriate test (aPTT when heparin is used). Fractionated low molecular weight heparin can also be used but requires special monitoring (19).

Replacement solutions

Circulating levels of albumin, the bulk protein and the main determinant of oncotic pressure should be kept constant to avoid potentially life threatening intracorporeal fluid shifts. To accomplish this, separated plasma has to be replaced isovolumetrically and isooncotically. Most centers prefer a solution as 4 to 5% human albumin solution). Attention must be paid to electrolyte in commercial albumin solutions. Calcium should be adjusted to a physiologic concentration to avoid hypocalcemic symptoms especially when citrate is used for anticoagulation. In large volume plasma exchanges with rapid reinfusion via a catheter placed in the superior caval vein, cardiac arrhythmias have been attributed to substitution fluid low in potassium (20). Colloid isooncotic replacement fluids (dextran, gelatin, hydroxyethyl starch) have been used in plasma exchange with the intention of cost reduction. This approach is best limited to replacement of the first 20% of the volume to be exchanged (e.g., first 500 ml in a 3 to 4 l plasma exchange). Synthetic colloidal substitutes are rapidly cleaved with a serum half-life of hours compared to 10 to 18 days for albumin.

In patients where a decrease of coagulation factors or other blood proteins (e.g., immunoglobulins, complement) might be clinically troublesome, fresh (frozen) plasma (FFP) is recommended for volume replacement However, FFP still has an intrinsic risk of transmitting (viral) infections: HIV 1:500,000–1:1 million; Hepatitis B about 1:50,000; Hepatitis C less than 1:5,000 (21). Furthermore, the incidence of immediate side reactions is highest with this type of volume replacement. Finally, as citrate is the anticoagulant in FFP, calcium must be replaced when FFP is infused.

Exchange volume and protein kinetics

Given the assumptions of a single pool model and no protein seiving by the membrane, the reduction in concentration of moeities not returned with the replacement fluid can be predicted by the following equation (22):

$$C = C0 \exp(-V/P) \qquad [4]$$

where C – protein concentration (g/l) after the volume, V, has been exchanged; C0 – initial protein concentration (g/l); P – total patient's plasma volume (l) and V – plasma volume actually exchanged (l) (see also Figure 6). The concentration of a particular protein at the end of a plasma exchange session depends on the plasma volume exchanged. As exchange volumes increase the overall removal efficiency decreases. As a result of redistribution and resynthesis the predicted protein concentration decrease is usually not completely reached (23). These removal kinetics have been validated experimentally for immunglobulins, coagulation factors, complement proteins and lipoproteins. However, circulating immune complexes demonstate a far more pronounced decrease than predicted by equation [4]. This phenomenon has been explained by 1) enhanced endogenous catabolism (24, 25), 2) formation of new immune complexes in the changed protein milieu which behave differently both biologically in the patient and biochemically in the assays used compared to the original ones, and 3) methodological problems with the detection of circulating immune complexes due to multiple interactions (26).

Plasma concentration of most proteins increases following a plasma exchange session. The first phase of this increment is governed primarily by a reequilibration of

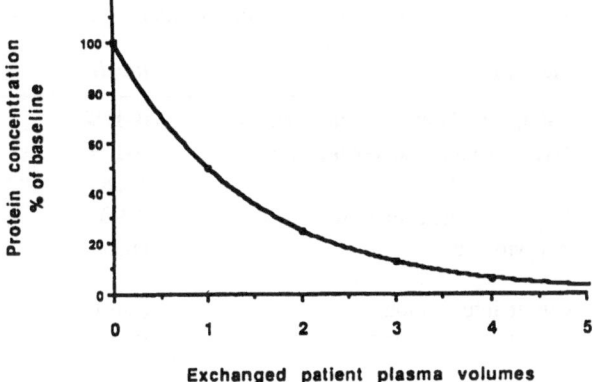

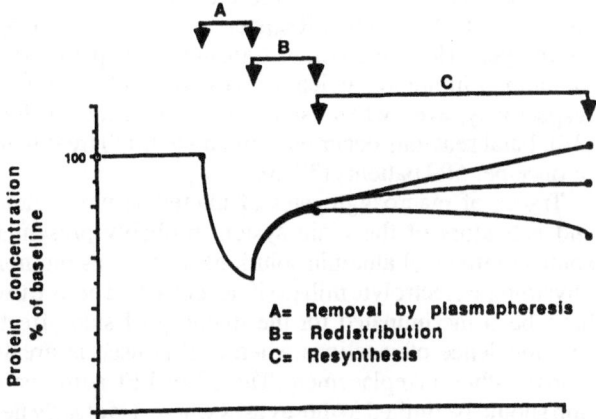

Figure 6. Protein kinetics in plasmapheresis. The upper panel demonstrates simple idealized first order pharmacokinetic removal. The lower panel includes the more clinically relevant phenomena of resynthesis and redistribution.

the plasma protein with that of the extravascular compartment (redistribution). This phase lasts about 6 to 12 h. Its amplitude depends on the distribution space of the particular protein within the body. For example only 25% of the total body IgM content is located extravascularly compared to about half of the total body IgG. Consequently, the post exchange increase of IgM is lower than that of IgG. The further time course of plasma protein concentrations primarily depends on the rate of resynthesis (Figure 6). In the case of (pathogenic) immunoglobulins (autoantibodies, paraproteins) synthesis can be reduced by cytotoxic drugs to deplete selectively B lymphocytes stimulated by the plasma exchange induced immunoglobulin depletion (27, 28).

Side effects and adverse reactions

Side effects observed in plasma exchange are caused by the substitution fluid, the anticoagulant, and the extra-

Table 2. Incidence and management of immediate side effects observed in therapeutic plasma exchange (20, 29–36)

Side effect	Incidence	Management
Allergic and quasiallergic reactions	0–12%	steroids, antihistamines, (calcium)
Hypotension, vaso-vagal rections	0–12%	atropine
Febrile reactions	1–18%	steroids, antipyretics
Hypocalcemic symptoms	0–9%	calcium
Arrhythmias	about 3%	depending on the type of arrhythmia, correction of electrolyte imbalances
Citrate intoxication	(rare)	calcium, decrease of citrate infusion rate

corporeal procedure itself, including technical failures. Common side effects of plasma exchange are summarized in Table 2 (20, 29–36). Severe side reactions are rare. According to the French Register for Plasma Exchange for the year 1985, the risk of transmitting hepatitis B or the human immunodeficiency virus was 0.4% or 0.09% respectively, even when using FFP as replacement fluid (34). Fatal reactons occur once in about 3,000 treatments or once per 500 patients (37, 38).

Traces of macroaggregates of altered serum proteins and activators of the kinin system probably present in some commercial albumin solutions, as well as the non-physiologic electrolyte milieu (if not corrected before use) have been incriminated for the majority of side effects. The incidence of reactions when FFP is used is greater than for albumin replacement. Therefore, FFP administration should be limited to those cases where it is clearly necessary. Administration of albumin at a far faster rate (10 to 40 ml/min) in plasma exchange than that recommended by the the pharmaceutical suppliers (8–10 ml/min) may explain the high incidence of side reactions seen in this treatment compared to the infusion of albumin in the common hospitalized population where albumin related side effects are rare (about 0.01%) (39). If plasma exchange is performed within 3 days prior to anaesthesia, the depletion of cholinesterase can cause prolonged post operative apnea requiring assisted ventilation (40).

Plasmapheresis, pharmacokinetics and concommitant medications

Few publications deal with the removal of therapeutic drugs during plasma exchange (41, 42). In general, the fractional removal of substances with a large volume of distribution is low regardless of the drug ratio bound to plasma proteins. An exchange of one patient plasma volume usually removes less than 1 to 3% of the total body store of a particular drug (Table 3). Consequently, an additional dose is usually not necessary. Nevertheless drug concentration should be directly monitored if possible, especially in drugs with a narrow therapeutic range as for example phenytoin. Samples should be drawn before and drugs administered after plasmapheresis. Plas-

Table 3. Volume of distribution (l/g) and protein binding (%) of some selected drugs (41, 42). The calculated volumes of distribution for a 70 kg person are included. For comparison, the volume of distribution for IgG is around 6–7 l and for IgM 4–5 l, respectively

Drug	Volume of distribution		Protein binding (%)
	l/kg	litres*	
Acetylsalicylic acid	0.1–0.2	7–14	50–90
Cyclophosphamide	0.79	55	12
Diazepam	0.95	67	97
Digoxin	6.8	476	2
Digitoxin	0.61	43	93
Paracetamol	1.1	77	2–3
Phenobarbital	0.7	49	51
Phenytoin	0.54	38	90
Prednisone	1	70	70–95
Theophylline	0.33–0.74	23–52	59

ma exchange is relatively ineffective at removing protein bound drugs or toxins and is used only for those intoxicants which exhibit high protein binding, small volume of distribution and prolonged biological half-life (43).

Alternative plasma exchange procedures

The application of (hollow fiber) membrane plasma separation modules is not necessarily limited to centers equipped with sophisticated hardware. These filters can be used in pumpless circuits either in a spontaneous arteriovenous pathway or in a one access set-up with gravity as the driving force for blood and plasma separation (44–46). Furthermore, both membrane-based and centrifugal plasma separation can also be combined with routine hemodialysis (47–49).

Plasma fractionation

Several procedures have been developed with the aim of selectively removing disease specific circulating macromolecular pathogens. Altogether these procedures are termed plasma fractionation or closed loop plasmapheresis. A few have become routine. The incentives for a procedure which removes only the pathogen and returns the 'normal proteins back to the patient are to minimize 1) side reactions (immediate reactions during the procedure and long term effects, e.g., infection) mostly related to the exogenous protein replacement, and 2) costs and sourcing of commercial plasma proteins (50). Existing plasma fractionation procedures employ routine laboratory protein separation techniques adapted to the requirements of an on line extracorporeal circuit. Currently, three strategies are used (50, 51).

Cascade filtration

With the help of a membrane filter the separated plasma is divided into a high and a low molecular weight fraction. The low molecular weight fraction containing most of the albumin is returned to the patient. The pathogen accumulates in the high molecular weight fraction retained by the filter. This process is called cascade filtration or double filtration and was first described by Agishi in 1980 (52). Withcurrently available filters, cascade filtration can be applied where the target pathogen has a molecular weight ten times higher than that of albumin. Hyperviscosity due to macroglobulinemia (IgM 970,000 Daltons) and familial hypercholesterolemia (β-lipoproteins, 2,400,000 Daltons) are clinical conditions in which cascade filtration is pefereable to unselective plasma exchange. Since many high molecular weight proteins are removed in addition to the pathogen, cascade filtration does not result in specific pathogen removal. It does, however, recover sufficient albumin to obviate exogenous replacement (53–55).

The efficacy of the plasma filtration process depends not only on the membrane but also on the design of the filtration process, which can be performed in a dead-end or in a single-pass format. Both configurations yield slightly different removal and recovery rates (55–57). Several techniques have been introduced to limit plugging of the secondary filters: reverse rinse at a rising TMP (58), backflushing of the filter (59), or pulsatile flow (60). None of the various secondary filters can separate IgG from albumin very well, and therefore the original promise of this approach remains unrealized, but has been reported at least by one group (61).

Adsorption techniques

In this approach, filtered plasma is processed through an adsorption column which contains a ligand capable of binding the target pathogen. This process is analogous to affinity chromatography. Three main types of ligands have been utilized for on-line plasma processing. In order to removeof antibodies of known specificity, the corresponding (multivalent) antigens are fixed to a solid matrix tp trap the antibodies from the perfusate. This has been described for DNA antibodies with a DNA-containing column in SLE (62). In other cases, the pathogenic protein's chemical affinity for another substance is employed for extraction. Low density lipoproteins (LDL), for example, which are known to bind to heparin or dextran sulfate can be removed from plasma by column perfusion using these ligands (63, 64). Other ligands under investigation are protein A (for binding of IgG 1, 2, 4 and IgG-based immune complexes), phenylalanine (for immune complexes) and tryptophan (for antiacetylcholine receptor antibodies in myasthenia gravis) (65). Immunoadsorption may also exploit specific polyclonal or monoclonal antibodies fixed to a solid matrix support. This technique offers a high degree of selectivity and specificity when compared with chemical affinity systems. Removal of human LDL with matrix fixed antibodies is already established (66–68). Currently, columns with antibodies directed against immunglobulins G or M (68) or against Lipoprotein (a) are are undergoing clinical evaluation. Some types of adsorption treatments, especially with protein A-silica columns produce side effects similar to acute phase reactions (69, 70).

Combination of physiochemical separation techniques

An excellent example of physiochemical separation and plasmapheresis is the removal of LDL from plasma by heparin precipitation. This technique, which has been introduced by Seidel and coworkers (71), employs the property of the LDL-heparin complex to form a precipitate at low pH, which then can be removed by filtration from the plasma. Following readjustment of pH and electroyte levels by dialysis and ultrafiltration, the processed plasma is recombined with the main bloodstream (71). This procedure has been termed Heparin induced Extracorporeal LDL-Precipitation (HELP). Its safety and efficacy in clinical application is well documented (72, 73). An advantage of the HELP procedure is that some other heparin-binding plasma proteins and lipoproteins are eliminated as well. This is the case with lipoprotein Lp(a) and fibrinogen (74, 75). The removal of fibrinogen by the HELP procedure induces acute and chronic improvements in hemorheological parameters (73, 76) which supports its application also in situations with a disturbed microcirculation.

Photopheresis

Photopheresis combines photochemotherapy and leucaplasmapheresis and was first described in 1987 for treatment of cutaneous T cell lymphoma (77). The patient is given an oral dose of 8 methoxypsoralen (8 MOP) and 1–2 h later after cell separation lymphocytes and plasma are exposed to ultraviolet long-wave irradiation. The low energy light activates the 8 MOP to become an alkylating agent that reverts to its inactive state when leaving the irradiation chamber (78). This immunomodulating therapy, which was widely used for treatment for cutaneous T-cell lymphomas in the early 1990s, is under clinical investigation for prevention of rejection in cardiac and other transplant patients (78, 79).

Application of plasma exchange in renal diseases

In the mid-1970s case reports of significant improvement from plasma exchange were published in diseases known to have poor prognoses (e.g., Goodpasture's syndrome, rapidly progressive glomerulonephritis, myasthenic crisis, thrombotic thrombocytopenic purpura) (80–83). These dramatic results stimulated widespread investigation of this new therapeutic approach for more than 200 different disease entities resulting in the publication of over 2,400 articles by 1984. These dealt primarily with the clinical results of plasma exchange (84). Several editorials and overview articles tried to summarize the overall clinical application of macromolecular separation (85–93). However, the recommendations provided were in part still controversial and the American Society for Apheresis, offers the following revised recommendations (93):

— Category I: Therapeutic hemapheresis is standard and acceptable but this does not imply that it is mandatory in all situations Evidence is usually derived from controlled and well-designed clinical studies.

— Category II: Therapeutic hemapheresis is generally accepted, however, it is considered to be supportive to other more definitive treatments rather than serving as primary therapy.

— Category III: Reported evidence is insufficient to establish the efficacy of therapeutic hemapheresis. Only anecdotal reports are available.

— Category IV: Available controlled trials have shown a lack of efficacy for therapeutic hemapheresis.

Table 4 contains the current classification of diseases into these categories (93). It must be stressed that patients with the same disease present with a quite heterogeneous clinical picture which leaves place for an individual treatment decision especially when conventional treatment has failed.

The rationale for the application of plasma exchange in renal diseases is the elimination of those circulating pathogenic proteins involved in the renal inflammatory process. These immune factors include circulating autoantibodies (anti-glomerular basement membrane [GBM] antibodies, anti-DNA antibodies, and C3 nephritic factor), circulating immune complexes and free antigens and antibodies capable of forming immune complexes *in situ* in the kidney. They also include paraproteins, unknown circulating factors responsible for microvascular lesions in hemolytic uremic syndrome and thrombotic thrombocytopenic purpura, anti-graft antibodies in vascular kidney transplant rejection, and mediators of inflammatory processes (e.g., fibrinogen and complement components).

Anti-glomerular basement membrane antibody mediated nephritis

This disorder is mediated by autoantibodies directed against a 26 kilodalton (kD) monomeric peptide (and a 48 kD dimeric aggregate) present in one of the two non-collagenous parts (NC I region) of type IV colla-

gen which is the main constituent of glomerular basement membrane (94, 95). Type IV collagen and hence the Goodpasture antigen is present not only in the kidney but also in other vascular regions (e.g., lungs). Because of the shared intramolecular location of the Goodpasture antgen in the extrarenal vessels, additional factors (such as cigarette smoke, viral infections) are necessary to enable the autoantibodies to obtain access to the normally cryptic antigen (96). Anti-GBM nephritis makes up but 5% of all glomerulonephritides. Usually, its clinical course is associated with a rapid decline of kidney function (rapidly progressive glomerulonephritis). In the early 1970s, poor prognosis of renal function was reported (97). In one series, onlyone of 39 untreated and only one of 29 patients treated with drugs retained adequate renal function (98). However, improved diagnostic tools (indirect immunofluorescence, anti-GBM antibody radioimmunoassay and ELISA, direct immunofluorescence of kidney biopsy specimens) have made it possible to identify early stages of this disease with a limited expression and more benign course. About 70% of cases with anti-GBM mediated nephritis present with pulmonary hemorrhage (Goodpasture's syndrome) (96, 99). In the mid-1970s an aggressive immunosuppressive regimen for patients with progressive renal failure due to anti-GBM nephritis was published and included daily plasma exchanges together with cytotoxic drugs (cyclophosphamide 3 mg/kg and azathioprine 1 mg/kg) as well as prednisone (starting dose 60mg/day) (100). This combined therapy resulted in improvement of renal function in 15 of 17 patients presenting with a serum creatinine below 600 mol/l. Patients with an advanced disease (serum creatinine exceeding 600 mol/l or oligo-anuric at presentation) exhibited a far poorer response with improvement in but one of 27 patients. Furthermore, most of the deaths occurred in this latter group. A similar response to treatment has susbsequently been reported by other centers (101, 102). Pulmonary hemorrhage can be readily controlled by plasmapheresis in about 90% of cases (100). As the lung infiltrates resolve there is parallel improvement in pulmonary gas exchange. In a controlled study with only a few patients, it was also possible to limit pulmonary hemorrhage with a high-dose steroid therapy (daily 1 g Methylprednisolone iv) (103). An inadequate response of pulmonary hemorrhage to plasmapheresis should make one suspect a superimposed infection or fluid overload both of which radiographically can enhance the appearance of the pulmonary lesions. Specific antibiotic treatment of the infection, volume reduction by diuretics or by ultrafiltration and, if necessary, positive pressure ventilation are the appropriate therapeutic measures in such cases. Circulating anti-GBM antibodies (measured by a sensitive radioimmunoassay rather than by indirect immunofluorescence) disappear in the shortest period in those patients most aggressively treated (daily plasma exchanges for 14 days, and immunosuppression as described above). In most of these individuals, antibody synthesis is switched

Table 4. Role of therapeutic hemapheresis for some selected disorders according to a categorization of the American Society for Apheresis (93). For details see text

Disorder	Therapeutic procedure	Category
Renal		
Cryoglobulinemia	Plasma exchange	I
Goodpasture's syndrome	Plasma exchange	I
Thrombotic thrombocytopenicpurpura (TTP)	Plasma exchange	I
Hemolytic uremic syndrome	Plasma exchange	II
Myeloma and paraproteinemias	Plasma exchange	II
Rapidly progressive nephritis (without anti-GBM)	Plasma exchange	II
Organ allograft rejection	Photopheresis	III
Renal allograft rejection	Plasma exchange	IV
Neurology		
Acute Guillain-Barré syndrome	Plasma exchange	I
Myasthenia gravis	Plasma exchange	I
Paraproteinemic peripheral neuropathy	Plasma exchange	II
Multiple sclerosis	Plasma exchange	III
Autoimmune		
HIV related syndromes		
Polyneuropathy	Plasma exchange	I
Hyperviscosity	Plasma exchange	I
TTP	Plasma exchange	I
Immune thrombocytopenia	Protein A adsorption	II
Systemic lupus erythematosus	Plasma exchange	II
Progressive systemic sclerosis	Plasma exchange	III
Rheumatoid arthritis	Plasma exchange	III
	Lymphacytapheresis	III
Metabolic		
Refsum's disease	Plasma exchange	I
Familial hypercholesterolemia	Plasma exchange	II
	Selective adsorption	I
Poisonings	Plasma exchange	II
Grave's disease (hyperthyroidism)	Plasma exchange	III
Hematology		
Cancer (non-hematologic)	Plasma exchange	III
	Protein A adsorption	III
Immune thrombocytopenia	Plasma exchange	III
	Protein A adsorption	III

off within 8 weeks. After the circulating antibody disappears, it does not usually reappear (104). With a less aggressive treatment the autoantibodies usually disappear as early as 7 weeks up to 1 year (104) compared to 1–2 years in those who received no treatment (105). During the later course of the disease, infections of the upper respiratory tract and the vascular access site (AV shunt)

may be associated with pulmonary and renal deterioration, however, without recurrence of the autoantibody (106). In these cases, the organs primarily involved in the disease process seem to be highly sensitive to all types of inflammatory lesions which mimic the original disorder. Pulmonary hemorrhage without renal relapse also has been observed in acutely overhydrated patients in whom the

Table 5. Results of a controlled trial of plasma exchange in patients with Wegener's granulomatosis, microscopic polyarteritis and idiopathic rapidly progressive glomerulonephritis as judged by number of patients with improvement of renal function at 1 month in relation to all patients in that group. The control group received prednisolone, azathioprine and cyclophosphamide, the study group additionally plasma exchanges (mean: nine 4-litre exchanges) (107)

Renal function at presentation	Control group	Study group
Creatinine < 500 μmol/l	7/8	9/9
Creatinine > 500 μmol/l	7/7	5/5
Dialysis-dependent*	3/8	10/11

*Significant ($p = 0.024$, Fisher's exact test).

antibody production had been controlled. As both types of relapses are not caused by autoimmunity, antibiotics and/or volume reduction or removal are the treatments of choice.

Pauci-immune crescentic glomerulonephritis

This entity represents those cases of rapidly progressive glomerulonephritis in which glomerular immunoglobulin deposits, either linear or granular, are absent. Circulating antibodies against neutrophil cytoplasmic antigens (ANCA) can be detected in up to 70–80% of these patients.. Pauci-immune rapidly progressive glomerulonephritis may either be idiopathic or part of a vasculitic disease with multi-system involvement (lungs, skin, nerves, muscles). In the absence of anti-GBM antibodies, the coexistence of pulmonary infiltrates (and hemorrhages), pauci-immune rapidly progressive glomerulonephritis and ANCA is typical for Wegener's granulomatosis. According to the classification of ANCAs, the diffuse cytoplasmatic immunofluorescence pattern is mostly associated with Wegener's granulomatosis, while the perinuclear immunofluorescence is typical for the microscopic variant of polyarteritis. Treatment decision in pauci-immune rapidly progressive glomerulonephritis can be based on results of a randomized controlled trial (107). Included were patients with Wegener's granulomatosis, microscopic polyarteritis, and idiopathic rapidly progressive glomerulonephritis but excluding those with defined other causes of crescentic glomerulonephritis, e.g., Henoch-Schönlein disease, SLE. Patients were randomized according to the renal functional status at beginning of treatment and received either prednisolone, cyclophosphamide, and azathioprine or additionally plasma exchange. Nine treatments were given with an exchange volume of 4 l per session. Table 5 summarizes the outcome at 1 month. It can be seen that those patients already requiring dialysis at the start of treatment showed a significantly better outcome in the plasma exchange group compared to the controls. No such difference was observed in the two groups with less severe renal involvement at the time of diagnosis in which the response rate approaches nearly 100% with both treatment regimens. In almost all patients, the improvement was maintained during the follow-up of one year (107). In contrast to patients with anti-GBM-mediated rapidly progressive glomerulonephritis and advanced renal involvement (dialysis-dependent at start of treatment), patients with pauci-immune rapidly progressive glomerulonephritis have a good change to experience an improvement of their renal function also when requiring dialysis at presentation. Plasma exchange must not be performed in all patients with pauci-immune rapidly progressive glomerulonephritis but it considerably improves the prognosis in those with advanced functional impairment at start of treatment.

Other types of glomerulonephritis

IgA nephropathy

The renal and extrarenal deposition of IgA 1 polymers in both primary and secondary IgA nephropathy appears to be the pathogenic event (108, 109) which initiates a chronic glomerular lesion that may lead to a less than favourable prognosis. About one quarter of such patients develops endstage renal disease within 6 years. Both immunosuppressive and phenytoin therapy have shown disappointing results of renal outcome. Plasma exchange has been performed with some success in those patients in whom primary IgA nephropathy (Berger's disease) or Henoch-Schönlein nephritis are associated with rapidly progressive deterioration of renal function (110, 111). Intermittent plasma exchange (initially intensive, later on once a week) combined in most patients with cyclophosphamide (1–1.5 mg/kg) and dipyridamole showed that the decline in renal function was significantly reduced in 10 of 13 patients when the 3-month treatment period was compared to the 3-month pre study time (112). Weekly intermittent plasma exchange may delay dialysis, especially in those patients with previous rapidly progressive course. It seems that plasma exchange does not cure IgA nephropathy but may delay the progression to endstage renal failure in about 50% of patients with progressive disease (112).

Membranoproliferative glomerulonephritis type II

C3 nephritic factor, an IgG autoantibody directed against the C3-B-complex stabilizing the C3 convertase activity of the alternative complement pathway, plays the central pathogenic role in membranoproliferative glomerulonephritis type II. Usually this disease progresses slowly to end-stage renal failure. Its course is uninfluenced by the use of cytotoxic drugs. Several anecdotal reports have been published showing moderate response to treatment with plasma exchange performed in patients with this form of glomerulonephritis (113).

Lupus nephritis

In situ immune complex formation (114) and the deposition of circulating immune complexes are involved in the renal lesions of lupus nephritis. Among the different types of glomerulonephritis, diffuse proliferative lupus nephritis has the poorest prognosis both in respect to renal function and to overall patient survival (22% 5-year survival) (115). The application of plasma exchange in systemic lupus erythematosus was first reported in 1976 (116). Since then hundreds of patients have undergone plasma exchange even though, in most cases, they were treated outside of randomized protocols. Logically there appear to be two reasons to justify the use of plasma exchange in patients with lupus erythematosus. Such therapy can be expected to remove circulating autoantibodies directed against nuclear constituents (e.g., dsDNA), peripheral blood cells and coagulation factors (117) or to remove circulating immune complexes present in lupus sera. Also deficient complement proteins, e.g., C3 and C4 are usually decreased in active disease and may be replaced by the use of fresh frozen plasma as substitution fluid. These considerations form the basis for applying plasma exchange in systemic lupus (117). Reported situations in which plasma exchange had been applied between 1975 and 1985 were: progressive renal and extrarenal organ involvement including leuko- and thrombocytopenia, and the requirement of high dose steroids to control disease activity.

Progressive renal failure responded to standard immunosuppression combined with plasma exchange in a mean of 69% in uncontrolled studies (117). Under controlled conditions, however, the additional use of plasma exchange has failed to confirm significant differences in the outcome when compared to standard treatment (118, 119). In a very large randomized controlled study published in 1992, a total of 86 patients with severe lupus nephritis were enrolled (120). In both groups (standard immunosuppressive drug treatment *vs* additional plasma exchange) 30–40% of the patients had a remission of their lupus nephritis. The frequency of negative outcomes (death or renal failure) was also the same in both groups. The authors concluded that the addition of plasma exchange to standard immunosuppression did not improve the outcome of lupus nephritis (120). In 1986, Austin et al. (121) published their study using high dose cyclophosphamide pulse therapy without plasma exchange in lupus. Because of the excellent results, this regimen became the treatment of choice for severe lupus nephritis. Another randomized multicenter study in severe lupus investigates whether the application of plasma exchange and subsequent pulse cyclophosphamide is more effective than repeated cyclophosphamide pulses alone (122). The administration of high-dose cyclophosphamide following a course of plasma exchanges has been referred to as the 'synchronization' concept (27, 123) and has been applied in small series of patients mostly with SLE with some success in the early 1980s (overview: 122). Results from the randomized international multicenter study can be expect-

ed not earlier than in 1996 (122). Despite the results from controlled studies, plasma exchange has its place in the management of individual cases with progressive disease, especially when not responding to standard treatment, and in life threatening complications of the systemic lupus erythematosus.

Polyarteritis nodosa and Churg–Strauss disease

Classic polyarteritis nodosa (PAN) is a multisystem necrotizing vasculitis of small and medium-sized arteries typically involving the renal and visceral but not pulmonary arteries. Some patients experience a rapid decline of renal function. Similar to classic PAN, allergic angiitis and granulomatosis is generally called Churg–Strauss-disease (CSD). CSD predominantly involves pulmonary arteries, capillaries and veins with additional granuloma formation. Leading clinical symptoms are asthmatic attacks and a striking eosinophilia. Other organs (skin, heart, kidneys, peripheral nerves, gastrointestinal tract) are also affected. The 5-year survival rates in untreated PAN and CSD are poor and do not exceed 13% and 25% respectively. With steroids the 5-year survival has been reported to be around 50% in both disorders, and the combined administration of prednisone and cyclophosphamide has resulted in (complete) remissions in up to 90%. A special aspect was analyzed in a French multicenter study in which 46 patients with PAN and CSD were randomly treated either with steroids and plasma exchange or with additional cyclophosphamide. Using cyclophosphamide showed no additional beneficial effect on 5-year survivals with 82% *vs* 77% (difference not significant) (124).

Hemolytic uremic syndrome; thrombotic thrombocytopenic purpura

Hemolytic uremic syndrome (HUS) and thrombotic thrombocytopenic purpura (TTP) represent expressions of an endotheliotropic hemolytic angiopathy with severe renal involvement (125). HUS is more common in children than in adults. Clinical presentation includes progressive renal failure associated with hemolytic anemia and thrombocytopenia. In addition to the above mentioned findings, fluctuating neurological symptoms and fever are characteristic for TTP. The typical histological lesions result from microthrombi consisting primarily of platelets. These can be found in the capillaries of virtually every tissue including skin and kidneys (125, 126). Both diseases develop as a result of extensive endothelial injury with not only renal (HUS, TTP) but also generalized (TTP) organ involvement. Etiology remains unknown in most cases. Triggering mechanisms include: preceding bacterial or viral infections, post partum and drug exposure (cyclosporine A, antineoplastic drugs, and contraceptives) (125, 126). Several mechanisms have been proposed to be operative in the pathogenesis of HUS and TTP (125–127): 1) lack of prostacyclin or a releasing factor from the vascular endothelium to prevent generalized intravascular coagulation, 2) lack of plasma factor necessary to degrade factor VIII: von Willebrand factor multimers (which potently trigger platelet agglutination under certain circumstances), 3) lack of plasma factor (probably an IgG) which inactivates a 'platelet aggregating factor', and 4) endothelial injury mediated by free radicals due to their reduced degradation (e.g., vitamin E deficiency).

In the late 1940s, the mortality rate of HUS in children was nearly 50%. It has decreased to 4 to 13% during recent years, primarily related to better supportive care (125). Generally, a favorable prognosis can be anticipated in children with either HUS or TTP. Plasma infusion therapy in children has influenced neither acute mortality nor long term prognosis (128). The prognosis of TTP has also improved in adults. Previously, patient survival rate was but 28% at 3 months (129). Recently, using different therapeutic regimens, remissions can be induced in 80 to 90% of the afflicted patients (129). Most published treatment regimens for HUS and TTP include infusion of fresh frozen plasma (FFP) or plasma exchange with FFP replacement. Each is combined with antiplatelet agents and/or corticosteroids. The replacement of a missing as yet undefined serum factor is the rationale for FFP infusions. In cases refractory to standard treatment (daily plasma exchanges using FFP as replacement), plasma from which the cryoprecipitate has been removed should be used (cryosupernatant plasma). All seven patients responding inadequately to intensive plasma exchange improved quickly when they were switched to receive cryosupernatant plasma in place of whole plasma (130). There are indications that very large von Willebrand factor (vWF) multimers may play a major role in causing the microthrombi in TTP (131) and that the largest vWF multimers are concentrated in cryoprecipitate. In a prospective randomized trial, the Canadian Apheresis Study Group compared plasma exchange therapy (7 treatments in the first nine days) with plasma infusion (30 ml per kg of body weight, daily for 9 days). Response rate and survival showed that plasma exchange is superior to plasma infusion in the treatment of TTP, both at the end of the first 9-day treatment cycle and after six months (133). Based on the results of this randomized study and from other published data, a polypragmatic therapeutic regimen including plasma exchange with FFP replacement, platelet aggregation inhibitors and corticosteroids is recommended for TTP as soon as the diagnosis is confirmed. In cases not responding to this treatment, cryosupernatant plasma should be used as replacement (130).

Renal involvement in paraproteinemia

About one half of the patients with multiple myeloma develop renal failure. These patients usually have a poor prognosis. Factors pathogenetically involved in myeloma renal failure include tubular and glomerular damage by light chains, amyloid deposition, hypercalcemia, hyperuricemia, hyperviscosity (rarely), interstitial infiltration by plasma cells, and acute renal failure following intravenous contrast media. The major fraction of the free light chains (22,000 Daltons) which are filtered by the glomeruli is readsorbed and catabolized by tubular cells. Precipitation of light chains in the distal tubules and a direct toxic effect on tubular cells are the pathogenetic mechanisms in paraproteinemic acute renal failure. Hypercalcemia, present in about 50% of these cases (134, 135), can also precipitate acute renal failure. Paraproteinemic acute renal failure is one of the few established indications for therapeutic plasma exchange. Of 142 patients suffering from this condition, 40% retained adequate renal function following plasma exchange (136). To reduce light chain synthesis, concomitant cytotoxic therapy should be administered. In a randomized controlled prospective study enrolling 29 patients with acute renal failure due to multiple myeloma, the patient group treated by plasma exchange, steroids, cyclophosphamide (and hemodialysis when necessary) had a better prognosis than the controls treated by steroids, cyclophosphamide and intermittent peritoneal dialysis if required (137). Statistically significant differences in favor of the plasma exchange group were found with respect to the number of patients in whom renal replacement therapy could be stopped; the serum creatinine at the end of the second month and the survival at one year. Overall survival was positively correlated with the recovery of renal failure (137). Renal failure in paraproteinemia, especially when light chains are involved, is an indication for plasma exchange and cytotoxic treatment.

If renal failure in these patients fails to respond to an adequate course of plasma exchange, factors other than light chain toxicity should be considered in kidney damage (e.g., amyloidosis, hypercalcemia, hyperuricemia) (137).

Mixed essential cryoglobulinemia

Mixed essential cryoglobulinemia is associated with a multisystem organ involvement primarily with skin rash, Raynaud's phenomenon, arthralgias, neuropathy and in half of the cases also secondary mesangiocapillary (membranoproliferative) glomerulonephritis (93, 138). Symptomatic relief of the purpuric rash and arthralgias is reported following plasma exchange, however, due to resynthesis of the cryoglobulins intermittent treatments are necessary to keep the patient free of symptoms. According to the underlying disorder of mixed essential cryoglobulinemia (e.g., lymphoma, Waldenström's disease, hepatitis B or C) plasmapheresis should be combined with an appropriate cytotoxic or immunomodulatory treatment to prevent rapid resynthesis. In cases with progressive renal involvement intermittent plasma exchange has been applied mostly combined with steroids and cytotoxic drugs resulting in stabilization or improvement of renal function in some patients (138). To maintain an adequate renal function, repeated plasma exchange treatment is necessary in intervals depending on the clinical response and the cryoglobulin resynthesis rate (138).

Plasmapheresis in renal transplantation

Removal of preformed lymphocytotoxic antibodies prior to transplantation

The presence of lymphocytotoxic antibodies against multiple HLA antigens may limit kidney transplantation in some dialysis patients. Plasma exchange has been performed in some highly sensitized individuals with the aim of removing these antibodies. To suppress further antibody synthesis, plasma exchange was combined with an immunosuppressive regimen. Nine of 18 patients showed a significant decrease in cytotoxic anti-HLA antibodies (139, 140) and were transplanted, six of them successfully. More recent studies with immunoadsorption using Protein-A-Sepharose columns to eliminate anti-HLA antibodies have reported both an appreciable reduction of these titers which enabled successful transplantation (141, 142) and a failure (143). Despite concomitant immunosuppressive treatment, rapid antibody resynthesis remains a major problem in this special situation.

Plasma exchange in renal transplant rejections

Plasma exchange has been used for treatment of acute and chronic rejection during post transplant course. The type of rejection (cellular or humoral/vascular) was confirmed by biopsy in but a few studies. According to a literature overview (144), 127 of 214 acute (59%) and five of 26 chronic (19%) rejections responded to plasma exchange. The response rate of 0 to 93% at different centers may be explained by differences in entry criteria and treatment protocols.

Controlled studies of acute rejections exhibited an overall successful outcome (61%) in the plasma exchange group compared to 51% in the controls (144). One prospective controlled trial used plasma exchange randomly in all acute transplant rejection episodes (85 patients). During the entire 4 year study period, the graft survival rate was better in the plasma exchange group than in the patients treated with conventional antirejection therapy (145). Paying special attention to anti-HLA antibodies an Italian group treated steroid resistant rejections in 44 patients in a randomized protocol, either by plasmapheresis or by pharmacological therapy alone. The rate of graft failures was lower in the plasma exchange group (7/23) than in the controls (17/21) (146).

In conclusion, some patients benefit from plasma exchange performed in acute kidney transplant rejection of either vascular or cellular variety. However, the data as a whole are derived from quite different entry and treatment protocols and do not yet allow a specification of subgroups for whom plasmapheresis can be recommended as standard therapy.

Recurrent glomerular disease in the transplanted kidney

A recurrence of primary renal disease in the transplanted organ was the reason for plasma exchange in occasional patients suffering from lupus nephritis, mesangial proliferative glomerulonephritis, anti-GBM nephritis, and focal segmental glomerulosclerosis (FSGS). In a few cases renal function or proteinuria improved (147, 148). This is especially true for recurrent FSGS where remissions have been reported. Thus, therapeutic plasma exchange can be attempted for those rare cases of recurrent primary renal disease in a transplant recipient (111).

CONCLUSIONS – PLASMA EXCHANGE

During the past two decades plasma exchange performed either by centrifugal or membrane-based equipment has become routine therapy in many hospitals. Its application is still accompanied by a certain risk posed by administration of substitution fluids. Plasma fractionation procedures offer more selective plasma manipulation especially in diseases with well characterized macromolecular circulating pathogens. The ability to remove specific pathogens still exceeds our knowledge of disease processes. This may, however, contribute to a more detailed understanding of disease pathogenesis.

Data are available from but a few conclusive controlled studies for some distinct situations in several disorders. Consequently, the physician's therapeutic decision must be influenced not only by published data but also by his experience with the disease process and extracorporeal immuno-modulating therapy.

HEMOPERFUSION

Hemoperfusion, the passage of blood over sorbent particles, has been used for the treatment of drug and chemical poisoning, uremia, hepatic encephalopathy and immunoadsorption. Other, less definitive, uses have been in schizophrenia and psoriasis – such uses having recently fallen into disfavor. In the area of uremia sorbent hemoperfusion has been used to increase the efficiency of the dialysis procedure, and its extension sorbent regeneration of dialysate is now fully accepted in the clinical management of uremia.

Principles of hemoperfusion

Hemoperfusion is the direct contact of blood with a sorbent system contained in devices which consist of plastic housings to incorporate the sorbent particulates within them. Blood usually flows in a laminar fashion over the sorbent particles which have been rendered biocompatible by the coating of the surface with a polymer membrane such as cellulose nitrate. The circuitry used for hemop-

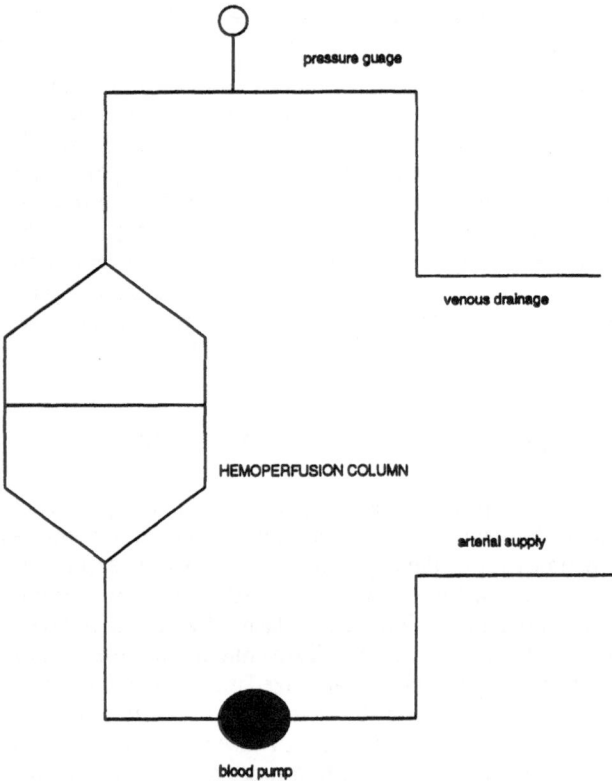

Figure 7. The circuitry used for hemoperfusion.

erfusion is similar to dialysis (Figure 7), and for blood contact anticoagulation is necessary with heparin and/or prostacyclin. Any coagulation occurring within the system is reflected in a rise in pressure in gauges placed on venous and arterial lines supplying and draining the device. Depending on the situation, blood flow through the devices ranges from 100 ml/min up to 300 ml/min. The systems can be combined with dialysis which can be used to warm the blood in patients who may be intoxicated and hypothermic, and also to increase the efficiency of the entire system.

Sorbents

Typical sorbents are activated carbons (charcoals), ion exchange resins, or non-ionic macroporous resins. Activated charcoals are available in many forms, but originally consisted of uncoated granular carbons in the loose-bed form, or fixed-bed form with particles attached to the backing (Becton Dickinson USA, now unavailable). Modern devices, however, use granular coated charcoal coated with albumin cellulose nitrate (collodion) (Chang's research model), or with acrylic hydrogel polymer (Hemocol) (Smith & Nephew, UK)), or heparinized co-polymer (Clark, USA). Further devices containing charcoals are prepared from extruded charcoal coated with cellulose acetate (AB Gambro, Sweden) or with

methacrylic hydrogel (Technologie, Biomediche, Italy and Organon Teknika, Netherlands). Other columns contain spherical charcoals derived from pyrolized macroporous resins or from petroleum and coated with albumin-collodion solutions (Hemosorba, Asahi Medical Inc, Japan). Other columns containing petroleum based charcoal coated with cellulose nitrate are now available in North America, (DiaKart (BioMicro-encapsulation Technology, Canada) and HemoKart or AluKart (Erika, USA). Two other cartridges containing cellulose nitrate (collodion) coated petroleum based spherical charcoal (Teijin Co, Ltd, Japan) or pitch-based polyhema coated spherical charcoal (Kuraray Co, Japan) are available The non-ionic resin XAD-4, which is a macroporous cross-lined polystyrene amberlite, is available in Europe (Braun, Germany). The latter contains 650 g (wet weight of washed heat sterilized pyrogen free XAD-4). Devices used in clinical studies contain between 70 g and 300 g of activated charcoal coated with polymer membranes ranging in thickness from 0.05 to 0.5 microns The details of each sorbent device are given below in the section on clinical studies of hemoperfusion in uremia and in Table 6.

Activated charcoals are in the main prepared from biological substances, for instance, coconut shells, sawdust, coal, peat, dust or molasses or from non-biological substances such as petroleum or pitch (149). While the physical properties are more influenced by the activation process, the choice of starting materials for activated carbons produces such characteristics as fine pore distribution. Activation is induced by controlled oxidation in air, carbon dioxide or steam, and a maximal adsorptive capacity is sought which will give a high surface porosity and large surface area (approximately 1,000 m^2/g). The pores are classified by the size of the radius which determines the efficiency of adsorption into micropores (< than 20 Å), transitional pores (20 to 500 Å) and macropores (radius equal to or greater than 500 Å). Some carbons also have the ability for chemisorption (which implies the formation of chemical bonds or chemical conversion of the compound under study). In general, non-polar solutes are better adsorbed from aqueous solution than are polar solutes. The rate limiting step for coated carbon is diffusion occurring through the polymer membrane, in contra-distinction to uncoated carbon where the rate limiting step is pore diffusion. For medical use in hemoperfusion devices activated carbons should possess the following qualities: freedom from microparticulates, washability, resistance to attrition, high adsorptive capacity, smooth surface morphology, low microparticle generation, minimal elution of toxic ions, high blood compatibility and easy sterilization, low toxicity and low pyrogenicity. These qualities which determine the manufacturer's choice of charcoal for hemoperfusion devices have been reviewed (149).

The macroporous resins are non-ionic gel type resins formed in beads by an agglomerate of microspheres cross-linked to a high degree, giving less swelling of the beads in solution. They have a high ability to adsorb organic solutes

Table 6. Available hemoperfusion devices

Manufacturer	Device	Sorbent type	Amount of sorbent	Polymer coating
Bioencapsulation Technology	DiaKart	Petroleum based charcoal	70 g	collodion
Clark	Biocompatible system	Charcoal	50, 100, 250 cc	heparinized polymer
Erika	Hemokart or Alukart	Petroleum based charcoal	60 or 155 g	collodion
Gambro	Adsorba	Norit	100 or 300 g	cellulose acetate
Organon-Teknika	Hemopur 260	Norit extruded charcoal	260 g	cellulose acetate
Smith and Nephew	Hemocol or Haemocol	Sucliffe Speakman charcoal	100 or 300 g	Acrylic Hydrogel
Braun	Haemoresin	XAD-4	350 g	none

Table 7. Putative uremic toxins removed by sorbents (molecular weight range 60 to 21,500 Daltons)

Adrenocorticotrophin	Middle molecule peaks[a]
(Aldosterone)[a]	Myoinositol
Amino acids[a]	Non-protein nitrogen
Calcium[a]	Norepinephrine
25,0H cholecalciferol[a]	Organic acids[a]
Creatinine[a]	Oxalate[a]
Cyclic AMP	Parathyroid hormone
Epinephrine	Phenols[a]
Folic acid[b]	(Phosphate)[a]
Fibronectin	Polyamino acids
Gastrin	(Renin)[a]
Glucagon	Ribonuclease
Glucose[a]	Serotonin
(Growth hormone)[a]	Guanidines
Trace metals: As, Co, Cr, Se (Magnesium)[a]	Indoles[a]
Triglycerides[a]	Insulin[a]
Thyroxine,[a] Triiodothyronine[a]	L-dopamine
(Urea)[a]	Lysozyme
Uric acid[a]	Vitamin B_{12}

[a] Studied during hemoperfusion in uremic patients.
[b] Unpublished. ( ) Incompletely removed.

on the surface with areas of 300 to 500 m^2/g. Uncharged macroporous resins, for example, XAD-4 and XAD-7, are similar to activated charcoal although they adsorb with less energetic forces. Consequently adsorption is more reversible than organic sorbents such as activated carbon. Elution of organic solutes from XAD-4 (e.g., barbiturates, methaqualone, and glutethimide) is more readily attained with the use of organic solutes such as methanol or ethanol than can be achieved with activated charcoal.

Solute spectrum adsorbed and the effects of coating adsorbents

Activated charcoal will absorb the uremic solutes shown in Table 7. The molecular weight of solutes being removed ranges from 60 to 21,500 Daltons, both *in vitro* and *in vivo*. For substances of low molecular mass, (creatinine (113 Daltons), uric acid (168 Daltons), hippuran (363 Daltons), vitamin B_{12} (1355 Daltons)), the cellulose coating reduces adsorption only slightly. At higher molecular weights, however, i.e., above 3550 Daltons, substantial reduction of adsorption occurs with polymer coating(150). Nevertheless, it is the capacity to adsorb molecules of 'middle molecular weight' size (300 to 1500 Daltons), that stimulated much interest in activated charcoal hemoperfusion in uremia, although this is less important now with the use of macroporous membranes used in dialysis such as polysulfone and polyacrylonitrile etc. Some biologically important small solutes are also adsorbed, such as, glucose, calcium, amino acids and middle molecules, all of which exhibit finite saturation rates for adsorption. Hormones have also been removed by charcoal hemoperfusion *in vivo* as have important trace metals, such as arsenic, cobalt, chromium and selenium.

Adverse effects of hemoperfusion

Particle embolization, a feature of the early poorly washed devices has been largely overcome by selecting charcoal resistant to attrition, using polymer coatings and by commercial washing procedures. The major side effect of early hemoperfusion devices with uncoated carbon was mainly related to platelet depletion. However, this has been reduced considerably with microencapsulation techniques (151, 152) to give mean platelet losses of 30%. Transient leukopenia similar to that observed during hemodialysis, also occurs during hemoperfusion in man, and may be a result of complement activation by surface contact in a similar manner to that observed during hemodialysis (153). Adsorption or activation of coagulation factors has also been observed during clinical hemoperfusion. The most significant change is a small reduction in fibrinogen concentration (and fibronectin) even with polymer coated activated charcoal devices (151, 152, 154). No appreciable changes in coagulation factors II to XII have been observed as a response to charcoal hemoperfusion in uremia (154). Although the side effects are minimal in nature, this has stimulated research for more biocompatible activated carbon adsorbents.

Hemostatic changes may be particularly severe in patients with hepatic failure (see below) and may be associated with production of platelet aggregates (155), although this has not been observed in uremic patients treated with charcoal hemoperfusion (154). Some observations suggest that vasoactive amines may be responsible for hypotension and may be released from platelet aggregates during hemoperfusion in hepatic coma (155). This led either to *in vitro* testing of pretreatment with sulfinpyrazone or aspirin (156), or prostacyclin (157) alone or in conjunction with heparin for patients undergoing hemoperfusion for hepatic coma; such treatment resulted in less platelet aggregation or depletion in such patients or a reduction in the degree of hypotension.

As mentioned above, hemoperfusion may also result in calcium or glucose removal, but this is transient since saturation of the devices occurs. Similarly, reduction in body temperature may occur during hemoperfusion by infusion of unheated blood products, but also as mentioned above, dialysis combined with hemoperfusion does result in blood warming and reverses this process. Pyrogenic reactions are not observed with modern devices but were seen with previous devices. In chronic use measured blood losses within devices are between 3.1 and 7 ml (158, 159).

Hemoperfusion and uremia

Historical background: Introduced in 1948 by Muirhead and Reid (160), and later by Schreiner in 1958 (161), ion exchange resins were used, in the former in uremia and in the latter in pentobarbital poisoning. These early studies were complicated by pyrogenic reactions, electrolyte disturbances and hemolysis and fell into disfavor. It was not until 1964 that Yatzidis reported that uncoated activated charcoal hemoperfusion in a device containing 200 g of charcoal derived from coconut shells, could absorb *in vitro*, barbital, phenobarbital, pentobarbital and salicylic acid, as well as glutethimide (162). Extension to uremia in man demonstrated that the uremic toxins, creatinine, uric acid, guanidine, indoles, phenolic compounds and organic acids, could be removed more efficiently than with the then current dialysis equipment. In 1965 Yatzidis and colleagues (163) demonstrated that uncoated charcoal hemoperfusion resulted in the recovery of consciousness in two patients with barbiturate poisoning after several sessions of hemoperfusion lasting one hour each. The side effects seen were, transient facial flushing and dyspnea and a burning sensation, along with platelet depletion and reduction of plasma fibrinogen concentrations. Later,

Dunea and Kolff (164) confirmed Yatzidis' observation on the removal of uremic toxins.

In 1966, Chang demonstrated that microencapsulation within polymers did not inhibit the adsorption on charcoal of uremic solutes, but did result in less platelet adsorption (151). He also confirmed that creatinine and urate clearances with hemoperfusion alone in man were greater than current and conventional hemodialysis of the time. These reports stimulated others to investigate, in short term studies, the solutes removed and the utility of using hemoperfusion in uremia (for full discussion of this particular aspect of hemoperfusion in uremia, see 3rd edition of this text). Table 8 gives data from selected short-term and long-term studies of charcoal hemoperfusion in uremia. Specifically, clinical improvements in 'well being', nerve conduction velocity in some but not in others, pericarditis, peripheral neuropathy and hypercoagulability, and reduction in dialysis time have been reported in the long term studies of charcoal hemoperfusion combined with dialysis in uremia. The major problem relates however, to the increased cost with the addition of hemoperfusion to standard hemodialysis, and to the availability now of highly efficient membranes which have increased the spectrum of solutes that can be removed with high efficiency/high flux dialysis.

In summary, hemoperfusion in uremia has some advantages but these have largely been overshadowed by modern dialyzers containing macroporous membranes. The devices used for hemoperfusion in uremia shown in Table 8, result in negligible urea clearance, and substantially increased creatinine, urate and middle molecule clearance with the addition of hemoperfusion to dialysis.

Potential clinical benefits

The potential clinical benefits relate to the wider spectrum of adsorptive qualities of charcoal and improvements in uremic symptomatology reported in various studies. The absence of urea, water, electrolyte and hydrogen ion removal however, renders it necessary to combine hemoperfusion with dialytic or ultrafiltration removal of water and solutes. The theoretical hybrid devices combining hemodialysis with hemoperfusion have not yet been devised. At present, the combination of charcoal hemoperfusion and hemodialysis improves upon the removal of iron-deferoxamine complex or aluminum-deferoxamine in patients with metal overload syndromes (170–173); at present this stands at the major reason for combined hemodialysis, hemoperfusion.

Hemoperfusion and drug intoxication

Of the large numbers of patients presenting with poisoning, only a minority of patients require intervention for drug removal. Data from the American Association of Poison Control Centers (174) indicate that a total of 1.75 million poisonings were reported in 1993. While the

Table 8. Selected short-term and long-term studies of hemoperfusion in uremia

First author (ref.)	System	Short-term (S) or long-term (L) (months)	Solutes removed and comments	Adverse effects
Yatzidis (162)	Uncoated Merck charcoal, 200 g, HP alone	S	U, Cr, UA, P, G, I, O	platelets fell 50%, fibrinogen fell, pyrexia, hypotension
Chang (165)	Fisher ACAC, 300 g, HP alone	S	Cr, UA	platelets fell 8%, pyrexia
Winchester (154)	Sutcliffe Speakman acrylic hydrogel coated, 300 g, HP alone or with HD	S	Cr, UA, MMs	platelets fell 30%, fibrinogen fell, aluminum encephalopathy unchanged
Asaba (166)	Norit cellulose acetate coated charcoal, 300 g, HP alone	S	MMs removed equal to PAN dialysis	–
Chang (158)	ACAC 300 g, with HD or UF, 1 session/week	L, 3 months	Cr, UA, MMs	NCV improved
Bonomini (167)	Norit hydroxymethacrylate coated, 150 g, 2 sessions/week	L, 1–36 (mean 7.5) months	Cr, UA, vitamin B_{12}	NCV and well-being improved, no fall in platelets, hypotension, pyrexia
Henderson (168)	Sutcliffe Speakman acrylic hydrogel coated, 300 g, HP/HD 3 sessions/week	L, 10 months	–	Improved well-being
Chang (169)	ACAC Diakart, 70 g, HP/HD 3 sessions/week	L, 6 month crossover, with 12 hours HD		no difference in biochemistry between HP/HD and HD alone

HP = hemoperfusion, HD = hemodialysis, U = urea, Cr = creatinine, UA = uric acid, P = phosphate, G = guanidines, Ca = calcium, I = indoles, O = organic acids, MMs = middle molecualr weight substances, AAs = amino acids, NCV = nerve conduction velocity

vast majority were treated at home, active intervention was used commonly, (749,371 by decontamination of the gastro-intestinal tract, 7,398 had alkalization of the urine. Hemodialysis was used in 646 patients, hemoperfusion in 64, and another extracorporeal procedure in 80.

Treatment of poisoned patients follows management guidelines which have been well tested and includes intensive and conservative supportive care (175). With this, mortality has dropped, e.g., in sedative poisoning from 25% in 1945 to less than 1% in 1966 (175). Mortality from severe sedative poisoning ranges from 8.3% to 34% (176), but these figures apply to drugs such as glutethimide and phenobarbital that are not widely used today. In very severely poisoned patients the guidelines proposed by Maher and Schreiner (177), apply to the use of dialytic techniques. Sorbent hemoperfusion has long been used in the treatment of severely drug intoxicated patients and has been reviewed in depth (178–181). Hemodialysis is more suitable for highly diffusible substances while hemoperfusion is more efficient for removal of lipid soluble drugs and protein bound drugs. The extraction ratio (the percent of drug removed in a single passage over a device) for

Table 9. Plasma drug extraction ratios with different hemodialysis/hemoperfusion devices[a]

	Standard hemodialysis charcoal	Coated or uncoated hemoperfusion	XAD-2 or XAD-4 resin hemoperfusion
Acetaminophen	0.4	0.5	0.7
Amobarbital	0.26	0.3	0.9
Acetylsalicylic acid	0.5	0.5	–
Carbromal	0.31	0.55	1.0
Digoxin	0.2	0.3–0.6	0.4
Ethchlorvynol	0.32	0.7	1.0
Glutethimide	0.16	0.65	0.8
Paraquat	0.5	0.6	0.9[b]
Phenobarbital	0.27	0.5	0.85
Theophylline	0.5	0.7	0.75
Tricyclics	0.35	0.35	0.8

[a] Calculated for blood flow rate 200 ml/min.
[b] Ion exchange resin.

certain drugs such as salicylates is similar for hemodialysis and hemoperfusion, while barbiturates and other lipid soluble drugs are more efficiently removed by hemoperfusion at the same blood flow rates and drug concentrations, than by dialysis (Table 9).

Clinical and laboratory studies

Table 10 gives a list of drugs removed by various hemoperfusion devices *in vitro* and *in vivo*. Most studies have dealt principally with activated charcoal hemoperfusion, less commonly with non-ionic macroporous resin hemoperfusion and rarely with ion exchange resin hemoperfusion. While XAD-4 resin is more specific for lipid soluble drugs, activated charcoal is less specific and can be used in a wide variety of clinical intoxications. Several *in vivo* studies in animals and clinical studies in man have shown that drug elimination can be substantially enhanced with hemoperfusion, while some studies have utilized pharmacokinetic principles to determine the efficiency of hemoperfusion (182–185).

Side effects seen with hemoperfusion in poisoning are similar to those in the treatment of uremia, and include thrombocytopenia, as well as adsorption of calcium and glucose (186). These side effects are usually transitory as well as mild. Repetitive hemoperfusion might be required in drug intoxication with drugs such as glutethimide, ethchlorvynol and other drugs which possess slow intercompartmental transfer rates and large volumes of distribution (187). Several have questioned the use of hemoperfusion on kinetic grounds for certain drugs arguing that conservative management alone is associated with a favorable clinical outcome (188).

These studies fail to account for the geographic variations in poisoning severity, such that consideration should be given to hemoperfusion or dialysis in severe cases with specific toxins. Small retrospective and prospective studies have suggested benefit from hemoperfusion, although it has not been possible to conduct large scale clinical trials (189). Therefore, reliance is based on clinical judgement and the guidelines in Table 11, sometimes combined with drug concentrations. (For the latter it is rare for single drug intoxications to occur, since most patients take mixed drug combinations. In this situation plasma levels of drugs are less reliable while combination of multiple agents may make the patient much more seriously ill).

Hemodialysis is more suited to the removal of poisons such as methanol, ethanol, ethylene glycol and salicylate poisoning since each of these drugs carries a risk of profound acidosis or formation of toxic metabolite(s). The primary goal is to correct the acidosis and remove the offending agent or metabolite (190).

Controversial areas where hemoperfusion remains of dubious benefit are in acetaminophen (191) and amitryptiline (192) poisoning, and unproven in paraquat poisoning (193–195). In regard to the latter, Okonek and others (194) have shown that it is possible to successfully treat patients with repetitive hemoperfusion and achieve

Table 10. Drugs and chemicals removed with hemoperfusion

Barbiturates	Antimicrobials/ anticancer	Cardiovascular
amobarbital	(adriamycin)[†]	digoxin
butabarbital	ampicillin	diltiazem
hexabarbital	carmustine[†]	(disopyramide)
pentobarbital	chloramphenicol	flecainide
phenobarbital	chloroquine	metoprolol
quinalbital	clindamycin	n-acetylprocainamide
secobarbital	dapsone	procainamide
thiopental	doxorubicin	quinidine
vinalbital	gentamicin	
	isoniazid	*Miscellaneous*
Nonbarbiturate	(methotrexate)	aminophylline
hypnotics, sedatives	thiabendazole	cimetidine
and tranquilizers	(5-fluorouracil)	(fluoroacetamide)
carbromal		(phencyclidine)
chloral hydrate	*Antidepressants*	phenols
chlorpromazine	(amitryptiline)	(podophyllin)
(diazepam)	(imipramine)	theophylline
diphenhydramine	(tricyclics)	
ethchlorvynol		
glutethimide		*Solvents, gases*
meprobamate	*Plant and animal*	carbon tetrachloride
methaqualone	*toxins, herbicides,*	ethylene oxide
methsuximide	*insecticides*	trichloroethane
methyprylon	amanitin	xylene
promazine	chlordane	
promethazine	demeton sulfoxide	*Metals*
(valproic acid)	dimethoate	(aluminum)*
	diquat	(iron)*
	methylparathion	
Analgesics,	nitrostigmine	
antirheumatic	(organophosphates)	
acetaminophen	phalloidin	
acetylsalicylic acid	polychlorinated biphenyls	
colchicine	paraquat	
d-propoxyphyene	parathion	
methylsalicylate		
phenylbutazone		
salicylic acid		

( ) Not well removed.
( )* Removed with chelating agent.
[†] Well removed in regional hemoperfusion.

survival of patients who would not otherwise survive (with serum concentrations of paraquat in relation to time exceeding the statistical cut-off point between survival and non-survival) (194). Animal studies in the removal of methotrexate and anthracycline antibiotics (doxorubicin) were initially encouraging for extension to clinical use (184, 196, 197). However, the plasma concentrations of the drugs in question are low and the volume of distribution is high, such that it is unlikely that reduction of

Table 11. Clinical and drug concentration* criteria for hemoperfusion in poisoning

Clinical	Drug Serum conc	(µg/ml)	(µmol/l)	Method of choice
1. Progressive deterioration despite intensive care.	Phenobarbital	100	430	HP > HD
	Other barbiturates	50	200	HP
	Glutethimide	40	180	HP
2. Severe intoxication with mid-brain dysfunction.	Methaqualone	40	160	HP
	Salicylates	800	5,000	HD
	Theophylline	400	2,200	HP > HD
3. Development of complications of coma.	Paraquat	0.1	0.5	HP > HD
	Trichloroethanol	50	335	HP > HD
	Meprobamate	100	460	HP
4. Impairment of normal drug excretory function.				
5. Intoxication with agents producing metabolic and/or delayed effects.				
6. Intoxication with an extractable drug which can be removed at a greater rate than endogenous elimination.				

*Suggested concentrations only: Clinical condition may warrant intervention at lower concentrations, e.g., in mixed intoxications.

tissue levels be achievable (the site of the toxicity of these drugs) unless very prolonged therapy was undertaken. These remarks do not apply to removal of drugs in the distribution phase, which has been associated with success in methotrexate removal (198), or to the successful removal of anticancer drugs from regional circulation (199, 200).

In digitalis poisoning, hemoperfusion has been used with success in both animals and in man, accompanied by increased drug elimination rates, reduction in plasma digitalis concentrations, and reduction in digitalis half-life (201–203). Other studies, however, have reported disappointing outcomes in digoxin poisoning (204), and it is our recommendation that hemoperfusion in digitalis poisoning be reserved for those end stage renal disease patients who become digitalis intoxicated. Administration of Fab fragments of digitalis antibodies, can reverse digitalis poisoning (205). In renal failure patients, however, while associated with initial success, recrudescence of poisoning some 24 to 48 hours later occurs (206). These remarks apply specifically to renal failure subjects in whom renal function is very important for the excretion of the digoxin by the dissociation of digoxin from its Fab binding protein.

Indications for hemoperfusion in intoxication

As mentioned above, patients who fit the criteria for severe progressive drug intoxication should be considered for hemoperfusion as well as dialysis. These criteria are given in Table 11. Drug concentrations may be a guide to determining severity of toxicity, but for some the toxic concentration may be unknown (diquat and amanita phalloides).

Aluminum overload as well as iron intoxication has also been treated with combined hemoperfusion and chelating agent therapy (170–173). Heavy metals and their

Table 12. Substances relevant to hepatic failure removed with sorbent hemoperfusion

Amino acids*	Fatty acids – oleic, hexanoic,
Aromatic > branched chain	octanoic N-valeric
(Ammonia)*	(Glucose)*
Bile acids*	Mercaptan
Bilirubin*	Middle molecules
(Calcium)*	Norepinephrine
Coagulation factors*	Octopamine
(Cyclic AMP)*	Phenols*
Dopamine	Protein bound molecules
Epinephrine	Inhibitor of Na/K ATPase*

*Studied in vivo.
( ) Ineffectively removed.

salts are not removed efficiently with dialysis or hemoperfusion alone (207–209), but removal may be enhanced with certain chelating agents such as n-acetylcysteine or cysteine (210, 211). Mercury and thallium removal with hemoperfusion appears modest at best (207–209). Chelating microspheres or chelate-metal groups for adsorption may prove useful for heavy metal removal (212, 213).

Hemoperfusion and hepatic encephalopathy

Hepatic encephalopathy like that of uremia is poorly understood and therapy directed at removing specific toxins has been limited. Current hypotheses on pathogenesis center around excessive production of octopamine, ammonia, false neurotransmitters, altered circulating plasma branched chain to aromatic amino acid ratio, and excessive production of gamma-aminobutyric acid which

Table 13. Effect of hemoperfusion in fulminant hepatic encephalopathy

Study (year) (ref)	# of patients	Recovery of consciousness	Survival	Biochemical changes, and comments	Device/ anticoagulant
Chang (1972) (217)	1	100%	100%	–	ACAC, heparin
Gazzard et al. (1974) (218)	31	48%	39%	amino acids removed	Hemocol 300, heparin
Chang et al. (1976) (219)	6	66%	16%	–	ACAC, heparin
Bartels et al. (1977, 1981) (220, 221)	19	–	28%	hormones removed	Hemocol 300, heparin
Silk & Williams (1978) (222)	71	–	23.9%	–	Hemocol 300, heparin
Gelfand et al. (1978) (223)	10	90%	40%	amino acid B/A ratio rose, csf cAMP rose	Hemocol 300, heparin
Gimson et al. (1980) (157)	12	nr	nr	–	Hemocol 100, heparin, prostacyclin
Gimson et al. (1982) (222)	31 Grade III 45 Grade IV	68% 22%	65% 20%	cerebral edema 49% cerebral edema 78%	Hemocol 100, heparin, prostacyclin
Cordopatri et al. (1982) (223)	2	100%	100%	BTG, platelets preserved	Adsorba 300C, prostacyclin
Williams (1983) (224)	as in (222)			MMS removed which inhibit Na/K ATPase	Hemocol 100, heparin, prostacyclin
Bihari et al. (1983) (225)	13 Grade IV 6 Grade III		42%		XAD-7 albumin coated resin 260 g
O'Grady (226) (1988)	75 Grade III 62 Grade III		51.3% vs 50% 39.3% vs 34.5%		5 hr vs 10 hr daily Hemocol 10 hr vs no daily HP

[a]Includes 5 patients in Stage III coma, BTG = beta-thromboglobulin, nr = not recorded.
[b]B/A ratio= branched chain-aromatic acid ratio.

contribute to neural inhibition (214–216). In 1972 Chang reported improvement in consciousness in a 50 year old woman treated with charcoal hemoperfusion for fulminant hepatic failure (217). Since that time, many studies of hemoperfusion in man in Stage IV or Stage III hepatic coma in small and in large clinical trials have given mixed results. The substances removed that might be relevant to hepatic failure are shown in Table 12. Selected clinical studies of hemoperfusion for hepatic encephalopathy are given in Table 13 (218–226). Recent work, however, has shown that intensive care alone may be the determining factor in survival or improvement of patients with hepatic coma; these authors the most experienced with hemoperfusion in hepatic coma have discontinued their studies (226). Attention more recently has turned to hybrid devices containing liver tissue (227, 228), high flux hemodialysis (229), and to extracorporeal liver perfusion (230, 231), and preparing the patient for liver transplantation.

Other uses of sorbent hemoperfusion

Schizophrenia and psoriasis

Although suggested as alternative therapies for treatment of these diseases (232, 233), controlled clinical trials of dialysis and/or hemoperfusion schizophrenia and psoriasis have shown little clinical benefit (234, 235).

Immunoadsorption

Antigen-coated or antibody-coated carrier particles enclosed in hemoperfusion devices for the specific adsorption of immune proteins have also been developed. It has been possible to remove antibodies to proteins or polypeptides such as bovine serum albumin, DNA and anti-glomerular basement membrane antibody from blood (236). DNA collodion coated charcoal in an extracorporeal device did remove significant quantities of single stranded anti-DNA antibodies and immune complexes from the circulating blood of a patient with systemic lupus erythematosus. Furthermore, comparison of pre and post treatment renal biopsy specimens revealed reduction in sub-endothelial glomerular deposits (237). Potential benefit in animal models of hyperacute xenograft rejection (238), using immunoadsorption on Protein-A sepharose columns has been used in renal transplant candidates (239). The sepharose beads have a high affinity for immunoglobulins and cause significant removal of circulating IgG antibodies and percent panelled reactive antibody (PRA) (239). This points to potential application for HLA removal in sensitized transplant candidates. Monoclonal LDL antibody sepharose column hemoperfusion has also been shown to reduce low density lipoprotein levels in patients with familial hypercholesterolemia, without significant reduction of HDL, albumin and other proteins, common adverse effects of plasma exchange (240). In animal models of digoxin poisoning (241) and in humans (242), hemoperfusion of blood through monoclonal anti-digoxin antibodies covalently coupled to sepharose, Bio-Gel, Affi-Gel, and Agarose Polyacrolein microsphere (APAM) beads achieved significant digoxin removal. In a canine spontaneous breast cancer model (243), staphylococcal-A protein hemoperfusion was associated with regression and complete disappearance of breast cancer. Studies in humans are awaited with interest (244, 245).

Miscellaneous

Hemoperfusion has also been used in the removal of bilirubin and in a variety of other conditions including sepsis. Its role in these conditions is not yet defined.

Future development

The continuing search for a 'bionic kidney' will likely involve the hybridization of sorbent technology, in conjunction with dialysis/hemofiltration techniques and perhaps also the use of renal tissue. At present several groups are working on the development of these technologies, but to date no devices have come to clinical use.

REFERENCES

1. Adam WS, Blahd WH, Bassett SH: A method of human plasmapheresis. *Proc Soc Exp Biol Med* 80: 377, 1952
2. Conway N, Walker JM: Treatment of macroglobulinaemia. *Br Med J* 2: 1296, 1962
3. Millward BL, Hoeltge GA: The historical development of automated hemapheresis. *J Clin Apheresis* 1: 25, 1982
4. Gloeckner WM, Sieberth HG: Plasma filtration, a new method of plasma exchange. *Proc Eur Soc Artif Organs* 4: 214, 1978
5. Gurland HJ, Samtleben W, Blumenstein M, Randerson DH, Schmidt B: Clinical applications of macromolecular separations. *Trans Am Soc Artif Intern Organs* 27: 356, 1981
6. Gurland HJ, Lysaght MJ, Samtleben W, Schmidt B: Comparative evaluation of filters used in membrane plasmapheresis. *Nephron* 36: 173, 1984
7. Lysaght MJ, Samtleben W, Schmidt B, Gurland HJ: Contemporary technical issues in membrane plasmapheresis: Controversies and reconciliation. in *Plasma Separation and Plasma Fractionation*, edited by Lysaght MJ, Gurland HJ, Basel, Karger, 1983, p 315
8. Beaudoin G, Jaffrin MY: Plasma filtration in Couette flow membrane devices. *Artif Organs* 13: 43, 1989
9. Nydegger UE, Pflugshaupt R: Quality control of blood plasma harvested by the flat-sheet filter system Autopheresis-C. *Plasma Ther Transfus Technol* 7: 57, 1986
10. Lysaght MJ, Schmidt B, Samtleben W, Gurland HJ: Transport considerations in flat sheet microporous membrane plasmapheresis. *Plasma Ther Transfus Technol* 4: 373, 1983
11. Colton CK, Henderson LW, Ford CA, Lysaght MJ: Kinetics of hemodiafiltration. I: *in vitro* transport characteristics of a hollow-fiber blood ultrafilter. *J Lab Clin Med* 85: 355, 1975
12. Nicholls AJ, Platts MM: Anaphylactoid reactions due to haemodialysis, haemofiltration, or membrane plasma separation. *Br Med J* 285: 1607, 1982
13. Klinkmann H, Schmitt E, Falkenhagen D, Schmidt R, Osten B, Ahrenholz P, Tessenow D: Reuse of membrane plasma filters. in *Plasmapheresis*, edited by Nosé Y, Malchesky PS, Smith JW, Krakauer RS, New York, Raven Press, 1983, p 107
14. Randerson DH, Blumenstein M, Samtleben W, Schmidt B, Gurland HJ: Reuse of membrane plasma separators. in *Plasmapheresis*, edited by Nosé Y, Malchesky PS, Smith JW, Krakauer RS, New York, Raven Press, 1983, p 161
15. Bosly A, Chatelain B, Doyen C, Moriau M: Plasma exchange in Waldenström's disease: efficacy and comparison of continuous centrifugation, discontinuous centrifugation, and filtration. *Plasma Ther* 5: 319, 1984
16. Grossman L, Benny WB, Buchanan J, Erickson RR, Buffaloe GW: Clinical evaluation of a flat-plate membrane plasma exchange system. *J Clin Apheresis* 1: 225, 1983
17. Randels J, Leitmann S, Strauss R, Nakayama S, Malchesky P: Questions and answers. *J Clin Apheresis* 7: 18, 1992
18. Gurland HJ, Lysaght MJ, Samtleben W, Schmidt B: A comparison of centrifugal and membrane-based apheresis formats. *Int J Artif Organs* 7: 35, 1984
19. Schinzel H, Berghoff K, Beuermann I, Blank R, Weileman LS: Anticoagulation with low molecular weight heparin (Fragmin) during plasmapheresis. First experience. *Ann Hematol* 68 (Suppl II): A72, 1994
20. Sutton DMC, Cardella CJ, Uldall PR, DeVeber GA: Complications of intensive plasma exchange. *Plasma Ther* 2: 19, 1981
21. Kubanek B: Risks of homologous blood transfusions. in *Erythropoietin. Molecular Physiology and Clinical Applications*, edited by Bauer C, Koch KM, Scigalla P, Wieczorek L, New York, Marcel Dekker, 1993, p 389
22. Roberts CG, Schindhelm K, Smeby LC, Farrell PC: Kinetic analysis of plasma separation: Use of an animal model. in *Plasma Separation and Plasma Fractionation*, edited by Lysaght MJ, Gurland HJ, Basel, Karger, 1983, p 25

23. Samtleben W, Randerson DH, Blumenstein M, Habersetzer R, Schmidt B, Gurland HJ: Membrane plasma exchange: principles and application techniques. *J Clin Apheresis* 2: 163, 1984

24. Frank MM, Hamburger MI, Lawley TJ, Kimberly RP, Plotz PH: Defective reticuloendothelial system Fc-receptor function in systemic lupus erythematosus. *N Engl J Med* 300: 518, 1979

25. Lockwood CM, Worlledge S, Nicholas A, Cotton C, Peters DK: Reversal of impaired splenic function in patients with nephritis or vasculitis (or both) by plasma exchange. *N Engl J Med* 300: 524, 1979

26. Samtleben W, Schmidt B, Bosch T, Gurland HJ: Are immune complex assays an appropriate tool for quantitation of plasma exchange? *Plasma Ther Transfus Technol* 6: 523, 1985

27. Schroeder JO, Euler HH, Loeffler H: Synchronization of plasmapheresis and pulse cyclophosphamide in severe systemic lupus erythematosus. *Ann Intern Med* 107: 344, 1987

28. Euler HH, Krey U, Schroeder O, Loeffler H: Membrane plasmapheresis technique in rats. Confirmation of antibody rebound. *J Immunol Methods* 84: 313, 1985

29. Aufeuvre JP, Morin-Hertel F, Cohen-Solal M, Lefloch A, Baudelot J: Hazards of plasma exchange. A nationwide study of 3431 exchanges in 592 patients. in *Plasma Exchange*, edited by Sieberth HG, Stuttgart, New York, Schattauer, 1981, p 149

30. Das PC, Smit Sibinga CT: Complications of therapeutic plasma exchange. *Lancet* 2: 455, 1983

31. Borberg H: Problems of plasma exchange therapy. in *Therapeutic Plasma Exchange*, edited by Gurland HJ, Heinze V, Lee HA, Berlin, Heidelberg, New York, Springer-Verlag, 1981, p 191

32. Bussel A, Sitthy X, Reviron J: Aspects technologiques et complications des exchanges plasmatiques. (Technical aspects and complications of plasma exchange). *Rev Fr Transfus Immunohematol* 25: 547, 1982

33. Fabre M, Andreu G, Mannoni P: Some biological modifications and clinical hazards observed during plasma exchange. in *Plasma Exchange*, edited by Sieberth HG, Stuttgart, New York, Schattauer, 1980, p 143

34. Gajdoŝ P, Pourrat J, Elkharrat D, Terre C: National register for plasma exchange – The French Society for Hemapheresis. Results for 1985. *Plasma Ther Transfus Technol* 8: 137, 1987

35. Samtleben W, Hillebrand G, Krumme D, Gurland HJ: Membrane plasma separation: clinical experience with more than 120 plasma exchanges. in *Plasma Exchange*, edited by Sieberth HG, Stuttgart, New York, Schattauer, 1980, p 175

36. Tindall RSA, Walker JE, Ehle AL, Near L, Rolins J, Becker D: Plasmapheresis in multiple sclerosis: prospective trial of pheresis and immunosuppression versus immunosuppression alone. *Neurology* 32: 739, 1982

37. Editorial: Hazards of apheresis. *Lancet* 2: 1025, 1982

38. Huestis DW: Mortality in therapeutic haemapheresis. *Lancet* 1: 1043, 1983

39. Ring J, Messmer K: Incidence and severity of anaphylactoid reactions to colloid colume substitutes. *Lancet* 1, 466, 1977

40. Evans RT, MacDonald R, Robinson EAE: Suxamethonium apnoea associated with plasmapheresis. *Anaesthesia* 35: 198, 1980

41. Jones JV, Parker WA, Sketris IS: The effect of plasmapheresis on therapeutic drugs. *Dial Transplant* 14: 225, 1985

42. Sketris IS, Parker WA, Jones JV: Plasmapheresis: Its effect on toxic agents and drugs. *Plasma Ther Transfus Technol* 5: 305, 1984

43. Sakellarious G: Plasmapheresis as a therapy in specific forms of acute renal failure. *Nephrol Dial Transplant* 9 (Suppl 4): 210, 1994

44. Schmidt B, Lysaght MJ, Samtleben W, Gurland HJ: Plasmapheresis without pumps for therapeutic and donor purposes. in *Plasma Separation and Plasma Fractionation*, edited by Lysaght MJ, Gurland HJ, Basel, Karger, 1983, p 188

45. Samtleben W, Lysaght MJ, Schmidt B, Gurland HJ: A very simple technique for spontaneous membrane plasma exchange without arterial access. *Blood Purif* 1: 90, 1983

46. Landini S, Coli U, Lucatello S, Fracasso A, Morachiello P, Righetto F, Scanferla F, Bazzato G: Spontaneous plasma exchange by gravity. *Int J Artif Organs* 7: 137, 1984

47. Samtleben W, Lysaght MJ, Banthien F, Hillebrand G, Gurland HJ: Simultaneous combined hemodialysis and membrane plasmapheresis. in *Plasma Separation and Plasma Fractionation*, edited by Lysaght MJ, Gurland HJ, Basel, Karger, 1983, p 213

48. Scheiner E, Reich L, Isaacs M, Vanamee P, Fombaum CD, van Strien S, Gulati SC: Simultaneous hemodialysis and plasmapheresis: ten years experience. (Abstract) *Kidney Int* 23: 160, 1983

49. Gross MLP, Baillod RA, Sweny P, Pearson RM: (Letter) *Plasma Ther* 2: 255, 1981

50. Lysaght MJ, Samtleben W, Schmidt B, Gurland HJ: Closed-loop plasmapheresis. in *Therapeutic Hemapheresis*, edited by MacPherson JL, Kasprisin DO, Boca Raton, CRC Press, 1985, Volume I, p 149

51. Samtleben W, Schindhelm K: Therapeutic plasmapheresis. (Editorial) *Biomed Pharmacother* 40: 281, 1986

52. Agishi T, Kaneko I, Hasou Y, Hayasaka Y, Sanaka T, Ota K, Abe M, Ono T, Kawai S, Yamane K: Double filtration plasmapheresis. *ASAIO Trans* 26: 406, 1980

53. Lysaght MJ, Samtleben W, Schmidt B, Gurland HJ: Technical assessment of membrane plasmapheresis in the treatment of a patient with IgM paraproteinemia. *Clin Hemorheology* 5: 27, 1985

54. Samtleben W, Schmidt B, Blumenstein M, Gurland HJ: Current status of membrane plasma separation and plasma filtration techniques. *Int J Artif Organs* 8 (Suppl 2): 33, 1985

55. Busnach G, Dal-Col A, Brando B, Capelleri A, Perrino ML, Bruncati C, Minetti L: Different cascade filtration operating modalities in clinical use. *Int J Artif Organs* 11: 493, 1986

56. Lysaght MJ, Samtleben W, Schmidt B, Gurland HJ: Contemporary technical issues in membrane plasmapheresis: Controversies and reconciliation. in *Plasma Separation and Plasma Fractionation – Current Status and Future Directions*, edited by Lysaght MJ, Gurland HJ, Basel, Karger, 1983, p 315

57. Kochinke F, von Baeyer H, Schwaner I, Schwerdtfeger R: Comparison of plasmafractionation filters and filtration techniques in the clinical practise of LDL-apheresis. *ASAIO Trans* 32: 389, 1986

58. Valbonesi M, Lercari S, Angelini G, Malfanti L, Ferrari M, Russo E, Nati S: Cascade filtration with reverse rinse of the secondary filter. *J Clin Apheresis* 3: 240, 1987

59. Bosch T, Gurland HJ: Overview: techniques and indications of LDL-apheresis. *Biomat Artif Cells Immobilization Biotechnol* 19: 1, 1991

60. Legallis C, Jaffrin MY: A process enhancing selectivity and limiting plugging in plasmafractionation for ApoB removal. *Int J Artif Organs* 16: 108, 1993

61. Yamazaki M, Asakura H, Jokoji H, Saito M, Uotani C, Kumabashiri I, Morishita E, Nakamura S, Naito T, Ohta H: Successful treatment of a patient with idiopathic factor VIII inhibitor with double filtration plasmapheresis and steroid administration. *Blood Coagul Fibrinolysis* 4: 491, 1993

62. Terman DS, Stewart I, Robinetti J, Carr R, Harbeck R: Specific removal of DNA antibodies *in vivo* with an extracorporeal immunoadsorbent. *Clin Exp Immunol* 24: 231, 1976

63. Lupien PJ, Moorjani S, Awad J: A new approach to the management of familial hypercholesterolemia: removal of plasma cholesterol based on the principle of affinity chromatography. *Lancet* 1: 1261, 1976

64. Yokoyama S, Hayashi R, Kikkawa T, Tani N, Takada S, Hatanaba K, Yamamoto A: Specific sorbent of apolipoprotein B-containing lipoproteins of plasmapheresis. Characterization and experimental use in hypercholesterolemic rabbits. *Arteriosclerosis* 4: 276, 1984

65. Ikonomov V, Samtleben W, Schmidt B, Blumenstein M, Gurland HJ: Adsorption profile of commercially available adsorbents: an *in vitro* evaluation. *Int J Artif Organs* 15: 312, 1992

66. Stoffel W, Borberg H, Greve V: Application of specific extracorporeal removal of low densitiy lipoprotein in familial hypercholesterolaemia. *Lancet* 2: 1005, 1981

67. Oette K, Borberg H: Variables involved in regression of atherosclerosis in familial hypercholesterolemic patients under long-term LDL-apheresis. *Plasma Ther Transfus Technol* 9: 17, 1988

68. du Moulin A, Müller-Derlich J, Bieber F, Richter WO, Frei U, Müller R, Späthe R: Antibody-based immunosorption as a therapeutic means. *Blood Purif* 11: 145, 1993

69. Samtleben W, Schmidt B, Gurland HJ: *Ex vivo* and *in vivo* Protein A perfusion: background, basic investigations, and first clinical experiences. *Blood Purif* 5: 179, 1987

70. Morrison FS, Huestis DW: Toxicity of the staphylococcal protein A immunoadsorption column. *J Clin Apheresis* 7: 171, 1992

71. Fuchs C, Windisch M, Wieland H, Armstrong VW, Rieger J, Koestering H, Scheler F, Seidel D: Selective continuous extracorporeal elimination of low-density lipoproteins from plasma by heparin precipitation without cations. in *Plasma Separation and Plasma Fractionation*, edited by Lysaght MJ, Gurland HJ, Basel, Karger, 1983, p 272

72. Seidel D, Armstrong VW, Schuff-Werner P and the HELP Study Group: The HELP-LDL-apheresis multicentre study, an angiographically assessed trial into the role of LDL-apheresis in the secondary prevention of coronary heart disease. I. Evaluation of safety and cholesterol-lowering effects during the first 12 months. *Eur J Clin Invest* 21: 375, 1991

73. Seidel D (ed): H E L P Report 1994. 10 Years of clinical experience. MMV Medizin Verlag Munich, 1994

74. Eisenhauer T, Armstrong VW, Wieland H, Fuchs C, Scheler F, Seidel D: Selective removal of low density lipoproteins (LDL) by precipitation at low pH: first clinical application of the HELP system. *Klin Wochenschr* 65: 161, 1987

75. Armstrong VW, Schleef J, Thiery J, Muche R, Schuff-Werner P, Eisenhauer T, Seidel D: Effect of the HELP-LDL-apheresis on serum concentrations of human lipoprotein(a): kinetic analysis of the post-treatment return to baseline levels. *Eur Clin J Invest* 19: 235, 1989

76. Schuff-Werner P, Schütz E, Seyde WC, Eisenhauer T, Jannings G, Armstrong VW, Seidel D: Improved haemorheology associated with a reduction in plasma fibrinogen and LDL precipitation (HELP). *Eur J Clin Invest* 19: 30, 1989

77. Edelson RL, Berger CL, Gasparro FP, Jegasothy BV, Heald PW, Wintroub B, Vonderheid E, Knobler R, Wolff K, Plewig G, McKiernan G, Christiansen I, Oster M, Honigsmann H, Wilford H, Kokoschka E, Rehle T, Perez M, Stingl G, Laroche L: Treatment of cutaneous T-cell lymphoma by extracorporeal photochemotherapy. *N Engl J Med* 316: 297, 1987

78. Christensen I, Heald P: Photopheresis in the 1990s. *J Clin Apheresis* 6: 216, 1991

79. Gurland HJ, Lysaght MJ: Future trends in renal replacement therapy. *Artif Organs* 17: 267, 1993

80. Lockwood CM, Rees AJ, Pearson TA, Evans DJ, Peters DK, Wilson CB: Immunosuppression and plasma-exchange in the treatment of Goodpasture's syndrome. *Lancet* 1: 711, 1976

81. Lockwood CM, Rees AJ, Pinching AJ, Pussell B, Sweny P, Uff J, Peters DK: Plasma-exchange and immunosuppression in the treatment of fulminating immune-complex crescentic nephritis. *Lancet* 1: 63, 1977

82. Pinching AJ, Peters DK, Newsom Davis J: Remission of myasthenia gravis following plasma-exchange. *Lancet* 2: 1373, 1976

83. Bukowski RM, King JW, Hewlett JS: Plasmapheresis in the treatment of thrombotic thrombocytopenic purpura. *Blood* 50: 413, 1977

84. Kambic H, Hyslop L, Nosé Y: *Topics in Plasmapheresis.* A Bibliography of Therapeutic Applications and New Techniques. Cleveland, ISAO Press, 1985

85. Conference report: Plasma exchange. *Ann Rheum Dis* 39: 95, 1980

86. Wysenbeck AJ, Smith JW, Krakauer RS: Plasmapheresis II: review of clinical experience. *Plasma Ther* 2: 61, 1981

87. Wenz B, Barland P: Therapeutic intensive plasmapheresis. *Sem Hematol* 18: 147, 1981

88. International Forum: What are the established clinical indications for therapeutic plasma exchange and how important is the choice of replacement for efficacy of therapeutic plasma exchange in these situations? *Vox Sang* 43: 270, 1982

89. Kennedy MS, Domen RE: Therapeutic apheresis: applications and future directions. *Vox Sang* 45: 261, 1983

90. Shumak KH, Rock GA: Therapeutic plasma exchange. *N Engl J Med* 310: 762 1984

91. Council on Scientific Affairs: Current status of therapeutic plasmapheresis and related techniques. Report of the AMA panel on therapeutic plasmapheresis. *JAMA* 253: 819, 1985

92. Klein HG, Balow JE, Dau PC, Hamburger MI, Leitmann SF, Pineda AA, Tindall RSA: Clinical applications of therapeutic apheresis. Report of the Clinical Applications Committee. American Society for Apheresis. *J Clin Apheresis* 3 (special issue), 1986

93. Strauss RG, Ciavarella D, Gilcher RO, Kasprisin DO, Kiprov DD, Klein HG, McLeod BC: An overview of current management. *J Clin Apheresis* 8: 189, 1993

94. Fish AJ, Lockwood MC, Wong M, Price RG: Detection of Goodpasture antigen in fractions prepared from collagenase digest of human glomerular basement membrane. *Clin Exp Immunol* 55: 58, 1984

95. Wieslander J, Byrgen P, Heinegard D: Isolation of the specific glomerular basement membrane antigen involved in Goodpasture syndrome. *Proc Natl Acad Sci USA* 81: 1544, 1984

96. Salant DJ: Immunopathogenesis of crescentic glomerulonephritis and lung purpura (Nephrology Forum). *Kidney Int* 32: 408, 1987

97. Wilson CB, Dixon FJ: Anti-glomerular basement membrane antibody-induced glomerulonephritis. *Kidney Int* 3: 74, 1973

98. Wilson CB, Dixon FJ: The renal response to immunological injury. in *The Kidney*, edited by Brenner BM, Rector FC, Philadelphia, London, Toronto, Saunders, 1981, p 1237

99. Rees AJ, Lockwood CM, Peters DK: Nephritis due to antibodies to GBM. in *Progress in Glomerulonephritis*, edited by Kincaid-Smith P, D'Apice AJF, Atkins RJ, New York, John Wiley, 1980, p 348

100. Lockwood CM, Pusey CD, Peters DK: Indications for plasma exchange: renal diseases. in *Plasma Separation and Plasma Fractionation*, edited by Lysaght MJ, Gurland HJ, Basel, Karger, 1983, p 145

101. Swainson CP, Winney RJ, Urbaniak SJ, Robinson JS: Plasma exchange in severe glomerulonephritis – who benefits? *Proc Eur Dial Transplant Assoc* 19: 732, 1982

102. Herody M, Bobrie G, Gouarin C, Grünfeld JP, Noel LH: Anti-GBM disease: Predictive value of clinical, histological and serological data. *Clin Nephrol* 40: 249, 1993

103. Johnson JP, et al.: Therapy of anti-glomerular basement membrane antibody disease: analysis of prognostic significance of clinical, pathologic and treatment factors. *Medicine* 64: 219, 1985

104. Peters DK, Pusey CD, Lockwood CM: Immunomodulation by plasma exchange: therapeutic objectives. in *Plasma Separation and Plasma Fractionating*, edited by Lysaght MJ, Gurland HJ, Basel, Karger, 1983, p 1

105. Flores JC, Savage COS, Lockwood CM, Taube D, Cameron JS, Williams DG, Ogg CS: Clinical and immunological evolution of oligoanuric anti-GBM nephritis by haemodialysis. *Lancet* 1: 5, 1986

106. Rees AJ, Lockwood CM, Peters DK: Enhanced allergic tissue injury in Goodpasture's syndrome by intercurrent infection. *Br Med J* 2: 723, 1977

107. Rees AJ, Pusey CD: Plasma exchange in systemic vasculitis. *Netherlands J Medicine* 36: 103, 1990

108. Kauffmann RH, van Es LA, Daha MR: The specific detection of IgA immune complexes. *J Immunol Meth* 40: 117, 1981

109. Valentijn RM, Kauffmann RH, De La Riviere GB, Daha MR, van Es LA: Presence of circulating macromolecular IgA in patients with hematuria due to primary IgA nephropathy. *Am J Med* 74: 375, 1983

110. Hene RJ, Kater L: Plasmapheresis in nephritis associated with Henoch-Schoenlein purpura and in primary IgA nephropathy. *Plasma Ther Transfus Technol* 4: 165, 1983

111. Samtleben W, Gurland HJ: Plasma exchange in nephrological diseases. in *Therapeutic Hemapheresis*, edited by Valbonesi M, Pineda AA, Biggs JC, Milano, Wichtig Editore, 1986, p 29

112. Nicholls K, Becker G, Walker R, Wright C, Kincaid-Smith P: Plasma exchange in progressive IgA nephropathy. *J Clin Apheresis* 5: 128, 199

113. Chalopin JM, Tanter Y, Wenning H: Immunosuppression and plasma exchange in dense deposit disease. *Abstracts Annales de Medicine Interne 135* (special issue): 31, 1984

114. Couser WG, Salant DJ: *In situ* immune complex formation and glomerular injury. *Kidney Int* 17: 1, 1980

115. Schwarzt RS: Immunologic and genetic aspects of systemic lupus erythematosus. *Kidney Int* 19: 474, 1981

116. Jones JV, Cumming RH, Bucknall RC, Asplin CM, Fraser ID, Bothamley J, Davis P, Hamblin TJ: Plasmapheresis in the management of acute systemic lupus erythematosus? *Lancet* 1: 709, 1976

117. Samtleben W, Lysaght MJ, Gurland HJ: Plasma exchange in lupus nephritis: Rationale and clinical experiences. *Dial Transplant* 14: 213, 1985

118. Austin HA, Klippel JH, Balow JE, Le Riche NGH, Steinberg AD, Plotz PH, Decker JL: Therapy of lupus nephritis. Controlled trial of prednisone and cytotoxic drugs. *N Engl J Med* 314: 614, 1986

119. Wei N, Kippel JH, Huston DP, Hall RP, Lawley TJ, Balow JE, Steinberg AD, Decker JL: Randomized trial of plasma exchange in mild systemic lupus erythematosus. *Lancet* 1: 17, 1983

120. Clark WF, Balfe JW, Cattran DC, Williams W, Koval JJ, Arnott M, Chodirker WB, Lindsay RM, Linton AL: Long-term plasma exchange in patients with systemic lupus erythematosus and diffuse proliferative glomerulonephritis. *Plasma Ther Transfus Technol* 5: 353, 1984

121. Lewis EJ, Hunsicker LG, Lan S-P, Rohde RD, Lachin JM: A controlled trial of plasmapheresis therapy in severe lupus nephritis. *N Engl J Med* 326: 1373, 1992

122. Euler HH, Schroeder JO, Zeuner RA, Teske E: A randomized trial of plasmapheresis and subsequent pulse cyclophosphamide in severe lupus: design of the LPSG trial. *Int J Artif Organs* 14: 639, 1991

123. Euler HH, Loeffler H, Chrisophers E: Synchronization of plasmapheresis and pulse cyclophosphamide in pemphigus vulgaris. *Arch Dermatol* 123: 1205, 1987

124. Guillevin L, Le Thi Huong Du, Godeau P, Jais P, Wechsler B: Clinical findings and prognosis of polyarteritis nodosa and Churg–Strauss angiitis: a study in 165 patients. *Br J Rheumatol* 27, 258, 1988

125. Remuzzi G: HUS and TTP: Variable expressions of a single entity. *Kidney Int* 32: 292, 1987

126. Neild G: The haemolytic uremic syndrome: a review. *Q J Med* 241: 367, 1987

127. Aster RH: Plasma therapy for thrombotic thrombocytopenic purpura. Sometimes it works, but why (Editorial retrospective). *N Engl J Med* 312: 985, 1985

128. Rizzoni G, Pavanelle L, Claris-Appiani A, Edefonti A, Facchin P, Ranchini F, Gussmano R, Imbasciati E, Perfumo F, Remuzzi G: Treatment of children with hemolytic uremic syndrome (HUS) with plasma: a multicenter controlled trial. (Abstract) *Helv Paediatr Acta* 41: 114, 1986

129. Stoffner D, Banthien FCA, Habersetzer R, Samtleben W, Clemm C, Unterburger P, Zaehringer J, Gurland HJ: Plasma exchange and concommitant therapy in TTP. *Int J Artif Organs* 7: 223, 1984

130. Byrnes JJ, Moake JL, Klug P, Periman P: Effectiveness of the cryosupernatant fraction of plasma in the treatment of refractory thrombotic thrombocytopenic purpura. *Am J Hematol* 34: 169, 1990

131. Moake JL, Rudy CK, Troll JH, Weinstein MJ, Colannio NM, Azocar J, Seder RH, Hong SL, Deykin D: Unusually large plasma factor VIII: von Willebrand factor multimers in chronic relapsing thrombotic thrombocytopenic purpura. *N Engl J Med* 307: 1432, 1982

132. Bell WR, Braine HG, Ness PM, Kickler TS: Improved survival in thrombotic thrombocytopenic purpura – hemolytic uremic syndrome. Clinical experience in 108 patients. *N Engl J Med* 325: 398, 1991

133. Rock GA, Shumak KH, Buskard NA, Blanchette VS, Kelton JG, Nair RC, Spasoff RA, and the Canadian Apheresis Study Group: Comparison of plasma exchange with plasma infusion in the treatment of thrombotic thrombocytopenic purpura. *N Engl J Med* 325: 393, 1991

134. Pourrat JP, Dueymes JM, Conte JJ, Pourrat O, Alcalay D, Touchard G, Patte D: Plasma exchange in myeloma renal failure. in *Plasmapheresis*, edited by Nosé Y, Malchesky PS, Smith JW, Krakauer RS, New York, Raven Press, 1983, p 349

135. Blumenstein M, Samtleben W, Gurland HJ: Die Behandlung des paraproteinämischen Nierenversagens mit Plasmapherese. (Plasma therapy for treatment of renal failure in patients with plasma cell diseases). *Nieren- und Hochdruck* 16: 140, 1987

136. Blumberg A, Buergi W, Marti HR: Plasmapheresebehandlung bei multiplem Myelom mit Niereninsuffizienz. (Plasmapheresis therapy for multiple myeloma with renal insufficiency). *Schweiz Med Wochenschr* 113: 398, 1983

137. Zucchelli P, Pasquali S, Cagnoli L, Ferrari G: Controlled plasma exchange trial in acute renal failure due to multiple myeloma. *Kidney Int* 33: 1175, 1988

138. Mason PD, Pusey CD: Plasma exchange in nephrological diseases. *Curr Stud Hematol Bllod Transfus* 57: 152, 1990

139. Hillebrand G, Castro LA, Samtleben W, Albert E, Scholz S, Illner WD, Land W, Gurland HJ: Removal of preformed cytotoxic antibodies in highly sensitized patients using plasma exchange and immunosuppressive therapy, azathioprine, or cyclosporine prior to renal transplantation. *Transplant Proc* 18: 1033, 1986

140. Minakuchi J, Takahashi K, Toma H, Teroaka S, Hayasaka Y, Ota K: Removal of preformed antibodies by plasmapheresis prior to kidney transplantation. *Transplant Proc* 18: 1083, 1986

141. Palmer A, Welsh K, Gjorstrup P, Taube D, Bewick M, Thick M: Removal of anti-HLA antibodies by extracorporeal immunoadsorption to enable renal transplantation. *Lancet* i: 10, 1989

142. Kupin WL, Venkat KK, Hayashi H, Mozes MF, Oh HK, Watt R: Removal of lymphocytotoxic antibodies by pretransplant immunoadsorption therapy in highly sensitized renal transplant recipients. *Transplantation* 51: 324, 1991

143. Swanepoel CR, Cassidy MJD, May M, Oudshoorn M, du Toit E, Wood L, Jacobx P: Reactivity of pretransplant cytotoxic antibodies to a selected HLA panel is not influenced by cyclosporin A, with or without plasma exchange. *J Clin Apheresis* 6: 28, 1991

144. Gurland HJ, Blumenstein M, Lysaght MJ, Samtleben W, Stoffner D: Plasmapheresis in renal transplantation. *Kidney Int* 23 (Suppl 14): S82, 1983

145. Cardella CJ, Sutton DMC, Uldall PR, Cook GT, deVeber GA: Factors influencing the effect of intensive plasma exchange on acute transplant rejection. *Transplant Proc* 17: 2777, 1985

146. Bonomini V, Vangelista A, Frasca GM, Di Felice A, Liviano D'Arcangelo G: Effects of plasmapheresis in renal transplant rejection. A controlled study. in *Therapeutic Plasma Exchange and Selective Plasma Separation*, edited by Bambauer R, Malchesky PS, Falkenhagen D, Stuttgart, New York, 1987, p 69

147. Li P, Lai F, Leung C, Lui S, Wang A, Lai K: Plasma exchange in the treatment of early recurrent focal glomerulosclerosis after renal transplantation. *Am J Nephrol* 13: 289, 1993

148. Glassock RJ: Therapy of idiopathic nephrotic syndrome in adults. *Am J Nephrol* 13: 422, 1993

149. Denti E, Walker JM: Activated carbon: properties, selection and evaluation. in *Sorbents and Their Clinical Applications*, edited by Giordano C, New York, Academic Press Inc, 1980, p 101

150. Denti E, Luboz MP, Tessore V: Adsorption characteristics of cellulose acetate coated charcoals. *J Biomed Mater Res* 9: 143, 1975

151. Chang TMS: Semipermeable aqueous microcapsules (artifical cells): with emphasis on experiments in an extracorporeal shunt system. *Trans Am Soc Artif Intern Organs* 12: 13, 1966

152. Chang TMS: Microcapsule artificial kidney in replacement of renal function. With emphasis on adsorbent hemoperfusion. in *Replacement of Renal Function by Dialysis*, First Edition, edited by Drukker W, Parsons FM, Maher JF. The Hague, Boston, London, Martinus Nijhoff, 1978, p 217

153. Craddock PR, Fehr J, Brigham KL, Kronenherg R, Jacobs HS: Complement and leukocyte-mediated pulmonary dysfunction in hemodialysis. *N Engl J Med* 296: 769, 1977

154. Winchester JF, Ratcliffe JG, Carlyle E, Kennedy AC: Solute, amino acid, and hormone changes with coated charcoal hemoperfusion in uremia. *Kidney Int* 14: 74, 1978

155. Weston MJ, Langley PG, Rubin MH, Hanid MA, Mellon P, Williams R: Platelet function in fulminant hepatic failure and effect of charcoal haemoperfusion. *Gut* 18: 897, 1977

156. Winchester JF, Forbes CD, Courtney JM, Reavey M, Prentice CRM: Effect of sulphinpyrazone and aspirin on platelet adhesion to activated charcoal and dialysis membranes *in vitro*. *Thromb Res* 11: 443, 1977

498   *Hans Gurland et al.*

157. Gimson AES, Langley PG, Hughes RD, et al.: Prostacyclin to prevent platelet activation during charcoal haemoperfusion in fulminant hepatic failure. *Lancet* 1: 173, 1980
158. Chang TMS, Chirito E, Barre B, Cole C, Hewish M: Clinical performance-characteristics of a new combined system for simultaneous hemoperfusion-hemodialysis-ultrafiltration in series. *Trans Am Soc Artif Intern Organs* 21: 502, 1975
159. Stefoni S, Coli L. Feliciangeli G, Baldrati L, Bonomini V: Regular hemoperfusion in regular dialysis treatment. A longterm study. *Int J Artif Organs* 3: 348, 1980
160. Muirhead EE, Reid AF: Resin artificial kidney. *J Lab Clin Med* 33: 841, 1948
161. Schreiner GE: The role of hemodialysis (artificial kidney) in acute poisoning. *Arch Intern Med* 102: 896. 1958
162. Yatzidis H: A convenient haemoperfusion microapparatus over charcoal for the treatment of endogenous and exogenous intoxications. Its use as an artificial kidney. *Proc Eur Dial Transplant Assoc* 1: 83, 1964
163. Yatzidis H, Voudiclari S, Oreopoulos D, Tsaparas N, Triantaphyllidis D, Gavras C, Stavroulaki A: Treatment of severe barbiturate poisoning. *Lancet* 2: 216, 1965
164. Dunea G, Kolff WJ: Clinical experience with the Yatzidis charcoal artificial kidney. *Trans Am Soc Artif Intern Organs* 11: 178, 1965
165. Chang TMS, Gonda A, Dirks JH, Malave N: Clinical evaluation of chronic intermittent and short term hemoperfusion in patients with chronic renal failure using semipermeable microcapsules (artificial cells) formed from membrane coated activated charcoal. *Trans Am Soc Artif Intern Organs* 17: 246, 1971
166. Asaba H: Uremic middle molecules. Accumulation, renal excretion and elimination by extracorporeal treatment. *Scand J Urol Nephrol* 67 (Suppl): 1, 1982
167. Bonomini V, Stefoni S, Feliciangeli G, Coli L, Scolari MP, Orsi C, Nanni Costa A, Prandini R, Galanti S: Shortened treatment time by combined hemodialysis and hemoperfusion. *Contrib Nephrol* 44: 57, 1985
168. Henderson IS, Kennedy AC: Long-term evaluation of charcoal haemoperfusion combined with dialysis for uraemic patients. in *Biomaterials in Artificial Organs*, edited by Paul JP, Gaylor JDS, Courtney JM, Gilchrist T, London, Basingstoke, The Macmillan Press Ltd, 1984, p 72
169. Chang TMS, Barre P, Kuruvilla S: Long-term reduced time hemoperfusion-hemodialysis compared to standard dialysis. A preliminary crossover analysis. *Trans Am Soc Artif Intern Organs* 31: 572, 1985
170. Chang TMS, Barre P: Effect of desferrioxamine on removal of aluminium and iron by coated charcoal haemoperfusion and haemodialysis. *Lancet* 2: 1051, 1983
171. Hakim RM, Schulman JM, Lazarus JM: Hemoperfusion in the treatment of aluminum (Al) and iron (Fe) induced bone disease. *Abstracts Am Soc Nephrol* 18: 65A, 1985
172. Winchester JF: Management of iron overload. *Semin Nephrol* 4 (Suppl 1): 22, 1986
173. Vasilakakis DM, D'Haese PC, Lamberts LV, Lemoniatou E, Digenis PN, De Broe ME: Removal of aluminoxamine and ferrioxamine by charcoal hemoperfusion and hemodialysis. *Kidney Int* 41: 1400, 1992
174. Litovitz TL, Clark LR, Soloway RA: 1993 Annual report of the American Association of Poison Control Centers

Toxic Exposure Surveillance System. *J Am Emerg Med* 12: 546, 1994
175. Clemmesen C, Nilsson E: Therapeutic trends in the treatment of barbiturate poisoning: the Scandinavian method. *Clin Pharmacol Ther* 2: 220, 1961
176. Winchester JF, Gelfand MC, Tilstone WJ: Hemoperfusion in drug intoxication – clinical and laboratory aspects. *Drug Metab Rev* 8: 69, 1978
177. Maher JF, Schreiner GE: The dialysis of poisons and drugs. *Trans Am Soc Artif Intern Organs* 13: 369, 1967
178. Winchester JF, Gelfand MC, Knepshield JH, Schreiner GE: Dialysis and hemoperfusion of poisons and drugs – update. *Trans Am Soc Artif Intern Organs* 23: 762, 1977
179. Cohan SL, Winchester JF, Gelfand MC: Treatment of intoxications by charcoal hemadsorption. *Drug Metab Rev* 13: 681, 1982
180. Rosenbaum JL, Kramer MS, Raja RM, Krug MJ, Boliday CG: Current status of hemoperfusion in toxicology. *Clin Toxicol* 17: 493, 1980
181. Cutler RE, Forland SC, Hammond PG, Evans JR: Extracorporeal removal of drugs and poisons by hemodialysis and hemoperfusion. *Annu Rev Pharmacol Toxicol* 27: 169, 1987
182. Winchester JF, Tilstone WJ, Edwards RO, Gilchrist T, Kennedy AC: Hemoperfusion for enhanced drug elimination – a kinetic analysis in paracetamol poisoning. *Trans Am Soc Artif Intern Organs* 20: 358, 1974
183. Verpooten GA, De Broe ME: Combined hemoperfusion-hemodialysis in severe poisoning: kinetics of drug extraction. *Resuscitation* 11: 275, 1984
184. Winchester JF, Rahman A, Tilstone WJ, Kessler A, Mortensen L, Schreiner GE, Schein PS: Sorbent removal of adriamycin *in vitro* and *in vivo*. *Cancer Treat Rep* 63: 1787, 1979
185. Pond S, Rosenberg J, Benowitz NL, Takki S: Pharmacokinetics of haemoperfusion in drug overdose. *Clin Pharmacokinet* 4: 329, 1979
186. Gelfand MC, Winchester JF, Knepshield JH, Hanson KM, Cohan SL, Strauch BS, Geoly KL, Kennedy AC, Schreiner GE: Treatment of severe drug overdose with charcoal hemoperfusion. *Trans Am Soc Artif Intern Organs* 23: 599, 1977
187. Gibson TP, Lucas SV, Nelson HA, Atkinson AJ, Okita GT, Ivanovich P: Hemoperfusion removal of digoxin from dogs. *J Lab Clin Med* 91: 673, 1978
188. Lorch JA, Garella S: Hemoperfusion to treat intoxications. *Ann Intern Med* 91: 301, 1979
189. Uldall PR: Controlled trial of resin hemoperfusion for the treatment of drug overdose at Toronto Western Hospital (TWH). *Trans Am Soc Artif Intern Organs* 28: 676, 1982
190. Winchester JF: Active Methods for Detoxification: oral sorbents, forced diuresis, hemoperfusion and hemodialysis. in *Clinical Management of Poisoning and Drug Overdose*, Second Edition, edited by Haddad LM, Winchester, JF, WB Saunders Co, Philadelphia, PA, 1990, p 148
191. Winchester JF, Gelfand MC, Helliwell M, Vale JA, Goulding R, Schreiner GE: Extracorporeal treatment of salicylate or acetaminiphen poisoning – is there a role? *Arch Intern Med* 141: 370, 1981
192. Diaz-Buxo JA, Farmer CD, Chandler TY: Hemopertusion in the treatment of amitriptyline poisoning. *Trans Am Soc Artif Intern Organs* 24: 699, 1978

193. Maini R, Winchester JF: Removal of paraquat from blood by haemoperfusion over sorbent materials. *Br Med J* 3: 281, 1975
194. Okonek S, Weilemann LS, Majdandzic H et al.: Successful treatment ofparaquat poisoning: Activated charcoal per os and 'continuous hemoperfusion'. *J Toxicol Clin Toxicol* 19: 807, 1982
195. Proudfoot AT: Predictive value of early plasma paraquat concentrations. in *Paraquat Poisoning, Mechanisms, Prevention, Management*, edited by C Bismuth, AH Hall, New York, Marcel Dekker, 1995, p 275
196. Winchester JF, Rahman A, Bregman H, Mortensen LM, Gelfand MC, Schein PS, Schreiner GE: Role of hemoperfusion in anticancer drug removal. in *Hemoperfusion, Kidney and Liver Support and Detoxification*, edited by Sideman S, Chang TMS, Washington DC, Hemisphere Publishing Corp, 1980, p 369
197. Hande KR, Balow JE, Draje JC, Rosenberg SA, Chabner BA: Methotrexate and hemodialysis. *Ann Intern Med* 87: 496, 1977
198. Molina R, Fahian C, Cowley B Jr: Use of charcoal hemoperfusion to reduce serum methotrexate levels in a patient with acute renal insufficiency. *Am J Med* 82: 350, 1987
199. Oldfield EH, Dedrick RL, Yeager RL, Clark WC, DeVroom HL, Chatterji DC, Doppman JL: Reduced systemic drug exposure by continuous intra-arterial chemotherapy with hemoperfusion of regional venous drainage. *J Neurosurg* 163: 726, 1985
200. Ku Y, Fukumoto T, Iwasaki T et al.: Clinical pilot study on high-dose intra-arterial chemotherapy with direct hemoperfusion under hepatic venous isolation in patients with advanced hepatocellular carcinoma. *Surgery* 117: 510, 1995
201. Shah G, Nelson HA, Atkinson AJ, Okita GT, Ivanovich P, Gibson TP: Effect of hemoperfusion on the pharmacokinetics of digitoxin in dogs. *J Lab Clin Med* 93: 370, 1979
202. Marbury T, Mahoney J, Juncos L, Conti R, Cade R: Advanced digoxin toxicity in renal failure – treatment with charcoal hemoperfusion. *South Med J* 72: 279, 1979
203. Hoy WE, Gibson TP, Rivero AJ, Jain JK, Talley TT, Bayer RM, Montondo DF, Freeman RB: XAD-4 resin hemoperfusion for digitoxic patients with renal failure. *Kidney Int* 23: 79, 1983
204. Slattery JR, Koup JR: Hemoperfusion in the management of digoxin toxicity. Is it warranted? *Clin Pharmacokinet* 4: 395, 1979
205. Wenger TL, Butler VP Jr, Haber E, Smith TW: Treatment of 63 severely digitalis-toxic patients with digoxin specific antibody fragments. *J Am Coll Cardiol* 5 (Isl Suppl A): 118A, 1985
206. Ujhelyi MR, Robert S, Cummings DM, Colucci RD, Sailstad JM, Vlasses PH, Findlay JWA, Zarowitz BJ: Disposition of digoxin immune Fab in patients with kidney failure. *Clin Pharmacol Ther* 54: 388, 1993
207. Worth DP, Davison AM, Lewins AM, Ledgerwood MJ, Taylor A: Haemodialysis and charcoal haemoperfusion in acute inorganic mercury poisoning. *Postgrad Med J* 60: 636, 1984
208. De Backer W, Zachee P, Verpooten GA, Majelyne W, Vanheule A, De Broe ME: Thallium intoxication treated with combined hemoperfusion-hemodialysis. *J Toxicol Clin Toxicol* 19: 259, 1982
209. De Groot, van Heijst AN, van Kesteren RG, Maes RA: An evaluation of the efficacy of charcoal haemoperfusion in the treatment of three cases of acute thallium poisoning. *Arch Toxicol* 57: 61
210. Lund ME, Banner W, Clarkson TW, Berlin M: Treatment of acute methylmercury ingestion by hemodialysis with n-acetylcysteine (Mucomyst) infusion and 2,3-dimercaptopropane sulfonate. *J Toxicol/Clin Toxicol* 22: 31, 1984
211. Al-Abassi AH, Kostyniak PJ, Clarkson TW: An extracorporeal complexing hemodialysis system for the treatment of methylmercury poisoning. III. Clinical applications. *J Pharmacol Exp Ther* 207: 249, 1978
212. Margel S: A novel approach for heavy metal poisoning treatment, a model. Mercury poisoning by means of chelating microspheres: hemoperfusion and oral administration. *J Med Chem* 24: 1263, 1981
213. Banner W, Koch M, Capin DM, Hopf SB, Chang S, Tong TG: Experimental chelation therapy in chromium. Iead and boron intoxication with n-acetylcysteine and other compounds. *Toxicol Appl Pharmacol* 83: 142, 1986
214. Zieve L, Doizeki WM, Zieve FJ: Synergism between mercaptans and ammonia or fatty acids in the production of coma; a possible role for mercaptans in the pathogenesis of hepatic coma. *J Lab Clin Med* 83: 16, 1974
215. James TH, Ziparo V, Jeppsson B, Fischer JE: Hyperammonaemia, plasma amino acid imbalance, and blood-brain amino acid transport: a unified theory of portal-systemic encephalopathy. *Lancet* 2: 772, 1979
216. Schafer DF, Jones EA: Hepatic encephalopathy and the gamma-aminobutyric-acid neurotransmitter system. *Lancet* 1: 18, 1982
217. Chang TMS: Haemoperfusion over microencapsulated adsorbent in a patient with hepatic coma. *Lancet* 2: 1371, 1972
218. Gazzard BG, Portmann BA, Weston MJ, Langley PG, Murray-Lyon IM, Dunlop EH, Flax H, Mellon PJ, Record CO, Ward MB, Williams R: Charcoal haemoperfusion in the treatment of fulminant hepatic failure. *Lancet* 1: 1301, 1974
219. Chang TMS: Hemoperfusion alone and in series with ultrafiltration or dialysis for uremia, poisoning and liver failure. *Kidney Int* 10 (Suppl 7): S305, 1976
220. Bartels O, Neidhardt B, Neidhardt M, Schellberger H, Issel W, Waldherr AM, Demling L: Untersuchungen und Entahrungen mit der Kohlehaemoperfusion bei Leberkoma. in *Entgiftung mit Hamoperfusion* (Investigation and experience with carbon hemoperfusion for liver coma. in *Detoxification by Hemoperfusion*), edited by Demling L, Bartels O, Freiburg, Bundernagel-Verlag, 1977, p 119
221. Bartels O, Neithardt M, Schellberger H: Hormone losses by charcoal haemoperfusion. in *Artificial Liver Support*, edited by Brunner G, Schmidt FW, Berlin, Springer-Verlag, 1981, p 121
222. Gimson AES, Braude S, Mellon PJ, Canalese J, Williams R: Earlier charcoal haemoperfusion in fulminant hepatic failure. *Lancet* 2: 681, 1982
223. Cordopatri F, Boncinelli S, Marsili M, Lorenzi P, Fabbri LP, Paci P, Salvadori M, Morhni M, Cinoti S, Casparini P: Effects of charcoal haemoperfusion with prostacyclin on the coagulation-fibrinolysis system and platelets

of patients with fulminant hepatic failure – preliminary observation. *Int J Artif Organs* 5: 243, 1982

224. Williams R: Fulminant hepatic failure. *Postgrad Med J* 59 (Suppl 4): 33, 1983

225. Bihari D, Hughes RD, Gimson AES, Langley PG, Ede RJ, Eder G, Williams R: Effects of serial resin haemoperfusion in fulminant hepatic failure. *Int J Artif Organs* 6: 299, 1983

226. O'Grady JG, Gimson AE, O'Brien CJ, Pucknell A, Hughes RD, Williams R: Controlled trials of charcoal hemoperfusion and prognostic factors in fulminant hepatic failure. *Gastroenterology* 94: 1186, 1988

227. Rozga J, Hozman MD, Ro MS, et al.: Development of a hybrid bioartificial liver. *Ann Surg* 217: 502, 1993

228. Rozga J, Podesta L, LePage E, et al.: Control of cerebral oedema by total hepatectomy and extracorporeal liver support in fulminant hepatic failure. *Lancet* 342: 898, 1993

229. Rozga J, Hozman MD, Ro MS et al.: Development of reliable artificial liver support (ALS) – plasma exchange in combination with hemodialfiltration using high-performance membranes. *Dig Dis Sci* 38: 469, 1993

230. Fix IJ, Langnas AN, Fristoe, LW et al.: Successful application of extracorporeal liver perfusion: a technology whose time has come. *Am J Gastroenterol* 88: 1876, 1993

231. Sussman NL, Gislason GT, Kelly JH: Extracorporelal liver support. Application to fulminant hepatic failure. *J Clin Gastroenterol* 18: 320, 1994

232. Maeda K, Asada H, Yamamoto Y, Ohta K: Psoriasis treatment with direct hemoperfusion. in *Hemoperfusion, Kidney and Liver Support and Detotification*, edited by Sideman S, Chang TMS, Washington DC, Hemisphere Publishing Corp, 1980, p 349

233. Kolff WJ: Dialysis of schizophrenics. Weird and novel applications of dialysis, hemofiltration, hemoperfusion, and peritoneal dialysis: Witchcraft? *Artif Organs* 2: 277, 1978

234. Schulz SC, VanKammen DP, Balow JE, Flye NW, Bunney WE: Dialysis in schizophrenia: a double blind evaluation. *Science* 211: 1060, 1981

235. Nissensson AB, Rapaport M, Gordon A, Narins RG: Controlled study demonstrates that psoriasis is not improved by hemodialysis. *Kidney Int* 14: 682, 1978

236. Terman DS: Extracorporeal immunoadsorbents for extraction of circulating immune reactants. in *Sorbents and Their Clinical Applications*, edited by Giordano C, New York, Academic Press Inc, 1980, p 470

237. Terman DS, Buffaloe G, Mattioli C, Cook G, Tillquist R, Sullivan M, Ayus JC: Extracorporeal immunoabsorption: initial experience in human systemic lupus erythematosus. *Lancet* 2: 824, 1979

238. Terman DS, Garcia-Rinaldi R, McCalman R, Crumb CC, Mattioli C, Cook G, Poser R: Modification of hyperacute renal xenograft rejection after extracorporeal immunoadsorption of heterospecific antibody. *Int J Artif Organs* 2: 35, 1979

239. Hakim, RM, Milford E, Himmelfarb J, Wingard R, Lazarus JM, Watt RM: Extracorporeal removal of anti-HLA antibodies in transplant candidates. *Am J Kidney Dis* 16: 423, 1990

240. Wingard, RL, Lee WO, Hakim RO: Extracorporeal treatment of familial hypercholesterolemia with monoclonal antibodies to low-density lipoproteins. *Am J Kidney Dis* 18: 559, 1991

241. Savin H, Marcus L, Margel S, Ofarim M, Ravid M: Treatment of adverse digitalis effects by hemoperfusion through columns with antidigoxin antibodies bound to agarose polyacrolein microsphere beads. *Am Heart J* 113: 1078, 1987

242. Brizgys, MV, Pincus S, Siebert CJ, Rollins DE. Removal of digoxin from circulation using immobilized monoclonal antibodies. *J Pharm Sci* 78: 393, 1989

243. Terman DS, Yamamoto T, Mattioli M, Cook G, Tillquis R, Henry J, Poser Daskal Y: Extensive necrosis of spontaneous canine mammary adenocarcinoma aftce extracorporeal perfusion over Staphylococcus aureus Cowans I. *J Immunol* 124: 795, 1980

244. Terman DS, Betram HJ: Antitumor effects of immobilized protein A and Staphylococcal products: linkage between toxicity and efficacy and tumoricidal reagents. *Eur J Cancer Clin Oncol* 121: 1115, 1985

245. Langone JJ, Das C, Bennett D, Terman DS: Generation of human C1, C3a, and C4a anaphylotoxin by protein A of Staphylococcus aureus and immobilized protein A reagents in serotherapy of cancer. *J Immunol* 133: 1057, 1984

PERITONEAL DIALYSIS ACCESS/PLACEMENT/CONNECTORS

BETH PIRAINO

INTRODUCTION

Remarkable advances have occurred in connection technology reducing peritonitis due to touch contamination. Less progress has been made in reducing catheter related problems (1). The peritoneal dialysis catheter, therefore, remains the 'Achilles' heel' of peritoneal dialysis (2). Catheter infections can lead to peritonitis, catheter loss, and transfer to hemodialysis (3–5). Catheter function may be inadequate requiring replacement. Considerable research has been focussed on designing and investigating new catheters that may decrease the risk of infection and mechanical failure.

PERITONEAL ACCESS

Types of peritoneal catheters

Palmer designed the first permanent catheter from silicone rubber with a long subcutaneous portion (6). Tenckhoff modified the catheter to include Dacron® felt subcutaneous cuffs (7). Since the Tenckhoff catheter can be left in place indefinitely, long term peritoneal dialysis became possible (8). This catheter or a variation of it is used in the majority of peritoneal dialysis patients today in the US (9–11).

Most peritoneal catheters have three portions: external, subcutaneous, and intra-abdominal (Figures 1, 2, 3). The subcutaneous portion has one or two cuffs. The superficial cuff is also referred to as the outer, subcutaneous, or external cuff while the deep cuff is sometimes called the epiperitoneal cuff since it is imbedded within the rectus muscle. A fibrous capsule forms around the subcutaneous

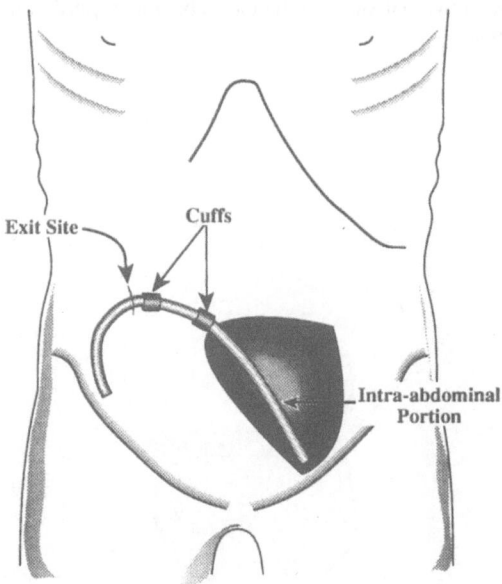

Figure 1. Diagram of a straight, double cuffed Tenckhoff catheter. The dark area indicates a portion of the abdominal cavity. The catheter between the exit site and the intra-abdominal portion is subcutaneous.

cuffs providing adherence to the surrounding tissue (12, 13). The subcutaneous tunnel between the exit site and the superficial cuff is the sinus tract, which is lined with epidermis (12, 13). The section between the cuffs, or intercuff segment, consists of a strong fibrous sheath. The intra-abdominal portion of the catheter contains multiple holes through which the dialysate flows. Most centers use

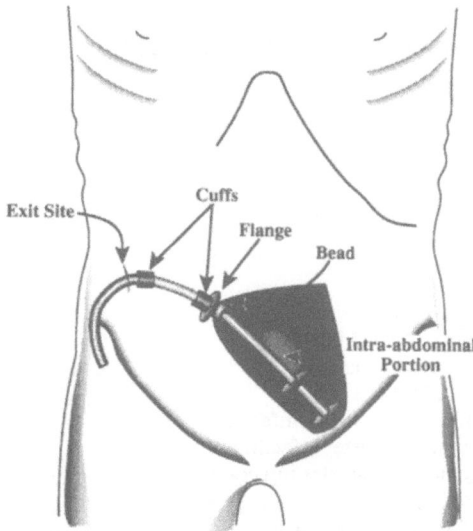

Figure 2. Diagram of the Toronto Western catheter. The dark area indicates a portion of the abdominal cavity. The catheter between the exit site and the intra-abdominal portion is subcutaneous.

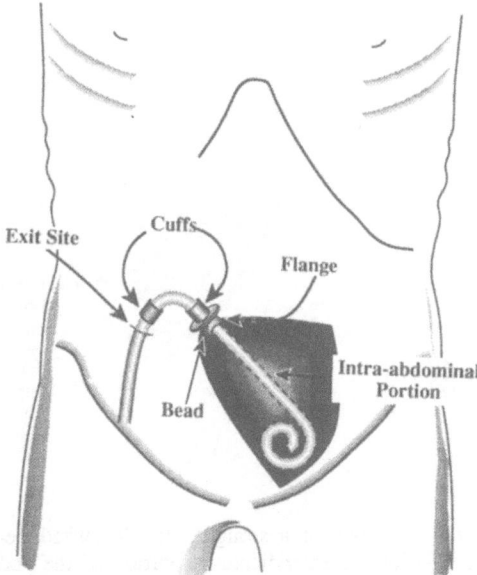

Figure 3. Diagram of the Swan neck Missouri catheter. The dark area indicates a portion of the abdominal cavity. The catheter between the exit site and the intra-abdominal portion is subcutaneous.

a short extension tubing (also called a transfer set) attached to the end of the catheter via a tight fitting adaptor. If the patient contaminates the transfer set at the time of an

Table 1. Commonly used catheter designs (11)

Tenckhoff silicone catheter
    Single or double cuffs
       Straight or curled intra-abdominal portion
       Straight or Swan neck tunnel portion
Swan neck Missouri catheter
Toronto Western Hospital catheter

exchange, the transfer set can be changed, leaving the catheter itself intact.

Currently there are many peritoneal catheter designs (14, 15). Those in common use are shown in Table 1. Most of the catheter styles are available with one or two subcutaneous cuffs (9). Leaks and exit site infections are as common using single versus double cuffed catheters (14), but double cuffed catheters, currently used in 72% of patients in the United States, have longer survival (16) and are associated with lower peritonitis rates than single cuff catheters (10).

The intra-abdominal portion of the peritoneal catheter may be straight or curled. A curled catheter, used in 40% of patients in the US may decrease outflow problems and infusion pain by decreasing the pressure from dialysate infusion against pelvic organs (10, 13, 17). Swartz et al. reported excellent (88%) two year catheter survival using a curled two cuff catheter (18). Only 4% of the catheters required replacement for drainage problems (18). However, in a randomized trial, mechanical complications and infusion pain occurred equally often with curled and straight Tenckhoff catheters (19).

The Toronto Western Hospital catheter, designed by Oreopoulos and Zellerman in 1976, has two flat silicone rubber discs on the intra-abdominal portion of the catheter to prevent migration of the catheter tip. In a further modification of this catheter a disc was placed at the base of the second cuff to decrease the risk of leaks (20) (Figure 2). One year catheter survival of 87% has been reported for the Toronto Western Hospital catheter, with outflow failure occurring in only 3% of catheters, all in patients who had previous abdominal surgery (20). However, in studies comparing the Toronto Western catheter with the Tenckhoff catheter, the proportions with drainage problems are similar (21, 22). Toronto Western catheter survival was the same in one study (21) and inferior to the Tenckhoff catheter in another (22). In a randomized prospective trial comparing the Toronto Western catheter, the double cuff straight Tenckhoff, and the coiled catheter, short term outcome was the same in all three groups (23).

The Swan neck Missouri catheter has a subcutaneous pathway which forms a curve over 180 degrees so that both the internal and external exit sites are downward (24–26). Theoretically, this design might minimize migration and exit site infections. The most recent modification has a curled intra-abdominal portion and two subcutaneous cuffs. The inner cuff has a flange (Figure 3). The Swan neck catheter, used in 12% of patients in the United Sates (10), has a one year catheter survival of 83% or better. The Swan neck catheter is somewhat more difficult to insert compared to the Tenckhoff catheter and may have a higher rate of accidental disconnections as the adaptor does not fit this catheter as well as the Tenckhoff catheter (27, 28). In a randomized trial comparing the single cuff Swan neck catheter to the single cuff straight Tenckhoff catheter there was no difference in 2 year catheter survival, peritonitis risk, or exit site infection between the two catheters (29). In two additional studies, exit site infections occurred as frequently with the Swan neck catheter as with the straight Tenckhoff catheter, although dislocation was less with the former (30, 31).

Many other catheters have been designed to decrease infection risk and mechanical problems but have not been widely adopted. The Cruz 'pail handle' catheter is made of polyurethane and allows rapid effluent outflow (32). Polyurethane, in contrast to silastic, may develop deformities of the external portion with repeated exposure to alcohol or local antibiotics such as mupirocin (1, 33, 34). The Gore-Tex® peritoneal catheter, with a silastic external and intra-abdominal portion and a transcutaneous section with a flange and cuff of polytetrafluoroethylene, was designed to decrease the incidence of tunnel infections, catheter cuff extrusions and exit site infection (35, 36). However, the converse proved true as exit site infection rate was high, frequently resulting in catheter removal (9, 37). Likewise the column disc catheter (Lifecath®), designed to increase outflow rate, minimize omental interference and prevent catheter migration (38), appears to have a higher risk of drainage failure requiring frequent replacement (22%) compared to the Tenckhoff catheter (5%) (39). The Dermaport® catheter, another polyurethane catheter with a subdermal flange, was designed to decrease catheter infections but was in practice found to have a high rate of catheter infections, often requiring catheter removal (40). The Valli® catheter, which has large holes at the end of the catheter surrounded by a silastic balloon with many holes, was designed to provide faster outflow but is seldom used (41).

Several new catheters, which have not yet been fully evaluated with clinical trials, are designed to solve a number of the problems associated with catheters, especially infection. The Moncrief–Popovich catheter is one such catheter (42). At the time of catheter insertion the entire external portion is placed into the subcutaneous tissue of the abdomen. After 3–5 weeks the end of the catheter is externalized via a small incision, which becomes the exit site (42, 43). In initial studies the peritonitis rate, but not the exit site infection rate, is reduced with use of this catheter; a randomized trial is in progress (44). Another newly designed catheter has a 3.5 cm outer cuff which is positioned half under the skin and half exposed allowing

for elimination of the sinus tract and formation of a barrier that may reduce infection (45). Twardowski et al. have suggested that a presternal Swan neck catheter may result in fewer exit site infections (46). Lastly, a silver impregnated catheter has been examined in animals as a method of reducing infection risk but trials in patients have not yet been done (47).

Catheter insertion

There are three techniques for insertion of the peritoneal catheter (1, 48): blind percutaneous, dissection, and percutaneous with peritoneoscopy. Historically, the peritoneal catheter was placed using a blind percutaneous approach (49, 50). This is the method used currently in only 8% of patients due to the risk of organ perforation, hemorrhage, and inadequate drainage (10, 18, 51). In most programs the catheters are placed in the operating room by a surgeon (10). The peritoneoscope, used in placing 6% of catheters in the United States, allows direct intra-abdominal visualization, which is ideal in patients with adhesions (10, 48). Catheter survival is the same with placement by an experienced nephrologist or surgeon (18).

Several principles apply regardless of the technique used for catheter insertion. Prior to catheter placement the physician or nurse should discuss with the patient the best location of the exit site for the patient's comfort and convenience. The belt-line should be avoided. Many patients would prefer to have the exit site below rather than above the waistline. Obese patients may require an exit site above the belt line to avoid fat folds (52). Avoidance of constipation in the peri-operative period is essential to obtain an adequately functioning catheter (1). The patient should void immediately prior to the procedure, and if a neurogenic bladder is present, catheterization of the bladder performed. Local anesthesia is acceptable for most patients if adequate sedation is provided, although some patients will require general anesthesia (53). The procedure requires a sterile environment, but the patient usually does not require admission. Prophylactic antibiotics are used in two thirds of dialysis centers (52, 54), but are not associated with a reduction in peritonitis or exit site infection rates (10, 55). However, the administration of gentamicin, 1.5 mg/kg, or vancomycin at the time of catheter insertion resulted in fewer exit site infections in the first month after catheter placement (56, 57).

The procedure for placing a peritoneal catheter using dissection is as follows (58). After the patient is prepped and draped, a small horizontal incision is made into the skin through the subcutaneous tissue and rectus abdominis muscle to expose the peritoneum. This incision for placement of the inner cuff should be paramedian, rather than midline, as a paramedian location of the deep cuff is associated with very low rates of both hernias and leaks (0.7%) (59). The catheter is immersed in sterile saline prior to insertion so that the cuff(s) become soaked, to promote fibrous ingrowth into the cuffs (52). Nonresorbable suture material is used to form a purse string in the peritoneum through which the catheter is passed using a catheter guide, which is then removed. The purse string is tied around the inner cuff. Fluid should be infused and drained from the catheter at this point to ensure adequate function (60). If this induces rectal or vaginal pain, the catheter is too deep and must be re-positioned. The subcutaneous tunnel is formed using a tunneler with the formation of a tight exit site around the catheter. No sutures are therefore required at the exit site. If the catheter has two cuffs, the superficial cuff should be 2 to 3 cm from the skin surface (1). The skin is closed with subcuticular sutures and Steristrips® (58).

In contrast to the above approach, in which the peritoneal cavity is minimally visualized, use of the peritoneoscope allows inspection of the abdominal cavity (48). Areas with adhesions can be avoided and the tip of the catheter properly positioned to allow optimal function. The procedure is described by Ash as follows. The abdomen is punctured with a cannula and internal trocar (48). The trocar is removed and the scope placed into the cannula so that the peritoneal surface can be examined. After 600 ml air is infused into the abdominal cavity, the scope is reinserted. Under direct visual inspection, the cannula is advanced to the desired position. The catheter is then advanced into position using a guide. The tunnel is formed as usual. In the hands of an experienced operator, early failure rate with this technique is as low as 3% (48). The risk of late catheter complications is similar with percutaneous placement using peritoneoscopy and with surgical placement using dissection (10). Success is dependent on the experience of the operator (61). In one series catheter leaks and/or poor dialysate flow subsequent to catheter placement using peritoneoscopy led to catheter removal in 11% of instances, but the cuff was not placed within the rectus muscle (62). Shyr achieved adequate catheter function in 96% of patients using dissection with blind placement, and reserved the laparoscope to reposition the catheter in the two patients whose catheters did not flow adequately when checked intra-operatively, thus eliminating the need for a second surgery (31). The use of the peritoneoscope is especially attractive in high risk patients with previous surgery in whom adhesions are suspected (54). Amerling and Cruz describe a variation of the peritoneoscopic placement described above, in which pneumoperitoneum (which can be uncomfortable) is optional and a scope which provides increased safety and a better view is used (64).

Blind percutaneous catheter placement was originally described by Tenckhoff. A small incision is made down to the level of the peritoneum. Generally, this is made in the infraumbilical area in the midline to avoid blood vessels, but this increases the risk of subsequent leak or hernia. A large bore needle (14 gauge) is placed into the abdominal cavity through which 2 liters of saline or dialysate are infused. A trocar is then pushed through the abdominal wall; a 'pop' tells the operator that the peritoneum has been entered. When the stylet is removed, fluid exits through the trocar informing the operator that the peritoneum has been entered. The catheter, reinforced by the obturator, is introduced through the trocar into the abdominal cavity. The trocar is angled to allow placement of the catheter tip into the pelvis. The catheter is advanced, the obturator is removed and the catheter is flushed to check fluid movement. The subcutaneous tunnel is then formed. An alternative percutaneous method for placing a peritoneal catheter is with the Seldinger technique (over a wire technique). This method is used currently at some institutions for placement of a catheter for acute renal failure, as catheter function is better and there are fewer dialysate leaks compared to the trocar technique (65, 66). Percutaneous blind catheter insertion is today the least desirable approach as the risk of organ perforation and drainage failure are increased compared to the other methods (51, 67, 68). Radiologists can place the catheter percutaneously using fluoroscopy to ensure proper positioning, but this technique is not widely practiced (69).

Post-operative management of the patient

Rapid healing of the catheter insertion site is associated with a small, tight fitting exit site, the use of Swan neck catheters, immobilization of the catheter, and the use of peri-operative vancomycin (57). Hematomas and dialysate leak lead to delayed healing. Most dialysis centers have dialysis personnel perform exit site care for up to 2 weeks post operatively as this may help reduce infection risk (54, 70, 71). The surgical dressing may be left intact for several days unless there is bleeding at the site. Povidone iodine solution is commonly used for postoperative cleaning of the exit site (54).

Peritoneal dialysis can be initiated immediately using low volumes with the patient in the supine position. This can be achieved by either automated peritoneal dialysis with rapid exchanges or manual exchanges in the evening and overnight for patients already familiar with the CAPD technique (72). Alternatively, the patient may be maintained on hemodialysis in the interim period while the catheter insertion site is healing. Patients temporarily on hemodialysis have similar catheter complications as patients temporarily on intermittent peritoneal dialysis during the catheter healing phase (73). If the patient does not need immediate dialysis, delaying CAPD for 10 days will minimize the risk of leak (74, 75). If the catheter is not to be utilized immediately, then the catheter should be flushed several times with 1 liter of dialysate (often with 500 units of heparin per liter added) until the effluent is clear, prior to capping the catheter until training is to begin (13, 73).

Insignificant hemoperitoneum is commonly seen shortly after peritoneal catheter insertion and generally clears quickly. Flushing the catheter with heparinized dialysate is useful to clear the catheter and prevent blockage

(76). Patients with previous abdominal surgery or non-peritoneal dialysis related peritonitis are at increased risk for hemorrhage serious enough to require transfusion (77). Injury to the inferior epigastric artery can also result in significant bleeding (76). Pain related to dialysate flow occurs in 3% of patients and usually resolves with time (53, 78). Decreasing the drain time to allow a larger residual of dialysate to accumulate is often helpful in decreasing the pain. More severe pain requires evaluation with an abdominal film and/or by placing contrast through the catheter and imaging the abdomen.

MECHANICAL COMPLICATIONS OF PERITONEAL CATHETERS

Catheter obstruction/inadequate drain

Slow and inadequate drainage is common and may occur shortly after catheter insertion or later in the course of dialysis (79). Both catheter inflow and outflow may be impeded or there may be inflow without outflow (80). The frequency of immediate failure of the catheter to drain is related to the expertise of the physician inserting the catheter and to adhesions secondary to previous abdominal surgery (59). Six to 7% of catheters have inadequate flow rates immediately after insertion, requiring replacement in one half (18, 53).

Migration of the tip of the peritoneal catheter, easily diagnosed by obtaining an abdominal film, causes late drainage problems in about 5% of straight catheters (18, 53, 81, 82). Ideally the tip of the catheter should be in one of the pelvic gutters, since this location results in the fastest rate of effluent outflow (83, 84). In contrast, location of the end of the catheter in the upper quadrants is often associated with inadequate drainage (83, 84). Migration of the end of the catheter from the pelvis to the upper quadrants may occur more often with the Tenckhoff than with the Toronto Western Hospital or Swan neck catheters (29, 85). Constipation, a common cause of decreased rate of effluent flow, generally resolves with laxatives unless the catheter position has shifted, in which case catheter replacement may be necessary. Therefore, it is important to avoid constipation in peritoneal dialysis patients. Although poor drainage due to malposition of the catheter occasionally resolves spontaneously, usually intervention with either a guide wire or surgery is necessary (29, 82, 86). Laparoscopic manipulation is successful in 50% of patients compared to a 33% success rate using a wire (86–89). If outflow obstruction is due to adherence of the end of the catheter to the peritoneum, a trocar inserted into the catheter to gently change the position may be successful (90). Placement of an omental cuff around the intra-abdominal portion of the catheter to hold the catheter in position has been described but is not widely used (91).

Two way obstruction may be due to clots or fibrin within the catheter (60, 78). Forcibly flushing the catheter with heparinized saline may resolve the obstruction. If this fails, fibrinolytic agents may be effective (92–96). The insertion of an endoscopy brush into the occluded catheter has been reported to successfully relieve catheter obstruction also (97).

Omentum can cause catheter obstruction (53, 60, 78). Omentectomy may be necessary, especially in children or with use of the Life-Cath® (53, 60, 98–101). Partial omentectomy as a routine procedure at the time of catheter placement improves catheter survival but is a much bigger surgical procedure (102). Unusual causes of catheter obstruction include fungus colonizing the catheter (103, 104), fallopian tubes obstructing the catheter (105, 106), catheter lithiasis (107), and fracture of the catheter (108).

Perforation and laceration of organs due to peritoneal catheters

Perforation of the bladder, bowel or laceration of the spleen may occur at the time of catheter insertion (101, 109). These are very uncommon events with either surgical or laparoscopic placement. Adhesions increase the risk of perforation (78). Perforation of an organ should be considered if the effluent is feculent or when watery diarrhea, polyuria or watery vaginal discharge occur with infusion of dialysate (78, 110). Voiding or placement of a urethral catheter (if the patient has a neurogenic bladder) prior to the procedure will help prevent bladder perforation (60). If bladder perforation occurs, the defect is surgically closed and a urethral catheter left in place (101). Perforation of the bowel from catheter placement may close without surgery but is more serious than bladder perforation and can lead to death (110, 111). A case of splenic laceration leading to shock from massive hemoperitoneum immediately subsequent to Tenckhoff catheter placement for acute renal failure has been reported (112).

Delayed injuries to intra-abdominal organs including bowel and bladder are uncommon but well recognized complications of peritoneal catheters (113–116). Splenic laceration from a translocated peritoneal catheter occurred in a patient previously stable on CAPD for 20 months (117). These complications may be due to necrosis resulting from pressure of the catheter against an organ (78). An unused peritoneal catheter is felt to be a cause of bowel perforation in transplant patients (118–121). Because of this unusual but serious complication, it is prudent to remove the peritoneal catheter soon after the renal transplant is deemed successful (78, 110).

Peritoneal catheter leaks

Peritoneal dialysate leaks may occur at several different locations, including the catheter exit site, inner cuff, sites of hernias and previous surgeries (58, 122, 123). Five to 10% of patients develop catheter leaks shortly after insertion of the catheter and a further 2 to 4% later in their course on peritoneal dialysis (18, 29, 39, 53, 58, 76, 124). Leaks are felt to be more common in association with steroids, obesity, multiparity, increased age and perhaps diabetes mellitus (1, 20).

Early leaks may present as clear dextrose-positive fluid from the exit site or as abdominal wall edema. Early leaks are often due to failure to anchor the deep cuff in the rectus muscle using nonabsorbable suture, the use of a midline rather than paramedian placement, and/or pressure on the insertion site by early initiation of CAPD (20, 60, 78, 128). Two to three purse string sutures around the inner cuff placed in a paramedian position in the rectus abdominalis muscle reduces the risk of leaks to ≤ 2% despite the institution of immediate dialysis using low volumes (59, 126).

A dialysate leak may resolve with temporary cessation of CAPD using either hemodialysis or supine peritoneal dialysis (58, 78, 127). Dialysate leaks from the exit site are often associated with infection, thus antibiotics should be given (128). If a leak occurring more than 1 month after catheter insertion does not resolve within 4 days of reduced volumes, or if it recurs after full volumes are resumed, surgical correction is generally required (129). Joffe has reported a unique method of correcting an exit site leak by instilling a fibrin sealant into the cuff and at the exit site (130).

The site of a subcutaneous dialysate leak, if not clinically obvious, may be located with scintigraphy or contrast imaging (131–133). Computerized tomography of the abdomen after 50 ml of contrast per liter of dialysate is instilled into the abdomen will often detect not only the site of the leak but other abnormalities such as hernias. Peritoneal scintigraphy, after dialysate containing 1 to 2 millicuries of either sulfur colloid or albumin colloid labelled with technetium-99m is infused into the abdominal cavity, is an alternative approach (132–134).

Edema of the scrotum or perineal area is usually due to a patent processus vaginalis or an inguinal hernia (132, 135–137). Scrotal edema develops in 10% of men on CAPD, while labial edema occurs in only 1.4% of women (132, 138). Temporarily this can be managed by supine peritoneal dialysis but surgical correction is generally required, certainly if a hernia is present (58, 127). Post operative management may include hemodialysis for 1 week or more (58).

Vaginal leakage of dialysate is rare but serious as it can lead to recurrent peritonitis, often with fungus (139–142). This complication should be suspected in any woman with watery vaginal discharge which is positive for glucose. A peritoneal-vaginal leak may be due to erosion of the catheter through the pouch of Douglas (in which case the catheter must be removed) or to dialysate leak through the fallopian tubes (corrected by tubal ligation) (143).

Acute hydrothorax occurs in 1.6% of CAPD patients (144). The interval between start of CAPD and presen-

Table 2. Commonly used connection methods

Straight system with attached bag
Ultraviolet irradiation
Manual exchange
Exchange assist device
Disconnect systems
Y-set with disinfectant
Y-set without disinfectant*
Y-set twin bag system
Automated peritoneal dialysis

*Can be used in conjunction with an ultraviolet irradiation device.

tation with the pleural effusion varies from 1 day to 8 years (144). The patient may be asymptomatic or complain of dyspnea (144, 145). The majority of these pleuro-peritoneal leaks are on the right side (144). The peritoneal fluid may enter the pleural cavity via diaphragmatic lymphatics or defects in the diaphragm (123, 146, 147). The diagnosis may be easily confirmed by thoracentesis and measurement of glucose (which will be generally but not invariably be elevated), LDH (which will be low) and/or D-lactate (as opposed to the natural occurring L-isomer) (145). Scintigraphy using 99 m Tc-sulfur colloid or computerized tomography with contrast also are useful to confirm the presence of the peritoneal pleural connection (145, 148). Treatment approaches include temporary cessation of CAPD (the effusion will spontaneously resorb), pleurodesis, surgical repair using teflon-felt patches, or permanent transfer to hemodialysis (144, 145, 149).

CONNECTION DEVICES

In contrast to peritoneal dialysis catheters, many important advances have occurred in connection techniques, resulting in a dramatic lowering of peritonitis rates. Early modifications included conversion from glass bottles to plastic bags and addition of an adaptor between the catheter and extension tubing to lessen the risk of accidental disconnections. For many years a straight line connection system, with the empty dialysate bag attached to the patient between dialysis exchanges, was the standard. The exchange was performed manually. The most important subsequent advances in connection technology have been the disconnect Y-set systems, in which there is a dialysate flush and drain prior to infusion, and the use of a chamber that provides ultraviolet light irradiation of the connection ports at the time of the exchange (150, 151). Other innovative techniques such as heat sealing devices which splice the tubing and fuse the new tubing to the old are not widely used (152, 153). The most common forms of connection systems used today are shown in Table 2.

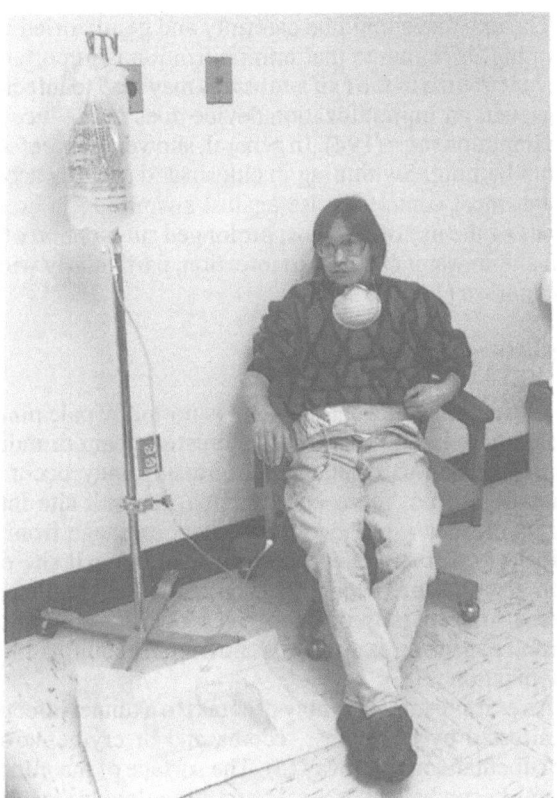

Figure 4. Photograph (taken by Wendy Hendricks) of a patient performing an exchange using a Y-set disconnect system. Patient has made her connection to the Y tubing. She will flush a small volume of dialysate from the full bag to the drain bag. Next she will drain the effluent within her abdominal cavity into the drain bag. In the third step she will close the line to the drain bag and infuse the fresh dialysate. Lastly, she disconnects from the Y tubing.

Disconnect technology

With the disconnect Y-set system, the patient connects his or her catheter to a Y set of tubing attached to a full dialysate bag and an empty bag (Figure 4). The patient flushes a small volume of dialysate from the fill bag through the line into the drain bag. Next, the patient drains the effluent from the peritoneum. Fresh dialysate is infused and the Y tubing disconnected, either by capping the catheter or snapping off the tubing. With this technique, therefore, the flush and drain remove bacteria present due to contamination, decreasing the risk of infection.

The disconnect Y-set systems are gradually replacing the manual straight spike system with the attached bag. In 1992 68% of European patients on CAPD used a disconnect Y system, although this percentage varied markedly from one country to another (154). In the United States, 37% of patients beginning CAPD during the first six months of 1989 used a disconnect system (10).

Table 3. Rates of staphylococcal peritonitis using the straight line system (1980–1984) and the disconnect Y-system (1985–1989) (124)

	Episodes/Patients/Year	
	1980–1984	*1985–1989*
Staphylococcus epidermidis	0.26	0.08
Staphylococcus aureus	0.10	0.09

Many studies document a decrease in peritonitis rates to 0.4–0.5/y using disconnect Y systems (155–166). In several randomized trials peritonitis rates were 0.4/y to 0.6/y using the Y-set versus 1.0/y to 1.2/y using the straight spike system (163, 164, 166). Patients switching from the straight spike to the Y set system also had a reduction in peritonitis rates from 1.2/y to $\leq$ 0.5/y (165, 167, 168). The decrease in peritonitis with the Y-set is primarily due to a reduction in peritonitis due to *S. epidermidis*, as shown in Table 3 (8, 124, 151, 169). *In vitro* studies confirm that the flush technique is more effective in removing contamination due to *S. epidermidis* than that due to other organisms (170, 171). In addition to the reduction in peritonitis rates, patients prefer the disconnect system for cosmetic reasons (172). For these reasons the disconnect systems have resulted in a reduction in peritoneal dialysis technique failure (164, 173, 174).

There are numerous forms of disconnect systems (Table 2). Some contain disinfectant within the lines while others do not. Peritonitis rates with use of a reusable Y tubing, which contains sodium hypochlorite between exchanges, are variably reported from 0.3 to 0.6/y (159, 166, 168, 175). Peritonitis rates appear to be similar with and without the use of disinfectant (176–179). The disadvantage of disinfectant is that accidental infusion of the disinfectant during performance of an exchange, although uncommon, causes severe abdominal pain. Reuse of the tubing for 8 weeks makes this an economical form of disconnect technology. The reusable disconnect system with disinfectant, when the reduction in peritonitis is considered, is cheaper than both the straight spike system and the ultraviolet box (179). Another economical disconnect system is a single use Y-set without disinfectant in which the fill bag is used for the drain bag in the subsequent exchange. A third cost-effective disconnect system uses straight reusable tubing (rather than Y tubing) which is disconnected between exchanges. With this system there is not a flush prior to infusion (180). Low peritonitis rates are produced by filling the caps and Luer lock connectors with iodine between exchanges (180).

More costly but convenient forms of the Y set have either pre-attached drain bag (with the patient attaching to the fill bag at the time of the exchange) or a Y set with pre-attached fill and drain bags, called the twin bag or integrated system. With the twin bag system the patient, therefore, only has to make the connection between the

Y tubing and the catheter (181). Peritonitis rates of 0.4/y have been reported with this technique, with very low rates of coagulase negative staphylococcus (181–184). In a center with relatively high peritonitis rates, conversion to the twin bag system resulted in a decrease in the rates which fell from 1.3/y to 0.7/y (185).

Ultraviolet light devices

Ultraviolet systems, in which the connection ports are irradiated within a chamber during each exchange, are used in 27% of patients beginning CAPD during the first 6 months of 1989 in the United States (10). Although the relative risk of peritonitis was reduced in comparison to the straight spike system (10), data for the effect of the ultraviolet system in reducing peritonitis rates are less convincing than for the disconnect systems. *In vitro* studies on the effectiveness of ultraviolet light in sterilizing hand contaminated spikes have conflicting results (186, 187). Nolph et al. in a multicenter trial was unable to show a decrease in peritonitis risk using ultraviolet irradiation compared to a straight spike system (151). Patients with impaired dexterity or vision have reduced peritonitis rates using a newer version of ultraviolet irradiation (using a xenon lamp) (188). A French study confirmed that the use of the xenon generated ultraviolet light device in the elderly, handicapped, and home bound patients resulted in peritonitis rates of 0.43/y with *S. epidermidis* rates of 0.05/y, indicating that touch contamination had been almost eliminated as a cause of peritonitis (182). The ultraviolet device, which can be used with either the straight spike system or the disconnect system, is an option to allow the handicapped patient to perform his/her own dialysis.

CATHETER EXIT SITE AND INFECTIONS

Chronic exit site care

The ideal approach to chronic exit site care is unknown. Studies are contradictory as to how the exit site should be cleaned and whether coverage is important (190, 191). Daily cleaning (often in the shower) with a bactericidal soap and water is effective, cheap and commonly used (54, 190). In a randomized trial comparing povidone iodine and a non-occlusive dressing to soap and water, there were more exit site infections in the soap and water group (191). *S. aureus* exit site infection rates were 0.22/y using povidone iodine and 0.47/y using soap and water. Jindal and Hirsch also reported very low exit site infections with an exit site care protocol that included occlusive dressings and cleaning of the exit site with povidone iodine every 5 days (192). Povidone iodine may lead to skin irritation (193). Hydrogen peroxide should not be routinely used for exit site care as it has been associated with increased exit site infection rates (190).

The exit site should be carefully and gently dried after cleaning. Most agree that immobilization is important to prevent trauma to the exit site as this may lead to infection. However, an immobilization device does not reduce exit site infection rates (194). In general, showers are preferred to tub bathing. Swimming in chlorinated pools is accepted but most centers advise against swimming in creeks, ponds or the use of hot tubs; prolonged submersion of the exit site in water can lead to infection, particularly with *P. aeruginosa* (13, 195).

Catheter infections

The skin around the catheter exit is normally pale pink or flesh colored, with no drainage, crusting, pain or induration (13). Serous drainage and crusting may occur but generally do not represent infection. An exit site infection is present when there is purulent drainage from the exit site or if there is erythema around the exit site or if both are present (196–199). The culture, if drainage is present, is generally positive, but a positive culture of a normal appearing exit site does not represent infection but colonization (200).

An exit site infection may progress to a tunnel infection, manifested by tenderness, edema and or erythema over the subcutaneous pathway (5). The surface of the infected tunnel becomes hemorrhagic and granulocytes accumulate (13). The cuffs do not prevent the spread of infection along the subcutaneous pathway and may become separated from the surrounding tissue (12, 13). A tunnel infection, especially with involvement of the inner cuff, may result in peritonitis, which is often refractory to antibiotic therapy requiring removal of the catheter for resolution of the infection (201). As a consequence, patients with a history of exit site infections are more likely to transfer to hemodialysis either temporarily or permanently (3, 5).

Rates of exit site infections vary widely, because differing definitions are used and because exit site infections and tunnel infections are not always separated (202,203). Many centers report exit site infection rates of 0.5 to 1/y (196, 204–206). Purulent exit site infections, approximately one-half of the total, are more likely to lead to peritonitis, recurrence, and catheter loss (196, 207).

The rate of clinically obvious tunnel infection is 0.19/y (204, 208). However, in contrast to exit site infections which are easily diagnosed, tunnel infections may be occult (209). When an exit site is present, ultrasound examination of the tunnel frequently demonstrates abnormal fluid collections around the subcutaneous catheter pathway (210, 211). Involvement of the tunnel, and especially the inner cuff as demonstrated by ultrasound, is an ominous sign as peritonitis frequently follows (211).

Micro-organisms causing exit site and tunnel infections are shown in Table 4. The most common organism causing exit site infections and tunnel infections is *Staphylococcus aureus*, with *Staphylococcus epidermidis* and *P. aeruginosa* the next most common (169, 196, 205, 208,

Table 4. Micro organisms causing peritoneal catheter infections (with a disconnect system) (169)

Micro-organism	Episodes per dialysis year	
	Exit site infection	Tunnel infection
S. aureus	0.34	0.07
S. epidermidis	0.12	0.01
Gram negative	0.12	0.03
No culture/sterile	0.10	0.02
Total	0.68	0.14

212). *S. aureus* exit site infection is frequently purulent while *S. epidermidis* and culture negative exit site infections are generally non-purulent (196). *Staphylococcus epidermidis* exit site infections are generally easily treated and seldom progress to tunnel infection and peritonitis, in contrast to exit site infections due to *Pseudomonas aeruginosa* or *S. aureus* (213–216).

S. aureus catheter infections are associated with a high rate of *Staphylococcus aureus* peritonitis and catheter loss due to infection (217). Patients with *S aureus* exit site infections had a *S. aureus* peritonitis rate of 0.5/y contrasted to those without *S. aureus* exit site infections who had a *S. aureus* peritonitis rate of 0.07/y (217). One half or more of patients presenting with *S. aureus* peritonitis will have a concomitant *S. aureus* catheter infection and many of the rest will have colonization of the exit site with *S. aureus* (213, 218–220). In addition to leading to peritonitis and catheter loss, *S. aureus* tunnel infection can cause toxic shock syndrome (221).

Risk factors for catheter infections

S. aureus nasal carriage is strongly associated with *S. aureus* exit site colonization, cathter and peritonitis (218, 222–225). The same subtype is found in the nares, colonizing the exit site and in the effluent when peritonitis is present (225, 227). *S aureus* nasal carriage can lead to *S. aureus* peritonitis by two routes: via exit site/tunnel infection and via touch contamination at the time of an exchange.

Forty five percent of patients starting CAPD will have *S. aureus* in their nares (222). With time on CAPD 30% of patients who were not initially *S. aureus* carriers will have one or more positive nose cultures (228). If carriage is defined as 2 of 3 positive nose cultures, 44% of peritoneal dialysis patients are carriers compared to 17% of the patients' partners (229). Approximately one third of peritoneal dialysis patients are chronic carriers with *S. aureus* in the nares or exit site in $\geq$ 75% of cultures, one third are intermittent carriers, and one third have zero or one positive nose cultures (225, 227). Age, sex, diabetes mellitus, and the use of subcutaneous erythropoietin are not known risk factors for *S. aureus* carriage (223, 228). Few risk factors for catheter infections other than *S. aureus* nasal carriage have been identified. Insulin dependent diabetes does not appear to be associated with an increased risk of catheter infection (230), although tunnel infection rates are higher in diabetic women than nondiabetic men (208). Black patients may have slightly higher catheter infection rates, but fewer *S. aureus* catheter infections than white patients (231). Obesity does not increase exit site infection rate but infections in such patients are more difficult to treat, increasing the probability of catheter loss (232).

Prevention of catheter infections

The most effective approaches to decreasing catheter infections have been directed at *S. aureus* carriage. Intranasal mupirocin, twice daily for 5 days each month, is effective in eliminating nasal carriage and reducing the catheter infection rate due to *S. aureus* (233, 234). Mupirocin applied daily to the exit site also is effective in reducing *S. aureus* catheter infections (235). Rifampin, highly effective in reducing *S. aureus* nasal carriage, reduced *S. aureus* catheter infections and peritonitis when given as 600 mg each day for 5 days every 3 months (236–240). Treatment of nasal carriage peri-operatively is also effective in reducing early *S. aureus* exit site infection, peritonitis and catheter loss from infections (241).

New catheter designs have been proposed to decrease the risk of catheter infections (242, 243). Pre-treating catheters with cationic surfactants allows bonding of anionic antibiotics to the surface, and thus theoretically a reduction in catheter infection rate (242). Although this approach is effective for intravascular catheters, pretreated peritoneal dialysis catheters bonded with cefoxitin had a similar rate of removal for catheter infections as untreated catheters (244, 245). Silver applied to the catheter exit site has also been reported to reduce infection rate (246).

Trauma to the exit site may predispose to catheter infections (70). Therefore, avoidance of trauma by avoiding the wasitline in placing the catheter exit site and immobilization of the catheter should help prevent infections, although little definitive evidence is available to support this common sense approach (194, 247). Twardowski et al. found that infections of downward directed exit sites required shorter treatment duration, thus, supporting the use of the Swan neck catheter design (24). Single cuffed catheters may be associated with catheter infections that require longer courses of antibiotics (24) and more frequent catheter removal for such infections (16).

Management of catheter infections

Exit site infections are generally treated with an oral antibiotic. The antibiotic is chosen to cover staphylococcus and then adjusted based on the culture and sensitivity results. For Gram positive infections, trimetho-prim/sulfamethoxazole is as effective as vancomycin with rifampin and more effective than vancomycin alone (207). The length of therapy is quite variable depending on the response and the micro-organism, but should be continued for 1 week after the exit site appears normal (13).

Local care of the exit site is generally intensified and in mild or equivocal exit site infections this may be the only therapy (54). Generally, povidone iodine, sodium hypochlorite, chlorhexidine, or antibacterial soap are used to clean the infected exit site (54). Hypertonic saline compresses applied to the infected exit site may hasten resolution (248). An application of silver nitrate to the exit site removes excessive granulation tissue (13, 249). For an equivocal exit site with serosanguinous drainage and crusting but without induration, erythema or purulence, local application of antibiotic ointment may be beneficial (13, 250).

Once prolonged antibiotic therapy fails to resolve the infection, revision of the tunnel with removal of the external cuff (in two cuffed catheters) may help to prolong the life of the catheter (205, 251) but often eventually results in peritonitis (251, 252). External cuff extrusion without infection does not require removal of the cuff (98). Cuff removal can be performed under local anesthesia with dissection and gentle traction to free the cuff, which is then shaved using a scalpel, carefully avoiding cutting the catheter itself (98). Some dissect the entire area of granulation tissue and cellulitis resulting in an open wound which is then packed until healing occurs (253, 254). Cuff shaving and tunnel revision are never effective if catheter related peritonitis is present (252).

Staphylococcus aureus catheter infections are difficult to treat successfully, thus long courses of antibiotics are given (214). Overall *S. aureus* exit site infections resolve approximately one half of the time with antibiotic therapy with most failures being due to relapses (255–257). Removal of the external cuff with excision of granulation tissue and the surrounding cellulitis cures another 23% of *S. aureus* catheter infections but most of the remainder develop peritonitis (257). When *S. aureus* peritonitis appears to have resolved with therapy but effluent cultures remain positive, a catheter infection is generally present; delay of catheter removal may result in the patient's death (258).

Most Gram negative exit site infections are due to *Pseudomonas aeruginosa* (207). Exit site infections due to *P. aeruginosa*, in contrast to infections with *Xanthomonas maltophilia*, frequently cause peritonitis and are difficult to treat successfully (207, 215, 216, 259). Ciprofloxacin, 250 to 500 mg bid for 4 weeks, is the drug of choice for *P. aeruginosa* catheter infections, but recurrence is common (260, 262). The addition of a second drug (ceftazidime or tobramycin) yields better results (207, 261). Recurrence is treated with further antibiotic therapy and removal of the external cuff of the catheter (261).

Catheter biofilm

Bacterial colonization of catheters without an exit site or tunnel infection is common (262). The rate of colonization depends on the degree of bacterial contamination at the time of implantation (263). Within 3 weeks of insertion most catheters are colonized and dialysis accelerates the process (263). Catheters removed after an average of 37 months (range 2–77 months) were covered with a biofilm, equally distributed between intra and extra-peritoneal segments (264). Scanning electron micrography of both used and unused Tenckhoff catheters indicates that all used catheters have microbial biofilm (265). Studies in rabbits have shown that bacterial biofilms rapidly develop on implanted peritoneal silastic disks that prevents clearing of *P. aeruginosa* from the peritoneal cavity (266). Colonization of silastic is related to quantity of bacteria as well as the micro-organism, with *S. epidermidis* and *P. aeruginosa* more likely to colonize silastic catheters than *E. coli* (267).

The relationship of biofilm to peritonitis is unclear. A proportion of patients with *S. epidermidis* peritonitis will have repeated episodes that rapidly respond to antibiotics but recur repeatedly. This problem is resolved by replacing the catheter and may be due to biofilm. However, colonization of the catheter does not inevitably result in peritonitis (268). Strains of coagulase negative Staphylococcus that are strongly adherent to silicone catheters *in vitro* are minimally altered by vancomycin (269). *S. epidermidis* in the fluid phase is invariably sensitive to rifampin and vancomycin but in the biofilm phase resistant to all antibiotics except rifampin (270). Thus, biofilm may make peritonitis difficult to eradicate.

CATHETER LOSS AND REPLACEMENT

The success of peritoneal dialysis is dependent on obtaining and maintaining a functional, non-infected catheter in the patient. This is not always easily accomplished; 18% of catheters require replacement by 1 year on CAPD, 30% by 2 years and 53% by 4 years with overall catheter replacement rates of 0.2/y (202, 203, 271). Malfunction accounts for the majority of catheters lost early after catheter placement while infections account for most of catheters lost later in the course of peritoneal dialysis (22, 273). Mechanical problems resulting in catheter removal include (in the order of frequency) drain failure, dialysate leak and pericatheter hernia (18). When a catheter is removed for mechanical reasons, a new catheter can be inserted immediately.

The rate of catheter removal for infections is 0.11 to 0.16/y (14, 18, 19, 69). Indications for catheter removal are shown in Table 5. Peritonitis episodes due to *S. aureus*, *P. aeruginosa*, and fungus often require catheter removal (1, 215, 258). Catheter related peritonitis accounts for approximately one third of the catheters removed, while

Table 5. Reasons for peritoneal catheter removal (1, 18, 272, 287–289)

Infectious reasons
    Refractory peritonitis[a]
    Recurrent peritonitis
    Peritonitis associated with GI pathology
    Refractory tunnel infection
Catheter malfunction
    Persistent leak
    Inadequate or no drain
    Pericatheter hernia
Structural abnormality of the catheter[b]
Sclerosing peritonitis
Transfer to hemodialysis or successful transplantation

---

[a]Frequently these peritonitis episodes are secondary to catheter infection.
[b]Uncommon cause of catheter loss.

the proportion and rate of catheter removal for isolated peritonitis has decreased with use of disconnect systems (18, 169). The timing of catheter removal for refractory tunnel infections varies from center to center. Traditionally, if catheters are removed due to infection, there is a waiting period to allow the infection to resolve prior to replacing the catheter. However, there are circumstances in which the infected catheter can be removed and a new catheter placed during the same procedure (274–277). This has been successfully done for recurrent (predominantly *S. epidermidis*) or relapsing peritonitis (predominantly *S. aureus*) (276, 277). Simultaneous catheter replacement is not warranted for peritonitis due to *Candida albicans* or *Pseudomonas aeruginosa*.

PERITONEAL CATHETERS IN CHILDREN

Peritoneal dialysis is a successful technique for maintaining children until transplantation can be performed (278, 279). Catheters are available in 3 lengths: neonatal (8–10 cm cuff to tip), juvenile (16 cm cuff to tip) and adult. Catheter length is chosen based on the size of the child (66). The Tenckhoff catheter is used in 93.4% of the children. Curled single cuffed catheters are used more often than straight catheters in children. Seventeen percent of the catheters have a Swan neck tunnel (278).

Special considerations in infants include the small length of the neonatal catheter and placement of the exit site above the diaper area to prevent contamination (99). Partial omentectomy is useful to prevent outflow problems. In male children exploration of the groins with herniotomy and ligation of patent processus vaginalis at the time of catheter placement diminishes subsequent inguinal hernia and hydrocele (99). Without these pre-

cautions complications of the catheters are very common (65).

Catheter problems in children have decreased with increasing experience. In 1982 Baum et al. reported a need for catheter replacement or re-positioning 19 times in 20 children for infection, obstruction, dislodgement, dialysate leaks, catheter perforation or hernia (279). A subsequent report noted catheter survival of 50% at 2 years with leaks in 26% and drain problems, primarily due to omentum, occurring 17% (280). In contrast, currently only ten percent of catheters in children require removal (278). Data obtained from the North American Pediatric Renal Transplant Cooperative Study show that catheter replacement was for mechanical malfunction (45%), leak (9%), peritonitis (18%) and exit site infections (13%) (278). Catheter survival is better with insertion of the catheter with a straight subcutaneous tunnel directed caudally toward the pelvis (1 year catheter survival 75%) as opposed to a slightly arcuate subcutaneous tunnel with a transverse orientation (1 year catheter survival 30%), due to high rates of outflow failure due to catheter migration or omentum with the second method (281). Hernias occur in 1/5 to 1/3 of children on CAPD (280, 282).

Exit site/tunnel infection rates in children are high: 1.1/y to 1.7/y (278, 283). Exit site infection in children, as with adults, is most often due to *S. aureus* (280, 283, 284). The rate of peritonitis associated with catheter infection in children is 0.23/y (285) to 0.48/y (260) and is predominately due to *S. aureus* or *P. aeruginosa*. Treatment of the child and dialysis provider (generally the parent) with rifampin for *S. aureus* carriage is effective in reducing *S. aureus* infectious complications (286).

ACKNOWLEDGEMENTS

The author thanks Judith Bernardini, BSN and James R. Johnston, MD for their helpful comments, Bill Brent for his art work, and Roberta Sheffler for allowing her photograph to be used.

REFERENCES

1. Gokal R, Ash SR, Helfrich GB et al.: Peritoneal catheters and exit-site practices: toward optimum peritoneal access. *Perit Dial Int* 13: 29, 1993
2. Copley JB: Common management errors in chronic PD. *Semin Dial* 6: 235, 1993
3. Piraino B, Bernardini J, Sorkin M: Catheter infections as a factor in the transfer of continuous ambulatory peritoneal dialysis patients to hemodialysis. *Am J Kidney Dis* 13: 365, 1989
4. Bernardini J, Holley JL, Johnston JR, Perlmutter JA, Piraino B: An analysis of ten-year trends in infections in adults on continuous ambulatory peritoneal dialysis (CAPD). *Clin Nephrol* 36: 29, 1991

5. Piraino B, Bernardini J, Sorkin M: The influence of peritoneal catheter exit site infections on peritonitis, tunnel infections, and catheter loss in patients on continous ambulatory peritoneal dialysis. *Am J Kidney Dis* 8: 436, 1986

6. Palmer RA, Newell JE, Gray EF, Quinton WE: Treatment of chronic renal failure by prolonged peritoneal dialysis. *N Engl J Med* 274: 248, 1966

7. Tenckhoff H, Schechter H: A bacteriologically safe peritoneal access device. *Trans Am Soc Artif Intern Organs* 14: 181, 1968

8. Lewis J, Abbott J, Crompton K, Fowler I, Smith B: CAPD disconnect systems: UK peritonitis experience. *Adv Perit Dial* 8: 306, 1992

9. Lindblad AS, Hamilton RW, Nolph KD, Novak JW: A retrospective analysis of catheter configuration and cuff type: a national CAPD registry report. *Perit Dial Int* 8: 129, 1988

10. Port FK, Held PJ, Nolph KD, Turenne MN, Wolfe RA: Risk of peritonitis and technique failure by CAPD connection technique: a national study. *Kidney Int* 42: 967, 1992

11. Nolph KD, Lindblad AS, Novak JW: Continuous ambulatory peritoneal dialysis. *N Engl J Med* 318: 1595, 1986

12. Twardowski ZJ, Dobbie JW, Moore HL et al.: Morphology of peritoneal dialysis catheter tunnel: macroscopy and light microscopy. *Perit Dial Int* 11: 237, 1991

13. Twardowski ZJ: Peritoneal dialysis catheter exit site infections: prevention, diagnosis, treatment, and future directions. *Semin Dial* 5: 305, 1992

14. Kim D, Burke D, Izatt S et al.: Single or double cuff peritoneal catheters? A prospective comparison. *Trans Am Soc Artif Intern Organs* 30: 232, 1984

15. Ash SR: Chronic peritoneal dialysis catheters: effects of catheter design, materials, and location. *Semin Dial* 3: 39, 1990

16. Diaz-Buxo JA, Geissinger WT: Single cuff versus double cuff Tenckhoff catheter. *Perit Dial Bull* 4 (Suppl): S100, 1984

17. Rottembourg J, Jacq D, Vonlanthen M, Issad B, El Shahat Y: Straight or curled Tenckhoff peritoneal catheter for continuous ambulatory peritoneal dialysis (CAPD). *Perit Dial Bull* 1: 123, 1981

18. Swartz R, Messana J, Rocher L, Reynolds J, Starmann B, Lees P: The curled catheter: dependable device for percutaneous peritoneal access. *Perit Dial Int* 10: 231, 1990

19. Akyol AM, Porteous C, Brown MW: A comparison of two types of catheters for continuous ambulatory peritoneal dialysis (CAPD). *Perit Dial Int* 10: 63, 1990

20. Khanna R, Izatt S, Burke D, Mathews R, Vas S: Oreopoulos DG Experience with the Toronto Western Hospital permanent peritoneal catheter. *Perit Dial Bull* 4: 95, 1984

21. Ponce SP, Peirratos A, Izatt S et al.: Comparison of the survival and complications of three permanent peritoneal dialysis catheters. *Perit Dial Bull* 2: 82, 1982

22. Flanigan MJ, Ngheim DD, Schulak J, Ullrich GE, Freeman RM: The use and complications of three peritoneal dialysis catheter designs: a retrospective analysis. *Trans Am Soc Artif Intern Organs* 33: 33, 1987

23. Scott PD, Bakran A, Pearson R et al.: Peritoneal dialysis access. Prospective randomized trial of 3 different peritoneal catheters – preliminary report. *Perit Dial Int* 14: 289, 1994

24. Twardowski ZJ, Nolph KD, Khanna R, Prowant BF, Ryan LP, Nichols WK: The need for a 'swan neck' permanently bent, arcuate peritoneal dialysis catheter. *Perit Dial Bull* 5: 219, 1985

25. Twardowski ZJ: Peritoneal catheter development. Currently used catheters: advantages/disadvantages/complications, and catheter tunnel morphology in humans. *Trans Am Soc Artif Intern Organs* 34: 937, 1988

26. Twardowski ZJ, Prowant BF, Nichols WK, Nolph KD, Khanna R: Six-year experience with Swan neck catheters. *Perit Dial Int* 12: 384, 1992

27. Ishizaki M, Suzuki K, Kurosawa K, Shishido Y, Takahashi H: Swan neck Sendai catheter: a modification of the swan neck Tenckhoff catheter. *Perit Dial Int* 8: 221, 1988

28. Perez JC, Caruana RJ, Wynn JJ, Hess C, Smith KL, Campbell HT: Connectology problems with swan neck peritoneal dialysis catheters. *Int J Artif Organs* 13: 521, 1990

29. Eklund BH, Hankanen EO, Kala A-R, Kyllonen LE: Catheter configuration and outcome in patients on continuous ambulatory peritoneal dialysis: a prospective comparison of two catheters. *Perit Dial Int* 14: 70, 1994

30. Nebel M, Marczewski K, Finke K: Three years of experience with the swan neck Tenckhoff catheter. *Adv Perit Dial* 7: 208, 1991

31. Shyr YM: Complications of peritoneal catheters placed by a single surgeon. *Perit Dial Int* 14: 401, 1994

32. Cruz C, Bonilla H, Melendez A, Faber MD, Dumler F: Flow dynamics in peritoneal dialysis; The search for optimal CAPD systems. *Perit Dial Int* 11 (Suppl 1): 54 (Abstract), 1991

33. Weaver ME, Dunbeck DC: Mupirocin (Bactroban) causes permanent structural changes in peritoneal dialysis catheters. *Perit Dial Int* 14 (Suppl 1): S20 (Abstract), 1994

34. Poisetti P, Bergonzi G, Ballocchi S, Fontana F, Scarpioni L: Aging of silastic peritoneal catheters. *Int J Artif Organs* 14: 765, 1991

35. Bay WH, Vaccaro PS, Powell SL, Erlich LF: The Gore-Tex peritoneal catheter: a clinical evaluation and comparison with the Tenckhoff catheter. *Am J Kidney Dis* 4: 268, 1984

36. Ogden DA, Benavente G, Wheeler D, Zukoski CF: Experience with the right angle GORE-TEX peritoneal dialysis catheter. in *Advances in Continuous Ambulatory Peritoneal Dialysis*, edited by Khanna R, Nolph KD, Prowant B, Twardowski ZJ, Oreopoulos DG, Toronto, Perit Dial Bull Inc, 1986, p 155

37. Boss HP, Ganger KH, Gluck A: Gore-tex versus Oreopoulos peritoneal catheters: clinical evaluation and comparison. *Int Artif Organs* 12: 369, 1989

38. Ash SR, Johnson H, Hartman J et al.: The column disc peritoneal catheter: a peritoneal access device with improved drainage. *Trans Am Soc Artif Intern Organs* 3: 109, 1980

39. Shah GM, Sabo A, Nguyen T, Juler GL: Peritoneal catheters: a comparative study of column disc and Tenckhoff catheters. *Int J Artif Organs* 13: 267, 1990

40. Hines WH, Smego DR, Longnecker RE: Failure of the Dermaport catheter as an access device in CAPD. *Am J Kidney Dis* 15: A10, 1990

41. Valli A, Crescimanno U, Midiri O et al.: Eighteen months experience with a new (Valli) catheter for peritoneal dialysis. *Perit Dial Bull* 3: 22, 1983

42. Moncrief JW, Popovich RP, Broadrick LJ, He AA, Simmons EE, Tate RA: The Moncrief–Popovich catheter. A new peritoneal access technique for patients on peritoneal dialysis. *ASAIO J* 39: 62, 1993

43. Moncrief JW, Popovich RP, Dasgupta M, Costerton JW, Simmons E, Moncrief B: Reduction in peritonitis incidence in continuous ambulatory peritoneal dialysis with a new catheter and implantation technique. *Perit Dial Int* 13 (Suppl 2): S329, 1993

44. Han DC, Cha HK, So IN et al.: Subcutaneously implanted catheters reduce the incidence of peritonitis during CAPD by eliminating infection by periluminal route. *Adv Perit Dial* 8: 298, 1992

45. Catizone L, Cantaluppi A, Peluso F, Zucchelli P: A new catheter to prevent exit site infection in peritoneal dialysis. *Adv Perit Dial* 8: 283, 1992

46. Twardowski ZJ, Nichols WK, Nolph KD, Khanna R: Swan neck presternal ('Bath tub') catheter for peritoneal dialysis. *Adv Perit Dial* 8: 316, 1992

47. Dasgupta MK, McKay S, Olsen M, Costerton JW: Siver-coated peritoneal catheter reduces colonization by *Staphylococcus aureus* in a rabbit model of peritoneal dialysis. *Perit Dial Int* 14 (Suppl 1): S86 (Abstract), 1994

48. Ash SR, Handt AE, Bloch R: Peritoneoscopic placement of the Tenckhoff catheter: further clinical experience. *Perit Dial Bull* 3: 8, 1983

49. Allon M, Soucie JM, Macon EJ: Complications with permanent peritoneal dialysis catheters: experience with 154 percutaneously placed catheters. *Nephron* 48: 8, 1988

50. Henao J, Mejia G, Arbelaez M et al.: A new approach for catheter placement and care in CAPD. *Perit Dial Bull* 5: 223, 1985

51. Nielsen PK, Hemmingsen C, Ladefoged J, Olgaard K: A consecutive study of 646 peritoneal dialysis catheters. *Perit Dial Int* 14: 170, 1994

52. Khanna R: Acute management of the patient requiring a chronic peritoneal catheter. *Semin Dial* 3: 93, 1990

53. Robison RJ, Leapman SB, Wetherington GM et al.: Surgical considerations of continuous ambulatory peritoneal dialysis. *Surgery* 96: 723, 1984

54. Prowant BF, Warady BZ, Nolph KD: Peritoneal dialysis catheter exit site care: results of an international survey. *Perit Dial Int* 13: 149, 1993

55. Lye WC, Lee EJC, Tan CC: Prophylactic antibiotics in the insertion of Tenckhoff catheters. *Scand J Urol Nephrol* 26: 177, 1992

56. Bennett-Jones DN, Martin J, Barratt AJ, Duffy TJ, Naish PF, Aber GM: Prophylactic gentamicin in the prevention of early exit site infections and peritonitis in CAPD. *Adv Perit Dial* 4: 147, 1988

57. Newman LN, Tessman M, Hanslik T, Schulak J, Mayes J, Friedlander M: A retrospective view of factors that affect catheter healing: four years of experience. *Adv Perit Dial* 9: 217, 1993

58. Schleifer CR, Morfesis FA, Cupit M, Chen C, Smink RD: Management of hernias and Tenckhoff catheter complications in CAPD. *Perit Dial Bull* 4: 146, 1984

59. Odor A, Alessio-Robles L, Leuchter JI et al.: Experience with 150 consecutive permanent peritoneal catheters in patients on CAPD. *Perit Dial Bull* 5: 226, 1985

60. Lovinggood JP: Peritoneal catheter implantation for CAPD. *Perit Dial Bull* 4 (Suppl 3): S106, 1984

61. Copley JB, Lindberg JS, Tapia NP, Back SN, Snyder PA: Peritoneoscopic placment of swan neck peritoneal dialysis catheters. *Perit Dial Int* 14: 295, 1994

62. Nahman NS, Middendorf DF, Bay WH, McElligott R, Powell S, Anderson J: Modification of the percutaneous approach to peritonal dialysis catheter placement under peritoneoscopic visualization: clinical results in 78 patients. *Am Soc Nephrol* 3: 103, 1992

63. Kimmelstiel FM, Miller RE, Molinelli BM, Lorch JA: Laparoscopic managment of peritoneal dialysis catheters. *Surg Gynec Obstet* 176: 565, 1993

64. Amerling R, Cruz C: A new laparoscopic method for implantation of peritoneal catheters. *ASAIO J* 39: M787, 1993

65. Lewis MA, Houston IB, Postlethwaite RJ: Access for peritoneal dialysis in neonates and infants. *Arch Dis Child* 65: 44, 1990

66. Lewis MA, Nycyk JA: Practical peritoneal dialysis – the Tenckhoff catheter in acute renal failure. *Pediatr Nephrol* 6: 470, 1992

67. Bullmaster JR, Miller SF, Finley RK, Jones LM: Surgical aspects of the Tenckhoff peritoneal dialysis catheter: a 7 year experience. *Am J Surg* 149: 339, 1985

68. Mellotte GJ, Ho CA, Morgan SH, Bending MR, Eisinger AJ: Peritoneal dialysis catheters: a comparison between percutaneous conventional surgical placement techniques. *Nephrol Dial Transplant* 8: 626, 1993

69. Jacobs IG, Gray RR, Elliott DS, Grosman H: Radiologic placement of peritoneal dialysis catheters: preliminary experience. *Radiology* 182: 251, 1992

70. Copley JB: Prevention of peritoneal dialysis catheter related infections. *Am J Kidney Dis* 10: 401, 1987

71. Copley JB, Smith BJ, Koger DM, Rodgers DJ, Fowler M: Prevention of postoperative peritoneal dialysis catheter related infections. *Perit Dial Int* 8: 195, 1988

72. Ash SR: Is a break-in period necessary following peritoneal catheter insertion? A break-in period is unnecessary. *Semin Dial* 5: 199, 1992

73. Lye WC, Giang MML, van der Straaten JC, Lee EJC: Breaking-in after the insertion of Tenckhoff catheters: a comparison of two techniques. *Adv Perit Dial* 3: 236, 1993

74. Khanna R: Is a break-in period necessary following peritoneal catheter insertion? A break-in period is recommended. *Semin Dial* 5: 197, 1992

75. Twardowski ZJ, Ryan LP, Kennedy JM: Catheter break-in for continuous ambulatory peritoneal dialysis – University of Missouri experience. *Perit Dial Bull* 4 (Suppl 3): S110, 1984

76. Francis DMA, Donnelly PK, Veitch PS et al.: Surgical aspects of continuous ambulatory peritoneal dialysis – 3 years experience. *Br J Surg* 71: 225, 1984

77. Levey AS, Simon GM, McCauley J, Smith TJ, Cho SI, Harrington JT: Outcome of peritoneal catheter placement in the high-risk patient. *Perit Dial Bull* 4 (Suppl 3): S112, 1984

78. Diaz-Buxo J: Mechanical complications of chronic peritoneal dialysis catheters. *Semin Dial* 4: 106, 1991

79. Gloor HJ, Nichols WK, Sorkin MK et al.: Peritoneal access and related complications in continuous ambulatory peritoneal dialysis. *Am J Med* 74: 593, 1983

80. Ward RA, Klein E, Wathen RL: Peritoneal catheters. *Perit Dial Bull* 3 (Suppl 2): S9, 1983

81. Yeh TJ, Wei CF, Chin TW: Catheter-related complicaitons of continuous ambulatory peritoneal dialysis. *Eur J Surg* 158: 277, 1992

82. Schleifer CR, Ziemek H, Teehan BP, Benz RL, Sigler MH, Gilgore GS: Migration of peritoneal catheters: personal experience and a survey of 72 other units. *Perit Dial Bull* 7: 189, 1987

83. Twardowski ZJ: Malposition and poor drainage of peritoneal catheters. *Semin Dial* 3: 57, 1990

84. Joffe P, Christensen AL, Jensen C: Peritoneal catheter tip location during non-complicated continuous ambulatory peritoneal dialysis. *Perit Dial Int* 11: 261, 1991

85. Oreopoulos DG, Izatt S, Zellerman G et al.: A prospective study of the effectiveness of three permanent peritoneal catheters. *Proc Clin Dial Transplant Forum* 6: 96, 1976

86. Moss JS, Minda SA, Newman GE et al.: Malpositioned peritoneal dialysis catheters: a critical reappraisal of correction by stiff-wire manipulation. *Am J Kidney Dis* 15: 305, 1990

87. Wilson JAP, Swartz RD: Peritoneoscopy in the management of catheter malfunction during continuous ambulatory peritoneal dialysis. *Digest Dis Sci* 30: 465, 1985

88. Gibson DH, Heasley RN, Price JH et al.: Laparoscopic repositioning of blocked peritoneal dialysis catheters in patients on CAPD. *Clin Nephrol* 33: 208, 1990

89. Smith DW, Rankin Ra: Value of peritoneoscopy for nonfunctioning continuous ambulatory peritoneal dialysis catheters. *Gastrointest Endosc* 35: 90, 1989

90. O'Regan S, Garel L, Patriquin H et al.: Outflow obstruction: whiplash technique for catheter mobilization. *Perit Dial Int* 8: 265, 1988

91. Hiltunen KM, Viranta M: One-way obstruction during continuous ambulatory peritoneal dialysis (CAPD) with Tenckhoff catheter. *Scand J Urol Nephrol* 19: 67, 1985

92. Benevent D, Peyronnet P, Brignon P, Leroux-Robert C: Urokinase infusion for obstructed catheters and peritonitis. *Perit Dial Bull* 5: 77, 1985

93. Wiegmann TB, Stuewe B, Duncan KA et al.: Effective use of streptokinase for peritoneal catheter failure. *Am J Kidney Dis* 6: 119, 1985

94. Palacios M, Schley W, Dougherty JC: Use of streptokinase to clear peritoneal catheters. *Dial Transplant* 11: 172, 1982

95. Bergstein JM, Andreoli SP, West KW, Grosfeld JL: Streptokinase therapy for occluded Tenckhoff catheters in children on CAPD. *Perit Dial Bull* 8: 137, 1988

96. Scalamogna A, Castelnovo C, Cataluppi A: Intraperitoneal infusion of streptokinase in the treatment of a total (inflow-outflow) peritoneal catheter obstruction. *Perit Dial Bull* 6: 41, 1986

97. Sharp J, Eastham EJ, Coulthard MG: Removal of a fibrin plug from within a Silastic peritoneal dialysis catheter: the Sheastard sweep. *Perit Dial Int* 10: 61, 1990

98. Helfrich GB, Winchester JF: What is the best technique for implantation of a peritoneal catheter? *Perit Dial Bull* 2: 132, 1982

99. Clark KR, Forsythe JLR, Rigg KM et al.: Surgical aspects of chronic peritoneal dialysis in the neonate and infant under 1 year of age. *J Pediatr Surg* 27: 780, 1992

100. Olcott C IV, Feldman CA, Coplon NS, Oppenheimer ML, Mehigan JT: Continuous Ambulatory Peritoneal Dialysis: technique of catheter insertion and management of associated surgical complications. *Am J Surg* 146: 98, 1983

101. Sanderson MC, Swartzendruber DJ, Fenoglio ME, Moore JT, Haun WE: Surgical complications of continuous ambulatory peritoneal dialysis. *Am J Surg* 160: 561, 1990

102. Nicholson ML, Burton PR, Donnelly PK: The role of omentectomy in continuous ambulatory peritoneal dialysis. *Perit Dial Int* 11: 330, 1991

103. DeVault GA, Brown ST, King JS: Tenckhoff catheter obstruction resulting from invasion by *Curvularia lunata* in the absence of peritonitis. *Am J Kidney Dis* 6: 165, 1985

104. Wegmann F, Heilesen AM, Horn T: Tenckhoff catheter penetrated by Aspergillus fumigatus: a case report. *Perit Dial Int* 8: 281, 1988

105. Abouljoud MS, Cruz C: Obstruction of PD catheters by Fallopian tubes. *Perit Dial Int* 14: 90, 1994

106. Macallister RJ, Morgan SH: Fallopian tube capture of chronic peritoneal dialysis catheters. *Perit Dial Int* 13: 74, 1993

107. Antonious S, Syreggelas D, Papadopoulos C, Dimitriadis A: Intraluminal lithiasis of a peritoneal catheter. *Perit Dial Int* 11: 358, 1991

108. Closkey GM, Zappacosta AR: CAPD drainage failure due to Tenckhoff catheter fracture: a case report. *Perit Dial Int* 12: 266, 1992

109. Valles M, Cantarell C, Vila J, Tovar JL: Delayed perforation of the colon by a Tenckhoff catheter. *Perit Dial Bull* 2: 190, 1982

110. Bustos E, Rotellar C, Mazzoni J, Rakowski TA, Argy WP, Winchester JF: Clinical aspects of bowel perforation in patients undergoing continuous ambulatory peritoneal dialysis. *Semin Dial* 7: 355, 1994

111. Fleisher AG, Kimmelstiel FM, Lattes CG, Miller RE: Surgical complications of peritoneal dialysis catheters. *Am J Surg* 149: 726, 1985

112. van der Niepen P, Sennesael JJ, Verbeelen DL: Massive hemoperitoneum due to spleen injury by a dislocated Tenckhoff catheter. *Perit Dial Int* 14: 90, 1994

113. Haj M, Kristal B, Shasha SM: Delayed laceratoin of intestinal wall by the permanent Tenckhoff peritoneal catheter. *Perit Dial Int* 8: 25, 1988

114. Korzets Z, Golan E, Ben-Dahan J, Neufeld D, Bernheim J: Decubitus small-bowel perforation in ongoing continuous ambulatory peritoneal dialysis. *Nephrol Dial Transplant* 7: 79, 1992

115. Vargemezis V, Pasadakis P, Thodis E, Ethimiadou A, Maltezos E, Kotsiou S: Late perforation of bladder as a complication of an unused straight Tenckhoff catheter. *Perit Dial Int* 8: 55, 1988

116. della Volpe M, Iberti M, Ortensia A, Veronesi GV: Erosion of the sigmoid by a permanent peritoneal catheter. *Perit Dial Bull* 4: 108, 1884

117. de los Santos AC, von Eye O, d'Avila D, Mottin CC: Rupture of the spleen: a complication of continuous ambulatory peritoneal dialysis. *Perit Dial Bull* 6: 203, 1986

118. Brady HR, Abraham G, Oreopoulos DG, Cardella CJ: Bowel erosion due to a dormant peritoneal catheter in immunosuppressed renal transplant recipients. *Perit Dial Int* 8: 163, 1988

119. Jansen GPPG, Gerlag PGG, Bruyninckx BCMA: Unusual presentation of bowel perforation by a CAPD catheter. *Perit Dial Int* 14: 181, 1994

120. Rambausek M, Zeier M, Weinreich T et al.: Bowel perforation with unused Tenckhoff catheters. *Perit Dial Int* 9: 82, 1989

121. Jamison MH, Fleming SJ, Ackrill P, Schofield PF: Erosion of rectum by Tenckhoff catheter. *Br J Surg* 75: 360, 1988

122. Kopecky RT, Frymoyer PA, Witanowski LS, Thomas FD: Complications of continuous ambulatory peritoneal dialysis: diagnostic value of peritoneal scintigraphy. *Am J Kidney Dis* 10: 123, 1987

123. Bargman JM: Complications of peritoneal dialysis related to increased intra-abdominal pressure. *Kidney Int* 43 (Suppl 40): S75, 1993

124. Lupo A, Tarchin R, Cancarini G et al.: Long-term outcome in continuous ambulatory peritoneal dialysis: a 10-year survey by the Italian cooperative peritoneal dialysis study group. *Am J Kidney Dis* 24: 826, 1994

125. Stegmayr BG, Hedberg B, Sandzen B, Wikdahl AM: Absence of leakage by insertion of peritoneal dialysis catheter through the rectus muscle. *Perit Dial Intern* 10: 53, 1990

126. Stegmayr BG: Paramedian insertion of Tenckhoff catheters with three purse-string sutures reduces the risk of leakage. *Perit Dial Int* 13 (Suppl 2): S124, 1993

127. Beaman M, Feehally J, Smith BA, Walls J: Anterior abdominal wall leakage in CAPD patients; management by intermittent peritoneal dialysis. *Perit Dial Bull* 5: 81, 1985

128. Holley JL, Bernardini J, Piraino B: Characteristics and outcome of peritoneal dialysate leaks and associated infections. *Adv Perit Dial* 9: 240, 1993

129. Hirsch DJ, Jindal KK: Late leaks in peritoneal dialysis patients. *Nephrol Dial Transplant* 6: 670, 1990

130. Joffe P: Peritoneal dialysis catheter leakage treated with fibrin glue. *Nephrol Dial Transplant* 8: 474, 1993

131. Schultz SG, Harmon TM, Nachtnebel KL: Computerized tomographic scanning with intraperitoneal contrast enhancement in a CAPD patient with localized edema. *Perit Dial Bull* 4: 253, 1984

132. Kopecky RT, Funk MM, Kreitzer PR: Localized genital edema in patients undergoing continuous ambulatory peritoneal dialysis. *J Urol* 124: 880, 1985

133. Mandel P, Faegenburg D, Imbriano LJ: The use of technetium-99m sulfur colloid in the detection of patent processus vaginalis in patients on continuous ambulatory peritoneal dialysis. 10: 553, 1985

134. Ducassou D, Vuillemin L, Wone C, Ragnaud JM, Brendel AJ: Intraperitoneal injection of technetium-99m sulfur colloid in visualization of a peritoneo-vaginalis connection. *J Nucl Med* 25: 68, 1984

135. Orfei R, Seybold K, Blumberg A: Genital edema in patients undergoing continuous ambulatory peritoneal dialysis (CAPD). *Perit Dial Bull* 14: 251, 1984

136. Schurgers MLC, Boelaert JRO, Daneels RFS, Robbens EJ, Vandelanotte MMJ: Open processus vaginalis. *Perit Dial Bull* 3: 30, 1983

137. Cooper JC, Nicholls AJ, Simms JM, Platts MM, Brown CB, Johnson AG: Genital oedema n patients treated by continuous ambulatory peritoneal dialysis: an unusual presentation of inguinal hernia. *Br Med J* 286: 923, 1983

138. Tzamaloukas AH, Gibel LJ, Eisenberg B et al.: Scrotal edema in patients on CAPD: causes, differential diagnosis and management. *Dial Transplant* 21: 581, 1992

139. Coward RA, Gokal R, Wise M et al.: Peritonitis associated with vagnial leakage of dialysis fluid in continuous ambulatory peritoneal dialysis. *Br Med J* 284: 1529, 1982

140. Diaz-Buxo JA, Burgess P, Walker PJ: Peritoneovaginal fistula-unusual complicaiton of peritoneal dialysis. *Perit Dial Bull* 3: 142, 1983

141. Khanna R, Oreopoulos DG, Vas S et al.: Fungal peritonitis in patients undergoing chronic intermittent or continuous peritoneal dialysis. *Proc Eur Dial Transplant Assoc* 17: 291, 1980

142. Swartz RD, Campbell DA, Stone D, Dickinson C: Recurrent polymicrobial peritonitis from a gynecologic source as a complication of CAPD. *Perit Dial Bull* 3: 32, 1983

143. Caporale N, Perez D, Alegre S: Vaginal leak of peritoneal dialysis liquid. *Perit Dial Int* 11: 284, 1991

144. Nomoto Y, Suga T, Nakajima K: et al.: Acute hydrothorax in continuous ambulatory peritoneal dialysis – a collaborative study of 161 centers. *Am J Nephrol* 9: 363, 1989

145. Abraham G, Shokker A, Blake P, Oreopoulos DG: Massive hydrothorax in patients on peritoneal dialysis: a literature review. *Adv Perit Dial* 4: 121, 1988

146. Boeschoten EW, Krediet RT, Roos CM, Kloek JJ, Schipper MEI, Arisz L: Leakage of dialysate across the diaphragm: an important complication of continuous ambulatory peritoneal dialysis. *Neth J Med* 29: 242, 1986

147. Grefberg N, Danielson BG, Benson L, Pitkanen P: Right sided hydrothorax complicating continuous ambulatory peritoneal dialysis. *Nephron* 34: 130, 1983

148. Mestas D, Wauquier JP, Escande G, Baguet JC, Veyr A: Diagnosis of hydrothorax-complicating CAPD and demonstration of successful therapy by scintigraphy. *Perit Dial Int* 11: 283, 1991

149. Green A, Logan M, Medawar W et al.: The management of hydrothorax in continuous ambulatory peritoneal dialysis (CAPD). *Perit Dial Int* 10: 271, 1990

150. Stegmayr BG, Granbom L, Tranaeus A, Wikdahl AM: Reduced risk for peritonitis in CAPD with the use of a UV connector box. *Perit Dial Int* 11: 128, 1991

151. Nolph KD, Prowant B, Serkes KD, Morgan LM et al.: A randomized multicenter clinical trial to evaluate the effects of an ultraviolet germicidal system on peritonitis rate in continuous ambulatory peritoneal dialysis. *Perit Dial Bull* 5: 19, 1985

152. Hamilton R, Charytan C, Kurtz S et al.: Reduction in peritonitis frequency by the Dupont sterile connector device. *Trans Am Soc Artif Intern Organs* 31: 651, 1985

153. Sharp J, Coulthard MG: A heat-sealing device to disconnect peritoneal dialysis lines. *Perit Dial Int* 8: 269, 1988

154. Geerlings W, Tufveson G, Ehrich HH et al.: Report on Management of renal failure in Europe, XXIII. *Nephrol Dial Transplant* 9 (Suppl 1): 6, 1994

155. Bazzato G, Coli U, Landini S et al.: The double bag system for CAPD reduces the peritonitis rate. *Trans Am Soc Artif Intern Organs* 30: 690, 1984

156. Bazzato G, Coli U, Landini S et al.: Closter: a new connection for a double-bag system to prevent exogenous peritonitis. *Perit Dial Bull* 6: 138, 1986

157. Buoncristiani U: Continuous ambulatory peritoneal dialysis connection systems. *Perit Dial Int* 13 (Suppl 2): S139, 1993

158. Burkart JM: Comparison of peritonitis rates using standard spike versus Y sets in CAPD. *Trans Am Soc Artif Organs* 34: 433, 1988

159. Cantaluppi A, Scalamogna A, Castelnovo C, Graziani G: Peritonitis prevention in continuous ambulatory peritoneal dialysis: long-term efficacy of a Y-connector and disinfectant. *Perit Dial Bull* 6: 58, 1986

160. Owen JE, Walker RG, Lemon J, Brett L, Mitrou D, Becker GJ: Randomized study of peritonitis with conventional versus O-set techniques in continuous ambulatory peritoneal dialysis. *Perit Dial Int* 12: 216, 1992

161. Diaz-Buxo JA: Comparison of peritonitis rates with CCPD, manual CAPD, Y-sets, O-sets, UV devices and sterile weld. *Adv Perit Dial* 5: 223, 1989

162. Fellin G, Gentile MG, Manna GM, Redaelli L, D'Amico G: Peritonitis prevention: a Y-connector and sodium hypochlorite. Three years' experience. Report of the Italian CAPD Study Group. in *Advances in Continuous Ambulatory Peritoneal Dialysis/1987*, edited by Khanna R, Nolph KD, Prowant B, Twardowski ZJ, Oreopoulos DG, Toronto, University of Toronto Press, 1987, p 114

163. Maiorca R, Cancarini GC, Broccoli R et al.: Prospective controlled trial of a Y-connector and disinfectant to prevent peritonitis in continuous ambulatory peritoneal dialysis. *Lancet* 2: 642, 1983

164. Maiorca R, Cancarini G, Manili L et al.: CAPD is a first class treatment: results of an eight-year experience with a comparison of patient and method survival in CAPD and hemodialysis. *Clin Nephrol* 30 (Suppl 1): S3, 1988

165. Rottembourg J, Brouard R, Issad B, Allouache M, Jacobs C: Prospective randomized study about Y-connectors in CAPD patients. in *Advances in Continuous Ambulatory Peritoneal Dialysis/1987*, edited by Khanna R, Nolph KD, Prowant B, Twardowski ZJ, Oreopoulos DG, Toronto, University of Toronto Press, 1987, p 107

166. Churchill DN, Taylor DW, Vas SI et al.: Peritonitis in continuous ambulatory peritoneal dialysis (CAPD): a multicentre randomized clinical trial comparing the Y connector disinfectant system to standard systems. *Perit Dial Int* 9: 159, 1989

167. Scalamogna A, De Vecchi A, Castelnovo C, Guerra L, Ponticelli C: Long-term incidence of peritonitis in CAPD patients treated by the Y set technique: experience in a single center. *Nephron* 55: 24, 1990

168. Bonnardeaux A, Ouimet D, Galarneau A et al.: Peritonitis in continuous ambulatory peritoneal dialysis: impact of a compulsory switch from a standard to a Y connector system in a single north American center. *Am J Kidney Dis* 19: 364, 1992

169. Holley JL, Bernardini J, Piraino B: Infecting organisms in continuous ambulatory peritoneal dialysis patients on the Y-set. *Am J Kidney Dis* 23: 569, 1994

170. Luzar MA, Slingeneyer A, Cantaluppi A, Pelusos FB: *In vitro* study of the flush effect in 2 reusable continuous ambulatory peritoneal dialysis disconnect systems. *Perit Dial Int* 9: 169, 1989

171. Orange GV, Henderson IS, Marshall EA: Effectiveness of the flush technique in CAPD disconnect systems. *Int J Artif Organ* 10: 185, 1987

172. Junor BJR: CAPD Disconnect Systems Current Concepts of CAPD. *Blood Purif* 7: 156, 1989

173. Tarchini R, Segoloni P, Gentile MG et al.: The role of experience and Y transfer set in preventing dropouts: a report from the Italian CAPD Study Group. in *Advances in Continuous Ambulatory Peritoneal Dialysis/1987*, edited by Khanna R, Nolph KD, Prowant B, Twardowski ZJ, Oreopoulos DG, Toronto, University of Toronto Press, 1987, p 192

174. Tarchini R, Segoloni GP, Gentile MG et al.: Long-term results of CAPD in Italy: a report from the Italian CAPD study Group. *Clin Nephrol* 30 (Suppl 1): S68, 1988

175. Swartz R, Reynolds J, Lees P, Rocher L: Disconnect during continuous ambulatory peritoneal dialysis (CAPD): retrospective experience with three different systems. *Perit Dial Int* 9: 175, 1989

176. Scalamogna A, Viglino G, Colombo A et al.: Controlled randomized trial between two Y-devices. in *Advances in Continuous Ambulatory Peritoneal Dialysis/1987*, edited by Khanna R, Nolph KD, Prowant B, Twardowski ZJ, Oreopoulos DG, Toronto, University of Toronto Press, 1988, p 288

177. Viglino G, Colombo A, Scalamogna A et al.: Prospected randomized study of two Y devices in continuous ambulatory peritoneal dialysis (CAPD). *Perit Dial Int* 9: 165, 1989

178. Ryckelynck JP, Verger C, Cam G, Faller B, Pierre D: Importance of the flush effect in disconnect systems. in *Advances in Continuous Ambulatory Peritoneal Dialysis*, edited by Khanna R, Nolph K, Prowant B, Twardowski Z, Oreopoulos D, Toronto, Toronto University Press, 1988, p 282

179. Cheng IKP, Chan CY, Cheng SW et al.: A randomized prospective study of the cost-effectiveness of the conventional spike, O-set, and UVXD techniques in continuous ambulatory peritoneal dialysis. *Perit Dial Int* 14: 255, 1994

180. Domrongkitchaiporn S, Karim M, Watson L, Moriarty M: The influence of continuous ambulatory peritoneal dialysis connection technique on peritonitis rate and technique survival. *Am J Kidney Dis* 24: 50, 1994

181. Balteau PR, peluso FP, Coles GA et al.: Design and testing of the Baxter integrated disconnect systems (IDS). *Perit Dial Int* 11: 131, 1991

182. Tielens E, Nube MJ, de Vet JA et al.: Major reduction of CAPD peritonitis after the introduction of the twin-bag system. *Nephrol Dial Transplant* 8: 1237, 1993

183. Honkanen E, Kala AR, Gronhagen-Riska C: Divergent etiologies of CAPD peritonitis in integrated double bag and traditional systems. *Adv Perit Dial* 7: 129, 1991

184. Grutzmacher P, Tsobanelis T, Bruns M, Kurz P, Hoppe D, Vlachojannis J: Decrease in peritonitis rate by integrated disconnect systems in patients on continuous ambulatory peritoneal dialysis. *Perit Dial Int* 13 (Suppl 2): S326, 1993

185. Dasgupta MK, Fox S, Gagnon D, Betcher K, Ulan RA: Significant reduction of peritonitis rate by the use of twin-bag system in a Canadian Regional CAPD program. *Adv Perit Dial* 8: 223, 1992

186. Jensen WM and Ahmad S: Evaluation of a germicidal device for peritoneal dialysis connectors. *Perit Dial Bull* 4: 219, 1984

187. Holmes CJ, Miyake C, Kubey W: *In-vitro* evaluation of an ultraviolet germicidal connection system for CAPD. *Perit Dial Bull* 4: 215, 1984

188. Nakamura Y, Hara Y, Ishida H, Moriwaki K, Shigemoto K: A randomized multicenter trial to evaulate the effects of UV-flash system on peritonitis rates in CAPD. *Adv Perit Dial* 8: 313, 1992

189. Durand PY, Chanliau J, Gamberoni J, Mariot A, Kessler M: UV-Flash: clinical evaluation in 97 patients; Results of a French Multicenter Trial. *Perit Dial Int* 14: 86, 1994

190. Prowant BF, Schmidt LM, Twardowski ZJ et al.: Peritoneal dialysis catheter exit site care. *ANNA J* 15: 219, 1988

191. Luzar MA, Brown CB, Balf D et al.: Exit site care and exit site infection in continuous ambulatory peritoneal dialysis: results of a randomized multicenter trial. *Perit Dial Int* 10: 25, 1990

192. Jindal KK, Hirsch DJ: Excellent technique survival on home peritoneal dialysis: results of a regional program. *Perit Dial Int* 14: 324, 1994

193. Hasbargen BJ, Rodgers DJ, Hasbargen JA, Quinn MJ, James MK: Exit site care – is it time for a change? *Perit Dial Int* 13 (Suppl 2): S313, 1993

194. Turner, Edgar D, Hair M, Uttley L, Sternland R, Hunt L, Gokal R: Does catheter immobilization reduce exit-site infections in CAPD patients? *Adv Perit Dial* 8: 265, 1992

195. Khanna R, Twardowski ZJ: Peritoneal catheter exit site. *Perit Dial Int* 8: 119, 1988

196. Abraham G, Savin E, Ayiomamitis A et al.: Natural history of exit-site infection in patients on continuous ambulatory peritoneal dialysis. *Perit Dial Bull* 8: 211, 1988

197. Gonthier D, Bernardini J, Holley FL, Piraino B: Erythema: does it indicate infection in a peritoneal catheter exit site? *Adv Perit Dial* 8: 230, 1992

198. Pierratos A: Peritoneal dialysis glossary. *Perit Dial Int* 4: 2, 1984

199. Twardowski ZJ: Recurrent peritoneal catheter exit-site infections: II. *Semin Dial* 6: 406, 1993

200. Luzar MA: Exit site infection in continuous ambulatory peritoneal dialysis: a review. *Perit Dial Int* 11: 333, 1991

201. Gibel LJ, Quintana BJ, Tzamaloukas AH, Garcia DL: Soft tissue complications of Tenckhoff catheters. *Adv Perit Dial* 5: 229, 1989

202. Vogt K, Binswanger U, Buchmann P, Baumgartner D, Keusch G, Largiader F: Catheter related complications during continuous ambulatory peritoneal dialysis: a retrospective study on sixty-two double-cuff tenckhoff catheters. *Am J Kidney Dis* 10: 47, 1987

203. Lindblad AS, Noval JW, Nolph KD (Eds): *Continuous Ambulatory Peritoneal Dialysis in the USA, Final Report of the National CAPD Registry 1981–1988*, Dordrecht, Kluwer Academic Publishers, 1989

204. Pollock CA, Ibels LS, Caterson RJ, Mahony JF, Waugh DA, Cocksedge B: Continuous ambulatory peritoneal dialysis Eight years of experience at a single center. *Medicine* 68: 293, 1989

205. Scalamogna A, Castelnovo C, De Vecchi A, Ponticelli C: Exit site and tunnel infections in continuous ambulatory peritoneal dialysis patients. *Am J Kidney Dis* 18: 674, 1991

206. Rotellar C, Black J, Winchester JF et al.: Ten years' experience with continuous ambulatory peritoneal dialysis. *Am J Kidney Dis* 17: 158, 1991

207. Flanigan MJ, Hochstetler LA, Langholdt D, Lim VS: Continuous ambulatory peritoneal dialysis catheter infections: diagnosis and management. *Perit Dial Int* 14: 248, 1994

208. Holley JL, Bernardini J, Piraino B: Risk factors for tunnel infections in continuous peritoneal dialysis. *Am J Kidney Dis* 18: 344, 1991

209. Diaz-Buxo JA, Black EB, Tyroler J: Ultrasonography in the diagnosis of peritoneal dialysis catheter tunnel abscess. *Perit Dial Int* 8: 218, 1988

210. Holley JL, Foulks CJ, Moss AH, Willard D: Ultrasound as a tool in the diagnosis and management of exit site infections in patients undergoing continuous ambulatory peritoneal dialysis. *Am J Kidney Dis* 14: 211, 1989

211. Plum J, Sudkamp S, Grabensee B: Results of ultrasound-assisted diagnosis of tunnel infections in continuous ambulatory peritoneal dialysis. *Am J Kidney Dis* 23: 99, 1994

212. Piraino B, Bernardini J, Sorkin M: A five year study of the microbiologic results of exit site infections and peritonitis in continuous ambulatory peritoneal dialysis. *Am J Kidney Dis* 4: 281, 1987

213. Kim D, Tapson J, Wu G, Khanna R, Vas SI, Oreopoulos DG: Staph aureus peritonitis in patients on continuous ambulatory peritoneal dialysis. *Trans Am Soc Artif Intern Organs* 30: 494, 1984

214. Piraino B: A review of *Staphylococcus aureus* exit-site and tunnel infections in peritoneal dialysis patients. *Am J Kidney Dis* 16: 89, 1990

215. Bernardini J, Piraino B, Sorkin M: Analysis of continuous ambulatory peritoneal dialysis related *Pseudomonas aeruginosa* infections. *Am J Med* 83: 829, 1987

216. Krothapalli R, Duffy B, Lacke C et al.: *Pseudomonas* peritonitis and continuous ambulatory peritoneal dialysis. *Arch Intern Med* 142: 1862, 1982

217. Zimmerman SW, O'Brien M, Wiedenhoeft FA, Johnson CA: *Staphylococcus aureus* peritoneal catheter related infections: a cause of catheter loss and peritonitis. *Perit Dial Bull* 8: 191, 1988

218. Davies SJ, Ogg CS, Cameron JS, Ponton S, Noble WC: *Staphylococcus aureus* nasal carriage, exit-site infection and catheter loss in patients treated with continuous ambulatory peritoneal dialysis (CAPD). *Perit Dial Int* 9: 61, 1989

219. West TE, Walshe JJ, Krol CP, Amsterdam D: Staphylococcal peritonitis in patients on continuous peritoneal dialysis. *J Clinical Microbiol* 23: 809, 1986

220. Swartz R, Messana J, Starmann B, Weber M, Reynolds J: Preventing *Staphylococcus aureus* infection during chronic peritoneal dialysis. *Am Soc Nephrol* 2: 1085, 1991

221. Sherbotie JR, Polise K, Costarino A, DiCarlo JV, Kaplan BS: Toxic shock syndrome with *Staphylococcus aureus* exit-site infection in a patient on peritoneal dialysis. *Am J Kidney Dis* 15: 80, 1990

222. Luzar MA, Coles G, Faller B et al.: *Staphylococcus aureus* nasal carriage and infection in patients on continuous ambulatory peritoneal dialysis. *N Engl J Med* 322: 505, 1990

223. Lye WC, Leong SO, Lee EJC: Methicillin-resistant *Staphylococcus aureus* nasal carriage and infections in CAPD. *Kidney Int* 43: 1357, 1993

224. Piraino B, Perlmutter JA, Holley JL, Bernardini J: *Staphylococcus aureus* peritonitis is associated with *Staphylococcus aureus* nasal carriage in peritoneal dialysis patients. *Perit Dial Int* 13 (Suppl 2): S332, 1993

225. Sesso R, Draibe S, Castelo A et al.: *Staphylococcus aureus* skin carriage and development of peritonitis in patients on continuous ambulatory peritoneal dialysis. *Clin Nephrol* 31: 264, 1989

226. Pignatari A, Pfaller M, Hollis R, Sesso R, Leme I, Herwaldt L: *Staphylococcus aureus* colonization and infection in patients on continuous ambulatory peritoneal dialysis. *J Clin Microbiol* 28: 1898, 1990

227. Sewell CM, Clarridge J, Lacke C, Weinman EJ, Young EJ: Staphylococcal nasal carriage and subsequent infection in peritoneal dialysis patients. *JAMA* 248: 1493, 1982

228. Selgas R, Castro MJ, Bajo MA et al.: *Staphylococcus aureus* nasal carrier status (SANCS) in CAPD patients; is it induced or favored by subcutaneous rHu-Erythropoietin? *Adv Perit Dial* 8: 253, 1992

229. Perez-Fontan M, Rosales M, Rodriguez-Carmona A et al.: Treatment of *Staphylococcus aureus* nasal carriers in CAPD with mupirocin. *Adv Perit Dial* 8: 242, 1992

230. Holley J, Bernardini J, Piraino B: Catheter infections in insulin-dependent diabetics on continuous ambulatory peritoneal dialysis. *Perit Dial Int* 11: 347, 1991

231. Holley JL, Bernardini J, Piraino B: A comparison of peritoneal dialysis related infections in black and white patients. *Perit Dial Int* 13: 45, 1993

232. Piraino B, Bernardini J, Centa PK, Johnston JR, Sorkin MI: The effect of body weight on CAPD related infections and catheter loss. *Perit Dial Int* 11: 64, 1991

233. Perez-Fontan M, Garcia-Falcon T, Roasles M et al.: Treatment of *Staphylococcus aureus* nasal carriers in continuous ambulatory peritoneal dialysis with mupirocin: long-term results. *Am J Kidney Dis* 22: 708, 1993

234. Coles GA for the Mupirocin Study Group: The effect of intranasal mupirocin on CAPD exit site infection (ESI). *Am Soc Nephrol* 5: 439 (Abstract), 1994

235. Piraino B, Bernardini J, Lutes R, Johnston J, Holley J: Randomized trial of mupirocin at exit site vs oral rifampin to prevent *S. aureus* infections. *Perit Dial Int* 14 (Suppl 1): S27 (Abstract), 1994

236. McAnally TP, Lewis MR, Brown DR: Effect of rifampin and Bacitracin on nasal carriers of Staphylococcus aureus. *Antimicrob Agents Chemother* 25: 422, 1984

237. Zimmerman SW, Ahrens E, Johnson CA et al.: Randomized controlled trial of prophylactic rifampin for peritoneal dialysis related infections. *Am J Kidney Dis* 18: 225, 1991

238. Sande MA, Mandell GL: Effect of rifampin on nasal carriage of Staphylococcus aureus. *Antimicrob Agents Chemother* 7: 294, 1975

239. Wheat LJ, Kohler RB, White AL, White A: Effect of rifampin on nasal carriers of coagulase-positive Staphylococci. *J Infect Dis* 144: 177, 1981

240. Oxton LL, Zimmerman SW, Roecker EB, Wakeen M: Risk factors for peritoneal dialysis related infections. *Perit Dial Int* 14: 137, 1994

241. Dryden MS, Ludlam HA, Wing AJ, Phillips I: Active intervention dramatically reduces CAPD-associated infection. *Adv Perit Dial* 7: 125, 1991

242. Trooskin SZ, Donetz AP, Baxter J, Harvey RA, Greco RS: Infection-resistant continuous peritoneal dialysis catheters. *Nephron* 46: 263, 1987

243. Gokal R: Continuous ambulatory peritoneal dialysis (CAPD) – ten years on. *Q J Med* 242: 465, 1987

244. Kamal GD, Pfaller MA, Rempe LE, Jebson PJR: Reduced intravascular catheter infection by antibiotic bonding. *JAMA* 265: 2364, 1991

245. Trooskin SZ, Harvey RA, Lennard TWJ, Greco RS: Failure of demonstrated clinical efficacy of antibiotic-bonded continuous ambulatory peritoneal dialysis (CAPD) catheters. *Perit Dial Int* 10: 57, 1990

246. Kahl AA, Grosse-Siestrup C, Khal KA et al.: Reduction of exit-site infections in peritoneal dialysis by local application of metallic silver: a preliminary report. *Perit Dial Int* 14: 1747, 1994

247. Piraino B, Bernardini J, Johnston JR, Sorkin MI: Exit-site location does not influence peritoneal catheter infection rate. *Perit Dial Int* 9: 127, 1989

248. Strauss FG, Holmes DL, Nortman DF, Friedman S: Hypertonic saline compresses: therapy for complicated exit-site infections. *Adv Perit Dial* 9: 248, 1993

249. Winchester JF: Recurrent peritoneal catheter exit site infections: I. *Semin Dial* 6: 405, 1993

250. Sherman RA: Ophthalmic antibiotic solutions for equivocal exit sites. *Semin Dial* 6: 327, 1993

251. Wadhwa NK, Cabralda T, Suh H, Kvilekval K, Mason R: Exit-site/tunnel infection and catheter outcome in peritoneal dialysis patients. *Adv Perit Dial* 8: 325, 1992

252. Piraino B, Bernardini J, Peitzman A, Sorkin M: Failure of peritoneal catheter cuff shaving to eradicate infection. *Perit Dial Bull* 7: 179, 1987

253. Nichols WK, Nolph KD: A technique for managing exit site and cuff infection in Tenckhoff catheters. *Perit Dial Bull* 3 (Suppl): S4, 1983

254. Andreoli SP, West KW, Grosfeld JL, Bergstein JM: A technique to eradicate tunnel infection without peritoneal dialysis catheter removal. *Perit Dial Bull* 4: 156, 1984

255. Eisele G, Bailie GR, Lamaestro B: Relationship between peritonitis and exit site infections in CAPD. *Adv Perit Dial* 8: 227, 1992

256. Fellin G, Gentile MG, Guerra L et al.: Exit-site infection: a randomized trial on topical vs parenteral therapy. in *Advances in Continuous Ambulatory Peritoneal Dialysis/1987*, edited by Khanna R, Nolph KD, Prowant B, Twardowski ZJ, Oreopoulos DG, Toronto, Toronto University Press, 1988, p 169

257. Scalamogna A, Castelnovo, De Vecchi A, Guerra L, Ponticelli C: Staphylococcus aureus exit site and tunnel infection in CAPD. *Adv Perit Dial* 6: 130, 1990

258. Tzamaloukas AH, Hartshorne MF, Gibel LJ, Murata GH: Persistence of positive dialysate cultures after apparent cure of CAPD peritonitis. *Adv Perit Dial* 9: 198, 1993

259. Dapena F, Munoz I, de Alvaro F et al.: Clinical significance of exit site infections due to *Xanthomonas maltophilia* in continuous ambulatory peritoneal dialysis (CAPD) patients: a comparison with Pseudomonas-related ESI. *Perit Dial Int* 14 (Suppl 1): S37, 1994

260. Kazmi HR, Raffone FD, Kliger AS, Finkelstein FO: Pseudomonas exit site infections in continuous ambula-

tory peritoneal dialysis patients. *Am Soc Nephrol* 2: 1498, 1992

261. Taber TE, Hegeman TF, York SM, Kinney RA, Webb DH: Treatment of Pseudomonas infections in peritoneal dialysis patients. *Perit Dial Int* 11: 213, 1991

262. Dasgupta MK, Kowalewaska-Grochowska K, Costerton JW: Biofilm and peritonitis in peritoneal dialysis. *Perit Dial Int* 13: S322, 1993

263. Read RR, Eberwein P, Dasgupta MK et al.: Peritonitis in peritoneal dialysis: bacterial colonization by biofilm spread along the catheter surface. *Kidney Int* 35: 614, 1989

264. Giangrande A, Allaria P, Torpia R, Baldassari L, Gelosia A, Donelli G: Ultrastructure analysis of Tenckhoff chronic peritoneal catheters used in continuous ambulatory peritoneal dialysis patients. *Perit Dial Int* 13 (Suppl 2): S133, 1993

265. Gorman SP, Mawhinney WM, Adair CG, Issouckis M: Confocal laser scanning microscopy of peritoneal catheter surfaces. *J Med Microbiol* 38: 411, 1993

266. Ward KH, Olson ME, Lam K, Costerton JW: Mechanism of persistent infection associated with peritoneal implants. *J Med Microbiol* 36: 406, 1992

267. Dasgupta MK, Ward K, Noble PA, Larabie M, Costerton JW: Development of bacterial biofilms on silastic catheter material in peritoneal dialysis fluid. *Am J Kidney Dis* 23: 709, 1994

268. Swartz R, Messana J, Holmes C, Williams J: Biofilm formation on peritoneal catheters does not require the presence of infection. *Trans Am Soc Artif Intern Organs* 37: 626, 1991

269. Finch RG, Edwards R, Filik R, Wilcox MH: Continuous Ambulatory Peritoneal Dialysis (CAPD) peritonitis: the effect of antibiotic on the adherence of coagulase-negative Staphylococci to silicone rubber catheter material. *Perit Dial Int* 9: 103, 1989

270. Richards GK, Prentis J, Gagnon RF: Antibiotic activity against *Staphylococcus epidermidis* biofilms in dialysis fluids. *Adv Perit Dial* 5: 133, 1989

271. Weber J, Mettang T, Hubel E, Kiefer T, Kuhlmann U: Survival of 138 surgically placed straight double-cuff tenckhoff catheters in patients on continuous ambulatory peritoneal dialysis. *Perit Dial Int* 13: 224, 1993

272. Wakeen MJ, Zimmerman SW, Bidwell D: Viscus perforation in peritoneal dialysis patients: diagnosis and outcome. *Perit Dial Int* 14: 371, 1994

273. Bierman MH, Kasperbauer J, Kusek A, Hammeke MD, Fitzgibbons RJ Jr, Egan JD: Peritoneal catheter survival and complications in end stage renal disease. *Perit Dial Bull* 5: 229, 1985

274. Schroder CH, Severijnen RSVM, de Jong MCJW, Monnens LAH: Chronic tunnel infections in children: removal and replacement of the continuous ambulatory peritoneal dialysis catheter in a single operation. *Perit Dial Int* 13: 198, 1993

275. Goldraich I, Mariano M, Rosito N, Goldraich N: One-step peritoneal catheter replacement in children. *Adv Perit Dial* 9: 325, 1993

276. Paterson AD, Bishop MC, Morgan AG, Burden RP: Removal and replacement of Tenckhoff catheter at a single operation: successful treatmetn of resistant peritonitis in continuous ambulatory peritoneal dialysis. *Lancet* 2: 1245, 1986

277. Swartz R, Messana J, Reynolds J, Ranjit U: Simultaneous catheter replacement and removal in refractory peritoneal dialysis infections. *Kidney Int* 40: 1160, 1991

278. Alexander SR, Sullivan EK, Harmon WE, Stablein DM, Tejani A for the NAPRTCS: Maintenance dialysis in North American children and adolescents: a preliminary report. *Kidney Int* 44 (Suppl 43): S104, 1993

279. Baum M, Powell D, Calvin S et al.: Continuous ambulatory peritoneal dialysis in children. *N Engl J Med* 25: 1537, 1982

280. Watson AR, Vigneux A, Hardy BE, Balfe JW: Six-year experience with CAPD catheters in children. *Perit Dial Bull* 5: 119, 1985

281. Hymes LC, Clowers B, Mitchell C, Warshaw BL: Peritoneal catheter survival in children. *Perit Dial Bull* 6: 185, 1986

282. Sieniawska M, Roszkowska-Blaim M, Jablczynska A, Korniszewska J, Wierzbowska-Lange B: Continuous ambulatory peritoena dialysis (CAPD) in children: a clinical report. *Perit Dial Int* 8: 159, 1988

283. Levy M, Balfe JW, Geary D, Fryer-Keene S, Bannatyne R: Exit site infection during continuous and cycling peritoneal dialysis in children. *Perit Dial Int* 10: 31, 1990

284. Chormann ML, Staccone M, Edd P, Andrus CH, Ornt DB: Experience with automated peritneal dialysis (APD) in a pediatric population. in *Advances in Peritoneal Dialysis*, edited by Khanna R, Nolph K, Prowant B et al., Peritoneal Dialysis Bulletin Inc, Toronto, 1987, p 66

285. Warady BA, Campoy SF, Gross SP, Sedman AB, Lum GM: Peritonitis with continuous ambulatory and continuous cycling peritoneal dialysis. *J Pediatr* 105: 726, 1984

286. Dabbagh S, Carroll K, Fleischmann L: Efficacy of rifampin prophylaxis in decreasing the rates of catheter-related infections in children on CCPD. *Perit Dial Int* 12 (Suppl 1): 109, 1992

287. Zappacosta AR, Perras ST: Role of catheter removal in therapy of bacterial peritonitis of continuous ambulatory peritoneal dialysis. *Trans Am Soc Artif Intern Organs* 35: 40, 1989

288. Tzamaloukas AH, Murata GH, Fox L: Peritoneal catheter loss and death in continuous ambulatory peritoneal dialysis peritonitis: correlation with clinical and biochemical parameters. *Perit Dial Int* 13 (Suppl 2): S338, 1993

289. The Ad Hoc Advisory Committee on Peritonitis Management: Peritoneal dialysis related peritonitis treatment recommendations 1993 update. *Perit Dial Int* 13: 14, 1993

SOLUTIONS FOR PERITONEAL DIALYSIS

MARIANO FERIANI, CLAUDIO RONCO and GIUSEPPE LA GRECA

INTRODUCTION

Solute removal in peritoneal dialysis is achieved both by diffusion and convection. The first mechanism takes place because of the concentration gradient between the blood of the peritoneal capillary and the peritoneal dialysis solution infused in the abdomen. The solution infused in the peritoneal cavity tends to equilibrate with plasma water over time and it is removed at the end of one exchange after partial or complete equilibration. The composition of the dialysis solution permits to remove, balance or even infuse solutes from and into the patient. The electrochemical concentration gradient is the driving force that allows such a passive diffusion (1, 2).

In addition, fluid movement across the peritoneal membrane may occur when a transmembrane pressure gradient is generated between the blood and the dialysate compartments.

Since a negative fluid balance is required in uremic patients, an osmotic agent is added to the dialysis solution to increase relative osmolality. In such condition, an osmotic pressure gradient is created and ultrafiltration occurs. As a consequence, solutes are moving across the membrane transported in the bulk flow and convective transport takes place (3, 4).

The composition of peritoneal dialysis solution is therefore the key factor that governes both diffusion and convection as well as the removal of the fluid excess from the body. In this way, utilizing different solutions, blood purification, acid-base control, electrolyte correction and body fluid balance can be adequately achieved in the patient (5, 6).

Table 1. Composition of the peritoneal dialysis fluid

		Boen (Ref (7))	Commercial CAPD
Na	mmol/l	135	132–134
K	mmol/l		0–2
Ca	mmol/l	1.5	1.25–1.75
Mg	mmol/l	0.75	0.25–0.75
Cl	mmol/l	107.5	95–106
Acetate	mmol/l	35	
Lactate	mmol/l		35–40
Glucose	Gm/dl	2.0 and higher	1.5–4.25

GENERAL ASPECTS

Several types of peritoneal dialysis solution are today produced for clinical use. The fluids are sterilized in varying volumes and glucose is added at various concentrations as an agent to vary dialysate osmolality. Solutions were originally provided in glass containers and subsequently in large plastic tanks. PD fluids are today supplied in collapsible plastic bags of different size.

Surprisingly enough, the composition of dialysis solutions today available for clinical use is very similar to that of the solution used in the late fifties in Seattle by Boen et al. (7) (Table 1).

Clinical studies however, have recently suggested that peritoneal dialysis solutions may be not completely adequate to achieve metabolic correction of the patient and may create various negative effects on the peritoneal membrane function and morphology (8–10). These observations have spurred new interest in possible improvements of PD fluids, in studying new constituents with lower degree of cellular toxicity, and in the clinical application of new buffers and osmotic agents with lower degree of side effects (11–13).

Therefore clinical trials on new peritoneal dialysis solutions have started in different countries and new developments are under technical and clinical evaluation.

In detail, more physiological concentrations of calcium and magnesium have been demonstrated to be of clinical benefit in several groups of patients (14).

Substances such as glycerol, gluconic acid, icodextrin and other glucose polymers have been studied as osmotic agents alternative to glucose (15–18). They have been chemically evaluated and clinically tested to elucidate possible advantages compared to glucose.

Acetate has been replaced by lactate as buffer and the physiological buffer, bicarbonate, has been recently proposed (19, 20).

Different types of sterilization have been evaluated and the noxious effects of glucose degradation products in heat sterilized solutions have been pointed out (21).

In conclusion, as the morphological and functional evaluation of the peritoneal mesothelium became possible thanks to *in vitro* cultured mesothelial cells and molecular biology studies of the various cells involved in the peritoneal membrane, subclinical damage of various structures have become evident. These lesions may be responsible for the short and long term damage of the peritoneal membrane and the need for a more physiologic and less irritating peritoneal dialysis solution apprears absolutely clear. The impact of peritoneal dialysis fluid on the living membrane of peritoneum is therefore the critical point of today's art of peritoneal dialysis.

ELECTROLYTE COMPOSITION

Electrolyte balance cannot fully be handled in end stage renal failure (22). Unphysiological values of serum electrolytes can result in life threatening complications in uremic patients (23). Hyperkalemia may frequently occur in uremic patients and the parallel disturbance of acid-base homeostasis may further contribute to a severe disequilibrium between intra and extracellular concentrations (24).

Sodium, potassium and magnesium must be removed or in some cases added to the patient, via the dialytic fluid in order to normalize the pools in the body and to achieve adequate homeostasis (25).

Calcium uptake from gastrointestinal tract is reduced and hypocalcemia is a common pattern in uremia if oral calcium and/or vitamin D supplementation is not provided during conservative therapy (26).

Peritoneal dialysis fluid composition is tailored to achieve adequate correction of these derangements and to obtain a restoration of the normal electrolyte composition of the body (27–30).

Sodium

Sodium concentration in peritoneal dialysis fluids ranges between 130 and 137 mmol/l. In addition, during industrial preparation procedures, 5% variation from the declared sodium concentration can be achieved.

Clinical studies have demonstrated that in CAPD different dialysate sodium concentrations (from 132 to 141 mmol/l) have no significant effect on serum sodium concentration (31). This could be explained by the peculiar characteristics of the electrolyte transport in CAPD.

Dialytic sodium balance is both a function of diffusion and a result of combined convective transport (32).

Sodium movement by diffusion across the peritoneal membrane may result in net uptake or removal depending on the concentration gradient between dialysis solution and plasma water (33). Peritoneal dialysis may also remove sodium by convection during ultrafiltration. However, the net sodium removal per liter of ultrafiltrate (about 70 mmol/l) is much less than one could expect from the extracellular fluid concentration. This effect seems to be due to the low sieving coefficient for sodium of the peritoneal membrane (34–37), even though the Donnan equilibrium may play an important additional role (38). In the clinical routine, the importance of convective transport of sodium may be such to render the concentration in the serum a negligible factor. Studies have demonstrated that when a wide range of drainage volumes, i.e., of ultrafiltration rates is observed, sodium removal does not correlate with the serum concentration (33). However, since in a stable patient the daily drainage volume is fairly constant, Nolph et al. have constructed nomograms to predict dialytic sodium balance at various serum and dialysate sodium concentrations (Figure 1). In such conditions, daily variations in net sodium balance are mostly function of serum concentration: an increase in dietary sodium intake will result in a parallel increase in serum sodium, that will consequently lead to an increase in dialytic sodium removal. These changes in net daily removal secondary to changes in serum concentration represent an intrinsic autoregulatory mechanisms for adjustment of removal rates (33).

On the other hand, if body fluid expansion is isonatric, due to positive balance of both sodium and water, the correction will be done in two steps. First, the increase of ultrafiltration by the increased number of hypertonic exchanges will result in a hyponatric dialysate with a net removal of water. Second, in this condition an increase of serum sodium concentration will progressively occur and this will lead to an increased dialytic sodium removal.

When dialysate sodium concentration is maintained at 132 mmol/l, a normal daily sodium intake of 150 mmol can be easily managed with 4 CAPD exchanges/day with

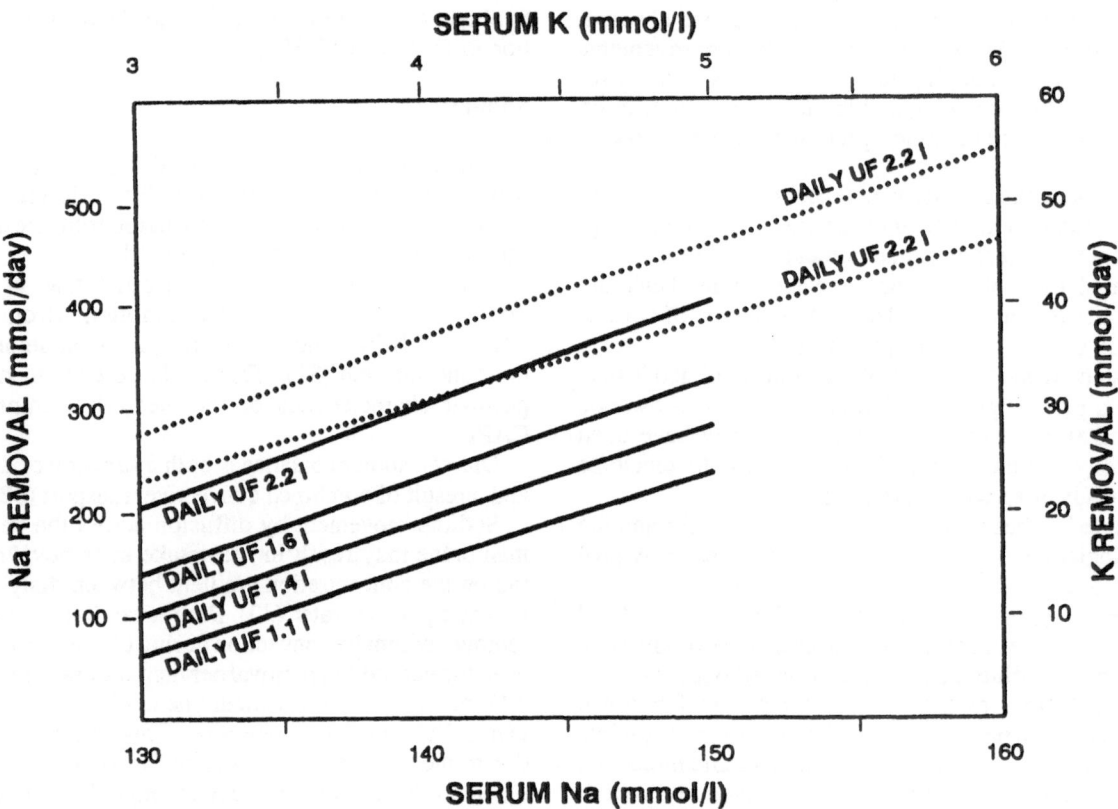

Figure 1.   Relationships between daily sodium (solid lines) and potassium (dotted lines) removals and their respective serum concentrations at different daily ultrafiltration rates (from Reference (33) modified).

about 1200 ml/day of ultrafiltration (33). When present, residual renal function can substantially contribute to sodium removal. It has been reported that, in absence of major hormonal derangements, urinary sodium content is rather constant at 70 mmol/l (39).

Since clinical studies have not reported specific side effects by using the currently available CAPD solutions with 132–134 mmol/l of sodium, few studies have been designed to explore the possible effects of variation of the sodium content in CAPD solutions.

Colombi (39) calculated the sodium removal at different urinary volumes and at different daily ultrafiltration rates using a 134 mmol/l sodium CAPD solution in presence of a serum concentration of 138 mmol/l. In these conditions a daily ultrafiltration of 1100 ml and a urinary volume of 500 ml should maintain constant the serum sodium concentration if the sodium intake is about 150 mmol/day. The author suggests that a reduction of dialysate sodium concentration to 130 mmol/l should be considered for patients without residual renal function.

De Vecchi et al. (40) used a dialysate sodium concentration of 137 mmol/l in 38 unselected patients to correct orthostatic hypotension. The average orthostatic systolic pressure increased from 129 to 139 mmHg without statistical significance. 3 patients required an increase of previous antihypertensive therapy while no significant changes in the sense of thirst or peripheral oedema were recorded.

In three hypotensive patients dialysate sodium concentration was increased to 142 mmol/l. One patient became hypertensive, one patient normotensive while no changes were reported in the last patient. The authors concluded that a 137 mmol/l sodium solution could enable a better control of mild symptomatic hypotension, while a 142 mmol/l sodium concentration is not always effective in the treatment of severe hypotension in CAPD patients.

Recently a solution with very low sodium concentration (98 mmol/l) has been proposed (41) to correct fluid overload in patients with insufficient ultrafiltration. The use of this solution led to a reasonable body weight reduction without hypotension or fatigue. However these data require further evaluation and need to be confirmed in a larger study.

Different sodium concentrations can also be proposed when the dialytic regimen is different as in the case of IPD, CCPD or ANPD.

During short dwell time exchanges convection plays a prime role, and an hyponatric ultrafiltrate is produced in the early phases of one exchange. Consequently, in rapid cycling techniques, water is removed faster than sodium and *hypernatremia* may occasionally occur (34–37). During rapid hypertonic exchanges, the use of solutions with 140 mmol/l of sodium resulted in severe thirst, hypertension a (42) and hypernatremia over 160 mmol/l (43).

Raja (35) suggests that hypernatremia can be avoided utilizing a sodium concentration of 115–120 mmol/l in a 7% dextrose dialysis solution or a concentration of 125–130 mmol/l in a 4.25% dextrose solution. In such conditions, an isonatric ultrafiltrate can be obtained.

Similar results have been reported by Ahearn et al. (37). More recently Shen et al. (44) proposed a sodium concentration of 118 for 2.5% glucose solutions and 109 mmol/l for 4.25% glucose solutions. However such solutions with lower sodium concentrations have never been commercially available. Furthermore, increased sense of thirst and difficult blood pressure control have been observed in patients on nightly automatic peritoneal dialysis by using dialysis solutions with 132 mmol/l of sodium (45).

Potassium

Hyperkaliemia is one of the most harmful complication in end stage renal failure. Dialysis treatment must therefore contribute to achieve and maintain an adequate potassium balance. Potassium balance in peritoneal dialysis is a function of several factors: among them, serum potassium concentration, insulin bioavailability, cell membrane Na/K pump activity, dialysate potassium concentration and acid-base correction.

The potassium concentration in the commercially available CAPD fluids ranges between 0 and 2 mmol/l. However, solutions without potassium are commonly used in the clinical routine.

Net potassium balance across the peritoneal membrane follows the same chemical-physical principles described for sodium. However, since potassium is absent in the dialysis solution, the gradient for diffusion is maximized. As the same time, since potassium concentration in extra-cellular fluid is low, the removal by convection is generally negligible and diffusion is the most important mechanism for net potassium removal (46).

Dialysate potassium should theoretically equilibrate with plasma faster than sodium because of the lower molecular weight and the smaller hydrated radius. However, even after long-dwell times, dialysate potassium does not completely equilibrate with serum (32). This is because several factors such as Donnan's equilibrium, membrane sieving and others may interfere with a complete equilibration. On the other hand, serum potassium measurements may be artifactually high because of leaching of potassium from red cells during serum separation (33).

Nomograms to predict daily potassium removal based on serum potassium concentration have been published (Figure 1). It can be seen that convection minimally increases net potassium removal as previously observed in IPD sessions with hypertonic dialysate (47).

In regular CAPD treatment (four 2 liters exchanges per day), about 30 mmol/day are lost in the dialysate (48). About 20 mmol per liter of urine are generally added to dialytic removal in case of preserved residual renal function (39). This overall amount is considerably lower than the usual daily intake of 70 to 80 mmol. Nevertheless, most patients have a normal serum potassium, which can be explained by an increased excretion in the stools (49). Increased intestinal excretion may become particularly important in patients with high potassium intake, since excretion in the stools is highly correlated with the levels of serum concentration (50). Insulin levels are also important since the activity of the hormone promotes cellular uptake and tends to restore intra-extra cellular gradients for the electrolyte.

In previous studies, a CAPD solution containing 4 mmol/l of potassium, induced hyperkalemia in about 50% of treated patients that required ionic exchange resin administration (51).

With the commonly used potassium free CAPD solutions, hypokaliemia is found in 10–36% of patients (52, 53), even though the intracellular muscle potassium (54) and total body potassium (55, 56) contents have been reported to be normal or slightly increased. It is not clear whether in such conditions, the hypokalemic state may be a consequence of an anabolic state or it may reflect a poor nutritional intake (57). A possible condition of hyperpolarization of the cells with increased transcellular potassium gradient might also contribute to explain this observation.

Magnesium

Magnesium is an important cation involved in several enzymatic reactions. The serum concentration of magnesium in dialysis patients depends on dietary intake and on the concentration of the cation in the dialysis solution.

Hypermagnesemia is a common finding in dialysis patients (58). While it is almost impossible to show abnormalities related to modestly elevated magnesium concentrations, hypomagnesemia has been associated with cardiac arrhythmias (59, 60) and various electrocardiographic abnormalities (61).

Normal values of total serum magnesium range from 0.65 to 0.98 mmol/l, while its diffusible fraction of is about 55%–60% of the total. Commercially available CAPD solutions contain 0.25–0.75 mmol/l of magnesium.

In such conditions, when 0.75 mmol/l magnesium and 1.5% glucose solutions are used in CAPD, a slight magnesium uptake from the dialysis solution usually occurs by diffusive gradient (62). Kwong et al. however, have reported a negative dialytic balance with the same solution (63).

When ultrafiltration is increased by a 4.25% dextrose solution, convective removal counteracts diffusive uptake yielding a negative magnesium mass transport in most patients (62).

524   *Mariano Feriani, Claudio Ronco and Giuseppe La Greca*

Not only is peritoneal transport of magnesium influenced by diffusion gradients and ultrafiltration rates, but also by dwell time and peritoneal permeability because of the large hydrated radius of the molecule (62).

In most papers (26, 64–66), the use of 0.75 mmol/l magnesium solutions resulted in elevated levels of magnesium in the serum. This, may lead to an excessive body burden and potentially inhibits bone remodelling (67, 68). Other authors pointed out that hypermagnesemia does not result in any clinical complication and, on the contrary, a protective role on soft tissue calcifications has been suggested (69). Despite such frequent hypermagnesemia the muscle content of magnesium is generally not altered (54). Therefore the relationship of serum magnesium to intracellular magnesium concentration and total body magnesium in CAPD patients is unclear. Dietary magnesium intake is a function of protein intake. On the other hand, magnesium removal with standard 0.75 mmol/l magnesium solutions is negligible. In spite of these observations, CAPD patients do not display a continuous increase of serum magnesium levels, and stool magnesium losses may probably play a regulatory function (31).

To achieve a correct balance, Nolph et al. suggested to lower dialysate magnesium to 0.25 mmol/l (64). The use of this solution did not cause hypomagnesemia, and most patients experienced a normalization of magnesium serum levels (64, 70).

The use of lower or zero magnesium dialysate has also been investigated to permit oral treatment of hyperphosphatemia with magnesium salts as a calcium free phosphate binder (71). This however, frequently results in a laxative effect, requiring carefull monitoring of compliance to therapy and serum magnesium levels (72, 73).

Calcium

Standard CAPD solutions contain 1.75 mmol/l of calcium. Since normal serum concentration of diffusible ionized calcium ranges from 1.15 to 1.29 mmol/l, calcium is absorbed from dialysate by diffusion (62). A significant correlation between positive calcium balance and dialysate/serum gradient for ionized calcium has been found (63). Blumenkrantz et al. have also reported that net dialytic calcium uptake inversely correlates with total serum calcium (49). In CAPD solutions, 30% of calcium is not ionized being 'chelated' by lactate (63). Ionized calcium probably crosses the peritoneum faster than chelated calcium. As a consequence, ionized calcium gradient is rapidly dissipated. The rapid increase in dialysate pH further contributes to this phenomenon decreasing calcium ionization in the solution (63).

When ultrafiltration increases in hypertonic exchanges, calcium uptake tend to decrease (62) or even to become negative (63, 74). Different rates of ultrafiltration may help to explain discrepancies among different studies. Convective removal counterbalance diffusive uptake and

decreases dialysate/serum gradient because of a dilution effect (67).

While a negative balance may result from the use of 1.5 mmol/l dialysate calcium (75), kinetic studies suggest that CAPD solutions with 1.75 mmol/l of calcium (3 exchanges with 1.5% glucose and 1 exchange with 4.25% glucose) generally lead to peritoneal calcium absorption and rapidly normalize total and ionized calcium levels in the serum (26, 62, 63, 74). This was suggested to be beneficial in order to prevent progression of osteodystrophy and calcium losses from the bone (66, 76). However, clinical studies did not confirm such positive effects (75, 77, 78).

Overall calcium mass-balance is also affected by gastrointestinal absorption. In CAPD patients an empirical relationship has been found between dietary intake and gastrointestinal absorption (49). 720 mg/day of dietary calcium intake resulted in an estimated average gastrointestinal absorption of 25 mg (49). If oral calcium supplementations are administered as phosphate binder, significantly greater amounts of calcium are absorbed from gastrointestinal tract. Assuming a daily phosphate intake of 1000 mg in CAPD patients (79), 70% of this should be bound in the intestinal tract to maintain the balance (74). This goal can be achieved with 6.25 g of calcium carbonate supplementation (2500 mg of elemental calcium), that leads to an average gastrointestinal calcium absorption of 700 mg/day (80, 81). Hence, in a standard patient, total calcium absorption from the diet and calcium carbonate is approximately 725 mg/day. In such condition, a large number of patients may encounter an increased risk of hypercalcemia and soft tissue calcification (82).

On the other hand aluminium-containing phosphate binders are the main source of aluminium in CAPD patients (83) and the dangers of aluminium toxicity in the form of bone disease and encephalopathy are now well recognized (84–86). A solution to this puzzle has been found in the use of lower dialysate calcium concentration. This approach has been suggested to avoid the risk of calcium carbonate-related hypercalcemia (62).

Martis et al. (87) have calculated on theoretical bases that a calcium concentration of 1.25 mmol/l in peritoneal fluid would lead to a calcium removal of 160 mg/day when serum ionized calcium is 1.3 mmol/l and to a greater removal in the case of hypercalcemia.

In a prospective clinical study, Hutchison et al. have demonstrated that a 1.25 mmol/l calcium dialysate allowed the administration of larger doses of calcium carbonate with good control of serum phosphate, and maintained serum ionized calcium near to the upper limit of the normal range. Parathyroid hormone was suppressed in the majority of patients and bone histology improved (70).

Similar results have been achieved in a large multicentric study in which 1 mmol/l calcium solution has been used and low dose of vitamin D and calcium carbonate as phosphate binder have been orally supplemented (88).

Low calcium PD fluids have been extensively studied by several investigators and the results confirm the benefit of this approach on uremic osteodystrophy (14, 89–92).

Long-term usage of lower calcium dialysate by large numbers of patients raises the question of safety in cases of poor compliance to oral calcium carbonate supplementation. In 12 patients treated with 1.5% glucose and 1.25 mmol/l calcium solution, a net gain of calcium was demonstrated when the serum ionized calcium level was less than 1.25 mmol/l. This observation seems to prove that a very low risk of hypocalcemia is present in these patients (70).

There is a much greater tendency to lose calcium regardless of the serum ionized calcium, in those patients treated with 4.25% glucose and low calcium solutions, On the other hand, a rapid exacerbation of hyperparathyroidism in some patients converted to low calcium dialysate without adequate oral calcium supplementation may be documented (93). Therefore in CAPD patients using two or more hypertonic bags per day and a low calcium solution, a careful surveillance of the mineral metabolism is needed.

The commercially available solutions for intermittent peritoneal dialysis treatments are substantially similar to those for CAPD. Adersen (94) reported that a positive calcium transfer from dialysis fluid can be obtained with a 2.16 mmol/l calcium concentration in dialysate both during 1.5% and 4% glucose 30-minute dwell-time exchanges.

A recent report suggests that, in automated peritoneal dialysis, the low calcium dialysis solution (1.25 mmol/l) could result in a negative calcium balance (95).

In summary, the use of solutions with lower calcium is nowadays observed in an increased number of dialysis units. This therapeutic approach is further confirmed in patients treated with oral administration of calcium carbonate as a phosphate binder.

OSMOTIC AGENTS

In peritoneal dialysis, net water removal is achieved by adding an osmotic agent to the solution and is directly proportional to the dialysate/plasma osmotic gradient (96). Low molecular weight solutes with high osmotic power [crystalloids] were firstly studied in animals (97). Only glucose appeared sufficiently safe, effective and readily metabolized. Lately glucose was used in the solutions for intermittent peritoneal dialysis and its reliability was clinically confirmed (98). However, peritoneal membrane is not completely impermeable to glucose, and a rapid decline in osmotic gradient, as a consequence of glucose absorption, is observed during long dwell time exchanges. This partially limits the osmotic power of glucose and creates the problem of carbohydrate load in CAPD patients (99).

Several substances have been examined as osmotic agents alternative to glucose. Low molecular weight agents [glycerol, sorbitol, amino acids, xylitol and fructose] have been utilized to overcome some of the metabolic problems caused by glucose. High molecular weight agents [glucose polymers, gelatin, polycations, dextrans and polypeptides] have also been proposed because of their slower absorption, and consequent sustained ultrafiltration in the prolonged dwells (100).

Osmotic power is dependent on the total number of osmotically active molecules in the solution. Therefore, a greater mass of substance is needed to obtain equivalent osmolality gradient, when high molecular weight agents are employed (101).

At high concentration these large molecules are less soluble, hyperviscous, non physiological and eventually allergenic. Nevertheless, high molar concentrations are not needed in dialysis fluid because these substances may equally provide a sustained slow ultrafiltration due to their lower or absent reabsorption. This effect is very similar to that exerted by albumin in biological systems ('colloid' osmotic pressure) and could be exploited in peritoneal dialysis to achieve sustained ultrafiltration at low molar concentration using dialysis solutions isosmotic to plasma (102).

The addition of a low molecular weight agent to an hypoosmolar solution containing a high molecular weight substance has been proposed to achieve a synergistic effect (103). In such condition, the crystalloid initiates a rapid phase of ultrafiltration which is then maintained by the slower and prolonged effect of the colloid.

By adjusting the proportion of the two agents, this bimodal ultrafiltration permits to optimize ultrafiltration kinetics during the exchange. It has been demonstrated that, in a 12 hour exchange, a 7.5% glucose polymer plus 0.35% glucose solution may provide greater ultrafiltration (+40%) compared to a 7.5% glucose polymer solution alone (103).

In summary small solutes yield high osmolality, but cross peritoneal membrane rapidly. Large solutes remain longer in the peritoneal cavity, but attract less water. While the smaller solutes should be favoured for short dwell time exchanges, the larger solutes should be suitable for exchanges with longer dwell times (101). Estimated ultrafiltration patterns with several small and large solutes at the same percentage concentration are depicted in Figure 2.

Low molecular weight osmotic agents

Glucose

At the time of this writing, glucose is the only commercially widely available osmotic agent in peritoneal dialysis solutions. Glucose content of commercial bags is expressed either as dextrose anhydrous or as dextrose monohydrate. Dextrose monohydrate concentrations of 1.5, 2.5 and 4.25% correspond to 1.36, 2.26 and 3.86%

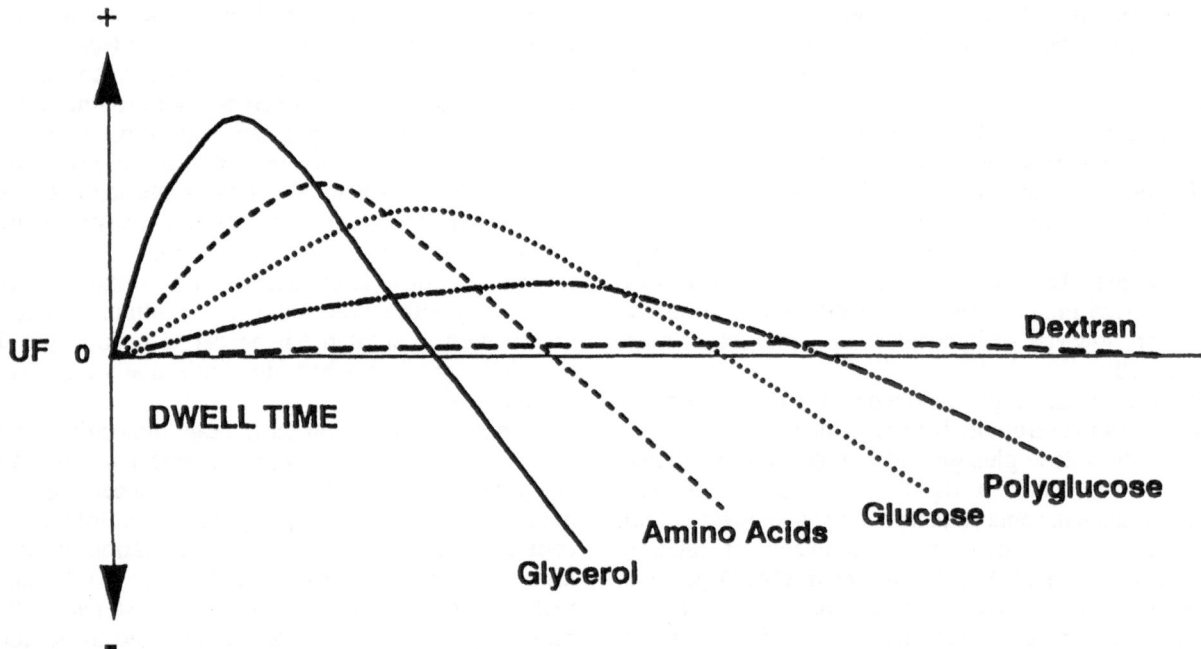

Figure 2. Estimate ultrafiltration patterns with osmotic agents of various molecular weights at the same percentage concentration (from Reference (101) with permission of Karger AG, Basel).

respectively of dextrose anhydrous. In this chapter, glucose concentrations are reported as dextrose monohydrate.

Since glucose is absorbed during the exchange, a progressive dissipation of osmotic gradient is observed (6, 31, 99, 101, 104–107). This determines the typical curve of the intraperitoneal volume (Figure 3). Ultrafiltration rate is maximal at the beginning of the exchange and the peritoneal volume reaches the maximal peak after 2–3 hours of dwell when the equilibration between dialysate and plasma osmolality occurs. After this point absorption becomes evident with a progressive reduction of the amount of fluid in the peritoneal cavity. The rate of fluid absorption is mainly dependent on the lymphatic flux (108, 109).

In short rapid exchanges, ultrafiltration is maintained throughout the exchange. In CAPD with 4 to 8 hour exchanges, a high rate of glucose absorption may result in a final positive fluid balance. Some patients absorb glucose so rapidly that adequate ultrafiltration can not be achieved even with more concentrated glucose solutions (101).

A significant correlation between the amount of glucose absorbed per day and the glucose concentration in the dialysate has been found in CAPD patients. The net daily glucose uptake can be therefore predicted from the empirical equation:

$$Gu \ (g/day) = [11.3 \times [G] - 10.9] \times V,$$

where Gu is glucose uptake in g/day; 11.3 and 10.9 are constants of correlation; [G] is the average dialysate glucose concentration and V is the dialysate inflow volume in liters (110). This relation has also been rejoined by others (111).

Since about 60–80% of the glucose instilled into the peritoneal cavity is absorbed during a 6 hour dwell time, 45–60 g of glucose are absorbed from 4.25% solution, 24–40 g from 2.5% and 15–22 g from 1.5% (112). Consequently a normal glucose uptake in CAPD patients ranges from 100 to 300 g per day (110–115).

This amount contributes to the total energy intake (20.3%) in CAPD patients and has been suggested to be beneficial for the caloric balance (110). However, the large amount of absorbed glucose may also result in several metabolic derangements.

A marked hyperglycemia has been observed in patients undergoing intermittent peritoneal dialysis (116, 117).

Although CAPD exchanges with 1.5% glucose dialysate have no significant effect on blood glucose and insulin levels (118, 119), a constant tendency towards hyperglycemia and hyperinsulinemia has been frequently reported (119, 120).

During hypertonic exchanges, glucose and insulin peak levels occur in patients after 45–90 minutes while glucagon slightly decreases (111, 118, 119, 121, 122). These effects are similar to those observed after an oral glucose load (122, 123).

It has been reported that some patients on CAPD developed *de novo* manifest diabetes mellitus due to the con-

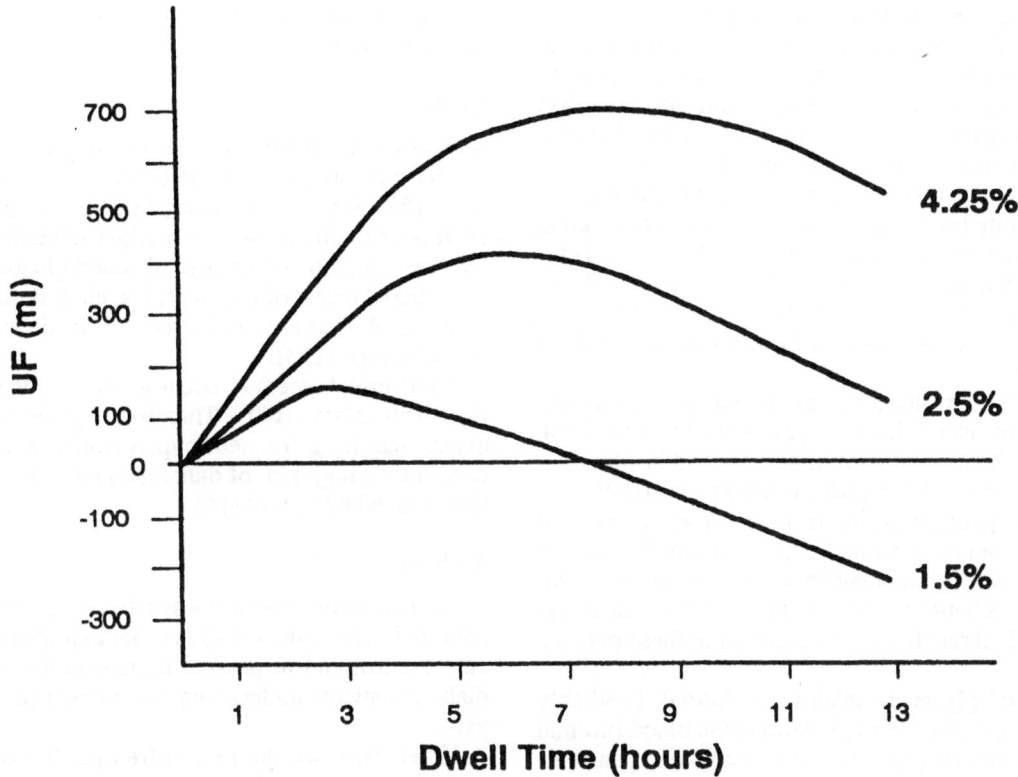

Figure 3.   Approximate ultrafiltration volumes related to dwell time with 1.5, 2.5 and 4.25% glucose concentration solutions (from Reference (101) with permission of Karger AG, Basel).

tinuous hyperglycemic stress (112). In addition, since sustained hyperinsulinemia may possibly increase athero-genesis, the elevated circulating insulin levels represent a potential risk factor for CAPD patients (112).

A hyperlipidemic effect of CAPD was demonstrated in several clinical studies. Hypertriglyceridemia and serum lipoprotein abnormalities were accentuated within the first months of treatment (113, 114, 124–129) and were attributed to continuous peritoneal absorption of glucose (130). These changes however, were at least in part transitory (131), suggesting an adaptation to peritoneal glucose load with a spontaneous reduction of the oral carbohydrate intake (112, 115).

Recent investigations in the field of the peritoneal fluid biocompatibility have raised the question of the long term toxicity of solutions containing glucose on peritoneal resident cells.

To prevent caramelization of glucose during heat sterilization, the pH of the solution is kept low (5–5.5). The high glucose concentration and the low pH of the commercially available solutions have been demonstrated to affect peritoneal cellular host defense mechanisms and peritoneal mesothelial cell viability (132–139). In addition, glucose is not entirely stable and some of its breakdown products can be detected in peritoneal dialysate especially when using fluids stored for long time. These degradation products of which 5-hydroxymethylfurfural (5-HMF) is the most easily measurable, have been found significantly elevated after 18 months of storage (140). A marked reduction of peritoneal ultrafiltration has been associated with the use of solutions which have been stored for more than 18 months. 5-HMF is relatively atoxic to biological tissues but combines readily with anions including lactate to form Schiff's bases and this compound may alter the characteristics of many tissue components (21).

High intraperitoneal glucose concentration has been associated with a non enzymatic glycosylation of proteins during severe peritonitis. Dobbie et al. (141) have demonstrated that repeated and severe episodes of peritonitis can remove the mesothelial layer, exposing the underlaying stroma to high concentrated glucose solutions. This condition can result in diabetes-like reduplication of the basement membrane of mesothelium and stromal blood vessels and in irreversible changes of exposed proteins (9).

Glycerol

Glycerol has been proposed as an alternative osmotic agent for CAPD solutions to overcome some metabolic effects of glucose, mainly in diabetic patients (15, 142). Glycerol containing solutions have a higher initial pH and therefore they should be more biocompatible (15).

Glycerol is a small molecular weight alcohol which does not require insulin to be metabolized. It is part of neutral fats and follows the carbohydrate metabolic pathway (143). Glycerol produces greater ultrafiltration than glucose during the early phase of the exchange because of its higher osmotic power. However, due to the low molecular weight, glycerol diffuses very rapidly into the blood providing lower amounts of total net ultrafiltration throughout the entire exchange (101, 144, 145). Thus, higher concentrations of glycerol are required to obtain adequate ultrafiltration in CAPD leading to a caloric load from the solution equivalent (146) or even higher (144) than glucose.

In non diabetics, no rise in blood glucose and insulin concentrations over a dialysis cycle was observed (146). However, in the long run, mean glucose and insulin concentrations rose steadily with the use of glycerol (146).

In diabetic patients the use of glycerol was associated with a decreased insulin requirement, but this favourable effect could not be maintained after 3–4 months (15). Nevertheless, a better control of glucose homeostasis and a better survival rate have been reported in these patients (143).

The use of glycerol-containing solutions inevitably leads to an accumulation of glycerol in the blood [normal value 0.12 mmol/l] (142, 147). The mean blood peak values with the 1.4% and 2.5% glycerol solutions have been reported to be 0.62 and 11.65 mmol/l respectively (147). In few cases, these high glycerol levels have been associated with hyperosmolar symptoms, even though mean plasma osmolality in the studied patients was similar to that observed in CAPD patients treated with standard glucose solution (147).

The long term studies have shown a dramatic increase of the blood fasting triglyceride concentrations after 6 months of treatment (143, 146). Since glycerol is measured together with triglycerides by the standard methodology, when triglyceride concentrations were corrected for free glycerol concentrations, the triglyceride increase appeared to be less dramatic (147). In conclusion there is a general agreement that glycerol solutions could be used in diabetic patients because of their better control on glucose homeostasis. However, special care should be paid to possible negative effects on other metabolic pathways (146–148).

In non diabetic CAPD patients the available evidence suggests that glycerol alone has little or no clinical advantage over glucose as an osmotic agent (101, 146, 149, 150).

There may be a role for glycerol in combination with amino acids. Recent experimental studies in rats have shown that this combination can be autoclaved and kept within a single solution without glucose caramelisation (151, 152). The mixture of amino acids and glycerol can reduce the carbohydrate absorption and improve the nutritional value of the CAPD solutions. The direct metabolism of both osmotic agents is independent from

insulin, making these solutions particularly suitable for diabetic patients.

Xylitol

Xylitol has been suggested as osmotic agent in diabetic CAPD patients since its metabolism is insulin independent (153). A preliminar study in 4 diabetic patients treated for 6 months showed a marked reduction in insulin requirement, a better control of blood glucose levels and normalized levels of triglycerides, cholesterol and HDL-cholesterol. However an increase of lactic and uric acids was observed (153).

Toxic effects seem to occur at absorption rates greater than 150 g/day (67). Therefore, patients with fluid excess requiring frequent hyperosmolar exchanges may encounter a high risk of dangerous metabolic abnormalities induced by xylitol (16).

Sorbitol

In the late sixties sorbitol was tried as substitute for glucose in dialysis fluid (154) in order to improve blood glucose control and to prevent hyperosmolar symptoms in diabetic patients undergoing intermittent peritoneal dialysis.

However, since the rate of transperitoneal absorption exceeds the metabolic capacity, this substance accumulates in blood causing hyperosmolar status with confusion, convulsion and coma (155, 156). Following this observation, the committee on peritoneal dialysis solution in 1973, did not recommend the use of sorbitol in dialysate (17).

Fructose

Fructose has the same molecular weight as glucose and similar osmotic power, but it is predominantly metabolized in the liver and it does not require insulin (157, 158).

Fructose does not appear to provide any advantage over glucose and it may be even more prone than glucose in producing hypertriglyceridemia (148) and hyperosmolar state (67).

Amino acids

In the late sixties Gjessing suggested to supplement peritoneal dialysis solutions with a mixture of amino acids to correct serum amino acid abnormalities and to prevent obligatory protein losses with dialysate (159).

More than 10 years later Oreopoulos et al. described the osmotic properties of different amino acid solutions for peritoneal dialysis in a uremic rabbit model (160). The author pointed out the advantage of substituting glucose in the solution and improving nutritional support.

Osmotic efficacy. Molecular weight of different amino acids range from 75 to 214 Daltons. Since amino acids mixtures for peritoneal dialysis usually contain a higher proportion of small molecular weight compounds, the average molecular weight represented in these solutions is approximately 100 Daltons (101) and therefore lower than that of glucose. In spite of that, absorption rate of aminoacids is not significantly faster than glucose. In fact, at neutral pH, aminoacids are electrically charged, and the consequent hydration shell increases the relative Einstein–Stokes radius of the molecules. As a consequence, diffusion coefficients are smaller in comparison to uncharged molecules with equivalent molecular weight, and absorption velocity is reduced (101).

Several studies have been performed to evaluate the ultrafiltration capacity of amino acid solutions. A 2% amino acid solution was compared to a 4.25% glucose solution in an acute study on 6 hour exchanges (161). The two solutions induced equivalent amounts of ultrafiltration and similar amounts of urea, creatinine and potassium removal. The initial dialysate osmolality was similar for the two solutions and similar dialysate osmolality changes during dwell time were observed. At the end of the exchange, 90% of the administered amino acids were absorbed.

Later, the same group (162) reported a short term study in which the ultrafiltration obtained with a 1% amino acid solution (osmolality 364 mmOsm/kg) was intermediate between that of 1.5% (osmolality 346 mmOsm/kg) and 2.5% (396 mmOsm/kg) standard glucose solution. Recently, Goodship et al. confirmed the observation of smaller but not statistically different ultrafiltrate volumes comparing a 1% amino acid solution with a 1.5% glucose solution (163).

A comparison of ultrafiltration profiles and solute mass transfer between a 4.25% glucose [478 mmOsm/kg] and a 2.76% amino acid (501 mmOsm/kg) solutions showed that intraperitoneal volume profiles were equal during the first 180 minutes of dwell. Later, the volume of amino acid solution tended to decrease more rapidly than that of glucose solution leading to a decreased net ultrafiltration at the end of the 6 hour dwell time exchange (164). These differences were not statistically significant.

Dialysate sodium, potassium, urea and total protein levels as well as dialysate-to-plasma concentration ratios (D/P) for these solutes were similar with the two solutions during dwell, although D/P after 360 minutes tended to be higher when using amino acids solutions. This difference was statistically significant for creatinine. In addition, the diffusive mass transport coefficient tended to be higher with amino acid solutions, but the difference was not statistically significant (164).

The conclusion was that the peritoneal permeability was not significantly altered by the use of amino acids instead of glucose (165).

In a more recent paper, Young et al. (166) studied ultrafiltration and D/P ratios of several proteins in an 8-hour dwell time exchange using a 1% amino acid solution in comparison with 1.5% glucose standard solution. Volumes of dialysate recovered at the end of the exchanges were significantly less after amino acid

exchanges although the osmolality decreased comparably during the dwell time. At the end of the study period (12 weeks) amino acids absorption and protein losses were increased as compared to the beginning of the study. The clearances of the studied proteins expressed as D/P ratios showed an 18 and 34% increase respectively at the beginning of the amino acid use and after 12 weeks. D/P ratios for creatinine showed increases of 7 and 10% respectively while no differences were observed for urea. The increase of the peritoneal permeability during the use of amino acid based solution was attributed to an activation of complement by amino acids or their metabolites to produce C5a (167) and the generation of prostaglandin E2 (168). The peritoneal permeability increase was reversed when standard glucose solutions were resumed (166).

Thus, there is clinical evidence that amino acid solutions can deliver ultrafiltration and small molecule clearances equivalent to those achieved with glucose solutions. The slight differences among various studies probably reflect the difference in concentration and composition of amino acids in the employed solutions. The osmotic power produced by different solutions is not only expressed by the osmolality, calculated or measured, but also depends on the degree of absorption and metabolization of each amino acid (169).

Nutritional efficacy. The nutritional value, the changes in serum amino acid profile, The effects on lipids and glucose metabolism of CAPD amino acid solutions have been evaluated in clinical studies. The amino acid composition of the commonly used CAPD solutions is reported in Table 2.

In the first long term study (162), 1% amino acid fluid (solution A in Table 1) was alternated with glucose exchanges for four weeks in 6 patients. A slightly improved nutritional status and an increase of total body nitrogen and serum transferrin were detected. Mean dietary protein intake (0.96 to 0.93 g/kg/day), energy intake (22 to 21.2 kcal/kg/day), anthropometric indexes, total body potassium and serum albumin, insulin and glucagon levels did not change during the study. Plasma triglycerides tended to decrease and HDL cholesterol to increase but after 4 weeks these changes were not statistically significant. BUN levels sharply increased (59%) and blood bicarbonate dropped although 33 mmol/l of lactate, 7 mmol/l of acetate and 4.5 mmol/l of bicarbonate were present in the solution. The low plasma concentrations of branch-chained amino acids valine, isoleucine and leucine observed before treatment remained unchanged, while glycine increased and alanine decreased.

The same group (170) found rather discouraging results by using a daily 2% amino acid solution exchange over 5 to 6 months in 3 patients. Only one patient, who was severely malnourished with low total body nitrogen and daily protein intake, improved during the study. In the remaining 2 patients, who had a normal total body nitrogen and an adequate protein intake, the benefits of amino

Table 2. Amino acids composition (mg/dl) of different studied solutions

		A *Ref(162, 170–172)*	B *Ref(174)*	C *Ref(175, 177–179)*	D *Ref(182)*
EBCAA	Valine	46	67	126	139.3
EBCAA	Leucine	62	82.6	92	101.9
EBCAA	Isoleucine	48	60.8	77	84.9
EAA	Threonine	42	46.8	59	64.5
EAA	Tyrosine	4	7.8	6	30
EAA	Phenylalanine	62	–	75	57
EAA	Lysine	58	60.8	86	95.5
EAA	Hystidine	44	37.4	65	71.4
EAA	Tryptophan	18	15.6	25	27
EAA	Methionine	58	29.6	77	84.9
NEAA	Arginine	104	51.4	97	107.1
NEAA	Serine	–	116.9	46	50.9
NEAA	Proline	42	126.3	54	59.5
NEAA	Glycine	213	32.7	46	50.9
NEAA	Alanine	213	46.8	86	95.1
NEAA	Aspartic acid	–	63.9	–	–
NEAA	Glutammic acid	–	140.3	–	–

EBCA: essential branch-chained amino acid; EAA: essential amino acid; NEAA: non essential amino acid.

acid supplementation were neutralized by loss of appetite associated with the use of these solutions.

The same results were obtained in a prospective randomized study (171) in which a 1% amino acid solution was evaluated for its ability to counteract the catabolic effect of peritonitis in CAPD patients. During 4 weeks 12 patients used the amino acid solution alternately with glucose solution, while 10 patients continued the regular dialysis with glucose-based solutions only. There was no improvement of nitrogen balance, plasma amino acid pattern or nutritional status. BUN increased by 50% and nine out of twelve patients lost their appetite. The mean dietary protein and energy intakes decreased during peritonitis.

The most recent study with solution A of Table 2 was published by Dombros et al. (172). 5 patients with low daily protein intake (< 0.8 g/kg/bw) and low serum albumin (< 35 g/l) received the 1% amino acid solution during the overnight exchange for 6 months. 3 patients, who received a 2% amino acid solution at the beginning of the study, developed symptoms of severe uremia such as anorexia, vomiting, malaise, pruritus, restlessness, abdominal cramps and a dramatic increase in BUN. The symptoms subsided upon reducing the amino acid concentrations from 2 to 1%. At the end of the study BUN slightly increased and total body nitrogen tended to decrease while oral total energy and protein intakes, cholesterol, triglycerides, albumin, transferrin, skinfold thickness, total body potassium and plasma amino acid levels remained basically unchanged. The authors concluded that the ineffective-

ness of the amino acid solution could be due to the amino acid composition of the fluid, the timing of administration or to a low caloric intake and/or that the patients were not severely malnourished. These studies used solutions not tailored to meet the needs of uremic patients (large amount of non essential amino acids) and with an inadequate amount of buffer. Therefore they were not able to normalize the amino acid pattern and contributed to acidosis. Furthermore the energy intake of the patients was low and consequently the intraperitoneal supply of amino acids was probably used as a source of energy (173). These disadvantages are well recognized by the authors and stimulated the search for an amino acid composition solution more suitable for CAPD patients.

The new solutions contain an increased amount of essential amino acids while non essential amino acid concentrations, namely glycine and alanine, are decreased.

Pedersen et al. (174) studied 6 patients for 3 months with a 1% amino acid solution (solution B in Table 2) used alternately with a 1.5% glucose solution. Patient protein intake at the beginning of treatment was 1.2–1.5 g/kg/day. During this study no detectable changes in the metabolism of glucose, lipids and proteins occurred. In particular serum triglycerides, cholesterol, albumin and transferrin were not different from the pre study values. Serum creatinine remained stable while serum BUN increased significantly during the study. Interestingly the serum branch-chained amino acids increased approaching the normal values. The increased amount of BCAA in the solution could explain this effect.

Young et al. (175) studied 8 hypoalbuminemic CAPD patients using only a morning exchange with a different amino acid solution for 12 weeks (solution C in Table 2). A modest nutritional benefit was recorded. Transferrin significantly increased and cholesterol and apolipoprotein B tended to decrease. No significant changes occurred in mean dietary protein and energy intakes, fasting amino acid, albumin, prealbumin and apolipoprotein A levels. BUN increased by 36% and bicarbonate decreased by 13% without signs of uremia and clinical acidosis. As a part of the same study a more detailed analysis (176) showed significant reduction of total and LDL cholesterol and apolipoprotein B. These parameters returned to baseline 2 weeks after returning the patients to glucose peritoneal fluid.

A more extended observation (6 months) in 6 non malnourished patients with one exchange per day of the same solution (177) showed an improved estimated nitrogen balance and serum amino acid profile, an increase of dietary protein and energy intakes and a decrease of serum cholesterol and triglycerides. Plasma protein concentrations remained unchanged, BUN increased by 29%, blood bicarbonate and pH decreased (the employed solution contained 35 mmol/l of lactate). When this solution was used twice a day in 7 patients for 8 weeks (178) the plasma essential amino acid concentrations increased (in particular branch-chained amino acids) as well as serum albumin. However BUN rose by 63% and blood bicarbonate dropped by 31% and a significant acidosis was developed by the patients. Other parameters such as anthropometry, total body potassium, dietary protein and caloric intakes, transferrin, insulin, glucagon, and lipids were unchanged.

The longest study available with the 1% amino acid solution describes 4 diabetic patients followed for more than 12 months (179). Serum albumin and cholesterol increased as compared with a control group. In addition the amount of insulin administered was reduced in the group receiving amino acids. As expected azotemia increased by 68% and bicarbonate decreased.

In summary the above mentioned studies using the improved 1% amino acid solution demonstrated more beneficial effects than the previous solution if patients with signs of protein malnutrition and low dietary protein intake were included. Energy intake should be sufficient to prevent diversion of absorbed amino acids as an energy source (180). Acidosis remained a commonly concern. This was most likely due to the acid load delivered by salts of basic amino acids (lysine hydrochloride) and that arising from metabolism of sulphur amino acids to sulphate (methionine) (181).

In order to further improve the clinical efficacy, a new formulation of the amino acid solution has been proposed and tested (solution D in Table 2). Essential amino acid concentrations were increased as well as lactate concentration (from 35 to 40 mmol/l). Total amino acid concentration was increased to 1.1% in order to provide the same osmotic effect as the 1.5% standard glucose solution.

An international multicentric study in CAPD patients with signs of protein malnutrition has been performed (182).

The preliminary results (180, 181) suggest that this solution improves nutritional status of the CAPD patients who have a low protein intake. Mean nitrogen balance increased significantly during the treatment period. Statistically significant increases were also observed in serum transferrin, total proteins and midarm muscle circumference over the 20-day treatment period. The pre exchange fasting amino acid pattern in plasma became more normal during the treatment phase. In conclusion in malnourished CAPD patients, dialysate with a more appropriate and recently introduced amino acid composition may improve their protein nutrition and metabolic status. However, increased BUN levels and the tendency toward acidosis remain problems to be solved. Finally, the cost of commercially available amino acid solutions is almost double of the standard glucose solution and this aspect must be considered as well.

High molecular weight osmotic agents

Albumin

Almost one hundred years ago albumin was shown to delay peritoneal fluid absorption (183). It is non toxic sistemically and does not cause biochemical or metabolic derangements thus representing an ideal osmotic agent (184). Because of its molecular weight (68,000 Daltons) albumin is absorbed slowly from the peritoneal cavity and exerts a sustained oncotic effect as evaluated in a rat model (185).

However it is currently too expensive to be considered as a substitute for glucose in clinical peritoneal dialysis and its use in humans has been restricted to study peritoneal fluid and solute transports (186).

Synthetic polymers

Polyacrylate, polyethylene-amine and dextran sulfate are the synthetic polymers which have been proposed and tried in an *in vitro* simulation of peritoneal dialysis, in rats and in rabbits (187–189). All obtained results showed high toxicity and possible clinical applicability was denied. Nevertheless, slow absorption and high osmotic driving forces in long dwell exchanges have been observed in animals.

Polyacrylate however, induced intraperitoneal bleeding, peritoneal membrane damage and cardiovascular instability (189). In addition, despite its high molecular weight (90,000 Daltons) polyacrylate crossed the peritoneal membrane.

Dextran sodium sulfate with a molecular weight of 500,000 Daltons exerts the osmotic effect because of sodium trapped in its glycosyl sulfate residue (188). Dextran was supposed to be non toxic since, if absorbed, it should be metabolized. However in animal models intraperitoneal bleeding occurred leading to the death of animals (189). Polyethylene-amine was even more toxic with the death of animals in one hour (189). Obviously the synthetic polymers are not suitable for clinical use.

Plasma substitutes

Gelatin, neutral dextran and hydroxyethyl starch are widely used in Europe as plasma substitutes to treat severe hypotensive episodes in hemodialysis. Crude gelatine (5%) was first used in the late forties as an osmotic agent during acute peritoneal dialysis (190). More recently (189) a 9% gelatin solution was tested in a rat model and was proved to yield an higher and more sustained ultrafiltration during a 7 hour dwell time as compared to a 4.25% glucose solution. There were not untoward effects on rats and no alterations of the peritoneal membrane as evaluated with light and scanning electron microscopy. However, high viscosity, gelation at room temperature and difficult sterilization were major problems. To avoid these technical problems, a cross-linked gelatin, gelatin isocyanate (Hemacel® 20,000–35,000 Daltons), was investigated (191). At 6-hour dwell time, the ultrafiltration volume of a 5.5% Hemacel solution was similar to that of a 4.25% glucose while 10% Hemacel yielded even higher ultrafiltration. Although gelatin is easily metabolized, the half-life of Hemacel is around 16 hours in hemodialyzed patient with minimal renal function and chronic toxicity is unknown (184). Anaphylactoid reactions in 0.038% of patients is the only adverse effect of gelatine when used as plasma substitute (192).

Neutral dextrans as osmotic agent in peritoneal dialysis were investigated in the late sixties (193). Very low osmotic driving force was exerted by a 6% dextran in saline and little ultrafiltration was achieved. These data were recently confirmed (194) while a 10% dextran solution showed a significant higher ultrafiltration (195). However, despite its high molecular weight (40,000 or 70,000 Daltons), 40 to 60% of dextran was absorbed over a six hour cycle time (194). Since accumulation of dextran in patients on maintenance hemodialysis has been demonstrated to yield reticuloendothelial system blockade, dextran does not seem to be a suitable alternative to glucose (196).

Hydroxyethyl starch (HES) is another synthetic substance in which starch has been modified by introducing an hydroxyethyl ether group and then hydrolyzed to yield a product with an average molecular weight of 480,000 Daltons. Studies in a rat model with 10 and 6% solutions have reported ultrafiltration profiles and absorption rates similar to those obtained with 6 and 10% dextran solutions (194, 195). In acute renal failure HES seemed to accumulate in the liver leading to a storage disease (197).

Glucose polymer

Glucose polymer (GP) or polyglucose is a mixture of polysaccharides consisting of linked glucose residues of varying chain length obtained by the hydrolysis of corn starch. More than 90% of the glucose bonds are 1–4 glucosidic linkages, the remaining 10% are 1–6 linkages.

A preparation of fractioned glucose oligosaccharides with chain length ranging from 2 to 15 glucose units (average molecular weight 710 Daltons) was first acutely used in man in concentrations ranging from 3 to 8% (12, 18).

When compared to a 4.25% glucose solution, an 8% GP solution produced similar ultrafiltration profile at 8 and 10 hour dwell times, despite a markedly lower initial osmolality (357 *versus* 485 mmOsm/kg). Solute clearances and D/P ratios for urea and creatinine were identical (12). 57 and 77% of glucose polymers were absorbed at 4 and 10 hours respectively. Although the solution was well tolerated by the patients, plasma oligosaccharide concentration (in particular G2 and G5) sharply increased during the GP exchange and even higher concentrations were recorded during the subsequent exchange with the standard glucose solution, thus indicating a very slow metabolism and clearance of absorbed oligosaccharides in patients with renal insufficiency. The calculated half life was about 20 hours (12).

Serum free glucose concentrations changed little after the exchanges using the GP solutions. However the potential energy load from a single exchange of a 8% GP solution was approximately two times that of 4.25% glucose solution. The authors suggested that a combination of higher molecular weight glucose polymer would be more suitable for CAPD patients (198).

A new GP solution composition with average molecular weight 7,000, (67% low molecular weight fraction – G1 to G12 – and 33% high molecular weight fraction – G < 12 – average length of polymers 5–6 units) was studied by Mistry et al. (199). A 5% GP solution was compared to a 1.5% glucose solution, while a 10% GP was to a 4.25% glucose solution.

Both isotonic and hypertonic GP solutions showed a significant increase in net ultrafiltration as compared to the corresponding glucose solutions at 6 hour dwell time. Significant increases in creatinine, uric acid and phosphate D/P ratios were observed with GP solutions and similarly, average clearances of solutes were also significantly greater with GP solutions at both concentrations suggesting that GP solutions may alter the peritoneum permeability.

The GP absorption from dialysate at 6 hour dwell time was 42.5% and 59% respectively for the iso and hyperosmotic GP solutions. However the caloric load was greater than that provided by the absorption of glucose from the standard solutions.

Fractions with 5 to 9 glucose units showed the highest intraperitoneal disappearance without concomitant rise in serum levels, whereas maltose (G2) and maltotriose (G3) with a slightly lower disappearance, produced a substantial rise in serum levels, suggesting considerable breakdown of intermediate molecules to smaller units.

In subsequent studies (102, 200, 201) a 5% solution of glucose polymer containing polymer fractions of variable chain length (ranging from 4 to 300 glucose units with average molecular weight 16,800) was compared with a commercially available 1.5% glucose solution. While the standard glucose solution is slightly hypertonic (332 mmOsm/kg), this GP solution was really isosmotic to uremic serum (302 mmOsm/kg).

A substantially greater net ultrafiltration was achieved at 6 hour dwell time. For the glucose solution, the prolonged exchange time to 12 hours led to absorption of fluid with a final drainage volume smaller than that infused. With the GP solution, ultrafiltration continued to increase without changes in dialysate osmolality throughout the 12 hour exchanges. At 6 and 12 hours, 14.4% and 28.1% of glucose polymer had been absorbed. Thus in term of total caloric load there was no difference between the two solutions, but GP solution provided less than 50% of caloric load of the glucose dialysate per unit of ultrafiltrate.

An enhanced peritoneal equilibration for solutes larger than urea was confirmed. A 7–9 fold increase in serum maltose with GP solution was also recorded.

The group of Manchester started in 1987 chronic clinical studies with an higher molecular weight (22,000) GP solution.

A short term (7 days) study did not show any side effects even with continuous use of a 5% GP solutions (202). Later, a 7.5% GP solution was used over a period of three months in 5 non diabetic patients (203). GP solution substituted the overnight glucose exchange (12 hours) and resulted in 500–1000 ml of net ultrafiltration. Serum biochemistry remained stable during the study period. There was a steady-state accumulation of maltose and maltotriose (30 fold higher than in uremic serum). No other side effects were recorded.

A long term randomized multicentric study in over 200 patients (106 with one 7.5% GP solution exchange) recently demonstrated no side effects and similar morbid events in both groups (204). Serum osmolality remained in the normal range and 15 diabetic patients included in the study tolerated the GP solution without problems.

These studies indicate that GP solution can be used during the overnight exchange as substitute for the glucose hypertonic solution because of its substained ultrafiltration over 12 hours. It could be also useful during the long diurnal exchange in patients undergoing CCPD. Moreover, GP solution could be beneficial for diabetic patients since it provides a caloric reduction per unit volume of ultrafiltration and does not yield insulin response.

Finally recent observations (13, 205) have suggested that the GP solution may be more biocompatible than glucose solution because of its lower osmolality.

The metabolism of the absorbed polymer is less than complete resulting in increased levels of its breakdown products maltose and maltotriose since the polymer is readily hydrolyzed by circulating amylase to disaccharide. Further metabolism from maltose to glucose is limited by the absence of maltase activity in human circulation (206). Even though substantial amounts of maltase have been demonstrated in a variety of extraintestinal tissues, the enzyme is most notably present in the kidneys. Therefore, in the absence of significant residual renal function, accumulation of maltose occurs (207).

Long term studies with GP solutions have demonstrated an increase of serum maltose during the first days of treatment until transperitoneal elimination of maltose during the three glucose exchanges ensured a steady-state level. This sustained and elevated level was not associated with any serious adverse effects over 6 months.

However long term effects of these levels are not known. In particular it should be excluded that a storage disease could occur. Since the accumulation within the macrophages leading to impairment of the phagocytic function (defined as reticulo-endothelial system blockade) has been documented for dextrans, HES, PVP and gelatin in mice (208), it should be excluded that glucose polymer could exert this effect in the long term.

Peptides

The first use in peritoneal dialysis of a mixture of peptides as osmotic agent in a rabbit model has been described by Klein et al. in 1986 (209).

A 5% solution of milk whey protein was hydrolized using a combination of trypsin and chymotrypsin in order to prepare a peptide mixture containing 3 to 10 amino acids. This preparation had an average molecular weight of 857 Daltons. The mixture contained approximately 2% free amino acids; 46% of essential amino acids was contained in the peptides.

As compared to a 2.5% glucose solution, peptide solution yielded twice net ultrafiltration after one hour of dwell time. Only 3% of the peptide mixture was absorbed from dialysate and no acute toxic effects were recorded.

Recently, a peptide solution containing 1.5% glucose and 1% peptides (molecular weight 600–700) with 381 mmOsm/kg of osmolality was compared to a standard 2.5% glucose solution (osmolality 404 mmOsm/kg) (210). The peptide solution was well tolerated in all patients and no differences were found in clearances and mass transfer area coefficient of urea, creatinine and glucose indicating that no irritating effect of peptide solution was present. Despite a lower osmolality of the peptide solution, no significant changes in ultrafiltration at 4 and 8 hour dwell time were recorded. No differences in plasma amino acid profile could be detected.

These preliminary data seem to indicate that peptides could have a potential use as an osmotic agent in peritoneal dialysis. A possible effect on nutritional status should be further evaluated.

In conclusion, several attempt have been done in recent years to find a possible alternative to the use of glucose as osmotic agent in PD solutions. *In vitro* studies and clinical trials are today going on and definite answers will be probably available in the coming future.

BUFFERS

One of the major results achieved by CAPD is the better correction of metabolic acidosis and the maintenance of a satisfactory acid-base status as compared to hemodialysis. This result appears to be stable over time and acid-base fluctuations, typical of intermittent treatments, are not observed. The steadiness of acid-base status depends on the continuous infusion of buffers in absence of significant losses into dialysate of bicarbonate and permits a good stability of blood gases and ventilation (211).

In intermittent peritoneal dialysis, acid base parameters fluctuate similarly to hemodialysis. At the end of a session blood bicarbonate and pH rise, while a slow decrease in these parameters is observed in the interdialytic period (212).

The effective correction of acidosis depends on the quantity of buffer really gained by the patient, on the patient's ability to metabolize the incoming buffer, and on bicarbonate and organic anions losses into the dialysate (212).

Bicarbonate was initially used in 1964 by Boen (213) in peritoneal dialysis fluid, but it was soon discovered that calcium carbonate was precipitating and the solution was becoming alkaline during autoclaving.

Sodium salts of several organic oxidizable anions (such as acetate, lactate, citrate, malate, pyruvate, succinate, etc) are able to consume H^+ derived from carbonic acid, causing the regeneration of bicarbonate (214). Consequently, acetate and lactate were introduced as alkaline agents in the clinical routine.

Acetate

Acetate was first described as buffer substance in peritoneal dialysis fluid by Boen in 1962 (215).

Bicarbonate is regenerated when acetate thiokinase activates the reaction between acetate and coenzyme A (CoA) to form acetyl-CoA and one hydrogen ion is captured in this process. Acetyl-CoA may enter different metabolic pathways such as decarboxylation in the Krebs cycle, condensation in ketone bodies or fatty acids and glucose generation via gluconeogenesis (216). The buffering effect is accomplished and hydrogen ion is transferred to the respiratory chain only when acetyl-CoA is decarboxylated.

Since only traces of acetate are normally produced by intermediate metabolism of fatty acids, the rate of the enzymatic reaction to acetyl-CoA is limited (211). In uremic patients treated with hemodialysis this rate is further decreased to a value of about 3 mmol/min (217). The buffer influx provided by a dialysate containing 40 mmol/l

of acetate during a IPD session at rate of 5 l/hour is 0.94 mmol/min. Although this influx is far less than the maximal rate of metabolization above described in uremics, a 4-fold increase of normal serum acetate levels has been recorded. These levels were fairly constant during each session and fell to normal value after the end of dialysis (212).

During CAPD with a 38.5 mmol/l acetate solution, the acetate mass transfer rate was 0.3 mmol/min but constantly high plasma levels were observed (218).

Acetate has been proved to correct uremic metabolic acidosis even better than lactate both in CAPD and in intermittent treatment.

However, these findings have today only an historical relevance since acetate has been abandoned when suspected to cause loss of peritoneal ultrafiltration and sclerosing peritonitis (219, 220).

Lactate

Lactate is the commonly used buffer in peritoneal dialysis. In nature two stereoisomeric forms of lactate exist: D- and L-lactate. Commercially available peritoneal dialysis fluids contain either L-lactate or a mixture of L- and D-lactate.

In humans small quantities of D-lactate are normally generated in the methylglyoxal pathway, while the predominant form is L-lactate. D-lactate is slowly metabolized by an aspecific enzyme (D-2-hydroxyacid-dehydrogenase) NAD (Nicotinaminde Adenine nucleotide) independent (221). L-lactate, on the contrary, is easily metabolized to pyruvate by lactic dehydrogenase, NAD dependent.

The buffering effect of lactate is accomplished by its complete metabolization via the Krebs cycle as for acetate, or via gluconeogenesis. With incomplete metabolism of lactate, the buffering effect does not take place. Searle et al. (222) demonstrated that 80–85% of the lactate produced in the normal metabolism is oxidized in the Krebs cycle, and only 15–20% is converted to glucose. While the oxidation takes place in all the cells with aerobic metabolism, gluconeogenesis is confined to the liver and renal cortex.

L-lactate turnover in normal subjects ranges 0.77 to 0.87 mmol/kg/hour (222). In patients with hepatic disease the rate of metabolism may be lower with consequent increase of lactate serum levels. In CAPD patients the lactate infusion is about 0.19 mmol/kg/h that is 25% of endogenous metabolic production (223). This lactate load does not represent a metabolic problem in patients with normal hepatic function as demonstrated by some studies reporting normal values of intermediate metabolites (223, 224).

In IPD (5 l/hour) the lactate infusion was 1 mmol/kg/hour [212) but lactate serum levels only occasionally slightly increased during the session and these data were confirmed by others (225, 226).

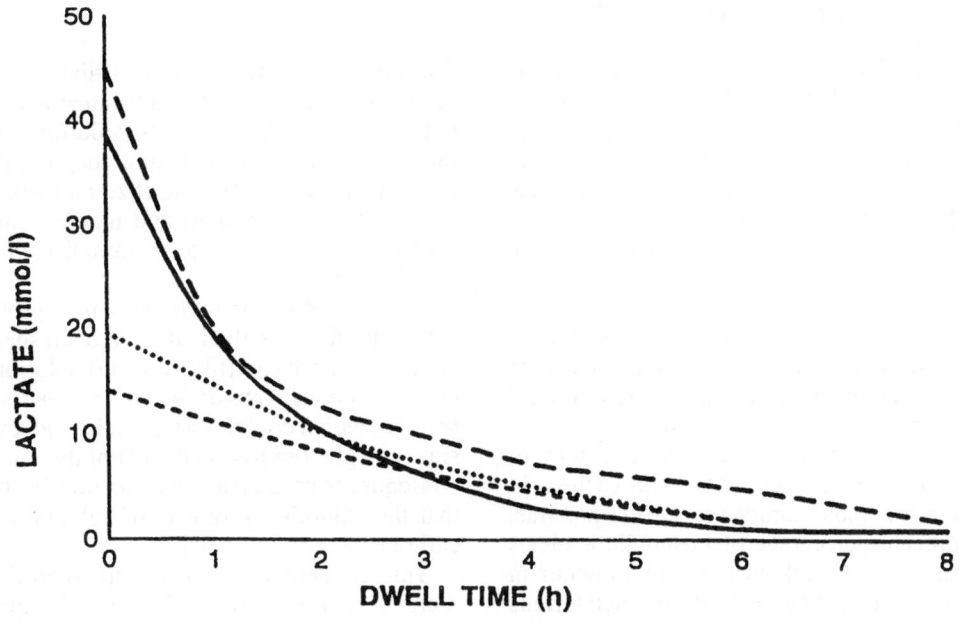

Figure 4. Disappearance rate of lactate from dialysate during dwell time (from Reference (211)).

The lactate disappearance rate from dialysate is depicted in Figure 4 (212, 227, 228). The rate of absorption is maximal in the first minutes of dwell while it subsequently approaches zero. This behaviour permits an adequate buffer transfer even when rapid exchanges are scheduled. It must be noted that D-lactate and L-lactate may have different rates of transport. Rubin et al. (228) demonstrated that the peritoneal membrane can operate a stereospecific selection in the process of lactate transport. L-lactate has an higher mass transfer rate and metabolization. D-lactate is very slowly metabolized, but the low mass transfer rate both in IPD and in CAPD seems to enable a complete metabolism since D-lactic acidosis has never been documented (229). Other studies have not confirmed different absorption rates between the two stereoisomers of lactate (225, 226).

In CAPD, long dwell times enables an almost complete transfer of buffer from the dialysis solution independently from the initial lactate solution concentration that, for this reason, represents the major determinant of base gain.

During dwell time bicarbonate back diffuses in the dialysate.

The major determinant of bicarbonate loss is the blood bicarbonate concentration. Several studies suggest a possible feed back mechanism between blood bicarbonate concentration and amount of bicarbonate lost in dialysate (19, 224, 225, 227). An increased blood bicarbonate level yields a parallel increase of bicarbonate loss that, in turn, results in a decrease of blood bicarbonate level. Inversely, in severe metabolic acidosis bicarbonate losses with dialysate are reduced so yielding a more favourable base balance.

Ultrafiltration also plays an important role. When dialysate/plasma equilibration occurs, an increase in drainage volume due to ultrafiltration, causes a greater loss of bicarbonate.

Finally organic anions, which are effective alkaline equivalents, are also lost in dialysate. Teehan et al. (224) have reported daily losses of 1 mmol of acetoacetate and 4.1 mmol of ß hydroxybutyrate. Other substances are lost in the dialysate such as tricarboxylic anions although they have never been quantified. Yet a significant anion gap (36 ± 17 mmol/day) was observed in the effluent dialysate (224).

Commercially available CAPD solutions contain 35 or 40 mmol/l lactate.

With a dialysis fluid lactate level of 35 mmol/l most patients display a chronic mild metabolic acidosis (48). Teehan et al. (224) have demonstrated that lactate uptake from the peritoneal dialysis fluid was often exceeded by the bicarbonate loss and metabolic acid production. Out of 10 patients only two had a normal acid base status the mean arterial blood bicarbonate being 20.6 mmol/l and total CO_2 (TCO_2) 22 mmol/l.

Other clinical observations have confirmed these findings (230). Nolph et al. (64) reported a mean venous TCO_2 of 23.8 mmol/l in 163 determinations (78 patients) 38% of values being below 22 mmol/l.

In order to correct the negative buffer balance and to improve acid base status, an increased lactate content to 40 mmol/l in the CAPD solutions has been suggested (64).

Neither buffer balance studies nor serum lactate levels have been measured with this solution. However significant better results on blood acid base status have been reported. Venous TCO_2 increased to 27.4 mmol/l after four months of treatment (mean baseline value 23.4 mmol/l) while pH and pCO_2 did not change (64).

However, since normal venous TCO_2 ranges between 26.7 and 30.3 mmol/l (mean value 28.4 mmol/l) (231), in this study (64), 16% of patients had TCO_2 values over the normal range, 52% under the normal range and 32% in the normal range, while the corresponding percentages in patients treated with the 35 mmol/l lactate solution were 3%, 75% and 22%.

Moreover a recent observation (232) in 8 stable patients treated with a solution containing 40 mmol/l of lactate showed a mean arterial blood bicarbonate of 21.6 mmol/l and an increased anion gap value (21.4 mmol/l).

In summary the increased lactate content to 40 mmol/l in the CAPD solution has been proved to improve the acid base status of a remarkable number of CAPD patients. However a significant percentage of metabolic acidosis still remains and metabolic alkalosis seems to occur in an increased number of patients. While the deleterious effects of metabolic acidosis on skeletal protein turnover is well demonstrated both in chronic renal failure rats and patients (233–235), the long term effects of chronic metabolic alkalosis in CAPD patients is unknown.

Some metabolic side effects of lactate have been suggested, although there is no clear evidence of their clinical relevance.

Lactate is a powerful peripheral vasodilator, affects myocardial contractility, reduces blood pressure and could play a role in the blood lipid disorders of the CAPD patients (236, 237).

In addition, the administration of large amounts of L-lactate without a proportionate amount of its redox partner pyruvate results in a lowering of the cellular redox state and the linked phosphorylation potential. This effect could impair many vital cellular functions including the distribution of inorganic ions between intracellular and extracellular fluid (236, 238, 239). Unbalanced ratios of L-lactate to pyruvate also favour the so-called catabolic state associated with the action of corticosteroid and other hormones potentiating the conversion of muscle protein into glucose (240).

The toxicity of D-lactate differs from that of L-lactate in that it is mainly observable in various forms of impaired cerebral function. Patients with blind loop syndrome and abnormal gut flora, producing sufficient of the D-isomer of lactic acid to elevate blood D-lactate to 3 mmol/l, developed clinically demonstrable encephalopathy (241). The use of CAPD dialysate containing 40 mmol/l D, L-lactate has been reported to result in repeated episodes of cerebral dysfunction characterized clinically by agitated confusion, depression and hyperventilation resulting in life-threatening metabolic alkalosis (242).

Bicarbonate

The ideal buffer for peritoneal dialysis would be sodium bicarbonate since this substance is the physiological buffer of the body. However, solutions containing mixtures of bicarbonate, calcium, magnesium and glucose are difficult to prepare, sterilize and store since, during the autoclaving, calcium and magnesium precipitate as carbonate salts and glucose caramelize, due to high pH of the solution.

In single pass hemodialysis this problem has been solved by the so called 'three-stream method' in which an acid and a basic (bicarbonate) solutions are continuously mixed with treated water. As a matter of fact the acid solution which contains an organic acid, calcium, magnesium and glucose lowers the pH of the final solution. As a consequence carbonate ion concentration becomes so low that the solubility products of calcium and magnesium carbonate is not exceeded.

This concept was adapted to intermittent peritoneal dialysis by Ing et al. (243) and subsequently modified to a 'two-stream method' in which equal volumes of an acid and basic (bicarbonate) solutions are simultaneously delivered by a roller pump to produce the final solution (244).

Later, these authors described (245) and used (246) during an IPD session a new method of producing a bicarbonate solution. The bicarbonate content of a glass syringe is added to an acid solution placed in a second container to yield two liters of the final dialysate. No problems were encountered during the clinical IPD session.

Independently, a single container, which is divided in two compartments (one containing the acid and one containing the basic solutions) by a partition wall, was developed for CAPD solutions (11). A breakable valve in the partition wall is broken by an external pressure just before the use thus allowing the mixing of the two solutions. The final dialysate pH value was around 7.4. One patient was treated for one week and 3 patients were treated for few exchanges with this solution containing 35 mmol/l of bicarbonate (19). The solution was well tolerated and no side effects occurred. The patient treated for one week increased the blood bicarbonate content until a plateau was achieved at about 29 mmol/l after a few days. In a subsequent study a solution containing 27 mmol/l of bicarbonate was employed in one patient for two months (247). No biochemical changes were observed but blood bicarbonate remained stable at pre study level (20 mmol/l).

In order to assess the safety and the optimal bicarbonate concentration for clinical use, *in vitro* stability tests, animal and kinetic studies have been performed.

No calcium carbonate precipitation has been demonstrated for up to 40 mmol/l of bicarbonate and 2 mmol/l of calcium concentration solutions over a clinical use range of temperatures (248).

In a rat model, repeated intraperitoneal injections of 100 ml/kg were not associated with histological lesions, crystal formation and fibrosis (249).

Kinetic studies demonstrated that changes in dialysate bicarbonate concentration at different dwell times were correlated to bicarbonate blood levels independently from the bicarbonate content of the fresh solution, thus suggesting a self-limited bicarbonate absorption (250).

A recent short term clinical evaluation (4 weeks) with a 34 mmol/l bicarbonate solution in 6 patients has shown an increase of blood bicarbonate, a slight but not statistically significant increase of ultrafiltration, a slight decrease of the creatinine D/P ratio and no changes of principal biochemical parameters and dialysis adequacy thus demonstrating that, at least in the short term, this solution is safe, well tolerated, does not affect peritoneal dialysis adequacy and is effective in the correction of uremic acidosis (251). The authors suggested that slight changes in ultrafiltration and creatinine equilibration could reflect a better biocompatibility of this solution. These findings were confirmed in several *in vitro* observations.

The bicarbonate solution did not result in peritoneal vasodilation as lactate solution did, showed less cytotoxic damages on mesothelial cells, did not affect phospholipid secretion of mesothelial cells (252) and eicosanoids and cytokines release from peripheral (13, 253) and peritoneal macrophages (254). However, in a recent study on a rabbit model, peritoneal membrane examinations did not reveal any microscopic or macroscopic differences among three animal groups in which the control group was not dialyzed and the other two groups performed peritoneal dialysis by using either a standard lactate solution or a bicarbonate buffered solution (255).

An alternative approach to provide a stable bicarbonate solution has been described by Yatzidis (20). A dipeptide, glycylglycine, has been added to a bicarbonate solution in order to stabilize the solution pH at about 7.35. This solution has been shown to be stable after 18 months in storage and has been tested in rabbits for up to 25 days with no pathological findings in the peritoneum. About 80% of glycylglycine was absorbed. In humans this substance is enzymatically degraded to glycine which is in turn metabolized to other non essential amino acids.

First clinical acute study demonstrated that glycylglycine-bicarbonate solution was well tolerated by patients and significantly increased net ultrafiltration as compared to a standard lactate solution (256). In addition, since the solution must be cold sterilized by filtration in order to avoid glucose caramelization, the concentration of glucose by-products were considerably reduced (257).

CONCLUSIONS

During the last ten years, several attempts have been made in order to improve the peritoneal dialysis solution.

Low calcium and magnesium solution has been the most extensively studied. Clinical results allow to define the range of utilization of this solution. It is now clear that a large majority of patients can benefit from its use. However, a careful surveillance of the mineral metabolism is needed.

The need for more physiological solutions in order to preserve the structure and function of the peritoneal membrane in the long term, has stimulated the search for alternative osmotic agents and buffers. Currently available solutions are hypertonic and have non bicarbonate bases and low pH values. Near isotonic solutions containing bicarbonate as a base at physiological pH would intuitively seem better. The preliminary results of multicentre trials on bicarbonate as a buffer and glucose polymers as osmotic agents seem to be encouraging.

Solutions containing amino acids are already available and will most likely receive increasing use in some patients. The expanded use of nutrient-containing solutions will depend much upon their cost.

The achievement of a better biocompatibility and the contribution to the improvement of the patients nutritional status will be the future goals for the peritoneal dialysis solutions.

REFERENCES

1. Boen ST: Peritoneal dialysis. A clinical study of factors governing its effectiveness. MD Thesis 1959, University of Amsterdam, Assen, van Gorcum and Comp NV – Dr HJ Prakke and HMG Prakke
2. Boen ST: *Peritoneal Dialysis in Clinical Medicine*, American Lecture Series, Springfield, IL, Charles C Thomas, 1964
3. Henderson LW: Peritoneal ultrafiltration dialysis. Enhanced urea transfer using hypertonic peritoneal dialysis fluid. *J Clin Invest* 45: 950, 1964
4. Henderson LW, Nolph KD: Altered permeability of the peritoneal membrane after using hipertonic peritoneal dialysis fluid. *J Clin Invest* 48: 992, 1969
5. Nolph KD, Miller FN, Pyle K, Popovich RP, Sorkin MJ: A hypothesis to explain the characteristics of peritoneal ultrafiltration. *Kidney Int* 20: 543, 1981
6. Ronco C, Feriani M, Chiaramonte S et al.: Pathophysiology of ultrafiltration in peritoneal dialysis. *Perit Dial Int* 10: 119, 1990
7. Boen ST. History of peritoneal dialysis. in *Peritoneal Dialysis*, edited by Noph KD, Dordrecht, Kluwer Academic Publishers, 1989, p 1
8. Dobbie JW, Zaki MA, Wilson LS: The morphology of the peritoneum with special reference to peritoneal dialysis. in *Renal Failure, Who Cares?*, edited by Parsons FM, Ogg CS Lancaster, MPT Press, 1982, p 3
9. Dobbie JW: Pathogenesis of peritoneal fibrosis syndromes (sclerosing peritonitis) in peritoneal dialysis. *Perit Dial Int* 12: 14, 1992
10. Di Paolo N, Sacchi G, De Mia M: Morphology of the peritoneal membrane during continuous ambulatory peri-

toneal dialysis. *Proc Eur Dial Transplant Assoc* 18: 199, 1981

11. Feriani M, Biasioli S, Borin D, Fabris A, Ronco C, La Greca G: Bicarbonate solutions for peritoneal dialysis: a reality. *Int J Artif Organs* 8: 57, 1985

12. Winchester JF, Stegink LD, Ahmad S et al.: A comparison of glucose polymer and dextrose as osmotic agents in CAPD. in *Frontiers in Peritoneal Dialysis*, edited by Maher JF, Winchester JF, New York, Field, Rich and Associates Inc, 1986, p 231

13. Jorres A, Gahl GM, Ludat K, Passlick-Deetjen J: CAPD dialysate inhibit cytokine production in PBMC activated with *Staph. Epidermidis (S. epi)*: partial restoration by alternative PD fluids. *Perit Dial Int* 13 (Suppl 1): S56, 1993

14. Hutchison AJ, Gokal R: Towards tailored dialysis fluids in CAPD the role of reduced calcium and magnesium in dialysis solution. *Perit Dial Int* 12: 199, 1992

15. De Paepe M, Matthijs E, Peluso F et al.: Experience with glycerol as the osmotic agent in peritoneal dialysis in diabetic and non-diabetic patients. in *Prevention and Treatment of Diabetic Nephropathy*, edited by Keen H, Legrain M, Boston, MTP Press Ltd, 1983, p 299

16. Wu G: Osmotic agents for peritoneal dialysis solutions. *Perit Dial Bull* 2: 151, 1982

17. Vidt DG: Recommendations on choice of peritoneal dialysis solutions. *Ann Intern Med* 78: 144, 1973

18. Higgins JT, Gross ML, Somani P: Patient tolerance and dialysis effectiveness of a glucose polymer-containing peritoneal dialysis solution. *Perit Dial Bull* 4: S131, 1984

19. Feriani M, Biasioli S, Borin D, La Greca G: Bicarbonate buffer for CAPD solution *Trans Am Soc Artif Intern Organs* 31: 668, 1985

20. Yatzidis H: A new stable bicarbonate dialysis solution for peritoneal dialysis: preliminary report. *Perit Dial Int* 11: 224, 1991

21. Henderson IS, Couper IA, Lumsden A: The effect of shelf-life of peritoneal dialysis fluid on ultrafiltration in CAPD. in *Peritoneal Dialysis*, edited by La Greca G, Chiaramonte S, Fabris A, Feriani M, Ronco C, Milan, Wichtig Editore, 1986, p 85

22. Merrill JP, Hampers CL: Uremia. *N Engl J Med* 282: 953, 1970

23. Lowrie EG, Steinberg SM, Galen MA et al.: Factors in the dialysis regimen which contribute to alterations in the abnormalities of uremia. *Kidney Int* 10: 409, 1976

24. Teschan PE: Electroencephalographic and other neurophysio-logical abnormalities in uremia. *Kidney Int* 7 (Suppl 2): S210, 1975

25. Popovich RP, Moncrief JW, Decherd JB, Bomar JB, Pyle WK: The definition of a novel portable/wereable equilibrium peritoneal dialysis technique. (Abstract) *ASAIO J* 5: 64, 1976

26. Gokal R, Fryer R, McHugh M, Ward MK, Kerr DNS: Calcium and phosphate control in patients on continuous ambulatory peritoneal dialysis. in *Continuous Ambulatory Peritoneal Dialysis*, edited by Legrain M, Amsterdam, Excerpta medica, 1980, p 283

27. Popovich RP, Moncrieff JW, Nolph KD, Ghods AJ, Twardowski Z, Pyle WK: Continuous ambulatory peritoneal dialysis. *Ann Intern Med* 88: 449, 1978

28. Winchester JF: CAPD systems and solutions. in *Continuous Ambulatory Peritoneal Dialysis*, edited by Gokal R, Edinburgh, Churchill Livingstone, 1986, p 94

29. Miller JH, Gipstein R, Maroules R, Swarz M, Rubini ME: Automated peritoneal dialysis: analysis of several methods of peritoneal dialysis. *Trans Am Soc Artif Intern Organs* 12: 98, 1966

30. Gokal R: Historical development and clinical use of continuous ambulatory peritoneal dialysis. in *Continuous Ambulatory Peritoneal Dialysis*, edited by Gokal R, Edinburgh, Churchill Livingstone, 1986, p 1

31. Nolph KD, Parker A: The composition of dialysis solution for continuous ambulatory peritoneal dialysis. in *Continuous Ambulatory Peritoneal Dialysis*, edited by Legrain M, Amsterdam, Excerpta medica, 1980, 341

32. Nolph KD, Twardowski ZJ, Popovich RP, Rubin J: Equilibration of peritoneal dialysis solutions during long dwell exchanges. *J Lab Clin Med* 93: 246, 1979

33. Nolph KD, Sorkin MJ, Moore H: Autoregulation of sodium and potassium removal during continuous ambulatory peritoneal dialysis. *Trans Am Soc Artif Intern Organs* 26: 334, 1980

34. Nolph KD, Hano JE, Teschan PE: Peritoneal sodium transport during hypertonic peritoneal dialysis: physiologic mechanisms and clinical implications. *Ann Intern Med* 70: 931, 1969

35. Raja RM, Cantor RE, Boreyco C, Bushchri H, Kramer MS, Rosenbaum JL: Sodium transport during ultrafiltration peritoneal dialysis. *Trans Am Soc Artif Intern Organs* 18: 429, 1972

36. Raja RM, Kramer MS, Rosenbaum JL, Manchanda R, Lazaro N: Evaluation of hypertonic peritoneal dialysis solutions with low sodium. *Nephron* 11: 342, 1973

37. Ahearn DJ, Nolph KD: Controlled sodium removal with peritoneal dialysis. *Trans Am Soc Artif Intern Organs* 18: 423, 1972

38. Bosch JP: Permeability characteristics of the peritoneal membrane. in *Peritoneal Dialysis*, edited by La Greca G, Chiaramonte S, Fabris A, Feriani M, Ronco C, Milan, Wichtig Editore, 1985, p 25

39. Colombi A: Fluid and electrolyte balance in CAPD patients. in *Peritoneal Dialysis*, edited by La Greca G, Chiaramonte S, Fabris A, Feriani M, Ronco C, Milan, Wichtig Editore, 1988, p 65

40. De Vecchi A, Paparella M, Scalamogna A, Guerra L, Castelnovo C: Effetti della variazione delle concentrazioni di sodio nel liquido di dialisi peritoneale. in *I liquidi nella dialisi*, edited by La Greca G, Petrella E, Cioni A, Milan, Ghedini Editore, 1991, p 93

41. Nakayama M, Yokoyama K, Kawaguchi Y, Sakai O: Effect of ultra low sodium concentration dialysate (ULNaD) in patients with UF loss. *Perit Dial Int* (Suppl 1): 187 (Abstract), 1991

42. Twardowski ZJ: New approaches to intermittent peritoneal dialysis therapies. in *Peritoneal Dialysis*, edited by Nolph KD, Dordrecht, Kluwer Academic Publishers, 1989, p 133

43. Gault MH, Ferguson EL, Sidhu JS, Corbin RP: Fluid and electrolyte complications of peritoneal dialysis. Choice of dialysis solutions. *Ann Intern Med* 75: 253, 1971

44. Shen FH, Sherrard DJ, Scollard D, Merrit A, Curtis FK: Thirst, relative hypernatremia and excessive weight gain

in maintenance peritoneal dialysis. *Trans Am Soc Artif Intern Organs* 24: 142, 1978

45. Twardowski ZJ, Nolph KD, Khanna R, Gluck Z, Prowant BF, Ryan LP: Daily clearances with continuous ambulatory peritoneal dialysis and nightly peritoneal dialysis. *Trans Am Soc Artif Intern Organs* 32: 575, 1986

46. Nolph KD: Kinetic of ultrafiltration and electrolyte transport during peritoneal dialysis. in *Peritoneal Dialysis*, edited by La Greca G, Chiaramonte S, Fabris A, Feriani M, Ronco C, Milan, Wichtig Editore, 1985, p 47

47. Brown ST, Ahearn DJ, Nolph KD: Potassium removal with peritoneal dialysis. *Kidney Int* 4: 67, 1973

48. Gokal R: Continuous ambulatory peritoneal dialysis. in *Replacement of Renal Function by Dialysis*, edited by Maher JF, Dordrecht, Kluwer Academic Publishers, 1989, p 590

49. Blumenkrantz MJ, Kopple JD, Moran JK, Coburn JW: Metabolic balance studies and dietary protein requirements in patients undergoing continuous ambulatory peritoneal dialysis. *Kidney Int* 21: 849, 1982

50. Sandle GI, Gaiger E, Tapster S, Goodship THJ: Evidence for large intestinal control of potassium homeostasis in uraemic patients undergoing CAPD. *Clin Sci* 73: 247, 1987

51. Lameire N, Ringoir S: Introductory remarks: an overview of peritonitis and other complications of continuous ambulatory peritoneal dialysis. in *Continuous Ambulatory Peritoneal Dialysis*, edited by Legrain M, Amsterdam, Excerpta medica, 1980, p 229

52. Oreopoulos DG, Khanna R, Williams P: Continuous ambulatory peritoneal dialysis. *Nephron* 30: 293, 1982

53. Spital A, Sterns RH: Potassium supplementation via the dialysate in continuous ambulatory peritoneal dialysis. *Am J Kidney Dis* 6: 173, 1985

54. Lindholm B, Alvestrand A, Hultman F, Bergstrom J: Muscle water and electrolytes in patients undergoing continuous ambulatory peritoneal dialysis. *Acta Med Scand* 219: 323, 1986

55. Heide B, Pierratos A, Khanna R et al.: Nutritional status of patients undergoing continuous ambulatory peritoneal dialysis. *Perit Dial Bull* 3: 138, 1983

56. Rubin J, Kirchner K, Barnes T, Teal N, Ray R, Bower JD: Evaluation of continuous ambulatory peritoneal dialysis. *Am J Kidney Dis* 3: 199, 1983

57. Schilling H, Wu G, Petit J et al.: Nutritional status of patients on long term CAPD. *Perit Dial Bull* 5: 12, 1985

58. Randall RE, Cohen MD, Spray CC, Rossmeisl EC: Hypermagnae-semia in renal failure: etiology and toxic manifestation. *Ann Intern Med* 61: 73, 1964

59. Whang R: Magnesium deficiency: pathogenesis, prevalence and clinical implications. *Am J Med* 82 (Suppl 3A): 24, 1987

60. Hollifield J: Magnesium depletion, diuretics and arrhythmias. *Am J Med* 82 (Suppl 3A): 30, 1987

61. Selling M: Electrocardiographic patterns of magnesium depletion appearing in alcoholic heart disease. *Ann NY Acad Sci* 162: 906, 1969

62. Parker A, Nolph KD: Magnesium and calcium mass transfer during continuous ambulatory peritoneal dialysis. *Trans Am Soc Artif Intern Organs* 26: 194, 1980

63. Kwong MBL, Lee JSK, Chan MK: Transperitoneal calcium and magnesium transfer during an 8-hour dialysis. *Perit Dial Bull* 7: 85, 1987

64. Nolph KD, Prowant B, Serkes KD et al.: Multicentric evaluation of a new peritoneal dialysis solution with a high lactate and low magnesium concentration. *Perit Dial Bull* 3: 63, 1983

65. Kohaut EC, Balfe JW, Potter D, Alexandre S, Lum G: Hypermagnesemia and mild hypocarbia in pediatric patients on CAPD. *Perit Dial Bull* 3: 41, 1983

66. Rahman R, Heaton A, Goodship T et al.: Renal osteodystrophy in patients on CAPD: a five year study. *Perit Dial Bull* 7: 1, 1987

67. Rubin J: Comments on dialysis solution, antibiotic transport, poisonings and novel uses of peritoneal dialysis. in *Peritoneal Dialysis*, edited by Nolph KD, Dordrecht, Kluwer Academic Publishers, 1989, p 199

68. Gonella M: Plasma and tissue levels of magnesium in chronically hemodialyzed patients: effects of dialysate magnesium levels. *Nephron* 34: 141, 1983

69. Meema HE, Oreopoulos DG, Rapoport A: Serum magnesium level and arterial calcification in end-stage renal disease. *Kidney Int* 32: 388, 1987

70. Hutchison AJ, Freemont AJ, Boulton HF, Gokal R: Low-calcium dialysis fluid and oral calcium carbonate in CAPD. A method of controlling hyperphosphataemia whilst minimizing aluminium exposure and hypercalcaemia. *Nephrol Dial Transplant* 7: 1219, 1992

71. Hutchison AJ, Gokal R: Improved solutions for peritoneal dialysis: physiological calcium solutions, osmotic agents and buffers. *Kidney Int* 42 (Suppl 38): S153, 1992

72. Breuer J, Moniz C, Baldwin D, Parsons V: The effects of zero magnesium dialysate and magnesium supplements on ionized calcium concentration in patients on regular dialysis treatment. *Nephrol Dial Transplant* 2: 347, 1987

73. Shan G, Winer R, Cutler R et al.: Effects of a magnesium-free dialysate on magnesium metabolism during continuous ambulatory peritoneal dialysis. *Am J Kidney Dis* 10: 268, 1987

74. Delmez JA, Slatopolsky E, Martin KJ, Gearing BN, Harter HR: Minerals, vitamin D, and parathyroid hormone in continuous ambulatory peritoneal dialysis. *Kidney Int* 21: 862, 1982

75. Digenis G, Khanna R, Pierratos A et al.: Renal osteodystrophy in patients maintained on CAPD for more than three years. *Perit Dial Bull* 3: 81, 1983

76. Gokal R, Ramos JM, Ellis HA et al.: Histological renal osteodystrophy and 25 hydroxycholecalciferol and aluminum levels in patients on continuous ambulatory peritoneal dialysis. *Kidney Int* 23: 15, 1983

77. Delmez JA, Fallon M, Bergfeld M, Gearing BN, Dougan C, Teitelbaum S: Continuous ambulatory peritoneal dialysis and bone. *Kidney Int* 30: 379, 1986

78. Bucciante G, Bianchi M, Valenti G: Progress of renal osteodystrophy during CAPD. *Clin Nephrol* 6: 279, 1984

79. Lindholm B, Bergstrom J: Nutritional aspects of CAPD. in *Continuous Ambulatory Peritoneal Dialysis*, edited by Edinburgh, Churchill Livingstone, 1986, p 228

80. Sheikh MS, Maguire JA, Emmett M et al.: Reduction of dietary phosphorus absorption by phosphorus binders. A theoretical, *in vitro*, and *in vivo* study. *J Clin Invest* 83: 66, 1989

81. Ramirez JA, Emmett M, White MG et al.: The absorption of dietary phosphorus and calcium in hemodialysis patients. *Kidney Int* 30: 753, 1986

82. Davenport A, Goel S, MacKenzie JC: Audit of the use of calcium carbonate as phosphate binder in 100 patients treated with continuous ambulatory peritoneal dialysis. *Nephrol Dial Transplant* 7: 632, 1992

83. Joffe P, Olsen F, Heaf J, Gammelgaard B, Pondephant J: Aluminium concentrations in serum, dialysate, urine and bone among patients undergoing continuous ambulatory peritoneal dialysis. *Clin Nephrol* 32: 133, 1989

84. Andreoli S, Briggs J, Junior B: Aluminium intoxication from aluminium containing phosphate binders in children with azotemia not undergoing dialysis. *N Engl J Med* 310: 1074, 1984

85. Ackrill P, Day J, Ahmed R: Aluminium and iron overload in chronic dialysis. *Kidney Int* 33 (Suppl 24): S163, 1988

86. Altmannn P, Dhanesha U, Hamon C, Cunningham J, Blair J, Marsch F: Disturbance of cerebral function by aluminium in hemodialysis patients without overt aluminium toxicity. *Lancet* ii: 7, 1989

87. Martis L, Serkes KD, Nolph KD: Calcium as a phosphate binder: is there a need to adjust peritoneal dialysate calcium concentration for patients using CaCO3. *Perit Dial Int* 9: 325, 1989

88. Weinreich T, Passlick-Deetjen J, Ziegelmayer C, Ritz E: Experience with low D-Calcium concentration in CAPD (LCa 1 mM) – randomized controlled multicenter trial. *Perit Dial Int* 13 (Suppl 1): S38, 1993

89. Cunningham J, Beer J, Coldwell RD, Noonan K, Sawyer N, Makin HLJ: Dialysate calcium reduction in CAPD patients treated with calcium carbonate and alfacalcidol. *Nephrol Dial Transplant* 7: 63, 1992

90. Ritz E, Weinreich T, Matthias S: Is it necessary to readjust dialysis calcium concentration. *J Nephrol* 5: 70, 1992

91. Brown CB, Hamdy NAT, Boletis J, Kanis JA: Rationale for the use of low calcium solution in CAP. in *Peritoneal Dialysis*, edited by La Greca G, Ronco C, Feriani M, Chiaramonte S, Conz P, Milan, Wichtig Editore, 1991, p 125

92. Piraino B, Perlmutter JA, Holley JL, Johnston JR, Bernardini J: The use of dialysate containing 2.5 mEq/l calcium in peritoneal dialysis patients. *Perit Dial Int* 12: 75, 1992

93. Beer J, Tailor D, Noonan K, Cunningham J: Rapid exacerbation of hyperparathyroidism in patients converted to low calcium dialysate without adequate calcium supplementation. *Perit Dial Int* 13 (Suppl 1): S30, 1993

94. Andersen KEH: Calcium transfer during intermittent peritoneal dialysis. *Nephron* 29: 63, 1981

95. Schmitt H, Ittel TH, Schafer L, Sieberth HG: Effect of a low calcium dialysis solution on serum parathyroid hormone in automated peritoneal dialysis. *Perit Dial Int* 13 (Suppl 1): S59, 1993

96. Putman J: The living peritoneum as a dialysis membrane. *Am J Physiol* 63: 548, 1923

97. Cunningham RS: Studies on absorption from serious cavities. III. The effect of dextrose upon the peritoneal mesothelium. *Am J Physiol* 53: 458, 1920

98. Palmer RA, Quinton WE, Gray JF et al.: Prolonged peritoneal dialysis for chronic renal failure. *Lancet* i: 700, 1964

99. Rubin J, Nolph KD, Popovich RP, Moncrief JW: Drainage volumes during continuous ambulatory peritoneal dialysis. *ASAIO J* 2: 54, 1979

100. Gokal R, Mistry CD: Glucose polymer as osmotic agent in CAPD. in *Peritoneal Dialysis*, edited by La Greca G, Ronco C, Feriani M, Chiaramonte S, Conz P, Milan, Wichtig Editore, 1991, p 119

101. Twardowski ZJ, Khanna R, Nolph KD: Osmotic agents and ultrafiltration in peritoneal dialysis. *Nephron* 42: 93, 1986

102. Mistry CD, Mallick NP, Gokal R: Ultrafiltration with an isosmotic solution during long peritoneal dialysis exchanges. *Lancet* ii: 178, 1987

103. Mistry CD, Gokal R: New osmotic agents for peritoneal dialysis: where we are and where we're going. *Semin Dial* 4: 9, 1991

104. Pyle WK, Moncrief JW, Popovich RP: Peritoneal transport evaluation in CAPD. in *CAPD Update*, edited by Moncrief JW, Popovich RP, New York, Masson Publishing USA Inc, 1981. p 35

105. Maher JF, Bennett RR, Hirszel P, Chakrabarti E: The mechanism of dextrose-enhanced transport rates. *Kidney Int* 28: 16, 1985

106. Krediet RT, Boeschoten EW, Zuyderhoudt FMJ, Arisz L: The relationship between peritoneal glucose absorption and body fluid loss by ultrafiltration during continuous ambulatory peritoneal dialysis. *Clin Nephrol* 27: 51, 1987

107. Maher JF: Peritoneal transport rate: mechanisms, limitation and methods for augmentation. *Kidney Int* 18: S117, 1980

108. Nolph KD, Mactier RA, Khanna R, Twardowski ZJ, Moore H, McGary T: The kinetics of ultrafiltration during peritoneal dialysis: the role of lymphatics. *Kidney Int* 32: 219, 1987

109. Mactier RA, Khanna R, Twardowski ZJ, Moore H, Nolph KD: Contribution of lymphatic absorption to loss of ultrafiltration and solute clearances in CAPD. *J Clin Invest* 80: 1311, 1987

110. Grodstein GP, Blumenkrantz MJ, Kopple JD, Moran JK, Coburn JW: Glucose absorption during continuous ambulatory peritoneal dialysis. *Kidney Int* 19: 564, 1981

111. DeSanto NG, Capodicasa G, Senatore R et al.: Glucose utilization from dialysate in patients on continuous ambulatory peritoneal dialysis. *Int J Artif Organs* 2: 119, 1978

112. Lindholm B, Bergstrom J: Nutritional management of patients undergoing peritoneal dialysis. in *Peritoneal Dialysis*, edited by Nolph KD, Dordrecht, Kluwer Academic Publishers 1989, p 230

113. Kreusch G, Bammatter F, Mordasini R, Binswanger U: Serum lipoprotein concentrations during continuous ambulatory peritoneal dialysis. in *Advances in Peritoneal Dialysis*, edited by Ghal GM, Kessel M, Nolph KD, Amsterdam, Excerpta medica, 1981, p 427

114. Lindholm B, Karlander SG, Norbek HE, Furst P, Bergstrom J: Carboyhdrate and lipid metabolism in CAPD patients. in *Peritoneal Dialysis*, edited by Atkins R, Thomson N, Farrell P, Edimburgh, Churchill Livingstone, 1981, p 198

115. Von Baeyer H, Gahl GM, Riedinger H et al.: Adaptation of CAPD patients to the continuous peritoneal energy upyake. *Kidney Int* 23: 29, 1983

116. Boyer J, Gill GN, Epstein FH: Hyperglycemia and hyperosmolality complicating peritoneal dialysis. *Ann Intern Med* 67: 568, 1967

117. Nolph KD, Rosenfeld PS, Powell JT, Danforth JR: Peritoneal glucose transport and hyperglycemia during peritoneal dialysis. *Am J Med Sci* 259: 272, 1970

118. Heaton A, Johnston DG, Burrin JM et al.: Carbohydrate and lipid metabolism during continuous ambulatory peritoneal dialysis: the effect of a single dialysis cycle. *Clin Sci* 65: 539, 1983

119. Amstrong VW, Creutzfeldt W, Ebert R, Fuchs C, Hilgers R, Scheler F: Effect of dialysis glucose load on plasma and glucoregulatory hormones in CAPD patients. *Nephron* 39: 141, 1985

120. Amstrong VW, Buschmann U, Ebert R, Fuchs C, Rieger J, Scheler F: Biochemical investigations of CAPD: plasma levels of trace elements and amino acids and impaired glucose tolerance during the course of treatment. *Int J Artif Organs* 3: 237, 1980

121. Oreopoulos DG, Marliss E, Anderson et al.: Nutritional aspects of CAPD and the potential use of amino acid containing dialysis solutions. *Perit Dial Bull* 3: 10, 1983

122. Wideroe TE, Smeby LC, Myking OL: Plasma concentrations and transperitoneal transport of native insulin and C-peptide in patients on continuous ambulatory peritoneal dialysis. *Kidney Int* 25: 82, 1984

123. Lindholm B, Bergstrom J, Karlander SG: Glucose metabolism in patients on continuous ambulatory peritoneal dialysis. *Trans Am Soc Artif Intern Organs* 17: 58, 1981

124. Lindholm B, Bergstrom J, Norbek HE: Lipoprotein (LP) metabolism in patients on continuous ambulatory peritoneal dialysis. in *Advances in Peritoneal Dialysis*, edited by Gahl GM, Kessel M, Nolph KD, Amsterdam, Excerpta medica, 1981, p 434

125. Lindholm B, Karlander SG, Norbek HE, Bergstrom J: Glucose and lipid metabolism in peritoneal dialysis. in *Peritoneal Dialysis* edited by La Greca G, Biasioli S, Ronco C, Milan, Wichtig Editore, 1982, p 219

126. Gokal R, Ramos JM, McGurk JG, Ward MK, Kerr DNS: Hyperlipidaemia in patients on continuous ambulatory peritoneal dialysis. in *Advances in Peritoneal Dialysis*, edited by Gahl GM, Kessel M, Nolph KD, Amsterdam, Excerpta medica, 1981, p 430

127. Roncari DAK, Breckenridge WC, Khanna R, Oreopoulos DG: Rise in high-density lipoprotein-cholesterol in some patients treated with CAPD. *Perit Dial Bull* 1: 136, 1981

128. Ramos JM, Heaton A, McGurk JG, Wark MK, Kerr DNS: Sequential changes in serum lipids and their subfractions in patients receiving continuous ambulatory peritoneal dialysis. *Nephron* 35: 20, 1983

129. Nolph KD, Ryan KL, Prowant B, Twardowski ZJ: A cross sectional assessment of serum vitamin D and triglyceride concentration in a CAPD population. *Perit Dial Bull* 4: 232, 1984

130. Lindholm B, Norbek HE: Serum lipids and lipoproteins during continuous ambulatory peritoneal dialysis. *Acta Med Scand* 220: 143, 1986

131. Khanna R, Breckenridge WC, Roncari DAK, Digenis G, Oreopoulos DG: Lipids abnormalities in patients undergoing continuous ambulatory peritoneal dialysis. *Perit Dial Bull* 3: S13, 1983

132. Duwe AK, Vas SI, Weatherhead JW: Effect of composition of peritoneal dialysis fluid on chemiluminescence, phagocytosis and bactericidal activity *in vitro*. *Infect Immun* 33: 130, 1981

133. Verbrug HA, Verkooyen RP, Verhoef J, Oe PL, van der Meulen J: Defective complement-mediated opsonization and lysis of bacteria in commercial peritoneal dialysis solution. in *Frontiers in Peritoneal Dialysis*, edited by Maher JF and Winchester JF, New York, Field, Rich and Associates Inc, 1986, p 559

134. Gallimore B, Gagnon RF, Stevenson MM: Cytotoxicity of commercial peritoneal dialysis solutions towards peritoneal cells of chronically uremic mice. *Nephron* 43: 283, 1986

135. Topley N, Alobaidi HM, Davies M et al.: The effect of dialysate on peritoneal phagocyte oxidative metabolism. *Kidney Int* 34: 404, 1988

136. Van Bronswijk H, Verbrugh HA, Bos HJ et al.: Cytotoxic effects of commercial continuous ambulatory peritoneal dialysis (CAPD) fluids and of bacterial exoproducts on human mesothelial cells *in vitro*. *Perit Dial Int* 9: 197, 1989

137. Manahan FJ, Ing BL, Chan JC et al.: Effect of bicarbonate containing versus lactate containing peritoneal dialysis solutions on superoxide production by human neutrophils. *Artif Organs* 13: 495, 1989

138. Topley N, Mackenzie R, Petersen MM et al.: *In vitro* testing of a potentially biocompatible continuous ambulatory peritoneal dialysis fluid. *Nephrol Dial Transplant* 6: 574, 1991

139. Jorres A, Jorres D, Topley N, Gahl GM, Mahiout A: Leukotriene release from peripheral and peritoneal leukocytes following exposure to solutions for peritoneal dialysis. *Nephrol Dial Transplant* 6: 495, 1991

140. Henderson IS, Couper IA, Lumsden A. Potentially irritant glucose in unused CAPD fluid. in *Frontiers in Peritoneal Dialysis* edited by Maher JF, Winchester JF, New York: Field, Rich and Associates Inc, 1986, p 261

141. Dobbie JW, Lloyd JK, Gall CA: Categorization of ultrastructural changes in peritoneal mesothelium, stroma and blood vessels in uremia and CAPD patients. in *Advances in Continuous Ambulatory Peritoneal Dialysis*, edited by Khanna R, Nolph KD, Prowant P, Twardowski ZJ, Oreopoulos DG, Toronto, Peritoneal Dialysis Bulletin Inc, 1990, p 3

142. Heaton A, Ward MK, Johnston DG, Nicholson DV, Alberti KGMM, Kerr DNS: Short-term studies on the use of glycerol as an osmotic agent in continuous ambulatory peritoneal dialysis. *Clin Sci* 67: 121, 1984

143. Matthys E, Dolkart R, Lameire N: Extended use of a glycerol-containing dialysate in diabetic CAPD patients. *Perit Dial Bull* 7: 10, 1987

144. Daniels FH, Leonard EF, Cortell S: Glucose and glycerol compared as osmotic agents for peritoneal dialysis. *Kidney Int* 25: 20, 1984

145. Lindholm B, Werynski A, Bergstrom J: Kinetic of peritoneal dialysis with glycerol and glucose as osmotic agents. *Trans Am Soc Artif Intern Organs* 33: 19, 1987

146. Heaton A, Ward MK, Johnston DG, Alberti KGMM, Kerr DNS: Evaluation of glycerol as an osmotic agent for continuous ambulatory peritoneal dialysis in end-stage renal failure. *Clin Sci* 70: 23, 1986

147. Matthys E, Dolkart R, Lameire N: Potential hazards of glycerol dialysate in diabetic CAPD patients. *Perit Dial Bull* 7: 16, 1987

148. Hain H, Kessel M: Aspects of new solutions for peritoneal dialysis. *Nephrol Dial Transplant* 2: 67, 1987

149. Gokal R, Mistry C: Osmotic agents in continuous ambulatory peritoneal dialysis. in *Peritoneal Dialysis*, edited

by La Greca G, Chiaramonte S, Fabris A, Feriani M, Ronco C, Milan, Wichtig Editore, 1988, p 61

150. Goodship THJ, Heaton A, Wilkinson R, Ward MK: The use of glycerol as an osmotic agent in continuous ambulatory peritoneal dialysis. in *Current Concepts in Peritoneal Dialysis*, edited by Ota K, Maher J, Winchester J, Hirszel P, Amsterdam, Excerpta Medica, 1992, p 143

151. Faict D, Lameire N, Kesteloot D, Peluso F: Evaluation of peritoneal dialysis solutions with amino acids and glycerol in a rat model. *Nephrol Dial Transplant* 6: 120, 1991

152. Faict D, Hartman JP, Lameire N, Kesteloot D, Peluso F: The evaluation of a peritoneal dialysis solution with amino acids and glycerol in a new rat model. *Perit Dial Int* 10 (Suppl 1): S60, 1990

153. Bazzato G, Coli U, Landini S et al.: Xylitol and low dosages of insulin: new perspectives for diabetic uremic patients on CAPD. *Perit Dial Bull* 2: 161, 1982

154. Yatuc W, Ward G, Shipetar G, Tenckhoff H: Substitution of sorbitol for dextrose in peritoneal irrigation fluid. A preliminary report. *Trans Am Soc Artif Intern Organs* 13: 168, 1967

155. Raja RM, Moros JG, Kramer MS, Rosenbaum JL: Hyperosmolal coma complicating peritoneal dialysis with sorbitol dialysate. *Ann Intern Med* 73: 993, 1970

156. Bischel MC, Barbour BH: Peritoneal dialysis with sorbitol versus dextrose dialysate: clinical findings and alterations of blood and cerebrospinal fluid. *Nephron* 12: 449, 1974

157. Robson MD, Levi J, Rosenfeld JB: Hyperglycemia and hyperosmolality in peritoneal dialysis. Its prevention by the use of fructose. *Proc Eur Dial Transplant Assoc* 6: 300, 1969

158. Raja RS, Kramer MS, Manchanda R, Lazaro N, Rosenbaum JL: Peritoneal dialysis with fructose dialysate. Prevention of hyperglycemia and hyperosmolality. *Ann Intern Med* 79: 511, 1973

159. Gjessing J: Addition of amino acids to peritoneal dialysis fluid. *Lancet* ii: 82, 1968

160. Oreopoulos DG, Crassweller P, Katirtzoglou A et al.: Amino acids as an osmotic agent (instead of glucose) in continuous ambulatory peritoneal dialysis. in *Continuous Ambulatory Peritoneal Dialysis*, edited by Legrain M, Amsterdam, Excerpta medica, 1980, p 335

161. Williams PF, Marliss EB, Harvey Anderson G et al.: Amino acid absorption following intraperitoneal administration in CAPD patients. *Perit Dial Bull* 2: 124, 1982

162. Oren A, Wu G, Harvey Anderson G et al.: Effective use of amino acid dialysate over four weeks in CAPD patients. *Perit Dial Bull* 3: 66, 1983

163. Goodship THJ, Lloyd S, McKenzie PW et al.: Short-term studies on the use of amino acids as an osmotic agent in continuous ambulatory peritoneal dialysis. *Clin Sci* 73: 471, 1987

164. Lindholm B, Werynsky A, Bergstrom J: Peritoneal dialysis with amino acid solutions: fluid and solute transport kinetics. *Artif Organs* 12: 2, 1988

165. Lindholm B, Traneus A, Werynski A, Osterberg T, Bergstrom J: Amino acids for peritoneal dialysis: technical and metabolic implications. in *Peritoneal Dialysis*, edited by La Greca G, Chiaramonte S, Fabris A, Feriani M, Ronco C, Milan, Wichtig Editore, 1986, p 149

166. Young GA, Dibble JB, Taylor AE, Kendall S, Brownjohn AM: A longitudinal study of the effects of amino acid-

167. Young GA, Dibble JB, Brownjohn AM: The use of amino acid based CAPD fluid in chronic renal failure. in *Amino Acids, Chemistry, Biology and Medicine*, edited by Lubec, Rosenthal, 1992, p 850

based CAPD fluid on amino acid retention and protein losses. *Nephrol Dial Transplant* 4: 900, 1989

168. Steinhauer HB, Lubrich-Birker I, Kluthe R, Horl WH, Schollmeyer P: Amino acid dialysate stimulates peritoneal prostaglandin E2 generation in humans. in *Advances in Peritoneal Dialysis*, edited by Khanna R, Nolph KD, Prowant BF, Twardowski ZJ, Oreopoulos DG, Toronto, Peritoneal Dialysis Bulletin Inc, 1988, p 21

169. Pedersen FB: Alternate use of amino acid and glucose solutions in CAPD. *Contrib Nephrol* 89: 147, 1991

170. Schilling H, Wu G, Pettit J et al.: Effects of prolonged CAPD with amino acid containing solutions in three patients. in *Advances in Continuous Ambulatory Peritoneal Dialysis*, edited by Khanna R, Nolph KD, Prowant BF, Twardowski ZJ, Oreopoulos DG, Toronto, University of Toronto Press, 1985, p 49

171. Schilling H, Wu G, Pettit J et al.: Use of amino acid containing solutions in continuous ambulatory peritoneal dialysis patients after peritonitis: results of a prospective controlled trial. *Proc Eur Dial Transplant Assoc-Eur Renal Assoc* 22: 421, 1985

172. Dombros NV, Prutis K, Tong M et al.: Six-month overnight intraperitoneal amino-acid infusion in continuous ambulatory peritoneal dialysis (CAPD) patients. No effect on nutritional status. *Perit Dial Int* 10: 79, 1990

173. Lindholm B, Bergstrom J: Amino acids in CAPD solutions: lights and shadows. in *Peritoneal Dialysis*, edited by La Greca G, Ronco C, Feriani M, Chiaramonte S, Conz P, Milan, Wichtig Editore, 1991, p 139

174. Pedersen FB, Dragsholt C, Laier E et al.: Alternate use of amino acid and glucose solutions in CAPD. *Perit Dial Bull* 5: 215, 1985

175. Young GA, Dibble JB, Hobson SM et al.: The use of an amino-acid-based CAPD fluid over 12 weeks. *Nephrol Dial Transplant* 4: 285, 1989

176. Dibble JB, Young GA, Hobson SM, Brownjohn AM: Amino-acid-based continuous ambulatory peritoneal dialysis (CAPD) fluid over twelve weeks: effects on carbohydrate and lipid metabolism. *Perit Dial Int* 10: 71, 1990

177. Bruno M, Bagnis C, Marangella M et al.: CAPD with an amino acid solution: a long-term, cross-over study. *Kidney Int* 35: 1189, 1989

178. Arfeen S, Goodship THJ, Kirkwood A, Ward MK: The nutritional/metabolic and hormonal effects of 8 weeks of continuous ambulatory peritoneal dialysis with a 1% amino acid solution. *Clin Nephrol* 33: 192, 1990

179. Scanziani R, Dozio B, Iacuitti G. CAPD in diabetics: use of amino acids. in *Current Concepts in Peritoneal Dialysis*, edited by Ota K, Maher J, Winchester J, Hirszel P, Amsterdam, Excerpta Medica, 1992, p 628

180. Lindholm B, Bergstrom J: Nutritional aspects on peritoneal dialysis. *Kidney Int* 42 (Suppl 38): S165, 1992

181. Jones MR, Martis L, Algrim CE et al.: Amino acid solutions for CAPD: rationale and clinical experience. *Miner Electrolyte Metab* 18: 309, 1992

182. Bernard D, Kopple JD, Brunori G et al.: Nutritional benefit of intraperitoneal (IP) amino acids (AA) in CAPD

patients. 6th Int Congr on Nutrition and Metabolism in Renal Disease, Harrogate, UK, 1991 (Abstract)

183. Lazarus-Barlow WS: Observations upon the initial rates of osmosis of certain substances in water and in fluids containing albumen. *J Physiol* 19: 140, 1895–6

184. Hain H, Ghal G: Osmotic agent. An update. *Contrib Nephrol* 89: 119, 1991

185. Daniels FH, Nedev ND, Cataldo T, Leonard EF, Cortell S: The use of polyelectrolytes as osmotic agent for peritoneal dialysis. *Kidney Int* 33: 925, 1988

186. Struijk DG, Bakker JC, Krediet RT, Koomen GCM, Stekkinger P, Arisz L: Effect of intraperitoneal administration of two different batches of albumin solutions on peritoneal solute transport in CAPD patients. *Nephrol Dial Transplant* 6: 198, 1991

187. Nolph KD, Hopkins C, Rubin J et al.: Polymer induced ultrafiltration in dialysis: high osmotic pressure due to impermeant polymer sodium. *Trans Am Soc Artif Intern Organs* 24: 162, 1978

188. Rubin J, Nolph KD, McGary TJ: Osmotic ultrafiltration with dextran sodium sulfate: potential for use in peritoneal dialysis. *J Dial* 3: 251, 1979

189. Twardowski ZJ, Moore HL, McGary TJ, Poskuta M, Stathakis C, Hirszel P: Polymers as osmotic agent for peritoneal dialysis. *Perit Dial Bull* 4 (Suppl 3): S125, 1984

190. Frank HA, Seligman AM, Fine J: Further experiences with peritoneal irrigation for acute renal failure. *Ann Surg* 128: 561, 1948

191. Twardowski ZJ, Hain H, McGary TJ, Moore HL, Keller RS: Sustained UF with gelatin dialysis solution during long dwell dialysis exchanges in rats. in *Frontiers in Peritoneal Dialysis*, edited by Maher JF, Winchester JF, New York, Field, Rich and Associates Inc, 1986, p 249

192. Ring J, Messmer K: Incidence and severity of anaphylactoid reactions to colloid substitutes. *Lancet* ii: 466, 1977

193. Gjessing J: The use of dextran as a dialysing fluid in peritoneal dialysis. *Acta Med Scand* 185: 237, 1969

194. Hain H, Schutte W, Pustelnik A, Gahl G, Kessel M: Ultrafiltration and absorption characteristics of hydroxyethylstarch and dextran during long dwell peritoneal dialysis exchanges in rat. in *Advances in Peritoneal Dialysis*, edited by Khanna R, Nolph KD, Prowant BF, Twardowski ZJ, Oreopoulos DG, Toronto, Peritoneal Dialysis Bulletin Inc, 1989, p 28

195. Hain H, Kempf D, Schnell P, Gahl G, Kessel M: Ultrafiltration patterns of dextran and hydroxyethylstarch during long dwell peritoneal dialysis exchanges in nonuremic rats. in *Ambulatory Peritoneal Dialysis*, edited by Avram MM, Giordano C, New York, Plenum Publishing Corporation, 1990, p 83

196. Bergonzi G, Paties C, Vassallo G et al.: Dextran deposit in tissues of patients undergoing hemodialysis. *Nephrol Dial Transplant* 5: 54, 1990

197. Dienes HP, Gerharz CD, Wagner R, Weber M, John HD: Accumulation of hydroxyethyl starch (HES) in the liver of patients with renal failure and portal hypertension. *J Hepatol* 3: 223, 1986

198. Winchester JF: Alternative osmotic agents to dextrose for peritoneal dialysis. in *Peritoneal Dialysis: Proceedings of Second International Course on Peritoneal Dialysis*, edited by La Greca G, Chiaramonte S, Fabris A, Feriani M, Ronco C, Milan, Wichtig Editore, 1986, p 135

199. Mistry CD, Gokal R, Mallick NP: Glucose polymer as an osmotic agent in CAPD. in *Frontiers in Peritoneal Dialysis*, edited by Maher JF, Winchester JF, New York, Field, Rich and Associates Inc, 1986, p 241

200. Mistry CD, Mallick NP, Gokal R: The advantage of glucose polymer as an osmotic agent in continuous peritoneal dialysis. *Proc Eur Dial Transplant Assoc* 22: 415, 1985

201. Mistry CD, Mallick NP, Gokal R: The use of large molecular weight polymer (MW 20,000) as an osmotic agent in continuous ambulatory peritoneal dialysis (CAPD). in *Advances in Peritoneal Dialysis*, edited by Khanna R, Nolph KD, Prowant BF, Twardowski ZJ, Oreopoulos DG, Toronto, Peritoneal Dialysis Bulletin Inc, 1986, p 7

202. Mistry CD, Gokal RL: The use of hyposmolar glucose polymer solution in continuous ambulatory peritoneal dialysis. in *Ambulatory Peritoneal Dialysis*, edited by Avram MM, Giordano C, New York, Plenum Publishing Corporation, 1990, p 83

203. Mistry CD, Walker M, Gokal R: Safe use of glucose polymer dialysate over three months in CAPD patients. *Nephrol Dial Transplant* 5: 299, 1990

204. Gokal R: Unpublished data. Personal communication

205. de Fijter CWH, Oe PL, Verbrugh HA et al.: Glucose polymers as osmotic agent in CAPD fluid: a more favorable effect on peritoneal macrophage (PMO) function than glucose-based solutions. *Kidney Int* 40: 978, 1991

206. Mistry CD, Gokal R: The use of glucose polymer in CAPD: essential physiological and clinical conclusions. in *Current Concepts in Peritoneal Dialysis*, edited by Ota K, Maher J, Winchester J, Hirszel P, Amsterdam, Excerpta medica, 1992, p 138

207. Mistry CD, Fox JE, Mallick NP, Gokal R: Circulating maltose and isomaltose in chronic renal failure. *Kidney Int* 32 (Suppl 22): S210, 1987

208. Schildt B, Bouveng R, Sollenberg M: Plasma substitute induced impairement of reticuloendothelial system function. *Acta Chir Scand* 141: 7, 1975

209. Klein E, Ward RA, Williams TE, Feldhoff PW: Peptides as substitute osmotic agent for glucose in peritoneal dialysis. *Trans Am Soc Artif Intern Organs* 32: 550, 1986

210. Imholz ALT, Lameire N, Faict D, Koomen GCM, Krediet RT, Martis L: Evaluation of short-chain polypeptides as an osmotic agent in CAPD patients. *Perit Dial Int* 13 (Suppl 1): S62, 1993

211. La Greca G, Fabris A, Feriani M, Chiaramonte S, Ronco C: Acid base homeostasis in clinical dialysis. in *Replacement of Renal Function by Dialysis*, edited by Maher JF, Dordrecht, Kluwer Academic Publishers, 1989, p 807

212. La Greca G, Biasioli S, Chiaramonte S et al.: Acid base balance on peritoneal dialysis. *Clin Nephrol* 16: 1, 1981

213. Boen ST: Kinetics of peritoneal dialysis. *Medicine* 40: 243, 1961

214. Preuss HG: Biochemistry of bicarbonate, lactate and acetate in man. *North Med Proc* 1: 1, 1977

215. Boen ST Mulinari AS, Dillard DH, Scribner BH: Periodic peritoneal dialysis in the management of chronic uremia. *Trans Am Soc Artif Intern Organs* 8: 256, 1962

216. Biasioli S, Feriani M, Chiaramonte S, La Greca G: Buffers in peritoneal dialysis. *Int J Artif Organs* 10: 3, 1987

217. Kveim M, Nesbakken R: Utilization of exogenous acetate during hemodialysis. *Trans Am Soc Artif Intern Organs* 21: 138, 1975

218. La Greca G, Biasioli S, Brendolan A et al.: Buffer balance in peritoneal dialysis. in *Peritoneal Dialysis*, edited by La Greca G, Biasioli S, Ronco C, Milan, Wichtig Editore, 1982, p 177

219. Faller B, Marichal JF: Loss of ultrafiltration in CAPD: a role for acetate. *Perit Dial Bull* 4: 10, 1984

220. Slingeneyer A, Mion C, Mourad G et al.: Progressive sclerosing peritonitis. A late and severe complication of maintenance peritoneal dialysis. *Trans Am Soc Artif Intern Organs* 29: 633, 1983

221. Brin M: The synthesis and metabolism of lactic acid isomers. *Ann NY Acad Sci* 119: 942, 1965

222. Searle GL, Cavalieri RR: Determination of lactate kinetics in the human analysis of data from single injection. *Proc Soc Exp Biol Med* 139: 1002, 1972

223. Fabris A, Biasioli S, Chiaramonte S et al.: Buffer metabolism in CAPD: relationship with respiratory dynamics. *Trans Am Soc Artif Intern Organs* 28: 270, 1982

224. Teehan BP, Schleifer CR, Reichard GA, Cupit MC, Sigler MH, Haff AC: Acid base studies in continuous ambulatory peritoneal dialysis. in *CAPD Update*, edited by Moncrief JW, Popovich RP, New York, Masson Publishing USA Inc, 1981, p 95

225. Richardson RMA, Roscoe JM: Bicarboante, L-lactate and D-lactate balance in intermittent peritoneal dialysis. *Perit Dial Bull* 6: 178, 1986

226. Nolph KD, Twardowski ZJ, Khanna R et al.: Tidal peritoneal dialysis with racemic or L-lactate solutions. *Perit Dial Int* 10: 161, 1990

227. Robson MD, Faivoseviz A, Malmoud H: Physiological transfer of acid base. in *Continuous Ambulatory Peritoneal Dialysis*, edited by Legrain M, Amsterdam, Excerpta medica, 1980, p 194

228. Rubin J, Adair C, Johnson B, Bower JD: Stereospecific lactate absorption during peritoneal dialysis. *Nephron* 31: 224, 1982

229. Fine A: Metabolism of D-lactate in the dog and in man. *Perit Dial Int* 9: 99, 1989

230. Nissenson AR: Acid base homeostasis in peritoneal dialysis patients. *Int J Artif Organs* 7: 175, 1984

231. Gennari FJ, Cohen JJ, Kassirer JP: Normal acid base values. in *Acid/Base*, edited by Cohen JJ, Kassirer JP, Boston, Little, Brown and Company, 1982, pp 107

232. Yamamoto T, Sakakura T, Yamakawa M et al.: Clinical effects of long-term use of neutralized dialysate for continuous ambulatory peritoneal dialysis. *Nephron* 60: 324, 1992

233. May RC, Kelly RA, Mitch WE: Mechanisms for defects in muscle protein metabolism in rats with chronic uremia. *J Clin Invest* 79: 1099, 1987

234. Williams B, Hattersley J, Layward E, Walls J: Metabolic acidosis and skeletal muscle adaptation to low protein diets in chronic uremia. *Kidney Int* 40: 779, 1991

235. Papadoyannakis NJ, Stefanidis CJ, McGeown M: The effect of the correction of metabolic acidosis on nitrogen and potassium balance of patients with chronic renal failure. *Am J Clin Nutr* 40: 623, 1984

236. Frohlich ED: Vascular effects of the Krebs intermediate metabolites. *Am J Physiol* 208: 149, 1965

237. Kirkendol PL, Devia CJ, Bower JD et al.: Comparison of the cardiovascular effects of sodium acetate, sodium bicarbonate and other potential sources of fixed base in hemodialysis solutions. *Trans Am Soc Artif Intern Organs* 23: 399, 1977

238. Veech RL: The untoward effects of the anions of dialysis fluid. *Kidney Int* 34: 587, 1988

239. Veech RL: The toxix impact of parenteral solutions on the metabolism of cells: a hypothesis for physiological parenteral therapy. *Am J Clin Nutr* 44: 519, 1986

240. Sistare FD, Haynes RC: The interaction between the cytosolic pyridine nucleotide redox potential and gluconeogenesis from lactate/pyruvate in isolated rat hepatocytes. *J Biol Chem* 23: 12748, 1985

241. Oh MS, Phelpo KR, Traube M et al.: D-lactic acidosis in a man with the short bowel syndrome. *N Engl J Med* 301: 249, 1979

242. Veech RL, Fowler RC: Cerebral dysfunction and respiratory alkalosis during peritoneal dialysis with D-lactate containing dialysis fluid. *Am J Med* 82: 572, 1986

243. Ing TS, Quon MJ, Daugirdas JT, Ghandi VC, Epstain MB: Preparation of bicarbonate containing peritoneal dialysate using an automated dialysate delivery system. *Int J Artif Organs* 4: 148, 1981

244. Ing TS, Quon MJ, Daugirdas JT, Liu P, Gandhi VC, Reid RR: On line preparation of bicarbonate containing dialysate for use in peritoneal dialysis. *Int J Artif Organs* 4: 308, 1981

245. Ing TS, Humayun HM, Daugirdas JT et al.: Preparation of bicarbonate-containing dialysate for peritoneal dialysis. *Int J Artif Organs* 6; 217, 1983

246. Ing TS, Ghandi VC, Daugirdas JT, Reid RW, Hunt J, Popli S: Peritoneal dialysis using bicarbonate buffered dialysate. *Int J Artif Organs* 7: 166, 1984

247. Feriani M, La Greca G: CAPD with bicarbonate solution. in *New Perspectives in Hemodialysis, Peritoneal Dialysis, Arterovenous Hemofiltration and Plasmaferesis*, edited by Horl WH, Schollmeyer PJ, New York, Plenum Publishing Corporation, 1989, p 139

248. Feriani M, Reinhard B, La Greca G: Calcium carbonate precipitation in oversatured bicarbonate containing CAPD solutions. in *Peritoneal dialysis*, edited by La Greca G, Ronco C, Feriani M, Chiaramonte S, Conz P, Milan, Wichtig Editore, 1991, p 145

249. Gretz N, Kraft E, Meisinger E, Lasserre J, Strauch M: Calcium deposits due to bicarbonate containing CAPD solutions? in *Advances in Peritoneal Dialysis*, edited by Khanna R, Nolph KD, Prowant BF, Twardowski ZJ, Oreopoulos DG, Toronto, Peritoneal Dialysis Bulletin Inc, 1988, p 220

250. Feriani M, Biasioli S, Barbacini S et al.: Acid base correction in bicarbonate CAPD patients. in *Advances in Peritoneal Dialysis*, edited by Khanna R, Nolph KD, Prowant BF, Twardowski ZJ, Oreopoulos DG, Toronto, Peritoneal Dialysis Bulletin Inc, 1989, p 191

251. Feriani M, Dissegna D, La Greca G, Passlick-Deetjen J: Short term clinical study with bicarbonate containing peritoneal dialysis solution. *Perit Dial Int* 1993. In press

252. Di Paolo N, Garosi G, Traversari L, Di Paolo M: Mesothelial biocompatibility of peritoneal dialysis solutions. *Perit Dial Int* 13 (Suppl 2): S109, 1993

253. Jorres A, Ghal GM, Ludat K, Muller C, Passlick-Deetjen J: *In vitro* biocompatibility testing of a new bicarbonate

buffered dialysis fluid for CAPD. *Perit Dial Int* 12: S2, 1992

254. Andre A, Egle B, Dobos GH, Lubrich-Birkner I, Schollmeyer P, Steinhauer HB. Comparison of lactate and bicarbonate buffered peritoneal dialysate (PD) fluids: effect on human peritoneal macrophages (PMO). *Perit Dial Int* 13 (Suppl 1): S24, 1993

255. Schambye HT, Flesner P, Pedersen RB et al.: Bicarbonate- versus lactate-based CAPD fluids: a bio-

compatibility study in rabbits. *Perit Dial Int* 12: 281, 1992

256. Slingeneyer A, Faller B, Michel C, Przybylski C, Rolland R, Mion C: Increased ultrafiltration capacity using a new bicarbonate CAPD solution. *Perit Dial Int* 13 (Suppl 1): S57, 1993

257. Slingeneyer A, Przybylski C, Rolland R, Mion C: A new bicarbonate buffered solution for CAPD. *Perit Dial Int* 13 (Suppl 1): S57, 1993

AUTOMATED PERITONEAL DIALYSIS

JOSE A. DIAZ-BUXO

HISTORIC OVERVIEW

Peritoneal dialysis (PD) was first used in clinical practice by Ganter in 1923 (1). The early experiences used a continuous flow and an intermittent technique with manual exchanges. Although the continuous technique gained popularity during the first two decades of clinical application, intermittent peritoneal dialysis (IPD) became the predominant method by the 1940's (2–13). The predilection for IPD was mostly due to the need for only one peritoneal catheter while the continuous technique required two. By the 1960's IPD was well established and markedly improved (14–19). Its use for the treatment of acute and chronic renal failure was well accepted. However, the manual procedures were time consuming and expensive since they required the supervision of medical personnel.

In 1962, Boen developed the first automated peritoneal delivery system (20). It consisted of a 40-liter 'carboy' container and a dispensing mechanism with solenoid-activated occluders capable of delivering a premeasured amount of sterile dialysate by gravity. This closed system reduced the rate of peritonitis and opened the doors for home dialysis.

In 1966, Lasker introduced a simple gravity-fed cycler (21). This device used sterile dialysate in 2-liter glass containers, plastic tubing for delivery, and a plastic bag for collection of spent dialysate. This new cycler could infuse variable volumes of warm dialysate. Mechanical timers were used to determine the length of infusion, dwell and drainage. The Lasker cycler was the forerunner of all modern cyclers. It further reduced the rate of peritonitis and simplified the IPD procedure. Its main disadvantages were the high cost of dialysate and the inconvenience of transporting and storing large volumes of solution.

In 1972, a new breed of delivery systems was introduced using reverse osmosis (RO) to supply sterile, pyrogen-free water in large volumes and dialysate concentrate in small containers (22). These devices used roller pumps or bellows to mix the RO-treated water with dialysate concentrate at a ratio of 19:1. The commercial concentrate mixed with water resulted in a dialysate glucose concentration of 1.5 to 3.0%. Additional glucose could be added to the concentrate according to the ultrafiltration (UF) needs of the patient. Other features of these systems were: safety monitors to evaluate the purity of water, resistivity monitors to ensure proper mixing of water and concentrate, variable dialysate temperature, pre-treatment devices to improve the quality of water and prolong the life of RO membranes (carbon filters, water softeners and bacterial filters), and automated disinfections of the RO modules and dialysate circuit (23–29). The clear advantage of RO systems was their ability to provide large volumes of dialysate at a lower cost. The many disadvantages included: the complexity of the equipment and its voluminous size, length of training in the use and sterilization of the equipment, cost and frequency of maintenance, and large volumes of drainage (dialysate effluent and unused tap water). The advent of continuous

PD (CPD) techniques and the use of smaller dialysate volumes resulted in virtual elimination of RO systems and adoption of cyclers.

In the late 1970's, Diaz-Buxo et al. and Suki et al. developed a new technique of automated PD (APD) called continuous cycling PD (CCPD) (30–33). This technique is based on the principles of equilibration PD (34) and consists of automated delivery of dialysate by a cycler while the patient rests at night, followed by infusion of a diurnal exchange in the morning that dwells undisturbed during the day until the next nocturnal session. CCPD is a virtual reversal of the exchanges used in continuous ambulatory PD (CAPD) since the shorter cycles occur at night and the prolonged cycle during the day.

Stephen et al. studied the use of 'reciprocating PD' in the late 1970's (35, 36). This technique used a fixed volume of dialysate constantly dwelling in the peritoneal cavity and an additional volume periodically infused and drained. The rationale for this technique was a better mixing of the dialysate and reduction of the wasted time during dialysate transit into and out of the peritoneal cavity. This technique was latter revived and referred to as tidal PD (TPD) (37, 38).

EQUIPMENT

Cyclers

The peritoneal cycler is the heart of the APD system. Progress in computer science and electronics has accelerated the evolution of the modern cycler. The primary functions of the cycler are:

- to deliver a measured volume of dialysate into the peritoneal cavity,
- to allow delivered dialysate to dwell in the peritoneal cavity for a specific period of time, and
- to drain the used or spent dialysate from the peritoneal cavity.

The target volume of dialysate can be attained by weighing or measuring the volume, or by timing the infusion of dialysate into the peritoneal cavity using a constant rate of delivery.

The secondary functions of a cycler include:

- warming of solutions to body temperature,
- calculation of fluid balance and net UF,
- safety monitors and alarms (temperature, fluid balance, power failure, dialysate flow obstruction and insufficient dialysate),
- built-in programs to determine modality of dialysis (IPD, CCPD, NPD or TPD),
- real time graphic displays of dialysate delivered and drained,
- automatic elimination of superfluous drain time and proportional increase in dwell time allotted for that cycle,

- selection of dialysate glucose concentration and volume for a particular cycle,
- data storage and telephone transmission of dialytic events (useful for determination of compliance with therapy and for calculation of dialysis prescription),
- use of large dialysate containers,
- direct drainage into a tray, drain or drainage bag,
- built-in kinetic programs,
- lockout features to restrict use of certain parameters and functions by unauthorized operators, and
- oversized visual displays and computerized voice recognition systems for the sight impaired.

The simplest cyclers use gravity for infusion and drainage of dialysate. These systems do not need pumps for fluid delivery and avoid the need for complex monitoring mechanisms to prevent accidental overdistention of the abdomen or suction of intraperitoneal contents. However, dialysis solutions must be hung above the peritoneal cavity and the end of the drain line below the patient's level in order to effect infusion and drainage. This feature demands a stand or tower which increases the size and weight of the system. The hanging of dialysate bags is often difficult to perform by debilitated patients. The addition of a pump to deliver dialysate from the ground to a level above the patient's abdomen can reduce the size of the cycler and facilitate the use of large dialysate containers.

Active infusion and drainage of dialysate is possible with the use of pumps to defy gravity and accelerate fluid flow. These systems can deliver and drain dialysate faster at a controlled rate of flow and are usually simpler and lighter by elimination of the cycler stand. Although several designs incorporating these features have been tried in the past, none have found clinical application until recently. A new cycler is being tested using pneumatic pressure pumps to transfer solutions from the container to the warming tray, to infuse solutions into the patient, and to drain the peritoneal cavity. This cycler also uses a disposable one-step set-up cassette to simplify the procedure. The potential disadvantages of these systems are the need for sensitive pressure monitoring devices to avoid accidental infusion of large volumes of dialysate and to avoid suction of the mesentery or other tissues during drainage of the spent dialysate. The sensitive monitors can also result in excessive alarms. Further clinical trials are needed with these devices.

A family of cyclers with limited features is being introduced. These systems are simple and inexpensive but lack many of the aforementioned capabilities and monitoring devices. They were designed to handle a limited number of exchanges at night in patients using hybrid modalities of PD (*vide infra*).

Tubing sets

Tubing sets are necessary to deliver the dialysis solution from the containers to the cycler, into the patient, and from the patient to the drain. Various materials have been used in their manufacturing always striving for biocompatibility, flexibility, durability and cost containment. The essential parts of the tubing kit are: connectors between tubing and bags, connector between tubing and patient's catheter, manifold between bag lines and cycler, patient line and drain line. Additional bags for dialysate weight or drainage are used according to the specific cycler design. The use of large dialysate containers has simplified the design of the tubing sets, reduced the number of connections to the bags and reduced manufacturing cost. Most tubing kits are disposable, while others have been approved for several uses. The clinical experience with multiple uses of tubing sets is favorable (39–41). Safe reuse of tubing sets could result in significant cost savings and reduction in the set-up time of the equipment.

Connectors

APD has shared the connectors developed for CAPD to effect connections between dialysis solution bags, transfer sets and the peritoneal catheter. The earliest of connectors were simple spikes. The ease of contamination during a connection and the high incidence of peritonitis stimulated the development of safer connectors. Newer connectors are characterized by having locking mechanisms to prevent accidental separation, outer sleeves to prevent contamination, outer shells containing disinfectant-saturated sponges, internal chambers filled with disinfectants or a combination of all these features (Safelock, Fresenius, Walnut Creek, CA). Connecting devices to assist the visual or neuromuscular impaired have also been used with some success. These systems automatically irradiate the connection site with UV light (Optum System, Abbott/Fresenius, Walnut Creek, CA) and performs the connection (UVXD, Baxter Healthcare Corp, Deerfield, IL). The influence of connectology in reducing the rate of peritonitis in CCPD is difficult to assess since the rates have been relatively low, even with the use of spikes, and many other factors, including 'flush before fill' flow patterns, may be of greater importance.

The disconnection procedure during APD can be performed using the standard methodology developed for CAPD or with external occlusion (42, 43) (DelClamp, Fresenius, Walnut Creek, CA). The device consists of a simple, disposable, plastic clamp to occlude the patient-cycler line distal to its connection with the peritoneal catheter (Figure 1). The line is then cut with unsterile scissors. The complete procedure takes a few seconds and prevents accidental contamination since the system remains closed.

DIALYSIS SOLUTIONS

The solutions used for APD are generally the same as those commercially available for CAPD (Table 1). A few

Table 1. Composition of standard solutions for APD

Dextrose	(%)	1.5–4.25
Sodium	(mEq/L)	132
Potassium	(mEq/L)	0
Calcium	(mEq/L)	2.5–3.5
Magnesium	(mEq/L)	0.5–1.5
Lactate	(mEq/L)	35–40

circumstances specific to APD techniques often influence solution selection.

Osmotic agents

Three standard concentrations of dextrose, 1.5, 2.5 and 4.25%, have been adopted for commercial dialysate. These percentages refer to the hydrated form of dextrose conventionally used in the USA. European solution concentrations are expressed for the non-hydrated molecule and are thus slightly lower. The use of higher dextrose concentrations (4.25%) is recommended for the long cycles of CCPD in order to maintain a certain degree of UF or to avoid excessive absorption of dialysate. Limited experience with amino acid-containing solutions suggests that UF is possible without affecting clearance of uremic toxins (44–46). However, it is possible that amino acid solutions may accomplish a lower net UF with prolonged cycles (> 8 hours) (46–49). Amino acid solutions have the potential to both reduce glucose absorption and provide nutritional supplementation during the long cycles of CCPD. Several concerns have been raised by recent investigations concerning the chronic use of amino acid solutions. Foremost are the possibilities of hypertonic amino acid solutions affecting peritoneal membrane transport properties (46, 48, 49); and, that these solutions may yield non-physiological high plasma levels of certain amino acids (46). Further research is necessary before adopting these solutions for clinical use. Other osmotic agents with potentially longer periods of osmotic gradients and high biocompatibility are being tested which may benefit CCPD (50–52).

Sodium

The only exception to the practice of a standard solution for APD and CAPD is the use of lower sodium concentrations for IPD with very high dialysate flows (> 3 liters/hour). Short, frequent exchanges with high glucose concentrations result in rapid UF with a disproportionate removal of extracellular water in relation to sodium. Since sodium removal depends on the plasma-dialysate concentration gradient, the degree of UF and the intravascular volume, this practice results in hypernatremia (53, 54). Under these circumstances a lower dialysate sodium concentration is recommended to avoid hypernatremia (53).

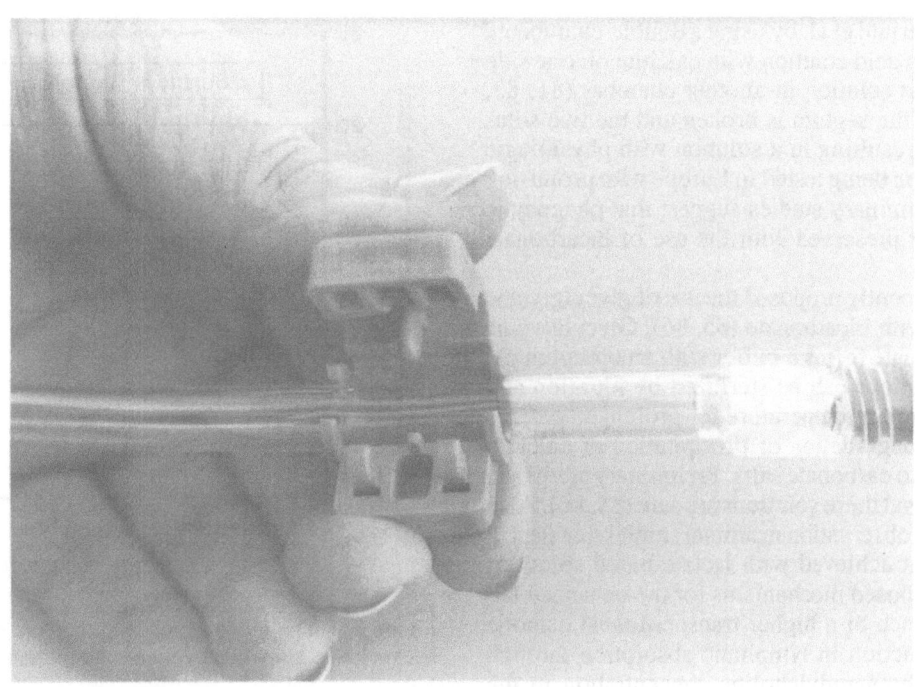

Figure 1. External occlusion device (Delclamp™). After occluding the transfer line completely with the device, the line can be cut with unsterile scissors to complete the disconnection procedure.

The adoption of CPD techniques have virtually eliminated high-flow IPD.

Potassium

All available solutions are potassium-free. The addition of potassium in appropriate doses to correct hypokalemia is recommended, but seldom necessary. Most patients can compensate for potassium losses by increasing dietary intake.

Calcium

Earlier solutions contained calcium in concentrations of 3 to 3.5 mEq/L in order to maintain calcium balance. Typical patients on a renal diet, in the absence of calcium salts supplementation, require these higher concentrations to maintain a neutral or positive calcium balance (55–57). In fact, with the use of 4.25% D solutions, negative calcium balance has been demonstrated (58–60). However, the introduction of calcium salts (carbonate and acetate) as phosphate binders has markedly increased calcium loads in dialysis patients and dictated the use of lower calcium concentrations in hemodialysis (HD) and PD solutions (61–65). The use of calcitriol in high doses has also increased calcium absorption. The most common calcium concentration available is 2.5 mEq/L. Lower concentrations, including a calcium-free solution, have been used in patients with extraosseous calcifications with some success (66). However, their use should be limited to patients with high calcium-phosphorus products and under very close supervision.

Magnesium

Magnesium concentrations of 0.5 to 1.5 mEq/L are available. The precise recommendation depends on the patient's magnesium stores and serum concentrations. Periodic serum magnesium concentration determinations are recommended to assess the potential need for a change in solution.

Buffer bases

Lactate is the standard buffer used in available dialysis solutions. The earlier use of acetate has been abandoned due to its implication in the development of peritoneal hyperpermeability, loss of peritoneal UF and peritoneal sclerosis (67–73).

Dialysis solutions containing lactate and dextrose have unphysiologically low pH values, have been shown to affect peritoneal membrane viability of mesothelial cells and resident peritoneal cells, and to interfere with phagocytic function (74–81). Lactate accumulation has also been shown to affect vital cellular function and to increase catabolism (82). The ideal buffer is bicarbonate since it is the natural base, does not need metabolism, and readily corrects metabolic acidosis. The main problem in the commercial production of bicarbonate has been the precipitation of calcium in an alkaline media. This problem has been solved by Feriani et al. by using a double-chambered bag containing an acid solution with calcium on one side and a bicarbonate solution in another chamber (81, 83, 84). Prior to use the septum is broken and the two solutions are mixed, resulting in a solution with physiologic pH. This product is being tested in Europe with promising results (81). Preliminary studies suggest that phagocytic function is better preserved with the use of bicarbonate solutions.

Yatzidis has recently proposed the use of glycylglycine in combination with bicarbonate (85, 86). Glycylglycine added to bicarbonate forms a buffer with an optimum pH of 7.35. The solutions can be sterilized by filtration and remain stable at room temperature for prolonged periods of time without degradation or precipitation of calcium or magnesium into carbonate salts. Preliminary studies in animals suggest that these solutions are safe (85, 86). Also noteworthy is the observation in animal studies that net UF is superior to that achieved with lactate-based solutions (86–88). The proposed mechanisms for the enhanced UF are the maintenance of a higher transperitoneal osmotic gradient and reduction in lymphatic absorption through an increase in phophatidylcholine concentration in the peritoneal cavity. The main limitation to the use of glycylglycine is that sterilization by filtration may not be adequate for commercial dialysate manufacturing.

Ing et al. devised a method of preparing peritoneal dialysate containing bicarbonate and glucose by using an automated dialysate delivery system that mixes water, acid concentrate and basic concentrate (89). This system has potential use for APD if proportioning systems become popular again to provide high flow PD therapy.

PHYSIOLOGIC AND KINETIC CONSIDERATIONS

Although the physiologic principles governing APD and CAPD are similar, special consideration must be given to specific circumstances that occur with the use of certain modalities of APD. Foremost is the fact that some modalities of APD are intermittent rather than continuous. Secondly, even with continuous modalities (CCPD and PD Plus) the shorter cycles do not achieve equilibrium between plasma and dialysate. Finally, most exchanges of APD occur with the patient in the supine position. The latter affects tolerance of intraperitoneal volume and peritoneal mass transfer rates.

Continuous *versus* intermittent therapy

CPD modalities share the advantages of providing a steady physiologic state, high clearances of solutes with molecular weights above 2000 as compared to HD and a relatively economical way of clearing small solutes through equilibration dialysis. Similar clinical outcomes for patients undergoing CAPD and HD have been observed despite

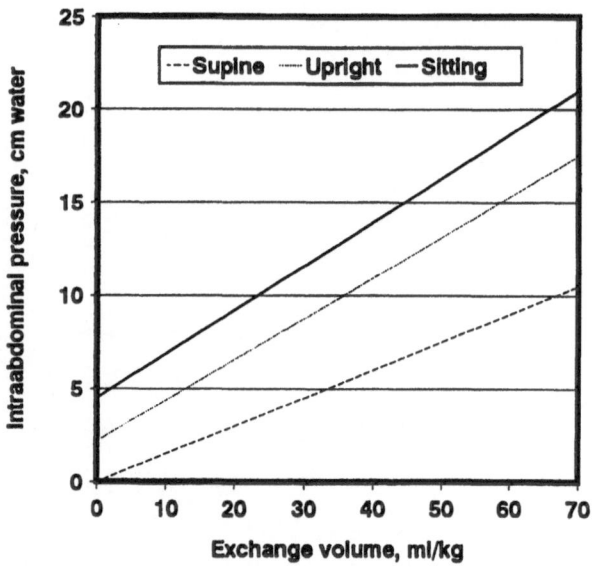

Figure 2.   The influence of body posture on the relationship between intraabdominal volume and intraabdominal pressure.

marked differences in their normalized urea clearances (KT/V) (90–107). This phenomenon has been explained on the basis of superior 'middle molecule' clearances with CAPD and the steady physiologic state it provides. The Peak Concentration Hypothesis has been proposed to explain this phenomenon (108). It states that the peak, rather than the time average concentration of urea (TACurea), relates to uremic toxicity. Thus, a higher KT/Vurea is required in HD to achieve a peak concentration at or below the steady state of CAPD. Based on this mathematical model, Gotch and others have proposed equivalency ratios for HD and CAPD KT/V (109, 110). A domain of adequacy of dialysis has been identified and is being validated with clinical studies (111). The present state of knowledge suggests that urea kinetic modeling (UKM) based on the Peak Concentration Hypothesis is valid for CAPD and probably for CCPD; however, it is likely that further adjustments to the model will be required for intermittent modalities such as IPD, NPD and TPD.

Intraabdominal pressure (IAP)

The infusion of dialysate into the peritoneal cavity results in an increase in IAP. A linear relationship between intraabdominal volume (Vip) and IAP has been demonstrated (112–114). Patient position affects the slope of the curve (113, 114). Assuming the same Vip, IAP is lowest with the patient supine, intermediate when standing and highest in the sitting position (Figure 2).

Increased IAP causes discomfort (IAP > 14 cm water) that is increased by bending, coughing and sneezing. Chronic exposure to high IAP results in various mechanical complications such as herniae, gastroesophageal reflux, back pain and hemorrhoids.

Most of the exchanges in APD occur with the patient in the supine position. Therefore the same or higher volumes as used for CAPD can be prescribed with a lower incidence of these complications. The practice of using larger Vip's is increasing and may have significant kinetic and economic implications (*vide infra*).

Effect of exchange volume (VIP) on solute transport

The plasma to dialysate (D/P) gradient is the diffusive driving force for solute transfer. This diffusive gradient can be increased by either increasing the dialysate flow rate while maintaining the same Vip or by increasing the Vip. The former is associated with a reduction in effective dialysis time as the flow increases due to an increasing ratio of inflow plus outflow time to total cycle time. The latter, however, increases the diffusive gradient without changing the effective dialysis time. Peritoneal clearance (Kp) is a function of dialysate flow rate and overall peritoneal permeability area product (KoA). Data are also accumulating to suggest that KoA or mass transfer area coefficient (MTAC) are strongly dependent on Vip (115–117). Although some studies initially suggested that TPD was approximately 20% more efficient than IPD when similar total dialysate inflow volumes were used over identical periods of time (38, 118–122), recent clinical studies have confirmed that the efficiency is the same or less (123–127). The earlier differences can be fully explained by the higher Vip's used with TPD as compared to IPD.

Effect of posture on solute transport

Body posture has also been implied as a significant factor affecting solute transport. Curatola et al. reported lower urea and creatinine clearances in the sitting as compared with the supine position (128). Fukodome et al. observed higher portal blood flows in CAPD patients in the supine position, suggesting more efficient mass transport of small solute with the patient supine (129). Schoenfeld et al. recently reported significantly higher KoA's in the supine position than in the standing position (117). Because the available information is limited and not all studies have confirmed these findings (130), further study is necessary.

AUTOMATED PD IN THE TREATMENT OF ACUTE RENAL FAILURE

PD was first used in the treatment of acute renal failure (ARF) and for many decades was the only method available. The availability of HD, and more recently of continuous arteriovenous hemofiltration (CAVH) and hemodialysis (CAVHD) has resulted in decreased utilization of PD

in most centers (131). Several advantages of PD, however, make it attractive for the therapy of ARF. PD can be performed in most hospital settings with a modicum of equipment or technical knowledge. Adequate access can be obtained at the bedside or in the surgical suite in a matter of minutes. Steady physiological state can be maintained without drastic changes in blood pressure, intravascular volume or body chemistries. Systemic anticoagulation is not required and blood loss is eliminated. A continuous infusion of glucose is provided through the absorption of glucose from dialysate. All of these features are desirable in the care of the patient with ARF who is often post-surgical, debilitated, malnourished and hemodynamically unstable.

Acute PD can also be used to correct electrolytic abnormalities in the post-surgical patient. Hypercalcemia can be easily corrected with the use of calcium-free dialysate. Severe metabolic acidosis can be treated by dialyzing with appropriately modified solutions which are available for IV use (i.e., 5% dextrose in one-half normal saline with added bicarbonate) or the treatment of metabolic alkalosis using 5% dextrose in normal saline. Acute PD offers definite advantages in patients at high risk for systemic anticoagulation or with thrombocytopenia secondary to heparin. Intraperitoneal heparin is recommended to avoid catheter obstruction from fibrin strands, but the use of intraperitoneal heparin does not result in systemic heparinization (132, 133). Finally, acute PD can be performed on the general medical ward or in the intensive care area with minimal training of the nursing personnel in contradistinction to methods requiring extracorporeal circulation.

The disadvantages of PD in the treatment of ARF must be considered as well. PD is relatively inefficient in removing small molecules as compared to HD or CAVHD. Patients who are septic, suffering from multiple trauma or post-surgical are usually hypercatabolic and in need of very efficient dialysis and aggressive nutrition. Although small solute clearance can be manipulated with the use of increased dialysate flows and higher volume exchanges, constant monitoring of the patient's nitrogenous waste product concentrations is essential and the institution of PD early in the course of ARF is recommended. Particular caution is necessary in patients who are immunocompromised in order to avoid peritonitis and additional co-morbid factors to a patient who is already critical. The presence of intraabdominal masses, intestinal ileus, pleuroperitoneal communications and abdominal drainages complicate fluid dynamics and may make PD impossible. Recent gastrointestinal or aortic surgery are also relative contraindications to the use of acute PD because of possible infection.

Multiple studies comparing loss of residual renal function (RRF) among HD and PD patients suggest that renal function is better preserved with PD. Among the many reasons proposed for this difference, the avoidance of drastic changes in intravascular volume, changes in solute concentrations and lower cytokine-mediated nephrotoxicity

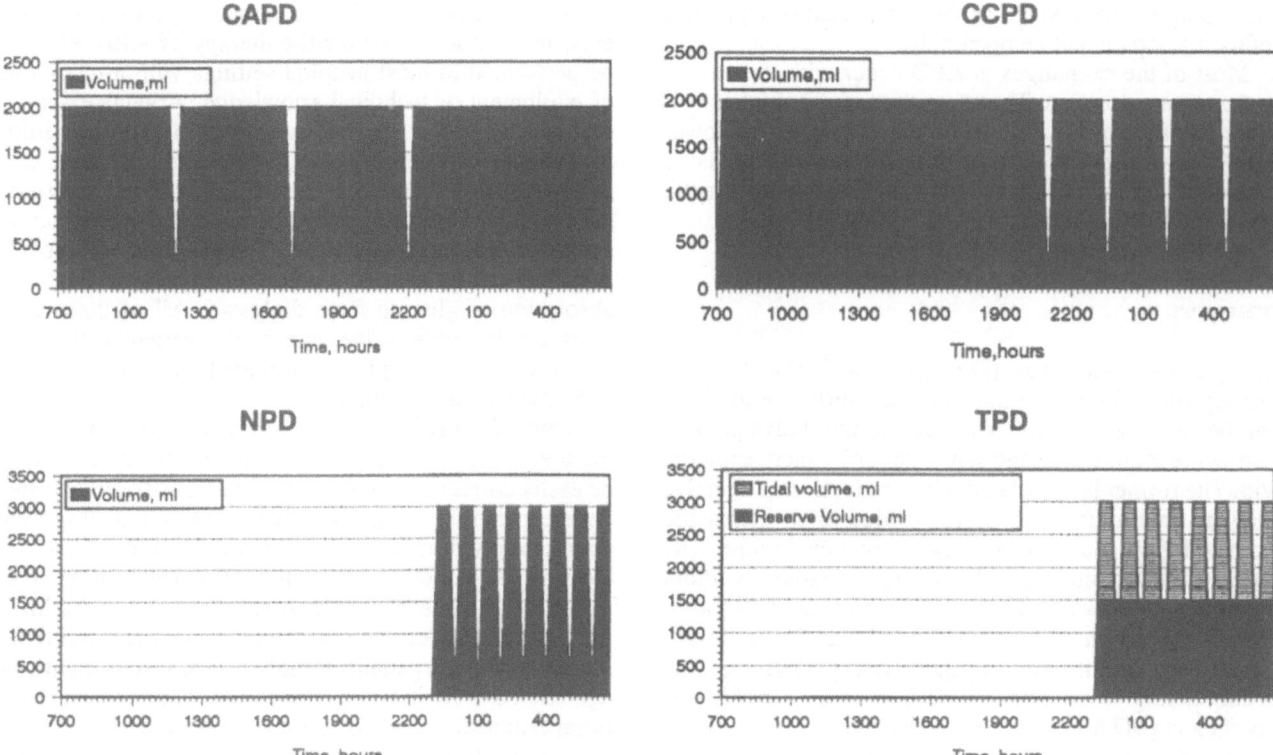

Figure 3. Dialysate flow patterns for CAPD, CCPD, NPD and TPD.

are most often quoted. Similar arguments can be made to propose PD for the treatment of ARF in an attempt to foster recovery of renal function.

Intermittent PD (IPD)

APD with the use of cyclers has many advantages over the manual infusion of dialysate into the peritoneal cavity for the treatment of ARF. A considerable reduction in the cost of delivery of therapy is achieved by minimizing nursing supervision with the use of APD. Modern systems have also reduced the incidence of peritonitis and have improved record keeping regarding fluid balance. Modern cyclers are capable of delivering IPD, TPD or CCPD in a simple manner with minimal human involvement.

The clinical experience with IPD in the treatment of ARF is extensive and has shown similar results to those obtained with HD (134, 135). The mortality rate in various series has been comparable of that of HD and the control of biochemical parameters has been acceptable, except in cases of extreme hypercatabolism. UF can be easily manipulated by varying the osmolality of the solution and the length of the dialysis exchanges.

Acute peritoneal access is usually much easier to obtain in small children than blood access, and hemodynamic fluctuations are easier to prevent with PD. A recent study on cost analysis of dialysis and modality of therapy for pediatric ARF revealed that APD provided good control of electrolyte imbalance and fluid overload while the cost was about one-third of that of HD and one-quarter of the cost of CAVHD (136).

Continuous equilibration PD (CEPD)

CEPD is a low-flow, continuous system that maintains stable levels of nitrogenous waste products and a steady hydration status similar to CAPD (137–140). Use of a cycler to administer dialysate exchanges is used instead of the manual exchanges of CAPD. A typical dialysis schedule for an adult consists of 2-liter dialysate exchanges using standard solutions for a total length of two to four hours. Variable UF can be achieved by adjusting the dialysate dextrose concentration and the length of dialysate dwell.

CEPD achieves lower small solute clearances than IPD because of the lower dialysate flows (141). However, its continuous nature is beneficial in hemodynamically unstable patients and provides higher clearances of larger molecules (142). UF can be programmed to accommodate the high UF needs of those patients requiring hyperalimentation, systemic antibiotic therapy and other high volume intravenous infusions. Because of the relatively low efficiency in clearing small solutes, CEPD should be initiated early in the course of ARF. Conversely, the patient can be aggressively dialyzed with IPD using high flows, followed by CEPD once the patient has stabilized.

AUTOMATED PD IN THE TREATMENT OF CHRONIC RENAL FAILURE

The incidence of treated end-stage renal disease (ESRD) has continued to increase worldwide during the past two decades (143). The main factors influencing this growth are the earlier diagnosis and treatment of uremia, the advancing age of the population, improved longevity of diabetic patients and advances in dialytic therapy. During the 1980's, the use of CAPD and CCPD showed a rapid increase. CCPD and other modalities of APD comprised a minuscule proportion of the ESRD population initially, but the growth has accelerated during the past few years in some countries. In the USA, the use of CCPD increased rapidly during the second half of the 1980's and now accounts for more than 10% of total PD population (144). The large majority of infants and younger pediatric patients undergo some type of APD. Similarly, APD is being used for the treatment of those requiring nursing home placement or constant help in performing the dialytic procedure by relatives. According to Viglino et al., 42% of home PD patients require the assistance of a partner (145). Likewise, 20% of all CAPD patients and one-third of the elderly in the USA need partner assistance (146).

The fastest growing segment of the ESRD population is diabetics (147). Multiple features of PD have made it a popular selection of therapy for diabetics. The proportion of diabetics in the ESRD population has grown from less than 10% in the 1970's to more than 30% in most industrialized nations in the 1990's. Better preservation of RRF with PD, improved control of glycemia and elimination of insulin injections, minimal fluctuations in intravascular volume, blood pressure and biochemical parameters, have increased the interest in PD for the treatment of diabetics. The high incidence of diabetic neuropathy and blindness has forced many diabetics to choose or transfer to APD in order to secure partner assistance.

The third major group of patients selecting APD are those gainfully employed and unable or unwilling to perform manual exchanges in the midst of a busy day, and full-time students. A common motivation of the latter is the improved self-image afforded by therapy in the privacy of their homes and the freedom to socialize for extended periods of time.

APD has been proposed for patients selecting or requiring PD, but plagued by frequent infections. Although the incidence of peritonitis with CCPD has been most favorable in most adult series, this indication should become infrequent in view of the improved results observed with disconnect CAPD systems.

Perhaps the most neglected but important indications for APD are inadequate dialysis and intolerance of high IAP. The improved longevity of CAPD patients has increased the proportion of anuric individuals who require higher solute removal and UF. The limitations of CAPD, combined with the undesirability of increasing the volume and number of manual exchanges has favored the growth of APD.

Intermittent PD (IPD)

IPD typically uses short exchanges with volumes of 2 to 3 liters, hourly dialysate flows of 2 to 6 liters, sessions lasting 8 to 10 hours and alternate day frequency. The total dialysate volume required to accomplish similar clearances to CAPD or CCPD is significantly higher, adding to the cost of therapy. The clearance of larger solutes with IPD is low as compared to CAPD/CCPD since it is mostly dependent on peritoneal surface area and time of contact between dialysate and the peritoneal membrane. Furthermore, IPD is an intermittent therapy and does not maintain the desirable steady physiologic state of CPD.

This therapy is seldom used today and is mostly reserved for patients with RRF, requiring supplemental dialysis; institutionalized patients; those with rapid peritoneal transport rates, incapable of achieving adequate UF with the longer exchanges of CAPD/CCPD, but enjoying higher rates of small solute removal; and, for patients mostly requiring UF due to extracellular fluid excess.

Peritonitis rates have been historically low with IPD. With the use of cyclers the peritonitis rate of IPD has been reported to be 0.14 episodes per year (148). Possible reasons for this low incidence of peritonitis are the lower number of connections and the rest period between procedures, favoring repopulation of peritoneal macrophages and its necessary immunoglobulins to combat infection (149). Catheter exit site infections are also lower and catheter life longer, probably a consequence of less trauma to the catheter anchor point during intermittent use. Catheter outflow obstruction has been reported to be higher than with continuous modalities of PD since catheter migration and omental wrapping of the catheter are more prone to occur when the peritoneal cavity is empty.

Although no controlled studies comparing the longevity of the peritoneal membrane between IPD and CAPD/CCPD have been performed, the reported incidence of UF failure and peritoneal sclerosis is low among large populations undergoing IPD. The intermittent, rather than constant, insult resulting from physical trauma during dialysate infusion, cytotoxic effects from plasticizers, acid and hypertonic solutions, and fewer infection rates may be responsible for these observations. A period of rest from temporary discontinuation of dialysis has been associated with restitution of normal peritoneal functional performance among CAPD patients suffering from UF failure (150). Thus, it is possible that the periodic rest provided by IPD allows sufficient time to partially heal peritoneal structures.

Nocturnal PD (NPD)

NPD is a variant of IPD used nightly or daily. The typical prescription for adults is a 2 to 3 liter exchange/hour for a total duration of 8 to 10 hours. Although the accumulation of extracellular fluid and the concentration of nitrogenous waste products steadily increase during the non-dialytic period, the fluctuations are lower than with IPD or HD. The complication rates and cost are similar to IPD.

The main indication for NPD is a state of high peritoneal transport. Adequate UF is possible as long as a reasonably high osmotic gradient can be maintained between dialysate and plasma. This can be easily determined by the use of the Peritoneal Equilibration Test (PET). Most patients with PET values within 2 standard deviations from the mean can remain on NPD. Due to the fast equilibration of small solutes, adequate peritoneal clearances can be obtained with the short, frequent exchanges of NPD in these patients.

In a small number of patients, a rapid peritoneal transport state has been observed prior to development of peritoneal sclerosis (151). Therefore, it is imperative to monitor these patients' peritoneal function with periodic PET's or other functional measures of peritoneal performance.

Continuous cycling PD (CCPD)

CCPD provides continuous PD in an automatic manner (31, 152). A variable number of exchanges are provided automatically with the use of a cycler over a period of 10 hours during the night, followed by a long diurnal exchange left in the abdomen during the day.

The shorter cycles of CCPD generally end before complete equilibration of small solutes is achieved, slightly reducing their clearance with similar dialysate flows as compared with CAPD. However, higher clearances of small solutes can be accomplished by increasing the flow by either adding exchanges or by increasing the exchange volume (Vip). The clearance of larger molecules is mostly dependent on time and peritoneal effective surface area and therefore is the same in CAPD and CCPD regardless of dialysate flow.

Some complications have been observed to occur less frequently than with CAPD. Peritonitis rates in adults have been relatively low since the inception of CCPD, regardless of the type of connectors or solutions used (33, 153, 154). *In-vitro* and clinical experiences suggest that the main reason for the lower rate of peritonitis is the direction of flow following a disconnection (155, 156). The first event to occur when the system is opened is outflow of spent dialysate. Verger and Luzar have demonstrated that this flush-before-fill is capable of eradicating most common contaminants with low adhesiveness such as Staph. epidermidis which accounts for most instances of peritonitis (155). The introduction of CAPD Y-sets has confirmed this hypothesis by significantly lowering the peritonitis rates for CAPD (157–160).

The long diurnal cycle of CCPD may also contribute to the prevention of peritonitis by allowing repopulation of the resident peritoneal macrophage population. We have observed a higher concentration of peritoneal cells during the long dwell of CCPD (43). Vlaanderen et al. have reported increased opsonic activity and IgG levels with prolonged dwell times (149). The number of phagocytes was also observed to increase with longer dwell times. Another factor that influences macrophage phagocytic activity is the dextrose concentration which is an indirect function of dwell time. De Fijter and coworkers demonstrated a depression of peritoneal macrophage phagocytic function with higher glucose concentrations (161). These macrophages exposed to high glucose concentrations were also less able to mount a respiratory burst. Since during the prolonged daytime dwell, the glucose concentrations in the peritoneal fluid fall to lower levels in CCPD than during the shorter dwells of CAPD, it is conceivable that macrophage function would be enhanced.

Other potential factors contributing to a lower rate of peritonitis are the reduced number of connections between the peritoneal catheter and the bags, the fact that all connections occur at one time and in a controlled environment, and that partners are often available for assistance. The latter is probably important in cases of visual and motor impairment and with children.

The incidence of catheter exit site infections has been similar to CAPD in most series. Burkart et al. reported a lower rate of peritonitis among patients using disconnect techniques such as Y-set CAPD and CCPD, but no difference in the incidence of exit site infections (162). However, Holley et al. observed the lowest rate of exit site infections among CCPD patients, followed by patients on CAPD Y-sets and those on standard CAPD (0.5, 0.8 and 1.2 episodes/patient-year, respectively) (163). The incidence of peritonitis was also lower for the disconnect systems.

Complications arising from increased IAP are also lower with CCPD. The CCPD prescription should be modified for patients at high risk for these complications by reducing the diurnal Vip by 25 to 35% since the IAP tends to be highest during the day when the patient is more likely to be standing or sitting. Elimination of the diurnal cycle is not recommended since it will significantly reduce the clearance of larger molecules and also result in intermittent therapy (NPD).

CCPD is the most commonly used modality of therapy for infants and small children in many countries. It is also popular among elderly and debilitated patients requiring assistance. In our experience, where all modalities of PD are equally offered to all patients, CCPD is often selected by students and actively employed patients. These groups benefit from the freedom from procedures CCPD provides during the day. Finally, the need for higher small solute clearances in larger patients and those with little or no RRF favor the use of CCPD and other automated modalities of PD (107, 164).

Although the optimal dose of PD has not been determined, the consensus of opinion, based on a wealth of clinical data, is that a minimum KT/Vurea of 0.25 per day should be provided in order to maintain a positive nitrogen balance and prevent uremic complications. While most patients starting dialysis have enough RRF to assure a total KT/Vurea exceeding 0.25 while on CAPD with four, 2-liter exchanges, most patients lose their RRF after three years and require significant modification of their PD prescription. Additional manual exchanges are not always possible or well accepted by patients on CAPD and increase in Vip during the day usually results in discomfort or complications. The logical alternatives under these circumstances are to increase Vip at night or to transfer to APD (also see hybrid systems).

Tidal PD (TPD)

The technique of TPD maintains a constant reserve volume (RV) of dialysis solution in the peritoneal cavity at all times and an additional tidal volume (TV) of dialysate which is intermittently cycled into and out of the peritoneal cavity. The RV is always in contact with the peritoneal membrane while the TV theoretically contributes to adequate mixing of the dialysate and restoration of the dialysate/plasma gradient which enhances peritoneal clearances. The technique uses a modified cycler which is regulated by volume rather than time.

Early reports suggested higher small solute clearances, surpassing those obtained with CAPD or CCPD (35, 37, 38). The likely explanation proposed for this phenomenon was a better mixing of dialysate and elimination of the unstirred layers between dialysate and plasma. However, recent reports suggest that the improved clearances were a function of higher exchange volumes (3 liters instead of the traditional 2 liters used for CAPD) rather than related to the tidal technique per se (116, 117, 165). Several clinical studies have confirmed that these differences in small solute clearances are the result of the higher Vip's used with TPD (127, 165–167).

During periods of high peritoneal dialysate flows, TPD has the advantage of eliminating the nondialytic period required for infusion and drainage of dialysate. The main disadvantages of this procedure are the need for a special volume controlled cycler and the very high dialysate flows which significantly increase the cost of therapy.

Hybrid systems

Hybrid systems based on CAPD and CCPD technology are undergoing clinical testing. These modalities of therapy have been designed to enhance clearance of small solutes for patients with large body mass and little or no RRF. The PD Plus system (Fresenius USA, Walnut Creek, CA) uses a simple, inexpensive cycler to provide

3 of 4 large volume exchanges during the night and a last exchange in the morning of 1.5 to 2.0 liters. A manual exchange is effected during the day using another 1.5 to 2.0 liters. Assuming three 3-liter Vip's at night and two 1.5-liter exchanges during the day, a total dialysate flow of 12 liters is used. However, the larger Vip's at night and the avoidance of long dwell times (exceeding equilibration time) maximize solute transport. The additional cost of dialysate is reduced by: 1) utilizing larger dialysate containers, 2) an inexpensive cycling device, and 3) reusing one of the empty dialysate bags for drainage of the first diurnal exchange. The main disadvantage of the system is the imposition of a manual exchange during the day.

CLINICAL EXPERIENCES

The clinical experience with CCPD is similar to that of CAPD in terms of maintenance of biochemical and hematologic parameters and mortality. The experience with selected complications such as peritonitis and IAP-related complications have been reviewed under the specific modalities. The management of certain population cohorts with APD deserves further discussion since APD either offers specific advantages or requires modification of therapy.

Patient selection, indications and contraindications

The specific advantages of the various modalities of APD have been discussed. In general, APD is favored whenever a partner is required, high dialysate flows are indicated or freedom from dialytic procedures is desired. Other advantages of APD are the lower IAP generated with similar volumes of dialysate as in CAPD with the patient supine and the lower rates of peritonitis observed with certain modalities. The few absolute contraindications for APD are: abnormally high or low peritoneal solute transport rates that will interfere with adequate solute removal and ultrafiltration; obliteration of the peritoneal cavity from adhesions or masses, interfering with dialysate flow; and, pleuroperitoneal or cutaneoperitoneal communications, causing leakage of dialysate.

Management of the diabetic patient

A large proportion of the adult APD population is diabetics. The main reasons for selection of APD are the frequent need for assistance due to blindness or peripheral neuropathy and unstable hemodynamics. Intraperitoneal insulin (ip) administration can achieve adequate glycemic control in most patients undergoing PD and has the following advantages: it provides a continuous infusion of insulin, similar to an insulin pump; eliminates all injections; and results in a more gradual and prolonged appearance of free insulin in the peripheral circulation.

The main disadvantages are: potential contamination of the dialysate during addition of insulin to the bags; the higher cost of additional insulin, since unabsorbed insulin is lost in the dialysate and some is absorbed in the bags; the occasional observation of hepatic subcapsular steatosis, and the potential for fibroblastic proliferation (168–170). After more than one decade experience with ip insulin administration in approximately 500 diabetic patients, we are pleased with diabetic control and have not observed any significant deleterious effects resulting from this practice. Preservation of peritoneal transport in our diabetic patients has not differed from nondiabetics, and the peritonitis rates have been similar between patients receiving ip insulin and those who do not. Glycemic control can be adequately maintained with subcutaneous injections, ip administration or insulin pumps. The patient's predilection and the medical team's expertise should be the main factor in the selection of therapy.

It is possible and relatively simple to control glycemia among patients on CCPD. However, dose adjustment through frequent monitoring is critical. Most patients require 50% of the dose during the day time and 50% for the nocturnal exchanges. The final total dose of insulin is usually two to three times the previous dose of injected insulin required for adequate control. We start with twice the total dose divided equally between the diurnal hypertonic bag and the nocturnal bags. Adjustments are made according to blood sugar concentrations determined four times per day and the number of hypertonic exchanges required. With this practice, the incidence of hypoglycemic reactions at night has been very infrequent and only 10% of patients have needed supplemental insulin injections.

Diabetic patients receiving IPD, NPD, TPD and other forms of intermittent PD are best managed with subcutaneous insulin injections and supplemental ip insulin to counteract the glucose load resulting from dialysate glucose absorption. The ip insulin dose must be adjusted according to the glucose concentration in the solution.

Management of the pediatric patient

The specific treatment of uremic children is discussed in another section.

Management of the geriatric patient

APD is being used more frequently among the very old because of the simplicity of care for patients in nursing homes and those who remain under the care of their families but require assistance with procedures (171–174). Despite the additional cost of supplies and equipment APD may prove cost effective for the elderly since it eliminates the high cost of transportation to dialysis centers, nursing homes or even hospitalization in some instances. The expanding geriatric population suffering from ESRD

has generated several reviews on this subject (171, 173, 175).

COST CONSIDERATIONS

The higher cost of therapy has affected the growth of APD and reserved it for special indications. The proportion of patients treated with APD varies significantly around the world depending on the national health structure and economy. Many centers of excellence use CAPD almost exclusively because of the lower cost (176). However, the cost of CAPD varies widely according to the specific system used, and the total cost of therapy is proportional with the incidence and severity of the complications. King et al. analyzed the total cost of CAPD and CCPD in the United Kingdom including the cost of treating infectious complications, supplies, cycler rental and maintenance (177). No significant differences were noted between the two modalities when total cost was considered.

The cost of APD can be effectively reduced by using larger dialysate containers, reutilizing tubing sets and by purchasing simple and reliable cyclers (39, 41). These practices have reduced the cost of care significantly without compromising the quality of care nor increasing the incidence of peritonitis.

REFERENCES

1. Ganter G: Ueber die Beseitigung giftiger Stoffe aus dem Blute durch Dialyse. *Munch Med Wochschr* 70–II: 1478, 1923
2. Rosenak S, Siwon P: Experimentelle Untersuchungen über die Peritoneale Ausscheidung harnpflichtiger Substanzen aus dem Blute. *Mitt a d Grenzgeb d Med u Chir* 39: 391, 1926
3. Heusser H, Werder H: Untersuchungen über Peritonealdialyse. *Bruns Beiträge z klin Chir* 141: 38, 1927
4. Bliss S, Kastler AO, Nadler SB: Peritoneal lavage. Effective elimination of nitrogenous wastes in the absence of kidney function. *Proc Soc Exp Biol Med* 29: 1078, 1932
5. Haam VE, Fine A: Effect of peritoneal lavage in acute uremia. *Proc Soc Exp Biol Med* 30: 396, 1932
6. Balázs J, Rosenak S: Zur Behandlung der Sublimaturie durch peritoneale Dialyse. *Wien Med Wochnschr* 47: 851, 1934
7. Wear JB, Sisk IR, Trinkle AJ: Peritoneal lavage in the treatment of uremia. *J Urol* 39: 53, 1938
8. Rhoads JE: Peritoneal lavage in the treatment of renal insufficiency. *Am J Med Sci* 196: 642, 1938
9. Abbott WE, Shea P: The treatment of temporary renal insufficiency by peritoneal lavage. *Am J Med Sci* 211: 312, 1946
10. Frank HA, Seligman AM, Fine J: Further experiences with peritoneal irrigation for acute renal failure. *Ann Surg* 128: 561, 1948
11. Odel HM, Ferris DO, Power MH: Peritoneal lavage as an effective means of extrarenal excretion. A clinical appraisal. *Am J Med* 9: 63, 1950

12. Grollman A, Turner LB, McLean JA: Intermittent peritoneal lavage in nephrectomized dogs and its application to the human being. *Arch Intern Med* 87: 379, 1951

13. Legrain M, Merrill JP: Short-term continuous transperitoneal dialysis: A simplified technique. *N Engl J Med* 248: 125, 1953

14. Ascari S, Morales P, Hotchkiss RS: Peritoneal dialysis. *NY State J Med* 59: 1981, 1959

15. Doolan PD, Murphy WP, Wiggins RA et al.: An evaluation of intermittent peritoneal lavage. *Am J Med* 26: 831–44, 1959

16. Maxwell MH, Rockney RE, Kleeman CR, Twiss MR: Peritoneal dialysis. I. Technique and applications. *JAMA* 170: 917, 1959

17. Boen ST: Kinetics of peritoneal dialysis. *Medicine* (Baltimore) 40: 243, 1961

18. Tenckhoff H, Ward G, Boen ST: The influence of dialysate volume and flow rate on peritoneal clearance. *Proc Eur Dial Transpl Assoc* 2: 113, 1965

19. Tenckhoff H, Schilipetar G, Boen ST: One year experience with home peritoneal dialysis. *Trans Am Soc Artif Intern Organs* 11: 11, 1965

20. Boen ST, Mulinari AS, Dillard DH, Scribner BH: Periodic peritoneal dialysis in the management of chronic uremia. *Trans Am Soc Artif Intern Organs* 8: 256, 1962

21. Lasker N, McCauley EP, Passarotti CT: Chronic peritoneal dialysis. *Trans Am Soc Artif Intern Organs* 12: 94, 1966

22. Tenckhoff H, Weston B, Shilipetar G: A simplified automatic peritoneal dialysis system. *Trans Am Soc Artif Intern Organs* 18: 436, 1972

23. Kabei N, Kolff WJ, Foux A: Evaluation of hollow-fiber reverse osmosis permeators for use in peritoneal dialysis. *Dial Transpl* 6: 59, 1977

24. Petersen NJ, Carson LA, Favero MS: Microbiological quality of water in an automatic peritoneal dialysis system. *Dial Transpl* 6: 38, 1977

25. Gutman RA, Shelburne JD: An outbreak of cryptogenic peritonitis: implications for reverse osmosis production of biologically safe water. *Dial Transpl* 6: 35, 1977

26. Karanicolas S, Oreopoulos DG, Pylypchuk G et al.: Home peritoneal dialysis: three years' experience in Toronto. *Can Med Assoc J* 116: 226, 1977

27. Diaz-Buxo JA, Chandler JT, Farmer CD, Smith DL: Chronic peritoneal dialysis at home – a comparison with hemodialysis. *Trans Am Soc Artif Intern Organs* 23: 191, 1977

28. Gutman RA: Automated peritoneal dialysis for home use. *Q J Med* 47: 261, 1978

29. Furman KI, Koornhof HJ, Frizelle K, Block C, VanWyck H, Allcock R: Unsafe automatic peritoneal dialysis in Johannesburg. (Abstract) *Kidney Int* 16: 86, 1979

30. Diaz-Buxo JA, Walker PJ, Farmer CD, Chandler JT, Holt KL, Cox P: Continuous cyclic peritoneal dialysis (CCPD). *Trans Am Soc Artif Intern Organs* 27: 51, 1981

31. Diaz-Buxo JA, Farmer CD, Walker PJ, Chandler JT, Holt KL: Continuous cyclic peritoneal dialysis–a preliminary report. *Artif Organs* 5: 157, 1981

32. Nakagawa D, Price C, Stinebaugh B, Suki W: Continuous cyclic peritoneal dialysis: a viable option in the treatment of chronic renal failure. *Trans Am Soc Artif Intern Organs* 27: 55, 1981

33. Price C, Suki W: New modifications of peritoneal dialysis: Options in the treatment of patients with renal failure. *Am J Nephrol* 1: 97, 1981

34. Popovich RP, Moncrief JW, Decherd JF, Bomar JB, Pyle WK: The definition of a novel portable/wearable equilibrium peritoneal dialysis technique. (Abstract) *Trans Am Soc Artif Intern Organs* 5: 64, 1976

35. Stephen RL: Reciprocating peritoneal dialysis with a subcutaneous peritoneal catheter. *Dial Transplant* 7: 834, 1978

36. Miller JH, Blumenkrantz MJ, Lewin AJ et al.: Optimizing low flow peritoneal dialysis. (Abstract) *Trans Am Soc Artif Intern Organs* 50, 1981

37. Twardowski Z, Nolph K, Khanna R et al.: Eight hr tidal peritoneal dialysis (TPD) matches 24 hr CAPD and surpasses 8 hr nightly intermittent peritoneal dialysis (NIPD) clearances (C). (Abstract) *Perit Dial Bull* 7: S79, 1987

38. Twardowski ZJ, Nolph KD, Khanna R et al.: Tidal peritoneal dialysis. in *Ambulatory Peritoneal Dialysis*, edited by Avram MM, Giordano C, New York, Plenum Publishing Corporation, 1990, p 145

39. Diaz-Buxo JA, Burgess WP, Farmer CD, Chandler JT, Walker PJ, Adcock A: Multiple tubing set (MTS) – making CCPD safe, simple and cost effective. (Abstract) *Perit Dial Bull* 7: S22, 1987

40. Strauss FG: CAPD connector technology. in *Dialysis Therapy*, 2nd Ed, edited by Nissenson AR, Fine RN, Philadelphia, Hanley & Belfus Inc, 1992, p 61

41. Wadhwa NK, Cabralda T, Suh H, Stratos J, Cascio C, Young N: Multiple use of cycler set in cycler peritoneal dialysis. in *Advances in Peritoneal Dialysis*, edited by Khanna R, Nolph KD, Prowant BF, Twardowski ZJ, Oreopoulos DG, Toronto, University of Toronto Press, 1992, p 192

42. Diaz-Buxo JA, Walker PJ, Farmer CD, Chandler JT, Holt KL: Continuous cyclic peritoneal dialysis (CCPD). (Abstract) *Kidney Int* 19: 145, 1981

43. Diaz-Buxo JA: Continuous ambulatory and continuous cycling peritoneal dialysis. in *Peritoneal Dialysis*, edited by La Greca G, Chiaramonte S, Fabris A, Feriani M, Ronco C, Milan, Wichtig Editore, 1985, p 257

44. Bruno M, Bagnis C, Marangella M, Rovera L, Cantaluppi A, Linari F: CAPD with an amino acid dialysis solution: a long-term, cross-over study. *Kidney Int* 35: 1189, 1989

45. Renzo S, Beatrice D, Giuseppe I: CAPD in diabetics: use of amino acids. in *Advances in Peritoneal Dialysis*, edited by Khanna R, Nolph KD, Prowant BF, Twardowski ZJ, Oreopoulos DG, Toronto, University of Toronto Press, 1989, p 12

46. Park MS, Heimbürger O, Bergström J, Waniewski J, Werynski A, Lindholm B: Peritoneal transport during dialysis with amino acid-based solutions. *Perit Dial Int* 13: 280, 1993

47. Hanning RM, Balfe JW, Zlotkin SH: Effectiveness and nutritional consequences of amino acid-based *vs* glucose-based dialysis solutions in infants and children receiving CAPD. *Am J Clin Nutr* 46: 22, 1987

48. Steinhauer HB, Lubrich-Birker I, Kluthe R, Hörl WH, Schollmeyer P: Amino acid dialysate stimulates peritoneal prostaglandin E$_2$ generation in humans. in *Advances in Peritoneal Dialysis*, edited by Khanna R, Nolph KD, Prowant BF, Twardowski ZJ, Oreopoulos DG, Toronto, University of Toronto Press, 1988, p 21

49. Young GA, Dibble JB, Taylor AE, Kendall S, Brownjohn AM: A longitudinal study of the effect of amino acid-based CAPD fluid on amino acid retention and protein losses. *Nephrol Dial Transplant* 4: 900, 1989

50. de Fijter CWH, Verbrugh HA, Oe LP et al.: Biocompatibility of a glucose-polymer-containing peritoneal dialysis fluid. *Am J Kidney Dis* 21: 411, 1993

51. Mistry CD, Gokal R: Single daily overnight (12-h dwell) use of 7.5% glucose polymer (Mw 18 700; Mn 7300) + 0.35% glucose solution: a 3-month study. *Nephrol Dial Transplant* 8: 443, 1993

52. Stein A, Peers E, Harris K, Feehally J, Walls J: Glucose polymer for ultrafiltration failure in CAPD. *Lancet* 341: 1159, 1993

53. Shen FH, Sherrard DJ, Scollard D, Merritt A, Curtis FK: Thirst, relative hypernatremia, and excessive weight gain in maintenance peritoneal dialysis. *Trans Am Soc Artif Intern Organs* 24: 142, 1978

54. Nolph KD, Sorkin ML, Moore H: Autoregulation of sodium and potassium removed during continuous ambulatory peritoneal dialysis. *Trans Am Soc Artif Intern Organs* 26: 334, 1980

55. Nolph KD, Parker A: The composition of dialysis solutions for continuous ambulatory peritoneal dialysis. in *Proceedings of the First International Symposium on CAPD*, edited by anonymous, Amsterdam, Excerpta medica, 1980, p 341

56. Parker A, Nolph KD: Magnesium and calcium net mass transfers during CAPD. *Trans Am Soc Artif Intern Organs* 26: 194, 1980

57. Frifelt JJ, Pedersen FB: CAPD using a high calcium concentration. in *Frontiers in Peritoneal Dialysis*, edited by Maher JF, Winchester JF, New York, Field, Rich and Assoc, 1986, p 265

58. Oreopoulos DG, Robson M, Faller B: Continuous ambulatory peritoneal dialysis: A new era in the treatment of chronic renal failure. *Clin Nephrol* 11: 125, 1979

59. Kwong MBL, Lee JSK, Chan MK: Transperitoneal calcium and magnesium transfer during an 8-hour dialysis. *Perit Dial Bull* 7: 85, 1987

60. Delmez JA: Bone and mineral metabolism in continuous ambulatory peritoneal dialysis. in *Contemporary Issues in Nephrology*, edited by Twardowski ZJ, Nolph KD, Khanna R, New York, Churchill Livingstone, 1990, p 191

61. Martis L, Serkes KD, Nolph KD: Calcium carbonate as a phosphate binder: is there a need to adjust peritoneal dialysate calcium concentrations for patients using $CaCO_3$?. *Perit Dial Int* 9: 325, 1989

62. Hamdy NAT, Boletis J, Charlesworth D et al.: Low calcium dialysate increase the tolerance to vitamin D in peritoneal dialysis. *Contrib Nephrol* 89: 190, 1991

63. Cunningham J, Beer J, Coldwell RD et al.: Dialysate calcium reduction in CAPD patients treated with calcium carbonate and alfacalcidol. *Nephrol Dial Transplant* 7: 63, 1992

64. Hutchison AJ, Merchant M, Boulton HF, Hinchcliffe R, Gokal R: Calcium and magnesium mass transfer in peritoneal dialysis patients using 1.25 mmol/L calcium, 0.25 mmol/L magnesium dialysis fluid. *Perit Dial Int* 13: 219, 1993

65. Montenegro J, Saracho R, Aguirre R, Martinez I: Calcium mass transfer in CAPD: the role of convective transport. *Nephrol Dial Transplant* 8: 1234, 1993

66. Cruz C, Schmidt R, Dumler F, VanDellen S, Duncan H, Kleerekoper M: Successful treatment of hypercalcemia and tumoral calcifications with calcium-free peritoneal dialysis. *Perit Dial Int* 12: 109, 1992

67. Gandhi VC, Ing TS, Jablokow JT et al.: Thickened peritoneal membrane in maintenance peritoneal dialysis patients. *Kidney Int* 14: 675, 1978

68. Vaziri ND, Ness R, Wellikson L, Barton C, Grup N: Bicarbonate buffered peritoneal dialysis – an effective adjunct in the treatment of lactic acidosis. *Am J Med* 67: 392, 1979

69. Vaziri ND, Warner AS: Peritoneal dialysis clearance of endogenous lactate. *J Dial* 3: 107, 1979

70. Gandhi VC, Humayun HM, Ing TS et al.: Sclerotic thickening of the peritoneal membrane in maintenance peritoneal dialysis. *Arch Intern Med* 140: 1201, 1980

71. Ing TS, Daugirdas JT, Gandhi VC: Peritoneal sclerosis in peritoneal dialysis patients. *Am J Nephrol* 4: 173, 1984

72. Nolph KD, Ryan L, Moore RH, Legrain M, Mion C, Oreopoulos DG: Factors affecting ultrafiltration in continuous ambulatory peritoneal dialysis. First report of an international cooperative study. *Perit Dial Bull* 4: 14, 1984

73. Faller B, Marichal JF: Loss of ultrafiltration in continuous ambulatory peritoneal dialysis: A role for acetate. *Perit Dial Bull* 4: 10, 1984

74. Dobbie JW, Zaki MA: The ultrastructure of the parietal peritoneum in normal and uremic man and in patients on CAPD. in *Frontiers in Peritoneal Dialysis*, edited by Maher JF, Winchester JF, New York, Field, Rich and Associates, 1986, p 3

75. Gallimore B, Gagnon RF, Stevenson MM: Cytotoxicity of commercial peritoneal dialysis solutions towards peritoneal cells of chronically uremic mice. *Nephron* 43: 283, 1986

76. Verbrug HA, Verkooyen RP, Verhoef J, Oe PL, van der Meulen J: Defective complement-mediated opsonization and lysis of bacteria in commercial peritoneal dialysis solution. in *Frontiers in Peritoneal Dialysis*, edited by Maher JF, Winchester JF, New York, Field, Rich and Associates, 1986, p 559

77. Van Bronswijk H, Verbrugh HA, Bos HJ: Cytotoxic effects of commercial continuous ambulatory peritoneal dialysis (CAPD) fluids and of bacterial exoproducts on human mesothelial cells *in vitro*. *Perit Dial Int* 9: 197, 1989

78. Manahan FJ, Ing BL, Chan JC: Effect of bicarbonate-containing *versus* lactate-containing peritoneal dialysis solutions on superoxide production by human neutrophils. *Artif Organs* 13: 495, 1989

79. Topley N, Mackenzie R, Petersen MM: *In vitro* testing of a potentially biocompatible continuous ambulatory peritoneal dialysis fluid. *Nephrol Dial Transplant* 6: 574, 1991

80. Jörres A, Jörres D, Topley N, Gahl GM, Mahiout A: Leukotriene release from peripheral and peritoneal leukocytes following exposure to solutions for peritoneal dialysis. *Nephrol Dial Transplant* 6: 495, 1991

81. Feriani M, Dissegna D, La Greca G, Passlick-Deetjen J: Short-term clinical study with bicarbonate-containing peritoneal dialysis solution. *Perit Dial Int* 13: 296, 1993

82. Veech RL: The untoward effects of the anions of dialysis fluid. *Kidney Int* 34: 587, 1988

83. Feriani M, Biasioli S, Borin D: Bicarbonate solutions for peritoneal dialysis. *Int J Artif Organs* 8: 57, 1985

84. Feriani M, Reinhard B, La Greca G: Calcium carbonate precipitation in oversaturated bicarbonate-containing CAPD solutions. in *Peritoneal Dialysis*, edited by La Greca G, Ronco C, Feriani M, Chiaramonte S, Conz P, Milan, Wichtig Editore, 1991, p 145

85. Yatzidis H: A new stable bicarbonate dialysis solution for peritoneal dialysis: Preliminary report. *Perit Dial Int* 11: 224, 1991

86. Yatzidis H: A new single bicarbonate CAPD solution. in *Peritoneal Dialysis*, edited by La Greca G, Ronco C, Feriani M, Chiaramonte S, Conz P, Milan, Wichtig Editore, 1991, p 151

87. Slingeneyer A, Faller B, Michel C, Pryzbylski C, Rolland R, Mion C: Increased ultrafiltration capacity using a new bicarbonate CAPD solution. (Abstract) *Perit Dial Int* 13: S57, 1993

88. Yatzidis H: Enhanced ultrafiltration in rabbits with bicarbonate glycylglycine peritoneal dialysis solution. *Perit Dial Int* 13: 302, 1993

89. Ing TS, Gandhi VC, Daugirdas JT, Hunt J, Quon MJ, Ropli S: Peritoneal dialysis using bicarbonate-containing dialysate produced by automated dialysate delivery machine. *Artif Organs* 6: 67, 1982

90. Mion CM, Mourad G, Canaud B: Maintenance dialysis: A survey of 17 years' experience in Languedoc-Roussillon with a comparison of methods in a standard population. *ASAIO J* 6: 205, 1983

91. Capelli JP, Camiscioli TC, Vallorani RD: Comparative analysis of survival on home hemodialysis, in-center hemodialysis and chronic peritoneal dialysis (CAPD-IPD) therapies. *Proc Eur Dial Transplant Assoc* 14: 38, 1985

92. Charytan C, Spinowitz BS, Galler M: A comparative study of continuous ambulatory peritoneal dialysis and center hemodialysis. *Arch Intern Med* 146: 1138, 1986

93. Burton PR, Walls J: Selection-adjusted comparison of life-expectancy of patients on continuous ambulatory peritoneal dialysis, haemodialysis, and renal transplantation. *Lancet* 1: 1115, 1987

94. Gokal R, Baillod R, Hunt L et al.: Multi-centre study on outcome of treatment in patients on continuous ambulatory peritoneal dialysis and haemodialysis. *Nephrol Dial Transplant* 2: 172, 1987

95. Gokal R, King J, Bogle S et al.: Outcome in patients on continuous ambulatory peritoneal dialysis and haemodialysis: 4-year analysis of a prospective multicentre study. *Lancet* 2: 1105, 1987

96. Posen G, Arbus G, Hutchinson T, Jeffery J: Survival comparison of adult non-diabetic patients treated with either hemodialysis or CAPD for end-stage renal failure. *Perit Dial Bull* 7: 78, 1987

97. Maiorca R, Vonesh E, Cancarini GC et al.: A six-year comparison of patient and technique survivals in CAPD and HD. *Kidney Int* 34: 518, 1988

98. Maiorca R, Cancarini G, Manili L et al.: CAPD is a first class treatment–results of an eight-year experience with a comparison of patient and method survival in CAPD and hemodialysis. *Clin Nephrol* 30: S3, 1988

99. Nolph KD: Comparison of continuous ambulatory peritoneal dialysis and hemodialysis. *Kidney Int* 33: S123, 1988

100. Piccoli G, Segoloni GP, Quarello F, Bonello F, Salomone M. CAPD in Italy: Data from two registries. in *Peritoneal Dialysis*, edited by La Greca G, Chiaramonte S, Fabris A, Feriani M, Ronco C, Milan, Wichtig Editore, 1988, p 217

101. Maiorca R, Cancarini GC, Camerini C et al.: Is CAPD competitive with haemodialysis for long-term treatment of uraemic patients? *Nephrol Dial Transplant* 4: 244, 1980

102. Diaz-Buxo JA: CAPD and hemodialysis-pride and prejudice. (editorial) *Perit Dial Int* 10: 5, 1990

103. Serkes KD, Blagg CR, Nolph KD, Vonesh EF, Shapiro F: Comparison of patient and technique survival in continuous ambulatory peritoneal dialysis (CAPD) and hemodialysis: A multicenter study. *Perit Dial Int* 10: 15, 1990

104. Wolfe RA, Port FK, Hawthorne VM et al.: A comparison of survival among dialytic therapies of choice: in-center hemodialysis *versus* continuous ambulatory dialysis at home. *Am J Kidney Dis* 15: 433, 1990

105. Disney APS: Dialysis in Australia, 1982 to 1988. *Am J Kidney Dis* 15: 402, 1990

106. Maiorca R, Vonesh EF, Cavalli PL et al.: A multicenter, selection-adjusted comparison of patient and technique survivals on CAPD and hemodialysis. *Perit Dial Int* 11: 118, 1991

107. Diaz-Buxo JA: Is CAPD adequate long-term therapy for ESRD? A critical assessment. (editorial review) *Am Soc Nephrol* 3: 1039, 1992

108. Keshaviah PR, Nolph KD, Van Stone JC: The peak concentration hypothesis: a urea kinetic approach to comparing the adequacy of continuous ambulatory peritoneal dialysis (CAPD) and hemodialysis. *Perit Dial Int* 9: 257, 1989

109. Gotch FA: Application of urea kinetic modeling to adequacy of CAPD therapy. in *Advances in Peritoneal Dialysis*, edited by Khanna R, Nolph KD, Prowant BF, Twardowski ZJ, Oreopoulos DG, Toronto, University of Toronto Press, 1990, p 178

110. Keshaviah P: Adequacy of CAPD: A quantitative approach. *Kidney Int* 42: S160, 1992

111. Gotch F, Gentile DE, Schoenfeld PY: CAPD prescription in current clinical practice. in *Advances in Peritoneal Dialysis*, edited by Khanna R, Nolph KD, Prowant BF, Twardowski ZJ, Oreopoulos DG, Toronto, University of Toronto Press, 1993, p 69

112. Gotloib LA, Garmizo L, Varak T, Mines M: Reduction of vital capacity due to increased intra-abdominal pressure during peritoneal dialysis. *Perit Dial Bull* 1: 63, 1981

113. Diaz-Buxo JA: CCPD is even better than CAPD. *Kidney Int* 28: S26, 1985

114. Twardowski ZJ, Prowant BF, Nolph KD, Martinez AJ, Lampton RN: High volume, low freqency continuous ambulatory peritoneal dialysis. *Kidney Int* 23: 64, 1983

115. Twardowski ZJ, Nolph KD, Khanna R et al.: Choice of peritoneal dialysis regimen based on peritoneal transfer rates. *Perit Dial Bull* 7: S79, 1987

116. Brandes J, Emerson P, Campbell D, Keshaviah P: The relationship between body size, fill volume and mass transfer area coefficient (MTAC) in PD. (Abstract) *Am Soc Nephrol* 3: 407, 1992

117. Schoenfeld P, Diaz-Buxo JA, Keen M, Gotch FA: The effect of body position (P), surface area (BSA), and

560   *Jose A. Diaz-Buxo*

intraperitoneal exchange volume (Vip) on the peritoneal transport constant (KoA). (Abstract) *Am Soc Nephrol* 4: 416, 1993

118. Twardowski ZJ: New approaches to intermittent peritoneal dialysis therapies. in *Peritoneal Dialysis*, edited by Nolph KD, Dordrecht, Kluwer Academic Publishers, 1989, p 133

119. Dobbie JW, Twardowski ZJ, Algrim C: Clinical evaluation of tidal PD (TPD) as a long-term dialysis therapy. (Abstract) *Perit Dial Int* 10: 50, 1990

120. Steinhauer HB, Keck I, Lubrich-Birkner I, Schollmeyer P: Increased dialysis efficiency in tidal peritoneal dialysis compared to intermittent peritoneal dialysis. *Nephron* 58: 500, 1991

121. Quellhorst E, Solf A, Hildebrand U: Tidal peritoneal dialysis (TPD) is superior to intermittent peritoneal dialysis (IPD) in long-term treatment of patients with chronic renal insufficiency (CRI). (Abstract) *Perit Dial Int* 11: 217, 1991

122. Lubrich-Birkner I, Wichary R, Schollmeyer P, Steinhauer HB: Ultrafiltration and solute clearances in tidal peritoneal dialysis (TPD) compared to intermittent peritoneal dialysis (IPD). (Abstract) *Perit Dial Int* 12: 138, 1992

123. Piraino B, Bernardini J, Bender F: Comparison of clearances (CL) on intermittent peritoneal dialysis (IPD) and tidal peritoneal dialysis (TPD). (Abstract) *Am Soc Nephrol* 2: 366, 1991

124. Flanigan MJ, Doyle C, Miller L: Tidal peritoneal dialysis: a pediatric experience. in *Advances in Peritoneal Dialysis*, edited by Khanna R, Nolph KD, Prowant BF, Twardowski ZJ, Oreopoulos DG, Toronto, University of Toronto Press, 1991, p 275

125. Doyle CL, Flanigan MJ, Mabe C: Tidal peritoneal dialysis *vs* continuous cyclic peritoneal dialysis: children's preference. *ANNA J* 19: 249, 1992

126. Aasarod K, Wideroe T, Flakne SC, Torgersen AK, Dahl K, Jorstad S: A comparison of solute and fluid transport between peritoneal dialysis (PD) strategies. *Perit Dial Int* 12: S10, 1992

127. Balaskas EV, Izatt S, Chu M, Oreopoulos DG: Tidal volume peritoneal dialysis *versus* intermittent peritoneal dialysis. in *Advances in Peritoneal Dialysis*, edited by Khanna R, Nolph KD, Prowant BF, Twardowski ZJ, Oreopoulos DG, Toronto, Multimed Inc, 1993, p 105

128. Curatola G, Zoccahi C, Cruccitti S, Siclani F, Maggionre Q: Effect of posture on peritoneal clearance. *Perit Dial Int* 8: 58, 1988

129. Fukudome Y, Ozawa K, Shoji T et al.: How is the portal vein flow in CAPD? Evaluation of postural change by colour flow-doppler ultrasound (CFDU). (Abstract) *Perit Dial Int* 12: S4, 1992

130. Otero A, Esteban J, Canovas L: Does posture modify solute transport in CAPD? (Correspondence) *Perit Dial Int* 12: 399, 1992

131. Ronco C: Continuous renal replacement therapies for the treatment of acute renal failure in intensive care patients. *Clin Nephrol* 40: 187, 1993

132. Furman KL, Gomperts ED, Hockley J: Activity of intraperitoneal heparin during peritoneal dialysis. *Clin Nephrol* 9: 15, 1978

133. Thayssen P, Pindborg T: Peritoneal dialysis and heparin. *Scand J Urol Nephrol* 12: 73, 1978

134. Stewart JH, Tuckwell LA, Sinnett PF, Edwards KDG, Whyte HM: Peritoneal and haemodialysis: A comparison of their morbidity and of their mortality suffered by dialysed patients. *Q J Med* 35: 406, 1966

135. Firmat J, Zucchini A: Peritoneal dialysis in acute renal failure. *Contrib Nephrol* 17: 33, 1979

136. Reznik VM, Randolph G, Collins CM, Peterson BM, Lemire JM, Mendoza SA: Cost analysis of dialysis modalities for pediatric acute renal failure. *Perit Dial Int* 13: 311, 1993

137. Katirzoglou A, Digenis G, Mayopoulou-Symvoulidis D, Zervaris D, Symvoulidis A, Komninos Z: Continuous equilibration peritoneal dialysis *versus* acute peritoneal dialysis. in *Advances in Peritoneal Dialysis*, edited by Gahl GM, Kessel M, Nolph KD, Amsterdam, Excerpta medica, 1981, p 122

138. Trevino-Becerra A, Munoz P, Avilez C: Equilibrium peritoneal dialysis (EPD) in acute renal failure (ARF) secondary to rhabdiomyolysis (sic). *Perit Dial Bull* 7: 244, 1987

139. Nolph KD: Continuous *versus* intermittent therapy for acute renal failure. *Trans Am Soc Artif Intern Organs* 34: 54–5, 1988

140. Steiner RW: Continuous equilibration peritoneal dialysis in acute renal failure. *Perit Dial Int* 9: 5, 1989

141. Nolph KD, Twardowski ZJ, Popovich RP: Equilibration of peritoneal dialysis solutions during long-dwell exchanges. *J Lab Clin Med* 93: 246, 1979

142. Moncrief JW, Nolph KD, Rubin J: Additional experience with continuous ambulatory peritoneal dialysis (CAPD). *Trans Am Soc Artif Intern Organs* 24: 476, 1978

143. USRDS 1993 Annual Data Report: International Comparisons of ESRD Therapy. *Am J Kidney Dis* 22: 85, 1993

144. USRDS 1993 Annual Data Report: Methods of ESRD Treatment. *Am J Kidney Dis* 22: 38, 1993

145. Viglino G, Grasso PG, Mariano F, Cavalli PL: Need of a partner on home peritoneal dialysis (HPD): incidence and an alternative choice. in *Advances in Peritoneal Dialysis*, edited by Khanna R, Nolph KD, Prowant BF, Twardowski ZJ, Oreopoulos DG, Toronto, University of Toronto Press, 1989, p 67

146. Nolph KD, Cutler SJ, Steinberg SM et al.: Special studies from the NIH USA CAPD Registry. *Perit Dial Bull* 1: 28, 1986

147. USRDS 1993 Annual Data Report: Incidence and causes of treated ESRD. *Am J Kidney Dis* 22: 30, 1993

148. Vas SI: Peritonitis. in *Peritoneal Dialysis*, 2nd Ed, edited by Nolph KD, Boston, Martinus Nijhoff Publishers, 1985, p 403

149. Vlaanderen K, de Fijter CW, Bos HJ et al.: The effect of dwell time on peritoneal phagocytic defense of chronic peritoneal dialysis patients. in *Advances in Peritoneal Dialysis*, edited by Khanna R, Nolph KD, Prowant BF, Twardowski ZJ, Oreopoulos DG, Toronto, University of Toronto Press, 1989, p 151

150. de Alvaro F, Castro MJ, Dapena F et al.: Peritoneal resting is beneficial in peritoneal hyperpermeability and ultrafiltration failure. in *Advances in Peritoneal Dialysis*, edited by Khanna R, Nolph KD, Prowant BF, Twardowski ZJ, Oreopoulos DG, Toronto, Multimed Inc, 1993, p 56

151. Diaz-Buxo JA: Peritoneal sclerosis in a woman on continuous cyclic peritoneal dialysis. *Semin Dial* 5: 317, 1992

152. Diaz-Buxo JA: Current status of CCPD. (Editorial) *Perit Dial Int* 9: 9, 1989
153. Diaz-Buxo JA, Walker PJ, Chandler JT, Farmer CD, Holt KL, Cox P: Continuous cyclic peritoneal dialysis. in *Advances in Peritoneal Dialysis*, edited by Gahl CM, Kessel M, Nolph KD, Amsterdam, Excerpta medica, 1981, p 126
154. Diaz-Buxo JA, Walker PJ, Burgess WP, Chandler JT, Farmer CD, Holt KL: Current status of CCPD in the prevention of peritonitis. in *Advances in Continuous Ambulatory Peritoneal Dialysis*, edited by Khanna R, Nolph KD, Prowant BF, Twardowski ZJ, Oreopoulos DG, Toronto, University of Toronto Press, 1986, p 145
155. Verger C, Luzar MA: *In vitro* study of CAPD Y-line system. in *Advances in Continuous Ambulatory Peritoneal Dialysis*, edited by Khanna R, Nolph KD, Prowant BF, Twardowski ZJ, Oreopoulos DG, Toronto: University of Toronto Press, 1986, p 160
156. Verger C, Faller B, Ryckelynck JPH, Cam G, Pierre D: Comparison between the efficacy of CAPD Y-lines without 'in-line' disinfectant and standard systems: A multicenter prospective controlled trial. *Perit Dial Bull* 7: S82, 1987
157. Bazzato G, Landini S, Coli U, Lucatello S, Francasso A, Moracchiello M: A new technique of continuous ambulatory peritoneal dialysis (CAPD): Double-bag system for freedom to the patient and significant reduction of peritonitis. *Clin Nephrol* 13: 251, 1980
158. Maiorca R, Cancarini GC, Broccoli R et al.: Prospective controlled trial of a Y-connector and disinfectant to prevent peritonitis in continuous ambulatory peritoneal dialysis. *Lancet* 2: 642, 1983
159. Suki WN, Walshe JJ, Ashebrook DW et al.: Multicenter evaluation of a bagless CAPD system. *Trans Am Soc Artif Intern Organs* 32: 572, 1986
160. Diaz-Buxo JA, Walshe JJ, Flanigan M: Multicenter experience with Y-set CAPD system (Freedom Set). (Abstract) *Perit Dial Bull* 7: S23, 1987
161. de Fijter CW, Verbrugh HA, Peters ED et al.: Another reason to restrict the use of a hypertonic glucose-bases peritoneal dialysis fluid: Its impact on peritoneal macrophage function *in vivo*. in *Advances in Peritoneal Dialysis*, edited by Khanna R, Nolph KD, Prowant BF, Twardowski ZJ, Oreopoulos DG, Toronto, University of Toronto Press, 1991, p 150
162. Burkart JM, Jordan JR, Durnell TA, Case LD: Comparison of exit-site infections in disconnect *versus* nondisconnect systems for peritoneal dialysis. *Perit Dial Int* 12: 317, 1992
163. Holley JL, Bernardini J, Piraino B: Continuous cycling peritoneal dialysis is associated with lower rates of catheter infections than continuous ambulatory peritoneal dialysis. *Am J Kidney Dis* 16: 133, 1990
164. Diaz-Buxo JA: Is peritoneal dialysis good for five years and maybe more? *Perit Dial Int* 13: S172, 1993
165. Shah J, Lane D, Shrivastava D, Berlyne GM, Barth RH: Isovolemic tidal technique does not increase clearances in intermittent peritoneal dialysis (IPD). (Abstract) *Am Soc Nephrol* 3: 419, 1992
166. Flanigan MJ, Doyle C, Lim VS, Ullrich G: Tidal peritoneal dialysis: preliminary experience. *Perit Dial Int* 12: 304, 1992
167. Flanigan MJ, Lim VS, Pflederer TA: Tidal peritoneal dialysis: kinetics and protein balance. *Am J Kidney Dis* 22: 700, 1993
168. Selgas R, Lopez-Rivas A, Alvaro F et al.: Insulin influence on the mitogenic-induced effect of the peritoneal effluent in CAPD patients. in *Advances in Peritoneal Dialysis*, edited by Khanna R, Nolph KD, Prowant BF, Twardowski ZJ, Oreopoulos DG, Toronto, University of Toronto Press, 1989, p 161
169. Wanless IR, Bargman JM, Oreopoulos DG et al.: Subcapsular steatosis in response to peritoneal insulin delivery: A clue to the pathogenesis of steatonecrosis in obesity. *Mod Pathol* 2: 69, 1989
170. Tzamaloukas AH, Oreopoulos DG: Subcutaneous *versus* intraperitoneal insulin in the management of diabetics on CAPD: a review. in *Advances in Peritoneal Dialysis*, edited by Khanna R, Nolph KD, Prowant BF, Twardowski ZJ, Oreopoulos DG, Toronto, University of Toronto Press, 1991, p 81
171. Diaz-Buxo JA, Adcock A, Nelms M: Experience with continuous cyclic peritoneal dialysis in the geriatric patient. in *Advances in Peritoneal Dialysis*, edited by Khanna R, Nolph KD, Prowant BF, Twardowski ZJ, Oreopoulos DG, Toronto, University of Toronto Press, 1990, p 61
172. Schleifer CR: Peritoneal dialysis in nursing homes. in *Advances in Peritoneal Dialysis*, edited by Khanna R, Nolph KD, Prowant BF, Twardowski ZJ, Oreopoulos DG, Toronto, University of Toronto Press, 1990, p 86
173. Diaz-Buxo JA: The place for cycler-assisted peritoneal dialysis in geriatric patients: comparison with hemodialysis. *Geriatric Nephrol Urol* 3: 7, 1993
174. Suh H, Wadhwa NK, Cabralda T, Sokunbi D, Solomon M: Peritoneal dialysis in elderly end-stage renal disease patients. in *Advances in Peritoneal Dialysis*, edited by Khanna R, Nolph KD, Prowant BF, Twardowski ZJ, Oreopoulos DG, Toronto, Multimed Inc, 1993, p 134
175. Nissenson AR: Peritoneal dialysis in the geriatric patient: overview and introduction. in *Advances in Peritoneal Dialysis*, edited by Khanna R, Nolph KD, Prowant BF, Twardowski ZJ, Oreopoulos DG, Toronto, Toronto University Press, 1990, p 1 (Suppl)
176. Oreopoulos DG: CAPD *vs* CCPD: Which is the right choice? *Nephrol News Issues* March: 16, 1983
177. King LK, Kingswood JC, Sharpstone P: Comparison of the efficacy cost and complication rate of APD and CAPD as long-term outpatient treatments for renal failure. in *Advances in Peritoneal Dialysis*, edited by Khanna R, Nolph KD, Prowant BF, Twardowski ZJ, Oreopoulos DG, Toronto, University of Toronto Press, 1992, p 123

22

CONTINUOUS PERITONEAL DIALYSIS

CHARLES M. MION

INTRODUCTION

In 1976, the concept of continuous ambulatory peritoneal dialysis (CAPD) was introduced by Popovich et al.. It was defined as a novel portable/wearable equilibrium peritoneal dialysis technique (1). Ironically, this new concept went unnoticed by a majority of clinicians in spite of its ingenious simplicity. The early clinical results reported two years later (2) attracted the interest of the nephrology community. These results validated the theoretical assumptions behind the principle of CAPD. Then, for the first time since the beginning of maintenance dialysis, a real practical method for a continuous dialytic therapy became available. As initially proposed, however, the technique had two major drawbacks: 1) the technical burden associated with the use of the dialysis fluid in two liter glass bottles which made this technique difficult to use; and 2) the high peritoneal infection rate due to the frequent openings of the dialysate delivery circuit.

In 1978, Oreopoulos et al. introduced the Toronto Western Hospital technique, which used dialysis solutions in plastic bags instead of glass bottles. The authors also discussed the use of a single administration tubing for one week (3). These two major technical improvements addressed these problems and transformed CAPD from an attractive theoretical concept to simplified procedures which could be easily and safely performed by the patients themselves. This new approach resulted in a decreased number of daily connections/disconnections required for dialysate infusion and drainage, and alleviated the ceaseless labor imposed upon the patient. As a consequence, the incidence of peritonitis was reduced to the acceptable level of one infection episode every ten to twelve patient treatment months.

Buoncristiani et al. (4) in 1980, introduced the Perugia connecting system, later identified as the 'Y set'. This new connecting device was shown both in uncontrolled (5) and in prospective randomized studies (6) to be the most effective in further reducing the risk of peritoneal infection. With the 'Y set', and the other developments described above, a new CAPD peritonitis rate was established, the average rate being about one episode every twenty-four patient treatment months.

Over the past eighteen years, CAPD has been established as one of the main treatment modalities for end stage renal disease (ESRD). An increasing number of ESRD patients received CAPD, not only in countries where the number of hemodialysis centers was restricted (7, 8), but also in countries where hemodialysis and transplantation were made available (9, 10). Extensive clinical experience demonstrated that mid-term survival on CAPD was similar to that on hemodialysis (HD), when comparing groups of patients with identical case-mix profile (11–15). However the technique survival has remained low. The CAPD patient fall out rate, higher than that of HD, does indicate the need to use both treatment modalities in an ESRD treatment program.

In parallel with the improvement in technique, which resulted in a decreased peritonitis incidence, the limitations of CAPD became an increasing concern (16–19). To overcome the multiple drawbacks of CAPD, continuous cyclic peritoneal dialysis (CCPD) was designed as an alternate therapy based on the continuous equilibrium dialysis concept (20). Since the introduction of this new technical approach, the term continuous peritoneal dialysis (CPD) includes by definition both CAPD and CCPD. Methods were developed to evaluate the functional characteristics of the peritoneal membrane (21, 22) and to quantify the dose of dialysis prescribed and delivered to the patients (23). Claims were made for individualizing the CAPD prescription (24). Malnutrition emerged as a major hazard for patients receiving this treatment modality (25, 26). Attempts were made to identify a relationship between the adequacy of CAPD and its outcome (27).

It is the aim of this chapter to present the most significant facts concerning the clinical use of CPD, the evaluation of dialysis adequacy and the outcome of patients receiving this treatment modality. Other chapters of this textbook deal with other important aspects of peritoneal dialysis and should be consulted according to the reader's interest.

CAPD AND CCPD TECHNIQUES

Continuous ambulatory peritoneal dialysis

CAPD is a simple manual procedure that entails several times a day the uninterrupted succession of instillation of a dialysis solution by gravity into the peritoneal cavity and of its drainage after a dwell period of variable duration.

The basic CAPD system consists of three main components: the permanent silastic peritoneal catheter; the transfer set which is permanently attached to the catheter; the plastic bags containing 0.5 to 3 liters of peritoneal dialysis fluid. Two main types of transfer sets are used in today's CAPD procedures:

— *the non-disconnect systems* made of a straight plastic tubing; after inflow, the bag still attached to the connecting tube, is carried rolled up in a waist purse under the clothing. At the end of the diffusion period, the dialysate is drained out into the same bag that is then discarded and replaced by a fresh bag (3). To prevent peritoneal infection with this type of connector, a variety of no-touch adaptors have been developped (28); these are made safer against infectious risks by the concommittent use of an ultraviolet light device (29);

— *the disconnect systems* utilising either a permanent Y-connector or a short straight connector with a double-bag system; in both cases, the bags are disconnected between exchanges, a feature that improves patient's comfort and esthetics (4). These systems have been shown to reduce the hazard of peritonitis (30, 31). Their efficiency rests with the fact that the connecting site between the bag and the transfer set is flushed by the peritoneal effluent during drainage and with a small (100 to 150 ml) volume of fresh dialysis solution before infusion (32). When a Y-connector is utilised, the inflow and outflow branches of the Y may be filled with sodium hypochlorite to decrease the risk of accidental contamination of the peritoneal cavity; at the time of bag exchange, the fresh bag is connected to the inflow branch and the disinfectant agent is completely flushed out through the outflow branch in the collecting bag of the peritoneal effluent (30). This procedure increases, however, hazard of introducing the disinfectant into the peritoneal cavity (33).

Whatever the type of connecting device utilised by the patient, the strict adhesion to careful aseptic procedures is a key factor in the prevention of peritonitis. Although non-touch aseptic techniques remain of major importance, the use of disinfecting solutions is mandatory during all connect/disconnect procedures required for peritoneal irrigation. In the absence of an ideal antiseptic, the use of 70% ethanol (containing 1% glycerol as an emollient when used as skin disinfectant) appears commendable because of a lower toxicity and a more reproducible efficacy than other disinfectants (34).

Due to these imperative precautions, the time required for a dialysis exchange will usually take as much as 30 to 45 minutes depending on the patient's manual ability and compliance with the recommended precautions. This loss of time with its inherent daily repetition is one of the major drawbacks of CAPD; as the dialysis solution exchanges occur during the active hours of the day, many patients oppose a strong resistance to an increased number of daily exchanges even if this modified prescription is justified by the occurrence of inadequate dialysis.

Continuous cyclic peritoneal dialysis

This technique provides three to five short dialysate exchanges at night, followed by a prolonged diurnal exchange. A simple peritoneal dialysis cycler delivers automatically all exchanges (20).

CCPD effectively reverses the schedule of CAPD and provides automated delivery of dialysate to the peritoneal cavity. This reversed schedule of peritoneal fluid delivery results in the following advantages: uninterrupted daytime activities; reduction in the number of connections/disconnections to two per day; increased flexibility of prescription by adding shorter exchanges during the night, which obtains higher clearances for small solutes and increased ultrafiltration; the assistance of a helper, if one is needed, with minimal time required on the helper's part since all technical manipulations take place before the patient retires for the night and early in the morning (35).

CAPD AND CCPD PRESCRIPTION

Frequency of exchanges

When CAPD was first clinically applied, the theory indicated that 10 liters of dialysis fluid daily would be required to maintain the blood urea level at 25 mmol/L (BUN 80 mg/dL) in an 80 kg man with an urea generation rate of 200 μmol/min (5 mg/min) (36). With the 2 liter bottles then available, five exchanges per day were required to supply the recommended amount of fluid. In clinical practice, this regimen was found to be cumbersome. The introduction of the 2 liter plastic bags led to the use of four 2 L exchanges/day (3). Since then, this regimen has become the standard prescription in most CAPD patients, irrespective of patients' height and weight or residual renal function. Other less frequent exchanges, still using 2 liters volume, have been proposed in an attempt both to improve the patient's quality of life and to lower the treatment costs (37). Three 2 L exchange protocols have been reported as giving short term satisfactory results, but this regimen is associated with a high risk of inadequate dialysis, particularly in the patient of large body built and/or with the progressive loss of residual renal function (38).

Volume of exchange

The standard use of an infusion volume of 2 L dialysis fluid during a CAPD exchange was mainly based on empirical routine derived from previous experience with intermittent PD. With a reduction in the number of daily exchanges, the use of larger volume infusion was explored (39, 40). The effect of fill volume and osmolality of dialysis solutions on ultrafiltration rates is shown in Figure 1. The increase in volume for each cycle maintains the total daily drainage volume at the desired level in spite of the

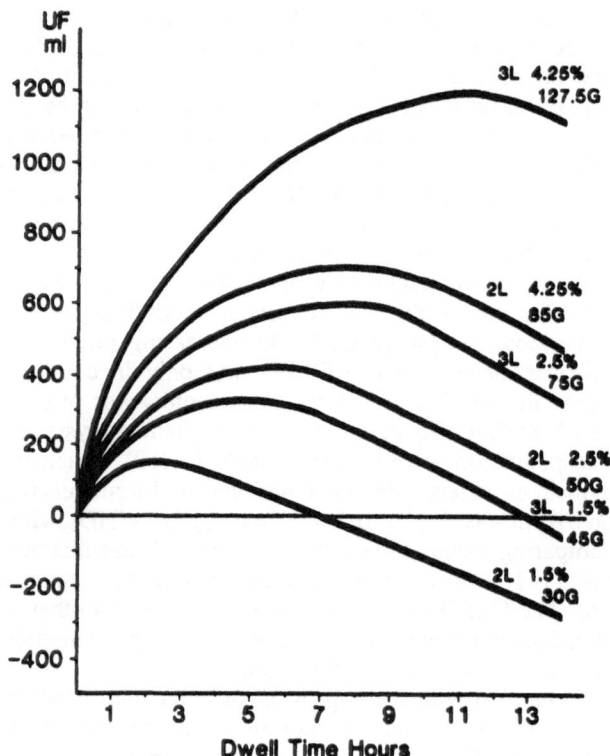

Figure 1. Approximate ultrafiltration volumes related to dwell time with 2- and 3-liter volumes, 1.5, 2.5, and 4.25% glucose concentrations (from Reference (88), with permission).

reduced number of exchanges. Consequently, the peritoneal clearances for small solutes, which depend on the dialysate flow rate, are preserved. Moreover, the protein losses are not increased since protein transperitoneal transport depends almost exclusively on membrane area and permeability (40, 41).

The relationship between fill volume and peritoneal function in terms of mass area coefficient (KoA) has been studied (42). The KoA is the product of the overall membrane permeability to a solute (such as urea, KoA-urea) and its surface area. In this study, 2.5% dextrose solution was used in varying volumes of 0.5, 1, 1.5, 2, 2.5 and 3 liters. The KoA-urea increased linearly with rising fill volume. A further increase above 3.0 liter was not associated with any further increase in KoA-urea. Similar results were obtained with KoA-creatinine and KoA-glucose. A linear relationship between increasing fill volume and KoA values for urea, creatinine and glucose was observed. It was also shown that the dialysate volume at which the urea KoA peaked correlated significantly with the patient's body surface area, as indicated in Figure 2. These data suggest that the KoA increases because of the recruitment of more effective peritoneal membrane surface area. Based on these observations, optimum volume for a patient can be estimated. Thus, for an average size

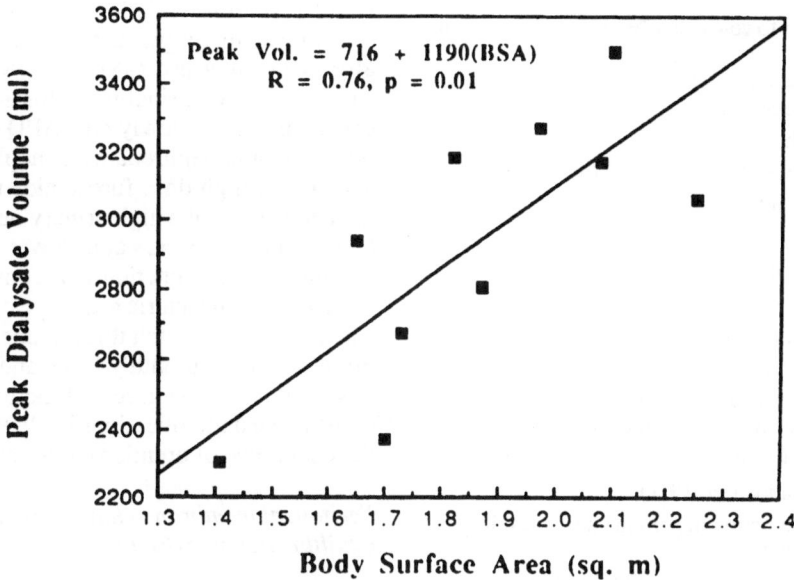

Figure 2. PD dialysate volume and mass transfer area coefficients (KoA). The dialysate volume at which the peak normalized KoA for urea occurred, based on the parabolic fit, is shown as a function of the patient's body surface area (from Reference (42), with permission).

adult with a BSA of 1.7 m^2 the optimum volume would be about 2.5 liters and for an individual with a BSA of 2 m^2 the optimum volume may be 3–3.5 liters. Another study comparing ultrafiltration rates with 2 and 3 L dialysate volumes in the same patients observed that the mean intraperitoneal volume change was lower with the 3 L than with 2 L solution. Increased lymphatic absorption was suggested as the presumed cause of increased water reabsorption rate during the 3 L exchanges (41). It should be stressed, however, that marked interindividual variations in ultrafiltration were noted in all these studies. The feasibility of higher volume CAPD is dictated by patient's tolerance; therefore, it should not be proposed to patients who feel the slightest discomfort with 2 L infusion volumes. The use of 2.5 or 3 L plastic bags is well tolerated by roughly 12 to 36% of patients (40, 43). The major determinant of the patient's tolerance is the alteration in forced vital capacity which decreases significantly in patients intolerant to larger volumes (40). In addition to pulmonary limitation, the increase in the intraperitoneal volume is a cause of more frequent dialysate leak and hernia formation, thus limiting the use of larger volumes. As the limitations of CAPD are more readily recognized, variations in dialysate volume should be an essential part of the individualised prescription. This should consider not only the daily dialysate volume for adequate dialysis, but also the degree of tolerance to abdominal distension and the benefits of less frequent daily exchanges (44).

Factors influencing CAPD prescription

The standard CAPD regimen recommending four 2 L exchanges every day is still used by a great majority of patients. This simplified approach, however, is far from giving the individual patient the adequate dose of dialysis; even though this standard prescription may be satisfactory when CAPD is initiated, the progressive loss of residual renal function will put the patient at a high risk of inadequate dialysis while treatment duration increases.

Short of definitely established rules, two empirical targets are currently recommended as a minimum for adequate therapy: a weekly creatinine clearance 50 liters per week and or a weekly urea index KT/V of 1.7 to 2.2 (45). They are discussed below in more details.

The main factors to take into account when writing orders for a CAPD patient are summarized in Table 1. Among these factors, the two major variables that will influence the overall CAPD efficiency are the daily drained dialysate volume and the residual renal function. On the other hand, the patient's size and the transport characteristics of the peritoneal membrane are fixed parameters that will only be altered by the metabolic or inflammatory side-effects of CAPD. Likewise, treatment times cannot be extended beyond 24 hours: in fact, the theoretical 24-hour-a-day of effective dialysis is reduced by 1 or 2 hours each day due to the time spent with a partially or completely empty abdomen during bag exchanges.

Table 1. Important factors to consider when prescribing continuous peritoneal dialysis

1. Patient's characteristics
    Size: height, weight
    Body mass index: weight (kg)/height^2 (m)
    Body surface area (m^2)
2. Dietary intake
    Protein and energy intake
    Sodium and water
    Inorganic phosphorus, potassium
3. Residual renal function
    Periodic assessment required to adjusting
    prescription (at least once every three months)
4. Peritoneal permeability characteristics
    Peritoneal equilibration test (PET)
    Periodic control: alteration in peritoneal permeability
    with duration of CPD
    Beware: acute changes in permeability during
    peritonitis
5. Prescription parameters
    Exchange volume (patient's tolerance)
    Frequency of daily exchanges
    Duration of dwell time per exchange
    Total daily drainage volume
    Selection of dialysis solution:
        Osmolality and type of osmotic agent
        (glucose, glucose polymers, aminoacids)
        Low (1.25) *vs* high (1.75)
        calcium content (mmol/L)
        Aminoacids for protein malnutrition
        Buffer: lactate *vs* bicarbonate

Residual renal function

When ESRD patients are starting maintenance therapy, they maintain some degree of renal function which declines at a variable pace depending on the nature of the nephropathy, the presence or absence of hypertension, the hydration state and the type of dialysis (48). In patients undergoing CAPD, this so-called residual renal function contributes an important part to the overall removal of uremic toxins (49–51). For example, in a patient with a total dialysate effluent volume of 10 liters per day producing a weekly urea peritoneal clearance of 70 liters (assuming a dialysate to plasma ratio of 1.0), a renal urea clearance of 2 to 5 ml/min will add approximately 20 to 50 liters of extra weekly clearance, amounting up to 78% of CAPD efficiency. When CAPD and HD were compared, however, the rate of decline of the CAPD patient was half that of HD patients (2.9 ± 0.3% per month for CAPD *versus* 5.8 ± 0.4% for HD) (51). The physiologic mechanisms for the less rapid fall-off of renal function on CAPD remains speculative: it could be related to the absence of extra-

cellular volume variations, maintaining a stable hemodynamic status; a permanent state of over-hydration has also been suggested (48). The type of nephropathy was shown to be a contributing factor in one study, the diuresis decreasing more slowly on CAPD than on HD in patients with interstial nephropathy or nephroangiosclerosis (50). The use of high dose furosemide may also contribute to the persistence of a high urinary output (49). On the other hand, even if it occurs at a slower rate than with HD, the decline in renal function is a constant finding and most patients become anuric after 3 years on CAPD. It is therefore essential to watch this parameter at regular intervals, preferably on a monthly basis and at least quarterly: the observed reduction in renal function will serve as a guide to the needed modifications in CAPD prescriptions before the occurence of uremic symptoms.

Peritoneal membrane characteristics: The peritoneal equilibration test (PET)

Since the early days of peritoneal dialysis, it has been recognized that the transport characteristics of the peritoneal membrane varied greatly among patients. These observations were confirmed by several studies determining mass transfer area coefficients (KoA) for various solutes (52, 53). This coefficient is an accurate measure of the maximal peritoneal clearance rates that would be realized in the absence of both ultrafiltration and solute accumulation in the dialysate. Several models of KoA have been developed: despite their experimental and theoretical interest, their use in clinical practice remained limited, presumably because of the complexity of the calculations (54). The stimulus for exploring the mechanisms of impaired peritoneal function in patients undergoing CAPD came from a study demonstrating the prognosis value of peritoneal equilibration curves (21). The PET was introduced (22) and has been widely accepted as a useful means to evaluate the peritoneal solute transport rate in the clinical setting (55, 56). The test consists of measuring the dialysate to plasma ratio (D/P) of creatinine and dialysate dextrose to baseline dextrose concentration (D/Do) at 0.5, 1, 2 and 4 hours; dialysate drainage volume (DV) at 4 hr is also determined by completely draining the dialysate. This protocol was later simplified with only the ratios and drainage volume at 4 hr measured and proposed as a useful alternative to the original PET (57). Excellent reproducibility was confirmed after standardizing the procedures for length of preceding exchange, times of inflow and drainage, patient's position and methods of obtaining and processing samples and laboratory assays. According to the 4-h D/P creatinine results, patients can be categorized into high (hi), high-average (ha), low-average (la) and low transporters (lo), as shown in Figure 3. The D/Do ratio can be used in a similar way. The test proved to be very useful for *dialysis regimen planning*, providing objective criteria to select the most appropriate CPD modality according to the patient's peritoneal characteristics (58). The high transporters usually have good solute

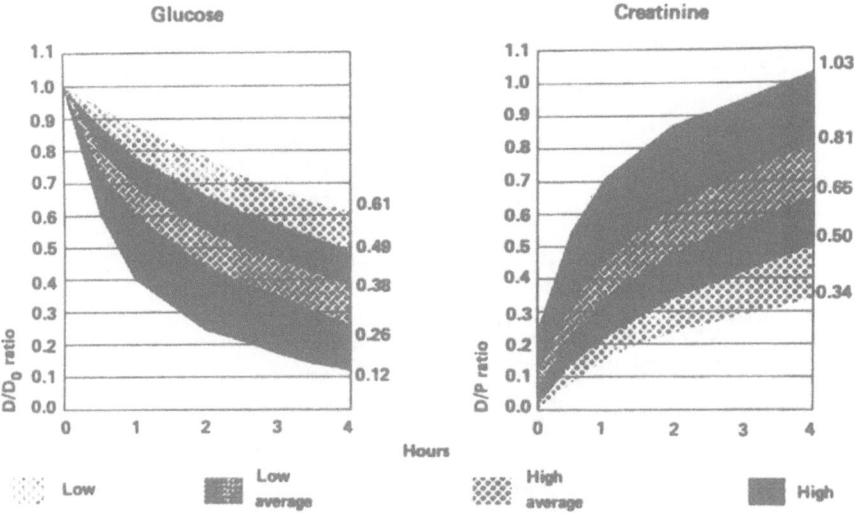

Figure 3. Peritoneal equilibration test: areas shaded in different patterns portray results representing high, high average, low average and low peritoneal transport rates (from Reference (21), with permission).

clearances but poor ultrafiltration if dwell time exceeds 4 hours: two hybrid systems between CAPD and CCPD may provide a practical therapeutic approach in this group of patients (59); the first adds one or two CAPD manual exchanges to a standard CCPD program, while the second adds one or two nocturnal exchanges administered by a simplified cycler to a standard CAPD program; intermittent automated dialysis offers another acceptable therapeutic alternative to high transporters, particularly in patients with significant residual renal function. The low transporters usually have good ultrafiltration, but low small solute clearances: the standard CAPD regimen is usually inadequate in the anuric patient. The ha and la transporters, particularly the former, usually have adequate clearances and ultrafiltration: standard CAPD or CCPD are suitable treatment modes in these patients. The PET is also used as a *diagnostic tool* in patients with apparent membrane failure (i.e., inadequate dialysis, loss of ultrafiltration). It should be noted, however, that the classification of patients hi, ha, la or lo transporters, does not affect the values of D/P urea measured in 24 hr dialysate collections: in a cross-sectional study, CAPD patients with different transport characteristics showed mean D/P urea values for all groups near 0.95, quite different from 4-hr PET evaluations where the lower margins of the range of D/P urea for hi, ha, la, and lo patients, respectively, were 1.0, 0.92, 0.85 and 0.75 (60). When using four 2-L exchanges over 24 hours, more time was available to approach near equilibration than with the 4-hr dwell time of the PET, erasing the differences between the 4 groups of transporters. On the other hand, mean drainage volumes (in liters) were approximately 9.0, 9.4, 10.0, and 10.0 per day for hi, ha, la, lo groups respectively, suggesting that restricted fluid intake and/or a greater diuresis

were required in hi transporters to maintain fluid balance despite a lower ultrafiltration. Finally, peritoneal transport characteristics may change with CAPD duration in a given patient. In a selected population of patients undergoing CAPD for at least two years on average, in whom two or more PET were performed, hi transporters showed a significant decrease in the mean D/P creatinine, while this ratio significantly increased in la and lo transporters. A significant increase of D/Do glucose was also observed in hi transporters. The change in D/P creatinine and D/Do were significantly and inversely correlated to each other, indicating an actual transport change. These changes may explain why patients with a longer duration of peritoneal dialysis are mostly ha transporters (61).

Other patient's characteristics

Two other major factors should be taken into consideration when prescribing a CAPD regimen: the *weight and height of the patient* and the *dietary protein intake* (DPI). Patients of high body weight, who have little or no residual renal function, cannot obtain adequate solute clearances on common starting protocols (60). The affect of patient's weight on CAPD efficiency using a standard dialysis regimen (four 2 L exchanges per day) was studied with reference to a target weekly KT/V urea of 1.7 or greater over a range of standard weights calculated as V/0.58 according to Watson (62). The following weight limitations were observed: anuric hi transporters will not meet a KT/V urea target above standard weights of 61 kg and anuric lo transporters will not reach the target at weights above 67 kg as shown in Figure 4 (60).

Concerning dietary proteins, nitrogen balance studies suggest that a daily protein intake in the range of 1.2–1.4 g/kg body weight per day is required to maintain a

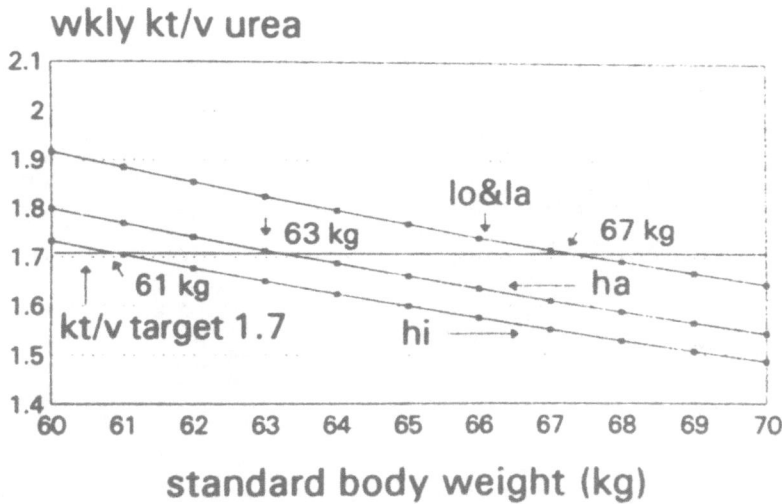

4 x 2 L CAPD in anephric pts, d/p urea 0.95, average DV

Figure 4. Weekly KT/V urea as related to standard body weight for high (hi), high average (ha), low average (la) and low (lo) transporters: la transporters have the same relationship as lo transporters. High average (ha) transporters have a maximum weight of 63 kg to meet the KT/V target (from Reference (60), with permission).

positive nitrogen balance (63, 64). As proteins are the main source of urea in a stable patient without intercurrent disease, the removal of this small molecule will be critically dependent on the amount of dialysis fluid drained per 24 hours. A relationship between the CAPD dose and the protein catabolic rate (PCR), which is the protein equivalent of the urea appearance rate (64), has been observed in several series: its significance is discussed in more details in the following section on nutrition (46, 61–69).

Quantitative prescription

One of the most difficult and controversial subject in clinical dialysis field has been the definition of adequacy of dialysis. It is our opinion that whether dialysis is adequate or not is a clinical question and must consider the overall clinical picture of the patient. When clinicians have limited their decision solely to numbers, problems have arisen (70). Various methods have been used for the quantification of dialysis treatment, but whether any dose is adequate or not must be decided in conjunction with other clinical parameters, such as nutritional status, uremic symptoms and control of extracellular volume.

Quantification of dose with CAPD
The definition of a dialysis index (24) and the use of weekly urea and creatinine clearances (46, 58, 71) were the earlier attempts to determine the dose of dialysis. The dialysis index for CAPD was defined as the ratio of the actual drainage volume to the prescribed volume, reflecting the fraction of urea clearance achieved; in practice,

this index has not received wide acceptance. The weekly creatinine clearance measured the peritoneal creatinine clearance plus the renal creatinine clearance: if the values were above 40 to 50 liters per week, the dose was deemed to be adequate, below these numbers as inadequate; in fact, the present trend is to consider that below a value of 50 liters, the dialysis dose is clearly inadequate (47, 72).

Urea kinetics concept
The wide use of the concept of urea kinetics (KT/V) to measure the dose of HD (73), led to the use of same concept in the calculation of CAPD dose (24, 71, 74, 75). In the equation KT/V, K is urea clearance, T time of dialysis and V volume of distribution of urea. For CAPD, the KT normally is equal to the volume of drainage volume plus the renal urea clearance: thus, in an anuric patient with a 24 hour drainage volume equal to 10 liters, the total clearance of urea is 10 liters. This is based on the assumption that dialysate urea concentration, with longer dwell time, is equal to plasma urea concentration. The volume of distribution of urea is equivalent to the total body water, which can be calculated from the body weight using Watson formula, i.e.: 0.58 × body weight. Thus if the above patient is anuric and weighs 70 kg, the V = 40.6 liters and daily KT/V = 0.24. In order to compare CAPD, which is a continuous therapy, with intermittent HD therapy, the daily KT/V is changed to weekly value by multiplying it with 7, or in the example 0.24 × 7 = 1.68. If a patient has a residual renal function, the renal

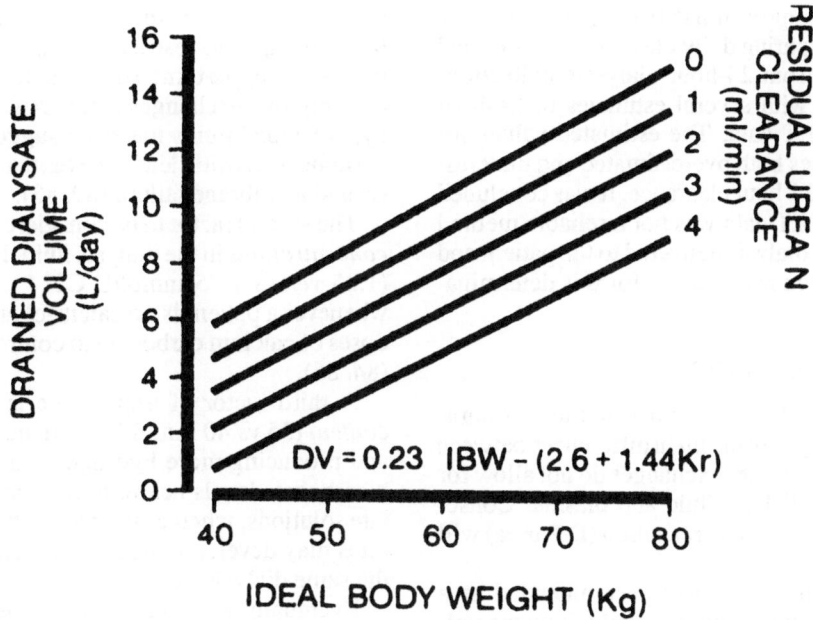

Figure 5. Relationship between ideal body weight and dialysate drainage volume for CAPD patients consuming 1.2 g/kg body weight per day of protein and with a target BUN of 70 mg/dL (blood urea 1.4 g/ L or 23.3 mmol/L) (from Reference (24), with permission).

urea clearance is to be added to the dialysis clearance to get KT.

How much KT/V is adequate is a matter of continued discussion (42, 72, 76, 77). From totally a theoretical consideration, in a patient with a daily protein intake of 1.2 g/kg/day (recommended intake), a daily KT/V of 0.34 will be needed in order to maintain a blood urea concentration of 25 mmol/L (1.5 g/L or BUN 75 mg/dL). Minimal adequate dose proposed by various investigators vary from 1.71, 1.28 to 1.21, whereas the target weekly KT/V was fixed at 2.29 in one study (24). The most important point to remember, however, is that the renal clearance of urea declines with time, as is was first described in patients receiving intermittent PD (77a). Although the loss of renal function occurs more slowly in CPD- than in IPD-treated patients (48–51), a sufficient increase in the peritoneal contribution should be provided to maintain at an adequate level the overall (i.e., peritoneal + renal) treatment dose (77). This reciprocal relationship between declining renal function and the daily drained dialysate volume required to maintain a stable dose of dialysis is shown in Figure 5 (24).

Weekly creatinine clearance concept
The concept of quantifying the dose of dialysis by total daily creatinine clearance was first proposed for intermittent PD. That concept was later applied to CAPD to calculate the dose of dialysis. The initial suggestion was that a weekly total creatinine clearance of 40–50 liters/week is adequate dialysis. At present, 50 liters/week/1.73 m^2

is recommended as a minimum for an adequate clearance (72). This value includes the contribution by the residual renal function. If this is measured as creatinine clearance, only the clearance achieved by the glomerular filtration should be included; this causes some confusion and uncertainty, since the tubular secretion of creatinine increases with advancing decline of GFR (45). Some investigators suggest using only three-eights of the value of measured creatinine clearance (45) or to measure simultaneous urea and creatinine renal clearances, and use the mean of these two measures as representing the GFR (78).

Other approaches
The concept of creatinine efficiency number (EN) has been proposed as an alternative method to measure the dose of dialysis (79). From PET, the D/P for creatinine can be measured and multiplying this value with the 24-hour instilled dialysate volume will give the daily peritoneal creatinine clearance. Next, the adjusted creatinine production is calculated from the daily peritoneal creatinine appearance and the creatinine degradation occurring via extrarenal pathways. The EN is calculated using the formula:

$$((D/P\ creat.) \times V24)/ACP,$$

where D/Pcreatinine – dialysate to plasma creatinine ratio, V24 – 24 hour dialysate volume, ACP – adjusted creatinine production.

With this method, the inconvenience of a 24-hour collection of effluent dialysis fluid is suppressed. However, the reliability of this approach has been questioned in a prospective study comparing daily clearances of urea and creatinine calculated from 24-hour dialysate collections by standard methods with several estimates of 24-hour clearance based on PET data. The estimated values for daily dialysis clearances both overestimated and underestimated the measured 24-hour clearance. It was concluded that extrapolation of PET data was not a reliable method to estimate the dose of dialysis delivered to the patient and that a 24-hour collection is necessary for this determination (80).

Quantification of dose with CCPD

Shorter duration of nightly dwell times and longer duration of daytime exchange are the main differences between CAPD and CCPD. The shorter exchanges do not allow for equilibration between dialysis fluid and plasma. Consequently, the dialysate to plasma urea ration (D/P urea) will be lower than one.

Urea kinetic modelling has been recommended as a useful tool to calculate the amount of daily drainage volume required to obtain a daily KT/V of 0.32 with CCPD (77). If the goals of this treatment modality include a neutral nitrogen balance at a protein intake of 1.2 g/kg/day and an average blood urea level of 25 mmol/L (1.5 g/L or BUN 75 mg/dL), the daily drainage volume can be easily calculated according to the following equation:

$$DDV = (0.23\ SBW - (2.7 + 1.44\ Kr))/D/P,$$

where DDV = daily drainage volume, in liter, SBW = standard body weight, in kg, Kr = residual renal urea clearance, in ml/min, D/P = dialysate to plasma urea ratio.

As Kr decreases, the volume of dialysis fluid necessary to maintain a stable CCPD efficiency will increase strikingly. For example, a patient with a SBW of 70 kg, with a D/P urea of 0.85 and a Kr of 3 ml/min, will require 10.68 L of DDV to reach the target KT/V. When Kr declines to reach zero, however, the same patient would require 15.76 L of dialysate drainage to achieve the same dose of dialysis. From this example, it is clear that the maintenance of a constant efficiency may induce a large increase in cost with CCPD (77).

Qualitative prescription

Prescribing the adequate dose of dialysis to correct or to prevent the relapse of uremic symptoms is of paramount importance. Choosing the dialysis solutions according to their formulation, however, is another important step to tailoring the dialysis prescription to the needs of the individual patient (81).

The first and most obvious factor to consider is the *osmolality of the dialysis solutions*: higher dextrose concentrations (25 and 40 g/L dextrose) should be used in adequate amount to maintain the dry weight. The need for hypertonic solutions will be greater in high transporters, whereas low transporters will obtain higher drain volumes

with a lesser use of those. The patient, however, should be encouraged to restrict fluid and sodium intake to limit the use of hypertonic solutions to no more than one or possibly two exchanges a day. An excessive use of these hyperosmolal fluids has been suggested as as a cause of peritoneal serositis leading eventually to peritoneal fibrosis and membrane failure (82, 83).

The second factor to be considered is the *divalent cation concentrations* in the dialysis fluid. Low calcium dialysate (1.25 *versus* 1.75 mmol/L Ca^{++}) should be prescribed whenever a patient is on calcitriol and/or has to take large doses of calcium carbonate to control hyperphosphatemia (84, 85).

A third factor of importance is the *dialysate lactate content* (35 *vs* 40 mmol/L): patients eating more proteins and producing more hydrogen ion, will maintain serum bicarbonate levels nearer to normal with 40 mmol/L lactate solutions, whereas patients with lower H$^+$ generation rates may develop a hazardous metabolic alcalosis using the same dialysis fluid (86).

Eventually, a fourth factor to consider is the *nutritional status* of the patient, particularly when revising the prescription of the long term CAPD patient in whom malnutrition can settle insidiously. The daily use of amino acid solutions (usually one mid-day exchange per 24 hours) may help restore a positive nitrogen balance in the patient with protein-calorie malnutrition (87).

In the near future, two new types of formulation will become commercially available and help tailoring an even more specific prescription to solve individual patients' problems. One group of these new formulae will replace dextrose by alternative osmotic agents, such as polypeptides, amino acids (88) or glucose polymers (89, 90). The other group will substitute the physiologic buffer bicarbonate to conventional lactate (91, 92). These promising new formulae are still at the stage of clinical evaluation.

UNDESIRABLE EFFECTS OF CAPD AND CCPD

Technically, CAPD presents itself as the simplest among the various dialysis therapies presently available. Using the peritoneal cavity as an artificial kidney, however, does not go without inherent undesirable effects. Although not life-threatening on the short term, some of these effects (e.g., protein losses, glucose load) are potentially harmful to the patient and to the peritoneal membrane on the long term. In spite of the extensive use of CAPD over the last decade, their clinical significance has not yet been fully elucidated.

The main undesirable effects of peritoneal dialysis are listed in Table 2. This list illustrates the numerous consequences of peritoneal dialysis which interfere locally with the physiology, the ultrastructure and the immunology of the peritoneum. Beyond its local actions, the irrigation of

Table 2. Undesirable side-effects of continuous peritoneal dialysis

1.	Bioincompatibility of peritoneal dialysis solutions (PDS)
1.1.	High osmolality
1.2.	High lactate concentration, low pH
1.3.	High dextrose concentration
1.3.1.	Non enzymatic glycosylation of proteins
1.3.2.	Glucose breakdown products (heat sterilization), 5-hydroxy-methylfurfural; aldehydes
1.3.3.	Plasticizers
2.	Volume effects of infused PDS in the peritoneal cavity
2.1.	Changes in intraabdominal pressure
2.1.1.	Abdominal distension
2.1.2.	Increased incidence of hernias
2.2.	Alteration in respiratory function
2.3.	Consequences on the cardiovascular system
2.4.	Interference with normal peritoneal physiology
2.4.1.	Suppression of normal peritoneal fluid circulation
2.4.2.	Lavage effect: removal of surfactant (phosphatidylcholine)
3.	Metabolic consequences of PDS
3.1.	Losses of protein and aminoacids
3.2.	Continuous transperitoneal glucose loading
3.3.	Dyslipidemia
3.4.	Increased atherogenic risk
3.5.	Losses of vitamins
4.	Digestive symptoms
4.1.	Decreased appetite
5.	Miscellaneaous
5.1.	Daily workload
5.1.1.	Patient and/or helper burnout
5.2.	Environmental problems
5.2.1.	Large volume of waste
5.2.2.	Viral contamination of dialysis fluid

the peritoneal cavity with unphysiologic dialysis solutions (e.g., hyperosmolar and acidic containing high dextrose concentrations), is also associated with metabolic disturbances while inducing subtle changes in cardiovascular and respiratory functions.

Bioincompatibility of peritoneal dialysis solutions

The term 'biocompatibility' as applied to peritoneal dialysis solutions (PDS) encompasses all the biological effects that these solutions exert on the normal functioning of the tissues and cells of the peritoneum during both uninfected and infected states (93). In fact, the name 'bioincompatibility' would be more appropriate to underscore the highly un-physiological composition of currently avail-

able commercial PDS, the toxic/inhibitory components of which are now well identified (94). These noxious factors include: a high glucose concentration, which is used as the osmotic agent, resulting in an increased fluid osmolality and the presence of glucose breakdown products generated during heat sterilization (e.g., aldehydes (95), 5-hydroxy-methyl furfural (96)); a low formulation pH 5.2 to 5.5, which is to prevent caramelization of glucose during the heat sterilization process; a high lactate concentration (35–40 mmol/L), which is used as the buffering system. The effects of PDS on various cellular functions and viability have been examined mostly *in vitro* on neutrophils or mononuclear cells, on mesothelial cells and on fibroblasts (93, 97). The results of these studies can be summarized as follows:

1. Simultaneous cell exposure to high lactate concentration and low pH results in additive inhibitory effects. In neutrophils, a marked decrease in respiratory burst was observed, phagocytosis fell by 30% whilst leukotriene B4 (LTB4) synthesis remained stable. In macrophages and mesothelial cells, cytokine release was inhibited in a pH dependent manner (98–103).

2. Hyperosmolar glucose based PDS have an adverse effect on cell function. In neutrophils, cytotoxicity causing LDH release was due to glucose *per se*, while LTB4 release and phagocytosis inhibition were related to osmolality rather than glucose. Furthermore, both osmolality and glucose were found to have independent inhibitory effects on cytokine release by monocytes and demonstrated significant cytotoxicity on mesothelial cell proliferation (104, 105).

3. Heat sterilized PDS containing glucose breakdown products (principally aldehydes) were shown to impair growth and inflammatory responses of cultured fibroblasts and human leucocytes more markedly than PDS of similar composition cold sterilized by filtration (106, 107).

4. The peritoneal mesothelium contribute to the control of peritoneal inflammation (108). Human peritoneal mesothelial cells (HPMC) secrete interleukin-1, interleukin-6 (109) and interleukin-8 (110); they also generate significant quantities of prostaglandins (PGE2, 6-keto PGF1 alpha) (111). An acute exposure of HPMC to PDS, followed by an extended *in vitro* recovery period, is sufficient to impair cytokine and prostaglandin synthesis by these cells (112).

Nonenzymatic glycosylation is another biological process relevant to the problem of bioincompatibility (113). Advanced glycosylation end products (AGEs) are formed as the result of the non-enzymatic glycosylation of proteins (114). *In vitro*, significant glycation of albumin incubated in PDS is observed at a rate related to the glucose concentration of the dialysate (115). Furthermore, increased levels of serum and dialysate glycated albumin have been found in CAPD patients: dialysate glycated albumin, however, was significantly higher than serum glycated albumin and the dialysate to serum glycated albu-

min ratio had a mean value of 1.14. This observation indicate that protein glycation occurs within the peritoneum
during CAPD (115). In this respect, it is noteworthy that
serum AGE levels are increased to a similar extent both in
CAPD and hemodialyzed patients without any apparent
influence of the peritoneal glucose load incurred by CPD
patients (116–118). By stimulating macrophages via a
receptor mediated process, AGEs could induce fibrogenic
cytokines such as tumor necrosis factor or interleukin-1.
No evidence exists as yet that dialysate glucose results
in glycosylation of peritoneal tissue in patients receiving
CAPD (83).

Plasticizers released into the dialysate from the
polyvinylchloride plastic bags may also be involved in the
bioincompatibility of CPD procedures. Incubating peripheral blood monocytes *in vitro* with diethylhexylphtalate
for 4 hours was shown to induce a significant increase in
IL-1 alpha and IL-1 beta, a process that could be involved
in the development of peritoneal sclerosis (119).

Permanent presence of dialysis fluid in the peritoneal cavity

When peritoneal dialysis solutions are infused into the
peritoneum, the peritoneal space is changed from a virtual to an actual cavity. The presence of two or more liters
of dialysis fluid (particularly during maximum ultrafiltration) in the abdomen may affect many cardiovascular and
respiratory functions, and results in deep disturbances of
peritoneal physiology.

Increased intraabdominal pressure

The intraabdominal pressure of the empty abdominal cavity ranges between 0.5 and 1.5 cm of water and it increases
linearly with the volume of dialysis fluid present in the
peritoneal cavity (40, 120, 121). Each liter of intraperitoneal fluid increases the intra-abdominal pressure by 2 to
3 cm of water and the abdominal girth by 1.81 cm. Coughing and straining generate the highest intra-abdominal
pressures in every position. The pressures, generally higher with greater dialysate volumes, vary with physical
activity; bicycle training produces lower pressure than
jogging or jumping. Intra-abdominal pressures are higher
with most maneuvers in obese patients and in the elderly (121). Raised intra-abdominal pressure is a major risk
factor in CAPD and CCPD; it may create dialysate leaks,
hernia, cardiopulmonary compromise and hemorrhoids. It
may also accentuate gastroesophageal reflux and urinary
incontinence. To reduce the risk of these complications,
useful recommendations to the patient include 1) a reduction in voluntary coughing, particularly after catheter
insertion; 2) careful prevention of constipation to prevent excessive straining; 3) emptying of the abdomen for
strenuous exercises (i.e., tennis, weight lifting) (121).

Alteration in respiratory function

Most studies of pulmonary function during peritoneal
dialysis, comparing data obtained with an empty or full
abdomen report a reduction in functional residual capacity (FRC) following dialysis fluid infusion, both in the
supine and sitting positions (122–124). A reduction in
vital capacity, however, is a less common finding (125,
126). In fact, when interpreting the results of pulmonary
function tests in patients receiving peritoneal dialysis, several parameters should be taken into account, including
the volume of infusate and the resulting intraperitoneal
pressure (126) as well as the patient's position (i.e., supine,
sitting or upright) and the compliance of the abdominal
wall (40). When 2 L dialysis solution were infused in
recumbent CAPD patients, a significant drop in FRC was
observed and resulted in airway closure as the FRC values
were lower than the closure capacity. The airway closure
induced a significant decrease in PaO2. This hypoxemia
was abolished a few months later, suggesting the development of compensatory mechanisms in long term CAPD
(124). This observation may account for the absence of
abnormalities in pulmonary function observed by one
group in CAPD patients studied in the sitting position
(127). In normal operating conditions, CPD procedures
do not induce respiratory distress. Severe discomfort or
dyspnea, however, can occur when the dialysate volume
is increased above 2 L, particularly when the patient is
lying flat in his bed (40). In practice, exchange volumes
and respiratory tolerance should be carefully monitored
in patients with borderline respiratory function.

Hemodynamic consequences

Instillation of 2 to 3 L of dialysis solution in the peritoneal
cavity induced a 98% increase in the inferior vena cava
pressure (128). Two hemodynamic studies conducted in
CAPD patients gave slightly divergent results (120, 129).
In one study, graded increases in exchange volume from
15 to 26 ml/kg/body weight in supine patients produced
a decreased cardiac output of 25% when intra-abdominal
pressure reached 15 cm of water. Simultaneously, heart
rate, mean arterial blood pressure and total peripheral
resistance showed significant increases, whereas a 35%
reduction in stroke volume was observed (120). In another
study, comparing hemodynamic changes induced by 2 L
of intraperitoneal dialysate in the standing *versus* supine
position, significant falls in blood pressure, stroke volume
and cardiac output, accompanied by an increase in heart
rate, were observed only in the upright position, with
no change in peripheral resistance (129). Differences in
methodology may account for the discrepancy observed
in these two studies.

The characteristics of cardiac structure and function
in CAPD patients have been studied with echocardiography (130–132). During acute intraperitoneal infusion
of increasing dialysate volumes, 1 or 2 liter infusion did
not affect either systolic function or cardiac output. On
the other hand, infusion of 3 liters or more of dialysis

fluid induced a significant decrease in left ventricular internal dimensions in diastole correlated to the rise in intraabdominal pressure. These effects were confined to a subgroup of patients with an increased left ventricular wall thickness (131). A high prevalence of left ventricular hypertrophy (LVH) was observed among CAPD patients, resulting from septal thickening (asymmetric LVH) in one series (131) and from concentric symmetric LVH in another study (132). Left atrial dilatation was also highly prevalent. An abnormal diastolic left ventricular filling was a common finding both in patients with and without LVH.

Interferences with the normal physiology of the peritoneum

The normal physiology of the peritoneum is markedly altered by the infusion of 2–3 liters of peritoneal dialysis fluid in the peritoneal cavity. This large volume of unphysiologic solution interferes with the functions of the normal peritoneal fluid and has a 'lavage effect' on the surfactant secreted by mesothelial cells.

Suppression of physiologic flow of normal peritoneal fluid

In healthy subjects, the peritoneum is a potential space containing about 50 ml of peritoneal fluid which provides lubrication of the abdominal viscera as they slide over one another (133). The normal peritoneal fluid, which contains phagocytic cells (mainly macrophages), immunoglobulins and complement (134, 135), flows continuously upwards from the pelvis to the subdiaphragmatic area, where it drains off into the lacunae of diaphragmatic lymphatics through small intercellular openings called the mesothelial stomata (136). This upward circulation of peritoneal fluid is induced by diaphragmatic contractions during respiration. This permanent flux sweeps the mesothelial surface and permits the rapid elimination from the peritoneal cavity of particulate matter up to 20 μm in size (including bacteria) through the diaphragmatic lymphatics and the thoracic duct to the systemic circulation (137). When the peritoneal cavity is filled with dialysate, the infused volume, 10 to 60 times larger than normal peritoneal fluid, presumably disrupts the physiologic intraperitoneal circulation. This disturbance may explain why bacteremia, a common finding in secondary bacterial peritonitis (133) is a rare observation among patients with CAPD peritonitis (138).

Removal of surfactants

Removal of surface-active material is another adverse effect of peritoneal dialysis (139). This material is composed of phospholipids, with a predominance of phosphatidylcholine. This substance, isolated from dialysate effluent was studied *in vitro*; it demonstrated a moderate degree of repellency and surface activity. In addition to surface-tension reduction, this surface-active material may have lubrication properties (139) and confers water

repellency to the mesothelial surface by its attachment to the anionic sites of the peritoneum (140). As shown in *in vitro* studies, the peritoneum is capable of synthesizing phosphatidylcholine in amounts equivalent to lung tissue (141). Mesothelial cells synthesize and secrete phospholipids from their apical portion by a process of exocytic extrusion of lamellar bodies similar to that established for type II pneumocytes (142). Furthermore, the rate of phospholipid synthesis by mesothelial cells *in vitro* can be manipulated in part by choline concentration in the culture medium (143). Among CAPD patients, phospholipid levels in the dialysis effluent were found to be lower in patients receiving CAPD for 8 to 48 months than in those starting treatment (144, 145). Phospholipid concentrations in spent dialysate were reported to be reduced in patients with decreased ultrafiltration in one series (144), but this fact was not confirmed in another study (145). Experimental studies in animals with normal renal function indicate that intraperitoneal phosphatidylcholine increases ultrafiltration rates in rats (146) and in sheep (147), but has no effect in rabbits (148).

Metabolic consequences

The non-selective process of peritoneal dialysis results in multiple complex metabolic disturbances. On the one hand, transperitoneal transport results in significant losses of proteins, aminoacids, vitamins and also of various hormones (a limited problem not discussed here). On the other hand, the high glucose content of peritoneal dialysis solutions induces a large daily load of glucose, accompanied by hormonal adaptation and abnormalities in lipid metabolism.

Protein losses

Protein losses are obligatory during CAPD and CCPD due to the high permeability of the peritoneal membrane. The transperitoneal transport of high molecular weight solutes such as proteins is dependent both on effective peritoneal surface area and the intrinsic permeability of the peritoneal membrane (149–151). Total protein losses range from 5 to 12 gm per 24 hours; albumin accounts for about 65% and IgG for 15% of the protein loss. IgA, IgM, transferrin, and C3 are also found in small quantities in the peritoneal effluent; the losses of IgG and IgM are correlated with the serum concentration of these immunoglobulins (152–154). During a single dialysate exchange, the amount of protein loss increases from 1.3 gm after a 4-hour dwell to 1.6 and 1.8 gm after 6- and 8-hour dwells respectively. Day-to-day variability of protein clearances has been reported: this phenomenon was attributed to alterations in the effective peritoneal surface area, because the restriction coefficient of the peritoneum for proteins had a low coefficient of variation (155). Large increases in protein losses occur during peritonitis and may persist for several weeks (156). In spite of external protein losses well within the nephrotic range, most CAPD patients maintain stable serum total protein and albumin levels that are only slightly reduced below normal. CAPD patients respond to the continuous loss of albumin via the peritoneal route with a decrease in both the absolute and fractional catabolic rates of albumin (157). An increase in albumin synthesis is also observed, which appears to be quantitatively determined by the rate of albumin loss in each patient. The total albumin mass and the distribution of albumin remain normal, an observation suggesting that the compensatory mechanisms are operating efficiently in these patients. Serum albumin concentration, however, does not fully return to normal level, because a combination of continuous albumin losses and expanded plasma volume maintains the patient in a constant state of 'catch up' (157, 158).

Amino acid losses

Amino acid losses in the peritoneal effluent of patients on CAPD is approximately 2 gm per day when patients drain a total dialysate volume of 10 liters, giving a weekly loss of 12 gm (159–161). CAPD does not correct the plasma amino acid abnormalities of uremia. During dialysis, the molar ratio of dialysate to plasma amino acids concentration approaches unity for most amino acids (with two notable exceptions of aspartic acid and tryptophan), suggesting a trend toward equilibrium due to a passive diffusion gradient (159–161).

Glucose loading

Glucose is continuously absorbed during CAPD with the daily absorption varying between 100 to 200 gm per 24 hours (162). This amount represents 70 to 75% of glucose supplied with the dialysate and 12 to 34% of total energy intake (162, 163). During a 6-hour cycle, 45 to 50 gm of glucose are absorbed from the 4.25 gm% dialysate, while 25 to 40 gm and 15 to 22 gm are absorbed respectively from 2.5 gm% and 1.5 gm% dialysis solutions. Large interindividual differences in the rate of glucose absorption exist between patients (21, 22). In the same patient, glucose absorption may increase with time on CAPD leading to poor ultrafiltration (164, 165). During CAPD a single dialysis cycle with hypertonic dialysate (glucose monohydrate 4.25 gm/dL) induces a rise in blood glucose and plasma insulin level to peak values within 45 to 90 minutes, whereas serum glucagon levels decrease only slightly (166). Glucose administered via the peritoneal route induces different kinetics of glucose oxydation rate compared to oral administration, but a given amount of glucose absorbed either by the peritoneum or by the gut contributes to a similar extent to glucose and energy balance (167). Studies on oral glucose tolerance after 6 and 12 months on CAPD show that blood glucose, serum insulin, and serum glucagon responses to an oral glucose load remain abnormal, but are not further impaired during CAPD in most patients (163). However, the insulin response to oral glucose has been reported to deteriorate with time in some patients, while de novo insulin dependent diabetes may complicate the course of CAPD due to the permanent hyperglycemic stress (166).

Hyperlipidemic effects

Dyslipidemia is an almost constant finding among chronic renal failure patients, with hypertriglyceridemia as the most common abnormality. To what extent this metabolic disorder is aggravated by CAPD is not fully established. The continuous glucose loading from dialysis solutions, the daily protein loss inducing an increased hepatic synthesis of lipoproteins, a greater loss of apolipoprotein A (apoA) over that of apolipoprotein B (apoB) via the peritoneal route and the reduced activity of tissue lipoprotein lipase and hepatic lipase together contribute to the development of lipid abnormalities in CPD patients. The most common lipid profile in CAPD patients includes a near normal or moderately increased level of total cholesterol (TC), reduced levels of apoA and high-density lipoprotein cholesterol (HDLC) and a marked elevation of low-density lipoprotein cholesterol (LDLC), triglycerides and apoB (168, 169). Increased plasma apoB levels are considered as the most prevalent dyslipoproteinemia in patients undergoing CAPD (170). An increased prevalence of high TC compared to HD patients has also been reported (171). During the first years of treatment, both serum triglycerides and serum cholesterol levels usually increase and show a later tendency to stabilize and even to return to predialysis values (172). Circulating triglyceride levels appear to be affected by energy intake and many centers recommend to their patients a restricted use of hypertonic dialysate as well as a decreased dietary energy intake (163). The fractional removal rate for exogenous triglyceride from the blood (K2) at intravenous fat tolerance tests appears to be an important factor because increasing K2 values were observed in patients with stable or decreasing triglyceride levels (173).

Plasma lipoprotein (a) [Lp(a)] levels show a two- to threefold increase by comparison to healthy controls in most series (174–177), with one remarkable exception (178). No correlation could be detected between elevated Lp(a) levels and various patient's characteristics (age, sex, presence or absence of diabetes, duration of dialysis) or other lipid-profile parameter, except in one series finding a correlation between Lp(a) concentrations and apoB levels (176).

Atherogenic risk

Potentially atherogenic changes are induced by CAPD, especially during the initial months of treatment. Atherogenic indices, such as the ratios between serum total cholesterol to HDLC and apoA1 to apoB, are significantly increased in CAPD patients (168). Other potential risk factors for atherosclerosis include hypertriglyceridemia, plasma Lp (a) greater than 30 mg/dL, sustained hyperinsulinemia, the accumulation of chylomicrons in the circulation with high postprandial chylomicron remnant plasma concentrations (179), and elevated plasma levels of advanced glycosylation end products (113). The long term effects of the abnormal lipid profile observed in CAPD patients have not been prospectively studied in large groups of patients. The incidence of cardiovascular deaths is said to be similar among CAPD and HD patient (11–15). In 1991, however, the Australia and New Zealand Dialysis and Transplantation Registry reported that cardiac deaths were significantly greater in nondiabetic CAPD patients than patients on HD; this difference was not found in diabetics (180). In one series, de novo symptomatic vascular disease developed in over 60% of patients undergoing CAPD: this observation was closely associated with hypercholesterolemia and increased systolic blood pressure (181). These findings increase the suspicion that CAPD is indeed atherogenic. Short-term therapeutic studies have demonstrated the efficacy of HMG CoA reductase inhibitors (182–184) or omega–3 fatty acids (185–187) in lowering serum triglyceride and total cholesterol levels in patients undergoing CAPD. Long-term clinical trials, however, will be required to evaluate the impact on the progression of atherosclerosis of these approaches proposed to correct the dyslipoproteinemia of CAPD patients.

Vitamin losses

Hydrosoluble vitamins are lost in significant amounts in the dialysate. This loss results in lower serum levels of vitamin B1, B6, folic acid, and vitamin C in some patients, while vitamins B2 and B12 remain normal in short-term studies (188–190). Daily supplementation with 30 mg vitamin B1, 10 mg vitamin B6 (190), 0.5 mg folic acid, and 100 mg vitamin C is advised (189). Decreasing serum vitamin B12 levels may also occur over longer periods of treatment, and supplementation with this vitamin appears warranted (189).

Liposoluble vitamin D metabolites are also lost via the peritoneal route in CAPD patients (191–193). The practical aspects concerning vitamin D supplementation in these patients is discussed below with the treatment of renal bone disease.

Digestive symptoms

A decreased appetite is not exceptional in patients undergoing CAPD, particularly during the early stages of the treatment, resulting in a selective reduction in dietary carbohydrate intake and in low protein consumption (194). In a study on eating behavior of dialyzed ESRD patients, those undergoing CAPD experienced less hunger and desire to eat and had a lower mean total food intake compared to a matched group of hemodialyzed subjects (195). The reason for the low eating drive in CAPD patients was not elucidated: measured intragastric pressures remained constant with or without dialysate in the abdomen (196). Poor appetite may result from the metabolic effects of the high sugar load from the dialysis fluid, gastric retention,

inadequate dialysis, or a combination of these factors. Obviously, inadequate dialysis as a cause of anorexia should be first ruled out before considering the loss of appetite as a side effect of CAPD, particularly when this symptom is associated with nausea and vomiting.

Workload and patient's burnout

One of the most prominent side effects of peritoneal dialysis, and also one of the most neglected, is the time spent in carrying out the daily dialysis procedures required to obtain adequacy of treatment with this dialysis modality. As four exchanges per day are usually required for treatment efficacy, the never ending manual labour of CAPD (197) is tantamount to about 2 to 2.5 h/day. It is no surprise, therefore, if weariness induced by repetition and time committment required for CAPD remains a cause of drop-out (14). In this respect, the schedule and technical characteristics of CCPD offer considerable advantages to certain patients (35).

Environmental concerns

CAPD, as a home dialysis procedure, generates a large amount of waste including plastic bags, spent dialysate contaminated with bacterias or viruses, and needles that raises serious and often neglected environmental issues (198, 199). Instructions should be given to the patient concerning dialysis waste: these recommendations should be made in accordance with local and national environmental conservation laws and regulations. Needles should be placed in a box and emptied bags should be sealed in a plastic bag prior to their disposal. The patients should be advised to drain their bags into the toilet. For patients infected with hepatitis B or HIV viruses, the use of bleach, poured into the toilet before draining the bag, is recommended to kill the viral particles that contaminate the spent dialysate (200). Dialysate contaminated with hepatitis B should be handled with great care as it represents a significant risk for the transmission of this virus (201). In HIV-infected patients, similar precautions should be taken as p24 HIV-1 antigen has been recovered from the peritoneal effluent of HIV carrier patients (202).

INDICATIONS AND CONTRAINDICATIONS

Indications

When CAPD was introduced in clinical practice, the continuous nature of this new modality made it an attractive alternative to HD. In the late seventies, acetate HD was still predominant. Cardiovascular instability was a major cause of morbidity during HD sessions in roughly 20–25% of hemodialyzed patients, particularly in those with coronary artery disease or cardiomyopathy, in diabetics, in the elderly and in low weight subjects. These so-called 'acetate intolerant' patients formed a heterogeneous population, in whom the benefits of CAPD with its slow continuous ultrafiltration were easy to demonstrate on the short-term. Today, progress in the technology of HD, particularly the introduction of bicarbonate dialysate and of accurate ultrafiltration monitors, have considerably reduced intra-dialytic morbidity. Furthermore, most series comparing survival in patients undergoing either CAPD or HD do not show any superiority to CAPD in that respect (11–15). This evolution makes it more difficult to define specific indications for CAPD except in HD patients with complete exhaustion of blood access sites. In fact, various non-medical factors interfere with the decision to use or not CAPD in a given patient (203). The striking variations in the deployment of CAPD among different countries indicate that the more or less extensive use of this treatment mode does not rest on well established and unanimously accepted prescription rules. In 1992, the percentage of ESRD patients undergoing CAPD ranged from 6% in Germany and in Japan to 17% in the United States, to 51% in the United Kingdom and to 93% in Mexico (204). The most common factors explaining these discrepancies are: the organization of health services in a given country, including the availability of in center HD, the price and payment practices; the nephrologist's experience and biases; the patient's will to gain the maximum independance in the conduct of his or her treatment; the distance between the patient's home and the dialysis center and the development of alternative home dialysis techniques (205).

Today, CPD is considered by most dialysis groups as one indispensable component of an ESRD treatment programme. The choice between HD and CPD may be based on specific medical indications or on patient's preference; it may also proceed from logistic reasons, when the priority is given to the development of home dialysis, or when center HD is not adequately developed (206). In adults, many groups including ours have preferentially used CAPD in the elderly (including patients over 80 years of age) and in patients with cardiovascular complications (18, 207–211). CAPD is also considered a satisfactory therapy in diabetic patients (212). Younger adults may choose CAPD as it fits a more independent lifestyle and makes travelling easier. CPD offers a simpler therapeutic approach in patients waiting for a transplant (213). However, the results obtained with renal transplantation in patients undergoing CAPD should be carefully watched in the light of a report suggesting that graft loss from renovascular thrombosis occurs more frequently among CAPD than HD patients (214). Finally, CAPD deserves consideration as a therapy for HIV-infected patients with ESRD, as comparable outcomes have been obtained with CAPD and HD in these patients (215, 216).

Specific indications for CCPD include poor biochemical profiles in the non-compliant CAPD patient, recurrent peritonitis and suppression of midday exchanges (a major benefit for working adults as well as for children (217,

218) and adolescents (219) attending school) (35, 59). CCPD may solve the problem of inadequate ultrafiltration in CAPD patients with an hyperpermeable peritoneal membrane (220). These patients require the use of frequent nocturnal exchange with shorter dwell times and the substitution of two diurnal exchanges to the usual long daytime cycle to prevent dialysate absorption; alternatively, they should be transferred to nocturnal PD or to HD. Continuous cyclic PD may also be preferred in patients with chronic low-back pain, recurrent catheter exit-site leakage, umbilical or inguinal hernias, diaphragmatic hernias and gastro-oesophageal reflux and hemorrhoids. These parietal complications of CAPD may benefit from the lower intra-abdominal pressure generated by CCPD, but the dialysate volume for the diurnal exchange should also be reduced (59).

Contraindications

CAPD should not be prescribed in patients with suspected low peritoneal urea clearance, particularly in those with prior extensive abdominal surgery (e.g., large bowel resection). Prior abdominal aortic graft aneurysm surgery is only a relative contraindication (221, 222). CPD should be discontinued early whenever low peritoneal clearance is confirmed in a given patient, lest the syndrome of inadequate dialysis develops. Patients of large body built are exposed at a high risk of inadequate dialysis and CPD becomes contraindicated once they are anuric (60).

Medical conditions carrying an increased risk of peritonitis (e.g., ileostomy, colostomy, ureterostomy) are contraindications to CAPD, as are those incompatible with self treatment (e.g., paralysis, severe mental retardation, psychosis or crippling arthritis of the hands). Abdominal hernias impede the use of CAPD, except if surgical repair is possible. By increasing intra-abdominal pressure, CAPD may decompensate severe obstructive lung disease and should be avoided in this setting. Peripheral vascular disease or diverticulosis of the bowel, where CAPD increases the risk of lower limb gangrene or of peritonitis are also considered relative contraindications to CAPD (203, 206). Certain patients will refuse CAPD because the bag exchange in the middle of the day cannot be done safely at work or because of body image concern: these patients may readily accept CCPD which eliminates the midday exchange, but some may still find the abdominal distension unacceptable (59). Finally, depression, social loneliness (particularly in the elderly) and poor motivation are unfavourable circumstances for the long term success of CAPD and should also be considered as relative contraindications.

CLINICAL RESULTS

Fifteen years after its introduction as another alternative to treat ESRD, the wealth of clinical studies reporting on the clinical efficiency of CPD are difficult to interprete objectively. The high drop out rates observed in most series obscure somewhat the issues when compared evaluations of CPD *vs* HD are attempted. Despite this difficulty, there is increasing evidence that CPD may be equivalent, when properly used, to center HD as regards the relief of uremic symptoms, the control of blood pressure, the quality of life and patient survival. CPD may be superior to HD, however, in improving anemia with a less frequent need to prescribe epoetin (human recombinant erythropoietin).

Control of uremia

The relief of uremic symptoms is usually observed soon after starting CPD, and many patient enjoy an increased sense of well being. Complaints of anorexia, tiredness, shortness of breath and inability to perform a job or household tasks were commonly noted with a greater frequency as CPD duration increased in early series (223, 224): these symptoms should always raise the suspicion of inadequate therapy. Clinical evaluation of CPD patients may be improved by the use of patient-reported symptom checklists (225) or nursing assessment scores (47, 71, 79). Stable serum biochemistries are readily obtained. Blood urea levels stabilize at about 25 to 30 mmol/L (blood urea nitrogen levels 70–90 mg/dL) and serum creatinine levels around 0.800 to 1.250 mmol/L (9.0 to 14 mg/dL). Serum potassium values remain in the normal range as well as serum bicarbonate levels particularly when a dialysis fluid with a lactate concentration of 40 mmol/L (40 mEq/L) is used (86). This state of equilibrium has been reported to persist in patients undergoing CAPD without interruption for 7 or more years (172, 226).

Blood pressure control

Since the early days of maintenance HD, the normalization of blood pressure by limitation of sodium dietary intake, adequate removal of excess extra-cellular volume, careful determination and maintenance of the patient's dry weight, has been shown to be the cornerstone for a successful treatment (227). The long term consequences of this factor, often neglected, have been convincingly demonstrated in a large cohort of long term HD patients; in this series, blood pressure control exclusively by careful monitoring of the dry weight was associated with the lowest cardiovascular mortality ever recorded in a dialysis population (228). It is the belief of the author of this chapter that this basic fact should hold true for CAPD even though no long-term study on the outcome of hypertension in CAPD patients is yet available, to allow for a fair comparison with HD.

CAPD, being a continuous process, facililitates sodium removal and extracellular volume reduction by osmotic ultrafiltration. This therapeutic modality readily allows for the daily removal of about 100 to 200 mmol of sodium without the hypotensive episodes often associated with the faster ultrafiltration of HD (229). Actually, when hypertensive ESRD patients are shifted from HD to CAPD, a decrease in blood pressure is obtained, most often associated with a significant weight loss (230). Several series have confirmed that hypertension is easily controlled in the early months of CAPD, when antihypertensive drugs may be progressively reduced in dosage and even be suppressed in many patients (230, 231). After one or more years, however, an apparent decline in efficiency of CAPD in controlling blood pressure is manifested by an increase in antihypertensive drug requirement and or an increased use of hypertonic dialysis solutions (172, 226, 230, 231). This problem may be related to liberalization in sodium and fluid intake by the patient, to the loss of residual renal function, or to the loss of ultrafiltration due to functional or structural changes in the peritoneal membrane such as peritoneal sclerosis or to increased lymphatic reabsorption. A report of the USA National CAPD Registry, studying the effect of this treatment modality on hypertension control in more than 200 patients, underscored the high prevalence of persisting hypertension in this population (232). The most important finding of this study was that 26% of previously controlled patients were uncontrolled hypertensives after one year on CAPD and that 24% of patients uncontrolled at baseline were still uncontrolled after one year. On the other hand, the persistence of a diurnal blood pressure pattern was observed in studies using ambulatory blood pressure monitoring (233–235). In a comparison of CAPD and HD patients, both groups exhibited similar diurnal blood pressure patterns, but CAPD patients had average lower systolic blood pressures and 'systolic loads' (percent systolic values > 140 mmHg) compared to HD patients (233). No differences in diastolic blood pressures, 'diastolic loads', mean arterial pressures, or heart rate were noted between the two dialysis modalities.

Another cause of persisting high blood pressure or of de novo hypertension is the use of epoetin to treat anemia (236). Before initiating epoetin therapy, attempts should be made to normalize the blood pressure by lowering the dry weight and, if necessary, by adjusting antihypertensive therapy (237). During the first weeks of epoetin administration, blood pressure should be carefully monitored to prevent severe complications, such as hypertensive encephalopathy (236).

When anti-hypertensive drugs are required, peritoneal transport may be affected as was shown for enalapril and nifepidine (238). Both these drugs were shown to increase significantly the peritoneal clearances of creatinine, beta-2-microglobulin, and glucose; the latter resulted in a decreased D/Do glucose with a decreased ultrafiltration volume (40% for enalapril, 22% for nifepidine), that could possibly justify an increased use of hyperosmolal solutions to maintain the dry weight.

Correction of anemia and the use of EPO

A rise in hematocrit and hemoglobin concentration occurs in most patients starting on CAPD, although the response can vary considerably (239, 240). The maximum rise in hematocrit appears in the first three to six months. There is some evidence, however, that an initial increase in hemoglobin levels may not be sustained with a tendency to stabilize to a pre-dialysis value (172). Patients on CAPD are characteristically less severely anemic and transfusion dependent than patients on hemodialysis (241). In fact, some patients switched from HD to CAPD have shown significant improvements in their anemia (242, 243). Several mechanisms are involved in the correction of anemia during CAPD. A reduction in plasma volume is partly responsible for the rise in hematocrit, but a well documented increase in red cell mass plays a major role in this improvement (239, 240, 244). A prolongation in red cell survival is also observed (245), but the reduced erythrocyte life span still persists (244, 246, 247). Ferrokinetic studies have brought direct evidence of improved erythropoiesis after starting CAPD: these observations suggest that red cell production is a major determinant of the total red cell mass (244, 246). The persistence of uremic anemia in patients on CAPD may result from a failure of erythropoiesis to catch up fully with the excessive red cell destruction. Improved erythropoiesis is accompanied by an increased proliferation of bone marrow erythropoietic progenitor cells (248, 249). This may relate to the removal of inhibitors of erythropoiesis by dialysis (249, 250). It should be noted, however, that the mere existence of such inhibitors has been questioned (237).

The improved erythropoiesis observed at the start of CAPD is also thought to be due to an increase in erythropoietin production. Serum erythropoietin concentrations in ESRD patients, who are not anephric, are in the normal range or slightly higher (244, 249), but the EPO concentration is always inadequately low for the severity of anemia. In one study, serum erythropoietin levels were significantly higher in patients on CAPD than those on HD (251). Three major factors have been proposed to explain the relative elevation of erythropoietin: 1) a better removal of uremic toxin inhibiting erythropoietin production; 2) an improved nutritional status; and, 3) the production of erythropoietin by peritoneal macrophages repeatedly stimulated by unphysiologic dialysis solution (252). In one study, patients with measurable levels of erythropoietin had higher hematocrits than those with undetectable or minimal levels of the hormone (242). In most cases, however, no relationship was found between serum erythropoietin levels and improved erythropoiesis (240, 244, 249). A better preservation of residual renal function of patients on CAPD compared to HD (48–51) could also affect erythropoiesis and EPO levels. A retrospective study, however, failed to show any significant correlation between the level of creatinine clearance and hematocrit (253). Although a few patients achieve normal hemoglobin levels during CAPD, in most of them, hematocrits stabilize in the range of 28 to 30% with hemoglobin concentrations around 95 to 100 g/L. About 30% of patients on CAPD will remain anemic with hematocrits of 27% or lower and hemoglobin levels below 90 g/L. Today, the problem of persisting anemia (in the absence of iron deficiency or other non-uremic factor) is easily resolved with the use of recombinant human erythropoietin (epoetin, EPO) (237, 254). The pharmacokinetics of EPO have been studied in patients on CAPD, comparing the intravenous (i.v.), subcutaneous (s.c.) and intraperitoneal (i.p.) routes of administration (255, 256). The results of these studies are more thoroughly discussed later. As previously noted in HD patients (257–259), the s.c. route of EPO administration requires about 20–50% less EPO than the i.v. route to maintain a similar hematocrit level. The use of the i.p. route for EPO has received considerable attention because it offers the possible advantage of simpler self administration to the CAPD patient (260–263). The bioavailability studies compared s.c. with i.p. EPO administered in 2 liter dialysate solution (diluted). The i.p. unit had a seven fold lower bioavailability (2.19% for i.p. *versus* 21.5% s.c routes) (255, 256). However, if dialysate containing EPO is infused in the dry, empty peritoneal cavity, the bioavailability increased nine fold to the same level as s.c. EPO (260). Another study compared i.p. route with s.c. route but added EPO to only one liter of dialysate: the rate of rise in hematocrit was slower with the i.p. route of administration (261). These studies show that the administration of EPO by the i.p. route is efficient but less cost-effective. However, the cost-effectiveness can be improved by adding EPO in a lower volume of dialysate or infusing the hormone into an empty peritoneal cavity. These approaches may reduce the cost of i.p. administration to that of s.c. level (263). Subcutaneous EPO is usually administered thrice-weekly (259, 264, 265), but twice-weekly dosing and even once-a-week administration have been successfully used in some patients (259, 266–269).

Patients responding to epoetin treatment report significant changes in energy level, social relationships and leisure activity (270). In one study, the improvement in quality of life was proportional to the target hemoglobin levels reached in a step-wise fashion. Energy improved significantly at hemoglobin levels of 110–115 g/L, but improvement in sleep and emotional well being were noted only when a target hemoglobin of 130–135 g/L was reached (265). An improved nutritional status has been reported in CAPD patients treated with epoetin, including a significant increase in serum total protein, serum albumin and absolute lymphocyte counts (271). Improved blood lipid profiles have been observed during epoetin induced correction of anemia in CAPD patients taking no lipid lowering agents; significant decreases of serum total cholesterol, triglycerides and lipoprotein B were noted (272).

Hypertension is the main adverse effect of epoetin in CAPD patients as observed in 30–50% of patients on EPO. This is defined as a rise in mean blood pressure, or in diastolic blood pressure of 10 mmHg or more, the need for higher doses of anti-hypertensive drugs or for initiating anti-hypertensive therapy (264–266, 273). A similar incidence of increased blood pressure is observed among HD patients (237, 254). Close monitoring of blood pressure is, therefore, recommended in CAPD patients receiving epoetin. Usually, hypertension can be adequately controlled by the use of appropriate anti-hypertensive medications (273).

Iron deficiency is the main cause of ineffectiveness of epoetin, while inflammation is the second most common cause of secondary epoetin failure (237). In contrast, peritonitis episodes complicating CAPD are associated with a non-significant decrease in hemoglobin concentration and restoration of hemoglobin levels to prior values was achieved with unchanged epoetin dose within a month of peritonitis episode (259, 274).

Effect of higher hematocrits on the efficiency of CAPD is controversial. A decrease in peritoneal transport was observed in some studies (250, 271), while other reports indicated increased peritoneal clearances sometimes associated with an increased ultrafiltration (250, 272). These findings have not been confirmed by other groups (277–280). In these studies, solute transport characteristics and ultrafiltration capacity remained stable after correction of anemia with epoetin. Likewise, serum biochemistries remained stable in all studies reported (254). These latter findings are consistent with the concept that peritoneal blood flow is not a rate limiting factor for the removal of small molecular weight solutes in patients on CAPD (36).

Renal osteodystrophy

The effects of CAPD on renal osteodystrophy remains controversial despite numerous studies on the control and development of this complication of chonic renal failure. Striking variations in the bone lesions assessed by repeated biopsies were shown among the patients, from complete healing of osteitis fibrosa to the persistence and aggravation of secondary hyperparathyroidism or the occurrence of aplastic bone disease (281, 282). The latter appears to be more prevalent in CAPD than in HD patients: this increased prevalence of non-aluminic adynamic/aplastic bone disease may be related to advanced age, diabetes mellitus, low parathyroid hormone concentration, and the use of calcium carbonate (282). They may also be due to differences in diagnostic approach and in management between renal units with regard to the use of bone biopsy, the degree of phosphate control, the type and amount of prescribed phosphate binders, and the use of vitamin D (282). In one series, bone histomorphometry detected osteitis fibrosa as the predominant bone disease (283). In this study, as significant positive

correlations were found between serum osteocalcin and bone formation parameters, it was suggested that serum osteocalcin is a valuable non-invasive index of metabolic bone disease, giving additional information to serum parathormone levels in patients undergoing CAPD (283). From the available data, there is no clear-cut evidence to suggest that renal bone disease is any different in CAPD than in HD.

Since the late eighties, the therapeutic approach aiming at the correction of the main calcium and phosphate metabolism abnormalities have followed major changes in CAPD patients. These changes concern the three parameters most commonly monitored in daily clinical practice: the correction of hyperphosphatemia, the maintenance of normal serum calcium levels and the prescription of active vitamin D3 metabolites (284–287).

The removal of inorganic phosphorus by CAPD is limited to about 300 mg per day, whereas the obligatory phosphate intake will be 1200 mg per day if the dietary protein intake is maintained at the recommended level of 1.2 g/kg body weight per day (63, 288). Therefore, to achieve a neutral phosphate balance, the gastrointestinal elimination of phosphorus should be in the range of 700 to 900 mg per day (284). Since the fraction of phosphate absorbed by patients with renal failure represents 40 to 80% of dietary phosphorus, gastrointestinal elimination should be enhanced by oral phosphate-binding agents (289). With the increasing awareness about the dangers of the aluminum salts prescribed to prevent phosphate absorption, calcium salts have replaced aluminum hydroxide as first line therapy for hyperphosphatemia in most renal units (290). Calcium carbonate has been shown to be equivalent in its efficacy to aluminum hydroxide (291, 292). By comparison with the latter, it has a beneficial effect on the progression of renal bone disease. The use of calcium carbonate as the sole phosphate binder is, also, associated with a steady decrease in serum aluminum levels in patients previously taking oral aluminum salts (290, 293, 294). Calcium-containing binders, however, are not without some problems, and calcium carbonate usage is a common cause of hypercalcemia (295, 296). To obviate this problem, a logical step was to reduce the concentration of calcium in peritoneal dialysis solutions in an attempt to decrease or reverse the peritoneal calcium flux (81, 284, 285, 297, 298). The three important determinants of transperitoneal flux are serum ultrafilterable calcium, dialysis fluid calcium and the volume of ultralfiltration. With standard CAPD fluids containing 1.75 mmol/L calcium, the patient gains about 30 mg of calcium during a 2-liter exchange with 15 g/L dextrose concentration. With a 40 g/L dextrose solution, the greater ultrafiltration results in a net convective loss from the patient of approximately 5 mg per exchange. If a patient performs four exchanges per day with three 15 g/L and one 40 g/L bags, the net calcium uptake will be approximately 85 mg (288). With 'low' calcium fluid, containing 1.25 mmol/L, a decrease in total body calci-

580   *Charles M. Mion*

um of 160 mg/L will be observed if the serum-ionized calcium reaches 1.3 mmol/L and greater decreases during episodes of hypercalcemia (284, 298). The use of 'low' calcium dialysis solution allowed the administration of larger doses of calcium carbonate: it resulted in improved phosphate control despite a decreased intake of aluminum-containing phosphate binders; the incidence of hypercalcemia was reduced (84, 85, 299). Low-calcium dialysate, however, may place the patients at higher risk for progression of hyperparathyroidism, if it is used without discrimination specially in the patient poorly compliant in taking calcium carbonate (300).

Levels of 1,25-dihydroxy-vitamin D3 (calcitriol) are low in CAPD patients as in others with chronic renal failure (286). However, 25-hydroxy-vitamin D3 [25(OH)-D3] levels, which are usually normal at the start of CAPD, may reach subnormal values with time or remain stable. This variation may be induced by different sunlight exposure among the study populations, the availability of adequate amounts of parent vitamin D2 and the duration of therapy. Although 25(OH)D3 and its binding protein are lost in the dialysate (191, 192), there is no universal agreement on a routine vitamin D supplement to replace these losses. This therapy is mainly indicated to control secondary hyperparathyroidism (286). Calcitriol or 1-alpha hydroxy-vitamin D3 are the appropriate replacement forms of vitamin D. Several routes of administration and timing intervals are available to the nephrologist contemplating the use of calcitriol in suppressing parathormone secretion in CPD patients: oral daily dosage (301), oral pulse therapy (302), the intraperitoneal (303) or subcutaneous routes (304, 305). No prospective study demonstrating the superiority of one of these modes of administration is yet available. Oral pulse therapy (2 to 5 μg of calcitriol three times a week) has been recommended as the preferable approach until more information is obtained (286). Giving calcitriol at bedtime instead of in the morning may reduce the incidence of hypercalcemia (306). The use of calcitriol in CAPD patients, however, is not without hazard: evidence for an increased frequency of low bone turnover or adynamic bone lesions during intermittent calcitriol treatment has been reported (307). Until more information is available, the aim of calcitriol therapy should be to maintain serum levels of intact parathormone (PTH) between 1.5 and 2.5 times the upper limit of normal. Bone formation, however, may decline despite persistently high serum levels of PTH and or alkaline phosphatase. This observation suggests that calcitriol may directly suppress osteoblastic activity in patients with secondary hyperparathyroidism when prescribed as oral pulse therapy in patients undergoing CPD (286).

Maintenance of good nutritional status

As with other modes of dialysis, a major aim of CPD is to improve nutritional status. Malnourished ESRD patients started on CPD have a 50 to 60% chance to return to a normal nutritional state during the first three months of treatment (25). In a large multi-centric cross-sectional study, almost 60% of the patients were classified as normal based on subjective global assessment after mean CAPD durations of 26 to 35 months (26). Metabolic studies have shown that nitrogen balance is neutral or positive in a majority of patients (63, 64, 308). A positive correlation was found between nitrogen balance (not corrected for 'unmeasured' nitrogen losses) and dietary protein intake and also with total energy intake in balance studies performed during the early months of treatment; when the balance was repeated after a year of CAPD, nitrogen balance correlated only to total energy intake (64). Although a protein intake below 1 g/kg body weight/day may be associated with a positive nitrogen balance in individual patients (64, 68, 163), clinically stable CAPD patients should have a diet with a protein content of about 1.2 g/kg body weight/day, to ensure a protein allowance large enough to satisfy the varied needs of individual patients. Protein requirements, however, may be increased in some protein-depleted patients who may benefit by eating 1.4 to 2.1 g protein/kg/day particularly during the initial months of treatment or following an episode of peritonitis (64). On the other hand, a number of studies have shown that there is a correlation between KT/V urea and protein intake, as assessed from the urea appearance rate (64–69, 309). The relationship between KT/V and the protein catabolic rate (PCR) was found to be different in CAPD patients compared to HD patients: at the same low KT/V levels, CAPD patients had higher protein intakes estimated from PCR than HD patients and the protein intake increased more for the same increase in KT/V in the CAPD than in the HD patients (310). This correlation has been interpreted as evidence that protein intake is related to the dialysis dose (65). As this relationship includes a mathematical component, however, its quantitative significance is not entirely clear (66, 309). The mathematical interrelationship is the consequence of using the same urea nitrogen appearance data in the calculation of both KT/V and PCR. Although the possibility that this relationship is a mathematical artifact still remains a matter of dispute (309, 311–314), the observation that a dissociation of KT/V urea and PCR is common, that the correlation between these two parameters is not linear and the fact that values of PCR for a given KT/V urea are influenced by the type of dialysis membrane, are cogent reasons to accept that the relationship between KT/V urea and PCR is physiological (311).

The best approach for assessing nutritional status in clinical routine remains a controversial issue. Anthropometric norms have been determined among a large group of HD patients in a study demonstrating the reliability and the reproducibility of anthropometric measurements (315). Similar data are not available for CAPD patients and the value of anthropometry in assessing nutritional status in this population is not well established (315, 316). Dietary history is often said to be of doubtful reliability:

however, the use of diaries kept by the patients on their diets and recall interviews provide accurate information on dietary protein and energy intake when evaluated by skilled dietitians (64). Several studies confirmed the accuracy of dietary protein intake evaluation by history, as a significant relationship was found between DPI and urea nitrogen appearance (UNA, calculated from the sum of urea nitrogen output in urine and dialysate, corrected for changes in total body urea nitrogen) or protein catabolic rate (PCR, the protein equivalent of UNA calculated as 6.25 UNA) (68). On the other hand, the estimation of dietary energy intake was more uncertain as it relies exclusively on dietary recall.

Methods to assess the nutritional status more objectively have been proposed, with a particular interest in analyzing body composition, as patients undergoing CAPD may lose muscle mass at the expense of fat or water gain and hence, remain at or above their ideal body weight. Besides the use of research tools such as total body nitrogen assessment by prompt neutron activation analysis (316, 317), muscle biopsy (318, 319) or total body potassium measurements (317, 318), clinically applicable methods have been proposed, including bioelectrical impedance analysis (320, 321), dual photon absorptiometry (322), total body electrical conductivity (323) and creatinine kinetics (324, 325). Bioelectrical impedance analysis measures total body water, fat mass and lean body mass, with a constant overestimation of the latter. Creatinine kinetics is based on the principle that creatinine production is proportional to muscle mass and that, in the stable patient, creatinine production is equal to the sum of creatinine excretion, in urine and dialysate, and metabolic degradation. The reliability and usefulness of these promising methods in the nutritional surveillance of CAPD patients are an area of active clinical research (316–329).

Serum albumin concentration is considered as a routine measure of visceral protein stores and is used as a guide for dietary protein intake in PD patients. Unfortunately, the various methods available to the determination of serum albumin concentration do not yield similar results (330). By comparison with immunoturbidimetry, which is accepted as the reference method, the most commonly used method utilizing the bromcresol green dye markedly overestimates the plasma albumin concentration, while the bromcresol purple method slightly underestimates it (330, 331). On average, CAPD patients are slightly hypoalbuminemic, but knowing the method of determination is of crucial importance for the interpretation of serum albumin values in individual patients as well as in studies analyzing the affect of serum albumin values on morbidity and mortality of dialysis patients (331). In CAPD patients, the serum albumin level is the net result of four dynamic processes: albumin synthesis, catabolism, body distribution of albumin and albumin losses in dialysate and in urine (in case of remaining residual renal function). Albumin homeostasis is maintained through successful compensatory mechanisms (see above

in section on protein losses) and nutrition is thought to be the most important factor promoting albumin synthesis in CAPD patients (157, 158). To what extent dietary protein intake (DPI) can influence serum albumin levels is still a matter of debate. In spite of conflicting results regarding this issue, it seems likely that a correlation exists between DPI (normalized to body weight) and serum albumin in CAPD patients, albeit this correlation may be weak (331). Furthermore, supplementing the diet with high protein nutrients has been shown to result in increased serum albumin levels in hypoalbuminemic CAPD patients (332). Many factors beside inadequate DPI, however, may induce a low serum albumin level among CAPD patients, including old age, comorbidity (e.g., diabetes mellitus), overhydration, increased dialysate albumin loss and intercurrent illness. Consequently, serum albumin levels do not always directly correlate to other measures of nutritional status. Some studies have reported a correlation between serum albumin *versus* other nutritional parameters such as subjective global assessment, anthropometric measurements, total body nitrogen, single-frequency body electrical impedance (BEI), nitrogen balance or total body potassium (331). On the other hand, other studies were unable to find any correlation between serum albumin *versus* lean body mass assessed by BEI (333) or dual energy x-ray absorptiometry (334), or *versus* total body nitrogen (335). In conclusion, serum albumin may be used as a good measure of short-term DPI and its level may fall more promptly in CAPD patients due to continued albumin loss. In the assessment of overall nutrition, however, albumin is not the most sensitive parameter and should not be used without reference to other nutritional markers such as body weight, body composition and the functional status of the patient (158).

Quality of life

The success of renal replacement therapy lies not only in patients' absolute survival time, but also in the quality of that survival (336). Many studies have approached this complex subject that encompasses such crucial areas as physical well-being, relations with other people, economic circumstances, social activities, personal development and recreation (337). In all areas explored in a large multicentric study, CAPD patients fared slightly better than patients undergoing in-center HD, whereas both groups of patients experienced a lesser quality of life than that observed in home HD and successful transplant patients (338). In another study, CAPD patients had lower scores for illness, modality-related stress and mood disturbances; they also had higher employment, higher community activities, better cognitive functions, a higher index of well-being and greater life satisfaction than patients receiving in-center HD (339, 340). Employment rates, however, varied considerably among the series and the loss of employment was one of the objective losses commonly identified by CAPD patients (338–342). As

Table 3. Complications of continuous peritoneal dialysis (excluding peritonitis and parietal complications)

1.	Inadequate dialysis
1.1.	Loss of residual renal function without adjustment of prescription
1.2.	Non-compliance
1.2.1.	Patient skipping out prescribed exchanges
1.2.2.	Patient reducing volume of exchanges or shortening dwell time (dumping)
2.	Malnutrition
2.1.	Inadequate protein intake
2.2.	Inadequate energy intake
2.3.	Low serum albumin
3.	Membrane failure (see Table 4)
4.	Cardiovascular complications
4.1.	Left ventricular diastolic dysfunction
4.2.	Cardiac arrhytmias
4.3.	Severe vasovagal syncope
4.4.	Deterioration of peripheral vascular disease: lower limb gangrene
4.5.	Chronic hypotension
5.	Miscellaneous
5.1.	Low back pain syndrome
5.2.	Obesity
5.3.	Beta-2 microglobulin associated amyloidosis
5.4.	Acquired renal cystic disease
5.5.	Chronic sleep disturbances
5.6.	Hyperosmolality states
5.7.	Oxalate kidney stones
5.8.	Eosinophilia

previously mentionned, epoetin treatment was shown to have a positive impact on several quality of life parameters in CAPD patients including energy, physical activity and sleep, but had no significant influence on vocational rehabilitation (270, 343).

COMPLICATIONS

The many complications that can plague the clinical course of CPD are listed in Table 3. The following discussion will be limited to the problems of inadequate dialysis, malnutrition, peritoneal membrane failure, cardiovascular complications and a few other less frequent conditions.

Inadequate dialysis

Inadequate dialysis is a cause of patient drop-out to HD in at least 10% of the patients undergoing CAPD (11, 344, 345), but this low percentage may reflect a gross underestimate (346). Anorexia, nausea or vomiting, persistent fatigue and weakness, decreasing hemoglobin level below 90 g/L in the absence of bleeding are all suggestive of inadequate dialysis, particularly if associated to a serum creatinine greater than 1200 μmol/L (12.5 mg/dL) in a small adult (less than 65 kilograms) or greater than 1350 μmol/L (15.0 mg/dL) in a larger adult (more than 65 kilograms) (23). Peripheral neuropathy or insomnia, less frequently pericarditis may also herald treatment inadequacy (163). Progressive wasting, occurring in the context of increasing blood pressure in a hitherto normotensive patient and requiring repeated downward adjustment of 'dry weight', is another clue to the diagnosis of underdialysis.

Progressive loss of residual renal function, not compensated for by an adequate increase in number of exchanges or instillation volumes, is the most frequent cause of inadequate dialysis. Poor compliance with the peritoneal dialysis prescription is also frequently observed, patients skipping out one or more exchanges per day, particularly when more than three daily exchanges are prescribed (347, 348). Noncompliance may easily be detected by comparing measured and calculated creatinine generation rates; using this approach, two studies reported non-compliance with the peritoneal dialysis prescription among 26 and 78% of CAPD patients, respectively (348, 349). Dialysate dumping in patients complaining of intolerable abdominal fullness is another cause of dialysis inadequacy: this practice consists in partial peritoneal drainage prior to the end of the prescribed dwell time or in flushing part of the fresh dialysis solution directly in the drain bag during infusion in patients using the requisite number of bags (350). Noncompliance and improper technique should always be suspected when inadequate dialysis is unexplained by significant changes in residual renal function or peritoneal permeability characteristics (as shown by stable PET test values). As non-compliance is a major reason for CAPD technique failure, the nephrologist should be keen at detecting those patients who do not comply with or modify prescriptions: the identification of the non-compliant patient should be taken as one opportunity either to adapt the prescription to a greater convenience (e.g., lesser frequency of exchanges with increased volume) or to teach again the patient about the importance of doing all prescribed exchanges (349). Severe alterations in peritoneal membrane transfer characteristics are not often reported as a cause of dialysis inadequacy, but this eventuality should be looked for by performing a PET test (55). If decreased peritoneal performances are confirmed, the patient should be transferred to HD.

Malnutrition

Protein-energy malnutrition is common among ESRD patients undergoing CAPD (25, 26). Several factors may contribute to the high prevalence of altered nutritional status in this population including the loss of protein and amino acids into the dialysis fluid, anorexia and declining appetite with time on dialysis, biochemical abnormalities, peritonitis and other intercurrent catabolic illnesses (351). Malnutrition in CAPD patients has been evaluated by subjective global assessment, a method based on history and physical examination, that characterizes the patients as normal or mildly to moderately or severely malnourished with excellent intra- and inter-observer reproducibility (352). In a cooperative cross-sectional study conducted in six CAPD centers in Europe and North America and including 224 patients, 8% of the patients were severely malnourished, 32.6% had signs of mild to moderate malnutrition and 59.4% were normal (26). Severely malnourished patients, 94% of whom had no residual renal function, had the following characteristics: they were receiving a lower total daily volume of dialysate by comparison with well-nourished patients with no residual renal function (who represented 41% of the latter); their actual body weights (ABW) were markedly less than their desirable body weights (DBW) due to recent losses of somatic protein and fat stores; if urea clearance was normalized to $0.58 \times$ DBW rather than to $0.58 \times$ ABW, this value was significantly lower than in well-nourished patients (309). These observations suggest that the failure to compensate for loss of residual renal function can lead to malnutrition. To what extent the plasma and free amino acid abnormalities observed in CAPD patients, particularly those of tryptophan and its metabolites, may facilitate the occurrence of malnutrition, has not yet been fully elucidated (353). In everyday practice, the nutritional status of patients undergoing CAPD should be closely monitored at regular intervals (e.g., twice yearly) using both clinical and biochemical parameters such as the subjective global assessment method, serial serum albumin measurements and periodic estimation of dietary protein intake from dietary recall or from urea generation rate (an approach that may be misleading in the catabolic patient) (64). The underdialyzed malnourished patient should be treated by an increase in total daily dialysate volume (23); he or she should also be offered dietetic counselling as well as protein and energy supplements (354). If these measures fail in restoring good nutrition, a trial with intraperitoneal amino acid solutions should be done, but the nutritional benefit remains uncertain (355–357). Eventually, the patient should be changed to HD if a clear improvement in the nutritional status is not obtained on the short-term.

Membrane failure

The development, either sudden or gradual, of an inability to adequately dialyze patients undergoing CAPD is often secondary to an alteration in peritoneal membrane function (358). The term 'membrane failure' has been coined to describe this condition that is due to a variety of pathophysiologic processes as shown in Table 4. The diagnosis of membrane failure should be considered in the presence of fluid overload associated or not with signs and symptoms of inadequate solute removal (i.e., uremia). Indeed, this entity has been initially described as permanent loss

Table 4. Main types, causes and differential diagnosis of membrane failure in continuous peritoneal dialysis

1.	Type I membrane failure
	Permanent loss of ultrafiltration capacity
	Good biochemical control
	PET high transporters
2.	Type II membrane failure
2.1.	Sclerosing peritonitis
	Permanent loss of ultrafiltration
	Poor biochemical control
	PET low transporter
	Malnutrition
2.2.	Peritoneal adhesion
	Loculation of PDS
	PET data: unreliable
2.3.	Peritoneal sclerosis
	UF preserved or increased
	Poor biochemical control
	PET low transporter
3.	Type III membrane failure
	Excessive lymphatic reabsorption (exclusion diagnosis)
4.	Differential diagnosis
4.1.	Peritoneal catheter dysfunction: abnormal outflow
4.1.1.	Constipation
4.1.2.	Catheter malposition
4.1.3.	Catheter displacement
4.1.4.	Omental entrapment
4.2.	Internal leak of peritoneal dialysis fluid
4.3.	Non-compliance with dietary recommendation
4.4.	Decreased 24-hr urinary volume
	Declining residual function

of ultrafiltration capacity (359). The use of the peritoneal equilibration test (PET) is of major importance to identify the underlying mechanisms of this disorder (55).

Several conditions mimicking 'membrane failure' should first be excluded before considering this diagnosis, including: patient's dietary indiscretion with excessive sodium and/or protein intake; patient's non-compliance with the dialysis prescription; the loss of residual renal function; malposition of the peritoneal catheter due to improper placement or migration from the pelvis; dialysate leaks from the peritoneal cavity to extra-abdominal tissues; increased lymphatic absorption due to increased intraperitoneal pressure. Peritonitis is also a cause of impaired ultrafiltration (UF), due to increased small solute peritoneal clearances with enhanced glucose absorption: peritoneal UF capacity returns promptly to normal with the cure of peritoneal infection (360).

The differential diagnosis of these various conditions will be guided by a medical history identifying a reduction in urinary output and seeking evidence of non-compliance with diet or dialysis (358, 361). The circumstances of fluid accumulation should also be described because malpositioned catheter or dialysate leaks have more acute presentation than membrane failure *per se*. A quick two liter exchange is helpful in rapidly recognizing mechanical problems with the catheter. The measurement of intraperitoneal pressure is a useful adjunct if increased lymphatic absorption is suspected (362). At this point, a standard PET should be performed if the diagnosis is still uncertain (55, 56).

Three types of membrane failure have been described according to the PET results: UF failure with high solute transport (type I failure); UF failure with low solute transport (type II failure); increased lymphatic absorption (occasionally referred to as type III failure) (358, 361).

Type I membrane failure is characterized by an increased diffusive mass transfer area coefficient for small solutes, without any change in the rate of protein transport. The increased net transport of glucose negatively influences ultrafiltration and results in fluid management problems, while biochemical control may improve due to the increased removal of other small solutes. According to PET results, these patients will be identified as high transporters. Type I membrane failure is responsible for about 80% of patients with permanent loss of UF capacity, with increased lymphatic absorption being responsible for the remainder (363, 364). The risk of UF capacity loss increases with time on CAPD and was found to be 2.6% after one year and 30.9% after six years of dialysis in one study (364). The frequent use of hypertonic dialysis solutions and peritonitis have been suggested as etiologic agents, but the relation between these factors and permanent UF failure remains unproven. In some cases, impaired UF capacity unrelated to peritonitis was found to be a reversible phenomenon: the PET values for solute transport and UF may return to their previous state after one or to months of interrupted CAPD, which can be successfully reinitiated (365). In the majority of patients, adequate UF will be restored by prescribing a regimen with shorter dwell times using various combinations of CAPD and automated PD (including CCPD with 4 exchanges during the day and 3 to 4 nightly exchanges). Short-term clinical studies suggest that oral or intraperitoneal phosphatidylcholine may improve ultrafiltration (144, 366, 367), but negative results have also been reported with this therapeutic approach (368, 369). Available clinical data do not allow suggesting guidelines about the use of phosphatidylcholine in patients with UF failure. Despite changes in PD prescriptions, some patients will fail PD and should be transferred to HD. Type I membrane failure has been shown to be an early manifestation of sclerosing peritonitis: the eventual occurrence of this dreadful complication following cessation of CAPD should be kept in mind (21, 370).

Type II membrane failure results from *sclerosing peritonitis*, a state of diffuse chronic inflammation of the peritoneum leading to a large reduction in membrane suface area and permeability (82, 371). The PET results in these patients will fall in the low transport category. The clinical presentation associates signs and symptoms of fluid overload, and uremia; with the progress of peritoneal sclerosis, symptoms of intestinal obstruction develop leading to severe protein-energy malnutrition and cachexia with a very poor prognosis (371–373). More information on this rare entity is presented in the chapter of this book dealing with the abdominal complications of CAPD. The formation of *peritoneal adhesions* may also be a cause of type II membrane failure either by reducing the intact mesothelial surface area available for diffusion through the peritoneum, or by limiting the dialysate flow throughout the abdominal cavity and compromising the contact between dialysate and the available surface area of the peritoneum through fluid trapping. In this context, the PET results should be interpreted with caution. Loculation of the dialysis fluid can be visualized with plain roentgenogram or computed tomography after the intraperitoneal infusion of a radiographic contrast material through the peritoneal catheter (374) or with peritoneal scintigraphy (375). If adhesions are localized, surgical lysis will improve dialysate flow and the patient may continue on CAPD. If adhesions are extensive, the surgical approach should be avoided and the patient be changed to HD.

Excessive lymphatic absorption, sometimes termed *type III membrane failure*, associates low UF rates and unchanged peritoneal solute transport as evaluated by the PET (376). Methods for measuring peritoneal lymphatic flow still pertain to the research setting (377, 378). The diagnosis of increased lymphatic absorption, therefore, remains a diagnosis of exclusion after eliminating other causes of UF failure that do not affect peritoneal membrane characteristics, such as peritoneal leaks, malpositioned catheter and increased intra-abdominal pressure (358, 361).

Cardiovascular complications

A high mortality due to cardiovascular disease is observed among ESRD patients treated by CAPD (10–15). Lethal cardiovascular events are said to occur with the same frequency in CAPD as in HD patients, although an increased risk of dying from atherosclerotic complications was reported among non-diabetic CAPD patients by comparison with hemodialyzed patients (180). In any event, cardiovascular diseases remain the leading cause of death in both groups of patients. Pre-existing heart and artery disease as well as a high prevalence of cardiovascular risk factors at the initiation of dialysis are held responsible for this observation. No specific pattern of cardiac disease has been ascribed to CAPD *per se* (379).

Left ventricular (LV) diastolic dysfunction was identified during the early months of CAPD, and was found to persist on the long term despite a significant increase in

LV mass and a decrease in LV volume/mass ratio. Both uncontrolled hypertension and inadequate dialysis were implicated in the persistence of this abnormality (380). In an echocardiographic analysis comparing surviving and non-surviving patients on CAPD, non-survivors had lower mean left ventricular (LV) ejection fraction, higher LV end-systolic volume indices and a shorter mean LV ejection time (381).

Cardiac arrhythmias, with an increased frequency of atrial and/or ventricular premature beats, have been reported in CAPD patients: preexisting left ventricular hypertrophy was identified as the main risk factor for their occurrence (382, 383).

Severe vaso-vagal reflex-inducing syncope related to dialysate infusion is a rare complication which was reported in patients initiating CAPD therapy (384, 385). Diabetic patients may be at higher risk for this complication. Antimuscarinic drugs should be used to prevent this reflex that tends to disappear spontaneously in a few weeks.

A high prevalence of *symptomatic vascular disease* has been observed in CAPD patients. While a significant number of patients may have the disease prior to the commencement of CAPD, peripheral vascular disease, either alone or in association with ischemic heart disease, has been shown to develop in a large number of patients during the course of CAPD (181). Hypercholesterolemia and systolic blood pressure were the factors most closely associated to vascular disease. Elevated levels of fibrinogen, factor VII coagulant activity and plasminogen activator inhibitor have also been found in CAPD patients suggesting a state of hypercoagulability and reduced fibrinolysis, which may promote the development of accelerated atherosclerosis (386). Symptomatic exacerbation of peripheral vascular disease should be of concern in patients starting CAPD, as limb perfusion may be compromised during hypotensive episodes induced by hypovolemia (387, 388).

Chronic hypotension may develop in some patients during the early months of CAPD (223, 229, 388). Blood pressure lowering is due to a combination of dialysate sodium loss and restricted sodium consumption leading to sodium depletion (389). Diabetic autonomic neuropathy or cardiac dysfunction are common predisposing factors. Liberalization of dietary sodium intake in such patients usually leads to the restoration of extracellular fluid volume and to an improved vascular pressure response, which result in blood pressure normalization (389).

Miscellaneous complications

The development or recurrence of a *low-back pain syndrome* has been reported in patients undergoing CAPD (390). This complication, which may lead to CAPD discontinuation, can effectively be prevented by training the patient to perform regularly proper exercises to reduce lumbar lordosis and to strengthen abdominal and lower extremity musculature (390).

Obesity is rarely observed in CAPD patients despite the daily glucose load absorbed from the dialysate. A moderate weight gain occurs in a majority of patients during the first year of treatment, with a tendency to stabilize around the ideal weight (172, 223, 226). In one study, however, a subgroup of patients weighing 110% or more of the ideal weight at start of CAPD were shown to be at risk to become very obese; in these patients, restriction of the total caloric intake was deemed necessary (390).

Beta-2 microglobulin (B2M) blood levels remain elevated despite an increased removal of this substance with CAPD compared to cuprophane HD (392–394). The use of an isoosmolar solution containing 5% glucose polymer enhanced 1.6 times the transperitoneal elimination of B2M, but did not affect serum concentrations during a 6-hour study (395). With both CAPD and HD, however, the residual renal function has a major impact on the total daily removal of B2M (392, 396). *Dialysis-associated amyloidosis* is seldom reported among CAPD patients, although a few cases of carpal tunnel syndrome have been observed (397, 398). The paucity of this complication, however, may be explained by the small number of patients receiving CAPD for five or more years (172, 226).

Acquired renal cystic disease was reported to have the same prevalence and severity in patients treated with CAPD as compared with those on HD (399, 400). The grade of cystic disease was found to correlate with the duration of CAPD and had no effect on hemoglobin levels (399).

Other complications include *chronic sleep disturbances* in relationship with the sleep apnea syndrome (401), *hyperosmolality states* leading to coma and convulsions (402), the occurrence of *kidney stones* in previously non-stone-forming patients (403) and the development of *eosinophilia* that appears more frequent in CCPD than in CAPD (404, 405).

CLINICAL OUTCOMES OF CONTINUOUS PERITONEAL DIALYSIS

Various parameters have been used to assess the outcomes of CAPD, including number of hospitalisation days per year (often referred to as morbidity), causes of death and patient and technique survival. Using these items, several series have analyzed outcomes comparatively in cohorts of CAPD and HD patients (11–15, 406–408). With CAPD, the number of days spent in the hospital per patient per year varied from 10.14 days (13) to 20 days (407), and peritonitis was the major cause of hospital admission (11, 407). Patient survival was similar among CAPD and HD patients, when the analysis used the Cox Proportional Hasards Model (409) with adjustment for various patient characteristics. Factors influencing adversely CAPD outcome included age, cardiovascular diseases, diabetes, malignancy and multisystem dis-

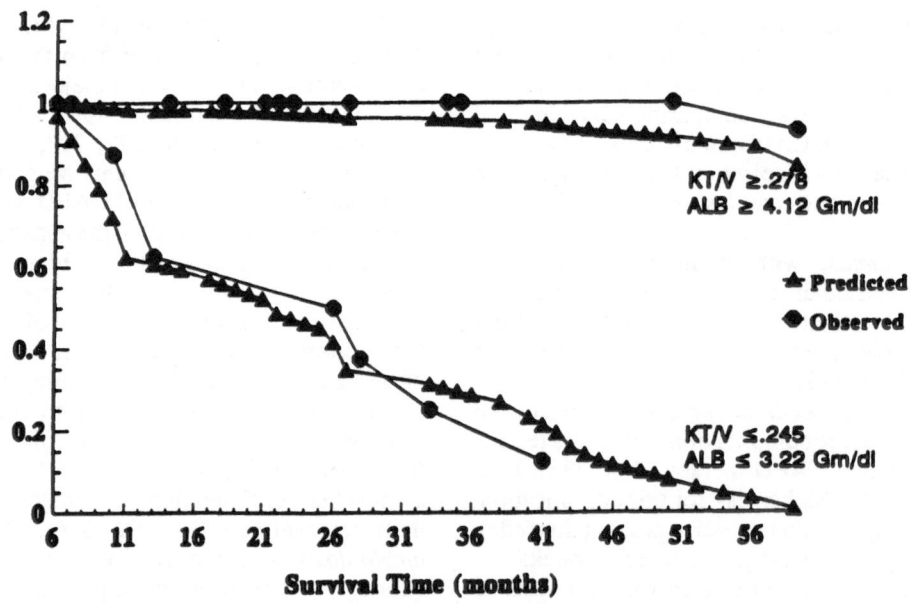

Figure 6. Estimated survival functions for selected covariate patterns, analyzed with the Cox Proportional Hazards Model. Serum albumin levels and KT/V values of 91 CAPD patients studied over 8.5 years combined as predictors of outcome in the statistical analysis (from Reference (77), with permission).

eases (12, 14, 406–408). In the elderly, however, an Italian series reported a better survival in CAPD than in HD patients (407), while the reverse was observed in an American study showing an increased mortality with CAPD among diabetics, particularly among elderly patients (408). The main causes of death on CAPD included cardiac, cerebral and/or peripheral vascular diseases, peritonitis (responsible for 7 to 10% of deaths) (12, 407), other infections, cachexia and malignancy. Technique survival was significantly lower in CAPD compared to HD, with peritonitis standing as the main cause for changing methods (40–47% of drop-outs), followed by loss of peritoneal function (15–19%) and catheter related problems (9–15%) (407). The relative risk of changing modality varied widely among the series (13, 14), but these differences in method survival could presumably be explained by differences in patient selection, availability of in center HD and/or physician's attitude when faced with clinical and technical problems.

Since 1990, several studies have attempted to determine to what extent treatment adequacy affects clinical CAPD outcomes (47, 71, 76, 77, 410–415). Such studies may eventually help answering the question: how much dialysis do CPD patients need? (416). Most of these studies, however, are retrospective, a fact that may limit the validity of their conclusions. In a longitudinal, 5 year survey of urea kinetic parameters, a significant negative correlation was observed between the mean KT/V urea index/year and the number of hospitalisation days/year (410). A similar correlation was found in another series, where patients with daily urea KT/V < 0.25 had more hospital admis-

sions per year than those with daily KT/V > 0.25 (411). In two retrospective studies using urea kinetics as a predictor of outcome, a lower probability of death was observed for weekly urea KT/V values at or above 1.89 (77, 413). In two other studies addressing the effect of adequacy of dialysis on a composite clinical outcome, good clinical outcomes were associated with weekly KT/V scores at or above 2.27, while poor outcomes were associated with values at or below 1.56 (412, 414). On the other hand, a lack of correlation between urea kinetic indices and clinical outcomes in CAPD patients was found in two other retrospective studies (69, 417). The weekly total creatinine clearance (TCC) has also been used as a predictor of outcome (47, 412, 414): a TCC lower than 50 liters per week was associated with poor clinical outcomes (412, 414) or an increased mortality (47). Finally, as previously observed in HD patients (418), many authors have confirmed the predictive value of a low serum albumin level in relation to mortality and/or hospitalisation in CAPD patients (419–424). In one study, when serum albumin levels and KT/V were combined as predictors of outcome, striking differences in survival were apparent as shown in Figure 6: survival was greater than 85% at 4.5 years when serum albumin was ≥ 4.12 g/dL and daily KT/V was > = 0.278, and mortality approached 90% at 3.5 years when serum albumin was ≤ 3.2 g/dL and daily KT/V was ≤ 0.245 (77).

Two retrospective studies used the large data base gathered during the years 1987, 1988 and 1989 to address the question of the relative risk (RR) of death on CPD *versus* HD (425) and to compare the causes of death between patients receiving either modality (426). A total of 42,372 deaths occurring over 170,700 patient years were reviewed. After adjusting for age, race, gender, diabetic status and duration of dialysis, the RR of death on CPD was 1.19 ($p < 0.001$) compared with that on HD; the risk was only significant after age 55 years, but the RR was significantly accentuated in patients with diabetes (1.38, $p < 0.001$) and in women *versus* men (1.30 *versus* 1.11; $p < 0.001$) (425). On the other hand, five causes of death were significantly higher in CPD- when compared to HD-treated patients. These causes included infection (RR: 1.42; $p < 0.001$), myocardial infarction (RR: 1.31; $p < 0.001$), withdrawal from dialysis (RR 1.21; $p < 0.001$), cerebrovascular disease (RR 1.2; $p < 0.002$), cardiac causes (RR 1.09; $p < 0.004$) and other causes (RR 1.19; $p < 0.001$) (426). Two major shortcomings characterised these studies: the comorbidity observed in the population studied was not identified and the dose of dialysis delivered in the two treatment modalities was unknown. Previous works from the USRDS suggest that there are few reasons to suspect major differences in the type of comorbidity in patients assigned to HD or CPD in the late 80's (408), whereas it is highly probable that CPD patients were delivered a low dialysis dose during this period (428). The reasons for the delivery of an inadequate dialysis dose in CPD from 1987 to 1989 include (427): the 'standard prescription' of four 2-L exchanges daily in a majority of patients (428); the common practice not to quantify treatment (416); the absence of monitoring to detect uncompliance (348, 349); the lack of concern about the progressive loss of residual renal function (48, 51). The contrast in outcomes between CPD and HD is further accentuated by another report using the same USRDS data base to examine the hospitalisation rates of CPD *versus* HD patients during the late 80's; after adjusting for age and comorbid conditions, these authors found a 14% higher rate of hospitalisation for CPD patients (429).

The results of a prospective multicenter study of a cohort of new CAPD patients in Canada and the United States have recently become available. A cohort of 698 patients commencing CPD was followed over a 3 year period (415). The clinical outcomes were patient survival, cause specific technique failure, cause specific hospitalisation and patient symptoms. When individually added to the model with age, cardiovascular disease, insulin dependent diabetes mellitus and serum albumin, KT/V and weekly creatinine clearance were found to be statistically significant predictors of survival. Patient survival was compared for those with a weekly weighted average KT/V ≥ 2.3 *versus* < 2.3. The probabilities of survival were 89 and 83% respectively at 18 months and 83 and 66% respectively at 36 months. In the same study, for any two patients with the same values on all other variables, the relative risk of death was 1.03 for a patient one year older, 0.95 for KT/V 0.1 unit greater, 0.85 for TCC 10 L/week greater, and 0.91 for serum albumin 1 gm/L greater (415).

In summary, increasing evidence suggests that the dose of dialysis is a significant independent predictor of clinical outcome in CPD (427). The theoretical data (67) as well as data on patient survival (77, 412, 413) and on morbidity (426) and mortality (425) of CPD patients lead to the conclusion that a minimum KT/V of 2.0 per week should be recommended for adequate CPD therapy (416). This value is in accordance with Popovich's original recommendation for an efficient CAPD regimen (36). Furthermore, studies including composite clinical indices suggest that a weekly KT/V value of 2.3 may result in added clinical benefit (412, 414). A KT/V of 2.3 per week is close to the target value initially proposed to quantify CAPD prescription (24): it may well correspond to the dose required to obtain optimal dialysis in CPD (i.e., a dose beyond which no further improvement in morbidity and mortality can be expected) (430). As the arguments for increasing the prescribed dose in CPD became more pressing, it was disappointing when the 1993 NIH Consensus Statement of Morbidity and Mortality of Dialysis retained a weekly KT/V urea of 1.7 as a reasonable minimal delivered dose for most functionally anephric patients (431). The increased morbidity and mortality observed in CPD treated patients was unveiled two years after the NIH Consensus Conference gave its conclusions. The observations obtained from the USRDS data bring an unequivocal message to the nephrologist. The sense of complacency that still prevailed in the early 90's toward practice patterns that result in the prescription of an inadequate dialysis dose (i.e., four 2-L exchanges daily) (12–14, 406, 407) should be abandonned. The dialysis dose should be quantified on an individual basis, and the patient's compliance and residual renal function should be closely monitored to prevent inadequate dialysis and its dismal consequences (24, 77, 425–427).

FUTURE OF CAPD

After more than fifteen years of extensive clinical use, Oreopoulos' prediction is confirmed: CAPD is here to stay (432)! The remarkable technical advances of the past decade have improved the safety and the technique survival of CAPD (433–435). This treatment modality has become an indispensable component of a comprehensive ESRD treatment programme besides HD and transplantation. However, as the limits of CAPD are better delineated, new problems have arisen for which solutions should be sought. With the decline in the incidence of peritonitis and a decrease in patient drop out, more cases of inadequate dialysis may complicate the course of CAPD in the future (67). Detecting malnutrition at an early stage should remain a major concern, since the available indicators of poor nutritional status are very crude (309, 316, 331). The methods to assess dialysis efficiency in CAPD should be standardized (436) and the selected outcomes be measured in a credible manner (416). Some aspects of current practice may be questioned: for instance, is it necessary to normalize the protein catabolic rate by patient size when this mathematical manipulation may change PCR in a flawed marker of nutrition in CAPD patients (437)? The validity of the 'Peak Concentration Hypothesis' (438), which states that the peak rather than the time average concentration of urea (TAC urea) relates to uremic toxicity, should be examined. Actually, the undiscriminating acceptance of this hypothesis should not become the justification for inadequate therapy (439). A thoughtful examination of the hypothesis concluded that, when the factors reducing the effectiveness of solute removal during intermittent HD are taken into account, both CAPD and HD begin to look and behave similarly (440). If this conclusion is confirmed, the need to define what is the optimal dose of CAPD will be even more pressing (416, 441). However, the required increase in dialysis prescription to compensate for declining renal function may be hampered by patient tolerance and/or compliance, and CAPD may be unable to provide adequate therapy on the long term in a large number of patients (442, 443). Trends to overcome these limitations by combining CPD with home automated PD are confronted with the high costs of this approach (427, 444). Finally, the problem of how long peritoneal dialysis can be safely used in a given patient remains unanswered. Dialysis-induced serositis is a common complication of CAPD, but its long-term consequences are unknown (83). Although a rare disease, sclerosing peritonitis is a serious threat to patients undergoing CPD as the incidence of this lethal complication increases with the overall duration of peritoneal dialysis (445). In practice, CAPD duration has been limited by low technique survival rates, as 50% of the patients were transferred to another treatment modality or died after 3 to 4 years on CAPD (446). The 1992 report of the Canadian Organ Replacement Registry indicated that the percentage of patients remaining on CPD after 4 years was 11.6% for age group 15–44 years, 12.9% for age group 45–64, and 8.8% for age group 65 years and over (447). Similarly, a large Italian multicenter study including 1990 patients studied over 10 years noted a mean observation period of 2.02 ± 1.86 per patient (448). Therefore, if one defined treatment duration as short-term for less than 2 years and long-term for more than 5 years, it seems fair to conclude that CAPD is a reasonable medium term treatment for a majority of ESRD patients (449).

After watching for 35 years the evolution of maintenance dialysis, the author of this chapter confirms his earlier view concerning the integration of therapies in the treatment of end stage renal disease (450). Over the past decade, an increasing number of patients have benefited of a sequential ESRD treatment utilizing successively CAPD, HD and renal transplantation (451). In this context, CAPD offers two specific advantages: 1) it involves actively the patient in the conduct of the treatment; 2) it is essentially a home dialysis technique. Because of its techical simplicity, CAPD/CCPD could be proposed as

the initial mode of dialysis to every new patient for a period of six months to one year, except to the handicapped, the very old or to those who would choose home HD. With such an approach, most patients could be trained in self-treatment with the possible advantage to maintain a more normal lifestyle. The patient would also learn the basics of maintenance dialysis (e.g., asepsy, dry weight, diet) through the training period and daily practice of CAPD. After this 'probatory' treatment stage, the status of the patient would be reevaluated taking into account his or her medical condition, the degree of compliance and autonomy, the spouse's opinion, the family impact and the quality of life. The patient could then choose to continue on CAPD, be transferred to in center HD for medical and/or social reasons or be offered more independent approaches to HD (i.e., home HD or self-dialysis) if his or her choice was to discontinue CAPD. During the whole period of CAPD trial and later on, the patients registered on a waiting list could benefit at any time from an available kidney transplant. This approach in initiating ESRD therapy would have the advantage to actively involve the patient in the choice of the definitive dialytic modality, starting with the simplest CAPD procedures to continue when needed with the more complex HD techniques. Furthermore this trial would not expose the patient to a major risk of inadequate dialysis, as the residual renal function is usually well preserved during the early months of CPD. In such a scheme, CAPD should be seen as a short term or medium term treatment modality with a duration of approximately one to five years. Obviously, to permit the 'free choice' of the patient initiated on CAPD, that will often mean a transfer to HD, both home and in-center HD should be adequately provisioned in the ESRD treatment programme.

ACKNOWLEDGEMENTS

I wish to thank Doctor Suhail Ahmad, MD, Assistant Professor of Medicine, University of Washington Medical School, Seattle, WA, USA, for his help during the preparation of this manuscript. His constructive criticisms and his practical advice, together with his king hospitality have strongly contributed to the completion of this chapter.

The extensive and excellent secretarial assistance of Mrs Maguy Elie is greatly appreciated.

REFERENCES

1. Popovich RP, Moncrief JW, Decherd JB, Bomar JB, Pyle WF: The definition of a novel portable/wearable equilibrium peritoneal dialysis technique. (Abstract) *Trans Am Soc Artif Intern Organs* 5: 64, 1976
2. Popovich RP, Moncrief JW, Nolph KD, Ghods AJ, Twardowski ZJ, Pyle WK: Continuous ambulatory peritoneal dialysis. *Ann Int Med* 88: 449, 1978

3. Oreopoulos DG, Robson M, Izatt S, Clayton S, de Veber GA: A simple and safe technique for continuous ambulatory peritoneal dialysis. *Trans Am Soc Artif Intern Organs* 24: 484, 1978
4. Buoncristiani U: The Y set with disinfectant is here to stay. *Perit Dial Int* 9: 149, 1989
5. Cantaluppi A, Scalamogna A, Castelnuovo C, Graziani G: Long term efficacy of a Y connector and disinfectant to prevent peritonitis in continuous ambulatory peritoneal dialysis. *Adv Perit Dial* 2: 182, 1986
6. Canadian CAPD clinical trials group: Peritonitis in continuous peritoneal dialysis: a multi-centre randomized clinical trial comparing the Y connector disinfectant system to standard systems. *Perit Dial Int* 9: 159, 1989
7. Trevino-Becerra A: The place of CAPD in the treatment of end stage renal disease in Mexico. *Perit Dial Bull* 1: 58, 1988
8. Anonymous: CAPD – The white Knight? *Lancet* 2: 1127, 1987
9. Geerlings W, Tufveson G, Ehrich JHH, Jones EHP, Landais P, Loirat C, Mallick NP, Margreiter R, Raine AEG, Salmela K, Selwood NH, Valderrabano F: Report on management of renal failure in Europe, XXIII. *Nephrol Dial Transplant* 9 (Suppl 1): 7, 1994
10. US Renal Data System, USRDS 1993: IV Methods of ESRD treatment. *Am J Kidney Dis* 22 (Suppl 2): 41, 1993
11. Gokal R, Baillod R, Bogle S, Hunt L, Jakubowski C, Marsh F, Ogg C, Oliver D, Ward M, Wilkinson R: Multicentre study on outcome of treatment in patients on continuous ambulatory peritoneal dialysis and haemodialysis. *Nephrol Dial Transplant* 2: 172, 1987
12. Burton PR, Walls J: Selection-adjusted comparison of life-expectancy of patients on continuous ambulatory peritoneal dialysis, haemodialysis, and renal transplantation. *Lancet* 1: 1115, 1987
13. Serkes KD, Blagg CR, Nolph KD, Vonesh EF, Shapiro F: Comparison of patient and technique survival in continuous ambulatory peritoneal dialysis and hemodialysis: a multicenter study. *Perit Dial Int* 10: 15, 1990
14. Maiorca R, Vonesh EF, Cavalli P, De Vecchi A, Giangrande A, La Greca G, Scarpioni LL, Bragantini L, Cancarini GC, Cantaluppi A et al.: A multicenter, selection-adjusted comparison of patient and technique survivals on CAPD and hemodialysis. *Perit Dial Int* 11: 118, 1991
15. Nelson CB, Port FK, Wolfe RA, Guire KE: Comparison of continuous ambulatory peritoneal dialysis and hemodialysis patient survival with evaluation of trends during the 1980s. *Am Soc Nephrol* 3: 1147, 1992
16. Friedman EA: Critical appraisal of continuous ambulatory peritoneal dialysis. *Ann Rev Med* 35: 233, 1984
17. Coles GA: Is peritoneal dialysis a good long term treatment? *Br Med J* 290: 1164, 1985
18. Mion C, Slingeneyer A, Canaud B, Mourad G, Chong G, Béraud JJ: The benefits and proper role of CAPD. *Contrib Nephrol* 44: 148, 1985
19. Diaz-Buxo JA: Continuous ambulatory peritoneal dialysis and hemodialysis: pride and prejudice. *Perit Dial Int* 10: 5, 1990
20. Diaz-Buxo JA, Farmer CD, Walker PJ, Chandler JT, Holt KL: Continuous cyclic peritoneal dialysis. *Artif Organs* 5: 157, 1981
21. Verger C, Larpent L, Dumontet M: Prognostic value of peritoneal equilibration curves in CAPD patients. in *Frontiers in Peritoneal Dialysis*, edited by Maher JF, Winchester JF, New York, Rich & Associates, 1986, p 88
22. Twardowski ZJ, Nolph KD, Khanna R, Prowant BF, Ryan LP, Moore HL, Nielsen MP: Peritoneal equilibration tests. *Perit Dial Int* 7: 138, 1987
23. Twardowski ZJ, Nolph KD: Peritoneal dialysis: how much is enough? *Semin Dial* 1: 75, 1988
24. Teehan BP, Schleifer CR, Sigler MH, Gilgore GS: A quantitative approach to CAPD prescription. *Perit Dial Bull* 5: 152, 1985
25. Fenton SSA, Johnston N, Delmore T: Nutritional assessment of continuous ambulatory peritoneal dialysis patients. *Trans Am Soc Artif Intern Organs* 33: 650, 1987
26. Young GA, Kopple JD, Lindholm B et al.: Nutritional assessment of continuous ambulatory peritoneal dialysis patients. An international study. *Am J Kidney Dis* 17: 462, 1991
27. Churchill DN: Adequacy of peritoneal dialysis and other outcome-related risk factors: a critical appraisal. *Semin Dial* 5: 142, 1992
28. Bargman JM: Peritoneal dialysis connection devices: what have we learned? *Perit Dial Int* 12: 9, 1992
29. Stegmayr BG, Granbom L, Tranaeus A, Wikdahl AM: Reduced risk of peritonitis in CAPD by the use of an UV-connector box. *Perit Dial Bull* 11: 128, 1991
30. Buoncristiani U, Quintiliani G, Cozzari M, Carobi C: Current status of the Y-set. *Adv Perit Dial* 2: 165, 1986
31. Viglino G, Colombo A, Scalamogna A, Cavalli PL, Guerra L, Renzetti G, Gandolfo C, De Vecchi A, Barzaghi V, Baltean P, Peluso F, Cantaluppi A: Prospective randomized study of two Y devices in continuous ambulatory peritoneal dialysis. *Perit Dial Int* 9: 165, 1989
32. Luzar MA, Slingeneyer A, Cantaluppi A, Peluso FP: *In vitro* study of the flush effect in two reusable continuous ambulatory peritoneal dialysis CAPD disconnect systems. *Perit Dial Int* 9: 169, 1989
33. De Vecchi A, Scalamogna A, Castlenovo C, Artuso K, Brancadoro A: Incidence, possible causes and social aspects of the symptomatic introduction of disinfectant into the peritoneal cavity in CAPD. *Int J Artif Organs* 17: 265, 1994
34. Werner HP: Disinfectants in dialysis: dangers, drawbacks and disinformation. *Nephron* 49: 1, 1988
35. Diaz-Buxo JA: Current status of continuous cyclic peritoneal dialysis. *Perit Dial Int* 9: 9, 1989
36. Popovich RP, Pyle WK, Moncrief JW: Kinetics of peritoneal transport. in *Peritoneal Dialysis*, 1st Ed, edited by Nolph KD, The Hague, Martinus Nijhoff Publishers, 1981, p 100
37. Henao JE, Mejia G, Arbelaez M, Arango JL, Garcia A, Sanchez J, Gil NE, Aramburo O: Six-and-a-half years of experience with three two-liter daily exchanges in CAPD. *Perit Dial Int* 8: 207, 1988
38. Moncrief JW, Popovich RP: A comparison of four *vs* three exchanges per day with continuous ambulatory peritoneal dialysis. in *Advances in Peritoneal Dialysis*, edited by Gahl GM, Kessel M, Nolph KD, Amsterdam, Excerpta medica, 1981, p 116

39. Twardowski Z, Janicka L: Three exchanges with a 2.5-liter volume for continuous ambulatory peritoneal dialysis. *Kidney Int* 20: 281, 1981

40. Twardowski ZJ, Prowant BF, Nolph KD, Martinez AJ, Lampton LM: High volume, low frequency continuous ambulatory peritoneal dialysis. *Kidney Int* 23: 64, 1983

41. Krediet RT, Boeschoten EW, Struijk DG, Arisz L: Differences in the peritoneal transport of water, solutes and proteins between dialysis in two- and with three-litre exchanges. *Nephrol Dial Transplant* 2: 198, 1988

42. Keshaviah P, Emerson PF, Vonesh EF, Brandes JC: Relationship between body size, fill volume, and mass transfer area coefficient in peritoneal dialysis. *Am Soc Nephrol* 4: 1820, 1994

43. Kim D, Khanna R, Wu G, Clayton S, Oreopoulos DG: Continuous ambulatory peritoneal dialysis with three-liter exchanges: a prospective study. *Perit Dial Bull* 4: 82, 1984

44. Twardowski ZJ, Burrows LM, Prowant BF: Individualization of exchange volume. *Perit Dial Bull*, 4 (Suppl 3): S134, 1984

45. Nolph KD: Quantitating peritoneal dialysis delivery: a required standard of care. *Semin Dial* 4: 139, 1991

46. Nolph KD, Moore HL, Prowant B, Meyer M, Twardowski ZJ, Khanna R, Ponferrada L, Keshaviah P: Cross sectional assessment of weekly urea and creatinine clearances and indices of nutrition in continuous ambulatory peritoneal dialysis patients. *Perit Dial Int* 13: 178, 1993

47. Blake PG, Balaskas EV, Izatt S, Oreopoulos DG: Is total creatinine clearance a good predictor of clinical outcomes in continuous ambulatory peritoneal dialysis? *Perit Dial Int* 12: 353, 1992

48. Rottembourg J: Residual function and recovery of renal function in patients treated by CAPD. *Kidney Int* 43 (Suppl 40): S106, 1993

49. Rottembourg J, Issad B, Callego JL, Degoulet P, Aime F, Gueffaf B, Legrain M: Evolution of residual renal function in patients undergoing maintenance haemodialysis or continuous ambulatory peritoneal dialysis. *Proc Eur Dial Transplant Assoc* 19: 397, 1982

50. Cancarini GC, Brunori G, Camerini C, Brasa S, Manili L, Maiorca R: Renal function recovery and maintenance of residual diuresis in CAPD and hemodialysis. *Perit Dial Bull* 6: 77, 1986

51. Lysaght MJ, Vonesh EF, Gotch F, Ibels L, Keen M, Lindholm B, Nolph KD, Pollock CA, Prowant B, Farrell PC: The influence of dialysis treatment modality on the decline of remaining renal function. *Trans Am Soc Artif Intern Organs* 37: 598, 1991

52. Randerson DH, Farrell PC: Mass transfer properties of the human peritoneum. *ASAIO J* 3: 140, 1980

53. Smeby LC, Wideroe T, Jorstad S: Individual differences in water transport during continuous peritoneal dialysis. *ASAIO J* 4: 17, 1981

54. Waniewski J, Werynski A, Heimburger O, Lindholm B: A comparative analysis of mass transport models in peritoneal dialysis. *Trans Am Soc Artif Intern Organs* 37: 65, 1991

55. Twardowski ZJ: Clinical value of standardized equilibration tests in CAPD patients. *Blood Purif* 7: 95, 1989

56. Davies SJ, Brown B, Bryan J, Russell GI: Clinical evaluation of the peritoneal equilibration test: a population-based study. *Nephrol Dial Transplant* 8: 64, 1993

57. Twardowski ZJ: The fast peritoneal equilibration test. *Semin Dial* 3: 141, 1990

58. Twardowski ZJ: PET – a simpler approach for determining prescriptions for adequate dialysis therapy. *Adv Perit Dial* 6: 186, 1990

59. Diaz-Buxo JA: Continuous cyclic peritoneal dialysis. in *Textbook of Nephrology*, 3rd Ed, edited by Massry SG, Glassock RJ, Baltimore, Williams and Wilkins, 1994, p 1584

60. Jensen RA, Nolph KD, Moore HL, Khanna R, Twardowski ZJ: Weight limitations for adequate therapy using commonly performed CAPD and NIPD regimens. *Semin Dial* 7: 61, 1994

61. Lo WK, Brendolan A, Prowant BF, Moore HL, Khanna R, Twardowski Z, Nolph KD: Changes in the peritoneal equilibration test in selected chronic peritoneal dialysis patients. *J Am Soc Nephrol* 4: 1466, 1994

62. Watson PE, Watson ID, Batt RD: Total body water volumes for adult males and females estimated from simple anthropometric measurements. *Am J Clin Nutr* 33: 27, 1980

63. Blumenkrantz MJ, Kopple JD, Moran JK, Coburn JW: Metabolic balance studies and dietary protein requirements in patients undergoing continuous ambulatory peritoneal dialysis. *Kidney Int* 21: 849, 1982

64. Bergström J, Fürst P, Alvestrand A, Lindholm B: Protein and energy intake, nitrogen balance and nitrogen losses in patients treated with continuous ambulatory peritoneal dialysis. *Kidney Int* 44: 1048, 1993

65. Lindsay RM, Spanner E: The protein catabolic rate is dependent upon the type and amount of treatment in dialyzed uremics. *Am J Kidney Dis* 5: 382, 1989

66. Lysaght MJ, Pollock CA, Hallet MD, Ibels LS, Farrell PC: The relevance of urea kinetic modeling to CAPD. *Trans Am Soc Artif Intern Organs* 35: 784, 1989

67. Keshaviah P: Adequacy of CAPD: a quantitative approach. *Kidney Int* 42 (Suppl 38): S160, 1992

68. Bergstrom J, Lindholm B: Nutrition and adequacy of dialysis. How do hemodialysis and CAPD compare? *Kidney Int* 43 (Suppl 40): S39, 1993

69. Goodship THJ, Passlick-Deetjen J, Ward MK, Wilkinson R: Adequacy of dialysis and nutritional status in CAPD. *Nephrol Dial Transplant* 8: 1366, 1993

70. Barth RH: Dialysis by the numbers: the false promise of Kt/V. *Semin Dial* 2: 207, 1989

71. Keshaviah PR, Nolph KD, Prowant B, Moore H, Ponferrada L, Van Stone J, Twardowski ZJ, Khanna R: Defining adequacy of CAPD with urea kinetics. *Adv Perit Dial* 6: 173, 1990

72. Nolph KD: Small solute clearances and clinical outcomes in CAPD. *Perit Dial Int* 12: 343, 1992

73. Gotch FA, Sargent JA: A mechanistic analysis of the national cooperative dialysis study (NCDS). *Kidney Int* 28: 526, 1985

74. Gotch FA: The application of urea kinetic modeling to CAPD. in *Peritoneal Dialysis: Proceedings of the 4th International Course on Peritoneal Dialysis*, edited by La Greca G, Ronco C, Feriani M, Chiaramonte S, Conz P, Milan, Wichtig Editore, 1991, p 47

75. Keshaviah P: Urea kinetic and middle molecule approaches to assessing the adequacy of hemodialysis and CAPD. *Kidney Int* 40: S28, 1993

76. Teehan BP, Schleifer CR, Brown JM, Sigler et al.: Urea kinetic analysis and clinical outcome on CAPD: a five-year longitudinal study. *Adv Perit Dial* 6: 181, 1990

77. Teehan BP, Schleifer CR, Brown J: Adequacy of CAPD. Morbidity and mortality in chronic peritoneal dialysis. *Am J Kidney Dis* 24: 990, 1994

77a. Ahmad S, Gallagher N, Shen F: Intermittent peritoneal dialysis: status reassessed. *Trans Am Soc Artif Intern Organs* 25: 86, 1979

78. Milutinovic J, Cutler RE, Hoover P, Heissen B, Scribner BH: Measurement of residual glomerular filtration rate in the patients receiving repetitive hemodialysis. *Kidney Int* 8: 185, 1975

79. Brandes JC, Piering WF, Beres JA: A method to assess efficacy of CAPD: preliminary results. *Adv Perit Dial* 6: 192, 1990

80. Burkart JM, Jordan JR, Rocco MV: Assessment of dialysis dose by measured clearance *versus* extrapolated data. *Perit Dial Int* 13: 184, 1993

81. Hutchinson AJ, Gokal R: Towards tailored dialysis fluids in CAPD. The role of reduced calcium and magnesium in dialysis fluids. *Perit Dial Int* 12: 199, 1992

82. Dobbie JW: Pathogenesis of peritoneal fibrosing syndromes (sclerosing peritonitis) in peritoneal dialysis. *Perit Dial Int* 12: 14, 1992

83. Dobbie JW: Serositis: comparative analysis of histological findings and pathogenetic mechanisms in nonbacterial serosal inflammation. *Perit Dial Int* 13: 256, 1993

84. Hutchison AJ, Freemont AJ, Boulton HF, Gokal R: Low-calcium dialysis fluid and oral calcium carbonate in CAPD. A method of controlling hyperphosphataemia whilst minimizing aluminium exposure and hypercalcaemia. *Nephrol Dial Transplant* 7: 1219, 1992

85. Cunningham J, Beer J, Coldwell RD, Noonan K, Sawyer N, Makin HLJ: Dialysate calcium reduction in CAPD patients treated with calcium carbonate and alfacalcidol. *Nephrol Dial Transplant* 7: 63, 1992

86. Nolph KD, Prowant B, Serkes KD, Morgan L, Baker B, Charytan C, Gham K, Hamburger R, Husserl F, Kleit S, McGuinness J, Moore H, Warren T: Multicenter evaluation of a new peritoneal dialysis solution with a high lactate and low magnesium concentration. *Perit Dial Bull* 3: 63, 1983

87. Bruno M, Bagnis C, Maragella M et al.: CAPD with an amino acid dialysis solution: a long-term cross-over study. *Kidney Int* 35: 1189, 1989

88. Twardowski ZJ, Khanna R, Nolph KD: Osmotic agents and ultrafiltration in peritoneal dialysis. *Nephron* 42: 93, 1986

89. Mistry CD, Mallick NP, Gokal R: Ultrafiltration with an isosmotic solution during long peritoneal dialysis exchanges. *Lancet* 330: 178, 1987

90. Mistry CD, Gokal R, Peers E, the MIDAS study group: A randomized multicenter clinical trial comparing isosmolar icodextrin with hyperosmolar glucose solutions in CAPD. *Kidney Int* 46: 496, 1994

91. Feriani M, Passlick-Deetjen J, Brown C, Buoncristiani U, Di Paolo N, Gahl G, Gotloib L, Hylander B, Lameire N, Montenegro J, Pedersen FB et al.: An open controlled randomized clinical trial with bicarbonate CAPD solutions: interim results. (Abstract) *J Am Soc Nephrol* 5: 414, 1994

92. Yatzidis H: A new stable bicarbonate dialysis solution for peritoneal dialysis: preliminary report. *Perit Dial Int* 11: 224, 1991

93. Holmes CJ: Biocompatibility of peritoneal dialysis solutions. *Perit Dial Int* 13: 88, 1993

94. Henderson IS: Composition of peritoneal dialysis solutions: potential hazards. *Blood Purif* 7: 86, 1989

95. Nilsson-Thorell CB, Huscalu N, Abdreb AHG, Kjellstrand PTT, Wieslander AP: Heat sterilization of peritoneal dialysis solutions gives rise to aldehydes. *Perit Dial Int* 13: 208, 1993

96. Henderson IS, Couper LA, Lumsden A: The effect of shelf-life of peritoneal dialysis fluid on ultrafiltration on CAPD. in *Peritoneal Dialysis: Proceedings of the 2nd International Course on Peritoneal Dialysis*, edited by La Greca G, Chiaramonte S, Fabris A, Feriani M, Ronco C, Milan, Wichtig Editore, 1986, p 85

97. Jörres A, Gahl GM, Frei U: Peritoneal dialysis fluid biocompatibility: does it really matter? *Kidney Int* 46 (Suppl 48): S79, 1994

98. Topley N, Alobaidi HM, Davies M, Coles GA, Williams JD, Lloyd D: The effect of dialysate on peritoneal phagocyte oxidative metabolism. *Kidney Int* 34: 404, 1988

99. Jörres A, Jörres D, Topley N, Gahl GM, Mahiout A: Leukotriene release from peripheral and peritoneal leucocytes following exposure to peritoneal dialysis solutions. *Nephrol Dial Transplant* 6: 495, 1991

100. Zhou XJ, Yu AW, Zhou FQ, Ryu J, Ing TS, Vaziri ND: Effects of an acidic, lactate-based peritoneal dialysis solution and its euhydric, bicarbonate-based counterpart on neutrophilic intracellular pH. *Int J Artif Organs* 16: 816, 1993

101. Ing TX, Yu AW, Podila PV, Zhou FQ, Kun EW, Strippoli P, Nawab ZM: Failure of neutrophils to recover their ability to produce superoxide after stunning by a conventional, acidic, lactate-based peritoneal dialysis solution. *Int J Artif Organs* 17: 194, 1994

102. Jörres A, Topley N, Steenweg L, Müller C, Köttgen E, Gahl GM: Inhibition of cytokine synthesis by peritoneal dialysate persists throughout the CAPD cycle. *Am J Nephrol* 12: 80, 1992

103. Dourlevani A, Rapoport J, Konforti A, Zlotnik M, Chaimovitz C: The effect of peritoneal dialysis fluid on the release of IL-1beta and TNF alpha by monocytes/macrophages. *Perit Dial Int* 13: 112, 1993

104. Liberek T, Topley N, Jörres A, Coles GA, Gahl GM, Williams JD: Peritoneal dialysis fluid inhibition of phagocyte function: effects of osmolality and glucose concentration. *J Am Soc Nephrol* 3: 1508, 1993

105. Breborowicz A, Podela H, Oreopoulos DG: Toxicity of osmotic solutes on human mesothelial cell *in vitro*. *Kidney Int* 41: 1280, 1992

106. Wieslander AP, Nordin MK, Hartinson E, Kjellstrand PTT, Boberg NC: Heat sterilized PD-fluids impair growth and inflammatory responses of cultured cell lines and human leucocytes. *Clin Nephrol* 39: 343, 1993

107. Wieslander AP, Nordin MK, Kjellstrand PTT, Boberg UC: Toxicity of peritoneal dialysis fluids on cultured fibroblasts. *Kidney Int* 40: 77, 1991

108. Topley N, Mack Enzie R, Jörres A, Coles GA, Williams JD: Cytokin networks in CAPD: interaction of resident cells during inflammation in the peritoneal cavity. *Perit Dial Int* 13 (Suppl 2): S282, 1993

592   *Charles M. Mion*

109. Topley N, Jörres A, Luttmann W, Petersen MM, Lang MJ, Thierauch KH, Müller C, Coles GA, Davies M, Williams JD: Human peritoneal mesothelial cells synthesize interleukin-6: induction by IL-1 beta and TNF alpha. *Kidney Int* 43: 226, 1993
110. Betjes MGH, Tuk CW, Struijk DG, Krediet RT, Arisz L, Hart M, Beelen RH: Interleukin-8 production by human peritoneal mesothelial cells in response to tumor necrosis factor alpha,interleukin-1, and medium conditioned by macrophages cocultured with *Staphylococcus epidermidis. J Infect Dis* 168: 1202, 1993
111. Topley N, Petersen MM, Mackenzie R, Neubauer A, Stylianou E, Kaever V, Davies M, Coles GA, Jörres A, Williams JD: Human peritoneal mesothelial cell prostaglandin synthesis: induction of cycloxygenase mRNA by peritoneal macrophages derived cytokines. *Kidney Int* 46: 900, 1994
112. Witowski J, Topley N, Jörres A, Liberek T, Coles GA, Williams JD: Effect of lactate buffered peritoneal dialysis fluids on human peritoneal mesothelial cell interleukin-6 and prostaglandin synthesis. *Kidney Int*, 47: 282, 1995
113. Vlassara H: Serum advanced glycosylation end products: a new class of uremic toxins? *Blood Purif* 12: 54, 1994
114. Brownlee M, Cerami A, Vlassara H: Advanced glycosylation end products in tissue and the biochemical basis of diabetic complications. *N Engl J Med* 318: 1315, 1988
115. Lamb E, Cattell WR, Dawnay A: Glycated albumin in serum and dialysate of patients on continuous ambulatory peritoneal dialysis. *Clin Sci Colch* 84: 619, 1993
116. Korbet SM, Makita Z, Firanek CA, Vlassara H: Advanced glycosylation end products in continuous ambulatory peritoneal dialysis patients. *Am J Kidney Dis* 22: 588, 1993
117. Makita Z, Bucala R, Rayfield EJ, Friedman EA, Kaufman AM, Korbet SM, Barth RH, Winston JA, Fuh H, Manogue KR, Cerami A, Vlassara H: Reactive glycosylation endproducts in diabetic uraemia and treatment of renal failure. *Lancet* 343: 1519, 1994
118. Papanastasiou P, Grass L, Rodela H, Patrikarea A, Oreopoulos D, Diamandis EP: Immunological quantification of advanced glycosylation end-products in the serum of patients on hemodialysis or CAPD. *Kidney Int* 46: 216, 1994
119. Fracasso A, Calo L, Landini S, Morachiello P, Righetto F, Scanferra F, Taffoletto P, Genchi R, Roncalli D, Cantaro S, De Silvestre G, Cavatton G et al.: Peritoneal sclerosis: role of plasticizers in stimulating interleukin-1 production. *Perit Dial Int* 13: S517, 1993
120. Gotloib L, Mines M, Garmizo L, Varka I: Hemodynamic effects of increasing intraabdominal pressure in peritoneal dialysis. *Perit Dial Bull* 1: 41, 1981
121. Twardowski ZJ, Khanna R, Nolph KD, Scalamogna A, Metzler MH, Schneider TW, Prowant B, Ryan LP: Intraabdominal pressures during natural activities in patients treated with continuous ambulatory peritoneal dialysis. *Nephron* 44: 129, 1986
122. Prefaut C, Monteil AL, Ramonatko M, Slingeneyer A, Chardon G, Mirouze J: Closing volume and pulmonary gas exchange during peritoneal dialysis. *Bull Europ Physiopath Resp* 14: 755, 1978
123. Ahluwalia M, Ishjikawa S, Gellman M, Shah T, Sekar T, MacDonnell KF: Pulmonary functions during peritoneal dialysis. *Clin Nephrol* 18: 251, 1982

124. Taveira da Silva AM, Davies WB, Winchester JF, Coleman DE, Weir CN: Peritonitis, dialysate infusion and lung function in continuous ambulatory peritoneal dialysis. *Clin Nephrol* 24: 79, 1985
125. Berlyne GM, Lee HA, Ralston AJ, Woolcock JA: Pulmonary complications of peritoneal dialysis. *Lancet* 2: 75, 1966
126. Goitloib L, Garmizo L, Varak I, Mines M: Reduction of vital capacity due to increased intra-abdominal pressure during peritoneal dialysis. *Perit Dial Bull* 1: 63, 1981
127. Epstein SN, Inouye T, Robson M, Oreopoulos DG: Effect of peritoneal dialysis fluid on ventilatory function. *Perit Dial Bull* 2: 120, 1982
128. Schurig R, Gahl G, Schartl M, Becker H, Kessel M: Central and peripheral hemodynamics in long term peritoneal dialysis patients. *Proc Eur Dial Transplant Assoc* 16: 165, 1979
129. Kong CH, Raval U, Thompson FD: Effect of 2 liters of intraperitoneal dialysate on the cardiovascular system. *Clin Nephrol* 26: 134, 1986
130. Franklin JO, Alpert MA, Twardowski ZJ, Khanna R, Nolph KD, Morgan RJ, Kelly DL: Effect of increasing intraabdominal pressure and volume on left ventricular function in continuous ambulatory peritoneal dialysis. *Am J Kidney Dis* 12: 291, 1988
131. Huting J, Kramer W, Reitinger J, Kuhn K, Wizemann V, Schutterle G: Cardiac structure and function in continuous ambulatory peritoneal dialysis: influence of blood purification and hypercirculation. *Am Heart J* 119: 334, 1990
132. Eisenberg M, Prichard S, Barre P, Patton R, Hutchinson T, Sniderman A: Left ventricular hypertrophy in end-stage renal disease on peritoneal dialysis. *Am J Cardiol* 60: 418, 1987
133. Hau T, Ahrenholz DH, Simmons RL: Secondary bacterial peritonitis: the biologic basis of treatment. *Curr Prob Surg* 16: 1, 1979
134. Haney AF, Muscato JJ, Weinberg JB: Peritoneal fluid cell populations in infertility patients. *Fertil Steril* 35: 696, 1981
135. Simberkoff MS, Moldover NH, Weiss G: Bactericidal and opsonic activity of cirrhotic ascites and non ascitic peritoneal fluid. *J Lab Clin Med* 91: 831, 1978
136. Allen L: The peritoneal stomata. *Anat Rec* 67: 89, 1936
137. Allen L, Wheatherford T: Role of fenestrated basement membrane in lymphatic absorption from peritoneal cavity. *Am J Physiol* 197: 551, 1959
138. Vas SI: Microbiologic aspects of chronic ambulatory peritoneal dialysis. *Kidney Int* 23: 83, 1982
139. Grahame GR, Torchia MG, Dankewich KA, Fergusson IA: Surface-active material in peritoneal effluent of CAPD patients. *Perit Dial Bull* 5: 109, 1985
140. Breborowicz A, Sombolos K, Rodela H, Ogilvie R, Bargman J, Oreopoulos DG: Mechanism of phosphatidylcholine action during peritoneal dialysis. *Perit Dial Bull* 7: 6, 1987
141. Dobbie JW, Pavlina T, Lloyd J, Johnson RC: Phosphatidylcholine synthesis by peritoneal mesothelium: its implications for peritoneal dialysis. *Am J Kidney Dis* 12: 31–36, 1988
142. Dobbie JW, Lloyd JK: Mesothelium secretes lamellar bodies in a similar manner to type II pneumocyte secretion of surfactant. *Perit Dial Int* 9: 215, 1989

143. Hjelle JT, Steidley KR, Pavlina TM, Dobbie JW: Choline incorporation into phospholipids in mesothelial cells *in vitro*. *Perit Dial Int* 13: 289, 1993

144. Di Paolo N, Buoncristiani U, Capotondo L, Gaggiotti E, De Mia M, Rossi P, Sansoni E, Bernini M: Phosphatidyl-choline and peritoneal transport during peritoneal dialysis. *Nephron* 44: 365, 1986

145. Beavis J, Harwood JL, Coles GA, Williams JD: Intraperitoneal phosphatidylcholine levels in patients on continuous ambulatory peritoneal dialysis do not correlate with adequacy of ultrafiltration. *J Am Soc Nephrol* 3: 1954, 1993

146. Mactier RA, Khanna R, Twardowski ZJ, Moore H, Nolph KD: Influence of phosphatidylcholine on lymphatic absorption during peritoneal dialysis in the rat. *Perit Dial Int* 8: 179, 1988

147. Yuan ZY, Rodela H, Hay JB, Oreopoulos DG, Johnston MG: Effect of phosphatidylcholine on lymphatic drainage and fluid loss from the peritoneal cavity of sheep. *Kidney Int* 46: 520, 1994

148. Di Paolo B, Chakrabarti E, Maher JF: Phosphatidylcholine does not affect peritoneal transport of intact rabbits. *Perit Dial Int* 9: 211, 1989

149. Henderson LW: The problem of peritoneal membrane area and permeability. *Kidney Int* 3: 405, 1973

150. Rippe B: Pathophysiological description of the ultrastructural changes of the peritoneal membrane during long term continuous ambulatory peritoneal dialysis. *Blood Purif* 12: 211, 1994

151. Krediet RT, Imholz ALT, Zemer D, Struijk DG, Koomen GCM: Clinical significance and detection of individual differences and changes in transperitoneal transport. *Blood Purif* 12: 221, 1994

152. Blumenkrantz MJ, Gahl GM, Kopple JD, Kamdar AV, Jones MR, Kessel M, Coburn JW: Protein losses during peritoneal dialysis. *Kidney Int* 19: 53, 1981

153. Dulaney JT, Hatch FE: Peritoneal dialysis and loss of proteins: a review. *Kidney Int* 26: 253, 1984

154. Young GA, Browjohn AM, Parsons FM: Protein losses in patients receiving continuous ambulatory peritoneal dialysis. *Nephron* 45: 196, 1987

155. Zemel D, Krediet RT, Koomen GCM, Struijk DG, Arisz L: Day-to-day variability of protein transport used as a method for analyzing peritoneal permeability in CAPD. *Perit Dial Int* 11: 217, 1991

156. Steinhauer HB, Schollmeyer P: Prostaglandin-mediated loss of proteins during peritonitis in continuous ambulatory peritoneal dialysis. *Kidney Int* 29: 584, 1986

157. Kaysen GA, Schoenfeld C: Albumin homeostasis in patients undergoing continuous ambulatory peritoneal dialysis. *Kidney Int* 25: 107, 1984

158. Schoenfeld PC: Albumin is an unreliable marker of nutritional status. *Semin Dial* 5: 218, 1992

159. De Santo NG, Capodicasa G, Di Leo VA, Di Serafino A, Cirillo D, Esposito R, Fiore R, Cucciniello E, Damiano M, Buonadonna L, Di Lorio R et al.: Kinetics of amino acids equilibration in the dialysate during CAPD. *Int J Artif Organs* 4: 23, 1981

160. Dombros N, Oren A, Marliss EB et al.: Plasma amino acid profiles and amino acid losses in patients undergoing CAPD. *Perit Dial Bull* 2: 27, 1982

161. Kopple JD, Blumenkrantz MJ, Jones MR et al.: Plasma amino acid levels and amino acid losses during contin-uous ambulatory peritoneal dialysis. *Am J Clin Nutr* 36: 395, 1982

162. Grodstein GP, Blumenkrantz MJ, Kopple JD, Moran JK, Coburn JW: Glucose absorption during continuous ambulatory peritoneal dialysis. *Kidney Int* 19: 264, 1981

163. Lindholm B, Bergström J: Nutritional aspects of CAPD. in *Continuous Ambulatory Peritoneal Dialysis*, edited by Gokal R, Edimburgh, Churchill Livingstone, 1986, p 228

164. Wideroe TE, Smeby LC, Mjaland S, Dahl K, Berg KJ, Aas TW: Long-term changes in transperitoneal water transport during continuous ambulatory peritoneal dialysis. *Nephron* 38: 238, 1984

165. Nolph KD, Ryan L, Moore H, Legrain M, Rottembourg J, Issad B, Montassine M, Mion C, Slingeneyer A, Bouzigues J, Oreopoulos DG: A survey of ultrafiltration in continuous ambulatory peritoneal dialysis. An international cooperative study. Second report. *Perit Dial Bull* 4: 137, 1984

166. Armstrong VW, Creutzfeldt W, Ebert R, Fuchs C, Hilgers R, Scheler F: Effect of dialysate glucose load on plasma glucose and glucoregulatory hormones in CAPD patients. *Nephron* 39: 141, 1985

167. Delarue J, Maingourd C, Lamisse F, Garrigue MA, Bagros P, Couet C: Glucose oxidation after a peritoneal and an oral glucose load in dialyzed patients. *Kidney Int* 45: 1147, 1994

168. Appel G: Lipid abnormalities in renal disease. *Kidney Int* 39: 169, 1991

169. Avram MM, Goldwasser P, Burrell DE, Antignani A, Fein PA, Mittman N: The uremic dyslipidemia: a cross-sectional and longitudinal study. *Am J Kidney Dis* 20: 324, 1992

170. Sniderman A, Cianflone K, Kwiterovich PO Jr, Hutchinson T, Barre P, Prichard S: Hyperbetalipoproteinemia. The major dylipoproteinemia in patients with chronic renal failure treated with contenous ambulatory peritoneal dialysis. *Atherosclerosis* 65: 257, 1987

171. Panarello G, Galianno G, De Baz H, Signori D, Cappeletti P, Tesio F: Does continuous ambulatory peritoneal dialysis induce hypercholesterolemia? *Perit Dial Int* 13 (Suppl 2): S421, 1993

172. Faller B, Lameire N: Evolution of clinical parameters and peritoneal function in a cohort of CAPD patients followed over 7 years. *Nephrol Dial Transplant* 9: 280, 1994

173. Chan MK, Varghese Z, Persaud JW, Baillod RA, Moorhead JF: Hyperlipidemia in patients on maintenance hemo- and peritoneal dialysis: the relative pathogenetic roles of triglyceride production and triglyceride removal. *Clin Nephrol* 17: 183, 1982

174. Thillet J, Faucher C, Issad B, Allouache M, Chapman J, Jacobs C: Lipoprotein(a) in patients treated by continuous ambulatory peritoneal dialysis. *Am J Kidney Dis* 22: 226, 1993

175. Anwar N, Bhatnagar D, Short D, Mackness MI, Durrington PN, Prais H, Gokal R: Serum lipoprotein (a) concentrations in patients undergoing continuous ambulatory peritoneal dialysis. *Nephrol Dial Transplant* 8: 71, 1993

176. Shozi T, Nishizawa Y, Nishitani H, Yamakawa M, Morii A: High serum lipoprotein (a) concentrations in uremic patients treated with continuous ambulatory peritoneal dialysis. *Clin Nephrol* 38: 271, 1992

177. Webb AT, Reaveley DA, O'Donnell M, O'Connor B, Seed M, Brown EA: Lipoprotein (a) in patients on main-

tenance haemodialysis and continuous ambulatory peritoneal dialysis. *Nephrol Dial Transplant* 8: 609, 1993

178. Kandoussi A, Cachera C, Pagniez D, Dracon M, Fruchart JC, Tacquet A: Plasma level of lipoprotein Lp(a) is high in predialysis or hemodialysis, but not in CAPD. *Kidney Int* 42: 424, 1992

179. Weintraub M, Burstein A, Rassin T, Liron M, Ringel Y, Cabili S, Blum M, Peer G, Iaina A: Severe defect in clearing postprandial chylomicron remnants in dialysis patients. *Kidney Int* 42: 1247, 1992

180. Atkins RC, Wood C: Hyperlipemia in CAPD. *Perit Dial Int* 13 (Suppl 2): S415, 1993

181. Webb AT, Brown EA: Prevalence of symptomatic arterial disease and risk factors for its development in patients on continuous ambulatory peritoneal dialysis. *Perit Dial Int* 13 (Suppl 2): S406, 1993

182. Dimitriadis A, Antoniou S, Hatzisavvas N, Pastore F, Kaldi I, Stangou M: The effect of simvastatin on dyslipidemia in continuous ambulatory peritoneal dialysis patients. *Perit Dial Int* 13 (Suppl 2): S434, 1993

183. Harangoni R, Civardi F, Masi F, Cimizio R, Maltagriati L, Longhena GR: Dyslipemia in patients undergoing continuous ambulatory peritoneal dialysis: pharmacological therapy (simvastatin) *versus* hemodialysis. *Perit Dial Int* 13 (Suppl 2): S431, 1993

184. Li PKT, Mak TWL, Lam CWK; Lai KN: Lovastatin treatment of dyslipoproteinemia in patients on continuous ambulatory peritoneal dialysis. *Perit Dial Int* 13 (Suppl 2): S428, 1993

185. Jones RG, Dibble JB, Gibson J, Tompkins L, O'Kane M, Hobson SM, Young GA, Grant AM, Turney JH, Brownjohn AM: Effect of dietary fish oil on lipid abnormalities in patients on continuous ambulatory peritoneal dialysis. *Perit Dial Int* 8: 203, 1988

186. Lempert KD, Rogers JS, Albrink MJ: Effects of dietary fish oil on serum lipids and blood coagulation in peritoneal dialysis patients. *Am J Kidney Dis* 11: 170, 1988

187. Fracasso A, Toffoletto P, Landini S, Morachiello P, Righetto F, Scanferla F, Genchi R, Roncali D, Bazzato G: Effect of hypertriglyceridemia correction by omega-3-fatty acids on peritoneal transport in continuous peritoneal dialysis. *Perit Dial Int* 13 (Suppl 2): S437, 1993

188. Blumberg A, Hanck A, Sander G: Vitamin nutrition in patients on continuous ambulatory peritoneal dialysis. *Clin Nephrol* 20: 244, 1983

189. Digenis GE, Dombros N, Charytan C, Oreopoulos DG: Supplements for the CAPD patients (vitamins, folic acid, zinc, iron and anabolic steroids). *Perit Dial Bull* 7: 219, 1987

190. Ross EA, Shah GM, Reynolds RD, Sabo A, Pichon M: Vitamin B6 requirements of patients on chronic peritoneal dialysis. *Kidney Int* 36: 702, 1989

191. Aloni Y, Shaby S, Chaimovitz C: Losses of 25-hydroxyvitamin D in peritoneal fluid: possible mechanism for bone disease in uremic patients treated with chronic ambulatory peritoneal dialysis. *Miner Electrolyte Metab* 9: 82, 1983

192. Shany S, Rapoport J, Goligorsky M, Yankowitz N, Zuici I, Chaimovitz C: Losses of 1,25- and 24,25-dihydroxycholecalciferol in the peritoneal fluid of patients treated with continuous ambulatory peritoneal dialysis. *Nephron* 36: 111, 1984

193. Shany S, Rapoport J, Zuili I, Yankowitz N, Chaimovitz C: Enhancement of 24,25-dihydroxyvitamin D levels in patients treated with continuous ambulatory peritoneal dialysis. *Nephron* 42: 141, 1986

194. Baeyer H, Gahl GM, Riedinger H, Borowzak R, Averdunk R, Schurig R, Kessel M: Adaptation of CAPD patients to the continuous peritoneal energy uptake. *Kidney Int* 23: 29, 1983

195. Hylander B, Barkeling B, Rossner S: Eating behavior in continuous ambulatory peritoneal dialysis and hemodialysis patients. *Am J Kidney Dis* 20: 592, 1992

196. Hylander BI, Dalton CB, Castell DO, Burkart J, Rossner S: Effect of intraperitoneal fluid volume changes on esophagal pressures: studies on patient on continuous ambulatory peritoneal dialysis. *Am J Kidney Dis* 17: 307, 1991

197. Shaldon S: A cynical critique of continuous ambulatory peritoneal dialysis. in *Continuous Ambulatory Peritoneal Dialysis*, edited by Legrain M, Amsterdam, Excerpta medica, 1980, p 137

198. Vas Si: Environmental protection and peritoneal dialysis garbage. *Perit Dial Int* 11: 12, 1991

199. Vas Si, Oreopoulos DG: Handle with care: hepatitis B antigen carrier in peritoneal dialysis units. *Nephron* 29: 105, 1981

200. Bailie GR, Kowalsky SF, Eisele G, Schwartzman MS: Disposal of CAPD waste in the community. *Perit Dial Int* 11: 72, 1991

201. Goodman W, Gallagher N, Sherrard DJ: Peritoneal dialysis fluid as a source of hepatitis antigen. *Nephron* 29: 107, 1981

202. Correa-Rotter R, Saldivar S, Soto LE, Ponce de Leon S, Ojeda F, Ruiz-Palacios G, Pena JC: Recovery of HIV antigen in peritoneal dialysis fluid. *Perit Dial Int* 10: 67, 1990

203. Gokal R: Who's for continuous ambulatory peritoneal dialysis. (Editorial) *Br Med J* 306: 1559, 1993

204. Nolph KD: What's new in peritoneal dialysis – an overview. *Kidney Int* 42: S148, 1992

205. Nissenson AR, Prichard SS, Cheng IKP, Gokal R, Kubota M, Maiorca R, Riella MC, Rottembourg J, Steward JH: Non-medical factors that impact on ESRD modality selection. *Kidney Int* 43: S120, 1993

206. Coles GA, Khanna R, Zimmermann SW, Wall J: When should chronic peritoneal dialysis be recommended over hemodialysis? *Semin Dial* 2: 213, 1989

207. Nissenson AR: Dialysis therapy in the elderly patient. *Kidney Int Suppl* 40: S51, 1993

208. Fenton SS, Desmeules M, Jeffery JR, Corman JL: Dialysis therapy among elderly patients; data from the Canadian Organ Replacement Register, 1981–1991. *Adv Perit Dial* 9: 124, 1993

209. Maiorca R, Cancarini G, Brunori G, Vonesh E, Manici L, Camerini C, Zusani R, Salomone M, Gaggiotti M, Cristinelli L: Continuous ambulatory peritoneal dialysis in the elderly. *Perit Dial Int* 13 (Suppl 2): S165, 1993

210. Gorban-Brennan N, Kliger AS, Finkelstein FO: CAPD therapy for patients over 80 years of age. *Perit Dial Int* 13: 140, 1993

211. Wizemann V, Timio M, Alpert MA, Kramer W: Options in dialysis therapy: significance of cardiovascular findings. *Kidney Int Suppl* 43 (Suppl 40): S85, 1993

212. Zimmermann SW: Diabetic patients on continuous ambulatory peritoneal dialysis: past, present and future. *Perit Dial Int* 13 (Suppl 2): S229, 1993
213. O'Donoghue D, Manos J, Pearson R, Scott P, Bakran A, Johnson R, Dyer P, Martin S, Gokal R: Continuous ambulatory peritoneal dialysis and renal transplantation: a ten-year experience in a single center. *Perit Dial Int* 12: 242, 1992
214. Murphy BG, Hill CM, Middleton D, Doherty CC, Brown JH, Nelson WE, Kernohan RM, Keane PK, Douglas JF, McNamee PT: Increased renal allograft thrombosis in CAPD patients. *Nephrol Dial Transplant* 9: 1166, 1994
215. Tebben JA, Rigsby MO, Selwyn PA, Brennan N, Kliger A, Finkelstein FO: Outcome of HIV infected patients on continuous ambulatory peritoneal dialysis. *Kidney Int* 44: 191, 1993
216. Kimmel PL, Umana WO, Simmens SJ, Watson J, Bosch JP: Continuous ambulatory peritoneal dialysis and survival of HIV infected patients with end-stage renal disease. *Kidney Int* 44: 373, 1993
217. Fine RN: Choosing a dialysis therapy for children with end stage renal disease. *Am J Kidney Dis* 4: 249, 1983
218. Fine RN: Nutritional status and growth in children undergoing CAPD/CCPD/APD. *Perit Dial Int* 13: S247, 1993
219. Fine RN: The adolescent with end-stage renal disease. *Am J Kidney Dis* 6: 81, 1985
220. Nolph KD, Moore HL, Prowant B, Twardowski ZJ, Khanna R, Gamboa S, Keshaviah P: Continuous ambulatory peritoneal dialysis with a high flux membrane. *ASAIO J* 39: 904, 1993
221. Gulanicar AC, Jindal KK, Hirsch DJ: Is chronic peritoneal dialysis safe in patients with intraabdominal prosthetic vascular grafts? *Nephrol Dial Transplant* 6: 215, 1991
222. Charytan C: CAPD after abdominal aortic graft surgery. *Perit Dial Int* 12: 227, 1992
223. Khanna R, Oreopoulos DG, Dombros N, Vas S, Williams P, Meema HE, Husdan M, Ogilvie R, Zellerman G, Roncari DAK, Clayton S, Izatt S: Continuous ambulatory peritoneal dialysis after three years: still a promising treatment. *Perit Dial Bull* 1: 24, 1981
224. Gilmour J, Wu G, Khanna R, Schilling H, Mitwalli A, Oreopoulos DG: Lont-term continuous ambulatory peritoneal dialysis. *Perit Dial Bull* 5: 112, 1985
225. Holley JL: Patient-reported symptoms and adequacy of dialysis as measured by creatinine clearance. *Perit Dial Int* 13 (Suppl 2): S219, 1993
226. Dombros NV, Digenis GE, Balaskas EV, Sombolos K, Abraham G, Oreopoulos DG: Long-term continuous ambulatory peritoneal dialysis. *Clin Nephrol* 39: 70, 1993
227. Hegstrom RM, Murray JS, Pendras JP, Burnell JM, Scribner BH: Two years' experience with periodic hemodialysis in the treatment of chronic uremia. *Trans Am Soc Artif Intern Organs* 8: 266, 1962
228. Charra B, Calemard E, Ruffet M, Chazot C, Terrat JC, Vanel T, Laurent G: Survival as an index of adequacy of dialysis. *Kidney Int* 41: 1286, 1992
229. Mion C, Slingeneyer A, Canaud B: Pathophysiology and management of hypertension in continuous ambulatory peritoneal dialysis. *Contrib Nephrol* 54: 202, 1986
230. Saldanha LF, Weiler EW, Gonick HC: Effect of continuous ambulatory peritoneal dialysis on blood pressure control. *Am J Kidney Dis* 21: 184, 1993
231. Hamburger RJ, Christ PG, Morris PA, Luft C: Hypertension in dialysis patients: does CAPD provide an advantage? *Adv Perit Dial* 5: 91, 1989
232. Stablein DN, Hamburger RJ, Lindblad AS, Nolph KD, Novak JW: The effect of CAPD on hypertension control: a report of the national CAPD registry. *Perit Dial Int* 8: 141, 1988
233. Rodby RA, Vonesh EF, Korbet SM: Blood pressures in hemodialysis and peritoneal dialysis using ambulatory blood pressure monitoring. *Am J Kidney Dis* 23: 401, 1994
234. Korzets Z, Erdberg A, Golan E, Bernheim J: Does diurnal variation in blood pressure exist in CAPD patients? *Nephrol Dial Transplant* 9: 274, 1994
235. Cheigh JS, Serur D, Paguirigan M, Stenzel KH, Rubin A: How well is hypertension controlled in CAPD patients? *Adv Perit Dial* 10: 55, 1994
236. Raine AEG, Roger SD: Effects of erythropoietin on blood pressure. *Am J Kidney Dis* 18: 76, 1991
237. Eschbach JW: Erythropoietin 1991 – an overview. *Am J Kidney Dis* 18 (Suppl 1): 3, 1991
238. Favazza A, Motanaro D, Messa P, Antonucci F, Gropuzzo M, Mioni G: Peritoneal clearances in hypertensive CAPD patients after oral administration of clonidine, enalapril, and nifepidine. *Perit Dial Int* 12: 287, 1992
239. De Paepe MBJ, Schelstraete KHG, Ringoir SM, Lameire NH: Influence on continuous ambulatory peritoneal dialysis on the anemia of end stage renal disease. *Kidney Int* 23: 744, 1983
240. Saltissi D, Coles GA, Napier JAE, Bentley P: The hematological response to continuous ambulatory peritoneal dialysis. *Clin Nephrol* 22: 21, 1984
241. Korbet SM: Comparison of hemodialysis and peritoneal dialysis in the management of anemia related to chronic renal disease. *Semin Nephrol* 9 (Suppl 1): 9, 1989
242. Zappacosta AR, Caro J, Erslev A: Normalization of hematocrit in patients with end-stage renal disease on continuous ambulatory peritoneal dialysis. The role of erythropoietin. *Am J Med* 72: 53, 1982
243. Chandra M, McVicar M, Clemons G, Mossey RT, Wilkes BM: Role of erythropoietin in the reversal of anemia of renal failure with continuous ambulatory peritoneal dialysis. *Nephron* 46: 312, 1987
244. Coles GA, Cavill I: Erythropoesis in the anemia of chronic renal failure: the response to CAPD. *Nephrol Dial Transplant* 1: 170, 1986
245. Lameire N, Matthys E, De Paepe M, Sys E, Schelstraete K, Ringoir S: Red-cell survival in patients on continuous ambulatory peritoneal dialysis. *Perit Dial Bull* 6: 65, 1986
246. Salahudeen AK, Keavy PM, Hawkins T, Wilkinson E: Is anaemia during continuous ambulatory peritoneal dialysis really better than during haemodialysis? *Lancet* 2: 1046, 1983
247. Hefti JE, Blumberg A, Marti HR: Red cell survival and red cell enzymes in patients on continuous ambulatory peritoneal dialysis. *Clin Nephrol* 19: 232, 1983
248. Lamperi S, Carozzi S, Icardi A: *In vitro* and *in vivo* studies of erythropoiesis during continuous ambulatory peritoneal dialysis. *Perit Dial Bull* 3: 94, 1983
249. McGonigle RJS, Husserl F, Wallin JD, Fisher JW: Hemodialysis and continuous ambulatory peritoneal dialysis effects on erythropoiesis in renal failure. *Kidney Int* 25: 430, 1984

250. Wideroe TE, Sanengen T, Halvorsen S: Erythropoietin and uremic toxicity during continuous ambulatory peritoneal dialysis. *Kidney Int* 24 (Suppl 16): S208, 1983

251. Chandra M, Clemons GK, McVicar M, Wilkes B, Bluestone PA, Mailloux LU, Mossey RT: Serum erythropoietin levels and hematocrit in end-stage renal disease: influence of the mode of dialysis. *Am J Kidney Dis* 13: 208, 1988

252. Chandra M, Clemons G, Sahdev I, McVicar M, Bluestone P: Intraperitoneal production of erythropoietin with continuous ambulatory peritoneal dialysis. *Pediatr Nephrol* 7: 281, 1993

253. Nolph KD, Prowant BF, Moore HL, Reyad SE: Hematocrit and residual renal creatinine clearance in patients undergoing continuous ambulatory peritoneal dialysis. *Perit Dial Int* 10: 279, 1990

254. Korbet SM: Anemia and erythropoietin in hemodialysis and continuous ambulatory peritoneal dialysis. *Kidney Int* 43 (Suppl 40): S111, 1993

255. Boelaert JR, Schurgers ML, Matthys EG, Belpaire FM, Daneels RF, De Cre MJ, Bogaert MG: Comparative pharmacokinetics of recombinant erythropoietin administered by the intravenous, subcutaneous, and intraperitoneal routes in continuous ambulatory peritoneal dialysis patients. *Perit Dial Int* 9: 95, 1989

256. MacDougall IC, Roberts DE, Neubert P, Dharmasena AD, Coles GA, Williams JD: Pharmacokinetics of recombinant human erythropoietin in patients on continuous ambulatory peritoneal dialysis. *Lancet* 1: 425, 1989

257. Bommer J, Santleben W, Koch KM, Baldamus CA, Grutzmacher P, Scigalla P: Variations of recombinant human erythropoietin applications in hemodialysis patients. *Contrib Nephrol* 76: 149, 1989

258. Besarab A, Flaharty KK, Erslev AJ, McCrea JB, Vlasses PH, Medina F, Caro J, Morris E: Clinical pharmacology and economics of recombinant human erythropoietin in end-stage renal disease: the case for subcutaneous administration. *J Am Soc Nephrol* 2: 1405, 1992

259. Eidemak I, Friedberg MO, Ladefoged SD, Lokkegaard H, Pedersen E, Skielboe M: Intravenous *versus* subcutaneous administration of recombinant human erythropoietin in patients on haemodialysis and CAPD. *Nephrol Dial Transplant* 7: 526, 1992

260. Bargman JM, Jones JE, Petro JM: The pharmacokinetics of intraperitoneal erythropoietin administered undiluted or diluted in dialysate. *Perit Dial Int* 12: 369, 1992

261. Frenken LA, Struijk DG, Coppens PJ, Tiggeler RG, Krediet RT, Koene RA: Intraperitoneal administration of recombinant human erythropoietin. *Perit Dial Int* 12: 378, 1992

262. Nasu T, Mitui H, Shinohara Y, Hayashida S, Ohtuka H: Effect of erythropoietin in continuous ambulatory peritoneal dialysis patients: comparison between intravenous and intraperitoneal administration. *Perit Dial Int* 12: 373, 1992

263. Nissenson AR: Erythropoietin and peritoneal dialysis: the efficacy of intraperitoneal dosing. *Perit Dial Int* 12: 350, 1992

264. Nissenson AR, Swartz R, Zimmerman SW, Watson A, and the Epogen study group: A double-blind, placebo-controlled study of recombinant human erythropoietin in peritoneal dialysis patients. (Abstract) *J Am Soc Nephrol* 1: 405, 1990

265. Stevens JM, Auer J, Strong CA, Hughes RT, Oliver DO, Winearls CG, Cotes PM: Stepwise correction of anaemia by subcutaneous administration of human recombinant erythropoietin in patients with chronic renal failure maintained by continuous ambulatory peritoneal dialysis. *Nephrol Dial Transplant* 6: 487, 1991

266. Macdougall IC, Davies ME, Hutton RD, Cavill I, Lewis NP, Coles GA, Williams JD: The treatment of renal anaemia in CAPD patients with recombinant human erythropoietin. *Nephrol Dial Transplant* 5: 950, 1990

267. Eisele G, Bailie GR, Clement C, Wong E: Erythropoietin in continuous ambulatory peritoneal dialysis: experience with subcutaneous administration. *Perit Dial Int* 12: 34, 1992

268. Hood VL, Ingraham A: Erythropoietin for chronic ambulatory peritoneal dialysis patients: once a week can be enough. *J Am Soc Nephrol* 2: 1545, 1992

269. Nomoto Y, Kawaguchi Y, Kubota M, Tagawa H, Kubo K, Ogura Y, Shoji T, Kawada Y, Koshikawa S, Mimura N, Maeda T: A multicenter study with once a week or once every two weeks high-dose subcutaneous administration of recombinant human erythropoietin in continuous ambulatory peritoneal dialysis. *Perit Dial Int* 14: 56, 1994

270. Auer J, Simon G, Stevens J, Griffiths P, Howarth D, Anastassiades E, Gokal R, Oliver D: Quality of life improvements in CAPD patients treated with subcutaeously administered erythropoietin for anemia. *Perit Dial Int* 12: 40, 1992

271. Balaskas EV, Melamed IR, Gupta A, Bargman J, Oreopoulos DG: Effect of erythropoietin treatment on nutritional status of continuous ambulatory peritoneal dialysis patients. *Perit Dial Int* 13 (Suppl 2): S544, 1993

272. Pollock CA, Wyndham R, Collett PV, Elder G, Field MJ, Kalowski S, Laurence JR, Waugh DA, George CRP: Effects of EPO therapy on the lipid profile in end stage renal failure. *Kidney Int* 45: 897, 1994

273. Balaskas EV, Melamed IR, Gupta A, Bargman J, Oreopoulos DG: Influence of erythropoietin on blood pressure in continuous ambulatory peritoneal dialysis patients. *Perit Dial Int* 13 (Suppl 2): S553, 1993

274. Meisl F, Manker W, Coisl U, Neyer U, Konig P: Peritonitis does not affect erythropoietin efficacy in patients on CAPD. (Abstract) *Kidney Int* 37: 332, 1990

275. Korbet SM, Vonesh EF, Firanek CA: The effect of hematocrit on peritoneal transport. *Am J Kidney Dis* 18: 573, 1991

276. Steinhauer HB, Lubrich-Birkner I, Dreyling KW, Horl WH, Schollmeyer P: Increased ultrafiltration after erythropoietin induced correction of renal anaemia in patients on continuous ambulatory peritoneal dialysis. *Nephron* 53: 91, 1989

277. Hutchison AJ, Ofsthun NJ, Howarth D, Gokal R: The effect of hemoglobin concentration on peritoneal mass transfer and drain volumes. *Perit Dial Int* 12: 230, 1992

278. Taylor JE, MacTier RA, Henderson IS, Belch JJ, Stewart WK: Dialysis efficiency in continuous ambulatory peritoneal dialysis patients treated with erythropoietin. *Perit Dial Int* 12: 221, 1992

279. Heimburger O, Barany P, Werynski A, Waniemski S, Tranaeus A, Lindholm B: The impact of anaemia correction with EPO on peritoneal transport kinetics. (Abstract) *Perit Dial Bull* 12: 125, 1992

280. Burkart JM, Freedman BI, Rocco MV: The effect of increasing hematocrit on peritoneal transport kinetics. *Am Soc Nephrol* 4: 1726, 1994

281. Brown CB, Hamdy NA, Boletis J, Boyle G, Beneton MN, Charlesworth D, Kanis JA: Osteodystrophy in continuous ambulatory peritoneal dialysis. *Perit Dial Int* 13 (Suppl 2): S454, 1993

282. Armstrong A, Cunningham J: The treatment of metabolic bone disease in patients on peritoneal dialysis. *Kidney Int* 46 (Suppl 48): S51, 1994

283. Joffe P, Heaf JG, Hyldstrup L: Osteocalcin: a noninvasive index of metabolic bone disease in patients treated by CAPD. *Kidney Int* 46: 838, 1994

284. Martis L, Serkes KD, Nolph KD: Calcium carbonate as a phosphate binder: is there a need to adjust peritoneal dialysate calcium concentrations for patients using $CaCO_3$? *Perit Dial Int* 9: 325, 1989

285. Weinreich T, Rambausek M, Ritz E: Is control of secondary hyperparathyroidism optimal with the currently used calcium concentration in the CAPD fluid? *Nephrol Dial Transplant* 6: 843, 1991

286. Delmez JA: Calcitriol and secondary hyperparathyroidism in continuous ambulatory peritoneal dialysis patients. *Perit Dial Int* 13: 95, 1993

287. Delmez JA: Removal of phosphorus by peritoneal dialysis. *Perit Dial Int* 13 (Suppl 2): S461, 1993

288. Delmez JA, Slatopolsky E, Martin KLJ, Gearing BN, Harter HR: Minerals, vitamin D and parathyroid hormone in continuous ambulatory peritoneal dialysis. *Kidney Int* 21: 862, 1982

289. Hercz G, Coburn J: Prevention of phosphate retention and hyperphosphatemia in uremia. *Kidney Int* 32 (Suppl 22): S215, 1987

290. Fournier A, Moriniere P, Sebert JL, Dkhissi H, Atik A, Leflon P, Renaud H, Gueris J, Gregoire I, Idrissi A, Garabedian M: Calcium carbonate, an aluminum-free agent for control of hyperphosphatemia, hypocalcemia and hyperparathyroidism in uremia. *Kidney Int* 29 (Suppl 18): S114, 1986

291. Ramirez JA, Emmett M, White MG, Fathi N, Santa Ana CA, Morawski SG, Fordtran JS: The absorption of dietary phosphorus and calcium in hemodialysis patients. *Kidney Int* 30: 753, 1986

292. Sheikh MS, Maguire JA, Emmett M, Santa Ana CA, Nicar MJ, Schiller LR, Fordtran JS: Reduction of dietary phosphorus absorption by phosphorus binders. *J Clin Invest* 83: 66, 1989

293. Hercz G, Kraut JA, Andress DA, Howard N, Roberts C, Shinaberger JH, Sherrard DJ, Coburn JW: Use of calcium carbonate as a phosphate binder in dialysis patients. *Mineral Electrolyte Metab* 12: 314, 1986

294. Tespersen B, Jensen JD, Nielsen HK, Lauridsen IN, Andersen HJF, Poulsen JH, Gammelgaard B, Pedersen EB: Comparison of calcium carbonate and aluminium hydroxide as phosphate binders on biochemical bone markers, PTA (1–94) and bone mineral content in dialysis patients. *Nephrol Dial Transplant* 6: 98, 1991

295. Stein HD, Yudis H, Sirota RA: Calcium carbonate and a phosphate binder. *N Engl J Med* 316: 109, 1987

296. Davenport A, Goel S, MacKenzie JC: Audit of the use of calcium carbonate as a phosphate binder in 100 patients treated with continuous ambulatory peritoneal dialysis. *Nephrol Dial Transplant* 7: 632, 1992

297. Piraino B: A review of clinical trials with 2.5 mEq/L calcium dialysate. *Perit Dial Int* 13 (Suppl 2): S464, 1993

298. Weinreich T, Colombi A, Echterhoff HH, Mielke G, Neber M, Ziegelmayer C, Passlick-Deetjen J: Transperitoneal calcium mass-transfer with a low calcium concentration (1.0 mM). *Perit Dial Int* 13 (Suppl 2): S467, 1993

299. Carozzi S, Nasini MG, Santoni O, Pietrucci A: Low- and high-turnover bone disease in continuous ambulatory peritoneal dialysis effects of low-Ca_2^+ peritoneal dialysis solution. *Perit Dial Int* 13 (Suppl 2): S473, 1993

300. Rotellar C, Kinsel V, Goggins M, Tarman G, Stull M, Mazzoni MJ, Mosher WF, Rakowski TA, Winchester JF: Does low-calcium dialysate accelerate secondary hyperparathyroidism in continuous ambulatory peritoneal dialysis patients? *Perit Dial Int* 13 (Suppl 2): S471, 1993

301. Salusky I, Fine RN, Kangarloo H, Gold R, Launier L, Goodman WG, Brill JE, Gilli G, Slatopolsky E, Coburn JW: 'High dose' calcitriol for control of renal osteodystrophy in children on continuous ambulatory peritoneal dialysis. *Kidney Int* 32: 89, 1987

302. Martin KI, Ballal HS, Domoto DT, Blalock S, Weinder M: Pulse oral calcitriol for the treatment of hyperparathyroidism in patients on continuous ambulatory peritoneal dialysis. *Am J Kidney Dis* 19: 540, 1992

303. Delmez JA, Dougan CS, Gearing BK, Rothstein M, Windus DW, Rapp N, Slatopolsky E: The effects of intraperitoneal calcitriol on calcium and parathyroid hormone. *Kidney Int* 31: 795, 1997

304. Rolla D, Paoletti E, Marsano L, Mulas D, Peloso G, Cannella G: Effects of subcutaneous calcitriol administration on plasma calcium and parathyroid hormone concentrations in continuous ambulatory peritoneal dialysis uremic patients. *Perit Dial Int* 13: 118, 1993

305. Selgas R, Martinez ME, Miranda B, Bajo MA, Romero JR, Ausejo M, Sanchez-Cabezudo MJ, Lopez-Revuelta K, Sanchez-Sicilia L: The pharmacokinetics of a single dose of calcitriol administered subcutaneously in continuous ambulatory peritoneal dialysis patients. *Perit Dial Int* 13: 122, 1993

306. Schaefer K, Umlauf E, Von Herrath D: Reduced risk of hypercalcemia for hemodialysis patients by administering calcitriol at night. *Am J Kidney Dis* 19: 460, 1992

307. Goodman WG, Ramirez JA, Belin TR, Chon Y, Gales B, Segre GV, Salusky IB: Development of adynamic bone in patients with secondary hyperparathyroidism after intermittent calcitriol therapy. *Kidney Int* 46: 1160, 1994

308. Buchwald R, Pena JC: Evaluation of nutritional status in patients on continuous ambulatory peritoneal dialysis. *Perit Dial Int* 9: 295, 1989

309. Jones MR: Etiology of severe malnutrition: results of an international cross-sectional study on continuous ambulatory peritoneal dialysis patients. *Am J Kidney Dis* 23: 412, 1994

310. Bergström J, Alvestrand A, Lindholm B, Tranaeus A: Relationship between Kt/V and protein catabolic rate is different in continuous peritoneal dialysis and hemodialysis patients. (Abstract) *J Am Soc Nephrol* 2: 358, 1991

311. Lindsay RM, Spanner E, Heidenheim P, Kortas C, Blake PG: PCR, Kt/V and membrane. *Kidney Int* 43 (Suppl 41): S268, 1993

312. Gotch FA: Dependence of normalized protein catabolic rate on Kt/V in continuous ambulatory peritoneal dialy-

598   *Charles M. Mion*

sis: not a mathematical artifact. *Perit Dial Int* 13: 173, 1993

313. Goldwasser P, Feldman JG: The observed correlation between PCRN and KT/V is not a mathematical artifact? (Letter) *Perit Dial Int* 14: 404, 1994

314. Blake PG: Dependence of normalized protein catabolic rate on Kt/V in CAPD: not a mathematical artifact. (letter) *Perit Dial Int* 14: 405, 1994

315. Nelson EE, Hong CD, Pesce AL, Peterson DW, Singh S, Pollak VE: Anthropometric norms in dialysis population. *Am J Kidney Dis* 16: 32, 1990

316. Pollock CA, Allen BJ, Warden RA, Caterson RJ,Blagojevic N, Cocksedge B, Mahony JF, Waugh DA, Ibels LS: Total body nitrogen by neutron activation in maintenance dialysis. *Am J Kidney Dis* 16: 38, 1990

317. Schilling H, Wu G, Pettit J, Harrison J, McNeill K, Siccion Z, Oreopoulos DG: Nutritional status of patients on longterm CAPD. *Perit Dial Bull* 5: 12, 1985

318. Panzetta G, Guerra U, D'Angelo A, Sandrini S, Terzi A, Oldrizzi L, Maiorca R: Body composition and nutritional status in patients on continuous ambulatory peritoneal dialysis. *Clin Nephrol* 23: 18, 1985

319. Lindholm B, Alvestrand A, Furst P, Bergstom J: Plasma and muscle free amino acids during continuous ambulatory peritoneal dialysis. *Kidney Int* 35: 1219, 1989

320. Schmidt RJ, Dumler F: Bioelectrical impedance analysis: a promising predictive tool for nutritional assessment in continuous ambulatory peritoneal dialysis patients. *Perit Dial Int* 13: 250, 1993

321. Chumlea WC, Guo SS, Kuczmarski RJ, Vellas B: Bioelectric and anthropometric assessments as reference data in the elderly. *J Nutr* 123: 449, 1993

322. Mazers RB: Dual-energy x-ray absorptiometry for total-body and regional bone-mineral and soft-tissue composition. *Am J Clin Nutr* 51: 1106, 1990

323. Fiorotto ML, Cochran WJ, Funk RC, Sheng HP, Klish WJ: Total body electrical conductivity measurements: effects of body composition and geometry. *Am J Physiol* 252: 794, 1987

324. Lo WK, Prowant BF, Moore HL, Gamboa SB, Nolph KD, Flynn MA, Londeree B, Keshaviah P, Emerson P: Comparison of different measurements of lean body mass in normal individuals and in chronic peritoneal dialysis patients. *Am J Kidney Dis* 23: 74, 1994

325. Keshaviah PR, Nolph KD, Moore HL, Prowant B, Emerson PF, Meyer M, Twardowski Z, Khanna R, Ponferrada L, Collins A: Lean body mass estimation by creatinine kinetics. *J Am Soc Nephrol* 4: 1475, 1994

326. Bhatla B, Moore AL, Prowant B, Nolph KD, Singh A: Lean body mass measurement in continuous ambulatory peritoneal dialysis patients using creatinine kinetics, bioimpedance and dual-energy x-ray absorptiometry. (Abstract) *J Am Soc Nephrol* 5: 488, 1994

327. Brooks MR, Brandes JC: Changes in lean body mass in chronic peritoneal dialysis patients. (Abstract) *J Am Soc Nephrol* 5: 488, 1994

328. Haraldsson B, Johansson AC, Attman PO: Creatinine generation rate: a blunt tool for assessments of lean body mass. (Abstract) *J Am Soc Nephrol* 5: 492, 1994

329. Lynn R, Ginsberg N, Stall S, Brignol YF, Zabetakis P, De Vita M, Wang J, Pierson R, Ma R: A comparison of four methods for estimating fat-free mass in dialysis patients. (Abstract) *J Am Soc Nephrol* 5: 497, 1994

330. Blagg CR, Liedtke RJ, Batjer JD, Racoosin B, Sawyer TK, Wick MJ, Lawson L, Wilkens K: Serum albumin concentration-related health care financing administration quality assurance cirterion is method-dependent: revision is necessary. *Am J Kidney Dis* 21: 138, 1993

331. Heimburger O, Bergström J, Lindholm B: Is serum albumin an index of nutritional status in continuous ambulatory peritoneal dialysis patients? *Perit Dial Int* 14: 108, 1994

332. Shimomura A, Tahara D, Azekura H: Nutritional improvement in elderly CAPD patients with additional high protein foods. *Adv Perit Dial* 9: 80, 1993

333. De Fitzer CWH, Oe LP, De Fitzer MW, Van den Meulen J, Donker AXM, De Vries PHJM: Is serum albumin a marker for nutritional status in dialysis patients. (Abstract) *J Am Soc Nephrol* 4: 402, 1993

334. Saxenhofer H, Horber FF, Jaeger P: Predictors of nutritional status in CAPD patients. (Abstract) *J Am Soc Nephrol* 4: 416, 1993

335. Heide B, Pierratos A, Khanna R, Pettit J, Ogilvie R, Harrison J, McNeil K, Siccion Z, Oreopoulos DG: Nutritional status of patients undergoing continuous ambulatory peritoneal dialysis. *Perit Dial Bull* 3: 138, 1983

336. Gokal R: Quality of life in patients undergoing renal replacement therapy. *Kidney Int* 43 (Suppl 40): S23, 1993

337. Churchill DN: The effect of treatment modality on the quality of life for patients with end-stage renal disease. *Adv Perit Dial* 4: 63, 1988

338. Evans RW, Manninen DL, Garrison LP, Hart LG, Blagg CR, Gutman RA, Hull AR, Lowrie EG: The quality of life of patients with end-stage renal disease. *N Engl J Med* 312: 553, 1985

339. Wolcott DL, Wellisch DK, Marsh JT, Schaeffer J, Landsverk J, Nissenson AR: Relationship of dialysis modality and other factors to cognitive function in chronic dialysis patients. *Am J Kidney Dis* 12: 275, 1988

340. Wolcott DL, Nissenson AR: Quality of life in chronic dialysis patients: a critical comparison of continuous ambulatory peritoneal dialysis and hemodialysis. *Am J Kidney Dis* 11: 402, 1988

341. Bremer BA, McCauley CR, Wrona RM, Johnson JP: Quality of life in end-stage renal disease: a reexamination. *Am J Kidney Dis* 13: 200, 1989

342. Julius M, Kneisley JD, Carpentier-Alting P, Hawthorne VM, Wolfe RA, Port FK: A comparison of employment rates of patients treated with continuous ambulatory peritoneal dialysis vs in-center hemodialysis. *Arch Intern Med* 149: 839, 1989

343. Evans RW: Recombinant human erythropoietin and the quality of life of end-stage renal disease patients: a comparative analysis. *Am J Kidney Dis* 18: 62, 1991

344. Nolph KD, Cutler SJ, Steinberg SM, Novak JW: Continuous ambulatory peritoneal dialysis in the United States: a three-year study. *Kidney Int* 28: 198, 1985

345. Finkelstein FO, Sorkin M, Cramton CW, Nolph KD: Initiatives in peritoneal dialysis: where do we go from here? (conference report). *Perit Dial Int* 11: 274, 1991

346. Banks JE, Langenohl KM, Brandes JC: Inadequate dialysis is a major reason for transfer from CAPD to hemodialysis. (Abstract) *Perit Dial Int* 12 (Suppl 1): 97, 1992

347. Tranaeus A, Heimburger O, Lindholm B, Bergstrom J: Six years' experience of CAPD at one centre: a survey of major findings. *Perit Dial Int* 8: 31, 1988

348. Keen ML, Lipps BJ, Gotch FA: The measured creatinine generation rate in CAPD suggests overall compliance with prescribed exchanges may be only 78%. *Perit Dial Int* 13: S16, 1993

349. Warren PJ, Brandes JC: Compliance with the peritoneal dialysis prescription is poor. *J Am Soc Nephrol* 4: 1627, 1994

350. Caruana RJ, Smith KL, Hess CP, Perez JC, Cheek PL: Dialysate dumping: a novel cause of inadequate dialysis in continuous ambulatory peritoneal dialysis patients. *Perit Dial Int* 9: 319, 1989

351. Bergström J: Protein catabolic factors in patients on renal replacement therapy. *Blood Purif* 3: 215, 1985

352. Detsky A, McLaighlin JR, Baker JP, Johnston N, Whittaker S, Mendelson RA, Jeejeebhoy KN: What is subjective global assessment of nutritional status? *J Parent Enter Nutr* 11: 8, 1997

353. Qureshi AR, Lindholm B, Garcia E, Groth CG, Bergström J: Tryptophan and its metabolites in patients on continuous ambulatory peritoneal dialysis and following renal transplantation. *Nephrol Dial Transplant* 9: 791, 1994

354. Heimburger O, Bergström J, Lindholm B: Maintenance of optimal nutrition in CAPD. *Kidney Int* 46 (Suppl 48): S39, 1994

355. Young GA, Dibble JB, Hobson SM, Tompkins L, Gibson J, Turney JH, Brownjohn AM: The use of amino acid based CAPD fluid over 12 weeks. *Nephrol Dial Transplant* 4: 285, 1989

356. Arfeen S, Goodship TH, Kirkwood A, Ward MK: The nutritional/metabolic and hormonal effects of 8 weeks of continuous ambulatory peritoneal dialysis with a 1% amino acid solution. *Clin Nephrol* 33: 192, 1990

357. Dombros NV: Chronic intraperitoneal administration of amino acids does not improve the nutritional status of malnourished continuous ambulatory peritoneal dialysis patients. *Perit Dial Int* 13 (Suppl 2): S487, 1993

358. Korbet SM, Rodby RA: Peritoneal membrane failure: differential diagnosis, evaluation, and treatment. *Semin Dial* 7: 128, 1994

359. Slingeneyer A, Canaud B, Mion C: Permanent loss of ultrafiltration capacity of the peritoneum in long term peritoneal dialysis: an epidemiological study. *Nephron* 33: 133, 1982

360. Krediet RT, Zuyderhoudt MJ, Boeschoten EW, Arisz L: Alterations in the peritoneal transport of water and solutes during peritonitis in continuous ambulatory peritoneal dialysis patients. *Eur J Clin Invest* 17: 43, 1987

361. Coles GA, Williams JD: The management of ultrafiltration failure in peritoneal dialysis. *Kidney Int* 46 (Suppl 48): S14, 1994

362. Durand PY, Chanliau J, Gamberoni J, Hestin D, Kessler M: Intraperitoneal pressure, peritoneal permeability, and ultrafiltration in CAPD. *Adv Perit Dial* 8: 22, 1992

363. Pollock CA, Ibels LS, Hallett MD, Cocksedge B, Caterson RJ, Mahony JF, Farrell PC: Loss of ultrafiltration in continuous ambulatory peritoneal dialysis. *Perit Dial Int* 9: 107, 1989

364. Heimburger O, Waniewski J, Werynski A, Tranaeus A, Lindholm B: Peritoneal transport in CAPD patients with permanent loss of ultrafiltration capacity. *Kidney Int* 38: 495, 1990

365. De Alvaro F, Castro MJ, Dapena F, Bajo MA, Bernandez-Reyes MJ, Romero JR, Jimenez C, Miranda B, Selgas R: Peritoneal resting is beneficial in peritoneal hyperpermeability and ultrafiltration failure. *Adv Perit Dial* 9: 56, 1993

366. Chan H, Abraham G, Oreopoulos DG: Oral lecithin improves ultrafiltration in patients on peritoneal dialysis. *Perit Dial Int* 9: 203, 1989

367. Krack G, Viglino G, Cavalli PL, Gandolfo C, Magliano G, Cantaluppi A, Peluso F: Intraperitoneal administration of phosphatidylcholine improves ultrafiltration in continuous ambulatory peritoneal dialysis patients. *Perit Dial Int* 12: 359, 1992

368. De Vecchi A, Castelnovo C, Guerra L, Scalamogna A: Phosphatidylcholine administration in continuous ambulatory peritoneal dialysis patients with reduced ultrafiltration. *Perit Dial Int* 9: 207, 1989

369. Chan PC, Tam SC, Robinson JD, Yu L, Ip MS, Chan CY, Cheng IK: Effect of phosphatidylcholine on ultrafiltration on patients on continuous ambulatory peritoneal dialysis. *Nephron* 59: 100, 1991

370. Krediet RT, Struijk DG, Boeschoten EW, Koomen GCM, Stouthard JML, Hoek FJ, Arisz L: The time course of peritoneal transport kinetics in continuous ambulatory peritoneal dialysis patients who develop sclerosing peritonitis. *Am J Kidney Dis* 13: 299, 1989

371. Mion C, Slingeneyer A: Sclerosing peritonitis: what is it? in *Peritoneal Dialysis*, edited by La Greca G, Chiaramonte S, Fabris A, Feriani M, Ronco C, Milan, Wichtig Editore, 1986, p 215

372. Slingeneyer A: Preliminary report on a cooperative international study on sclerosing encapsulating peritonitis. *Contrib Nephrol* 57: 239, 1987

373. Lo WK, Chan KT, Leung AC, Pang SW, Tse CY: Sclerosing peritonitis complicating prolonged use of chlorhexidine in alcohol in the connection procedure for continuous ambulatory peritoneal dialysis. *Perit Dial Int* 11: 166, 1991

374. Korzets A, Korsets Z, Peer G, Papo J, Stern D, Bernheim J, Blum M: Sclerosing peritonitis. Possible early diagnosis by computerized tomography of the abdomen. *Am J Nephrol* 8: 143, 1988

375. Kopecky RT, Grymoyer PA, Witanowski LS, Thomas FD, Wojtazsek J, Reinitz CR: Prospective peritoneal scintigraphy in patients begining continuous ambulatory peritoneal dialysis. *Am J Kidney Dis* 15: 228, 1990

376. Mactier RA, Khanna R, Twardowski ZJ, Nolph KD: Ultrafiltration failure in continuous ambulatory peritoneal dialysis due to excessive peritoneal cavity lymphatic absorption. *Am J Kidney Dis* 10: 461, 1987

377. Krediet RT, Struijk DG, Koomen GCM, Arisz L: Peritoneal fluid kinetics during CAPD measured with intraperitoneal dextran 70. *Trans Am Soc Artif Intern Organs* 37: 662, 1991

378. Waniewski J, Heimburger O, Park MS, Werynski A, Lindholm B: Methods for estimation of peritoneal dialysate volume and reabsorption rate using macromolecular markers. *Perit Dial Int* 14: 8, 1994

379. Lameire N, Bernaert P, Lambert MC, Vijt D: Cardiovascular risk factors and their management in patients on continuous ambulatory peritoneal dialysis. *Kidney Int* 46 (Suppl 48): S31, 1994

380. Huting J, Alpert MA: Course of left ventricular diastolic dysfunction in end-stage renal disease on long-term con-

600   *Charles M. Mion*

tinuous ambulatory peritoneal dialysis. *Clin Nephrol* 39: 81, 1993

381. Huting J, Schutterle G: Cardiovascular factors influencing survival in end-stage renal disease treated by continuous ambulatory peritoneal dialysis. *Am J Cardiol* 69: 123, 1992

382. Peer G, Korzets A, Hochhauzer E, Eschbar Y, Blum M, Aviram A: Cardiac arrhythmia during chronic ambulatory peritoneal dialysis. *Nephron* 45: 192, 1987

383. Canziani ME, Saragoça MA, Draide SA, Barbieri A, Ajzen H: Risk factors for the occurrence of cardiac arrythmias in patients on continuous ambulatory peritoneal dialysis. *Perit Dial Int* 13 (Suppl 2): S409, 1993

384. Caravaca F, Dominguez C, Machado V, Arrobas M: Vasovagal syncope related to peritoneal dialysate infusion. *Perit Dial Int* 13: 63, 1993

385. Handa SP: Vasovagal syncopy related to peritoneal dialysate infusion. (letter) *Perit Dial Int* 13: 240, 1993

386. Cavagna R, Schiavon R, Tessarin E, Paca N, Scorrano D, Casol D, De Silvestro L: Risk factors of ischemic cardiac disease in patients on continuous ambulatory peritoneal dialysis. *Perit Dial Int* 13 (Suppl 2): S402, 1993

387. Brown PM, Johnston KN, Fenton SS, Cattran DC: Symptomatic exacerbation of peripheral vascular disease with chronic ambulatory peritoneal dialysis. *Clin Nephrol* 16: 258, 1981

388. Khanna R, Wu G, Vas S, Oreopoulos DG: Mortality and morbidity on continuous ambulatory peritoneal dialysis. *ASAIO J* 6: 197, 1983

389. Leenen FHH, Shah P, Boer WH, Khanna R, Oreopoulos DG: Hypotension on CAPD: an approach to treatment. *Perit Dial Bull* 3 (Suppl 1): S33, 1983

390. Goodman CE, Husserl FE: Etiology, prevention and treatment of back pain in patients undergoing continuous ambulatory peritoneal dialysis. *Perit Dial Bull* 1: 119, 1981

391. Boeschoten EW, Zuyderhoudt FMJ, Krediet RT, Arisz L: Changes in weight and lipid concentrations during CAPD treatment. *Perit Dial Int* 8: 19, 1988

392. Canaud B, Assounga A, Flavier JL, Slingeneyer A, Aznar R, Robinet-Lévy M, Mion C: Beta–2 microglobulin serum levels in maintenance dialysis. What does it mean? *Trans Am Soc Artif Intern Organs* 34: 923, 1988

393. Di Raimondo CR, McCarley P, Stone WJ: Beta-2 microglobulin in peritoneal dialysis patients: serum levels and peritoneal clearances. *Perit Dial Int* 8: 43, 1988

394. Lysaght MJ, Pollock CA, Moran JE, Ibels LS, Farrell PC: Beta-2 microglobulin removal during continuous ambulatory peritoneal dialysis. *Perit Dial Int* 9: 29, 1989

395. Mistry CD, O'Donoghue DJ, Nelson S, Gokal R, Ballardie FW: Kinetic and clinical studies of beta-2 microglobulin in continuous ambulatory peritoneal dialysis: influence of renal enhanced peritoneal clearances using glucose polymer. *Nephrol Dial Transplant* 5: 513, 1990

396. Catizone L, Cocchi R, Fusaroli M, Zucchelli P: Relationship between plasma beta 2-microglobulin and residual diuresis in continuous ambulatory peritoneal dialysis and hemodialysis patients. *Perit Dial Int* 13 (Suppl 2): S523, 1993

397. Colombi A, Wegmann W: Beta-2 microglobulin amyloidosis in a patient on long-term continuous ambulatory peritoneal dialysis. *Perit Dial Int* 9: 321, 1989

398. Buoncristiani U, Cancarini GC, Giangrande A, Catizone L, Ferrara R, Carobi C, Di Paolo N: Carpal tunnel syndrome in CAPD patients. in *Current Concepts in Peritoneal Dialysis*, edited by Ota K, Maher J, Winchester J, Hirszel P, Amsterdam, Elsevier Science Publishers, Excerpta medica, International Congress series No 974, 1992, p 729

399. Thomson BJ, Jenkins DAS, Allan PL, Elton RA, Winney RJ: Acquired cystic disease of the kidney in patients with end-stage chronic renal failure: a study of prevalence and aetiology. *Nephrol Dial Transplant* 1: 38, 1986

400. Ishikawa I: Acquired renal cystic disease and its complications in continuous ambulatory peritoneal dialysis patients. *Perit Dial Int* 12: 292, 1992

401. Wadhwa NK, Seliger M, Greenberg HE, Bergofsky E, Mendelson WB: Sleep related respiratory disorders in end-stage renal disease patients on peritoneal dialysis. *Perit Dial Int* 12: 51, 1992

402. Tzamaloukas AH, Kapsner CO: Diagnosis and management of hypertonicity in peritoneal dialysis. *Perit Dial Int* 8: 225, 1988

403. Oren A, Husdan H, Cheng PT, Khanna R, Pierratos A, Gigenis G, Oreopoulos DG: Calcium oxalate kidney stones in patients on continuous ambulatory peritoneal dialysis. *Kidney Int* 25: 534, 1984

404. Backenroth R, Spinowitz BS, Galler M, Golden RA, Rascoff JH, Charytan C: Comparison of eosinophilia in patients undergoing peritoneal dialysis and hemodialysis. *Am J Kidney Dis* 8: 186, 1986

405. Patterson R, Lerner C, Roberts M, Moel D, Grammer LC: Ethylene oxide (ETO) as a possible cause of an allergic reaction during peritoneal dialysis and immunologic detection of ETO from dialysis tubing. *Am J Kidney Dis* 8: 64, 1986

406. Gentil MA, Carriazo A, Pavon MI, Rosado M, Castillo D, Ramos B, Algarra GR, Tejuca F, Banasco VP, Milan JA: Comparison of survival in continuous ambulatory peritoneal dialysis and hospital haemodialysis: a multicentric study. *Nephrol Dial Transplant* 6: 444, 1991

407. Maiorca R, Cancarini GC, Brunori G, Camerini C, Manili L: Morbidity and mortality of CAPD and hemodialysis. *Kidney Int Suppl* 43 (Suppl 40): S4, 1993

408. Held PJ, Port FK, Turenne MC, Gaylin DS, Hamburger RJ, Wolfe RA: Continuous ambulatory peritoneal dialysis and hemodialysis: comparison of patient mortality with adjustment for comorbid conditions. *Kidney Int* 45: 1163, 1994

409. Cox D: Regression models and life tables. *J Roy Stat Sc* 34: 187, 1972

410. Lameire NH, Vanholder R, Veyt D, Lambert MC, Ringoir S: A longitudinal, five year survey of urea kinetic parameters in CAPD patients. *Kidney Int* 42: 426, 1992

411. Tattersall JE, Doyle S, Greenwood RN, Farrington K: Kinetic modelling and underdialysis in CAPD patients. *Nephrol Dial Transplant* 8: 535, 1993

412. Brandes JC, Piering WF, Berez JP, Blumenthal SS, Fritsche C: Clinical outcome of continuous ambulatory peritoneal dialysis predicted by urea and creatinine kinetics. *J Am Soc Nephrol* 2: 1430, 1992

413. Selgas R, Bajo MA, Fernandez-Reyes MJ, Bosque E, Lopez-Revuelta K, Jimenez C, Borrego F, De Alvaro F: An analysis of adequacy of dialysis in a selected population on CAPD for over 3 years: the influence of urea

and creatinine kinetics. *Nephrol Dial Transplant* 8: 1244, 1993

414. Arkouche W, Delawari E, My H, Caville M, Abdullah E, Traeger J: Quantification of adequacy of peritoneal dialysis. *Perit Dial Int* 13 (Suppl 2): S215, 1993

415. Churchill DN, Thorpe K, Taylor DW, Keshaviah P, for the Canada-USA study of peritoneal dialysis adequacy: Adequacy of peritoneal dialysis. (Abstract) *J Am Soc Nephrol* 5: 439, 1994

416. Churchill DN: Adequacy of dialysis: how much dialysis do we need? *Kidney Int* 46 (Suppl 48): S2, 1994

417. Blake PG, Sombolos K, Abraham G, Weissgarten J, Pemberton R, Chu GL, Oreopoulos DG: Lack of correlation between urea kinetic indices and clinical outcomes in CAPD patients. *Kidney Int* 39: 700, 1991

418. Lowrie EG, Lew NL: Death risk in hemodialysis patients: the predictive value of commonly measured variables and an evaluation of death rate differences between facilities. *Am J Kidney Dis* 15: 458, 1990

419. Blake PG, Flowerdew G, Blake RM, Oreopoulos DG: Serum albumin in patients on continuous ambulatory peritoneal dialysis-predictors and correlations with outcomes. *J Am Soc Nephrol* 3: 1501, 1993

420. Spiegel DM, Anderson M, Campbell U, Hall K, Kelly G, McClure E, Breyer JA: Serum albumin: a marker for morbidity in peritoneal dialysis patients. *Am J Kidney Dis* 21: 26, 1993

421. Rocco MV, Jordan JR, Burkart JM: The efficacy number as a predictor of morbidity and mortality in peritoneal dialysis patients. *J Am Soc Nephrol* 4: 1184, 1993

422. Spiegel DM, Breyer JA: Serum albumin: a predictor of long-term outcome in peritoneal dialysis patients. *Am J Kidney Dis* 23: 283, 1994

423. Avram MM, Goldwasser P, Erroa M, Fein PA: Predictors of survival in continuous ambulatory peritoneal dialysis patients: the importance of prealbumin and other nutritional and metabolic markers. *Am J Kidney Dis* 23: 91, 1994

424. Struijk DG, Krediet RT, Koomen GCM, Boeschoten EW, Arisz L: The effect of serum albumin at the start of continuous ambulatory peritoneal dialysis treatment on patient survival. *Perit Dial Int* 14: 121, 1994

425. Bloembergen WE, Port FK, Mauger EA, Wolfe RA: A comparison of mortality between patients treated with hemodialysis and peritoneal dialysis. *J Am Soc Nephrol* 6: 177, 1995

426. Bloembergen WE, Port FK, Mauger EA, Wolfe RA: A comparison of causes of death between patients treated with hemodialysis and peritoneal dialysis. *J Am Soc Nephrol* 6: 184, 1995

427. Teehan BP, Hakim R: Continuous ambulatory peritoneal dialysis – Quo vadis? *J Am Soc Nephrol* 6: 139, 1995

428. United States Renal Data System, USRDS 1992 Annual Data Report: V. Characteristics of dialysis prescriptions in the US 1986–1987. *Am J Kidney Dis* 20 (Suppl 2): 39, 1992

429. Habach G, Bloembergen WE, Mauger EA, Wolfe RA, Port FK: Hospitalisation among United States dialysis patients: hemodialysis *versus* peritoneal dialysis. *J Am Soc Nephrol* 5: 1940, 1995

430. Hakim RM, Depner TA, Parker III TF: Adequacy of hemodialysis. *Am J Kidney Dis* 20: 107, 1992

431. Morbidity and Mortality of Dialysis. An NIH Consensus Conference Statement. *Ann Intern Medicine* 121: 62, 1994

432. Oreopoulos DG: Peritoneal dialysis is here to stay. *Nephron* 24: 7, 1979

433. Maiorca R, Cancarini GC, Manili L, Camerini C, Brunor I: Peritonitis rates and CAPD results. in *Peritoneal Dialysis: Proceedings of the 4ths International Course on Peritoneal Dialysis*, edited by La Greca G, Ronco C, Feriani M, Chiaramonte S, Conz P, Milan, Wichtig Editore, 1991, p 223

434. Jindal KK, Hirsch DJ: Excellent technique survival on home peritoneal dialysis: results of a regional programme. *Perit Dial Int* 14: 324, 1994

435. Nolph KD: Technique survival in CAPD. *Perit Dial Int* 14: 322, 1994

436. Krediet RT, Koomen GR, Struijk DG, Van Olden RW, Inholz ALT, Boeschoten EN: Practical methods for assessing dialysis efficiency during peritoneal dialysis. *Kidney Int* 46 (Suppl 48): S7, 1994

437. Harty JC, Boulton H, Curwell J, Heelis N, Uttley L, Venning MC, Gokal R: The normalized protein catabolic rate is a flawed marker of nutrition in CAPD patients. *Kidney Int* 45: 103, 1994

438. Keshaviah PR, Nolph KD, Vanstone JC: The peak concentration hypothesis: a urea kinetic approach to comparing the adequacy of continuous ambulatory peritoneal dialysis and hemodialysis. *Perit Dial Int* 9: 257, 1989

439. Sherman RA: The peak concentration hypothesis – a justification for inadequate therapy? *Semin Dial* 7: 318, 1994

440. Depner TA: Quantifying hemodialysis and peritoneal dialysis: examination of the peak concentration hypothesis. *Semin Dial* 7: 315, 1994

441. Ronco C, Bosch JP, Lew SQ, Feriani M, Chiaramonte S, Conz P, Brendolan A, La Greca G: Adequacy of continuous ambulatory peritoneal dialysis: comparison with other dialysis techniques. *Kidney Int* 46 (Suppl 48): S18, 1994

442. Tattersall JE, Doyle S, Greenwood, Farrington K: Maintaining adequacy in CAPD by individualizing the dialysis prescription. *Nephrol Dial Transplant* 9: 749, 1994

443. Harty JC, Boulton H, Uttley L, Venning MC, Gokal R: Limitations of modelling dialysis therapy. (Abstract) *J Am Soc Nephrol* 5: 516, 1994

444. Brunkhorst R, Wrender E, Krautzig S, Ehlerding G, Mahiout A, Koch KM: Clinical experience with home automated peritoneal dialysis. *Kidney Int* 46 (Suppl 48): S25, 1994

445. Campbell S, Clarke P, Hawley C, Wigan M, Kerlin P, Butler J, Wall D: Sclerosing peritonitis: identification of diagnostic, clinical and radiological features. *Am J Kidney Dis* 24: 819, 1994

446. Diaz-Buxo JA: Is continuous ambulatory peritoneal dialysis good for five years and may be more? *Perit Dial Int* 13 (Suppl 2): S172, 1993

447. Canadian Organ Replacement Registry: 1992 Report, Canadian Institution for Health Information, Don Mills (ON) 1994, March, p 210

448. Viglino G, Cancarini G, Catizone L, Cocchi R, De Vecchi A, Lupo A, Segoloni GP, Giangrande A: Ten years of continuous ambulatory peritoneal dialysis: analysis of

patient and technique survival. *Perit Dial Int* 13 (Suppl 2): S175, 1993

449. Heaton A, Rodger RSC, Sellars L, Goodship THJ, Fletcher K, Nikolakakis N, Ward MK, Wilkinson R, Kerr DNS: Continuous ambulatory peritoneal dialysis after the honeymoon: review of experience in Newcastle 1979–84. *B Med J* 293: 938, 1986

450. Mion C: Integration of peritoneal dialysis in a regional end stage renal disease programme: a French experience in Languedoc-Roussillon. in *Peritoneal Dialysis*, edited by Atkins RC, Thompson NM, Farrell PC, Edinburgh, Churchill Livingstone, 1980, p 395

451. Wing AJ: Survival on integrated therapies: what asumptions should we make? *Am J Kidney Dis* 4: 224, 1994

INDICATIONS FOR, LONG TERM RESULTS AND LIMITATIONS OF PERITONEAL DIALYSIS

DAVID N. CHURCHILL

INTRODUCTION

Historical perspective

The technique of peritoneal lavage was first described as a novel treatment for recurrent ascites in 1744 (1). Mr Warrick, a surgeon from Cornwall, England drained large volumes of ascitic fluid from a 50 year old woman and replaced it with a bloodwarm mixture of equal parts of fresh Bristol water and a Bordeaux wine. Although the ascites disappeared for at least 1 month, the treatment had been associated with considerable pain. The Reverend Stephen Hales wrote a letter (2) suggesting a modification of this procedure which would cause less pain. This modification involved the use of two trochars, one for infusion and one for withdrawal of fluid, and is the first description of continuous peritoneal lavage.

Ganter is generally credited with the first use of peritoneal dialysis in humans. He had performed experimental peritoneal dialysis by injecting saline into the peritoneal cavity of rabbits and guinea pigs made uremic by bilateral ureteric ligation. Among his observations were an equilibration of the non-protein nitrogen concentration in the peritoneal fluid with the blood concentration within 3 hours of infusion of the saline. He also noted that 40–80% of the infused fluid was absorbed. Two uremic humans treated with 1.5–3.0 infusions of saline into the peritoneal cavity had a temporary clinical improvement. These observations were published in 1923 (3). Necheles (4) attempted to replicate Ganter's findings using bilaterally nephrectomized dogs and cats. Although there was removal of non-protein nitrogen, the animals did not survive very long.

There were 2 reports of unsuccessful attempts to use peritoneal dialysis for the treatment of acute renal failure due to mercury bichloride in 1927 and 1934 (5, 6). Although removal of protein and mercury was documented, the patients did not survive. In 1938, Wear and associates (7) treated 5 patients with acute renal failure with 2–5 hours of dialysis and observed a fall in serum creatinine and non-protein nitrogen. One patient improved and recovered following surgical removal of bladder stones. Also in 1938, Rhoades (8) treated 2 uremic patients with an intermittent peritoneal dialysis technique involving instillation of 1.5 litres of dialysate through a single catheter and drainage through that catheter following a 15 minute dwell.

The technique of peritoneal dialysis as a treatment for renal failure gained considerable credibility from the reports of Frank, Seligman and Fine in 1946–1948 (9–12). In uremic dogs, using the continuous flow technique described by others, they demonstrated urea clearances of 5–11 ml/min using a dialysate flow of 25–50 ml/min. The dogs died, not from uremia, but from peritoneal catheter related infection.

In the early 1950's peritoneal dialysis was still considered an experimental procedure. Death from peritonitis was a major complicating factor. In 1959, Maxwell et al. (13) described a technique which made peritoneal dialysis more feasible. They suggested the use of commercially prepared dialysate in litre infusion flasks. The dialysate was an idealized potassium free extracellular solution with dextrose added to give an osmolality of 372 mOsm/litre. The base was lactate. In order to decrease the probability of infection, 25 mg tetracyclene was added to each litre of fluid. Two sets of Y tubing were used. The dialysis procedure involved infusion of 2 litres of fluid over 5–10 minutes, an hour dwell and drainage by siphon over 10 minutes. Each dialysis treatment would last 12–36 hours. They described 76 mechanically successful treatments and 6 failures. Five of the six failures had intra-abdominal adhesions from previous surgery.

The use of repeated intermittent peritoneal dialysis for chronic renal failure required reliable access to the peritoneal cavity. Repeated placement of a stiff stylet catheter for each dialysis was associated with pain, risk of bowel perforation and peritonitis. Jacob and Deane described a technique in which a Teflon rod, attached to a retainer disc, is inserted into the sinus track left following removal of the stylet catheter. Subsequent dialyses involved removal of the prosthesis and placement of the peritoneal dialysis catheter without puncture (14). The first indwelling Silastic catheter for maintenance peritoneal dialysis was developed by Palmer in 1964 (15). The Tenckhoff catheter, introduced in 1968, added Dacron felt cuffs to promote tissue ingrowth and provided reliable long term access to the peritoneal cavity (16). The many permanent peritoneal catheters now available are modifications of this basic catheter design.

Despite these advances, peritoneal dialysis did not become popular as a mode of chronic dialysis until the concept of continuous ambulatory peritoneal dialysis (CAPD) was introduced by Popovich et al. (17) and Moncrief et al. (18). Initially, the method was cumbersome in that the solutions were available only in glass 2 litre containers. The commercial availability of dialysate in plastic bags increased the popularity of this technique.

Recurrent peritonitis was very common but the use of the flush-before-fill technique has dramatically reduced this problem (19, 20).

Current status

In 1992, over 65,000 patients were receiving peritoneal dialysis as treatment for chronic renal failure (21). This is about 14% of the worldwide dialysis population. The percentage of patients on peritoneal dialysis ranges from 6% in Japan to 51% in the United Kingdom to 93% in Mexico. About 85% are on CAPD. Among the explanations for the observed differences are availability of hemodialysis facilities, re-imbursement schedules, environmental factors, cultural differences and physician attitudes.

INDICATIONS FOR ACUTE PERITONEAL DIALYSIS

Acute renal failure

The treatment modalities available for the treatment of acute renal failure include hemodialysis, hemofiltration and peritoneal dialysis. These can be used intermittently or continuously. The continuous forms of treatment include continuous arterio-venous hemofiltration (CAVH), continuous veno-venous hemofiltration (CVVH) with or without slow continuous dialysis (e.g., continuous veno-venous hemofiltration-dialysis or CVVHD) and CAPD. The role of intermittent peritoneal dialysis in this setting is limited.

The treatment modality selected will depend on the circumstances. There have been no formal controlled trials comparing either intermittent or continuous peritoneal dialysis treatment to hemodialysis or hemofiltration for acute renal failure.

Acute renal failure in small children is preferentially treated by peritoneal dialysis (22). For neonates and infants, vascular access difficulties and intra-dialytic blood flow problems make hemodialysis difficult. The infant's peritoneal surface area is, per unit weight, about twice that of an adult and this is reflected in more efficient clearance of urea and creatinine. Latta et al. (23) reported on 48 children, median age 1.8 years, treated with continuous peritoneal dialysis between 1985–1991. Peritoneal access was by a surgically implanted Tenchkoff catheter. Treatment was complicated by peritonitis in 11 patients and leakage occurred at the catheter site in 5 patients. Twenty-two had hemolytic uremic syndrome; 21 recovered renal function. Among the remaining 26 patients were 7 with acute renal failure post cardiac surgery. These 7 patients experienced difficulties with ultrafiltration and similar patients may be better treated with CAVH or CVVH (24).

Posen and Luisello (25) have described the use of continuous equilibration peritoneal dialysis for 20 adults with acute renal failure and have suggested it to be a viable alternative to hemodialysis. Access was via a surgically implanted Tenchkoff peritoneal catheter. The dialysis had to be discontinued in 4 patients; one due to a hypercatabolic state and 3 due to peritoneal catheter malfunction. In 7 cases, there was a transient dialysate leak. Eleven of 20 patients survived. None of the patients developed peritonitis. Compared to conventional intermittent hemodialysis, the advantages of continuous peritoneal dialysis include avoidance of acute intra-dialytic volume and blood pressure changes, absence of systemic heparinization and the use of a bio-compatible dialysis membrane. Heparin free dialysis and use of bio-compatible hemodialysis membranes diminishes the relative advantage of continuous peritoneal dialysis. The disadvantages of continuous peritoneal dialysis include the unpredictability of ultrafiltration and solute clearance, dialysate leaks, the danger of peritonitis, possible adverse effects on respiratory function and inadequate clearance for hypercatabolic patients. For patients with active intra-abdominal problems, with the possible exception of acute pancreatitis, use of peritoneal dialysis may complicate the management. For patients who can tolerate anti-coagulation, the use of CAVH and CVVH, with or without dialysis, provides efficient continuous renal replacement therapy.

In summary, continuous peritoneal dialysis appears to be the treatment of choice for most small children with acute renal failure. For complicated cases, CAVH or CVVH with or without dialysis is a viable alternative. For adults, selected indications for acute peritoneal dialysis treatment of acute renal failure have been published by the American College of Physicians (26). These are hemodynamic instability, gastrointestinal bleeding, head trauma or danger of central nervous system bleeding. If the alternative is conventional intermittent hemodialysis with standard heparin anti-coagulation, continuous equilibration peritoneal dialysis is a viable option. However, for patients with bleeding problems, hemodialysis can be accomplished without anticoagulation (e.g., saline flushes) and for patients with hemodynamic instability, CVVH with or without dialysis should be considered.

Congestive heart failure

The decreased renal blood flow associated with severe congestive heart failure results in increased proximal tubular re-absorption of salt and water. These patients become unresponsive to the potent loop diuretics. Bargman has recently reviewed the non-uremic indications for peritoneal dialysis (27). Among the indications is congestive heart failure. Intermittent peritoneal dialysis has been used as a temporary support for patients awaiting valve replacement (28) or during the recovery from acute myocardial infarction (29). The peritoneal dialysis also corrects the dilutional hyponatremia associated with severe congestive heart failure. However, intermittent peritoneal dialysis shares with intermittent hemodialysis, the problems

associated with interdialytic re-accumulation of fluid and intra-dialytic hypotension. Theoretically, CAPD would be superior in view of the gentle continuous nature of this therapy.

Other indications

Acute pancreatitis

During acute pancreatitis, toxic substances from the pancreas are released into the peritoneal cavity. The enzymes contained in this exudate can produce systemic hypotension, histamine release and increased vascular permeability. Peritoneal dialysis for acute pancreatitis in humans was first reported by Wall in 1965 (30). He used peritoneal dialysis for 3 patients with renal failure in association with clinically severe acute pancreatitis and observed dramatic improvement. Two of the 3 patients survived. Ransom et al. (31) treated 5 patients with severe acute pancreatitis with peritoneal dialysis and compared outcomes to those in 5 similar patients treated without peritoneal dialysis. For the peritoneal dialysis group, there were fewer days in the Intensive Care Unit (mean 8.4 vs 17.4) and fewer days hospitalized (mean 33 vs 40). In 1978, Ransom and Spencer compared a cohort of 18 patients with severe acute pancreatitis treated with 48–96 hours of peritoneal dialysis to a cohort of 61 similar patients treated without peritoneal dialysis (32). The peritoneal dialysis was started within 48 hours of diagnosis. The overall survival was not different between the groups; 83% for those treated with peritoneal dialysis and 84% for those treated conservatively. The timing and cause of death differed between the groups. The group treated conservatively had an excess of early cardiovascular and respiratory deaths while those treated with peritoneal dialysis had more late deaths due to sepsis, mostly related to late peripancreatic abscesses. In an effort to evaluate the effect of short compared to long peritoneal dialysis on late abscess formation and abscess related deaths, Ranson and Berman systematically assigned 29 patients to either 2 or 7 days of peritoneal dialysis (33). The results suggested a decrease in abscess formation and abscess related deaths with short dialysis but the change was not statistically significant. There was no difference in overall mortality. In 1980, Stone and Fabian studied the effect of peritoneal dialysis in patients with acute alcoholic pancreatitis (34). Patients considered to have severe acute pancreatitis were systematically, based on hospital number, assigned to receive either conventional treatment or at least 24 hours of peritoneal dialysis in addition to conventional treatment. Thirty-six patients were assigned to conventional care and 34 to peritoneal dialysis. In the peritoneal dialysis group, there was a decided improvement in 29/34 within the first 24 hours of treatment compared to 13/36 patients in the control group. Seventeen of the control group were then switched to peritoneal dialysis. Application of an intention to treat analysis to these data indicates a mortality of 14.7% for those assigned to peritoneal dialysis and 25% for those assigned to conventional care. This difference is statistically significant. In a multicentre study 90 patients with acute severe pancreatitis were randomly allocated to either conventional care or conventional care plus at least 72 hours of peritoneal dialysis (35). Forty-five patients were allocated to each treatment. The mortality rate was 28% in the control group and 27% in the peritoneal dialysis group. Major complications occurred in 35% of the control and 38% of the comparison group. Peritoneal dialysis did not appear to modify the incidence of pancreatic collections or plasma amylase concentration.

The use of peritoneal dialysis for acute pancreatitis appears to produce early clinical improvement but, with the exception of one study (34), has not improved patient survival.

Hypo and hyperthermia

For patients with hypothermia, use of external rewarming without concurrent core rewarming is associated with more central chilling and peripheral vasodilation. Successful use of peritoneal dialysis as a technique for core rewarming for accidental hypothermia has been reported by several groups (36–38). For patients with heat stroke, iced peritoneal lavage has been recommended (39).

Poisoning

Peritoneal dialysis, as a technique to enhance removal of drugs and poisons, has been replaced by hemodialysis and hemoperfusion (40). However, if these are not available, peritoneal dialysis can be used.

Plasmapheresis

Popovich et al. (41) have described a novel process called 'peritoneal membrane plasmapheresis'. This involves application of vasoactive agents to the peritoneal membrane in order to remove plasma proteins at a rate comparable to conventional extracorporeal plasmapheresis. Conventional CAPD is associated with protein loss of 5–20 gm/day. The effect of different vasoactive drugs and peritoneal dialysis schedules in dogs was evaluated. Alternating hypertonic dialysate containing histamine with hypotonic dialysate containing norepinephrine removed 40% of the total serum protein each day. This is roughly equivalent to conventional extra-corporeal plasmapheresis every other day.

It has been suggested that the loss of immunoglobulin in dialysate would make peritoneal dialysis preferable to hemodialysis for the treatment of renal failure associated with multiple myeloma and other protein disorders (42). However, plasma exchange is far more effective than conventional peritoneal dialysis for the removal of these proteins (43) and is the treatment of choice for paraproteinemia associated with acute renal failure (44). Application of the techniques described by Popovich et al. (41) to human protein mediated disease may be an alternative to conventional plasmapheresis. However, further research in animal models is required.

Inborn errors of metabolism

Acute peritoneal dialysis has been successfully used in the emergency treatment of the metabolic crises associated with several inborn errors of metabolism. These include neonatal hyperammonemia due to urea cycle defects, propionic acidemia, methylmalonic acidemia and maple syrup urine disease (45–48). Neu et al. have recently reviewed the treatment alternatives for these inborn errors of metabolism (49). Exchange transfusion is inefficient in removing molecules distributed in total body water and is ineffective in the treatment of urea cycle disorders. The clearance with hemofiltration is about 10% of that achieved with hemodialysis. The clearance with peritoneal dialysis is also about 10% of hemodialysis clearance (15). Although hemodialysis is considered the treatment of choice (49), technical difficulties may cause a delay in commencement of therapy. Peritoneal dialysis can be used as an alternative to hemodialysis if the latter is not available or if a significant delay is anticipated.

INDICATIONS FOR CHRONIC PERITONEAL DIALYSIS

Chronic renal failure

General comparison to hemodialysis

The choice between peritoneal dialysis and hemodialysis must weigh the advantages against the disadvantages for individual patients. Compared to conventional intermittent hemodialysis with cuprophane membranes, the clinical advantages include the continuous nature of CAPD treatment, the biocompatibility of the peritoneal membrane and better clearance of higher molecular weight solutes (e.g., beta-2-microglobulin). The continuous nature of CAPD treatment avoids the acute volume changes seen with intermittent hemodialysis. The biocompatible peritoneal membrane does not activate the alternate complement pathway. The better clearance of higher molecular weight solutes is thought to reduce the incidence of dialysis related amyloid and also to reduce the severity of anemia. The latter is reflected in the greater proportion of hemodialysis patients (50%) than peritoneal dialysis patients (32%) prescribed recombinant human erythropoietin (EPO) as reported in Canada in 1991 (50). There is no need for a vascular access. There is no exposure to the increase in cardiac output associated with this structure nor to the risk of infection of the access. In general, blood pressure control is better than with intermittent hemodialysis (51) and this may partly explain reports of stable or decreasing left ventricular mass in peritoneal dialysis patients (52) in contrast to the increases reported for hemodialysis patients (53). Among the disadvantages are the risks of peritoneal catheter exit site infection and peritonitis.

There are life style advantages and disadvantages. Among the advantages are fewer dietary and fluid restrictions for those on CAPD and the ability to perform dialysis at home or while travelling. This is particularly important for those who live significant distances from hemodialysis centres. On the other hand, the disadvantages include the need to perform these dialysis exchanges 4 times daily every day. The former is particularly important for patients with vocational and life-style commitments which interfere with the scheduled exchange times. For these patients, continuous cyclic peritoneal dialysis (CCPD) uses an automatic cycler to perform 3–4 exchanges at night with 1 exchange during the day. The shorter dwell times during the evening exchanges decreases the 24 hour clearance of urea and creatinine. In view of concern about these diminished clearances, the use of more frequent exchanges using cyclers has become more popular. While this approach maintains the clinical and life-style advantages of CCPD and can increase clearance, there is an increase in cost involved.

Special patient groups

There are specific patient groups for whom peritoneal dialysis has been considered the preferred treatment modality. These include children, the elderly, those with cardiovascular disease and those with diabetes mellitus.

Peritoneal dialysis for children
There is general agreement that peritoneal dialysis is preferred to hemodialysis for children. The relatively high ratio of the peritoneal membrane surface area to body weight increases the efficiency of CAPD relative to adults. Creation of a vascular access for hemodialysis is often difficult and the repeated needling required is a particularly unpleasant experience for children. Additionally, the rapid fluid shifts associated with intermittent hemodialysis are poorly tolerated by small children. For these patients, continuous peritoneal dialysis avoids these problems and provides additional dietary freedom. The disadvantage of peritonitis is increased by the danger of fecal soiling in infants. The constant pressure of performing CAPD may be associated with provider 'burnout'. Use of CCPD or APD may diminish this stress.

Peritoneal dialysis for the elderly
In 1987, 12% of the population of the United States was > age 65 and this is expected to increase to 21% by 2020 (54). In the United States, the percentage of ESRD patients in this age group is expected to grow from 47% to 60% by the end of the 20th century.

The theoretical medical indications for peritoneal dialysis are common in the elderly. These include cardiovascular disease and diabetes mellitus. The psychosocial advantages compared to hemodialysis include increased mobility, independence, better control over illness and better psychological adaptation (55). However, the elderly are under-represented in the population of patients treated by peritoneal dialysis. While physician bias may be partly responsible, elderly patients may have physical and cognitive deficits which prevent them from learning and performing self care peritoneal dialysis. For those who commence peritoneal dialysis, treatment may be complicated by malnutrition, bowel dysfunction and poor wound healing (55).

Evaluation of the efficacy of peritoneal dialysis in the elderly requires comparison to treatment with hemodialysis. In the absence of randomized controlled clinical trials, comparison must be between cohorts of patients treated with hemodialysis and peritoneal dialysis. The Canadian Organ Replacement Registry (50) has reported data on patients > age 64 treated by hemodialysis (N = 2621) and peritoneal dialysis (N = 1766). The 1 year patient survival probability was 73% for those treated with peritoneal dialysis compared to 68% for those treated with hemodialysis. After 3 years, the survival probability was 30% for both groups. However, these data are not adjusted for other factors which determine survival and which might not be equally distributed between these patient groups. Maiorca et al. (56) have described clinical outcomes for 480 CAPD patients and 373 hemodialysis patients in Italy. The CAPD patients differed from the hemodialysis patients in that the average was 6 years greater, there were relatively more females and there were more co-morbid risk factors. Increased age was associated with an increased risk of death for both groups. With statistical adjustment for other risk factors, there was a difference between CAPD and hemodialysis for the risk of death associated with increasing age. Above the age of 53.5 years, patients treated with hemodialysis had a greater risk of death than those treated with CAPD and the magnitude of the difference increased with age. Although these results suggest a survival advantage for those elderly patients treated with peritoneal dialysis, statistical adjustment is limited to the variables entered. The CAPD patients differed from the hemodialysis patients in that the former group were capable of self care while many of the latter group were not. A combination of cognitive, physical and motivational factors may be responsible for the self-care capability and also influence survival.

Maiorca et al. (57) have also examined the hospitalization rate for 493 patients > age 65 years treated with CAPD or hemodialysis. Those treated with CAPD had fewer hospital admissions than those treated with hemodialysis (1.67 *vs* 1.71 per patient-year) but more days hospitalized (22.2 *vs* 16.0 per patient-year). In another study (58) comparing 30 CAPD and 31 hemodialysis patients aged > 65 years, there were more days hospitalized for the CAPD patients (18.5 *vs* 13.8). In neither of these studies (57, 58) was there adjustment for maldistribution of other factors likely to affect hospitalization. A cross-sectional study of the nutritional status of 170 patients > 65 years old was reviewed by Maiorca et al.

608 *David N. Churchill*

(57). For CAPD, 50% of the women and 57% of men were well nourished compared to 50% and 53% for hemodialysis. However, severe malnutrition was present in 8% of women and 15% of men on CAPD compared to 3% and 6% for those on hemodialysis. The duration of dialysis and adequacy of dialysis was not discussed.

In summary, compared to hemodialysis, elderly patients appear to have a slightly higher survival probability but are hospitalized more and there may be more severe malnutrition. These conclusions are subject to the biases inherent in the study designs producing these data.

Evaluation of clinical outcomes more relevant to peritoneal dialysis (e.g., technique survival and peritonitis) requires comparison between the elderly and those < 65 years old. In Italy, there was no difference in technique survival between these groups (57) while Canadian data indicate better technique survival for the elderly (50). Data from the National CAPD Registry in the United States (59) indicates a relative risk of 1.12 for peritonitis for patients aged > 60 years compared to younger patients. Thus, elderly patients, compared to younger patients, have a slightly higher risk of peritonitis (59) but technique survival is equal (57) or superior (50).

Peritoneal dialysis and diabetes mellitus

The potential advantages of CAPD over hemodialysis are improved glycemic control through the use of intra-peritoneal insulin; improved cardiovascular outcomes through better blood pressure control; less retinopathy related to better glycemic control, avoidance of heparin and better blood pressure control; less neuropathy due to better glycemic control and better removal of middle molecular weight substances.

In the absence of randomized controlled clinical trials, cohorts of patients with diabetes mellitus treated with either peritoneal dialysis or hemodialysis must be compared. The Canadian Organ Replacement Registry (50) indicates that, over 5 years, there is no difference between peritoneal and hemodialysis with respect to patient survival. The 1 year survival is 80% for peritoneal dialysis and 75% for hemodialysis. At 2 years, the survival is 58 and 55% respectively while at 3 years the probability of survival is 40% for both treatment modalities. Zimmerman (60) has reviewed recent publications addressing diabetic patient survival and morbidity. For 759 patients reported in 11 studies from Europe and the United States, the 1 and 2 year survivals were 84 and 69% respectively. Survival differs for Type I and Type II diabetes. Those with Type I diabetes have 1 and 2 years survival probabilities of 89 and 76% compared to 71 and 50% for type II diabetes (60). These data are univariate analyses without adjustment for other important clinical factors (e.g., age). Data from the US Renal Data System indicates suggests a general trend towards better survival of elderly diabetic patients on hemodialysis (61).

Other studies have addressed the issues of technique survival and peritonitis rates for diabetic patients compared to non-diabetic patients treated with CAPD. In the Canadian Organ Replacement Registry, the 5 year technique survival for diabetic patients was 50% compared to 35% for non-diabetic patients aged 45–64 years (50). Studies comparing peritonitis rates in patients with diabetes are difficult to interpret in that the effect of different types of connectors has not been controlled. There is little convincing evidence that the peritonitis rate differs from that reported for non-diabetic patients. There is a theoretical increased risk for Staphylococcus aureus exit site infection and peritonitis. Luzar et al. (62) have reported a 70% prevalence of nasal colonization with this organism among those with diabetes compared to 36% for non-diabetics.

Insulin can be administered either sub-cutaneously or intra-peritoneally as described by Flynn and Nanson (63). The latter more closely resembles physiologic insulin secretion with absorption into the portal vein. There is considerable debate regarding the efficacy of this mode of administration but there are few comparative studies (64, 65). Among the concerns related to intra-peritoneal insulin is the development of hepatic subcapsular steatosis (66); the clinical significance is uncertain. In a small randomized clinical trial, Selgas et al. (67) found slightly higher hemoglobin$_{AIC}$ levels among those using the intra-peritoneal method.

In summary, there are several theoretical advantages for CAPD compared to intermittent hemodialysis for diabetic patients. There does not appear to be any difference in survival although there is some concern about worse survival in Type II diabetes mellitus patients treated with CAPD. There are no randomized trials comparing these treatment modalities with respect to other clinical outcomes. Patients with diabetes mellitus appear to have better technique survival than non-diabetic patients on CAPD while the peritonitis rates are similar. The most efficacious route for insulin administration has not been resolved.

Congestive heart failure

The success reported for the short term treatment of congestive heart failure has been extended to longer term treatment of these patients (68–71). CAPD appears to be effective in preventing volume overload in patients with congestive heart failure and some have even reported an improvement in cardiac function (69–71). Among the possible explanations are reduction in right ventricular overload with an improvement in left ventricular performance, ultrafiltration induced improvement in cardiac contractility due to a reversal of the downslope of the Frank-Starling curve and improvement in cardiac afterload. If there was co-existent renal dysfunction, removal of uremic metabolites might improve cardiac function as has been demonstrated for high-flux hemodialysis (72). Shilo et al. have reported an improvement in renal plasma flow and inulin clearance, probably secondary to improved cardiac function (73). The long term prognosis for these patients is determined by the underlying cardiac disease. Among 8 patients reported by Rubin and Ball (70), the median survival was less than 1 year and there was no decrease in morbidity as estimated from hospitalization. Except for patients with remediable causes for the congestive heart failure, CAPD is limited to symptomatic control of fluid overload and correction of dilutional hyponatremia. Long term survival is limited.

Other indications

Psoriasis

Bargman has reviewed the data addressing the use of peritoneal dialysis for the treatment of severe psoriasis (27). Most of the studies are uncontrolled (74–77) and cannot exclude a placebo effect of the treatment nor can they exclude an effect of co-intervention. The effect of hemodialysis on psoriasis was evaluated in a small crossover study (78) of seven patients, 4 with generalized psoriatic exfoliative dermatitis and 3 with extensive plaque type psoriasis. The membranes used were low-flux and relatively bio-incompatible. The treatments were for 6 hours daily for 4 consecutive days. The subjects were randomly allocated to either true dialysis or sham dialysis and then received the alternate treatment 4 weeks later. The outcome was evaluated by a dermatologist who was unaware of the treatment order. All patients had a temporary improvement for 1 week after the first therapy, either true or sham. This effect disappeared within 1 week and was not repeated for the second treatment and the authors concluded that hemodialysis was ineffective for the treatment of psoriasis. The effect of peritoneal dialysis was evaluated by Whittier et al. (79) in a cross-over study of 5 patients with plaque type psoriasis. Each patient was treated once weekly with 48 hours of either true or sham peritoneal dialysis. The alternative treatment was received after a 4 week period of observation. Follow-up was continued for another 2 months. Photography and clinical evaluation by dermatologists blinded to treatment order was used as the outcome measure. Four of 5 patients improved on real dialysis; none improved on the sham dialysis.

The results of small cross-over studies must be interpreted with caution. In the case of the hemodialysis study (78), would the results have been different if all patients had plaque type psoriasis or membranes with better clearance or adsorption of higher molecular weight solutes had been used? For the CAPD study (79), could the results have been explained by an order effect? Three of the 4 patients who responded to real dialysis did so during the second phase of the cross-over. The small sample size did not permit statistical evaluation of that possibility.

In an editorial, Anderson commented that plaque type psoriasis appeared to be more responsive than those with pustular psoriasis (80). The mechanism for this improvement is unclear. Peritoneal dialysis would have to remove a pro-psoriatic factor which was either too large to be filtered by the glomerulus or which was filtered and reabsorbed with little catabolism.

However, the use of peritoneal dialysis for the treatment of severe resistant psoriasis has not gained much popularity. It is an invasive treatment and involves nephrologists and dialysis nurses. The single controlled trial had a sample size of only 5 patients and this prevented statistical evaluation of an order effect.

Chemotherapy

The use of intraperitoneal chemotherapy for the treatment of ovarian cancer has been reviewed by Myers (81). The ideal drug for intraperitoneal use would have a large peritoneal to plasma concentration gradient, a steep dose-response relationship over the peritoneal fluid concentration range, no local peritoneal toxicity and no cross resistance with agents used for systemic treatment. In order to avoid the danger of bowel perforation associated with repeated puncture of the abdominal wall and peritoneum, placement of a permanent Tenckhoff peritoneal catheter has been recommended. Use of small volumes of intraperitoneal fluid will not produce adequate exposure of all peritoneal contents to the chemotherapeutic agent. Volumes of approximately 2 litres are required. Hypokalemia and hypomagnesemia must be considered and prevented by the addition of these electrolytes to the dialysate. No net fluid movement is desired and normal saline has been suggested rather than standard dialysis fluids. The concentration of drug is chosen to provide blood levels similar to those attained with intravenous administration and peritoneal fluid levels 10–2000 times greater. The limited clinical experience prior to 1984 has been reviewed by Meyer (81).

LONG TERM RESULTS

The long term results of peritoneal dialysis must be compared to those obtained with hemodialysis. The outcomes of interest are patient survival, technique survival, morbidity, hospitalization, patient symptoms and quality of life. A credible comparison requires a randomized controlled clinical trial. In the absence of such a trial cohorts of patients treated with these 2 major treatment modalities have been compared with the use of statistical techniques to adjust for major differences in factors thought likely to influence the clinical outcomes. Among these factors are age, cardiovascular disease and diabetes mellitus.

Patient survival

Patient survival, when adjusted for age, diabetes mellitus and other co-morbidity appears to be equivalent for hemodialysis and CAPD (50, 56, 82, 83). In Canada, the probability of survival for 5 years was 80%, 50% and 20% for non-diabetic patients aged 15–44, 45–64 and > 64 years old respectively for both hemodialysis and peritoneal dialysis (50). For patients with diabetes mellitus, all ages, the overall survival probability was 20% at 5 years for both hemodialysis and peritoneal dialysis (50). Gokal et al. (82) compared patient survival for 610 new CAPD and 329 hemodialysis patients in 7 renal units in England. Patients starting CAPD were older and more likely to have diabetes mellitus or cardiovascular disease. The patient survival estimates at 4 years were 74% for hemodialysis and 62% for CAPD but the role of treatment modality versus age and co-morbidity was unexplained. Burton and Walls (83), in a study of 389 patients accepted for renal replacement therapy, identified 9 factors which had a significant effect on patient survival. Adverse factors were increased age, amyloidosis, ischemic heart disease, convulsions and acute presentation. Favourable factors were male sex, parenthood and local residence. Statistical adjustment for these factors results in survival curves which are not different from each other. The predicted 10 year patient survival was 53% for CAPD and 45% for hemodialysis. Maiorca et al. (56) reported actual 6 year patient survivals of about 60% for hemodialysis and 40% for CAPD. Adjustment for important prognostic factors removed this difference. There appeared to be a survival advantage for those aged > 53.5 years treated with CAPD. Others have reported similar results indicating that survival does not differ according to treatment modality (84, 85).

In summary, patients starting CAPD tend to be older and to have more co-morbidity. Comparisons which do not adjust for these prognostic factors will favour hemodialysis. Following adjustment, there appears to be no difference in patient survival. However, these results may be biased in that patients experiencing clinical problems are more likely to be transferred from peritoneal dialysis to hemodialysis than the reverse. Deaths which occur after transfer are attributed to the modality at the time of death and this may favour peritoneal dialysis.

Technique survival

Studies addressing technique survival must be evaluated critically. In many of the early technique survival studies, death and transplantation were considered technique failures. The phrase, alive and still on CAPD allowed death and transplantation to be considered technique failures. Clearly, transplantation is not a technique failure. Death is a patient survival failure, not a technique failure. Comparisons between hemodialysis and peritoneal dialysis technique failure almost always will show the former to be superior.

Peritonitis was the dominant cause for technique failure during the early experience with CAPD. In 1983, Maiorca et al. (86) demonstrated a dramatic decrease in the incidence of peritonitis with the use of a Y connector-disinfectant set. These findings were replicated in a Canadian multicentre study (87). In Canada (50), about 47% of technique failures were due to infective complications in 1984. This proportion had decreased to 26% by 1991. The majority of infection related technique failure appears related to Staphylococcus aureus and gram negative organisms. Neither appears to be diminished by the flush-before-fill techniques which decrease infections due to coagulase negative staphylococci. Other factors which may decrease technique survival include inadequate dialysis, progression of co-morbid disease, technical problems with the peritoneal dialysis catheter, hernias and patient fatigue.

Many reports addressing technique failure contain patients who commenced dialysis prior to the introduction of the flush before fill technology. This technique has been extensively used in Italy since the report of Maiorca et al. in 1983 (86). The Italian experience may be predictive of the rate of technique survival which might now be expected. The 3 year technique survival rate reported by Maiorca et al. (56) in 1991 was 80% while the 5 year rate was 70%.

In the United States, black race and prior hemodialysis were associated with a greater probability of transfer from CAPD to hemodialysis (88). For new CAPD patients in England, Gokal et al. (82) could find no factors which predicted transfer to hemodialysis. Technique survival was evaluated among 1990 patients over 10 years in 30 Italian centres (89). The probability of technique survival at 7 years was 50.1%. Age > 65 years was associated with better technique survival than in younger patients. Prior treatment with hemodialysis predicted worse technique survival. The most common causes of technique failure were peritonitis (30%), clinical complications (18.2%) and peritoneal membrane failure (16.4%).

The rate of technique failure remains a cause for concern. Although peritonitis remains as an important problem, failure of ultrafiltration and inadequate dialysis may become the limiting factors for conventional CAPD.

Morbidity

Morbidity among patients treated with dialysis is difficult to measure. One approach is deal with organ system specific morbidity (e.g., cardiac, gastroenterologic, musculoskeletal etc); another is to use hospitalization as a surrogate estimate of overall morbidity. The organ system specific approach will be used in the section describing limitations of peritoneal dialysis. For this section, hospitalization will be used as an estimate of morbidity.

Few studies compare the hospitalization rates between those treated with hemodialysis and peritoneal dialysis. Gokal et al. (82) found that those treated with hemodialysis were hospitalized 12.4 days per patient year compared to 14.8 days for those treated with CAPD. Non-dialysis related causes were responsible for 8.4 days in the CAPD group compared to 9.3 for the hemodialysis group. Peritonitis and catheter related problems required 5.7 days for the CAPD group; vascular access problems accounted for 3.1 days for the hemodialysis group. After the first year, the vascular access related admissions declined but those related to peritonitis did not. This comparison did not adjust for the effect of differences in the distribution of factors which might also determine hospitalization. In 1986, Charytan et al. (90) found that non-diabetic patients had similar hospitalization rates whether treated with hemodialysis or CAPD; 19.0 vs 17.1 days per patient-year. Patients with diabetes had more hospital days but there was no difference between hemodialysis and CAPD; 48.0 vs 40.3 days. For hemodialysis, the following factors were associated with an increased probability of hospitalization: synthetic graft for vascular access, renal failure due to diabetes or vascular disease, a lower serum albumin level and history of cardiovascular disease (91). For CAPD, age < 20 years was the strongest predictor of hospitalization with lesser effects of diabetes mellitus, age > 60 years, black race and prior ESRD therapy (88). Teehan et al. (92) found an increase in number of days hospitalized with a lower serum albumin value and with a longer time on CAPD.

Adequacy of dialysis

The long term results of CAPD are ultimately dependent on the adequacy of dialysis. The most commonly used estimates of adequacy of dialysis are the fractional clearance of urea or Kt/V and the clearance of creatinine. For CAPD, both are conventionally expressed as a weekly value. For CAPD, theory suggests that 1.7–2.25 represents an adequate weekly Kt/V (93–96). Clinical experience suggests that a weekly creatinine clearance of > 50 litres per 1.73 m^2 represents adequate dialysis (97).

Teehan et al. studied 51 patients over 5 years and found, using multivariate statistical techniques, that low Kt/V was associated with a lower survival probability (92). However, the effect was less than that of the average serum albumin value, age and duration of CAPD treatment. Other studies using univariate statistical analysis suggest that patient survival is significantly decreased if the weekly Kt/V value was < 1.5 and that values > 1.9 were associated with improved survival (98–102). Studies using a composite of patient symptoms, nursing observation and biochemical indices suggest poor outcomes with weekly Kt/V values < 1.5 and good outcomes with values > 2.3 (103–105). The corresponding weekly creatinine clearance values, uncorrected for tubular secretion of creatinine were 52 and 87 litres; 35 and 71 litres corrected (104, 105).

Lameire et al. (102) have studied 16 patients who had been on CAPD for 5 years. Although there is a less rapid loss of residual renal function with CAPD than with hemodialysis (106), the loss is complete after 3–5 years on CAPD treatment. A report of 16 patients surviving 5 years on CAPD suggests that this is an unusual occurrence. In the Canada, there were 223 patients who had survived 5 years on CAPD in 1991 (50).

The multicentre Canada–USA (CANUSA) peritoneal dialysis study used a prospective cohort design to enroll 680 incident continuous peritoneal dialysis patients between 1990 and 1992. The multivariate analysis controlled for demographic factors, clinical factors and nutritional status. Adequacy of dialysis, estimated from combined residual renal and peritoneal clearance, had a statistically significant and clinically important association with patient survival, technique survival and hospitalization. An increase of 0.1 Kt/V unit per week was associated with a 5% decrease in the relative risk of death; an increase in creatinine clearance of 5 L/week/1.73 m^2 was associated with a 7% decrease in the relative risk of death. A weekly Kt/V of 2.1 and a weekly creatinine clearance of 70 L/week/1.73 m^2 were each associated with a predicted 2 year patient survival of 78% (107). However, over the dose range in this study there appeared to be increased survival associated with increased dose. There was no plateau effect with Kt/V to 2.3 or creatinine clearance to 95 L/week/1.73 m^2.

LIMITATIONS OF PERITONEAL DIALYSIS

Peritoneal dialysis catheter problems

Access to the peritoneal cavity requires the placement of a foreign body. The problems associated with these catheters include leakage of peritoneal fluid at the insertion site, migration of the catheter from the pelvis, omental wrapping around the catheter and infection. The standard peritoneal dialysis catheter is the Tenchkoff catheter but there have been many modifications developed in an effort to correct these problems. The incidence of leaks may vary with the experience of the physician inserting the catheter, the time between insertion and first use and the nutritional status of the patient. Rubin et al. (108) compared the effect of insertion site (midline or lateral rectus) and intraperitoneal catheter segment (straight or spiral) on catheter function. There were 85 patients studied. There was no difference among the groups with respect to leakage around the catheter or with respect to catheter malfunction. Overall, the incidence of leakage was 11% with 44% requiring removal; 11% had catheter obstruction with 78% requiring removal. The probability of catheter survival for 1 year was 51–56% for all groups. In 1990, Twardowski et al. (109) described long term experience with the Swan Neck catheter and compared it to the retrospective experience with Tenchkoff and Toronto Western catheters. The probability of leak during the first year was 1% for the Swan neck compared to 4.6% for the others. For catheter malfunction, the probabilities were 4.1% and 16.2%. The overall survival probabilities were 81.8% and 60.9% respectively. In a small randomized controlled clinical trial, Eklund et al. (110) randomized 40 patients to a straight Tenchkoff catheter or a Swan neck catheter. There was no difference in catheter survival probability. Leakage occurred in only 1 patient and catheter migration occurred in only 3 patients but all 4 were in the Tenchkoff group. Recently, Moncrief et al. (111) have developed a new catheter and implantation technique which includes leaving the catheter segment normally brought out through the skin completely buried in a sub-cutaneous tunnel. Four to six weeks later, the distal segment of the catheter is brought out through the skin. Controlled clinical trials will be required to evaluate the efficacy of this approach.

The 50–60% probability of catheter survival for 1 year is a complication which diminishes the appeal of peritoneal dialysis as a treatment for ESRD and may contribute to the technique failure rate. The development of the Swan Neck catheter appears to have diminished the problems related to leak and migration. Whether the Moncrief–Popovich catheter will decrease the incidence of infection mediated catheter loss is unknown.

Peritonitis

The use of the flush before fill technique, with or without disinfectant, has dramatically reduced the incidence of peritonitis due to coagulase negative organisms (19, 20). The incidence of Staphylococcus aureus and gram negative peritonitis remains unchanged. Most of the former are associated with the nasal carrier state (62). Strategies devised to eradicate the nasal carrier state and the associated exit site infections have been reviewed by Herwaldt (112). The results have been inconclusive. There are no effective strategies to prevent gram negative peritonitis. Despite the advances in peritonitis prevention, this complication remains a most serious limitation to peritoneal dialysis.

Cardiovascular disease

The theoretical advantages of CAPD compared to hemodialysis for cardiovascular disease appear to outnumber the disadvantages (113). The advantages include better control of blood pressure, higher hemoglobin values with a decreased requirement for EPO, regression of left ventricular mass and avoidance of an arteriovenous fistula for vascular access. The disadvantage is a less favourable lipoprotein profile. The magnitude of these favourable and unfavourable factors is unknown and therefore the net effect cannot be determined.

In the absence of a randomized controlled clinical trial comparing hemodialysis to peritoneal dialysis treatment, the effect of treatment modality on cardiovascular outcome will be difficult to evaluate. There is no difference between these treatment modalities with respect to death due to cardiac causes (114). However, patients with pre-existent risk factors will be more likely to have cardiac events than those without those risk factors. Comparisons between cohorts of hemodialysis and peritoneal dialysis patients must statistically control for imbalance in the

distribution of these risk factors. In a prospective study of new CAPD patients in Canada and the United States, the preliminary results indicated that 25% had prior cardiovascular disease and that 28% had diabetic nephropathy (115). The impact of prior cardiovascular disease on patient survival for hemodialysis patients is considerable. Those with prior cardiovascular disease had a 1 year survival probability of 74% compared to 88% for those without this risk factor. The relative risk for non-fatal cardiac events was 3.15 (91). Among peritoneal dialysis patients, those with more cardiac risk factors had a worse survival probability (116). Concern regarding the adverse effect of hyperlipidemia in CAPD patients has produced the recommendation that this disorder be treated vigorously with dietary advice and lipid lowering drugs. However, evidence for clinical efficacy has not been established in this particular patient population (117).

Musculoskeletal disorders

The major musculoskeletal disorders affecting long-term dialysis patients are renal osteodystrophy and amyloidosis. Pei et al. have reported bone biopsy data from 117 patients treated with hemodialysis, 116 treated with CAPD and 26 treated with intermittent peritoneal dialysis (118). Compared to hemodialysis patients, those treated with peritoneal dialysis had a much lower prevalence of hyperparathyroid bone disease (13% vs 44%), less aluminum bone disease (22% vs 33%) and a much higher prevalence of adynamic bone disease (50% vs 18%). Explanations for the lower prevalence of hyperparathyroid bone disease include better clearance of PTH and better suppression of PTH via higher serum ionized calcium and higher levels of 1,25 dihydroxycholecalciferol. The clinical significance of the adynamic bone disease is unclear. Bone pain was present in 55% of those with hyperparathyroid bone disease, 68% of those with aluminum bone disease and only 10% of those with adynamic bone disease. Pathologic fractures had occurred in 22, 13 and 1% respectively. The available evidence suggests that the bone disease most prevalent in CAPD patients is adynamic bone disease and that there are few symptoms associated with this disorder. Longer follow-up is required to define the natural history for adynamic bone disease.

The amyloid syndromes associated with hemodialysis have been classified as carpal tunnel syndrome, arthropathy and skeletal manifestations (119). These problems are present in most patients treated with conventional hemodialysis for > 10 years. The presence of beta-2 type amyloid in the articular and peri-articular tissues of patients with arthropathy suggests a pathogenetic role for amyloid. There have been few reports of amyloid clinical syndromes among patients treated by CAPD. This was attributed to lower serum levels of beta-2-microglobulin (B2M) due to better peritoneal clearance of B2M and better preservation of residual renal function. Recent reports indicate that the prevalence of clinical amyloid syndromes increases with the duration of treatment with CAPD and may not differ substantially from hemodialysis treatment (120, 121).

Malnutrition

Nutritional aspects of treatment with peritoneal dialysis have been reviewed by Lindholm and Bergstrom (122, 123). Peritoneal dialysis will correct the nutritional abnormalities associated with untreated renal failure but causes new metabolic and nutritional problems. Among the problems are loss of appetite, dialysate loss of 5–15 grams protein daily and dialysate loss 2–4 grams amino acid daily. The continuous supply of glucose and lactate provides an energy load which may induce or worsen hyperglycemia, hyperinsulinemia or hypertriglyceridemia.

Although there appears to be net anabolism during the first year of dialysis (122), protein-calorie malnutrition is common with longer term follow-up. During the first 3 months of CAPD, clinically apparent malnutrition is present in 18% compared to 42% of those treated for more than 3 months (124). Most studies show an increase in total body weight over the first 12–18 months of CAPD treatment (125, 126). During the first year of CAPD treatment there was a decrease in total body nitrogen and this was greatest for patients with a higher initial total body nitrogen (126, 127). The changes in total body weight and total body nitrogen appear to stabilize after 12–18 months treatment (127). However, these results were observed in a small number of patients who had remained on CAPD for 24–36 months and exclude those who had died or had been transferred to hemodialysis. The increased total body weight and decreased total body nitrogen occurs coincident with an increase in total body fat (128).

The progression of malnutrition has been attributed to the synergistic effects of loss of residual renal function, anorexia and inadequate dietary intake. The recommended dietary intake of protein for CAPD patients is 1.2 gm/kg body weight while the energy requirement for inactive persons is 35–40 kcal/kg body weight per day (122). However, the actual protein intake is about 0.91 gm/kg body weight daily (129). Heide et al. (126) observed a decrease in protein intake from 1.37 gm/kg/day early in CAPD treatment to 0.98 after 18 months. Caloric intake decreased from 33.1 to 28.8 kcal/kg/day over the same time period.

With progressive loss of residual renal function, there is considerable concern that anorexia may worsen nutritional status in patients treated with long-term CAPD.

Other complications

Hernias

Intra-abdominal pressure increases with increased volumes of instilled dialysate. The higher intra-abdominal pressure and increased volume will together increase ten-

sion on the abdominal wall and predispose the patient to hernia formation. In a review of this subject, Bargman has indicated that hernias develop in 10–25% of the CAPD population (130). O'Conner et al. (131) reported that the risk of hernia formation was about 20% per year and that the risk was increased for those > age 40 years, multiparity, previous hernia repair and > 3 laparotomies. Others have shown that female sex and post catheter insertion leak were associated with the development of hernias (130). The hernias commonly occur at the site of catheter insertion, at other incision sites and the processus vaginalis. The appropriate strategy, for most patients, is hernia repair followed by a period of small volume supine intermittent peritoneal dialysis or hemodialysis.

Genital edema

This complication occurs in a small percentage of peritoneal dialysis patients. There are at least 2 mechanisms by which this complication can occur. Dialysate may track along a soft-tissue plane from the catheter incision site or through a patent processus vaginalus to the labia or scrotum. Strategies to deal with this problem include bedrest and the use of low volume intermittent peritoneal dialysis while supine or temporary cessation of peritoneal dialysis.

Hydrothorax

The leakage of dialysate from the peritoneal cavity to the thorax occurs in < 5% of CAPD patients. Although most occur early in CAPD treatment, others may be delayed for years. Females are more at risk than males (132). Right sided effusions are more common than left sided ones. The leak is thought to occur through the tendinous part of the diaphragm and that the defect on the left side is covered by the pericardium (133). If the pleural effusion is large, there may be respiratory distress. Diagnostic strategies include thoracocentesis to identify the high glucose content or instillation of radio-isotopes into the peritoneal cavity for later detection in the thorax. For most patients with this complication, temporary transfer to hemodialysis is the appropriate strategy. The hydrothorax should respond spontaneously. If it recurs, operative repair (134) or one of several techniques for obliteration of the pleural space can be attempted (130).

Respiratory complications

Concern has been expressed about possible adverse effects of peritoneal dialysis on respiratory function. In 1966, Berlyne et al. reported atelectasis, pneumonia and pleural effusion in association with acute intermittent peritoneal dialysis (135). However, CAPD differs significantly from intermittent peritoneal dialysis. An important difference is the lower intra-abdominal pressure in CAPD patients due to the continuous distension of the abdominal wall. A study of 10 ESRD patients, without respiratory disease, treated with CAPD showed that when the dialysate was drained, these patients had a maximal inspiratory pressure less than that of control subjects (136). This was considered indicative of respiratory muscle dysfunction due to chronic renal failure. Infusion of 2 litres of dialysate produced, in both the supine and sitting positions, a decrease in functional residual capacity. However, there was a compensatory increase in inspiratory capacity such that there was no change in vital capacity. Similar findings were reported for patients with respiratory and cardiac disease (137). The explanation for this increased inspiratory capacity is that as the diaphragm is displaced upwards by the increased intra-abdominal pressure, it becomes more curved and, according to Laplace's law, generates more pressure for a given tension in the muscle (138). The diaphragmatic muscles also produce an increased isometric force when the muscle fibres lengthen (139). Reports addressing changes in arterial oxygen saturation indicate either no change or transient decrease (130). CAPD does not appear to be associated with significant undesirable changes in pulmonary function, even in patients with respiratory disease.

Sclerosing encapsulating peritonitis

This syndrome is characterized by malnutrition, intermittent bowel obstruction and a decreased peritoneal transport of water and solutes. The small intestine is encapsulated by a thick fibrous layer. Usually the bowel appears normal, although the diffuse sclerosing process has been reported to infiltrate the bowel wall (140, 141). This syndrome is associated with a 50% mortality rate (142). The etiology is uncertain. Among the causes suggested are the use of acetate rather than lactate as the dialysate buffer, recurrent peritonitis, repeated exposures to chlorhexidine and use of beta-blockers (142). This syndrome, primarily reported from Europe, has diminished with the removal of acetate from dialysate and chlorhexidine from exchange techniques. Treatment of this established syndrome is generally unsuccessful.

Back pain

The presence of 2 litres of dialysate in the abdominal cavity tends to exaggerate the normal lumbar lordosis. This is more pronounced in those with weak abdominal musculature in whom anterior protuberance is greater. Many patients with ESRD are elderly and malnourished and are therefore susceptible to this problem. Moreover, pre-existent disease of the vertebral column may be worsened. Persistent back pain may significantly decrease the quality of life for these patients. The use of lower exchange volumes will require an increased frequency of exchange to maintain adequate dialysis and this may be unacceptable from the patient's perspective. The other alternatives include automated nightly peritoneal dialysis or transfer to hemodialysis.

CONTRAINDICATIONS TO PERITONEAL DIALYSIS

There are few absolute contraindications for peritoneal dialysis. The decision to select peritoneal dialysis as a treatment modality must be determined by weighing the advantages and disadvantages for a given clinical situation and by patient preference. The relative contraindications range from very strong to minor contraindications. For self care peritoneal dialysis, the patient should have the physical and cognitive skills required and must be reasonably compliant. For those with physical limitations (visual handicaps, severe arthritis, tremor), assist devices are available for those who must be self reliant.

RELATIVE CONTRAINDICATIONS

Extensive abdominal surgery

Peritoneal clearance may be considerably diminished in patients who have had large mesenteric resection (e.g., following bowel infarction) or who have multiple adhesions and are likely to have loculation of peritoneal fluid. These anatomical abnormalities result in reduced peritoneal surface area and/or poor dialysate flow characteristics.

Severe obesity

The thickness of the subcutaneous tissue makes catheter implantation difficult and dialysate leakage is more common (143). The tendency for patients to gain weight, mostly fat, will worsen the pre-existent obesity.

Enterostomies

The presence of enterostomies probably increases the risk of peritoneal infection and is generally considered a strong relative contraindication for peritoneal dialysis. On the other hand, there are no published data indicating that the risk is truly increased.

Severe chronic obstructive lung disease

The available evidence suggests that instillation of 2 litres of intra-peritoneal fluid is associated with a decrease in functional residual volume and a compensatory increase in inspiratory capacity in those with normal respiratory function and those with mild-moderate respiratory disease (136, 137). However, there are few data for patients with severe chronic obstructive lung disease and it appears prudent to use hemodialysis rather than CAPD for those patients.

Abdominal aortic grafts

The presence of an abdominal aortic graft has been considered a strong contraindication to long term peritoneal dialysis because of the danger of infection. In 1992, ten of 23 centres responded to a questionnaire addressing this issue (144). Eleven patients with abdominal aortic grafts had been treated with CAPD; only one developed peritonitis and this resolved with antibiotic treatment. An additional 6 patients were described in a letter (145). The 2 patients who developed peritonitis responded to antibiotics. The favourable experience with 17 patients (144, 145) does not remove the concern regarding the danger of infection of the aortic graft. On the other hand, patients treated with hemodialysis have an annual probability of septicemia of 11.5% and the relative risk for those with a synthetic vascular access compared to a native fistula is 5.85 (91). The decision regarding choice of dialysis modality must incorporate these data.

Diverticular disease

The presence of diverticular disease may predispose to fecal peritonitis and it has been suggested that this might be a relative contraindication to CAPD. However, there is no convincing evidence that fecal peritonitis is more common in patients with diverticular disease nor is there an increased incidence of this complication in elderly patients with a presumed higher prevalence of diverticular disease.

Hernias

Pre-existent hernias should be repaired prior to the institution of CAPD. If a hernia develops while on CAPD, repair should be followed by either temporary hemodialysis or low volume supine intermittent peritoneal dialysis.

REFERENCES

1. Warrick Ch: An improvement on the process of tapping; by which that operation instead of a relief for symptoms, becomes an absolute cure for ascites. *Philos Trans R Soc Lond (Biol)* 43: 5, 1744–1745
2. Hales S: A method of conveying liquors into the abdomen during the operation of tapping. *Philos Trans R Soc Lond (Biol)* 43: 8, 1744–1745
3. Ganter G: Uber die Beseitigung giftiger Stoffe aus dem Blute durch Dialyse (On the elimination of toxic substances from the blood by dialysis). *Munch Med Wochenschr* 50: 1478, 1923
4. Necheles H: Uber dialysieren des stromenden Blutes am Lebenden (On dialysis of the circulating blood *in vivo*). *Klin Wochenschr* 2: 1257, 1923
5. Heusser H, Werder H: Untersuchungen uber die Peritoneal-dialyse (Investigations on peritoneal dialysis). *Brun's Beitr Klin Chir* 141: 38, 1927
6. Balazs J, Rosenak S: Zur behandlung der sublimatanurie durch peritoneale Dialyse (On the treatment of anuria caused by mercury bichloride with peritoneal dialysis). *Wien klin Wochenschr* 47: 851, 1934
7. Wear JB, Sisk IR, Trinkle AJ: Peritoneal lavage in the treatment of uremia. *J Urol* 39: 53, 1938
8. Rhoads JE: Peritoneal lavage in the treatment of renal insufficiency. *Am J Med Sci* 196: 642, 1938
9. Fine J, Frank HA, Seligman AM: The treatment of acute renal failure by peritoneal irrigation. *Ann Surg* 124: 857, 1946
10. Frank HA, Seligman AM, Fine J: Treatment of uremia after acute renal failure by peritoneal irrigation. *JAMA* 130: 703, 1946
11. Seligman AM, Frank HA, Fine J: Treatment of experimental uremia by peritoneal irrigation. *J Clin Invest* 25: 211, 1946
12. Fine J, Frank HA, Seligman AM: Further experiences with peritoneal irrigation for acute renal failure. *Ann Surg* 128: 561, 1948
13. Maxwell MH, Rockney RE, Kleeman CR, Twiss MR: Peritoneal dialysis. *JAMA* 170: 917, 1959
14. Jacob GB, Deane N: Repeated peritoneal dialysis by the catheter replacement method. Description of a technique and a replaceable prosthesis for chronic access to the peritoneal cavity. *Trans Eur Dial Transplant Assoc* 4: 136, 1964
15. Palmer RA, Quinton WE, Gray JE: Prolonged peritoneal dialysis for chronic renal failure. *Lancet* 1: 700, 1964
16. Tenchkoff H, Schechter H: A bacteriologically safe peritoneal access device. *Trans Am Soc Artif Intern Organs* 14: 181, 1968
17. Popovich RP, Moncrief JW, Dechard JB, Bomar JB, Pyle WK: The definition of a novel portable/wearable equilibrium peritoneal dialysis technique. *Abstracts Trans Am Soc Artif Intern Organs* 5: 64, 1976
18. Popovich, Moncrief JW, Nolph KD, Ghods AJ, Twardowski ZJ, Pyle WK: Continuous ambulatory peritoneal dialysis. *Ann Intern Med* 88: 449, 1978
19. Maiorca R, Cantaluppi A, Cancarini GC et al.: Prospective controlled trial of a Y connector and disinfectant to prevent peritonitis in continuous ambulatory peritoneal dialysis. *Lancet* 2: 642, 1983
20. Canadian CAPD Clinical Trials Group: Peritonitis in continuous ambulatory peritoneal dialysis; a multi-centre randomized clinical trial comparing the Y connector disinfectant system to standard systems. *Perit Dial Int* 9: 159, 1989
21. Nolph KD: Update on peritoneal dialysis worldwide. *Perit Dial Int* 13 (Suppl 2): S15, 1993
22. Steele BT: Infant and neonatal peritoneal dialysis, in *Dialysis Therapy*, edited by Nissenson AR, Fine RN, Philadelphia, Hanley & Belfus Inc, 1993, p 368
23. Latta K, Offner G, Brodehl: Continuous peritoneal dialysis in children. *Adv Perit Dial* 8: 406, 1992
24. Ronco C, Brendolan A, Bragantini L et al.: Treatment of acute renal failure in newborns by continuous arteriovenous hemofiltration. *Kidney Int* 29: 908, 1986
25. Posen GA, Luisello J: Continuous equilibration peritoneal dialysis in the treatment of acute renal failure. *Perit Dial Bull* 1: 6, 1980
26. American College of Physicians: Clinical competance in acute peritoneal dialysis. (Position paper) *Ann Intern Med* 108: 763, 1988
27. Bargman JM: Non-uremic indications for peritoneal dialysis. *Perit Dial Int* 13 (Suppl 2): S159, 1993
28. Cairns KB, Porter GA, Kloster FE, Bristow JD, Griswold HE: Clinical and hemodynamic results of peritoneal dialysis for severe cardiac failure. *Am Heart J* 76: 227, 1968
29. Malach M: Peritoneal dialysis for intractable heart failure in myocardial infarction. *Am J Cardiol* 29: 61, 1972

30. Wall AJ: Peritoneal dialysis in the treatment of severe acute pancreatitis. *Med J Aust* 2: 281, 1965

31. Ranson JHC, Rifkind KM, Turner JW: Prognostic signs and non-operative peritoneal lavage in acute pancreatitis. *Surg Gynecol Obstet* 143: 209, 1976

32. Ranson JHC, Spenser FC: The role of peritoneal lavage in severe acute pancreatitis. *Ann Surg* 187: 565, 1978

33. Ranson JHC, Berman RS: Long peritoneal lavage decreases peitoneal sepsis in acute pancreatitis. *Ann Surg* 211: 708, 1990

34. Stone HH, Fabian TC: Peritoneal dialysis in the treatment of acute alcoholic pancreatitis. *Surg Gynecol Obstet* 150: 878, 1980

35. Mayer AD, McMahon MJ, Corfield AP et al.: Controlled clinical trial of peritoneal lavage for the treatment of severe acute pancreatitis. *N Engl J Med* 312: 399, 1985

36. Lash RF, Burdette JA, Ozdil T: Accidental profound hypothermia and barbiturate intoxication: a report of rapid core rewarming by peritoneal dialysis. *JAMA* 201: 269, 1967

37. Davis FM, Judson JA: Warm peritoneal dialysis in the treatment of accidental hypothermia: report of five cases. *N Z Med J* 94: 207, 1981

38. Troelsen S, Rybro L, Knudsen F: Profound accidental hypothermia treated with peritoneal dialysis. *Scand J Urol Nephrol* 20: 221, 1986

39. Horowitz BZ: The golden hour in heat stroke; use of iced peritoneal lavage. *Am J Emerg Med* 7: 616, 1989

40. Wogan JM: Enhancement of elimination. in *Manual of Toxicologic Emergencies*, edited by Noji EK, Kelen GD, Chicago, London, Boca Raton, Year Book Medical Publishers Inc, 1989

41. Popovich R, Zengzhi H, Moncrief J: Peritoneal membrane plasmapheresis. *Perit Dial Int* 13 (Suppl 2): S82, 1993

42. Rosansky SJ, Richards FW: Use of peritoneal dialysis in the treatment of patients with renal failure and paraproteinemia. *Am J Nephrol* 5: 361, 1985

43. Russell JA, Fitzharris BM, Corringham D, Darcy DA, Powles RL: Plasma exchange versus peritoneal dialysis for removing Bence Jones proteins. *Br Med J* 2: 1397, 1978

44. Zucchelli P, Pasquali S, Cagnoli L, Ferrari G: Controlled plasma exchange trial in acute renal failure due to multiple myeloma. *Kidney Int* 33: 1175, 1988

45. Wiegand C, Thompson T, Bock GH, Mathis RK, Kjellstrand CM, Mauer SM: The management of life-treatening hyperammonemia: a comparison of several therapeutic modalities. *J Pediatr* 96: 142, 1980

46. Robert MF, Schultz DJ, Wolf B, Cochran WD, Schwartz AL: Treatment of a neonate with propionic acidemia and severe hyperammonemia by peritoneal dialysis. *Arch Dis Child* 54: 962, 1979

47. Moreno-Vega A, Govantes JM: Methylmalonic acidemia treated by continuous ambulatory peritoneal dialysis. *N Engl J Med* 312: 1641, 1985

48. Clow CL, Reade TM, Scriver CR: Outcome of early and long-term management of classical maple syrup urine disease. *Pediatrics* 68: 856, 1981

49. Neu AM, Christenson MJ, Brusilow SW: Hemodialysis for inborn errors of metabolism. in *Clinical Dialysis*, edited by Nissenson AR, Fine RN, Philadelphia, Hanley & Belfus Inc, p 341

50. Canadian Organ Replacement Registry: 1991 Annual Report, Hospital Medical Records Institute, Don Mills, Ontario, April, 1993

51. Hamburger RJ, Christ PG, Morris PA, Luft FC: Hypertension in dialysis patients: Does CAPD provide an advantage? *Adv Perit Dial* 5: 91, 1989

52. Leenen FHH, Smith DL, Khanna R, Oreopoulos DG: Changes in left ventricular hypertrophy and function in hypertensive patients started on continuous ambulatory peritoneal dialysis. *Am J Heart* 110: 102, 1985

53. Parfrey PS, Harnett JD, Griffiths SM et al.: The clinical course of left ventricular hypertrophy in dialysis patients. *Nephron* 55: 114, 1990

54. Nissenson AR: Peritoneal dialysis in the geriatric patient: overview and introduction. *Adv Perit Dial* 6 (Suppl 1): 1, 1990

55. Ross CJ, Rutsky EA: Dialysis modality selection in the elderly patient with end-stage renal disease: Avantages and disadvantages of peritoneal dialysis. *Adv Perit Dial* 6 (Suppl 1): 11, 1990

56. Maiorca R, Vonesh EF, Cavalli PL et al.: A multicentre, selection adjusted comparison of patient and technique survivals on CAPD and hemodialysis. *Perit Dial Int* 11: 118, 1991

57. Maiorca R, Cancarini G, Brunori G et al.: Continuous ambulatory peritoneal dialysis in the elderly. *Perit Dial Int* 13 (Suppl 2): S165, 1993

58. O'Brien M, Zimmerman S: Comparison of peritoneal dialysis and hemodialysis in the elderly. *Adv Perit Dial* 6 (Suppl 1): 65, 1990

59. Nolph KD, Lindblad AS, Novak JW, Steinberg SM: Experiences with the elderly in the National CAPD registry. *Adv Perit Dial* 6 (Suppl 1): 33, 1990

60. Zimmerman SW: Diabetic patients on continuous ambulatory peritoneal dialysis: past, present and future. *Perit Dial Int* 13 (Suppl 2): S229, 1993

61. US Renal Data System: USRDS 1991 Annual Data Report, The National Institute od Diabetes and Digestive and Kidney Diseases. *Am J Kidney Dis* 18 (Suppl 2): 49, 1991

62. Luzar MA, Coles GA, Faller B et al.: Staphylococcus aureus nasal carriage and infection in patients on continuous ambulatory peritoneal dialysis. *N Engl J Med* 322: 505, 1990

63. Flynn CT, Nanson JA: Intra-peritoneal insulin with CAPD: an artificial pancreas. *Trans Am Soc Artif Intern Organs* 25: 14, 1979

64. Tzamaloukas AH, Oreopoulos DG: Subcutaneous *versus* intraperitoneal insulin in the management of diabetics on CAPD. *Adv Perit Dial* 7: 81, 1991

65. Rottembourg J, Issad B, Allouache M: Insulin prescription, glycemic control and diabetic complications in diabetics treated by continuous ambulatory peritoneal dialysis. *Perit Dial Int* 13 (Suppl 2): S232, 1993

66. Wanless JR, Bargman JM, Oreopoulos DG, Vas SI: Subcapsular steatosis in response to peritoneal insulin delivery: a clue to the pathogenesis of steatonecrosis in obesity. *Modern Pathology* 2: 69, 1989

67. Selgas R, Diez JJ, Monoz J et al.: Comparative study of 2 different routes for insulin administration in CAPD patients. A multicentre study. *Adv Perit Dial* 5: 181, 1989

68. McKinnie JJ, Bourgeois RJ, Husserl FE: Long term thera-

py for heart failure with continuous anbulatory peritoneal dialysis. *Arch Intern Med* 145: 1128, 1985

69. Kim D, Khanna R, Wu G et al.: Successful use of continuous ambulatory peritoneal dialysis in refractory heart failure. *Perit Dial Bull* 5: 127, 1985

70. Rubin J, Ball R: Continuous ambulatory peritoneal dialysis treatment for severe congestive heart failure in the face of chronic renal failure. *Arch Intern Med* 146: 1533, 1986

71. Konig PS, Lhotta K, Kronenberg F, Joannidis M, Herold M: CAPD: a successful treatment for patients suffering from therapy-resistant congestive heart failure. *Adv Perit Dial* 7: 97, 1991

72. Churchill DN, Taylor DW, Tomlinson CW, Beecroft ML, Gorman J, Stanton E: Effect of high-flux hemodialysis on cardiac structure and function among patients with end-stage renal failure. *Nephron* 65: 573, 1993

73. Shilo S, Slotki IN, Iaina A: Improved renal function following acute peritoneal dialysis in patients with intractable congestive heart failure. *Isr J Med Sci* 23: 821, 1987

74. Twardowski ZJ, Nolph KD, Rubin J, Anderson PC: Peritoneal dialysis for psoriasis. an uncontrolled study. *Ann Intern Med* 88: 345, 1978

75. Halevy S, Halevy J, Boner G, Rosenfeld JB, Feuerman EJ: Dialysis therapy for psoriasis. Report of three cases and review of the literature. *Arch Dermatol* 117: 69, 1981

76. Twardowski ZB, Lempert KD, Lankhorst BJ et al.: Continuous ambulatory peritoneal dialysis for psoriasis. A report of 4 cases. *Arch Intern Med* 146: 1177, 1986

77. Sobh MA, Abdel Rasik MM, Moustafa FE et al.: Dialysis therapy of severe psoriasis: a random study of 40 cases. *Nephrol Dial Transplant* 2: 351, 1987

78. Nissenson AR, Rapaport M, Gordon A et al.: Hemodialysis in the treatment of psoriasis: a controlled trial. *Ann Intern Med* 91: 218, 1979

79. Whittier FC, Evans DH, Anderson PC, Nolph KD: Peritoneal dialysis for psoriasis: a controlled study. *Ann Intern Med* 99: 165, 1983

80. Anderson PC: Dialysis treatment of psoriasis. *Arch Dermatol* 117: 67, 1981

81. Myers C: The use of intraperitoneal chemotherapy in the treatment of ovarian carcinoma. *Semin Oncol* 11: 275, 1984

82. Gokal R, Jakubowski C, King J et al.: Outcome in patients on continuous ambulatory peritoneal dialysis and hemodialysis: 4-year analysis of a prospective multicentre study. *Lancet* 2: 1105, 1987

83. Burton PR, Walls J: Selection-adjusted comparison of life-expectancy of patients on continuous ambulatory peritoneal dialysis, hemodialysis and renal transplantation. *Lancet* 1: 1115, 1987

84. Lunde Nm, Port FK, Wolfe RA, Guire KE: Comparison of mortality risk by choice of CAPD versus hemodialysis among elderly patients. *Adv Perit Dial* 7: 68, 1991

85. Gentil MA, Carriazo A, pavon MI et al.: Comparison of survival in continuous ambulatory peritoneal dialysis and hospital hemodialysis. A multicentric study. *Nephrol Dial Transplant* 6: 444, 1991

86. Maiorca R, Cantaluppi A, Cancarini GC et al.: Prospective controlled trial of a Y connector disinfectant system to prevent peritonitis in continuous ambulatory peritoneal dialysis. *Lancet* 2: 642, 1983

87. Canadian Clinical Trials group: Peritonitis in continuous ambulatory peritoneal dialysis; a multicentre randomized clinical trial ccomparing the Y connector disinfectant system to standard systems. *Perit Dial Int* 9: 159, 1989

88. Nolph KD, Cutler SJ, Steinberg SM, Novak JW, Hirschman GH: Factors associated with morbidity and mortality among patients on CAPD. *Trans Am Soc Artif Intern Organs* 33: 57, 1987

89. Viglino G, Cancarini G, Catizone L et al.: Ten years of continuous ambulatory peritoneal dialysis: analysis of patient and technique survival. *Perit Dial Int* 13 (Suppl 13): S175, 1992

90. Charytan C, Spinowitz BS, Galler M: A comparative study of continuous ambulatory peritoneal dialysis and centre hemodialysis. *Arch Intern Med* 146: 1138, 1986

91. Churchill DN, Taylor DW, Cook RJ et al.: Canadian hemodialysis morbidity study. *Am J Kidney Dis* 19: 214, 1992

92. Teehan BP, Schleifer CR, Brown JM, Sigler MH, Raimondo J: Urea kinetic analysis and clinical outcome on CAPD. A five year longitudinal study. *Adv Perit Dial* 6: 181, 1990

93. Popovich RP, Moncrief JW: Kinetic modeling of peritoneal transport. *Contrib Nephrol* 17: 59, 1979

94. Teehan BP, Schleifler CR, Sigler MH, Gilgore GS: A quantitative approach to the CAPD prescription. *Perit Dial Bull* 5: 152, 1985

95. Keshaviah PR, Nolph KD, Van Stone JC: The peak urea concentration hypothesis: a kinetic approach to comparing the adequacy of continuous ambulatory peritoneal dialysis and hemodialysis. *Perit Dial Int* 9: 257, 1989

96. Gotch FA: Application of urea kinetic modeling to adequacy of CAPD therapy. *Adv Perit Dial* 6: 178, 1990

97. Twardowski ZJ, Nolph KD: Peritoneal dialysis: How much is enough? *Semin Dial* 1: 75, 1988

98. Blake PG, Balaskas E, Blake R, Oreopoulos DG: Urea kinetics has limited relevance in assessing adequacy of dialysis in CAPD. *Adv Perit Dial* 8: 65, 1992

99. Blake PG, Somolos K, Abraham G, Weissgarten J, Pemberton R, Chu GL, Oreopoulos DG: Lack of correlation between urea kinetic indices and clinical outcomes in CAPD patients. *Kidney Int* 39: 700, 1991

100. Teehan BP, Schleifer CR, Brown J: Urea kinetic modeling is an appropriate assessment of adequacy. *Semin Dial* 5: 189, 1992

101. DeAlvaro F, Bajo MA, Alvarez-Ude F et al.: Adequacy of peritoneal dialysis: does Kt/V have the same predictive value as in HD? A multicentre study. *Adv Perit Dial* 8: 93, 1992

102. Lameire NH, Vanholder R, Veyt D, Lambert MC, Ringoir S: A longitudinal five year survey of kinetic parameters in CAPD patients. *Kidney Int* 42: 426, 1992

103. Keshaviah PR, Nolph KD, Prowant B et al.: Defining adequacy of peritoneal dialysis with urea kinetics. *Adv Perit Dial* 6: 173, 1990

104. Brandes JC, Piering WF, Beres JA, Blumenthal SS, Fritsche C: Clinical outcome of continuous ambulatory peritoneal dialysis predicted by urea and creatinine kinetics. *Am Soc Nephrol* 2: 1430, 1992

105. Arkouche W, Delawari E, My H et al.: Quantification of adequacy of peritoneal dialysis. *Perit Dial Int* 13 (Suppl 13): S215, 1993

106. Lysaght MJ, Vonesh EF, Gotch F et al.: The influence of dialysis treatment modality on the decline of remaining

renal function. *Trans Am Soc Artif Intern Organs* 37: 598, 1991

107. Churchill DN, Thorpe K, Taylor DW, Keshaviah P for the CANUSA Study of Peritoneal Dialysis Adequacy: Adequacy of peritoneal dialysis. *J Am Soc Nephrol* 5: 439, 1994

108. Rubin J, Didlake R, Raju S, Hsu H: A prospective randomized evaluation of chronic peritoneal catheters. *Trans Am Soc Artif Intern Organs* 36: M497, 1990

109. Twardowski ZJ, Prowant BF, Khanna R, Nichols WK, Nolph KD: Long-term experience with Swan Neck Missouri catheters. *Trans Am Soc Arif Intern Organs* 36: M491, 1990

110. Eklund BH, Honkanen EO, Kala AR, Kyllonen LE: Catheter configuration and outcome in patients on continuous ambulatory peritoneal dialysis: a prospective comparison of two catheters. *Perit Dial Int* 14: 70, 1994

111. Moncrief JW, Popovich RP, Dasgupta M et al.: Reduction in peritonitis incidence in continuous ambulatory peritoneal dialysis with a new catheter and implantation technique. *Perit Dial Int* 13 (Suppl 13): S329, 1993

112. Herwaldt LA: Staphylococcus aureus nasal carriage: role in continuous ambulatory peritoneal dialysis-associated infections. *Perit Dial Int* 13 (Suppl 2): S301, 1993

113. Churchill DN: Comparative morbidity among hemodialysis patients and continuous ambulatory peritoneal dialysis patients. *Kidney Int* 43 (Suppl 40): S16, 1993

114. Maher JF: Cardiovascular disease and risk factors in patients treated by continuous ambulatory peritoneal dialysis. *Perit Dial Int* 13 (Suppl 2): S389, 1993

115. CANUSA Peritoneal Dialysis study Group: Canada-USA multicentre study of peritoneal dialysis adequacy: Description of the study population and preliminary results. *Adv Perit Dial* 1990

116. Lameire N: Cardiovascular risk factors and blood pressure control in continuous ambulatory peritoneal dialysis patients. *Perit Dial Int* 13 (Suppl 2): S394, 1993

117. Atkins RC, Wood C: Hyperlipidemia in CAPD. *Perit Dial Int* 13 (Suppl 2): S415, 1993

118. Pei Y, Hercz G, Greenwood C et al.: Non-invasive prediction of aluminum bone disease in hemo and peritoneal dialysis patients. *Kidney Int* 41: 1374, 1992

119. Kleinman KS, Coburn JW: Amyloid syndromes associated with hemodialysis. *Kidney Int* 35: 567, 1980

120. Cornelius F, Bardin T, Faller B et al.: Rheumatic syndromes and B-2-M amyloidosis in patients receiving long term peritoneal dialysis. *Arthr Rheum* 32: 785, 1989

121. Benz RL, Siegfried JW, Teehan BP: Carpal tunnel syndrome in dialysis patients; comparison between continuous ambulatory peritoneal dialysis and hemodialysis populations. *Am J Kidney Dis* 11: 473, 1988

122. Lindholm B, Bergstrom J: Nutritional aspects on peritoneal dialysis. *Kidney Int* 42 (Suppl 42): S165, 1992

123. Bergstrom J, Lindholm B: Nutrition and adequacy of dialysis. How do hemodialysis and CAPD compare? *Kidney Int* 43 (Suppl 40): S39, 1993

124. Young GA, Kopple JD, Lindholm B et al.: Nutritional assessment of CAPD patients. An international study. *Am J Kidney Dis* 17: 462, 1991

125. Bouma SF, Dwyer JT: Glucose absorption and weight change in 18 months of continuous ambulatory peritoneal dialysis. *J Am Diet Assoc* 84: 194, 1984

126. Heide B, Pierratos A, Khanna R et al.: Nutritional status

127. Schilling H, Wu G, Pettit J et al.: Nutritional status of patients on long-term CAPD. *Perit Dial Bull* 5: 12, 1985

128. Soreide R, Dracup E, Svarstad E, Iversen BM: Increased total body fat during PD treatment. *Adv Perit Dial* 8: 173, 1992

129. Lysaght MJ, Pollock CA, Hallet MD, Ibels LS, Farrell PC: The relevance of urea kinetic modeling to CAPD. *Trans Am Soc Artif Intern Organs* 35: 784, 1989

130. Bargman JM: Complications of peritoneal dialysis related to increased intra-abdominal pressure. *Kidney Int* 43 (Suppl 40): S75, 1993

131. O'Conner JP, Rigby RJ, Hardie IR et al.: Abdominal hernias complicating continuous ambulatory peritoneal dialysis. *Am J Nephrol* 6: 271, 1986

132. Benz RL, Schleifer CR: Hydrothorax in continuous ambulatory peritoneal dialysis: Successful treatment with intrapleural tetracycline and a review of the literature. *Am J Kidney Dis* 5: 136, 1985

133. Boeschoten EW, Krediet RT, Roos CM et al.: Leakage of dialysate across the diaphragm. An important complication of continuous ambulatory peritoneal dialysis. *Neth J Med* 29: 242, 1986

134. Pattison CW, Rodger DSC, Adu D, Michael J, Mathews HR: Surgical treatment of hydrothorax complicating continuous ambulatory peritoneal dialysis. *Clin Nephrol* 21: 191, 1984

135. Berylne GM, Lee HA, Ralston AJ, Woolcock JA: Pulmonary complications of peritoneal dialysis. *Lancet* 2: 75, 1966

136. Gomez-Fernandez P, Sanchez Agudo L, Calatrava JM et al.: Respiratory muscle weakness in uremic patients under continuous ambulatory peritoneal dialysis. *Nephron* 36: 219, 1984

137. Beasley CRW, Ripley JM, Smith DA, Neale TJ: Pulmonary function in chronic renal failure patients managed by continuous ambulatory peritoneal dialysis. *New Zeal Med J* 99: 313, 1986

138. Rebuck AS: Peritoneal dialysis and the mechanics of the diaphragm. *Perit Dial Bull* 2: 109, 1982

139. Pengally LD, Alderson AM, Milic-Emili J: Mechanics of the diaphragm. *J Appl Physiol* 30: 797, 1971

140. Slingeneyer A, Canaud B, Mourad G et al.: Progressive sclerosing peritonitis, a late and severe complication of maintenance peritoneal dialysis. *Trans Am Soc Artif Intern Organs* 12: 633, 1983

141. Rottenbourg J, Gahl GM, Poignet JL et al.: Severe abdominal complications in patients undergoing continuous ambulatory peritoneal dialysis. *Proc Eur Dial Transpl Assoc* 20: 236, 1983

142. Rottenbourg J, Issad B, Langois P et al.: Loss of ultrafiltration and sclerosing encapsulating peritonitis during CAPD; Evaluation of the potential risk factors. *Perit Dial Bull* 4: 556, 1984

143. Ponce PE, Pierratos A, Izatt S et al.: Comparison of the survival and complications of three permanent peritoneal dialysis catheters. *Perit Dial Bull* 2: 82, 1982

144. Charytan C: Continuous ambulatory peritoneal dialysis after abdominal aortic graft surgery. *Perit Dial Int* 12: 227, 1992

145. Gulanikar AC, Jindal KK, Hirsch DJ: CAPD after aortic graft surgery. *Perit Dial Int* 12: 399, 1992

of patients undergoing continuous ambulatory peritoneal dialysis. *Perit Dial Bull* 3: 138, 1983

QUANTIFICATION AND PRESCRIPTION
GENERAL PRINCIPLES

PETER BLAKE and JOHN DAUGIRDAS

INTRODUCTION

The quantification and prescription of dialysis have received enormous attention in recent years. There has been increasing evidence that higher doses of dialysis are associated with better patient survival and superior clinical outcomes. Measurement of dialytic dose has therefore become almost routine in many centers. It has become apparent, however, that there are many methodological and practical problems associated with both quantification and prescription of both hemodialysis (HD) and peritoneal dialysis (PD). This chapter will review this important subject and related topics in detail.

QUANTIFICATION AND PRESCRIPTION FOR HEMODIALYSIS

In the formative years of hemodialysis, empirically derived treatment protocols evolved, which resulted in most patients being dialyzed for $3 \times$/week, 6–8 hours per dialysis session. As equipment improved and as more efficient dialyzers and higher blood flows became available, average dialysis session length in many countries was shortened to approximately 4 hours. The manufacture of very highly efficient dialyzers and the ability to routinely use blood flows in the 400–500 ml/min range led to even further shortening of the dialysis session length. In the United States, reduced funding for ESRD therapy also generated economic pressure to shorten dialysis time. Concomitantly, patient acceptance of dialysis session lengths greater than 4 hours has declined. In some

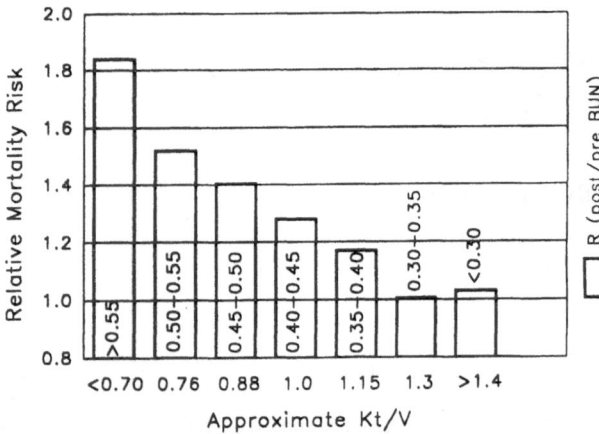

Figure 1. Relationship between the urea reduction ratio (1-post SUN/pre SUN) and case-mix and laboratory-mix adjusted mortality. (Modified with permission from Reference (4).)

instances, short dialysis times have been used in combination with low efficiency dialyzers and relatively low blood flow rates. Thus, today there exists large variation in the dialysis prescriptions being offered to dialysis patients. The minimum amount of dialysis as well as the optimal dialysis regimen continue to be a matter of controversy.

UREA

At present the quantification and prescription of hemodialysis focus on measures of urea removal. Urea is only a 'mild' uremic toxin, in that elevated plasma levels of urea (in the 100–200 mg/dl range) per se cause no demonstrable toxic effects (1, 2). However, urea, MW 60, is a surrogate for other water soluble, poorly protein-bound compounds of similar molecular weight which are hypothesized to accumulate in uremia and have noxious effects (3).

Indices of urea removal

Post/predialysis urea ratio and the urea reduction ratio

The simplest measure of urea removal in hemodialysis patients is the ratio of the postdialysis (Cpost) to the predialysis (Cpre) serum urea level (R), where R = Cpost/Cpre. Variants of this are the urea reduction ratio (URR), which is equal to 1 − R, and the percent reduction in urea (PRU), where PRU = 100 × URR. For example, if the predialysis serum urea nitrogen level (SUN) is 50 mg/dl and the postdialysis SUN is 20, then R will be 0.4, URR will be 0.6, and PRU will be 60. The best data linking simple indices of urea removal to outcome in dialysis patients is that of Owen et al. (4) in a set of approximately 15,000 patients. In that study, case-mix

adjusted mortality rate declined in an exponential fashion as the URR increased up to about 65% (Figure 1).

Urea rebound

When R, URR, or PRU are measured, the first impulse is to equate the numbers with an actual solute removal index; i.e., if the URR is 0.60, one would might assume that dialysis has removed 60% of the urea from the body. In actual fact, a lesser amount of urea has been removed, due to the occurrence of postdialysis urea rebound (5). Despite some early evidence that urea rebound may be due to heightened catabolism (6, 7) it now is generally accepted that increased catabolism plays little role in this phenomenon (8). When the postdialysis blood specimen is taken from the arterial line, urea rebound is caused primarily by three factors, each with its own time constant: access recirculation, cardiopulmonary recirculation, and urea compartmentalization. *Access recirculation*, if present, lowers the dialyzer inflow line urea concentration throughout dialysis due to dilution of arterial line blood with dialyzer outflow venous blood coursing retrograde through the vascular access (9). In patients with access recirculation, as soon as dialysis is stopped, retrograde flow through the access ceases. The urea concentration measured from a sampling port on the inflow blood line increases promptly once the 'dead space' in the line has been cleared of recirculated blood. This usually is done by reducing blood flow to 50 ml/min and running the pump for 15–20 sec (when the dead space volume is about 10 ml). *Cardiopulmonary recirculation* (10, 11) occurs when blood which has just left the dialyzer outlet port returns to the dialyzer inlet port via the heart and lungs without first having traversed a major systemic capillary bed. Cardiopulmonary recirculation occurs only when a dialyzer is being fed from the arterial side of the circulation. When the dialyzer is connected to the patient via a venovenous access, although an arteriovenous gradient is established during dialysis, all blood leaving the dialyzer outlet port must first traverse systemic capillaries before returning to the dialyzer. Thus, with a venovenous access, the dialyzer 'rides' the venous intradialytic urea profile, whereas with an arteriovenous access the dialyzer 'rides' the arterial intradialytic urea profile. As a result, with an arteriovenous access, the efficiency of dialysis is reduced by a factor equal to the ratio of the arterial to venous urea concentrations during dialysis. Prior to dialysis, venous and arterial urea concentrations will be identical. Once dialysis is initiated, return of blood that has been cleared of urea from the access to the heart will cause a rapid stepdown in the arterial urea concentration, which will persist throughout the dialysis session. After dialysis is stopped, the dialyzer no longer returns cleared blood to the heart and the effect of cleared blood on the areriovenous gradient dissipates within 1–2 min (11). In patients with an arteriovenous acess, the mixed venous postdialysis urea concentration can be estimated from a sample obtained from the·dialyzer inlet line 2 min after having slowed the blood flow rate to 50 ml/min. *'Compartment' effects* are due to lack of complete equilibration of urea between blood and tissues during dialysis. Whereas some interpretations suggest that urea sequestration during dialysis is due to delayed removal from intracellular stores (12–15), a regional blood flow model predicts that urea sequestration occurs in tissues that are relatively poorly perfused but which contain substantial amounts of urea, notably muscle, and perhaps also skin (depending on dialysate and ambient temperature), and bone (16, 17). Urea concentration in such tissues is theorized to remain higher than that of mixed venous blood during dialysis. After dialysis has ceased, equilibration between blood and poorly perfused tissues (and perhaps other compartments where urea was sequestered) continues, causing the third phase of postdialysis rebound, lasting 30, sometimes as much as 60, minutes (5, 18). The time courses for rebound due to access recirculation, cardiopulmonary recirculation, and compartment effects are shown in Figure 2. Accordingly, to avoid the effects of access recirculation, one should sample blood about 15–20 sec after slowing the blood flow to 50 ml/min. To avoid the effects of cardiopulmonary recirculation, one should sample 2 min after slowing the blood flow rate to 50 ml/min (11). To avoid compartment effects due to blood flow related or anatomic sequestration of urea, one should sample 30–60 min after the end of dialysis (18). When blood is sampled at 30–60 min after dialysis, the solute removal index and the urea reduction ratio become nearly identical (except for solute removed due to ultrafiltration) (19–21).

Effect of rebound on indices of urea removal

There are two methods of expressing urea rebound: either as a percent of the post-dialysis urea level, or as a percent of the intradialytic fall in urea. For example, if the predialysis SUN is 60 mg/dl, the immediate postdialysis value is 20 mg/dl, and the value 30 min later is 24 mg/dl, the rebound can be (24–20)/20 = 20%, or (24–20)/(60–20) = 10%. The second method is preferred, as the first is highly affected by the actual value of the immediate postdialysis SUN. In the example given, the value for URR would be (1–20/60) = 0.67 based on immediate postdialysis sampling, but URR would be (1–24/60) = 0.60, based on 30 min postdialysis sampling.

Urea rebound is not necessarily a large problem when assessing dialysis adequacy. provided that one waits at least 20 sec after dialysis (depending on the inflow line dead space volume) to sample blood, to obviate the effects of access recirculation which can be quite large. Most studies examining the relationship between indices of urea removal and mortality have used post-dialysis blood specimens taken shortly after the cessation of dialysis. When assessing the adequacy of dialysis in a given patient, it is reasonable to make therapeutic decisions based on URR values taken in the same way as in most published mortal-

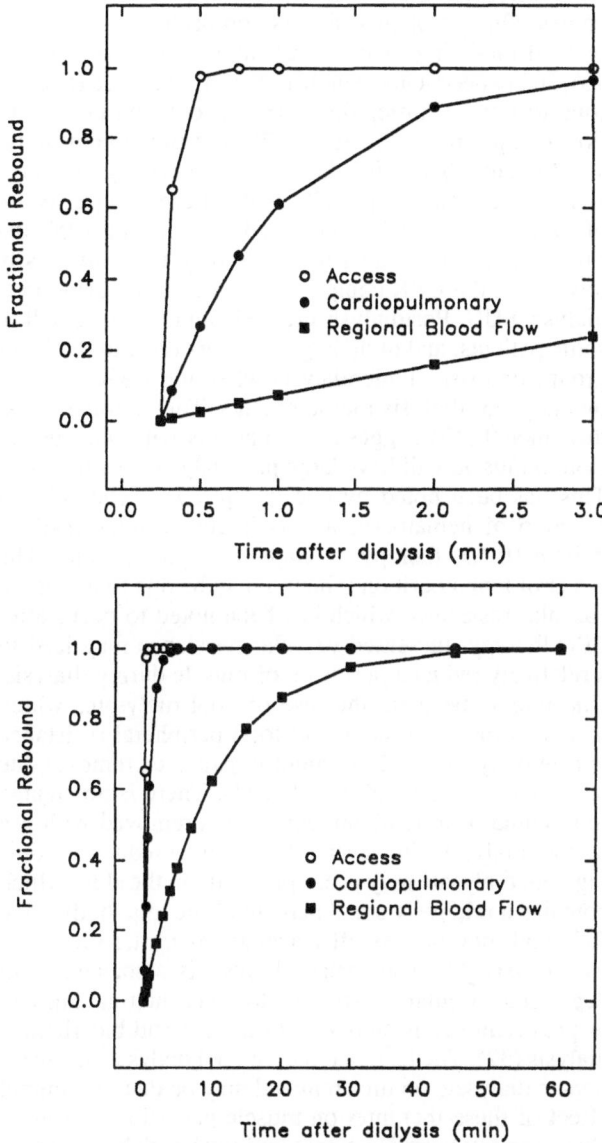

Figure 2. The time courses of the three type of postdialysis urea rebound, shown over a time interval of 0–3 min (Figure 2a) and 0–60 min (Figure 2b). As shown in Figure 2a, in a patient with access recirculation, after showing the blood flow to 50 ml/min, once the dead space in the lines between the tip of the artificial needle and sampling port has been cleared of recirculated blood (this usually takes about 15 sec), the urea concentration at the sampling site should rise promptly. For this reason, when the dead space volume is about 10 ml, and flow is reduced to 50 ml/min, a time delay of about 20 sec is recommended to ensure that postdialysis blood is not contaminated by recirculated blood. The effects of cardiopulmonary recirculation become prominent soon thereafter, and hence sampling should be done within 30 sec of slowing the blood pump in patients with A-V access unless one wishes to obtain a sample reflecting the mixed venous urea concentration post-dialysis. In contrast, the effects of urea sequestration due to compartment and/or regional blood flow effects require 30–60 min to dissipate.

ity studies: i.e., using near-immediate post-dialysis SUN values. One problem with this approach is, that mathematical modeling of urea (see below) predicts (17, 22, 23), and experiments demonstrate (24), that urea rebound (due to either cardiopulmonary recirculation (11) or to flow/compartment effects (17, 22) is a function of dialysis efficiency. Thus, in adult patients receiving high efficiency treatments, especially when those treatments are of short duration (18), and in pediatric patients (25), the true 'equilibrium' value for URR may be substantially lower than the URR computed based on immediate postdialysis SUN. Postdialysis urea rebound may be small in some patients, and quite large in others (26). In the latter group, one risks underdialysis when the URR is based on early postdialysis measurements. The regional blood flow model (17) suggests that patients with poor perfusion to muscle will have large postdialysis urea rebound. This has been noted by one group (27). Rebound is a function of hematocrit, and is increased after erythropoietin (EPO) therapy at 'high' hematocrits (28). The effect of hematocrit on rebound may be due to increased vascular resistance which has been noted to occur after EPO therapy. Increased vascular resistance may lead to a relatively reduced perfusion of muscle during dialysis. One might speculate that use of cool dialysate, which increases blood pressure and total peripheral resistance during dialysis (29, 30), might impair urea removal due to reduction in flow to muscle beds. There is no change in rebound or in total amount of urea removed with use of cool dialysate, however (31), and flow reductions during cool dialysate may occur primarily in the skin, which contains a relatively small percent of the total body urea. Rebound may be less after acetate than after bicarbonate dialysis, because acetate dialysis is associated with decreased vascular resistance. However the total amount of urea removed is similar with acetate and bicarbonate dialysis (32). The lack of effect of cool dialysate or bicarbonate dialysate on urea removal may be due to minimal effect of these therapies on muscle perfusion, despite a change in total cardiac output and total peripheral vascular resistance. Patients with chronically high TPR (i.e., due to congestive heart failure) are at high risk for a high post-dialysis urea rebound (27, 33), as may be patients who suffer frequent hypotensive episodes during dialysis (24).

THE FRACTIONAL REMOVAL OF UREA, Kt/V

Despite the simplicity of measures such as the URR, most published studies of dialysis adequacy have used a slightly more complex measure of urea removal, the Kt/V, where K is the clearance of urea by the dialyzer, t is the dialysis session length, and V is the volume of distribution of urea. This measure of urea removal was popularized by Gotch and Sargent in a reanalysis of the National Coop-

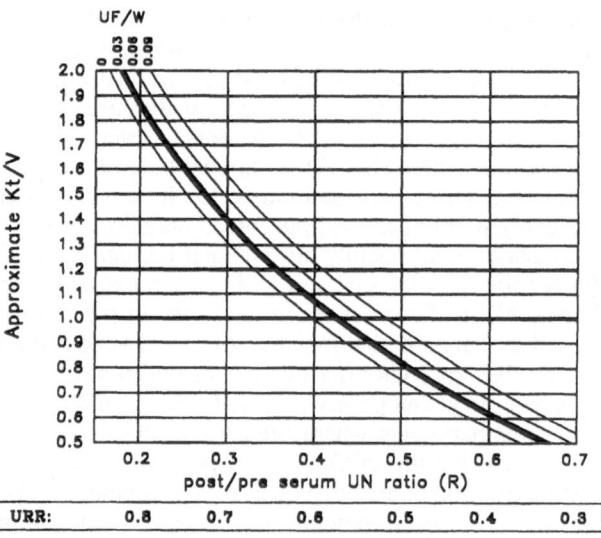

Figure 3. Relationship between R or URR and Kt/V. (Modified with permission from Reference (38).) This nomogram can be used with immediate postdialysis samples (20 sec or 2 min slow flow sampling technique) to extimate single-pool arterial or mixed venous Kt/V, respectively, or with measured or predicted equilibrated post-dialysis SUN values to derive an effective or whole body Kt/V.

erative Dialysis Study (34). The National Cooperative Dialysis Study was the first large prospective randomized trial designed to study the effect of dialysis adequacy on morbidity. The emphasis of the NCDS was to compare the benefits of removal of urea *vs* middle molecules. Morbidity in four groups of dialysis patients were compared. In two groups the dialysis dose was adjusted to achieve a time averaged urea concentration of about 50 mg/dl. One group was dialyzed for an average of about 3.25 hours, and another an average of 4.5 hours. In two other groups the dialysis session lengths were the same, but dialyzer clearances and blood flow rates were altered to keep TAC close to 100 mg/dl (actually about 89 mg/dl). Morbidity was much lower in the two groups dialyzed to a low TAC urea level, and the effect of dialysis session length on morbidity was significant only when hospitalizations were taken into account (35). Gotch and Sargent reanalyzed the data from this study in terms of the fractional urea removal rate, Kt/V, and found that Kt/V values of 0.8 and lower were associated with a markedly increased probability of adverse events (34).

Relationship between Kt/V and the post/pre dialysis SUN ratio, R

To compute the value for Kt/V in the NCDS patients, Gotch and Sargent used a variable volume single-pool urea kinetic model (36, 37). In this model, which is described in detail elsewhere in this volume, the Kt/V is calculated from the ratio of the post/predialysis SUN level, with corrections based on estimated urea generation rate and volume change due to ultrafiltration. A simplified equation showing the link between Kt/V, the post/pre SUN ratio (R), the volume of ultrafiltrate removed (UF), and the postdialysis weight is (38):

$$Kt/V = -\ln(R - 0.008t) + (4 - 3.5R)UF/W.$$

The relationship is graphed in Figure 3 for different amounts of ultrafiltration volume to weight (UF/W). If the urea distribution volume is known, the above formula's accuracy can be further increased by using (0.55)UF/V instead of UF/W for the ultrafiltration term. Other formulas relating Kt/V to R or to the percent urea reduction (PRU) have been proposed (39, 40) but are not as accurate. A recent formula proposed by Garred is generally accurate (41), but overestimates Kt/V when Kt/V is less than 0.9. An even more recent formula proposed by Garred eliminates the overestimation problem at low values of Kt/V and is quite accurate (Garred, personal communication).

Modeled Kt/V and morbidity/mortality

From Figure 3 we see that the critical Kt/V level of 0.8 determined from the NCDS data set corresponds to a urea reduction ratio of 0.50. However, according to data from Owen et al. (4) (Figure 1), the relative mortality risk with a urea reduction ratio of 0.50 is 1.4 times higher than that associated with a urea reduction ratio of 0.70 (which corresponds to a Kt/V of 1.3). Thus, conclusions pertaining to dialysis adequacy reached by the NCDS, which studied short-term morbidity only and which excluded elderly patients and diabetics, cannot be generalized to mortality in the dialysis population of the 1990s. An interesting observation partially reconciling the differences between the minimum dialysis doses suggested by the NCDS (Kt/V > 0.9) (34) and the large study of Owen et al. (Kt/V ≥ 1.2) (4) was made by Collins et al. (42). In a retrospective trial these investigators examined the relationship between dialysis dose and mortality in the context of co-morbidity. In non-diabetic patients with few co-morbid factors, a dialysis dose greater than Kt/V = 1.0 was not associated with further reductions in mortality. In non-diabetic patients with a number of co-morbid factors, mortality continued to decrease until a dialysis dose of Kt/V = 1.2 was reached, and in diabetic patients with co-morbid conditions, mortality did not level off until a Kt/V of 1.4 was attained (42).

Although there have been no randomized prospective studies since the NCDS to address the question of dialysis adequacy, several interesting non-randomized trials have been reported. Such studies suggest that hospitalizations decrease (43), and that nPCR, hematocrit (44), and survival (45) increase, when the Kt/V is raised to 1.3 or higher. Charra et al. reported on a cohort of 445 patients dialyzed to a mean single-pool Kt/V of about 1.8 (46). Patient survival, computed for up to 20 years, was much

improved in all age groups *vs* age-matched US/European patients, and survival was improved in a subgroup of patients receiving a Kt/V of 2.0 *vs* a subgroup receiving a Kt/V of 1.4 (46). The need for a benchmark Kt/V level higher than that proposed by the NCDS is also supported by data from at least three additional groups of investigators (42, 47, 48) and from analysis of large dialysis patient registries in both the United States and in Japan (49, 50). Nevertheless, there continues to be the need for a prospective, randomized study in this area, to more firmly establish the benefits of increasing Kt/V well above 1.2; there is no guarantee in crossover trials that Kt/V assignment was random, and there is also no guarantee in retrospective time control trials that aspects of dialysis other then Kt/V were not changed along with the level of Kt/V.

Whether the beneficial effects of increasing Kt/V level off when Kt/V reaches 1.2 is not known. As noted above, Charra et al. reported superbly low mortality with much higher Kt/V values (46). In the Japanese registry, with mortality not corrected for comorbidity, mortality continues to decrease as Kt/V is increased above 1.5 (49). In a recent analysis of data from the United States Renal Data Systems, Held et al. also found no evidence of a plateau effect at high Kt/V levels (50). Because the relationship between Kt/V and URR is exponential, large increases in Kt/V above 1.5 result in only a small amount of additional urea removal. For example, increasing the Kt/V from 1.5 to 2.0 is associated with an increase in the URR from 73% to only 82%. Thus, if levels of Kt/V above 1.5 do provide additional clinical benefit, it is logical to surmise that the added results may be due to removal of solutes other than those represented by urea, or to some other factor.

Effect of residual renal function on dialysis adequacy

The additional clearance of urea during dialysis due to residual renal function (usually 2–7 ml/min) has little effect on either the URR or the Kt/V. However, the time-averaged effect of residual renal function is important, and, on a weekly basis, can account for a substantial amount of both solute and fluid removal. Mathematical methods have been devised by Gotch to add the residual renal urea clearance to the dialysis session Kt/V (22). The formula proposed (for 3 ×/week dialysis only) is:

$$Kt/V(corrected) = Kt/V + (5.5)Kru/V,$$

where Kru is in ml/min and V is in liters. If V is about 40 liters, 2 ml/min of residual renal function will be equivalent to about (5.5)(2)/40 = 0.27 Kt/V units. If one believes that the delivered Kt/V should be 1.3, in such a patient, one might justifiably reduce the dialysis Kt/V by 0.3, as this amount is being supplied by residual renal function. However, the trend has been to ignore residual renal function in the dialysis prescription, given that residual renal function is time-consuming to measure and may deteriorate rapidly in hemodialysis patients. If dialysis therapy is reduced based on the presence of residual renal function, and then a fall in renal function occurs which is not detected promptly, underdialysis may result. Furthermore, if a reduced dose of dialysis is prescribed initially for patients with substantial residual renal function, the session length will most likely need to be lengthened in the future once residual renal function falls; it is difficult to lengthen the dialysis session once a patient has become accustomed to a particular regimen.

The effect of residual renal function on morbidity/mortality has not been well studied. Theoretically, the contributions of the residual nephron to middle molecule clearance, removal of protein-bound uremic toxins, and maintenance of euvolemia should be very important. Because the rate of fall in residual renal function depends to some extent on the primary renal diagnosis (51), and because primary renal diagnosis is related to mortality (51), the presence of confounding variables in such an analysis is likely.

Post-dialysis urea rebound and Kt/V

The comments applying to urea reduction ratio and urea rebound apply to Kt/V as well. At present, most centers calculate Kt/V from samples immediately after the end of dialysis when an arteriovenous access is being used. Using such a technique fails to correct for effects of access and cardiopulmonary recirculation, and for the third phase rebound believed to be due to regional blood flow/compartment effects. If access recirculation is excluded, the effects of cardiopulmonary recirculation and regional blood flow/compartment effects are to decrease the single-pool arterial Kt/V (defined as that obtained postdialysis 20 sec after slowing the blood pump to 50 ml/min) by about 0.15–0.25 Kt/V units, depending on the efficiency (K/V) of dialysis. Kt/V computed on the basis of an equilibrated (30–60 min postdialysis) SUN sample is really a measure of 'effective' or 'whole body' Kt/V (eKt/V), and correlates very well with the Kt/V derived from dialysis quantification (see below). When a Kt/V of about 1.0–1.2 is delivered over 4 hours, eKt/V will be in the range of 0.95 (23, 24, 31). If a high efficiency dialysis regimen is used, and about 1.6 Kt/V units are given over 4 hours, eKt/V will be about 1.35–1.4. (52). With high efficiency dialysis regimens such that a Kt/V of about 1.4 is given over 2.5–3.0 hours, eKt/V will be about 1.1 (18, 24). In pediatric dialysis patients, and in small adult patients undergoing high efficiency dialysis, eKt/V may be more than 0.25 Kt/V units less than single pool Kt/V (25). In adult patients it is reasonable to allow for a 0.20 Kt/V unit overestimation of Kt/V due to urea rebound (when the postdialysis sample is obtained 20 sec after dialysis). Tattersall and colleagues have proposed one estimate of rebound based on observational data (23). Their recommendation is to calculate Kt/V based on single-pool modeling, and to add 30 min of additional dialysis time. Thus, with a 2-hour dialysis, the added

30 min would provide an additional 25% Kt/V, whereas with 4-hour dialysis, the added 30 min would provide 12.5% additional Kt/V. Recently, a prediction equation for effective Kt/V has been derived based on the regional blood flow urea kinetic model (53). The equation is:

$$eKt/V = Kt/V - 0.6 \times K/V + 0.03,$$

that is, effective Kt/V (eKt/V) is equal to single-pool arterial Kt/V (Kt/V calculated in the usual fashion using 20 sec slow flow postdialysis samples) minus $0.6 \times (K/V) + 0.03$. The K/V value is calculated by dividing the single-pool arterial Kt/V by the number of hours of dialysis. According to the regional blood flow model, this equation will predict effective Kt/V when the cardiac index is 2.8, the access blood flow is 800 ml/min, and the flow fraction to muscle, skin, and bone is 15% of the total cardiac output. For higher levels of cardiac output or flow fractions to muscle, skin, and bone, the slope of the correction equation changes. However, it appears that this relationship will predict effective Kt/V for the great majority of dialysis patients (53). An important confounder is access recirculation. If a slow flow technique is not used to obtain the postdialysis blood sample, the above formula may grossly overestimate the eKt/V in patients with access recirculation, in whom the eKt/V can easily be 0.6 Kt/V units lower than that measured immediately after dialysis!

If Kt/V is computed using 2 min slow flow postdialysis samples, then we are in effect computing a 'mixed venous' single-pool Kt/V. In this case, the amount of postdialysis rebound is reduced by approximately 30%. To compute the eKt/V from the 'mixed venous' single-pool Kt/V, one should first compute the arterial single-pool Kt/V as follows (53):

$$Kt/V \text{ spart} = Kt/V \text{ spven} \div (1 - 0.17/h),$$

where h is the dialysis session length in hours. Then one can use the estimation equation for eKt/V based on the single pool arterial Kt/V described above. Because almost all morbidity (NCDS) and mortality data have been obtained using postdialysis samples obtained soon after the end of dialysis (with at least one notable exception (47)), one should not use such data directly to interpret measurements of eKt/V.

Kt/V vs URR as measures of solute extraction

Statistically, Kt/V and URR are mathematically tightly coupled, to the extent that neither one of these measures is more predictive than the other of dialysis patient mortality (Held PJ, personal communication). Indeed, the NCDS morbidity data were reanalyzed by Lowrie in terms of URR instead of Kt/V, with no loss of predictive power (Lowrie E, personal communication). The principal benefit of following Kt/V is the relatively large amount of data concerning morbidity/mortality that has accumulated using this measure, the ability to compute the normalized

Table 1. Effect of access recirculation, cardiopulmonary recirculation, and regional blood flow 'compartment' effects on the accuracy of the modeled urea distribution volume and delivered Kt/V

'Recirculation'[a]	Time of post-sample	Effect on Kt/V	Effect on V
Access Recirc	0'	Overestimated	Unchanged or decreased
Access Recirc	> 20 sec post	None	Overestimated[c]
CPR[b]	20 sec post	Overestimated	Unchanged or decreased
	2 min post	None	Overestimated[d]
Regional blood	2 min	Overestimated	Unchanged or decreased
flow/compartment	30–60' post	None	Overestimated[e]

[a]Each recirculation effect is assessed singly, as if the others were not present.
[b]No CPR correction required when dialyzer is fed from a venovenous access.
[c]Correct V by multiplying Kd by the ratio of inlet to arterial SUN (assuming that the degree of access recirculation is constant throughout dialysis).
[d]Correct V by multiplying K by the ratio of arterial to venous blood SUN.
[e]No easy correction method; see Reference (54).

protein catabolic rate or nPCR, the ability to rationally plan changes in therapy, and the advantages of serial monitoring of the computed urea distribution volume (V) in a given patient. A sudden change in the calculated value of V can reflect improper postdialysis sampling, laboratory error, development of access recirculation, alteration of expected clearance of the dialyzer, or errors in blood flow or dialysis time.

MONITORING THE UREA DISTRIBUTION VOLUME (V)

Although a detailed discussion of modeling is beyond the scope of this chapter, a simplified analysis is as follows: Kt/V is computed primarily from the ratio of the postdialysis to predialysis SUN ratio corrected for urea generation and ultrafiltration (for example, Figure 3). Once Kt/V is known, K is then estimated or measured and V can be solved for because t is known.

Effect of K and V on Kt/V

For a given post/pre SUN ratio, variations in K or V have only a small effect on Kt/V (a 10% error in K or V will usually cause only a 0.02 Kt/V unit error in Kt/V). The values for K and V will, however, affect one another in tandem. An overestimation of K will result in a proportional overestimation of V, and underestimation of K (which is unusual) will cause underestimation of V.

Effect of rebound on computed values for V

Errors in Kt/V due to postdialysis urea rebound (access, cardiopulmonary, or flow/compartment effects) may not be reflected by errors in V if the postdialysis blood sample is drawn before that particular rebound occurs. For

example, in patients with access recirculation, if the postdialysis blood is sampled immediately postdialysis without clearing the dead space volume from the inlet blood line, the postdialysis SUN will be artefactually low, and the Kt/V will be artefactually high; however, the value for V may be similar to the patient's usual value and to the anthropometric V because, with access recirculation, K also is overestimated (54).

When samples are obtained postdialysis to compute Kt/V by the 2 min slow flow method in patients dialyzed via an arteriovenous access, the effects of cardiopulmonary recirculation need to be accounted for to obtain a proper V. Because effective dialyzer clearance is reduced by a factor equal to the arterial/mixed venous urea concentration during dialysis (the A/V gradient), the estimated K must be multiplied by this factor (usually about 0.95) to arrive at an accurate value for V. Most currently available urea kinetic modeling programs do not automatically make this correction. For a detailed discussion of access and cardiopulmonary recirculation effects on the value for V, see (54).

An appropriate value for V does not guarantee that a particular patient does not have a substantial amount of rebound due to regional blood flow/compartment effects. Again, this is due to offsetting errors in V and Kt/V (54, 55). Thus, in patients with substantial rebound due to regional blood flow/compartment effects, when the postdialysis sample is obtained soon after dialysis, the value for V (single pool V) is close to the patient's true V because of the same offsetting errors in Kt/V and V discussed above for access recirculation. On the other hand, in patients with substantial rebound, whenever postdialysis samples are obtained AFTER rebound has occurred (i.e., 30–60 min postdialysis) to compute an equilibrated Kt/V or eKt/V, if this value is divided by the dialyzer clearance K, the computed value for V will be artefactually increased (11, 54). This is because factors producing urea rebound also proportionately lower the SUN profile during dialysis (25). In this case, the single-pool urea kinetic model estimates the SUN profile from the pre and post SUN concentrations, and under these conditions the true intradialytic SUN profile is markedly overestimated. This causes an overestimation of K. When the Kt/V derived from equilibrated postdialysis SUN samples (or eKt/V) is divided by the artefactually inflated value for K, there is a proportionate overestimation in the value for V (Table 1).

Effect of dialyzer outlet sampling on computed value for V

When blood is mistakenly sampled from the dialyzer outlet line, there will be an artefactual decrease in the post-dialysis SUN by about 70%, because the outlet/inlet SUN concentration ratio is usually about 0.3. This error usually will cause an increase in calculated Kt/V by about 1.2 units. The modeled Kt/V will be 2.2 instead of 1.2, and the computed V will be 100% of body weight instead of about 55% of body weight.

Effect of errors in blood flow, treatment time, and dialyzer performance on V

Errors in blood flow, undocumented shortening of treatment time (or slowing of the blood flow rate), or loss of dialyzer performance due to partial clotting or batch variation will not cause much of an error in the Kt/V, because the latter depends primarily on the post/pre SUN ratio. However, K or t is overestimated, and division of Kt/V by an inflated K or t causes overestimation of V.

ESTIMATING UREA REBOUND FROM UREA INBOUND

The three factors that cause post-dialysis rebound, access recirculation, cardiopulmonary recirculation, and regional blood flow/'compartment' effects also cause a proportional alteration in the intradialytic SUN profile in the arterial blood line, lowering it compared to that expected from an exponential plot connecting the predialysis and the postdialysis values. We have defined the degree of this lowering as intradialytic urea 'inbound'. In the case of access or cardiopulmonary recirculation, the reasons for the lowering of arterial blood line intradialytic SUN profile (urea inbound) are obvious. In the case of regional blood flow/'compartment' effects, urea is being removed during dialysis from a smaller effective compartment; hence, there is a more rapid initial decline in the plasma SUN than predicted. Because it is impractical to routinely have patients wait 30–60 min after dialysis for postdialysis SUN sampling, efforts have been made to predict the amount of rebound from the degree of 'inbound'. The methods of using urea inbound to pre-

dict rebound, first popularized by Smye et al. (25) are beyond the scope of this chapter and are discussed elsewhere in this volume. All of the methods need to make the assumption that the degree of access recirculation, cardiopulmonary recirculation, or 'compartment' effect is constant throughout dialysis, and that the same degree of urea compartmentalization exists after dialysis as during dialysis. Also, because the amount of urea inbound during dialysis is relatively small, it is markedly affected by even slight errors in the measurement of the predialysis and the intradialytic urea concentrations. Perhaps for all of these reasons, preliminary results suggest that urea inbound is not a very accurate predictor of postdialysis urea rebound for a given dialysis treatment (56). In our own hands, the Smye technique works rather well in predicting urea rebound. However, care must be taken in how the blood samples are drawn. In the presence of access recirculation, the degree of urea inbound can underestimate the degree of urea rebound, because the severity of access recirculation often increases during the course of a dialysis session (57). The confounding effect of access recirculation can be avoided by taking both the inbound sample and the postdialysis sample in such a way that both samples are not contaminated with dialyzer outflow blood (e.g., 20 sec slow flow method).

2×/WEEKLY HEMODIALYSIS SCHEDULES

Virtually all studies examining the relationship between dialysis adequacy and morbidity/mortality have focused on patients being dialyzed 3×/week. Obviously patients being dialyzed twice weekly and 3×/weekly using the same level of URR or Kt/V per treatment are receiving vastly different amounts of dialysis. Because of the lack of morbidity/mortality data for 2×/week patients, the only guidelines for prescription for 2×/week patients are theoretical. Based on a mathematical analysis, Gotch has proposed that a Kt/V of about 1.8–2.0 delivered twice weekly is roughly equivalent to a Kt/V of 1.0 delivered 3×/week (22). In most centers, 2×/week dialysis regimens are used only for patients with very substantial amounts of residual renal function or for patients who for some reason will not or cannot be dialyzed 3×/week. The general consensus appears to be, that a 2×/week dialysis regimen should be primarily a transitional strategy for patients with large amounts of residual renal function.

4–7×/WEEKLY HEMODIALYSIS SCHEDULES

The practice of 3×/week dialysis undoubtedly was based on the structure of the American/European workweek. It would make more sense to dialyze patients every other day, but this would require patients being dialyzed on different days of the week on alternate weeks, and also being dialyzed on alternate Sundays. The adequacy of 3×/week dialysis schedules was initially questioned by Twardowski and others, who proposed 4×/week or 5×/week dialysis for patients who required more intensive dialysis (58–61). Buoncristiani and colleagues have championed a daily dialysis schedule (62), and claim both excellent control of biochemical measures, as well as superior control of hypertension. However, a randomized controlled trial comparing 3×/weekly dialysis with more frequent dialysis has not yet been done.

UREA REMOVAL INDICES FOR DIALYSIS IN ACUTE RENAL FAILURE

In acutely uremic patients, relatively short, low-intensity dialysis sessions have been advocated for the first one or two hemodialysis sessions to limit the risk of precipitating disequilibrium syndrome (63, 64). The optimal intensity of subsequent therapy is completely unknown. Many patients with acute renal failure require daily dialysis to assist in fluid removal. Because many such patients have high urea generation rates due to elevated protein catabolism, a rather intensive dialysis regimen is often necessary for adequate control of the serum UN level. Nevertheless, no experimentally validated guidelines for therapy in this situation are available. Continuous forms of dialysis or hemofiltration such as CAVH, CVVH, CAVHD and CVVHD have become increasingly popular in the acute renal failure setting, but controlled trials comparing outcome with intermittent dialysis and continuous modes of therapy are few. In one such randomized trial, no significant difference in survival between continuous and intermittent therapy was found (65).

OTHER MEASURES OF UREA REMOVAL

The URR and Kt/V are measures of urea removal that are grounded in measurement of pre and postdialysis serum concentrations. The confounding effects of intradialytic urea inbound and postdialysis urea rebound have been discussed above. Alternative methods of measuring solute removal involve measuring urea in samples of collected dialysate (20, 66, 67). Dialysate collection allows one to compute accurately the number of grams of urea removed in a given treatment. This information is not particularly useful per se: For example, knowing that one removed 15 g of urea during dialysis by itself says little as to whether that treatment was adequate or not. Removal of 15 g of urea from a small patient with a predialysis SUN of 60 mg/dl has different implications than removal of the same amount from a large patient in whom the predialysis SUN was 120 mg/dl. Ultimately, pre and postdialysis SUN levels must be measured or inferred in order to arrive at some type of solute removal index or Kt/V. One ingenious device samples the urea concentration of the spent dialysate continually during dialysis via a urea sensor attached to the dialysate outlet stream. This allows for measurement of total urea removed. Predialysis SUN is determined by performing isolated ultrafiltration for a 10 minute period at the outset of dialysis. Postdialysis SUN is estimated from an analysis of the dialysate SUN profile over time (68). Another method is to perform intermittent or continuous sampling of the spent dialysate (69, 70), resulting in collection of a representative aliquot, the UN concentration of which can be measured.

Much ado has been made about apparent differences in the urea distribution volumes calculated from blood and dialysate side modeling, implying that there is something inherently erroneous about blood-sided measures of urea solute removal (67). In fact, when one takes all phases of rebound into account, and obtains 'equilibrated' postdialysis SUN samples 30–60 min after dialysis, and when one corrects for the amount of urea in the spent dialysate due to urea generation and to ultrafiltration, including urea generation during the rebound time period, the values for urea distribution volumes derived by blood and dialysate-sided modeling are not significantly different (19–21).

PRACTICAL ISSUES RELATING TO UREA QUANTIFICATION

Achieving the desired URR or Kt/V

Assuming one decides to target a URR of 65–70% (based on a 20 sec or a 2 min postdialysis sample), which is equivalent to a Kt/V of 1.2 to 1.4, it is not a difficult task to select the proper dialyzer and blood flow rate to achieve this goal in most patients. In large male patients the dialysis session length may need to be extended well beyond 4 hours, or else a dual dialyzer system (71) may need to be employed. The first several times that a patient is dialyzed, his or her urea distribution volume V will not be known. V can, however, be estimated from anthropometric equations. Either the Hume–Weyers equations, which do not use the patient's age (72), or the Watson equations (73), which do, can be used. The Hume-Weyers equations are conveniently available as nomograms (74, 75). The next step is to estimate the dialyzer clearance (K), that will be delivered. The expected dialyzer clearance K can be derived from the mass transfer area coefficient KoA of the dialyzer that will be used and the blood flow rate. The mass transfer area coefficient, KoA, which has units of ml/min, is simply the maximum theoretical urea clearance of that dialyzer at infinite blood and dialysate flow rates. Typically, KoA values of dialyzers range from 350 to 1100 ml/min. Dialyzers with KoA values greater than 700 ml/min can be thought of as high efficiency dialyzers and should always be used in larger patients. An argument can be made to use high efficiency dialyzers for all patients, as in this manner one will be providing for the maximum amount of dialysis possible. There is no evidence that high efficiency dialysis is associated with more symptoms than lower efficiency dialysis, provided that bicarbonate dialysate and volumetric ultrafiltration controllers are employed. Some dialyzer companies do not routinely publish KoA values for their products. Lists of KoAs derived from manufacturer-supplied dialyzer specifications are available (76). Alternatively, one can compute the KoA from published *in vitro* urea clearance data that is found in dialyzer specification charts, using either an equation or a nomogram (74, 75).

Once the K_0A of a dialyzer is known, the *in vitro* urea clearance at any blood and dialysate flow rate can be computed using the equation (77, 78):

$$Z = (K_0A/Q_b)(1 - Q_b/Q_d)$$
$$K = Q_b(e^Z - 1)/(e^Z - Q_b/Q_d)$$

Clearance should be corrected for blood water content, and also for blood flow errors due to deformation of the blood tubing at high blood flow rates, particularly when prepump negative pressure is marked (79). Clearance should also be corrected for cardiopulmonary recirculation if the dialyzer is being fed from an arteriovenous access and postdialysis samples equivalent to mixed venous blood (2 min slow flow method) are used. Again, a convenient nomogram has been validated for this purpose (74). The effect of these corrections is to reduce the theoretical value for dialyzer clearance K by about 18% when the cardiopulmonary recirculation correction is included. Once V and K have been estimated, Kt/V is known, and the required dialysis session length t can be solved for algebraically. Using this method to estimate the initial dialysis prescription will give mean values of Kt/V that are not much different from modeled Kt/V values (80). In some patients, the initial prescription will yield Kt/V values substantially different from those predicted. This is because anthropometric estimates of V have a relatively large standard deviations of about 20% (72). After several dialyses where both pre and postdialysis SUNs have been measured, V can be determined algebraically from the estimated K and the Kt/V (see comments about errors in modeled V above, however). Subsequent adjustments to dialysis therapy can be made using this modeled value for V. Of course the same computations are made easily by many commercially available urea kinetic modeling programs.

MONITORING DELIVERED THERAPY

Predialysis and postdialysis SUN values should be monitored monthly. Kt/V can be computed using either simplified equations or using a urea kinetic modeling program. Decisions about whether or not the desired Kt/V is being delivered should be based on the average of several measurements, as there will be a certain amount of variability due to laboratory measurement of SUN and to treatment related factors (dialyzer clearance, blood flow, and session length).

LABORATORY MEASUREMENT OF UREA

There are four techniques in current use to measure urea concentrations. In one method, urea reacts directly with diacetyl monoxime to form a colored product (Fearon reaction). In the other three techniques, urea is first converted to ammonia by reacting it with urease. Ammonia is a charged ion and will increase the conductivity of the reaction mixture. In one urease method the amount of generated ammonia is assessed directly by conductivity measurements. In a second technique, the ammonium reacts with phenol or salicylate to form a blue or green dye (Berthelot reaction). In a third method, widely used in autoanalyzers, the generated ammonia is used to drive the enzymatic conversion of alpha-ketoglutarate to glutamate in a reaction that involves oxidation of NADH to NAD. The concentration of NAD that is generated is assessed by UV spectroscopy, using either an endpoint or a kinetic method (for a review of all of these methods, see (81)). There have been no studies comparing the accuracy of these methods in measuring urea in dialysis patients, and, in particular, whether the change in other plasma constituents accompanying dialysis creates a bias in these methods when measuring pre *vs* postdialysis specimens. We have encountered difficulty in measuring low SUN values (e.g., < 10–15 mg/dl) accurately with an automated machine based on the urease-conductivity method. Also, predialysis SUN values measured by the Berthelot reaction tend to give slightly lower values than those obtained by the urease-conductivity method or the coupled enzyme technique (Daugirdas, unpublished observations).

Although urea is thought to be quite stable in frozen plasma samples, stability over more prolonged frozen storage has not been assessed. In particular, we have seen a fall in the urea concentrations of samples subjected to several freezing/thawing cycles. We have found that dialysate machine drain tubings often are heavily contaminated with urea-splitting micro-organisms. When dialysate samples are collected in a non-sterile fashion, the dialysate urea concentration can quickly diminish on storage, probably due to contamination with such organisms (82). Another problem is encountered when analyzing frozen urea samples. After thawing, there may be layering of the protein and solute components of the specimen. Intense and repeated vortexing, more than one would assume necessary, or ideally repeated inversion of the thawed sample tube, is required to assure proper mixing of previously frozen specimens.

COMPLIANCE ISSUES

In an important subgroup of patients, the delivered Kt/V or URR regularly falls short of the prescribed amount, even after adjustments for urea distribution volume have been made. In general, these patients fall into two categories. In the first, the desired blood flow cannot be maintained because of vascular access dysfunction, because of frequent symptoms, or because of dialysis staff error. Lowering the blood flow without good reason should be avoided. When the patient is being treated by volumetric dialysis machines and bicarbonate dialysate is being used, the blood flow rate need not be lowered as a first line of therapy for hypotension unless hypotension is severe. Rather, lowering the UF rate to zero and administration of volume expanders or hypertonic saline should be sufficient initial therapy in most situations. In the second group of patients, the prescribed therapy is not delivered because of chronic non-compliance. Either the patient arrives habitually late, expecting to end treatment at the previously targeted finish time, or else the patient demands to be removed from the dialysis machine before the required dialysis session length has elapsed. Periodically, such patients often fail to report for a dialysis treatment altogether (83). Sometimes dialysis unit staff cause dialysis session length to be shortened because they take patients off dialysis prematurely to maximize their own convenience. Studies designed to identify and treat causes of such non-compliance are urgently needed.

TIME-AVERAGED UREA CONCENTRATION (TAC-UREA)

The weekly profile of SUN *vs* time in hemodialysis patients has a sawtooth shape. With $3 \times$/week schedules, the highest tooth occurs on Monday or Tuesday with teeth of progressively lesser height prior the midweek and end-week sessions. The time-averaged urea concentration, or TAC-urea, is the height of a rectangle having the same area as the surface created by this sawtooth pattern. A relatively simple method of estimating TAC-urea from the pre and postdialysis SUN and other parameters has been proposed (84); alternatively, TAC-urea is easily derived from most urea kinetic modeling programs.

It is presumed that a number of uremic toxins are nitrogenous, as dietary restriction of protein will improve signs and symptoms of uremia (85). Urea is an especially good surrogate for low molecular weight (and minimally protein-bound) uremic toxins derived from protein catabolism, as the generation rates of both urea and nitrogenous uremic toxins should vary in tandem. High and low serum urea levels should then appropriately mirror high and low serum levels of such uremic toxins. If the toxicity of such compounds is proportional to their plasma concentration, TAC-urea should be an important parameter for dialysis adequacy.

The use of the TAC-urea to monitor dialysis therapy gained popularity after publication of the NCDS, where the TAC-urea was the primary independent variable (35). The NCDS found that therapy targeting a TAC urea of about 50 mg/dl was associated with far less morbidity than therapy achieving a TAC urea of about 90 mg/dl. Based on that study, the concept has been advanced that urea

kinetic modeling should be used to ensure that TAC does not exceed the region of 50 mg/dl. For example, based on the results of the NCDS study, one treatment strategy that was advocated by Gotch and Sargent was to target a Kt/V value of about 1.05, but to increase this Kt/V value in those patients with high predialysis SUN values, in order to keep the TAC-urea close to 50 mg/dl (22). However, the recent trend is to recommend a target Kt/V value of ≥ 1.2 for all patients. Once a baseline Kt/V of ≥ 1.2 is being given, the need to increase Kt/V even further in patients in whom TAC-urea remains high is not documented by experimental evidence. There are patients who do ingest very high protein diets and in whom the predialysis SUN level will be quite high. If such patients are already being dialyzed to a Kt/V of 1.4, dietary counseling to limit protein intake appears to be the most reasonable way of controlling TAC-urea. In a large cross-sectional study by Lowrie, mortality did not increase until the predialysis SUN exceeded 110 mg/dl (in patients being dialyzed to an average Kt/V of about 1.0) (86).

Certainly a low TAC-urea in and of itself does not testify to the adequacy of the dialysis regimen. The TAC-urea is the result of the balance between urea removal and generation. There may well be important uremic toxins the production rates of which are not tied to the protein catabolic rate. The serum urea level would not necessarily reflect serum levels of such toxins, even if removal of such toxins and removal or urea were similar, because the generation rates of these toxins would not be proportional to the urea generation rate. In patients with liver disease or low dietary protein intake, for example, the SUN (expressed as TAC-urea) might underestimate the serum level of such toxins, whereas in hypercatabolic patients or in patients with very high dietary protein intake, the SUN would tend to overestimate the serum levels of such toxins. As further evidence for the lack of usefulness of a low TAC-urea in predicting mortality, we have the study of Lowrie, cited above, where mortality rate was studied in relation to the predialysis SUN (86). Mortality was increased both in those with a predialysis SUN > 110 mg/dl, and in those with predialysis SUN values < 60 mg/dl. Those with low predialysis SUN values most likely had a poor outcome due to poor nutritional status and low protein (and probably also low energy) intake. The cause of poor protein and energy intake is undoubtedly multifactorial, but it is reasonable to provide such patients with a large amount of dialysis, also.

THE UREA GENERATION RATE AND THE NORMALIZED PROTEIN CATABOLIC RATE (nPCR)

Urea as a marker solute has an advantage over other potential marker solutes because the serum level of urea reflects the balance between urea removal and urea generation. Urea production by the liver serves to contain nitrogen generated during catabolism of body proteins and food in a relatively non-toxic form. Although a fixed proportion of nitrogen derived from net protein catabolism is metabolized to compounds other than urea, there is a direct linear relationship between the urea generation rate (g) and the net protein catabolic rate (PCR). The experimentally observed relationship (87) is:

$$g = 0.154 \times PCR - 1.7,$$

where both g and PCR are expressed as g/day. Thus, by following serum levels of urea, *vs* other solutes, one can, through use of kinetic modeling, estimate a patient's net protein catabolic rate. In patients who are not markedly catabolic or anabolic, the net protein catabolic rate, which is the balance between anabolism and catabolism, will correlate closely with the dietary protein intake. Based on balance studies in hemodialysis patients, when protein intake is adjusted for body size, protein intake levels at about 1.1 g/kg/day tend to be associated with non-negative nitrogen balance provided that caloric intake is above 35 kcal/kg/day (63). Thus, following urea as a marker solute, which allows us to compute the urea generation rate (g), gives important nutritional information relating to dietary protein intake in non-catabolic patients.

The NCDS found that a high normalized protein catabolic rate (nPCR), presumably reflective of a high protein intake, was associated with reduced morbidity (34). The findings of the NCDS pertaining to nPCR were supported by the data of Acchiardo et al. (88) showing that morbidity and mortality in dialysis patients were inversely related to nPCR. Preliminary data reported by Dumler et al. suggest that, using a Cox proportional hazard model, a low protein intake (estimated as nPCR) is an important, independent risk factor for survival on hemodialysis (89). The utility of the nPCR as an important marker for dialysis mortality has been questioned, however. In an analysis of mortality in a large dataset, Lowrie and colleagues failed to find that nPCR was an important predictor of mortality once the data were adjusted for URR (90). Moreover, a high nPCR may not always be a sign of good health and a high protein intake, but may be evidence for increased catabolism. For example, it is now widely held that dialysis patients have functional deficiency of insulin-like growth factor activity, and treatment with recombinant human growth hormone lowers the predialysis SUN and the nPCR by either reducing catabolism or enhancing anabolism (91). Moreover, nPCR is rather difficult to measure, as it requires a knowledge of residual renal function and is subject to errors inherent in single-pool modeling (see below).

Instead, Lowrie and colleagues have emphasized the relationship between serum albumin and mortality in dialysis patients. An increase in the mortality rate was found in patients with even minor decreases in the serum albumin level, and mortality rate was lowest when the serum albumin level was 4.0 g/dl or greater (4). In an earlier analysis from the same group, the serum albumin level was the most important predictor of mortality (using a logistic regression model) in a large sample of dialysis patients (90). The predictive value of the serum albumin results for mortality was confirmed by Held et al. in a sample of 3,000 patients from the USRDS data set (92). The relationship between serum albumin level and mortality in dialysis patients is not surprising given that most deaths other than sudden deaths are preceded by a period of wasting illness during which a reduction in protein/caloric intake and perhaps hypercatabolism occur. In many nondialysis patient populations a similar inverse correlation between serum albumin level and subsequent mortality is found (93–96).

There appears to be an interaction between nPCR and Kt/V. When the Kt/V is increased deliberately, an increase in nPCR is observed (97). The presumption is, that once patients are given larger amounts of dialysis, they feel better, perhaps are more active, and ingest more food, and more protein in particular. One group of investigators has alleged that the interaction between Kt/V and nPCR is a mathematical artefact (98), but this view is not widely shared. The relationship between modeled PCR and DPI certainly is present when careful dietary histories are taken (99). In contrast to the weak albeit demonstrable relationship between nPCR and Kt/V, the relationship between the predialysis serum albumin level and Kt/V is more tenuous (90). The extent to which the serum albumin is a general marker of poor health or comorbidity, the extent to which low serum albumin levels can be corrected using intensive nutritional therapy, and the extent to which normalizing low serum albumin levels reduces mortality risk are all areas that require further investigation. Two technical problems to note: (a) serum albumin levels can differ by about 0.5 g/dl, depending on whether the bromcresol green or purple method is used (100), and (b) the serum albumin levels may be artefactually low in some patients with high interdialytic weight gains due to excessive hemodilution (101).

MEASUREMENT OF THE nPCR

Urea kinetic modeling is used to estimate the nPCR, utilizing the relationship between the urea generation rate and the net protein catabolic rate described at the outset of this discussion. In one method, the rise in SUN over the interdialytic interval is used to calculate g, using the urea distribution volume calculated from Kt/V and K during the dialysis session. Residual renal function must also be measured when present, as urea lost in the urine will not otherwise be taken into account. Another method, popularized by Depner (102), but first described by Gotch (103), is to model the sawtooth pattern in SUN for the entire week using a computer, and continuing to generate weeks of urea sawtooths until the serum UN levels stabilize. At steady-state, the predialysis 'points' of the sawtooth will settle at a unique level that depends on the balance between urea removal (Kt/V and residual renal function) and urea generation. If Kt/V and Kru are known, the urea generation rate can be inferred from the level of the predialysis SUN (104). Recent analysis suggests that the corrections for Kru previously advocated need to be modified for accurate prediction of the nPCR (104).

When using modeling methods to estimate urea generation and nPCR, one should keep in mind that dietary intake of both energy and protein fluctuates markedly from day to day. When using the 3-point interdialytic interval method to estimate nPCR, the values obtained are highly dependent on what the patient had to eat during that interdialytic interval. When using the 2-point method, the values depend on the protein intake during the 48 or 72-hour period immediately preceding the predialysis SUN used in the computations. Depner has argued that the 2-point method is less affected by variations in protein intake, as an untypical rise or fall in the SUN will have more effect on a method that is based on the difference of two SUN measurements than on a method which is based on a single SUN value (55, 102). Nevertheless, one should look at the average of a number of modeling sessions when trying to ascertain g or nPCR in a given patient. Both the 3-point and 2-point methods of measuring nPCR will give somewhat inflated results when single-pool modeling is used. In the 3-point method, an artefactually low, unequilibrated postdialysis SUN increases the magnitude of the interdialytic rise in SUN, inflating the estimate of g. In the 2-point method, because Kt/V is overestimated, a higher than actual g is computed to arrive at the observed predialysis SUN. Recently available 2-pool urea modeling programs automatically correct for these errors.

The value of nPCR can be obtained using a simplified approach, using nomograms or equations based on 2-point variable volume single-pool modeling (74, 104). Using one nomogram or equation (38), the Kt/V is obtained from the post/pre SUN, ultrafiltrate volume, and postdialysis weight. A second nomogram or equation (74, 104) is used to estimate nPCR from the Kt/V (to which residual renal function has been added, if present) and the predialysis SUN. Because the height of the predialysis sawtooth points in a given week is different for each treatment, separate nomograms or equations need to be used depending on whether the predialysis specimen being analyzed is obtained prior to a first-of-the-week or a mid-week dialysis. When using the nPCR nomograms or equations (74, 104) in patients receiving high efficiency dialysis, the Kt/V value should ideally be reduced before to correct for rebound. Otherwise nPCR will be overestimated. Effective Kt/V can be computed by the equation described earlier in the chapter. Parenthetically, there are differences in published nomograms to estimate the nPCR. In the midweek nomogram published by Gotch (22), which has been widely disseminated, an underestimation bias of about 8% is present (105). If this nomogram is used, no correction for effective Kt/V is necessary.

MIDDLE MOLECULES

If removal of middle molecules (substances with molecular weights in the range of 350 to 10,000 daltons) is of importance to the control of uremic symptoms, one would expect better results in patients being dialyzed with high-flux membranes and with techniques which favor removal of such substances because of enhanced convective removal such as hemodiafiltration and hemofiltration. A comparison of the vitamin B12 index to measure dialysis adequacy (B12 being a middle molecule with a MW of about 1355) and Kt/V urea was reviewed by Gotch et al., including most published studies as of about 1991 (22). The data suggested that a good outcome depended first and foremost on adequate removal of urea. Treatment regimens with high vitamin B12 indexes did not appear to offer any well documented advantage, and when the vitamin B12 index was high and Kt/V was less than 0.8, outcome appeared to be poor (22). The NCDS, which was designed primarily to assess the role of urea-like solutes *vs* that of middle molecules, came to the same conclusion, i.e., that removal of urea appeared to be the most important predictor of treatment success (35). Although removal of urea-like solutes appears to be of prime importance in assuring adequacy of dialysis, a role for middle molecules or a role for protein-bound uremic toxins cannot be excluded.

EFFECT OF MEMBRANE ON MORBIDITY/MORTALITY

The issue of membrane effects on dialysis adequacy and morbidity/mortality is complex, because the dimension of flux (i.e., removal of high molecular weight solutes) is intermingled with that of biocompatibility. The most popular low-flux membranes in use today, made of unsubstituted cellulose (Cuprophan, cuprammonium rayon, regenerated cellulose, saponified cellulose ester) are associated with a high degree of complement activation and complement fragment release during dialysis, whereas almost all high-flux membranes have very little complement fragment releasing potential. Thus, if treatment with a high-flux *vs* a low-flux membrane is shown to have some beneficial effect on morbidity or survival, the reason may not necessarily be related to better removal of middle molecules by the high-flux membrane; the better result may be related more to biocompatibility issues.

There are at least four mechanisms whereby choice of a dialysis membrane may affect morbidity and mortality. With each mechanism, flux and biocompatibility issues are intertwined. The four mechanisms are: nutritional, infectious/immune, nephrotoxic, and cardiovascular. *Nutritional*: Use of high-flux membranes has been associated with an increased nPCR, which has been interpreted to be due to increased dietary protein intake (106). Low-flux, unsubstituted cellulose membranes have been

632 Peter Blake and John Daugirdas

associated with post-dialysis catabolism in normal volunteers (107). The mechanism for this has been inferred to be biocompatibility, as similar post-dialysis catabolism does not occur with low-flux cellulose acetate membranes (108). *Infectious, immune*: A number of adverse effects on the immune system, including impaired neutrophil phagocytic function and ability to generate superoxide, impaired natural killer cell function and altered thymocyte IL-2 receptor density, have been associated with dialysis using a unsubstituted cellulose membranes (109). *Nephrotoxic*: In rats made acutely uremic using an ischemic renal failure model, injection of complement-activated serum or exposure of blood to unsubstituted cellulose membranes during sham dialysis prolongs the duration of renal failure (110). In humans being treated for acute renal failure, preliminary data suggests that oliguria and mortality are increased when an unsubstituted cellulose membrane is used (111). *Cardiovascular*: Several studies suggest that use of a high-flux membrane is associated with an increased serum HDL concentration and decreased serum triglyceride values (112, 113). Lipid peroxidation, which has been linked to atherosclerosis, may be increased in patients dialyzed with unsubstituted cellulose membranes (114).

There are several non-randomized, retrospective trials of ESRD patients now either published (115, 116) or reported in abstract form (117–120) in which annual mortality rate decreased concomitant with a switch from low-flux, complement-fragment releasing membranes to high-flux membranes with little complement fragment releasing ability. Whether the decreases in mortality in these retrospective trials represents a membrane effect is not clear, as in all of the studies a number of changes were made in dialysis delivery between the two observation periods, and in most of the trials the amount of delivered Kt/V and the use of EPO were different among the two study periods. In contrast, a recently reported prospective, randomized, relatively large (n = 638) Spanish trial found no difference between synthetic and CU membranes on the number of hospitalization days (mortality was not assessed) (121). Two very recent analyses suggest that beneficial effects of synthetic membranes on morbidity and/or mortality may exist, and that they may be due more to biocompatibility than to clearance of middle molecules: In one analysis using information collected by the United States Renal Data Systems, mortality was increased in patients being dialyzed with unsubstituted cellulose membranes compared to those dialyzed with high-flux synthetic membranes (122). The mortality risk with low-flux 'semi-synthetic' membranes (primarily cellulose acetate) was lower than mortality with unsubstituted cellulose membranes and similar to mortality with high-flux membranes. These results suggest that membrane biocompatibility may be a major factor affecting mortality. In another trial, which is an ongoing, randomized comparison of low flux polymethylmethacrylate (PMMA) *vs* unsubstituted cellulose membranes, patients randomized to the low-flux biocompatible synthetic membrane (PMMA) demonstrated increased weight gain compared to those dialyzed with an unsubstituted cellulose membrane (123).

PROTEIN-BOUND UREMIC TOXINS

Whereas a number of protein-bound compounds are removed well by conventional and high-flux hemodialysis, the serum concentration of other, tightly-bound ligands changes little if at all as a result of dialysis (124). Some protein-bound ligands are normally removed from albumin by endothelial cells (125). In patients with normal renal function, presumably a similar mechanism is active in cells lining the capillary network surrounding the renal tubules (126). Some other protein-bound ligands probably are catabolized and disposed of by the renal tubules after being passed into the urine through the glomerular capillary wall along with their carrier low molecular weight proteins.

It has been shown that such protein-bound ligands are removed more efficiently by peritoneal dialysis than by hemodialysis, as a certain amount of protein is lost along with the peritoneal effluent. Indeed, peritoneal effluent has been shown to contain numerous protein-bound ligands which are absent from ultrafiltrates of uremic blood (127). Better removal of protein-bound toxins may be one reason why peritoneal dialysis shows relatively good outcomes despite much poorer control of the serum urea level compared to hemodialysis.

Extracorporeal methods of removing protein-bound ligands from uremic patients are few. The use of activated charcoal in combination with dialysis has been tried by some investigators, with some demonstrable benefits in patients with hyperparathyroidism (128). A new method, being developed primarily for treatment of liver failure or jaundice, involves adding albumin to the dialysate to help remove protein bound toxins from the blood (129). This aspect of dialysis adequacy must be relegated to future study.

LENGTH OF THE DIALYSIS SESSION

The report of extremely good survival in a group of patients treated in Tassin, France with 24 hours/week of dialysis focused attention on the length of the dialysis session as an important factor in dialysis adequacy. What made this data more impressive was, that patients obtained very high survival times despite being treated with acetate dialysate and with cuprophan membranes (46). A number of potential explanations for high survival in this population have been advanced. Initially, it was assumed that patient selection may have accounted partially for the increased survival, but subsequent subgroup analysis refuted this concept (130). Increased removal of large molecular weight uremic toxins, which is primarily a function of membrane surface area and dialysis session length (square meter-hour hypothesis (131)) might be invoked; however, the dialysis membranes used at the center involved had modest B12 clearances. In their initial report, the investigators from this group emphasized the good control of blood pressure in their patients. Recent data in which the effect of 24 hr/week dialysis was evaluated on new patients and transients, it was found that postdialysis dry weight decreased substantially, as did blood pressure and the requirement for anti-hypertensive therapy, after several weeks of 24 hr/week dialysis therapy (130, 132). Ultrasound measurements of inferior vena caval diameter confirmed that, 24 hours after dialysis (to allow complete equilibration) the Tassin patients were relatively less fluid overloaded and had a lower vascular resistance than patients undergoing more standard regimens (133). In contrast to the data from Tassin, when shorter (< 4.5 hour) dialysis session lengths are analyzed, the dialysis session length does not appear to be an independent predictor of mortality (4).

The implications of the Tassin data are great. For example, with new dialysis methods involving two high flux dialyzers connected in series and hemodiafiltration, extremely large clearance of both small molecular weight uremic toxins and larger molecules can be achieved in a very short time (134). Even after rebound, effective Kt/V values for urea in the neighborhood of 1.5 can be delivered over 1.5–3 hours in many patients (71). If, however, according to interpretation of the Tassin data, patients undergoing 3–4 hour dialysis sessions often remain fluid overloaded after dialysis (133), then ultrashort dialysis may not be the best option, and either new strategies of dialysis need to be considered, or additional methods of removing excess salt and water from these patients may need to be developed. There may not, on the other hand, be much of a difference in fluid balance between 2.5 and 4 hour dialysis sessions; a recent report suggests that the incidence of hypertension was similar in patients being dialyzed with a variety of regimens where the session length was between 2.5 and 4 hours (135).

CONTROL OF ACIDOSIS

Because of the acid-ash diet eaten by the overwhelming majority of dialysis patients, some degree of acidosis commonly is present, despite its intermittent neutralization by bicarbonate or acetate absorbed during the hemodialysis session. In patients being dialyzed with 38 mM acetate dialysis solutions, predialysis serum bicarbonate typically is in the range of 16–20 mEq/L, somewhat lower than that (20 mEq/L) in patients being dialyzed using bicarbonate solutions (136). The mortality rate of ESRD patients is increased in patients with moderate acidosis or moderate alkalosis (86). The acid load of the diet is tied to protein intake, and is higher in patients with high protein

intakes. Bicarbonate delivery to the patient is increased with increasing amounts of Kt/V, but bicarbonate delivery from dialysate is impeded when patients require high amounts of ultrafiltration. Thus, patients with high interdialytic weight gains and/or high protein intakes may require higher dialysate bicarbonate concentrations (137). Kinetic modeling programs designed to predict bicarbonate concentrations have been developed (138), but have not been widely tested and are not commonly used. Because acidosis might have adverse effects on bone metabolism (139) and certainly has adverse effects on protein synthesis (140), it is important to keep the predialysis serum HCO_3 level in the range of 20–24 mEq/L. Recently, an increase in the dialysate HCO_3 level from 38–42 mM has been advocated (141), in order to limit the occurrence of predialysis acidosis. A theoretically more attractive approach is to avoid swings in the serum HCO_3 level altogether by administration of sodium bicarbonate or sodium acetate throughout the interidalytic interval.

SUMMARY – HEMODIALYSIS

In summary, the 3×/week dialysis schedule continues to be the most widely used, with dialysis session lengths commonly ranging from 2.5–4 hours in the United States, 4–5 hours in Japan. The possible beneficial effects of longer (8 hr) dialysis sessions reported from one center (46) are unlikely to result in such regimens being used elsewhere due to lack of patient acceptability and the economic structure of center-based hemodialysis. The benefits of short dialysis sessions being given 4–7×/week are again being considered, but may be practical only in a home dialysis setting.

Although removal of middle molecules and protein-bound substances is undoubtedly of some importance, evidence from the only prospective randomized trial, and evidence from an increasing number of cross-sectional studies, suggest that the extent of urea removal during a representative dialysis treatment (in a 3×/week schedule) is highly correlated with both morbidity and survival. When urea removal is assessed from samples taken shortly after dialysis, a urea reduction ratio of 0.65 to 0.70, corresponding to a Kt/V of 1.2–1.4, is a reasonable target urea removal value. Even higher fractional urea removal values may be of benefit, although this is a matter for further study. Because the amount of urea rebound with dialysis regimens commonly used in the United States translates into approximately a 0.20 Kt/V unit reduction in effective Kt/V value, the target equilibrated Kt/V value (derived from urea samples taken predialysis and 30–60 min after dialysis) should be in the range of 1.0–1.2. One alternative to obtaining equilibrated postdialysis blood samples is to estimate the amount of rebound and effective Kt/V from an intradialytic sample obtained about 1/3 of the way into dialysis (25, 56, 142). Another is to use a prediction equation based on a regional blood flow model of urea kinetics and population-derived hemodynamic indices of perfusion (53).

We believe that monitoring TAC-urea concentrations in patients being dialyzed according to the above specifications is of secondary importance, although the amount of dialysis being given may need to be increased above even 1.2–1.4 Kt/V units in patients who are ingesting very large amounts of protein, to prevent TAC-urea from substantially exceeding 50 mg/dl. Computation of the protein catabolic rate may be of some usefulness, as is it an indirect measure of protein intake in stable patients, although the serum albumin level may be a more appropriate nutritional marker to follow if the desire is to predict future morbidity or mortality. Control of hypertension and prevention of covert fluid overload is an important feature of an adequate dialysis prescription, as hypertension and presence of left ventricular hypertrophy impact adversely on the survival (132, 143, 144). Control of hypertension may be superior in patients undergoing ultralong dialysis sessions. Control of acidosis by provision of adequate levels of base during dialysis and possibly, during the interdialytic interval, is also an important feature of adequate dialysis therapy.

QUANTIFICATION AND PRESCRIPTION OF PERITONEAL DIALYSIS

Background

With the worldwide increase in use of PD, and especially of continuous ambulatory peritoneal dialysis (CAPD), in the 1980s, it was inevitable that the principles of dialytic quantification and prescription learned from the NCDS (145) and other HD studies would be applied to PD. As early as 1978, Boen had defined a PD index based on creatinine clearance (146), but it was not until Teehan, in a seminal paper published in 1985, described a Dialysis Index based on urea kinetics that the debate on adequacy of dialysis in PD began in earnest (147).

Teehan's Dialysis Index was based on the concept that an appropriate target in CAPD was a SUN of 25 mmol/l (70 mg/dl), in association with a protein intake of 1.2 g/kg/d. The choice of the latter was based on nitrogen (N) balance studies done by Blumenkrantz et al. (148) showing that this intake was required to achieve positive N balance in most patients but the choice of the former was somewhat arbitrary, being based on clinical impression. When applied in practice, it became apparent that few patients without residual function could achieve the target Dialysis Index of 1.0.

Teehan's Dialysis Index was soon displaced by Kt/V urea as the most popular index of dialytic dose, principally because Kt/V was familiar to the dialysis community and facilitated comparison with HD. Indeed, with the latter point in mind, Kt/V was initially expressed as a weekly value divided by 3, but this was somewhat contrived

and, more recently, it has been expressed as a weekly or daily value (147–151). The problem with Kt/V in CAPD became apparent when values were compared to those achieved with HD and found to be 30–50% lower in spite of the numerous comparative studies showing similar mortality and morbidity rates for the two dialytic modalities. Keshaviah attempted to resolve this paradox with his 'peak concentration hypothesis' which proposed that peak rather than time averaged urea levels determined uremic toxicity so that a Kt/V of 2.0/week in CAPD corresponded to 3.0/week in HD (152).

During the early 1990s the first studies attempting to validate Kt/V and other measures of dialytic dose in CAPD by seeking correlations with patient outcomes appeared (153–158). Results have been variable and controversial so that there is still no clear consensus as to what are appropriate targets. Much has been learned from these studies, however, and larger prospective trials are now underway to seek more definitive conclusions.

Clearly, no model or yardstick for measuring dialytic dose should be accepted unless it is convincingly validated by clinical studies showing an ability to predict important patient outcomes such as death, hospitalisation or quality of life. The ability of any single yardstick to achieve this will likely be limited by the fact that uremia is a syndrome mediated not by a single toxin but rather by excesses and deficiencies of multiple substances, many of which may be uncharacterized. Also, much of the morbidity and mortality that occurs in dialysis patients is related to vascular disease and to access problems and it is unclear how much these can be influenced by dialytic therapy *per se*.

MEASUREMENT OF UREA KINETIC INDICES IN PD

Just as in HD, there are measurement problems with Kt/V in PD. The Kt component is easily calculated as collecting dialysate and urine for measurement of urea content is simpler in PD than in HD. The urea content of a 24 hour collection of dialysate and urine is divided by the blood urea concentration, which is of course relatively constant, to give a daily Kt (Table 2). Strictly speaking, the blood urea should first be corrected for plasma water by dividing by 0.93 but this is not done in practice. An even simpler method of estimating Kt is to measure the renal component as above but to consider the daily dialysate Kt as exactly equal to the daily drain volume. This method presumes full equilibration for urea between blood and dialysate which is a reasonable approximation for most, but not all, patients. Blake et al. have shown that this method leads, on average, to a 4.3% overestimate of peritoneal Kt but, in individual patients, the error may be much greater so that direct urea quantification is preferable (159).

An important technical point is that the increasing use of peritoneal dialysis fluid administration sets based on

Table 2. Formulae for calculation of Kt/V and dialysis index

$$\text{Kt [daily]} = \frac{\text{(Dialysate urea) (DDDV)}}{\text{Blood urea}} + \frac{\text{(Urinary urea) (Daily urine volume)}}{\text{Blood urea}}$$

$$\text{DDDV} = \text{Daily Dialysate Drain Volume}$$

V Watson

$$= 2.447 - 0.09516\,A + 0.1704\,H + 0.3362\,W \qquad \text{[in males]}$$

$$= -2.097 + 0.1069\,H + 0.02466\,W \qquad \text{[in females]}$$

V Hume Weyers

$$= 0.194786\,H + 0.296785\,W - 14.012934 \qquad \text{[in males]}$$

$$= 0.344547\,H + 0.193809\,W - 35.270121 \qquad \text{[in females]}$$

$$A = \text{Age [years]}$$
$$H = \text{Height [cms]}$$
$$W = \text{Weight [kg]}$$

$$\textit{DIALYSIS INDEX} = \frac{\textit{Actual DDDV}}{\textit{Required DDDV}}$$

$$\textit{Required DDDV (litres)} = 0.23\,(IBW) - (2.6 + 1.44\,Kr)$$

$$\text{IBW} = \text{target weight [kg] for that patient}$$
$$\text{Kr} = \text{Residual renal urea clearance [ml/min]}$$
$$\text{DDDV} = \text{Daily dialysate drain volume [litres]}$$

---

the 'flush before fill' principle can lead to inaccuracies in measurement of dialysate Kt. The flush volume, which should be less than 100 ml, may be much greater in some patients and goes directly into the drain bag so that the patient receives less dialysis fluid volume than prescribed and the drain volume appears greater than it actually is. Direct measurement of dialysate urea content will of course still give an accurate Kt value but estimates based on presumption of full urea equilibration will be particularly unreliable and dialysate to plasma urea concentration ratios will be misleadingly low.

The measurement of V in CAPD is problematic, especially because back calculation using urea kinetic modeling, as is done in HD, is not possible. Early studies used fixed fractions of actual body weight such as 50–55% for females and 58–60% for males to estimate V, but these are obviously crude approximations. This is especially so because body fat tends to increase, relative to other tissue components, with time on CAPD (160). Nomograms such as those of Watson and Hume-Weyers, using height, weight, age and sex, have been used to estimate V (72, 73). The Watson V is on average 5% lower than the fixed fraction V and the discrepancy increases with time on CAPD (159). These nomograms have however been derived from normal people and are not validated for dialysis patients. Keshaviah has recently reported that, in HD, V by Watson is 10% greater than V by kinetic modeling (161) and it is likely that the overestimation is even greater

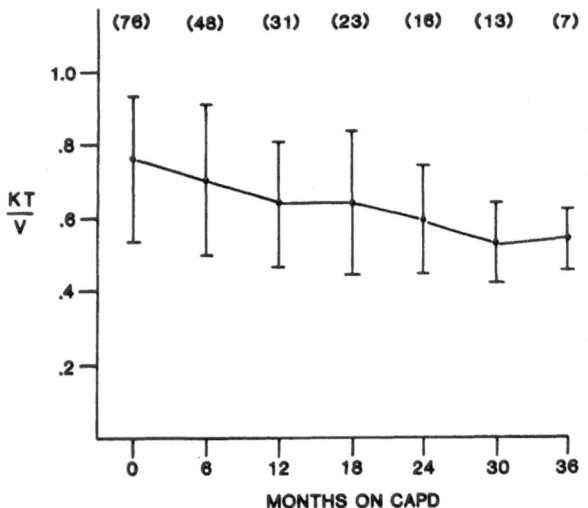

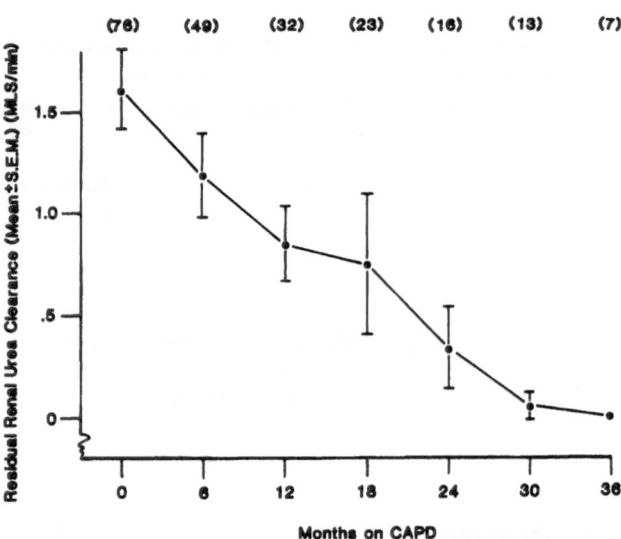

Figure 4. Changes in Kt/V with time on CAPD. Figures in brackets show number of patients at each six month interval. Points and bars represent mean values and standard deviations. With permission from Reference (154).

Figure 5. Change in residual renal function with time on CAPD. Figures in brackets show number of patients at each six month interval. Points and bars represent mean values and errors of the mean. With permission from Reference (154).

in PD because of the higher proportion of body fat. Obviously, overestimation of V leads to underestimation of Kt/V. Methods based on bioelectric impedance (162) or antipyrine dilution (163) have not been validated and, at present, the Watson nomogram is preferred.

It has been suggested that estimates of peritoneal Kt/V in CAPD can be extrapolated from measurements derived from one standardized 4 hour dwell (164). The theory is that, if the degree of urea, or creatinine, equilibration after 4 hours is known, then that after longer periods can be predicted and a total clearance value can be deduced. Burkart has, however, shown that clearance values extrapolated in this way differ substantially from actual measured values in at least 50% of patients and these abbreviated methods are therefore not reliable (165). This discrepancy likely relates to changes in effective peritoneal surface area and permeability with activity, posture, drugs, alterations in blood flow and other factors.

Typical values for the peritoneal component of Kt/V on standard CAPD regimens are 1.3 to 1.8 per week (0.18 to 0.25 per day) and are obviously very dependent on V and, therefore, on body weight (154, 158). Kt/V values are difficult to alter in individual patients because of the relative inflexibility of CAPD schedules. The residual renal component is much more variable, averaging about 20% of the total Kt/V in patients starting CAPD and usually falling to zero over about 2 years (153, 154, 157). Clearly, most variation in Kt/V values between patients is related to residual function and this is important to consider when evaluating clinical studies in this area.

Kt/V falls with time on CAPD and this relates mainly to declining residual function but also to the tendency for body weight, and hence V, to increase and for ultrafil-

tration (UF) volumes to decrease, in many patients (154, 158) (Figures 4 and 5).

Teehan's Dialysis Index is also based on urea kinetics but is now probably only of historical interest (147). It represents a ratio between the actual daily dialysate drainage volume and the volume that would be required to maintain that patient's blood urea nitrogen at 25 mmol/l (70 mg/dl) if the protein intake was an ideal 1.2 g/kg/day. The formula used to calculate the required volume takes into account residual function and body weight and presumes full urea equilibration (see Table 2).

MEASUREMENT OF nPCR

As in HD, urea kinetic modeling allows the normalized protein catabolic rate (nPCR) to be calculated in PD. In the stable patient, nPCR is thought to reflect dietary DPI. Different formulae, some of which have been adapted from HD, have been used to measure nPCR (Table 3). An important point to emphasize is that protein and other non-urea N losses are a greater proportion of total N losses in PD than in HD (148, 166). These extra losses in PD include obligatory dialysate protein losses which are very variable but average about 8 g daily. They also include non-protein, non-urea, N losses which are about 20 mg/kg/day greater in PD than in non-dialyzed uremic patients. This difference is mainly accounted for by dialysate losses of amino acids and of other uncharacterized nitrogenous compounds and is equivalent to 6 to 10 g of additional protein losses daily (166). Also, according to calculations by Bergstrom et al., PD patients appear

Table 3. Formulae for calculations of protein catabolic rate (PCR) or protein equivalent of nitrogen appearance (PNA)

$$G \text{ [urea N appearance rate]} = \frac{\text{[Dialysate urea] [DDDV]} + \text{[urine urea] [daily urine volume]}}{1440} \text{ [mg/min]}$$

                       DDDV =   **daily dialysate drain volume**

PCR [Randerson]   =   *10.76 [G + 1.46]*
[g/day]

PCR [Modified Borah]   =   *9.35 G + .294 V + daily dialysate protein losses [grams]*
[g/day]   **V = volume of urea distribution in litres**

PCR [Teehan]   =   *6.25 [daily dialysate and urine urea content (grams) +*
[g/day]   *1.81 + .031 BW]*
                           BW = body weight in kg

PCR [Modified Teehan]   =   *6.25 [daily dialysate + urine urea content (grams) + 0.5 + .031 BW]*
[g/day]   *+ daily dialysate and urine protein losses (grams)*

PCR [Kjelldahl]   =   *6.25 [total daily N losses (directly measured) in dialysate*
[g/day]   *and urine]*

PROTEIN NITROGEN APPEARANCE [PNA]:

PNA   =   *19 + 7.62 [daily dialysate + urine urea content (grams)]*
[g/day]
                    or

PNA   =   *13 + 7.31 [daily dialysate + urine urea content (grams)] + daily*
[g/day]   *dialysate and urine protein losses (grams)*

NORMALIZED PCR [or PNA]   = $\dfrac{\textit{PCR [or PNA]}}{\textit{Actual body weight [kg]}}$

           or $\dfrac{\textit{PCR [or PNA]}}{\textit{1.72 V Watson}}$ *or* $\dfrac{\textit{PCR [or PNA]}}{\textit{Normal body weight [kg]}}$

         Actual body weight   =   **Patient's edema-free body weight**
         V Watson   =   **Total body water by Watson's formula**
         Normal body weight   =   **appropriate weight for that patient from NHANES**
                                  tables

---

to have unmeasured N losses, via the lungs, the skin and other routes, equivalent to as much as 9 g of protein daily (166). This is thought to be greater than in HD patients and may relate to the higher time averaged blood urea levels in those on PD. Formulae for estimating PCR that do not take these extra losses into account will underestimate protein intake in PD relative to HD patients.

The Randerson and Borah methods of measuring PCR involve estimating the urea generation rate (g) from dialysate and urinary urea content in a given period (167, 168). Both then apply formulae derived from clinical studies showing a linear relationship between g and estimated DPI (Table 3). In Randerson's formula this relationship was derived from HD and confirmed in CAPD patients but, in only taking g into account, it does not allow for

the substantial interpatient variation that exists in protein and other non-urea N losses (167). The Borah formula was originally derived from HD but has been modified for CAPD in that it requires dialysate protein losses to be measured and added. It does not take into account other non-urea N losses however (167). Teehan's method is based on measuring urea removed by dialysate and urine and then adding an estimate for protein and other non-urea N losses (Table 3) (147). This formula again does not allow for interpatient variability in non-urea N losses but a widely used modified version does incorporate an actual measurement of protein losses. The Kjelldahl method directly measures actual N losses in dialysate and urine and is theoretically more accurate but does not include losses by other routes and is not widely available in clin-

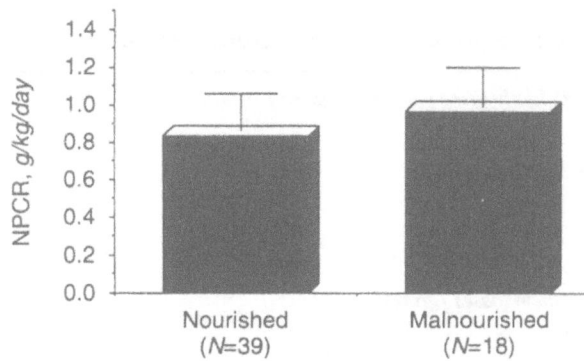

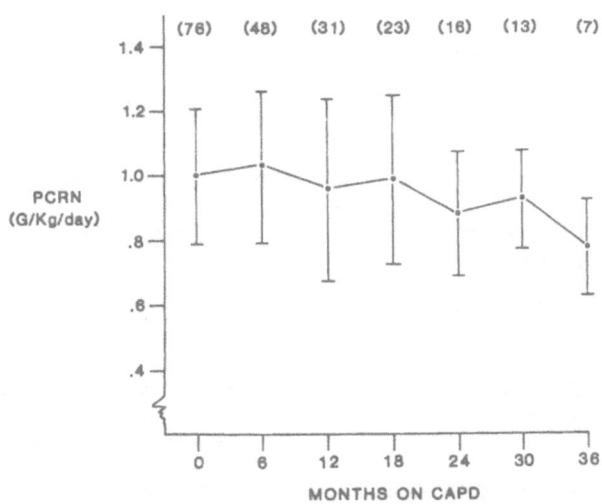

Figure 6. Comparison of mean NPCR values between values between nourished and severely malnourished groups in patients receiving a homogeneous 4 × 2 litre dialysis prescription. $P = 0.0007$. With permission from Reference (171).

Figure 7. Change in PCRN with time on CAPD. Figures in brackets show number of patients at each six month interval. Mean values and standard deviations are represented by points and bars. With permission from Reference (154).

ical laboratories (169). A recent study comparing these methods showed that all gave reasonably similar values for PCR with about 8% difference between the lowest (Borah) and highest (Kjelldahl) estimates (170). There is, of course, no gold standard for comparison but all formulae gave average results similar to the average DPI based on three day diet histories. The correlation between PCR and DPI in this study was under 0.6, however, and there were significant discrepancies in both directions in many patients.

The replacement of the term PCR by protein nitrogen appearance (PNA) has recently been proposed and Bergstrom has developed new formulae to calculate this PNA (166) (Table 3). These are the first formulae relating total N appearance and PCR (PNA) to urea appearance that have been independently derived from CAPD patients and they may eventually become standards. As already noted, Bergstrom states that, because of N losses unmeasured in balance studies, even these formulae may underestimate true protein intake by about 9 g daily (166).

The use of PCR as an index of DPI can be a problem for other reasons. It assumes that the patient is in steady state but this is often not the case and intercurrent illnesses can, therefore, give misleading impressions of DPI. nPCR has also been criticized because it entails normalization to actual body weight. Harty et al. have shown that nPCR is actually higher in malnourished than in well nourished CAPD patients, presumably because weight has fallen faster than protein intake in the former group (171) (Figure 6). To avoid this absurdity, they suggest that PCR should either be left uncorrected or, alternatively, be normalized to ideal or 'normal' body weight obtained from the National Health and Nutrition Evaluation Survey (NHANES) tables. These tables give the median body weights of normal Americans of the same age, sex, height and frame as the patient and are regularly updated. An alternative approach is to use an estimate of obesity-free or standardized body weight for normalization. V is cal-

culated using the Watson nomogram and multiplied by 1.72 (1/0.58) on the presumption that it is 58% of obesity free body weight (159, 171). Given that CAPD patients often have increased body fat, this normalization leads to higher nPCR values than when actual body weight is used. There is obviously a need to standardize the measurement of PCR and its normalization in CAPD.

If normalization is to actual body weight, typical values for nPCR in CAPD patients are 0.7 to 1.1 g/kg/day with only a small minority achieving the recommended 1.2 g/kg/day (153, 158). Some studies suggest that nPCR falls with time on CAPD (154) (Figure 7). If normalization is to obesity-free or standardized body weight, nPCR is 7% higher on average and the discrepancy increases with time, presumably due to increasing body fat (159).

PARADOXES OF UREA KINETICS IN PD

It will now be apparent that there are two major paradoxes when standard urea kinetics are applied to CAPD. Firstly, Kt/V values are 30–50% lower than those for HD. Secondly, nPCR values are 10–20% lower than in HD and 20–40% lower than the target recommended to achieve N balance. Despite this, no differences in mortality and morbidity have been shown in numerous studies and registry reports comparing the two modalities (172–177). Attempts to resolve these paradoxes have been central to the debate on urea kinetics in CAPD.

Keshaviah's 'peak concentration hypothesis' was formulated to address the first of these paradoxes (152). Basically, this states that peak rather than time averaged urea levels determine uremic toxicity and that therefore it is more appropriate to compare the pre-dialysis BUN

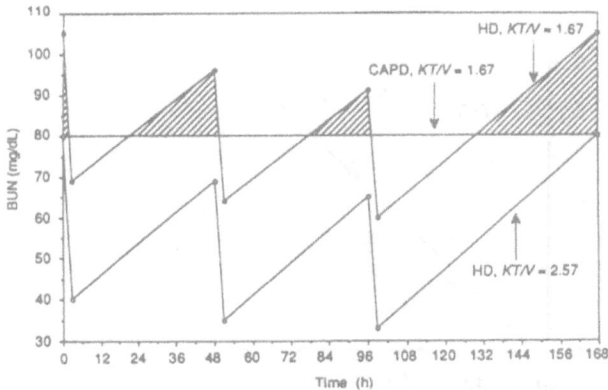

Figure 8. Weekly BUN profiles for hemodialysis and CAPD. At the same Kt/V of 1.67, the TAC$_{urea}$ for hemodialysis and the steady-state BUN for CAPD are almost identical. However, because of the intermittent nature of hemodialysis, BUN levels on hemodialysis exceed the CAPD level for 88 out of 168 h in the week. Reprinted from Keshaviah PR, Nolph KD, Van Stone JC: The peak concentration hypothesis: A urea kinetic approach to comparing the adequacy of continuous ambulatory peritoneal dialysis (CAPD) and hemodialysis, ©(1989), 257–260, with kind permission from Elsevier Science Ltd, The Boulevard, Langford Lane, Kidlington OX5 1GB, UK.

in HD with the constant BUN in CAPD (Figure 8). By this hypothesis, a Kt/V on HD of 3.0/week is equivalent to about 2.0/week in CAPD. Depner has recently argued that the inherent inefficiencies, in terms of solute removal and compartment disequilibria, of any form of clearance delivered intermittently, as distinct from continuously, are sufficient to explain the discrepancies between the required Kt/V in HD and CAPD and that it is not, therefore, necessary to invoke the 'peak concentration hypothesis' (178).

A related argument is that the generally more stable metabolic and biochemical milieu in CAPD compensates for the inferior urea clearances. In particular, stable hydration status may be more favorable from a cardiovascular point of view than the swings from volume expansion to depletion that occur in HD. Another factor favouring CAPD is the better preservation of residual function that has been demonstrated in a number of studies (179, 180). This may relate to the more stable volume status and lower protein intake in PD and to the apparently nephrotoxic effects of the blood hemodialyzer interaction in HD (149). Residual function is important, not just because it gives extra Kt/V but, also, because it adds disproportionately to larger molecule clearance and because it may be associated with better maintenance of non-solute clearance related renal functions. It has also been argued that CAPD may compensate for its inferior clearances of small molecules with its superior clearance of so called middle and larger molecules and of possible protein-bound uremic toxins. The clinical significance of this is difficult to resolve without identification of uremic toxins in that molecular

weight range. One candidate is beta-2 microglobulin and there is a suggestion that dialysis amyloidosis is less common in PD (181). It has recently been pointed out that, in contrast to conventional cellulosic membranes, modern high flux dialyzers have large molecule clearances that are superior even to PD, so complicating this argument further (182). Finally, some of the Kt/V paradox may be explained by the relative overestimates of V in CAPD compared to HD, as discussed above.

The nPCR paradox has also led to speculation, particularly in view of the belief that CAPD patients require more and not less protein than those on HD (148). Again, as reviewed above, nPCR in CAPD may be underestimated relative to HD, both because of the normalization process and because of the greater non-urea N losses. At least three other factors may account for lower, rather than higher, protein requirements in CAPD relative to HD. Firstly, Mitch and others have shown that acidosis has a direct catabolic effect in uremia (183). Significant acidosis is uncommon in CAPD and so may reduce protein requirements. Secondly, HD with its membrane induced activation of complement and cytokines, is itself catabolic in a way that PD is not (184). Thirdly, the obligatory glucose absorption in PD often leads to patients having a greater total energy intake than those on HD and work by Bergstrom and others has shown that energy intake has a protein sparing effect and is actually more predictive of N balance than protein intake in long-term PD patients (166) (Figure 9). Finally, as pointed out earlier, estimates of nPCR in HD are often based upon single-pool modeling and so are falsely inflated.

The validity of Blumenkrantz et al.'s original suggestion that CAPD patients may require 1.2 g/kg/day to achieve N balance has also been questioned (148). This work was based on young, middle aged males and may not be valid for older, less active patients. Indeed, Lindholm et al. have now shown that some CAPD patients achieve N balance at protein intakes as low as 0.7 g/kg/day (185). It is not clear if achieving balance is the endpoint that matters or whether the level of intake at which it is achieved is also important.

In summary, some progress has been made on resolving the paradoxes of urea kinetics in CAPD but it has to be pointed out that many of the proposed explanations represent intriguing but unvalidated speculations. The possibility that the whole urea kinetic model is simply not as helpful in CAPD as in HD has to be entertained. Indeed the protean nature of the uremic syndrome makes it unlikely that morbidity will be accounted for by disturbances in clearance of one solute only.

CLINICAL OUTCOME STUDIES AND UREA KINETICS IN CAPD

For urea kinetic indices to be validated as clinically useful in CAPD, they must be shown to be predictive of impor-

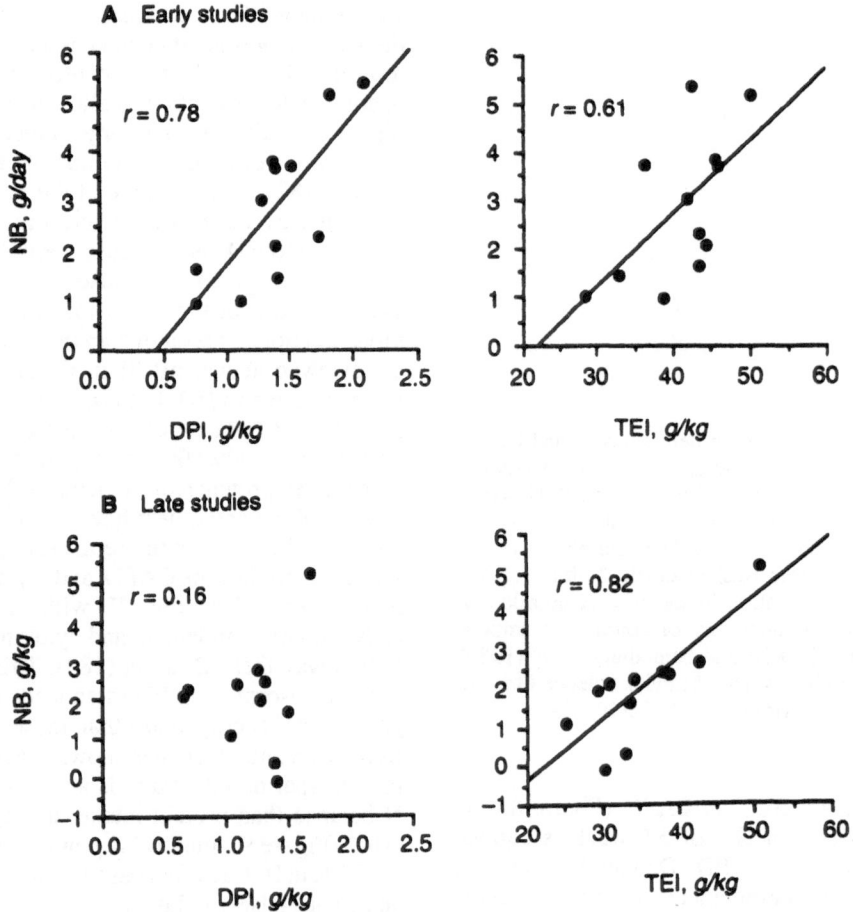

Figure 9. Relationships between nitrogen balance (NB) not corrected for 'unmeasured' nitrogen losses and dietary protein intake (DPI) and total energy intake (TEI) during the early and late studies. With permission from Reference (166).

tant patient outcomes. There has, as yet, been no randomized study analogous to the NCDS in HD to resolve this issue. There have, however, been a number of clinical studies yielding conflicting results, some of which may be explained by the logistic problems involved in long term follow up of urea kinetic indices in CAPD (186).

The methodological issues in measuring Kt/V and nPCR have already been discussed. Patient drop out and adequate duration of follow up are also problems in a modality where patient retention at 2 years is typically less than 40%. The fact that residual function is so significant and is constantly changing makes randomization to distinct Kt/V regimens difficult and means that any analysis has to take into account that Kt/V is itself a 'moving target'. There is also the associated concern that differences in Kt/V primarily represent differences in body weight and residual function, rather than in actual dialytic dose, and that only a tightly controlled, randomized study can separate out these factors. Morbidity in CAPD is also problematic in that much of it is access related and might not be expected to be dependent on dialytic dose (186).

All of the existing studies are imperfect. Some are cross-sectional or have only short follow up while others use relatively 'soft' end points. The best evidence for urea kinetics comes from Teehan's work which shows superior survival after 3 years for patients with an average Kt/V over 1.89/week but, due to drop out, the numbers after 3 years are small and Kt/V is a less powerful predictor than serum albumin (153, 186) (Figure 10). Selgas et al. report similar findings but only studied patients on CAPD for more than 3 years (150). Lameire et al., in a select group of patients on CAPD for 5 years, also found hospitalisation and, surprisingly, peritonitis to be inversely proportional to Kt/V (158). Blake et al. found no correlations between Kt/V and morbidity but did detect excess mortality when Kt/V was less than 1.5/week (154, 159). With regard to nPCR, there is no good evidence of an association with mortality and only weak evidence for an association with hospitalisation (153). Two recent studies, interestingly, have found no correlation between nPCR and other nutritional indices (171, 188).

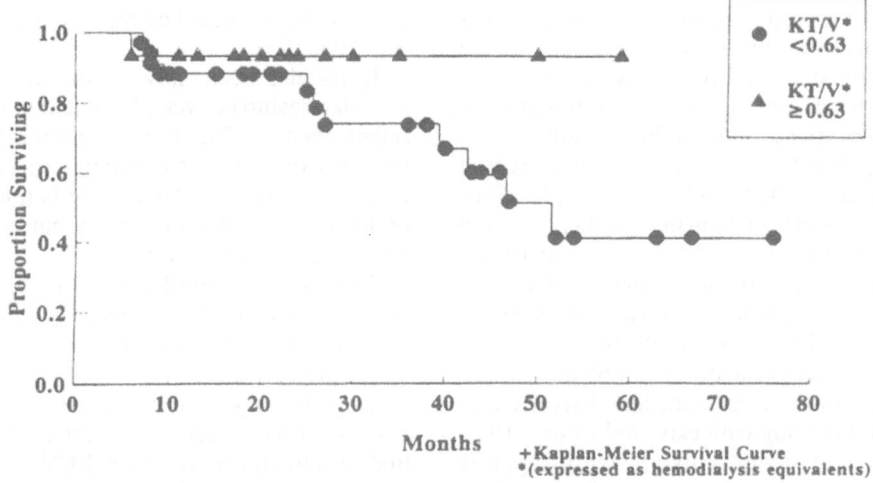

Figure 10. Survival on CAPD as a function of Kt/V. With permission from Reference (187).

Preliminary results from a large multicentre prospective cohort study by Churchill et al. suggest that Kt/V is a significant predictor of mortality, even after correction for age, diabetic status, cardiovascular disease and serum albumin, and that higher Kt/V values are associated with better survival (189). In particular, patients with Kt/V > 2.3/week appear to have 10% better survival at two years than those with lower Kt/V values. Kt/V values above 2.3/week are rarely achieved on standard CAPD without residual renal function and, so, there is a risk of a confounding effect here as better residual function is also associated with better large molecule clearance, volume regulation and endocrine function. It is difficult, therefore, to know how these findings would impact on the management of CAPD patients who have little or no residual renal function. Nevertheless, this study does appear to strengthen the case for quantifying dialytic dose and is likely to have a major influence on prescription of PD in the years ahead.

A reasonable consensus, pending prospective randomised studies, is that low levels of Kt/V (< 1.5/week) are associated with excess mortality and that intermediate levels (1.5–1.9/week) may also be, after longer periods on CAPD, but that this is not so easily demonstrated because less than half of patients remain on the modality after 3 years. Also, there may be some confounding in that higher Kt/V values are usually associated with retention of residual function which may be associated with better outcomes for other reasons. nPCR is an unreliable index of nutritional status and a poor predictor of patient outcome.

Table 4. Weight limits for CAPD with various Kt/V targets and prescriptions in anepheric patients

Target Kt/V	> 1.5/week	> 1.7/week	> 1.9/week	> 2.3/week
Daily regimen				
4 × 2 L	< 66 kg	< 58 kg	< 52 kg	< 43 kg
4 × 2.5 L	66–81 kg	58–71 kg	52–64 kg	43–53 kg
4 × 3 L	81–96 kg	71–84 kg	64–75 kg	53–62 kg

Assumes 1 L UF, V = 60% WT and D/P Ur 0.95.

INCREASING DIALYTIC DOSE IN PD

If low Kt/V values are an adverse risk factor in CAPD, the question that arises is how they can be increased. Once residual function is lost, patients weighing more than 66 kg are unlikely to achieve values above 1.5/week with conventional 8 liters a day regimens. In these situations, the first option is to increase dwell volumes to 2.5 liters but not all patients tolerate this. An alternative strategy is to use a fifth exchange but few patients find this acceptable. If 1.5/week is a minimum target, then 3 liter exchanges will be required once weight exceeds 81 kg and CAPD will not be feasible above 96 kg, without a fifth exchange. If the target is raised to 1.7/week, as has been suggested, then the respective cut off points become 58, 71 and 84 kg respectively (Table 4). Clearly, if even higher targets are used, most patients will need more than the conventional prescription once they lose residual function and many will be unable to be dialyzed 'adequately' on CAPD at all.

New CAPD assist devices make a fifth exchange at night more feasible (190) and this will make it possible routinely to achieve Kt/V targets as high as 1.9, even in anephric patients. At present, however, to achiever higher Kt/V many patients would need to go to automated or cycler PD and use significantly greater dialysate volumes to allow for the shorter equilibration times and the relatively more intermittent nature of the therapy.

When increasing dialytic dose in CAPD, the increased risk of patient 'burn out' and of mechanical complications such as hernias, leaks and back pain must be kept in mind and balanced against the expected benefits of increased clearance. This is especially true in the older patient.

The issue of poor compliance with exchanges in PD is rarely raised and is likely a bigger problem than suspected. Keen et al. have suggested that compliance can be monitored by measuring 24 hour urine and dialysate creatinine losses and comparing with expected values (191). If the measured value is significantly greater, it suggests that the patient has missed exchanges and is now playing 'catch up'. On this basis, it was suggested that 22% of exchanges were being missed in the population studied. Similar results have been reported by Warren et al. (192).

THE Kt/V AND nPCR CORRELATION

Lindsay et al. have described a correlation between Kt/V and nPCR in both HD and CAPD patients (97) and this was subsequently confirmed in a larger study by Blake et al. (154) (Figure 11). Bergstrom has pointed out that the regression lines for the individual modalities are such that CAPD patients have a greater nPCR and, by implication, protein intake, for a given Kt/V, than those on HD (193) (Figure 12). This relationship has led to the suggestion that there is a homeostatic mechanism operating in uremia by which the body protects itself from the accumulation of toxic byproducts of N metabolism by limiting appetite for protein.

The nature of this relationship has however recently been questioned, especially in CAPD (194–196). Firstly, it has been pointed out that both Kt/V and nPCR are calculated from the same data points. These are the daily dialysate and urine urea contents and the body weight. The only item directly used to calculate Kt/V, but not nPCR, is the blood urea. Accordingly, any errors in data collection and any distortion introduced in normalization of Kt and PCR by factors such as increased body fat or overhydration, will introduce a systematic unidirectional bias that will artefactually increase the correlation between Kt/V and nPCR by correlating two identical errors (149, 159). This is the most likely explanation for the finding that the correlation coefficient for the relationship decreases when apparently more accurate methods such as the Watson nomogram are used to estimate V (159, 197). The correlation still exists but is less close when normalization is avoided altogether and Kt and PCR are directly compared (197). Harty et al. suggest that the relationship,

both in HD and CAPD, is a fallacy based on the phenomenon of mathematical coupling but this has been disputed (98, 194, 195).

It has also been shown, both in HD and CAPD, that the relationship between Kt/V and nPCR is not linear but, rather, tends to flatten out at higher Kt/V values so that there is a diminishing return in terms of nPCR for further increases in Kt/V (198–200). It is not clear at what level of Kt/V this flattening occurs but it may be as low as 1.8/week in CAPD (200).

The clinical significance of this relationship also remains controversial, especially as nPCR is proving to be a poor marker of nutritional status and a weak predictor of patient outcome. There is no doubt however that inadequate dialysis, regardless of how it is measured, is associated with poor protein intake and malnutrition and that an attempt to increase Kt/V is indicated if this is perceived to be a problem.

CREATININE CLEARANCE IN PD

Creatinine kinetics have also been used to measure dialytic dose in PD. This dates from Boen's original PD index which targeted 4–5 ml/min total creatinine clearance (TCC) for patient well-being on intermittent PD (146). Twardowski and Nolph later recommended a target of 40–50 liters/week normalized to 1.73 sq. m body surface area and this has been widely used in clinical practice although it is not well validated (201). Interest in TCC has persisted, in part because of the problems with urea kinetics in PD.

There are a number of problems with measurement of TCC in PD. The large quantities of glucose in dialysate interfere with creatinine assays based on the Jaffe reaction (202). This can result in a 5–7% overestimate of creatinine levels and each laboratory should develop its own correction factor using creatinine measurements from fresh dialysate bags containing different concentrations of glucose (203). Newer enzymatic colorimetric assays do not require these corrections to be made (64).

The measurement of the residual renal component of TCC also raises issues. It is well known that, in the failing kidney, creatinine clearance significantly overestimates glomerular filtration because of tubular secretion. It is therefore argued that, if renal creatinine clearance is used to calculate TCC, the value will be misleadingly high and that, instead, an average of renal urea and creatinine clearance, which is thought to approximate more closely to actual glomerular filtration, should be used (205). A purist might however argue that when urea kinetics are being applied, no such manipulation of renal urea clearance is carried out and that, with TCC, the same principles should apply (203). The consensus, however, is that an average residual clearance should be used. Correction for surface area is done using the nomogram of du Bois and du

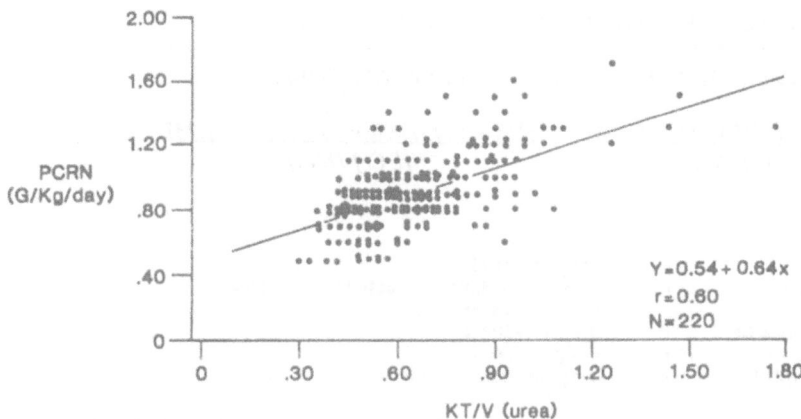

Figure 11. Plot of PCRN values against Kt/V values for 220 studies. With permission from Reference (154).

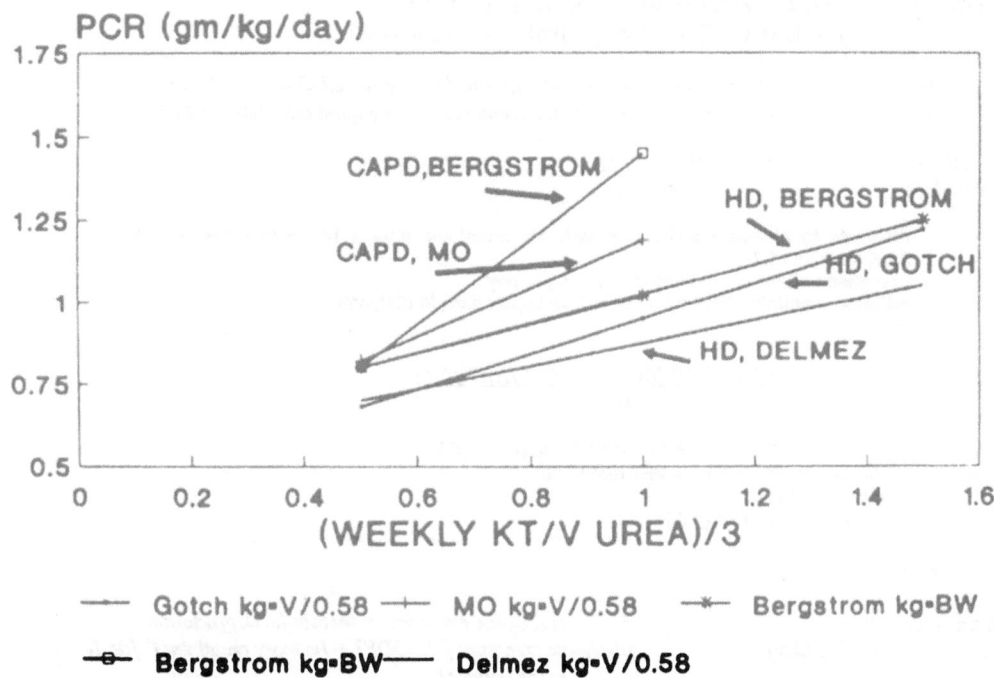

Figure 12. PCR and Kt/V urea in HD and CAPD. PCR is related to weekly (Kt/V urea)/3 in 2 CAPD populations and 3 HD populations. With permission from *Perit Dial Int* 13: 178–183, 1993.

Bois which takes into account height and weight but which is not validated for dialysis patients (206) (Table 5).

Typical values of TCC on starting CAPD are 55–110 liters/week/1.73 sq m with a mean of 89 liters/week/1.73 sq m and are about 10% lower if an average of urea and creatinine clearance is used for the renal component (203). The renal component accounted for 45% of TCC at the onset of CAPD as against 25% after 1 year, 12% after 2 years and zero at 3 years in one study (203). On standard regimens, most patients initially achieve the target of 50 liters/week but, by 2 years, only a minority do (Figure 13). Creatinine equilibration tends to increase with time, so

improving peritoneal clearance (Figure 14), but this varies greatly between patients and is offset by the tendency for ultrafiltration volumes to decrease (203).

Creatinine excretion can be followed over time as an index of muscle mass. Significant decreases occur but some of this may be accounted for by increased non-renal, non-peritoneal creatinine clearance (203). Keshaviah et al. have proposed that creatinine kinetics can be used to estimate lean body mass (LBM), an index of somatic protein content, in both HD and PD patients (207). The theory is that, in dialysis patients, LBM is proportional to creatinine excretion plus metabolic degradation. Excretion can

Table 5. Formulae for calculation of total creatinine clearance and related indices

	DIALYSATE COMPONENT	RENAL COMPONENT*

$$\text{TOTAL CREATININE CLEARANCE [corr. for 1.73 m}^2\text{ BSA]} = \frac{[D\,Cr]\,[DDDV]\,[1.73]}{[SCr]\,[BSA]} + \frac{[Urine\,Cr]\,[Daily\,urine\,volume]\,[1.73]}{[S\,Cr]\,[BSA]}$$

S Cr	=	Serum creatinine
D Cr	=	Dialysis creatinine corrected for dialysate glucose concentration
Urine Cr	=	Urine creatinine
BSA	=	Body surface area [m²]
DDDV	=	Daily dialysate drain volume

* *Alternatively renal component is given as the average of the residual renal clearances of urea and creatinine [corrected for 1.73 m² BSA]*

BSA [duBois]:   Log A = .425 Log W + .725 Log H + 1.8564
A = BSA [cm²], W = weight [kg], H = height [cms]

Corrected Dialysate Creatinine   =   *measured dialysate creatinine - [c.f.] [measured dialysate glucose]*
c.f. = correction factor which each laboratory must calculate for itself

$$\text{EFFICACY NUMBER [L/g of creatinine/day]} = \frac{[D/P\,Cr]\,[V]}{ACP_{PD}}$$

D/P Cr	=	dialysate to plasma equilibration ratio for creatinine after 4 hours of a standard 2 litre 2.5% glucose PET test
V	=	precribed volume of exchanges in litres per day
ACP$_{PD}$	=	adjusted creatinine production based on appearance in dialysate

$$ACP_{PD} = \frac{[D\,Cr]\,[V]\,[6] + [S\,Cr]\,[BW]\,[0.4]}{1000}$$

D Cr	=	dialysate creatinine after a 4 hour PET test [in mg/dL]
V	=	drain volume after a 4 hour PET test in dL
BW	=	body weight in kg
S Cr	=	serum creatinine [in mg/dL]

CREATININE KINETICS:

Creatinine production	=	*creatinine excretion + metabolic degradation*
Creatinine excretion [mg/day]	=	[dialysate creatinine]* [DDDV] + [urinary creatinine]* [daily urine volume]
Creatinine degradation [mg/day]	=	[0.38] [serum creatinine]* [body weights (kg)] * all in mg/dL
Lean body mass [kg]	=	7.38 + [0.029] [creatinine production]

be measured by adding dialysate and urinary creatinine content and degradation is calculated from body weight and serum creatinine, using the formula derived by Mitch et al. (208) (Table 5). In CAPD patients, LBM by this method was lower than, but correlated well with, LBM by techniques such as bioimpedance and near infrared. Values were below normal for sex and age in 66% of PD patients and averaged only 59% of body weight, suggesting significant depletion of somatic protein (207).

An alternative creatinine based index of dialytic dose is the Efficacy Number (EN), devised by Brandes et al., which has the advantage of requiring only data from a peritoneal equilibration test (PET) rather than 24 hour urine and dialysate collections (209) (Table 5). However, clinical studies have not supported the use of the EN, with mortality being more associated with high than low values (210). This paradox is probably due to creatinine production, which is an index of nutritional status, being part of the denominator.

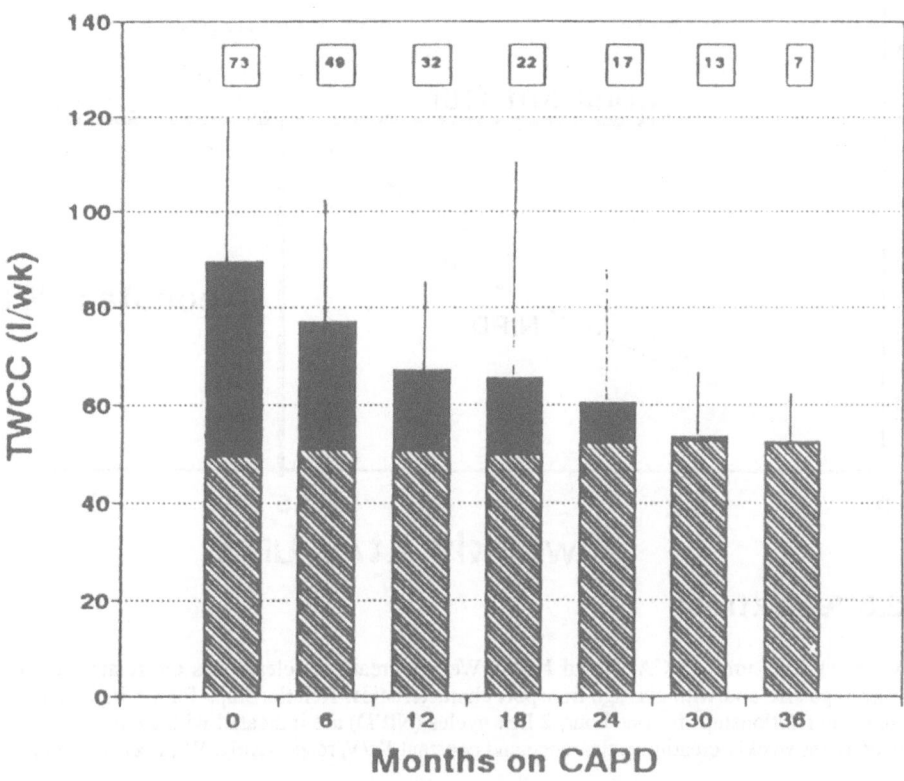

Figure 13. Change in the total weekly creatinine clearance with time. The hatched and shaded areas indicate the proportion of total clearance accounted for by peritoneal and residual renal clearance, respectively. The bars represent standard deviations. The figures in the boxes refer to the number of patients at each six-month interval. With permission from Reference (203).

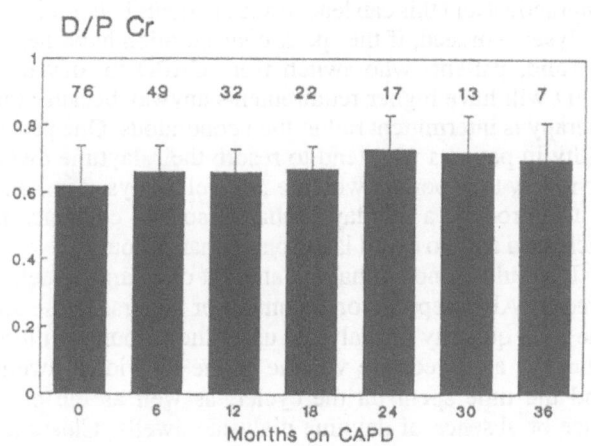

Figure 14. Change in D/P creatinine with time on CAPD. The bars represent standard deviations, and the figures above the columns refer to the number of patients at each six-month interval. With permission from Reference (203).

Studies looking at TCC have shown varied results with regard to predicting adverse outcomes. Blake et al.

showed an association between mortality and TCC values under 48 liters/week but otherwise no correlation with morbidity (203). Brandes et al. showed that creatinine kinetics were better than urea kinetics in distinguishing patients with different degrees of uremic morbidity (155), but Selgas et al. found the opposite in a study with longer follow up (151). Again preliminary results from the large prospective cohort multicentre study by Churchill et al. suggest that TCC is at least as good a predictor of mortality as Kt/V and that values greater than 80 liters a week may be associated with superior survival (189). Again, however, such values are only likely to be achieved in those with significant residual renal function and, as discussed earlier, this makes interpretation more difficult. As is the case with urea kinetics, the exact importance of TCC in CAPD remains unclear.

AUTOMATED PD (APD)

There is almost no clinical data on the dialytic clearances achieved or the appropriate targets to be aimed for in

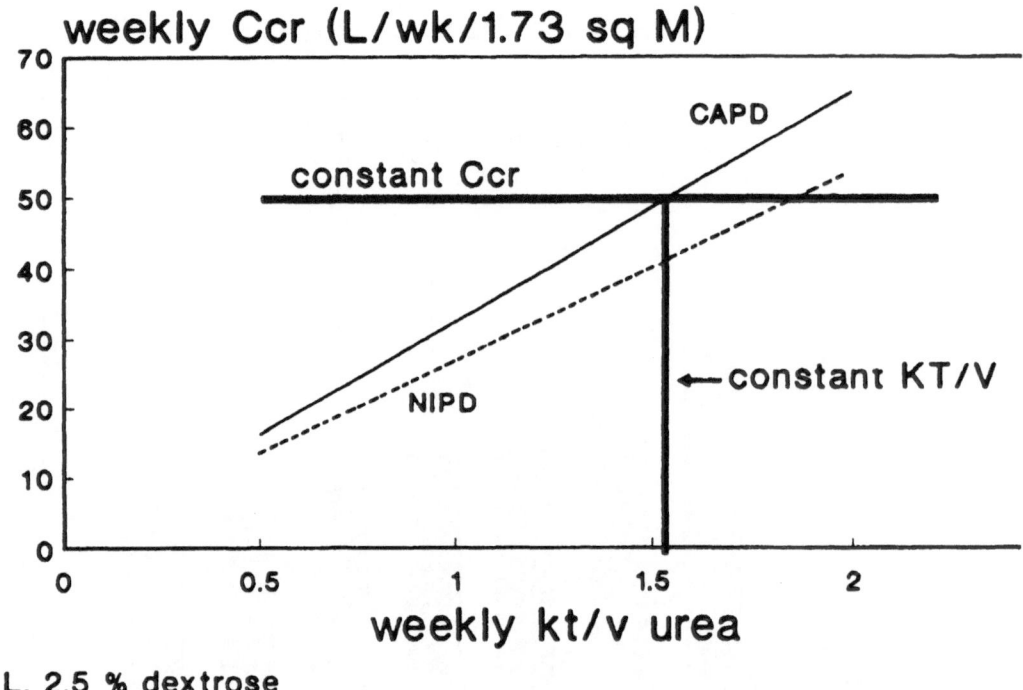

2 L, 2.5 % dextrose

Figure 15. Weekly Ccr *vs* Kt/V urea on CAPD and NIPD. Weekly creatinine clearances are related to weekly Kt/V urea in a theoretical patient of average size and with average transport characteristics. Relationships for six hour, 2 litre cycles (CAPD) are indicated by a solid line and relationships for one hour, 2 litre cycles (NIPD) are indicated with a dashed line. Thick horizontal and vertical lines indicate constant weekly creatinine clearance and constant Kt/V, respectively. With permission from Reference (211).

patients on home APD. Measurement of dialysate clearances are clumsy because of the need to collect large dialysate volumes. Some units have taught patients to sample proportionately from drain bags according to their weight but this increases the potential for errors. The choice of a blood urea or creatinine for calculation of clearance is also an issue as a steady state no longer exists. An average of pre- and post-cycling values is probably best but, if APD is done each night, a midday value is more feasible and almost as accurate.

Typical regimens involve 4 to 7, two liter dwells nightly and lead to urea reduction ratios of 10–20%, but some centres use greater volumes. If a daytime dwell is also done the regimen is called continuous cycler PD (CCPD) and, if not, it is called nightly PD (NPD). With the shorter dwell times in APD, equilibration is not as complete as in CAPD and this discrepancy is greater with larger molecules such as creatinine than with urea. Nolph et al. have pointed out that, for this reason, keeping Kt/V constant leads to a decrease in TCC in patients who switch from CAPD to APD (211) (Figure 15). Since it is unclear whether Kt/V or TCC is more important, it is suggested that the more demanding TCC be monitored during such switches. It should be noted that, if patients are not prescribed a daytime dialysis fluid dwell, it may require much greater volumes of fluid to be delivered by the cycler to achieve equivalent clearances to conventional CAPD (212). This

is especially so in low transporters in whom it may be impossible to achieve adequate dialysis without a daytime dwell. Some APD patients do not tolerate daytime dwells or resorb them to such a degree that their prescription is impractical and this can lead to such patients being 'underdialysed'. Indeed, if the 'peak concentration hypothesis' is valid, patients who switch from CAPD to 'day dry' APD will have higher requirements anyway because the therapy is intermittent rather than continuous. One possibility in patients who tend to resorb their daytime dwell or in low transporters who are not well dialysed in APD is to introduce a midday exchange so that clearance is increased and no dwell lasts longer than 7 hours.

It should be noted that the amount of clearance delivered by APD depends on a number of factors. These are the total quantity of dialysate used, the amount of ultrafiltration achieved, the volume of the individual dwells and the time spent on the cycler, as well as the presence or absence of daytime dialysate dwells. Clearance is also affected by the patient's peritoneal transport to a much greater degree than is the case in CAPD where the longer dwell times allow for more complete equilibration to occur, especially in the case of urea.

The use of tidal PD (TPD) has been advocated to improve clearances on APD regimens. The theory is that, if a constant reserve volume of dialysate is maintained throughout the treatment time, there is continuous con-

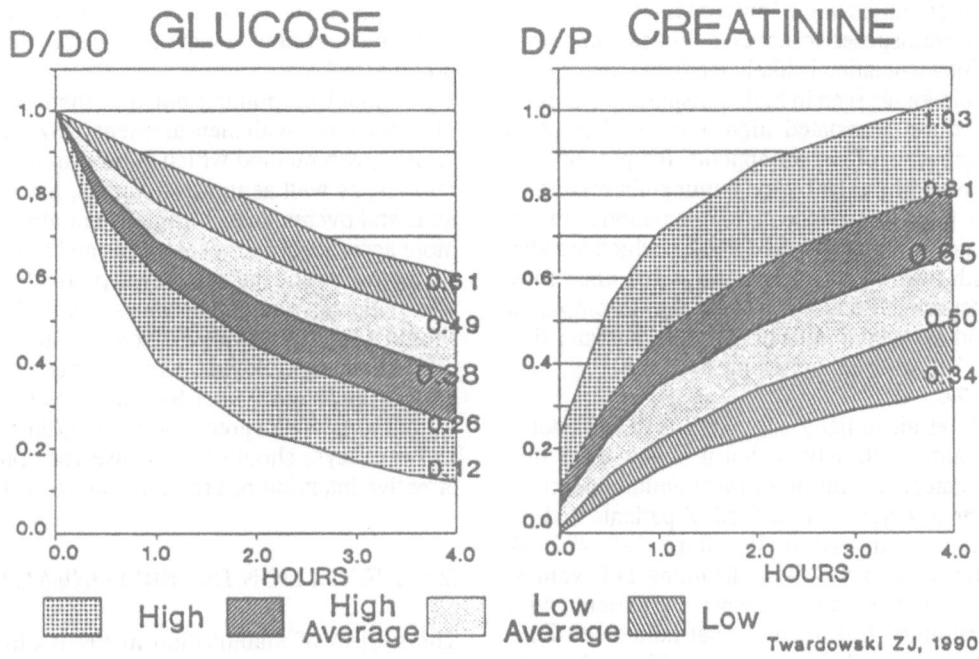

Figure 16. PET results. Ranges of values for D/Do glucose and D/P creatinine (corrected) in standard Peritoneal Equilibration Test. With permission from Reference (202).

tact of significant volumes of dialysate with the peritoneal membrane, allowing uninterrupted clearance to occur. In contrast, in standard APD, there is a 'down time' late in the drain cycle and early in the fill cycle, during which there is minimal dialysate contact with the membrane and a consequent decrease in clearance. In practice, clearances have not been much higher with TPD in most comparative studies, perhaps due to incomplete mixing of of solutes between the tidal and reserve volumes of dialysate (213, 214).

THE PERITONEAL EQUILIBRATION TEST (PET) AND ADEQUACY OF DIALYSIS

The PET was first described by Verger et al. and subsequently popularised by Twardowski et al. as a simple, reproducible method of estimating peritoneal transport (202, 215). Patients were classified into low, low average, high average and high transporters on the basis of their degree of dialysate to plasma creatinine and urea equilibration (D/P Cr and D/P Ur) and of glucose absorption (D/Do G) after four hours of a 2.5 % dextrose 2 liter dwell under standard conditions (Figure 16). It was suggested that average transporters would do well on standard CAPD but that high transporters would do best on short dwell regimens such as NPD because of their tendency to have poor ultrafiltration (UF). Low transporters would do best with high volume cycling at night supplemented by a daytime dwell, as in CCPD, because of their tendency to achieve lower peritoneal clearances (202). Just as in the calculation of TCC, dialysate creatinine values should be corrected for dialysate glucose levels. Despite their simplicity, D/P ratios correlate very well with mass transfer area coefficients, which are a more sophisticated measure of peritoneal transport (216).

The PET is widely performed and has greatly increased awareness of peritoneal transport but the idea that it should be used to direct patients to NPD and CCPD is not widely followed in practice. One problem is that high D/P Cr values are not always good predictors of net daily UF. This is probably because other factors such as lymphatic absorption influence UF volumes. Also, when smaller molecules like urea are being considered, even low transporters achieve high degrees of equilibration on CAPD and Kt/V values are not greatly affected. Levels of TCC in CAPD are however influenced by D/P Cr and, should this index prove to be more significant than Kt/V, there may be a greater tendency to direct low transporters to CCPD. At present, the decision to use cyclers is more likely to be made for lifestyle reasons or when actual clinical evidence of inadequate UF or dialysis is seen. Once a patient is actually on APD, as discussed earlier, dwell times are much shorter and the peritoneal transport status is a critical determinant of the amount of clearance that will be achieved. It is therefore particularly important to monitor PET status in these patients.

An important point about the PET is that a number of groups have now described a correlation between being a high transporter and having a low serum albumin (SA), which in turn predisposes to adverse clinical outcomes (217, 218). This association is likely mediated by the high dialysate protein losses seen in high transporters but other factors may be the associated high glucose absorption having a suppressive effect on appetite for protein and a degree of hemodilutional hypoalbuminemia related to poor UF. Also, there is evidence of an association between high D/P Cr and both old age and diabetes, which are also associated with low SA (219). It is suggested, therefore, that high transporters be monitored for the development of low SA and associated nutritional problems and that consideration be given to switching to HD if these are refractory (217).

Twardowski et al. initially suggested that PET status was stable in almost all patients but it is now clear that many change category with time. Most authors describe a drift upwards in a quarter to a third of patients and, in extreme cases, this can lead to UF failure (220–222). A smaller number of patients show declining D/P values, and perhaps the most extreme of these are patients with sclerosing peritonitis. It is unclear what influences these alterations but it is unlikely that peritonitis is the sole factor. Rocco et al. have shown that D/P values acutely increase in the first few weeks after commencing PD, perhaps due to a dialysate induced increase in effective peritoneal surface area (223). If the initial PET is not done early, this increase may be missed and this may explain some of the discrepancies in the literature regarding trends in equilibration ratios and other transport indices.

It should also be emphasized that the PET protocol includes a requirement for patients to roll side to side that is not always observed. Gotch et al. have shown that this rolling can increase D/P ratios by as much as 10% (224).

SERUM ALBUMIN

It is now apparent from numerous studies that low SA is a powerful predictor of mortality and morbidity in both HD and CAPD (151, 187, 217) (Figure 17). This raises the question of whether low SA is primarily a nutritional issue which may be influenced by protein intake and dialytic dose or whether it is mainly a marker of comorbidity and, as such, is not easily amenable to change. Blake et al. found that the strongest predictor of low SA in CAPD was a high D/P Cr, as has been discussed above, and that other factors were older age, diabetes and shorter time on CAPD, but that neither nPCR nor dialytic dose were predictive (217). Other groups have also found absent or weak associations between low SA and Kt/V and nPCR values (5, 10, 12, 28) but a number of investigators did detect a relationship (150, 155, 157, 171), leaving the issue controversial. Interestingly, Harty et al. have found that uncorrected PCR is correlated, to some degree, with SA, raising again the issue of appropriate normalization

of this parameter (171). All this suggests that SA may not easily be modified by increases in dialytic dose or even in protein intake.

It should be pointed out that there are also methodological issues with measurement of SA (226). The bromcresol green method which is used in most clinical laboratories, as well as in most studies, has specificity problems and overestimates SA substantially compared to the more accurate bromcresol purple and immunoturbidimetric methods. The discrepancy is particularly great in dialysis patients, ranging between 5 and 8 g/liter and this should be kept in mind when comparing studies using the different methodologies. A reasonable consensus from the present literature is that SA values below 30–33 g/liter, using bromocresol green, or 25–28 g/liter, using the alternative assays, should be a cause for concern, although effective interventions remain elusive (226).

MALNUTRITION IN PERITONEAL DALYSIS

The subject of malnutrition in PD is closely associated with that of adequacy of dialysis. Poor nutrition is quite prevalent in CAPD as reflected by a multicenter study of 224 CAPD patients which showed that 8% were severely malnourished and that a further 33% had mild to moderate malnutrition (227).

The importance of malnutrition is indicated by studies showing that indices of nutrition such as serum albumin and subjective global assessment are predictive of survival and other clinical outcomes (187, 217, 228). As already stated, it is unclear how much these indices reflect comorbidity rather than just inadequate nutritional intake. Similarly, it is not clear how easily they can be modified by therapeutic interventions.

Initial management of malnutrition in the PD patient should include dietary assessment and counselling, treatment of any comorbidity, especially upper gastrointestinal disorders, dentition problems and depression. Attention should also be given to cultural and socio-economic issues and, where relevant, oral nutritional supplements should be considered although objective evidence for their benefit is lacking. In view of the already described relationship between protein intake and Kt/V, dialysis dose should be significantly increased if malnutrition persists, especially if there are other symptoms and signs suggestive of inadequately controlled uremia.

Two other more expensive options are intraperitoneal amino acids and administration of recombinant human growth hormone. Intraperitoneal amino acids in CAPD have been studied for over a decade but they are still not much used in clinical practice (229). The quantities that can be administered have been limited, not just by expense, but also by the associated increases that occur in acidosis and degree of uremia (230). The latter problem, in particular, suggests the existence of an anabolic defect in patients with renal failure. Efforts to deal with these

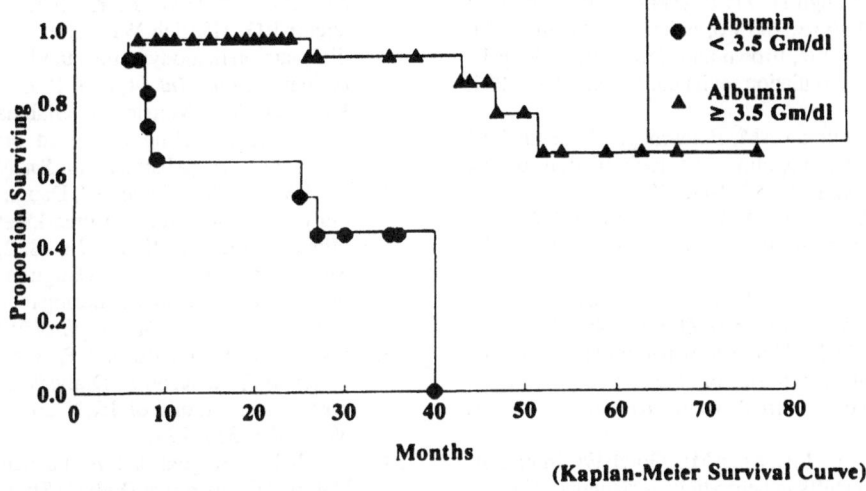

Figure 17. Survival on CAPD as a function of serum albumin. With permission from Reference (187).

problems have included concomitant increases in the dialytic prescription, alterations in the amino acid mixture, and the co-administration of calories to prevent diversion of the amino acids for use as an immediate energy source (230–233). Nutritional and clinical outcomes with intraperitoneal amino acids have been variable and their use continues to be limited (230–233).

More promising is the administration of growth hormone which has now been shown to have a profound anabolic effect in CAPD, as well as in HD patients (91, 234, 235). Uremia is associated with a state of growth hormone resistance which leads to inappropriately low serum levels of insulin-like growth factor (236, 237). In addition there are rises in the levels of insulin-like growth factor binding proteins which further decrease insulin-like growth factor bioavailability. This, in turn, leads to an unfavourable imbalance between protein anabolism and catabolism in uremic patients (236, 237). Growth hormone resistance in these patients can be effectively overcome by pharmacological doses of recombinant growth hormone and, just as this has been shown to enhance growth in uremic children (238), it can also increase anabolism in adults on dialysis (234). Although preliminary reports on the use of this intervention in CAPD patients are promising, studies to date have been relatively short term and issues such as long-term side effects and expense will need to be dealt with.

Thus a strategy for treating malnutrition based on optimising dialytic dose, providing appropriate supplements, and stimulating anabolism may improve management of this problem which is at present is often intractable in CAPD patients.

SUMMARY – PERITONEAL DIALYSIS

The quantification of dialytic dose in PD is still in its infancy. Existing models are not well validated and there is a lack of randomised prospective trials on which to base recommendations. Some minimum standards are being accepted for CAPD but almost nothing is established for APD. Dietary requirements remain unclear in view of the apparent discrepancies between recommendations and patients' actual intakes and a more effective approach to the problem of malnutrition in PD is required. Resolution of these issues may help to decrease morbidity and mortality and improve patient retention on PD.

REFERENCES

1. Johnson WJ, Hagge WW, Wagoner RD, Dinapoli RP, Rosevear JW: Effects of urea loading in patients with far-advanced renal failure. *Mayo Clin Proc* 47: 21, 1972
2. Merril JP, Legrain M, Hoigne R: Observations on the role of urea in uremia. *Ann Intern Med* 14: 519, 1953
3. Bergstrom J: Uraemic toxins. This edition
4. Owen WF Jr, Lew NL, Liu Y, Lowrie EG, Lazarus JM: The urea reduction ratio and serum albumin concentration as predictors of mortality in patients undergoing hemodialysis. *N Engl J Med* 329: 1001, 1993
5. Pedrini LA, Zereik S, Rasmy S: Causes, kinetics and clinical implications of post-hemodialysis urea rebound. *Kidney Int* 34: 817, 1988
6. Ward RA, Shirlow MJ, Hayes JM, Chapman GV, Farrell PC: Protein catabolism during hemodialysis. *Am J Clin Nutr* 32: 2443, 1979
7. Farrell PC, Hone PW: Dialysis-induced catabolism. *Am J Clin Nutr* 33: 1417, 1980
8. Lim VS, Bier DM, Flanigan MJ, Sum-Ping ST: The effect of hemodialysis on protein metabolism: A leucine kinetic study. *J Clin Invest* 91: 2429, 1993

9. Van Stone JC, Daugirdas JT: Physiologic Principles. in *Handbook of Dialysis*, 2nd Ed, edited by Daugirdas JT, Ing TS, Boston: Little, Brown and Company, 1994, p 13

10. Sherman RA: Recirculation revisited. *Semin Dial* 4: 221, 1991

11. Schneditz D, Kaufman AM, Polaschegg H, Levin NW, Daugirdas JT: Cardiopulmonary recirculation during hemodialysis. *Kidney Int* 42: 1450, 1992

12. Shackman R, Chisholm GD, Holden AJ, Pigott RW: Urea distribution in the body after haemodialysis. *Br Med J* 34: 817, 1962

13. Schindhelm K, Farrell PC: Patient-hemodialyzer interactions. *Trans Am Soc Artif Intern Organs* 24: 357, 1978

14. Frost TH, Kerr DNS: Kinetics of hemodialysis: A theoretical study of the removal of solutes in chronic renal failure compared to normal health. *Kidney Int* 12: 41, 1977

15. Heineken FG, Evans MC, Keen ML, Gotch FA: Intercompartmental fluid shifts in hemodialysis patients. *Biotechnol Progr* 3: 69, 1987

16. Schneditz D, Van Stone JC, Daugirdas JT: A regional blood circulation alternative to in-series two-compartment urea kinetic modeling. *ASAIO J* 39: M573, 1993

17. Schneditz D, Daugirdas JT: Formal analytical solution to a regional blood flow and diffusion-based urea kinetic model. *ASAIO J* 1994. In press

18. Depner TA, Cheer A, Vedantham R: Is two-compartment modeling required for high-flux hemodialysis? (Abstract) *Am Soc Nephrol* 1: 354, 1990

19. Cappello A, Grandi F, Lamberti C, Santoro A: Comparative evaluation of different methods to estimate urea distribution volume and generation rate. *Int J Artif Organs* 1994. In press

20. Bosticardo GM, Alloatti S: Classical urea kinetic model and direct dialysis quantification agreement. *ASAIO J* 41: 14798, 1995

21. Tattersall JE, Aldridge C, Greenwood RN, Farrington K. How good is the dialysate collection method for determination of V? (Abstract) *Am Soc Nephrol* 5: 530, 1994

22. Gotch FA: Kinetic modeling in hemodialysis. in *Clinical Dialysis*, 2nd Ed, edited by Nissenson AR, Fine RN, Gentile DE, Norwalk, Appleton & Lange, 1990, p 118

23. Tattersall JE, Greenwood RN, Farrington K: Intercompartmental diffusion and cardiopulmonary recirculation in long and short dialyses. (Abstract) *Am Soc Nephrol* 1995

24. Spiegel DM, Paker PL, Babcock S, Contiguglia R, Klein M: Hemodialysis urea rebound: the effect of increasing dialysis efficiency. *Am J Kidney Dis* 25: 26, 1995

25. Smye SW, Evans JHC, Will E, Brocklebank JT: Paediatric haemodialysis: estimation of treatment efficiency in the presence of urea rebound. *Clin Phys Physiol Meas* 13: 51, 1992

26. Star RA, Hootkins R, Thompson JR, Poole T, Toto RD: Variability and stability of two pool urea mass transfer coefficient. *Am Soc Nephrol* 3: 395, 1992

27. Tsang HK, Leonard EF, LeFavour GS, Cortell S: Urea dynamics during and immediately after dialysis. *ASAIO J* 8: 251, 1985

28. Keshaviah P, Hanson G, Abraham P, Collins A: Erythropoietin and cell membrane permeability. (Abstract) *Kidney Int* 37: 304, 1990

29. Jost CMT, Agarwal R, Khair-El-Din K, Grayburn PA, Victor RG, Henrich WL: Effects of cooler temperature dialysate on hemodynamic stability in 'problem' dialysis patients. *Kidney Int* 44: 606, 1993

30. Kaufman AM, Morris AT, Glabman MB et al.: Effect of dialysate cooling on blood pressure and effective dialysate dose. (Abstract) *Am Soc Nephrol* 5: 517, 1994

31. Yu AW, Ing TS, Zabaneh RI, Daugirdas JT: Effect of cold dialysate temperature on urea kinetics during moderate efficiency dialysis. *Kidney Int* 48: 237, 1995

32. Yu AW, Ing TS, Ejaz AA, Daugirdas JT: Effect of acetate dialysate on urea kinetics during moderate efficiency dialysis. (Abstract) *Am Soc Nephrol* 5: 533, 1994

33. Kjellstrand C, Kjellstrand P, Skroder R, Cederlof IO, Ericsson F, Jacobson S: Dialysis kinetics using pre- and post-concentrations of BUN are not accurate. *Am Soc Nephrol* 3: 375, 1992

34. Gotch FA, Sargent JA: A mechanistic analysis of the National Cooperative Dialysis Study (NCDS). *Kidney Int* 28: 526, 1985

35. Lowrie EG, Laird NM, Parker TF, Sargent JA: Effect of the hemodialysis prescription on patient morbidity. *N Engl J Med* 305: 1176, 1981

36. Sargent JA, Gotch FA: Mathematical modeling of dialysis therapy. *Kidney Int* 18: S2, 1980

37. Sargent JA: Control of dialysis by a single-pool urea model: the National Cooperative Dialysis Study. *Kidney Int* 23: S13, 1983

38. Daugirdas JT: Second generation logarithmic estimates of single-pool variable volume Kt/V: an analysis of error. *Am Soc Nephrol* 4: 1205, 1993

39. Jindal KK, Manuel A, Goldstein MB: Percent reduction in blood urea concentration during hemodialysis (PRU). *Trans Am Soc Artif Intern Organs* 33: 286, 1987

40. Basile C, Casino F, Lopez T: Percent reduction in blood urea concentration during dialysis estimates Kt/V in a simple and accurate way. *Am J Kidney Dis* 15: 40, 1990

41. Garred LJ, McCready W: A theory based, simple formula for Kt/V calculation from pre/post urea. *Abstr Am Soc Artif Intern Organs* 70, 1992

42. Collins AJ, Ma JZ, Umen A: Urea index (Kt/V) and other predictors of hemodialysis patient survival. *Am J Kidney Dis* 23: 272, 1994

43. Ahmad S, Cole JJ: Lower morbidity associated with higher Kt/V in stable hemodialysis patients. (Abstract) *Am Soc Nephrol* 1: 346, 1990

44. Loon NR, Pinevich AJ, Banic S, Anderson C: Improved adequacy of hemodialysis (Kt/V) does not improve nutritional status. (Abstract) *Am Soc Nephrol* 2: 336, 1991

45. Shen FH, Hsu KT: Lower mortality and morbidity associated with higher Kt/V in hemodialysis patients. (Abstract) *Am Soc Nephrol* 1: 377, 1990

46. Charra B, Calemard E, Ruffet M et al.: Survival as an index of adequacy of dialysis. *Kidney Int* 41: 1286, 1992

47. Hakim RM, Breyer J, Ismail N, Schulman G: Effects of dose of dialysis on morbidity and mortality. *Am J Kidney Dis* 23: 661, 1994

48. Parker TF, Husni L, Huang W, Lew N, Lowrie EG: Survival of hemodialysis patients in the Unites States is improved with a greater quantity of dialysis. *Am J Kidney Dis* 23: 670, 1994

49. Maeda K: Preliminary Report, Japanese Dialysis Society Registry, 1991

50. Held PJ, Port FK: Relationship between Kt/V and mortality. *Am Soc Nephrol* 5: 37P, 1994

51. Lysaght MJ, Vonesh EF, Gotch F et al.: The influence of dialysis treatment modality on the decline of remaining renal function. *Trans Am Soc Artif Intern Organs* 37: 598, 1991

52. Pflederer BJ, Torrey C, Lau AH, Daugirdas JT: Postdialysis urea rebound after 'long' session length (3.5–4.5 hour) hemodialysis. (Abstract) *Am Soc Nephrol* 4: 377, 1993

53. Daugirdas JT, Schneditz D: Overestimation of hemodialysis dose (DKt/V) depends on dialysis efficiency (K/V) by regional blood flow but not by conventional 2-pool UKM. *ASAIO J* 41: 14719, 1995

54. Daugirdas JT, Schneditz D: Effect of access and cardiopulmonary recirculation on the modeled urea distribution volume. *Am J Kidney Dis* 1996. In press

55. Depner TA: *Prescribing Hemodialysis: A Guide to Urea Modeling,* Dordrecht/Boston/London, Kluwer Academic Publishers, 1990

56. MMHD Study Group, Levin NW, Agodoa LY et al.: Comparisons of Smye algorithm with double pool model solution for estimating e(Kt/V). (Abstract) *Am Soc Nephrol* 5: 519, 1994

57. Pflederer BJ, Torrey C, Daugirdas JT: Use of the inlet Smye technique in patients with vascular access recirculation. *Kidney Int* 48: 832, 1995

58. Twardowski Z: Effect of long-term increase in the frequency and/or prolongation of dialysis duration on certain clinical mainfestations and results of laboratory investigations in patients with chronic renal failure. *Acta Med Pol* 116: 31, 1975

59. Snyder D, Louis BM, Gorfien P, Mordujovich J: Clinical experience with long-term, brief, 'daily' haemodialysis. *Proc Eur Dial Transplant Assoc,* 11: 128, 1975

60. Hombrouckx R, Bogaert AM, Leroy F et al.: Limitations of short dialysis are the indications for ultrashort daily auto dialysis. *Trans Am Soc Artif Intern Organs* 35: 503, 1989

61. Marichal JF, Brignon P, Faller B: Experience d'hémodialyse quotidienne ultra-courte avec abord vasculaire atraumatique. A propos de deux cas. *Nephrologie* 11: 135, 1990

62. Buoncristiani U, Giombini L, Cozzari M, Carobi C, Quintaliani G, Brugnano R: Daily recycled bicarbonate dialysis with polyacrylonitrile. *Trans Am Soc Artif Intern Organs* 29: 669, 1983

63. Harris CP, Townsend JJ: Dialysis disequilibrium syndrome. *West J Med* 151: 52, 1989

64. Daugirdas JT: Acute hemodialysis prescription. in *Handbook of Dialysis,* 2nd Ed, edited by Daugirdas JT, Ing TS, Boston, Little, Brown and Company, 1994, p 78

65. Simpson K, Allison MEM: Dialysis and acute renal failure: Can mortality be improved? (Abstract) *Proc Eur Dial Transplant Assoc* 160, 1993

66. Malchesky PS, Ellis P, Nosse C, Magnusson M, Lankhorst B, Nakamoto S: Direct quantification of dialysis. *Dial Transplant* 12: 694, 1983

67. Buur T, Larsson R: Accuracy of hemodialysis urea kinetic modeling. Comparison of different models. *Nephron* 59: 358, 1991

68. Keshaviah P, Ebben J, Luhring D, Emerson P, Collins A: Clinical evaluation of a new on-line monitor of dialysis adequacy. *Am Soc Nephrol* 3: 374, 1992

69. Garred LJ, DiGiuseppe B, Chand W, McCready W, Canaud B: Kt/V and protein catabolic rate determination from serial urea measurement in the dialysate effluent stream. *Artif Organs* 16: 248, 1992

70. Ing TS, Yu AW, Tiwari P et al.: Collection of a spent hemodialysate aliquot the composition of which reflects that of total spent dialysate. *Am J Kidney Dis* 1995. In press

71. von Albertini B, Garcia-Valdecasas J, Barlee V, Lew SQ, Bosch JP: Solute rebound in highly efficient dialysis: impact on quantification of therapy. (Abstract) *Am Soc Nephrol* 4: 393, 1993

72. Hume R, Weyers E: Relationship between total body water and surface area in normal and obese subjects. *J Clin Pathol* 24: 234, 1971

73. Watson PE, Watson ID, Batt RD: Total body water volumes for adult males and females estimated from simple anthropometric measurements. *Am J Clin Nutr* 33: 27, 1980

74. Daugirdas JT, Depner TE: A nomogram approach to hemodialysis urea modeling. *Am J Kidney Dis* 23: 33, 1994

75. Daugirdas JT: Chronic hemodialysis prescription. in *Handbook of Dialysis, 2nd Ed,* edited by Daugirdas JT, Ing TS, Boston, Little, Brown and Company, 1994, p 92

76. Van Stone JC: Hemodialysis apparatus. in *Handbook of Dialysis,* 2nd Ed, edited by Daugirdas JT, Ing TS, Boston, Little, Brown & Company, 1994, p 32

77. Gotch F: Hemodialysis: Technical and kinetic considerations. in *The Kidney,* edited by Brenner B, Rector FC Jr, Philadelphia, WB Saunders Co, 1976, p 1972

78. Sargent J, Gotch F: Principles and biophysics of dialysis. in *Replacement of Renal Function by Dialysis,* 2nd Ed, edited by Drukker W, Parsons F, Maher J, The Hague, Martinus Nijhoff Publishers, 1985, p 53

79. Depner TA, Rizwan S, Stasi TA: Pressure effects on roller pump blood flow during hemodialysis. *Trans Am Soc Artif Intern Organs* 36: M456, 1990

80. Matzke GR, Rault R, Joy M, Freed B: Can delivered dialysis Kt/V be accurately predicted from the dialysis prescription? (Abstract) *Am Soc Nephrol* 5: 522, 1994

81. Taylor AJ, Vadgama P: Analytical reviews in clinical biochemistry: the estimation of urea. *Ann Clin Biochem* 29: 245, 1992

82. Daugirdas JT, Ing TS, Humayun HM et al.: Two-hour, high-surface-area hemodialysis: a feasibility study. *Int J Artif Organs* 4: 13, 1981

83. Schiff M, Parker E, Carlson C et al.: Too little, too long: why do patients remain underdialyzed? (Abstract) *Am Soc Nephrol* 5: 527, 1994

84. Leypoldt JK, Kablitz C, Gregory MC, Senekjian HO, Cheung AK: Prescribing hemodialysis using a weekly urea mass balance model. *Biochem Pharmacol* 9: 271, 1991

85. Giovannetti S, Maggiore Q: A low nitrogen diet with proteins of high biological value for severe chronic uremia. *Lancet* 1: 1000, 1964

86. Lowrie EG, Lew NL: Death risk in hemodialysis patients: the predictive value of commonly measured variables and

an evaluation of death rate differences between facilities. *Am J Kidney Dis* 5: 458, 1990

87.   Borah MF, Schoenfeld PY, Gotch FA, Sargent JA, Wolfson M, Humphreys MH: Nitrogen balance during intermittent dialysis therapy of uremia. *Kidney Int* 14: 491, 1978

88.   Acchiardo SA, Moore LM, Latour PA: Malnutrition as the main factor in morbidity and mortality of hemodialysis patients. *Kidney Int* 24 (Suppl 16): S199, 1983

89.   Dumler F, Zasuwa G: Factors influencing protein catabolic rate in chronic maintenance hemodialysis patients. *Kidney Int* 37: 294, 1990

90.   Lowrie EG, Lew NL, Liu Y: The effect of differences in urea reduction ratio (URR) on death risk in hemodialysis patients: a preliminary analysis, Memo to National Medical Care DSD Medical Directors, 1991, November 5: 1

91.   Schulman G, Wingard RL, Hutchison RL, Lawrence P, Hakim RM: The effects of recombinant human growth hormone and intradialytic parenteral nutrition in malnourished hemodialysis patients. *Am J Kidney Dis* 21: 527, 1993

92.   Held PJ, Port FK, Garcia J, Gaylin DS, Levin NW, Agodoa L: Hemodialysis prescription and delivery in the US: results from USRDS Case Mix Study. (Abstract) *Am Soc Nephrol* 2: 328, 1991

93.   Herrmann FR, Safran C, Levkoff SE, Minaker KL: Serum albumin level on admission as a predictor of death, length of stay, and readmission. *Arch Intern Med* 152: 125, 1992

94.   Murray MJ, Marsh HM, Wochos DN, Moxness KE, Offord KP, Callaway CV: Nutritional assessment of intensive-care unit patients. *Mayo Clin Proc* 63: 1106, 1988

95.   Pollak AJ, Strong RM, Gribbon R, Shah H: Lack of predictive value of the APACHE II score in hypoalbuminemic patients. *J Parent Ent Nutr* 15: 313, 1991

96.   Gentric A, Cledes J: Immediate and long-term prognosis in acute renal failure in the elderly. *Nephrol Dial Transplant* 6: 86, 1991

97.   Lindsay RM, Spanner E: A hypothesis: The protein catabolic rate is dependent upon the type and amount of treatment in dialyzed uremic patients. *Am J Kidney Dis* 13: 382, 1989

98.   Venning MC, Faragher EB, Harty JC et al.: The relationship between Kt/V and nPCR in haemodialysis patients in cross sectional studies is mathematical coupling. (Abstract) *Am Soc Nephrol* 4: 393, 1993

99.   Poignet JL, Chauveau P, Desassis JF, Puget J: Adequacy of hemodialysis and nutrition: evaluation of an on-line urea monitor. (Abstract) *Am Soc Nephrol* 5: 525, 1994

100.   Mabuchi H, Nakahashi H: Underestimation of serum albumin by the bromcresol purple method and a major endogenous ligand in uremia. *Clin Chim Acta* 167: 89, 1993

101.   Gault MH, Campbell N, Purchase L, Longerich L: Interdialysis weight gain with low predialysis concentrations of proteins and lipids and high end-dialysis values after weight removal. (Abstract) *Am Soc Nephrol* 4: 347, 1993

102.   Depner TA, Cheer AY: Modeling urea kinetics with two *vs* three BUN measurements: A critical comparison. *Trans Am Soc Artif Intern Organs* 35: 499, 1989

103.   Gotch FA, Keen ML: Care of the patient on hemodialysis. in *Introduction to Dialysis*, edited by Cogan MG, Garovoy MR, New York, Churchill Livingstone, 1985, p 73

104.   Depner TA, Daugirdas JT: Formulas for prediction of normalized protein catabolic rate. *J Am Soc Nephrol* 1996. In press

105.   Daugirdas JT: The post:pre-dialysis plasma urea nitrogen ratio to estimate Kt/V and NPCR: validation. *Int J Artif Organs* 12: 420, 1989

106.   Lindsay RM, Spanner E, Heidenheim P, Lindsay S, LeFebvre JMJ: The influence of dialysis membrane upon protein catabolic rate. *Trans Am Soc Artif Intern Organs* 37: M134, 1991

107.   Gutierrez A, Alvestrand A, Wahren J, Bergstrom J: Effect of *in vivo* contact between blood and dialysis membranes on protein catabolism in humans. *Kidney Int* 38: 487, 1990

108.   Gutierrez A, Bergstrom J, Alvestrand A: Protein catabolism in sham-hemodialysis: the effect of different membranes. *Clin Nephrol* 38: 20, 1992

109.   Himmelfarb J: Infection in hemodialysis patients: do dialysis membranes play a role? *Semin Dial* 5: 108, 1992

110.   Schulman G, Fogo A, Gung A, Badr K, Hakim R: Complement activation retards resolution of acute ischemic renal failure in the rat. *Kidney Int* 40: 1069, 1991

111.   Hakim RM, Wingard RL, Lawrence P, Parker RA, Schulman G: Use of biocompatible membranes improves outcome and recovery from acute renal failure. (Abstract) *Am Soc Nephrol* 3: 367, 1992

112.   Seres DS, Strain GW, Hashim SA, Goldberg IJ, Levin NW: Improvement of plasma lipoprotein profiles during high-flux dialysis. *Am Soc Nephrol* 3: 1409, 1993

113.   Josephson MA, Fellner SK, Dasgupta A: Improved lipid profiles in patients undergoing high-flux hemodialysis. *Am J Kidney Dis* 20: 361, 1992

114.   Parthasarathy S, Steinberg D, Witztum JL: The role of oxidized low-density lipoproteins in the pathogenesis of atherosclerosis. *Annu Rev Med* 43: 219, 1992

115.   Chanard J, Brunois JP, Melin JP, Lavaud S, Toupance O: Long-term results of dialysis therapy with a highly permeable membrane. *Artif Organs* 6: 261, 1982

116.   Hornberger JC, Chernew ME, Petersen J, Garber AM: A multivariate analysis of mortality and hospital admissions with high-flux dialysis. *Am Soc Nephrol* 3: 1227, 1992

117.   Levin NW, Dumler F, Zasuwa G, Stalla K: Mortality comparison between conventional and high flux dialysis. (Abstract) *Am Soc Nephrol* 1: 365, 1990

118.   Levin NW, Zasuwa GA, Dumler F: Effect of membrane type on causes of death in hemodialysis patients. (Abstract) *Am Soc Nephrol* 2: 335, 1991

119.   Pollak VE, Kant S, Pesce A: A recent decrease in the dialysis case fatality rate: Is there an explanation? (Abstract) *Am Soc Nephrol* 2: 345, 1991

120.   DeOreo PB: Analysis of time, nutrition, and Kt/V as risk factors for mortality in dialysis patients. (Abstract) *Am Soc Nephrol* 2: 321, 1991

121.   Martin-Malo A, Castillo D: Adequacy of dialysis: is it really determined by the type of membrane and buffer? (Abstract) *Proc Eur Dial Transplant Assoc* 147, 1993

122.   Hakim RM, Stannard D, Port FK, Held PJ: The effect of the dialysis membrane on mortality of chronic hemodialysis patients. (Abstract) *Am Soc Nephrol* 5: 451, 1994

123. Hakim RM, Wingard RL, Ikizler TA et al.: Interrelationships of dialyzer biocompatibility with nutritional parameters. (Abstract) *Am Soc Nephrol* 5: 451, 1994

124. Vanholder RC, DeSmet RV, Ringoir SM: Assessment of urea and other uremic markers for quantification of dialysis efficacy. *Clin Chem* 38: 1429, 1992

125. Bassingthwaighte JB, Noodleman L, van der Vusse G, Little SE, Glatz JFC, Reneman RS: Albumin-facty-acid-endothelial membrane interactions and fatty acid transport in the heart. *Fed Proc* 46: 686, 1987

126. Besseghir K, Mosig D, Roch-Ramel F: Facilitation by serum albumin of renal tubular secretion of organic anions. *Am J Physiol* 256: F475, 1989

127. Gulyassy PF, Depner TA, Shearer GC: Comparison of binding by concentrated peritoneal dialysate and serum. *ASAIO J* 39: M569, 1993

128. Morachiello P, Ladini S, Fracasso A et al.: Combined hemodialysis-hemoperfusion in the treatment of secondary hyperparathyroidism of uremic patients. *Biochem Pharmacol* 9: 148, 1991

129. Stange J, Ramlow W, Mitzner S, Schmidt R, Klinkmann H: Dialysis against a recycled albumin solution enalbes the removal of albumin-bound toxins. *Artif Organs* 17: 809, 1993

130. Charra B: Importance of hypertension to survival on long dialysis. Personal communication, 1994

131. Babb AL, Popovich RP, Christopher TC, Scribner BH: The genesis of the middle molecule hypothesis. *Trans Am Soc Artif Intern Organs* 17: 81, 1971

132. Charra B, Laurent G, Calemard E et al.: Survival in dialysis and blood pressure control. *Contrib Nephrol* 106: 179, 1994

133. Luik A, Charra B, Katzarski K et al.: Blood pressure control and fluid state in patients on long treatment time dialysis. (Abstract) *Am Soc Nephrol* 5: 521, 1994

134. von Albertini B, Miller JH, Gardner PW, Shinaberger JH: Performance charactreristics of high flux haemodiafiltration. *Proc Eur Dial Transplant Assoc* 21: 447, 1985

135. Velasquez MT, von Albertini B, Lew SQ, Moore J, Bosch JP: Shorter treatment time with adequate highly efficient hemodialysis is not associated with higher incidence of hypertension in ESRD patients. (Abstract) *Am Soc Nephrol* 5: 532, 1994

136. Gennari FJ, Rimmer JM: Acid-base disorders in end-stage renal disease. *Semin Dial* 3: 81, 1990

137. Heineken FG: Brady-Smith M, Haynie J, Van Stone JC: Prescribing dialysate bicarbonate concentrations for hemodialysis patients. *Int J Artif Organs* 11: 45, 1988

138. Thews O, Hutten H: A comprehensive model of the dynamic exchange processes during hemodialysis. *Med Prog Technol* 16: 145, 1990

139. Bushinsky DA, Lam BC, Nespeca R, Sessler NE, Grynpas MD: Decreased bone carbonate content in response to metabolic, but not respiratory, acidosis. *Am J Physiol* 265: F530, 1993

140. Mitch WE, May RC, Maroni BJ, Druml W: Protein and amino acid metabolism in uremia: influence of metabolic acidosis. *Kidney Int* 27 (Suppl): S205, 1989

141. Oettinger CW, Oliver JC: Normalization of uremic acidosis in hemodialysis patients with a high bicarbonate dialysate. *Am Soc Nephrol* 3: 1804, 1993

142. Schneditz D, Holzer H, Daugirdas JT: A nomogram approach to estimate equilibrated post-dialysis BUN and whole-body (2-pool) Kt/V in hemodialysis. *Proc Eur Dial Transplant Assoc-Eur Renal Assoc* 213, 1994

143. Foley RJ et al.: Left ventricular hypertrophy in dialysis patients. *Semin Dial* 5: 34, 1992

144. Zager P, Campbell M, Skipper B et al.: Effect of blood pressure on mortality in hemodialysis patients. (Abstract) *Am Soc Nephrol* 5: 534, 1994

145. Lowrie EG, Laird NM: Cooperative dialysis study. *Kidney Int* 23: S1, 1983

146. Boen ST, Haagsman-Schouten WAG, Birnie RJ: Long-term peritoneal dialysis and a peritoneal dialysis-index. *Dial Transplant* 7: 377, 1978

147. Teehan BP, Schleifer CR, Sigler MH, Gilgore GS: A quantitative approach to the CAPD prescription. *Perit Dial Bull* 5: 152, 1985

148. Blumenkrantz MJ, Kopple HD, Moran JK: Coburn JW: Metabolic balance studies and dietary protein requirements in patients undergoing continuous ambulatory peritoneal dialysis. *Kidney Int* 21: 849, 1982

149. Lysaght MJ, Pollock CA, Hallet MD, Ibels LS, Farrell PC: The relevance of urea kinetic modeling to CAPD. *Trans Am Soc Artif Intern Organs* 35: 784, 1989

150. Tattersall JE, Doyle S, Greenwood RN, Farrington K: Kinetic modelling and underdialysis in CAPD patients. *Nephrol Dial Transplant* 8: 535, 1993

151. Selgas R, Bajo MA, Fernandez-Reyes MJ, Bosque E, Lopez-Revuelta K, Jimenez C, Borrego F, de Alvaro F: An analysis of adequacy of dialysis in a selected population on CAPD for over 3 years: the influence of urea and creatinine kinetics. *Nephrol Dial Transplant* 8: 1244, 1993

152. Keshaviah PR, Nolph KD, Van Stone JC: The peak concentration hypothesis: a urea kinetic approach to comparing the adequacy of continuous ambulatory peritoneal dialysis (CAPD) and hemodialysis. *Perit Dial Int* 9: 257, 1989

153. Teehan BP, Schleifer CR, Brown JM, Sigler MH, Raimondo J: Urea kinetic analysis and clinical outcome on CAPD. A five year longitudinal study. *Adv Perit Dial* 6: 181, 1990

154. Blake PG, Sombolos K, Abraham G, Weissgarten J, Pemberton R, Chu GL, Oreopoulos DG: Lack of correlation between urea kinetic indices and clinical outcomes in patients on continuous ambulatory peritoneal dialysis. *Kidney Int* 39: 700, 1991

155. Brandes JC, Piering WF, Beres JA, Blumenthal SS, Fritsche C: Clinical outcome of continuous ambulatory peritoneal dialysis predicted by urea and creatinine kinetics. *Am Soc Nephrol* 2: 1430, 1992

156. Keshaviah PR, Nolph KD, Prowant B, Moore H, Ponferrada L, Van Stone J, Twardowski ZJ, Khanna R: Defining adequacy of CAPD with urea kinetics. *Adv Perit Dial* 6: 173, 1990

157. Goodship THJ, Ward MK, Wilkinson R: Urea kinetic modelling (UKM) and nutritional status in CAPD. *Am Soc Nephrol* 2: 361, 1991

158. Lameire NH, Vanholder R, Veyt D, Lambert MC, Ringoir S: A longitudinal, five year survey of urea kinetic parameters in CAPD patients. *Kidney Int* 42: 426, 1992

159. Blake PG, Balaskas E, Blake R, Oreopoulos DG: Urea kinetics has limited relevance in assessing adequacy of dialysis in CAPD. *Adv Perit Dial* 8: 65, 1992

654   *Peter Blake and John Daugirdas*

160. Soreide R, Dracup B, Svarstad E, Iversen BM: Increased total body fat during PD treatment. *Adv Perit Dial* 8: 173, 1992

161. Keshaviah PR: Presentation at 14th Annual Conference on Peritoneal Dialysis, Orlando, January 1994

162. Schmidt R, Dumler F, Cruz C: Indirect measures of total body water may confound precise assessment of peritoneal dialysis adequacy. *Perit Dial Int* 13 (Suppl 2): S224, 1993

163. Odar-Cederlof I, Ericsson F, Eriksson CG, Kjellstrand CM: Oral antipyrin, a simple, accurate and non-bloody way of measuring total body water in hemodialysis patients. *Am Soc Nephrol* 2: 342, 1991

164. Dumler F, Schmidt R, Cruz C: Abbreviated method for urea kinetic modeling in continuous ambulatory peritoneal dialysis patients. *Perit Dial Int* 13 (Suppl 2): S50, 1993

165. Burkart JM, Jordan JR, Rocco MV: Assessment of dialysis dose by measured clearance *versus* extrapolated data. *Perit Dial Int* 13: 184, 1993

166. Bergstrom J, Furst P, Alvestrand A, Lindholm B: Protein and energy intake, nitrogen balance and nitrogen losses in patients treated with continuous ambulatory peritoneal dialysis. *Kidney Int* 44: 1048, 1993

167. Randerson DH, Chapman GV, Farrell PC: Amino acid and dietary status in long-term CAPD patients. in *Peritoneal Dialysis*, edited by Atkins RC, Farrell PC, Thomson N, Edinburgh, Churchill-Livingstone, 1981, p 171

168. Borah MH, Schoenfeld PY, Gotch FA, Sargent JA, Wolson M, Humphreys MH: Nitrogen balance during intermittent dialysis therapy of uremia. *Kidney Int* 14: 491, 1978

169. Kjeldahl J: Neue Methode zur Bestimmung des Stickstoffs in organischen Körpers. *Z Analyt Chem* 22: 366, 1883

170. Keshaviah PR, Nolph KD: Protein catabolic rate calculations in CAPD patients. *Trans Am Soc Artif Intern Organs* 37: M400, 1991

171. Harty JC, Boulton H, Curwell J, Heelis N, Uttley L, Venning MC, Gokal R: The normalized protein catabolic rate is a flawed marker of nutrition in CAPD patients. *Kidney Int* 45: 103, 1994

172. Burton PR, Walls J: Selection-adjusted comparison of life expectancy of patients on continuous ambulatory peritoneal dialysis, haemodialysis and renal transplantation. *Lancet* 1: 1115, 1997

173. Posen G, Arbus G, Hutchinson T, Jeffery J: Survival comparison of adult non diabetic patients treated with either hemodialysis or CAPD for end-stage renal failure. *Perit Dial Bull* 7: 78, 1987

174. Maiorca R, Cancarini G, Manili L, Camerini C, Brunori G: Life table analysis of patient and method survival in continuous ambulatory peritoneal dialysis and hemodialysis after six years' experience. in *Advances in CAPD*, edited by Khanna R, Nolph KD, Prowant B et al., Toronto, University of Toronto Press, 1986, p 27

175. US Renal Data System: USRDS 1991 Annual Data Report, The National Institute of Health, National Institutes of Diabetes and Digestive and Kidney Diseases, Bethesda, MD, 1991

176. Lunde NM, Port FK, Wolfe RA, Guire KE: Comparison of mortality risk by choice of CAPD *versus* hemodialysis among elderly patients. *Adv Perit Dial* 7: 68, 1991

177. Nelson CB, Port FK: Dialysis patient survival: evaluation of CAPD vs HD using 3 techniques. *Perit Dial Int* (Suppl 1): 144, 1992

178. Depner TA: Quantifying hemodialysis and peritoneal dialysis: examination of the Peak Concentration Hypothesis. *Semin Dial* 7: 315, 1994

179. Rottembourg J, Issad B, Gallego JL et al.: Evolution of residual renal functions in patients undergoing maintenance hemodialysis or continuous ambulatory peritoneal dialysis. *Proc Eur Dial Transplant Assoc* 19: 397, 1982

180. Cancarini GC, Brunori G, Camerini C, Brasa S, Manili L, Maiorca R: Renal function recovery and maintenance of residual diuresis in CAPD and hemodialysis. *Perit Dial Bull* 6: 76, 1986

181. Ballardie F, Kerr D, Tennent G et al.: Haemodialysis *versus* CAPD: equal predisposition to amyloidosis? *Lancet* 1: 793, 1986

182. Keshaviah P: Urea kinetic and middle molecule approaches to assessing the adequacy of hemodialysis and CAPD. *Kidney Int* 43 (Suppl 40): S28, 1993

183. Mitch WE, Jurkovita C, England BK: Mechanisms that cause protein and amino acid metabolism in uremia. *Am J Kidney Dis* 91, 1993

184. Hakim RM: Clinical implications of hemodialysis membrane biocompatibility. *Kidney Int* 44: 484, 1993

185. Lindholm B, Bergstrom J: Nutritional aspects of peritoneal dialysis. *Kidney Int* 42 (Suppl 38): S165, 1992

186. Blake PG: Problems predicting continuous ambulatory peritoneal dialysis outcomes with small solute clearances. *Perit Dial Int* 13 (Suppl 2): S209, 1993

187. Teehan BP, Schleifer CR, Brown J: Urea kinetic modeling is an appropriate assessment of adequacy. *Semin Dial* 5: 189, 1992

188. Goodship THJ, Passlick-Deetjen J, Ward MK, Wilkinson R: Adequacy of dialysis and nutritional status in CAPD. *Nephrol Dial Transplant* 8: 1366, 1993

189. Churchill DN, Thorpe K, Taylor DW, Keshaviah P: Adequacy of peritoneal dialysis. *Am Soc Nephrol* 5: 439, 1994

190. Cruz C, Dumler F, Schmidt R, Gotch F: Enhanced peritoneal dialysis delivery with PD-Plus™. *Adv Perit Dial* 8: 288, 1992

191. Keen M, Lipps B, Gotch F: The measured creatinine generation rate in CAPD suggests only 78% of prescribed dialysis is delivered. *Adv Perit Dial* 9: 73, 1993

192. Warren PJ, Brandes JC: Compliance with the peritoneal dialysis prescription is poor. *Am Soc Nephrol* 4: 1627, 1994

193. Bergstrom J, Alvestrand A, Lindholm B, Tranacus A: Relationship between KT/V and protein catabolic rate is different in continuous peritoneal dialysis and haemodialysis patients. *Am Soc Nephrol* 2: 358, 1991

194. Harty JC, Farragher B, Boulton H et al.: Is the correlation between the normalised protein catabolic rate (NPCR) and Kt/V the result of mathematical coupling? *Am Soc Nephrol* 4: 407, 1993

195. Gotch FA: Dependence of normalized protein catabolic rate on Kt/V in continuous ambulatory peritoneal dialysis: not a mathematical artifact. *Perit Dial Int* 13: 173, 1993

196. Stein A, Walls J: The correlation between Kt/V and protein catabolic rate — a self-fulfilling prophecy. *Nephrol Dial Transplant* 9: 743, 1994

197. Blake PG: Dependence of normalized protein catabolic rate on Kt/V in CAPD: not a mathematical artifact. *Perit Dial Int* 14: 405, 1994

198. Lindsay RM, Spanner E, Heidenheim P, Kortas C, Blake PG: PCR, Kt/V and membrane. *Kidney Int* 43 (Suppl 1): S268, 1993

199. Blake PG, Lindsay RM, Spanner E, Heidenheim P, Baird J, Allison M, Oreopoulos DG: Factors modifying the relationship between Kt/V urea and normalized protein catabolic rate (PCRN) in CAPD. *Am Soc Nephrol* 4: 398, 1993

200. Ronco C, Conz P, Agostini F, Bosch JP, Lew SQ, La Greca G: The concept of adequacy in peritoneal dialysis. *Perit Dial Int* 14: S93, 1994

201. Twardowski ZJ, Nolph KD: Peritoneal dialysis: how much is enough? *Semin Dial* 1: 75, 1988

202. Twardowski ZJ, Nolph KD, Khanna R et al.: Peritoneal equilibration test. *Perit Dial Bull* 7: 138, 1987

203. Blake PG, Balaskas EV, Izatt S, Oreopoulos DG: Is total creatinine clearance a good predictor of clinical outcomes in continuous ambulatory peritoneal dialysis? *Perit Dial Int* 12: 353, 1992

204. Larpent L, Verger C: The need for using an enzymatic colorimetric assay in creatinine determination of peritoneal dialysis solutions. *Perit Dial Int* 10: 89, 1990

205. Nolph KD, Moore HL, Twardowski ZJ et al.: Cross-sectional assessment of weekly urea and creatinine clearances in patients on continuous ambulatory peritoneal dialysis. *Trans Am Soc Artif Intern Organs* 38: M139, 1992

206. du Bois D, du Bois EF: A formula to estimate the approximate surface area if height and weight be known. *Arch Intern Med* 17: 863, 1916

207. Keshaviah PR, Nolph KD, Moore HL, Prowant B, Emerson PF, Meyer M, Twardowski ZJ, Khanna R, Ponferrada L, Collins A: Lean body mass estimation by creatinine kinetics. *Am Soc Nephrol* 4: 1475, 1994

208. Mitch WE, Collier VU, Walser M: Creatinine metabolism in chronic renal failure. *Clin Sci* 58: 327, 1980

209. Brandes JC, Piering WF, Beres JA: A method to assess efficacy of CAPD: preliminary results. *Adv Perit Dial* 6: 192, 1990

210. Rocco MV, Burkart JM: The efficacy number as a predictor of morbidity and mortality in peritoneal dialysis patients. *Am Soc Nephrol* 4: 1184, 1993

211. Nolph KD, Twardowski ZJ, Keshaviah PR: Weekly clearances of urea and creatinine on CAPD and NIPD. *Perit Dial Int* 12: 298, 1992

212. Holley JL, Piraino B: Careful patient selection and dialysis prescription are required for effective nightly intermittent peritoneal dialysis. *Perit Dial Int* 14: 155, 1994

213. Piraino B, Bender F, Bernardini J: A comparison of clearances on tidal peritoneal dialysis and intermittent peritoneal dialysis. *Perit Dial Int* 24: 145, 1994

214. Balaskas E, Izatt S, Chu M, Oreopoulos DG: Tidal volume peritoneal dialysis (TVPD) *versus* intermittent peritoneal dialysis. *Perit Dial Int* 3 (Suppl): S65, 1993

215. Verger C, Larpent L, Dumontet M: Prognostic values of peritoneal equilibration curves in CAPD patients. in *Frontiers in Peritoneal Dialysis*, edited by Maher JF, Winchester JF, New York, Field, Rich and Assoc Inc, 1986, p 88

216. Heimburger O, Waniewski J, Werynski A, Sun Park M, Lindholm B: Dialysate to plasma solute concentration (D/P) *versus* peritoneal transport parameters in CAPD. *Nephrol Dial Transplant* 9: 47, 1994

217. Blake PG, Flowerdew G, Blake RM, Oreopoulos DG: Serum albumin in patients on continuous ambulatory peritoneal dialysis – predictors and correlations with outcomes. *Am Soc Nephrol* 3: 1501, 1993

218. Nolph KD, Moore HL, Prowant B, Twardowski ZJ, Khanna R, Camboa S, Keshaviah P: Continuous ambulatory peritoneal dialysis with a high flux membrane. *ASAIO J* 39: 904, 1993

219. Blake PG, Sombolos K, Izatt S, Oreopoulos DG: A highly permeable membrane is an adverse risk factor in CAPD. *Clin Invest Med* 14 (Suppl): 792, 1991

220. Blake PG, Abraham G, Sombolos K, Izatt S, Weissgarten J, Ayiomamitis A, Oreopoulos DG: Changes in peritoneal membrane transport rates in patients on long term CAPD. *Adv Perit Dial* 5: 3, 1989

221. Passlick-Deetjen J, Chlebowski H, Koch M, Grabensee B: Changes of peritoneal membrane function during long-term CAPD. *Adv Perit Dial* 6: 35, 1990

222. Lo W-K, Brendolan A, Prowant BF, Moore HL, Khanna R, Twardowski ZJ, Nolph KD: Changes in the peritoneal equilibration test in selected chronic peritoneal dialysis patients. *Am Soc Nephrol* 4: 1466, 1994

223. Rocco JR, Burkart JM: Changes in peritoneal tansport during the first month of peritoneal dialysis. *Perit Dial Int* 13: S77, 1993

224. Gotch F, Schoenfeld P, Gentile D: The peritoneal equilibration test is not a realistic measure of peritoneal clearance. *Am Soc Nephrol* 3: 361, 1992

225. Lindsay RM, Spanner E: The lower serum albumin does reflect nutritional status. *Semin Dial* 5: 215, 1992

226. Heimburger O, Bergstrom J, Lindholm B: Is serum albumin an index of nutritional status in continuous ambulatory peritoneal dialysis patients? *Perit Dial Int* 14: 108, 1994

227. Young GA, Kopple J, Lindholm B et al.: Nutritional assessment of CAPD patients: an international study. *Am J Kidney Dis* 17: 462, 1991

228. Fenton SA, Johnston N, Delmore T et al.: Nutritional assessment of continuous ambulatory peritoneal dialysis patients. *Trans Am Soc Artif Intern Organs* XXXIII: 650, 1987

229. Oreopoulos DG, Crassweller P, Katirtzoglou A et al.: Amino acids as an osmotic agent in CAPD. in *Continuous Ambulatory Peritoneal Dialysis*, edited by Legrain M, Amsterdam, Excerpta medica, 1979, p 335

230. Jones MR, Martis L, Algrim CE et al.: Amino acid solutions for CAPD; rationale and clinical experience. *Miner Electrolyte Metab* 18: 309, 1992

231. Bruno M, Bagnis C, Marangella M et al.: CAPD with an amino acid dialysis solution: a long-term, cross-over study. *Kidney Int* 35: 1189, 1989

232. Dombros NV, Prutis K, Tong M et al.: Six-month overnight intraperitoneal amino-acid infusion in continuous ambulatory peritoneal dialysis (CAPD) patients – no effect on nutritional status. *Perit Dial Int* 10: 79, 1990

233. Kalil R, Jones MR, Martis L, Blake P, Anderson H, Oreopoulos DG: Modification of amino acid peritoneal dialysis fluid to decrease risk of acidosis. *Perit Dial Int* 14: S14, 1994

234. Ikizler TA, Wingard RL, Breyer JA et al.: Short-term effects of recombinant human growth hormone in CAPD patients. *Kidney Int* 46: 1178, 1994

235. Kang DH, Lee SW, Kang SW et al.: Recombinant human growth hormone improved nutritional status of under-nourished adult CAPD patients. *Am Soc Nephrol* 5: 494, 1994

236. Kopple JD: The rationale for the use of growth hormone or insulin-like growth factor I in adult patients with renal failure. *Miner Electrolyte Metab* 18: 269, 1992

237. Blake PG: Growth hormone and malnutrition in dialysis patients. *Perit Dial Int* 15: 210, 1995

238. Fine RN: Stimulating growth in uremic children. *Kidney Int* 42: 188, 1992

PERITONEAL INFECTIONS, HERNIAS AND RELATED COMPLICATIONS

RAM GOKAL

Ever since the introduction of peritoneal dialysis in the management of renal failure, complications related to the technique, in particular peritonitis and access related problems, have bedevilled its wider use and acceptance. Even after the introduction of CAPD in 1976 (1) and the subsequent technical and other advances, these problems still remain the Achilles heel of peritoneal dialysis therapy. They account for considerable morbidity, hospitalisation and therapy change to haemodialysis and indeed remain pre-eminent areas of research to try and minimise these complications. This chapter addresses the topic of peritoneal infections (peritonitis, exit site and tunnel infections, sclerosing peritonitis) and hernia and related complications. Problems related to peritoneal access are addressed in a related chapter.

PERITONITIS

The frequent occurrence of peritonitis remains the major complication of peritoneal dialysis and up until very recently has hindered its development and acceptance. In the mid 40s Seligman and colleagues (2) reported a method of continuous peritoneal lavage for the treatment of acute renal failure; high incidence of infection and technical difficulties discouraged its use. Subsequent workers drew attention to the value of peritoneal dialysis in treatment of acute renal failure but it was not until the introduction of a nylon catheter, which allowed safe access to the peritoneal cavity (3, 4) that intermittent peritoneal dialysis became possible with infection rates of 5.2–7.5 episodes of peritonitis per patient year of treatment (5, 6). In 1964 Palmer et al. (7) tried to provide longterm intermittent peritoneal dialysis employing an indwelling silicon rubber irrigating catheter device, which Tenckhoff (8) later modified to its present form. This technique further reduced infection rates to 0.23 to 1.3 episodes of peritonitis per patient year (9–12).

Since the introduction of CAPD in 1976 and its subsequent dramatic increase in use, the problems of peritonitis became even more apparent. Employing bottled dialysate the pioneering workers initially reported incidence of peritonitis of 4.6 episodes per patient year (13). This technique was subsequently modified and the development of a simplified method utilising PD fluid in plastic bags by Oreopolous et al. contributed to a marked decrease in the frequency of peritonitis (14). This arrangement was more convenient for the patients and substantially reduced the number of manipulations of the catheter and therefore the infection rate. Subsequently, many workers using this technique reported rates of peritonitis varying from 1.2–6.3 episodes per patient year (15–17). However, these high rates of infection have been the major criticism of the procedure (18, 19), but with increasing control of infection, this technique has now become an accepted method for treating patients with endstage renal failure. This has been aided by changes in the connecting technique and of the transfer sets to catheter (titanium connector), long life tubing which requires less frequent tube changes and the introduction of the so called 'Y set' or disconnect systems (20, 21). The latter was first introduced in Italy with reported rates of peritonitis of an episode every 24–36 patient months. A multicentre study in Canada confirmed the results (22). This flush before fill method has now become widely accepted in its many variations (23) making it possible for the average unit to report an episode of peritonitis every two years. The United States Renal Data System (USRDS) reports that the time to first peritonitis of patients on a Y set was 20.6 months compared to the standard connection system where it was 11.4 months (24).

In spite of this, peritoneal infection still occurs at a rate 3–5 times higher than that observed amongst patients receiving intermittent peritoneal dialysis (IPD) (25). The reason for this difference is not quite clear but may be related to the decreased number of connections, and periods during the week when the abdomen is free of fluid with IPD, thus allowing host defence mechanisms to return back to 'normal'. Continuous cycling peritoneal dialysis (CCPD) and other automated peritoneal dialysis techniques (APD) have peritonitis rates in between CAPD and IPD (26).

Pathogenesis of peritonitis

The clinical aspects of peritonitis complicating the course of CAPD have been thoroughly analysed. Several features distinguish peritoneal infection from the classic picture of acute surgical peritonitis. First, peritoneal infection is a rare complication of abdominal surgery in spite of a constant contamination of the peritoneum by microorganisms. By contrast, peritonitis occurs readily amongst peritoneal dialysis patients, following apparently minor episodes of contamination (27). Secondly, due to the permanent bathing of the peritoneal dialysis fluid infection diffuses readily to the entire peritoneal cavity even though the initial process might seem localised. Toxic manifestations are unusual, fever is often lacking or moderate and early signs and symptoms may be mild and difficult to identify by the patients. In this respect very few blood cultures are positive in CAPD peritonitis whereas this may be so in up to 35% of episodes of surgical peritonitis. Finally, the repeated drainage of the peritoneal fluid offers a unique opportunity for the early detection of peritoneal inflammation and turbidity of the drain bag can be easily recognised by the patient and remains the earliest detector of a probable peritoneal infection. The direct access of the peritoneal cavity allows antibiotics to be given so as to act at the very site of the infection by adding antibiotics in adequate concentrations to the PD fluid. CAPD peritonitis certainly has a more benign prognosis than surgical peritonitis.

Improved bacteriological methods have permitted a better analysis of the microbiological aspects of peritoneal infections amongst CAPD patients (27). Predominance of skin commensals, particularly staphylococcus epidermidis, has been confirmed and progress in culture techniques has resulted in decreased incidence of 'sterile' or culture negative peritonitis. This has unmasked the pathogenic role of opportunistic organisms, providing the clinician with invaluable information as to the most appropriate decision concerning therapeutic strategies.

An increasing number of studies have approached the effect of CAPD on the local host defence mechanisms of the peritoneal cavity. The consequences of hyperosmolar acidic dialysis solution on the phagocytic function of intraperitoneal neutrophils and macrophages have been elucidated (28). These studies have deeply modified our approach to the management of peritonitis (29). A deficiency of opsonins in the peritoneal fluid was also shown to facilitate the occurrence of bacterial peritonitis in some patients (30).

Thus a better understanding of the pathophysiology of peritoneal infections during CAPD has led to the development of more effective measures for the prevention of peritonitis.

Definitions and clinical diagnosis of peritonitis in peritoneal dialysis

The constant presence of fluid in the peritoneal cavity has certainly modified the definition and clinical features of peritonitis in CAPD. A practical definition (31) of peritonitis requires the presence of two of the following criteria in any combination:

a: Presence of organisms on gram stain or subsequent culture of PD fluid.
b: Cloudy fluid (WBC greater than 100 cells, with greater than 50% neutrophils).
c: Symptoms of peritoneal inflammation.

In episodes of peritonitis, cloudiness of the dialysate effluent is almost invariably present (32). For practical purposes it should be seen as the earliest detector of peritoneal infection, which can be readily identified by the patient even in the absence of abdominal pain. Turbidity can be seen with cell counts greater than 100 mm^3. The patients are usually told to report to the dialysis unit as soon as this is detected.

Signs and symptoms

Several series have now reported the presenting signs and symptoms of peritonitis (25, 32, 33). Cloudy dialysate effluent is almost invariably present (90% of patients) whilst abdominal pain was present in 80–95% of cases. It is mainly an acute pain, diffuse in nature but it sometimes is subtle and insidious, described as an abdominal discomfort, mild gas pain or muscle cramping. The gastrointestinal symptoms (nausea, vomiting, diarrhoea) range from 7–36% whilst chills were present in 12–23% of the cases.

Fever was often lacking and was recorded in only about one third of the cases whilst abdominal tenderness was present in 4 out of 5 cases, together with rebound tenderness in 60% of the patients. Other signs and symptoms include anorexia, malaise, the occurrence of drainage problems (about 15% of the cases), increased protein catabolic rate and dialysate protein losses (34, 35).

Cloudy bag

Among the various manifestations of peritonitis, a cloudy peritoneal effluent is almost a constant finding. This modification of the appearance of a drained dialysate is usually sudden; it is observed without gradation from one exchange draining clear fluid to the next showing a cloudy effluent. The turbidity of the peritoneal effluent may not be easy to recognise at a glance. The patient should learn how to identify even the slight opalescence of the drain bag by bringing it before a light. As shown in Table 1, which lists the causes of a cloudy dialysate drainage, the observation of a cloudy dialysate is not synonymous with peritonitis. The differential diagnosis should be made with peritoneal eosinophilia, neutrophilia, intraperitoneal bleeding and the presence of fibrin in the peritoneal effluent.

Table 1. Causes of a cloudy bag

Infectious peritonitis
Peritoneal fluid eosinophilia
Blood tinged dialysate
Fibrin filaments
Chylous
Intra-abdominal pathologies (Cholecystitis, pancreatitis, appendicitis, saplingitis)
Diarrhoea

Absolute cell count

The use of routine absolute and differential cell count has been advocated as a useful tool in the clinical diagnosis and management of peritonitis during CAPD (25). Several studies on the cellularity of the peritoneal effluent collected in asymptomatic, uninfected CAPD patients demonstrate few cells, the mean count ranging from 11–36/mm^3. With white cell counts higher than 50/mm^3, a slight degree of opalescence is usual and cloudiness is invariably found when the cell count is greater than 100 cell/mm^3 (25). Occasionally, in the patients who complain of abdominal pain and present with clear peritoneal fluid and cell count between 50 and 100 mm, it has been found that the fluid can subsequently become cloudy and that the fluid can be positive for organisms (25). This confirms the fact that bacteria may be present in the peritoneal cavity 24–48 hours before the development of a cloudy dialysate and this has been shown elegantly by prospective studies from Betjes et al. (37), who in addition shows that malfunctioning of phagocytosis by peritoneal macrophages may contribute to the development of CAPD peritonitis.

Differential diagnosis

Peritoneal eosinophilia syndrome. The syndrome of peritoneal eosinophilia is not frequent, is observed in the early stages of CAPD (39) and by definition, cloudy fluid is always present. In contrast with infectious peritonitis, peritoneal eosinophilia is not associated with abdominal pain and is relatively asymptomatic (38). Dialysate white cell count gives values ranging from 10%, reaching values of 95%. Repeated cultures of the peritoneal fluid dialysis are persistently negative. The clinical course is characterised by the rapid clearing of the dialysis effluent after a few days. There appears to be a close association of eosinophils with hypersensitivity reactions which suggests a role for some allergenic substances brought into the peritoneal cavity by CAPD procedures (40). Specific therapy is not indicated although at times intraperitoneal hydrocortisone is necessary (41).

Other diagnoses that need to be considered are listed in Table 1.

Clinical course of peritonitis

The incubation period of peritonitis is not well known but it is estimated from touch contamination incidents as well as prospective studies that this is usually 24–48 hours. The appearance of the symptoms may be very rapid (27). In most cases of peritonitis the symptoms decrease rapidly after the initiation of therapy and disappear within two to three days. During this period the cell counts decrease and the bacterial cultures become negative. In the majority of the cases, positive peritoneal cultures are present only for three to four days (25). Persistence of symptoms is indicative of a complicated cause or a possible resistant organism which is not responding well to antibiotics used; these require further investigation and possible catheter removal.

Relapse, recurrence or reinfection

These concepts are not well defined in the peritoneal dialysis population. *Relapse* is the reappearance of symptoms, the appearance of positive cultures after cultures have become negative or an increase of neutrophils in the peritoneal dialysis fluid after they have declined. It indicates either inadequate treatment or possibly the opening of an abscess cavity which was previously inaccessible to treatment. *Recurrence* is the term used of reappearance of symptoms of infection, after the therapy has been stopped within a four week period. It indicates either inadequate therapy or the presence of an endogenous focus (like exit site or tunnel infection) from which seeding has occurred. *Reinfection* is a new peritonitis episode beyond the four week period either with the same organism or a different organism. If reinfection happens with the same organism as before an internal focus should be suspected. The debate about what constitutes reinfection or relapse continues even after clinical criteria and typing methods are used (301).

Portals for entry of organisms to peritoneal cavity

There exists a delicate balance between the invaders that gain access into the peritoneal cavity and the host defence mechanisms that are present to counteract such invasion. In the intact abdomen the occasional penetrations of organisms are appropriately dealt with by such mechanisms; this is probably a frequent event but only rarely does it lead to major infections. The situation is different for peritoneal dialysis patients. It is well known that penetration of infectious organisms into the peritoneal cavity is more frequent than the episodes of peritonitis (42, 43). The host defence mechanisms are thought to be impaired in peritoneal dialysis and hence peritonitis rates will be much higher in patients undergoing peritoneal dialysis. Since the conditions that lead to peritonitis are not known, all portals of entry have to be considered seriously in order to reduce peritonitis incidence.

Surveillance cultures from abdominal skin site, throat and hands done on peritoneal dialysis patients before they

Table 2. Routes of infection in CAPD patients

Route	Organism	%
Exogenous		
Transluminal (Endoluminal catheter contamination)	S. Epidermidis Acinetobacter	3–40
Perluminal (skin exit of tunnel)	S. Epidermidis S. Aureus Pseudomonas Yeasts	20–30
Endogenous		
Transmural (bowel perforation)	Enteric gram negative Anaerobes	25–30
Haematogenous	Streptococcus Anaerobes	5–10
Ascending (female genital tract)	Yeasts Lactobacillus	2–5

enter a dialysis programme have been undertaken (33). These are the areas from which incidental contamination of peritoneal dialysis patients can occur. Such studies show that the patients are at high risk from their own flora rather than acquiring infections from the environment or other people (44). It is therefore possible to generate a probable listing which estimates the probable route of entry from the type of organisms isolated (Table 2). The main pathways for the introduction of infecting organisms to the peritoneal cavity are listed in Table 3.

Exogenous infections

Transluminal or endoluminal contamination through the catheter lumen is the most common portal of entry for organisms in peritoneal dialysis. Most of these develop after accidental touch contamination of the connector site or disconnection of the dialysis tubing, which based on three to four exchanges per day, have to be done up to 1500 times each year. Contamination even in the best trained patient must occur (45). Airborne contamination by infected skin scales has also been suggested, skin scales contain viable bacteria and are attracted to plastic surfaces by electrostatic charges, the chances of contamination increasing with the exposure time (46, 47). Other cases are given in Table 3.

Exogenous contamination across the abdominal wall usually entails infection of the catheter exit site or tunnel. The

Table 3. Possible portals of entry for infection of the peritoneal cavity

---

1. Exogenous – through lumen of catheter (Transluminal)
   Bag exchange (25, 33, 44, 45)
   Transfer set exchange (25, 33, 36)
   Injection of drugs
   Airborne contamination (40, 47)
   Defective PD systems (53)
   Accidental disconnections
   Infected PD fluid (54)
   Water borne infection (52)

2. Exogenous – through abdominal wall (Perluminal)
   Exit site infection (48, 55)
   Cuff and tunnel infection (48, 55)
   Water borne infections (52)

3. Endogenous
   Transcolonic migration of bacteria (50)
   Intra-abdominal infected viscera (51, 56)
   Haematogenous (36, 57)
   Female genital tract (58, 59, 60, 61)

4. Other routes
   ?Lymphatics

---

silastic catheter never forms a completely sealed junction with the skin or subcutaneous tissue and the cuffs (the purpose of which is to reduce the penetration of bacteria around the catheter) do not always achieve this goal. It is probably necessary for an infectious process to establish itself in the tissues of the exit site or subcutaneous tunnel to produce a peritoneal infection. Morphological studies on exit sites by Twardowski *et al.* (48) have raised many interesting possibilities on the development of exit site infections and subsequent peritonitis. Catheter infections occur in 9–20% of patients and the estimated incidence of peritonitis secondary to catheter infection ranges from 2–9% of peritonitis episodes (25, 49).

Endogenous infections

Transmural or intestinal infections are the major cause of most gram negative peritoneal infections. There is some evidence that bacteria may migrate through intact intestinal wall (50). Pre-existing diverticulosis in these patients may well be a constant source of intestinal leak (51). Environmental infections and factors may be important. Peritonitis from acinitobacter and other environmental bacteria has been observed (52). It is possible that these infections develop by contact with portals, either entering through the exit site or contamination of the catheter during exchange procedures.

Endogenous contamination via the blood stream as well as through the female genital tract is a well recognised but not a frequent cause of peritoneal infections. Streptococcal peritonitis has been described following dental treatment (57), while the female genital tract can be a source through retrograde menstruation (58), fluid leaks (59, 60) or intrauterine contraceptive devices (61).

Microbiological aspects

Infectious peritonitis during peritoneal dialysis results mainly from contamination of the peritoneal cavity by bacteria and, with lesser frequency, by fungi. The use of adequate bacteriologic techniques permits the isolation and identification of infecting organism in most cases of peritoneal infection and reduces the incidence of so called sterile or culture negative peritonitis. Most of peritonitis episodes are due to well recognised pathogens, but there is a growing list of peritoneal infections due to bacteria and fungi previously considered as part of the normal skin and digestive flora or as non-pathogenic environmental saprophytes (62).

Microbiological diagnosis of peritonitis

The two major steps for the identification of the causative agents of peritonitis are the microscopic examination of gram stain smears of the dialysis effluent and inoculation of culture media with the peritoneal fluid. Several studies deal with the conditions necessary for improved diagnosis in peritoneal dialysis peritonitis (27, 63, 67, 100). All these studies point to the importance of early cultures as soon as peritonitis is suspected, and the need for large volumes to be concentrated for improving the recovery rate as is the need to inject blood culture bottles. Finally identification and sensitivity testing needs to be done as soon as possible to achieve rational antibiotic therapy (67). Figure 1 depicts the standard diagnostic procedures to be performed in the bacteriological department to the infected fluid.

Gram stain and culture procedure

The gram stain from the sediment of the peritoneal dialysate bag establishes the presence of microorganisms in only about 20–30% of the cases. This is not a sufficiently sensitive test to permit rational therapy. However, gram staining may be helpful for the establishment of fungal peritonitis.

The microbiological culturing of peritoneal dialysis samples is of utmost importance in establishing a proper infective agent and hence appropriate antibiotic therapy (68). Both concentration methods and inoculation of blood culture media are important. Several reports have suggested the use of limulus lysate test for the diagnosis of gram negative peritonitis (69, 70), based on a sensitive demonstration of endotoxin which appears to correlate with gram negative peritonitis cases but it does

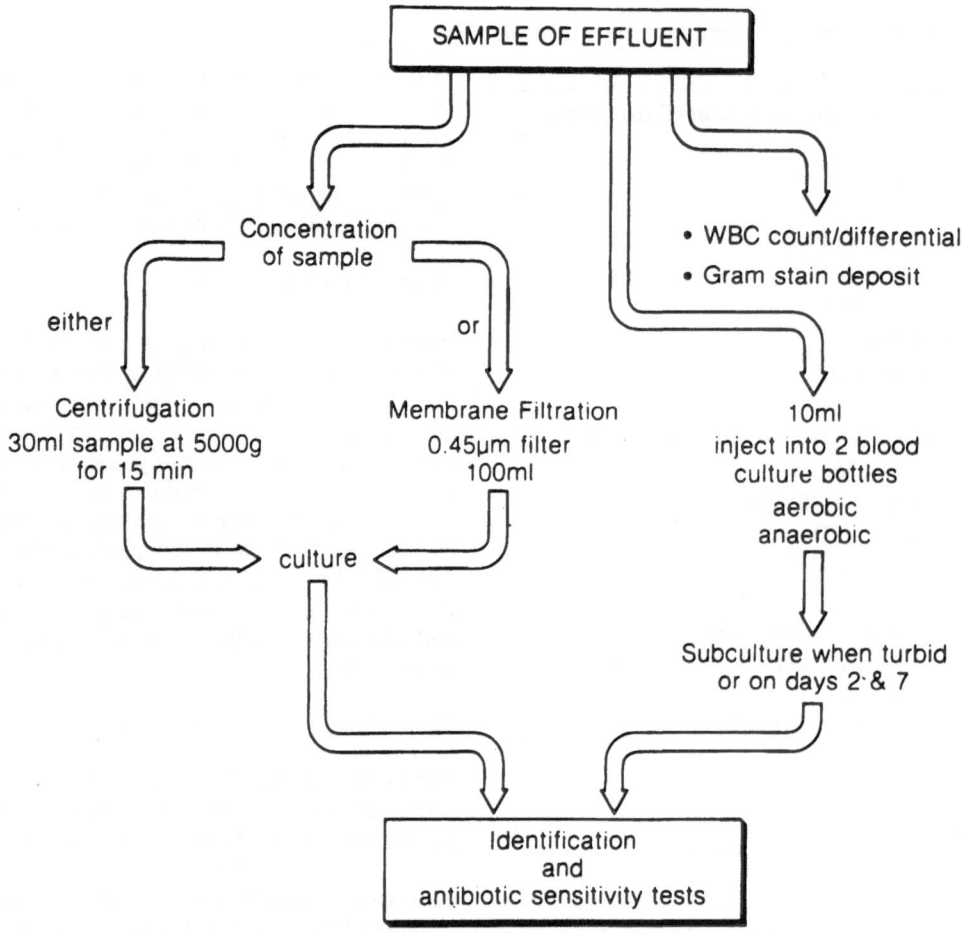

Figure 1. Flow diagram for bacteriological isolation of a causative organism in a sample of PD effluent. (From Ref. (25) with permission)

not seem to have made any roads into clinical practice. For concentration procedures the Addichek filtration, or Bactec methods are being used to good effect in many laboratories (71). The use of distilled water or Triton X to increase the yield by releasing intracellular organisms appear to show no advantage over the blood culture techniques (64). Antibiotic sensitivity testing is an essential part of the microbiological work up. It is important to be informed of local antibiotic sensitivity patterns of organisms since these vary from hospital to hospital.

Cell counts
Cell counts are routinely obtained from the first dialysis fluid and at regular intervals thereafter to follow the efficiency of therapy (72). Cytospin smears for differential cell counts help in judging the clinical course of peritonitis.

Causative organisms of peritoneal infection

The various micro-organisms isolated from infected peritoneal fluids are listed in Table 4. The most common organisms are gram positive (up to 70% of all episodes), gram negative bacteria (about 20% of all episodes) and yeasts (up to 5%). Anaerobic bacteria are less commonly involved and mycobacteria, higher bacteria and filamentous fungi are seldom encountered.

Gram positive organisms
Staphylococcus epidermidis is the most common coagulase negative staphylococcus isolated from these episodes although other biotypes have been identified (73). Staphylococcus epidermidis, one of 12 species of coagulase negative staphylococci is part of the normal skin flora. These may shed from various parts of the body, and the organism contaminates the air and the environmental surfaces.

Table 4. Bacteria isolated from infected peritoneal effluent in patients with peritonitis complicating CAPD

	Isolated bacteria	
	Common	*Uncommon*
I. Gram positive species bacteria	*Staphylococcus epidermis*	*Corynebacterium*
	Staphylococcus aureus	*Listeria monocytogenes*
	Streptococcus 'viridans'	
	Streptococcus fecalis (Group D Enterococcus)	
	Streptococcus species	
II. Gram negative bacteria	*Escherichia coli*	*Agrobacterium species*
	*Klebsiella/*Enterobacter*/ Serratia species*	*Alcaligenes species*
	Pseudomonas species	*Alteromonas purefaciens*
	Acinetobacter species	*Branhamella catarrhalis*
	Citrobacter species	*(Neisseria species)*
		Bordatella bronchiseptica
		Camptylobacter species
		Flavobacterium species
		Gardnerella vaginalis
		Haemophilis influenzae
		Pasteurella multocida
		Vibrio alginoliticus
III. Anaerobic bacteria	*Bacterioides fragilis*	*Clostrodium species*
		Fusobacterium species
		Proptionibacterium species
IV. Mycobacteria	*Mycobacterium tubercolis*	*Mycobacterium chelonei*
		Mycobacterium avisintracellulare
		Mycobacterium fortuituim
V. Yeasts	*Candida species*	*Rhodotorula rubra*
		Torulopsis glabatra
		Pytyrosporum species
		Cryptococcus neoformans
VI. Other fungi	*Fusarium species*	Alternaria alternata
		Aspergillus fumigatus
		Coccidioides immitis
		Dreschlera spicifera
		Exophiala jeanselmi
		Malassezia furfur
		Mucor species
		Penicillium species
		Trichosporum species

It remains viable for an extended time because of its resistance to drying and temperature changes. It seems uniquely adapted to adhere to smooth surfaces such as plastic and silastic where it produces a mucoid extra cellular polysaccharide slime substance (biofilm) that appears to facilitate the colonisation of plastic surfaces (74, 75). The main portal of entry into the peritoneal cavity is via the catheter lumen as tunnel infection with staphylococcus epidermidis is infrequent.

Staphylococcus aureus is a cause of about 10% of peritonitis and indeed a much more serious infliction than coagulase negative staphylococcus. Patients who develop this infection can be hypotensive, or in septic shock. Frequently they complain of extensive abdominal pain. Typically the clinical improvement is much slower than with staph epidermidis and sometimes residual abscesses are found (76). Staphylococcus aureus produces a host of toxins, a factor responsible for the most severe form of the infection in these patients (77, 78). Streptococcus species are isolated in 10–15% of bacterial peritonitis. The predominant species is Streptococcus viridans and it is speculated that they reach the peritoneum by haematogenous spread (27, 57).

Diptheroids are increasingly recognised in CAPD (79, 80). Corynebacterium species are commonly present on the skin and mucus membranes of normal subjects. No specific clinical or laboratory approach distinguishes these peritonitis episodes from other forms of peritoneal infection, except for a common association with inflammation and discharge of catheter skin exit site (80). The diagnosis and timely determination of antibiotic sensitivity are often delayed by the slow growth of the organisms.

Gram negative bacteria
Two major groups of gram negative bacteria are responsible for up to 20% of peritonitis episodes: the Enterobacteriacae and pseudomonas species. The latter are responsible for about 4–5% of peritoneal infections and can be associated with severe infections which are difficult to eradicate because like staphylococcus aureus there is a tendency to abscess formation and they are frequently resistant to common antibiotics (81). Pseudomonas peritonitis is also associated with the loss peritoneal cavity as well as ultrafiltration (82). The association of an exit site infection and peritonitis with pseudomonas has a bad prognosis and catheter removal is advocated (83). Anaerobic bacteria are held responsible for infection in up to 5% of peritonitis episodes (27). In spite of its rarity, anaerobic peritonitis deserves special mention because of its important diagnostic and therapeutic implications. Bowel perforation and faecal leakage is almost certain, whenever the peritoneal fluid is infected with bacteroides and/or clostridium species (25).

Mycobacterium tuberculosis is a rare cause of peritonitis among patients receiving peritoneal dialysis (84, 85). It necessitates a high index of suspicion for diagnosis and timely institution of adequate therapy (86). Non-tuberculous mycobacteria also cause peritonitis in peritoneal dialysis patients. Mycobacterium chelonei-like organisms, avis-intracellularis, and fortuitium were found to be the cause in peritonitis episodes in CAPD patients (25).

Fungi
Initially, considered as an uncommon cause of peritonitis, fungi are recognised today as an aetiological factor in about 5% of peritonitis episodes (27, 87, 88). A list of the varieties of yeasts and filamentous fungi isolated during fungal peritonitis is given in Table 4. Yeasts are the predominant organism, candida species being the most frequently encountered. They probably enter the peritoneal cavity intraluminally or periluminally, though in a few cases vaginal infection was considered the source. These infections are difficult to treat with anti fungal antibiotics (88) as these organisms are resistant to normal mechanism like phagocytic killing. Filamentous fungi rarely contaminate a catheter and cause peritoneal infection (87, 89). Since most filamentous fungi are resistant to anti fungal antibiotics, early catheter removal is necessary.

Host defence mechanisms of the peritoneal cavity

In order for contamination to progress to peritonitis, the first lines of host defence have to be overwhelmed. The macrophage is classically considered the primary component of first line defence. However, the concentration of macrophages, may not be sufficient to eradicate bacteria, especially if contamination is a result of a large inoculant. Besides the low number of cells in the peritoneal effluent, the unphysiological nature of peritoneal dialysis fluid, with its low pH and high osmolality, may interfere with white cell function (90, 91). If contamination of the peritoneal cavity goes unchecked, a dynamic process is set in motion, resulting in clinical peritonitis. Following microbial induced injury, a variety of chemotactic factors are released. These interactions cause white cells to emigrate out of circulation into the area of injury. Neutrophils from the peripheral blood arrive at the site of injury with a usual maximum response within hours, following the microbial insult.

Before a phagocyte can ingest bacteria, recognition must occur. Opsonisation of an antigenic surface involves C3b (complement aviation) and IgG antibody. Once coated with the opsonin, the micro-organism can therefore be recognised by binding to specific receptors for C3B or the FC fragment present on the cell surface of neutrophils or monocytes. Uninfected peritoneal dialysis effluent has about 1% of IgG and C3 levels as compared to serum (30). During episodes of peritonitis these levels increase secondary to the enhanced permeability of the peritoneal membrane.

Several studies have suggested that level of opsonic activity or IgG in dialysate are lower in patients with high incidence of peritonitis in particular due to staph epidermidis (30, 92, 93). These studies strongly implied that subjects with low levels of opsonin represent a high risk group. Similar results were obtained when measures of opsonic activity or C3 levels were assessed (92). However, more than half the patients classified into a high risk group did not develop this complication. Not all studies have been able to confirm these findings (94, 95). Anwar et al., in a prospective longitudinal study found no relationship to opsonin levels with respect to peritonitis episodes, the levels in a non-infected patients were variable and were not affected by an episode of peritonitis (95). It is thus not possible at start of CAPD to predict with any accuracy those that are more prone to peritonitis based on overnight effluent opsonic levels (98, 99).

Effect of dialysate on host defence is considerable. Firstly, there is a marked dilution effect on the number of macrophages and IgG concentrations such that there may be insufficient amounts of antibody, complement and cells present to act as effective combatant to the invading bacteria. In addition, to this dilutional effect, dialysate is directly toxic to phagocytes as well as mesothelial cells (28, 91, 96). A number of cell functions are affected which include cell viability, depression of phagocytic capacity, suppression of oxygen uptake and superoxide generation by macrophages and neutrophils. Several investigators have attempted to delineate the factors in commercial dialysate responsible for the depressed phagocytic function. Possible toxic constituents include the low pH, lactate, osmolality, glucose itself and any compounds produced by the heat sterilisation process (90). However, the full clinical significance of the deleterious effects of unused dialysate on cells *in vitro* remains uncertain, as *in vivo* the effect of pH and lactate are transient (96). It is more likely that impaired phagocytosis occurs for almost the entire CAPD cycle, particularly so if hyperosmolar fluids are being used (97). Though there is no doubt that unused dialysate can seriously impair a variety of host defences *in vitro*, the *in vivo* evidence is not conclusive.

Treatment of peritonitis

When peritonitis occurs in a patient on peritoneal dialysis, treatment should be started immediately after completion of the appropriate microbiological work up. However, treatment has to be initiated in the absence of appropriate diagnostic information and therefore certain arbitrary decisions have to be taken on the appropriateness of the antibiotic treatment based on the considerations presented above on causative organisms. Many protocols for antibiotic treatments have been proposed; however, there is an increasing consensus towards a standardised approach combining the continuation of CAPD with intraperitoneal administration of antibiotics (67, 100, 101).

Peritoneal lavage

The evidence of detrimental effect of fresh dialysis solution on local host defence mechanisms (28, 102) have convinced most Nephrologists to abandon prolonged rapid exchange peritoneal lavage in the management of peritoneal infection. However, after a few in and out exchanges, that remove inflammatory products and often relieve abdominal pain, CAPD is resumed with long dwell exchanges. In a study by Ejlersen et al. (103) the findings of poorer outcome in patients treated with 24 hours of initial lavage vindicates this policy. The dwell time has to be shortened in cases of difficulty with ultrafiltration as there is recognised increased permeability during an episode of peritonitis. Peritoneal lavage however, remains indicated in cases of faecal peritonitis with the presence of faeces in the peritoneal fluid.

Antibiotic regimes

The antibiotic selected for initial treatment should be effective against most frequently occurring organisms observed in peritonitis. The antibiotic sensitivity pattern of the organisms isolated from peritonitis episodes should be based on sensitivity of organisms prevalent in the hospital and hence close liaison with the microbiology department is essential.

Various modes of antibiotic administration have been recommended including intraperitoneal, intravenous, or oral routes. The intraperitoneal route is the most preferred one and if antibiotics are added to the dialysis fluid in each exchange, then the levels in the serum become equivalent to the dialysate concentration based on the 'steady state' principle. However, an alternative intraperitoneal approach is to use the antibiotics in an intermittent fashion which could be anything from alternate exchanges, to once a day, to once a week. Vancomycin administration of 1–2 g per exchange which is allowed to dwell for up to six hours is appropriate when administered once a week. This dosage provides adequate levels for the length of required treatment (104, 105). For aminoglycosides the principle of intermittent therapy is based on the fact that bactericidal action of aminoglycoside is proportionate to its concentration. In addition, after the application of the appropriate concentrations of the antibiotic, the majority of susceptible bacteria are killed while the remaining ones have an increased susceptibility to the antibiotic–'post antibiotic' effect (106). Based on this, once a day aminoglycoside therapy for a localised infection is feasible. This approach is more convenient and cheaper and reduces toxic side effects (107, 108).

Many antibiotics have been utilised in the management of CAPD patients. Whilst not all are utilised regularly the need to use some uncommon ones does occasionally arise. Hence a full list of antibiotics with their dosage as modified for peritoneal use is listed in Table 5.

Since no microbiological information is usually available at the start of treatment the first choice of antibiotics should cover the most frequent organism causing these infections. Most centres use Vancomycin as initial choice for gram positive cover, though Cepheloxin in appropriate dosage is still widely used. In addition, to cover the more threatening intestinal organisms the addition of an aminoglycoside or Ceftazidime is utilised. After the organisms have been identified and antibiotic sensitivity is available appropriate adjustments are made to the therapy.

Several expert committees have met and reviewed therapeutic recommendations (67, 100, 102). The Ad Hoc Advisory Committee on Peritonitis Management (67) reported recently on treatment recommendations. The recommendations are given in Figures 2, 3 and 4 representing management on clinical presentation of peritonitis (Figure 2). For *gram positive organisms* (Figure 3), staph aureus peritonitis is more serious and if identified and clinical improvement is not seen within 4–5 days, rifampicin should be added to the regimen and therapy continued for

Table 5. Pharmacokinetics of antibiotics in CAPD patients and proposed regimens for the treatment of CAPD peritonitis. (From Ref. (67) with permission)

	Half-life (H)				Dose (per 70 kg adult)[a] Maintenance dose	
	Normal	ESRD	CAPD	Initial dose (mg/2-L bag)	Intermittent mg/2-l bag per dosing interval	Continuous (mg/2-L bag)
Aminoglycosides						
Amikacin	1.6	39	40	500	120/d	12–24
Gentamicin	2.2	53	32	70–140	40/d	8–16
Netilmicin	2.1	42	18	70–140	40/d	8–16
Tobramycin	2.5	58	36	70–140	40/d	8–16
CeDnalosoorins						
First generation						
Cefazolin	2.2	28	30	500–1000	1000/d	250–500
Cefonicid	4.0	68	50	250	ND	50
Cephalothin	0.2	3.7	ND	1000	ND	200
Cephradine	0.9	12	ND	500	ND	250
Cephalexin	0.8	19	9	1000 PO	500/QID PO	NA
Second generation						
Cefamandole	1.0	10	8.0	1000	1000/d	500
Cefmenoxime	1.3	11.3	6.0	2000	1000/d	100
Cefoxitin	0.8	20	15	1000	ND	200
Cefuroxime	1.3	18	15	1000	400/d IV/PO	150–400
Third generation						
Cefixime	3.2	11.5	15	400 PO	400/d PO	NA
Cefoperazone	1.8	2.3	2.2	2000	ND	400–1000
Cefotaxime	0.9	2.5	2.4	2000	2000/d	500
Cefsulodin	0.8	11	11	1000	500/d	50
Ceftazidime	1.8	26	13	1000	1000/d	250
Ceftizoxime	1.6	28	11	1000	1000/d	250
Ceftriaxone	8.0	15	12	1000	1000/d	250–500
Moxalactam	2.2	20	16	1000	1000/d	350
Penicillins						
Aziocillin	0.9	5.1	ND	500	ND	500
Meziocillin	1.0	4.3	ND	3000 IV	3000/BID IV	500
Piperacillin	1.2	3.9	2.4	4000 IV	4000/BID IV	500
Ticarcillin	1.2	15	ND	1000–2000	2000/BID	250
Quinolones						
Ciprofloxacin	4.0	8.0	11	500 PO	500/TIP PO	50
Fleroxacin	13	27	27	800 PO	400/d PO	NA
Ofoxacin	7.0	30	25	400 PO	200/d PO	NA

three weeks (67, 109). For enterococci which are gram positive aminoglycoside in one exchange daily should be used in addition to the Vancomycin. However, for enterococcal infections, an intra-abdominal pathology should be sought and the possibility of the presence of other fas- tidious organism in the dialysate should also be considered. For the culture negative episodes (should not exceed more than 10% of all episodes) antibiotics at the initiation of the peritonitis episode are continued if there is clini-

Table 5. (Continued)

	Half-life (H)			Initial dose (mg/2-L bag)	Dose (per 70 kg adult)[a] Maintenance dose		
	Normal	ESRD	CAPD		Intermittent mg/2-l bag per dosing interval	Continuous (mg/2-L bag)	
Vancomycin and others							
Vancomycin	6.9	161	92	1000–2000	1–2000/7d	30–50	
Teicoplanin	50	260	260	400	400/BID	40°	
Aztreonam	2.0	7.0	9.3	1000	1000/d	500	
Clindamycin	2.8	2.8	ND	300	ND	300	
Erythromycin	2.1	4.0	ND	ND	500/QID PO	50	
Metronidazole	7.9	7.7	11	500 PO/IV	500/TID PO/IV	ND	
Minocycline	15.5	20	ND	NA	100/BID PO	NA	
Rifampin	4.0	8.0	ND	600 PO	600/d PO	NA	
Antifungal agents							
Amphotericin B	360	360	ND	NA	20–30/d IV	2–8	
Flucytosine	4.2	115	ND	2000–3000 PO	1000/d PO	NA	
Fluconazole	22	125	72	NA	150 mg g 2d	ND	
Ketoconazole	2.0	1.8	2.4	400 PO	200–800/d PO	NA	
Miconazole	24	25	ND	200	ND	100–200	

cal improvement. Duration of therapy should be for two weeks.

For gram negative micro-organisms outcome is usually reasonably good for E coli, Klebsiella and proteus (101): in these situations aminoglycoside alone or Ceftazidime alone should be used. Recently the use of fluoroquinolones has been advocated for either initial or gram negative peritonitis (110). However, the experience of this is not entirely satisfactory and certainly response to oral Ciprofloxacillin is not favourable nor is its efficacy against a number of gram positive infections (111, 112). If anaerobic organisms are isolated, either alone or in combination with other gram negative organisms, serious consideration should be given to surgical intervention, because of the likelihood of perforation.

If pseudomonas aeroginosa or xanthomonas organisms are identified, therapy with at least two agents that have activity against the micro-organisms should be used (Figure 4). Piperacillin, if used, needs to be used intravenously in order to minimise the effect of inactivation of the aminoglycoside by this class of semisynthetic penicillin. Clinical experience has shown that pseudomonas peritonitis in CAPD patients is extremely difficult to cure particularly when this develops as a result of exit site or tunnel related infection (113). Chan et al. (81) found in the 25 episodes of peritonitis from pseudomonas that Ceftazidime in combination with aminoglycosides was an effective regimen; oral ofloxicallin was not useful. Five of these patients required catheter removal. Taber et al. reported on the successful use of a combination of Ceftazidime and oral Ciprofloxacilin in the small case study of eleven exit site and seven peritonitis episodes with pseudomonas (115). They found this combination successful in conjunction with debridement of the external cuff. Whatever the antibiotic regime utilised, therapy is recommended for three to four weeks if the patient is clinically improving. Consequence of persistent gram negative peritonitis, particularly pseudomonas, on peritoneal membrane integrity over the long term is considerable; hence consideration of early catheter removal is vital to preserve peritoneal function. In addition avoidance of longterm treatment with potentially toxic antibiotics is also important (108, 116).

Fungal Organisms. Whilst initial reports suggested that catheter removal was the treatment of choice once these organisms were identified (100, 102), recent experience with newer imidazoles/triazoles and flucytosine have suggested that these agents can be reasonably efficacious without the need to resort immediately to catheter removal (Figure 2). Hence, the initial approach would be to manage yeast peritonitis with imidazole/triazoles and flucytosine combination and if clinical improvement does not occur after 4–7 days of therapy the catheter should be removed. Therapy with these agents should be continued after catheter removal orally with flucytosine and fluconazole for an additional 10 days (67). However, reports continue to show the outcome of fungal peritonitis is not particularly good (88, 101, 117). Successful prophylaxis for fungal peritonitis in CAPD patients has been described (114).

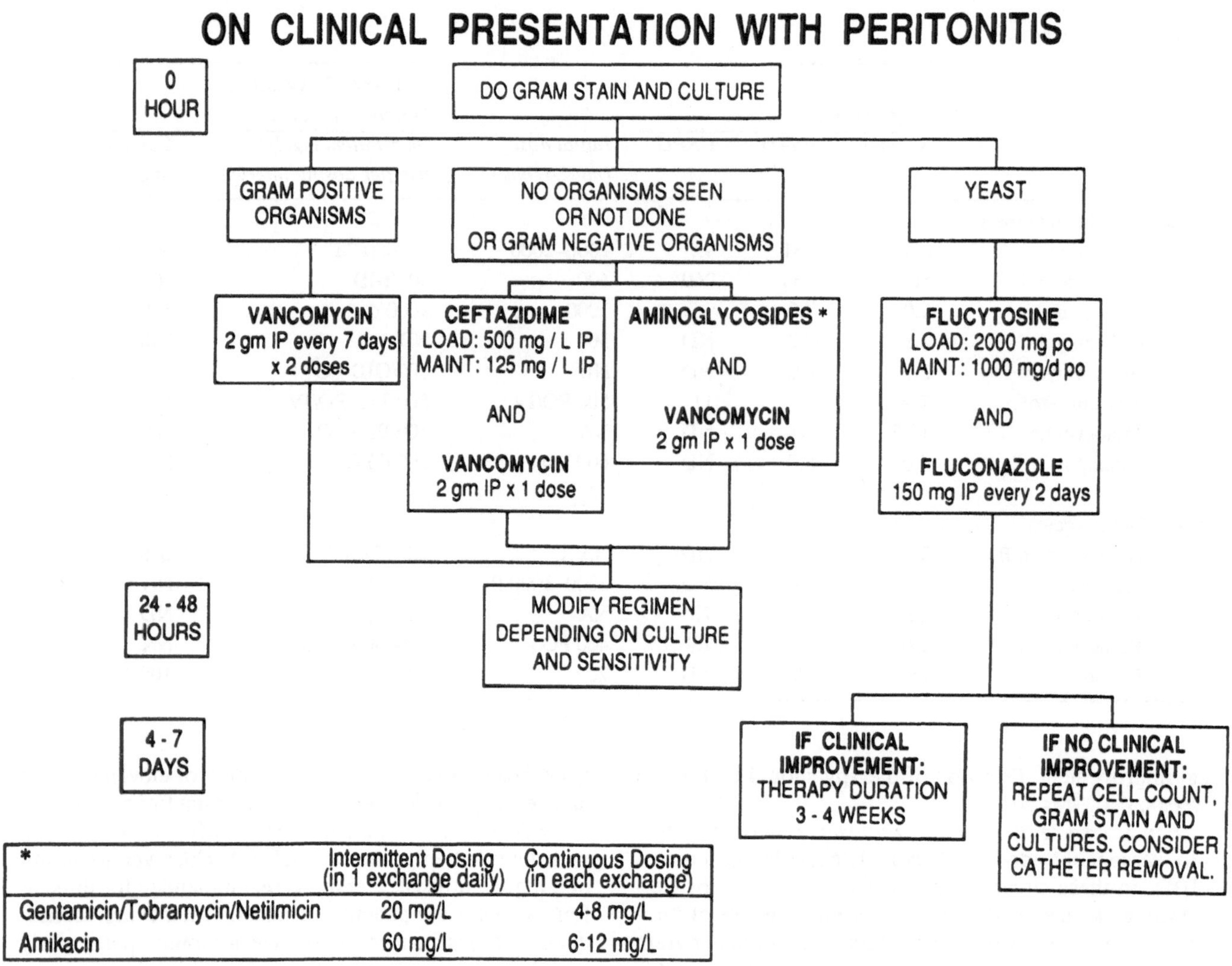

ON CLINICAL PRESENTATION WITH PERITONITIS

Figure 2. Treatment outline for managing Peritoneal Dialysis peritonitis on presentation – initial antibiotic selection. (From Ref. (67) with permission)

Other therapeutic approaches to peritonitis

Relapsing peritonitis

Relapsing infections with coagulase positive organisms should be treated with Vancomycin and Rifampicin for approximately four weeks. It enterococci are recultured Vancomycin and aminoglycosides should be used. Consideration here should also be given to an intra-abdominal abscess. Catheter removal is indicated if there is no improvement after 96 hours of therapy. If the patient responds clinically but subsequently relapses an additional time, catheter removal and replacement are recommended. Two relapses is an indication for catheter removal. If the relapsing peritonitis is caused by gram negative organisms an intra-abdominal abscess should be suspected and catheter removal and surgical exploration should be strongly considered.

Catheter removal and reinsertion

In certain circumstances of peritoneal infection, continuation of CAPD may become a hazard to the patient and catheter removal is essential. The indications for catheter removal during peritonitis are shown in Table 6. The optimum time between catheter removal for infection and reinsertion of a new catheter is not known and still controversial. A minimum of three weeks is recommended (67).

Recently several reports have indicated that refractory peritoneal dialysis infections or recurrent ones could be managed by catheter removal and insertion of a new one during the same operation (118, 119). Overall the success rate is reasonable but still leaves about 30–40% of cases requiring prolonged peritoneal rest after catheter removal. Some reports have advocated temporary discontinuation of peritoneal dialysis either in resistant or mild episodes of peritonitis (120, 121). This certainly has not

TREATMENT OF PERITONITIS — 1993 UPDATE

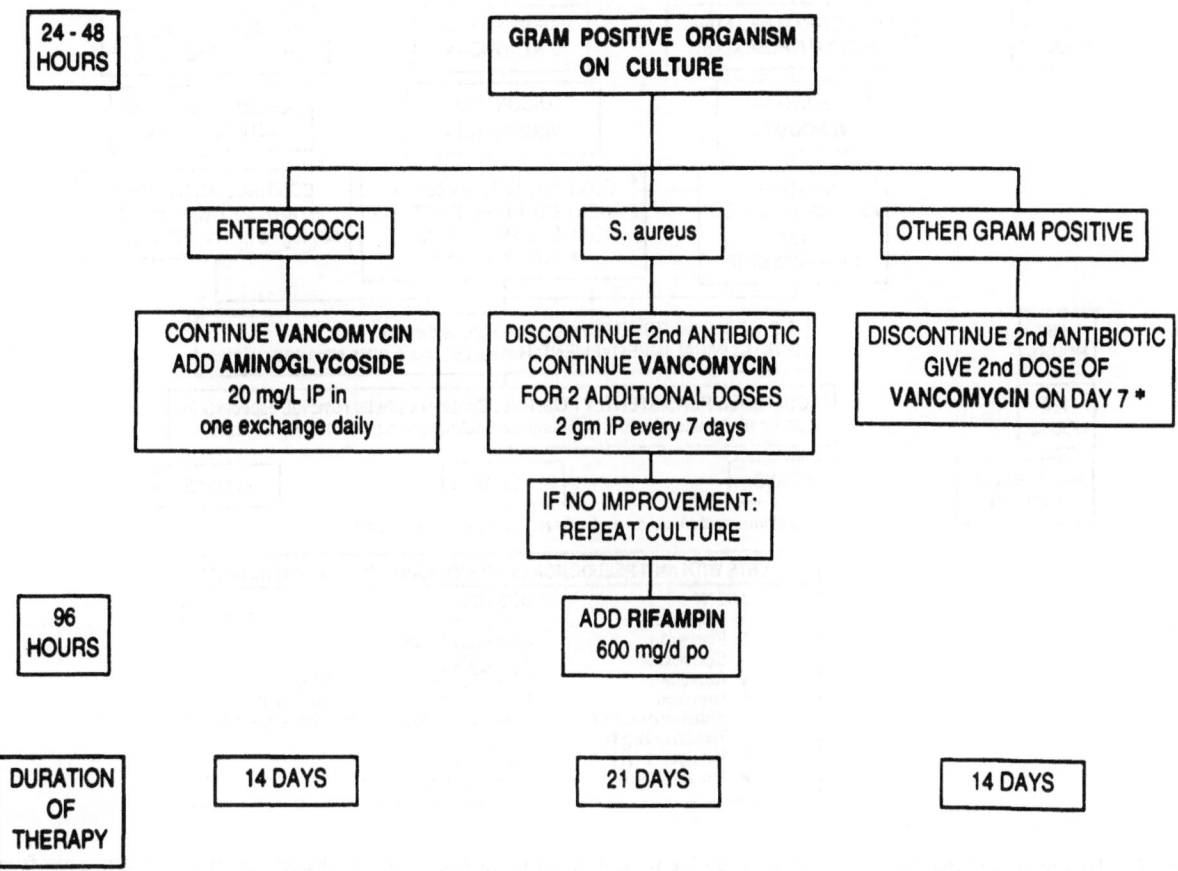

Figure 3.   Treatment and management of gram positive peritonitis in peritoneal dialysis. (Reproduced with permission from Ref. (67)

met with much favour but it is difficult to decide what a mild episode of peritonitis is. Hence immediate reinsertion after catheter removal may well be a useful adjustment to therapy in some patients; this is yet not a proven approach.

Use of thrombolytic agents for recurring peritonitis
Thrombolytic agents such as Streptokinase and Urokinase have been used in the setting of recurrent peritonitis, or if the infection is failing to respond to appropriate antibiotics (122–125). The success of this regime may well be related to 'removal' of the catheter biofilm (126–127). Evidence would suggest that fibrinolytics should be reserved for those infections where no other cause or complication is evident and probably should be limited to coagulase negative staphylococci or culture negative infection. In a prospectively randomised study looking at fibrinolytic therapy with simultaneous catheter removal and replace-

ment the results were dramatically in favour of catheter replacement (recurrence rate of only 5% with this as compared to 41% with fibrinolytic therapy) (128). Fibrinolytics are associated with symptoms of pain, fever and a peritonitis like syndrome (122). Thrombolytic agents are not advocated for routine use in recurrent peritonitis.

Length of antibiotic treatment

No clinical trials have established the optimum length of therapy for peritonitis. Regimes vary from antibiotics for seven days after the last positive culture or 5–7 days after the fluid has cleared (129, 130). This amounts roughly to a treatment of 10–14 days. The recommendations from the adhoc committee on peritonitis (67) appear in Figures 3 and 4.

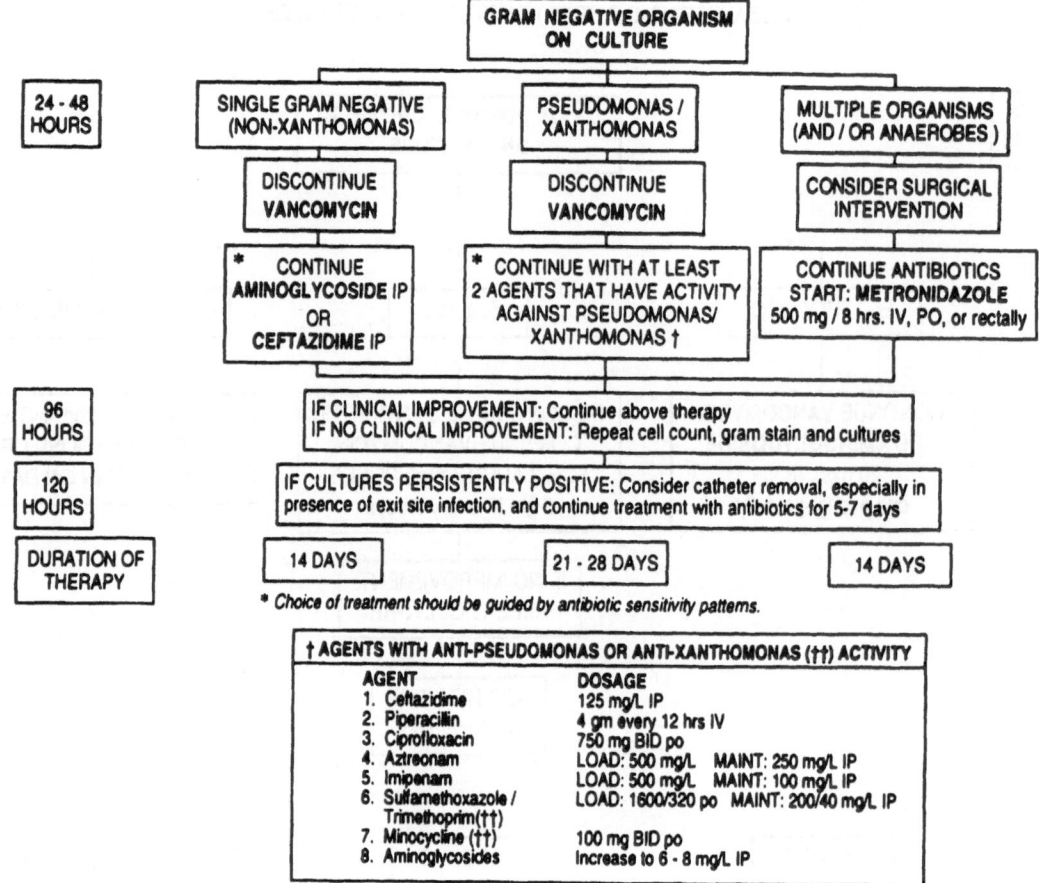

Figure 4. Treatment and management of gram negative peritonitis in peritoneal dialysis. (Reproduced with permission from Ref. (67)

Table 6. Indications for peritoneal catheter removal during peritonitis

Absolute Indication
Frequent recurrence of peritonitis
Relapse with same organism
Peritonitis persisting after 5–7 days of adequate therapy
Tunnel infection with peritonitis
Intraperitoneal abscess
Faecal peritonitis

Relative Indications
Fungal peritonitis
Tuberculous peritonitis

Outcome of peritonitis

Complications

Although rare, complications are not exceptional particularly in the elderly. In the acute stage of the disease several complications can be observed; pulmonary oedema, basal atelectasis and pneumonia, intercurrent cardiovascular events, severe protein malnutrition and muscle wasting, and intestinal perforation from diverticulitis (25, 51). Clostridium difficile related colitis was an important treatment sequel of peritonitis requiring total colectomy in two patients and bleeding to death in one patient (82). At a later stage, the formation of adhesions or the development of peritoneal fibrosis may result in progressive peritoneal failure leading to inadequate dialysis and loss of ultrafiltration (81, 131). Initially the phase of peritoneal deterioration can go unrecognised for weeks and months; peritoneal mass transfer coefficients subsequent to attacks of peritonitis for periods ranging from 6–18 months, have shown declining values in up to one quarter of the patients (132, 133). The precise role of peritonitis in peritoneal failure cannot be determined from these studies but Dobbie has proposed a series of outcomes related to peritoneal damage (see peritoneal fibrosis). Undoubtedly, there are alterations in the peritoneal transfer acutely during peritonitis (134) associated with increased protein losses. This, combined with decreased protein intake and increased catabolism, usually leads to an overall negative nitrogen balance (135). In severe cases, nutritional support may well be needed to meet the daily requirements of calorics and protein.

Mortality

Even though CAPD peritonitis is considered to be a benign illness, it is reported as a cause of death in up to 12% of patients receiving this mode of treatment (35, 101, 136–138). Wide variations in the incidence of peritonitis related deaths may reflect some bias in the analyses of causes of death particularly if the terminal event is related to patients' existing comorbidity. Factors that increase the risk of death from peritonitis include unresolving and protracted course, intra-abdominal abscess formation, infection with Staphylococcus aureus, multiple organism, fungi and the presence of bowel perforation (138).

Impact of peritonitis on morbidity

There is considerable morbidity related to peritonitis. Hospitalisation rates are variable and dependent on the policy of managing peritoneal infections. Some units have in the past managed all episodes as in patients thus increasing the hospitalisation rate. Where a minimal hospitalisation policy is practised then rates related to peritonitis alone can amount to five days per patient year of therapy (139, 140). The impact of peritonitis on CAPD results again show that up to 20% of patients changing therapy to haemodialysis are for reasons of peritonitis (101, 140, 141). Both these factors mean that to run a reasonable CAPD programme there must be adequate back up, which includes haemodialysis and in-patient facilities to cater for permanent as well as temporary changes of therapy (140).

Role of peritoneal solutions in peritonitis

Carozzi and Lamperi (142) first advocated that the dialysate calcium concentration may well have an impact on peritonitis rates. Calcium is an important intracellular ion for final bacterial killing within macrophages and neutrophils. Piraino et al. (143) reported a higher incidence of Staph epidermidis peritonitis in the group of patients treated with low dialysate calcium (1.25 mmol/l). However, there was no increase in overall peritonitis rates; this was substantiated by a study from Japan (14). However, from our unit (145) the use of 1.25 mmol calcium solution showed no difference in peritonitis rates when compared to patients using the 1.75 mmol fluid. In this study the probability to the first episode of peritonitis as well as the second episode were no different when all the factors were controlled (145). Currently therefore there is no evidence that lowering the dialysate calcium in any way enhances the peritonitis risk.

Presently used dialysis solutions are not ideal since they allegedly decrease defence mechanisms against infection (28). Research into solutions containing alternate buffer-

Table 7. Factors implicated in the development of peritonitis

CAPD systems	*Renal unit*	*Patients*
Connectors	Training programme	Compliance
Catheter	Enthusiasm	Motivation
Lines	Adequate staff	Depression
Fluid	Training area	Social support
	Back up HD/Beds	Host defence
	Surgical expertise	
	Microbiology	

ing agents to reverse the pH factor (146) or the osmolality factor (e.g., isosmolar solution using glucose polymer (147)) continues.

Prevention of peritonitis

Whilst CAPD is considered a simple technique this apparent simplicity masks the persisting difficulty in preventing peritonitis. Any sensible approach to peritonitis prevention must be cogniscent of the many factors that are implicated in its pathogenesis (Table 7). There are patient, unit and system related factors which all combine to create the risk of peritonitis.

CAPD programme

The proper organisation and implementation of a CAPD programme is of prime importance for the success of the therapy (148, 149). Furthermore, a dedicated group of experienced nurses should manage the patients and train them appropriately. The observance of strict sterile conditions during connections and disconnections, use of disinfectant on areas exposed to possible contamination are all important facets in a training programme. The single most important approach for prevention is development of appropriate procedural protocols and a careful training of patients (150). An example of this very intensive training is reflected in long training periods in Japan (anything up to 4–5 weeks); peritonitis rates in Japan are reported to be extremely low in comparison to Western results (151).

Connectology

Various connecting devices and technical improvements over the last decade and half have had a major impact on peritonitis rate (5). Initially the luer lock replaced the spike system which enabled the connection to be made between transfer set and the peritoneal dialysis bag. To avoid contamination, the use of ultraviolet devices as well as the sterile connection device did decrease the peritonitis rate but not substantially (152–154). These devices are expensive and this limited the use to those regarded to be of high risk for peritonitis.

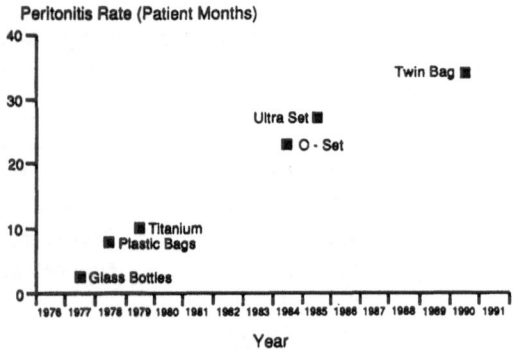

Figure 5. Decline incidence of peritonitis over the last 15 years related to technological improvements.

Development of a 'disconnect' connection also resulted in the reduction of peritonitis episodes in high risk patients. A randomised controlled study comparing conventional spike system with the 'O' system showed the superiority of the latter (155), as did the results obtained when patients were switched from a standard to an 'O' disconnect system (156). The widespread use of disconnect systems (flush before fill, Y set with or without disinfectant) has certainly reduced the incidence of peritonitis (157–161). The most commonly used disconnect system is the double bag or twin bag system, where both full bag and drainage bag are disconnected after each exchange. These systems have reduced the peritonitis rate further (162, 163), but have been reported to reduce mainly the incidence of gram positive peritonitis with no effect on gram negative ones (22).

Antibiotic prophylaxis

The role of antibiotic prophylaxis to prevent CAPD peritonitis has not resulted in any improvement in peritonitis rates. One double blind prospective study failed to show any benefit for oral cephalexin on peritonitis (164) and similarly the oral Septrin for prophylaxis was also unsuccessful (165). There have been no studies prospectively looking at the role of prophylactic antibiotics at the time of catheter insertion. The study from Sweden using prophylatic Cefazolin and Gentamicin prior to surgery did not show any reduction in exit site infection or peritonitis after the insertion (166). However, based on other surgical experience, it has been considered acceptable to give prophylatic antibiotics at the time of catheter insertion and the advocated antibiotic appears to be Vancomycin at a dose of 500 mg given intravenously just prior to surgery. A controlled trial of prophylactic Rifampicin for peritoneal dialysis related infections did not show any major advantages (167). Schwarz et al. (168) have outlined the strategy for preventing Staphylococcus aureus infection during chronic peritoneal dialysis. They studied prophylaxis in a randomised controlled trial of septrin from time of insertion of the catheter. Prophylaxis had a lower rate

of peritonitis, but only for those who were carriers of staphylococcus aureus at entry into the study and this was only during the first three months. They felt that efforts had to be found on general technology and specific microorganisms causing infection.

In order to prevent possible contamination and peritonitis following surgical or dental procedures prophylatic antibiotics have been advocated. Certainly peritonitis has been reported following colonoscopy (169, 170). Diverticular disease of the colon is regarded as a risk factor for peritonitis in peritoneal dialysis (171). In this situation a gram negative antibiotic cover may well be appropriate. Penicillin cover for dental treatment may also be appropriate (57).

Peritoneal dialysis can be undertaken without the risk of peritonitis in patients who have had prosthetic vascular graft or intra-aortic surgery. Here there is no need for prophylatic antibiotics (172, 173).

Enhancing host defence

Even though the evidence is not entirely conclusive that diminished host defence mechanisms significantly increase the risk of peritonitis attempts have been made to improve the opsonic activity intraperitoneally with the addition of IgG into the peritoneum (174). This work has not been substantiated by others and this at present remains an invalidated means to enhance host defence. Vaccination for prevention of CAPD associated Staphylococcal infection has also been studied. Poole-Warren et al. (175) found in a prospective multicentre clinical trial that vaccination against Staphylococcus infection did not in fact prevent peritonitis. Overall therefore the role of enhancing host defence remains limited.

EXIT SITE INFECTION AND ITS MANAGEMENT

Catheter related infections represent a significant complication of peritoneal dialysis therapy. These infections may be associated with patient morbidity in the form of peritonitis or catheter loss. They require hospitalisation and tend to be refractory to treatment (176, 177). Data from the NIH CAPD Registry document an occurrence rate of 0.7 exit site and tunnel infection per patient year with a 40% risk of infection by the end of twelve months of treatment (178). The problem is of major concern, and may even supplant peritonitis as the 'Achilles heel' of chronic peritoneal dialysis therapy.

Tunnel morphology

A detailed description of the peritoneal catheter tunnel morphology has been reported by Twardowski et al. (48). In this the exit site is defined as the most external part (0.5–1 cm) of the sinus tract and the skin surrounding the exit site of the tunnel. In the majority, the epidermal cells penetrate only a few millimetres from the skin exit and may reach the cuff located less than 15 mm from the exit. Close to the exit the surface of the sinus tract is covered with wrinkled epidermis, containing all layers of epidermis including a horny layer. Deeper, the epidermis looses the horny layer and becomes similar to the mucosal epithelium and the surface becomes glistening and white. The rest of the sinus tract is covered by granulation tissue which is yellowish in appearance. Twardowski (176) states that the most important factors influencing the healing process and early infections are tissue perfusion, sinus bacterial colonisation, epithelialisation, use of local cleaning agents and exit direction. Of these epithelialisation appears to be an important factor. Epidermal cells grow over the granulation tissue beneath the scab. If the scab is forcibly removed during cleansing the epidermal layer is broken thus prolonging this epithelialisation process. The other factor is bacterial colonisation of the sinus; there is a constant struggle between the colonising bacteria and defence mechanism of the sinus tract. The part of the sinus tract covered with epidermis seems to respond to bacteria in the same ways as the rest of the body integument but the part covered with granulation tissue appears to respond by constant exudation of serum with white blood cells to suppress bacterial proliferation and curb their penetration deeper into the sinus. As the number of bacteria increases and the amount of exudates increases, granulation tissue proliferates and becomes more vascularised. Defence mechanisms are best in undamaged epidermis and to a lesser extent granulation tissue; trauma to these structures may tilt the balance towards attacking micro-organisms and allow the rapid multiplication necessary for an exit site infection.

Definition of exit site infection

The most widely accepted definition is "redness or skin induration or purulent discharge from the exit site. Formation of the crust around the exit may not indicate infection. Positive cultures from the exit site in the absence of inflammation do not indicate infection" (31). However, Twardowski disagrees with this simplistic, "infected and not infected" definition and has elaborated five categories of exit site appearances each with its clinical features and management. These are: acutely inflamed, chronically inflamed, equivocal, good and perfect (179).

The perfect exit site he characterises as being mature, strong, with mature epithelium in the sinus which is usually dry. Crust forms no more frequently than every seven days and the exit cover is natural or dark. There is an absence of pain, induration, red colour around the exit, external drainage, and visible granulation tissue.

An acutely inflamed exit site has the following features: pain, induration, redness with a diameter greater than 13 mm, liquid external drainage, exuberant granu-

lation tissue on exit and in the sinus. This is the exit site that needs immediate systemic antibiotics, regular dressing change, catheter immobilisation and prevention from trauma is essential. Exuberant granulation tissue needs to be cauterised with a silver nitrate stick.

Treatment of exit site infections

There is at present a paucity of information regarding the therapeutic efficacy of any agent in patients with exit site infection. However, if gram positive organisms are present either oral Cephalexin or parenteral Vancomycin is indicated. Figure 6 details an algorithm for treatment of exit site infections as set out by the Ad Hoc Committee (67). For gram negative organisms, Ciprofloxacin or Ceftazidime is indicated. If there are no clinical signs of improvement then Rifampicin is added for gram positive infection. If after a further two to three weeks of therapy there is still persisting infection with drainage and erythema, exploration of the tunnel and the removal of the external cuff should be considered. If this manoeuvre fails then removal of the catheter is the only option. Similar strategies apply for gram negative exit site infections. If a pseudomonas exit site infection is demonstrated it is unlikely that the infection will respond to antimicrobial therapy and early catheter removal should be considered.

Outcome of exit site and tunnel infection

Staph aureus exit site and tunnel infections are a source of considerable morbidity for peritoneal dialysis patients. These infections are difficult to resolve, can lead to peritonitis and often require removal of the peritoneal catheter (180). Piraino advocates controlled prospective studies designed to investigate methods of preventing and treating Staph aureus exit site infections. In an extensive study of exit and tunnel infections by Scalamogna et al. (181) an incidence of one episode every 23.7 patient months was found in patients with a history of exit site infection, the overall CAPD incidence was one episode every 48.7 patient months. In 3 of the 27 Staph aureus exit site infections unresponsive to antibiotic and local care, deroofing and outer cuff shaving completely resolved the infection. Despite this treatment catheters of the remaining 14 patients had to be removed because of the peritonitis associated with the tunnel infection. These authors conclude that shaving the cuff can act as a rescue treatment in about half of the resistant cases but the outlook is still not good. The use of disconnect systems does not seem to impact any protection against exit site infections despite a reduction in peritonitis rates (182). Pseudomonas exit site infections usually have a poor prognosis with enormous difficulty experienced in eradicating the infection. However, Kazmi et al. (183) reported an experience of 18 episodes of pseudomonas aeroginosa exit site infections in 17 patients on CAPD. The treatment consisted of

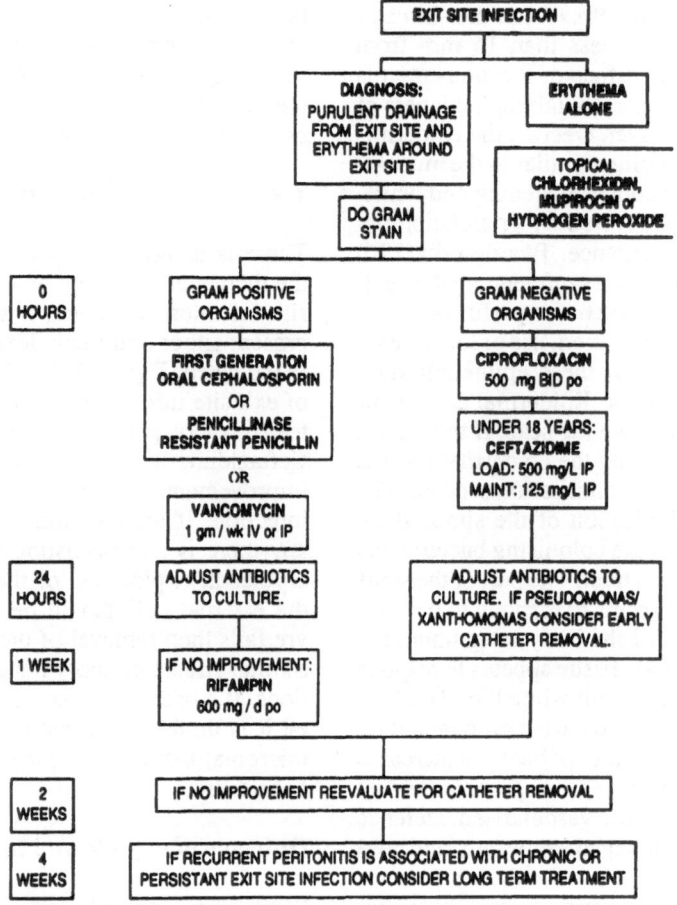

Figure 6. Management of exit site infections. (Reproduced with permission from Ref. (67)

oral Ciprofloxacin and local exit site care with antiseptic agents. 83% of these infections resolved with therapy and three required catheter removal. However four of the 15 patients whose exit site infections resolved developed pseudomonas peritonitis 2–9 months after the clinical resolution. Piraino et al. (184) found that exit site location did not influence peritoneal catheter infection rate contrary to the view by Twardowski (176).

Exit site care

This has a considerable bearing on exit site infections. In a randomised multicentre trial (185) a protective dressing with a disinfectant was associated with significantly less exit site infections than minimum care which entailed cleansing the exit site with non-disinfectant soap and water. Exit site and tunnel infections have a bearing on catheter outcome in peritoneal dialysis patients and anything up to 55% of patients transfer to haemodialysis because of catheter infections (186–190). There is a well held view that immobilisation of the catheter, especially after catheter insertion may well reduce catheter exit site infection. Whilst this is still the view held and rec-

ommended by the Ad Hoc Committee (55) some studies do not support this although the immobilisation technique and devices may be ineffective rather than the actual principle (191).

Nasal carriage and exit site infections and peritonitis

Staph aureux exit site infections have a poor outcome; Piraino et al. (192) reported that exit site infections independent of peritonitis were responsible for 57% of cannulas removed during a five year period. Zimmerman et al. (193) reported similar outcomes. Also the high rate of recurrence associated with Staph aureus infection (194) indicates that more information is needed about the predisposition of Staph aureus invasion in patients undergoing CAPD. Several investigations among patients undergoing CAPD suggested a possible link between nasal carriage of Staph aureus and exit site infection (194–196). However, it was Luzar et al. (96) who established that in patients beginning CAPD the nasal carriage of Staph aureus was associated with an increased risk of catheter exit site infections and that the identification of nasal carriage before the implantation of the catheter, can identify patients at high risk of subsequent morbidities. The question that remains unanswered is what constitutes nasal carriage. In the study of Luzar et al. (197) a positive culture indicated a carrier state. Indeed if this carriage is associated with an increased risk then eradicating the carriage will have potential benefit. Small studies have pointed to this and treatment of nasal carriage of Staphylococcus aureus with Mupirocin or Naseptin have been promising (197). Currently, a double blind multicentre trial of the effect of Mupirocin on exit site infection is being conducted and should provide a definite answer. Sesso et al. (198) looked at nasal carriage of Staphylococcus aureus by doing nasal swabs every two months. They based the classification on Sewell et al. (195). Chronic carriers have positive cultures from the nose or from the skin peri-catheter, 75% or more of the time; intermittent carriers have positive cultures more than once but less than 75% of the time and non-carriers either never had a positive culture or had only one isolate. Recently, a prospective study on Methicillin-resistant Staph aureus (MRSA) nasal carriage was reported to showing an increased risk of CAPD related infections (exit site and peritonitis) and catheter losses and technique failure (199). Whether frequent use of antibiotics predispose to the MRSA situation is unknown but this is a worrying development.

PERITONEAL FIBROSIS AND SCLEROSING ENCAPSULATING PERITONITIS

The peritoneum has a remarkable ability to heal by total resolution of any inflammatory exudate that may result from insults that are inflicted during peritonitis. On most occasions this healing leaves the peritoneal cavity in its pristine premorbid condition (200). Even chronic inflammation may resolve with minimal local residual damage. Such is the vital nature of maintaining a mobile alimentary tube that, in man and animals, diffuse or widespread chronic peritoneal inflammation resulting in a global fibrosis is a most unusual and uncharacteristic peritoneal reaction. However, the development of CAPD has been associated with the appearance of a new form of iatrogenic fibrosis which is remarkable both for the aggressiveness of its fibrogenesis and a global nature of its peritoneal involvement (201).

CAPD associated fibrosis of the peritoneum covers a wide spectrum, from simple opacification through to formation of new fibrous sheets and plaques resulting in the notorious and serious sclerosing encapsulating peritonitis (SEP). Peritoneal opacification is something that most surgeons with any experience observe in patients treated by CAPD. Whilst there are not studies to correlate the degree of opacification with microscopic appearances, Dobbie has observed that normally orientated collagen fibres are disorganised together with the expansion of the matrix ground substance (202). Dobbie goes on to further

describe a 'tanned' peritoneal syndrome which comprises at operation a peritoneum which is dry, wrinkled and light brown in colour. The peritoneum thus exhibits a thick, leathery appearance implying as it were that the membrane has been 'tanned' *in situ*. This is associated histologically with the outer portion of the peritoneum being replaced by an acellular rind of hyalinised collagen (cellular desert) (201, 203). Here the mesothelium is absent and there is a sparse, monocellular infiltrate. The next stage histologically is the formation of mural fibrosis, an aggressive process which may subsequently develop in the underlying serosa following on from the tanned peritoneal syndrome. Mural fibrosis represents a pathological progression of the tanned peritoneal syndrome, where the bowel is stiffened and apparently thickened. Although the patient presents with symptoms of bowel obstruction, adhesions are not present and SEP is never found (204).

Sclerosing encapsulating peritonitis

This is the most frequently used and familiar term used to describe the process of peritoneal fibrosis associated with peritoneal dialysis (200, 205, 206). 'Sclerosing' implies progressive formation of dense collagenous tissue, encapsulating refers to the cocooning of the small bowel by a sheet of new fibrous tissues, while peritonitis acknowledges the histologically reality that this new tissue is invariably permeated by mononuclear inflammatory infiltrates. SEP is the endstage of an intra-abdominal inflammatory process resulting in the formation of sheets of new fibrous tissue which cover, bind and restrict, thereby compromising the mobility of the bowel. At surgery it is possible to peel off the membrane from the bowel relatively easily (207) and the bowel exposed may appear normal.

Causes of SEP

There are numerous possibilities and the causes are by and large by association rather than definitively proven. These are shown in Table 8. The original reports came from centres where the dialysate buffer was primarily acetate rather than lactate (207, 212, 213). However, SEP has also been reported in patients dialysing with lactate (207, 227). Recurrent peritonitis (56, 214, 220, 222) or subclinical peritonitis (224) has been suggested as a cause of this distressing syndrome, although clearly many patients had never had peritonitis, or had a relatively low incidence of peritonitis (214). Recurrent infection and/or severe episodes of peritonitis, characterised by a duration of greater than 10 days, preceded the reintroduction of CAPD in most cases. A quarter of these infections were due to Staph aureus (222); this observation is of particular relevance if one counts the number of toxins produced by Staph aureus, some of which are more important stimulators of IL1 production by macrophages. It is possible however, that one severe episode of peritonitis may con-

Table 8. Factors associated with the occurrence of SEP in peritoneal dialysis patients

1. *CAPD procedures*
   Acetate-containing dialysate (207, 212, 213)
   In line bacterial filter (25, 208, 212)
   Hypertonic dialysis solution (214)
   Plasticizer (214, 215, 228)
   Chlorhexidine (216, 217, 221)
   Glucose breakdown products (218)
   Catheter (214, 219)

2. *Infectious peritonitis*
   Recurrent episodes (56, 214, 220, 222)
   Severe episode leading to PD cessation (220, 222)
   Staph aureus/Pseudomonas peritonitis (222)
   Unrecognised low grade episode with fastidious
       bacteria (224)

3. *Drugs*
   Betablockers (214, 225, 225)
   ?intraperitoneal antibiotics (56)

4. *Others*
   Multiple abdominal surgeries (227)
   High interdialytic peritoneal content of fibrinogen (207)

dition the peritoneum for the development of this syndrome. Certainly, the use of Chlorhexidine used as part of the spray to disinfect the connector system has been implicated (216, 217, as has formalin (223) and this has certainly been proven in animal studies (221).

Pathogenesis

Shaldon and colleagues (208) have suggested that the peritoneal macrophage being similar to the blood monocyte, is in a highly irritated state in CAPD. This results in a progressive inflammatory change resulting in release of IL1 and PG2. Interleukin I has several local peritoneal actions including the stimulation of fibroblast proliferation to increase collagen production and stimulation of endothelial cells to release Prostacyclin. Of particular interest is the observation that acetate is an important stimulator of IL1 release (209). However, Dobbie suggests that the large molecular weight of IL1 would impede the transport through or around the mesothelium to affect the deeply situated fibroblasts. In addition, histologically, loss of normal cellular constituents appear to be more important than fibroblast proliferation in the pathogenesis of peritoneal sclerosis (210). Rather than the fibroblast proliferation, it may be the loss of plasminogen activation from the damaged mesothelial cells that impairs normal fibrinolysis and allows fibrosis. In support of this is the observation of elevated levels of type I and type III procollagen peptides which have been found in the peritoneal fluid of a patient who subsequently developed peritoneal fibrosis (211). Dobbie (210) has put forward a composite pathogenetic outline for SEP; he concludes that fibrin deposition and fibrinolysis, hyalinisation of the superficial stromal collagen, probably tanned through non-enzymatic glycosylation by dialysate glucose and the proliferative potential of mesothelial stem cells play an important role triggered by various factors shown in Table 8.

Signs and symptoms

The clinical manifestation of SEP ranges from insidious symptomatology, consisting of loss of ultrafiltration, usually compensated for by an increased use of hypertonic dialysis solution to the state of inadequate dialysis that eventually leads to CAPD cessation and transfer to haemodialysis. Krediet et al. (229) studied the time course of peritoneal transport kinetics in CAPD patient who developed sclerosing peritonitis and found that in some it was related to increased peritoneal glucose absorption (increased surface area) and other decreased surface area – extensive formation of collagen); in one patient this was not influenced by phosphatidylcholine (230). Most commonly, however, the patients clinical status deteriorates as digestive symptoms develop, including nausea, intermittent vomitting, vague abdominal pain and anorexia that result in progressive wasting (20, 222). At a more advanced stage, manifestations of small bowel obstruction progresses from acute intermittent crisis of colicky pain to a state of permanent complete obstruction (214). Malnutrition becomes obvious with muscle wasting, and peripheral oedema due to inadequate ultrafiltration.

Radiological investigation

Plain abdominal radiograph shows evidence of small bowel intestinal obstruction and barium studies are more informative with characteristic radiological features which show marked dilatation of the duodenum and small bowel, with regular rounded projections of the bowel resulting in a 'concertina like deformity'. Ultrasound changes that have been reported in SEP include increased small bowel peristalsis, tethering of the bowel to the posterior abdominal wall, intraperitoneal echogenic strands and new membrane formation (231). With CT scanning the advanced picture is characteristic (232). In the early stages, loculated ascites, adherent bowel loops, narrowing of the bowel lumen and thickening of the peritoneal membrane, may be markers of the subsequent developing SEP, although these changes may also represent those seen with peritoneal fibrosis.

Treatment and outcome

In the absence of small bowel obstruction SEP, may become asymptomatic following removal of the peritoneal catheter and switching over to HD (205). However, at a late stage when intestinal obstruction predominates, abdominal surgery becomes a necessity to free the small bowel loops from the constricting fibrosis. Two surgical procedures have been used; the first aims at stripping away completely the fibrous membrane that surrounds the bowel thus exposing the normal intestine from duodenum to terminal ileum (233). This operation is not without its problems (214). The second approach is a simpler procedure which aims at releasing the encased and shortened small intestine from the constricting tissue by making multiple incisions adequately dimensioned and positioned. Surgical treatment is fraught with hazard and in cases of life threatening obstruction, post operative mortality is high. If possible the bowel should be "put to rest" and patient receive parenteral alimentation (234, 235). Use of IP Prednisolone, irrigation of the peritoneal cavity with heparinised lactate have remained unsuccessful (214). A recent report suggests that Prednisolone and Azathioprine led to improved bowel function (236).

The outcome of SEP is generally poor. A mortality of 8–20% was observed when the patients were transferred to HD in the presence of an acute problem such as difficulty of dialysis drainage or persisting infection. On the other hand a mortality of 55–78% was observed when CAPD was ceased following more insidious clinical manifestation such as reduced capacity of the peritoneum to ultrafiltrate with progression of the disease to a stage of complete small bowel obstruction (217, 222, 235).

HERNIAS, GENITAL OEDEMA AND HYDROTHORAX

These are fairly common complications of peritoneal dialysis with anything up to 11% of CAPD patients developing hernias during a five year follow up with the risk increasing for each year on CAPD beyond the first year (237, 238). This high incidence of hernia is really not surprising. The presence of dialysis fluid in the peritoneal cavity leads to increased intra-abdominal pressure. Pressure within the abdomen rises in proportion to the volume of dialysate instilled (239, 240). The supine patient generates the lowest intraperitoneal pressure for a given volume of fluid and patients who are older and those who are more obese generate higher intra-abdominal pressures for any given activity (240). Increased abdominal pressure and abdominal wall tension lead to hernia formation in those with congenital or acquired defects in or around the abdomen. The areas of weakness are probably very important in the pathogenesis of hernias especially in the peritoneal dialysis environment. Indeed the intra-abdominal pressure in patients with hernias is no different from the pressure measured in those without hernias (241).

Large variety of hernias have been described in peritoneal dialysis patients (Table 9). The most common forms of hernias are incisional or through the catheter placement site (237, 238), inguinal (237–246) or umbilical (246,

Table 9. Types of hernias in patients on peritoneal dialysis. (Reproduced with permission from Ref. (220)

Umbilical (204, 246, 247, 253)
Inguinal (237–246, 252, 253, 254)
Catheter incision site (237, 238, 250, 252, 253)
Ventral (242, 244, 246, 253)
Catheter exit site (220)
Epigastric (237, 238, 245)
Incisional (237–240, 251)
Cystocele (238)
Foramen of Morgagni (262)
Richters (250, 255)
Enterocoele (238, 259)
Spigelian (260)
Obturator (261)

247). Asymptomatic hernias are probably quite common and may not be detected until some complications such as bowel strangulation occurs (237). It is the older female multiparus patient, as well as those who have experienced a high frequency of post operative leaks at the time of catheter insertion who tend to have hernias. In addition patients with polycystic kidney disease may also be predisposed to hernia formation because of higher intra-abdominal pressure or a manifestation of the generalised disorder of collagen (248).

Weakness in the abdominal wall

A major potential area of weakness is the abdominal incision for the implantation of the dialysis catheter. Midline incisions have a greater propensity for incisional hernia as this is anatomically a weak area (237, 242, 244, 247, 249, 250). Certainly the policy now advocated and generally practised of a paramedian incision through the rectus muscle has resulted in less perioperative leaks and hernia formation (55, 251). The processus vaginalis, which normally undergoes obliteration after the migration of the testes in foetal life is another potential weakness for herniation. When this does not occur the increased abdominal pressure during CAPD may push bowel into the processus vaginalis resulting in an indirect inguinal hernia. Paediatric patients are particularly predisposed to this complication and develop unilateral inguinal hernia or a fluid leak through them. Tank and Hatch (252) reported that 7 of 19 children developed this on starting CAPD. Von Lillen et al. (253) found that 40% of 93 children developed 60 hernias (36 ventral, 14 inguinal, 7 umbilical, 3 scrotal); the rate of development was higher in the first three months. Similar experiences have been reported by others (254).

Management of hernias

Hernias can present in various ways: painless swellings (238), herniation of bowel through the hernia (which can result in incarceration and strangulation), Richters hernia presenting as a tender lump (250, 255), recurrent gram negative peritonitis bowel obstruction and perforation (238, 256).

Hernias in PD patients, need to be repaired even though they may not carry a high risk of complication, e.g. large ventral hernias. It is also possible to repair hernias at the time of catheter insertion without fluid leaks or other complications (257). Management of patients post operatively could be by the use of low volume intermittent peritoneal dialysis to allow time for wound healing or PD could be discontinued and intermittent haemodialysis instituted if the surgical repair has been very extensive or post operatively there is a fluid leak through the wound incision. Inguinal herniorrhaphy can be successfully undertaken with commencement of CAPD immediately post operatively and with a very low risk of recurrence (257). If hernias recur, other options include changing the patient to night time cycler dialysis (NIPD) where the patient dialyses supine and hence there is a lower intra-abdominal pressure or using low volumes of dialysate but with more frequent exchanges. This may indeed be more pertinent in paediatric cases (253, 254).

Genital and abdominal wall oedema

The incidence of genital oedema varies considerably from a few percent to 10% of CAPD patients; recent reports suggest that the incidence may be declining (261–268). Women have a much lower incidence of genital oedema compared to men but whenever this occurs it is a distressing complication of peritoneal dialysis. Abdominal wall oedema related to fluid leaks into the abdominal wall are more difficult to detect, may be insidious and may sometimes only come to light because of a drop in drainage ultrafiltrate volume.

Several mechanisms have been suggested to explain the oedema (263). However, two predominant mechanisms have found favour. Firstly, dialysate can track through the soft tissue planes from the catheter insertion site, from a soft tissue defect within a hernia or a peritoneo-facial defect. In any of these cases genital oedema may be associated with oedema of the anterior abdominal wall (262). Secondly, dialysis fluid can travel through a patent process vaginalis to the labial scrotum where it may leak into the surrounding soft tissue. Indeed, there may be an associated inguinal hernia (268).

The presence of abdominal wall oedema suggests that the origin of the peritoneal leak is present at the potential sites mentioned above. At times this is difficult to diagnose (268). Occasionally, the dialysis leak is accompanied by a coolness related to the PD fluid and it may even look paler than usual. There is usually skin indentation from the pressure of the elastic waist band on underwear; sometimes this is difficult to differentiate from the gross fluid overload that some patients have. Abdominal leaks in CAPD may also present as a reduction in the volume of dialysate effluent (269).

Treatment

Management of oedema of the genital area of abdominal wall usually requires bedrest, scrotal elevation and the dialysis continued with use of frequent low volume exchanges. In addition cessation of peritoneal dialysis for a week or two may allow the defect causing the leak to seal on its own. However, there may be a need for period of prolonged haemodialysis, if the site of leak is not apparent. Radiological and isotopic diagnosis may help to localise the point of leak and thereby appropriate repair undertaken. Many patients can resume CAPD after cessation for a period or surgical repair (262).

Radiological and isotopic diagnosis of hernias and genital oedema

Abdominal scintigraphy with Technetium 99 as well as the use of other different radioligands (DTPA, albumin, radiocolloid) have been utilised successfully to identify hernias and leaks (262, 263, 270–275). It has been suggested that these may be used prospectively (275) but this has not found to be useful. Position (patient sitting up or leaning forward) (276), delayed images after ambulation (277, 278) may enhance the diagnostic yield.

Computerised tomographic (CT) scanning. This can be helpful in diagnostic leaks and a cause of genital oedema and the peritoneal instillation of radio-contrast dye with CT scanning detects more leaks and hernias compared to plain peritoneaography without CT scanning (279–282). Hollet et al. (280) reviewed 60 consecutive CT studies in 48 patients over a five year period 29 dialysate leaks were detected as were loculated, unopacified PD fluid collections, adhesions and hernias. Similar results were reported by others (279, 280) who all support the value of the investigation in patient management.

HYDROTHORAX

This is defined as the accumulation of dialysis fluid in the pleural cavity. It is not clear what the incidence of this complication is but most studies estimate that this is less than 5% (283–287).

Pathogenesis

A defect in the diaphragm must be present to allow dialysis fluid from the peritoneum into the pleural cavity. When hydrothorax has been investigated by surgery or pleuroscopy 'blisters or burns' have sometimes been noted on the pleural surface of the diaphragm (287). Presumably this represents areas of deficiency in the usual support structures of the diaphragm described at autopsy. With the installation of dialysis fluid into the peritoneal cavity, these blebs can be seen to swell, weep and rupture thus providing a pathway for the movement of dialysate into the pleural space. The extent of the deficiency in the hemidiaphragm which will vary in patients is not entirely clear. Whilst hydrothorax can develop at any time, certainly those patients in whom it does so months to years after starting peritoneal dialysis, there is attenuation of tissue separating a pleural from peritoneal space and may 'give way' in response to repeated exposure to raised intra-abdominal pressure or an episode of peritonitis.

Diagnosis of hydrothorax

This is relatively straightforward in cases that present with marked respiratory embarrassment. However, small effusions may be more difficult to pick up and could be thought to be related to congestive heart failure. Chest X-ray usually shows a pleural effusion which occurs predominantly on the right side in most patients. There is a paramount need for other causes of pleural effusion to be ruled out but the patient who develops a large right sided effusion with the first few dialysis exchanges is strongly suggestive of hydrothorax. Pleural tapping of the effusion to establish the glucose concentration of the fluid which will have a lower protein concentration, is diagnostic. Investigators have pointed out that the dextro-isomer of lactate is present in dialysis fluid but not in endogenous pleural effusions and this is another way of identifying dialysate in the pleural cavity (288).

Whilst the use of methylene blue dye has been suggested, this is not recommended and it can lead to chemical peritonitis. Technicium- labelled micro-aggravated albumin or sulphur colloid have been instilled into the peritoneal cavity along with the usual volume of dialysis fluid to try and elicit the site of peritoneal pleural communications. This method is convenient but not absolute foolproof. Defects have been found in the diaphragm at surgery, in patients in whom isotope scanning was negative (240, 290).

Treatment of hydrothorax

Thoracocentesis is a recommended approach for the immediate treatment of the hydrothorax if there is respiratory embarrassment. Discontinuing peritoneal dialysis often leads to a rapid and dramatic resolution of the pleural effusion (285, 291, 292). Subsequently, management depends on whether the patient is going to continue on peritoneal dialysis. Several options are available to managing these patients, which include temporary haemodialysis for up to four weeks with subsequent return to CAPD (293). This is unlikely to work for early leaks soon after CAPD. Another approach is temporary haemodialysis

with return to low volume intermittent PD (294). Several studies have reported on the successful obliteration of the pleural cavity. Agents used for pleurodesis are Oxytetracycline, talc and these can be administered by a thoracotomy tube (285, 291, 295, 296). Instillation of 40 ml of autologous blood in the pleural cavity has also resulted in obliteration of the pleural cavity (297). Combination of aprotin–calcium chloride-thrombin and 'fibrin glue' in the pleural cavity was reported to successfully prevent recurrent hydrothorax in previously failed treatment with another agent (298). During operative repair, a communication between peritoneal and pleural spaces may be visualised. If this approach is taken then it is recommended that 2–3 litres of dialysate be infused into the peritoneal cavity through the dialysis catheter. The diaphragm is impeded from the pleural side for seepages of dialysate through holes and blisters (299, 300).

REFERENCES

1. Popovich RP, Moncrief JW, Decherd JB, Bomar JB, Pyle WK: The definition of a novel portable/wearable equilibrium peritoneal dialysis technique. *Abstr Am Soc Artif Intern Organs* 5: 64, 1976
2. Seligman AM, Frank HA, Fine J: Treatment of experimental uremia by means of peritoneal irrigation. *J Clin Invest* 25: 11, 1946
3. Doolan PD, Murphy WP, Wiggins RA et al.: An evaluation of intermittent peritoneal lavage. *Am J Med* 26: 831, 1959
4. Weston RE, Roberts M: Clinical use of stylet-catheter for peritoneal dialysis. *Arch Intern Med* 115: 659, 1965
5. Cohen SL, Percival A: Prolonged peritoneal dialysis in patients awaiting renal transplantation. *Br Med J* 1: 409, 1968
6. Leigh DA: Peritoneal infections in patients on long term peritoneal dialysis before and after human cadaveric renal transplantation. *J Clin Path* 22: 539, 1959
7. Palmer RA, Quinton WE, Gray JE: Prolonged peritoneal dialysis for chronic renal failure. *Lancet* 1: 700, 1964
8. Tenckhoff H, Schecter H: A bacteriologically safe peritoneal access device. *Trans Am Soc Artif Intern Organs* 14: 181, 1968
9. Tenckhoff H, Curtis FK: Experience with maintenance peritoneal dialysis in the home. *Trans Am Soc Artif Intern Organs* 16: 90, 1970
10. Brewer TE, Caldwell FT, Patterson RM, Flanigan WJ: Indwelling peritoneal dialysis catheter – experience with 24 patients. *JAMA* 219: 1001, 1972
11. Lankisch PG, Tonnis HJ, Fernandez-Redo E et al.: Use of Tenckhoff catheter for peritoneal dialysis in terminal renal failure. *Br Med J* 4: 712, 1973
12. Devine H, Oreopoulos DG, Izatt S, Mathew R, deVeber GA: The permanent Tenckhoff catheter for chronic peritoneal dialysis. *Can Med Assos J* 113: 219, 1975
13. Popovich RP, Moncrief JW, Nolph KD, Ghods AJ, Twardowski ZJ, Pyle WK: Continuous ambulatory peritoneal dialysis. *Ann Intern Med* 88: 449, 1978
14. Oreopoulos DG, Robson M, Izatt S, Clayton S, deVeber GA: A simple and safe technique for continuous ambu-

latory peritoneal dialysis (CAPD). *Trans Am Soc Artif Intern Organs* 24: 84, 1978

15. Oreopoulos DG: CAPD in Canada. *Can Med Assos J* 120: 16, 1979

16. Rubin J, Rodgers WA, Taylor HM et al.: Peritonitis during continuous ambulatory peritoneal dialysis. *Ann Intern Med* 92: 7, 1980

17. Gokal R, McHugh M, Fryer R, Ward MK, Kerr DNS: CAPD: one years experience in a UK dialysis unit. *Br Med J* 280: 474, 1980

18. Editorial: Peritoneal dialysis in chronic renal failure. *Lancet* 2: 303, 1978

19. Shaldon S: A cynical critique of CAPD. in *Continuous Ambulatory Peritoneal Dialysis*, edited by Legrain M, Amsterdam, Excerpta Medica, 1980, p 137

20. Buoncristiani C, Bianci P, Cozzani M et al.: A new safe simple connection system for CAPD. *Int J Urol Nephrol* 1: 45, 1980

21. Maiorca R, Cantaluppi A, Cancarini GC et al.: Prospective controlled trial of a Y connector and disinfectant to prevent peritonitis in CAPD. *Lancet* 2: 642, 1983

22. Canadian CAPD Clinical Trials Group: Peritonitis in CAPD: a multi-center randomised clinical trial comparing the Y connector disinfectant system to standard systems. *Perit Dial Int* 9: 159, 1989

23. Viglino G, Cantaluppi A, Gandolfo C, Peluso F, Cavalli PL: Y-set evolution. in *Peritoneal Dialysis*, edited by La Greca G et al., Milan, Wichtig Editore, 1991, p 281

24. VI Catheter related factors and peritonitis risk in CAPD patients. USRDS 1992 Annual Report. *Am J Kidney Dis* 20 (Suppl 2): 48, 1993

25. Mion C, Slingeneyer A, Canuad B: Peritonitis. in *Continuous Ambulatory Peritoneal Dialysis*, edited by Gokal R, Edinburgh, Churchill Livingstone, 1986, p 163

26. Diaz-Buxo JA, Suki WN: Automated peritoneal dialysis. in *The Textbook of Peritoneal Dialysis*, edited by Gokal R, Nolph KD, Dordrecht, Kluwer Academic Publishers, 1994, p 399

27. Vas SI: Microbiological aspects of chronic ambulatory peritoneal dialysis. *Kidney Int* 23: 83, 1983

28. Vas SI, Duwe A, Weatherhead J: Natural defence mechanisms of the peritoneum: the effect of peritoneal dialysis fluid on polymorphonuclear cells. in *Peritoneal Dialysis*, edited by Atkins R, Thomson N, Farrell PC, Edinburgh, Churchill Livingstone, 1981, p 41

29. Williams P, Khanna R, Vas SI et al.: The treatment of peritonitis in CAPD patients: to lavage or not? *Perit Dial Bull* 1: 12, 1980

30. Keane W, Comty CM, Verbrugh HA, Peterson PK: Opsonic deficiency of peritoneal dialysis effluent in CAPD. *Kidney Int* 25: 539, 1984

31. Pierratos A: Peritoneal dialysis glossary. *Perit Dial Bull* 4: 2, 1984

32. Fenton SS, Wu G, Cattran D, Wadgymar A, Allen RF: Clinical aspects of peritonitis in patients on CAPD. *Perit Dial Bull* 1 (Suppl 1): S4, 1981

33. Keane WF, Vas SI: Peritonitis. in *The Textbook of Peritoneal Dialysis*, edited by Gokal R, Nolph KD, Dordrecht, Kluwer Academic Publishers, 1994, p 473

34. Grodstein GP, Blumenkrantz MJ, Kopple JD: Effect of intercurrent illnesses on nitrogen metabolism in uremic patients. *Trans Am Soc Artif Intern Organs* 25: 438, 1979

35. Slingeneyer A, Mion C, Beraud JJ, Oules R, Branger B, Balmes M: Peritonitis, a frequently lethal complication of intermittent and continuous ambulator peritoneal dialysis. *Proc EDTA* 18: 212, 1981

36. Vas SI: Peritonitis during CAPD: a mixed bag. *Perit Dial Bull* 1: 47, 1981

37. Betjes MGH, Tuk CW, Zemel D, Krediet RT, Arisz L, Beelen, RH: Analysis of the peritoneal cellular system during CAPD shortly before a clinical peritonitis. *Nephrol Dial Transplant* 9: 684, 1994

38. Gokal R, Ramos JM, Ward MK, Kerr DNS: 'Eosinophilic peritonitis' in CAPD, *Clin Nephrol* 15: 328, 1981

39. Digenis GE, Khanna R, Pantalony D: Eosinophilia after implantation of the peritoneal catheter. *Perit Dial Bull* 2: 98, 1982

40. Nassberger L: Eosinophilic peritonitis – hypothesis. *Nephron* 46: 103, 1987

41. Salgia P, Manos J, Gokal R: Cutaneous manifestations heralding eosinophilic peritonitis. *Perit Dial Bull* 4: 265, 1984

42. Sombolos K, Vas S, Rifkin O et al.: Propioni-bacteria isolates and asymptomatic infections of the peritoneal effluent in CAPD patients. *Nephrol Dial Transplant* 1: 175, 1986

43. Williams PS, Hendry MS, Ackeril P: Routine daily surveillance cultures in the management of CAPD patients. *Perit Dial Bull* 7: 183, 1987

44. Eisenberg ES, Ambalu M, Szylagi G, Aning V, Soeiro R: Colonisation of skin and development of peritonitis due to coagulase negative staphylococci in patients undergoing peritoneal dialysis. *J Inf Dis* 156: 478, 1987

45. Leahy TJ, Sullivan MJ, Slingeneyer A, Mion C: The efficiency of microbial retention by peritoneal dialysis filters. *Trans Am Soc Artif Int Organs* 26: 225, 1980

46. Davies RR, Noble WC: Dispersal of bacteria on desquamated skin. *Lancet* 2: 1295, 1962

47. Parsons F, Ahmed-Jusuf IH, Brownjohn AM et al.: CAPD peritonitis. *Lancet* 1: 348, 1983

48. Twardowski ZJ, Dobbie JW, Moore HL et al.: Morphology of peritoneal dialysis catheter tunnel. 1. Macroscopy and light microscopy. *Perit Dial Int* 11: 152, 1991

49. Gloor HJ, Nichols WK, Sorkin MI et al.: Peritoneal access and related complications in CAPD. *Am J Med* 74: 593, 1983

50. Schweinburg FB, Seligman AM, Fine J: Transmural migration of intestinal bacteria. A study based on the use of radioactive E Coli. *N Eng J Med* 242: 747, 1950

51. Wu G, Khanna R, Vas S, Oreopoulos DG: Is extensive diverticulosis of the colon a contraindication to CAPD? *Perit Dial Bull* 3: 180, 1983

52. Abrutyn E, Goodhart GI, Roos K, Anderson R, Buxton A: Acinetobacter outbreak associated with peritoneal dialysis. *Am J Epidemiol* 107: 328, 1985

53. Gokal R, Manos J, Walker C, Mallick N: Peritonitis related to defective CAPD equipment. *Lancet* 2: 382, 1982

54. Stewart WK, Anderson DC, Wilson MI: Hazards of peritoneal dialysis: contaminated fluid. *Brit Med J* 254: 606, 1967

55. Gokal R, Ash S, Helfrich GB et al.: Peritoneal catheters and exit site practices: towards optimum peritoneal access. *Perit Dial Int* 13: 29, 1993

56. Rottembourg J, Gahl GM, Poignet JL et al.: Severe abdominal complications in patients undergoing CAPD. *Proc EDTA* 20: 457, 1983

57. Kiddy K, Brown PP, Michael J, Adu J: Peritonitis due to streptococcus viridans in patients receiving CAPD. *Brit Med J* 290: 969, 1985

58. Coronel F, Maranjo P, Torrente J, Prats D: The risk of retrograde menstruation in women undergoing CAPD. *Perit Dial Bull* 4: 190, 1984

59. Coward RA, Gokal R, Wise M, Mallick NP, Warrell D: Peritonitis associated with vaginal leak of dialysis fluid in CAPD. *Brit Med J* 284: 1529, 1982

60. Diaz-Buxo J, Burgess P, Walker PJ: Peritoneo-vaginal fistula: an unusual complication of peritoneal dialysis. *Perit Dial Bull* 3: 142, 1983

61. Stuck A, Seiler A, Frey FJ: Peritonitis due to an intrauterine contraceptive device in a patient on CAPD. *Perit Dial Bull* 7: 105, 1986

62. Young JB, Ahmed-Yusuf IH, Brownjohn AH et al.: Opportunistic peritonitis in CAPD. *Clin Nephrol* 22: 268, 1984

63. Fenton P: Laboratory diagnosis in patients undergoing CAPD. *J Clin Path* 35: 1181, 1982

64. Gould IM, Casewell MW: The laboratory diagnosis of peritonitis during CAPD. *J Hosp Infect* 7: 155, 1986

65. Ludlam H, Dickens A, Simpson A, Phillips I: A comparison of four culture methods for diagnosing infection in CAPD. *J Hosp Infect* 16: 263, 1990

66. Ludlam HA, Price TN, Berry AJ, Phillips I: Laboratory diagnosis of peritonitis in patients on CAPD. *J Clin Microbiol* 26: 1757, 1988

67. Keane WF, Everett ED, Golper TA et al.: Peritoneal dialysis related peritonitis – treatment recommendations 1993 update. *Perit Dial Int* 13: 14, 1993

68. Von Graevenitz A, Amsterdam D: Microbiological aspects of peritonitis associated with CAPD. *Clin Microbiol Rev* 5: 26, 1992

69. Peer G, Serban I, Blum M, Cabili S, Iaina A: Early diagnosis of gram-negative peritonitis in CAPD patients with the Lymulus amebocyte lysate assay. *Am J Nephrol* 12: 19, 1992

70. Bowman RA, Medley AS, Karthigasu KT: Limulus amoebocyte lysate assay in the diagnosis of peritonitis in patients receiving CAPD. *J Clin Path* 45: 72, 1992

71. Males BM, Walshe JJ, Garringer L, Koscinski D, Amsterdam D: Addi-Chek filtration, Bactec, and 10ml culture methods for the recovery of microorganisms from dialysis effluent during episodes of peritonitis. *J Clin Microbiol* 23: 350, 1986

72. Williams P, Pantalony D, Vas SI, Khanna R, Oreopoulos DG: The value of dialysate cell count in the diagnosis of peritonitis in patients on CAPD. *Perit Dial Bull* 1: 59, 1981

73. Gruer LD, Bartlett R, Aycliffe AJ: Species identification and antibiotic sensitivity of coagulase negative staphyloccoci from CAPD peritonitis. *J Antibiotic Chemother* 13: 577, 1984

74. Read RR, Eberwein P, Dasgupta MK et al.: Peritonitis in peritoneal dialysis: bacterial colonisation by biofilm spread along the catheter surface. *Kidney Int* 35: 614, 1989

75. Dasgupta MK, Costerton JW: Significance of biofilm-adherent bacterial microcolonies on Tenckhoff catheters of CAPD patients. *Blood Purif* 7: 144, 1989

76. Kapral FA, Goodwin JR, Dye ES: Formation of intraperitoneal abscesses by staphylococcus aureus. *Infec Immun* 30: 204, 1980

77. Gregory MC, Duffy DP: Toxic shock following staphylococcal peritonitis. *Clin Nephrol* 20: 101, 1983

78. Kim D, Tapson J, Wu G et al.: Staphylococcus aureus peritonitis in patients on CAPD. *Trans Am Soc Artif Int Organs* 30: 494, 1984.

79. Pierard D, Cauwers S, Mouton MC, Sennasael J, Verbeelen D: Group JK Corynebacterium peritonitis in a patient undergoing CAPD. *J Clin Microbiol* 18: 1111, 1983

80. Leung ACT, Orange G, Henderson IS, Kennedy AC: Diphteroid peritonitis associated with CAPD. *Clin Nephrol* 22: 200, 1984

81. Chan MK, Chan PC, Cheng IP, Chan CY, Ng WS: Pseudomonas peritonitis in CAPD patients: characteristics and outcome of treatment. *Nephrol Dial Transplant* 4: 814, 1989

82. Gokal R, Ramos M, Francis D et al.: Peritonitis in CAPD. *Lancet* 2: 1388, 1982

83. Piraino B, Bernadini J, Sorkin M: A five-year study of the microbiologic results of exit site infections and peritonitis in CAPD. *Am J Kidney Dis* 10: 281, 1987

84. Ahijado F, Luno J, Soto I et al.: Tuberculous peritonitis in patients on CAPD. *Contrib Nephrol* 89: 79, 1991

85. Cheng IK, Chan PC, Chan MK: Tuberculous peritonitis complicating long term peritoneal dialysis. Report of 5 cases and review of the literature. *Am J Nephrol* 9: 155, 1989

86. Morfurd DW: High index of suspicion for tuberculous peritonitis in CAPD patients. *Perit Dial Bull* 2: 189, 1982

87. Kerr CM, Perfect JR, Craven PC et al.: Fungal peritonitis in patients on CAPD. *Ann Intern Med* 99: 334, 1983

88. Tapson JS, Mansy H, Freeman R, Wilkinson R: The high morbidity of CAPD fungal peritonitis – description of 10 cases and review of treatment strategies. *Quart J Med* 61: 1047, 1986

89. Khanna R, McNeely DJ, Oreopoulos DG, Vas SI, McCready W: Treating fungal infections: fungal peritonitis in CAPD. *Brit Med J* 280: 1147, 1980

90. Coles GA, Lewis SL, Williams JD: Host defence and effects of solutions on peritoneal cells. in *The Textbook of Peritoneal Dialysis*, edited by Gokal R, Nolph KD, Dordrecht, Kluwer Academic Publishers, 1994, p 503

91. Van Bronswijk H, Verbrugh HA, Heezius EZ et al.: Host defence in CAPD treatment: the effect of the dialysate on cell function. *Contrib Nephrol* 85: 67, 1990

92. Coles GA, Alobaidi H, Topley N, Davies M: Opsonic activity of dialysis effluent predicts those at risk of staphylococcal peritonitis. *Nephrol Dial Transplant* 2: 359, 1987

93. Stein S, Brenchleyy P, Manos J, Pumphrey R, Gokal R: Opsonising capacity of peritoneal fluid and the relationship to peritonitis in CAPD patients. in *Frontiers in Peritoneal Dialysis*, edited by Maher JF, Winchester JF, New York, Field Rich, 1986, p 565

94. De Vecchi A, Castelnovo C, Failla N, Scalamonga A: Clinical significance of peritoneal dialysate IgG levels in CAPD patients. *Adv Perit Dial* 6: 98, 1990

682   *Ram Gokal*

95. Anwar N, Hutchison A, Manos J, Uttley L, Brenchley P, Gokal R: Peritoneal dialysate IgG/C3 levels do not predict peritonitis. *Perit Dial Int.* In press
96. Alobaidi HM, Coles GA, Davies M, Lloyd D: Host defence in CAPD: the effect of the dialysate on phagocyte function. *Nephrol Dial Transplant* 1: 16, 1986
97. de Fijter CWH, Verbrugh HA, Peters ED et al.: *In vivo* exposure to the currently available peritoneal dialysis fluids decreases the function of peritoneal macrophages in CAPD. *Clin Nephrol* 39: 75, 1993
98. Lewis SL, Young SA, Wood BJ, Morgan KS, Erickson DG, Holmes CJ: Relationship between frequent episodes of peritonitis and altered immune status. *Am J Kidney Dis* 22: 456, 1993
99. Coles GA, Minors SJ, Horton JK, Fifield R, Davies M: Can the risk of peritonitis be predicted for new CAPD patients? *Perit Dial Int* 9: 69, 1989
100. Report of a Working Party of the BSAC: Diagnosis and management of peritonitis in CAPD. *Lancet* 1: 845, 1987
101. Tranaeus A, Heimburger O, Lindholm B: Peritonitis during CAPD: risk factors, clinical severity and pathogenetic aspects. *Perit Dial Int* 8: 253, 1988
102. Keane W, Everett ED, Fine RD et al.: CAPD peritonitis – Treatment recommendations (1988 update). *Perit Dial Int* 9: 247, 1989
103. Ejlersen E, Brandi L, Lokkegard H, Ladefoged J, Kopp R, Haarh P: Is initial (24 hours) lavage necessary in treatment of CAPD peritonitis? *Perit Dial Int* 11: 38, 1991
104. Harford AM, Sica DA, Tartaglione T, Polk RE, Dalton HP, Poynor W: Vancomycin pharmcokinetics in CAPD patients with peritonitis. *Nephron* 43: 217, 1986
105. Bastani B, Freer K, Read D et al.: Treatment of gram positive peritonitis with two intraperitoneal doses of vancomycin in CAPD patients. *Nephron* 45: 283, 1987
106. Levison ME: New dosing regimens for aminoglycoside antibiotics. *Ann Int Med* 117, 693, 1992
107. Nikolaidis P, Vas S, Lawson V et al.: Is intraperitoneal tobramycin ototoxic in CAPD patients? *Perit Dial Int* 11: 156, 1991
108. Were AJ, Marsden A, Tooth A, Ramsden R, Mistry CD, Gokal R: Netilmycin and vancomycin in the treatment of peritonitis in CAPD patients. *Clin Nephrol* 37: 209, 1992
109. Zimmerman SW, Johnson CA: Rimfampicin use in peritoneal dialysis. *Perit Dial Int* 9: 241, 1989
110. Janknegt R: CAPD peritonitis and fluoroquinolones: a review. *Perit Dial Int* 11: 53, 1991
111. Waite NM, Johnson MD, Webster NR, Fong IW: Poor response to oral ciprofloxacin in the treatment of peritonitis in patients on intermittent peritoneal dialysis. *Perit Dial Int* 13: 50, 1993
112. Perez-Fontan M, Rosales M, Fernandes F et al.: Ciprofloxacin in the treatment of gram-positive bacterial peritonitis in patients undergoing CAPD. *Perit Dial Int* 11: 233, 1991
113. Millikan SP, Matze GR, Keane WF: Antimicrobial treatment of peritonitis associated with CAPD. *Perit Dial Int* 11: 252, 1991
114. Zaruba K, Peters J, Jungbluth H: Successful prophylaxis for fungal peritonitis in patients on CAPD: six years experience. *Am J Kidney Dis* 17: 43, 1991
115. Taber TE, Hegeman TF, York SM, Kinney RA, Webb DH: Treatment of pseudomonas infections in peritoneal dialysis patients. *Perit Dial Int* 11: 213, 1991

116. Chong TK, Piraino B, Bernardini J: Vestibular toxicity due to gentamicin in peritoneal dialysis patients. *Perit Dial Int* 11: 152, 1991
117. Cheng IPK, Fang GX, Chan TM et al.: Fungal peritonitis complicating peritoneal dialysis: report of 27 cases and review of treatment. *Q J Med* 71: 407, 1989
118. Swartz R, Messana J, Reynolds J, Ranjit U: Simultaneous catheter replacement and removal in refractory peritoneal dialysis infections. *Kidney Int* 40: 1160, 1991
119. Paterson AD, Bishop M, Morgan AG, Burden RP: Removal and replacement of Tenckhoff catheter at a single operation: successful treatment of resistant peritonitis in CAPD. *Lancet* 2: 1245, 1986
120. Pagniez DC, MacNamara E, Fortin F et al.: Withdrawal of CAPD to treat mild peritonitis. *Br Med J* 297: 1174, 1988
121. Cairns HS, Becket J, Rudge CJ, Thompson FD, Mansell MA: Treatment of resistant CAPD peritonitis by temporary discontinuation of peritoneal dialysis. *Clin Nephrol* 32: 27, 1989
122. Nankivell BJ, Lake N, Gillies A: Intracatheter streptokinase for recurrent peritonitis in CAPD. *Clin Nephrol* 35: 20, 1991
123. Pickering SJ, Fleming SJ, Bowley JA et al.: Urokinase: a treatment for relapsing peritonitis due to coagulase-negative staphylococci. *Nephrol Dial Transplant* 4: 62, 1989
124. Jones BF, Lake N: Intraperitoneal streptokinase in the treatment of recurrent peritonitis. *Perit Dial Bull* 9: 352, 1989
125. Tzamaloukas AH: Peritoneal fluid cell counts and cultures in CAPD patients receiving intraperitoneal streptokinase (urokinase) for relapsing peritonitis. *Perit Dial Int* 9: 143, 1989
126. Dasgupta MK: Use of streptokinase or urokinase in recurrent CAPD peritonitis. *Adv Perit Dial* 7: 169, 1991
127. Dasgupta MK, Kowalewska-Grochowska K, Larabie M, Costerton JW: Catheter biofilm and recurrent CAPD peritonitis. *Adv Perit Dial* 7: 165, 1991
128. Williams AJ, Boeltis I, Johnson BF et al.: Tenckhoff catheter replacement or intraperitoneal urokinase: a randomised trial in the management of recurrent CAPD peritonitis. *Perit Dial Int* 9: 65, 1989
129. Anwar N, Gokal R: Experience with vancomycin, aminoglycosides and newer B lactam antibiotics in CAPD peritonitis. *Dial Transplant* 33: 134, 1993
130. Digenis OE, Khanna R, Pierratos A, Vas S: Morbidity and mortality after treatment of peritonitis with prolonged exchanges and intraperitoneal antibiotics. *Perit Dial Bull* 2: 45, 1982
131. Wu, G and The Toronto Coll Dialysis Group: A review of peritonitis episodes that caused interruption of CAPD. *Perit Dial Bull* 3 (Suppl 1): S11, 1983
132. Selgas R, Rodrigues-Carmona A, Martinez ME et al.: Peritoneal mass transfer in patients on long term CAPD. *Perit Dial Bull* 4: 153, 1984
133. Ota K, Mineshima M, Watanabe N, Naganuma S: Functional deterioration of the peritoneum: does it occur in the absence of peritonitis? *Nephrol Dial Transplant* 2: 30, 1987
134. Krediet R, Zuyderhoudt FM, Boeschoten EW, Arisz L: Alterations in the peritoneal transport of water and solutes during peritonitis in CAPD. *Eur J Clin Invest* 17: 43, 1987

135. Bannister DK, Acciardo SR, Moore LW, Kraus AP: Nutritional effects of peritonitis in CAPD patients. *J Am Diet Assoc* 87: 53, 1987

136. Khanna R, Wu G, Vas S, Oreopolous D: Mortality and morbidity on CAPD. *ASAIO J* 6: 197, 1983

137. Digenis GE, Abraham G, Savin E et al.: Peritonitis-related deaths in CAPD patients. *Perit Dial Int* 10: 45, 1990

138. Fenton SSA: Peritonitis related deaths among CAPD patients. *Perit Dial Bull* 3 (Suppl 3): S9, 1983

139. Gokal R, King J, Jakubowski C et al.: Peritonitis-still a major problem in CAPD: results of multicentre study. *Journal of Nephrology* 2: 95, 1990

140. Gokal R, King J, Jakubowski C et al.: Outcome in patients on CAPD and haemodialysis: 4-year analysis of a prospective multicentre study. *Lancet* 2: 1105, 1987

141. Viglino G, Cancarini G, Gatizone L et al.: The impact of peritonitis on CAPD results. *Adv Perit Dial* 8: 269, 1992

142. Carozzi S, Nasini M, Schelotto C et al.: Peritoneal macrophage antimicrobial activity modulation by peritoneal dialysis fluid CA++ and 1,25(OH)2D3 in CAPD patients. in *Current Concepts in Peritoneal Dialysis*, edited by Ota K et al., Amsterdam, Excerpta Medica, 1992, p 250.

143. Piraino B, Perlmutter J, Holley JL, Johnston J, Bernardini J: Use of dialysate containing 2.5meq/l Ca in peritoneal dialysis patients. *Perit Dial Int* 12: 76, 1992

144. Suga H, Honda H, Naganuma S et al.: A low Ca++ level in effluent as a risk factor for the peritonitis in CAPD patients. *Adv Perit Dial* 6: 102, 1990

145. Hutchinson AJ, Turner K, Gokal R: Effect of long-term therapy with 1.25mmol/l calcium peritoneal dialysis fluid on the incidence of peritonitis in CAPD. *Perit Dial Int* 12: 321, 1992

146. Hutchison AJ, Gokal R: Improved solutions for peritoneal dialysis: development and use of physiological calcium solutions, osmotic agents and buffers. *Kidney Int* 42 (Suppl 38): S153, 1992

147. Mistry CD, Mallick NP, Gokal R: Ultrafiltration with an isosmotic solution during long peritoneal dialysis exchanges. *Lancet* 2: 178, 1987

148. Oreopoulos DG: Requirements for the organisation of a CAPD programme. *Nephron* 24: 261, 1979

149. Gokal R: CAPD. in *Renal Failure Who Cares?*, edited by Parsons F, Ogg C, Lancaster, MTP Press, 1982, p 137

150. Oreopoulos DG, Vas S, Khanna R: Prevention of peritonitis during CAPD. *Perit Dial Bull* 3 (Suppl 3): S18, 1983

151. Ota K, Kawaguchi Y: Peritoneal dialysis in Japan. in *Current Concepts in Peritoneal Dialysis*, edited by Ota K et al., Amsterdam, Excerpta Medica, 1992, p 849

152. Nolph KD: Randomised multicentre clinical trial to evaluate the effects of an ultraviolet germicidal system on peritonitis rates in CAPD. *Perit Dial Bull* 5: 19, 1985

153. Holmes CJ, Miyake C, Kubey W: *In vitro* evaluation of an ultraviolet germicidal connection system for CAPD. *Perit Dial Bull* 4: 215, 1984

154. Feriani M, La Greca G, Kriger FL, Winchester JF: CAPD systems and solutions. in *The Textbook of Peritoneal Dialysis*, edited by Gokal R, Nolph KD, Dordrecht, Kluwer Academic Publishers, 1994, p 233

155. Owen JE, Walker RG, Lemon J, Brett L, Mitrou D, Becker GJ: Randomised study of peritonitis with conventional versus O-set techniques in CAPD. *Perit Dial Int* 12: 216, 1992

156. Bonardeaux A, Ouimet D, Galarneau A et al.: Peritonitis in CAPD: impact of a compulsory switch from a standard to a Y-connector system in a single North American Centre. *Am J Kidney Dis* 19: 364, 1992

157. Port PK, Held PJ, Nolph KD et al.: Risk of peritonitis and technique failure by CAPD connection technique: a national study. *Kidney Int* 42: 967, 1992

158. Junor BJR: CAPD disconnect systems. *Blood Purif* 7: 156, 1989

159. Piraino B, Bernardini J, Sorkin MI: The effect of the Y-set on catheter infection rates in CAPD patients. *Am J Kidney Dis* 16: 46, 1990

160. Buoncristiani U: The Y set with disinfectant is here to stay. *Perit Dial Int* 9: 149, 1989

161. Luzar MA, Slingeneyer A, Cantaluppi A, Peluso FP: *In vitro* study of the flush effect in two reusable CAPD disconnect systems. *Perit Dial Int* 9: 169, 1989

162. Geerlings W, Tufveson G, Ehrich JH et al.: Report on management of renal failure in Europe XIII. *Nephrol Dial Transplant* 9 (Suppl 1): 6, 1994

163. Dasgupta MK, Fox S, Gagnon D, Ettcher K, Ulan RA: Significant reduction of peritonitis rate by the use of twin-bag system in a Canadian regional CAPD programme. *Adv Perit Dial* 8: 223, 1992

164. Low DE, Vas SI, Oreopoulos DG et al.: Randomised clinical trial of prophylactic cephalexin in CAPD. *Lancet* 2: 753, 1986

165. Churchill DN, Oreopoulos DG, Taylor DW et al.: Peritonitis in CAPD patients – a randomised clinical trial of trimethoprimsulfamethoxazole prophylaxis. *Abstracts Am Soc Nephrol* 97A, 1987

166. Lye WC, Lee EJ, Tan CC: Prophylatic antibiotics in the insertion of Tenckhoff catheters. *Scand J Urol Nephrol* 26: 177, 1992

167. Zimmerman SW, Ahrens E, Johnson CA et al.: Randomised controlled trial of prophylactic rifampin for peritoneal dialysis-related infections. *Am J Kidney Dis* 18: 225, 1991

168. Swartz R, Messana J, Starman B, Weber M, Reynolds J: Preventing Staphylococcus aureus infection during chronic peritoneal dialysis. *J Am Soc Nephrol* 2: 1085, 1991

169. Ray SM, Piraino B, Holley J: Peritonitis following colonoscopy in a peritoneal dialysis patient. *Perit Dial Int* 10: 97, 1990

170. Peterson JH, Weesner RE, Giannella RA: E Coli peritonitis after left-sided colonoscopy in a patient on CAPD. *Am J Gastroenterol* 82: 171, 1987

171. Tranaeus A, Heimburger O, Granqvist S: Diverticular disease of the colon: a risk factor for peritonitis in CAPD. *Nephrol Dial Transplant* 5: 141, 1990

172. Gulanikar AC, Jindal KK, Hirsch DJ: Is chronic peritoneal dialysis safe in patients with intra-abdominal prosthetic vascular grafts? *Nephrol Dial Transplant* 6: 215, 1991

173. Schmidt RJ, Cruz C, Dumler F: Effective CAPD following abdominal aortic aneurysm repair. *Perit Dial Int* 13: 40, 1993

174. Lamperi S, Carozzi S: Immunological defences in CAPD. *Blood Purif* 7: 126, 1989

175. Poole-Warren LA, Farrell PC: The role of vaccination in the prevention of staphylococcal peritonitis in CAPD. *Perit Dial Int* 13: 176, 1993

176. Twardowski ZJ, Khanna R: Peritoneal dialysis access and exit site care. in *The Textbook of Peritoneal Dialysis*, edited by Gokal R, Nolph KD, Dordrecht, Kluwer Academic Publishers, 1994, p 271

177. Copley JB: Prevention of PD catheter related infections. *Am J Kidney Dis* 10: 401, 1987

178. Nolph KD, Cutler SJ, Steinberg S et al.: CAPD in the US – a 3 year study. *Kidney Int* 28: 198, 1985

179. Twardowski ZJ: Peritoneal catheter exit site infections: prevention, diagnosis, treatment, and future directions. *Seminar Dial* 5: 305, 1992

180. Piraino B: A review of Staphlococcus aureus exit-site and tunnel infections in peritoneal dialysis patients. *Am J Kidney Dis* 16: 89, 1990

181. Scalamogna A, Castelnovo C, De Vecchi A, Ponticelli C: Exit-site and tunnel infections in CAPD patients. *Am J Kidney Dis* 18: 674, 1991

182. Burkart JM, Jordan JR, Durnell TA, Case LD: Comparison of exit-site infections in disconnect versus nondisconnect systems for peritoneal dialysis. *Perit Dial In* 12: 317, 1992

183. Kazmi HR, Raffone FD, Kliger AS, Finkelstein FO: Pseudomonas exit site infections in CAPD patients. *J Am Soc Nephrol* 2: 1498, 1992

184. Piraino, B, Bernadini J, Johnson JR, Sorkin MI: Exit-site location does not influence peritoneal catheter infection rate. *Perit Dial Int* 9: 127, 1989

185. Luzar MA, Brown CB, Balf D et al.: Exit-site care and exit-site infection in CAPD: results of a randomised multicentre study. *Perit Dial Int* 10: 25, 1990

186. Piraino B, Bernardini J, Sorkin M: Catheter infections as a factor in the transfer of CAPD patients to hemodialysis. *Am J Kidney Dis* 13: 365, 1989

187. Wadhwa NK, Cabralda T, Suh H, Kvilekval K, Mason R: Exit-site/tunnel infection and catheter outcome in peritoneal dialysis patients. *Adv Perit Dial* 8: 325, 1992

188. Bernardini J, Holley JL, Johnston JR, Perlmutter JA, Piraino B: An analysis of ten year trends in infections in adults on CAPD. *Clin Nephrol* 36: 29, 1991

189. Holley JL, Bernardini J, Piraino B: Risk factors for tunnel infections in continuous peritoneal dialysis. *Am J Kidney Dis* 18: 344, 1991

190. Luzar MA: Exit-site infections in CAPD: a review. *Perit Dial Int* 11: 333, 1991

191. Turner K, Edgar D, Hair M et al.: Does catheter immobilisation reduce exit-site infections in CAPD patients? *Adv Perit Dial* 8: 265, 1992

192. Piraino B, Bernardini J, Sorkin M: The influence of peritoneal catheter exit-site infections on peritonitis, tunnel infections, and catheter loss in patients on CAPD. *Am J Kidney Dis* 8: 436, 1986

193. Zimmerman SW, O'Brien M, Wiedenhoeft FA, Johnson CA: Staphylococcus aureus peritoneal-catheter related infections: a cause of catheter loss and peritonitis. *Perit Dial Int* 8: 191, 1988

194. Davies SJ, Ogg CS, Cameron JS, Poston S, Noble WC: Staphylococcus aureus nasal carriage, exit-site infection and catheter loss in patients treated with CAPD. *Perit Dial Int* 9: 61, 1989

195. Sewell CM, Clarridge J, Lacke C, Weineman EJ, Young EJ: Staphylococcus nasal carriage and subsequent infection in peritoneal dialysis patients. *JAMA* 248: 1493, 1982

196. Luzar MA, Cloes GA, Faller B et al.: Staphylococcus aureus nasal carriage and infection in patients on CAPD. *N Engl J Med* 322: 505, 1990

197. Perez-Fontan M, Rosales M, Rodrigues-Carmona A et al.: Treatment of Staphylococcus aureus nasal carriers in CAPD with mupirocin. *Adv Perit Dial* 8: 242, 1992

198. Sesso R, Draibe S, Castelo A et al.: Staphylococcus aureus skin carriage and development of peritonitis in patients on CAPD. *Clin Nephrol* 31: 264, 1989

199. Lye WC, Leong SO, Lee EJC: Methicillin resistant staphylococcus aureus nasal carriage and infections in CAPD. *Kidney Int* 43: 1357, 1993

200. Dobbie JW: Pathology of the peritoneum. in *The Peritoneum and Peritoneal Access*, edited by Bengmark S, London, Wright, 1989, p 42

201. Gotloib L, Bar Sella P, Shostak A: Reduplicated basal lamina of small venules and mesothelium of human parietal peritoneum: ultrastructural changes of reduplicated peritoneal basal membrane. *Perit Dial Bull* 5: 212, 1985

202. Dobbie JW: Morphology of the peritoneum. *Blood Purif* 7: 74, 1989

203. Dobbie JW: New concept in molecular biology and ultrastructural pathology of the peritoneum: their significance for peritoneal dialysis. *Am J Kidney Dis* 15: 97, 1990

204. Hauglustaine D, Monballyu J, van Meerbeek J et al.: Sclerosing peritonitis with mural bowel fibrosis in a patient on long term CAPD. *Clin Nephrol* 22: 158, 1984

205. Gandhi VC, Humayan HM, Ing TS et al.: Sclerotic thickening of the peritoneal membrane in maintenance peritoneal dialysis patients. *Arch Int Med* 140: 1201, 1980

206. Dobbie JW: Ultrastructure and pathology of the peritoneum in peritoneal dialysis. in *The Textbook of Peritoneal Dialysis*, edited by Gokal R, Nolph KD, Dordrecht, Kluwer Academic Publishers, 1994, p 17

207. Ing TS, Daugirdas JT, Ghandi VC: Peritoneal sclerosis in peritoneal dialysis patients. *Am J Nephrol* 4: 173, 1984

208. Shaldon S, Koch K, Quellhorst E, Dinarello CA: Pathogenesis of sclerosing peritonitis in CAPD. *Trans Am Soc Artif Int Organs* 30: 193, 1984

209. Shaldon S: Peritoneal macrophage – the first line of defence. in *Peritoneal Dialysis*, edited by La Greca G, Ronco C, Ferriani M *et al*, Milan, Wichtig Editore, 1986, p 201

210. Dobbie JW: Pathogenesis of peritoneal fibrosing syndromes (sclerosing peritonitis) in peritoneal dialysis. *Perit Dial Int* 12: 14, 1992

211. Joffe P, Jensen LT: Type I and III procollagens in APD: markers of peritoneal fibrosis. *Adv Perit Dial* 8: 158, 1991

212. Rottembourg J, Issad B, Langloes P et al.: Loss of ultrafiltration and sclerosing encapsulating peritonitis during CAPD. Evaluation of the potential risk factors. *Adv Perit Dial* 1: 109, 1985

213. Faller B, Marichal JF: Loss of UF in CAPD: role of acetate. *Perit Dial Bull* 4: 10, 1984

214. Slingeneyer A, Mion C, Mourad G et al.: Progressive sclerosing peritonitis: a late and severe complication of maintenance peritoneal dialysis. *Trans Am Soc Artif Int Organs* 29: 633, 1983

215. Lasker N, Burke J, Patschfsky A: Peritoneal reactions to particulate matter in peritoneal dialysis solutions. *Trans Am Soc Artif Intern Organs* 21: 342, 1975

216. Junor B, Briggs JD, Forwell M, Dobbie J, Henderson I: Sclerosing peritonitis – the contribution of chlorhexidine in alcohol. *Perit Dial Bull* 5: 101, 1985

217. Lo WK, Chan KT, Leung ACT, Pang SW, Tse CY: Sclerosing peritonitis complicating CAPD with the use of chlorhexidine in alcohol. *Adv Perit Dial* 6: 79, 1990

218. Henderson IS, Couper IA, Lumsden A: The effect of shelf-life of peritoneal dialysis fluid on the ultrafiltration in CAPD. in *Peritoneal Dialysis*, edited by La Greca G, Ronco C, Ferriani M et al., Milan, Wichtig Editore, 1986, p 85

219. Novello A, Port F: Sclerosing encapsulating peritonitis. *Int J Artif Organs* 9: 393, 1986

220. Bargman JM: Non-infectious complications of peritoneal dialysis. in *The Textbook of Peritoneal Dialysis*, edited by Gokal R, Nolph KD, Dordrecht, Kluwer Academic Publishers, 1994, p 555

221. Mackow RC, Winchester JF, Argy WP et al.: Sclerosing encapsulating peritonitis in the rat; an experimental study with intraperitoneal antiseptics. *Contr Nephrol* 57: 213, 1987

222. Slingeneyer A: Preliminary report on a cooperative international study on sclerosing encapsulating peritonitis. *Contr Nephrol* 57: 239, 1987

223. Karatson A, Buzogany I, Wagner G, Racz L: Sclerosing peritonitis caused by disinfectant in a patient on CAPD. *Int Urol Nephrol* 23: 185, 1991

224. Ing T, Daugirdas J, Gandhi VC, Leehey D: Sclerosing peritonitis after peritoneal dialysis. *Lancet* 2: 1080, 1983

225. Grefberg N, Nillson P, Andreen T: Sclerosing obstructive peritonitis, beta blockers and CAPD. *Lancet* 2: 733, 1983

226. Oreopoulos DG, Khanna R, Wu G: Sclerosing obstructive peritonitis after CAPD. *Lancet* 2: 409, 1983

227. Daugirdas J, Gandhi VC, McShane A et al.: Peritoneal sclerosis in CAPD dialysed exclusively with lactate-buffered dialysate. *Int J Artif Organs* 9: 416, 1986

228. Sabatini S, Fracasso A, Bazzato G, Kurtzman A: Effect of phthalate acid esters on transport in toad bladder membrane. *J Pharmacol Exp Ther* 250: 910, 1989

229. Krediet RT, Struijk DG, Boeschoten EW et al.: The time course of peritoneal transport kinetics in CAPD patients who develop sclerosing peritonitis. *Am J Kidney Dis* 13: 299, 1989

230. Struijk DG, van der Reijden HJ, Krediet RT, Koomen GC, Arisz L: Effect of phosphatidylcholine on peritoneal transport and lymphatic absorption in a CAPD patient with sclerosing peritonitis. *Nephron* 51: 577, 1989

231. Hollman AS, McMillan MA, Briggs D, Junor B, Morley P: Ultrasound changes in sclerosing peritonitis following CAPD. *Clin Radiol* 43: 176, 1991

232. Korezs A, Kortezs Z, Peer G et al.: Sclerosing peritonitis – possibly early diagnosis by computerised tomography of the abdomen. *Am J Nephrol* 8: 143, 1988

233. Jackson BT: Surgical treatment of sclerosing peritonitis caused by practalol. *Brit J Surg* 64: 255, 1977

234. Kittur DS, Korpe SW, Raytch RE, Smith GW: Surgical aspects of sclerosing encapsulating peritonitis. *Arch Surg* 125: 626, 1990

235. Pusatiri R, Ross R, Marshall R, Meredith JH, Hamilton RW: SEP: report of a case with small bowel obstruction managed by long term parenteral hyperalimentation, and a review of the literature. *Am J Kidney Dis* 8: 56, 1986

236. Junor B, McMillan MA: Immunosuppression in sclerosing peritonitis. *Perit Dial Int* 13 (Suppl 1): S64, 1993

237. O'Connor J, Rigby R, Hardie I et al.: Abdominal hernias complivating CAPD. *Am J Nephrol* 6: 271, 1986

238. Gigenis G, Khanna R, Mathews R, Oreopoulos DG: Abdominal hernias in patients undergoing CAPD. *Perit Dial Bull* 2: 115, 1982

239. Gotloib L, Mines M, Garmizo L, Varka I: Hemodynamic effects of increasing intra-abdomina pressure in peritoneal dialysis. *Perit Dial Bull* : 41, 1981

240. Twardowski Z, Khanna R, Nolph KD et al.: Intra-abdominal pressures during natural activities in patients treated with CAPD. *Nephron* 44: 129, 1986

241. Durand PY, Chanliau J, Gamberoni J, Hestin D, Kessler M: Routine measurement of hydrostatic intraperitoneal pressure. *Adv Perit Dial* 8: 108, 1992

242. Rubin J, Raju S, Teal N, Hellems E, Bower J: Abdominal hernias in patients undergoing CAPD. *Arch Intern Med* 142: 1453, 1982

243. Kauffman H, Adams M: Indirect inguinal hernia in patients undergoing peritoneal dialysis. *Surgery* 99: 254, 1986

244. Rocco M, Stone W: Abdominal hernias in chronic peritoneal dialysis patients: a review. *Perit Dial Bull* 5: 171, 1985

245. Engeset J, Youngson G: Ambulatory peritoneal dialysis and hernial complications. *Surg Clin North Am* 64: 385, 1984

246. Wetherington G, Leapman S, Robinson R, Filo RS: Abdominal wall and inguinal hernias in CAPD. *Am J Surg* 150: 357, 1985

247. Wise M, Manos J, Gokal R: Small umbilical hernias in patients on CAPD. *Perit Dial Bull* 4: 270, 1984

248. Modi KB, Grant AC, Garret A, Rodger RSC: Indirect inguinal hernia in CAPD patients with polycystic kidney disease. *Adv Perit Dial* 5: 84, 1989

249. Apostolodis NS, Tzardis PJ, Manouras AJ, Kosinidou MD, Katirtzoglou AN: The incidence of post-operative hernia as related to the site of insertion of permanent peritoneal catheter. *Am Surgeon* 54: 318, 1988

250. Griffin P, Coles G: Strangulated hernias through Tenckhoff cannula sites. *Brit Med J* 284: 1937, 1982

251. Spence P, Mathews R, Khanna R, Oreopulos DG: Improved results with a paramedian technique for the insertion of peritoneal dialysis catheters. *Surg Gynecol Obstet* 161: 585, 1985

252. Tank ES, Hatch DA: Hernias complicating CAPD in children. *J Pediatr Surg* 21: 41, 1986

253. von Lilien T, Salusky IB, Yap HK, Fonkalsrud EW, Fine RN: Hernias: a frequent complication in children treated with continuous peritoneal dialysis. *Am J Kidney Dis* 10: 356, 1987

254. Khoury AE, Charendoff J, Balfe JW, McLorie GA, Churchill BM: Hernias associated with CAPD in children. *Adv Perit Dial* 7: 279, 1991

255. Power D, Edward N, Catto G et al.: Richter's hernia: an unrecognised complication of CAPD. *Brit Med J* 283: 528, 1981

256. Steiner RW, Halasz NA: Abdominal catastrophes and other unusual events in CAPD. *Am J Kidney Dis* 15: 1, 1990

257. Pauls DG, Basinger BB, Shield CF: Inguinal herniorrhaphy in the CAPD patient. *Am J Kidney Dis* 20: 497, 1992
258. Nassberger L: Enterocele due to CAPD. *Acta Obstet Gynecol Scand* 63: 283, 1984
259. Francis D, Schofield I, Veitch P: Abdominal hernias in patients treated with CAPD. *Br J Surg* 69: 409, 1982
260. Lee A, Waffle C, Trebbin W: Clostridial myonecrosis. Origin from an obturator hernia in a dialysis patient. *J Am Med Assoc* 246: 1232, 1983
261. Ramos J, Burke D, Veitch P: Hernia of Morgagni in patients on CAPD. *Lancet* 1: 161, 1982
262. Beaman M, Feehally J, Smith B, Walls J: Anterior abdominal wall leakage in CAPD patients: management by intermittent peritoneal dialysis. *Perit Dial Bull* 5: 81, 1985
263. Kopecky R, Funk M, Kreitzer P: Localised genital oedema in patients undergoing CAPD. *J Urol* 134: 880, 1985
264. Orfei R, Seybold K, Blumberg A: Genital edema in patients treated by CAPD. *Perit Dial Bull* 4: 251, 1984
265. Twardowski Z, Tully R, Nichols W, Sunderrajam S: Computerised tomography (CT) in the diagnosis of subcutaneous leak sites during CAPD. *Perit Dial Bull* 4: 163, 1984
266. Tzamaloukas AH, Gibel LJ, Eisenberg B et al.: Scrotal edema in patients on CAPD: causes, differential diagnosis and management. *Dial Transplant* 21: 581, 1992
267. Abraham G, Blake PG, Mathews RE, Bargman JM, Izatt S, Oreopoulos DG: Genital swelling as a surgical complication of CAPD. *Surg Gynecol Obstet* 170: 306, 1990
268. Singal K, Segel DP, Bruns FJ, Fraley DS, Adler S, Julian TB: Genital edema in patients on CAPD. Report of 3 cases and review of the literature. *Am J Nephrol* 6: 471, 1986
269. Litherland J, Gibson M, Sambrook P et al.: Investigation and treatment of poor drains of dialysate fluid associated with anterior abdominal leaks in patients on CAPD. *Nephrol Dial Transplant* 7: 1030, 1992
270. Mandel P, Faegenburg D, Imbriano L: The use of technetium-99m colloid in the detection of patent processus vaginalis in patients on CAPD. *Clin Nucl Med* 10: 553, 1985
271. Dubin L, Froelich L: Evaluation of scrotal edema in a patient on peritoneal dialysis. *Clin Nucl Med* 10: 173, 1985
272. Eisenberg B, Arrington ER, Hartshorne MF et al.: Intraperitoneal radiocolloid imaging in dialysate leaks. *Am J Physiol Imaging* 4: 155, 1989
273. Kopecky RT, Frymore PA, Witanowski LS, Thomas FD: Complications of CAPD: diagnostic value of peritoneal scintigraphy. *Am J Kidney Dis* 10: 123, 1987
274. Kopecky RT, Frymore PA, Witanowski LS et al.: Prospective peritoneal scintigraphy in patients beginning CAPD. *Am J Kidney Dis* 15: 228, 1990
275. Johnson J, Baum S, Smink RD: Radionuclide imaging in the diagnosis of hernias related to peritoneal dialysis. *Arch Surg* 12: 952, 1987
276. Johnson BF, Segasby CA, Holroyd AM et al.: A method for demonstrating subclinical inguinal herniae in patients undergoing peritoneal dialysis: the isotope 'periotneoscrotogram'. *Nephrol Dial Transplant* 2: 254, 1987
277. Berman C, Velchik MG, Shusterman N, Alavi A: The clinical utility of the Tc-99m SC intraperitoneal scan in CAPD patients. *Clin Nucl Med* 14: 405, 1989
278. Sissons GRJ, Meecham-Jones SM, Evans C, Richards AR: Scintigraphic detection of abdominal hernias associated with CAPD. *Br J Rad* 53: 1158, 1991
279. Scanziani R, Dozio B, Caimi F, De-Rossi N, Magri F, Surian M: Peritoneography and peritoneal computerized tomography: a new approach to non-infectious complications of CAPD. *Nephrol Dial Transplant* 27: 1035, 1992
280. Hollett MD, Marn CS, Ellis JH, Francis IR, Swartz RD: Complications of CAPD: evaluation with CT peritoneography. *Am J Roentgenol* 159: 983, 1992
281. Twardowski Z, Tully RJ, Ersoy FF, Dedhia NM: CT with and without intraperitoneal contrast for determination of intra-abdominal fluid distribution and diagnosis of complications in peritoneal dialysis patients. *Trans Am Soc Artif Intern Organs* 36: 95, 1990
282. Caimi F, Roveroe G, Phillipson M, Battaglia E: Contribution of peritoneography combined with CT, in the assessment of abdominal complications in patients undergoing CAPD. *Radiologia Medica* 81: 189, 1991
283. Bunchman T, Wood E, Lynch R: Hydrothorax as a complication of peritoneal dialysis. *Perit Dial Bull* 7: 237, 1987
284. Scheldewaert R, Bogaerts Y, Pauwels R et al.: Management of a massive hydrothorax in a CAPD patient: a case report and a review of the literature. *Perit Dial Bull* 2: 69, 1982
285. Nomoto Y, Suga T, Nakajima K et al.: Acute hydrothorax in CAPD – a collaborative study of 161 centres. *Am J Nephrol* 9: 363, 1989
286. Grefberg N, Danielson B, Benson L et al.: Right-sided hydrothorax complicating peritoneal dialysis. *Nephron* 34: 130, 1983
287. Boeschoten E, Krediet R, Roos CM et al.: Leakage of dialysate across the diaphragm: an important complication of CAPD. *Neth J Med* 29: 242, 1986
288. Benz R, Schleifer CR: Hydrothorax in CAPD: successful treatment with intrapleural tetracycline and a review of the literature. *Am J Kidney Dis* 2: 136, 1985
289. Gibbons G, Baumert J: Unilateral hydrothorax complicating peritoneal dialysis: use of radionuclide image. *Clin Nucl Med* 3: 83, 1983
290. Kennedy J: Procedures used to demonstrate a pleuroperitoneal communication: a review. *Perit Dial Bull* 5: 168, 1985
291. Green A, Logan M, Medawar W et al.: The management of hydrothorax in CAPD. *Perit Dial Int* 10: 271, 1990
292. Vezina D, Winchester JF, Rakowski TA: Spontaneous resolution of a massive hydrothorax in a CAPD patient. *Perit Dial Bull* 7: 212, 1987
293. Ing A, Rutland J, Kalowski S: Spontaneous resolution of hydrothorax in CAPD. *Nephron* 61: 247, 1992
294. Townsend R, Fragola JA: Hydrothorax in a patient receiving CAPD-successful treatment with intermittent peritoneal dialysis. *Arch Int Med* 142: 1571, 1982
295. Chow CC, Sung JY, Chueng CK, Hamilton-Wood C, Lai KN: Massive hydrothorax in CAPD: diagnosis, management and review of the literature. *New Zealand Med J* 101: 475, 1988
296. Posen G, Sachs H: Treatment of recurrent pleural effusions in dialysis patients by talc insufflation. *Am Soc Artif Int Organs* (abstract) 1979, p 75

297. Catizone L, Zuchelli A, Zuchelli P: Hydrothorax in a PD patient: successful treatment with intrapleural autologous blood instillation. *Adv Perit Dial* 7: 221, 1991

298. Vlachojannis J, Boettcher I, Brandt L, Schoeppe W: A new treatment for unilateral recurrent hydrothorax during CAPD. *Perit Dial Bull* 5: 180, 1985

299. Pattison C, Rodger R, Adu J et al.: Surgical treatment of hydrothorax complicating CAPD. *Clin Nephrol* 21: 191, 1984

300. Allen S, Matthews HR: Surgical treatment of massive hydrothorax complicating CAPD. *Clin Nephrology* 36: 299, 1991

301. Brown AL, Stephenson JR, Baker LR, Tabaqchali S: Recurrent CAPD peritonitis caused by coagulase-negative staphyloccocci: reinfection or relapse determined by clinical criteria and typing methods. *J Hosp Infect* 18: 109, 1991

ACUTE COMPLICATIONS OF HEMODIALYSIS AND THEIR PREVENTION AND TREATMENT

SALIM K. MUJAIS, TODD ING and CARL KJELLSTRAND

INTRODUCTION

Hemodialysis is the most successful and most commonly used form of organ replacement therapy. Its success and widespread worldwide use attest to its safety. The latter is based on a combination of factors primordial among which is the vigilance and attention to detail of health-care workers providing the therapy. Advances in dialysis technology (both machinery and disposables) contribute significantly to the safety of this therapeutic modality. Awareness of the potential complications of the procedure should facilitate preventive and remedial interventions. The present chapter offers a discussion of the most common complications and their therapies.

FREQUENCY OF PROBLEMS

The largest study of acute hemodialysis problems included 44,000 dialyses in France (1). The most common symptom was hypotension, occurring in 24.3% of the dialyses followed by cramps in 12.8%, vomiting in 4.2% and headache in 3.2%. In this study, conducted during the early 70's, women had more side-effects than men. A smaller but more detailed analysis found a higher incidence, with hypotension being reported in 46%, hypertension in 17%, nausea in 15%, vomiting in 6% and cramps in 4% (2). On average, every dialysis was associated with one or another of these symptoms. The symptoms were much more common during the early part of a dialysis session than during the later part. During the first three or four dialysis runs, there was a mean of three symptoms per dialysis but this incidence fell as patients adjusted to the dialysis procedure. It took, however, one full month or 15 hemodialyses for the symptoms of the treatment to fall to the overall mean. From this point on, the frequency of symptoms did not change.

These studies were done with longer acetate-based dialysis treatments and with machines that could not perform programmed linear ultrafiltration. With the arrival of newer machines and of bicarbonate-based and higher-sodium dialysates, there has been a marked decline in the incidence of these symptoms. In a recent review of problems during 1,890 dialyses in 135 patients, hypotension occurred in 16%, cramps in 5%, vomiting in 4%, headaches in 2.4% and arrhythmia and angina in 1% of the dialyses (Kjellstrand, unpublished observation). Although much improvements have been obtained over the years, hemodialysis obviously remains a procedure that can be very uncomfortable for patients.

PATHOGENESIS, PATHOPHYSIOLOGY AND MEDIATORS

An overview of the possible factors causing the most common and dangerous symptom, dialysis hypotension, is outlined in Figure 1. It must be understood that interrelationships are speculative, and controversial from study to study. However, it is important to clearly separate out the pathogenesis from the mediator to the final pathophysiology that in turn is dependent on underlying patient pathology. For example, as a hypothetical illustration, as osmolality falls during dialysis it is known that vasopressin concentration in blood appropriately decreases. The *pathogenesis* (osmolality decrease) affects the *mediator* (vasopressin), and this will in turn lead to the pathophysiology (decreased total peripheral resistance). If the patient then has either vessel disease or underlying autonomic nervous dysfunction he may not be able to recruit appropriate counter measures with vasoconstrictors, and the *symptom* hypotension develops. Unless these relations are understood manipulations of the dialysis procedure or of the patient, will be hopelessly empirical.

HYPOTENSION

Clinical features

Intradialytic hypotension is one of the most common complications observed during hemodialysis. Cross sectional studies suggest that it occurs in about a third of patients. Prospective longitudinal studies placed the incidence closer to 15% of all treatments (3). Its occurrence is closely correlated with other symptoms such as cramps, nausea and vomiting (3). Predisposing factors appear to be a low body mass (women in particular), advanced age and the presence of a cardiovascular disease (3). While intuitively one would expect intradialytic hypotension to occur more in elderly patients (over 65 years of age) compared to younger patiens (under 45 years of age) (3), Capuana et al. (4), however, found the incidences to be similar between the 2 groups. This observation may be related to the fact that the dialysis conditions in the elderly are already adjusted (lower blood flow, slower ultrafiltration, etc.) to control for their increased risk. The incidence of symptomatic hypotensive episodes is particularly high in patients who have normal or low blood pressure at the initiation of dialysis and in patients who have large interdialytic weight gains (5). The development of hypotension does not seem to be influenced by the type of hemodialysis membrane used (6).

Some authors have distinguished between two types of intradialytic hypotension based on the temporal behavior of blood pressure (7, 8). In one type (gradual hypotension), blood pressure declines gradually during hemodialysis with eventual appearance of symptoms. The other type is more acute (sudden hypotension) characterized by an abrupt and sharp fall in blood pressure along with the appearance of symptoms. While some mechanistic differences have been proposed to distinguish between the two types (7), notably a role for adenosine in sudden hypotension (8), it is unclear at present whether these types tend to

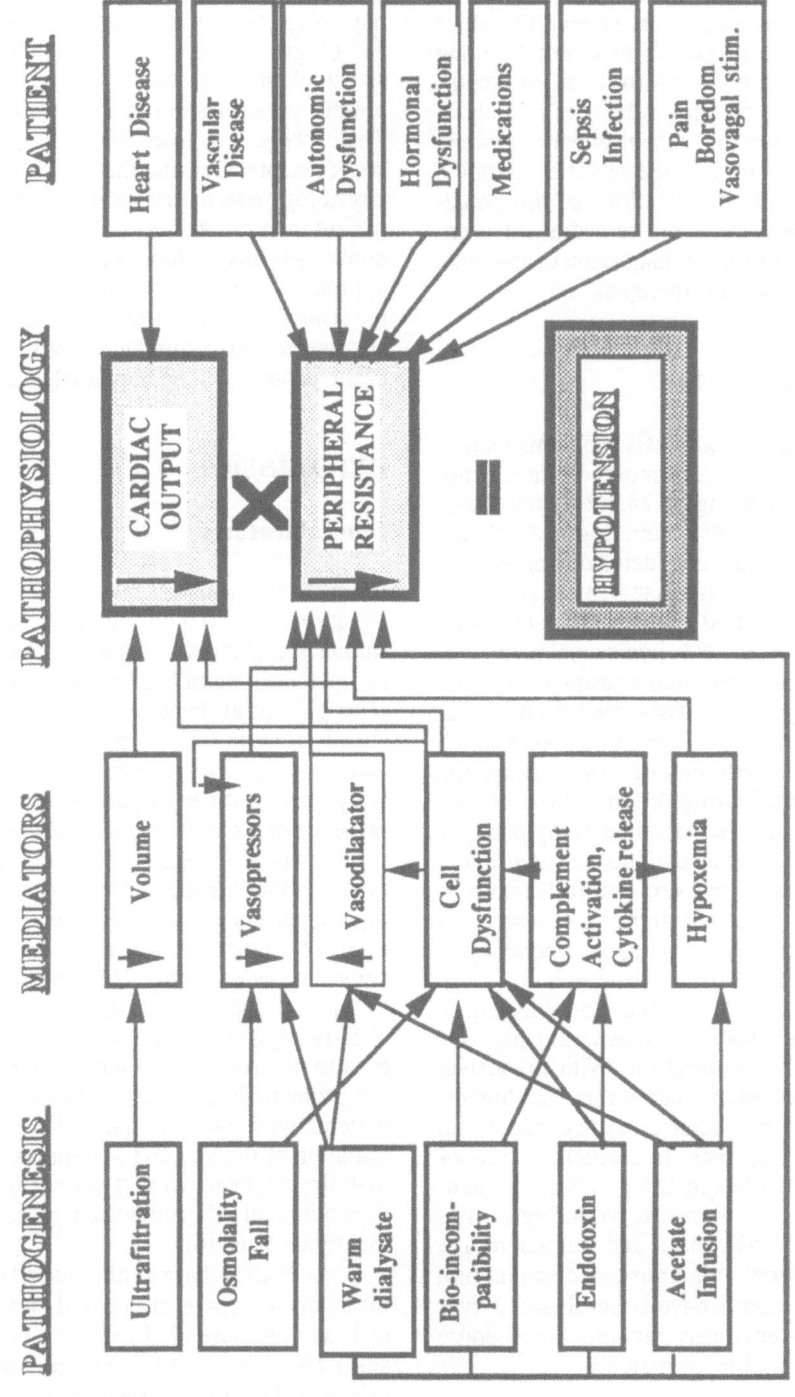

Figure 1. Scheme of the mechanisms underlying dialysis induced hypotension. Many pathogenic factors may operate simultaneously. They activate the mediators that directly, or through other mediators in turn, will decrease cardiac output on peripheral resistance or both. Pathology in patients may then interfere with the defence against the dialysis induced decrease in cardiac output or peripheral resistance and thus hypotension ensues.

occur in distinct subsets of patients and whether separate predisposing factors can be identified.

Subtyping of dialysis-induced hypotension has also been done on the basis of hemodynamic behavior. Santoro et al. (9) observed two types of collapse on the basis of heart rate behavior: the classic 'tachycardiac' collapse with an elevation in heart rate and a reduction in stroke volume, and the so-called 'bradycardiac' collapse with a paradoxical reduction in heart rate and an increase in stroke volume. 'Bradycardiac' collapses were observed in 54% of the cases. The development of bradycardia and hypotension during hemodialysis appears to be related to a sudden parasympathetic vagal overactivity and could be attributed to the Bezold–Jarisch reflex (9).

Pathophysiology

Volume-dependent factors

Since fluid is initially withdrawn from the intravascular compartment, blood volume will decline rapidly. A fluid shift (refill) from the overhydrated interstitium into the intravascular compartment counteracts hypovolemia. Under-estimation of postdialytic dry weight will cause interstitial dehydration and consequently a low refill capacity. The relation between the hydration status of the patient and changes in blood volume during treatment has recently been examined by de Vries et al. (10). Hemodialysis patients were divided into three groups according to their postdialytic extracellular fluid volume measured by means of the non-invasive conductivity method. Blood volume reduction was greater in the dehydrated than in the normohydrated and overhydrated groups. In the dehydrated group, the frequency of hypotensive episode (48%) was significantly greater compared to the normohydrated (20%) or overhydrated (6%) group. In this regard, Sherman et al. (11) also have shown that transfusions of red blood cells in anemic subjects reduces the short-term frequency of hypotensive episodes.

Intradialytic volume changes

While fluid removal during hemodialysis occurs from the intravascular space, refilling from interstitial fluid is effective enough that by the end of a typical dialysis treatment there is a greater reduction in interstitial fluid volume than in plasma volume (12). Vascular refilling depends on the rate and degree of ultrafiltration by hemodialysis as well as on other patient-related factors such as body size, fluid status, regional blood flow distribution, plasma osmolality and plasma protein concentration (13). Refilling takes place during ultrafiltration and continues after cessation of fluid removal (14). While conceptualizing these fluid shifts between fluid spaces, it is important to keep in mind that patients with ESRD have altered body composition. In ESRD, total body water (TBW) constitutes from 48.5 to 51.0% of body weight (15). The extracellular fluid (ECF) constitutes from 41.8 to 46.3% of the total body water. The ratio of plasma volume (PV) to interstitial fluid (ISF) volume approximates 1.1 to 1.2:3 (15). Salt and water alterations (under condition of ultrafiltration with normal-sodium or high-sodium dialysate) are restricted mostly to the ECF component of the TBW (16). In the ECF, it is principally the ISF that buffers salt and water depletion. The ISF is therefore, the buffer zone which maintains the proper balance and relationship between vascular capacity and volume. In ESRD, interstitial colloid osmotic pressure is reduced and transcapillary colloid osmotic gradient is raised, conditions that would favor refilling (17). After hemodialysis, interstitial colloid osmotic pressure tends to rise indicating fluid loss, but the transcapillary gradient remains in favor of refilling (17).

The dependence of refilling on interstitial hydration would imply that overhydration was associated with better refilling. Moreover, as ultrafiltration proceeds and the interstitial volume gradually contracts, one would expect a progressive drop in refilling rate over the course of a hemodialysis session. This formulation is consonant with the observation that hypotension occurs usually during the latter half of a hemodialysis run.

Maneuvers that are aimed at enhancing vascular refilling would be expected to have a salutary effect on the occurrence of vascular instability during dialysis. Sodium modeling (16, 18–22) and hypertonic hemodiafiltration (23) have been shown to be effective in this regard. The effect of dialysate base composition on refilling was evaluated by Hsu et al. (24). The cumulative decline in plasma volume after dialysis was significantly less during low sodium-bicarbonate dialysis than during low sodium-acetate dialysis. High sodium-acetate dialysis also resulted in less net fall in plasma volume than low sodium-acetate dialysis, with similar cumulative refilling rates for low sodium-bicarbonate and high sodium-acetate dialyses (24). Improved hemodynamic stability utilizing sodium-bicarbonate dialysis may be due, in part, to a greater plasma refilling and a better preservation of plasma volume.

Hypotension often develops in the latter half of dialysis. This point in time does not always correspond to the maximal reduction in plasma volume. At or before the time that dialysis-induced hypotension takes place, there is usually no sharp fall in blood volume nor any change in the plasma refilling rate (25). This observation suggests that hypotension is caused by a sudden breakdown of the blood pressure support mechanism compensating for a contracted blood volume.

Vascular tone-related factors

During hemofiltration and sequential ultrafiltration, the patient's ability for vasoconstrictive counterregulation is better maintained than during conventional hemodialysis (26). Hemodynamic studies have repeatedly shown that while significant reduction of cardiac output, stroke volume, pulmonary artery pressure and plasma volume are observed during hemodialysis, only a minimal elevation in peripheral resistance is observed (26).

Inappropriate peripheral venodilatation has been proposed as an important contributor to the development of dialysis-induced hypotension (27–31). Bradley et al. (29) found that while vascular resistance in the forearm rose during dialysis with acetate and with bicarbonate (more so with the latter), the venous bed of the forearm dilated. Maeda et al. (28) in a hemodynamic study found a sharp drop in cardiac output during dialysis-induced hypotension, along with concomitant sudden drops in the mean pulmonary arterial pressure and in the mean right atrial pressure. These changes have been attributed to a reduction in venous return (31). Since there was no recognizable alteration in blood volume with the sharp fall in blood pressure, this curtailment in venous return is believed to be caused by a relocation of circulating blood, possibly associated with a sudden decrease in venous tone (28). The significance of the reduction in venous return is highlighted by the effort of Rozich et al. (32) to determine whether hemodialysis results in alterations in left ventricular diastolic filling that might contribute to dialysis-induced hypotension. Following hemodialysis there was a significant prolongation in left ventricular isovolumetric relaxation time, as well as a significant drop in the rate and extent of early rapid ventricular filling. In contrast, late atrial-assisted filling did not change significantly (32). Rozich et al. also demonstrated a significant independent inverse relationship between the frequency of dialysis-related hypotensive episodes and the duration of early left ventricular filling. Such results suggest that hemodialysis leads to discrete alterations in early left ventricular filling, with no significant compensatory rise in late atrial-assisted ventricular filling. Moreover, patients with the shortest early left ventricular filling times appeared to have the greatest predilection for becoming hemodynamically unstable during dialysis (31, 32).

Converse et al. (33) likened the development of sudden hypotension during hemodialysis to that encountered in hemorrhage-induced hypovolemia. The latter can trigger a sudden fall in sympathetic activity resulting in bradycardia and vasodilatation. A similar type of vasodepressor reaction developing during dialysis would exacerbate the volume-dependent decline in blood pressure. Furthermore, Converse et al. compared the hemodynamic and sympathetic nerve activity (using intraneural microelectrodes for measurement) responses during hemodialysis in patients with and in those without a history of hemodialysis-induced hypotension (33). While progressive rises in vascular resistance and sympathetic activity were observed in the hypotension-resistant patients, in the hypotension-prone patients, however, the precipitous fall in blood pressure was accompanied by reductions in sympathetic activity, vascular resistance, and heart rate as well as symptoms of vasodepressor syncope. On an interdialysis day, both groups of patients raised vascular resistance normally during unloading of cardiopul-

monary baroreceptors using a lower-body negative pressure, and increased heart rate normally during unloading of arterial baroreceptors using an infusion of nitroprusside. These findings indicate that in some hemodialysis patients, hemodialysis-induced hypotension is not caused by a chronic uremic impairment in arterial or cardiopulmonary baroreflexes but rather by an acute, paradoxical withdrawal of sympathetic vasoconstrictor drive. Such a withdrawal often engenders a vasodepressor syncope (33).

Autonomic neuropathy

Abnormalities of autonomic function have been observed in patients with chronic renal failure both before and after initiation of maintenance dialytic therapy. The cold pressor test, response to sudden loud noise and mental arithmetic maneuvers were normal in non-dialyzed patients with chronic renal failure, suggesting an intact efferent sympathetic pathway (34). Expiration/inspiration ratio, lying/standing ratio, Valsalva ratio and the baroreceptor sensitivity slope were significantly abnormal in non-dialyzed patients. These results indicate a defective efferent parasympathetic pathway and a depressed baroreceptor sensitivity (34). The heart rate response to standing and the baroreceptor sensitivity are significantly lower in patients who develop hypotension during hemodialysis (34). Lower baroreflex sensitivity could contribute to hypotension during dialysis. Similarly, Heber et al. (35) found that day/night blood pressure variations were significantly reduced in patients with chronic renal failure when compared with a control population. Hemodialysis patients had a 'square wave' response to the Valsalva maneuver. In this group of patients, the hypotension was not due to left ventricular dysfunction, but to a failure of the baroreceptor response to volume depletion during hemodialysis. Lilley et al. (36) have suggested that hemodialysis-induced hypotension may result from a lesion in the baroreceptors, cardiopulmonary receptors, or visceral afferent nerves. Furthermore, the usual elevated mean non-dialysis blood pressures in patients with hemodialysis hypotension (and in other ESRD patients as well (37)) may be neurogenic in origin, akin to the hypertension that follows baroreceptor deafferentation in experimental animals (36).

Role of dialysate

Intradialytic hypotension is more common during acetate dialysis compared to bicarbonate dialysis, particularly in elderly subjects (38–40). This phenomenon has been attributed to a slower metabolism of acetate as reflected in lower post-dialysis plasma bicarbonate concentrations (38). These observations have encouraged the examination of the role of acetate in the genesis of intradialytic hypotension. DiBello et al. (41), in an echocardiographic study in patients receiving acetate dialysis, found no evidence of myocardial suppression related to the use of acetate. Wizemann et al. (42) demonstrated that acetate

Table 1. Vasoactive substances during hemodialysis

Peptide	Sham HD	Isolated UF	Isovolemic HD	Standard HD
Vasoconstrictors				
Noradrenaline	increase	increase	decrease	unchanged
Renin activity	increase	increase	unchanged	increase
Vasopressin	unchanged	increase	decrease	unchanged
Neuropeptide Y	unchanged	increase	unchanged	increase
Gamma 2-MSH		increase	decrease	increase
Vasodilators				
ANP	decrease			
Substance P	increase	unchanged	decrease	increase
VIP	increase	unchanged	decrease	decrease
Motilin	decrease	unchanged	unchanged	variable
CGRP	unchanged	unchanged	unchanged	unchanged
Beta endorphin	unchanged	increase	decrease	variable

MSH = melanocyte-stimulating hormone, ANP = atrial natriuretic peptide, VIP = vasoactive intestinal peptide, CGRP = calcitonin gene-related peptide.

infusions had no effect on myocardial contractility. Hyperacetatemia, however, did result in a decrease in preload (42), a finding compatible with the venodilatatory effect of acetate (43). Indeed, Bradley et al. (29) had already shown in 1988 that the rate of fall of blood pressure was significantly greater during dialysis using acetate compared with that using bicarbonate. In addition, acetate dialysis led to a smaller rise in vascular resistance and a greater venodilatation.

As variations in dialysate calcium concentration may be required in some subjects, and as calcium may have a significant effect on myocardial contractility and vascular reactivity, it is important to determine whether such variations may adversely impact on hypotension-prone patients. Sherman et al. (44) found a lower blood pressure throughout dialysis with a low-calcium (2.5 mM) bath, compared to a high-calcium (3.5 mM) one. The difference, however, was clinically minor (less than 5 mmHg) and individuals prone to intradialytic hypotension were not adversely affected.

Vasoactive peptides

Several studies have evaluated the effects of hemodialysis on vasoactive peptides and the changes in these substances that may supervene during intradialytic hypotension (45, 46). Hegbrant et al. (47–49) examined the effects of sham dialysis, isolated ultrafiltration, isovolemic hemodialysis and standard hemodialysis on a variety of vasoactive peptides. Their results are shown in Table 1.

Sham hemodialysis was associated with variable changes in these vasoactive substances, changes that are likely to be related to membrane interaction, heparinization, or cooling of the blood during the procedure (47).

These findings suggest that the extracorporeal circulation per se affects plasma levels of vasoactive substances and influences vascular stability. Isolated ultrafiltration resulted in a uniform increase in all vasoconstrictor substances assayed while a less uniform decline was observed during isovolemic hemodialysis (48). Not unexpectedly, standard hemodialysis manifested a summation effect of its separate components (namely, diffusion dialysis and ultrafiltration during dialysis), with rises in the levels of several vasoconstrictors (49). The levels of vasodilator substances showed minimal variations during all three modalities (47–49).

Niwa et al. (50) suggested that the levels of vasoactive substances may be altered during hemodialysis in a membrane-dependent fashion. While differences were shown among the various membranes as far as the levels of vasoactive substances are concerned, there was no correlation between the dialysis-induced changes in blood pressure and the observed alterations in the concentrations of these substances (50). Moreover, it is doubtful whether opioid peptides play any role in intradialytic hypotension as premedication with naloxone has no preventive or therapeutic value (51).

Management: Prevention

The treatment of dialysis hypotension is outlined in Table 2.

Patient factors

As at least one type of dialysis hypotension is dependent on the volume of fluid removed, it is important that the patients should strive to gain as little weight as possible

694   *Salim K. Mujais, Todd Ing and Carl Kjellstrand*

between dialysis treatments. It is doubtful that this limitation in weight gain can be accomplished with restrictions of fluid intake as almost all patients present with a normal pre-dialysis serum sodium value on the day of dialysis. The underlying mechanism, therefore, appears to be related to the development of thirst as a result of sodium intake. Consequently, in order to curtail weight gain, sodium intake must be restricted. Patient education is a very time-consuming process and the return on the effort is often regretably meager. Most dialysis patients gain about 1 kg of weight daily. This must mean that the patient's sodium intake is close to 9 g of sodium chloride (154 mmol), a value approximating a normal intake in most of the developed world. Nevertheless, limiting sodium intake is the key to a successful treatment.

Meticulous blood sugar control in diabetics is clearly desirable and mandatory as these patients otherwise will be exposed to thirst and will drink as a consequence. Some patients have abnormal thirst and present with hyponatremia. ACE-inhibitors have only been partially useful as antidipsogenic agents.

Patients should also be told not to eat shortly before dialysis if they are prone to hypotension. This is because, in some patients, eating can lead to more hypotension as blood is shunted to the splanchnic area (52, 53). It is also prudent to withhold blood pressure medications shortly before dialysis. The same holds true for other drugs that influence the regulation of the blood pressure by the nervous system (54). An example of such drugs is phenothiazine.

Dialysis procedure

Slower, ultrafiltration-controlled, sodium-ramped dialysis

A longer dialysis session which curbs the amount of ultrafiltration per time unit may be beneficial In some patients simply reducing the dialyzer clearance by slowing the blood flow may be helpful. Over-zealous dialyzer clearance may be the reason why in the French study, women with their smaller body weights had much more hypotension than men; therefore, the dialyzer clearance for each individual should be adjusted to the individual's body weight (1). The use of linear or modeled ultrafiltration using volume controllers may be of help; so may sodium modeling with a higher sodium dialysate level during the early part of dialysis (55). Raising the dialysate concentration of calcium has also helped some patients (56, 57). Sequencing dialysis with separation of ultrafiltration and hemodialysis is not uniformly successful and the logistic burden may preclude its applicability (58, 59).

Dialysate cooling

The greater cardiovascular stability encountered during isolated ultrafiltration has been related to the cooling of blood in the extracorporeal circuit by as much as two degrees Celsius (60). This observation lends support to the suggestion that lowering blood temperature during

Table 2. Treating dialysis hypotension

PREVENTION
Patient
    Low weight gain
        Low Na – Diet
        Meticulous diabetes control
    No food during dialysis
    Hold BP – MEDS
Dialysis procedure
    Slower, longer dialysis
    UF-controller/modulated dialysis
    Non-linear UF
    High (ramped) sodium
    Higher dialysate calcium
    Sequencing (Alt. days)
    Lower dialysate temperature
    Bicarbonate
    CAPD
Pharmacological
    Hyper-oncotic albumin
    Nasal oxygen
    Mannitol
    L-carnitine
    L-DOPA/L-DOPS
    Mineral/gluco-corticoids
    PG-Inhibition (NSAIDS)
    Ace-inhibitors
Other
    Elevate legs
    Compression legs
    Higher HCT (Erythropoietin/transfusion)
    Stimulation
ACUTE TREATMENT
Volume
    Super-saturated sodium   . . . 10 mL 23%
    Mannitol   . . . 50 mL 20%
    Dextran 70   . . . 100–500 mL 6%
Vasoconstrictors
    Metaramine
    Phenylepinephrine
    NOR-epinephrine
    Lysine vasopressin
    Caffeine
    Midodrine
    Amezinium
Nasal oxygen

hemodialysis may afford a similar advantage (60). Lowering dialysate temperature from 37° to 35°C significantly reduces the incidence of intradialytic hypotension (3, 5, 60, 61). While the decline in incidence has been reported to be dramatic in short-term studies (5, 62), the overall reduction in incidence in prospective long-term studies has been modest (3, 63, 64). Moreover, the possibility of having a placebo effect has also been raised (63). The effect of a lower dialysate temperature is unrelated to any changes in biocompatibility behavior as these parameters are not altered by the cooling (61). Greater elevations in peripheral vascular resistance and higher post-dialysis catecholamine levels suggest that dialysate cooling may enhance vasoconstrictor mechanisms (5). In one study, dialysate cooling brought about a greater incidence of cramps (64).

Modulated dialysis

Determination of blood volume changes by continuous monitoring has allowed the development of blood volume-controlled ultrafiltration. Such measures have resulted in a lower incidence of symptomatic hypotension (65). Methods of modulated dialysis such as the above diverge from the usual constant ultrafiltration scheme and may link the period of highest ultrafiltration to modifications in dialysate sodium level (66).

Bicarbonate, membrane, CAPD

Should acetate be used as the buffer base, it should be replaced by bicarbonate, a base that causes lesser vasodilatation. Large studies have found no effect of membrane type on blood pressure values during dialysis (67–70). Should a patient have excessive hypotension, dialytic therapy should be switched to CAPD.

Pharmacological manipulation

Hyperoncotic albumin 20–25% may prevent hypotension and allow more ultrafiltration to take place. If given, albumin should be infused rapidly during the first 15 to 30 minutes of dialysis to promote mobilization of any edematous fluid that may be present. The excessive fluid can then be removed by ultrafiltration. Nasal oxygen has also enabled some patients to maintain blood pressure; so have mannitol infusions. These infusions, however, cannot be given for more than 3 or 4 dialyses because of the problem of accumulation. L-carnitine, DOPA and L-DOPA have been reported to prevent dialysis hypotension (71, 72) as has treatment with mineralocorticoids and glucocorticoids, particularly in patients with high predialysis serum potassium levels. Non-steroidal antiinflammatory drugs, perhaps by reducing circulating and released prostaglandins during dialysis have also led to higher blood pressures (73).

Miscellaneous treatment

Elevating the legs or using compressive bandages may facilitate mobilization of the edema and allow more ultrafiltration to proceed with less blood pressure problems. Similarly, raising the hematocrit by transfusions or by erythropoietin therapy has curtailed the incidence of dialysis-related hypotension in some patients. It is also important to provide patients with appropriate stimulation since simply the boredom of lying and waiting may worsen hypotensive episodes.

Management: Acute treatment

Volume administration

The management of intradialytic hypotension has relied on volume expansion irrespective of the underlying mechanism in each particular patient. Volume expansion has frequently been done by infusions of normal saline, a practice that frustrates attempts to attain dry weight by increasing the fluid burden, thus necessitating greater ultrafiltration and further hypotension. As a consequence, a vicious cycle is created. The volume overload present in between dialysis sessions gives rise to hypertension that necessitates the use of antihypertensive agents. Such use aggravates the hypotension occurring during dialysis.

Hypertonic saline solutions safely and effectively treat dialysis-induced hypotension and may offer a better alternative. As these solutions are available in distinct concentrations, the relevance of the total osmotic load administered *versus* the specific concentration of sodium in the administered solution have been debated. Gong et al. (74) compared the efficacy of three hypertonic saline solutions for treating dialysis-induced hypotension in a randomized, blinded, crossover clinical trial Dialysis-induced hypotension was treated with an intravenous bolus of either 10 mL of a 23% saturated hypertonic saline, 30 mL of a 7.5% hypertonic saline, or 30 mL of a 7.5% saline with 6% dextran 70, each containing osmolar loads of 80, 80, and 100 mOsm, respectively. When a patient is given equal osmolal loads (e.g., the first 2 hypertonic saline boluses above-mentioned), the more concentrated solutions produced a greater increase in systolic blood pressure. The addition of an oncotic agent such as dextran may prolong the blood pressure response beyond 10 minutes (74).

Dextrans are useful plasma expanders to employ in the management of hypotension. Recent autopsy and biopsy reports (75, 76), however, have documented the intracellular deposition of dextrans in various tissues such as lymph nodes, the heart, adrenals, the bone marrow and others. The deposits are a PAS-positive, birefringent material with an unusual ultrastructure (75). These deposits were not present in the macrophages of dialysis patients who had not been administered dextrans. The presence and intensity of depositions were related to the cumulative amount of dextrans received by the patients (75, 76). A similar problem may be encountered with mannitol as the fate of this non-metabolizable alcohol is also unclear.

Vasoconstrictors

As at least some of the pathophysiology of dialysis hypotension appears to be due to vasodilatation, simply giving the patient vasoconstrictors such as metaramine, phenylepinephrine, norepinephrine, midodrine, amezinium, vasopressin or caffeine, has been associated with better maintenance of blood pressure (8, 77–80).

HYPOXEMIA

Clinical features

Patients maintained on intermittent hemodialysis harbor a continuously changing acid-base internal environment. In the interdialytic period, the progressive accumulation of non-volatile acids leads to a compensatory hyperventilation. During dialysis, re-titration of the retained acids takes place along with a gain of alkali and an abatement of the hyperventilation, only to have the acidosis recur as the acid burden progressively rises postdialysis (81). The intradialytic period is more complex and involves changes in both oxygen and carbon dioxide levels.

Hypoxemia of variable degrees and duration occurs in the intradialytic period. In some subjects it occurs early and is of short duration, while in others it may have a late onset and be prolonged (82). The latter pattern has been associated with a heightened release of tissue plasminogen activator (82). The hypoxemia is especially pronounced in patients with preexisting pulmonary abnormalities (83) in that it may persist postdialysis (84). Continuous measurements of oxygen saturation reveal a drop in saturation of 1 to 4% coinciding with the observed hypoxemia (85). The hypoxemia is usually innocuous except when severe in patients with underlying respiratory decompensation, or in subjects with partially compensated ischemic heart disease who may experience anginal episodes necessitating oxygen supplementation for prevention. There is no relationship between dialysis-induced hypoxemia and hypotension (86).

Pathophysiology

Effects of dialysate

Most studies agree that acetate dialysis is associated with a more severe hypoxemia than bicarbonate dialysis or isolated ultrafiltration (38, 81, 83, 86–96). The role of dialysate composition in the genesis of hypoxemia has been elegantly illustrated by the study of Francos et al. (87). Patients were studied with both polyacrylonitrile (PAN) and cuprophan membranes containing different priming solutions. Despite leukopenia and complement activation, hypoxemia did not occur during membrane

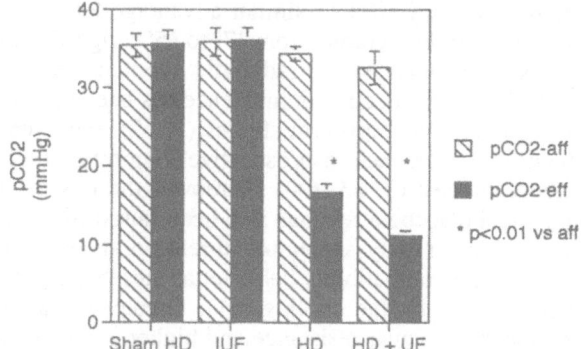

Figure 2. Effect of differing modalities of extracorporeal therapy on blood P_{CO_2}. Abreviations: sham HD: blood circulation with no ultrafiltration and no dialysate; IUF: isolated ultrafiltration; HD: acetate hemodialysis with no ultrafiltration; HD + UF: acetate hemodialysis with ultrafiltration; aff: afferent (arterial) line; eff: efferent (venous) line. Data from 29 patients using a parallel plate dialyzer and 200 mL/min blood flow. (Mujais SK, unpublished observations).

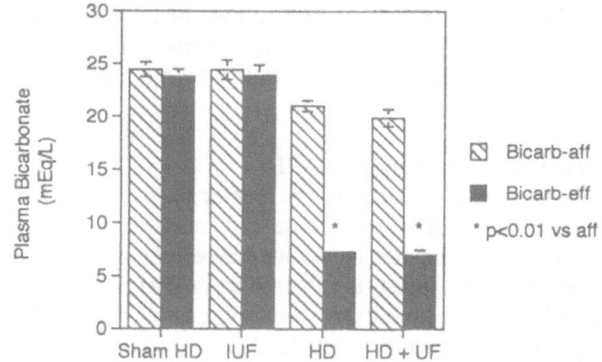

Figure 3. Effect of differing modalities of extracorporeal therapy on plasma bicarbonate. Abreviations: sham HD: blood circulation with no ultrafiltration and no dialysate; IUF: isolated ultrafiltration; HD: acetate hemodialysis with no ultrafiltration; HD + UF: acetate hemodialysis with ultrafiltration; aff: afferent (arterial) line; eff: efferent (venous) line. Data from 29 patients using a parallel plate dialyzer and 200 mL/min blood flow. (Mujais SK, unpublished observations).

contact only. After 15 minutes of subsequent acetate dialysis, significant hypoxemia occurred with both membranes (87). Significantly less hypoxemia was noted during bicarbonate dialysis (87).

While there is general agreement that carbon dioxide unloading is a primary factor in the genesis of the hypoventilation and the associated hypoxemia, the mechanisms of carbon dioxide unloading remain a subject of debate. During acetate dialysis, a significant loss of carbon dioxide and bicarbonate takes place across the dialyzer (Figures 2 and 3). The resultant hypocapnea has been assumed to give rise to hypoventilation and subsequent hypoxemia (90, 92). Another possible cause for the hypocapnea has been advanced by Oh et al. (93). These authors suggested that the loss of carbon dioxide was too small to alter significantly carbon dioxide balance and that greater carbon dioxide consumption occurs with metabolism of the acetate acquired during dialysis (93).

Hypoxemia has also been observed with bicarbonate dialysis, albeit of a much milder degree. In this setting, hypoxemia has been related to the degree of alkalinization induced by a high-bicarbonate bath. In favor of this postulate is the demonstration by Ganss et al. (88) that a low-bicarbonate dialysate (29 mM) prevented the hypoxemia observed with a high-bicarbonate dialysate (36 mM). Alkalinization occurs in both bicarbonate and acetate dialyses, being somewhat delayed in the latter form of dialysis as time is required to metabolize acetate to bicarbonate. By raising the affinity of hemoglobin for oxygen, such alkalinization would reduce tissue oxygen delivery and thereby magnify the clinical effects of dialysis-induced hypoxemia (95).

Effect of membrane

If pulmonary leukosequestration plays a role in dialysis-induced hypoxemia, then membranes with differing complement-activating potentials and varying ability to induce neutropenia would be expected to cause disparate degrees of hypoxemia in proportion to their neutropenic effects. Under conditions of acetate dialysis, however, no differences in the degree of hypoxemia have been observed between membranes (83, 90, 92, 96). These observations may be explained by the different time courses of pulmonary leukosequestration and hypoxemia. Ross et al. (94), using [111]indium-radiolabelled leukocytes, found similar degrees of pulmonary leuko-sequestration with both acetate and bicarbonate dialyses. However, hypoxemia developed later in the course of dialysis and was seen only with acetate dialysis.

Mechanisma proposed for the explanation of pulmonary leukosequestration include: (1) complement-dependent leukocyte activation with expression of adhesion molecules, (2) actin polymerization with enhanced stiffness of the leukocytes and trapping in the pulmonary capillary bed, and (3) the formation of platelet-leukocyte microaggregates with heightened endothelial interaction (97). The role of complement activation or other mechanisms mediating the leukosequestration and hypoxemia during cuprophan dialysis has to be evaluated against the background of disparate time profiles of the phenomena observed. Dissociations between the occurrence of complement activation and the appearance of leukopenia have been observed (87, 96). Complement activation across the dialyzer persists throughout dialysis, whereas late in dialysis, both the leukopenia and the hypoxemia resolve (87). A similar disparity has been demonstrated between the persistence of actin polymerization and the formation of platelet-leukocyte aggregates on the one hand and leukosequestration on the other (97).

While complement-dependent leukocyte activation and actin polymerization are membrane-dependent, the formation of platelet-leukocyte aggregates occurs in the same manner with all the membranes (97).

Taken together, these observations suggest that the main mechanism of dialysis-induced hypoxemia is carbon dioxide unloading with minor contributions from other mechanisms, and that difference between membranes are not clinically significant.

MUSCLE CRAMPS

Clinical profile

Muscle cramps represent a vexing and persistent problem plaguing a significant number of patients maintained on hemodialysis. Such cramps develop repeatedly in about 25% of all hemodialysis patients (98). While benign in its biological significance, the clinical and emotional toll of the condition can frustrate the most stoic of patients. Painful cramps, usually of the lower extremities, occur in the second half of a dialysis session and are sometimes preceded by hypotension. A delayed course is also observed and cramps can recur over several hours after the end of a dialysis run. Cramps are commonly observed in the setting of rapid ultrafiltration (even if all the excess fluid has not yet been completely removed), or when a patient's volume status falls below the empirically determined 'dry weight'.

Pathophysiology

There have been very few studies examining the mechanisms underlying the appearance of muscular cramps during or after hemodialysis. Since cramps take place in a setting of relative hypovolemia developing as a result of the discrepancy between the magnitude of the ultrafiltration and the vascular refilling rate, a role for volume contraction in their genesis has been entertained. This assertion is supported by the common observation that volume expansion with hypertonic solutions frequently brings relief. Electromyographic measurements in cramp-prone subjects during dialysis demonstrated a progressive rise in tonic activity during the second half of hemodialysis culminating in the paroxysm of the cramp (99).

Vasoconstrictor mechanisms activated by volume removal are plausible mediators of reduced muscle blood flow. The success of nifedipine in alleviating established cramps may be considered adjunctive evidence for a role of vasoconstrictor mechanisms (99). Cramps, however, can continue to take place in hemodialysis patients treated with chronic calcium-channel blocker therapy. Piergies et al. (100) have shown that activation of the renin-angiotensin system has no role in the causation of skeletal muscle cramps during hemodialysis. The activation of the renin-angiotensin system was not unusually enhanced in patients with frequent cramps, nor did angiotensin converting enzyme inhibition reduce the frequency or severity of the cramps. In a follow-up study, the same investigators suggested that cramps were prone to develop during hemodialysis in patients whose sympathetic nervous system response to volume stress was partially intact since a greater ratio of tilt/recumbent norepinephrine levels was demonstrated in patients with frequent cramps than in those who cramped infrequently (101). This assertion is consistent with the observation that more frequent cramps were seen in subjects who had been on dialysis for a shorter period (101). However, it is not consonant with a higher incidence in diabetics as described in the above follow-up study, unless one is to invoke a mechanism similar to that of hyperadrenergic syncope that has been described in diabetics by Cryer et al. (102). The role for a more marked sympathetic nervous system response to volume stress in patients who have cramps is supported by the observation that small doses of prazosin given at the beginning of a dialysis session significantly reduce the frequency of cramps when compared to administering a placebo (103). The use of prazosin, however, was associated with an increase in the incidence of hypotension making the intervention not clinically useful.

Tissue hypoxia has been suggested as a cause for dialysis-induced cramps. This hypothesis posits that declines in 2,3-diphosphoglycerate levels observed in uremia and the transient alkalosis of hemodialysis combine to raise the affinity of hemoglobin for oxygen and consequently reduce tissue oxygen delivery (96). Further research is needed before this hypothesis can be established. Cramping, however, is not usually a feature of extremity ischemia and the relief of the pain with maneuvers that do not alter oxygen delivery, makes this hypothesis less likely. The observation that carnitine supplementation is associated with a reduced incidence of muscle cramps has led to the formulation of the hypothesis that uremic cramps may be due to carnitine deficiency (71). The latter, however, causes myopathy rather than cramps, and when carnitine deficiency-related cramps develop, they usually take place during exercise and not at rest.

It is clear from the above that while many of the conditions associated with cramps are known, a definitive pathophysiologic scheme relating cramping to one or several of such conditions, is at present lacking.

Cramps can be encountered in some patients with no clear-cut underlying plausible mechanism at all. It is important to realize that well-performed studies have shown a strong correlation between affect and somatic symptoms particularly cramps. Improvement of affect may in some patients have an important impact on the development of this somatic complaint (104).

The occurrence of cramps has been implicated (105) as a cause for a rise in creatine kinase levels in some hemodialysis patients. Other more serious causes for such elevations need to be evaluated, however, before ascrib-

ing raised values to muscle cramps in any individual patient.

Management

Hypertonic solutions

Hypertonic solutions of dextrose, mannitol, and saline are effective treatments for hemodialysis-associated muscle cramps. The concern that post-dialysis retention of mannitol and saline may lead to increased thirst, interdialytic weight pain, and elevated blood pressure has not been validated. In a prospective, randomized, double-blind crossover study the safety and efficacy of the three solutions have been found to be equivalent (106). Cramps can be treated with 50 mL (126 mOsm) 50% dextrose water, 100 mL (138 mOsm) 25% mannitol, and 10–15 mL (126 mOsm) 23.5% saline. Saline solutions of lower concentrations can also be used. Mild postdialysis hyperglycemia and hypernatremia during administration of dextrose and saline, respectively, are the only significant laboratory abnormalities observed (106).

Drug therapy

Both quinine (325 mg orally at bedtime) and vitamin E (400 IU orally at bedtime) are effective in reducing the incidence and severity of leg cramps in hemodialysis patients. The effect of these drugs is observed early (within 2 weeks of therapy) and has been found to be sustained in short-term studies (up to 2 months) (107). The two drugs have similar efficacy, but it is not known whether their effects are additive or whether subjects unresponsive to one agent would respond to the other. Quinine reduces the excitability of the motor endplate to nerve stimulation and enhances the muscle refractory period. The drug is cleared primarily by the liver and toxicities, while serious, are very rare with the usually prescribed dosages (99). Variability in response among patients may be related to the drug's variable bioavailability.

There is anecdotal evidence that administration of chloroquine phosphate (a drug effective in alleviating ordinary cramps) may reduce the frequency of cramps during hemodialysis (108). Similarly, nifedipine has been found by some to relieve established dialysis-induced cramps (99). The frequent occurrence of simultaneous hypotension, however, makes the routine use of nifedipine unpractical

L-carnitine supplementation

Several studies have suggested that correction of the carnitine deficiency of uremia may have a salutary effect on the musculoskeletal symptoms associated with hemodialysis (71). A double-blind, placebo-controlled, and randomized study in a large sample of long-term hemodialysis patients, showed a decrease in the incidence in intradialytic cramps with L-carnitine supplementation given intravenously at the end of a dialysis session. This improve-

Table 3. Proposed causes of intradialytic hypoxemia

Hypoventilation secondary to CO_2 unloading during acetate dialysis

Hypoventilation due to correction of acidosis and developing alkalosis

Hypoventilation due to changes in respiratory quotient with acetate

Central effects of acetate

Pulmonary microembolization

Pulmonary microcirculatory damage

Table 4. Sterilizability of different membranes

Membrane	ETO	Steam	Gamma irradiation	Comment
Cuprophan	+	+	+	
Hemophan	+	+	+	
Cellulose acetate	+	–	+	Glass point 45°C
Polysulphone	+	+	+	
PAN	+	–	+	Glass point 80°C
PMMA	–	–	+	ETO-reservoir
Polycarbonate	+	–	+	Hydrolysis
Polyamide	+	–	+	Hydrolysis
EVAL	+	–	+	Glass point 66°C

Data for this table are courtesy of Dr J Vienken, Wuppertal, Germany.
PAN = polyacrylonitrile, PMMA = polymethylmethacrylate, EVAL = ethylene-vinylalcohol copolymer, ETO = ethylene oxide.

ment was observed in association with a reduction in the incidence in intradialytic hypotension, which frequently accompanies cramping, and improvement in muscle mass and several biochemical parameters (71). The relationship of this symptomatologic improvement and the trophic effect of carnitine therapy on skeletal muscle integrity remains to be clarified.

Modulated dialysis

The frequent association of hypotensive episode and the development of cramps has encouraged the examination of the effects of maneuvers aimed at alleviating hypotension on the incidence of cramps. Sodium modeling and blood volume-controlled ultrafiltration have reduced the incidence of hypotension and cramps in parallel (54, 65).

ACUTE ALLERGIC REACTIONS

Clinical features

Allergic reactions occurring immediately after the initiation of dialysis using fresh dialyzers (also known as the 'first-use syndrome') consist of a constellation of many of the following symptoms: burning retrosternal pain, burning sensation along the arterio-venous fistula, sensation of diffuse heat, cold perspiration, urticaria, pruritus, periorbital and facial edema, flushing, laryngeal stridor, bronchial hypersecretion, bronchospasm, dyspnea, hypotension, bradycardia, and loss of consciousness (109–114). Death can occur (109, 112).

In patients who are dialyzed in a dialyzer-reuse program, allergic reactions have been reported to develop often on the days when fresh dialyzers are used but not on the days when re-used dialyzers are employed (115).

Pathophysiology

Sterilant-related

Initially, acute allergic reactions occurring when fresh dialyzer were used, were claimed to be due to cupro-

phan, but subsequently were linked to the sterilant ethylene oxide. Such reactions were more common with the use of hollow-fiber dialyzers than with the use of parallel-plate and coil dialyzers (111, 114). All hollow-fiber dialyzers and some parallel-plate dialyzers contain, at their ends, potting material in the form of polyurethanes for the anchoring of the hollow fibers and of the parallel plates respectively. Other parallel-plate dialyzers and all coil dialyzers do not possess potting material at all. Hollow-fiber dialyzers vary widely in the method of sterilization employed. This latter is related to membrane structure as well as to manufacturer preference. Some types of membranes are versatile enough to be suitable for all forms of sterilization while others are more restricted in their suitability for certain sterilization methods. Such methods are summarized in Table 4.

Being one of the most commonly used agents for sterilization, ethylene oxide (ETO) has been clearly implicated in the causation of a majority of cases of acute anaphylactic reactions to new dialyzers (112, 113, 115–123). In addition, ETO residuals in clinically used dialyzers have been found to be neurotoxic *in vitro* and a role for ETO in the peripheral neuropathy of ESRD patients has been proposed on the basis of these experimental observations (124, 125). The higher incidence of the first-use syndrome in the case of hollow-fiber dialyzers is believed to be related to the universal presence of the polyurethane potting material which functions as a reservoir for ethylene oxide (126, 127). Removal of ETO from dialyzers is directly related to the volume of rinse, the temperature of the rinsing solution, and the duration of storage of the dialyzers prior to use. Priming solutions that have remained within the blood compartment of a dialyzer for a substantial length of time should be discarded and not be given to the patient. This is because ETO can diffuse from the potting material into the priming solution to reach an inordinately high level (126). The amount of ETO is less in dialyzers in which a portion of the potting compound has been replaced with a polycarbonate ring (126). In patients who reuse dialyzers, the occurrence of the first-use syndrome on the days when fresh, ETO-sterilized dialyzers are used (115) is consistent with the assertion that the patients are exposed, and reacting, to a high concentration of ETO on those particular days (reuse rids dialyzers of ETO). There has been a progressive drop in the use of ETO sterilization by European manufacturers from 88% in 1986 to 70% in 1992, and ETO sterilization has been completely abandoned by Japanese manufacturers.

Specific ETO-related IgE antibodies are found in patients with hypersensitivity reactions to the sterilant (113, 117–121, 123, 128–133). IgG antibodies, in contrast, are demonstrated in many hemodialysis patients who have never suffered from any hypersensitivity reactions. The presence of these antibodies denotes mere exposure (128). Both cutaneous testing and ELISA testing for assessing reactivity to ethylene oxide-human serum albumin can be carried out in hemodialysis patients with anaphylactic reactions. Cutaneous testing, while clinically simpler, offers no real advantage as the sensitivity, specificity, and negative predictive values of the two methods are similar (132).

In the majority of patients with anaphylaxis to dialysis, ethylene oxide has been identified as the etiologic agent. However, in a significant minority of patients sustaining such reactions, the responsible agent remains unidentified (130, 131). Conflicting results have been published with regard to identifying isocyanates as a possible antigen. Grammer et al. (118) found equal incidence of having IgE antibodies directed against toluene diisocyanate-human serum albumin in hemodialysis patients with anaphylaxis in whom IgE against ethylene oxide-human serum albumin was not identified and in peritoneal dialysis patients without anaphylaxis. Complement activation has been proposed as a mechanisms in some of the subjects with no identifiable antigen(s). No correlations between the time of onset of symptoms (if any symptoms were present) and the degree of complement activation were detected, however, among patients suffering from severe, moderate, or no hypersensitivity reactions (119), suggesting that complement activation plays no role in these reactions. Moreover, as above-mentioned, hollow-fiber, parallel-plate and coil dialyzers of comparable surface areas activate complement to a similar extent (135). If the complement activation were responsible for the dialyzer reactions, why should only hollow-fiber dialyzers be associated with a high incidence of the 'first-use syndrome'? Anaphylaxis to formaldehyde during reuse has been reported (136, 137). In a few unique cases, allergic reactions continued to occur irrespective of modifications in dialyzer choice, in sterilization methods and in prophylactic measures (138, 139). Symptoms reminiscent of the first-use reactions have also been encountered during reuse. However, it has been suggested that the development of such reactions is not related to the type of disinfectant product, the reprocessing method (manual or automated), or the type of dialysate (bicarbonate, acetate, or both) (140). Finally, anaphylactoid reactions have also been reported in patients who were dialyzed with reused dialyzers and receiving ACE inhibitors at the same time (141).

Membrane-related

Recently, however, acute allergic reactions have been reported when AN69 (a type of polyacrylonitrile membrane) dialyzers were used in patients taking angiotensin converting enzyme inhibitors (142, 143). There is convincing evidence that this reaction is related to an early and vigorous production of bradykinin induced by the contact of blood (via the contact pathway (144)) with the negatively charged AN69 membrane (142, 143). In the setting of using the AN69 membrane along with an ACE-inhibitor, bradykinin accumulates in the blood because ACE-inhibitors block the action of the enzyme kininase II which is responsible for the destruction of bradykinin.

PRURITUS

Clinical features

In the predialysis era, the incidence of pruritus was in the neighborhood of 13% (145). This low incidence is likely to be due to the overshadowing of this disorder by the more protean manifestations of the uremic syndrome. At present, at least 50% of patients maintained on dialysis suffer from itching (146–148) and the prevalence is similar with both hemodialysis and peritoneal dialysis (146). The prevalence of pruritus seems to rise with the duration of dialysis (149). This finding has led to the postulate that either the dialytic procedure contributes to the development of itching, or, the longer survival made possible by dialysis and the failure of dialysis to correct the uremic state fully, combine to allow pruritogenic mechanisms to become more manifest.

Continuous monitoring studies (148, 149) in hemodialysis patients suffering from pruritus reveal that itching peaks at night after two days without dialysis, occurs relatively more often during dialysis treatment and the least often on the day following dialysis. These observations are consistent with the notion that the condition is improved by dialysis, suggesting that the accumulation of pruritogenic substances is of major importance in the pathogenesis of uremic pruritus. Contrary to this postulate, there have been reports (150) of pruritus occurring mostly during or soon after hemodialysis in some 25% of patients, and becoming more severe during dialysis in an additional 40% of subjects. This disparity in clinical behavior highlights an underlying heterogeneity in the clinical manifestations and in the pathophysiology of the disorder.

Pathophysiology

Although subjected to intense study, the mechanism(s) underlying pruritus in subjects treated with renal replacement therapy continues to elude a unifying formulation. Several mechanisms have been proposed that may be responsible, singly, or in combination, for the development of this condition. It is clear, however, from the variance in the literature that a great deal of individual variations may be present and that a search for major contributory factors should be individualized. While uremic subjects are not immune to the myriad of conditions that induce pruritus in the general population (151, 152), the following discussion is restricted to the pathophysiology of the itching that is peculiar to the uremic state.

Dryness or xerosis has been investigated as a possible cause of uremic pruritus. In xerosis, the stratum corneum epidermidis becomes devoid of water. Being very dry, the most superficial layer functions like a foreign body. Scratching removes this superficial layer and relieves itching. Evidence for and against this mechanism has been advanced (146, 153). Whether the skin changes of aging are additive to the effects of uremia in the genesis of pruritus is a plausible consideration.

The landmark observation that severe pruritus disappeared 2 to 7 days after subtotal parathyroidectomy in maintenance hemodialysis patients, suggested that either parathyroid hormone (PTH) or derangements in calcium or phosphate metabolism may be responsible for the pruritus (153–156). Several lines of evidence favor a role for PTH in the genesis of pruritus in uremia. Patients with pruritus have significantly higher serum concentrations of PTH than those without (148). Moreover, reduction of PTH values by control of hyperphosphatemia or by charcoal hemoperfusion brings about a reduction in pruritus. It is noteworthy that not all uremic patients with secondary hyperparathyroidism, even when severe enough to warrant subtotal parathyroidectomy, suffer from pruritus. These observations have led to the contention that additonal factors may be operative in uremic pruritus.

Histamine has been implicated to play a major role in the pathogenesis of uremic pruritus. Plasma histamine values are higher in patients with chronic renal failure compared to those in controls (157). Since histamine and its metabolites are normally excreted in the urine, the higher concentrations of histamine may be a consequence of its retention in renal failure. Furthermore, plasma histamine values were, in a few studies, shown to be significantly higher in hemodialysis patients with pruritus than in those without (157, 158).

As mast cells and monocytes are known to be the main source of histamine production, several studies have investigated the relationship of these cells to pruritus in uremia. In some studies, the number of mast cells was found to be raised in patients undergoing maintenance hemodialysis (159, 160); and, in addition, patients with pruritus were discovered to have, in their skin, many, diffusely scattered and degranulated mast cells. Consequently the high plasma level of histamine might be a result of degranulation of the mast cells and the basophils. In contrast, Mettang et al. (147) found no relationship between the level of plasma histamine, the number of skin mast cells and the extent of pruritus in uremic patients. Moreover, Cohen et al. (161) showed that the number of mast cells was the same in itching dialysis patients and in controls who happened to be living-related kidney donors. Francos et al. (158) demonstrated that ketotifen, a mast cell stabilizer, was effective in reducing itching without causing any significant change in histamine level, histaminase activity or skin histamine content. Such an observation suggests that mast cell activation, separate from histamine release, may contribute to the pruritus in uremia.

It is clear from this survey of possible etiologies that a unitary etiology or mechanism for the pruritus of uremia is not discernible. It is very likely that different factors may be operative in different subjects and while some common elements may be evident, individualization of evaluation needs to be observed.

Management

Since pruritus appears to be multifactorial in its pathogenesis, several modalities of treatment have been suggested. In some patients, dialysis is enough to relieve the itching; in others, however, pruritus starts during dialysis or is even exacerbated by dialysis. Some have suggested that pruritus may be alleviated by an improvement in the dialysis prescription as judged by urea kinetic modeling (162). Subtotal parathyroidectomy has been found to be successful in patients with secondary hyperparathyroidism who suffered from pruritus. However, this treatment is not effective in all cases, and not all uremic patients with secondary hyperparathyroidism suffer from pruritus either.

Sun exposure is known to relieve the pruritus associated with several unrelated dermatoses and sunburn doses of ultraviolet light from artificial sources are effective in treating uremic pruritus. In an extensive literature search focusing on the most effective treatment for uremic pruritus, Tan et al. (163) found that ultraviolet B (UVB) phototherapy is the treatment of choice in moderate to severe uremic pruritus. The response occurs more rapidly in patients treated two or three times weekly than in those treated once weekly. Recurrences can come about, but usually respond to new UVB treatments. Being rare and mild, side effects mainly consist of localized sunburn. The mechanism of action of UVB is unclear. Since many patients with generalized pruritus respond to half body phototherapy, it has been suggested that UVB can inactivate a circulating pruritogenic substance or induce the formation of an antipruritic substance that relieves the pruritus. UVB irradiation might inhibit mast cell granule release or might relieve pruritus by damaging the cutaneous nerves.

Several drugs have been used in the treatment of uremic pruritus, but all have met with varying degrees of success and of failure. Topical emollients are hydrophilic compounds that hydrate the skin and form an occlusive film that reduces evaporation. These medications are helpful in alleviating pruritus caused by dryness of the stratum corneum epidermidis. Although histamine is a major itch mediator, use of antihistamines is not consistently successful.

Capsaicin (Zostrix) which is used topically for the temporary relief of pain from rheumatoid arthritis and osteoarthritis, and for the relief of neuralgias such as the pain associated with shingles or with diabetic neuropathy, has been shown to be safe and efficacious in the treatment of localized pruritus in hemodialysis patients (164). Capsaicin is known to deplete substance P from primary sensory afferent neurons of small, non-myelinated type which are associated with the transmission of pain sensation. However, if the drug is chronically applied, it may cause these neurons to degenerate.

De Marchi et al. (165) found that therapy with erythropoietin induced a fall in plasma histamine concentrations in uremic patients with pruritus and in those without, and resulted in a marked improvement of the pruritus if this symptom had been present to begin with. Itching, however, continues to be observed frequently even with the almost universal use of EPO in hemodialysis.

It is likely that pruritus will continue to plague patients and their physicians, and unless more definitive and practical therapeutic regimens are discovered, the management of this condition will remain problematic.

HEMOLYSIS

A mild degree of hemolysis manifested by the presence of detectable free hemoglobin in blood is commonly observed during dialysis. This finding, however, is of minimal clinical significance and can be attributed to a variety of factors including mechanical trauma to the red blood cells and possibly complement activation (166). The method of dialysis has a significant bearing on the development of hemolysis as it is observed more frequently with single-needle dialysis than with the double-needle one (167). Inherent changes in the red blood cells of uremic subjects which are thought to contribute to the mild chronic hemolysis observed in uremia (168), may predispose to this hemolysis. These inherent changes include increased red blood cell rigidity and fragility, and reduced deformability secondary to oxidative damage (169–173).

Clinically significant hemolysis is observed with technical problems related to the dialysis procedure itself. Kinked blood lines (174), contamination of dialysis fluid with hydrogen peroxide because of inadequate rinsing of the water treatment system after disinfection (175), residual formaldehyde in reused dialyzers (176), and accidental hypochlorite infusion (177), have all been reported to be associated with serious life-threatening hemolysis. Clinically, the affected patients complain of malaise, nausea, headache and severe abdominal pain. Death due to hyperkalemia may also occur. Undetected excessive ultrafiltration with major hemolysis has also been described (178). Other rare causes of dialysis-associated hemolysis are described in the latter part of this chapter.

ARRHYTHMIAS

Arrhythmias are frequent occurrences in patients on hemodialysis with reported incidences varying from 30 to 48% of patients (179–184). These abnormalities can span from supraventricular (184, 185) to severe ventricular arrhythmias (179, 182–184, 186). There is an increased frequency of occurrence clustering around dialysis time (179, 180, 183–186). Identified predisposing factors include increased left ventricular mass (182, 187), advanced age (183, 184), pre-existing ischemic heart disease (183, 186), potassium depletion (179, 181, 186) and the duration of end-stage renal disease (182).

Left ventricular mass is increased in the majority of dialysis patients, both normotensive and hypertensive (182, 187), and, as in patients with normal renal function, represents a major risk factor for ventricular arrhythmias. In uremics, however, the cardiac hypertrophy is not correlated with the hypertension. In addition, in these patients, intermyocardiocytic fibrosis is present, a finding not observed in similarly hypertensive non-uremic subjects (187). How these changes augment electrical instability in uremics is not completely understood at present. The wide electrolytic and volume changes taking place during dialysis may create a window of vulnerability leading to serious arrhythmic consequences. Independently, however, arrhythmias do not seem to predict mortality, with age and ischemic heart disease being better correlated with survival (182). The presence of pericarditis is also associated with a heightened frequency of supraventricular arrhythmias (188). Computer-modulated potassium lowering during dialysis seems to offer an advantage in lowering the frequency of ventricular arrhythmias in susceptible patients (179). The elevation of plasma calcium concentration during hemodialysis might induce either reentry-activity or triggered-activity types of arrhythmias during treatment (189). Use of dialysate with a lower calcium concentration reduces the incidence of arrhythmias in certain subjects (189).

Fantuzzi et al. (186) compared the arrhythmogenic effects of acetate dialysis with those of bicarbonate dialysis. A higher frequency of ventricular arrhythmias was encountered during acetate dialysis than during bicarbonate dialysis. Classes III and IV ventricular arrhythmias (classification of Lown and Graboys) were more often seen with acetate dialysis than with bicarbonate dialysis (186). The quicker and more regular correction of acidosis with bicarbonate dialysis and the consequent difference in ionic flows between the intra- and extracellular spaces, as demonstrated by changes in the intraerythrocytic potassium value at the end of the session, could account for the seemingly less arrhythmogenic effect of bicarbonate dialysis (186).

BLEEDING DURING DIALYSIS

The bleeding tendency of uremia is considered to represent an acquired defect in primary hemostasis. The most common clinical manifestations of uremic bleeding are the least severe, and include ecchymoses, purpura, epistaxis, gingival bleeding, and bleeding from venipuncture sites. Major hemorrhages, from gastrointestinal, retroperitoneal, pericardial, or intracranial sites, seldom develop spontaneously and frequently reflect underlying pathology.

Pathophysiology

Investigations to date have revealed a multiplicity of defects that may underlie this bleeding diathesis. However, a precise pathogenetic framework continues to be elusive. While defects in blood coagulation factors, alterations of the fibrinolytic system, and vascular abnormalities have been considered to be contributory, platelet dysfunction has been the most consistently described hemostatic abnormality in patients with ESRD (190, 191). Uremic platelets exhibit reduced adhesion to vascular subendothelium and impaired aggregation response to various stimuli such as ADP, epinephrine, collagen, and thrombin. Abnormal platelet aggregation does not appear to correlate with the severity of renal failure, but the abnormalities seem to improve after hemodialysis. Platelet function studies have shown that platelet spreading on glass surfaces and platelet adhesiveness are abnormal Biochemical studies revealed an impaired dense-granule release of ATP and serotonin, reduced synthesis of thromboxane A2, elevated cytosolic cAMP and calcium in uremic platelets (190, 191). Altered interaction of adhesive macromolecules such as fibrinogen and von Willebrand factor (vWf), with platelet membrane glycoproteins have been suggested to contribute to the aggregation and adhesion defects.

Uremia results in a defect in platelet adhesion to subendothelial structures, thus contributing to the increased bleeding tendency. Fibrinogen receptor (QPllb-llla) function of platelets from chronic renal failure patients is impaired. This impairment is most likely to be related to a conformational change and a fibrinogen-ligand-binding defect of GP11b-llla. Hemodialysis improves fibrinogen-ligand-binding of GP11b–111a, indicating removal of a uremic inhibitor by dialysis treatment. The defect is repro-

duced in normal platelets when they are incubated in predialysis uremic plasma, but not with post-dialysis plasma. Chronic renal failure patients treated with erythropoietin for correction of anemia show an increased GPllb-llla expression, implying that the erythropoietin treatment could ameliorate platelet dysfunction in uremic patients. Platelets of patients with chronic renal failure reveal an aggregation defect, that is, partially at least, related to an intrinsic GPllb-llla dysfunction and to the presence of a putative uremic toxin which inhibits fibrinogen binding to GPllb-llla (190, 191).

Management

Dialysis

Both peritoneal dialysis and hemodialysis can lead to correction, often only partial, of the uremic hemostatic defect. Moreover, adequacy of dialysis has been suggested to be an important factor in the improvement in bleeding tendency. Platelet fibrinogen receptor function is ameliorated after dialysis, the amelioration likely to be due to the removal of a dialyzable toxic product that accumulates in uremia (190, 191). Thus, adequate dialysis treatments may improve platelet aggregation and lower bleeding tendency by removing substances that interfere with fibrinogen-platelet binding and, therefore, platelet aggregation. Removal of toxic products may also improve platelet adhesion to the subendothelium. The often partial character of the response to dialysis implies that patients with high bleeding risk may require further pharmacological therapy.

Erythropoietin

The hemostatic defect of uremia improves after treatment with recombinant human erythropoietin. Erythropoietin transiently raises platelet counts, shortens skin bleeding time, and improves platelet aggregation. Moreover, platelets from patients receiving erythropoietin therapy appear to be more activated during hemodialysis; such activation could pose problems in terms of dialyzer clotting and arterio-venous fistula thrombosis. Erythropoietin treatment augments the number of GP11b–111a molecules found on the platelet plasma membrane (190, 191). Administration of erythropoietin to uremic patients might, therefore, have an impact on thrombopoiesis in addition to erythropoiesis. Consequently, uremic patients with a high frequency of bleeding complications may benefit from appropriate erythropoietin therapy.

Cryoprecipitate

Cryoprecipitate shortens or normalizes bleeding time in patients with renal failure. The peak effect appears several hours after infusion and persists for 12 to 24 hours. Factor VIII/von Willebrand factor complex (FVIII/vWf) has been shown to play an important role in the pathophysiology of uremic bleeding and it is this component of cryoprecipitate that is postulated to give rise to improved platelet functions in uremia. The delayed onset of action, the short duration of effect, and the risk of contracting infections may limit its application.

Desmopressin

The importance of FVIII/vWf for uremic platelet dysfunction is substantiated by the fact that 1-deamino-8-D arginine vasopressin (dDAVP) which causes the release of autologous, preformed FVIII/vWf from endothelial storage sites, is effective in the treatment of the bleeding tendency present in patients with acute or chronic renal failure. Bleeding time is improved or normalized one hour after the infusion while the effect of the infusion lasts approximately 4 to 6 hours. The treatment is very well tolerated and has been said to prevent bleeding complications when given prophylactically. Von Willebrand activities rise after d-DAVP therapy in the responders but not in the non-responders.

Estrogen

Being well tolerated, estrogen therapy appears to be effective in improving the bleeding tendency in uremia, although the mechanism of action is unclear. Between two and five days after beginning estrogen therapy, bleeding time improves or normalizes in patients with chronic renal failure. After discontinuation of the therapy, the bleeding time remains normal for 3 to 10 days. Although the duration of action compared to that of cryoprecipitate or of dDAVP is longer, the absolute magnitude of the effect on bleeding time may be less.

DIALYSIS ACCIDENTS

Erroneous temperatures

Dialysate temperature, normally set at 37°C, is regulated by a thermostat, a component of the dialysate temperature monitoring system. Malfunctions of the thermostat or of the other components of the monitoring system can result in abnormal dialysate temperatures. Although a cool dialysate (e.g., 34.5°C) (192) has been used to promote vasoconstriction to maintain an adequate blood pressure during dialysis, too low a temperature can bring about shivering and increased secretion of catecholamines (193). In addition, an augmentation in transfusion requirement as a result of the use of a dialysate whose temperature is less than 38 °C has been reported (194). This higher requirement was believed to be a consequence of the activation of the cold agglutinin, anti N.

Should the dialysate temperature be too high, cutaneous vasodilatation, sweating, and a sensation of warmth will occur. For the conscious patient, overheating is often detected before a dangerous elevation in body temperature makes its appearance. If dialysate temperature is allowed to rise to 55°C or higher, massive hemolysis with resultant hyperkalemia (195) and death can take place. In those instances in which dialysate temperature reaches only 50–51°C, the onset of hemolysis can be delayed for up to 2 days (196). This delay is related to splenic trapping and peripheral destruction of the damaged erythrocytes (197).

Treatment for hemolysis requires the immediate cessation of dialysis, the discard of blood present in the extracorporeal circuit and the transfusion of blood in case anemia is severe. Hyperkalemia should be treated by the usual means, not the least of which is another dialysis treatment using functional equipment and potassium-poor or potassium-free dialysate.

Air embolism

Air embolism is one of the dreaded complications of hemodialysis and the extracorporeal system is designed with redundant safeguards to avoid its occurrence. It is important, however, to maintain vigilance as human and technical failures are always possible. It can occur either as a result of the manipulation of the extracorporeal circuit, or as a complication of a temporary vascular access placement procedure. Venous air embolism, however, remains an infrequent complication. The cardiovascular, pulmonary, and central nervous systems may all be affected, with severity ranging from absence of symptoms to immediate cardiovascular collapse. Symptoms and signs attributable to air embolism can take place with small volumes of air entering the patient's circulation. While it is difficult to quantitate the amount of air in clinical settings, experimental studies suggest that the introduction of 1 mL/kg may be fatal.

The manifestations of air embolism depend on the posture of the patient and the flow of air obeys the law of gravity. In the sitting position, air will flow along the venous system to reach the central circulation and then will backflow into the cerebral venous system. The patient will transiently be aware of the sound of the air in his vessels and then will lose consciousness and develop seizures. In recumbent patients, air will reach the right atrium and the right ventricle, with the developing air-blood foam occluding the right ventricular outflow tract and the pulmonary vascular bed. Chest pain and shortness of breath appear, followed by cardiovascular collapse.

Venous air embolism can occur during the insertion, the disconnection or the removal of a central venous catheter (198, 199). Air embolization through a residual track after removal of a central venous catheter, particularly after long-term catheterization or repeated use of the same puncture site, is an elusive mechanism that while rare, can be recognized only if searched for carefully (200).

Venous air embolism induces rapid hemodynamic changes, most notably a sharp increase in central venous pressure (201). In addition to the obstructive element, pulmonary vasoconstriction modulated by the action of the platelet activating factor, also takes place (202). Pulmonary edema can set in (203). Entry of air into the pulmonary arterial tree causes physical obstruction of the microvasculature and leads to permeability changes, release of mediators, and injury to lung tissues (204). Both thromboxane B2 and endothelin concentrations also rise, suggesting their involvement in the raised pulmonary arterial resistance (204). Moreover, there might be a possible role for activated leukocytes in the pathogenesis of lung injury induced by air emboli (204).

In addition to its hemodynamic consequences, air in the circulating blood activates complement in a dose-dependent fashion (205). Platelet activation is also induced by air in the circulation (206).

Air in blood vessels can be visualized by real time ultrasonography (207) and air volume, estimated by a doppler (208, 209).

Therapeutic interventions include mechanical measures, such as positioning, withdrawal of air from the right atrium (210, 211), and means aimed at reducing bubble size (212, 213). Speed in therapy is essential The blood lines should be clamped and the patient rapidly positioned in the Trendelenburg position with the left side down. This posture reduces the movement of air to the brain and traps the air bubbles in the right ventricle. This air trapping minimizes foaming which ordinarily takes place also mainly in the right ventricle. In this position, air may even migrate to the periphery; such air migration can be detected by the development of patchy cyanosis over the lower extremities. While migration of the air may affect the distal sites, it is clearly less catastrophic than having air in the central circulation or in the cerebral vessels.

Hyperbaric oxygen therapy holds some promise in accomplishing reduction of air bubble size (214). Even after a prolonged delay, patients with cerebral air embolism may still benefit from hyperbaric oxygen therapy (214). Even normobaric oxygen may be useful, particularly if mechanical ventilation is employed. Experimental studies suggest that the removal rate of air from cerebral vessels is dramatically enhanced by mechanical ventilation at an FiO_2 of 1.0 (215). The prompt application of mechanical ventilation with an FiO_2 of 1.0 is recommended when air embolism is suspected particularly in centers where facilities for administering hyperbaric oxygen therapy are not available.

While prevention and early diagnosis represent the cornerstones of management, definitive therapy of a massive air embolus may require aspiration of the air through an appropriately located multi-orifice catheter. Currently, the most common method for accurately positioning a multi-orifice catheter in the high right atrium depends on the use of an intravenous electrocardiogram. Alternatively, a right ventricular waveform on a pressure recording can be used as a marker for accurate and reliable catheter localization (217) Throughout management, the patient should be moved as little as possible.

Dialyzer rupture or clotting

Dialyzer rupture is a rare event in hemodialysis. It is usually detected by an alarm which is triggered by the presence of very low concentrations of blood in the dialysate. A variety of factors predisposes to this complication; such factors include faulty construction, high venous pressures secondary to clotting or kinking of blood lines, and improper priming. While most ruptures result in the loss of only a small amount of blood and may seal spontaneously, the potential for massive blood loss requires that immediate remedial measures be taken. Septicemia is also a risk. The blood lines should be clamped, the patient disconnected from the extracorporeal circuit and the latter completely changed. Moreover, the dialysate circuit and the blood leak detector will need to be cleaned.

Dialyzer clotting is a more common event and is usually due to inadequate heparinization. This, however, cannot be the sole cause as hemodialysis without anticoagulation is readily performed with either intermittent or continuous saline rinsing. Additional factors include a high venous pressure, a low blood flow, a low dialysate pH (218), a large amount of air in the drip chambers or in the dialyzer headers because of poor attention to proper rinsing procedures prior to starting dialysis. Furthermore, rapid connection of the patient to the extracorporeal circuit immediately after heparin administration without allowing for systemic anticoagulation to begin taking effect may be contributory.

PERICARDITIS WITH PERICARDIAL EFFUSION

Pericarditis in ESRD patients can be categorized into two varieties, namely, uremic pericarditis and dialysis pericarditis (219). Uremic pericarditis, a manifestation of renal failure, occurs in individuals who have never received dialytic therapy and often responds to intensive dialysis, e.g., daily 4-hour dialysis runs for 2 to 3 weeks. Dialysis pericarditis, on the other hand, occurs in patients who have already been treated with maintenance dialysis for a period of time. Although most authorities believe that dialysis pericarditis is a manifestation of inadequate dialytic therapy, this form of pericarditis may not readily respond to intensive dialysis (only about 40% of patients respond (219)). Because of this peculiar characteristic, it has been suggested that this form of pericarditis might be of viral origin (220).

Patients with pericarditis often present with precordial pain, hypotension, dyspnea, fever and rapid weight gain due to fluid overload (221). A pericardial friction rub may be heard. A large percentage of pericarditis patients may develop pericardial effusion. Patients with significant pericardial effusion tend to be intolerant of fluid removal by ultrafiltration (221), presumably because a high venous pressure is required to maintain adequate cardiac filling and cardiac output (222). When this high venous pressure is lowered by fluid removal during ultrafiltration, reductions in venous return, cardiac output and blood pressure are the consequences. Should fluid removal by ultrafiltration be excessive for the degree of pericardial effusion, cardiac tamponade characterized by tachycardia, hypotension and a rising venous pressure may result. Death from cardiac tamponade is not uncommon. Noteworthy is the fact that in many patients suffering from cardiac tamponade, a pulsus paradoxus may not be demonstrable (223).

Since patients with pericardial effusion are prone to develop hypotension during ultrafiltration (221), large volumes of saline are frequently administered intravenously to combat this untoward effect. As a consequence, an already substantial state of overhydration is often aggravated.

It should be noted that the amount of fluid necessary to produce tamponade may be as little as 250 mL when the fluid accumulates quickly, or over 2 liters in slowly developing effusions when the pericardial sac has had the opportunity to stretch and adapt to the increasing volume of fluid. In addition, a pericardial effusion accumulating in a previously healthy distensible pericardial sac has less hemodynamic effect than that of an effusion developing in a previously diseased, non-compliant pericardial sac (221). Finally, certain dialysis patients have a small amount of fluid in their pericardial sacs. These small effusions have no clinical significance (224).

Diagnosis of pericardial effusion is based on a high index of suspicion and best confirmed by echocardiography. Once the diagnosis is established, further dialysis should be performed with a heparin-free or a citrate-anticoagulation technique to minimize the risk of developing hemopericardium. Intensive dialysis should be carried out daily for 2 to 3 weeks, using a higher dialysate potassium value than normal (e.g., 3.5 mM or so instead of 2 mM if removal of potassium by the daily dialysis is excessive), and a lower dialysate buffer base level than usual (e.g., 26 mM or so instead of 35 mM if metabolic acidosis begins to be replaced by metabolic alkalosis). Should dialysis-induced hypophosphatemia appear likely, dialysate can be enriched prophylactically with phosphate salts (225).

In order to avoid the risks associated with intensive dialysis such as cardiac tamponade, and cardiac arrhythmias secondary to dialysis-induced electrolyte imbalances, and since dialysis pericarditis with effusion responds less readily to intensive dialysis, prompt surgical drainage of moderately large (e.g., 250 mL) or very large effusions has been recommended (226). With regard to surgical drainage, we prefer the subxiphoid pericardiostomy approach utilizing local anesthesia and a large-bore drainage tube (226), with or without the topical instillation of non-absorbable steroids (227, 228). The pericardial fluid is allowed to drain until it dwindles to less than 50 mL a day over a period of several days. Should local

drainage fail, pericardiectomy or pericardial fenestration is usually required (221, 229).

DIALYSIS DISEQUILIBRIUM

Clinical features

This dialysis-induced syndrome consists of manifestations in the form of mental confusion or agitation, nausea, vomiting, headache, drowsiness, lassitude, confusion, muscle twitching, delirium, seizures and coma. In severe cases, there is an rise in blood pressure, pulse rate and respiratory rate. Occasionally, death can occur (230–232). In addition, characteristic electroencephalographic abnormalities in the form of high-voltage rhythmic delta waves are commonly encountered (233).

The syndrome is more likely to take place when the initial plasma urea level is markedly elevated and correction of the azotemia is rapid (230). Therefore, the syndrome is encountered mostly in the early stages of dialysis therapy when plasma urea level often is highest, but may recur even after many months of dialysis should the patient raise his protein intake. In addition, the syndrome is frequently seen toward the end of a dialysis and usually transient, lasting for 24 hours after the termination of dialysis (230, 234). Finally, it should be noted that a predisposing factor for the development of the syndrome is a pre-existing neurologic disorder (231).

Pathophysiology

The exact pathogenetic mechanism for the dialysis disequilibrium syndrome is not fully understood at present. What is known for certain is that there is evidence of cerebral swelling as a consequence of entry of water into the brain cells. The presence of cerebral swelling was substantiated by: (a) the finding of a swollen brain flap during dialysis (235), (b) the post-mortem demonstration of brain swelling in fatal cases (231, 236), and (c) experimental observations of a raised intracranial pressure in uremic dogs during dialysis (237).

There are several theories concerning the pathogenesis of the dialysis disequilibrium syndrome, the most popular being the 'reverse urea effect' theory. In this theory, the intracellular water gain is believed to be a result of a dialysis-induced lowering of the plasma urea level in the presence of a lesser fall in intracellular urea concentration (230–234). Support for this theory has been lent by the demonstration of a higher cerebrospinal fluid urea level than its plasma counterpart at the end of a dialysis session when plasma urea value has been substantially reduced over a relatively short period of time. The demonstration of this urea gradient implies the slower passage of urea out of brain tissue and the consequent transfer of water from the blood to the brain. Furthermore, the suppression of dialysis-induced electroencephalographic abnormalities by the use of a urea-enriched dialysate adds weight to the 'reverse urea effect' contention (233). In a similar vein, clinical manifestations associated with the dialysis disequilibrium syndrome can be ameliorated by maintaining plasma osmolality with the use of a high-sodium dialysate (238). Recently, the concept of the 'reverse urea effect' has received additional support from the finding of an elevation in brain water and a rise in the brain-to-plasma urea ratio in azotemic rats subjected to acute hemodialysis treatments (239).

Acidosis of the cerebrospinal fluid and brain has been proposed as a possible cause for the disequilibrium syndrome seen in experimental animals (240). However, such an acidosis has not been found in uremic patients as a result of dialysis (234).

Management

The syndrome is rarely seen when a moderately elevated plasma urea nitrogen level (e.g., 29 mM (80 mg/dL)) is substantially lowered by conventional or high-efficiency dialysis (e.g., to 15 mM (40 mg/dL)). Moreover, it should be remembered that it is best to initiate dialysis long before azotemia becomes extreme. For example, ordinarily, it would appear prudent to begin dialytic therapy before the plasma urea nitrogen concentration is in excess of 36 mM (100 mg/dL). In the event that dialysis is required in a patient with an extremely raised plasma urea nitrogen value (e.g., 89 mM (250 mg/dL)), in order to discourage the development of the dialysis disequilibrium syndrome, an inefficient dialysis treatment can be delivered by shortening the duration of a dialysis run to 25 to 40% of the normal, by lowering dialyzer blood or dialysate flow rates, or by using a less efficient dialyzer. If no untoward effects appear, the efficacy of the subsequent daily dialysis treatments can be lengthened in a step-wise manner over the next several days until regular dialysis treatments can be safely delivered.

Prophylactic administration of osmotic agents such as glucose, fructose, glycerol, mannitol, urea and sodium chloride either intravenously or via the dialysate route, with the aim of reducing the incidence of the dialysis disequilibrium syndrome has been recommended (238, 241, 242). However, more research is required before one can identify the osmotic agent of choice. Since modern dialysis machines can raise dialysate sodium levels readily, use of a high-sodium dialysate may be the most convenient approach. Once the dyequilibrium syndrome sets in, treatment will be symptomatic. Seizures can be treated with intravenous diazepam (Valium), with effects lasting 30 to 60 minutes. When compared to barbiturates, diazepam causes less respiratory depression. Short-acting barbiturates can also be given but are more dangerous since they can cause more respiratory depression. It should be noted that even though diazepam and some related drugs are metabolized by the liver, great care should be exercised in their use since many renal failure patients cannot toler-

ate the dosages ordinarily recommended for patients with normal liver and renal functions.

ELECTROLYTE ABNORMALITIES

Metabolic alkalosis

Metabolic alkalosis as a consequence of intensive dialysis (e.g., daily dialysis) using a dialysate with a high level of buffer base (e.g., 40 mM), is rarely described. What is more often encountered, however, is metabolic alkalosis developing as a complication of hemodialysis employing sodium citrate as a means of regional anticoagulation (243–245). The infused citrate is converted into bicarbonate by the body. In some regional anticoagulation regimens, citrate concentrations of 7 mM have been found in afferent blood, resulting in severe metabolic alkalosis (243). Prevention requires employing as small an amount of citrate as possible. Should reduction in citrate administration be impossible, the level of buffer base in the dialysate can be curtailed (245). Severe metabolic alkalosis can be treated, if desired, by hemodialysis using a low buffer-base and high chloride dialysate.

Metabolic acidosis

Metabolic acidosis can develop if the delivery of buffer base to the dialysate in the form of sodium acetate or sodium bicarbonate is defective (246–249). For instance, the single 'acetate concentrate' meant for dilution with water to form an acetate-based dialysate can be accidentally replaced by the 'acid concentrate' component of a two-component, bicarbonate-based dialysate generating system (246). This 'acid concentrate' contains sodium, potassium, calcium, magnesium, chloride, glucose and acetic acid. Since this concentrate is devoid of buffer base, its use would bring about metabolic acidosis as a result of the removal of bicarbonate from the blood by dialysis. Another way for metabolic acidosis to set in during dialysis involves the faulty delivery of a buffer base-containing concentrate. For example, the tube responsible for the siphoning off of a 'bicarbonate concentrate' can be damaged (247). A third way for metabolic acidosis to develop centers on the presence, in the dialysate, of too much water in relation to the available buffer base (an example of dilution acidosis) (248). A fourth way to produce metabolic acidosis is to use a chloride-rich and acetate-poor infusate, in conjunction with the employment of a low-bicarbonate dialysate, in the course of a sorbent system hemodialysis. In this instance, an inadequate amount of buffer base is transferred into the blood across the dialyzer membrane (249). Finally, metabolic acidosis has been described in hemodialysis patients suffering from the cytotoxic effects of fluoride poisoning (250), or afflicted with acute copper intoxication as a result of oxidative release of copper from copper heating coils or copper pipes present in a dialysate delivery system in association with a fall in pH following exhaustion of a de-ionizer (251).

Many patients who experienced metabolic acidosis were found to feel ill (246). Either hypertension or hypotension has been reported (246). Treatment of the acidosis comprises the administration of sodium bicarbonate, or of a properly performed acetate- or bicarbonate-based dialysis session using appropriate and functional equipment. Finally, for the prevention of equipment-related metabolic acidosis developing during dialysis, the use of dialysis machines equipped with pH sensors is recommended.

Hyponatremia

Inadvertent use of a markedly hyponatric dialysate during dialysis can occur if conductivity limits of the dialysis machine are not adjusted appropriately such that abnormal proportioning among concentrate(s) and product water are left undetected (248, 252). Use of such hyponatric dialysates can bring about hyponatremia as a result of the removal of sodium from, and the introduction of water into, the body. The resultant plasma hypoosmolality causes water to enter the intracellular space leading to water intoxication, cerebral edema and hemolysis. Hypervolemia may occur due to entry of water into the blood from the hyponatric dialysate although extracellular water is also being lost into the cells at the same time. Clinical manifestations include cramping abnormal pain, diarrhea, leg cramps, hypertension, Kussmaul's breathing, apprehension, coma, and other neurological disturbances (248, 252). Hyperkalemia can occur because of the hypoosmolality-induced hemolysis while metabolic acidosis can take place because of dilution of plasma bicarbonate by dialysate water and loss of plasma bicarbonate into the dialysate (248). Treatment consists of cessation of the current dialysis run, initiation of another dialysis treatment using sound equipment and proper dialysate (e.g., dialysate sodium level can be from 120–130 mM; as desired, potassium-free or potassium-poor dialysate should be used if hyperkalemia is present). Since the onset of the hyponatremia is abrupt, rapid correction of the hyponatremia with hypertonic saline infusion, is justified in order to reduce the degree of cerebral edema (253). However, serum sodium level should not be brought back to a level higher than 120–125 mM or so initially. Blood transfusion should be given if the anemia is severe. Prevention of dialysis-associated hyponatremia depends on meticulous attention to details in the preparation of dialysate and the frequent monitoring of dialysate conductivity value.

Hypernatremia

Dialysate sodium concentrations can be abnormally raised if water and dialysate concentrate pumps are faulty (254) and, at the same time, the conductivity sensor is also either defective or not adjusted properly. In addition, malfunction of a cationic exchange resin water softener (255) has been found to lead to hypernatremia. The resultant hypernatremia can abstract water into the extracellular space from the intracellular compartment causing cellular (including cerebral) dehydration. In those situations in which a hypernatric dialysate is used, extracellular fluid volume may not be elevated because water is also being lost to the dialysate. Central nervous system manifestations such as headache, disorientation, seizures, spasticity and coma are frequently encountered (255, 256). Other symptoms include nausea, vomiting, hot flushes, weakness, and profound thirst. Death can result.

Treatment consists of discontinuation of the current dialysis session, drinking of water, intravenous administration of 5% glucose water, and dialysis with a dialysate containing appropriate levels of sodium. The rate of fall of plasma sodium permitted should be guided by the clinical response. It is also better not to have the plasma sodium level drop below, for example, 145 mM initially so that cerebral edema can be averted.

Hypokalemia

Renal failure patients who are dialyzed against a very low-potassium or a potassium-free dialysate can develop hypokalemia and intracellular potassium depletion due to loss of potassium into the dialysate (257, 258). This complication can take place even in the patient with pre-dialysis hyperkalemia. Patients who are hypokalemic are at risk of developing cardiac arrhythmias, including premature ventricular contractions and ventricular fibrillation. In addition, hypotension, fatigue, muscular weakness and paralysis can occur. These manifestations are mainly the result of an impaired neuromuscular transmission (259).

Acute lowering of serum potassium engenders a high ratio between intracellular fluid potassium concentration and extracellular fluid potassium level, resulting in a more negative resting membrane potential and, hence, a hyperpolarization block (259). Predisposing to this hypokalemia-induced cardiac arrhythmia is the presence of coronary artery disease, hypertensive cardiovascular disease, digitalis therapy, hypercalcemia, hypomagnesemia and metabolic alkalosis. Affected patients often give a history of nausea, vomiting, diarrhea, naso-gastric aspiration and diuretic therapy.

It should be noted that a patient's serum potassium level may fall during dialysis even if dialysate potassium concentration is considerably higher than the pre-dialysis serum potassium value (260, 261). The cause of this hypokalemia is believed to be a rapid shift of potassium from the extracellular to the intracellular space as a result of the correction of systemic metabolic acidosis by dialysis and, as is often the case, by supplemental sodium bicarbonate therapy (260, 261) (although whether bicarbonate therapy can lower the serum potassium value in dialysis patients is at present controversial (262)). Patients entering dialysis with a history suggestive of prolonged potassium loss, marked metabolic acidosis, moderate hypokalemia or normokalemia (e.g., 2.5–4.0 mM range) are especially vulnerable to this complication. The use of a dialysate potassium level higher than that in plasma under such circumstances may provide a false sense of security so much so that a vigilant watch for the development of dialysis-associated hypokalemia is neglected. As a matter of fact, it has been surmised that a number of sudden deaths occurring during the initial dialysis of acutely ill patients may be the consequence of such hypokalemia.

Intensive dialysis in an average dialysis patient without severe metabolic acidosis can bring about a metabolic alkalosis with resultant hypokalemia even if a normal-potassium dialysate is used. This phenomenon occurs because of the high level of buffer base used in standard dialysate (e.g., 35 to 40 mM). The resultant systemic metabolic alkalosis produced fosters the entry of extracellular fluid potassium into cellular stores.

Prevention of dialysis-induced hypokalemia due to loss of potassium into dialysate centers on the use of appropriate levels of potassium in the dialysate so that excessive removal by dialysis is prevented. In those patients who develop hypokalemia due to shift of potassium into cells, a high-potassium (e.g., 6.0–6.5 mM) dialysate can be used and potassium salts can be given intravenously during dialysis if necessary. In these latter patients, if possible, the use of a high-glucose dialysate should be avoided so that cellular uptake of potassium will not be excessive (260, 261).

In patients who develop metabolic alkalosis-induced hypokalemia as a result of intensive dialysis, the dialysate buffer base level should be lowered appropriately. In all patients who might develop dialysis-induced hypokalemia, frequent monitoring of serum electrolyte and acid-base values and of EKG's should be carried out during dialysis.

With regard to patients who are prone to have dialysis-associated cardiac arrhythmias, special precautions are necessary. It has been found that raising dialysate potassium value from 2.0 to 3.5 mM reduced the frequency of arrhythmias in those patients who suffered from arrhythmias while being dialyzed with the lower-potassium dialysate. This reduction was, however, bought at the expense of a higher pre-dialysis serum potassium value of the succeeding dialysis treatment (258). Furthermore, in dialysis patients who are receiving digitalis preparations, use of a low-potassium dialysate is associated with an increased incidence of arrhythmias (258).

Hyperkalemia

Hyperkalemia occurs commonly in dialysis patients who have not adhered to their diets. However, hyperkalemia developing as a complication of dialysis is infrequent.

A noteworthy cause of dialysis-induced hyperkalemia is hemolysis. Intradialytic hemolysis has been reported following accidental exposure to overheated (195–197) or hypotonic dialysate (248–252), chloramine (263), formaldehyde (264), nitrate (265), copper (251), and sodium hypochlorite (266). Another rare cause for the development of hyper-kalemia is dialysis with fluoride-contaminated dialysate (267). Of course, hyperkalemia could occur if a dialysate with an inordinately high-potassium level were inadvertently used.

Prevention of dialysis-induced hyperkalemia centers on the proper preparation of dialysate. Treatment of hyperkalemia is best done by dialyzing against a potassium-poor or potassium-free dialysate.

Hypophosphatemia

Hyperphosphatemia is almost a universal finding in ESRD patients because the ability of hemodialysis to remove phosphorus from the blood is limited. However, one may encounter situations in which dialysis-induced hypophosphatemia develops. These situations are exemplified by: (1) Intensive (e.g., daily) dialysis for patients suffering from dialysis pericarditis; (2) Thrice weekly regular dialysis treatments in those maintenance dialysis patients who do not consume enough phosphorus-containing food because of an intercurrent illness. In the first instance, hypophosphatemia is the result of excessive removal by dialysis. In the second instance, hypophosphatemia develops because the regular removal of phosphorus by dialysis is now coupled with a reduced intake.

Dialysis-induced hypophosphatemia can also be seen in patients with normal renal function who are dialyzed because of intoxications with poisons such as lithium. Therapy of such intoxications often focuses on prolonged and repeated dialysis treatments. Such intensive dialytic therapy is necessary because any dialysis-induced lowering of the serum level of the poison is frequently followed soon by a rebound, suggesting that the transfer between intracellular and extracellular compartments is slow (268). Hypophosphatemia may develop in these patients because of the removal, by dialysis, of phosphorus from their bodies whose phosphorus contents are not elevated to start with on account of the presence of normal renal function (225).

Hypophosphatemia causes dysfunction of erythrocytes, leukocytes, platelets, the central nervous system, skeletal and cardiac muscles as well as the skeleton (269). However, hypophosphatemic manifestations are usually mild unless serum phosphorus level falls below 0.33 mM (1.0 mg/dL). Treatment of hypophosphatemia centers on the ingestion of phosphorus-rich food (such as skim milk) and of phosphorus salts (such as sodium or potassium phosphate), and, in severe cases, the intravenous administration of sodium or potassium phosphate (270).

Dialysis-related hypophosphatemia can be prevented by the use of a phosphorus-enriched dialysate. For instance, sodium phosphates (in the form of Fleet Phospho-soda™ saline laxative) can be added to either the 'acid concentrate' or the 'base concentrate' of a two-concentrate, bicarbonate-based dialysate generating system to produce a dialysate containing 1.3 to 2.6 mM (4–8 mg/dL) of phosphorus (225).

Hypercalcemia and hypermagnesemia

Dialysis against a conventional 1.32 mM calcium dialysate can raise plasma calcium concentrations of dialysis patients from a pre-dialysis value of 2.28 mM to a post-dialysis level of 2.45 mM (271). This dialysis-induced hypercalcemia is partly due to an increase in plasma protein concentrations brought about by the loss of a protein-free fluid from plasma as a result of ultrafiltration. The rise in plasma protein level is accompanied by a corresponding increase in the protein-bound fraction of plasma calcium (272). Another cause for the development of hypercalcemia is the liberation of calcium from bone, consequent to the removal of phosphorus by dialysis (271). In addition, the small intradialytic gain of calcium by the body from the dialysate also contributes to the hypercalcemia.

Dialysis-induced hypercalcemia is transient in nature and does not lead to symptoms. No treatment is required. However, its clinical significance is at present unknown.

In the recent past, a dialysate calcium level of 1.75 mM was the standard dialysate calcium concentration used in most dialysis centers. Since aluminum hydroxide preparations were universally employed as phosphorus-binders at that time, the use of such a high dialysate calcium value was appropriate. With the replacement of aluminum hydroxide by calcium salts (such as calcium acetate or carbonate) as phosphorus-binders and the widespread use of calcitriol and related compounds to combat renal osteodystrophy, hypercalcemia is not uncommonly encountered if a dialysate calcium level of 1.75 mM is used (273). Another predisposing factor for the development of hypercalcemia is aluminum toxicity. Aluminum poisoning causes defective bone mineralization, thus impairing bone uptake of calcium and fostering the occurrence of hypercalcemia (274). Because of the above reasons, dialysate calcium level is nowadays often lowered to 1.0–1.25 mM to discourage the development of hypercalcemia.

Treatment for this type of hypercalcemia consists of ingesting calcium-containing phosphorus-binders only during meals so that the calcium administered will combine with the phosphorus present in food to form insoluble calcium phosphates. As a consequence, absorption of ingested calcium is curbed. In addition, vitamin D therapy should be discontinued. Aluminum toxicity, if present, should be promptly treated. A dialysate containing an appropriately low level of calcium should be employed. Pamidronate, a drug that reduces osteoclast-induced resorption of bone and curtails transformation of

osteoclast precursors into mature osteoclasts, has been used successfully to control the present variety of hypercalcemia (275). However, whether therapy with this drug is superior to dialysis using a low-calcium dialysate remains to be determined. At present, it would appear that the use of a low-calcium dialysate is the simpler of the two methods.

Inadvertent addition of excessive amounts of calcium (without those of magnesium) to dialysate with resultant development of acute hypercalcemia (plasma calcium level as high as 3.45 mM) has been described (276). Apart from mental changes, abnormal movements and seizures, the affected patients often exhibited diffusely slow background activity and paroxysms of slow waves in their electro-encephalograms.

In many parts of the world, water intended for consumption often has very high concentrations of calcium and magnesium (277–281). Specifically, the levels of calcium and magnesium in such water have been found to reach values as high as 2.0 and 0.95 mM respectively (277). Should the means of purification of such water (e.g., water softener or deionizer) for the purpose of dialysis be faulty, a patient could be exposed to inordinately elevated dialysate levels of the divalent cations, resulting in what is known as the 'hard-water syndrome' (277–281).

Post-dialysis plasma levels of calcium and magnesium as high as 4.9 and 3 mM respectively have been recorded (277) (the plasma values were greater than those in the water because divalent cations had been added to the water also to make the dialysate that was used).

Patients suffering from the 'hard-water syndrome' often complain of nausea, vomiting, general malaise, somnolence, weakness, sweating, warm skin sensation, abdominal pain, tachycardia, hypertension or hypotension. In addition, neurological manifestations in the form of headaches, dysarthria, seizures and myoclonic jerks are common. Mental abnormalities such as hallucinations, confusion, memory loss and judgment defects can occur (277–281). Moreover, pancreatitis has also been encountered (279).

Many of the above symptoms can be caused by either hypercalcemia or hyper-magnesemia, or by both. A burning sensation in the skin is a characteristic symptom in many hypermagnesemic states (277, 282). The simultaneous rise in both calcium and magnesium levels is probably responsible for the dearth of more severe and possible fatal complications. Comparable degrees of hypercalcemia in other diseases have resulted in much more serious manifestations such as coma, cardiac arrhythmias and cardiac arrest. The relative lack of severe complications may be related to the fact that calcium and magnesium have many antagonistic physiologic effects (277).

Accidental use of a high-magnesium dialysate (7.5 mM) has been reported (282). Symptoms observed included warm skin sensation of the face, nausea, blurring of vision, muscular weakness, ataxia, inability to stand and hypotension.

Table 5. Contaminanats in dialysis water

Contaminant	Toxic manifestation
Chloramines	Hemolysis, anemia
Calcium/magnesium	Hard water syndrome
Copper	Hemolysis, hepatic damage
Iron	Hemosiderosis
Fluoride	Osteomalacia and osteoporosis
Sulfate	Metabolic acidosis
Zinc	Anemia
Aluminum	Encephalopathy, bone disease etc
Nitrates	Methemoglobulinemia
Microorganisms	Febrile reactions
Hydrocarbons	Potential carcinogenesis

Treatment for hypercalcemia or hypermagnesemia as a consequence of the inadvertent use of high-calcium and/or high-magnesium dialysate centers on the use of a dialysate containing appropriate amounts of the divalent cations.

CONTAMINATION OF DIALYSATE WATER (TABLE 5)

Fluoride

Dialysis patients are particularly susceptible to fluoride intoxication due to their repeated exposures to the large volumes of water in the course of dialysis (120 L per dialysis session; 19,000 L per year of maintenance hemodialysis) and to their lack of the usual renal route of fluoride excretion (250). Since fluoride has a molecular weight of only 19 daltons, it is readily transferable into the blood from the dialysate (283). Although municipal water generally contains in the realm of 53 micromolar fluoride (284), product water used for preparing dialysate should have a fluoride level less than 11 micromolar (i.e., < 0.2 parts per million) (285). In general, properly reverse-osmosis-treated and deionized water can more than meet this requirement. Faulty reverse-osmosis and deionization systems can result in contamination of product water by fluoride (250, 284, 286, 287). Many of the deionization systems are of the 'mixed bed' variety in which both cationic and anionic resins are intermingled within a single vessel (285, 286). Cationic resins exchange hydrogen ions for other cations and anionic resins exchange hydroxyl ions for other anions (285, 286). The liberated hydrogen and hydroxyl ions then combine to form water. As exchange sites on the resins become depleted, fewer ions are removed from the incoming water, the ion content of the effluent rises, and the resistivity of the effluent falls (288). Continued use of the exhausted resins to treat municipal water causes low-affinity anions, such as fluo-

ride, already bound to the resins, to be displaced into the effluent by higher-affinity anions, such as nitrate, sulfate, and chloride (285, 286). As a consequence, a patient can be exposed to a dialysate fluoride level as high as 1,000 micromolar (287). Finally, a rare cause for a high level of fluoride in dialysate is the accidental gross contamination of municipal water with fluoride-containing compounds while reverse osmosis and de-ionization equipment is not being utilized (289).

The toxicity of fluoride is related to its ability to oxidize other chemicals and to combine with organic compounds, resulting in a direct interference with various cellular metabolic processes. In addition, fluoride, being the most electronegative element, can readily bring down the serum levels of calcium and magnesium because of its tight binding with these cations (267).

Because a period of fluoride accumulation is necessary to incite patient responses, the onset of clinical manifestations can be anticipated to take place late into, or soon after dialysis (250, 287). Many patients in the same dialysis unit (if they share the same source of product water) are likely to demonstrate similar signs and symptoms at approximately the same time (250, 287). Early symptoms include nausea, vomiting, pruritus, burning or feverish feeling, headache, syncope, back or abdominal pain, diarrhea, chest pressure or pain, cardiac irritability and bradycardia (250, 287). Later on, binding of blood calcium by fluoride can bring about generalized muscle twitching, tetany, petechiae and bleeding from vascular access puncture sites. Still later, respiratory failure, hypotension, seizure, coma, cardiac arrest, and death can occur (250, 267, 289). Laboratory investigations may reveal metabolic acidosis of the high anion gap type, primary respiratory acidosis, low ionized serum calcium concentration, hyperkalemia and prolonged clotting time (250, 267). Serum levels of fluoride in affected patients have reached levels as high as 700 micromolar (287) (serum fluoride levels in normal subjects and in chronically hemodialyzed patients are in the realm of 0.7 and 1.3 micromolar respectively (290, 291). Treatment of acute fluoride poisoning entails the immediate cessation of the current dialysis; intravenous administration of calcium salts, sodium bicarbonate, glucose and insulin (for the therapy of hyperkalemia, acidosis and hypocalcemia if these abnormalities are present); and prompt dialysis using a bicarbonate-based, zero-to-normal potassium and fluoride-undetectable dialysate. Multiple or prolonged dialysis treatments may be required to remove adequate amounts of fluoride from the body (292). Should hemodialysis using fluoride-undetectable dialysate be unavailable, peritoneal dialysis should be instituted. Prevention of fluoride toxicity involves the meticulous purification of product water, frequent measurement of the fluoride concentration in product water and the ensuring of proper functioning of the reverse-osmosis and the de-ionization systems.

Methemoglobinemia

When the ferrous ion that is attached to the heme of hemoglobin is oxidized to the ferric form by an oxidizing agent, a derivative of hemoglobin known as methemoglobin, is produced. Methemoglobin is without function because its heme molecule cannot bind oxygen (293).

Patients suffering from mild methemoglobinemia are usually asymptomatic. At a level of methemoglobin up to 40%, symptoms of fatigability, malaise and giddiness have been described. In severe acute methemoglobinemia with levels of methemoglobin higher than 60 to 70%, collapse, coma, and death have been reported (293).

Signs suggestive of methemoglobinemia are comprised of the sudden onset of cyanosis in the presence of a normal blood Po_2 and without physical findings of a cardiac, pulmonary, or intracranial disorder, a characteristic chocolate-brown discoloration of the venous blood which does not become bright red when exposed to oxygen, and failure of the cyanosis to improve with oxygen therapy (293, 294).

Dialysis-associated methemoglobinemia can occur as a result of exposure to oxidizing agents such as:

Nitrate

Patients who are dialyzed with nitrate-rich well water can develop methemoglobinemia (294). Wells that are poorly constructed or poorly located may have a high level of nitrates in their water due to seepage of wastes. It should be noted that production of methemoglobin secondary to ingestion of nitrate in man depends on the conversion of the chemical to nitrite by intestinal microorganisms. Absorption of the nitrite thus produced from the intestines leads to direct oxidation of hemoglobin to methemoglobin. However, in patients dialyzed with nitrate-rich well water, it is surmised that the nitrate that has been transferred into the blood gains access to the lumen of the large intestines and is then converted into nitrite by intestinal bacteria. The nitrite so formed is then absorbed back into the circulation to cause methemoglobinemia (294). Prevention of the present methemoglobinemia depends on the removal of nitrites from product water by means of a de-ionizer (295). The Association for the Advancement of Medical Instrumentation (AAMI) recommends that the nitrate (as N) level in product water should be less than 2 mg/L (296). For treatment of the methemoglobinemia, one should stop using the nitrate-containing dialysate. When the methemoglobinemia is mild, no treatment is necessary since the methemoglobin will be spontaneously reduced to hemoglobin by the body over 2 to 3 days. For severely affected patients, 1 to 2 mg/kg of a 1% solution of methylene blue in saline is administered intravenously over 10 minutes (293). A second dose can be repeated in an hour if an adequate response is wanting. The rationale for the use of methylene blue is based on its ability to activate the NADH-methemoglobin reductase enzyme system in the erythrocytes (297).

Chloramine

Chlorine is often used as a disinfectant for municipal water supplies. However, chloramines, compounds composed of chlorine and ammonia, are increasingly considered to be environmentally safer alternatives to chlorine for disinfecting water supplies (298). This is because chloramines are less volatile and have a less objectionable smell and taste than chlorine (299). Furthermore, unlike chlorine, chloramines do not react with naturally occurring organic compounds to form chloroform (300). For the purpose of dialysis, municipal water treated with chloramines is ordinarily purged of these disinfectants by passage through charcoal filters (also known as carbon filters) containing granular activated carbon particles (299). These particles possess numerous pores whose surfaces are covered with active sites that can reduce mono-chloramine to ammonia and dichloramine to molecular nitrogen (301). Should the charcoal filters be defective, chloramines in municipal water can escape into product water.

In case the delivery of municipal water to a charcoal filter is excessive in relation to the capacity of the filter to remove chloramines, that particular filter can become prematurely exhausted and allow chloramines to enter and contaminate the product water (298). Also noteworthy is the fact that drought conditions require the use of larger amounts of chloramines because drought-induced stagnation of water encourages bacterial and fungal growth. The greater quantity of chloramines added may tax the capacity of existing filters to remove these disinfectants (302).

The problem of high chloramine levels is more complicated for home dialysis patients. Chloramine levels may vary, depending on the distance of the patient's home from the municipal water source, and on the age and composition of the water pipes. If the pipes are old and made of iron, then the farther the home is from the water source, the lower the chloramine level. This is because oxidized iron pipes have the ability to convert chloramine to chlorine and ammonia (299).

According to AAMI standards, product water geared for dialysis should not have a chloramine level higher than 0.1 mg/L (0.1 ppm) (303). High blood levels of chloramines can oxidize the hemoglobin in the blood to form methemoglobin and Heinz bodies, the latter being intracellular precipitates of denatured hemoglobin (293, 304, 305). In addition, high blood levels can induce damage to the hexose monophosphate shunt of erythrocytes, thereby impairing the capacity of these cells to defend themselves against oxidant damage (e.g., that due to drugs). Because of the aforementioned reasons, red cells affected by chloramines are very susceptible to hemolysis and a hemolytic anemia, sometimes called Heinz body-positive hemolytic anemia, is readily encountered (304, 305). On the contrary, chlorine does not appear to have any of these untoward effects.

The treatment of methemoglobinemia has previously been discussed. The hemolytic anemia due to exposure to chloramines can be severe enough to warrant blood transfusion therapy (298, 302). Prevention consists of routing municipal water through appropriate charcoal filters (298, 303), with the realization that chloramines are not removed by reverse-osmosis (305). The Food and Drug Administration of the USA recommends that two charcoal filters be used in series for a water treatment system. A systemic plan for replacing the filters as they become exhausted should be established. With the filters in series, the exhausted first filter can be replaced with the second, and a new filter placed in the second position. Whenever a charcoal filter is replaced, the filter housing should be disinfected and thoroughly rinsed before the new filter is installed (303). Exhausted charcoal filters should be replaced with fresh ones, and should not be rejuvenated by backwashing (backwashing may loosen the packed carbon particles and restore surface area); however, backwashing does not remove previously aggregated material from the charcoal and, therefore, does not regenerate the filter (298). Whether chloramines are removed by de-ionization is controversial; both effective (306) and ineffective (307) removal have been reported. It has been suggested that de-ionization systems do indeed remove some chloramines, probably through reaction with the structural part of the resin molecules but not with the cationic or anionic sites (308). In order to ensure the absence of chloramines, product water should be tested for the chemicals at least once per patient shift to ensure patient safety (303).

Addition of vitamin C, a reducing agent, to a dialysate at a concentration of 17–34 mg/L has also been found to be effective in converting dialysate chloramines to the relatively innocuous ammonium chloride, whether the batch method or the proportioning method of producing dialysate is used (305, 308, 309). It should be emphasized that patients who are dialyzed with vitamin C-enriched dialysate should not take oral vitamin C supplements. This approach of enriching dialysate with vitamin C will only result in serum levels approximating those seen in maintenance dialysis patients taking standard oral vitamin supplements (308). Because of such non-excessive serum levels, the occurrence of vitamin C-induced deposition of oxalate crystals in tissues is very unlikely in patients dialyzed with a vitamin C-enriched dialysate. Some centers employ both charcoal filters and vitamin C enrichment at the same time (308).

MISCELLANEOUS COMPLICATIONS

Febrile episodes and endotoxin

Pyrogenic episodes associated directly with hemodialysis treatments are infrequent (310) and their presence should always elicit a search for underlying bacterial infections (311, 312). Occasionally, clustering of febrile episodes (313), particularly after any mechanical work on the water supply system, raises the possibility of contamination. Bicarbonate dialysate concentrates can support bacterial growth with endotoxin production. Endotoxins or bacteria may cross or interact at the membranes of high-flux dialyzers, triggering the release of endogenous pyrogens (e.g., certain cytokines) by peripheral blood mononuclear cells to cause pyrogenic reactions. Pyrogenic reactions occur at a rate of 0.7 reaction per 1,000 hemodialysis treatments (314). This incidence is not different between conventional, and high-flux or high-efficiency modalities of dialysis (314).

Pyrogenic reactions occurring in clusters are more frequently reported in centers that reuse conventional dialyzer membranes compared to centers that do not. This enhanced risk is evidenced only in centers that use Renalin™ (an acetic acid/peracetic acid/hydrogen peroxide mixture) or glutaraldehyde (but not formaldehyde) for reprocessing and occurred with both automated and manual reprocessing systems (315–317). Use of dialyzers with detachable components such as headers has been associated with an increased incidence of infections (e.g., 'header sepsis') with a variety of organisms including Xanthomonas, and other slow-growing organisms, a problem that can be solved with proper disinfections of the O rings and other components of the header (318, 319). Improper preparation of the disinfectant has also been associated with clusters of infection with Pseudomonas species (313, 320). Nontuberculous mycobacteria are ubiquitous in muncipal water and outbreaks of infection with these organisms during reuse have been reported (321). Because of the organisms' greater germicide resistance compared to that of most other naturally occurring water bacteria, attention to the quality and concentration of disinfectants is mandatory.

The importance of dialysate contamination with endotoxin is paramount under conditions of backfiltration that may occur with high-flux dialysis. The minimal dose of endotoxin necessary to induce fever in man (5 ng/kg; 1 ng corresponds to 10 endotoxin units) can be readily achieved in some contaminated dialysates (322). Levels higher than 100 EU/mL have been found in up to ten percent of German dialysis units surveyed (323). The actual occurrence of endotoxin transfer into patients is documented by the determination of anti-endotoxin antibodies. Yamagami et al. (324) observed a low incidence of such antibodies in patients maintained on low-flux dialysis (26% compared to 19% in controls, not statistically different), but a significantly higher prevalence in patients treated with high-flux dialysis (60% $p < 0.05$ *vs* low-flux dialysis). Vanholder et al. (325) have documented the absence of in-vivo endotoxin transfer during hemodialysis with small-pore dialyzer membranes, but a rise in limulus amebocyte lysate (LAL) reactivity during hemodialysis with membranes possessing larger pores. The LAL activity presumably mirrors the occurrence of backdiffusion/filtration when the latter membranes are used (325).

Endotoxin transfer may contribute to cytokine induction. While the clinical significance of the latter phenomenon remains unknown, the use of ultrapure water has been reported to result in a reduction in the prevalence of the carpal tunnel syndrome (326). In examining for endotoxemia in dialysis patients, care should be taken to use the proper test. The limulus amebocyte lysate-reactive material (LAL-RM) is cellulose-derived and cross-reacts with LAL via factor G. Using the conventional chromogenic limulus test, all patients treated with regenerated cellulose dialyzers will show elevated values. In this setting, a specific endotoxin assay with factor G-free LAL should be used (312).

Seizures

A variety of causes for seizure in dialysis patients have been described. A detailed description of the different etiologies and management strategies are beyond the scope of this chapter. (See chapter of Neurological Problems.)

In children and adolescents, hemodialysis is associated with a significant incidence of seizures (9% of all children treated with hemodialysis in one series (327)). The risk of hemodialysis-associated seizures among those with a prior history of seizure (29%) was significantly higher than among those with no such history (8%) (327). In view of the prevalence of underlying bone diseases, metabolically induced seizures can be associated with bone fractures (328).

Bowel ischemia

Mesenteric ischemia manifesting as abdominal pain and possibly acute diarrhea occurring with or shortly after an episode of dialysis-induced hypotension, is a dreaded complication that is associated with a high mortality (329, 330). Both occlusive (329) and non-occlusive infarctions (330) have been described, and afflicted patients often have associated guaiac-positive stools and leukocytosis (329). Occasionally, cecal necrosis and perforation may occur, particularly if constipation and colon distension are present at the time of the hypotensive episode (331).

Ocular changes

During hemodialysis, minor fluctuations in intraocular pressure (usually a slight rise) occur; such fluctuations may have some significance in subjects with underlying glaucoma (332). Isolated ultrafiltration often causes a fall in intraocular pressure. Sudden blindness secondary to leukoembolization of retinal arterioles (333) (Purtscher's-like retinopathy) has been described in hemodialysis patients. Accompanied by varying reversible neurological signs and symptoms, this retinopathy usually manifests

as sudden but reversible loss of vision during hemodialysis. In addition, various reversible neurological signs and symptoms are frequently present. Leukoembolization is an uncommon occurrence during dialysis. Moreover, while transient pulmonary leuko-sequestration is common, distal ischemic manifestations are exceedingly rare. Another cause of painless sudden loss of vision is ischemic optic neuropathy (334), an entity associated with many systemic processes, including shock. The condition has been reported to occur in association with recurrent hemodialysis-associated hypotension. Although serious, these manifestations are rare enough to be considered mere curiosities.

Complication of thrombolytic therapy

Localized thrombolytic therapy is frequently used to insure patency of clogged or partially clogged dialysis access catheters or grafts. This therapy may occasionally be associated with bleeding complications, particularly in subjects with underlying predisposing conditions (335). Systemic thrombolytic therapy has been advocated as an alternative to 'blind' surgical intervention in subjects with recently clotted vascular access (336). Careful screening of patients is clearly necessary prior to use of this modality.

Priapism

Priapism is a rare and peculiar occurrence observed in approximately 0.5% of male dialysis patients during or a few hours after dialysis (337). Androgen therapy is a common association, and the condition is observed twice as frequently in black as in white patients (337). Hypoxemia is a possible contributing factor as it induces priapism in patients with sickle cell disease. The latter disease was also present in a few black subjects experiencing priapism. The condition is relatively innocuous and resolves spontaneously.

Hypertensive emergencies

Sometimes during dialysis and ultrafiltration a paradoxical hypertensive response occurs. In one study hypertension occurred in 17% of dialyses (2). With new equipment and anti-hypertensive treatment this may have decreased to approximately 9%. Occasionally, however, a patient is encountered who has an uncorrected severe hypertension despite correction of fluid overload, or as a response to fluid removal (Figure 4). The latter hypertensive response to hemodialysis may be due to exaggerated vasoconstrictor responses to fluid removal In some patients, we have observed a dramatic rise in plasma catecholamines in parallel with the increment in blood pressure, and an abrogation of the hypertensive response with phentolamine administration. Alternatively, activation of the renin-angiotensin system as a result of volume deple-

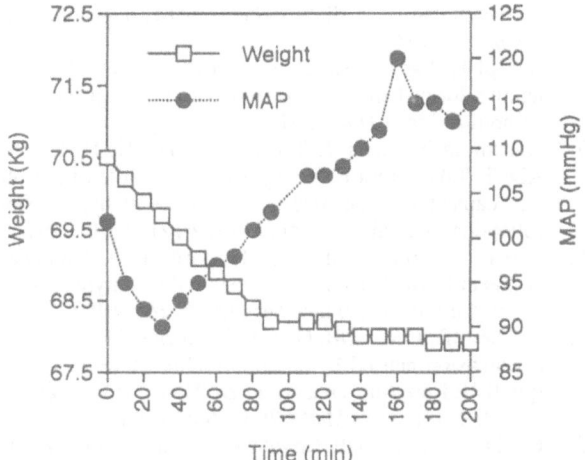

Figure 4. Patient with paradoxical hypertension induced by fluid removal during dialysis. After an initial drop, blood pressure rises to baseline and overshoots, remaining high at 'dry weight'. In this particular patient, the hypertensive response was associated with pronounced elevations of plasma catecholamines and was abrogated by phentolamine administration. (Mujais, SK, unpublished observations).

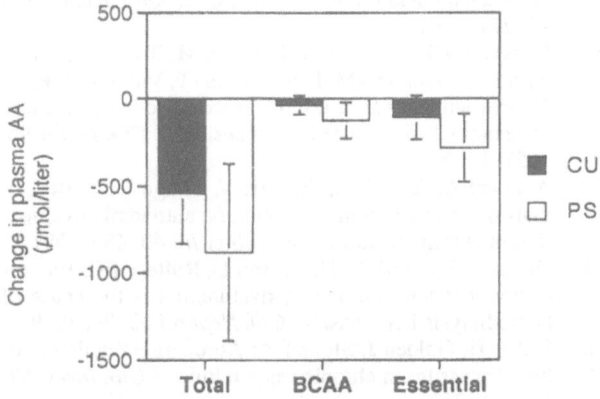

Figure 5. Effect of a cellulosic (cuprophan (CU)) and a synthetic (polysulphone (PS)) membranes on plasma amino acids. Data from Reference (340). The differences between CU and PS are significant at $p < 0.05$.

tion may be contributory. However, since the paradoxical hypertension has been observed both in the absence of changes in sympathetic activity and in anephric subjects, the above mechanisms cannot be claimed to occur uniformly in all subjects with the condition. The occurrence of this hypertensive response to fluid removal does not appear to be related to the dialysate calcium level. Hypertensive patients are usually instructed to withhold their antihypertensive medications on the day of dialysis to avoid intradialytic hypotension. The persistent elevation of blood pressure at the end of dialysis may represent a rebound of antihypertensive withdrawal which should

respond promptly to resumption of medications. Under conditions when the physician considers that such delays may be injurious to the patient, immediate therapy is in order. Both sublingual captopril and nifedipine administrations are useful in this setting and appear to be equally effective (338). The response to nifedipine is brisker, but associated with more side effects. The real need for institution of urgent antihypertensive therapy has to be clearly established particularly as a delayed hypotensive response to hemodialysis may be observed. The simple resumption of the patient's established antihypertensive regiment may be sufficient in the majority of cases.

Dialysis-associated catabolism

Hemodialysis is considered to be a catabolic event, increasing urea generation rate during dialysis and leading to a negative nitrogen balance. A major contributory factor to this event is the loss of amino acids during dialysis ranging between 6 to 13 g per dialysis session. This loss in amino acids via the dialysate leads to a decline in arterial amino acid concentrations and a concomitant rise in efflux of amino acids from tissue, mainly skeletal muscle. This phenomenon does not appear to be related to the presence or absence of glucose in the dialysate (or conversely the gain or loss of glucose) (339). This effect appears to be dialyzer membrane-dependent, being greater with high-flux membranes, and still greater with the reuse of such membranes (Figure 4). Reuse of high-flux dialyzer membranes also appears to augment albumin losses during dialysis. After the 20th reuse, the loss of albumin can reach 10 g per session (340).

REFERENCES

1. Degoulet P, Roulx J-P, Aime F: Programme dialyse-informatique III. Données epidemiologiques stratégies de dialyse et resultats biologiques. *J Urol Nephrol* (Paris) 82: 1001, 1976
2. Rosa AA, Fryd DS, Kjellstrand CM: Dialysis symptoms and stabilization in long-term dialysis. Practical application of the cusum plot. *Arch Intern Med* 140: 804, 1980
3. Orofino L, Marcen R, Quereda C, Villafruela J, Sabater J, Matesanz R, Pascual J, Ortuño J: Epidemiology of symptomatic hypotension in hemodialysis: is cool dialysate beneficial for all patients? *Am J Nephrol* 10: 177, 1990
4. Capuano A, Sepe V, Cianfrone P, Castellano T, Andreucci VE: Cardiovascular impairment, dialysis strategy and tolerance in elderly and young patients on maintenance haemodialysis. *Nephrol Dial Transplant* 5: 1023, 1990
5. Jost CM, Agarwal R, Khair, Grayburn PA, Victor RG, Henrich WL: Effects of cooler temperature dialysate on hemodynamic stability in 'problem' dialysis patients. *Kidney Int* 44: 606, 1993
6. Anonymous: Acute intradialytic well-being: results of a clinical trial comparing polysulfone with cuprophan. Bergamo Collaborative dialysis Study Group. *Kidney Int* 40: 714, 1991

7. Shinzato T, Nakai S, Odani H, Nakane K, Takai I, Maeda K: Relationship between dialysis induced hypotension and adenosine released by ischemic tissue. *ASAIO J* 38: 286, 1992

8. Shinzato T, Milwa M, Nakai S, Morita H, Odani H, Inove I, Maeda K: Role of adenosine in dialysis-induced hypotension. *Am Soc Nephrol* 4: 1987, 1994

9. Santoro A, Mancini E, Spongano M, Rossi M, Paolini F, Zucchelli P: A haemodynamic study of hypotension during haemodialysis using electrical bioimpedance cardiography. *Nephrol Dial Transplant* (Suppl 1): 147, 1990

10. de Vries PJ, Kouw PM, vanderMeer N, Olthof CG, Oe LP, Donker AJ, de Vries PM: Non-invasive monitoring of blood volume during hemodialysis: its relation with post-dialytic dry weight. *Kidney Int* 44: 851, 1993

11. Sherman RA, Torres F, Cody RP: The effect of red cell transfusion on hemodialysis-related hypotension. *Am J Kidney Dis* 11: 33, 1988

12. Lins LE, Hedenborg G, Jacobson SH et al.: Blood pressure reduction during hemodialysis correlates to intradialytic changes in plasma volume. *Clin Nephrol* 37: 308, 1992

13. Schneditz D, Roob J, Oswald M, Pogglitsch H, Moser M, Kenner T, Binswager U: Nature and rate of vascular refilling during hemodialysis and ultrafiltration. *Kidney Int* 42: 1425, 1992

14. Di Maggio A, Basile C, Scatizzi A: Plasma volume changes induced by sequential ultrafiltration-hemodialysis and sequential hemodialysis-ultrafiltration. *Int J Artif Organs* 10: 291, 1987

15. Bauer JH, Brooks CS: Body fluid composition in chronic renal failure. *Clin Nephrol* 16: 114, 1981

16. Van SJ, Bauer J, Carey J: The effect of dialysate sodium concentration on body fluid compartment volume, plasma renin activity and plasma aldosterone concentration in chronic hemodialysis patients. *Am J Kidney Dis* 2: 58, 1982

17. Fauchald P: Transcapillary colloid osmotic gradient and body fluid volumes in renal failure. *Kidney Int* 29: 895, 1986

18. Fleming SJ, Wilkinson JS, Greenwood RN, Aldridge C, Baker LR, Cattell WR: Effect of dialysate composition on intercompartmental fluid shift. *Kidney Int* 32: 267, 1987

19. Kimura G, Van SJ, Bauer JH: Model prediction of plasma volume change induced by hemodialysis. *J Lab Clin Med* 104: 932, 1984

20. Martin MA, Perez R, Gomez J, Burdiel LG, Andres E, Castillo D, Moreno E, Aljama P: Sequential hypertonic dialysis. *Nephron* 40: 458, 1985

21. Po CL, Afolabi M, Raja RM: The role of sequential ultrafiltration and varying dialysate sodium on vascular stability during hemodialysis. *ASAIO J* 39: 798, 1993

22. Swartz RD, Sommermeyer MG, Hsu CH: Preservation of plasma volume during hemodialysis depends on dialysate osmolality. *Am J Nephrol* 2: 189, 1982

23. Basile C, Coates JE, Ulan RA: Plasma volume changes induced by hypertonic hemodiafiltration and standard hemodialysis. *Am J Nephrol* 7: 264, 1987

24. Hsu CH, Swartz RD, Sommermeyer MG, Raj A: Bicarbonate hemodialysis: influence on plasma refilling and hemodynamic stability. *Nephron* 38: 202, 1984

25. Maeda K, Morita H, Shinzato T, Vega BV, Kobayakawa H, Ishihara T, Inagaki H, Igarashi I, Kitano T: Role of hypovolemia in dialysis-induced hypotension. *Artif Organs* 12: 116, 1988

26. Hampl H, Paeprer H, Unger V, Kessel MW: Hemodynamics during hemodialysis, sequential ultrafiltration and hemofiltration. *J Dial* 3: 51, 1979

27. Nakamura Y, Ikeda T, Takata S, Yokoi H, Hirono M, Abe T, Takazakura E, Kobayashi K: The role of peripheral capacitance and resistance vessels in hypotension following hemodialysis. *Am Heart J* 121: 1170, 1991

28. Maeda K, Fujita Y, Shinzato T, Morita H, Kobayakawa H, Takai I: Mechanism of dialysis-induced hypotension. *Trans Am Soc Artif Intern Organs* 35: 245, 1989

29. Bradley JR, Evans DB, Gore SM, Cowley AJ: Is dialysis hypotension caused by an abnormality of venous tone? [published erratum appears in *Br Med J* (*Clin Res Ed*) 297: 330, 1988]. *Br Med J* 296: 1634, 1988

30. Bradley JR, Evans DB, Cowley AJ: Comparison of vascular tone during combined haemodialysis with ultrafiltration and during ultrafiltration followed by haemodialysis: a possible mechanism for dialysis hypotension. *Br Med J* 300: 1312, 1990

31. Kooman JP, Gladziwa U, Bocker G, van BL, van HJ, Leunissen KM: Role of the venous system in hemodynamics during ultrafiltration and bicarbonate dialysis. *Kidney Int* 42: 718, 1992

32. Rozich JD, Smith B, Thomas JD, Zile MR, Kaiser J, Mann DL: Dialysis-induced alterations in left ventricular filling: mechanisms and clinical significance. *Am J Kidney Dis* 17: 277, 1991

33. Converse RJ, Jacobsen TN, Jost CM, Toto RD, Grayburn PA, Obregon TM, Fouad-Tarazi F, Victor RG: Paradoxical withdrawal of reflex vasoconstriction as a cause of hemodialysis-induced hypotension. *J Clin Invest* 90: 1657, 1992

34. Agarwal A, Anand IS, Sakhuja V, Chugh KS: Effect of dialysis and renal transplantation on autonomic dysfunction in chronic renal failure. *Kidney Int* 40: 489, 1991

35. Heber ME, Lahiri A, Thompson D, Raftery EB: Baroreceptor, not left ventricular, dysfunction is the cause of hemodialysis hypotension. *Clin Nephrol* 32: 79, 1989

36. Lilley JJ, Golden J, Stone RA: Adrenergic regulation of blood pressure in chronic renal failure. *J Clin Invest* 57: 1190, 1976

37. McGrath BP, Tiller DJ, Bune A, Chalmers JP, Korner PI, Uther JB: Autonomic blockade and the Valsalva maneuver in patients on maintenance hemodialysis: a hemodynamic study. *Kidney Int* 12: 294, 1977

38. Hakim RM, Pontzer MA, Tilton D, Lazarus JM, Gottlieb MN: Effects of acetate and bicarbonate dialysate in stable chronic dialysis patients. *Kidney Int* 28: 535, 1985

39. Diamond SM, Henrich WL: Acetate dialysate *versus* bicarbonate dialysate: a continuing controversy. (Review) *Am J Kidney Dis* 9: 3, 1987

40. Malberti F, Surian M, Colussi G, Minetti L: The influence of dialysis fluid composition on dialysis tolerance. *Nephrol Dial Transplant* 2: 93, 1987

41. DiBello V, Bianchi AM, Caputo MT et al.: Fractional shortening/end-systolic stress correlation in the evaluation of left ventricular contractility in patients treated by acetate dialysis and lactate haemofiltration. *Nephrol Dial Transplant* (Suppl 1): 115, 1990

42. Wizemann V, Soetanto R, Thormann J, Lubbecke F, Kramer W: Effects of acetate on left ventricular function in hemodialysis patients. *Nephrol* 64: 101, 1993

43. Daugirdas JT: Dialysis hypotension: a hemodynamic analysis. *Kidney Int* 39: 233, 1991

44. Sherman RA, Bialy GB, Gazinski B, Bernholc AS, Eisinger RP: The effect of dialysate calcium levels on blood pressure during hemodialysis. *Am J Kidney Dis* 8: 244, 1986

45. Kjellstrand CM: Vasodilatory hormones in hemodialysis. *Int J Artif Organs* 13, 1990

46. Odar CI, Kjellstrand CM, Theodorsson E: Is calcitonin gene-related peptide (CGRP) a regulator of blood pressure in hemodialysis patients? *Int J Artif Organs* 13: 134, 1990

47. Hegbrant J, Martensson L, Thysell H, Ekman R, Boberg U: Effects of sham hemodialysis on plasma levels of vasoactive peptides in patients wtih uremia. *ASAIO J* 38: 197, 1992

48. Hegbrant J, Thysell H, Martensson L, Ekman R, Boberg U: Changes in plasma levels of vasoactive peptides during sequential bicarbonate hemodialysis. *Nephron* 63: 309, 1993

49. Hegbrant J, Thysell H, Martensson L, Ekman R, Boberg U: Changes in plasma levels of vasoactive peptides during standard bicarbonate hemodialysis. *Nephron* 63: 303, 1993

50. Niwa T, Fujishiro T, Uema K et al.: Effect of hemodialysis on plasma levels of vasoactive peptides: endothelin, calcitonin gene-related peptide and human atrial natriuretic peptide. *Nephron* 64: 552, 1993

51. Sturani A, Degli EE, Chiarini C, Spongano M, Santoro A, Zucchelli P: Failure of naloxone in reversal hemodialysis-induced hypotension. *Blood Purif* 3: 184, 1985

52. Sherman RA, Torres F, Cody RP: Postprandial blood pressure changes during hemodialysis. *Am J Kidney Dis* 12: 37, 1988

53. Barakat MM, Nawab ZM, Yu AW, Lau AH, Ing TS, Daugirdas JT: Hemodynamic effects of intradialytic food ingestion and the effects of caffeine. *Am Soc Nephrol* 3: 1813, 1993

54. DeFremont JF, Coevert B, Andrejak M, Makdassi R, Quichaud J, Lambrey G, Gueris J, Caillens C, Harichaux P, Alexandre JM, Fournier A: Effects of antihypertensive drugs on dialysis-resistant hypertension, plasma renin and dopamine betahydroxylase activities, metabolic risk factors and calcium phosphate homeostasis. Comparison of metoprolol, alphamethyldopa and clonidine in a crossover trial. *Clin Nephrol* 12: 198, 1979

55. Sadowski RH, Allred EN, Jabs K: Sodium modeling ameliorate intradialytic and interdialytic symptoms in young hemodialysis patients. *Am Soc Nephrol* 4: 1192, 1993

56. Zawada ET, Bennett EP, Steinson JB, Ramirez G: Serum calcium in blood pressure regulation during hemodialysis. *Arch Intern Med* 141: 657, 1981

57. Maynar J, Cruz C, Kleerekope RM, Levin N: Blood pressure response to changes in serum ionized calcium during hemodialysis. *Ann Intern Med* 104: 358, 1986

58. Pierides AM, Kurts SB, Johnson W: Ultrafiltration followed by hemodialysis. A longterm trial and acute studies. *J Dial* 2: 325, 1978

59. Jones EO, Ward MK, Hoenich NA, Kerr DN: Separation of dialysis and ultrafiltration – does it really help? *Proc Eur Dial Transplant Assoc* 14: 160, 1977

60. Maggiore Q, Pizzarelli F, Zoccali C, Sisca S, Nicolo F: Influence of blood temperature on vascular stability during hemodialysis and isolated ultrafiltration. *Int J Artif Organs* 8: 175, 1985

61. Quereda C, Marcen R, Lamas S et al.: Hemodialysis associated hypotension and dialysate temperature. *Life Support Systems* 1: 18, 1985

62. Sherman RA, Rubin MP, Cody RP, Eisinger RP: Amelioration of hemodialysis-associated hypotension by the use of cool dialysate. *Am J Kidney Dis* 5: 124, 1985

63. Kerr PG, van BC, Dawborn JK: Assessment of the symptomatic benefit of cool dialysate. *Nephron* 52: 166, 1989

64. Marcen R, Quereda C, Orofino L et al.: Hemodialysis with low-temperature dialysate: a long-term experience. *Nephron* 49: 29, 1988

65. Stiller S, Wirtz D, Waterbar F, Gladziwa U, Dakshinamurty KV, Mann H: Less symptomatic hypotension using blood volume controlled ultrafiltration. *Trans Am Soc Artif Intern Organs* 37: 138, 1991

66. Sturniolo A, Costanzi S, Barbera G, Ruffini MP, Passalacqua S, Fulignati P, Splendiani G: Computerised monitoring of sodium and fluid during haemodialysis. *Nephrol Dial Transplant* 1: 162, 1990

67. Skroeder NR, Jacobson SH, Lins K, Kjellstrand CM: Biocompatibility of dialysis membranes is of no importance for objective or subjective symptoms during or after hemodialysis. *Trans Am Soc Artif Intern Organs* 36: M637, 1990

68. Anonymous, Bergamo Collaborative Dialysis Study Group: Acute intradialytic well-being: results of a clinical trial comparing polysulfone with cuprophan. *Kidney Int* 40: 714, 1991

69. Branger B, Deschodt G, Oules R, Balducchi JP, Granolleras C, Aisabadani B, Fourcade J, Shaldon S: Biocompatible membranes and hemodynamic tolerance to hemodialysis. *Kidney Int* 24: S196, 1988

70. Collins DM, Lambert MB, Tannenbaum JS, Oliverio M, Schwab SJ: Tolerance of hemodialysis: a randomized prospective tiral of high-flux *versus* conventional high-efficiency hemodialysis. *Am Soc Nephrol* 4: 148, 1993

71. Ahmad S, Robertson HT, Golper TA et al.: Multicenter trial of L-carnitine in maintenance hemodialysis patients. II. Clinical and biochemical effects. *Kidney Int* 38: 912, 1990

72. Iida N, Tscubakihara Y, Shirai D, Imada A, Suzuki M: Treatment of dialysis-induced hypotension with L-threo-3, 4-dihydroxyphenylserine. *Nephrol Dial Transplant* 9: 1130, 1994

73. Borges HF, Kjellstrand CM: On the effect of prostaglandin inhibition on the clinical course of chronic hemodialysis. *Nephron* 42: 120, 1986

74. Gong R, Lindberg J, Abrams J, Whitaker WR, Wade CE, Gouge S: Comparison of hypertonic saline solutions and dextran in dialysis-induced hypotension. *Am Soc Nephrol* 3: 1808, 1993

75. Stejskalova A, Stejskal J, Elleder M: Iatrogenic generalized storage of dextran in patients on regular dialysis. *Czech Med* 10: 201, 1987

76. Bergonzi G, Paties C, Vassallo G, Zangrandi A, Poisetti PG, Ballochi S, Fontana F, Scarpioni L: Dextran deposits

718   *Salim K. Mujais, Todd Ing and Carl Kjellstrand*

in tissues of patients undergoing haemodialysis. *Nephrol Dial Transplant* 5: 54, 1990

77. Warren SE, Olshan A, Beck CHJ: Use of phenylephrine HCl for treatment of refractory dialysis-aggravated hypotension. *Nephrol Dial Transplant* 9: 492, 1980

78. Shimoyama H, Suwata J, Saitoh H, Oguchi K, Kobayashi S, Kawada Y: Changes in catecholamine level in hypotensive patients subjected to dialysis. *Nipon Jinzo Gakkai Shi* 31: 165, 1989

79. Lindberg JS, Copley JB, Melton K. Wade CE, Abrams J, Goode D: Lysine vasopressin in the treatment of refractory hemodialysis-induced hypotension. *Am J Nephrol* 10: 269, 1990

80. Flynn JJ, Mitchell MC, Caruso FS, McElligott MA: A pilot evaluation of midodrine to treat patients with hemodialysis hypotension. (Abstract) *Am Soc Nephrol* 4: 345, 1993

81. De Broe M, DeBacker W: Pathophysiology of hemodialysis-associated hypoxemia. (Review) *Adv Nephrol Necker Hosp* 18: L297, 1989

82. Ozdemir O, Arik N, Ozcebe O, Arinsoy T, Sungur C, Dundar S, Turgan C, Yasauul U, Caglar S, Kiragli S: Evidence for the role of dialysis hypoxemia in the pathogenesis of hemodialysis-induced rise in tissue-type plasminogen activator. *Thromb Res* 67: 697, 1992

83. Pitcher WD, Diamond SM, Henrich WL: Pulmonary gas exchange during dialysis in patients with obstructive lung disease. *Chest* 96: 1136, 1989

84. Cardoso M, Vinay P, Vinet B, Léveillé M, Prud'homme M, Téjédor A, Courteau M, Gougoux A, St. Louis G, Lapierre L, Piette Y: Hypoxemia during hemodialysis: a critical review of the facts. (Review) *Am J Kidney Dis* 11: 281, 1988

85. Gilli Y, Binswanger U: Continuous pulse-oxymetry during haemodialysis. *Nephron* 44: 368, 1990

86. Fujiwara Y, Hagihara B, Yamauchi A, Shirai D: Hypoxemia and hemodialysis-induced symptomatic hypotension. *Clin Nephrol* 24: 9, 1985

87. Francos GC, Besarab A, Burke F, Peters J, Tahamont MV, Gee MH, Flynn JT, Gzesh D: Dialysis-induced hypoxemia: membrane dependent and membrane independent causes. *Am J Kidney Dis* 5: 191, 1985

88. Ganss R, Aarseth HP, Nordby G: Prevention of hemodialysis associated hypoxemia by use of low-concentration bicarbonate dialysate. *ASAIO J* 38: 820, 1992

89. Germain MJ, Burke EJ, Braden GL, Fitzgivvons JP: Amelioration of hemodialysis-induced fall in PaO2 with exercise. *Am J Nephrol* 5: 351, 1985

90. Igarashi H, Kioi S, Gejyo F, Arakawa M: Physiologic approach to dialysis-induced hypoxemia. Effects of dialyzer material and dialysate composition. *Nephron* 41: 62, 1985

91. Jones JG, Bembridge JL, Sapsford DJ, Turney JH: Continuous measurements os oxygen saturation during haemodialysis. *Nephrol Dial Transplant* 7: 110, 1992

92. Kishimoto T, Tanaka H, Maekawa M, Ivanovich P, Levin N, Bergstrom J, Klinkmann H: Dialysis-induced hypoxaemia. *Nephrol Dial Transplant* 2: 25, 1993

93. Oh MS, Uribarri J, Del Monte ML, Heneghan WF, Kee CS, Friedman EA, Carroll H: A mechanism of hypoxemia during hemodialysis. Consumption of CO_2 in metabolism of acetate. *Am J Nephrol* 5: 366, 1985

94. Ross EA, Tashkin D, Chenoweth D, Webber MM, Nissenson AR: Pulmonary leukosequestration without hypoxemia during hemodialysis. *Int J Artif Organs* 10: 367, 1987

95. Soliani F, Davoli V, Franco V, Lindner G, Lusanti T, Parisoli A, Brini M, Borgatti PP: Intradialytic changes of the oxyhaemoglobin dissociation curve during acetate and bicarbonate haemodialysis. Possible interactions with haemodialysis-associated hypoxaemia. *Nephrol Dial Transplant* 1: 119, 1990

96. Wiegmann TB, MacDougall ML, Diederich DA: Dialysis leukopenia, hypoxemia, and anaphylatoxin formation: effect of membrane, bath, and citrate anticoagulation. *Am J Kidney Dis* 11: 418, 1988

97. Gawaz M, Mujais SK, Schmidt B, Gurland HJ: Platelet-leukocyte aggregation during hemodialysis. *Kidney Int* 46: 489, 1994

98. Chou CT, Wasserstein A, Schumacher HJ, Fernandez P: Musculoskeletal manifestations in hemodialysis patients. *J Rheumatol* 12: 1149, 1985

99. McGee SR: Muscle cramps. *Arch Intern Med* 150: 511, 1990

100. Piergies AA, Atkinson AJ, Hubler GL, Del GF: Activation of renin-angiotensin system does not cause skeletal muscle cramps during hemodialysis. *Int Journal Clin Pharmacol Ther Toxicol* 28: 405, 1990

101. Kaplan B, Wang T, Rammohan M, Del GF, Molteni A, Atkinson AJ: Response to head-up tilt in cramping and noncramping hemodialysis patients. *Int J Clin Pharmacol Ther Toxicol* 30: 173, 1992

102. Cryer PE, Silverberg AB, Santiago JV, Shan SD: Plasma catecholamines in diabetes. The syndrome of hypoadrenergic and hyperadrenergic postural hypotension. *Am J Med* 64: 407, 1978

103. Sidhom O, Odeh Y, Krumlovsky F, Budris WA, Wamg Z, Pospisil PA, Atkinson AJ Jr: Low-dose prazosin in patients with muscle cramps during hemodialysis. *Clin Pharmacol Ther* 56: 445, 1994

104. Barrett BJ, Vavasour HM, Major A, Parfrey PS: Clinical and psychological correlates of somatic symptoms in patients on dialysis. *Nephron* 55: 10, 1990

105. Hernando P, Caramelo C, Lopez GD, Hernando L: Muscle cramps: a cause of elevated creatine kinase levels in hemodialysis patient [see comments]. *Nephron* 55: 231, 1990

106. Canzanello VJ, Hylander RB, Sands RE, Morgan TM, Jordan J, Burkart JM: Comparison of 50% dextrose water. 25% mannitor, and 23.5% saline for the treatment of hemo-dialysis-associated muscle cramps. *Trans Am Soc Artif Intern Organs* 37: 649, 1991

107. Roca AO, Jarjoura D, Blend D, Cugino A, Rutecki GW, Nuchikat PS, Whittier FC: Dialysis leg cramps. Efficacy of quinine *versus* vitamin E. *ASAIO J* 38: 481, 1992

108. Sever MS, Kocak N: Chloroquine phosphate reduces the frequency of muscle cramps during maintenance hemodialysis. (Letter) *Nephron* 56, 1990

109. Popli S, Ing TS, Daugirdas JT, Kheirbek AO, Viol GW, Vilbar RM, Gandhi VC: Severe reactions to cuprophan capillary dialyzers. *Artif Organs* 6: 312, 1982

110. Ing TS, Daugirdas JT, Popli S, Gandhi VC: First-use syndrome with cuprammonium cellulose dialyzers. *Int J Artif Organs* 6: 235, 1983

111. Nicholls A: Ethylene oxide and anaphylaxis during haemodialysis. *Br Med J* 292: 1221, 1986

112. Daugirdas JT, Ing TS, Roxe DM, Ivanovich PT, Krumlovsky F, Popli S, McLaughlin MM: Severe anaphylactoid reactions to cuprammonium cellulose hemodialyzers. *Arch Intern Med* 145: 489, 1985

113. Daugirdas JT, Ing TS: First-use reactions during hemodialysis: a definition of subtypes. *Kidney Int* 33 (Suppl 24): 537, 1988

114. Rockel A, Thiel C, Abdelhamid S, Fiegel P, Walb D: Three cases of hemodialysis-associated hypersensitivity reactions. *Int J Artif Organs* 8: 179, 1985

115. Villarroel F, Ciarkowski AA: A survey on hypersensitivity reactions in hemodialysis. *Artif Organs* 9: 231, 1985

116. Caruana RJ: First-use reactions: a potential hazard for referral centers. *Int J Artif Organs* 12: 688, 1989

117. Cavaillon JM, Poignet JL, Fitting C, Delons S, David B: Reduction of allergice reactions in patients undergoing long-term hemodialysis. *J Allergy Clin Immunol* 92: 355, 1993

118. Grammer LC, Harris KE, Shaughnessy MA, Dolovich J, Patterson R, Evans S: Antibodies to toluene diisocyanate in patients with and without dialysis anaphylaxis. *Artif Organs* 15: 2, 1991

119. Lemke HD, Heidland A, Schaefer RM: Hypersensitivity reactions during haemodialysis: role of complement fragments and ethylene oxide antibodies. *Nephrol Dial Transplant* 5: 264, 1990

120. Levin NW, Zasuwa G: Relationship between dialyzer type and signs and symptoms. *Nephrol Dial Transplant* 8 (Suppl 2): 30, 1993

121. Masin G, Polenakovic M, Ivanovski N, Atanasov N. Olivera S, Cakalaroski K: Hypersensitivity reactions to ethylene oxide: clinical experience. *Nephrol Dial Transplant* 3: 50, 1991

122. Tielemans C, Goldman M, Vanherweghem JL: Immediate hypersensitivity reactions and hemodialysis. (Review) *Adv Nephrol Necker Hosp* 22: 401, 1993

123. Walter J, Taraba I: Dialysis hypersensitivity. *Nephrol Dial Transplant* 3: 47, 1991

124. Lemke HD: Mediation of hypersensitivity reactions during hemodialysis by IgE antibodies against ethylene oxide. *Artif Organs* 11: 104, 1987

125. Windebank AJ, Blexrud MD: Residual ethylene oxide in hollow fiber hemodialysis units is neurotoxic *in vitro*. *Ann Neuro* 26: 63, 1989

126. Garnaas KR, Windebank AJ, Blexrud MD, Kurtz SB: Ultrastructural changes produced in dorsal root ganglia *in vitro* by exposure to ethtylene oxide from hemo-dialysis. *J Neuropathol Exp Neurol* 50: 256, 1991

127. Ansorge W, Pelger M, Dietrich W, Baurmeister U: Ethylene oxide in dialyzer rinsing fluid: effect of rinsing technique, dialyzer storage time, and potting compound. *Artif Organs* 11: 118, 1987

128. Ing TS, Daugirdas JT: Extractable ethylene oxide from cuprammonium cellulose plate dialyzers. *Trans Am Soc Artif Intern Organs* 21: 108, 1986

129. Wass U, Belin L, Delin K: Longitudinal study of specific IgE and IgG antibodies in a patient sensitized to ethylene oxide through dialysis. *J Allergy Clin Immunol* 82: 679, 1988

130. Grammer LC, Paterson BF, Roxe D et al.: IgE against ethylene oxide-altered human serum albumin in patients with anaphylactic reactions to dialysis. *J Allergy Clin Immunol* 76: 511, 1985

131. Grammer LC, Patterson R: IgE against ethylene oxide-altered human serum albumin (ETO-HSA) as an etiologic agent in allergic reactions of hemodialysis patients. *Artif Organs* 11: 97, 1987

132. Grammer LC, Roberts M, Wiggins CA, Fitzsimmons RR, Ivanovich PT, Roxe DM, Patterson R: A comparison of cutaneous testing and ELISA testing for assessing reactivity to ethylene oxide-human serum albumin in hemodialysis patients with anaphylactic reactions. *J Allergy Clin Immunol* 87: 674, 1991

133. Marshall CP, Pearson FC, Sagona MA, Lee W, Wathen RL, Ward RA, Dolovich J: Reactions during hemodialysis caused by allergy to ethylene oxide gas sterilization. *J Allergy Clin Immunol* 75: 563, 1985

134. Bousquet J, Maurice F, Rivory JP, Skassa-Brociek W, Florence P, Chouzenoux R, Mion C, Michel FB: Allergy in long-term hemodialysis. II. Allergic and atopic patterns of a population of patients undergoing long-term hemodialysis. *J Allergy Clin Immunol* 81: 605, 1988

135. Daugirdas JT, Potempa LD, Dinh N, Gandhi VC, Ivanovich PJ, Ing TS: Plate, coil, and hollow-fiber cuprammonium cellulose dialyzers: discrepancy between incidence of anaphylactic reactions and degree of complement activation. *Artif Organs* 11: 140, 1987

136. Maurice F, Rivory JP, Larsson PH, Johansson SG, Bousquet J: Anaphylactic shock caused by formaldehyde in a patient undergoing long-term hemodialysis. *J Allergy Clin Immunol* 77: 594, 1986

137. Kessler M, Cao HT, Mariot A, Chanliau J: Hemodialysis-associated complications due to sterilizing agents ethylene oxide and formaldehyde. *Contrib Nephrol* 62: 13, 1988

138. Wenzel SK, Sharma AM, Keller F: Repeated dialysis anaphylaxia. *Nephrol Dial Transplant* 5: 821, 1990

139. Rault R, Silver MS: Severe reactions during hemodialysis. *Am J Kidney Dis* 5: 128, 1985

140. Update: Acute allergic reactions associated with reprocessed hemodialyzers – United States, 1989–90. *MMWR* 40: 147, 153, 1991

141. Pegues DA, Consuelo M, Beck-Sague, Woollen SW, Greenspan B, Burns SM, Bland LA, Arduino MJ, Favero MS, Mackow RC, Jarvis WR: Anaphylactoid reactions associated with reuse of hollow fiber hemodialyzers and ACE inhibitors. *Kidney Int* 42: 1232, 1992

142. Parnes EL, Shapiro WB: Anaphylactoid reactions in hemodialysis patients treated with the AN69 dialyzer. *Kidney Int* 40: 1148, 1991

143. Schulman G, Hakim R, Arias R, Silverberg M, Kaplan AP, Arbeit L: Bradykinin generation by dialysis membranes: possible role in anaphylactic reaction. *Am Soc Nephrol* 3: 1563, 1993

144. Vaziri ND: Is contact activation of the coagulation system involved in the genesis of the first-use syndrome. *Artif Organs* 11: 163, 1987

145. Chargin K: Skin disease in non-surgical renal disease. *Arch Dermatol Syphilol* 26: 314, 1932

146. Balaskas EV, Chu M, Uldall RP, Gupta A, Oreopoulos DG: Pruritus in continuous ambulatory peritoneal dialysis and hemodialysis patients. *Perit Dial Int* 13: S527, 1993

147. Mettang T, Fritz P, Weber J, Machleidt C, Hubel E, Kuhlmann U: Uremic pruritus in patients on hemodialysis or continuous ambulatory peritoneal dialysis (CAPD). The role of plasma histamine and skin mast cells. *Clin Nephrol* 34: 136, 1990

148. Stahle-Backdahl M: Uremic pruritus. Clinical and experimental studies. *Acta Derm Venereol* 145 (Suppl): 1, 1989

149. Stahle-Backdahl M., Wahlgren CF, Hagermark O: Computerized recording of itch in patients on maintenance hemodialysis. *Acta Derm Venereol* 69: 410, 1989

150. Gilchrest BA, Stern RS, Steinman TI, Brown RS, Arndt KA, Anderson WW: Clinical features of pruritus among patients undergoing maintenance hemodialysis. *Arch Dermatol* 118: 154, 1982

151. Lempert KD, Baltz PS, Welton WA, Whittier FC: Pseudouremic pruritus: a scabies epidemic in a dialysis unit. *Am J Kidney Dis* 5: 117, 1985

152. Pascual J, Medina S, Teruel JL, Freire P, Ortuno J: Captopril-induced lichenoid eruption in an uremic patient. (Letter) *Nephron* 56: 110, 1990

153. Stahle-Backdahl M: Stratum corneum hydration in patients undergoing maintenance hemodialysis. *Acta Derm Venereol* 68: 531, 1988

154. Grosshans E, Maleville J, Jahn H, Frankhauser J: Pruritus during repeated hemodialysis in chronic renal insufficiency. Etiological and histopathological data. *Bulletin de la Société française de Dermatologie et de Syphiligraphie* 77: 828, 1970

155. Massry SG, Kleeman CR: Calcium metabolism in patients treated with maintenance haemodialysis. *Triangle* 10: 147, 1971

156. Parfitt AM, Massry SG, Winfield AC, DePalma JR, Gordon A: Disordered calcium and phosphorus metabolism during maintenance hemodialysis. Correlation of clinical, roentgenographic and biochemical changes. *Am J Med* 51: 319, 1971

157. Stockenhuber F, Kurz RW, Sertl K, Grimm G, Balcke P: Increased plasma histamine levels in uraemic pruritus. *Clin Sci* 79: 477, 1990

158. Francos GC, Kauh YC, Gittlen SD, Schulman ES, Besarab A, Guyal S, Burke JF Jr: Elevated plasma histamine in chronic uremia. Effects of ketotifen on pruritus. *Int J Dermatol* 30: 884, 1991

159. Dimkovic N, Djukanovic L, Radmilovic A, Bojic P, Juloski T: Uremic pruritus and skin mast cells. *Nephron* 61: 5, 1992

160. Matsumoto M, Ichimaru K, Horie A: Pruritus and mast cell proliferation of the skin in end stage renal failure. *Clin Nephrol* 23: 285, 1985

161. Cohen EP, Russell TJ, Garancis JC: Mast cells and calcium in severe uremic itching. *Am J Med Sci* 303: 360, 1992

162. Masi CM, Cohen EP: Dialysis efficacy and itching in renal failure. *Nephron* 62: 257, 1992

163. Tan JK, Haberman HF, Coldman AJ: Identifying effective treatments for uremic pruritus. *J Am Acad Dermatol* 25: 811, 1991

164. Breneman DL, Cardone JS, Blumsack RF, Lather RM, Searle EA, Pollack VE: Topical capsaicin for treatment of hemo-dialysis-related pruritus. *J Am Acad Dermatol* 26: 91, 1992

165. De Marchi S, Cecchin E, Villalta D, Sepiacci G, Santini G, Bartoli E: Relief of pruritus and decreases in plasma histamine concentrations during erythropoietin therapy in patients with uremia [see comments]. *N Engl J Med* 326: 969, 1992

166. Schaefer RM, Rauterberg EW, Deppisch R, Vienken J: Assembly of terminal SC5b–9 complement complexes: a new index of blood-membrane interaction. *Miner Electrolyte Metab* 16: 73, 1990

167. Brunner J, Seidel D: Comparative hemolysis studies of various dialysis technics. *Z Urol Nephrol* 78: 381, 1985

168. Blumberg A: Pathogenesis of anemia due to kidney disease. *Nephron* 1: 15, 1989

169. Taccone GM, Lubrano R, Belli A, Meloni C, Morosetti M, Meschini L, Elli M, Boffo V, Pisani F, Giardini O: Disappearance of oxidative damage to red blood cell membranes in uremic patients following renal transplant. *Trans Am Soc Artif Intern Organs* 35: 533, 1989

170. Durak I, Akyol O, Basesme E, Canbolat O, Kavutcu M: Reduced erythrocyte defense mechanisms against free radical toxicity in patients with chronic renal failure. *Nephron* 66: 76, 1994

171. Lubrano R, Taccone GM, Mazzarella V, Bandino D, Citti G, Elli M, Gardino O, Casciani C: Relationship between red blood cell lipid peroxidation, plasma hemoglobin, and red blood cell osmotic resistance before and after vitamin E supplementation in hemodialysis patients. *Artif Organs* 10: 245, 1986

172. Peuchant E, Salles C, Vallot C, Wone C, Jensen R: Increase of erythrocyte resistance to hemolysis and modification of membrane lipids induced by hemo-dialysis. *Clin Chim Acta* 178: 271, 1988

173. Zachee P, Ferrant A, Daelemans R, Coolen L, Goosens W, Lins RL, Couttenye M, DeBroe ME, Boogaerts MA: Oxidative injury to erythrocytes, cell reigiity and splenic hemolysis in hemodialyzed patients before and during erythropoietin treatment. *Nephron* 65: 288, 1993

174. Gault MH, Duffett S, Purchase L, Murphy J: Hemodialysis intravascular hemolysis and kinked blood lines. *Nephron* 62: 267, 1992

175. Gordon SM, Bland LA, Alexander SR, Newman HF, Arduino MJ, Jarvis WR: Hemolysis associated with hydrogen peroxide at a pediatric dialysis center. *Am J Nephrol* 10: 123, 1990

176. Ng YY, Chow MP, Lyou JY, Huh Y, Yung CH, Fan CD, Huang TP: Resistance to erythropoietin: immunohemolytic anemia induced by residual formaldehyde in dialyzers. *Am J Kidney Dis* 21: 213, 1993

177. Klein E: Effects of disinfectants in renal dialysis patients. *Environ Health Perspect* 69: 45, 1986

178. Hudson S, Taylor JE, Stewart WK: Undetected excessive ultrafiltration and serious haemolysis during maintenance haemodialysis. *Nephrol Dial Transplant* 8: 477, 1993

179. Ebel H, Saure B, Laage C, Dittmar A, Keucher M, Stellwaag M, Lange H: Influence of computer-modulated profile haemodialysis on cardiac arrhythmias. *Nephrol Dial Transplant* 1: 165, 1990

180. Kinoshita O, Kamakura S, Kimura G, Omae T: Increased ventricular vulnerability during haemodialysis. (Letter) *Lancet* 338: 1333, 1991

181. Rombola G, Colussi G, De FM, Frontini A, Minetti L: Cardiac arrhythmias and electrolyte changes during haemodialysis. *Nephrol Dial Transplant* 7: 318, 1992

182. Saragoca MA, Canziani ME, Cassiolato JL, Gil MA, Andrade JL, Draibe SA, Martinez EE: Left ventricular

hypertrophy a risk factor for arrhythmias in hemodialysis patients. *J Cardiol Pharma* 17 (Suppl 2): S136, 1991

183. Sforzini S, Latini R, Mingardi G, Vincenti A, Redaelli B: Ventricular arrhythmias and four-year mortality in haemodialysis patients. Gruppo Emodialisi e Patologie Cardiovascolari [see comments]. *Lancet* 339: 212, 1992

184. Shapira OM, Bar KY: ECG changes and cardiac arrhythmias in chronic renal failure patients on hemodialysis. *J Electrocardiol* 25: 273, 1992

185. Krivoshiev S, Antonov S, Koteva A, Kirijakov Z: Paroxysmal atrial fibrillation during haemodialysis. (Letter) *Nephrol Dial Transplant* 5: 474, 1990

186. Fantuzzi S, Caico S, Amatruda O, Cervini P, Abu-Turky H, Baratelli L, Donati D, Gastaldi L: Hemo-dialysis-associated cardiac arrhythmias: a lower risk with bicarbonate? *Nephron* 58: 196, 1991

187. Ritz E, Rambausek M, Mall G: Cardiac changes in uremia and the possible relation to cardiovascular instability on dialysis. *Contrib Nephrol* 78: 221, 1990

188. Rostand SG, Rutsky EA: Pericarditis in end-stage renal disease. (Review) *Cardiol Clin* 8: 701, 1990

189. Nishimura M, Nakanishi T, Yasui A, Tsuji Y, Kunishige H, Hirabayashi M, Takahashi H, Yoshimura M: Serum calcium increases the incidence of arrhythmias during acetate hemodialysis. *Am J Kidney Dis* 19: 149, 1992

190. Gawaz M, Mujais SK: Platelet membrane glycoprotein abnormalities and uremic bleeding. *J Nephrol* 1995. In press

191. Gawaz MP, Dobos G, Mujais SK: Impaired function of platelet glycoprotein GPllb/llla in end stage renal disease. *Am Soc Nephrol* 5: 36, 1994

192. Maggiore Q, Pizzarelli F, Zoccali C, Sisca S, Nocolo F, Parlongo S: Effect of extracorporeal blood cooling on dialytic arterial hypotension. *Proc Eur Dial Transplant Assoc* 18: 587, 1981

193. Ganong WF: *Review of Medical Physiology*, 15th Ed, Norwalk, Connecticut, Appleton E Lange, 1991, p 234

194. Harrison P, Jansson K, Kronenberg H, Mahony J, Tiller D: Cold agglutinin formation in patients undergoing haemodialysis. A possible relationship to dialyser re-use. *Aust NZ J Med* 5: 195, 1975

195. Fortner R, Nowakowski A, Carter C, King L, Knepshield J: Death due to overheated dialysate during dialysis. *Ann Intern Med* 73: 443, 1970

196. Berkes S, Kahn S, Chazan J, Garella S: Prolonged hemolysis from overheated dialysate. *Ann Intern Med* 83: 363, 1975

197. Ham T, Shen S, Fleming E, Castle WB: Studies on the destruction of red blood cells. IV. *Blood* 3: 373, 1948

198. Mennim P, Coyle CF, Taylor J: Venous air embolism associated with removal of central venous catheter. *Br Med J* 305: 171, 1992

199. Halliday P, Anderson DN, Davidson AI, Page JG: Management of cerebral air embolism secondary to a disconnected central venous catheter. *Br J Surg* 81, 1994

200. Phifer TJ, Bridges M, Conrad SA: The residual central venous catheter trace-an occult source of lethal air embolism: case report. *J Trauma* 31: 1558, 1991

201. Aibiki M, Ogura S, Seki K, Honda K, Omegaki O, Shirakawa Y, Ogli K: Role of vagal afferents in hypotension induced by venous air embolism. *Am J Physiol* 266: R790, 1994

202. Ohno S, Suzuki N, Kitamura S: The roles of platelet-activating factor (PAF) in pulmonary vasoconstriction during venous air embolism in anesthetized mongrel dogs. *J Lipid Mediat* 5: 187, 1992

203. Lam KK, Hutchinson RC, Gin T: Severe pulmonary edema after venous air embolism (Review) *Can J Anaesth* 40: 964, 1993

204. Wang D, Li MH, Hsu K, Shen CY, Chen HI, Lin YC: Air embolism-induced lung injury in isolated rat lungs. *J Appl Physiol* 72: 1235, 1992

205. Bergh K, Hjelde A, Iversen OJ, Brubakk AO: Variability over time of complement activation induced by air bubbles in human and rabbit sera. *J Appl Physiol* 74: 1811, 1993

206. Thorsen T, Klausen H, Lie RT, Holmsen H: Bubble-induced aggregation of platelets: effects of gas species, proteins, and decompression. *Undersea Hyperbar Med* 20: 101, 1993

207. Brenton BC, Mittelstaedt CA, Curnes JT, Scatliff JH: Real-time ultrasonographic visualization of intra-cranial air embolism. *J Ultrasound Med* 1: 379, 1982

208. Bunegin L, Wahl D, Albin MS: Detection and volume estimation of embolic air in the middle cerebral artery using transcranial Doppler sonography. *Stroke* 25: 595, 1994

209. Markus H: Transcranial Doppler detection of circulating cerebral emboli. A review. (Review) *Stroke* 24: 1246, 1993

210. Artru AA: Modification of a new catheter for air retrieval and resuscitation from lethal venous air embolism: effect of nitrous oxide on air retrieval. *Anesth Analg* 75: 226, 1992

211. Hanna PG, Gravensein N, Pashayan AG: *In vitro* comparison of central venous catheters for aspiration of venous air embolism: effect of catheter type, catheter tip position, and cardiac inclination [see comments]. *J Clin Anesth* 3: 290, 1991

212. Dudney TM, Elliott CG: Pulmonary embolism from amniotic fluid, fat, and air. *Prog Cardiovasc Dis* 36: 447, 1994

213. Orebaugh SL: Venous air embolism: clinical and experimental considerations. *Crit Care Med* 20: 1169, 1992

214. Weiss LD, Van MK: The applications of hyperbaric oxygen therapy in emergency medicine [see comments]. (Review) *Am J Emerg Med* 10: 558, 1992

215. Dunbar EM, Fox R, Watson B, Akrill P: Successful late treatment of venous air embolism with hyperbaric oxygen. *Postgrad Med J* 66: 469, 1990

216. Annane D, Troche G, Delisle F, Devauchelle P, Paraire F, Raphael JC, Gajdos P: Effects of mechanical ventilation with normobaric oxygen therapy on the rate of air removal from cerebral arteries. *Crit Care Med* 22: 851, 1994

217. Mongan P, Peterson RE, Culling RD: Pressure monitoring can accurately position catheter for air embolism aspiration. *J Clin Monit* 8: 121, 1992

218. Schwarzbeck A, Wagner L, Squarr HU, Strauch M: Clotting in dialyzers due to low pH of dialysis fluid. *Clin Nephrol* 7: 125, 1977

219. Renfrew R, Buselmeier TJ, Kjellstrand CM: Pericarditis and renal failure. *Ann Rev Med* 31: 345, 1980

220. Osanloo E, Salhoub RJ, Cioffi RF, Parker RH: Viral pericarditis in patients receiving hemodialysis. *Arch Intern Med* 139: 301, 1979

722   *Salim K. Mujais, Todd Ing and Carl Kjellstrand*

221. Comty CM, Shapiro FL: Cardiac complications of regular dialysis treatment. in *Replacement of Renal Function*, edited by Drukker W, Parsons FM, Maher JF, The Hague, Martinus Nijhoff Medical Division, 1978, p 519
222. Cooper FW Jr, Stead EA, Warren JV: The beneficial effect of intravenous infusions in acute pericardial tamponade. *Ann Surg* 120: 822, 1944
223. Watson AJJ, Finn MMR, Keaugh JAB: Cardiac tamponade without demonstrable pulsus paradoxus in hemodialysis patients. *Irish J Med Sci* 150: 78, 1981
224. Horton JD, Gelfand Mc, Sherber HS: Natural history of asymptomatic pericardial effusions in patients on maintenance hemodialysis. *Proc Dial Transplant Forum* 7: 76, 1977
225. Zabaneh RI, Ejaz AA, Khan AA, Nawab ZM, Leehey DJ, Ing TS. Use of a phosphorus-enriched dialysis solution to hemodialyze a patient with lithium intoxication. *Artif Organs* 19: 94, 1995
226. Leehey DJ, Daugirdas JT, Ing TS: Early drainage of pericardial effusion in patients with dialysis pericarditis. *Arch Intern Med* 143: 1673, 1983
227. Buselmeier TJ, Simmons RL, Najarian JS, von Hartitzch B, Dietzman RH, Kjellstrand CM: Intractable uremic pericardial effusion. *Proc Eur Dial Transplant Assoc* 10: 289, 1973
228. Daugirdas JT, Leehey DK, Popli S, McCray GM, Gandhi VC, Pifarre R, Ing TS: Subxiphoid pericardiotomy for hemodialysis-associated pericardial effusion. *Arch Intern Med* 146: 1113, 1986
229. Ghavamian M, Gutch CF, Hughes RK, Kopp KF, Kolff WJ: Pericardial tamponade in chronic-hemodialysis patients: Treatment by pericardiectomy. *Arch Intern Med* 131: 249, 1973
230. Kennedy AC, Linton AL, Eaton JC: Urea levels in cerebrospinal fluid after haemodialysis. *Lancet* 1962, 1: 410
231. Peterson H de C, Swanson AG: Acute encephalopathy occurring during hemodialysis – the reverse urea effect. *Arch Intern Med* 113: 877, 1964
232. Kleeman CR: Metabolic coma. *Kidney Int* 36: 1142, 1989
233. Kennedy AC, Linton AL, Luke RG, Renfrew S: Electroencephalographic changes during haemodialysis. *Lancet* 1: 408, 1963
234. Rosen SM, O'Connor K, Shaldon S: Haemodialysis disequilibrium. *Br Med J* 2: 672, 1964
235. Scribner BH: *Trans Am Soc Artif Intern Organs* 8: 195, 1962
236. Kerr DNS, Edwards EC: Discussion in acute renal failure, edited by Shaldon S, Cook GC, Oxford, Blackwell Scientific Publications, 1964, p 78
237. Sitprija V, Holmes JH: Preliminary observations on the change in intracranial pressure and intraocular pressure during hemodialysis. *Trans Am Soc Artif Intern Organs* 8: 300, 1962
238. Port FK, Johnson WJ, Klass DW: Prevention of dialysis disequilibrium syndrome by use of high sodium concentration in the dialysate. *Kidney Int* 3: 327, 1973
239. Silver SM, DeSimone JA Jr, Smith DA, Sterns RH: Dialysis disequilibrium syndrome (DDS) in the rat: role of the 'reverse urea effect'. *Kidney Int* 42: 161, 1992
240. Arieff AI, Guisado R, Massry SG, Lazarowitz VC: Central nervous system pH in uremia and the effects of hemodialysis. *J Clin Invest* 58: 306, 1976
241. Kennedy AC, Linton AL, Luke RG, Renfrew S, Dinwoodie A: The pathogenesis and prevention of cerebral dysfunction during dialysis. *Lancet* 1: 790, 1964
242. Rodrigo F, Shideman J, McHugh R, Buselmeier T, Kjellstrand C: Osmolality changes during hemodialysis. *Ann Intern Med* 86: 554, 1977
243. Kelleher SP, Schulman G: Severe metabolic alkalosis complicating regional citrate hemodialysis. *Am J Kidney Dis* 9: 235, 1987
244. Silverstein FJ, Oster JR, Perez GO, Materson BJ, Lopez RA, Al-Reshaid K: Metabolic alkalosis induced by regional citrate hemodialysis. *Trans Am Soc Artif Intern Organs* 35: 22, 1989
245. van der Meulen J, Janssen MJ, Langendijk PN, Bouman AA, Oe PI: Citrate anticoagulation and dialysate with reduced buffer content in chronic hemodialysis. *Clin Nephrol* 37: 36, 1992
246. Brueggemeyer CD, Ramirez G: Dialysate concentrate: a potential source for lethal complications. *Nephron* 46: 397, 1987
247. Hartmann A, Reisaeter A, Holdaas H, Rolfsen B, Fauchald P: Accidental metabolic acidosis during hemodialysis. *Artif Organs* 18: 214, 1994
248. Said R, Quintanilla A, Levin N, Ivanovich P: Acute hemolysis due to profound hypo-osmalality. A complication of hemodialysis. *J Dial* 1: 447, 1977
249. Brezis M, Brown RS: An unsuspected cause for metabolic acidosis in chronic renal failure: sorbent system hemodialysis. *Am J Kidney Dis* 6: 425, 1985
250. Wathen RL, Burcham CW Jr: Understanding the dangers of fluoride during dialysis. *Nephrol News Issues* (Sept): 32, 1993
251. Klein WJ Jr, Metz EN, Price AR: Acute copper intoxication. A hazard of hemodialysis. *Arch Intern Med* 129: 578, 1972
252. Schuett H, Port FK: Hemolysis in hemodialysis patients. *Dial Transplant* 9: 345, 1980
253. Sterna RH, Ocdol H, Schrier RW, Narins RG: Hyponatremia: pathophysiology, diagnosis, and therapy. in *Clinical Disorders of Fluid and Electrolyte Metabolism*, 5th Ed, edited by Narins RG, New York, McGraw-Hill Inc, 1994, p 585
254. Bluemle LW Jr: Current status of chronic hemodialysis. *Am J Med* 44: 749, 1968
255. Nickey WA, Chinitz VL, Kim KE, Onesti G, Swartz C: Hypernatremia from water softener malfunction during home dialysis. *JAMA* 214: 915, 1970
256. Lindner A, Moskovtchenko JF, Traeger J: Accidental mass hypernatremia during hemodialysis. *Nephron* 9: 99, 1972
257. Lazarus JM: Complications in hemodialysis: an overview. *Kidney Int* 18: 783, 1980
258. Morrison G, Michelson EL, Brown S, Morganroth J: Mechanism of prevention of cardiac arrhythmias in chronic hemodialysis patients. *Kidney Int* 17: 811, 1980
259. Seldin DW, Carter NW, Rector FC Jr: Consequences of renal failure and their management, in *Diseases of the Kidney*, 2nd Ed, edited by Strauss MB, Welt LG, Boston, Little, Brown and Company, Boston, 1971, p 211
260. Wiegand C, Davin T, Raij L, Kjellstrand C: Life-threatening hypokalemia during hemodialysis. *Trans Am Soc Artif Intern Organs* 25: 416, 1975

261. Wiegand CF, Davin TD, Raij L, Kjellstrand CM: Severe hypokalemia induced by hemodialysis. *Arch Intern Med* 141: 167, 1981

262. Blumberg A, Weidmann P, Ferrari P: Effect of prolonged bicarbonate administration on plasma potassium in terminal renal failure. *Kidney Int* 41: 369, 1992

263. Kjellstrand CM, Eaton JW, Yawata Y, Swofford H, Kolpin CF, Buselmeier TJ, von Hartitzsch B, Jacob HS: Hemolysis in dialysed patients caused by chloramines. *Nephron* 13: 247, 1974

264. Orringer EP, Mattern WD: Formaldehyde-induced hemolysis during chronic hemodialysis. *N Engl J Med* 294: 1416, 1976

265. Carlson DJ, Shapiro FL: Methemoglobinemia from well water nitrates: a complication of home dialysis. *Ann Intern Med* 73: 757, 1970

266. Hoy RH: Accidental systemic exposure to sodium hypochlorite (Clorox) during hemodialysis. *Am J Hosp Pharm* 38: 1512, 1981

267. McIvor M, Baltazar RF, Beltran J, Mower MM, Wend R, Lustgarten J, Salomon J: Hyperkalemia and cardiac arrest from fluoride exposure during hemodialysis. *Am J Cardiol* 51: 901, 1983

268. Winchester JF, Gelfand MC, Knepshield JH, Schreiner GE: Dialysis and hemoperfusion of poisons and drugs – update. *Trans Am Soc Artif Intern Organs* 23: 762, 1977

269. Popovtzer MM, Knochel JP, Kumar R: Disorders of calcium, phosphorus, vitamin D, and parathyroid hormone activity, in *Renal and Electrolyte Disorders*, 4th Ed, edited by Schrier RW, Boston, Little, Brown and Company, 1992, p 287

270. Lentz RD, Brown DM, Kjellstrand CM: Treatment of severe hypophosphatemia. *Ann Intern Med* 89: 941, 1978

271. Tamm HS, Nolph KD, Maher JF: Factors affecting plasma calcium concentration during hemodialysis. *Arch Intern Med* 128: 769, 1971

272. Carney SL, Gillies AHB: Acute dialysis hypercalcemia and dialysis phosphate loss. *Am J Kidney Dis* 11: 377, 1988

273. Argiles A, Kerr PG, Canaud B, Flavier JL, Mion C: Calcium kinetics and the long-term effects of lowering dialysate calcium concentration. *Kidney Int* 43: 630, 1993

274. Ott SM, Maloney NA, Coburn JW, Alfrey AC, Sherrard DJ: The prevalence of bone aluminum deposition in renal osteodystrophy and its relation to the response to calcitriol therapy. *N Engl J Med* 307: 709, 1982

275. Davenport A, Goel S, Mackenzie JC: Treatment of hypercalcaemia with pamidronate in patients with end-stage renal failure. *Scand J Urol Nephrol* 27: 447, 1993

276. Rivera-Vasquez AB, Noriega-Sanchez A, Ramirez-Gonzales R, Martinez-Maldonado M: Acute hypercalcemia in hemodialysis patients: distinction from 'dialysis dementia'. *Nephron* 25: 243, 1980

277. Freeman RM, Lawton RL, Chamberlain MA: Hard-water syndrome. *N Engl J Med* 276: 113, 1967

278. Drukker W: The hard water syndrome: a potential hazard during regular dialysis treatment. *Proc Eur Dial Transplant Assoc* 5: 284, 1968

279. Evans DB, Slapak M: Pancreatitis in the hard water syndrome. *Br Med J* 5: 284, 1968

280. Mulloy AL, Mulloy LL, Weinstein RS: Hypercalcemia due to hard water used for home dialysis. *South Med J* 85: 1131, 1992

281. Tzamaloukas AH: Hypercalcemia due to hard well water in a home hemodialysis patient. *South Med J* 86: 844, 1993

282. Govan JR, Porter CA, Cook JGH, Dixon B, Trafford JAP: Acute magnesium poisoning as a complication of chronic intermittent haemodialysis. *Brit Med J* 2: 278, 1968

283. Taves DR, Freeman RB, Kamm DE, Ramos CP, Scribner BH: Hemodialysis with fluoridated dialysate. *Trans Am Soc Artif Intern Organs* 14: 412, 1968

284. Johnson WJ, Taves DR: Exposure to excessive fluoride during hemodialysis. *Kidney Int* 5: 451, 1974

285. Keshaviah PR et al.: Investigation of the Risks and Hazards Associated with Hemodialysis Devices, Technical Report, Rockville, Maryland, U.S. Food and Drug Administration, Department of Health, Education and Welfare, 1980

286. Keshaviah PR: Pretreatment and preparation of city worker for hemodialysis, in: *Replacement of renal function by dialysis*, 3rd Ed, edited by Maher JF, Dordrecht, Kluwer Academic Publishers, 1989, p 189

287. Arnow PM, Bland LA, Garcia-Houchins S, Fridkin S, Fellner SK: An outbreak of fatal fluoride intoxication in a long-term hemodialysis unit. *Ann Intern Med* 131: 339, 1994

288. Clifford DA: Ion exchange and inorganic adsorption, in *Water Quality and Treatment: A Handbook of Community Water Supplies*, edited by Pontius FW, New York, McGraw-Hill, 1990, p 561

289. Anderson R, Beard JH, Sorley D: Fluoride intoxication in a dialysis unit-Maryland. *MMWR Morb Mortal Wkly Rep* 29: 134, 1980

290. Taves DR: Normal human serum fluoride concentrations. *Nature* 211: 192, 1966

291. Chaleil D, Sinon P, Tessier B, Cartier F, Allain P: Blood plasma fluoride in haemodialysed patients. *Clin Chim Acta* 156: 105, 1986

292. Berman L, Taves D, Mitra S, Newmark K: Inorganic fluoride poisoning: treatment by hemodialysis. *N Engl J Med* 189: 922, 1973

293. Wyngaarden JB, Smith LH JR, Bennett JC: *Cecil Textbook of Medicine*, 19th Ed, W.B. Saunders Co, Philadelphia, 1992, pp 862, 879

294. Carlson DJ, Shapiro FI: Methemoglobinemia from well water nitrates: a complication of home dialysis. *Ann Intern Med* 73: 757, 1970

295. Salvadori M, Martinelli F, Comparini L, Bandini S, Sodi A: Nitrate induced anaemia in home dialysis patients. *Proc Eur Dial Transplant Assoc-Eur Renal Assoc* 21: 321, 1984

296. Luehmann DA, Keshaviah PR, Ward RA, Klein E: *A Manual on Water Treatment for Hemodialysis*, US Department of Health and Human Services, Public Health Service, Food and Drug Administration, Center for Devices and Radiological Health, Rockville, Maryland, 1989, p 10

297. Jaffe ER, Heller P: Methemoglobinemia in man. *Progr Hemat* 4: 48, 1964

298. Tipple MA, Shusterman N, Bland LA, McCarthy MA, Favero MS, Arduino MJ, Reid MH, Jarvis WR: Illness in hemodialysis patients after exposure to chloramine contaminated dialysate. *Trans Am Soc Artif Organs* 37: 588, 1991

724   *Salim K. Mujais, Todd Ing and Carl Kjellstrand*

299. Meyer MA, Klein E: Granular activated carbon usage in chloramine removal from dialysis water. *Artif Organs* 7: 484, 1983

300. Symons J, Bellor T, Carswell J, Demarco J, Kropp K, Robeck G, Seeger D, Slocum C, Smith B, Stevens A: National organics reconnaissance survey for halogenated organics. *J Am Water Works Assoc* 7: 634, 1975

301. Bauer RC, Snoeyink VL: Reactions of chloramines with active carbon. *J Water Pollut Control Fed* 45: 2290, 1973

302. Caterson RJ, Savdie E, Raid E, Coutts D, Mahoney JF: Heinz-body haemolysis in haemodialyzed patients caused by chloramines in Sydney tap water. *Med J Aust* 2: 367, 1982

303. FDA safety alert: Chloramine contamination of hemodialysis water supplies. *Am J Kidney Dis* 11: 447, 1988

304. Eaton JW, Kolpin CF, Swofford HS, Kjellstrand CM, Jacob HS: Chlorinated urban water: a cause of dialysis-induced hemolytic anemia. *Science* 181: 463, 1973

305. Kjellstrand CM, Eaton JW, Yawata Y, Swofford H, Kolpin CF, Buselmeier TJ, von Hartitzsch B, Jacob HS: Hemolysis in dialized patients caused by chloramines. *Nephron* 13: 427, 1974

306. Favero MS, Petersen NJ, Carson LA, Bond WW, Hindman SH: Gram-negative water bacteria in hemodialysis systems. *Health Lab Sci* 12: 321, 1975

307. Comty C, Luehmann D, Wathen R, Shapiro F: Prescription water for chronic hemodialysis. *Trans Am Soc Artif Intern Organs* 20: 189, 1974

308. Ward DM, Minch K, Bahr TE: The use of ascorbic acid in water treatment for hemodialysis. *Contemp Dial Nephrol* 2: 33, 1985 and 3: 35, 1985

309. Neilan BA, Ehlers SM, Kolpin CF, Eaton JW: Prevention of chloramine-induced hemolysis in dialyzed patients. *Clin Nephrol* 10: 105, 1978

310. Gaynes R, Friedman C, Maclaven C, Foley K, Swartz R: Hemodialysis-associated febrile episodes: surveillance before and after major alteration in the water treatment system. *Int J Artif Organs* 13: 482, 1990

311. Goldman M, Vanherweghem JL: Bacterial infections in chronic hemodialysis patients: epidemiologic and pathophysiologic aspects. *Adv Nephrol Necker Hosp* 19: 315, 1990

312. Taniguchi T, Katsushima S, Lee K, Hidaka A, Konishi J, Ideguchi H, Kawaguchi Y: Endotoxemia in patients on hemodialysis. *Nephron* 56: 44, 1990

313. Vanholder R, Vanhaecke E, Ringoir S: Waterborne Pseudomonas septicemia. *Trans Am Soc Artif Intern Organs* 36, 1990

314. Gordon SM, Oettinger CW, Bland LA, Olivier JC, Ardvino WJ, Aquero SM, McAllister SK, Favero MS, Jarvis WR: Pyrogenic reactions in patients receiving conventional, high-efficiency, or high-flux hemodialysis treatments with bicarbonate dialysate containing high concentrations of bacteria and endotoxin. *Am Soc Nephrol* 2: 1436, 1992

315. Alter MJ, Favero MS, Miller JK, Moyer LA, Bland LA: National surveillance of dialysis-associated diseases in the United States, 2987. *Trans Am Soc Artif Intern Organs* 35: 820, 1989

316. Alter MJ, Favero MS, Moyer LA, Miller JK, Bland LA: National surveillance of dialysis-associated diseases in

the United States, 1988. *Trans Am Soc Artif Intern Organs* 36: 107, 1990

317. Alter MJ, Favero MS, Moyer LA, Bland LA: National surveillance of dialysis-associated diseases in the United States, 1989. *Trans Am Soc Artif Intern Organs* 37: 97, 1991

318. Flaherty JP, Garcia-Hutchins S, Chudy R, Arnow PM: An outbreak of gram-negative bacteremia traced to contaminated O-rings in reprocessed dialyzers. *Ann Intern Med* 119: 1072, 1993

319. Roberts B, Alvarado N, Garcia, Solis Y, Lopez O, Dukes C: Header sepsis syndrome: waterborne Xanthomonas-induced fevers. *Dial Transplant* 23: 464, 1994

320. Vanholder R, Vanhaecke E, Ringoir S: Pseudomonas septicemia due to deficient disinfectant mixing during reuse. *Int J Artif Organs* 15: 19, 1992

321. Bland L, Alter M, Favero M, Carson L, Cusick L: Hemodialyzer reuse: practices in the United States and implication for infection control. *Trans Am Soc Artif Intern Organs* 31: 556, 1985

322. Klinkmann H, Ebbighausen H, Uhlenbusch I, Vienken J: High-flux dialysis, dialysate quality and backtransport, in: *Evolution in Dialysis Adequacy*, Contributions in Nephrology, Vol 3, edited by Bonomini V, Basel, Karger, 1993, p 89

323. Bambauer R, Schauer M, Vienken J: Contamination of dialysis water and dialysate. *Blood Purif* 9: 32, 1991

324. Yamagami S, Adachi T, Sugirmura T, Wada S, Kishimoto T, Mackawa M. Yoshimura R, Niwa M, Terano Y, Shaldon S: Detection of endotoxin antibody in longterm dialysis patients. *Int J Artif Organs* 13: 205, 1990

325. Vanholder R, Van HE, Veys N, Ringoir S: Endotoxin transfer through dialysis membranes: small- *versus* large-pore membranes. *Nephrol Dial Transplant* 7: 333, 1992

326. Baz M, Durand C, Jaber K, Marzouk T, Berland Y: The impact of 12 years ultrapure dialysate use in hemodialysis related amyloidosis. *Int J Artif Organs* 547: 1990

327. Glenn CM, Astley SJ, Watkins SL: Dialysis-associated seizures in children and adolescents. *Pediatr Nephrol* 6: 182, 1992

328. Berman AT, Lorio R, Brelin J: Three central acetabular fracture-dislocations secondary to metabolically induced seizures in ESRD patients. *Orthopedics* 16: 1265, 1993

329. Dahlberg PJ, Kisken WA, Newcomer KL, Yutuc WR: Mesenteric ischemia in chronic dialysis patients. *Am J Nephrol* 5: 327, 1985

330. Diamond SM, Emmett M, Henrich WL: Bowel infarction as a cause of death in dialysis patients. *JAMA* 256: 2545, 1986

331. Friedell ML: Cecal necrosis in the dialysis-dependent patient. *Am Surgeon* 51: 621, 1985

332. Leiba H, Oliver M, Shimshoni M, Bar-Khayim Y: Intraocular pressure fluctuations during regular hemodialysis and ultrafiltration. *Acta Ophthalmol* 68: 320, 1990

333. Arora N, Lambrov FH Jr, Stewart MW, Vidrine-Parks L, Sandroni S: Sudden blindness associated with central nervous symptoms in a hemodialysis patient. *Nephron* 59: 490, 1991

334. Servilla KS, Groggel GC: Anterior ischemic optic neuropathy as a complication of hemodialysis. *Am J Kidney Dis* 8: 61, 1986

335. Quittenbaum S, Grefberg N: Massive bladder haemorrhage after thrombolytic therapy in a haemodialysis

patient with secondary amyloidosis. *Nephrol Dial Transplant* 8: 1174, 1993

336. Matuszkiewicz RJ, Billip-Tomecka Z, Rowinski W, Sicinski A: Systemic streptokinase infusion for declotting of hemodialysis arteriovenous fistulas. *Nephron* 66: 67, 1994

337. Singhal PC, Lynn RI, Scharschmidt LA: Priaprism and dialysis. *Am J Nephrol* 6: 358, 1986

338. Wu SG, Lin SL, Shiao WY, Huang HW, Lin CF, Yang YH: Comparison of sublingual captopril, nifedipine and prazosin in hypertensive emergencies during hemo-dialysis. *Nephron* 65: 284, 1993

339. Gutierrez A, Bergstrom J, Alvestrand A: Hemodialysis associated protein catabolism with and without glucose in the dialysis fluid. *Kidney Int* 46: 814, 1994

340. Ikizler TA, Flakoll PJ, Parker RA, Hakim RM: Amino acid and albumin losses during hemodialysis. *Kidney Int* 46: 830, 1994

REPLACEMENT OF RENAL FUNCTION BY DIALYSIS

GERHARD LONNEMANN and KARL M. KOCH

INTRODUCTION

In this review we will discuss the importance of bacterial contamination of dialysate fluid and the associated risk of pyrogenic reactions for patients on hemodialysis therapy. The degree of bacterial contamination of dialysate, relevant bacterial species and pyrogenic substances released from these microorganisms will be described. In addition, information about bacteriological methods to determine bacterial growth as well as assays to measure the pyrogenic activity of bacteria-derived substances will be given. Furthermore, we will describe *in vitro* studies testing the permeability of dialyzer membranes to pyrogenic substances derived from dialysate-born bacteria. We will discuss recent investigations suggesting that bacterial contamination of dialysate may cause repeated stimulation of immuno-competent cells including monocytes, lymphocytes and neutrophils, resulting in increased production of inflammatory mediators in end-stage renal disease (ESRD) patients. Finally, we will describe an effective approach to reduce the bacterial contamination of dialysis and the associated risk of pyrogenic reactions during hemodialysis.

PYROGENIC REACTIONS DURING HEMODIALYSIS

Since the beginning of routine hemodialysis therapy bacterial contamination of the dialysate fluid has been a major concern (1, 2). In spite of multiple technical improvements including the introduction of reverse osmosis units to clean water for the preparation of dialysate and the use of manufactured single-use dialyzers, the frequency of pyrogenic reactions associated with hemodialysis is still approximately 1–5 pyrogenic reactions per 1000 hemodialysis sessions, as it has been reported in several studies conducted in the United States (3).

It is still under debate which hemodialysis-dependent factors cause pyrogenic reactions. The national surveillance of hemodialysis associated diseases by the Center for Disease Control (CDC) in the United States of America analyzed the influence of bicarbonate dialysate versus acetate dialysate, the use of high-flux dialyzer versus low-flux dialyzers, performance of single use versus reuse of dialyzers, as well as various reuse procedures and combinations of all these factors on the frequency of pyrogenic reactions in hemodialysis. For 1989 the CDC report states that dialysis centers using high-flux dialyzers in combination with bicarbonate dialysate were more likely to report pyrogenic reactions, particularly when dialyzers were reused (4). In 1990 and 1991, the use of bicarbonate dialysate was no longer associated with a higher risk of pyrogenic reactions compared to acetate dialysate (5, 6). In centers performing only single use of dialyzers, the frequency of pyrogenic reactions in patients treated with high-flux dialyzers was not significantly different from that found in patients treated with low-flux dialyzers (5). In 1991, the number of dialysis centers reporting more than two pyrogenic reactions per year was higher in centers using any high-flux dialyzer membranes compared to those using none (16% versus 10%, $p < 0.05$) as well as in the centers performing reuse compared to no reuse (15% versus 7%, $p < 0.05$) (6). Because most of the centers using high-flux dialyzers also performed reuse, it is not clear from the raw data which of the two factors, high-flux membranes or reuse, is more likely associated with the occurrence of pyrogenic reactions. Statistical analysis using stepwise logistic regression with adjustment for confounding factors was applied to describe the role of reuse and high-flux dialyzers separately (6). This analysis revealed that the dialysis practice most significantly associated with the reporting of pyrogenic reactions was dialyzer reuse (6). Comparing various reuse techniques, renalin manual reuse was most highly associated with an increased number of reported pyrogenic reactions. Only formaldehyde manual reuse was not significantly associated with pyrogenic reactions (6).

In summary, the surveillance data indicate that hemodialysis-dependent pyrogenic reactions are mainly associated with the performance of reuse. When reuse is avoided, the risk of pyrogenic reactions is not significantly increased in high-flux dialysis compared to low-flux dialysis.

BACTERIAL GROWTH IN DIALYSATE

The degree of bacterial contamination in reverse-osmosis water and dialysate exceeds the upper limits of the standards recommended by the American Association of Medical Instrumentation (AAMI) in a high percentage. The standards were set for water and dialysate at 200 colony forming units (CFU) per ml and 2000 CFU/ml, respectively. Klein et al. reported from a multi center study conducted in the United States of America that 35% of water samples and 19% of dialysate samples exceeded the AAMI standards (7). The degree of bacterial contamination of dialysate in the United States as well as in Europe was very variable (10^2–10^5 CFU/ml) between hemodialysis centers but also in the same center over time (8, 9). World wide estimates are that approximately 20% of dialysate samples contain more than 2000 CFU/ml of bacteria.

Several investigations were performed to characterize microorganisms growing in dialysate. Klein et al. (7) reported that bacteria grown from dialysate were almost exclusively Gram-negative and that *Pseudomonas species* are most commonly found. In addition, fungi are found occasionally and Gram-positive microorganisms are very rare in dialysate. Harding et al. (10) showed that adequate culture conditions are required to determine bacterial growth in dialysate correctly. Gram-negative bacteria isolated from dialysate grow better in salt containing but nutritient poor culture medium such as R2A as compared to standard media such as Tryptic Soy Agar (TSA) (10). Furthermore, growth of these microorganisms was enhanced when cultures were incubated at room temperature as compared to 37°C. In order to improve the sensitivity of the bacterial cultures, incubations were prolonged to 96 hours (7, 10). As these special culture conditions have not been used in most of the previous studies testing bacterial growth in dialysate, one may speculate that the degree of bacterial contamination may be even higher than reported.

PYROGENIC BACTERIAL SUBSTANCES

Fever in response to Gram-negative infection is caused by pyrogenic substances released from bacterial debris or actively secreted from growing bacteria. Substances released from bacterial debris include cell wall components such as lipopolysaccharides (LPS), peptidoglycans and muramyl peptides (11). In addition, Gram-negative bacteria produce peptides such as exotoxin A derived from *Pseudomonas species* (12), or hemolysin secreted from *E.*

Table 1. Bacteria-derived pyrogens

	Molecular weight (Kilo Dalton)
Cell wall components	
Lipopolysaccharide (LPS):	> 100
Lipid A-related LPS fragments:	2–4
other LPS fragments:	< 8
Peptidoglycans:	1–20
Muramylpeptides:	0.4–1
Actively secreted toxins	
exotoxin A:	66
exotoxin A fragments:	< 5
other exotoxins:	20–50

coli (13). All these bacterial products are called exogenous pyrogens because they are of foreign origin, invade the host and induce the production of endogenous pyrogens in circulating mononuclear cells (PBMC). In addition to the induction of fever, endogenous pyrogens have been shown to be important mediators of the host response to inflammation and infection (14). As endogenous pyrogens such as interleukin-1 (IL-1) and tumor necrosis factor (TNFα) are peptide messengers between various cells they are also called cytokines (15).

In order to induce cytokines during hemodialysis, bacterial substances contaminating dialysate need to get into contact with circulating mononuclear cells on the other side of the dialyzer membrane. Therefore, the molecular sizes of bacterial substances contaminating dialysate are important to estimate whether these pyrogens could penetrate dialyzer membranes (Table 1). LPS are large molecules with molecular weights of > 100,000 Dalton. The pyrogenic subunit of LPS, lipid A, is small (4000 Dalton) but does only exist in small quantities in its monomeric form in water. Evidence was provided that low molecular weight LPS fragments (< 2000 Dalton) and other small pyrogens may appear in contaminated dialysate which are different from lipid A, and possibly derived from the polysaccharide part of the LPS molecule (16). Like LPS, peptidoglycans are components of the bacterial cell wall with molecular sizes of approximately 25,000 Dalton. Subunits of peptidoglycans, the muramylpeptides can be as small as 1000 Dalton (11). Enzymatic activity (e.g., lysozym) produced by neutrophils is required to release small molecular weight muramyl peptides from the parent peptidoglycan molecule (17). More recent data by A. Mahiout suggest that exotoxins from Gram-negative bacteria are secreted from growing microorganisms in contaminated dialysate. Although exotoxin A from *P. aeruginosa* is a relatively large molecule, 66000 Dalton (12),

Mahiout et al. reported that pyrogenic fragments of exotoxin A as small as < 5000 Dalton are present in bicarbonate dialysate contaminated with *P. aeruginosa* (18). These data suggest that contaminated dialysate may contain low molecular size pyrogens which are small enough to penetrate intact dialyzer membranes.

PYROGEN PERMEABILITY OF DIALYZER MEMBRANES

As the molecular size exclusion of dialyzes membranes is between 5000 Dalton for low-flux and 25,000–30,000 Dalton for high-flux membranes, one may speculate that low-flux membranes are less permeable for small pyrogens than high-flux membranes. This question was addressed by several *in vitro* studies investigating the permeability of dialyzer membranes to bacterial substances. The results of these studies are difficult to compare because of the lack of standardization of *in vitro* test conditions (e.g., the absence or presence of blood or plasma in the blood compartment), the challenge material, the challenge dose, and the assays used to measure bacterial substances.

A variety of different challenge materials were used including purified LPS (19–22), synthetic LPS fragments (23), and bacterial culture filtrates (19, 24, 25). The strength of the challenge material as measured by the Limulus amebocyte lysate (LAL) assay was also very variable with LPS concentrations between 0.2 and 250 μg/ml (26). However, it has to be emphasized that bacterial culture filtrates contain pyrogens such as exotoxins which are not detected by the LAL assay. Thus, LAL measurements are likely to underestimate the entire pyrogenic activity of the challenge material.

In several studies, bacterial products were measured by the LAL assay which detects only LPS and lipid A containing subunits of LPS. Other studies used the *in vitro* incubation of human peripheral blood mononuclear cells (PBMC) with the subsequent measurement of pyrogen-induced cytokines in PBMC culture supernatants by radioimmunoassay (27) to detect the entire pyrogenic activity of all bacterial substances present in the challenge material.

Using purified LPS from *E. coli* to contaminate the dialysate and the LAL test to measure LPS in the blood compartment, studies failed to show LPS-permeability of low-flux regenerated cellulosic as well as high-flux polysulfone dialyzer membranes (19, 20). In contrast, when the *in vitro* incubation of PBMC was used to determine the cytokine-inducing activity, pyrogens were detected in the blood side of low-flux regenerated cellulosic membranes after the dialysate was challenged with purified LPS from *E. coli* (19). However, the presence of whole heparinized donor blood or a solution containing 10% plasma in saline in the blood compartment were required to demonstrate penetration of pyrogens derived from *E.*

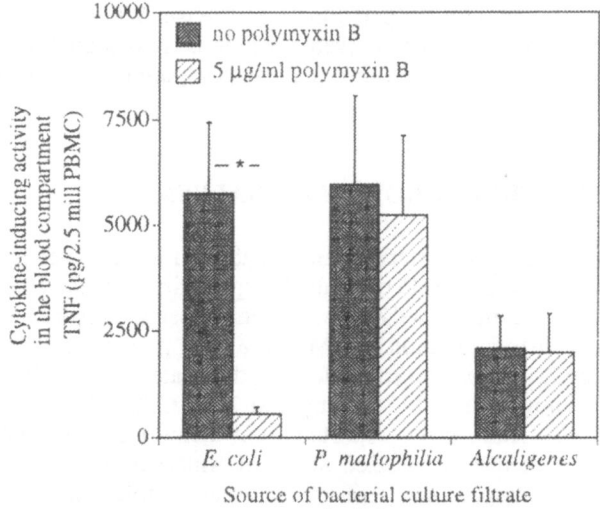

Figure 1. Effect of polymyxin B on cytokine-inducing substances derived from *E. coli* ($n = 5$), *P. maltophilia* ($n = 8$) or *Alcaligenes* ($n = 3$) penetrating cellulosic dialyzer membranes. After contamination of the dialysate of an *in vitro* dialysis system with the indicated bacterial culture filtrate, samples from the blood compartment were incubated with PBMC in the presence and absence of 5 μg/ml polymyxin B. TNFα-inducing activity is expressed as picogram per 2.5 $\times$ 10^6 PBMC and 18 hours of incubation. Mean $\pm$ SEM. *$p < 0.05$ compared to samples without polymyxin B.

coli across dialyzer membranes. The pyrogenic activity in the blood side was significantly inhibited by polymyxin B, a cationic antibiotic which specifically binds to the lipid A subunit of LPS (Figure 1) (19). The reason why plasma is required to demonstrate pyrogens in the blood compartment is still not fully understood. We speculate that specific LPS-binding proteins (such as LBP) and non-specific carrier-proteins for LPS (such as α2 macroglobulin) bind LPS fragments and present them to the PBMC.

Using radiolabeled low molecular weight fragments of LPS, low-flux regenerated cellulose, high flux AN69 and polysulfone were shown to be permeable when radioactivity or the cytokine-inducing activity was measured in the blood compartment (22, 23). In these studies, the LAL assay failed to detect the LPS-derived fragments in the blood side.

These data indicate that when purified LPS was used to challenge dialyzer membranes, the LAL test did not detect pyrogens on the other side of the membrane. However, there are pyrogens released from purified LPS during *in vitro* dialysis which are negative in the LAL assay but highly active in inducing cytokine production in the PBMC assay. Reasons for the failure of the LAL test to detect these LPS-derived subunits remain speculative. It had been suggested that these fragments are either too small (< 4000 Dalton) to be detected by the LAL assay

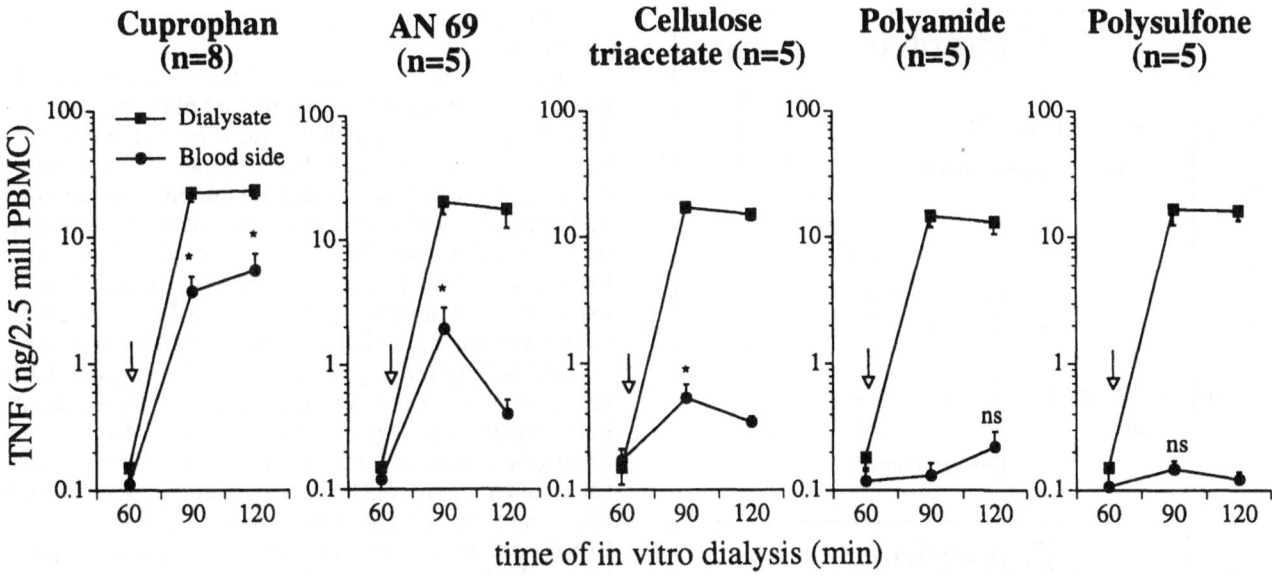

Figure 2. Permeability of dialyzer membranes to *P. maltophilia*-derived TNFα-inducing substances under the conditions of *in vitro* dialysis with 10% plasma in the blood compartment. The dialysate was sterile for 60 minutes and subsequently contaminated with *P. maltophilia* culture filtrate (LPS 200 ng/ml), indicated by the arrow. TNFα-inducing activity is expressed as nanogram per 2.5×10^6 PBMC and 18 hours of incubation. Mean ± SEM. $^*p < 0.05$ compared to 60 minute samples, ns = not significant.

(23) or do not contain the LAL-reactive lipid A subunit of LPS.

As *E. coli* are not routinely found in dialysate, further studies were performed using culture filtrates from dialysate-born bacteria such as *P. maltophilia*, *P. aeruginosa*, *P. testosteroni*, *Alcaligenes*, and others (23–25). All studies used the PBMC assay to measure the cytokine-inducing activity of the bacterial filtrates. In general it has to be concluded from these *in vitro* studies that every dialyzes membrane can be demonstrated to be permeable to pyrogens.

There were, however, quantitative differences in the pyrogen-permeability of dialyzes membranes depending on the experimental design as well as the challenge material and the challenge dose. Under comparable *in vitro* conditions with plasma present in the blood compartment and the use of *Pseudomonas* culture filtrate as challenge material, the TNFα-inducing activity increased significantly in the blood compartments of low-flux Cuprophan, high-flux cellulose triacetate and the synthetic high-flux membrane AN69. In contrast, there was no significant increase of TNFα-inducing activity in the blood side of the other synthetic high-flux membranes polyamide and polysulfone (Figure 2) (25). When whole donor blood instead of plasma was recirculated in the blood compartment of low-flux Cuprophan and high-flux polysulfone (Figure 3), there was a significant increase in the blood compartments of both dialyzers (28). However, after 120 minutes of *in vitro* dialysis, the blood side activity in polysulfone dialyzers was less ($p < 0.03$) than that in Cuprophan dialyzers. This tendency of reduced pyrogen permeability

of the polysulfone membrane compared to Cuprophan is in agreement with the results of the experiments using 10% plasma. It has to be emphasized that in the presence of whole blood, polysulfone appeared to be permeable to IL-1-inducing substances derived from *P. aeruginosa* whereas in the former study using 10% plasma, TNFα-inducing substances derived from *P. maltophilia* were not detectable in the blood compartment of the same dialyzer membrane. These data indicate, again, that variables in the experimental design including the challenge material, the solution in the blood compartment and the type of cytokine measured in PBMC cultures influence the results of experiments testing the permeability of dialyzer membranes to cytokine-inducing bacterial substances.

In spite of multiple differences in experimental designs of the *in vitro* studies, it can be concluded that all dialyzer membranes are permeable to pyrogenic substances of bacterial origin and that high-flux membranes in general are not more permeable than low-flux membranes. Thus, the controversial issue of whether pyrogens are able to penetrate intact dialyzer membranes is solved: the answer is yes. It remains controversial, however, whether there are differences in the pyrogen permeability of the various dialyzer membranes due to their chemical composition. For example the differences between the synthetic high-flux membrane polysulfone and the cellulose-derived high-flux cellulose-triacetate shown in Figure 2 could not be confirmed when saline instead of plasma was recirculated in the blood compartments. Under protein-free conditions, the polysulfone membrane appeared to be more permeable than a modified cellulose triacetate membrane (29).

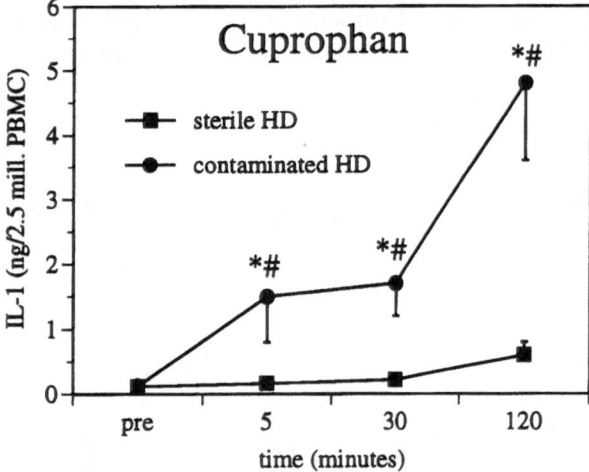

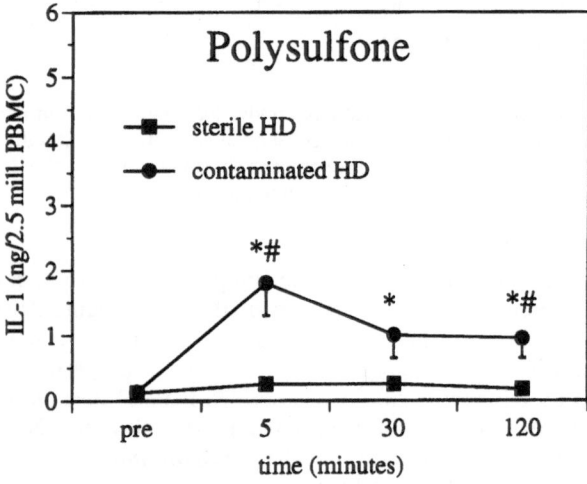

Figure 3. Appearance of IL-1β-inducing substances in the blood compartment during whole blood circulation. Samples were drawn from the blood compartment containing heparinized donor blood, centrifuged and an equal volume of plasma was added to PBMC separated from non-circulated blood of the same donor. After 20 hours of incubation, total IL-1β production (cell-associated plus secreted) was determined by radioimmunoassay. Dialysate was either sterile saline or saline contaminated with *P. aeruginosa* filtrate. Experiments were performed using blood from the same donor for both dialyzers. Results are mean ± SEM, $n = 6$; *$p < 0.05$ versus pre dialysis; #$p < 0.05$ versus sterile dialysis. The difference between both membranes was statistically significant ($p < 0.03$) at 120 minutes.

When these two membranes were pre-coated with plasma, the permeability of polysulfone but not that of modified cellulose triacetate was significantly reduced (29). These data indicate that plasma components influence the permeability of dialyzer membranes to pyrogens differently. Depending on the interaction of plasma components with bacterial products and the specific dialyzer membrane material, plasma may enhance, reduce or not influ-

ence the permeability of dialyzer membranes to bacterial substances.

Additional characterization of the *Pseudomonas* culture filtrate (filtration through 300 kD filter) revealed that the cytokine-inducing activity was provided in only 50% by LAL-positive material. The remaining 50% were not detected by the LAL assay and not inhibited by polymyxin B or bactericidal/permeability increasing protein (BPI), two LPS inhibitors (25, 30). An additional important finding was that although the challenge material in the dialysate side consisted in 50% of LPS-like material, the cytokine-inducing activity in the blood side was not at all inhibited by polymyxin B (Figure 1) (25), and LAL-negative (19). These data indicate, that predominantly LAL-negative pyrogens derived from *Pseudomonas* and *Alcaligenes* bacteria penetrate dialyzer membranes. These small molecular pyrogens have not yet been identified. In addition to the previously described LAL-negative small LPS fragments, a recent study suggests that LAL-negative bacterial substances may, at least in part, represent peptide fragments of exotoxin A [18]. These exotoxin fragments are only detectable by the PBMC/cytokine assay. A specific assay is not available.

In conclusion, the LAL test which is a standard assay to determine the amount of endotoxin (LPS) contamination in water and dialysate fluid, is unable to detect small molecular weight cytokine-inducing pyrogens which are able to penetrate all dialyzer membranes. In order to measure pyrogen permeability of dialyzer membranes the PBMC/cytokine assay is recommended. According to the *in vitro* studies discussed, low-flux dialyzer membranes are not protective against the challenge of contaminated dialysate and are not less permeable than high-flux dialyzer membranes for pyrogenic bacterial substances.

PYROGEN ADSORPTION TO DIALYZER MEMBRANES

The adsorptive capacity for pyrogens of the specific dialyzer membrane material itself (31–33) as well as the formation of a pyrogen-adsorbing protein layer on the dialyzer membrane may reduce the permeability of dialyzer membranes to bacterial products (22, 29). *In vitro* studies showed that the adsorptive capacity is higher for synthetic high-flux membranes than for cellulosic low-flux membranes (23). Because of the presence of small pyrogens (molecular weight below the cutoff of low-flux membranes) in contaminated dialysate, low-flux dialyzer membranes do not prevent permeation of pyrogens into the patients blood. This assumption is in agreement with the surveillance data form the CDC report demonstrating that in single use dialysis the frequency of pyrogenic reactions is similar in low-flux and high-flux dialysis (5).

The increased adsorptive capacity of synthetic high-flux membranes for pyrogens has been used to test these membranes as ultrafilters to reduce the pyrogen content of contaminated dialysate. Polysulfone and polyamide ultrafilters were challenged with bacterial culture filtrates derived from *E. coli* or *P. aeruginosa*. Culture filtrates were used in a concentration containing approximately 250 ng/ml of endotoxin (LAL assay) derived from approximately 5×10^6 organisms/ml. Compared to routine dialysate this is a very high degree of contamination. Both ultrafilters completely removed cytokine-inducing pyrogens from the *E. coli* filtrate. Using four liters of *P. aeruginosa* filtrate with the endotoxin contents indicated above, pyrogens appeared on the filtrate side of both ultrafilters. When decreased challenge concentrations were used, pyrogens were retained. In summary, polysulfone ultrafilters reduce the cytokine-inducing activity of highly contaminated dialysate containing *E. coli* or *P. aeruginosa*-derived pyrogens by a factor of 100–1000 (Figure 4) (33, 34). Similar results were obtained when polyamide ultrafilters were used (31, 32).

EFFECT OF ULTRAFILTERED DIALYSATE ON THE PBMC CYTOKINE CONTENT IN ESRD PATIENTS

The results of the *in vitro* studies described above suggest that measurement of the pyrogen-induced cytokine production in PBMC may be the best way to determine whether pyrogens derived from contaminated dialysate penetrate dialyzer membranes *in vivo*. We studied the cytokine content in PBMC isolated from the blood of ESRD patients under the conditions of low-flux hemodialysis with regenerated cellulosic membranes and either regular bicarbonate dialysate or ultrafiltered bicarbonate dialysate (35). Whereas in non filtered dialysate the median of the bacterial count was 148 CFU/ml (range 61–400 CFU/ml) there were no CFU detectable in ultrafiltered dialysate. The cytokine content of PBMC, in this case interleukin-1 receptor antagonist (IL-1Ra), fell significantly from an averaged value of 1.467 ng/2.5×10^6 PBMC to 1.166 ng/2.5×10^6 PBMC ($p = 0.016$) in ESRD patients (Figure 5) (35). Although IL-1Ra is a functional antagonist of IL-1, production of IL-1Ra by PBMC is one log higher than that of IL-1 itself, parallels IL-1 and is the most sensitive marker of PBMC activation (36). In order to reduce hemodialysis-associated pyrogendependent PBMC activation which may contribute to chronic inflammatory processes in long-term hemodialysis patients (37) we recommend the use of ultrafiltered dialysate.

SUMMARY

Pyrogenic reactions occur in a frequency of approximately 1 per 1000 hemodialysis treatments. Surveillance data from the Center of Disease Control, USA, do not prove a higher risk of pyrogenic reactions when sin-

E. coli challenge

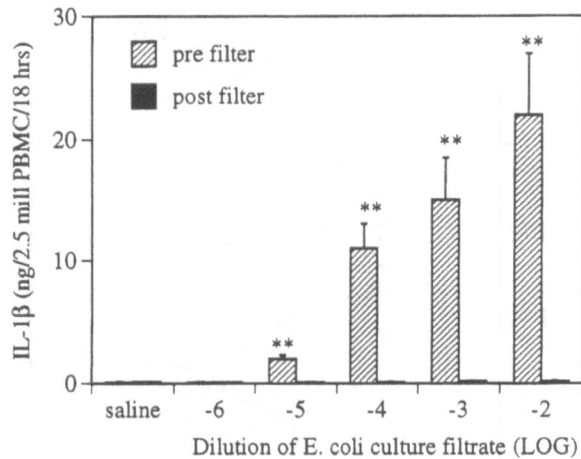

P. aeruginosa challenge

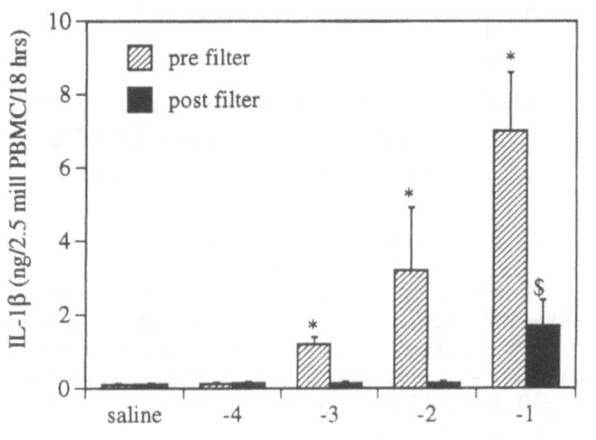

Figure 4. Ultrafiltration of *E. coli* and *P. aeruginosa* culture filtrates using polysulfone filters. Ultrafilters were challenged with 4 liter of water containing the indicated dilutions of bacterial culture filtrate. *E. coli* ($n = 4$); *P. aeruginosa* ($n = 3$); mean ± SEM. $^{**}p < 0.02$, $^{*}p < 0.05$ compared to unstimulated PBMC (saline). $^{\$}p < 0.05$ compared to all other post filter samples.

gle use high-flux dialyzers are used compared to single use low-flux dialyzers. Bacterial contamination of dialysate is common and exceeds the recommended standards (< 2000 CFU/ml) in about 20% of all tested samples. Gram-negative *Pseudomonas* species are predominantly found in dialysate. *Pseudomonas*-derived toxins include lipopolysaccharides (LPS), peptidoglycans and exotoxins as well as small molecular weight fragments of these so called exogenous pyrogens. In spite of the lack of standardization of experimental conditions, evidence accumulated over the past ten years that small molecular weight pyrogens derived from contaminated dialysate are

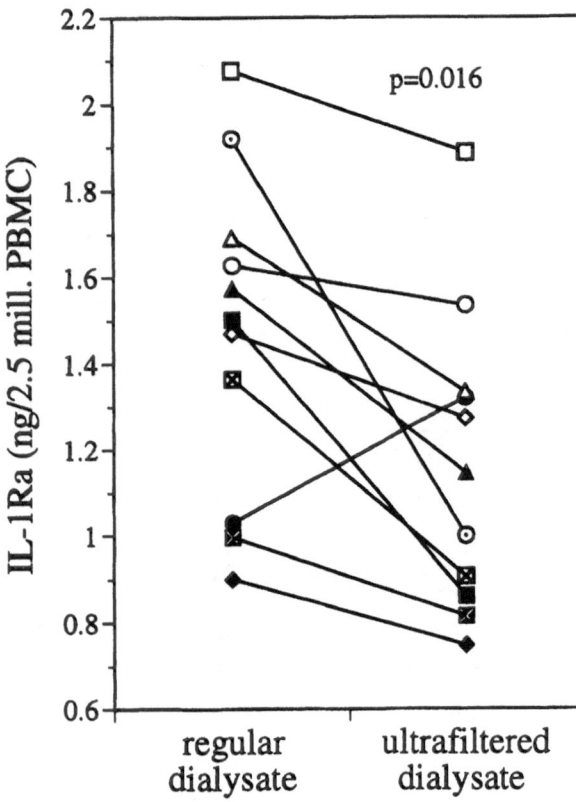

Figure 5. Effect of ultrafiltered dialysate on the IL-1Ra content in PBMC from ESRD patients on hemodialysis. IL-1Ra content in PBMC in 11 patients dialyzed with and without ultrafiltered dialysate. Each data point represents the average of 3–6 weekly values for IL-1Ra in each treatment period. Means are 1.467 ± 0.113 ng/2.5×10^6 PBMC without and 1.166 ± 0.104 ng/2.5×10^6 PBMC with filter ($p = 0.016$).

able to penetrate low-flux as well as high-flux dialyzer membranes and induce cytokine production in circulating mononuclear cells. On the other hand, the employment of pyrogen-adsorbing ultrafilters in the dialysate circuit reduces the pyrogen content of contaminated dialysate by a factor of 100–1000.

Because of new experimental approaches including the use of PBMC cultures to detect the cytokine-inducing activity of bacterial products, the former controversial issue of whether dialyzer membranes are permeable to pyrogens is solved; the answer is yes. The question whether there are differences in the pyrogen permeability of different dialyzer membranes remains controversial because of multiple factors influencing the appearance of bacterial substances in the patients' blood. Those factors include the microorganism-dependent variability in the composition of pyrogens in the dialysate, mechanisms of adsorption of pyrogens to the dialyzer membrane as well as blood components influencing the responsiveness of blood leukocytes to bacterial substances. Measurement of the *ex vivo* cytokine production by PBMC from

ESRD patients offers a sensitive test system to investigate dialyzer-dependent differences in pyrogen permeability *in vivo*.

There is evidence from *in vitro* as well as *in vivo* studies that cytokines such as IL-1 and TNFα are induced in activated PBMC during hemodialysis. Although it remains to be clinically proven that increased cytokine production contributes to chronic inflammatory processes associated with long-term hemodialysis, PBMC activation due to bacterial contamination of dialysate should be minimized for example by the use of ultrafiltered dialysate.

REFERENCES

1. Favero MD, Petersen NJ, Boyer KM, Carson LA, Bond WW: Microbial contamination of renal dialysis and associated health risk. *Trans Am Soc Artif Internal Organs* 20:175, 1974
2. Kolmos HI: Hygienic problems in dialysis. Factors determining bacterial contamination of fluids and equipment used for haemo- and peritoneal dialysis, associated health risks, and methods of prevention. *Dan Med Bull* 32: 338, 1985
3. Gordon SM, Oettinger CW, Bland LA, Oliver JC, Arduino MJ, Aguero SM, McAllister SK, Favero MS, Jarvis WR: Pyrogenic reactions in patients receiving conventional, high-efficiency, or high-flux hemodialysis treatments with bicarbonate dialysate containing high concentrations of bacteria and endotoxin. *J Am Soc Nephrol* 2: 1436, 1992
4. Alter MJ, Favero MS, Moyer LA, Bland LA: National surveillance of dialysis-associated diseases in the United States, 1989. *Asaio Trans* 37: 97, 1991
5. Tokars JI, Alter MJ, Favero MS, Moyer LA, Bland LA: National surveillance of hemodialysis associated diseases in the United States, 1990. *ASAIO J* 39: 71, 1993
6. Tokars JI, Alter MJ, Favero MS, Moyer LA, Bland LA: National surveillance of dialysis associated diseases in the United States, 1991. *ASAIO J* 39: 966, 1993
7. Klein E, Pass T. Harding GB, Wright R. Million C: Microbial and endotoxin contamination in water and dialysate in the central United States. *Artif Organs* 14: 85, 1990
8. Bambauer R. Meyer S. Jung H. Goehl H. Nystrand R.: Sterile versus non-sterile dialysis fluid in chronic hemodialysis treatment. *Asaio Trans* 36: 317, 1990
9. Pegues DA, Oettinger CW, Bland LA, Oliver JC, Arduino MJ, Aguero SM, McAllister SK, Gordon SM, Favero MS, Jarvis WR: A prospective study of pyrogenic reactions in hemodialysis patients using bicarbonate dialysis fluids filtered to remove bacteria and endotoxin. *J Am Soc Nephrol* 3: 1002, 1992
10. Harding GB, Klein E, Pass T, Wright R, Million C: Endotoxin and bacterial contamination of dialysis center water and dialysate; a cross sectional survey. *Int J Artif Organs* 13: 39, 1990
11. Takahashi I, Kotani S, Takada H, Shiba T, Kusumoto S: Structural requirements of endotoxic lipopolysaccharides and bacterial cell walls in induction of interleukin-1. *Blood Purif* 6: 188, 1988
12. Misfeldt ML, Legaard PK, Howell SE, Fornella MH, Le Grand RD: Induction of interleukin-1 from murine peri-

toneal macrophages by Pseudomonas aeruginosa exotoxin A. *Infect Immun* 58: 978, 1990

13. Bhakdi S, Muhly M, Korom S, Schmidt G: Effects of Escherichia coli hemolysin on human monocytes. *J Clin Invest* 85: 1746, 1990

14. Dinarello CA, Wolff SM: The role of interleukin-1 in disease. *N Engl J Med* 328: 106, 1993

15. Dinarello CA: Interleukin-1 and tumor necrosis factor and their naturally occurring antagonists during hemodialysis. *Kidney Int Suppl* 38: S68, 1992

16. Haeffner-Cavaillon N, Caroff M, Cavaillon JM: Interleukin-1 induction by lipopolysaccharides: structural requirements of the 3-deoxy-D-manno-2-octulosonic acid (KDO). *Mol Immunol* 26: 485, 1989

17. Dinarello CA: Pathogenesis of fever during hemodialysis. *Contrib Nephrol* 36: 90, 1983

18. Mahiout A, Shaldon S, Koch KM: Production of exotoxin and its related subfragments in contaminated bicarbonate dialysate. *J Am Soc Nephrol* 2: 337, 1991

19. Lonnemann G. Bingel M, Floege J, Koch KM, Shaldon S, Dinarello CA: Detection of endotoxin-like interleukin-1-inducing activity during *in vitro* dialysis. *Kidney Int* 33: 29, 1988

20. Bommer J, Becker KP, Urbaschek R, Ritz E, Urbaschek B: No evidence for endotoxin transfer across high flux polysulfone membranes. *Clin Nephrol* 27: 278, 1987

21. Bingel M, Lonnemann G, Shaldon S, Koch KM, Dinarello CA: Human interleukin-1 production during hemodialysis. *Nephron* 43: 161, 1986

22. Urena P, Herbelin A, Zingraff J, Lair M, Man NK, Descamps LB, Drueke T: Permeability of cellulosic and non-cellulosic membranes to endotoxin subunits and cytokine production during *in-vitro* haemodialysis. *Nephrol Dial Transplant* 7: 16, 1992

23. Laude-Sharp M, Caroff M, Simard L, Pusineri C, Kazatchkine MD, Haeffner-Cavaillon N: Induction of IL-1 during hemodialysis: transmembrane passage of intact endotoxins (LPS). *Kidney Int* 38: 1089, 1990

24. Evans RC, Holmes CJ: *In vitro* study of the transfer of cytokine-inducing substances across selected high-flux hemodialysis membranes. *Blood Purif* 9: 92, 1991

25. Lonnemann G, Behme TC, Lenzner B, Floege J, Schulze M, Colton CK, Koch KM, Shaldon S: Permeability of dialyzer membranes to TNF alpha-inducing substances derived from water bacteria. *Kidney Int* 42: 61, 1992

26. Lonnemann G: Dialysate bacteriological quality and the permeability of dialyzer membranes to pyrogens. *Kidney Int Suppl* 41: 195, 1993

27. Duff GW, Atkins E: The detection of endotoxin by *in vitro* production of endogenous pyrogen: Comparison with Limulus amebocyte lysate gelation. *J Immunol Method* 52: 323, 1982

28. Schindler R, Lufft V, Lonnemann G, Mahiout A, Marra MN, Shaldon S, Koch KM: Induction of interleukin-1 and interleukin-1 receptor antagonist during contaminated in vitro dialysis with whole blood. 1994. Submitted

29. Lonnemann G, Schindler R, Lufft V, Mahiout A, Shaldon S, Koch KM: The role of plasma coating on the permeation of cytokine-inducing substances through dialyzer membranes. *Nephrol Dial Transplant* 10: 207, 1995

30. Marra MN, Wilde CG, Griffith JE, Snable JL, Scott RW: Bactericidal/permeability-increasing protein has endotoxin-neutralizing activity. *J Immunol* 144: 662, 1990

31. Dinarello CA, Lonnemann G, Maxwell R, Shaldon S: Ultrafiltration to reject human interleukin-1-inducing substances derived from bacterial cultures. J Clin Microbiol 25: 1233, 1987

32. Lonnemann G, Mahiout A, Schindler R, Cotton CK: Pyrogen retention by the polyamide membranes. *Contrib Nephrol* 96: 47, 1992

33. Schindler R, Dinarello CA: Ultrafiltration to remove endotoxins and other cytokine-inducing materials from tissue culture media and parenteral fluids. *Bio Techniques* 8: 408, 1990

34. Lonnemann G, Schindler R: Ultrafiltration using the polysulfone membrane to reduce the cytokine-inducing activity of contaminated dialysate. *Clin Nephrol* 42: S37, 1994

35. Schindler R, Lonnemann G, Schaffer J, Shaldon S, Koch KM, Krautzig S: The effect of ultrafiltered dialysate on the cellular content of interleukin-1 receptor antagonist in patients on chronic hemodialysis. *Nephron* 68: 229, 1994

36. Pereira BJ, Poutsiaka DD, King AJ, Strom JA, Narayan G, Levey AS, Dinarello CA: *In vitro* production of interleukin-1 receptor antagonist in chronic renal failure, CAPD and HD. *Kidney Int* 42: 1419, 1992

37. Dinarello CA: Cytokines: agents provocateurs in hemodialysis? [clinical conference]. *Kidney Int* 41: 683, 1992

BIOCOMPATIBILITY – CLINICAL ASPECTS

H.-D. LEMKE, A. GRASSMANN, J. VIENKEN and S. SHALDON

Such laboured nothings, in so strange a style, Amaze the unlearned, and make the learned smile.

Be not the first by whom the new are tried, Nor yet the last to lay the old aside.

Alexander Pope, Essay on Criticism

INTRODUCTION

The clinical aspects of biocompatibility require a clear definition as the title could be misleading. We shall discuss the meaning of biocompatibility in its current usage in haemodialysis therapy and the clinical associations claimed to relate in part or toto from bioincompatible events derived from haemodialysis therapy.

Historically, the initial observation of neutropenia in the early phase of haemodialysis (1) and the subsequent suggestion by Craddock et al. (2) that activation of the alternative pathway of complement would lead to granulocytic clumping in the pulmonary capillaries and contribute to the early reduction in PaO_2 seen during haemodialysis, stimulated considerable interest in the mechanisms controlling these observations. The demonstration that the chemical structure of the dialysis membrane, regenerated cellulose, could have an effect on the activation of the alternate pathway to produce the anaphylatoxins C3a and C5a opened the gates to the production of membranes that did not have this effect or had a reduced effect thereon ((3), Figure 1). Since that time a variety of lesser or non-C5a-activating membranes have been studied in haemodialysis and collectively called biocompatible membranes as opposed to regenerated cellulose that is called bioincompatible. Indeed, the paradigm of today suggests that such a membrane is outdated and may indeed be unethical to use. It will be the function of this review to critically judge the

Complement Activation and Leukopenia

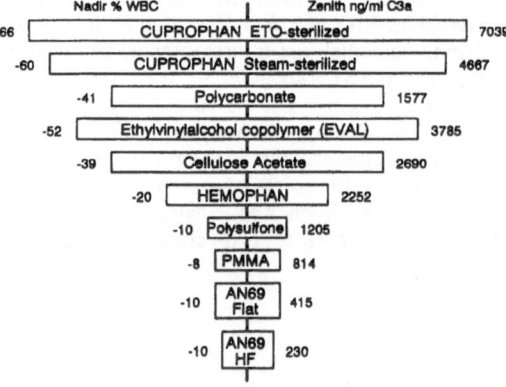

Figure 1. Dialysis membranes induce different levels of complement activation and different degrees of leukopenia depending on their chemical composition. Adapted from (3).

evidence available to justify this paradigm and to suggest that at this moment in time the evidence is too superficial and incomplete to permit a comprehensive scientific analysis of the pathophysiology sequelae of biocompatibility.

BIOCOMPATIBILITY: EFFECTOR SYSTEMS

Biocompatibility has been defined as the ability of a material or device or system to perform without a clinically significant host response (4, 5). Although several biological systems undergo activation during extracorporeal circulation, discussions on biocompatibility of the haemodialysis treatment have centered around complement activation only. It is only recently that the contact activation-dependent generation of bradykinin has also been considered as a parameter of biocompatibility. Furthermore, the possible consequences of microbial contamination of dialysate are increasingly associated with clinical consequences of haemodialysis.

While there is no doubt about the biochemical events associated with each of these three effector systems occurring during haemodialysis, their clinical implications are far from certain. It is therefore, the intention in this chapter, to consider how the biochemical data available with regard to the following areas might relate to clinical observations during the treatment:

- Complement activation and generation of the anaphylatoxins C3a and C5a
- Activation of the contact system and the release of bradykinin
- Microbial contamination of dialysate.

After a brief overview of the main biochemical reactions of these systems the following criteria will be discussed to establish a relationship between a single biochemical entity as suspected cause for an observed clinical effect.

- Is the suspected pathway or substance known and chemically defined in sufficient detail?
- Is a dose/response between cause and clinical effect established?
- Is the observed clinical effect reproducible?
- Can the involved pathways and/or activities be blocked and thus abolish the clinical effects?

Complement activation and generation of C3a and C5a

Activation of the complement system results in the generation of a number of split products cleaved off proteolytically from their parent molecules in a cascade of biochemical reactions. The fragments, in particular of C3 and C5, as well as the terminal complement complex (TCC) have been implicated in the biochemical reactions associated with biocompatibility of devices used in extracorporeal blood circulation. Both C3 and C5 can interact with several cell types via specific receptors and are thus able to transfer the signal of activation to this level.

Clinical consequences of biocompatibility parameters have been associated only with the anaphylatoxins C3a and C5a. For instance, they are considered to cause allergic reactions, because when injected into animals, they induce a response resembling to anaphylaxis (6). The

chemistry of these molecules is reasonably well defined (7). Virtually every blood cell type, with the exception of perhaps erythrocytes, responds either directly via receptors, or indirectly via secondary mediators to the anaphylatoxins C3a and C5a. However, in the past decade, it has been the interaction of the anaphylatoxins with the neutrophil cell that has led to the central hypothesis of biocompatibility. In this context, a causal interaction between complement activation at the dialyzer membrane surface and neutrophil activation, trapping of neutrophils in the lung and the symptoms of hypoxemia was established. The evidence for such a causal relationship will now be reviewed.

Dose/reponse effects of the anaphylatoxins C3a and C5a have been studied in detail widh respect to vascular permeability and contractile responses in *in vitro* and in animal models (7). As studied in rabbits, vascular permeability changes are in part mediated by histamine as well as by prostaglandin E_2 (PGE$_2$) and other prostaglandins, whereas in the guinea pig lung prostaglandins and leukotrienes serve as secondary mediators (8). The transfer and association of these data to effects on the human organism are more difficult to acertain, since several species related differences exist with regard to the potency and the stability of C3a and C5a. This is true in particular with regard to their conversion to the desArg derivatives by carboxypeptidase N_1 (7) which abolishes anaphylatoxin activity (6).

No specific inhibitor, such as a receptor antagonist interfering with anaphylatoxin activity is known. This renders it fairly difficult to determine the contribution of anaphylatoxins, generated during dialysis, to clinical signs of inflammation at present (9). C5a and its desArg-derivative are equivalent with regard to monocyte chemotaxis and polarization (10). This effect may be clinical meaningful, if C5a generation would result in cytokine release. The *in vitro* effects of C3a and C5a, however, which might have been contaminated with endotoxins during their isolation from plasma, are controversially discussed. C3a and C5a isolated from human plasma were found to induce the release of IL-1β from monocytes (11, 12). This was contradicted by a report showing that no IL-1 release was found when purified plasma-C5a was used (13). These data are in agreement with further experiments using recombinant C5a which induced only transcription of the IL-1 gene into mRNA and not synthesis of the protein (14). The differences between recombinant and isolated C5a might be due to the oligosaccharide moiety which is missing on the recombinant C5a peptide (7). Since this conclusion is derived from two separate reports (13, 14), further studies are justified to clarify the issue. The problem is complicated further since direct induction of IL-1 protein synthesis by C5a can be influenced by tiny amounts of endotoxins in the range of even below 1 pg/ml introduced with the C5a preparation or buffers. However, *in vitro* and *in vivo* studies (15, 16) using Cuprophan® dialyzers showed only an increase in IL-1β PBMC-mRNA but no increase in IL-1β-protein leaving the dialyzers. Thus, in the clinical situation, there appears to be no contribution of a membrane alone to the increase in cytokine protein synthesis.

Contact activation and the generation of kinins

The contact system of plasma which includes the proteins Hageman factor (factor XII), high-molecular weight kininogen (HMWK) and prekallikrein has been postulated to be involved in thrombogenicity since it can be activated by (negatively charged) biomaterial surfaces (17, 18). Activation leads to the cleavage of HMWK by kallikrein and release of kinins, in particular bradykinin, into the circulation. Beside the plasmatic system a glandular kallikrein-kinin system is also known. Bradykinin is a nonapeptide which is normally inactivated within seconds in plasma by kininase I which is carboxypeptidase N_1, the same enzyme inactivating C5a and C3a, and kininase II (angiotensin-converting enzyme, ACE). It must be noted that only the degradation products of kininase II are completely inactive. The *in vivo* activities of kinins include vasodilation with consecutive reduction in blood pressure, diuresis, natriuresis, stimulation of vascular permeability, and induction of inflammatory hyperemia, edema and pain (19). The dose of bradykinin which is needed to decrease blood pressure by approximately 20% can be reduced by two orders of magnitude in the presence of an ACE-inhibitor, like Captopril or Lisinopril (19). Therefore, bradykinin is believed to be involved in regulation of the blood pressure. Its generation during haemodialysis has been suggested to play a role in hypersensitivity reactions during haemodialysis and might be particularly dangerous for patients receiving ACE-inhibitors. This issue will be discussed in greater detail in a later section. Bradykinin acts through binding to β2-receptors whereas the degradation product of kininase I, desArg9-bradykinin binds to β1-receptors. In recent years, although specific β2-receptor antagonists have been developed (19), no β1-receptor antagonists are available. As discussed in (19) several studies on the effects of β2-receptor antagonists have been published without providing conclusive evidence on the role of bradykinin in endotoxin shock.

Cytokine-inducing, bacteria-derived products

A number of microbial products may have clinical relevance for the outcome of the haemodialysis therapy. They may enter the patient's blood stream via the vascular access or through the dialyzer membrane. Endotoxin is the best described class of products of microbial origin. Its outstanding clinical importance comes from the property to act as the prime initiator of sepsis (20). Endotoxins can be encountered by the host in several forms, e.g., as whole bacteria, bacterial fragments, or in the form of aggregated or monodispersed molecules, resulting in a variety of sizes and molecular masses. Endotoxins are lipopolysaccha-

rides (LPS) derived from the outer membranes of Gram-negative bacteria. They are a class of substances having a well defined structure which can, nevertheless, be highly complex and variable depending on the bacterial strain it is derived from. The simplest LPS-structures contain lipid A linked to a diglucosamine (2-keto-3-deoxyoctonic acid or KDO). More complex LPS-molecules also contain other complex oligosaccharide structures linked to KDO. Further information on LPS-structures can be found in (21). LPS is known to activate monocytes, neutrophils, platelets, endothelial cells, epithelial cells and B-cells (22).

Probably the key-consequence of the action of LPS is the release of cytokines, e.g., of TNF-alpha and IL-1 from monocytes and endothelial cells mediating a number of clinical relevant events, such as fever and hypotension. Several possibilities exist to block the effects of either endotoxins or of subsequent mediators, such as IL-1β. They include lipid A antagonists and LPS-binding protein (like the bactericidal/permeability-increasing protein (BPI)), inhibitors of IL-1 synthesis, inhibitors of enzymes involved in intracellular IL-1 processing or IL-1-release from cells, such as the IL-1β converting enzyme (ICE), anti-IL-1 antibodies or soluble IL-1 receptors and anti-IL-1 receptor antibodies or IL-1 receptor antagonists (22, 23). Unlike agents reducing IL-1 activity, the use of endotoxin antagonists would provide a more direct proof of the pathological role of endotoxins in morbid conditions and in infections of haemodialysis patients.

CLINICAL ASPECTS – ACUTE EFFECTS

Immediate symptomatology

Patients on haemodialysis are frequently symptomatic. Symptoms include cramps, nausea and vomiting, headache, chest pain, back pain, itching, pruritus, fever and chills. Their etiology is multifactorial and often in so far unclear, as symptoms may be caused by several different modalities associated with the dialysis procedure.

Hypersensitivity reactions are acute and dangerous complications of haemodialysis. They can best be characterized by the fact that they occur within minutes after the onset of dialysis. As a general rule, immediate symptomatology can be related to anaphylaxis and allergy, whereas symptoms occurring much later during the dialysis procedure are less obviously of an allergic nature. Immediate symptoms may involve symptoms of variable severity, involving several organs. Severe reactions are often associated with hypotension, tachycardia, heavy dyspnea, shock, respiratory and cardiac arrest.

Role of IgE-antibodies

A series of mechanisms need to be considered to explain hypersensitivity reactions during haemodialysis. First, the involvement of classical type I or IgE-mediated type of reactions was clearly identified. IgE-antibodies against the common sterilant for medical products, ethylene oxide (ETO), have been found in many patients on dialysis (24–28). As a rough estimation, 70% of severe reactions are associated with a high titer of IgE-antibodies against ethylene oxide (25). Severe reactions are associated, among others, with one of the following symptoms: bronchospasm, cyanosis, laryngeal edema, shock, respiratory arrest, cardiac arrest. Hypotension, as a consequence of type I reactions, has been observed relatively often, in some other cases hypertension. Further studies, which were focused on specific IgE, have found only a minor role of potential allergens other than ETO, like isocyanates, phthalates, etc (25, 29, 35).

Role of complement fragments

Since most of the reactions reported in the 1980s were observed with dialyzers containing new membranes made from unmodified regenerated cellulose, complement activation, and the anaphylatoxins C5a and C3a were therefore made responsible for the so-called 'first-use syndromes', in particular since re-used cellulosic membranes did not show complement activation (30). In 1980, it was proposed that elevated plasma-C5a is associated with acute respiratory distress syndrome (ARDS) and the measurements of C5a had a diagnostic value (31). In contrast to the aforementioned recommendation, it was concluded in a follow-up study that measurement of anaphylatoxins does not provide additional information relating to the status or prognosis of the patients' injury (32).

In a later study, the cardiopulmonary effects of C5adesArg were studied in a swine model (33). Animal studies in general and swine in particular are very problematic because of pronounced species-related differences in the activities of anaphylatoxins. Porcine-C5a is approximately 10-fold more active than human C5a (7). Human-C5a is about 1000-fold more active compared to human C5adesArg, whereas porcine C5adesArg is about 1000-fold more active than human C5adesArg (7). These differences may be explained by the structure of the oligosaccharide moiety of the C5a-molecule, pig-C5a being highly glycosylated compared to human-C5a. The oligosaccharide moiety may protect the peptide chain from the attack of the anaphylatoxin-inactivating enzyme carboxypeptidase N_1. It is of note that in man the permeability and anaphylatoxic effects of the C5a molecule are believed to be more rigorously controlled by this protease than in animals (7, 34).

Support for the role of anaphylatoxins in hypersensitivity reactions came from a clinical study of Hakim (30). Patients experiencing symptoms had higher levels of C3a and C5a after 10–15 minutes of beginning haemodialysis with new cellulosic membranes comparet to patients without symptoms dialyzed with the same material. However, this study examined only 6 patients with symptoms, 2 patients during cardiopulmonary collapse and 10 patients without symptoms. Although it is impossible to perform a controlled prospective study of anaphylactic reactions, based on the number of patients involved, there is some justification to consider this study being of limited value. It is of note that all dialyzers in this study, including new ones, were stored in 2% formaldehyde and rinsed with a minimal volume of saline before use, resulting in the possibility that a formaldehyde allergic effect might have been involved (35). In addition, whereas the C3a concentration increased from controls for case patient-1 with severe symptoms (collapse), the C3a-value was below the mean of the symptomatic group for case patient-2 with severe symptoms. Moreover, the maximal C5a-value of case 1 was 78.8 ng/ml in contrast to 19.5 ng/ml for case 2, which was even below the mean value of the group without symptoms. It was not entirely clear where the blood from these patients was sampled since in the methods section arterial sampling was described for case 1 and venous sampling for case 2. In the results section, on the other hand, venous sampling is indicated for both. Thus, arteriovenous differences cannot be excluded for the different anaphylatoxin data reported on case patients 1 and 2.

Another inherent weakness of the study is that the possibility of an IgE-mediated reaction was not excluded by measuring IgE-antibodies. A subsequent report suggested that symptomatic, as well as non-symptomatic patients show a wide scatter in response to the complement system seen both by arterial and venous C3a- and C5a-values during dialysis with cellulose membranes (36). This variability, however, was unrelated to symptoms, when 13 patients with a history of anaphylactic reactions were compared with control patients. Furthermore, activities of carboxypeptidase N_1 were found to be comparable in both patient groups. Given the paramount importance of this enzyme for the control of anaphylatoxin-activity of both C3a and C5a (7), it is very difficult to attribute a key role in hypersensitivity reactions to these peptides during haemodialysis. An additional peptidase which may have a role in anaphylatoxin breakdown, namely angiotensin converting enzyme (ACE) will be discussed in more detail below. It is clear, however, that cellulosic membranes do not have an increased rate of hypersensitivity reactions in patients receiving ACE-inhibitors. Thus, ACE does not play a major role in the inactivation of C3a and C5a generated with cellulosic membranes.

In a third clinical study, generation of C3a and C5a in allergic and non-allergic patients ($n = 7$ each) was compared during haemodialysis (37). However, the choice of the patients in this study differed from those in the two other studies mention above. Only patients with mild intradialytic symptoms were included. Atopic patients were selected based on a positive IgE-RAST (RAST: radio-allergo-sorbent test) against three common allergens not related to dialysis and studied with respect to complement activation. Complement activation was more pronounced in atopic compared to non-atopic patients whereas no difference in complement activation between symptomatic and non-symptomatic haemodialysis patients was found.

Thus, this study cannot be used at all to explain allergic symptoms during haemodialysis by complement activation since patients were selected based on laboratory data (IgE-levels) and not on clinical symptomatology. In the earlier studies mentioned (30, 36) patients were selected based on symptoms and patients with severe and less severe reactions were included in both studies. Thus, no further conclusion with regard to severity and reaction mechanisms can be drawn based on these studies. Since both anaphylatoxins are well known to release histamine from basophils (38–40), which in part mediates the systemic effects of anaphylatoxins in animal models a study of histamine release during haemodialysis comparing complement with non-complement activating membranes would be appropriate.

Recently, several hypersensitivity reactions have been described to occur relatively often with re-used membranes as well (41–43). Thus, the basic premise associating new cellulosic membranes as complement-activating materials with symptoms and re-used cellulosic membranes as non-complement-activating membranes with no symptoms, no longer holds. In addition, the incidence of hypersensitivity reactions observed with ethylene-oxide sterilized parallel-plate dialyzers containing a cellulosic membrane was far below the reaction rate of ethylene-oxide sterilized hollow-fiber dialyzers (44, 45). Although both configurations generate comparable amounts of anaphylatoxins (46), but hollow-fiber dialyzers contain large storage pools for ethylene oxide in the potting material (47). These findings can best be explained by allergy against ethylene oxide and not by complement activation.

In conclusion, the majority of severe hypersensitivity cases is mediated by IgE antibodies against ethylene oxide. Since specific inhibitors of anaphylatoxin action are not available, no conclusive proof of their role as mediators of hypersensitivity has been provided. Given the wide distribution of complement activating membranes and since the initial report implicating an involvement of the anaphylatoxins could not be confirmed even by indirect studies, the proof in favor the hypothesis claiming an active role of C3a and C5a in hypersensitivity reactions should be regarded as obsolete.

Role of bradykinin

In 1990, a series of hypersensitivity reactions were described occurring immediately after the first passage of blood through the extracorporeal circuit up to 5 minutes after onset of dialysis (48, 49). Symptoms including nausea, vomiting, severe swelling of the face and laryngeal mucosae, edema, flushing, abdominal cramps, shock, bronchospasm were observed together with severe hypotension. Antibodies of the IgE-type and specifically against ethylene oxide could not be found, thereby excluding the possibility of an IgE-mediated reaction. There was no increase observed in C3a or histamine levels across the dialyzer (50). Common to all of these reports

and subsequent ones (51, 52) was the combined use of an AN69 membrane dialyzer. Symptoms did not occur when the PAN dialyzer was changed to another membrane (e.g., Hemophag® (49)) or when the intake of ACE inhibitors was discontinued (52). Recently, in contrast to earlier reports with ETO-sterilized dialyzers similar reactions have been described with gamma-sterilized polymethylmethacrylate (PMMA) membranes (53). With regard to the ACE-inhibitor it was a class-specific effect including drugs with low and high half life since reactions were reported to occur with both types. Originally two explanations were postulated for the reactions, namely contamination of dialysate with microbial products (48) and the bradykinin-hypothesis as follows (49). After contact activation at the negatively charged membrane surface, bradykinin is released from high-molecular weight kininogen by kallikrein. Normally, bradykinin is rapidly inactivated by kininase I and kinase II (ACE) but not in the presence of an ACE-inhibitor. Several arguments speak against dialysate-derived endotoxin as cause of these reactions. Against initial findings, reactions were not only observed during haemodialysis but also during haemofiltration, when no dialysate is in contact with membrane (52, 54, 55).

Second, endotoxins are not known to induce hypersensitivity reactions of the immediate type (56). In addition, in these hypersensitivity episodes, no febrile reactions were demonstrated. Certain technical maneuvers have been described to avoid this reaction. A particular rinsing procedure (57) separating the first contact with blood from dialysate theoretically allows protein coating of the membrane to occur prior to a possible transfer of endotoxins across the membrane. The protein coating would then protect the blood from the endotoxin by preventing its passage through the membrane. Finally, it was reported that reactions can be prevented by alkaline rinsing (58), or by the use of a calcium concentration of 3.5 mEq/l in the dialysate (62). At present, it is too early to draw any conclusions with regard to the clinical practice or reaction mechanisms based on these reports.

Several lines of evidence, including *in vitro* (59), animal (60) and clinical work (50, 61), support the bradykinin hypothesis. It was found in *in vitro* experiments that upon incubation of several membranes with blood or plasma, bradykinin can be generated. Generation is dependent on membrane type and on the presence of an ACE-inhibitor (59). *In vitro* low amounts of bradykinin are measured with AN69 in the absence of an ACE-inhibitor. Presence of an ACE-inhibitor leads to a concentration dependent increase of bradykinin observed (Figure 2) (59).

During dialysis with PAN-membranes (AN69) in sheep receiving ACE-inhibitors, four of six animals had anaphylactic reactions and a fall in blood pressure was observed within 10 minutes after onset (60). Increased plasma levels of bradykinin with a peak at 5 minutes were measured in the presence and absence of ACE-inhibitors (Figure 3) (60). The higher bradykinin-levels in the presence of an

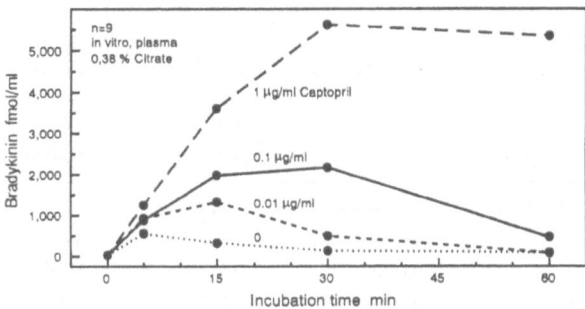

Figure 2. *In vitro* bradykinin accumulation in plasma induced by AN69 membranes depends on the dose of ACE-inhibitors. Data are means of 9 measurements.

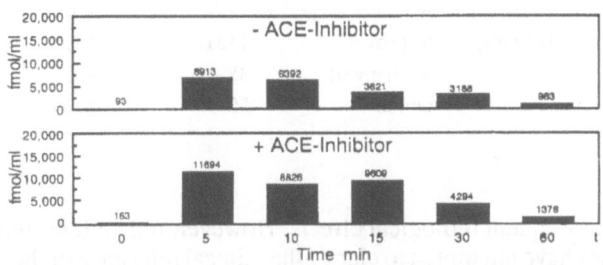

Figure 3. Bradykinin generation observed in an animal model with sheep ($n = 6$) during haemodialysis with AN69 membranes. Bradykinin levels can be attributed to anaphylactoid reactions associated with a fall in blood pressure within 10 minutes. Bradykinin concentrations rise even in the absence of an ACE-inhibitor, as it has to be postulated, if the mechanism follows the contact phase cascade initiated by negatively charged surfaces. In the presence of ACE-inhibitors, bradykinin degradation is reduced, consequently of higher plasma levels are observed (adapted from (60)).

ACE-inhibitor are explained by a reduced degradation rate of this peptide following ACE-inhibition. A control PAN-membrane in the presence of ACE-inhibition neither led to hypersensitivity reactions nor to the generation of bradykinin in these animal studies. Further studies are planned to block the symptoms observed in sheep by a bradykinin receptor antagonist.

In clinical dialysis plasma bradykinin concentrations were measured during the time course of reactions, they were elevated and correlated with symptoms (50, 61). Moreover, patients having a reaction associated with severe hypotension displayed higher bradykinin plasma levels compared to reactive patients without a fall in blood pressure. Membrane differences could be established *in vivo* with patients not treated with ACE-inhibitors (50). Episodes of hypersensitivity were also observed in patients treated with an AN69 dialyzer without ACE-inhibition and high concentrations of plasma-bradykinin were measured (48, 51, 61). Hypersensitivity reactions have been described during single use and during reuse of dialyzers with either hypochlorite, hydrogen peroxide or

peracetic acid (41, 48). Six reactions were associated with the use of ACE-inhibitors and polysulfone membranes, whereas three reactions were observed with patients on cellulose acetate membranes and ACE-inhibitor therapy (41). When reuse practice was discontinued hypersensitivity reactions disappeared. In a demographic survey, 32 of 1290 centers reported hypersensitivity reactions during re-use. The etiology of the reaction was clearly multifactorial. Since no information on ACE-inhibitor intake of these patients was available, the possible mechanism of these reactions remains uncertain. Probably the most intriguing feature of the hypersensitivity reactions described is their sporadic incidence which suggests the complete mechanism explaining the 'bradykinin-hypersensitivity reaction' still remains to be elucidated. Similar reactions have been reported incriminating bradykinin as a mediator involved in reactions on LDL-apheresis with negatively charged dextran sulfate columns (63–64) and during venom immunotherapy (65).

Role of endotoxins

Hypersensitivity reactions have also been observed with non-cellulosic membranes e.g. made from polyacrylonitrile (66–68) or polysulfone (69). Permeation of endotoxins has been implicated in the etiology of these reactions (48, 57, 67–69). Indeed, epidemiological data indicate a strong relationship between the use of high-flux membranes and pyrogenic reactions (70). As outlined above at least the reactions with negatively charged polyacrylonitrile membranes can alternatively be explained by a bradykinin-mediated mechanism. In addition, it is hardly possible that the hypothetical endotoxin effect is mediated by IL-1 since release of this cytokine by monocytes and other cell types requires protein synthesis, i.e., at least 30–60 minutes. Therefore, a mediation of anaphylactic shock on a time scale of minutes by endotoxins and IL-1 remains speculative and not in line with the complete lack of reports involving endotoxins or other microbial products in hypersensitivity reactions (56). However, chronic effects of these substances are well possible, as can be concluded from the observation that antibodies against endotoxin were found in patients dialyzed with high-flux membranes (71). Some publications relate the chronic effect of amyloidosis to contaminated dialysate (72, 73). According to these findings, β2-m serum levels can be reduced (72) and amyloidosis at least postponed by the use of ultrapure dialysate (73). In addition, vascular stability and related blood pressure effects can be related to the presence of endotoxins in dialysate, as proposed by the interleukin hypothesis (74).

Recent data have proven the validity of this hypothesis in showing that the systemic vascular resistance index decreases during haemodialysis with high-flux AN69 membranes, whereas it remained constant during haemofiltration with the same membrane (Figure 4, (75)). It was concluded that it is unlikely that a direct

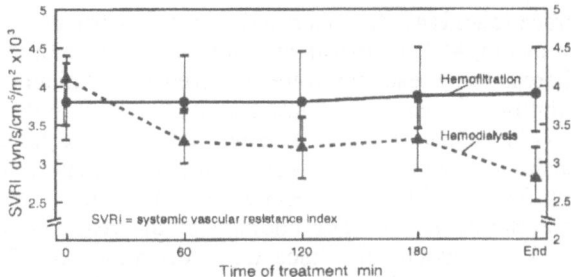

Figure 4. Systemic vascular resistance index (SVRI) observed during haemofiltration and haemodialysis with high-flux PAN (AN69) membranes. Levels of SVRI fall during haemodialysis and not during haemofiltration. This finding possibly indicates a transfer of dialysate contaminants to the blood stream. Following the interleukin hypothesis (74), the generation of cytokines due to stimulation of monocytes and granulocytes by bacterial products may result in hypotension (adapted from (75)).

Table 1. Frequency of symptoms produced by chronic hemodialysis treatments in various studies. Modified from (80)

Symptoms	% of treatments $n = 185,227$	% of patients $n = 709$
Hypotension	31.3	58.7
Muscle cramps	12.5	63.0
Nausea	8.8	23.7
Itching	1.3	25.3
Vomiting	3.8	16.0
Headache	5.5	36.0
Restlessness	0.3	7.7
Chest pain	0.8	11.3
Back pain	0.4	4.3
Fever	0.1	2.3
Chills	0.1	2.7
Hypertension	4.3	19.0
Tiredness	11.0	

blood-membrane contact could account for the disparate haemodynamic responses. It remained plausible, however, that exposure of blood cells to dialysate contaminants may generate vasoactive mediators, such as IL-1, thereby contributing to haemodynamic instability during haemodialysis (75, 76). An adequate measure to improve both, vascular stability and the occurence of amyloidosis, would therefore be the use of an ultrafilter for cleaning up dialysate (76–79).

General intradialytic symptomatology

As reviewed in detail in the previous section, numerous studies have shown that bioincompatible membranes activate the alternative pathway of complement with possible

Table 2. Symptoms scored after dialysis compared to pre-dialysis rating (number of patients). Modified from (83)

Symptoms		% of patients $(n = 709)$	
		Cuprophan	Polysulfone
Headache	improved	3.7	7.9
	unchanged	81.1	81.7
	worse	15.2	10.4
Pruritus	improved	5.5	9.2
	unchanged	82.3	75.6
	worse	12.2	15.2
Nausea	improved	3.1	0.6
	unchanged	95.1	96.3
	worse	1.8	3.1
Well-being	improved	11.0	11.6
	unchanged	38.4	26.8
	worse	50.6	81.6

consequent biological effects. However, only a few studies have attempted to clarify the clinical relevance of these phenomena. The pathophysiology of intradialytic symptomatology has recently been reviewed (80). Acute symptoms are common with a mean frequency of one symptom per patient per dialysis treatment (81). Typical symptoms and their frequency of occurrence are listed in Table 1 (80). Several authors claimed that there is an increase in dialysis hypotension and intradialytic symptomatology when complement activating membranes are used (e.g., 30, 82). However, more controlled prospective studies have failed to confirm these earlier claims. In a multicenter, double-blind clinical study conducted by the Bergamo collaborative dialysis study group (83) 428 chronic haemodialysis patients were divided into two matching groups. High-flux polysulfone and low-flux Cuprophan® dialyzers were manufactured to look alike and were compared regarding their effects on the occurrence of acute clinical symptoms. The main focus of this study was the number of episodes of intradialytic hypotension, defined as a blood pressure fall of at least 25 mmHg systolic and 10 mmHg diastolic accompanied by general discomfort and requiring some form of therapeutic intervention. The second focus was the occurrence of subjective symptoms, such as headache, nausea, pruritus and worsening of general well-being. These symptoms were scored by the patients on a scale from 1 to 10. Overall 71 hypotensive episodes occurred, 32 in the Cuprophan® group and 39 in the polysulfone group. Table 2 (83) summarizes the subjective symptoms scored after dialysis compared to the pre-dialysis rating. No statistically significant difference was observed in the distribution of scores or in the pre-post dialysis changes. Another similar study addressed the same topic in a randomized, prospective, crossover clinical study with large surface area dialyzers

(84). Here, PAN membranes were used as the high-flux alternative to Cuprophan®. Once again focus was put on hypotension and other acute symptoms. The incidence of hypotension and of intradialytic symptoms did not differ with the membrane type. The authors concluded that biocompatible membranes do not reduce the acute complications of dialysis (84). Similar findings have been reported in acute studies of chronic patients dialyzed with Cuprophan® and high-flux, non-complement activating membranes (85). Thus, in summary, it would appear that the use of a biocompatible membrane does not influence clinical effects. These observation reinforce the doubt that complement activation via the alternative pathway plays a major role in acute dialysis symptomatology.

Hypoxemia

Routine haemodialysis with either bicarbonate or acetate buffered dialysate is accompanied by the development of a certain degree of hypoxemia (86–88). Arterial oxygen tension (PaO$_2$) begins to decrease within minutes after the onset of dialysis and persists for as long as dialysis is continued (86, 89, 90). As one underlying mechanism for this effect it was suggested that complement activating cellulosic membranes induce transient leukopenia with leukoctyes trapped in the microvasculature of the lungs (2). Intrapulmonary leukostasis followed by the release of lysosomal enzymes and vasoactive mediators from activated granulocytes is then made responsible for the increase in alveolar arterial oxygen gradient and hypoxemia (88). However, kinetics of leukopenia and hypoxemia differ, as leukopenia is transient and cell-counts return to nearly normal within 60 minutes of dialysis (2, 91, 92). In addition, a reflux of leukocytes from the lungs to the blood circulation was found when analyzing leukocytes, which had been labeled with 111-Indium prior to haemodialysis (91, 92).

Hypoxemia is also observed with non-complement activating membranes, such as polyacrylonitrile (PAN, (90)), polymethylmethacrylate (PMMA, (89)) and polysulfone (PSu, (93)). These membranes induce either a limited or no leukopenia, but hypoxemia is observed, if they are simultaneously used with acetate dialysate. Alternatively to dialysis membranes, the major cause of hypoxemia can therefore be attributed to alveolar hypoventilation, subsequent to the loss of carbondioxide in the dialysate (CO$_2$-unloading) during acetate-buffered dialysis (94–96). This is supported by findings showing that hypoxemia is absent independent of the type of membrane used, if the loss of CO$_2$/HCO$_3^-$ in the dialysate is prevented, e.g., by using HCO$_3^-$ (bicarbonate) dialysate (89, 90, 93). Therefore, the effect of hypoxemia as a consequence of dialyzer biocompatibility must be considered to be overestimated in the past.

Acute renal failure and dialysis membranes

Exposure to complement-activating cellulosic dialysis membranes was claimed to adversely affect the course of acute renal failure (ARF), both in animals (97) and in dialysis patients (98, 99). Thus, the controversy of the ideal dialysis membrane is transposed from chronic renal failure into the acute form of the disease. Such a transposition should be met with vehement skepticism, as a subtle and pervasive change in dialysis prescription during therapy of ARF is observed. Furthermore, relating patient outcome in ARF solely to a single factor such as the membrane, overestimates membrane consequences, and implies a wide spectrum of simplifications. The limitations of the single parameter model are particularly true when its evaluation is fraught with methodological problems.

This may be supported by analysing a recent paper related to ARF in rats. Whilst comparing Cuprophan® with PAN (AN69) membranes the authors concluded that the use of Cuprophan® delays the resolution of the acute renal failure (98). Although the aim of this animal trial was to study the effects of blood exposure to differing dialysis membranes during treatment of ARF, dialysis *per se* is never performed, rather blood conditioned by incubation in minidialyzers is injected. Further, the time of injection does not correspond to real clinical situations as the conditioned blood is injected during the induction phase of ARF, a situation clearly different from the clinical use of the therapy. Recent studies, using real dialysis in rats after induction of acute renal failure, have proven that dialysis had no effect on the severity or degree and rates of recovery from ARF (100). In this study three different complement and non-complement activating membranes were used and no difference was found between the various membrane groups and a control group of undialyzed animals.

A preliminary clinical study report claims to support the hypothesis that synthetic membranes improve patient survival and shows a reduced hospitalization compared to cellulosic membranes (98). This report uses the APACHE II system to assure clinical comparability, although this score does not correct for different etiologies in ARF, nor does it adequately cover all indices presumed to have prognostic value in the syndrome (101). The raw APACHE II score is only one factor in an exponential equation which must be solved prior to determining a given mortality risk. One must conclude therefore that the validity of studies which support equal randomization by the use of the unadjusted APACHE II score must be reevaluated.

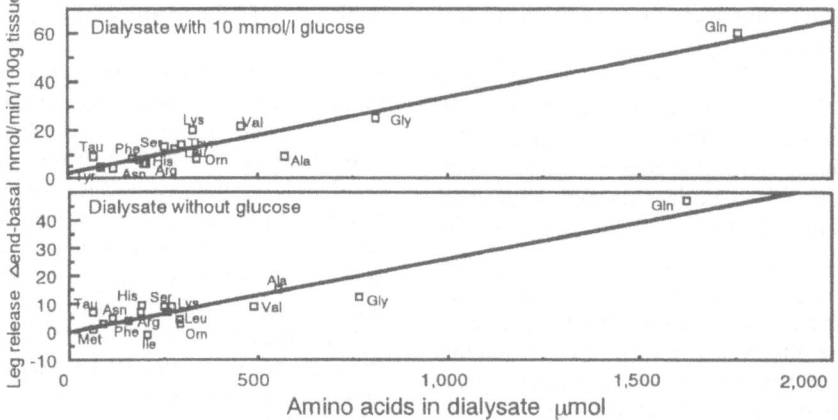

Figure 5. Loss of amino acids into the dialysate. Under conditions of clinical dialysis in chronic dialysis patients, protein catabolism, as judged by amino acid leg muscle release, correlated with amino acid-loss in the dialysate. About 8 g of free amino acids were found in the dialysate independent of its glucose content. Thus, a substantial amount of amino acids must have been released from the tissues to compensate for the gradual decline in the extracellular amino acid levels due to its loss into dialysate (adapted from (117)).

CLINICAL ASPECTS – CHRONIC EFFECTS

Protein catabolism and dialysis membranes

Malnutrition is an important risk factor for haemodialysis patients (102, 103) and a strong association between low serum levels of albumin and increased mortality has been established (103). The most important and convincing evidence for the role of membrane bioincompatibility and its clinical relevance has related to the observation that in the normal subject exposed to a Cuprophan® dialysis membrane without dialysate (sham-dialysis), there was a significant increase in leg muscle protein catabolism, investigated as such by the release of the branched chain essential amino acids, tyrosine, phenylalanine and 5-methylhistidine into the femoral venous blood stream (104, 105).

It has been demonstrated that interaction between blood and cellulosic membranes induces release of elastase and other granulocytic enzymes (106, 107). However, since catabolic granulocytic enzymes are rapidly inactivated in plasma (106), it is doubtful that they can have a generalized effect on protein turnover. In addition, apart from complement C5a-formation, blood-membrane interaction during sham-dialysis is considered to cause the release of other factors which directly or indirectly may induce catabolism of muscle protein. One such factor is interleukin-1 (IL-1). The induction of protein catabolism due to interleukin-1 seems to take place by way of a local release of prostaglandin E_2 in skeletal muscle, which in turn stimulates lysosomal protein degradation (108), this effect being blocked by the administration of indomethacin.

Interleukin-1 is synthesized and released by monocytes after stimulation by pyrogens (109). Furthermore, recent observations have shown that the concentrations of IL-1 are elevated in dialysis patients treated with either acetate dialysate (110) or dialysate contaminated with endotoxins (111, 112). Exotoxins derived from Pseudomonas aeruginosa bacteria are also able to induce interleukin-1 production in macrophages (113). However, during sham-dialysis no dialysate flow is used, such that here, endotoxins or acetate from this source could not have contributed to monocyte activation. Utilizing partially purified human interleukin-1, Baracos et al. (108) showed that IL-1 induces protein breakdown, which could not be reproduced in later experiments with recombinant interleukin-1 (114). This casts doubt on the impact of interleukin-1 on protein breakdown and favors the influence of complement C5a. The notion is further supported by the finding in a rat model that zymosan-activated serum and endotoxin injections, each of which may activate the alternate pathway of complement, produced a dramatic increase in dialysate protein concentration (115). Furthermore, C5a does not induce interleukin-1 generation in human monocytes in the absence of endotoxin contamination (13). Such an increased amino acid release was not seen in sham dialysis with non-C5a-generating, socalled biocompatible membranes, made from PAN or PSu (116). However, when similar studies were repeated in chronic haemodialysis patients under conditions of clinical dialysis and with the passage of dialysate, protein catabolism, as judged by amino acid leg muscle release, correlated with amino acid-loss in the dialysate during dialysis with a cellulose acetate membrane (Figure 5, (117)). About 8 g of free amino acids were found in the dialysate independent of its glucose content. Thus, a substantial amount of amino acids must have been released from the tissues to compensate for the gradual decline in the extracellular amino acid levels due to its loss into dialysate.

Similar results we reported using ^{13}C-leucine as a marker for protein metabolism during Cuprophan® haemodialysis in chronic dialysis patients (118, 119). These studies also showed that the protein breakdown in chronic dialysis patients was not different from that in controls. As the studies of Gutierrez et al. (117) and Lim et al. (119) show a direct relationship between low molecular weight amino acid-loss and protein catabolism, it seems difficult to impute a specific role of a complement activating membrane to the situation in the dialysis patient. One explanation for the apparent absence of a measurable C5a-related effect in the chronic dialysis patient, as compared to the healthy normal, is the known blockage or down-regulation effect for C5a-receptors following chronic repeated stimulus of cells by C5a (120). These observations cast doubt on the meaningfulness of the limited observations of reduced protein catabolic rates seen with PAN-membrane compared to Cuprophan® in a small number of chronic haemodialysis patients (121).

Infection

Numerous studies have adressed an increased infection rate in haemodialysis and its relation to death (122). Excellent and recent reviews are available which summarise the data available on infection in extracorporeal circulation (123–127). Apart from the epidemiological data, the mechanisms relating death on haemodialysis to sepsis as a consequence of membrane involvement are uncertain. The problem underlying the analysis of a single variable suggests that the membrane in the complex field of the ESRD patient on dialysis and his susceptibility of infection permits bias to dominate.

For instance, the recent reports of a prospective study on white blood cell function in two populations dialyzed with either Cuprophan® or polysulfone dialyzers noted in a single paragraph that three out of eight patients on the Cuprophan® membrane developed an episode of sepsis over a follow-up period of 20 weeks. On the other hand, none of the control group of 8 patients on polysulfone showed similar effects after the same period. No further details are given. However, this poorly detailed regime is held to be the clinical evidence for the predisposition of Cuprophan® to facilitate sepsis in haemodialysis patients. Epidemiological studies on large numbers of patients (122, 128) have not adressed the impact of dialysis membranes on infection as a cause of death till today, further prospective studies are, therefore, needed to draw a clearcut conclusion.

Dialysis membranes and β2-microglobulin (β2-m)

The pathogenesis of β2-microglobulin amyloidosis remains uncertain. Elevated β2-m serum levels due to chronic retention of this protein in the presence of renal failure is probably the main causative factor. The role, played by the dialysis membrane in the pathogenesis of β2-m amyloidosis, however, is controversial. In *vivo* evidence has suggested that PAN-membranes (129–131) may delay the clinical onset of amyloidosis. However, the mechanism underlying this finding is completely unknown. Therefore, in the absence of precise diagnostic methodology and the lack of causal mechanisms the clinical asertion of a dialyzer membrane superiority must remain scientifically in doubt until prospective studies are available.

Attempts in *vitro* to incriminate the cellulosic membrane as a causative factor for β2-m amyloidosis by suggesting an increase in β2-m generation originate from the observation that the uncorrected plasma levels of this protein rise during a Cuprophan® dialysis (132). This phenomenon has been completely explained as an artifact neglecting the differential shift of water during haemodialyis with weight loss. Correction for this effect has shown that there is no real increase in circulating β2-m mass during a haemodialysis with Cuprophan® (133) or other low-flux, β2-m impermeable membranes. Furthermore, no increase in synthetic rate for β2-m was found in patients dialyzed with Cuprophan® dialyzers compared to high-flux polysulfone (F60), PAN (AN69) dialyzers, CAPD-patients or normal controls (134–136, 144, Table 3).

The failure to demonstrate an in *vivo* effect from cellulosic membranes has not deterred research in *vitro* from attempting to show a stimulatory effect of the cellulosic membrane on a white cell production of β2-m. Zaoui et al. (137) reported on an increased synthesis of β2-m in cell cultures of peripheral blood mononuclear cells (PBMNC) which were obtained from patients after dialysis with cellulosic membranes. Membrane-induced cytokine-or complement C5a-generation were considered to act as a stimulus on PBMNCs. Similar data were observed (138) when mononuclear cells were contacted with cellulosic membranes. In these experiments, increased synthesis of β2-m was related to the generation of the late complement complex, C5b-9 by cellulosic membranes. Finally, it was claimed that lymphocytes from healthy donors, incubated with Cuprophan®, showed an increase in β2-m mRNA (139).

However, other work has not confirmed these claims (140–143), as an incubation of PBMNCs with Cuprophan® did not increase β2-m production. It is possible that poorly controlled endotoxin contamination of the cell incubation media in the positive reports could explain the discrepancy. It may be concluded that in the absence of prospective studies, there is a lack of evidence to confirm the role of a membrane dependent mechanism for β2-m amyloidosis.

Mortality

It has recently been suggested that an improved survival rate for ESRD patients can be obtained with the use of dia-

Table 3. *In vivo* data on the synthetic rate of β2-microglobulin in normal, CAPD and end stage renal disease patients. Adapted from (129)

Subjects		Treatment	HD Membrane	β2-m Synthetic rate		Authors
				Median	Range	
Normals	$(n = 6)$	–	–	3.0	2.6 to 4.3	Karlson 1980
Normals	$(n = 2)$	–	–	1.9	1.6 and 2.2	Vincent 1980
Normals	$(n = 5)$	–	–	2.5	1.7 to 3.4	Floege 1991
Normals	$(n = 5)$	–	–	4.0	2.2 to 5.7	Vincent 1992
Uraemics	$(n = 2)$	HD	?	2.7	2.5 and 2.8	Odell 1991
Uraemics	$(n = 5)$	HD	Cuprophan	2.9	2.5 to 4.4	Floege 1991
Uraemics	$(n = 5)$	HD	Cuprophan	5.8	3.0 to 9.1	Vincent 1992
Uraemics	$(n = 5)$	HD	Cuprophan	3.3	2.8 to 4.9	Odell 1991
Uraemics	$(n = 5)$	HD	PAN	6.2	1.2 to 7.0	Vincent 1992
Uraemics	$(n = 1)$	HD	PMMA	–	4.5	Floege 1991
Uraemics	$(n = 5)$	HD	PSu	2.6	2.2 to 3.2	Floege 1991
Uraemics	$(n = 4)$	HF	PSu	2.1	1.9 to 3.4	Vincent 1992
Uraemics	$(n = 3)$	CAPD	–	3.0	2.2 to 8.9	Vincent 1992

All differences in the studies of Floege and Vincent not significant by ANOVA. HD: haemodialysis; HF: haemofiltration; PSu: polysulfone; PAN: polyacrylonitrile (AN69); PMMA: polymethylmethacrylate; β2-m Synthetic rate in mg/kgBW/day.

lyzers with non-complement activating membranes such as polysulfone and AN69 (145–148). In addition there has been a suggestion that there is a better survival from acute renal failure when non-complement activating membranes were used for dialysis (98). The possibility that the improvement in survival for chronic dialysis relates more to removal of larger molecular weight toxins rather than to less complement activation is suggested by use of the term high-flux dialyzer (145). In so far as membrane properties are being associated with outcome paramenters such as mortality, it seems appropriate to discuss the scientific correctness of these associations. The majority of reports are still in abstract form (98, 145, 146, 149) and hence hard to evaluate in detail. Nevertheless, the following criticisms seem applicable. Most of the studies were retrospective and the control group of patients was historical. This design necessitates caution in accepting the results uncritically. An historical control does not allow for a center learning effect with the newer test group and for the benefits from advances in technology particular to that group. Thus the comparison of high-flux therapy with a low-flux historical control (145) never evaluated the role of dialysate buffer. The most important uncontrolled variable could be the nutritional status of the patient which is a key factor in survival (150). The historical control group was mainly dialyzed with acetate and the high-flux group received bicarbonate dialysis. The better correction of acidosis achieved with bicarbonate reduces the net efflux of essential branched chain amino acids from the muscle and thus improves the nutritional status of the patient by reducing protein catabolism (151).

In addition, the improved vascular stability resulting from the use of volumetric controlled dialysate delivery systems for high-flux dialysis in addition to bicarbonate dialysate might well improve the tolerence to dialysis and ultimately survival. The improvement in appetite reported with erythropoietin therapy would also help the nutritional status of the patient.

The prospective studies on the membrane effect on survival are limited. One recent study quoted an annual mortality of 7% for patients treated with high-flux dialysis compared to 20% for conventional dialysis patients (148). However, patients with extreme interdialytic weight gains were excluded from the high-flux group only suggesting that a biased selection criteria may have influenced the outcome. A planned prospective study sponsored by the National Institute of Health (NIH, (152)) will compare mortality in high and low-flux membrane groups. However, the design of this study can be critised as reuse of the membranes will be permitted and it is known that chemical reprocessing of certain high-flux membranes affects the removal rates of large molecules in a variable fashion (153–155). Furthermore, the design of the study fails to distinguish between the hypothesis that low mortality rates are associated with increased removal of large molecular weight substances and the hypothesis that they are associated with activation of the complement system. The same critism applies to another planned prospective study with similar aims, but putting more emphasis on bicompatibility (the complement system) (156). The design of this study can be further criticised as it will cover a period of only 18 months which may not be sufficient to allow conclusions about mortality. Results on the role of complement activation are additionally compromised due to the fact that again all dialyzers will be reused, and a distinction between complement activating and non-complement activating membranes is then very difficult (81, 157).

The suggestion that membrane characteristics play a role in recovery from acute renal failure stems from a clinical study whose results have as yet only been published in abstract form (98), and is cowry to the established view that mortality in acute renal failure usually depends on the course of the underlying disease. The preliminary nature of these results does not permit a detailed critical evaluation. However, use of the uncorrected APACHE II score to assure comparability of the two groups is inadequate as it does not correct for different etiologies or cover all indices presumed to have prognostic value in acute renal failure (101).

The best longterm survival data in the world for haemodialysis have been reported by Tassin. The patient survival rate was 87% at five years, 75% at ten years, 55% at fifteen years and 43% at twenty years (158). The authors attribute their outstanding survival rates to long hours of dialysis with excellent blood pressure control without the use of anti-hypertensive drugs. It is of interest that they use exclusively the complement activating bioincompatible membrane Cuprophan®. This suggests that the membrane is less important than the dose of dialysis which includes urea removal capacity and the time of dialysis. Similar, results emphasising improved survival by increasing the dose of dialysis with Cuprophan® membranes has been reported (159). These data contradict the assertion that Cuprophan® complement activation membranes are associated with an increased mortality (160).

CONCLUSIONS

If it is accepted that haemodialysis therapy for end-stage renal disease still requires an empirical approach, even after 30 years of experience, it is clear that the proof of clinical relevance of biochemical changes occurring as the consequence of blood-dialyzer interaction will continue to remain controversial. Furthermore, although survival by haemodialysis now exceeds thirty years, the long-term survivors are not normal. Indeed, they give the impression of having lost body mass and perhaps have aged too fast. In addition, acute intradialytic symptomatology continues to hinder rehabilitation and often affects the quality of life of the patient. Thus, there is no doubt that haemodialysis needs to be improved. The questions raised by considering the effects of particular membranes on complement and kinin activation, suggest that while neither is proven on balance it may be desirable to avoid the activation of both systems. In addition, it is clearly desirable to reduce or eliminate the bacterial content of dialysate. The easi-

est way to do this is with an ultrafilter. Finally, a realistic approach would suggest that all three effector systems can be minimised. However, as long as economical questions are relevant, the cost benefit of justifying the ultimate in biocompatibility, namely high-flux dialyzers with ultrafiltered dialysate, will remain controversial. In addition, the clinical relevance of these goals still largely remains to be proven.

REFERENCES

1. Kaplow LS, Geoffinet JA: Profound neutropenia during the early phase of haemodialysis. *JAMA* 203: 1135, 1968
2. Craddock PR, Fehr J, Dalmasso AP, Brigham KL, Jakob HS: Hemodialysis leukopenia: pulmonary vascular leukostasis resulting from complement activation of dialyzer cellophane membranes. *J Clin Invest* 59: 979, 1977
3. Foret M, Hachache T, Maftahi H, Milongo R, Kuentz F, Christollet M et al.: The long-term evaluation of the biocompatibility of nine different hemodialysis membranes. *Life Support Systems* 5: 203, 1987
4. Williams DF, ed: *Definitions in Biomaterials*. Elsevier. Amsterdam, 1987.
5. Gurland HJ, Davison AM, Bonomini V et al.: Definitions and terminology in biocompatibility. *Nephrol Dial Transplant* 9 (Suppl 2): 4, 1994
6. Frank MM, Fries LF: The role of complement in inflammation and phagocytosis. *Immunol Today* 12: 322, 1991
7. Hugli TE: Structure and function of the anaphylatoxins. *Springer Seminar Immunopathol* 7: 193, 1984
8. Jose PJ, Forrest MJ, Williams TJ: Human C5a desarg increases vascular permeability. *J Immunol* 127: 2376, 1981
9. Stimler-Gerard NP: Role of the complement anaphylatoxins in inflammation and hypersensitivity reactions in the lung. *Surv Synth Path Res* 4: 423, 1985
10. Marder SR, Chenoweth DE, Goldstein IM et al.: Chemotactic responses of Human Peripheral Blood Monocytes to complement-derived peptides C5a and C5a desarg. *J Immunol* 134: 3325, 1985
11. Haeffner-Cavaillon CN, Cavaillon JM, Laude M, Kazatchkine MD: C3a(C3adesArg) induces production and release of interleukin 1 by cultured human monocytes. *J Immunol* 139: 794, 1987
12. Okusawa S. Dinarello CA, Yancey KB et al.: C5a induction of human interleukin 1. Synergistic effect with endotoxin or interferon-gamma. *J Immunol* 139: 2635, 1987
13. Arend WP, Massoni JR, Niemann MA, Giclas PC: Absence of induction of IL-1 production in human monocytes by complement fragments. *J Immunol* 142: 173, 1989
14. Schindler R, Gelfand JA, Dinarello CA: Recombinant C5a stimulates transcription rather than translation of IL-1 and TNF; translational signal provided by LPS or IL-1 itself. *Blood* 76: 1631, 1990
15. Schindler R, Linnenweber S, Schulze M, Oppermann M, Dinarello C, Shaldon S, Koch KM: Gene expression of interleukin-1S during hemodialysis. *Kidney Int* 43: 712, 1993

16. Schindler R, Lonnemann G, Shaldon S, Koch KM, Dinarello C: Transcription, not synthesis, of interleukin-1 and tumor necrosis factor by complement. *Kidney Int* 37: 85, 1990

17. Cochrane CG, Griffin JH: The biochemistry and pathophysiology of the contact system of plasma. *Adv Immunol* 33: 241, 1982

18. Matsuda T: Biological responses at non-physiological interfaces and molecular design of biocompatible surfaces. *Nephrol Dial Transplant* 4 (Suppl 2): 60, 1989

19. Bönner G: Kallikrein-Kinin systems in shock. in *Handbook of Mediators in Septic Shock*, CRC, Boca Raton, 1993

20. Glauser MP, Zanetti G, Baumgartner JD, Cohen J: Septic shock: pathogenesis. *Lancet* 338: 732, 1991

21. Raetz CRH: Biochemistry of endotoxins. *Ann Rev Biochem* 59: 129, 1990

22. Lynn WA, Golenbrock DT: Lipopolysaccharide antagonists. *Immunol Today* 13: 271, 1992

23. Dinarello CA: Modalities for reducing interleukin 1 activity in disease. *Immunol Today* 14: 260, 1993

24. Dolovich J, Bell B: Allergy to a product(s) of ethylene oxide gas: demonstration of IgE and IgG antibodies and hapten specificity. *J Allergy Clin Immunol* 62: 30, 1978

25. Lemke HD: Mediation of hypersensitivity reactions during hemodialysis by IgE antibodies against ethylene oxide. *Artif Organs* 11: 104, 1987

26. Bommer J, Ritz E: Ethylene oxide (ETO) as a major cause of anaphylactoid reactions in dialysis. *Artif Organs* 11: 111, 1987

27. Rumpf KW, Seubert S, Seubert A et al.: Association of ethylene oxide-induced IgE antibodies with symptoms in dialysis patients. *Lancet* 2 (8469–70): 1385, 1985

28. Grammer LC, Paterson BF, Roxe D et al.: IgE against ethylene oxide-altered human serum albumin in patients with anaphylactic reactions to dialysis. *J Allergy Clin Immunol* 76: 511, 1985

29. Grammer LC, Harris KE, Shaughnessy A et al.: Antibodies to toluene diisocyanate in patients with and without dialysis anaphylaxis. *Art Organs* 15: 2, 1991

30. Hakim RM, Breillatt J, Lazarus M, Port FK: Complement activation and hypersensitivity reactions to dialysis membranes. *N Engl J Med* 311: 878, 1984

31. Hammerschmidt DE, Weaver LJ, Hudson LD, Craddock PR, Jakob HS: Association of complement activation and elevated plasma-C5a with adult respiratory distress syndrome: pathophysiological relevance and possible prognostic value. *Lancet* i: 947, 1980

32. Weinberg PF, Mathay MA, Webster RO, Roskos KV, Goldstein IM, Murray JF: Biological active products of complement and acute lung injury in patients with the sepsis syndrome. *Am Rev Resp Dis* 130: 791, 1984

33. Cheung AK, LeWinter M, Chenoweth DE et al.: Cardiopulmonary effects of cuprophan-activated plasma in the swine. *Kidney Int* 29: 799, 1986

34. Schulman ES, Post TJ, Henson PM, Giclas PC: Differential effects of the complement peptides, C5a and C5a desArg on human basophil and lung mast cell histamine release. *J Clin Invest* 81: 918, 1988

35. Bousquet J, Michel FB: Allergy to formaldehyde and ethylene oxide. *Clin Rev Allergy* 9: 357, 1991

36. Lemke HD, Heidland A, Schaefer RM: Hypersensitivity reactions during hemodialysis: role of complement

37. Röckel A, Klinke B, Hertel J et al.: Allergy to dialysis materials. *Nephrol Dial Transplant* 4: 646, 1989

38. Siraganian RP, Hook WA: Complement-mediated release of histamine from human basophils. II. Mechanism of the histamine release reaction. *J Immunol* 116: 639, 1976

39. Grant JA, Settle L, Whorton EB, Dupree E: Complement-mediated release of histamine from human basophils. III. Biochemical characterization of the reaction. *J Immunol* 117: 450, 1977

40. Farnam J, Grant JA, Lett-Brown MA, Hunt C, Thueson DO, Giclas PC: Complement and IgE-mediated release of histamine from basophils *in vitro*. V. Differential effects of drugs modulating arachidonic acid metabolism. *J Immunol* 134: 541, 1985

41. Pegues DA, Beck-Sague CM, Woollen SW et al.: Anaphylactoid reactions associated with reuse of hollow-fiber hemodialyzers and ACE-inhibitors. *Kidney Int* 42: 1232, 1992

42. US Centers for disease control: Update: acute allergic reactions associated with reprocessed hemodialyzers in the United States, 1989–1990. *Morbid Mortal Weekly Rep* 40: 147, 1991

43. Schmitter L, Sweet S: Anaphylactoid reactions with the addition of hypochlorite to reuse in patients maintained on reprocessed polysulfone hemodialyzers and ACE inhibitors. (Abstract) *ASAIO Transactions* 95, 1993

44. Villaroel F: Incidence of hypersensitivity in hemodialysis. *Artif Organs* 8: 278, 1984

45. Daugirdas JT, Potempa LD, Dinh N, Gandhi VC, Ivanovitch PT, Ing TS: Plate, coil, and hollow-fiber cuprammonium cellulose dialyzers: discrepancy between incidence of anaphylactic reactions and degree of complement activation. *Artif Organs* 11: 140, 1987

46. Schaefer RM, Heidland A, Hörl WH: Effect of dialyzer geometry on granulocyte and complement activation. *Am J Nephrol* 7: 121, 1987

47. Ansorge W, Pelger M, Dietrich W, Baurmeister U: Ethylene oxide residuals in dialyzers after a simulated clinical rinsing procedure. *Artif Organs* 11: 118, 1987

48. Verresen L, Waer M, Vanrentergem Y, Michielsen P: Angiotensin-converting-enzyme inhibitors and anaphylactoid reactions to high-flux membrane dialysis. *Lancet* 336: 1360, 1990

49. Tielemans C, Madhoun P, Lenaers M, Schandene L, Goldman M, Vanherweghem JL: Anaphylactoid reactions during hemodialysis on AN69 membranes in patients receiving ACE inhibitors. *Kidney Int* 38: 982, 1990

50. Verresen L, Fink E, Lemke HD, Vanrenterghem Y: Bradykinin is a mediator of anaphylactoid reactions during hemodialysis with AN69 membranes. *Kidney Int* 45: 1497, 1994

51. Parnes EL, Shapiro WB: Anaphylactoid reactions in hemodialysis patients treated with the AN69 dialyzer. *Kidney Int* 40: 1148, 1991

52. Brunet P, Jaber K, Berland Y, Baz M: Anaphylactoid reactions during hemodialysis and hemofiltration: role of associating AN69 membrane and angiotensin I converting enzyme inhibitors. *Am J Kidney Diseases* 19: 444, 1992

53. Schwarzbeck A, Wittenmeier KW, Hällfritzsch U: Anaphylactoid reactions, angiotensin-converting enzyme inhibitors and extracorporeal hemotherapy. *Nephron* 65: 499, 1993

54. Jadoul M, Struyven J, Stragier A, van Ypersele de Strihou C: Angiotensin-converting-enzyme inhibitors and anaphylactoid reactions to high-flux membrane dialysis. *Lancet* 337: 112, 1991

55. Petrie JJB, Campbell Y, Hawley CM, Hogan PG: Anaphylactoid reactions in patients on hemofiltration with AN69 membrane whilst receiving ACE inhibitors. *Clin Nephrol* 36: 264, 1991

56. Dinarello CA: ACE inhibitors and anaphylactoid reactions to high-flux membrane dialysis. *Lancet* 337: 370, 1991

57. Bigazzi R, Atti M, Baldari G: High-permeable membranes and hypersensitivity-like reactions: role of dialysis fluid contamination. *Blood Purif* 8: 190, 1990

58. Lacour F, Maheut H: AN69 membrane and conversion enzyme inhibitors: prevention of anaphylactic shock by alkaline rinsing. *Nephrol* 13: 135, 1992

59. Lemke HD, Fink E: Accumulation of bradykinin formed by the AN69- or PAN DX-membrane is due to the presence of an ACE inhibitor *in vitro*. (Abstract) *J Am Soc Nephrol* 3: 376, 1992

60. Krieter DH, Lemke HD, Fink E, Bönner G, Grassmann A, You HM, Eisenhauer T: Hemodialysis related anaphylactoid reactions in sheep pretreated with captopril. *Nephrol Dial Transplant* 10: 509, 1995

61. Schaefer RM, Fink E, Schaefer L, Barkhausen R, Kulzer P, Heidland A: Role of bradykinin in anaphylactoid reactions during hemodialysis with AN69 membranes. *Am J Nephrol* 13: 473, 1993

62. Van der Niepen P, Sennesael JS, Verbeelen DL, Van Ingelgem D: Prevention of anaphylactoid reactions to high-flux membrane dialysis and ACE inhibitors by calcium. *Nephrol Dial Transplant* 9: 87, 1993

63. Kojima S, Harada-Shiba M, Nomura S et al.: Effect of nafamostat mesilate on bradykinin generation during low-density lipoprotein apheresis using a dextran sulfate column. *Trans ASAIO* 27: 644, 1991

64. Olbricht CJ, Schaumann D, Fischer D: Anaphylactoid reactions, LDL apheresis with dextrane sulfate, and ACE inhibitors. *Lancet* 340: 908, 1992

65. Tunon-de-Lara J, Villanueva P, Marcos M, Taytard A: ACE inhibitors and anaphylactoid reactions during venom immunotherapy. *Lancet* 340: 908, 1992

66. Man NK, Cianconi C, Faivre JM et al.: Dialysis-associated adverse reactions with high-flux membranes and microbial contamination of liquid bicarbonate concentrate. *Contr Nephrol* 62: 24, 1988

67. Bouvier P, Barnouin F, Briat C et al.: Choc anaphylactique en hemodialyse: à propos de deux observations. *Nephrol* 10: 40, 1990

68. Montagnac R, Schillinger F, Milcent T et al.: Réaction d'hypersensibilité en cours d'hémodialyse. Roles de la haute perméabilité, de la rétrofiltration et de la contamination bactérienne du dialysat. *Nephrol* 9: 29, 1988

69. Nicholls AJ, Platts MM: Anaphylactoid reactions due to hemodialysis, haemofiltration, or plasma separation. *Br Med J* 285: 1607, 1982

70. Tokars JI, Alter MJ, Favero MS, Moyer LA, Bland LA: National surveillance of hemodialysis associated diseases in the United States, 1990. *ASAIO J* 39: 71, 1993

71. Yamagami S, Adachi T, Sugimura T et al.: Detection of endotoxin antibody in long-term dialysis patients. *Int J Artif Organs* 13: 205, 1990

72. Quellhorst E, Schünemann B: Beta-2 amyloidosis and haemofiltration. in *Dialysis Amyloidosis*, edited by Geijo F, Brancaccio D, Bardin Y, Wichtig Editore, 1989, p 123

73. Baz M, Durand C, Ragon A, Jaber K, Andrieu D, Merzouk T et al.: Using ultrapure water in hemodialysis delays carpal tunnel syndrome. *Int J Artif Organs* 14: 681, 1991

74. Shaldon S, Deschodt G, Branger B, Granolleras C, Baldamus C, Koch K, Lysaght M, Dinarello C: Haemodialysis hypotension: the interleukin hypothesis restated. *Proc EDTA-ERA* 22: 229, 1985

75. Fox S, Henderson LW: Cardiovascular response during hemodialysis and hemofiltration: thermal, membrane and catecholamine influences. *Blood Purif* 11: 224, 1993

76. Bambauer R, Walther J, Meyer S, Ost S, Schauer M, Jung W, Gohl H, Vienken J: Bacteria and endotoxin-free dialysis fluid for use in chronic hemodialysis. *Artif Organs* 18: 188, 1994

77. Bambauer R, Walther J, Jung W: Ultrafiltration of dialysis fluid to obtain a sterile solution during hemodialysis. *Blood Purif* 8: 309, 1990

78. Erley C, von Herrath D, Hartenstein-Koch K, Kutschera D, Amir-Moazami B, Schaefer K: Easy production of sterile, pyrogen-free dialysate. *Trans ASAIO* 34: 205, 1988

79. Frinak S, Polaschegg HD, Levin N, Pohlod D, Dumler F, Saravolatz L: Filtration of dialysate using an on-line dialysate filter. *Int J Artif Organs* 14: 691, 1991

80. Abuelo JG, Shemin D, Chazan JA: Acute symptoms produced by hemodialysis: a review of their causes and associations. *Seminars in Dialysis* 6: 59, 1993

81. Rosa AA, Fryd DS, Kjellstrand CM: Dialysis symptoms and stabilization in long-term dialysis. *Arch Intern Med* 140: 804, 1980

82. Dumler F, Zasuwa G, Lewin NW: Effect of dialyzer reprocessing methods on complement activation and hemodialyzer-related symptoms. *Artif Organs* 11: 128, 1987

83. Bergamo collaborative dialysis study group Acute intra-dialytic well-being: results of a clinical trial comparing polysulfone with cuprophan. *Kidney Int* 40: 714, 1991

84. Collins DM, Lambert MB, Tannenbaum JS, Oliverio M, Schwab SJ: Tolerance of hemodialysis: a randomized prospective trial of high-flux versus conventional high-efficiency hemodialysis. *J Am Soc Nephrol* 4: 148, 1993

85. Skroeder NR, Jacobson SH, Lins LE, Kjellstrand CM: Biocompatibility of dialysis membranes is of no importance for objective or subjective symptoms during or after hemodialysis. *Trans ASAIO* 36: M637, 1990

86. Garella S, Chang B: Hemodialysis-associated hypoxemia. *Am J Nephrol* 4: 273, 1984

87. Duarte R: Blood pressure, ventilation and lipid imbalance during hemodialysis: effect of dialysate composition. *Blood Purif* 3: 199, 1985

88. De Broe M: Hemodialysis-induced hypoxemia. *Nephrol Dial Transplant* 9 (Suppl 2): 173, 1994

89. Igarashi H, Kioi S, Geijo F, Arakawa A: Physiologic approach to dialysis-induced hypoxemia: effects of dialyser material and dialysate composition. *Nephron* 41: 62, 1985

90. De Backer W, Verpooten G, Borgonjon D, Vermeire P, Lins R,. DeBroe M: Hypoxemia during hemodialysis: effects of different membranes and dialysate composition. *Kidney Int* 23: 738, 1983

91. Becker W, Schaefer R, Börner W: *In vivo* viability of 111-In-labelled granulocytes demonstrated in a sham dialysis. *Br J Radiol* 62: 462, 1989

92. Dodd N, Gordge M, Tarrant J, Parsons V, Weston M: A demonstration of neutrophil accumulation in the pulmonary vasculature during haemodialysis. *Proc EDTA* 20: 186, 1983

93. Flaherty K, Cheung A, Marshall E, Munger M: Cardiopulmonary events during hemodialysis using various membranes and dialysate. *J Am Soc Nephrol* 4: 345, 1993

94. Sherlock J, Ledwith J, Letteri J: Hypoventilation and hypoxemia during hemodialysis: reflex response to removal of CO_2 across the dialyzer. *Trans ASAIO* 23: 406, 1977

95. Dumler F, Levin N: Leucopenia and hypoxemia, unrelated effects of hemodialysis. *Arch Intern Med* 139: 1103, 1979

96. Dolan M, Whipp B, Davidsons W, Weitzman R, Wasserman K: Hypnea associated with acetate hemodialysis: carbon dioxide-flow dependent ventilation. *New Engl J Med* 305: 72, 1981

97. Schulman G, Fogo A, Gung A, Badr K, Hakim R: Complement activation retards resolution of ischemic renal failure in the rat. *Kidney Int* 40: 1069, 1991

98. Hakim RM, Wingard RL, Lawrence P, Parker RA, Schulman G: Use of biocompatible membranes improves outcome and recovery from acute renal failure. (Abstract) *J Am Soc Nephrol* 3: 367, 1992

99. Hakim RA: Clinical implications of hemodialysis membrane biocompatibility. *Kidney Int* 44: 484, 1993

100. Kränzlin B, Reuss A, Gretz N, Kirschfink M, Ryan CJ, Mujais S: Recovery of renal function following acute ischemic renal failure. *Nephrol Dial Transplant* 1995. Submitted

101. Kaplan A: What are the important considerations in the care of critically ill patients with acute renal failure? *Seminars in Dialysis* 7: 103, 1994

102. Teehan B, Schleifer C, Brown J, Sigler M, Raimondo J: Urea kinetic analysis and clinical outcome on CAPD. A five year longitudinal study. *Adv Perit Dial* 6: 181, 1991

103. Lowrie E, Lew N: Death risk in hemodialysis patients: the predictive value of commonly measured variables and an evaluation of death rate differences between facilities. *Am J Kidney Dis* 15: 458, 1990

104. Gutierrez A, Alvestrand A, Wahren J, Bergström J: Effect of *in vivo* contact between blood and dialysis membranes on protein catabolism in humans. *Kidney Int* 38: 487, 1990

105. Gutierrez A, Alvestrand A, Bergström J: Membrane selection and muscle protein catabolism. *Kidney Int* 42 (Suppl 38): S86, 1992

106. Hoerl WH, Schaefer R, Heidland A: Effect of different dialyzers on proteinases and proteinase inhibitors during hemodialysis. *Am J Nephrol* 5: 320, 1985

107. Hoerl W, Heidland A: Evidence for the participation of granulocyte proteinases on intradialytic catabolism. *Clin Nephrol* 21: 314, 1984

108. Baracos V, Rodeman H, Dinarello C, Goldberg A: Stimulation of muscle protein degradation and prostaglandin E2 release by leukocyte pyrogen (interleukin-1). *N Engl J Med* 308: 553, 1983

109. Dinarello CA, Wolff SM: Molecular basis of fever in humans. *Am J Med* 72: 799, 1982

110. Bingel M, Lonnemann G, Koch KM, Dinarello C, Shaldon S: Enhancement of *in vitro* human interleukin-1 production by sodium acetate. *Lancet* i: 14, 1987

111. Haeffner-Cavaillon N, Jahns G, Poignet JL, Kazatchkine D: Induction of interleukin-1 during hemodialysis. *Kidney Int* 43 (Suppl 39): 139, 1993

112. Lonnemann G, Bingel M, Floege J, Koch KM, Shaldon S, Dinarello C: Detection of endotoxin-like interleukin-1 inducing activity during *in vitro* dialysis. *Kidney Int* 33: 29, 1988

113. Misfeldt M, Legaard P, Howell S, Fornella M, LeGrand R: Induction of interleukin-1 from murine peritoneal macrophages by Pseudomonas aeruginosa Exotoxin A. *Infect Immun* 58: 978, 1990

114. Goldberg AL, Kettelhut IC, Furuni K, Fagan JM, Baracos V: Activation of protein breakdown and prostaglandin E_2 production in rat skeletal muscle in fever is signaled by a macrophage product distinct from interleukin-1 or other known cytokines. *J Clin Invest* 81: 1378, 1988

115. Miller F, Hammerschmidt D, Anderson G, Moore J: Protein loss induced by complement activation during peritoneal dialysis. *Kidney Int* 25: 480, 1984

116. Gutierrez A, Bergström J, Alvestrand A: Protein catabolism in sham-hemodialysis: the effect of different membranes. *Clin Nephron* 38: 20, 1992

117. Gutierrez-Martones A: Protein catabolism and bioincompatibility in hemodialysis. PhD Thesis, Karolinska Institute, Huddinge University Hospital, Stockholm, Sweden, 1993

118. Berkelhammer C, Baker J, Leither L, Uldall P, Whitall R, Salter A, Wolman S: Whole body protein turnover in adult hemodialysis patients as measured by ^{13}C-leucine. *Am J Clin Nutr* 46: 778, 1987

119. Lim V, Bier D, Flanigan J, Sum-Ping S: The effect of hemodialysis on protein metabolism: a leucine kinetic study. *J Clin Invest* 91: 2429, 1993

120. Lewis S, Van Epps D, Chenoweth D: Leukocyte C5a receptor modulation during hemodialysis. *Kidney Int* 31: 112, 1987

121. Lindsay R, Bergström J: Membrane biocompatibility and nutrition in patients on maintenance hemodialysis. *Nephrol Dial Transplant* 9 (Suppl 2): 150, 1994

122. Parfrey P, Harnett J: Cardiac disease in chronic uremia. Pathophysilogy and clinical epidemiology. *ASAIO J* 40: 121, 1994

123. Ward RA: Phagocytic cell function as an index of biocompatibility. *Nephrol Dial Transplant* 9 (Suppl 2): 46, 1994

124. Vanholder R, Van Bliesen W, Ringoir S: Contributing factors to the inhibition of phagocytosis in hemodialyzed patients. *Kidney Int* 44: 208, 1993

125. Moran J, Blumenstein M, Gurland HJ: Immunodefiencies in chronic renal failure. *Contrib Nephrol* 86: 91, 1990

126. Haag-Weber M, Hörl WH: Uremia and infection: mechanisms of impaired cellular host defense. *Nephron* 63: 125, 1993
127. Vanholder R: Biocompatibility issues in hemodialysis. *Clinical Materials* 10: 87, 1992
128. United States Renal Data System: United States Renal Data System 1991 Annual Report, Bethesda. The National Institute of Diabetes and Digestive and Kidney Diseases 1991
129. Van Ypersele de Strihou Ch, Floege J, Jadoul M, Koch KM: Amyloidosis and its relationship to different dialysers. *Nephrol Dial Transplant* 9 (Suppl 2): 156, 1994
130. Miura Y, Ishiyama T, Inomata A, Takeda T, Senma S, Okuyama K, Suzuki Y: Radiolucent bone cysts and the type of dialysis membrane used in patients undergoing longterm hemodialysis. *Nephron* 60: 268, 1992
131. Van Ypersele de Strihou Ch, Jadoul M, Malghem J, Maldague J, Jamart J: Effect of dialysis membrane and patients age on signs of dialysis-related amyloidosis. *Kidney Int* 39: 1012, 1991
132. Hauglustaine D, Waer M, Michielson P: Haemodialysis membranes, serum β2-microglobulin, and dialysis amyloidosis. *Lancet* i: 1211, 1986
133. Bergström J, Wehle B: No change in corrected β2-m concentration after Cuprophan® hemodialysis. *Lancet* i: 628, 1987
134. Floege J, Bartsch A, Schulze M, Shaldon S, Koch KM, Smeby L: Turnover of 131-β2-microglobulin in hemodialysed patients. *J Lab Clin Med* 118: 153, 1991
135. Vincent C, Chanard J, Caudwell V, Lavoud S, Wong T, Revillard J: Kinetics of ^{125}I-β2-microglobulin turnover in dialysed patients. *Kidney Int* 42: 1434, 1992
136. Odell R, Slowiaczek P, Moran J, Schindhelm K: β2-microglubulin kinetics in end stage renal failure. *Kidney Int* 39: 909, 1991
137. Zaoui P, Stone W, Hakim R: Effects of dialysis membranes on β2-microglobulin production and cellular expression. *Kidney Int* 38: 962, 1990
138. Schoels M, Jahn B, Hug F, Deppisch R, Ritz E, Hänsch G: Stimulation of mononuclear cells by contact with Cuporphan membranes: further increase of β2-microglobulin synthesis by activated late complement components. *Am J Kidney Dis* 21: 394, 1993
139. Jahn B, Betz M, Deppisch R, Janssen O, Hänsch GM, Ritz E: Stimulation of β2-microglobulin synthesis in lymphocytes after exposure to cuprophan dialyzer membranes. *Kidney Int* 40: 285, 1991
140. Knudsen P, Leon J, Ng A, Shaldon S, Floege J, Koch KM: Hemodialysis-related induction of β2-m and interleukin-1 and release by mononuclear phagocytes. *Nephron* 53: 188, 1989
141. Campistol J, Molina R, Bernard D, Rodriguez R, Mirapeix E, Munoz-Gomez J, Revert L: Synthesis of β2-m in lymphocyte culture: role of hemodialysis, dialysis membranes, dialysis amyloidosis and lymphokines. *Am J Kidney Dis* 22: 691, 1993
142. Paczek L, Schäfer R, Heidland A: Dialysis membranes inhibit *in vitro* release of β2-m from human lymphocytes. *Nephron* 56: 267, 1990
143. Campistol J, Molina R, Rodriguez R, Mirapeix E, Munoz-Gomez J, Revert L: Dialysis membranes inhibit synthesis and release of β2-m in lymphocyte culture. *Nephron* 56: 691, 1991
144. Karlsson F, Groth T, Sege K, Wibell L, Peterson P: Turnover in humans of β2-microglobulin: the constant chain of HLA-antigens. *Eur J Clin Invest* 10: 293, 1980
145. Levin NW, Dumler F, Zasuwa G, Stalla K: Mortality comparison between conventional and high flux dialysis. *J Am Soc Nephrol* 1: 365, 1990
146. Levin NW, Zasuwa GA, Dumler F Effect of membrane type on causes of death in hemodialysis patients. *J Am Soc Nephrol* 1: 365, 1990
147. Chanard J, Brunoios JP, Melin JP, Lavaud S, Toupance O: Longterm results of dialysis therapy with a highly permeable membrane. *Artif Organs* 6: 261, 1982
148. Hornberger JC, Chernew ME, Petersen J, Garber AM: A multivariate analysis of mortality and hospital admissions with high-flux dialysis. *Am Soc Nephrol* 3: 1227, 1992
149. Simpson K, Allison MEM: Dialysis and acute renal failure: can mortality be improved? (Abstract) *Nephrol Dial Transplant* 8: 946, 1993
150. Owen WF, Lew NL, Liu Y, Lowrie EG, Lazarus JM: The urea reduction ratio and serum albumin concentration as predictors of mortality in patients undergoing hemodialysis. *N Engl J Med* 329: 1001, 1993
151. Bergström J, Alvestrand A, Fürst P: Plasma and muscle free amino acids in maintainance hemodialysis patients without protein malnutrition. *Kidney Int* 38: 108, 1990
152. Kusek JW, Agodoa LY, Dixon NC, coordinators: *Mortality and Morbidity in Hemodialysis Study*. Presented at the NIH consensus development conference; 1993 Nov 1–3; Bethesda, Maryland
153. Diaz RJ, Washburn S, Cauble L, Siskind MS, Van Wyck D: The effect on dialyzer reprocessing on performance and β2-microglobulin removal using polysulfone membranes. *Am J Kidney Dis* 21: 405, 1993
154. Goldman M, Lagmiche M, Dhaene M, Amraoui Z, Thayse C, Vanherweghem JL: Adsorption of β2-microglobulin on dialysis membranes: comparison of different dialyzers and effects of reuse procedures. *Int J Artif Organs* 12: 373, 1989
155. Graeber CW, Halley SE, Lapkin RA, Graeber CA, Kaplan AA: Protein losses with reused dialyzers. *J Am Soc Nephrol* 4: 349, 1993
156. Parker TF, Hakim RM: Interrelationships of dialysis prescription, protein catabolic rate and morbidity/mortality with dialyzer biocompatibility. *Blood Purif* 11: 341, 1993
157. Kuwahara T, Markert M, Wauters JP: Biocompatibility aspects of dialyzer reprocessing: a comparison of 3 reuse methods and 3 membranes. *Clin Nephrol* 32: 139, 1989
158. Charra B, Calemard E, Ruffet M, Chazot C, Terrat JC, Vanel T, Laurent G: Survival as an index of adequacy of dialysis. *Kidney Int* 41: 1286, 1992
159. Parker TF, Husni L, Huang W, Lew N, Lowrie EG, Dallas Nephrology Associates: Survival of hemodialysis patients in the United States is improved with a greater quantity of dialysis. *Am J Kidney Dis* 23: 670, 1994
160. Hakim RM, Breyer J, Ismail N, Schulman G: Effects of dose of dialysis on morbidity and mortality. *Am J Kidney Dis* 23: 661, 1994

REPLACEMENT OF RENAL FUNCTION BY DIALYSIS

Fourth edition

Library of Congress Cataloging in Publication Data

Replacement of renal function by dialysis / edited by Claude Jacobs
  ... [et al.]. -- 4th ed.
      p.   cm.
  Includes bibliographical references and index.

  1. Hemodialysis.   I. Jacaobs, Claude.
  [DNLM: 1. Hemodialdsis.   WJ 378 R425 1995]
RC901.7.H45R46 1995
617.4'61059--dc20
DNLM/DLC
for Library of Congress   95-31081

ISBN 978-94-017-4178-1   ISBN 978-0-585-36947-1 (eBook)
DOI 10.1007/978-0-585-36947-1

Printed on acid-free paper

Cover illustration:

The illustration on the cover is meant to visualize a blood contacting biomaterial by an artistic concept of molecular modelling.
The colours indicate the hydrophilicity of the functional groups ranging from deep blue (hydrophilic) to reddish (hydrophobic).
It shows a Hemophan® hemodialysis membrane, with its hydrophobic DEAE substituents evolving
from the hydrophilic cellulose backbone.
Copyright by C. Hahn and M. Diamantoglou, Akzo Nobel Central Research

DRUKKER, PARSONS and MAHER

REPLACEMENT OF RENAL FUNCTION BY DIALYSIS

Fourth edition

Edited by

C. JACOBS

C. M. KJELLSTRAND

K. M. KOCH

J. F. WINCHESTER (editor-in-chief)

Springer-Science+Business Media, B.V.

FOREWORD TO THE FOURTH EDITION

BELDING H. SCRIBNER

Within these pages the reader will find detailed descriptions of dialysis techniques and equipment whose excellence is to this old timer almost unbelievable. The question that has bothered me more and more these past few years is whether or not we nephrologists are making the best use of all this largess. On the basis of disappointing survival data, especially in the United States, the answer is 'No.' Of course there are outstanding exceptions and I will discuss some of these below.

Why have survival results, especially among patients on dialysis in the United States, been so disappointingly poor? Some of the answers will be found in the pages of this long overdue 4th edition. However, 2 factors seem to stand out above all others The first cause of shortened survival is gross underdialysis of large numbers of patients. Gotch was among the first to identify this serious problem in a classic paper in which he studied visitors to his unit in San Francisco (1). Since then this fact of widespread underdialysis has been repeatedly documented.

I believe that underdialysis is caused mainly by the widespread misuse of the technique of high efficiency *shortened time* hemodialysis. This misuse results from the fact that it is very easy to shorten dialysis time because everybody is in favor of it – especially the patients and the 'bottom liners.' In sharp contrast it is extremely difficult to increase hemodialysis efficiency, unless special equipment is used and special precautions are taken. Most hemodialysis units simply do not have the equipment and/or the know-how to increase dialysis efficiency. In this connection it is important to remember that whenever a dialysis technique is pushed toward the upper limit of performance, as it must be in high efficiency dialysis, the chances of error and malfunction increase exponentially. Therefore those readers who do get involved with high efficiency/shortened time dialysis should study very carefully the chapters in this volume that deal with this subject.

Even when properly carried out, I believe that high efficiency/shortened time dialysis has very limited application. It should be used only on the minority of patients who can maintain normal blood pressure despite the marked reduction in dialysis time. Two to three hours of dialysis simply does not allow sufficient time to remove the salt water accumulated since the last dialysis. This fact brings me to a brief discussion of the second major factor responsible for the low survival among hemodialysis patients, namely failure to control blood pressure.

Despite the fact that the classic paper by Haire and Sherrard on the adverse effect of hypertension (and smoking) on survival of patients on dialysis was published back in 1978 (2), surprisingly few papers and presentations at meetings have dealt with this all important subject. Important exceptions are the publications of Charra and his colleagues from Tassin in France (3, 4). Indeed their 1992 paper (4) sets the gold standard for survival on dialysis. Because they were using a very long low efficiency dialysis technique, they were able to deliver a very large dose of dialysis and provide a large protein intake to the 445 patients in their series thereby eliminating these two important factors that could adversely affect survival. That made it possible to pinpoint excellent control of blood pressure as the major factor that accounted for their outstanding survival data. Readers of this volume should pay particular attention to the chapters that deal with control of blood pressure both during the years before starting dialysis as well as control while on dialysis and after transplantation if survival figures among patients on renal replacement therapy are to improve significantly in the future.

As this is being written in the spring of 1994, studies are in progress on Charra's patients to try and determine whether or not the long 8 hour dialysis also lowers blood pressure by removing a uremic toxin that increases blood pressure, as suggested in a recent publication by Ritz (5). If Ritz's postulate is correct, this toxin must behave during dialysis like a middle molecule, whose removal, unlike urea, is mainly a function of time on dialysis (6). For a more general discussion of this topic of uremic toxins, see Chapter 1 by Vanholder.

Of emerging importance is the observation that nutritional parameters may also affect survival. Several analytic studies in hemodialysis (7), and in CAPD (8) and confirmed by the US Renal Data System (9), show that a serum albumin lower than normal increases the relative risk of death on dialysis. This deserves further study, and attention to detail in nutritional management of dialysis patients.

The experience we have had over the years with some of our original patients sheds additional light on matters under discussion here. Patient #2 in our series, who began dialysis on March 20, 1960, survived 28 years and died suddenly of an acute myocardial infarction while playing golf at Palm Springs, California in the winter of 1989. This death probably was due to the accelerated atherosclerosis (10) that he may have developed during his early years on dialysis when we did not understand the importance of blood pressure control. Patient #5, who began dialysis in the summer of 1960, currently is in his 34th year of hemodialysis and as such is the longest survivor in the world. He has had a very successful career in academia as a Professor of Physics. In January of 1963 we accepted for temporary treatment a young medical student from Guy's Hospital in London. Now 30 years later this patient is a world renowned dermatologist on the faculty of the University of London. His health is good, having received a cadaveric transplant, which was performed by Mr Peter Morris at Oxford in 1991. This patient has provided a fascinating account of what it was like to be a chronic hemodialysis patient during the early years (11). Even though they are anecdotal, these early successful outcomes stand in sharp contrast to what is being reported today in terms of survival and quality of life among dialysis patients. These outcomes are all the more remarkable when one takes into account the fact that by today's standards, all 3 of these early patients received very poor care during their first decade on renal replacement therapy because we simply did not know what constituted good dialysis care.

Finally, a word about quality of life among dialysis patients. The recent literature reports that quality of life on dialysis is good in only a minority of patients. These poor results are encountered despite the fact that the improvement in anemia with erythropoietin promised a considerable improvement in quality of life. The reasons for the disappointing quality of life are multifactorial. There is no question that the modern dialysis patient not only is older, but has more intercurrent conditions (diabetes, cardiac disease, drug addiction, aids, etc) and complications of those conditions (blindness, amputations, etc) than his/her early dialysis predecessor. The disabilities entailed by aging or non-renal complications cannot be overcome by dialysis itself, and demand much from the practicing nephrologist. Such patients present a medical challenge to the modern dialysis practitioner, and consequently place more demands on the medical community for adequate training. It is my observation that there may be a serious deficiency in the training that we nephrologists have received over the years. During fellowships, most nephrologists learn about dialysis by taking care of patients with acute potentially reversible renal failure and with rare exceptions get very little exposure to the day to day care of chronic dialysis patients. Recently there are indications that this neglected area of training may be corrected. If and when this task is undertaken, I believe it is important to keep in mind the often overlooked fact that patients with chronic renal failure suffer from a *chronic disease*. This fact in turn means that nephrologists must be taught the same skills used in the care of chronic illness that are taught routinely to fellows in rehabilitation medicine and rheumatology. Perhaps if that is done, then the quality of life of dialysis patients will improve and thereby indicate that the best use is being made of the marvelous knowledge and technology presented in this volume.

References

1. Gotch FA, Yarian S, Keen M: A kinetic survey of US hemodialysis prescriptions. *Am J Kidney Dis* 5: 511, 1990
2. Haire HM, Sherrard DJ, Scarpadane O, Curtis FK, Brunzell JD: Smoking, hypertension and mortality in a maintenance dialysis population. *Cardiovasc Med* 3: 1163, 1978
3. Charra B, Calemard E, Laurent G: Control of hypertension and prolonged survival on maintenance hemodialysis. *Nephron* 33: 96, 1983
4. Charra B, Calemard E, Ruffet M, Chazot C, Terrat JC, Vanel T, Laurent G: Survival as an index of adequacy of dialysis. *Kidney Int* 41: 286, 1992
5. Ritz E: Hypertension and cardiac death in dialysis patients – should target blood pressure be lowered? *Semin Dial* 6: 227, 1993
6. Babb AL, Farrell P, Uvelli D, Scribner BH: Hemodialyzer evaluation by examination of solute molecular spectra. *Trans Am Soc Artif Intern Organs* 18: 98, 1972
7. Lowrie EG, Lew NL: Death risk in hemodialysis patients: The predictive value of commonly measured variables and an evaluation of death rate differences between facilities. *Am J Kidney Dis* 15: 458, 1990
8. Teehan BT, Schleifer C, Brown J, *et al*: Urea kinetic analysis and in CAPD. A five year longitudinal study. *Adv Peritoneal Dial* 6: 181, 1990
9. US Renal Data System, USRDS 1992 Annual Data Report, The National Institutes of Health, National Institute of Diabetes and Digestive and Kidney Diseases, Bethesda, MD, August 1992.
10. Lindner A, Charra B, Sherrard DJ, Scribner BH: Accelerated atherosclerosis in prolonged maintenance hemodialysis. *N Engl J Med* 290: 697, 1974
11. Eady RAJ: A patient's experience of over one thousand haemodialyses. *Proc Eur Dial Transplant Assoc* 8: 50, 1971

INTRODUCTION AND TRIBUTE TO DRUKKER, PARSONS AND MAHER

CLAUDE JACOBS, CARL M. KJELLSTRAND, KARL M. KOCH and JAMES F. WINCHESTER

The years 1978, 1983, and 1989 were the publication dates for the three previous editions of this book, the first two editions having all three editors in place, while the last was edited by Jack Maher alone. This book has been a global resource and considered as the prime textbook for information on dialysis for many years. As Maher wrote in his introduction in 1989, they were all 'first generation nephrologists', and in our opinion at the leading edge of clinical and research nephrology of the times. Sadly, we cannot call on them for advice, as all have passed away. However, we have gleaned knowledge from them in the past in person, and by their written word. We have also been aided in having the same publisher, Boudewijn Commandeur, for this edition as in all previous. He has served as a lynchpin for the project. Therefore, during the construction of this book we have as much as possible tried to keep the same flavor, of first outlining the principles of a subject, and then its clinical application.

First, we asked is there a need for this book? Despite our cumulative nephrology experience of at least a century, we were unanimous in our affirmative answer. There, of course, are other books related to dialysis available, but what made the previous editions unique, were the careful eye to detail, in theory and in application, the introduction of topics never previously discussed in a single text (e.g. in this text, dialysis in developing countries), and finally the comprehensive nature of all previous editions, and hopefully this edition as well. We strived to make this book a repository of information, as a reference text, as well as a practical clinical tool. We want this book to become familiar to seasoned nephrologists, nephrology trainees, dialysis nurses and technicians, and perhaps to students as well – it is our wish to see this book used – even torn and tattered. We have, therefore, gathered together, those whom we consider leaders in this subject, be it theoretical, or be it practical.

In acute renal failure, we have become more cognizant of the fact that multi-organ involvement is associated with a poor outcome. This has led to continuous therapies, such as arterio-venous and veno-venous hemodialysis and hemofiltration, to automated machines to accomplish these tasks, to the use of biocompatible membranes, to citrate anticoagulation, and to intensive nutritional support. All of these subjects are covered in detail. Similarly, the infrastructure necessary to perform acute or chronic hemodialysis and peritoneal dialysis is covered – namely, water preparation, dialysate composition, bacterial contamination, and machine design. Today's dialysis machines are largely automated and have built in safety controls, blood pressure monitors, continuous anticoagulation, programmable sodium delivery, in-line solute measurement. The fledgling nephrologist might easily by-pass the theory and the nuances of dialysis understanding. We hope that this text will be used to overcome and give understanding of the complexities of modern dialysis apparatus, whose starting point was the simple physical process discovered by Thomas Graham in 1861, that solutes travel down a concentration gradient.

We have tried to address the current problems in dialysis practice today. Over half a million patients receive dialysis world-wide. There appears to be no shortage of patients, nor trends towards a global decrease in patients reaching end-stage renal disease from the most common diseases, such as diabetes, hypertension, glomerulonephritis, or inherited renal disorders. Despite demonstrations that control of hypertension, and control of diabetes may slow the progress of, or prevent, end-stage kidney disease, and the identification of genetic abnormalities, any effect on prevalence of patients requiring dialysis has yet to filter down to the nephrology community at large. We must not forget that, while life span has increased in the modern world this brings with it reduction in renal function, and intercurrent conditions which make the application of dialysis that much more difficult (mostly related to vascular disease), as well as diabetes and severe hypertension. For these reasons we have added sections specifically to address these issues. How do we as specialists assess the effect of dialysis? After all it is a substitute only for the solute excretory component of renal function. Yes, we can now replace the renal hormones erythropoietin and 1,25 dihydroxycholecalciferol, but what of the other hormonal derangements, the lipid disorders, the impaired immunological function, etc. Most importantly, perhaps, how do we know if we are prescribing enough, or if the patient is receiving enough, dialysis – these issues are at the forefront of investigation and clinical application. Each of these topics and more are dealt with in detail.

Continuous ambulatory peritoneal dialysis is now the preferred home dialysis therapy throughout the world, and we have concentrated on discussion of its application, its amplification by machine delivered peritoneal fluid, its limitations and its complications. Like the problems facing the hemodialysis patient with angioaccess, also described in this book, the peritoneal dialysis patient also faces problems with access to the peritoneal cavity. These topics are addressed in a special section. Because of renewed interest in home hemodialysis, we have added a section to cover that topic.

How does the patient feel about dialysis? Can he/she work? Can he/she play? Is dialysis long-term survival or outcome the same all over the world? When should we let our patients tell us that it is time to stop, and let them die? These issues are real ones, and we may have been remiss in the past by not addressing them in detail. For that reason we have added sections on quality of life, and a new section on outcome analysis, lacking in the previous editions.

What other 'new' problems face the dialysis patient, and perhaps dialysis staff in the late 1990s. We are all familiar with the hepatitis B outbreaks and deaths of the 1970s, and the often observed bacteremia in hemodialysis patients. But what of the diseases of the 1990s – human immunodeficiency virus, hepatitis C, and tuberculosis. Each has unique characteristics, management problems, complications and affects to a great extent staffing and organization of dialysis units. Currently, the Centers for Disease Control, in Atlanta, Georgia, does not recommend isolation of patients with HIV nor hepatitis C, yet for the latter the debate may not be definitively closed.

Tuberculosis has its own 1990s uniqueness, drug resistance and association with recent immigration or HIV. All these topics can be found in this text.

We have also striven to make sure that all the topics covered are correct in detail, but we wish the reader to make judgements as to validity of concept, a prescription, a formula, a diagram, and to use such judgement to adjust therapy in clinical application. Due to the ever changing nature of medicine, and technology, differences of opinion are to be found in this book, and the publisher and editors assume no responsibility for these differences of opinion, rather publishing them as written to improve the academic impact of our text.

Finally, what have we left and what have we taken away. We felt that the previous chapter on the history of dialysis as written by Drukker could not be bettered, and in deference to him we omitted it. We have changed many of the authors in this text, not for changes sake, but to bring in new and younger, and perhaps the fourth or fifth generation nephrologists. This is a changing field, steeped in tradition, and to honor that tradition it was our decision to retain the name of the text as Drukker, Parsons and Maher, our first generation nephrology colleagues and friends. In keeping with the changing nature of investigation, to molecular biology, we have replaced the familiar cover diagram of middle molecule peak 7c, with a schematic of molecular modeling of a well known cellulosic dialysis membrane.

Claude Jacobs, Paris
Carl M. Kjellstrand, Edmonton
Karl M. Koch, Hannover
James F. Winchester, Washington

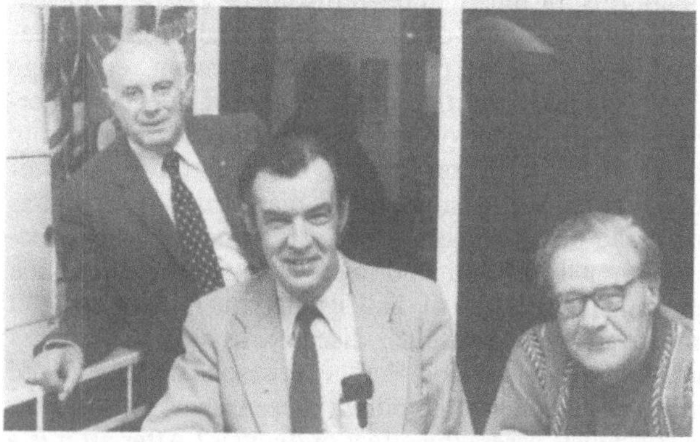

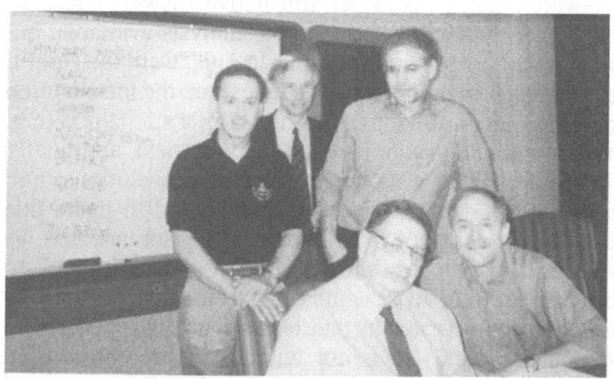

Figure 1. William Drukker, Jack Maher, Frank Parsons.

Figure 2. Jim Winchester, Boudewijn Commandeur (Publisher), Karl Koch, Claude Jacobs, Carl Kjellstrand.

CONTRIBUTING AUTHORS

T. Agishi, M.D.
Kidney Center
Tokyo Women's Medical College
Department of Surgery
8-1 Kawada-Cho, Shinjuku-ku
Tokyo 162, Japan
Chapter 58C

J. Ahlmén, M.D., Ph.D.
Department of Nephrology
Central Hospital
S-541 85 Skövde, Sweden
Chapter 62B

Alfred C. Alfrey, M.D.
Veterans Affairs Medical Center
1055 Clermont Street
Denver, CO 80220, USA
Chapter 51

G.S. Arbus, M.D.
Department of Nephrology
Hospital for Sick Children
555 University Avenue
Toronto, ON, Canada M5G 1X8
Chapter 58F

R.S. Barsoum, M.D.
The Cairo Kidney Center
P.O. Box 91
Bab-el-Louk
Cairo 11513, Egypt
Chapter 60

Robert H. Barth, M.D.
Hemodialysis Unit
VA Medical Center
800 Poly Place
Brooklyn, NY 11209, USA
Chapter 16

William M. Bennett, M.D., Ph.D.
Division of Nephrology and Hypertension
Oregon Health Sciences University
3181 SW Sam Jackson Park Road
L 455 Portland, OR 97201, USA
Chapter 29

Christopher Blagg, M.D.
Northwest Kidney Centers
700 Broadway
Seattle, WA 98122, USA
Chapter 56

Peter Blake, M.D.
University of Western Ontario
Victoria Hospital Corp.
P.O. Box 5375, 375 South Street
London, Ontario N6A 4G5, Canada
Chapter 24

Marcel Broyer, M.D.
Department of Pediatric Nephrology
Hospital for Sick Children
Paris, France
Chapter 31

C.E. Butler, M.D.
Brigham & Women's Hospital
Department of Surgery
Boston, MA 02115, USA
Chapter 10

Bernard J.M. Canaud, M.D.
Division of Nephrology
Lapeyronie University Hospital
F-34295 Montpellier, France
Chapter 8

Cyril Chantler, M.D.
Evelina Children's Department
Guy's and St. Thomas' Hospital
Guy's Hospital
London, England
Chapter 31

D.N. Churchill, M.D.
Division of Nephrology
McMaster University
Hamilton, Ontario, Canada L8N 4A6
Chapter 23

Allan J. Collins, M.D.
Regional Kidney Disease Program
914 S. 8th Street
Minneapolis, MN 55404, USA
Chapters 46, 61

C.K. Colton, Ph.D.
Department of Chemical Engineering
Massachusetts Inst. of Technology
25 Amnes St., Room 66-452
Cambridge, MA 02139, USA
Chapter 3

P.F. Copleston, M.D.
Canadian Organ Replacement Register
Canadian Institute for Health Information
Box 3900
Don Mills, Ontario, Canada M3C 2T9
Chapter 58F

Ronald Cranford, M.D.
Hennepin County Medical Centre
701 Park Ave S
Minneapolis Minnesota 55415, USA
Chapter 63

John Daugirdas, M.D., Ph.D.
University of Illinois at Chicago
Department of Research (151)
Westside VA Medical Center
820 South Damen Avenue
Chicago, Illinois 60612, USA
Chapter 24

Alex M. Davison, M.D., Ph.D.
Department of Renal Medicine
St. James's University Hospital
Beckett Street
Leeds LS9 7TF, England
Chapter 54

R. De Smet, M.D.
Nephrology Department
University Hospital
De Pintelaan 185
B-9000 Ghent, Belgium
Chapter 1

Wilfried A. De Backer, M.D.
Department of Pulmonary Medicine
University Hospital Antwerp
Wilrijkstraat 10
B-2650 Edegem-Antwerpen, Belgium
Chapter 41

Marc E. De Broe, M.D., Ph.D.
Department of Nephrology-Hypertension
University Hospital Antwerp
Wilrijkstraat 10
B-2650 Edegem-Antwerpen, Belgium
Chapter 41

Françoise Degos, M.D.
Service d'Hépato-Gastro-Entérologie 2
Hôpital Beaujon
100 Boulevard du Gen. Leclerc
92110 Clichy, France
Chapter 47B

Barbara G. Delano, M.D.
Department of Medicine
State University of New York
Health Science Center Brooklyn
450 Clarkson Ave, Box 52
Brooklyn, NY 11203, USA
Chapter 55A

B. Descamps-Latscha, M.D., Ph.D.
INSERM U.25
GH Necker-Enfants Malades
161 rue de Sèvres
75015 Paris, France
Chapter 45

Marie Desmeules, M.D.
Laboratory Centre for Disease Control
LCDC Building, Rm22-c
Tunney's Pasture
Ottawa, ON, Canada K1A 0L2
Chapter 58F

J.A. Diaz-Buxo, M.D.
Metrolina Nephrology Associates P.A.
928 Baxter Street
Charlotte, NC 28204-2879, USA
Chapter 21

A.P.S. Disney, M.D.
The Queen Elizabeth Hospital
28 Woodville Road
Woodville South
Adelaide, South Australia 5011
Chapter 58E

Raymond Donckerwolcke, M.D.
Department of Nephrology
Alberta Children's Hospital
1820 Richmond Road SW
Calgary, Alberta
Canada T2T 5C7
Chapter 31

Jochen H.H. Ehrich M.D.
Charité University Hospital
Humboldt University
Berlin, Germany
Chapter 33

Joseph W. Eschbach, M.D.
Department of Medicine
University of Washington
515 Minor Ave.
Seattle, WA 98104, USA
Chapter 43

Aldo Fabris, M.D.
Department of Nephrology
St. Bortolo Hospital
Via Rodolfi
I-36100 Vicenza, Italy
Chapters 9, 40

S.A. Fenton, M.D.
Toronto Hospital-General Division
200 Elizabeth Street, EN13-232
Toronto, Ontario, Canada M5G 2C4
Chapter 58F

Mariano Feriani, M.D.
Department of Nephrology
St. Bortolo Hospital
Via Rodolfi
I-36100 Vicenza, Italy
Chapters 9, 20, 40

M.J. Flanigan, M.D.
Department of Internal Medicine, W336-16
University of Iowa Hospitals and Clinics
200 Hawkins Drive
Iowa City, IA 52246, USA
Chapter 49

R.N. Foley, M.D.
Division of Nephrology
The Health Sciences Center
Memorial University
St. Johns, Newfoundland, Canada A1B 3V6
Chapter 38

Denis Fouque, M.D.
Department of Nephrology
Hôpital Edouard Herriot
University Claude Bernard
69437 Lyon Cédex 03, France
Chapter 52

Ulrich Frei, M.D.
Virchow-Klinikum of Humboldt-University
Medical Clinic and Policlinic
Department of Internal Medicine and Nephrology
Augustenburger Platz 1
13353 Berlin, Germany
Chapter 34

Eli A. Friedman, M.D.
SUNY Health Science Center
450 Clarkson Ave, Box 52
Brooklyn, NY 11203, USA
Chapters 17, 35

Daniel H. Froment, M.D.
Service de Néphrologie
Hôpital Notre Dame
Université du Montréal
Montréal, Québec, Canada
Chapter 58F

Ram Gokal, M.D.
Manchester Royal Infirmary
Department of Renal Medicine
Oxford Road
Manchester M13 9WL, England
Chapter 25

Thomas A. Golper, M.D.
University of Arkansas
College of Medicine, Mail Slot 501
Department of Internal Med./Div. of Nephrology
4301 West Markham Street
Little Rock, AR 72205, USA
Chapter 29

Frank A. Gotch, M.D.
University of California
45 Castro Street # 227
San Francisco, CA 94114, USA
Chapter 2

E. Grapsa, M.D.
Division of Nephrology
Toronto Hospital – Western Division
399 Bathurst Street
Toronto, Ontario, Canada M5T 2S8
Chapter 32

A. Grassmann, Ph.D.
AKZO Nobel Faser AG
Business Unit Membrana
Öhder Strasse 28
D-42289 Wuppertal, Germany
Chapter 28

A.P. Guérin, M.D.
Nephrology and Hemodialysis Department
Center Hospitalier Manhès
8 Grande Rue
91700 Fleury Mérogis, France
Chapter 37

Rolf W. Günther, M.D.
Department of Diagnostic Radiology
University of Technology
Pauwelsstrasse
D-52057 Aachen, Germany
Chapter 11

Hans Gurland, M.D.
Nephrology Division
Medical Department I
Klinikum Grosshadern
Marchioninistrasse 15
D-8000 Munich 70, Germany
Chapter 18

Raymond M. Hakim, M.D., Ph.D.
Renal Division
S-3307 MCN, VUMC
1161 21st Avenue S. and Garland
Nashville, TN 37232-2372, USA
Chapter 6

J.D. Harnett, M.D.
Division of Nephrology
The Health Sciences Center
Memorial University
St. Johns, Newfoundland, Canada A1B 3V6
Chapter 38

Philip J. Held, Ph.D.
Department of Health Services Management and Policy
University of Michigan
Ann Arbor, MI 48103, USA
Chapter 58B

Lee W. Henderson, M.D.
Baxter Healthcare Corp.
1620 Waukegan Rd
McGaw Park, IL 60085-6730, USA
Chapter 4

J. Himmelfarb, M.D.
Maine Nephrology Associates P.A.
1600 B Congress Street
Portland, ME 04102, USA
Chapter 6

Nicholas A. Hoenich, Ph.D.
Department of Medicine, Medical School
University of Newcastle upon Tyne
Newcastle-upon-Tyne NE2 4HH, England
Chapter 7

C. Hsu, M.D., Ph.D.
Nephrology Division
Department of Medicine
University of Michigan Medical School
Ann Arbor, MI 48103, USA
Chapter 1

Todd Ing, M.D.
Loyola University, Chicago
Stritch School of Medicine
Maywood, IL 60153, USA
Chapter 26

I. Ishikawa, M.D.
Department of Internal Medicine
Kanazawa Medical University
1-1 Daigaku, Uchinada-Machi
Kahoku-gun, Ishikawa-ken, 920-02 Japan
Chapter 58C

Katsumi Ito, M.D.
Department of Surgery
Kidney Center
Tokyo Women's Medical College
8-1 Kawada-Cho-Shinjuku-Ku
Tokyo 162, Japan
Chapter 58F

Claude Jacobs, M.D.
Service de Néphrologie
Hôpital de La Pitié
83, Blvd. de l'Hôpital
75013 Paris, France
Chapter 57

John J. Jeffery, M.D.
Section of Nephrology
Health Sciences Center
820 Sherbrook Street
Room GE-441
Winnipeg, MB, Canada
Chapter 58F

Paul Jungers, M.D.
Department of Nephrology
GH Necker-Enfants Malades
161 rue de Sèvres
75015 Paris, France
Chapters 45, 47B

A.A. Kaplan, M.D.
University of CT Health Center
Division of Nephrology, MC 1405
Farmington, CT 06030, USA
Chapter 15

B.L. Kasiske, M.D.
Hennepin County Medical Center
Div. of Nephrology
701 Park Ave. S.
Minneapolis, MN 55415, USA
Chapter 36

Michael Kaye, M.D.
Montreal General Hospital
2650 Cedar Ave
Montreal Quebec H3G 1A4, Canada
Chapter 63

William F. Keane, M.D.
University of Minnesota
Division of Nephrology
Department of Medicine
Hennepin County Medical Center
701 Park Avenue
Minneapolis, MN 55415, USA
Chapter 46

Carl M. Kjellstrand, M.D., Ph.D.
Department of Medicine
2E3-31 W. McKenzie
University of Alberta Hospital
Edmonton, Alberta, Canada T6G 2B7
Chapters 26, 30, 58F, 63

Saul Klahr, M.D.
Department of Medicine
The Jewish Hospital of St. Louis
216 South Kingshighway
St. Louis, Missouri 63110, USA
Chapter 59

Karl M. Koch, M.D.
Department of Nephrology
Medizinische Hochschule Hannover
Postfach 610180
D-3000 Hannover 61, Germany
Chapters 27, 53

Joe D. Kopple, M.D.
Harbor-UCLA Medical Center
1000 W. Carson Street
Torrance, CA 90509, USA
Chapter 52

S. Koshikawa, M.D.
Department of Internal Medicine
Showa University Fujigaoka Hospital
1-30 Fujigaoka, Midori-ku
Yokohama-Shi, 227 Japan
Chapter 58C

Raymond T. Krediet, M.D., Ph.D.
Renal Unit, F4-215
Academic Medical Center
Meibergdreef 9
1105 AZ Amsterdam, The Netherlands
Chapter 5

Giuseppe La Greca, M.D.
Department of Nephrology
St. Bortolo Hospital
Via Rodolfi
I-36100 Vicenza, Italy
Chapters 20, 40

J.M. Lazarus, M.D.
Brigham and Women's Hospital
Nephrology Department
75 Francis Street
Boston, MA 02215, USA
Chapter 42

H. Lemke, M.D.
AKZO Nobel
D-63785 Obernburg, Germany
Chapter 28

N.W. Levin, M.D.
Division of Nephrology
Beth Israel Medical Center
1st Avenue at 16th Street
New York, NY 10003, USA
Chapter 13

V.S. Lim, M.D.
Department of Internal Medicine
W336-16
University of Iowa Hospitals and Clinics
200 Hawkins Drive
Iowa City, IA 52246, USA
Chapter 49

Robert MacGregor Lindsay, M.D.
University of Western Ontario
375 South Street
London, Ontario N6A 4G5, Canada
Chapter 44

Robert R. Lins, M.D., Ph.D.
Department of Nephrology
A.Z. Stuivenberg
Lange Beeldekensstraat 267
B-2060 Antwerpen, Belgium
Chapter 41

Francisco Llach, M.D.
Beth Israel Medical Center
201 Lyons Avenue
Newark, NJ 07112, USA
Chapter 48

Gérard London, M.D., Ph.D.
Nephrology and Hemodialysis Department
Center Hospitalier Manhès
8 Grande Rue
91700 Fleury Mérogis, France
Chapter 37

G. Lonnemann, M.D.
Department of Nephrology
Medizinische Hochschule Hannover
Postfach 610180
D-3000 Hannover 61, Germany
Chapter 27

Michael J. Lysaght, Ph.D.
Division of Biology and Medicine
Brown University
Providence, RI, USA
Chapters 3, 18

Netar P. Mallick, M.D.
Manchester Royal Infirmary
Department of Renal Medicine
Oxford Road
Manchester M13 9WL, England
Chapters 58A, 58D

D.A. Mandelbrot, M.D.
250 Longwood Ave.
Seeley Mudd Bldg, Rm 504
Boston, MA 02115, USA
Chapter 42

S. Marchais, M.D.
Nephrology and Hemodialysis Department
Center Hospitalier Manhès
8 Grande Rue
91700 Fleury Mérogis, France
Chapter 37

M.A. Marx, Ph.D.
Asst. Professor of Pharmacy Practice
College of Pharmacy
University of Arkansas for Med. Sciences
Little Rock, AR 72205, USA
Chapter 29

Anne Marie V. Miles, M.D.
SUNY-Health Science Center at Brooklyn
450 Clarkson Avenue-Box 52
Brooklyn, NY 11203, USA
Chapters 17, 35

Charles M. Mion, M.D.
Division of Nephrology
Lapeyronie University Hospital
F-34259 Montpellier Cédex, France
Chapters 8, 22

Salim K. Mujais, M.D.
Northwestern University School of Medicine
Section of Nephrology
Chicago, IL 60153, USA
Chapter 26

Iraj Nadjafi, M.D.
Nephrology-Dialysis-Transplant Unit
Dr Shariaty Hospital
University of Tehran
Kargar Avenue
Tehran, Iran
Chapter 61

H. Nihei, M.D.
Kidney Center
Tokyo Women's Medical College
Department of Surgery
8-1 Kawada-Cho, Shinjuku-ku
Tokyo 162, Japan
Chapter 58C

M. Nowicki, M.D.
Department Nephrology
Silesian School of Medicine
Katowice, Poland
Chapter 39

Dimitrios G. Oreopoulos, M.D.
Division of Nephrology
Toronto Hospital – Western Division
399 Bathurst Street
Toronto, Ontario, Canada M5T 2S8
Chapter 32

K. Ota, M.D.
Kidney Center
Tokyo Women's Medical College
Department of Surgery
8-1 Kawada-Cho, Shinjuku-ku
Tokyo 162, Japan
Chapter 58C

Patrick S. Parfrey , M.D., Ph.D.
Division of Nephrology
The Health Sciences Center
Memorial University
St. Johns, Newfoundland, Canada A1B 3V6
Chapter 38

Beth Piraino, M.D., Ph.D.
Medical Center
F1159 Presbyterian University Hospital
200 Lothrop Street
Pittsburgh, PA 15213, USA
Chapter 19

Hans D. Polaschegg, Ph.D.
Grünswiesenweg 9
D-61440 Oberursel, Germany
Chapter 13

Frederick K. Port, M.D.
University of Michigan
Kidney Epidemiology and Cost Center
315 W. Huron St., Suite 240
Ann Arbor, MI 48103. USA
Chapter 58B

Eduard A. Quellhorst, M.D.
Nephrology Center Niedersachsen
Vogelsang 105
D-34346 Hannover-Münden, Germany
Chapter 14

V.E. Quijada, M.D.
Department of Nephrology
Georgetown University Medical Center
3800 Reservoir Road
Washington, DC 20007, USA
Chapter 44

T.K. Sreepada Rao, M.D.
SUNY Health Science Center at Brooklyn
450 Clarkson Ave., Box 52
Brooklyn, NY 11203-2098, USA
Chapter 47A

Giuseppe Remuzzi, M.D.
Division of Nephrology and Dialysis
Ospedali Riuniti di Bergamo
I-24100 Bergamo, Italy
Chapter 12

Ann Rinehart, M.D.
Hennepin County Medical Center
Department of Medicine/Div. of Neprohology
701 Park Avenue
Minneapolis, MN 55415, USA
Chapter 46

Severin Ringoir, M.D., Ph.D.
Nephrology Department
University Hospital
De Pintelaan 185
B-9000 Ghent, Belgium
Chapter 1

E. Ritz, M.D., Ph.D.
Ruperto Carola University
Department of Internal Medicine
Bergheimerstr. 58
D-69115 Heidelberg, Germany
Chapter 39

Gianfranco Rizzoni, M.D.
Division of Nephrology and Dialysis
Department of Pediatric Research and Teaching
Ospedale Bambino Jesu
Rome, Italy
Chapter 31

Claudio Ronco, M.D.
Department of Nephrology
St. Bortolo Hospital
Via Rodolfi
I-36100 Vicenza, Italy
Chapters 7, 9, 20, 40

G. Said, M.D.
Service de Neurologie
Center Hospitalier Universitaire
Bicêtre
78, Ave. de Général Leclerc
94275 Le Kremlin
Bicêtre Cédex, France
Chapter 50

Walter Samtleben, M.D.
Nephrology Division
Medical Department I. Klinikum Grosshadern
University of Munich
München, Germany
Chapter 18

John A. Sargent, Ph.D.
5901 Christie Avenue
Suite 201
Emeryville, CA 94608, USA
Chapter 2

J. Schaeffer, M.D.
Division of Nephrology – 6840
Hannover Medical School
D-30623 Hannover, Germany
Chapter 53

A. Schieppati, M.D.
Mario Negri Inst. for Pharmacol. Res.
Clinical Res.Cntr. for Rare Diseases 'Aldo e Cele Dacco'
Villa Camozzi
I-24020 Ranica, Italy
Chapter 12

Belding H. Scribner, M.D.
Division of Nephrology
University of Washington
Mailstop Rm 11
Seattle, WA 98195, USA
Foreword

Neville H. Selwood, Ph.D.
UK Transplant Service
Southmead Hospital
Bristol, England
Chapter 57

Stanley Shaldon, M.D.
86, Rue de Grezac
F-34100 Montpellier, France
Chapter 28

A. Shinoda, M.D.
Department of Internal Medicine
Kanazawa Medical University
1-1 Daigaku, Uchinada-Machi
Kahoku-gun, Ishikawa-ken, 920-02 Japan
Chapter 58C

C. Shuler, M.D.
Division of Nephrology and Hypertension
Oregon Health Sciences University
3181 SW Sam Jackson Park Road
L 455
Portland, OR 97201, USA
Chapter 29

Heinz-Günther Sieberth, M.D.
Department Internal Medicine II
University of Technology
Pauwelsstrasse
D-52057 Aachen, Germany
Chapter 11

Kim Solez, M.D.
Department of Laboratory Medicine
5B4.02 W. MacKenzie Center
University of Alberta Hospitals
Edmonton, Alberta, Canada T6G 2R7
Chapter 61

B.P. Teehan, M.D.
Lankenau Medical Center # 135
100 Lancaster Avenue
Wynnewood, PA 19096, USA
Chapter 30

S. Teraoka, M.D., Ph.D.
Kidney Center
Tokyo Women's Medical College
8-1 Kawada-Cho, Shinjuku-ku
162 Tokyo, Japan
Chapter 58C

Nicholas L. Tilney, M.D.
Division of Transplant Surgery
Brigham and Women's Hospital
75 Francis Street
Boston, MA 02115, USA
Chapter 10B

H. Toma, M.D.
Kidney Center
Tokyo Women's Medical College
Department of Surgery
8-1 Kawada-Cho, Shinjuku-ku
Tokyo 162, Japan
Chapter 58C

Sato Tsuyoshi, M.D.
Tokai University School of Medicine
Department of Transplantation I, Boseidai, Isehara-shi
Kanagawa-ken, 269-11 Japan
Chapter 58F

M.N. Turenne, M.D.
Department of Medicine and Epidemiology
University of Michigan
Ann Arbor, MI 48103, USA
Chapter 58B

R. Uldall, M.D. (deceased)
Wellesley Hospital
Room 372
160 Wellesley Str., Bruce Wing 3-372
Toronto, Ontario M4Y 1J3, Canada
Chapter 10A

Raymond Vanholder, M.D., Ph.D.
Nephrology Department
University Hospital
De Pintelaan 185
B-9000 Ghent, Belgium
Chapter 1

Claude Verger, M.D.
Hôpital René Dubos
Unité de Dialyse
Avenue de l'Ile de France
F-95301 Pontoise, France
Chapter 55B

Jorg Vienken, M.D.
Fresenius AG
Medical Department
Borkenberg 14
D-61440 Oberursel, Germany
Chapter 28

G. Vigano, M.D.
Mario Negri Inst. for Pharmacol. Res.
Clinical Res.Cntr. for Rare Diseases 'Aldo e Cele Daccò'
Villa Camozzi
I-24020 Ranica, Italy
Chapter 12

P. Vogeleere
Nephrology Department
University Hospital
De Pintelaan 185
B-9000 Ghent, Belgium
Chapter 1

Dierk Vorwerk, M.D.
Department of Diagnostic Radiology
University of Technology
Pauwelsstrasse
D-52057 Aachen, Germany
Chapter 11

A. Wiecek, M.D.
Department of Nephrology
Silesian School of Medicine
Francuska 20
40-027 Katowice, Poland
Chapter 39

P.G. Wilson, M.D.
Department of Psychiatry
Cornell University Medical Center
525 68th Street
New York, NY 10021, USA
Chapter 62A

James F. Winchester, M.D.
Department of Nephrology
Georgetown University Medical Center
3800 Reservoir Road
Washington, DC 20007, USA
Chapters 18, 44

Antony J. Wing, M.D.
Department of Renal Medicine
St. George's Hospital
Blackshaw Road, Tooting
London SW17 0QT, England
Chapter 33

C. Woffindin, M.D.
Renal Unit
Royal Victoria Infirmary
Queen Victoria Road
Newcastle upon Tyne, NE1 4LP, England
Chapter 7

Ali-Reze Atef Zafarmand, M.D.
Nephrology-Dialysis-Transplant Unit
Dr Shariaty Hospital
University of Tehran
Kargar Avenue
Tehran, Iran
Chapter 61

TABLE OF CONTENTS

SECTION I
Pathophysiology of the uremic syndrome.
Principles and biophysics of dialysis

SECTION II
Technology of dialysis and associated methods

SECTION III
Quantification and prescription of dialysis

SECTION IV
Complications of dialysis

SECTION VIII
Organization and results of chronic dialysis

DRUG DOSAGE IN DIALYSIS PATIENTS

THOMAS A. GOLPER, MICHAEL A. MARX, CATHRYN SHULER and WILLIAM M. BENNETT

The elimination of most drugs and their metabolites is completely or partially dependent on renal excretion. Pharmacologic action is related to free drug concentration achieved at tissue receptor sites. To avert drug accumulation and possible toxicity, proper consideration must be taken when prescribing dosage regimens for patients with renal failure. Awareness of basic pharmacokinetic and pharmacodynamic principles is necessary to understand the alterations in drug metabolism and elimination that occur in uremia (1, 2). Typically, dialysis patients receive more than eight different medications (2). Adverse drug reactions occur more frequently in patients with renal insufficiency compared to nonazotemic hospitalized patient (3). This chapter addresses the principles relating to rational drug therapy in dialysis patients.

PHARMACOLOGIC AND PHARMACODYNAMIC CONSIDERATIONS IN UREMIA

Bioavailability

Conceptually, bioavailability is defined as the fraction (F) of an administered dose that reaches the systemic circulations (4). Practically, bioavailability is determined by two processes. Initially, there is liberation of the drug from its dosage form, and subsequently, there is entry into the systemic circulation. Drug efficacy is determined by both the rate and quantity of drug input into the body. The rate of input dictates the duration of drug effect and the quantity of input dictates the intensity of the effect. Bioavailability is usually determined by measuring the peak plasma level and plasma appearance rate after a single dose. A drug's absorption is affected by the character of the membranes it must cross to reach the circulation, the blood flow at the site of absorption, absorptive surface area, and contact time between the drug and the absorptive surface area. Local pH affects drug release from the dosage form and physicochemical properties of the drug such as pK_a molecular size, and lipid solubility influence the rate and extent (quantity) of drug absorption.

Since most drugs are administered orally, bioavailability is predominantly related to gastrointestinal function. Factors impacting on bioavailability of drugs absorbed through the gastrointestinal system include the dosage form of the drug, membrane permeability, gut lumenal metabolism of the drug, metabolism in the gut wall, and enterohepatic recycling of drug. The semipermeable nature of gastrointestinal membranes allow absorption of nutrients while excluding the entry of other compounds. For low molecular weight and highly lipid soluble drugs, absorption is generally passive, characterized by drug movement down an electrochemical or concentration gradient. No energy is required for this movement and it is not retarded by metabolic inhibitors. For many drugs metabolized in the liver there is substantial hepatic extraction after oral administration. This is referred to as 'first pass' effect. For drugs with low hepatic extraction, bioavailability is not much affected by the 'first pass' through the liver. However, for drugs with a high hepatic extraction ratio, the first pass may have profound effects on drug availability to the systemic circulation. The major impact of this phenomenon is seen when liver dysfunction develops. Reduction of first pass effect leads to greatly increased serum concentrations and often drug toxicity. Hepatic 'first pass' effects are greatly reduced when *shallow* rectal administration is employed (the inferior rectal vein empties directly into the *vena cava*) and eliminated altogether by sublingual, buccal, transdermal, and parenteral administration (5).

Edema can slow the absorption of drugs from the site of an intramuscular injection. This generalization is applicable following oral administration to dialysis patients. Gastrointestinal manifestations of uremia (nausea, vomiting, diarrhea, bowel edema) may contribute to drug malabsorption. Certain drugs, for example, nonsteroidal antiinflammatory agents (NSAIDs), may add to gastrointestinal symptoms by local irritative effects. Pancreatic exocrine dysfunction is now recognized as a major contributor to the malabsorptive syndromes noted in uremic patients (6). Drug absorption is probably also adversely affected.

Gastric pH is frequently altered in uremic patients. Dialysis patients have an increased salivary urea concentration which is converted to ammonia by gastric ure-

ases. This results in the buffering of gastric hydrochloric acid (HCl), raising gastric pH. Phosphate-binding antacids have a similar effect on pH. Drugs requiring an acidic milieu for optimal absorption (iron, antidepressants, and antihistamines) may exhibit decreased absorption in the uremic setting. Further reduction of stomach acidity from H_2 blocker use impairs absorption of such agents as ketoconazole. Antacids may also form nonabsorbable chelation products with certain drugs, for example digoxin, tetracycline, and fluoroquinolones such as ciprofloxacin.

Distribution

Individual drugs distribute themselves through the body in a characteristic manner. The apparent volume of distribution (V_d) is the amount of drug in the body divided by the plasma concentration of the drug when plasma and tissue equilibrium is reached and before any elimination occurs. The V_d does not correspond to a specific anatomic compartment but denotes a mathematical relationship. V_d assumes that the body is a homogenous reservoir. The apparent V_d is that volume in which the administered dose must have been dissolved to give the observed plasma concentration.

Many of the same factors that affect the absorption of a drug also influence the dispersion of drug into various compartments. These include physicochemical properties such as pK_a and lipid solubility, and important drug-body interactions such as protein binding and tissue binding. These drug-body interactions may be modified by patient specific factors such as age, gender, disease (CHF, thyroid status), body composition (edema, fat), regional blood flow compromise, and miscellaneous factors such as environmental conditions and concomitant drug therapy.

Disease states often produce deviations from the V_d observed in normal subjects. Alterations in fluid compartments as evidenced by edema and ascites tend to increase V_d for hydrophilic drugs, whereas volume depletion or dehydration reduce it. Infection may lead to changes in fluid compartments through fever, vomiting or diarrhea. Infection may also effect changes in the V_d by altering the extent of protein or tissue binding (e.g., vancomycin in peritonitis). Uremia alters the V_d of a number of drugs (clofibrate, digoxin, naproxen, phenytoin), through various mechanisms. In the case of phenytoin, the change in V_d in uremia is secondary to alterations in protein binding. Endogenous inhibitors to binding are retained in renal failure and lead to a larger V_d. Drugs minimally bound to plasma proteins, for example aminoglycosides, have the same V_d in uremia that is observed in healthy subjects. Systemic acidosis associated with uremia allows the increased penetration of salicylates and phenobarbital into the central nervous system (CNS).

Digoxin is highly bound to cardiac and other tissue Na/K transport enzymes accounting for its large V_d of 300–500 liters and very low plasma concentrations measured in units of ng/ml. Transport inhibitors accumulating in uremic patients may displace digoxin from its tissue binding sites, reducing V_d (7). In fact, some of these inhibitors may cross react with the anti-digoxin antibody used in therapeutic drug monitoring assays producing 'therapeutic' digoxin levels in patients not even taking the drug. Renal failure decreases the V_d of digoxin such that smaller loading doses are necessary to produce comparable plasma concentrations. Changes in V_d as the result of disease are usually of clinical importance only when the V_d is small under normal circumstances. This is true for drugs which have distribution volumes corresponding to the size of the total body water compartment or less (< 0.7 l/kg). Highly protein bound drugs are restricted to the intravascular space and have a small V_d. A drug that is more than 90% protein bound and poorly tissue bound will usually have a V_d of ≈ 0.2 l/kg. Highly lipid soluble drugs easily cross cellular membranes and have a large V_d. Drugs that bind with high affinity to specific tissue sites, for example digoxin, have a large V_d that may even exceed total body water (8). The larger the V_d, the smaller the proportion of drug remaining in circulation and hence the lower the delivery of the drug to the dialysis membrane. Therefore, dialytic drug removal will be insignificant for such agents.

Protein binding

As seen above, protein binding helps determine where a drug is distributed once in the body. The degree of protein binding also has a significant impact on pharmacologic effects (9). It is the unbound (free) drug that is responsible for both therapeutic efficacy and toxicity. Drugs highly bound to plasma proteins remain confined to the vasculature, and may not reach extravascular tissue receptor sites. Unbound drugs are available for distribution, but also for excretion. Protein binding is an equilibrium reaction, and distribution and excretion are inexorably tied to the association and dissociation of the drug-protein complex. Protein binding essentially acts as a storage pool for the drug, with the drug-protein complex equilibrium controlling drug effect and elimination. Routine analytical methods for determining blood, plasma, or serum drug levels usually measure bound plus unbound (total drug) concentrations. Sera from many patients with renal disease demonstrate decreased binding of various drugs when compared to sera from normal individuals. Albumin is the most prevalent plasma protein, and as such, drugs that bind primarily to albumin (acidic drugs) are more profoundly affected by uremia. These binding alterations (decreased binding) have generally been attributed to a combination of decreased serum albumin concentration and a reduction in albumin affinity for the drug, likely the result of accumulation of binding inhibitors in uremia (10–12). However, qualitative changes in the albumin of uremic subjects has also been an explanation for altered protein binding in uremia (13). This decrease in albu-

Table 1. Drugs with clinically relevant binding decreases in renal failure

Acids	Bases	Tissue binding
Barbiturates	Diazepam	Cardiac glycosides
Clofibrate	Mexilitine	Methotrexate
Diazoxide	Triamterene	
Digitoxin		
Furosemide		
Methotrexate		
Metolazone		
Penicillins		
Phenytoin		
Probenecid		
Salicylates		
Sulfonamides		
Warfarin		

min binding results in an increase in V_d and usually a lower total plasma drug concentration for a given dose (assuming that extravascular distribution and metabolism occur). Changes in protein binding may result in changes in the clearance and V_d for an agent. The intensity of the pharmacologic effect may be different than expected for a given plasma concentration because the ratio of free to total drug concentration may be altered. Due to changes in V_d and clearance with altered protein binding, it is difficult to predict accurately the clinical consequences in a particular patient.

Malnutrition and proteinuria lower serum protein levels. This increases the free fraction of drug due to saturation of the reduced number of available protein binding sites (14). Uremic toxins may decrease the affinity of albumin for a variety of drugs (Table 1) (10, 11, 15). Acidic drugs (e.g., cephalosporins, imipenem, vancomycin, and ciprofloxacin) have a larger free fraction than do basic drugs such as tobramycin due to the chronic organic acidemia that accompanies renal failure (16). Organic acids compete with acidic drugs for certain protein binding sites.

Uremia and albumin abnormalities are not the only conditions affecting drug-protein binding (17). Basic drugs bind avidly to serum proteins other than albumin (16, 18). Some of these proteins, such as α_1, acid glycoprotein, are acute phase reactans (16, 19). Myocardial infarction and stressors such as surgery can increase the availability of these proteins, enhancing drug binding and decreasing the quantity of free drug at receptor sites (20). Uremia decreases the protein binding of penicillins, digitoxin, phenobarbital, phenytoin, warfarin, morphine, primidone, salicylates, theophylline, and sulfonamides (Table 1). Factors contributing to this include pH, molar concentrations of drug and protein, competition for binding sites by retained inhibitors, other displacing drugs (e.g., heparin),

Table 2. Pharmacologically active metabolites of common drugs accumulated in renal failure

Parent drug	Metabolite	Pharmacologic action of metabolite
Acetohexamide	Hydroxyhexamide	Hypoglycemic
Allopurinol	Oxypurinol	Same as parent drug; enhanced desquamative skin eruptions due to xanthine oxidase inhibition
Azathioprine	6-mercaptopurine	Immunosuppressive
Clofibrate	Chlorophenoxyisobutyric acid	Increased skeletal muscle damage
Diazepam	Oxazepam	Anxiolytic
Lidocaine	Glycinexlidide	CNS reactions including seizures
Meperidine	Normeperidine	Seizures
Nitroprusside	Thiocyanate	CNS toxicity
Procainamide	N-acetyl procainamide	Antiarrhythmic
Propanolol	4-hydroxypropanolol	Beta-blocker
Rifampicin	Desacetylrifampin	Antibiotic
Sulfonamides	Acetylated metabolites	Nausea, vomiting, skin reactions

elevated free fatty acids, and probably other as yet unidentified factors. Clinical problems related to altered binding include the muscle toxicity noted with clofibrate use, the CNS effects of theophylline, phenytoin, the penicillins, and phenobarbital, and the many toxic effects of salicylates.

Metabolism

Metabolism is the biochemical conversion of a drug to another chemical form, which occurs primarily in the liver. The result is a more polar, less lipid-soluble, and more easily excreted metabolite. Metabolites usually possess different activity and toxicity profiles than the parent compound. Some metabolites possess pharmacologic activity similar to but usually less intense than the parent compound. While the desired pharmacologic property of the metabolite may be less than the parent compound, the toxicities may be more pronounced. When these metabolites are retained due to renal insufficiency, they accumulate and may cause adverse effects (Table 2).

In general, drugs that undergo hepatic metabolism by microsomal oxidation have similar elimination time profiles in patients with normal or diminished renal function (21). Some drugs (phenytoin and antipyrine) actually demonstrate accelerated metabolism because inducers of the hepatic enzyme systems have accumulated in the uremic patient.

Drug metabolism by reduction (cortisol), peptide hydrolysis (insulin, glucagon, parathyroid hormone (PTH)), or ester hydrolysis (diflunisal, procaine) is often slowed in uremia, necessitating dosage adjustment and individualization of therapy. This is attributable to decreases in nonhepatic (especially renal) metabolism. Drug metabolism by hepatic acetylation and glucuronide or sulfate conjugative synthesis are usually normal in uremia, an exception being isoniazid.

Elimination

Clearance is defined as the rate of elimination of a substance by all routes relative to the concentration of the substance in the sampled medium (usually plasma) (4). As used clinically, clearance implies the volume of plasma from which a drug or solute has been completely removed per unit time. Clearances by different routes are additive. Systemic or total body clearance is the sum of regional clearances (hepatic, renal, respiratory, biliary, extracorporeal). Hepatic drug clearance was discussed in the previous section and involves a biochemical transformation of the parent compound. Renal clearance is a reflection of the usual renal excretory processes (filtration and secretion), and renal metabolism, countered by reabsorption. In renal failure, accumulated organic acids may compete with acidic drugs for the same transport system and interfere with the secretion of other solutes.

Most drugs are eliminated from the body by first-order kinetics. This means that the elimination rate is directly proportional to the amount of drug in the body at that time, its concentration time course will yield a straight line if plotted on semilog graph paper, and its elimination reflects a nonsaturable process (2, 4, 22). Drug removal rate is often expressed as the elimination half-life, $t_{1/2}$, the time required to decrease total body drug burden and serum concentration by 50%. The $t_{1/2}$ for any drug is dependent on its clearance and its volume of distribution. The relationship is given by the formula $t_{1/2} = (0.693 \times V_d)/\text{clearance}$. Thus, for any given clearance, the $t_{1/2}$ will be longer when the V_d is larger. A reduction in clearance will prolong $t_{1/2}$ if the V_d remains constant. Since in each half-life 50% of the drug burden is eliminated, after five half-lives only 3% remains. For most drugs, total body clearance is determined by a combination of metabolic transformation and renal excretion. As previously mentioned, metabolism may be enhanced for some drugs in uremia, increasing clearance and decreasing $t_{1/2}$. In renal impairment a drug usually cleared by renal mechanisms will have a prolonged $t_{1/2}$. Increases in V_d because of renal dysfunction or decreased protein binding further complicates this relationship.

Excretion

Most drugs are excreted by the kidneys, usually after some metabolic transformation. Some are eliminated via the biliary system and a very few by other routes. With renal excretion virtually unavailable to dialysis patients, drug removal is often dependent on extracorporeal methods (dialysis). Generally, drugs ordinarily eliminated by glomerular filtration will be at least partially dialyzable. Those drugs eliminated ordinarily by tubular secretion may or may not be dialyzable.

DRUG ADMINISTRATION IN END STAGE RENAL DISEASE

Assessment of renal function

This chapter specifically addresses the clinical situation of ESRD and, as such, patients are dialysis dependent. Therefore creatinine clearance is presumed to be less than 10 ml/min. Patients with substantial urine output may have a significant degree of residual renal function and a 24-hour creatinine clearance determination may be helpful. However, as renal function deteriorates, creatinine clearance measurements, even when performed carefully, become increasingly subject to error as a surrogate measurement of glomerular filtration rate (GFR). This is due to the contribution of tubular secretion of creatinine in the filtrate. Radioisotope or nonradioactive clearance methods (iothalamate or iohexol) may be preferred in this setting as they correlate well with traditional inulin studies. The drug dosing tables which appear later in this chapter specifically address dosage adjustments for patients whose GFR is low enough to require dialysis.

The rationale for dosage adjustment

Drugs eliminated primarily by the kidneys or those that have active or toxic metabolites which are renally excreted are candidates for dosage adjustment in renal failure. Safety, then, is the primary impetus for making dosage adjustments. Other legitimate considerations are ease of administration (convenience) and cost. Knowledge of the drug's pharmacologic properties is essential to rational prescribing of these agents. This is especially true for drugs with a low therapeutic index (efficacy to toxicity ratio) such as cardiac glycosides, antiarrhythmics, and aminoglycoside antibiotics. In situations in which the clinician is in doubt about the need for dosage modification, it is important to review the usual pharmacologic handling

of the compound or to follow specific recommendations as we attempt later in this chapter.

DOSAGE ADJUSTMENT

Loading doses

Loading doses are administered to quickly attain desired concentrations of an agent. Typically, patients receive multiple doses of a medication at short, regularly spaced intervals. Complete elimination of one dose does not occur before the next dose is administered. Hence, drug accumulation occurs. This accumulation continues until steady state is reached. Renal failure may prolong the elimination half life more than ten fold. If dosage is simply adjusted for a prolonged half life in renal failure and attainment of effective concentrations is dependent on this accumulation, effective therapy may be unnecessarily delayed. Therefore, a loading dose is recommended. The size of the loading dose is dependent on the desired concentration and the volume of distribution of that drug in that patient. As discussed previously, factors that help determine V_d may be altered in the dialysis patient. Such considerations must be taken when determining the loading dose. Calculation of loading doses is discussed in the section on Drug Concentration Monitoring.

Maintenance doses

Two major approaches to dosage adjustment are employed in patients with renal failure. One can either extend the time between doses while maintaining the usual dose size (interval extension method) or the size of the dose can be reduced while maintaining the usual dosing interval (dosage reduction method). Occasionally, both approaches may be used together. The choice of dosing strategy is governed by the pharmacokinetic and pharmacodynamic relationships of the particular agent. We follow these principles in our specific recommendations appearing later in this chapter.

The interval extension method has the advantages of generating normal drug concentrations, using standard or normal dose size, and offering ease of calculation. The major disadvantages are (1) there may be prolonged periods where the drug concentration may be subtherapeutic if no loading dose is given, and (2) the dosing interval may require an odd dosing schedule. Odd dosing schedules lead to more frequent dosing errors and decreased compliance with the prescribed regimen. The amount of time above the minimum effective concentration is a function of both drug half-life and the magnitude (height) of the peak concentration (the area under the drug concentration-time curve). This is, in turn, dependent on the amount given (dose size) and the V_d. Thus, the amount of time spent above the effective concentration is dependent on the total dose given. The limiting factor for this approach will be the therapeutic index (relationship between effective therapeutic concentration and toxic concentration). The interval extension method is particularly practical for drugs with a relatively long serum half-life. The interval extension method is strongly encouraged for agents which exhibit concentration dependent killing, such as aminoglycoside antibiotics.

For therapeutic regimens where it is desired to minimize fluctuation in serum concentrations (bronchodilators, antiarrhythmics, cardiac glycosides, some antibiotics, antidepressants), the dosage reduction method is more appropriate. This method utilizes a reduction of the size of an individual dose prescribed at the same dosing interval as in patients without renal impairment. The advantages of the dosage reduction method are the constancy of drug concentrations, ease of calculation, and the convenient dosing intervals. Periods of subtherapeutic concentrations are minimized. The disadvantages are that the unusual dose sizes invite medication errors and there are circumstances where stable serum concentrations may not always be desirable (nephrotoxicity and ototoxicity from aminoglycosides).

DRUG CONCENTRATION MONITORING

Relatively few drugs used in clinical practice are routinely monitored by determining their concentration in serum, plasma, or whole blood. Drugs are dosed to obtain a specific clinical outcome and dosage adjustments are made empirically or guided by intermediate endpoints (blood pressure, lipid concentrations, symptom amelioration). In order to justify drug concentration monitoring as the basis for dosage adjustment, relationships have to have been established between concentration and effect or outcome. Few such relationships have been firmly established. The widest acceptance exists for drugs with a low therapeutic index, where therapeutic efficacy is balanced against avoidance of toxicity.

Most drug concentrations are determined in serum or plasma; whole blood is used occasionally. Serum and plasma concentrations are usually similar because differences between serum or plasma and whole blood are simply a reflection of drug distribution into erythrocytes (e.g., meperidine, cyclosporine). Reported drug concentrations generally represent total (protein bound + free drug) concentration, thus, confounding attempts to establish concentration-effect relationships in disparate patient populations.

Drug concentrations can only be properly interpreted if one knows the context surrounding the reported concentration. Important and relevant facts pertaining to the dosing regimen include the dose size, the time of administration, the route, the dosing interval, steady state versus nonsteady state conditions, and the time of sampling relative to the dose administration. In order to make dosage modifications based upon the drug concentrations the patient must be under 'stable' conditions – that is, the V_d and clearance must be constant. If one has two concentrations drawn after the drug's distribution phase, one can easily calculate the elimination rate and half life. Knowing the $t_{1/2}$ is useful because one can estimate the time required to attain steady state ($\approx$ 3 to 5 half lives), the time to completely remove a drug (> 5 half lives), and a reasonable dosing interval (usually 2 to 3 half lives).

When the clinician knows what drug concentrations are desirable and which concentrations are associated with toxicity, drug concentration monitoring can be an indispensable tool to individualizing drug therapy. Both loading and maintenance doses can be calculated. Table 3 describes these processes. The currently observed concentration (current concentration or level) is subtracted from the concentration one wishes to achieve (desired concentration or level), leaving the difference level, all in the same units. The difference level times the V_d times the body weight in kilograms will give the amount of drug needed to boost the current level to the desired level. For loading doses the current level is zero. For maintenance doses the trough concentration can be used as the current level. This approach can be applied to the administration of any drug whose concentration is available and whose V_d is known. It is particularly suitable for the setting of renal insufficiency when the exact drug clearance is not known because of changing conditions (e.g., changing clinical status, hemodynamics, dialysis).

UNIQUE PHARMACOLOGIC PROBLEMS IN DIALYSIS PATIENTS

Altered drug sensitivity in uremia

Drug sensitivity is the relationship between drug concentration at its receptor and the drug effect. Distinguishing between altered V_d and drug sensitivity is often difficult. Uremia and/or its associated acidosis can change V_d by modifying the drug-barrier or drug-protein interactions. Decreased protein binding of phenytoin and thiopental and the increased blood-brain barrier penetration of salicylates and barbiturates are examples of altered V_d. Examples of altered sensitivities in uremia include the CNS effects of benzodiazepines and opiates and resistance to the pressor effects of catecholamines. Uremia-associated electrolyte and acid-base abnormalities can predispose patients to altered drug sensitivity. Hyperkalemia potentiates the conduction system effects of cardiac glycosides, quinidine, procainamide, phenothiazines, and tricyclic antidepressant (1). Alkalosis, hypokalemia, and hypomagnesemia predispose patients to dysrhythmias in the presence of digitalis . Uremia, through its contribution to dysautonomia, may accentuate bradycardia from β-adrenergic blocking agents. Titration to clinical end points is the prudent approach to dosing these agents in the patient with ESRD.

Table 3. Calculation of loading and supplemental doses

Loading dose (mg/kg)	= Desired serum concentration × volume of distribution (mg/l) (l/kg)
Actual dose size (mg)	= Desired serum concentration × V_d × body wt. (kg)

Example for gentamicin where the desired peak concentration is 6 mg/l; V_d of 0.25 l/kg

Loading dose	= 6 mg/l × 0.25 l/kg = 1.5 mg/kg
Supplemental dose (mg/kg)	= Difference concentration (mg/l) × V_d (l/kg)
Where difference concentration	= Desired minus current concentration

Example for gentamicin when trough concentration is 1.5 mg/l and the desired concentration is 6 mg/l

Difference concentration	= 6 mg/l minus 1.5 mg/l = 4.5 mg/l
Supplemental dose	= 4.5 mg/l × 0.25 l/kg = 1.125 mg/kg

Urinary tract infections

When renal function is significantly impaired, it is difficult to attain adequate antibiotic concentrations in the renal parenchyma or urine. Therefore, despite adequate serum concentrations a urinary tract infection may not be eradicated. Aminoglycosides, which enter the urine solely through glomerular filtration, may not reach adequate concentrations in a patient with a very low GFR (23). Drugs that enter the urine by tubular secretion (penicillins, sulfonamides, trimethoprim, and cephalosporins) are effective in eradicating urinary tract infections in uremic patients infected with sensitive organisms. Similar doses to those used in nonuremic patients should be employed to ensure adequate urine concentrations. This will result in modest drug accumulation in the serum, but these agents are usually well tolerated with little associated toxicity from the increased serum concentrations (24).

Renal cyst infections

One complication suffered by patients with polycystic kidney disease is the development of infected cysts. These may result from upper urinary tract infections. Antibiotics may not penetrate cyst walls and eradication of the infecting organism may not occur without surgical drainage. Antibiotics that have demonstrated some clinical efficacy in treating renal cyst infections include trimethoprim-sulfamethoxazole, chloramphenicol, and fluoroquinolones (25, 26). Other drugs commonly used to treat urinary infections (penicillins, cephalosporins) do not penetrate into cysts well and must be given for prolonged periods in high doses even in patients with renal failure. Aminoglycosides exhibit poor penetrance into renal cysts and there is reduced activity of aminoglycosides in the acidic environment within many cysts. Patients may present with constitutional symptoms, fever, and acute or chronic flank pain, or hematuria. Cyst infection may be present in patients with sterile urine. Ultrasound or computed tomography examination may reveal thickened cyst walls and provide diagnostic clues in difficult cases.

Muscle paralysis

The accumulation of aminoglycoside antibiotics in patients with renal failure can potentiate the effects of neuromuscular blocking agents. Respiratory dysfunction may result, often manifested as failure to recover spontaneous respirations in the immediate postoperative period. Most of the clinically available neuromuscular blocking agents can have profound and delayed effects on patients with impaired renal function (27). Anesthesiologists, surgeons, and other clinicians involved in the patient's care must be cognizant of these interactions in order to anticipate potential problems when patients receiving aminoglycosides require surgery.

Metabolic loads

Many commonly employed drugs contain accompanying substances (sodium, potassium) that may not be adequately excreted in patients with renal failure. Other drugs may alter normal metabolism in uremia such that the endogenous load of waste products is enhanced (antianabolic

Table 4. Drugs with significant metabolic loads

Metabolic load	Examples
Acid	Acetazolamide, NH_4Cl, aspirin, methenamine mandelate, ethanol, paraldehyde
Alkali	Antacids, carbenicillin, plasma protein concentrates, licorice, oral hyperalimentation, tobacco
Creatinine	Anabolic and androgenic steroids
Magnesium	Laxatives, antacids
Potassium	Potassium penicillin (3 mEq per million units, Pen G 1.7 mEq/million units), salt substitutes
	K-sparing diuretics, neuromuscular blocking agents, blood transfusion, oral hyperalimentation fluid
Sodium	Ampicillin (3.0 mEq/g), Azlocillin (2.7 mEq/g), Carbenicillin (4.7 mEq/g), Cephalothin (2.4 mEq/g), Kayexalate (1.5 mEq/g), Mezlocillin (1.9 mEq/g), Moxalactam (3.8 mEq/g), Piperacillin (1.9 mEq/g), Ticarcillin (5.2 mEq/g), Antacids, oral hyperalimentation fluids
Urea	Glucocorticosteroids, tetracyclines, hyperalimentation, protein
Water	Nonsteroidal antiinflammatory drugs, oral hypoglycemics, clofibrate, cyclophosphamide, carbamazepine, vincristine, narcotics

Table 5. Drug-laboratory test interactions: effect on creatinine determinations

Drug	Effect
Ascorbic acid	Elevates total chromogen; false increase in creatinine measurement
p-Aminohippurate	Elevates total chromogen; false increase in creatinine measurement
Methyldopa/levodopa	Reducing agents interfere with autoanalyzer measurement; increases measured creatinine when blood level of methyldopa > 2 mg/ml
Trimethoprim	Competition for tubular secretion causes true increase in serum creatinine
Acetylsalicylic acid	Competition for tubular secretion causes true increase in serum creatinine
Cefoxitin	False increase in creatinine measurement by interference with Jaffe reaction
Cimetidine	Competition for tubular secretion causes true increase in serum creatinine

agents). The metabolic loads inherent with several drugs are categorized in Table 4.

Aggravation of uremia

Medications should always be suspect when there is some change in the clinical status of the patient. Many agents cause vomiting and gastrointestinal upset, mimicking uremic symptoms. This is especially so for drugs having a direct effect on the gastric mucosa, such as NSAIDs, but is also true of antihypertensives drugs and antibiotics. Resultant volume depletion may aggravate existing renal blood flow compromise and lead to loss of residual function. This may necessitate more aggressive dialysis or dietary restriction. Tetracyclines, androgenic agents, and glucocorticosteroids increase protein catabolism and azotemia (28). Aspirin and other NSAIDs, dipyridamole, and sulfinpyrazone impair platelet function; this may be difficult to distinguish from the platelet functional defect of uremia. The differentiation of drug toxicity from uremia is critical in the evaluation of CNS depression, gastrointestinal bleeding, bone marrow suppression, hemolysis, peripheral neuropathies, and seizures.

Laboratory abnormalities

Uremia and certain medications may affect the results of certain laboratory tests. For instance, metabolites of propranolol in the serum of the uremic patient will often falsely elevate the serum bilirubin if performed by the automated diazo technique (SMA 12/60, Technicon Instruments) (29). When the Bilirubinometer is used this effect does not occur. Ketone bodies (20), acetohexamide (31), methyldopa (32), and some cephalosporins (33) have been reported to cause a laboratory artifact, which results in falsely high serum creatinine levels. Cimetidine (34) and trimethoprim (35) interfere with the renal tubular secretion of creatinine. This results in an elevated serum creatinine and lower creatinine clearance, but inulin clearance is not affected. Potassium-sparing diuretics also interfere with the serum measurement of creatinine (1). Table 5 summarizes these observations.

Table 6. Drug properties which affect dialytic clearance

Molecular weight
Protein binding
Volume of distribution
Charge
Water or lipid solubility
Membrane binding
Alternative excretory pathway

DRUG DIALYZABILITY

Most studies of drug removal during dialysis were performed utilizing conventional hemodialysis techniques. Specific data describing drug removal with highly permeable membranes were until very recently almost exclusively based on observations noted during continuous hemofiltration or continuous hemodialysis. Drug removal with these therapies is discussed later. Some recommendations will be based upon extrapolation from data known about specific drugs which have been tested and from known clearance data of middle molecular markers such as vitamin B_{12} and inulin. To this end, drugs are considered solutes of variable water solubility, for which the principles for dialytic clearance apply. Table 6 summarizes the unique properties of drugs which affect their removal by dialysis.

DRUG PROPERTIES WHICH AFFECT DIALYZABILITY (TABLE 6)

Molecular weight

Drug molecular weight is a reliable predictor of drug dialyzability (36, 37). Drugs larger than 1000 Daltons depend less upon diffusion and more upon convection for dialytic clearance. This is the circumstance where high flux membranes will dialyze larger quantities of this drug. Molecular volume is determined by the weight, shape, stearic hindrance and charge of the species in question. If a drug cannot fit through a dialysis membrane pore because of its geometric proportions, it is reflected and not cleared by the dialyzer. There is an inverse semilogarithmic relationship between dialysis clearance and molecular weight (38).

Protein binding

The binding of drugs to circulating plasma proteins is another reliable predictor of a drug's dialyzability. Many factors including uremia may influence the extent of drug-protein binding. Drugs which are highly protein bound will have a low proportion of the drug available for removal by dialysis.

Heparin administration during dialysis stimulates lipoprotein lipase, which increases levels of free fatty acids (18, 39, 40). Free fatty acids compete with tryptophan, sulfonamides, salicylates, phenylbutazone, phenytoin, thiopentone, and valproic acid for albumin binding sites, causing an increase in the free fraction of drug during and after the heparin exposure. To illustrate the complexity of drug-protein interactions, free fatty acid may displace cefamandole, but may enhance the binding of cephalothin or cefoxitin (41). Golper and associates have shown that free fatty acids increase the free fraction of phenytoin, a highly protein bound drug (42). Thus, greater clearances by dialysis would be anticipated.

Volume of distribution

For dialytic removal of a drug to be clinically significant, the fraction of the total body burden of drug that is removed must be substantial. Even if the extraction of the drug across the dialyzer is 100%, if the amount of drug in the blood is small relative to the body's total amount, dialytic removal will be insignificant (e.g., digoxin). When the drug's V_d is large, the drug is highly bound to tissue and its availability to the circulation and to the dialyzer is minimal (18). Compared to drugs with a larger V_d but the same molecular weight and protein binding, drugs with $V_d < 1$ l/kg will be more readily dialyzed. Drugs with V_d between 1–2 l/kg have marginal dialytic clearances, and substantial drug removal is unlikely if the V_d is > 2 l/kg.

Despite rapid extracellular solute clearances with short time high flux or high efficiency dialysis, intracellular equilibration with extracellular fluid can be slow, especially with larger molecules (43). This is probably related to lipid solubility of the drug and tissue compartmentalization. Post-dialysis intracellular concentrations may vary by only 1–2% (44). Consequently, there is a drug concentration gradient between intracellular and extracellular fluid. There may be a post-hemodialysis rebound of 10–25% with intercompartmental equilibration (45). Higher ultrafiltration rates will aggravate this phenomenon. Vancomycin's rebound was 50% higher than the initial post-dialysis drug concentration and highly variable regarding the time to reach a peak (46). Thus, it is difficult to predict this phenomenon for a specific situation. We recommend that you follow drug levels closely.

Drug-RBC binding

Drugs may partition into red blood cells (RBCs). Whole blood clearance can be measured by multiplying blood flow rate times the pre-dialyzer and post-dialyzer concentration difference. Ultrafiltration during dialysis raises hematocrit, complicating the determination of intradialytic drug clearance by this method (47). The proper reference value is either the whole blood concentration or the plasma concentration. This is particularly relevant to the clearance of ethambutol, a drug known to partition into the RBC (48). Drugs which have a partition coefficient (whole blood to plasma concentration ratio) exceeding unity (e.g., procainamide, glutethimide, and acetaminophen), may have decreased clearances due to hemoconcentration at the end of dialysis (18). Thus, for drugs that partition into RBC, total dialytic clearance may be reduced in these hemoconcentrated states. Furthermore, the issue of rapid re-equilibration between RBC drug and plasma drug becomes more important.

These observations were made prior to the routine use of erythropoietin. Higher pre-dialysis hematocrits will result in greater RBC partitioning and in less free drug, with the potential consequences described above. Even for a drug with low RBC partitioning, clearance may also be decreased in the setting of higher hematocrits because, like all plasma solutes, dialytic clearance is dependant on delivery of plasma to the dialyzer. Therefore, one must be cautious when interpreting *in vivo* dialyzer clearances of solutes with RBC partitioning. For drugs, measuring whole body (total) clearance during dialysis is more helpful than dialytic clearance.

Miscellaneous drug properties

For drugs to be dialyzable, the free drug must be in equilibrium with plasma water. Since dialysate is aqueous, drugs poorly soluble in water will not be dialyzable. Thus, drug *water solubility* is a factor. Drugs that are *charged* are not as dialyzable as uncharged drugs. This is partly related to charge repulsion at the membrane surface but may also relate to *drug binding to the membrane*. These issues are discussed in more detail in the section below on drug-membrane interactions. Lastly, as a rule of thumb, if dialytic clearance can increase total body clearance by 30%, this regional clearance by dialysis is considered clinically important (49, 50). Thus, the nondialytic clearance is a major factor in determining the overall significance of the dialytic clearance. Uremia may impair, stimulate or have no effect on the nonrenal or nondialytic clearance of a drug. For many drugs this is known and must be considered.

DIALYTIC PROPERTIES WHICH AFFECT DRUG CLEARANCE

Properties which affect drug clearance could be divided into three categories: properties of the dialyzer, the dialysate, and the technique of dialysis. The disadvantage of a categorization such as this is that these properties are interdependent and stand alone only during experimental conditions. Nonetheless, as one reads the following comments, it may be helpful to think in terms of these three categories which are summarized in Table 7.

Table 7. Dialysis properties which affect drug clearance

Hemodialyzer properties
Pore size (membrane materials)
Blood flow rate (operating conditions)
Surface area
Membrane binding

Dialysate Properties
Dialysate flow rate (operating conditions)
Solute concentration (operating conditions)
pH
Temperature (operating conditions)

Convection versus Diffusion

Properties of the dialyzer

Membrane materials

The development of membranes with a wide range of solute permeabilities was in part related to the concern over the importance of larger molecular weight uremic toxins. Dialysis membranes are generated from natural and synthetic polymers, including cellulose, cellulose acetate, polysulfone, polyamide, polyacrylonitrile (PAN, e.g. AN69) and polymethylmethacrylate (PMMA).

With re-used polysulfone membranes trace quantities of albumin appear in the dialysate (51), especially when the dialyzers are reprocessed for re-use with bleach and formaldehyde (52, 53). Clearances of vancomycin vary with different membranes (45, 54–56). AN69 and polysulfone membranes yield the greatest clearance, while Cuprophan® has minimal clearance of vancomycin under similar conditions (54, 56). Gentamicin clearance is greater with a cuprammonium rayon membrane compared to a saponified cellulose ester membrane (57). Thus, membranes vary in permeability because of their own composition, but also because of altered composition after they are manufactured.

Surface area

Small solute dialyzability is dependent upon the concentration gradient between blood and dialysate. This is maximized by increasing flow rates and/or by increasing surface area, dispersing the undialyzed blood to areas of fresh dialysate. These principles are applied to high flux and high efficiency dialysis. As molecular size increases, diffusivity is limited by the membrane's pore size, and the clearance of the molecule becomes more dependent upon convection. The hydraulic permeability of high flux membranes exceeds that of conventional membranes, enhancing the clearances of larger molecules because of the greater contribution from convection. When hydraulic permeability limits are achieved, a larger surface area becomes the most influential factor. For PAN, PMMA and polysulfone dialyzers, surface area and ultrafiltration have major effects on the clearances of beta₂ microglobulin and phosphate, two poorly dialyzable species (58). This is not a new concept. For example, the amount of vancomycin removed by high flux dialysis was correlated to membrane surface area (54). Furthermore, surface area is a major determinant of the ultrafiltration rate. Increasing surface area has been the mainstay of several clearance enhancing techniques (59, 60).

Drug-membrane charge interaction and membrane binding

The PAN membrane's negative charge causes interactions with solutes such as gentamicin and doxycycline (61). Theoretical estimates of gentamicin clearance did not correlate well with clinical observations during dialysis with PAN filters (62). It is possible that the negative charge of the membrane retarded gentamicin clearance. The other possible explanation for decreased aminoglycoside clearance could be drug adsorption to the dialysis membrane (63–65). Drug-membrane binding has also been demonstrated in the absence of proteins during experimental conditions of continuous arteriovenous hemofiltration (42, 66–68).

Diffusion

Drug diffusivity decreases as molecular size increases (69). Diffusive clearance through conventional dialysis membranes is negligible for molecules larger than 1000 Daltons. Very few commonly used drugs are this large. Most drugs are of the size that the membrane diffusive cutoffs play a role in determining dialyzability. Countercurrent flow, and high blood and dialysate flow augment the concentration gradient between blood and dialysate, enhancing the efficiency of diffusion. This is particularly important for drugs in the lower of middle molecular weight ranges, for example aminoglycosides at around 600 Daltons. Small solute clearances increase considerably as dialysate and blood flow increase. This is referred to as flow rate limited clearance (14). For larger molecules, their size limits the rate of diffusion through the membrane pores. Thus, the blood to dialysate concentration gradient remains high. Flow rates of either dialysate or blood have less influence for the diffusion of middle or larger weight molecules. However, under those conditions the surface area and hydraulic permeability become important, allowing convective removal (see below). While convective removal occurs, the addition of high ultrafiltration rates during high flux hemodialysis causes mixing of the ultrafiltrate and the dialysate. Under certain conditions this diminishes the concentration gradient and the diffusive clearance of solutes(16, 70–72).

Convection

Convection is defined as the ultrafiltration bulk flow from the blood to the dialysate. Within the convected fluid is solute at the same concentration as in the water component of plasma. Convection of solute ceases when (1) the permeability of the membrane is reached, or (2) the negative transmembrane pressure causes collapse of the dialysate compartment, or (3) the membrane ruptures. Ultrafiltration affects all sizes of molecules, but its effect is more evident with large molecules because of their poor diffusion. Henderson and associates have demonstrated that convection removes larger molecules more readily than does diffusion (69, 73–75). Utilizing conventional low flux cellulosic membranes, removal of solutes greater than 1000 Daltons generally requires ultrafiltration. Depending on the membrane, even during ultrafiltration, molecules greater than 2000 Daltons are partially reflected by the membrane (76).

Diffusion dominates convection in most cases of solute removal during dialysis. This is especially noted for small molecular sized substances, and less so for middle and large molecules, whose clearance is dependent on convection. Increasing blood flow does not influence the clearance of middle weight or larger molecules (76).

The binding of proteins to the membrane decreases ultrafiltration. Vincent et al. have shown predictable deterioration of ultrafiltration secondary to protein binding to the membrane (77). This is probably related to alteration in the porosity of the membrane by protein binding or reduction in the surface area. Protein layering against the dialysis membrane (protein concentration polarization) creates a physical barrier which 'widens the membrane'. Protein at the membrane surface results in increased osmotic and oncotic activity on the blood side that ultimately retard convection.

Operating conditions (conventional, high efficiency and high flux HD)

For patients on dialysis the artificial kidney dialyzer is an important route of drug removal. High efficiency, high flux and conventional hemodialysis differ because of membrane porosity, surface area, and the flow rates of blood and dialysate. All these factors influence drug handling to greater or lesser degrees. High efficiency dialysis utilizes conventional 'tight' membranes with a large surface area and high blood and dialysate flow rates. This strategy was designed to improve small solute clearance so that the duration of treatment could be reduced. However, under these operating conditions, clearance is average to poor for middle and large molecular sized species and is far more dependent upon the duration of dialysis.

Membranes with greater diffusive properties allow substantial diffusive clearance of molecules in the middle to large molecular size range. In general clinicians do not make a distinction between membranes that have greater diffusive properties and 'high flux' membranes, which are usually defined simply by high hydraulic permeabilities.

Because of the high hydraulic permeability intrinsic to these more 'open' membranes, high flux dialysis utilizes greater ultrafiltration rates to achieve maximum convective solute removal of middle and large molecules. That property rather than greater diffusion probably explains the greater clearance of middle molecules with high flux membranes.

Modification of clearances across a broad spectrum of molecular sizes is of particular interest to a discussion of drug clearance, since most drugs have molecular weights falling in the small to middle molecular weight range. Adjustments made with short time high efficiency dialysis suggest that drug clearance may not vary from longer time conventional dialysis. Depending on the size of the drug, there may be significant differences in drug removal with high flux dialysis. Very large drugs may be removed only by convection, and that can only occur substantially with high flux dialyzers.

CLINICAL APPLICATION OF THESE PRINCIPLES

Example – vancomycin

Bastani et al. first compared vancomycin and urea clearances through dialyzers of different membrane material but with equal surface areas and flow rates (55). Unlike urea, vancomycin clearance was highest with AN69 membranes, intermediate with cellulose acetate and lowest with Cuprophan®. These results have been corroborated (56). Torras et al. demonstrated similar results and further showed that by increasing blood flow rates from 250 to 350 ml/min through an AN69 dialyzed vancomycin clearance increased another 50% (78). Up to 200 mg of vancomycin was removed during a high flux hemodialysis session. However, De Bock et al. removed a similar quantity utilizing a cellulose acetate dialyzer under standard operating conditions (45).

Lanese et al. examined the relationship between vitamin B_{12} clearance and the removal of vancomycin with other variables including membrane surface area and ultrafiltration coefficients (hydraulic permeability) (54). A tight linear correlation between vitamin B_{12} clearance and vancomycin clearance was demonstrated. They concluded that the correlation between the clearance of vitamin B_{12} and the percent of vancomycin removed may be the best available data in the absence of specific dialyzer vancomycin removal rates. They derived the following expression for vancomycin removal during dialysis:

$$\% \text{ vancomycin removal during dialysis}$$
$$= (0.09 \times Cl_{B12} - 1.5)$$
$$\times (0.75 + 0.001 \times Q_B) \times (\text{time, hr})$$

where Cl_{B12} is the manufacturer's reported vitamin B_{12} clearance, Q_B is dialyzer blood flow and time is duration of dialysis in hours. Such a mathematical approach is possible for other medications.

Conclusions

Certain generalizations seem valid. High efficiency dialysis utilizes 'tight' membranes. Urea clearance is high because flow rates and surface areas are increased above those seen in conventional dialysis. These adjustments allow for shortened dialysis time while overall dialysis delivery is probably unchanged from conventional dialysis. Therefore, drug dosing recommendations for conventional dialysis will probably apply reliably to high efficiency dialysis. This will need to be confirmed in clinical trials. For high flux dialysis there are several variables which make generalizations less reliable. For example, while the 'open' membranes utilized in high flux may demonstrate greater diffusivity and convectivity (and thus, clearance) for middle molecular weight species, the shortened dialysis time may reduce overall clearance. The larger the molecule, the longer it takes to remove it, no matter what membrane is utilized. Even though most drugs are either small molecules (< 500 Daltons), or in the lowest ranges of 'middle molecular weight', this principle of time and clearance applies. In addition, any technique that utilizes shortened dialysis times jeopardizes the clearance of molecules that have a substantial degree of tissue binding or intracellular deposition. Rapid depletion through the dialyzer of unbound or extracellular drug cannot be replaced rapidly from protein bound, tissue bound or intracellular stores. Therefore, the openness of the membrane and the shortening of dialysis time may counteract each other regarding overall drug clearance. Some membranes, particular AN69, bind drugs more readily than other high flux membranes. Therefore, until the actual studies are performed to define drug removal during high flux dialysis, we must be cautious in our predictions.

DRUG REMOVAL DURING CONTINUOUS RENAL REPLACEMENT THERAPIES

Continuous renal replacement therapies include hemofiltration, hemodialysis, and the blend of these two, called hemodiafiltration. Since these therapies are generally reserved for critically ill patients, knowledge of drug disposition in this setting is imperative to avoid pharmacologic errors.

Since peritoneal dialysis is often performed in a continuous manner, we have included it in this section, although the patients treated by peritoneal dialysis are clinically different from those treated by continuous hemofiltration, continuous hemodialysis, or continuous hemodiafiltration.

Hemofiltration (HF)

Solute removal during pure HF is convective. The sieving coefficient (S) is defined as the solute concentration in the ultrafiltrate divided by the solute concentration in plasma. S is the mathematical expression of the solute's ability to convectively permeate a membrane. An S of 1 states that the solute freely passes through the membrane with the bulk flow of the solvent, while an S of 0 describes complete rejection of the solute, despite flow of the solvent. Colton et al. have shown that a reasonable approximation is:

$$S = \frac{UF}{(A + V)/2} = \frac{2UF}{A + V}$$

where A, V, and UF represent the arterial, venous and ultrafiltrate concentrations, respectively (79). Golper et al. have further shown that under continuous HF conditions, S = UF/A, which eliminates the need for a venous sample (80). Under conditions of continuous HF, S is usually constant (42, 81). Furthermore, sieving is independent of blood flow (42, 82). During HF clearance is the product of S times the ultrafiltration rate (UFR). Since S is constant, clearance is linearly related to UFR.

Thus, the most important way to describe drug handling in HF is to determine its S. This is applicable for continuous or intermittent HF.

Kronfol et al. have demonstrated that in the absence of proteins, there are drug-membrane interactions during HF (66–68). Sieving coefficients for several drugs through PAN and polyamide membranes were significantly different from those through polysulfone. Drug charge can affect either convective or diffusive transport, depending on the nature of the drug-membrane charge interaction (discussed above). In an aqueous solution the polycationic antibiotic gentamicin had an S through Amicon polysulfone of only 0.94 (42). From its molecular weight, one would expect an S of 1.0. For some reason, interaction between the drug and the membrane prevent complete sieving. Lysaght has shown that even a cation as small as sodium has an S less than unity (83). The introduction of a negative charge on macromolecules can cause a major decrease in sieving during HF (84). However, small anions such as chloride and bicarbonate have S's greater than unity (85, 86), thought to be secondary to the Gibbs–Donnan effect of circulating proteins. Penicillins and cephalosporins are anionic antibiotics which may demonstrate this phenomenon during hemofiltration (Table 8).

Drugs bind to dialysis membranes as discussed above (61). When aminoglycosides bind to membranes, S is very low for the first few minutes after exposure, but as the binding sites saturate, S rises. A Biospal 0.5 m^2 PAN filter binds 10 to 20 mg of tobramycin (65).

Binding to nonultrafilterable plasma proteins will play a dominant role in determining a drug's convective transport. Protein-bound drug will not be filtered. As discussed

Table 8. Drug-sieving coefficients (S) in HF compared to unbound fraction (UF)

Antibiotics			Other		
Drug	S	Alpha	Drug	S	Alpha
Amikacin	0.9	0.9	Bromide	1.0	1.0
Amphotericin B	0.3	0.1	Chlordiazepoxide	0.05	0.05
Ampicillin	0.7	0.8	Cisplatin	0.1	0.1
Cefoperazone	0.3	0.1	Clofibrate	0.06	0.04
Cefotaxime	0.62	0.6	Cyclosporine	0.6	0.1
Cefoxitin	0.6	0.5	Diathybarbital	1.0	0.9
Ceftazidime	0.9	0.9	Diazepam	0.02	0.02
Ceftriaxone	0.8	0.1	Digitoxin	0.1	0.1
Cephapirin	1.5	0.6	Digoxin	0.9	0.8
Cilastin	0.8	0.6	Famotidine	0.7	0.8
Ciprofloxacin	0.76	0.7	Glibencamide	0.6	0.01
Clindamycin	0.5	0.4	Glutethimide	0.02	0.5
Doxycycline	0.4	0.2	Lidocaine	0.2	0.4
Erythromycin	0.4	0.3	Metamizole	0.4	0.4
Gentamicin	0.8	0.9	NAPA	0.9	0.9
Imipenem	1.0	0.8	Nitrazepam	0.08	0.1
Metronidazole	0.8	0.8	Nomifensin	0.7	0.4
Mezlocillin	0.7	0.7	Oxazepam	0.1	0.1
Nafcillin	0.5	0.2	Phenobarbital	0.8	0.6
Netilmicin	0.9	0.9	Phenytoin	0.4	0.2
Oxacillin	0.02	0.05	Procainamide	0.9	0.9
Penicillin	0.7	0.5	Pyrithyldione	0.4	–
Streptomycin	0.3	0.6	Ranitidine	0.8	0.85
Sulfamethoxazole	0.3	0.6	Theophylline	0.9	0.45
Tobramycin	0.8	0.9			
Vancomycin	0.8	0.9			

earlier many factors affect drug-protein binding. As proteins collect along the membrane (protein concentration polarization) the molar concentrations of drug and proteins are changed, contributing to altered protein binding. The unbound drug is the pharmacologically active moiety. If there is displacement, the pharmacologic effect, metabolism, and removal will be enhanced.

Table 8 displays the S and unbound fraction (alpha) of drugs whose S has been determined either from our experience or the literature (80, 87). There is a statistically significant correlation between S and alpha. Kroh et al. have shown that an even tighter correlation occurs when S is defined as AUCuf/AUCp, where AUCuf and AUCp represent the areas under the time-drug concentration curves for ultrafiltrate (uf) and plasma (p), respectively (88).

The role of molecular size (weight and stearic hindrance) on membrane transport has been extensively studied and was discussed above. For most drugs in clinical use, molecular size will not be an issue for removal during HF. The membrane molecular weight cutoffs exceed the molecular weight of the drugs. During hemodialysis molecular weight is even more important.

Drug removal during hemofiltration

Inulin readily traverses polysulfone hemofilter membranes (82, 89, 90). Since virtually all therapeutic agents have a molecular weight less than that of inulin, one can reasonably assume that these drugs will permeate these membranes limited mostly by the extent of their protein binding. Protein binding data are available, usually from studies of healthy people (91). Slight discrepancies may arise when comparing those data to critically ill patients.

One can measure the removal of drug during HF by multiplying the ultrafiltrate (UF) drug concentration by the filtration rate. Since 'arterial' plasma levels are usually required for clinical management, one could calculate the UF concentration from the arterial concentration (A) by the formula:

$$UF = A \times alpha$$

where the protein binding is *assumed* to be normal (91). The following schema summarizes the technique to determine drug removal from CAVH:

1. Determine steady-state arterial conc. (A).
2. Determine fraction *not* bound to protein (alpha) (91).
3. Determine filtration rate.
4. Amount removed = A × unbound fraction × filtration rate.

The arterial sample should represent a steady-state level. The ideal time to obtain it is halfway between maintenance doses after at least 3 half-lives. The $t_{1/2}$ data are also available (91).

Drug removal during continuous hemodialysis (HD)

During continuous hemodialysis drug removal occurs mostly by diffusion. Protein binding still plays a role in that unbound drug is more diffusible than bound drug. Drug diffusivity was discussed above. Vincent et al. have shown that a drug's diffusive mass transfer coefficient through 'open' membranes during continuous dialysis is dependent on molecular weight according to the formula:

$$Kd/Kdc = (MW/113)^{-0.42}$$

where Kd and Kdc are the diffusive mass transfer coefficients for the drug and creatinine, respectively, and MW is the drug's molecular weight (36).

During continuous therapies performed with venovenous access and blood flows of 125–250 ml/min, urea and creatinine clearances are 20–30 ml/min, corresponding to a GFR of 20–30 ml/min. Since the therapy is continuous, one should empirically dose drugs for a GFR of 20–30 ml/min.

Supplemental doses

Drug levels may be a useful tool for determining supplemental doses for continuous therapies when the desired level is known. The currently observed level (current level) is subtracted from the level one wishes to achieve (desired level) leaving the *difference level*. all in the same units. The difference level times the volume of distribution times the body weight in kilograms will give the amount of drug needed to boost the current level to the desired level. This was discussed in detail in the section on Drug Concentration Monitoring and summarized in Table 3.

This method is useful for administering any drug whose level is available and whose V_d is known. It is especially applicable to the setting of continuous therapies when the amount of drug removed is not clearly known and the clinician has only drug levels to assess the pharmacologic status of the patient. V_d data are readily available (91).

This is the recommended approach. Proper management of critically ill ICU patients demands the rapid availability of drug levels for most agents employed in this setting that are not managed by titration or have narrow therapeutic indices. For those agents whose levels are not available, the above principles should help the clinician approximate losses.

DRUG REMOVAL BY PERITONEAL DIALYSIS (PD)

Overall, peritoneal dialysis is not very efficient for removing most solutes and, consequently, drug clearance by PD is quite low (92). Many of the same drug properties which affect removal by hemodialysis also apply to peritoneal dialysis, but the latter is considerably more inefficient. In order for significant removal to occur, the drug generally must have a low volume of distribution, low protein binding and minimal removal by alternate routes of drug elimination. Several factors influence the transperitoneal transport of drugs and they are categorized in Table 9 (93). There is an inverse semilogarithmic relationship between clearance and molecular weight (94). According to this relationship, if the physico-chemical characteristics of the drug are typical, the peritoneal dialysis clearance of the unbound drug can be estimated by multiplying urea clearance (20 ml/min) by the ratio of the square root of the weight of urea (60 Daltons) over the square root of the drug's molecular weight (38).

The clearance rate of small molecules is essentially dependent on dialysate flow rate, whereas the clearances of middle and large molecular weight species are relatively independent of either dialysate or blood flow rates (94, 95). As for virtually all biological membranes, the diffusion of charged species across the peritoneal membrane is much slower than for neutral species. However, once in the peritoneal dialysate, ionized drugs tend to exhibit less back diffusion into blood. By compromising

Table 9. Factors affecting transperitoneal transport

Drug Properties
Molecular weight
Charge
Lipid or water solubility
V_d (tissue binding)
Protein binding
Other forms of stearic hindrance
Rapid excretion by another pathway
Red blood cell partitioning

Intrinsic Peritoneal Membrane Properties
Surface blood flow
Surface area
Loculation
Sclerosis
Pore size
Vascular disease
Fluid films

Dialysate Properties
Flow rate
Volume
Chemical composition
Distribution
Temperature

Miscellaneous Properties
Ultrafiltration
Clearance-raising additives

Table 10. Intraperitoneal antibiotic dosing for the treatment of peritonitis in CAPD patients

	Loading dose	Continuous	Intermittent
Aminoglycosides			
Amikacin	–	6–12 mg/l	60 mg/l/d
Gentamicin	–	4–8 mg/l	20 mg/l/d
Netilmicin	–	4–8 mg/l	20 mg/l/d
Tobramycin	–	4–8 mg/l	20 mg/l/d
Cephalosporins			
Cefazolin	–	125–250 mg/l	500 mg/l/d
Cephalothin	500 mg/l	100 mg/l	No data
Cephradine	–	125 mg/l	No data
Cefoxitin	500 mg/l	100 mg/l	No data
Cefotaxime	1,000 mg/l	250 mg/l	1,000 mg/l/d
Ceftazidime	500 mg/l	125 mg/l	500 mg/l/d
Ceftriaxone	500 mg/l	125–250 mg/l	500 mg/l/d
Penicillins			
Azlocillin	–	250 mg/l	No data
Mezlocillin	–	250 mg/l	No data
Piperacillin	–	250 mg/l	No data
Ticarcillin	–	125 mg/l	No data
Quinolones			
Ciprofloxacin	500 mg po	50 mg/l	No data
Ofloxacin	400 mg po	200 mg/d po	No data
Miscellaneous			
Aztreonam	500 mg/l	250 mg/l	500 mg/l/d
Imipenem	1,000 mg	100 mg/l	250 mg/l/d
Sulfamethoxazole/ trimethoprim	1,600/320 po	200/40 mg/l	No data
Vancomycin	–	15–25 mg/l	1–2,000 mg/l/week
Antifungal Agents			
Fluconazole	–	No data	150 mg q 2d

mesenteric blood flow, vascular disease or hypotension will decrease drug removal via peritoneal dialysis. Larger volume exchanges and alternating hypertonic with isotonic exchanges will enhance solute removal (96, 97). Small solute clearances are maximized at dialysate flow rates of 4 l/h (96, 98). During rapid exchange peritoneal dialysis, raising dialysate temperature from room temperature to body temperature will increase small solute clearances (99). This may be particularly relevant to tidal or other forms of aggressive automated peritoneal dialysis. However, with longer dwells as during continuous ambulatory peritoneal dialysis, the warming of dialyzate will not affect drug clearances (100). Although various pharmacological maneuvers have been attempted to increase solute clearance during peritoneal dialysis, no practical method for routine use has yet appeared. Thus, utilizing peritoneal dialysis for the removal of excess drug burden is not often of value.

For most drugs in clinical use there is little evidence of substantial drug removal during chronic peritoneal dialysis (93, 101, 103). A reasonable generalization is that if hemodialysis does not remove a drug, peritoneal dialysis will not either. The converse is clearly not true. Hemodialysis can remove drugs that peritoneal dialysis cannot. For example, one hemodialysis treatment usually removes about two thirds of the body burden of aminoglycoside antibiotics, whereas 24 hours of CAPD may remove only one fourth to one third of the body burden. Even aggressive cycler or other forms of rapid exchange peritoneal dialysis will not remove substantial drug burdens in the same time interval that hemodialysis will. With aggressive peritoneal dialysis over an entire day, some drugs will be dialyzable, i.e. 30% of the total body clearance can be attributed to the dialysis. These will usually be drugs with low protein binding and small volumes of distribution.

It is clear that peritoneal drug transport is predominantly unidirectional, from peritoneal dialysate to blood (104, 106). The reason for this is that one can achieve high drug concentrations in dialysate, creating a large concentration gradient from dialysate to blood. Also, peritoneal lymphatic absorption of drugs is active. Lastly, the dialysate can act is a protein-free reservoir for slow delivery of drug. This is the basis for the administration of drugs through the peritoneum. The addition of regular insulin to the dialysate is very effective in the stabilization of blood glucose levels in diabetic patients undergoing CAPD. The insulin is absorbed directly into the portal circulation, where there appears to be a distinct physiological advantage over the traditional subcutaneous route of administration. An initial dose per bag is about one fourth of the previous daily requirement, with a nighttime reduction of another 50% (107).

Immediately after the insertion of a peritoneal dialysis catheter or during dialysis-associated peritonitis, protein clearances into the dialysate increase such that fibrinous material forms that may plug the catheter. Intraperitoneal heparin is administered under these conditions, usually in doses ranging from 100 to 1000 units/l of dialysate. Systemic coagulation is rarely affected, because the strong positive electrostatic charge of the heparin molecule prevents its absorption (108).

Peritoneal dialysis-associated peritonitis is often treated by administering antibiotics in the dialysate (109, 110). Table 10 describes appropriate loading and maintenance doses for such administration and this is discussed in more detail in describing Table 11 below. Most antibiotics are stable (retain at least 80% of their original activity) in peritoneal dialysate (111). The additives heparin and insulin do not affect the stability or clinical activity of these antibiotics when employed in usual doses. Furthermore, loading and maintenance doses of a commonly used combination of antibiotics, cephapirin (or equivalent) plus tobramycin (or equivalent), are also stable in dialysate in the presence of insulin and heparin (111).

The tabulated drug dosing recommendations found later in this chapter address drug administration to dialysis patients and include information on whether peritoneal dialysis removes enough of the drug such that a supplemental dose is needed.

Supplemental dose for dialysis removal

Supplemental doses may be required if significant removal of the drug occurs with dialysis. As discussed earlier in this chapter, drugs with molecular weights of less than 500 Daltons, minimal protein binding and a small volume of distribution may have significant elimination by the various dialytic modalities. In general, dialysis clearance must increase plasma clearance in a particular patient by 30 to 50% to be clinically significant (49, 50). The need for supplemental dosing can often be eliminated if consideration is given during the construction of the patient's drug administration regimen such that drugs significantly removed by intermittent dialysis (aminoglycosides, penicillins, most cephalosporins) are scheduled to be given at times corresponding to the end of the dialysis session.

THE DOSING TABLES

We have utilized the preceding concepts to generate the dosing recommendations in Tables 11 through 20. Absent from Tables 11–20 are drugs that we think are not appropriate for patients requiring dialysis, such as diuretics, uricosurics, and some urinary tract antibiotics (e.g., nalidixic acid, nitrofurantoin). For agents not listed which may be administered to patients with end-stage renal disease, one can approximate dosing guidelines by using the principles described above (e.g., molecular weight, volume of distribution, protein binding, charge), available blood drug concentrations, accurate time recordings, and stable conditions.

Under the heading 'Major Elimination Route' the major organ responsible for clearance of the drug is listed. *H* refers to hepatic, i.e., drugs whose major elimination/metabolism is by the liver. *R* refers to renal, i.e., drugs whose major elimination/metabolism is by the kidney. The first letter notation is the major system, while the letter appearing in parenthesis refers to a minor pathway of elimination/metabolism, but still significant enough to be mentioned.

The *Adjustment for GFR* addresses only an adjustment recommended for patients whose renal function is poor enough to require dialysis on a routine basis. Because certain continuous renal replacement therapies may generate a prolonged GFR of 10–50 ml/min, we included these adjustments. The *Method* of adjustment could be *interval extension*, noted as the letter *I*, or *dosage reduction*, noted as the letter *D*. When the method is interval extension, adjustment refers to how many hours should transpire between doses (e.g., q6h means every six hours). When the method is dosage reduction, the adjustment refers to the percent of the dose that would be given to a patient with normal kidney function at the usual dosing interval (e.g., 50% means give to the ESRD patient a dose equal to 50% of the dose given a normal patient and the dosing interval is as if the patient had normal renal function). Although both methods are frequently combined, Tables 11 through 20 usually recommend one method or the other. When interval extension is recommended, the dosage should be the amount given to a patient with normal renal function. When the dosage reduction method is recommended, normal dosing intervals should be employed. When the methods are combined the adjustment is given as milligrams (or other dosage units) per interval.

Table 11. Antimicrobial agents

Drug, toxicity, notes	Major elimination route	Dose for normal renal function	Method	Adjustment for GFR, ml/min		Supplements for dialysis
				10–50	< 10	
Amikacin (212–124)	R	5 mg/kg q 8h	D, I	30–70% q 12 h	20–30% q 24–48 h	Hemo: 2/3 normal dose after dialysis CAPD: 30% q 24 h CAVH: Dose for GFR 10–50
Gentamicin (115–117) Concurrent penicillins may result in subtherapeutic blood levels	R	1 mg/kg q 8 h	D, I	30–70% q 12 h	20–30% q 24–48 h	Hemo: 2/3 normal dose after dialysis CAPD: 30% q 24 h CAVH: Dose for GFR 10–50
Kanamycin (118)	R	5 mg/kg q 8 h	D, I	30–70% q 12 h	20–30% q 24–48 h	Hemo: 2/3 normal dose after dialysis CAPD: 30% q 24 h CAVH: Dose for GFR 10–50
Netilmicin (119–121)	R	5 mg/kg q 8 h	D, I	30–70% q 12 h	20–30% q 24–48 h	Hemo: 2/3 normal dose after dialysis CAPD: 30% q 24 h CAVH: Dose for GFR 10–50
Streptomycin (91, 122)	R	1 gm/d	I	q 24–72 h	q 72–96 h	Hemo: 1/2 normal dose after dialysis CAPD: Dose for GFR 10–50 CAVH: Dose for GFR 10–50
Tobramycin (123, 124) Concurrent penicillins may result in subtherapeutic blood levels	R	1 mg/kg q 8 h	D, I	30–70% q 12 h	20–30% q 24–48 h	Hemo: 2/3 normal dose after dialysis CAPD: 30% q 24 h CAVH: Dose for GFR 10–50

Aminoglycoside Antibiotics

Ototoxic, nephrotoxic; rare respiratory paralysis; check serum concentrations to ensure efficacy.

Post hemodialysis dose is 2/3 of normal maintenance dose or 1/2 of a loading dose.

Larger supplement may be required for highly permeable membranes.

Volume of distribution larger with obesity, edema, or ascites.

Table 11. (Continued)

Drug, toxicity, notes	Major elimi-nation route	Dose for normal renal function	Method	Adjustment for GFR, ml/min		Supplements for dialysis
				10–50	< 10	
Cefaclor (125, 126)	R	250 mg tid	D	50–100%	50%	Hemo: Dose after dialysis CAPD: 250 mg q 8–12 h CAVH: Unknown
Cefadroxil (127)	R	0.5–1 gm q 12 h	I	q 12–24 h	q 24–48 h	Hemo: Dose after dialysis CAPD: Unknown CAVH: Unknown
Cefamandole (128, 129)	R	0.5–1 gm q 4–8 h	I	q 6–8 h	q 12 h	Hemo: Dose after dialysis CAPD: Dose GFR 10–50 CAVH: Dose for GFR 10–50
Cefazolin (130)	R	0.5–1.5 gm q 6 h	I	q 12 h	q 24–48 h	Hemo: Dose after dialysis CAPD: None CAVH: None
Cefixime (131)	R (H)	200 mg q 12 h	D	75%	50%	Hemo: None CAPD: None CAVH: Unlikely
Cefmenoxime (132, 134)	R (H)	1 gm q 6 h	D, I	1 gm q 12–24 h	750 mg q 24 h	Hemo: 750 mg after dialysis CAPD: None CAVH: Unknown
Cefmetazole (135, 136)	R	2 gm q 8 h	I	q 12–24 h	q 48 h	Hemo: Dose after dialysis CAPD: Unknown CAVH: Unknown
Cefonicid (137, 138)	R	1 gm q 24 h	D, I	0.25–0.5 gm q 24 h	0.25 gm q 48 h	Hemo: None CAPD: None CAVH None
Cefoperazone (139, 140)	H	1–2 qm q 12 h	D	100%	100%	Hemo: None CAPD: None CAVH: None
Ceforanide (141, 142)	R	0.5–1 gm q 12	I	q 24–48 h	q 48–72 h	Hemo: 0.5–1 gm after dialysis CAPD: None CAVH: None
Cefotaxime (143, 144)	R (H)	1 gm q 6 h	I	q 8–12 h	q 24 h	Hemo: 1 gm after dialysis CAPD: None CAVH: None

Cephalosporin Antibiotics
Rare allergic interstitial nephritis; absorbed well when administered intraperitoneal, may cause bleeding in patients with renal failure.

Table 11. (Continued)

Drug, toxicity, notes	Major elimination route	Dose for normal renal function	Method	Adjustment for GFR, ml/min		Supplements for dialysis
				10–50	< 10	
Cefotetan (145, 146)	R (H)	1–2 gm q 12 h	D	50%	25%	Hemo: 1 gm after dialysis CAPD: None CAVH: None
Cefoxitin (147, 148) May raise creatinine by interference with assay	R (H)	1–2 gm q 6–8 h	I	q 8–12 h	q 24–48 h	Hemo: 1 gm after dialysis CAPD: Dose GFR 10–50 CAVH: Dose GFR 10–50
Ceftazidime (149–152)	R (H)	1 gm q 8–12 h	I	q 24–48 h	q 48–72 h	Hemo: 1 gm after dialysis CAPD: Dose GFR 10-50 CAVH: Dose GFR 10–50
Ceftizoxime (153–156)	R (H)	1–2 gm q 8–12 h	I	q 24–48 h	q 48–72 h	Hemo: Dose after dialysis CAPD: Dose GFR 10–50 CAVH: Dose GFR 10–50
Ceftriaxone (157–159)	H (R)	1 gm q 12 h	D	100%	100%	Hemo: None CAPD: None CAVH: None
Cefuroxime (160–162)	R	0.75–1.5 gm q 8 h	I	q 8–12 h	q 24 h	Hemo: Dose after dialysis CAPD: None CAVH: Likely to be removed dose for GFR 10–50
Cephalexin (163)	R	250–500 mg q 6 h	I	q 6 h	q 8–12 h	Hemo: 250 mg after dialysis CAPD: Dose for GFR 10–50 CAVH: Dose for GFR 10–50
Cephalothin (164)	R (H)	0.5–2.0 g q 6 h	I	q 6–8 h	q 12 h	Hemo: Dose after dialysis CAPD: Dose for GFR 10–50 CAVH: Dose for GFR 10–50
Cephapirin (165)	R (H)	0.5–2 g q 6 h	I	q 6–8 h	q 12 h	Hemo: Dose after dialysis CAPD: Dose for GFR 10–50 CAVH: Dose for GFR 10–50

Table 11. (Continued)

Drug, toxicity, notes	Major elimination route	Dose for normal renal function	Method	Adjustment for GFR, ml/min		Supplements for dialysis
				10–50	< 10	
Cephradine (147)	R	0.25–2 g q 6 h	D	50%	25%	Hemo: Dose after dialysis CAPD: Dose for GFR 10–50 CAVH: Dose for GFR 10–50
Moxalactam (167–169)	R (H)	1–2 g q 8–12 h	I	q 12–24 h	q 24–48 h	Hemo: Dose after dialysis CAPD: Dose for GFR 10–50 CAVH: Dose for GFR 10–50
Macrolide Antibiotics						
Azithromycin (170, 171)	H	250 mg q 24 h	D	100%	100%	Hemo: None CAPD: None CAVH: Unlikely
Clarithromycin (172)	H	250–500 mg bid	D	50–100%	50%	Hemo: Unlikely CAPD: Unlikely CAVH: Unlikely
Erythromycin (173, 174) Ototoxicity with high doses in ESRD	H	250–500 mg q 6–12 h	D	100%	50–75%	Hemo: None CAPD: None CAVH: Unlikely
Penicillins						
Amoxicillin (175–177)	R (H)	500 mg q 8 h	I	q 8–12 h	q 12 h	Hemo: Dose after dialysis CAPD: Dose for GFR 10–50 CAVH: Dose for GFR 10–50
Ampicillin (178)	R (H)	250–2000 mg q 6 h	I	q 6–12 h	q 12–24 h	Hemo: Dose after dialysis CAPD: Dose GFR 10–50 CAVH: Dose for GFR 10–50
Azlocillin (179, 180) Sodium – 2.7 mEq/g	R (H)	2–3 g q 4 h	I	q 6–8 h	q 6–8 h	Hemo: Dose after dialysis CAPD: Dose for GFR < 10 CAVH: Dose for GFR 10–50
Dicloxacillin (91, 122)	R (H)	250–500 mg q 6 h	D	100%	100%	Hemo: None CAPD: None CAVH: None

Table 11. (Continued)

Drug, toxicity, notes	Major elimination route	Dose for normal renal function	Method	Adjustment for GFR, ml/min		Supplements for dialysis
				10–50	< 10	
Methicillin (91, 122)	H (R)	1–2 g q 4 h	D	q 6–8 h	q 8–12	Hemo: None CAPD: None CAVH: None
Mezlocillin (181, 182) Sodium – 1.9 mEq/g	R (H)	1.5–4 g q 4–6 h	I	q 6–8 h	q 8 h	Hemo: None CAPD: None CAVH: None
Nafcillin (91, 122) Coagulopathy may develop	H (R)	1–2 g q 4–6 h	D	100%	100%	Hemo: None CAPD: None CAVH: None
Penicillin G (91, 183) Potassium 1.7 mEq/million units Risk of seizures with high doses in renal insufficiency (Six million units/d upper limit dose in ESRD)	R (H)	0.5–4 million units q 6 h	D	75%	25–50%	Hemo: Dose after dialysis CAPD: Dose GFR < 10 CAVH: Dose for GFR < 10
Piperacillin (184, 186) Sodium 1.9 mEq/g	R (H)	3–4 g q 4 h	I	q 6–8 h	q 8 h	Hemo: Dose after dialysis CAPD: Dose GFR < 10 CAVH: Dose for GFR < 10
Ticarcillin (187) Sodium 5.2 mEq/g	R	3 g q 4 h	D, I	1–2 g q 8 h	1 g q 12 h	Hemo: 3 gm after dialysis CAPD: Dose for GFR < 10 CAVH: Dose for GFR < 10
Quinolones						
Ciprofloxacin (188–190) Poorly absorbed with antacids	R (H)	500–750 mg q 12 h	D	50%	33%	Hemo: 250 mg CAPD: Dose for GFR 10–50 CAVH: Dose for GFR 10–50
Enoxacin (191–193)	R (H)	200–400 mg q 12 h	D	50%	50%	Hemo: None CAPD: None CAVH: Unlikely
Fleroxacin (194)	R (H)	400 mg q 12 h	D	50%	50%	Hemo: Dose after dialysis CAPD: None CAVH: None
Norfloxacin (195)	H (R)	400 mg q 12 h	I	q 12–24 h	q 24 h	Hemo: None CAPD: Unlikely CAVH: Unlikely

Table 11. (Continued)

Drug, toxicity, notes	Major elimination route	Dose for normal renal function	Method	Adjustment for GFR, ml/min		Supplements for dialysis
				10–50	< 10	
Ofloxacin (196)	R (H)	400 mg/d	D	50%	25%	Hemo: Dose after dialysis CAPD: None CAVH: Dose for GFR 10-50
Tetracycline Antibiotics Potentiate acidosis. Hyperphosphatemia. Increase BUN, antianabolic.						
Doxycycline (197) Tetracycline of choice in patients with renal insufficiency. Not associated with antianabolic syndrome.	H (R)	100–200 mg/d	D	100%	100%	Hemo: None CAPD: None CAVH: Unlikely
Minocycline (198)	H	100 mg q 12 h	D	100%	100%	Hemo: None CAPD: None CAVH: Unlikely
Tetracycline (198)	R (H)	250–500 mg qid	I	q 12–24 h	Avoid	Hemo: None CAPD: Unlikely CAVH: Unlikely
Miscellaneous Antibacterial Antibiotics						
Aztreonam (199, 200)	R (H)	1–2 g q 8–12 h	D	50–75%	25%	Hemo: 0.5 gm after dialysis CAPD: Dose for GFR < 10 CAVH: Dose for GFR 10–50
Chloramphenicol (201)	H	12.5 mg/kg q 6 h	D	100%	100%	Hemo: None CAPD: Unlikely CAVH: Unlikely
Cilastatin (202–205) Given with Imipenem	R (H)	(see Imipenem)	D	100%	100%	Hemo: Dose after dialysis CAPD: None CAVH: Dose for GFR 10–50
Clindamycin (206)	H	150–300 mg q 6 h	D	100%	100%	Hemo: None CAPD: Unlikely CAVH: Unlikely
Imipenem (202–205)	H (R)	0.25–1 g q 6 h	D	50%	25%	Hemo: Dose after dialysis CAPD: None CAVH: Dose for GFR 10–50

Table 11. (Continued)

Drug, toxicity, notes	Major elimination route	Dose for normal renal function	Method	Adjustment for GFR, ml/min		Supplements for dialysis
				10–50	< 10	
Metronidazole (207–209) Metabolites accumulate	H	75 mg/kg q 6 h	D	100%	50%	Hemo: Dose after dialysis CAPD: None CAVH: Likely to be removed Dose for GFR 10–50
Sulfisoxazole (210) Protein binding decreased in ESRD Use normal dosing for UTI in ESRD	R (H)	1–2 g q 6 h	I	q 8–12 h	q 12–24 h	Hemo: 2 gm after dialysis CAPD: Dose for GFR 10–50 CAVH: Dose for GFR 10–50
Teicoplanin (211, 212)	R (H)	6 mg/kg/d	I	q 48 h	q 72 h	Hemo: None CAPD: None CAVH: None
Trimethoprim/ sulfamethoxazole (213) Use normal dosing for UTI in ESRD Trimethoprim component interferes with secretion of creatinine	R (H)	160 mg trimethoprim and 800 mg sulfamethoxazole q 12 h	D, I	100% q 12–24 h	50% q 24 h	Hemo: 1/2 dose after dialysis CAPD: None CAVH: Likely to be removed, dose for GFR 10–50
Vancomycin (46, 54, 214, 215) Ototoxicity Monitor serum levels	R	1 g q 12 h	I	q 2–7 days	q 7–10 days	Hemo: Conventional – None Permeable membranes – Dose for GFR 10–50 CAPD: Dose for CFR 10–50 CAVH: Dose for GFR 10–50
Antifungal Agents						
Amphotericin B (216–220) Nephrotoxicity proportional to total dose. Renal tubular acidosis, hypokalemia, hypomagnesemia, nephrogenic diabetes insipidus	H	0.3–0.5 mg/k/d	D	100%	100%	Hemo: None CAPD: Unlikely CAVH: Unlikely

Table 11. (Continued)

Drug, toxicity, notes	Major elimi- nation route	Dose for normal renal function	Method	Adjustment for GFR, ml/min 10–50	< 10	Supplements for dialysis
Fluconazole (221–225)	R (H)	50–200 mg/d	D	50%	25%	Hemo: Dose after dialysis CAPD: Dose for GFR < 10 CAVH: Dose for GFR < 10
Flucytosine (226–228) Hepatic dysfunction Bone marrow suppression more common in azotemic patients Adjust dose to maintain peak serum concentrating between 40–60 mg/l	R	150 mg/kg/d in 3–4 divided doses	D, I	25–50 mg/kg q 12–24 h	50 mg/kg q 24–48 h	Hemo: Dose after dialysis CAPD: Dose for GFR 10–50 CAVH: Dose for GFR 10–50
Griseofulvin (216–217)	H	125–250 mg q 6 h	D	100%	100%	Hemo: None CAPD: None CAVH: Unlikely
Itraconazole (221, 229, 230)	H (R)	100–200 mg q 12 h	D	100%	100%	Hemo: None CAPD: None CAVH: Unlikely
Ketoconazole (221, 224)	H	200–400 mg/d	D	100%	100%	Hemo: None CAPD: Unlikely CAVH: Unlikely
Miconazole (232)	H	200–1200 mg q 8 h	D	100%	100%	Hemo: None CAPD: Unlikely CAVH: Unlikely
Antiparasitic Antibiotic Chloroquine (233, 234)	R (H)	1.5 gm over 3 days	D	100%	50%	Hemo: None CAPD: None CAVH: Unlikely
Mebendazole (234, 235)	H	100 mg bid × 3 days Pinworm infection: 100 mg one dose)	D	100%	100%	Hemo: None CAPD: Unlikely CAVH: Unlikely
Mefloquine (237)	H (R)	Non-immune pts: 1250–1500 mg total in 2–3 doses over 24 hrs Semi-immune pts: 750–1000 mg total in 2–3 doses over 24 hrs	D	100%	50%	Hemo: Unlikely CAPD: Unlikely CAVH: Unlikely

Table 11. (Continued)

Drug, toxicity, notes	Major elimination route	Dose for normal renal function	Method	Adjustment for GFR, ml/min		Supplements for dialysis
				10–50	< 10	
Pentamidine (238, 239)	H	4 mg/kg/d	I	q 24–36 h	q 48 h	Hemo: Unlikely CAPD: Unlikely CAVH: Unlikely
Praziquantel (240)	H	Dose varies	D	100%	100%	Hemo: None CAPD: Unlikely CAVH: Unlikely
Pyrimethamine (233, 234)	H (R)	50–75 mg/d	D	100%	100%	Hemo: Unknown CAPD: Unknown CAVH: Unknown
Quinine (233, 234)	H	10 mg/kg q 8 h	I	q 8–12 h	q 24 h	Hemo: Unlike CAPD: None CAVH: Unlikely
Antituberculous Agents Capreomycin (241)	R (H)	1 g qd	D, I	100% q 48–72 h	25–50% q 48–72 h	Hemo: Dose after dialysis CAPD Unknown CAVH: Likely to be removed Dose for GFR 10–50
Cycloserine (91, 122) CNS toxicity	R (H)	250 mg q 12 h	I	q 12–24 h	q 24 h	Hemo: Unknown CAPD: Unknown CAVH: Unknown
Ethambutol (242) Ocular toxicity Peripheral neuritis	R (H)	15 mg/kg q 24 h	D	50–100%	25–50%	Hemo: Dose after dialysis CAPD: Dose for GFR 10–50 CAVH: Dose for GFR 10–50
Ethionamide (91, 122)	H	250–500 mg q 12 h	D	100%	50%	Hemo: Unknown CAPD: Unknown CAVH: Unknown
Isoniazid (243)	H (R)	5 mg/kg q 24 h	D	75–100%	50%	Hemo: Dose after dialysis CAPD: Dose for GFR 10–50 CAVH: Dose for GFR 10–50

Table 11. (Continued)

Drug, toxicity, notes	Major elimination route	Dose for normal renal function	Method	Adjustment for GFR, ml/min		Supplements for dialysis
				10–50	< 10	
PAS (Para-aminosalicyclic acid) Significant sodium load	R (H)	50 mg/kg q 8 h	D	50–75%	50%	Hemo: Dose after dialysis CAPD: Unknown CAVH: Unknown
Pyrazinamide (244, 245) Impairs urate excretion. Can precipitate gout.	H	15–30 mg/kg q 24 h	I	q 24 h	q 48–72 h	Hemo: Dose after dialysis CAPD: Unknown CAVH: Likely to be removed Dose for GFR 10–50
Rifampin (246)	H (R)	600 mg q 24 h	D	100%	100%	Hemo: None CAPD: None CAVH: None
Antiviral Agents						
Acyclovir (247, 249) Neurotoxic in patients with renal failure, may cause acute renal failure if injected IV rapidly	R (H)	5 mg/kg q 8 h	D, I	5 mg/kg q 12–24 h	2.5 mg/kg q 24 h	Hemo: Dose after dialysis CAPD: Same as for GFR < 10 CAVH: 3.5 mg/kg/d
Amantadine (250–252)	R	100 mg q 12 h	I	q 48–72 h	q 168 h	Hemo: None CAPD: Unlikely CAVH: Unlikely
Didanosine (253, 254)	H (R)	200–300 mg q 12 h	D	50–75%	50%	Hemo: Dose after dialysis CAPD: Unknown CAVH: Likely to be removed Dose for GFR 10–50
Foscarnet (255) Nephrotoxicity common	R	60–100 mg/kg q 8–12 h	D	10–50%	Avoid	Hemo: Dose after dialysis CAPD: Unknown CAVH: Likely to be removed. Dose for GFR 10–50
Ganciclovir (256)	R	2.5 mg/kg q 8 h	I	q 24 h	q 48–96 h	Hemo: Dose after dialysis CAPD: Unknown CAVH: 3.5 mg/kg/d

Table 11. (Continued)

Drug, toxicity, notes	Major elimination route	Dose for normal renal function	Method	Adjustment for GFR, ml/min		Supplements for dialysis
				10–50	< 10	
Ribavirin (257) Loading dose required	H (R)	200 mg q 8 h	D	100%	50%	Hemo: None CAPD: Unlikely CAVH: Unlikely
Vidarabine (258)	R (H)	15 mg/kg infusion q 24 h	D	100%	75%	Hemo: Give after dialysis CAPD: None CAVH: Dose GFR 10–50
Zidovudine (AZT) (260–262)	H (R)	200 mg q 4 h	D	100%	50%	Hemo: Dose after dialysis CAPD: None CAVH: Likely to be removed. Dose for GFR 10–50

Supplement for dialysis

Refers to whether or not a supplemental maintenance dose should be administered after a dialysis treatment. In parentheses are the forms of dialysis referred to by the words 'Yes' or 'No'. Hemodialysis is abbreviated as *H*, and peritoneal dialysis as *P*. 'Yes' or 'No' specifically refer to known data. The absence of specific data regarding either type of dialysis is indicated by the absence of the H or P abbreviation in parentheses. No data at all is indicated by a question mark. Some drugs with reasonable dialysis clearance are designated by 'No' because the amount removed does not necessitate supplemental postdialysis doses. The designation 'No' does not preclude the use of dialysis for drug overdoses.

Guidelines for prescribing specific drugs in renal disease

As discussed previously, the adjustment of drug dosages for patients with uremia is predicated on the complex pharmacokinetic and pharmacodynamic alterations which may occur in this population. The dosage reduction method, the interval extension method, or a combination of the two are utilized to produce the most favorable kinetic and dynamic relationship, thus maximizing the opportunity for a positive therapeutic outcome. Drug removal by dialysis complicates these relationships. This section addresses specific agents or classes of drugs for which additional consideration is warranted when prescribing them to ESRD patients.

The removal of drugs by dialysis is dependent on numerous factors including both drug properties (molec-ular weight, protein binding, volume of distribution, etc) and dialytic properties (modality, duration, membrane characteristics, etc). For a more detailed explanation of these factors, please refer to the section entitled Drug Dialyzability.

Supplemental dosing after hemodialysis and special dosing considerations for peritoneal dialysis and continuous renal replacement therapies may be found in the Tables 11–20. Unless otherwise noted, the need for supplemental dosing after hemodialysis is based on the use of conventional membranes. Relatively few drugs are significantly removed by peritoneal dialysis (92). If significant removal occurs, increasing the dose (or decreasing the interval) to that recommended for patients with a GFR of 10 to 50 ml/min is recommended. Most of the data for drug removal with continuous renal replacement therapies is derived from studies done on patients undergoing continuous arterio-venous hemofiltration (80, 87, 586, 587). For continuous veno-venous hemodialysis, empiric dosing for a GFR of 20 to 30 ml/min is reasonable as urea and creatinine clearance are within this range at blood flows of 125 to 250 ml/min. For many agents, extensive data are not available on the effect of dialysis on drug removal. If data are not available, the likelihood of removal depends on the degree of protein binding and volume of distribution.

ANTIMICROBIAL AGENTS (TABLE 11)

Infectious complications represent an important source of morbidity and mortality in dialysis patients (588, 589). Early recognition of infection and prompt attainment of therapeutic plasma antibiotic concentrations are necessary for optimal antimicrobial treatment. Many antibiotics exhibit significant alterations in their pharmacokinetics in the uremic patient which necessitates dosage modification. Accumulation of the parent drug or its metabolites may dispose the patient to a greater risk of toxicity (590). Specific dosing guidelines for individual antimicrobial agents are found in Table 11. Several areas which require emphasis or further explanation are discussed below.

The initial selection of antimicrobial agents is often empiric. It is based on the type of infection and the likely infecting pathogens. Other considerations when choosing empiric therapy are knowledge of the potential toxicities of the agent, possible interactions with other drugs, the patient's allergy history, local antimicrobial susceptibility patterns, and cost. Culture results are key as antibiotic coverage can often be narrowed to more specific or less toxic agents once a firm identification and sensitivity pattern have been established.

Depending on the agent(s) chosen, one or more pharmacokinetic parameters may be altered in the patient with uremia. Some agents have decreased absorption (tetracycline 198 or ciprofloxacin 188) when administered concurrently with antacids or phosphate binders. Decreased protein binding may contribute to the increased risk of neurotoxicity for the beta-lactam antibiotics (590). The majority of antimicrobial agents are excreted at least partially by the kidneys. In addition to glomerular filtration, antibiotics such as trimethoprim-sulfamethoxazole (213) or ciprofloxacin (188), as well as the penicillins, reach the tubular lumen via tubular secretion, achieving high urinary concentrations even though the glomerular filtration rate is decreased.

Generally, the loading dose will be the same as that for the patient with normal renal function. Significant alterations in extracellular fluid volume may necessitate small adjustments. Rapid achievement of therapeutic drug concentrations are particularly critical for life threatening infections such as bacterial pneumonia where there is often a direct relation between drug concentration and antimicrobial efficacy. As discussed earlier in this chapter, the maintenance dose may be modified by extending the interval between doses, decreasing the dose or some combination of the two. Agents which exhibit concentration dependent killing (aminoglycosides, fluoroquinolones, penems, and newer macrolides) should be dosed utilizing the interval extension method. More recently, it has become recognized that several classes of antibiotics demonstrate a significant post antibiotic effect (591, 592). This phenomenon of persistent inhibition of bacterial growth for intervals when serum concentrations are below the minimum inhibitory concentration (MIC) may be utilized for therapeutic advantage. Thus, it may not be necessary to maintain levels above the MIC throughout the duration of the dosing interval. Convenient dosing intervals utilizing the interval extension method may be used in these antibiotics without compromising therapeutic efficacy.

The intraperitoneal administration of antibiotics is widely employed for the treatment of peritonitis in peritoneal dialysis patients (593, 594). For most antibiotics, significant systemic absorption occurs due to the small volume of distribution in the peritoneal cavity and low availability of proteins for binding (92). Additionally, increased permeability of the peritoneum during peritonitis further increases systemic absorption. Antibiotics administered orally or intravenously may have slow penetration into the peritoneum depending on molecular size, extent of protein binding, and volume of distribution. For this reason, the intraperitoneal route is preferred for the treatment of peritonitis. Guidelines for intraperitoneal dosing of commonly administered antibiotics for the treatment of peritonitis are provided in Table 10. The reader is referred to Keane et al. for a more comprehensive listing of intraperitoneal dosing of antibiotics (594).

The nephrotoxicity of antimicrobial agents remains an important issue even in dialysis dependent patients. Some dialysis patients, particularly those on PD, may have enough residual renal function to allow them a more lenient diet or less intense dialysis regimen. It is important to guard against a further infringement on their lifestyle through unnecessary nephrotoxic exposures. Appropriate dosing and monitoring of drug concentrations is crucial for minimizing the nephrotoxicity of agents such as the aminoglycosides (595). Attention to other risk factors such as volume depletion and hypokalemia prior to instituting therapy are also important to consider. Acute interstitial nephritis occurs sporadically with certain antibiotics (classically with methicillin), however there are no identified risk factors or preventive measures for this complication (596). Tetracyclines, through their anti-anabolic effects result in an increase in the blood urea nitrogen (BUN) and should probably be avoided if possible in the dialysis patient. Trimethoprim, through its competition for secretory transport sites, raises serum creatinine concentration (597). Certain cephalosporins such as cefoxitin, cause interference with the creatinine assay (33). A variety of electrolyte disturbances have been described such as magnesium and potassium wasting with amphotericin therapy and hypokalemia with large doses of carbenicillin. These are not usually a major problem in the ESRD patient. The clinician should be aware that a significant potassium or sodium load is conferred by treatment with certain agents, particularly the penicillins (183). These are delineated in Table 4.

Other complications may occur with increased frequency in the patient with renal disease (590). Ototoxicity and vestibular toxicity may develop with the aminoglycosides, vancomycin and erythromycin. The cumulative dose appears to play a role, in addition to other risk factors found in the dialysis patient such as underlying uremic neuropathy affecting the eighth cranial nerve and accumulation of the parent drug or its metabolites. Bleeding

Table 12. Analgesics and agents utilized by anesthesiologists

Drug, toxicity, notes	Major elimination route	Dose for normal renal function	Method	Adjustment for renal failure, GFR ml/min		Supplements for dialysis
				10–50	< 10	

Narcotics and Narcotic Antagonists

All agents in this group may cause excessive sedation and respiratory depression (263)

Drug, toxicity, notes	Major elimination route	Dose for normal renal function	Method	10–50	< 10	Supplements for dialysis
Alfentanil (264)	H	Anesthetic induction	D	100%	100%	Hemo: Not applicable (NA) CAPD: NA CAVH: NA
Butorphanol (265)	H	2 mg q 3–4 h	D	75%	50%	Hemo: Unlikely CAPD: Unlikely CAVH: Unlikely
Codeine (266)	H	30–60 mg q 4–6 h	D	75%	50%	Hemo: Unknown CAPD: Unknown CAVH: Unknown
Fentanyl (267)	H	Anesthetic induction	D	75%	50%	Hemo: NA CAPD: NA CAVH: NA
Meperidine (268) Normeperidine, an active metabolite, accumulates in ESRD and may cause seizures	H	50–100 mg q 3–4 h	D	75%	50%	Hemo: None CAPD: None CAVH: Unlikely
Methadone (269)	H	2.5–10 mg q 6–8 h	D	100%	50–75%	Hemo: None CAPD: None CAVH: Unlikely
Morphine (270, 271) Metabolites may accumulate	H	20–25 mg po q 4 h or 2–10 mg IV	D	75%	50%	Hemo: None CAPD: Unlikely CAVH: Unlikely
Naloxone (263, 264)	H	2 mg	D	100%	100%	Hemo: NA CAPD: NA CAVH: NA
Pentazocine (263, 264)	H	50 mg q 4 h	D	75%	50%	Hemo: None CAPD: Unlikely CAVH: Unlikely
Propoxyphene (272) Active metabolite norpropoxyphene accumulates in ESRD	H	65 mg po tid-qid	D	100%	Avoid	Hemo: None CAPD: None CAVH: Unlikely
Sufentanil (263, 264)	H	Anesthetic induction	D	100%	100%	Hemo: NA CAPD: NA CAVH: NA

Non-Narcotic Analgesics

Drug, toxicity, notes	Major elimination route	Dose for normal renal function	Method	10–50	< 10	Supplements for dialysis
Acetaminophen (273, 274) Metabolites may accumulate in renal insufficiency Drug is major metabolite of phenacetin	H	650 mg q 4h	I	q 6 h	q 8 h	Hemo: 1/2 dose CAPD: None CAVH: Unknown

Table 12. (Continued)

Drug, toxicity, notes	Major elimi- nation route	Dose for normal renal function	Method	Adjustment for renal failure, GFR ml/min		Supplements for dialysis
				10–50	< 10	
Salicylate (275) May decrease GFR when blood flow is prostaglandin-dependent Excretion enhanced in alkaline urine May add to uremic gastrointestinal symptoms and platelet dysfunction Protein binding reduced	H (R)	650 mg q 4 h	I	q 4–6 h	Avoid	Hemo: Dose after dialysis CAPD: None CAVH: Likely to be removed
Neuromuscular Agents (276)						
Atracurium (277–280)	H	0.4–0.5 mg/kg load, then 0.08–0.1 mg/kg q 15–25 min	D	100%	100%	Hemo: Unknown CAPD: Unknown CAVH: Unknown
Etomidate (273)	H	0.2–0.6 mg/kg	D	100%	100%	Hemo: Unknown CAPD: Unknown CAVH: Unknown
Gallamine (281) Recurarization may occur up to 24 h after dose. If blockade not responsive to neostigmine, dialysis may be useful.	R	0.5–15 mg/kg	D	Avoid	Avoid	Hemo: NA CAPD: NA CAVH: NA
Ketamine (278)	H	1–4.5 mg/kg	D	100%	100%	Hemo: Unknown CAPD: Unknown CAVH: Unknown
Metocurine (282)	H (R)	0.2–0.4 mg/kg	D	Avoid	Avoid	Hemo: Unknown CAPD: Unknown CAVH: Unknown
Neostigmine (283)	R (H)	15–375 mg/d	D	50%	25%	Hemo: Unknown CAPD: Unknown CAVH: Unknown
Pancuronium (284) Recurarization may occur up to 24 h after dose.	H (R)	0.04–0.1 mg/kg	D	50%	Avoid	Hemo: Unknown CAPD: Unknown CAVH: Unknown
Propofol (285)	H	2.0–2.5 mg/kg load then 6–12 mg/kg/h	D	100%	100%	Hemo: Unknown CAPD: Unknown CAVH: Unknown
Pyridostigmine (286) Renal excretion decreased by basic drugs.	(R) H	60–1500 mg/d	D	35%	20%	Hemo: Unknown CAPD: Unknown CAVH: Unknown

Table 12. (Continued)

Drug, toxicity, notes	Major elimination route	Dose for normal renal function	Method	Adjustment for renal failure, GFR ml/min		Supplements for dialysis
				10–50	< 10	
Succinylcholine (287) Hyperkalemia in ESRD	H	0.3–1.1 mg/kg load, then 0.04–0.07 mg/kg prn	D	100%	100%	Hemo: Unknown CAPD: Unknown CAVH: Unknown
Tubocurarine (288) Large or repetitive doses may result in prolonged effect. Recurarization may occur.	H (R)	0.1–0.2 mg/kg	D	50%	Avoid	Hemo: Unknown CAPD: Unknown CAVH: Unknown
Vecuronium (289)	R (H)	0.08–0.1 mg/kg load, then 0.01–0.05 mg/kg	D	100%	100%	Hemo: Unknown CAPD: Unknown CAVH: Unknown

diatheses due to antibiotic therapy may also occur with increased frequency due to underlying platelet dysfunction and heparin exposure during hemodialysis.

The antiviral agents acyclovir, ganciclovir, valacyclovir, famciclovir, and foscarnet also possess potential for adverse effects when used in the dialysis patient. The clinician must be aware of and attentive to the development of bone marrow suppression, central nervous system toxicity, and nephrotoxicity, and adjust doses accordingly to minimize these events.

ANALGESICS AND AGENTS UTILIZED BY ANESTHESIOLOGIST (TABLE 12)

Most analgesics are hepatically metabolized and usually require little dose adjustment for renal failure. However, the presence of renal failure tends to increase the sensitivity to the therapeutic and toxic effects of drugs in this category (263). The reasons for this include altered pharmacokinetics and the additive effects of retained uremic toxins. Profound narcosis can occur even when modest dosages are prescribed. For this reason, it is wise to start most analgesics at a reduced dose and then titrate cautiously according to clinical response. Chronic administration of meperidine results in the accumulation of normeperidine, a metabolite which has central nervous system excitatory properties (268). A higher incidence of seizures has been observed in patients with renal failure receiving meperidine chronically. For this reason, use of this agent should be avoided in the dialysis patient.

Surgical procedures are frequently required in dialysis patients. As such, the anesthesiologist must be familiar with the pharmacokinetics of various agents utilized for the induction and maintenance of anesthesia in uremic patients. Many of the neuromuscular blocking agents are excreted at least to some degree by the kidney and as a result may display prolonged action and recurarization as the effect of the antagonist wears off (276). For this reason, use of neuromuscular blockers with little dependence on renal excretion such as atracuronium or vecuronium may be preferred in uremic patients. Succinylcholine, a depolarizing muscle relaxant, results in potassium movement out of cells. Although this results in only a minor rise in serum potassium concentration in normal subjects, the dialysis patient may have life threatening hyperkalemia. A summary of recommendations for analgesics and agents utilized by anesthesiologists is found in Table 12.

ANTIHYPERTENSIVE AND CARDIOVASCULAR AGENTS (TABLE 13)

Cardiovascular disease frequently accompanies renal disease and continues to be the most common cause of death in the ESRD population (598). Not surprisingly, antihypertensive and cardiovascular agents are widely prescribed in this population. Considerable overlap exists in the drugs utilized for the treatment of arrhythmias, coronary artery disease, congestive heart failure and hypertension. Beta-blockers have proven effective for the treatment of hypertension, angina and arrhythmias and the ACE inhibitors are beneficial for both hypertension and congestive heart failure. But both β-blocking drugs and angiotensin-converting enzyme inhibitors can cause hyperkalemia in dialysis patients. Thus, concomitant medical conditions are important factors when choosing cardiovascular drugs.

Table 13. Antihypertensive and cardiovascular agents

Drug, toxicity, notes	Major elimination route	Dose for normal renal function	Method	Adjustment for renal failure, GFR ml/min		Supplements for dialysis
				10–50	< 10	
Adrenergic Modulators						
Clonidine (290, 291) Rebound hypertension if drug is suddenly withdrawn	H (R)	0.1–0.6 mg bid	D	100%	100%	Hemo: None CAPD: None CAVH: Unlikely
Doxazosin (292, 293)	H	1–15 mg/d	D	100%	100%	Hemo: None CAPD: Unlikely CAVH: Unlikely
Guanabenz (294)	H	8–16 mg bid	D	100%	100%	Hemo: Unlikely CAPD: Unlikely CAVH: Unlikely
Guanadrel (295, 296)	H (R)	10–50 mg bid	I	q 12–24 h	q 24–48 h	Hemo: Unknown CAPD: Unknown CAVH: Unknown
Guanethidine (91, 122)	H (R)	10–100 mg/d	I	q 24 h	q 48 h	Hemo: Unlikely CAPD: Unlikely CAVH: Unlikely
Guanfacine (297, 298)	H (R)	1–2 mg/d	D	100%	100%	Hemo: None CAPD: Unlikely CAVH: Unlikely
Methyldopa (299)	H (R)	250–500 mg tid	I	q 8–12 h	q 12–24 h	Hemo: 250 mg CAPD: None CAVH: Significant removal likely. Dose for GFR 10–50
Prazosin (300, 301)	H	1–15 mg bid	D	100%	100%	Hemo: None CAPD: Unlikely CAVH: Unlikely
Reserpine (302) Excessive sedation	H	0.05–0.25 mg/d	D	100%	100%	Hemo: Unlikely CAPD: Unlikely CAVH: Unlikely
Terazosin (303)	H (R)	1–20 mg/d	D	100%	100%	Hemo: Unlikely CAPD: Unlikely CAVH: Unlikely
Angiotensin Converting Enzyme Inhibitors Hypotensive effects exacerbated by diuretics or sodium depletion May cause hyperkalemia, metabolic acidosis Acute renal dysfunction with bilateral or transplant renal artery stenosis Dry cough in 5–10%						
Benazepril (304, 305)	H	10–40 mg qd	D	50–75%	25–50% (Maximum dose 10 10 mg/d)	Hemo: Unlikely CAPD: Unlikely CAVH: Unlikely
Captopril (306–308) Rare nephrotic syndrome, granulocytopenia. Increases serum digoxin levels.	H (R)	25–50 mg q 8 h	D, I	75% q 12 h	50% q 24 h	Hemo: Dose after dialysis CAPD: None CAVH: Likely to be removed. Dose for GFR 10–50

Table 13. (Continued)

Drug, toxicity, notes	Major elimi- nation route	Dose for normal renal function	Method	Adjustment for renal failure, GFR ml/min		Supplements for dialysis
				10–50	< 10	
Enalapril (309, 310)	H (R)	5–10 mg q 12 h	D	75–100%	50%	Hemo: Dose after dialysis CAPD: None CAVH: Likely to be removed. Dose for GFR 10–50
Fosinopril (311–313)	H	10–40 mg qd	D	100%	100%	Hemo: Dose after dialysis CAPD: None CAVH: Unlikely
Lisinopril (314, 315)	R (H)	5–40 mg qd	D	50–75%	25–50%	Hemo: Dose after dialysis CAPD: Unknown CAVH: Likely to be removed. Dose for GFR 10–50
Quinapril (316)	H (R)	10–20 mg qd	D	100%	75–100%	Hemo: Dose after dialysis CAPD: Unlikely CAVH: Unlikely
Ramipril (317, 318)	H	10–20 mg qd	D	50–75%	25–50%	Hemo: Dose after dialysis CAPD: None CAVH: Likely to be removed. Dose for GFR 10–50

Antiarrhythmic Agents
Blood levels and clinical response best guide to therapy; t-1/2 may be prolonged in heart failure or with reduced hepatic blood flow.

Drug, toxicity, notes	Major elimi- nation route	Dose for normal renal function	Method	Adjustment for renal failure, GFR ml/min		Supplements for dialysis
Amiodarone (319) Thyroid dysfunction; peripheral neuropathy; pulmonary fibrosis.	H	800–1200 mg load 200–600 g mg/d	D	100%	100%	Hemo: None CAPD: None CRRT: Unlikely
Bretylium (320, 321)	R (H)	5–30 mg/kg load 5–10 mg IV q 6 h	D	25–50%	25%	Hemo: None CAPD: Unlikely CRRT: Unlikely
Disopyramide (322–324) Urinary retention. Variable V_D and extrarenal elimination mandates individualized dosing.	H (R)	100–200 mg q 6 h	I	q 12–24 h (GFR > 50: q 6–8 h)	q 24–48 h	Hemo: None CAPD: None CRRT: Unlikely
Encainide (325, 326) Active metabolites may accumulate in renal failure.	R (H)	25 mg q 8 h to 50 mg q 6 h	D	75%	50%	Hemo: Unlikely CAPD: Unlikely CRRT: Unlikely
Flecainide (327, 328) Excretion enhanced in acid urine.	R (H)	100–200 mg q 12 h	D	100%	50–75%	Hemo: None CAPD: Unlikely CRRT: Unlikely

Table 13. (Continued)

Drug, toxicity, notes	Major elimi- nation route	Dose for normal renal function	Method	Adjustment for renal failure, GFR ml/min		Supplements for dialysis
				10–50	< 10	
Lidocaine (329) T-1/2 dependent on hepatic bloodflow; active metabolite	H	Load I mg/kg IV bolus, then 0.5 mg/kg bolus q 8–10 min up to a total of 3 mg/kg Maint: 1–4 mg/min IV infusion	D	100%	100%	Hemo: None CAPD: Unlikely CAVH: Unlikely
Lorcainide (330)	H	100 mg bid	D	100%	100%	Hemo: Unlikely CAPD: Unlikely CAVH: Unlikely
Mexiletine (331, 332)	H	100–300 mg q 6–8 h	D	100%	100%	Hemo: None CAPD: None CAVH: Unlikely
Moricizine (333, 334)	H	200–300 mg q 8 h	D	100%	100%	Hemo: Unlikely CAPD: Unlikely CAVH: Unlikely
N-Acetyl procainamide (335, 336)	R (H)	500 mg q 6–8 h	D, I	50% q 8–12 h	25% q 12 h	Hemo: None CAPD: None CAVH: Replace by blood level
Procainamide (335–337)	R (H)	350–400 mg q 3–4 h	I	q 6–12 h	q 12–24 h	Hemo: 200 mg CAPD: None CAVH: Replace by blood level
Propafenone (338, 339)	H	150–300 mg q 8 h	D	100%	100%	Hemo: None CAPD: Unlikely CAVH: Unlikely
Quinidine (340, 341) Active metabolite, increases plasma digoxin and digitoxin; excretion enhanced in acid urine	H	200–400 mg q 4–6 h	D	100%	75%	Hemo: None CAPD: None CAVH: Unlikely
Tocainide (342, 344)	H (R)	400–600 mg q 8 h	D	100%	50%	Hemo: 200 mg CAPD: None CAVH: Unknown
Beta Blockers						
Acebutolol (345–349) Active metabolites with long half-life	R (H)	400–600 mg/d or bid	D	50%	30–50%	Hemo: Dose after dialysis CAPD: Unknown CAVH: Probably removed. Dose for GFR 10–50.

Table 13. (Continued)

Drug, toxicity, notes	Major elimi- nation route	Dose for normal renal function	Method	Adjustment for renal failure, GFR ml/min		Supplements for dialysis
				10–50	< 10	
Atenolol (350, 351) Significant accumulation in ESRD	R	50–100 mg/d	D	50%	25%	Hemo: 25–50 mg CAPD: None CAVH: Probably removed. Dose for GFR 10–50.
Betaxolol (352)	R (H)	10–20 mg/d	D	100%	50%	Hemo: Dose after dialysis CAPD: Unknown CAVH: Probably removed. Dose for GFR 10–50.
Carteolol (353, 354)	R (H)	5–20 mg/d	D	50%	25%	Hemo: Unknown CAPD: Unknown CAVH: Unknown
Dilevolol (355, 356)	H	200–800 mg po qd	D	100%	100%	Hemo: None CAPD: Unknown CAVH: Unknown
Esmolol (357, 358)	H	50–150 μg/kg/min infusion	D	100%	100%	Hemo: None CAPD: None CAVH: Unknown
Labetalol (359, 360)	H	200–600 mg bid	D	100%	100%	Hemo: None CAPD: None CAVH: Unknown
Metoprolol (361)	H	50–100 mg bid	D	100%	100%	Hemo: Dose after dialysis CAPD: Unknown CAVH: Likely to be removed. Dose for GFR 10–50.
Nadolol (362, 363)	R	80–320 mg/d	D	50%	25%	Hemo: 40 mg CAPD: None CAVH: Likely to be removed. Dose for GFR 10–50.
Penbutolol (364)	H	10–40 mg/d	D	100%	100%	Hemo: Unlikely CAPD: Unlikely CAVH: Unlikely
Pindolol (365)	H (R)	10–40 mg bid	D	100%	100%	Hemo: Unlikely CAPD: Unlikely CAVH: Unlikely
Propranolol (366, 367) Metabolites may accumulate; hypoglycemia reported in ESRD	H	80–160 mg bid	D	100%	100%	Hemo: None CAPD: Unlikely CAVH: Unlikely
Sotalol (368, 369)	R (H)	160–480 mg/d	D	30%	15–30%	Hemo: Dose after dialysis CAPD: None CAVH: Likely to be removed. Dose for GFR 10–50.

Table 13. (Continued)

Drug, toxicity, notes	Major elimination route	Dose for normal renal function	Method	Adjustment for renal failure, GFR ml/min		Supplements for dialysis
				10–50	< 10	
Timolol (345, 346)	R	10–20 mg/bid	D	100%	100%	Hemo: None CAPD: None CAVH: Unlikely
Calcium Channel Blockers						
Amlodipine (370, 371)	H	5 mg/qd	D	100%	100%	Hemo: None CAPD: Unlikely CAVH: Unlikely
Diltiazem (372–374)	H	30–90 mg q 8	D	100%	100%	Hemo: None CAPD: Unlikely CAVH: Unlikely
Felodipine (375–377)	H	10 mg bid	D	100%	100%	Hemo: None CAPD: Unlikely CAVH: Unlikely
Isradipine (378–380)	H	5–10 mg/day	D	100%	100%	Hemo: None CAPD: Unlikely CAVH: Unlikely
Nicardipine (381)	H	20–30 mg tid	D	100%	100%	Hemo: None CAPD: Unlikely CAVH: Unlikely
Nifedipine (382, 383) Nifedipine XL	H	10–30 mg q 8 h (XL: 30–120 mg qd)	D	100%	100%	Hemo: None CAPD: Unlikely CAVH: Unlikely
Nimodipine (370)	H	30 mg q 8 h	D	100%	100%	Hemo: None CAPD: Unlikely CAVH: Unlikely
Nisoldipine (370)	H	10 mg bid	D	100%	100%	Hemo: None CAPD: Unlikely CAVH: Unlikely
Nitrendipine (384, 385)	H	20 mg bid	D	100%	100%	Hemo: None CAPD: Unlikely CAVH: Unlikely
Verapamil (386–388) Verapamil SR	H	80 mg q 8 h (SR: 180 mg qd– 240 mg q 12)	D	100%	100%	Hemo: None CAPD: Unlikely CAVH: Unlikely

Cardiac Glycosides

Add to uremic gastrointestinal symptoms; serum levels guide therapy; toxicity enhanced by dialysis potassium and magnesium removal.

Drug, toxicity, notes	Major elimination route	Dose for normal renal function	Method	10–50	< 10	Supplements for dialysis
Digitoxin (389, 390) Protein binding decreased by dialysis; volume of distribution reduced by uremia.	H (R)	0.1–0.2 mg/d	D	100%	100%	Hemo: None CAPD: None CAVH: None

Table 13. (Continued)

Drug, toxicity, notes	Major elimination route	Dose for normal renal function	Method	Adjustment for renal failure, GFR ml/min		Supplements for dialysis
				10–50	< 10	
Digoxin (7, 391–393) Radioimmunoassay may overestimate serum levels in uremia; clearance reduced by spironolactone, quinidine, verapamil; hypokalemia, hypomagnesemia enhance toxicity.	R (H)	1–1.5 mg load 0.25–0.5 mg/d	D, I	25–75% q 24 h	10–25% q 48 h	Hemo: None CAPD: None CAVH: Unlikely
Ouabain (91, 122)	H (R)	0.25 mg load 0.1 mg q 12 h	I	q 24 h	q 48 h	Hemo: None CAPD: None CAVH: Unlikely
Diuretics Natriuretic drugs may cause volume depletion.						
Acetazolamide (394–396) May potentiate acidemia Ineffective in ESRD	R	250 mg q 6–12 h	I	q 12 h	Avoid	Hemo: Unlikely CAPD: Unlikely CAVH: Unlikely
Amiloride (397) Hyperkalemia Hyperchloremic metabolic acidosis	H (R)	5–10 mg q 24 h	D	50%	Avoid	Hemo: NA CAPD: NA CAVH: NA
Bumetanide (398, 399) Ototoxicity in combination with aminoglycosides Protein binding reduced in renal failure	R (H)	1–2 mg q 8–12 h	D	100%	100%	Hemo: Unlikely CAPD: Unlikely CAVH: Unlikely
Chlorthalidone (400) Ineffective with low GFR	H (R)	25 mg/d	D	100%	Avoid	Hemo: NA CAPD: NA CAVH: NA
Ethacrynic acid (401) Otoxicity	H (R)	50 mg tid	I	q 8–12 h	Avoid	Hemo: NA CAPD: NA CAVH: NA
Furosemide (402–404) Otoxocity	R (H)	40–80 mg bid	D	100%	100%	Hemo: None CAPD: None CAVH: NA
Indapamide (405) Hypotensive effect independent of diuretic effect	H	2.5–5 mg/d	D	100%	100%	Hemo: None CAPD: Unlikely CAVH: Unlikely
Metolazone (394, 395)	R (H)	5–10 mg/d	D	100%	100%	Hemo: Unlikely CAPD: Unlikely CAVH: Unlikely
Piretanide (406, 407) Ototoxicity	H (R)	6–12 mg/d	D	100%	100%	Hemo: Unlikely CAPD: Unlikely CAVH: Unlikely

Table 13. (Continued)

Drug, toxicity, notes	Major elimination route	Dose for normal renal function	Method	Adjustment for renal failure, GFR ml/min		Supplements for dialysis
				10–50	< 10	
Spironolactone (408) Hyperkalemia common when GFR < 30 Hyperchloremic acidosis Active metabolites with long half-life	H (R)	25–50 mg tid	I	q 12–24 h	Avoid	Hemo: NA CAPD: NA CAVH: NA
Thiazides (409) Ineffective when GFR < 30 ml/min Hyperuricemia	R	12.5 mg qd 50 mg bid	D	100%	Avoid	Hemo: NA CAPD: NA CAVH: NA
Triamterene (410) Hyperkalemia common when GFR < 30 Crystalluria in acid urine can cause acute renal failure Active metabolite with long half-life	H	25–50 mg bid	D	100%	Avoid	Hemo: NA CAPD: NA CAVH: NA
Inotropic Agents						
Amrinone (411, 412)	H (R)	5–10 μg/kg min Daily < 10 mg/kg	D	100%	50–75%	Hemo: Unknown CAPD: Unknown CAVH: Unknown
Dobutamine (413, 414)	H	2.5–15 μg/kg/min	D	100%	100%	Hemo: Unknown CAPD: Unknown CAVH: Unknown
Milrinone (415, 416)	R (H)	2.5–15 mg q 6 h	D	100%	50–75%	Hemo: Unknown CAPD: Unknown CAVH: Unknown
Nitrates						
Isosorbide (417–419)	H	10–20 mg tid	D	100%	100%	Hemo: Dose after dialysis CAPD: None CAVH: Unknown
Nitroglycerin (417)	H	Many methods and routes of dosing	D	100%	100%	Hemo: Unknown CAPD: Unknown CAVH: Unknown
Vasodilators						
Diazoxide (420) Decreased protein binding in renal failure	H (R)	150–300 mg bolus	D	75–100%	50%	Hemo: None CAPD: None CAVH: None
Hydralazine (421) Drug induced lupus	R (H)	25–50 mg tid	I	q 8 h	q 12 h	Hemo: None CAPD: None CAVH: Unlikely

Table 13. (Continued)

Drug, toxicity, notes	Major elimination route	Dose for normal renal function	Method	Adjustment for renal failure, GFR ml/min		Supplements for dialysis
				10–50	< 10	
Minoxidil (422) Fluid retention, pericardial effusion	H	5–30 mg bid	D	100%	100%	Hemo: Dose after dialysis CAPD: Unknown CAVH: Unknown
Nitroprusside (423, 424) Toxic metabolite, thiocyanate, accumulates causing seizures, coma. Thiocyanate is hemodialyzable	H	0.25–8 µg/kg/min infusion	D	100%	100%	Hemo: None CAPD: None CAVH: Unlikely

Hypertension is present in the majority of patients with ESRD and has important adverse consequences on the progression of and risk for cardiovascular events (599, 600). Although many of the antihypertensive agents are renally excreted, the dosage is generally titrated to the blood pressure response. Nevertheless, the clinician should be aware of those antihypertensive agents primarily excreted renally. Nadolol and atenolol accumulate in uremia and must be used with caution. It is prudent to initialize therapy with low doses and slowly titrate upward until blood pressure control is achieved, side effects develop or the maximal dose is reached.

Prescribing antihypertensive therapy in dialysis patients is similar to patients with normal renal function, however several comments on selected drugs should be made. Hypertension in ESRD patients is largely volume mediated so the use of diuretics in controlling blood pressure is essential when patients can produce significant amounts of urine. Loop diuretics are required as thiazides are not effective for volume reduction once the GFR has declined below 30 ml/min. Potassium sparing diuretics should be avoided in because of the risk of hyperkalemia. Beta-blockers are useful in selected patients, particularly those with angina or recent myocardial infarction. Those with low lipid solubility are primarily renally excreted and therefore generally require a decrease in the starting dose. ACE inhibitors are attractive for patients with concomitant heart failure or patients with high renin activity mediated hypertension. The ACE inhibitors are excreted renally with the exception of fosinopril which demonstrates dual hepatic and renal elimination. In general, the starting dose for ACE inhibitors should be low and titrated with monitoring of potassium concentrations and blood pressure response. Calcium channel blockers and the majority of the vasodilators and adrenergic modulators do not require dosage adjustment for renal failure.

Many agents used to treat cardiac arrhythmias are at least partially renally excreted. Initiation of treatment at low doses is appropriate as outlined in Table 13. In general, subsequent adjustment is then tailored to arrythmia suppression and the development of side effects. Several of these agents have active metabolites which may accumulate in renal failure.

Management of angina usually involves the use of nitrates, beta-blockers or calcium blockers either alone or in combination. With the exception of the renally excreted beta-blockers, major dose adjustments for renal failure are not required. Table 13 summarizes dosing recommendations for antihypertensive and cardiovascular agents.

ANTINEOPLASTIC AGENTS (TABLE 14)

Renal failure frequently complicates the course of malignancy. A variety of mechanisms may be involved including urinary tract obstruction, tumor lysis syndrome, tumor associated glomerulonephritis and drug related nephrotoxicity (601, 602). As the ESRD population increases in age, the frequency of malignancy may be anticipated to rise. For this reason, knowledge of the renal handling of chemotherapeutic agents and appropriate dosage adjustment is essential.

The majority of chemotherapeutic agents are myelosuppressive and may compound the platelet dysfunction, anemia and immune suppression associated with uremia. Several agents, such as cisplatinum and methotrexate, are excreted primarily by the kidney and require significant dose adjustment. Significant magnesium wasting and salt wasting may occur in those patients substantial residual renal function. Table 14 summarizes dosing recommendations for antineoplastic agents.

Table 14. Antineoplastic agents

Drug, toxicity, notes	Major elimination route	Dose for normal renal function	Method	Adjustment for renal failure, GFR ml/min		Supplements for dialysis
				10–50	< 10	
Bleomycin (425)	R (H)	10–20 u/m^2	D	75%	50%	Hemo: None CAPD: Unlikely CAVH: Unknown
Busulfan (426)	H	4–8 mg/d	D	100%	100%	Hemo: Unknown CAPD: Unknown CAVH: Unknown
Carboplatin (427–429)	R (H)	400–500 mg/m^2	D	50–75%	50%	Hemo: Unknown CAPD: Unknown CAVH: Unknown
Chlorambucil (430)	H	0.1–0.2 mg/kg/d	D	Unknown	Unknown	Hemo: Unknown CAPD: Unknown CAVH: Unknown
Cisplatin (431, 432)	H (R)	20–120 mg/m^2	D	75%	50%	Hemo: Yes CAPD: Unknown CAVH: Unknown
Cyclophosphamide (433–435) Hemorrhagic cystitis Bladder fibrosis and bladder cancer (SIADH)	H	1–5 mg/kg/d	D	100%	75%	Hemo: Dose after dialysis CAPD: Unknown CAVH: Unknown
Cytarabine (436) Increased risk of neurotoxicity with high dose therapy (2–3 g/m^2) in patients with renal insufficiency	H	100–200 mg/m^2	D	100%	100%	Hemo: Unknown CAPD: Unknown CAVH: Unknown
Daunorubicin (437)	H	30–45 mg/m^2	D	100%	100%	Hemo: Unknown CAPD: Unknown CAVH: Unknown
Doxorubicin (438)	H	60–75 mg/m^2	D	100%	100%	Hemo: None CAPD: Unlikely CAVH: Unlikely
Etoposide (439)	H (R)	35–100 mg/m^2/d	D	75%	50%	Hemo: None CAPD: Unlikely CAVH: Unlikely
Fluorouracil (440)	H	12 mg/kg/d	D	100%	100%	Hemo: Dose after dialysis CAPD: Unknown CAVH: Unknown
Formostane (122)	H	250 mg/m^2 q 2 weeks	D	100%	100%	Hemo: Unknown CAPD: Unknown CAVH: Unknown
Hydroxyurea (91, 122)	R (H)	20–30 mg/kg/d	D	50%	20%	Hemo: Unknown CAPD: Unknown CAVH: Unknown
Idarubicin (441)	H (R)	12 mg/m^2	D	100%	100%	Hemo: Unknown CAPD: Unknown CAVH: Unknown
Melphalan (442, 443)	H	6 mg/d	D	75%	50%	Hemo: Unlikely CAPD: Unlikely CAVH: Unlikely

Table 14. (Continued)

Drug, toxicity, notes	Major elimi-nation route	Dose for normal renal function	Method	Adjustment for renal failure, GFR ml/min		Supplements for dialysis
				10–50	< 10	
Methotrexate (444–446)	R (H)	low dose 15–30 mg/d high dose 12 g/m² (with leucovorin rescue)	D	50%	Avoid	Hemo: None CAPD: None CAVH: Unlikely
Mitomycin C (447) Hemolytic uremic syndrome	H	20 mg/m² q 6–8 wks	D	100%	75%	Hemo: Unknown CAPD: Unknown CAVH: Unknown
Nitrosureas (446–448)	R (H)	Varies	D	75%	25–50%	Hemo: None CAPD: Unlikely CAVH: Unlikely
Plicamycin (450)	R (H)	25–30 μg/kg/d	D	75%	50%	Hemo: Unknown CAPD: Unknown CAVH: Unknown
Streptozocin (451)	H	500 mg/m²/d	D	75%	50%	Hemo: Unknown CAPD: Unknown CAVH: Unknown
Tamoxifen (452)	H	10–20 mg bid	D	100%	100%	Hemo: Unknown CAPD: Unknown CAVH: Unknown
Teniposide (91, 122)	H	50–250 mg/m²	D	100%	100%	Hemo: None CAPD: Unlikely CAVH: Unlikely
Vinblastine (453)	H	3.7 mg/m²	D	100%	100%	Hemo: Unknown CAPD: Unknown CAVH: Unknown
Vincristine (91, 122)	H	1.4 mg/m²	D	100%	100%	Hemo: Unknown CAPD: Unknown CAVE: Unknown

ENDOCRINE AND METABOLIC AGENTS (TABLE 15)

Peripheral resistance to the action of insulin and decreased metabolism of insulin by the kidney occur in uremia (603–605). Diabetes is a leading cause of end-stage renal disease, and as such it is not surprising that hypoglycemic agents are frequently prescribed in patients with renal failure. In uremia, sulfonylureas that are excreted primarily by the kidney should be avoided as prolonged hypoglycemia may result from drug accumulation. Chronic peritoneal dialysis offers the unique opportunity to administer insulin into the peritoneal cavity. Intraperitoneal insulin therapy has been shown to result in better overall control of plasma glucose as compared to standard insulin therapy (606).

An increased incidence of hyperlipidemia is associated with renal failure and may contribute to the increased risk of cardiovascular disease in this population (607–609). Although dietary modification remains the mainstay of treatment, many patients require drug therapy for adequate control of lipid levels (610, 611). Bile acid sequestrants require a significant volume of fluid for dilution and may worsen acidemia (460). Several of the hypolipidemic agents, including lovastatin and clofibrate, have been associated with the development of rhabdomyolysis (464). Rhabdomyolysis may also occur in the setting of a variety of drug combinations which include antilipemic agents and cyclosporine. Antithyroid agents and thyroid replacement therapy generally do not require significant dose adjustment in renal failure. Dosing requirements for drugs utilized in the treatment of endocrine and metabolic disorders are summarized in Table 15.

Table 15. Endocrine and metabolic agents

Drug, toxicity, notes	Major elimination route	Dose for normal renal function	Method	Adjustment for renal failure, GFR ml/min		Supplements for dialysis
				10–50	< 10	
Hypoglycemic Agents						
Acarbose (454)	Not Absorbed	50–200 mg tid	D	100%	100%	Hemo: Unlikely CAPD: Unlikely CAVH: Unlikely
Acetohexamide (455) Has diuretic effects. May falsely elevate serum creatinine level. Prolonged hypoglycemia in azotemic patients	H	250–1500 mg/d	D	Avoid	Avoid	Hemo: Unknown CAPD: Unknown CAVH: Unknown
Chlorpropamide (455) Impairs water excretion Prolonged hypoglycemia in azotemic patients	H (R)	100–500 mg/d	D	Avoid	Avoid	Hemo: Unlikely CAPD: Unlikely CAVH: Unlikely
Gliclazide (456)	H	160–320 mg/d	D	100%	100%	Hemo: Unlikely CAPD: Unlikely CAVH: Unlikely
Glipizide (457)	H	2.5–15 mg/d	D	100%	100%	Hemo: Unlikely CAPD: Unlikely CAVH: Unlikely
Glyburide (458)	H (R)	1.25–20 mg/d	D	Avoid	Avoid	Hemo: Unlikely CAPD: Unlikely CAVH: Unlikely
Insulin (459) Renal metabolism of insulin decreases in renal insufficiency May be given intraperitoneal route in CAPD patients	H	Variable	D	75%	50%	Hemo: None CAPD: Unlikely CAVH: Unlikely
Tolazamide (455)	H	100–250 mg/d	D	100%	100%	Hemo: Unlikely CAPD: Unlikely CAVH: Unlikely
Tolbutamide (455)	H	1–2 g/d	D	100%	100%	Hemo: Unlikely CAPD: Unlikely CAVH: Unlikely
Hypolipidemic Agents						
Bezafibrate (460) Monitor CK levels	H (R)	200 mg tid	D	50%	25%	Hemo: Unlikely CAPD: Unlikely CAVH: Unlikely
Choleslyramine (460) Hyperchloremic acidosis Requires fluids for dilution	Not Absorbed	4 qm 4–6 h	D	100%	100% (Use with caution)	Hemo: None CAPD: None CAVH: None
Clofibrate (461)	H (R)	500 1000 mg bid	I	q 12–24 h	Avoid	Hemo: Unlikely CAPD: Unlikely CAVH: Unlikely
Colestipol (460) Hyperchloremic acidosis Requires fluids for dilution	Not Absorbed	13–30 g/d	D	100%	100%	Hemo: None CAPD: None CAVH: None

Table 15. (Continued)

Drug, toxicity, notes	Major elimi- nation route	Dose for normal renal function	Method	Adjustment for renal failure, GFR ml/min		Supplements for dialysis
				10–50	< 10	
Fenofibrate (461)	H	300 mg/d	D	25–50%	Avoid	Hemo: None CAPD: Unlikely CAVH: Unlikely
Fluvastatin (462)	H	20–40 mg/d	D	100%	100%	Hemo: None CAPD: None CAVH: None
Gemfibrozil (463)	H	600 mg bid	D	100%	100%	Hemo: None CAPD: Unknown CAVH: Unknown
Lovastatin (464, 465) Risk of rhabdomyolysis with concurrent use of cyclosporine	H	20–80 mg/d	D	100%	100%	Hemo: Unlikely CAPD: Unlikely CAVH: Unlikely
Nicotinic acid (466) Aspirin may attenuate flushing	H	1–2 gm tid	D	50%	25%	Hemo: Unknown CAPD: Unknown CAVH: Unknown
Pravastatin (467)	H (R)	10–40 mg/d	D	Unknown (probably decreased)	Unknown (probably decreased)	Hemo: Unknown CAPD: Unknown CAVH: Unknown
Probucol (468)	H	500 mg bid	D	100%	100%	Hemo: Unknown CAPD: Unknown CAVH: Unknown
Simvastatin (469)	H	5–40 mg/d	D	100%	100%	Hemo: Unknown CAPD: Unknown CAVH: Unknown
Thyroid Medications						
L-thyroxine (122) Adjust dose according to thyroid function tests	H	100–200 mcg/d	D	100%	100%	Hemo: Unlikely CAPD: Unlikely CAVH: Unlikely
Methimazole (470, 471)	H	5–20 mg tid	D	100%	100%	Hemo: Unknown CAPD: Unknown CAVH: Unknown
Propylthiouracil (470)	H	5–20 mg tid	D	100%	100%	Hemo: Unlikely CAPD: Unlikely CAVH: Unlikely

GASTROINTESTINAL DRUGS (TABLE 16)

Gastrointestinal disorders, particularly uremic gastritis and peptic ulcer disease, occur with increased frequency in patients with ESRD. Prior to the development of the Histamine-2 receptor antagonists (H-2 blockers), antacids were the mainstay of therapy for peptic ulcer disease and related disorders. They are still widely used and are readily available to the patient without a prescription. Their action is to neutralize gastric acid with the active ingredients including aluminum, calcium, magnesium or sodium bicarbonate salts. Systemic absorption of these constituents may result in a variety of metabolic complications including hypermagnesemia, hypercalcemia and metabolic alkalosis. Excessive intake of calcium carbonate in normal individuals may result in the development of the milk-alkali syndrome characterized by the triad of hypercalcemia, metabolic alkalosis and acute renal failure (612). Significant absorption and accumulation of aluminum may occur with chronic ingestion of aluminum containing antacids in the absence of adequate renal function. The development of aluminum toxicity may manifest as bone disease, anemia or neurologic impairment. Patients should be counseled to avoid their use without

Table 16. Gastrointestinal agents

Drug, toxicity, notes	Major elimi-nation route	Dose for normal renal function	Method	Adjustment for renal failure, GFR ml/min		Supplements for dialysis
				10–50	< 10	
Antiemetics, Antidiarrheals, Motility Agents						
Cisapride (122)	H	5–10 mg qid	D	100%	100%	Hemo: None CAPD: Unlikely CAVH: Unlikely
Diphenoxylate (122) (Each tablet contains 2.5 mg dipheoxylate and 0.025 mg of atropine)	H	2 tabs qid	D	50–100%	Avoid	Hemo: Unknown CAPD: Unknown CAVH: Unknown
Granisetron (122)		40–160 μg/kg as 5–30 min IV infusion	D	100%	100%	Hemo: Unknown CAPD: Unknown CAVH: Unknown
Metoclopramide (472, 473) Extrapyramidal reactions increased in ESRD		10–15 mg qid	D	75%	50%	Hemo: None CAPD: Unlikely CAVH: Unlikely
Odansetron (474)	H	0.15 mg/kg as a 15 min infusion	D	100%	100%	Hemo: Unlikely CAPD: Unlikely CAVH: Unlikely
Prochlorperazine (122)	H	5–10 mg po tid-qid 25 mg pr bid	D	100%	100%	Hemo: Unknown CAPD: Unknown CAVH: Unknown
H-2 Antagonists						
Cimetidine (475–479) Increases serum creatinine by inhibition of tubular creatinine secretion	R (H)	400 mg bid or 400–800 mg	D	50–75%	25–50%	Hemo: None CAPD: None CAVH: Unlikely
Famotidine (480–483)	R (H)	20–40 mg qhs	D	25–50%	10%	Hemo: None CAPD: None CAVH: None
Nizatidine (484, 485)	R (H)	150–300 mg qhs	D, I	50%	50% qod	Hemo: Unknown CAPD: Unknown CAVH: Unknown
Ranitidine (486–489)	R (H)	150–300 mg qhs	D	50%	25%	Hemo: 1/2 dose CAPD: None CAVH: Dose for GFR 10–50
Roxatidine (480)	R (H)	150 mg qhs	D	50%	25%	Hemo: Unknown CAPD: Unknown CAVH: Unknown

first consulting their physician. Sucralfate, a locally acting agent, contains a significant quantity of aluminum which may be absorbed and may lead to toxicity with chronic use in the dialysis patient. Short term use appears to be safe.

H-2 blockers are frequently prescribed for patients with ESRD. The drugs in this group have significant renal excretion, however the therapeutic index is high making their use relatively safe. A significant amount of the renal elimination occurs by tubular secretion. Dosage reductions in dialysis patients reduces the CNS effects which may occur with these agents. Other agents used in the treatment of peptic disease include prostaglandin analogues, and the proton pump inhibitors. Significant

Table 16. (Continued)

Drug, toxicity, notes	Major elimi- nation route	Dose for normal renal function	Method	Adjustment for renal failure, GFR ml/min		Supplements for dialysis
				10–50	< 10	

Other Drugs Used for Peptic Disease

Antacids

Calcium, magnesium and aluminum salts all have absorption of constituent cations which have reduced elimination in renal failure producing hypercalcemia, hypermagnesemia and elevated aluminum levels respectively. Protracted use may cause nephrolithiasis, metabolic alkalosis and milk alkali syndrome. Calcium salts now drugs of choice as phosphate binders. For these reasons, other agents are preferred in the treatment of peptic disease in patients with renal failure.

Drug, toxicity, notes	Major elimination route	Dose for normal renal function	Method	10–50	< 10	Supplements for dialysis
Enprostil (122)	H (R)	35 μg bid	D	100%	100%	Hemo: Unknown CAPD: Unknown CAVH: Unknown
Lansoprazole (490)	H	30 mg qd	D	100%	100%	Hemo: Unlikely CAPD: Unlikely CAVH: Unlikely
Misoprostol (491)	H	100–200 pg qid	D	100%	100%	Hemo: Unlikely CAPD: Unlikely CAVH: Unlikely
Omepxazole (492, 493)	H	20–40 mg/d	100%	100%	Hemo: None	CAPD: Unlikely CAVH: Unlikely
Sucralfate (494, 495) Contains aluminum which may be absorbed to produce dementia, renal osteodystrophy and anemia. Less than 5% of dose absorbed.	Not Absorbed	1 g qid	D	100%	100% CAPD: NA	Hemo: NA CAVH: NA

dosage reductions are not required for these drugs in renal failure.

The majority of the antiemetic and motility agents do not require dosage adjustment in the dialysis patient. The dose of metoclopramide, however, should be decreased as significant renal clearance does occur and the risk of extrapyramidal side effects appears to be increased in ESRD. A variety of laxatives are readily available without prescription. Proper patient education is essential since preparations such as magnesium containing laxatives and phosphate containing enemas may result in significant accumulation of magnesium or phosphorus. Suggested guidelines for prescribing gastrointestinal agents are outlined in Table 16.

NEUROLOGIC AGENTS (TABLE 17)

Seizures occur with increased frequency in patients with end-stage renal disease (613). Although often attributed to reversible precipitating metabolic events, in some cases a specific etiology is not identified and long term anticonvulsant therapy is undertaken. Phenytoin is one of the most frequently prescribed anticonvulsants. In renal failure, the volume of distribution of this agent is increased and the degree of protein binding is markedly reduced (499). Although dosage adjustment is not generally made for renal insufficiency, the clinician should be aware that the proportion of free or active drug will be increased. Thus, a low total plasma phenytoin level may not necessarily be subtherapeutic. Serum concentration monitoring is best accomplished in uremia by directly measuring the free serum phenytoin concentration. Anti-Parkinson agents and drugs utilized for the treatment of migraine headaches generally do not require dosage adjustment for renal failure. Recommendations for dosing neurologic drugs are outlined in Table 17.

RHEUMATOLOGIC AGENTS (TABLE 18)

NSAIDs are widely prescribed for musculoskeletal pain. Although dose adjustment is generally not required for renal insufficiency, several precautions should be noted. The first applies to patients not yet dialysis dependent. Under conditions of diminished renal perfusion such as

Table 17. Neurologic agents

Drug, toxicity, notes	Major elimination route	Dose for normal renal function	Method	Adjustment for renal failure, GFR ml/min		Supplements for dialysis
				10–50	< 10	
Anticonvulsants. Monitor serum levels						
Carbamazepine (496–498)	H	200 mg to 1200 mg/d	D	100%	100%	Hemo: None CAPD: Unlikely CAVH: Unlikely
Ethosuximide (499)	H (R)	500–1500 mg/d	D	75–100%	50%	Hemo: 250 mg CAPD: Unknown CAVH: Dose for GFR 10–50
Oxcarbazepine (122)	H	200–400 mg tid	D	100%	100%	Hemo: Unknown CAPD: Unknown CAVH: Unknown
Phenytoin (500, 501) Protein binding decreased and distribution volume increased in renal failure. Monitor free dilantin levels	H	1000 mg load, then 300–400 mg/d	D	100%	100%	Hemo: None CAPD: None CAVH: Unlikely
Primidone (502) Partially converted to phenobarbital and other metabolites with long half-life	H (R)	200–500 mg qid	I	q 8–12 h	q 12–24 h	Hemo: 1/3 dose CAPD: Unknown CAVH: Likely to be removed Dose for GFR 10–50
Trimethadione (91, 122)	H	300–600 mg tid-qid	I	q 8–12	q 12–24 h	Hemo: Unknown CAPD: Unknown CAVH: Unknown
Valproic acid (503, 504) Decreased protein binding in uremia Concurrent phenytoin, phenobarbital and primidone shorten half-life	H	15–60 mg/k/d	D	100%	100%	Hemo: None CAPD: Unlikely CAVH: Unlikely
Vigabatrin (91, 122)	R (H)	24 g/d	D	50%	25–50%	Hemo: Unknown CAPD: Unknown CAVH: Unknown
Anti-Parkinson Agents						
Bromocriptine (505) Orthostatic hypotension	H	1.25 mg bid	D	100%	100%	Hemo: Unlikely CAPD: Unlikely CAVH: Unlikely
Carbidopa (506)	H (R)	1 tab tid to 6 tabs daily	D	100%	100%	Hemo: Unknown CAPD: Unknown CAVH: Unknown
Levodopa (506)	H	250–500 mg bid to 8 g/d	D	100%	100%	Hemo: Unknown CAPD: Unknown CAVH: Unknown
Trihexyphenidyl (507)	R (H)	1–2 mg/d to 6–10 mg/d	D	Unknown	Unknown	Hemo: Unknown CAPD: Unknown CAVH: Unknown

Table 17. (Continued)

Drug, toxicity, notes	Major elimination route	Dose for normal renal function	Method	Adjustment for renal failure, GFR ml/min		Supplements for dialysis
				10–50	< 10	
Agents used for the treatment of migraine headaches						
Ergotamine (122) (Ergotamine 1 mg caffeine 100 mg)	H	Acute attack: 1 tab q 30 min (maximum 6 tabs)	D	100%	100%	Hemo: Unknown CAPD: Unknown CAVH: Unknown
Dihydroergotamine (122)	H	Acute attack: 1 mg IM or IV q 1 h (maximum 3 mg)	D	100%	100%	Hemo: Unknown CAPD: Unknown CAVH: Unknown

congestive heart failure or cirrhosis with ascites, vasodilatory prostaglandins (PGE_2, PGI_2) become critical in maintaining renal blood flow. Administration of NSAIDs in this setting may cause an acute reversible decline in renal function through interference with prostaglandin synthesis. Other renal effects of NSAIDs include impairment of potassium excretion and interference with sodium and water excretion (614). Additionally, a hypersensitivity reaction may rarely occur characterized by acute interstitial nephritis in conjunction with a minimal change glomerular lesion. Gastrointestinal complications such as gastritis and peptic pain may limit the use of these agents in many patients. ESRD patients are particularly susceptible to gastrointestinal irritation from these agents. Occult or overt gastrointestinal bleeding may occur with these agents. NSAIDs should be used cautiously and with careful monitoring for electrolyte disturbances, blood loss, and blood pressure control.

Appropriate dose reduction must be taken in prescribing anti-gout agents to minimize side effects. Allopurinol reduces the production of uric acid and is commonly prescribed for the treatment of hyperuricemia and gout. Accumulation of its metabolite (oxipurinol) occurs with renal insufficiency and may explain the development of exfoliative dermatitis in a subset of patients (508). Patients with renal failure appear to be at greater risk for developing myopathy and polyneuropathy with the use of colchicine (510). In addition to dose reduction, patients should be monitored closely for symptoms of muscle weakness with chronic use of the agent. In general, uricosuric drugs are ineffective when the GFR is decreased. Dosing guidelines for rheumatologic agents are summarized in Table 18.

SEDATIVES, HYPNOTICS AND PSYCHIATRIC AGENTS (TABLE 19)

The majority of drugs in this category are lipid soluble, highly protein bound and excreted primarily by hepatic transformation to inactive or less active metabolites. Increased sensitivity to the sedative side effects may occur in the dialysis patient. Recognition of side effects may be delayed as malaise and somnolence are common in the uremic population. Benzodiazepines are widely prescribed for anxiety. Several of these agents including diazepam, flurazepam and chlordiazepoxide, have active polar metabolites which accumulate and cause prolonged sedation. For this reason, chronic use of these agents should be avoided. Depression is common in patients with chronic illness such as renal failure, occasionally requiring treatment with antidepressant medications. Although dose reduction generally is not required, increased sensitivity to the side effects of tricyclic antidepressants warrants caution when prescribing these agents. The initial dose should be low and titrated according to clinical response and side effects. Side effects due to phenothiazines such as extrapyramidal symptoms and changes in mental status may be accentuated in renal failure. Therefore, the lowest effective dose should be prescribed.

In contrast to most psychotropic drugs, lithium is water soluble and renally excreted. Lithium may have several renal effects including the development of renal failure with acute lithium overdose and nephrogenic diabetes insipidus in patients on chronic treatment (557). Lithium levels should be monitored closely. Volume depletion and concomitant diuretic therapy should be avoided if possible as lithium reabsorption in the kidney increases in sodium avid states. Significant removal of lithium occurs with hemodialysis and may be used for the treatment of lithium overdose. Table 19 summarizes dosing recommendations for agents utilized in psychiatry.

Table 18. Rheumatologic agents

Drug, toxicity, notes	Major elimination route	Dose for normal renal function	Method	Adjustment for renal failure, GFR ml/min		Supplements for dialysis
				10–50	< 10	
Gout Agents						
Allopurinol (508, 509) Active metabolite	H (R)	300 mg/d	D	50%	25%	Hemo: 1/2 dose CAPD: Unknown CAVH: Unknown
Colchicine (510, 511) Increased risk of myopathy and neuropathy in renal failure. Monitor CK values.	H	Acute: 2 mg, then 0.5 mg q 6 h Chronic: 0.5–1 mg/d	D	50%	25%	Hemo: None CAPD: Unlikely CAVH: Unlikely
Probenicid (512) Ineffective at decreased GFR	H	500 mg bid	D	Avoid	Avoid	Hemo: Unlikely CAPD: Unlikely CAVH: Unlikely

Non-steroidal Antiinflammatory Drugs

Drugs in this group may be associated with renal dysfunction secondary to prostaglanding inhibition; prostaglandin inhibitors may increase uremic bleeding and gastrointestinal symptoms; nephrotic syndrome; interstitial nephritis, and hyperkalemia reported.

Drug	Route	Dose	Method	10–50	< 10	Supplements
Diclofenac (513, 514)	H	25–75 mg bid	D	100%	100%	Hemo: None CAPD: None CAVH: None
Diflunisal (515)	H	250–500 mg bid	D	100%	50%	Hemo: None CAPD: None CAVH: None
Etodolac (516)	H	200–600 mg bid	D	100%	100%	Hemo: None CAPD: None CAVH: None
Flurbiprofen (517)	H	100 mg bid-tid	D	100%	100%	Hemo: None CAPD: None CAVH: None
Ibuprofen (518)	H	800 mg tid	D	100%	100%	Hemo: None CAPD: None CAVH: None
Indomethacin (519)	H (R)	25–50 mg tid	D	100%	100%	Hemo: None CAPD: None CAVH: None
Ketoprofen (520)	H	25–75 mg tid	D	100%	100%	Hemo: None CAPD: None CAVH: None
Ketorolac (521)	H	5–30 mg qid	D	100%	100%	Hemo: None CAPD: None CAVH: None
Meclofenamic acid (513)	H	50–100 mg tid-qid	D	100%	100%	Hemo: None CAPD: None CAVH: None
Mefenamic acid (513)	H	250 mg qid	D	100%	100%	Hemo: None CAPD: None CAVH: None
Naproxen (522)	H	500 mg/bid	D	100%	100%	Hemo: None CAPD: None CAVH: None

Table 18. (Continued)

Drug, toxicity, notes	Major elimination route	Dose for normal renal function	Method	Adjustment for renal failure, GFR ml/min		Supplements for dialysis
				10–50	< 10	
Phenylbutazone (513)	H	100 mg tid-qid	D	100%	100%	Hemo: None CAPD: None CAVH: None
Piroxicam (523)	H	20 mg/d	D	100%	100%	Hemo: None CAPD: None CAVH: None
Sulindac (524) Active sulfide metabolite; relatively renal sparing.	H	200 mg/bid	D	100%	100%	Hemo: None CAPD: None CAVH: None
Tolmetin (513)	H	400 mg tid	D	100%	100%	Hemo: None CAPD: None CAVH: None
Other Agents Utilized in the Treatment of Arthritis						
Auranofin (525) Rarely nephrotic Proteinuria common, rarely progresses to nephrotic syndrome	H (R)	6 mg/d	D	Avoid	Avoid	Hemo: Unlikely CAPD: Unlikely CAVH: Unlikely
Gold sodium thiomalate (526) Nephrotoxic, proteinuria, membranous nephritis	R (H)	25–50 mg	D	Avoid	Avoid	Hemo: Unlikely CAPD: Unlikely CAVH: Unlikely
Penicillamine (91, 122)	H (R)	250–1000 mg/d	D	Avoid	Avoid	Hemo: Unknown CAPD: Unknown CAVH: Unknown

MISCELLANEOUS AGENTS (TABLE 20)

A wide variety of agents are included in the table of miscellaneous agents. Although most of the information is self explanatory, a few comments are appropriate. Uremic platelet dysfunction may increase the risk of bleeding in patients receiving anticoagulants and requires close monitoring. Streptokinase and urokinase should probably only be utilized for local thrombolytic therapy because of the preexisting hemostatic defect in uremia. Antihistamines may cause excessive sedation in some patients. Once again, the initial dose should be low and increased slowly until the lowest effective dose is found. Immunosuppressive agents may be utilized as treatment for a primary renal disease or for an autoimmune disorder. There is no dosage adjustment required for steroids or cyclosporine as hepatic metabolism is the primary route of elimination. Table 20 summarizes dosing recommendations for miscellaneous agents.

CONCLUSIONS

Prescribing drugs for the patient with ESRD poses a difficult challenge for the clinician. Drug pharmacokinetics and pharmacodynamics are frequently altered in the uremic setting. In addition, multiple medical problems frequently exist and result in the need for multiple medications in most patients. The risk of adverse drug reactions is increased in this population and contributes significantly to patient morbidity, prolongation of hospital stays and financial costs of drug therapy. In order to minimize toxicity and maximize efficacy, it is essential that the clinician be aware of these issues and adjust drug dosages appropriately.

Table 19. Sedative, hypnotics, drugs used in psychiatry

Drug, toxicity, notes	Major elimi- nation route	Dose for normal renal function	Method	Adjustment for renal failure, GFR ml/min		Supplements for dialysis
				10–50	< 10	
Antidepressants						
Amoxapine (527)	H	75–200 mg/d	D	100%	100%	Hemo: Unlikely CAPD: Unlikely CAVH: Unlikely
Bupropion (528)	H	100 mg q 8 h	D	100%	100%	Hemo: Unlikely CAPD: Unlikely CAVH: Unlikely
Fluoxetine (529, 530)	H	20 mg/d	D	100%	100%	Hemo: None CAPD: Unlikely CAVH: Unlikely
Maprotiline (91, 122)	H	75–150 mg/d	D	100%	50–75%	Hemo: Unlikely CAPD: Unlikely CAVH: Unlikely
Barbiturates May cause excessive sedation.						
Pentobarbitol (91, 122)	H	30 mg tid-qid	D	100%	100%	Hemo: Dose after dialysis CAPD: Unknown CAVH: Unknown
Phenobarbital (91, 122)	H (R)	50–100 mg bid-tid	D, I	100% q 8–12	50% q 12 h	Hemo: Dose after dialysis CAPD: 75% q 12 h CAVH: Unknown, likely to be removed.
Secobarbital (91, 122)	H	30–50 mg tid-qid	D	100%	100%	Hemo: Dose after dialysis CAPD: Unknown CAVH: Unknown
Thiopental (531)	H	Anesthesia induction	D	100%	75%	Hemo: Unlikely CAPD: Unlikely CAVH: Unlikely
Benzodiazepines						
Alprazolam (532, 533)	H	0.25–5 mg tid	D	100%	100%	Hemo: Unlikely CAPD: Unlikely CAVH: Unlikely
Clorazepate (534) Active metabolite.	H (R)	15–60 ng/d	D	100%	100%	Hemo: Unknown CAPD: Unknown CAVH: Unknown
Chlordiazepoxides (535) Active metabolite.	H	15–100 mg/d	D	100%	50%	Hemo: Unlikely CAPD: Unlikely CAVH: Unlikely
Clonazepam (532)	H	1.5 mg/d	D	100%	100%	Hemo: Unknown CAPD: Unknown CAVH: Unknown
Diazepam (91, 122)	H	540 mg/d	O	100%	100%	Hemo: Unlikely CAPD: Unlikely CAVH: Unlikely

Table 19. (Continued)

Drug, toxicity, notes	Major elimi-nation route	Dose for normal renal function	Method	Adjustment for renal failure, GFR ml/min		Supplements for dialysis
				10–50	< 10	
Flurazepam (532) Active metabolite.	H	15–30 mg hs	D	100%	100%	Hemo: Unlikely CAPD: Unlikely CAVH: Unlikely
Lorazepam (536)	H	1–2 mg bid-tid	D	100%	100%	Hemo: None CAPD: Unlikely CAVH: Unlikely
Midazolam (537)	H	1.25 mg IV initial, titrate to response	D	100%	100%	Hemo: Unlikely CAPD: Unlikely CAVH: Unlikely
Nitrazepam (535)	H	5–10 mg hs	D	100%	100%	Hemo: Unknown CAPD: Unknown CAVH: Unknown
Oxazepam (539)	H	30–120 mg/d	D	100%	100%	Hemo: None CAPD: Unlikely CAVH: Unlikely
Prazepam (532) Active metabolite	H (R)	20–60 mg hs	D	100%	100%	Hemo: Unlikely CAPD: Unlikely CAVH Unlikely
Quazepam (540)	H	15 mg hs	D	100%	100%	Hemo: Unlikely CAPD: Unlikely CAVH: Unlikely
Temazepam (532)	H	30 mg hs	D	100%	100%	Hemo: Unlikely CAPD: Unlikely CAVH: Unlikely
Triazolam (541, 542) Protein binding correlates with alpha-1 acid glycoprotein glycoprotein concentration	H	0.125–0.5 mg hs	D	100%	100%	Hemo: Unlikely CAPD: Unlikely CAVH: Unlikely

Phenothiazines
Anticholinergic, urinary retention, orthostatic hypotension, confusion.

| Chlorpromazine (543) | H | 300–800 mg/d | D | 100% | 100% | Hemo: Unlikely CAPD: Unlikely CAVH: Unlikely |
| Promethazine (544) | H | 20–100 mg/d | D | 100% | 100% | Hemo: Unlikely CAPD: Unlikely CAVH: Unlikely |

Tricyclic Antidepressants
Anticholinergic urinary retention orthostatic hypotension excessive sedation.

Amitriptyline (545–547)	H	25 mg tid	D	100%	100%	Hemo: None CAPD: None CAVH: Unlikely
Clomipramine (548)	H	25–50 mg bid-tid	D	100%	100%	Hemo: Unlikely CAPD: Unlikely CAVH: Unlikely
Desipramine (549) Active metabolites	H	75–150 mg/d	D	100%	100%	Hemo: Unlikely CAPD: Unlikely CAVH: Unlikely

Table 19. (Continued)

Drug, toxicity, notes	Major elimination route	Dose for normal renal function	Method	Adjustment for renal failure, GFR ml/min		Supplements for dialysis
				10–50	< 10	
Doxepin (550) Protein binding decrease in ESRD	H	25 mg tid	D	100%	100%	Hemo: None CAPD: Unlikely CAVH: Unlikely
Imipramine (551) Active metabolite	H	25 mg tid	D	100%	100%	Hemo: Unlikely CAPD: Unlikely CAVH: Unlikely
Nortriptyline (552)	H	25 mg tid-qid	D	100%	100%	Hemo: None CAPD: Unlikely CAVH: Unlikely
Protriptyline (553)	H	15–60 mg/d	D	100%	100%	Hemo: Unlikely CAPD: Unlikely CAVH: Unlikely
Miscellaneous Agents						
Buspirone (554) Active metabolite accumulates	H	5–10 mg tid	D	100%	50%	Hemo: Unlikely CAPD: Unlikely CAVH: Unlikely
Clozapine (555)	H	150–200 mg bid	D	100%	100%	Hemo: Unlikely CAPD: Unlikely CAVH: Unlikely
Chloral hydrate (91, 122) Active metabolite. Excessive sedation.	H	250 mg tid	D	Avoid	Avoid	Hemo: None CAPD: Unlikely CAVH: Unlikely
Ethchlorvynol (91, 122) Excessive sedation.	H	500 mg q hs	D	Avoid	Avoid	Hemo: Avoid CAPD: Avoid CAVH: Avoid
Haloperidol (555) Hypotension, excessive sedation.	H	1–2 mg bid-tid	D	100%	100%	Hemo: Unlikely CAPD: Unlikely CAVH: Unlikely
Lithium carbonate (525, 555, 556) Nephrogenic diabetes insipidus Nephrotoxic, monitor serum levels Toxicity enhanced by volume depletion, diuretics and NSAIDs	R	900–1200 mg total dose/d	D	50–75%	25–50%	Hemo: Dose after dialysis CAPD: None CAVH: Likely to be removed, follow levels
Meprobamate (91, 122)	H (R)	300–400 mg q 6 h	D, I	q 8–12 h	50% q 12 h	Hemo: 200–400 mg CAPD: Unknown CAVH: Likely to be removed
Phenelzine (91, 122)	H	20–30 mg tid	D	100%	100%	Hemo: Unknown CAPD: Unknown CAVH: Unknown

Table 20. Miscellaneous agents

Drug, toxicity, notes	Major elimination route	Dose for normal renal function	Method	Adjustment for renal failure, GFR ml/min		Supplements for dialysis
				10–50	< 10	

Anticoagulants and Antiplatelet Agents

Agents in this group should be carefully titrated to achieve therapeutic effects; may potentiate uremic bleeding.

Drug, toxicity, notes	Major elimination route	Dose for normal renal function	Method	10–50	< 10	Supplements for dialysis
Dipyridamole (559)	H	50 mg tid	D	100%	100%	Hemo: Unlikely CAPD: Unlikely CAVH: Unlikely
Heparin (560) t-1/2 increases with dose	H	75 U/kg load then 0.5 U/kg/min	D	100%	100%	Hemo: Unlikely CAPD: Unlikely CAVH: Unlikely
Streptokinase (561)	H	250,000 U load, then 100,000 u/h		100%	100%	Hemo: NA CAPD: NA CAVH: NA
Sulfinpyrazone (562)	H (R)	200 mg bid		100%	Avoid	Hemo: Unlikely CAPD: Unlikely CAVH: Unlikely
Ticlopidine (563)	H	500 mg bid	D	100%	100%	Hemo: Unknown CAPD: Unknown CAVH: Unknown
Tissue-type plasminogen (564) activator	H	100 mg total over 3 hours	D	100%	100%	Hemo: Unlikely CAPD: Unlikely CAVH: Unlikely
Urokinase (122)	H	4400 u/kg load, then 4400 u/kg/h	D	100%	100%	Hemo: Unknown CAPD: Unknown CAVH: Unknown
Warfarin (565) Follow prothrombin time	H	10–15 mg load, then 2–10 mg/d	D	100%	100%	Hemo: Unlikely CAPD: Unlikely CAVH: Unlikely

Antihistamines

May cause excessive sedation

Drug, toxicity, notes	Major elimination route	Dose for normal renal function	Method	10–50	< 10	Supplements for dialysis
Astemizole (566, 567)	H	10 mg/d	D	100%	100%	Hemo: Unlikely CAPD: Unlikely CAVH: Unlikely
Brompheniramine (566)	H	4 mg q 4–6 h	D	100%	100%	Hemo: Unknown CAPD: Unknown CAVH: Unknown
Chlorpheniramine (566)	H	4 mg q 4–6 h	D	100%	100%	Hemo: None CAPD: Unlikely CAVH: Unlikely
Diphenhydramine (566) Anticholinergic effects may cause urine retention	H	25 mg tid-qid	D	100%	100%	Hemo: Unlikely CAPD: Unlikely CAVH: Unlikely
Flunarizine (91, 122)	H	Unknown	D	None	None	Hemo: Unlikely CAPD: Unlikely CAVH: Unlikely
Hydroxyzine (91, 122)	H	50–100 mg qid	D	Unknown	Unknown	Hemo: Unknown CAPD: Unknown CAVH: Unknown
Orphenadrine (566)	H	100 mg bid	D	100%	100%	Hemo: Unknown CAPD: Unknown CAVH: Unknown

Table 20. (Continued)

Drug, toxicity, notes	Major elimination route	Dose for normal renal function	Method	Adjustment for renal failure, GFR ml/min		Supplements for dialysis
				10–50	< 10	
Oxatomide (568)	H	Unknown	D	100%	100%	Hemo: Unlikely CAPD: Unlikely CAVH: Unlikely
Promethazine (566)	H	12.5–25 mg qd-qid	D	100%	100%	Hemo: Unlikely CAPD: Unlikely CAVH: Unlikely
Terfenadine (569)	H	60 mg bid	D	100%	100%	Hemo: Unlikely CAPD: Unlikely CAVH: Unlikely
Tripelennamine (566)	H	25–50 mg tid-qid	D	Unknown	Unknown	Hemo: Unknown CAPD: Unknown CAVH: Unknown
Triprolidine (566)	H	2.5 mg q 4–6 h	D	Unknown	Unknown	Hemo: Unknown CAPD: Unknown CAVH: Unknown
Bronchodilators						
Albuterol (570)	R (H)	2–4 mg tid-qid aerosol: 100–200 mg tid-qid	D	75%	50%	Hemo: Unknown CAPD: Unknown CAVH: Unknown
Bitolterol (571)	R (H)	Aerosol: 2 inhalations q 8 h	D	100%	100%	Hemo: Unknown CAPD: Unknown CAVH: Unknown
Dyphylline (572)	R	15 mg/kg/d	D	50%	25%	Hemo: 1/3 dose CAPD: Unknown CAVH: Likely to be removed
Ipratropium (570)	H	2 inhalations qid	D	100%	100%	Hemo: Unlikely CAPD: Unlikely CAVH: Unlikely
Terbutaline (570)	R (H)	2.5–5 mg tid	D	50%	Avoid	Hemo: Unknown CAPD: Unknown CAVH: Unknown
Theophylline (573, 574)	H	200–400 mg q 12 h	D	100%	100%	Hemo: 1/2 dose CAPD: Unknown CAVH: Likely to be removed, monitor levels
Immunosuppressive Drugs						
Azathioprine (575, 576)	H	1.5–2.5 mg/kg/d	D	75%	50%	Hemo: Dose after dialysis CAPD: Unknown CAVH: Unknown

Table 20. (Continued)

Drug, toxicity, notes	Major elimination route	Dose for normal renal function	Method	Adjustment for renal failure, GFR ml/min		Supplements for dialysis
				10–50	< 10	
Corticosteroids						
May aggravate azotemia, sodium retention, glucose intolerance, and hypertension						
Betamethasone (91, 122)	H	0.5–9 mg/d	D	100%	100%	Hemo: Unknown CAPD: Unknown CAVH: Unknown
Cortisone (91, 122)	H	25–500 mg/d	D	100%	100	Hemo: None CAPD: Unlikely CAVH: Unlikely
Dexamethasone (577)	H	0.75–9 mg/d	D	100%	100%	Hemo: Unknown CAPD: Unknown CAVH: Unknown
Hydrocortisone (91, 122)	H	20–500 mg/d	D	100%	100%	Hemo: Unknown CAPD: Unknown CAVH: Unknown
Methylprednisolone (578)	H	4–48 mg/d	D	100%	100%	Hemo: Yes CAPD: Unknown CAVH: Likely to be removed
Prednisone (579)	H (R)	5–60 mg/d	D	100%	100%	Hemo: None CAPD: Unlikely CAVH: Unlikely
Triamcinolone (91, 122)	H	4–48 mg/d	D	100%	100%	Hemo: Unknown CAPD: Unknown CAVH: Unknown
Cyclosporine (580) Nephrotoxic. Hypertension, seizures, tremor. Inhibitors of hepatic metabolism increase blood levels	H	3–10 mg/kg/d	D	100%	100%	Hemo: Unknown CAPD: Unknown CAVH: Unknown
Miscellaneous						
Acetohydroxamic acid (581) May accumulate in ESRD	R (H)	10–15 mg/kg/d	D	100%	Avoid	Hemo: Unknown CAPD: Unknown CAVH: Unknown
Desferrioxamine (582, 583) Fungal infections in ESRD Used in treatment for iron or aluminum overload	H (R)	Chronic Fe overload 0.5–1 g/d	D, I	50% qd	5–10 mg/k/week (Avoid if possible	Hemo: Chelation product removed CAPD: Chelation product removed CAVH: Chelation product removed
Pentoxifylline (584, 585)	H	400 mg tid	I	bid-tid	q 24 h	Hemo: Unknown CAPD: Unknown CAVH: Unknown

REFERENCES

1. Golper TA, Bennett WM: Altering drug dose in liver and kidney diseases. in *Handbook of Drug Therapy in Liver and Kidney Disease*, edited by Schrier R, Gambertoglio J, Boston, Little Brown, 1991, p 1

2. Bennett WM: Adjustment of drug dosage in patients with renal insufficiency. in *Textbook of Internal Medicine*, edited by Kelley WM, New York, Lippincott, 1991, p 763

3. Jick H: Adverse drug effects in relation to renal function. *Am J Med* 62: 514, 1977

4. Benet LZ, Massoud N: Pharmacokinetics. in *Pharmacokinetic Basis for Drug Treatment*, edited by Benet LZ, Massoud N, Gambertoglio JG, New York, Raven, 1984, p 1

5. Ritschel WA: *Handbook of Basic Pharmacokinetics – Including Clinical Applications*, 3rd Edition. Hamilton, Drug Intelligence Press Inc, 1986, p 163

6. Sachs EF, Hurwitz FJ, Bloch HM, Milne FJ: Pancreatic exocrine hypofunction in the wasting syndrome of end-stage renal disease. *Am J Gastroenterol* 78, 170, 1983

7. Ochs HR, Greenblatt DJ, Bodem G, Dengler HJ: Disease-related alterations in cardiac glycoside disposition. *Clin Pharmacokinet* 7: 434, 1982

8. Gibaldi M: Drug distribution in renal failure. *Am J Med* 62: 471, 1977

9. Reidenberg MM: The binding of drugs to plasma proteins and the interpretation of measurements of plasma concentrations of drugs in patients with poor renal function. *Am J Med* 62: 466, 1977

10. Gulyassy PF, Depner TA: Impaired binding of drugs and endogenous ligands in renal disease. *Am J Kidney Dis* 2: 578, 1983

11. McNamara PJ, Lalka D, Gibaldi M: Endogenous accumulation products and serum protein binding in uremia. *J Lab Clin Med* 98: 730, 1981

12. Vanholder R, Van Landschoot N, De Smet R, Schoots A, Ringoir S: Drug protein binding in chronic renal failure: evaluation of nine drugs. *Kidney Int* 33: 996, 1988

13. Boobis SW: Alteration of plasma albumin in relation to decreased drug binding in uremia. *Clin Pharmacol Ther* 22: 147, 1977

14. Maher JF: Principles of dialysis and dialysis of drugs. *Am J Med* 62: 475, 1977

15. Golper TA, Bennett WM: Drug visage in dialysis patients. in *Clinical Dialysis*, 2nd Edition, edited by Nissenson A, Fine R, Gentile D, Norwalk, Appleton-Lange, 1988, p 608

16. Vos MC, Vincent HH, Yzerman EPF, Vogel M, Mouton JW: Drug cleared by continuous hemodiafiltration (CAVHD): results with the AN69 capillary hemofilter and recommended dose adjustments for seven antibiotics. *Drug Invest* 1994. In press

17. Tillement JP, Lhoste F, Findicelli TF: Diseases and drug protein binding. *Clin Pharmacokinet* 3: 144, 1978

18. Lee CS, Marbury TC: Drug therapy in patients undergoing haemodialysis. Clinical pharmacokinetical considerations. *Clin Pharmacokinet* 9: 42, 1984

19. Piafsky KM: Disease induced changes in the serum binding of basic drugs. *Clin Pharmacokinet* 5: 246, 1980

20. Garfinkel D, Mamelok RD, Blaschke TF: Altered therapeutic range for quinidine after myocardial infarction an cardiac surgery. *Ann Intern Med* 107: 48, 1987

21. Reidenberg MM: The biotransformation of drugs in renal failure. *Am J Med* 62: 482, 1977

22. Aronoff GR, Luft FC: Antimicrobial therapy in patients with impaired renal function. *Dial Transplant* 8: 14, 1979

23. Bennett WM, Hartnett MN, Craven R, Gilbert DN, Porter GA: Gentamicin concentrations in blood, urine and renal tissue of patients with end-stage renal disease. *J Lab Clin Med* 90: 389, 1977

24. Bennett WM, Craven R: Urinary tract infections in patients with severe renal disease: treatment with ampicillin and trimethoprim-sulfamethoxazole. *JAMA* 236: 946, 1976

25. Elzinga L, Golper TA, Rashad AL, Carr ME, Bennett WM: Trimethoprim-sulfamethoxazole activity in cyst fluid from autosomal dominant polycystic kidneys. *Kidney Int* 32: 884, 1987

26. Elzinga LW, Golper TA, Rashad AL, Carr ME, Bennett WM: Ciprofloxacin activity in cyst fluid from polycystic kidneys. *Antimicrob Agents Chemother* 32: 844, 1988

27. Miller RD, Cullen DJ: Renal failure and post-operative respiratory failure: recurarization? *Br J Anaesth* 48: 253, 1976

28. Phillips ME, Eastwood JB, Curtis JR, Gower PC, De Wardener HE: Tetracycline poisoning in renal failure. *Br Med J* 2(911): 149, 1974

29. Al-Damluji S, Meek JH: Interference of a propranolol metabolite with serum bilirubin estimation in chronic renal failure. *Br Med J* 280(6229): 1414, 1980

30. Molitch ME, Rodman E, Hirsch CA, Dubinsky E: Spurious serum creatinine elevations in ketoacidosis. *Ann Inter Med* 93: 280, 1980

31. Baba S, Baba T, Iwanga T: Effect of acetohexamide (a sulfonylurea hypoglycemic agent) in blood plasma on creatinine assay in clinical laboratory tests. *Chem Pharmacol Bull* 27: 139, 1979

32. Maddocks J, Hann S, Hopkins M, Coles GA: The effect of methyldopa on creatinine estimation. *Lancet* 1(795): 157, 1973

33. Ayneck ML, Berardi RR, Johnson RM: Interference of cephalosporins and cefoxitin with serum creatinine determination. *Am J Hosp Pharm* 38: 1348, 1981

34. Burgess E, Blair A, Krichman K, Cutler RE: Inhibition of renal creatinine secretion by cimetidine in humans. *Renal Physiol* 5: 27, 1982

35. Rainer G, Rosenberg AR: Effect of co-trimoxazole on the glomerular filtration rate of healthy adults. *Chemotherapy* 27: 229, 1981

36. Vincent HH, Vos MC, Akcahuseyin E, Goessens WHF, van Duyl WA, Schalekamp MADH: Drug clearance by continuous haemodiafiltration (CAVHD). Analysis of sieving coefficients and mass transfer coefficients of diffusion. *Blood Purif* 11: 99, 1993

37. Keller F, Wilms H, Schultze G, Offerman G, Molzahn M: Effect of plasma protein binding, volume of distribution, and molecular weight on the fraction of drugs eliminated by hemodialysis. *Clin Nephrol* 19: 201, 1983

38. Maher JF: Pharmacokinetics in patients with renal failure. *Clin Nephrol* 21: 39, 1984

39. Dromgoole SH: The effect of hemodialysis on the binding capacity of albumin. *Clinica Chim Acta* 46: 269, 1973

40. Rutstein DD, Castelli WP, Nickerson, R: Heparin and human lipid metabolism. *Lancet* i(603): 1003, 1969

41. Suh B, Craig WA, England AC, Elliott RL: Effect of free fatty acids on protein binding of antimicrobial agents. *J Infect Dis* 143: 609, 1981

42. Golper TA, Saad AM: Gentamicin and phenytoin sieving through hollow-fiber polysulfone hemofilters. *Kidney Int* 30: 937, 1986

43. Fabris A, La Greca G, Chiaramonte S et al.: Total solute extraction versus clearance in the evaluation of standard and short hemodialysis. *Trans Am Soc Artif Intern Organs* 34: 627, 1988

44. Sprenger KGB, Stephan H, Kratz W, Huber K, Franz HE: Optimizing of hemodiafiltration with modern membranes? *Contrib Nephrol* 46: 43, 1985
45. De Bock V, Verbeelen D, Maes V, Sennesael J: Pharmacokinetics of vancomycin in patients undergoing hemodialysis and hemofiltration. *Nephrol Dial Transplant* 4: 635, 1989
46. Matzke GR, O'Connell MB, Collins AJ, Keshaviah PR: Disposition of vancomycin during hemofiltration. *Clin Pharmacol Ther* 40: 425, 1986
47. Marbury TC, Lee CS, Perchalski RJ, Wilder BJ: Hemodialysis clearance of ethosuximide in patients with chronic renal disease. *Am J Hosp Pharm* 38: 1757, 1981
48. Lee CS, Marbury TC, Benet LZ: Clearance calculations in hemodialysis: application to blood, plasma, and dialysate measurements for ethambutol. *J Pharmacokinet Biopharm* 8: 69, 1980
49. Levy G: Pharmacokinetics in renal disease. *Am J Med* 62: 461, 1977
50. Gibson TP: Problems in designing hemodialysis drug studies. *Pharmacotherapy* 5: 23, 1985
51. Brunner H, Mann H, Stiller S, Sieberth HG: Permeability for middle and higher molecular weight substances. *Contrib Nephrol* 46: 33, 1985
52. Donahue PR, Ahmad S: Dialyzer permeability alteration by reuse. (Abstract) *J Am Soc Nephrol* 3: 363, 1992
53. Graeber CW, Halley SE, Lapkin RA, Kaplan AA: Protein losses with reused dialyzers. (Abstract) *J Am Soc Nephrol* 4: 349, 1993
54. Lanese DM, Alfrey PS, Molitoris BA: Markedly increased clearance of vancomycin during hemodialysis using polysulfone dialyzers. *Kidney Int* 35: 1409, 1989
55. Bastani R, Spyker DA, Minocha A, Cummings R, Westervelt FB Jr: *In vivo* comparison of three different hemodialysis membranes for vancomycin clearance: cuprophan, cellulose acetate, and polyacrylonitrile. *Dial Transpl* 17: 527, 1988
56. Barth RH, DeVincenzo N, Zara AC, Berlyne GM: Vancomycin pharmacokinetics in high-flux hemodialysis. (Abstract) *J Am Soc Nephrol* 1: 348, 1990
57. Agarwal R, Toto RD: Gentamicin clearance during hemodialysis: a comparison of high-efficiency cuprammonium rayon and conventional cellulose ester hemodialyzers. *Am J Kidney Dis* 22: 296, 1993
58. Jindal K, McDougall J, Goldstein M: High flux dialyzers: impact of ultrafiltration and surface area on clearance of small and large molecular weight substances. (Abstract) *Nat Kidney Found* p A10, 1987
59. Von Albertini B, Miller JH, Gardner PW, Shinaberger JH: Performance characteristics of high flux haemodiafiltration. *Proc Eur Dial Transplant Assoc* 21: 447, 1984
60. Surian M, Malberti F, Corradi B et al.: Adequacy of haemodiafiltration. *Nephrol Dial Transplant* 4: 32, 1989
61. Rumpf KW, Rieger J, Doht B, Ansorg R, Scheler F: Drug elimination by hemofiltration. *J Dialysis* 1: 677, 1977
62. Ernest D, Cutler DJ: Gentamicin clearance during continuous arteriovenous hemodiafiltration. *Crit Care Med* 20: 586, 1992
63. Rumpf KW, Rieger J, Ansorg R et al.: Binding of antibiotics by dialysis membranes and its clinical relevance. *Proc Eur Dial Transpl Assoc* 14: 607, 1978
64. Kraft D, Lode H: Elimination of ampicillin and gentamicin by hemofiltration. *Klin Wochenschr* 57: 195, 1979
65. Kronfol NO, Lau AH, Barakat MM: Aminoglycoside binding to polyacrylonitrile hemofilter membranes during continuous hemofiltration. *Trans Am Soc Artif Intern Organs* 33: 300, 1987
66. Kronfol N, Lau AH, Colon-Rivera J, Libertin CL: Effect of CAVH membrane types on drug sieving coefficients and clearances. *Trans Am Soc Artif Intern Organs* 32: 85, 1986
67. Lau AH, Kronfol NO, Jaber N, Libertin CL: Determinants of drug removal by continuous arteriovenous hemofiltration. (Abstract) *Drug Intell Clin Pharm* 20: 467, 1986
68. Kronfol N, Lau A, Jaber N, Libertin CL: Effect of membrane properties on drug clearances by CAVH. (Abstract) *Nat Kidney Found* A10, 1986
69. Henderson LW: Hemodialysis: rationale and physical principles. in *The Kidney*, 1st Edition, edited by Brenner BM, Rector FC, Philadelphia, WB Sanders Company, 1976, p 1643
70. Husted FC, Nolph KD, Vitale FC, Maher JF: Detrimental effects of ultrafiltration on diffusion in coils. *J Lab Clin Med* 87: 435, 1976
71. Nolph KD, New DL: Effects of ultrafiltration on solute clearances in hollow fiber artificial kidneys. *J Lab Clin Med* 88: 593, 1976
72. Nolph KD, Hopkins C, Van Stone J: Effects of ultrafiltration on solute clearances in parallel plate dialyzers. *Clin Nephrol* 8: 453, 1977
73. Henderson LW, Silverstein ME, Ford CA, Lysaght MJ: Clinical response to maintenance hemodiafiltration. *Kidney Int* (Suppl 2): S58, 1975
74. Hamilton R, Ford C, Colton C, Cross R, Steinmuller S, Henderson L: Blood cleansing by diafiltration in uremic dog and man. *Trans Am Soc Artif Intern Organs* 17: 259, 1971
75. Henderson LW, Ford C, Colton CK, Bluemle LW, Bixler HJ: Uremic blood cleansing by diafiltration using hollow-fiber ultrafilter. *Trans Am Soc Artif Intern Organs* 16: 107, 1970
76. Jaffrin MY, Ding L, Laurent JM: Simultaneous convective and diffusive mass transfers in a hemodialyzer. *J Biomech Eng* 112: 212, 1990
77. Vincent HH, van Ittersum FJ, Akcahuseyin E, Vos MC, Van Duyl WA, Schalekamp MA: Solute transport in continuous arteriovenous hemodiafiltration: a new mathematical model applied to clinical data. *Blood Purif* 8: 149, 1990
78. Torras J, Cao C, Rivas MC, Cano M, Fernandez E, Montoliu J: Pharmacokinetics of vancomycin in patients undergoing hemodialysis with polyacrylonitrile. *Clin Nephrol* 36: 35, 1991
79. Colton CK, Henderson LW, Ford CA, Lysaght MJ: Kinetics of hemodiafiltration. I. *In vitro* transport characteristics of a hollow fiber blood ultrafilter. *J Lab Clin Med* 85: 355, 1975
80. Golper TA, Wedel SK, Kaplan AA, Saad AM, Donta ST, Paganini EP: Drug removal during CAVH: theory and clinical observations. *Intern J Artif Organs* 8: 307, 1985
81. Ronco C, Brendolan A, Borin D et al.: Permeability characteristics of polysulfonic membranes in CAVH. in *Continuous Arteriovenous Hemofiltration (CAVH)*, edited by Sieberth HG, Mann H, Basel, Karger, 1985, p 59
82. Frigon RP, Leypoldt JK, Alford MF, Uyeji S, Henderson LW: Hemofilter solute sieving is not governed by

dynamically polarized protein. *Trans Am Soc Artif Intern Organs* 30: 486, 1984

83. Lysaght MJ: An experimental model for the ultrafiltration of sodium ion from blood or plasma. *Blood Purif* 1: 25, 1983

84. Leypoldt JK, Frigon RP, Henderson LW: Macromolecular charge affects hemofilter solute sieving. *Trans Am Soc Artif Intern Organs* 32: 384, 1986

85. Kaplan AA, Longnecker RE, Folkert VW: Continuous arteriovenous hemofiltration – a report of 6 months' experience. *Ann Intern Med* 100: 358, 1984

86. Paganini EP, Flague J, Whitman G, Nakamoto S: Amino acid balance in patients with oliguric renal failure undergoing slow continuous ultrafiltration (SCUF). *Trans Am Soc Artif Intern Organs* 28: 615, 1982

87. Golper TA, Vincent HH, Kroh U: Drug use in critically ill patients with acute renal failure. in *Acute Renal Failure in the Critically Ill*, edited by Bellomo R, Ronco C, Heidelberg, Springer-Verlag, 1995. In press

88. Kroh U, Hofmann W, Dehne M, el Abed K, Lennartz H: Dosisanpassung von pharmaka während kontinuierlicher hämofiltration. *Anaesthesist* 38: 225, 1989

89. Leypoldt JK, Frigon RP, Henderson LW: Dextran sieving coefficients of hemofilter membranes. *Trans Am Soc Artif Intern Organs* 29: 678, 1983

90. Dodd NJ, O'Donovan RM, Bennett-Jones DN et al.: Arteriovenous hemofiltration: a recent advance in the management of renal failure. *Br Med J* 287: 1008, 1983

91. Bennett WM, Aronoff GR, Golper TA, Morrison G, Brater DC, Singer I: *Drug Prescribing in Renal Failure: Dosing Guidelines for Adults*, 3rd Edition. Philadelphia, American College of Physicians, 1994

92. Keller E, Reetze P, Schollmeyer P: Drug therapy in patients undergoing continuous ambulatory peritoneal dialysis. *Clin Pharmacokinet* 18: 104, 1990

93. Golper TA: Drugs and peritoneal dialysis. *Dial Transplant* 8: 41, 1979

94. Lasrich M, Maher JM, Hirszel P, Maher JF: Correlation of peritoneal transport rates with molecular weight: a method for predicting clearances. *ASAIO J* 2: 107, 1979

95. Nolph KD, Popovich RP, Ghods AS, Twardowski Z: Determinants of low clearances of small solutes during peritoneal dialysis. *Kidney Int* 13: 117, 1978

96. Robson M, Oreopoulos DG, Izatt S, Olivie R, Rapaport R, deVeber GA: Influence of exchange volume and dialysate flow rate on solute clearance in peritoneal dialysis. *Kidney Int* 14: 486, 1978

97. Zelman A, Gisser D, Whitlam PJ, Parsons RH, Shuyler R: Augmentation of peritoneal dialysis efficiency with programmed hyper/hypoosmotic dialysates. *Trans Am Soc Artif Intern Organs* 23: 203, 1977

98. Rubin J, Adair C, Barnes T, Bower J: Dialysate flow rate and peritoneal clearance. *Am J Kidney Dis* 4: 260, 1984

99. Gross M, McDonald HP: Effect of dialysate temperature and flow rate on peritoneal clearance. *JAMA* 202: 363, 1967

100. Indraprasit S, Namwongprom A, Sooksriwongse C, Buri PS: Effect of dialysate temperature on peritoneal clearances. *Nephron* 34: 45, 1983

101. Manuel MA, Paton TW, Cornish WR: Drugs and peritoneal dialysis. *Perit Dial Bull* 3: 117, 1983

102. Janknegt R, Koks CH: Pharmacologic aspects during continuous ambulatory peritoneal dialysis: a literature review. *Pharmaceutisch Weekblad* 6: 229, 1984

103. Paton TW, Cornish WR, Manuel MA, Hardy BG: Drug therapy in patients undergoing peritoneal dialysis: clinical pharmacokinetic considerations. *Clin Pharmacokinet* 10: 404, 1985

104. Smithivas T, Hyams PJ, Matalon R, Simberkoff MS, Rahal JJ Jr: The use of gentamicin in peritoneal dialysis. I. Pharmacologic results. *J Infect Dis* 124 (Suppl): S77, 1971

105. Singlas E, Colin JN, Rottenbourg J et al.: Pharmacokinetics of sulfamethoxazole-trimethoprim combination during chronic peritoneal dialysis: effect of peritonitis. *Eur J Clin Pharmacol* 21: 409, 1982

106. Bunke CM, Aronoff GR, Brier ME, Sloan RS, Luft FC: Cefazolin and cephalexin kinetics in continuous ambulatory peritoneal dialysis. *Clin Pharmacol Ther* 33: 66, 1983

107. Roscoe JM: Practices of insulin administration in CAPD. *Perit Dial Bull* 2 (Suppl 2): S27, 1982

108. Furman KI, Gomperts ED, Hockley J: Activity of intraperitoneal heparin during peritoneal dialysis. *Clin Nephrol* 9: 15, 1978

109. Golper TA, Bennett WM, Jones SR: Peritonitis associated with chronic peritoneal dialysis: a diagnostic and therapeutic approach. *Dial Transplant* 7: 282, 1978

110. Millikin SP, Matzke GR, Keane WF: Antimicrobial treatment of peritonitis associated with continuous ambulator peritoneal dialysis. *Perit Dial Int* 11: 252, 1991

111. Sewell DL, Golper TA, Brown SD, Nelson E, Knower M, Kimbrough RC: Stability of single and combination antimicrobial agents in various peritoneal dialysates in the presence of insulin and heparin. *Am J Kidney Dis* 3: 209, 1983

112. Blaser J, Rüttimann S, Bhend H, Luthy R: Increase of amikacin half-life during therapy in patients with renal insufficiency. *Antimicrob Agents Chemother* 23: 888, 1983

113. Lanao JM, Dominguez-Gil A, Tabernero JM, Sanchez Tomero JA: Pharmacokinetics of amikacin (BB-K8) in patients undergoing hemodialysis. *Int J Clin Pharmacol Biopharm* 17: 357, 1979

114. Smeltzer BD, Schwartzman MS, Bertino JS: Amikacin pharmacokinetics during continuous ambulatory peritoneal dialysis. *Antimicrob Agents Chemother* 32: 236, 1988

115. Goetz DR, Pancorbo S, Hoag S, Bloom P: Prediction of serum gentamicin concentrations in patients undergoing hemodialysis. *Am J Hosp Pharm* 37: 1077, 1980

116. Gyselynck AM, Forrey A, Cutler R: Pharmacokinetics of gentamicin: distribution and plasma and renal clearance. *J Infect Dis* 124 (Suppl): S70, 1971

117. Zarowitz BJ, Anandan JV, Dumler F et al.: Continuous arteriovenous hemofiltration of aminoglycoside antibiotics in critically ill patients. *J Clin Pharmacol* 26: 686, 1986

118. Healy JK, Drum PJ, Elliott AJ: Kanamycin dosage in renal failure. *Aust N Z J Med* 3: 474, 1973

119. Campoli-Richards DM, Chaplin S, Sayce RH, Goa KL: Netilmicin: a review of its antibacterial activity, pharmacokinetic properties and therapeutic use. *Drugs* 38: 703, 1989

120. Herrero A, Rius Alarcó F, García Díez JM, Mahiques E, Domingo JV: Pharmacokinetics of netilmicin in renal insufficiency and hemodialysis. *Int J Clin Pharmacol Ther Toxicol* 26: 84, 1988

121. Pechére JC, Dugal R, Pechére MM: Pharmacokinetics of netilmicin in renal insufficiency and haemodialysis. *Clin Pharmacokinet* 3: 395, 1978

122. Seyffart G (ed): *Drug Dosage in Renal Insufficiency.* Dordrecht, The Netherlands, Kluwer Academic Publishers, 1991

123. Brogden RN, Pinder RM, Sawyer PR, Speight TM, Avery GS: Tobramycin: a review of its antibacterial and pharmacokinetic properties and therapeutic use. *Drugs* 12: 166, 1976

124. Pechere JC, Dugal R: Pharmacokinetics of intravenously administered tobramycin in normal volunteers and in renal-impaired and hemodialyzed patients. *J Infect Dis* 134 (Suppl): S118, 1976

125. Wise R: The pharmacokinetics of the oral cephalosporins – a review. *J Antimicrob Chemother* 26 (Suppl E): 13, 1990

126. Gartenberg G, Meyers BR, Hirschman SZ, Srulevitch E: Pharmacokinetics of cefaclor in patients with stable renal impairment, and patients undergoing haemodialysis. *J Antimicrob Chemother* 5: 465, 1979

127. Leroy A, Humbert G, Godin M: Pharmacokinetics of cefadroxil in patients with impaired renal function. *J Antimicrob Chemother* 10 (Suppl B): 39, 1982

128. Bliss M, Mayersohn M, Arnold T, Logan J, Michael UF, Jones W: Disposition kinetics of cefamandole during continuous ambulatory peritoneal dialysis. *Antimicrob Agents Chemother* 29: 649, 1986

129. Brogard JM, Kopferschmitt J, Spach MO, Grudet O, Lavillaureix J: Cefamandole pharmacokinetics and dosage adjustments in relation to renal function. *J Clin Pharmacol* 19: 366, 1979

130. Bergan T, Brodwall EK, Ørjavik Ø: Pharmacokinetics of cefazolin in patients with normal and impaired renal function. *J Antimicrob Chemother* 3: 453, 1977

131. Guay DRP, Meatherall RC, Harding GK, Brown GR: Pharmacokinetics of cefixime (CL 284,635; FK027) in healthy subjects and patients with renal insufficiency. *Antimicrob Agents Chemother* 30: 458, 1986

132. Campoli-Richards DM, Todd PA: Cefmenoxime. A review of its antibacterial activity pharmacokinetic properties and therapeutic use. *Drugs* 34: 188, 1987

133. Evers J, Borner K, Koeppe P: Elimination of cefmenoxime during continuous haemofiltration. *Eur J Clin Pharmacol* 44 (Suppl 1): S31, 1993

134. Konishi K: Pharmacokinetics of cefmenoxime in patients with impaired renal function and in those undergoing hemodialysis. *Antimicrob Agents Chemother* 30: 901, 1986

135. Halstenson CE, Guay DR, Opsahl JA et al.: Disposition of cefmetazole in healthy volunteers and patients with impaired renal function. *Antimicrob Agents Chemother* 34: 519, 1990

136. Schentag JJ: Cefmetazole sodium: pharmacology, pharmacokinetics, and clinical trials. *Pharmacotherapy* 11: 2, 1991

137. Blair AD, Maxwell BM, Forland SC, Jacob L, Cutler RE: Cefonicid kinetics in subjects with normal and impaired renal function. *Clin Pharmacol Ther* 35: 798, 1984

138. Saltiel E, Brogden RN: Cefonicid. A review of its antibacterial activity, pharmacological properties and therapeutic use. *Drugs* 32: 222, 1986

139. Greenfield RA, Gerber AU, Craig WA: Pharmacokinetics of cefoperazone in patients with normal and impaired hepatic and renal function. *Rev Infect Dis* 5 (Suppl): S127, 1983

140. Hodler JE, Galeazzi RL, Frey B, Rudhardt M, Seiler AJ: Pharmacokinetics of cefoperazone in patients undergoing chronic ambulatory peritoneal dialysis: clinical and pathophysiological implications. *Eur J Clin Pharmacol* 26: 609, 1984

141. Campoli-Richards DM, Lackner TE, Monk JP: Ceforanide. A review of its antibacterial activity, pharmacokinetic properties and clinical efficacy. *Drugs* 34: 411, 1987

142. Hess JR, Berman SJ, Boughton WH et al.: Pharmacokinetics of ceforanide in patients with end stage renal disease on hemodialysis. *Antimicrob Agents Chemother* 17: 251, 1980

143. Matzke GR, Abraham PA, Halstenson CE, Keane WF: Cefotaxime and desacetyl cefotaxime kinetics in renal impairment. *Clin Pharmacol Ther* 38: 31, 1985

144. Todd PA, Brogden RN: Cefotaxime. An update of its pharmacology and therapeutic use. *Drugs* 40: 608, 1990

145. Ohkawa M, Hirano S, Tokunaga S: Pharmacokinetics of cefotetan in normal subjects and patients with impaired renal function. *Antimicrob Agents Chemother* 23: 31, 1983

146. Ward A, Richards DM: Cefotetan. A review of its antibacterial activity, pharmacokinetic properties and therapeutic use. *Drugs* 30: 382, 1985

147. Greaves WL, Kreeft JH, Ogilvie RI, Richards GK: Cefoxitin disposition during peritoneal dialysis. *Antimicrob Agents Chemother* 19: 253, 1981

148. Humbert G, Fillastre JP, Leroy A, Godin M, Van Winzum C: Pharmacokinetics of cefoxitin in normal subjects and in patients with renal insufficiency. *Rev Infect Dis* 1: 118, 1979

149. Nikolaidis P, Tourkantonis A: Effect of hemodialysis on ceftazidime pharmacokinetics. *Clin Nephrol* 24: 142, 1985

150. Richards DM, Brogden RN: Ceftazidime. A review of its antibacterial activity, pharmacokinetic properties and therapeutic use. *Drugs* 29: 105, 1985

151. Tourkantonis A, Nikolaidis P: Pharmacokinetics of ceftazidime in patients undergoing peritoneal dialysis. *J Antimicrob Chemother* 12 (Suppl A): 263, 1983

152. Welage LS, Schultz RW, Schentag JJ: Pharmacokinetics of ceftazidime in patients with renal insufficiency. *Antimicrob Agents Chemother* 25: 201, 1984

153. Burgess ED, Blair AD: Pharmacokinetics of ceftizoxime in patients undergoing continuous ambulatory peritoneal dialysis. *Antimicrob Agents Chemother* 24: 237, 1983

154. Gross ML, Somani P, Ribner BS, Roeader R, Freimer EH, Higgins JT Jr: Ceftizoxime elimination kinetics in continuous ambulatory peritoneal dialysis. *Clin Pharmacol Ther* 34: 673, 1983

155. Kowalsky SF, Echols RM, Venezia AR, Andrews EA: Pharmacokinetics of ceftizoxime in subjects with various degrees of renal function. *Antimicrob Agents Chemother* 24: 151, 1983

156. Richards DM, Heel RC: Ceftizoxime. A review of its antibacterial activity, pharmacokinetic properties and therapeutic use. *Drugs* 29: 281, 1985

157. Patel IH, Sugihara JG, Weinfeld RE, Wong EG, Siemsen AW, Berman SJ: Ceftriaxone pharmacokinetics in patients with various degrees of renal impairment. *Antimicrob Agents Chemother* 25: 438, 1984

158. Ti TY, Fortin L, Kreeft JH, East DS, Ogilvie RI, Somerville PJ: Kinetic disposition of intravenous ceftriaxone in normal subjects and patients with renal failure on hemodialysis or peritoneal dialysis. *Antimicrob Agent Chemother* 25: 83, 1984

159. Yuk JH, Nightingale CH, Quintiliani R: Clinical pharmacokinetics of ceftriaxone. *Clin Pharmacokinet* 17: 223, 1989

160. Höffler D, Koeppe P, Schleith A: Pharmacokinetics of cefuroxime-axetil in patients undergoing haemodialysis therapy. *Acta Therapeutica* 17: 107, 1991

161. Konishi K, Suzuki H, Hayashi M, Saruta T: Pharmacokinetics of cefuroxime axetil in patients with normal and impaired renal function. *J Antimicrob Chemother* 31: 413, 1993

162. Weiss LG, Cars O, Danielson BG, Grahnen A, Wikstrom B: Pharmacokinetics of intravenous cefuroxime during intermittent and continuous arteriovenous hemofiltration. *Clin Nephrol* 30: 282, 1988

163. Bailey RR, Gower PE, Dash CH: The effects of impairment of renal function and haemodialysis on serum and urine levels of cephalexin. *Postgrad Med J* 46 (Suppl): 60, 1970

164. Venuto RC, Plaut M: Cephalothin handling in patients undergoing hemodialysis. *Antimicrob Agents Chemother* 10: 50, 1970

165. McCloskey RV, Terry EE, McCracken AW, Sweeney MJ, Forland MF: Effect of hemodialysis and renal failure on serum and urine concentrations of cephapirin sodium. *Antimicrob Agents Chemother* 1: 90, 1972

166. Solomon AE, Briggs JD: The administration of cephradine to patients in renal failure. *Br J Clin Pharmacol* 2: 443, 1975

167. Bolton WK, Scheld WM, Spyker DA, Overby TL, Sande MA: Pharmacokinetics of moxalactam in subjects with various degrees of renal dysfunction. *Antimicrob Agents Chemother* 18: 933, 1980

168. Carmine AA, Brogden RN, Heel RC, Romankiewicz JA, Speight TM, Avery GS: Moxalactam. A review of its antibacterial activity, pharmacokinetic properties and therapeutic use. *drugs* 26: 279, 1983

169. Srinivasan S, Neu HC: Pharmacokinetics of moxalactam in patients with renal failure and during hemodialysis. *Antimicrob Agents Chemother* 20: 398, 1981

170. Cooper MA, Nye K, Andrews JM, Wise R: The pharmacokinetics and inflammatory fluid penetration of orally administered azithromycin. *J Antimicrob Chemother* 26: 533, 1990

171. Foulds G, Shephard RM, Johnson RB: The pharmacokinetics of azithromycin in human serum and tissues. *J Antimicrob Chemother* 25 (Suppl A): 73, 1990

172. Peters DH, Clissold SP: Clarithromycin: a review of its antimicrobial activity, pharmacokinetic properties and therapeutic potential. *Drugs* 44: 117, 1992

173. Disse B, Gundert-Remy U, Weber E, Andrassy K, Sietzen W, Lang A: Pharmacokinetics of erythromycin in patients with different degrees of renal impairment. *Int J Clin Pharmacol Ther Toxicol* 24: 460, 1986

174. Kanfer A, Stamatakis G, Torlotin C, Fredj G, Kenouch S, Mery JP: Changes in erythromycin pharmacokinetic induced by renal failure. *Clin Nephrol* 27: 247, 1987

175. Francke EL, Appel GB, Neu HC: Kinetics of intravenous amoxicillin in patients on long-term dialysis. *Clin Pharmacol Ther* 26: 3, 1979

176. Humbert G, Spyker DA, Fillastre JP, Leroy A: Pharmacokinetics of amoxicillin: dosage nomogram for patients with impaired renal function. *Antimicrob Agents Chemother* 15: 28, 1979

177. Todd PA, Benfield P: Amoxicillin/clavulanic acid: an update of its antibacterial activity, pharmacokinetic properties and therapeutic use. *Drugs* 39: 264, 1990

178. Blum RA, Kohli RK, Harrison NJ, Schentag JJ: Pharmacokinetics of ampicillin (2.0 grams) and sulbactam (1.0 gram) coadministered to subjects with normal and abnormal renal function and with end-stage renal disease on hemodialysis. *Antimicrob Agents Chemother* 33: 1470, 1989

179. Leroy A, Humbert G, Godin M, Fillastre JP: Pharmacokinetics of azlocillin in subjects with normal and impaired renal function. *Antimicrob Agents Chemother* 17: 344, 1980

180. Whelton A, Stout RL, Delgado FA: Azlocillin kinetics during extracorporeal haemodialysis and peritoneal dialysis. *J Antimicrob Chemother* 11 (Suppl B): 89, 1983

181. Aronoff GR, Sloan RS, Luft FC, Nelson RL, Maxwell DR, Kleit SA: Mezlocillin pharmacokinetics in renal impairment. *Clin Pharmacol Ther* 28: 523, 1980

182. Kampf D, Schurig R, Weihermüller K, Forester D: Effects of impaired renal function, hemodialysis, and peritoneal dialysis on the pharmacokinetics of mezlocillin. *Antimicrob Agents Chemother* 18: 81, 1980

183. Baron DN, Hamilton-Miller JM, Brumfitt W: Sodium content of injectable β-Lactam antibiotics. *Lancet* i(8386): 1113, 1984

184. Holmes B, Richards DM, Brogden RN, Heel RC: Piperacillin: a review of its antibacterial activity, pharmacokinetic properties and therapeutic use. *Drugs* 28: 375, 1984

185. De Schepper PJ, Tjandramage RB, Mullie A et al.: Comparative pharmacokinetics of piperacillin in normals and in patients with renal failure. *J Antimicrob Chemother* 9 (Suppl B): 1982

186. Welling PG, Craig WA, Bundtzen RW, Kwok FW, Gerber AU, Madsen PO: Pharmacokinetics of piperacillin in subjects with various degrees of renal function. *Antimicrob Agents Chemother* 23: 881, 1983

187. Parry MF, Neu HC: Pharmacokinetics of ticarcillin in patients with abnormal renal function. *J Infect Dis* 133: 46, 1976

188. Vance-Bryan K, Guay DR, Rotschafer JC: Clinical pharmacokinetics of ciprofloxacin. *Clin Pharmacokinet* 19: 434, 1990

189. Davies SP, Azadian BS, Kox WJ, Brown EA: Pharmacokinetics of ciprofloxacin and vancomycin in patients with acute renal failure treated by continuous haemodialysis. *Nephrol Dial Transplant* 7: 848, 1992

190. Kowalsky SF, Echols M, Schwartz MT, Baile GR, McCormick E: Pharmacokinetics of ciprofloxacin in subjects

with varying degrees of renal function and undergoing hemodialysis or CAPD. *Clin Nephrol* 39: 53, 1993

191. Neuman M: Clinical pharmacokinetics of the newer antibacterial 4-quinolones. *Clin Pharmacokinet* 14: 96, 1988

192. Henwood JM, Monk JP: Enoxacin. A review of its antibacterial activity, pharmacokinetic properties and therapeutic use. *Drugs* 36: 32, 1988

193. Nix DE, Schultz RW, Frost RW et al.: The effect of renal impairment and haemodialysis on single dose pharmacokinetics of oral enoxacin. *J Antimicrob Chemother* 21 (Suppl B): 87, 1988

194. Weidekamm E: Pharmacokinetics of fleroxacin in renal impairment. *Am J Med* 94: 70S, 1993

195. Holmes B, Brogden RN, Richards DM: Norfloxacin. A review of its antibacterial activity, pharmacokinetic properties and therapeutic use. *Drugs* 30: 482, 1985

196. Lameire N, Rosenkranz B, Malerczyk V, Lehr KH, Veys N, Ringoir S: Ofloxacin pharmacokinetics in chronic renal failure and dialysis. *Clin Pharmacokinet* 21: 357, 1991

197. Saivin S, Houin G: Clinical pharmacokinetics of doxycycline and minocycline. *Clin Pharmacokinet* 15: 355, 1988

198. Siegel D: Tetracyclines: new look at old antibiotic. I. Clinical pharmacology, mechanism of action, and untoward effects. *N Y State J Med* 78: 950, 1978

199. Fillastre JP, Leroy A, Baudoin C et al.: Pharmacokinetics of aztreonam in patients with chronic renal failure. *Clin Pharmacokinet* 10: 91, 1985

200. Gerig JS, Bolton ND, Swabb EA, Scheid WM, Bolton WK: Effect of hemodialysis and peritoneal dialysis on aztreonam pharmacokinetics. *Kidney Int* 26: 308, 1984

201. Ambrose PJ: Clinical pharmacokinetics of chloramphenicol and chloramphenicol succinate. *Clin Pharmacokinet* 9: 222, 1984

202. Buckley MM, Brogden RN, Barradell LB, Goa KL: Imipenem/Cilastatin. A reappraisal of its antibacterial activity, pharmacokinetic properties and therapeutic efficacy. *Drugs* 44: 408, 1992

203. Gibson TP, Devetriades JL, Bland JA: Imipenem/cilastatin: pharmacokinetic profile in renal insufficiency. *Am J Med* 78 (Suppl 6A): 54, 1985

204. Konishi K, Suzuki H, Saruta T et al.: Removal of imipenem and cilastatin by hemodialysis in patients with end stage renal failure. *Antimicrob Agents Chemother* 35: 1616, 1991

205. Vos MC, Vincent HH, Yzerman EP: Clearance of imipenem/cilastatin in acute renal failure patients treated by continuous hemodiafiltration (CAVHD). *Intensive Care Med* 18: 282, 1992

206. Roberts AP, Eastwood JB, Gower PE, Fenton C, Curtis J: Serum and plasma concentrations of clindamycin following a single intramuscular injection of clindamycin phosphate in maintenance haemodialysis patients and normal subjects. *Eur J Clin Pharmacol* 14: 435, 1978

207. Guay DR, Meatherall RC, Baxter H, Jacyk WR, Penner B: Pharmacokinetics of metronidazole in patients undergoing continuous ambulatory peritoneal dialysis. *Antimicrob Agents Chemother* 25: 306, 1984

208. Kreeft JH, Ogilvie RI, Dufresne LR: Metronidazole kinetics in dialysis patients. *Surgery* 93: 149, 1983

209. Lau AH, Lam NP, Piscitelli SC, Wilkes L, Danzinger LH: Clinical pharmacokinetics of metronidazole and other nitroimidazole anti-infectives. *Clin Pharmacokinet* 23: 328, 1992

210. Shermantine M, Gambertoglio J, Amend W, Vincenti F, Oie S: Pharmacokinetics of sulfisoxazole in renal transplant patients. *Antimicrob Agents Chemother* 28: 535, 1985

211. Bonati M, Traina GL, Villa G et al.: Teicoplanin pharmacokinetics in patients with chronic renal failure. *Clin Pharmacokinet* 12: 292, 1987

212. Campoli-Richards DM, Brogden RN, Faulds D: Teicoplanin. A review of its antibacterial activity, pharmacokinetic properties and therapeutic potential. *Drugs* 40: 449, 1990

213. Paap CM, Nahata MC: Clinical use of trimethoprim/sulfamethoxazole during renal dysfunction. *DICP, Ann Pharmacother* 23: 646, 1989

214. Moellering RC, Krogstad DJ, Greenblatt DJ: Vancomycin therapy in patients with impaired renal function: a nomogram for dosage. *Ann Intern Med* 94: 343, 1981

215. Nielsen HE, Sorensen I, Hansen HE: Peritoneal transport of vancomycin during peritoneal dialysis. *Nephron* 24: 274, 1979

216. Daneshmend TK, Warnock DW: Clinical pharmacokinetics of systemic antifungal drugs. *Clin Pharmacokinet* 8: 17, 1983

217. Lyman CA, Walsh TJ: Systemically administered antifungal agents. A review of their clinical pharmacology and therapeutic applications. *Drugs* 44: 9, 1992

218. Craven PC, Ludden TM, Drutz DJ, Rogers W, Haegele KA, Skrdlant HB: Excretion pathways of amphotericin B. *J Infect Dis* 140: 329, 1979

219. Morgan DJ, Ching MS, Raymond K et al.: Elimination of amphotericin B in impaired renal function. *Clin Pharmacol Ther* 34: 248, 1983

220. Janknegt R, de Marie S, Bakker-Woudenberg IA, Crommelin DJ: Liposomal and lipid formulations amphotericin B. *Clin Pharmacokinet* 23: 279, 1992

221. Cleary JD, Taylor JW, Chapman SW: Imidazoles and triazoles in antifungal therapy. *Ann Pharmacother* 26: 502, 1992

222. Bailey EM, Krakovsky DJ, Rybak MJ: The triazole antifungal agents: a review of itraconazole and fluconazole. *Pharmacotherapy* 10: 146, 1990

223. Toon S, Ross CE, Gokal R, Rowand M: An assessment of the effects of impaired renal function and haemodialysis on the pharmacokinetics of fluconazole. *Br J Clin Pharmacol* 29: 221, 1990

224. Oono S, Tabei K, Tetsuka T, Asano Y: The pharmacokinetics of fluconazole during haemodialysis in uraemic patients. *Eur J Clin Pharmacol* 42: 667, 1992

225. Debruyne D, Ryckelynck JP: Clinical pharmacokinetics of fluconazole. *Clin Pharmacokinet* 24: 10, 1993

226. Bennet JE: Flucytosine. *Ann Intern Med* 86: 319, 1977

227. Cutler RE, Blair AD, Kelly MR: Flucytosine kinetics in subjects with normal and impaired renal function. *Clin Pharmacol Ther* 24: 333, 1978

228. Eisenberg ES: Intraperitoneal flucytosine in the management of fungal peritonitis in patients on continuous ambulatory peritoneal dialysis. *Am J Kidney Dis* 11: 465, 1988

229. Boelaert J, Schurgers M, Matthys E et al.: Itraconazole pharmacokinetics in patients with renal dysfunction. *Antimicrob Agents Chemother* 32: 1595, 1988

230. Grant SM, Clissold SP: Itraconazole: a review of its pharmacodynamic and pharmacokinetic properties, and therapeutic use in superficial and systemic mycoses. *Drugs* 37: 310, 1989

231. Daneshmend TK, Warnock DW: Clinical pharmacokinetics of ketoconazole. *Clin Pharmacokin* 14: 13, 1988

232. Lewi PJ, Boelaert J, Daneels R et al.: Pharmacokinetic profile of intravenous miconazole in man. *Eur J Clin Pharmacol* 10: 49, 1976

233. White NJ: Clinical pharmacokinetics of antimalarial drugs. *Clin Pharmacokinet* 10: 187, 1985

234. White NJ: Antimalarial pharmacokinetics and treatment regimens. *Br J Clin Pharmacol* 34: 1, 1992

235. Edwards G, Breckenridge AM: Clinical pharmacokinetics of anthelmintic drugs. *Clin Pharmacokinet* 15: 67, 1988

236. Keystone JS, Murdoch JK: Mebendazole. *Ann Intern Med* 91: 582, 1979

237. Palmer KJ, Holliday SM, Brogden RN: Mefloquine. A review of its antimalarial activity, pharmacokinetic properties and therapeutic efficacy. *Drugs* 45: 430, 1993

238. Goa KL, Compoli-Richards DM: Pentamidine Isethionate. A review of its antiprotozoal activity, pharmacokinetic properties and therapeutic use in *Pneumocystis carinii* pneumonia. *Drugs* 33: 242, 1987

239. Conte JE Jr: Pharmacokinetics of intravenous pentamidine in patients with normal renal function or receiving hemodialysis. *J Infect Dis* 163: 169, 1991

240. King CH, Mahmoud AA: Drugs five years later: praziquantel. *Ann Intern Med* 110: 290, 1989

241. Lehmann CR, Garrett LE, Winn RE et al.: Capreomycin kinetics in renal impairment and clearance by hemodialysis. *Ann Rev Respir Dis* 138: 1312, 1988

242. Varughese A, Brater DC, Benet LZ, Lee CS: Ethambutol kinetics in patients with impaired renal function. *Am Rev Respir Dis* 134: 34, 1986

243. Weber WW, Hein DW: Clinical pharmacokinetics of isoniazid. *Clin Pharmacokinet* 4: 401, 1979

244. Lacroix C, Hermelin A, Guiberteau R et al.: Haemodialysis of pyrazinamide in uraemic patients. *Eur J Clin Pharmacol* 37: 309, 1989

245. Stamatikis G, Montes C, Trouvin JH et al.: Pyrazinamide and pyrazinoic acid pharmacokinetics inpatients with chronic renal failure. *Clin Nephrol* 30: 230, 1988

246. Acocella G: Clinical pharmacokinetics of rifampicin. *Clin Pharmacokinet* 3: 108, 1978

247. Burgess ED, Gill MJ: Intraperitoneal administration of acyclovir in patients receiving continuous ambulatory peritoneal dialysis. *J Clin Pharmacol* 30: 997, 1990

248. Laskin OL, Longstreth JA, Whelton A et al.: Acyclovir kinetics in end-stage renal disease. *Clin Pharmacol Ther* 31: 594: 1982

249. O'Brien JJ, Campoli-Richards DM: Acyclovir: an updated review of its antiviral activity, pharmacokinetic properties and therapeutic efficacy. *Drugs* 37: 233, 1989

250. Aoki FY, Sitar DS: Clinical pharmacokinetics of amantadine hydrochloride. *Clin Pharmacokinet* 14: 35, 1988

251. Horadam VW, Sharp JG, Smilack JD, McAnalley BH, Garriott JC, Stephens MK: Pharmacokinetics amantadine hydrochloride in subjects with normal and impaired renal function. *Ann Intern Med* 94: 454, 1981

252. Wu MJ, Ing TS, Soung LS, Daugirdas JT, Hano JE, Gandhi VC: Amantadine hydrochloride pharmacokinetics patients with impaired renal function. *Clin Nephrol* 17: 19, 1982

253. Morse GD, Shelton MJ, O'Donnell AM: Comparative pharmacokinetics of antiviral nucleoside analogues. *Clin Pharmacokinet* 24: 101, 1993

254. Faulds D, Brogden RN: Didanosine: a review of its antiviral activity, pharmacokinetic properties and therapeutic potential in human immunodeficiency virus infection. *Drugs* 44: 94, 1992

255. Chrisp P, Clissold SP: Foscarnet: a review of its antiviral activity, pharmacokinetic properties and therapeutic use in immunocompromised patients with cytomegalovirus retinitis. *Drugs* 41: 104, 1991

256. Faulds D, Heel RC: Ganciclovir: a review of its antiviral activity, pharmacokinetic properties and therapeutic efficacy in cytomegalovirus infections. *Drugs* 39: 597, 1990

257. Kramer TH, Gaar GG, Ray CG, Minnich L, Copeland JG, Connor JD: Hemodialysis clearance of intravenously administered ribavirin. *Antimicrob Agents Chemother* 34: 489, 1990

258. Aronoff GR, Szwed JJ, Nelson RL, Marcus RL, Kleit SA: Hypoxanthine-arabinoside pharmacokinetics after adenine arabinoside administration to a patient with renal failure. *Antimicrob Agents Chemother* 18: 212, 1980

259. Collins JM, Unadkat JD: Clinical pharmacokinetics of zidovudine. An overview of current data. *Clin Pharmacokinet* 17: 1, 1989

260. Gallicano KD, Tobe S, Saha J et al.: Pharmacokinetics of single and chronic dose zidovudine in two HIV positive patients undergoing continuous ambulatory peritoneal dialysis (CAPD). *J Acquir Immune Defic Syndr* 5: 242, 1992

261. Garraffo R, Cassuto-Viguier E, Barillon J, Changlet L, Lapalus P, Duplay H: Influence of hemodialysis on zidovudine (AZT) and its glucuronide (GAZT) pharmacokinetics: two case reports. *Int J Clin Pharmacol Ther Toxicol* 27: 535, 1989

262. Gleason JR, Brier ME: Zidovudine in renal failure. *Semin Dial* 3: 101, 1990

263. Chan GL, Matzke GR: Effects of renal insufficiency on the pharmacokinetics and pharmacodynamics of opioid analgesics. *Drug Intell Clin Pharm* 21: 773, 1987

264. Horton MW, Byerly WG: Opioid analgesics. *Semin Dial* 3: 187, 1990

265. Heel RC, Brogden RN, Speight TM, Avery GS: Butorphanol: a review of its pharmacological properties and therapeutic efficacy. *Drugs* 16: 473, 1978

266. Barnes JN, Williams AJ, Tomson MJ, Toseland PA, Goodwin PJ: Dihydrocodeine in renal failure: further evidence for an important role of the kidney in the handling of opioid drugs. *Br Med J* 290(6470)L 740, 1985

267. Mather LE: Clinical pharmacokinetics of fentanyl and its newer derivatives. *Clin Pharmacokinet* 8: 422, 1983

268. Szeto HH, Inturrisi CE, Houde R, Saal S, Cheigh J, Reidenberg MM: Accumulation of normeperidine, and active metabolite of meperidine, in patients with renal failure or cancer. *Ann Intern Med* 86: 738, 1977

269. Kreek MJ, Schecter AJ, Gutjahr CL, Hecht M: Methadone use in patients with chronic renal disease. *Drug Alcohol Depend* 5: 197, 1980

270. Chauvin M, Sandouk P, Scherrmann JM, Farinotti R, Strumza P, Duvaldestin P: Morphine pharmacokinetics in renal failure. *Anesthesiology* 66: 327, 1987

271. Säwe J, Odar-Cederlöf I: Kinetics of morphine in patients with renal failure. *Eur J Clin Pharmacol* 32: 377, 1987

272. Giacomini KM, Gibson TP, Levy G: Effect of hemodialysis on propoxyphene and norpropoxyphenne concentrations in blood of anephric patients. *Clin Pharmacol Ther* 27: 508, 1980

273. Clissold SP: Paracetamol and phenacetin. *Drugs* 32 (Suppl 4): 46, 1986

274. Prescott LF, Speirs GC, Critchley JA, Temple RM, Winney RJ: Paracetamol disposition and metabolite kinetics in patients with chronic renal failure. *Eur J Clin Pharmacol* 36: 291, 1989

275. Needs CJ, Brooks PM: Clinical pharmacokinetics of the salicylates. *Clin Pharmacokinet* 10: 164, 1985

276. Agoston S, Vandenbrom RH, Wierda JM: Clinical pharmacokinetics of neuromuscular blocking drugs. *Clin Pharmacokinet* 22: 94, 1992

277. Davis PJ, Cook DR: Clinical pharmacokinetics of the newer intravenous anaesthetic agents. *Clin Pharmacokinet* 11: 18, 1986

278. Pollard BJ: Editorial: neuromuscular blocking drugs and renal failure. *Br J Anaesth* 68: 545, 1992

279. Gramstad L: Atracurium, vecuronium and pancuronium in end-stage renal failure. Dose-response properties and interactions with azathioprine. *Br J Anaesth* 59: 995, 1987

280. Mongin-Long D, Chabrol B, Baude C et al.: Atracurium in patients with renal failure. Clinical trial of a new neuromuscular blocker. *Br J Anaesth* 58 (Suppl): 44S, 1986

281. Ramzan MI, Shanks CA, Triggs EJ: Gallamine disposition in surgical patients with chronic renal failure. *J Clin Pharmacol* 12: 141, 1981

282. Brotherton WP, Matteo RS: Pharmacokinetics and pharmacodynamics of metocurine in humans with and without renal failure. *Anesthesiology* 55: 273, 1981

283. Aquilonius SM, Hartvig P: Clinical pharmacokinetics of cholinesterase inhibitors. *Clin Pharmacokinet* 11: 236, 1986

284. McLeod K, Watson MJ, Rawlins MD: Pharmacokinetics of pancuronium in patients with normal and impaired renal function. *Br J Anaesth* 48: 341, 1976

285. Kirvelä M, Olkkola KT, Rosenberg PH, Yli-Hankala A, Salmela K, Lingren L: Pharmacokinetics of propofol and haemodynamic changes during induction of anaesthesia in uraemic patients. *Br J Anaesth* 68: 178, 1992

286. Cronnelly R, Stanski DR, Miller RD, Sheiner LB: Pyridostigmine kinetics with and without renal function. *Clin Pharmacol Ther* 28: 78, 1980

287. Bishop M, Hornbein TF: Prolonged effect of succinylcholine after neostigmine and pyridostigmine administration in patients with renal failure. *Anesthesiology* 58: 384, 1983

288. Matteo RS, Nishitateno K, Pua EK, Spector S: Pharmacokinetics of d-tubocurarine in man: effect of an osmotic diuretic on urinary excretion. *Anesthesiology* 52: 335, 1980

289. Lynam DP, Cronnelly R, Castagnoli KP et al.: The pharmacodynamics and pharmacokinetics of vecuronium in patients anesthetized with isoflurane with normal renal function or with renal failure. *Anesthesiology* 69: 227, 1988

290. Hulter HN, Licht JH, Ilnicki LP, Singh S: Clinical efficacy and pharmacokinetics of clonidine in hemodialysis and renal insufficiency. *J Lab Clin Med* 94: 223, 1979

291. Lowenthal DT, Matzek KM, MacGregor TR: Clinical pharmacokinetics of clonidine. *Clin Pharmacokinet* 14: 287, 1988

292. Carlson RV, Bailey RR, Begg EJ, Cowlishaw MG, Sharman JR: Pharmacokinetics and effect on blood pressure of doxazosin in normal subjects and patients with renal failure. *Clin Pharmacol Ther* 40: 561, 1986

293. Young RA, Brogden RN: Doxazosin. A review of its pharmacodynamic and pharmacokinetic properties, and therapeutic efficacy in mild or moderate hypertension. *Drugs* 35: 525, 1988

294. Holmes B, Brogden RN, Heel RC, Speight TM, Avery GS: Guanabenz. A review of its pharmacodynamic properties and therapeutic efficacy in hypertension. *Drugs* 26: 212, 1983

295. Finnerty FA, Brogden RN: Guanadrel. A review of its pharmacodynamic and pharmacokinetic properties and therapeutic use in hypertension. *Drugs* 30: 22, 1985

296. Halstenson CE, Opsahl JA, Abraham PA et al.: Disposition of guanadrel in subjects with normal and impaired renal function. *J Clin Pharmacol* 29: 128, 1989

297. Carchman SH, Sica DA, Davis J et al.: Steady-state plasma levels and pharmacokinetics of guanfacine in patients with renal insufficiency. *Nephron* 53: 18, 1989

298. Sorkin EM, Heel RC: Guanfacine. A review of its pharmacodynamic and pharmacokinetic properties, and therapeutic efficacy in the treatment of hypertension. *Drugs* 31: 301, 1986

299. Myhre E, Rugstad HE, Hansen T: Clinical pharmacokinetics of methyldopa. *Clin Pharmacokinet* 7: 221, 1982

300. Lameire N, Gordts J: A pharmacokinetic study of prazosin in patients with varying degrees of chronic renal failure. *Eur J Clin Pharmacol* 31: 333, 1986

301. Vincent J, Meredith PA, Reid JL, Elliot HL, Rubin PC: Clinical pharmacokinetics of prazosin – 1985. *Clin Pharmacokinet* 10: 144, 1985

302. Zsoter TT, Johnson GE, DeVeber GA, Paul H: Excretion and metabolism of reserpine in renal failure. *Clin Pharmacol Ther* 14: 325, 1973

303. Jungers P, Ganeval D, Pertuiset N, Chaveau P: Influence of renal insufficiency on the pharmacokinetics and pharmacodynamics of terazosin. *Am J Med* 80 (Suppl 5B): 94, 1986

304. Hoyer J, Schulte KL, Lenz T: Clinical pharmacokinetics of angiotensin converting enzyme (ACE) inhibitors in renal failure. *Clin Pharmacokinet* 24: 230, 1993

305. Balfour JA, Goa KL: Benazepril. A review of its pharmacodynamic and pharmacokinetic properties, and therapeutic efficacy in hypertension and congestive heart failure. *Drugs* 42: 511, 1991

306. Brogden RN, Todd PA, Sorkin EM: Captopril. An update of its pharmacodynamic and pharmacokinetic properties, and therapeutic use in hypertension and congestive heart failure. *Drugs* 36: 540, 1988

307. Duchin KL, Pierides AM, Heald A, Signhvl HM, Rommel AAJ: Elimination kinetics of captopril in patients with renal failure. *Kidney Int* 25: 942, 1984

308. Fujimura A, Kajiyama H, Ebihara A, Iwashita K, Nomura Y, Kawahara Y: Pharmacokinetics and pharmacodynamics of captopril in patients undergoing continuous ambulatory peritoneal dialysis. *Nephron* 44: 324, 1986

309. Fruncillo RJ, Rocci ML Jr, Vlasses PH et al.: Disposition of enalapril and enalaprilat in renal insufficiency. *Kidney Int* 31 (Suppl 20): S117, 1987

310. Todd PA, Goa KL: Enalapril. A reappraisal of its pharmacology and therapeutic use in hypertension. *Drugs* 43: 346, 1992

311. Gehr TW, Sica DA, Grasela DM, Fakhry I, Davis J, Duchin KL: Fosinopril pharmacokinetics and pharmacodynamics in chronic ambulatory peritoneal dialysis patients. *Eur J Clin Pharmacol* 41: 165, 1991

312. Hui KK, Duchin KL, Kripalani KJ, Chan D, Kramer PK, Yanagawa N: Pharmacokinetics of fosinopril in patients with various degrees of renal function. *Clin Pharmacol Ther* 49: 457, 1991

313. Murdoch D, McTavish D: Fosinopril. A review of its pharmacodynamic and pharmacokinetic properties, and therapeutic potential in essential hypertension. *Drugs* 43: 123, 1992

314. Lancaster SG, Todd PA: Lisinopril. A preliminary review of its pharmacodynamic and pharmacokinetic properties, and therapeutic use in hypertension and congestive heart failure. *Drugs* 35: 646, 1988

315. van Schaik BA, Geyskes GG, van der Wouw PA, van Rooij HH, Porsius AJ: Pharmacokinetics of lisinopril in hypertensive patients with normal and impaired renal function. *Eur J Clin Pharmacol* 34: 61, 1988

316. Halstenson CE, Opsahl JA, Rachael K et al.: The pharmacokinetics of quinapril and its active metabolite quinaprilat in patients with varying degrees Rnal function. *J Clin Pharmacol* 32: 344, 1992

317. Schunkert H, Kindler J, Gassmann M et al.: Pharmacokinetics of ramipril in hypertensive patients with renal insufficiency. *Eur J Clin Pharmacol* 37: 249, 1989

318. Todd PA, Benfield P: Ramipril. A review of its pharmacological properties and therapeutic efficacy in cardiovascular disorders. *Drugs* 39: 110, 1990

319. Gill J, Heel RC, Fitton A: Amiodarone: an overview of its pharmacological properties, and review of its therapeutic use in cardiac arrhythmias. *Drugs* 43: 69, 1992

320. Josselson J, Narang PK, Adir J, Yacobi A, Sadler JH: Bretylium kinetics in renal insufficiency. *Clin Pharmacol Ther* 33: 144, 1983

321. Rapeport WG: Clinical pharmacokinetics of bretylium. *Clin Pharmacokinet* 10: 248, 1985

322. Brogden RN, Todd PA: Disopyramide: a reappraisal of its pharmacodynamic and pharmacokinetic properties, and therapeutic use in cardiac arrhythmias. *Drugs* 34: 151, 1986

323. Burk M, Peters U: Disopyramide kinetics in renal impairment: determinants of interindividual variability. *Clin Pharmacol Ther* 34: 331, 1983

324. Haughey DB, Kraft CJ, Matzke GR, Keane WF, Halstenson CE: Protein binding of disopyramide and elevated alpha-1-acid glycoprotein concentrations in serum obtained from dialysis patients and renal transplant recipients. *Am J Nephrol* 5: 35, 1985

325. Bergstrand RH, Wang T, Roden DM et al.: Encainide disposition in patients with renal failure. *Clin Pharmacol Ther* 40: 64, 1986

326. Brogden RN, Todd PA: Encainide: a review of its pharmacological properties and therapeutic efficacy. *Drugs* 34: 519, 1987

327. Forland SC, Burgess E, Blair AD et al.: Oral flecainide pharmacokinetics in patients with impaired renal function. *J Clin Pharmacol* 28: 259, 1988

328. Forland SC, Cutler RE, McQuinn RL et al.: Flecainide pharmacokinetics after multiple dosing in patients with impaired renal function. *J Clin Pharmacol* 28: 727, 1988

329. Bennett PN, Aarons LJ, Bending MR, Steiner JA, Rowland M: Pharmacokinetics of lidocaine and its deethylated metabolite: dose and time dependency studies in man. *J Pharmacokinet Biopharm* 10: 265, 1982

330. Eiriksson CE, Brogden RN: Lorcainide: a preliminary review of its pharmacodynamic properties and therapeutic efficacy. *Drugs* 27: 279, 1984

331. Monk JP, Brogden RN: Mexiletine: a review of its pharmacodynamic and pharmacokinetic properties, and therapeutic use in the treatment of arrhythmias. *Drugs* 40: 374, 1990

332. Wang T, Wuellner D, Woosley RL, Stone WJ: Pharmacokinetics and nondialyzability of mexiletine in renal failure. *Clin Pharmacol Ther* 37: 649, 1988

333. Fitton A, Buckley MT: Moricizine: a review of its pharmacological properties, and therapeutic efficacy in cardiac arrhythmias. *Drugs* 40: 138, 1990

334. Pieniaszek HJ, McEntegart CM, Mayersohn M, Michael UF: Moricizine pharmacokinetics in renal insufficiency: reevaluation of elimination half-life. *J Clin Pharmacol* 32: 412, 1992

335. Stec GP, Atkinson AJ, Nevin MJ et al.: N-actylprocainamide pharmacokinetics in functionally anephric patients before and after perturbation by hemodialysis. *Clin Pharmacol Ther* 26: 618, 1979

336. Harron DW, Brogden RN: Acecainide (N-acetylprocainamide): a review of its pharmacodynamic and pharmacokinetic properties, and therapeutic potential in cardiac arrhythmias. *Drugs* 39: 720, 1990

337. Raehl CL, Moorthy AV, Beirne GJ: Procainamide pharmacokinetics in patients on continuous ambulatory peritoneal dialysis. *Nephron* 44: 191, 1986

338. Bryson HM, Palmer KJ, Langtry HD, Fitton A: Propafenone: a reappraisal of its pharmacology, pharmacokinetics and therapeutic use in cardiac arrhythmias. *Drugs* 45: 85, 1993

339. Burgess E, Duff H, Wilkes P: Propafenone disposition in renal insufficiency and renal failure. *J Clin Pharmacol* 29: 112, 1989

340. Crevasse L: Quinidine: an update on therapeutics, pharmacokinetics and serum concentration monitoring. *Am J Cardiol* 62: 221, 1988

341. Kessler KM, Perez GO: Decreased quinidine plasma protein binding during hemodialysis. *Clin Pharmacol Ther* 30: 121, 1981

342. Holmes B, Brogden RN, Heel RC, Speight TM, Avery GS: Tocainide: a review of its pharmacological properties and therapeutic efficacy. *Drugs* 26: 93, 1983

343. Rachl CL, Beirne GJ, Moorthy AV, Patel AK: Tocainide pharmacokinetics during continuous ambulatory peritoneal dialysis. *Am J Cardiol* 60: 747, 1987

344. Wiegers U, Hanrath P, Kuck KH et al.: Pharmacokinetics of tocainide in patients with renal dysfunction and during haemodialysis. *Eur J Clin Pharmacol* 24: 503, 1983

345. Borehard U: Pharmacokineties of beta-adrenoceptor blocking agents: clinical significance of hepatic and/or renal clearance. *Clin Physiol Biochem* 8 (Suppl 2): 28, 1990

346. Riddell JG, Harron DW, Shanks RG: Clinical pharmacokinetics of β-adrenoceptor antagonists. An update. *Clin Pharmacokinet* 12: 305, 1987

347. Kirch W, Köhler H, Berggren G, Braun W: The influence of renal function on plasma levels and urinary excretion of acebutolol and its main N-acetyl metabolite. *Clin Nephrol* 18: 88, 1982

348. Roux A, Aubert P, Guedon J, Flouvat B: Pharmacokineties of acebutolol in patients with all grades of renal failure. *Eur J Clin Pharmacol* 17: 339, 1980

349. Singh BN, Thoden WR, Ward A: Acebutolol: a review of pharmacological properties and therapeutic efficacy in hypertension, angina pectoris and arrhythmia. *Drugs* 29: 531, 1985

350. Kirch W, Kohler H, Mutschler E, Schafer M: Pharmacokinetics of atenolol in relation to renal function. *Eur J Clin Pharmacol* 19: 65, 1981

351. Wadworth A, Murdoch D, Brogden RN: Atenolol: a reappraisal of its pharmacological properties, and therapeutic use in cardiovascular disorders. *Drugs* 42: 468, 1991

352. Beresford R, Heel RC: Betaxolol: a review of its pharmacodynamic and pharmacokinetic properties, and therapeutic efficacy in hypertension. *drugs* 31: 6, 1986

353. Amemiya M, Tabei K, Furuya H, Sakairi Y, Asano Y: Pharmacokinetics of carteolol in patients with impaired renal function. *Eur J Clin Pharmacol* 43: 417, 1992

354. Hasenfub G, Schafer-Korting M, Knauf H, Mutschler E, Just H: Pharmacokinetics of carteolol in relation to renal function. *Eur J Clin Pharmacol* 29: 461, 1985

355. Chrisp P, Goa KL: Dilevalol: a review of its pharmacodynamic and pharmacokinetic properties, and therapeutic potential in hypertension. *Drugs* 30: 234, 1990

356. Kelly JG, Laher MS, Donohue J, Doyle GD: The pharmacokinetics of dilevalol in renal impairment. *J Hum Hypertens* 4 (Suppl 2): 59, 1990

357. Benfield P, Sorkin EM: Esmolol: a preliminary review of its pharmacodynamic and pharmacokinetic properties, and therapeutic efficacy. *Drugs* 33: 392, 1987

358. Flaherty JF, Wong B, LaFollette G, Warnock DG, Hulse JD, Gambertoglio JG: Pharmacokinetics of esmolol and ASL-8123 in renal failure. *Clin Pharmacol Ther* 45: 321, 1989

359. Goa KL, Benfield P, Sorkin EM: Labetalol: a reappraisal of its pharmacology, pharmacokinetics and therapeutic use in hypertension and ischemic heart disease. *Drugs* 37: 583, 1989

360. Halstenson CE, Opsahl JA, Pence TV et al.: The disposition and dynamics of labetalol in patients on dialysis. *Clin Pharmacol Ther* 40: 462, 1986

361. Regardh CG, Johnsson G: Clinical pharmacokinetics of metoprolol. *Clin Pharmacokinet* 5: 557, 1980

362. Dreyfuss J, Griffith DL, Singhvi SM et al.: Pharmacokinetics of nadolol, a beta-receptor antagonist: administration of therapeutic single- and multiple-dosage regimens to hypertensive patients. *J Clin Pharmacol* 19: 712, 1979

363. Frishman WH: Nadolol: a new B-adrenoceptor antagonist. *N Engl J Med* 305: 678, 1981

364. Bernard N, Cuisinaud G, Pozet N, Zech PY, Sassard J: Pharmacokinetics of penbutolol and its metabolites in renal insufficiency. *Eur J Clin Pharmacol* 29: 215, 1985

365. Ohnhaus EE, Heidemann H, Meier J, Maurer G: Metabolism of pindolol in patients with renal failure. *Eur J Clin Pharmacol* 22: 423, 1982

366. Stone WJ, Walle T: Massive propranolol metabolite retention during maintenance hemodialysis. *Clin Pharmacol Ther* 28: 449, 1980

367. Wood AJ, Vestal RE, Spannuth CL, Stone WJ, Wilkinson GR, Shand DG: Propranolol disposition in renal failure. *Br J Clin Pharmacol* 10: 561, 1980

368. Blair AD, Burgess ED, Maxwell BM, Cutler RE: Sotalol kinetics in renal insufficiency. *Clin Pharmacol Ther* 29: 457, 1981

369. Singh BN, Deedwania P, Koonlawee N, Ward A, Sorkim EM: Sotalol: a review of its pharmacodynamic and pharmacokinetic properties, and therapeutic use. *Drugs* 34: 311, 1987

370. Kelly JG, O'Malley K: Clinical pharmacokinetics of calcium antagonists. An update. *Clin Pharmacokinet* 22: 416, 1992

371. Laher MS, Kelly JG, Doyle GD et al.: Pharmacokinetics of amlodipine in renal impairment. *J Cardiovasc Pharmacol* 12 (Suppl 7): S60, 1988

372. Buckley MM, Grant SM, Goa KL, McTavish D, Sorkin EM: Diltiazem. A reappraisal of its pharmacological properties and therapeutic use. *Drugs* 39: 757, 1990

373. Grech-Bélangér O, Langlois S, LeBoeuf E: Pharmacokinetics of diltiazem in patients undergoing continuous ambulatory peritoneal dialysis. *J Clin Pharmacol* 28: 477, 1988

374. Pozet N, Brazier JL, Aïssa AH et al.: Pharmacokinetics of diltiazem in severe renal failure. *Eur J Clin Pharmacol* 24: 635, 1983

375. Buur T, Larsson R, Regårdh CG, Aberg J: Pharmacokinetics of felodipine in chronic hemodialysis patients. *J Clin Pharmacol* 31: 709, 1991

376. Edgar B, Regårdh CG, Attman PO, Aurell M, Herlitz H, Johnsson G: Pharmacokinetics of felodinine in patients with impaired renal function. *Br J Clin Pharmacol* 27: 67, 1989

377. Todd PA, Faulds D: Felodipine. A review of the pharmacology and therapeutic use of the extended release formulation in cardiovascular disorders. *Drugs* 44: 251, 1992

378. Chandler MH, Schran HF, Cutler RE, Smith AJ, Gonasun LM, Blouin RA: The effeets of renal function on the disposition of isradipine. *J Clin Pharmacol* 28: 1076, 1988

379. Fitton A, Benfield P: Isradipine. A review of its pharmacodynamic and pharmacokinetic properties, and therapeutic use in cardiovascular disease. *Drugs* 40: 31, 1990

380. Schonholzer K, Marone C: Pharmacokinetics and dialysability of isradipine in chronic haemodialysis patients. *Eur J Clin Pharmacol* 42: 231, 1992

381. Sorkin EM, Clissold SP: Nicardipine. A review of its pharmacodynamic and pharmacokinetic properties, and therapeutic efficacy, in the treatment of angina pectoris, hypertension and related cardiovascular disorders. *Drugs* 33: 296, 1987

382. Martre H, Sari R, Taburet AM, Jacobs C, Singlas E: Haemodialysis does not affect the pharmacokinetics of nifedipine. *Br J Clin Pharmacol* 20: 155, 1985

383. Sorkin EM, Clissold SP, Brogden RN: Nifedipine. A review of its pharmacodynamic and pharmacokinetic properties, and therapeutic efficacy, in ischaemic heart disease, hypertension and related cardiovascular disorders. *Drugs* 30: 182, 1985

384. Goa KL, Sorkin EM: Nitrendipine. A review of its pharmacodynamic and pharmacokinetic properties, and therapeutic efficacy in the treatment of hypertension. *Drugs* 33: 123, 1987

385. Mikus G, Mast V, Fischer C, Machleidt C, Kuhlman U, Eichelbaum M: Pharmacokineties, bioavailability, metabolism and acute and chronic antihypertensive effects of nitrendipine in patients with chronic renal failure and moderate to severe hypertension. *Br J Clin Pharmacol* 31: 313, 1991

386. Hanyok JJ, Chow MS, Kluger J, Izard MW: An evaluation of the pharmacokinetics, pharmacodynamics, and dialyzability of verapamil in chronic hemodialysis patients. *J Clin Pharmacol* 28: 831, 1988

387. McTavish D, Sorkin EM: Verapamil. An updated review of its pharmacodynamic and pharmacokinetic properties and therapeutic use in hypertension. *Drugs* 38: 19, 1989

388. Mooy J, Schols M, van Baak M, van Hooff M, Muytens A, Rahn KH: Pharmacokinetics of verapamil in patients with renal failure. *Eur J Clin Pharmacol* 28: 405, 1985

389. Graves PE, Fenster PE, MacFarland RT, Marcus FI, Perrier D: Kinetics of digitoxin and the bis- and monodigitoxosides of digitoxigenin in renal insufficiency. *Clin Pharmacol Ther* 36: 607, 1984

390. Vohringer HF, Rietbrock N: Digitalis therapy in renal failure with special regard to digitoxin. *Int J Clin Pharmacol Ther Toxicol* 19: 175, 1981

391. Gibson TP, Nelson HA: The question of cumulation of digoxin metabolites in renal failure. *Clin Pharmacol Ther* 27: 219, 1980

392. Keller F, Molzahn M, Ingerowski R: Digoxin dosage in renal insufficiency: impracticality of basing it on the creatinine clearance, body weight and volume of distribution. *Eur J Clin Pharmacol* 18: 433, 1980

393. Sonnenblick M, Abraham AS, Meshulam Z, Eylath U: Correlation between manifestations of digoxin toxicity and serum digoxin, calcium, potassium, and magnesium concentrations and arterial pH. *Br Med J* 286: 1089, 1983

394. Lant A: Diuretics. Clinical pharmacology and therapeutic use (Part I). *Drugs* 29: 57, 1985

395. Lant A: Diuretics. Clinical pharmacology and therapeutic use (Part II). *Drugs* 29: 162, 1985

396. Chapron DJ, Gomolin IH, Sweeney KR: Acetazolamide blood concentrations are excessive in the elderly: propensity for acidosis and relationship to renal function. *J Clin Pharmacol* 29: 348, 1989

397. Spahn H, Reuter K, Mutschler E, Gerok W, Knauf H: Pharmacokinetics of amiloride in renal and hepatic disease. *Eur J Clin Pharmacol* 33: 493, 1987

398. Pentikäinen PJ, Pasternack A, Lampainen E, Neuvonen PJ, Pentilla A: Bumetanide kinetics in renal failure. *Clin Pharmacol Ther* 37: 582, 1985

399. Ward A, Heel RC: Bumetanide. A review of its pharmacodynamic and pharmacokinetic properties and therapeutic use. *Drugs* 28: 426, 1984

400. Mulley BA, Parr GD, Rye RM: Pharmacokinetics of chlorthalidone. *Eur J Clin Pharmacol* 17: 203, 1980

401. Pillay VK, Schwartz FD, Aimi K, Kark RM: Transient and permanent deafness following treatment of ethacrynic acid in renal failure. *Lancet* 1(585), 77, 1969

402. Brater DC, Anderson SA, Brown-Cartwright D: Response to furosemide in chronic renal insufficiency: rationale for limited doses. *Clin Pharmacol Ther* 40: 134, 1986

403. Ponto LL, Schoenwald RD: Furosemide (Frusemide). A pharmacokinetic/pharmacodynamic review (Part I). *Clin Pharmacokinet* 18: 381, 1990

404. Traeger A, Stein G, Sperschneider H, Keil E: Pharmacokinetic and pharmacodynemic effects of furosemide in patients with impaired renal function. *Int J Clin Pharmacol Ther Toxicol* 22: 481, 1984

405. Acchiardo SR, Skoutakis VA: Clinical efficacy, safety, and pharmacokinetics of indapamide in renal impairment. *Am Heart J* 106: 237, 1983

406. Clissold SP, Brogden RN: Piretanide. A preliminary review of its pharmacodynamic and pharmcokinetic properties, and therapeutic efficacy. *Drugs* 29: 489, 1985

407. Marone C, Reubi FC, Perisic M, Lahn W: Pharmacokinetics of high doses of piretanide in moderate to severe renal failure. *Eur J Clin Pharmacol* 27: 589, 1984

408. Skluth HA, Gums JG: Spironolactone: a re-examination. *DICP Ann. Pharmacother* 24: 52, 1990

409. Niemeyer C, Hasenfub G, Wais U, Knauf H, Shafer-Korting M, Mutschler E: Pharmacokinetics of hydrochlorothiazide in relation to renal function. *Eur J Clin Pharmacol* 24: 661, 1983

410. Fairley KF, Woo KT, Birch DF, Leaker BR, Ratnaike S: Triamterene-induced crystalluria and cylinduria: clinical and experimental studies. *Clin Nephrol* 26: 169, 1986

411. Bottorff MB, Rutledge DR, Pieper JA: Evaluation of intravenous amrinone: the first of a new class of positive inotropic agents with vasodilator properties. *Pharmacotherapy* 5: 227, 1985

412. Ward A, Brogden RN, Heel RC, Speight TM, Avery GS: Amrinone: a preliminary review of its pharmacological properties and therapeutic use. *Drugs* 26: 468, 1983

413. Majerus TC, Dasta JF, Bauman JL, Danzinger LH, Ruffolo RR: Dobutamine; ten years later. *Pharmacotherapy* 9: 245, 1989

414. Sonnenblick EH, Frishman WH, LeJemtel TH: Dobutamine; a new synthetic cardioactive sympathetic amine. *N Engl J Med* 300: 17, 1979

415. Larsson R, Liedholm H, Andersson KE, Keane MA, Henry G: Pharmacokinetics and effects on blood pressure of a single oral dose of milrinone in healthy subjects and in patients with renal impairment. *Eur J Clin Pharmacol* 29: 549, 1986

416. Young RA, Ward A: Milrinone: a preliminary review of its pharmacological properties and therapeutic use. *Drugs* 36: 158, 1988

417. Bogaert MG: Clinical pharmacokinetics of glyceryl trinitrate following the use of systemic and topical preparations. *Clin Pharmacokinet* 12: 1, 1987

418. Evers J, Bonn R, Boertz A et al.: Pharmacokinetics of isosorbide-5-nitrate during haemodialysis and peritoneal dialysis. *Eur J Clin Pharmacol* 32: 503, 1987

419. Evers J, Krakamp B, Klimkait W et al.: Pharmacokinetics of isosorbide-5-nitrate in renal failure. *Eur J Cl Pharmacol* 30: 349, 1986

420. Pearson RM: Pharmacokinetics and response to diazoxide in renal failure. *Clin Pharmacokinet* 2: 198, 1977

421. Ludden TM, McNay JL, Shepherd AM, Lin MS: Clinical pharmacokinetics of hydralazine. *Clin Pharmacokinet* 7: 185, 1982

422. Halstenson CE, Opsahl JA, Wright CE et al.: Disposition of minoxidil in patients with various degrees of renal function. *J Clin Pharmacol* 29: 798, 1989

423. Rindone JP, Sloane EP: Cyanide toxicity from sodium nitroprusside: risks and management. *Ann Pharmacother* 26: 515, 1992

424. Schulz V: Clinical pharmacokinetics of nitroprusside cyanide thiosulphate and thiocyanate. *Clin Pharmacokinet* 9: 239, 1984

425. Crooke ST, Comis RL, Einhorn LH, Strong JE, Broughton A, Prestayko AW: Effects of variations in renal function on the clinical pharmacology of bleomycin administered as an IV bolus. *Cancer Treat Rep* 61: 1631, 1977

426. Ehrsson H, Hassan M, Ehrnebo M, Beran M: Busulfan kinetics. *Clin Pharmacol Ther* 34: 86, 1983

427. Elferink F, van der Vijgh WJ, Klein I, ten Bokkel Huinink WW, Dubbelman R, McVie JG: Pharmacokinetics of carboplatin after intraperitoneal administration. *Cancer Chemother Pharmacol* 21: 57, 1988

428. Motzer RJ, Niedzwiecki D, Isaacs M et al.: Carboplatin-based chemotherapy with pharmacokinetic analysis for patients with hemodialysis-dependent renal insufficiency. *Cancer Chemother Pharmacol* 27: 234, 1990

429. Van der Vijgh WJ: Clinical pharmacokinetics of carboplatin. *Clin Pharmacokinet* 21: 242, 1991

430. Newell DR, Calvert AH, Harrap KR, McElwain TJ: Studies on the pharmacokinetics of chlorambucil and prednimustine in man. *Br J Clin Pharmacol* 15: 253, 1983

431. Blachley JD, Hill JB: Renal and electrolyte disturbances associated with cisplatin. *Ann Intern Med* 95: 628, 1981

432. Corden BJ, Fine RL, Ozols RF, Collins JM: Clinical pharmacology of high-dose cisplatin. *Cancer Chemother Pharmacol* 14: 38, 1985

433. Juma FD, Rogers HJ, Trounce JR: Effect of renal insufficiency on the pharmacokinetics of cyclophosphamide and some of its metabolites. *Eur J Clin Pharmacol* 19: 443, 1981

434. Moore MJ: Clinical pharmacokinetics of cyclophosphamide. *Clin Pharmacokinet* 20: 194, 1991

435. Wang LH, Lee CS, Majeske BL, Marbury TC: Clearance and recovery calculations in hemodialysis: application to plasma, red blood cell, and dialysate measurements for cyclophosphamide. *Clin Pharmacol Ther* 29: 365, 1981

436. Damon LE, Mass R, Linker CA: The association between high-dose cytarabine neurotoxicity and renal insufficiency. *J Clin Oncol* 7: 1563, 1989

437. Goto M, Yoshida H, Honda A et al.: Delayed disposition of adriamycin and its active metabolite in haemodialysis patients. (Letter) *Eur J Clin Pharmacol* 44: 301, 1993

438. Speth PA, vanHoesel QG, Haanen C: Clinical pharmacokinetics of doxorubicin. *Clin Pharmacokinet* 15: 15, 1988

439. Henwood JM, Brogden RN: Etoposide: a review of its pharmacodynamic and pharmacokinetic properties, and therapeutic potential in combination chemotherapy of cancer. *Drugs* 39: 438, 1990

440. Diasio RB, Harris BE: Clinical pharmacology of 5-fluorouracil. *Clin Pharmacokinet* 16: 215, 1989

441. Hollingshead LM, Faulds D: Idarubicin: a review of its pharmacodynamic and pharmacokinetic properties, and therapeutic potential in the chemotherapy of cancer. *Drugs* 42: 690, 1991

442. Alberts DS, Chen HG, Benz D, Mason NL: Effect of renal dysfunction in dogs on the disposition and marrow toxicity of melphalan. *Br J Cancer* 43: 330, 1981

443. Österborg A, Ehrsson H, Eksborg S, Wallin I, Mellstedt H: Pharmacokinetics of oral melphalan in relation to renal function in multiple myeloma patients. *Eur J Cancer Clin Oncol* 25: 899, 1989

444. Sand TE, Jacobsen S: Effect of urine pH and flow on renal clearance of methotrexate. *Eur J Clin Pharmacol* 19: 453, 1981

445. Jolivet J, Cowan KH, Curt GA, Clendeninn NJ, Chabner BA: The pharmacology and clinical use of methotrexate. *N Engl J Med* 309: 1094, 1983

446. Shen DD, Azarnoff DL: Clinical pharmacokinetics of methotrexate. *Clin Pharmacokinet* 3: 1, 1978

447. Den Hartigh J, McVie JG, Van Oort WS, Pinedo HM: Pharmacokinetics of mitomycin C in humans. *Cancer Res* 43: 5017, 1983

448. Ellis ME, Weiss RB, Kuperminc M: Nephrotoxicity of lomustine: a case report and literature review. *Cancer Chemother Pharmacol* 15: 174, 1985

449. Oliverio VT: Toxicology and pharmacology of the nitrosoureas. *Cancer Chemother Rep* 413, 1973

450. Kennedy BJ: Metabolic and toxic effects of mithramycin during tumor therapy. *Am J Med* 49: 494, 1970

451. Hall-Craggs M, Brenner DE, Vigorito RD, Sutherland JC: Acute renal failure and renal tubular squamous metaplasia following treatment with streptozocin. *Hum Pathol* 13: 597, 1982

452. Buckley MM, Goa KL: Tamoxifen: a reappraisal of its pharmacodynamic and pharmacokinetic properties, and therapeutic use. *Drugs* 37: 451, 1989

453. Owellen RJ, Hartke CA, Hains FO: Pharmacokinetics and metabolism of vinblastine in humans. *Cancer Res* 37: 2597, 1977

454. Clissold SP, Edwards C: Acarbose. A preliminary review of its pharmacodynamic and pharmacokinetic properties, and therapeutic potential. *Drugs* 35: 214, 1988

455. Ferner RE, Chaplin S: The relationship between the pharmacokinetics and pharmacodynamic effects of oral hypoglycaemic drugs. *Clin Pharmacokinet* 12: 379, 1987

456. Palmer KJ, Brogden RN: Gliclazide. An update of its pharmacological properties and therapeutic efficacy in non-insulin-dependent diabetes mellitus. *Drugs* 46: 92, 1993

457. Lebovitz HE: Glipizide: a second-generation sulfonylurea hypoglycemic agent. *Pharmacotherapy* 5: 63, 1985

458. Feldman JM: Glyburide: a second-generation sulfonylurea hypoglycemic agent. *Pharmacotherapy* 5: 43, 1985

459. Brogden RN, Heel RC: Human insulin. A review of its biological activity, pharmacokinetics and therapeutic use. *Drugs* 34: 350, 1987

460. Guba EA, Abel SR, Golper TA: Practical guidelines for drug therapy in dialysis: lipid lowering agents. *Semin Dial* 2: 186, 1989

461. Sherrard DJ, Goldberg AB, Haas LB, Brunzell JD: Chronic clofibrate therapy in maintenance hemodialysis patients. *Nephron* 25: 219, 1980

462. Tse FL, Jaffe JM, Troendle A: Pharmacokinetics of fluvastatin after single and multiple doses in normal volunteers. *J Clin Pharmacol* 32: 630, 1992

463. Manninen V, Malkonen M, Esailo A: Gemfibrozil treatment of dyslipidaemias in renal failure with uraemia or in the nephrotic syndrome. *Res Clin Forums* 4: 113, 1982

464. Corpier CL, Jones PH, Suki WN et al.: Rhabdomyolysis and renal injury with lovastatin use. Report of two cases in cardiac transplant recipients. *JAMA* 260: 239, 1988

465. Henwood JM, Heel RC: Lovastatin. A preliminary review of its pharmacodynamic properties and therapeutic use in hyperlipidaemia. *Drugs* 36: 429, 1988

466. Figge HL, Figge J, Souney PF, Mutnick AH, Sacks F: Nicotinic acid: a review of its clinical use in the treatment of lipid disorders. *Pharmacotherapy* 8: 287, 1988

467. McTavish D, Sorkin EM: Pravastatin. A review of its pharmacological properties and therapeutic potential in hypercholesterolaemia. *Drugs* 42: 65, 1991

468. Buckley MM, Goa KL, Price AH, Brogden RN: Probucol. A reappraisal of its pharmacological properties and therapeutic use in hypercholesterolaemia. *Drugs* 37: 761, 1989

469. Mauro VF: Clinical pharmacokinetics and practical applications of simvastatin. *Clin Pharmacokinet* 24: 195, 1993

470. Kampmann JP, Hansen JM: Clinical pharmacokinetics of antithyroid drugs. *Clin Pharmacokinet* 6: 401, 1981

471. Jansson R, Lindstrom B, Dahlberg PA: Pharmacokinetic properties and bioavailability of methimazole. *Clin Pharmacokinet* 10: 443, 1985

472. Lauritsen K, Laursen LS, Rask-Madsen J: Clinical pharmacokinetics of drugs used in the treatment of gastrointestinal diseases (Part I). *Clin Pharmacokinet* 19: 11, 1990

473. Harrington RA, Hamilton CW, Brogden RN, Linkewich JA, Romankiewicz JA, Heel RC: Metoclopramide: an updated review of its pharmacological properties and clinical use. *Drugs* 25: 451, 1983

474. Milne RJ, Heel RC: Ondansetron: therapeutic use as an antiemetic. *Drugs* 41: 574, 1991

475. Lin JH: Pharmacokinetic and pharmacodynamic properties of histamine H_2-receptor antonists. Relationship between intrinsic potency and effective plasma concentrations. *Clin Pharmacokinet* 20: 218, 1991

476. Somogyi A, Gugler R: Clinical pharmacokinetics of cimetidine. *Clin Pharmacokinet* 8: 463, 1983

477. Larsson R, Bodemar G, Norlander B: Oral absorption of cimetidine and its clearance in patients with renal failure. *Eur J Clin Pharmacol* 15: 153, 1979

478. Larsson R, Erlanson P, Bodemar G et al.: The pharmacokinetics of cimetidine and its sulphoxide metabolite in patients with normal and impaired renal function. *Br J Clin Pharmacol* 13: 163, 1982

479. Bjaeldager PA, Jensen JB, Nielsen LP, Larsen NE, Hvidberg EF: Pharmacokinetics of cimetidine in patients undergoing hemodialysis. *Nephron* 34: 159, 1983

480. Krishna DR, Klotz U: Newer H_2-receptor antagonists. Clinical pharmacokinetics and drug interaction potential. *Clin Pharmacokinet* 15: 205, 1988

481. Echizen H, Ishizaki T: Clinical pharmacokinetics of famotidine. *Clin Pharmacokinet* 21: 178, 1991

482. Gladziwa U, Klotz U, Krishna DR, Schmitt H, Glockner WM, Mann H: Pharmacokinetics and dynamics of famotidine in patients with renal failure. *Br J Clin Pharmacol* 26: 315, 1988

483. Halstenson CE, Abraham PA, Opsahl JA, Chremos AN, Keane WF, Matzke GR: Disposition of famotidine in renal insufficiency. *J Clin Pharmacol* 27: 782, 1987

484. Price AH, Brogden RN: Nizatidine: a preliminary review of its pharmacodynamic and pharmacokinetic properties, and its therapeutic use in peptic ulcer disease. *Drugs* 36: 521, 1988

485. Saima S, Echizen H, Yoshimoto K, Ishizaki T: Hemofiltrability of histamine H_2-receptor antagonist, nizatidine, and its metabolites in patients with renal failure. *J Clin Pharmacol* 33: 324, 1993

486. Comstock TJ, Sica DA, Harford A, Eshelman F: Ranitidine bioavailability and disposition kinetics in patients undergoing chronic hemodialysis. *Nephron* 52: 15, 1989

487. Grant SM, Langtry HD, Brogden RN: Ranitidine: an updated review of its pharmacodynamic and pharmacokinetic properties, and therapeutic use in peptic ulcer disease and other allied diseases. *Drugs* 37: 801, 1989

488. Meffin PJ, Grgurinovich N, Brooks PM, Miners JO, Cochran M, Stranks G: Ranitidine disposition in patients with renal impairment. *Br J Clin Pharmacol* 16: 731, 1983

489. Zech PY, Chau NP, Pozet N, Labeeuw M, Hadj-Aissa A: Ranitidine kinetics in chronic renal impairment. *Clin Pharmacol Ther* 34: 667, 1983

490. Barradell LB, Faulds D, McTavish D: Lansoprazole: a review of its pharmacodynamic and pharmacokinetic properties, and its therapeutic efficacy in acid-related disorders. *Drugs* 44: 225, 1992

491. Jones JB, Bailey RT: Misoprostol: a prostaglandin E_1 analog with antisecretory and cytoprotective properties. *DICP, Ann Pharmacother* 23: 276, 1989

492. Howden CW: Clinical pharmacology of omeprazole. *Clin Pharmacokinet* 20: 38, 1991

493. Naesdal J, Andersson T, Bodemar G et al.: Pharmacokinetics of [^{14}C]omeprazole in patients with impaired renal function. *Clin Pharmacol Ther* 40: 344, 1986

494. Burgess E, Muruve D, Audette R: Aluminum absorption and excretion following sucralfate therapy in chronic renal insufficiency. *Am J Med* 92: 471, 1992

495. Roxe DM, Mistovich M, Barch DH: Phosphate-binding effects of sucralfate in patients with chronic renal failure. *Am J Kidney Dis* 13: 194, 1989

496. Eadie MJ: Anticonvulsant drugs. An update. *Drugs* 27: 328, 1984

497. Bertilsson L, Tomson T: Clinical pharmacokinets and pharmacological effects of carbamazepine and carbamazepine-10,11-epoxide: an update. *Clin Pharmacokinet* 11: 177, 1986

498. Lee CS, Wang LH, Marbury TC, Bruni J, Peschalski RJ: Hemodialysis clearance and total body elimination of carbamazepine during chronic hemodialysis. *Clin Toxicol* 17: 429, 1980

499. Marbury TC, Lee CS, Perchalski RJ, Wilder BJ: Hemodialysis clearance of ethosuximide in patients with chronic renal disease. *Am J Hosp Pharm* 38: 1757, 1981

500. Dasgupta A, Abu-Alfa A: Increased free phenytoin concentrations in predialysis serum compared to postdialysis

818   *Thomas A. Golper, Michael A. Marx and Cathryn Shuler*

serum in patients with uremia treated with hemodialysis. *Am J Clin Pathol* 98: 19, 1992

501. Czajka PA, Anderson WH, Christoph RA, Banner W Jr: A pharmacokinetic evaluation of peritoneal dialysis for phenytoin intoxication. *J Clin Pharmacol* 20: 565, 1980

502. Lee CS, Marbury TC, Perchalski RT, Wilder BJ: Pharmacokinetics of primidone elimination by uremic patients. *J Clin Pharmacol* 22: 301, 1982

503. Brewster D, Muir NC: Valproate plasma protein binding in the uremic condition. *Clin Pharmacol Ther* 27: 76, 1980

504. Zaccara G, Messori A, Moroni F: Clinical pharmacokinetics of valproic acid-1988. *Clin Pharmacokinet* 15: 367, 1988

505. Cedarbaum JM: Clinical pharmacokinetics of antiparkinsonian drugs. *Clin Pharmacokinet* 13: 141, 1987

506. Yeh KC, August TF, Bush DF et al.: Pharmacokinetics and bioavailability of sinemet CR: a summary of human studies. *Neurology* 39 (Suppl 2): 25, 1989

507. Burke RE, Fahn S: Pharmacokinetics of trihexyphenidyl after short-term and long-term administration to dystonic patients. *Ann Neurol* 18: 35, 1985

508. Hande K, Noone RM, Stone WJ: Severe allopurinol toxicity: description and guidelines for prevention in patients with renal insufficiency. *Am J Med* 76: 47, 1984

509. Murrel GA, Rapeport WG: Clinical pharmacokinetics of allopurinol. *Clin Pharmacokinet* 11: 343, 1986

510. Wallace SL, Singer JZ, Duncan GJ, Wigley FM, Kuncl RW: Renal function predicts colchicine toxicity: guidelines for the prophylactic use of colchicine in gout. *J Rheumatol* 18: 264, 1991

511. Levy M, Spino M, Read SE: Colchicine: a state of the art review. *Pharmacotherapy* 11: 196, 1991

512. Cunningham RF, Israili ZH, Dayton PG: Clinical pharmacokinetics of probenecid. *Clin Pharmacokinet* 6: 135, 1981

513. Verbeeck RK, Blackburn JL, Loewen GR: Clinical pharmacokinetics of non-steroidal anti-inflammatory drugs. *Clin Pharmacokinet* 8: 297, 1983

514. Todd PA, Sorkin EM: Diclofenac sodium: a reappraisal of its pharmacodynamic and pharmacokinetic properties, and therapeutic efficacy. *Drugs* 35: 244, 1988

515. Eriksson LO, Wahlin-boll E, Odar-Cederlof I, Lindholm L, Melander A: Influence of renal failure, rheumatoid arthritis and old age on the pharmacokinetics of diflunisal. *Eur J Clin Pharmacol* 36: 165, 1989

516. Balfour JA, Buckley MM: Etodolac. A reappraisal of its pharmacology and therapeutic use in rheumatic diseases and pain states. *Drugs* 42: 274, 1991

517. Cefali EA, Poynor WJ, Sica D, Cox S: Pharmacokinetic comparison of flurbiprofen in end-stage renal disease subjects and subjects with normal renal function. *J Clin Pharmacol* 31: 808, 1991

518. Albert KS, Gernaat CM: Pharmacokinetics of ibuprofen. *Am J Med* 77: 40, 1984

519. Skoutakis VA, Acchiardo SR, Carter CA, Wojciechowski NJ, Straun AB, Meyer MC: Dialyzability and pharmacokinetics of indomethacin in adult patients with end-stage renal disease. *Drug Intell Clin Pharm* 20: 956, 1986

520. Williams RL, Upton RA: The clinical pharmacology of ketoprofen. *J Clin Pharmacol* 28 (Suppl 12): S13, 1988

521. Brocks DR, Jamali F: Clinical pharmacokinetics of ketorolac tromethamine. *Clin Pharmacokinet* 23: 415, 1992

522. Todd PA, Clissold SP: Naproxen. A reappraisal of its pharmacology, and therapeutic use in rheumatic diseases and pain states. *Drugs* 40: 91, 1990

523. Verbeeck RK, Richardson CJ, Blocka KL: Clinical pharmacokinetics of piroxicam. *J Rheumatol* 13: 789, 1986

524. Ravis WR, Diskin CJ, Campagna KD, Clark CR, McMillan CL: Pharmacokinetics and dialyzability of sulindac and metabolites in patients with end-stage renal failure. *J Clin Pharmacol* 33: 527, 1993

525. Chaffman M, Brogden RN, Heel RC, Speight TM, Avery GS: Auranofin: a preliminary review of its pharmacological properties and therapeutic use in rheumatoid arthritis. *Drugs* 27: 378, 1984

526. Blocka KL, Paulus HE, Furst DE: Clinical pharmacokinetics of oral and injectable gold compounds. *Clin Pharmacokinet* 11: 133, 1986

527. Levy NB: Psychopharmacology in patients with renal failure. *Int J Psychiatr Med* 20: 325, 1990

528. Preskorn SH, Othmer SC: Evaluation of bupropion hydrochloride: the first of a new class of atypical antidepressants. *Pharmacotherapy* 4: 20, 1984

529. Aronoff GR, Bergstrom RF, Pottratz ST, Sloan RS, Wolen RL, Lemberger L: Fluoxetine kinetics and protein binding in normal and impaired renal function. *Clin Pharmacol Ther* 36: 138, 1984

530. Benfield P, Heel RC, Lewis SP: Fluoxetine. A review of its pharmacodynamic and pharmacokinetic properties, and therapeutic efficacy in depressive illness. *Drugs* 32: 481, 1986

531. Christensen JH, Andreasen F, Jansen J: Pharmacokinetics and pharmacodynamics of thiopental in patients undergoing renal transplantation. *Acta Anaesthesiol Scand* 27: 513, 1983

532. Garzone PD, Kroboth PD: Pharmacokinetics of the newer benzodiazepines. *Clin Pharmacokinet* 16: 337, 1989

533. Schmith VD, Piraino B, Smith RB, Kroboth PD: Alprazolam in end-stage renal disease: I. Pharmacokinetics. *J Clin Pharmacol* 31: 571, 1991

534. Ochs HR, Rauh HW, Greenblatt DJ: Clorazepate dipotassium and diazepam in renal insufficiency: serum concentrations and protein binding of diazepam and desmethyldiazepam. *Nephron* 37: 100, 1984

535. Greenblatt DJ, Shader RI, MacLeod SM, Sellers EM: Clinical pharmacokinetics of chlordiazepoxide. *Clin Pharmacokinet* 3: 381, 1978

536. Morrison G, Chiang ST, Koepke HH, Walker BR: Effect of renal impairment and hemodialysis on lorazepam kinetics. *Clin Pharmacol Ther* 35: 646, 1984

537. Vinik HR, Reves JG, Greenblatt DJ, Abernethy DR, Smith LR: The pharmacokinetics of midazolam in chronic renal failure patients. *Anesthesiology* 59: 390, 1983

538. Ochs HR, Oberem U, Greenblatt DJ: Nitrazepam clearance unimpaired in patients with renal insufficiency. *J Clin Psychopharmacol* 12: 183, 1992

539. Greenblatt DJ, Murray TG, Audet PR, Locniskar A, Koepke HH, Walker BR: Multiple-dose kinetics and dialyzability of oxazepam in renal insufficiency. *Nephron* 34: 234, 1983

540. Ankier SI, Goa KL: Quazepam. A preliminary review of its pharmacodynamic and pharmacokinetic properties, and therapeutic efficacy in insomnia. *Drugs* 35: 42, 1988

541. Kroboth PD, Smith RB, Sorkin MI et al.: Triazolam protein binding and correlation with alpha-1 acid glycoprotein concentration. *Clin Pharmacol Ther* 36: 379, 1984

542. Roth T, Roehrs TA, Zorick FJ: Pharmacology and hypnotic efficacy of triazolam. *Pharmacotherapy* 3: 137, 1983

543. Loo JC, Midha KK, McGilveray IJ: Pharmacokinetics of chlorpromazine in normal volunteers. *Communications in Psychopharmacology* 4: 121, 1980

544. Taylor G, Houston JB, Shaffer J, Mawer G: Pharmacokinetics of promethazine and its sulphoxide metabolite after intravenous and oral administration to man. *Br J Clin Pharmacol* 15: 287, 1983

545. Lieberman JA, Cooper TB, Suckow RF et al.: Tricyclic antidepressant and metabolite levels in chronic renal failure. *Clin Pharmacol Ther* 37: 301, 1985

546. Sandoz M, Vandel S, Vandel B et al.: Metabolism of amitriptyline in patients with chronic renal failure. *Eur J Clin Pharmacol* 26: 227, 1984

547. Tasset JJ, Singh S, Pesce AJ: Evaluation of amitriptyline pharmacokinetics during peritoneal dialysis. *Ther Drug Monit* 7: 255, 1985

548. McTavish D, Benfield P: Clomipramine. An overview of its pharmacological properties and a review of its therapeutic use in obsessive compulsive disorder and panic disorder. *Drugs* 39: 136, 1990

549. DeVane CL, Savett M, Jusko WJ: Desipramine and 2-hydroxy-desipramine pharmacokinetics in normal volunteers. *Eur J Clin Pharmacol* 19: 61, 1981

550. Faulkner RD, Senekjian HO, Lee CS: Hemodialysis of doxepin and desmethyldoxepin in uremic patients. *Artif Organs* 8: 151, 1984

551. Potter WZ, Calil HM, Sutfin TA et al.: Active metabolites of imipramine and desipramine in man. *Clin Pharmacol Ther* 31: 393, 1982

552. Dawling S, Lynn K, Rosser R, Braithwaite R: Nortriptyline metabolism in chronic renal failure: metabolite elimination. *Clin Pharmacol Ther* 32: 322, 1982

553. Ziegler VE, Biggs JT, Wylie LT et al.: Protriptyline kinetics. *Clin Pharmacol Ther* 23: 580, 1978

554. Caccia S, Vigano GL, Mingardi G et al.: Clinical pharmacokinetics of oral buspirone in patients with impaired renal function. *Clin Pharmacokinet* 14: 171, 1988

555. Fitton A, Heel RC: Clozapine. A review of its pharmacological properties, and therapeutic use in schizophrenia. *Drugs* 40: 722, 1990

556. Froemming JS, Lam YW, Jann MW, Davis CM: Pharmacokinetics of haloperidol. *Clin Pharmacokinet* 17: 396, 1989

557. Singer I: Lithium and the kidney. *Kidney Int* 19: 374, 1981

558. Luisier PA, Schultz P, Dick P: The pharmacokinetics of lithium in normal humans: expected and unexpected observations in view of basic kinetic principles. *Pharmacopsychiatry* 20: 232, 1987

559. Mahoney G, Wolfram KM, Cochetto D, Bjorsson TD: Dipyridamole kinetics. *Clin Pharmacol Ther* 31: 330, 1982

560. Kandrotas RJ: Heparin pharmacokinetics and pharmacodynamics. *Clin Pharmacokinet* 22: 359, 1992

561. Grierson DS, Bjornsson TD: Pharmacokinetics of streptokinase in patients based on amidolytic activator complex activity. *Clin Pharmacol Ther* 41: 304, 1987

562. Pedersen AK, Jakobsen P, Kampmann JP, Hansen JM: Clinical pharmacokinetics and potentially important drug interactions of sulphinpyrazone. *Clin Pharmacokinet* 7: 42, 1982

563. McTavish D, Faulds D, Goa KL: Ticlopidine. An updated review of its pharmacology and therapeutic use in platelet-dependent disorders. *Drugs* 40: 238, 1990

564. Collen D, Lijnen HR, Todd PA, Goa KL: Tissue-type plasminogen activator. A review of its pharmacology and therapeutic use as a thrombolytic agent. *Drugs* 38: 346, 1989

565. Holford NH: Clinical pharmacokinetics and pharmacodynamics of warfarin. Understanding the dose-effect relationship. *Clin Pharmacokinet* 11: 483, 1986

566. Paton DP, Webster DR: Clinical pharmacokinetics of H1-receptor antagonists (The antihistamines). *Clin Pharmacokinet* 10: 477, 1985

567. Krstenansky PM, Cluxton RJ: Astemizole: a long-acting, nonsedating antihistamine. *Drugs Intell Clin Pharm* 21: 947, 1987

568. Richards DM, Brogden RM, Heel RC, Speight TM, Avery GS: Oxatomide: a review of its pharmacodynamic properties and therapeutic efficacy. *Drugs* 27: 210, 1984

569. Carter CA, Wojciechowski NJ, Hayes JM, Skoutakis VA, Rickman LA: Terfenadine, a nonsedating antihistamine. *Drug Intell Clin Pharm* 19: 812, 1985

570. Morgan DJ: Clinical pharmacokinetics of beta-agonists. *Clin Pharmacokinet* 18: 270, 1990

571. Friedel HA, Brogden RN: Bitolterol. A preliminary review of its pharmacological properties and therapeutic efficacy in reversible obstructive airways disease. *Drugs* 35: 22, 1988

572. Lee CCU, Wang LH, Majeske BL, Marbury TC: Pharmacokinetics of dyphylline elimination by uremic patients. *J Pharmacol Exp Ther* 217: 340, 1981

573. Bauer LA, Bauer SP, Blouin RA: The effect of acute and chronic renal failure on theophylline clearance. *J Clin Pharmacol* 22: 65, 1982

574. Kradjan WA, Martin TR, Delaney CJ, Blair AD, Cutler RE: Effect of hemodialysis on the pharmacokinetics of theophylline in chronic renal failure. *Nephron* 32: 40, 1982

575. Chan GL, Canafax DM, Johnson CA: The therapeutic use of azathioprine in renal transplantation. *Pharmacotherapy* 7: 165, 1987

576. Salemans J, Hoitsma AJ, De Abreu RA et al.: Pharmacokinetics of azathioprine and 6-mercaptopurine after oral administration of azathioprine. *Clin Transplant* 1: 217, 1987

577. Kawai S, Ichikawa Y, Homma M: Differences in metabolic properties among cortisol, prednisolone, and dexamethasone in liver and renal diseases: accelerated metabolism of dexamethasone in renal failure. *J Clin Endocrinol Metal* 60: 848, 1985

578. Sherlock JE, Letteri JM: Effect of hemodialysis on methylprednisolone plasma levels. *Nephron* 18: 208, 1977

579. Frey BM, Frey FJ: Clinical pharmacokinetics of prednisone and prednisolone. *Clin Pharmacokinet* 19: 126, 1990

580. Follath F, Wenk M, Vozeh S et al.: Intravenous cyclosporine kinetics in renal failure. *Clin Pharmacol Ther* 34: 638, 1983

581. Putcha L, Griffith DP, Feldman S: Pharmacokinetics of acetohydroxamic acid in patients with staghorn renal calculi. *Eur J Clin Pharmacol* 28: 439, 1985

582. Boelaert JR, Fenves AZ, Coburn JW: Deferoxamine therapy and mucormycosis in dialysis patients: report of international registry. *Am J Kidney Dis* 18: 660, 1991

583. Verpooten GA, D'Haese PC, Boelaert JR, Becaus I, Lamberts LV, De Broe ME: Pharmacokinetics of aluminoxamine and ferrioxamine and dose finding of desferrioxamine in haemodialysis patients. *Nephrol Dial Transplant* 7: 931, 1992

584. Silver MR, Kroboth PD: Pentoxifylline in end-stage renal disease. *Drug Intell Clin Pharm* 21: 976, 1987

585. Ward A, Clissold SP: Pentoxifylline. A review of its pharmacodynamic and pharmacokinetic properties, and its therapeutic efficacy. *Drugs* 34: 50, 1987

586. Reetze-Bonorden P, Böhler J, Keller E: Drug dosage in patients during continuous renal replacement therapy. *Clin Pharmacokinet* 24: 362, 1993

587. Kroh UF, Dehne M, El Abed K, Feubner KD, Hofmann W, Lennartz H: Drug dosage during continuous hemofiltration: pharmacokinetics and practical implications. in *Contrib Nephrol*, Vol 93, edited by Sieberth HG, Mann H, Stummvoll HK, Basel, Karger, 1991, p 127

588. Goldman M, Vanherweghem J: Bacterial infections in chronic hemodialysis patients: epidemiologic and pathophysiologic aspects. *Adv Nephrol Necker Hosp* 19: 315, 1990

589. Mailloux LU, Bellucci AG, Wilkes BM et al.: Mortality in dialysis patients: analysis of the causes of death. *Am J Kidney Dis* 18: 326, 1991

590. Manian FA, Stone WJ, Alford RH: Adverse antibiotic effects associated with renal insufficiency. *Rev Infect Dis* 12: 236, 1990

591. Gilbert DN: Once-daily aminoglycoside therapy. *Antimicrob Agents Chemother* 35: 399, 1991

592. Wood CA, Norton DR, Kohlhepp SJ et al.: The influence of tobramycin dosage regimens on nephrotoxicity, ototoxicity, and antibacterial efficacy in a rat model of subcutaneous abscess. *J Infect Dis* 158: 13, 1988

593. Johnson CA, Zimmerman SW, Rogge M: The pharmacokinetics of antibiotics used to treat peritoneal dialysis-associated peritonitis. *Am J Kidney Dis* 4: 3, 1984

594. Keane WF, Everett ED, Golper TA et al.: Peritoneal dialysis-related peritonitis treatment recommendations. 1993 update. *Perit Dial Int* 13: 14, 1993

595. Humes HD: Aminoglycoside nephrotoxicity. *Kidney Int* 33: 900, 1988

596. Cameron JS: Allergic interstitial nephritis: clinical features and pathogenesis. *Q J Med* 66: 97, 1988

597. Shouval D, Ligumsky M, Ben-Ishay D: Effect of cotrimoxazole on normal creatinine clearance. *Lancet* i(8058): 244, 1978

598. Agodoa LY, Held PJ, Port FK: Causes of death. in *US Renal Data System, USRDS 1993 Annual Data Report*, Bethesda, The National Institutes of Health, National Institute of Diabetes and Digestive and Kidney Disease, 1993, p 49

599. Parving HH, Smidt UM, Hommel E et al.: Effective antihypertensive treatment postpones renal insufficiency in diabetic nephropathy. *Am J Kidney Dis* 22: 188, 1993

600. Castelli WP: Epidemiology of coronary heart disease: The Framingham Study. *Am J Med* 76: 4, 1984

601. Fer MF, McKinney TD, Richardson RL, Hande KR, Oldham RK, Greco FA: Cancer and the kidney: renal complications of neoplasms. *Am J Med* 71: 704, 1981

602. Narins RG, Carley M, Bloom EJ, Harrison DS: The nephrotoxicity of chemotherapeutic agents. *Semin Nephrol* 10: 556, 1990

603. Adrogué HJ: Glucose homeostasis and the kidney. *Kidney Int* 42: 1266, 1992

604. Alvestrand A, Mujagic M, Wajngot A, Efendic S: Glucose intolerance in uremic patients: the relative contributions of impaired β-cell function and insulin resistance. *Clin Nephrol* 31: 175, 1989

605. Hager SR: Insulin resistance of uremia. *Am J Kidney Dis* 14: 272, 1989

606. Wideröe TE, Smeby LC, Berg KJ, Jorstad S, Svartas TM: Intraperitoneal (^{125}I) insulin absorption during intermittent and continuous peritoneal dialysis. *Kidney Int* 23: 22, 1983

607. Attma PO, Samuelsson O, Alaupovic P: Lipoprotein metabolism and renal failure. *Am J Kidney Dis* 21: 573, 1993

608. Cheung AK, Wu LL, Kablitz C, Leypoldt JK: Atherogenic lipids and lipoproteins in hemodialysis patients. *Am J Kidney Dis* 22: 271, 1993

609. Joven J, Vilella E, Ahmad S, Cheung MC, Brunzell JD: Lipoprotein heterogeneity in end-stage renal disease. *Kidney Int* 43: 410, 1993

610. Golper TA: Therapy for uremic hyperlipidemia. *Nephron* 38: 217, 1984

611. D'Amico G, Gentile MG: Treatment of hyperlipidemia in human renal disease. *Miner Electrolyte Metab* 19: 196, 1993

612. Orwoll ES: The milk-alkali syndrome: current concepts. *Ann Intern Med* 97: 242, 1982

613. Fraser CL, Arieff AI: Nervous system complications in uremia. *Ann Intern Med* 109: 143, 1988

614. Clive DM, Stoff FS: Renal syndromes associated with nonsteroidal antiinflammatory drugs. *N Engl J Med* 310: 563, 1984

ACUTE RENAL FAILURE

CARL M. KJELLSTRAND and BRENDAN P. TEEHAN

INTRODUCTION

The introduction of the artificial kidney into clinical practice in 1943 by Kolff in the Netherlands, and in 1947 by Alwall in Sweden and Murray in Canada was an astounding technical breakthrough in modern medicine (1–3). Subsequently, the most frequent abnormality for which dialysis has been used acutely has been acute tubular necrosis. It is the diagnosis in approximately two-thirds of all patients dialyzed for acute renal failure.

Since 1950, many groups have presented their clinical experiences with large series of patients (4–10). (The his-

torical development of dialysis is described in Chapters 3 and 22.)

Unfortunately, the mortality rate in patients with acute tubular necrosis, except for some early gains (11), has not improved. It remains between 30% and 80% depending mainly on the severity of the underlying precipitating event. On the other hand, the one year mortality rate of patients dialyzed for chronic renal failure has decreased from 50 to 15% over the last 20 years. The lower mortality rate in patients treated by dialysis for chronic renal failure reflects technical improvements of the dialysis procedure. The lack of improvement of mortality in patients with acute renal failure has two explanations: the patients are now much sicker than those treated in the early days of hemodialysis. Many milder cases of acute tubular necrosis are now treated with improved fluid management, cardiovascular monitoring and potent diuretics (5–7). Secondly, the causes of death in most instances are infections and multi-organ failure, and these causes are not amenable to improvements in dialysis technology.

This chapter touches upon the major causes of acute renal failure and both conservative and dialysis treatments. The focus however will be on the technical aspects of dialysis. This has become more complicated, as the new methods of continuous hemofiltration and/or hemodialysis have come of age. The clinical situations where the relative advantage of each method is best utilized are presently being established.

INCIDENCE OF ACUTE RENAL FAILURE, NEED FOR DIALYSIS

The largest effort to establish the incidence was the European Dialysis and Transplant Association survey from 32 countries. It found a mean of 28.9 (range was 0.4 to 177.1) patients per million population per year that required dialysis for acute renal failure (11). The highest incidence occurred in countries in war conditions. As only centers performing chronic dialysis were questioned the true incidence is probably higher. Several individual teams investigating the need for dialysis for acute renal failure have concluded that 30–60 patients per million population need dialysis yearly (12–17).

For every patient with acute renal failure that requires dialysis there are 10–12 patients with milder forms of renal insufficiency, manageable by conservative treatment (17). A recent survey from England found an overall incidence of acute renal failure of 140 per million population per year, 18 of whom needed dialysis (14).

The clinical course of these patients is swift, typically requiring only four dialyses (10) before either death or recovery occurs, almost always within one month. Thus, in industrialised countries there is a need of 100–200 dialyses per million population per year for acute renal failure.

CAUSES OF ACUTE RENAL FAILURE, GENERAL WORKUP OF PATIENTS

The most common disease, leading to acute renal failure is acute tubular necrosis, responsible for about 80% of such cases. Of these one-quarter are an acute exacerbation of underlying chronic renal disease. Approximately 12% of these patients have primary parenchymal disease (glomerulonephritis, vasculitis, other immunological diseases, hemolytic–uremic syndrome, interstitial nephritis). Five percent of the patients have post-renal obstruction (Figure 1) (4–15).

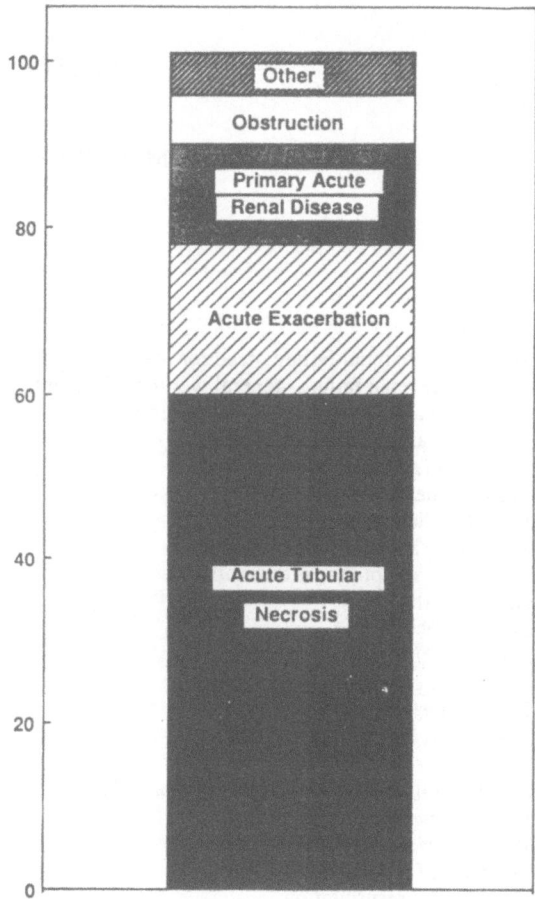

Figure 1. The most common cause of acute renal failure is acute tubular necrosis either in patients with normal renal function or also commonly in those with underlying chronic renal failure. This syndrome makes up approximately 80% of all cases of acute renal failure.

Over the five decades acute dialysis has been available there has been little change in the relative frequency of the diseases causing acute renal failure. However, with time there has been a marked change in the causes of acute tubular necrosis (Figure 2). Before the mid-1970s, surgery and trauma were the most common cause of acute tubular necrosis (18). Now the disease is usually secondary to medical disorders (volume contraction and decreased cardiac output) and from iatrogenic toxins: antibiotics, ACE-inhibitors, non-steroidal anti-inflammatory drugs, contrast media, diuretics and antihypertensives (17, 18).

Symptomatic and supportive treatments are usually all that can be offered to patients with acute renal failure. Despite suggestions that early treatment of tubular necrosis may change its natural course, the main-stay of treatment is supportive while awaiting spontaneous recovery of renal function. The same is true for most patients with an acute exacerbation of chronic renal failure. When urinary obstruction occurs, urinary flow must be re-established,

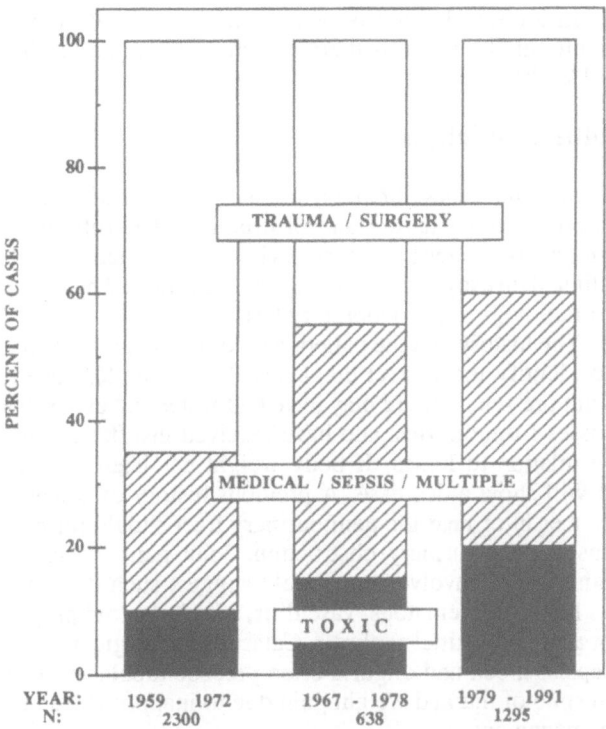

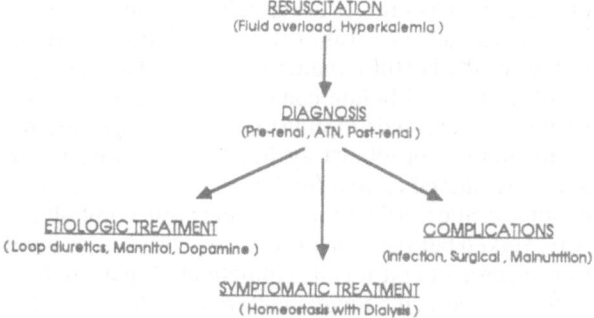

Figure 3. Schedule of approach to management of patients with acute renal failure.

Figure 2. The underlying problem leading to acute tubular necrosis. These causes have changed from trauma and surgery to increasingly being due to toxic iatrogenic renal disease or acute renal failure occurring in the setting of medical disease, sepsis, and often with multiple contributory causes combining ischemia and renal toxins.

e.g., through surgery, in order to achieve return of renal function. Similarly, when the kidney is under-perfused, this abnormality must be corrected. Renal cortical necrosis exemplifies lesions that begin acutely, require considerable supportive management, do not respond to any treatment and result in severe persistent impairment of renal function.

Patients who suffer from such parenchymal renal diseases as glomerulonephritis, Goodpasture's syndrome, hemolytic-uremic syndrome, acute interstitial nephritis or vasculitis, pose a particularly difficult and unresolved dilemma. All etiologic treatments of these disorders, such as immunosuppression, corticosteroids, anticoagulation, plasmapheresis and intravenous gammaglobulin, carry considerable risk in both morbidity and mortality. There is as yet no satisfactory answer of what treatment is best for most of these patients. In the rare patient who suffers from systemic disease with life threatening involvement of other organs systems, the solution is easy. Almost any form of treatment that may benefit the patient, should be tried.

When the manifestations of the disease are only renal however, a dilemma arises. The benefits and dangers of combinations of immunosuppression, prednisone, antico-

agulation and plasma and cyta-pheresis must be weighed against the low mortality rate in patients with chronic renal failure treated by dialysis. Astounding successes have been achieved in individual cases but mortability has also resulted from the treatment.

The rest of this chapter will be devoted to acute tubular necrosis. However, the sections regarding symptomatic and supportive treatment apply to all patients with acute renal failure.

Figure 3 outlines the basic approach when a patient develops acute renal failure. Immediate dangers in such patients include fluid overload with pulmonary edema and hyperkalemia with cardiac arrest. After guarding against these, diagnosis takes place differentiating pre- and post-renal failure from acute tubular necrosis. Treatment with fluid or cardiotonics or both in the patients with pre-renal failure, removal of obstruction in those with post-renal failure, and possibly a trial of renal vasodilator-diuretics in the patient with acute tubular necrosis is then undertaken. Should these efforts fail, homeostasis is maintained with dialysis, and a constant watch for specific complications is instituted.

PATHOGENESIS, PATHOPHYSIOLOGY, AND DIFFERENTIAL DIAGNOSIS OF ACUTE RENAL FAILURE

Experimental studies

The etiology, pathogenesis and pathophysiology of acute tubular necrosis are of interest in experimental research. Ideally, an animal model should meet several criteria. The initiating factors should be identical to those operating in acute tubular necrosis in humans, a situation where multiple factors are usually involved. Secondly, it should be possible to determine the transition point from subclinical renal illness to clinical acute renal failure, the point of no return. Five models presently used frequently are: renal artery constriction, intrarenal norepinephrine, intramuscular glycerol, mercuric chloride and uranyl nitrate. None of these models mimics accurately most situations causing acute tubular necrosis in humans and the interpretation of the results is still a matter of debate. The pathogenesis of acute renal failure could involve perpetuated renal ischemia, decreased filtration through a changed glomerular membrane, or tubular dysfunction with a backleak of normally filtered tubular fluid, alone or in various combinations. Acute renal failure can occur with morphologically preserved but functionally damaged tubules, or involve frank necrosis of the tubular epithelium. When tubular cell necrosis occurs, the tubular cell may be shed of its basement membrane and potentially cause obstruction with increased intraluminal hydrostatic pressure. Almost any of these events can be found at one point or another in the various models described above. It has become clear that none of them very faithfully mimic the human situation that seems to evolve through many stages (19–25). However, at least two animal models combine ischemia and nephrotoxicity and both show a synergistic detrimental effect on renal function (26, 27).

Clinical studies

Figure 4 summarizes factors precipitating and perpetuating acute tubular necrosis. There may be two principal initiating events, ischemia and nephrotoxicity. Clinically, there is almost always a mixture of these factors. Thus, nephrotoxic proteins such as myoglobin and hemoglobin may cause both direct tubular damage and ischemia or obstruction. Conversely, factors that cause ischemia may lead to release of nephrotoxic substances such as myoglobin or nephrotoxic drugs may be given to the patient.

A number of factors cause renal ischemia without necessarily decreasing systemic blood pressure. These include dehydration secondary to burns, edema into non-traumatized tissue, diarrhea, vomiting and sequestration of extracellular fluid due to ileus, or retroperitoneally in such conditions as acute pancreatitis or after surgery. Similarly, any reduction in cardiac output following myocardial dysfunction or reduction of the circulating blood volume or the ratio of blood volume to capacitance of the vascular system such as may occur in bacterial gram negative sepsis, endotoxemia or anaphylactic reactions, can also cause acute tubular necrosis. Surgery and general anaesthesia uniformly decrease renal blood flow.

Almost no critically ill patients escape being treated with drugs that are potentially nephrotoxic. Aminoglycoside and cephalosporin antibiotics are used especially frequently in this circumstance. Increasingly, diagnostic procedures also cause problems such as nephropathy following contrast radiography (28). Self-inflicted intoxication with such substances as ethylene glycol and carbon tetrachloride is less frequent. Certain endogenously produced substances such as uric acid, calcium, myoglobin and hemoglobin, are also potentially nephrotoxic.

In a clinical analysis of 145 patients who developed acute tubular necrosis there was more than one insult in 74% (29).

Differential diagnosis

In most instances, tubular necrosis is easily distinguished from pre-renal failure and obstruction. The differential diagnosis is made by history, review of the patient's charts, clinical investigation, and frequently confirmed by a series of radiological and laboratory tests.

The history and the patient's records often reveal clues to identify the correct diagnosis. For example, patients with pre-renal failure may have had water and electrolyte losses from diarrhea and have received insufficient fluid in relation to losses. If body weight has been recorded it will show a decrease. A previous history of stones or cancer in or near the genitourinary tract should raise the suspicion of urinary obstruction. Joint pain, rashes, or other organ involvement should suggest such diagnoses as lupus erythematous, vasculitis, anaphylactoid purpura or acute interstitial nephritis. Catastrophic surgical events, sepsis, shock and oliguria often precede tubular necrosis in spite of marked weight gain due to inappropriate fluid management.

It used to be believed that urinary volume was a good indicator of kidney function and that acute tubular necrosis was usually signalled by oliguria. It has been increasingly recognized however that polyuria is common in acute tubular necrosis, particularly when caused by antibiotics. Even more confusing is the finding that patients with severe dehydration and pre-renal failure may continue to make large amounts of urine (30). Patients with partial urinary tract obstruction may also have normal or increased urinary output. However, absolute anuria, particularly when interspersed with episodes of polyuria, suggests obstruction.

On physical examination, the patient with marked pre-renal failure shows sunken eyes, central venous and pulmonary wedge pressures are low, skin turgor is decreased and orthostatic hypotension is present. These classical findings of extracellular fluid volume depletion may be absent however in some patients who have pre-renal azotemia due to a decreased cardiac output (with markedly increased total body water because of edema). This is most commonly encountered in patients with heart failure secondary to myocardial infarction or after heart surgery for valve replacement or coronary artery bypass. A septic patient also may suffer from a sudden decrease in effective blood volume secondary to decreased tone of capacitance vessels without a decrease in total body fluid volume.

There is no typical physical finding in patients with acute tubular necrosis. Many such patients however have signs of fluid overload (edema, fluid lung or frank pulmonary edema) secondary to inappropriate fluid management. Patients with urinary obstruction may have a large urinary bladder and (or) a pelvic mass.

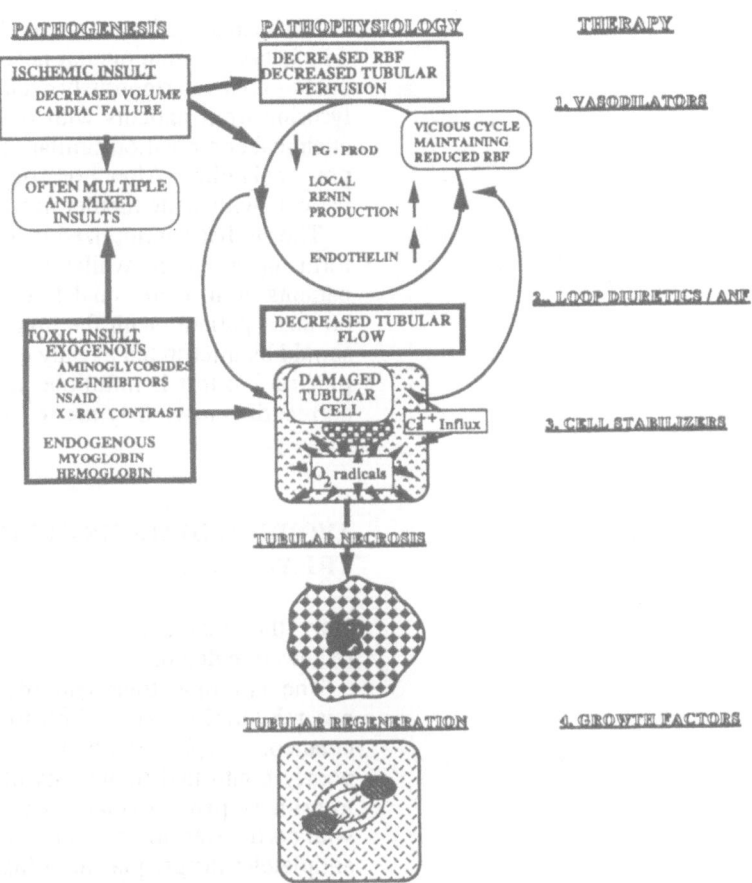

Figure 4. Summary of the pathogenical pathophysiologic events that follow ischemic or nephrotoxic insult to the kidneys in the clinical situation. Several vicious feedback loops perpetuate or aggravate decreased tubular flow, renal ischemia and tubular cell injury. With either an ischemic insult or a toxic insult there is decresed tubular flow. Prostaglandin production decreases and the transport of vasodilatory prostaglandin back to the juxta-glomerula apparatus decreases. Local renin production continuous further to renal ischemia as does the local release of endothelin. Even when the tubular cell damage by a toxic or ischemic insult is over, these mechanisms continue to further damage the tubular cells. This in turn results in calcium influx and release of oxygen radicals that finally leads to full-blown tubular necrosis. Simultaneously with these mechanisms tubular regeneration from still viable cells starts to take place.

Radiological procedures are often helpful, particularly in the diagnostic of obstruction. Thus, ultrasonography, computerized axial tomography or radioisotope renography, with or without furosemide administration, demonstrate a dilated renal pelvis.

Ultrasonography of the obstructed kidney gives particularly accurate diagnostic information. It has a low incidence of false positive and false negative findings. Some cases, however, will require cystoscopy and retrograde or antegrade pyelography for a definitive diagnosis (31–33).

Radiologic tests are less useful in differentiating between pre-renal failure and acute tubular necrosis. The kidneys tend to be small in pre-renal failure and enlarged in acute tubular necrosis, but these are unreliable signs. Radiologic examination of the chest is very important however for the diagnosis of fluid overload in the lungs.

Some patients have a low cardiac output but marked increase in total body water so that paradoxically they suffer both the fluid excess and pre-renal failure.

The numerous diagnostic tests used to differentiate pre-renal failure from acute tubular necrosis are listed in Table 1. The physiologic hypotheses is that with pre-renal failure, glomerular filtrate is modified considerably by the intact tubules under maximum ADH and aldosterone stimulation. To the contrary, with acute tubular necrosis or urinary tract obstruction the renal tubule modifies the glomerular filtrate very little.

The literature regarding the accuracy of these tests is confusing and has recently been summarized (34, 35). When first described, many of these tests were considered highly accurate, but later were found to be of very limited or no use, a frequent fate of medical tests (36). There is also no unanimity regarding the values that differentiate

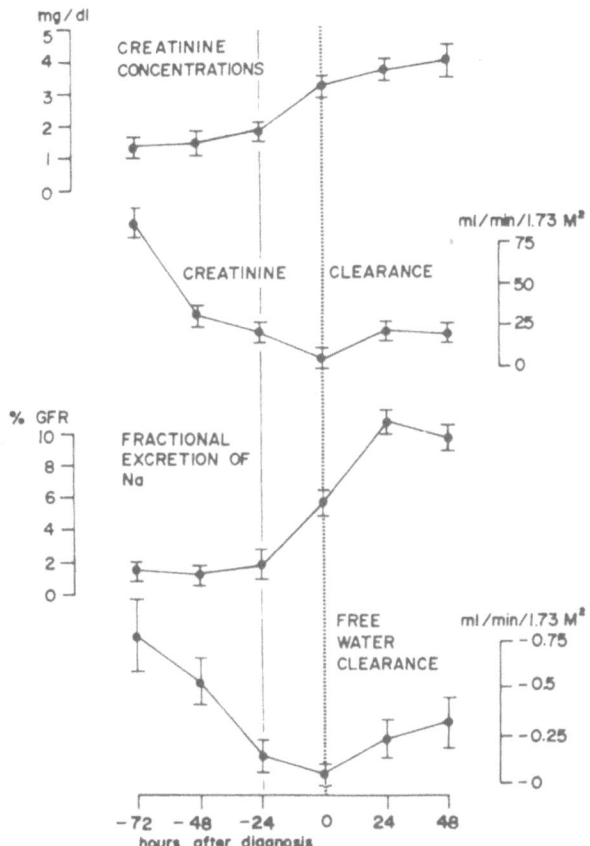

Figure 5. Serial changes in tests of renal function in 13 patients followed prospectively and who developed acute renal failure. The dotted vertical line indicate a time when 3 of the 4 criteria for renal failure were met (free water clearance higher than 0 ml/min, creatinine clearance < 30 ml/min, FeNa > 3% and persistently rising serum creatinine). The solid vertical line indicates a time, 24 hours earlier, when the diagnosis of renal failure was established by changes in creatinine clearance and free water clearance. These two latter parameters change earlier than FeNa or serum creatinine concentrations. One must do a repeated test for the earliest possible diagnosis. Figure reproduced from (37) with permission.

acute tubular necrosis from pre-renal failure. For example, the urine sodium concentration or the urine to plasma creatinine concentration ratio, reported to be suggestive of acute tubular necrosis, varies almost ten-fold.

The fractional excretion of sodium (FENa) is not even accurate. Serial free water and creatinine clearances may be the best tests differentiating pre-renal failure from acute tubular necrosis (Figure 5) (37). Pre-renal failure is a very common precursor of acute tubular necrosis. Pre-renal failure and acute tubular necrosis may succeed each other or even co-exist in a patient (35). Often therefore, a specific diagnosis of either tubular necrosis or pre-renal failure cannot be made definitively; many patients have findings that fluctuate between the two entities.

The urinary sediment should be a good test to differentiate between acute tubular necrosis and pre-renal failure but has not been rigorously evaluated in recent years. Early urine from patients with obstruction tends to have a chemical composition similar to urine from patients with pre-renal failure. After 2 or 3 days it resembles urine from patients with acute tubular necrosis (34).

The studies summarized in Table 1 are all easy to perform and should be available in any hospital dealing with patients with acute renal failure. They should be done on these patients with the understanding that the results should be interpreted as only one part of the total clinical picture. No test is infallible: most are only clues to the correct diagnosis, they are most reliable when employed serially.

AVOIDING DIALYSIS – ETIOLOGIC TREATMENT

Only the treatment of acute tubular necrosis will be reviewed in detail.

The etiologic treatment of dehydration is a vigorous rehydration, and of obstruction, operative or percutaneous nephrostomy drainage. The dangerous and poorly controlled treatments of acute renal failure due to primary parenchymal renal disease include treatment with corticosteroids, various cytostatics, anticoagulation, antiplatelet drugs, plasma infusion, plasmapheresis and cytapheresis will not be further examined.

The aim of the treatment of acute tubular necrosis is to stop the progress of the renal failure and inhibit the feedback loops and should restore renal bloodflow, increase tubular flow of urine, and repair ongoing intracellular injury.

Figure 4 summarizes a possible scheme for the etiology, pathogenesis and pathophysiology of acute tubular necrosis. In the clinical situation, as noted above, there are almost always several factors operative. The first step in treatment is to review the patients' medications. If possible, those that are potentially nephrotoxic should be discontinued.

The key element in the ischemic pathway leading to acute tubular necrosis is decreased renal blood flow and a final common pathway for acute renal failure, independent of nephrotoxicity or ischemia, is a decrease in tubular fluid flow.

Changes in the rate of delivery of salt and water to the distal tubuli, sensed at the macula densa, also can stimulate renin release, causing renal ischemia. A decrease in renal medullary vasodilator prostaglandin activity can also contribute to the decrease in renal blood flow. These factors may perpetuate renal ischemia. Drugs that increase renal blood flow and/or tubular flow, could thus theoretically influence the development of acute tubular necrosis. Finally, drugs that stabilize the intracellular mileau could be beneficial.

Table 1. Differential diagnosis between pre-renal failure and acute tubular necrosis

Test	Pre-renal failure	Acute tubular necrosis
Urinary specific gravity	> 1.030	< 1.020
Urinary osmolality	> 400 mOsm/kg/H$_2$O	< 350 mOsm/kg/H$_2$O
Urine/plasma osmolal ratio	> 1.4	< 1.1
Urine/plasma creatinine ratio	> 30	< 20
Urine/plasma urea ratio	> 7	< 5
Serum urea N/creatinine ratio	> 10	< 10
Urinary sodium concentration	< 30 mmol/l	> 30 mmol/l
Excreted/filtered sodium	< 1%	> 2%
Renal failure index	< 1	> 1
Free water clearance	Negative	Rising to 0
2 h creatinine clearance	Stable	Falling
Urinary sediment	Hyaline or finely granular casts	Tubular cell casts Coarse granular casts
Proteinuria	0+ to 1+	1+ to 2+

Loop diuretics increase both renal blood flow and tubular fluid flow rates. Mannitol, ethacrynic acid and furosemide have each been used clinically a) prophylactically, b) as a treatment for aborting incipient acute tubular necrosis or shortening its clinical course, and c) to change oliguria to non-oliguria. Several clinical trials of these drugs have been undertaken; few of these have been controlled or randomized. Controlled trials have shown that furosimide, particularly when combined with dopamine in daily dose up to 4,000 mg, can change oliguric acute tubular necrosis to non-oliguria, thus easing management or will appreciably shorten both the anuric period and perhaps the time it takes for the plasma creatinine concentration to fall to normal values. These drugs are potentially effective only when used early during the development of acute renal failure. In many patients they induce diuresis. Investigators, reviewing the reports of treatment of acute tubular necrosis with diuretics and mannitol, have found suggestive evidence that many patients respond by changing from oliguria to a diuresis, but that mortality rates are not decreased. The data have recently been reviewed (38, 39).

Clinical and experimental data suggest that low-dose intravenous dopamine, infused at a rate of 1 μg/kg/min, may also change oliguria to diuresis (40, 41). Experimental studies suggest that a combination of dopamine and furosemide may be more effective (42). Recent experiments also indicate that atrial natriuretic factor, a potent diuretic and vasodilator of the renal bed, is of benefit in renal ischemic injury (43). A large multi-institutional study will soon be completed. Finally, damage can theoretically be repaired by the use of xanthine oxidase inhibitors, calcium channel blockers, free oxygen radical scavengers, and the infusions of intracellular substances, particularly magnesium, nucleotides, and amino acids (44–51). Both the experimental and clinical studies of this approach are controversial. Many drugs cannot be used in patients because of the risk of toxicity. One exception is the use of intravenous amino acids. Some have found that they decrease the creatinine elevation and lower the mortality rate in patients with acute tubular necrosis. Others have found them useless (52, 53). Amino acids in experimental acute renal failure have been reported both to improve and worsen renal function and to lower and increase mortality.

Recently, two new groups of substances Calcitonin Gene Related Peptide and growth factors have been found to ameliorate acute renal failure in animals. (54, 55).

The clinical management of acute tubular necrosis is also obviously controversial. Some nephrologists believe there is no true etiologic treatment and will do nothing further after fluid volumes have been restored and cardiac output maximized. Others will use dopamine, mannitol, and furosamide alone or in combination. We suggest that patient with a creatinine of less than 5 mg/dl should be treated with dopamine infused at a rate of 1 mcg/kg/minute and with rapidly increasing doses of furosemide, approximately 2–5–10 mg/kg infused at hourly intervals over a 15–20 minute period to decrease the oto-toxicity of a high peak level. If diuresis occurs it can often be maintained by continued infusion of mannitol and furosemide. A 60 kg adult will be infused with 500 ml, 20% mannitol to which has been added the furosemide dose to which the patient responded, at a rate of 20 ml/h. This often maintains diuresis and sometimes creatinine levels also decreases. Even without a fall in creatinine, the diuresis makes the conservative management of such a patient much easier. Osmolality must frequently be checked by determinations of actual and calculated blood osmolality to avoid manni-

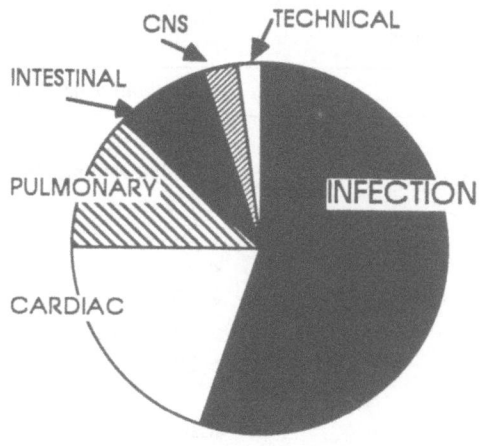

Figure 6. Summary of causes of death in approximately 2,000 reported patients dialyzed for acute renal failure.

tol intoxication (56). Rare side effects of furosemide are pancreatitis and deafness.

Some cases of acute renal failure resolve if an increased abdominal pressure is reduced to normal (57, 58).

CAUSE OF DEATH AND PROGNOSTIC FACTORS

Cause of death

The cause of death in patients dialyzed for acute renal failure is depicted in Figure 6. Infections are the most common cause of death in almost all reports. Infection is often complicated by progressive sequential system failure. Cardiac disease is the next most common cause of death. Death occurs secondary to acute myocardial infarction or irreversible cardiac failure in the old patient with degenerative vascular disease. Gastrointestinal disease (hemorrhage or perforation) and pulmonary insufficiency come next but intestinal hemorrhage has decreased with early more frequent dialysis. Some patients die from irreversible central nervous disease, secondary to bleeding, brain edema or unexplained coma. This general problem shows only slight variation with geographical location and clinical setting (59–66). A few patients die from hyperkalemia, digitalis intoxication, and technical dialysis mishaps. Although these latter tend to be underreported (67) they should occur then less in 1 of 50,000 dialyses (68, 69). Thus, most patients die of infections, organ system failure or irreversible, underlying diseases. The exact role of each is poorly understood. Infection often seems complicated by organ system failure.

Prognostic factors

Patients with acute renal failure are often extremely ill and need high technology medicine in an intensive care setting. This treatment is often extremely uncomfortable to patients, frightening to relatives, expensive and the beds in the intensive care units are limited. Exact prognosis, so one could avoid to unnecessarily treat patients, who are invariably going to die of their acute illness, would thus be of great benefit to all. In spite of many attempts, there is confusion as to what factor is of prognostic importance for survival in those who need dialysis. Age, sex, infections, organ failure, degree of renal failure and a number of treatment variables have all been alternatively accepted as important variables or been shown to be useless in prognostication. Mortality is thus very high and prognostic variables are unknown and disputed in acute renal failure.

Demographic factors

Sex has not been found to influence the outcome in patients dialyzed for acute renal failure.

The influence of age is controversial. Some have found a direct relationship between age and mortality (4, 66). In one series the mortality in patients below age 29 was 39% and rose to almost 80% in patients over the age of 80. Some groups reported a U-shaped relationship between survival and age: the lowest survival was encountered in the youngest and the very oldest patients (10, 70). Most have found age to be of no importance for survival in patients dialyzed for acute renal failure (17, 71).

The time period of dialysis is of no importance (4, 7, 17, 71–73). There has been no improvement in survival in war-induced acute renal failure.

Co-morbid condition

Most have found a history of pre-existing disease to be of no importance (71, 74, 75).

Basic underlying disease

The basic disease causing acute tubular necrosis is one of the most important factors in determining survival. Gastrointestinal and cardiovascular surgery have particularly high mortality rates, around 80%. The mortality in patients with underlying medical disease is now also high. Acute renal failure, secondary to obstruction and urological surgery, usually carries a low mortality rate (4, 7–10, 70, 72).

Type and degree of renal failure

Survival after toxic and ischemic acute tubular necrosis is similar (17). A higher survival has been reported by some in non-oliguric renal failure. A 26% mortality rate occurred in non-oliguric patients compared to 50% in those with oliguria. The figures were 58% and 82% in another study (66, 74, 76). Others have found no difference in mortality between oliguric or non-oliguric patients when stratifying for age and underlying disease (71, 75).

In one study, there was a direct, linear correlation between the degree of creatininemia and mortality in non-dialyzed patients with acute renal failure. It was the most important factor associated with death, of six factors studied (17).

Signs of infections

Infections are the most common cause of death in acute renal failure. A direct relation between the number of infections and mortality has been observed. Survival was 80% in the non-infected patient and less than 30% in patients with four or more infections (70). In 50 patients with acute renal failure after aortic aneurysm surgery, there was decreased survival in patients who had a temperature over 100°F, or a white cell count over 10,000 WBCs per mm^3, if persisting two weeks after the onset of renal failure. No patient with positive blood cultures during antibiotic coverage survived (71). Many others have similar findings of a dismal outcome in septic patients (77–80), but in others it was of no importance (75, 81).

Complicating disorders, 'organ system failure'

'Organ system failure' is a poor prognostic sign in patients dialyzed for acute renal failure. It is often secondary to severe infection (80–83). In one study, over 90% of the patients survived if no other organ system than the kidneys failed, but less than 30% of those with more than seven organs failing, survived (70, 73). Pulmonary complications and central nervous system dysfunction (66, 71, 74, 75, 78–80) in particular occur more often in patients who die than in those who survive. The influence on survival by cardiac problems or gastrointestinal problems is less certain. It is difficult to know whether 'organ system failure' is due to primary incurable disease, or occurs secondary to infections. The data have recently been reviewed (80).

Type and quantity of dialysis

Since the introduction of early start and the use of daily or every-other-day dialysis, there is no difference in pre-dialysis chemistries between survivors and patients who die (17, 84). There was no difference in survival at any time between comparable patients who had immediate renal function, and those who needed dialysis for acute renal failure following transplantation (85).

In the most thorough, recent comparison of daily to every-other-day dialysis, survival was equivalent, 41% in daily, 53% in the every-other-day group. BUN was 60 mg/dl, creatinine 5.3 mg/dl, bicarbonate 23 m Mol/l, PO$_4$ 4.3 mg/dl, and pH 7.42 in the daily versus 101 mg/dl, 9.1 mg/dl, 18 mmol/l, 6.7 mg/dl and 7.35 respectively (86). Thus, dialysis *per se*, is almost never a cause of death and present every-other-day treatment schedules seem to achieve maximal survival.

In several comparisons of peritoneal dialysis to hemodialysis for acute renal failure, there is no difference in survival, nor is there any dramatic difference in survival between continuous and intermittent hemodialysis (5, 86–89).

Multifactorial prognostic formulae

Using multifactorial statistical analysis, several teams have tried to create formulas predicting death and survival. In one study of 17 factors influencing survival in 300 patients with post-operative acute renal failure, a linear discriminant function was derived. It included 7 factors (age, transfusions, cardiac surgery, cardiac failure, sex, vascular surgery and interval to dialysis). The only variable that could be influenced was the creatinine level before the first dialysis. It was 6.6 ± 1.7 mg/dl in survivors and 8.6 ± 7.8 mg/dl in patients who died (81).

The combination of sepsis, respiratory failure and oliguria in 151 patients was associated with almost no survival (79). In another study of 58 dialyzed patients, CNS dysfunction, the use of inotropic drugs and old age were bad prognosticators (75). In a third study of 148 patients, seen by a nephrologist, 10 factors (acute cardiac illness, cancer, oliguria, pancreatitis, trauma, pre-existing renal- and heart disease, CNS and respiratory failure and surgery) could be used for an accurate discriminatory score predicting death.

Summary of prognostic factors

No group has derived a perfect predictive index in patients who develop acute renal failure. However, the combination of sepsis, CNS and respiratory failure in patients with acute renal failure, particularly if the patient is elderly and post-operative, should make one strongly consider using only conservative management. Unfortunately, the created instruments of prediction appears useful only in the institution where they were created. A large international, multi-institutional study of prognostic factors is being planned (Solez K, personal communication).

TREATMENT EARLY: RESUSCITATION

Patients with acute renal failure are frequently very ill, often suffer iatrogenic disease and half of them will die. Time is running out and there is little margin for error. The differential diagnosis maybe impossible without an extended time to evaluate the situation and the psychological pressure on the nephrologist is heavy. It is therefore necessary to approach and solve the problems in a logical order described in Figure 3.

First, immediate dangers to the patient's life must be removed. Then the differential diagnosis resolved and etiological treatment tried, as outlined in the section on 'Avoiding dialysis – Etiologic Treatment'. If this fails, one must decrease the chance of complications, particularly

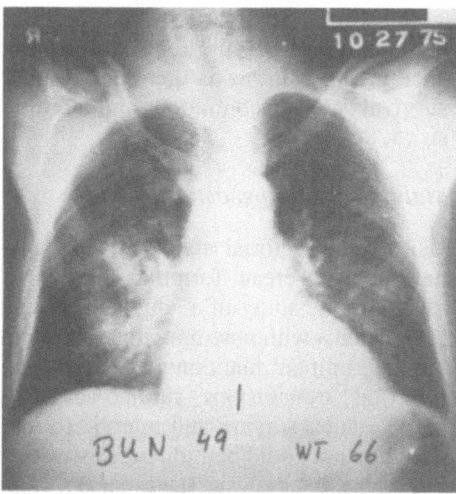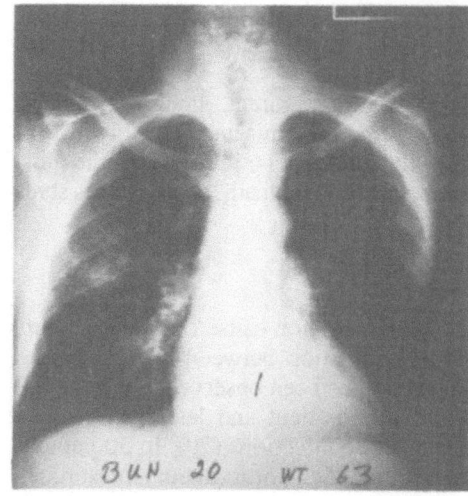

Figure 7. Classical appearance of fluid overload in a uremic patient. Note the occurrence of the central (butterfly or bat-wing pattern) pulmonary edema. The infiltration rapidly clears with fluid removal by ultrafiltration in this patient. The first chest x-ray taken in the morning before dialysis, the second one the evening of the same day after dialysis with a 3 kg fluid removal. From (92) with permission.

infectious and metabolic, by conservative and dialysis treatment.

Immediately after the onset of acute renal failure, two main threats to the patient's life arise. One is fluid overload, almost always iatrogenic, as excessive fluids are often used to treat real or imagined dehydration. The second problem is hyperkalemia, due both to the release of potassium from traumatized, damaged tissue and hematoma, as well as from shifts from the intracellular to the extracellular space, because of the acidosis that is almost uniformly present in such patients.

Fluid overload

Assessment of a patient's fluid state requires daily measurements of bodyweight, an accurate review of intake and output and continuous monitoring of fluid balance. Even when all these data are available it is difficult to deal with such patients because of the impossibility of quantifying third spaced (sequestered) fluid volume accurately. See also the section on 'Differential diagnosis'.

The most dangerous complication of fluid overload is fluid lung (pulmonary edema, uremic 'pneumonitis').

Patients with acute renal failure frequently have a decreased plasma oncotic pressure, an increased hydrostatic pressure in pulmonary capillaries because of fluid overload, and subtle capillary injury in their lungs, particularly in the perihilar region. All these factors make such patients susceptible to pulmonary edema (4, 90, 91). Figure 7 shows the typical perihilar x-ray localization of fluid. The edema is rarely atypical but may then be difficult to differentiate from infections or pulmonary emboli (4, 92, 93) and may cause hemoptysis. The x-rays of one

such patient with lobar pulmonary edema, indistinguishable from pneumonia, are shown in Figure 8.

During the acute restoration phase, invasive monitoring of blood pressure, central venous pressure (CVP), cardiac output and pulmonary arterial and wedge pressures are often necessary to maximise volumes without causing pulmonary edema (94, 95).

A mild degree of fluid overload can sometimes be treated simply by not replacing ongoing output. In more urgent situations, oral sorbitol (70% solution, 2 ml/kg) or rectal sorbitol (20% solution, 10 ml/kg) can be used, provided that the gastrointestinal tract is functional (4, 96). Up to 5 kg per day of fluid can be removed this way. Furosemide may contribute to clearing of the pulmonary edema even in oliguric patients by increasing venous capacitance (96). Severe fluid overload is one of the classical indications for emergency dialysis with ultrafiltration.

Hyperkalemia

The second lethal threat to a patient with acute renal failure is hyperkalemia. It is frequently associated with acidosis and necrosis of large organs or muscle (97). It is disproportionally high in acute renal failure caused by non-steroidal anti-inflammatory drugs (98). Hyperkalemia causes cardiac conduction defects, leading to ectopic rhythms ending in ventricular fibrillation or asystole. Figure 9 illustrates the electro-cardiographic changes encountered in hyperkalemia and the approximate plasma potassium levels at which they occur. Rarely, electro-cardiographic changes are indistinguishable from those of myocardial infarction in extreme hyperkalemia (99). The treatment of hyperkalemia consists of antagonizing the effects on the

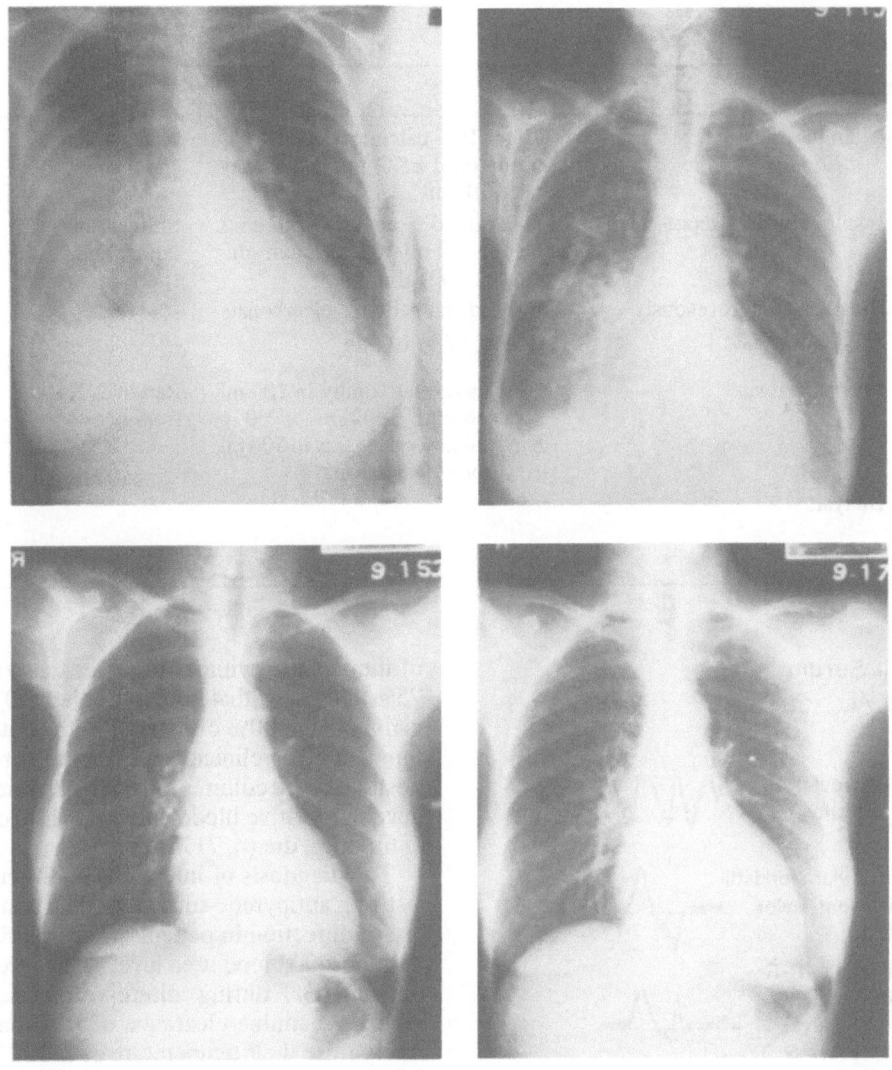

Figure 8. Lobar pulmonary edema in a patient with renal failure. Top left picture was taken immediately before dialysis; the second top right picture 5 hours later after 5 kg fluid removal with dialysis. The lower left picture was taken the next morning with a further 1 kg weight loss induced by diarrhea. The bottom right picture was taken 3 days after dialysis with no further fluid removal.

myocardium, shifting potassium to the intracellular space and removing it (92).

Both calcium and sodium ions directly antagonize the cardiotoxic effect of potassium. Calcium should be infused under electro-cardiographic monitoring. In less urgent situations, infusion of a mixture of glucose, insulin, calcium is started. This promoted flux of the potassium ion from the extracellular to the intracellular space. β-adrenergic stimuli also facilitates movement of K^+ to the intracellular space. An infusion of 0.5 mg albuterol sulphate will decrease the K^+ approximately 1 mmol/l in 20 minutes (100). Removal of potassium is achieved through the oral or rectal administration of exchange resins or by dialysis. Table 2 summarizes the treatment for hyperkalemia and Figure 10 exemplifies the use of all treatment modalities.

TREATMENT LATE: CONSERVATIVE

Once the restoration phase in a patient with acute tubular necrosis is over, treatment directed against commonly occurring complications and problems, is instituted. Included are prophylaxis against infections, a watch for surgical complications and bleeding.

Table 2. Treatment of hyperkalemia

Urgency	Treatment	Dose	Mechanism	Time for effect
Hyperacute	Calcium intravenously	10 ml 10% calcium gluconate/1–5 min until EKG improves. May need 100 ml	Antagonism	Immediate
Acute	A. Insulin-glucose-lactate-calcium	500 ml 30% dextrose 30 units insulin. 30 ml 10% calcium gluconate; 100 ml in 1st hr	Shifts K+ to intracellular space	30 min
	B. Bicarbonate intravenously	Depends on patient's bicarbonate	–"–	Uncertain
	C. Albuterol sulfate	0.5 mg IV in 10 min	–"–	30 min
Less urgent	A. Exchange resin	30 g Kayexalate orally in 100 ml 20% sorbitol solution or 60 g Kayexalate as an enema in 500 ml 10% sorbitol solution	Removes K+ from body	1 to 2 hours
	B. Dialysis			Depends on dialysis units' readiness

K⁺ in Serum
mEq./L

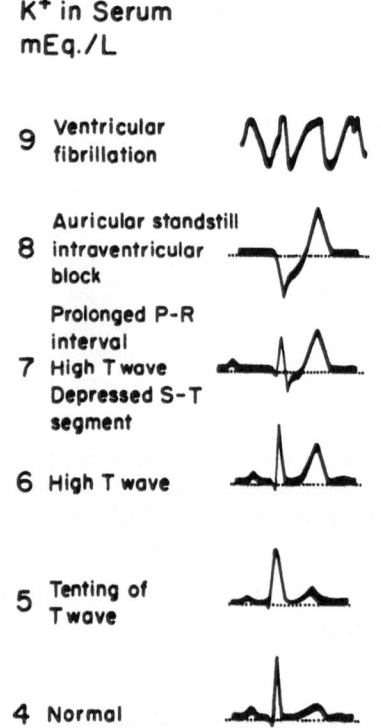

Figure 9. Electrocardiographic changes seen at various plasma potassium levels. Note that the plasma levels are only approximate and the electrocardiographic changes only roughly correlate to the plasma potassium level. From (92) with permission.

Avoiding infections

The number of infections that occur in a patient with acute renal failure is directly correlated to mortality. While 85%

of the patients without infections survived in one series, 75% of those with 4 infections died (70). The urinary tract is infected in 80% of patients with acute renal failure, the lungs in 60%, clinical septicemia is present in 30%, and positive blood cultures in 15% (4). Almost all patients who develop positive blood cultures while on broad-spectrum antibiotics, die (4, 71, 84).

The diagnosis of infections is difficult because urea is a strong antipyretic substance. The temperature increases less in infection in patients with uremia. While a patient with normal blood urea level, will develop a temperature of over 103°F during culture-verified septicemia, patients with a creatinine clearance of less than 30 ml/min will rarely raise their temperature over 102°F (101).

The white blood cell response to culture-verified septicemia, is also decreased. Only 5/17 patients on chronic dialysis raised their segmented neutrophils count to over 5,000 cells/mm³. Nonsegmented neutrophils/mm³ may be more accurate, as 13/17 patients had a count of more than 400 non-segmented neutrophils/mm³ during septicemia (102, 103).

Most patients with acute tubular necrosis are oliguric or develop oliguria when started on dialysis. An indwelling urinary catheter is not necessary and can be very dangerous in oliguric patients. As soon as it is clear that the patient is oliguric, the catheter should be removed and the bladder palpated and percussed daily. Straight catheterization can be performed if retention of urine is suspected. If a catheter is deemed necessary, a condom catheter should be tried. A closed system should always be utilized. Almost all bladders with indwelling catheters are infected after 4 days. Pyelonephritis and sepsis may result (104).

As soon as the restoration phase is over, all intravascular catheters, not absolutely necessary for hemodynamic

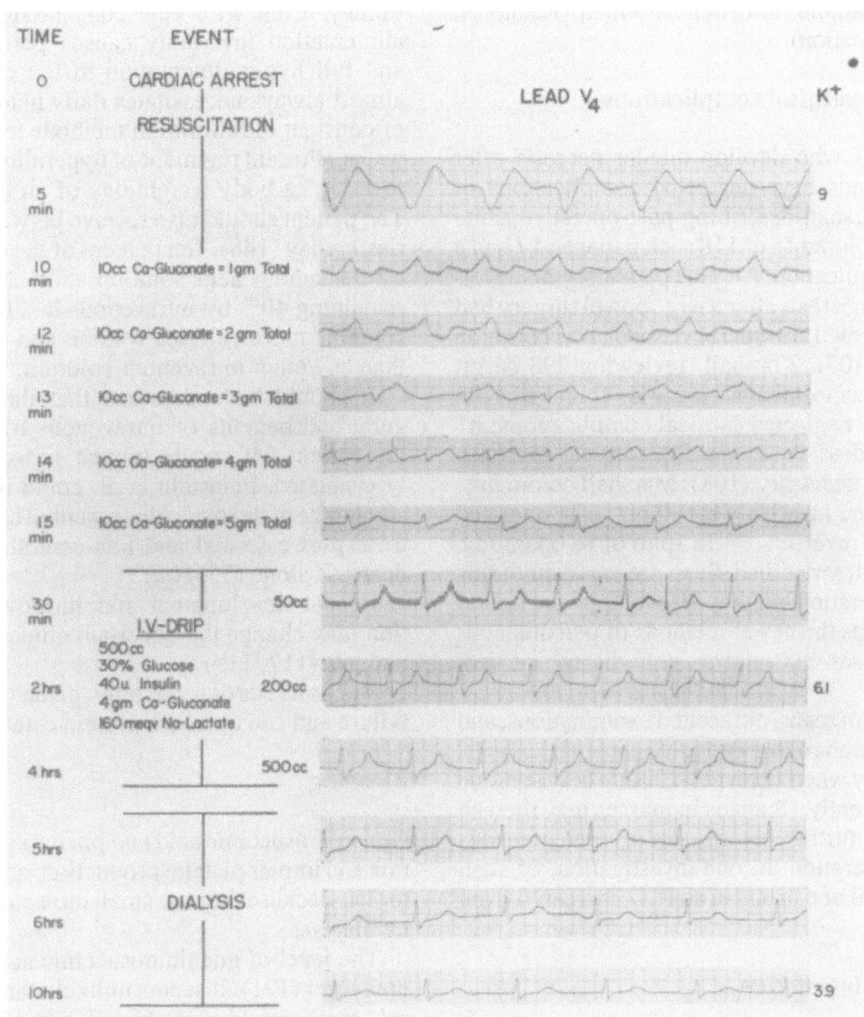

Figure 10. Electrocardiographic changes in a patient with hyperkalemia treated with rapid infusion of calcium gluconase, antagonizing potassium toxicity, followed by shifting of potassium into intracellular space through insulin, glucose, calcium and lactate infusion, and finally by dialysis. From (92) with permission.

monitoring, should be removed. There is almost never a reason to measure intra-arterial blood pressure in any patient. Nor should there be any need for continued measurements of central venous or wedge pressures. Clinical examination and chest x-ray suffice. Intravascular catheters become infected with increased frequency beyond the 4th day. Of patients with flow-directed pulmonary artery catheters, 53% showed endocardial lesions, 19% of the catheter tips had positive cultures and 7% of the patients developed infective endocarditis after 1–2 weeks (105). A central catheter may be necessary for hyperalimentation, but it may be safer to administer hyperalimentation fluids through an arteriovenous shunt. We have successfully hyperalimented many patients through their shunts and believe infections are infrequent and easier to diagnose with this approach.

As the lungs so often become the site of infection, patients should be extubated as soon as possible and mobilized. Physical therapy, breathing and coughing exercises are instituted, although the value of these is controversial.

Indwelling catheters and treatment with broad spectrum antibiotics are often complicated by fungal infections, particularly Candida. Prophylaxis is indicated with nystatin or clotrimazole, swish and swallow, every 4 hours or administered through a nasogastric tube. Specimens for culture should be obtained frequently. Isolation of the patient is probably of little help.

A small trial comparing high dose intravenous IgG to placebo found a lower mortality among the IgG treated patients (106). Unfortunately preliminary analysis from a larger study has found no beneficial effect (Keane W, personal communication).

Re-operation and surgical complications

Almost all patients who develop tubular necrosis after abdominal operations have neglected complications of surgery. Thus, Marshall describing post-operative acute renal failure, re-explored 18 of 118 such patients; 17 had a gross surgical complication. All nine patients, who developed acute tubular necrosis after a large bowel surgery had developed a fecal leak. Post-operative shock was common in these patients (107). Kornhall, reviewing 298 surgical patients with acute tubular necrosis, found that 98 patients (33%) had neglected surgical complications; 81 of these 98 (83%) died. An aggressive surgical approach to these patients is necessary (108). Marshall comments: '... these patients are invariably too ill not to be operated on, rather than the reverse ...'. In spite of re-operation, most patients in both series died. Such patients cannot survive without re-operation but they also tolerate the operations poorly. Perhaps the newer methods of percutaneous drainage of abscesses can improve this dismal survival rate.

Gallium or Indium scans, ultrasound examinations, and CAT-scan examinations of the operative areas of the body, should be done early when acute renal failure develops and then repeated frequently. Changes in masses may then be detected early and further investigated by percutaneous aspirations or exploration. In one investigation, of such an approach survival of patients in an ICU, increased from 19 to 31% (109).

Nutrition, hyperalimentation

Many patients with acute tubular necrosis are critically ill and under maximal stress. They may utilize 5,000 calories and 200 g of protein per day (110).

Malnourished patients suffer from increased post-operative complications including deficient wound healing, immunological defects and increased rates of infections. It is therefore important to supply adequate calories and protein to such patients (111–113).

For feeding, the gastrointestinal route is much safer than intravenous hyperalimentation and should be used whenever possible. New techniques include small diameter soft nasogastric tubes, operative and percutaneous gastrostomy and ileostomy. An elemental oral diet is no more effective than regular homogenized high calorie, high quality protein, normal food. To the contrary, use of the elemental diet, because of the higher osmotic load, is complicated by diarrhea more often (114–117).

Intravenous hyperalimentation causes a number of clinical problems. Plasma electrolyte concentrations may change rapidly and need to be measured frequently. Hypoglycemia and hyperglycemia can occur, contributing to water shifts and intracellular edema or dehydration.

Finally, even with new concentrated solutions, hyperalimentation invariably causes periodic fluid overload and full hyperalimentation in the oliguric patient, and almost always necessitates daily hemodialysis or the use of constant ultrafiltration methods to remove the 'carrier water'. Present regimens of hyperalimentation include 0.5 to 1.5 g/kg body weight/day of an amino acid solution. The patient should also receive between 40 and 100 calories/kg/day (148). Ten percent of the calories are supplied by the amino acid solution, 50% by dextrose and the remaining 40% by intravenous fat. The 20% fat solution contains more calories/volume and less osmoles/calorie than any other intravenous solution.

It should be understood that the exact needs, dangers, and benefits of intravenous hyperalimentation for the patient with acute tubular necrosis are not yet fully evaluated. Feinstein et al. could not find any definite advantage of dextrose plus essential amino acids over dextrose plus essential and non-essential amino acids over dextrose alone (55, 106).

Recent development and improvement in alimentation may change the uncertain clinical approach to these patients (117, 119).

Anabolic steroids are often given to patients with renal failure and can decrease protein catabolic rate (120).

Bleeding

Guanidinosuccinic acid and phenolic acid increase in uremia and impair platelet production, adhesiveness, and factor III. Because they are small molecules they are removed by dialyses.

The level of guanidinosuccinic acid level is related to urea level (121). It seems unlikely that guanidinosuccinic acid level should cause bleeding at a BUN level less than 60 mg/dl, but is a problem if the blood urea nitrogen level exceeds 100 mg/dl (120b). Platelet levels fall mean of 30%, but sometimes more during dialysis and this may cause significant bleeding (122, 123).

Some defects in the clotting cascade are not improved by dialysis. Sometimes prolonged bleeding can be normalized through the use of cryoprecipitate, approximately 10 units (124). Deamino-arginine vasopressin 0.3 μg/kg can rapidly improve bleeding time in some uremic patients (125). Progesterone in high doses (10–30 mg daily), for several days, may also help (126). Bleeding is more common if the hematocrit is less than 30% (127, 128). Other post-operative complications are also increased if hematocrit is below this level (127, 128). Prostacyclin is increased in blood vessel walls in patients on dialysis (129). It is unknown if this contributes to bleeding. The best clinical tests for bleeding include: platelet count, Ivy bleeding time, thrombin time and prothrombin time. If they are abnormal and surgery is planned, vitamin K deficiencies and thrombocytopenia should be corrected, the hematocrit be over 30%, and the patient's BUN decreased to less than 60 mg/dl. If bleeding parameters still are abnormal, the use of cryoprecipitate, deamino-arginine-vasopressin and progesterone may normalize them.

Other metabolic problems

Although gastrointestinal bleeding is now less common, patients with acute renal failure are stressed and the gastrin level is elevated. The exact treatment remains controversial as the customary prevention with either aluminium hydroxide suspension and histamine receptor inhibitors can lead to change in bowel flora and perhaps nosocomial pneumonia (130). It may be best to use these drugs only on indication.

The onset of acute uremia causes several endocrine-metabolic problems. Peripheral insulin sensitivity is decreased in uremia and many such patients have hyper-insulinemia. Furthermore, glucose metabolism tends to be decreased. If septicemia occurs, hyperglycemia often occurs. Glycose levels, therefore must be carefully monitored to prevent marked fluid shifts (117).

Shortly after the onset of acute renal failure, plasma calcium levels start to decrease. This is not due to increased excretion but reflects a shift of calcium out of the extracellular space (see also Chapter 35). Calcitonin increases to extremely high levels (131), and secondary to the decline in plasma calcium concentration, parathyroid hormone levels rise (132). Calcium and magnesium levels in the brain increase which may contribute to the stupor and confusion often observed in such patients (133). Plasma phosphorus levels usually rise and may also contribute to the secondary hyperparathyroidism, the decline in plasma calcium concentration and the increase in calcitonin levels. The hypocalcemia and hyperphosphatemia can be particularly marked in patients with rhabdomyolysis and acute renal failure. When uremia subsides, some patients with acute renal failure, develop marked hypercalcemia; this is also particularly pronounced in patients who suffered from rhabdomyolysis (134–136). Many other hormonal abnormalities occur, but are insufficiently studied. Plasma gastrin levels increase and may contribute to the stress ulcers that patients develop.

Anemia develops quickly, secondary to a decreased erythropoietin level (137) and perhaps decreased peripheral sensitivity to erythropoietin. As mentioned above, these patients should be transfused to a hematocrit of approximately 30% (127, 128). The use of erythropoietin in acute renal failure has not been systematically studied. Plasma uric acid levels rise; particularly high levels are seen in patients with neoplasms or rhabdomyolysis. Excess uric acid may perpetuate the acute renal failure by precipitating in renal tubules (138, 139). In such patients, the ratio of uric acid to creatinine in urine exceeds 1.0 (140). Many of these metabolic problems, e.g., plasma calcium, phosphorus and uric acid levels, improve with dialysis. They rarely need special treatment (141, 142).

USE / METHOD	INTERMITTENT	CONTINUOUS
HEMODIALYSIS HD	STANDARD	COMPLICATED EXPERIENCE ACCUMULATING
HEMOFILTRATION HF	LITTLE EXPERIENCE	COMPLICATED. SPONTANEOUS CLEARENCE TOO LOW. NEEDS TO BE PUMPDRIVEN
COMB HD + HF	COMPLICATED NOT USED	COMPLICATED. GAINING POPULARITY EXPERIENCE ACCUMULATING
PERITONEAL D. PD	CLEARANCE TOO LOW	SIMPLE BORDERLINE CLEARANCE BUT RESULT APPEAR EQUAL TO IHD

Figure 11. Outline of the methods for toxin removal in acute renal failure: hemodialysis hemofiltration, combined hemodialysis, hemofiltration, and peritoneal dialysis. Each can be used intermittently or continuously. Most experience, now exceeding 40 years, is with intermittent hemodialysis to which the others should be compared.

Use of drugs

The elimination of most drugs is modified in patients with acute renal failure and by dialysis treatment, necessitating adjustment of normal dosages. Many drugs are normally excreted in urine, many are removed by dialysis and protein binding drugs, and hepatic metabolism may change in patients with uremia and sepsis. Excellent monographs and frequently updated reviews should be consulted (143).

TREATMENT WITH ACUTE DIALYSIS

Overview of methods

Although the mortality rate in acute renal failure remains high there is considerable variability in clinical outcome in recent reports (144–149) and these suggest that there may be cause for cautious optimism as new treatment options are explored (150–166). Any hope for improved clinical outcome in this group of patients however must be tempered by the clinical impression that their mean age seems to be increasing, co-morbidity is increasing and acute renal failure is more frequently complicated by multiple organ failure syndrome. Nevertheless, the variety of clinical strategies and technical improvements developed in recent years provide the clinician with a broad array of therapeutic options for dialysis. Practically any patient is now dialyzable and uremic solute removal and fluid balance can be achieved safely and effectively even

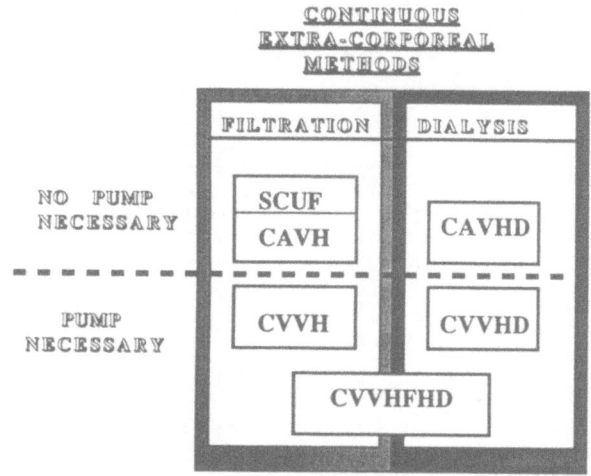

METHOD / CLINICAL PROBLEM	INTERMITTENT HEMODIALYSIS	CONTINOUS PERITONEAL DIAL.	SLOW COMBINED HEMO-DIAL/FILTR
UNSTABLE	−	+	+
STABLE	+	0	−
BLEEDING	0	++	−
HEAD-INJURY	− −	++	0
CATABOLIC	+	−	0
HYPERALIMENTATION	−	0	+
CAN BE MOBILISED	++	−	− −

Figure 12. Outline of the various continuous extracorporeal method, the need or not of pump on the bloodlines and their combinations. SCUF = slow continuous ultrafiltration; CAVH = continuous arteriovenous hemofiltration; CAVHD = continuous arteriovenous hemodialysis; CVVH = continuous venovenous hemofiltration; CVVHD = continuous venovenous hemodialysis; CVVHFHD = continuous venovenous hemofiltration hemodialysis.

Figure 13. Outline of the commonly applied dialysis procedure, intermittent hemodialysis, continuous peritoneal dialysis and combined hemodialysis/hemofiltration, and the clinical situation where they may be best applied. Minus sign means the method is unsuitable, 2+ method probably best, zero means no particular advantage or disadvantage. For example, in the cardiovascular unstable patient the slow continuous methods cause less stress than does intermittent hemodialysis. On the other hand, in the stable patient who can be mobilized, intermittent hemodialysis allows a patient to be up and around. This is impossible with slow continuous hemodialysis/hemofiltration and more difficult in a peritoneal dialysis patients with a catheter that has not healed in completely. In the patient with bleeding head injury continuous peritoneal dialysis is by far the best method because it gives rise to no brain edema and no anticoagulation is necessary. The relative indications are undergoing continuous evaluation.

in hemodynamically unstable patients with mean arterial pressure as low as 50 mmHg. There are now three different types of extracorporeal dialysis available: hemodialysis, hemofiltration, combined hemodialysis and hemofiltration, and one intracorporeal treatment – peritoneal dialysis. All four methods can be done either intermittently or continuously. The treatments are outlined in Figure 11 as well as their approximate clinical status at this time. The continuous extracorporeal methods can also be connected to the vascular system, either in an arteriovenous configuration where it is not absolutely necessary to use a blood pump, or a veno-venous where a blood pump is necessary. The various combinations are outlined in Figure 12 with commonly used abbreviations.

A summary of the dialytic technique available is presented in Table 3. Each option can be used alone or in combination with another, as a clinical situation may require. No method is 'best' under all circumstances. Although a complete centre dealing with acute dialysis should have all options available this is not the case or possible everywhere. Technical familiarity is important when selecting a method. Depending on the clinical situation, each of the principal methods that presently are in widespread use, i.e., intermittent hemodialysis, continuous peritoneal dialysis and continuous hemodialysis and/or hemofiltration, have their advantages. The clinical situations and the relative merits of the methods are outlined in Figure 13.

The main advantage of intermittent hemodialysis is its high clearance, and the fact that it frees the patients up for other therapeutic or rehabilitative efforts. There is also less manipulation of the blood accesses, anticoagula-

tion is needed less than in any continuous extracorporeal method and the blood is not continuously exposed to a foreign surface. The intermittency however has unavoidable disadvantages. The method may induce cardiovascular instability and unavoidably introduce some degree of brain edema with a number of symptoms headed under the general term of 'disequilibrium' with nausea, vomiting, confusion, cramps, and in extreme cases seizures, coma, with increased cranial pressure. It may also be difficult to remove large amounts of volume in borderline stable patients. Finally, electrolytes and waste levels oscillate up and down in an unphysiologic manner.

All the disadvantages mentioned for hemodialysis are avoided by the slow continuous hemodialysis/hemofiltration methods. There is practically no cardiovascular embarrassment, and brain edema and large amounts of fluid can easily be removed by this method. There are however also unavoidable disadvantages continuous anticoagulation may be necessary, there is much manipulation with blood lines as filters have to be changed, it is somewhat difficult to keep track of the large fluid volumes that are necessary if filtration is applied and the method is personnel-demanding for supervision

Table 3. Dialytic techniques for treatment of acute renal failure

Type of therapy	Transport mechanism	Urea clearance (ml/min)	Ultrafiltration rate (l/day)
Intermittent hemodialysis	Diffusion and convection	200–400	~4–6
Continuous arteriovenous hemofiltration (CAVH)	Convection	7–10	0–12
Continuous venovenous hemofiltration (CVVH)	Convection	15–17[a]	0–12
Continuous venovenous hemodialysis (CAVHD)	Diffusion and convection	16–39	4–12
Continuous venovenous hemodialysis (CVVHD)	Diffusion and convection	16–39	4–12
Continuous peritoneal dialysis	Diffusion and convection	12–17	~1–3

[a] Although CAVH and CVVH are very similar conceptually, the higher area nitrogen clearance achieved with CVVH is due to the greater reliability of continuous blood flow with the latter technique.

of fluid balance or complicated and potentially dangerous machinery needs constant supervision. With the new volume-controlled dialysis machines, whereby the same membranes as previously could be used only for hemofiltration can also be used for hemodialysis, it is uncertain whether the filtration methods offers any advantages over dialysis with an open biocompatible membrane.

Continuous peritoneal dialysis has borderline clearance and the disadvantage of an intraperitoneal catheter in the patients who are susceptible to infections. However, it offers the smoothest of all, uremia control methods. There is no foreign membrane and no anticoagulation is necessary. This makes it particularly suitable in bleeding patients and particularly in those patients who have head injury.

Comparison of dialysis methods; intermittent and continuous hemodialysis; peritoneal dialysis

While it remains true that there are still no published prospective trials comparing clinical outcome using the various forms of dialytic support in acute renal failure, several themes are emerging from a number of retrospective studies. For example, these reports suggest that survival or return of renal function may be enhanced by continuous hemodialysis therapies (160, 164) or by the use of more biocompatible membranes (165). The various forms of continuous hemodialysis are undergoing rapid evolutionary changes and the technology for this modality has not yet been optimized. Nevertheless, a variety of dialysis delivery systems for this modality are being used with increasing frequency, already exceeding 50% in some countries (164). The appeal of the continuous therapies is derived from two observations: first, acute renal failure patients often demonstrate both hemodynamic instability and the need for significant levels of fluid intake as inotropes and parenteral nutrition; and, second, they tend to be hypercatabolic as a result of infection, trauma or the post-operative state. Managing these factors with intermittent hemodialysis, even on a daily basis can be very challenging. Use of the continuous therapies is not only

easier (159) but may also be more effective in terms of clinical outcome (163, 164).

The contrast between continuous versus intermittent therapies, in terms of controlling urea levels, is graphically displayed in Figure 14. Three levels of dialytic control are displayed. In each case a urea generation rate of 13.79 mg/min (or a protein catabolic rate of 2 g/kg/day in a 70 kg patient) is assumed. The solute profile curves in this figure are based on the urea kinetic modelling equations of Gotch (167). Curve A describes the typical sawtooth profile of urea nitrogen levels in a patient on daily intermittent hemodialysis. Dialysis time is 4 hours and average urea nitrogen clearance is 216 ml/min. In this case, peak urea nitrogen concentration approaches a stable level of 60 mg/dl after four daily dialysis treatments. This is an optimal scenario in terms of controlling uremic solute levels but, in practice, the initial dialysis for a patient with acute renal failure should probably not be designed to reduce the BUN level from 100 mg/dl to 35 mg/dl since this may induce symptoms of disequilibrium in these fragile patients. Curve C represents the urea nitrogen concentration profile in a patient treated with high efficiency continuous veno-venous hemodialysis, i.e., dialyzer clearance $(K_D) = 39$ ml/min. In this case, the urea nitrogen level approaches a constant level just below 40 mg/dl after about 96 hours of continuous hemodialysis, in spite of a high urea generation rate and a high average urea volume of distribution. If the peak concentration of uremic solutes, using urea as a surrogate, is an indicator of uremic toxicity as suggested by the peak concentration hypothesis (168) this level of CVVHD therapy may be more efficacious than daily intermittent hemodialysis in this patient group, since the steady state level of BUN is far below the peak levels in daily IHD. Finally, curve B in Figure 14 indicates the solute profile over time when $K_D = 26$ ml/min. This is not an arbitrary clearance level. In terms of the urea kinetic model it represents a level of dialyzer clearance which maintains a urea nitrogen level comparable to the peak levels found in daily IHD. On a practical level, however, this level of continuous clearance is representative of what happens when optimal CVVHD can be delivered

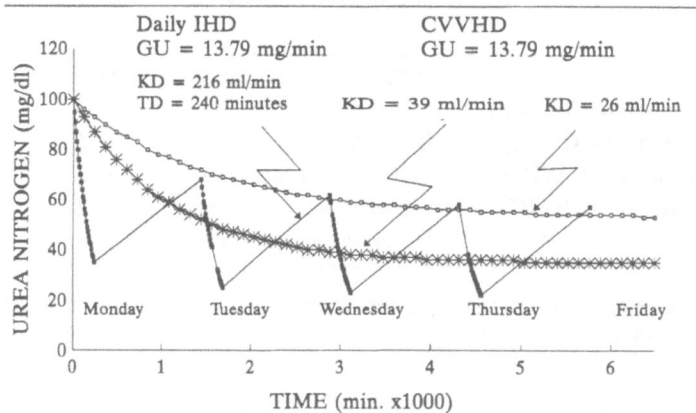

Figure 14.   Blood urea nitrogen profile in a hypothetical 70 kg patient with a protein catabolic rate of 2 g/kg/day. BUN levels are constructed from a solution of the function $C = C_0e - KT/V + G/K(1 - eKT/V)$ at hourly intervals. Control of azotemia is contrasted between daily intermittent hemodialysis (IHD) and two levels of continuous venovenous dialysis. See text for further details. KD = dialysis urea clearance. TD = dialysis duration with intermittent hemodialysis (IHD).

for only 16 h/day because of clotting or malfunction of the CVVHD system. This therapeutic scenario has been characterized, somewhat ironically, as 'intermittent' continuous venovenous hemodialysis. However, even in this reduced operating capacity the level of azotemia (BUN) is comparable to that of the peak levels achieved by daily intermittent hemodialysis. It should be noted that the dialysis disequilibrium syndrome is not a consideration with the continuous therapies.

These theoretical models of azotemia control in acute renal failure strongly suggest that continuous methods surpass even the most intensive intermittent hemodialysis therapies. Clark et al. (179) have recently validated these theoretical constructs with clinical data derived from patients treated with intermittent and continuous hemodialysis therapies. They concluded that for equivalent amounts of therapy, the continuous therapies achieve better control of BUN levels than intermittent hemodialysis.

In addition to improved control of azotemia, the continuous hemodialysis therapies represent a major advance in volume control. The desired ultrafiltration rate can be adjusted virtually on a minute to minute basis from 0 to 500 ml/h. There is no longer the need to remove 3–4 litres during a typical 4 hour acute hemodialysis procedure in a patient who may already be on pressors because of hemodynamic instability. While certain technical advances in hemodialysis delivery systems (controlled ultrafiltration, sodium modelling, bicarbonate dialysate and even cooler dialysate) have improved hemodynamic stability during acute intermittent hemodialysis, management of fluid balance and maintenance of a stable mean arterial pres-

sure with this modality are still major concerns with each treatment.

The continuous therapies, however, are not without problems of their own as indicted in Table 3 and Figure 15. For example, if we assume a 70 kg patient with a protein catabolic rate of 2 g/kg/day, as a typical patient, we see that continuous arteriovenous hemofiltration (A) not only fails to control azotemia, the BUN would actually increase over time in severely catabolic patients with this modality. In addition, both CAVH and CAVHD require prolonged cannulation of an artery, and dialytic efficiency is dependent on mean arterial pressure levels which are frequently below 90 mm Hg in this patient group. Continuous peritoneal dialysis (B) is also limited, even at a relatively high clearance of 17 ml/min. The BUN level will plateau at 81 mg/dl after about 5 days of continuous operation. The limited and less predictable rate of ultrafiltration with this modality is also problematic. Finally, the 'continuous equivalent' of two levels of urea clearance for intermittent hemodialysis (200 and 300 ml/min) supplied on alternate days is also shown in Figure 15. The 'continuous equivalents' would be 19 (C) and 28.6 (D) ml/min, respectively. The average urea nitrogen level reaches a plateau of 72 mg/dl after 6.5 days when urea clearance is 200 ml/min for 4 hour, alternate day dialysis sessions. Only at a urea clearance of 300 ml/min, supplied at the same frequency and duration does the average level plateau below 50 mg/dl after about 4 days. CVVHD at a clearance of 33.3 ml/min (E) is also shown for comparison. With this modality, the BUN is reduced below 50 mg/dl in less than 2 days and a steady state BUN = 41 mg/dl is achieved in 4 days. Continuous urea nitrogen

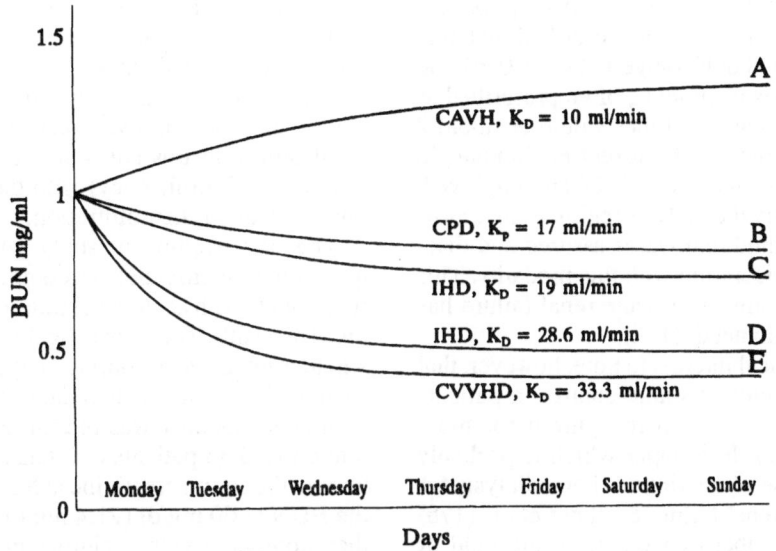

Figure 15. Blood urea nitrogen profile in a hypothetical 70 kg patient with a protein catabolic rate of 2 g/kg/day. Five profiles are depicted, each reflecting the theoretical level of azotemia control achieved by either an intermittent or a continuous therapy. The concentration of urea nitrogen at any point is based on the same predictions as the equation in Figure 14.

clearance values of 33 ml/min are readily achieved with a variety of dialyzers in CVVHD (169).

Although the continuous renal replacement therapies (CRRT) vary widely in terms of overall efficiency, it is clear that some forms of CRRT, especially CVVHD, provide superior control of azotemia, when compared to a broad variety of alternate therapies. Nevertheless, there are no prospective trials to support the choice of one of these therapies above others, and various authors have supported (170) and criticized (171) the use of CRRT in the treatment of acute renal failure. Actually, prospective trials comparing IHD and CRRT are currently under way but their results may not be available for several years. In the meantime, each center dealing with acute renal failure patients may prefer to select the modality with which they are most proficient.

ACUTE DIALYSIS

Start, frequency and speed of dialysis

While it is easy to define the extreme levels of uremic toxicity at which dialysis should be started in patients with acute renal failure, it is more difficult to define the optimal point at which dialytic support is appropriate. For example, no one would deny dialysis to an otherwise healthy patient with oliguric acute renal failure with a serum potassium approaching 7 mEq/l, a BUN above 100 mg/dl, a serum creatinine above 10 mg/dl and a serum bicarbonate level below 15 mmol/l. Yet, recognizing that several major complications of acute renal failure, infec-

tions and bleeding, are a function of the level of azotemia, most would view these as excessive levels at which to start dialysis. In fact, it now seems prudent to start dialytic support long before azotemic solutes reach these levels. In many cases, the main reason for starting dialysis in this clinical setting is actually not the level of azotemia, but the need to maintain fluid balance. In critically ill oliguric patients supported by multiple inotropes and various levels of parenteral alimentation, volume overload may precede significant azotemia by several days. Nevertheless, whether dialysis is started earlier for control of volume status or for better control of azotemia, the common wisdom is that this is the preferred approach to patients with acute renal failure. Even in patients with non-oliguric acute renal failure, once the diagnosis is established, it is probably better to err on the side of starting dialysis early, rather than later. This principle was first introduced by Teschan et al. (172) during the Korean War. When dialysis was started based only on clinical indications, such as coma or severe electrolyte and fluid disturbances, mortality was over 70%. in contrast, when dialysis was started prophylactically to maintain the pre-dialysis BUN below 120 mg/dl (42.9 mmol/l), the mortality rate was reduced to 30%. In these important early studies, however, major covariates such as Apache scores were not available.

When nephrologic consultation for patients with acute renal failure is delayed to the point that azotemia is advanced, it is important to modify the dose of dialysis if acute intermittent dialysis is used, in order to avoid symptoms of disequilibrium (hypotension, cramps, seizures, etc). Daugirdas offers a prudent approach, based on the level of reduction of urea nitrogen level with each treatment (173). He suggests that for the typical 70 kg patient the urea nitrogen clearance should be prescribed such that the post/pre-BUN ratio should range between 0.70 and 0.65 in the first 3 dialysis treatments, often prescribed as daily dialysis. Typical treatment times would be about 2 hours for the first 2–3 days with current equipment. In contrast, when various methods of CRRT are employed, there is no need to modify the dialysis regimen since slow continuous solute and fluid removal is assured and disequilibrium is not a consideration with this modality. This approach to dialytic treatment of acute renal failure has recently been reviewed in detail (174).

It is more than historical interest to note, however, that the need for improved uremic solute control in patients with acute renal failure has been recognized for more than 30 years (175–177). In a paper which is probably the first to report the use of continuous hemodialysis for the treatment of acute renal failure Scribner et al. (178) state "An increasing number of workers in the field of hemodialysis are becoming convinced of the validity of the principle that it is dangerous for critically ill patients to develop the uremic syndrome." They go on to describe a pumpless hemodialysis system which is conceptually identical to that developed by Geronemus and Schneider (179) more than 20 years later and now referred to as continuous arteriovenous hemodialysis. In the technique described by Scribner et al., non-protein nitrogen removal rates equalled or exceeded 20 g/day. This is equivalent to a protein catabolic rate (PCR) of about 2 g/kg/day, the same normalized PCR (PCRN) as shown in Figure 15. In effect, the ability to control azotemia (and volume) on a continuous basis in azotemic patients with acute renal failure has been available for more than 30 years, but has only been exploited gradually over the past decade.

A number of studies in recent years have suggested that clinical outcome is improved with continuous therapies (153–155, 158–164). However, virtually all of these studies are retrospective and usually rely on historical controls. In the report of Barton et al. (163), for example, 250 patients were studied between 1981 and 1991. Over this decade continuous venovenous hemofiltration became the preferred treatment for patients with acute renal failure in their dialysis unit. In a logistic regression analysis for mortality, eight variables were found to be the most significant predictors; these were: age, ventilator-dependency, use of inotropes, elevated bilirubin, elevated serum creatinine, oliguria, level of base deficit, and quintile of accession number to the study, i.e., at what point over the decade of this study the patient entered the study. In this analysis, the quintile of the accession number was the most significant ($p < 0.0001$) predictor of mortality in this study. However, for practical purposes, the authors concluded that, in rank order, the following factors predicted outcome in patients with acute renal failure; age, ventilator-dependency, inotrope use, urine output and bilirubin level. While the authors discounted the significance of the accession number, the predictive value of this factor was emphasized in an editorial comment on this report. The odds ratio for mortality for the first 50 patients entering this study was defined as 1.00. For the last 50 patients, the odds ratio was markedly reduced to 0.195. It was concluded that the improved survival in patients with acute renal failure in this study was due to the increased use (and implied proficiency) with the technique of continuous venovenous hemofiltration.

The only significant study which has addressed the question of intense dialysis compared to standard dialysis for patients with acute renal failure was reported by Guillium et al. (180). These investigators addressed the question whether intensive or routine dialysis could reduce mortality in patients with acute renal failure. In both groups, the treatment modality was intermittent hemodialysis. They randomized 34 patients to intensive daily dialysis, maintaining the serum creatinine at 5.3 mg/dl (469 μmol/l) and the BUN at 60 mg/dl (21.4 mmol/l). These patients were then compared with a similar group of patients treated with 'ordinary dialysis.' In this group, the mean comparable values of pre-dialysis serum creatinine was 9.1 mg/dl (805 μmol/l) and BUN, 101 mg/dl (36.1 mmol/l). The mortality rate and the complication rate in the intensively dialyzed groups (58.5%) were not significantly different than in the 'ordinary dialysis' group (47.1%). The authors conclude that there is no advantage to intensive dialysis in the management of acute renal failure. Similar observations have been made by others (181, 182). In one study, 236 patients requiring dialysis for post-operative acute renal failure following renal transplantation were compared to matched controlled patients with good renal function. There was no difference in mortality, indicating that dialysis, which was used every other day, had maximally lowered mortality (183).

Although a variety of methods may be used to prescribe hemodialysis in acute renal failure, it is common practice to make daily adjustments based on the assessment of volume status and level of azotemia. The gold standard is formal urea kinetic analysis (167) but there are alternatives. The following method is based on simplified urea kinetics. Since the level of BUN is directly proportional to urea generation rate (Gu) and inversely proportional to urea nitrogen clearance (KT_{urea}), the relation among these variables can be expressed as follows; $BUN \approx Gu/KT_{urea}$. This expression can be easily rearranged to yield, $KT = Gu/BUN$. KT equals the sum of dialyzer and residual renal clearance of urea nitrogen, in ml/min. (The latter is often negligible in acute renal failure and, therefore, KT reduces to K_D, which is dialyzer clearance). The value for BUN should be the time average value being targeted, usually 50 mg/dl or less. For our purposes here, BUN should be expressed in mg/ml for our purposes; therefore, 0.5 mg/ml. The value for Gu may be calculated from $Gu = 0.107 PCR - 0.031V$ (see (167)), where PCR equals the amount of protein the patient is receiving, in g/day. This is known from the parenteral nutrition prescribed. V is an estimation of urea volume of distribution, in litres.

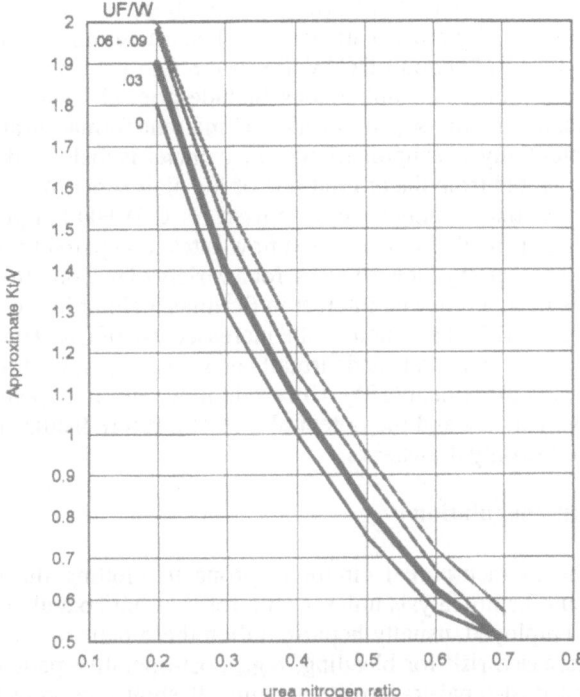

Figure 16. The level of KT/V may be estimated from the ration of post- and pre-dialysis BUN levels and the ratio of ultrafiltration and body weight, UF/W. See text for details. Adapted from Daugirdes and Depener (147) with permission.

A 70 kg patient receiving 2 g of protein/kg/day or 140 g of protein would have a value for Gu = 13.68 mg/min and a continuous K_D = 27.36 ml/min to maintain a BUN = 0.5 mg/dl, i.e., K_{Dc} = 13.68/0.5. This is close to the value of 26 ml/min which was derived by formal urea kinetic analysis in Figure 14, curve B. The conversion of a continuous value for K_{Dc} into its intermittent equivalent (K_{Di}) is simple; K_{Di} = (K_{Dc} × M)/T_D, where M is the number of minutes during which K_{Dc} would be operating – e.g., 1440 min for daily dialysis, 2880 for alternate day dialysis; T_D is the duration of the intermittent dialysis, expressed in minutes. For example, the intermittent equivalent of K_{Dc} = 27.36 ml/min for an alternate day regimen of acute intermittent dialysis of 4 hours duration would be (27.36 × 2880)/240 = 328 ml/min.

Having calculated a urea removal rate based on a known value of protein intake, a rising BUN level would suggest endogenous protein catabolism or an effective dialyzer clearance which is less than the amount prescribed. This simplified method is intended for clinical purposes only. It is an estimate of K_D. It ignores intradialytic urea generation and ultrafiltration effects.

Another simplified approach to prescribing intermittent hemodialysis has been proposed by Daugirdas and Depner (184). This is based on values of KT/V, ultrafiltration rates and urea reduction ratios as well as normalized

protein catabolic rates for both initial and subsequent dialyses. Since adequate doses of dialysis for stable chronic ESRD patients are in the range of KT/V = 1.2–1.4 Collins, (185) it is likely that target values for KT/V in acute renal failure should be higher. However, there are no prospective, randomized trials to support this recommendation. Figure 16, taken from the study of Daugirdas and Depner, can be used to derive a KT/V value, based on measured values of pre- and post-dialysis BUN levels, and the ultrafiltration rate. In a preliminary report Garred has recently presented a simplified method for calculating PCR from known values of KT/V and the pre- and post-dialysis BUN levels (186). PCR = 0.0076 [KT/V][Cpre + Cpost] + 0.17. Cpre and Cpost are the pre- and post-dialysis levels of BUN, expressed in mg/dl. In 540 simulations the maximum error was < 5%. In effect, estimates of the important dialytic parameters, KT/V and PCR, can be derived from pre- and post-dialysis levels of BUN and the validated nomogram of Daugirdas and Depner.

In summary: It is preferable to start dialysis early, especially in those patients where a prolonged course of acute renal failure may be expected (post-operative open heart surgery) or patients who are already septic and catabolic. Fluid overload or the threat thereof should also provoke early dialysis. The frequency of dialysis treatments pertains only to intermittent hemodialysis and this will be a function of the patient's need and the resources of the dialysis unit. Although daily or alternate day dialysis seems prudent, intensive dialysis has not been shown to be superior to the conventional three times per week schedule (180). The solute and volume shifts typical of acute hemodialysis have led some to question whether this may lead to renal ischemia and possibly delayed recovery from acute renal failure (196). Nevertheless, control of volume status without hypotension and maintaining uremic solutes at acceptable levels (BUN $\leq$ 50 mg/dl) are reasonable goals. Finally, there can be little doubt that these acutely ill patients require more dialysis than stable chronic outpatients, for whom weekly KT/V values of 3.6–4.2 are now recommended (185). The duration and speed of dialysis are of concern only for intermittent hemodialysis. While the goals of dialysis, volume and uremic solute control should be achieved, disequilibrium must be avoided. This will be discussed further below. Disequilibrium results from rapid reduction of extracellular solutes and subsequent cerebral edema. To avoid this, it is recommended that the reduction of BUN during the first three dialysis treatment be no more than 30–35% and the duration of these initial treatments should be about 2 hours, probably on a daily basis (173).

Vascular access

Access to the circulation for acute hemodialysis should be easy to achieve, provide adequate blood flow rates and be free of complications. The dual lumen femoral catheter has generally met these criteria. It is easily inserted percutaneously over a guide wire, using a modified Seldinger technique. Blood flow rates of 300–400 ml/min can be achieved and recirculation is minimized if the distal perforations are separated by about 2 cm in each limb of the catheter. The catheters are manufactured from a variety of plastics which tend to be somewhat rigid at room temperature, thereby facilitating insertion, but more pliable at body temperature, thereby minimizing vessel wall trauma over time. While it was once common practice to remove femoral catheters after 24–36 hours (187), now they are often left in place for 3–5 days (188). Daily care of these catheters includes cleaning the exit site using aseptic technique and often applying a small gel of povidone iodine. Prolonged use of femoral catheters probably occurred as a result of more intensive (daily) intermittent hemodialysis or the increasing popularity of the continuous hemodialysis techniques. In ambulatory patients, however, femoral vein catheters should be removed after use. Complications of femoral vein catheterization include femoral arterial puncture, groin hematoma formation and pulmonary emboli (189). Rarely, inadvertent puncture of the femoral or iliac vein can result in a large retroperitoneal hematoma.

Alternate sites for dual lumen catheter insertion include the subclavian and internal jugular veins. Each of these sites has a greater potential for complications. Subclavian vein catheterization can result in pneumothorax, subclavian artery puncture with hemothorax, and cardiac tamponade secondary to hemopericardium if the superior vena cava is punctured (190, 192). Internal jugular vein catheterization carries the risk of carotid artery puncture, but a lower risk of pneumothorax. Radiographic localization of the catheter is often recommended prior to use. Typically, these catheters are left in place for 2–3 weeks, but latter two sites have been associated with central venous thrombosis. This may be asymptomatic and compensated by collateral channels until one attempts to place a chronic vascular access in the ipsilateral arm. At that time massive edema of the extremity may occur, secondary to the high flow and pressure imposed on a compromised venous drainage system.

Complications common to virtually all catheters used for acute hemodialysis include infection and thrombosis. Infection seems to correlate with prolonged use and lack of daily care as described above. Skin flora (Staphylococcus and Streptococcus species) are usually involved. Bacteremia, and rarely, seeding of distal sites may occur. Infection almost always warrants removal of the catheter (193). Thrombosis may be minimized by filling the volume of each limb of the catheter with heparin (1,000 units/ml) after dialysis is completed. If thrombosis does occur, thrombolytic therapy with urokinase is often successful (194). The volumes of the catheter lumen should be filled with urokinase (5,000 units/ml). This is allowed to set for 20 minutes and is then withdrawn. Alternatively, this may be allowed to set over night.

Prolonged femoral artery cannulation, often with a number 11 French catheter, has been a limiting factor in the application of CAVHD to the treatment of acute renal failure. Complications include arterial laceration, distal ischemia or embolization, hematoma formation and, potentially, exsanguination if the catheter is dislodged or separated from the arterial line of the dialyzer (174).

Scribner shunts have been used for CAVHD but generally provide inferior blood flow rates, compared to the femoral artery. Nevertheless, for a variety of reasons, there has been a renewed interest in Scribner's shunt in recent years; (187) these include the increased use of CAVHD, a lower infection rate and virtually no serious complications during placement (195). Uncertain flow rates in hypotensive patients and the potential loss of a future fistula site are the only drawbacks.

Anticoagulation

The extracorporeal circuit is prone to clotting during acute hemodialysis unless some form of anticoagulation is employed, usually heparin. Often these patients are at increased risk for bleeding, e.g., post-operative patients and post-renal transplant patients. It should be kept in mind that patients with renal failure already have a defect in platelet function resulting in altered platelet-vessel wall interaction. Standard heparinization for patients not at risk of bleeding would involve a constant infusion of 800–1,000 units of heparin per hour. The dose is adjusted to keep the partial thromboplastin time between 1.5 and 2 times normal. Finally, it should be pointed out that in patients with serious coagulopathies, e.g., DIC, no anticoagulation is necessary.

In patients at risk of bleeding, a variety of strategies have been devised to minimize this risk. The most common strategy is heparin-free dialysis, (197, 198) which may be successful in more than 95% of acute intermittent hemodialysis treatments (199). The technique is simple. The dialyzer and lines are primed with normal saline containing 2,000–5,000 units of heparin. The heparinized saline is flushed from the lines and dialyzer with normal saline prior to use. Once dialysis is started, blood flow rate is increased to 250–350 ml/min as quickly as possible. (This manoeuvre to prevent clotting should be balanced against the possibility of rapid reductions in BUN levels and provoking the disequilibrium syndrome.) Every 15–30 min after dialysis is under way, the blood circuit is flushed (pre-dialyzer) with 50–100 ml of normal saline. This is intended to minimize hemoconcentration in the dialyzer. The net ultrafiltration volume for the treatment must take these saline flushes into account. The high success rate associated with changing the lines and dialyzer during the treatment (199) suggests that some fibrin must be forming in the system and that removing this is an important step in assuring a system clotting rate as low as 3%. However, the high cost, in terms of time, equipment and personnel to achieve this marginal increase in success rate, i.e., 95 versus 97%, is questionable. It was initially thought that no heparin dialysis was most successful with cellulose acetate hollow fiber dialyzers, (197) but comparable success has been achieved with a variety of membranes (197, 198). As a result, this technique is the preferred method of anticoagulation for patients who would be at risk of bleeding if exposed to systemic heparinization.

The second most common approach to anticoagulation in patients at risk of bleeding is referred to as minimal heparinization. This technique has been shown to decrease the incidence of bleeding in high risk patients to 19 versus 10% (200) when compared to patients treated with traditional regional heparinization (201). This technique also requires high blood flow rates but small doses of heparin are added, usually as a bolus of about 500 units/30–60 min. A typical 4 hours acute dialysis may be completed with a total of 2,000–3,500 units of heparin. A small dose of protamine equal to half the dose of heparin may be given to reduce the risk of bleeding following dialysis. When the heparin dialysis method fails, this approach is a reasonable alternative but risks some degree of systemic heparinization.

Traditional regional anticoagulation of the extracorporeal circuit involves a constant infusion of heparin into the arterial line and a neutralizing dose of protamine into the venous line (201). The aim of this technique is to maintain the PTT in the extracorporeal system between 1.5 and 2 times baseline, but return the PTT to baseline, via protamine, post-dialyzer, as blood is returned to the patient. This technique remained a standard for several years but when it was recognized that bleeding may occur several hours after dialysis when the reticuloendothelial system released heparin from the heparin-protamine complex (202) this technique gradually fell into disuse. Currently, it has been displaced by regional citrate anticoagulation.

This elegant but complicated technique has been applied to both acute intermittent hemodialysis (203, 204) and continuous hemodialysis (205). The basis of the regional citrate anticoagulation technique is the fact that the calcium-dependent coagulation cascade is interrupted by citrate-calcium complexing when trisodium citrate (102 mmol/l) is infused, pre-dialyzer, into the extracorporeal circuit. Although the calcium-citrate complex is removed by dialysis the dialysate must be adjusted for the sodium content of the citrate infusion and the loss of calcium cleared with the citrate complex must be replaced, usually distal to the venous limb of the system. If the dialysate calcium level or the infusion level of calcium must be increased to compensate for dialysate losses, serum phosphate levels should be monitored also in order to avoid tissue deposition of calcium-phosphate complexes.

This regional anticoagulation technique requires a carefully designed dialysate composition, frequent monitoring to prevent hypo- or hypercalcemia and one-on-one nursing to monitor this therapy. Its principle application may

be in the continuous therapies where the no heparin technique is impractical since clotting is likely at the lower blood flow rates ($\leq$ 200 ml/min) typical of these modalities, even with periodic saline flushes. Low dose heparin also tends to be unsuccessful in the continuous therapies (174).

Another technique involves prostacyclin, a product of arachidonic acid metabolism. Prostacyclin functions as a regional anticoagulant because of its very short half-life (3–5 min). It acts by inhibiting platelet aggregation and is effective at doses of 4–8 ng/kg/min infused into the extracorporeal circuit. Since it is also a vasodilator, however, it can cause hypotension (63). This latter property will greatly limit its use in critically ill patients.

Dialyzers and dialysis machines, biocompatibility

A wide variety of dialyzers and dialysate delivery systems are available for the treatment of acute renal failure. Previously, dialyzers have usually been selected based on safety, efficiency and cost. Biocompatibility (BC) was often a secondary consideration. In recent years, however, a large body of evidence has been accumulated (217) detailing the consequences of dialyzer membrane bioincompatibility (BIC) and suggesting, from both animal (218) and human studies (165) that the use of BIC membranes may delay recovery from acute renal failure. For example, Hakim et al. (165) prospectively randomized 83 patients with acute renal failure into two treatment groups. One was dialyzed with BIC cellulosic hollow fibre dialyzers; the second group was dialyzed with BC polymethylmethacrylate hollow fibre dialyzers. The groups were matched for age, APACHE II scores and prevalence of oliguria at the start of dialysis. Recovery of renal function was significantly higher in the BC group (62%) than in the BIC group (37%) $p = 0.022$. Overall survival was not significantly different between the two groups; 57% for those dialyzed with BC membranes and 37% for those dialyzed with BIC membranes, $p = 0.069$. However, when only those patients who were not oliguric at the initiation of dialysis were considered survival was significantly higher in the BC group, $p = 0.010$. Hakim (165) cites animal studies which suggest that the adverse effect of BIC membranes may be mediated by activating the complement cascade, followed by activation of neutrophils and monocytes (218). With respect to complement activation, this is more likely to occur with cellulosic membranes, compared to dialyzers fabricated with synthetic polymers. So called BC membranes, however, are not without problems of their own. For example, polyacrylonitrile membranes (AN69) are negatively charged and, therefore, more likely to activate the contact pathway, ultimately leading to the release of various kinins. This, in turn, poses the threat of anaphylactoid reactions (212) in patients simultaneously treated with angiotensin converting enzyme inhibitors (which also inhibit kininases). Recently, Schaefer et al. (213) described an episode of anaphylaxis in a patient dialyzed on an AN69 membrane but not on an ACE inhibitor. In two additional patients, there was a greater than two-fold increase in bradykinin levels in the venous effluent of AN69 dialyzers. Neither patient was on ACE inhibitors. It appears, therefore, that on rare occasions, a negatively charged membrane alone may be sufficient to cause symptomatic activation of the contact pathway. It is of interest that virtually every dialyzer commonly used in the continuous hemodialysis therapies (Table 4) is fabricated with biocompatible polymers (174). Finally, repeated exposure to cuprophane membranes is known to induce defects in neutrophil function and, thereby, exposure of the patient to increased risk of infection, the most common cause of mortality in acute renal failure. In conclusion, it would seem prudent to consider these properties of dialysis membranes when dealing with critically ill patients.

This more discriminating approach to selecting a dialyzer in the treatment of patients with acute renal failure is now being applied to the selection of the dialysate delivery system or dialysis equipment, but with considerably less scientific rationale. For example, many clinicians would agree that recent technical advancements in these systems, including controlled ultrafiltration, sodium modelling, bicarbonate dialysate and cooler dialysate all improve hemodynamic stability in this clinical setting, yet no prospective, randomized trials have been conducted to address these questions in patients with acute renal failure.

The rate of fluid and solute removal during dialysis appear to be the major determinants of hemodynamic stability during dialysis, while dialysate composition and temperature (*vide infra*) are subordinate, but still important, considerations. Modern equipment permits both constant and variable fluid removal which can be adjusted to the unique hemodynamic status of each patient. Plasma osmolality can also be individualized, primarily by sodium modelling, thereby preventing vascular volume contraction as the lag (hours) in urea movement from the intra- to the extracellular space draws fluid from the vascular to the intracellular space. The rise in serum sodium concentration, achieved by dialysate sodium modelling, especially in the first hour of hemodialysis, prevents this osmotic shift while permitting an on-going optimal rate of urea clearance. When sodium modelling is not available, improved strategies for maintaining plasma osmolality during urea clearance can be used. Gong and colleagues (214) have recently compared equal osmolar (80, 80, 100 mOsm) doses of 23% saturated hypertonic saline (10 ml), 7.5% hypertonic saline (3.0 ml) and 7.5% saline with 6% dextran 70 × (30 ml). All three solutions raised systolic blood pressure compared to pre-treatment values within 5 min ($p < 0.05$). However, the magnitude of the increase was greater with saturated hypertonic saline (15 mm Hg) and dextran (17 mmHg), compared to hypertonic saline (9 mmHg) $p > 0.05$. The authors concluded that, given equal osmolar loads, the more concentrated solutions produced a greater increase in systolic pressure

and that the addition of an oncotic agent such as dextran may prolong the blood pressure response. Since automated sodium modelling may achieve these same goals in a much less labour intensive fashion, it is likely that these computerized sodium modelling techniques will replace the use of bolus doses of various osmotic agents in the prevention/treatment of hypotension in patients with acute renal failure. The role of dialysate sodium concentration will be discussed hereafter.

Although there are a number of systems designed for hemofiltration (BSM22, and AK-10, CGH Medical, and the BM11, Baxter Health Care), there is no system designed specifically for the most efficient of the continuous therapies, CVVHD. Nevertheless, the BSM22 is easily converted to a dialysate delivery system for CVVHD by using the fluid replacement pump (left, in Figure 17) for dialysate outflow and adding an independent infusion pump for dialysate inflow. Urea clearances of 33–39 ml/min are easily achieved at dialysate inflow rates of 2 l/h. Flow rates are reliable for prolonged periods after pump calibration and pump segments show little evidence of wear after 48 hours of continuous use. It would seem prudent, however, to change tubing and filter at 48 hours intervals. This table-top device, measuring 30 × 23 × 60 cm has been readily accepted by ICU nurses once they have been in-serviced by the dialysis staff. Its main shortcoming is the fact that the dialysate inflow (Q_{Di}) and outflow (Q_{Do}) pumps are completely independent and, therefore, one may operate while the other is off. For example, it is theoretically possible to have Q_{Do} = zero and Q_{Di} = 2 l/h, leading to some degree of reverse ultrafiltration. Over time, the volume consequences of this could be considerable. On a practical level, however, with one-on-one ICU nursing, the problem is easily recognized and corrected. Since the dialysate is sterile, small amounts of reverse ultrafiltration are inconsequential. In the opposite situation, i.e., Q_{Do} set at 2 l/h and Q_{Di} = 0, the potential for volume loss is probably closer to 500 ml/h with the dialyzers commonly used for CVVHD (Table 4). This problem is also easily recognized and corrected. An improved version of this device, the BSM32, is available in Europe but this problem has not been corrected in the latest model. It is likely, however, that as the continuous therapies, and especially CVVHD, gain popularity (and scientific validity) truly integrated delivery systems for these modalities will be developed.

Dialysis solutions-intermittent hemodialysis

Sodium

There is a general consensus that the dialysate composition used for stable chronic outpatients may not be appropriate for critically ill patients with acute renal failure (195) but there is some uncertainty about just what the optimal composition should be. Palmer (215) has recently reviewed the effects of various dialysate components on systemic hemodynamics. As early as 1979, Dum-

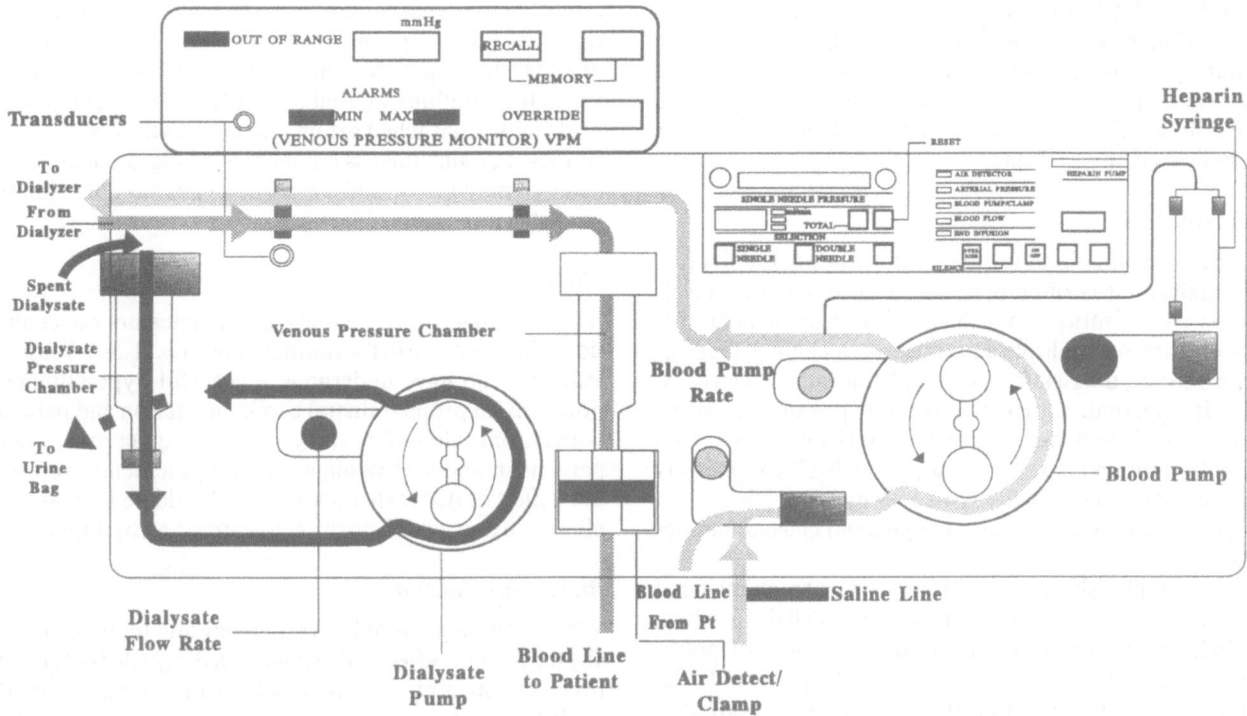

Figure 17. The blood and dialysate flow patterns and pressure monitors are shown for the BSM-22 dialysis system. This is one of several systems which may be adapted to continuous hemodialysis.

Table 4. Selected dialyzers in current use for continuous hemodialysis therapies and slow continuous ultrafiltration (SCUF)

Brand name	Membrane	Surface area (m^2)	Priming volume
Hemospal	Polyacrylonitrile	0.50	60
PAN-50-p	Polyacrylonitrile	0.50	50
Diafilter-10	Polysulfone	0.20	25
Diafilter-20	Polysulfone	0.25	27
Ultraflux-400	Polysulfone	0.50	48
FH-55	Polyamide	0.60	43
FH-66	Polyamide	0.60	43
HF-250	Polysulfone	0.25	27
HF-500	Polysulfone	0.50	39

PP = parallel-plate. The others are hollow fiber designs.

ler et al. (216) showed that there were fewer episodes of symptomatic hypotension and a more stable systolic blood pressure when dialysate sodium was maintained at 150 mEq/l for the first 3 hours of dialysis, but then reduced to 130 mEq/l to avoid thirst, weight gain and worsening hypertension in the interdialytic interval. Henrich et al. (217) confirmed the improved hemodynamic stability of higher dialysate sodium (144 mEq/l) compared to low dialysate sodium (132 mEq/l). These investigators also demonstrated that there was no significant increase in interdialytic blood pressure and that any increase in interdialytic weight gain was easily removed in this more stable dialysis mode.

These and other studies (218) have led to the manufacture of increasingly sophisticated sodium modelling techniques (Century 3, CGH Medical, CD-1000 Althin; 2008-E, Fresenius, among others). However, there are other studies which raise questions concerning the cost-benefit ratio of sodium modelling. For example, Daugirdas et al. (219) was unable to find a significant difference in blood pressure stability or dialysis-related symptoms when patients were dialyzed with sodium modeled between 160 → 133 mEq/l, compared to patients dialyzed with constant dialysate sodium levels of 135 or 143 mEq/l. Studying a more narrow and perhaps more practical range of sodium modelling (145 → 135 mEq/l, Raja et al. (220) were unable to demonstrate any difference in overall hemodynamic stability when compared to dialysis with a fixed dialysate sodium of 140 mEq/l. It is not clear, therefore, that hemodynamic stability is further improved with dialysate sodium is already in the range of 140–145 mEq/l. It should be remembered, however, that most of these studies were done in stable chronic renal failure patients. Therefore, it is still quite possible that there is a subset of critically ill patients in whom sodium modelling will yield some additional advantage in terms of hemodynamic stability.

Potassium

In order to maintain serum potassium levels below 6 mEq/l pre-dialysis, it is often necessary to use dialysate levels as low as 2–3 mEq/l. In patients with ischemic heart disease, those on multiple inotropes or receiving digitalis preparations, the risk for a hypokalemia-induced arrhythmia is apparent. Other effects of hypokalemia during hemodialysis include an increase in resistance in skeletal muscle, skin and coronary vascular beds (215), possibly by enhancing the sensitivity of vascular smooth muscle to endogenous (and perhaps exogenous) catecholamines (221).

These high risk patients warrant frequent monitoring of serum potassium during intermittent hemodialysis when, as Palmer (215) points out, the usual amount of potassium removed over 4 hours (50–80 mEq) exceeds the entire amount in the extracellular space. The continuous therapies achieve the same level of potassium removal (222) but over a longer time period, thereby avoiding the recurrent episodes of hyper- and hypokalemia typical of intermittent hemodialysis.

Calcium

Just as low dialysate sodium is inappropriate for treating patients, with acute renal failure, the same is true for calcium. Dialysate calcium concentrations of 2.5 mEq/l in chronic renal failure were designed to avoid dialysis-induced hypercalcemia and permit optimal doses of calcitriol to suppress parathormone and control osteodystrophy. This rationale has no place in the treatment of acute renal failure. Several studies have shown that hemodynamic stability is improved at high (3.5–3.75 mEq/l) compared to low (2.25–2.5 mEq/l) dialysate calcium levels (223–224). Felner et al. (225) explored a broader range of dialysate calcium concentrations (1.0, 3.5 and 5.0 mEq/l) and found that serum calcium concentrations correlated directly with systolic, diastolic and mean arterial blood pressure. Various non-invasive measures of left ventricular function suggested that the improved blood pressure profile at high calcium levels was related to improved left ventricular stroke volume rather than increased peripheral vascular resistance. The benefits of higher dialysate calcium levels appear to be enhanced by hypokalemia. Wizemann et al. (226) studied myocardial contractility as a function of the calcium/potassium ratio. They found that improvement in myocardial function was related to both an increase in serum calcium and a decrease in serum

potassium. When serum potassium remained constant, their was no benefit.

We may conclude from these studies that in the setting of acute renal failure dialysate calcium levels in the range of 3.5 mEq/l are preferred. The only exceptions would be those patients with acute renal failure secondary to such conditions as rhabdomyolysis and treatment of acute leukemias when serum phosphorus may be markedly elevated and this, combined with elevated dialysate calcium may lead to diffuse tissue deposition of calcium-phosphorus complexes (195).

Magnesium

It is customary to use a dialysate magnesium concentration which is close to the normal range, i.e., 1.5–1.7 mEq/l. Patients who have undergone successful hyperalimentation without proper mineral supplementation and patients with chronic alcoholism may be hypomagnesemic. These patients should receive magnesium supplements to correct the deficit or dialysate magnesium should be increased to eliminate any pre-disposition to cardiac arrhythmias.

Bicarbonate/acetate

With increasing use of high efficiency and high flux dialysis, the adverse effects of acetate as a dialysate buffer have become apparent. The metabolism of acetate normally leads to the generation of a bicarbonate molecule in addition to CO_2 and H_2O. However, this process may be slower in patients with renal failure (227). Thus, when large amounts of acetate enter the blood stream and the rate of metabolic disposal is exceeded several adverse effects may be seen, especially vasodilation, hypoxemia and acidosis. Acetate is a potent vasodilator and can increase splanchnic blood flow significantly; (228) in addition, it may have a direct negative effect on myocardial contractility (229, 230). These effects, especially in the presence of ongoing ultrafiltration, are likely to result in hypotension. The relative effects of acetate versus dialysate sodium concentration on cardiovascular stability during hemodialysis have not been thoroughly studied and there are reports which suggest that at a dialysate sodium concentration of 140 mEq/l or more, there is no benefit of bicarbonate over acetate, except in patients who may be acetate intolerant (~10% of dialysis patients) (215). In a double-blind, cross-over study of 120 dialyses in 30 patients with acute renal failure, Borges et al. (231) found no significant difference in maintenance of blood pressure or clinical symptoms between the use of acetate or bicarbonate dialysate.

Two mechanisms appear to account for the hypoxemia seen during acetate dialysis. Dissolved CO_2 in blood is lost into dialysate resulting in decreased ventilatory drive and hypoxemia. In addition, metabolism of acetate results in a significant amount of oxygen consumption (215, 232). A moderate degree of acidosis may occur with acetate dialysate due to the loss of bicarbonate into dialysate and inadequate generation of new bicarbonate because of the

Table 5. Dialysate composition* for use in continuous hemodialysis

Solute	Baxter CAV-HD dialysis fluid	Dianeal (1.5%) (Baxter, Inc)
Sodium	140	132
Calcium	3.5	3.5
Potassium	2.0	0
Magnesium	1.5	1.5
Chloride	117	102
Lactate	30	35
D-glucose	100 mg/dl	1,360 mg/dl
Unit volume	3 litres	2, 2.5, 3 & 5 litres

CAV-HD = continuous arteriovenous hemodialysis.
* All solutes except D-glucose measured in mEq/litre.

lowered rate of acetate metabolism. Although the available studies appear to be inconclusive, there has been an overall trend toward bicarbonate dialysate, especially in the setting of acute renal failure. Since many of these patients are critically ill, it would be preferable not to expose them to some of the potential adverse effects of acetate and, therefore, this trend is probably prudent.

Dextrose

When dextrose is not added to dialysate, the dialysis treatment can result in a negative nitrogen balance, suggesting gluconeogenesis (235). This is undesirable at any time but especially during acute renal failure. In addition, there are more subjective complaints and more episodes of hypotension when patients undergo dialysis with dextrose-free dialysate (234). The minimum level of dialysate should probably be 100 mg/dl (195). Slightly high dextrose concentrations such as 250 mg/dl will supply some calories during dialysis while causing only modest increases in blood glucose (~20–30 mg/dl) (235).

Phosphorus

Although hyperphosphatemia is the rule in acute renal failure, it is not rare to see hypophosphatemia develop during successful hyperalimentation in this clinical setting. Hypophosphatemia may also be seen in certain disorders such as heat stroke and some burn cases (236, 237).

Chloride

The chloride concentration simply makes up the difference between the cations and other anions. It is determined primarily by the choice of sodium level and buffer base concentration. In some alkalemic patients, such as those on prolonged or high volume nasogastric suction, a lower level of buffer base and a higher than normal chloride concentration may be beneficial (238).

Dialysis solutions – continuous hemodialysis

The composition of the two most common dialysate preparations used in continuous hemodialysis is displayed in Table 5. Both solutions are sterile and supplied in plastic bags of various volumes, as shown. The first solution was specifically formulated for continuous hemodialysis while the second, Dianeal, was designed to meet the needs of peritoneal dialysis patients. The first solution takes advantage of those features which tend to promote hemodynamic stability in intermittent hemodialysis patients, i.e., Na = 140 mEq/l, Ca = 3.5 mEq/l, Mg – 1.5 mEq/l and D-glucose – 100 mg/dl. A small amount of potassium (K = 2.0 mEq/l) is added as an extra precaution against hypokalemia. This solution requires no modification before use in most patients. In contrast, Dianeal requires at least the addition of hypertonic saline (usually 10 ml of 23.4% saline, i.e., 40 mEq of sodium/5 litre bag or 8 mEq of sodium/litre). This will increase dialysate sodium to 140 mEq/l. The higher glucose concentration in Dianeal results in the uptake of about 700 kcal/day. Occasionally, this results in significant hyperglycemia and insulin administration may be necessary. Potassium may be added to either solution depending on serum K levels. The only other difference between the two preparations is cost; Dianeal is significantly less expensive.

Complications of hemodialysis and their treatment

These are dealt with in detail in Chapter 26 and will only be outlined here.

Blood pressure problems

The most common and dangerous problem occurring during acute hemodialysis is hypotension. A fall in blood pressure exceeding 25% of baseline occurs in 20–50% of all acute hemodialysis treatments (231, 239–241). The pathogenesis of hypotension during dialysis has recently been reviewed (238). While the mechanisms are not completely understood it is clear that ultrafiltration, *per se*, is not the cause. This was demonstrated by Bergstrom et al. (242). They showed that a given amount of ultrafiltration would provoke hypotension during standard dialysis, but was well-tolerated during isolated ultrafiltration. The mechanism underlying this difference relates to the decrease in plasma osmolality (relative to intracellular osmolality) due to diffusive loss of small molecules during dialysis. This results in the shift of fluid from the vascular to the intracellular space, thereby adding to the volume lost by ultrafiltration. In the absence of diffusion (i.e., isolated ultrafiltration) this intracellular fluid shift does not occur.

In a recent review of dialysis-induced hypotension, Zucchelli and Santoro emphasized the role of plasma refilling time in the pathogenesis of hypotension (243). They used a continuous on-line optical technique to esti-

848   *Carl M. Kjellstrand and Brendan P. Teehan*

mate blood volume from hematocrit level during dialysis with ultrafiltration. Even at constant ultrafiltration rates, patients showed considerable variation in blood volume during dialysis, a finding best explained by differences in plasma refilling times from one patient to another. Those with slower refill times were designated as hypotension-prone while those with rapid refill times were considered to be hypotension-resistant. It is not clear from the data presented whether dialysate sodium concentration and serum protein levels, two major determinants of plasma refill time, were comparable in the two groups of patients. In a preliminary report using a similar optical technique, Steuer et al. (244) were able to relate three intradialytic morbid events, mean arterial pressure less than 75 mmHg, cramping and lightheadedness to either a patient-specific level of hematocrit or an estimated level of circulating blood volume. They found that the critical level of blood volume at which morbid events occurred during dialysis was 46 ± 7 ml/kg, compared to a normal value of 68 ml/kg. They also confirmed the finding of Zucchelli and Santoro that blood volume changes were greater in patients with intradialytic morbid events ($-12.2 \pm 5.5\%$/h) compared to those who remained asymptomatic during dialysis ($5.6 \pm 3.6\%$/h). If these optical devices are validated, they may become a useful adjunct to acute intermittent hemodialysis in critically ill patients. If intradialytic hypotension can be predicted and avoided, it may be possible to prevent the development of hypotension-related events such as arrhythmias and perhaps even improve recovery time in acute renal failure (195). To optimize the role of these devices in acute hemodialysis, the circulating blood volume sensor should be detected by the ultrafiltration control system in a feedback control system which would decrease fluid removal as the sensor recognizes a critical value of circulating volume is approached.

A variety of pathogenetic factors resulting in hypotension during dialysis, along with matching therapeutic options, are listed in Table 6. One of the simplest approaches to patients with recurrent hypotension on dialysis is the use of cool dialysate, i.e., 35°C compared to the normal 37°C. In a recent study, Jost et al. (245) compared the effects of cool versus normal temperature dialysate in patients with frequent episodes of hypotension. Significant increases in blood pressure and vascular resistance were found in the cool dialysate group while all of the hypotensive episodes were limited to the normal temperature dialysate patients. Both increased left ventricular contractility and increased vascular resistance have been demonstrated with cooler dialysate, perhaps mediated by cold-activation of the autonomic nervous system (246). Body temperature may fall by about one degree centigrade with this technique, but this is generally well-tolerated. Since temperature regulation is available on most modern dialyzers, this therapeutic option may be used alone or with others listed in Table 6.

In the continuous hemodialysis therapies room temperature (25°C) dialysate or replacement solutions are often

Table 6. Treatment of dialysis hypotension

Pathogenic factors	Treatment
Ultrafiltration	Frequent, short dialysis
	Continuous methods
	Constant ultrafiltration
	Separate dialysis and ultrafiltration
Osmolality fall	Slow dialysis efficiency
	Frequent short dialysis
	Higher Na-dialysate
	Infuse: Na, mannitol, other osmolar agents
Bio-incompatibility	New membranes
Acetate infusion	Bicarbonate dialysis
Endotoxin infusion	Clean dialysate
	Tighter membranes
Mediators	
Volume	Smaller dialyzers
	Osmolar agents
	Hyperoncotic albumin
Vasopressors	Vasoactive amines
Vasodilators	Dialysate temperature
	Prostaglandin inhibition
	Higher dialysate calcium
Patient factors	
Heart disease	Beta-agonist
Medications	Discontinue
Vascular disease	?
Autonomic dysfunction	Vasoactive amines
Hormonal dysfunction	Steroids
Infection	Cure
Pain	Ameliorate
Vasovagal	Atropine

used. In addition to the slow ultrafiltration rate and the absence of significant acute osmolar changes, this may be another element which promotes hemodynamic stability with these dialytic techniques. However, in about 30–50% of patients dialyzed against room temperature dialysate persistent chills may be seen and some method of warming the dialysate (usually a temperature-controlled heating pad) may be needed.

The role of biocompatible membranes in preventing intradialytic morbid events has already been emphasized above (205–209). In general, biocompatible membranes tend to activate both the complement, and the contact pathway, ultimately leading to the release of prostaglandins, various kinins and a series of cytokines which, in aggregate, promote hypotension and hypoxemia both of which predispose critically ill patients to arrhythmias and cardiovascular instability. Use of biocompatible membranes should be the standard practice in these patients.

In some patients, notably the elderly and those with prior cardiac surgery or heart disease, myocardial dysfunction may impair their ability to increase cardiac output in response to the fall in peripheral vascular resistance that occurs during dialysis, especially with acetate dialysate. In this regard Raine et al. (247) have shown in animal experiments, that renal failure induces myocardial dysfunction by interfering with cellular calcium utilization and that this defect may be partially overcome by correction of hypocalcemia. These findings further emphasize the role of higher dialysate calcium concentrations in acute hemodialysis and probably in the continuous hemodialysis therapies.

It should also be kept in mind that some of these patients may be on medications which lower blood pressure. An intravenous nitroglycerin drip is a typical example. Occasionally, patients are on inotropic support with dopamine while also being sedated with haloperidol, a dopamine receptor antagonist. It is apparent, therefore, that a review of all medications which the patient may be on is a prudent step prior to undertaking acute dialysis.

Finally, septic patients with circulatory parameters characterized by elevated cardiac output but low peripheral vascular resistance, are especially prone to intradialytic hypotension. Treatment with appropriate antibiotics should be started as soon as possible and pressor support may be necessary. In those patients with persistently low mean arterial pressures in spite of these maneuvers, an efficient continuous therapy such as CVVHD may be necessary since these patients also tend to be quite catabolic and, therefore, not easily managed with peritoneal dialysis.

Cardiac arrhythmias

In the acutely ill patient undergoing intermittent hemodialysis there are numerous factors which may predispose to cardiac arrhythmias; these include underlying heart disease, the concurrent use of multiple inotropes, rapid changes in serum electrolytes (especially potassium) and osmolality, hypotension and hypoxemia. Hypokalemia should be carefully avoided in patients who are on digitalis preparations. Because of these multiple risk factors for arrhythmias, it has been standard practice to use continuous cardiac rhythm monitoring during acute hemodialysis – for both the intermittent and the continuous therapies. This allows prompt recognition and treatment of the arrhythmia as well as monitoring the response to various interventions. When serious arrhythmias do not respond to therapy and threaten circulatory stability, it is often prudent to discontinue dialysis until this problem has been resolved.

Electrolyte abnormalities

Significant electrolyte changes during dialysis, especially acute hypokalemia, are usually due to mistakes in formulating the dialysate composition. This has been discussed above in the section on dialysis solutions. Another potential cause of acute and possibly severe electrolyte abnormalities during hemodialysis is the use of regional citrate anticoagulation (204). Unless carefully designed and monitored, this technique can result in hypernatremia, hypocalcemia and alkalosis.

Disequilibrium

Dialysis disequilibrium is a neurologic disorder, presenting with varying degrees of severity, which appears to arise from the osmotic shift of water into brain cells during dialysis. The patients most at risk have the following characteristics; those just starting on dialysis, especially with a high pre-dialysis BUN, the elderly and the pediatric age groups, those with preceding brain damage, including ischemia or a pre-existing seizure disorder and those with severe metabolic acidosis (248). In its mildest form, symptoms of this syndrome may be limited to headache and nausea but these findings may progress to restlessness, confusion, disorientation, blurred vision, seizures, coma and death. In recent years, severe disequilibrium is rare in adults because the clinical setting in which it occurs is well-recognized and preventive measures are routinely employed, especially in the acute dialysis setting. However, in children and adolescents an incidence of dialysis-associated seizures as high as 7% has been reported (249).

The pathophysiology of this syndrome has recently been studied. The role of urea in promoting the osmotic shift of water into brain cells and causing cerebral edema has been reconfirmed in uremic rats (250). In these studies, rapid dialysis resulted in a decrease in blood urea nitrogen from 200 to 95 mg/dl over a 90 minute period. While the blood urea nitrogen decreased by 53%, brain urea nitrogen fell by only 13%, reflecting the fact that movement of urea out of brain cells is a relatively slow process, probably taking hours to complete and, therefore, acting as an effective osmolar force throughout the period of a typical acute hemodialysis treatment. These rats developed cerebral edema while those dialyzed against a high urea dialysate, and control rats which were not dialyzed, did not.

As indicated above dialysis disequilibrium may become a serious condition. It should be anticipated in patients at risk, and avoided by appropriate interventions. If intermittent dialysis is to be used, the efficiency of the initial treatments should be low, yielding a urea reduction ratio of URR perhaps 0.3, where URR = (Pre-BUN − Post-BUN/Pre-BUN). Daily treatments may be necessary to achieve control of azotemia for the first 5 to 7 days. It should be noted that the continuous therapies, including peritoneal dialysis, are ideal in preventing this syndrome because of their inherent low efficiency in urea removal compared to standard hemodialysis. Finally, when disequilibrium is suspected, the infusion of osmotically active agents, such as mannitol (one ampule) or hypertonic saline (10 ml of 23.4% saline) should help to reduce cerebral edema.

Cell destruction

Hemodialysis may have an effect on the formed elements of the blood. After 15 minutes of hemodialysis on a cellulosic dialyzer, when complement activation is at a maximum, (251) the leukocyte count typically falls to very low values (252–259). The mechanism of this leukopenia has been attributed to complement activation followed by increased leukocyte margination and sequestration in pulmonary capillaries, which, in turn, may result in hypoxemia. This theory, however, has been challenged because some membranes vigorously activate complement but do not cause leukopenia, whereas the reverse is true of other membranes (259). Although there may not be a fully satisfactory explanation for this leukopenia, the vast majority of recent studies support the choice of biocompatible membranes for the treatment of patients with acute renal failure (165, 107–211).

A decrease in platelet count of about 15% can be expected during hemodialysis. Parallel plate dialyzers may cause more thrombocytopenia than hollow fibre dialyzers. The cause of this thrombocytopenia is unknown (260). In the setting of disseminated intravascular coagulation or in cases of heparin-associated antibody more dramatic degrees of thrombocytopenia may be seen.

Red cell life span is normal in well-dialyzed patients (261). Evidence of hemolysis, especially acute hemolysis, should provoke a detailed review of the dialysis procedure to exclude those risk factors associated with major errors in the formulation of dialysate composition, including over-heated dialysate, exposure to chloramines, zinc, copper, formaldehyde, hydrogen peroxide-peracetic acid or bleach.

Hypoxemia

During hemodialysis P_aO_2 will fall 10–20 mmHg. In a patient with normal oxygen tension prior to dialysis this drop is of no consequence since it changes the blood oxygen saturation very little. However, in seriously ill patients with baseline hypoxemia pre-dialysis, the further drop in P_aO_2 can be catastrophic, provoking arrhythmias and possibly hypotension even before the dialysis treatment is well under way. Use of supplemental oxygen is mandatory in these patients.

As indicated above, the cause of hypoxemia on dialysis is multifactorial but two factors stand out – first is the use of bioincompatible membranes and the second is acetate dialysate. In part, the decrease in P_aO_2 is due to complement activation followed by complement-mediated leukostasis in pulmonary capillaries (255–259, 262). These effects appear to be triggered by some cellulosic membranes (165, 217–221) and, therefore, these should be avoided in critically ill patients. It should be emphasized, however, that not all cellulosic membranes are potent complement activators. For example, in one study (263) the use of a cellulose triacetate membrane resulted in little or no neutropenia, small transient increases in thromboxane and no rise in mean pulmonary pressure.

The choice of acetate dialysate may also provoke hypoxemia (215, 232). At least two mechanisms may be involved; the first is the loss of pCO_2 and, therefore, ventilatory drive; the second is increased oxygen consumption in the metabolism of acetate to bicarbonate.[72] This latter point is somewhat controversial, however, since others have found no difference in oxygen consumption during acetate versus bicarbonate dialysis (264). In the case of bicarbonate dialysate, the pCO_2 of the dialysate tends to be in the 50–60 mmHg range and there may be a net uptake of CO_2 during the dialysis treatment. Nevertheless, arterial pCO_2 does not increase, even in patients with chronic obstructive lung disease and elevated pre-dialysis levels of PCO_2.

Finally, in critically ill patients who may already have some degree of hypoxia pre-dialysis, it would be prudent to use supplemental oxygen and avoid the use of bioincompatible membranes and acetate dialysate.

PERITONEAL DIALYSIS

Peritoneal dialysis is discussed in detail in other chapters. Although previous studies (265–268) have shown no difference in the mortality rate of acute renal failure whether the patients were treated with peritoneal or hemodialysis, there have been major changes in hemodialysis technology since then, while peritoneal dialysis technology has been relatively static, except for the development of more reliable automated peritoneal dialysis machines and the more widespread use of the Tenckhoff catheter. Moreover, peritoneal dialysis is inherently inefficient and, as indicated in Figure 15, it cannot achieve adequate control of azotemia in catheter patients, even during the optimal condition of continuous operation. It cannot be used in patients who have undergone major abdominal surgery such as emergency repair of an abdominal aortic aneurysm. Patients with colostomies, ileostomies or feeding gastroscopy tubes are probably better handled by hemodialysis. And, at least in the rat, an intraperitoneal catheter close to an intestinal suture line impairs healing (269). Nevertheless, peritoneal dialysis offers several major advantages; it does not provoke hemodynamic instability, significant disequilibrium or hypoxemia and it does not require anticoagulation. Therefore, it is still well-suited for patients with head trauma (182, 270) marked cardiovascular instability (271) and those at high risk of bleeding, especially if these patients are not highly catabolic. Finally, it may be used as initial therapy in patients who already have a high urea inventory (BUN

> 150 mg/dl) when first referred for dialysis. The BUN should gradually come down over a period of days if the rate of catabolism is not high and, therefore, the risk of disequilibrium will be avoided (272).

Access to the peritoneum

Peritoneal access can be obtained either with a stiff Teflon or a soft silastic catheter. Either can be placed percutaneously at the bedside over a guide wire. The silastic catheter, with its larger lumen, may require the use of 1 or 2 graded dilators or a minilaparotomy for insertion. This catheter has the advantages of improved drainage, less risk of infection due to a cuff and a subcutaneous tunnel, and prolonged function for those patients with protracted acute renal failure. The choice of catheter and insertion technique will depend on the skill of the operator. However, in patients with ileus, mechanical bowel distension or bowel ischemia, it is often wise to place a soft silastic catheter under the condition of direct surgical vision.

Choice of fluids and additives

Presently available commercial peritoneal dialysis solutions contain electrolytes in their usual extracellular concentrations. The exceptions are potassium, which can be added as the clinical situation requires, and lactate which is used instead of bicarbonate. The dextrose monohydrate concentration is varied between 1.5 and 4.25 g/dl (76–215 mmol/l). The lower dextrose concentration often induces little net fluid removal from the patient, especially during the relatively short dwell times (30 min) typical of acute peritoneal dialysis. The more concentrated solution will remove up to 250–500 ml/exchange depending on the cycling techniques. The desired ultrafiltration rate is often achieved by alternating the dextrose content of the exchanges.

Practice patterns vary with respect to the use of heparin in peritoneal dialysis. Some add heparin only when fibrin strands are present in the dialysate or when peritonitis develops. The rationale in each case is to prevent fibrin from blocking the catheter, since blockage frequently results in catheter replacement. Others use heparin routinely in acute peritoneal dialysis based on the observation that fibrin strands are frequently seen in these bed-bound acutely ill patients. Doses of heparin up to 1,000 units per litre of dialysate generally have no systemic effect and will not alter the baseline PTT. If higher doses are used, however, it would be prudent to monitor the PTT. Since low doses of heparin are safe and may prevent blockage of the catheter, this regimen appears to be justified.

Antibiotics are of no value prophylactically. They should be added to the dialysate and also used systematically, however, in patients with pre-existing peritonitis or those who develop peritonitis. Peritoneal lavage with antibiotics improves survival in patients with peritonitis. Antibiotics are added to the dialysis fluid to achieve a level

Table 7. Complications of peritoneal dialysis

I.	Mechanical:	Pain
		Hemorrhage
		Puncture of intra-abdominal organ
		Leakage
		Inadequate drainage
		Dissection of fluid
		Wound/bowel suture problems
		Intraperitoneal catheter loss
II.	Metabolic:	Hypo/hyperglycemia
		Hypo/hypernatremia
		Hypo/hyperkalemia
		Acidosis/alkalosis
		Protein/amino acid loss
III.	Cardiovascular/ pulmonary:	Fluid overload/pulmonary edema
		Hypotension
		Hypertension
		Arrhythmia/cardiac arrest
		Atelectasis
		Pneumonia
		Aspiration
		Hydrothorax
IV.	Infectious complications:	Abscess at puncture site
		Bacterial/fungal peritonitis
		(Sterile peritonitis)

equal to the desired plasma water concentration. Once the patient has received a loading dose there is often no need to give more systemic antibiotics. Plasma levels obviously should be measured, especially in patients on continuous hemodialysis.

A number of vasodilating pharmacological agents can be added to peritoneal dialysis fluid to increase the efficiency of the procedure. They include dopamine, glucagon, isoproterenol, tolazoline, nitroprusside, dipyridamole, prostaglandins precursors. Moderate increases in dialysis efficiency can be achieved but none have been widely used clinically. The most frequently used agent for this purpose is probably nitroprusside, in a dialysis fluid concentration of 4 to 5 μg/l (15 to 19 mmol/l). It has little or no systemic effect when used in this fashion (273).

Complications of peritoneal dialysis

The complications of peritoneal dialysis are outlined in Table 7. They have been described by several authors and are discussed in other chapters. They will be only briefly discussed here.

Technical problems

The first technical problems of peritoneal dialysis include perforation of the intestine or bladder. Most authors suggest that when the intestine is perforated, the catheter should be replaced. Peritoneal dialysis with antibiotics added to the dialysis solution should then be instituted as it augments cleaning of the abdominal cavity and decreases the risk of peritonitis. Most such puncture wounds of the intestine heal spontaneously (274, 275).

Drainage problems during peritoneal dialysis are ordinarily due to positional problems or plugging of the catheter. Sometimes the problem can be solved by the use of a Fogarty embolectomy catheter to remove a fibrin plug from the peritoneal catheter. Changing the patient's position sometimes improves drainage. Unfortunately, if the problem is fibrin blockage, the catheter must be replaced.

Metabolic complications

Hyperglycemia can occur with any form of peritoneal dialysis as large amounts (100 to 200 g/day) of dextrose are absorbed from the solution. This problem is exaggerated in patients on hyperalimentation, especially if they also have diabetes mellitus. Frequent glucose determinations are then necessary. The addition of small amounts of regular insulin to the peritoneal dialysis solution (such as 20 units to the 1.5% solution and two to three times that amount to the 4.25% solution) may stabilize the glucose levels even in diabetic patients (276, 277).

Hypernatremia may occur during osmotic ultrafiltration because water traverses the peritoneum more easily than sodium. The addition of furosemide to the dialysate has been suggested to increase sodium transport (278) Hyponatremia is a rare complication of peritoneal dialysis, usually due to inappropriate composition of dialysis solution.

Hypokalemia may occur because of potassium removal or an intracellular shift, resulting from correction of acidosis or cellular uptake of glucose.

Some patients with lactic acidosis cannot be dialyzed using solutions containing lactate as they do not metabolize it rapidly enough to correct their acidosis. Special solutions containing bicarbonate must be used in such patients (279).

Large amounts of protein and amino acids may be lost in the dialysate, particularly when peritonitis exists. Plasma concentrations of these substances should be monitored and intravenous repletion is often necessary (280, 281).

Cardiovascular and pulmonary complications

Arrhythmias and hypotension can occur during the instillation of the dialysis solution. This should be avoided by slowing the inflow rate or decreasing the infusion volume. Atelectasis and hypostatic pneumonia may complicate peritoneal dialysis, but can be partially counteracted by physical therapy. Hydrothorax occurs in 5 to 10% of patients with acute renal failure treated by peritoneal dialysis. It can obviously be a disastrous complication in an acutely ill patient.

Infectious complications

The most common complication of any form of peritoneal dialysis is peritonitis. The incidence should decrease when a long subcutaneous tunnel with a soft peritoneal dialysis catheter and a closed system of dialysis fluid delivery are used. Peritonitis can be diagnosed promptly by inspecting the dialysate for turbidity and by daily microscopic examination and culture. It is important, however, to recognize that with the short dwell times typical of acute peritoneal dialysis, turbidity of fluid may not be apparent at the onset of peritonitis since the protein and cell count is diluted by the volume of each hourly exchange. Therefore, both quantitative and objective measures are needed to establish a diagnosis of peritonitis in these patients. In this setting, the daily culture of dialysate is probably a prudent practice. More than 500 leukocytes/μl signifies peritonitis. A test-strip for leukocyte esterase has also been used. When peritonitis is suspected, antibiotics should be added to the dialysate after fluid has been sent for culture. Sometimes parenteral administration of antibiotics is also necessary, although peritonitis in this setting rarely results in bacteremia. Daily cultures of peritoneal fluid in such patients may detect an infection early.

IMPROVING SURVIVAL

It is clear that the outcome of acute renal failure depends on the underlying disease. For example, patients who are otherwise well may develop acute renal failure from administration of radiocontrast media. But even though their serum creatinine may increase by 2 mg/dl or more, they are usually asymptomatic, non-oliguric and rarely require dialysis (282). However, in patients who undergo dialysis for primary renal disease, mortality increases to 24% and when acute tubular necrosis is due to multiple medical or surgical insults, mortality may approach 70% (163, 283, 284). Patients most at risk are those with multiple organ failure syndrome, a condition in which inflammatory mediators such as tumour necrosis factor play a part in the ongoing catabolic stress (285). Mortality rates may increase to 80% when acute renal failure follows major cardiovascular or gastrointestinal surgery.

Given these high mortality rates in acute renal failure and the fact that only a limited number of studies suggest ways to improve survival (163–165), it would appear that prevention of acute renal failure and treatment of the underlying disease(s), should be the main goals of management. The major cause of death in this setting is not uremia but infection and the underlying disease (such as hypotension following cardiac surgery). A high degree of suspicion, frequent cultures and careful, selective use of antibiotics should help to minimize the impact of infectious complications. It should be recognized in this regard that repeated exposure to nephrotoxins, such as aminoglycosides, may be a critical factor in delaying recovery of renal function (286). In patients who respond poorly, become jaundiced, remain catabolic and febrile or develop a disproportionate acidosis, underlying conditions such as ischemic hepatitis, acalculous cholecystitis, ischemic bowel or ischemic extremities should be considered.

Pharmacologic treatment of acute renal failure offers some promise but the majority of studies are limited to experimental animals. For example, it has been shown in several animal models that the administration of insulin-like growth factor or epidermal growth factor can accelerate tubular regeneration and recovery of renal function in both ischemic and nephrotoxic models of acute renal failure (287–290). In the norpinephine model of post-ischemic acute renal failure, Conger et al. (291) studied the effects of infusing atrial natriuretic peptide (ANP) plus dopamine in established acute renal failure. Saline-infused animals were used as controls. They found that by day 4 of ATN serum creatinine began to decrease in the treated rats but continued to increase in the controls. There was also a significant increase in renal blood flow and GFR in the treated animals. Based on these results, Rahman et al. (292) have studied the role of ANP in the treatment of established acute renal failure in humans. They randomized 53 patients to either ANP infusion or the control group. At 24 hours after the ANP infusion, mean creatinine clearance increased from 10 to 20 ml/min and the rate of progression to dialysis was 23 versus 53% for the control group. A large (> 500 patients) study of ANP in patients with ARF has just been concluded and is under analysis. These results, as well as those achieved with growth factors offer some hope for improved survival in patients with acute renal failure. It is probably only a matter of time before these agents, all of which are experimental, become available to the clinician.

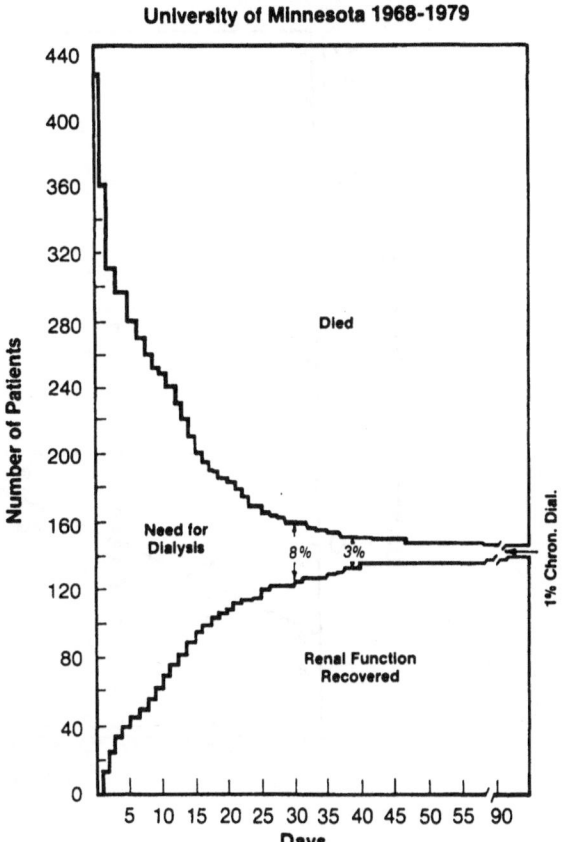

**Acute Tubular Necrosis
University of Minnesota 1968-1979**

Figure 18. Clinical course of 432 patients with acute tubular necrosis who needed dialysis. The median time for patients who recovered renal function is approximately 12 days, for those who die 5 days. By 30 days 92% of the patients recovered renal function or died. At 40 days only 3% of the patients remained on dialysis. Ultimately only 1% of the patients who started on dialysis (4% of those who survive) need chronic dialysis. From (10) with permission.

RECOVERY OF RENAL FUNCTION: NEED FOR CONTINUOUS DIALYSIS

The clinical course of acute tubular necrosis is rapid. This is illustrated in Figure 18. In patients dialyzed for acute renal failure at the University of Minnesota, the median interval between initiation of dialysis and recovery of renal function of the survivors was 12 days. The median time between start of dialysis and death was 5 days. By 1 month 92% and by 1 1/2 months 97% of the patients had either regained renal function or died. After 45 days of acute renal failure 1/3 of the remaining patients died. Another 1/3 recovered renal function and 1/3 needed regular dialysis. The longest time a patient was dialyzed and recovered renal function was 88 days (293).

The usual duration of acute renal failure is 7 to 21 days, provided the patient is not subjected to repeated exposure

to nephrotoxins or episodes of hypotension (294). Thus, these patients have a swift clinical course and although they require an enormous investment in care and equipment, few patients require dialysis and intensive care for more than 4 weeks. Renal function usually continues to improve for approximately one month after the last dialysis. Approximately 1/3 of the patients are left with moderate renal dysfunction (plasma creatinine level 1.5 to 3 mg/dl [133 to 265 μmol/l]) and 10% have residual chronic renal failure with plasma creatinine concentration exceeding 3 mg/dl (265 μmol/l) (293, 295–301). The duration of dialysis for acute tubular necrosis does not correlate with the ultimate plasma creatinine concentration. Thus, patients who were dialyzed only once eventually had the same plasma creatinine concentration (more than 1 month after the last dialysis) as those who needed dialysis for more than 1 month (293). One patient needed dial-

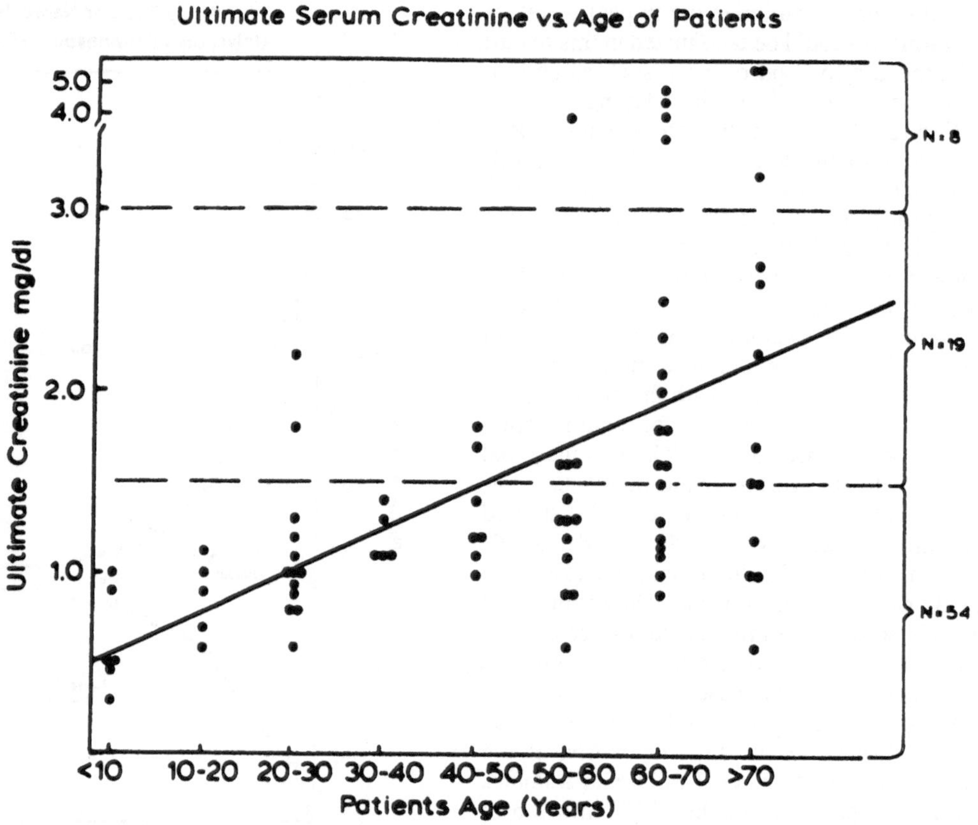

Figure 19.   Ultimate serum creatinine versus age of patients who needed dialysis for acute tubular necrosis. There is a direct relation of the ultimate serum creatinine level to age. Severe chronic renal failure occurs only in patients over the age of 50 years. From (10) with permission.

ysis for almost 3 months but ultimately reached a serum creatinine level of 1.2 mg/dl (106 μmol/l). Age, however, is directly related to the final serum creatinine concentration (Figure 19). Older patients progress to chronic renal failure, more often than younger patients do.

Chronic renal failure requiring ongoing dialysis after acute renal failure is uncommon but may occur when one or more of the following factors are present; prolonged acute renal failure (> 8 weeks), repeated episodes of hypotension and recurrent exposure to nephrotoxins (286). Prolonged acute renal failure is seen in patients with persistent sepsis and a high catabolic rate (286, 294). Thus, the major factors which predict failure to recover renal function are avoidable or treatable. Attention to these factors may further reduce the 5% or so of patients with acute renal failure who go on to chronic dialysis (293).

CONCLUSIONS

Most patients with acute renal failure have acute tubular necrosis. The mortality rate in these patients remains between 20 to 80% and has shown little improvement over time. Prevention should be the mainstay in the management of patients at risk for acute renal failure. Once renal function is lost, prompt treatment of infection and avoiding hypotensive insults are essential. While intermittent therapy (acute intermittent hemodialysis) is prone to provoking hemodynamic instability, the continuous therapies, especially those relying primarily on diffusive, as opposed to convective solute removal, may be less prone to recurring episodes of hypotension. The use of biocompatible membranes which avoid the activation of complement and the induction of cytokine and kinin release appears to improve outcome in intermittent dialysis and should probably be standard practice in the treatment of acute renal failure for the continuous therapies also. However, both of these approaches should be confirmed in larger studies. Finally, the use of specific growth factors (insulin-like growth factor 1 and epidermal growth factor) show some promise in animal studies, while the use of atrial natriuretic factor plus dopamine have shown some benefit in both animal models and human studies of established acute renal failure. Although promising, these agents are still classified as experimental at the present time.

REFERENCES

1. Kolff WJ: First clinical experience with the artificial kidney. *Ann Intern Med* 62: 608, 1965
2. Alwall N: On the artificial kidney. I. Apparatus for dialysis of the blood *in vivo*. *Acta Med Scand* 128: 31, 1947
3. Murray G: Development of an artificial kidney: experimental and clinical experiences. *Arch Surg* 55: 505, 1947
4. Alwall N: *Therapeutic and Diagnostic Problems in Severe Renal Failure*, Copenhagen, Munksgaard, 1963
5. Kennedy AC, Burton JA, Luke RG, Briggs JD, Lindsay RM, Allison MEM, Edward N, Dargie HJ: Factors affecting the prognosis in acute renal failure. A survey of 251 causes. *Q J Med* 42: 73, 1973
6. Alexopoulos E, Vakianis P, Kokolina E, Koukoudis P, Sakellariou G, Memmos D, Papadmimtriou M: Acute renal failure in a medical setting: changing patterns and prognostic factors. *Renal Failure* 16: 273, 1994
7. Biesenbach G, Zazgornik J, Kaiser W, Grafinger P, Stuby L, Necek S: Improvement in prognosis of patients with acute renal failure over a period of 15 years: an analysis of 710 cases in a dialysis center. *Am J Nephrol* 12: 319, 1992
8. Kirkland K, Edwards KDG, Whyte HM: Oliguric renal failure. A report of 400 cases including classification, survival and response to dialysis. *Aust Ann Med* 14: 275, 1965
9. Druml W, Lax F, Grimm G, Schneeweiss B, Lenz K, Laggner AN: Acute renal failure in the elderly 1975–1990. *Clin Nephrol* 41: 342, 1994
10. Kjellstrand CM, Ebben J, Davin T: Time of death, recovery of renal function, development of chronic renal failure and need for chronic hemodialysis in patients with acute tubular necrosis. *Trans Am Soc Artif Intern Organs* 27: 45, 1981
11. Teschan PE, Baxter CR, O'Brien TF, Freuhof JN, Hall WH: Prophylactic hemodialysis in the treatment of acute renal failure. *Ann Intern Med* 53: 992, 1960
12. Lundberg M: Dialysbehandling vid akut njurinsufficiens (Dialysis treatment in acute renal insufficiency). *Lakartidningen* 67: 487, 1970
13. Eliahou HA, Boichis H, Bott-Kanner G, Barell V, Bar-Noach N, Modan B: An epidemiologic study of renal failure. II. Acute renal failure. *Am J Epidemiol* 101: 281, 1975
14. Feest TG, Round A, Hamad S: Incidence of severe acute renal failure in adults: results of a community based study. *BMJ* 306: 481, 1993
15. Lachlein L, Kielstein R, Sauer K, Reinschke P, Muller V, Krumhaar I, Falkenhagen D, Schmidt R, Klinkmann H: Evaluation of 433 cases of acute renal failure. *Proc Eur Dial Transplant Assoc* 14: 628, 1977
16. Wing AJ, Broyer M, Brunner FP, Brynger H, Challa S, Donckerwolke RA, Gretz N, Jacobs C, Kramer P, Selwood NH: Combined report on regular dialysis and transplantation in Europe, XIII, 1982. *Proc Eur Dial Transplant Assoc* 20: 5, 1983
17. Hou S, Bushinsky DA, Wish JB, Cohen JJ, Harrington JT: Hospital-acquired renal insufficiency: A prospective study. *Am J Med* 74: 243, 1983
18. Porter GA, Bennett WM: Nephrotoxic-induced acute renal failure. in *Acute Renal Failure*, edited by BM Brenner and JH Stein, New York, Churchill-Livingstone, 1980
19. Hermreck AS, Ruiz-Ocana FM, Proberts KS, Meisel RL, Crawford DG: Mechanisms for oliguria in acute renal failure. *Surgery* 82: 141, 1977
20. Levinsky NG: Pathophysiology of acute renal failure. *N Engl J Med* 296: 1453, 1977
21. Solez K, Morel-Maroger L, Sraer JD: The morphology of 'acute tubular necrosis' in man: analysis of 57 renal biopsies and a comparison with the glycerol model. *Medicine* 58: 362, 1979
22. Myers BD, Carrie BJ, Yee RR. Hilberman M, Michaels AS: Pathophysiology of hemodynamically mediated acute renal failure in man. *Kidney Int* 18: 110, 1980
23. Olbricht CHJ: Experimental models of acute renal failure. *Contrib Nephrol* 42: 603, 1980
24. Conger JD, Schrier RW: Renal hemodynamics in acute renal failure. *Ann Rev Physiol* 42: 603, 1980
25. Richmond JM, Walker JF, Avila A, Petrakis A, Finely RJ, Sibbald WJ, Linton AL: Renal and cardiovascular response to nonhypotensive sepsis in a large animal model with peritonitis. *Surgery* 97: 205, 1985
26. Zager RA, Sharma HM, Johannes GA: Gentamicin increases renal susceptibility to an acute ischemic insult. *J Lab Clin Med* 101: 670, 1983
27. Fink MP, MacVittie TJ, Casey LC: Effects of non-steroidal anti-inflammatory drugs on renal function in septic dogs. *J Surg Res* 36: 516, 1984
28. Harkonen S, Kjellstrand C: Contrast nephropathy. *Am J Nephrol* 1: 69, 1981
29. Rasmussen HH, Lloyd SI: Acute renal failure. *Am J Med* 73: 211, 1984
30. Miller PD, Krebs RA, Neal BJ, McIntyre DO: Polyuric pre-renal failure. *Arch Intern Med* 140: 907, 1980
31. Ellenbogen P, Schieble F, Talner L: Sensitivity of gray scale ultrasound in detecting urinary tract obstruction. *Am J Roentgenol* 130: 731, 1978
32. Rascoff JH, Golden RA, Spinowitz BS, Charytan C: Non-dilated obstructive nephropathy. *Arch Intern Med* 143: 696, 1983
33. McClennan B: Current approaches to the azotemic patient. *Radiol Clin North Am* 17: 314, 1979
34. Wilson DR: Renal function during and following obstruction. *Ann Rev Med* 28: 329, 1977
35. Pru C, Kjellstrand CM: Indices and urinary chemistries in the differential diagnosis of pre-renal failure and acute tubular necrosis. *Semin Nephrol* 5: 224, 1985
36. Ransohoff DR, Feinstein AR: Problems of spectrum and bias in evaluating the efficacy of diagnostic tests. *N Engl J Med* 299: 926, 1978
37. Brown R, Babcock R, Tablert J, Gruenberg J, Czurak C, Campbell M: Renal function in critically ill postoperative patients: sequential assessment of creatinine, osmolar and free water clearance. *Crit Care Med* 8: 68, 1980
38. Shilliday I, Allison ME: Diuretics in acute renal failure. *Renal Failure* 16: 3, 1994
39. Mann HJ, Fuhs DW, Hemstrom CA: Acute renal failure. *Drug Intell Clin Pharm* 20: 421, 1986

40. Henderson IS, Beattie TJ, Kennedy AC: Dopamine Hydrochloride in oliguric states. *Lancet* 2: 827, 1980

41. Neiberger RE, Passmore JC: Effects of dopamine on canine intrarenal blood flow distribution during hemorrhage. *Kidney Int* 15: 219, 1979

42. Lindner A: Synergism of dopamine and furosemide in diuretic-resistant, oliguric acute renal failure. *Nephron* 33: 121, 1983

43. Rahman SN, Kim GE, Mathew AS, Goldberg CA, Allgren R, Schrier RW, Conger JD: Effects of atrial natriuretic peptide in clinical acute renal failure. *Kidney Int* 45: 1731, 1994

44. Paller MS: Free radical scavengers in mercuric chloride-induced acute renal failure in the rat. *J Lab Clin Med* 105: 459, 1985

45. Paller MS, Hoidal JR, Ferris TF: Oxygen free radicals in ischemic acute renal failure in the rat. *J Clin Invest* 74: 1156, 1985

46. Siegel NJ, Glazier WB, Chaudry IH, Gaudio KM, Lytton B, Baue AE, Kashgarian M: Enhanced recovery from acute renal failure by the post-ischemic infusion of adenine nucleotides and magnesium chloride in rats. *Kidney Int* 7: 338, 1980

47. Sumpio BE, Chaudry IH, Baue AE: Reduction of the drug-induced nephrotoxicity by ATP – MgCl$_2$, I. Effects on the cis-diamminedicholoroplatinum-treated isolated perfused kidneys. *J Surg Res* 38: 429, 1985

48. Oken DE, Sprinke FM, Kirschbaum BB, Landwehr DM: Amino acid therapy in the treatment of experimental acute renal failure in the rat. *Kidney Int* 17: 14, 1980

49. Loutzenhiser R, Epstein M: Calcium antagonists and the kidney. *Hospital Practice* Jan 15: 63, 1987

50. Wagner K, Albrech S, Neumayer HH: Prevention of delayed graft function in cadaveric kidney transplantation by a calcium antagonist. Preliminary results of two prospective randomized trials. *Transplant Proc* 18: 510, 1986

51. Wagner K, Schultze G, Molzahn M, Neumayer H-H: The influence of long-term infusion of the calcium antagonist diltiazem on postischemic acute renal failure in conscious dogs. *Klin Wochenschr* 64: 135, 1986

52. Abel RM, Beck CH, Abbott WM, Ryan JA, Barnett GO, Fisher JE: Improved survival from acute renal failure after treatment with intravenous essential L-amino acids and glucose. *N Engl J Med* 288: 695, 1973

53. Baek SM, Makabali GG, Bryan-Brown CW, Kusek J, Shoemaker WC: The influence of parenteral nutrition on the course of acute renal failure. *Surg Gynecol Obstet* 141: 405, 1975

54. Bergman AS, Fäit K, Odar-Cederlöf, Westman L, Rakolander R: Calcitonin gene-elated peptide attentuates experimental ischemic renal failure in a rat model of reversible renal ischemic insult. *Renal Failure* 16: 351, 1994

55. Hammer MR, Miller SB: Therapeutic use of growth factors in renal failure. *J Am Soc Nephrol* 5: 1, 1994

56. Borges H, Hocks J, Kjellstrand CM: Mannitol intoxication in patients with renal failure. *Arch Intern Med* 142: 63, 1982

57. Smith JH, Merrell RC, Raffin TA: Reversal of postoperative anuria by decompressive celiotomy. *Arch Intern Med* 145: 553, 1985

58. Gehrig JJ: Oliguria and increased intra-abdominal pressure. *JAMA* 253: 39, 1985

59. Chugh KS: Clinicopathological spectrum of acute renal failure in India. in *Proc First Asian Pacific Congr Nephrol Hihol Univ Dept of Med Tokyo* 1979, p 133

60. Chugh KS, Pal Y, Chakravarty RN, Datta DB, Mehta R, Sakhuja V, Mandal AK, Sommers SC: Acute renal failure following poisonous snakebite. *Am J Kidney Dis* 4: 30, 1984

61. Sitprija V: The kidney in acute tropical disease. *Abstracts 8th Int Congress Nephrol* 8: 279, 1981

62. Lordon RE, Burton JR: Post-traumatic renal failure in military personnel in Southeast Asia: experience at Clark USAF Hospital. Republic of the Philippines. *Am J Med* 53: 137, 1972

63. Fischer RP: High mortality of post-traumatic renal insufficiency in Vietnam: a review of 96 cases. *Am Surg* 40: 172, 1974

64. Stone WJ, Knepshield JH: Post-traumatic renal insufficiency in Vietnam. *Clin Nephrol* 2: 186, 1974

65. Barsoum RS, Rihan ZEB, Baligh OK, Hozayen A, El-Ghonaimy EHG, Ramzy MF, Ibrahuim AS: Acute renal failure in the 1973 Middle East War; Experience of a specialized base hospital: Effect of the site of injury. *J Trauma* 20: 303, 1980

66. Bullock ML, Umen AJ, Finkelstein M, Keane WR: The assessment of risk factors in 462 patients with acute renal failure. *Am J Kidney Dis* 5: 97, 1985

67. Plough AL, Salem S: Social and contextual factors in the analysis of mortality in end-stage renal disease patients: implications for health policy. *Am J Public Health* 7: 1293, 1982

68. Avram MM, Pahilan A, Altman E, Gan A, Iancu M: A 15-year experience with intradialytic treatment mortality. *Abstracts Am Soc Artif Intern Organs* 11: 41, 1982

69. Friedman EA, Manis T, Delano BG, Rao TKS, Levits CS, Lundin AP III: Extraordinary safety of hemodialysis. *Abstracts Am Soc Artif Intern Organs* 11: 48, 1982

70. McMurray SD, Luft FC, Maxwell DR, Hamburger RJ, Futty D, Swed JJ, Lavelle KJ, Kleit SA: Prevailing patterns and predictor variables in patients with acute tubular necrosis. *Arch Intern Med* 138: 950, 1978

71. Gornick CC Jr, Kjellstrand CM: Acute renal failure complicating aortic aneurysm surgery. *Nephron* 35: 145, 1983

72. Wheeler DC, Feehally J, Walls J: High risk acute renal failure. *Quart J Med* 61: 977, 1986

73. Abreo K, Moorthy V, Osborne M: Changing patterns and outcome of acute renal failure requiring hemodialysis. *Arch Int Med* 146: 1338, 1986

74. Rasmussen HH, Pitt EA, Ibels LS, McNeil DR: Prediction of outcome in acute renal failure by discriminant analysis of clinical variables. *Arch Int Med* 145: 2015, 1985

75. Lien J, Chan V: Risk factors influencing survival in acute renal failure treated by hemodialysis. *Arch Intern Med* 145: 2067, 1985

76. Anderson RJ, Linas SL, Berns AS, Henrich WL, Miller TR, Gabow PA, Schrier RW: Non-oliguric acute renal failure. *New Engl J Med* 296: 1134, 1977

77. Kunz A, Glinz W, Keusch G, Binswanger U: Akutes Nierenversagen bei polytraumatisierten Patienten (Acute renal failure in multiple traumatized patients). *Schweiz Med Wochenschr* 114: 876, 1984

78. Wagner DP, Knaus WA, Draper EA: Physiologic abnormalities and outcome from acute disease. *Arch Intern Med* 146: 1389, 1986
79. Corwin HL, Teplick RS, Schreiber MJ, Fang LST, Bonventre JV, Coggina CH: Prediction of outcome in acute renal failure. *Am J Nephrol* 7: 8, 1987
80. Wardle EN: Acute renal failure and multiorgan failure. *Nephrol* 66: 380, 1994
81. Cioffi WG, Ashikaga T, Gamelli RL: Probability of surviving postoperative acute renal failure. *Ann Surg* 2: 205, 1984
82. Polk HC Jr, Shields CL: Remote organ failure: A valid sign of occult intra-abdominal infection. *Surgery* 81: 310, 1977
83. Fry DE, Pearlstein L, Fulton RL, Polk HC Jr: Multiple system organ failure. *Arch Surg* 115: 136, 1980
84. Matas AJ, Payne WD, Simmons RL, Buselmeier TJ, Kjellstrand CM: Acute renal failure following blunt civilian trauma. *Ann Surg* 185: 301, 1977
85. Mentzer SJ, Fryd DS, Kjellstrand CM: Why do patients with postsurgical acute tubular necrosis die? *Arch Surg* 120: 907, 1985
86. Gillum DM, Dixon BS, Yanover MJ, Kelleher SP, Shapiro MD, Benedetti RG, Dillingham MA, Paller MS, Goldberg JP, Tomford RC, Gordon JA, Conger JD: The role of intensive dialysis in acute renal failure. *Clin Nephrol* 25: 249, 1986
87. Liano F: Severity of acute renal failure: The need of measurement. *Nephrol Dial Transplant* 9: 229, 1994
88. Marshall VC: Acute renal failure in surgical patients. *Br J Surg* 58: 17, 1971
89. Ronco C: Continuous renal replacement therapies in the treatment of acute renal failure in intensive care patients. Part I. Theoretical aspects and techniques. *Nephrol Dial Transplant* 9: 191, 1994
90. Zimmerman JE: Respiratory failure complicating post-traumatic acute renal failure: etiology, clinical features and management. *Ann Surg* 174: 12, 1971
91. Lucas CE, Ledgerwood AM, Shier MR, Bradley VE: The renal factor in the post-traumatic fluid overload syndrome. *J Trauma* 17: 667, 1977
92. Kjellstrand CM, Davin TJ, Matas AJ, Buselmeier TJ: Post-operative acute renal failure: diagnosis, etiologic and symptomatic treatment and prognosis, in *Clinical Surgical Care*, edited by Najarian JS, Delaney JP, New York, Stratton Intercontinental Med Book Corp, 1977, p 309
93. Kohen JA, Opsahl JA, Kjellstrand CM: Deceptive patterns of uremic pulmonary edema. *Am J Kidney Dis* 7: 456, 1986
94. Bland R, Shoemaker WC, Shabot MM: Physiologic monitoring goals for the critically ill patient. *Surg Gynecol Obstet* 147: 833, 1978
95. Holliday RL, Doris PJ: Monitoring the critically ill surgical patient. *Can Med Assoc J* 121: 931, 1979
96. Anderson CC, Shahravi MBG, Simmerman JE: The treatment of pulmonary edema in the absence of renal function – a role for sorbitol and furosemide. *JAMA* 241: 1008, 1979
97. Bercovitch DD, Davidman M, Lichter M: Hyperkalemia provoked by acute hepatic necrosis. *Am J Nephrol* 6: 296, 1986
98. Galler M, Folkert VW, Schlondorff D: Reversible acute renal insufficiency and hyperkalemia following indomethacin therapy. *JAMA* 246: 155, 1981
99. Hylander B: Survival of extreme hyperkalemia. *Acta Med Scand* 221: 121, 1987
100. Montoliu J, Lens XM, Revert L: Potassium-lowering of albuterol for hyperkalemia in renal failure. *Arch Intern Med* 147: 713, 1987
101. Wolk PJ, Apicella MA: The effect of renal function on the febrile response to bacteremia. *Arch Intern Med* 138: 1084, 1978
102. Goldblum SE, Reed WP: Host defenses and immunologic alterations associated with chronic hemodialysis. *Ann Intern Med* 93: 597, 1980
103. Peresecerschi G, Blum M, Aviram A, Spirer ZH: Impaired neutrophil response to acute bacterial infection in dialyzed patients. *Arch Intern Med* 141: 1301, 1981
104. Turck M, Stamm W: Nosocomial infection of the urinary tract. *Am J Med* 70: 651, 1981
105. Rowley KM, Clubb KS, Walker Smith GJ, Cabin HS: Right-sided infective endocarditis as a consequence of flow-directed pulmonary-artery catheterization. *N Engl J Med* 311: 1152, 1984
106. Keane WF, Hirata-Dulas CA, Bullock ML, Ney AL, Guay DR, Roberto S, Kalil N, Dinarello A, Halstenson CE, Peterson PK: Adjunctive therapy with intravenous human immunoglobulin G improves survival of patients with acute renal failure. *J Am Soc Nephrol* 2: 841, 1991
107. Marshall V: Secondary surgical intervention in acute renal failure. *Aust NZ J Surg* 44: 96, 1974
108. Kornhall S: Acute renal failure in surgical disease with special regard to neglected complications. *Acta Chir Scand* 419: 3, 1971
109. Sinanan M, Maier RV, Carrico CJ: Laparatomy for intra-abdominal sepsis in patients in an Intensive Care Unit. *Arch Surg* 119: 652, 1984
110. Feinsten EI, Blumenkrantz MJ, Healy M: Clinical and metabolic response to parenteral nutrition in acute renal failure. A controlled double blind study. *Medicine* 60: 124, 1981
111. Daly JM, Dudrick SJ, Copeland EM: Intravenous hyperalimentation: effect on delayed cutaneous hypersensitivity in cancer patients. *Ann Surg* 192: 587, 1980
112. Dionigi R, Zonta A, Dominioni L, Gnes F, Ballabio A: The effects of total parenteral nutrition on immunodepression due to malnutrition. *Ann Surg* 185: 467, 1977
113. Mullen JL, Buzby GP, Matthews DC, Smale BF, Rosato EF: Reduction of operative morbidity and mortality by combined preoperative and postoperative nutritional support. *Ann Surg* 192: 604, 1980
114. Michel L, Serrano A, Malt RA: Nutritional support of hospitalized patients. *N Engl J Med* 304: 1147, 1981
115. Editorial: Current status of peripheral alimentation. *Ann Intern Med* 95: 114, 1981
116. Padberg FT, Ruggiero J, Blackburn GL, Bistrian BR: Central venous catheterization of parenteral nutrition. *Ann Surg* 193: 264, 1981
117. Abel RM: Acute renal failure, role of parenteral nutrition. *Contemp Surg* 13: 21, 1987
118. Fan S-T, Lo C-M, Edward CS, Lai MS, Chu K-M, Liu C-L, Wong J: Perioperative nutritional support in patients undergoing hepatectomy for hepatocellular carcinoma. *New Eng J Med* 331: 1547, 1994

119. Cerra FB: Hypermetabolism, organ failure, and metabolic support. *Surgery* 1: 1, 1987

120. Blagg CR, Parsons FM: Earlier dialysis and anabolic steroids in acute renal failure. *Am Heart J* 61: 287, 1961

121. Kopple JD, Gordon SI, Wang M, Swendseid ME: Factors affecting serum and urinary guanidinosuccinic acid levels in normal and uremic subjects. *J Lab Clin Med* 90: 303, 1977

122. Lynch RE, Bosl RH, Streifel AJ, Ebben JP, Ehlers SM, Kjellstrand CM: Dialysis thrombocytopenia: parallel plate vs hollow fiber dialyzers. *Trans Am Soc Artif Intern Organs* 24: 704, 1978

123. Vicks SL, Gross ML, Schmitt GW: Massive hemorrhage due to hemodialysis-associated thrombocytopenia. *Am J Nephrol* 3: 30, 1983

124. Janson PA, Jubelirer S, Weinsten M, Deykin D: Treatment of the bleeding in uremia with cryoprecipitate. *New Engl J Med* 303: 1318, 1980

125. Mannucci PM, Remuzzi G, Pusineri F, Lombardi R, Valsecchi C, Mecca G, Zimmerman TS: Deamino-8-arginine vasopressin shortens bleeding in uremia. *N Engl J Med* 308: 8, 1983

126. Liu YK, Kosfeld RE, Marcum SG: Treatment of uraemic bleeding with conjugated oestrogen. *Lancet* 2: 887, 1984

127. Czer LSC, Shoemaker WC: Optimal hematocrit value in critically ill postoperative patients. *Surg Gynecol Obset* 147: 463, 1978

128. Livio M, Marchesi D, Remuzzi G, Gotti E, Mecca G, Gaetano G: Uraemic bleeding: role of anaemia and beneficial effect of red cell transfusions. *Lancet* 2: 1013, 1982

129. Remuzzi G. Marchesi D, Cavenaghi AE, Livio M, Donati MB, de Gaetano G, Mecca G: Bleeding in renal failure: a possible role of vascular prostacyclin (PGI$_2$). *Clin Nephrol* 12: 127, 1979

130. Ben-Menachem T, Fogel R, Patel RV, Touchette M, Zarowitz BJ, Hadzijahic N, Divine G, Verter J, Bresalier RS: Prophylaxis for stress-related gastric hemorrhage in the medical intensive care unit. *Ann Intern Med* 121: 568, 1994

131. Ardaillou R, Beaufils M, Nivers M-P, Isaac R, Mayaud C, Sraer J-D: Increased plasma calcitonin in early acute renal failure. *Clin Sci Mol Med* 49: 301, 1985

132. Weinstein RS, Hudson JB: Parathyroid hormone and 25-hydroycholecalciferol levels in hypercalcemia of acute renal failure. *Arch Intern Med* 140: 410, 1980

133. Arieff AI, Massry SG: Calcium metabolism of brain in acute renal failure: effects of uremia, hemodialysis and parathyroid hormone. *J Clin Invest* 53: 387, 1974

134. de Torrente A, Berl T, Cohn PD, Kawamoto E, Hertz P, Schrier RW: Hypercalcemia of acute renal failure: clinical significance and pathogenesis. *Am J Med* 61: 119, 1976

135. Feinstein EI, Akmal M, Telfer N, Massry SG: Delayed hypercalcemia with acute renal failure associated with non-traumatic rhabdomyolysis. *Arch Intern Med* 141: 753, 1981

136. Chugh KS, Nath IVS, Ubroi HS, Singhal PC, Pareek SK, Sarkar AK: Acute renal failure due to non-traumatic rhabdomyolysis. *Postgrad Med J* 55: 386, 1979

137. Schiller WR, Long CL, Blakemore WS: Creatinine and nitrogen excretion in seriously ill and injured patients. *Surg Gynecol Obstet* 149: 561, 1979

138. Kjellstrand CM, Campbell DC, von Hartizsch B, Buselmeier TJ: Hyperuricemic acute renal failure. *Arch Intern Med* 133: 349, 1974

139. Nielsen OJ, Thaysen JH: Erythropoietin deficiency in acute tubular necrosis. *J Intern Med* 227: 373, 1990

140. Kelton J, Kelley WN, Holmes EW: A rapid method for the diagnosis of acute uric acid nephropathy. *Arch Intern Med* 138: 612, 1978

141. Zaloga GP, Chernow B: Hypocalcemia in critical illness. *JAMA* 10: 924, 1986

142. Zaloga GP, Rainey TG: Hypocalcemia in the critically ill: when to suspect and what to do. *J Crit Illness* 1: 12, 1986

143. Bennett WM, Aronoff GR, Golper TA, Morrison G, Singer I, Brater DC: *Drug Prescribing in Renal Failure*, Am College Physicians, Philadelphia PA, 1991

144. Woodrow G, Turney J: Cause of death in acute renal failure. *Nephrol Dial Transplant* 7: 230, 1992

145. Bullock M, Umen A, Finkelstein N, Keane W: The assessment of risk factors in 462 patients with acute renal failure. *Am J Kid Dis* 5: 97, 1985

146. Pascual J, Orofino L, Liano F, Marcen R, Naya M, Orte L, Ortuno J: Incidence and prognosis of acute renal failure in older patients. *J Am Geriatr Soc* 38: 25, 1990

147. Schaefer JH, Jochimsen F, Keller F, Wegscheider K, Distler A: Outcome prediction of acute renal failure in medical intensive care. *Intensive Care Med* 17: 19, 1991

148. Corwin H, Teplick R, Schreiber M, Fang L, Bonventre J, Coggins C: Prediction of outcome in acute renal failure. *Am J Nephrol* 7: 8, 1987

149. Lohr J, McFarlane M, Grantham J: A clinical index to predict survival in acute renal failure patients requiring dialysis. *Am J Kid Dis* 11: 254, 1988

150. Bellomo R, Ernst D, Love J, Parkin G: Continuous arteriovenous haemodiafiltration: Optimal therapy for acute renal failure in an intensive care setting? *Aust NZ J Med* 20: 237, 1990

151. Stevens PE, Rainford DJ: Isovolemic hemodialysis combined with hemofiltration in acute renal failure. *Renal Failure* 122: 205, 1990

152. Storck M, Hartl WH, Zimmerer E, Inthorn D: Comparison of pump-driven and spontaneous continuous hemofiltration in post-operative acute renal failure. *Lancet* 337: 452, 1991

153. McDonald BR, Mehta RL: Decreased mortality in patients with acute renal failure undergoing continuous arteriovenous hemodialysis. *Contrib Nephrol* 93: 51, 1991

154. Biesenbach G, Zazornick J, Kaiser W, Grafinger P, Stuby U, Nacek S: Improvement in prognosis of patients with acute renal failure over a period of 15 years: an analysis of 710 cases in a dialysis center. *Am J Nephrol* 12: 319, 1992

155. Bellomo R, Mansfield D, Rumble S, Shapiro J, Parkin G, Boyce N: Conventional dialysis *vs* acute continuous hemodiafiltration. *J Am Soc Artif Intern Organs* 38: M654, 1992

156. Bellomo R, Parkin G, Love J, Boyce N: Use of continuous haemofiltration: an approach to the management of acute renal failure in the critically ill. *Am J Nephrol* 12: 240, 1992

157. Ronco C: Continuous renal replacement therapies in the treatment of acute renal failure in intensive care patients. *Clin Nephrol* 40: 187, 1993

158. Kruczynski K, Irvine-Bird K, Toffelmire EB, Morton AR: A comparison of continuous arteriovenous hemofiltration in intermittent hemodialysis in acute renal failure patients in the intensive care unit. *J Am Soc Artif Intern Organs* 39: M778, 1993

159. Davenport A, Will EH, Davidson AM: Improved cardiovascular stability during continuous modes of renal replacement therapy in critically ill patients with acute hepatic and renal failure. *Crit Care Med* 21: 328, 1993

160. Bellomo R, Boyce N: Continuous venovenous hemodiafiltration compared with conventional dialysis in critically ill patients with acute renal failure. *J Am Soc Artif Intern Organs* 39: M794, 1993

161. Alarabi AA, Danielson BG, Wilkstrom B: Continuous arteriovenous hemodialysis: Outcome in intensive care acute renal failure patients. *Nephron* 64: 58, 1993

162. Bellomo R, Mansfield D, Rumble S, Shapiro J, Parkin G, Boyce N: A comparison of conventional dialytic therapy and acute continuous hemodiafiltration in the management of acute renal failure in the critically ill. *Renal Failure* 15: 595, 1993

163. Barton IK, Hilton PJ, Taub NA, Warburton FG, Swan AV, Dwight J, Mason JC: Acute renal failure treated by haemofiltration: Factors affecting outcome. *Q J Med* 86: 81, 1993

164. Firth JD: Renal replacement therapy on the intensive care unit. *Q J Med* 86: 75, 1993

165. Hakim RM, Wingrad RL, Parker RA: The effect of the dialysis membrane on outcome of acute renal failure. *N Engl J Med* 331: 1338, 1994

166. Clark WR, Alaka KJ, Macias WL, Mueller BA: A comparison of metabolic control by continuous and intermittent therapies in acute renal failure. *J Am Soc Nephrol* 4: 1413, 1994

167. Gotch F: Urea kinetic modeling in hemodialysis. in *Clinical Dialysis* 2nd Edition, edited by Nissenson A, Fine R, Gentile D, East Norwalk, CT, Appleton and Lange, 1990, p 118

168. Keshaviah PR, Nolph KD, VanStone J: The peak concentration hypothesis: a urea kinetic approach to comparing the adequacy of continuous ambulatory peritoneal dialysis (CAPD) and hemodialysis. *Peritoneal Dial Int* 9: 257, 1989

169. Ifediora O, Teehan BP, Sigler MH: Solute clearance in continuous venovenous hemodialysis: a comparison of cuprophane, polyacrylonitrile and polysulfone membranes. *Trans Am Soc Artif Intern Organs* 38: M697, 1992

170. Paganini E: Continuous renal replacement is the preferred treatment for all acute renal failure patients receiving intensive care. *Semin Dial* 7: 176, 1993

171. Henrich W: Arteriovenous or venovenous continuous therapies are not superior to standard hemodialysis in all patients with acute renal failure. *Semin Dial* 6: 174, 1993

172. Teschan PE, Baxter CR, O'Brien TF, Freehof HN, Hall WH: Prophylactic hemodialysis in the treatment of acute renal failure. *Ann Intern Med* 53: 992, 1960

173. Daugirdas JT: Acute hemodialysis prescription. in *Handbook of Dialysis*, 2nd Edition, edited by Daugirdas JT, Ing TS, Little Brown, 1994, p 78

174. Sigler MH, Teehan BP: Continous renal replacement therapy. in *Clinical Dialysis*, 3rd Edition, edited by Nissenson AR, Fine RN, Gentile DE, East Norwalk, CT, Appleton and Lange, 1994. In press

175. Salisbury PF: Timely versus delayed use of the artificial kidney. *Arch Int Med* 101: 690, 1958

176. Scribner BH: Role of the artificial kidney in management of acute renal failure. *Northwest Med* 58: 555, 1959

177. Scribner BH, Magid GJ, Burnell JM: Prophylactic hemodialysis in the management of acute renal failure. *Clin Research* 8: 136, 1960

178. Scribner BH, Caner JE, Buri R, Quinton W: The technique of continuous hemodialysis. *Trans Am Soc Artif Intern Organs* 6: 88, 1960

179. Geronemus R, Schneider N: Continuous arteriovenous hemodialysis: A new modality for treatment of acute renal failure. *Trans Am Soc Artif Intern Organs* 30: 610, 1984

180. Guillam DN, Dixon BS, Yanover MJ, Kelleher SP, Schapiro MD, Beneditti RG, Dillingham MA, Paller MS, Goldberg JP, Tomford RC, Gordon JA, Conger JD. The role of intensive dialysis in acute renal failure. *Clin Nephrol* 25: 249, 1986

181. Gornick CC, Kjellstrand CM: Acute renal failure complicating aortic aneurysm surgery. *Nephron* 35: 145, 1983

182. Matas AJ, Payne WD, Simmons RL, Buselmeier TJ, Kjellstrand CM: Acute renal failure following blunt civilian. *Ann Surg* 185: 301, 1977

183. Mentzer SJ, Fryd DS, Kjellstrand CM: Why do patients with post-surgical acute tubular necrosis die? *Arch Surg* 120: 907, 1985

184. Daugirdas JT, Depner TA: A nomogram approach to hemodialysis urea modeling. *Am J Kidney Dis* 23: 33, 1994

185. Collins AJ, Ma JZ, Umen A, Keshaviah R: Urea index and other predictors of hemodialysis patient survival. *Am J Kidney Dis* 23: 272, 1994

186. Garred LJ, Barichello D, Canaud B, McCready W: Simple formulas for protein catabolic rate calculation from pre- and post-dialysis urea. (Abstract) *J Am Soc Artif Intern Organs* 71, 1994

187. Kjellstrand CM, Mevino GE, Mauer SM, Casali R, Busselmeir TJ: Complications of percutaneous femoral vein catheterizations for hemodialysis. *Clin Nephrol* 4: 37, 1975

188. Fan PY, Schwab SJ: Vascular access: concepts for the 1990s. *J Am Soc Nephrol* 3: 1, 1992

189. Raja RM, Fernandes M, Kramer MS et al.: Comparison of subclavian vein with femoral vein with femoral vein catheterization for hemodialysis. *Am J Kidney Dis* 2: 474, 1983

190. Vanholder R, Lamiere N, Verbank J et al.: Complications of subclavian catheters for hemodialysis: a 5 year prospective study in 257 consecutive patients. *Int J Artif Organs* 2: 297, 1982

191. Edwards RW, King TC: Cardiac tamponade from central venous catheters. *Arch Surg* 117: 965, 1982

192. Bernard RW, Stahl WM: Subclavian vein catheterization: a prospective study of non-infectious complications. *Ann Surg* 173: 184, 1971

193. Cheesbrough JS, Finch AJ, Burder RP: A prospective study of the mechanisms of infection associated with hemodialysis catheters. *J Infect Dis* 154: 579, 1986

194. Schwab SJ, Buller GL, McCann RL, Bollinger RR, Stickel DL: Prospective evaluation of a Dacron cuffed

hemodialysis catheter for prolonged use. *Am J Kidney Dis* 11: 166, 1988

195. Kjellstrand CM, Jacobson S, Lins LE: Acute renal failure. in *Replacement of Renal Function by Dialysis*, Third ed, edited by Maher, JF, Dordrecht, Kluwer Academic Publishers, 1989, p 616

196. Conger JD: Does hemodialysis delay recovery from acute renal failure? *Semin Dial* 3: 146, 1990

197. Caruana RJ, Raja RM, Bush VG et al.: Heparin free dialysis: comparative data and results in high risk patients. *Kidney Int* 31: 1351, 1987

198. Schwab SJ, Onorato JJ, Sharar LR, Dennis PA: Hemodialysis without anticoagulation. One year prospective trial in hospitalized patients at risk for bleeding. *Am J Med* 83: 405, 1987

199. Preushof L, Keller F, Seemann J, Offermann G: Heparin-free hemodialysis with prophylactic change of dialyzer and blood lines. *Int J Artif Organs* 11: 255–258, 1988

200. Swartz RD, Port FK: Preventing hemorrhage in high risk hemodialysis. Regional versus low-dose heparin. *Kidney Int* 16: 513, 1979

201. Maher JF, Lapierre L, Schreiner GE, Geiger M, Westervelt FB: Regional heparinization for hemodialysis. *N Eng J Med* 268: 451, 1963

202. Blaufox MD, Hampers CL, Wallin JD: Rebound anticoagulation after regional heparinization for hemodialysis. *Trans Am Soc Artif Intern Organs* 12: 207, 1966

203. Pinnick E, Wiegmanson TE, Dieherich DA: Regional citrate anticoagulation for hemodialysis in the patient at high risk for bleeding. *N Engl J Med* 308: 258, 1983

204. Flanigan MJ, Von Brecht JH, Freeman RM, Lim VS: Reducing the hemorrhagic complications of dialysis: a controlled comparison of low-dose heparin and citrate anticoagulation. *Am J Kidney Dis* 9: 147, 1987

205. Mehta RL, McDonald BR, Aguilar MM, Ward DM: Regional citrate anticoagulation for continuous arteriovenous hemodialysis in critically ill patients. *Kidney Int* 38: 976, 1990

206. Swartz RD, Flamenbaum W, Dubrow A, Hall JC, Crow JW, Cato A: Epoprostenol (PG12 prostacyclin) during high risk hemodialysis – preventing further bleeding complications. *J Clin Pharmacol* 28: 818, 1988

207. Hakim RM: Clinical implications of hemodialysis membrane biocompatibility. *Kidney Int* 44: 484, 1993

208. Schulman G, Fogo A, Gung A, Badr K, Hakim RM: Complement activation retards resolution of acute renal failure in the rat. *Kidney Int* 40: 1069–1074, 1991

209. Harris K, Schreiner G, Klahr S: Effect of leukocyte depletion on the function of the postobstructed kidney in the rat. *Kidney Int* 36: 210–215, 1989

210. Badr, Schreiner G: Preservation of the glomerular capillary ultrafiltration coefficient during rat nephrotoxic serum nephritis by a specific leukotriene D_4 receptor antagonist. *J Clin Invest* 81: 1702, 1988

211. Linas S, Whittenberg D, Parsons P, Repine J: Mild renal ischemia activates primed neutrophils to cause acute renal failure. *Kidney Int* 42: 610, 1992

212. Parnes EL, Shapiro WB: An aphylactoid reactions in hemodialysis patients treated with AN69 dialyzers. *Kidney Int* 40: 1148, 1991

213. Schaefer RM, Fink E, Schaefer L, Barkhausen R, Kulzer P, Heidland A. Role of bradykinin in anaphylactoid

reactions during hemodialysis with AN69 dialyzers. *Am J Nephrol* 13: 473, 1993

214. Gong R, Lindberg J, Abrams J, Whitaker WR, Wade CE, Gouge S: Comparison of hypertonic solutions and dextran in dialysis-induced hypotension. *J Am Soc Nephrol* 3: 1808, 1993

215. Palmer BF: The effect of dialysate composition on systemic hemodynamics. *Semin Dial* 5: 54, 1992

216. Dumler F, Grondin G, Levin NW: Sequential high/low hemodialysis: an alternative to ultrafiltration. *Trans Am Soc Artif Intern Organs* 25: 351, 1979

217. Henrich WL, Woodard TD, McPhaul JJ: The chronic efficacy and safety of high sodium dialysate: double-blind cross-over study. *Am J Kidney Dis* 2: 349, 1982

218. Bihaphala S, Bell AJ, Bennett CA, Evans SM, Dawborn JK: Comparison of high and low sodium and acetate dialysis in stable chronic hemodialysis patients. *Clin Nephrol* 23: 179, 1985

219. Daugirdas JT, Al-Kudsi RR, Ing TS, Norusis MJ: A double-blind evaluation of sodium gradient hemodialysis. *Am J Nephrol* 5: 163, 1985

220. Raja R, Kramer M, Barber K, Chen S: Sequential changes in dialysate (D_{Na}) during hemodialysis. *Trans Am Soc Artif Intern Organs* 29: 649, 1983

221. Linas SL: The role of potassium in the pathogenesis and treatment of hypertension. *Kidney Int* 39: 771, 1991

222. Sigler MH, Teehan BP, VanValkenburgh D: Solute transport in continuous hemodialysis: a new treatment for acute renal failure. *Kidney Int* 32: 562, 1987

223. Maynard JC, Cruz C, Kleerekoper M, Levin NW: Blood pressure response to changes in serum ionized calcium during hemodialysis. *Ann Int Med* 104: 358, 1986

224. Sherman RA, Bialy GB, Gazinski B, Bernholc AS, Eisinger RP: The effect of dialysate calcium levels on blood pressure during hemodialysis. *Am J Kidney Dis* 8: 244, 1986

225. Fellner SK, Lang RM, Neumann A, Spencer KT, Bushinsky DA, Borow KM: Physiologic mechanisms for calcium-induced changes in systemic arterial pressure in stable dialysis patients. *Hypertension* 13: 213, 1989

226. Wizemann V, Kramer W, Bechthold A, Thormann J: Acute effects of dialysis on myocardial contractility: influence of cardiac status and calcium/potassium ratio. *Contrib Nephrol* 52: 60, 1986

227. Henrich WL: Hemodynamic instability during hemodialysis. *Kidney Int* 30: 605, 1986

228. Daugirdas JT: Dialysis hypotension: a hemodynamic analysis. *Kidney Int* 39: 233, 1991

229. Cizawa Y, Ohmori T, Imai K, Nara Y, Matsuoka M, Hirasawa Y: Depressant action of acetate upon the human cardiovascular system. *Clin Nephrol* 8: 477, 1977

230. Kirkendol PL, Devia CJ, Bower JD, Holbert RD: A comparison of the cardiovascular effects of sodium acetate, sodium bicarbonate and other potential sources of fixed base in hemodialysis solutions. *Trans Am Soc Artif Intern Organs* 23: 399, 1978

231. Borges HF, Fryd DA, Rosa AA, Kjellstrand CM: Hypotension during acetate and bicarbonate dialysis in patients with acute renal failure. *Am J Nephrol* 1: 24, 1981

232. Wolff J, Pendersen T, Rossen M, Cleeman-Rasmussen K: Effects of acetate and bicarbonate dialysis on cardiac

performance, transmural myocardial perfusion and acid-base balance. *Int J Artif Organs* 9: 105, 1986

233. Wathen R, Keshaviah P, Hommeyer P, Cadwell K, Comty C: Role of dialysate glucose in preventing gluconeogenesis during hemodialysis. *Trans Am Soc Artif Intern Organs* 23: 393, 1977

234. Leski M, Neithammer T, Wyss T: Glucose enriched dialysate and tolerance to maintenance hemodialysis. *Nephron* 24: 271, 1979

235. Rodrigo R, Shideman J, McHugh R, Buselmeier T, Kjellstrand CM: Osmolality changes during hemodialysis. Natural history, clinical correlations and influence of dialysate glucose and intravenous mannitol. *Ann Intern Med* 86: 554, 1977

236. Knochel JP, Caksey JH: The mechanism of hypophosphatemia in acute heat stroke. *JAMA* 238: 425, 1977

237. Nordstrom H, Lennquist S, Lindell B, Sjoberg HE: Hypophosphatemia in severe burns. *Acta Chir Scand* 143: 395, 1977

238. Cyrus JC, Olivero JJ, Adrogue HJ: Alkalemia associated with renal failure. *Arch Intern Med* 140: 513, 1980

239. Rosa AA, Fryd DS, Kjellstrand CM: Dialysis symptoms and stabilization in long-term dialysis: practical application of the CUSUM plot. *Arch Intern Med* 140: 804, 1980

240. Degoulet P, Roulx J-P, Aime F, Berger C, Bloch P, Goupy F, Legrain M: Programme dialyse-informatique III. Donnees epidemiologiques strategies de dialyse et resultats biologiques (Dialysis program information. Epidemiologic data of different dialysis strategies and biologic results). *J Urol Nephrol* (Paris) 82: 1001, 1976 (in French)

241. Kjellstrand CM: Can hypotension during dialysis be avoided? *Controv Nephrol* 2: 12, 1980

242. Bergstrom J, Asaba H, Furst P: Dialysis ultrafiltration and blood pressure. *Proc Eur Dial Transplant Assoc* 13: 293, 1976

243. Zucchelli P, Santoro A: Dialysis-induced hypotension: a fresh look at pathophysiology. *Blood Purif* 11: 85, 1993

244. Steuer RR, Leypoldt JK, Cheung AK, Harris DH, Conis JM: (Abstract) *J Am Soc Artif Intern Organs* 84, 1994

245. Jost CM, Agarwal R, Khair-el-din T, Grayburn PA, Victor RG, Henrich WL: Effects of cooler temperature dialysate on hemodynamics stability in 'problem' dialysis patients. *Kidney Int* 44: 606, 1993

246. Levy FL, Grayburn PA, Foulks CJ, Brickner ME, Henrich WL: Improved left ventricular contractility with cool temperature hemodialysis. *Kidney Int* 41: 961, 1992

247. Raine AE, Seymour AM, Roberts AF, Radda GK, Ledingham JG: Impairment of cardiac function and energetics in experimental renal failure. *J Clin Invest* 92: 2934, 1993

248. Arieff AI: Dialysis disequilibrium syndrome: current concepts on pathogenesis. in *Controversies in Nephrology*, edited by Schreiner GE, Winchester JF, Washington DC, Georgetown University Press, 1982, p 367

249. Glenn CM, Astley SJ, Watkins SL: Dialysis-associated seizures in children and adolescents. *Pediatr Nephrol* 6: 182, 1992

250. Silver SM, DiSimone JA, Smith DA, Sterns RH: Dialysis disequilibrium syndrome (DDS) in the rat: role of 'reverse urea effect'. *Kidney Int* 42: 161, 1992

251. Hakim RM, Fearon DT, Lazarus JM: Biocompatibility of dialysis membranes: effects of chronic complement activation. *Kidney Int* 26: 192, 1984

252. Hoenich NA, Levett D, Fawcett S, Woffindin C, Kerr DNS: Biocompatibility of haemodialysis membranes. *J Biomed Eng* 8: 3, 1986

253. Shaldon S, Deschodt G, Branger B, Granolleras C, Baldamus CA, Koch KM, Lysaght MJ, Dinarello CA: Hemodialysis hypotension. The interleukin hypothesis restated. *Proc Eur Dial Transplant Assoc* 22: 229, 1985

254. Branger B, Deschodt G, Oules R, Granolleras C, Alsabadani N, Baudin G, Balducchi J-P, Fourcade J, Shaldon S: Can vascular stability be improved with short acetate hemodialysis if biocompatible membranes are used? *Proc Int Symp, Trondheim*, Basel, Karger AG, 1985, p 214

255. Craddock PR, Fehr J, Daimasso AP, Brigham Kl, Jacob HS: Hemodialysis leukopenia: pulmonary vascular leukostasis resulting from complement activation by dialyzer cellophane membranes. *J Clin Invest* 59: 878, 1977

256. MacGrigor RR: Granulocyte adherence changes induced by hemodialysis. Endotoxin, epinephrine and glucocorticoids. *Ann Intern Med* 86: 35, 1977

257. Craddock PR, Fehr J, Brigham KL, Kronenberg RS, Jacob HS: Complement and leukocyte mediated pulmonary dysfunction in hemodialysis. *N Engl J Med* 296: 769, 1977

258. Agar JW, Hull JD, Kaplan M, Letka PG: Acute cardiopulmonary decompensation and complement activation during hemodialysis. *Ann Intern Med* 94: 792, 1981

259. Aljama P, Bire PAE, Ward MK, Feest TG, Walker W, Tamboga H, Sussman M, Kerr DNS: Hemodialysis-induced leucopenia and activation of complement: effect of different membranes. *Proc Eur Dial Transplant Assoc* 15: 144, 1978

260. Lynch RE, Bosl RH, Streifel AJ, Ebben JP, Ehlers SM, Kjellstrand CM: Dialysis thrombocytopenia: parallel plate vs hollow fiber dialyzers. *Trans Am Soc Artif Intern Organs* 24: 704, 1978

261. von Hartitzsch B, Carr D, Kjellstrand CM, Kerr DNS: Normal red cell survival in well-dialyzed patients. *Trans Am Soc Artif Intern Organs* 19: 471, 1973

262. Aurigemma NM, Feldman NT, Gottlieb M, Ingram RH, Lazarus JM, Lowrie EG: Arterial oxygenation during hemodialysis. *N Engl J Med* 297: 871, 1977

263. Burhop KE, Johnson RJ, Simpson J, Chenoweth DE, Borgia J: Biocompatibility of hemodialysis membranes: Evaluation in an ovine model. *J Lab Clin Med* 121: 276, 1993

264. Mault JR, Dechert RE, Bartlett RH, Swartz RD, Ferguson SK: Oxygen consumption during hemodialysis for acute renal failure. *Trans Am Soc Artif Organs* 28: 510, 1982

265. Kleinknecht D, Junger P, Chanard J, Barbanal C, Ganeval D: Uremic and non-uremic complications in acute renal failure: evaluation of early and frequent dialysis on prognosis. *Kidney Int* 1: 190, 1972

266. Marshall VC: Acute renal failure in surgical patients. *Br J Surg* 58: 17, 1971

267. Stott RB, Ogg CS, Cameron JS, Bewick M: Why the persistent high mortality in acute renal failure? *Lancet* 2: 75, 1972

268. Marshall V: Secondary surgical intervention in acute renal failure. *Aust NZ J Surg* 44: 96, 1974

269. Tolhurst Cleaver CL, Hopkins AD, Kee Kwong KC NG, Rafiery AT: The effect of postoperative peritoneal lavage

on survival, peritoneal wound healing and adhesion formation following fecal peritonitis: an experimental study in the rat. *Br J Surg* 61: 601, 1974

270. Sipkins JH, Kjellstrand CM: Severe head trauma and acute renal failure. *Nephron* 28: 36, 1981

271. Casali R, Simmons RL, Najarian JS, von Hartizsch B, Buselmeier TJ, Kjellstrand CM: Acute renal insufficiency complicating major cardiovascular surgery. *Ann Surg* 181: 370, 1975

272. Posen GA, Luiselto J: Continuous equilibration peritoneal dialysis in the treatment of acute and chronic renal failure. *Proc Clin Dial Transplant Forum* 9: 50, 1979

273. Nolph KD, Ghods AJ, Van Stone J, Brown PA: The effects of intraperitoneal vasodilators on peritoneal clearances. *Trans Am Soc Artif Intern Organs* 22: 586, 1976

274. Rubin J, Oreopoulos DG, Lio TT, Mathews R, de Verber GA: Management of peritonitis and bowel perforation during chronic peritoneal dialysis. *Nephron* 15: 220, 1968

275. Simkin EP, Wright FK: Perforating injuries of the bowel complicating peritoneal catheter insertion. *Lancet* 1: 64, 1968

276. Grodstein GP, Blumenkrantz MH, Kopple JD, Moran JK, Coburn JW: Glucose absorption during continuous ambulatory peritoneal dialysis. *Kidney Int* 19: 564, 1981

277. Crossley K, Kjellstrand CM: Intraperitoneal insulin for control of blood sugar in diabetic patients during peritoneal dialysis. *Br Med J* 1: 269, 1971

278. Maher JF, Hahnadel DC, Shea C, DiSanzo F, Cassetta M: Effect of intraperitoneal diuretics on solute transport during hypertonic dialysis. *Clin Nephrol* 7: 96, 1977

279. Vaziri ND, Ness R, Wellikson L, Barton C, Greep N: Bicarbonate buffered peritoneal dialysis an effective adjunct in the treatment of lactic acidosis. *Am J Med* 67: 392, 1979

280. Blumekrantz MJ, Gahl GM, Kopple JD, Kamdar AV, Jones MR, Kessel M, Coburn JW: Protein losses during peritoneal dialysis. *Kidney Int* 19: 593, 1981

281. Rubin J, McFarland S, Hellems EW, Bower JD: Peritoneal dialysis during peritonitis. *Kidney Int* 19: 460, 1981

282. Lautin EM, Freeman NJ, Schoenfeld AH Bakal CW, Haramati N, Friedman AC, Lautin JL, Braha S, Kadish EG, Sprayregen S, Belizon I: Radiocontrast-associated renal dysfunction: incidence and risk factors. *AJR Am J Roentgenol* 157: 49, 1991

283. Turney JH, Marshall DH, Brownjohn AM, Ellis CM, Parsons FM: The evolution of acute renal failure, 1956–1988. *Q J Med* 74: 83, 1990

284. Lange HW, Aeppli DM, Brown DC: Survival of patients with acute renal failure requiring dialysis after open heart surgery: early prognostic indicators. *Am Heart J* 113: 1138, 1987

285. Beal AL, Cerra FB: Multiple organ failure syndrome in the 1990's. Systemic inflammatory response and organ dysfunction. *JAMA* 171: 226, 1994

286. Spurney RF, Fulkerson WJ, Schwab SJ: Acute renal failure in critically ill patients: prognosis for recovery of kidney function after prolonged dialysis support. *Crit Care Med* 19: 8, 1991

287. Humes HD, Cieslinski DA, Coimbra TM, Messana JM, Galvao C: Epidermal growth factor enhances renal tubule cell regeneration and repair and accelerates the recovery of renal function in postischemic acute renal failure. *J Clin Invest* 84: 1757, 1989

288. Coimbra TM, Cieslinski DA, Humes HD: Epidermal growth factor accelerates renal repair in mercuric chloride nephrotoxicity. *Am J Physiol* 259: F438, 1990

289. Miller SB, Martin DR, Kissane J, Hammerman MR: Insulin-like growth factor accelerates recovery from ischemic acute tubular necrosis in the rat. *Proc Natl Acad Sci USA* 89: 11876, 1992

290. Ding H, Kopple JD, Cohen A, Hirschberg R: Recombinant human insulin-like growth factor-I accelerates recovery and reduces catabolism in rats with ischemic acute renal failure. *J Clin Invest* 91: 2281, 1993

291. Conger JD, Falk SA, Hammond WS: Atrial natriuretic peptide and dopamine in established acute renal failure in the rat. *Kidney Int* 40: 21, 1991

292. Rahman N, Kim G, Mathews A: Atrial natriuretic peptide increases creatinine clearance and reduces need of dialysis in patients with established acute renal failure. (Abstract) *J Am Soc Nephrol* 4: 323, 1993

293. Kjellstrand CM, Ebben J, Davin T: Time of death, recovery of renal function, development of chronic renal failure and need for chronic hemodialysis in patients with acute tubular necrosis. *Trans Am Soc Artif Intern Organs* 27: 45, 1981

294. Myers BD, Moran SM: Hemodynamically mediated acute renal failure. *N Engl J Med* 314: 97, 1986

295. Ing TS, Daugirdas JT, Bregman H, Leehey DJ: Continuous arteriovenous hemodialysis. *Int J Artif Organs* 3: 117, 1985

296. Finkenstaedt JT, Merrill JP: Renal function after recovery from acute renal failure. *N Engl J Med* 254: 1023, 1956

297. Price JDE, palmer RA: A functional and morphological follow-up study of acute renal failure. *Arch Intern Med* 105: 90, 1960

298. Briggs JD, Kennedy AC, Young LN, Luke RG, Gray M: Renal function after acute tubular necrosis. *Br J Med* 3: 513, 1967

299. Hall JW, Johnson WJ: Maher JF, Schreiner GE: Immediate and long-term prognosis in acute renal failure. *Ann Intern Med* 73: 515, 1970

300. Lewers DT, Mathew TH, Maher JF, Schrener GE: Long-term follow-up of renal function and histology after acute tubular necrosis. *Ann Intern Med* 73: 523, 1970

301. Fuchs JH, Thelen M, Wibrandt R: Die Nierenfunktion nach akutem Nierenversagen – Eine Langzeitstudie an 70 Patienten (Renal function after acute renal failure – a long-term study). *Dtsch Med Wochenschr* 99: 1641, 1974 (in German)

RENAL REPLACEMENT THERAPY IN CHILDREN

R. DONCKERWOLCKE, M. BROYER, C. CHANTLER and G. RIZZONI

INTRODUCTION

Renal function in infants and children

Successful management of acute renal failure (ARF) in children, particularly infants, requires knowledge of the functional characteristics of the kidney during development and understanding of the metabolic balance of the growing child. The newborn kidney is immature containing only 17% of its adult cellular complement; at 6 months postnatally cell division is complete and further growth is due to an increase in cell size. Nephron for-mation is complete before birth but superficial cortical nephrons are not functionally mature; at birth the more mature juxtamedullary nephrons contribute a greater proportion of total glomerular filtration than in the adult. There is a proportional increase in juxtamedullary blood flow but total renal blood flow is low because of the high renal vascular resistance. Glomerular filtration rate (GFR) at birth averages about 20 ml/min/1.73 m^2 body surface area but the rapid postnatal increase in renal blood flow is associated with a rapid rise in GFR to 48 ml/min/1.73 m^2 at one month and to 80 ml/min/1.73 m^2 by 6 months of age (1).

Table 1. Causes of acute renal failure related to age in 42 children seen at Guy's Hospital in 1983

Cause	Neonates (birth to 4 wk)	Infants (5 wk to 1 yr)	Children 1 yr to 14 yr)
Pre-renal			3
Poor renal perfusion	12	4	7
Infection	1		
Haemolytic-uraemic syndrome			3
Glomerulonephritis			6
Acute on chronic	1		1
Other	1		2
Total	15	4	23

It is likely that the low GFR is controlled by the immaturity of tubular function thus preventing over-perfusion of nephrons and wasting of salt and water (2, 3); fractional reabsorption of filtered sodium in the proximal tubule is reduced with greater reabsorption in the distal tubule to maintain sodium balance. Excessive urinary sodium loss is present in very immature infants between 28 and 32 weeks gestation (3) and sodium wasting is also common in infants with obstructive uropathy and distal tubular damage. The low GFR, the low blood flow, the high renal vascular resistance and the immaturity of the tubules suggest that functional reserve of the neonatal kidney is small and it is not surprising that further impairment of blood flow can lead to acute renal failure. The high haematocrit at birth also reduces renal blood flow and anoxia from birth asphyxia is common. Hence, minor degrees of renal impairment occur in the newborn and acute renal failure occurs more frequently that at any other time during childhood (Table 1).

METABOLIC AND FLUID BALANCE

Water requirement is directly proportional to energy expenditure and it is fortuitously convenient that the expenditure of one kilocalorie requires the consumption of one millilitre (ml) of water. Basal metabolic rate is about 1,000 kcal/m^2 body surface area, thus the basal water requirement is 1,000 ml/m^2. Conditions in hospital, increase energy consumption by 50%. Therefore, the normal water intake is about 1,500 ml/m^2 of which 400 ml/m^2 is utilised by insensible losses. The water requirements increases by 12%/1°C that body temperature exceeds 37°C.

Metabolic rate and energy requirement correlate closely with body surface area (4). Thus both the energy intake and water requirement can be calculated from the child's surface area. In the anuric child the daily water requirement may be taken as 400 ml/m^2 plus measured losses.

Infants and to a lesser extent children have a much higher metabolic rate in relation to body mass than adults (4) and, given the relation between body surface area and metabolic rate, the ratio of surface area to weight is increased. Thus, the energy requirement per kilogram body weight of an infant is 3 to 4 times higher than for an adult. Expressed per unit body weight the energy requirement may be calculated as 100 kcal/kg up to 10 kg body weight plus 50 kcal for each kg between 10 and 20 kg, plus 20 kcal/kg for each kg over 20 kg. Babies between 5 and 10 kg require 120 kcal/kg and those between 2.5 and 5 kg need 150 kcal/kg. Insensible water loss and water turnover in relation to body weight is five times higher in an infant compared to an adult. Consequently, serious derangements of fluid and electrolyte metabolism such as acidosis, uraemia and hyperkalaemia occur rapidly in infants with acute renal failure. The problem is compounded by the absence of normal thirst control because a baby is unable to make known his need for more water when depleted of fluid or overloaded with sodium.

GFR per surface area is comparable in children and adults from the age of one year and food intake is, as noted, roughly comparable when related to body surface area but not to weight. The intake of nutrients such as protein, or salts, is determined by the amount of food consumed which, in turn, depends on the energy intake. These other nutrients are all consumed in excess of need and this excess is excreted in the urine. The relationship between GFR and surface area means that GFR is higher in relation to body mass in a child which helps to preserve body composition. Obviously this advantage is lost in renal failure emphasising the importance of careful management of the intake of energy and other nutrients. These considerations also affect the amount of dialysis required by an anuric child and the size of the dialyzer which can be used, as will be discussed later.

Blood pressure rises steadily throughout childhood from an upper limit of 100/65 at birth to 130/80 mm Hg at 18 years. (Figures 1 and 2) (5). Care must be taken to use a blood pressure cuff of sufficient size to avoid erroneously high readings; the inflatable bladder should be centred over the brachial artery encircling at least three quarters of the circumference of the arm and the width of the cuff should be at least two-thirds of the length of the upper arm. Stiff cuffs fastened with velcro should be avoided.

ACUTE RENAL FAILURE IN INFANCY AND CHILDHOOD

Aetiology

The incidence and causes of acute renal failure (Table 2) vary in different countries depending on the general quality of health care and environmental conditions. Table 1 shows the diagnosis in 42 children referred to Guy's Hos-

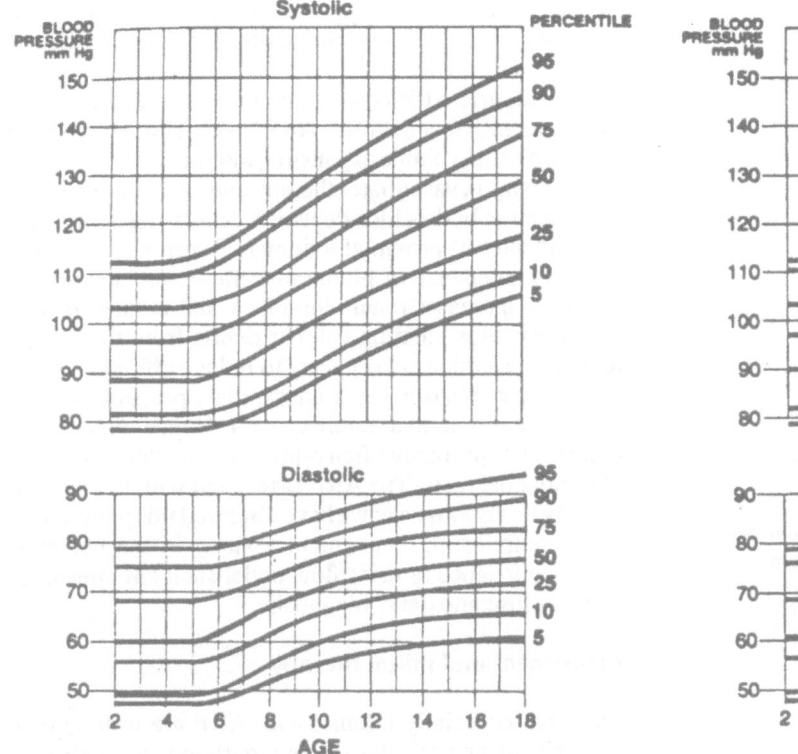

Figure 1. Percentiles of blood pressure measurement in boys (5).

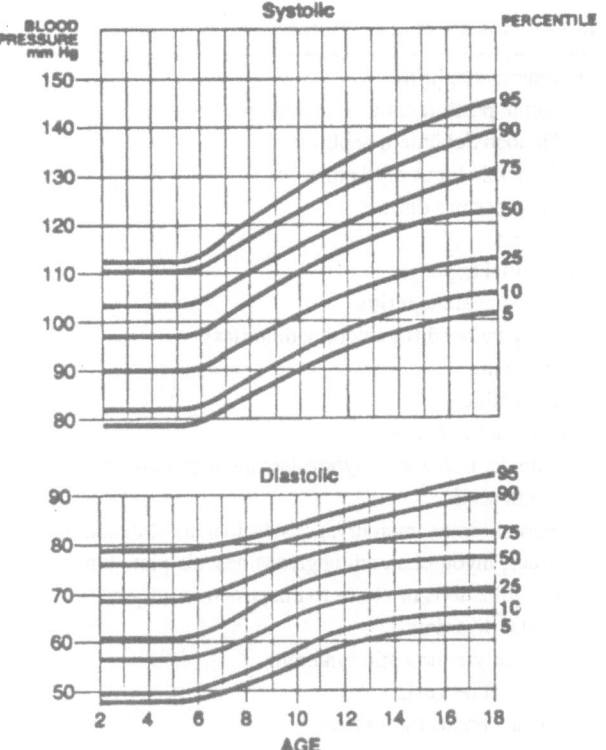

Figure 2. Percentiles of blood pressure measurement in girls (5).

pital over one year; 30% were less than 4 weeks old. Poor renal perfusion accounted for nearly half of all referrals; the cause is usually obvious and includes gastroenteritis, pyloric stenosis, cardiac failure, post-surgery especially after cardiovascular operations (6), burns and renal vascular catastrophies in the newborn. Sudden relapse of nephrotic syndrome may be associated with hypovolaemia due to the rapid loss of salt and water into the extracellular space as the plasma albumin concentrations falls. This occasionally leads to ARF and may also be associated with circulatory collapse or, in association with the hypercoagulability state of nephrotic syndrome, with vascular thrombosis. The best test to detect haemoconcentration is the haemoglobin concentration because pulse and blood pressure may be surprisingly well maintained by peripheral vasoconstriction which is reflected by a wide gap between the rectal and peripheral temperature.

As previously noted, the newborn kidney is especially susceptible to vascular damage. Medullary or papillary necrosis may accompany severe acute tubular necrosis. Hyperosmolar solutions used for contrast renal radiology may cause medullary damage. Cortical necrosis occurs after severe fluid loss, birth asphyxia, haemorrhage, or burns; focal necrotising lesions in other organs are com-

mon. Renal venous thrombosis is especially common in infants: 70% of cases present in the first month of life (7, 8). Antecedent events include shock, perinatal asphyxia, cyanotic heart disease and hyperosmolar dehydration and frequently disseminated intravascular coagulation is found.

Urinary tract infection in the newborn is often complicated by septicaemia perhaps because of the low concentration of circulating immunoglobulin at this age; accordingly, it may present with generalized symptoms and signs such as vomiting, lethargy and jaundice. Congenital obstructive uropathy is complicated by inability to concentrate the urine and by sodium wasting due to distal nephron damage. Hence, these infants may present severely fluid depleted. ARF following extensive and complicated surgery is now less common perhaps because of improved anaesthesia and awareness of fluid and electrolyte requirements. But, it is still frequent after prolonged cardiopulmonary bypass (9) or following vascular surgery in the neonate (6). More careful attention to the need to maintain or restore circulatory blood volume with more liberal use of plasma expanders and physiological saline, rather than dextrose in water, during and after surgery is likely to reduce the incidence further (10).

Table 2. Causes of acute renal failure

Glomerulonephritis
    Acute postinfectious glomerulonephritis
    Henoch Schönlein nephritis
    Systemic lupus erythematosus
    Goodpasture disease
    Others
Interstitial nephritis
    Acute pyelonephritis
    Drug induced (methicillin, diuretics)
    Post viral
    Idiopathic
Acute tubular necrosis
    Anoxia, ischaemia, hypovolaemia, hypotension
    Septicaemia
    Nephrotoxins, mercury, nonsteroidal anti-inflammatory
    drugs, myoglobin, aminoglycosides, cis-platinum
    Combinations of above (burns, trauma, surgery)
Vascular disorders
    Haemolytic uraemic syndrome
    Cortical necrosis
    Renal venous thrombosis
    Disseminated intravascular coagulation
Crystalluria
    Uric acid (following anti tumour therapy)
    Sulphonamides
Acute on chronic
    e.g., infection with obstructive uropathy; dehydration
    with IgA nephropathy
Miscellaneous (rare) cases
    e.g., oxalic acid (ingestion of polyethylene glucol)

Pathogenesis

The pathophysiology of ARF has been extensively reviewed (9, 11). Injury to the tubules is central to the oliguria though the mechanisms by which tubular damage reduces urine flow are not entirely clear. Back leak of filtrate through damaged tubules, and tubular obstruction from necrotic cell debris may occur. Increased solute delivery to the macula densa because of reduced reabsorption by damaged tubules is thought to stimulate renin release in the juxtaglomerular apparatus, which by increasing the intrarenal production of angiotensin II constricts the afferent arteriole thus reducing GFR (2). This prevents overperfusion of damaged nephrons and the considerable loss of salt and water that would occur.

As already noted, the mature neonate despite tubular immaturity has a well developed capacity to conserve sodium suggesting that the low GFR results from suppression of superficial nephron filtration by tubular glomerular feedback. Thus even a small further impairment of tubular function might lead to suppression of glomerular filtration and ARF; simply stated, the neonate is born halfway to ARF.

Nonoliguric ARF now occurs more commonly. Many measures used to ameliorate ARF in experimental animals such as plasma volume expansion, inotropic stimulation of cardiac output, vasodilator therapy and particularly the use of dopamine hydrochloride which causes renal vasodilation and inhibits proximal sodium reabsorption contribute to the maintenance of glomerular filtrate and urine flow. Mannitol increases renal blood flow and induces osmotic diuresis thus clearing cellular debris from the tubular lumen. Frusemide also appears to reduce afferent arteriolar resistance restoring the transcapillary pressure gradient across the glomerular capillary wall. Hence, nonoliguric renal failure probably often represents an attenuated form of tubular necrosis. The ARF associated with tubular toxins may be nonoliguric; we have observed this pattern with ARF complicating gentamicin toxicity in the newborn. The maintenance of urine flow under such circumstances may confuse and delay diagnosis.

Assessment and initial therapy

Children, especially infants, with ARF are usually dangerously ill and for the reasons outlined the metabolic derangements are rapid in onset and severe. Therefore, treatment and investigation must proceed simultaneously. Whilst the indications for dialysis are similar to those for adults, the increased metabolism and energy demands necessitate more frequent dialysis for it is difficult to manage an anuric catabolic infant conservatively. The initial assessment includes clinical evaluation of the degree of fluid loss, blood pressure measurement, if necessary using oscillometry (12), central and peripheral temperature measurement to gauge tissue perfusion (10), haemoglobin and plasma and urine electrolytes. Urine sodium and urea concentrations are especially useful to determine the adequacy of renal perfusion: fractional excretion of sodium is less than 2% with pre-renal failure (13). From these determinations the amount of intravenous fluid required to restore extracellular volume can be calculated, but careful continuous monitoring is essential to prevent overload. The blood volume of a child can be calculated as 80 ml/kg. Thus, an initial transfusion 20 ml/kg of whole blood or plasma in a shocked child is usually safe. An obviously saline-depleted infant will have lost about 10% of body weight as water, so the rapid infusion of 20 ml/kg of physiological saline can be given whilst more precise calculations are being undertaken. If peripheral circulation is not restored by adequate fluid replacement, even though blood pressure and venous pressure are normal, then the use of peripheral vasodilator (hydralazine, or chlorpromazine 0.1 mg/kg intravenously [IV]) often restores urine flow. Hypernatraemia should be corrected only slowly over 48 h to avoid neurological damage; the calculated water deficit being supplied by sodium solutions of 25 to

Table 3. Composition of energy feed for renal failure

Glucose polymer	200 g
Arachis oil emulsion	130 ml
Water	400 ml

Flavour to taste with chocolate or milk shake flavourings. Provides 1385 kcal in 464 ml water, protein as clinifeed (Laboratories Sopharga Puteaux France) may be added.

40 mmol/l providing not more than 100 ml/kg of free water per 24 h. Hypertension usually responds to oral nifidepin 0.25 to 1.0 mg/kg, IV hydralazine 0.5 to 1.0 mg/kg or to the infusion of labetolol 1 to 3 mg/kg/h. Hyperkalaemia, if life-threatening, should be treated with 2.5% calcium gluconate 2 ml/kg. Acidosis should be corrected and calcium-potassium exchange resin (1 g/kg orally and rectally) can be administered. Recently the intravenous infusion of salbutamol (0.5 mg/15 min) has been shown to lower plasma potassium significantly in children with hyperkalaemia complicating renal failure (14). Hypocalcaemia in the neonate presents with jittery movements or convulsions and should be treated with IV calcium gluconate. Hypoglycaemia requires IV dextrose (1 g/kg). Metabolic acidosis can be corrected with 8.4% sodium bicarbonate (1 mmol/ml) diluted before use; 2 mmol/kg will raise plasma bicarbonate by about 6 mmol/l in the infant. It is not advisable to correct the acidosis completely because of the risk of hypokalaemia, decrease of ionized calcaemia, and the sodium load involved in the treatment. Intensive treatment of possible septicaemia should be undertaken after blood cultures have been obtained. Care must be exercised when drugs whose excretion depends on renal function are used; the dose should be reduced accordingly and the plasma concentration measured at intervals.

Traumatic investigations involving renal radiology, or renal biopsy should only be undertaken when the condition of the child has been stabilised if necessary by dialysis. Nonetheless, urgency is imperative because an obstructed infected urinary tract may require immediate surgery to establish adequate drainage. The most useful investigation is sonography of the kidneys and urinary tract undertaken by a skilled operator (15). Not only can this demonstrate obstruction but the patency of the renal vasculature can often be confirmed. If however the child is anuric the obstructed urinary tract may not be dilated and the dilation will only become apparent when urine flow recommences (16). The next most useful investigations in an emergency are bladder catheterisation to exclude obstruction of bladder outflow, and micturation cystography to determine the presence of vesico-ureteral reflux.

Conservative management

Whilst dialysis is usually resorted to at an early stage, careful control of fluid, electrolyte and nutritional intake is required. After the fluid deficit has been corrected, intake should be reduced to the level of insensible loss plus an allowance for pyrexia, abnormal losses, urine output and loss by ultrafiltration during dialysis. Electrolyte requirements are difficult to estimate and intake should be kept as low as possible with sodium and potassium intake not exceeding 2 mmol/kg/24 h unless the child receives dialysis. An adequate calcium intake of 500 mg/24 h should be ensured, if necessary by feeding supplements. The high energy intake of infants has been mentioned and at least 150 kcal/kg/day is required at birth. About 2 g/kg of first class protein should be provided at birth falling to 1 g/kg at 1 year and thereafter. Suitable oral feeds which take account of all these requirements can be made by using low solute or humanised cows milk preparations (SMA, S$_{26}$, Ostermilk new, Cow and Gate baby milk plus) but unmodified cows milk or evaporated milk is not suitable. Extra energy can be provided with double cream (4 kcal/ml), or arachis oil emulsion (Prosparol) and with a glucose polymer such as caloreen or calonutrin. A high energy low water feed can be made up using energy supplements (Table 3). Alkali can be added as sodium bicarbonate (1 to 2 mmol/kg/24 h). The osmolality of the feed should be measured and the concentration slowly increased to prevent diarrhoea and vomiting. With older children the help of an experienced dietitian is essential so that account can be taken of the child's taste preferences. The important point is to ensure that the diet prescribed is actually eaten and this can only be done with the child's cooperation. Alternatively, an adequate intake can be ensured by nasogastric tube feeding.

Maintaining adequate nutrition in infants with renal failure who cannot be maintained on an oral intake is extremely difficult and even with the most concentrated IV feeding regimes frequent dialysis is essential to remove the excess water involved. Continuous arteriovenous haemofiltration is especially valuable in the management of ARF allowing much better control of fluid balance than peritoneal dialysis (see below).

Renal replacement therapy in acute renal failure

Indications for the treatment of acute renal failure by renal replacement therapy are: fluid overload refractory to diuretics and associated with hypertension or congestive heart failure, a hypercatabolic state, or the requirement of large amounts of fluids for parenteral nutrition or for sustaining systemic circulation. Also patients with prolonged oliguria require dialysis.

In ARF due to primary kidney disease either peritoneal or haemodialysis may be used. In newborns and infants peritoneal dialysis is the treatment of choice, because of its simplicity, availability, relative safety and effectiveness. Children weighing more than 20 kg with a prolonged oliguria are often treated with haemodialysis after one or two peritoneal dialyses. Available facilities and expertise often determine the choice between peritoneal dialysis and haemodialysis in older children. There is no evidence that outcome is better with either technique. For critically ill patients when ARF complicates severe infections or major operations, either mode of dialysis is often inadequate. Continuous arteriovenous or venovenous haemofiltration allows considerable fluid intake for administration of nutrients and drugs without the danger of fluid overload and therefore may provide a safer alternative in these patients.

Peritoneal dialysis in acute renal failure

The technique and equipment used for acute dialysis are similar to those used for chronic intermittent peritoneal dialysis in children. If dialysis has to be performed urgently a plastic disposable peritoneal catheter or a Tenckhoff catheter may be inserted at the bedside instead of surgical insertion of a Silastic catheter requiring a laparotomy. In critically ill newborns or infants it is generally recommended to control respiratory movements by a respirator with endotracheal intubation before inserting a peritoneal catheter.

Procedure of stylet catheter insertion
Premedication with diazepam (0.25 mg/kg IV) chlorpromazine (0.5 mg/kg IM) or chloral hydrate (30 mg/kg rectally) is recommended in an anxious child. After local anaesthesia with procaine, the abdomen should be primed with 20 ml dialysis solution/kg through a small bore needle or cannula prior to inserting the peritoneal catheter. This is necessary to avoid the catheter penetrating an intra-abdominal organ such as the inferior vena cava for the small infant is unable to tense the abdominal muscles when the catheter is inserted. A special paediatric plastic peritoneal catheter (available from McGaw, Vygon, Wallace) with stylet is then inserted through a small skin incision, a few centimeters below the umbilicus in the midline; when the peritoneum is entered, the stylet is removed and the catheter advanced to the left side of the pelvis. The introduction of silastic cannulae utilizing a Seldinger wire (Cook Co) has improved the safety of the procedure (see below). When midline insertion is not possible, the catheter can be inserted in the flank, outside the line of the inferior epigastric artery. After insertion, it is better to dialyse for a few days and then remove the catheter, allowing a period on conservative management before reinsertion than to leave the same catheter in place indefinitely.

Complications related to insertion of stylet catheters
These include catheter malfunction, perforation of a viscus and bleeding. Obstruction of the catheter may be caused by omental fat, fibrin or blood clots. Extravasation of fluid into the abdominal wall frequently compli-

cates peritoneal dialysis in children. The use of a suitable catheter, which should be correctly inserted with all perforations inside the peritoneal cavity will avoid this problem. The cannula must be removed when any leakage occurs in the abdominal wall. Perforation of a viscus (bowel or bladder) is a rare complication. The catheter should be removed and reinserted; usually the perforation closes spontaneously. Bleeding after insertion of the catheter, continuing during the first cycles, is not uncommon. Exceptionally the haemorrhage is considerable, leading to hypotension and shock.

Procedure of Tenckhoff catheter insertion
Following sedation and desinfection of the abdominal wall, the area for incision is anaesthetised with lidocaine solution containing adrenaline. The best place for incision is at the level of the umbilicus, 1–5 cm lateral to the rectus sheath on the left hand side. Following incision and exposure of the external oblique muscle, a needle is inserted into the peritoneum and the abdomen is primed with dialysate solution. Subsequently a guide wire is introduced through the needle and advanced towards the rectovesical pouch. After removal of the needle, a dilator with peel away sheath over it, is advanced over the wire into the peritoneum. With the sheath in place in the abdomen, dilator and guide wire are removed. An adapted catheter with Dacron cuff is then advanced through the sheath (neonatal size 8–10 cm, paediatric 16 cm). Following removal of the sheath, the opening around the catheter is tied by a purse string and the cuff attached to the external oblique fascia and muscle. The catheter is tunnelled through the fascial layers, an exit side is made 3–5 cm proximal of the incision and fascia and skin are closed (17).

Complications related to Tenckhoff catheters
The problems with the Tenckhoff are similar to those described for the stylet catheters. However Tenckhoff catheter survival is longer and also offers a better flow than the stylet catheter. However if prolonged peritoneal dialysis is envisaged surgical insertion of a cuffed Silastic catheter is preferred.

Haemodialysis in acute renal failure

Vascular access
For emergency haemodialysis a simple immediately usable vascular access is required. Methods for cannulation of the superior and inferior vena cava have been developed. Superior vena cava catheterisation is effected through the subclavian or jugular vein (see vascular access chronic haemodialysis). Acute haemodialysis using one or two percutaneous femoral vein catheters is possible even in small children and a single needle device allows dialysis through a single femoral vein catheter. When two catheters are to be inserted in small children, it is easier to catheterise each femoral vein instead of insertion of both catheters on the same side. Femoral catheterization is

useful when only a few dialyses are necessary but for prolonged treatment subclavian cannulation is preferred.

Technique of haemodialysis
The technique of haemodialysis in acute renal failure does not differ from that in chronic renal failure. However, patients with ARF often have an unstable cardiovascular system, making dialysis more hazardous.

In acute dialysis vigorous ultrafiltration is often required. To avoid circulatory collapse, a dialyzer allowing careful regulation of ultrafiltration and without compliance during application of negative pressure for ultrafiltration is preferred.

Using a dialyzer with restricted efficiency (urea clearance less than 2.0 ml/kg/min), bicarbonate containing dialysate and infusion of mannitol during dialysis may enhance haemodynamic stability.

Continuous blood purification systems

Continuous arteriovenous and venovenous haemofiltration (CAVH, CVVH) and diahaemofiltration (CAVHD, CVVHD) are methods for extracorporeal blood treatment in which fluid and nonprotein plasma solutes are removed in a continuous process. The system consists of a haemofilter connected to an artery and a vein or to (one or) two veins. In CAVH and CVVH plasma water and dissolved solutes are filtered through the membrane and collected into a bag and blood purification is based solely on convective transport; CAVHD and CVVHD combines both diffusive and convection transport by adding dialysate perfusion through the ultrafiltrate compartment (18).

Slow continuous ultrafiltration without fluid substitution can be used to remove excess fluid. If large volumes of uraemic ultrafiltrate are removed and replaced by substitution fluid or if combined with dialysis the procedure can be used as a renal replacement. These methods are applicable in newborns, infants and children.

Indications
These techniques are indicated whenever haemodialysis or peritoneal dialysis is precluded, because of technical problems or because of the unstable clinical condition of the patient. They are ideally suited for critically ill patients with ARF who have multiple organ failure or are haemodynamically unstable. This may be the case in patients who develop ARF following septic shock or after cardiopulmonary bypass surgery. In patients with pulmonary complications they decrease the risk of complications associated with increased abdominal pressure, and peritoneal pleural leaks. They also may be used in patients with life-threatening edema resistant to diuretic therapy or peritoneal dialysis (19, 20).

Technical aspects
In CAVH(D) the driving force for blood flow through the circuit is the gradient between arterial and venous pressures, while in CVVH(D) a blood pump is used.

CAVH(D) requires arterial as well as venous cannulation. This can be obtained with catheters or an arteriovenous shunt. In neonates catheterization of the umbilical vessels using a 3.5–5 French umbilical arterial catheter and a 5–8.5 French umbilical venous catheter may provide an efficient access. In infants and children catheters are placed in femoral or brachial arteries as arterial access, while jugular or femoral veins are used for the return of the blood (18). Peripheral cannulation should be avoided because of the high risk of thrombosis due to haemoconcentration and the infusion of hypertonic replacement solutions. To avoid unnecessary pressure loss, short cannulas (25 to 33 mm) of 18 to 20 gauge should be used. Thereby blood flow rates 15 to 50 ml/min may be achieved. A shunt can be placed either in an arm or a leg. Blood flow is higher when femoral artery cannulation is performed than when a peripheral shunt is used. For CVVH(D) access either by a dual lumen venous catheter or two separate venous catheters can be utilized. In smaller children cannulation of the femoral vein (dual lumen 6.5 or 7 French) and in older children both subclavian or femoral veins (dual 9 French) can be utilized.

For CAVH(D) special short paediatric blood lines with low blood volumes (8 ml) are commercially available (Amicon, Gambro). The arterial line has a port for the infusion of replacement fluids and a sampling port. At the inlet and outlet of the circuit three way stopcocks are placed allowing lavage of the filter or replacement of the filter after clotting. A long ultrafiltration line connects the ultrafilter and a collection bag. Adaptation of the height between filter and collection bag allows modification of negative pressure within the filter and thereby of transmembrane pressure and ultrafiltrate production. Constant ultrafiltration rates may be obtained by suction with a pump on the ultrafiltration port but requires a stable blood flow through the filter to avoid haemoconcentration and clotting. The use of pumps draining into a volumetric collection bag is preferred to allow better control of the system. For CVVH the blood monitor component of a haemodialysis machine and blood lines for haemodialysis can be used. This allows to maintain a constant blood flows by the pump and a better control of the extracorporeal blood compartment. Early detection of venous resistance is possible by the venous pressure monitor and the airleak detector avoids the potential risk of air emboli. The commercial available haemodialysis blood lines have also sufficient blood ports for sampling and fluid infusion. There are commercially available haemofilters suitable for CAVH(D) and CVVH(D) in infants and children (Table 4).

Heparinised saline is used to prime the blood lines and filter, but to prevent clotting of the filters heparinisation must be maintained throughout treatment. A loading dose

Table 4. Paediatric haemofilters

Haemofilters	Membrane nature	Surface (m^2)	Fiber length (mm)	Fiber diameter (mm)	Haemofilter volume (ml)	Ultrafiltration range (ml/min)
Amincon Minifilter	PS[a]	0.005	10.0	570	6	0.5–1.5
Plus	PS[a]					
Diafilter 20	PS[a]	0.25	12.7	200	20	5–17
Gambro FH22H	PA[b]	0.20	11.5	220	13	8–17
Sorin HFT02	PS[a]	0.24	12.0	200	15	5–15

[a]PS = Polysulfone.
[b]PA = Polyamide.

of heparin (50 U/kg) is administered followed by continuous infusion of heparin at 10 to 20 U/kg/h. Activated clotting time (ACT) is measured every 3 h and the heparin dose is adjusted to maintain ACT between 150 to 200 seconds (normal: 80 to 120 seconds).

Strict control of all intake and output of fluids is required to maintain body fluid balance. When the main objective is to control fluid balance the amount of fluid given is determined by the needs for parenteral nutrition and intravenous drug administration. When CAVH or CVVH are used to prevent uraemia large amounts of ultrafiltrate (more than 15% of body weight) must be removed and replaced by a solution that achieves electrolyte and acid-base balance. Ringer-lactate or normal saline with appropriate additions of calcium and magnesium and separate infusion of bicarbonate may be used. Also commercially available substitution fluids may be used (Table 5).

Dialysate used in CAVD and CVVHD is that used in peritoneal dialysis. Because the ultrafiltration that occurs with the haemofilter is not glucose dependent, a 1.36% glucose concentration is commonly used. In both methods relatively slow dialysate flow rates (1 l/h) are used, while in CAVHD also blood flow rates are low. Therefore clearances are low and effective blood purification is depending on the continual nature of these techniques.

Clinical experience
Continuous renal replacement systems have been successfully used in premature babies, in infants and in children for the following clinical indications.

Fluid overload
Precise control of the rate and volume of ultrafiltrate formation made CA(V)VH a safe method of fluid removal in infants and children. Weight losses up to 15% of body weight were well tolerated without side effects (18). Hypotension was noted if the rate of ultrafiltration exceeded 0.5 ml/kg/min; but was not related to the volume of plasma water removed.

Renal replacement therapy (19, 20)
Due to the identical composition of ultrafiltrate and plasma water, CA(V)VH is limited in removing uraemic waste products by the ultrafiltrate volume. Ultrafiltrate formation and administration of substitution fluids in excess of 15% of body weight are required to obtain sufficient solute clearances (16). In highly catabolic patients with high rates of urea generation, the treatment is insufficient in removing waste products. In those patients CAVHD or preferably CVVHD must be used to enhance clearances.

Parenteral nutrition in acute renal failure
CA(V)VH allows administration of large quantities of fluids in anuric patients without the risk of fluid overload. Besides administration of glucose, lipids and amino acids the intravenous fluids must also compensate for the loss of electrolytes with the ultrafiltrate.

Complications

The complications and cause of death in ARF relate primarily to the underlying cause of renal failure and to the complications of the renal replacement technique most of which can be avoided.

Convulsions are common especially in infants and are usually attributed to a combination of factors such as uraemia, hyponatraemia, hypocalcaemia and hypertension, though the primary disorder causing the renal failure e.g. haemolytic uraemic syndrome may be implicated. Again, good management can minimise the risk. Hyperglycaemia is not uncommon especially when peritoneal dialysis solutions with a high dextrose concentration are used for fluid removal. In this respect it is usually not necessary to use a concentration greater than 3 g/dl (3%). The hyperglycaemia is also related to the glucose intolerance associated with the overall catabolic state of uraemia and infection. There is some evidence that extra insulin in these circumstances will reduce net protein catabolism as well as lower the blood glucose. Certainly, blood glucose must be carefully monitored because high levels will increase plasma osmolarity and rapid change will

Table 5. Replacement fluids

Company	Composition (mmol/l)							
	Na^+	K^+	Ca^{2+}	Mg^{2+}	Cl^-	Lact.	HCO_3^-	Glucose
Fresenius HF 11	140	1	1.63	0.75	101	45.0	0	10.9
Schiwa SH-35hep	140	0	1.75	0.50	10	2.9	31.4	5.6
Gambro Haemofiltrasol 23	140	1	1.80	0.75	100	45.0	0	11.1
Fresenius HF 21	135	2	1.88	0.75	109	33.8	0	8.3

increase the risk of cerebral complications. Careful control of IV hypertonic dextrose infusions is also very important; unfortunately it is often not possible to substitute IV fat emulsions for dextrose as an alternative source of energy because of the reduced clearance of plasma lipids in uraemia.

Complications of CAVH(D) and CVVH(D) are hypotension, risk of air emboli, and errors in fluid and electrolyte balance. To avoid the risk of artery thrombosis CVVH(D) is often preferred to CAVH(D) (18).

Conclusion

The prognosis of acute renal failure in childhood is relatively good and a majority of children if properly managed make a full recovery. The services required to achieve this are, however, formidable, requiring skilled paediatric nursing, chemical pathology and haematology, paediatric radiology and nuclear medicine, paediatric dietitians and social workers, nephrologists familiar with paediatric problems, and experienced paediatric urologists as well as the general nephrology and dialysis expertise. Accordingly, such services tend to be concentrated in a few units serving a large population.

CHRONIC RENAL FAILURE IN INFANCY AND CHILDHOOD

Incidence and age of onset

The incidence of end stage renal disease (ESRD) in children less than 15 is now much better known than previously. The annual collection of data by international and national registries gives a good concept of this incidence.

The annual incidence of ESRD can be estimated by the acceptance rate of new patients reported by the European Dialysis and Transplant Association (EDTA) Registry (21) for the years 1965 to 1991; it increased slowly but steadily until 1989 and decreased thereafter (Figure 3). For the five major European Countries the number of new patients accepted for renal replacement therapy ranged between 4 and 6 new patients per million child population (below age 15) in 1991.

However the incidence of ESRD can be overestimated due to acceptance of patients from abroad. A realistic figure in the late 1980s is approximately 6 new children per million child population per year. This is confirmed by the data from the Canadian Registry (22) which collects the totality of the paediatric cases in that country. It is difficult to foresee whether the incidence and acceptance rate and, therefore, the need for renal replacement therapy will further increase in the future or not. The increase in the acceptance of younger children will raise this figure, while the decrease in the natality rate and also a better comprehensive conservative treatment during the predialysis period might decrease it.

The annual acceptance rate, of children less than 5 also increased in the last decade and does not differ much from that observed in older children varying between 2 and 6 per million population under age 5 (23).

The age distribution of children accepted for treatment of ESRD changed during recent years. In a total of 430 new paediatric patients starting renal replacement therapy (RRT) in 1991, 11.6% were under age 2, 16.6% were between 2 and 5 and 71.8% were 6 to 14 years old. The proportion of younger children (between 5 and 10 and less than 5) substantially increased during the last 5 years (21) and will probably increase even more in the future.

Primary renal disease in children

The incidence of different primary renal diseases (PRD) which caused ESRD in 2,735 children aged less than 15 in the period 1987 to 1991 is shown in Table 6 (21).

Glomerulonephritis account approximately for 26% while pyelonephritis and congenital hypoplasia-dysplasia represent, altogether, 36% of PRD. Multisystem diseases account for 7.8% of all PRDs while only 7.8% of the patients reached ESRD because of uncertain cause. The examination of the incidences of different PRD groups from 1972 to 1991 confirms the tendency of GN to decrease as a cause of ESRD while the other groups of PRD, remain rather stable (Figure 4).

In the group of glomerulonephritis (GN), steroid resistant nephrotic syndrome with focal glomerulosclerosis (FSGS) accounts for approximately 36%, dense deposits membranoproliferative GN for 5.7% and IgA nephropathy for 8.4% (21).

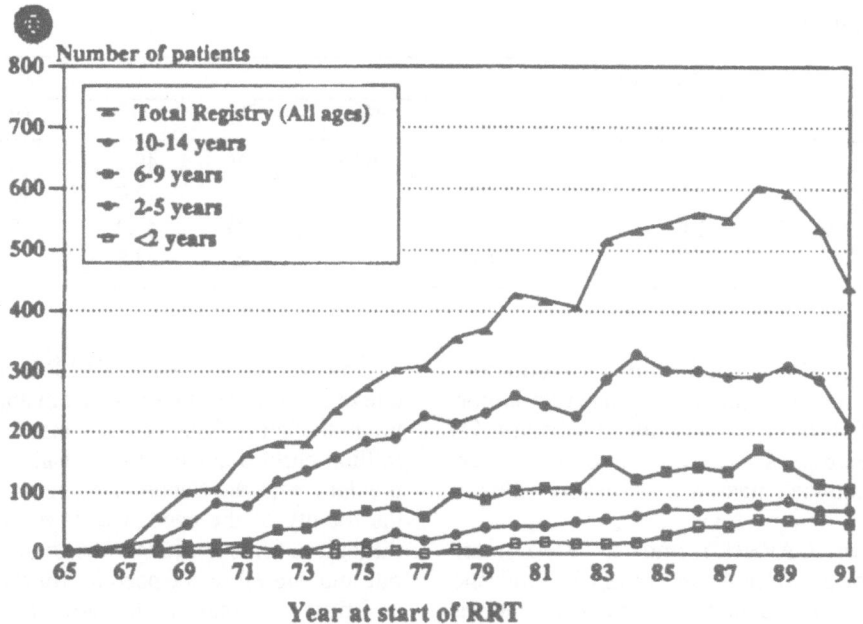

Figure 3. Number of new patients reported at commencing renal replacement therapy before the age of 15 years, between the years 1965 and 1991 (21).

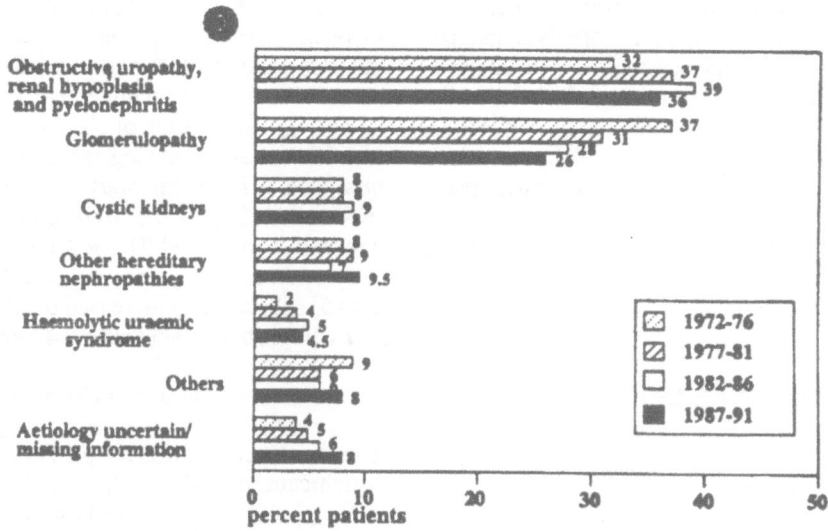

Figure 4. Primary renal disease groups in patients starting renal replacement therapy in 1972–1976, 1977–1981, 1982–1986 and 1987–1991 (21).

Organisation of services and facilities required for children

The relatively small number of children starting dialysis each year results in logistics that differ from those in adults. It has been suggested that a limited number of specialised children's centres should be established to cope with the problem rather than treat the occasional child who presents with chronic renal failure in a local

adult centre. Treatment of children in adult centres often results in complications due to inappropriate dialysis technique; moreover treatment of children on an adult ward may create additional psychological problems in both categories.

One paediatric centre per million child population per country was considered sufficient to provide treatment for all children with end stage renal disease. But to avoid too long distance travel more centres have been created in

Table 6. Distribution of primary renal diseases in children who started RRT before the age of 15 years from 1987 to 1991 EDTA Report 1992 (21)

Primary Renal Disease		Percent	Patients
Obstructive uropathy and/or renal hypoplasia-dysplasia and/or pyelonephritis		36	
Glomerulopathy		26	
Nephrotic syndrome with focal sclerosis			9.4
IgA nephropathy			
* idiopathic (Berger)			0.5
* Henoch-Schönlein purpura			1.7
Membrano-proliferative GN	type I		1.2
	type II		1.5
Membranous GN			0.5
Rapidly progressive GN without systemic disease			0.7
Lupus erythematosus			0.7
Goodpasture's syndrome			0.4
Cystic kidneys		7.8	
Polycystic kidneys			
dominant type			0.6
recessive type			1.5
Medullary cystic disease, nephronophtisis			4.7
Other, unspecified			1.3
Other hereditary familial nephropathies		9.5	
Alport			1.5
Cystinosis			3.5
Oxalosis			1.6
Haemolytic-uraemic syndrome		4.5	
Others		7.8	
Insulin dependent diabetes			0.3
Amyloid			0.6
Nephropathies due to drugs			0.2
Kidney tumor			0.9
Aetiology, unknown		7.8	

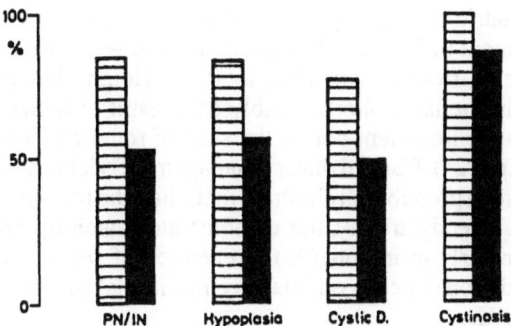

Figure 5. Proportion of children with height at start of treatment lower than −3SD. Children commencing treatment in ▤ 1976–1980 are compared with those commencing treatment in ▮ 1981–1985. PN/IN: pyelonephritis; interstitial nephritis. Cystic D: cystic disease.

to dietary noncompliance. A teacher should be attached to the hospital team to provide tutoring during dialysis and to establish a direct liaison between the hospital and the school in order to achieve the best possible educational program for each child. Instruction during dialysis also emphasises the importance of a proper educational program. The role of social worker and psychologist are obvious for helping families to cope with all the problems generated by dialysis. Paediatric surgery and urology, and the support of a general paediatric unit are also required.

A paediatric specialised unit must be capable of offering all modes of treatment for ESRD, not only hospital haemodialysis but also continuous ambulatory peritoneal dialysis (CAPD) and home haemodialysis. Above all, a kidney transplantation has to be planned for the child as soon as possible, either in the same hospital or in another. When a specialised paediatric unit is not available in the vicinity for a child with ESRD it is recommended at least to start dialysis in the nearest specialised centre and to continue afterwards a regular clinical assessment in this unit as the child undergoes maintenance dialysis in a nonspecialised centre.

Medical problems

Growth failure and endocrine disorders

Growth retardation is a common though not an inevitable consequence of chronic renal failure. During conservative treatment growth is particularly vulnerable during times of rapid growth, such as in the first year of life and during puberty, while during mid-childhood growth velocity can be normal. Height is below the third percentile for age in approximately 40% of the children by the time dialysis is initiated (25).

Figure 5 shows the proportion of children with selected primary renal diseases whose height at the start of treatment was lower than 3SD of normal in the EDTA

some countries. Paediatric units, which should be separated from adult treatment areas, are usually small (less than 20 patients on dialysis) with a relatively high staff to patient ratio. They have to be run by a paediatric nephrologist fully trained in both specialities. Nurses of such units must be experienced with children and dialysis. Several facilities not required for adult patients are needed in a paediatric specialised unit including a full time dietician, social worker, teacher and a psychologist. A dietician is all the more important as dietary prescription is of major interest in children. One out of seven deaths reported in the paediatrics EDTA registry in children on dialysis in the period 1981–1985 was caused by hyperkalaemia and cardiovascular overload, both complications related

paediatric registry. In this figure children commencing treatment in 1976 to 1980 are compared with those commencing treatment in 1981 to 1985. Height deficit was less in the last cohort possibly as a result of better conservative treatment before the start of renal replacement therapy (24). Careful dietary management of chronic renal failure in prepubertal children, including the prevention of renal osteodystrophy, has demonstrated catch-up growth particularly in infants (25). Prevention of severe growth retardation depends on intensive nutritional support prior to ESRD.

The very greatest attention must be paid to growth in children with renal failure. Height should be measured accurately using precise apparatus, and both height and weight should be recorded every 3 months (26). Inadequate nutrition is indicated if the weight is less than expected for height and correlates with poor growth (27). Measurements of triceps and subscapular skinfold thickness also provide useful indicators of nutritional adequacy. Skeletal maturation is often retarded by 2 years or more and should be assessed regularly (28, 29). Radiographs for bone age should be carefully inspected for evidence of osteomalacia and secondary hyperparathyroidism. Serum parathyroid hormone levels should be measured regularly. Pubertal development is delayed by chronic renal failure and should be charted; pubertal delay correlates with the retardation in bone age (29). The delay in bone age is of practical importance because affected individuals continue to grow beyond the ages of normal growth, sometimes up to the age of 20 years or more. However, this late growth is generally limited and as a result many reach adult life severely stunted which causes considerable psychological disturbance both to the children and to their parents. Nutritional and metabolic consequence of renal failure in children have been recently reviewed (30). All nutrients other then energy are normally ingested in excess of requirement and the excess is excreted in the urine. A balance between intake and output is maintained in chronic renal failure, otherwise progressive changes in body composition would occur rapidly leading to death.

The severity of chronic renal failure is characterised by the extent of the changes in body composition that are necessary in order to maintain the balance between intake and output. Dialysis is required when the renal capacity for excretion is so limited that the changes in body composition become incompatible with life. It is obvious that control of intake by altering diet is fundamental in the management of chronic renal failure and in determining the need for dialysis.

Anorexia, which is a frequent characteristic of renal insufficiency, naturally lowers the intake of nutrients such as protein and electrolytes, normally consumed excessively and therefore reduces the alterations in body composition that would otherwise occur. However, the reduced intake frequently leads to energy malnutrition which increases the tendency to catabolism and the risk of intercurrent infection from reduced immune competence. The energy content of the diet should be increased to maintain normal energy intake, whilst reducing the intake of all other nutrients as necessary to limit the changes in body composition.

The reduced energy intake characteristic of chronic renal failure is exacerbated by abnormal energy metabolism, with a reduced peripheral consumption of glucose for energy in spite of secondary hyperinsulinaemia (31). In addition, the pancreatic response to hyperglycemia is inhibited by secondary hyperparathyroidism (32). Uraemic alterations in energy metabolism necessarily affect protein metabolism. Hence, protein malnutrition occurs despite an adequate dietary intake of protein. Reductions in cell mass, plasma protein concentration, plasma branched chain amino acid concentrations, the protein content of muscle, and protein turnover and muscle protein synthesis have all been observed in patients with chronic renal insufficiency (30). In addition, a dialysable constituent of uraemic plasma has a direct inhibitory effect on protein synthesis *in vitro* (33). Reduction of nitrogen intake in uraemic children sufficient to maintain the blood urea between 20–30 mmol/l has improved growth as well as glucose metabolism during hyperglycaemia with a reduction in insulin resistance (34).

Sodium retention with an increase in total body sodium content is common in chronic renal failure, but is not invariable. Some individuals, particularly children with obstructive uropathy or a renal dysplasia, may-be salt depleted and in some the syndrome of hyporeninaemic hypoaldosteronism develops and reduces growth (35).

Many disturbances of endocrine function have been described in chronic renal failure. In children with chronic renal failure the 24-hour growth hormone profile can vary substantially (36). One study reported normal 24-hour GH profile in 70% of the children, while 15% had low profiles and 15% elevated GH profile, with GH peaks on top of the elevated baseline levels. The type of treatment (conservative or dialysis) did not influence GH secretion (37). In a study of adolescents, the amplitudes of GH peaks were higher than normal, but the number of peaks was not affected (38). In children with chronic renal failure various levels of plasma IGF-I and II have been found (36). IGF-I concentrations may be normal or elevated, while IGF-II concentrations are above normal. An increase of IGF-binding proteins is found. The excess of IGF-binding protein 3 causes a decrease in IGF bioactivity. A significant negative correlation exists between the glomerular filtration rate and serum IGF-BP3 levels. Many clinical studies with the use of biosynthetic growth hormone have been reported. GH therapy accelerates growth in children with chronic renal failure. Increment of height velocity between 3–5 cm/year were reported. Bone age did not show an inappropriate advance during GH treatment. There was no significant effect on body composition and muscle strength. Side effects were benign. A deterioration of kidney function was not observed, glucose tolerance was unchanged, but in patients with osteodystrophy an increase in bone abnormalities was noticed (39). Data on final height following long term treatment are not yet available. Hyperprolactinaemia occurs in chronic renal failure, levels are unaffected by dialysis, and may be partly responsible for the delay in pubertal development. Testosterone levels are normal in prepubertal boys, but may be reduced after puberty. High basal levels of luteinising hormone with loss of the normal pulsatile pattern of secretion have been demonstrated in men with chronic renal failure. Plasma cortisol concentrations are normal in children with chronic renal failure. Thyroid function is within the low normal range with depressed TSH levels except in children with cystinosis who frequently develop hypothyroidism with increased plasma TSH concentrations (40).

Renal osteodystrophy

Osteodystrophy is common in children with chronic renal failure (41). Its occurrence is probably stimulated by the rapid turnover rate of bone associated with remodelling and growth. In addition to the changes which occur in adults (see Chapter 44) the metaphyseal growth zone is affected and abnormalities similar to nutritional rickets are seen on radiographs. Osteodystrophy is especially common in children with congenital renal disease leading to renal insufficiency early in life (42). Whilst evidence of osteomalacia and osteitis fibrosa may not be apparent on radiographs until renal failure is well advanced, early changes can be detected in bone biopsies (42). Raised levels of parathyroid hormone are found in children when the GFR falls below 45 ml/min/1.73 m^2 (43). Decreased mean circulating plasma 1,25 dihydroxyvitamin D (1,25 [OH]$_2$D$_3$) concentrations occur when the GFR falls below 50 ml/min/1.73 m^2) (41).

Subperiostial resorption zones and changes at the metaphyses are the most usual signs of renal osteodystrophy on radiography. Both, however, may be due to osteitis fibrosa and there is no single sign which is specific for osteomalacia (41). Children with severe osteomalacia and slipped epiphyses also have more severe osteitis fibrosa (41). Unless recognized early, bone deformities can appear with alarming rapidity in the young infant. Soft tissue and vascular calcification are less common though corneal and conjunctival calcification sometimes occur. Epiphyseolysis is a severe complication of renal osteodystrophy in children and is associated with the accumulation of woven bone and fibrous tissue in the radiolucent zone between ossification centres (44). The osteodystrophy should be treated medically before orthopaedic surgery is undertaken to correct any deformity. Attempts to stabilise slipped epiphyses e.g. by screws should be discouraged even though the epiphyses, especially in the femoral region, may consolidate outside the normal position (44).

Avascular necrosis of bone, especially in the head of the femur, is a well recognised complication occurring after transplantation but can also occur in children on dialysis. It is undesirable to perform femoral head replacement operations in small children, but a femoral osteotomy is often successful in alleviating pain and abolishing the limp in symptomatic children. Early mobilisation after surgery is desirable and the operation is tolerated well as long as it is undertaken after the osteodystrophy has been suppressed medically. Hyperparathyroid bone disease (osteitis fibrosa) is the predominant skeletal lesions in children, while aplastic lesions (low turnover bone disease) are found in a minority (10%) of these patients (45). Following the introduction of calcium salts as phosphate-binders the prevalence of aluminium accumulation in bone has significantly decreased. However, young children probably absorb more aluminium from the intestine than adults and aluminium accumulates in the body when renal function is reduced. Therefore, it is advisable to check the aluminium content of solute and food preparations used in infants with renal failure. Normal or slightly elevated aluminium levels do not exclude aluminium intoxication. Plasma aluminium levels probably reflect aluminium intake and do not accurately indicate body aluminium content. A rise of plasma aluminium concentration of more than 150 μg/l after deferoxiamine is a useful predictor of an increased total bone aluminium content (46). Prevention of renal osteodystrophy in children with chronic renal insufficiency should be considered early in the course of the disease. We routinely monitor bone radiographs and parathyroid hormone concentrations when the GFR is below 35 ml/min/1.73 m^2. Treatment of renal osteodystrophy requires regular supplementation with vitamin D derivates to suppress hyperparathyroidism and phosphate absorption should be reduced by restricting dietary phosphate intake and using agents that bind phosphate in the intestines. The preparation of vitamin D used for prophylaxis and treatment depends on availability and compliance (Table 6). We tend to use 1 alpha (OH) D$_3$ or 1-25 (OH)$_2$ D$_3$. Supplement of vitamin D are only prescribed after the plasma phosphate concentrations has been reduced to within the normal range. The plasma calcium concentration is raised to the upper limit of normal, but it is vitally important that the level is monitored regularly to prevent hypercalcaemia which can lead to further deterioration in renal function. The plasma phosphate concentration is reduced towards, but not below the lower

Table 7. Vitamin D preparations for use in the treatment of renal osteodystrophy in children

	Dose (μg/day)		*Half-life*
	prophylaxis	*treatment*	
25(OH)D$_3$	12.5–25	50–50	2 weeks
dihydrotachysterol	120–150	500–2000	weeks
1α(OH)D$_3$	0.25–0.5	1–4	hours
1,25(OH)$_2$D$_3$	0.12–0.25	0.5–2.0	4–6 hours

Table 8. Comparison of phosphate binding capacity of calcium salts

	Ca Carbonate	Ca Acetate	Ca Citrate
mg Phosphate bounded per mg Ca ingested	0.57	1.04	0.43

limit of normal by restricting the intake of dairy products, particularly milk, cheese and yoghurt. Phosphate binders are administered with meals as necessary to achieve the desired plasma phosphate concentration. Calcium salts are the phosphate binders of choice. The phosphate binding capacity of different calcium salts is given in Table 8. $CaCO_3$ is often preferred because the simultaneous correction of acidosis. Simultaneous administration of calcium salts and the active metabolite of vitamin D may result in hypercalcaemia. If hypercalcaemia develops and is associated with hyperphosphataemia, combined treatment of calcium and magnesium salts as phosphate binding agents is possible. Persistent hypercalcaemia despite temporarily withholding of calcium supplement and calcitriol may develop. Hypercalcaemia associated with high turnover bone disease indicate secondary hyperparathyroidism. The diagnosis can be made by measurements of the intact PTH molecule by the immunoradiometric assay (IRMA) or by bone biopsy. Pulse therapy with either intravenous or oral high dose of calcitriol may allow suppression of PTH secretion. If not and hypercalcaemia persists parathyroidectomy is required. Hypercalcaemia with low bone turnover (adynamic bone disease) is associated with low alkaline phosphatase and low (intact) PTH (less than 55 pg/ml) levels. If aluminium intoxication is excluded, the dialysate calcium concentration is lowered (to 1.25 mmol/l) and low doses of calcitriol are administered. When aluminium toxicity is present, administration of the chelating agent, deferoxamine during dialysis is indicated (47).

The following recommendations for the treatment of renal osteodystrophy can be made:

1. Restrict dietary phosphate intake, but an adequate intake of protein is required.
2. If hypercalcaemia develops a differentiation between high and low bone turnover disease should be made. Low bone turnover requires lowering of dialysate calcium concentration from 1.75 to 1.25 mmol/l.
3. Serum PTH levels should be measured regularly during calcium salts and vitamin D administration. Reducing PTH levels to relatively low values contributes to subnormal rates of bone formation and "aplastic" bone disease. PTH levels should not be reduced below 2 times normal values.
4. Plasma aluminium levels should be monitored and the use of aluminium containing phosphate binders should be omitted.

Anaemia

Children with end stage renal disease are usually profoundly anaemic; in one study the mean haematocrit levels were 19.3% ± 9.9% (48). Prepubertal children are more anaemic than pubertal. Many factors contribute to severe anaemia, including blood loss, decreased red cell survival, iron, folic acid and erythropoietin deficiency and a depression of bone marrow. Anaemia is more severe in haemodialysis than in CAPD patients, probably as a result of a larger blood loss in haemodialysis patients (49).

Administration of recombinant human erythropoietin (rHuEPO) has proved to be highly effective in correcting the anaemia of predialysis and dialysis patients. It may be administered intravenously (i.v.), subcutaneously (s.c.) and in patients on CAPD intraperitoneally (i.p.). Different doses and dosing intervals are required according to the route of administration. For the i.v. route also age differences were found. In a large multicenter study, including 142 paediatric haemodialysis patients, three times weekly administration of rHuEPO resulted in an increase of the Hct from 20 to 30%, elimination of transfusion requirements and reduction of iron overload. The main maintenance dose was respectively 320, 230, 158 and 136 IU/kg BW per week in the age groups less than 5 years, between 5 and 10, between 10 and 15 and over 15 years old (50). In children on CAPD, i.p. administration of a weekly dose of 300 IU/kg BW divided over three doses and administered in a reduced dialysate volume (20 ml/kg) during a long dwell period (8–10 h) resulted in correction of the anaemia (51).

Because of the risk of peritonitis s.c. administrations in CAPD patients is often preferred. Maintenance of haematocrit over 30% can be achieved with s.c. administration of 100 IU/kg BW once a week or divided in two weekly doses (52).

Maintaining adequate iron stores is critical, when treating patients with rHuEPO. Serum ferritin is the best predictor of the development of iron deficiency. Treatment with high doses oral iron (5 mg/kg/day) or i.v. iron should be started if serum ferritin is less than 60 μg/l (53). Possible side effects are hypertension, seizures, access clotting and reduced efficiency of dialysis.

Patients receiving the drug by s.c. administration sometimes complain of pain and irritation at the side of injection. The pain is mainly caused by the citrate component of the rHuEPO vehicle of the available commercial product. Increased blood pressure is the most important side effect associated with rHuEPO. It occurs in the first months of treatment and is not related to dose or rate of increase of haematocrit (54).

Cardiovascular complications

Hypertension in children on regular haemodialysis usually responds to increased salt and water removal by ultrafiltration during dialysis. Inadequate dialysis with dialyzers that are too small or too large (leading to hypotension during dialysis and hypertension after washback) is the commonest cause of persistent hypertension in children treated by regular haemodialysis.

Some children persistently develop hypotension during conventional haemodialysis which necessitates saline or plasma infusion to stabilise blood pressure and leads to hypertension after dialysis. Sequential ultrafiltration and dialysis in such patients usually allows sufficient fluid removal during dialysis without hypotension.

A vicious circle of hypertension between dialyses, hypotension on dialysis and therefore inadequate dialysis, high blood urea concentrations, anorexia with poor food intake leading to malnutrition and hypercatabolism can easily develop. This requires extra attention to nutrition using energy supplements and even nasoenteric feeding combined with frequent short dialyses until the patient's condition stabilises. Rapid weight gain between dialysis with hypertension is generally due to excessive sodium intake increasing thirst rather than being due to simply drinking too much water, for these children are rarely hyponatraemic.

In occasional children severe hypertension is due to hyperrennininaemia. This is especially common in children with renal failure due to haemolytic uraemic syndrome or focal glomerular sclerosis. In such children excessive salt and water removal during dialysis does not control blood pressure but results in nausea, anorexia and lethargy. The introduction of angiotensin converting enzyme inhibitors such as captopril or enalapril will usually control the hypertension and improve the child's health, appetite and activity; bilateral nephrectomy is now required only rarely. However in children with hypertension related to hyperreninemia, severe hypertension may develop following transplantation. Therefore, left nephrectomy is performed during dialysis and the right kidney will be removed during the transplant procedure.

Chronic hypertension, uraemia, and malnutrition all contribute to impaired cardiac performance in children on haemodialysis but anaemia and, in some children increased cardiac output caused by large arteriovenous fistulae are of a special importance. Echocardiography may reveal impaired left ventricular performance and a uraemic cardiomyopathy in some children (58). Cardiac arrest and pulmonary oedema are among the causes of death in children on dialysis; frequent cardiac assessment is an important part of management.

Neurological complications

Neurological complications (see Chapter 46) are rare in children in chronic renal failure who are being properly dialysed. Nonetheless neurological development is often below normal in children with severe chronic renal failure dating from infancy. Developmental delay has been detected in over 60% of such cases and particularly affects gross motor and language development (56). There is some evidence that early transplantation may improve development in such children (57). The cause of this developmental delay and the long term prognosis are not yet determined. Malnutrition, poor electrolyte control with wide swings in plasma osmolality in early life, and aluminium toxicity from the ingestion of aluminium have been implicated (56).

REGULAR HAEMODIALYSIS IN CHILDREN

The basic principles and procedures of haemodialysis in children are the same as in adults. However, haemodialysis of (small) children is associated with complications such as access failures, hypotension, nausea, vomiting, abdominal pain and encephalopathy during dialysis and hypertension, cardiac failure and pulmonary oedema following dialysis when equipment and methods designed for adults are used. Several modifications in techniques and equipment are required for paediatric purposes.

Vascular access

Angioaccess is a major problem in paediatric patients. Although external arteriovenous cannulae have been used extensively for chronic dialysis in children, the short functional life of shunts and the frequent complications (thrombosis, infections) has led to abandonment of this type of vascular access.

A better temporary vascular access is achieved by a percutaneously placed indwelling catheter in the jugular or subclavian vein. A silicone rubber catheter (Hickman) is positioned into the right atrium and fixed subcutaneously with a Dacron cuff. Depending on the size of the patient catheters with an internal diameter of 1.6 or 2.6 mm can be used. Both double and single lumen catheters are available. After dialysis 3 ml heparinised saline is injected into the catheter and a cap is placed at the external end. A longer life span is noticed than with Scribner shunts (58, 59), but thrombosis of a major vessel is a common complication. Therefore the only acceptable access for long term haemodialysis are arteriovenous fistulae. Brescia-Cimino radiocephalic fistulae at the wrist have a low complication rate in children. The side (artery) to end (vein) anastomosis should be preferred to the end to end anastomosis because of better flow through the hand when the distal portion of the artery remains patent. In small children, weighing less than 15 kg, the use of microsurgical techniques or secondary superficialisation of a deep vein or both allows construction of arteriovenous fistulae (60, 61). Shortness of the puncturable part of the vein often requires the use of single needle technique in children. It should be pointed out that this technique reduces dialysis efficiency. Maximizing arterial inflow volume decreases recirculation but requires a compliance chamber in the dialysis circuit to avoid increased hydrostatic pressure and thereby excessive ultrafiltration and increases extracorporeal blood volume (62).

A saphenous vein autograft is an efficient alternative if the forearm vessels are not suitable for fistula creation.

Excellent results were obtained in children with autogenous saphenous vein grafts inserted in a loop configuration in the forearm (63). A common complication of these grafts placed between the brachial artery and cephalic vein is the enormous dilatation of the vessel and aneurysm formation after long term use. Moreover, the high blood flow through the fistula may induce congestive heart failure. Polytetrafluoroethylene (PTFE) grafts (Goretex, Impra) may also be used for vascular access in children. When this graft is inserted in the thigh between the superficial femoral artery and the proximal saphenous vein, attention should be given not to place the graft too deeply into the subcutaneous tissue to avoid cannulation problems. Although efficient dialysis with PTFE grafts has been reported, a higher complication rate (thrombosis, infection) was noticed than with Brescia-Cimino fistulas or saphenous vein grafts (64).

Choice of dialyzer and blood lines

The dialyzer should be carefully adapted to the size of the patient. Selection relates to the blood volume of the dialyzer and blood lines and to the efficiency of the dialyzer. The volume of the extracorporeal blood circuit should never exceed 10% of the patient's blood volume (80 ml/kg/body weight). Calculation of extracorporeal blood volume should include increases of dialyzer blood volume during application of negative pressure for ultrafiltration. Special paediatric blood lines with volumes varying between 20 and 80 ml are commercially available. Paediatric blood lines with 1.5–3.0 mm internal diameter tubing will restrict blood flow to less than 30–75 ml/min. If higher blood flows are required special short blood lines with larger inner diameter will reduce extracorporeal blood volume. Although blood flow rates must be individually determined for each patient, general guidelines are proposed based on the patient's weight. Blood flow rates of 5 ml/kg BW may provide efficient BUN clearances. In children weighing less then 10 kg blood flow rates should not exceed 75 ml/min, and in children weighing more than 40 kg rates up to 250 ml/min can be used (65).

Several disposable hollow fibre and flat plate dialyzers are suitable for the treatment of children. The patient's body weight and surface area and clinical condition should determine the clearance characteristics of the dialyzer to be used (Table 9).

To avoid dialysis disequilibrium it is safer to start treatment with a urea clearance not exceeding 3 ml/min/kg. Subsequently the choice of the dialyzer should be adapted to the individual tolerance of the patient, but dialyzers with urea clearances ranging between 6 and 8 ml/min/kg are required for regular short dialysis.

Fluid removal during haemodialysis is a function of transmembrane hydrostatic pressure and osmotic gradients. The rate of fluid removal depends on the dialyzer membrane surface area and hydraulic permeability. A dialyzer that accurately predicts ultrafiltration is required unless special devices for regulation of ultrafiltration are used.

Management of regular dialysis in children

The dialysis should be adjusted to the individual need of the child as determined not only by the size of the patient but also by individual variations in dialysis tolerance. Therefore, careful observation of the patient during dialysis is necessary. In small children critical changes in vital signs may appear. Regular control of vital signs is extremely important.

Especially in small children careful control of ultrafiltration is mandatory. Special devices for accurate control of ultrafiltration should be used; if not available continuous weight recording is imperative. Weight readings should be unaffected by normal movements of the patient or by the dialysis equipment.

General heparinisation can be effected by administration of a bolus of 50 U heparin/kg body weight at the beginning of dialysis, followed by infusion of 25 U heparin/kg/h. When low molecular weight heparin is used sufficient anticoagulation is obtained by administration of only a bolus at the beginning of dialysis. Advised doses of fragmin are in patients less then 15 kg: 1500 anti-Factor Xa units, in patients between 15 and 30 kg: 2500 U and in patients between 30 and 50 kg: 5000 U.

In patients weighing 8 to 15 kg and without marked fluid retention (less than 2.5% of body weight) between dialysis, the priming fluid is often transfused into the patient at the beginning of the procedure. In very small children, weighing less than 8 kg, transfusion of the priming fluid into the patient is always required. In larger children the priming fluid is discharged unless the patient did not gain weight during the interdialytic period. At the end of dialysis the extracorporeal blood is transfused back to the patient. Only small amounts of saline (less than 100 ml) are used for the dialyzer washback procedure.

Ultrafiltration should be planned carefully and any excessive fluid loss should be replaced throughout dialysis. Ultrafiltration combined with dialysis has to be reduced to less than 5% of body weight in order to avoid severe hypotension during dialysis. Treatment of hypotension requires administration of 0.9% saline, or albumen solution.

The requirement for dialysis is proportional to the metabolic rate, because the intake of all nutrients is proportional to metabolic rate. Metabolic rate is proportional to body surface area (BSA) which for a child is greater in relation to body weight than for an adult. Due to the high need for calories, protein and fluids relative to body weight, the child will accumulate metabolic waste products faster than adults do. Therefore, paediatric patients need more dialysis in relation to their body weight than adults. Children without significant residual kidney function are often dialysed thrice weekly. Children weighing

Table 9. Characteristics of some disposable paediatric dialyzers

Dialyzers	Membrane		Priming volume ml	Ultrafiltration coefficient (ml/h/mm Hg TMP)	Urea clearance at Q_B (ml/min)				
	Nature	Surface area (m²)			50	75	100	150	200
Asahi AM 0.3	Cuprammonium	0.30	30	1.4	45	59	64	68	–
Asahi AM 0.6	Cuprammonium	0.60	60	2.1		69	88	100	
Gambro Pro 100	Polycarbonate	0.30	19	2.2	51	60	54	66	
Gambro Pro 200	Polycarbonate	0.50	43	3.5	47		73	88	94
Fresenius F3	Polysulfone	0.40	30	1.7	45	63	78	98	120
Fresenius F4	Polysulfone	0.70	44	2.8					155
Biospal 1200 S	PAN	0.50	60	23.0		70	84	98	99
Filtral 8	PAN	0.70	53	19.0				127	148
Filtral 6	PAN	0.55	48	15.0		72	91	117	136
Cobe HG-100	Hemophan	0.22	18	2.0	50		80	102	
Nipro FB-30 U	Cellulose acetate	0.30	25	5.7			88		126
Nipro FB-50 U	Cellulose acetate	0.50	35	9.6			97		158
Nipro FB-70 U	Cellulose acetate	0.70	45	11.0			99		175

less than 8 kg will need four dialyses per week because the increase of body fluid will lead to circulatory overload when subsequent dialyses are not performed within 48 h (65). The duration of dialysis is determined by the time required for adequate fluid and solute removal. In patients with a moderately restricted protein intake (below 1.5 g/kg/day) adequate solute removal is achieved with a 3 to 5 h dialysis three times weekly.

Because most paediatric dialyzers have small ultrafiltration coefficients, dialysis time is often determined by fluid removal requirements. Shortening dialysis time is achieved by the use of dialyzers with highly permeable membranes or by haemodiafiltration.

Complications

Side effects related to the "unphysiology" of dialysis may develop. These include nausea, vomiting, headache, hypotension and convulsions (disequilibrium syndrome). Convulsions occur in 10% of dialysed children but EEG abnormalities are found more often if continuously registered during dialysis (66). A rapid decline in plasma osmolality with shifting of water into the cells, a reduction of peripheral vascular resistance by acetate, high ultrafiltration rates and blood volume shifts to the dialyzer may contribute to these side effects.

If symptoms persist despite restriction of the efficiency of the dialyzer and avoidance of dialyzers with poor compliance characteristics, other measures must be taken. Dissociation of the dialysis and ultrafiltration procedure will allow ultrafiltration without the development of hypotension. During sequential ultrafiltration and dialysis a period of ultrafiltration precedes or follows standard dialysis, using the same dialyzer. Ultrafiltration is effected by an increase in transmembrane pressure. This is generated by application of a negative pressure across the non-blood side of the dialyzer's membrane or a positive pressure on the blood side of the membrane. During this procedure dialysate bypasses the dialyzer. Transmembrane pressure differences up to 500 mm Hg have to be used (67).

Intravenous infusion of mannitol at 1 g/kg will also reduce the decrease in serum osmolality during dialysis. However, mannitol will accumulate and reach a steady state level within a few dialyses with infusions. At this level an amount equal to that infused will be removed during each dialysis and it will be inefficient in preventing the decrease in osmolality. To avoid accumulation mannitol should be administered only once weekly (68).

The substitution of bicarbonate for acetate has significantly improved dialysis tolerance in children (69, 70). In the absence of a special device for the preparation of bicarbonate dialysate the use of biofiltration may result in a similar improvement in dialysis tolerance (74). Biofiltration is a haemodiafiltration technique performed with an acetate-free dialysate using dialyzers with highly permeable membranes and carefully controlled ultrafiltration. Substitution fluids containing bicarbonate are used (71). In children ultrafiltration rates of 2,000 ml/1.73 m² per dialysis were achieved. Ultrafiltered fluids in excess of required net ultrafiltrate were replaced by isotonic bicarbonate. Improvement of dialysis tolerance similar to that achieved by bicarbonate dialysis was found.

Modification in composition of the dialysate will also affect symptoms associated with dialysis. Improved tolerance to haemodialysis can be obtained using 400 mg/dl dextrose enriched dialysate, which reduces the fall in serum osmolality during dialysis (72). However, high dialysate dextrose concentrations increase the risk of bacterial proliferation and endotoxin release. Another way to increase plasma osmolality is to use dialysate with a high

Table 10. Fistula creation and start of dialysis

Age (yr)	Fistula creation at serum creatinine	Start of dialysis at serum creatinine
1–5	350–550 μmol/l	650–700 μmol/l
5–10	450–650 μmol/l	700–800 μmol/l
10–15	550–700 μmol/l	800–900 μmol/l

sodium concentration (145 mmol/l). High sodium levels may be maintained at a constant level but also a progressive decrease in dialysate sodium concentration throughout dialysis has been used to avoid chronic volume expansion, hypertension and heart failure (73). Excessive ultrafiltration during dialysis will induce intolerance. Accurate assessments of dry weight may be achieved by measurements of inulin distribution volume (IDV). In children developing hypotension during ultrafiltration an IDV less than 22% of body weight was found (74). Hypotension between dialyses sometimes occurs in nephrectomised patients, despite salt and fluid retention (75). The use of hypertonic dialysate may increase blood pressure in these patients. Persistence or increase of hypertension during dialysis, despite adequate ultrafiltration, is occasionally seen. If in those patients hypertension resists treatment with inhibitors of converting enzyme (captopril, enalapril) bilateral nephrectomy may be required. Recurrent pericarditis despite adequate dialysis occasionally occurs in children. These children are mostly hypertensive and usually overhydrated. If clinical assessment of fluid overload is difficult in these patients, IDV determination may be useful. In fluid overloaded patients IDV in excess of 29% of body weight was found (74). Excessive interdialytic weight gain related to dietary noncompliance increases mortality rate in dialysed children (76). Hyperkalaemia occurs more frequently in small children than in adults during catabolic states or from high intakes and also represents a vital risk.

Hypersensitivity reactions related to dialysis material (first use syndrome) have been reported in children and may occur at any time after the start of treatment by dialysis (77). Symptoms resembling anaphylaxis start within 1 to 60 min following the onset of the dialysis procedure and range from urticaria to cardiopulmonary collapse. Their severity may require interruption of the dialysis procedure and emergency treatment.

Practical directives for haemodialysis in children

Preparation for dialysis

Before its initiation, dialysis has to be explained to the child by drawings and by attending a dialysis session of other children.

For blood access an arteriovenous fistula is created several months prior to the start of dialysis. Serum creatinine

is quantified frequently to determine the time of fistula creation and subsequently the start of dialysis (Table 10). The rate of deterioration of renal function must also be considered when deciding on the time of fistula creation. Preparations for home dialysis are initiated at the time of fistula creation if the patient and his family are willing to perform the treatment at home.

Dietary prescriptions and controls for adequate nutrition are essential. Cumulative interdialytic weight gain from excessive fluid intake should be distinguished from real weight gain from an increase of the child's body mass. The child should have his own responsibility for his interdialytic weight increase. Calorie and protein intakes are assessed by diet surveys recorded during similar interdialytic periods at monthly intervals. Calculation of the urea generation rate can be used to check adherence to the prescribed protein intake (78).

Dialysis technique

Fistula needles of gauge 18 to 14 are required for adequate blood flow. Single needle technique allows adequate dialysis even in small children with only a short vessel area available for needle insertion (2 to 3 cm).

Primary nursing improves the quality of care for paediatric patients. Individual nurse-patient allocation not only provides more efficient technical work, but also improves patient's adaptation to treatment.

The play-leader and teacher have to plan a playing and educational programme for each patient during the time spent on dialysis. Adequate cooperation between home school and the dialysis teaching team is required to obtain optimal schooling.

A basic rule is to adjust each dialysis according to the individual requirement of each child. Estimation of 'dry or ideal' body weight is essential. Percentile cards should be used to determine the ideal weight according to the child's body height and build. If the patient thrives and grows and the muscle mass increases, the ideal body weight also increases.

The choice of the dialyzer should be individually adapted to each patient. A special procedure has to be applied for the first sessions including the use of a less effective dialyzer (urea clearance less than 3 ml/kg), a shorter duration of dialysis (1.5 to 2 h), prophylactic use of diazepam (2 to 5 mg IV) and administration of mannitol IV during dialysis (1 g/kg). Subsequently the dialyzer and duration of dialysis should be adapted to individual tolerance and requirements. The blood volume of the extracorporeal circuit (volumes of blood lines and dialyzer, including the additional volume due to compliance of the dialyzer) should not exceed 10% of the child's circulating blood volume.

The prescribed amount of ultrafiltration during dialysis depends on the interdialytic weight gain. Excessive weight gain between dialyses is usually due to high sodium intake with secondary excessive water intake; limitation of dietary sodium should be encouraged. Fluid

Table 11. Proposed combinations of dialysis time, dialyzer size and blood flow rates according to patient's size

Patient				Dialyzer				
age (yr)	weight (kg)	BSA (m^2)	blood volume (ml)	DSA (m^2)	Extracorporeal blood volume (ml)	blood flow (ml/min)	Cl_{BUN} dialysis	time (h)
2	11	0.50	770	0.37	75	125	44	3–5
4	17	0.75	1190	0.56	115	145	68	3–5
9	28	1.00	1960	0.75	190	170	112	3–5
14	43	1.30	3010	0.98	300	190	172	3–5

loss by ultrafiltration during dialysis in excess of 5% of body weight will induce symptoms of hypotension. Precise and continuous monitoring and regulation of ultrafiltration is mandatory in paediatric patients. Continuous weight recording is less reliable. Weight changes may be caused by food and fluid intake, fluid loss by vomiting and by shifting of blood into (or out of) the dialyzer, due to volume changes caused by compliance of the membrane. If ultrafiltration in excess of 5% of body weight is required sequential ultrafiltration and dialysis should be applied. Small amounts of saline usually correct hypotension during dialysis.

Individual differences in dialysis tolerance are often observed. To obviate regular recurrence of headache, dizziness, nausea, abdominal pain and vomiting during dialysis the following modifications in treatment may be considered (79): withdrawal of antihypertensive drugs prior to dialysis, reconsider the choice of the dialyzer, infusion of mannitol (1 g/kg) during the first dialysis of the week, substitution of acetate by bicarbonate as the alkalinising buffer in the dialysate, and sequential hypertonic dialysis (use of decreasing dialysis fluid sodium concentrations during dialysis).

In paediatric patients dialysis twice a week may allow satisfactory rehabilitation but three dialyses a week are recommended allowing a more liberal dietary and fluid intake and reducing the side-effects during dialysis with vigorous ultrafiltration. In young children (< 5 years) the higher metabolic rate and poor compliance to the diet requires three dialyses per week. Infants less than 8 kg require four dialyses per week. Measurements of protein catabolic rate and normalized whole body urea clearance will allow individualised prescription of dialysis and thereby prevent overdialysis. Although no guidelines for target range of Kt/V in children are available, a value between 0.9 and 1.5 is considered acceptable (80). In Table 11 the proposed combinations of dialysis time, dialyzer size and blood flow rates according to patient's size are given.

Close supervision of the patient is required during dialysis. Careful observation will reveal agitation, color changes and abdominal pain. These clinical signs often precede hypotension. Regular determination of body weight and blood pressure pre- and postdialysis is required.

Treatment of complications during dialysis

Institution of dialysis often improves hypertension markedly, but many children remain hypertensive despite dialysis with ultrafiltration. Hypertensive emergencies are treated by diazoxide (5 mg/kg IV) or labetalol (0.5 mg/kg.hr IV). For prolonged treatment of hypertension beta-adrenergic blocking agents are preferred to methyldopa because of less frequent adverse reactions. In cases of refractory hypertension the administration of captropril or enalapril is usually effective.

Ultrafiltration with an inappropriate dialyzer is the most common cause of hypotension during dialysis. Saline and albumen solutions are commonly used to treat hypotension. Convulsions during dialysis should be treated by administration of diazepam (5 to 10 mg according to body weight). Recurrent convulsions are either due to cerebral abnormalities or inappropriate dialysis technique.

REGULAR PERITONEAL DIALYSIS

Regular peritoneal dialysis has been extensively used in the treatment of ESRD in children and has been shown as effective as regular haemodialysis for control of uremia and its complications. Since the introduction of CAPD an increasing number of paediatric patients have undergone peritoneal dialysis. In 1992, 38% of all children on regular dialysis in Europe were undergoing CAPD (21).

Types of peritoneal dialysis

There are three types of chronic peritoneal dialysis (CPD): intermittent peritoneal dialysis (IPD), continuous ambulatory peritoneal dialysis (CAPD) and automated peritoneal dialysis (APD). The latter includes continuous cyclic peritoneal dialysis (CCPD), nightly intermittent peritoneal dialysis (NIPD) and tidal peritoneal dialysis (TPD).

Intermittent peritoneal dialysis

In IPD, dialysis is performed two or three times per week with a duration of 40 to 60 h/week. This technique has been replaced in most instances by the continuous technique of PD (CAPD) or nightly intermittent peritoneal dialysis (NIPD) (21).

Continuous ambulatory peritoneal dialysis (CAPD)

Technique

CAPD is performed through an indwelling Silastic catheter, tailored to the size of the child. The adult size (intraperitoneal portion: 15 cm) is used for children weighing more than 30 kg. The paediatric size (12 cm) for those between 10 and 30 kg, and the neonatal size (10 cm) in smaller children.

Straight and curled catheters with one or two Dacron cuffs are used. Catheter placement technique is similar in children and adults. Modifications proposed in children are the insertion of the catheter beneath the body of the rectus muscle instead of a midline entry site in order to have more tissue in which to bury the cuff. Also omentectomy is performed at the time of cannula insertion in small children because they are more susceptible to obstruction of the catheter by omental fringes (81).

Immediately following insertion, the patient is dialyzed with an automatic cycling machine for 4 to 6 days, while gradually dwell time (10 min to 4 h) and the volume of dialysate (10 to 50 ml/kg) are increased. Prophylactic antibiotics are administered before surgery (tobramycin 1.5 mg/kg IV and cephalotin 20 mg/kg IV). During the period of 'break in' heparin (500 IU/l) and cephalotin (250 mg/l) are added to the dialysis solution. Subsequently CAPD is started on the basis of four exchanges per day with 50 ml/kg of dialysis solution. After commencing regular CAPD, the patients and their parents are trained to perform CAPD at home. Children 10 years of age or older are able to learn the technique themselves. Teaching of parents or patients includes such aspects as bag change, dressing change, measurements of blood pressure and recognition of signs of peritonitis. They are advised about correct 'dry weight' and the type of dialysis fluid required to maintain that weight. Once the patient is discharged from the hospital, close contact is maintained by telephone. Regular attendances, at least once a month, at the dialysis centre are required (82).

Indications

The choice to perform CAPD should be a collective decision of the patient, his family and the nephrology team. CAPD may be a better alternative in the treatment of ESRD in infants in whom haemodialysis is difficult to perform, in children living a long distance from the dialysis centre, in patients with no vascular access sites available for haemodialysis and for patients at risk for increased intracranial pressure. Also patients with poor haemodialysis tolerance and children with severe psychological prob-

lems related to the haemodialysis should benefit from conversion to CAPD. Children whose parents are afraid or unwilling to accept responsibility to perform the treatment at home, are regarded as unsuitable for CAPD.

Results

Clearances of small and middle molecules with CAPD are higher than with IPD, but BUN and plasma creatinine values are higher than in patients on regular haemodialysis. Patients on CAPD use less phosphate binders and exchange resins than those on haemodialysis. Normal growth was not different in patients on CAPD compared to those on haemodialysis (90). Rehabilitation of children on CAPD is excellent and fulltime school attendance is frequently achieved. Physical activity could be almost normal, but some limitations, in order to protect the cutaneous exit site of the catheter, are recommended.

Continuous cycling peritoneal dialysis and nightly intermittent peritoneal dialysis

Technique

CCPD and NIPD consist of multiple nocturnal exchanges of variable duration. In children four to five, 2-h exchanges with an automatic cycler delivering up to 50 ml/kg of dialysate are performed during the night. In NIPD none and CCPD only one daytime dwell lasting 12 to 15 h and using a smaller dialysate volume is effected.

Indications

Patients who require more than four daily exchanges to control the biochemical abnormalities of uremia or to obtain adequate ultrafiltration, and those who are unable to tolerate the dialysate volume required to achieve adequate dialysis, because of hydrothorax, repeated hernia or dialysate leak, may benefit from conversion to CCPD. CCPD may be primarily chosen over CAPD by parents who are unavailable to perform the daytime exchanges and by patients attending school who are unable to perform the procedure at school (92).

Results

CCPD is as efficient as CAPD in biochemical control of uremia. Procedural difference between CAPD and CCPD may lead to a lower rate of peritonitis with the latter (93). In small children the shorter dwell time of CCPD will increase ultrafiltration.

Tidal peritoneal dialysis

Tidal peritoneal dialysis (TPD) is a dialytic therapy in which the peritoneal cavity always remains in contact with dialysate fluid, because only a portion of the initial fill volume is repetitively exchanged.

Indications

Maximizing dialysis transport by minimizing the time spent with an empty peritoneum, is the most important indication for TPD. It may also be of benefit in patients with poor ultrafiltration characteristics due to high peritoneal glucose permeability and to shorten overnight dialysis time in adolescents. This technique has also been used to avoid haemoperitoneum in patients with peritoneal calcifications (83).

Clinical management of children on peritoneal dialysis

Peritoneal dialysis prescription

The appropriate peritoneal dialysis prescription in children should be based on patient's size, peritoneal membrane function, residual renal function and metabolic need.

Prescription for CAPD

The aims of CAPD are to maintain stable concentrations of solutes within the body and water balance. Blood urea levels are often used as indications of uraemic toxicity and therefore dialytic therapy is adapted to maintain BUN at 20 mmol/l. However, BUN values are dependent on protein intake and acceptable BUN values may be found in patients with malnutrition, irrespective of dialysis efficiency. Quantification of dialysis by measured weekly dialytic KT/V urea (weekly urea clearance/total body water) and creatinine clearance (weekly CrCl/surface area) has been used in adults (84). Weekly urea KT/V of at least 1.7 and weekly CrCl of 50 l/1.73 m^2 BSA were reported to represent adequate dialysis. A wide range for both values were found in children and reference values are still to be determined (85). The peritoneal equilibration test (PET) may be used to characterise peritoneal solute transport and to determine the cause of inadequate dialysis. Several modifications of the test originally described by Twardowski were used in children (85–87). Modifications were related to fill volumes used and glucose concentration of the dialysate (86). Data collected in different studies suggest that children are more rapid transporters of glucose and have a more rapid equilibration of creatinine. To avoid erroneous conclusions fill volumes should be determined on body surface area (86). The PET is performed after an overnight dwell. Following infusion of 1,100 ml/m^2 SA of 2.5% glucose dialysate, dialysate samples are obtained at 0, 120 and 240 min and a blood sample at 120 min.

The D/P rates for creatinine at 2 and 4 h and reabsorption of glucose are calculated. Although KT/V urea and CrCl can be estimated using data obtained from the PET, these data are more important to assess changes in membrane characteristics over time and to determine optimal dwell times.

The amount of body water that needs to be ultrafiltered should be calculated on the basis of 'dry weight'. Dry weight is determined on clinical symptoms but in hypertensive children measurements of extracellular fluid volume may be required. Ultrafiltrate volumes depend on dextrose concentrations of the dialysate, exchange volumes and duration of the exchange. Drainage volumes after a 4 h exchange exceed infused volumes of dialysate containing dextrose monohydrate in concentrations of 1.5% and 4.25% by approximately 15 to 25% and 30 to 40% respectively (88).

It should be noted that in small children ultrafiltrate volumes are usually less; this is probably due to enhanced lymphatic absorption (89). Dialysis and ultrafiltration requirements as well as individual peritoneal membrane characteristics will determine the number of exchanges, dwell time and dextrose concentration used.

Nutrition

In addition to the recommendations given later, calculation of energy intake should include glucose uptake (3.75 kcal/g) from the dialysate. In children less than 6 years old glucose absorption (2.74 ± 1.05 g/kg/day) is higher than in older children (1.49 ± 0.72 g/kg/day) (90).

The recommended protein intake for children on CAPD is 1.5 to 2.0 g/kg, whereas in infants 2.5 to 3.0 g/kg is proposed. Also protein loss into the dialysate is higher in younger patients (0.24 ± 0.04 g/kg/day) compared to older children (0.17 ± 0.06 g/kg/day) (91).

In children undergoing CAPD high serum levels of triglycerides and cholesterol were found. The hypertriglyceridemia was related to impaired clearance of triglycerides (90). The uptake of glucose from the dialysate may also increase triglyceride production.

To improve protein metabolism dialysate dextrose has been replaced by aminoacid solutions. Although aminoacid dialysis is equally effective in ultrafiltration and therefore may be of benefit by decreasing glucose supplementation, its effect on protein metabolism and nutritional state is not yet well established (91).

Increases in cholesterol and triglycerides were also more pronounced in younger children, who also had higher protein losses in the dialysate (92). Dietary fat should provide about 50% of dietary energy intake with a ratio of polyunsaturated to saturated fatty acid of 1.5 to 1.0. This fatty acid ratio may reduce serum triglyceride levels.

Mineral metabolism

Despite stable serum Ca levels, worsening of renal osteodystrophy in children treated with CAPD has been reported. During CAPD vitamin D binding protein and 25-hydroxy vitamin D are lost into the dialysate. Using a dialysate with 1.75 mmol/l of calcium, losses of calcium into the dialysate are minimal. Salusky et al. (93) reported that higher doses of calcitriol (0.25 to 2.25 µg/day), than those commonly used in haemodialysis patients, should be used to treat secondary hyperparathyroidism.

Complications of peritoneal dialysis

The most common complications of PD are peritonitis, hernia, catheter related complications such as exit-site infection, leakage, obstruction of the catheter, outer cuff extrusion and catheter dislocation. Reported survival time ranged from 14 to 17 months (94).

Peritonitis

Peritonitis is a major complication of peritoneal dialysis. The incidence of peritonitis in patients on CAPD is about one episode every 19.8 patient months, but more than 50% of the patients are still peritonitis-free after 24 months of treatment. In the majority of cases peritonitis is caused by failure in technique, but may be associated with exit site infections or tunnel infections. Two thirds of the organisms isolated are gram positive (Staph aureus, Staph epidermidis, Strept viridans) and one third is gram negative. Fungal infections are occasionally found. An incidence of 'culture negative' peritonitis in up to 50% of cases was reported (95). Abdominal pain, fever and cloudy dialysate are the most consistent clinical signs of peritonitis. Peritonitis with clear fluid and low dialysate cell count (less than 100 cell/μl) is unusual in patients on CAPD but may be found in patients on intermittent peritoneal dialysis.

Treatment of peritonitis

On CAPD the patient or his parents are told to call the hospital if signs of peritonitis occur. Unless they can reach the dialysis unit quickly, they are instructed to start treatment at home. After drainage of the abdominal cavity, the dialysate is saved for gram staining, cell count and culture. Thereafter three rapid exchanges with the usual volumes are performed, and CAPD is then resumed on a 6-h schedule with antibiotics and heparin added to each bag of dialysate. If no result of gram stain is available, a loading dose of 500 mg of cephalotin per liter of dialysate and of 1.7 mg/kg of tobramycin and 500 IU of heparin is added to the first exchange. Thereafter, 250 mg of cephalotin per liter is added to the dialysate. If a gram positive organism is identified, cephalothin treatment alone is continued, while if a gram negative organism is found, tobramycin alone is used (10 mg/l). In the presence of no growth both antibiotics are continued. Treatment is continued for 12 days with repeated cultures on day 5 and 10. Afterwards treatment is prolonged if clinically required. Antibiotic treatment is modified according to bacteriologic examination if dialysate fluid has not become clear after 48 h of treatment (dosage see Table 12). Heparin is added to the dialysate until the fluid is clear and fibrin clots disappear (82).

With peritonitis, CCPD patients are switched to CAPD for at least one week and treatment is similar to that in patients on CAPD. For patients treated by IPD, after the diagnosis of peritonitis is made, three rapid exchanges, are performed. Following these three exchanges, an exchange

Table 12. Recommended doses of intraperitoneal antibiotics in the treatment of peritonitis in patients on CAPD

	Loading dose	Maintenance dose
Cephalothin	500 mg/l	250 mg/l
Cephradine	250 mg/l	125 mg/l
Tobramycine	1.7 mg/kg/bag	8 mg/l
Gentamicin	1.5 mg/kg/bag	10 mg/l
Ampicillin	500 mg/l	50 mg/l
Cloxacillin	1000 mg/l	100 mg/l
Vancomycin	10 mg/kg/bag	30 mg/l
Clindamycin	300 mg/l	50 mg/l
Amikacin	250 mg/l	50 mg/l

with a loading dose of 500 mg of cephalothin per liter, tobramycin 1.7 mg/kg and 500 IU of heparin is effected. This exchange is left in the abdomen for 6 h. Continuous peritoneal lavage containing a maintenance dose of antibiotics (cephalothin 100 mg/l and tobramycin 10 mg/l) is initiated for 2 days followed by daily dialysis for 3 days. Antibiotics are added to the dialysis fluid for 2 weeks. Also oral antibiotics are added to the treatment.

Outcome of peritonitis

Early treatment results in improvement of symptoms after 24 h. Recurrent or persistent peritonitis may develop despite appropriate antibiotic treatment in patients with skin-exit site or tunnel infection. With persistent bacterial infection for more than 5 days, in the presence of fungal peritonitis and in severe skin-exit or tunnel infections, the peritoneal catheter should be removed.

Hernia

Children may develop inguinal or ventral (incisional) hernias. Commonly these hernias appear within the first months of dialysis and are more frequent in young children. Incisional hernias at the site of catheter insertion are more often found in patients with a midline incision and in those who developed dialysate leak in the postoperative period.

Hydrothorax complicating peritoneal dialysis was also reported in children (96). The use of CCPD with small dialysate volumes may prevent recurrence of hydrothorax. No data regarding adhesion pleurodesis with talc or tetracycline have been reported in children.

Electrolyte abnormalities

Hypernatraemia may occur from more rapid removal of water than sodium and can be caused by dialysis solutions containing high dextrose concentration during treatment with IPD. Treatment consists of prolonging dialysis cycles or the substitution of the dialysis fluid by a solution with a sodium concentration of 130 mmol/l. Hyponatraemia has been reported in infants treated with CAPD requiring significant ultrafiltration. In this situation dialysate sodium loss may exceed oral sodium intake. Symptomatic hypotension may complicate such sodium loss (97).

Changes of peritoneal membrane characteristics

A permanent loss of ultrafiltration associated with increased glucose reabsorption, while peritoneal clearances remained unaltered, has been noted (98). In one series membrane failure was reported to be 16.2% (99). Multiple adhesions with partial or even total obliteration of the peritoneal cavity is found in some of these patients. In patients with sclerosing encapsulating peritonitis the peritoneal membrane may incarcerate the small bowel and lead to bowel obstruction. Several factors such as peritonitis, particularly peritonitis caused by pseudomonas aeruginosa and streptococcal organisms, dialysate containing acetate buffer, use of chlorexidine as antiseptic agent during exchanges, and the use of beta blockers, have been related to the development of membrane alterations (100).

Peritoneal dialysis in infants

Indications

Indications for CAPD in infants are replacement of renal function for end-stage renal disease or following bilateral nephrectomy. Indications for beginning peritoneal dialysis include fluid and electrolyte abnormalities or failure to thrive despite optimal medical management. Bilateral nephrectomy may be required in infants with massive urinary protein loss due to steroid resistant nephrotic syndrome and in patients with bilateral Wilm's tumor.

Technical aspects

The peritoneal membrane of infants is relatively larger and more permeable than that of children and adults. Peritoneal diffusion rates for urea, glucose, middle molecules and protein are higher when related to body size. The rapid absorption of glucose dissipates the osmotic gradient, decreasing ultrafiltration capacity. However, dialysate volume is a major determinant of ultrafiltration, and adequate ultrafiltration may be obtained if dialysate volumes of 1,200 ml/m^2 are used (97).

The technique of CAPD is similar in infants and larger children. The availability of 250 and 275 ml dialysate containers has made application of CAPD in infants possible. However, to improve ultrafiltration shorter dwell times are often used. In infants at least five exchanges a day are performed. Different modifications in technique were proposed to avoid frequent disconnection procedures required by shorting dwell times. Conley et al. (101) used two bags adapted to a Y connector that allowed multiple exchanges a day while entering the system only once. Warady et al. (105) used recirculating dialysis with a 2 l dialysate bag. Exchange volumes of 40 ml/kg, determined

by weighing the bag of dialysate on a bedside scale, were infused into the peritoneal cavity and after completion of a 1-h dwell the peritoneal effluent drained back into the same bag. Once connected the system was not broken until completion of dialysis (8 h/day) (102).

Nutrition

Energy intake should at least equal recommended dietary allowances (RDA). Protein intake should meet RDA (2.5 to 3 g/kg/day) plus replace protein lost in the dialysate (0.25 g/kg/day). Carbohydrate, fat and protein supplements must be added to the formula, if fluid restriction is required because of anuria.

In infants with minimal residual urine production, dialysate sodium losses due to ultrafiltration will exceed intake, requiring oral sodium chloride supplementation (97). These nutritional requirements are often not met with *ad lib* intake. Frequently intermittent nasogastric or continuous transpyloric tube feedings will be necessary.

Burn-out

Burn-out or treatment fatigue has been reported in both children and parents during CAPD. Behavior patterns indicative of burn-out are: failure to maintain accurate home records, failure to take medications, frequent episodes of infections, neglect of appointments and inability to make decisions (103). Measures for dealing with burn-out are regular contact and home visits by the nursing staff, contact with other families and children on CAPD, personal attention by one of the team members, retraining, and involving more family members in the treatment. Conversion to CCPD has been a major mode of dealing with CAPD burn-out, especially in families of very young children and adolescents.

KIDNEY TRANSPLANTATION IN CHILDREN

Kidney transplantation is the treatment of choice in children with end stage renal disease while dialysis is usually considered as a means for awaiting transplant surgery, or an interlude between two grafts after an initial failure.

Although this principle is agreed upon by the majority of nephrologists, transplantation is not always possible when needed, which explains why all children with ESRD do not have a functioning graft. On December 31, 1991, out of 2084 patients with ESRD less than 15 years of age recorded to be alive in the registry of EDTA, only 1191 had a functioning graft, but the proportion of grafted children varied from country to country from 6% in Spain to 61% in Nordic Countries, between 1986–1991 (21). Another way of presenting transplantation strategy is to consider the proportion of patients surviving by the means of a graft at different times after starting renal replacement therapy. Using this mode of analysis, more than 50% of children had a functioning graft after one year in Nordic Countries, while the 50% mark was reached by 2 years in UK, 3 years in FRG and 4 years in France. Thus, the mean waiting time on dialysis is very variable according to country and longer for a cadaver than for a living related graft. Both sources are used for transplanting kidneys in children. In spite of the current controversy about transplanting a kidney from a living donor, all agree to use such donation for paediatric patients. Nevertheless, here again marked differences in policy are noted between countries. In Europe in 1991 out of 346 transplantations, 16% were performed from living related donors. This proportion was much higher in North America reaching 80% of transplantations in some single centre reports (104).

Some children are transplanted directly without even a short period on dialysis. According to the data of the EDTA registry, the percentage of preemptive grafts has increased in almost all countries during recent years, but it remained limited to 8–16% in countries like Spain, France, Germany and Benelux; 23% percent of new paediatric patients in the United Kingdom and 27% in Nordic countries were transplanted before dialysis was required in 1986–1991 (21). Another trend is to perform the second graft when the first fails without passage again on dialysis.

Preparation of children for transplantation

The preparation protocol may be different according to the center, but for children, several points have to be carefully considered. Blood transfusions continue to be considered as useful preoperatively by many groups. The severity of anaemia of children with ESRD usually will indicate transfusion as well. Recently the treatment with recombinant human erythropoietin (rHuEPO) has became available for uraemic patients. The goals of this treatment are to decrease the risk of viral infections, iron overload, sensitization and to improve the quality of life in these children. Even if rHuEPO reduced to great extent the need for transfusions, the crucial points is to look for cytotoxic antibodies after each transfusion in order to stop administering blood containing sensitising HLA antigens if sensitisation appears with only the use of frozen-thawed or especially with filtered blood. Some centres use blood of the kidney donor. Recent reports do not seem to confirm the need of such a protocol when using cyclosporine after grafting. Although definitive answers may not be given, such protocols are now controversial and, probably, the risk directly linked to transfusions is not justified by the results on graft survival. Evaluation and repair of low urinary tract abnormalities is mandatory. A voiding cystogram is part of the check list before grafting. Massive reflux may be an indication for nephroureterectomy. A small pathological bladder may be enlarged with a segment of gut. Moreover, a Bricker neocystostomy may be performed as a first step in patients without any blad-

der available e.g. those with spina bifida or neurological bladder.

Immunizations have to be updated, especially those using a living attenuated virus such as varicella and measles, immunization should be performed at least 2 months before grafting. Severe hypertension caused by native kidneys require left nephrectomy during dialysis and a right nephrectomy at the time of transplantation. The same approach may be applied for children with persisting nephrotic syndrome and massive proteinuria.

For children who had convulsions and receive phenobarbital or hydantoins, it is recommended to try and switch to other anticonvulsivant drugs such as valproic acid or clonazepam which do not induce hepatic microsomial catabolism of corticosteroid and cyclosporine.

Perioperative management

At the time of transplantation, with a cadaver transplant, the best HLA matching is sought since the best results continue to be observed in well matched grafts, even in patients receiving cyclosporine (106).

An adult kidney can be grafted in a young patient, as was shown in several series (107), but below 10 to 12 kg it would be better to use a paediatric cadaver kidney. In this case the prevalence of renal artery thrombosis raises to be the second cause of graft loss (108). This may be at least in part prevented by using low molecular weight heparin in the first three weeks after transplantation (109). According to some authors one-year first cadaveric graft survival is predicted to be 53% for a 2-year-old-patient, 72% for a 10-year-old-patient and 78% for an 18-year-old-patient (110). It has been demonstrated that youngest recipients experienced better survival when they matched with adult donors (110).

Operative and post-operative management have to be very careful in children. Haemodynamic stability must be maintained at the time of declamping the graft renal artery. The best way for succeeding on this point is to check continuously pulmonary artery pressure by means of a Swan Ganz catheter and maintain pressure between 20 and 25 mm Hg. Vital parameters and difference between peripheral and central temperature are also used postoperatively as basic guides for the management (107, 111).

Medical treatment and follow up

The immunosuppressive regimen after grafting is similar in children and in adult patients, except for adapted doses of drugs according to body size. But the incrimination of corticosteroids in growth retardation mandates selection of immunosuppressive protocols for children using the lowest corticosteroid dosage as possible.

Immunosuppressive treatment has to be continued indefinitely and part of the follow up is to monitor and encourage compliance to the medical prescription, since noncompliance is a major cause of graft failure in adolescents (112, 113). The conventional treatment consists of azathioprine and prednisone. The dose of azathioprine is usually adjusted to body weight (2 to 3 mg/kg). This is decreased with renal insufficiency down to 1 to 2 mg/kg. Azathioprine is stopped at least briefly in case of viral infection. Some patients develop a cholestatic hepatotoxicity with this drug leading to its termination. Prednisone is progressively tapered down to a daily dose defined by the transplant unit between 5 and 10 mg/m^2. Many paediatric patients are switched to alternate day therapy receiving twice this every other day.

CsA is now the basis of most of the immunosuppressive protocols in children. Patients receiving cyclosporine have a dose generally adjusted at the start according to the blood or plasma through level; the aim is currently to maintain a blood level between 150 and 400 ng/ml or a plasma level between 50 and 150 ng/ml. This is obtained usually with a dose of 4 to 10 mg/kg. Some authors have recommended administering cyclosporine on the basis of body surface area giving a initial dose of 500 mg/m^2 (114).

A new formulation of CsA is becoming now available. It shows a greater bioavailability and has a significantly improved correlation between AUC and both through level and dose. Furthermore, it exhibits a reduced variability regarding AUC, Coin, Cmax and Tmax, thus leading to an improved predictability of systemic drug exposure. Studies on clinical safety and on immunosuppressive effects are on going (115).

Among the other immunosuppressive molecules presently on study, the most promising is FK506 (104).

There are many different protocols using cyclosporine, with and without corticosteroids, associated with low dose azathioprine (triple therapy) or not, prescribed from the day of grafting or after 1 to 6 weeks, prescribed indefinitely to conventional treatment. None of these protocols has definitely proved its superiority; all need a careful follow up of the patient looking for the side effects of cyclosporine, mainly nephrotoxicity suspected by an increase of plasma creatinine but sometimes only discovered on systemic transplant biopsy (110).

Recently, some authors have proposed that maintaining high doses of CsA may reduce the incidence of chronic rejection (116).

Other prescriptions in transplanted children include antihypertensive agents or anticonvulsivants (preferably valproic acid or clonazepam). Prevention of corticosteroid effects on bone is attempted by calcium or vitamin D supplements with a careful follow up of calciuria and calcaemia.

Diagnosis of rejection. The main complication of transplantation remains rejection, consequently the main objective of the follow up is to detect rejection as early as possible. The classical acute rejection crisis includes symptoms as fever, graft tenderness, oliguria and decrease of GRF. In fact after the first month such symptoms are rather rare and rejection is only marked by biochemical symptoms such as a slight increase in plasma creatinine,

slight proteinuria (of glomerular and tubular origin), acidosis and lower haemoglobin. Echography of the graft may detect obvious findings such as increase in the size of the graft, decreased echogenicity of the renal pyramids, thickening of the renal cortex and nonhomogenous regional loss of cortical echogenicity with overall increase or decrease in cortical thickness. Doppler ultrasound has been proposed as a more reliable tool for an early detection of rejection (117). Its use is however still debated (118). Transplant biopsy is often needed to ascertain the diagnosis and direct treatment. This treatment consists usually in IV high dose methylprednisolone (1 g/1.73 m^2) followed or not by a temporary increase of daily prednisone. Rejection crisis may also be treated with success by antilymphocyte or antithymocyte globulins.

Other causes of impairment of GRF and increase of plasma creatinine are also sometimes detected. These include obstruction of the urinary tract by lithiasis or secondary stenosis usually shown by graft echography, stenosis of the renal artery of the graft always associated with severe hypertension and nephrotoxicity of cyclosporine which is the main problem in patients receiving this drug. Nephrotoxicity may be proved by immediate improvement of renal function after stopping cyclosporine for 1 or 2 days; in dubious cases a renal biopsy may be useful.

The follow up of a child with a functioning graft has to cope with two difficulties. On one hand follow up should not interfere too much with the day to day life and especially the school attendance and the planned vacations and on the other hand it is important not to miss any problem at its beginning especially rejection. This follow up is mainly the responsibility of the transplant unit where the graft was performed, but individual solutions may be found involving a local physician or laboratory or both, previously informed to react to any 10 to 20% increase in plasma creatinine concentration and to slight proteinuria. The frequency of biological checkings, at first weekly, can be spaced to every 3 weeks or month after 1 year, and to every 2 months after 3 or 5 years. Any change in the immunosuppressive protocol indicates more frequent monitoring. Regular outpatient consultations are mandatory to check all biological data, to detect any complications related or not to the treatment, to note growth velocity and last but not least to check the drug compliance.

Results and causes of failure

The general results of transplantation in children improved clearly in recent years, probably due to the new immunosuppressive agents. Actuarial first cadaver graft survival in patients transplanted under 15 years of age in the EDTA registry in the years 1981 to 1985 was 75% at 6 months, 68% at 1 year and 60% at 2 years. Children transplanted in 1983 to 1985 receiving cyclosporine (*n* at start = 274) had a better graft survival: 80% at 6 months and 75% at 1 year versus respectively 74% and 68% in others (n at start = 350). Monocentric studies reported higher survival rates, for example 80% at 1 year and 69% at 3 years under conventional treatment (112) while with cyclosporine graft survival was reported high as 93% at 1 year and 78% at 3 years (114).

Long term results are only known for patients having received conventional immunosuppression; graft survival was 40% at 10 years in a monocentric report (112).

Live related donor (LRD) transplantation leads to better results. In the EDTA registry of the 267 LRD grafts performed in 1981 to 1985 actuarial graft survival was 87% at 6 months, 82% at 1 year and 79% at 2 years. Here again data from monocentric studies are even better.

The major cause of graft failure remains rejection accounting for two thirds of failures in the paediatric EDTA registry, but other causes in children include postoperative vascular thrombosis and also recurrence of primary renal diseases such as nephrotic syndrome with focal sclerosis and oxalosis.

Growth after transplantation

Growth is very variable after a kidney graft; a catch up curve is reported in only 20 to 50% of the cases while one third of patients continue to be stunted (119–121) even in the presence of a good glomerular filtration rate.

A number of factors may interfere with growth after transplantation. The most important are renal function of the graft and corticosteroid therapy: Renal function has to be normal or almost normal for catch up growth which was rarely observed in patients with a plasma creatinine above 120 μmol/l, in contrast to observations in patients with chronic renal failure under conservative treatment. Corticosteroids are known to limit growth velocity at doses above 5 or 6 mg/m^2/day, and this is the case of most children under conventional treatment. Giving corticosteroids every other day may improve growth velocity and is recommended in children whenever possible especially at puberty (119). New immunosuppressive regimens using cyclosporine are generally associated with less corticosteroids and reportedly allow a better growth rate (122). Children under 7 years were reported to grow better, but a catch up curve may also be observed in older patients. There is an inverse relationship between growth velocity after transplantation and statural stunting at the start; the smaller for age the child is, the better the standard deviation score after grafting (119). Bone maturation is also important to follow since a pubertal growth spurt, observed in 1/3 of patients, was reported for a bone age of 11 in girls and of 13 in boys, earlier than in normal subjects, but occurring with a delay of 1 to 5 years considering chronological age (119). Adult height was analysed in 185 females and 191 males recorded in the EDTA registry as having started RRT under age 15. It was 154.3 cm in females and 161.3 in males ranging from 135 to 180 cm in both sexes. Patients grafted under the age of 15 did not

have a higher ultimate height, but those who were never grafted were shorter than other patients.

Recently recombinant human growth hormone (rhGH) has became a new treatment for short children with preterminal chronic renal failure, dialysis and after renal transplant. During first-year of treatment prepubertal children nearly double their height velocity (123–125) while in pubertal children the result of treatment is not similarly good. A decline in renal function is described by some authors during rhGH treatment in renal transplant patients. The deterioration of renal function could be the result of a progressive glomerulosclerosis and tubulointerstitial scarring (124). Finally, some authors suggested that immunologic mechanisms may have some role in the progressive decline of renal graft function in patients who have chronic rejection (126–128).

Complications after transplantation

A number of complications may occur after kidney transplantation. In the postoperative period acute tubular necrosis is frequently observed and when severe may lead to a permanent reduction in nephron mass. Thrombosis of the transplant renal artery or vein is a cause of primary anuria, more frequent in young children than in adults, leading to the loss of the graft (129). Surgical complications such as urinary leak also can occur.

Acute rejection crisis, as already mentioned, is the main complication; it is sometimes irreversible, especially in the first weeks after transplantation, but is usually controlled by adequate treatment. Chronic rejection is most often the sequela of an acute crisis, but may also develop insidiously. Transplant biopsy is useful for the precise diagnosis of the lesions.

Recurrence of primary diseases accounts for 5–15% of graft losses in paediatric series. Most of the recurrences are due to steroid resistant nephrotic syndrome with focal sclerosis. Less frequently, membranoproliferative glomerulopathy, IgA nephropathy and haemolytic-uraemic syndrome may also relapse leading to graft loss (129). Hypertension is also a major cause of concern in transplanted children with a high risk of encephalopathy and neurological sequelae (130, 131). Blood pressure has to be checked frequently and hypotensive drugs have to be administrated and adjusted as necessary. Transplant angiography must be performed if there is any doubt about a renal artery stenosis.

In case of stenosis, this may be successfully treated in nearly half of the patients with angioplasty; surgical repair should therefore be used only if this method revealed to be inadequate (132).

Infections are also a permanent risk in children under immunosuppression. In the early postoperative period they are especially vulnerable to septicaemia and cytomegalovirus infection. The prognosis of infectious complications depends on early diagnosis and specific treatment.

Complications related to steroids are also possible; gastroduodenal haemorrhage, psychiatric disturbances and diabetes mellitus are quite rare and only observed in the first few weeks post grafting. Aseptic bone necrosis was a major complication of high dose steroid protocol, but its prevalence has dramatically decreased in the recent years (112). Osteoporosis may also develop in the long term.

Late surgical complications as urinary lithiasis, secondary stenosis of urinary tract anastomosis or lymphocoele are quite rare and usually do not affect graft survival.

SURVIVAL AND CAUSES OF DEATH

Survival of patients on renal replacement therapy (RRT) has been studied widely, especially based on the experience of individual centres. For this reason the results reported by different authors vary widely, depending not only on the quality of care but also on the selection criteria and, therefore, on the characteristics of children accepted for RRT. Data obtained from the EDTA registry provide the average survival for children treated in many centres in all European countries. The 3-year survival of children after first RRT increased from 80% in those who started RRT in 1976 to 1978 to 86% in those who reached ESRD in 1982 to 1984 (23). This improvement with time in the 3-year survival rate is also apparent for each of the age groups 0 to 4, 5 to 9 and 10 to 14. It is noteworthy that younger children (0 to 4 years old) have a worse 3-year survival (73%) than those aged 5 to 9 (83%) and 10 to 14 (84%) respectively (23).

The comparison of patient survival on different modes of RRT has to be made with caution, because the populations are not necessarily comparable, but can be selected according to different criteria. Furthermore the patients are assigned to a given group only depending on their last mode of renal replacement therapy. With these limitations, home haemodialysis provides a 5-year survival of 85% compared to 74% for hospital haemodialysis (133).

It is well known that cardiovascular abnormalities are the main causes of death in children on chronic dialysis treatment. A recent survey by the Paediatric Registry of the EDTA on all causes of death occurring from 1981 to 1985 showed that hyperkalaemia accounted for 7.2% of all deaths, hypertensive cardiac failure for 6.0%, fluid overload for 9.7% and cerebrovascular accident for 6.9%. Excess weight gain, defined as a gain exceeding 8% of body weight at least once a week between two haemodialysis sessions, appeared to be a problem in children aged 5 to 10 (76). From that study it appeared very clearly that mortality during 1983 was higher among children with excess weight gain (7.5%) than in those without it (2.5%).

The second most frequent group of causes are infections (approximately 17% of all deaths) (134). Finally 4% of the deaths were due to malignant disease. Causes of death on chronic dialysis do not differ substantially in children and in patients over 15, except for myocardial ischemia and infarction which are much more frequent in adults.

PSYCHOSOCIAL PROBLEMS

Optimal functioning of a dialysis programme for children not only requires appropriate medical and technical knowledge but simultaneous attention must also be paid to the emotional and social impact of the treatment on the juvenile patients and their families (135). A team including physicians, nurses, social workers, teachers and a psychologist should be available to cope with the problems relating to the child and his disease as discussed in the section on organization of services and facilities for treatment of children.

The child and his disease

Even before beginning regular dialysis treatment the behaviour of young patients is influenced by their long-standing disease. At this stage the children are invariably depressed. Mutilation in conception and representation of their body image frequently prevail. The children are preoccupied with their illness and show evidence of a clear consciousness of death. They resent having their lives full of unpleasant restrictions. The relationships of these children are characterised by withdrawal from social contacts and increasing dependence on their parents. Dialysis adds another important stress to the patient and adaptation at the beginning of treatment is often difficult. Anxiety, that may be either obvious or repressed will influence adaptation to the treatment. When the child's health improves, drastic changes in attitudes and behaviour are frequently seen. The child becomes more active and less frightened. However, during the following months frequently recurring patterns of maladjustment emerge characterised by passivity, refuge in sleep, inaccessibility to others, anorexia and vomiting. Some children react with excessive dependence, other become overdemanding or react with aggressive behaviour. Complications and necessary surgical procedures will influence the incidence of these setbacks.

The families

The parents, depressed by the problems of a child with chronic life threatening disease, often put too high expectations on the effect of dialysis. Therefore, if problems increase or even persist important reactions may occur such as aggressive behaviour to the staff, lack of cooperation and unreasonable demands on the medical team. Faced with the problems of repetitive dialysis, the entire family is confronted with a series of stresses and demands that influence the relationships both within and beyond

the family. Daily life is disturbed by the demanding programme: dialysis, diet, medication, restrictions of activity
and hospitalizations of the child. The stresses and burdens that this situation places upon the family accentuate
personal problems of members of the family such as psychosomatic diseases, danger of family breakdown and
relational problems of the parents at their work. The other
children in the family may experience various degrees of
emotional deprivation.

The dialysis team

The dialysis team participates with parents and children in
all emotional problems generated during treatment. The
demands of meeting the emotional needs of the patients
and their families, however, often extend beyond the
capacity of the team members. This sometimes leads to
reactions of withdrawal into regressive patterns in members of the team and disruption of communications within
the group. Assistance by a paediatric psychiatrist will be
necessary in crisis situations. Team discussions may be
helpful to place problems in perspective and allow team
members to support each other at times of stress.

REHABILITATION

The aim of regular dialysis treatment of paediatric patients
is not only to prolong life but also to provide a basis
for normal, physical, social and intellectual development.
Rehabilitation should already be initiated during conservative treatment of the youthful chronic renal failure
patient. Successful rehabilitation during dialysis largely
depends on the previous support, and can only be obtained
by a harmonious team as in a specialised paediatric unit.
Proper school facilities and arrangements for leisure times
and holidays should be provided. A normal school programme should be attained whenever possible. However,
the time lost on recurrent dialysis may be a hindrance. In
this respect home or peritoneal dialysis should be encouraged.

Physical activities need not be restricted during leisure
time. Normal leisure times should be encouraged within
the child's own possibilities to overcome the natural resistance of overprotective relatives. School attendance has to
be assessed regularly.

According to EDTA data, 20–50% of the children have
school problems. The proportion of children under 10
years of age who achieve full time schooling is slightly
lower than in older children. Schooling in children on
dialysis is worse than in transplant children (full time
schooling in 52% versus 86%). Full time schooling is
better in patients treated with CAPD than in those on
hospital haemodialysis.

The reported long term rehabilitation has been excellent in young adults who started renal replacement therapy as children and who have been successfully graft-

Table 13. Recommended daily allowances for children

Age	Height	Energy (kcal/day)		Minimum protein (g/day)		Calcium
(yr)	(cm)	A	B	A	B	(g)
0.5–1	72	100/kg	100/kg	1.8/kg	1.8/kg	0.6
1–2	81	1100	1170	18/day	21	0.7
2–4	96	1300	1330	22	25	0.8
4–6	110	1600	1800	29	30.5	0.9
6–8	121	2000	2100	29	33	0.9
8–10	131	2200	2460	31	35	1.0
10–12	141	2450	2600	36	41.5	1.2
12–14 (M)	151	2700	2720	40	45	1.4
12–14 (F)	154	2300	2190	34	46	1.3

ed (137). Social failures were especially related to poor
school attendance in the primary school period (138),
which emphasizes that adequate attention to teaching and
education should have high priority and should be undertaken at an early stage.

DIETARY PRESCRIPTION

The high energy requirements relative to body weight in
children have been discussed and the impact of uraemia
on the nutritional status of a child is more drastic because
the energy deficit caused by the anorexia of renal failure is
greater. It is important to ensure an adequate food intake
for children on dialysis. It has been shown the difference in
growth between prepubertal children on dialysis in whom
weight was normal for height compared with children who
were undernourished.

Energy intake should at least satisfy the recommended daily allowances for children as set out in Table 13.
Energy supplements taken with meals consisting of fat
(double cream, polyunsaturated oil emulsions) and carbohydrate (glucose polymer) flavoured to taste are useful
to increase total energy intake. This also serves to reduce
the intake of other foods containing nutrients, such as
protein and electrolytes, normally consumed in excess of
need. If anorexia is severe, particularly when associated with catabolic stress from intercurrent infection, then
nasoenteric feeding through indwelling soft cannulae can
be useful in breaking the vicious circle of anorexia and
malnutrition.

Protein intake should be controlled so that the pre-
dialysis blood urea concentration does not exceed 25 to
35 mmol/l. Minimum protein requirements should, however, be satisfied (Table 13). If high quality protein is
given, the intake can probably be reduced as necessary
so that protein supplies not more than 4 to 6% of total
calories in the diet. By comparison human milk or human
milk substitutes provide about 8% of total calories from

protein whereas the normal intake can exceed 12%. Very low protein diets can be supplemented by feeding essential amino or keto acids but this is expensive and rarely required (139–141). Too severe a restriction of protein intake can lead to protein malnutrition and plasma albumin or transferrin levels should be monitored to detect this.

Phosphate intake should be reduced by limiting or removing dairy products in the diet as discussed above. Calcium intake should be maintained, if necessary by feeding calcium supplements, and in this respect calcium from calcium carbonate, given as a phosphate binder, is absorbed. Sodium supplements are rarely required in children on dialysis though they may be necessary in some children with residual renal function, especially in case of nephronophthisis. Similarly, bicarbonate supplements are rarely required in children on dialysis to prevent metabolic acidosis. An adequate intake of all vitamins should be given because of losses in the dialysate and the restricted nutritional intake. Pyridoxine deficiency occurs in chronic renal failure and supplements of pyridoxine hydrochloride (10 mg daily) should be provided (142–143). Folate deficiency can occur even in the presence of normal serum folate acid concentrations owing to alterations in folate metabolism (143), but excessive accumulation of folic acid has been also reported in patients on dialysis (144).

Iron, zinc, copper, manganese, chromium, cobalt, selenium, iodine and fluoride are essential or beneficial to man. The accumulation of aluminium and iron has already been mentioned, but copper toxicity can also occur and may be associated with anaemia. Tissue zinc levels are usually increased but low levels of plasma zinc have been observed. A number of abnormalities in patients with renal failure such as anorexia impaired taste acuity and poor growth have been attributed to zinc deficiency.

Children do not respond well to special diets and it is usually better to influence their consumption of normal foods rather than to prescribe special foods; nevertheless, low protein noodles or bread may be useful. Above all tension over eating must be avoided otherwise a refusal to eat may develop. An experienced dietician working with the child and family can do much to encourage a good diet in accordance with the child's own preferences.

Food intake should be monitored regularly by the dietician and evaluated in relation to the nutritional status of the child. As well as the usual and regular biochemical determinations plasma lipids should be monitored. A raised plasma cholesterol is an indication to reduce the content of cholesterol and saturated fat in the diet whilst raised plasma triglyceride levels can be treated by reducing the carbohydrate, especially the sucrose content, and increasing the polyunsaturated fat content of the diet. Fluid intake is usually limited to the level of insensible loss plus urinary volume but excessive weight gain between dialysis is often due to excessive sodium intake rather than primarily due to drinking too much water though this

can occur. This excess of weight gain was found to be associated with an excess of mortality rate in children on dialysis.

REFERENCES

1. Arant BS: Postnatal development of renal function during the first year of life. *Pediatr Nephrol* 1: 308, 1987
2. Thurau K, Boylan JW: Acute renal success: the unexpected logic of oliguria in acute renal failure. *Am J Med* 61: 308, 1976
3. Al-Dahhan JA, Haycock GB, Chantler C, Stimmler L: Sodium homeostasis in mature and immature neonates I. Renal aspects. *Arch Dis Child* 58: 335, 1983
4. Holliday MA: Body composition, metabolism and growth. in *Pediatric Nephrology*, edited by Holliday MA, Barratt TM, Vernier R, Baltimore, Williams & Wilkins, 1987, p 3
5. Recommendations of the task force on blood pressure control in children. *Pediatrics* 59: 797, 1977
6. Rigden SPA, Barratt TM, Dillon MG, De Leval M, Stark J: Acute renal failure complicating cardiopulmonary bypass surgery. *Arch Dis Child* 57: 425, 1982
7. Arneil GL, MacDonald AM, Murphy AV, Sweet RM: Renal venous thrombosis. *Clin Nephrol* 1: 119, 1973
8. Clark AGB, Saunders A, Bewick M, Haycock GB, Chantler C: Neonatal inferior vena cava and renal venous thrombosis treated by thrombectomy and nephrectomy. *Arch Dis Child* 60: 1076, 1985
9. Myers BD, Moran SM: Hemodynamically mediated acute renal failure. *N Eng J Med* 314: 97, 1986
10. Judd BA, Haycock GB, Dalton N, Chantler C: Hyponatraemia in premature babies and following surgery in older children. *Acta Paediatr Scand* 76: 385, 1987
11. Bird JE, Blantz RC: Acute renal failure: the glomerular and tubular connection. *Pediatr Nephrol* 1: 348, 1987
12. Elseed AM, Shinebourne EA, Joseph MC: Assessment of techniques for measurement of blood pressure in infants and children. *Arch Dis Child* 48: 932, 1973
13. Matthew OP, Jones AS, James E, Bland H, Groshong T: Neonatal renal failure; usefulness of diagnostic indices. *Pediatrics* 65: 57, 1980
14. Murdoch IA, Dos Anjos R, Haycock GB: Treatment of hyperkalaemia with intravenous salbutamol. *Arch Dis Child* 66: 527, 1991
15. Gordon I, Barratt TM: Imaging the kidneys and urinary tract in the neonate with acute renal failure. *Pediatr Nephrol* 1: 321, 1987
16. Barratt TM, Dillon MJ, Gordon I, Ransley PG: Clinical Quiz, *Pediatr Nephrol* 1: 379, 1987
17. Lewis MA, Nycyk JA: Practical peritoneal dialysis – the Tenckhoff catheter in acute renal failure. *Pediatr Nephrol* 6: 470, 1992
18. Bunchman TE, Donckerwolcke RA: Continuous arterialvenous diahemofiltration and continuous venovenous diahemofiltration in infants and children. *Pediatr Nephrol* 8: 96, 1994
19. Ronco C: Continuous arteriovenous hemofiltration in infants. in *Acute Continuous Renal Replacement Therapy*, edited by Paganini EP, Den Haag, Martinus Nijhoff, 1986, p 201

20. Lieberman KV: Continuous arteriovenous hemofiltration in children. *Pediatr Nephrol* 1: 330, 1987
21. Loirat C, Ehrich JHH, Geerlings W, Jones EHP, Landais P, Mallick NP, Margreiter R, Raine AEG, Salmela K, Selwood NH, Tufveson G, Valderrabano F: Report on management of renal failure in children in Europe, XXII, 1992. *Nephrol Dial Transplant* (Suppl 1): 26, 1994
22. Arbus GS: 1985 report on pediatric patients. in *Canadian Renal Failure Register*, Kidney foundation of Canada 1986
23. Rizzoni G, Broyer M, Brunner FP, Brynger H, Challah S, Fassbinder W, Guillou PJ, Oules R, Selwood NH, Wing AJ: Combined report on regular dialysis and transplantation of children in Europe, XVI, 1985. (Personal communication)
24. Broyer M, Chantler C, Donckerwolcke R, Ehrich JHH, Rizzoni G, Schärer K: The paediatric registry of the European Dialysis and Transplant Association: 20 years' experience. *Pediatr Nephrol* 7: 758, 1993
25. Rees L, Rigden SPA, Chantler C, Haycock GB: Growth and methods of improving growth in chronic renal failure managed conservatively. in *Karger Symposium on Endocrine Abnormalities in Chronic Renal Failure*, edited by Schärer K, 1987
26. Barratt TM, Broyer M, Chantler C, Gilli G, Guest G, Marti Henneburg C, Preece MA, Rigden SPA: Assessment of growth. *Am J Kidney Dis* 7: 340, 1986
27. Jones RWA, Rigden S, Barratt TM, Chantler C: The effects of chronic renal failure in infancy on growth nutritional status and body composition. *Pediatr Res* 16: 784, 1982
28. Tanner JM, Whitehouse RH, Marshall WA, Healy MJR, Goldstern H: *Assessment of Skeletal Maturity and Prediction of Adult Height TW2 Method*, London, Academic Press, 1975
29. Broyer M, Kleinknecht C, Loirat C, Marti-Henneberg C, Roy MP: Maturation osseuse et développement pubertaire chez l'enfant et l'adolescent en dialyse chronique. (Osseous maturation and pubertal development in infants and children on chronic dialysis.) *Proc Eur Dial Transplant Assoc* 9: 181, 1972
30. Chantler C, Holliday MA: Chronic renal insufficiency. in *Pediatric Nephrology*, edited by Holliday MA, Barratt TM, Vernier R, Baltimore, Williams & Wilkins, 1987
31. Mak RHK, Turner C, Thompson T, Haycock GB, Chantler C: Glucose metabolism in children with uremia; effect of dietary phosphate and protein. *Kidney Int* 32 (Suppl 22): 206, 1987
32. Mak RHK, Haycock GB, Thompson T, Turner C, Chantler C: The role of secondary hyperparathyroidism in the glucose intolerance of chronic renal failure. *J Clin Endocrinol Metab* 60: 229, 1985
33. Delaporte C, Gros F, Anagnostopoulos T: Inhibitory effects of plasma dialysate on protein synthesis *in vitro*, influence of dialysis and transplantation. *Am J Clin Nutr* 33: 1407, 1980
34. Mak RHK, Turner C, Thompson T, Haycock GB, Chantler C: The effects of a low protein diet with amino/keto acid supplements on glucose metabolism in children with uraemia. *J Clin Endocrinology Metab* 63: 985, 1986
35. Rodriguez-Soriano J, Arant BS, Brodehl J, Norman ME: Fluid and electrolyte imbalances in children with chronic renal failure. *Am J Kidney Dis* 7: 268, 1968
36. Mehls O: Growth hormone and IGF-1 in chronic renal failure: pathophysiology and rationale for growth hormone treatment. *Acta Paediatr Scand* 370 (Suppl 28), 1990
37. Hokken-Koelega ACS, Hackeng WHL, Stijnen T, Wit JM, de Muinck Keizer-Schrama SMPF, Drop SLS: 24 hours plasma GH profiles, urinary GH excretion and plasma IGF-I and II levels in prepubertal children with chronic renal insufficiency and severe growth retardation. *J Clin Endocrinol Metab* 71: 688, 1990
38. Schaefer F, Hammill G, Stanhope R, Preece MA, Schärer K: Pulsatile growth hormone secretion in peripubertal patients with chronic renal failure. *J Pediatr* 119: 568, 1991
39. Hokken-Koelega ACS, Stijnen T, de Muinck Keizer-Schrama SMPF, Wit JM, Wolff ED, de Jong MCJW, Donckerwolcke RA, Abbad NCB, Bot A, Blum WF, Drop SLS: Placebo controlled double blind cross over trial of growth hormone treatment in prepubertal children with chronic renal failure. *Lancet* 338: 585, 1991
40. Burke J, El-Bishti M, Maisy MN, Chantler C: Hypothyroidism in children with cystinosis. *Arch Dis Child* 53: 947, 1978
41. Mehls O, Salusky IB: Recent advances and controversies in childhood renal osteodystrophy. *Pediatr Nephrol* 1: 212, 1987
42. Broyer M: Chronic renal failure. in *Paediatric Nephrology*, edited by Royer P, Habib R, Mathieu H, Broyer M, Philadelphia, WB Saunders Co, 1974, p 358
43. Norman ME, Mazin AT, Borden S, Gruskin A, Anast C, Baren R, Rasmussen H: Early diagnosis of renal osteodystrophy. *J Pediatr* 97: 226, 1980
44. Mehls O, Ritz E, Krempien B, Gilli G, Lush K, Wulich E, Schärer K: Slipped epiphyses in renal osteodystrophy. *Arch Dis Child* 50: 545, 1975
45. Salusky IB, Goodman WG: Renal bone disease in pediatric patients receiving treatment with maintenance peritoneal dialysis. *Child Nephrol Urol* 11: 165, 1991
46. Milliner DS, Ottsin Nebeker HG, Andress DL, Sherrard DJ, Alfrey AC, Slatopolsky E, Coburn JW: Deferoxamine infusion test for the diagnosis of aluminium related osteodystrophy. *Ann Intern Med* 101: 775, 1984
47. Coburn JW: Mineral metabolism and renal bone disease: effects of CAPD versus hemodialysis. *Kidney Int Suppl* 40: S 92, 1993
48. Muller-Wiefel D, Sinn H, Gilli G, Schärer K: Hemodialysis and blood loss in children with chronic renal failure. *Clin Nephrol* 8: 481, 1977
49. Schärer K, Muller-Wiefel D: Complications of renal failure: haematological complications. in *Pediatric Nephrology*, edited by Holliday MA, Barratt TM, Vernier R, Baltimore, Williams & Wilkins, 1987, p 880
50. Scigalla P, Bonzel KE, Bulla M, Geisert J, Leumann E, van Lilien T, Muller-Wiefel DE, Offner G, Piston K, Zoellner K: Therapy of renal anemia with recombinant human erythropoietin in children with end stage renal disease. *Contrib Nephrol* 76: 227, 1989
51. Reddingius RE, Schröder CH, Monnens LAH: Intraperitoneal administration of erythropoietin once per week

instead of three times per week. *Nephrol Dial Transplant* 8: 280, 1993

52. Navarro M, Alonso A, Avilla JM, Espinosa L: Anemia of chronic renal failure: treatment with erythropoietin. *Child Nephrol Urol* 11: 146, 1991

53. Morris KP, Watson S, Reid MM, Hamilton PJ, Coulthard MG: Assessing iron status in children with chronic renal failure: which measurements should we use? *Pediatr Nephrol* 8: 51, 1994

54. Franken LAM, van Lier HJ, Gerlag PGG, den Hartog M, Koene RAP: Assessment of pain after subcutaneous injection of erythropoietin in patients receiving haemodialysis. *BMJ* 303: 288, 1991

55. Ullmer HE, Greiner H, Schuler HW, Schrer K: Cardiovascular impairment and physical working capacity in children with chronic renal failure. *Acta Paediatr Scand* 67: 43, 1978

56. Polinsky MS, Kaiser RA, Stover JB, Frankenfield M, Baluarte HJ: Neurologic development of children with severe chronic renal failure from infancy. *Pediatr Nephrol*: 157, 1987

57. Nevins TE: Transplantation in infants less than 1 year of age. *Pediatr Nephrol* 1: 154, 1987

58. Mahan ID, Mauer SM, Nevins T: The Hickman catheter: a new hemodialysis device for infants and small children. *Kidney Int* 24: 694, 1983

59. Weiss M, Sutherland DE: Percutaneous subclavian catherization for hemodialysis in small children. *Surgery* 95: 353, 1984

60. Bourquelot P, Wolfeler L, Lamy L: Microsurgery for hemodialysis distal arteriovenous fistulae in children weighing less than 10 kg. *Int J Microsurg* 3: 187, 1981

61. Gagnadoux MF, Pascal B, Bronstein M, Bourquelot P, Broyer M: Arteriovenous fistulae in small children. *Dial Transplant* 9: 318, 1980

62. Blumenthal SS, Ortiz MA, Kleinman JC, Piering WF: Inflow time and recirculation in single needle hemodialysis. *Am J Kidney Dis* 8: 202, 1986

63. D'Apuzzo VC, Gruskin CM, Brennan CP, Stiles GR, Fine RN: Saphenous vein autograft arteriovenous fistula for extended hemodialysis in children. *Acta Paediatr Scand* 62: 28, 1973

64. Applebaum K, Shaskikumar VL, Somers LA, Baluarte HJ, Gruskin AB, Grossman M, McGarvey MJ, Weintraub WK: Improved hemodialysis access in children. *J Pediatr Surg* 15: 764, 1980

65. Donckerwolcke RA, Bunchman TE: Hemodialysis in infants and small children. *Pediatr Nephrol* 8: 103, 1994

66. Ford DM, Portman RJ, Hurst DL, Lum GM: Unsuspected seizures during hemodialysis = effect of dialysate prescription. *Pediatr Nephrol* 1, 1987

67. Ing IS, Vilbar RM, Skin RD: Predialytic isolated ultrafiltration. *Dial Transplant* 7: 557, 1978

68. Swamy AP, Cestero RVM: Mannitol and maintenance hemodialysis. *Artif Organs* 3: 116, 1979

69. Chantler C, Trompeter R, Rigden S, Dalton N, Haycock G: Vascular stability during haemodialysis. in *Pediatric Nephrology*, edited by Brodehl J. Ehrich JHH, Berlin, Springer Verlag, 1984, p 96

70. Broyer M, Antignac C: Advances in dialysis treatment in children – an overview. in *Recent Advances in Pediatric Nephrology*, edited by Murakami K, Kitagawa T, Yabuta K, Sakai T, Amsterdam, Elsevier, 1987, p 175

71. Panzetta G, Tissitore N, Valvo E, Lupo A, Loschiavo G, Fabris A, Oldrizzi L, Gammaro L, Rugin C, Bellotti Z, Maschio G: Biofiltration in the treatment of patients with acetate intolerance. *Clin Nephrol* 26: 33, 1986

72. Nevins TE, Kjellstrand CM: Hemodialysis for children: a review. *Int J Pediatr Nephrol* 4: 155, 1983

73. Martin Malo A, Perez R, Gomez J, Burdiel LG, Andres E, Castillo D, Morena E, Aljano P: Sequential hypertonic dialysis. *Nephron* 40: 458, 1985

74. Leroy M, Dechaux M, Guest G: Extracellular volume and blood pressure in 82 hemodialysed children. *Proc Eur Dial Transplant Assoc – Eur Ren Assoc* 22: 847, 1985

75. Broyer M, Gagnadoux MF, Bacri JL, Laborde K: Problems of long term dialysis in children. in *Pediatric Nephrology*, edited by Gruskin AB, Norman ME, The Hague, Martinus Nijhoff, 1981, p 185

76. Rizzoni G. Broyer M, Brunner FP, Brynger H, Challah S. Kramer P, Oules RE, Selwood NH, Wing AJ, Balas EA: Combined report on regular dialysis and transplantation of children in Europe, XIV, 1983. *Proc Eur Dial Transplant Assoc – Eur Ren Assoc* 21: 69, 1984

77. Villaroel F: Incidence of hypersensitivity in hemodialysis. *Artif Organs* 8: 278, 1984

78. Harmon WE, Spinozzi N, Meyer A, Grupe WE: The use of protein catabolic rate to monitor pediatric hemodialysis. *Dial Transplant* 10: 324, 1981

79. Henrich WL: Hemodynamic instability during hemodialysis. *Kidney Int* 30: 605, 1985

80. Evans JHC, Smye SW, Brocklebank JT: Mathematical modelling of haemodialysis in children. *Pediatr Nephrol* 6: 349, 1992

81. Alexander SR, Tank ES, Corneil AT: Five year's experience with CAPD/CCPD catheters in infants and children. in *CAPD in Children*, edited by Fine RN, Schärer K, Mehls O, Berlin, Springer Verlag, 1985, p 174

82. Balfe JW, Stefanidis CJ, Steele BI, Hewitt IK: Continuous ambulatory peritoneal dialysis: clinical aspects. in *End Stage Renal Disease in Children*, edited by Fine RN, Gruskin AB, Philadelphia, WB Saunders Co, 1984, p 135

83. Warady BA, Bohl V, Alon U, Hellerstern S: Symptomatic peritoneal calcification in a child: treatment with tidal peritoneal dialysis. *Perit Dial Int* 14: 26, 1994

84. Nolph KD: Update on peritoneal dialysis worldwide. *Perit Dial Int* 13 (Suppl 2): 15, 1993

85. Mendley SR, Umans JG, Majkowski NL: Measurement of peritoneal dialysis delivery in children. *Pediatr Nephrol* 7: 284, 1993

86. Morgenstern BZ: Equilibration testing: close but not quite right. *Pediatr Nephrol* 7: 290, 1993

87. Henna JD, Foreman JW, Gehr TWB, Chan JCM, Wolfrum J, Ruddley J: The peritoneal equilibration test in children. *Pediatr Nephrol* 7: 731, 1993

88. Gruskin AB: The peritoneal dialysis prescription in children. *Persp Peritoneal Dial* 3: 42, 1985

89. Reddingius RE, Schröder CH, Willems HL, van den Brandt FCA, Koomen GCM, Krediet RT, Monnens LAH: Measurement of peritoneal fluid handling in children on continuous ambulatory peritoneal dialysis using autologous hemoglobin. *Perit Dial Int* 14: 42, 1994

90. Salusky IB, Fine RN: Nutritional recommendations for children undergoing continuous peritoneal dialysis. *Persp Peritoneal Dial* 2: 18, 1984

91. Canepa A, Perfumo F, Carrea A, Giallongo F, Verina E, Cantaluppi A, Gusmano R: Longterm effect of aminoacid dialysis solution in children on continuous ambulatory peritoneal dialysis. *Pediatr Nephrol* 5: 215, 1991

92. Drachman R, Niaudet P, Dartois AM, Broyer M: Protein losses during peritoneal dialysis in children. in *CAPD in Children*, edited by Fine RN, Schärer K, Mehls O, Berlin, Springer Verlag, 1985, p 78

93. Salusky IB, Paunier L, Coburn JW, Kangarloo H, Slatopolsky E, Fine RN: Protein losses during peritoneal dialysis in children. in *CAPD in Children*, edited by Fine RN, Schärer K, Mehls O, Berlin, Springer Verlag, 1985, p 144

94. Verrina E and the Italian Registry of Paediatric Chronic Peritoneal Dialysis: Chronic peritoneal dialysis in paediatrics: experience of a national registry. *Pediatr Nephrol* 6: 78, 1992

95. Leichter HE, Salusky IB, Davidson M, Wilson M, Hall T, Fine RN: Peritonitis in children undergoing CAPD versus CCPD. in *CAPD in Children*, edited by Fine RN, Schärer K, Mehls O, Berlin, Springer Verlag, 1985 p 190

96. Lorentz WB: Acute hydrothorax during peritoneal dialysis. *J. Pediatr* 94: 417, 1979

97. Kohaut EC, Alexander SR, Mehls O: The management of the infant on CAPD. in *CAPD in Children*, edited by Fine RN, Schärer K, Mehls O, Berlin, Springer Verlag, 1985, p 97

98. Niaudet P, Drachman R, Gubler MC, Broyer M: Loss of ultrafiltration and peritoneal membrane alterations on CAPD. in *CAPD in Children*, edited by Fine RN, Schärer K, Mehls O, Berlin, Springer Verlag, 1985, p 158

99. Andreoli SP, Langefeld CD, Stadler S, Smith P, Sears A, West K: Risk of peritoneal membrane failure in children undergoing longterm peritoneal dialysis. *Pediatr Nephrol* 7: 543, 1993

100. Niaudet P, Berard E, Revillon Y, Lothon M, Broyer M: Sclerosing encapsulating peritonitis in children. *Contrib Nephrol* 57: 230, 1987

101. Conley SB, Brewer ED, Grady S: Normal growth in very small children on peritoneal dialysis. *Abstracts Natl Kidney Found* 12: 8A, 1982

102. Warady BA, Stall C, Paulsen J, Johnson CB, Sedman A, Lum GM: A unique approach to peritoneal dialysis in infants. *Am J Kidney Dis* 7: 235, 1985

103. Hall IL, Wilson M, Davidson D, Foley J: The importance of the CAPD nurse in dealing with patient/family burnout. in *CAPD in Children*, edited by Fine RN, Schärer K, Mehls O, Berlin, Springer Verlag, 1985, p 207

104. Ellis D, Shapiro R, Jordan ML, Scantlebury VP, Gilboa N. Hopp L, Wichler N, Tzakis AG, Simmons RL: Comparison of FK-506 and cyclosporine regimens in pediatric renal transplantation. *Pediatr Nephrol* 8: 193, 1994

105. Potter DE, Portale AA, Melzer JS, Feduska NJ, Garovoy MR, Husing RM, Salvatierra O: Are blood transfusions beneficial in the cyclosporine era? *Pediatr Nephrol* 5: 168, 1991

106. Opelz G.: Effect of HLA matching in 10,000 cyclosporine treated cadaver kidney transplantation. *Transplant Proc* 19: 641, 1987

107. Broyer M, Gagnadoux MF, Beurton D, Pascal B. Louville J: Transplantation in children: technical aspects drug therapy and problems related to primary renal disease. *Proc Eur Dial Transplant Assoc* 18: 313, 1981

108. Gagnadoux MF, Niaudet P, Broyer M: Non immunological risk factors in pediatric renal transplantation. *Pediatr Nephrol* 7: 89-95, 1993

109. Broyer M, Gagnadoux MF, Sierro A, Fischer AM, Revillon Y, Jan D, Beurton D, Niaudet P: Prevention des thromboses vasculaire après transplantation rénale par un héparine de bas poids moleculaire. *Ann Pediatr (Paris)* 38(6): 397, 1991

110. Arbus GS, Rochon J, Thompson D: Survival of cadaveric renal transplant grafts from young donors and in young recipients. *Pediatr Nephrol* 5: 152, 1991

111. Haycock GB: Intra-operative and immediate post-operative care in the management of the paediatric transplant recipient. in *Pediatric Nephrology*, edited by Brodehl J, Ehrich JHH, Berlin, Heidelberg, Springer Verlag, 1984, p 146

112. Broyer M, Gagnadoux MF, Guest G, Beurton D, Niaudet P, Habib R, Busson M: Kidney transplantation in children. Results of 383 grafts performed at Enfants Malades Hospital from 1973 to 1984. *Adv Nephrol* 16: 307, 1987

113. Korsch B, Fine RN, Negrette VR: Non compliance in children with renal transplant. *Pediatrics* 61: 872, 1978

114. Offner G, Hoyer PF, Brodehl J, Pichlmayr R: Cyclosporin A in paediatric kidney transplantation. *Pediatr Nephrol* 1: 125, 1987

115. Neumayer HH, Farber C, Haller P, Koch C, Kohnen R, Maibucher A, Mayer I, Oberdorf E, Schmieder R, Schuster M, Vollmer J, Wauser J, Werner M: Conversion from Sandimmun to Sandimmune-Neoral. Experience in 300 patients after renal transplantation. Third International Congress on Cyclosporine. Seville 29–13: p 131, 1994 (abstract)

116. Almond PS, Matas A, Gilligham K, Dunn DL, Payne WD, Gores R, Gruessner R, Najarian JS: Risk factors for chronic rejection in renal allograft recipient. *Transplantation* 55: 752, 1992

117. Rigsby CM, Burns PM, Weltin GG, Chen B, Bia M, Taylor KJ: Doppler signal quantification in renal allografts: comparison in normal on rejection transplant's with pathologic correlation radiology. *Radiology* 162: 39, 1987

118. Fitzpatrick MM, Gleeson FV, De Broyn R, Trompeter RJ, Gordon I: The evolution of paediatric renal transplants using resistive index and renal blood flow. *Pediatr Nephrol* 6: 172, 1992.

119. Broyer M, Guest G: Croissance après transplantation rénale. in *Journées Parisiennes de Pédiatrie*, Paris, Flammarion Medicine Sciences, 1987, p 135

120. Van Diemen-Steenvoorde R, Donckerwolcke R, Brackel H, Wolff ED, De Jong JW: Growth and bone maturation in children after kidney transplantation. *J Pediatr* 110: 351, 1987

121. Fennell RS, Love JT, Carter RL, Hudson TM, Pfaff WW, Howard RJ, Van Densen W, Garin EH, Iravani A, Walker RD, Richard OA: Statistical analysis of staturnal growth following transplantation. *Eur J Pediatr* 145: 377, 1986

122. Brodehl J, Offner G, Hoyer PF: Cyclosporine in pediatric kidney transplantation. *Adv Nephrol* 16: 335, 1987

123. Benfield MR, Parker KL, Waldo FB, Overstreet L, Kohaut C: Growth hormone in the treatment of growth failure in children after renal transplantation. *Kidney Int* 44 (Suppl 43): 62, 1993

124. Jabs K, Van Dop C, Harmon WE: Growth hormone treatment of growth failure among children with renal transplants. *Kidney Int* 44 (Suppl 43): 71, 1993.

125. Wühl E, Haffner D, Tönshoff B, Mehls O and the German Group Study: Predictors of growth response to rhGH in short children before and after renal transplantation. *Kidney Int* 44 (Suppl 43): 76, 1993

126. Johansson G, Sietnieks A, Janssens F, Proesmans W, Vanderschueren-Lodeweyckx M, Holsberg C, Sipila I, Broyer M, Rappaport R. Albertsson-Wikland K, Berg U, Jodal U, Rees L, Rigden SPA, Preece MA: Recombinant human growth hormone treatment in short children with chronic renal disease, before transplantation or with functioning renal transplants. *Acta Pediatr Scand* (Suppl) 370: 36, 1989

127. Schwartz ID, Warady BA: Cadaveric renal allograft rejection after treatment with recombinant human growth hormone. *J Pediatr* 121: 664, 1992

128. Tyden G, Berg U, Reinholt F: Acute renal graft rejection after treatment with human growth hormone. *Lancet* 336: 1455, 1990

129. Gagnadoux MF, Niaudet P, Broyer M: Non immunological risk factors in pediatric renal transplantation. *Pediatr Nephrol* 7: 89, 1993

130. Broyer M, Guest G. Gagnadoux MF, Beurton D: Hypertension following renal transplantation in children. *Pediatr Nephrol* 1: 16, 1987

131. Tejani A: Post transplant hypertension and hypertensive encephalopathy in renal allograft recipient. *Nephron* 34: 73, 1983

132. Benoit G, Moukarrel M, Hiesse C, Verdelli G, Charpentier B, Fries D: Transplant renal artery stenosis: experience and comparative results between surgery and angioplasty. *Transplant Int* 3: 137, 1990

133. Broyer M, Donckerwolcke RA, Brunner FP, Brynger H, Challah S, Gretz N, Jacobs C, Kramer P, Selwood NH, Wing AJ: Combined report on regular dialysis and transplantation of children in Europe, XIII, 1982. *Proc Eur Dial Transplant Assoc – Eur Ren Assoc* 20: 79, 1983

134. Rubin RH: Infections disease complications of renal transplantation. *Kidney Int* 44: 221, 1993

135. Korsch B: Current issues in comprehensive care for children with chronic illness. in *Pediatric Nephrology*, edited by Brodehl J, Ehrich JHH, Berlin, Heidelberg, Springer Verlag, 1984, p 179

136. Ehrich JHH, Rizzoni G, Broyer M, Brunner FP, Brynger H, Fassbinder W, Geerlings W, Selwood NH, Tufveson G, Wing AJ: Rehabilitation of young adults during renal replacement therapy in Europe. II Schooling, employment and social situation. *Nephrol Dial Transpl* 7: 579, 1992

137. Chantler C, Broyer M, Donckerwolcke R, Brynger H, Brunner FP, Jacobs C, Kramer P, Selwood NH, Wing A: Growth and rehabilitation of the long term survivous of treatment for end stage renal failure in childhood. *Proc Eur Dial Transplant Assoc* 18: 329, 1981

138. Andre JL, Picon G.: Aspects psychosociaux du traîtement de l'insuffisance rénale terminale. (Psychological aspects of treatment of terminal renal insufficiency). in *26e Congrès des Pédiatres de Langue Française*, edited by Regnier, Toulouse, Fournié, 1981, p 611

139. Jones RWA, Dalton N, Start K, El Bishti M, Chantler C: Oral essential amino acid supplements in children with advanced chronic renal failure. *Am J Clin Nutr* 33: 1696, 1980

140. Counahan R, El Bishti M, Chantler C: Oral essential amino acids in children on regular haemodialysis. *Clin Nephrol* 9: 11, 1978

141. Jones RWA, Dalton N, Turner C, Start K, Haycock GB, Chantler C: Oral essential amino acid and keto acid supplements in children with chronic renal failure. *Kidney Int* 24: 95, 1983

142. Kopple JD: Abnormal amino acid and protein metabolism in uremia. *Kidney Int* 14: 340, 1978

143. Kopple JD, Swendseid ME: Vitamin nutrition in patients undergoing maintenance hemodialysis. *Kidney Int* 7 (Suppl 2): S-79, 1975

144. Leung AC, Henderson IS, Maharai D, Thomson G: Excessive accumulation of folic acid in uremic patients on dialysis. *Dial Transplant* 14: 575, 1985

DIALYSIS IN THE ELDERLY

EIRINI GRAPSA and DIMITRIOS G. OREOPOULOS

INTRODUCTION

The aged are a heterogeneous group and an individual's chronological age does not necessarily reflect his or her physiological status. The commonly used cut off of 65 years to designate an individual as elderly is arbitrary; Bismark in Germany first used this milestone to identify those individuals who would be entitled to social benefits. In 1900 only 4% of the Western world's population was over 65 years of age, but now this fraction is 12% and rising (1). This progressive increase in the ranks of the elderly and the success of dialysis have produced a dramatic increase in the numbers of elderly dialysis patients worldwide. Thus in the United States 47% of those on dialysis are over 65, and this fraction is expected to increase to over 60% by the end of this century (2). In Canada in 1989, 35% of end-stage renal disease (ESRD) patients were over the age 65, compared to 25% in 1981 (3). A similar trend has been reported by the European Renal Association Registry; in 1980, only 11% of patients starting renal replacement therapy were older than 65 years whereas by 1987 this proportion had increased to nearly 30% (4). In a UK dialysis center that provides the sole nephrological service for a population of 1.2 million, those over 65 constitute more than 25% of all new patients accepted for dialysis (5). It is noteworthy that, in the United Kingdom in 1987, 44% of all new patients accepted for renal replacement therapy were placed on continuous ambulatory peritoneal dialysis (CAPD) (6).

Of the systemic diseases that lead to ESRD in elderly patients, hypertension and diabetes taken together account for 40–65% (7, 8). Tubulointerstitial disorders, obstructive uropathy, glomerular disease and polycystic kidney disease, respectively, account for 13.5, 10.9, 10.6 and 2% (8). In most series, in a percentage that varies from 10 to 46% (average 24%), the etiology of renal disease is unknown (5, 9–12). The incidence of comorbid chronic illness increases with advancing age. Thus 78% of the individuals older than 65 years of age have chronic ill-

nesses and 30% have 3 or more (13). Chronic peritoneal dialysis (PD), while used extensively in some countries like Canada and the UK, has been systematically neglected in others such as the US. Similarly, home hemodialysis is underused in the elderly. As a mode of treatment in the elderly renal transplantation remains limited and controversial (14–16).

HEMODIALYSIS

In most countries hemodialysis is the principal form of renal replacement in the elderly with ESRD (14, 15). As in the young, double-lumen subclavian catheters and permanent jugular catheters are used in the elderly patients, either temporarily or permanently (17–19). Regarding permanent access, reports vary concerning the success of the arteriovenous (A-V) fistula in the elderly. Wing et al. (20) reported a high success rate (82%) using the Brescia–Cimino fistula in patients over 65 years while others have reported less satisfactory results (25–30%) with the same technique (8, 21). The major threat to the A-V fistulae is lesions of the vessels due to hypertensive vascular disease or diabetes, which is frequent in these patients (21, 22). Despite this theoretical risk, results of vascular access for chronic hemodialysis in elderly patients are similar to those in younger ones (22, 25).

Hinsdale et al. reviewed the experience of vascular access in 119 elderly patients with a mean age of 63.5 years (47% over 65). Of these, 75% had polytetrafluoroethylene (PTFE) grafts and 25% Brescia–Cimino fistulae. All fistulaes in patients over 65 years had failed at one year (21). In a retrospective review (over a 4 year period) with 435 angioaccess procedures in patients with ESRD aged 29 to 81 years, Ballard et al. (18) found a higher use of PTFE grafts in elderly patients than of Brescia–Cimino fistulaes. When stratified for age, those older than 60 who had a major angioaccess complication had a statistically significantly higher mortality rate than did those younger than 60. Overall death occurred in 20% of patients over 50, 45% in those over 60 and 43% in those over 70 (statistically not significant) (18). In 79 patients (all of whom had a PTFE graft) older than 65 (range 65–87 years) when compared to 55 patients younger than 65, Didlake et al. (22) noted no difference in the frequency of thrombosis, infections, flow problems, or pseudoaneurysm formation. The only difference between the two age groups was minor wound and skin complications, due to age related changes in skin physiology.

In the United States, hemodialysis vascular access morbidity was analysed in patients with ESRD from 1984 to 1986. The elderly (> 64 years) experienced more access-related hospital stays than any other age group. At two years of follow-up, of those > 64, 24% were hospitalized compared to 19% for age 45–64 and 15% for age 20–44. The elderly had a higher rate of access morbidity even after the investigators controlled for the differential survival, transplant and peritoneal dialysis experience (26).

Vascular-access thrombosis associated with recombinant human erythropoietin (rHEPO) therapy was more common in the elderly individuals. Among patients ≥ 50 years old, thrombosis was found in 17% of those with native-vein fistulaes and 67% of those with PTFE grafts; among those < 50 years, thrombosis was seen in 12% with native-vein fistulas and 42% in those with PTFE grafts (27).

Complications of hemodialysis

Disequilibrium syndrome: Both young and elderly patients may develop this syndrome after rapid hemodialysis (28), and experience headaches, nausea, lethargy, seizures and abnormal electroencephalograms (29–31). It has been suggested that rapid hemodialysis may increase intracranial pressure and produce cerebral edema that may be responsible for these symptoms (32). After an experimental study in dogs, Wakim (33) suggested that hyponatremia is the main cause of this syndrome. Others suggest that rapid hemodialysis in uremic animals induces a fall in cerebrospinal-fluid pH and accumulation of idiogenic osmoles in the brain; this produces an osmotic gradient between brain and plasma, which causes cerebral edema, increased intracranial pressure and seizures (34).

Hypotension: This is a frequent complication during hemodialysis for both young and elderly patients. Some investigators have reported a higher incidence in the elderly (35, 36) while others have found no difference (8, 37).

The elderly may develop hypotension even after minimal loss of fluid volume; this may be difficult to correct because elderly patients have autonomic dysfunction and a low cardiac reserve and their response to volume removal is more sluggish than in younger patients. The sequelae may include seizures, cerebral infarction, myocar-

dial ischemia, aspiration pneumonia and vascular access thrombosis (38–41).

Hypoxemia: Hypoxemia develops 15 minutes after the initiation of hemodialysis. Its overall frequency is 70%. The PAO_2 drops by 5–35 Sarrhythmias mmHg and it increases 60–120 minutes after hemodialysis (42). This fall in PAO_2 is critical in the elderly patient who has decreased cardiac or pulmonary reserve, and is prominent after dialysis that uses acetate dialysate and cellulosic membranes (42).

Arrhythmias: Some studies (43–46) have stressed the arrhythmogenic effect of hemodialysis but others (47–49) have not.

Of 127 hemodialysis patients from 13 centres, studied with 48-hour Holter monitoring 76% had ventricular arrhythmias (43). The risk factors for ventricular arrhythmias were age ≥ 55 years and left ventricular dysfunction. In a study of 321 uremic patients on hemodialysis aged from 16 to 77 years, Niwa et al. (50) found that 43.8% of patients over 50 years had high-grade arrhythmias but only 17.9% of patients under 50 years had this disturbance. They concluded that the incidence of dangerous arrhythmias increases progressively with the duration of hemodialysis and the age of the patients; this fact may be responsible for the high incidence of cardiac deaths in these patients. Ebel et al. (44), who studied hemodialysis patients aged 66.9 ± 6.2 years found a high correlation between the number of ventricular extrasystoles in the last hour of dialysis and the difference between pre- and postdialysis serum potassium concentration. Finally, among 292 elderly and young patients, Capuano et al. found that, during dialysis, 15% of the elderly and 9% of young patients had detectable arrhythmias; 11 older patients developed persistent arrhythmias (in most cases atrial fibrillation) but none of the young patients did ($p > 0.05$) (51).

Infections: Infection remains an important cause of morbidity and mortality in dialysis patients. In a recent multicenter French study the frequency of infection-related deaths was low (6.3%), and the mean age of those who died from it was 67.5 years; the fatal bacteremias were vascular access – related and were caused by *S. aureus* (52). Berman et al. reported an increased infection-related mortality in those over 60 years of age; in their experience, bacteremia was not related to the vascular access site. Pneumonia was more frequent in older individuals. The incidence of pneumonia was 1.4 episodes per 100 months of hemodialysis for patients over 70 years, compared to 0.4 episodes per 100 months of hemodialysis for patients under 50 years. Death from pneumonia occurred only in patients over 65 years (53). Dobkin et al. reported a four-fold increase in deaths due to vascular access-related infections and a nine-fold increase in non-vascular access site related infections in elderly individuals (54).

Septicemia and pulmonary infections are the second-leading cause of death in US hemodialysis patients over the age of 64 (55). Recently the Canadian Organ Replacement Register reported that the infection mortality rate for dialysis patients age 45–64 years was 9.8% and 8.9% for those 65 years old and over. Among patients aged 65 and over, deaths from infection were significantly more frequent in those on PD (10.4%) than in those on HD 7.5% (56).

Subdural hematoma: This relatively uncommon complication of hemodialysis was described as early as 1969, in both young and elderly patients (57–61). The estimated incidence of subdural hematoma is 3.3% and the mortality rate is 85% (60).

Gastrointestinal bleeding: Gastritis, duodenal ulceration and angiodysplasia are common in patients with end stage renal failure, particularly in elderly dialysis patients (62, 63). In the elderly on dialysis hemorrhagic gastritis is due mainly to uremia and to the use of non-steroidal antiinflammatory drugs (NSAIDS) (3, 64).

In the elderly the sources of GI bleeding are often multiple and occasionally are undiagnosed; its high incidence and the desire to mitigate the anemia of chronic renal failure in the elderly, partly explain the increased transfusion rate. Thus elderly patients received a mean of 6.9 ± 1.2 units of blood/yr/patient compared to 3.4 ± 0.6 units/yr for young controls ($p < 0.02$) (65). More severe bleeding occurs in those with angiodysplasia (63) – the second most common cause of gastrointestinal bleeding in elderly ESRD patients (8).

Colonic angiodysplasia may cause lower intestinal hemorrhage in elderly hemodialysis patients (66). Perforation of colonic diverticulosis, which may complicate the clinical course of older ESRD patients, may be related to the constipating effects of aluminum based phosphate binders. Vague abdominal pain in the elderly with low-grade fever, which may be the only initial presenting symptom, should be pursued aggressively to rule out a perforated colon (67, 68). While, in hemodialysis patients a small colonic perforation may have a benign course, in elderly CAPD patients, it usually presents as fecal peritonitis and often requires catheter removal.

CONTINUOUS AMBULATORY PERITONEAL DIALYSIS (CAPD)

CAPD is now an established method in the treatment of ESRD patients. CAPD has a particular place in the treatment of elderly ESRD patients; in some countries (69–73) a high percentage of the elderly are treated with this modality while in others, such as the US, there are fewer elderly patients on CAPD than on hemodialysis (14). Among the geriatric ESRD patients who live in US nursing homes, only 10% are on CAPD (74). CAPD has, for the elderly, various medical advantages (75), such as reduced cardiovascular instability and arrhythmias, better maintenance of residual renal function, good control of hypertension and anemia, no need of vascular access,

efficacy of intraperitoneal insulin therapy and removal of B2-microglobulin and middle molecules; many however may not choose this mode because of psychosocial factors such as inadequate family and social support, physical and mental impairment (76).

Complications in elderly patients on CAPD

1. Peritonitis: This infection is the main reason for hospitalization of patients on CAPD (9, 10, 14, 77–87). In elderly patients on CAPD the incidence of peritonitis varies among centers from 0.42 to 2.8 episodes/pt/year depending on the system used (77–80, 88–91), and whether the patients themselves are able to do the exchanges (92). Several authors (14, 80, 92–94) have reported no difference in the incidence of peritonitis between young and elderly patients. Among 3188 patients (United States Renal Data System) on various connection systems Port et al. (91) found a significantly higher relative risk (RR) for peritonitis among younger and black patients. Similarly Nebel et al. (84) had better results in the elderly, but others (90, 95) had worse results.

The elderly showed a distribution of organisms responsible for peritonitis that was similar to that in young patients (80). In a small number ($n = 10$) of CAPD patients 65 years or older, Joglar and Saade (96) found a high incidence of fungal peritonitis (33.3%). Piccoli et al. (12) found that as a cause of dropout, peritonitis was similar (21% vs 20%) among the young and elderly CAPD patients ($n = 231$). As a cause of death, peritonitis was more common among elderly patients (2.3% under 65 years and 3.2% over 74), compared with those younger than 65 years (1.4%).

Catheter related complications: Among CAPD patients many complictions are related to the catheter – early or late pericatheter leak, exit-site infection, cuff extrusion or hernia at the peritoneal tunnel (97). Holley et al. found no differences in age and race among 411 CAPD patients with and without tunnel infections (98); others (95) have reported similar tunnel infection rates in young and elderly CAPD patients. Recently, Holley et al. (94) compared 103 CAPD elderly patients 60 years old or older with 103 younger CAPD patients (18–40 years old) and found a lower tunnel infection rate in the elderly (0.15 vs 0.25 episode per patient year). Similarly Nissenson et al. (80) found that only 9% of his elderly CAPD patients required catheter replacement compared to 20% of younger patients; 7% of the elderly had tunnel infection vs 13% of the younger. Contrary to these findings Tzamaloukas et al. (99) analyzed 120 episodes of peritonitis and found that advanced age was one of the variables associated with catheter removal, along with prolonged duration of peritonitis and coexisting exit-site and tunnel infection.

Hernias: Frequently CAPD patients develop one or more of several types of hernias (14, 83, 95). Gentile et al. (14) reported a similar frequency of hernia between younger and older patients (7.8% *vs* 9.9%). Ross and Rutsky (95) also reported similar frequencies.

Hyperlipidemia: This is common among patients on CAPD (100–102). Maiorca et al. reported that, in both women and men, blood cholesterol was significantly higher in elderly patients on CAPD compared to those on HD; however, they found no significant differences in triglyceride levels between patients on the two dialysis methods (92). Panarello et al. (102) reported similar results.

CHRONIC COMPLICATIONS IN ELDERLY PATIENTS ON CAPD AND HD

Cardiovascular Complications: Cardiovascular disease is the most frequent cause of death in ESRD patients (103–105). Older age is an independent risk factor for congestive heart failure in those on dialysis (40, 41). Uremic pericarditis and uremic cardiomyopathy also are associated with heart failure. The ages of those with early or late pericarditis did not differ from the mean age of patients without such complications (106). Asymptomatic pericardial effusions were found in both young and elderly hemodialysis patients. The likelihood of an effusion was not influenced significantly by the patient's weight, urea nitrogen (BUN), age, sex or duration of dialysis (107). Capuono et al. (51) found that cardiovascular impairment was more common in older (35%) than in younger (16%) hemodialysis patients. This difference was present even before dialysis (27% for the elderly and 10% for the young patients). Hypertension, angina or myocardial infarction is associated with an above-average mortality for young and older patients on peritoneal dialysis (CAPD). Three-year survival was 57% in young patients (< 55 years) and 35% in older patients with cardiac risk factors (108). A comparative study of elderly patients (65 years and above) on hemodialysis and continuous ambulatory peritoneal dialysis showed that ischemic heart disease and congestive cardiac failure was associated with a significant increase in mortality. Thus ischemic heart disease was present in 56% of CAPD patients and 47% of HD patients, while congestive cardiac failure was present in 50% of CAPD patients and 47% of HD patients (83); these differences are not statistically significant.

Neurological Complications: Patients with chronic renal failure often have peripheral and central neurological abnormalities. Chronic hemodialysis may produce slight improvement, stabilization or deterioration of neuropathy (109–111).

Bazzi et al. (111) studied uremic polyneuropathy in 135 short- and long-term hemodialysis patients (age range 21–72 years). Selective analysis demonstrated that, in those who have had up to 10 years of dialysis, nervous-system impairment is mild and requires the use of sensitive electrophysiological parameters for its detection; older patients or those with more prolonged treatment have more significant and clinically apparent signs of such

impairment. Dialysis encephalopathy syndrome (dialysis dementia), that almost uniformly has been fatal, has been described in ESRD patients from several units (112–116). Several workers (112, 117–119) have implicated increased aluminum load as the cause of dialysis dementia. Although typically confined to patients on long term chronic hemodialysis, the syndrome may be seen in patients with chronic renal failure before dialysis (120), or in those on peritoneal dialysis (121, 122). Sporadic cases of dialysis dementia encountered in centers using a water supply low in aluminum, and in units that have reduced dialysate aluminum to minimal levels (123), suggests that this syndrome may be related to the ingestion of aluminum given for phosphate binding. No relationship was demonstrated with age, race, sex, diet, blood pressure or cause of renal failure (116, 119).

Osteodystrophy: Renal osteodystrophy is a major concern among patients receiving long term dialysis. Bone and joint pain, history of fractures and disability are the main findings (124–126). The degree of disability is significantly correlated with bone aluminum, but there is no correlation with age, time on dialysis, serum calcium, alkaline phosphatase, parathyroid hormone (PTH) levels, type of bone disease or histomorphometric parameters (124). Schaab et al. (127) reported 11 femoral-neck fractures in nine patients receiving long-term dialysis, mean age 67 years (52–82). Seven of these were on hemodialysis and one was on peritoneal dialysis, from 0.5 to 15.4 years. The histologic and clinical picture was consistent with aluminum related osteodystrophy.

Faugere et al. (128) in 120 HD and PD patients consisting of females 2–77 years old and males, 13 to 73 years old, found that the aluminum accumulation in bone may be associated not only with disturbed mineralization but also with loss of bone mass. Patients receiving long-term dialysis – both those with and without deposition of aluminum in bone – still show the bone loss associated with advanced age. It is of interest that the negative correlation between age and bone mass is more pronounced in patients with stainable bone aluminum suggesting that aluminum deposition may enhance the age related bone loss in patients with renal failure. Bone-mineral density (BMD) was measured in 25 elderly HD patients with a mean age of 68 ± 10 years and from 1 to 156 months on HD. In these patients, loss of BMD was not uniform in the various parts of the axial skeleton, for example femoral-neck BMD loss was greater than loss in lumbar vertebrae. Sex and age were not independent correlates of BMD in this study (129).

β₂-Microglobulin-Related Amyloid Bone Disease: Accumulation of β_2-microglobulin (β_2M), an 11,800 dalton protein, is a potentially crippling complication of long-term dialysis. The clinical manifestations include carpal-tunnel syndrome, swollen painful joints and pathologic fractures (130–132). Some workers have postulated a potential synergism between aluminum, iron and β_2-microglobulin (β_2M)-related amyloid deposits, but others, have not confirmed this (130, 131). CAPD patients may have serum levels of β_2-microglobulin lower (133, 134) or similar to those of HD patients (135, 136). Van Ypersele et al. (137) who studied the effect of dialysis membrane and age on deposits and other signs of dialysis-related amyloidosis among patients from 12 centers (221 patients) found that age at onset of dialysis showed a striking correlation with the development of carpal tunnel syndrome and bone amyloidosis, but that hyperparathyroidism, sex or year of dialysis had no significant effect. Also they have reported increased prevalence of β_2M amyloidosis with age, and use of cellulosic membranes for more than 5 years (137). The risk of dialysis related amyloidosis in patients treated with peritoneal dialysis is unknown. Patients on CAPD have developed cystic lesions, carpal tunnel syndrome and amyloid deposits; all of these were elderly and had been on CAPD for up to 7 years (138–141).

Malnutrition: Malnutrition is a common complication in patients with uremia (142–144). In hemodialysed patients, factors affecting nutritional status are inadequate dialysis, as measured by kinetic modelling of urea with a Kt/V < 1.0, with poorly biocompatible membranes, loss of amino acids and peptides in dialysate, acidosis, high parathyroid-hormone levels, low hematocrit, low insulin-like growth factor (IgF1), advanced age, and general loss of independence (143). Malnutrition increases with advancing age; Ross and Rutsky reported a frequency of 20% for the elderly and 2% for the young CAPD patient (95). Similarly cachexia as the cause of death increases with age (12). Increased malnutrition and cachexia among elderly dialysis patients may reflect a lower protein intake by this group compared to younger patients (144, 145). Many investigators (146–148) have confirmed an inverse correlation between normalized protein catabolic rate (NPCR) and age. Serum albumin was similar in older and younger patients (149) and did not change as age increased (147). They observed that neither serum albumin nor serum transferrin changed significantly after four years of CAPD, and after 8 years in a subgroup of eight patients (147). In 95 HD patients, Movilli et al. (146) found that serum albumin was lowest in patients $\geq$ 75 years old. Among patients with low time averaged concentration of blood urea (TAC), Simon et al. (150) found that the incidence of morbidity was significantly increased in those over 50 years of age. Comparing the two forms of dialysis, Maiorca et al. (92) found that in both CAPD and HD, the percentage of malnourished patients increased with age.

Psychological Problems: The elderly are not a homogeneous group but vary widely in their physiologic and psychosocial characteristics as well as in the number and severity of their diseases (76). More than 10% of elderly persons living in the community show significant symptoms of depression (151) and in most instances, such symptoms are related to physical disability such as ESRD or other life stresses (95). End-stage renal disease is a severe illness that requires changes in lifestyle by both the patient and family. Common handicaps are a decrease in socioeconomic status, changes in family roles, restriction of social activities, sexual problems, psychological symptoms, and eventually withdrawal from dialysis (95, 152–155). Approximately 8% of dialysis patients have major depressive episodes (156).

Psychiatric morbidity has been observed in 52% of elderly patients on both CAPD and HD; 29% are mild, 16% are moderate and 7% are severe (157). Among elderly dialysis patients 60–70 years old, McKevitt et al. found that 62% showed symptoms of depression as measured by the Beck Depressive Inventory (158).

However, age is not significantly related to the severity of the patient's depression (159) nor to the severity of depressive symptoms (153). Rodin et al. reported that the two groups of dialysis patients – depressed and non-depressed – did not differ significantly in age (160). Older patients in either dialytic modality perceived life stresses in a way similar to age-matched controls (161). Iordanidis et al. (157) found no significant relationship between psychiatric morbidity and method of dialysis. Depression was significantly related to mortality at a 2 year follow-up (162). In another study of 78 ESRD patients over 70 years of age, Husebye et al. (163) found that 54% had died by 3 years, 43% through withdrawal from dialysis. Those who died had a lower Karnofsky scale (78 *vs* 85).

Quality of life

The term quality of life subsumes several concepts including personal experiences and objective medical, psychological and social factors (164–167). In a comparative study of 349 elderly dialysis patients and 354 controls, Kutner and Brogan (168) found that the dialysis patients were more functionally disabled, had a decreased ability to do things they would like to do, and had a lower level of perceived mastery of their lives. The significantly higher number of health problems, and significantly lower mean income among the dialysis patients might have been responsible for the difference. Kjellstrand et al. (169) reported good quality of life among their elderly dialysis patients; most of them were doing well, were at home (73%), had good contacts with other people (90%), spent much time outdoors (86%), enjoyed life (71%) and ranked high on the Karnofky scale (73% Karnofky > 80). Horina et al. (170) found that their elderly HD patients had low Karnofsky scores (20–90%) but had adapted satisfactorily to their disease and resulting disabilities. Similarly among 159 patients on CAPD and HD, Stout et al. (161) found that those < 60 appeared less satisfied with life on several scales of assessment. The elderly group (> 60) with and without risk factors perceived life to be less stressful than did younger patients and these workers concluded that the elderly had a good perceived-quality of life even when they had added risk factors. Moody et al. (171) reported good results for the elderly: their young patients appreciated dialysis the least, older patients (50–69 years) appreciated dialysis the most. Patients older than 75 were less active and less outgoing, but, perceived their health as quite good and took life in better stride than did younger dialysis patients; these very old subjects were neither particularly happy or unhappy.

Other workers have reported worse results with regards to quality of life among the elderly. Wolcott et al. (172) who studied the quality of life of a small number ($n = 66$) of ESRD patients (22–65 years old), found that, compared to the younger group (< 51), those over 50 had fewer years of education, lower Karnofsky scores, and higher fatigue scores. They also participated significantly less frequently in community activity, and their psychological status was more variable than younger individuals. Despite these differences the elderly perceived their quality of life to be similar to that of younger people. Similarly in Muthny and Koch's (165) study of the quality of life of HD/CAPD and transplant patients, on average, the elderly reported more marked complaints, had a lower overall life satisfaction, but, had a higher satisfaction with partnership and family. Similarly Barany et al. (173) found that their elderly patients had less satisfaction with their health, had more sleep disturbances and more physical symptoms, such differences disappearing after the correction of anemia. According to Kutner and Brogan (174) a poorer social support network may be responsible for these differences. Diaz-Buxo (11) found lower scores among elderly patients on all modalities but those on CCPD and home HD had higher scores than those on center HD. In an effort to compare elderly and younger dialysis patients, Denistron et al. (1989) (175) studied the quality of life of 742 dialysis patients aged 20–89 years. Analysis by age group (20–40), (41–60) and (61–89) showed a decreasing quality of life with increasing age, in certain indices (ADL Index and positive affect scales). In other measures such as (Index of General Affect, the 'life is free' and 'good days' items) the 41–60 age group had highest scores. The middle age group reported less satisfaction with sexual life than either the younger or the older group, and the General Well Being Index score was lowest in the younger group and equal to that in the older group. There were no statistically significant differences between any of the quality of life measures, nor in age or sex distribution between home and center dialysis patients. In other studies, age had no value as a predictor of quality of life (176, 177).

Morbidity: Hospitalization, a common expression of morbidity in elderly ESRD patients, is due to cardiovascular disease, infections (pneumonia or peritonitis), diabetic complications, fluid overload and angioacccess clotting (92, 178–182). Furthermore, the elderly who have a variety of comorbid conditions may require additional hospitalization. Many workers report a greater number of hospitalization days per year for the elderly hemodialysis patient (182–183). The same difference has been described in elderly CAPD compared to younger patients (22.2 *vs* 16.9 days/year) (184). When the elderly cannot do their own dialysis fluid exchanges, these differences become greater (43.7/days/patient year *vs* 7.6 day/patient year) (178), however, Wadhwa et al. (185) have reported lower hospitalization rates and duration of stay (one admission/6 patient months) for elderly disabled CAPD patients with home nurses, than for patients without such assistance (one admission/4 patients months). Maiorca et al. (92) reported that the elderly on CAPD required slightly fewer admissions than those on HD (1.67 *vs* 1.71 per patient per year). White elderly patients on dialysis (CAPD-HD) used the hospital approximately 25% more than black patients, both in number of admissions and total hospital days (180).

Mortality: The risk of death in ESRD patient increases with age (55, 180, 184, 186) and coexisting disease (187). After a study of 842 patients on HD and 272 patients on CAPD, Gentil et al. (188) found that age, diabetes and cardiovascular disease were associated with a shorter survival. Early mortality (within 90 days) among the elderly on dialysis increased significantly from 15% for those patients 65–75 years old, to 20% for those 75–84, and 30% for those over 84 years old, these deaths were associated with high risk comorbid conditions (189). Survival on dialysis of elderly patients with ESRD is shown in Tables 1, 2 and 3.

Held et al. (204) who compared 5-year survival for ESRD patients between 1982 and 1987 in US, Europe and Japan, found that for ages 65–74 and 75–84, survival was 19% and 10% respectively in the US, and 32% and 19% in Europe. For the age groups 60–74 and 75–84, the 5-year survival in the US was 22% and 10% respectively, compared to 38% and 18% in Japan.

Elderly who were 'forced' to begin on CAPD had a worse survival (25% at two years) compared to those who chose CAPD (25% at five years) (82). Many workers report that cardiovascular disease is the main or second cause of death in the elderly dialysis patients (55, 56, 184, 189, 205). Cachexia, which accounts for 10% of the deaths in patients aged < 65, rises to 36% in those over 65 and to 44% in patients over 75 (12). Infection (20–50%), multisystem failure and/or withdrawal from dialysis (30%), are other frequent causes of death for the elderly on dialysis (189, 205). Withdrawal from dialysis was the most common cause of death in 239 patients on dialysis over 70 years old (192) or was the second cause (55). Deaths from social causes (suicide or withdrawal from treatment) are more frequent among the elderly, (15.4% of all deaths among patients aged 65 and over 10% for those aged 46–64) (56). Hirsch reported that between 1982–1987, 6% of all patients discontinued dialysis (16% of all deaths). The mean age of these deaths was 67 ± 5 years (206). Some workers have reported that withdrawal from dialysis was more common among the elderly receiving in-centre hemodialysis (205, 206). Other important factors associated with the decision to withdraw from dialysis were cancer, malnutrition, hypercatabolic state and dissatisfaction with life (205).

Table 1. Survival during maintenance hemodialysis in elderly patients in selected centers. Adapted and reprinted with permission (3)

Source	Age (yr) range	No. of patients	Survival (%)						
			1 yr	2 yr	3 yr	5 yr	6 yr	7 yr	10 yr
Westlie et al. (193)	70–87	157	78	47	–	22	–	–	
Chester et al. (65)	70–85	45	–	42	23	–	–	–	
Husebye and Kjellstrand (192)	71–84	239	–	–	–	–	–	17	
Schaefer et al. (194)	68–78	180	90	80	67	50	–	30	
	> 75	45	–	–	–	50	–	–	
	> 80	11	–	–	50	–	–	–	
Laurent et al. (190)	> 55	90	95	92	88	85	80	78	75
Panarello et al. (195)	60–78	35	92	85	70	52	28	–	
Mion et al. (196)	65–69	33	–	–	77	65 (4y)			
Park and Lee (197)	> 60	22	75	·	52	–		–	
Port et al. (191)	60–95	1,831	65	46	35	20	–	10	
Tapson et al. (69)	60–76	–	–	–	–	53	–	–	
Wall (5)	65–74	28	77	68	46	–	–	–	
Rotellar et al. (183)	65–85	–	70	50	31	15	–	–	
Loew (198)	60–70	–	–	–	–	45	–	–	
	70–80					25			
Benevent (77)	65–79	31	82	55	45	–	–	–	
Lupo et al. (87)	> 65	263					30 (4y)		

Table 2. Survival during maintenance hemodialysis in elderly patients in national and international registries. Reproduced with permission (3)

Source	Age (yr)	Survival (%)			Comments
		1 yr	2 yr	5 yr	
Renal Data System (55)	65–69	73.4(a)	54.9(b)	22.4(c)	(a) From day 91 to 1 year + 90 d year of incidence 1989
	70–74	68.2	47.4	16.9	
	75–79	64.8	40.6	12.0	(b) From day 91 to 2 years + 90 d year of incidence 1988
	80–84	59.8	34.1	9.3	
	85+	53.6	27.6	3.5	(c) From day 91 to 5 years + 90 d
Odaka (199)	60–74	73	63	38	Japan 1980–1988
	75–89	54	40	18	
Brunner and Selwood (200)	65–74	81	66	35	EDTA Registry 1980–1987
	75–84	75	55	20	
Posen (201)	65+	65	50	20	Canadian Renal Failure Registry 1981–1987
Disney (202)	65–74	77	65	34	Australia, 1982–1988 # patients aged
	75–84	68	55	< 10%	75–84 too small (< 30)

ADEQUACY OF DIALYSIS

Various workers have estimated adequacy of dialysis through clinical findings such as insomnia, asthenia, pruritus, hypertension, anorexia, nausea, anemia, rate of hospitalization, and mortality, or through biochemical parameters such as kinetic modelling of urea (Kt/V), protein catabolic rate, serum albumin, and prealbumin (207–210). Delmez et al. (211) have performed kinetic modeling of urea (Kt/V) in 291 male and 326 female HD patients of mean age 60.4 ± 15.5 years and duration of dialysis 43.3 ± 42.8 months. They found that 55% of the patients did not reach a Kt/V of 1.0, i.e., the minimal value indicating adequate dialysis. There was a significant correlation

Table 3. Patient survival (%) of elderly patients on continuous ambulatory peritoneal dialysis. Adapted and reprinted with permission (3)

	No. of patients	3-year survival	5-year survival
Canadian Registry (203)	1,348	35	15
Segoloni et al. (9)	514	40	16
Nissenson et al. (80)	492	49	32
Gokal (82)	192	–	25 (6yr)
Piccoli et al. (12)	134	30	–
Walls (5)	85	46	–
Williams et al. (83)	49	38	–
Benevent et al. (77)	39	35	–
Nebel and Finke (84)	26	42	–
Panarello et al. (97)	19	49	–
Lupo et al. (87)	249	40(4yr)	–
Vlachojannis et al. (108)	29	55	–
Range		30–49	15–32

between protein catabolic rate (PCR) and Kt/V, but no correlation between age and PCR or Kt/V. HD patients with Kt/V > 1.0 and PCR > 1.0 had fewer hospitalizations although they were older (mean age 66 ± 4) (212). Movilli et al. (146), who studied 85 patients on HD, found no correlation between Kt/V and NPCR nor between Kt/V and patients' age; however, there was a strong inverse correlation between age and NPCR; the lowest values of NPCR were found in patients ≥ 75 years old. De Alvaro et al. (213) who carried out the Kt/V kinetic modelling of urea for 102 CAPD patients, mean age 54.4 ± 14.8 years, found a significant correlation between PCR and Kt/V ($p < 0.05$) and between normalized protein catabolic rate (NPCR) with serum BUN. Patients who died, had a Kt/V and NPCR significantly lower than patients who were alive at the end of follow up but the former were older (60.7 ± 8.2 *vs* 54.0 ± 15) and had a higher frequency of co-morbidity. Studies among CAPD patients found no significant differences in age between groups with good, intermediate, or poor indices of adequacy of dialysis or clinical outcome such as fatigue, weakness, poor appetite, nausea, vomiting, uremic symptoms, mortality, hospital days, biochemical indices (207, 208, 214); however, there was a good correlation between clinical scores and dialysis dose (208). Shimomura et al. (215) found that a large number of elderly CAPD patients were assigned to the 'poor group' with no definite differences in the urea kinetic parameters, compared with the fairly good and good groups. Nolph et al. (149) studied 71 patients on CAPD (30–75 years old) and found that older patients increased their NPCR with increased Kt/V urea in a fashion similar to that of younger patients. Older patients with reduced creatinine production rates and serum creatinine values, when well dialysed, will have much lower serum

creatinine concentrations than those in younger patients (149).

COMPARISON OF HEMODIALYSIS AND PERITONEAL DIALYSIS IN ELDERLY PATIENTS

Hemodialysis and peritoneal dialysis have been used as equivalent replacement therapies for elderly ESRD patients. Many studies have compared outcomes of the two methods using mortality rates, hospitalization days, technique survival, complications, biochemical status, clinical status and life satisfaction (77, 83, 86, 92, 216, 217). All studies showed that increased age was accompanied by an increased death rate. While the majority of the studies showed no difference in mortality between CAPD and HD (5, 12, 77, 82, 188), some have reported better results for CAPD than for HD in elderly patients (87, 92, 218). Age and comorbid conditions seem to have a statistically significant impact on patient survival but the type of dialytic treatment does not (87). Elderly diabetic patients on CAPD appear to have a higher relative death rate than diabetic HD patients but the difference was not statistically significant (219). Analysis of the USRDS data showed that, in younger diabetic patients, mortality rates tended to be higher for HD than for CAPD, while the opposite was true among older patients (55). The mortality among older diabetics on HD was reported to be lower in Southern Europe but not in Northern Europe (220).

Gentil et al. (188) have reported that the elderly (> 60) and diabetics on center hemodialysis have a higher probability of changing to CAPD, compared to those on CAPD. Hospitalization rate (days per year) was similar in elderly patients on HD and on CAPD (31 HD and 30 CAPD) (93). Benevent et al. (77) reported that elderly CAPD patients had fewer days in hospital per month of treatment (4.74 ± 0.53 days) but more (2.29 per year) admissions than those on HD (6 ± 2.72 days per month, 1.48 admissions per year). Brunori et al. (216) reported fewer hospital days per patient year for 51 patients on HD > 65 years (17.6 days/patient year) and 24.0 days/patient year for 109 patients on CAPD > 65 years old. The number of admissions per patient per year was 1.8 for HD and 1.7 for CAPD patients > 65 years old.

Peritonitis was the primary cause of hospitalization (31.2%) in the CAPD group; other causes were cardiovascular diseases (22.5%), neurological symptoms (11.2%) and technique – related complications other than peritonitis (9.4%). In the HD group, the main cause of hospitalization was cardiovascular diseases (25.9%), while other causes were thrombosis of vascular access (15.2%), technique related difficulties other than vascular access (12.5%) and neurological problems 8% (77). Cardiovascular complications (23%) and access-related difficulties (18.5%) were the most common causes of hospitalization among 2319 older dialysis patients in Georgia and South

Carolina from 1982–1986 (180). Geriatric HD patients required more access procedures than did those on CAPD (93), but more elderly CAPD patients (16.5%) were transferred to HD than HD patients transferred to CAPD (12%) (5).

Clinical and Biochemical Status: The incidence of hypertension was similar in the two groups (HD-CAPD) (92) but was greater in the HD elderly (93), arrythmias were more frequent in the elderly on HD than in those on CAPD (92) and the incidence of malnutrition was similar (12, 92). There were no significant differences in levels of blood urea nitrogen, serum creatinine, calcium or phosphorus (93). Cholesterol levels were lower and serum albumin levels higher in HD elderly HD patients (92, 93, 102). Elderly patients on CAPD were reported to have a better quality of life than those on HD (77); others report this feature to be similar (193). Diaz-Buxo reported higher scores in elderly patients on CAPD and home HD than in those on center HD (11).

ETHICAL ISSUES

The worldwide increase in the acceptance rate of elderly patients for dialysis suggests that in the early years when dialysis was limited, these persons were excluded. However now that health-care resources are becoming limited, the elderly are considered to be expendable, as demonstrated by the response of 452 directors of nephrology units to Kilner's survey (221). In his famous book, Setting Limits (222), Daniel Callahan provides the rationalization necessary to those who want to save the heath care system from bankruptcy by restricting services to the elderly. He recommends that society provide only minimal services to persons above a certain age. Callahan writes: "Dialysis represents precisely the kind of technology that should not be sought or developed in the future. It does not greatly increase the life expectancy (an average of only five years), and for most the gain is at the price of a doubtful or poor quality of life and an inability to achieve earlier levels of functioning" (222).

Those who propose to use age as a criterion upon which to base life-and-death decisions such as withholding or withdrawing dialysis, ignore the important differences between chronological and physiological age. The elderly are a heterogenous group and our failure to consider them as individuals constitute the discrimination of ageism. In its 1991 report, the Institute of Medicine (USA) supported the position that age should never be a criterion when it concluded, "... Chronological age was considered and explicitly rejected by the committee as a criterion of patient acceptance, since it does not measure the ability of individuals to benefit from a treatment" (223). The elderly stand to lose more than any other group in society when resources such as dialysis become restricted. Seniors and ESRD support groups do not lobby vigorously against the bias of ageism and elderly patients usually are passive. Nephrologists, as their patients' advocates, have an obligation to fight for the needs of the elderly.

REFERENCES

1. Oreopoulos DG: Who are the elderly? *Perit Dial Int*, 1994. In press
2. Nissenson AR: Peritoneal dialysis in geriatric patient: an overview and introduction. *Adv Perit Dial* 6 (Suppl): 1, 1990
3. Ismail N, Hakim RM, Patrikarea A, Oreopoulos DG: Renal replacement therapies in the elderly. *Am J Kidney Dis* 22: 759, 1993
4. Geerlings W, Tufveson G, Brunner FP, Ehrich JHH, Fassbinder W, Landais P, Mallick N, Margreiter R, Raine AEG, Rizzoni G, Selwood NC: Combined report on regular dialysis and transplantation in Europe XXI 1990. *Nephrol Dial Transplant* 6 (Suppl 4): 5, 1991
5. Walls J: Dialysis in the elderly. Some UK experience. *Adv Perit Dial* 6 (Suppl): 82, 1990
6. Brunner FP, Fassbinder W, Broyer M, Brynger H, Dykes SR, Ehrich JHH, Geerlings W, Rizzoni G, Selwood NH, Tufveson G, Wing AJ: Combined Report on Regular Dialysis and Transplantation in Europe XVIII 1987. *Nephrol Dial Tranplant* 4 (Suppl 2): 5, 1989
7. Blagg CR: Chronic renal failure in the elderly. in *Geriatric Nephrology*, edited by Oreopoulos DG, Boston, Martinus, Nijhoff, 1986, p 117
8. Porush JG, Faubert PF: Chronic renal failure. in *Renal Diseases in the Aged*, edited by Porush JG, Faubert PF, Boston Mass, Little Brown Co, 1991, p 285
9. Segoloni GP, Salomone M, Piccoli GB: CAPD in the elderly: Italian multicenter study experience. *Adv Perit Dial* 6 (Suppl): 41, 1990
10. Posen GA, Fenton SA, Arbus GS, Churchill DN, Jeffery JR: The Canadian experience with peritoneal dialysis in the elderly. *Adv Perit Dial* 6 (Suppl): 47, 1990
11. Diaz-Buxo JA, Adcock A, Nelms M: Experience with continuous cyclic peritoneal dialysis in the geriatric patient. *Adv Perit Dial* 6 (Suppl): 61, 1990
12. Piccoli G, Quarello F, Salomone M, Bonello F, Pacitti A, Beltrame G, Piccoli GB, Vercellone A: Dialysis in the elderly: comparison of different dialytic modalities. *Adv Perit Dial* 6 (Suppl): 72, 1990
13. Williams P, Ruch Dr: Geriatric polypharmacy. *Hosp Prac* 21: 104, 1986
14. Gentile DE and the Geriatric Advisory Committee: Peritoneal dialysis in geriatric patients: a survey of clinical practices. *Adv Perit Dial* 6 (Suppl): 29, 1990
15. Nissenson AR: Chronic peritoneal dialysis in the elderly. *Geriatric Nephrol Urol* 1: 3, 1991
16. Mattern WD, McGaghie WC, Rigby RJ, Nissenson AR, Dunham CB, Khayrallah MA: Selection of ESRD treatment: an international study. *Am J Kidney Dis* 13: 457, 1989
17. Schwab SJ, Buller GL, McCann RL, Bollinger RR, Stickel DL: Prospective evaluation of a Dacron cuffed hemodialysis catheter for prolonged use. *Am J Kidney Dis* XI: 166, 1988
18. Ballard JL, Bunt TJ, Malone JM: Major complications of angioaccess surgery. *Am J Surg* 164: 229, 1992

19. Winsett OE, Wolma FJ: Complications of vascular access for hemodialysis. *Southern Med* 78: 513, 1985

20. Wing AJ, Brunner FP, Brynger H: Combined report on regular dialysis and transplantation in Europe, IX 1978. *Proc Eur Dial Transplant Assoc* 13: 2, 1979

21. Hinsdale JG, Lipcouritz GS, Hoover EL: Vascular access in the elderly: results and perspectives in a geriatric population. *Dial Transplant* 14: 560, 1985

22. Didlake R, Raju S, Rhodes RS, Bower J: Dialysis access in patients older than 65 years. in *Vascular Access for Hemodialysis – II*, edited by Sommer BG, Henry ML, Boston, Mass, WL Gore and Assoc, Inc, 1991, p 166

23. Ghantous WN, Bailey GL, Zschaeck D, Hampers CL, Merrill JP: Long-term hemodialysis in the elderly. *Trans Am Soc Artif Intern Organs* 17: 125, 1971

24. Rathaus M, Bernheim JL: Are your elderly patients good candidates for dialysis? *Geriatrics* 33: 56, 1978

25. Pourchez T, Moriniere P, St Priest A: Outcome of vascular access for hemodialysis in the elderly (> 75 years). (Abstract) *Proc Eur Dial Transplant Assoc* 27: 160, 1990

26. Feldman HI, Held PJ, Hutchinson JT, Stoiber E, Hartigan MF, Berlin JA: Hemodialysis vascular access morbidity in the United States. *Kidney Int* 43: 1091, 1993

27. Tang IY, Vrahnos D, Valaitis D, Lau AH: Vascular access thrombosis during recombinant human erythropoietin therapy. *ASAIO J* 38: M528, 1992

28. de Peterson H, Swanson AG: Acute encephalopathy occurring during hemodialysis. *Arch Intern Med* 113: 877, 1964

29. Kennedy AC Linton AL, Eaton JC: Urea levels in cerebrospinal fluid after hemodialysis. *Lancet* 1: 410, 1962

30. Kennedy AC, Linton AL, Luke RG, Renfrew S, Dinwoodie A: Electro-encephalographic changes during haemodialysis. *Lancet* 1: 790, 1964

31. Rosen SM, O'Connor K, Shaldon S: Haemodialysis disequilibrium. *Br Med J* 2: 672, 1964

32. Maher JF, Schreiner GE: Hazards and complications of dialysis. *N Engl J Med* 273: 370, 1965

33. Wakim KG: Predominance of hyponatremia over hypoosmolality in simulation of the dialysis disequilibrium syndrome. *Mayo Clin Proc* 44: 433, 1969

34. Arieff AI, Massry SG, Barrientos A, Kleeman CR: Brain water and electrolyte metabolism in uremia: effects of slow and rapid hemodialysis. *Kidney Int* 4: 177, 1973

35. Bernard DR: Hypotension, bradycardia, and syncope during hemodialysis. *ASAIO J* 2: 42, 1979

36. Rathaus M, Kortets Z, Bernheim J: Results of regular hemodialysis treatment in the elderly: a retrospective study. *Dial Transplant* 9: 1015, 1980

37. Jacobs C, Diallo A, Bales EH, Nectoux M, Etienne S: Maintenance haemodialysis treatment in patients aged over 60 years. Demobrahic Profile, clinical aspects and outcome. *Proc Eur Dial Transplant Assoc* 21: 477, 1984

38. Walker PJ, Ginn HE, Johnson HK, Stone WJ, Teschan PE, Latos D, Stouder D, Lamberth EL, O'Brien K: Long-term hemodialysis for aptients over 50. *Geriatrics* 31: 55, 1976

39. Henrich WL: Dialysis considerations in the elderly patient. *Am J Kidney Dis* 16: 339, 1990

40. Parfrey PS, Harnett JD, Griffiths SM, Gault MH, Barre P: Congestive heart failure in dialysis patients. *Arch Intern Med* 148: 1519, 1988

41. Harnett JD, Parfrey PS, Griffiths SM, Gault MH, Barre P, Gutmann RD: Left ventricular hypertrophy in end-stage renal disease. *Nephron* 48: 107, 1988

42. Ross EA, Nissenson AR: Dialysis-associated hypoxemia: insights into pathophysiology and prevention. *Semin Dial* 1: 33, 1988

43. Gruppo Emodialisi e Pathologie Cardiovascolari: Multicentre, cross-sectional study of ventricular arrhythmias in chronically haemodialysed patients. *Lancet* 305, 1988

44. Ebel H, Saure B, Laage Ch, Dittmar A, Keuchel M, Stellwaag M, Lange H: Influence of computer-modulated profile haemodialysis on cardiac arrhythmias. *Nephrol Dial Transplant* Suppl 1: 165, 1990

45. Kimura, K, Tabei K, Asano Y, Hosoda Saichi: Cardiac arrhythmias in hemodialysis patients. *Nephron* 53: 201, 1989

46. Fantuzzi S, Caico S, Amatruda O, Cervini P, Abu-Turky H, Baratelli L, Donati D, Gastaldi L: Hemodialysis-associated cardiac arrhythmias: a lower risk with bicarbonate. *Nephron* 58: 196, 1991

47. Wizemann V, Kramer W, Funke T, Schutterle G: Dialysis-induced cardiac arrhythmias: fact or fiction? *Nephron* 39: 356, 1985

48. Weber H, Schwarzer C, Stummvoll HK, Joskowics, Wolf A, Steinback K, Kaindl F: Chronic hemodialysis: high risk patients for arrhythmias? *Nephron* 37: 180, 1984

49. Marzegalli M, Bernasconi M, Potenza S, Caprari M, Regalia F, Fiorista F, Vendemia F: Incidence, prognosis and therapy of cardiac arrhythmias in dialysis patients. *Contrib Nephrol* 61: 181, 1988

50. Niwa A, Taniguchi K, Ito H, Nakagawa S, Takeuchi J, Sasaoka T, Kanayama M: Echocardiographic and Holter findings in 321 uremic patients on maintenance hemodialysis. *Japan Heart J* 26: 403, 1985

51. Capuano A, Sepe V, Cianfrone P, Castellano T, Andreucci VE: Cardiovascular impairment, dialysis strategy and tolerance in elderly and young patients on maintenance haemodialysis. *Nephrol Dial Transplant* 5: 1023, 1990

52. Kessler M, Hoen B, Mayeux D, Hestin D, Fontenaille C: Bacteremia in patients on chronic hemodialysis: a multicenter prospective survey. *Nephron* 64: 95, 1993

53. Berman SJ, Hess JR, Burns JA, Sugihara JG, Wong ECG, Wong AW, Siemsen AW: Morbidity of infection in chronic hemodialysis. *Dial Transplant* 8: 324, 1979

54. Dobkin JF, Miller MH, Steigbigel NH: Septicemia in patients on chronic hemodialysis. *Annals Intern Med* 88: 28, 1978

55. USRDS Annual Data Report 1991: III. Incidence and causes of treated ESRD, IV. methods of ESRD treatment, V. survival probabilities and causes of death. *Am J Kidney Dis* 18 (Suppl 2): 30, 1991

56. Fenton SSA, Desmeules M, Jeffery JR, Corman JL: Dialysis therapy among elderly patients; data from the Canadian Organ Replacement Register, 1981–1991, edited by Khanna R, Nolph KD, Prowant B, Twardowski ZJ, Oreopoulos, *Adv Perit Dial* 9: 124, 1993

57. Talalla A, Halbrook H, Barbour BH, Kurze T: Subdural hematoma associated with long-term hemodialysis for chronic renal disease. *JAMA* 212: 1847, 1970

58. Weber DL, Reagan T, Leeds M: Intracerebral hemorrhage during hemodialysis. *New York State J Med* Jul 15: 1853, 1972.

59. Tietjen DP, Moore J, Gouge SF: Hemodialysis-associated acute subdural hematoma. *Am J Nephrol* 7: 478, 1987

60. Leonard CD, Shapiro FL: Subdural hematoma in regularly hemodialized patients. *Ann Intern Med* 82: 650, 1975

61. Stein MF, Cimino JE, Brescia MJ: Subdural hematoma during hemodialysis. *New York State J Med* 70: 2022, 1970

62. Shepherd AMM, Stewart WK, Wormsley KG: Peptic ulceration in chronic renal failure. *Lancet* I: 1357, 1973

63. Zuckerman GR, Cornette GL, Clouse RE, Harter HR: Upper gastrointestinal bleeding in patients with chronic renal failure. *Ann Intern Med* 102: 588, 1985

64. Doherty CC: Gastrointestinal bleeding in dialysis patients. *Nephron* 63: 132, 1993

65. Chester AC, Rakowski TH, Argy WP, Ciacalone A, Schreiner GE: Hemodialysis in the eight and ninth decades of life. *Arch Intern Med* 139: 1001, 1979

66. Thomas Flynn C, Chandran PKG: Renal failure and angiodysplasia of the colon. *Ann Intern Med* 103: 154, 1985

67. Lipschutz DE, Easterling RE: Spontaneous perforation of the colon in chronic renal failure. *Arch Intern Med* 132: 758, 1973

68. Stacy W, Sica D: Dialysis of the elderly patient. in *Geriatric Nephrology and Urology*, edited by Zawada ET, Sica DA, Littleton, MA, PSG Publishing, 1985, p 229

69. Tapson JS, Rodger RSC, Mansy H, Elliot RS, Ward MK, Wilkinson R: Renal replacement therapy in patients aged over 60 years. *Postrad Med J* 63: 1071, 1987

70. Oreopoulos DG: Geriatric Nephrology. (Editorial) *Perit Dial Bull* 4: 197, 1984

71. Kaye M, Pajel PA, Somervile PJ: Four year's experience with CAPD in the elderly. *Perit Dial Bull* 3: 17, 1983

72. Nissenson AR, Diaz-Buxo JA, Adcock A, Nelms M: Peritoneal dialysis in the geriatric patients. *Am J Kidney Dis* 16: 335, 1990

73. Nissenson AR, Gentile DE, Soderblom RE, Brax C: Peritoneal dialysis in the elderly. in *Geriatric Nephrology*, edited by Oreopoulos DG, The Netherlands, Dordrecht, Martinus Nijhoff, 1986, p 147

74. Schleifer CR: Peritoneal dialysis in nursing homes. *Adv Perit Dial* 6 (Suppl): 29, 1990

75. Maiorca R, Cancarini GC, Camerini C, Manili L, Brunori G: Modality selelction for the elderly: medical factors. *Adv Perit Dial* 6 (Suppl): 18, 1990

76. Rowe JW: Health care of the elderly. *N Engl J Med* 312: 827, 1985

77. Benevent D, Benzakour M, Peyronnet P, Legarde C, Leroucx-Robert C, Charmes JP: Comparison of continuous ambulatory peritoneal dialysis and hemodialysis in the elderly. *Adv Perit Dial* 6 (Suppl): 68, 1990

78. Gorben-Brennan N, Kliger AS, Finkelstein FO: CAPD therapy for patients over 80 years of age. *Perit Dial Int* 13: 140, 1993

79. Soreide R, Svarstad E, Versen BM: CAPD in patients above 70 years of age. *Adv Perit Dial* 7: 73, 1991

80. Nissenson AR, Gentile DE, Soderblom R: CAPD in the elderly: Southern California/Southern Nevada experience. *Adv Perit Dial* 6 (Suppl): 51, 1990

81. Nolph KD, Lindblad AS, Novak JW, Steinberg SM: Experiences with the elderly in the National CAPD Registry. *Adv Perit Dial* 6 (Suppl): 33, 1990

82. Gokal R: CAPD in the elderly-European and UK experience. *Adv Perit Dial* 6 (Suppl): 38, 1990

83. Williams AJ, Nicholl JF, El-Nahas AM, Moorehead PS, Plant MJ, Brown CB: Contiuous ambulatory peritoneal dialysis and haemodialysis in the elderly. *Q J Med* 274: 215, 1990

84. Nebel M, Finke K: CAPD in patients over 60 years of age. *Adv Perit Dial* 6 (Suppl): 56, 1990

85. Ramos J, Gokal R, Siamopoulos K, Ward MK, Wilkinson R, Kerr DNS: CAPD: three years experience. *Q J Med* 52: 165, 1983

86. Maiorca R, Cancarini GC, Camerini C, Brunori G, Manili L, Movilli E, Feller P, Mombelloni S: Is CAPD competitive with haemodialysis for long term treatment of uraemic ptients? *Nephrol Dial Transpl* 4: 244, 1989

87. Lupo A, Cancarini G, Catizone L, Cocchi R, de Vecci A, Viglino G, Salomone M, Segoloni G, Giangrande A, Limido A, Conte F, Lonati F, Piccoli G, Quarrelo F: Comparison of survival in CAPD and haemodialysis: a multicenter study. *Adv Perit Dial* 8: 136, 1992

88. de Fitjter CWH, Oe PL, Nauta JJP, van der Meulen J, ter Wee PM, Snoek FJ, Donker AJM: A prospective, randomized study comparing the peritonitis incidence of CAPD and Y-connector (CAPD-Y) with continuous cyclic peritoneal dialysis (CCPD). *Adv Perit Dial* 7: 186, 1991

89. Strauss FG, Holmes DL, Dennis RL, Nortman DF: Pre-spiking dialysate bags: improved peritonitis prevention in patients on CAPD. *Adv Perit Dial* 7: 193, 1991

90. Grutzmacher P, Tsobanelis T, Bruns M, Kurz P, Hoppe D, Vlachojannis J: Decrease in peritonitis rate by integrated disconnect system in patients on continuous ambulatory peritoneal dialysis. *Perit Dial Int* 13 (Suppl 2): S326, 1993

91. Port FK, Held PH, Nolph KD, Turenne MN, Wolfe RA: Risk of peritonitis and technique failure by CAPD connection technique: a national study. *Kidney Int* 42: 967, 1992

92. Maiorca R, Cancarini G, Brunori G, Vonesh E, Manili L, Camerini C, Zubani R, Salomone M, Gaggiotti M, Cristinelli L: Continuous ambulatory peritoneal dialysis in the elderly. *Perit Dial Int* 13 (Suppl 2): S165, 1993

93. O'Brien M, Zimmerman S: Comparison of peritoneal dialysis and hemodialysis in the elderly. *Adv Perit Dial* 6 (Suppl): 65, 1990

94. Holley JL, Bernardini J, Perlmutter JA, Piraino B: A comparison of infection rates among older and younger patients on continuous peritoneal dialysis. *Perit Dial Int* 14: 77, 1994

95. Ross C, Rutsky EA: Dialysis modality selection in the elderly patient with end-stage renal disease: advantages and disadvantages of peritoneal dialysis. *Adv Perit Dial* 6 (Suppl): 11, 1990

96. Joglar F, Saade M: Improved overall survival of elderly patients on peritoneal dialysis. *Adv Perit Dial* 7: 63, 1991

97. Shah GM, Sabo A, Nguyen T, Juler GL: Peritoneal catheter: a comparative study of column disk and Tenckhoff catheters. *Artif Kidney Dialysis* 13: 267, 1990

98. Holley JL, Bernardini J, Piraino B: Risk factors for tunner infections in continuous peritoneal dialysis. *Am J Kidney Dis* 18: 344, 1991

99. Tzamaloukas AH, Murata GH, Fox L: Peritoneal catheter loss and death in continuous ambulatory peritoneal dial-

ysis peritonitis: correlation with clinical and biochemical parameters. *Perit Dial Int* 13 (Suppl 2): S338, 1993

100. Atkins R, Wood C: Hyperlipedemia in CAPD. *Perit Dial Int* 13 (Suppl 2): S415, 1993

101. Nakagawa S, Ozawa K: Protective aspects for atherogenesis and lipid abnormalities in CAPD patients. *Perit Dial Int* 13 (Suppl 2): S418, 1993

102. Panarello G, Calianno G, De Baz H, Signori D, Capelletti P, Tesio F: Does CAPD induced hypercholesterolemia? *Perit Dial Int* 13 (Suppl 2): S421, 1993

103. Pafrey S, Harnett JD, Barre PE: The natural history of myocardial disease complications in renal failure. *J Am Soc Nephrol* 2: 2, 1991

104. Rostand SG, Brunzell JD, Cannon RO III, Victor RG: Cardiovascular complication in renal myopathy. *J Am Soc Nephrol* 2: 1053, 1991

105. London GM, Guerin AP, Marchais SJ, Metivier F: Cardiomyopathy in end-stage renal failure. *Semin Dial* 2: 102, 1989

106. Drueke T, Le Pailleur C, Zingraff J, Jungers P: Uremic Cardiomyopathy and Pericarditis. *Adv Nephrol* 9: 33, 1980

107. Horton JDF, Gelfand MC, Sherber HS: Natural history of asymptomatic pericardial effusions in patients on maintenance hemodialysis. *Proc Dial Transplant* 7: 76, 1977

108. Vlachojannis J, Kurz P, Hoppe D: CAPD in elderly patients with cardiovascular risk factors. *Clin Nephrol* 30: S13, 1988

109. D'Amour ML, Dufresne LR, Morin C, Slaughter D: Sensory nerve conduction in chronic uremic patients during the first six months of hemodialysis. *Can J Neurol Sci* 11: 269, 1984

110. Knoll O, Dierker E: Detection of uremic neuropathy by reflex response latency. *J Neurol Sci* 47: 305, 1980

111. Bazzi C, Pagani C, Sorgato G, Albonico G, Fellin G, D'Amico G: Uremic polyneuropathy: a clinical and electrophysiological study in 135 short and long term hemodialyzed patients. *Clin Nephrol* 35: 176, 1991

112. Alfrey AC, LeGendre GR, Kaehny WD: The dialysis encephalopathy syndrome. *N Engl J Med* 29: 184, 1976

113. Arieff AI, Cooper JD, Armstrong D, Lazarowitz VC: Dementia, renal failure, and brain aluminum. *Ann Intern Med* 90: 741, 1979

114. Dewberry FL, McKinney TD, Stone WJ: The dialysis dementia syndrome: report of fourteen cases and review of the literature. *ASAIO J* 3: 102, 1980

115. Alfrey AC, Mishell JM, Burks J, Contiguglia SR, Rudolph H, Lewin E, Holmes JH: Syndrome of dyspraxia and multifocal seizures associated with chronic hemodialysis. *Trans Am Soc Artif Int Organs* 18: 257, 1972

116. Chui HC, Damasio AR: Progressive dialysis encephalopathy ('dialysis dementia'). *J Neurol* 222: 145, 1980

117. Ladurner G, Wawschinek O, Pogglitsch H, Petek W, Urlesberger H, Holzer H: Neurophysiological findings and serum aluminum in dialysis encephalopathy. *Eur Neurol* 21: 335, 1982

118. Schreeder MT, Favero MS, Hughes JR, Petersen NJ, Bennett PH, Maynard JE: Dialysis encephalopathy and aluminum exposure: an epidemiologic analysis. *J Chronic Dis* 36: 581, 1983

119. Mach JR, Korchik WP, Mahowald MW: Dialysis dementia. *Clin Geriatric Med* 4: 853, 1988

120. Mehta R: Encephalopathy in chronic renal failure appearing before the start of dialysis. *Canad Med Assoc J* 120: 1112, 1979

121. Oreopoulos DG: Chronic peritoneal dialysis. *Clin Nephrol* 9: 165, 1978

122. Smith DB, Lewis JA, Burks JS et al.: Dialysis encephalopathy in peritoneal dialysis. *JAMA* 244: 365, 1980

123. Alfrey AC: Dialysis encephalopathy. *Kidney Int* 29: S53, 1986

124. Piraino BM, Rault R, Dominguez JH, Puschett JB: Renal Osteodystrophy in patients on hemodialysis for more than 10 years. *Mineral Electrolyte Metab* 12: 390, 1986

125. Sherrard DJ, Hercz G, Pei Y, Maloney NA, Greenwood C, Manuel A, Saiphoo C, Fenton SS, Segre GV: The spectrum of bone disease in end-stage renal failure. An evolving disorder. *Kidney Int* 43: 436, 1993

126. Piraino B, Chen T, Cooperstein L, Segre G, Puschett J: Fractures and vertebral bone mineral density in patients with renal osteodystrophy. *Clin Nephrol* 30: 57, 1988

127. Schaab PC, Murphy G, Tzamaloukas AH, Hays MB, Merlin TL, Eisenberg B, Avasthi PS, Worrell RV: Femoral neck fractures in patients receiving long-term dialysis. *Clin Orthopaedics Related Res* 260: 224, 1990

128. Faugere MC, Arnala IO, Ritz E, Malluche HH: Loss of bone resulting from accumulation of aluminum in bone of patients undergoing dialysis. *J Lab Clin Med* 107: 481, 1986

129. Eisenberg B, Tzamaloukas AH, Murata GH, Elliott TM, Jackson JE: Factors affecting bone mineral density in elderly men receiving chronic in-center hemodialysis. *Clin Nucl Med* 16: 30, 1991

130. Onishi S, Andress DL, Maloney NA, Coburn JW, Sherrard DJ: Beta$_2$-microglobulin deposition in bone in chronic renal failure. *Kidney Int* 39: 990, 1991

131. Kleinman KS, Coburn JW: Amyloid syndromes associated with hemodialysis. *Kidney Int* 35: 567, 1989

132. Koch KM: Dialysis-related amyloidosis. *Kidney Int* 41: 1416, 1992

133. Di Raimondo CR, Stone WJ: Beta-2-microglobulin in peritoneal dialysis patients. (Abstract) *Kidney Int* 31: 197, 1987

134. Tielemans C, Dratwa M, Bergmann P, Goldman M, Flamion B, Collart F, Wens R: Continuous ambulatory peritoneal dialysis *vs* haemodialysis: a lesser risk of amyloidosis? *Nephrol Dial Transplant* 3: 291 1988

135. Gagnon RF, Somerville P, Thomson DMP: Circulating form of Beta-2-microglobulin in dialysis patients. *Am J Nephrol* 8: 379, 1988

136. Mistry CD, O'Donoghue DJ, Nelson S, Gokal R, Ballardie FW: Kinetic and Clinical Studies of B2-microglobulin in continuous ambulatory peritoneal dialysis: influence of renal and enhanced peritoneal clearances using glucose polymer. *Nephrol Dial Transplant* 5: 513, 1990

137. Van Ypersele De Strihou C, Jadoul M, Malghem J, Maldague B, Jamart J, The Working Party on Dialysis Amyloidosis. Effect of dialysis membrane and patient's age on signs of dialysis-related amylouidosis. *Kidney Int* 39: 1012, 1991

138. Brown E, Soldano L, Hendler E: Dialysis-related amyloidosis during peritoneal dialysis. *Trans Am Soc Artif Intern Organ* 36: 17, 1990

139. Jadoul M, Noel H, van Ypersele de Strihou C: B₂-microglobulin amyloidosis in a patient treated exclusively by continuous ambulatory peritoneal dialysis. *Am J Kidney Dis* 15: 86, 1990

140. Gagnon RF, Lough JO, Bourgouin PA: Carpal tunnel syndrome and amyloidosis associated with continuous ambulatory peritoneal dialysis. *Canad Med Assoc J* 139: 753, 1988

141. Digenis GE, Davidson G, Dombros NV, Katz A et al.: Destructive spondyloarthropathy in a patient on continuous ambulatory peritoneal dialysis for 13 years. *Perit Dial Int* 13: 228, 1993

142. Mitch WE: Uremia and the control of protein metabolism. *Nephron* 49: 89, 1988

143. Hakim RM, Levin NL: Malnutrition in hemodialysis patients. *Am J Kidney Dis* 21: 125, 1993

144. Piccoli G, Bonello F, Massara C, Salomone M et al.: Death in conditions of cachexia: The price for the dialysis treatment of the elderly? *Kidney Int* 43: S282, 1993

145. Shimomura A, Tahara D, Azekura H: Nutritional improvement in elderly CAPD patients with additional high protein foods. *Adv Perit Dial* 9: 80, 1993

146. Movilli E, Mombelloni S, Gaggiotti M, Maiorca R: Effect of age on protein catabolic rate, morbidity, and mortality in uraemic patients with adequate dialysis. *Nephrol Dial Transplant* 8: 735, 1993

147. Cancarini G, Costantino E, Brunori G et al.: Nutritonal status in long-term CAPD patients. *Adv Perit Dial* 8: 84, 1992

148. Abdo F, Clemente L, Davy J et al.: Nutritonal status and efficiency of dialysis in CAPD and CCP patients. *Adv Perit Dial* 9: 76, 1993

149. Nolph KD, Moore HL, Prowant B et al.: Age and indices of adequacy and nutrition in CAPD patients. *Adv Perit Dial* 9: 87, 1993

150. Simon PO, Ang KS, Cam G et al.: Indices of adequate dialysis in paitents hemodialyzed with AN 69 membrane. *Kidney Int* 43: S291, 1993

151. Blazer D: Depression in the elderly. *N Engl J Med* 320: 164, 1989

152. Soskolne V, De-Nour AK: The psychosocial adjustment of patients and spouses to dialysis treatment. *Soc Sci Med* 29: 497, 1989

153. Rideout EM, Rodin GM, Littlefield CH: Stress, social support, and symptoms of depression in spouses of the medically ill. *Int J Psychiatr Med* 20: 37, 1990

154. Holley JL, Finucane TE, Moss AH: Dialysis patients' attitudes about cardiopulmonary resuscitation and stopping dialysis. *Am J Nephrol* 9: 245, 1989

155. Fukunishi I: Psychosomatic aspects of patients on hemodialysis. 1. With special reference to aged patients. *Psychother Psychosom* 52: 51, 1989

156. Kennedy SH, Craven JL, Roin GM: Major depression in renal diaysis patients: an open trial of antidepressant therapy. *J Clin Psychiatr* 50: 60, 1989

157. Iordanidis P, Alivanis P, Iakovidis A et al.: Psychiatric and psychosocial status of elderly patients undergoing dialysis. *Perit Dial Int* 13 (Suppl 2): S192, 1993

158. McKevitt PM, Jones JF, Marion RR: The elderly on dialysis: physical and psychosocial functioning. *Dial Transplant* 15: 130, 1986

159. Carney RM, Wetzel RD, Hagberg J, Goldberg AP: The relationship between depression and aerobic capacity in hemodialysis patients. *Psychosom Med* 48: 143, 1986

160. Rodin G, Voshart K: Depressive symptoms and function impairment in the medically ill. *Gen Hosp Psychiatr* 9: 251, 1987

161. Stout JP, Gokal R, Hillier VF et al.: Quality of life of high-risk and elderly dialysis patients in the UK. *Dial Transplant* 16: 674, 1987

162. Peterson RA, Kimmel PL, Sacks CR et al.: Depression, perception of illness and mortality in patients with end-stage renal disease. *Int J Psychiatr Med* 21: 343, 1991

163. Husebye DG, Westlie L, Styrvoky TJ, Kjellstrand CM: Psychological, social, and somatic prognostic indicators in old patients undergoing long-term dialysis. *Arch Intern Med* 147: 1921, 1987

164. Koch U, Muthny FA: Quality of life in paitents with end-stage renal disease in relation to the method of treatment. *Psychother Psychosom* 54: 161, 1990

165. Muthny FA, Koch U: Quality of life of patients with end-stage renal failure: a comparison of hemodialysis, CAPD, and transplantation. *Contrib Nephrol* 89: 265, 1991

166. Gokal R: Quality of life in patients undergoing renal replacement therapy. *Kidney Int* 43: S23, 1993

167. Fox E, Peace K, Neale TJ, Morrison RBI, Hatfield PJ, Mellsop G: 'Quality of life' for patients with end-stage renal failure. *Renal Failure* 13: 31, 1991

168. Kutner NG, Brogan DJ: Assisted survival, aging, and rehabilitation needs: comparison of older dialysis patients and age-matched peers. *Arch Phys Med Rehabil* 73: 309, 1992

169. Kjellstrand C, Koppy K, Umen A, Nestrud S, Westlie L: Hemodialysis of the elderly. in *Geriatric Nephrology*, edited by Oreopoulos DG, Boston, Martinus Nijhoff, 1986, p 135

170. Horina JH, Holzer H, Reisinger EC, Krejs GJ, Neugebauer JS: Elderly patients and chronic haemodialysis. *Lancet* 339: 183, 1992

171. Moody H, Moody C, Szabo E, Kjellstrand C: Are old dialysis patients happy and can they fend for themselves or not? (Abstract) *XIIth Int Congr Nephrol* 518: 1993

172. Wolcott DL, Nissenson AR, Landsverk J: Quality of life in chronic dialysis patients: factors unrelated to dialysis modality. *Gen Hosp Psychiatr* 10: 267, 1988

173. Barany P, Pettersson E, Konarski-Svensson JK: Long-term effects on quality of life in haemodialysis patients of correction of anaemia with erythropoietin. *Nephrol Dial Transplant* 8: 426, 1993

174. Kutner NG, Brogan D: Expectations and psychological needs of elderly dialysis patients. *Int Aging Human Devel* 31: 239, 1990

175. Deniston OL, Carpentier-Alting P, Kneisley J, Hawthorne VM, Port FK: Assessment of quality of life in end-stage renal disease. *Hlth Serv Res* 24: 555, 1989

176. Seedat YK, Machintosh CG, Subban JV: Quality of life for patients in an end-stage renal disease programme. *S Afric Med J* 71: 500, 1987

177. Morgan BW: The relationship between chronological age and perceived quality of life of hemodialysis patients. *Am Nephrol Nurs Assoc J* 17: 63, 1990

178. Tsai TJ, Tsai HF, Chen YM, Hsieh BS, Chen WY, Yen TS: CAPD in patients unable to do their own bag change. *Perit Dial Int* 11: 356, 1991

179. Gutman RA, Blumenkrantz MJ, Chan YK, Barbour GL, Gandhi VC, Shen FH, Tucker T, Murawski B, Coburn JW, Kurtis FK: Controlled comparison of hemodialysis and peritoneal dialysis: veterans administration multicenter study. *Kidney Int* 26: 459, 1984

180. Brogan D, Kutner NG, Flagg E: Survival differences among older dialysis aptients in the Southest. *Am J Kidney Dis* 20: 376, 1992

181. Chazan JA, Shemin D, London MR, Pono L: The clinical course of 62 octagenarians on chronic hemodialysis (CHD): when is old too old? (Abstract) *J Am Soc Nephrol* 4: 339, 1993

182. US Renal Data System, 1991: VII Hospitalization for dialysis patients. *Am J Kidney Dis* 18 (Suppl 2): 74, 1991

183. Rotellar E, Lubelza RA, Rotellar C, Martinez-Camps E, Alea MV, Valls R: Must patients over 65 be haemodialyzed. *Nephron* 41: 152, 1985

184. Suh H, Wadhwa NK, Cabralda T, Sokunbi D, Solomon M: Peritoneal dialysis in elderly end-stage renal disease patients. *Adv Perit Dial* 9: 134, 1993

185. Wadhwa NK, Suh H, Cabralda T, Sokol E, Sokumbi D, Solomon M: Peritoneal dialysis with trained home nurses in elderly and disabled end-stage renal disease patients. *Adv Perit Dial* 9: 130, 1993

186. Verbeelen D, De Neve W, Van der Niepen P, Sennesael J: Dialysis in patients over 65 years of age. *Kidney Int* 43: S27, 1993

187. Khan IH, Catto GRD, Edward N, Fleming LW, Henderson IA, MacLeod AM: Influence of coexisting disease on survival on renal-replacement therapy. *Lancet* 341; 415, 1993

188. Gentil MA, Carriazo A, Pavon MI, Rosado M, Castillo D, Ramos B, Algarra GR, Tejuca F, Banasco VP, Milan JA: Comparison of survival in continuous ambulatory peritoneal dialysis and hospital haemodialysis: a multicentric study. *Nephrol Dial Transplant* 6: 444, 1991

189. Michael C, Khayat R, Viron B, Siohan P, Mignon F: Early mortality during renal replacement therapy (RRT) in ESRD patients 65 years and over. (Abstract) *J Am Soc Nephrol* 4: 369, 1993

190. Laurent G, Calemard E, Charra B: Long dialysis: a review of 15 years in one center, 1968–1983. *Proc Eur Dial Transplant* 20: 122, 1983

191. Port FK, Novello AC, Wolfe RA: Outcome of treatment modalities for geriatric end-stage renal disease. in *Geriatric Nephrology*, edited by Michelis MF, Davis BB, Preuss HG, New York, NY, Field Rich and Associates, 1986, p 149

192. Husebye DG, Kjellstrand CM: Old patients and uremia. Rates of acceptance to and withdrawal for dialysis. *Int J Artif Organs* 10: 166, 1987

193. Westlie L, Umen A, Nestrud S, Kjellstrand C: Mortality morbidity and life satisfaction in the very old dialysis patient. *Trans Am Soc Artif Intern Organs* 30: 21, 1984

194. Schaefer K, Asmus G, Quellhorst E, Pauls A, von Herrath D: Optimum dialysis treatment for patients over 60 years with primary renal disease. Survival data and clinical results from 242 patients treated either by hemodialysis or hemofiltration. *Proc Eur Dial Transplant Assoc Eur Renal Assoc* 21: 510, 1985

195. Panarello G, De Baz H, Cecchin E, Tesis F: Dialysis for the elderly: survival and risk factors. *Adv Perit Dial* 5: 49, 1989

196. Mion C, Oules R, Canaud B, Mourad G, Slingeneyer A, Branger B, Granolleras C, Al Sabadani B, Florena P, Chouzenoux R, Maurice F, Issautier R, Flavier JL, Polito C, Saumier F, Marty L, Fontanier P, Emond C, Ramtoolah H, de Cornellissen F, Huchard G, Fitte H, Boudet R: Maintenance dialysis in the elderly: a review of 15 years' experience in Languedoc-Roussilon. *Proc Eur Dial Transplant Assoc Eur Renal Assoc* 21: 490, 1984

197. Park MS, Lee HB: Outcome of dialysis in the elderly. *Geriatr Nephrol Urol* 1: 173, 1992

198. Loew H: Die dauerdialysebehandlung in hoheren lebensalter (Long-term dialysis treatment in advanced age). *Z Gerontol* 20: 52, 1987

199. Odaka M: Mortality in chronic dialysis aptients in Japan. *Am J Kidney Dis* 15: 410, 1990

200. Brunner FP, Selwood NH: Results of renal replacement therapy in Europe 1980–1987. *Am J Kidney Dis* 15: 384, 1990

201. Posen GA, Jeffrey JR, Fenton SSA, Arbus GS: Results from the Canadian Renal Failure Registry. *Am J Kidney Dis* 15: 397, 1990

202. Disney APS: Dialysis treatment in Aurstralia, 1982–1988. *Am J Kidney Dis* 15: 384, 1990

203. Canadian Organ Replacement Register: 1989 Report Kidney Foundation of Canada

204. Held PJ, Brunner F, Odaka M, Garcia JR, Port FK, Gaylin DS: Five-year survival for end-stage renal disease patients in the United States, Europe and Japan 1982 to 1987. *Am J Kidney Dis* 15: 451, 1990

205. Mailloux LU, Bellucci AG, Napolitano B, Mossey RT, Wilkes BM, Bluestone PA: Death by withdrawal from dialysis: a 20 years clinical experience. *J Am Soc Nephrol* 3: 1631, 1993

206. Hirsch DJ: Death from dialysis termination. *Nephrol Dial Transplant* 4: 41, 1989

207. Holley JL: Patient-reported symptoms and adequacy of dialysis as measured by creatinine clearance. *Perit Dial Int* 13 (Suppl 2): S219, 1993

208. Arkouche W, Delawari E, My H, Laville M, Abdullah E, Traeger J: Quantification of adequacy of peritoneal dialysis. *Perit Dial Int* 13 (Suppl 2): S215, 1993

209. CANUSA Peritoneal Dialysis Study Group. Canada-USA (CANUSA) multicentre study of peritoneal dialysis adequacy: description of the study population and preliminary results. *Adv Perit Dial* 8: 88, 1992

210. Held Philip, Levin NW, Bovbjerg RR, Mauly MV, Diamond LH: Mortality and duration of hemodialysis treatment. *JAMA* 265: 871, 1991

211. Delmez JA, Windus DW, The St. Louis Nephrology Study Group: Hemodialysis prescription and delivery in a metropolitan community. *Kidney Int* 41: 1023, 1992

212. Raja RM, Ijelu G, Goldstein M: Influence of Kt/V and protein catabolic rate on hemodialysis morbidity. *ASAIO J* 38: M179, 1992

213. De Alvaro F, Bajo MA, Alvarez-Ude F, Vigil A, Molina A, Coronel F, Selgas R: Adequacy of peritoneal dialysis: Does KT/V have the same predictive value as in HD? A multicenter study. *Adv Perit Dial* 8: 93, 1992

214. Brandes JC, Plering WF, Beres JA, Blumenthal SS, Fritsche C: Clinical outcome of continuous ambulatory peritoneal dialysis predicted by urea and creatinine kinetics. *J Am Soc Nephrol* 2: 1430, 1992

215. Shimomura A, Tahara D, Azekura H, Matsuo H, Kamo M: Key factors to improve survival of elderly patients on CAPD. *Adv Perit Dial* 8: 166, 1992

216. Brunori G, Camerini C, Cancarini G, Manili L, Sandrini S, Movilli E, Galvani G, Maiorca R: Hospitalization: CAPD versus hemodialysis and transplant. *Adv Perit Dial* 8: 71, 1992

217. Gokal R, Jakubowski C, King J, Hunt L, Bogle S, Baillod R: Outcome in aptients on continuous ambulatory peritoneal dialysis and hemodialysis: 4-year analysis of a prospective multicenter study. *Lancet* 2: 1105, 1987

218. Maiorca R, Vonesh E, Cancarini GC, Cantaluppi A, Manili L, Grunori G, Camerini C, Feller P, Strada A: A six-year comparison of patient and technique survivals in CAPD and HD. *Kidney Int* 34: 518, 1988

219. Lunde NM, Port FK, Wolfe RA, Guire KE: Comparison of mortality risk by choice of CAPD versus hemodialysis among elderly patients. *Perit Dial* 7: 68, 1991

220. Fassbinder FP, Brunner FP, Brynger H et al.: Combined report of regular dialysis and transplantation in Europe, XX, 1989. *Nephrol Dial Transplant* 6 (Suppl 1): 5, 1991

221. Kilner JF: Selecting patients when resources are limited: a study of US medical directors of kidney dialysis and transplantation facilities. *Am J Public Health* 78: 144, 1988

222. Callahan D: *Setting Limits: Medical Goals in an Aging Society*, New York, Simon and Schuster, 1987

223. Rothenberg LS: Withholding and withdrawing dialysis from elderly ESRD patients: Part 1 – a historical view of the clinical experience. *Geriatr Nephrol Urol* 2: 109, 1992

PREGNANCIES IN WOMEN ON RENAL REPLACEMENT THERAPY

ANTONY J. WING and JOCHEN H.H. EHRICH

INTRODUCTION

Successful pregnancy in a woman on renal replacement therapy (RRT) is an impressive demonstration of physiological well-being and emotional rehabilitation. It has been reported on more than a thousand occasions in women with functioning transplants, but far less frequently in those on haemodialysis and peritoneal dialysis.

Although women with renal failure have reduced fertility, many are capable of conception. Their physicians will need to know about the risks for mother and foetus so that they can give balanced advice about contraception and about termination of any pregnancy which occurs. Fortunately, there is now a consistent literature on the experience of pregnancy in patients on treatment for end-stage renal failure. In this chapter we review available reports, making particular use of those prepared by the EDTA-ERA Registry and, in the light of these, we discuss the appropriate management of women who are unfortunate enough to have end-stage renal failure during their reproductive years.

DEMOGRAPHY

Historical

Early anecdotal reports in single and groups of patients established that successful pregnancy could occur in the patient with a renal transplant. The first report was by Murray et al. in 1963 (1). The mother was the recipient of a renal graft donated by an identical twin and was not receiving immunosuppressive drugs. Delivery was by Caesarean section on 10 March 1958. In April and September 1966, two recipients of related but non-twin living donor transplants, receiving Azathioprine and Prednisolone as immunosuppression gave birth to normal infants by spontaneous vaginal delivery (2, 3). The following year the first successful pregnancy following transplantation of a cadaver kidney occurred in Canada (4). Subsequently, individual cases in Europe were documented (5–8) and a few small series presented (9–12). Golby reviewed experiences of centres reporting to the Human Kidney Transplant Registry in 1970 (13) and Nolan et al. (14) published information on 23 patients including two of their own and Rifle and Traeger presented an international survey in 1975 (15). Larger series of cases have now strengthened the information, highlighting the problems and trumpeting the successes (16, 17).

The first description of conception and successful delivery in a patient on chronic haemodialysis was by Confortini et al. (18) and further individual case reports followed (19–21). However, although pregnancy regularly occurs in dialysis patients, it is not so likely to reach a successful conclusion as in those with well functioning transplants.

The Registry of the EDTA-ERA has collected information on patients on RRT in 34 countries since 1965 and has, since its inception, recorded successful pregnancies. Annual reports have usually contained an update on the demography of cyesis in dialysed and transplanted women in Europe. Reports augmented by data from special pregnancy questionnaires have punctuated the regular updates. The early demography was summarised in 1980 (22), extended in 1986 (23) and reviewed with a case control study into the effects of pregnancy on transplant function in 1992 (24).

Conception in women on renal replacement therapy

In the early years of the EDTA Registry, a question on therapeutic and spontaneous abortion was asked on the individual patient questionnaire. In reviewing this data up till 1978, it was concluded that 0.9% of the 13,000 registered women of child-bearing age became pregnant at some time after commencing renal replacement therapy. However, therapeutic and spontaneous abortion rates were thought to be under-reported and not reliable, and the conception rate was probably much higher (22). A report from Saudi Arabia, drawn from 50% of the country's dialysis patients, found that 7.3% of married women aged less than 50 became pregnant during the time they were being treated with chronic dialysis (25). Hou reported a recent survey of American dialysis units and found that 1.5% of women of child-bearing age became pregnant over a two year period (26).

Successful pregnancies in women on dialysis

The outcome of pregnancy in women on dialysis has not been good. According to Hou (27) spontaneous abortion, stillbirth and neonatal death end 75–80% of pregnancies. In 1991 Davison reviewed 2,309 gestations in 1,594 transplanted patients and found that 40% of the pregnancies did not go beyond the first trimester. Rates of spontaneous abortion were similar to that in the population at large (approximately 16%), therapeutic abortions accounting for the rest.

Diagnosis of pregnancy is often delayed because of irregularity of the menstrual cycle in women on RRT and sometimes because the patient is reluctant to report a possible pregnancy to the physician, possibly fearing advice to terminate or remonstration because of failed contraception. Nausea and abdominal pain are not infrequent in dialysis patients and, for all these reasons, mean time of diagnosis has been reported at 16.5 weeks gestation (28). Urine pregnancy tests are useful in transplanted patients but not reliable in patients on dialysis. Serum level of the beta sub-unit of HCG may be borderline in dialysis patients who are not pregnant and may be elevated above the level usually commensurate with gestational age. Once the diagnosis is made or seems likely, ultrasound should be carried out to confirm it and to get a more reliable indication of gestational age.

In the first EDTA Registry report on this subject, only 23% of pregnancies that were not spontaneously or therapeutically terminated resulted in a surviving baby (22). Amongst the Saudi Arabian patients the rate was slightly higher at 26% (25). Successful outcome amongst the US patients was 21% but, when only those pregnancies occurring after 1990 are considered, then 52% of the babies survived (26). This suggests that either there was under-reporting of unsuccessful pregnancies or that results had improved, hopefully indicating better management.

Many of the patients who have been reported as delivering live children while on dialysis have either had some degree of residual renal function or have developed renal failure and commenced dialysis during their pregnancy. Acute renal failure in pregnancy was reviewed by Gruenfeld et al. (29) and Cattanes et al. (30) drew attention to the particular dangers of acute complications, such as cortical necrosis or haemolytic uraemic syndrome occurring in apparently healthy women during the last trimester of pregnancy. Naik et al. (31) reported a case of acute crescentic glomerulonephritis causing acute renal failure in pregnancy and successfully treated by haemodialysis and the development of acute on chronic renal failure is exemplified in the report by Leader et al. (32).

Case reports of dialytic support of acute renal failure which permitted the successful delivery of a live infant began to appear in the late '70s (33–35) and the first survey reported from the EDTA Registry emphasised that, in all the 16 successful pregnancies up till 1978 in women on dialysis, the mothers had some residual renal function (22).

Continuous ambulatory peritoneal dialysis has been performed successfully during pregnancy (36) and has also been shown to succeed in a pregnant diabetic (37). This mode of dialysis has been recently recommended as the primary approach in the management of severe renal insufficiency in pregnancy (38).

SUCCESSFUL PREGNANCIES IN WOMEN WITH RENAL TRANSPLANTS

Following successful kidney transplantation, renal, endocrine and sexual functions return and a large proportion of young female adults menstruate normally. About one in 50 women of child-bearing age, with a functioning graft, becomes pregnant (39). A large proportion of pregnancies end in spontaneous abortion or therapeutic termination, both of which are most likely in patients with hypertension, unstable or deteriorating graft function or ureteric obstruction. Successful pregnancies reported to the registries are, therefore, selected amongst patients with normal blood pressure, stable graft function and satisfactory urinary tract. Patients with live donor grafts are over-represented; 26% of births occurred in recipients of living donor grafts although these comprised only 14% of all transplants in women aged 15–44 (22).

Table 1 shows the number of successful pregnancies reported to the EDTA-ERA Registry up to the close of 1991. Births prior to 1979 and between 1979 and 1982 have been previously reported (22, 23) and are therefore aggregated. Births in the years 1983 to 1991 are shown separately. So far 1057 successful pregnancies have been confirmed by receipt of completed special questionnaires following initial announcement on the centre questionnaire. Only 95 pregnancies occurred in women on dialysis

Table 1. Successful pregnancies reported to the EDTA-ERA Registry up to the end of 1991, shown according to treatment status of mother

Mode of Treatment	Number of successful pregnancies											
	1965–1978 (22)	*1965–1982 (23)*	1983	1984	1985	1986	1987	1988	1989	1990	1991	Total 1965–1991
Transplanted	109	275	58	59	64	79	87	84	83	69	80	938
Dialysed	16	35	8	6	9	11	5	5	2	3	11	95
Not recorded			2	2	0	3	1	1	6	7	2	24
Total	125	310	68	67	73	93	93	90	91	79	93	1057

Table 2. Number and gender of children born alive to mothers on the EDTA-ERA Registry up to the end of 1991

Gender of Child	Number of children born alive											
	1965–1978 (22)	*1965–1982 (23)*	1983	1984	1985	1986	1987	1988	1989	1990	1991	Total 1965–1991
Male	54	142	40	33	40	45	51	40	48	44	48	531
Female	63	159	27	30	30	45	40	50	41	32	42	496
Not recorded	14	16	1	4	3	4	3	2	3	3	3	43
Total	131	317	68	67	73	94	94	92	92	80	93	1070

and, in 24 cases, the mode of treatment was not reported.

The 1057 pregnancies resulted in the births of 1070 children: there were five sets of twins and one of triplets. The gender was not recorded for 43 babies but, amongst those in whom it was, there was a marginal preponderance of male children (1.07:1.0) as shown in Table 2 (23).

Table 3 shows pregnancies reported to the Registry by country of birth. The UK, with 338 successful pregnancies, accounts for one-third of the total: other countries with active transplant programmes contribute an increasing percentage to the total. However, the proportion of transplanted females in the child bearing years (17–40) who gave birth varied between countries, being highest in the UK at 3%. Between 1977–86 it was about 0.5% in Western Germany, Italy, Denmark and France, between 0.5 and 1.0% in Sweden, Finland and Belgium, and 1.3% in Spain. When the two periods 1977–81 and 1982–86 were compared, these proportions remained unchanged in each respective country (Figure 1) and it was only in the period 1987–91 that the proportion of women having successful pregnancies increased in almost all countries.

In the United States of America, a National Transplantation Pregnancy Registry was established in 1991 to study pregnancy outcome in transplant recipients; an analysis of 325 pregnancies was reported in 1992 (41) and the outcomes of 154 pregnancies in cyclosporin treated female kidney transplant recipients was published in 1994 (17).

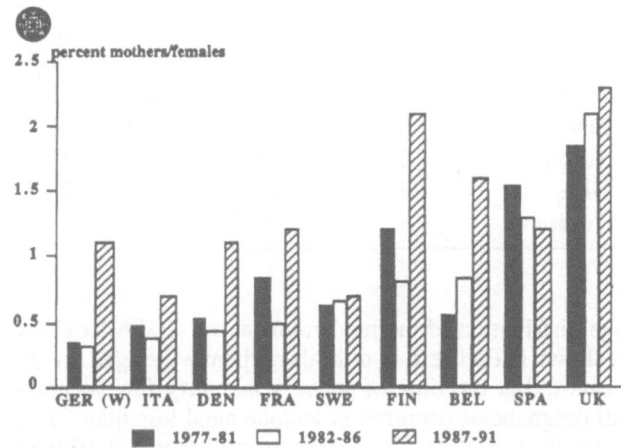

Figure 1. Successful pregnancies in Europe in 1977–81, 1982–86 and 1987–91 as a proportion of all females with a functioning graft aged 17–40 at the end of 1981, 1986 or 1991. EDTA-ERA Registry.

PREGNANCY

Maternal characteristics

Linking the pregnancy data with the corresponding EDTA patient questionnaire made it possible to study age, primary renal disease and time interval from grafting. The

Table 3. Successful pregnancies notified to the EDTA-ERA Registry up to the end of 1991, shown according to the country of treatment of the mother

Country	Number of successful pregnancies											Total 1965–1991
	1965–1978 (22)	1965–1982 (23)	1983	1984	1985	1986	1987	1988	1989	1990	1991	
Austria	1	3	0	1	0	1	4	2	2	1	1	15
Belgium	5	11	3	2	4	4	4	2	9	5	4	48
Cyprus	0	0	0	0	1	0	1	0	0	0	2	4
Czechoslovakia	3	7	0	0	0	2	1	1	3	5	1	20
Denmark	4	10	0	0	0	1	2	0	1	1	2	17
Egypt	0	0	0	1	0	2	1	0	0	0	0	4
Finland	9	12	0	3	1	1	2	2	1	3	5	30
France	14	42	16	4	7	11	10	15	11	12	16	144
Germany: East	2	6	1	0	3	4	3	1	0	0	2	20
Germany: West	3	13	2	3	11	· 2	6	10	12	6	7	72
Greece	2	9	0	2	0	0	0	1	0	1	0	13
Hungary	0	0	0	0	1	2	0	1	1	1	0	6
Ireland	3	3	1	1	1	2	2	3	2	2	1	18
Israel	2	2	0	0	1	5	2	1	1	0	0	12
Italy	7	17	2	4	2	3	3	9	4	3	3	50
Netherlands	1	5	2	0	0	1	0	4	4	1	1	18
Norway	1	4	1	0	1	2	5	2	2	1	3	21
Poland	0	1	0	0	1	1	2	3	0	2	8	18
Portugal	0	0	0	0	0	3	2	1	0	2	1	9
Spain	4	18	7	6	6	14	14	7	11	7	8	98
Sweden	9	15	2	2	6	2	3	0	0	5	0	35
Switzerland	4	6	0	1	0	0	1	1	2	1	2	14
Tunisia	0	0	0	1	0	1	1	0	1	0	1	5
Turkey	0	0	0	1	0	0	2	0	0	0	0	3
UK	47	116	25	33	27	29	23	23	23	18	21	338
Yugoslavia	4	6	1	2	0	0	0	1	1	1	4	16

age distribution of the mothers from the EDTA Registry is shown in Figure 2; two-thirds of them were aged 24–32 years old at the time of delivery and very few successful pregnancies occurred in women aged less than 21 or more than 40 (24). The youngest mother was a 19 year old transplant patient and the oldest a 42 year old woman on dialysis (23).

Comparison of the frequency of the main primary renal disease groups in 445 transplanted mothers and that in all transplanted women of child-bearing age (16–40) on the Registry files did not reveal any striking differences (Figure 3).

Some 40% of all deliveries took place during the third and fourth year after transplantation, with a small percentage reported during the first year and as late as nine or more years after transplantation (Figure 4). Similar findings are reported by the US Registry in which the mean age of conception was 26.8 ± 4.7 years amongst 264 pregnancies in 186 female kidney transplant recipients (42). The mean interval from date of transplant to conception was 4.0 ± 3.5 years (range < 1 year to 16.3 years). The data concerning outcomes suggest that shorter intervals from graft to pregnancy were associated with an increased risk to the live born infants who had a greater tendency towards very low birth weight and neonatal deaths.

The 1978 EDTA-ERA survey reported on clinical problems during pregnancies (22). A quarter of the mothers took anti-hypertensive drugs and the management of hypertension appeared to be particularly difficult in patients on dialysis. Extra haematinics were widely prescribed and the dialysis patients in those days, prior to the availability of erythropoietin, required frequent supportive blood transfusions. The early literature reported pre-eclampsia in about 30% of transplant patients compared with only 8% of healthy subjects (43). Some of

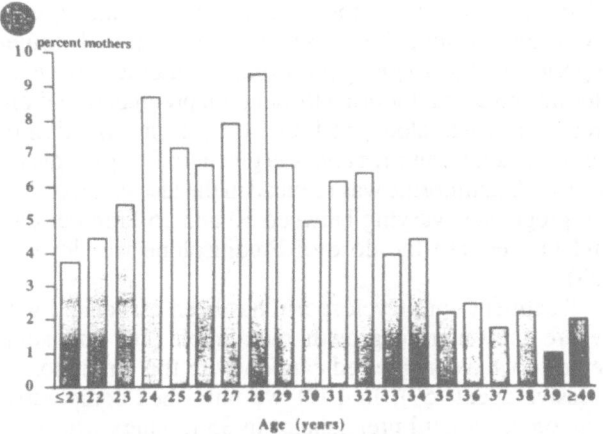

Figure 2. Proportional distribution of women with successful pregnancies according to age at delivery. EDTA-ERA Registry.

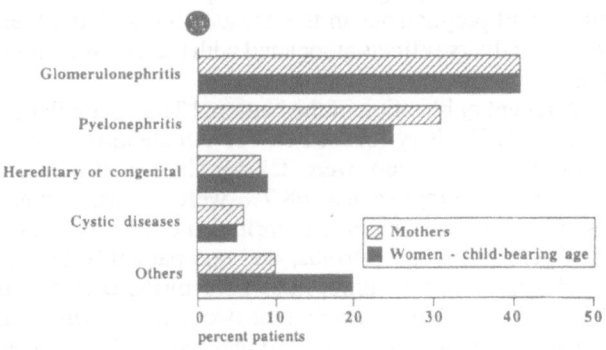

Figure 3. Primary renal diseases reported in patient questionnaire for 445 mothers who had at least one successful pregnancy whilst on renal replacement therapy; the prevalence of different primary renal diseases in this population is compared with that in all women of child bearing age (17–40 years) recorded alive on RRT. EDTA-ERA Registry.

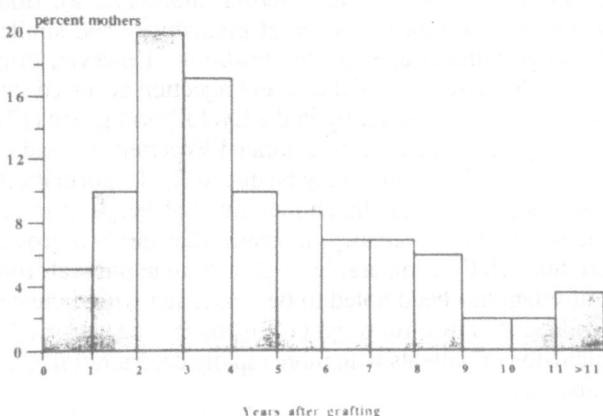

Figure 4. Time in years from graft to delivery shown as a proportion of transplanted women who had successful pregnancies. Nearly half of the deliveries occurred between 2 and 5 years after grafting. EDTA-ERA Registry.

the early series emphasised the common occurrence of respiratory and urinary infections (12).

Management of pregnancy in dialysis patients

Hou recommends that patients should monitor their own blood pressure since increases can occur abruptly and malignant hypertension may require intensive treatment (28). The patient must be dialysed to her dry weight, after which front line medications are alpha-methyldopa, which has been used for the longest time in pregnancy, beta-blockers and Labetalol. Hydralazine may be added to a regime containing a beta-blocker and is effective when given parenterally during hypertensive crisis prior to delivery. Although Nifedipine has been controversial, it undoubtedly works in pregnant women with resistant hypertension (44, 45). ACE inhibitors should not be used because of risk of increased foetal loss, bone deformities and neonatal oliguria (46, 47).

Many authors conclude that erythropoietin should be used for the treatment of anaemia (48, 49) in order to avoid all need for blood transfusions because of the risk of exacerbating hypertension and causing circulatory overload (50). A target haemoglobin of over 10 g/dl is thought desirable. Increased dose may be required during pregnancy (51, 52). Iron saturation should be monitored monthly and daily folate increased to 1.8 mg (53). Although teratogenicity has been noted in animals (54) the doses used were higher than those in clinical practice and erythropoietin is thought not to cross the placenta (53).

Intensive dialysis, with haemodialysis patients treated daily, has frequently been practised (19, 20), the rationale being that optimum dialytic control of the biochemistry must confer an advantage. Uraemia may be a contributory factor in the onset of premature labour, and in the development of pre-eclampsia (43). Dialysis patients with significant residual renal function certainly feature amongst those reported to have done well (22), and this is probably because they have the most liberal diet allowing adequate foetal nutrition. Daily haemofiltration might be the best of all possible regimens but would place heavy demands on the time of patients and staff. We are not aware whether it has ever been used in a pregnant woman with end-stage renal failure.

CAPD has the theoretical advantage over intermittent haemodialysis of metabolic stability and gradual fluid shifts. Until the third trimester the peritoneum is not embarrassed by the size of the gravid uterus. Small volume exchanges, best carried out by an automatic cycler, provide a satisfactory answer to the patient's difficulty in tolerating the increased intra-abdominal volume. Peritonitis must be avoided for it may precipitate delivery. Blood stained effluent may herald spontaneous abortion or abruptio placentae. Peritoneal changes can be interrupted for 24 hours while an extra peritoneal Caesarean section is carried out. Despite the theoretical advantages of peritoneal dialysis, the worldwide reported experience

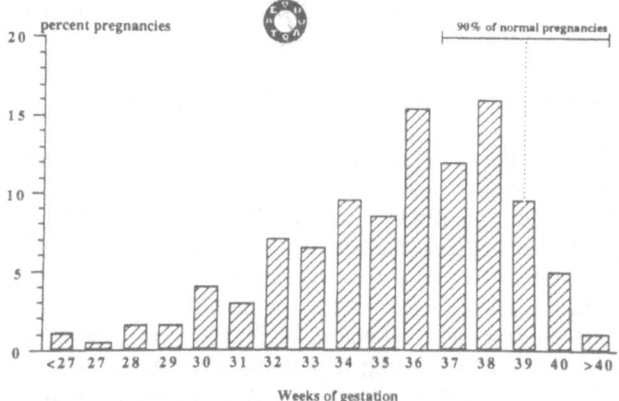

Figure 5. Length of gestation in weeks shown as a proportion of women on renal replacement therapy who had successful pregnancies. EDTA-ERA Registry.

of pregnancy on CAPD amounts to only 18 pregnancies in 17 women with an overall success of 67%, which is better than that reported for haemodialysis patients (27). Nevertheless, any assessment of results between the two methods of dialysis must take account of the tendency to report successes rather than failures.

It is rare for any pregnancy in a patient on RRT to go to term and, particularly in dialysed patients, there is always a risk of premature labour. Early home contraction monitoring is recommended from the mid second trimester. Premature labour can be controlled by beta-agonists, provided the patient is not hypertensive. Alternatively, Indomethacin may be given but, if use must be prolonged, then the foetus must be monitored by regular ultrasound to detect right heart dilatation (53). Magnesium has also been used but has its risks (55).

Management of pregnancy in transplanted patients

The EDTA-ERA Registry documents that the length of gestation for babies born to women on RRT was much shorter than in the normal population. Our first report gave an average duration of pregnancy of 35.6 weeks (range 24–43 weeks) in 103 pregnancies in transplanted women and 33.2 weeks (range 25–42 weeks) in 16 pregnancies in dialysed women (22). The length of gestation in 490 pregnancies reported to the end of 1986 is shown in Figure 5; only 50% of babies had a pregnancy of the normal 37 or more weeks duration compared to 90% in the general population.

The potential risk of foetal abnormality due to immunosuppressive drugs has encouraged some authors to reduce the dose of drugs. However, rejection episodes do not appear to have been a particular problem (43). The mothers of most of the babies born before the mid '80s were taking Prednisolone and Azathioprine. In 1982 the EDTA-

ERA Registry collected information on immunosuppressive drugs. Among the 44 pregnancies in grafted women reported to the Registry in 1982, 39 mothers were on steroids plus Azathioprine throughout pregnancy and one was on steroids alone; in four cases, no information on immunosuppressive regime was given. In five patients the dose of Azathioprine was reduced in the last six months of the pregnancy, varying between 50 and 150 mg per day; and in one case the dose of Prednisolone was lowered (23).

Treatment with Cyclosporin has been associated with severe intra-uterine growth retardation (56) and some reviewers have suggested caution with this immunosuppressive agent (57). In 1991 we published comparative data on successful pregnancies in 35 mothers who were treated with Cyclosporin alone ($n = 6$) or Cyclosporin combined with steroids ($n = 29$), and in 40 mothers on combinations of Azathioprine and steroids. Birth weight and duration of pregnancy both improved compared to successful pregnancies in the decade 1977–87 and there were no adverse effects associated with use of Cyclosporin (58).

A recent publication of the National Transplant Patient Pregnancy Registry focused on 115 female kidney transplant recipients who were taking Cyclosporin. Of a total of 154 pregnancies, 68.7% were on triple therapy with Cyclosporin, Azathioprine and steroids; 30.4% on Cyclosporin and steroids; and one patient (0.9%) on Cyclosporin and Azathioprine. Live births occurred in 68.6% of 156 babies (including two sets of twins) and the infants had a mean gestational age of 35.6 weeks (range 37–42 weeks) and a mean birth weight of 2407 g. Maternal risk factors for significantly lower birth weight infants were pre-pregnancy drug treated hypertension; a pre-pregnancy creatinine $\geq$ 1.5 mg/dl (130 μmol/l); and diabetes. The Cyclosporin recipients were contrasted retrospectively with 146 non-Cyclosporin recipients who were treated with Azathioprine and steroids (90.4%), Azathioprine alone (2.1%) and steroids alone (7.5%). Both groups had a high incidence of prematurity and similar mean gestational ages in the newborns. However, drug treated hypertension, diabetes and rejection occurred significantly more frequently in the Cyclosporin group (17). The high incidence of drug treated hypertension and of diabetes, both of which may be due to Cyclosporin itself, taken together with the shorter interval between transplantation and pregnancy, indicates that the two groups are not strictly comparable. A shorter time interval from transplant has been noted to be associated with a greater tendency to low birth weight (42), possibly because of the inclusion of patients with more rapidly deteriorating graft function.

Does pregnancy damage the renal transplant?

Early reports of changes in transplant function associated with pregnancy gave cause for concern. Damage to the transplant kidney appeared to occur both towards the end of pregnancy and also post-partum (59). Post-partum loss of transplant function may be acute due to haemolytic uraemic syndrome of which we know of two cases (22, 60) or a gradual remote consequence, difficult to dissociate from chronic rejection.

The increase in glomerular filtration rate characteristic of early pregnancy has also been shown to occur in transplant recipients (61) and it is conceivable that this could mask deterioration in graft function. Furthermore, hyperfiltration in a nephron population which is smaller than normal (because the graft is a single kidney) has a potential for glomerular damage and adverse effects on long-term graft function (57).

Some work on experimental animals is reassuring. Baylis and Reckelhoff (1991) documented that renal hyperfiltration induced in the pregnant rat was accompanied by parallel vasodilatation of both afferent and efferent arterioles so that glomerular pressure remains unaltered (62). Hyperfiltration maximised to enhance the insult did not cause any glomerular morphological damage or renal functional decrement (63).

Early attempts to study this problem in humans found a reduction in glomerular filtration rate in the third trimester with return to normal after delivery, while others found no change in graft function (2, 3). Case reports of permanent impairment of transplant function associated with pregnancy (6) and of progressive loss of function added to the concern over this issue. Twenty-one (17%) of the 125 mothers included in our first report (22) had some evidence of damage to their transplant during the pregnancy.

More recently, the Helsinki group have again emphasised that there may be considerable risks. They reported that they had 905 out of 2,248 patients transplanted between 1964–89 who had a potential for parenthood, 22 of the women gave birth to 30 children. In five patients, pregnancy accelerated the rate of decline of graft function, resulting in a loss of three grafts (64). The same authors have also reported a retrospective case control study to evaluate the long-term effects of pregnancy on graft function. For each of 24 patients who had 31 successful pregnancies, they chose as controls the two nearest female transplant recipients matched as to kidney disease, type of graft, immunosuppression, time from grafting, but non-pregnant. Mean increase in creatinine in patients was 44 ± 27 μmol/l at three months after delivery (one graft lost within one month) and 58 ± 31 μmol/l at one year after delivery. On the other hand, in controls the changes in creatinines were minimal (-3 ± 2 and $+5 \pm 4$ μmol/l respectively) and no grafts were lost. They conclude that the usual slow decline in transplant function with time is exemplified by their controls and that a rapid decline in function is not likely in stable transplants. Pregnancy was associated with loss of one graft and an "indisputably negative influence on serum creatinine in the surviving grafts" (65).

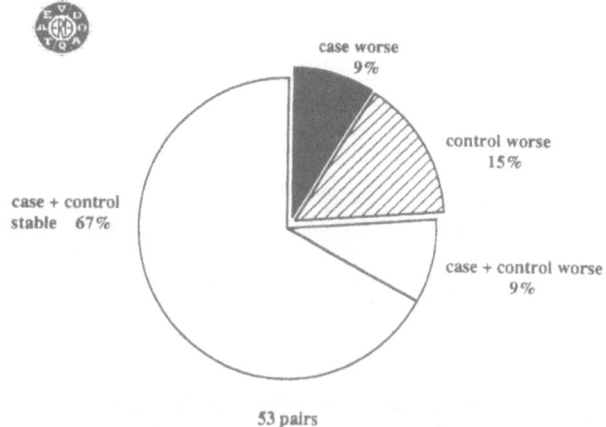

Figure 6.   Graft function according to creatinine level after successful pregnancy for cases and in controls as compared to graft function prior to pregnancy. EDTA-ERA Registry.

Sturgess and Davison (66) have recently reported a further single centre retrospective case control study to investigate the effect of pregnancy on long-term function of renal allografts. In their index group there were 34 pregnancies among 18 women; 24 of these pregnancies went beyond the first trimester. For each subject a control case was identified matched for date of transplantation ($\pm$ six months), age and primary renal disease. Plasma creatinine, its reciprocal or measured inulin clearance were used as parameters of renal function and were studied over a follow-up period of between 4 and 23 years. At outset, plasma creatinine was lower in the index group (94 ± 26 μmol/l) than in the controls (118 ± 31 μmol/l). By the end of follow-up, these increased by 19 and 8% respectively and were not significantly different; GFR in the index group and the controls decreased by 18 and 7% respectively. Mean arterial pressure in the pregnancy group decreased by 1% and in the controls increased by 5%. The authors concluded that there was no evidence of an adverse effect of pregnancy in renal allograft recipients on long-term renal function or the development of hypertension.

Our own contribution to this debate was another retrospective case control study (24). With the huge number of cases available on the Registry database, we were able to restrict our study to transplanted mothers with a successful pregnancy between November 1984 and January 1987; each test case was matched by computer with a control which had to come from the same country, to have been transplanted within the same year and from the same type of donor and to have identical code for plasma creatinine concentration prior to date of pregnancy. There were 40 pairs of fully matched controls and, by the inclusion of six pairs mismatched for sex and seven pairs mismatched for primary renal disease, the study eventually comprised 53 case control pairs. Since the Registry records plasma creatinine at the end of each year, the time intervals between

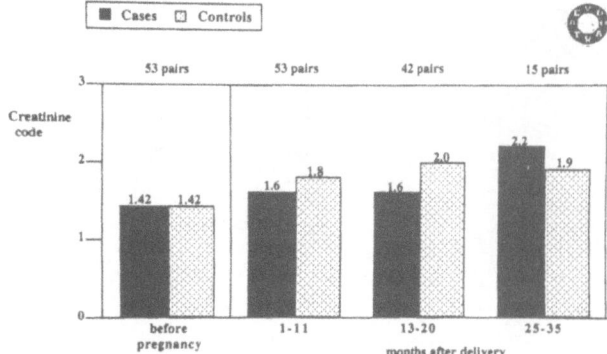

Figure 7. Mean of creatinine codes before and after successful pregnancy and in controls with a functioning graft. Graft failure was recorded for one case 31 months after delivery and for 5 controls 7–31 months after their respective case's date of delivery. EDTA-ERA Registry.

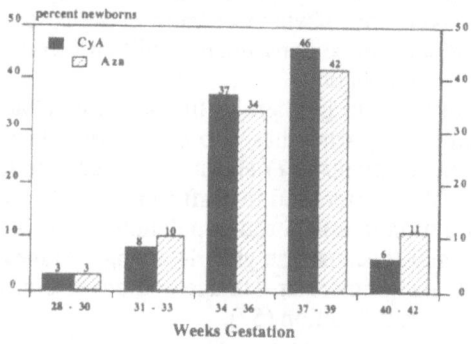

GESTATIONAL AGE
73 NEWBORNS OF TRANSPLANTED MOTHERS IN 1988

Figure 8. Gestational age of 73 newborns born to transplanted mothers in 1988, shown according to whether the mother received Cyclosporin or Azathioprine. EDTA-ERA Registry.

measurements and pregnancies were not all the same. Creatinine codes indicated improved or stable graft function in both test and control cases in 67% of the pairs. In 9% of the pairs the test case became worse but the control did not; in 15% the control deteriorated but the test case did not; in the remaining 9% renal function in both test and control cases deteriorated (Figure 6). A long-term effect of pregnancy on renal function was studied by calculating the average creatinine codes in test cases and controls at 1–11 months (53 pairs), 13–20 months (42 pairs) and 25–35 months (15 pairs) (Figure 7). Average value increased (i.e., deteriorated) with time but test cases did not do so more rapidly than controls.

In conclusion, the early anecdotal reports contained conflicting messages of gloom and triumph; these have been reinforced by three retrospective attempts at case control studies, each with its own defects and not all concurrent in their results. One suspects that at least one conflicting variable is escaping the analyses. Could this be the severity of hypertension? Hypertension has been shown to be associated with adverse perinatal outcome whether or not it was apparently satisfactorily controlled (67). Pregnancy causes an increase in GFR which, in the renal allograft, is super-imposed on the hyperfiltration already occurring in a single kidney (68). Hyperfiltration is partly the consequence of glomerular hypertension and it is this, rather than increased flow, which causes glomerular sclerosis (69).

Whether or not pregnancy aggravates primary glomerular disease has been one of the more enduring controversies in nephrology. Katz and Lindheimer summarised the data in 1985 and their conclusions have general relevance to this discussion: firstly, normotensive women with glomerular disease which is not part of a multi-system illness and with only mildly decreased renal function tolerate pregnancy well. Secondly, in gravidas with moderate degree of renal insufficiency at conception (e.g. serum

creatinine 1.5–2.5 mg/dl, 130–220 μmol/l) it appears that the prognosis for the foetus is reasonably good but renal function and blood pressure deteriorate in a substantial proportion and that in perhaps a third of them this is not reversible after the delivery. Thirdly, for women with more advanced renal failure (e.g., serum creatinine ≥ 3 mg/dl, 260 μmol/l), the likelihood of conception and of successful pregnancy is low, maternal risk and hazard to the foetus are both high. The long-term prognosis of the putative mother must be carefully considered. Fourthly, in any woman with kidney disease with hypertension at conception or early in pregnancy, this tends to follow an unpredictable course and must be treated particularly aggressively. Fifthly, the suggestion that some forms of glomerular disease are particularly vulnerable in pregnancy is unproven (with the probable exception of mesangiocapillary glomerulonephritis) (70).

DELIVERY

Pre-term delivery

Pre-term delivery (i.e., before week 37 of gestation) occurred in 52% of successful pregnancies in European patients up till the end of 1982 (23). Of births recorded by the Registry, 66% were premature (i.e., less than 37 weeks of gestation and yielding an infant of less than 2,500 g). Intervention for obstetric reasons is common in this group of patients, premature labour being more likely in patients with hypertension and renal insufficiency, and foetal distress due to placental insufficiency arising in patients with some degree of arterial disease.

Pregnancies managed in recent years have included fewer of short duration and there is no adverse effect of Cyclosporin. In 1988, 4% of European pregnancies lasted less than 31 weeks compared to 10% in 1984–86. The

⊙BIRTH WEIGHT

64 NEWBORNS OF TRANSPLANTED MOTHERS IN 1988

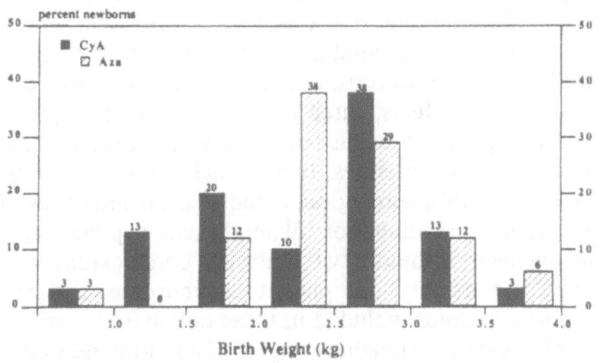

Figure 9. Birth weight of 64 babies born to transplanted mothers in 1988, shown according to whether the mother received Cyclosporin or Azathioprine. EDTA-ERA Registry.

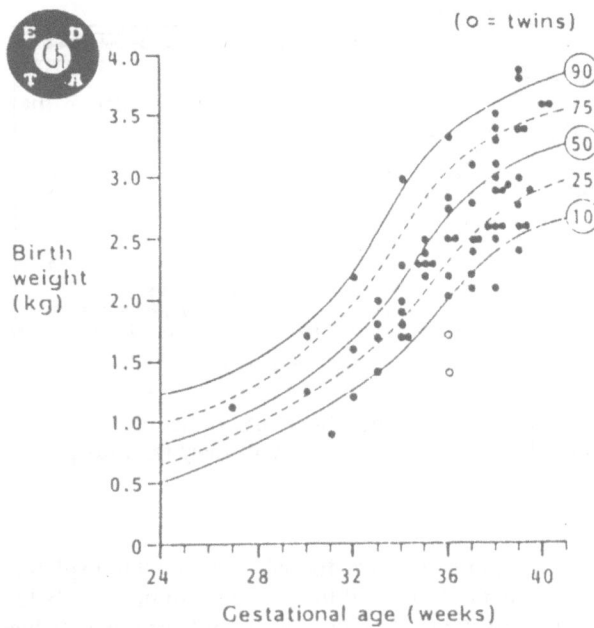

Figure 10. Birth weights of babies born to mothers on renal replacement therapy in 1983 according to gestational age. EDTA-ERA Registry.

gestational age of 73 babies born to mothers on RRT in 1988 is shown in Figure 8 according to whether the mothers received Azathioprine or Cyclosporin and it will be seen that the proportional distribution of the two groups shows no significant difference.

Caesarean section

A large survey of early American experience reported a Caesarean section rate of 25% (71); in the 1980 EDTA Registry review, 47% of recorded deliveries in transplant patients were by this method (22). A recent single centre report from California recorded 20 Caesarean sections in 25 deliveries (72). The indications were foetal distress in three, cephalopelvic disproportion in one, presumed pelvic outlet obstruction by the allograft in two, and the presence of active genital herpes in one. Repeat Caesarean sections were used in seven patients who had had one for their first delivery. For six cases no clear indication was recorded. However, according to one recent reviewer, spontaneous labour and vaginal delivery are generally considered to be the aim, albeit not commonly achieved (73). The transplanted kidney in the iliac fossa does not obstruct the birth canal, nor is ureteric compression by the descending foetal head a major problem.

INFANTS

Birth weights

The 1986 EDTA-ERA Registry review recorded a mean birth weight of 2.6 kg in 265 babies born to transplanted mothers, and of 1.8 kg in 30 babies born to dialysed mothers. These mean values have shown no trend to increase (23). Amongst babies born in 1988 in Europe the mean

birth weight was 2.6 kg ± 0.6 SD in 41 babies born to mothers on Azathioprine and 2.3 kg ± 0.7 SD in 36 babies born to mothers on Cyclosporin (74) (Figure 9). This difference was not significant.

Observations collected by the National Transplant Pregnancy Registry in the United States were similar (17). Mean birth weight amongst live born infants of Cyclosporin treated mothers was 2407 g and amongst those of Azathioprine treated mothers it was 2684 g. The proportion of babies with a low birth weight (< 2500 g) was 49.5% in Cyclosporin treated mothers and 39.1% in Azathioprine treated mothers. Maternal hypertension and diabetes appeared to be risk factors contributing to significantly lower birth weights.

The EDTA-ERA Registry determined the relationship between gestational age and birth weight for all babies born in 1983 (Figure 10); almost all fell between the 10th and 90th percentile for the normal population (75), suggesting that the newborns were small mainly because they were premature (24).

Neonatal mortality

Of the 500 newborns reported to the EDTA-ERA Registry between 1977 and 1986, nine died in the first month of life (1.8%); eight of these had a birth weight of less than 1.8 kg. The reported causes of death were acute respiratory distress syndrome (3), sudden unexplained death (2), malformation (2), intracerebral haemorrhage (1) and prolapsed cord (1). Elsewhere (76) neonatal mor-

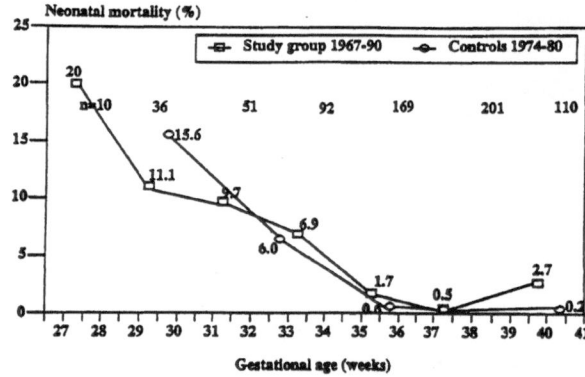

Figure 11. Neonatal mortality of 669 babies born to mothers on renal replacement therapy (control study from Koops et al. 1982 (78)).

tality is reported as 2.8% for babies from all transplanted mothers but only 1.2% if the serum creatinine was below 160 μmol/l, 5.5% if above 160 μmol/l. Amongst babies of dialysed mothers it is estimated at 10% (76).

Neonatal mortality in 669 first children reported to the EDTA-ERA Registry was related to prematurity (Figure 11) (77), falling to its minimum at 37 weeks and being very close to neonatal mortality rates for gestational age in the general population (78). High neonatal mortality in various reported series of babies is due to the excess proportion of infants who are pre-term.

Congenital abnormalities

Between 1982 and 1986, the Registry requested information on the follow-up pregnancy mini questionnaire about any chromosome studies which had been performed. Two cases were reported: one child had a translocation abnormality also present in the mother (23). In the 1978 survey, 16 children had undergone chromosomal analysis and chromatid breaks were discovered in two. Of 16 children studied elsewhere, 11 were found to have structural chromosome abnormalities (5, 79, 80), which had usually disappeared by one year of age.

Azathioprine in large doses has been shown to be teratogenic in some experimental animals (81). In Europe, prior to 1986, 12 heterogeneous congenital abnormalities were recorded in babies born to transplant mothers taking Azathioprine and two in offspring of dialysed mothers (23). Transplanted mothers who gave birth to babies with malformations included in the 1978 survey were taking a significantly greater dose of Azathioprine than those who had normal children (22).

Cyclosporin in high dose has also been shown to induce fetotoxicity in the rat, but does not appear to be associated with an increased risk of congenital abnormality in clinical studies. Preliminary data from the EDTA-ERA Registry on 35 babies was reassuring (24). In the USA there was a lower incidence of complications and

neonatal death reported in 107 newborns of Cyclosporin recipients compared with 207 non-Cyclosporin recipients (17). There is no over representation of any particular abnormality in either the American or European reports. Twenty-seven congenital abnormalities were reported in 500 European newborns, amongst which were five congenital heart defects, three urinary tract malformations, two hypospadias, four gastrointestinal tract abnormalities, three CNS abnormalities, two cranial abnormalities and single cases of haemangioma frontalis, medullary cystic disease, bilateral club foot, bilateral cataract, pigeon chest and agenesis of thumb, two umbilical cord vessels, 'congenital cytomegaly' and phenytoin syndrome. The large number of babies included in these collaborative studies permit the conclusion that congenital abnormalities occur with no more than a marginally increased frequency in children born to mothers on renal replacement therapy compared with the general population (24).

Steroids in the doses given to women with stable transplants have negligible risk to the foetus although lymphoid, thymic and adrenal hypoplasia are recorded (23). Congenital viral infections with cytomegalovirus (82) and hepatitis B (83) are also a hazard.

Breast feeding

The concentration of Azathioprine and its metabolites in breast milk is low (84). Information on breast feeding was collected by the EDTA-ERA Registry between 1979 and 1982. Twenty-nine of 186 (16%) babies were breast fed and no adverse comments were recorded. Cyclosporin passes into the breast milk to at least the same level as in the mother's blood and, therefore, mothers taking Cyclosporin should not breast feed their infants.

Multiple pregnancies

There was some suggestion in earlier literature that multiple pregnancies might occur with increased frequency in transplanted patients (23). Twin pregnancies were included in relatively small series reported by Sciarra et al. (12) and Lower et al. (85). There was one set of twins among 86 births collected by Rifle and Traeger (15) and four in the series reported by Rudolph et al. (43). The EDTA-ERA Registry has recorded six multiple pregnancies in 1057 successful pregnancies between 1967 and 1991 (Tables 1 and 2) including one triple pregnancy which has been separately reported (86). This represents a multiple pregnancy rate of one in 176 pregnancies, no different from that in the general population.

Repeated pregnancies

The 820 successful pregnancies in 718 women on renal replacement therapy reported by the EDTA-ERA Registry until 1989 includes 99 mothers who had two, and three who had three successful pregnancies. Of these 102 mothers, 96 went through all their pregnancies on the same graft, 87 being first grafts and nine being second. The others were re-transplanted after their first pregnancy. The mean age of the women was 21 years ± 5 SD at start of renal replacement therapy, 23 years ± 5 SD at first transplantation and 27 ± 5 SD at time of first delivery. 22% of them had live donor grafts (77).

There seems to be no greater risk to mother or foetus in subsequent pregnancies compared to the first. One mother has had five pregnancies and one abortion after transplantation without deterioration of graft function (87). However, neonatal mortality was calculated at 3.8% for repeated pregnancies in transplanted mothers.

CONCLUSIONS

More than 100 reports have been published in international literature concerning pregnancies in women on renal replacement therapy. Over 1000 babies have been born, mostly to women with functioning transplants. This is the best possible proof of physiological well being and psychological rehabilitation from end-stage renal failure. However, data on unsuccessful pregnancies that terminate in miscarriage or therapeutic abortion are incomplete.

Women of child-bearing age should be given appropriate counsel. If they wish to avoid the disturbance and sadness of uncompleted pregnancies, they must take contraceptive precautions. Because of coincident hypertension, it is probable that mechanical rather than hormonal methods will be advised. Failure to raise this issue with female patients leaves them vulnerable to accidental pregnancy.

If a woman treated by dialysis or transplantation is anxious to have a child, then her best opportunity arises following successful transplantation, and particularly if live donor transplantation is available. Only 2.3% of successful pregnancies in women in Europe have occurred on dialysis. Organisation of optimum dialysis represents a considerable 'tour de force' and many of the successes have occurred in patients with significant residual renal function, conception often antedating the need for dialysis. The baby is likely to be premature and has a high risk (10%) of neonatal death.

However, following transplantation the opportunity for successful pregnancy is greater. Most nephrologists would advise that pregnancy should not be embarked upon until two years of good transplant function have been achieved. If the plasma creatinine is below 160 μmol/l, the patient does not have diabetes or hypertension requiring drug therapy, then the outcome so far as mother's transplant function and the infant's birth weight and neonatal survival are concerned is close to normal. Risk of congenital abnormality is no more than marginally increased compared to the normal population.

The risk of pregnancy to graft function cannot be totally discounted. Two out of the three case control studies were reassuring; the third was not, and there are uncomfortable anecdotes. The long-term impact requires further study. Kidney grafts deteriorate with time and it is difficult to be certain that this long-term graft loss rate has not been accelerated by pregnancy. When the mother returns to dialysis or requires re-transplantation or dies, the child she bore so courageously is disadvantaged.

We have observed a striking but consistent difference between countries in the frequency of pregnancies in transplanted women. One third of the pregnancies reported in Europe have occurred in the UK. The proportions of transplanted women of child-bearing age in each country who had a successful pregnancy did not substantially increase from the mid seventies to the mid eighties. This suggests that the advice given by doctors and nurses differs from country to country. There could be more consistency in professional wisdom.

ACKNOWLEDGEMENTS

We gratefully acknowledge the collaboration of the directors of European renal units for the return of their data without which the EDTA-ERA Registry could not function. Financial support of the Registry is listed in our annual reports published in *Nephrology Dialysis and Transplantation* and we thank the Editor of this journal for permission to reproduce Figures 1–10.

REFERENCES

1. Murray JE, Reid DE, Harrison JH, Merrill JP: Successful pregnancies after human renal transplantation. *New Engl J Med* 269: 341, 1963
2. Board JA, Lee HM, Draper DA, Hume DM: Pregnancy following kidney homo-transplantation from a non-twin. *Obstet Gynecol* 29: 318, 1967
3. Kaufman JJ, Dignam W, Goodwin WE, Martin DC, Goldman R, Maxwell MH: Successful normal childbirth after kidney homo-transplantation. *JAMA* 200: 162, 1967
4. Caplan RM, Dossetor JB, Maughan GB: Pregnancy following cadaver kidney homo-transplantation. *Am J Obstet Gynecol* 106: 644, 1970
5. Gevers RH, Hintzen AHJ, Kalff MW et al.: Pregnancy following kidney transplantation. *Eur J Obstet Gynaecol* 1: 147, 1971
6. Horbach J, Van Liebergen F, Mastboom J, Wijdeveld P: Pregnancy in a patient after cadaveric renal transplantation. *Acta Med Scand* 194: 237, 1973
7. Robertson JG, Cockburn F, Woodruff M: Successful pregnancy after cadaveric renal transplantation. *J Obstet Gynaecol Br Commonw* 81: 777, 1974
8. Jacob ET, Grunstein S, Shapira Z, Berant M, Better OS, Boner G: Successful pregnancy in a recipient of a cadaver kidney allograft. *Isr J Med Sci* 10: 206, 1974
9. Merkatz IR, Schwartz GH, David DS, Stenzel KH, Riggio RR, Whitsell JC: Resumption of female reproductive

function following renal transplantation. *JAMA* 216: 1949, 1971

10. Merrill LK, Board JA, Lee HM: Complications of pregnancy after renal transplantation including a report of spontaneous uterine rupture. *Obstet Gynecol* 41: 270, 1973

11. Penn I, Makowski EL, Harris P: Parenthood following renal transplantation. *Kidney Int* 18: 221, 1980

12. Sciarra JJ, Toledo-Preyra LH, Bendel RP, Simmons RL: Pregnancy following renal transplantation. *Am J Obstet Gynecol* 123: 411, 1975

13. Golby M: Fertility after renal transplantation. *Transplantation* 10: 201, 1970

14. Nolan GH, Sweet RL, Laros RK, Roure CA: Renal cadaver transplantation followed by successful pregnancies. *Obstet Gynecol* 43: 732, 1974

15. Rifle G, Traeger J: Pregnancy after renal transplantation: an international survey. *Transplant Proc* 7 (Suppl 1): 723, 1975

16. Davison JM: Renal transplantation and pregnancy. *Am J Kidney Dis* 9: 374, 1987

17. Armenti VT, Ahlswede KM, Ahlswede BA, Jarrell BE, Moritz MJ, Burke JF: National Transplant Registry: outcomes of 154 pregnancies in Cyclosporine-treated female kidney transplant recipients. *Transplantation* 57: 502, 1994

18. Confortini P, Galanti G, Ancona G, Giongo A, Bruschi E, Lorenzini E: Full term pregnancy and successful delivery in a patient on chronic haemodialysis. in *Proceedings of the European Dialysis and Transplant Association*, edited by Cameron JS, Pitman Medical, London, 1971, p 74

19. Unzelman RF, Alderfer GR, Chojnacki RE: Pregnancy and chronic hemodialysis. *Trans Am Soc Artif Intern Organs* 19: 144, 1973

20. Ackrill P, Goodwin FJ, Marsh FP, Stratton D, Wagman H: Successful pregnancy in patients on regular dialysis. *Br Med J* 2: 172, 1975

21. Rigenbach M, Renger B, Beauvais P, Imbs JF, Eschbach J, Frey G: Grossesse et accouchement d'un enfant vivant chez une patiente traitée par hémodialyse iterative. *J Urol Nephrol (Paris)* 84: 360, 1978

22. Registration Committee of the European Dialysis and Transplant Association: Successful pregnancies in women treated by dialysis and kidney transplantation. *Br J Obstet Gynaecol* 87: 839, 1980

23. Challah S, Wing AJ, Broyer M, Rizzoni G: Successful pregnancies in women on regular dialysis treatment and women with a functioning transplant. in *The Kidney in Pregnancy*, edited by Andreucci VE, Amsterdam, Martinus Nijhoff, 1986, p 185

24. Rizzoni G, Ehrich JH, Broyer M et al.: Successful pregnancies in women on renal replacement therapy: report from the EDTA Registry. *Nephrol Dial Transplant* 7: 279, 1992

25. Souqiyyeh MZ, Huraib SO, Mohd. Saleh AG et al.: Pregnancy in chronic hemodialysis patients in the kingdom of Saudi Arabia. *Am J Kidney Dis* 19: 235, 1992

26. Hou SH: Frequency and outcome of pregnancy in women on dialysis. *Am J Kidney Dis* 23: 60, 1994

27. Hou S: Pregnancy and birth control in dialysis patients. *Dial Transplant* 23: 22, 1994

28. Hou S, Grossman SD: Pregnancy in chronic dialysis patients. *Seminars in Dialysis* 3: 224, 1990

29. Gruenfeld JP, Ganeval D, Bournerias F: Acute renal failure in pregnancy. *Kidney Int* 18: 179, 1980

30. Cattaneo AA, Belghiti D, Milliez J, Plovin PF, Sobel AT: Renin, hypertension et grossesse, III: risque des néphropathies au cours de la grossese. *Nouv Presse Med* 11: 1791, 1982

31. Naik RB, Clark AD, Warren DT: Acute proliferative glomerulonephritis with crescents and renal failure in pregnancy successfully managed by intermittent haemodialysis: case report. *Brit J Obstet Gynaecol* 86: 819, 1979

32. Leader L, Strasburg ER, Baillie P, Keeton RD: Haemodialysis in pregnancy: a case report. *S African Med J* 53: 871, 1978

33. Cole EH, Bear RA, Steinberg W: Acute renal failure at 24 weeks of pregnancy: a case report. *Can Med Assoc J* 122: 1161, 1980

34. Hensel A, Pauls A, von Herrath D, Schaefer K: Successful hemodialysis for acute renal failure in late pregnancy. *Am J Nephrol* 2: 98, 1982

35. Kopsa H, Schmidt P, Friedrich F et al.: Spontangeburt eines lebensfähigen Kindes bei erfolgreicher Haemodialysebehandlung einer Schwangerschafts-pyelonephritis mit akuter Oligo-anurie. *Schweiz Med Wochenschr* 108: 999, 1978

36. Cattran DC, Benzie RJ: Pregnancy in a continuous ambulatory peritoneal dialysis patient. *Peritoneal Dial Bull* 3: 13, 1983

37. Kioki EM, Shaw KM, Clarke AD et al.: Successful pregnancy in a diabetic patient treated with continuous ambulatory peritoneal dialysis. *Diabetes Care* 6: 298, 1983

38. Jakobi P, Ohel G, Szylman P et al.: Continuous ambulatory peritoneal dialysis as the primary approach in the management of severe renal insufficiency in pregnancy. *Obstet Gynecol* 79: 808, 1992

39. Lau J, Scott JR: Pregnancy following renal transplantation. *Clin Obstet Gynecol* 28: 339, 1985

40. Geerlings W, Tufveson G, Brunner FP et al.: Combined report on regular dialysis and transplantation in Europe, XXI, 1990. *Nephrol Dial Transplant* 6 (Suppl 4): 5, 1991

41. Armenti VT, Ahlswede KM, Ahlswede BA, Mortiz MJ, Jarre BE, Burke JF: The National Transplantation Pregnancy Registry: an analysis of 325 pregnancies in female kidney recipients. *J Am Soc Nephrol* 3: 851, 1992

42. Armenti VT, Ahlswede BA, Moritz MJ, Jarrell BE: The National Transplantation Pregnancy Registry: analysis of pregnancy outcomes of female kidney recipients with relation to time interval from transplant to conception. *Transplant Proc* 25: 1036, 1993

43. Rudolph JE, Schweizer RT, Bartus SA: Pregnancy in renal transplant patients. *Transplantation* 26: 27, 1979

44. Walters BNJ, Redman CWG: Treatment of severe pregnancy-associated hypertension with the calcium antagonist nifedipine. *Br J Obstet Gynaecol* 91: 330, 1984

45. Constantine G, Beevers DG, Reynolds AL et al.: Nifedipine as a second line antihypertensive drug in pregnancy. *Br J Obstet Gynaecol* 94: 1136, 1987

46. Ferris TF, Weir EK: Effect of captopril on uterine blood flow and prostaglandin E synthesis in the pregnant rabbit. *J Clin Invest* 71: 809, 1983

47. Anon: Are ACE inhibitors safe in pregnancy? *Lancet* 2: 482, 1989

48. Conrad M, Barton JC: Factors affecting iron balance. *Am J Hematol* 10: 199, 1991

49. Mitwalli A, Malik GH, Fayed H et al.: Erythropoietin therapy in a pregnant woman on maintenance haemodialysis. *Saudi J Kidney Dis Transplant* 5(4): 489, 1994

50. Davison JM: Dialysis, Transplantation and pregnancy. *Am J Kidney Dis* 17: 127, 1991

51. Fujumi S, Hori K, Mijima C, Shigematsu M: Successful pregnancy and delivery in a patient following r-HuEPO therapy and on long term dialysis. *J Am Soc Nephrol* 1: 397, 1990

52. Yankowitz J, Piraino B, Laifer SA et al.: Erythropoietin in pregnancies complicated by severe anemia of renal failure. *Obstet Gynecol* 80: 485, 1992

53. Hou S, Orlowski J, Pahl M, Ambrose S, Hussey M, Wong D: Pregnancy in woman with end stage renal disease: treatment of anemia and premature labour. *Am J Kidney Dis* 21: 16, 1993

54. Anon: Erythropoietin for anemia. *Med Lett Drugs Ther* 31: 85, 1989

55. Redrow M, Cherem L, Elliot J et al.: Dialysis in the management of patients with renal insufficiency. *Medicine* 67: 199, 1988

56. Pickrell MD, Sawyers R, Michael J: Pregnancy after renal transplantation: severe intrauterine growth retardation during treatment with cyclosporin A. *Br Med J* 296: 825, 1988

57. Lindheimer MD, Katz AI: Pregnancy in the renal transplant patient. *Am J Kidney Dis* 19: 173, 1992

58. Raine AEG, Margreiter R, Brunner FP et al.: Report on management of renal failure in Europe, XXII, 1991. *Nephrol Dial Transplant* 7 (Suppl 2): 7, 1993

59. Legrain M: Transplantation renalé et grossesse. *Gynecologie* 27: 535, 1976

60. Wing AJ, Davies DV: Acute post-partum renal failure in a renal transplant recipient. Unpublished

61. Davison JM: The effect of pregnancy on kidney function in renal allograft recipients. *Kidney Int* 27: 74, 1985

62. Baylis C, Reckelhoff JF: Renal hemodynamics in normal and hypertension pregnancy: lessons from micropuncture. *Am J Kidney Dis* 17: 98, 1991

63. Baylis C, Rennke HG: Renal hemodynamics and glomerular morphology in repetitive pregnant ageing rats. *Kidney Int* 28: 140, 1985

64. Salmela K, Kylloenen L, Holmberg C: Renal transplantation and parenthood. *Transplantation Proceedings* 24: 1744, 1992

65. Salmela K, Kylloenen L, Holmberg et al.: Influence of pregnancy on kidney graft function. *Transplant Proc* 25: 1302, 1993

66. Sturgiss SN, Davison JM: Effect of pregnancy on long-term function of renal allografts. *Am J Kidney Dis* 19: 167, 1992

67. Sturgiss SN, Davison JM: Perinatal outome in renal allograft recipients: prognostic significance of hypertension and renal function before and during pregnancy. *Obstet Gynecol* 78: 573, 1991

68. Davison JM: The effect of pregnancy on kidney function in renal allograft recipients. *Kidney Int* 27: 74, 1985

69. Brenner BM, Meyer TW, Hostetter TH: Dietary protein intake and the progressive nature of kidney disease: the role of hemodynamically mediated glomerular injury in the pathogenesis of glomerular sclerosis in ageing, renal ablation and intrinsic renal disease. *N Engl J Med* 307: 652, 1982

70. Katz AI, Lindheimer MD: Does pregnancy aggravate primary glomerular disease? *Am J Kidney Dis* 6: 261, 1985

71. Davison JM: Pregnancy in renal transplant recipients: clinical perspectives. *Contrib Nephrol* 37: 170, 1984

72. Pahl MV, Vaziri ND, Kaufman DJ et al.: Childbirth after renal transplantation. *Transplant Proc* 25: 2727, 1993

73. Gallery ED: Pregnancy in women with renal transplants. (Editorial) *Int J Artif Organs* 12: 141, 1989

74. Ehrich JHH, Rizzoni G, Broyer et al.: Combined report on regular dialysis and transplantation of children in Europe, 1987. *Nephrol Dial Transplant* 4 (Suppl 2): 33, 1989

75. Lubchenco LO, Hansman C, Dressler M, Boyd E: Intrauterine growth as estimated from liveborn birthweight: data at 24 to 42 weeks of gestation. *Pediatrics* 32: 793, 1963

76. Ehrich JHH, Rizzoni G, Brunner FP et al.: Combined report on regular dialysis and transplantation of children in Europe, 1989. *Nephrol Dial Transplant* 6 (Suppl 1): 37, 1991

77. Ehrich JHH, Loirat C, Rizzoni G et al.: Repeated successful pregnancies after kidney transplantation in 102 women; report by the EDTA-ERA Registry. Unpublished

78. Koops B, Morgan L, Battaglia F: Neonatal mortality risk in relation to birth-weight and gestational age. *J Pediatr* 101: 969, 1982

79. Price HV, Salaman JR, Laurence KM, Langmaid H: Immunosuppressive drugs and the foetus. *Transplantation* 21: 294, 1976

80. Leb DE, Weisskopf B, Kawovitz BS: Chromosome aberrations in the child of a kidney transplant recipient. *Arch Intern Med* 128: 441, 1971

81. Githens JH, Rosenkrantz JG, Tunnock SM: Teratogenic effects of azathioprine (Imuran). *J Pediatr* 66: 959, 1965

82. Evans TJ, McCollum JPK, Valdimarsson H: Congenital cytomegalovirus infection after maternal renal transplantation. *Lancet* 1: 1359, 1975

83. Skinhoj P, Cohn J, Bradburne AF: Transmission of hepatitis type B from healthy HBs Ag-positive mothers. *Br Med J* 1: 10, 1975

84. Verco CJ, Hawkins DF: Pregnancy after renal transplantation. *Br J Obstet Gynaecol* 3: 29, 1982

85. Lower GD, Stevens LE, Najarian JS, Reemtsma K: Problems from immunosuppressives during pregnancy. *Am J Obstet Gynecol* 111: 1120, 1971

86. MacLean AB, Briggs JD, Sharp F, Macpherson SG: Successful triplet pregnancy in renal transplant recipient. *Scot Med J* X: 320, 1980

87. Scott JR, Branch DW, Kochenour NK et al.: The effect of repeated pregnancies on renal allograft function. *Transplantation* 42: 694, 1985

THE DIALYSIS PATIENT AND TRANSPLANTATION

ULRICH FREI

INTRODUCTION

The availability of regular dialysis as renal replacement therapy is not only an essential prerequisite for the performance of renal transplantation but also still offers the sole possibility of survival for a large percentage of patients with end-stage renal disease. The rising cost of keeping the steadily growing population of patients with end-stage renal disease alive by regular dialysis challenges the health economies and the commitments of even the developed countries. Renal transplantation offers the potential to slow this cost explosion and to eventually stabilize the population on regular dialysis as well as to provide the best personal rehabilitation in the treatment of terminal renal failure (1). The consequence therefore is to offer the chance of renal transplantation to each suitable dialysis patient as substantial part of an integrated treatment framework. Unfortunately this possibility is only a theoretical one because of the limited availability of suitable organs for transplantation in most countries. Religious, social, political and educational constraints do not allow to use all available cadaver donors or to perform transplants from living related or unrelated donors. This influences the selection of recipients as well as organ allocation. The nephrologist is urged to make a balanced decision between the demand of the society to achieve best results with the limited resources available and the wish of the individual patient to be relieved of his personal suffering. During the last decade the increase of transplants performed was outweighed by the faster increase of the waiting list due to the possibility to perform transplantation successfully in spite of extended selection criteria. To provide all suitable patients with grafts within an acceptable time span major efforts are necessary in two directions: 1. to increase the number of available grafts; 2. to improve the survival time of grafts and thereby reduce the need for regrafts.

EXPECTATIONS AND RESULTS

Renal transplantation nowadays is a standard procedure carried out in more than 500 institutions round the world. Nevertheless the individual dialysis patient needs to get precise information about results and risks of this treatment. The most optimistic scenario is as follows: The patients expects to be put on a waiting list (I) early after commencement of regular dialysis. After a short waiting time (II) he wants to get a graft of good quality (III): that is well matched (IIIa), from a donor with normal renal function (IIIb), without hypertension and viral disease (IIIc), to be transplanted within a short ischemia time (IV), with immediate postoperative function (V), under use of nontoxic and effective immunosuppressive agents (VI), with limited or treatable rejection episodes (VII) and a long-standing firm graft function (VIII) without serious long-term complications (IX). Although to meet all of those criteria is not possible, they set the goals of a well functioning transplant program. This paragraph should address these criteria in detail and put them into relation to the present clinical practice and the results achieved.

(I) The acceptance rate to a waiting list varies widely in different countries depending upon the acceptance rate for renal replacement therapy (RRT), donor availability, from the proportion of living donor transplants and the overall pool size of patients on RRT. There are major regional differences, between and within countries. The acceptance rate is sometimes influenced by a socioeconomic bias as well as by a bias to the disadvantage of minorities (2–5). Unequivocal criteria for the acceptance of patients as transplant candidates are lacking as demonstrated exemplarity by a survey of the policy in US transplant centers (6).

(II) Time spent on a waiting list depends upon the relation of the number of patients waiting to the number of transplants performed per year as well as upon the organ allocation procedure. If compatibility is to be of low significance than the 'first come, first serve' principle

(III) Good graft quality is an increasing matter of concern. Due to donor shortage more and more questionable donors are accepted (7–12) of debatable value in particular in terms of donor age (less than 5 years or older than 55/60 years). It has been demonstrated that these organs have inferior short and long-term results if compared to grafts from donors between 20 and 45 years of age (13). This has been explained by a yet lower or a diminished number of functioning nephrons. The same applies for grafts from donors with preexisting hypertension (died for cerebrovascular accident). Such kidneys most often have inferior results and carry also the risk of induction of hypertension (14). In spite of careful examination of the donors there is still a risk of infection by viral disease present in the donor tissue such as HIV, HCV, HBV, CMV and Herpes viruses. Whereas the risk of transmitting HIV after bad experiences in the eighties is now negligible low, there is substantial risk to attract HCV, and there is no way to omit CMV if not a substantial percentage of the donor organs should be discarded.

(IV) Cold ischemia time (CIT) clearly influences initial graft function and short term results. Whether there is a long-term effect after the first postoperative year is still controversial. Most consistently the duration of CIT is correlated positively with the percentage of initially nonfunctioning grafts. Efforts to reduce the impact of CIT by introducing new preservations solutions such as the UW (University of Wisconsin) solution (15, 16) or the HTK-solution (Histidin–Tryptophan–Ketoglutarat buffer) (17) improved the situation only moderately, CIT still is affecting initial graft function. In addition to CIT also warm ischemia time may become more relevant since due to donor shortage the use of non-heart-beating donors is now proposed. Most of them die of cardiac arrest by coronary artery diseases and have substantial warm ischemia times.

(V) Initially nonfunctioning grafts have 10–20% inferior short-term results compared to grafts with immediate function. It has been shown however that initial nonfunction with a duration of more than one week may also have a poor long-term prognosis. Attempts have been made to reduce the percentage of INF by fluid loading, administration of drugs such as calcium channel blockers (18), prostaglandin analogs (19) or atriopeptins (20).

(VI) During the last decade for postoperative immunosuppression only few standardized protocols were applied and evaluated. More than 90% of the transplants have been performed under use of a cyclosporine A (CyA) based protocols. Nearly identical populations received cyclosporine alone, CyA + steroids or CyA + steroids + azathioprine. In rare cases cyclosporine + azathioprine or steroids + azathioprine were used, the latter combination mostly because of economic reasons. The potential nephrotoxicity of CyA was recognized very soon after its introduction and is taken into account in today recommended protocols. Under these precautions there is no certain proof for a progressive cyclosporine nephrotoxicity after long-term application.

(VII) The most important proof for the efficacy of an immunosuppressive protocol is the incidence of acute rejections and the number of rejection episodes per patient. With the today's usual protocols it is possible to reduce the incidence of acute rejection episodes within the first year to around 50%. The occurrence of so called 'late' acute rejections after 30 or 60 days posttransplant is of specific prognostic relevance, since it has been shown that late acute rejection carry an inferior long-term prognosis for the graft (21).

(VIII) It is generally accepted that the 1-year survival rate of renal allografts has improved during the last decade. Most transplant centers currently report a 90% 1-year graft survival for cadaveric allografts. The improvement in 1-year survival rates has been attributed to advances in tissue typing, refinements in patient care and more effective immunosuppressive treatment. Only limited data are available about the course of graft function over time because most registries are analyzing graft failure instead of graft function.

(IX) Although in most centers the short-term mortality after kidney transplantation has dropped to percentages clearly below 5%, death of the recipient is the cause of 30–50% of late graft losses. Serious long-term complications are accelerated coronary and peripheral vessel disease, myocardial infarction and heart failure, an increasing number of de-novo malignant disease with a limited prognosis and chronic infections, in particular the late consequences of viral hepatitis with liver failure (22).

SELECTION AND PREPARATION OF THE RECIPIENT

During the seventies the selection of suitable recipients for a kidney transplant was influenced by the fear of fatal complications. Therefore, an age limit of 45–50 years was applied. In addition normal cardiovascular status and good cooperation was mandatory. During the last 15 years the criteria for recipient selection widened regarding age, concomitant diseases, personal behavior and ability for cooperation. This was due to the introduction of less dangerous immunosuppressive regimens with less steroids and better medication for intestinal and infectious complications. In the past there was no uniform concept how to evaluate and how to consider preexisting disease. At least in US transplant centers there was a heterogeneous approach for evaluating patients for renal transplantation particularly in the regard to viral hepatitis, cardiovascular disease and noncompliance (6). Recently an excellent work-up protocol was published by Kasiske et al. (23). The assessment of a candidate for the waiting list should consist of a medical history, a physical examination, defined laboratory tests, radiological examinations as well as the testing of immunological parameters. It is absolutely necessary that the patient presents himself personally in the transplant center. A reference laboratory should perform the immunological investigations, whereas the referring nephrologist carries out the remaining examination. Table 1 gives a list of the mandatory assessment and investigations.

The RRT population has changed during the last decade. More elderly patients and more patients with severe concomitant diseases ask for transplantation. In pediatric transplantation there is a tendency to younger recipients. Nevertheless only some contraindications remain. Incurable malignant disease, active infections, liver failure and surgical obstacles as severe calcifications of the abdominal and pelvic vessels and extended radiation in the pelvic area are still contraindications. If there are – as in most cases – no contraindications certain risk factors have to be considered. Two different aspects are addressed: First: Is there an increased risk to loose the graft significantly earlier than in the general transplant population (Example: Hyperoxaluria of the considered recipient)? This is a question related to the problem of allocation of grafts from inadequate resources. Second: Is there a risk for the patient to die significantly earlier after transplantation than on continued dialysis (Example: severe chronic heart failure (CHF) of the recipient)?

Main risk related to the underlying primary renal disease is the risk of its recurrence in the graft (24, 25). Certain entities of primary glomerular disease have a higher tendency to recur. Most often this is the case in focal glomerulosclerosis (26–29). Membranous nephropathy also tends to recur but less often. It also may develop de-novo as manifestation of chronic rejection (transplant glomerulopathy). Other glomerular diseases with the risk of recurrence are membranoproliferative GN, IgA-nephropathy and anti glomerular basement membrane nephritis (AGBM-nephritis). Also in systemic diseases with renal involvement such as primary hyperoxaluria, Fabry's disease, amyloidosis, lupus erythematodes, Wegener's granulomatosis and diabetic nephropathy recurrence of renal manifestation has to be considered. Other risk factors arise from concomitant diseases such as cardiovascular, pulmonary and gastrointestinal disease (30, 31). There is still debate whether patients with coronary or valvular disease are acceptable and whether patients with CHF should be transplanted (32–34). Our policy is to consider each dialysis patient for cardiac surgery as it would be indicated in a nonuremic patient. After successful angioplasty, bypass grafting or valvular repair there is no contraindication for transplantation. CHF and persistent valvular disease, at least if the potential recipient (with a low ejection fraction) is highly volume intolerant, are contraindications. However it has been reported that left ventricular function may improve after kidney transplantation in some cases of CHF (35).

Gastrointestinal disease plays a decreasing role as a risk factor due to better prophylaxis for peptic ulcers. Colon perforations due to diverticel are the most serious complications. Therefore it is mandatory to ask for a history of diverticulitis, to perform a contrast enema and in cases with proven history and diverticel suspicious for infection or perforation to operate prophylactically. Furthermore preexisting viral hepatic disease plays an important role as a long-term risk factor (see below). There is still debate whether to accept patients with hepatitis B or C or not. Several authors propose to perform a liver biopsy and to reject patients with active inflammation. In hypercalcemic medically not well controlled cases of secondary hyperparathyroidism parathyroidectomy is mandatory. Persistent hyperparathyroidism after kidney transplantation in most cases regress very slowly. But only a small percentage of cases need surgery within the following years.

Although urinary tract anomalies in general do not represent contraindication, thorough evaluation is mandatory for a careful planning of transplant surgery. The acceptance of patients with a history of a malignancy is a matter of debate. The usual policy asking for a tumor free interval of 2 years has to be considered as a compromise with limitations (36).

The recipient should be evaluated concerning increased immunological risk to adjust immunosuppressive protocols. This is the case in patients with a previous failed graft due to rejection (37), with sensitization due to HLA-antibodies (38, 39), with homozygosity for HLA-antigens, in children or in blacks (40, 41) and concomitant medication which does influence the availability of immunosuppressive drugs such as rifampicin, hydantoins or ketokonazol (42–44).

The patient himself as an individual also carries some risk such as age, reduced compliance and drug abuse. For many years elderly people were considered unsuitable as graft recipient. It has been proven by several groups, that kidney transplantation in recipients up to 70 years of age is not accomplished by excess mortality (when compared to dialysis) and if death with a functioning graft was censored a very low rate of graft losses due to rejection because of the reduced immune response in the elderly was observed (45, 46). In addition drug compliance is a serious individual factor for graft outcome. Graft losses due to noncompliance are reported in significant numbers. The reason may be the individual inability to follow prescription plans but also socioeconomic factors (47–50).

ORGAN ALLOCATION

In most countries there is severe shortage of available grafts for transplantation. Therefore it was debated for many years how to allocate available grafts in a fair and equitable way considering the individual needs, the outcome probability and economic aspects of the society (51–64). Not only the access to but also the waiting time for a transplant is of concern (65). Some attempts were made to equalize waiting time by sophisticated computer programs

Table 1. Assessment for the waiting list

Medical history: Renal history – underlying renal disease, duration, onset and duration of hypertension, urinary tract abnormalities, infections, previous grafts
Family history, inherited renal disease
Concomitant diseases: cardiovascular disease, MI, stroke, gastrointestinal, hepatitis, diverticel, diabetes mellitus, onset
Operations: urinary tract operations, nephrectomy, PTX, splenectomy, iliac vessels
Actual treatment data
Blood pressure (24h ABPM)
Residual renal function
Mode of dialysis, hours, dialyzer, exchange volume
Transfusion history, pregnancies
Drugs, erythropoietin, vitamin D

Laboratory assessment
Hematological parameters, Hb, Hct, Leucocyte/Platelet count
Liver enzymes, calcium, phosphate, alkaline phosphatase, PTH, Hepatitis serology, HBs antigen, HBs antibodies, HCV antibodies, CMV antibodies, HIV antibodies, VZV, EBV

Radiological assessment
Chest film, plain film of abdomen and pelvic area (vessel wall calcifications) in case of peripheral artery disease: angiography

Others
ultrasound abdomen, native kidneys
cardiac evaluation: ECG, echocardiography, stress testing (exercise, thallium or stress echo)
urological examination (if applicable)
urinary culture, cytology

Immunological investigations
Blood group, tissue typing, if necessary family typing
antibody screening for immunization and specificity

such as proposed by Wujciak and Opelz (66). There is no doubt concerning the major impact of HLA-matching on short and long-term graft and patient survival (67–69). In large population analyses, this effect exceeds by far the impact of other factors such as ischemia time, graft quality, center effect or mode of immunosuppression. However in the individual case the graft quality, which depends upon donor factors such as age, donor blood pressure, number of functioning nephrons and preexisting renal disease as well as upon ischemia time and mode of preservation, influences the individual graft outcome to an important extent. Proof for that are data of transplants from nonrelated living donors, which are totally mismatched, but of proven good graft quality and transplanted under optimal conditions. Under these circumstances the 3 year graft survival is superior to well matched cadaver grafts (70, 71). Nevertheless most of the recipients must rely on cadaver grafts harvested under suboptimal conditions. For these patients graft allocation according to HLA-matching seems mandatory with some adjustments for children, for long waiting time, low match probability and sensitiza-

tion. Equitable organ allocation is an increasing matter of concern, because of donor shortage many attempts have been observed to overrule allocation principles by influence, power and finances. In most countries there is no doubt that nobody owns cadaver grafts, neither the harvesting transplant center nor the relatives. Therefore the public of each country has to ascertain a equitable and fair allocation procedure giving everybody a comparable chance to get a suitable graft in an acceptable time.

MANAGEMENT OF THE RECIPIENT

The perioperative management of the recipient cannot be reviewed in detail in this chapter but a number of issues are of major interest:

(I) Because initial graft function has a crucial impact on short term survival prophylactic measures should be taken. The cold ischemia time should be kept as short as possible. The pre- and postoperative fluid balance is of utmost importance for initial graft function. Therefore by

Table 2. Recurrence of original diseases (23, 25, 125)

	Recurrence %	Graft losses %
I. Recurrence of primary glomerular disease		
Focal-segmental-glomerulosclerosis	20–30%	30–40%
Membranous Nephropathy	3–7%	rare
Membranoproliferative GN Type I	20–30%	30–40%
MPGN type II	> 80%	10%
IgA-Nephropathy	50%	10%
Anti-GBM-Nephritis	12%	rare
II. Recurrence of secondary glomerular diseases		
Hennoch–Schoenlein	10–15%	10–20%
Lupus-Nephritis	< 1%	rare
Hemolytic uremic syndrome	13–25%	40–50%
Diabetic-Nephropathy	100%	< 5%
Amyloidosis	5–30%	rare
M Wegener	single cases	
III. Recurrence of nonglomerular diseases		
Hyperoxaluria	90–100%	90–100%
Cystinosis	10%	rare
M Fabry	rare	?
Scleroderma	?	?
Alport-Syndrom	< 10%	rare by AGBM-nephritis

taking into account the history of interdialysis weight gain it should be determined which fluid load the patient is able to tolerate without becoming critically volume overloaded. Preoperative dialysis to achieve 'dry' weight should be avoided. A central venous pressure of 12–15 cm H_2O during surgery is mandatory. The use of calcium channel blockers to reduce the percentage of initially nonfunctioning grafts is worthwhile. Positive data exist for diltiazem as adjunct to the preservation fluid as well for prophylactic treatment of the recipient (18).

(II) Perioperative a short course of prophylactic antibiotic treatment is indicated. The duration depends upon the presence of indwelling venous lines or bladder catheters and should be kept as short as possible.

(III) Prophylactic anticoagulation is recommended to avoid arterial or venous graft thrombosis, fistula thrombosis and deep vein thrombosis. At least in cases of critical grafts (poor reperfusion) and anastomoses (multiple vessels, atherosclerosis) or high hematocrit prophylactic application of heparin is encouraged.

(IV) There is no standardized policy with regard to initial prophylactic immunosuppressive protocols after kidney transplantation round the world and not even within countries.

In principle there is no controversy regarding the use of cyclosporine. Differing protocols exist concerning dosage, route of administration (oral *vs* intravenously) and the time of institution (preoperative, postoperative, after start of graft function).

Overall agreement exists regarding the use of corticosteroids although some centers – particular in the UK – prefer cyclosporine monotherapy. It is still under discussion how long corticosteroids should be used (72, 73). Uncertain and matter of a continuous change of policy is the use of azathioprine. Whereas a number of centers have added azathioprine during the last years to exploit its synergistic immunsuppressive effect and to avoid cyclosporine toxicity, prospective and retrospective studies have failed to prove its value. Except for regrafts and immunized patients it appears to be of no advantage. There also are differing opinions regarding the value of prophylactic application of antilymphocytic preparations. They are more often used for this indication in the US than in Europe, perhaps because of inferior histocompatibility accepted in the US.

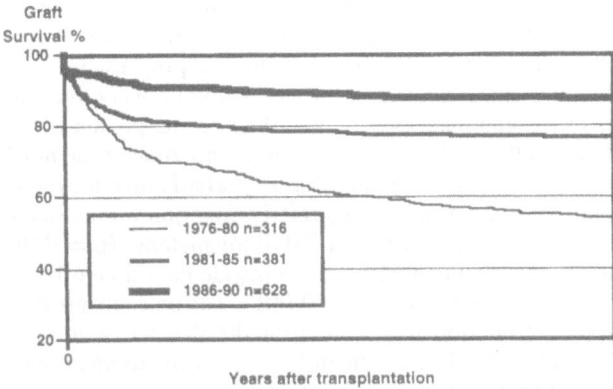

Figure 1. 1-year survival for first cadaver grafts transplanted in three different time periods.

Corticosteroids play a pivotal role for therapeutic immunosuppression in rejection treatment. But again there is no agreement with regard to the mode of application (oral *vs* parenteral), dosage and duration of treatment. In case there is no response within a short time and rejection persists in a graft biopsy than the rejection is determined 'steroid resistant'. Steroid resistant rejections are treated by the use of poly- or monoclonal antilymphocytic sera most often by the anti-TAC-antibody OKT3. There exists convincing evidence that OKT3 is capable to suppress 90% of steroid resistant rejections.

LONG-TERM ASPECTS OF RENAL TRANSPLANTATION

Acute graft survival, defined as the one year survival of a first cadaver graft, has markedly improved during the last 15 years (74). Figure 1 shows single center (75) data given for three time periods: 1) the period between 1976–1980 in which the immunosuppression mostly consisted of steroids, azathioprine and prophylactic polyclonal antilymphocyte sera, 2) the period between 1981–1985, in which centers had to learn how to use cyclosporine A and 3) the period between 1986–1990. Whereas the one year graft survival in the first period was only 56%, it improved in the next period to 76% and reached 87% between 1986–1990. Similar improvement of one year survival was demonstrated by other single centers, organ exchange networks as well as by international collaborative studies (74). Results were analyzed in detail with respect to the influence of HLA-matching (76), donor organ quality (age), ischemic damage (11, 77, 78), and recipient sensitization status (39). Optimal matching was in favor for improved short-term results, increasing donor age was accompanied by inferior results, extended ischemia times resulted in an increased number of initially nonfunctioning grafts and higher graft losses within the first year. The effect of combinations of immunosuppressive drug

therapy was surprisingly small (79–81). The main interest has focused on graft survival, only in rare instances the quality of graft function in terms of glomerular filtration rate was analyzed (82, 83). In more recent years it has become increasingly difficult to prove the superiority of newly developed drugs or drug regimens over the already used regimens because of the high standard already achieved.

The introduction of cyclosporine A was the most important contribution to this improvement. However also ample data exist to prove the increasing influence of HLA-typing and matching on the one year graft outcome irrespective of the immunosuppressive regimen used and irrespective of other factors such as ischemia times, sensitization or number of grafts (67, 68, 84, 85). This effect is even much more obvious if typing for HLA-splits (86) and improved HLA-DR determination by DNA typing was performed (87). In spite of the dramatic improvement in the one year survival of first grafts no comparable improvement was made in patients at risk for immunological complications such as patients with early rejected grafts or with presensitization for HLA-antigens. The results in this group of patients is still 10–15% inferior when compared to first grafts (84).

Fortunately one year graft survival is affected only to a minor extent by one year patient survival which has steadily improved over the years and which now reaches numbers greater than 95% in most of the centers. These favorable results were obtained in spite of extended recipient selection criteria regarding age and severity of secondary diseases. Patients with cardiomyopathy, after coronary bypass grafting and aortic repair are now accepted for kidney transplantation (88, 89). Mean recipient age in adults (> 16 years) did increase in our population from 38.24 ± 10.7 years (mean ± SD) in 1980 to 42.76 ± 11.4 in 1985 and 44.56 ± 12.9 in 1991. The percentage of patients older than 55 years increased from 3.6% 1980, to 11.8% 1985 and 23.9% 1991.

Because of the favorable results achieved during the first year after transplant the main focus in survival data analysis has now been extended to the long-term results regarding graft survival and graft function as well as for patient morbidity and survival (90, 91). There is some influence of HLA-compatibility, but not as strong as during the first year. In contrast to first year analysis, in the long term HLA-DR matching appears to be less important than matching for HLA-B and especially HLA-A (92). A commonly used method to describe long term results is the calculation of graft half-life after the first postoperative year for different time periods, matches and patient groups. The Collaborative Transplant study with a data base of more than 100,000 grafts as well as Terasaki et al. demonstrated an effect of the degree of HLA-mismatching on graft half-life time; 10-year graft survival was estimated by projection and was found to be the shorter the greater the number of HLA-mismatches were (68, 93, 94). We analyzed survival data for our center by comparing the

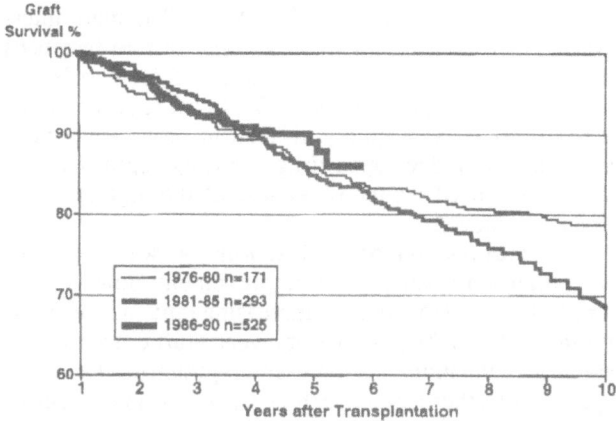

Figure 2. Long-term survival after the first postoperative year of first cadaver grafts transplanted in three different time periods. Grafts already functioning after the first year = 100%.

identical time periods mentioned above (Figure 1) for all grafts that were functioning after one year (counted as 100% in the Kaplan–Meyer-analysis). In contrast to the improvement in 1-year graft survival, there was no improvement in long-term graft survival for the later time periods (Figure 2). A comparable number of grafts were lost during the years 2–10 after transplant in all three time periods studied.

Chronic graft losses are supposed to be mainly due to chronic rejection. However other possible factors such as hypertensive nephropathy, chronic cyclosporine nephrotoxicity due to high doses, recurrence of original disease and hyperfiltration injury may also play an important role. Profound improvement of graft function was observed after switching from cyclosporine A to azathioprine (95), strict blood pressure control has stopped the deterioration of graft function (96) and protein restriction was discussed to be of some value (97, 98). Recurrence of the original renal disease damaged grafts irrespective of compatibility and mode of immunosuppression (99). Until now only very limited tools for the differential diagnosis of chronic allograft dysfunction are available. Furthermore, the best treatment to stop chronic rejection still is under discussion (100–103).

From the survival curves (Figure 2) one might speculate that function of all grafts is deteriorating at the same rate. In the literature there are only scarce data available describing the natural course of glomerular function in long-term grafted patients. To identify risk factors for chronic progressive renal allograft dysfunction, we conducted a retrospective study in 639 patients transplanted between 1983 and 1990 (104). Graft function was assessed by the slope of individual 1/creatinine regression lines and chronic progressive graft dysfunction was defined as a slope of the 1/creatinine line of > 0.1 dl/mg/year, indicating a loss of glomerular filtration rate of > 10 ml/min/year regardless of the initial serum

creatinine value. A number of possible risk factors were determined and analyzed by linear regression analysis. 106 patients (16.6%) showed chronic progressive graft dysfunction. No correlation was found between the rate of functional deterioration and the age and gender of the donor or the recipient, the total ischemia time or the number of kidneys from female donors grafted into male recipients. Chronic progressive graft dysfunction was associated with the number of HLA-B/DR mismatches ($p = 0.04$) and with a first acute rejection episode later than 60 days after transplantation ($p < 0.001$). Chronic progressive graft dysfunction also occurred in the absence of an acute rejection episode. Significantly ($p < 0.001$) more patients with chronic progressive graft dysfunction were hypertensive not only 12 months after transplantation, but also at the time of transplantation, indicating that hypertension may not only be secondary to deteriorating graft function, but that hypertension *per se* leads to graft damage and initiates chronic progressive graft dysfunction.

CHRONIC PATIENT SURVIVAL

Death of patients with a functioning graft has emerged as an increasingly important factor in the analysis of long-term survival. Death after kidney transplantation is mainly due to cardiovascular disease, infections, malignancies and liver disease. The contributions of these causes to the overall mortality has markedly changed during the last 15 years. The incidence of infectious causes has markedly decreased whereas cardiovascular disease and malignancies have increased to 2/3 of the causes. In an analysis done by Kasiske et al. preexisting cardiovascular disease is the strongest prognostic indicator for posttransplant death (105). Well known cardiovascular risk factors such as hypertension, hypercholesterinemia, diabetes mellitus, obesity and corticosteroid therapy accumulate in grafted patients. Cyclosporine therapy has been reported to worsen blood pressure (106) and cholesterol levels (107, 108). Corticosteroids may cause a diabetic state. It was shown that strict control of cardiovascular risk factors such as bilateral nephrectomy to normalize blood pressure and intervention in life style and smoking habits was able to achieve superior long-term results.

It is well known that immunosuppressive therapy after organ transplantation increases the risk for malignant disorders (109, 110). However only few studies are available in which the occurrence of malignancies is correlated to the total number of patient years treated and time after transplantation, and only a few studies compared their results to a nontransplanted general population. Except for some series of patients with overimmunosuppression which caused a high incidence of consecutive lymphoproliferative disorders (111) the number of malignancies seems to be approximately 3–4 fold compared to general cancer registries (112, 113). The results are comparable for Europe and for Australia with the exception of skin malignancies, which are more frequent in Australia (114). The expected *vs* observed numbers of malignancies in our own population stratified for gender and age and according to the numbers of patients and the observed patient years were 3–4 fold (115).

A further matter of concern is the high number of deaths due to liver failure. This was observed after kidney transplantation in earlier years and also more recently (116, 117). However the underlying reason may have changed. In earlier years hepatotoxicity of azathioprine played an important role whereas today an increasing number of patients die for liver cirrhosis due to chronic viral hepatitis (B and C) acquired years before renal transplantation (118, 119).

BACK ON DIALYSIS: THE PATIENT WITH THE FAILED GRAFT

There is only very limited information in the literature concerning the patient with a failed graft. In most of the transplant registries no firm data about patients with a failed graft are available except if they are registered for a retransplantation. The same applies for the fate of retained failed grafts. Also few data are available regarding specific medical question arising after graft failure: How has the immunosuppression to be reduced? Is a specific dialysis regimen necessary and is erythropoietin as efficacious as before transplantation (120, 121)?

In most cases, chronic allograft failure is characterized by a steadily progressive decline in function. If there is no clear information on the underlying process a graft biopsy should be taken to differentiate chronic rejection, late acute rejection, recurrent disease or hypertensive/hyperfiltration nephropathy. This is of high importance to avoid useless immunosupressive therapy during a preuremic state which will increase significantly the risks the patient with a failing graft is facing. If graft function has ceased one has to decide how to reduce or stop immunosuppression and whether the graft should be removed (120, 122, 123). Concerning graft nephrectomy it has been suggested that symptomatic rejection after cessation of immunosuppressive therapy may increase the risk for antibody formation substantially. Thus, immunosuppression must be tapered cautiously to prevent symptomatic rejection. If symptomatic rejection occurs, one has to consider removal of the graft. However, there is ample experience – at least after chronic rejection – that grafts remain asymptomatic after stopping immunosuppressive drugs (123). After having returned to hemodialysis, a certain number of patients may experience a long-lasting steroid withdrawal syndrome with fever, arthralgias and stiffness. Tapering with very low doses over months may be necessary (124). Our advice is after return on dialysis to stop cyclosporine immediately and to taper steroids very slowly. If there are any signs for a symptomatic rejecting graft, such as tenderness, fever, hematuria and unexplained anemia graft nephrectomy should be performed as soon as possible.

REFERENCES

1. Koch KM, Halloran PF: Dialysis and transplantation. (Editorial) *Curr Opin Nephrol Hypertens* 1: 3, 1992
2. Singer PA: A review of public policies to procure and distribute kidneys for transplantation. *Arch Intern Med* 150: 523, 1990
3. Groenewoud AF, Persijn GG, Hendriks GF, D'Amaro J, Cohen B: Influence of HLA matching, donor age, and cyclosporine on unrelated pediatric renal allograft survival. *Transplant Proc* 19: 699, 1987
4. Ellison MD, Breen TJ, Guo TG, Cunningham PR, Daily OP: Blacks and whites on the UNOS renal waiting list: waiting times and patient demographics compared. *Transplant Proc* 25: 2462, 1993
5. Edwards EB, Guo T, Breen TJ, Bowen GR, Daily OP: The UNOS OPTN waiting list from 1988 to 1993. *Clin Transpl* 71, 1993
6. Ramos EL, Kasiske BL, Alexander SR, Danovitch GM, Harmon WE, Kahana L et al.: The evaluation of candidates for renal transplantation. The current practice of US transplant centers. *Transplantation* 57: 490, 1994
7. Rosenthal JT: Expanded criteria for cadaver organ donation in renal transplantation. *Urol Clin North Am* 21: 283, 1994
8. Creagh TA, McLean PA, Donovan MG, Walshe JJ, Murphy DM: Older donors and kidney transplantation. *Transpl Int* 6: 39, 1993
9. Rao KV, Kasiske BL, Odlund MD, Ney AL, Andersen RC: Influence of cadaver donor age on posttransplant renal function and graft outcome. *Transplantation* 49: 91, 1990
10. Foster MC, Wenham PW, Rowe PA, Blamey RW, Bishop MC, Burden RP et al.: Use of older patients as cadaveric kidney donors. *Br J Surg* 75: 767, 1988
11. Ploeg RJ, Visser MJ, Stijnen T, Persijn GG, van Schilfgaarde: Impact of donor age and quality of donor kidneys on graft survival. *Transplant Proc* 19: 1532, 1987
12. Orloff MS, Reed AI, Erturk E, Kruk RA, Paprocki SA, Cimbalo SC et al.: Nonheartbeating cadaveric organ donation. *Ann Surg* 220: 578, 1994
13. Terasaki PI, Koyama H, Cecka JM, Gjertson DW: The hyperfiltration hypothesis in human renal transplantation. *Transplantation* 57: 1450, 1994
14. Ratner LE, Joseph V, Zibari G, Patel S, Maley WR, Kittur D et al.: Transplantation of kidneys from hypertensive cadaveric donors. *Transplant Proc* 27: 989, 1995
15. Kalayoglu M, Sollinger HW, Stratta RJ, D'Alessandro AM, Hoffmann RM, Pirsch JD et al.: Extended preservation of the liver for clinical transplantation. *Lancet* 1: 617, 1988
16. Ploeg RJ, Goossens D, Vreugdenhil P, McAnulty JF, Southard JH, Belzer FO: Successful 72-hour cold storage kidney preservation with UW solution. *Transplant Proc* 20: 935, 1988
17. Kallerhoff M, Blech M, Kehrer G, Kleinert H, Siekmann W, Helmchen U et al.: Post-ischemic renal function after

kidney protection with the HTK-solution of Bretschneider. *Urol Res* 14: 271, 1986

18. Frei U, Margreiter R, Harms A, Bosmuller C, Neumann KH, Viebahn R et al.: Preoperative graft reperfusion with a calcium antagonist improves initial function: preliminary results of a prospective randomized trial in 110 kidney recipients. *Transplant Proc* 19: 3539, 1987

19. Neumayer HH, Kunzendorf U, Schreiber M: Protective effects of diltiazem and the prostazycline analogue iloprost in human renal transplantation. *Ren Fail* 14: 289, 1992

20. Klein HG, Dimitrov D, Atanasova I, Hohenfellner RM, Schmausser U, Natcheff N et al.: Atrial natriuretic factor infusion following acute renal ischemia in anesthetized dogs. *Renal Physiol Biochem* 15: 73, 1992

21. Almond PS, Gillingham KJ, Sibley R, Moss A, Melin M, Leventhal J et al.: Renal transplant function after ten years of cyclosporine. *Transplantation* 53: 316, 1992

22. Kliem V, Ringe B, Holhorst K, Frei U: Kidney transplantation in hepatitis B surface antigen carriers. *Clin Investig* 72: 1000, 1994

23. Kasiske BL, Ramos EL, Gaston RS, Bia MJ, Danovitch GM, Bowen PA et al.: The evaluation of renal transplant candidates: Clinical Practice Guidelines. *J Am Soc Nephrol* 6: 1, 1995

24. Cameron JS: Recurrent disease in renal allografts. *Kidney Int* 43 (Suppl): S91, 1993

25. Ramos EL, Tisher CC: Recurrent diseases in the kidney transplant. *Am J Kidney Dis* 24: 142, 1994

26. Artero M, Biava C, Amend W, Tomlanovich S, Vincenti F: Recurrent focal glomerulosclerosis: natural history and response to therapy. *Am J Med* 92: 375, 1992

27. Tejani A, Stablein DH: Recurrence of focal segmental glomerulosclerosis posttransplantation: a special report of the North American Pediatric Renal Transplant Cooperative Study. *J Am Soc Nephrol* 2: S258, 1992

28. Dantal J, Bigot E, Bogers W, Testa A, Kriaa F, Jacques Y et al.: Effect of plasma protein adsorption on protein excretion in kidney-transplant recipients with recurrent nephrotic syndrome. *N Engl J Med* 330: 7, 1994

29. Li PK, Lai FM, Leung CB, Lui SF, Wang A, Lai KN: Plasma exchange in the treatment of early recurrent focal glomerulosclerosis after renal transplantation. Report and review. *Am J Nephrol* 13: 289, 1993

30. Soderdahl G, Tyden G, Groth CG: Incidence of gastrointestinal complications following renal transplantation in the cyclosporin era. *Transplant Proc* 26: 1771, 1994

31. Benoit G, Moukarzel M, Verdelli G, Hiesse C, Buffet C, Bensadoun H et al.: Gastrointestinal complications in renal transplantation. *Transpl Int* 6: 45, 1993

32. Kasiske BL: Risk factors for accelerated atherosclerosis in renal transplant recipients. *Am J Med* 84: 985, 1988

33. Braun WE: Long-term complications of renal transplantation (clinical conference). *Kidney Int* 37: 1363, 1990

34. Reis G, Marcovitz PA, Leichtman AB, Merion RM, Fay WP, Werns SW et al.: Usefulness of dobutamine stress echocardiography in detecting coronary artery disease in end-stage renal disease. *Am J Cardiol* 75: 707, 1995

35. Burt RK, Gupta-Burt S, Suki WN, Barcenas CG, Ferguson JJ, Van Buren C: Reversal of left ventricular dysfunction after renal transplantation. *Ann Intern Med* 111: 635, 1989

36. Penn I: Effect of immunosuppression on preexisting cancers. *Transplant Proc* 25: 1380, 1993

37. Thorogood J, van Houwelingen JC, Persijn GG, van Rood JJ: The contribution of failure time of first kidney graft to predicting failure of regrafts. *Transplant Proc* 22: 15, 1990

38. Taube D: Immunoadsorption in the sensitized transplant recipient (clinical conference). *Kidney Int* 38: 350, 1990

39. Rankin GW Jr, Wang XM, Terasaki PI: Sensitization to kidney transplants. *Clin Transpl* 417, 1990

40. Cecka JM, Gjertson DW, Cho Y, Terasaki PI: HLA polymorphisms, ethnicity, and graft survival: united network for organ sharing. UNOS Scientific Renal Transplant Registry. *Transplant Proc* 25: 2446, 1993

41. Gaston RS, Shroyer TW, Hudson SL, Deierhoi MH, Laskow DA, Barber WH et al.: Renal retransplantation: the role of race, quadruple immunosuppression, and the flow cytometry cross-match. *Transplantation* 57: 47, 1994

42. Sketris IS, Methot ME, Nicol D, Belitsky P, Knox MG: Effect of calcium-channel blockers on cyclosporine clearance and use in renal transplant patients. *Ann Pharmacother* 28: 1227, 1994

43. Sorenson AL, Lovdahl M, Hewitt JM, Granger DK, Almond PS, Russlie HQ et al.: Effects of ketoconazole on cyclosporine metabolism in renal allograft recipients. *Transplant Proc* 26: 2822, 1994

44. Peschke B, Ernst W, Gossmann J, Kachel HG, Schoeppe W, Scheuermann EH: Antituberculous drugs in kidney transplant recipients treated with cyclosporine. *Transplantation* 56: 236, 1993

45. Tesi RJ, Elkhammas EA, Davies EA, Henry ML, Ferguson RM: Renal transplantation in older people. *Lancet* 343: 461, 1994

46. Velez RL, Brinker KR, Vergne-Marini PJ, Nesser DA, Long DL, Trevino G et al.: Renal transplantation with cyclosporine in the elderly population. *Transplant Proc* 23: 1749, 1991

47. Kalil RS, Heim-Duthoy KL, Kasiske BL: Patients with a low income have reduced renal allograft survival. *Am J Kidney Dis* 20: 63, 1992

48. Sketris I, Waite N, Grobler K, West M, Gerus S: Factors affecting compliance with cyclosporine in adult renal transplant patients. *Transplant Proc* 26: 2538, 1994

49. Siegal BR: Postrenal transplant compliance: report of 519 responses to a self-report questionnaire. *Transplant Proc* 25: 2502, 1993

50. Kiley DJ, Lam CS, Pollak R: A study of treatment compliance following kidney transplantation. *Transplantation* 55: 51, 1993

51. Terasaki PI, Gjertson DW, Cecka JM, Takemoto S: HLA matching for improved cadaver kidney allocation. *Curr Opin Nephrol Hypertens* 3: 585, 1994

52. Braun WE: Allocation of cadaver kidneys: new pressures, new solutions. *Am J Kidney Dis* 24: 526, 1994

53. Cohen DJ, Benvenisty AI, Benstein JA, Reed EF, Ho E, Suciu-Foca N et al.: Influence of HLA matching on kidney allograft survival: UNOS allocation system greatly improves the outcome. *Transplant Proc* 27: 805, 1995

54. Takemoto S, Terasaki PI, Gjertson DW, Cecka JM: Equitable allocation of HLA-compatible kidneys for local pools and minorities. *N Engl J Med* 331: 760, 1994

55. Yuan Y, Gafni A, Russell JD, Ludwin D: Development of a central matching system for the allocation of cadaveric kidneys: a simulation of clinical effectiveness versus equity. *Med Decis Making* 14: 124, 1994

56. Davies DB, Breen TJ, Guo T, Ellison MD, Daily OP, Harmon WE: Waiting times to pediatric transplantation: an assessment of the August 1990 change in renal allocation policy. *Transplant Proc* 26: 30, 1994

57. Matas AJ: Is MHC matching as a primary criterion in kidney allocation justified? (News) *Nat Genet* 5: 210, 1993

58. Gaston RS, Ayres I, Dooley LG, Diethelm AG: Racial equity in renal transplantation. The disparate impact of HLA-based allocation (see comments). *JAMA* 270: 1352, 1993

59. Sanfilippo F: Organ allocation: current problems and future issues. *Transplant Proc* 25: 2467, 1993

60. Rosenberg JC, Beyersdorf TM, Derbyshire N, Fortunato R, Manley G, Williams T: Retrieval and allocation of organs for transplantation: the Michigan experience. *Clin Transpl* 335, 1993

61. Lazda VA: Access to the kidney donor pool for racial minority population is maximized by a variance of the UNOS point system – a regional experience. Regional Organ Bank of Illinois. *Clin Transpl* 325, 1993

62. Harris JS, De Lone PA: Allocation of cadaver kidneys. *ANNA J* 19: 47, 1992

63. Gjertson DW, Terasaki PI, Takemoto S, Mickey MR: National allocation of cadaveric kidneys by HLA matching. Projected effect on outcome and costs. *N Engl J Med* 324: 1032, 1991

64. Takemoto S, Terasaki PI, Cecka JM, Cho YW, Gjertson DW: Survival of nationally shared, HLA-matched kidney transplants from cadaveric donors. The UNOS Scientific Renal Transplant Registry. *N Engl J Med* 327: 834, 1992

65. Sanfilippo FP, Vaughn WK, Peters TG, Shield CF 3rd, Adams PL, Lorber MI, et al.: Factors affecting the waiting time of cadaveric kidney transplant candidates in the United States. *JAMA* 267: 247, 1992

66. Wujciak T, Opelz G: A computer model for improved cadaver kidney allocation. *Transplant Proc* 25: 31, 1993

67. Opelz G: The benefit of exchanging donor kidneys among transplant centers. *N Engl J Med* 318: 1289, 1988

68. Takiff H, Cook DJ, Himaya NS, Mickey MR, Terasaki PI: Dominant effect of histocompatibility on ten-year kidney transplant survival. *Transplantation* 45: 410, 1988

69. Held PJ, Kahan BD, Hunsicker LG, Liska D, Wolfe RA, Port FK et al.: The impact of HLA mismatches on the survival of first cadaveric kidney transplants. *N Engl J Med* 331: 765, 1994

70. Wyner LM, Novick AC, Streem SB, Hodge EE: Improved success of living unrelated renal transplantation with cyclosporine immunosuppression. *J Urol* 149: 706, 1993

71. Sankari BR, Wyner LM, Streem SB: Living unrelated donor renal transplantation. *Urol Clin North Am* 21: 293, 1994

72. Schulak JA, Hricik DE: Steroid withdrawal after renal transplantation. *Clin Transplant* 8: 211, 1994

73. Hricik DE, Whalen CC, Lautman J, Bartucci MR, Moir EJ, Mayes JT et al.: Withdrawal of steroids after renal transplantation – clinical predictors of outcome. *Transplantation* 53: 41, 1992

74. Terasaki PI: Overview. in: *Clinical Transplants 1988*, edited by Terasaki PI, Cecka JM, Takemoto S, Yuge J, Mickey MR, Park MS et al., Los Angeles, UCLA Tissue Typing Laboratory, 1988, p 409

75. Frei U, Brunkhorst R, Schindler R, Bode U, Repp H, Pichlmayr R et al.: Present status of kidney transplantation. *Clin Nephrol* 38 (Suppl 1): S46, 1992

76. Opelz G: The benefit of exchanging donor kidneys among transplant centers. *N Engl J Med* 318: 1289, 1988

77. Donnelly P, Veitch P, Bell P, Henderson R, Oman P, Proud G: Donor-recipient age difference – an independent risk factor in cyclosporin-treated renal transplant recipients. *Transpl Int* 4: 88, 1991

78. Donnelly PK, Simpson AR, Milner AD, Nicholson ML, Horsburgh T, Veitch PS, et al.: Age-matching improves the results of renal transplantation with older donors [see comments]. *Nephrol Dial Transplant* 5: 808, 1990

79. Soulillou JP, Cantarovich D, Le Mauff B, Giral M, Robillard N, Hourmant M et al.: Randomized controlled trial of a monoclonal antibody against the interleukin-2 receptor (33B3.1) as compared with rabbit antithymocyte globulin for prophylaxis against rejection of renal allografts. *N Engl J Med* 322: 1175, 1990

80. Frey DJ, Matas AJ, Gillingham KJ, Canafax D, Payne WD, Dunn DL et al.: MALG *vs* OKT3 following renal transplantation: a randomized prospective trial. *Transplant Proc* 23: 1048, 1991

81. Hoitsma AJ, Tiggeler RG, Wetzels JF, Berden JH, Koene RA: Comparison of 10-day and 21-day ATG-antirejection treatment in renal transplant patients treated with either cyclosporine or azathioprine as basic immunosuppression. *Transplant Proc* 21: 1732, 1989

82. Palmer BF, Dawidson I, Sagalowsky A, Sandor Z, Lu CY: Improved outcome of cadaveric renal transplantation due to calcium channel blockers. *Transplantation* 52: 640, 1991

83. Hoyer PF, Offner G, Brodehl J, Ringe B, Bunzendahl H, Pichlmayr R: Renal function and donor age: five years' experience with cyclosporin A. *Transplant Proc* 21: 30, 1989

84. Thorogood J, Houwelingen JC, Persijn GG, Zantvoort FA, Schreuder GM, van Rood JJ: Prognostic indices to predict survival of first and second renal allografts. *Transplantation* 52: 831, 1991

85. Opelz G: Influence of HLA matching on survival of second kidney transplants in cyclosporine-treated recipients. *Transplantation* 47: 823, 1989

86. Opelz G: Importance of HLA antigen splits for kidney transplant matching. *Lancet* 2: 61, 1988

87. Opelz G, Mytilineos J, Scherer S, Dunckley H, Trejaut J, Chapman J et al.: Analysis of HLA-DR matching in DNA-typed cadaver kidney transplants. *Transplantation* 55: 782, 1993

88. Gouny P, Lenot B, Decaix B, Rondeau E, Kitzis M, Lacave R et al.: Aortoiliac surgery and kidney transplantation. *Ann Vasc Surg* 5: 26, 1991

89. Wright JG, Tesi RJ, Massop DW, Henry ML, Durham JR, Ferguson RM et al.: Safety of simultaneous aortic reconstruction and renal transplantation. *Am J Surg* 162: 126, 1991

90. Langle F, Muhlbacher F, Steininger R, Kovarik J, Derfler K, Balcke P et al.: Long-term outcome in renal patients

beyond five years after kidney transplantation. *Transplant Proc* 21: 2176, 1989

91. Olivari M-T, Kubo SH, Braunlin EA, Bolman RM, Ring WS: Five-year experience with triple-drug immunosuppressive therapy in cardiac transplantation. *Circulation* 82 (Suppl 4): IV276, 1990

92. Thorogood J, Persijn GG, Schreuder GM, D'Amaro J, Zantvoort FA, van Houwelingen JC et al.: The effect of HLA matching on kidney graft survival in separate posttransplantation intervals. *Transplantation* 50: 146, 1990

93. Gjertson DW: Multifactorial analysis of renal transplants reported to the United Network for Organ Sharing Registry. *Clin Transpl* 299, 1992

94. Takiff H, Mickey MR, Cicciarelli J, Terasaki PI: Factors important in ten-year kidney graft survival. *Transplant Proc* 19: 666, 1987

95. Hall BM, Tiller DJ, Hardie I, Mahony J, Mathew T, Thatcher G et al.: Comparison of three immunosuppressive regimens in cadaver renal transplantation: long-term cyclosporine, short-term cyclosporine followed by azathioprine and prednisolone, and azathioprine and prednisolone without cyclosporine. *N Engl J Med* 318: 1499, 1988

96. Vanrenterghem Y, Roels L, Lerut T, Waer M, Gruwez J, Michielsen P: Long-term prognosis after cadaveric kidney transplantation. *Transplant Proc* 19: 3762, 1987

97. Fujimori K, Satomi S, Okazaki H, Taguchi Y, Mori S: The effect of protein intake on creatinine clearance in transplanted kidneys. *Transplant Proc* 21: 2048, 1989

98. Windus DW, Lacson S, Delmez JA: The short-term effects of a low-protein diet in stable renal transplant recipients. *Am J Kidney Dis* 17: 693, 1991

99. Fabrega AJ, Lopez-Boado M, Gonzalez S: Problems in the long-term renal allograft recipient. *Crit Care Clin* 6: 979, 1990

100. Rao KV: Mechanism, pathophysiology, diagnosis, and management of renal transplant rejection. *Med Clin North Am* 74: 1039, 1990

101. Rao KV, Andersen RC: Long-term results and complications in renal transplant recipients. Observations in the second decade. *Transplantation* 45: 45, 1988

102. Rosenblum ND, Harmon WE, Levey RH: Treatment of chronic renal allograft rejection with cyclosporine and prednisone. *Transplantation* 45: 232, 1988

103. Mennander A, Tiisala S, Halttunen J, Yilmaz S, Paavonen T, Hayry P: Chronic rejection in rat aortic allografts. An experimental model for transplant arteriosclerosis. *Arterioscler Thromb* 11: 671, 1991

104. Frei U, Schindler R, Wieters D, Grouven U, Brunkhorst R, Koch KM: Pre-transplant hypertension – a major risk factor for chronic progressive renal allograft dysfunction? *Nephrol Dial Transplant* 10: 1206, 1995

105. Wright JG, Tesi RJ, Massop DW, Henry ML, Durham JR, Ferguson RM et al.: Safety of simultaneous aortic reconstruction and renal transplantation. *Am J Surg* 162: 126, 1991

106. Schorn TF, Frei U, Brackmann H, Lorenz M, Vogt P, Wiese B et al.: Cyclosporine-associated posttransplant hypertension incidence and effect on renal transplant function. *Transplant Proc* 20: 610, 1988

107. Isoniemi H, Tikkanen M, Hayry P, Eklund B, Hockerstedt K, Salmela K et al.: Lipid profiles with triple drug immunosuppressive therapy and with double drug combinations after renal transplantation and stable graft function. *Transplant Proc* 23: 1029, 1991

108. Schorn TF, Kliem V, Bojanovski M, Bojanovski D, Repp H, Bunzendahl H et al.: Impact of long-term immunosuppression with cyclosporin A on serum lipids in stable renal transplant recipients. *Transpl Int* 4: 92, 1991

109. Penn I: Cancer in the immunosuppressed organ recipient. *Transplant Proc* 23: 1771, 1991

110. Penn I: Occurrence of cancers in immunosuppressed organ transplant recipients. *Clin Transpl* 53, 1990

111. Cockfield SM, Preiksaitis J, Harvey E, Jones C, Hebert D, Keown P et al.: Is sequential use of ALG and OKT3 in renal transplants associated with an increased incidence of fulminant posttransplant lymphoproliferative disorder? *Transplant Proc* 23: 1106, 1991

112. Vogt P, Frei U, Repp H, Bunzendahl H, Oldhafer K, Pichlmayr R: Malignant tumours in renal transplant recipients receiving cyclosporin: survey of 598 first-kidney transplantations. *Nephrol Dial Transplant* 5: 282, 1990

113. Walz MK, Albrecht KH, Niebel W, Eigler FW: De novo malignant tumors during drug immunosuppression. The findings following 1245 cadaveric kidney transplants in 1080 patients. *Dtsch Med Wochenschr* 117: 927, 1992

114. Sheil AG, Disney AP, Mathew TH, Amiss N: De novo malignancy emerges as a major cause of morbidity and late failure in renal transplantation. *Transplant Proc* 25: 1383, 1993

115. Frei U, Bode U, Repp H, Schindler R, Brunkhorst R, Vogt P et al.: Malignancies under cyclosporine after kidney transplantation: analysis of a 10-year period. *Transplant Proc* 25: 1394, 1993

116. Pol S, Debure A, Degott C, Carnot F, Legendre C, Brechot C et al.: Chronic hepatitis in kidney allograft recipients. *Lancet* 335: 878, 1990

117. Parfrey PS et al.: The impact of transplantation on the course of hepatitis B liver disease. *Transplantation* 39: 610, 1985

118. Toussaint C, Kinnaert P, Vereerstraeten P: Late mortality and morbidity five to eighteen years after kidney transplantation. *Transplantation* 45: 554, 1988

119. Rao KV, Kasiske BL, Anderson WR: Variability in the morphological spectrum and clinical outcome of chronic liver disease in hepatitis B-positive and B-negative renal transplant recipients. *Transplantation* 51: 391, 1991

120. Kiberd BA, Belitsky P: The fate of the failed renal transplant. *Transplantation* 59: 645, 1995

121. Almond MK, Tailor D, Marsh FP, Raftery MJ, Cunningham J: Increased erythropoietin requirements in patients with failed renal transplants returning to a dialysis programme. *Nephrol Dial Transplant* 9: 270, 1994

122. Cattran DC, Fenton SS: Contemporary management of renal failure: outcome of the failed allograft recipient. *Kidney Int* 41 (Suppl): S36, 1993

123. Hansen BL, Rohr N, Svendsen V, Birkeland SA: Graft failure and graft nephrectomy without severe complications. *Nephrol Dial Transplant* 2: 189, 1987

124. Verresen L, Vanrenterghem Y, Waer M, Hauglustaine D, Michielsen P: Corticosteroid withdrawal syndrome in dialysis patients. *Nephrol Dial Transplant* 3: 476, 1988

125. Ramos EL: Recurrent diseases in the renal allograft. *J Am Soc Nephrol* 2: 109, 1991

DIALYTIC MANAGEMENT OF DIABETIC UREMIC PATIENTS

ELI A. FRIEDMAN and ANNE MARIE V. MILES

INTRODUCTION

Diabetic nephropathy is the most prevalent cause of end-stage renal disease (ESRD) in the United States. According to the 1994 United States Renal Data System (USRDS) report, diabetes accounted for 17,882 of 49,909 (35.8%) incident cases (Figure 1) and 48,274 of 186,261 (24.9%) prevalent cases of ESRD in the US in 1991 (1). The lower prevalence than incidence of diabetic ESRD patients in the US is a consequence of their higher mortality during uremia therapy. This point is illustrated in Figure 2 which plots relative survival for diabetic versus the entire population of hemodialysis and peritoneal dialysis patients.

Prior to the 1980s, diabetics were nearly uniformly excluded from ESRD programs because of their excessive mortality and morbidity attributed to blindness, coronary, cerebrovascular and peripheral artery vasculopathy. Illustrating this reality, Avram reported in 1966, in Brooklyn, that no diabetic on maintenance hemodialysis lived for longer than six months (2). A subsequent early series of 32 diabetics started on hemodialysis had only 8 survive as long as 3 months (3). Most pioneer reports of dialysis in diabetics (mainly insulin dependent patients) from the United States, recounted a two year survival ranging from 25–40% (4–6). In Europe, only 34% of diabetics survived after 3 years of dialysis (7).

Continuous growth in the number of diabetics treated for ESRD over the past 20 years is illustrated by their increased prevalence from 6,362 in 1981 (10% of the ESRD population) to 41,034 in 1990 (24.5% of the ESRD population). Registry statistics similarly document diabetes as the leading cause of treated renal failure in Canada (8). Throughout Europe, Japan, and Australia/New Zealand, diabetes ranks first among causes of ESRD. At least three interrelated reasons explain the dominance of

ESRD INCIDENCE: USA, 1991

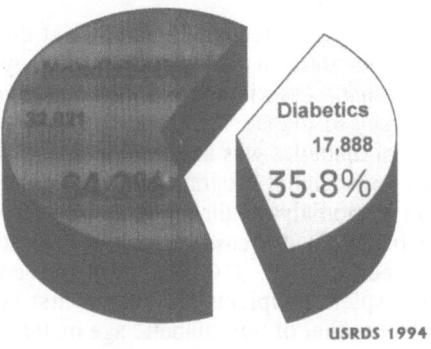

Figure 1. In the United States, more than a third of newly treated ESRD patients have diabetes. Although not clearly documented, the large majority of those ESRD patients who are diabetic developed renal failure because of diabetic nephropathy. The proportion of ESRD patients who are diabetic is increasing more than 1% each year. Data from USRDS 1994 report.

diabetes as the preeminent cause of ESRD in the industrialized world: 1) Extended life expectancy results in an older population bearing a greater risk of non-insulin dependent diabetes (NIDDM). 2) After World War II, better access to food – associated with a greater prevalence of obesity – heightened expression of clinical diabetes in those carrying a genetic predisposition to NIDDM. 3) Realization that onset of uremia in diabetic patients need not end useful life promotes their increased acceptance into renal replacement programs. Establishment in the US of Medicare reimbursement for ESRD therapy

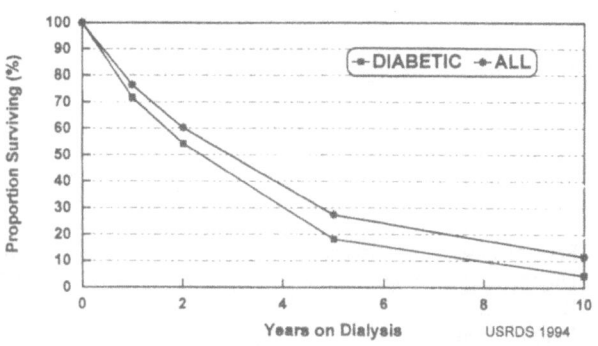

Figure 2. Diabetic dialysis patients (both peritoneal dialysis and hemodialysis treated) have substantially lower survival than do non-diabetic dialysis patients. Note that at two years, about half of diabetics have died. Fewer than one in twenty diabetic patients on dialysis are alive ten years after starting dialysis. Data from USRDS 1994 report.

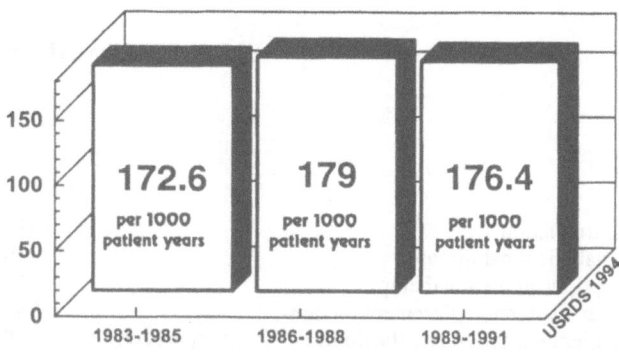

Figure 3. Although the mean age and proportion of diabetics have increased progressively in incidence, the mortality of ESRD treatment in the US has not decreased. Indeed, survival in age matched subsets of diabetic and non-diabetic patients actually improved. Data from USRDS 1994 report.

in 1972, stimulated expansion of long-term ESRD care including diabetics.

Medical-surgical team collaboration at the University of Minnesota initiated trials of dialytic therapy and kidney (and later, pancreas-kidney) transplants encouraging dialytic therapy of diabetics. By the early 1980s, improved survival of diabetics was achieved in the US and Europe in renal replacement programs. By the mid-1990s, mortality in hemodialyzed diabetics though greater than in non-diabetics (9), decreased to a one year death rate ranging between 11–30% (10–13). Diabetic cadaver donor renal transplant recipients may attain first year survival equivalent to that of non-diabetic age matched recipients (14).

DIABETIC RENAL DISEASE

Consensus thinking by nephrologists – inferred by the authors – holds that both renal disease and ESRD are more prevalent in patients with insulin-dependent diabetes mellitus (IDDM) than in NIDDM. Due to the greater than 10 to 1 higher prevalence of NIDDM over IDDM, however, the majority of diabetics in US hemodialysis programs have NIDDM. Before life extension for diabetic patients was the rule, there was a misperception that only 3–10% of patients with NIDDM developed ESRD (15), compared to 30–45% of those with IDDM (16). Contemporary reports (17, 18) indicate that the rate of renal disease is similar in NIDDM and IDDM. Humphrey et al.'s longitudinal study in Rochester, Minnesota (17) found that in 1,832 individuals with NIDDM and 136 with IDDM, followed for 30 years, there were equivalent rates of renal failure (133 per 100,000 person years in NIDDM, and 170 per

100,000 person years in IDDM). This finding was echoed in Heidelberg, Germany, in patient cohorts with IDDM and NIDDM followed for 20 years who developed nearly identical rates of renal impairment (serum creatinine level < 1.4 mg/dl) of 59% in IDDM, and 63% in NIDDM (18). As a generalization from surveys of NIDDM in diverse ethnic groups (American Pima Indians (19), Blacks, and Hispanics (20)), NIDDM and ESRD are more prevalent than has been previously appreciated.

Mainly due to selective attack rates – by gender and race – in NIDDM, diabetic nephropathy afflicts 20% more women than men (21), and is three to seven times more prevalent in Blacks (22); Mexican Americans and Native Americans (23, 24) compared to other racial subgroups. Black women between 55–74 years of age have the highest attack rate of NIDDM explaining their disproportionate number of new cases of diabetic ESRD in the US.

In IDDM, nephropathy progresses through stages described by Mogensen (25); typically, in those destined to develop renal complications, ESRD occurs within 15–30 years of the initial diagnosis of diabetes, usually about three years after the onset of a nephrotic syndrome. Recent epidemiologic familial studies indicate that only a distinct subset – probably genetically predetermined – of those with IDDM are at risk for nephropathy (26). Less precision surrounds efforts to detail the natural history of NIDDM, mainly because of ambiguity in defining a specific date of onset which as extrapolated from retinal photographs is usually 7–9 years earlier than thought based on first recognition of hyperglycemia (27). Door to door surveys of random glucose levels from Alaska to Hawaii show that about one-half of those with NIDDM in the US are undiagnosed (28). The older the age at onset of NIDDM the more rapid the development of ESRD (29). Renal failure has been most frequently reported (48–59%)

Uremia Therapy: USA, 1991

USRDS 1994

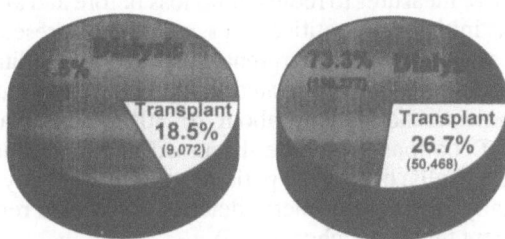

DIABETICS   ALL ESRD

Figure 4. Diabetic ESRD patients are less likely to receive a kidney transplant than are non-diabetic ESRD patients. The explanation for this difference is inferred to be the older age and greater rate of comorbid extrarenal disease in diabetics, though this presumption is not carefully documented. Data from USRDS 1994 report.

Table 1. Options in uremia therapy for diabetic ESRD patients

1. Passive suicide which is the consequence of declining dialysis or kidney transplantation
2. Hemodialysis
    Facility hemodialysis
    Home hemodialysis
3. Peritoneal dialysis
    Intermittent peritoneal dialysis (IPD)
    Continuous ambulatory peritoneal dialysis (CAPD)
    Continuous cyclic peritoneal dialysis (CCPD)
4. Renal transplantation
    Cadaver donor kidney
    Living donor kidney
5. Pancreas plus kidney transplantation
    IDDM
    ?NIDDM

in IDDM diagnosed before the age of 20 years (30); in this subset of diabetics (before the application of ESRD therapy), mean survival is only seven months once the serum creatinine reaches 8 mg/dl.

OPTIONS IN UREMIA THERAPY

Misrepresentation of the US ESRD program has portrayed an inordinately high mortality compared to death rates in Europe and Japan. More critical assessment of US and world ESRD survival statistics, however, supports the inference that US mortality actually improved despite a case mix which has progressively aged and contains more diabetics (31). Figure 3 shows the constant US overall mortality rate in ESRD patients from 1983 to 1991, despite the growing acceptance of older and sicker patients.

As depicted in Figure 4, assignment to therapy results in a greater proportion (81.5%) of diabetics receiving maintenance hemodialysis and a lesser proportion given a renal transplant (18.5%) (1). When compared with the previous USRDS report (1993) the proportion of diabetic patients relegated to maintenance hemodialysis rose from 80%, underscoring the growing dominance of hemodialysis as the most applied ESRD regimen for diabetics (32).

Determination of which treatment option is 'best' for a particular diabetic ESRD patient, however, is an individualized judgment (Table 1) depending on the patient's age, education, geographic location, family and social support systems, and the extent of co-morbid conditions, most importantly, cardiovascular integrity. Major subjects which must be appraised when devising a long-term plan for ESRD management include anticipated patient compliance and potential to participate in self treatment. Each ESRD treatment option must be explained in understand-

able terms covering probable survival rate, degree of rehabilitation, and expected stabilization of extrarenal diabetic complications. Ideally, what has been termed a 'life plan' should be constructed for every ESRD patient after consultation between the health care team, patient, and members of the patient's social support system.

Few reports document the comparative fate of ESRD treatment by type of diabetes. In a German population of 196 diabetics admitted to 28 dialysis centers, actuarial survival three years after beginning maintenance hemodialysis was equivalent in 67 patients with IDDM (40%) to that in 129 with NIDDM (43%) even though the median age of the IDDM cohort was 15 years younger (49 years) than the NIDDM cohort (64 years) (33). While the best rehabilitation of diabetic ESRD patients is achieved in recipients of living related donor renal transplants, this superior outcome may reflect a selection bias in which younger, healthier patients are chosen for a transplant leaving a residual pool of more morbid dialysis patients. Morbidity from blindness and neuropathy (but not coronary artery or peripheral vascular disease) is decreased in diabetic kidney transplant recipients (34). Lacking randomized prospective trials of diabetics treated by dialytic therapy versus a kidney transplant, controlled for age, race, gender, and severity of extrarenal complications, caution must be exercised when assessing one ESRD therapy against another. A reasonable policy can be based on the premise that while the best rehabilitation is effected by renal transplantation, there is no distinctly superior treatment for the uremic diabetic, and therefore, assessment and treatment of diabetics with ESRD must be highly individualized.

Table 2. Diabetic complications which persist and/or progress during ESRD

1. Retinopathy, glaucoma, cataracts
2. Coronary artery disease. Cardiomyopathy
3. Cerebrovascular disease
4. Peripheral vascular disease: limb amputation
5. Motor neuropathy. Sensory neuropathy
6. Autonomic dysfunction: diarrhea, constipation, hypotension
7. Myopathy
8. Depression

STARTING RENAL REPLACEMENT THERAPY

Realization that ESRD support therapy, most often maintenance hemodialysis, must be initiated is usually resisted by the patient despite weeks to months of preparatory discussions between doctor and patient. Patients trapped by a decision that cannot be avoided may become hostile, depressed and non-compliant to their medical regimen. Patient support groups and collaboration with a diabetes nurse educator aid in supporting patients through this time of despair and threat.

PATIENT EDUCATION AND THE MULTIDISCIPLINARY APPROACH

Patient education should begin as soon as it is evident that renal failure is probable. During the pre-ESRD stages of diabetic nephropathy, the benefits of blood pressure control, glucose regulation, and dietary protein restriction in retarding loss of renal function should be explained. Admittedly, the value – in terms of preserving renal function – of enhancing glycemic control in 'established' nephropathy is unproven. Clinical observation, however, suggests that well being, resistance to infection, and stability of retinopathy are maximized by the closest approximation to euglycemia that can be attained. Sodium and fluid restriction become components of the regimen in diabetic nephropathy when a nephrotic syndrome or congestive heart failure become symptomatic.

Management of diabetic patients with deteriorating renal function can be tricky because of potentially progressive multiple extrarenal comorbid complications reflecting system wide micro- and macrovasculopathy (Table 2). Particularly vexing is loss of vision. Ophthalmologic evaluation must be obtained at least three to four times per year once proliferative retinopathy is detected. Skilled retina surgeons applying panretinal photocoagulation are usually able to halt what previously was thought an inexorable march toward blindness (35). Like preservation of sight,

a foot care regimen is vital to forestall lower limb amputation. Daily inspection of the feet, wearing heel booties when confined to bed, plus surveillance by a podiatrist are effective measures to reduce limb loss before and after dialysis is initiated. Repetitive assessment of the presence and extent of comorbid extrarenal disorders is facilitated by a rating scale as illustrated in Table 3. As residual creatinine clearance falls to about 20–30 ml/min, available ESRD options should be discussed and a selection made. Practically, bias by the patient's most trusted physician usually is the major factor determining which renal replacement therapy is chosen (36).

For the 80% of uremic diabetics selecting hemodialysis, construction of a vascular access is of great importance. Predialysis management should preserve forearm cutaneous veins by avoiding intravenous catheters or cutdowns. Once it is clear that uremia is a near-term probability (less than one year) an arteriovenous access should be constructed. Creation of vascular access for diabetic hemodialysis patients can be difficult in arm vessels calcified or occluded by atherosclerosis. First choice in hemodialysis access in diabetics is an autologous arteriovenous fistula of the Cimino-Brescia type. When vessels are not suitable, a Dacron or polytetraflouroethylene (PTFE) graft can be inserted. Mean three year survival of arteriovenous fistulae in diabetics is about 80%, while arteriovenous grafts remain viable for 47% after three years (37). Enthusiasts for newer PTFE grafts suggest that they last as long as endogenous fistulae (38). For many diabetics surviving more than one year on hemodialysis, repetitive access revision, often requiring partial or total graft replacement is the rule.

The pros and cons of peritoneal dialysis versus hemodialysis for diabetic ESRD patients are presented in Table 4. When peritoneal dialysis is selected, advance planning should ensure that a suitable peritoneal catheter is *in situ* 2–4 weeks before starting dialysis. Referral to a nearby training facility while the patient is free of uremic complications facilitates easy initiation of dialytic therapy. Opting for a kidney or a kidney plus pancreas transplant obviously demands referral to and evaluation by a transplant team. In the case of an intended living related donor transplant, interim dialysis can be avoided by proper planning, performing the transplant at an early stage of uremic symptoms. A long wait, two or more years, is usual for a cadaver kidney in New York City. Accordingly, patients should be entered on waiting lists when the creatinine clearance is about 10–15 ml/min.

TIMING THE START OF DIALYTIC THERAPY

The decision to discontinue conservative management of renal insufficiency in diabetic nephropathy in favor of dialysis or a kidney transplant is a judgement call in most cases. There is no doubt that ESRD care is urgently required

Table 3. Variables in morbidity in diabetic kidney transplant recipients. The Co-Morbidity Index*

1.	Persistent angina or myocardial infarction.
2.	Other cardiovascular problems, hypertension, congestive heart failure, cardiomyopathy.
3.	Respiratory disease.
4.	Autonomic neuropathy (gastroparesis, obstipation, diarrhea, cystopathy, orthostatic hypotension).
5.	Neurologic problems, cerebrovascular accident or stroke residual, transient ischemic attacks, monoplegias from motor neuropathy, dialysis dementia (aluminum poisoning).
6.	Musculoskeletal disorders, including all varieties of renal bone disease.
7.	Infections including AIDS but excluding vascular access-site or peritonitis.
8.	Hepatitis, hepatic insufficiency, enzymatic pancreatic insufficiency.
9.	Hematologic problems other than anemia, leukopenia, purpura.
10.	Spinal abnormalities, lower back problems or arthritis.
11.	Vision impairment (minor to severe – decreased acuity to blindness) loss.
12.	Limb amputation (minor to severe – finger to lower extremity).
13.	Mental or emotional illness (neurosis, depression, psychosis).

*To obtain a numerical Co-Morbidity Index for an individual patient, rate each variable from 0 to 3 (0 = absent, 1 = mild – of minor import to patient's life, 2 = moderate, 3 = severe). By proportional hazard analysis, the relative significance of each variable can be isolated from the other 12.

when agonal signs of uremia (pericardial rub, asterixis, gastrointestinal hemorrhage, advancing motor neuropathy) are discovered in a newly evaluated diabetic patient. Similarly, a carefully performed creatinine clearance of less than 5 ml/min or a serum creatinine concentration greater than 10 mg/dl are clear objective signs of the need for ESRD support. At the other extreme, minimally symptomatic azotemic diabetic patients, with a creatinine clearance greater than 15 ml/min, or a serum creatinine concentration below 4 mg/dl, require neither dialytic therapy nor renal transplantation. Because diabetics develop symptomatic uremia and volume overload at creatinine clearances which are higher than in non-diabetics, however, exceptions to these indications may be appropriate – especially in patients who are nephrotic, elderly, and/or in congestive heart failure.

In such patients, dialysis is started at creatinine clearances as high as 15–20 ml/min, at serum creatinine levels as low as 3–5 mg/dl. Though no randomized trial comparing early versus late initiation of dialysis in diabetics has been reported, the authors believe that earlier institution of therapy is one factor which has improved survival and reduced morbidity of diabetics in dialysis programs over the past 15–20 years. Kjellstrand, in 1972 (39), observed that retinopathy in diabetics progresses rapidly during the one to two year period prior to the initiation of dialysis. It follows that early institution of dialysis may eliminate the adverse effects on retinopathy of hypertension and volume overload while correcting the hemorrhagic diathesis of uremia, thereby retarding its progression. Starting dialysis when substantive renal function persists may also retard acceleration of uremic neuropathy in patients with concurrent diabetic autonomic neuropathy. Survival of dialyzed diabetics improved over the past decade. No single factor

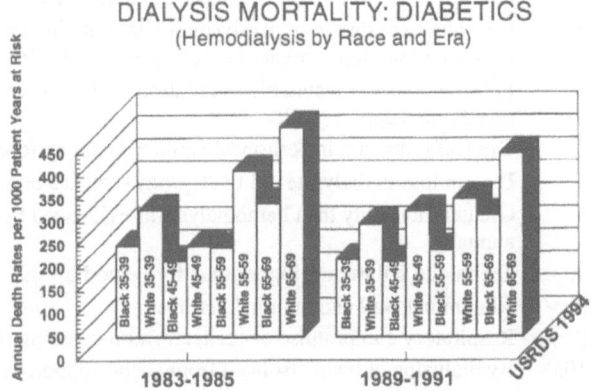

Figure 5. Between 1983 and 1991 mortality of hemodialysis and peritoneal dialysis treated diabetic patients improved in both Black and White patients. Selected age subsets are compared for both races and both therapies. Note that Blacks have survival superior to Whites and hemodialysis survival is superior to that on peritoneal dialysis (CAPD/CCPD). Younger patients have better survival than older patients. Data from the USRDS by special request in 1994.

is credited with reducing the death rate of hemodialyzed diabetics though better control of hypertension, reduction in intravascular volume overload, better nutrition, and better vascular access surgery have contributed.

HEMODIALYSIS IN DIABETICS

Overcoming unfavorable initial reports of the efficacy of hemodialysis in diabetics cited above, hemodialysis

Table 4. Opting for CAPD/CCPD in diabetic ESRD patients

Pros:

1. Widely available.
2. Performed at home after short training period. Not preempted by bad weather.
3. Avoids precipitous periodic hypotension complicating hemodialysis.
4. Stable internal milieux without chemical peaks and valleys.
5. Easy insulin administration when added to dialysate.
6. Liberal diet, minimized fluid restriction.
7. Transportable therapy to work place or vacation.
8. Higher hematocrit than on hemodialysis.
9. Avoids need for vascular access – no painful needle sticks – escaping threat of hand ischemia and gangrene.
10. No arm cosmetic disfigurement from dilated vessels.
11. Escapes highly prevalent 'under dialysis' consequent to prescription of too short hemodialyses by busy facilities attempting to maximize utilization of dialysis stations.
12. Hypertension typically managed by fluid extraction (hyperosmolar dialysate) rather than resort to antihypertensive medications.
13. Bypasses maintenance hemodialysis requirement for adherence to facility scheduled treatments that impose travel and inconvenience especially in rural areas where few dialysis units exist.

Cons:

1. Requires nearly total preoccupation of patient with self-treatment delivering four tedious dialysate exchanges daily, risking ennui, 'burn out,' and lapse in compliance.
2. Constant exposure to hyperglycemic dialysate induces hyperlipidemia and higher level of glycated proteins imposing long-term threat of accelerated atherosclerosis.
3. Peritonitis nearly inevitable as duration of therapy extends beyond one year. Abdominal distension and hernia mandating support girdle.
4. Gradual reduction in peritoneal surface area may force transfer to hemodialysis.
5. Protein loss in dialysate – 8 to 20 g/day – makes muscle preservation tenuous.
6. Greater morbidity than hemodialysis as evidenced by more frequent hospitalizations and more days hospitalized annually.
7. Technique failure rate higher than for hemodialysis.
8. Abdominal wall and inguinal herniae.
9. Respiratory compromise or bradyarryhtmias during fluid instillation.
10. By dialyzing at home, isolated from social support system, thereby misses benefit of staff morale boosting and patient support groups.
11. Storage of supplies (boxed dialysate) cumbersome. Travel necessitates loading heavy cartons of dialysate, tubing and intravenous saline.
12. Mortality greater than hemodialysis whether compared by equivalent subsets matched by age, race, or gender.

emerged as the most common treatment for all forms of renal failure including diabetic nephropathy (Figure 4). Diabetics on hemodialysis die at a rate of 11–30% per year (11–14, 40), but their death rate when adjusted for age is decreasing in Blacks and Whites (Figure 5). Heart disease, stroke, infection, and withdrawal from treatment are the most common causes. Death from macrovascular disease (atherogenesis) in diabetics is the consequence of hypertension, hypertriglyceridemia, hypercholesterolemia (particularly in nephrosis), arterial calcification, and cigarette smoking.

Surveys in Germany, Japan, and the US concur in finding heart disease, principally coronary artery disease and congestive failure, the major cause of death in diabetics treated by hemodialysis or peritoneal dialysis (Figure 6). Weinrauch et al. suggest that a finding of abnormal motion of the left ventricular wall, detected by echocardiography, is the most important determinant of survival as compared with an abnormal standard electrocardiogram at baseline, or history of angina pectoris or myocardial infarction (41). In an autopsy study of 106 consecutive ESRD patients, cardiovascular pathology was present in 36% with acute myocardial infarction accounting for the death of 15% (42). Death from cardiovascular disease was predicted by diabetes and hypertension in this series. Cardiovascular disease causes death in 23–54% of diabetics on dialysis (10). A 19.2% yearly incidence of myocardial infarction or congestive heart failure, and a 10% incidence of

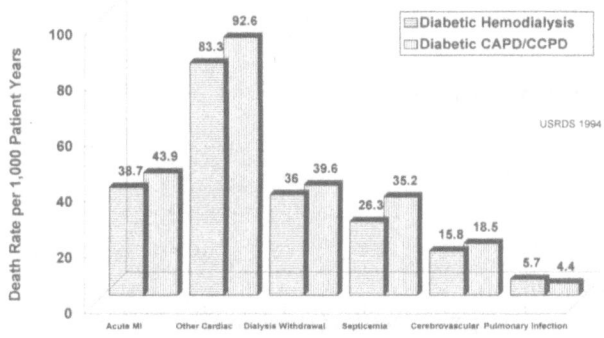

Extrarenal Mortality: Diabetic Dialysis Patients US 1989-1991

Figure 6. In hemodialysis treated as in peritoneal dialysis treated diabetic patients, cardiac disease is the greatest cause of death. Note that for each identified cause of death – except pulmonary infection – peritoneal dialysis has a death rate higher than does hemodialysis. Data from the USRDS 1994 report.

cerebral hemorrhage or thrombosis in diabetics on dialysis was reported in 1977 (43). Cardiovascular mortality was 4.8 times higher in IDDM and 3.0 times higher in NIDDM than in non-diabetic hemodialysis patients in a retrospective study of 200 age and sex-matched diabetic and non-diabetic hemodialysis patients treated between 1972 and 1983 (44). Death in this series was attributed to 'Sudden Death' in 80%, myocardial infarction in 13%, and stroke in 7%. Strong predictors of death were: systolic blood pressure over 160 mmHg at the start of dialysis, cardiomegaly on chest Xray – associated with electrocardiographic evidence of left ventricular hypertrophy. Coronary artery disease though severe, may be silent. With no prior expression of coronary artery disease, IDDM patients subjected to coronary angiography when starting treatment for ESRD had a 42–55% prevalence of significant (> 50% stenosis) coronary artery disease (45). Comorbidity in diabetics on hemodialysis limits rehabilitation and results in excess number of hospitalizations and longer stays in hospital than in non-diabetic patients. No clear advantage, in terms of progression of neuropathy, retinopathy and/or peripheral vascular disease can be credited to hemodialysis, peritoneal dialysis or renal transplantation (46). Blindness in diabetics on hemodialysis can be prevented by preventive eye care. Wantanabe et al. followed 268 Japanese diabetics on hemodialysis who had a 50% survival at 60 months and demonstrated stabilization of visual acuity in 364/418 eyes (87.1%) with 20/418 eyes improved and only 34/418 eyes (8.1%) worse (47).

Complications arising during dialysis

1. Hypotension. Hypotension is more prevalent in diabetic than in non-diabetic hemodialysis patients. Episodic hypotension is at least 20% greater in incidence while nausea and vomiting are three times more prevalent (48). A linkage between hypotension and antecedent nausea and vomiting is common in diabetic dialysis patients despite obvious clinical volume overload and edema. Severe or sustained hypotension may precipitate angina pectoris culminating in acute myocardial infarction.

Predisposing to this sequence is decreased left ventricular compliance and filling caused by ischemic heart disease, or hypertensive diastolic dysfunction components of diabetic cardiomyopathy (4). Magnifying the impact of diabetic cardiomyopathy, conjoint diabetic plus uremic autonomic diabetic neuropathy abolishes reflex increase in heart rate and peripheral vascular resistance (producing decreased venous compliance hence increased preload, as well as increased systemic vascular resistance) which prevents hemodialysis-induced hypotension. Also predisposing to dialysis induced hypotension is hypoalbuminemia resulting from both nephrotic protein loss and malnutrition, that reduces colloid oncotic pressure retarding the plasma refilling rate (49). Uremic anemia aggravates diabetics susceptibility to intradialytic hypotension. In anemic patients, hypoviscosity of plasma and reduced peripheral vascular resistance impairs blood volume maintenance during ultrafiltration. Additionally, anemia may contribute to dialysis-related angina pectoris; a recent fall in hematocrit should always be sought in the diabetic patient who develops chest pain on dialysis.

Gotch postulates that thermal amplification (50) may contribute to dialysis associated hypotension. He theorizes that increased core heat during hemodialysis (51), combined with reduced heat loss due to cutaneous vasoconstriction in response to hypovolemia early in dialysis, results in reflex vasodilation of cutaneous blood vessels and sudden hypotension near the end of dialysis. Dialysis-related hypotension responds to measures listed in Table 5. For diabetic patients prone to angina during dialysis, a combination of nasal oxygen and sublingual nitroglycerin is usually efficacious. Cutaneous application of 2% nitroglycerin ointment 30–60 min before dialysis usually prevents anginal episodes. Failure to preempt hemodialysis-induced angina in diabetic patients is reason to attempt a trial of peritoneal dialysis.

2. Hypertension. Ritz and others report that hypertension is more prevalent in diabetic than in non-diabetic hemodialysis patients. About one-half of hemodialyzed diabetics require antihypertensive medications, compared to 27.7% of non-diabetics (44). The course of hypertension in diabetics during dialysis is variable, improvement is typical in volume dependent hypertension after intradialytic fluid extraction. Other diabetics continue to require antihypertensive medications following initiation of hemodialysis, and some may, in addition, experience progressive elevation in blood pressure during or after hemodialysis. Activation of the renin-angiotensin system by ultrafiltration-induced reduced intravascular volume may explain intradialytic hypertension in some diabetics.

Table 5. Minimizing hemodialysis-induced hypotension in diabetics

1. Bicarbonate rather than acetate dialysate.
2. High sodium concentration (140–145 mmol/l) in dialysate.
3. Slow rate of ultrafiltration.
4. Schedule sequential ultrafiltration and dialysis in patients who are grossly edematous.
5. Prime dialysis circuit with hypertonic albumin solution.
6. Maintain hematocrit at or above 30 vol % with erythropoietin.
7. Omit antihypertensive medications on morning of dialysis.
8. Restrict meals immediately before or during hemodialysis.
9. Leg toning exercises to improve venous return.
10. Decrease dialysate temperature (particularly near conclusion of treatment).
11. Explore potential benefits of: alpha agonists (phenylephrine); indirect sympathomimetics (amezinium).

In this instance, treatment with angiotensin-converting enzyme inhibitors as part of an antihypertensive regimen, or at the start of, or during dialysis, is beneficial. Calcium channel blockers and central vasodilators such as clonidine may reduce hypertensive pressures unresponsive to volume depletion. Very rarely (< 1%), recalcitrant hypertension forces resort to minoxidil and its consequent side effects. Beta blockers should be not be used in diabetics as they exacerbate hypertriglyceridemia, worsen glucose control and mask symptoms of severe hypoglycemia.

3. High interdialytic weight gain. Diabetics gain a mean 30% more weight between hemodialyses than do non-diabetics. Excess interdialytic weight gain in diabetic hemodialysis patients is well recognized (53, 52). Ifudu, Dulin, and Friedman have shown that increased interdialytic weight gain correlates with glycemic control, age, duration of ESRD, continuing urine output, dry weight, or duration of diabetes (52). In diabetes, high intracellular sodium content increases thirst (53). Noncompliance with sodium, fluid and caloric restrictions in diabetic hemodialysis patients causes interdialytic weight increments of 10–20 lbs. Intensified metabolic control facilitated by dietary counselling plus sodium modelling of dialysis, and sequential ultrafiltration curtails weight swings and their deleterious consequences.

Metabolic control

Diet, activity, extent of correction of uremia, intercurrent illness, corticosteroid and other drugs, and concomitant use of oral antihyperglycemic agents all affect insulin requirements during maintenance hemodialysis (54). 'Tight' metabolic control – a key component in diabetic management – risks potentially fatal hypoglycemic episodes in hemodialysis patients (55). As endogenous catabolism of insulin decreases, diabetic patients with progressive renal insufficiency experience reduction in insulin requirement. Effective hemodialysis returns appetite in some diabetics increasing insulin need over predialysis doses. Delayed gastric emptying result-

ing from diabetic gastroparesis (discussed below) causes poor metabolic regulation and so-called 'brittle' diabetes (56).

Hypertriglyceridemia, observed in 30–50% of ESRD patients is more prevalent in diabetic than non-diabetic patients. As shown by Koch et al., the serum lipid level is the strongest predictor of sudden death or myocardial infarction in diabetics starting maintenance hemodialysis (33). It follows that in addition to glucose regulation, hyperlipidemia must be treated in diabetic hemodialysis patients by, at first, dietary restriction of simple sugars and saturated fats in association with weight optimization and appropriate exercise. Persistent hyperlipidemia is strong indication for prescription of hypolipidemic drugs. For any program of metabolic regulation of diabetes to succeed, education of the patient (57) to become a participating member of the health care team is a necessity that cannot be over emphasized. We find the input of a nurse educator, dedicated to diabetic ESRD patients, invaluable in gaining patient cooperation, understanding, and successful participation.

Retinopathy

Retinopathy in diabetes ranks first as a cause of blindness in those aged 20–74 years in the United States (58). Of freshly evaluated diabetic ESRD patients, about 97% have significant retinopathy (59) and 25–30% are blind or have severe vision loss (60, 61). Macular edema and proliferative retinopathy with associated vitreous hemorrhage and retinal detachment most frequently induce vision loss in diabetics. Glaucoma, cataracts and corneal disease must also be considered in diabetics facing blindness. Onset and severity of proliferative retinopathy correlates with duration of diabetes, gender (women > men), and severity of hypertension. Between 1966 and 1971, in Minneapolis, 44% of newly treated IDDM patients on hemodialysis experienced progressive visual loss culminating in blindness, the high rate of visual loss fell to 20% between 1972–1975 and to 4% since 1976 (9). Credit for retention of sight is assigned to better blood pressure control, improved hemodialysis techniques of hemodialysis, and aggressive ophthalmologic intervention (35).

Laser surgery of the retina – focal or panretinal laser photocoagulation – halts previously inexorable proliferative retinopathy. Vitrectomy may restore vision after extensive vitreous hemorrhage. Routine collaboration with an ophthalmologist skilled in diabetic retinal disorders removes the pall of impending and inevitable blindness from the diabetic ESRD patient. Eye care is vital to comprehensive management of ESRD in diabetics (62). Koch, Tschope, and Ritz make the important observation that only 98 of 208 diabetic dialysis patients in Germany had examination by an ophthalmologist in the 12 months preceding their first dialysis (63). Prevention of blindness in diabetic ESRD patients is contingent in large part in getting practicing nephrologists to obtain assistance from an eye surgeon when intervention is likely to prove effective.

Problems related to vascular access

1. Radial steal syndrome: Diabetic hemodialysis patients risk compromised blood flow to the hand when the radial artery is anastomosed side to side with the cephalic vein in an arteriovenous fistula. In this circumstance, termed a steal, radial arterial blood no longer provides adequate blood flow to the fingers, the fistula provides a low pressure 'run off' system bypassing the ulnar and interosseous arterial blood supply through the palmar arch, a system which is often compromised by medial arterial calcification (64). Suggestive of a steal syndrome is a swollen, painful, numb hand discolored by livido with ischemia and gangrene of the fingers. Ligation of the distal radial artery segment to prevent retrograde flow of blood from the ulnar arterial system into the fistula avoids a steal syndrome. Alternatively, the primary anastomosis can be an *end*-artery to side or end-vein fistula.

2. Venous hypertension: In diabetics, an arteriovenous access may cause chronic hand swelling and a 'sore thumb' syndrome, due to hypertension in the distal vein segment (65). Venous hypertension occurs in association with venous stenosis of the access, or proximal stenosis of the subclavian vein which may have been previously catheterized for temporary vascular access. Correction requires ligature of the distal venous limb of the fistula or graft.

3. Infection/thrombosis: Three of four diabetics on hemodialysis require revision or replacement of their graft vascular access within 3 years, only 20% with a primary fistulae need operative intervention (38). Patency was equivalent in diabetics and non-diabetics at one year (35) in 324 arteriovenous accesses in 256 patients of whom 34 were diabetic with 22 Cimino fistulae and 27 PTFE grafts surviving. Our experience indicates that diabetic and non-diabetic hemodialysis patients have equivalent length of hospitalization for problems related to vascular access (66). Others, however, note that diabetic hemodialysis patients have more frequent and longer hospitalizations than do non-diabetics.

Arteriovenous grafts sustain more infections that do Cimino fistulae. Perigraft hematomas and graft thrombosis predispose to local and then systemic infection. Signs of impending access failure include a venous pressures in excess of 250 mmHg, and a progressively weakening arterial pulse. Angiography of the access locates the site for application of corrective balloon angioplasty of the stenosed segment of vein – typically immediately distal to the venous anastomosis – performed before thrombosis supervenes. Correction of graft stenosis requires a patch or a jump graft.

4. Ischemic monomelic neuropathy. Diabetics may manifest multiple distal mononeuropathies in the upper limb after creation of a proximal arteriovenous access (67). Abrupt onset of painful weakness of the forearm and hand muscles developing hours after creation of an access is caused by peripheral nerve ischemia due to sudden diversion of blood flow to a proximal brachio-cephalic fistula. Cessation of the pain results from closure of the fistula or removal of the graft.

Peripheral vascular disease

Rehabilitation of patients falters after amputation of a lower extremity – a complication afflicting 5–25% of diabetic hemodialysis patients each year (68). Awareness of potential limb disease, patient education, and surveillance forestall irreversible complications. By daily washing, drying, and examination of the nails, soles and interdigital creases of the feet; the wearing of comfortable, non-constricting shoes with socks or stockings; use of heel booties when confined to bed, the informed diabetic practices defensive medicine. A further beneficial practice entails routine visits to a podiatrist for nail and callus care. Diabetic ESRD patients are instructed not cut their own toenails because of difficulty in seeing with precision; a small cut risks infection, retarded healing, and eventual limb amputation. Collaboration with a vascular surgeon prevents symptoms or signs of limb ischemia from progressing without considering vascular bypass surgery or limb-preserving minimal amputation.

Diabetic neuropathy

Diabetics on hemodialysis become invalids because of diabetic sensorimotor and/or autonomic neuropathy. Uremic and diabetic neuropathy share similar histopathology; indeed, the two are indistinguishable. Peripheral neuropathy progresses less frequently in diabetic ESRD patients treated with renal transplantation (46): over a 6 year observation, 53% of 43 IDDM hemodialysis patients had mild or moderate neuropathy progressed; while none of 15 patients with similar clinical severity of neuropathy treated by renal transplantation had worsening of neuropathy. Purportedly, motor neuropathy is less severe in diabetics treated with CAPD. The inability to halt progression of motor neuropathy on hemodialysis is a reason to switch to peritoneal dialysis, an ESRD technique in which extraction of middle molecular weight neurotoxins – speculated to be responsible for clinical neuropathy – are more efficiently removed. A target glycosylated hemoglobin level below 7.5%, and aggressive hemodialysis are tools to ameliorate of symptoms.

Autonomic neuropathy expressed as gastropathy, cystopathy, and orthostatic hypotension, is a frequently overlooked, highly prevalent disorder impeding life quality in the diabetic. Diabetic cystopathy, though common, is frequently unrecognized and confused with worsening diabetic nephropathy and is sometimes interpreted as allograft rejection in diabetic kidney transplant recipients. In 22 diabetic patients who developed renal failure – 14 men and 8 women of mean age 38 years – an air cystogram detected cystopathy in 8 (36%) manifested as detrusor paralysis in 1 patient; severe malfunction in 5 patients (24%); and mild impairment in 1 patient. Gastroparesis, afflicts one-quarter to one-half of azotemic diabetic persons when initially evaluated for renal disease (69). Clark and Nowak provide a helpful review of diagnostic and therapeutic options in diabetic gastroparesis (70). Other expressions of autonomic neuropathy – obstipation and explosive nighttime diarrhea – often coexists with gastroparesis (71). Obstipation responds to daily doses of cascara, while diarrhea is treated with psyllium seed dietary supplements one to three times daily, plus loperamide (72) in repetitive 2 mg doses to a total dose of 18 mg daily.

Bone disease

Adynamic bone disease characterized by low bone turnover without accumulation of unmineralized osteoid afflicts in diabetic hemodialysis patients (73). In diabetic rats, decreased osteoblast proliferation and defective mineralization contribute to a low rate of bone formation (74). Reduced bone formation allows time for deposition of aluminum on the ossification front. After a year of hemodialysis, aluminum deposition (related to use of aluminum-containing phosphate binders) on bone surfaces in diabetics is detected, and bone pain and fractures related to aluminum bone diseases may start as early as 2 years after initiation of hemodialysis (75). Aluminum bone disease is also unmasked or accelerated following parathyroidectomy. Diabetics on hemodialysis should not be given aluminum-containing phosphate binders. Bone pain and/or fractures signal the need to measure plasma aluminum levels before and after a single infusion of desferrioxamine. Aluminum associated bone disease in hemodialyzed diabetics responds to a regimen of vitamin D, calcium and desferrioxamine.

Malnutrition

Malnutrition in diabetic hemodialysis patients is pervasive, resulting from: intercurrent illnesses, poor glycemic control promoting gluconeogenesis and muscle catabolism, gastroparesis, diabetic diarrhea, and underdialysis (76). Owen et al. advise that in hemodialysis patients, solute clearance during dialysis and nutritional adequacy are determinants of mortality (77). There is clear correlation between the risk of death and both a low urea reduction ratio (% decrease in blood urea nitrogen concentration in a single dialysis) and the serum albumin concentration. Diabetics have lower urea reduction ratios and lower serum albumin concentrations – markers of higher risks of death. Increased prealbumin and increased lipoprotein(a) concentrations, in 125 hemodialysis patients observed for 14 months, are independently associated with patient and vascular access survival in diabetic and non-diabetic hemodialysis patients (78).

Satisfactory nutrition in diabetic hemodialysis patients calls for a diet of 25–30 kcal/kg/day, with 50% of the calories coming from complex carbohydrates; and protein content of 1.3–1.5 gm/kg/day (54). During and after the catabolic stress of intercurrent illness – especially sepsis – diabetic hemodialysis patients require early and intensive nutritional support with resort to enteral or peripheral parenteral nutrition, if necessary. Dialysate should contain at least 200 mg/dl of glucose. Glucose-free dialysate promotes rapid glucose loss, hypoglycemia, and acute starvation with acidosis and hyperkalemia. Metoclopramide in divided dosages, ranging from 10–40 mg/day, or cisapride as an alternative, before meals, improves delayed gastric emptying in the more than 50% of diabetic hemodialysis patients whose nutrition is impeded by gastroparesis (79). Unremitting diarrhea – an expression of autonomic neuropathy – may respond to broad spectrum antibiotics to decrease bacterial overgrowth in adynamic bowel segments. We find prophylactic daily doses of loperamide break the enervating and embarrassing cycle of unremitting diarrhea.

Psychosocial problems

Without exception, diabetic patients who develop ESRD are depressed either intermittently or constantly. Coping with failing vision and the omnipresent threat of limb loss add to the burden of compliance with often conflicting and incomprehensible instructions on dietary and fluid restrictions. The tendency to become hypotensive during hemodialysis leads to missed or shortened treatments, and all of the adverse effects of insufficient correction of uremia. Recognition of depression, counselling, involvement in patient support groups, and antidepressant therapy – in selected patients – improves but does not eliminate the stress of ESRD.

CAPD/CCPD

Peritoneal dialysis is the treatment elected for in approximately 12% of diabetic ESRD patients in the US. CAPD proffers advantages of freedom from a machine, performance at home, rapid training, minimal cardiovascular stress and avoidance of heparin (80). To permit CAPD, an intraperitoneal catheter is implanted one or more days before CAPD is begun. Even blind diabetic patients learn to perform CAPD at home within 10 to 30 days. As reviewed elsewhere in this text, CAPD requires exchange of 2 to 3 l of sterile dialysate, containing insulin, antibiotics, and other drugs, 3 to 5 times daily. Mechanical cycling of dialysate, termed continuous cyclic peritoneal dialysis (CCPD) can be performed during sleep. CAPD and CCPD pose the constant risk of peritonitis as well as a gradual decrease in peritoneal surface area. Some clinicians characterize CAPD as 'a first choice treatment' for diabetic ESRD patients (81). Peritoneal dialysis may be the only life line available for some uremic diabetics: patients in whom vascular access sites have been exhausted, or patients with severe hemodialysis-associated hypotension or angina related to atherosclerotic heart disease. Slower ultrafiltration, and less rapid removal of urea produce smaller shifts in serum osmolality accounting for the absence of significant hypotension on CAPD. Hypotension may be induced by repeated use of hypertonic (4.25%) exchanges. A claimed advantage for CAPD is the absence of cytokine-mediated toxic responses provoked by contact of blood with biomaterials in the extracorporeal circuit and membranes used in hemodialysis (82).

Regular insulin (83), in higher than prior subcutaneous doses (60–130 U/day) is added to each bag of dialysate or injected through the connecting tubing (to avoid adsorption of insulin to the polyvinylchloride of the bag) just before each exchange. Insulin requirements increase during peritonitis. Insulin given intraperitoneally is best absorbed when the abdominal cavity is free of fluid, and is predominantly taken up by the portal circulation, a more physiologic route than subcutaneously administered insulin. A target 2 hour post prandial glucose level of between 150–250 mg/dl is advised (68).

When insulin requirements exceed 100 U per exchange, and blood glucose control is erratic, a subcutaneous long acting insulin preparation is added. Although intraperitoneal insulin achieves better glucose control, reducing the amplitude of glycemic excursions (84), high glycosylated hemoglobin levels – in the presence of acceptable glucose control – are usual. What is measured in this circumstance is carbamylated hemoglobin – increased in uremia – which cannot be distinguished from glycosylated hemoglobin by usual chromatographic assays. Elevated levels of glycosylated hemoglobin are also found in non-diabetics on CAPD, hence measurement of glycosylated hemoglobin as a measure of glucose control is unreliable in uremic diabetics (85). Insulin can be effectively admin-

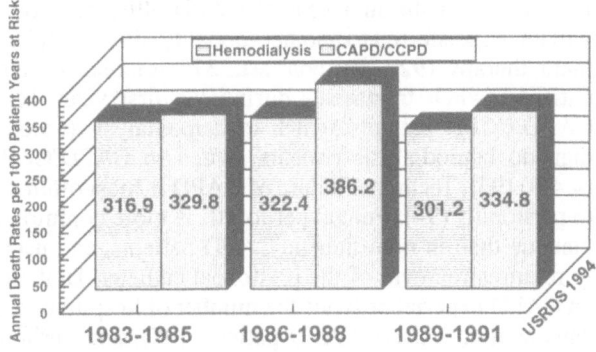

Figure 7. By era, over eight years, peritoneal dialysis has a higher death rate than does hemodialysis. Patients are grouped by treatment modality. Note that over the eight years depicted, mean age of treated patients increased meaning that a stable death rate actually reflects improvement in outcome. Data from the USRDS by special request in 1994.

istered by either the subcutaneous or intraperitoneal route in diabetic CAPD patients. Initial regulation should first be attempted by adding insulin to dialysate (86). Rubin et al. were not enthusiastic about CAPD in a largely black diabetic population treated with CAPD in Jackson, Mississippi (87). Only 34% of patients remained on CAPD after two years, and at three years, only 18% continued on CAPD. By objective measures of death or hospitalization rates, CAPD fares less well than hemodialysis for diabetic ESRD patients (Figures 6 and 7). Assignment of an individual patient to CAPD, demands reflection on the variables listed in Table 4. Distinction between physician bias and patient preference means that the patient must weigh the benefits of CAPD, including freedom from a machine and electrical outlets, and facile travel against the disadvantages of unremitting attention to fluid exchange, constant risk of peritonitis, and disappearing exchange surface, and greater probability of hospitalization and death. The authors concur with a Lancet editorial which concluded: "Until the frequency of peritonitis is greatly reduced, most patients can expect to spend only a few years on CAPD before requiring a different form of treatment, usually haemodialysis" (88).

Though no prospective, controlled studies have been reported, diabetic retinopathy often stabilizes during peritoneal dialysis (89, 90). Preservation and even improvement of vision is attributed to less rapid changes in intravascular volume with less potential for exacerbation of retinal ischemia. More effective blood pressure and blood glucose control are also major factors in stabilizing retinopathy. Even blind diabetics can be successfully taught blind CAPD protocols. Blind diabetics on CAPD, in one report, survived longer than sighted diabetic patients (91).

DISADVANTAGES OF CAPD

By the end of the first year of CAPD, 49% of patients will have transferred to another modality of renal replacement therapy (92). By contrast, 37% of hemodialysis patients switch treatments during the first year. More CAPD/CCPD patients switch to hemodialysis (15.6%), than do hemodialysis patients switch to CAPD/CCPD (4.4%) (93). Technical failure of CAPD is most often due to peritonitis (94). Fungal peritonitis is more common in diabetic than in non-diabetic CAPD patients, and usually requires removal of the peritoneal catheter. Diabetics on CAPD experience twice the number of hospitalization days as non-diabetic CAPD patients (95), and peritonitis accounts for 30–50% of the hospitalization days (96). Despite the longer duration of each episode of peritonitis, the overall risk of peritonitis is no greater in diabetics than in non-diabetics (97). Resort to a Y-set dialysate drainage system lowers the incidence of peritonitis.

Kinetic modelling has been applied to peritoneal dialysis (98). To maintain the same level of blood urea nitrogen in a CAPD patient and a hemodialysis patient, the KT/v (K = dialyzer clearance, T = time on dialysis, v = volume of distribution of urea) must be maintained at a higher level in the CAPD patient. The amount of dialysis delivered on CAPD may have to be increased with time as residual renal function is lost, and peritoneal clearance decreases due to advanced vascular disease or to recurrent episodes of peritonitis. Whether hemodialysis or peritoneal dialysis is better for diabetics is intensely debated. In selected series, the death rate in patients younger than 60 years old is similar or lower in CAPD patients than in hemodialysis patients (99). A recent analysis by the USRDS, however, shows that in every age subset, the death rate of hemodialysis patients is lower than that in CAPD/CCPD patients (Figure 7).

As is true for diabetics on hemodialysis, malnutrition may also afflict CAPD patients (100). Rotellar et al. reviewed a decade of experience with CAPD patients noting that 8% were severely malnourished, 33% were moderately malnourished, while 59% had no evidence of malnutrition (101). Serious malnutrition in CAPD patients was also described in 43 with IDDM (26 on hemodialysis and 17 on CAPD) followed for a mean of 11.6 months, of whom 26% were below the 85th percentile of ideal body weight, and 41% had a serum albumin below 3.5 mg/dl (102). CAPD-treated diabetics become malnourished because of: a) reduced appetite caused by glucose infusion from dialysate, or early satiety due to increased intra-abdominal pressure, b) large protein losses (8–10 g per day) in dialysate (103). Dialysate protein loss in diabetics on CAPD increases with time due to generalized increase in permeability related to diabetic microangiopathy involving the peritoneal vessels (104). For adequate nutrition, CAPD patients should ingest at least 1.5 g/kg of protein per day, and between 130–150 g

of carbohydrates per day. Malnourished CAPD patients may benefit from intraperitoneal amino acids (105).

RENAL TRANSPLANTATION IN PATIENTS WITH DIABETIC NEPHROPATHY

Early in their management of ESRD, diabetics should be asked about the possibility of using an intrafamilial living kidney donor; rehabilitation is best after a live donor kidney transplant. Furthermore, renal transplantation is the least expensive form of renal replacement therapy. As predicted by Sutherland et al. (106), following a renal transplant, patient survival at one and two years is now equivalent in diabetic and non-diabetic recipients (107), though graft survival remains marginally lower in diabetic persons (Figure 8). Statistical superiority in survival after a renal transplant, compared with dialytic therapy, does not tell the whole story as rehabilitation is incomparably better. The enhanced life quality effected prompts selection of a kidney transplant as the distinctly favored treatment presented to newly evaluated diabetic persons with ESRD under the age of 60 (Table 6). More than half of diabetic kidney transplant recipients in most series live for at least three years: many survivors return to occupational, school and home responsibilities. Though regarded as investigational by some (108) and, even when successful, applicable to no more than 8% of uremic diabetic patients (who have IDDM), a combined pancreas and kidney transplant for the diabetic ESRD patient is growing in acceptability and technical success (109). In the best series, survival one year post-renal transplant, in 995 diabetic kidney recipients who also received a pancreas, transplant renal allograft survival was a remarkable 84% (110). World-

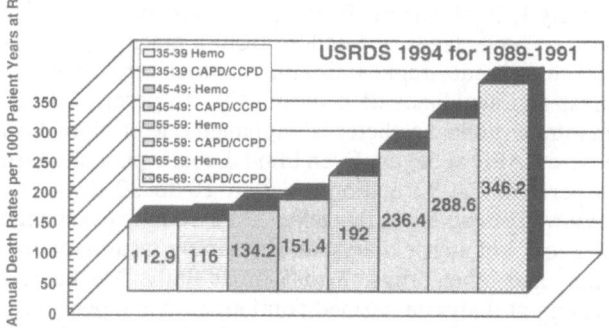

Figure 8. Specific death rates for diabetic ESRD patients treated by peritoneal dialysis or hemodialysis for age subsets chosen by the author from a special USRDS study done in 1994. In each age group, peritoneal dialysis is more likely to end in death than is hemodialysis over the two year study interval. Data from the USRDS by special request in 1994.

Table 6. Treatment options for ESRD in diabetes

Variable	Peritoneal dialysis	Hemodialysis	Kidney transplant
Extensive extrarenal disease	No limitation	No limitation except for hypotension	Excluded in cardiovascular insufficiency
Older patients (over age 60 years)	No limitation	No limitation	Arbitrary exclusion as determined by program
Complete rehabilitation	Rare, if ever	Very few individuals	Common so long as graft functions
Relative death rate	Higher than for non-diabetics and greater than in hemodialysis	Higher than for non-diabetics and for diabetic transplant recipients	Equal to non-diabetics for two years then higher. Less than on dialysis.
First year survival	Approx. 75%	Approx. 75%	>90%
Survival beyond 10 years	Almost never	Few than 5%	Approx. 1 in 5
Further complications	Usual and unremitting. Hyperglycemia and hyperlipidemia accentuated. Late amputation and blindness.	Usual and unremitting. Late limb amputation and blindness.	Slowed by correction of azotemia. Hypertension in majority. May be blocked by pancreas transplant.
Special advantage	Can be self-performed. Avoids swings in solute and intravascular volume level.	Can be self-performed Efficient extraction of solute and water in hours.	Cures uremia. Freedom to travel.
Disadvantage	Peritonitis. Hyperinsulinemia, hyperglycemia, hyperlipidemia. Long hours of treatment. More days hospitalized than either hemodialysis or transplant.	Blood access a hazard for clotting, hemorrhage and infection. Cyclical hypotension, weakness. Aluminum toxicity, amyloidosis.	Cosmetic disfigurement from steroids and cyclosporine, hypertension, personal expense for cytotoxic drugs. Induced malignancy. HIV transmission.
Patient acceptance	Variable, usual compliance with passive tolerance for regimen. Depressed and enervated after repetitive complications.	Variable, often noncompliant with dietary, metabolic, or antihypertensive component of regimen. Depressed over long-term.	Enthusiastic so long as renal allograft function is satisfactory. A rising creatinine heralds depression. Exalted when pancreas proffers euglycemia.
Relative cost.	Most expensive than hemodialysis over long run.	Less expensive than kidney transplant in first year, subsequent years more expensive.	Pancreas + kidney engraftment most expensive uremia therapy for diabetic. After first year, kidney transplant – alone – lowest cost option.

wide results in simultaneous kidney-pancreas transplants show that more than 90% of recipients were alive at 1 year, more than 80% had functioning kidney grafts, and more than 70% no longer required insulin (111).

Combining pancreas and kidney transplants does not raise perioperative mortality; but perioperative morbidity is greatly increased, mainly due to mechanical and inflammatory problems diverting pancreatic exocrine secretions into the urinary system. A great expectation for pancreatic transplantation is the interdiction of diabetic micro and macrovascular extrarenal complications. Several reports of kidney biopsies in patients who have received sequential kidney and later pancreas allografts indicate that a functioning pancreas does impede progression or recurrence of diabetic nephropathy. Likewise, the course of diabetic neuropathy following combined pancreas and kidney transplantation underscores stabilization and, in some patients, improvement in diabetic motor neuropathy

(112). Unfortunately, pancreas transplantation in patients with extensive extrarenal disease, has neither arrested nor reversed diabetic retinopathy, diabetic cardiomyopathy, or extensive peripheral vascular disease (113, 114). Nevertheless, a functioning pancreas transplant frees patients from the dreaded daily sentence of balancing diet, exercise, and insulin dosage (115). In 1994, consensus of clinical nephrologists is that the ESRD patient with IDDM should consider a simultaneous kidney and pancreas transplant as at least a temporary cure of inexorable disease (116). There is no absolute age cutoff for renal transplantation in diabetics (our oldest transplanted diabetic was 72 years old), but generally patients over the age of 65 years are not considered for transplantation.

Diabetic ESRD patients with a history of angina pectoris, previous myocardial infarction, or heart failure should have preoperative coronary angiography, with angioplasty or bypass grafting of significant occlusive lesions. Since diabetics often have clinically silent coronary artery disease, some form of preoperative cardiac assessment is necessary even in diabetics with no symptoms of cardiac disease. A treadmill exercise stress test ± a thallium stress test should be done routinely in asymptomatic diabetic ESRD patients being considered for renal transplantation. Routine coronary angiography for patients without cardiac symptoms is unnecessary. Only 31 of 151 IDDM patients screened with coronary angiography pretransplantation had angiographically significant lesions (117).

Comparisons (retrospective and prospective) of the fate of diabetic ESRD patients by different modalities lack balanced treatment groups adjusted for age, race, gender, diabetes type, severity of complications, and degree of metabolic control. Reported prospective studies of renal transplantation compared with peritoneal or hemodialysis do not overcome biases introduced by patient and physician refusal to permit random assignment to one treatment over another. As a generalization, younger patients with fewer complications are assigned to renal transplantation while residual older, sicker patients are treated by dialysis. Furthermore, combined kidney/pancreas transplants have been virtually restricted to Caucasian IDDM patients younger than age 50.

REHABILITATION

An optimistic view of rehabilitation during maintenance hemodialysis was projected by a state-wide longitudinal prospective study of 979 ESRD patients in Minnesota in which the Karnofsky scoring system (118) was employed to assess patient well being (119). Initial Karnofsky scores showed that 50% of all patients were able to care for themselves when starting treatment. After two years of maintenance hemodialysis, 78% of patients maintained or improved their functional status. Kidney transplant recipients, however, had higher initial Karnofsky scores than did those relegated to long-term dialysis. Selection for a kidney transplant gleaned the most functional patients leaving a residual population of less functional patients. Thereafter, comparisons of relative rehabilitation in transplant and dialysis groups – like comparisons of survival – are flawed by selection bias favoring kidney transplant recipients.

At the opposite extreme, Gutman, Stead and Robinson measured functional assessment in 2,481 dialysis patients irrespective of location or type of dialysis (120). Diabetic patients achieved minimal rehabilitation; only 23% of diabetic patients (versus 60% of non-diabetic patients) were capable of physical activity beyond caring for themselves. A decade later, Lowder et al. found an equivalent very low level of rehabilitation in diabetics on hemodialysis in Brooklyn (121). Further confirmation of this point was afforded by Ifudu et al. who documented dismal rehabilitation in a multicenter studies of diabetic and non-diabetic

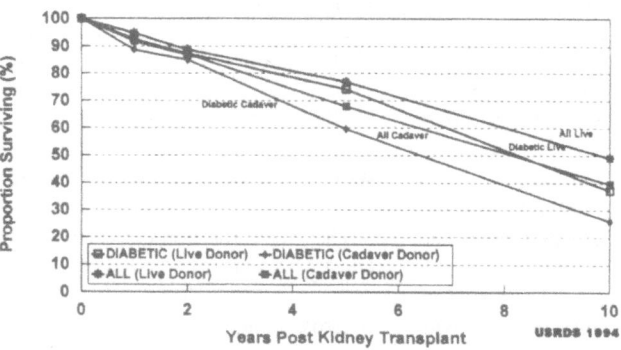

Figure 9. Whether recipients of live donor kidneys or cadaver donor kidneys are compared, diabetics have inferior survival to non-diabetics. Note, however, that compared with survival on hemodialysis (Figure 2), diabetic kidney transplant recipients have better survival. At two years, for example, more than 80% of diabetics are alive after a kidney transplant while only about 50% of dialysis treated diabetics survive. How much of this superior survival is the result of selection bias favoring renal transplantation is unestablished. Data from USRDS 1994 report.

(122), and elderly inner-city (123) hemodialysis patients. An unhappy, unescapable conclusion drawn from the literature detailing rehabilitation in diabetic ESRD patients treated by hemodialysis is that – as presently practiced – rehabilitation is unlikely and assistance is required to complete daily chores associated with routine living.

FUTURE DIRECTIONS OF THERAPY

During progressive loss of renal function, diabetic patients accumulate advanced glycosylated end-products (AGEs) in 'toxic' amounts that are not decreased to normal by hemodialysis, but fall sharply, to within the normal range, within days after renal transplantation (124). AGEs may be a major cause of tissue and organ damage in long-term diabetes. Experimental evidence supports this thesis. For example, Vlassara et al. injected AGEs to non-diabetic rats and rabbits and showed that physiologic and morphologic changes typical of diabetes resulted (125). As reasoned by Brownlee, glycosylation of proteins leads to diabetic microangiopathy through formation of advanced glycosylation end-products (AGEs) (126). If Brownlee's conjecture as to the importance of AGEs to diabetic complications is correct, a fresh approach to prevention of nephropathy and other diabetic complications – blocking formation of AGEs – may be devised. Evidence rapidly being accumulated suggests that aminoguanidine hydrochloride, a nucleophilic hydrazine derivative, is capable of interdicting synthesis of AGEs. The chemical structure, empirical formula, and molecular weight of aminoguanidine are shown below:

$$H_2C\!-\!C\!-\!NHNH_2$$
$$\|$$
$$NH$$

Empirical formula: $CH6N4.HCl$, molecular weight: 110.5 Daltons.

Aminoguanidine hydrochloride is a white, crystalline powder, which is very soluble in water, soluble in ethanol, and practically insoluble in ether. When administered to streptozotocin-induced diabetic rats in a 9 month trial from onset of experimental diabetes, aminoguanidine prevented widening of the glomerular basement membrane typical of diabetes (127). Experimental diabetic retinopathy was also prevented in rats by treatment with aminoguanidine which blocked retinal capillary closure, the principal pathophysiologic abnormality underlying diabetic retinopathy (128). Further evidence of the potential value of aminoguanidine is the finding that experimental diabetic neuropathy in the rat is minimized as judged by motor nerve conduction velocity and the accumulation of AGEs in nerves (129). The rationale for preventing AGE formation as a means of impeding development of diabetic complications is compelling (130, 131).

The mechanism by which aminoguanidine blocks diabetic complications is unclear. It is established that aminoguanidine prevents NO activation. Corbett et al. speculate that aminoguanidine inhibits interleukin-1 beta-induced nitrite formation (an oxidation product of NO) (132). In a derivative study (133), aminoguanidine but not methylguanidine, inhibited AGE formation from L-lysine and glucose-6-phosphate while both guanidine compounds are equally effective in normalizing albumin permeation in induced-diabetic rats. Relative or absolute increase in NO production in the pathogenesis of early diabetic vascular dysfunction is also inferred. Inhibition of diabetic vascular functional changes by aminoguanidine could reflect inhibition of NO synthase activity rather than, or in addition to, prevention of AGE formation. An alternative role for aminoguanidine is that of a glucose competitor for the same protein-to-protein bond (134), links formation and accumulation of irreversible and highly reactive advanced glycation end-products over long-lived fundamental molecules such as the constituents of arterial wall collagen, glomerular basement membranes, nerve myelin, DNA and others. Whatever the mechanism by which aminoguanidine prevents renal, eye, nerve, and other microvascular complications in diabetic animals, clinical trials now in progress proffer a new means of addressing the enormous burden imposed by ESRD in diabetes (135, 136).

REFERENCES

1. United States Renal Data System: USRDS 1994 Annual Data Report. The National Institutes of Health, National Institute of Diabetes and Digestive Diseases, Bethesda, MD, September 1994
2. Avram MM: Use of special hemodialysis methods in diabetic uremia. *Proc Conf on Dialysis as a Practical Workshop*, National Union Catalogue, NY, 1966, p 15
3. Chazan BI, Rees SB, Balodimus MS et al.: Dialysis in diabetics. A review of 44 patients. *J Am Med Assoc* 1969; 209: 2026–2030.
4. Comty CM, Leonard A, Shapiro FL: Management and prognosis of diabetic patients treated by chronic hemodialysis. (Abstract) *Am Soc Nephrol* 5: 15, 1971
5. Comty CM, Kjellsen D, Shapiro FL: A reassessment of the prognosis of diabetic patients treated by chronic hemodialysis. *Trans Am Soc Artif Intern Organs* 22: 404, 1976
6. Ghavamian M, Gutch CF, Kopp KF et al.: The sad truth about hemodialysis in diabetic nephropathy. *J Am Med Assoc* 222: 1386, 1972
7. Jacobs C, Broyer M, Brunner FP et al.: Combined report on regular dialysis and transplantation in Europe, XI, 1980. Presented at the 17th Congress of the European Dialysis and Transplantation Association, Paris, July 5–8th, 1981
8. Canadian Organ Replacement Register: New and registered patients in 1989. Toronto, 1989, p 35
9. Shapiro FL, Comty CM: Hemodialysis in diabetics – 1981 update. in *Diabetic Renal Retinal Syndrome*, edited by Friedman EA, L'Esperance FA, New York, Grune and Stratton, 1981, p 309
10. Ma KW, Master DS, Brown DC: Hemodialysis in diabetic patients with chronic renal failure. *Ann Intern Med* 53: 215, 1975
11. Kjellstrand CM, Whitley K, Comty CM et al.: Dialysis in patients with diabetes mellitus nephropathy. *Diabetic Nephropathy* 2: 15, 1983
12. Whitley KY, Shapiro FL: Hemodialysis for end-stage diabetic nephropathy. in *Diabetic Renal Retinal Syndrome*, edited by Friedman EA, L'Esperance FA, New York, Grune and Stratton, 1986, p 349
13. Zander E, Schultz B, Beckert R et al.: Clinical course in insulin-dependent diabetics undergoing hemodialysis. *Exp Clin Endocrinol* 85: 105, 1985
14. Kjellstrand CM: A comparison of dialysis and transplantation in patients with end-stage renal failure of diabetes. in *Diabetic Renal Retinal Syndrome*, edited by Friedman EA, L'Esperance FA, New York, Grune and Stratton, 1986, p 333
15. Balodimus MC: Diabetic nephropathy. in: *Joslin's Diabetes*, edited by Marbel A, White P, Bradley RF et al., Philadelphia: Lea and Febiger, 1971, p 526
16. Marks HH: Longevity and mortality of diabetics. *Am J Public Health* 55: 416, 1965
17. Humphrey LL, Ballard DJ, Frohnert PP et al.: Chronic renal failure in non-insulin dependent diabetes mellitus. *Ann Intern Med* 111: 788, 1989

18. Hasslacher CH, Ritz E, Wahl P et al.: Similar risks of nephropathy in patients with type I or type II diabetes mellitus. *Nephrol Dial Transplant* 4: 859, 1989

19. Nelson RG, Newman JM, Knowles WC et al.: Incidence of end-stage renal disease in type 2 (non-insulin dependent) diabetes mellitus in Pima Indians. *Diabetologia* 31: 730, 1988

20. Cowie CC, Port FK, Wolfe RA et al.: Disparities in incidence of diabetic end-stage renal disease according to race and type of diabetes. *N Engl J Med* 321: 1074, 1989

21. James E, Knowles WC, Bennett PH: Incidence and risk factors for non-insulin dependent diabetes. Diabetes in America. Washington DC, US Govt Printing Office, 1985, IV–I, NIH Publication No 85-1468.

22. Nostrand SG, Kirk RA, Rutsky EA et al.: Racial differences in the incidence of treatment for end stage renal disease. *N Engl J Med* 306: 1276, 1982

23. Pugh JA, Stern MP, Haffner Fl et al.: Excess incidence of end stage renal disease in Mexican Americans. *Am J Epidemiol* 127: 135, 1988

24. Waring GO: The sequelae of diabetes in mid-Western American Indians. *Diabetes* 19: 403, 1970

25. Mogensen CE, Christensen CK, Vittinghus E: The stages of diabetic renal disease with emphasis on the stage of incipient diabetic nephropathy. *Diabetes* 32: 64, 1983

26. Earle K, Viberti GC: Familial, hemodynamic and metabolic factors in the predisposition to diabetic kidney disease. *Kidney Int* 45: 434, 1994

27. Harris MI, Klein R, Welborn TA, Knuiman MW: Onset of NIDDM occurs at least 4–7 yr before clinical diagnosis. *Diabetes Care* 15: 815, 1992

28. Harris MI: Impaired glucose tolerance in the US population. *Diabetes Care* 12: 464, 1989

29. Nolph KD, Lundblad AS, Novak JW: Current concepts: continuous Ambulatory Peritoneal Dialysis. *N Engl J Med* 318: 1595, 1988

30. Kussman MJ, Goldstein HH, Gleason RE: The clinical course of diabetic nephropathy. *J Am Med Assoc* 236: 1861, 1976

31. Friedman EA (Ed): *Death on Hemodialysis: Preventable or Inevitable?*, Dordrecht, The Netherlands, Kluwer Academic Publishers, 1994

32. US Renal Data System: USRDS 1993 Annual Data Report, The National Institutes of Health, National Institute of Diabetes and Digestive and Kidney Diseases, Bethesda, MD, August 1993

33. Koch M, Thomas B, Tschope W, Ritz E: Survival and predictors of death in dialysed diabetic patients. *Diabetologia* 36: 1113, 1993

34. Legrain M, Rottemburg J, de Groc F et al.: Selecting the best uremia therapy. in *Diabetic Renal Retinal Syndrome*, edited by Friedman EA, L'Esperance FA, New York, Grune and Stratton, 1986, p 453

35. Berman DH, Friedman EA, Lundin AP: Aggressive ophthalmological management in diabetic ESRD: a study of 31 consecutively referred patients. *Am J Nephrol* 12: 344, 1992

36. Friedman EA: Physician bias in uremia therapy. *Kidney Int* Suppl A: S38, 1985

37. Ortega-Gayton M, Hong JH, Shirani K et al.: Angioaccess for maintenance hemodialysis in end stage diabetic nephropathy. *Proc Clin Dial Transplant Forum* 9: 99, 1979

38. Palder SB, Kirkman RL, Whittemore AD: Vascular access for hemodialysis. Patency rates and results of revision. *Ann Surg* 202: 235, 1985

39. Kjellstrand CM, Simmons RL, Goetz FC et al.: Mortality and morbidity in diabetic patients accepted for renal transplantation. *Proc Eur Dialysis Transplant Assoc* 9: 345, 1972

40. Matson M, Kjellstrand CM: Long term followup of 369 diabetic patients undergoing dialysis. *Arch Intern Med* 148: 600, 1988

41. Weinrauch LA, Delia JA, Gleason RE, Hampton LA, Smith-Ossman S, DeSilva RA, Nesto RW: Usefulness of left ventricular size and function in predicting survival in chronic dialysis patients with diabetes mellitus. *Am J Cardiol* 70: 300, 1992

42. Ansari A, Kaupke CJ, Vaziri ND, Miller R, Barbari A: Cardiac pathology in patients with end-stage renal disease maintained on hemodialysis. *Int J Artif Organs* 16: 31, 1993

43. Rubin JE, Friedman EA: Dialysis and transplantation of diabetics in the United States. *Nephron* 18: 309, 1977

44. Ritz E, Strumpf C, Katz F et al.: Hypertension and cardiovascular risk factors in hemodialyzed diabetic patients. *Hypertension* 7 (Suppl II): 118, 1985

45. Herman WH, Teutsch SM: Kidney Disease associated with diabetes. Diabetes in America. Washington DC, US Govt Printing Office, 1985, XIV.1–31 (NIH publication No 85-1468)

46. Khauli RB, Novick AC, Steinmuller DR et al.: Comparison of renal transplantation and dialysis in rehabilitation of diabetic end stage renal disease patients. *Urology* 27: 521, 1986

47. Watanabe Y, Yuzawa Y, Mizumoto D, Tamai H, Itoh Y, Kumon S, Yamazaki C: Long-term follow-up study of 268 diabetic patients undergoing haemodialysis, with special attention to visual acuity and heterogeneity. *Nephrol Dial Transplant* 8: 725, 1993

48. Shideman JR, Buselmeier TJ, Kjellstrand CM: Hemodialysis in diabetics. *Arch Intern Med* 136: 1126, 1976

49. Daugirdas JT: Dialysis hypotension: a hemodynamic analysis. *Kidney Int* 39: 223, 1991

50. Gotch FA, Keen ML, Yarian SR: An analysis of thermal regulation in hemodialysis with one and three compartment models. *Trans Am Soc Artif Intern Organs* 35: 622, 1989

51. Maggiore Q, Pizzarelli F, Zocalli C et al.: Effect of extracorporeal blood cooling on dialytic arterial hypotension. *Proc Eur Dial Transplant Assoc* 28: 597, 1981

52. Ifudu O, Dulin AL, Friedman EA: Interdialytic weight gain correlates with glycosylated hemoglobin in diabetic hemodialysis patients. *Am J Kidney Dis* 23: 686, 1994

53. Jones R, Poston R, Hinestrota A et al.: Weight gain between dialysis in diabetics. Possible significance of raised intracellular sodium content. *Br Med J* 1: 153, 1980.

54. Davis M, Comty C, Shapiro F: Dietary management of patients with diabetes treated by hemodialysis. *J Am Diet Assoc* 75: 265, 1979

55. Tzamaloukas AH, Murata GH, Eisenberg B, Murphy G, Avasthi PS: Hypoglycemia in diabetics on dialysis with poor glycemic control: hemodialysis versus continuous ambulatory peritoneal dialysis. *Int J Artif Organs* 15: 390, 1992

56. Hackelsberger N, Piwernetz K, Renner R, Gerhards W, Hepp KD: Postprandial blood glucose and its relation to diabetic gastroparesis – a comparison of two methods. *Diabetes Res Clin Pract* 20: 197, 1993

57. McLaughlin S: Nutritional considerations for other complications of diabetes. *Diabetes Educ* 18: 527, 1992

58. Klein R, Klein BEK: Vision disorders in diabetes. Diabetes in America. Washington DC, US Govt Printing Office, 1985, XIII.1–36 (NIH publication No 85-1468)

59. Blagg CR: Visual and vascular problems in dialyzed diabetic patients. *Kidney Int* 6: S27, 1974

60. Goldstein DA, Massry SG: Diabetic nephropathy: clinical cause and effect on hemodialysis. *Nephron* 20: 286, 1978

61. Jacobs C, Rottemburg J, Frantz P et al.: Treatment of end-stage renal failure in the insulin-dependent diabetic patient. *Adv Nephrol* 8: 101, 1979

62. Berman DH, Friedman EA, Lundin AP: Aggressive ophthalmological management in diabetic ESRD: a study of 31 consecutively referred patients. *Am J Nephrol* 12: 344, 1992

63. Koch M, Tschope W, Ritz E: Does the care of diabetic patients with renal failure in the predialysis phase need improvement? *Dtsch Med Wochensch* 116: 1543, 1991

64. Tzamaloukas AH, Murata GH, Harford AM et al.: Hand gangrene in diabetic patients on chronic dialysis. *Trans Am Soc Artif Intern Organs* 37: 638, 1991

65. Butt KMH, Friedman EA, Kountz SL: Angioaccess. *Curr Probl Surg* 12: 9, 1976

66. Mayers JD, Markell MS, Cohen LS et al.: Vascular access surgery for maintenance hemodialysis. Variables in hospital stay. *ASAIO J* 38: 113, 1992

67. Riggs JE, Moss AH, Labosky DA et al.: Upper extremity ischemic monomelic neuropathy: a complication of vascular access procedures in uremic diabetic patients. Neurology 1989; 39: 997–998.

68. Legrain M, Rottemburg J, Bentchikou A et al.: Dialysis treatment of insulin-dependent diabetic patients. Ten years experience. *Clin Nephrol* 21: 72, 1984

69. Clark DW, Nowak TV: Diabetic gastroparesis. What to do when gastric emptying is delayed. *Postgrad Med* 95: 195, 1994

70. Clark DW, Nowak TV: Diabetic gastroparesis. What to do when gastric emptying is delayed. *Postgrad Med* 95: 201, 1994

71. Battle WM, Cohen JD, Snape WJ Jr: Disorders of colonic motility in patients with diabetes mellitus. *Yale J Biol Med* 56: 277, 1983

72. Lux G: Disorders of gastrointestinal motility – diabetes mellitus. *Leber Magen Darm* 19: 84, 1989

73. Vincenti F, Arnaud SB, Recker R et al.: Parathyroid and bone response of the diabetic patient to uremia. *Kidney Int* 25: 677, 1984

74. Weiss RE, Reddi AH: Influence of experimental diabetes and insulin on matrix-induced cartilage and bone differentiation. *Am J Physiol* 238: E200, 1980

75. Andress DL, Kopp JB, Maloney NA et al.: Early deposition of aluminum in bone in diabetic patients on hemodialysis. *N Engl J Med* 316: 292, 1987

76. Cheigh J, Raghavan J, Sullivan J et al.: Is insufficient dialysis a cause for high morbidity in diabetic patients. (Abstract) *J Am Soc Nephrol* 2: 317, 1991

77. Owen WF Jr, Lew NL, Liu Y, Lowrie EG, Lazarus JM: The urea reduction ratio and serum albumin concentration as predictors of mortality in patients undergoing hemodialysis. *N Engl J Med* 329: 1001, 1993

78. Goldwasser P, Michel MA, Collier J, Mittman N, Fein PA, Gusik SA, Avram MM: Prealbumin and lipoprotein(a) in hemodialysis: relationships with patient and vascular access survival. *Am J Kidney Dis* 22: 215, 1993

79. Dremth JP, Engels LG: Diabetic gastroparesis. A critical reappraisal of new treatment strategies. *Drugs* 44: 537, 1992

80. Lindblad AS, Nolph KD, Novak JW, Friedman EA: A survey of the NIH CAPD Registry population with end-stage renal disease attributed to diabetic nephropathy. *J Diabetic Complications* 2: 227, 1988

81. Legrain M, Rottembourg J, Bentchikou A et al.: Dialysis treatment of insulin dependent diabetic patients. Ten years experience. *Clin Nephrol* 21: 72, 1984

82. Nolph KD: Is residual renal function preserved better with CAPD than with hemodialysis? *AKF Nephrol Lett* 7: 1, 1990

83. Flynn CT, Nanson JA: Intraperitoneal insulin with CAPD – An artificial pancreas. *Trans Am Soc Artif Intern Organs* 25: 114, 1979

84. Scarpioni LL, Ballocchi S, Castelli A et al.: Continuous ambulatory peritoneal dialysis in diabetic patients. *Contrib Nephrol* 84: 50, 1990

85. Fluckiger R, Harmon W, Meier W et al.: Hemoglobin carbamylation in uremia. *N Engl J Med* 304: 823, 1981

86. Tzamaloukas AH, Oreopoulos DG: Subcutaneous versus intraperitoneal insulin in the management of diabetics on CAPD: a review. *Adv Perit Dial* 7: 81, 1991

87. Rubin J, Hsu H: Continuous ambulatory peritoneal dialysis: ten years at one facility. *Am J Kidney Dis* 17: 165, 1991

88. Anonymous editorial: Prevention of peritonitis in CAPD. *Lancet* 337: 22, 1991

89. Tzamaloukas AH, Oreopoulos DG: Subcutaneous versus intraperitoneal insulin in the management of diabetics on CAPD: a review. *Adv Perit Dial* 7: 81, 1991

90. Mitchell JC, Frohnert PP, Kurtz SB et al.: Chronic peritoneal dialysis in juvenile-onset diabetes mellitus. A comparison with hemodialysis. *Mayo Clin Proc* 53: 775, 1978

91. Levin ME: Peripheral vascular disease in the person with diabetes. in *Diabetes Mellitus*, edited by Rifkin, H, New York, Elsevier, 1990, p 768

92. Held PJ, Port FK, Blagg CR et al.: The United States Renal Data Systems' Annual Data Report. *Am J Kidney Dis* 16 (Suppl 2): 34, 1990

93. Yuan ZY, Balaskas E, Gupta A et al.: Is CAPD or hemodialysis better for diabetic patients? CAPD is more advantageous. *Semin Dial* 5: 181, 1992

94. Nolph KD: Continuous ambulatory peritoneal dialysis as long term treatment for end stage renal disease. *Am J Kidney Dis* 17: 154, 1991

95. Khanna R, Oreopoulos DG: Continuous ambulatory peritoneal dialysis in diabetics with end stage renal disease. A combined experience of 2 North American centers. in *Diabetic Renal Retinal Syndrome*, edited by Friedman EA, L'Esperance FA, New York, Grune and Stratton, 1986, p 363

96. Rottemburg J: Peritoneal dialysis in diabetics. in *Peritoneal Dialysis*, edited by Nolph KD, Boston, Martinus Nijhoff, 1985, p 365

97. Rubin J, Oreopoulos DG, Blair RDG et al.: Chronic peritoneal dialysis in the management of diabetics with terminal renal failure. *Nephron* 19: 265, 1977

98. Gotch F: The application of urea kinetic modelling to CAPD. in *Peritoneal Dialysis*, edited by LaGreca G, Ronco C, Feriani M et al., Milano, Wichtig Editore, 1991, p 47

99. Gokal R, Jakubowski C, Hunt L: Multicenter study of outcome of CAPD and hemodialysis patients. *Nephrol Dial Transplant* 1: 111, 1986

100. Young GA, Kopple JD, Lindholm B et al.: Nutritional assessment of chronic ambulatory peritoneal dialysis patients: an international study. *Am J Kidney Dis* 17: 462, 1991

101. Rotellar C, Black J, Winchester JF et al.: Ten years experience with continuous ambulatory peritoneal dialysis. *Am J Kidney Dis* 17: 158, 1991

102. Miller DG, Levine S, Bistrian B et al.: Diagnosis of protein calorie malnutrition in diabetic patients on hemodialysis and peritoneal dialysis. *Nephron* 33: 127, 1983

103. Blumenkrantz MJ, Gahl GM, Kopple JD et al.: Protein losses during peritoneal dialysis. *Kidney Int* 19: 593, 1981

104. Krediet RT, Zuyderhoudt FMJ, Boeschoten EW et al.: Peritoneal permeability to protein in diabetic and non-diabetic continuous ambulatory dialysis patients. *Nephron* 42; 133, 1986

105. Oreopoulos DG, Yuan ZY: CAPD in diabetics. Presented at the American Society of Nephrology Annual Meeting, November, 1991, Baltimore, MD

106. Sutherland DER, Morrow CE, Fryd DS, Ferguson R, Simmons RL, Najarian JS: Improved patient and primary renal allograft survival in uremic diabetic recipients. *Transplantation* 34: 319, 1982

107. Sollinger HW, Ploeg RJ, Eckhoff DE, Stegall MD, Isaacs R, Pirsch JD, D'Alessandro AM, Knechtle SJ, Kalayoglu M Belzer FO: Two hundred consecutive simultaneous pancreas-kidney transplants with bladder drainage. *Surgery* 114: 736, 1993

108. Robertson RP: Pancreas transplantation in humans with diabetes mellitus. *Diabetes* 40: 1085, 1991

109. Diagnostic and therapeutic technology assessment (DATTA). Pancreatic transplantations. *JAMA* 265: 510, 1991

110. Cecka JM, Terasaki PI: 1991. The UNOS Scientific Renal Transplant Registry – 1991. *Clinical Transplants 1991*, edited by Terasaki PI, UCLA Tissue Typing Lab, Los Angeles CA, 1992, p 1

111. Sutherland D, Gruessner A, Moudry-Munns K: International Pancreas Transplant Registry report. *Transplant Proc* 26: 407, 1994

112. Kennedy WR, Navarro X, Goetz FC et al.: Effects of Pancreatic Transplantation on Diabetic Neuropathy. *N Engl J Med* 322: 1031, 1990

113. Ramsay RC, Goetz FC, Sutherland DE, Mauer SM, Robison LL, Cantril HL, Knobloch WH, Najarian JS: Progression of diabetic retinopathy after pancreas transplantation for insulin-dependent diabetes mellitus. *N Engl J Med* 318: 208, 1988

114. Remuzzi G, Ruggenenti P, Mauer SM: Pancreas and kidney/pancreas transplants: experimental medicine or real improvement? *Lancet* 353: 27, 1994

115. Katz H, Homan M, Velosa J et al.: Effects of pancreas transplantation on postprandial glucose metabolism. *N Engl J Med* 325: 1278, 1991

116. Taylor RJ, Bynon JS, Stratta RJ: Kidney/pancreas transplantation: a review of the current status. *Urol Clin North Am* 21: 343, 1994

117. Manske CL, Wang Y, Rector T et al.: Coronary revascularization in insulin-dependent diabetic patients with chronic renal failure. *Lancet* 340: 998, 1992

118. Karnofsky DA, Burchenal JH: The clinical evaluation of chemotherapeutic agents in cancer. in *Evaluation of Chemotherapeutic Agents*, edited by MacLeod CM, New York, Columbia University Press, 1949, p 191

119. Carlson DM, Johnson WJ, Kjellstrand CM: Functional status of patients with end-stage renal disease. *Mayo Clin Proc* 62: 338, 1987

120. Gutman R A, Stead WW, Robinson RR: Physical activity and employment status of patients on maintenance dialysis. *N Engl J Med* 304: 309, 1981

121. Lowder GM, Perri NA, Friedman EA: Demographics, diabetes type, and degree of rehabilitation in diabetic patients on maintenance hemodialysis in Brooklyn. *J Diabetic Complications* 2: 218, 1988

122. Ifudu O, Paul H, Mayers JD, Cohen LS, Brezsynyak WF, Herman AI, Avram MM, Friedman EA: Pervasive failed rehabilitation in center-based maintenance hemodialysis patients. *Am J Kidney Dis* 23: 394, 1994

123. Ifudu O, Mayers J, Matthew J, Tan CC, Cambridge A, Friedman EA: Dismal rehabilitation in geriatric inner-city hemodialysis patients. *JAMA* 271: 29, 1994

124. Makita Z, Radoff S, Rayfield EJ, Yang Z, Skolnik E, Delaney V, Friedman EA, Cerami A, Vlassara H: Advanced glycosylation end products in patients with diabetic nephropathy. *N Engl J Med* 325: 836, 1991

125. Vlassara H, Fuh H, Makita Z, Krungkrai S, Cerami A, Cucala R: Exogenous advanced glycosylation end products induce complex vascular dysfunction in normal animals: a model for diabetic and aging complications. *Proc Natl Acad Sci USA* 89: 12043, 1992

126. Brownlee M: Glycosylation of proteins and microangiopathy. *Hosp Pract* (Off Ed) 27 (Suppl 1): 46, 1992

127. Ellis EN, Good BH: Prevention of glomerular basement membrane thickening by aminoguanidine in experimental diabetes mellitus. *Metabolism* 40: 1016, 1991

128. Hammes HP, Martin S, Federlin K, Geisen K, Brownlee M: Aminoguanidine treatment inhibits the development of experimental diabetic retinopathy. *Proc Natl Acad Sci USA* 88: 11555, 1991

129. Yagihashi S, Kamijo M, Baba M, Yagihashi M, Nagai K: Effect of aminoguanidine on functional and structural abnormalities in peripheral nerve of STZ-induced diabetic rats. *Diabetes* 41: 47, 1992

130. Brownlee M: Pharmacological modulation of the advanced glycosylation reaction. *Prog Clin Biol Res* 304: 235, 1989

131. Nicholls K, Mandel TE: Advanced glycosylation endproducts in experimental murine diabetic nephropathy: effect of islet isografting and of aminoguanidine. *Lab Invest* 60: 486, 1989

132. Corbett JA, Tilton RG, Chang K, Hasan KS, Ido Y, Wang JL, Sweetland MA, Lancaster JR Jr, Williamson JR, McDaniel ML: Aminoguanidine, a novel inhibitor of nitric oxide formation, prevents diabetic vascular dysfunction. *Diabetes* 4: 552, 1992

133. Tilton RG, Chang K, Hasan KS, Smith SR, Petrash JM, Misko TP, Moore WM, Currie MG, Corbett JA, McDaniel

ML et al.: Prevention of diabetic vascular dysfunction by guanidines. Inhibition of nitric oxide synthase versus advanced glycation end-product formation. *Diabetes* 42: 221, 1993

134. Sensi M, Pricci F, Andreani D, DiMario U: Advanced nonenzymatic glycation endproducts (AGE): their relevance to aging and the pathogenesis of late diabetic complications. *Diabetes Res* 16: 1, 1991

135. Edelstein D, Brownlee M: Mechanistic studies of advanced glycosylation end product inhibition by aminoguanidine. *Diabetes* 41: 26, 1992

136. Eika B, Levin RM, Longhurst PA: Collagen and bladder function in streptozotocin-diabetic rats: effects of insulin and aminoguanidine. *J Urol* 148: 167, 1992

DIALYSIS IN SPECIAL CLINICAL SITUATIONS: ANESTHESIA

BERTRAM L. KASISKE

INTRODUCTION

The number of patients with chronic renal failure who undergo surgery is not likely to decrease in the near future. In the United States, for example, there have been notable demographic trends in the end stage renal disease patient population over the past several years that will ensure a continued need for surgical interventions. Not only has the size of the population grown, but the number and complexity of complications among patients with end stage renal disease has also grown. This is in large part due to the fact that increasingly greater proportions of patients with end stage renal disease are older and have diabetes (1). As a result of these trends, the need for surgery in patients with chronic renal failure is unlikely to diminish any time soon.

A survey of major surgeries performed at the Regional Kidney Disease Program, Minneapolis, Minnesota, over the past five years shows that a large number of procedures were carried out (Table 1). From 1989 through 1993 the number of dialysis patients treated in this program increased from 657 to 910, but averaged 810 patients over this period. During this time, the most common major surgical procedure was renal transplantation. The high number of amputations reflected the high incidence of peripheral vascular disease and diabetes in this population. Similarly, there was a large number of other surgeries performed to treat complications of peripheral vascular and coronary artery disease. It is clear from these data that the number of major surgeries performed in a dialysis population is high, and that the risk of surgery is also likely to be high due to the number of procedures carried out in individuals with atherosclerotic vascular disease.

This chapter will review major aspects of the anesthesia care that a surgical patient with chronic renal failure requires. This care begins in the preoperative period with an assessment of risk for surgery and anesthesia. Under-

standing the risks is important for helping patients make informed choices and for directing attention to steps that will help to prevent major complications. After assessing risk, the next step is to prepare the patient in a manner that will minimize the number and severity of complications. It is beyond the scope of this chapter to review the general management of patients who undergo major surgery, and there are many other comprehensive reviews of general preoperative care (2–5). Rather emphasis will placed on the management of clinical conditions that are particularly common in the dialysis patients. These include electrolyte disorders, blood pressure and intravascular volume alterations, bleeding abnormalities, and anemia. Most, but not all of these abnormalities, can be managed by timely preoperative dialysis. Like preoperative patient preparation, the selection and judicious use of pharmacologic agents during anesthesia and surgery also requires special attention in hemodialysis patients, and this will be discussed in detail. Finally, several potentially life-threatening complications can be anticipated and dealt with at the time of surgery and in the immediate postoperative period. These include hyperkalemia, hypotension, hypertension, pulmonary edema, bleeding, and sepsis.

PREOPERATIVE PATIENT MANAGEMENT

The risk of surgical complications in dialysis patients

Most would agree that the risk of major surgery for a hemodialysis patient is greater than that for an age- and sex-matched individual with normal renal function. However, there have been few systematic studies of sufficient size to precisely define the risk of anesthesia and surgery in the hemodialysis population. To better assess this risk, I have combined data from reported series of

Table 1. The ten most common major surgical procedures performed during a five year period in a large dialysis population[a]

Procedure	Total number of procedures	Average number of procedures per year
1. Kidney transplantation	417	83.4
2. Amputation (digit, leg, etc)	217	43.4
3. Abdominal (cholecystectomy, colectomy, etc)	150	30.0
4. Vascular (aortic aneurysm, femoral bypass, etc)	130	26.0
5. Cardiac (bypass or valve replacement)	54	10.8
6. Orthopedic (laminectomy, arthroplasty, etc)	47	9.4
7. Native kidney nephrectomy	28	5.6
8. Transplant nephrectomy	13	2.6
9. Parathyroidectomy	10	2.0
10. Pericardiectomy	9	1.8

[a]Data from the Regional Kidney Disease Program at Hennepin County Medical Center, Minneapolis, Minnesota, where there was an average annual census of 810 (range 657–910) dialysis patients from 1989–93.

Table 2. Perioperative mortality in dialysis patients who underwent open heart surgery

Center	Year	Number (bypass)	Age mean (range)	HYHA class 3 or 4 (%)	Months of dialysis mean (range)	Number who died (%)	Causes of death (number)			
							Cardiac	Bleeding	Sepsis	Other
Brussels (6)	1991	10 (10)	53 (41–66)	80	44 (9–180)	2 (20)	0	2	0	0
Chicago, IL (7)	1989	21 (16)	61 (32–72)	86	26 (1–60)	2 (10)	0	0	2	0
Rochester, MN (8)	1991	25 (25)	57 (27–77)	96	46 (1–120)	5 (20)	3	0	0	2
Philadelphia, PA (9)	1989	16 (16)	62 (52–72)	83	–	1 (6)	0	0	1	0
Minneapolis, MN (10)	1988	39 (39)	60 (33–79)	85	19 (1–142)	1 (3)	0	0	1	0
Birmingham, AL (11)	1988	20 (20)	52 (30–73)	–	30 (–)	4 (20)	3	0	0	1
Nashville, TN (12)	1986	10 (9)	57 (42–74)	100	41 (1–124)	1 (10)	0	0	1	0
Iowa City, IA (13)	1986	12 (12)	61 (51–67)	100	30 (0–101)	1 (8)	1	0	0	0
Total		153 (147)	58 (27–79)	90	34 (0–180)	17 (11)	7	2	5	3

coronary artery bypass surgery in patients on maintenance hemodialysis (Table 2). To minimize publication bias, I included only series reporting ten or more patients. Literature was located by carrying out a Medline search and by reviewing bibliographies in pertinent publications. A number of reports were excluded because they had fewer than ten patients, or failed to provide adequate information on perioperative mortality.

Of the eight reports reviewed (6–13), a total of 153 patients underwent open heart surgery (Table 2). While all but six of these patients had coronary artery bypass surgery, some also underwent simultaneous valve replacement. Overall, 90% were at least New York Heart Association Class 3. There were seven perioperative deaths, with an overall mortality rate of 12%. The most common causes of death were cardiac, bleeding and infection. In comparison, in a large series of unselected patients under-

going open heart surgery, perioperative mortality was only 2.9% (14). The most common cause of early death was cardiac (82% of deaths), while only 2% of deaths were from infection and 2% were due to bleeding complications (14). Even among unselected patients over 65 years of age the perioperative mortality in another large series was only 5.2%, while that of patients who were less than 65 years old was only 1.9% (15).

These data suggest that the perioperative mortality associated with cardiovascular surgery is increased in patients with chronic renal disease. More over, this increase may be due to a greater frequency of hemorrhagic and infectious complications. Otherwise, from the little information given in these reports, it is difficult to determine how end stage renal disease *per se* may have affected mortality and morbidity in patients undergoing cardiac surgery. The incidence of perioperative deaths caused by myocardial infarction and arrhythmias could have been influenced by hemodynamic instability and electrolyte abnormalities common in the dialysis population. Several patients died of infection, a known complication associated with end stage renal disease. In one report, three patients had major intrathoracic hemorrhage resulting in two deaths (6). Certainly, end stage renal disease may have contributed to this complication. Thus, these data indicate that the risk of major surgery could indeed be increased as a result of abnormalities directly attributable to end stage renal failure.

It is also interesting that the reported incidence of death in hemodialysis patients undergoing open heart surgery varied substantially from center to center. It is possible that this variability reflected differences in patient populations or small sample sizes. However, it is also possible that these differences reflected variability in patient management, and that careful management strategies may reduce the risk of major surgery in dialysis patients.

Anecdotal reports suggest that the risk of other major, non-cardiovascular surgical procedures may be increased in hemodialysis patients as well (16). Although it is difficult to compare renal transplantation with other surgical procedures in dialysis patients or in patients with normal renal function, the incidence of perioperative deaths does not appear to be increased after renal transplantation (17, 18). Nevertheless, the morbidity associated with renal transplantation, as with other major surgical procedures in dialysis patients, appears to be relatively high. Non-fatal complications have included prolonged neuromuscular blockade, infections and bleeding (16–19).

Preoperative risk assessment

Although the morbidity and mortality of major surgery is increased in patients with end stage renal disease, this increased risk is not shared equally by all patients. Thus, it is important to assess risk in each individual patient. This will help the patient make an informed choice regarding therapy options and may help target specific preventive measures. Methods for assessing risk that have been developed in non-dialysis populations can be applied to patients on dialysis. The most commonly used index of overall risk is the American Society of Anesthesiologists (ASA) physical status index (20). In this system patients are assigned one of five classes: I. healthy, II. mild disease without functional limitations, III. severe disease with definite functional limitations, IV. severe disease that is a constant threat to life, and V. expected to die within 24 hours.

Several studies have shown that overall death rates and deaths related to anesthesia are roughly proportional to the ASA class. In particular, overall mortality and deaths due to anesthesia are increased in class III and IV patients compared to class I and II (21–23). Most dialysis patients probably fall in class II–III. The overall risk of death is less than 0.5% for patients in class II, 2–4% in class III,

10–20% in class IV and 10–50% in class V (22, 23). Of course, these risks were not determined for dialysis patients, *per se*. Thus, any additional risk associated with dialysis would likely increase the risk associated with ASA physical status.

The incidence of coronary artery disease is increased in dialysis patients compared to the general population (24, 25). Thus, an assessment of risk in a dialysis patient facing surgery should include an assessment of risk attributable to cardiovascular disease complications. Probably the most widely used index of cardiovascular risk is that of Goldman et al. (26). The index assigns points based on age, history of myocardial infarction, physical findings of heart failure, arrhythmias, routine laboratory tests (including potassium bicarbonate, urea nitrogen and creatinine) and the type of surgery. Although subsequent investigations have confirmed that this index roughly predicts patients who develop major cardiac complications from surgery (27, 28), others have failed to confirm this finding (29–31). Although there are no data confirming the usefulness of such an index in dialysis patients, it is likely that the findings used in the composite index indicate increased risk in most dialysis patients.

Other factors that are common in dialysis patients, but are not unique to this population, may increase the risk of anesthesia and surgery. Patients who are malnourished are at increased risk when faced with surgery (32, 33), and inadequate nutrition is a common complication associated with dialysis. Indeed, serum albumin levels have recently been shown to be a predictor of overall mortality in hemodialysis patients (34). Thus, it is likely that dialysis patients with low serum albumin and other findings suggestive of poor nutrition are at increased risk for anesthesia and surgery. Since an increasingly greater proportion of dialysis patients have hypertension and diabetes, attention should also be given to the effect of diabetes, hypertension and their complications on surgical risk (35, 36).

Electrolyte disorders

The most life-threatening electrolyte complication faced by dialysis patients undergoing surgery is hyperkalemia. A number of factors, in addition to the absence of renal potassium excretion, contribute to the risk of hyperkalemia in this setting. Tissue trauma and blood transfusions, for example, can increase the potassium load in the perioperative period. Acute acidemia and succinylcholine infusion (see below) can shift potassium from the intra-cellular to the extra-cellular space and thereby raise serum potassium levels. Lack of insulin and a decrease in adrenergic activity associated with autonomic neuropathy may also exacerbate hyperkalemia in dialysis patients with diabetes. Due to the high incidence of cardiovascular disease in the dialysis population a large number of patients are also receiving therapy with digitalis which can contribute to hyperkalemia.

In general, serum potassium should be in the low-normal range at the time of induction. A possible exception to this rule is the patient treated with digitalis, in whom a low potassium can potentiate digitalis-associated cardiac arrhythmias. In such a patients potassium should be maintained in the normal range. When possible, an optimal pre-induction potassium should be achieved by measures that remove potassium from the body, and not by measures effecting temporary trans-cellular shifts. This can usually best be accomplished by ensuring adequate preoperative dialysis. However, in some patients in whom this is not possible, preoperative administration of cation exchange resins (sodium polystyrene sulfonate) can be used effectively. Such resins can be given either orally or rectally.

Metabolic acidosis should also be treated prior to induction. It is not enough to know that the blood pH is not too low. If, for example, the pH is being compensated for by an increased ventilatory rate, then the pH is at risk to fall suddenly and precipitously the moment ventilation is slowed or interrupted. Such an occurrence can lead to arrhythmias and cardiac arrest at the time of induction. Therefore, it is important to be sure that the serum bicarbonate level is adequate, so that there is enough buffering capacity to prevent a sudden, life-threatening drop in blood pH. Ideally the bicarbonate level should be 20 mEq/l or greater at the time of induction. This can best be achieved by adequate preoperative dialysis. If this is not possible, judicious use of intravenous sodium bicarbonate can be used if intravascular volume status is monitored closely.

Occasionally, hyponatremia can be a problem in a dialysis patient undergoing surgery. This is usually easily remedied with well-timed, preoperative dialysis. Other electrolyte problems commonly encountered in dialysis patients rarely cause major problems in the perioperative period. Hypocalcemia is most often seen in association with low serum albumin and high serum phosphorous, and ionized calcium levels in this setting are usually not low enough to cause symptoms. Similarly, hyperphosphatemia is rarely of clinical consequence in the perioperative period.

Blood pressure and intravascular volume abnormalities

Markedly elevated preoperative blood pressure can pose a substantial perioperative risk to patients with end stage renal disease. Hypertension in the dialysis population is most often volume-dependent, and adequate preoperative fluid removal with dialysis can be used to reduce elevated blood pressure before surgery. However, since anesthesia usually reduces blood pressure, mild preoperative hypertension probably poses little risk. The utility of continuing antihypertensive medications until the time of surgery was demonstrated in a study where blood pressure and hemodynamic changes were prospectively monitored in 81 patients undergoing renal transplantation (37). Patients

with hypertension were maintained on beta-blockers and vasodilating agents until surgery. After induction, blood pressure was similar in hypertensive and normotensive patients, and none had serious complications. These data confirm that antihypertensive medications should be continued up to the time of surgery.

Although adequate dialysis can reduce the risk of developing pulmonary edema in the perioperative period, that risk is in fact small. On the other hand, preoperative intravascular volume contraction from over-zealous fluid removal can increase the risk of hypotension at induction or during surgery. Indeed, hypotension has been found to be a more frequent complication than hypertension during surgery in dialysis patients (17, 18). Thus, it is probably best to use preoperative dialysis to achieve normal or near-normal intravascular volume, and not to induce hypovolemia. In occasional high-risk patients it may be wise to monitor preoperative and intra-operative intravascular volume status with a central venous or right heart catheter.

Bleeding abnormalities

Patients with renal failure have a well-described, but not completely understood bleeding tendency, and major perioperative bleeding complications are probably more frequent in dialysis patients than in patients with normal renal function (6, 16, 19). This bleeding tendency is not reflected by abnormalities in standard coagulation screening tests. Indeed, prothrombin time, partial thromboplastin time, and platelet counts are not affected by uremia *per se*. Rather the bleeding tendency seems to correlate best with abnormalities in platelet function. Although there are few published data, a prolonged bleeding time may best correlate with an increased risk of major bleeding in a dialysis patient undergoing surgery. The accuracy of the bleeding time is arguably low, but a very prolonged value should probably prompt efforts at correction.

A number of measures have been found to effectively reduce the bleeding time in small clinical trials. Oral or intravenous conjugated estrogens can correct the bleeding time after five to seven days (38–40). A more rapid correction can be achieved by giving cryoprecipitate or 1-deamino–8-D-arginine vasopressin (41, 42). To what extent correcting the bleeding time prior to surgery reduces the risk of major bleeding complications in dialysis patients is unknown. However, adverse effects from these agents are few, and their preoperative use is probably warranted in high risk individuals with a very prolonged bleeding time.

Anemia

Severe anemia is now less of a problem in chronic dialysis patients than it was before the introduction of recombinant erythropoietin. Most dialysis patients who have a serum hematocrit level that is less than 30% receive erythropoietin therapy. Since this level of hematocrit is probably adequate for most routine surgeries, the need for preoperative blood transfusions has diminished. At the same time there are reasons not to give unnecessary blood transfusions. In the United States there is and will continue to be a small but ineradicable risk of transmission of viruses through transfused blood. For dialysis patients waiting for a kidney transplant, there is also a small risk that the patient will form antibodies that will make it more difficult to find a cross-match negative kidney in the future. For all of these reasons, the routine use of preoperative blood transfusions in dialysis patients has diminished. Should transfusion be deemed necessary, blood can best be given during a pre-operative dialysis treatment to minimize the risk of hyperkalemia.

Hemodialysis

It goes without saying that hemodialysis is an important part of the management of chronic renal failure patients who undergo surgery. Ideally, patients should be well-dialyzed prior to surgery, and hemodialysis should be available at any time during the perioperative period. An adequate dialysis access site should also be available for use at any time in the perioperative period. All too frequently hemodialysis access devices thrombose during surgery or during the immediate postoperative period. Care should be taken to prevent external pressure and interruption of access blood flow during and immediately after surgery.

When possible patients should undergo hemodialysis within a day of surgery. This will permit optimal control of electrolytes, blood pressure, and intravascular volume. Dialysis carried out just prior to surgery also decreases the chances that additional dialysis will be required intra-operatively or in the immediate postoperative period when the patient may be unstable. In addition, preoperative dialysis provides an opportunity to administer blood safely if a transfusion is required. The amount of heparin given on the preoperative dialysis run can usually be minimized. More over, blood levels of heparin decline rapidly after dialysis, so that residual effects of anticoagulation should usually not preclude the use of preoperative dialysis. Regional anticoagulation can also be used to obviate concerns about post-run bleeding. Occasionally, it may not be possible to delay surgery long enough to prepare the patient with dialysis. Such patients can usually be managed safely, although the chances that intra-operative, or early post-operative dialysis may be needed are increased. The increased catabolic demand associated with major surgery may not be adequately met by peritoneal dialysis. In anticipation of this, peritoneal dialysis patients may also need to undergo hemodialysis prior to major surgery.

THE SELECTION AND USE OF AGENTS IN ANESTHESIA

Regional *vs* general anesthesia

Many minor surgical procedures can be safely and effectively carried out using local or regional anesthesia. Procedures to place or repair hemodialysis access devices, for example, are routinely performed with local or regional anesthesia. It has been reported that the duration of regional block is shorter in patients with chronic renal failure (43). However, more recent data suggest that both latency and duration of regional anesthesia are similar in patients with chronic renal failure compared to patients with normal renal function (44). There have been isolated reports of toxicity from the use of epinephrine and bivucaine with regional anesthesia in patients with chronic renal disease (45, 46). However, the careful use of regional blocks for minor surgical procedures in dialysis patients is generally safe and effective.

Occasionally, major surgical interventions have been carried out in dialysis patients using regional anesthesia. Indeed, the routine use of regional anesthesia has even been advocated for renal transplantation (47). There are theoretical advantages for using regional anesthesia for high risk dialysis patients. Potential problems with the use of muscle relaxants in dialysis patients can be avoided. The risks associated with endotracheal intubation can also be avoided. However, the use of regional anesthesia for major surgical procedures has not generally been adopted for several reasons. First, the sometimes lengthy duration of the procedure can necessitate the use of large amounts of intravenous sedative hypnotics. Second, high blocks or continuous catheter techniques may be necessary, and the bleeding tendency found in some dialysis patients can increase the risk of potentially dangerous hematoma formation. Epidural and spinal anesthesia can also cause hemodynamic instability, and the vasodilation associated with their use can lead to significant hypotension. Intra-operative hypotension may be more difficult to manage in dialysis patients because intravenous fluid administration must be judicious. For all of these reasons, regional techniques are rarely used for major surgical procedures in dialysis patients.

Antimuscarininc agents

Atropine and other anticholinergic compounds such as glycopyrrolate are largely dependent on renal excretion for their elimination (48, 49). Thus, repetitive doses of these agents may result in their accumulation in dialysis patients. However, use of a single dose is generally safe. Although scopalamine is less dependent on renal excretion than atropine, the use of scopalamine should also be limited to a single dose prior to induction in patients with end stage renal disease due to the risk of possible adverse central nervous system effects.

Intravenous analgesics and tranquilizers

Most narcotic analgesics such as codeine, morphine, and meperidol, are metabolized almost exclusively by the liver (50). Nevertheless, alterations in protein binding and tissue distribution, renal excretion of active metabolites, and the affects of uremia on liver metabolism can all contribute to altered pharmacodynamic activity of narcotic analgesics in dialysis patients (51). Indeed, there have been clinical reports of prolonged central nervous system depression following the use of narcotic analgesics in patients with chronic renal failure (52). Therefore, all of these agents should be used with caution in dialysis patients. As a general rule, doses of narcotic analgesics should be reduced by up to 50% and the dosing interval should be prolonged (53). Naloxone can be successfully used to antagonized and reverse the effects narcotic analgesics in patients with renal disease (52).

In single doses, the duration of action of the newer opioid analgesic fentanyl is largely dependent on tissue redistribution (54, 55). Only about 10% of a dose of fentanyl is excreted by the kidneys, and any effect of renal failure on plasma protein binding probably has little clinical relevance (56, 57). The newer fentanyl derivatives have also been examined in patients with renal failure. In general, the pharmacokinetic and pharmacodynamic activities of both sufentanil and alfentanil have been found to be similar in patients with renal failure compared to normal controls (58–62). However, prolonged postoperative respiratory depression has been reported in at least one chronic renal failure patient who had high blood levels of sufentanil (63). Hence, as with other narcotic analgesics, the possibility of over-sedation should not be overlooked, especially when repetitive doses of these agents are used in dialysis patients.

There is little information on the use of droperidol in patients with renal disease. In one series of 176 patients who underwent renal transplantation using neuroleptanesthesia, droperidol was used successfully for induction, but was felt to be less desirable than thiomebutol (64). Although barbiturates are predominately metabolized by the liver, the effects of short-acting barbiturates may be prolonged in patients with chronic renal disease (65). Whether this is due to altered plasma protein binding or to other effects is unclear (66–68). Although the plasma clearance of most benzodiazepines is not altered in patients with chronic renal failure, there may be alterations in plasma protein binding and active metabolites may be dependent on renal excretion (69, 70). Nevertheless, single doses of short-acting benzodiazepines have been used successfully as premedication in patients with chronic renal failure undergoing surgery.

Given the safety of inhalational agents, few would advocate the exclusive use of intravenous agents for general anesthesia in patients with chronic renal failure. Nevertheless, intravenous agents can be used for induction in patients with renal disease. Reduced doses of thiopental, fentanyl, or the combination of fentanyl and droperidol have all been used successfully for induction in dialysis patients (17, 18). Most potential problems these agents can cause in dialysis patients can be obviated by avoiding repetitive doses and prolonged infusions.

Inhalational agents

Some metabolic products of inhaled anesthetics are excreted by the kidney. Nevertheless, altered renal function does not appear to affect the pharmacodynamic activity of any of these agents. Therefore, inhaled anesthetic agents are theoretically well-suited for general anesthesia in patients with renal disease. It is important, however, to select the agent that is least toxic.

Much has been written about the nephrotoxic potential of several inhaled anesthetic agents. It is tempting to disregard the issue of nephrotoxicity in choosing an agent for a dialysis patient. However, there are two clinical situations in which nephrotoxicity may have significant adverse consequences for a dialysis patient undergoing general anesthesia. First, a newly transplanted kidney may be particularly vulnerable to drug-induced nephrotoxicity due to the effects of underlying ischemia. Thus, it is prudent to avoid the use of nephrotoxic agents in dialysis patients undergoing renal transplantation. Second, some dialysis patients still derive substantial benefit from residual renal function. Residual urine volume may decrease the amount of fluid that needs to be removed at the time of dialysis, thus reducing the incidence of hypotension and other untoward effects of aggressive ultrafiltration. Residual renal excretion of metabolic waste products may also augment the benefits of delivered dialysis therapy. Since an increasing amount of data has correlated small differences in renal replacement therapy to survival, preserving residual renal function may be more important than previously thought (71). Thus, it may be wise to avoid using nephrotoxic anesthetic agents in dialysis patients with residual renal function or in patients undergoing renal transplantation.

The metabolism of many inhaled anesthetic agents can result in the renal accumulation of toxic inorganic fluorides. Indeed, the relative nephrotoxicity of an inhaled agent is proportional to its fluoride content (72–75). Thus, methoxyflurane was found to be the most nephrotoxic, and it is no longer in use (75). Less inorganic fluoride is produced from the metabolism of enflurane, and even less is produced from isoflurane. Nevertheless, the nephrotoxic threshold for inorganic fluorides in dialysis patients with residual renal function or in patients undergoing renal transplantation is unclear. Thus, it is probably best to avoid these agents when there are other suitable alternatives. Neither halothane or nitrous oxide appear to exert significant nephrotoxicity, and both of these agents have been used successfully in patients with chronic renal failure (17, 18, 76). Since, even with the advent of erythropoietin, anemia is common in end stage renal dis-

960   *Bertram L. Kasiske*

ease patients, attention should be given to maintaining adequate oxygenation when using high concentrations of nitrous oxide.

Muscle relaxants

The depolarizing agent succinylcholine has a rapid onset of action that is particularly useful at the time of endotracheal intubation. It is rapidly hydrolyzed by cholinesterases. Levels of cholinesterase do not appear to be different in dialysis patients compared to patients with normal renal function (77–79), and elimination of succinylcholine does not appear to be appreciably dependent on renal excretion. However, increases in succinic acid and choline after succinylcholine administration may lead to higher levels of the precursor succinylmonocholine. Succinylmonocholine is a non-depolarizing blocker and is excreted by the kidney (80). Thus, decreased renal function may indirectly lead to prolonged paralysis, and continuous intravenous infusion of succinylcholine should probably be avoided in dialysis patients.

The rapid onset and short duration of action, as well as the fact that it is well tolerated and does not cause histamine release, make the use of succinylcholine particularly attractive. Unfortunately, succinylcholine typically increases serum potassium levels by about 0.5 mEq/l (81, 82). Although the increase in potassium from succinylcholine is comparable in dialysis patients and in patients with normal renal function (82, 83), hyperkalemia is more often a clinical problem in patients with chronic renal failure. Thus, succinylcholine should only be used in well-dialyzed patients whose serum potassium is in the low normal range.

The effect of decreased renal function on the elimination of nondepolarizing muscle relaxants has been extensively studied (Table 3). The older nondepolarizing muscle relaxants are dependent on renal excretion (84–92). Prolonged paralysis has been reported in patients with chronic renal failure, especially with the use of gallamine (91, 92). Indeed, gallamine is contraindicated in patients with chronic renal failure. Some of the newer muscle relaxants may be less dependent on renal excretion. Atracurium, for example, is eliminated through nonrenal pathways, and this agent appears to be ideally suited for use in dialysis patients (93–98). In contrast, vecuronium appears to be more dependent on renal excretion and the effects of vecuronium may be prolonged in patients with renal failure (94–103). Indeed a recent meta-analysis of the pharmacodynamic activity of vecuronium concluded that the duration of action of vecuronium was prolonged in patients with renal failure (100). Among other new agents, preliminary data suggest that renal failure has little effect on doxacurium and rocurium (104–106). In contrast the effects of mivacurium were prolonged in nine patients undergoing renal transplantation (107).

Of all the non-depolarizing muscle relaxants that have been well studied in renal failure patients, atracurium

Table 3. The use of muscle relaxants in dialysis patients

Agent	Suitability in dialysis patients[a]	Elimination half-life prolonged
Depolarizing muscle relaxant		
Succinylcholine (77–83)	+	Minimal
Nondepolarizing muscle relaxants		
Atracurium (93–98)	++	Minimal
Vecuronium (94–103)	+	1.5-fold
d-Tubocurarine (84–87)	–	1.5-fold
Pancuronium (88, 89)	–	2-fold
Metocurine (90)	–	2-fold
Gallamine (91, 92)	– –	5-fold
Cholinesterase Inhibitors		
Neostigmine (112)	+	2-fold
Pyridostigmine (113)	+	3-fold
Edrophonium (111)	+	2-fold

[a] +/- indicate relative degree of suitability in dialysis patients.

seems to be the most suitable. However, atracurium, like other agents in this class, can cause histamine release (94). In addition, prolonged paralysis can sometime result from interactions with other drugs. For example, in patients treated with atracurium postoperative respiratory failure was more common in those who also received cyclosporine compared to those who did not (108). Prolonged neuromuscular blockade with pancuronium has also been reported when used it was used concomitantly with cyclosporine (109). Studies in animal models have shown that some of the interaction between intravenous cyclosporine and muscle relaxants may be due to the cremophor vehicle (110).

Cholinesterase inhibitors used to reverse the effects of nondepolarizing muscle relaxants are to a large extent excreted by the kidney (Table 3) (111–114). As a result, recurarization after reversal of muscle relaxants in dialysis patients has been relatively uncommon. Indeed, when recurarization occurs in this setting, it is most likely the result of interactions between muscle relaxants and other medications.

Intraoperative and postoperative complications

Many complications can be avoided by following preventive measures outlined above. More over, careful perioperative monitoring of high-risk dialysis patients can also help to prevent complications. Electrolytes, oxygenation, and cardiovascular status should all be monitored closely. In some high-risk patients intravascular volume status may need to be monitored with a central venous or right heart catheter. Neuromuscular blockade can be effective-

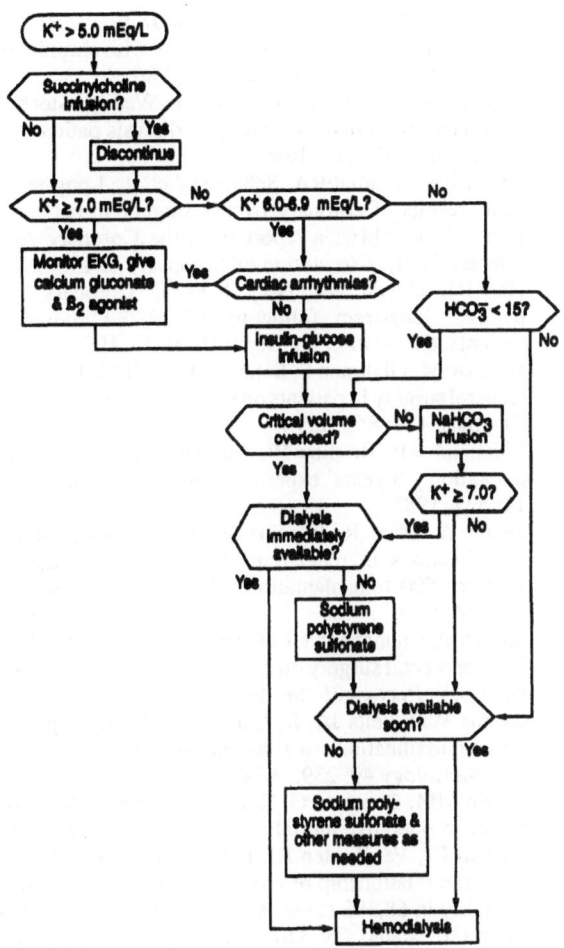

Figure 1. One possible approach to the treatment of hyperkalemia in patients with chronic renal failure undergoing surgery. See text for details and for suggested doses of specific medications.

mias. Nebulized or intravenous beta-2 adrenergic agonists have been shown to effectively shift potassium into cells and immediately lower serum potassium levels in chronic dialysis patients. Beta-2 agonists may be less effective in patients taking a beta-blocker, but adverse effects have been few. Nebulized salbutamol (20 mg), nebulized albuterol (10–20 mg), intravenous salbutamol (4 micrograms/kg over 20 minutes), intravenous epinephrine (0.01 microgram/kilogram/min), and other approaches have all been shown to be safe and effective in dialysis patients (115–120).

An intravenous infusion of regular insulin (20 units) and glucose (50 g) should be infused over 30–60 minutes. If the patient is not in pulmonary edema, an infusion of sodium bicarbonate (50–100 mEq) should be administered slowly. Both of these measures will shift potassium into cells and temporarily lower serum potassium levels. Ultimately, however, it is critical to remove potassium from the body. If dialysis is immediately available, and if the potassium level is still 7.0 mEq/l or greater, the patient should undergo hemodialysis. Alternatively, sodium polystyrene sulfonate (Kayexalate, 25–50 g) can be given rectally with sorbitol, and dialysis arranged as soon as possible.

As previously noted, intra-operative hypotension is more common than hypertension in dialysis patients undergoing major surgery (17, 18). Hypotension can be treated with the judicious use of intravenous fluids and with adrenergic agents. That intravenous fluids need not be unduly restricted was illustrated by a study in which fluid replacement was carefully monitored in 14 dialysis patients undergoing pre-transplant nephrectomy (121). Patients were all dialyzed one day before surgery. The average amount of perioperative fluid replacement was just slightly less than 6 liters. Patients dialyzed again within 29 hours of completing surgery, and no major complications were encountered (121). Although most would advocate that fluids be used cautiously in dialysis patients, this report illustrates that moderate amounts of intravenous fluids can usually be given safely.

Intra-operative hypertension in dialysis patients can be treated with intravenous antihypertensive agents. If hypertension is severe or life-threatening, sodium nitroprusside can be used. Nitroprusside is effective, easy to titrate, and can be used until other longer acting agents take effect. However, prolonged infusions of nitroprusside can lead to thiocyanate toxicity in patients with chronic renal failure, and a nitroprusside infusion should be replaced as soon as possible with other agents. A vasodilator such as hydralazine is effective in hypertensive dialysis patients. Combined alpha- and beta-blockers such as labetalol, or intravenous calcium antagonists are also effective parenteral antihypertensive agents in the perioperative period (122, 123). Recently, there has been much interest in the use of calcium channel blockers in renal transplant recipients. Indeed, some investigators have suggested that these agents may reduce allograft reperfusion injury and pos-

ly monitored with nerve stimulation. However, even with close monitoring and efforts directed at prevention, major complications are more frequent in patients with end stage renal disease. These include hyperkalemia, hypertension, hypotension, pulmonary edema, bleeding, and sepsis.

Hyperkalemia-induced cardiac arrhythmias are a potentially lethal complication of surgery and anesthesia in dialysis patients. Fortunately, fatal hyperkalemia is rare. Serum potassium levels should be monitored frequently, and increased levels should be treated. In general, treatment should be tailored to the severity of the potassium elevation and electrocardiographic changes (Figure 1). If succinylcholine is being continuously infused, this should be immediately stopped. If serum potassium is 7.0 mEq/l or higher, and/or if the hyperkalemia is associated with cardiac arrhythmias, 10–30 ml of calcium gluconate (10%) should be given intravenously over 3–5 minutes to antagonize the cardiac membrane effects of hyperkalemia and reduce the risk of fatal arrhyth-

sibly antagonize the renal toxicity of cyclosporine (124–126).

Acute pulmonary edema in dialysis patients can be treated in the usual manner, with the exception that immediate dialysis must replace diuresis. Standard measures aimed at reducing central venous pressure by tourniquets, raising the upper body, and increasing venous capacitance with morphine are effective short-term measures. Treating severe hypertension, delivering adequate oxygen and airway pressure with mechanical ventilation, and using of bronchodilators can also be life-sustaining until fluid can be removed with ultrafiltration. Bleeding often complicates surgery in a dialysis patient. Measures to correct a uremic bleeding tendency, as described for use in the preoperative period above, can also be effective in reducing postoperative bleeding. Finally, infection is a common postoperative complication in patients with chronic renal failure. Generally, the use of prophylactic antibiotics is not helpful. However, removing central venous access lines as soon as possible can help reduce the incidence of postoperative sepsis.

REFERENCES

1. US Renal Data System, USRDS 1993 Annual Data Report, Bethesda, MD: The National Institutes of Health, National Institute of Diabetes and Digestive, 1993
2. Collins VJ: Preanesthetic evaluation and preparation. in *Principles of Anesthesiology*, 3rd Edition, Philadelphia, Lea & Febiger, 1993, p 207
3. Roizen MF: Preoperative evaluation. in *Anesthesia*, 3rd Edition, edited by Miller RD, New York, Churchill Livingstone, 1990, p 743
4. Gluck R, Munoz E, Wise L: Preoperative and postoperative medical evaluation of surgical patients. *Am J Surg* 155: 730, 1988
5. Houston MC, Ratcliff DG, Hays JT, Gluck FW: Preoperative medical consultation and evaluation of surgical risk. *South Med J* 80: 1385, 1987
6. De Meyer M, Wyns W, Dion R, Khoury G, Pirson Y, van Ypersele de Strihou C: Myocardial revascularization in patients on renal replacement therapy. *Clin Nephrol* 36: 147, 1991
7. Blakeman BM, Pifarre R, Sullivan HJ, Montoya A, Bakhos M: Cardiac surgery for chronic renal dialysis patients. *Chest* 95: 509, 1989
8. Batiuk TD, Kurtz SB, Oh JK, Orszulak TA: Coronary artery bypass operation in dialysis patients. *Mayo Clin Proc* 66: 45, 1991
9. Deutsch E, Bernstein RC, Addonizio VP, Kussmaul WG, III: Coronary artery bypass surgery in patients on chronic hemodialysis. *Ann Intern Med* 110: 369, 1989
10. Opsahl JA, Husebye DG, Helseth HK, Collins AJ: Coronary artery bypass surgery in patients on maintenance dialysis: long-term survival. *Am J Kidney Dis* 12: 271, 1988
11. Rostand SG, Kirk KA, Rutsky EA, Pacifico AD: Results of coronary artery bypass grafting in end-stage renal disease. *Am J Kidney Dis* 12: 266, 1988
12. Laws KH, Merrill WH, Hammon JW Jr, Prager RL, Bender HW Jr: Cardiac surgery in patients with chronic renal disease. *Ann Thorac Surg* 42: 152, 1986
13. Marshall WG Jr, Rossi NP, Meng RL, Wedige–Stecher T: Coronary artery bypass grafting in dialysis patients. *Ann Thorac Surg* 42: S12, 1986
14. Gersh BJ, Kronmal RA, Schaff HV et al.: Long-term (5 year) results of coronary bypass surgery in patients 65 years old or older: a report from the Coronary Artery Surgery Study. *Circulation* 68 (Suppl II): II-190, 1983
15. Hall RJ, Elayda MA, Gray A et al.: Coronary artery bypass: long-term follow-up of 22,284 consecutive patients. *Circulation* 68 (Suppl II): II-20, 1983
16. Haimov M, Glabman S, Schupak E, Neff M, Burrows L: General surgery in patients on maintenance hemodialysis. *Ann Surg* 179: 863, 1974
17. Marsland AR, Bradley JP: Anaesthesia for renal transplantation – 5 years' experience. *Anaesth Intensive Care* 11: 337, 1983
18. Heino A, Orko R, Rosenberg PH: Anaesthesiological complications in renal transplantation: a retrospective study of 500 transplantations. *Acta Anaesthesiol Scand* 30: 574, 1986
19. Sheikh F, Khubchandani IT, Rosen L, Sheets JA, Stasik JJ: Is anorectal surgery on chronic dialysis patients risky? *Dis Colon Rectum* 35: 56, 1992
20. Owens WD, Felts JA, Spitznagel EL Jr: ASA physical status classifications: a study of consistency of ratings. *Anesthesiology* 49: 239, 1978
21. Cohen MM, Duncan PG, Tate RB: Does anesthesia contribute to operative mortality? *JAMA* 260: 2859, 1988
22. Vacanti CJ, VanHouten RJ, Hill RC: A statistical analysis of the relationship of physical status to postoperative mortality in 68,388 cases. *Anesth Analg* 49: 564, 1970
23. Marx GF, Mateo CV, Orkin LR: Computer analysis of postanesthetic deaths. *Anesthesiology* 39: 54, 1973
24. Greaves SC, Sharpe DN: Cardiovascular disease in patients with end-stage renal failure. *Aust N Z J Med* 22: 153, 1992
25. Parfrey PS: Cardiac and cerebrovascular disease in chronic uremia. *Am J Kidney Dis* 21: 77, 1993
26. Goldman L, Caldera DL, Nussbaum SR et al.: Multifactorial index of cardiac risk in noncardiac surgical procedures. *N Engl J Med* 297: 845, 1977
27. Goldman L: Assessment of the patient with known or suspected ischaemic heart disease for non-cardiac surgery. *Br J Anaesth* 61: 38, 1988
28. Goldman L: Multifactorial index of cardiac risk in noncardiac surgery: ten-year status report. *J Cardiothorac Anesth* 1: 237–244, 1987
29. Jeffrey CC, Kunsman J, Cullen DJ, Brewster DC: A prospective evaluation of cardiac risk index. *Anesthesiology* 58: 462, 1983
30. Carliner NH, Fisher ML, Plotnick GD et al.: Routine preoperative exercise testing in patients undergoing major noncardiac surgery. *Am J Cardiol* 56: 51, 1985
31. Gerson MC, Hurst JM, Hertzberg VS et al.: Cardiac prognosis in noncardiac geriatric surgery. *Ann Intern Med* 103: 832, 1985
32. Meguid MM, Mughal MM, Meguid V, Terz JJ: Risk-benefit analysis of malnutrition and perioperative nutritional support: a review. *Nutrition International* 3: 25, 1987

33. Hensle TW, Askanazi J: Metabolism and nutrition in the perioperative period. *J Urol* 139: 229, 1988

34. Lowrie EG, Lew NL: Commonly measured laboratory variables in hemodialysis patients: relationships among them and to death risk. *Semin Nephrol* 12: 276, 1992

35. Charlson ME, MacKenzie CR, Gold JP, Ales KL, Topkins M, Shires GT: Preoperative characteristics predicting intraoperative hypotension and hypertension among hypertensives and diabetics undergoing noncardiac surgery. *Ann Surg* 212: 66, 1990

36. Goldman L, Caldera DL. Risks of general anesthesia and elective operation in the hypertensive patient. *Anesthesiology* 50: 285, 1979

37. Pouttu J: Haemodynamic responses during general anaesthesia for renal transplantation in patients with and without hypertensive disease. *Acta Anaesthesiol Scand* 33: 245, 1989

38. Livio M, Mannucci PM, Vigano G et al.: Conjugated estrogens for the management of bleeding associated with renal failure. *N Engl J Med* 315: 731, 1986

39. Vigano G, Gaspari F, Locatelli M, Pusineri F, Bonati M, Remuzzi G: Dose-effect and pharmacokinetics of estrogens given to correct bleeding time in uremia. *Kidney Int* 34: 853, 1988

40. Shemin D, Elnour M, Amarantes B, Abuelo JG, Chazan JA: Oral estrogens decrease bleeding time and improve clinical bleeding in patients with renal failure. *Am J Med* 89: 436, 1990

41. Janson PA, Jubelirer SJ, Weinstein MJ, Deykin D: Treatment of the bleeding tendency in uremia with cryoprecipitate. *N Engl J Med* 303: 1318, 1980

42. Mannucci PM, Remuzzi G, Pusineri F et al.: Deamino-8-D-arginine vasopressin shortens the bleeding time in uremia. *N Engl J Med* 308: 8, 1983

43. Bromage PR, Gertel M: Brachial plexus anesthesia in chronic renal failure. *Anesthesiology* 36: 488, 1972

44. Martin R, Beauregard L, Tétrault JP: Brachial plexus blockade and chronic renal failure. *Anesthesiology* 69: 405, 1988

45. Rooke NT, Milne B: Acute pulmonary edema after regional anesthesia with lidocaine and epinephrine in a patient with chronic renal failure. *Anesth Analg* 63: 363, 1984

46. Gould DB, Aldrete JA: Bupivacaine cardiotoxicity in a patient with renal failure. *Acta Anaesthesiol Scand* 27: 18, 1983

47. Linke CL, Merin RG: A regional anesthetic approach for renal transplantation. *Anesth Analg* 55: 69, 1976

48. Gosselin RE, Gabourel JD, Wills JH: The fate of atropine in man. *Clin Pharmacol Ther* 1: 597, 1960.

49. Tønnesen M: The excretion of atropine and allied alkaloids in urine. *Acta Pharmacol Toxicol* 6: 147, 1950.

50. Verbeeck RK, Branch RA, Wilkinson GR: Meperidine disposition in man: influence of urinary pH and route of administration. *Clin Pharmacol Ther* 30: 619, 1981

51. Olsen GD, Bennett WM, Porter GA: Morphine and phenytoin binding to plasma proteins in renal and hepatic failure. *Clin Pharmacol Ther* 17: 677, 1975

52. Don HF, Dieppa RA, Taylor P: Narcotic analgesics in anuric patients. *Anesthesiology* 42: 745, 1975

53. Aweeka FT: Drug dosing in renal failure. in *Applied Therapeuties – The Clinical Use of Drugs*, 5th Edition, edited by Koda-Kimble MA, Young LY, Kradjan WA, Gugliel-

mo BJ, Vancouver, Applied Therapeutics, Inc, 1992, p 26-1

54. Hug CC Jr, Murphy MR: Tissue redistribution of fentanyl and termination of its effects in rats. *Anesthesiology* 55: 369, 1981

55. McClain DA, Hug CC Jr: Intravenous fentanyl kinetics. *Clin Pharmacol Ther* 28: 106, 1980

56. Mather LE: Clinical pharmacokinetics of fentanyl and its newer derivatives. *Clin Pharmacokinet* 8: 422, 1983

57. Bower S: Plasma protein binding of fentanyl: the effect of hyperlipoproteinaemia and chronic renal failure. *J Pharm Pharmacol* 34: 102, 1982

58. Sear JW: Sufentanil disposition in patients undergoing renal transplantation: influence of choice of kinetic model. *Br J Anaesth* 63: 60, 1989

59. Fyman PN, Reynolds JR, Moser F, Avitable M, Casthely PA, Butt K: Pharmacokinetics of sufentanil in patients undergoing renal transplantation (see comments). *Can J Anaesth* 35: 312, 1988

60. Davis PJ, Stiller RL, Cook DR, Brandom BW, Davin-Robinson KA: Pharmacokinetics of sufentanil in adolescent patients with chronic renal failure. *Anesth Analg* 67: 268, 1988

61. Chauvin M, Lebrault C, Levron JC, Duvaldestin P: Pharmacokinetics of alfentanil in chronic renal failure. *Anesth Analg* 66: 53, 1987

62. Van Peer A, Vercauteren M, Noorduin H, Woestenborghs R, Heykants J: Alfentanil kinetics in renal insufficiency. *Eur J Clin Pharmacol* 30: 245, 1986

63. Wiggum DC, Cork RC, Weldon ST, Gandolfi AJ, Perry DS: Postoperative respiratory depression and elevated sufentanil levels in a patient with chronic renal failure. *Anesthesiology* 63: 708, 1985

64. Lindahl-Nilsson C, Lundh R, Groth CG: Neurolept anaesthesia for the renal transplant operation. *Acta Anaesthesiol Scand* 24: 451, 1980

65. Dundee JW, Richards RK: Effect of azotemia upon the action of intravenous barbiturate anesthesia. *Anesthesiology* 15: 333, 1954.

66. Ghoneim MM, Pandya HB, Kelley SE, Fischer LJ, Corry RJ: Binding of thiopental to plasma proteins: effects on distribution in the brain and heart. *Anesthesiology* 45: 635, 1976

67. Ghoneim MM, Pandya H: Plasma protein binding of thiopental in patients with impaired renal or hepatic function. *Anesthesiology* 42: 545, 1975

68. Burch PG, Stanski DR: Decreased protein binding and thiopental kinetics. *Clin Pharmacol Ther* 32: 212, 1982

69. Vinik HR, Reves JG, Greenblatt DJ, Abernethy DR, Smith LR: The pharmacokinetics of midazolam in chronic renal failure patients. *Anesthesiology* 59: 390, 1983

70. Ochs HR, Rauh HW, Greenblatt DJ, Kaschell HJ: Clorazepate dipotassium and diazepam in renal insufficiency: serum concentrations and protein binding of diazepam and desmethyldiazepam. *Nephron* 37: 100, 1984

71. Collins AJ, Ma JZ, Umen A, Keshaviah P: Urea index and other predictors of hemodialysis patient survival. *Am J Kidney Dis* 23: 272, 1994

72. Mazze RI, Cousins MJ, Barr GA: Renal effects and metabolism of isoflurane in man. *Anesthesiology* 40: 536, 1974

73. Mazze RI: Metabolism of the inhaled anaesthetics: implications of enzyme induction. *Br J Anaesth* 56: 27S, 1984

74. Wickström I: Enflurane anesthesia in living donor renal transplantation. *Acta Anaesthesiol Scand* 25: 263, 1981

75. Cousins MJ, Mazze RI: Methoxyflurane nephrotoxicity – a study of dose response in man. *JAMA* 225: 1611, 1973

76. Mazze RI, Sievenpiper TS, Stevenson J: Renal effects of enflurane and halothane in patients with abnormal renal function. *Anesthesiology* 60: 161, 1984

77. Desmond JW, Gordon RA: The effect of haemodialysis on blood volume and plasma cholinesterase levels. *Can J Anaesth* 16: 292, 1969.

78. Ryan DW: Preoperative serum cholinesterase concentration in chronic renal failure. *Br J Anaesth* 49: 945, 1977

79. Thomas JL, Holmes JH: Effect of hemodialysis on plasma cholinesterase. *Anesth Analg* 49: 323, 1970.

80. Sirotzky L, Lewis EJ: Anesthesia related muscle paralysis in renal failure. *Clin Nephrol* 10: 38, 1978

81. Gronert GA, Theye RA: Pathophysiology of hyperkalemia induced by succinylcholine. *Anesthesiology* 43: 89, 1975

82. Koide M, Waud BE: Serum potassium concentrations after succinylcholine in patients with renal failure. *Anesthesiology* 36: 142, 1972

83. Miller RD, Way WL, Hamilton WK, Layzer RB: Succinylcholine-induced hyperkalemia in patients with renal failure? *Anesthesiology* 36: 138, 1972

84. Sheiner LB, Stanski DR, Vozeh S, Miller RD, Ham J: Simultaneous modeling of pharmacokinetics and pharmacodynamics: application to *d*-tubocurarine. *Clin Pharmacol Ther* 25: 358, 1979

85. Miller RD, Matteo RS, Benet LZ, Sohn YJ: The pharmacokinetics of *d*-tubocurarine in man with and without renal failure. *J Pharmacol Exp Ther* 202: 1, 1977

86. Matteo RS, Nishitateno K, Pua EK, Spector S: Pharmacokinetics of *d*-tubocurarine in man: effect of an osmotic diuretic on urinary excretion. *Anesthesiology* 52: 335, 1980

87. Gibaldi M, Levy G, Hayton WL: Tubocurarine and renal failure. *Br J Anaesth* 44: 163, 1972

88. Somogyi AA, Shanks CA, Triggs EJ: The effect of renal failure on the disposition and neuromuscular blocking action of pancuronium bromide. *Eur J Clin Pharmacol* 12: 23, 1977

89. McLeod K, Watson MJ, Rawlins MD: Pharmacokinetics of pancuronium in patients with normal and impaired renal function. *Br J Anaesth* 48: 341, 1976

90. Brotherton WP, Matteo RS: Pharmacokinetics and pharmacodyanmics of metocurine in humans with and without renal failure. *Anesthesiology* 55: 273, 1981

91. Ramzan MI, Shanks CA, Triggs EJ: Gallamine disposition in surgical patients with chronic renal failure. *Br J Clin Pharmacol* 12: 141, 1981

92. Feldman SA, Levi JA: Prolonged paresis following gallamine: A case report. *Br J Anaesth* 35: 804, 1963.

93. Fahey MR, Rupp SM, Fisher DM et al.: The pharmacokinetics and pharmacodynamics of atracurium in patients with and without renal failure. *Anesthesiology* 61: 699, 1984

94. Orko R, Heino A, Björkstén F, Scheinin B, Rosenberg PH: Comparison of atracurium and vecuronium in anaesthesia for renal transplantation. *Acta Anaesthesiol Scand* 31: 450, 1987

95. Link J, Papadopoulos G, Heine P, Wolter J: The action of atracurium and vecuronium in chronically hemodialyzed patients. *Anaesthesist* 42: 34, 1993

96. Bach A, Layer M: Muscle relaxants for kidney transplantation. A comparison between vecuronium and atracurium. *Anaesthesist* 39: 96, 1990

97. Lepage JY, Malinge M, Cozian A, Pinaud M, Blanloeil Y, Souron R: Vecuronium and atracurium in patients with end-stage renal failure. A comparative study. *Br J Anaesth* 59: 1004, 1987

98. Gramstad L: Atracurium, vecuronium and pancuronium in end-stage renal failure. Dose-response properties and interactions with azathioprine. *Br J Anaesth* 59: 995, 1987

99. Lynam DP, Cronnelly R, Castagnoli KP et al.: The pharmacodynamics and pharmacokinetics of vecuronium in patients anesthetized with isoflurane with normal renal function or with renal failure. *Anesthesiology* 69: 227, 1988

100. Beauvoir C, Peray P, Daures JP, Peschaud JL, D'Athis F: Pharmacodynamics of vecuronium in patients with and without renal failure: a meta-analysis. *Can J Anaesth* 40: 696, 1993

101. Takita K, Goda Y, Kawahigashi H, Okuyama A, Kubota M, Kemmotsu O: Pharmacodynamics of vecuronium in the kidney transplant recipient and the patient with normal renal function. *Masui* 42: 190, 1993

102. Lagasse RS, Katz RI, Petersen M, Jacobson MJ, Poppers PJ: Prolonged neuromuscular blockade following vecuronium infusion. *J Clin Anesth* 2: 269, 1990

103. Vanacker BF, Van de Walle J: The neuromuscular blocking action of vecuronium in normal patients and in patients with no renal function and interaction vecuronium-tobramycin in renal transplant patients. *Acta Anaesthesiol Belg* 37: 95, 1986

104. Cashman JN, Luke JJ, Jones RM: Neuromuscular block with doxacurium (BW A938U) in patients with normal or absent renal function. *Br J Anaesth* 64: 186, 1990

105. Khuenl-Brady KS, Pomaroli A, Puhringer F, Mitterschiffthaler G, Koller J: The use of rocuronium (ORG 9426) in patients with chronic renal failure. *Anaesthesia* 48: 873, 1993

106. Szenohradszky J, Fisher DM, Segredo V et al.: Pharmacokinetics of rocuronium bromide (ORG 9426) in patients with normal renal function or patients undergoing cadaver renal transplantation. *Anesthesiology* 77: 899, 1992

107. Cook DR, Freeman JA, Lai AA et al.: Pharmacokinetics of mivacurium in normal patients and in those with hepatic or renal failure. *Br J Anaesth* 69: 580, 1992

108. Sidi A, Kaplan RF, Davis RF: Prolonged neuromuscular blockade and ventilatory failure after renal transplantation and cyclosporine (see comments). *Can J Anaesth* 37: 543, 1990

109. Crosby E, Robblee JA: Cyclosporine-pancuronium interaction in a patient with a renal allograft. *Can J Anaesth* 35): 300, 1988

110. Gramstad L, Gjerløw JA, Hysing ES, Rugstad HE: Interaction of cyclosporin and its solvent, cremophor, with atracurium and vecuronium. *Br J Anaesth* 58: 1149, 1986

111. Morris RB, Cronnelly R, Miller RD, Stanski DR, Fahey MR: Pharmacokinetics of edrophonium in anephric and renal transplant patients. *Br J Anaesth* 53: 1311, 1981

112. Cronnelly R, Stanski DR, Miller RD, Sheiner LB, Sohn YJ: Renal function and the pharmacokinetics of neostigmine in anesthetized man. *Anesthesiology* 51: 222, 1979

113. Cronnelly R, Stanski DR, Miller RD, Sheiner LB: Pyridostigmine kinetics with and without renal function. *Clin Pharmacol Ther* 28: 78, 1980

114. Aquilonius SM, Hartvig P: Clinical pharmacokinetics of cholinesterase inhibitors. *Clin Pharmacokinet* 11: 236, 1986

115. Leanza HJ, Rivarola G, Graciela Garcia M, Najun Zaraza-ga CJ, Casadei D: Rapid correction of acute hyperkalemia with nebulized salbutamol. *Medicina* 52: 99, 1992

116. Velaszuez L, Munoz R: The treatment of hyperkalemia with salbutamol. *Bol Med Hosp Infant Mex* 48: 775, 1991

117. Murdoch IA, Dos Anjos R, Haycock BB: Treatment of hyperkalaemia with intravenous salbutamol. *Arch Dis Child* 66: 527, 1991

118. Allon M, Takeshian A, Shanklin N: Effect of insulin-plus-glucose infusion with or without epinephrine on fasting hyperkalemia. *Kidney Int* 43: 212, 1993

119. Salem MM, Rosa RM, Batlle DC: Extrarenal potassium tolerance in chronic renal failure: implications for the treatment of acute hyperkalemia. *Am J Kidney Dis* 18: 421, 1991

120. Allon M, Dunlay R, Copkney C: Nebulized albuterol for acute hyperkalemia in patients on hemodialysis. *Ann Intern Med* 110: 426, 1989

121. Sheinfeld J, Linke CL, Talley TE, Linke CA: Selective pre-transplant nephrectomy: indications and perioperative management. *J Urol* 133: 379, 1985

122. Ruegg PC, Karmann U, Keller H: Management of perioperative hypertension using intravenous isradipine. *Am J Hypertens* 4: 203S, 1991

123. Hogenson KD: Acute postoperative hypertension in the hypertensive patient. *J Post Anesth Nurs* 7: 38, 1992

124. Chrysostomou A, Walker RG, Russ GR, d'Apice AJF, Kincaid-Smith P, Mathew TH: Diltiazem in renal allograft recipients receiving cyclosporine. *Transplantation* 55: 300, 1993

125. Neumayer H-H, Kunzendorf U, Schreiber M: Protective effects of calcium antagonists in human renal transplantation. *Kidney Int* 41 (Suppl 36): S-87, 1992

126. Harper SJ, Moorhouse J, Veitch PS et al.: Improved immediate graft function with nifedipine in cyclosporine-treated renal allograft recipients – a randomized prospective study. *Transplantation* 54: 742, 1992

BLOOD PRESSURE CONTROL IN CHRONIC HEMODIALYSIS PATIENTS

G. LONDON, S. MARCHAIS and A.P. GUERIN

INTRODUCTION

Cardiovascular complications are the leading cause of mortality and morbidity in the population of end-stage renal disease (ESRD) patients on renal replacement therapy (1). Hypertension, either as a primary cause, or consequence of renal failure, is a major risk factor contributing to the high cardiovascular morbidity and mortality in uremic patients and has been found in approximately 80% of patients developing ESRD (2, 3). The prevalence of hypertension in ESRD varies somewhat according to the different etiologies of renal failure. Patients with glomerulonephritis, diseases involving small vessels (vasculitis, scleroderma) or diabetic nephropathy have hypertension more often than those with tubulointerstitial disease (4). Once dialysis is begun, 5 to 50% remain hypertensive on the basis of casual blood pressure (BP) measurements (5). Continuous BP monitoring has shown that the proportion of ESRD patients with uncontrolled hypertension is much higher than that whose BP is adequately controlled (85 versus 15%) (6). Hypertension increases the severity and incidence of left ventricular hypertrophy (LVH) (7, 8) and atherosclerosis (9), implying that the treatment of hypertension and the maintenance of a normal BP are mandatory in ESRD patients. Hypertension is a complex hemodynamic abnormality and the understanding of basic mechanisms controlling BP is a prerequisite to proper management of hypertension in ESRD patients on hemodialysis.

GENERAL PRINCIPLES AND CONTROL OF BLOOD PRESSURE

Blood pressure is the product of the mechanical energy imparted to the blood by ventricular ejection and the opposition of the systemic arterial system. Because ventricular contraction is intermittent, BP is recorded as a pressure oscillation during cardiac cycles, i.e. in the form of an arterial pulse pressure (PP) curve. Using Fourier analysis of oscillatory phenomena, the pulse pressure curve can be decomposed into its component sine waves of increasing frequency (10), with harmonic zero (zero frequency, i.e. sine wave of infinite period) reflecting the value of mean BP (MBP), and the first (heart rate frequency) and subsequent harmonics the values of oscillatory components around the mean (Figure 1). Therefore, an arterial pressure curve has two distinct components: 1) a steady component, i.e. MBP, determined exclusively by cardiac output (CO) and total peripheral resistance (TPR) (11), and 2) an oscillation around this mean the pulse pressure, i.e. (PP, whose limits during a cardiac cycle are the systolic and diastolic BP) (12) determined by the pattern of ventricular ejection, arterial distensibility, and the intensity and timing of arterial wave reflections (10).

CONTROL OF MEAN BLOOD PRESSURE AND ITS ALTERATIONS IN ESRD

The driving force for the systemic blood flow from the aorta through tissues back to the right atrium is the difference between the MBP and right atrial pressure (RAP). By analogy with Ohm's law, the systemic blood flow can be calculated as MBP − RAP/TPR, where TPR is the total peripheral resistance. Systemic blood flow is equal

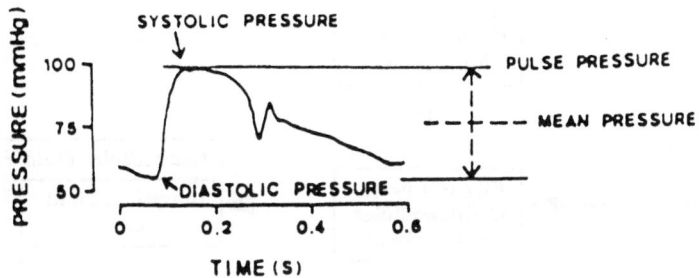

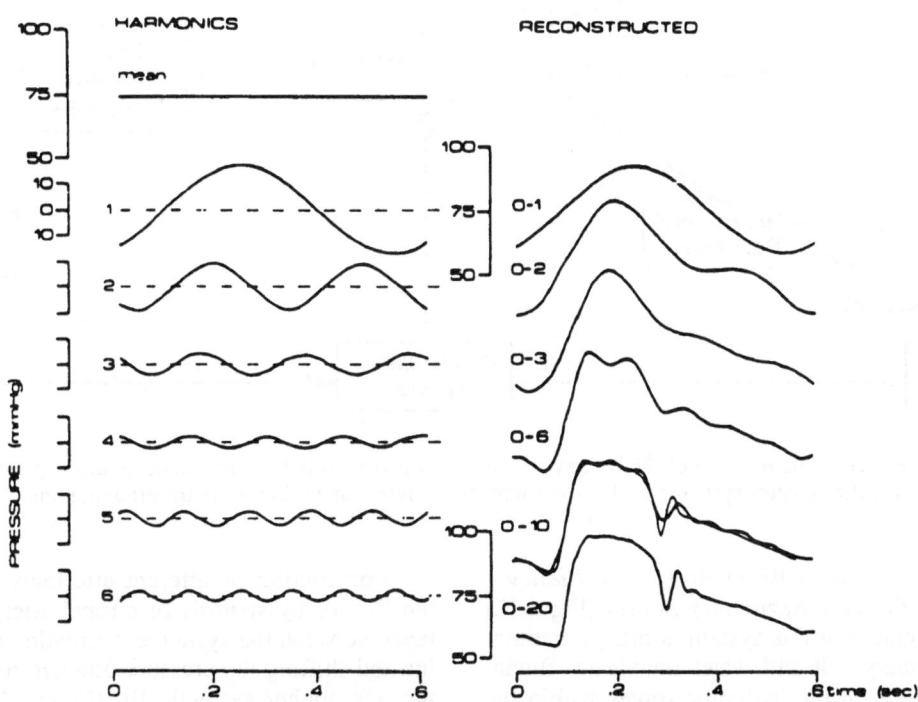

Figure 1. The top panel represents the recorded arterial pressure wave with its two components – mean blood pressure and the pulse pressure. The principle of Fourier's analysis is represented in the lower panel. Left: for the analysis of pressure, the signal is decomposed into a mean value plus a number of sine waves of increasing frequency (first harmonic with heart rate frequency f and higher harmonics with frequencies $2f$, $3f$, etc.). Right: individual harmonics are added to reproduce the original signal (using the first 6 (0–6), or first 20 (0–20) harmonics). (Adapted with permission from Westerhof N, Sipkema P, Elzinga G, Murgo JP, Giolma JP: Arterial impedance, in *Quantitative Cardiovascular Studies, Clinical and Research Applications of Engineering Principles*, edited by Hwang NHC, Gross DR, Patel DJ, University Park Press, Baltimore, 1979)

to cardiac output (CO), and since RAP is small, the usual expression of these relations becomes: MBP = CO × TPR. Thus, an increase in MBP must be accounted for by an increase in TPR or CO or both. Although chronic hypertension is most frequently characterized by normal CO and increased TPR, CO is elevated in several types of hypertension (13, 14). Nevertheless, even in hypertension associated with high CO, it is not clear whether the high BP is directly related to the increased systemic blood flow. In primary hyperaldosteronism, BP and CO were found to be inversely related (14), and acute reduction of CO with propanolol in borderline, renovascular and essential hypertension did not decrease BP (15). Arteri-

al pressure is in fact maintained by a hierarchy of control systems including: 1) a long-term BP control system which determines the BP's set-point over long periods of time, and 2) a short- or intermediate-term control system preventing excessive pressure fluctuations around the set-point. The short-term control systems react almost immediately, within seconds (baroreflexes and chemoreflexes), or within minutes and hours (capillary fluid shift, stress relaxation, hormonal controls involving the renin-angiotensin-aldosterone system and vasopressin), but cannot correct pressure changes completely (11). The long-term control react in hours, is long-acting, and capable of an almost complete correction of pressure changes.

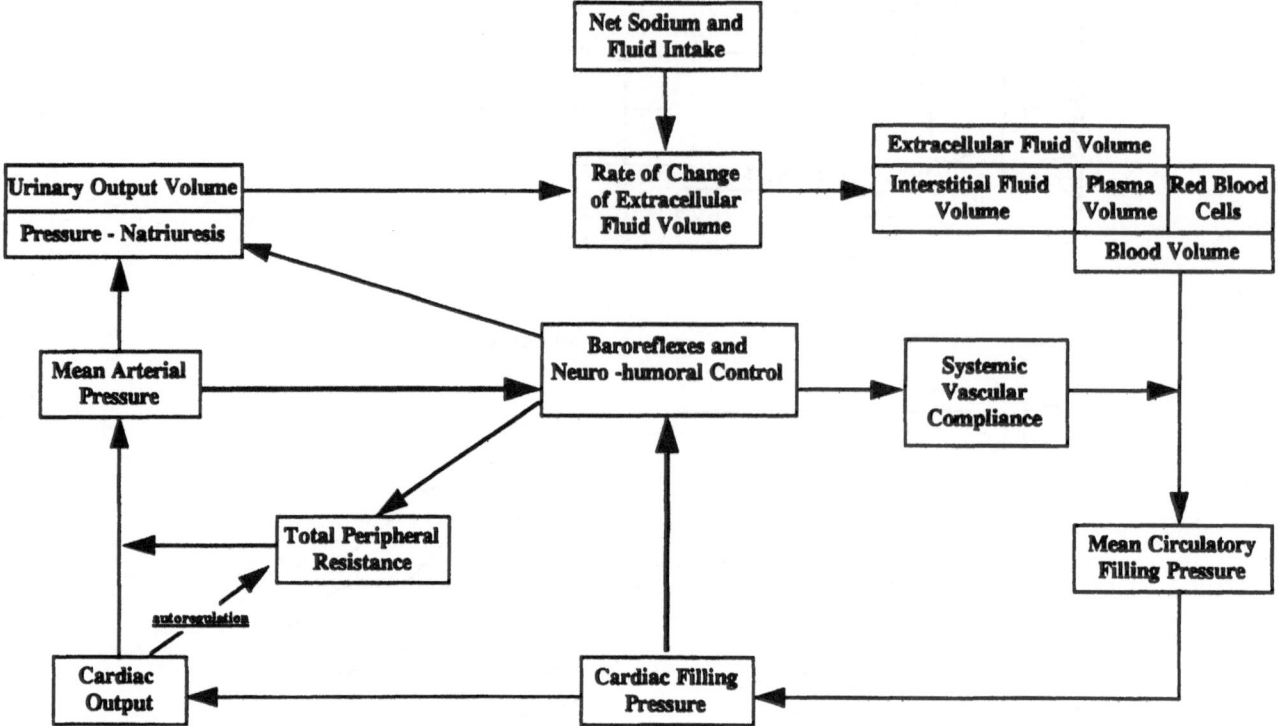

Figure 2. Simplified schematic diagram of the Kidney – Volume – Pressure relationship and mean blood pressure regulation and the neurohumoral and reflex control systems; thick arrows represent afferent and thin arrows the efferent parts of control loops).

The keystone of long-term BP control is the *Kidney – Blood Volume – Pressure Regulatory System* (Figure 2) (16). The key element of this system is that glomerular filtration and urinary salt and water output are fundamentally dependent on the hydraulic forces within the vascular system, i.e. MBP. This relationship is known as the pressure-natriuresis relationship (Figure 3). This system operates as follows: if the amount of salt and water entering the extracellular and vascular space exceeds the amount excreted, the extracellular fluid volume and blood volume increase, increasing mean circulatory filling pressure and venous return. The cardiac pump is normally able to pump all volume returning to it and CO increases, increasing the MBP and hence urinary salt and water excretion until normal levels are attained. Increased filling pressure in the vascular segments activates low and high pressure stretch-sensitive baroreflexes, with consequent decreases in sympathetic outflow to vasculature and the kidneys (17, 18), renin-angiotensin-aldosterone system activity (19–21) and vasopressin release (22), and increased release of atrial natriuretic peptides (23) and Na/K-ATPase inhibitor (24), increasing the effect of the pressure-natriuresis mechanisms. An abnormal pressure-natriuresis relationship is the fundamental alteration in any type of hypertension. There are three sites where the pressure-natriuresis relationship can be altered: 1) the preglomerular site, which can be influenced by diffuse vasoconstriction of afferent arterioles (essential hypertension) or by stenosis of a renal artery, creating resistance between the systemic circulation and the glomerulus and shifting the pressure-diuresis curve in parallel to the new higher systemic BP (Figure 3); 2) glomerular filtration, which may be altered by various diseases; and 3) tubular reabsorption of Na and water, influenced by catecholamines, angiotensin, vasopressin, atrial natriuretic factors, Na/K-ATPase inhibitors, etc. Factors which influence the glomerular filtration and tubular reabsorption depress the slope of renal function curve and shift it to higher pressure levels (Figure 3) (25).

However it was found that in essential hypertension and several forms of secondary hypertension the extracellular fluid volume and CO could be either normal or low, and elevation of TPR appeared to be the only hemodynamic variable characteristic of sustained hypertension (26, 27). Mechanisms which could transform an initial increase in CO into a high TPR are generally considered as part of a whole-body autoregulatory response (28). According to this concept, expansion of body fluid volumes with elevation of CO results in overperfusion of peripheral organs, which in turn vasoconstrict to normalize tissue flow. Peripheral resistance therefore increases and CO returns to normal following blood volume contraction secondary to renal pressure diuresis. This sequence from increased CO to increased peripheral resis-

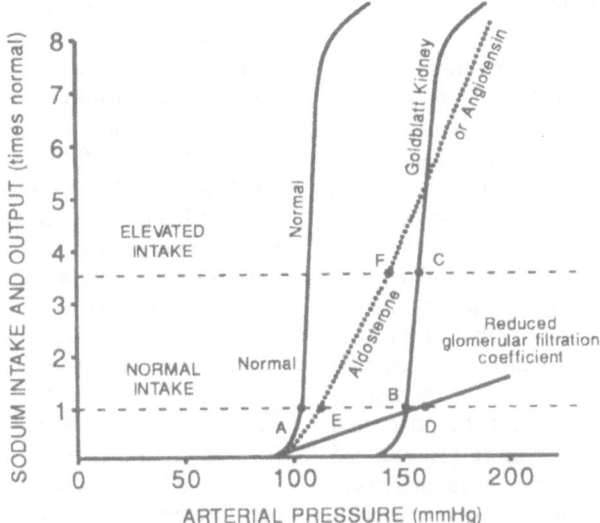

Figure 3. Renal function curves and pressure-natriuresis mechanism in normal and in different pathophysiological conditions. A–E equilibrium points where the renal function curves and the sodium intake curves cross. (Adapted with permission from reference (19))

tance has been shown to occur in essential hypertension and following fluid overload in anephric humans (29), as well as in experimental renal, mineralocorticoid or essential hypertension (30). The underlying mechanisms of the increase in TPR are poorly understood. The increase in blood flow triggers an acute autoregulatory response in various tissues through myogenic and metabolic mechanisms and factors intrinsic to vessel wall function (such as prostanoids, endothelium-derived substances, etc.). Autoregulation related to hypertension develops slowly over days and months (28) and involves gradual structural alteration of vascular architecture, with an increased arteriolar wall-to-lumen ratio due to vessel wall hypertrophy or remodeling and anatomical vessels rarefaction (31–33). It is these slowly developing structural changes that largely contribute to the changes observed in TPR during the development of volume-induced types of hypertension. Structural changes also involve the venous system, resulting in a decrease in the systemic compliance of the circulation (34). Reduced systemic venous compliance maintains normal or increased mean circulatory filling pressure and sensitizes the blood volume/cardiac output/pressure diuresis system, with cardiac filling pressure and cardiac output being more sensitive to blood volume variations (35, 36).

Cross-sectional studies in patients with non-uremic parenchymatous renal diseases have shown that hypertension is usually maintained by an increase in TPR while the CO remains normal (13). Longitudinal studies in patients with mild and moderate non-anemic renal insufficiency nevertheless suggested that an increase in CO precedes the increase in TPR. Brod et al. (13) sequentially measured hemodynamic changes during a 2 to 8-year follow-up period in 97 patients with parenchymal renal disease. On initial examination, 12 from 32 normotensive patients had a hyperkinetic circulation with high CO, expanded blood volume and low TPR. At the end of follow-up, 11 out of 12 of these patients had developed hypertension with a normal CO and a sustained increase in TPR. Patients initially with W.H.O. stage I–II hypertension had contemporaneous increased CO and normal TPR. Their blood volume was normal but they had reduced venous compliance. Patients initially with W.H.O. stage III hypertension had contemporaneous normal CO output and increased TPR. These data support the concept that early in the course of renal hypertension, increased BP results from expanded blood volume and increased CO, whereas later hypertension is maintained by increased TPR. In patients on dialysis, the principal hemodynamic pattern is an increased CO (29, 37–39) due to anemia, arteriovenous shunts, volume expansion, and decreased systemic venous compliance (40). CO is increased in both normotensive and hypertensive patients, the only difference being 'normal' or increased TPR in hypertensive patients. Serial transfusions of packed red cells with an increase in hematocrit to at least 40% produced a linear decrease in CO with a parallel increase in BP and TPR, clearly demonstrating that the hypertension in ESRD is sustained by high TPR (41). The increased TPR in ESRD patients results from the increased body salt and water and from a resetting of the extracellular volume-vasopressor feedback control mechanisms, with increased activity of the vasopressor systems.

SALT AND VOLUME OVERLOAD

Volume-dependent hypertension is the most common type of hypertension in ESRD, and about 80% of hypertensive ESRD patients have their BP controlled by ultrafiltration and achievement of 'dry weight'. The plasma volume (42, 43), extracellular fluid volume (ECFV) (44) and exchangeable sodium (39, 42, 44, 45) are increased in most patients with terminal renal failure. Moreover, for the same effect on ECFV as in control subjects, salt administration to ESRD patients increased plasma volume to a greater extent (46). This preferential distribution of ECF to the intravascular compartment was also demonstrated in anephric rats and was attributed to the decreased compliance of interstitial gel (47). As renal function declined the abnormal ECFV distribution was more pronounced and the effects of salt loading on BP were increased (48). Nevertheless, in several studies the direct correlations between BP and exchangeable sodium or plasma volume were weak or absent (42,49). The basic mechanism of volume overload is renal inability to maintain appropriate salt and water excretion. In chronic parenchymatous renal diseases, the pressure-natriuresis curve has a reduced slope and is shifted to a higher pressure range; this curve is completely abolished in anephric patients (Figure 3). ECFV expansion and reduced venous compliance increase circulatory filling pressure and CO, resulting in a long-term 'autoregulatory' increase in TPR (28). While this sequence of hemodynamic events has been demonstrated in anephric patients by some authors (29, 30), it has been challenged by others (38). In a study of anephric patients who were normotensive prior to nephrectomy, salt and water loading increased exchangeable sodium and induced hypervolemia but not hypertension (50). These authors also studied the sequential hemodynamic changes in response to salt and water loading in dialysis patients and found that the sequence of 'whole-body autoregulation' was observed in only one of ten patients studied – they concluded that mechanisms other than autoregulation played a role (38). The concept of whole-body autoregulation also seems contradicted by the persistence of high CO in hypertensive hemodialysis patients. In normotensive uremic patients, the TPR is low. The high CO and decreased TPR is a normal response to anemia and decreased oxygen delivery, and does not induce a whole-body autoregulatory response, which occurs only in conditions of overperfusion, i.e., when the CO is increased and the system responsible for oxygen delivery normal. In hypertensive dialysis patients the TPR can be normal or elevated – in either case, this represents a failure of vasodilation in the presence of anemia, i.e., a relative or absolute 'vasoconstriction'. These patients usually have a long-standing history of hypertension in the pre-uremic stage of the disease and a tendency to increase TPR and BP to a greater extent during correction of anemia (41). Hypertension in ESRD is associated with both morphological and functional abnormalities of resistance vasculature, similar to those observed in essential hypertensive patients, i.e., an increased media thickness/lumen ratio (33). This structural alteration in essential hypertension is associated with decreased maximal vasodilation (31) and impaired endothelium-mediated vasodilation (51). The presence of asymmetric dimethylarginine, a competitive inhibitor of NO synthesis from L-arginine, in the circulation of uremic animals (52) and of high levels of endothelin in plasma of uremic patients (53) support the possibility of 'impaired vasodilation' in hypertensive uremic patients.

Autoregulation is not the only mechanism which can increase TPR. An alternative view is that volume expansion increases the plasma Na/K-ATPase inhibitory activity (24,54) due to release of ouabain or ouabain-isomer (55). This inhibitor induces widespread inhibition of Na/K-ATPase, acting on renal tubules as well as on non-renal tissues such as vascular smooth muscle, depolarizing cell membranes and causing a rise in intracellular sodium. It was proposed that reduction of the sodium gradient across the cell membrane would decrease calcium extrusion from the cell via the Na/Ca exchanger; in consequence, intracellular Ca would rise, increasing the vascular reactivity and contractility that underlies the increased vascular tone and TPR (57). In addition, the inhibition of the Na/K pump at synaptic neuronal clefts would lead to decreased norepinephrine reuptake prolonging vascular smooth muscle activation (57). Uremic serum contains high concentrations of ouabain-like substances, inducing defective Na/K-ATPase activity and increased intracellular Na^+ in erythrocytes of uremic patients (58–60). Moreover, in some cases the Na/K-ATPase activity correlates inversely with TPR and MBP in ESRD patients (61). However, others have found erythrocyte sodium to be decreased or normal in uremia because of reduced sodium influx with no evidence of changes in active sodium pumps (62, 63). Nevertheless, the hypothesis that 'hypervolemia – defective Na/K-ATPase – Na/Ca exchange' is one of the mechanisms of hypertension in ESRD is supported by clinical observations of increased dihydropyridine calcium channel blocker antihypertensive efficacy is increased in overhydrated dialysis patients (64, 65). Increased free calcium has been shown in platelets of patients with chronic renal failure, and a direct relationship between cytosolic Ca and MBP has been observed in uremic patients (66). The Na/K-ATPase inhibition is not the only mechanism which would increase intracellular calcium. Gafter et al. (67) found an increased in cytosolic calcium of erythrocytes from ESRD patients in association with a decreased calcium/ATPase activity. The inhibition of calcium/ATPase activity seems to be due to a dialyzable and heat-stable circulating inhibitor (68). Finally, the direct association between platelets cytosolic Ca and parathormone (PTH) levels in uremic patients suggests that PTH could exert an effect on TPR and hypertension in these subjects (66). The role of PTH is supported by the observation of greater dihydropyridine calcium blocker antihypertensive efficacy in dialysis patients with secondary hyperparathyroidism (69).

HYPERACTIVITY OF VASOPRESSOR SYSTEMS

In contrast to the majority of patients whose BP is favorably influenced by salt and volume depletion, in about 20% of patients, hypertension is not controlled by maintenance of 'dry weight'. In these patients increased TPR and hypertension result from a relative or absolute hyperactivity of neural and humoral vasomotor systems.

The renin-angiotensin system

Patients whose hypertension is not controlled by maintenance of dry weight have increased plasma renin activity (PRA) and demonstrate a dramatic improvement in BP control after interruption of the renin-angiotensin axis (RAA) by bilateral nephrectomy. In a study by Del Greco et al. (70), bilateral nephrectomy improved BP control in almost 80% of patients, the response being dependent on pre-nephrectomy renin activity: those with high activity responded more frequently than those with low activity. In dialysis patients with severe and malignant hypertension, direct correlations were observed between PRA and BP or TPR (39, 41). Bilateral nephrectomy decreased TPR, with a sharp decrease in PRA to low or undetectable levels, even in the absence of blood volume changes or changes in exchangeable sodium (41). Bilateral nephrectomy also decreased BP in patients with volume-dependent hypertension (71). Safar et al. (39) have shown that in hypertensive ESRD patients, high blood volume is the fundamental cause of the high BP. In non-nephrectomized hypertensive patients, the slope of the curve relating BP to blood volume was steeper and reset to higher pressures – the slope was less steep in nephrectomized subjects, indicating that, when present a functional RAA acts mainly by increasing the sensitivity of the BP-blood volume relationship. However, in ESRD patients with mild and moderate hypertension, high PRA was found in only about 30% of subjects, and the PRA and Angiotensin II levels varied widely from low to high values (42, 43, 72, 73). The function of the RAA is preserved in ESRD (72–76), and PRA increases with volume contraction, orthostasis (77) and after angiotensin II blockade (2, 73, 78). Nevertheless, its responsiveness to ECFV changes is blunted, and the PRA in dialysis patients seems inappropriately increased relative to blood volume, ECFV and exchangeable Na levels (42, 44, 45). Weidmann et al. (42) demonstrated that at any given level of exchangeable Na and blood volume, the PRA was higher in uremic patients, and two fold higher in hypertensives than in normotensives. Moreover in this study BP correlated more closely with the 'exchangeable Na-renin' product than with Na or renin considered separately. Finally, the participation of the RAA in BP

regulation in uremic patients is also demonstrated by the antihypertensive effects of angiotensin antagonists and ACE inhibitors (73, 78, 79). This antihypertensive effect is also observed in patients with low PRA activity and is not correlated with baseline plasma PRA levels – it could therefore be associated with blockade of the tissular renin-angiotensin system (80). Tissue angiotensin may exert autocrine and paracrine functions, stimulating vasoconstriction by activating receptors on vascular smooth muscle, or by facilitating catecholamine release from nerve endings. Angiotensin can also act as a growth factor, inducing vascular wall hypertrophy and increased peripheral resistance (80).

Sympathetic nervous system and catecholamines

The role of the sympathetic nervous system in hypertension in ESRD is in many aspects controversial. In most studies, basal plasma norepinephrine (NE) and dopamine were found to be increased (76, 81–84), but normal (85, 86) or even low (87) values have been reported. The elevated plasma levels concern the free and sulfoconjugated NE and dopamine, while the glucuroconjugated metabolites are at normal levels (84, 88). Contradictory results were published concerning dopamine β-hydroxylase levels, found to be low (89) or normal (87). The effect of hemodialysis on plasma catecholamine concentrations was studied by several authors, with contradictory results: some found increases (82, 87, 90), while others found no change (84, 85, 91) or a decrease (92). Plasma volume contraction and negative Na balance induce an increase in plasma catecholamine levels. This was also shown in ESRD patients undergoing isolated ultrafiltration (91, 93). Catecholamines are small dialyzable molecules, and their removal during hemodialysis could be responsible for the 'non-response' observed by some authors during standard dialysis (84, 91). It is still a matter of debate whether the changes in plasma catecholamines result from decreased metabolic clearance (94, 95), decreased neuronal reuptake (96, 97), or increased release (82) secondary to increased sympathetic nerve discharge. Using a direct recording of post-ganglionic sympathetic-nerve discharge (obtained by microneurography), Converse et al. (98) found no correlation between the rate of sympathetic nerve discharge and plasma NE or PRA levels. In the same study, they showed that the increased sympathetic nerve discharge in patients undergoing hemodialysis was constant throughout the interdialytic intervals, despite large variations in volume and pressure. These results could be interpreted as suggesting that in ESRD patients the increased sympathetic nerve firing is due to alteration of the reflex control of the vasomotor center, via abnormal functioning of the high- and low-pressure baroreceptor systems (17, 18, 85, 99, 100). However, the fact that alterations in autonomic function are acutely improved by dialysis (100) while the increased sympathetic-nerve discharge is not (98) do not favor this conclusion. Studies in animals and humans have shown that the kidney is a sensory organ containing sensitive afferent nerves causing reflex activation of the sympathetic nervous system on exposure to ischemic or uremic metabolites (101, 102). Converse et al. (98) showed that bilateral nephrectomy abolishes the increased sympathetic-nerve discharge and that the kidney might be the principal and direct source of the sympathetic nervous system activation in ESRD. The interpretation of the role of the sympathetic nervous system must take into account the relationship between sympathetic-nerve activity, catecholamine concentrations and the end-organ responsiveness to the stimulation. In experimental uremia, both increased (103) and decreased (96, 104) responsiveness to NE infusion have been observed. Zimlichman et al. (103) showed in a rat model of chronic uremia that the systemic pressor response to infused NE was increased. This hypersensitivity was abolished by parathyroidectomy, suggesting that elevated intracellular Ca content potentiated the vasopressor effect. In contrast, using a similar rat model Iseki et al. (104) demonstrated a decreased response to infused NE which could be prevented by prior parathyroidectomy and abolished by administration of indomethacin. A similar decreased response, sensitive to indomethacin but not to parathyroidectomy, was shown by Rascher et al. (96). The decreased response could be related to down-regulation of α- and β-receptors, to increased occupancy of receptors, or to a post-receptor defect. Animal and human studies of the number and responses of lymphocyte β-2 receptors after stimulation have shown that both down-regulation and a post-receptor defect (with blunted cAMP formation in response to receptor stimulation) are present in the uremic state (105). Despite all the contradictions and the absence of a direct relationship between the alterations in the sympathetic nervous system and systemic BP, sympathetic overactivity appears to play an important role in the maintenance of hypertension, as demonstrated by the dramatic reduction in TPR and BP after administration of debrisoquine (106) to hypertensive ESRD patients.

Arginine vasopressin (AVP) and endothelial factors

Experimental data suggest that AVP play a role in BP homeostasis in animals with subtotal renal ablation or bilateral nephrectomy (107). AVP was found increased in dialysis patients, mostly in relation to plasma osmolarity (108, 109). The results concerning the effect of dialysis procedures on plasma AVP are contradictory, with blood volume reduction inducing either an increase (110) or no change (108). Decreased plasma AVP levels during dialysis were observed in relation to changes in osmolarity (108). Increased AVP was observed during acute hypotensive episodes in some dialysis patients, and decreased BP was observed during AVP inhibition in humans with chronic renal failure, suggesting that in hypotensive con-

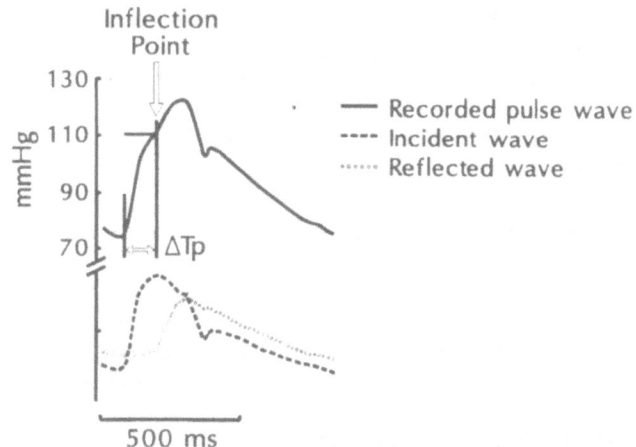

Figure 4. Analysis of arterial pressure wave and its component incident and reflected waves. ΔTp is the travel time of the pressure wave from the heart to the reflecting site(s) and back.

ditions AVP could participate in BP maintenance (108, 111).

The endothelium plays an important role in the regulation of vasomotor tone (112). When stimulated by vasoactive agents such as acetylcholine (112) or by increased shear stress (113), endothelial cells produce endothelial relaxing factor, identified as nitric oxide (NO) (114), which relaxes the underlying vascular smooth muscle. The endothelial cells produce NO from L-arginine, under the action of NO-synthases which cleave L-arginine into citrulline and NO (114). The role of these factors in the hemodynamic alterations in ESRD patients is unknown. Vallance et al. (52) demonstrated that NO synthesis can be inhibited by an endogenous substance identified as asymmetrical dimethylarginine (ADMA). Normally excreted in the urine, ADMA accumulates in patients with ESRD, impairing NO synthesis. These results seem contradictory with those of Noris et al. (115) who found increased NO synthesis in uremic subjects. Endothelial cells also produce endothelin which causes smooth muscle cells to constrict, and the alterations in endothelium-dependent vasomotor control in ESRD patients could be potentiated by an increase in plasma endothelin levels (53, 116).

Atrial natriuretic peptide

Basal levels of atrial natriuretic peptides (ANP) are increased in both mild to moderate renal insufficiency and in ESRD (117-120). A positive feedback control loop was observed in dialysis patients between ANP secretion and (i) blood volume level, and (ii) atrial dimensions, with ANP concentration increasing with ECFV expansion and decreasing after dialysis ultrafiltration. ANP inhibits the reflex sympathetic activity by either sensitizing cardiopulmonary mechanoreceptors or by central and ganglionic sympathoinhibition, inhibits the release of renin,

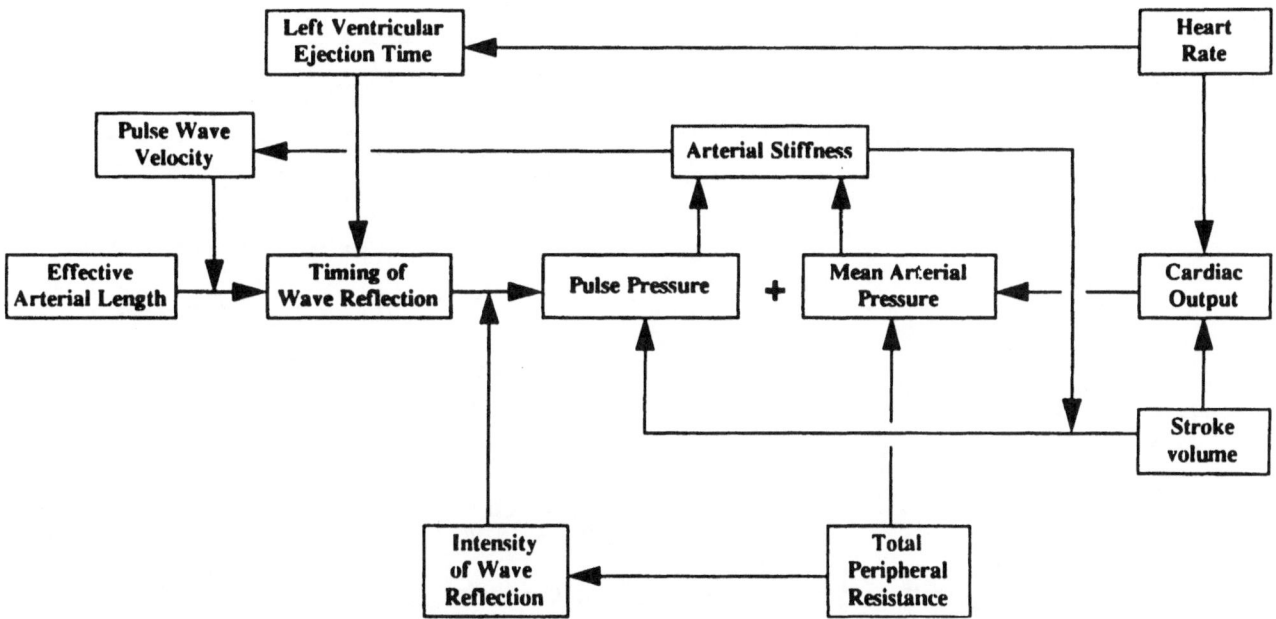

Figure 5. Schematic representation of major determinants of arterial pressure considered in terms of its steady (mean blood pressure) and oscillatory (pulse pressure) components.

aldosterone and AVP, and also directly relaxes smooth muscle Sells (121–124). It is likely that the increased ANP in ESRD patients modulates the vasoconstrictor action of the vasomotor systems directly, or, as already mentioned, by central or ganglionic sympathoinhibitory action. The kidney produces several vasodilating substances such as kinins, prostaglandins, or antihypertensive neutral renomedullary lipid (125), and decreased production and activity of these substances could play a role in the pathogenesis of the hypertension. Indeed, decreased blood levels of vasodilating prostaglandin PgE2 have been observed in hypertensive ESRD patients (126), and a negative correlation between the prostacyclin metabolite 6-keto-PgFlα (127) and BP has been observed in ESRD.

PULSATILE COMPONENT OF BLOOD PRESSURE AND ITS ALTERATIONS IN ESRD

Analytical studies of arterial function treat BP as a periodic phenomenon that has two components: a steady component (Mean BP) determined exclusively by CO and TPR (10), and a pulsatile component (Pulse Pressure – PP) consisting of the oscillation around this mean and determined by the interaction of a pressure wave generated by heart contraction with one or more reflected waves generated by the arterial system (128) (Figures 4–5). Ventricular contraction generates a pressure wave (incident or forward wave) which is propagated along the arterial tree at a speed of 5–15 m/sec (pulse wave velocity-PWV) (129). As the pressure wave moves away from the heart, part of the energy is reflected back at various sites of the arterial tree in the form of a reflected or backward wave representing a natural 'counterpulsation' (128). Reflections are caused by the changes in character of the vessels along which the wave passes and are generated wherever there is discontinuity of arterial caliber or vessel distensibility, or any mismatch of vascular impedances (128, 130). Under normal circumstances the major sites of wave reflections are in the peripheral circulation where small peripheral conduit arteries terminate in high-resistance arterioles (128). The high PWV ensures that the reflected waves return towards the aorta during the same heart contraction in which they were generated, merging with the incident wave. As the pressure wave travels at a finite velocity, the timing and the final characteristics of the pressure wave depend on the arterial site where the pressure wave is recorded (131, 132). Peripheral arteries are stiffer than the aorta, generating local reflections (128). Moreover, peripheral arteries are closer to peripheral reflecting sites and incident and reflected waves merge almost instantaneously with a resulting pressure wave amplitude that is the summation of the two waves (131, 132). Aorta is distant from peripheral reflecting sites and, due to finite PWV, it takes a certain time (Δtp on Figure 4) for the reflected wave to return from these sites. When the PWV is high, the reflected wave returns to the aorta during systole, merging with the incident wave and increasing aortic systolic and pulse pressures to the same extent as in peripheral arteries. When the PWV is low, the reflected wave returns to the aorta later, during early diastole. The incident and reflected waves are not in phase and the reflected wave does not influence the aortic systolic and pulse pressures which are lower than in the peripheral arteries (Figure 6)

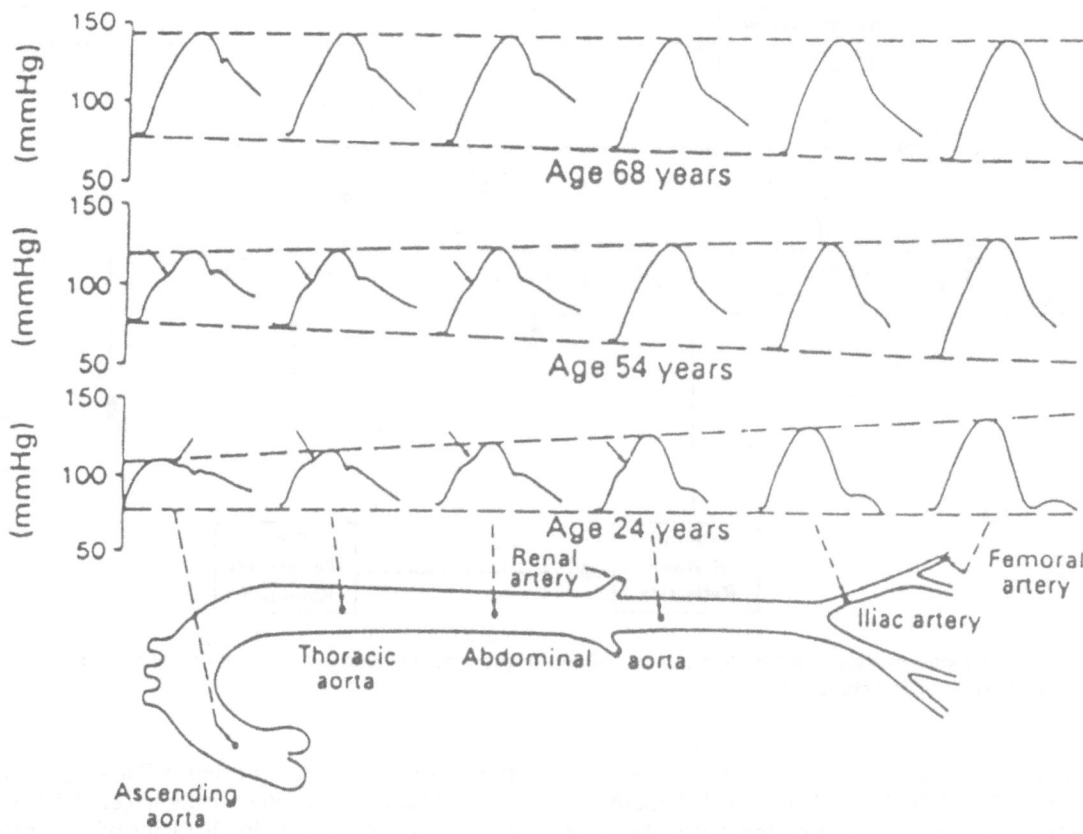

Figure 6. Arterial pressure waves recorded at different sites along the arterial tree in three adult subjects aged 24, 54 and 68 years. In the youngest subject the pressure wave is amplified during its travel from the aorta to the peripheral arteries. In the oldest subject the amplification during wave transmission has disappeared. (Reproduced with permission from reference (136))

(128, 131–134). The amplitude of pressure waves and the timing of wave reflections are critically dependent on the arterial stiffness, a stiffer artery requiring a higher distending pressure for a given diameter increase (or intra-arterial volume increase) (135). The relative proportion of elastin, collagen and smooth muscle cells in the media of an artery determine its physical properties. Due to the non-uniformity of arterial wall elasticity, the diameter-distending pressure relation is non-linear, with tension at low distending pressure being borne by elastin fibers, and at high pressure by less extensible collagen fibers. Stiffness is determined from the tangent of the diameter (or volume)/pressure curve at any given distending pressure and is expressed as Ep (Peterson's Elastic modulus) or E (Young's modulus) according to the following formulae: $Ep = (\Delta P/\Delta D) \cdot D$ or $E = (\Delta P/\Delta D) \cdot (D/h)$ (135), where ΔP and ΔD are the changes in pressure and diameter (or volume) about a mean diameter D in an artery with wall thickness h. These are measures of stiffness, and 'compliance' or 'distensibility' are the reciprocal of stiffness ($1/Ep$ or $1/E$). Due to the non-linear pressure-diameter relationship, an artery becomes stiffer as pressure increases and this is one of the reasons for

higher arterial stiffness in hypertension. Arterial stiffening increases systolic and pulse pressures directly by increasing the amplitude of the incident pressure wave generated by a given flow impulse from the heart, and indirectly by increasing pulse wave velocity so that wave reflection occurs early in the systolic period (135, 136). Arterial PWV is a well accepted index of arterial stiffness and is related to Young's modulus by the Moens–Korteweg equation: $PWV^2 = E \cdot h/D \cdot \rho$, where E is Young's modulus, h wall thickness, D diameter, and ρ blood density (129, 135, 136). The physiological aging process is the principal cause of arterial stiffening, increasing the amplitude of pressure waves and arterial PWV. This causes an early return of wave reflections from the periphery to the aorta, with a boosting effect on aortic peak- and end-systolic pressures, and an equalization of pressures along the arterial tree (136). In young subjects with compliant arteries, pressure wave amplitude is smaller and PWV lower. The return of reflected waves is delayed to early diastole and the aortic systolic and pulse pressures are lower than in the peripheral arteries (Figure 6), where the systolic and pulse pressures can be amplified by 15–30% in comparison to those in the aorta (128, 131–134). The transit time of wave reflections from the aorta to reflecting sites and back is not only influenced by the PWV, but also by the distance of the reflecting sites from the heart. This distance, called 'effective length' of the arterial tree, depends on body length (130, 134, 137, 138). Thus, for any given PWV, the transit time is decreased in small subjects, and the effect of wave reflections in the aorta and central arteries is increased (134, 137–139).

Increased arterial pulsatility has serious ill effects on the heart and arteries. Several studies have shown that PP is an independent cardiovascular risk factor (140, 141), and systolic BP a better predictor of end-organ damage than diastolic BP (142). The role of pressure pulsatility is particularly important in the aorta and central arteries. An increased pulsatile component of BP causes an impedance mismatch between the left ventricle and the systemic arterial system, leading to greater pulsatile energy losses, increased systolic pressure and total heart work, increased myocardial oxygen consumption, impaired ventricular ejection, ventricular hypertrophy and a relative decrease in the diastolic pressure-time index (mean diastolic pressure), compromising the coronary blood flow (136).

Clinical and epidemiological studies have shown a high prevalence of systolic hypertension in ESRD (1, 6, 129, 134, 143, 144). According to the EDTA report (1) only 30% of males and 36% of females had a pre-dialysis systolic BP below 140 mmHg, and 32% of both males and females had a pre-dialysis BP over 160 mmHg. This contrasted with the median diastolic pressure in both males and females which was in the normal range of 80–89 mmHg. While the post-dialysis systolic BP distribution was shifted to a lower pressure range, 42% of males and 35% of females still had a systolic BP above 140 mmHg. In contrast with the gradual decline in the prevalence of systolic-diastolic hypertension after a few years of dialysis, that of borderline-systolic or isolated systolic hypertension increases over the years (143). Forty-eight-hour BP monitoring in ESRD patients has shown that the systolic load is higher than the diastolic load, and that the systolic BP is more difficult to control during the interdialytic interval despite antihypertensive treatment (6).

The principal factor responsible for increased systolic and pulse pressures in ESRD patients is increased arterial stiffness (with increased arterial PWV) (129, 134, 145, 146). This is more pronounced in the aorta than in peripheral arteries (129) but the mechanisms responsible are not clear. Increased arterial stiffness is not related to the metabolic and hormonal disturbances commonly observed in terminal uremia (129). Weak correlations were observed in non-uremic controls and ESRD patients between aortic PWV and the presence of arterial calcifications and a low level of HDL-Cholesterol (129). Several studies, including in ESRD patients, indicate that Na may act on the arterial wall independently of other factors, including BP (147–149). In ESRD patients a positive relationship between interdialytic body weight gain and aortic PWV was observed, supporting the potential role of Na^+ excess (148). Furthermore it has been shown that the improvement of aortic compliance in ESRD patients taking calcium channel blockers was dependent on Na^+ and volume balance, the effect of treatment being superior in overhydrated subjects (149). The dialysis procedure itself does not improve the compliance of large arteries, even in the presence of decreased BP. This is in part due to the increased ionized Ca during hemodialysis, and the effect of hypercalcemia on the vasomotor tone of large arteries (150). Besides the increase in peripheral arterial systolic and pulse pressures, the most obvious consequence of increased arterial stiffness and PWV in ESRD patients is an alteration in the timing of wave reflections in central arteries and the aorta (134, 146). These alterations are responsible for equalization of pressure between the aorta and peripheral arteries, with an abnormal increase in end-systolic stress and development of left ventricular hypertrophy independently of the BP recorded in peripheral arteries (146). Besides the role of increased PWV, the second factor associated with an early return of wave reflections and abnormal pressure amplification in central arteries in ESRD patients is a shorter 'effective length' of the arterial tree (134, 146). This is related to their lower body size, principally shorter body height, resulting from the malnutrition and growth retardation frequently observed in azotemic children and adults with nephropathies starting in childhood (134, 146). Nevertheless, the influence of body height on timing and amplitude of pressure waves in central arteries is not restricted to ESRD patients and is observed in the general population (138).

HYPERTENSION ASSOCIATED WITH ERYTHROPOIETIN THERAPY

Early reports indicated that the incidence of hypertension in erythropoietin (EPO)-treated dialysis patients was 30–35% (151, 152). For some authors, the BP increase was more frequently observed in patients with pre-existing hypertension (152, 153), a positive family history of hypertension (154), rapid correction of anemia, or with more severe anemia (155). Nevertheless, the most recent reports indicate that hypertension associated with EPO therapy frequently remits in the long-term (156) and is then less common, involving 10–12% of treated patients (157).

Hemodynamic surveillance during treatment with EPO have shown that CO decreases and TPR increases with the increase in hemoglobin level (156, 158, 159). The decrease in CO is due either to a decrease in stroke volume or to a lower heart rate or both. The increase in red blood cell mass is compensated by a decrease in plasma (and extracellular fluid) volume (160), so that the blood volume does not change (161) or decreases only slightly. Hence the principal reason for the increase in BP is an increased TPR, even if in some cases the CO can remain inappropriately elevated (162). Blood viscosity increases in proportion to the hematocrit, and according to Poiseuille's law directly influences TPR. Increased blood viscosity and the resulting increase in shear stress have often been invoked as the principal reasons for the effect of EPO on TPR and BP (152, 163–165). However, the increase in TPR cannot totally account for the increased BP. Indeed, for the same changes in hematocrit and blood viscosity, BP increases in some patients and not in others; the same viscosity changes obtained with transfusion do not induce BP elevation (41, 50); and finally the blood viscosity of normal subjects is higher than that of EPO-treated patients and is not associated with hypertension. The second mechanism by which TPR may increase with correction of the anemia is via the reversal of hypoxic vasodilation following improved tissue oxygenation (166). The reversal of anemia-related hypoxia vasodilation was demonstrated in ESRD patients breathing 60% oxygen (167), and was greater in patients whose BP increased during treatment with EPO.

The observation that erythropoietin therapy can induce hypertension without raising the hematocrit (168) supports the view that EPO can exert a direct vasoconstrictor effect. Indeed, EPO has been shown to increase venomotor tone in normotensive dialysis patients (158), and to be efficacious in the treatment of orthostatic hypotension in non-uremic patients with autonomic neuropathy. Against this hypothesis, however, is that EPO does not induce vasoconstriction directly in human subcutaneous resistance arterioles (169). Experimental studies are also controversial, since a direct vasopressor effect of EPO on resistance vessels was observed by Heidenreich et al. (170), but not by Pagel et al. (171). There is some evidence that EPO may increase agonist-stimulated platelet cytosolic free-calcium, and calcium uptake of cultured vascular smooth muscle cells (162). This raises the possibility of a calcium-mediated increase in vascular tone or in reactivity to vasoactive substances (172), but there are no convincing arguments for the activation of vasopressor systems with EPO (161, 164, 173). Intravenous EPO injection has been shown to increase endothelin levels and arterial pressure in dialysis patients (174). Endothelial cells have receptors for erythropoietin, which has mitogenic and chemotactic effects on these cells (175) and increases endothelin-1 release (176). Furthermore, EPO may function as a vascular smooth muscle cell growth factor, contributing to vascular hypertrophy and functional alterations (177). These changes could alter the release of nitric oxide consecutive to increase in shear stress during the erythropoietin-mediated increase in blood viscosity (178). In uremic patients, the increased levels of asymmetric dimethylarginine, an endogenous inhibitor of NO-synthase, could also contribute the abnormal increase in TPR (52). Free hemoglobin is an inhibitor of NO *in vitro*, and inhibits endothelium-dependent coronary artery relaxation in response to acetylcholine *in vivo* (179),

but there is no evidence that increases in red blood cell hemoglobin affect vascular tone.

The extensive use of EPO could increase the incidence of intra- and post-dialytic hypertension, typically occurring during of after the second half of dialysis. While this hypertension could be explained in some treated hypertensive patients by the dialytic elimination of their antihypertensive drugs, in the majority of patients it represents an exaggerated vascular response to neurohumoral alterations secondary to volume depletion (increased sympathetic nerve discharge, plasma catecholamine levels, and PRA). The abnormal vascular reactivity could be potentiated by the dialysis-induced increase in serum ionized calcium. The ionized calcium directly increases TPR and the vasomotor tone of the arterial system and increases myocardial contractility, stroke volume, cardiac output, and the sensitivity of the cardiovascular system to neurohumoral stimulation (180–182).

THERAPY OF ARTERIAL HYPERTENSION IN ESRD

The goal of antihypertensive therapy in ESRD is to adequately control BP levels, in order to prevent or improve end-organ damage such as atherosclerosis or left ventricular hypertrophy (LVH). The choice of antihypertensive therapy is important, since for similar antihypertensive efficacy not all drugs are equally effective in causing regression of LVH (183). Unfortunately, few quality controlled intervention studies have been undertaken in dialysis patients and the impact of the various antihypertensive drugs on end-organ damage in the dialysis population is virtually unknown (184). There are several indications that pressures lower than the generally admitted upper limits of 140/90 mmHg would be optimal in ESRD (185), but no controlled epidemiological studies have been conducted to verify this hypothesis. In the absence of controlled studies specifically concerning dialysis patients, the general principles of treatment of hypertensive ESRD patients are similar to those used in essential hypertension, with ultrafiltration and maintenance of an appropriate dry weight replacing the use of diuretics to control salt and volume balance (3) and respect of drugs dosage related to renal function and dialysis elimination (Table 1).

The first steps consist of appropriate limitation of dietary salt and fluid intake, control of volume homeostasis by ultrafiltration and achievement of correct dry weight. Dry weight should be attained gradually over a period of 2 to 3 months. Long, slow hemodialysis procedures allow better control of sodium balance than aggressive techniques associated with high hourly ultrafiltration rates (186, 187). Studies have indicated that BP control is better in patients on peritoneal dialysis (188), due to the slow, continuous and smooth ultrafiltration achieved with continuous ambulatory or intermittent use of this procedure. In some hypertensive patients, the conventional

Table 1. Pharmacokinetics of commonly antihypertensive agents in hemodialysed patients

	Elimin. metab.	T 1/2 (hrs) NML/ESRD	Plasma Protein Binding %	Dosing	Supplem. require with dialysis	Miscellaneous
Diuretics						
Thiazides/chlortalidone	R			AVOID		
K+ sparing: Sphronolacione	R			AVOID		*K+ sparing: risk of Hyperkalemia*
Triamterene	H(R)			AVOID		*Accumulate in uremia*
Amiloride	R			AVOID		
Acetazolamide	R			AVOID		May potentiate acidosis
Loop agents						
Furosemide	R(H)			Useful in high doses	NO	*Ototoxicity and may augment*
Butetanide	R(H)			Useful in high doses	?	*aminoglycoside toxicity*
Etacrynic acid	H(R)			AVOID		
B-blockers						
Acebutolol	H(R)	8–9/7	10–20	25–50% of nml dose	NO	Active metabolites accumulation
Atenolol	R	6–9/15–35	< 5	25–50% after dialysis	YES	Removed by dialysis
Labetalol	H	3–8/3–8	50	Unchanged	NO	
Metoprolol	H	3–4/3–4	10	Unchanged	NO	
Nadolol	R	14–17/36	20–30	50% of nml dose	YES	Removed by dialysis
Pindolol	H(R)	3–4/3–4	40–55	Unchanged	NO	
Propranolol	H	3.5–6/2.3	90–96	Unchanged	NO	Active metabolites accumulation interfere with bilirubin dosage
Sotalol	R	5–8/40–50	< 10	30% of nml dose	YES	Class 3 antirrhythmic properties
Tertatolol	R	3/?	95	Unchanged	NO	Active metabolites accumulation
Timolol	H	3–4/4	10	Unchanged	NO	Inactive metabolites accumulation
Anti-adrenergic modulators						
Centrally acting						
methyl Dopa	R(H)	1,4–5,8/3—16	< 20	Interval extension of dosage adjustment: 12–24 h	YES	Active metabolites accumulation risk of prolonged hypotension
Clonidine	R	6–23/39–42	20–30	50% of nml dose	NO	Risk of rebond hypertension
Peripherally acting						
Prazosin	H(R)	2–3/?	> 90	Unchanged	NO	First dose effect. Renal failure ↓ the amount of protein bound-chemical
Urapidil	H(R)	3/?	80	Unchanged	NO	Inactive metabolites accumulation
ACE inhibitors						*Anemia: Anaaphylactoid reactions*
Benazepril	R(H)	3/12	95	50% of nml dose	NO	Non-renal clearance of Benazeprilate
Captopril	R	2–3/20–30	25–30	25–50% of nml dose	YES	Active metabolites accumulation
Cilazapril	R(H)	3–60/> 60	25–30	25% of nml dose	YES	
Enalapril	R(H)	7/35	50–60	50% of nml dose	YES	Patent drug accumulation
Fosinopril	R and H	4/20	> 95	Unchanged	NO	ACEI undergoes 50% of hepatic elimination
Lisinopril	R	5–7/> 5	10	25% of nml dose	YES	
Perindopril	R(H)	5/27	20	25–50% of nml dose	YES	
Quinapril	R(H)	2/17.5	97	25–50% of nml dose	NO	
Ramipril	R(H)	5/15	60	50% of nml dose	?	
Trandolapril	R(H)	16–24/?	> 80	50% of nml dose	?	Trandolaprilat is further metabolised prior to excretion
Calcium-channel blockers						
Amlodipine	H	45/45	97	Unchanged	NO	
Diltiazem	H	2–8/2–8	80–86	Unchanged	NO	Risk of conduction disturbance
Felodipine	H	20–25/?	97	Unchanged	NO	
Isradipine	H	2–8/8,5–14	95	Minimal dose available	?	
Lacidipine	H					
Nicardipine	H	1/1	95–98	Unchanged	NO	
Nifedipine	H	4–5,5/4–5,5	92–98	Unchanged	NO	
Nitrendipine	H	12/12	98	Unchanged	NO	
Verapamil	H	3–7/2,4–4	85–95	50–75 Active metabolites accumulation	NO	Negative inotropic effect
Vasodilators						
Diazoxide	R(H)	17–31/20–53	90	Unchanged	YES	Smaller doses or slof infusion to avoid ↓ BP. ↓ of protein binding
Hydralazine	H(NR)	7–4,5/7—16	87	Dosing interval prolonged 12–24 h	NO	Induction of tupus-like syndrome Prolonged activity in slow acetylators
Minoxidil	H	2,8–4,2/3–4	0	Unchanged	YES	Active metabolites accumulation
Nitroprusside	NR	< 10mm/sam	0	Titrate by blood pressure	YES	Accumulation of Thiocyanate: need to monitor levels to keep < 10 mg/dL Thiocyanate is dialysable.

hemodialysis/ultrafiltration procedure is poorly tolerated and the isolated ultrafiltration or sequential hemofiltration/dialysis procedures with dissociation of blood volume and plasma osmolar changes, are frequently better tolerated (189). Diuretics should be used with caution in ESRD patients, since the high doses necessary to obtain a limited increase in urinary output, carry the risk of ototoxicity. With the exception of ethacrynic acid (which carries a higher risk of ototoxicity), only loop diuretics can be used. Maintenance of dry weight controls BP in 80% of dialysis patients; when this fails to control BP, antihypertensive medication must be added (3). The general principle is to start monotherapy with one of the first-line agents (calcium channel blockers, β-blockers, or angiotensin converting enzyme inhibitors), or bitherapy associating first-line agents or a second-line drug: central sympathoinhibitors or vasodilators (3). According to the EDTA report, calcium entry blockers are the agents most frequently employed, followed in decreasing order by β-blockers, ACE inhibitors, centrally acting agents, α-1-antagonists and vasodilators (1).

Calcium channel blockers

These agents block the voltage-dependent calcium channels in cardiac and vascular smooth muscle cells. Comparing the two types of calcium channel blockers, verapamil and diltiazem have greater chronotropic, inotropic and dromotropic effects and a more potent action on myocardial cells than on arterial smooth muscle. Dihydropyridines are peripheral vasodilators with less pronounced cardiac effects. All are extensively metabolized, their half-life is not altered by renal failure, they are not eliminated by dialysis and dosage adjustment is not required (190). The dihydropyridines are the most widely studied and used agents in ESRD patients. In a long-term, placebo-controlled study, nitrendipine was effective in controlling BP in dialysis patients with a minimum of adverse effects (65). The antihypertensive effect of dihydropyridines has been shown to be more pronounced in overhydrated patients (64, 65) and in those with secondary hyperparathyroidism (66, 69). Nitrendipine was more effective in improving arterial stiffness in patients with extensive arterial calcifications (191). Nitrendipine decreased the intensity and improved the timing of arterial wave reflections in central arteries (192), but, in a controlled study, did not reduce LVH in ESRD patients (65).

Beta-blockers

β-blockers are widely used in dialysis patients for their multiple cardiovascular properties, including their antiarrhythmic and antianginal effects. They decrease renin release and modulate central adrenergic activity. β-blockers could be classified according to their water or lipid solubility, intrinsic sympathomimetic activity, cardioselectivity or additive direct vasodilating properties

(dilevalol). Water-soluble blockers (nadolol, atenolol), excreted unchanged by the kidney, have a prolonged elimination in these patients requiring dosage reduction (190). Lipid-soluble β-blockers are metabolized in the liver, to give water-soluble metabolites and a dose reduction is also necessary. β-blockers decrease arterial PWV and increase the compliance of large arteries in proportion to the BP decrease (192). With the exception of dilevalol, β-blockers increased the intensity of arterial wave reflections and did not improve their timing (192, 193). Regression of LVH with β-blockers in ESRD patients has not been demonstrated in controlled studies.

ACE inhibitors

Converting enzyme inhibitors block the generation of angiotensin II and the degradation of bradykinin, and control BP effectively in dialysis patients (73, 78, 79). ACE inhibitors are only the third most commonly prescribed agents in these patients in Europe (1). This is probably because of the higher frequency of side effects and the possibility of anaphylactoid reactions with these drugs in some dialysis patients (194). The most probable explanation for these effects could be inappropriate dosage. The recommended dose is usually 25–50% of the normal dose, with or without an increased time interval between two doses (190). Pharmacokinetic studies of perindoprilat after long-term perindopril administration therapy have shown that 10–20% of a normal dose controls BP adequately (79). ACE inhibitors increase aortic and large artery compliance in dialysis patients independently of BP changes, and this increase is accompanied by a decrease in the intensity, and an improvement in the timing, of wave reflections (195). A controlled study in ESRD patients showed that perindopril monotherapy for a period of 12 months was effective in reducing LVH (195). ACE inhibitors are especially useful in ESRD patients with heart failure, improving clinical symptoms and cardiac function.

Centrally acting sympatholytic agents and α-blockers

Clonidine and α-methyldopa are effective antihypertensive agents in ESRD patients (3, 196). It is recommended that the dose of clonidine be reduced and the dosing interval for α-methyldopa be increased (with posthemodialysis dosing) in these patients (190). However, side effects with these drugs are often troublesome, with frequent intradialytic hypotension making these agents second-line drugs. LVH regression with these agents has been observed in essential hypertension but not in ESRD. Prazosin is an α1-blocker not requiring dosage adjustment which has been shown to be effective in hemodialysis patients (197). It has no deleterious metabolic effects, including on plasma lipids. Prasozin-related regression of ESRD patients end-organ damage has not been demonstrated in controlled studies. Labetalol is a combined α- and β-blocker which has been shown effective in the treatment of acute hypertensive episodes in dialysis patients (198).

Vasodilators

This group includes several drugs (hydralazine, minoxidil, diazoxide, nitroprussiate) acting directly on the arterial wall and decreasing TPR. Inducing reflex stimulation of sympathetic activity, they require concomitant use of sympatholytic agents (3). They are not effective in reducing LVH, and moreover dialysis patients receiving minoxidil are at higher risk of developing pericardial effusions (3). These drugs are used as second-line therapy in subjects with resistant hypertension, or for hypertensive emergencies. Minoxidil is the most frequently used in uncontrolled resistant hypertension and is effective in the majority of cases, making bilateral nephrectomy unnecessary. Bilateral nephrectomy is indicated for the control of resistant and malignant hypertension; however, it is now performed infrequently given the number of effective antihypertensive drugs currently available. The prevalence of this operation in different European countries is 0–7%; this figure includes those subjects whose bilateral nephrectomy was done for reasons other than uncontrolled hypertension (1).

VASCULAR INSTABILITY AND DIALYSIS-HYPOTENSION

Severe symptomatic hypotension (unrelated to antihypertensive therapy), remains a major problem in the treatment of hemodialysis patients. Hypovolemia with a fall in circulatory filling pressure and cardiac output, and/or a defect in the regulation of vascular tone with an inappropriate increase in peripheral resistance, are the primary but not exclusive causes of hypotension (199). The better tolerance of isolated ultrafiltration, which also reduces blood volume, indicates that the hemodialysis procedure itself can cause hypotension, via the vasodilatory action of dialysate or membrane biocompatibility (200, 201).

The critical function of ECFV and blood volume control is to ensure the adequacy of the circulation, i.e. to maintain perfusion pressure and tissue blood flow. The adequacy of the circulation depends on its filling pressure, especially the cardiac filling pressure (202). Besides directly influencing cardiac performance (Frank–Starling effect), changes in cardiac filling activate stretch-sensitive receptors in the heart and cardiopulmonary system which initiate reflexes controlling ECFV distribution, renal excretion of Na^+ and water, and peripheral vascular motricity (17–22, 203).

The filling pressure of the circulation depends on the relationship between the blood volume and the holding capacity of the vascular space, its capacitance (202–204).

Capacitance is determined by two parameters: (i) the compliance ($C = \Delta V / \Delta P$), defining the change in vascular volume (ΔV) due to change in transmural pressure (ΔP), and (ii) the unstressed volume, i.e. the volume of blood in the vasculature at zero transmural pressure (135, 205). Since the compliance of the arterial system represents only 2–3% of the systemic compliance, this parameter is mainly determined by the viscoelastic properties and smooth muscle activity of the low-pressure venous system which holds 80–85% of blood volume (205). The venous compliance determines the cardiac filling pressure and the distribution of blood volume between the systemic and cardiopulmonary circulations and that of ECFV between plasma and interstitial spaces (34, 36). In normal conditions, reciprocal variations of blood volume and venous compliance enable the filling pressure to be kept constant (34). This equilibrium results from the monitoring of filling pressure by cardiopulmonary receptors. During hypovolemia, the reduced cardiopulmonary blood volume and cardiac filling pressure decrease the activity of stretch-sensitive cardiopulmonary receptors, disinhibiting vasomotor centers (17–22). Sympathetic activation produces arteriolar and venous constriction with decreases in venous compliance and 'unstressed' volume, resulting in a translocation of blood from systemic veins to the cardiopulmonary compartment, thereby maintaining cardiac filling (206–208). The changes in venous capacitance are the result of active venoconstriction and passive venous recoil as a consequence of arteriolar vasoconstriction, which reduces regional postcapillary flow and venous pressure (the DeJager–Krogh phenomenon) (209). The precapillary arteriolar constriction also reduces the capillary hydrostatic pressure, favoring vascular system refilling from the interstitium. Finally, blood volume is also progressively restored, in normal conditions, via the contributions of RAA activation, catecholamine release and reduced atrial natriuretic peptide secretion (18–22). The two vascular beds most involved in the adjustment of circulatory capacitance during hypovolemia are the splanchnic and cutaneous circulations (206–208). In severe hypovolemia, the abovementioned mechanisms are insufficient to maintain cardiac output and arterial pressure falls, activating aortic and carotid high-pressure baroreflexes which produce a further increase in the resistance of the cutaneous and splanchnic circulations, an increase in muscular vascular resistance, and increases in heart rate and myocardial contractility with shifts of the Frank–Starling curve towards a lower pressure range (17, 18, 210–212).

The changes in blood volume during dialysis are determined by the ratio between fluid removal by ultrafiltration and the refilling rate from the interstitium. In normal circumstances the refilling depends on the Starling capillary forces, i.e. on the equilibrium between oncotic and hydrostatic pressure, the later determined by systemic arterial pressure and the pre- to post-capillary resistance ratio (213). Fluid removal during dialysis results in a decrease in capillary hydrostatic pressure and increased plasma oncotic pressure, promoting an inward shift of fluid (214) from the interstitium whose volume and pressure are increased in the overhydrated state (214). The decreased capillary hydrostatic pressure is the consequence of pre-capillary arteriolar vasoconstriction and of the decrease in postcapillary venous pressure. Several factors can alter the refilling rate in dialysis patients, leading to hypovolemia and hypotension. A high ultrafiltration rate will lead to a rapid fall in plasma volume which cannot be entirely compensated immediately, since a certain time lag exists between removal and refilling (214–216). Acetate is a direct vasodilator (217, 218) which decreases the precapillary arteriolar vasoconstriction and thus increases the capillary hydrostatic pressure opposing refilling. A rapid fall in plasma osmolarity during dialysis induces fluid shifts from the interstitium to the intracellular compartment, decreasing the interstitial hydrostatic pressure (219). The interstitial tissue pressure also depends on the state of hydration, and when the dry weight is underestimated, refilling from the interstitium is hampered, leading to a rapid fall in plasma volume (214, 216). The recommendations which have been made to ensure better volume stability during hemodialysis include: (i) use of bicarbonate instead of acetate as buffer (220, 221); (ii) limitation of ultrafiltration rate and lengthening of dialysis sessions (186); (iii) maintenance of stable plasma osmolality using high- or variable-sodium dialysis and isolated or sequential ultrafiltration (219,222); and (iv) determination and monitoring of optimal post-dialysis dry weight (223) and optimal ultrafiltration rate (224, 225).

The consequences of hypovolemia on cardiac filling pressure depend on the capacitive properties of the venous system. When venous compliance is reduced, the baseline, steady-state filling pressure can be maintained in the normal range even with lower blood volume. Nevertheless, due to the steeper slope of the volume/pressure relationship, the reduction in venous compliance increases the sensitivity of cardiac filling pressure to changes in blood volume, with a steeper decrease during acute hypovolemia. On the other hand, reduction of venous compliance increases the post-/pre-capillary resistance ratio, altering the capillary hydrostatic pressure and the rate of vascular refilling. Reduced venous compliance in baseline conditions has been observed in dialysis patients, resulting from structural alterations of the venous walls (40, 226, 227). As already stressed, hypovolemia normally induces venoconstriction and decrease in venous compliance and resistance to venous return resulting in translocation of blood towards the cardiopulmonary circulation, which maintains the cardiac filling pressure (205). The reaction of the peripheral venous system to an efferent sympathetic stimulus is preserved in hemodialysis patients (40). In dialysis patients, venous tone increases significantly during isolated ultrafiltration and less so during combined ultrafiltration/bicarbonate dialysis (226, 227). An inadequate increase in venous tone and venous pooling

was observed during acetate dialysis (227, 228). Acetate may increase venous capacitance by a direct venorelaxant effect or through arteriolar vasodilation and the DeJager–Krogh effect. The capacitance system also includes the cardiac ventricles in diastole, and the compliance of the left ventricle is an important determinant of stroke volume (229). In the case of a stiff, noncompliant ventricle, a small decrease in venous return and ventricular volume induces an important fall in cardiac filling pressure and stroke volume. Left ventricular hypertrophy with reduced left ventricular compliance is typical in ESRD patients (7, 146, 230) and is associated with recurrent intradialytic hypotension (187). Indeed, dialysis-induced hypovolemia and decreased venous return is accompanied by a sharp decline in cardiac filling and cardiac output. In extreme conditions, the cardiac underfilling may induce profound sympathoinhibition (231) through the Bezold–Jarisch reflex, a vagal reflex initiated by the stimulation of cardiac mechanoreceptors by vigorous contraction of an underfilled left ventricle (232). In patients with ventricular hypertrophy and diastolic dysfunction, as well as in aged subjects and patients with hyperkinetic left ventricular function, the rate of ultrafiltration must be reduced and rapid fluid removal and short dialysis avoided (233). The sympathetic activation usually accompanying hypovolemia increases myocardial contractility, shifting the Frank–Starling curve to the left along the pressure axis. In patients with normal cardiac function, the changes in left ventricular function produced by dialysis are the result of decreased load and increased myocardial contractility through sympathetic stimulation and increased ionized calcium (181, 182, 234, 235). In patients with cardiomyopathies and decreased cardiac reserve, this effect can be absent or decreased. Whether the acetate exerts clinically important cardiodepressant effects is controversial, since both decreased (236) and normal cardiac performance have been seen during acetate hemodialysis (237, 238).

Under normal conditions, the decrease in arterial and cardiac filling pressures is detected by mechanoreceptors which reflexly augment the efferent sympathetic discharge, thereby increasing the heart rate and arterial vasoconstriction. Decreased response to baroreflex activation has been observed during aging, in atherosclerosis and cardiac hypertrophy, and as a consequence of autonomic dysfunction (17, 18, 239). A defect in the afferent limb of the baroreflex arc, with abnormal response to the Valsalva maneuver or amyl nitrate inhalation, was reported in varying proportions of ESRD patients (85, 99, 100, 240–243). Early reports indicating that such autonomic dysfunction with an inadequate increase in heart rate was more commonly observed in patients with dialysis-hypotension (240, 241) were contradicted by later studies (242–244). On the other hand, an inadequate increase in peripheral resistance has been shown to be an important cause of dialysis hypotension (244). Most dialysis patients exhibit normal postural blood pressure and heart rate responses, an appropriate increase in plasma catecholamines with head-up tilt or standing (81, 245), and a normal response to the cold pressor test (40, 242, 243). Abnormal secretion and control of vasoactive hormones during dialysis hypovolemia has been implicated, but the results are contradictory. Isolated ultrafiltration stimulated catecholamine release and increased plasma norepinephrine concentration (91, 93, 246), this response being identical (247, 248), less pronounced (82, 87, 90) or absent (84, 85) during conventional dialysis/ultrafiltration. In hypotensive dialysis patients, the catecholamine response to blood volume reduction displayed a wide interindividual variance with blunted and reduced response in some patients (76, 249). Renin-angiotensin response to hypovolemia is occasionally reduced in dialysis patients (76, 248, 249), although this is also controversial (90, 246). Dialysis patients with chronic hypotension have an activated renin-angiotensin-aldosterone system in the absence of hypovolemia and display a significantly blunted pressor response to AII infusion (250, 251) and reduced number of AII receptors on their platelets (250). Plasma arginine vasopressin levels have been shown to increase (96, 110) or not change (108, 109) in response to dialysis ultrafiltration, and in hypotensive dialysis patients, the response of plasma vasopressin was either normal (110) or blunted (249). Plasma levels of calcitonin gene-related peptide, a potent vasodilator, have been shown to be increased in uremic patients (252), and its plasma levels were increased during ultrafiltration or isovolemic hemodialysis (246), but the clinical implications of these abnormal levels are not known.

Besides the already mentioned vasodilating effect of acetate, several physiological mechanisms could be responsible for an insufficient increase in peripheral resistance. Maggiore et al. (253) suggested that an increase in body temperature could cause dialysis hypotension. Standard dialysis produces a small elevation of central temperature, necessitating heat dissipation through increased cutaneous blood flow (254). This has several consequences: hypovolemia-induced cutaneous vasoconstriction is hampered, blood is sequestrated in the cutaneous veins, and cutaneous flow is increased at the expense of flow in the more vital circulatory beds. Previous studies have shown that cool temperature dialysis decreased the frequency of dialytic hypotension and increased the tolerance of ultrafiltration (253, 255–258). The advantages of cool temperature dialysis have been ascribed to increased peripheral vasoconstriction (258), improvement of ventricular contractility (235) and increased catecholamine release (255, 258). Consumption of meals during dialysis can alter the arterial pressure control and has been associated with dialysis hypotension (259, 260). Food ingestion induces splanchnic vasodilation and redistribution of cardiac output towards mesenteric and hepatic circulations causing splanchnic blood sequestration, increased cardiac output and decreased peripheral resistance (261). This hemodynamic response to food ingestion can interfere with the vasoconstriction response to hypovolemia, there-

by hampering efforts to achieve blood pressure stability. Caffeine has been shown to attenuate the postprandial hypotension in subjects with autonomic failure (262).

Hypovolemia is certainly not the only cause of dialysis hypotension since isovolemic hemodialysis can also result in hypotension. In this condition dialysis hypotension results from an inappropriately high venous capacitance for the given (normal) blood volume, and/or from abnormal peripheral arteriolar vasodilation. It has been suggested that the inflammatory cytokines interleukin-1 (IL-1) and tumor necrosis factor (TNF) mediate this hypotension (201). IL-1 and TNF are chronically elevated in dialysis patients and have been shown to increase further during dialysis (263) due to activation of monocyte/macrophages by contact with bioincompatible dialysis membranes (264), acetate (265) or endotoxins (266) in the dialysate. It has been proposed that the vasodilating action of cytokines is mediated through the accumulation of inducible Nitric Oxide-synthase mRNA and large amounts of nitric oxide in vascular smooth muscle cells (267).

REFERENCES

1. Raine AEG, Margreiter R, Brunner FP, Ehrich JHH, Geerlings W, Landais P, Loirat C, Mallick NP, Selwood NH, Tufveson G. Valderrabano F: Report on management of renal failure in Europe, XXII, 1991. *Nephrol Dial Transplant* 7 (Suppl 2):7, 1992
2. Acosta JH: Hypertension in chronic renal disease. *Kidney Int* 22: 702, 1982
3. Paganini EP, Fouad FM, Tarazi RC: Systemic hypertension in chronic renal failure. in *The Heart and Renal Disease*, edited by O'Rourke RA, Brenner BM, Stein JH, New York, Churchill Livingstone, 1984 , p 127
4. Blythe WB: Natural history of hypertension in renal parenchymal disease. *Am J Kidney Dis* 5: A50, 1985
5. White RP, Rubin AL: Blood pressure control in chronic dialysis patients, in *Replacement of Renal Function by Dialysis*, edited by Drukker W, Parsons FM, Maher JF, Boston, Martinus Nijhoff Publishers, 1983, p 575
6. Cheigh JS, Milite C, Sullivan JF, Rubin AL, Stenzel KH: Hypertension is not adequately controlled in hemodialysis patients. *Am J Kidney Dis* 19: 453, 1992
7. Parfrey PS, Harnett JD, Griffiths SM, Gault MH, Barre P: Congestive heart failure in dialysis patients. *Arch Intern Med* 148: 1519, 1988
8. London GM, Fabiani F: Left ventricular dysfunction in end-stage renal disease: echocardiographic insights. in *Cardiac Dysfunction in Chronic Uremia*, edited by Parfrey PS, Harnett JD, Boston, Kluwer Academic Publishers, 1992, p 17
9. Vincenti F, Amend WJ, Abele J, Feduska NJ, Salvatierra O: The role of hypertension in hemodialysis-associated atherosclerosis. *Am J Med* 68: 363, 1980
10. Nichols WW, O'Rourke MF: Pulsatile pressure/flow relations, in *McDonald's Blood Flow in Arteries: Theoretical, Experimental and Clinical Principles*, 3rd edition, London, Edward Arnold, 1990, p 125

11. Guyton AC: The body's approach to arterial pressure regulation. in *Circulatory Physiology III – Arterial Pressure and Hypertension*, Philadelphia, WB Saunders Company, 1980, p 1

12. Gallagher DE, O'Rourke MF: What is the arterial pressure? in *Arterial Vasodilation, Mechanisms and Therapy*, edited by O'Rourke M, Safar M, Dzau V, London, Edward Arnold, 1993, p 134

13. Brod J, Bahlman J, Cachovan M, Pretschner P: Development of hypertension in renal disease. *Clin Sci* 64: 141, 1983

14. Tarazi RC, Ibrahim MM, Bravo EL, Dustan HP: Hemodynamic characteristics of primary aldosteronism. *N Engl J Med* 289: 1330, 1973

15. Ulrych M, Frohlich EC, Dustan HP, Page IH: Immediate hemodynamic effects of beta-adrenergic blockade with propranolol in normotensive and hypertensive man. *Circulation* 37: 411, 1968

16. Guyton AC, Hall JE, Jackson TE: The basic kidney-blood volume-pressure regulatory system: he pressure diuresis and natriuresis phenomena, in *Circulatory Physiology III – Arterial Pressure and Hypertension*, Philadelphia, WB Saunders Company, 1980, p 87

17. Mancia G, Mark AL: Arterial baroreflexes in humans. in *Handbook of Physiology*, Section 2: The Cardiovascular System – Peripheral Circulation and Organ Blood Flow, edited by Shepherd JT, Abboud FM, Geiger SR, Am Physiol Soc, Bethesda, 1983, p 755

18. Mark AL, Mancia G: Cardiopulmonary baroreflexes in humans. in *Handbook of Physiology*, Section 2: The Cardiovascular System – Peripheral Circulation and Organ Blood Flow, edited by Shepherd JT, Abboud FM, Geiger SR, Am Physiol Soc, Bethesda, 1983, p 795

19. Powis DA, Donald DE: Involvement of renal α- and β-adrenoreceptors in release of renin by carotid baroreflex. *Am J Physiol* 236: H580, 1979

20. Epstein M, Pins DS, Sancho J, Haber E: Suppression of plasma renin and plasma aldosterone during water immersion in normal man. *J Clin Endocrinol Metab* 411: 618, 1975

21. London GM, Guerin AP, Bouthier JD, London AM, Safar ME: Cardiopulmonary blood volume and plasma renin activity in normal and hypertensive humans. *Am J Physiol* 249 (*Heart Circ Physiol* 18): H807, 1985

22. Epstein M, Preston S. Weitzman RE: Isoosmotic central blood volume expansion suppresses plasma arginine vasopressin in normal man. *J Clin Endocrinol Metab* 52: 256, 1981

23. Rodeheffer RJ, Tanaka I, Imada T, Hollister AS, Robertson D, Inagami T: Atrial pressure and secretion of atrial natriuretic factor into the human central circulation. *J Am Coll Cardiol* 8: 18, 1986

24. de Wardener HE, MacGregor GA, Clarkson EM, Alaghband-Zadeh J, Bitensky L, Chayen J: Effect of sodium intake on ability of human plasma to inhibit renal Na^+-K^+-adenosine triphosphatase *in vitro*. *Lancet* i: 411, 1981

25. Guyton AC, Norman RA, Cowley AW Jr, DeClue JW: The renal function curve and its significance in long-term arterial pressure regulation, in *Circulatory Physiology III: Arterial Pressure and Hypertension*, Philadelphia, WB Saunders Company, 1980, p 100

26. Tarazi RC, Conway J: The hemodynamics of hypertension. in *Hypertension: Physiopathology and Treatment*, 2nd ed., edited by Genest J, Kuchel O, Hamet P, Cantin M, New York, McGraw-Hill Inc., 1983, p 15

27. Safar ME, London GM, Simon ACh, Chau NP: Volume factors, total exchangeable sodium, and potassium in hypertensive disease. in *Hypertension: Physiopathology and Treatment*, 2nd ed., edited by Genest J, Kuchel O, Hamet P, Cantin M, New York, McGraw-Hill Inc., 1983, p 43

28. Guyton AC, Granger JH, Coleman TG: Autoregulation of the total systemic circulation and its relation to control of cardiac output and arterial pressure. *Circ Res* 28 (Suppl I): I93, 1971

29. Coleman TG, Bower JD, Langford HG, Guyton AC: Regulation of arterial pressure in the anephric state. *Circulation* 42: 509, 1970

30. Ferrario CM, Page IH: Current view concerning cardiac output in the genesis of experimental hypertension. *Circ Res* 43: 821, 1978

31. Folkow B: Cardiovascular structural adaptation: its role in the initiation and maintenance of primary hypertension. The fourth Volhard lecture. *Clin Sci Mol Med* 55 (Suppl): s3, 1978

32. Harper RN, Moore MA, Marr MC, Watts LE, Hutchings PM: Arteriolar rarefaction in the conjunction of human essential hypertensives. *Microvasc Res* 16: 369, 1978

33. Aalkjaer C, Pedersen EB, Danielsen H, Fjeldborg O, Jespersen B, Kjaer T, Sorensen SS, Mulvany MJ: Morphological and functional characteristics of isolated resistance vessels in advanced uremia. *Clin Sci* 71: 657, 1986

34. London GM, Safar ME, Simon AC, Alexandre JM, Levenson JA, Weiss YA: Total effective compliance, cardiac output and fluid volumes in essential hypertension. *Circulation* 57: 995, 1978

35. Safar ME, London GM, Levenson JA, Simon AC, Chau NP: Rapid dextran infusion in essential hypertension. *Hypertension* 1: 615, 1979

36. London GM, Levenson JA, London AM, Simon AC, Safar ME: Systemic compliance, renal hemodynamics, and sodium excretion in hypertension. *Kidney Int* 26: 342, 1984

37. Kim KE, Onesti G, Schwartz AB, Chinitz JL, Swartz C: Hemodynamics of hypertension in chronic end-stage renal disease. *Circulation* 46: 456, 1972

38. Kim KE, Onesti G, Del Guercio ET, Greco J, Fernandes M, Eidelson B, Swartz C: Sequential hemodynamic changes in end-stage renal disease and the anephric state during volume expansion. *Hypertension* 2: 102, 1980

39. Safar ME, London GM, Weiss YA, Milliez PL: Overhydration and renin in hypertensive patients with terminal renal failure: a hemodynamic study. *Clin Nephrol* 5: 183, 1975

40. Kooman JP, Wijnen JAG, Draaijer P, van Bortel LMAB, Gladziwa U, Peltenburg HG et al.: Compliance and reactivity of the peripheral venous system in chronic intermittent hemodialysis. *Kidney Int* 41: 104, 1992

41. Kim KE, Onesti GL, Swartz CD: Hemodynamics of hypertension in uremia. *Kidney Int* 8: S155, 1975

42. Weidmann P, Beretta-Piccoli C, Steffen F, Blumberg A, Reubi FC: Hypertension in terminal renal failure. *Kidney Int* 9: 294, 1976

43. Schultze G, Piefre S, Molzahn M: Blood pressure in terminal renal failure. Fluid spaces and the renin angiotensin system. *Nephron* 25: 12, 1980

44. Davies DL, McElroy K, Atkinson AB, Brown JJ, Cumming AMM, Fraser R et al.: Relationship between exchangeable sodium and blood pressure in different forms of hypertension in man. *Clin Sci Mol Med* 57: 69S, 1979

45. Schalekamp MA, Beevers AG, Briggs JD, Brown JJ, Davies DL, Fraser R et al.: Hypertension in chronic renal failure. An abnormal relation between sodium and the renin-angiotensin system. *Am J Med* 55: 379, 1973

46. Koomans HA, Geers AB, Boer P: A study on the distribution of body fluid after rapid saline expansion in normal subjects and in patients with renal insufficiency: preferential intravascular deposition in renal failure. *Clin Sci* 64: 153, 1983

47. Lucas J. Floyer MA: Renal control of changes in the compliance of the interstitial space; factor in the aetiology of renoprival hypertension. *Clin Sci* 44: 397, 1973

48. Koomans HA, Roos JC, Dorhout Mees EJ, Delawi IMK: Sodium balance in renal failure: a comparison of patients with normal subjects under extremes of sodium intake. *Hypertension* 7: 714, 1985

49. Kornerup HJ: Hypertension in end-stage kidney disease. *Acta Med Scand* 200: 257, 1976

50. Onesti G, Kim KE, Greco JA, Del Guercio ET, Fernandes M, Swartz C: Blood pressure regulation in end-stage renal disease and anephric man. *Circ Res* 36&37 (Suppl I): I145, 1975

51. Panza JA, Quyyumi AA, Brush JE, Epstein SE: Abnormal endothelium-dependent vascular relaxation in patients with essential hypertension. *N Engl J Med* 323: 22, 1990

52. Vallance P, Leone A, Calver A, Collier J, Moncada S: Accumulation of an endogenous inhibitor of nitric oxide synthesis in chronic renal failure. *Lancet* 339: 572, 1992

53. Koyama H, Nishzawa Y, Morii H, Tabata T, Inoue T, Yamaji T: Plasma endothelin levels in patients with uremia. *Lancet* i: 99, 1989

54. Gonick HC, Kramer HJ, Paul W, Lu E: Circulating inhibitor of sodium-potassium activated adenosine triphosphatase after expansion of extracellular fluid volume in rats. *Clin Sci Mol Med* 53: 329, 1977

55. Ludens JH, Clark MA, DuCharme DW, Harris DW, Lutzke BS, Mandel F et al.: Purification of an endogenous digitalis-like factor from human plasma for structural analysis. *Hypertension* 7: 923, 1991

56. de Wardener HE, MacGregor GA: Dahl's hypothesis that a saluretic substance may be responsible for a sustained rise in arterial pressure: its possible role in essential hypertension. *Kidney Int* 18: 1, 1980

57. Blaustein MP, Hamlyn JM: Sodium transport inhibition, cell calcium and hypertension. The natriuretic hormone/Na$^+$-Ca^{++} exchange/Hypertension hypothesis. *Am J Med* 77: 45, 1984

58. Graves SW, Brown B, Valdes R Jr: An endogenous digoxin-like substance in patients with renal impairment. *Ann Intern Med* 99: 604, 1983

59. Cheng JT, Kahn T, Kaji DM: Mechanisms of alteration of sodium potassium pump of erythrocytes from patients with chronic renal failure. *J Clin Invest* 74: 1811, 1984

60. Bisordi JE, Holt S: Digitalis-like immunoreactive substances and extracellular fluid volume status in chronic hemodialysis patients. *Am J Kidney Dis* 13: 396, 1989

61. Boero R, Guarena C, Berto IM, Deabate MC, Rosati C, Quarello F, Piccoli G: Erythrocyte Na, K pump activity and arterial hypertension in uremic dialysed patients. *Kidney Int* 34: 691, 1988

62. Izumo H, Izumo S, De Luise M, Flier JS: Erythrocyte Na K pump in uremia. Acute correction of a transport defect by hemodialysis. *J Clin Invest* 74: 581, 1984

63. Thomas TH, Mansy H, Wilkinson R: Erythrocyte sodium and sodium flux in relation to hypertension in chronic renal failure. *Nephrol Dial Transplant* 4: 21, 1989

64. Salvetti A, Bozzo MV, Graziola M, Abdel-Haq B: Acute hemodynamic effect of nifedipine in hypertension with chronic renal failure: the influence of volume status. *J Cardiovasc Pharmacol* 10 (Suppl 10): 143, 1987

65. London GM, Marchais SJ, Guerin AP, Metivier F, Safar ME, Fabiani F et al.: Salt and water retention and calcium blockade in chronic uremia. *Circulation* 82: 105, 1990

66. Raine AEG, Bedford L, Simpson AWM, Ashley CC, Brown R, Woodhead JS, Ledingham JGG: Hyperparathyroidism, platelet intracellular free calcium and hypertension in chronic renal failure. *Kidney Int* 43: 700, 1993

67. Gafter U, Malachi T, Barak H, Djaldeti M, Levi J: Red blood cell calcium homeostasis in patients with end-stage renal disease. *J Lab Clin Med* 114: 222, 1989

68. Lindner A, Gagne E-R, Zingraff J, Jungers P, Dracke TB, Hannaert P, Garay R: A circulating inhibitor of the RBC membrane calcium pump in chronic renal failure. *Kidney Int* 42: 1328, 1992

69. Guerin AP, London GM, Marchais SJ, Metivier F, Safar ME, Sassano P: Parathyroid hormone and cardiovascular effects of dihydropyridines in chronic renal failure. *Am J Hypertens* 3: 566, 1990

70. DelGreco F, Davies WA, Simon NM, Huang C, Krumlovsky FA: Hypertension of chronic renal failure: role of sodium and renal pressor system. *Kidney Int* 7: S176, 1975

71. Bianchi G, Ponticemi C, Bardi V, Redae MB, Campolo L, De Ponti CZ et al.: Role of the kidney in salt- and water-dependent hypertension of end-stage renal disease. *Clin Sci Mol Med* 42: 47, 1972

72. Weidmann P, Maxwell MH: The renin-angiotensin-aldosterone system in terminal renal failure. *Kidney Int* 8: S219, 1975

73. Fadem SZ, Lifschitz MD: Use of saralasin in end-stage renal disease. *Kidney Int* 15: S93, 1979

74. Henrich WL, Katz FH, Molinoff PB, Schrier RW: Competitive effects of hypokalemia and volume depletion on plasma renin activity, aldosterone and catecholamines. *Kidney Int*, 12: 279, 1977

75. Wehle B, Asaba H, Castenfors J, Farst P, Gunnarsson B, Shaldon S et al.: Hemodynamic changes during sequential ultrafiltration and dialysis. *Kidney Int* 15: 411, 1979

76. Textor SC, Gavras H, Tifft CP, Bernard DB, Idelson B, Brunner HR: Norepinephrine and renin activity in chronic renal failure. *Hypertension* 3: 294, 1981

77. Leenen FH, Galla SJ, Redmon DP, Vagnucci AH, McDonald RH, Shapiro AP: Relationship of the renin-angiotensin-aldosterone system and sodium balance to blood pressure regulation in chronic renal failure of polycystic kidney disease. *Metabolism* 24: 589, 1975

78. Brunner HR, Wauters JP, McKinstry D, Waeber B, Turini G, Gavras H: Inappropriate renin secretion masked by captopril in hypertension of chronic renal failure. *Lancet* 2: 704, 1978

79. Guerin A, Resplandy G, Marchais S, Taillard F, London G: The effect of haemodialysis on the pharmacokinetics of perindoprilat after long-term perindopril. *Eur J Clin Pharmacol* 44: 183, 1993

80. Dzau VJ: Tissue renin-angiotensin system in myocardial hypertrophy and failure. *Arch Int Med* 153: 937, 1993

81. McGrath BP, Ledingham JGG, Benedict CR: Catecholamines in peripheral venous plasma in patients on chronic hemodialysis. *Clin Sci Mol Med* 55: 89, 1975

82. Izzo JL Jr, Izzo MS, Sterns RH, Freeman RB: Sympathetic nervous system hyperactivity in maintenance hemodialysis patients. *Trans Am Soc Artif Intern Organs* 28: 604, 1982

83. Elias AN, Vaziri ND, Maksy M: Plasma norepinephrine, epinephrine and dopamine levels in end-stage renal disease. *Arch Intern Med* 145: 1013, 1985

84. Cuche JL, Prinseau J, Selz F, Ruget G, Baglin A: Plasma free-, sulfo- and glucuro-conjugated catecholamines in uremic patients. *Kidney Int* 30: 566, 1986

85. Campese V, Romoff MS, Levitan D, Lane K, Massry SG: Mechanisms of autonomic nervous system dysfunction in uremia. *Kidney Int* 20: 246, 1981

86. Kettner A, Goldberg A, Hagberg J, Delmez J, Harter H: Cardiovascular and metabolic responses to submaximal exercise in hemodialysis patients. *Kidney Int* 26: 66, 1984

87. Corder CN, Sharma J, McDonald RH Jr: Variable levels of plasma catecholamines and dopamine-beta-hydroxylase in hemodialysis patients. *Nephron* 23: 267, 1980

88. Corneille L, Lachance S, Demassieux S, Carrier S: Turnover of free and conjugated serum catecholamines during hemodialysis. *Clin Invest Med* 6: 12, 1983

89. Spohr U, Schneider HW, Streicher E, Schrack R, Ritz E: Hemofiltration and plasma dopamine-beta-hydroxylase activity. *Nephron* 25: 121, 1980

90. Ratge D, Augustin R, Wisser H: Catecholamines, renin, aldosterone and arterial pressure in patients on chronic hemodialysis treatment. *Int J Artif Organs* 6: 255, 1983

91. Baldamus CA, Ernst W. Frei U, Koch KM: Sympathetic and hemodynamic response to volume removal during different forms of renal replacement therapy. *Nephron* 31: 324, 1982

92. Frewin DB, Bartholomeusz FDL, Cummings MF, Clarkson AR, Barry LA, Furber B et al.: Changes in plasma catecholamine levels during hemodialysis. *Aust NZ J Med* 14: 31, 1974

93. Zucchelli P, Catizone L, Degli Esposti E, Fusaroli M, Ligabue A, Zuccala A: Influence of ultrafiltration on plasma renin activity and adrenergic system. *Nephron* 21: 31, 1978

94. Atuk NO, Bailey CJ, Turner S, Peach MJ, Westervelt FB: Red blood cell catechol-0-methyl transferase, plasma catecholamines and renin in renal failure. *Trans Am Soc Artif Intern Organs* 22: 195, 1976

95. Ziegler MG, Kennedy B, Morrissey E, O'Connor DT: Norepinephrine clearance, chromogranin A and dopamine-13-hydroxylase in renal failure. *Kidney Int* 37: 1357, 1990

96. Rascher W. Schömig A, Kreye VA, Ritz E: Diminished vascular response to noradrenaline in experimental chronic uremia. *Kidney Int* 21: 20, 1982

97. Smogorzewski M, Campese VM, Massry SG: Abnormal norepinephrine uptake and release in brain synaptosomes in chronic renal failure. *Kidney Int* 36: 458, 1989

98. Converse RL Jr, Jacobsen TN, Toto RD, Jost CMT, Cosentino F, Fouad-Tarazi F et al.: Sympathetic overactivity in patients with chronic renal failure. *N Engl J Med* 327: 1912, 1992

99. Lazarus JM, Hampers HD, Lowrie EG, Merril JP: Baroreceptor activity in normotensive and hypertensive uraemic patients. *Circulation* 47: 1015, 1973

100. Grassi G, Parati G, Pomidossi G, Giannattasio C, Casadei R, Bolla G; et al.: Effects of haemodialysis and kidney transplantation on carotid and cardiopulmonary baroreflexes in uraemic patients. *J of Hypertension* 5 (Suppl 5): S367, 1987

101. DiBona GF: The function of the renal nerves. *Rev Physiol Biochem Pharmacol* 94: 76, 1982

102. Faber JE, Brody MJ: Afferent renal nerve-dependent hypertension following acute renal artery stenosis in the conscious rat. *Circ Res* 57: 676, 1985

103. Zimlichman RR, Chaimovitz C, Chaichenco Y, Goligorsky M, Rapoport J, Kaplansky J: Vascular hypersensitivity to noradrenaline: a possible mechanism of hypertension in rats with chronic uremia. *Clin Sci* 67: 161, 1984

104. Iseki K, Massry SG, Campese VM: Evidence for a role of PTH in the reduced pressor response to norepinephrine in chronic renal failure. *Kidney Int* 28: 12, 1985

105. Brodde O-E, Daul A: Alpha- and beta-adrenoreceptor changes in patients on maintenance hemodialysis. *Contr Nephrol* 41: 99, 1984

106. Shohn D, Weidmann P, Jahn H, Beretta-Piccoli C: Norepinephrine-related mechanism in hypertension accompanying renal failure. *Kidney Int* 28: 814, 1985

107. Manning RD, Guyton AC, Coleman TG, McCaa RE: Hypertension in dogs during antidiuretic hormone and hypotonic saline infusion. *Am J Physiol* 236: H314, 1979

108. Fasanella D'Amore T, Wauters JP, Waeber B, Nussberger J, Brunner HR: Response of plasma vasopressin to changes in extracellular volume and/or plasma osmolality in patients on maintenance hemodialysis. *Clin Nephrol* 23: 299, 1985

109. Jawadi MH, Ho LS, Dipette D, Ross DL: Regulation of plasma arginine vasopressin in patients with chronic renal failure maintained on hemodialysis. *Am J Nephrol* 6: 175, 1986

110. Zoccali C, Mallamaci F, Ciccarelli M, Parlongo S, Salnitro F, Curatola A: The reflex control of vasopressin in haemodialysis patients. *Nephrol Dial Transplant* 6: 631, 1991

111. Gavras H, Ribeiro AB, Kohlmann O. Saragoca M, Mulinari RA, Ramos OZ et al.: Effects of a specific inhibitor of the vascular action of vasopressin in human. *Hypertension* 6 (Suppl I): I156, 1984

112. Furchgott RF, Zawadski JW: The obligatory role of endothelial cells in the relaxation of arterial smooth muscle by acetylcholine. *Nature* 288: 373, 1980

113. Griffith TM, Edwards DH, Davies RL, Harrion TJ, Evans RT: EDRF coordinates the behaviour of vascular resistance vessels. *Nature* 329: 442, 1987

114. Palmer RMJ, Ferrige AG, Moncada S: Nitric oxide accounts for the biological activity of endothelium-derived relaxing factor. *Nature* 327: 524, 1987

115. Noris M, Benigni A, Boccardo P, Aiello S, Gaspari F, Todeschini M et al.: Enhanced nitric oxyde synthesis in uremia: implications for platelet dysfunction and dialysis hypotension. *Kidney Int* 44: 445, 1993

116. Warrens AN, Cassidy MJD, Takahashi K, Ghatei MA, Bloom SR: Endothelin in renal failure. *Nephrol Dial Transplant* 5: 418, 1990

117. Rascher W, Tulassy T, Lang RE: Atrial natriuretic peptide in plasma of volume-overloaded children with chronic renal failure. *Lancet* ii: 303, 1985

118. Saxenhofer H, Gnädinger MP, Weidmann P, Shaw S, Schohn D, Hess C et al.: Plasma levels and dialysance of atrial natriuretic peptide in terminal renal failure. *Kidney Int* 32: 554, 1987

119. Cannella G, Albertini A, Assanelli D, Ghielmi S, Poiesi C, Gaggiotti M et al.: Effects of changes in intravascular volume on atrial size and plasma levels of immunoreactive atrial natriuretic peptide in uremic man. *Clin Nephrol* 4: 187, 1988

120. Leunissen KML, Menheere PPCA, Cheriex EC, van den Berg BW, Noordzij TC, van Hooff JP: Plasma alpha-human atrial natriuretic peptide and volume status in chronic haemodialysis patients. *Nephrol Dial Transplant* 4: 382, 1989

121. Thoren P, Mark AL, Morgan DA, O'Neill TP, Needleman P, Brody MJ: Activation of vagal depressor reflexes by atriopeptins inhibits renal sympathetic nerve activity. *Am J Physiol* 251: H1252, 1986

122. Imaizumi T, Takeshita A, Higashi H, Nakamura M: a-ANP alters reflex control of lumbar and renal sympathetic nerve activity and heart rate. *Am J Physiol* 253: H1136, 1987

123. Takeshita A: Effects of atrial natriuretic factor on baroreceptor reflexes. *Hypertension* 15: 168, 1990

124. Floras JS: Sympathoinhibitory effects of atrial natriuretic factor in normal humans. *Circulation* 81: 1860, 1990

125. Muirhead EE, Pitcock J, Nasjletti A, Brown P, Brooks B: The antihypertensive function of the kidney. *Hypertension* 7 (Suppl I): I127, 1985

126. Losonczy Gy, Walter J, Mucha I, Taraba I: Changes of arterial prostaglandin E2 during haemodialysis. *Nephrol Dial Transplant* 5: 937, 1990

127. Kishimoto T, Terada T, Okahara T, Abe Y, Yamagami S, Meakawa M: Correlations between blood prostaglandins and blood pressure in chronic renal failure. *Nephron* 47: 49, 1987

128. O'Rourke MF: *Arterial Function in Health and Disease*, Edinburgh, Scotland, Churchill Livingstone Publisher, 1982, pp 94, 185

129. London GM, Marchais SJ, Safar ME, Genest AF, Guerin AP, Metivier F et al.: Aortic and large-artery compliance in end-stage renal failure. *Kidney Int* 37: 137, 1990

130. Latham RD, Westerhof M, Sipkema P, Rubal BJ, Reuderink P, Murgo JP: Regional wave travel and reflections along human aorta: a study with six simultaneous micromanometric pressures. *Circulation* 72: 1257, 1985

131. Kroeker EJ, Wood EH: Comparison of simultaneously recorded central and peripheral arterial pressure pulses during rest, exercise and tilted position in man. *Circ Res* 3: 623, 1955

132. Burattini R. Knowlen GG, Campbell KB: Two arterial reflecting sites may appear as one to the heart. *Circ Res* 68: 85, 1991

133. Kelly R, Hayward C, Avolio A, O'Rourke M: Noninvasive determination of age-related changes in the human arterial pulse. *Circulation* 80: 1652, 1989

134. London GM, Guerin AP, Pannier B, Marchais SJ, Benetos A, Safar ME: Increased systolic pressure in chronic uremia: role of arterial wave reflections. *Hypertension* 20: 10, 1992

135. Gow BS: Circulatory correlates: vascular impedance, resistance and capacity. in *Handbook of Physiology* Section 2, *The Cardiovascular System*, Vol. 2, edited by Bohr DF, Somlyo AP, Sparks HV Jr, Geiger SR, Amer Physiol Soc, Bethesda, 1980, p 353

136. Nichols WW, Avolio AP, Kelly RP, O'Rourke MF: Effects of age and hypertension on wave travel and reflections. in *Arterial Vasodilation: Mechanisms and Therapy*, edited by O'Rourke M, Safar M, Dzau V, Edward Arnold Publisher, London, 1993 p 22

137. Gow BS, O'Rourke MF: Comparison of pressure and flow in the ascending aorta of different mammals. *Proceedings, Australian Physiol and Pharmacol Soc* 1970, p 1

138. London GM, Guerin AP, Pannier BM, Marchais SJ, Metivier F: Body height as a determinant of carotid pulse contour in humans. *J Hypertens* 10 (Suppl 6): S93, 1992

139. Hsieh KY, O'Rourke MF, Avolio AP, Doherty JB, Kelly RP, Chen YT: Pressure wave contour in the ascending aorta of children: paradoxical similarity to the elderly. *Aust NZ J Med* 19: 55, 1989

140. Christensen KL: Reducing pulse pressure in hypertension may normalize small artery structure. *Hypertension* 18: 722, 1990

141. Darne B, Girerd X, Safar M, Cambien F, Guize L: Pulsatile versus steady component of blood pressure: a cross-sectional and prospective analysis of cardiovascular mortality. *Hypertension* 13: 392, 1989

142. SHEP cooperative research group: Prevention of stroke by antihypertensive drug treatment in older persons with isolated systolic hypertension: final results of the systolic hypertension in the elderly program. *J Am Med Assoc* 17: 308, 1990

143. Piccoli G, Bonello F, Salomone M, Boero R. Piccoli GB, Bergia R et al.: Epidemiology of arterial blood pressure and hypertension in maintenance hemodialysis. in *La Pression Arterielle chez l'Uremique*, IX Symposium Gambro, Marseille, France, September 23–26, 1988, p 177

144. Simon P, Ang KS, Benziane A: Hypertension artérielle systolique isolée chez l'urémique chronique hémodialysé. *Arch Mal Coeur* 84: 1205, 1991

145. Barénbrock M, Spieker C, Laske V, Baumgart P, Hoeks APG, Zidek W, Rahn KH: Effect of long-term hemodialysis on arterial compliance in end-stage renal failure. *Nephron* 65: 249, 1993

146. Marchais SJ, Guerin AP, Pannier BM, Levy BI, Safar ME, London GM: Wave reflections and cardiac hypertrophy in chronic uremia: Influence of body size. *Hypertension* 22: 876, 1993

147. Avolio AP, Deng FQ, Li DQ, Luo YF, Huang ZD, Xing LF, O'Rourke MF: Effects of aging on arterial distensibility in populations with high and low prevalence of

hypertension: comparison between urban and rural communities in China. *Circulation* 71: 202, 1985

148. Safar ME, Asmar RG, Benetos A, London GM, Levy BI: Sodium, large arteries and diuretic compounds in hypertension. *J of Hypertens* 10 (Suppl 6): S133, 1992

149. London GM, Safar ME, Levy BI: Arterial compliance and effect of calcium antagonists. in *Calcium Antagonists in Clinical Medicine*, edited by Epstein M, Hanley & Belfus, Inc., Philadelphia, 1992, p 89

150. Marchais S, Guerin A, Safar M, London G: Arterial compliance in uraemia. *J of Hypertens* 7 (Suppl 6): S84, 1989

151. Eschbach JW, Abdulhadi MH, Browne JK, Delano BG, Downing MR, Egrie JC et al.: Recombinant human erythropoietin in anemic patients with end-stage renal disease: results of a phase III multicentre clinical trial. *Ann Intern Med* 111: 992, 1989

152. Samtleben W, Baldamus CA, Bommer J, Fassbinder W, Nonnast-Daniel B, Gurland HJ: Blood pressure changes during treatment with recombinant human erythropoietin. *Contrib Nephrol* 66: 114, 1988

153. Sundal E, Kaeser U: Correction of anemia of chronic renal failure with recombinant human erythropoietin: safety and efficacy of one year's treatment in a European multicentre study of 150 haemodialysis-dependent patients. *Nephrol Dial Transplant* 4: 979, 1989

154. Ishimitsu T, Tsukada H, Ogawa Y, Numabe A, Yagi S: Genetic predisposition to hypertension facilitates blood pressure elevation in hemodialysis patients treated with erythropoietin. *Am J Med* 94: 401, 1993

155. Raine AEG: Seizures and hypertension events. *Semin Nephrol* 10 (Suppl 1): 40, 1990

156. Nonnast-Daniel B, Deschodt G, Brunkhorst R, Creutzig A, Bahlmann J, Shaldon S, Koch KM: Long-term effects of treatment with recombinant human erythropoietin on haemodynamics and tissue oxygenation in patients with renal failure. *Nephrol Dial Transplant* 5: 444, 1990

157. Pascual J, Teruel JL, Liano F, Ortuno J: Decreased blood pressure after a year of erythropoietin. *Nephron* 58: 374, 1991

158. London GM, Zins B, Pannier B, Naret C, Berthelot JM, Jacquot C et al.: Vascular changes in hemodialysis patients in response to human recombinant erythropoietin. *Kidney Int* 36: 878, 1989

159. Silberberg US, Racine N, Barre PE, Sniderman AD: Regression of left ventricular hypertrophy in dialysis patients following correction of anemia with recombinant human erythropoietin. *Can J Cardiol* 6: 1, 1990

160. Abraham PA, Opsahl JA, Keshavian PR, Collins AJ, Whalen JJ, Asinger RW et al.: Body fluid spaces and blood pressure in hemodialysis patients during amelioration of anemia with erythropoietin. *Am J Kidney Dis* 14: 438, 1990

161. Hori K, Onoyama Y, Iseki K, Fujimi S, Fujishima M: Hemodynamic and volume changes by recombinant human erythropoietin (rHuEPO) in the treatment of anemic hemodialysis patients. *Clin Nephrol* 6: 293, 1990

162. Raine AEG, Roger SD: Effects of erythropoietin on blood pressure. *Am J Kidney Dis* 18 (Suppl 1): 76, 1991

163. Raine AEG: Hypertension, blood viscosity, and cardiovascular morbidity in renal failure: implications of erythropoietin therapy. *Lancet* 1: 97, 1988

164. Steffen HM, Brunner R, Muller R Degenhardt S, Pollok M, Lang R, Baldamus CA: Peripheral hemodynam-

ics, blood viscosity and renin-angiotensin system in hemodialysis patients under therapy with recombinant human erythropoietin. *Contrib Nephrol* 66: 114, 1988

165. Schaefer RM, Leschke M, Strauer BE, Heidland A: Blood rheology and hypertension in hemodialysis patients treated with erythropoietin. *Am J Nephrol* 8: 449, 1988

166. Nonnast-Daniel B, Creutzig A, Kuhn K, Bahlmann J, Reimers E, Brunkhorst R et al.: Effect of treatment with human erythropoietin on peripheral hemodynamics and oxygenation. *Contr Nephrol* 66: 185, 1988

167. Roger SD, Grasty MS, Baker LRI, Raine AEG: Effects of oxygen breathing and erythropoietin on hypoxic vasodilation in uremic anemia. *Kidney Int* 42: 975, 1992

168. Gill ML, Anderson JL: Erythropoietin-induced hypertension without raising haematocrit. *Nephrol Dial Transplant* 8: 1264, 1993

169. Bund SJ, Heagerty A, Edmunds M, Walls J: Erythropoietin does not induce vasoconstriction directly in human subcutaneous resistance arterioles. *Nephron* 53: 173, 1989

170. Heidenreich S, Rahn KH, Zidek W: Direct vasopressor effect of recombinant human erythropoietin on renal resistance vessels. *Kidney Int* 39: 259, 1991

171. Pagel H, Jelkmann W, Weiss C: Erythropoietin and blood pressure. *Horm Metab Rev* 21: 224, 1989

172. Jandeleit K, Heintz B, Gross-Heitfeld E, Kindler J, Sieberth HG, Kirsten R, Nelson K: Increased activity of the autonomic nervous system and increased sensitivity to angiotensin II infusion after therapy with recombinant human erythropoietin. *Nephron* 56: 220, 1990

173. Roger SD, Baker LRI, Raine AEG: Autonomic dysfunction and the development of hypertension in patients treated with recombinant human erythropoietin (rHuEPO). *Clin Nephrol* 39: 103, 1993

174. Carlini R, Obialo Ci, Rothstein S: Intravenous erythropoietin (rHuEPO) administration increases plasma endothelin and blood pressure in hemodialysis patients. *A J Hypertens* 6: 103, 1993

175. Anagnostou A, Lee ES, Kessimian N, Levinson R, Steiner M: Erythropoietin has a mitogenic and positive chemotactic effect on endothelial cells. *Proc Natl Acad Sci USA* 87: 5978, 1990

176. Carlini RG, Dusso AS, Obialo CI, Alvarez UM, Rothstein M: Recombinant human erythropoietin (rHuEPO) increases endothelin-1 release by endothelial cells. *Kidney Int* 43: 1010, 1993

177. Gogusev J, Zhu DL, Marche P, Drucke T: Recombinant human erythropoietin (rHuEPO) stimulates rat vascular smooth muscle cell (VSMC) growth in culture. *J Am Soc Nephrol* 4: 512, 1993 (abstract)

178. Wilcox CS, Deng X, Doll AH, Snellen H, Welch WJ: Nitric oxide mediates renal vasodilation during erythropoietin-induced polycythemia. *Kidney Int* 44: 430, 1993

179. Collins P, Burman J, Chung HI, Fox K: Hemoglobin inhibits endothelium-dependent relaxation to acetylcholine in human coronary arteries *in vivo. Circulation* 87: 80, 1993

180. Maynard JC, Cruz C, Kleerkoper M, Levin NW: Blood pressure response to changes in serum ionized calcium during hemodialysis. *Ann Intern Med* 104: 358, 1986

181. Lang RM, Fellner SK, Neumann A, Bushinsky DA, Borow KM: Left ventricular contractility varies direct-

ly with blood ionized calcium. *Ann Int Med* 108: 524, 1988

182. Fellner SK, Lang RM, Neumann A, Spencer KT, Bushinsky DA, Borow KM: Physiological mechanisms for calcium-induced changes in systemic arterial pressure in stable dialysis patients. *Hypertension* 13: 213, 1989

183. Koren MJ, Devereux RB: Mechanisms, effects and reversal of left ventricular hypertrophy in hypertension. *Current Opinion in Nephrol and Hypertension* 2: 87, 1993

184. Parfrey PS: Cardiac and cerebrovascular disease in chronic uremia. *Am J Kidney Dis* 21: 77, 1993

185. Ritz E, Fliser D: Hypertension and the kidney – an overview. *Am J Kidney Dis* 21 (Suppl 3): 3, 1993

186. Charra B, Calemard E, Cuche M, Laurent G: Control of hypertension and prolonged survival on maintenance hemodialysis. *Nephron* 33: 96, 1983

187. Ritz E, Rambausek M, Mall G, Ruffmann K, Mandelbaum A: Cardiac changes in uraemia and their possible relationship to cardiovascular instability on dialysis. *Nephrol Dial Transplant* (Suppl 1): 93, 1990

188. Hamburger RJ, Christ Pg, Morris PA, Luft FC: Hypertension in dialysis patients: Does CAPD provide an advantage? *Adv Perit Dial* 5: 91, 1989

189. Wehle B, Asaba H, Castenfors J, Furst P, Gunnarsson B, Shaldon S, Bergstrom J: Hemodynamic changes during sequential ultrafiltration and dialysis. *Kidney Int* 14: 411, 1979

190. Maher JF: Pharmacological considerations for renal failure and dialysis. in *Replacement of Renal Function by Dialysis*, 3rd ed., edited by Maher J, Kluwer Academic Publishers, Dordrecht, 1989, p 1018

191. Marchais SJ, Boussac I, Guerin AP, Delavaux G, Metivier F, London GM: Arteriosclerosis and antihypertensive response to calcium antagonists in end-stage renal failure. *J Cardiovasc Pharmacol* 18 (Suppl 1): S74, 1991

192. Guerin AP, Pannier BM, Marchais SJ, Metivier F, Safar M, London GM: Effects of antihypertensive agents on carotid pulse contour in humans. *J of Human Hypertens* 6 (Suppl 2): S37, 1992

193. Ting CT, Chou CY, Chang MS, WAng SP, Chiang BN, Yin FCP: Arterial hemodynamics in human hypertension: effects of adrenergic blockade. *Circulation* 84: 1049, 1991

194. Tielemans C, Madhoun P, Lenaers M, Schandene l, Goldman M, Vanherweghem JL: Anaphylactoid reactions during hemodialysis on AN69 membranes in patients receiving ACE inhibitors. *Kidney Int* 38: 982, 1990

195. Pannier BM, Guerin AP, Marchais SJ, Cuche JL, Vicaut E, London GM: Amelioration pression independante de la distensibilite aortique chez l'hemodialyse hypertendu. *Arch Mal Coeur* 87: 1059, 1994

196. Hulter HN, Licht JH, Ilnicki LP, Singh S: Clinical efficacy and pharmacokinetics of clonidine in hemodialysis and renal insufficiency. *J Lab Clin Med* 94: 223, 1979

197. Harter HR, Delmez JA: Effects of prazosin on the control of blood pressure in hypertensive dialysis patients. *J Cardiovasc Pharmacol* (Suppl 1): S43, 1979

198. Keusch G, Schiffl H, Binswanger U: Diazoxide and labetalol in acute hypertension during hemodialysis. *Eur J Clin Pharmacol* 25: 523, 1983

199. Daugirdas JG: Dialysis hypotension: A hemodynamic analysis. *Kidney Int* 39: 233, 1991

200. Bergström J, Asaba H, Furst P: Dialysis ultrafiltration and blood pressure. *Proc Eur Dial Transplant Assoc* 13: 293, 1976

201. Henderson LW, Koch KM, Dinarello CA, Shaldon S: Hemodialysis hypotension: the interleukin hypothesis. *Blood Purif* 1: 3, 1988

202. Guyton AC, Coleman TG, Granger HJ: Circulation: Overall regulation. *Ann Rev Physiol* 34: 13, 1972

203. Gauer OH, Henry JP: Neurohumoral control of plasma volume. in *Cardiovascular Physiology II, International Review of Physiology*, edited by Guyton AC, Cowley AW Jr, Baltimore, University Park Press, 1976 vol 9, p 145

204. Echt M, Duweling J, Gauer OH, Lange L: Effective compliance of the total vascular bed and the intrathoracic compartment derived from changes in central venous pressure induced by volume changes in man. *Circ Res* 34: 61, 1974

205. Rothe CF: Venous system: physiology of the capacitance vessels. in *Handbook of Physiology*, Section 2 *Cardiovascular System*, Vol. 3, *Peripheral Circulation and Organ Blood Flow*, edited by Shepherd JT, Abboud FM, Am Physiol Soc, Bethesda, 1983, p 397

206. Greenway CV, Seaman KL, Innes IR: Effect of Norepinephrine on venous compliance and unstressed volume in cat liver. *Am J Physiol* 248: H468, 1985

207. Bennett TD, Wyss CR, Scher AM: Changes in vascular capacity in awake dogs in response to carotid sinus occlusions and administration of catecholamines. *Circ Res* 55: 440, 1984

208. Hirsch AT, Levenson DJ, Cuttler SS, Dzau VJ, Creager MA: Regional vascular responses to prolonged lower body negative pressure in normal subjects. *Am J Physiol* 257: H219, 1989

209. Rothe CF: Reflex control of veins and vascular capacitance. *Physiol Rev* 63: 1281, 1983

210. Johnson JM, Rowell LB, Niederberger M, Eisman MM: Human splanchnic and forearm vasoconstrictor response to reductions in right atrial and aortic pressure. *Circ Res* 34: 515, 1974

211. Abboud FM, Eckberg DL, Johannsen UJ, Mark AL: Carotid and cardiopulmonary baroreceptor control of splanchnic and forearm vascular resistance during venous pooling in man. *J Physiol* 286: 173, 1979

212. Victor RG, Leimbach WN Jr: Effects of lower body negative pressure on sympathetic discharge to leg muscle in humans. *J Appl Physiol* 63: 2558, 1987

213. Michel CC: Fluid movements through capillary walls. in *Handbook of Physiology*, Section 2, *The Cardiovascular System*, Vol. 4 *Microcirculation*, Am Physiol Soc, Bethesda, 1984, p 375

214. Koomans HA, Geers AB, Dorhout Mees EJ: Plasma volume recovery after ultrafiltration in patients with chronic renal failure. *Kidney Int* 26: 848, 1984

215. Geers AB, Koomans HA, Roos JC, Dorhout Mees EJ: Preservation of blood volume during edema removal in nephrotic subjects. *Kidney Int* 28: 652, 1985

216. Leunissen KML, Noordzij TC, van Hoff JP: Pathophysiologic aspects of plasma volume preservation. *Contrib Nephrol* 78: 201, 1990

217. Daugirdas JT, Nawab ZM: Acetate relaxation in isolated vascular smooth muscle. *Kidney Int* 32: 39, 1987

218. Nutting CW, Islam S, Ye M, Batlle DC, Daugirdas JT: The vasorelaxant effects of acetate: role of adenosine,

glycolysis, Iyotropism, and pHi and Cai^{++}. *Kidney Int* 41: 166, 1992

219. Fleming SJ, Wilkinson JS, Greenwood RN, Aldridge C, Baker LRI, Cattel WR: Effect of dialysate composition on intercompartment fluid shift. *Kidney Int* 32: 267, 1987

220. Graefe U, Milutinovitch J, Follette WC, Vizzo JE, Babb AL, Scribner BH: Improved tolerance to rapid ultrafiltration with the use of bicarbonate in dialysate. *Proc Eur Dial Transplant Assoc* 14: 153, 1977

221. Hsu CH, Swartz RD, Somermeyer MG, Raj A: Bicarbonate hemodialysis: influence on plasma refilling and hemodynamic stability. *Nephron* 38: 202, 1984

222. de Vries PMJM, Olthof CG, Solf A, Schuenemann B, Oe PL, Quellhorst E et al.: Fluid balance during haemodialysis and haemofiltration: the effect of dialysate sodium and a variable ultrafiltration rate. *Nephrol Dial Transplant* 6: 257, 1991

223. Kouw PM, Olthoff CG, ter Wee PM, Oe LP, Donker AJM, Schneider H, de Vries PMJM: Assessment of post-dialysis dry weight: an application of the conductivity measurement method. *Kidney Int* 41: 440, 1992

224. Schneditz D, Roob J, Oswald M, Pogglitsch H, Moser M, Kenner T, Binswanger U: Nature and rate of vascular refilling during hemodialysis and ultrafiltration. *Kidney Int* 42: 1425, 1992

225. de Vries JPPM, Kouw PM, van der Meer NJM, Olthof CG, Oe LP, Donker AJM, de Vries PMJM: Non-invasive monitoring of blood volume during hemodialysis: its relation with post-dialytic dry weight. *Kidney Int* 44: 851, 1993

226. Kooman JP, Gladziwa U, Bocker G, van Bortel LMAB, van Hoof JP, Leunissen KML: Role of the venous system in hemodynamics during ultrafiltration and bicarbonate dialysis. *Kidney Int* 42: 718, 1992

227. Bradley JR, Evans DB, Cowley AJ: Comparison of vascular tone during combined haemodialysis with ultrafiltration and during ultrafiltration followed by haemodialysis: a possible mechanism for dialysis hypotension. *Br Med J* 300: 1312, 1990

228. Nakamura Y, Ikeda T, Takata S, Yokoi H, Hirono M, Abe T et al.: The role of peripheral resistance and capacitance vessels in hypotension following hemodialysis. *Am Heart J* 121: 1170, 1991

229. Grossman W, McLaurin LP: Diastolic properties of the left ventricle. *Ann Intern Med* 84: 316, 1991

230. Hutting J, Kramer W, Schutterle G, Wizemann V: Analysis of left-ventricular changes associated with chronic hemodialysis: a noninvasive follow-up study. *Nephron* 49: 284, 1988

231. Sanders JS, Ferguson DW: Profound sympathoinhibition complicating hypovolemia in humans. *Ann Intern Med* 111: 439, 1989

232. Mark AL: The Bezold–Jarisch reflex revisited: clinical implications of inhibitory reflexes originating in the heart. *J Am Coll Cardiol* 1: 90, 1983

233. Vizemann V, Kramer W: Choice of ESRD treatment strategy according to cardiac status. *Kidney Int* 33 (Suppl 24): S191, 1988

234. Nixon JV, Mitchell JH, McPhaul JJ, Henrich WL: Effect of hemodialysis on left ventricular function. Dissociation of changes in filling volume and in contractile state. *J Clin Invest* 71: 377, 1983

235. Levy FL, Grayburn PA, Foulks CJ, Brickner ME, Henrich WL: Improved left ventricular contractility with cool temperature hemodialysis. *Kidney Int* 41: 961, 1992

236. Hakim RM, Pontzer MA, Lazarus MJ, Gottlieb M: Effects of acetate and bicarbonate dialysate in stable chronic dialysis patients. *Kidney Int* 28: 535, 1985

237. Mehta BR, Fischer D, Ahmad M, Dubose TD: Effects of acetate and bicarbonate hemodialysis on cardiac function in chronic dialysis patients. *Kidney Int* 24: 782, 1983

238. Anderson LE, Nixon JV, Henrich WL: Effects of acetate and bicarbonate dialysate on left ventricular performance. *Am J Kidney Dis* 10: 350, 1987

239. Trimarco B, Lembo G, Deluca N, Volpe M, Ricciardelli B, Condorelli G et al.: Blunted sympathetic response to cardiopulmonary receptor unloading in hypertensive patients with left ventricular hypertrophy. A possible compensatory role of atrial natriuretic factor. *Circulation* 80: 883, 1989

240. Soriano G, Eisinger R: Abnormal response to Valsalva manoeuvre in patients on chronic haemodialysis. *Nephron* 9: 251, 1972

241. Kersh E, Kronfield J, Unger A, Popper R, Cantor S, Cohn K: Autonomic insufficiency as a cause of haemodialysis-induced hypotension. *New Engl J Med* 290: 650, 1974

242. Nies A, Robertson D, Stone W: Haemodialysis hypotension is not the result of uraemic peripheral neuropathy. *J Lab Clin Med* 94: 395, 1979

243. Zoccali C, Ciccarelli M, Maggiore Q: Defective reflex control of heart rate in dialysis patients. Evidence for an afferent autonomic lesion. *Clin Sci* 63: 285, 1982

244. Chaignon M, Chen WT, Tarazi RC, Nakamoto S, Bravo EL: Blood pressure response to hemodialysis. *Hypertension* 3: 333, 1981

245. Nakashima Y, Fouad FM, Nakamoto S, Textor CS, Bravo EL, Tarazi RC: Localization of autonomic nervous system dysfunction in dialysis patients. *Am J Nephrol* 7: 735, 1987

246. Odar-Cederlof I, Theodorsson E, Eriksson E, Hamberger B, Tidgren B, Kjellstrand CM: Vasoactive agents and blood pressure regulation in sequential ultrafiltration and hemodialysis. *Int J Artif Organs* 16: 662, 1993

247. Fox SD, Henderson LW: Cardiovascular response during hemodialysis and hemofiltration – thermal, membrane, and catecholamine influence. *Blood Purificat* 11: 224, 1993

248. Heintz B, Konigs F, Dakshinamurty KV, Kierdorf H, Gladziwa U, Kirsten R et al.: Response of vasoactive substances to intermittent ultrafiltration in normotensive hemodialysis patients. *Nephron* 65: 266, 1993

249. Heintz B, Reiners K, Gladziwa U, Kirsten R, Nelson K, Wieland D et al.: Response of vasoactive substances to reduction of blood volume during hemodialysis in hypotensive patients. *Clin Nephrol* 39: 198, 1993

250. Sorensen SS, Danielsen H, Jespersen B, Pedersen EB: Hypotension in end-stage renal disease: effect of postural changes, exercise and angiotensin II infusion on blood pressure and plasma concentrations of angiotensin II, aldosterone and arginine vasopressin in hypotensive patients with chronic renal failure treated by dialysis. *Clin Nephrol* 26: 288, 1986

251. Moore TJ, Lazarus M, Hakim RM: Reduced angiotensin receptors and pressor response in hypotensive hemodialysis patients. *Kidney Int* 26: 288, 1986

252. Odar-Cederlof I, Theodorsson E, Eriksson CG, Kjellstrand CM: Plasma concentrations of calcitonin gene-related peptide increase during haemodialysis: relation to blood pressure. *J Intern Med* 226: 177, 1989

253. Maggiore Q, Pizzarelli F, Zoccali C, Sisca S, Nicolo F, Parlongo S: Effect of extracorporeal blood cooling on dialytic arterial hypotension. *Proc Eur Dial Transplant Assoc* 18: 597, 1981

254. Roddie IA: Circulation to skin and adipose tissue. in *Handbook of Physiology*, Section 2, *The Cardiovascular System*, Vol. 3, *Peripheral Circulation and Organ Blood Flow*, edited by Shepherd JT, Abboud FM, Geiger SR (eds), Am Physiol Soc, Bethesda, 1983, p 285

255. Mahida BH, Dumler F, Zasuwa G, Fleig G, Levin NW: Effect of cooled dialysate on serum catecholamine and pressure stability. *Trans Am Soc Artif Intern Organs* 29: 384, 1983

256. Maggiore Q, Pizzarelli F, Sisca S, Catalano G, Delfino D: Vascular stability and heat in dialysis patients. *Clin Nephrol* 41: 398, 1984

257. Sherman RA, Rubin MP, Cody RP, Eisinger RP: Amelioration of hemodialysis-associated hypotension by the use of cool dialysate. *Am J Kidney Dis* 5: 124, 1986

258. Jost CMT, Agarwal R, Khair-el-Din T, Grayburn PA, Victor RG, Henrich WL: Effects of cooler temperature dialysate on hemodynamic stability in 'problem' dialysis patients. *Kidney Int* 44: 606, 1993

259. Sherman RA, Torres F, Cody RP: Postprandial blood pressure changes during hemodialysis. *Am J Kidney Dis* 12: 37, 1988

260. Zoccali C, Mallamaci F, Ciccarelli M, Maggiore Q: Postprandial alterations in arterial pressure control during hemodialysis in uremic patients. *Clin Nephrol* 31: 323, 1989

261. Donald DE: Splanchnic circulations. in *Handbook of Physiology*, Section 2, *The Cardiovascular System*, Vol. 3, *Peripheral Circulation and Organ Blood Flow*, edited by Shepherd JT, Abboud FM, Geiger SR, Am Physiol Soc, Bethesda, 1983, p 219

262. Onrot J, Goldberg MR, Biagioni I, Hollister AS, Kingaid D, Robertson D: Hemodynamic and humoral effects of caffeine in autonomic failure. Therapeutic implications for postprandial hypotension. *New Engl J Med* 313: 549, 1985

263. Herbelin A, Nguyen AT, ZingraffJ, Urena P, Descamps-Latcha B: Influence of uremia and hemodialysis on circulating interleukin-1 and tumor necrosis factor α. *Kidney Int* 37: 116, 1990

264. Chenoweth DE, Cheung AK, Henderson LW: Anaphylatoxin formation during hemodialysis. Effects of different hemodialyzer membranes. *Kidney Int* 24: 764, 1983

265. Bingel N, Lonnemann G, Koch KM, Dinarello CA, Shaldon S: Enhancement of *in-vitro* human interleukin-1 production by sodium acetate. *Lancet* 1: 14, 1987

266. Laude-Sharp M, Caroff M, Simard L, Pusineri C, Kazatchkine MD, Haeffner-Cavaillon N: Induction of IL-1 during hemodialysis: transmembrane passage of intact endotoxin (LPS). *Kidney Int* 38: 1089, 1990

267. Beasley D, Brenner BM: Role of nitric oxide in hemodialysis hypotension. *Kidney Int* 42 (Suppl 38): S96, 1992

ORGAN AND METABOLIC COMPLICATIONS: CARDIAC

P.S. PARFREY, R.N. FOLEY and J.D. HARNETT

INTRODUCTION

The burden of illness due to cardiac disease in chronic uremia is high. Cardiac disease is the major cause of death in dialysis patients, accounting for about 40% of deaths in dialysis patients (1). When compared to a non-renal cohort aged 45–64 years the death rate in a dialysis cohort of similar age was 3.5 times higher (2). Indices of morbidity are also high. The prevalence of clinical manifestations of cardiac disease on initiation of ESRD therapy is high (3) (Table 1). The probability of having a myocardial infarction or angina requiring hospitalization in hemodialysis patents is 10%/year (4). There is a similar probability of developing pulmonary edema requiring hospitalization or additional ultrafiltration (4). The prevalence of persistent or recurrent congestive heart failure in patients established on dialysis is 10% (5), ischemic heart disease 17–34% (6), and complex premature ventricular complexes 18% (7).

UNDERLYING CARDIAC DISEASES

The clinical consequences of cardiac disease usually result from cardiomyopathy or ischemic heart disease. Cardiomyopathy may be the consequence of dilated cardiomyopathy with systolic failure, LV hypertrophy with diastolic dysfunction and/or ischemic heart disease (Figure 1). The relative contribution of each of these disorders

Table 1. The prevalence of clinical and echocardiographic manifestations of cardiac disease in 433 patients on initiation of end stage renal disease therapy. (Derived from Foley et al., Ref (3))

Clinical manifestations	%
Ischemic heart disease	22
Cardiac failure	31
Dysrhythmia	7
Echocardiographic manifestations	
Systolic failure	15
Left ventricular hypertrophy with normal systolic function	76
Left atrial dilatation	30
Left ventricular dilatation	23

to uremic cardiomyopathy varies from patient to patient. Ischemic symptoms result from coronary artery disease or non-atherosclerotic ischemic disease (8, 9). Coronary artery disease predisposes to diastolic dysfunction and to systolic failure. LV hypertrophy is present nearly always in dilated cardiomyopathy, but also causes diastolic dysfunction with or without normal systolic function.

Systolic failure is an adverse prognostic indicator in non-renal patients with ischemic heart disease or congestive heart failure (10–12). In the Framingham Heart Study

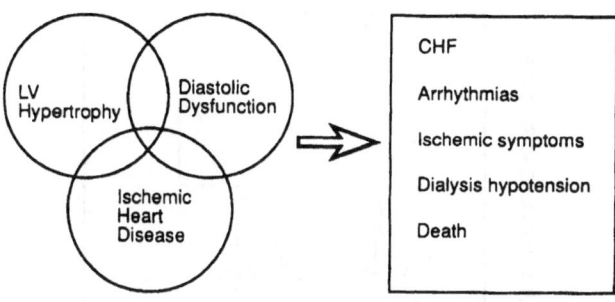

Figure 1. The clinical consequences of cardiomyopathy in chronic uremia.

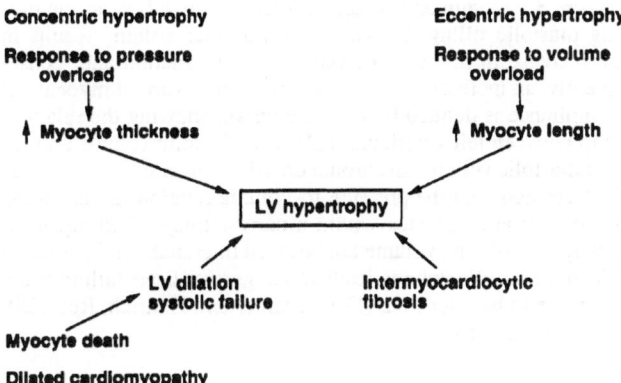

Figure 2. Causes of left ventricular hypertrophy. (From Parfrey and Harnett, *ASIO J* 40: 121–129, 1994 (with permission)

systolic dysfunction, measured by left ventricular fractional shortening, was infrequent, but when present was a more powerful predictor of mortality than left ventricular hypertrophy (13). In non-renal populations echocardiographic left ventricular hypertrophy is an adverse prognostic indicator, independent of age, diabetes, hypertension, hyperlipidemia and smoking (14–16). Left ventricular geometry, as indicated by the presence of concentric as opposed to eccentric hypertrophy, may also have prognostic implications (16). In a cohort of 90 patients starting end stage renal disease therapy left ventricular hypertrophy was shown to adversely and independently influence outcome (17).

PATHOLOGY (FIGURE 2)

At autopsy of dialysis patients a prominent and frequent manifestation is the presence of a big, heavy heart. Myocardial hypertrophy has two components: hypertrophy of the myocytes and hyperplasia of the non-myocyte elements (18).

Myocardial hypertrophy

Myocytes are unable to replicate and consequently enlarge in hypertrophic conditions. Three patterns of LV hypertrophy are recognized: concentric, eccentric and asymmetric (19).

In concentric hypertrophy myocytes increase in thickness. The increased LV mass is associated with increased thickness of both the interventricular septum and the LV free (or 'posterior') wall. The overall volume of the ventricle remains normal so that, relative to the left ventricular end diastolic diameter, wall thickness is increased. Concentric hypertrophy is thought to be an adaptive mechanism to chronic pressure overload, as in uncontrolled hypertension.

In eccentric hypertrophy myocytes grow longer. The increased LV mass is associated with increased LV volume and some increase of LV posterior wall thickness: relative to the LV end diastolic diameter, wall thickness is lower than in concentric hypertrophy. Eccentric hypertrophy is thought to be an adaptive mechanism to states of chronic volume overload in which LV end diastolic pressure tends to normalize at the expense of increased end diastolic volume.

In asymmetric hypertrophy the septal wall is disproportionately enlarged in relation to the posterior LV wall. This may result from increased afterload, which exposes the septum to a greater stress than the free wall (20), or from stimulation of the sympathetic nervous system (21).

In dilated cardiomyopathy compensatory hypertrophy occurs secondary to ventricular dilation, which may result from myocyte death. In the late stages of dilated cardiomyopathy hypoperfusion is caused by the maximally hypertrophied myocardium's inability to further increase energy transfer to the intraventricular blood during systole, the energy of contraction being largely consumed in developing pre-ejection mural tension.

In chronic uremia conditions predisposing to both concentric and eccentric hypertrophy are present. Nonetheless the degree of hypertrophy relative to the volume of the left ventricle may be inadequate (22). This inadequate hypertrophy may predispose to the development of systolic failure.

Interstitial fibrosis

The interstitium constitutes 25% of the normal myocardium and it retains this proportion in even the largest hearts, through a proliferation of the cellular, vascular and connective tissue elements normally present (18). This produces the histological appearance of a marked fibrosis, especially in the peri-vascular areas.

Irrespective of the inducing factor(s), in LV hypertrophy there is a proliferation of fibroblasts with an increase in the amount of collagen matrix. The cardiac myocytes remain normal in number, but as a result of the disproportionate increase in collagen matrix, abnormal alignment of myocytes occurs, which may lead to abnormal interdigitation in systole, and limitation of slippage during diastole (23). The predominant effect of LV hypertrophy appears to be on diastolic function.

Intermyocardiocytic fibrosis has been demonstrated at autopsy in uremic patients. From animal and autopsy studies it appears that uremia is an important factor related to intermyocardiocytic fibrosis, independent of hypertension, diabetes mellitus, anemia, heart weight and dialysis procedure (24).

In non-uremic patients with LV hypertrophy, a close correlation has been reported between impaired LV compliance measured invasively and interstitial fibrosis on endomyocardial biopsy (25). Interstitial fibrosis may provide high resistance sites to electrical conductivity, and this may predispose to re-entry tachycardia and severe arrhythmias (26).

Coronary artery disease

This condition is highly prevalent in dialysis patients, because of the demographic characteristics of the patient population and the underlying diseases, such as hypertension and diabetes mellitus (6). However it is likely that atherosclerotic coronary artery disease is not accelerated in chronic uremia, as it is neither more intense nor more prevalent than in the general population (27).

PATHOPHYSIOLOGY

Congestive heart failure

This clinical manifestation of cardiac disease may result from systolic failure, usually caused by dilated cardiomyopathy, or from diastolic dysfunction, usually caused by LV hypertrophy. In fact diastolic dysfunction is almost as frequent a cause of recurrent or persistent congestive heart failure in dialysis patients as is dilated cardiomyopathy (5).

Among patients with diastolic dysfunction congestive heart failure results from impaired ventricular relaxation, which leads to an exaggerated increase in LV end diastolic pressure for a given increase in LV end diastolic volume (Figure 3) (28). As a result, a relatively small excess of salt and water can lead rapidly to a large increase in LV end diastolic pressure, culminating in pulmonary edema.

In dilated cardiomyopathy cardiac output is maintained at the expense of an increase in both the end diastolic fiber length and end diastolic volume (i.e. through the Frank–Starling mechanism). As ventricular volume increases, however, a constant wall stress requires (by Laplace's law) a proportionate increase in LV end diastolic pressure. This increase in LV end diastolic pressure leads to increased pulmonary capillary pressure and dyspnea.

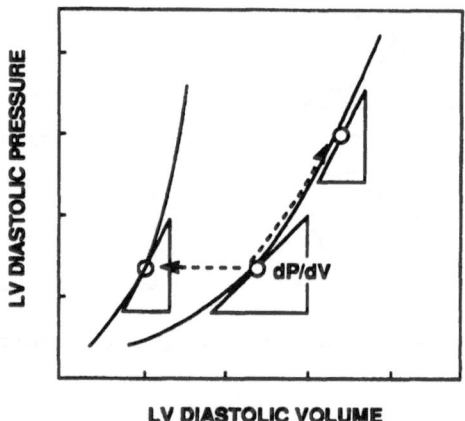

Figure 3. Compliance characteristics of the left ventricle during diastolic filling. Increase in ventricular volume results in an increase in the force of ventricular contraction and, consequently, an increase in ventricular pressure. Normal myocardial compliance is defined by the right curve, showing the relationship between left ventricular (LV) end diastolic volume and LV end diastolic volume. In chronic uremia, myocardial compliance is decreased, and the pressure-to-volume relationship is shifted to the left and operates within a narrow range. Consequently, changes in plasma volume are not well tolerated. An increase in LV end diastolic volume leads to congestive heart failure and a decrease to hypotension. (From Palmer and Henrich, Ref. (28), with permission)

Ischemic heart disease

Myocardial infarction and angina results from decreased perfusion of the myocardium. Although symptoms of ischemic heart disease are most often due to the presence of coronary artery disease, they may also result from non-atherosclerotic disease, in which a reduction in coronary vasodilator reserve, and altered myocardial oxygen delivery and use, predispose to ischemic symptoms. In dialysis patients the presence of LV hypertrophy and anemia predisposes to non-atherosclerotic ischemic disease. As the demand for oxygen increases, the coronary vasculature dilates above baseline, and a further increase in myocardial oxygen requirement may not be met with adequate increase in coronary flow, especially if there are pathologic changes in the large coronary arteries or in the small coronary vessels (Figure 4). Small vessel smooth muscle hypertrophy and endothelial abnormalities have been described in LV hypertrophy which would further predispose to ischemia (6).

Dialysis hypotension

The pathophysiology of this clinical manifestation is multifactorial and not fully understood (29). It may occur in the presence of systolic failure, diastolic dysfunction or ischemic disease. Usually in the latter condition, whether it be atherosclerotic or non-atherosclerotic in ori-

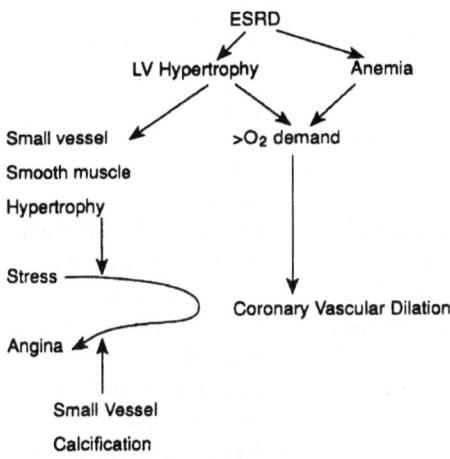

Figure 4. The pathogenesis of non-atherosclerotic ischemic heart disease in chronic uremia. (From Parfrey and Harnett, *ASAIO J* 40: 121–129, 1994 (with permission)

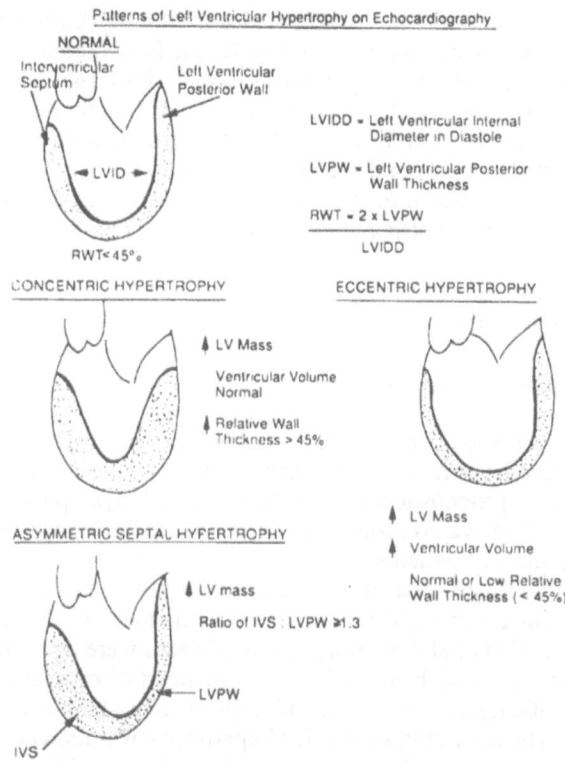

Figure 5. Patterns of left ventricular hypertrophy observed on echocardiography in patients with normal systolic function. LVID: left ventricular end diastolic internal diameter; RWT: relative wall thickness; IVS: interventricular septal wall thickness in diastole; LVPW: left ventricular posterior wall thickness in diastole. (From Foley, Parfrey and Harnett, Ref. (19) with permission)

gin, hypotension is usually associated with chest pain. In dilated cardiomyopathy hypotension during dialysis will only occur in patients who are unable to augment intrinsic myocardial contractility in response to plasma volume depletion. Such patients usually have very severe systolic failure, as the dialysis procedure actually improves myocardial performance in most patients with depressed LV function (30, 31).

LV hypertrophy may also be a contributing factor to dialysis hypotension. Because of diminished LV compliance, the relationship between LV end-diastolic pressure and volume is exaggerated (Figure 3) (28). As a result, during dialysis, relative hypovolemia may lead to disproportionately large decrease in LV end diastolic pressure, which in turn leads to a decreased stroke volume and hypotension, if a compensatory increase in peripheral resistance does not occur. A number of investigators have documented an excess prevalence of LV hypertrophy among dialysis patients prone to dialysis hypotension (32).

CARDIAC STRUCTURE AND FUNCTION IN CHRONIC UREMIA

Assessment

Echocardiography provides a non-invasive assessment of left ventricular structure and function. Systolic dysfunction, diagnosed by low fractional shortening or ejection fraction can be determined, as can LV geometry and LV hypertrophy. The degree of hypertrophy can be identified by increased LV wall thickness or by calculating left ventricular mass index according to various formulas. Figure 5 demonstrates the various types of LV hypertrophy recognizable on echocardiography.

Although LV mass measurement using echocardiography is highly reproducible between observers, its measurement varies over the course of a hemodialysis session by as much as 25 g/m² (33). This occurs because LV internal diastolic diameter increases as the patients blood volumes increases, as a result of fluid ingestion. A concomitant decrease in LV wall thickness is not observed. Consequently the LV mass index measured predialysis is higher than the post-dialysis measurement, although the actual LV mass has not changed. Therefore where possible, imaging should be carried out when the patient has achieved 'dry weight', the weight below which hypotension or symptoms such as muscle cramps occur.

Prevalence (Table 1)

We have recently completed a prospective cohort study of 433 patients, who survived at least 6 months on dialysis and were followed for a mean of 41 months from the start of ESRD therapy. Only 12.4% had a normal echocardiogram on initiation of ESRD therapy. The prevalence of indices of poor myocardial contractility was relatively high: 63 of 408 (15.4%) had a fractional shortening ≤ 25% on echocardiography (3). By the Framingham criteria, only 64 of 256 males (25%) and 18 of 147 (12%) females whose left ventricular mass index could be calculated, had normal left ventricular mass index (3). In patients with normal systolic function and LV hypertrophy nearly two-thirds had concentric hypertrophy and the remainder eccentric hypertrophy.

PROGNOSIS

Baseline cardiac disease

In a retrospective study age, diabetes mellitus, and congestive heart failure have been identified as independent adverse prognostic indicators for death in dialysis patients (34) We have confirmed this in our prospective study of 433 dialysis patients (3).

When age, diabetes, ischemic heart disease, systolic dysfunction and LV hypertrophy were included in a Cox's regression model the relative risk of death were age > 60 years; 2.54, diabetes; 2.32, ischemic heart disease; 2.14, systolic dysfunction: 1.8, and high LV mass index: 1.31 (3). The modest impact of LV hypertrophy was unexpected, but may be related to confounding effects of LV mass and LV volume. In patients with normal cavity volume, we observed that patients with a high mass to volume ratio had a significantly worse prognosis than those with a lower ratio (35). By contrast in patients with high cavity volume, patients with a low mass to: volume ratio had a worse prognosis than those with a higher ratio (35). It appears that in concentric hypertrophy the extent of hypertrophy is adverse, whereas in eccentric hypertrophy the lack of hypertrophy is associated with a poor prognosis.

Uremia related risk factors

In our Canadian cohort we measured monthly blood pressure, weight gains between dialysis, hemoglobin, serum creatinine, urea, electrolytes, calcium, phosphorus, alkaline phosphatase, albumin, and less frequently we measured serum ferritin, cholesterol, parathyroid hormone and aluminum levels. After taking into account baseline adverse prognostic factors (age, diabetes and cardiovascular disease) the following were identified as further independent, significant adverse prognostic factors: low hemoglobin, low blood pressure, low serum creatinine, and low serum albumin (36).

In our cohort the level of mean hemoglobin during follow-up on dialysis did not predict death on univariate analysis. However a disproportionately high number of patients with mean hemoglobins > 100 g/dl had ischemic heart disease and congestive heart failure, suggesting that physicians were trying to keep the hemoglobin level high in this subgroup of patients, either by blood transfusions or

Table 2. Potential risk factors for cardiac disease in chronic uremia

Non-uremia	Uremia
Age	Anemia
Diabetes	A-V fistula
Cigarette smoking	Changes in blood volume
Hypertension	Acquired valvular disease
LV hypertrophy	Hyperparathyroidism
Hyperlipoproteinuria	Increased calcium × phosporus product
Family history	Aluminium overload
	Iron overload
	B₂ microglobulinemia deposition
	Malnutrition
	Inadequate dialysis

erythropoietin. This confounding effect of cardiovascular disease on the adverse impact of anemia was revealed by the multivariate analysis. The prognostic effect of anemia was also independent of age, diabetes, mean blood pressure during follow-up, mean serum albumin and serum creatinine levels (37).

None of our patients had a mean diastolic blood pressure ≥ 100 mmHg during follow-up. Consequently it would be difficult to demonstrate an adverse effect of high blood pressure. However low blood pressure was an independent adverse predictor of mortality. Although low blood pressure was itself correlated with age and cardiovascular disease, nonetheless its prognostic effect was independent of these risk factors. It is unclear whether low blood pressure is an added marker for more severe cardiovascular disease or whether the blood pressure is low because of iatrogenic reasons. This is an important question for investigation, as its answer will determine the target blood pressure during therapy.

Low serum creatinine and hypoalbuminemia have been reported as adverse prognostic indicators by others (38, 39). It is likely that the low serum creatinine reflects deficient muscle protein and low production of creatinine, together with poor dietary intake. Hypoalbuminemia is usually considered to be an indicator of malnutrition. Whether or not low serum creatinine and hypoalbuminemia induce an adverse cardiac effect is unclear.

ETIOLOGY

Potential risk factors for cardiac mortality include those identified by the Framingham study in a non-renal population and those associated with uremia (Table 2). The degree of risk associated with many of the Framingham derived variables in dialysis patients is unclear, and the additional impact of risk factors related to uremia is even less clear.

Ischemic heart disease

The Framingham study demonstrated that hypertension is a more important predictor of coronary heart disease than blood sugar, level of cholesterol, or cigarette smoking (40). Nonetheless the risk of heart disease bore a strong relationship to baseline serum cholesterol. It is likely that a better predictor of cardiac risk is the ratio of total cholesterol to HDL cholesterol (41). In an elderly cohort from Framingham the presence of LV hypertrophy was also a predictor for subsequent development of coronary artery disease (42).

Most uremic individuals have a normal lipid profile, although various abnormal lipoprotein phenotypes can occur (43). The most common is hypertriglyceridemia, especially in CAPD patients. The atherogenicity of this abnormality is uncertain. Total serum cholesterol is either slightly elevated or normal, but the most atherogenic lipids, LDL cholesterol, are usually increased. In patients receiving continuous ambulatory peritoneal dialysis the lipid profile is similar to that observed in nephrotic syndrome. Together with low serum albumin, mean values for total cholesterol and apolipoprotein B are significantly higher than for patients on hemodialysis (44).

In dialysis patients age, white race, hypertension and hypercholesterolemia have been identified as risk factors for symptomatic ischemic heart disease (45). LV hypertrophy, as a risk for the subsequent development of coronary disease, in dialysis patients has not yet been demonstrated, but it is highly likely that the increased myocardial demands associated with hypertrophy would predispose to non-atherosclerotic ischemic heart disease.

Twenty-seven percent of dialysis patients with symptoms of ischemic heart disease do not have significant coronary stenosis at angiography (8). This observation may partly reflect the high percentage of dialysis patients with cardiac hypertrophy, a condition that requires a high level of oxygen delivery. When this is combined with intraventricular compressive forces which reduce small vessel perfusion, subendocardial ischemia may result. Acute ischemia is more likely to occur during episodes of tachycardia. Among non-ESRD patients studied with 24-hour continuous electrocardiography significantly more silent ischemia was seen among elderly patients with LV hypertrophy than among elderly patients without LV hypertrophy (45).

Congestive heart failure

Independent predictors of congestive heart failure on initiation of ESRD therapy include systolic dysfunction, older age, diabetes mellitus, and ischemic heart disease (46). In a cohort of patients without congestive heart failure at baseline independent risk factors for the development of new congestive heart failure in dialysis patients include older age, systolic dysfunction at baseline, low mean hemoglobin during follow-up, low serum albumin during follow-up, hypertension and LV hypertrophy at baseline (46).

Systolic failure

In our cohort followed from the initiation of ESRD therapy 15% already had systolic failure (fractional shortening < 25%), implying that its etiologic factors were present during the pre-ESRD period (3). Independent predictors of the presence of systolic failure at the initiation of ESRD in this group were ischemic heart disease, current cigarette use, and a low serum creatinine (< 11.3 mg/dl). A further 15% developed systolic failure following the initiation of dialysis, during which time factors related to chronic uremia could be pathogenic. The nature of these factors has not yet been clarified.

In a cross-sectional study the best clinical predictors of dilated cardiomyopathy were age, a high serum alkaline phosphate (which probably reflects hyperparathyroidism) and smoking (5). The observation that some patients with severe heart failure and dilated cardiomyopathy without coronary artery disease recover after renal transplantation is suggestive that some factor(s) associated with uremia is/are cardiotoxic (47).

Inadequate cardiac hypertrophy, in which the LV wall thickness fails to hypertrophy in response to an increase in LV diameter (22), may predispose to dilated cardiomyopathy. This may be due to hyperparathyroidism, which may exert important myocardial effects in hemodialysis patients (48). The other important factor associated with inadequate hypertrophy was hypertension. When ESRD and control subjects were analyzed by the presence or absence of hypertension, inadequate LV mass/volume ratio was observed only in hypertensive ESRD patients (49).

LV hypertrophy

Independent predictors of LV hypertrophy present on starting dialysis were anemia at baseline, hypoalbuminemia, older age and a history of hypertension for 10 years or longer (3).

In chronic uremia the correlation between blood pressure and LV mass, obtained in cross-sectional studies, is weak or absent. However hypertension has been associated with severe LV hypertrophy, although a substantial proportion of the LV hypertrophy was not explicable on the basis of hypertension alone (50). To more accurately determine the role of hypertension in causing LV hypertrophy a group of dialysis patients with normal LV mass has been followed prospectively for several years (51). The two risk factors independently associated with the development of hypertrophy were systolic hypertension and age. The mean systolic blood

Table 3. Known, potentially reversible, risk factors for cardiac disease in chronic uremia

LV hypertrophy	Dilated cardiomyopathy	Ischemic heart disease
Anemia	Coronary artery disease	Coronary artery disease
Hypertension	Smoking	Hyperlipoproteinemia
Uremia	Hyperparathyroidism	Hypertension
Aluminium	Uremia	LV hypertrophy
		Anemia

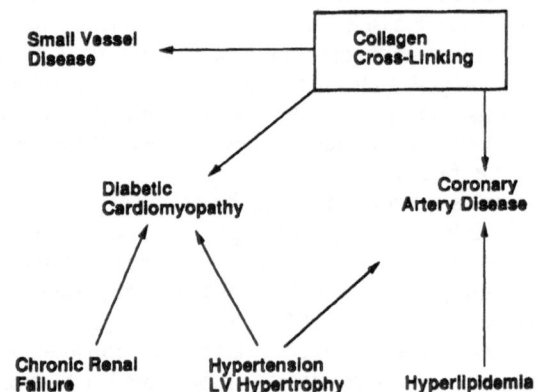

Figure 6. The pathogenesis of cardiomyopathy in diabetic renal disease (From Parfrey and Harnett, *ASAIO J* 40: 121–129, 1994 with permission)

pressure in the group who developed hypertrophy was 150 ± 13 mmHg and in the group who remained normal it was 137 ± 16 mmHg. A recent paper demonstrated that control of blood pressure in a small group of hypertensive hemodialysis patients induced a substantial regression of LV hypertrophy (52). In the control group of normotensive hemodialysis patients no change in LV mass occurred. However it is not likely that hypertension is the entire explanation. After renal transplantation two-thirds of dialysis patients had substantial regression of hypertrophy despite maintenance of blood pressure at similar levels before and after transplantation (53). This implies that some factor(s), other than hypertension, associated with uremia, is/are maintaining hypertrophy.

The treatment of anemia with erythropoietin demonstrates that both increased LV dilatation and mass can be attributed to anemia (54–62). On treatment with erythropoietin left atrial and ventricular chamber volumes decreased, as did LV mass. However in some patients, treated with erythropoietin, LV mass changed little, probably because blood pressure had increased and prevented the regression of LV hypertrophy (62, 63).

Table 3 summarizes the known, potentially reversible, risk factors for cardiac disease in chronic uremia. Further research is required to expand this list further.

The effect of diabetes mellitus

Glycation of collagen may induce cross-linking of collagen fibres (64). This may cause large and small vessel disease and myocardial dysfunction (Figure 6). However the diabetic with chronic uremia has multiple other risk factors for cardiomyopathy including hyperlipidemia, hypertension, LV hypertrophy and chronic uremia.

Diabetes mellitus is an independent risk factor for the development of heart failure and coronary artery disease (65). Diabetic patients have more widespread coronary artery disease than do age- and sex-matched controls (66). Some diabetic patients with ESRD have impairment of LV function despite normal coronary arteries, perhaps because of a diabetic cardiomyopathy (67). Echocardiographic LV hypertrophy is probably a more frequent finding in hypertensive diabetic patients than in hypertensive non-diabetic patients (68). In diabetic patients, this increased LV mass seems closely related to the level of blood pressure. A comparison of the pathologic spectrum of hypertensive, diabetic and hypertensive–diabetic heart disease shows that the latter group had a significantly higher heart weight and a higher total fibrosis score than either of the other two groups (69).

MANAGEMENT

Risk factor intervention has probably reduced cardiovascular mortality in the general population during the past 3 decades. Between 1950 and 1980 there has been a 30% decrease in cardiovascular deaths in the United States, two-thirds of which has occurred since 1970 (70). This has not occurred in chronic uremia.

In an attempt to clarify the causes of the decline in cardiovascular mortality in non-renal patients, a recent report from Framingham compared males who were 50 to 59 years of age on January 1, 1950 with a similar cohort from 1970 (70). Among those initially free of heart disease, a reduction in ten-year mortality of 60% was noted. This reduction was not due to a reduced prevalence of cardiovascular disease at baseline or to a change in disease severity. A decline in incidence of new disease of 19%, from 190 to 154 per 1000 per ten years, was noted. A marked decrease in case-fatality rate was observed, with a reduction from 26 to 13% in ten-year mortality from new disease. Significant improvements in risk factors were noted among those men initially free of heart disease, including a reduction in serum cholesterol from 5.90 to 5.72 mmol per liter, a reduction in systolic blood pressure from 139 to 135 mmHg, better management of hypertension (22%, as opposed to 0%, on antihypertensive medication), and reduced cigarette smoking (from 56 to 34%).

The Framingham risk factor approach is usually applied to dialysis patients, although there are no studies to demonstrate that the traditional risk factors have the same impact in dialysis patients as they do in the

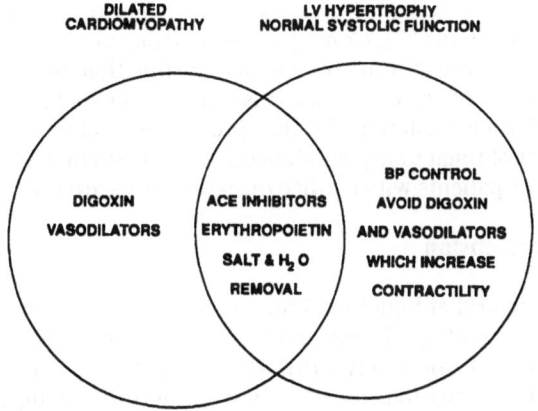

Figure 7. The effect of the underlying echocardiographic disease on the management of congestive heart failure in chronic uremia. (From Parfrey and Harnett, *Blood Purif* 12: 267–276, 1994 with permission)

general population. It is unclear how uremia related risk factors such as anemia, weight gains between dialyses, volume removal during dialysis, fistula, hyperparathyroidism, divalent ion abnormalities, aluminum, iron, acidosis, etc. impact on cardiac prognosis, and how they interact with the traditional risk factors such as hypertension, LV hypertrophy, diabetes mellitus, hyperlipidemia, obesity and smoking. Furthermore the dialysis population is substantially different from the general population, having a high prevalence of cardiac disease at the start of dialysis, and a higher proportion with multiple cardiac risk factors. Although further accurate data on the most important, reversible, cardiac risk factors on dialysis patients is required from quality epidemiological studies, some clinical trials to determine the most effective interventions in dialysis patients with cardiac disease should be initiated.

Congestive heart failure

Echocardiography should be undertaken in patients who present with congestive heart failure to differentiate between dilated cardiomyopathy with systolic failure and those with LV hypertrophy, who have diastolic dysfunction but normal systolic function, particularly as the treatment for these two disorders is different (Figure 7). Recent studies demonstrate that ACE inhibitors induce an improvement in clinical outcome in both symptomatic and asymptomatic non-renal patients with systolic failure (71, 72). The data from several well-designed studies suggest that non-renal patients with congestive heart failure benefit from digoxin therapy (73, 74). It may be that this benefit is confined to those patients with more severe heart failure who have evidence of systolic dysfunction with dilated left ventricles. Digoxin should not be prescribed to patients with congestive heart failure due to diastolic dysfunction, as the increased contractibility

could cause increased diastolic dysfunction. Patients with congestive heart failure due to diastolic dysfunction may benefit from ACE inhibitors, calcium channel blockers or beta blockers. However vasodilators which induce compensatory increase in cardiac contractibility should not be prescribed when congestive heart failure is caused by diastolic dysfunction.

Correction of anemia

The number of dialysis patients entered in studies of the effect of erythropoietin on cardiac structure and function have been small (54–62). These studies, only one of which is a randomized clinical trial, include a total of 128 subjects and show a beneficial effect of erythropoietin on LV mass, with an average decrease in mass of > 20%. Therefore it is likely that partial correction of anemia will induce regression of hypertrophy, but it does not normalize mass. Furthermore irreversible myocardial fibrosis is probably responsible for some increase in LV mass (24), and is likely to persist despite amelioration of anemia. If so correction of anemia may not prevent all the clinical consequences of LV hypertrophy.

This beneficial effect of rHuEPO on LVH depends also on careful attention to blood pressure control. We studied 20 dialysis patients with echocardiography before and after a mean of 22 months of rHuEPO therapy (63). We found no beneficial effect on LVH but noted a significant rise in systolic blood pressure from 138 to 150 mmHG ($p = 0.007$). We concluded that even this modest elevation in blood pressure was probably sufficient to prevent the beneficial effect of rHuEPO on LVH. This observation was also reported by Zehnder et al. (62) who has shown failure of regression of LVH in 5 hypertensive patients on rHuEPO compared to 7 normotensive controls also given rHuEPO. Both of these studies serve to reiterate the importance of careful blood pressure control in dialysis patients receiving rHuEPO.

The impact of erythropoietin on other subsets of dialysis patients with other cardiac diseases, especially ischemic heart disease and cardiac failure is not well studied. Rationally one would expect an improvement in coronary reserve if anemia is improved, with a consequent improvement in ischemic symptoms. Amelioration of anemia by erythropoietin in dialysis patients with significant coronary artery disease reduced exercise induced myocardial ischemia (75). It is also possible that the decrease in cardiac output and increase in LV end diastolic diameter may improve dilated cardiomyopathy. If dilated cardiomyopathy has an ischemic component improvement in coronary reserve should also produce symptomatic improvement.

It appears that the intuition of nephrologists is to raise hemoglobin levels in patients with cardiac disease, as we have observed in our cohort study that patients with hemoglobin levels > 10 g/d have a substantially higher prevalence of clinical manifestations of cardiac disease than those with lower hemoglobins (37) i.e. nephrologists have pushed the hemoglobin level of patients with symptomatic cardiac disease to a higher level with blood transfusions or erythropoietin. The question that persists however is what is the optimal level of hemoglobin for such patients. Will normalization of hematocrit provide a better outcome than partial correction in various groups with cardiac disease? Consequently we await with interest studies that investigate these questions.

Uremia therapy

There is no evidence that CAPD is better than hemodialysis in prolonging life in those with cardiac diseases, or in predisposing to the development of cardiac disease. CAPD has potential advantages in that there is no necessity for an arteriovenous fistula, there are no rapid fluctuations in blood volume, and middle molecules are better dialyzed than in hemodialysis. However it has disadvantages in that lipid abnormalities and hypoalbuminemia are more frequent, and the high glucose load may predispose to a hyperinsulinemic state. It is difficult to imagine a randomized trial of CAPD *vs* hemodialysis being undertaken, but prospective cohort studies may be able to identify subgroups of patients who may benefit for one or other of the major dialysis modalities.

It is clear that indices of malnutrition, such as low serum albumin, have adverse prognostic significance, and that inadequate dialysis, as reflected by low serum urea reduction, also limits longevity (39). It is not clear that these adverse indicators exert their pathogenetic effect through cardiac dysfunction, although we have demonstrated that a low mean serum albumin predisposes to the development of new congestive heart faiure during dialysis therapy (46). Several questions require study in patients with cardiac disease: is prescription of a high KT/V (> 1.4) better than a lower KT/V? Are high flux dialysis membranes better than cupraphane membranes? Are aggressive interventions to prevent and treat malnutrition better than little intervention? Is longer time on hemodialysis better than the minimum necessary to provide the prescribed KT/V? Do these changes in prescription of dialysis therapy exert their effect through improvement in cardiac structure or function? Unfortunately trials to examine these questions would require sample sizes of over 1200 patients and follow-up of 4–5 years to demonstrate clinically relevant improvement in mortality. Nonetheless the crucial questions currently being asked concerning the provision of the best type of hemodialysis are not answerable without them.

Transplantation

Renal transplantation often improves systolic function in patients with dilated cardiomyopathy (47, 53), presumably through the removal of adverse cardiac factors associated with chronic uremia. Transplantation also will induce regression of concentric LV hypertrophy and of LV dilatation (53). Consequently patients who are symptomatic from systolic or diastolic dysfunction, that is not the result of coronary artery disease, should not be denied renal transplantation. Further prospective studies of the effect of renal transplantation on clinical outcome in subsets of patients with cardiac diseases are necessary.

Hypertension

It is clear that high blood pressure predisposes to stroke, coronary artery disease and LV hypertrophy, and should be treated effectively (76). Blood pressure control has become easier to achieve in dialysis units during the past decade. Despite one report of poor overall blood pressure control in dialysis patients (77), in our study we have observed that the mean blood pressure during the duration of the study was infrequently greater than systolic of 160 mmHg or diastolic greater than 95 mmHg. In fact we observed that low blood pressure was an independent significant adverse prognostic indicator. At present it is unclear whether the lower blood pressure is a marker for poor cardiac function or overzealous antihypertensive therapy. It is certainly possible that some antihypertensive agents have detrimental effect in dialysis patients, particularly if blood pressure is controlled too tightly. The paucity of high quality randomized clinical trials comparing the efficacy of antihypertensive agents in dialysis patients is surprising, given the high prevalence of hypertension in this group and the 'captive' nature of their medical care. The advent of 24 hour blood pressure monitoring (78), the abnormal circadian rhythms of blood pressure in dialysis patients (79, 80), the adverse prognostic implications of LV hypertrophy (3, 17), the high prevalence of LV hypertrophy in dialysis patients (3, 81), all suggest that good quality intervention studies of antihypertensive agents are urgently required using control of 24 hour blood pressure, regression of LV hypertrophy, and clinical events as outcomes to be assessed.

Regression of LV hypertrophy

In essential hypertension a recent meta-analysis revealed that ACE inhibitors were associated with a 16% regression of LV hypertrophy and calcium channel blockers with an 8% regression (82). Whether such regression will occur in dialysis patients with multiple other risk factors present is not at all clear.

Although hypertension predisposes to LV hypertrophy it is likely that several other factors are also important. LV hypertrophy may be a normal physiologic response to several factors associated with uremia. Attempts to induce regression of such hypertrophy may consequently be harmful, particularly in patients with eccentric hypertrophy and low mass to volume ratio. Identification of the causative factors of such hypertrophy with appropriate treatment of these factors, would be the most logical approach. For example anemia may cause LV dilation, which induces a compensatory hypertrophic response. Correction of the anemia should correct both the LV dilation and hypertrophy. Hyperparathyroidism maybe responsible for inadequate hypertrophy. Correction of hyperparathyroidism may permit further appropriate hypertrophy to occur. In concentric hypertrophy and high mass to volume ratio efforts to directly induce regression of hypertrophy may improve prognosis.

Systolic failure

Factors associated with the presence of systolic failure in dialysis patients probably include smoking, hyperparathyroidism and ischemic heart disease. These patients should stop smoking and coronary artery disease should be investigated appropriately and treated.

Our current armentarium of Vitamin D analogues, phosphate binders, and high flux dialyzers should diminish the incidence of hyperparathyroidism. The increased acceptance of early parathyroidectomy in those with non-responsive hyperparathyroidism should reduce the duration of time that the heart is exposed to high levels of this cardiotoxic hormone. Thus it is likely that the impact of hyperparathyroidism as a potentially important cardiac toxin will diminish. Our current decreased use of aluminum phosphate binders should have a similar result on the potentially toxic effect of aluminum on the heart (49).

Although prospective studies are necessary to define the most important factors involved in the development of systolic failure in chronic uremia, nonetheless the effect of erythropoietin, modalities of dialysis therapy and ACE inhibitors on systolic failure could be studied immediately. Initial trials could examine their effect on indices of systolic function using echocardiography or radionuclide angiography.

Hyperlipidemia

Aggressive pharmacological treatment of dyslipidemia in end stage renal failure must be considered experimental. In non-renal patients lipid lowering agents reduce serum cholesterol (83) and have been shown to reduce plaques in coronary arteries (84). Although these agents may reduce mortality, this has not yet been conclusively shown. The relationship between various lipid abnormalities and clinical outcome in dialysis patients have not been reported. In view of the increased risk of side effects in patients with renal impairment, the efficacy of lipid lowering agents needs to be demonstrated in controlled trials in dialysis patients, initially to show whether they reduce atherogenic lipids to normal levels, and then to demonstrate whether they reduce adverse clinical outcomes. Recently improvement of lipoprotein profiles has been reported during high-flux dialysis (85). The effect of dialysis prescription on atherogenic lipids needs further study.

Diabetes

Glycation of collagen may be prevented by drugs which prevent cross-linking of collagen fibres. Trials of this intervention in the prevention and treatment of diabetic cardiac disease may be undertaken in the future. It is possible that in dialysis patients the effect of the intervention may be obscured by the presence of multiple other risk factors unrelated to cross-linked such as hyperlipidemia, hypertension, LV hypertrophy and chronic uremia.

CONCLUSIONS

The burden of cardiac disease in dialysis patients is high. The major cardiac diseases predisposing to adverse clinical manifestations include concentric and eccentric hypertrophy, dilated cardiomyopathy and ischemic heart disease. Risk factors for each of these disorders have been identified, but the most appropriate interventions to treat these disorders require further study.

REFERENCES

1. US Renal Data System, USRDS 1991 Annual Report, Bethesda, Maryland: The National Institute of Diabetes and Digestive and Kidney Diseases, 1991
2. Greaves SC, Sharpe DN: Cardiovascular disease in patients with end stage renal failure. *Aust NZ J Med* 22: 153, 1992
3. Foley RN, Parfrey PS, Harnett JD, Kent G, Martin CJ, Murray D, Barre PE: Clinical and echocardiographic cardiovascular disease in patients starting end-stage renal disease therapy: prevalence, associations and prognosis. *Kidney Int* 47: 186, 1995
4. Churchill DN, Taylor DW, Cook RJ et al.: Canadian hemodialysis morbidity study. *Am J Kidney Dis* 19: 214, 1991
5. Parfrey PS, Harnett JD, Griffiths SM, Gault MH, Barre PE: Congestive heart failure in dialysis patients. *Arch Int Med* 148: 1519, 1988
6. Rostand SG, Rutsky EA: Ischemic heart disease in chronic renal failure: demography, epidemiology and pathogenesis. in *Cardiac Dysfunction in Chronic Uremia*, edited by Parfrey PS, Harnett JD, Kluwer Academic Publishers, Boston, 1992, p 53
7. Wizemann V, Kramer W: Cardiac arrhythmias in end stage renal disease: prevalence, risk factors and management. in *Cardiac Dysfunction in Chronic Uremia*, edited by Parfrey PS, Harnett JD, Kluwer Academic Publishers, Boston, 1992, p 67
8. Rostand SG, Kirk KA, Rutsky EA: Dialysis-associated ischemic heart disease: insights from coronary angiography. *Kidney Int* 25: 653, 1984
9. Rostand SG, Kirk KA, Rutsky EA: Relationship of coronary risk factors to hemodialysis-associated ischemic heart disease. *Kidney Int* 22: 304, 1982
10. The Multicenter Postinfarction Research Group: Risk stratification and survival after myocardial infarction. *N Engl J Med* 309: 331, 1983

11. White HD, Norris RM, Brown MA, Brandt PWT, Whitlock RML, Wild CJ Left ventricular end-systolic volume as the major determinant of survival after recovery from myocardial infarction. *Circulation* 76: 44, 1987

12. Keough AM, Baron DW, Hickie JB: Prognostic guides in patients with idiopathic or ischemic dilated cardiomyopathy assessed for cardiac transplantation. *Am J Cardiol* 65: 903, 1990

13. Lauer MJ, Evans JC, Levy D: Prognostic implications of subclinical left ventricular dilatation in men free of overt cardiovascular disease (The Framingham Heart Study). *Am J Cardiol* 70: 1180, 1992

14. Levy D, Garrison RJ, Savage DD, Kannel WR, Castelli WP: Prognostic implications of echocardiographically determined left ventricular mass in the Framingham Heart Study. *N Engl J Med* 322: 1561, 1990

15. Casale PN, Devereaux RB, Milner M et al.. Value of echocardiographic measurement of left ventricular mass in predicting cardiovascular morbid events in hypertensive men. *Ann Intern Med* 105: 173, 1986

16. Koren MJ, Devereux RB, Casale PN, Savage DD, Laragh JH: Relation of left ventricular mass and geometry to morbidity and mortality in uncomplicated essential hypertension. *Ann Intern Med* 114: 345, 1991

17. Silberberg JS, Barre P, Prichard S, Sniderman AD: Left ventricular hypertrophy: an independent determinant of survival in end stage renal failure. *Kidney Int* 36: 286, 1989

18. Hutchins GM: Cardiac pathology in chronic renal failure. in *Cardiac Dysfunction in Chronic Uremia*, edited by Parfrey PS, Harnett JD, Kluwer Academic Publishers, Boston, 1992, p 85

19. Foley RN, Parfrey PS, Harnett JD: Left ventricular hypertrophy in dialysis patients. *Seminars in Dialysis* 5: 34, 1992

20. Heng MK, Janz RF, Jobin J: Estimation of regional stress in the left ventricular septum and free wall: an echocardiographic study suggesting a mechanism for asymmetric septal hypertrophy. *Am Heart J* 110: 84, 1985

21. Bernardi D, Bernini L, Cini G, Ghione S, Bonechi I: Asymmetric septal hypertrophy and sympathetic overactivity in normotensive hemodialyzed patients. *Am Heart J* 109: 539, 1985

22. London GM, Fabiani F, Marchais SJ, de Vernejoul M-C, Guerin AP, Safar ME, Metivier F, Llach F: Uremic cardiomyopathy: an inadequate left ventricular hypertrophy. *Kidney Int* 31: 973, 1987

23. Wever KT: Cardiac interstitium in health and disease: the fibrillar Collagen Network. *J Am Coll Cardiol* 13: 1637, 1989

24. Mall G, Huter W, Schneider J, Lundin P, Ritz E: Diffuse intermyocardiocytic fibrosis in uremic patients. *Nephrol Dial Transplant* 5: 39, 1990

25. Hess OM, Schneider J, Koch R, Bamert C, Grimm J, Krayenbuehl HP: Diastolic function and myocardial structure in patients with myocardial hypertrophy. *Circulation* 63: 360, 1981

26. McLenachan JM, Henderson E, Dargie HJ: A possible mechanism of sudden death in hypertensive left ventricular hypertrophy. *J Hypertension* 5 (Suppl 5): 630, 1987

27. Rostand SG, Rutsky EA: Ischemic heart disease in chronic renal failure: management considerations. *Semin Dial* 2: 98, 1989

28. Palmer BF, Henrich WL: The effect of dialysis on left ventricular contractibility. in *Cardiac Dysfunction in Chronic Uremia*, edited by Parfrey PS, Harnett, JD, Kluwer Academic Publishers, Boston, 1992, p 171

29. Daugirdas JT: Dialysis hypotension: a hemodynamic analysis. *Kidney Int* 39: 233, 1991

30. Madsen BR, Alpert MA, Shiting RB, Van Stone J, Ahmad M, Kelly DL: Effect of hemodialysis on left ventricular performance. Analysis of echocardiographic subsets. *Am J Nephrol* 4: 86, 1984

31. Hung J, Harris PJ, Uren RF, Tiller DJ, Kelly DT: Uremic cardiomyopathy – effect of hemodialysis on left ventricular function in end-stage renal failure. *N Engl J Med* 302 (10): 547, 1980

32. Ruffmann K, Mandelbaum A, Bowmer J et al.: Doppler echocardiographic findings in dialysis patients. *Nephrol Dial Transplant* 5: 426, 1990

33. Harnett JD, Murphy B, Collingwood P, Purchase L, Kent G, Parfrey PS: The reliability and validity of echocardiographic measurement of left ventricular mass index in hemodialysis patients. *Nephron* 65: 212, 1993

34. Hutchinson TA, Thomas CD, MacGibbon B: Predicting survival in adults with end stage renal failure: an age-equivalence index. *Ann Intern Med* 96: 417, 1982

35. Foley RN, Parfrey PS, Harnett JD, Kent GM, Murray DC, Barre PE: Left ventricular geometry: a critical prognostic variable in ESRD patients. *J Am Soc Nephrol* 5: 2024, 1995

36. Foley RN, Parfrey PS, Harnett JD, Kent G, Barre PE: Uremia related prognostic factors in dialysis patients: a cohort study from the start of dialysis therapy. *JASN* 4: 346, 1993

37. Harnett JD, Parfrey PS, Foley RN, Kent GM, Barre PE: Anemia: an important risk factor for cardiovascular morbidity and mortality in dialysis patients. *JASN* 4: 346, 1993

38. Iseki K, Kawazoe N, Fukiyama K: Serum albumin is a strong predictor of death in chronic dialysis patients. *Kidney Int* 44: 115, 1993

39. Owen OF, Lew NL, Liu Y, Lowrie EG, Lazarus JM: The urea reduction rato and serum albumin concentration as predictors of mortality in patients undergoing hemodialysis. *N Engl J Med* 329: 1001, 1993

40. Levy D, Wilson PWF, Anderson KM et al.: Stratifying the patient at risk from coronary disease: new insights from the Framingham Heart Study. *Am Heart J* 119: 712, 1990

41. Gordon T, Kannel WB: Multiple risk factors for predicting coronary heart disease: the concept, accuracy and application. *Am Heart J* 103: 1031, 1982

42. Levy D, Garrison RJ, Savage DD, Kannel WB, Castelli WP: Left ventricular mass and incidence of coronary heart disease in an elderly cohort. The Framingham Heart Study. *Ann Intern Med* 110: 105, 1989

43. Shapiro RJ: Atherogenesis in chronic renal failure. in *Cardiac Dysfunction in Chronic Uremia*, edited by Parfrey PS, Harnett JD, Kluwer Academic Publishers, Boston, 1992, p 187

44. Lal SM: Hyperlipidemia in continuous ambulatory peritoneal dialysis patients. *ASAIO J* 39: 87, 1993

45. Aronow WS, Epstein S, Koengsberg M: Usefulness of echocardiographic left ventricular hypertrophy and silent ischemia in predicting new cardiac events in elderly patients with systemic hypertension and coronary artery disease. *Angiology* 41: 189, 1990

46. Harnett JD, Foley RN, Kent GM, Murray DC, Barre PE, Parfrey PS: Congestive heart failure in dialysis patients: prevalence, incidence, prognosis and risk factors. *Kidney Int* 47: 884, 1995

47. Burt RK, Gupta-Burt S, Suki WN et al.: Reversal of left ventricular dysfunction after renal transplantation. *Ann Intern Med* 111: 635, 1989

48. London GM, De Vernejoul MC, Fabiani F et al.: Secondary hyperparathyroidism and cardiac hypertrophy in hemodialysis patients. *Kidney Int* 32: 900, 1987

49. London GM, Fabiani F: Left ventricular dysfunction in end-stage renal disease: echocardiographic insights. in *Cardiac Dysfunction in Chronic Uremia*, edited by Parfrey PS, Harnett JD, Kluwer Academic Publishers, Boston, 1992, p 125

50. Harnett JD, Parfrey PS, Griffiths SM, Gault MH, Barre P, Guttman RD: Left ventricular hypertrophy in end stage renal disease. *Nephron* 48: 107, 1988

51. Harnett JD, Kent GM, Barre PE, Taylor R. Parfrey PS: The development of left ventricular hypertrophy in dialysis patients: a nested case control study. *J Am Soc Nephrol* 4: 1486, 1994

52. Cannella G, Paoletti E, Delfino R et al.: Regression of left ventricular hypertrophy in hypertensive dialysed uremic patients on long-term antihypertensive therapy. *Kidney Int* 44: 881, 1993

53. Parfrey PS, Harnett JD, Foley RN, Kent GM, Murray DC, Barre PE, Guttmann RD: Impact of renal transplatation on uremic cardiomyopathy. *Transplatation* 1995. (In press)

54. London GM, Zins B, Pannier B et al.: Vascular changes in hemodialysis patients in response to recombinant human erythropoietin. *Kidney Int* 36: 878, 1989

55. MacDougall IC, Lewis NP, Saunders MJ et al.: Long-term cardiorespiratory effects of amelioration of renal anaemia by erythropoietin. *Lancet* 335: 489, 1993

56. Silberberg J, Racine N, Barre P, Sniderman AD: Regression of left ventricular hypertrophy in dialysis patients following correction of anemia with recombinant human erythropoietin. *Can J Card* 6: 1, 1990

57. Cannella G, LaCanna G, Sandrini M et al.: Reversal of left ventricular hypertrophy following recombinant human erythropoietin treatment of anemia dialysed uremic patients. *Nephrol Dial Transplant* 6: 31, 1993

58. Low-Friedrich I, Grutzmacher P, Marz W, Bergman M, Schoeppe W: Therapy with recombinant human erythropoietin reduces cardiac size and improves heart function in chronic hemodialysis patients. *Am J Nephrol* 11: 54, 1991

59. Pascual J, Teruel JL, Moya JL, Liano F, Jimenez-Mena M, Ortuno J: Regression of left ventricular hypertrophy after partial correction of anemia with erythropoietin in patients on hemodialysis: a prospective study. *Clin Nephrol* 35: 280, 1991

60. Goldberg N, Lundin AP, Delano B, Friedman EA, Stien RA: Changes in left ventricle size, wall thickness, and function in anemic patients treated with recombinant human erythropoietin. *Am Heart J* 124(2): 424, 1992

61. Martinez-Vea A, Bardaji A, Garcia C, Ridao C, Richart C, Oliver JA: Long term myocardial effects of correction of anemia with recombinant human erythropoietin in aged patients on hemodialysis. *Am J Kidney* XIX(4): 353, 1992

62. Zehnder C, Zuber M, Sulzer M, Meyer B, Straumann F, Jenzer HR, Blumberg A: Influence of longterm amelioration of anemia and blood pressure control on left ventricu-

lar hypertrophy in hemodialyzed patients. *Nephron* 61: 21, 1992

63. Harnett JD, Le H, Parfrey PS: The importance of blood pressure control in dialysis patients receiving erythropoietin. *JASN* 3(3): 426, 1992 Abstract

64. Bromlee M, Cerami A, Vlassara H: Advanced glycosylation end products in tissue and biochemical basis of diabetic complications. *N Engl J Med* 318: 1315, 1988

65. Kannel WB, McGee DL: Diabetes and cardiovascular disease. The Framingham Study. *JAMA* 241: 2035, 1979

66. Valsania P, Zarich SW, Kowalchuk GJ, Kosinski E, Warram JH, Krolewski AS: Severity of coronary artery disease in young patients with insulin-dependent diabetes mellitus. *Am Heart J* 122: 695, 1991

67. Galderisi M, Anderson KM, Wilson PWF, Levy D: Echocardiographic evidence for the existence of a distinct diabetic cardiomyopathy (The Framingham Heart Study). *Am J Cardiol* 68: 85, 1991

68. Grossman E, Shemesh J, Shamiss A, Thaler M, Carroll J, Rosenthal T: Left ventricular mass in diabetes-hypertension. *Arch Intern Med* 152: 1001, 1992

69. van Hoeven KH, Factor SM: A comparison of the pathological spectrum of hypertensive, diabetic, and hypertensive-diabetic heart disease. *Circulation* 82: 848, 1990

70. Sytkowski PA, Kannel WB, D'Agostino RB: Changes in risk factors and the decline in cardiovascular mortality. The Framingham Study. *N Engl J Med* 311: 1144, 1990

71. The SOLVD investigators: Effect of enalapril on survival in patients with reduced left ventricular ejection fractions and congestive heart failure. *N Engl J Med* 325: 293, 1991

72. The SOLVD investigators: Effect of enalapril on mortality and the development of heart failure in asymptomatic patients with reduced left ventricular ejection fractions. *N Engl J Med* 327: 685, 1992

73. Jaeschke R, Oxman AD, Guyatt GH: To what extent do congestive heart failure patients in sinus rhythm benefit from Digoxin therapy? A systematic overview and meta-analysis. *Am J Med* 88: 279, 1990

74. Pacrer M, Cheorghiade M, Young JB et al. for the RADIANCE Study: Withdrawal of digoxin from patients with chronic heart failure treated with antiotension-converting-enzyme inhibitors. *N Engl J Med* 329: 1, 1993

75. Wizemann V, Kaufmann J, Kramer W: Effect of erythropoietin on ischemia tolerance in anemia hemodialysis patients with confirmed coronary artery disease. *Nephron* 62: 161, 1992

76. Ritz E, Koch M: Morbidity and mortality due to hypertension in patients with renal failure. *Am J Kid Dis* 21: 113, 1993

77. Cheigh JS, Milite C, Sullivan JF, Rubin AL, Stenzel KH: Hypertension is not adequately controlled in hemodialysis patients. *Am J Kid Dis* 14: 453, 1992

78. American College of Physicians: Automated ambulatory blood pressure and self-measured blood pressure monitoring devices: their role in the diagnosis and management of hypertension. *Ann Int Med* 118: 889, 1993

79. Baumgart P, Walger P, Gerke M, Dorst KG, Vetter H, Rahn KH: Nocturnal hypertension in renal failure, hemodialysis and after renal transplantation. *J Hypertens* 7: S70, 1989

80. Van de Bourne P, Tielemans C, Collart F, Vanherweghem J-L, Degaute J-P: Twenty-four hour blood pressure and heart rate patterns in chronic hemodialysis patients. *Am J Kid Dis* 22: 419, 1993

81. Parfrey PS, Harnett JD, Griffiths SM: The clinical course of left ventricular hypertrophy in dialysis patients. *Nephron* 55: 114, 1990

82. Daholf B, Pennert K, Hansson L: Reversal of left ventricular hypertrophy in hypertensive patients. A metaanalysis of 109 treatment studies. *Am J Hypertens* 5: 95, 1992

83. Lovastatin Pravastatin Study Group: A multicenter comparative trial of lovastatin and prevastatin in the treatment of hypercholesterolemia. *Am J Cardiol* 71: 810, 1993

84. Brown G, Albert JJ, Fisher LD et al.: Regression of coronary artery disease as a result of intensive, lipid-lowering therapy in men with high levels of apolipoprotein B. *N Engl J Med* 323: 1289, 1990

85. Seres DS, Strain GW, Haskim SA, Goldberg IJ, Levin NW: Improvement of lipoprotein profiles during high-flux dialysis. *J Am Soc Nephrol* 3: 1409, 1993

ORGAN AND METABOLIC COMPLICATIONS: LIPIDS/ATHEROSCLEROSIS

EBERHARD RITZ, MICHAL NOWICKI and ANDRZEJ WIECEK

INTRODUCTION

The incidence of and mortality from atherosclerotic complications, particulary coronary atherosclerosis, is strikingly increased in dialysed patients. One of the factors involved is dyslipoproteinemia. The main cause of dyslipoproteinemia is reduced activity of enzymes catabolising lipoproteins (hepatic triglyceride lipase, lipoprotein lipase), but additional abnormalities clearly contribute. Specific patterns of dyslipoproteinemia are present in patients with the nephrotic syndrome, diabetes mellitus and with immunosuppression (steroids, cyclosporin A). A paradoxical inverse relationship is noted between several lipid indicators and cardiac mortality in dialysis patients. This is presumably due to the confounding effect of malnutrition. Lipid indicators like Lp(a) and apolipoprotein ratios (AI/CIII) are predictive of atherosclerotic vascular disease, however, particularly in the high risk population of diabetics.

Strategies to interfere with dyslipoproteinemia are dietary intervention (high carbohydrate, low saturated fat), physical exercise and pharmacological intervention, particularly statines and (more problematical) fibrates. Apart from lipids a number of other factors in uremia may contribute to or interfere with atherogenesis.

HISTORICAL COMMENTS

In 1974 Lindner et al. (1) reported an alarming incidence of cardiovascular and coronary death in dialysed patients. At the end of a 13 year follow-up period, overall mortality was 56.4% and 14 out of 23 deaths were of cardiovascular origin, myocardial infarction accounting for eight fatalities. Subsequent investigators confirmed the high cardiovascular mortality and high rate of cardiac death, although the magnitude tended to be somewhat less than in the original study. The most recent analysis of the EDTA registry (2) confirmed that the incidence of cardiac death in dialysed patients is higher by a factor of 5–20 compared to the general population. This difference is consistently found, irrespective of the baseline risk in the respective non-uremic population, e.g. when male or female hemodialysis patients are compared to male or female individuals in the general population and when uremic patients and normal subjects are compared in high risk areas (like the UK) and in low risk areas (Italy) (Figure 1). Only a proportion of cases of cardiac death are due to myocardial infarction (3). Nevertheless the overall rate of cardiac deaths of dialysis patients is comparable in magnitude to that of survivors of myocardial infarction and markedly higher than for instance that of diabetics, a known high risk population, where the relative risk of cardiac death is increased by a factor of 3.

In their seminal report Lindner et al. (1) proposed the hypothesis that atherogenesis was accelerated in endstage renal failure and this was thought to result from dyslipidemia and hypertension. The issue has remained moot. While there is no doubt that the prevalence of atheroma in the dialysis population is excessive, acceleration of plaque formation has not been directly documented. The incidence of cardiovascular death does not rise progressively with time on dialysis as one would anticipate if atherogenesis were accelerated. On the contrary, cardiovascular death is highest in the first years of dialysis, presumably as a result of coronary disease acquired prior to dialysis.

To this day it remains uncertain whether the classical risk factors mainly hypertension, dyslipidemia and smoking are sufficient to account for the high prevalence of coronary atherosclerosis in the dialysed patient (4, 5). While the issues of blood pressure and its control will be dealt with elsewhere in this volume, this chapter will primarily focus on dyslipidemia and its potential role in atherogenesis of the uremic patient.

per 1000 patient years

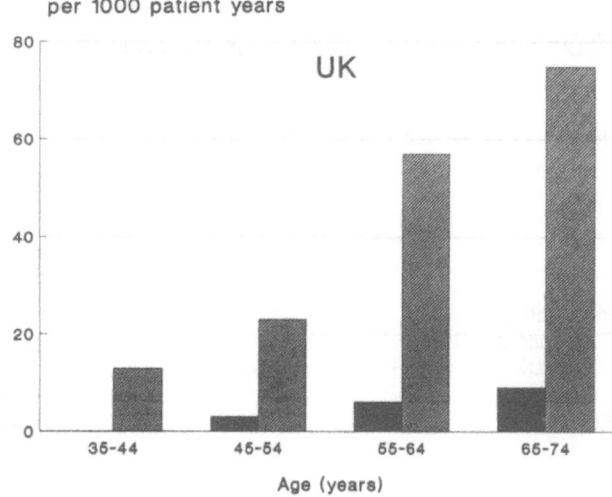

per 1000 patient years

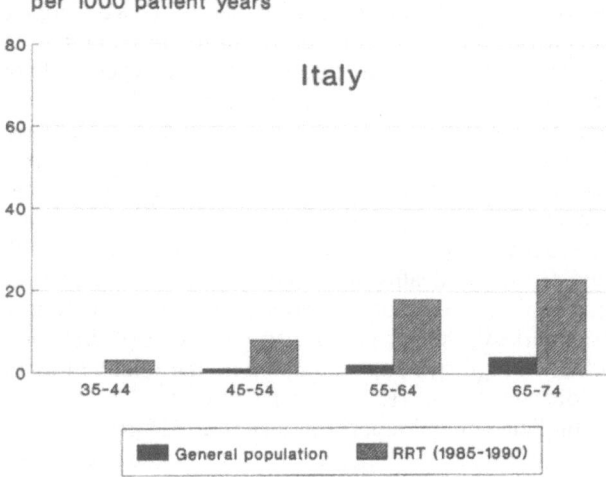

Figure 1. Age-specific death rate from myocardial ischemia and infarction in males commencing RRT between 1985 and 1990 in the United Kingdom and in Italy compared to that of males in the general population (WHO 1988). After ref. (2).

DYSLIPIDEMIA

Lactescence of the serum of uremic patients was known even to Richard Bright (6) and for many decades hyperlipoproteinemia has been a well known feature of renal failure (7). Following the work of Bagdade (8) the dyslipoproteinemia of renal failure has recently been intensively investigated. Some alterations of lipid parameters are noted very early in renal failure (9, 10) and particularly abnormalities of lipoprotein lipase activity and apolipoprotein composition may be found even in normolipidemic patients. The pattern of dyslipidemia in the uremic patients is modified by conditions like the nephrotic syndrome (11) and diabetes mellitus (12) (Figure 2). Specific lipoprotein abnormalities also exist in the trans-

Table 1. Lipid and lipoprotein abnormalities in renal failure

Parameter	Abnormality
Total lipids	Hyperlipoproteinemia, type IV
Lipid classes	Increased VLDL and IDL, decreased HDL
	Increased Lp(a)
Lipoprotein composition	Elevated TG in VLDL, IDL, LDL
	Elevated CHOL in VLDL and late prebeta lipoprotein (β-VLDL)
	Diminished CHOL in HDL
Apolipoproteins	Diminished apo-A1, apo-A2, increased apo-4 and apo-B-48
	Diminished apo-C2 and increased apo-C3 in HDL and VLDL
	Abnormal distribution of apo-A1
Enzymes	Diminished HDL, diminished (tissue level of) LPL, diminished LCAT

VLD: very low density lipoprotein; IDL: intermediate density lipoprotein; HDL: high density lipoprotein; TG: triglycerides; CHOL: cholesterol; apo: apolipoprotein; HTGL: hepatic triglyceride lipase; LPL: lipoprotein lipase; LCAT: lecithincholesterylacyl-transferase; LDL: low density lipoprotein.

planted patients as a result of steroid treatment and presumably also of cyclosporin A (13).

Dyslipoproteinemia can be categorized into abnormalities (i) of the lipid spectrum, (ii) of lipid subclasses according to flotation characteristics and (iii) apolipoprotein content (Table 1). In the fasting patient, one usually notes an increase in VLDL and IDL and decrease of HDL, suggesting delayed catabolism of endogenous lipoprotein particles. More recently, delayed clearance of exogenous lipoprotein particles, i.e., chylomicrons, with accumulation of chylomicron remnants has also been well documented (14). This is indicated by the presence of intestinal apolipoproteins AIV and B_{48}, which are not normally present in the fasting plasma (15).

Hepatogenic endogenous lipoprotein particles of intermediate density with abnormally slow migration on electrophoresis, so called late prebeta-particles, are the most common finding (16). Delayed interconversion of VLDL into IDL and finally LDL results also in low concentrations of HDL. Such abnormal interconversion and clearance of lipoprotein particles is the result of diminished activities of lipases including (i) consistently hepatic triglyceride lipase (16), (ii) somewhat less consistently tissue and circulating LPL (17, 18) and (iii) plasma lecithin:cholesterol-acyl-transferase activity (LCAT) (18).

Apart from such deficient enzymatic remodelling of circulating lipoprotein particles, tissue level handling of lipoprotein particles via LDL receptors (19) is reduced and conversely disposal of modified particles via the scavenger receptor, an important step in atherogenesis, is pre-

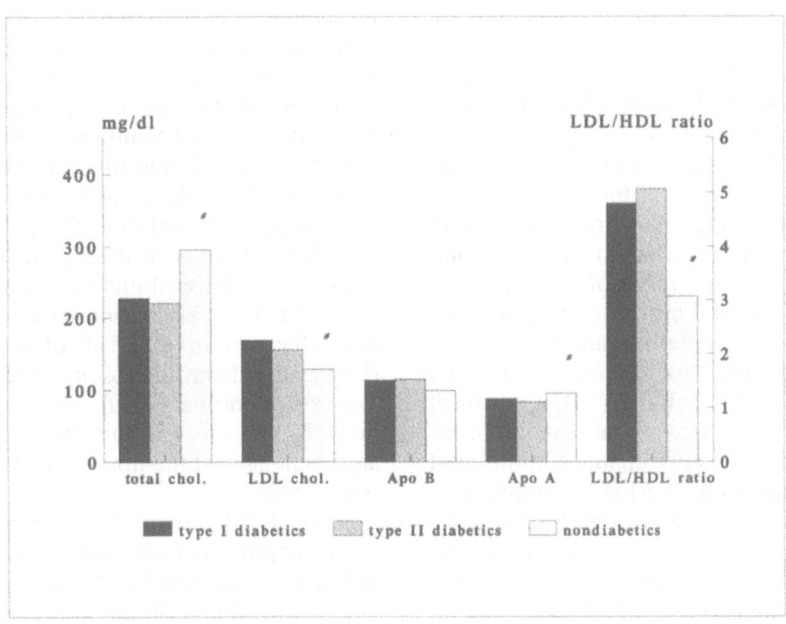

Figure 2. Lipid parameters in dialysis patients with type I or type II diabetes and in non-diabetic dialysis patients (after Tschöpe et al., ref. (12)). (# Significant difference between diabetic vs. non-diabetic patients)

sumably increased. It is of note that apolipoproteins are covalently modified in uremic patients, e.g., by carbamylation (20) and by glycosylation forming advanced glycosylation endproducts (21) and leads to diminished LDL uptake (18). In addition, further steps distal to lipoprotein lipase are altered as suggested by diminished fatty acid incorporation into adipose tissue of uremic subjects (22). Such tissue level abnormalities, not necessarily reflected in circulating lipid profile, may contribute importantly the atherogenic risk in uremia.

Apolipoproteins solubilize insoluble lipids and determine size, density and electrophoretic mobility of lipid particles. Apolipoproteins also determine the metabolic fate of particles by providing specific signals for interaction with cell surface receptors, thus regulating cellular uptake. Abnormal apolipoprotein composition is therefore of key importance for the understanding of the metabolic fate of lipoprotein particles in uremia. The main abnormalities of apolipoprotein composition are (i) diminution of apo-A_I and apo-A_{II} levels, (ii) variably diminished levels of apo-C_{II} (an activator of LPL) and elevation of apo-C_{III} (an inhibitor of LPL), (iii) variable concentrations of apo-E, some authors reporting increased levels (15) and abnormal partitioning between lipoprotein fractions (23), (iv) normal or slightly diminished concentrations of apolipoprotein B.

Of eminent importance is the recent demonstration that Lp(a), is consistently elevated in renal failure (24), independent of apo-a (25). This lipoprotein particle plays a major role in atherogenesis as documented by its highly atherogenic effects in transgenic animals (26). Lp(a) has

been shown to be an independent predictor of cardiac risk in uremic patients (27).

It is well established that oxidized lipoproteins are more atherogenic than native lipoproteins. It is therefore of note that, at least when measured with the thiobarbiturate method, high concentrations of oxidatively modified VLDL are found in dialysis patients (28, 29). The extent to which oxidative modification is favoured by diminished antioxidative capacity in renal failure (Selenium, Vitamin E, etc.) is currently under investigation. For further details several recent reviews in this field are recommended (30–34).

It has not been clearly established which (major) primary abnormality is responsible for delayed clearance and catabolism of endogenous and exogenous lipoprotein particles in renal failure. It is likely that the well known insulin resistance of renal failure, i.e. diminished peripheral action of insulin, is involved, since insulin is known to activate the lipoprotein lipase (35). In several studies a correlation was noted between immunoreactive insulin (IRI) levels and lipoprotein abnormalities (10). In some studies, PTH was also shown to be related to lipid disturbances (10, 36). Abnormal regulation of intracellular calcium in some target cells of lipid metabolism, as postulated by Mak and DeFronzo (37) is an attractive possibility to provide a mechanism for insulin resistance and dyslipidemia. Insulin resistance is improved by hemodialysis and several low molecular weight inhibitors of insulin-mediated (46) and non-insulin-mediated (47) glucose uptake have been recently recognized. In addition to such suggestive evidence for underlying hormonal disturbances, there is also some past (38) and more recent (39) evidence for circulating inhibitors of lipoprotein lipase.

Uncontrolled (40) and controlled (41) studies showed significant amelioration of dyslipidemia when high flux membranes were used, but the primary hypothesis, i.e., that postheparin LPL activity was improved, could not be directly proven (41). Other facets of the dialysis procedure do also impact on the lipid profile. Some (42) but not all (43) low molecular weight heparins ameliorate dyslipidemia in the dialysis patient as a result of their effect on lipoprotein lipase. Regional and systemic heparinisation had similar effects on lipid metabolism and heparin-free dialysis (with a proteinase inhibitor as anticoagulant) did not alter postheparin lipolytic activity (34). Controlled trials also documented that acetate as compared to bicarbonate hemodialysis, did not cause changes in the lipid spectrum (44, 45). Furthermore, CAPD, presumably as a consequence of glucose and calory overload and the ensuing stimulation of hepatic VLDL synthesis, aggravates hypertriglyceridemia. Total triglyceride and cholesterol values tend to be higher on CAPD/CCPD than on hemodialysis (46). Another feature may be peritoneal protein loss, although we found no correlation of lipid levels with protein loss or glucose uptake (34).

ATHEROGENESIS

A high prevalence of atherosclerosis of coronary and peripheral, i.e., carotid and iliac, arteries has been noted in several autopsy studies (49) and was also documented by examination of iliac artery specimens obtained at the time of transplantation (50) and by examination of dialysed patients by coronary angiography (51–54). Angiographic information is available (i) mainly from patients considered for transplantation and subjected to coronary arteriography irrespective of symptoms and (ii) from dialysis patients studied because of angina pectoris. Ikram et al. (51) found significant coronary artery disease in 10/32 patients, 31% of whom had double vessel and Z triple vessel disease. Hässler et al. (54) examined 100 patients prior to renal transplantation and found coronary heart disease in 64 patients; coronary artery stenosis (narrowing 70%) was found in 35 patients. The sensitivity (52%) and specificity (64%) of clinical symptoms was poor and this is also confirmed by observations of Rostand et al. (55, 56). Kramer et al. (52) performed coronary angiography in 29 dialysis patients considered for renal transplantation who had angina like chest pain and found coronary artery disease in only 7/29 patients. Although for obvious reasons systematic studies in asymptomatic patients are not available, it appears that the prevalence of significant coronary artery disease in non-diabetic dialysis patients in general is around 20–30%. The prevalence is significantly higher in diabetic patients (57, 58).

Less information is available concerning atheroma of iliac (50) and carotid arteries, although recent technolog-

ical advances in sonographic techniques have shown consistent and considerable abnormalities of carotid artery architecture in dialysed patients (59).

An important aspect is the question at what time in the course of renal failure such atheromas develop. Rostand et al. (55) found that a considerable proportion of dialysed patients developed ischemic heart disease during the first two years of dialysis. This is in agreement with our observations that of 89 patients with moderate renal failure 17 developed endstage renal failure over a three year period of observation while 12 died, most of them of cardiac causes (60). This observation suggest that the risk to suffer from atherosclerotic disease is high early on. The rate of coronary death does not increase with time on dialysis, however (5), this observation provides a strong argument against the notion of accelerated atherogenesis (see above).

Several risk factors for atherosclerotic disease have been recognized in dialysed patients particularly age (50) and diabetes mellitus (57, 58). Recently, Manske (61) provided clinical algorithms to predict the coronary risk in dialysed patients with type I diabetes. Similar algorithms in the non-diabetic patient are sorely needed.

The above epidemiological observations of a high prevalence of atheroma in the dialysis population raises the issue of other specific acceleration of atherogenesis exists which is related to uremia. Interestingly, despite the occurrence of dyslipoproteinemia in uremic animals, atherosclerotic lesions are not a consistent feature, but interpretation must be cautious in view of potential species differences. Horsch et al. (62) examined subtotaled nephrectomized rats the endothelial cells of which had been subjected to immunological injury. The animals were on an atherogenic diet. Despite severe hyperlipoproteinemia aortic wall lipid content was not elevated and no lesions in the aorta were found by histology. Similarly, Kamstrup et al. (63) found no intimal lesions and no cholesterol accumulation in uremic rabbits with long-term uremia. Aortic calcification, but no net cholesterol accumulation, was noted. In another study, coronary but not aortic lesions, were found in uremic rabbits (64).

It would be naive to consider atherogenesis only as the passive direct result of insulation of lipid loaden serum into the vessel wall. In its genesis functional or structural injury to endothelial cells and interactions between monocytes or platelets and the vessel wall play major roles. Subsequently, local cell proliferation and matrix deposition occur, and the ultimate result is the complicated exulcerating plaque. It is important to have in mind the complete evolution of the atherosclerotic lesion, because – at least in principle – renal failure may affect the early and the advanced (complicated) lesion in a different fashion. For instance atherosclerotic coronary lesions appear to be more frequently calcified in uremic compared non-uremic patients (65). Calcifying atherosclerotic coronary lesions are related not only to lipid concentrations, but also to the Ca-P product (unpublished observations). After PTCA

Table 2. Proatherogenic and antiatherogenic features of the uremic syndrome

Proatherogenic
- Dyslipoproteinemia incl. elevated Lp(a)
- Oxidized lipoproteins
- Modified apolipoproteins (carbamylation, glycosylation)
- Elevated insulin
- Homocysteinemia
- AGE (advanced glycosylation end)-products
- Inhibition of NO-synthase
- Local complement activation (cumulation of factor D)

Antiatherogenic
- Diminished platelet, macrophage and granulocyte function
- Increased prostacyclin, diminished thromboxane synthesis
- Reduced concentration of active vitamin D

the one year reocclusion rate is 70% in uremic patients (66), worse than in any other high risk category including diabetes. This observation is consistent with the presence of progressive advanced lesions in uremia.

The dialysed uremic patient is exposed to a number of potentially proatherogenic insults which shall not be discussed in detail (Table 2). These include, apart from dyslipoproteinemia and particularly elevated Lp(a) (see above) the following: (i) the presence of oxidized lipoproteins (28, 29), (ii) the presence of apolipoproteins modified by carbamylation (20) or glycosylation (21), (iii) elevated levels of insulin, a vascular growth factor, (iv) elevated levels of homocystein (67), injurious to vascular integrity as shown by accelerated atherosis in since congenital hyperhomocysteinemia promotes atherogenesis, (v) accumulation of AGE peptides and proteins, which not only cross-link structural proteins in the vessel wall, but also activate endothelial cells and induce cytokine formation, glycosylated AGE products are removed by hemofiltration, but not by hemodialysis (70), (vi) inhibition of NO synthase by asymmetric dimethyl-L-arginin (68), a novel uremic toxin. This may be relevant for atherogenesis, because NO is inhibitory to vascular smooth muscle cell proliferation, a key step in atherogenesis (5). The situation may even be more complex: the observation of reduced responsiveness to NO, at least in some vascular beds, raises the possibility of additional NO resistance (69). (vii) Finally factor D of the complement system cumulates in renal failure (5); it is removed by hemofiltration, but not by hemodialysis (71). Factor D causes continuous subthreshold activation of the complement system and amplifies complement-mediated injury. This may be important because local complement activation is known to occur in atherosclerotic lesions (72). (viii) Although the

evidence for increased atherosclerotic risk from smoking in dialysis patients is not perfectly clear (73), it deserves mentioning that the half life of nicotine is prolonged in renal failure (74).

In order to avoid oversimplification and expose the complexity of the situation in uremia, it should be pointed out that several features might counterbalance low proatherogenetic stimuli in renal failure, e.g., disturbed platelet, macrophage and granulocyte function or increased prostacyclin (PGI$_2$) and diminished thromboxane synthesis by platelets of uremic patients (75). Calcium and calcium-dependent steps play a key role in the development of the atherosclerotic plaque (34) and low concentrations of the active metabolite of vitamin D, a known proatherogenic agent, may be partially protective.

IS THERE A CORRELATION BETWEEN HIGH LIPID CONCENTRATIONS AND CARDIOVASCULAR DEATH?

In view of the potential atherogenicity of dyslipidemia, as discussed above, it is surprising to see that several authors found no relation between dyslipidemia and cardiac death (50, 55); even a paradoxically inverse relation was noted by others (76–79). As shown in Table 3 the French Diaphane Study (77) found that with increasing cholesterol concentration total and cardiovascular mortality was paradoxically decreased. This observation has recently been confirmed by Avram et al. (78) who found that in survivors on hemodialysis total cholesterol and apolipoprotein B concentrations were significantly higher than in patients dying from cardiac causes. That the expected relation between lipidemia and cardiac (or coronary) death is not present may be explained by a confounding factor. Recently, the overriding importance of malnutrition has been well documented for survival in dialysis patients (80, 81). It is therefore of note that in the New York patient sample a positive relation was found between S-albumin and cardiac death and an inverse one between cholesterol and cardiac death (79).

Lower total and cardiovascular mortality in patients with higher cholesterol levels do of course not negate a deleterious effect of high lipid levels. First, in dialysis patients more sophisticated indices of dyslipidemia, e.g., Lp(a) (27) and apolipoprotein A I/C III ratios (23) are correlated to cardiac survival and vascular disease respectively. Furthermore, in an segment of the dialysis population with excessive cardiac risk, i.e., in diabetic patients, Tschöpe et al. (12) found in a prospective study that lipid levels at the start of dialysis were highly predictive of subsequent myocardial infarction in type I and type II diabetics and sudden death in type II diabetics (Table 4).

The pathway(s) through which the effect of malnutrition on mortality (and presumably also cardiac mortality), is mediated are currently unknown. It has recently been

Table 3. Lipid values in diabetic patients dying from cardiac causes (myocardial infarction/sudden death) and in survivors. After Tschöpe et al., ref. (12)

	Type I diabetes		Type II diabetes	
	MI (n = 8)	survivors (n = 38)	MI (n = 10)	survivors (n = 64)
Total cholesterol	278[a] (224–293)	228 (148–329)	253 (126–300)	221 (66–372)
LDL-cholesterol	197 (156–243)	163 (89–322)	168 (91–256)	153 (43–295)
LDL/HDL cholesterol ratio	6.0[a] (5.3–8.6)	4.4 (2.4–8.3)	4.4 (3.1–9.1)	4.9 (1.5–11.9)

[a] $p < 0.05$ (difference between respective group and survivors).

Table 4. Therapeutic strategies to treat dyslipidemia

Non-pharmacological
– diet, physical exercise

Pharmacological
– fibrates (prodrugs)
– statines
– nicotinic acid derivatives
– bile acid sequesterants, e.g. cholestyramine
– omega-3-eicosapentenic acid (fish oil)

Other
– LDL apheresis

Table 5. Strategies to reduce atherosclerotic target organ damage

– Ischemia tolerance (CEI, CCB)
– Reversal of anemia (Epo)
– Pharmacological modification of aortic elasticity (CEI, CCB)
– Pre- and afterload reduction (volume control, antihypertensive treatment, CEI)
– Exercise
– Aspirin

proposed (82) that the effect is mediated, at least in part, through an adverse effect of low substrate concentration, i.e., low L-arginine levels on generation of NO via NO synthase. In uremia, the activity of NO synthase is inhibited by a circulating inhibitor and such competitive inhibition may render the enzyme activity more susceptible to changes in substrate concentration (68). NO inhibits, and its absence may favour, proliferation of cells in the vessel wall.

INTERVENTION

Here we discuss separately (i) prevention of atherogenesis by modulating dyslipidemia (Table 5); the potential roles of controlling blood pressure and eliminating other risk factors like smoking shall not be discussed here; and (ii) mitigation of the effects of atherosclerosis on target organ damage (Table 6). Interventions to restore paten-

cy of the coronary and other vascular beds by PTCA or bypass surgery are discussed elsewhere in this volume.

Diet and drug therapy

Both in experimental (83) and clinical studies (84–87) serum lipids were found to respond to dietary manipulation in hyperlipidemic uremic animals and humans respectively. Lowering of fasting or postprandial plasma triglycerides in response to diets with low carbohydrate, low cholesterol content and a high polyunsaturated/saturated fat (P/S) ratio (84) and in response to diets with selectively low carbohydrate content (85) was described by San Felippo et al. in non-dialysed and dialysed patients respectively. Similar observations by Cattran (86) and Yasugi (87) also document a decrease of VLDL and LDL and an increase of HDL in response to low carbohydrate high P/S diets. After institution of a low carbohydrate diet, a significant reduction in serum triglycerides with no change of extrahepatic and hepatic postheparin lipolytic activity was further demonstrated in Japanese patients with renal failure (88).

While the above dietary intervention trials document the efficacy of dietary intervention, they do not answer

Table 6. Factors increasing the susceptibility of the heart to ischemic injury in renal failure

- Left ventricular hypertrophy (LVH)
- Aortic stiffness
    * pulsatile LV workload
    * diastolic coronary perfusion
- Coronary reserve
    * LV
    * anemia
    * compromised microcirculation (arterioles, capillaries)
    * impaired vasodilatation (autocaoids)
- Metabolism
    * insulin mediated glucose uptake
    * creatine phosphate
    * intracellular calcium
- Automatic innervation
    * sympathetic overactivity
    * autonomic imbalance

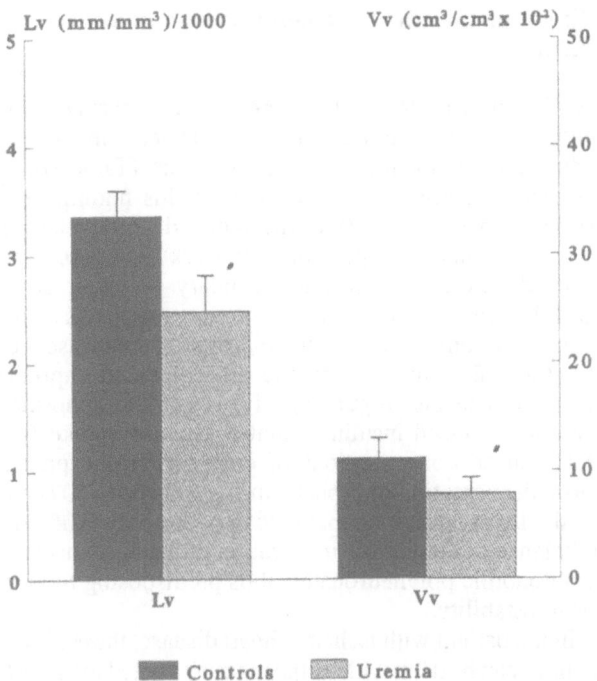

Figure 3. Reduced capillary density in the myocardium of uremic rats (after Amann et al., ref (106)). Note induced length density (LV), i.e., total capillary length per unit volume, and volume density of capillary lumina, e.g., capillary volume per unit volume of heart, in uremic animals vs. controls. Analogous changes were not seen in animals hypertensive from other causes and comparable LV hypertrophy.

the crucial question whether the hypothetical benefit on atherogenesis outweighs costs and potential hazards of such diets. Uremic patients are frequently anorectic and easily become malnourished when put on restricted diets. Longterm palatability and acceptability of modified diets are difficult to achieve in uremic patients (89) and clinical nephrologists have been decidedly non-enthusiastic to prescribe such modified diets. A particular point of concern is that malnutrition has recently been shown to be a potent predictor of death on dialysis (90), adding weight to the argument that avoidance of malnutrition must be absolutely ensured if dietary intervention is considered.

Another non-pharmacological approach to lower plasma lipids is exercise training (91). Twelve months of endurance training, e.g. cycling, walking and jogging increased glucose disappearance rate by 18%, lowered fasting insulin levels by 52% and decreased plasma triglycerides by 23% with a concomitant increase in HDL cholesterol.

When should one consider pharmacological intervention? The consideration of the pathogenesis of dyslipidemia in renal failure, i.e., impaired catabolism of lipoprotein particles, would argue for the use of fibrates. Clofibrate (92), bezafibrate, gemfibrocil (93) and clinofibrate (94) have been used in renal patients. Enthusiasm for their use has been tempered by the fact that fibrates, with the exception of clinofibrate (94) are prodrugs. The active metabolites are excreted via the kidney and cumulation in renal patients may cause myotoxicity (95).

Nicotinic acid derivatives are notoriously poorly tolerated and cholestyramine, though very effective, causes a high rate of gastro-intestinal side effects particularly in uremic patients. Recently, Wanner et al. (96) showed that

statines, i.e. HMG-CoA-reductase inhibitors are remarkably safe in hypercholesterolemic patients on hemodialysis (96) and this observation has been confirmed (97, 98). It is reasonable to administer statines in patients who have elevated total cholesterol, e.g., above 250 mg/dl and particularly elevated LDL cholesterol, e.g., above 160 mg/dl. Decision thresholds for drug intervention should even be lower if patients have additional risks, e.g., excessive Lp(a) concentrations, familial history of coronary heart disease, preexistent ischemic heart disease etc. Patients should be monitored for muscle enzymes (CK-aldolase) and hepatic enzymes (gamma-GT) to avoid toxicity.

Fish oil has repeatedly been recommended for the treatment of dyslipidemia in renal failure (99). These compounds are not inert and do have considerable side effects. They are easily oxidized and provide considerable caloric intake (99, 100).

In exceptional cases of severe hyperlipoproteinemia, unresponsive to other measures, LDL apheresis may be considered (101).

Mitigating the effect of atherosclerosis on target organs

As discussed in detail elsewhere (4), high cardiac mortality in the dialysis patient is due, at least in part, to reduced ischemia tolerance of the heart (Table 6). A number of factors are responsible for this finding, e.g., (i) LV hypertrophy (102), (ii) reduced aortic elasticity causing increased pulsatile LV work load (103) and reduced coronary perfusion secondary to lower aortic diastolic pressure, (iii) reduced coronary reserve as a consequence of anemia (104) and microvascular disease, i.e., structural abnormalities on the arteriolar and capillary (105, 106) levels (Figure 3), (iv) metabolic abnormalities like reduced insulin-mediated glucose uptake (46) and reduced concentrations of energy-rich phosphates, particulars creatine-phosphate during ischemia (107) and (v) finally excessive sympathetic nerve activity (108) and imbalance of autonomic innervation of the heart because of autonomic polyneuropathy, thus predisposing to electrical instability.

In the patient with ischemic heart disease, these abnormalities can be dealt with by the measures listed in Table 6. In addition, in view of disturbed autonomic innervation one should consider administration of betablockers.

REFERENCES

1. Lindner A, Charra B, Sherrard D, Scribner BM: Accelerated atherosclerosis in prolonged maintenance hemodialysis. *N Engl J Med* 290: 697, 1974
2. Combined Report on Regular Dialysis and Transplantation in Europe XXII, 1991: *Nephrol Dial Transplant* 7 (Suppl 2): 5, 1992
3. Ritz E, Strumpf C, Katz F, Wing AJ, Quellhorst E: Hypertension and cardiovascular risk factors in hemodialyzed diabetic patients. *Hypertension* 7 (Suppl II): II-118, 1985
4. Ritz E, Wiecek A, Rambausek M: Cardiovascular death in patients with end-stage renal failure; strategies for prevention. *International Yearbook Nephrol Dial Transplant* 9 (Suppl): 120, 1994
5. Ritz E, Deppisch R, Stier E, Hansch G: Atherogenesis and cardiac death: are they related to dialysis procedures and biocompatibility? *Nephrol Dial Transplant* 9 (Suppl 2): 165, 1994
6. Bright R: *Response of Medical Cases Selected with a View of Illustrating the Symptoms and Cures of Diseases by Reference to Morbid Anatomy*, London, Longman, Rus Orme, Brown and Greene, 1827
7. Bloor WR: The blood lipids in nephritis. *J Biol Chem* 31: 575, 1917
8. Bagdade JD, Shafrir E, Wilson D: Mechanism(s) of hyperlipidemia in chronic uremia. *Trans Am Soc Artif Organs* 22: 42, 1976
9. Gnasso A, Haberbosch W, Augustin J, Ritz E: Abnormal lipoprotein metabolism in incipient renal failure. *Proc EDTA-ERA* 22: 1129, 1985
10. Attman PO, Alaupovic P: Lipid and apolipoprotein profiles of uremic dyslipoproteinemia – relation to renal function and dialysis. *Nephron* 57: 401, 1991
11. Kaysen GA, Pan XM, Couser WG, Staprans I: Defective lipolysis persists in hearts of rats with Heymann nephritis in the absence of nephrotic plasma. *Am J Kidney Dis* 22: 128, 1993
12. Tschöpe W. Koch M, Thomas B, Ritz E: Serum lipids predict cardiac death in diabetic patients on maintenance hemodialysis (results of a prospective study). *Nephron* 64: 354, 1993
13. Vathsala A, Weinberg RB, Schoenberg L et al.: Lipid abnormalities in cyclosporine-prednisone treated renal transplant recipients. *Transplantation* 48: 37, 1989
14. Weintraub M, Burstein A, Rassin T et al.: Severe defect in clearing postprandial chylomicron remnants in dialysis patients. *Kidney Int* 42: 1247, 1992
15. Nestel PJ, Fidge NH, Tan MH: Increased lipoprotein-remnant formation in chronic renal failure. *N Engl J Med* 307: 329, 1982
16. Mordasini R, Frey F, Flury W, Klose G, Greten H: Selective deficiency of hepatic triglyceride lipase in uremic patients. *N Engl J Med* 297: 1362, 1977
17. Druml W, Zechner R, Magometschnigg D: Post-heparin lipolytic activity in acute renal failure. *Clin Nephrol* 23: 289, 1985
18. Gonen B, Goldberg AP, Harter HR, Schonfeld G: Abnormal cell-interactive properties of low-density lipoproteins isolated from patients with chronic renal failure. *Metabolism* 34: 10, 1985
19. Takemura T, Yoshioka K, Aya N: Apolipoproteins and lipoprotein receptors in glomeruli in human kidney diseases. *Kidney Int* 43: 918, 1993
20. Hörkko S, Savolainen MJ, Kervinen K, Kesäniemi YA: Carbamylation-induced alterations in low-density lipoprotein metabolism. *Kidney Int* 41: 1175, 1992
21. Ritz E, Deppisch R, Nawroth P: Toxicity of uraemia – does it come of AGE. *Nephrol Dial Transplant* 9: 1, 1994
22. Walidius G, Norbeck JE: Effective fatty acid incorporation into adipose tissue (FIAT) in uremic subjects with hypertriglyceridemia. *Eur J Clin Invest* 8: 346, 1978
23. Attman PO, Alaupovic P, Gustafson A: Serum apolipoprotein profile of patients with chronic renal failure. *Kidney Int* 32: 368, 1987
24. Webb AT, Reaveley DA, O'Donnell M, O'Connor B, Seed M, Brown EA: Lipoprotein (a) in patients on maintenance haemodialysis and continuous ambulatory peritoneal dialysis. *Nephrol Dial Transplant* 8: 609, 1993
25. Dieplinger H, Lackner C, Kronenberg F et al.: Elevated plasma concentrations of lipoprotein (a) in patients with end-stage renal disease are not related to the size polymorphism of apolipoprotein (a). *J Clin Invest* 91: 397, 1993
26. Scott J: Arterial hardening in mice. *Nature* 360: 631, 1992
27. Cressman MD, Heyka RJ, Paganini EP, O'Neil J, Skibinski CI, Hoff HF: Lipoprotein (a) is an independent risk factor for cardiovascular disease in hemodialysis patients. *Circulation* 86: 475, 1992
28. Daerr WH, Windler ETE, Greten H: Peroxidative modification of very-low density lipoproteins in chronic hemodialysis patients. *Nephron* 63: 230, 1993
29. Paul JL, Sail ND, Soni T et al.: Lipid peroxidation abnormalities in hemodialyzed patients. *Nephron* 64: 106, 1993

30. Guijarro C, Keane WF: Lipid abnormalities and changes in plasma proteins in glomerular diseases and chronic renal failure. *Curr Opinion in Nephrol Hypertens* 2: 372, 1993

31. Kasiske BL, O'Donnell MP, Cowardin W, Keane WF: Lipids and the kidney. *Hypertension* 15: 443, 1990

32. Walli AK, Gröne E, Miller B. Gröne HJ, Thiery J, Seidel D: Role of lipoproteins in progressive renal disease. *Am J Hypertens* 6: 358S, 1993

33. Maggi E, Bellazzi R, Falaschi F et al.: Enhanced LDL oxidation in uremic patients: an additional mechanism for accelerated atherosclerosis. *Kidney Int* 45: 876, 1994

34. Ritz E, Querfeld U: Atherosclerosis – is it accelerated in uremia? *Semin Dial* 2: 246, 1989

35. Attman PO, Nyberg G, William-Olsson T, Knight-Gibson C, Alaupovic P: Dyslipoproteinemia in diabetic renal failure. *Kidney Int* 42: 1381, 1992

36. Massry SG, Akmal M: Lipid abnormalities, renal failure and parathyroid hormone. *Am J Med* 87 (Suppl 5): 42N, 1989

37. Mak RHK, DeFronzo RA: Glucose and insulin metabolism in uremia. *Nephron* 61: 377, 1992

38. Cattran DC, Fenton SA, Wilson DR, Steiner G: Defective triglyceride removal in lipemia associated with peritoneal dialysis and hemodialysis. *Ann Intern Med* 85: 29, 1976

39. Chan MK, Persaud J, Varghese Z, Moorhead JF: Pathogenic roles of post-heparin lipases in lipid abnormalities in hemodialysis patients. *Kidney Int* 25: 812, 1984

40. Josephson MA, Fellner SK, Dasguptam A: Improved lipid profiles in patients undergoing high-flux hemodialysis. *Am J Kidney Dis* 20: 361, 1992

41. Blankestijn PJ, Vos PF, Rabelink AJ, van Rijn H, Jansen H, Koomans HA: High-flux dialysis membranes improve lipid profiles in hemodialysis patients. *J Am Soc Nephrol* 4: 334A, 1993

42. Akiba T, Tachibana K, Ozawa K et al.: Long-term use of low molecular weight heparin ameliorates hyperlipidemia in patients on hemodialysis. *ASAIO J* 38: M326, 1992

43. Schrader J, Stibbe W, Armstrong VW et al.: Comparison of low-molecular weight heparin to standard heparin in hemodialysis/hemofiltration. *Kidney Int* 33: 890, 1988

44. Heuck CC, Ritz E: Hyperlipoproteinemia in renal insufficiency. *Nephron* 25: 1, 1980

45. Kluge R, Heuck CC, Ritz E: Lipidstoffwechsel unter Bikarbonatdialyse. *Nieren Hochdruckkrankheiten* 13: 143, 1984

46. DeFronzo RA, Tobin JD, Rowe JW, Adres R: Glucose intolerance of uremia. Quantification of pancreatic beta cell sensitivity to glucose and tissue sensitivity to insulin. *J Clin Invest* 62: 425, 1978

47. Maloff B, Lockwood D: Cellular basis for insulin resistance in uremia. *Diabetes* 30 (Suppl 1): 28, 1981

48. Ramos JM, Hetaon A, McGurk JG, Ward MK, Kerr DNS: Sequential changes in serum lipids and their subfractions in patients receiving continuous ambulatory peritoneal dialysis. *Nephron* 33: 20, 1983

49. Clyne N, Lind LE, Pehrsson K: Ischemic heart disease in uremia. *Proc EDTA-ERA* 20: 25A, 1983

50. Vincenti F, Amend WJ, Abele J, Feduska NJ, Salvatierra O: The role of hypertension in hemodialysis-associated atherosclerosis. *Am J Med* 68: 363, 1980

51. Ikram H, Lynn KL, Bailey RR, Littel PJ: Cardiovascular changes in chronic hemodialysis patients. *Kid Int* 24: 371, 1983

52. Kramer W, Thormann J, Kindler M, Müller K, Wizemann W: Uramische Herzkrankheit. II. Ventrikeldynamik bei terminaler Niereninsuffizienz im Vergleich zur idiopathisch-dilatativen Kardiomyopathie. *Med Welt* 36: 1317, 1985

53. Braun WE, Phillips D, Vidt DG et al.: Coronary artery disease in terminal renal failure. *Transplant Proc* 113: 128, 1981

54. Hässler R, Hofling B, Castro L et al.: Koronare Herzkrankheit und Herzklappenerkrankung bei Patienten mit terminaler Niereninsuffizlenz. *Dtsch Med Wschr* 112: 714, 1987

55. Rostand SG, Kirk KA, Rutsky EA: Dialysis-associated ischemic heart disease: insights form coronary angiography. *Kidney Int* 25: 653, 1984

56. Rostand SG, Rutsky EA: Ischemic heart disease in chronic renal failure. *Sem Dial* 2: 98, 1989

57. Bennet WM, Kloster F, Rosch J et al.: Natural history of asymptomatic coronary arteriographic lesions in diabetic patients with end-stage renal disease. *Am J Med* 15: 779, 1978

58. Braun WE, Phillips DF, Vidt DT et al.: Coronary disease in 100 diabetics with end-stage renal failure. *Transplant Proc* 16: 603, 1984

59. Ansari A, Kaupke CJ, Vaziri ND, Miller R, Barbari A: Cardiac pathology in patients with end-stage renal disease maintained on hemodialysis. *Int J Artif Organs* 16: 31, 1993

60. Fliser D, Schweizer C, Ritz E: How many patients with renal insufficiency survive until end-stage renal failure (letter). *Nephrol Dial Transplant* 6: 600, 1991

61. Manske CL, Thomas W, Wang Y, Wilson RF: Screening diabetic transplant candidates for coronary artery disease: identification of a low risk group. *Kidney Int* 44: 617, 1993

62. Horsch A, Ritz E, Heuck CC, Hofmann W, Kuhne E, Bisson M: Atherogenesis in experimental uremia. *Atherosclerosis* 40: 279, 1981

63. Kamstrup P, Tyedegaard E, Stender S: Effect of chronic uremia on plasma lipids and the aortic accumulation of cholesterol in hypercholesterolemic rabbits. *Nephron* 26: 280, 1980

64. Kamstrup O, Tvedegaard E: Increased uptake of cholesterol and increased mineral content in the aorta of long-term uremic rabbits. *Nephron* 33: 267, 1983

65. Fiegel P, Abdelhamid S, Meves M, Walb D, Thomas L: HDL- und LDL-Cholesterin und Gefäßverkalkungen bei Dialysepatienten. Dialysenarztetreffen Innsbruck, 1982

66. Rinehart AL, Herzog CA, Collins AJ, Flack JM, Ma JZ, Opsahl JA: Greater risk of cardiac events after coronary angioplasty (PTCA) than bypass grafting (CABG) in chronic dialysis patients. *J Am Soc Nephrol* 3: 389, 1992

67. Chauveau P, Chadefaux B, Coude M et al.: Hyperhomocysteinemia, a risk factor for atherosclerosis in chronic uremic patients. *Kidney Int* 43 (Suppl 41): S72, 1993

68. Vallance P, Leone A, Calver A, Collier J, Moncada S: Accumulation of an endogenous inhibitor of nitric oxide synthesis in chronic renal failure. *Lancet* 339: 572, 1992

69. Wystrychowski A, Strauss H, Wagner J, Haufe CC, Ganten D, Ritz E: Decreased responsiveness of the renal vasculature to inhibition of nitric oxide (NO) after subtotal nephrectomy. *J Am Soc Nephrol* 3: 557A, 1992

70. Makita Z, Bucala R, Raufield EJ et al.: Efficiency of removal of circulating advanced glycosylation end products and mode of treatment in patients with ESRD. *J Am Soc Nephrol* 4: 335A, 1992

71. Kaiser JP, Götze O, Göhl H, Asmus G, Schäfer K: Hemofiltration but not hemodialysis leads to an impressive reduction of factor D in uremia. *J Am Soc Nephrol* 3: 372A, 1992

72. Seifert PS, Messner M, Roth J, Bhakdi S: Analysis of complement C3 activation product in human atherosclerotic lesions. *Atherosclerosis* 91: 155, 1991

73. Freemen DJ, Griffin BA, Murray E et al.: Smoking and plasma lipoproteins in man: effects on low-density lipoprotein cholestrol levels and high density lipoprotein subfraction distribution. *Eur J Clin Invest* 23: 630, 1993

74. Davis JW, Arnold J, Wiegemann T: Cigarette smoking affects platelet and endothelium in chronic hemodialysis patients. *Nephron* 64: 359, 1993

75. Remuzzi G, Benigni A, Dodesini P et al.: Reduced platelet thromboxane formation in uremia. *J Clin Invest* 71: 762, 1983

76. Koch M, Thomas B, Tschöpe W, Ritz E: Survival and predictors of death in dialysed diabetic patients. *Diabetologia* 36: 1113, 1993

77. Degoulet P, Legrain M, Reach J, Aime F, Devries C, Rojas P, Jacobs C: Mortality risk factors in patients treated by chronic hemodialysis. Report of the Diaphane collaborative study. *Nephron* 31: 103, 1982

78. Avram MM, Goldwasser P, Burrell DE, Antignani A, Fein PA, Mittman N: The uremic dyslipidemia: a cross-sectional and longitudinal study. *Am J Kidney Dis* 10: 324, 1992

79. Goldwasser P, Michel MA, Collier J: Prealbumin and lipoprotein (a) in hemodialysis: relationships with patients and vascular access survival. *Am J Kidney Dis* 22: 215, 1993

80. Lowrie EG, Lew NL, Huang WH: Race and diabetes as death risk predictors in hemodialysis patients. *Kidney Int* 42: 22, 1992

81. Held P, Blagg C, Liska DW, Port FK, Hakim R, Levin N: The dose of hemodialysis according to dialysis prescription in Europe and the United States. *Kidney Int* 42: 16, 1992

82. Ritz E, Vallance P, Nowicki M: The effect of malnutrition on cardiovascular mortality in dialysis patients: is L-arginine the answer? *Nephrol Dial Transplant* 9: 129, 1994

83. Heuck CC, Ritz E, Liersch M, Mehls O: Serum lipids in renal insufficiency. *Am J Clin Nutr* 31: 1547, 1978

84. Sanfelippo ML, Swenson RS, Reaven GM: Reduction of plasma triglycerides by diet in subjects with chronic renal failure. *Kidney Int* 11: 54, 1977

85. Sanfelippo ML, Swenson RS, Reaven GM: Response of plasma triglycerides to dietary change in patients on hemodialysis. *Kidney Int* 14: 180, 1978

86. Cattran DC, Steiner G, Fenion SSA, Ampil M: Dialysis hyperlipemia: response to dietary manipulation. *Clin Nephrol* 13: 177, 1980

87. Yasugi T: Effect of dietary treatment on lipolytic activities and lipids and lipoproteins in patients with uremia. in *Atherosclerosis*, edited by Schettler G, Goho AM, Habernicht AGR, Gjuricka KR, Springer Verlag, Berlin, 1983, p 251

88. Okubo M, Tsukamoto Y, Yoneda T, Hommma Y, Nakamura H, Marumo F: Deranged fat metabolism and the lowering effect of carbohydrate poor diet on serum triglycerides in patients with chronic renal failure. *Nephron* 25: 8, 1980

89. Ritz E, Augustin J, Bommer J, Gnasso A, Haberbosch W: Should hyperlipemia of renal failure be treated? *Kidney Int* 28: S84, 1985

90. Goldwasser P, Mittman N, Antignati A et al.: Predictors of mortality in hemodialysis patients. *J Am Soc Nephrol* 3: 1613, 1993

91. Goldberg AP, Geltman EM, Gavin JR et al.: Exercise training reduces coronary risk and effectively rehabilitates hemodialysis patients. *Nephron* 42: 311, 1986

92. Pierides AM, Alverez-Ude F, Kerr DNS: Clofibrate induced muscle damage in patients with chronic renal failure. *Lancet* 2: 1279, 1975

93. Pasternack A, Vänttinen T, Solakivi T, Kuusi T, Korte T: Normalization of lipoprotein lipase and hepatic lipase by gemfimbrozil results in correction of lipoprotein abnormalities in chronic renal failure. *Clin Nephrol* 27: 163, 1987

94. Nishizawa Y, Shoji T, Nishitani H et al.: Hypertriglyceridemia and lowered apolipoprotein C-II/CC-III ratio in uremia, effect of a fibric acid, clinofibrate. *Kidney Int* 44: 1352, 1993

95. Kijima Y, Sasaoka T, Kanayama M, Kubota S: Untoward effects of clofibrate in hemodialyzed patients. *N Engl J Med* 296: 515, 1977

96. Wanner C, Hörl W, Luley CH, Wieland H: Effects of HMG-CoA reductase inhibitors in hypercholesterolemic patients on hemodialysis. *Kidney Int* 39: 754, 1991

97. Grundy SM: Management of hyperlipidemia of kidney disease. *Kidney Int* 37: 847, 1990

98. Fiorini F, Patrone E, Ardu F, Castellucio A: Efficacy and safety of simvastatin in the treatment of hyperlipidemia in uremic patients undergoing hemodialysis. *Minerva Urol Nephrol* 44: 165, 1992

99. Bilo HJG, Homan van der Heide JJ, Gans ROB, Donker AJM: Omega-3 polyunsaturated fatty acids in chronic renal insufficiency. *Nephron* 57: 385, 1991

100. Scharchmidt LA, Gibbons NB, McGarry L et al.: Effects of dietary fish oil on renal insufficiency in rats with subtotal nephrectomy. *Kidney Int* 32: 700, 1987

101. Bosch T, Thiery J, Gurland HJ, Seidel D: Long-term efficiency, biocompatibility, and clinical safety of combined simultaneous LDL-apheresis and haemodialysis in patients with hypercholesterolaemia and end-stage renal failure. *Nephrol Dial Transplant* 8: 1350, 1993

102. Silberberg JS, Barre PE, Pichard SS, Sniderman AD: Impact of left ventricular hypertrophy on survival in end-stage renal disease. *Kidney Int* 36: 286, 1989

103. London G, Guerin A, Pannier B, Marchais S, Benetos S, Safar M: Increased systolic pressure in chronic uremia. Role of arterial wave reflections. *Hypertension* 20: 10, 1992

104. Wizemann V, Kaufmann J, Kramer W: Effect of erythropoietin on ischemia tolerance in anemic hemodialysis

patients with confirmed coronary artery disease. *Nephron* 62: 161, 1992

105. Amann K, Wiest G, Irzyniec T, Neusüß R, Ritz E, Mall G: Changes of vascular architecture independent of blood pressure in experimental uremia. *J Hypertens* In press

106. Amann K, Wiest G, Zimmer G, Gretz N, Ritz E, Mall G: Reduced capillary density in the myocardium of uremic rats. A stereological study. *Kidney Int* 42: 1079, 1992

107. Cleminson WG, Manchester KL, Diesel WJ, Margolins LP: Adenine nucleotide concentrations and energy charge in muscle of chronic haemodialysis patients. *Nephron* 60: 232, 1992

108. Bigazzi R, Kosogov E, Campese VM: Increased sympathetic nervous system activity and hypertension in rats with chronic renal failure. *J Am Soc Nephrol* 4: 507A, 1994

ORGAN AND METABOLIC COMPLICATIONS: ACID-BASE

MARIANO FERIANI, CLAUDIO RONCO, ALDO FABRIS and GIUSEPPE LA GRECA

INTRODUCTION

Since the earliest experiences with hemodialysis, the correction of uremic acidosis has represented a complex problem still not completely resolved.

Kolff in 1943 (1), and later Scribner (2) et al., used a dialysis solution with 27 mmol/l of bicarbonate as a buffer. Bicarbonate containing dialysate was prepared in large containers before the dialysis session thus creating problems related to calcium and magnesium precipitation, easy bacterial contamination and, finally, to the rate of delivery, limited to 500 ml/min.

In 1964, in Seattle, Mion et al. (3) introduced the use of acetate as alkaline equivalent in the dialysis fluid. Acetate containing solutions were easily prepared, chemically stable and microbiologically safe. Rapidly, acetate solutions became widely applied in clinical dialysis being used world wide for more than 20 years. The low cost, the equimolar conversion to bicarbonate in the body and the bacteriostatic effect in the solution, made acetate a first choice substrate for the correction of acid-base derangements in hemodialysis. Acetate solutions rendered hemodialysis more simple thus stimulating the proliferation of renal replacement therapy.

In the late 1970s, new dialytic strategies, based on more efficient dialyzers and highly permeable membranes, that increased dialysis efficiency and shortened treatment time uncovered technical and clinical limitations imposed by acetate. Hence, the use of bicarbonate in clinical dialysis has been reintroduced recently, supported by new procedures of dialysate preparation, mixing and delivery. The high clinical tolerance and the new technological advances, made bicarbonate dialysis more and more popular. Today, more than 70% of hemodialysis in North America, Western Europe and Japan are treated with bicarbonate dialysis (4).

METABOLIC ACIDOSIS AS UREMIC TOXIN

Acidosis is a characteristic feature of chronic renal insufficiency. Irrespective of the nature of the underlying disease, the acid-base disturbance always reflects a failure of tubular function to keep pace with the body's normal demands for bicarbonate reabsorption, net acid excretion, or both (5).

Experimental studies on animals and clinical observations suggest that metabolic acidosis affects several organs and physiological functions (6). Cardiac function is affected both directly and indirectly. *In vitro* studies of cardiac muscle contractility show a depressant effect of the acidosis due to a decrease in myocardial response to circulating catecholamines (7). In addition this disturbance could reflect the influence of intracellular pH on contractile proteins. Intracellular acidification also depresses the response of myocardium to calcium and decreases the performance of ischemic muscle; these effects probably reflect the displacement of calcium by hydrogen ion from critical binding sites (8).

The carbonate content of bone is an important buffer reservoir in the defense against chronic metabolic acidosis. Several reports have documented that uremic acidosis may have a role in worsening uremic osteodystrophy (9). The hydrogen ion increase can be buffered by release of alkali from bone in order to maintain a stable blood bicarbonate level (10).

The involvement of the bone in buffering an acid load has been demonstrated both in humans (9) and in animal experimental models (11). Lemann et al. in 1966 (10) demonstrated that, after an ammonium chloride load, mineral bone may participate in the overall buffering process. With chronic acidosis, different buffer systems are activated in the following sequence: 1) extracellular buffers, 2) extracellular and intracellular buffers, 3) intracellular and bone buffers and 4) bone buffers alone. When an acid load ceases, extracellular and intracellular buffers are completely repleted while the calcium lost from the bone is not completely restored and the amount of acid given is not completely excreted. Lemann et al. suggested that this observation may demonstrate the interaction between bone calcium and hydrogen ions when chronic acidosis is present.

Moreover, low pH stimulates cell-mediated bone reabsorption (12) and increases circulating PTH activity (13).

In patients on dialysis, the participation of extracellular, intracellular and bone buffers should depend on the weekly acid-base balances of the patient. When negative base balances occur devastating effects on bone mineralization would be expected in the long run. On the contrary, when base balance is near zero without a progressive accumulation of hydrogen ions in the body and a mild stable metabolic acidosis is present, severe bone disease should be less likely. The latter condition would mimic, as suggested by Gennari (14), the clinical setting of proximal renal tubular acidosis where a resetting of plasma bicarbonate at a lower level is present and no bone disease is observed.

However in acetate dialysis the base balance may frequently be negative and a continuous administration of oral alkaline supplementations may be required (15). When complete correction of acidosis was achieved by using bicarbonate dialysate, the plasma osteocalcin levels and the bone formation rate increased in patients with a previous reduction of the bone formation, while in patients with high bone formation rate the progressive increase of the osteocalcin levels was retarded. The correction of acidosis also resulted in lower PTH levels, thus demonstrating a reduction of the hyperparathyroidism and of the osteodystrophy (16).

There is increasing evidence that metabolic acidosis is an important stimulus of net protein catabolism.

Acidosis rather then uremia *per se* has been proved to enhance protein breakdown (17). Acidosis was also accompanied by an increase in glucocorticoid production and glucocorticoids were necessary for the muscle proteolysis stimulated by acidosis (18).

In addition metabolic acidosis also affects branched-chain amino-acid (BCAA) metabolism (19). Leucine stimulates muscle protein synthesis, while the keto acid of leucine inhibits protein degradation (20). In acidotic rats,

plasma and muscle BCAA levels are low and the activity of branched-chain keto acid dehydrogenase is increased thus leading to an increase of BCAA breakdown (19).

Clinical studies have demonstrated that correction of uremic metabolic acidosis with bicarbonate supplementation improves nitrogen balance (21) and protein breakdown is inversely correlated to arterial bicarbonate concentration (22).

The plasma levels of urea and uric acid were significantly reduced when the acidosis was corrected in chronic renal failure patients on protein-restriction diet (23).

In another study (24), when the urinary excretion of 3-methylhistidine was used as a simple indicator of muscle turnover, the restriction of dietary protein intake resulted in a reduction of nitrogen excretion and slight improvement of plasma bicarbonate. However, the increase of 3-methylhistidine release indicated an enhanced protein degradation. When metabolic acidosis was corrected by oral bicarbonate supplementation, both the excretion of nitrogen and 3-methylhistidine were reduced thus demonstrating the role of acidosis in protein wasting.

Recently Bergstrom et al. (25) have reported that the intracellular valine concentration in muscle is low in patients treated with hemodialysis. The valine concentration was correlated with the pre dialysis blood standard bicarbonate which varied from 18 to 24 mmol/l, demonstrating that even slight and intermittent acidosis might have stimulated the catabolism of valine in muscle.

Therefore full correction of acidosis to normal plasma bicarbonate levels is needed in dialyzed patients to prevent disturbances in BCAA metabolism and to prevent protein breakdown.

In conclusion, since metabolic acidosis is up to now about the only uremic toxin that has been clearly proved to have a number of clinically relevant detrimental effects, all efforts should be made in order to provide the best possible correction of it.

ACID BASE BALANCE IN CLINICAL DIALYSIS

Mechanism of acid-base correction

Correction of metabolic acidosis in the uremic patients represents one of the fundamental aims of dialysis. In patients on maintenance hemodialysis, the physiological restoration of body buffer content normally accomplished by the kidneys, should be replaced by the buffer administration through the dialysis membrane. Base gain during dialysis simulates the bicarbonate regeneration process by the normal kidneys.

Diet and metabolism are potential source of fixed non volatile acids. Sulphur of the sulphuric containing amino acids is oxidized to sulphuric acid; phosphate of proteins and phospholipids is metabolized to phosphoric acid and, finally, organic acids can be produced in excess of the metabolic elimination capacity (26).

Because these acids can not exist as free dissociated ions in the body fluids, they are instantaneously buffered, mostly by bicarbonate with a consequent production of the corresponding sodium salts and carbonic acid. Carbonic acid is then transformed into H_2O and CO_2, the latter being excreted by the lungs. By this buffering, the net loss of one alkaline equivalent occurs for each hydrogen ion neutralized.

In patients without renal function the maintenance of acid-base balance will only be achieved when the dialytic base gain equals the patient's metabolic acid production.

Acid production and removal

Endogenous acid production in uremic patients ranges between 0.7 and 1.2 mmol/kg/24 h. These values, mostly depending on diet and metabolism, appear similar to those observed in normal subjects. However the precise evaluation of the daily acid production in a single patient, would require metabolic balance studies. Since this procedure may be extremely complex, easier methods of calculation have to be used clinically. It has been pointed out by Gotch et al. (27) that in normal subjects the ratio between net acid excretion in the urine and protein catabolic rate is constant and equal to 0.77. The normal daily acid production is, therefore, calculated as

$$H^+G_{24h} = PCR \times 0.77. \quad [1]$$

Assuming a similar rate of production in hemodialysis patients without residual renal function (27), the hydrogen ion accumulation between two dialysis sessions can be calculated as:

$$H^+G_x = PCR \times 0.77 \times N \quad [2]$$

where: H^+G_x is the interdialytic hydrogen ion generation (mmol), PCR is the protein catabolic rate (g/kg/24 h), and N is the number of days between two dialysis sessions. Furthermore, in addition to bicarbonate, other alkaline equivalents lost through dialysis must be considered as an additional source of acids (H^+G_d) (28).

The overall weekly acid production in hemodialysis patients without residual renal function can therefore be calculated as follows:

$$H^+G_w = (PCR \times 0.77 \times 7) + (H^+G_d \times n) \quad [3]$$

where: H^+G_w is the weekly acid generation in the body, H^+G_d represents the amount of acid equivalents generated in the body during each dialysis session due to bicarbonate and other alkali losses in the dialysate and n is the number of dialysis sessions in a week.

Hemodialysis cannot remove large quantities of free hydrogen ion because of its low concentration in the blood. As hydrogen ions are produced, they are rapidly buffered by plasma bicarbonate and other body buffers

thus remaining at very low concentration in the plasma water (27).

In hemodialysis, therefore, H^+ removal from the blood is mainly achieved by the flux of alkaline equivalents from dialysate into the blood, with replacement of the depleted buffers. Hence, during dialysis fixed acids are converted to volatile acids.

To achieve adequate correction of metabolic acidosis the amount of buffers administered with dialysis should at least equal overall acid production in the patient. Base transfer across the dialysis membrane, is generally achieved in clinical dialysis by using acetate or bicarbonate containing dialysate.

Once acetate has entered the body, it is rapidly metabolized in the Krebs cycle and almost totally converted into bicarbonate. Of this bicarbonate 20% repletes body stores while 80% is lost across the membrane in the dialysate (27).

According to the formula

$$CO_2 + H_2O \leftrightarrows H_2CO_3 \leftrightarrows H^+ + HCO_3^- \quad [4]$$

the bicarbonate loss during dialysis causes a significant CO_2 removal by a shift to the right of the equilibrium.

Not only is CO_2 removed as bicarbonate, but also as a dissolved gas. However since plasma CO_2 concentration as a dissolved gas is very low (about 1 mmol/l) the losses under this form are small (0.2–0.3 mmol/min). Furthermore, while dissolved CO_2 is neutral and does not affect the acid base balance, CO_2 losses as bicarbonate influence acid-base balance considerably creating an equimolar accumulation of H+ in the body (29).

Hence, in acetate dialysis, the overall dialytic mass transfer rate of CO_2, averages 3 mmol/min and takes place in two ways: a) transport of dissolved CO_2 as a neutral gas, and b) transport of CO_2 as bicarbonate. These two forms represent respectively 2 and 24% of the overall CO_2 metabolic production (11 ± 3 mmol/min) (29).

In the dialytic transport of CO_2 the participation of red blood cells has also been postulated.

Bosch et al. (30) demonstrated that the amount of total CO_2 found in the dialysate exceeds the amount calculated to have left the blood in the same period. They suggested that CO_2 may be generated in the red cells during passage through the dialyzer. As CO_2 is lost in the dialysate, a concentration gradient is created between red cells and plasma. This gradient operates as a diffusive driving force for CO_2 through the red cell wall.

Since CO_2 diffuses faster than bicarbonate, intracellular pH increases stimulating the pentose-phosphate pathway which leads to further intracellular CO_2 production. As a consequence, the total CO_2 appearing in the dialysate may exceed the amount that has left the blood. Of course, such a phenomenon might influences total CO2 mass balance calculations.

During dialysis there is additional source of acid generation caused by the flux across the membrane of anions of organic acids such as lactate, β-hydroxybutirate and acetoacetate. Under normal conditions these substances and

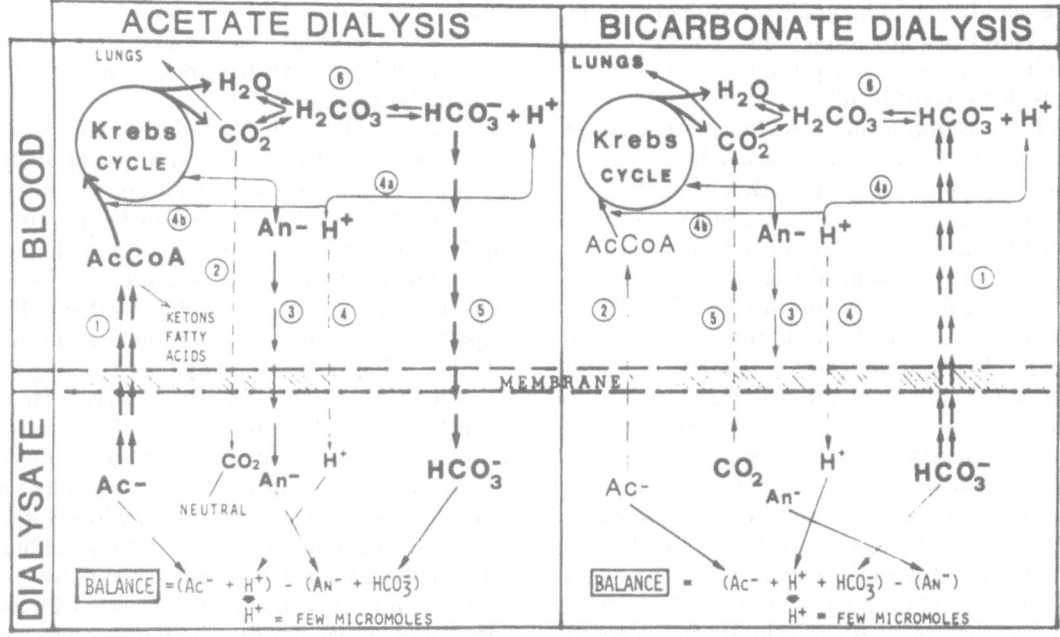

Figure 1. Mechanisms of acid-base correction in acetate and bicarbonate hemodialysis. Acetate dialysis: the final balance depends on the base gain (acetate infused in the blood and hydrogen ions lost in the dialysate) minus the base loss (anions of organic acids and bicarbonate). Bicarbonate dialysis: the final balance depends on the base gain (bicarbonate + small amounts of acetate and the hydrogen ions lost in the dialysate) minus the base loss (anions of organic acids) (see text).

their relative acids are neutralized by oxidation to CO_2 and H_2O. If the anions are removed by dialysis, the oxidation does not take place with a consequent net accumulation of hydrogen ions (31). A similar phenomenon occurs when other Krebs cycle intermediates, such as fumarate, succinate and glutarate, are lost in the dialysate, although the amount of these compounds lost across the membrane is very low.

A significant increase in blood levels of intermediates such as acetoacetate and β-hydroxybutirate and therefore an increased loss in the dialysate is observed when glucose free dialysis solutions are used. Under these conditions glucose is also lost in the dialysate and its plasma level falls causing a parallel decrease of insulin concentration. Low plasma levels of insulin may limit the rate of acetate metabolism in the Krebs cycle, increasing metabolic intermediates, or ketone and fatty acid via alternative pathways (32).

When dialysis fluid containing bicarbonate is used, bicarbonate losses do not occur; base losses are mostly due to the flux of organic anions in the dialysate. Under these conditions however organic anion loss in the dialysate is less than in acetate dialysis because of their lower production. The final bicarbonate balance will mainly depend on the dialysate/plasma concentration gradient. Bicarbonate containing solutions generally have a very high pCO_2; this may depend on the CO_2 insufflation in a closed system or on the chemical reaction with small quantities of acetic acid. Both these processes are utilized to maintain

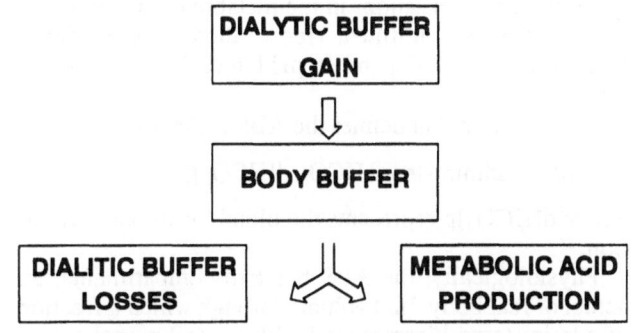

Figure 2. Acid base balance in dialyzed patients.

the dialysis solution chemically stable. Because of the difference in pCO_2 between plasma and dialysate, some dissolved CO_2 is administered to the patient during dialysis. However, since dissolved CO_2 is neutral this does not interfere with acid-base balance, and the excess CO_2 is finally excreted by the lungs (Figure 1).

Buffer balance

The general concept of the acid-base balance in dialyzed patients is summarized in Figure 2.

In order to maintain an optimum patient's acid-base status, the result of this balance should be zero. If the hydrogen ion production exceeds the buffer gain from dialysis, the acidity would be continuously buffered by intracellular buffers leading to undesired clinical consequences, while, if the buffer gain prevails, an extracellular metabolic alkalosis would result.

However patients starting dialysis often present a large buffer deficit due to the long term positive hydrogen ion balance during the pre dialysis period. The analysis of the distribution volume for bicarbonate could be useful in order to quantify the base deficit in these patients.

Applying the pharmacological concept of volume of distribution, a distribution volume for bicarbonate, or apparent bicarbonate space (ABS), is defined as the ratio of administered bicarbonate to the observed change in the plasma bicarbonate concentration. Extracellular bicarbonate system not only modulates the hydrogen ion concentration (pH) in the extracellular space but also exerts a buffering effect on the intracellular buffer systems that regulate the intracellular pH. Therefore, ABS normally ranges between 40 and 50% of the total body weight, i.e., almost twice of the extracellular volume where the bicarbonate is really present (33). Clinical observations have highlighted that ABS increases in acidosis and decreases in alkalosis, suggesting that pH would be the major determinant of the ABS (34).

However more recently experimental findings (35) demonstrated that ABS decreases in the respiratory acidosis (lower pH, higher bicarbonate) and increases in the respiratory alkalosis (higher pH, lower bicarbonate), while the previous observations in the metabolic acid-base disturbances were confirmed. Hence, there is an evidence that ABS does not depend on pH but on blood bicarbonate.

The equation that defines the ABS is the following:

$$ABS = administered\ HCO_3/d[HCO_3]p$$

where $d[HCO_3]p$ represents the blood bicarbonate variation.

Physiologically, the ABS has two compartments, an actual or real body fluid volume through which a fraction of administered bicarbonate is diluted (dilutional space, DS) and a bicarbonate sink in which the remaining fraction of administered bicarbonate is titrated by non-bicarbonate buffers. This titration takes place in a body space that will be called the titration space (TS). Thus it can be written:

$$Administered\ HCO_3 = HCO_3\ over\ DS$$
$$+ HCO_3\ titrated\ in\ TS.$$

DS and TS are purely functional terms, and not actual physical spaces corresponding to any body fluid compartments (33).

By using the chemical laws of the buffering power it was possible to extrapolate the following equation:

$$ABS = (0.4 + 2.6/blood\ HCO_3) \times body\ weight$$

that can predict the distribution volume for bicarbonate in any clinical condition (33). This equation was utilized in some mathematical models in order to predict post dialysis blood bicarbonate values and dialytic base gain (36). Several clinical studies have dealt with buffer balance in hemodialysis.

Vreman et al. (37) measured a total infusion of acetate per dialysis of 1165 ± 49 mmol, using dialyzers with surface areas varying between 1 and 2.5 m². Tolchin et al. (38) reported total acetate infusion per dialysis varying from 788 ± 45 to 1048 ± 100 mmol. These results were obtained with 2.5 m² dialyzers and two different dialysis solutions containing 30 and 40 mmol/l of acetate respectively. Gotch et al. (27) found an average acetate infusion of 780 ± 61 mmol/dialysis utilizing dialyzers of 1.3 and 1.8 m². Kishimoto (39) observed a total infusion of acetate per dialysis of 819 ± 125 mmol with 1.1 m² dialyzers. In those studies bicarbonate losses varied from 550 to 900 mmol/dialysis. The additional loss of alkaline equivalents such as lactate and β-hydroxibutirate ranged from 50 to 100 mmol/dialysis (27). Some of these authors calculated weekly net base balances slightly positive or at least near zero. This however, contrasts with the frequent observation of patients undergoing chronic acetate dialysis with a pre dialytic plasma bicarbonate ranging from 14 to 18 mmol/l (40).

The buffer balance in bicarbonate dialysis has not yet been studied extensively. Gotch et al. (27) reported a weekly balance in 8 patients undergoing bicarbonate dialysis with 1.3 to 1.8 m² dialyzers, blood flow of 200 ml/min, dialysate flow of 400 ml/min and 36 mmol/l of bicarbonate in the dialysate. In this study the net base gain was calculated taking into account other factors such as ultrafiltration, net H⁺ generation and lactate and β-hydroxibutirate losses during dialysis. The average weekly H⁺ generation was 352 mmol; β-hydroxybutirate and lactate losses were 37 and 55 mmol/week respectively. Bicarbonate mass transfer was 618 mmol/week (206 mmol/dialysis). The final net base gain was +175 mmol/week. Such a positive balance might even be higher considering the patients uptake of acetate derived from the acid part of the dialysis concentrate. In case of body buffer depletion this positive balance may help to restore the acid-base equilibrium and to replenish the buffer stores. However when the acid-base status is near normal only small amounts of base are required and excessive base administration can cause alkalosis.

Controlled studies of patients treated with bicarbonate dialysis for more than 12 weeks demonstrated the high risk of postdialytic alkalosis with plasma bicarbonate levels exceeding 30 mmol/l and blood pH higher than 7.55. This acute alkalosis may cause headache, nausea, vomiting and letargia and such chronic effects as calcium deposition in soft tissues. On the basis of these observations Ward et al. (41) suggested progressive reduction of dialysate bicarbonate concentration over time. On the other hand, studies carried out with dialysate solutions containing 31 mmol/l of bicarbonate and 5 mmol/l of

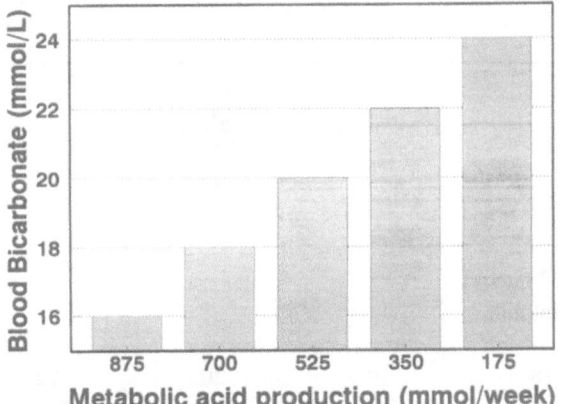

Figure 3. Relationship between weekly metabolic acid production and pre dialysis blood bicarbonate in acetate dialysis. (Modified from Reference (14).)

acetate, have shown insufficient correction of metabolic acidosis and no significant differences from the results achieved with acetate dialysis (40).

However, it has been argued that, after regular dialysis treatment is started, retention of acid or depletion of buffer does not occur any further and the constant mild acidosis observed in these patient represents a balanced state.

Gennari (14) pointed out that, during acetate dialysis, acetate delivery is constant if dialytic schedule (i.e. blood and dialysate flows, acetate concentration in the bath, dialyzer and ultrafiltration) is constant, while bicarbonate loss across the dialysis membrane varies inversely with the blood bicarbonate concentration. Net alkali gain is the difference between acetate entry and bicarbonate loss; therefore more alkali are gained when plasma bicarbonate concentration is low and *vice versa*. An hypothetical example is reported in Table 1 in order to illustrate in a quantitative fashion the effect of this feedback system on pre dialysis bicarbonate concentration. If the patient has a low pre dialysis plasma bicarbonate level, the base balance should be positive and consequently, the bicarbonate concentration should be higher at the time of the next dialysis. On the contrary, if the pre dialysis plasma bicarbonate concentration is 22 mmol/l, only 161 mmols of net alkali will be gained; this amount is less than that required to maintain balance. Thus, unneutralized, retained hydrogen ion will causes the next pre dialysis bicarbonate concentration to be lower. With time, pre dialysis bicarbonate concentration will be maintained at somewhere between 19 and 20 mmol/l. At this level, net alkali gain will equal acid production and long-term acid balance will be zero.

This hypothesis (14) suggests that, with constant dialysis characteristic, pre dialysis bicarbonate concentration is inversely related to endogenous acid production (Figure 3).

This feedback hypothesis could be applied to bicarbonate dialysis as well. Table 2 reports the same example

of Table 1 but parameters are calculated for bicarbonate dialysate treatments.

From the viewpoint of acid balance it makes little difference. In a system with these specification, plasma bicarbonate concentration before dialysis will hover at approximately 21 mmol/l (14).

Oral base supplements

Although several studies of dialysis patients demonstrate that the net weekly base influx may compensate for daily H^+ production (27), before each dialysis metabolic acidosis is characteristic.

For this reason some authors (15, 41) have suggested the use of oral alkaline supplements in the interdialytic period.

However, although these substances generally correct uremic acidosis, their participation in the final acid-base status is not easy to evaluate because of many variants. Among these, the most important are the individual differences on intestinal absorption, the distribution volume for bicarbonate, which relates to the interdialytic weight gain, and the possible interference with other drugs.

All these factors must be taken into account to assess the acid-base balance of the individual patient which does not depend only on the dialytic base gain.

FACTORS AFFECTING BUFFER BALANCE IN CLINICAL DIALYSIS

Mass transfer of buffers across dialysis membrane is achieved as for other solutes via diffusive or convective transport or both. However the rapid conversion into other metabolites and the equilibration in a wide distribution space make mass balance calculations for these substances more complex and difficult.

Diffusive transport

The amount of acetate that diffuses across the membrane is a function of the concentration gradient between dialysate and blood and the membrane surface area. Other factors influencing acetate mass transfer are the temperature and a constant, defined as diffusivity, which depends on the membrane material and its interface with the solute and solvent under consideration. Since the latter factors are fairly stable in clinical dialysis, the concentration gradient and the surface area of the membrane are the major determinants of acetate transport. Once the surface area of the dialyzer has been established, acetate mass transfer rate (AcMTR) will depend on acetate dialysance (AcD) and on its average concentration gradient between dialysate and plasma during dialysis (Cd_i-Cp_i): Since Dialysance = $MTR/(Cd_i$-$Cp_i)$, therefore MTR = $D(Cd_i$-$Cp_i)$. A simplified weekly mass balance calculation

$$H^+G_w = AcMTR \times n \times dt = D(Cd_i - Cp_i) \times n \times dt \quad [5]$$

Table 1. Theoretic acid-base balance in acetate dialysis

Metabolic acid production (mmol/week)	420
Organic anion loss during dialysis (mmol/week)	<u>300</u>
Weekly base required (mmol/week)	720
Dialytic base gain required (mmol/dialysis)	240
3 dialysis/week	

Dialysis duration = 4 hours; Acetate concentration in the bath = 37 mmol/l
Acetate dialysance = 120 ml/min; Bicarbonate dialysance = 150 ml/min

Blood Bicarbonate (mmol/l)	16	18	19	20	22
Bicarbonate lost (mmol/session)	576	648	684	720	792
Acetate gain (mmol/session)	953	953	953	953	953
Dialytic base gain (mmol/session)	377	305	269	233	161
Base gain – 240 (mmol/session)	137	65	29	-7	-79

Table 2. Theoretic acid-base balance in bicarbonate dialysis

Metabolic acid production (mmol/week)	420
Organic anion loss during dialysis (mmol/week)	<u>300</u>
Weekly base required (mmol/week)	720
Dialytic base gain required (mmol/dialysis)	240
3 dialysis/week	

Dialysis duration = 4 hours; Bicarbonate concentration in the bath = 32 mmol/l
Bicarbonate dialysance = 150 ml/min

Blood Bicarbonate (mmol/l)	16	18	20	22	24
Bicarbonate gain (mmol/session)	360	315	270	225	180
Base gain – 240 (mmol/session)	120	75	30	-15	-60

where H^+G_w is the weekly acid production, n is the number of dialyses sessions in a week, and dt is the duration of the dialysis session, would define the exact amount of buffer to administer in a week to balance the overall acid production:

$$H^+G_w - NBG_w = 0 \qquad [6]$$

where NBG_w is the net base gain during the week.

This amount of buffer could be achieved varying the dialysate concentration of acetate, the blood flow, the dialyzer surface area, the number of dialysis per week or the duration of each session. From equation [5] it would be theoretically possible to predict the dialysate concentration of acetate adequate for this purpose. The average concentration of acetate in dialysis solutions is 35–38 mmol/l while the blood acetate concentration at the beginning of the session is only 0.1 mmol/l. This gradient is the driving force moving acetate across the membrane. With 1 m² dialyzers a countercurrent blood/dialysate flow ratio of 250/500 guarantees an average acetate clearance of 125 ml/min, i.e., an average mass transfer rate of 4.75 mmol/min. Several techniques have been used to increase the acetate MTR during dialysis. Increasing blood flow results in a parallel increase in acetate dialysance until the curve reaches a plateau which is determined by the limiting effect of the membrane permeability and surface area (Figure 4). Higher mass transfer rates were achieved by Bjaeldager et al. (42) by increasing acetate concentration in the bath from 32.6 to 38.2 mmol/l. Mansell et al. (43) however, demonstrated that significant variations of blood acetate levels in patients undergoing acetate dialysis do not result in parallel changes of acetate fluxes across the membrane. As patients passed from 2.4 to 4.5 mmol/l of acetatemia during dialysis the acetate flux changed from 202 to 191 mmol/h/1.73 m² while in patients passing from 5.5 to 15.6 mmol/l the acetate flux changed from 195 to 229 mmol/h/1.73 m². It is still controversial whether small variations in the dialysate/blood concentration gradient may influence significantly the rate

Acetate Dialysance

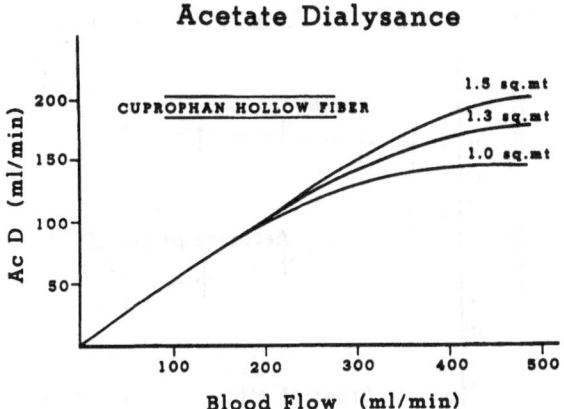

Figure 4. Acetate dialysance versus blood flow with cuprophan hollow fiber dialyzers of different surface area.

of acetate transport. Furthermore, the rate of acetate transport is lower than one would predict by its molecular weight. The negative charges and the large hydration mantle of the molecule may in fact reduce the final diffusivity coefficient.

The rate of conversion of acetate into bicarbonate has been demonstrated to vary from 2.5 to 5.5 mmol/min with a mean value of 5 mmol/min in normals and 3 mmol/min in the uremic population. This conversion prevents dissipation of the gradient between dialysate and blood that would take place with accumulation of infused acetate. Accumulation may occur, however, as demonstrated by Tolchin et al. (38), when high blood flows and large surface areas are utilized, and highly efficient treatments are performed. Under those conditions the high mass transfer of acetate across the membrane may exceed the maximal metabolic capacity (44–47). In this situation the plasma concentration of acetate may reach values above 10 mmol/l, which are considered dangerous and life threatening. Since clearances of acetate and urea are linked, it appears that urea clearance can not be increased in acetate dialysis over a certain limit lest dangerously high mass transfer of acetate occur. In highly efficient treatments, another limitation derives from the high total CO_2 clearance and the consequent bicarbonate losses which may even be greater than the amount of acetate administered and may worsen the metabolic acidosis (48).

When bicarbonate containing dialysate is used a concentration gradient of 6 to 20 mmol/l between dialysate and blood is the driving force moving the buffer across the membrane. This gradient must be adequate to generate a bicarbonate flux into the blood sufficient to restore the body buffer stores without inducing alkalosis at the end of dialysis. A bicarbonate concentration in the dialysate varying from 30 to 38 mmol/l may generate in a 240 min a mass transfer of buffer ranging from 150 to 250 mmol depending on pre dialysis serum bicarbonate concentration. Sargent and Gotch (29) found that bicarbonate flux

across the membrane is a function of the inlet concentration gradient ($Cd_i - Cp_i$). For a gradient between 18 and 23 mmol they reported a bicarbonate MTR of 2.0 to 2.7 mmol/min with an average dialysance of 118 ml/min. These results, however, are highly influenced by the blood and dialysate flows and by the geometry of the dialyzer and cannot be assumed as constant values. The bicarbonate concentrations now used clinically were not derived from kinetic studies but came mostly from empirical evaluations of their clinical adequacy. However, since the individual requirement of buffer administration varies among patients, it is difficult to propose a universally adequate fixed concentration; the personalization of the dialysis bath would be useful in answering the individual needs. The bicarbonate concentration should be also adapted to the state of body buffer depletion; when a full restoration of the body stores is required, higher concentrations of bicarbonate may be required to achieve a remarkably positive base balance, while lower concentrations (30 mmol/l) may be enough to maintain serum levels under adequate control after repletion is achieved. Ward and Wathen (49) have also recommended varying the concentration of bicarbonate in the dialysate during the dialysis session to avoid post dialytic alkalaemia.

Furthermore, other substances move through the membrane governed by a concentration gradients and affect the final "net base gain". In bicarbonate dialysis small amounts of acetic acid are in the dialysate (3 to 5 mmol/l) creating a flux of acetate into the blood ranging from 0.2 to 0.8 mmol/min. Because of its conversion to bicarbonate, acetate can produce a further base gain during bicarbonate dialysis varying from 50 to 200 mmol/session. Finally the mass transfer rate of organic anions generally ranges between 0.2 and 0.5 mmol/min while only a few micromoles of free hydrogen ions cross the membrane in response to very low concentration gradients.

Convective transport

Base transfer across the dialysis membrane can also be achieved by convection. While the reciprocal influence of diffusion and convection is a complex process, extremely difficult to evaluate, the kinetic of buffers in exclusively convective therapies such as hemofiltration or ultrafiltration is quite easily understood. During standard hemodialysis dry weight is achieved via ultrafiltration of plasma water. This process leads to a certain bicarbonate loss that cannot be precisely evaluated because of the continuous interference of diffusion. In this condition, convective transport is present but it is not a pure and separate process. Its influence on the final bicarbonate balance can more precisely be evaluated by collecting the total spent dialysate and measuring the bicarbonate concentration (50).

The base balance in mixed diffusive-convective treatments, such as hemodiafiltration, is further complicated by the reinfusion of replacement solutions. Large amounts of bicarbonate are lost by convection in the ultrafiltrate and

FACTORS AFFECTING DIALYTIC ACID–BASE BALANCE

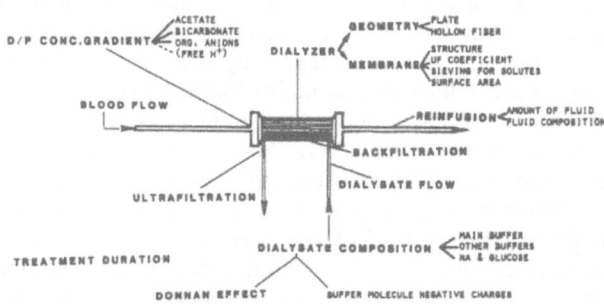

Figure 5. Factors affecting dialytic acid-base balance in clinical dialysis (see text).

ACID-BASE in ACETATE DIALYSIS

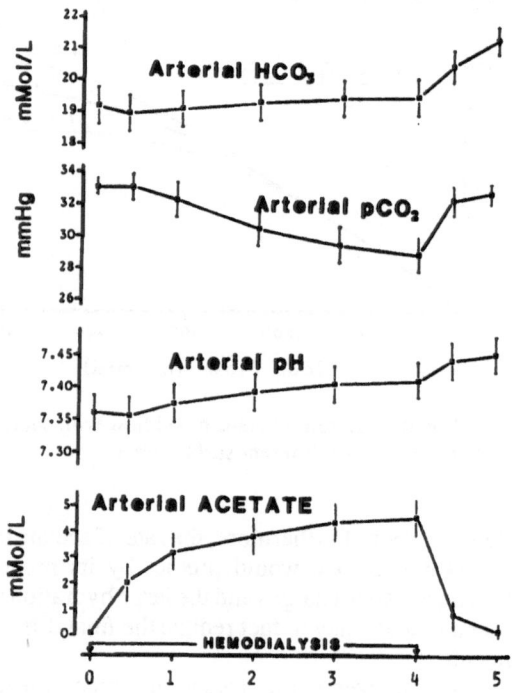

Figure 6. Blood gases and acid-base behaviour during acetate dialysis.

again the precise evaluation can only be made by collecting the entire pool of dialysate. The reinfusion of commercially prepared buffer containing solutions allows a substitution of the bases lost via ultrafiltration and increases plasma bicarbonate concentration.

The average buffer concentration in the replacement solutions (acetate, lactate or bicarbonate) varies from 35 to 60 mmol/l. This amount of alkaline equivalents infused directly helps to restore the body buffer content and offsets the base losses via ultrafiltration. In these treatments the final balance therefore depends on the same diffusive parameters as in hemodialysis plus the convective component which is linked to the number of liters of fluid exchanged per session.

The base balance calculation is easier in hemofiltration where a pure convective mechanism operates and solute transport is mostly governed by the permeability of the membrane (51–53). Since non diffusible anions, such as proteins, are present on one side of the membrane, the concentration of bicarbonate in the ultrafiltrate will be determined by the Donnan equilibrium which will provide for the electroneutrality on both sides of membrane. Therefore the bicarbonate concentration in the ultrafiltrate is generally higher than in plasma water and sieving values range between 1.10 and 1.15 depending on plasma protein concentration at the inlet of the filter and the filtration fraction. In this case, the product of the bicarbonate concentration in the ultrafiltrate times the volume of ultrafiltrate produced will equal the amount of base losses in a session. The buffers infused via replacement solution will balance these losses and will also give the excess amount of alkaline equivalents necessary to balance the metabolic acid production.

The net base balance in different types of substitutive therapy therefore depends on several factors that may affect the kinetics of buffers during the treatment (Figure 5).

ACETATE DIALYSIS

The use of acetate in dialysis may influence the patient's clinical conditions both during treatment and in the interdialytic period. Specific effects on acid-base equilibrium, ventilation, cardiovascular activity and endogenous metabolism can be observed.

Effects on acid base

Acetate dialysis is characterized by a flux of acetate into the blood and concurrent losses of bicarbonate in the dialysate. In the first 30 minutes of a dialysis, acetate metabolism may not be so fast enough to balance bicarbonate losses and a fall of HCO_3 and pH can be observed. This effect may even worsen the metabolic acidosis in this period (46). Subsequently, the rate of acetate utilization increases counterbalancing bicarbonate losses; patients therefore show a progressive decrease of pCO_2, an increase of blood pH and a relative stability of plasma bicarbonate (Figure 6). Plasma acetate levels rise during the session reaching at the end an average value of 5 mmol/l (37, 47). After dialysis has ceased pH and HCO_3 rapidly increase while pCO_2 returns to predialytic values (37). These effects depend on the sudden decrease of bicarbonate losses through the dialyzer and on the complete metabolism of acetate accumulated in the body. These observations are typical of a standard dialysis session carried out with blood flow of 250 ml/min, dialysate flow of 500 ml/min and cuprophan dialyzers for 240 minutes. When high surface area dialyzers are utilized (38, 54) acetate and bicarbonate fluxes across the membrane are greater and the consequent effects on acid-base equilibrium are more considerable. In these conditions the maximal acetate metabolic rate is exceeded with a consequent accumulation of the buffer in the blood. This substantially decreases plasma bicarbonate and pCO_2, while variations of pH are either slight (54) or towards alkalaemia (38). At the end of the session a remarkable increase of pH, pCO_2 and bicarbonate is observed leading to metabolic alkalosis (54). These observations suggest the possible limitations imposed by acetate dialysis in increasing the efficiency of the treatment and reducing treatment time.

In between two dialysis sessions, blood pH and bicarbonate progressively decrease in accord with the metabolic acid production and its accumulation in the body. In a 60 kg patient, with a theoretical HCO_3 distribution space of 35 l, plasma bicarbonate should decrease by about 2 mmol/24 h when daily acid production is about 70 mmol and it is completely buffered by the bicarbonate system. Based on these calculations, one could predict the plasma bicarbonate concentration at the beginning of the subsequent session, to be 4 to 6 mmol lower than that observed at the end of the previous dialysis. However, the calculation is only theoretical and an extreme variability of the pre dialytic bicarbonate concentrations can be noted in patients on regular dialysis treatment. This variability may depend on the intervention of buffers other than bicarbonate, on different daily acid productions and on variations of the interdialytic weight gain.

Effects on ventilation

Acetate dialysis significantly decreases arterial pO_2 during the entire duration of the treatment. This fall of pO_2 occurs in about 90% of patients ranging between 5 and 35 mmHg (average value 14 mmHg) (55). After the treatment, pO_2 values return to the pre dialytic values within one or two hours. Some authors have suggested that this dialysis induced hypoxemia might be important in the genesis of some intradialytic symptoms especially hypotension particularly evident in patients with compromised cardio-pulmonary function.

This hypoxemia has a multifactorial origin and its pathophysiology has not yet been totally clarified. Dialytic hypoxemia has been ascribed to a possible Bohr effect (56). The pH increase during dialysis might lead to a parallel increase in hemoglobin affinity for O_2. In this setting, although a stable pO_2 and blood oxygen content are maintained, the O_2 delivery to the tissues decreases significantly. However, it has been pointed out by Hirtsel et al. (57) that the variations of blood pH and 2,3-diphosphoglycerate inside the red cells, as well as other

intracellular phosphates, are not sufficient to explain completely the dialysis induced hypoxemia.

Bischel et al. (58) have suggested that hypoxia may depend on a microembolisation in the lungs due to circulating micro-aggregates of platelets, leucocytes or fibrin deriving from the blood/membrane interaction. In other studies, however (59), the microfiltration of venous blood was not able to prevent hypoxemia during dialysis. Craddox et al. (60) have suggested that the blood interaction with cuprophan membranes may activate complement via the alternative pathway with a consequent leucocyte agglutination and pulmonary trapping of the microaggregates and a final effect of neutropenia. This might lead to an impairment of gas diffusion in the lungs and consequent hypoxia.

Two observations, however, are in contrast with this hypothesis:

1. hypoxemia also occurs with more biocompatible membranes such polyacrylonitrile or polysulphon in which complement activation does not take place and neutropenia is blunted (61);

2. during isolated ultrafiltration with cellulosic membranes the neutropenic effect is present but hypoxemia does not occur (62).

Sherlock et al. (63) and Aurigemma et al. (59) have proposed that the CO_2 losses across dialysis membrane could be the main cause of hypoventilation and hypoxemia. The reduced CO_2 excretion with increased O_2 consumption, without any alteration of A-a O_2 gradient, determines a significant fall of RQ. RQ, however, is in the normal range when its calculation takes into account CO_2 losses through the dialyzer. As a further proof of this hypothesis, these authors demonstrated that hypoventilation and hypoxemia can be avoided by bubbling CO_2 in the dialysate. Dolan et al. (64) demonstrated the occurrence of hypoventilation-hypoxemia in acetate but not in bicarbonate dialysis where CO_2 losses do not take place. The importance of hypoventilation in inducing hypoxemia during dialysis has also been confirmed by Bouffard et al. (65). These authors have demonstrated that hypoxemia does not take place in patients with acute renal failure dialyzed with mechanical ventilatory support.

A different approach to the problem has been proposed by Oh et al. (66). They suggest that acetate metabolism may be the main cause of increased O_2 consumption and decreased CO_2 production with a consequent RQ reduction. This reduction will be proportional to the amount of acetate administered to the patient as observed by Raya et al. (67) who noted more hypoxemia during dialysis carried out with higher acetate concentration in the dialysate. In conclusion (68) dialysis induced hypoxemia appears to be a multifactorial phenomenon and, although it has not yet been completely clarified, two major determinants are generally considered: acetate infusion and metabolism, and CO_2 losses through the dialyzer. An important contribution of the latter process already pointed out in the early seventies (69), is supported by the occurrence of hypoxemia in bicarbonate dialysis without bubbling CO_2 in the dialysate (67) and by the absence of hypoxemia when CO_2 is bubbled in the dialysate both in acetate dialysis (70), and in bicarbonate dialysis (63).

Cardiovascular effects

When cardiovascular effects of acetate dialysis are considered, it is important to distinguish the specific effects determined by acetate from the general effects generated by dialysis treatment. It is well known that acetate infusion in man has a vasodilatory effect (71, 72). It has, therefore, been suggested that in some patients acetate could be the main cause of hypotension and other cardiovascular effects recorded during dialysis. Kirkendol et al. (73), studying the effects of an intravenous bolus of acetate in anesthetized dogs, concluded that acetate produces a dose-dependent reduction of the myocardiac performance and of arterial blood pressure thus suggesting a cardiodepressant action of the buffer. The same finding was reported by Aizawa et al. (74). However, in a subsequent study carried out at a constant rate of acetate infusion, Kirkendol et al. (75) found an increase in cardiac output and a decrease of total peripheral resistance and mean arterial pressure. These effects on cardiac output were later confirmed by Chen et al. (76) using echocardiography. Studies carried out in normal anesthetized dogs infused with increasing doses of acetate (77) showed an increase of cardiac output, heart rate, stroke volume and a decrease of peripheral resistance suggesting that acetate may have a positive inotropic effect on the myocardium. Metha et al. (78) later confirmed these findings excluding a myocardio-depressant action of acetate in patients undergoing dialysis therapy. Finally in a recent study carried out in healthy volunteers treated with isovolemic acetate dialysis, Danielsson et al. (79) demonstrated with invasive techniques that a systemic vasodilation is produced during dialysis, compensated by a heart rate dependent increase of cardiac output. Thus, it has been widely demonstrated that acetate has a direct vasodilatory effect although its pathogenesis is not clear. A possible interaction of acetate with ionized calcium necessary for the contraction of the vascular musculature (72) or a direct vasodilatory effect induced by acetate metabolites such as adenosine or adenine nucleotides (77) have been suggested. The myocardiac response to this vasodilation is an increase in cardiac output in the attempt to maintain a stable blood pressure. This response however may be altered during dialysis because of a remarkable autonomic nerve dysfunction or a borderline cardiomyopathy.

Hence, dialysis induced hypotension is probably due to different mechanisms and several factors. One of them could be an insufficient increase in cardiac output in response of the vasodilation induced by acetate. Hypoxemia, altered serum osmolality, ultrafiltration and hypovolemia with a consequent reduction of the vascular filling

pressure may also contribute to this pathological event during acetate dialysis (80).

Metabolic effects

Acetate represents an important substrate for different metabolic pathways. During its metabolism via AcCoA, acetate can be partially shifted to lipids synthesis probably contributing to the hyperlipidemia and accelerated atherosclerosis of patients on regular dialysis treatment. However, Rorke et al. (81) demonstrated, using labelled acetate on dialyzed dogs, that only 1% or less of the infused acetate is incorporated in the plasma lipids. This amount represents the regular metabolic turnover and it does not imply increased lipids production or deposition in the tissues. Other studies carried out in humans on acetate dialysis and in animals fed with atherogenic diet supplemented with acetate or bicarbonate (82), have also concluded that there is no evidence for a significant lipidogenic effect of acetate. Morin et al. (83) in a cross-over study on patients on acetate and bicarbonate dialysis, could not detect significant differences between the two dialysis treatment periods; hyperlipidemia of dialyzed patients depends more on a reduced lipid removal than on increased production. Acetate, therefore, is not an important source of lipids and this metabolic pathway might only become critical when other lipogenic factors coexist.

Although acetate represents the main caloric substrate during dialysis, it is not a relevant caloric source overall, generating only 200 Cal/mol (38). Since the total amount of acetate given per session is about 1 mol, the caloric load from acetate metabolism represents less than 5% of the weekly caloric intake in a standard patient.

Biocompatibility

Acetate has been supposed to be one of the component of hemodialysis which stimulates monocytes to produce interleukin-1 (IL-1), according to interleukin hypothesis (84). IL-1 biological activities include the ability to cause fever and sleep, induce local inflammation, activate lymphocytes, stimulate catabolism in muscle, bone and cartilage, induce fibroblast and endothelial cell proliferation as well as hepatic acute phase protein synthesis, stimulate interleukin-2 production and increase the expression of major histocompatibility class 1 antigens on cell surfaces (85). This last phenomenon may be associated with release of beta2-microglobulin into the extracellular fluid.

In accordance with the so-called incubator model (86), monocytes located near or on the dialysis membrane will be exposed to the highest concentration of component of the dialysate which permeate across the membrane (87). Some studies have demonstrated that concentrations of sodium acetate comparable to those found in dialysate can enhance IL-1 production and act in a synergistic manner with endotoxin to stimulate IL-1 production (88, 89).

BICARBONATE DIALYSIS

The mechanism of correction of metabolic acidosis operating in bicarbonate dialysis differs from that of acetate dialysis (Figure 1). This results in different effects on acid-base balance, ventilation, cardiovascular function and metabolism.

Effects on acid-base status

In bicarbonate dialysis, blood pH and plasma bicarbonate progressively increase throughout the session while pCO_2 shows stable values (90, 91) or a moderate increase (54). At the end of dialysis a moderate metabolic alkalosis can be observed; its degree depends on the total bicarbonate balance and on the pre-dialytic acid-base status. Thereafter, blood pH and plasma bicarbonate progressively decrease until the subsequent dialysis. This behaviour contrasts with acetate dialysis where, at the end of dialysis session, the rapid metabolism of the infused acetate in absence of bicarbonate losses temporarily increases pH and plasma bicarbonate. Patients treated by bicarbonate dialysis generally present for subsequent dialysis with an acid-base status close to normal, but some have an acidotic status similar to that observed in acetate dialysis (92), despite a positive buffer balance (27).

Effects on ventilation

The effects of bicarbonate dialysis on ventilation and in particular on the possible occurrence of dialysis induced hypoxemia ar still controversial. Some authors (93, 94) have observed no differences in patients treated alternatively with bicarbonate and acetate dialysis. Others (38, 91) could not observe hypoxemia in patients undergoing bicarbonate dialysis. The observation of dialysis induced hypoxemia in some patients treated with bicarbonate dialysis might depend on the bicarbonate concentration in the dialysate. In fact, dialysate concentrations of bicarbonate higher than 37 mmol/l might be responsible for a rapid alkalinization of the patient with a consequent compensatory hypoventilation (95).

Cardiovascular effects

Several studies report a better clinical tolerance of bicarbonate dialysis in terms of incidence of hypotensive episodes and intradialytic symptomatology such as nausea, vomiting, headache and cramps (54, 96). Unanimous agreement on this point has not yet been reached, however (Table 3).

Patients on bicarbonate hemodialysis respond hemodynamically quite differently from those on acetate dialysis.

Under similar conditions of ultrafiltration, bicarbonate dialysis achieves better stability of mean arterial pressure due to the maintenance of systemic vascular resistance, cardiac output and heart rate within adequate ranges (96). This hemodynamic response observed in bicarbonate dialysis, may be explained by the absence of the vasodilatory effect of acetate, or a favourable effect of alkalosis on vascular reactivity (97). Furthermore, myocardial contractility and left ventricular function may be improved in this condition (98), despite a possible reduction in myocardial reactivity due to variations of ionized calcium related to alkalosis (99). Mansell et al. (100), comparing acetate and bicarbonate dialysis, showed a significant increase of heart rate only with acetate, while blood pressure and peripheral resistance were similar. They attributed the beneficial effects of bicarbonate dialysis more by a steadiness of the arterial pO_2 during the treatment, than to the absence of adverse cardiovascular effects of acetate. Furthermore, when high sodium dialysate solutions are used, the differences in vascular stability between acetate and bicarbonate dialysis seem to be cancelled. Comparative studies could not show significant advantages of bicarbonate versus acetate dialysis when high sodium dialysis fluid was used (101). Moreover, Henrich et al. (102) reported similar hemodynamic responses with acetate and bicarbonate dialysis when dialysis fluid with higher osmolality was used, although with bicarbonate dialysis the number of therapeutic interventions was significantly less. But the constant use of high sodium concentrations in the dialysis fluid may increase the incidence of hypertension, thirst and excessive interdialytic weight gain. Hence, it is still controversial whether bicarbonate dialysis may directly benefit vascular stability during dialysis; although the vasodilatory effects of acetate are avoided, bicarbonate dialysis cannot really eliminate other causes of hypotension such as ultrafiltration and preload reduction with a consequent reduction of the vascular filling pressure.

Effects on metabolism

Bicarbonate has not significant metabolic effects, *per se*, and therefore does not interfere with biochemical processes such as gluconeogenesis or lipid synthesis. Morin et al. (83) have demonstrated that no significant differences in cholesterol, triglycerides, LDL, VLDL and HDL can be noted between acetate and bicarbonate dialysis.

HEMOFILTRATION

Few acid-base studies have been carried out in patients treated by hemofiltration (HF). The net base balance in post dilutional HF is obtained by the difference between the base losses in the ultrafiltrate (bicarbonate, organic anions and part of the buffer infused intravenously) and the amount of base administered to the patient via the substitution fluid. The buffers utilized in the replacement

Table 3. Comparison of clinical tolerance between acetate and bicarbonate dialysis

Ref.	Year	Author	Hypotension	Nausea	Vomiting	Headache	Cramps
74	1977	Aizawa	−	0	0	0	0
54	1978	Graefe	+	0	+	+	+
103	1978	Whele (Na 145)	+	0	0	0	0
	1978	Whele (Na 135)	−	0	0	0	0
96	1980	Iseki	+	0	0	0	0
94	1981	Borges	−	−	−	−	−
105	1982	Hampl	+	0	0	0	0
107	1982	Pagel	+	+	−	−	0
104	1983	Chen	+	0	0	0	0
106	1984	Vanholder	−	+	+	−	−
101	1984	Velez (Na (141)	−	0	0	0	0
92	1995	Hakim	+	−	−	0	−
40	1987	La Greca	+	−	−	−	−
100	1987	Mansell	−	0	0	0	0

+ = Significantly better with bicarbonate.
− = No difference with acetate.
0 = Not studied.

solutions are acetate and lactate at an average concentration of 40 mmol/l.

Comparative studies have demonstrated that in HF pO_2, pCO_2, pH and bicarbonate have a behaviour similar to that observed in acetate dialysis (109). Specifically, pO_2 shows a moderate decrease, pCO_2 remains stable and pH and bicarbonate progressively increase during the session. However, pCO_2 and plasma bicarbonate concentrations are significantly higher in HF. Comparing the two techniques in the long run, HF appears to correct acid-base status better than acetate dialysis does.

Similar results have been achieved by Schaefer et al. (110), who compare acetate dialysis with hemofiltration using lactate as the substitution fluid buffer. HF patients show less alterations in pO_2, a stability of pCO_2 which is slightly higher than with acetate dialysis and a significantly higher bicarbonate concentration when the session was stopped. In both groups pH increased, but more so in HF patients after the end of the treatment; however HF patients experienced a significant initial drop of pH accompanied by a decrease in bicarbonate concentration, probably related to accumulation of lactate in plasma at this time.

Better control of pH in HF have been observed by Kishimoto et al. (39). In studies comparing HF and acetate dialysis they noted that although the net load of acetate was comparable with HF and hemodialysis (660 *vs* 819 mmol respectively), acetate conversion into bicarbonate was significantly greater in HF.

The use of bicarbonate as a buffer in the substitution fluid has been proposed some years ago (108). The main problem, i.e., the bicarbonate stability in a preformed solution, was solved by dividing the substitution fluid bag in two compartment with a septum. The two separated solutions, one alkaline containing bicarbonate and the other acid containing calcium and magnesium, were mixed just before the use by breaking a valve in the partition wall.

Recently this solution has been commercially developed and a feasibility study has been performed (111). Three different solutions containing 30, 35 and 40 mmol/l of bicarbonate were investigated and the influence of these solutions on acid-base balance was evaluated. The end treatment blood bicarbonate concentration was directly correlated with the bicarbonate concentration in the substitution fluid and with the apparent bicarbonate space. A statistical model in order to predict the base gain during the session was presented.

In conclusion, several schedules of hemofiltration have been proposed. They mainly differ in the number of liters exchanged per session and in the composition of substitution fluid. On line production of replacement fluid has also been proposed to avoid the problems related to the wide variability of the commercially prepared solutions in Europe. All these new treatments present different buffer balances and the final acid-base status therefore relates to the technique used.

HEMODIAFILTRATION AND RAPID DIALYSIS

Since blood purification in hemodiafiltration (HDF) is achieved with a mixed diffusive-convective transport, base balance calculations are extremely complex. The net buffer fluxes depend on the interaction between driving force (diffusive parameter) and ultrafiltration (convective parameter).

If diffusive and convective transports for a particular buffer are in the same direction a higher negative net flux would result (29). Convective flux is always negative for any buffer and any treatment because ultrafiltration brings from patient to dialysate all the buffers contained in the patient's plasma.

A negative diffusive flux occurs when the studied buffer is more concentrated in blood than in dialysate and consequently the driving force is negative.

If diffusive and convective fluxes are in the opposite directions (such as when driving force is positive, i.e., when the studied buffer is more concentrated in dialysate than in blood), a decrease in the expected positive net flux would be seen (29). Perhaps some solvent-solute interactions occur which limits diffusive entry of small molecules against a high convective current. The type of interactions determines the dialytic buffer fluxes and consequently allows to optimize the type and the concentration of the buffer in the substitution fluid, the time session and the ultrafiltration rate to be applied.

The classic HDF proposed by Leber in 1978 (112), utilized a dialysis fluid containing acetate as a buffer and 9 liters of substitution fluid containing lactate at a concentration of 40 mmol/l. Some authors later (113, 114) reported a better cardiovascular stability in HDF when bicarbonate replaces acetate in the dialysis solution. Others (115) suggested that bicarbonate substitution fluid may maintain a satisfactory acid-base status in patients on chronic HDF.

These preliminary observations suggest that bicarbonate should be preferred in HDF both for dialysis fluid and replacement solutions (116). The use of acetate containing dialysis solution may promote bicarbonate loss and induce an acetate load greater than the maximal metabolic capacity. On the other hand, substitution fluid containing lactate might progressively increase plasma lactate concentrations with consequent metabolic problems.

A base balance in HDF using bicarbonate both in dialysate (31 mmol/l) and in substitution fluid (41 mmol/l) (114) suggested that bicarbonate losses correlate with the amount of ultrafiltrate produced during the treatment. But the amount of buffer administered via the substitution fluid is generally sufficient to maintain an adequate base balance. Bicarbonate losses during an HDF session carried out exchanging 9 liters of fluid averages 300 mmol. Under these conditions, the reinfusion of 9 liters of substitution fluid containing 41 mmol/l of bicarbonate allows for a slightly positive dialytic bicarbonate balance. Furthermore, blood gases remain fairly stable during treatment with a general steadiness of cardiovascular function and ventilation.

A more recent study (117) demonstrated that in a HDF session with a bicarbonate dialysis fluid, bicarbonate flux is negative even associated with a positive driving force. Multiple linear regression allowed to predict that dialytic bicarbonate flux only becomes positive when the driving force is greater than 17.5 mmol/l (implying a clinical mean blood bicarbonate concentration of less than 17.5 mmol/l if a 35 mmol/l bicarbonate containing dialysate is used) at 50 ml/min of ultrafiltration. This surprising result depends on the opposite directions of diffusive and convective fluxes.

Adding substitution buffer flux to dialytic bicarbonate flux, the buffer balance in this HDF conditions could be predicted. Either lactate (2 mmol/min) or bicarbonate (2.5 mmol/min) containing substitution fluid could lead to an optimum positive buffer balance at clinically utilized ultrafiltration rates for HDF (60–80 ml/min). However lactate containing substitution fluid provided an optimum buffer gain when the mean blood bicarbonate was around 20 mmol/l. These blood bicarbonate values mean that uremic acidosis is not fully correct by this HDF setting. In contrast, when bicarbonate was employed both in dialysis and substitution fluids an optimum buffer balance was reached at a blood bicarbonate concentration of about 25 mmol/l. Therefore this HDF setting would seem the most physiologically appropriate and therapeutic choice (117).

The introduction in the clinical routine of highly permeable membranes and equipments with ultrafiltration control systems has stimulated new interest in HDF and several new techniques have been developed. In Europe HDF is carried out utilizing variable amounts of substitution fluid. Hence, the buffer concentration must be adapted to the amount of fluid exchanged per session. When low volumes of fluid are utilized and a lower convective component is present as in Biofiltration (3 liters/session), higher buffer concentrations are used in the substitution fluid (60–100 mmol/l) (50). Even higher quantities of bicarbonate are reinfused when acetate is completely eliminated from dialysate such as in Acetate Free Biofiltration (AFB) (145–167 mmol/l of bicarbonate) (118). This method of treatment has generated an increased interest because of the high intradialytic tolerance, the simple procedures and the good correction of metabolic acidosis (119).

Since in AFB there is only one directional flow across the dialysate membrane, both convective and diffusive, from the blood to the dialysis bath, a modeling approach in order to optimize the base balance in the individual patient has been proposed (36, 120). The bicarbonate gain may be planned by changing the hourly infusion of the bicarbonate substitution fluid in order to personalize acidosis correction. However, in term of accuracy, these models display a broad range of data dispersion. It has been suggested that the dialytic bicarbonate loss is not a linear function of bicarbonate blood levels and ultrafiltration rate (121). When an AFB schedule with a large connective component is applied, the higher ultrafiltration rate seems to reduce the negative bicarbonate flux. The explanation of this very interesting phenomenon could be that when a high ultrafiltration rate is applied, an higher reinfusion rate is needed. Since the available commercial solutions contain a high bicarbonate concentration, a rapid increase of blood bicarbonate levels is usually seen during the dialytic session. Consequently, large amounts of ultrafiltrate with a high bicarbonate concentration will cross the filter toward the dialysate so that in some part of the dialyzer, dialysate could no longer be 'bicarbonate free', and bicarbonate diffusive flux will be reduced (121). This observation was later confirmed by others (120).

Finally the replacement process is not always carried out utilizing commercially prepared solutions. New techniques have been proposed (48) in which the replacement of fluid lost via ultrafiltration is achieved by backfiltration of sterile dialysate through the hemodiafilter.

In all these new techniques the acid-base balance has not yet been studied even though a satisfactory correction of metabolic acidosis is frequently achieved. A final problem to be clarified concerns the use of highly efficient treatments that allow for a marked reduction of dialysis treatment time. While it is clear that bicarbonate is the only possible buffer for highly efficient treatments, it is still controversial whether acid-base balance can be maintained within acceptable ranges with these rapid techniques.

CONTINUOUS THERAPIES

Continuous arteriovenous hemofiltration (CAVH) and derived techniques are widely used to treat acute renal failure in the critically ill patients. Metabolic acidosis is frequently observed in these patients and an adequate correction is achieved from the buffer balance between ultrafiltration losses and substitution fluid infusion (122).

Bicarbonate loss during CAVH can easily be measured directly in the ultrafiltrate or predicted using the formula:

$$HCO_3\ (f) = UF \times HCO_3\ (p) \times 1.124$$

where HCO_3 (f) and HCO_3 (p) = bicarbonate concentration in the ultrafiltrate and in the plasma; UF = total amount of ultrafiltrate and 1.124 = average bicarbonate sieving coefficient.

When CAVH is applied without fluid substitution in order to reduce the patient's fluid overload, bicarbonate losses are compensated by the reduction of the distribution volume for bicarbonate and the serum concentration does not change significantly. On the contrary, when replacement solutions are infused to maintain the body fluid balance, the same amount of bicarbonate lost in the ultrafiltrate must be administered to achieve stable serum levels of the buffer. Finally, when CAVH is utilized to correct metabolic acidosis, the amount of HCO_3 in the replacement fluid must exceed the amount lost in the ultrafiltrate, providing a positive balance of buffer (123). In some cases lactate can be administered as a buffer without major

problems; this, however, has to be carefully monitored to avoid any risk of lactic acidosis.

In continuous dialysis (CAVHD) the buffer in the dialysate provides an adequate base balance and smaller fluctuations of the acid-base status can be observed with a remarkable clinical stability. Lactate or bicarbonate containing dialysate are generally used in these treatment. Acetate dialysate could be used as well but the possible hemodynamic side effects or the slowed acetate metabolism may increase the risk of intolerance to treatment.

PERITONEAL DIALYSIS

Although intermittent peritoneal dialysis (IPD) has been for years an alternative treatment in patients with end stage renal disease, this type of treatment has now been almost abandoned and continuous ambulatory peritoneal dialysis (CAPD) represents the most common intracorporeal dialysis treatment.

One of the major results achieved with CAPD is the good correction of metabolic acidosis and the maintenance of a satisfactory acid-base status. This is confirmed by an average plasma bicarbonate concentration in patients on CAPD ranging between 22 and 25 mmol/l (124). This result appears to be stable over time and acid-base fluctuations typical of intermittent treatments are not observed. The steadiness of acid-base status probably depends on the continuous infusion of buffers in absence of significant losses of bicarbonate and permits a certain stability of blood gases and ventilation.

Lactate is the commonly used buffer in CAPD. Acetate has also been used in the past but it has been subsequently abandoned when suspected to be responsible for long term side effects such as ultrafiltration loss, severe anatomical alterations of peritoneal membrane and sclerosing peritonitis (125, 126). Furthermore it has been pointed out that acetate levels in the blood may reach dangerous high concentrations with consequent undesired effects (127).

Weekly buffer balance in patients on CAPD can be calculated as follows:

$$NBG_w = n[Binf - (HCO_3 + OA)lost - TAd] - H^+G_w$$

where NBG_w is net base gain per week; n is number of exchanges in a week; Binf is the Buffer infused in each exchange; $(HCO_3 + OA)$ lost is the bicarbonate and organic acid anions lost in the dialysate in each exchange; TAd is the titratable acidity of the inlet dialysis solution (128); and H^+G_w is the weekly metabolic acid production.

In CAPD, long dwell times, permit an almost complete transfer of the buffer from the dialysis solution into the blood. As shown in Figure 7, the buffer disappearance rate is maximal in the first few minutes of the exchange while it subsequently approaches zero. This behaviour is important because it also permits an adequate buffer transfer when rapid exchanges are scheduled. Since in CAPD

LACTATE DISAPPEARANCE FROM DYALISATE

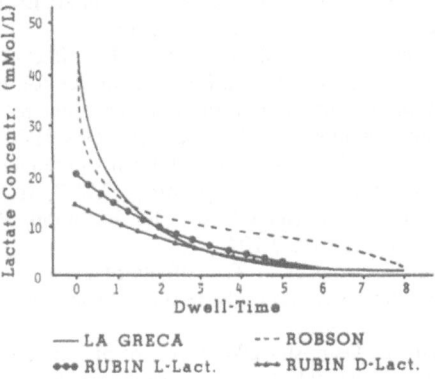

Figure 7. Disappearance of lactate from dialysate (123, 125, 127).

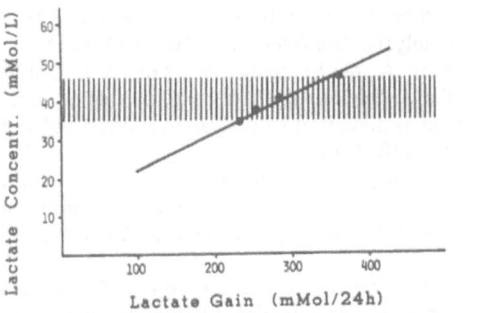

Figure 8. Mass transfer of lactate in relation with lactate concentration in the dialysis solution (123, 125, 127, 128).

the buffer diffuses almost completely from dialysate, the major determinants of net base gain are the concentration of the buffer in the inlet dialysis solution and dwell time.

Figure 8 reports the correlation between the daily buffer gain and the concentration of the buffer in the dialysis solution. Accordingly it would be possible to predict the daily buffer gain in a given patient on the basis of the buffer concentration in the dialysis solution. It must be noted that D-lactate and L-lactate may have different rates of transport. Rubin et al. (129) demonstrated that the peritoneal membrane can operate a stereospecific selection in the process of lactate transport. L-lactate has an higher mass transfer rate (MTR) and it is rapidly metabolized in the body. D-lactate is metabolized more slowly, but the very low MTR permits complete metabolism of this stereoisomeric compound as well.

During dialysis, bicarbonate back diffuses in the dialysate. However, bicarbonate losses in peritoneal dialysis are not easy to quantify because of specific problems related to ultrafiltration, plasma bicarbonate concentra-

tion and methodology of measurement of bicarbonate in the dialysate.

Ultrafiltration is the major determinant of bicarbonate losses in the dialysate. It is evident that when dialysate/plasma equilibration takes place, an increase in drainage volume due to ultrafiltration, causes a greater loss of bicarbonate. The same effect is determined by higher HCO_3 plasma concentrations although several studies suggest a possible feed back mechanism between plasma bicarbonate concentration and amount of bicarbonate lost in the dialysate (130, 131). An increased plasma bicarbonate level causes a parallel increase of bicarbonate losses until the dialysate/plasma equilibration is reached and no more bicarbonate diffuses. It may also be argued that a Donnan equilibrium could cause bicarbonate losses greater than expected from the plasma concentration because of the presence of non diffusable anions such as plasma proteins in the blood compartment, but this phenomenon is too small for any clinical relevance.

A further problem concerns the method of measurement of the carbonic acid/bicarbonate system in the peritoneal dialysis solution. It does not have the same pK as in blood so the measurements cannot be correctly done with the commonly used analyzers.

Finally we must consider the losses in the dialysate of metabolizable anions of organic acids. These substances represent effective alkaline equivalents since their metabolism produces bicarbonate. Among these substrates, only acetoacetate and β-hydroxybutirate have quantitative relevance. Teehan et al. (132) have reported daily losses in the dialysate of 1.0 ± 0.3 mmol of acetoacetate and 4.1 ± 1.9 of β-hydroxybutirate. Other substances are lost in the dialysate such as tricarboxylic anions although they have never been quantified. Yet a significant anion gap (36 ± 17 mmol/24 h) is observed in the effluent dialysate (132).

For all these reasons a remarkable difference among the various acid-base balance studies can be noted, although there is a general agreement that CAPD corrects metabolic acidosis quite well (124, 127, 131). The different results of acid-balance studies depend on the several variables mentioned above. But the major determinant of the net base gain is the concentration of the buffer in the dialysis solution.

Bicarbonate has been recently proposed as a buffer for CAPD (130, 133). Experimental and clinical pilot studies (134, 135) demonstrated that, in the short term period, the solution is safe, well tolerated, does not affect peritoneal adequacy and is effective in the correction of metabolic acidosis. Larger multicentre studies are still in progress.

FINAL REMARKS

Review of the literature and the clinical experience confirm that correction of metabolic acidosis in uremic patients with dialysis is not yet optimized and still presents some controversies. Acetate dialysis has been almost totally substituted by bicarbonate dialysis being supported by several experimental and clinical observations. Bicarbonate is the physiological buffer, it does not require metabolic conversion and it does not cause any known side effect except for possible alkalosis deriving from excessive administration. Technological problems concerning dialysis equipments and solutions have been overcome and treatment costs are not significantly higher using bicarbonate dialysate. Finally, the excellent clinical tolerance of bicarbonate dialysis, makes this treatment a first choice therapy today.

This trend assumes more and more importance in relation to the widening application in clinical practice of highly efficient treatments with a consistent reduction of dialysis treatment time. Bicarbonate in fact becomes mandatory as a buffer for hemodialysis when high surface area dialyzers and highly permeable membranes are utilized in conjunction with high blood and dialysate flows.

A final consideration concerns the necessity to achieve a good acid-base status in dialysis patients and the need to make great efforts at metabolic correction with dialysis treatment. Some authors (14) suggested that this is a negligible problem which does not cause any long term clinical effect. We believe that all possible efforts must be made to achieve, together with an adequate blood purification, the best possible correction of metabolic acidosis in uremic patients. This concept derives from the conviction that acidosis may interfere with several functions of the body such as ventilation, cardiovascular activity, skeletal metabolism and finally chemical and enzymatic reactions.

REFERENCES

1. Kolff WJ: Le rein artificiel: un dialyseur a grande surface. *Presse Medicale* 52: 103, 1944
2. Scribner BH, Caner JEZ, Buri R: The technique of continuous hemodialysis. *Trans Am Soc Artif Intern Organs* 6: 88, 1960
3. Mion CM, Hegstrom RM, Boen ST, Scribner BH: Substitution of sodium acetate for sodium bicarbonate in the bath fluid for hemodialysis. *Trans Am Soc Artif Intern Organs* 10: 110, 1964
4. Ledebo I: Bicarbonate in high-efficiency hemodialysis. in *Hemodialysis. High-Efficiency Treatments*, edited by Bosch JP, New York, Churchill Livingstone, 1993, p 9
5. Schwartz WB, Hall PV, Hays RM, Relman AS: On the mechanism of acidosis in chronic renal disease. *J Clin Invest* 38: 39, 1959
6. Zucchelli P, Santoro A: Correction of acid balance by dialysis. *Kidney Int* 43 (Suppl 41): 179S, 1993
7. Marsiglia JC, Cingolani HE, Gonzales NC: Relevance of beta receptor blockade to the negative inotropic effect induced by metabolic acidosis. *Cardiovasc Res* 7: 336, 1973
8. Harrington JT, Cohen JJ: Metabolic acidosis. in *Acid/Base*, edited by Cohen JJ, Kassirer JP, Boston, Little, Brown and Company, 1982, p 121
9. Lemann J Jr, Litzow JR, Lennon EJ: The effect of chronic acid loads in normal man: further evidence for the partecipation of bone mineral in the defence against chronic metabolic acidosis. *J Clin Invest* 45: 1608, 1966
10. Massry SG: Divalent ion metabolism and renal osteodystrophy. in *Textbook of Nephrology*, Vol 2, 1st Edition, edited by Massry SG, Glassock RJ, Baltimore, Williams & Wilkins, 1983, p 7.104
11. Barzel US, Jowsey J: The effects of chronic acid and alkali administration on bone turnover in adult rat. *Clin Sci* 36: 517, 1969
12. Arnett TR, Dempster DW: Effect of pH on bone resorption by rat osteoclasts *in vitro*. *Endocrinology* 119: 119, 1986
13. Bichara M, Mercier O, Borensztein P, Paillard M: Acute metabolic acidosis enhances circulating parathyroid hormone, which contributes to renal response against acidosis in the rat. *J Clin Invest* 86: 430, 1990
14. Gennari FJ: Acid-base balance in dialysis patients. *Kidney Int* 28: 678, 1985
15. Van Stone JC: Oral base replacement in patients on hemodialysis. *Ann Intern Med* 101: 199, 1984
16. Lefebvre A, de Verneoul MC, Gueris J, Goldfarb B, Graulet AM, Morieux C: Optimal correction of acidosis changes progression of dialysis osteodystrophy. *Kidney Int* 36: 1112, 1989
17. May RC, Kelly RA, Mitch WE: Mechanisms for defects in muscle protein metabolism in rats with chronic uremia: the influence of metabolic acidosis. *J Clin Invest* 79: 1099, 1987
18. May RC, Kelly RA, Mitch WE: Metabolic acidosis stimulates protein degradation in rat muscle by a glucocorticoid-dependent mechanism. *J Clin Invest* 77: 614, 1986
19. Hara Y, May RC, Kelly RA, Mitch WE: Acidosis, not azotemia, stimulates branched-chain amino acid catabolism in uremic rats. *Kidney Int* 32: 808, 1987
20. Mitch WE, Clark AS: Specificity of the effect of leucine and its metabolites on protein degradation in skeletal muscle. *Biochem J* 222: 579, 1984
21. Papadoyannakis NJ, Stefanides CJ, McGeown M: The effect of the correction of metabolic acidosis on nitrogen and protein balance of patients with chronic renal failure. *Am J Clin Nutr* 40: 623, 1984
22. Garibotto G, Russo R, Sala MR et al.: Muscle protein turnover and amino acid metabolism in patients with chronic renal failure. *Miner Electrolyte Metab* 18: 217, 1992
23. Jenkins D, Burton PR, Bennet SE, Baker F, Walls J: The metabolic consequences of the correction of acidosis in uraemia. *Nephrol Dial Transpl* 4: 92, 1989
24. Williams B, Hattersley J, Layward E, Walls J: Metabolic acidosis and skeletal muscle adaptation to low protein diets in chronic uremia. *Kidney Int* 40: 779, 1991
25. Bergstrom J, Alvestrand A, Furst P: Plasma and muscle free amino acids in maintenance hemodialysis patients without protein malnutrition. *Kidney Int* 38: 108, 1990
26. Lennon EJ, Lemann J Jr, Litzow JR: The effects of diet and stool composition on the net external acid balance of normal subjects. *J Clin Invest* 45: 1601, 1966

27. Gotch FA, Sargent JA, Keen ML: Hydrogen ion balance in dialysis therapy. *Artif Organs* 6: 388, 1982
28. Assomull VM, Vreman HJ, Weiner MW: Mass balance of base equivalents during hemodialysis: importance of organic acid anions. *Proc Clin Dial Transplant Forum* 8: 137, 1978
29. Sargent JA, Gotch FA: Bicarbonate and carbon dioxide transport during hemodialysis. *ASAIO J* 2: 61, 1979
30. Bosch JP, Glabman S, Moutoussis G, Belledonne M, von Albertini B, Kahn T: Carbon dioxide removal in acetate hemodialysis: effects on acid base balance. *Kidney Int* 25: 830, 1984
31. Christensen HN: General concepts of neutrality regulation. *Am J Surg* 103: 286, 1962
32. Wathen RL, Ward RA: Disturbances in fluid, electrolyte, and acid base in the dialysis patient. in *Textbook of Nephrology*, Vol 2, 1st Edition, Massry SG, Glassok RJ, Baltimore, Williams & Wilkins, 1983, p 7.98
33. Fernandez PC, Cohen RM, Feldman GM: The concept of bicarbonate distribution space: the crucial role of body buffers. *Kidney Int* 36: 747, 1989
34. Garella S, Dana CL, Chazan JA: Severity of metabolic acidosis as a determinant of bicarbonate requirements. *N Engl J Med* 289: 121, 1973
35. Androgué HJ, Brensilver J, Cohen JJ, Madias NE: Influence of steady-state alterations in acid-base equilibrium on the fate of administered bicarbonate in the dog. *J Clin Invest* 71: 867, 1983
36. Pacitti A, Atti M, Alloatti A et al.: Computer modeled bicarbonate kinetic in acetate free biofiltration. in *Blood Purification in Perspective: New Insights and Future Trends*, Vol 2, edited by Man NR, Botella J, Zucchelli P, Cleveland, Icaot Press, 1992, p 191
37. Vreman HJ, Assomull VM, Kaiser BA, Blaschke TF, Weiner MW: Acetate metabolism and acid-base homeostasis during hemodialysis: influence of dialyzer efficiency and rate of acetate metabolism. *Kidney Int* 18 (Suppl 10): 62S, 1980
38. Tolchin N, Roberts JL, Hayashi J, Lewis EJ: Metabolic consequences of high mass-transfer hemodialysis. *Kidney Int* 11: 366, 1977
39. Kishimoto T, Yamamoto T, Yamamoto K et al.: Acetate kinetics during hemodialysis and hemofiltration. *Blood Purif* 2: 81, 1984
40. La Greca G, Feriani M, Bragantini L, Petrosino L, Santoro A, Altieri P: Effects of acetate and bicarbonate dialysate on vascular stability: a prospective multicentric study. *Int J Artif Organs* 10: 157, 1987
41. Ward RA, Wathen RL, Williams TE: Effects of long-term bicarbonate hemodialysis (BHD) on acid-base status. *Trans Am Soc Artif Intern Organs* 28: 295, 1982
42. Bjaeldager PAL, Christiansen E, Jensen HAE, Paulev PEK: Improved effect of hemodialysis on acidemic patients from an acetate concentration of 38 mmol/l. *Nephron* 27: 142, 1981
43. Mansell MA, Nunan TO, Laker MF, Boon NA, Wing AJ: Incidence and significance of rising blood acetate levels during hemodialysis. *Clin Nephrol* 12: 22, 1979
44. Richards RH, Vreman HJ, Zager Ph, Feldman C, Blaschke T, Weiner MW: Acetate metabolism in normal human subject. *Am J Kidney Dis* 11: 47, 1982

45. Lewis EJ, Tolchin N, Roberts JL: Estimation of the metabolic conversion of acetate to bicarbonate during hemodialysis. *Kidney Int* 18 (Suppl 10): 51, 1980
46. Kveim M, Nesbakken R: Utilisation of exogenous acetate during hemodialysis. *Trans Am Soc Artif Intern Organs* 21: 138, 1975
47. Kaiser BA, Potter DE, Bryant RE, Vreman HJ, Weiner MW: Acid-base changes and acetate metabolism during routine and high efficiency hemodialysis in children. *Kidney Int* 19: 70, 1981
48. von Albertini B, Miller JH, Gardner PW, Shinaberger JH: High-flux hemodiafiltration: under six hours/week treatment. *Trans Am Soc Artif Intern Organs* 30: 227, 1984
49. Ward RA, Wathen RL: Utilization of bicarbonate for base repletion in hemodialysis. *Artif Organs* 6: 369, 1982
50. Feriani M, Bragantini L, Dell'Aquila R et al.: Buffer kinetics in biofiltration. *Int J Artif Organs* 9 (Suppl 3): 1S, 1986
51. Sprenger KBG, Kratz W, Lewis AE, Stadtmüller U: Kinetic modeling of hemodialysis, hemofiltration, and hemodiafiltration. *Kidney Int* 24: 143, 1983
52. Colton CK, Henderson LW, Ford CA, Lysaght MJ: Kinetic of hemodiafiltration. I. *In vitro* transport characteristics of a hollow-fiber blood ultrafilter. *J Lab Clin Med* 85: 355, 1975
53. Henderson LW, Colton CK, Ford CA: Kinetics of hemodiafiltration. II. Clinical characterization of a blood cleansing modality. *J Lab Clin Med* 85: 372, 1975
54. Graefe U, Milutinovich J, Follette WC, Vizzo JE, Babb AL, Scribner BH: Less dialysis-induced morbidity and vascular instability with bicarbonate in dialysate. *Ann Int Med* 88: 332, 1978
55. Nissenson AR, Kraut JA, Shinaberger JH: Dialysis-associated hypoxemia: pathogenesis and prevention. *ASAIO J* 7: 1, 1984
56. Wathen RL, Ferris FZ, Nagar D, Keshaviah P: An alternative explanation for dialysis-induced arterial hypoxemia. (Abstract) *Kidney Int* 14: 689, 1978
57. Hirtzel P, Maher JF, Tempel GE, Mengel CE: Effect of hemodialysis on factors influencing oxygen transport. *J Lab Clin Med* 85: 978, 1975
58. Bischel MD, Scoles BG, Mohler JG: Evidence for pulmonary microembolization during hemodialysis. *Chest* 67: 335, 1975
59. Aurigemma NM, Feldman NT, Gottlieb M, Ingram RH, Lazarus JM, Lowrie EG: arterial oxygenation during hemodialysis. *N Engl J Med* 297: 871, 1977
60. Craddock PR, Fehr J, Brigham KL, Kronenberg RS, Jacob HS: Complement and leukocyte-mediated pulmonary dysfunction in hemodialysis. *N Engl J Med* 296: 770, 1977
61. Jacob AI, Gavellas G, Zarco R, Perez G, Bourgoignie JJ: Leucopenia, hypoxia and complement function with different hemodialysis membranes. *Kidney Int* 18: 105, 1980
62. Brautbar N, Shinaberger JH, Miller JH, Nachman M: Hemodialysis hypoxemia: evaluation of mechanism utilizing sequential ultrafiltration-dialysis. *Nephron* 26: 96, 1980
63. Sherlock J, Ledwith J, Letteri J: Hypoventilation and hypoxemia during hemodialysis: reflex response to

removal of CO2 across the dialyzer. *Trans Am Soc Artif Intern Organs* 23: 406, 1977

64. Dolan MJ, Whipp BJ, Davidson WD, Weitzman RE, Wasserman K: Hypopnea associated with acetate hemodialysis: carbon dioxide flow-dependent ventilation. *N Engl J Med* 305: 72, 1981
65. Bouffard Y, Viale JP, Annat G et al.: Pulmonary gas exchange during hemodialysis. *Kidney Int* 30: 920, 1986
66. Oh MS, Uribarri J, Del Monte ML, Friedman EA, Carroll HJ: Consumption of CO2 in metabolism of acetate as an explanation for hypoventilation and hypoxemia during hemodialysis. *Proc Clin Dial Transplant Forum* 9: 226, 1979
67. Raja RM, Kramer MS, Rosenbaum JL, Bolisay CG, Krug MJ: Hemodialysis associated hypoxemia. Role of acetate and pH in etiology. *Trans Am Soc Artif Intern Organs* 27: 180, 1982
68. Garella S, Chang BS: Hemodialysis-associated hypoxemia. *Am J Nephrol* 4: 273, 1984
69. Graziani G, Ponticelli C, Di Filippo G, Radaelli B: Acid-base changes in hemodialysis. *Br Med J* 3: 163, 1970
70. Romaldini H, Stabile C, Faro S, Lopes Dos Santos M, Ramos OL, Ribeiro Ratto O: Pulmonary ventilation during hemodialysis. *Nephron* 32: 131, 1982
71. Bauer W, Richards JW: A vasodilator action of acetate. *J Physiol* 66: 371, 1928
72. Frohlich ED: Vascular effects of the Krebs intermediate metabolites. *Am J Physiol* 208: 149, 1965
73. Kirkendol PL, Devia CJ, Bower JD, Holbert RD: A comparison of the cardiovascular effects of sodium acetate, sodium bicarbonate and other potential sources of fixed base in hemodialysate solutions. *Trans Am Soc Artif Intern Organs* 23: 399, 1977
74. Aizawa Y, Ohmori T, Imai K, Nara Y, Matsuoka M, Hirakawa Y: Depressant action of acetate upon the human cardiovacsular system. *Clin Nephrol* 8: 477, 1977
75. Kirkendol PL, Robie NW, Gonzalez FM, Devia CJ: Cardiac and vascular effects of infused sodium acetate in dogs. *Trans Am Soc Artif Intern Organs* 24: 714, 1978
76. Chen TS, Friedman HS, Del Monte M, Smith AJ: Hemodynamic changes during dialysis. *Proc Clin Dial Transplant Forum* 9: 66, 1979
77. Liang CS, Lowenstein JM: Metabolic control of the circulation effects of acetate and pyruvate. *J Clin Invest* 62: 1029, 1978
78. Metha BR, Fischer D, Ahmad M, Dubose TD Jr: Effects of acetate and bicarbonate hemodialysis on cardiac function in chronic dialysis patients. *Kidney Int* 24: 782, 1983
79. Danielsson A, Freyschuss U, Bergström J: Cardiovascular function and alveolar gas exchange during isovolemic hemodialysis with acetate in healthy man. *Blood Purif* 5: 41, 1987
80. Kinet JP, Soyeur D, Balland N, Saint-Remy M, Collignon P, Godon JP: Hemodynamic study of hypotension during hemodialysis. *Kidney Int* 21: 868, 1982
81. Rorke SJ, Davidson WD, Guo SS, Morin RJ: Metabolic fate of C-Acetate during dialysis. *Proc Eur Dial Transpl Assoc* 13: 394, 1976
82. Assomull VM, Vreman HJ, Weiner MW: Evidence that acetate in dialysate does not stimulate lipid synthesis. *Proc Dial Trasplant Forum* 9: 73, 1979

83. Morin RJ, Srikanraiah MV, Woodley Z, Davidson WD: Effect of acetate *vs* bicarbonate on plasma lipid and lipoprotein levels in uremic patients. *J Dial* 4: 9, 1980
84. Henderson LW, Koch KM, Dinarello CA, Shaldon S: Hemodialysis hypotension: The interleukin hypothesis. *Blood Purif* 1: 3, 1983
85. Colton CK: Analysis of membrane process for blood purification. *Blood Purif* 5: 202, 1987
86. Shaldon S, Deschodt G, Branger B et al.: Hemodialysis hypotension: the interleukin hypotesis restated. *Proc Eur Dial Transpl Assoc* 22: 229, 1985
87. Dodd NJ, Parson V, Weston MJ: Leukocyte occlusion of cuprophane membrane as a cause of reduced hemodialysis efficiency. *Int J Artif Organs* 5: 275, 1982
88. Koch KM, Shaldon S, Baldamus CA, Lysaght MJ, Lonnemann G, Bingel M, Dinarello CA: Convective mass transport in dialysis. *Proc Eur Dial Transpl Assoc* 22: 467, 1985
89. Bingel M, Koch KM, Dinarello CA, Shaldon S: Human interleukin-1 production is enhanced by sodium acetate. *Lancet* i: 14, 1987
90. Man NK, Fournier G, Thireau P, Gaillard JL, Funk-Brentano JL: Effect of bicarbonate-containing dialysate on chronic hemodialysis patients: A comparative study. *Artif Organs* 6: 421, 1982
91. Nissenson AR: Prevention of dialysis-induced hypoxemia by bicarbonate dialysis. *Trans Am Soc Artif Intern Organs* 26: 339, 1980
92. Hakim RM, Pontzer MA, Tilton D, Lazarus JM, Gottlieb MN: Effects of acetate and bicarbonate dialysis in stable chronic dialysis patients. *Kidney Int* 28: 535, 1985
93. Abu-Hamdan DK, Mahajan SK, Desai S et al.: Hypoxemia during bicarbonate dialysis. (Abstract) *Am Soc Nephrol* 13: 33, 1980
94. Borges H, Fryd DS, Rosa AA, Kjellstrand CM: Hypotension during aceta and bicarbonate dialysis in patients with acute renal failure. *Am J Nephrol* 1: 24, 1981
95. Eiser AR, Jayammane D, Kokseng C, Che H, Slifkin RF, Neff MS: Contrasting alterations in pulmonary gas exchange during acetate and bicarbonate hemodialysis. *Am J Nephrol* 2: 123, 1982
96. Iseki K, Onoyama K, Maeda T et al.: Comparison of hemodynamics induced by conventional acetate hemodialysis, bicarbonate hemodialysis and ultrafiltration. *Clin Nephrol* 14: 294, 1980
97. Mitchell J, Wildenthal K, Johnson R: The effects of acid-base disturbances on cardiovascular and pulmonary function. *Kidney Int* 1: 375, 1972
98. Ruder MA, Alpert MA, Van Stone J et al.: Comparative effects of acetate and bicarbonate hemodialysis on left ventricular function. *Kidney Int* 27: 768, 1985
99. Henrich W, Hunt J, Nixon J: Increased ionized calcium and left ventricular contractility during hemodialysis. *N Engl J Med* 310: 19, 1983
100. Mansell MA, Morgan SH, Moore R, Kong KH, Laker MF, Wing AJ: Cardiovascular and acid-base effects of acetate and bicarbonate hemodialysis. *Nephrol Dial Transpl* 1: 229, 1987
101. Velez RL, Woodard TD, Henrich WL: Acetate and bicarbonate hemodialysis in patients with and without autonomic dysfunction. *Kidney Int* 26: 59, 1984
102. Henrich WL, Woodard TD, Meyer BD, Chappell TR, Rubin LJ: High sodium bicarbonate and acetate

hemodialysis: double-blind crossover comparison of hemodynamic and ventilatory effects. *Kidney Int* 24: 240, 1983

103. Whele B, Asaba H, Casterfors J et al.: The influence of dialysis fluid composition on the blood pressure response during dialysis. *Clin Nephrol* 10: 62, 1978

104. Chen T, Friedman H, Smith A, Del Monte M: Hemodynamic changes during hemodialysis role of dialysate. *Clin Nephrol* 20: 190, 1983

105. Hampl H, Wolfquiler M, Pustelruk A, Schiller R, Hanefeld F, Kessel M: Advantage of bicarbonate hemodialysis. *Artif Organs* 6: 410, 1982

106. Vanholder R, Piron M, Ringoir S: Absence of a beneficial haemodynamic effect of bicarbonate *vs* acetate haemodialysis. *Proc Eur Dial Transpl Assoc* 21: 195, 1984

107. Pagel MD, Ahmad S, Vizzo JE, Scribner BH: Acetate and bicarbonate fluctuations and acetate intolerance during dialysis. *Kidney Int* 21: 513, 1982

108. Feriani M, Biasioli S, Fabris A et al.: Calcium and bicarbonate containing solutions for peritoneal dialysis and hemofiltration. in *Progress in Artificial Organs*, edited by Nosè Y, Kjellstrand C, Ivanovich P, Cleveland, ISAO Press, 1986, p 277

109. Bosch JP, Lauer A: Acid-base balance in hemofiltration. in *Hemofiltration*, edited by Henderson LW, Quellhorst EA, Baldamus CA, Lysaght MJ, Berlin, Springer-Verlag, 1986, p 147

110. Schaefer K, Ryzlewicz T, Sandri M, von Bernewitz S, von Herrath D: Effect of hemofiltration on acid-base status and ventilation. *Contrib Nephrol* 32: 69, 1982

111. Santoro A, Ferrari G, Bolzani R, Spongano M, Zucchelli P: Regulation of base balance in bicarbonate hemofiltration. *Int J Artif Organs* 17: 27, 1994

112. Leber HW, Wizemann V, Goubeand G, Rawer P, Schütterle G: Simultaneous hemofiltration/hemodialysis: an effective alternative to hemofiltration and conventional hemodialysis in the treatment of uremic patients. *Clin Nephrol* 9: 115, 1978

113. Scheider H, Liornin E, Streicher E: Haemodinamyc studies of diffusive and convective procedures using a polysulphone membrane. *Contrib Nephrol* 46: 134, 1985

114. Feriani M, Biasioli S, Bragantini L et al.: Buffer balance in bicarbonate hemodiafiltration. *Trans Am Soc Artif Intern Organs* 32: 422, 1986

115. Arisi L, Calderini C, David S, Manari A, Mancuso S, Cambi V: Acid base balance in hypertonic hemodiafiltration. in *Uremic Acidosis*, editd by Petrella E, Milano, Wichtig editore, 1983, p 71

116. Biasioli S, Feriani M, Chiaramonte S et al.: Different buffers for hemodiafiltration: a controlled study. *Int J Artif Organs* 12: 25, 1989

117. Feriani M, Ronco C, Biasioli S, Bragantini L, La Greca G: Effect of dialysate and substitution fluid buffer on buffer flux in hemodiafiltration. *Kidney Int* 39: 711, 1990

118. Bene B, Beruard M, Perrone B, Simon P: Simultaneous dialysis and filtration with buffer-free dialysate. (Abstract) *Blood Purif* 2: 217, 1985

119. Santoro A, Ferrari G, Spongano M, Badiali F, Zucchelli P: Acetate-Free Biofiltration: a viable alternative to bicarbonate hemodialysis. *Artif Organs* 13: 476, 1989

120. Santoro A, Spongano M, Ferrari G et al.: Analysis of the factors influencing bicarbonate balance during acetatefree biofiltration. *Kidney Int* 43 (Suppl 41): 184S, 1993

121. Feriani M, Bragantini L, Milan M et al.: Bicarbonate kinetics in Acetate-Free Biofiltration. in *Blood Purification in Perspective: New Insights and Future Trends*, Vol 2, edited by Man NR, Botella J, Zucchelli P, Cleveland, Icaot Press, 1992, p 164

122. Ronco C: Continuous renal replacement therapies for the treatment of acute renal failure in intensive care patients. *Clin Nephrol* 40: 187, 1993

123. Raimondi F, Bianchi T, Emmi V: Use of continuous arteriovenous hemofiltration (CAVH) in lactic acidosis: a case report. in *CAVH*, edited by La Greca G, Fabris A, Ronco C, Milano, Wichtig Editore, 1986, p 135

124. Fabris A, Biasioli S, Chiaramonte S et al.: Buffer metabolism in CAPD: Relationship with respiratory dynamics. *Trans Am Soc Artif Intern Organs* 28: 270, 1982

125. Faller B, Marichal JF: Loss of ultrafiltration in CAPD a role for acetate. *Perit Dial Bull* 4: 10, 1984

126. Slingeneyer A, Mion C, Mourad G, Canaud B, Faller B, Beraud JJ: Progressive sclerosing peritonitis. A late and severe complication of maintenance peritoneal dialysis. *Trans Am Soc Artif Intern Organs* 29: 633, 1983

127. La Greca G, Biasioli S, Chiaramonte S et al.: Acid-base balance on peritoneal dialysis. *Clin Nephrol* 16: 1, 1981

128. Pedersen FB, Ryttof N, Deleuran P, Dragsholt C, Kildeberg P: Acetate *vs* lactate in peritoneal dialysis solutions. *Nephron* 39: 55, 1985

129. Rubin J, Adair C, Johnson B, Bower JD: Stereospecific lactate absorption during peritoneal dialysis. *Nephron* 31: 224, 1982

130. Feriani M, Biasioli S, Borin D et al.: Bicarbonate buffer for CAPD solution. *Trans Am Soc Artif Intern Organs* 31: 668, 1985

131. Robson MD, Faivoseviz A, Malmoud H: Physiological transfer of acid base. in *Continuous Ambulatory Peritoneal Dialysis*, Legrain M, Amsterdam, Excerpta Medica, 1980, p 194

132. Teehan BP, Schleifer CR, Reichard GA, Cupit MC, Siglar MH, Haff AC: Acid-base studies in CAPD. in *CAPD Update*, edited by Moncrief JW, Popovich RP, New York, Masson Publishing, 1981, p 95

133. Yatzidis H: A new stable bicarbonate dialysis solution for peritoneal dialysis: preliminary report. *Perit Dial Int* 11: 224, 1991

134. Feriani M, Biasioli S, Barbacini S et al.: Acid base correction in bicarbonate CAPD patients. *Adv Perit Dial* 5: 191, 1989

135. Feriani M, Dissegna D, La Greca G, Passlick-Deetjen J: Short term clinical study with bicarbonate containing peritoneal dialysis solution. *Perit Dial Int* 13: 296, 1993

PULMONARY ASPECTS OF DIALYSIS PATIENTS

MARC E. DE BROE, ROBERT L. LINS and WILFRIED A. DE BACKER

INTRODUCTION

Patients with acute or end-stage chronic renal failure, whether treated by dialysis or not, frequently develop pulmonary complications such as edema, pleural effusion and infection (1). In addition, hemodialysis treatment is always accompanied with a variable degree of hypoxemia at the start or towards the end of the treatment session. Respiratory failure secondary to hyperkalemia is a life threatening, fortunately rare complication, in chronic hemodialysis.

UREMIC LUNG

Radiologists first described the characteristic butterfly or batwing appearance in anteroposterior X-rays of the lung. The periphery of the lung remains normally translucent, while more central areas are opaque and display a waist-like constriction of the shadow. As this entity frequently complicates end-stage renal failure, it was referred to as 'uremic lung'. Later on, it was also recognized in other conditions as in acute rheumatic fever and chronic left ventricular failure. In patients with chronic renal failure, the pressure forces in the Starling equation often favor secondary pulmonary edema. Hydrostatic pressures in the central circulation may be high because of increased intravascular volume or congestive heart failure or both.

Intravascular oncotic pressure may also be low because of hypoproteinemia, predisposing to pulmonary edema at lower hydrostatic pressures (2). For these reasons alone, butterfly infiltrates of pulmonary edema on chest radiograph would be expected. Uremic lung thus is a form of pulmonary edema which can eventually result in fibrotic interstitial changes.

In the early phase the alveoli fibrinous edema fluid and the interlobular septa are very edematous and swollen. Usually the edema fluid is completely absorbed, but in more chronic persistent cases the exudate organizes and fibrotic changes occur in the interstitium.

The characteristic distribution of the edematous exudate found in 'uremic lung' is largely explained by diversion of flow to more central parts of the lung which are supplied by the shortest arterial pathway. Indeed, the raised pulmonary venous pressure due to left ventricular failure causes reflex vasoconstriction in the pulmonary arteries especially of the longer arterial pathways resulting in diversion of the blood flow through more central parts of the lung.

It is now generally agreed that uremic lung is a form of pulmonary edema caused primarily by left ventricular failure and pulmonary engorgement, but in which in addition a local capillary toxic factor and possibly deficient fibrinolysis also play a part. This toxic factor, still unknown and most probably the same as mentioned in the occurrence of uremic pleuritis, increases the permeability of alveolar capillaries resulting in leakage of macromolecular proteins and even red blood cells.

The most important cause of lung edema in dialysis patients is noncompliance with fluid restriction, a rather frequent condition especially in patients with no or negligible residual diuresis. Patients with acute renal failure are also highly susceptible to pulmonary edema. Indeed, they frequently have decreased plasma oncotic pressure, an increased hydrostatic pressure in pulmonary capillaries because of fluid overload and changes in alveolar capillaries due to their uremic state. Severe fluid overload in patients with acute renal failure not responding to high doses of loop diuretics, is a classical indication for emergency dialysis with ultrafiltration or continuous slow ultrafiltration.

PLEURAL EFFUSION IN DIALYSIS

Richard Bright noted that in patients who died of nephritis 'of all the membranes the pleura has decidedly been most often diseased' (3). Uremic patients have an increased susceptibility to many causes of transudative or exudative pleural effusion such as congestive heart failure, nephrotic syndrome, salt and water retention and infection (4). In addition there exists an idiopathic uremic pleural effusion.

Furthermore, dialysis patients may develop pleural effusion directly related to their type of treatment such as a catheter related superior *vena cava* obstruction or subclavian venous catheter leak (5). With peritoneal dialysis a leakage of dialysate through a small, often congenital diaphragmatic defect may result in a small pleural effusion relieved by erect posture, up to a massive usually right-sided hydrothorax within hours to days after starting this type of treatment.

Idiopathic pleural involvement in uremia and in dialysis patients results from necrotizing fibrinous inflammation and often results in a serous serosanguineous or even hemorrhagic effusion (6, 7). This type of pleural reaction may occur without concomitant overhydration and without apparent cause; gradual spontaneous resolution often occurs sometimes followed by recurrences (6). One should search carefully for evidence of coexisting pericardial effusion in these cases. A few patients have progressive disease wherein the pleural fluid becomes gelatinous and a thick fibrous peel develops (8, 9). Fibrous uremic pleuritis causes progressive restriction of pulmonary function with restricted lung volumes and disabling dyspnea of increasing severity until relieved by surgical decortication (8).

The etiology and/or pathogenesis of uremic pleuritis remains unknown and has been the subject of numerous speculations (4). It must be emphasized that the finding of bloody pleural effusion in an uremic patient (dialyzed or not) requires the exclusion of all causes of hemorrhagic pleural effusion before it is concluded to be due to uremia.

DIALYSIS ASSOCIATED HYPOXEMIA

The dialysis patient, being treated intermittently on a three times weekly schedule, is exposed during the short dialysis period (4 h) to abrupt changes in the internal milieu.

The patient slowly accumulates H^+ ions during the 44 h interdialytic period and is in a respiratory compensated (hyperventilation) metabolic acidosis at the start of dialysis. Indeed, a HCO_3^- level between 17 and 23 mEq/l and a rather low $PaCO_2$ of 33 to 36 mmHg is observed. Four hours later, using a biocompatible (polyacrylonitrile, PAN) or bioincompatible membrane (cuprophane, CP) and a bicarbonate or acetate dialysis bath, he ends up with a slight degree of metabolic alkalosis, mild to moderate hypoventilation, with or without breathing irregularities (Figures 1A, B). Defined in another way: the dialysis patient is an acid accumulator for 44 h followed by a 4 h efficient period of retitration which can be accompanied by a variable degree of hypoxemia.

The latter phenomenon has been the subject of numerous investigations during the last 15 years (for review see (10–13)). As happens with complex biological processes, the conclusions reached by different investigators are conflicting depending on their viewpoint and the variables they examined. Since Johnson and colleagues in 1970 (14) showed that patients dialyzed with an acetate containing dialysate developed hypoxemia and attributed it to the hypoventilation following CO_2 losses through the dialyzer a number of other mechanisms have been proposed, defended by some, questioned by others. The various proposed mechanisms will be critically evaluated and the respective role of the two most important ones i.e., 'CO_2 unloading' and the 'complement-activation-hypoxemia' cascade will be defined.

Pulmonary microembolization

Bishel et al. (15) suggested that microemboli of particulate material (platelets, leucocytes, fibrin) originating from the interaction between blood and the extracorporeal circuit might be responsible for decrease in arterial oxygen tension (PaO_2). This hypothesis could not be confirmed by others (16) since hypoxemia occurred despite microfiltration of venous blood.

Changes in oxygen transport (Bohr effect) and ventilation due to correction of acidosis

The small increase in pH which is usually observed in the course of hemodialysis (17) (Figure 1B) could theoretically lead to hypoxemia on the basis of an alkalosis-induced central respiratory center depression, or the alkalinization of the blood can result in greater oxygen-hemoglobin affinities (Bohr effect) (18).

Dialysis induced hypoxemia however can be temporally dissociated from the change in systemic pH (19). Hemodialysis with bicarbonate-containing dialysate can

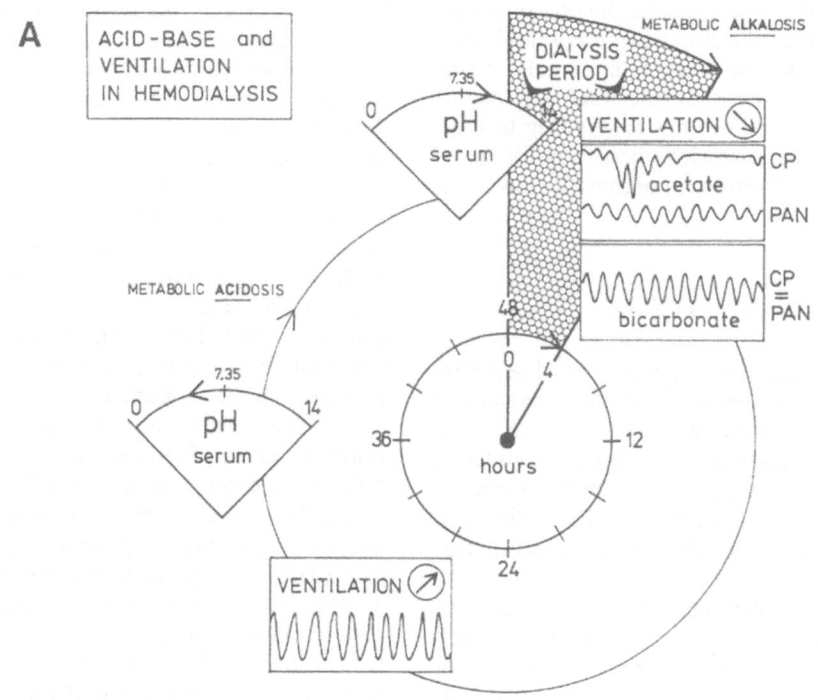

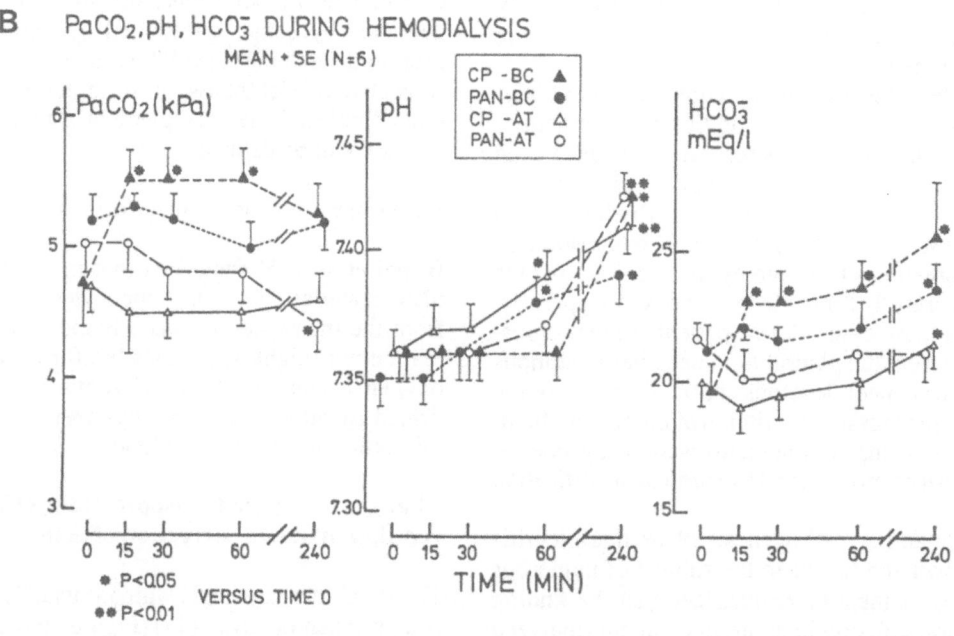

Figure 1. (A) Acid base, ventilation, (B) PaCO₂, systemic pH, and arterial HCO₃⁻ during hemodialysis. Abbreviations: CP, cuprophane membrane; PAN, polyacrylonitrile membrane; AT, acetate-containing dialysate; BC, bicarbonate containing dialysate; PaCO₂, arterial carbon dioxide tension. ∿ = regular, ⋀⋁⋀ = irregular breathing pattern. Figure 1B reprinted from (21) with permission.

Table 1. Gas exchange during acetate infusion in dialysis patients between two dialysis sessions (28)

	Before	*15 min*	*30 min*	*60 min*
pH	7.37 ± 0.02	7.40 ± 0.02	$7.43^b \pm 0.02$	$7.47^b \pm 0.01$
PaO$_2$ (mmHg)	92.6 ± 6.0	87.2 ± 4.6	91.4 ± 8.2	86.4 ± 9.2
PaCO$_2$ (mmHg)	38.4 ± 1.7	39.0 ± 1.3	39.2 ± 1.3	40.2 ± 1.3
HCO$_3$ (mmol/l)	22.6 ± 1.6	$24.6^a \pm 0.9$	$26.2^b \pm 1.3$	$29.6^b \pm 1.4$
RQ	0.78 ± 0.05	0.72 ± 0.04	$0.71^b \pm 0.05$	$0.63^b \pm 0.04$
VO$_2$ (ml/min)	264 ± 30	248 ± 19	271 ± 24	272 ± 30
VCO$_2$ (ml/min)	217 ± 41	180 ± 22	197 ± 27	175 ± 30

pH; arterial oxygen tension, (PaO$_2$); arterial carbon dioxide tension, (PaCO$_2$); arterial bicarbonate concentration, (HCO$_3^-$); respiratory exchange ratio, (RQ); oxygen consumtpion, (VO$_2$); and carbon dioxide production, (VCO$_2$), expressed as mean $\pm$ SEM of five patients before and during acetate infusion.
$^a p > 0.05$; $^b p > 0.01$. Both p values are versus those obtained before the start of the infusion.

be performed in the absence of clear changes in ventilation and PaO$_2$ despite a systemic alkalosis particulary when a low concentration (29 mmol/l) of bicarbonate is used in stead of the classical 36 mmol/l (20). On the other hand dialysis hypoxemia has been shown to occur even in the absence of changes in systemic pH (21, 22). Such discordant responses suggest a minor role for the correction of acidosis observed in the course of hemodialysis and indicate that additional factors dependent on the dialysate composition or the membrane used or both account for the dialysis hypoxemia.

Hypoventilation from lower respiratory quotient during acetate metabolism

Another possible explanation for the observed decreased ventilation during hemodialysis has been sought in the metabolism of acetate gained (3 to 4 mmol/min) during a dialysis session using dialysis fluid containing acetate (23). As proposed the metabolism of acetate results in a higher oxygen consumption (VO$_2$) and a decreased CO$_2$ production (VCO$_2$), leading to a substantial reduction in respiratory quotient (RQ), therefore resulting in hypoventilation and consequently hypoxemia (24, 25). Although this explanation seems attractive, some arguments weaken this possibility. Firstly, Romaldini et al. (26, 27) showed no hypoxemia and decrease in RQ in the course of dialysis with an acetate containing dialysate in which CO$_2$ was bubbled. If the metabolism of acetate plays an important role in the hemodialysis-induced hypoxemia, the bubbling of CO$_2$ into the bath should not affect this mechanism. Consequently, a decrease in RQ due to acetate metabolism would still occur.

Secondly, Oh et al. (25) used the dialysate flow rate and PCO$_2$ difference between dialysate inflow and outflow for the estimation of HCO$_3^-$ and CO$_2$ losses into the dialysate. They were unable to calculate the total CO$_2$ content following the Henderson-Hasselbach equation, since they take into account only the dissolved CO$_2$ in gaseous

form. This leads to a substantial underestimation of the total amount of CO$_2$ lost into the dialysate.

Thirdly, we could show (28) that acetate infusion in hemodialysis patients (4 mmol/min) given 24 h after a dialysis session (a nondialysis day) has no significant effect on ventilation, blood gases and breathing patterns (Table 1). This contrasts with previous observations by Oh et al. (25), who studied the effect of acetate metabolism in volunteers with normal renal function. The small decrease in ventilation we observed can totally be accounted for by the abrupt increase in pH resulting in metabolic alkalosis (28). The respiratory center is known to be very sensitive to changes in H$^+$ ion concentration and this marked increase in systemic pH causes some decrease in alveolar ventilation and sometimes a small fall in PaO$_2$.

The metabolism of acetate resulted in a decreased VCO$_2$ production and an unchanged or slightly increased VO$_2$ (22) and a low RQ. Despite acetate metabolism as indicated by the steadily increase in plasma bicarbonate concentration and in pH hypoxemia did not occur. In view of all these arguments, it is difficult to maintain the hypothesis of metabolism of acetate as a cause of hypoventilation and hypoxemia during hemodialysis with acetate containing dialysate.

Direct effect of acetate on the central respiratory center and myocard

Nissenson (29) and others (30, 31) suggested that ventilation decreases secondarily to a direct effect of acetate on the central respiratory center. Our findings (28) with acetate infusion in chronic dialysis patients between two dialysis sessions, could not confirm this hypothesis. Indeed, we could not find any effect of acetate infusion on ventilation, blood gases and breathing patterns, the latter measured using respiratory inductance plethysmography (32). In a recent experimental study, the hypothesis of the acetate induced hemodynamic instability through periph-

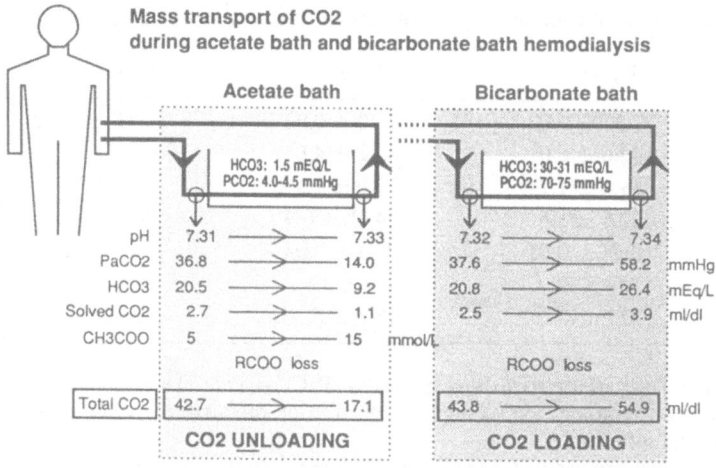

Figure 2. Mass transport of CO₂ during acetate bath and bicarbonate bath hemodialysis.

eral vasodilation and reduced myocardial contractility was discussed again (33).

Hypoventilation from 'CO₂ unloading' and/or membrane bioincompatibility

Literature survey

It is appropriate to discuss these two mechanisms in the same section since they are strongly interrelated and the main determinants of hemodialysis associated hypoxemia. Over the years, there have been strong supporters and opponents for one of the two concepts. It turned out, however, that both can play a role in the development of the hemodialysis hypoxemia (21). In 1968 Kaplow and Goffinet (34) first reported the occurrence of a significant decrease in the white blood cell count, mainly granulocytes between 2 and 15 min after the start of hemodialysis. Craddock et al. (36) suggested that this transient granulocytopenia was due to intrapulmonary leucostasis resulting from the activation of the alternative pathway of the complement system. These authors found a decrease in PaO_2 soon after the start of hemodialysis and an increase in the calculated alveolar-arterial oxygen tension difference $(AaDO_2)$. They suggested that the parallel course of the early leucopenia and hypoxemia soon after the start of hemodialysis were indicative of a causal relationship.

This concept gained further support by reports that the interaction between plasma and the dialyzer membrane generated a small-molecular-weight cleavage fragment of the fifth component of complement, i.e., C5a, modulating an increased expression of MO1, a granulocyte adhesion promoting surface glycoprotein (37), or β2 integrin adhesion receptors (CD11b, CD18-CD116, CD18) (38–40). These aggregated activated granulocytes adhere to each other and also to the first microcirculation they encounter, i.e., the pulmonary microcirculation (9, 22) where they

liberate lysosomal enzymes (41) such as elastase, vasoactive mediators, and oxygen radicals (42) causing endothelial damage releasing into the serum, proteins localized specifically at this microcirculation (e.g., human placental alkaline phosphatase (43)) and thromboxane from the lungs (44). This results in a local inflammatory reaction, pulmonary hypertension and some degree of hypoxemia. The transience of this phenomenon is due to selective down-regulation of the cellular response to C5a (C5a receptor desensitization). The absence of the stimulus for transendothelial migration (45), which limits the deleterious effect of adherent granulocytes on the endothelium (17). Alternatively Sherlock et al. (46), Aurigemma et al. (16) and Dumler and Levin (47) attributed the major cause of hypoxemia to alveolar hypoventilation subsequent to the loss of carbon dioxide in the dialysate (CO₂-unloading, Figure 2). This was supported by their finding that no hypoxemia occurred if the decrease of PCO_2 in the dialysate was prevented. These results were only partially confirmed by Tolchin et al. (48), since in their 'constant PCO_2 dialysate' set-up they still found a small decrease in PaO_2.

Recently, Dolan et al. (22) proposed once more that hypoventilation secondary to CO₂ losses through the dialyzer is the most important mechanism of hypoxemia observed with acetate dialysis. In this well-designed and controlled set of experiments, hypoxemia developed when acetate-containing dialysate was used; the fall in PaO_2 was accompanied by decreased ventilation and maintenance of normal $PaCO_2$. By contrast, neither hypoxemia nor decreased ventilation were seen when bicarbonate-containing dialysate (CO₂ loading, Figure 2) was used.

Whereas the respiratory quotient remained unchanged in the course of bicarbonate dialysis, it dropped from approximately 0.80 to approximately 0.64 in the course of acetate dialysis; these values were calculated from the amounts of CO₂ excreted and of oxygen taken up by the lungs. Brautbar et al. (49) showed that improved hemodynamic function and removal of excess interstitial fluid during ultrafiltration must be taken into account in the interpretation of hemodialysis hypoxemia. The absence of hypoxemia during bioincompatible membrane dialysis using prostacyclin can also be interpreted in this context (50).

Respective role of CO_2 unloading and complement activation-pulmonary inflammation in dialysis associated hypoxemia

To unravel the respective roles of the two main proposed mechanisms of dialysis associated hypoxemia we studied the same group of patients, selected to be clinically stable and having comparable predialysis PaO_2 values, submitted in a randomized order to a dialysis session using a biocompatible (polyacrylonitrile, PAN) or bioincompatible (cuprophane, CP) membrane, and acetate (AT) of bicarbonate (BC, PCO_2 = 35 mmHg) in the dialysate.

We found (Figures 3A, B, C) that the worst pair of experimental conditions was CP membrane and AT containing dialysate. Indeed, both complement activation-leucopenia and subsequent increase in $AaDO_2$ together with reduction in alveolar PO_2, respiratory quotient (RQ) and mean inspiratory flow resulting in the most striking decrease in PaO_2 was observed.

The best combination without any effect on leucocytes, PAO_2, RQ, ventilation and PaO_2 was dialysis with a biocompatible membrane (PAN) and BC in the dialysate. When a CP membrane and BC in the dialysate was used, leucopenia together with an early reversible increase in $AaDO_2$ and decrease in PaO_2 was observed. With a PAN membrane and AT in the dialysate a delayed sustained decrease in PAO_2, RQ and PaO_2 was seen, $AaDO_2$ remained unchanged. It is striking to note that the increase in $AaDO_2$ with CP membrane dialysis was sustained or transient depending respectively on AT or BC in the dialysate. The 'scavenger' function of BC offers a possible explanation for this intriguing observation.

In summary, the two types of membranes have a markedly different effect upon leucocyte count, $AaDO_2$ and PaO_2 shortly after the start of hemodialysis. Furthermore, independent of the type of membrane used, dialysis solution containing acetate always induces a sustained striking decrease in alveolar PO_2 (hypoventilation) RQ and PaO_2.

It was concluded that both mechanisms may occur separately or simultaneously depending on the dialysis setup.

Intrapulmonary leucostasis with mediator release and inflammation at the level of the pulmonary microcirculation is an early event depending upon the biocompatibility of the dialyzer membrane used and has a measurable but rather limited effect upon the PaO_2.

Alveolar hypoventilation depends upon the CO_2 unloading capacity of the hemodialysis set-up, is independent of the dialyzer membrane and can have an impor-

tant effect on PaO_2. This hypoventilation can be due to extracorporeal losses of CO_2 or (and) due to changes in the endogenous production of carbon dioxide (VCO_2) and consumption of oxygen (VO_2) secondary to the metabolism of acetate (the latter mechanism was discussed earlier in the text). To us it seems most likely that the loss of CO_2 into the dialysate with PCO_2 in the blood returning to the patient decreasing to as low as 10 to 15 mmHg causes alveolar hypoventilation and hypoxemia. The observed hypoventilation, unaccompanied by CO_2-retention, resulting in a rather small decrease in PaO_2 (see Figure 3B), is characterized by a decreased respiratory drive (decrease in VT/Ti). Phillipson, Duffin and Cooper (51) have demonstrated the critical dependence of respiratory drive and rhythmicity on the metabolic carbon dioxide load by causing complete cessation of breathing at normal arterial blood gases in adult sheep, when CO_2 was removed from the blood at a rate equal to its metabolic production. The suggestion that this hypoventilation could be mediated through slowly adapting chemoreceptors in the venous circulation or in the lungs reacting to a low venous PCO_2 (Figure 2) is an attractive possibility (52) necessitating however, pulmonary venous blood sampling in strictly controlled condition. Recently, more experimental evidence has been presented for the presence in dogs and cats of CO_2 sensitive pulmonary chemoreceptors that interact with the nonpulmonary chemoreceptors in the control of minute ventilation (53, 54). Wasserman et al. (55) demonstrated in dogs that when venous CO_2 is artificially increased, ventilation increased proportionally providing additional evidence for the existence of pre- or pulmonary chemoreceptors sensitive to PCO_2.

Role of the early-limited-complement-activation-induced hypoxemia in the generation of irregular breathing

As mentioned earlier, intrapulmonary leucostasis, mediator release and inflammation at the level of the pulmonary microcirculation are early dialyzer membrane dependent effects with a measurable but rather limited influence on the PaO_2. On the other hand, the CO_2 unloading results in alveolar hypoventilation and may have an important effect on PaO_2. To gain more insight into the mechanism of this alveolar hypoventilation, ventilation and breathing patterns were studied using respiratory inductance plethysmography (RIP). This method indeed allows (32) both qualitative and quantitative measurements and avoids the important artefacts caused by breathing through a mouthpiece (56).

As in our previous studies, we used a biocompatible (PAN) or bioincompatible (CP) dialyzer membrane in combination with an acetate (AT) or bicarbonate (BC) bath. Comparable results to our previous studies (21) were obtained for the different ventilation parameters. However, we were surprised by the marked irregularities in the breathing pattern during CP-AT dialysis. Whereas in the three other dialysis modes, an almost regular breathing pattern was observed (Figure 4D), recently confirmed by

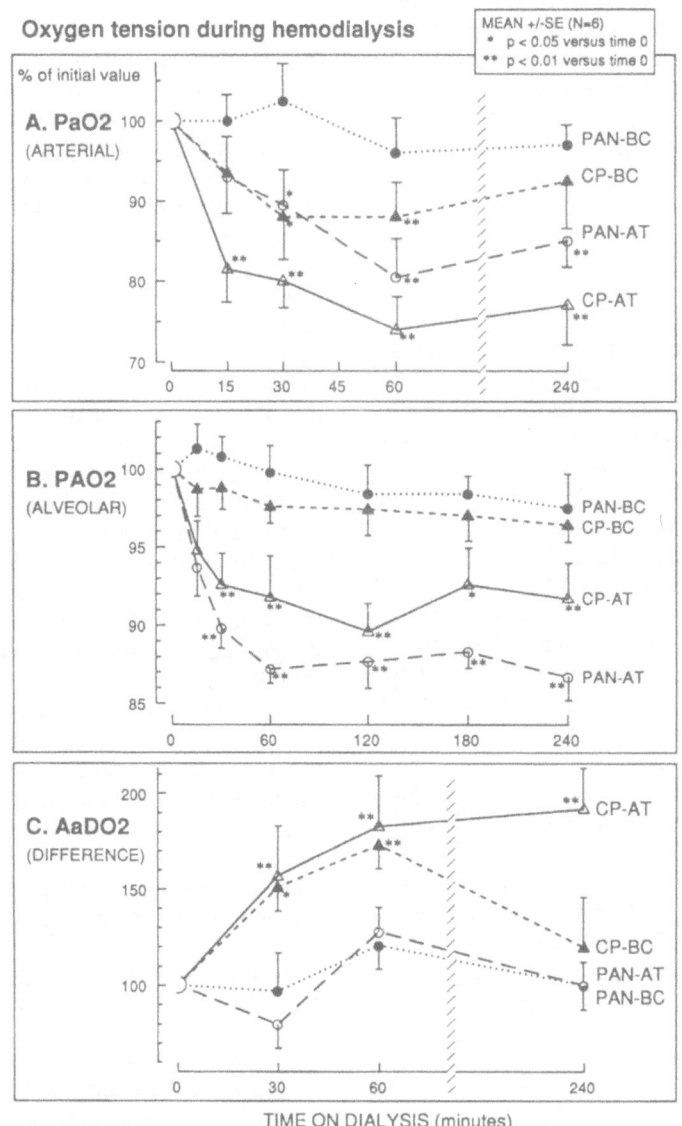

Figure 3. Arterial oxygen tension (PaO₂) (A), alveolar oxygen tension (PaO₂) (B) and alveolar-arterial oxygen tension difference during hemodialysis (AaDO₂) (C) using a bioincompatible (CP) and biocompatible (PAN) membrane and an acetate (AT) or bicarbonate (BC) dialysate in six patients. $*p > 0.05$, $**p > 0.01$; both values are versus time 0. Figures 3A and B reprinted from (21) with permission.

others (57), in the CP-AT mode important variation in the tidal volume from breath to breath (Figure 4A), apneas exceeding 10 sec (Figure 4B, Figure 5) and real periodic breathing were observed (Figure 4C).

The intriguing observation here was that the important irregular breathing pattern observed in the CP-AT dialysis was not, or almost not, seen in the other dialysis modes, especially the PAN-AT mode which is also accompanied by an important CO₂ unloading. This suggested strongly the important role of the early 'complement activated' hypoxemia, being the most striking difference between the CP-AT and PAN-AT dialysis, in the generation of the irregular breathing patterns.

A number of our observations and some reported data support our concept that hypoxemia is necessary in the pathogenesis of irregular breathing seen during extracorporeal CO₂ unloading.

Firstly, in some patients dialyzed with the CP-AT set up with negligible leucopenia and subsequently no hypoxemia due to very limited complement activation, as has been described also by others (58), no irregular breathing was observed.

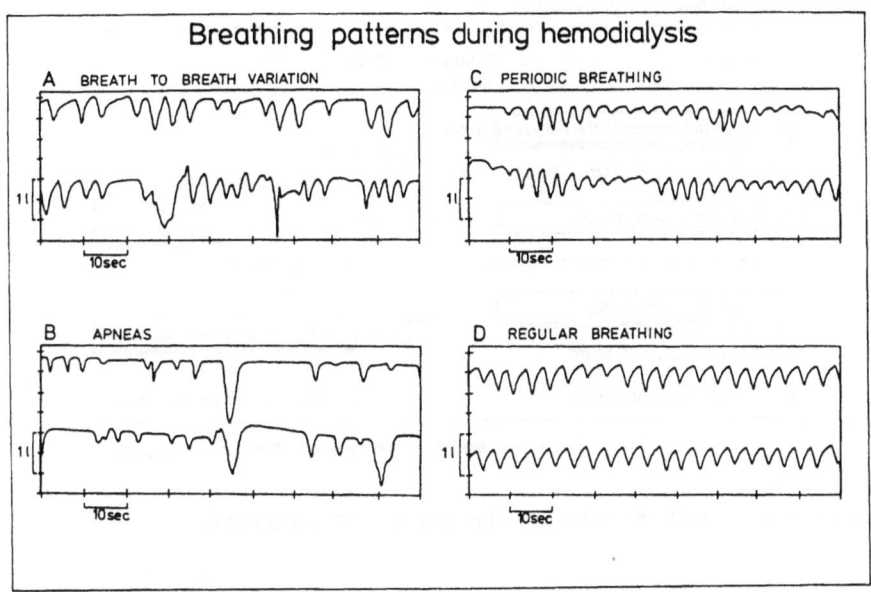

Figure 4. Breathing patterns obtained during different dialysis modes. A, B, C, were seen during the CP-AT dialysis. During PAN-BC, PAN-AT, CP-BC dialysis, an almost constant regular breathing pattern was observed (D). For abbreviation see legend of Figure 1. Reprinted from (63) with permission.

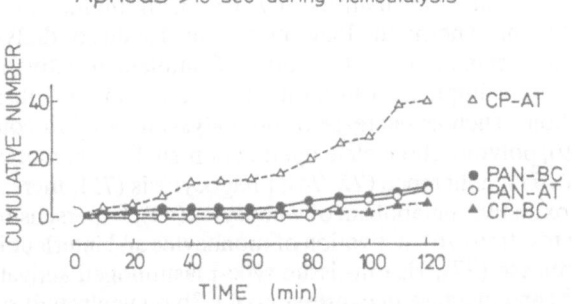

Figure 5. Cumulative number of apneas lasting more than 10 seconds expressed as a total number at a given time in 5 patients using different dialysis modes. For abbreviations see legend of Figure 1.

Secondly, administration of oxygen to patients presenting abnormal breathing patterns during CP-AT dialysis almost immediately turned this irregular breathing into a regular one without changes in the minute ventilation (59). Thirdly, using the biofiltration technique (60) which allows a gradual progressive controlled CO_2 unloading, we observed irregular breathing only when CO_2 unloading was accompanied by a certain degree of hypoxemia induced by the use of a bioincompatible membrane.

Finally, the observed irregularities in breathing during bioincompatible hemodialysis with CO_2 unloading can be compared to those observed at high altitude. At high altitude, lowlanders hyperventilate to compensate for the decreased inspiratory oxygen tension. This hyperventilation, however, does not prevent hypoxemia at extreme altitudes and at the same time makes the lowlanders hypocapnic. In this situation irregular breathing and especially periodic breathing is observed (61). Oxygen breathing again promptly eliminates this periodic breathing.

Several mechanisms can account for the observed breathing irregularities. Correction of acidosis is highly unlikely since during the first hour no significant differences in pH were observed during CP-AT dialysis although irregular breathing is already present.

It could be argued that the patients were sleeping. In such a clinical setting the controlling role of the cortex is diminished rendering ventilation mediated by the peripheral chemical control systems and resulting in irregular breathing patterns (62). We could rule out this sleeping hypothesis by measuring body movements using 'Actigraphy' (63).

The direct effect of acetate as a cause of irregular breathing was also excluded by our observation in dialysis patients infused with acetate outside a dialysis session (28).

The CO_2 unloading combined with mild hypoxemia itself thus clearly seems to be the most obvious cause of the breathing irregularities during CP-AT dialysis. The values of $PaCO_2$ of approximately 33 mmHg found in AT bath dialysis is the one known to be the critical point for switch-off of central CO_2 chemoreceptors (29, 51).

When this point is reached in hypoxic conditions, ventilation became at least partly dependent on the output of the peripheral chemoreceptors which are stimulated by

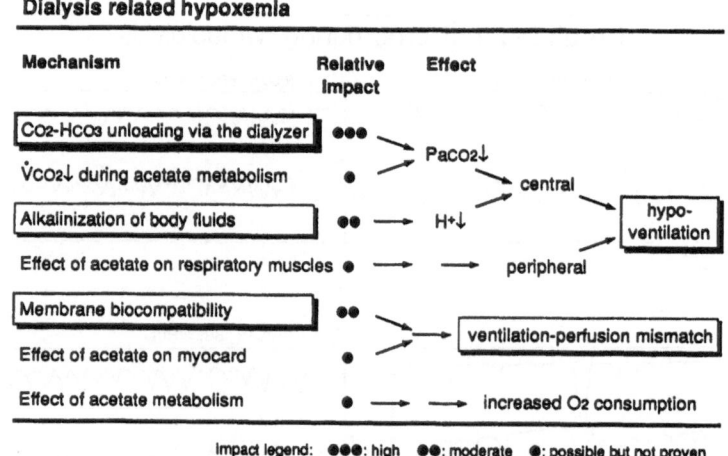

Figure 6. Mechanisms: their effects and their relative impact in dialysis related hypoxemia.

hypoxemia (64, 65). In other words, in hypoxic conditions the peripheral chemoreceptors react briskly to changes in $PaCO_2$ which is immediately reflected in the breathing pattern.

Without hypoxemia CO_2 unloading itself, such as seen during PAN-AT, does not result in irregular breathing. The observed rather important hypoventilation in this setting could be mediated through slowly adapting chemoreceptors in the venous circulation or in the lungs reacting to a low PCO_2 in the blood returning to the patient. Several experimental observations fit with this hypothesis (26, 52, 54, 55).

In summary (Figure 6), the pathophysiology of the hemodialysis associated hypoxemia depends highly on the dialysate composition and to some extend to the alkalinization of body fluids and on the type of membrane used. The latter effect is determined by the capacity of the membrane to activate complement with its subsequent cascade of biological events.

During PAN-BC, CP-BC dialysis the decrease in alveolar ventilation in the absence or negligible decrease in PaO_2 is due to the sensitivity of the central respiratory center to the increased systemic pH and HCO_3^-. During PAN-AT dialysis an important CO_2 unloading occurs (low PCO_2 in the blood returning to the patient) which added to the previous effects results in a more pronounced decrease in VE and VT. During CP-AT dialysis the complement activation induced early hypoxemia superimposed on the CO_2 unloading results in hypoventilation and irregular breathing (Table 2).

Clinical implication of dialysis associated hypoxemia

The clinical implication of this dialysis-induced hypoxemia is of immediate importance to those dialyzed patients with an already compromised cardiopulmonary function. They represent 10 to 15% of an average dialysis population who have predialysis PaO_2 values below 80 mmHg. The additional 25% decrease of PaO_2 after the start of dialysis using a bioincompatible membrane and acetate in the dialysis solution results in desaturation (66). These patients should be dialyzed with a noncomplement-activating membrane and a dialysis system in which loss of CO_2 is prevented.

The exact role of a thrice weekly complement activation or alternative mechanisms (67, 68) using bioincompatible membranes in the long-term clinical status of dialysis patients remains to be determined. Complement activation has been implicated in an impressive number of observations, such as decrease of predialysis neutrophil count (69); polymorphonuclear dysfunction, such as chemotaxis (70, 71); adherence (72–74); phagocytosis (75); increase in oxidative metabolism of leucocytes (42); hypersensitivity reaction (76); activation of monocytes and interleukin-1 release (77); rise in tissue type plasminogen activator (78) and increase in expression of C3b on neutrophil surface (79). Pulmonary fibrosis (80, 81), joint problems, and amyloidosis (82, 83) may all be related to this mechanism as we recently proposed for beta-2-microglobulin amyloidosis (43). Indirect evidence also suggests that chronic dialysis with complement activating surfaces may be associated with increased morbidity of dialysis patients (10, 84–87).

THE LUNG IN THE CHRONICALLY DIALYSED PATIENT

Changes in lung mechanics and lung hemodynamics occur even without overt signs or symptoms in patients with end stage chronic renal failure. Lee and Stretton (81) studied the pulmonary function of 55 patients with chronic renal failure, 10 of them undergoing chronic dialysis treatment. These patients had no clinical nor radiographic evidence of lung disease.

Table 2. A summary of the important events related to the hemodialysis associated hypoxemia (see also text). The meanings of the abbrevations are in the legend to Figure 1

	Early hypoxemia	CO_2 unloading	Hypoventilation	Irregular breathing
PAN-BC	−	−	±	±
CP-BC	+	−	±	±
PAN-AT	−	++	++	±
CP-AT −	+	++	++	++

They found a defect in gas transfer (decrease in carbon monoxide diffusing capacity (DLCO)) due to a reduction in the diffusing capacity across the alveolar capillary membrane, vital capacities were decreased indicative of mild restriction, while forced vital capacity and the ratio of the forced vital capacity in the first second to the vital capacity ruled out obstructive disease.

In a study dealing with the long term survival of regular dialysis treatment patients, over 10 years on dialysis, Avram (88) found that eight out of 11 of these patients had severe restrictive lung function. The effects of hemodialysis on pulmonary function appear attributable to changes in fluid volume. Dialysis causes an increase in the diffusing capacity (89), decrease in closing capacity (90), increased ventilation to basilar areas of the lung (89), and in patients with edema an increase in vital capacity (91). All these changes can be explained by a decrease in lung water content (92). The new technique for recording and analysing continuous measurement of oxygen saturation by pulse oximeter in dialysis patients seems promising to identify patients at risk to clinically relevant hypoxemia (93).

In addition to these limited observations concerning the functional pulmonary changes in end-stage renal failure (with or without dialysis) patients, there are also some important pathological observations. Soft tissue calcification was identified in 79% of dialysis patients and 44%, 60% in nondialysis patients with chronic renal failure (80, 94, 95). Lesions were severe in 36% of the dialysis population and were most frequently found in heart, lungs and stomach. Serum calcium levels were slightly higher in patients with calcifications, but there was no measurable association with the duration of dialysis, serum phosphorus concentration, calcium x phosphorus product, serum bicarbonate level or arterial pH. A critical assessment of the role of parathyroid hormone in the pathogenesis of this pulmonary calcification is still required. Pulmonary clinical symptoms were scarce, X-ray findings were absent except in a single patient.

The calcific lesion consists in deposits occurring as linear bands occasionally as granular humps in alveolar septal walls. Varying degree of thickening and fibrosis of the alveolar walls accompanying the deposits. Calcium was found frequently located within the walls of pulmonary vessels and smaller bronchi. In general vascular calcifications in the lungs paralleled those of the pulmonary parenchyma. By X-ray diffraction a whitlockite crystal pattern $(CaMg)_3 (PO_4)_2$ was found predominantly, with calcium pyrophosphate in these pulmonary calcifications. Jarara and colleagues (96) found pulmonary calcifications in 40% of their hemodialysis patients detected by Technetium-99m diphosphonate scanning.

Pulmonary function tests showed a close relation between changes in vital capacity, DLCO and the severity of lung calcifications. However, the limitation of significant abnormalities of vital capacity and diffusion to those with the severest histopathological changes suggests that the degree of septal thickening and fibrosis rather than the mere presence of calcium deposits determined the magnitude of the functional changes.

The available biochemical data are not sufficient to evaluate adequately either the cause or pathogenesis of these metabolic calcifications, fibrosis and alveolar septal thickening.

Several hypotheses (80) have been put forth but none of these would explain all aspects of this disorder(s), although the variable degree of secondary hyperparathyroidism present in almost all patients with severe renal failure, whether treated by dialysis or not has to be taken into account. It remains speculative to link the thrice weekly complement activation, observed in the majority of patients dialyzed with bioincompatible membranes, accompanied by an acute inflammatory reaction at the level of the pulmonary microcirculation, with the morphological lung lesions observed in the majority of the chronically hemodialyzed subjects.

PULMONARY FUNCTION DURING PERITONEAL DIALYSIS

From the beginning of its use, peritoneal dialysis has been associated with significant alterations in pulmonary function and gas exchange (97–100).

Atelectasis, pneumonia, purulent bronchitis, chronic pleural effusion and acute hydrothorax are among the various complications which may occur during peritoneal dialysis (97, 101).

In a severely ill patient the level of consciousness may be diminished, causing impaired cough reflex. Bronchial secretions may pool in the basal atelectic segments predisposing to purulent bronchitis or pneumonia or both (101). Pleural effusions mostly right-sided, are also a well-known complication of CAPD and rarely massive hydrothorax may occur. In most instances of this complication, peritoneal dialysis has to be discontinued. In a few cases successful pleurodesis has been described (102).

Atelectasis of the basal segments of the lung is considered as the consequence of the upward displacement of the diaphragm following overdistention of the peritoneal cavity with dialysate. The effect on pulmonary function is attributed to the increased intraperitoneal pressure. This leads to an elevated and lengthened diaphragm, a reduced functional residual capacity, possible hypoxemia, and altered respiratory muscle function (99, 100). Distention of the abdomen with 2 and with 3 liter dialysate causes significant reduction of total lung capacity, vital capacity, functional residual capacity, and a reduction in PaO_2 and in $A\text{-}aO_2$ (Alveolar-arterial gradient) (98, 103–105). In patients on chronic peritoneal dialysis, adaptations may occur that limit the reductions in lung volumes, PaO_2 (100, 106). On the other hand there is an increase in respiratory muscle strength due to a rightward shift in the force-length relationship of the diaphragm during CAPD (104). During the periods of peritonitis, however, a 25–30% drop in vital capacity and a 11.7 mmHg drop in PaO_2 was observed (106). The most likely explanation is altered mobility of the diaphragm because of pain. Casuistic data showed also a respiratory acidosis in patients with ventilatory limitation. Excess CO_2 production resulted from high glucose loads and was reversed by decreasing the glucose concentration in the dialysate (107).

Although all these effects are limited in extent and time, we can conclude from these results that it is important not to forget the pulmonary function, when considering peritoneal dialysis for patients with limited pulmonary capacity.

CONTRIBUTION OF HEMODIALYSIS TO BASIC LUNG PHYSIOLOGY

Pulmonary gas exchange

Activation of the alternative pathway of the complement system and subsequent inflammatory processes have been thought to be involved in the pathogenesis of several pulmonary diseases. One of them is the Adult Respiratory Distress Syndrome (ARDS) which remains a problem without effective treatment. This is partly due to the lack of good models in the human.

We felt that the phenomena occurring in hemodialysis patients may at least partly mimic the pathogenetic pathway of ARDS. Indeed, it could be well demonstrated that the activation of the alternative pathway of the complement system by some dialysis membranes results in leucoaggregation, trapping of the activated leucocytes in the

first microcirculation they encounter, i.e., the pulmonary microcirculation, releasing mediators and inducing acute inflammation, increasing the alveolar-arterial oxygen gradient and subsequent hypoxemia. Furthermore, the use of bicarbonate in the dialysis solution showed a modulating effect on this inflammatory reaction suggesting a scavenger effect of bicarbonate. In dialysis with membranes considered to be biocompatible (i.e., not activating complement) disturbances in pulmonary gas exchanges are absent. These observations can be considered as a clinical proof of the local pulmonary inflammation in humans during extracorporeal circulation. In addition some preliminary data obtained in the well controllable hemodialysis model with prostacyclin give some hope for the development of pharmacological inhibition of these phenomena.

Ventilation during venous CO_2-unloading

The study of the chemical control of ventilation in humans has been faced with several problems. One of them is the ventilatory adaptation during CO_2-unloading. Until now, only studies dealing with 'ventilatory-unloading' due to induced hyperventilation have been available. They have the disadvantage that measurements can only be performed during a very short period of time and simultaneous control of the inspiratory oxygen concentration is difficult to obtain. Hemodialysis and biofiltration allows us to study in humans the ventilatory adaptations to controllable degrees of venous CO_2-unloading.

Although ventilation decreases due to the correction of the acidosis it could be demonstrated that the CO_2-unloading in itself is associated with a degree of hypoventilation that cannot be accounted for by the acid-base changes. In addition to the overall decrease in ventilation, the breathing pattern in hypoxic patients undergoing CO_2-unloading becomes irregular with episodes of apnea. We believe that this is due to a dysrhythmogenic effect of the stimulated peripheral chemoreceptors since oxygen breathing eliminates the irregularities in breathing.

Nevertheless, the decrease in ventilation does not prevent a small but very reproducible and significant decrease in $PaCO_2$. This observation seems to be the first indication in humans for a weaker interdependence between ventilation and $PaCO_2$ in the hypocapnic range of the ventilatory-PCO_2 response curve. It is a first argument to accept that also in man the CO_2 response curve becomes shaped as a dog-leg in this hypocapnic area, in other words that ventilation became less dependent on changes in $PaCO_2$.

Further studies with biofiltration will allow us to detect more accurately the cut-off value of $PaCO_2$ where the CO_2 response curve becomes alinear (or dog-leg shaped). We believe that these observations will add to our understanding of the ventilatory adaptations in man in situations where chemical control is important such as at high altitude and during sleep.

CONCLUSION

The lung is the target organ predisposed to suffer from the important disturbances in the water and electrolyte balance characteristic for the patient with end stage renal failure.

Dialysis associated hypoxemia is multifactorial in origin as is now generally accepted (108–110). Part of this hypoxemia is determined by biocompatibility of the membrane used, part is due to CO_2 unloading and its consequent hypoventilation. Correction of acidosis (increase of systemic pH) goes along with a depression of the central respiratory center contributing to a limited extent to the dialysis-associated hypoxemia.

The long term effect of thrice weekly complement activation on pulmonary function is not known. It is striking to note that the literature does not contain a prospective study of the lung function during chronic hemo- or peritoneal dialysis. Based on present knowledge it is recommended that elderly patients, those with compromised cardiopulmonary function, patients who have experienced hypersensitivity to cellulose based membranes, and those with acute renal failure, should be dialyzed with a biocompatible membrane and bicarbonate-containing dialysate.

ACKNOWLEDGEMENTS

This study was partly supported by grants of the Belgian National Fund for Scientific Medical Research (FGWO, FRSM) Grant 3.0069.82 (MEDB) and by the Scientific Planning of the Belgian Government, Contract 82-87/47.MEDB. The secretarial work of Erik Snelders is once more greatly appreciated.

REFERENCES

1. Bush A, Gabriel R: Pulmonary function in chronic renal failure: effects of dialysis and transplantation. *Thorax* 46: 424, 1991
2. Guyton A, Linsey A: Effect of elevated left atrial pressure and decreased plasma protein concentration on the development of pulmonary edema. *Circ Res* 7: 649, 1959
3. Bright R: Tabular view of the morbid appearance in 100 cases connected with albuminous urine, with observations. *Guys Hosp Rep* 1: 380, 1836
4. Maher JF: Uremic pleuritis. *Am J Kidney Dis* 10: 19, 1987
5. Criado A, Mena A, Figuerdo R, Reige E, Avello F: Late perforation of superior vena cava and effusion caused by central venous catheter. *Anaesth Intensive Care* 9: 286, 1981
6. Berger HW, Rammohan G, Neff MS, Buhain WJ: Uremic pleural effusion. A study in 14 patients on chronic dialysis. *Ann Intern Med* 82: 362, 1975
7. Galen MA, Steinberg SM, Lowrie FG, Lazarus JM, Hampers CL, Merrill JP: Hemorrhagic pleural effusion in patients undergoing chronic hemodialysis. *Ann Intern Med* 82: 359, 1975
8. Rodelas R, Rakowski TA, Argy WP, Schreiner GE: Fibrosing uremic pleuritis during hemodialysis. *JAMA* 243: 2424, 1980
9. Brown CM, Sloan DF, Berns AS, Kanter A: Fibrosing uremic pleuritis during hemodialysis. *JAMA* 245: 705, 1981
10. Cheung AK, Henderson LW: Effects of complement activation by hemodialysis membranes. *Am J Nephrol* 6: 81, 1986
11. Duarte R: Blood pressure, ventilation and lipid imbalance during hemodialysis: effect of dialysate composition. *Blood Purif* 3: 199, 1985
12. Eiser A: Pulmonary gas exchange during hemodialysis and peritoneal dialysis: interaction between respiration and metabolism. *Am J Kidney Dis* 6: 131, 1985
13. Garella S, Chang BS: Hemodialysis-associated hypoxemia. *Am J Nephrol* 4: 273, 1984
14. Johnson NR, Bischel KD, Boylen CT: Hypoxia and hypoventilation in chronic hemodialysis. *Clin Res* 19: 145, 1970
15. Bischel MD, Scoles BG, Mohler JG: Evidence for pulmonary microembolization during hemodialysis. *Chest* 67: 335, 1975
16. Aurigemma NM, Feldman NT, Gottlieb M, Ingram RH, Lazarus JM, Lowrie FG: Arterial oxygenation during hemodialysis. *N Engl J Med* 297: 871, 1977
17. Skubitz KM, Craddock PR: Reversal of hemodialysis granulocytopenia and pulmonary leukostasis. A clinical manifestation of selective downregulation of granulocyte response to C5a desarg. *J Clin Invest* 67: 1383, 1981
18. Wathen RL, Ferris FZ, Nagar D, Keshaviah P: An alternative explanation for dialysis-induced arterial hypoxemia. *Kidney Int* 14: 689, 1978
19. Hampl H, Paeper H, Unger V, Fischer CH, Resa I, Kessel M: Hemodynamic changes during hemodialysis, sequential ultrafiltration and hemofiltration. *Kidney Int* 18: 83S, 1980
20. Ganss R, Aarseth HP, Norby B: Prevention of hemodialysis associated hypoxemia by use of low-concentration bicarbonate dialysate. *ASAIO J* 38: 820, 1992
21. De Backer WA, Verpooten GA, Borgonjon DA, Vermeire PA, Lins RR, De Broe ME: Hypoxemia during hemodialysis: effects of different membranes and dialysate compositions. *Kidney Int* 23: 738, 1983
22. Dolan MJ, Whipp BJ, Davidson WD, Weitzman RE, Wasserman K: Hypopnea associated with acetate hemodialysis: carbon dioxide-flow dependent ventilation. *N Engl J Med* 305: 72, 1981
23. Ikeda T, Hirasawa Y, Aizawa Y, Shibita A, Gejyo F, Ei K: Effect of acetate upon arterial gases. *J Dialysis* 3: 135, 1979
24. Eiser AR, Jayamanne D, Kokseng C, Che H, Slifkin RF, Neff MS: Contrasting alterations in pulmonary gas exchange during acetate and bicarbonate hemodialysis. *Am J Nephrol* 2: 123, 1982
25. Oh MS, Uribarri J, Del Monte MI, Heneghan WF, Kee CS, Friedman EA, Carroll HJ: A mechanism of hypoxemia during hemodialysis: consumption of CO_2 in metabolism of acetate. *Am J Nephrol* 5: 366, 1985
26. Romaldini H, Rodriguez-Roisin R, Lopez FA, Ziegler TW, Bencowitz HZ, Wagner PD: The mechanism of arte-

1046 *Marc E. De Broe, Robert L. Lins and Wilfried A. De Backer*

rial hypoxemia during hemodialysis. *Am Rev Respir Dis* 129: 780, 1984

27. Romaldini H, Stabile C, Faro S, Lopes Dos Santos M, Ramos OL, Ribeiro Ratto O: Pulmonary ventilation during hemodialysis. *Nephron* 32: 131, 1982

28. Heyrman RM, De Backer WA, Van Waeleghem JP, Wittesaele WM, De Broe ME: The effect of acetate on ventilation in hemodialysis patients. *Nephrol Dial Transplant* 4: 1060, 1989

29. Nissenson A: Prevention of dialysis induced hypoxemia by bicarbonate dialysis. *Trans Am Soc Artif Intern Organs* 26: 339, 1980

30. Raja R, Kramer M, Rosenbaum JL, Bolisay C, Krug M: Prevention of hypotension during isoosmolar hemodialysis with bicarbonate dialysate. *Trans Am Soc Artif Intern Organs* 26: 375, 1980

31. Vanstone J, Bauer J, Carey J: The effect of dialysate sodium concentration on body fluid distribution during hemodialysis. *Trans Am Soc Artif Intern Organs* 26: 283, 1980

32. Cohn MA, Rao AS, Broudy M, Birch S, Watson H, Atkins N: The respiratory inductive plethysmograph: a new noninvasive monitor of respiration. *Bull Eur Physiopathol Resp* 18: 643, 1983

33. Herrero JA, Trobo JI, Torrente J, Torralbo A, Tornero F, Cruceyra A, Coronel F, Barrientos A: Hemodialysis with acetate, DL-lactate and bicarbonate: a hemodynamic and gasometric study. *Kidney Int* 46: 1167, 1994 1994.

34. Kaplow LS, Goffinet JA: Profound neutropenia during the early phase of hemodialysis. *JAMA* 203: 1135, 1968

35. Craddock PR, Fehr J, Brigham KL, Kronenberg R, Jacobs HS: Complement and leukocyte-medicated pulmonary dysfunction in hemodialysis. *N Engl J Med* 296: 769, 1977

36. Craddock PR, Fehr J, Dalmasso AP, Brigham KL, Jacobs HS: Hemodialysis leucopenia: pulmonary vascular leucostasis resulting from complement activation by dialyzer cellophane membranes. *J Clin Invest* 59: 879, 1977

37. Amin Arnaout M, Hakim RM, Todd RF, Dana N, Colten HR: Increased expression of an adhesion-promoting surface glycoprotein in the granulocytopenia of hemodialysis. *N Engl J Med* 312: 457, 1985

38. Alvarez V, Pulido R, Campanero MR, Paraiso V, de Landázuri MO, Sánchez-Madrid F: Differentially regulated cell surface expression of leukocyte adhesion receptors on neutrophils. *Kidney Int* 40: 899, 1991

39. Himmelfarb J, Zaoui P, Hakim R: Modulation of granulocyte LAM-1 and MAC-1 during dialysis. A propsective, randomized controlled trial. *Kidney Int* 41: 388, 1992

40. Thylén P, Lundahl J, Fernvik E, Hed J, Svenson SB, Jacobson SH. Mobilization of an intracellular glycoprotein (Mac-1) on monocytes and granulocytes during hemodialysis. *Am J Nephrol* 12: 393, 1992

41. Horl WH, Jochum M, Heidland A, Fritz H: Release of granulocyte proteinases during hemodialysis. *Am J Nephrol* 3: 213, 1983

42. Ritchey EE, Wallin JD, Shah SV: Chemiluminescence and superoxide anion production by leukocytes from chronic hemodialysis patients. *Kidney Int* 19: 349, 1981

43. De Broe ME, Nouwen EJ, Van Waeleghem JP: On the mechanism and site of production of B2 microglobulin during hemodialysis. *Nephrol Dial Transplant* 2: 124, 1987

44. Cheung AK, Baranowski RL, Wayman AL: The role of thromboxane in cuprophan-induced pulmonary hypertension. *Kidney Int* 31: 1072, 1987

45. Ward RA: Phagocytic cell function as an index of biocompatibility. *Nephrol Dial Transplant* 9 (Suppl 2): 46S, 1994

46. Sherlock J, Ledwith JK, Letteri J: Hypoventilation and hypoxemia during hemodialysis: reflex response to removal of CO_2 across the dialyzer. *Trans Am Soc Artif Intern Organs* 23: 406, 1977

47. Dumler F, Levin NW: Leucopenia and hypoxemia, unrelated effects of hemodialysis. *Arch Intern Med* 139: 1103, 1979

48. Tolchin N, Roberts JL, Lewis EJ: Respiratory gas exchange by high efficiency hemodialyzer. *Nephron* 21: 137, 1978

49. Brautbar N, Shinaberger JH, Miller JH, Nachman M: Hemodialysis hypoxemia: evaluation of mechanisms utilizing sequential ultrafiltration dialysis. *Nephron* 26: 96, 1980

50. De Broe ME, De Backer WA, Verpooten GA, Vermeire PA, Van Waeleghem JP, Herman AG: Leucopenia and hypoxemia during hemodialysis with different types of membranes: effect of prostacyclin. *Contrib Nephrol* 36: 26, 1983

51. Phillipson EA, Duffin J, Cooper JD: Critical dependence of respiratory rhythmicity on metabolic CO_2 load. *J Appl Physiol* 50: 45, 1981

52. Kotobow T, Gattonini L, Tomlinson TA, Pierce JE: Control of breathing using an extracorporeal membrane lung. *Anesthesiology* 46: 138, 1977

53. Ponte J, Purves MJ: CO_2 and venous return and their interaction as stimuli to ventilation in the cat. *J Physiol* 274: 455, 1978

54. Sheldon ML, Green JF: Evidence for pulmonary CO_2 chemosensitivity: effects on ventilation. *J Appl Physiol* 52: 1192, 1982

55. Wasserman K, Whipp BJ, Casaburi R, Hutsman DJ, Dastagna J, Lugliani R. Regulation of arterial PCO_2 during intravenous CO_2 loading. *J Appl Physiol* 38: 651, 1975

56. Rodenstein DO, Mercenier C, Stanescu DC: Influence of the respiratory route on the resting breathing pattern in humans. *Am Rev Respir Dis* 131: 163, 1985

57. Navarro J, Serrano C, Donna E, Perez GO: Disordered breathing patterns during bicarbonate hemodialysis in COPD. Effect of cuprophane versus polysulfone membranes. *ASAIO J* 38: 811, 1992

58. Abu-Hamdan DK, Desai SG, Mahajan SK, Muller BF, Briggs WA, Lynne-Davies P, McDonald FD: Hypoxemia during hemodialysis using acetate versus bicarbonate dialysate. *Am J Nephrol* 4: 248, 1984

59. Heyrman RM, De Backer WA, Van Waeleghem JP, Willemen MJ, Vermeire PA, De Broe ME: Effect of oxygen administration on the breathing pattern during hemodialysis in man. *Eur Resp J* 2: 972, 1989

60. Panzetta G, Tessitore N, Valvo E, Lupo A, Loschiavo C, Fabris A, Oldrizzi L, Gammaro L, Rugiu C, Bellotti Z, Maschio G: Biofiltration in the treatment of patients with acetate dialysis intolerance. *Clin Nephrol* 26: 33, 1986

61. West JB: Man at extreme altitude. *J Appl Physiol* 52: 1393, 1982

62. Berssenbrugge A, Dempsey J, Iber C, Skatrud J, Wilson P: Mechanisms of hypoxia-induced periodic breathing during sleep in humans. *J Physiol* 343: 507, 1983

63. De Backer WA, Heyrman RM, Wittesaele WM, Van Waeleghem JP, Vermeire PA, De Broe ME: Ventilation and breathing patterns during hemodialysis induced carbon dioxide unloading. *Am Rev Respir Dis* 136: 406, 1987

64. Berkenbosch A, Van Beek JHGM, Olievier CN, De Goede J, Quanjer PH: Central respiratory CO_2, sensitivity at extreme hypoxapnia. *Respir Physiol* 55: 95, 1984

65. Lahiri S, Hsiao C, Zheng R, Mokashi A, Nishino T: Peripheral chemoreceptors in respiratory oscillations. *J Appl Physiol* 58: 1901, 1985

66. Peres-Serrano A, Fernandez-Vega F, Alvarez-Grande J: Hypoxemia during hemodialysis in patients with impairment in pulmonary function. *Nephron* 42: 14, 1986

67. Camussi G, Segolini G, Rotunno M, Vercellone A: Mechanism involved in acute granulocytopenia in hemodialysis: cell-membrane direct interactions. *Int J Artif Organs* 1: 123, 1978

68. Danielson BG, Hallgren R, Benge P: Neutrophil and eosinophil degranulation by hemodialysis membrane. *Contrib Nephrol* 37: 83, 1984

69. Hakim RM, Fearon DAT, Lazarus JM, Perzanowski CS: Biocompatibility of dialysis membranes: effect of chronic complement activation. *Kidney Int* 26: 194, 1984

70. Greene WH, Casann RS, Mauer M, Quie P: The effect of hemodialysis on neutrophil chemotactic responsiveness. *J Lab Clin Med* 88: 971, 1976

71. Henderson LW, Miller ME, Hamilton RW, Norman ME: Hemodialysis leukopenia and polymorph random mobility – a possible correlation. *J Lab Clin Med* 85: 191, 1975

72. Chenoweth PE, Cheung AK, Henderson LW: Anaphylatoxin formation during hemodialysis: effects of different dialyzer membranes. *Kidney Int* 24: 764, 1983

73. Lespier-Dexter LE, Guerra C, Ojeda W, Martinez-Maldonado M: Granulocyte adherence in uremia and hemodialysis. *Nephron* 24: 64, 1979

74. McGregor RR: Granulocyte adherence changes induced by hemodialysis, endotoxin, epinephrine, and glucocorticoids. *Ann Intern Med* 86: 35, 1977

75. Hallgren R, Fjellstrom KE, Hakansson L, Venge P: Kinetic studies of phagocytosis. II. The serum-independent uptake of IgG-coated particles by polymorphonuclear leukocytes from uremic patients on regular dialysis treatment. *J Lab Clin Med* 94: 277, 1979

76. Hakim RM, Breillatt J, Lazarus JM, Port RK: Complement activation and hypersensitivity reaction to dialysis membranes. *N Engl J Med* 311: 878, 1984

77. Dinarello CA: The biology of interleukin-1 and its relevance to hemodialysis. *Blood Purif* 1: 197, 1983

78. Ozdemir O, Arik N, Ozcebe O, Arinsoy T, Sungur C, Dundar S, Turgan C, Yasavul U, Caglar S, Kirazli S: Evidence for the role of dialysis hypoxemia in the pathogenesis of hemodialysis-induced rise in tissue-type plasminogen activator. *Thromb Res* 67: 697, 1992

79. Lee J, Hakim RM, Fearon DT: Increased expression of the C3b receptor by neutrophils and complement activation during hemodialysis. *Clin Exp Immunol* 56: 205, 1984

80. Conger JD, Hammond WS, Alfrey AC, Contiguglia SR, Stanford RE, Huffer WE: Pulmonary calcification in chronic dialysis patients. *Ann Intern Med* 83: 330, 1975

81. Lee HY, Stretton TB, Barnes AM: The lungs in renal failure. *Thorax* 30: 46, 1975

82. Schwarz A, Keller F, Seyfert S, Poll W, Molzahn M, Distler A: Carpal tunnel syndrome, a late complication in chronic hemodialysis. *Dtsch Med Wochenschr* 109: 285, 1984

83. Allieu Y, Asencio G, Mailhe D, Baldet P, Mion C: Carpal tunnel syndrome in chronic hemodialysis patients. *Rev Chir Orthop* 69: 233, 1983

84. Bok DU, Pascular L, Herberger C, Sawyer R, Levin NW: Effect of multiple use of dialyzers on intradialytic symptoms. *Proc Clin Dial Transplant Forum* 10: 92, 1980

85. Kant KS, Pollak VE, Cathey M, Goetz D, Berlin R: Multiple use of dialyzers: safety and efficacy. *Kidney Int* 19: 728, 1981

86. Man NK, Fournier G, Thireau P, Gaillard JL, Funck Brentano JL: The effect of bicarbonate containing dialysate on chronic hemodialysis patients: a comparative study. *Artif Organs* 6: 421, 1982

87. Chanard J, Brunois JP, Melin JP, Lavaud S, Toupance O: Long-term results of dialysis therapy with a highly permeable membrane. *Artif Organs* 6: 261, 1982

88. Avram MM: The Long Island College Hospital experience with the decade or longer hemodialysis patient. in *Prevention of Kidney Disease and Long-Term Survival*, edited by Avram MM, New York, London, Plenum Pub Co, 1982, p 165

89. Zidulka A, Despas PJ, Millic-Emili J, Anthonisen NR: Pulmonary function with acute loss of excess lung water by hemodialysis in patients with chronic uremia. *Am J Med* 55: 134, 1973

90. Craig DB, Wahba WM, Don HF, Couture JG, Becklake MB: Closing volume and its relationship to gas exchange in seated and supine positions. *J Appl Physiol* 31: 717, 1971

91. Robson M, Levin A, Ravid M: Serial measurement of vital capacity in patients on chronic hemodialysis. *Nephron* 19: 60, 1977

92. Brigham KL, Bernard G: Pulmonary complications of chronic renal failure. *Semin Nephrol* 1: 188, 1981

93. Jones JG, Bembridge JL, Sapsford DJ, Turney JH: Continuous measurements of oxygen saturation during haemodialysis. *Nephrol Dial Transplant* 7: 110, 1992

94. Kuzela DC, Huffer WE, Conger JD, Winter SD, Hammond WS: Soft tissue calcification in chronic dialysis patients. *Am J Pathol* 86: 403, 1977

95. Milliner DS, Zinsmeister AR, Lieberman E, Landing B: Soft tissue calcification in pediatric patients with end-stage renal failure. *Kidney Int* 38: 931, 1990

96. Jarava C, Marti V, Gurpegui ML, Merello JI, Rdez-Quesada B, Palma A: Pulmonary calcification in chronic dialysis patients: *Nephrol Dial Transplant* 8: 673, 1993

97. Berlyne GM, Lee HA, Ralston AJ, Woodlock JA: Pulmonary complications of peritoneal dialysis. *Lancet* 2: 75, 1966

98. Goggin MJ, Joekes AM: Pulmonary gas exchange during peritoneal dialysis. *Br Med J* 2: 247, 1971

99. Ahluwalia M, Ishikawa S, Gellman M, Shah T, Sekar T, MacDonnel KF: Pulmonary functions during peritoneal dialysis. *Clin Nephrol* 18: 251, 1982

100. Prezant DJ: Effect of uremia and its treatment on pulmonary function. *Lung* 168: 1, 1990

101. Khanna R, Oreopoulos DG: Complications of peritoneal dialysis other than peritonitis. in *Peritoneal Dialysis*, Nolph KD, The Hague, Martinus Nijhoff, 1985, p 441

102. Scheldewaert R, Bogaerts Y, Pauwels R, Van der Straeten M, Ringoir S, Lameire N: Management of a massive hydrothorax in a CAPD patient: a case report and a review of the literature. *Perit Dial Bull* 2: 69, 1982

103. Freedman S, Maberly DJ: Pulmonary gas exchange during dialysis. *Br Med J* 3: 48, 1971

104. Prezant DJ, Aldrich TK, Karpel JP, Lynn RI: Adaptations in the diaphragm's *in vitro* force-length relationship in patients on continuous ambulatory peritoneal dialysis. *Am Rev Respir Dis* 141: 1342, 1990

105. O'Brien AA, Power J, O'Brien L, Clancy L, Keogh JA: The effect of peritoneal dialysate on pulmonary function and blood gasses in CAPD patients. *Irish J Med Sci* 159: 215, 1990

106. Taveira Da Silva AM, Davis WB, Winchester JF, Coleman DE, Wei CW: Peritonitis, dialysate infusion and lung function in continuous ambulatory peritoneal (CAPD). *Clin Nephrol* 24: 79, 1985

107. Cohn J, Balk RA, Bone RC: Dialysis-induced respiratory acidosis. *Chest* 98: 1285, 1990

108. Kishimoto T, Tanaka H, Maekawa M, Ivanovich P, Levin N, Bergstrom J, Klinkmann H: Dialysis-induced hypoxaemia. *Nephrol Dial Transplant* 8 (Suppl 2): 25S, 1993

109. De Broe ME: Haemodialysis-induced hypoxaemia. *Nephrol Dial Transplant* 9 (Suppl 2): 173S, 1994

110. Salem M, Ivanovich PT, Ing TS, Daugirdas JT: Adverse effects of dialyzers manifesting during the dialysis session. *Nephrol Dial Transplant* 9 (Suppl 2): 127S, 1994

GASTROINTESTINAL COMPLICATIONS IN DIALYSIS PATIENTS

DIDIER A. MANDELBROT and J. MICHAEL LAZARUS

INTRODUCTION

Long before the routine use of dialysis, patients dying of uremia were found to have a high incidence of gastrointestinal abnormalities (1). This chapter will address issues relating to the digestive system in dialysis patients, with an emphasis on conditions that affect these patients more commonly than the general population. Improvements in dialysis technique and changes in the patient population undergoing dialysis have modified the spectrum of gastrointestinal diseases seen in patients with end-stage renal disease (ESRD), so the more recent literature will be emphasized.

A variety of non-specific gastrointestinal symptoms are commonly encountered in patients with advanced renal insufficiency. These include nausea, vomiting, anorexia, metallic taste and loss of taste. The uremic breath associated with renal failure, sometimes described as 'fishy', is caused by secondary and tertiary amine compounds (2). These advanced uremic symptoms were encountered more commonly in the past, but can still be seen in cases where dialysis is unavailable or delayed. Furthermore, they are useful guides both for the need to initiate dialysis and for the presence of inadequate dialysis.

UPPER GASTROINTESTINAL DISEASE

Peptic ulcer disease and inflammation

Early radiologic contrast studies in patients with renal failure documented an increased prevalence of thickened mucosal folds, involving both stomach and duodenum (3, 4), that are consistent with inflammation. Subsequent endoscopic and histologic studies confirmed this finding (5, 6), with histologic gastritis found in as many as 89% of dialysis patients, compared to 21 percent of controls (7). Most studies have found gastritis in approximately one half of dialysis patients (8).

On autopsy, uremic patients who had never been dialyzed had gastritis more frequently than a comparison group on chronic hemodialysis (9). Similarly, the prevalence of gastritis in a group of patients with advanced renal insufficiency was notably reduced after they initiated dialysis (10). It is also interesting to compare a 1934 series of patients dying of uremia (1) with a more recent autopsy study of dialysis patients (11). While both found frequent mucosal inflammation, only the earlier study of untreated uremics found hemorrhagic, ulcerative and pseudomembranous changes. These findings suggest the importance of adequate dialysis in minimizing the tendency for gastritis.

Some early reports suggested an increased incidence of peptic ulcer in dialysis patients (12–14), and one noted an increase in gastric but not duodenal ulcers (15). However, most larger and more recent studies have found no increase in either type of peptic ulcer (3, 5, 16–18). Unlike those on dialysis, patients with renal tranplants have a significantly increased risk of peptic ulcer, often with complications and high mortality (19).

Several factors may be responsible for the increase in gastritis seen in dialysis patients. Studies on the role of acid secretion are sometimes contradictory, but important conclusions can be drawn. Some early studies suggested that excess acid secretion contributes to gastritis, and found increased basal (14) and pentagastrin-stimulated (20, 21) gastric acid production. In part because of decreased renal metabolism of gastrin (22), gastrin levels are increased in patients with renal failure (23–30), sometimes to levels in the range associated with gastrinomas (23, 25). Therefore, some investigators concluded that increased gastrin levels are responsible for both acid hypersecretion and mucosal abnormalities (6).

However, the increased pentagastrin response in dialysis patients was not reproducible in several studies (25, 28). Rather than being the cause of gastric hypersecretion, the elevated gastrin levels are more likely the result of negative feedback from undersecretion of acid, for example because of atrophic gastritis (29, 30). Atrophic gastritis has in fact been estimated to occur in 15% of dialysis patients compared with 2% in the normal population (7). Several studies have even found that gastrin and acid secretion are negatively correlated (18, 30). One of these studies further noted a negative correlation between gastrin levels and mucosal lesions, suggesting that decreased acid production leads to both increased gastrin levels and less mucosal damage (30). Other investigators have noted that some dialysis patients have hypochlorhydria while other patients have hyperchlorhydria (28), suggesting that solely analyzing mean values might miss important individual abnormalities.

The interpretation of changes in gastrin levels in dialysis patients is further complicated by the fact that many other gastrointestinal hormone concentrations are also increased in renal failure (26, 31, 32). Some of these hormones, such as gastrin-releasing peptide, could increase levels of gastrin, while others could have the opposite effect. Some of these hormones could also be expected to have direct effects on acid secretion; for example, increased levels of gastric inhibitory polypeptide would decrease acid production.

Despite an extensive body of work on gastrin and other gastrointestinal hormones, most investigators have concluded that gastrin elevation does not explain the mucosal lesions in patients with ESRD. The routine measurement of gastrin has no clinical role, but the literature documenting gastrin elevations in renal failure should be kept in mind if searching for a gastrinoma in a dialysis patient.

Several other mechanisms may contribute to the mucosal abnormalities in ESRD. For example, biliary reflux can worsen gastroduodenal inflammation. Since gastrin can decrease pyloric sphincter tone, high gastrin levels may worsen biliary reflux, thus worsening mucosal injury (33). Also, high urea levels may promote increased proton back diffusion (34). For duodenal ulcers, impaired pancreatic bicarbonate secretion (35, 36) and increased pepsinogen release (36, 37) in renal failure might also play a role. Several studies have also noted that upper gastrointestinal hemorrhage in dialysis patients is often associated with the use of ulcerogenic drugs such as steroids, iron and especially non-steroidal anti-inflammatory agents (15, 38), but this is also true in the general population.

Although *Helicobacter pylori* infection is clearly important in causing gastroduodenal lesions in all patients, the infection rates have not been found to be increased in patients with renal failure (39–41).

Esophageal disease

Although less extensively studied than gastroduodenal disease, esophagitis has also been reported to be more prevalent in dialysis patients (5). Erosive esophagitis has been found to be a more common cause of upper gastrointestinal bleeding in dialysis patients than in the general population (42). Mallory–Weiss tears seem to have a prevalence that is independent of renal function, while esophageal varices may be less frequent in the dialysis population (42). Patients with renal transplants are at increased risk of esophagitis from opportunistic infections such as candida, cytomegalovirus and herpes simplex. Therefore, dialysis patients still tapering immunosuppressive therapy after failed allograft should be carefully watched for these infections.

Gastric emptying

While uremic patients not on dialysis may have delayed gastric emptying (43), end stage renal disease itself generally does not cause delayed emptying (44, 45). However, slower gastric emptying has been documented in peritoneal dialysis patients studied acutely during a dialysis fluid dwell period (46). Furthermore, gastrointestinal symptoms related to decreased motility are common in diabetic patients (47), a group which comprises a large proportion of many dialysis populations. Therefore, dialysis patients with gastrointestinal neuropathy are frequently encountered in practice. Standard treatment is with promotility agents such as metoclopramide, and some have suggested a role for intravenous erythromycin (48), but delayed gastric emptying remains a difficult problem to manage.

LOWER GASTROINTESTINAL DISEASE

Ischemia

Several characteristics of dialysis patients predispose them to mesenteric ischemia and infarction. They have accelerated atherosclerosis (49) which affects the mesenteric circulation, and they are also more likely to have a variety of cardiac diseases which can produce a low flow state, including coronary artery disease, valvular disease and arrythmias. Furthermore, many are diabetic and have the vascular abnormalities associated with diabetes. Several medications have also been associated with decreased mesenteric perfusion. Beta blockers reduce cardiac output, while other medications, including digoxin and vasodilators, can produce a 'steal' syndrome in which blood flow is redirected away from the intestines (50). Most specific to hemodialysis patients is the need for repetitive ultrafiltration, which is often associated with severe hypotension, especially in patients with autonomic neuropathy or large fluid gain between dialysis treatments.

These episodes of hypotension can precipitate ischemia and infarction in predisposed patients (51). Other causes of volume loss such as vomiting and diarrhea are also associated with bowel infarction (50, 52). Principles of diagnosis and management of mesenteric ischemia are essentially unchanged in dialysis patients, and include volume repletion, angiography and consideration for surgery.

A therapeutic intervention that has received particular attention as a cause of intestinal necrosis is sodium polystyrene (kayexalate) given in a sorbitol enema. Studies in animals have suggested that uremia is a significant predisposing factor (53) and that sorbitol alone can cause intestinal necrosis (53, 54). In humans, however, many of the reported cases have been transplant patients, suggesting that some aspect of the postoperative course, such as the immunosuppressive regimen or intestinal dysmotility, may also predispose patients to necrosis from these enemas (54, 55). As the utility of adding sorbitol to kayexalate enemas is questionable, such enemas should be given only in saline, and caution should be used. Although not extensively studied, it is also prudent to use lactulose rather than sorbitol as an oral osmotic laxative, especially in patients with a history of intestinal ischemia.

Obstruction

Obstruction and pseudo-obstruction also seem to occur more frequently in hemodialysis patients. Chronic constipation and the use of aluminum-containing antacids are common, and constitute major risk factors for impaction (56, 57) and perforation (58). Other constipating agents commonly used in the dialysis population include narcotics, ferrous sulfate and certain antihypertensive agents. Bowel motility may also be impaired by advanced age, electrolyte disturbances and autonomic neuropathies. Perforation is associated with a mortality of 5% in dialysis patients (58).

Constipation is a frequent and potentially serious problem in dialysis patients, and if predisposing medications can not be avoided, dietary measures, stool softeners and laxatives should be considered. Among these, a high fiber diet and the osmotic laxative lactulose can be safely recommended. Physical activity also promotes intestinal motility. Enemas are occasionally useful, but those containing phosphate (Fleets enemas) should be avoided in renal failure because of the risk of excessive phosphate absorption. Similarly, laxatives containing magnesium should be avoided because of the danger of hypermagnesemia. As with all patients, those on dialysis should be watched particularly carefully for fecal impaction when they are bedridden or in a perioperative period.

Diverticular disease

Although most dialysis patients have no predisposition for diverticulosis or diverticulitis, those with polycystic kidney disease have a significant increase in diverticular disease. Diverticulosis has been reported in 83% of polycystic dialysis patients, more than twice the frequency in controls (59). Perforation from diverticulosis can occur, often with a delay in diagnosis because of the mild symptoms (60). Diverticulitis is also more frequent in polycystic dialysis patients, and in one series, those with this diagnosis all progressed to intestinal perforation (59). The symptoms of diverticulitis, including abdominal pain, fever and leukocytosis, can be confused with bleeding or infection of a cyst, so both diagnoses should be seriously considered in dialysis patients with polycystic kidney disease.

Perforation

In addition to the more common causes of intestinal perforation, including ischemia, obstruction and diverticular disease, several rare causes of perforation have been reported in patients with end-stage renal disease. Colonic ulcers are often associated with conditions such as ischemia and cytomegalovirus infection, but several cases of idiopathic ulcers of the large intestine have been reported in dialysis patients (61, 62). These patients presented with bleeding or peritoneal signs, and had a high mortality. Spontaneous idiopathic perforation of the colon has also been reported in patients with renal failure (63, 64), and pathologic criteria to distinguish stercoral (due to fecaloma) perforation and spontaneous perforation have been described (65). These unusual causes of perforation also seem to be associated with severe constipation, use of aluminum-based antacids, and other causes of impaired intestinal motility. Perforation is also a potential complication of the indwelling peritoneal catheter used by patients on peritoneal dialysis (66). Finally, transplantation increases the risk of perforation, especially from diverticular disease and ischemia, as well as predisposing patients to infectious colitis (19).

Clostridium difficile infection

The contagious nature of *C difficile* infection has been well documented on general hospital wards as well as dialysis units, making isolation procedures essential (66, 68). Although controlled studies are lacking, impaired immune function and decreased gastrointestinal motility in patients with renal failure may predispose them to *C difficile* infection (68), and large outbreaks have been reported in patients with renal failure (69). These patients often have explosive diarrhea, but can also be asymptomatic. Because of the risk of spread among patients in a dialysis unit, nephrologists should have a low threshold for sending stool for *C difficile* toxin in patients with diarrhea.

DISEASES AFFECTING BOTH UPPER AND LOWER TRACTS

Angiodysplasia

Angiodysplasia has a significantly increased prevalence in chronic renal failure (70–75). In one study, angiodysplasia was the cause of over 20% of upper gastrointestinal bleeds in patients with chronic renal failure, compared to 5% in those with normal renal function; in this series, angiodysplasia was also the most frequent source of recurrent bleeding in patients with renal failure (42). The increased prevalence of angiodysplasia affects the entire length of the digestive system, including the stomach, small intestine and colon. Proposed explanations for this predisposition in dialysis patients include vascular calcification, constipation, and chronic venous congestion from fluid overload, but the mechanism is still poorly understood.

Amyloidosis

Patients on dialysis for many years develop widespread manifestations of a specific type of amyloidosis caused by the accumulation of beta 2 microglobulin. The amyloid fibrils found in the joints of dialysis patients are also present throughout the intestine (76, 77). Visceral involvement has been reported in as many as 58% of long term hemodialysis patients (78). Amyloidosis can either cause bleeding or massive diarrhea (76), and less commonly can produce intestinal infarction (79). Diagnosis is typically made by biopsy, but an imaging procedure using a radio-labeled amyloid component has been proposed as a non-invasive diagnostic technique (80). No specific treatment is available, so supportive care must be directed towards symptoms such as bleeding, diarrhea and pain.

GASTROINTESTINAL BLEEDING

Dialysis patients have an increased incidence of bleeding from the gastrointestinal tract, both because of their predisposition for certain lesions (Table 1), and because of their coagulopathies. Furthermore, recurrence of bleeding is more likely in dialysis patients (42), and bleeding in these patients may be associated with greater morbidity (15). A study using chromium-labelled red blood cells showed that even renal failure patients without gastrointestinal symptoms have increased blood loss. Normal volunteers averaged 0.83 ml blood lost per day, azotemic patients not yet on dialysis lost 3.15 ml/day, and dialysis patients lost 6.27 ml/day (81). The authors estimated that a typical dietary intake of iron is 400 mg per month, of which dialysis patients lose 250 mg each month. Therefore, iron depletion is a common problem and aggressive repletion is important even in asymptomatic patients.

Table 1. Causes of gastrointestinal bleeding in dialysis patients

Upper GI
Gastritis*
Duodenitis
Peptic ulcer
Esophagitis*
Esophageal varices
Mallory–Weiss tear

Lower GI
Ischemic colitis*
Obstruction*
Diverticular disease*
Colonic ulcer
Spontaneous perforation
Inflammatory bowel disease
Hemorrhoids

Both upper and lower GI
Angiodysplasia*
Amyloidosis*
Infection
Neoplasm

*Indicates conditions more frequent in dialysis patients than the general population

The more frequent blood loss in dialysis patients makes a positive test for occult blood in the stool relatively common. One study found that 15% of dialysis patients had positive tests, and that the incidence of colon cancer was much lower among this group than the hemoccult-positive general population, but some occult malignancies were identified (82). No direct studies of this issue are available, but it may be reasonable to raise the threshold for aggressive evaluation of dialysis patients with trace blood in the stool. For example, in asymptomatic younger patients in low risk groups, such as those with no family history of polyps or malignancy, invasive testing may be even less appropriate than in the population at large.

In many respects, the diagnosis of gastrointestinal abnormalities is the same whether or not a patient is on dialysis. However, because of the increased prevalence of angiodysplasia in dialysis patients, both upper and lower endoscopy are more appropriate than barium studies in evaluating gastrointestinal bleeding. Endoscopic procedures should be avoided immediately after systemic heparinization for dialysis, either by waiting several hours, or by minimizing the heparin dose and limiting its administration to early during the dialysis treatment.

Once a diagnosis is made, several management issues unique to dialysis patients must be kept in mind. If gastric lavage is performed, water rather than normal saline should be used to avoid volume overload. Similarly, to avoid volume and potassium excess, blood transfusions should be administered during the time of dialysis, although they occasionally must be given emergently. The mainstay of peptic ulcer disease treatment continues to be histamine antagonists, given at reduced doses appropriate for renal failure. Although the experience with cimetidine in hemodialysis patients now extends over 15 years (83), newer agents in this class are usually favored because they have fewer drug interactions and side effects. Antacids play an important role too, but because of the risk of aluminum (84) and magnesium toxicity, antacids containing these two elements should be avoided. The use of sucralfate is also limited by the risk of aluminum toxicity (85). Finally, omeprazole is the most potent agent in reducing gastric acid, but experience in dialysis patients is more limited. Available evidence also suggests that a reduced dose should be used in patients on dialysis (86, 87).

Because of the platelet dysfunction in uremia, and its partial correction with dialysis (88), maintaining adequate dialysis is particularly important during an episode of gastrointestinal bleeding. Desmospressin (DDAVP) (89) and cryoprecipitate (90) both appear to improve the function of uremic platelets by increasing serum levels of von Willebrand factor. Chronic administration of erythropoietin also improves platelet function and bleeding times, both by direct effects on platelets and by the indirect benefit of increased erythrocyte mass on thrombosis (91, 92).

Several studies have reported that the use of oral estrogens improves both bleeding times and clinical bleeding in dialysis patients (93), and in particular, bleeding from angiodysplasia (94, 95). The use of estrogens is especially appealing for the treatment of angiodysplasia because these lesions are usually multiple and cannot all be identified, lesions of the distal small intestine are generally inaccessible to endoscopy, and other attempted techniques such as electrocautery, heater probe and sclerotherapy have been relatively ineffective (94).

One of several available options should be used to minimize the systemic anticoagulation from heparin during dialysis. These include dialysis without heparin, regional heparinization, fractional heparinization, and the use of citrate as an anticoagulant (modalities discussed in Section II, Chapter 6).

PANCREATIC DISEASE

Several pancreatic abnormalities are more frequent in dialysis patients. An autopsy study found that more than 50% of hemodialysis patients had histologic abnormalities of the pancreas, including ductal ectasia, metaplasia or proliferation, and interstitial inflammation or fibrosis. These changes were of uncertain clinical significance, but were found in only 12% of controls (96). Pancreatitis in particular seems to occur more frequently in dialysis patients, with an autopsy prevalence of 28% (97). Based on a

clinical diagnosis, the 10 year incidence of pancreatitis in dialysis patients was found to be 2.3%, compared to 0.5% in controls (98). Pancreatic pseudocysts were also found to occur more frequently, and the mortality from pancreatitis in this study was 20%. Peritoneal dialysis patients seem to have a higher incidence of pancreatitis than hemodialysis patients. A potential complication of pancreatic disease is exocrine insufficiency. This insufficiency can contribute to the wasting syndrome of end-stage renal disease, and pancreatic supplementation can occasionally improve nutritional status (99). The cause of pancreatic disease in dialysis patients remains unclear, but atherosclerosis of the pancreatic arterioles (96) and the hyperparathyroidism of renal failure may contribute (100, 101). Several factors complicate the diagnosis of pancreatitis in dialysis patients. The classic symptoms of abdominal pain, nausea and vomiting can be produced by several of the conditions that are frequently seen in such patients, such as gastritis and intestinal ischemia. Furthermore, serum amylase and lipase are frequently elevated in renal failure (102–104). Several factors could contribute to the increased enzymes, including oversecretion due to subclinical pancreatitis, overproduction related to uremia but without any inflammation, and underexcretion due to decreased renal clearance. Since amylase is excreted by the kidneys (105), it is not surprising that many asymptomatic dialysis patients have persistently elevated serum amylase. In general, the upper limit of normal for amylase and lipase in dialysis patients should be considered to be two to three times higher than the level in patients with intact renal function. Transient elevation of enzymes above this level associated with classic symptoms strongly suggests the diagnosis of pancreatitis.

Several investigators have tried to increase the accuracy of diagnosis by using amylase isoenzyme levels, but no clear benefit has emerged, because the pancreatic isoenzyme is elevated in renal failure too (103, 106). In peritoneal dialysis patients, as in any patient with ascites, the presence of pancreatic enzymes in the peritoneal fluid is helpful in the diagnosis of pancreatitis (102).

HEPATOBILIARY DISEASE

Hepatic abnormalities

A variety of conditions affect the liver in dialysis patients. The frequent blood transfusions required by these patients place them at high risk for hepatitis B and C. Viral hepatitis (addressed in detail in Section VII, Chapter 10) is a major factor in the frequent elevation of liver function tests. One autopsy study found that 90% of dialysis patients had some histologic abnormality of the liver, including periportal fibrosis, fatty changes and hemosiderosis (107). This study also noted that 50% had hepatomegaly, often due to hepatic congestion from volume overload or cardiac failure. However, some of the cases of hepatomegaly had no discernible cause, and another series reported dialysis patients with hepatomegaly but otherwise normal liver function tests and histology. These investigators postulated that accumulation of an unknown growth factor in dialysis patients may be responsible (108).

The frequent blood transfusions in dialysis patients also predispose them to the hepatic accumulation of iron and the eventual risk of cirrhosis, although hemochromatosis is rare (109). Before the advent of serologic tests for hepatitis C, hepatic hemosiderosis could mascarade as non-A, non-B hepatitis, because both can elevate hepatic transaminases (110) . Iron overload should generally be suspected in patients with serum ferritin over 1,000 g/ml, and diagnosis is by liver biopsy. Although deferoxamine was used in the past to chelate iron, problems with its efficacy (111) and the advent of erythropoietin greatly limit the current use of chelation therapy. Erythropoietin has both reduced the need for transfusion, thereby reducing the risk of iron overload, and has been successfully combined with phlebotomy to mobilize and remove excess iron stores (112).

Other compounds have also been found to accumulate in the liver of dialysis patients. The liver is one of the sites of greatest accumulation of aluminum, an important cause of encephalopathy, but toxic effects of hepatic aluminum have not been clearly identified (113). The toxicity of silicone is also poorly defined, but the presence of silicone particles in the liver is well described. These particles have been reported to be associated with inflammation, fibrosis and in some cases, granuloma formation in the liver (114). The source of the particles was localized to siliconized tubing in the roller pump of the dialysis machine. Silicone particles can be difficult to clear, since they were found as long as four years after successful kidney tranplantation (115). However, other studies found that although the prevalence of these particles increases with time on hemodialysis, there is no association between silicone and the presence of histologic liver disease (116). High occlusion force within the dialysis blood pump increases release of silicone (117), so it is important that manufacturer's recommendations for settings on the dialysis system be followed to minimize detachment of silicone particles.

Hepatic toxicity from medications in dialysis patients can also occur, and the viral hepatitis frequently seen in these patients seems to lower the threshold for drug toxicity, but end-stage renal disease itself does not seem to be a major predisposing factor (118).

Ascites

Since the first reports in 1970 (119, 120), several case series have described idiopathic ascites in dialysis patients, without any evidence of liver disease or other known cause of ascites. Most reports of ascites were clustered between 1974 and 1976, and the incidence of this condition may be reduced in recent years, suggesting that improved dialysis techniques and nutritional counseling have allowed better control of volume or toxic substances that may contribute to ascites. However, the presence of ascites seems to be a poor prognostic sign (121).

Several factors are likely to contribute to the formation of ascites in dialysis patients. Some of the reported cases of dialysis ascites were in fact due to known causes such as cardiac failure, pericarditis or unrecognized liver cirrhosis. A comprehensive review of 138 cases reported before 1987 found that 15% had such identifiable causes of ascites (121). Volume overload is an important factor, and was found in approximately two-thirds of patients. However, many of the patients had minimal peripheral edema, suggesting some degree of ascitic compartmentalization (122, 123). This is partly due to the slower maximum rate of fluid mobilization from the peritoneum compared to fluid from peripheral edema (121). Some have suggested that ESRD-related hypoalbuminemia contributes to ascites formation, but the protein concentration in the ascites seems to be more important. Unlike cirrhotics, dialysis patients usually have a high ascitic protein concentration (124, 125), which exerts an oncotic pressure to increase the volume of ascites. Similarly, a phenomenon termed osmotic disequilibrium may be important. In one study, the osmolality of ascites before dialysis was similar to that of serum, but by the end of the dialysis treatment was significantly higher, producing an osmolal gradient for the reaccumulation of ascitic fluid (126).

Unknown uremic factors may also contribute to ascites by modifying vascular and peritoneal membrane permeability (127, 128) or promoting inflammation (125). Several studies found that the majority of patients with dialysis ascites had previously been on peritoneal dialysis (127–129), although this finding was not universal (130). Of all the cases reported until 1987, 69% had previously been on peritoneal dialysis, and almost one-half of available peritoneal biopsies showed some inflammatory changes. These findings suggest a role for an abnormal peritoneal cavity in maintaining ascites, but the precise mechanism for this is unclear (121).

Because the mass effect of ascites can produce anorexia and severe cachexia, and successful treatment can improve nutrition, dialysis ascites should be managed aggressively. Correction of volume overload is central to the management. Reduced salt and water ingestion is essential (122, 124), and psychotherapy has been suggested to play a potential role in making these dietary changes (123). Diet is particularly important because large volume ultrafiltration during dialysis is often poorly tolerated. Isolated ultrafiltration, however, can be useful, since it induces fewer hypotensive complications (131).

Peritoneo-venous shunts have been placed for dialysis ascites (121), but given the effectivenes of conservative measures and the general decline in the use of these shunts because of severe side effects (132), this modality has a limited role. The most definitive treatment of dialysis ascites is renal transplantation, and the response has been essentially universal (122, 123, 125, 128, 133).

REFERENCES

1. Jaffe RH, Laing DR: Changes of the digestive tract in uremia: pathologic anatomic study. *Arch Intern Med* 53: 851, 1934
2. Simenhoff ML, Burke JF, Saukkonen JJ et al.: Biochemical profile of uremic breath. *N Engl J Med* 297: 132, 1977
3. Weiner SN, Vertes V, Shapiro H: The upper gastrointestinal tract in patients undergoing chronic dialysis. *Radiology* 92: 110, 1969
4. King AY, Schneider HJ, King LR: The roentgen appearance of the small bowel during long-term hemodialysis for chronic renal disease. *Radiology* 99: 331, 1971
5. Margolis DM, Saylor JL, Geisse G, Deschryver-Kecskemeti K, Harter HR, Zuckerman GR: Upper gastrointestinal disease in chronic renal failure: a prospective evaluation. *Arch Intern Med* 138: 1214, 1978
6. Franzin G, Musola R, Mencarelli R: Morphological changes of the gastroduodenal mucosa in regular dialysis uraemic patients. *Histopathology* 6: 492, 1982
7. Milito G, Taccone-Gallucci M, Brancaleone C et al.: The gastrointestinal tract in uremic patients on long-term hemodialysis. *Kidney Int* 28 (Suppl 17): 157S, 1985
8. Wee A, Kang JY, Ho MS, Choong HL, Wu AY, Sutherland IH: Gastroduodenal mucosa in uraemia: endoscopic and histological correlation and prevalence of helicobacter-like organisms. *Gut* 31: 1093, 1990
9. Chachati A, Godon JP: Effect of haemodialysis on upper gastrointestinal tract pathology in patients with chronic renal failure. *Nephrol Dial Transplant* 1: 233, 1987
10. Ala-Kaila K: Upper gastrointestinal findings in chronic renal failure. *Scand J Gastroenterol* 22: 372, 1987
11. Vaziri ND, Dure-Smith B, Miller R, Mirahmadi MK: Pathology of gastrointestinal tract in chronic hemodialysis patients: an autopsy study of 78 cases. *Am J Gatroenterol* 80: 608, 1985
12. Goldstein H, Murphy D, Sokol A, Rubini ME: Gastric acid secretion in patients undergoing chronic dialysis. *Arch Intern Med* 120: 645, 1967
13. Boner G, Berry EM: Gastrointestinal hemorrhage complicating chronic hemodialysis. *Isr J Med Sci* 4: 66, 1968
14. Shepherd AMM, Stewart WK, Wormsley KG: Peptic ulceration in chronic renal failure. *Lancet* 1: 1357, 1973
15. Boyle JM, Johnston B: Acute upper gastrointestinal hemorrhage in patients with chronic renal disease. *Am J Med* 75: 409, 1983
16. Musola R, Franzin G, Mora R, Manfrini C: Prevalence of gastroduodenal lesions in uremic patients undergoing dialysis and after renal transplantation. *Gastrointest Endosc* 30: 343, 1984
17. Andriulli A, Malfi B, Recchia S, Ponti V, Triolo G, Segoloni G: Patients with chronic renal failure are not at a risk of developing chronic peptic ulcers. *Clin Nephrol* 23: 245, 1985
18. Kang JY, Wu AY, Sutherland IH, Vathsala A: Prevalence of peptic ulcer in patients undergoing maintenance hemodialysis. *Dig Dis Sci* 33: 774, 1988
19. Kang JY: The gastrointestinal tract in uremia. *Dig Dis Sci* 38: 257, 1993
20. McConnell JB, Stewart WK, Thjodleifsson B, Wormsley KG: Gastric function in chronic renal failure: Effects of maintenance haemodialysis. *Lancet* 2: 1121, 1975
21. Ventkateswaran PS, Jeffers A, Hocken AG: Gastric acid secretion in chronic renal failure. *Br Med J* 4: 22, 1972
22. Clendinnen BG, Davidson WO Reeder DO, Jackson BM, Thompson JC: Renal uptake and excretion of gastrin in the dog. *Surg Gynecol Obstet* 132: 1039, 1971
23. Maxwell JG, Moore JG, Dixon J, Stevens LE: Gastrin levels in anephric patients. *Surg Forum* 127: 305, 1971
24. Korman MG, Laver MC, Hansky J: Hypergastrinaemia in chronic renal failure. *Br Med J* 1: 209, 1972
25. Falcao HA, Wesdorp IC, Fischer JE: Gastrin levels and gastric acid secretion in anephric patients and in patients with chronic and acute renal failure. *J Surg Research* 18: 107, 1975
26. Owyang C, Miller LJ, DiMagno EP, Brennan LA, Go VW: Gastrointestinal hormone profile in renal insufficiency. *Mayo Clin Proc* 54: 769, 1979
27. Doherty CC, Buchanan KD, Ardill J, McGeown MG: Gut hormones and renal failure. *Dial Transplant* 9: 245, 1980
28. Gold CH, Morley JE, Viljoen M, Tim LO, de Fomseca M, Kalk WJ: Gastric acid secretion and serum gastrin levels in patients with chronic renal failure on regular hemodialysis. *Nephron* 25: 92, 1980
29. Muto S, Murayama N, Asano Y, Hosoda S, Miyata M: Hypergastrinemia and achlorhydria in chronic renal failure. *Nephron* 40: 143, 1985
30. Ghonaimy E, Barsoum R, Soliman M et al.: Serum gastrin in chronic renal failure: morphological and physiological correlation. *Nephron* 39: 86, 1985
31. Sirinek KR, O'Dorisio TM, Gaskell HV, Lefine BA: Chronic renal failure: effect of hemodialysis on gastrointestinal hormone. *Am J Surg* 148: 732, 1984
32. Hegbrant J, Thysell H, Ekman R: Plasma levels of gastrointestinal regulatory peptides in patients receiving maintenance hemodialysis. *Scand J Gastroenterol* 26: 599, 1991
33. Fisher RS, Lipshutz W, Cohen S: The hormonal regulation of pyloric sphincter function. *J Clin Invest* 52: 1289, 1973
34. Mitchell CJ, Jewell DP, Lewin MR et al.: Gastric function and histology in chronic renal failure. *J Clin Path* 32: 208, 1979
35. Bartos V, Melichar J, Erben J: The function of the exocrine pancreas in chronic renal disease. *Digestion* 3: 33, 1970
36. Dinoso VP Jr, Murthy SN, Saris AL et al.: Gastric and pancreatic function in patients with end-stage renal disease. *J Clin Gastroenterol* 4: 321, 1982
37. Swamy AP, Mangla JC, Cestero VM, Guarasci G: Serum pepsinogens and gastrins in chronic hemodialysis patients. *Biochem Med* 25: 227, 1981
38. Alvarez L, Puleo J, Balian JA: Investigation of gastrointestinal bleeding in patients with end stage renal disease. *Am J Gatroenterol* 88: 30, 1993
39. Shousha S, Arnout AH, Abbas SH, Parkins RA: Antral Helicobacter pylori in patients with chronic renal failure. *J Clin Pathol* 43: 397, 1990

40. Ali-Kaila K, Vaajalahti P, Karvonen AL, Kokki M: Gastric Helicobacter and upper gastrointestinal symptoms in chronic renal failure. *Ann Med* 23: 403, 1991

41. Gladziwa U, Haase G, Handt S et al.: Prevalence of helicobacter pylori in patients with chronic renal failure. *Nephrol Dial Transplant* 8: 301, 1993

42. Zuckerman GR, Cornette GL, Clouse RE, Harter HR: Upper gastrointestinal bleeding in patients with chronic renal failure. *Ann Intern Med* 102: 588, 1985

43. McNamee PT, Moore GW, McGeown M, Doherty CC, Collins BJ: Gastric emptying in chronic renal failure. *Br Med J* 291: 310, 1985

44. Wright RA, Clemente R, Wathen R: Gastric emptying in patients with chronic renal failure receiving hemodialysis. *Arch Intern Med* 144: 495, 1984

45. Soffer EE, Geva B, Helman C, Avni Y, Bar-Meir S: Gastric emptying in chronic renal failure patients on hemodialysis. *J Clin Gastroenterol* 9: 651, 1987

46. Brown-Cartwright D, Smith HJ, Feldman M: Gastric emptying of an indigestible solid in patients with end-stage renal disease on continuous ambulatory peritoneal dialysis. *Gastroenterology* 95: 49, 1988

47. Feldman M, Schiller LR: Disorders of gastrointestinal motility associated with diabetes mellitus. *Ann Intern Med* 98: 378, 1983

48. Janssens J, Peeters TL Vantrappen G et al.: Improvement of gastric emptying in diabetic gastroparesis by erythromycin. *N Engl J Med* 322: 1028, 1990

49. Lindner A, Charra B, Sherrard DJ, Scribner BH: Accelerated atherosclerosis in prolonged maintenance hemodialysis. *N Engl J Med* 290: 697, 1974

50. Diamond SM, Emmett M, Henrich WL: Bowel infarction as a cause of death in dialysis patients. *JAMA* 256: 2545, 1986

51. Margolis DM, Etheredge EE, Garza-Garza R, Hruska K, Anderson CB: Ischemic bowel disease following bilateral nephrectomy or renal tranplant. *Surgery* 82: 667, 1977

52. Dahlberg PJ, Kisken WA, Newcomer KL, Yutuc WR: Mesenteric ischemia in chronic dialysis patients. *Am J Nephrol* 5: 327, 1985

53. Romolo JL, Williams GM: Effect of kayexalate and sorbitol on colon of normal and uremic rats. *Surg Forum* 30: 369, 1979

54. Lillemoe KD, Romolo JL, Hamilton SR, Pennington LR, Burdick JF, Williams GM: Intestinal necrosis due to sodium polystyrene (Kayexalate) in sorbitol enemas: Clinical and experimental support for the hypothesis. *Surgery* 101: 267, 1987

55. Wootton FT, Rhodes DF, Lee WM, Fitts CT: Colonic necrosis with kayexalate-sorbitol enemas after renal transplantation. *Ann Intern Med* 111: 947, 1989

56. Townsend CM Jr, Remmers AR Jr, Sarles HE, Fish JC: Intestinal obstruction from medication bezoar in patients with renal failure. *N Engl J Med* 288: 1058, 1973

57. Welch JP, Schweizer RT, Bartus SA: Management of antacid impactions in hemodialysis and renal transplant patients. *Am J Surg* 139: 561, 1980

58. Adams PL, Rutsky EA, Rostand SG, Han SY: Lower gastrointestinal tract dysfunction in patients receiving long-term hemodialysis. *Arch Intern Med* 142: 303, 1982

59. Scheff RT, Zuckerman G, Harter H, Delmez J, Koehler R: Diverticular disease in patients with chronic renal failure due to polycystic kidney disease. *Ann Intern Med* 92: 202, 1980

60. Galbraith P, Bagg MN, Schabel SI, Rajagopalan PR: Diverticular complications of renal failure. *Gastrointest Radiol* 15: 259, 1990

61. Mills B, Zuckerman G, Sicard G: Discrete colon ulcers as a cause of lower gastrointestinal bleeding and perforation in end-stage renal disease. *Surgery* 89: 548, 1981

62. Brown KM: Isolated ascending colon ulceration in a patient with chronic renal insufficiency. *J Natl Med Assoc* 84: 185, 1992

63. Lipschutz DE, Easterling RE: Spontaneous perforation of the colon in chronic renal failure. *Arch Intern Med* 132: 758, 1973

64. Bartolomeo RS, Calabrese PR, Taubin HL: Spontaneous perforation of the colon: A potential complication of chronic renal failure. *Digestive Dis* 22: 656, 1977

65. Gekas P, Schuster MM: Stercoral perforation of the colon: Case report and review of the literature. *Gastroenterology* 80: 1054, 1981

66. Krebs RA, Burtis BB: Bowel perforation. A complication of peritoneal dialysis using a permanent peritoneal cannula. *JAMA* 198: 486, 1966

67. Bruce D, Ritchie C, Jennings LC, Lynn KL, Bailey RR, Cook HB: Clostridium difficile-associated colitis: cross infection in predisposed patients with renal failure. *N Z Med J* 95: 265, 1982

68. Leung AC, Orange G, McLay A, Henderson IS: Clostridium difficile-associated colitis in uremic patients. *Clin Nephrol* 24: 242, 1985

69. Barany P, Stenvinkel P, Nord CE, Bergstrom J: Clostridium difficile infection – a poor prognostic sign in uremic patients? *Clin Nephrol* 38: 53, 1992

70. Cunningham JT: Gastric telangiectasias in chronic hemodialysis patients: a report of six cases. *Gastroenterology* 81: 1131, 1981

71. Dave PB, Romeu J, Antonelli A, Eiser AR: Gastrointestinal telangiectasias: a source of bleeding in patients receiving haemodialysis. *Arch Intern Med* 144: 1781, 1984

72. Clouse RE, Costigan DJ, Mills BA, Zuckerman GR: Angiodysplasia as a cause of upper gastrointestinal bleeding. *Arch Intern Med* 145: 458, 1985

73. Marcuard SP, Weinstock JV: Gastrointestinal angiodysplasia in renal failure. *J Clin Gastroenterol* 10: 482, 1988

74. Navab F, Masters P, Subramani R, Ortego TJ, Thompson CH: Angiodysplasia in patients with renal insufficiency. *Am J Gatroenterol* 84: 1297, 1989

75. Gheissari A, Rajuagur V, Kumashiro R, Matsumoto T: Gastrointestinal hemorrhage in end stage renal disease patients. *Int Surg* 75: 93, 1990

76. Maher ER, Hamilton Dutoit S, Baillod RA, Sweny P, Moorhead JF: Gastrointestinal complications of dialysis related amyloidosis. *Br Med J* 297: 265, 1988

77. Takahashi S, Morita T, Koda Y, Murayama H, Hirasawa Y: Gastrointestinal involvement of dialysis-related amyloidosis. *Clin Nephrol* 30: 168, 1988

78. Campistol JM, Sole M, Munoz-Gomez J, Lopez-Pedret J, Revert L: Systemic involvement of dialysis-amyloidosis. *Am J Nephrol* 10: 389, 1990

79. Choi HS, Heller D, Picken MM, Sidhy GS, Kahn T: Infarction of intestine with massive amyloid deposition in

two patients on long-term hemodialysis. *Gastroenterology* 6: 230, 1989

80. Nelson SR, Hawkins PN and Richardson S et al.: Imaging of haemodialysis-associated amyloidosis with 123I-serum amyloid P component. *Lancet* 338: 335, 1991

81. Rosenblatt SG, Drake S, Fadem S, Welsch R, Lifschitz MD: Gastrointestinal blood loss in patients with chronic renal failure. *Am J Kidney Dis* 1: 232, 1982

82. Ajam M, Ramanujam LS, Gandhi VC et al.: Colon-cancer screening in dialysis patients. *Artif Organs* 14: 95, 1990

83. Doherty CC, O'Connor FA, Buchanan KD, McGeown MC: Cimetidine for duodenal ulceration in patients undergoing hemodialysis. *Br Med J* 2: 1506, 1977

84. Salusky IB, Foley J, Nelson P, Goodman WG: Aluminum accumulation during treatment with aluminum hydroxide and dialysis in children and young adults with chronic renal disease. *N Engl J Med* 324: 527, 1991

85. Robertson JA, Salusky IB, Goodman WH, Norris KC, Coburn JW: Sucralfate, intestinal aluminum absorption and aluminum toxicity in a patient on dialysis. *Ann Intern Med* 111: 179, 1989

86. Howden A, Payton CD, Meredith PA et al.: Antisecretory effect and oral pharmacokinetics of omeprazole in patients with chronic renal failure. *Eur J Clin Pharmacol* 28: 637, 1985

87. Roggo A, Filippini L, Colombi A: The effect of hemodialysis on omeprazole plasma concentrations in the anuric patient: a case report. *Int J Clin Pharmacol Ther Toxicol* 28: 115, 1990

88. DiMinno G, Martinez J, McKean ML, DeLaRosa J, Burke JF: Platelet dysfunction in uremia: multifaceted defect partially corrected by dialysis. *Am J Med* 79: 552, 1985

89. Mannucci PM: Desmopressin: a nontransfusional form of treatment of congenital and acquired bleeding disorders. *Blood* 72: 1449, 1988

90. Janson PA, Jubelirer SJ, Weinstein MJ, Deykin D: Treatment of the bleeding tendency in uremia with cryoprecipitate. *N Engl J Med* 303: 318, 1980

91. Roger SD, Piper J, Tucker B, Raine AE, Baker LR, Kovacs IB: Enhanced platelet reactivity with erythropoietin but not following transfusion in dialysis patients. *Nephrol Dial Transplant* 8: 213, 1993

92. Cases A, Escolar G, Reverter JC et al.: Recombinant human erythropoietin treatment improves platelet function in uremic patients. *Kidney Int* 42: 668, 1992

93. Shemin D, Elnour M, Amarantes B, Abuelo JG, Chazan JA: Oral estrogens decrease bleeding time and improve clinical bleeding in patients with renal failure. *Am J Med* 89: 436, 1990

94. Bronner MH, Pate MB, Cunningham JT, Marsh WH: Estrogen-progesterone therapy for bleeding gastrointestinal telangiectasisias in chronic renal failure: An uncontrolled trial. *Ann Intern Med* 105: 371, 1986

95. Richardson JD, Lordon RE: Gastrointestinal bleeding caused by angiodysplasia: a difficult problem in patients with chronic renal failure receiving hemodialysis therapy. *Am Surg* 59: 636, 1993

96. Avram MM: High prevalence of pancreatic disease in chronic renal failure. *Nephron* 18: 68, 1977

97. Vaziri ND, Dure-Smith B, Miller R, Mirahmadi M: Pancreatic pathology in chronic dialysis patients-an autopsy study of 78 cases. *Nephron* 46: 347, 1987

98. Rutsky EA, Robards M, Van Dyke JA, Rostand SG: Acute pancreatitis in patients with end-stage renal disease without transplantation. *Arch Intern Med* 146: 1741, 1986

99. Sachs EF, Hurwitz FJ, Bloch HM, Milne FJ: Pancreatic exocrine hypofunction in the wasting syndrome of end-stage renal disease. *Am J Gatroenterol* 78: 170, 1983

100. Robinson DO, Alp MG, Grant AK, Lawrence JR: Pancreatitis and renal disease. *Scand J Gastroenterol* 12: 17, 1977

101. Avram RM, Iancu M: Pancreatic disease in uremia and parathyroid hormone excess. *Nephron* 32: 60, 1982

102. Royse VL, Jensen DM, Corwin HL: Pancreatic enzymes in chronic renal failure. *Arch Intern Med* 147: 537, 1987

103. Bastani B, Mifflin TE, Lovell MA, Westervelt FB, Bruns DE: Serum amylases in chronic and end-stage renal failure: effects of mode of therapy, race, diabetes and peritonitis. *Am J Nephrol* 7: 292, 1987

104. Vaziri ND, Chang D, Malekpour A, Radhat S: Pancreatic enzymes in patients with end-stage renal disease maintained on hemodialysis. *Am J Gatroenterol* 83: 410, 1988

105. Blainey JD, Northam BE: Amylase excretion by the human kidney. *Clin Sci* 32: 377, 1967

106. Berk JE, Fridhandler L, Ness RL: Amylase and isoamylase activities in renal insufficiency. *Ann Intern Med* 90: 351, 1979

107. Pahl MV, Vaziri ND, Dure-Smith B, Miller R, Mirahmadi MK: Hepatobiliary pathology in hemodialysis patients : an autopsy study of 78 cases. *Am J Gatroenterol* 91: 783, 1986

108. Blum M, Tchetchik M, Schujman E, Aviram A: Liver enlargemtent in long-term hemodialysis patients. *Arch Intern Med* 140: 343, 1980

109. Ali M, Fayemi AO, Rigolosi R, Frascino J, Marsden T, Malcolm D: Hemosiderosis in hemodialysis patients. An autopsy study of 50 cases. *JAMA* 244: 343, 1980

110. Stanbaugh GH, Gillit DM, Holmes AW: Dialysis hemosiderosis mimicking non-A, non-B hepatitis. *Trans Am Soc Artif Intern Organs* 30: 217, 1984

111. Roxe DM, Krumlovsky FA, Del Greco F, Fitzsimons E: Failure of deferoxamine to improve iron overload in chronic hemodialysis patients. *Int J Artif Organs* 13: 211, 1990

112. Lazarus JM, Hakim RM, Newell J: Recombinant human erythropoietin and phlebotomy in the treatment of iron overload in chronic hemodialysis patients. *Am J Kidney Dis* 16: 101, 1990

113. Alfrey AC, Hegg A, Craswell P: Metabolism and toxicity of aluminum in renal failure. *Am J Clin Nutr* 33: 1509, 1980

114. Leong AS, Disney AP, Gove DW: Spallation and migration of silicone from blood-pump tubing in patients on hemodialysis. *N Engl J Med* 306: 135, 1982

115. Hunt J, Farthing MJ, Baker LR, Crocker PR, Levison DA: Silicone in the liver: possible late effects. *Gut* 30: 239, 1989

116. Laochapand T, Osman EM, Morley AR, Ward MK, Kerr DN: Accumulation of silicone elastomer in regular dialysis. *Proc Eur Dial Transplant Assoc* 19: 143, 1983

117. Bommer J, Pwenicka E, Kessler J, Ritz E: Reduction of silicone particle release during haemodialysis. *Proc Eur Dial Transplant Assoc Eur Ren Assoc* 21: 287, 1985

118. Simon P, Meyrier A, Brissot P: Uremia and the liver. II: Drugs and the liver in the uremic patient. *Nephron* 29: 7, 1981

119. Cinque TJ, Letteri J: Idiopathic ascites – complication of chronic extracorporeal dialysis. *Abstr Am Soc Nephrol* 4: 16, 1970

120. Mahoney JF, Gutch CF, Holmes JH: Intractable ascites in chronic hemodialysis patients. *Abstr Am Soc Nephrol* 4: 51, 1970

121. Gluck Z, Nolph KD: Ascites associated with end-stage renal disease. *Am J Kidney Dis* 10: 9, 1987

122. Wang F, Pillay VKG, Ing TS, Armbruster KFW, Rosenberg JC: Ascites in patients treated with maintenance hemodialysis. *Nephron* 12: 105, 1974

123. Gotloib L, Sevadio C: Ascites in patients undergoing maintenance hemodialysis. *Am J Med* 61: 465, 1976

124. Gutch CF, Mahony JF, Pingerra W, Holmes JH, Ramirez G, Ogden DA: Refractory ascites in chronic dialysis patients. *Clin Nephrol* 2: 59, 1974

125. Craig R, Sparber M, Ivanovich P, Rice L, Dordal E: Nephrogenic ascites. *Arch Intern Med* 134: 276, 1974

126. Fajardo B, Gonzalez G, Tannenberg AM: Osmotic disequilibrium causing ascites during chronic hemodialysis. *Trans Am Soc Artif Intern Organs* 34: 617, 1988

127. Cinque TJ, Letteri JM: Idiopathic ascites in chronic renal failure. *NY State J Med* 73: 781, 1973

128. Singh S, Mitra S, Berman LB: Ascites in patients on maintenance hemodialysis. *Nephron* 12: 114, 1974

129. Rodriquez HJ, Walls J, Slatopolsky E, Klahr S: Recurrent ascites following peritoneal dialysis. *Arch Intern Med* 134: 283, 1974

130. Arismendi GS, Izard MW, Hampton WR, Maher JF: The clinical spectrum of ascites associated with maintenance dialysis. *Am J Med* 60: 46, 1976

131. Shin KD, Ing TS, Popli S et al.: Isolated ultrafiltration in the treatment of dialysis ascites. *Artif Organs* 3: 120, 1979

132. Conn HO: Complications of peritoneovenous shunts. *Trans Am Soc Artif Intern Organs* 35: 176, 1989

133. Popli S, Chen WT, Nakamoto S, Daugirdas JT, Cespedes LE, Ing TS: Hemodialysis ascites in anephric patients. *Clin Nephrol* 15: 203, 1981

HEMATOLOGICAL PROBLEMS OF RENAL FAILURE

JOSEPH W. ESCHBACH

INTRODUCTION

Renal failure, whether acute or chronic, adversely affects a number of hematological parameters. Red cell production and destruction, granulocyte and lymphocyte function, platelet function and coagulation are affected to various degrees. These changes result in anemia, and an increased susceptibility to infection and hemorrhage. This chapter will deal primarily with the pathogenesis of the anemia of chronic renal failure, erythropoietin (Epo) metabolism, the treatment of this anemia with recombinant human Epo (epoetin), and the benefits of this therapy. Infection, immunological dysfunction and bleeding disorders are reviewed in Chapters 7B, 8 and 9.

PATHOGENESIS OF THE ANEMIA OF RENAL FAILURE

Acute renal failure

Anemia develops in most cases of acute renal failure regardless of the cause. Erythropoiesis is markedly suppressed as indicated by the virtual absence of erythroid cells on marrow examination (1) and few circulating reticulocytes. Presumably this is because of a marked decrease in renal Epo secretion by the acutely injured kidneys. Red cell survival is also shortened (2), presumably due to inflammation, infection, cytokines and possibly 'uremia', although anemia may be present prior to marked elevation in uremic solutes. Frank hemolysis usually is not present. Therefore, a severe hypoproliferative anemia exists. Hemodilution, due to saline excess, may accentuate the anemia (3).

An unusual form of acute renal failure is observed in the Hemolytic-Uremic Syndrome. This syndrome is characterized by the triad of microangiopathic hemolytic anemia, thrombocytopenia, and acute renal failure. Epo production is initially increased resulting in erythroid hyperplasia on marrow examination and reticulocytosis; hemolysis results in a decreased or absent plasma haptoglobin and fragmentation of red cells on peripheral smear; and mechanical trauma to the red cells and platelets, induced by the disrupted endothelial lining of the renal arteriolar and glomerular capillary bed, results in thrombocytopenia.

Chronic renal failure

It has long been assumed that the pathogenesis of the anemia of chronic renal failure was multifactorial with Epo deficiency, shortened red cell survival, uremic inhibition and bleeding due to uremic platelet dysfunction being the major factors (4). It is now apparent that relative erythropoietin deficiency is the single most important cause of the anemia, since administration of epoetin can completely correct the anemia (5–7). Red cell life span (normally approximately 120 days) may vary from 60 to 90 days, but occasionally may be normal (8–10). However, this mild hemolysis does not seem to prevent epoetin from being effective and there appears to be no correlation between the amount of epoetin required for therapy and the degree of shortening in red cell survival (11). Inhibition of red cell production by retained uremic solutes has been assumed to play a significant role in this anemia, particularly since many *in vitro* studies have shown that uremic plasma suppresses the stimulating action of Epo on red cell progenitor growth (12–14). Myeloid and megakaryocyte growth are also suppressed by uremic plasma *in vitro* (15). Since leukopenia and thrombocytopenia are uncommon in human chronic renal failure, the *in vitro* uremic inhibition of erythropoiesis must be considered non-specific. Furthermore, these *in vitro* studies utilized canine or murine erythroid progenitor cells. However, when human, autologous marrow cells were cultured and incubated with uremic plasma and Epo, there was no inhibition in erythroid progenitor cell growth (16), nor was there inhibition in the growth of erythroid progenitor cells from uremic or normal sheep when incubated with uremic sheep plasma (17). *In-vivo* studies with the infusion of Epo-rich sheep plasma into normal and uremic, hemodialyzed sheep (18), and with the infusion of epoetin into normal subjects and hemodialysis patients (19), indicate that erythropoiesis, as quantitated by ferrokinetics, reticulocyte response, and transferrin receptor levels, is not blunted in subjects with chronic renal failure. Hence, uremic inhibition plays a minimal role, if any, in the pathogenesis of this hypoproliferative anemia. The fact that almost all patients with chronic renal failure, if iron replete, and without inflammation or infection, will have an appropriate erythropoietic response to epoetin, also implies that uremic inhibition, plays a minor, if any, role in the pathogenesis of this anemia. However, there is the impression that 'better' hemodialysis results in less anemia, as indicated by higher hematocrit and hemoglobin levels and less transfusion requirements of home hemodialysis patients prior to the use of epoetin (20), and by less severe anemia in patients dialyzed by continuous ambulatory peritoneal dialysis (20). The latter phenomenon has been theorized as due to the removal of uremic erythroid inhibitors by the peritoneal membrane which allows for diffusion of larger molecular weight solutes than regular hemodialysis membranes. Prior to the use of epoetin, European and Middle Eastern patients that hemodialyzed for 15 or more hours per week had a mean hemoglobin of approximately 9.5 g/dl, whereas those that had 12 or less hours of hemodialysis per week had a mean hemoglobin of less than 8.5 g/dl (20). However, the iron status, presence of infection or inflammation, and the ingestion of androgenic steroids (i.e., other factors that could effect the erythroid response) in these patients was not disclosed.

ERYTHROPOIETIN METABOLISM

Erythropoietin is a glycoprotein hormone of 30,400 Dalton molecular weight containing 165 amino acids and 4 carbohydrate side chains which terminate with a sialic acid residue (21). The existence of an erythropoietic hormone was first postulated by Carnot and Deflandre in 1906 (22), but their experiment could not be confirmed until Erslev, in 1953, demonstrated an 'erythropoietic stimulating factor' in the plasma of anemic rabbits (23). The kidney was found to be the source of Epo by Jacobson and colleagues in 1957 (24). Measuring Epo by bioassay utilizing ^{59}Fe uptake in post-hypoxic polycythemic mice, Adamson demonstrated an inverse relationship between urinary and plasma Epo levels and hematocrit, indicating that there is feedback control of erythropoiesis dependent on oxygen delivery to the site of renal Epo production (25). This was subsequently confirmed in 1974 by Erslev who showed that the perfusion of hypoxic rabbit kidneys *in vitro* with a serum-free solution resulted in the production of intact Epo (26).

A major breakthrough occurred in 1977 when Miyake, Kung and Goldwasser were able to purify Epo from human urine (27). This information, and the utilization of oligonucleotide probes derived from these purification studies, allowed Lin et al. in 1983 to isolate and clone the Epo gene from a human fetal liver genomic library (28). Jacobs et al. (29), and Powell et al. (30) also subsequently isolated the Epo gene, which is located on chromosome 7. This gene encompasses about 3,000 base pairs and contains 5 exons and 4 introns and codes for a 193 amino acid polypeptide. A 27 amino acid leader sequence at the N-terminal part and a carboxy-terminal arginine molecule are cleaved off during secretion, resulting in the circulating Epo molecule containing 165 amino acids.

The site of Epo production in the hypoxic mouse kidney has been shown to be the renal peritubular capillary endothelial cell, based on *in situ* hybridization techniques with ^{35}S for Epo-specific messenger ribonucleic acid (mMRA) (31, 32). However, Epo mRNA has also been localized to renal interstitial fibroblasts utilizing a double immunohistochemical labelling (33, 34). The liver can also produce Epo, but the percent of total Epo production is debatable. Ablation studies suggest that the liver contributes 10–20% (35), but up to 30–40% of total circulating Epo in severe anemia or hypoxia can be accounted by hepatic Epo mRNA (36). Most of the hepatic Epo is produced by centrilobular hepatocytes (37). Despite normal liver function, only rarely in the anephric state can there be enough Epo production to provide for significant erythropoiesis (38) suggesting that the liver is less sensitive than the kidney to hypoxic stimuli. However, hepatitis may result in a transient increase in hematocrit levels as noted in some anephric dialysis patients (39, 40).

How hypoxia stimulates Epo secretion in the kidney is incompletely understood. The Epo secretory cell in the anemic rat is not located in the renal medulla, where hypoxia is the greatest due to the renal countercurrent exchange of oxygen, but in the renal cortex and outer medulla (41). However, tissue pO_2 levels are also decreased in the renal cortex (42). Another mechanism for hypoxic stimulation to the Epo secreting cell, whether it is a cortical peritubular capillary endothelial cell or a cortical interstitial fibroblast, could be due to the differential hypoxia that occurs due to the marked oxygen consumption by the proximal tubule for solute transport of the majority of the glomerular filtrate. Epo production is reduced when proximal tubular function is altered in hypoxic mice following the administration of the diuretic acetazolamide (43), and when glomerular filtration is reduced in the isolated rat kidney perfused with hyperoncotic bovine serum albumin (44). This suggests, but does not prove, that improved renal oxygenation accounts for the reduced Epo secretion. While the mechanisms for the effect of changes in renal oxygenation on renal Epo secretion remain to be clarified, it seems likely that a reduction in the number of Epo-secreting renal cells due to progression of intrinsic renal disease, of whatever variety, will lead to reduced Epo secretion even with maximal hypoxic stress.

The subcellular mechanism(s) by which the kidney recognizes altered oxygen availability are also unknown. However, studies utilizing the Hep 3B human hepatoma cell line suggest that the oxygen-sensing mechanism is dependent on a heme protein that binds oxygen reversibly (45). In addition to hypoxia, cobalt, nickel, and manganese stimulate Epo mRNA production in the Hep 3B cell and lock the heme protein in the de-oxy form, suggesting that the ferrous ion in the porphyrin ring is critical for this oxygen sensor (45). Carbon monoxide does the opposite: it reduces Epo gene expression by mimicking oxygen in liganding the heme protein (46).

Hypoxia to the rat kidney results in the release of increased Epo mRNA within an hour (47) and secretion ceases approximately one-two hours after the hypoxic stimulus abates. The number of interstitial cells that produce Epo mRNA, as shown by *in situ* hybridization, increases with progressive anemia in the plebotomized rat (48). This suggests that these renal Epo producing cells act in an on/off manner, and are not able to increase the amount of Epo produced per cell.

Epo circulates in minute amounts, varying in normal subjects between 3 to 18 milliUnits/ml as quantitated by a bioassay utilizing a plasma concentration technique (49), 16.5 ± 3.4 mU/ml by radioimmunoassay (50), and 3.3–13.5 mU/ml by enzyme-linked immunoabsorbent assay (ELISA) (51). The wide range in the normal Epo plasma levels suggest that there is an equally wide range in the secretory rate and erythroid response to Epo. Plasma levels of Epo determined by radioimmunoassay, in anemic, non-dialyzed subjects with progressive renal failure, and in those dialyzed with or without their native kidneys, were similar: 14.3 ± 2.6, 15.3 ± 4.2 and 15.2 ± 3.4 mU/ml, respectively, similar to normal, non-anemic

subjects (50). Using ^{125}I labelled rHuEpo in a steady-state infusion, the secretion rate of native Epo is similar in anemic, hemodialysis patients (not receiving epoetin as therapy) and normal subjects (255 pg/kg/h, range 68–1,101 for patients; 190 pg/kg/h, range 52–382 for normal subjects) (52). When converted to mU, this is equivalent to 25.5 and 19 mU/kg/h, respectively (52). Others have found that uremic subjects, when compared to normal subjects, have lower plasma Epo levels (20.0 *vs* 26.3 mU/ml), reduced production of Epo (146 *vs* 290 U/day per 1.73 m²) and reduced terminal elimination half-life of Epo (8.31 *vs* 4.9 hours) (53). The three N-linked glycosolated side chains of the Epo molecule (the other glycosolated side chain is O-linked) are responsible for *in-vivo* activity of Epo (54), which allow it to remain in the circulation for a half-life of 4.5 ± 0.9 (55) or 5.4 ± 1.7 hours (56) if epoetin is given IV, or 25 ± 12 hours if given SC (55). The pharmacokinetics of IV or SC epoetin in chronic renal failure may (57) or may not (53) be similar to that of normal subjects, but the site of Epo degradation is neither the kidney nor the marrow. Anephric patients and patients with hypoproliferative erythroid marrows do not have higher serum levels of Epo after infusion of epoetin, and mice with hypo or hyperplastic marrows have normal epoetin half-lives (58).

Epo exerts its effect on erythropoiesis by binding to a surface receptor on the erythroid progenitor cells: burst-forming unit-erythroid (BFU-E), colony-forming unit-erythroid (CFU-E) and early proerythroblasts, resulting in proliferation and differentiation of these cells (59, 60). The Epo receptor has been cloned (61), the site of the Epo-Epo receptor ligand in the mouse has been identified (62), but the mechanism for the signal transduction is still being elucidated. Epo is a survival factor for the erythroid progenitor cells, preventing apoptosis or programmed cell death of these cells (63). Epo therefore allows these cells to differentiate and proliferate resulting in increased production of new red blood cells as reticulocytes, which are subsequently released into the circulation. Epo also results in the premature release, or shift of immature reticulocytes into circulation (64).

The normal hormonal feedback mechanism is completed by the level of circulating red cells (the red cell mass). This sensing mechanism of the Epo-producing renal interstitial cells results in the fine-tuning of Epo production and subsequent red cell production required for the daily production of 2×10^{11} red cells in the normal individual.

EPOETIN TREATMENT OF THE ANEMIA OF CHRONIC RENAL FAILURE

Background

Epoetin was first produced after the human Epo gene was isolated and cloned by Lin and colleagues in 1983 at Amgen, Thousand Oaks, CA (28). This feat was sub-

1062 Joseph W. Eschbach

sequently followed by Jacobs et al. of Genetics Institute, Cambridge, MA (29) and Powell et al. at the University of Washington, Seattle (30). The human gene is inserted into the nucleus of the chinese hamster ovary cell by genetic engineering methods. As a result of the usual intracellular transcription and translation processes, a glycosolated polypeptide hormone is secreted from the cell. The hormone-containing fluid is purified of all foreign protein and has been shown to be equivalent immunologically, biologically, and chemically to the natural hormone (21). The Amgen product, epoetin-alfa, is marketed in the United States for dialysis patients by Amgen and for predialysis patients and for patients with other Epo-responsive anemias by Johnson & Johnson's Ortho Biotech, in Canada by J & J's Ortho-Biotech, and in Europe, the Middle East, Asia, Australia and South America by J & J's Cilag and Jansson divisions. Amgen's product is produced in Japan by the Kirin Brewery Company, Pharmaceutical Division. Genetic Institute's epoetin-beta, which is physiologically identical to epoetin-alfa in its action and pharmacokinetics, is marketed in Europe by Boehringer-Mannhein and in Japan by Chugai Pharmaceutical Company. Epoetin is also produced by Elanex.

rHuEpo was first given to hemodialysis patients as part of a Phase I-II Clinical Trial in early December, 1985, but its efficacy was not apparent until the dosage was increased to 50 U/kg, IV, three times a week (6). Subsequently a pilot study was initiated in the United Kingdom (5). These studies, plus the many subsequent multicenter studies in the United States, Europe, Canada, Asia, and Japan using either epoetin-alfa or epoetin-beta, confirmed the efficacy and relative safety of this recombinant hormone (66–70).

The significance of the anemia of chronic renal failure is greater than formerly appreciated and contributes extensively to the increased morbidity, and possibly the increased mortality, of patients treated with long-term dialysis. Prior to the advent of epoetin therapy, approximately 75% of dialysis patients had hematocrit values less than 30, many had values less than 20, and approximately 15–25% required periodic red cell transfusions. In the United States prior to 1989, when epoetin was released for the treatment of the anemia of chronic renal failure, there was no data for the entire dialysis population as to the mean hematocrit, but in Europe in 1987, the mean hemoglobin for 6869 dialysis patients was 89 ± 2 g/dl (CAPD, 96.1, home hemodialysis, 95.1, and in-center hemodialysis 87.4 g/dl). Sixteen and one-half percent of patients required red cell transfusions (20).

Patients symptomatic from the hypoproliferative anemia associated with progressive renal failure, dialysis, or chronic transplant rejection are candidates for epoetin therapy. Usually symptoms develop when the hematocrit decreases to 30 or less, but therapy is indicated at a higher hematocrit if angina or other anemic symptoms develop, as may occur in older individuals. Younger patients often adjust better to anemia. Before hormone replacement ther-

apy is initiated, other causes of anemia must be excluded. Iron deficiency is the most common factor that can exacerbate the hypoproliferative anemia of chronic renal failure. It is not necessary to obtain a serum erythropoietin level to confirm the diagnosis assuming the patient is anemic, has azotemia, and a normal to decreased reticulocyte count or index. Because epoetin therapy requires the concomitant need for iron to synthesize new hemoglobin, and because approximately 20% of dialysis patients will have a significant elevation in blood pressure during the induction or acute phase of therapy, it is essential that adequate iron stores be available and that diastolic pressures be normal before initiating epoetin. Ideally, the serum ferritin should be > 100 ng/ml, with a percent transferrin saturation in excess of 20.

Principles of epoetin therapy

The erythroid response is dose-dependent, but variable between patients

The increasing reticulocytosis and rate of rise in hematocrit that occurs with epoetin doses greater than 15 units/kg, up to a maximum of 1500 units/kg, IV, three times a week, was first shown in the Phase I-II clinical trial in the USA (6). The variability of patient response has been noted in the bell-shaped distribution pattern of the doses required to maintain a stable hematocrit in iron replete, stable dialysis patients, and in the increasing percent of patients that will attain a target hematocrit when the dose is increased between a range of 25 (25%) to 150 (96%) units/kg, IV, three times a week. Although factors that may blunt the action of epoetin could contribute to this variable response, most observations have failed to detect obvious reasons why some patients respond to 25 units/kg, IV, three times a week, whereas others may require as much as 100–150 units/kg (11). It is most likely that this bell-shaped responsiveness is consistent with normal biological variability.

Route and frequency of administration

Epoetin responsiveness is dependent not only on an adequate dose, but also on appropriate frequency of administration, which in turn may vary depending upon the route of administration. The pharmacokinetics of epoetin alfa and beta are similar. The intravenous administration results in a T 1/2 of 4–9 hours requiring dosing every other or every third day, since Epo levels, which quickly peak within several hours, return to baseline within 24–36 hours, depending on the amount given. Subcutaneous (SC) administration results in a slower increase in blood levels, a maximum level approximately 1/10th that achieved by IV administration of the same dose, but maintenance of a stable level for hours, so that dosing can be less frequent than if given IV, as long as serum Epo levels are greater than 50–100 mU/ml. Epoetin can also be given intraperitoneally (IP), which may be preferable to SC administration for small children or infants treated with peritoneal dialysis. However, the epoetin must be given into a dry peritoneum and allowed to remain in the abdomen for up to 12 hours without dilution from peritoneal dialysate exchange. This may be practical for CCPD but not for CAPD. In one study, approximately 100 U/kg was given to 8 stable peritoneal dialysis patients, comparing the IV, SC, and IP routes of administration (71). Maximum serum concentrations were similar following SC and IP administration, but were only about 5% of that achieved by the IV route. However, there was more bioavailability from SC than IP administration (21.8 ± 11% *vs* 11.4 ± 6.6%) (71).

Most studies have shown that SC administration three times a week requires less epoetin than if it is given IV to elicit an erythroid response (7) or to maintain a stable hematocrit or hemoglobin (72), despite the fact that there is only 10–49% bioavailability when given SC (73–74). Although there is 100% bioavailability when given IV, most of the IV administered dose is probably wasted since once the relatively small number of Epo receptors on the erythroid progenitor cells are saturated, the remaining epoetin is rapidly cleared. Because of the longer maintenance of elevated serum levels of epoetin following SC dosing, the frequency can usually be lengthened to twice a week, weekly, or even occasionally every other week. However, approximately 20% of patients will not have a more efficacious utilization of epoetin with SC dosing, and will need it three times a week, either IV or SC. Although an initial report suggested that daily, SC administration was even more efficacious than every other day administration (75), another study failed to substantiate any advantage to daily dosing with Epo (76).

Maintain epoetin therapy

Occasionally the hematocrit exceeds the target goal for the patient and a lower maintenance dose of epoetin is appropriate. In the past, epoetin doses have been temporarily discontinued until the hematocrit fell below a certain value. This policy developed for several reasons. In the USA reimbursement for epoetin is paid by the Health Care Financing Administration, which has decreed that dialysis centers will not be reimbursed if a patient's hematocrit exceeds 36, unless a medical exception is requested. Hence, if the hematocrit reaches this level, or a predetermined level set by the dialysis center, epoetin is discontinued so that the hematocrit will not exceed the reimbursement level. Another reason for discontinuing therapy is related to the fear that if hypertension developed or worsened during the induction phase of epoetin therapy, hypertensive encephalopathy might occur: therefore, epoetin was discontinued until the blood pressure was controlled. Discontinuing epoetin in this setting is appropriate since controlling blood pressure to prevent its complications takes precedence over acutely increasing the hematocrit. However, a rise in blood pressure during epoetin therapy develops in only 20% of newly treated dialysis patients (and a marked rise in blood pressure

is much less frequent), but some units have maintained a policy of discontinuation of epoetin for a rise in blood pressure even after the target hematocrit has been attained. Since blood pressure varies greatly in dialysis patients, it makes little since to discontinue epoetin for blood pressure changes in the patient with a stable hematocrit, otherwise, the roller coaster pattern for the hematocrit will be common.

In order to maintain a fairly constant hematocrit with epoetin therapy, erythroid progenitor cell receptors for Epo should be constantly stimulated. Discontinuation of epoetin for up to1 week results in suppression of erythropoiesis to a level less than existed prior to initiation of epoetin, as measured by ferrokinetics (77). Therefore, resumption of epoetin will require a period of time before there is a maximal reticulocyte response and attainment of a stable level of erythropoiesis. For the patient receiving IV epoetin, doses should not be reduced to less than twice a week, therefore the individual dose should be reduced, not discontinued (unless there is a medical emergency such as prospective hypertensive encephalopathy). A 25–50% dose reduction should maintain receptor stimulation without a marked reduction in hematocrit. The dose can subsequently be adjusted further, if necessary. For the patient receiving SC epoetin, the dose can either be reduced by 25–50% or the frequency can be lengthened (i.e., from twice a week to once a week).

Maintain iron stores

Normally, three-quarters of body iron is present in circulating red blood cells, and one-quarter exists as storage iron, mainly in the liver and marrow. As anemia develops in patients with progressive renal insufficiency, the iron that previously existed in circulating red cells shifts into storage iron, unless lost by bleeding. In the pre-epoetin era, the normal pattern of iron storage was reversed in advanced renal failure associated with its hypoproliferative anemia: one-quarter of the body iron was in circulating red cells and three-quarters existed as storage iron, resulting in iron overload. If transfusions had been given, then there was even a greater degree of iron overload. In the absence of blood loss, and even in the absence of transfusions and inflammation, the serum ferritin, a marker of storage iron, was usually elevated when patients initiated dialysis. One of the major reasons why most of the hemodialysis patients initially treated with epoetin responded so dramatically in the clinical trials is that most patients were iron overloaded. Since the widespread use of epoetin, iron overload is now uncommon, whereas iron deficiency has become quite common. Actually, iron deficiency was more common that appreciated in the pre-epoetin era, especially in those hemodialysis patients who did not require or receive red cell transfusions.

In addition to erythropoietin, erythropoiesis is dependent upon the nutrients iron and folate. Folate depletion is uncommon since most dialysis patients take folic acid supplements and dietary intake usually replaces what is dialyzed out of the body. Iron deficiency, on the other hand, is very common because of the repetitive blood loss (1 ml of red blood cells contains 1 mg of iron) remaining in the hemodialyzer at the end of dialysis, the routine sloughing of iron-containing gastrointestinal cells, menstrual losses in women, the periodic phlebotomies for analysis of blood chemistries, the relatively iron-restricted diet and non-compliance for oral iron salts. Fortunately, iron absorption is physiologic in patients with chronic renal failure (78), but since the erythroid marrow is usually stimulated with pulsed, extra-physiologic doses of erythropoietin when epoetin is given IV, more iron is needed to meet these erythropoietic demands than can be provided by diet, or in many instances from consuming 150–200 mg of elemental iron as iron salts. Therefore, intravenous iron (as iron dextran in North America, iron gluconate in Europe) is often necessary to maintain iron stores to maximize the action of epoetin.

Almost all patients treated with epoetin should be ingesting oral iron salts, 150–200 mg of elemental iron daily, unless iron overloaded. If the serum ferritin is less than 100 ng/ml when epoetin therapy is initiated, IV iron is recommended since iron deficiency will rapidly develop. Iron stores range from approximately 800 mg in the adult female to 1200 mg in the adult male. Therefore, approximately 500 mg, either given in a divided or a single dose, should be given. Serial determinations of serum iron, transferrin (measured as total iron binding capacity) and serum ferritin should be determined every 2–3 months in order to monitor iron stores. The percent transferrin saturation (serum iron divided by the TIBC × 100) indicates how much transferrin bound iron is available for erythropoiesis. Sixteen percent or less is indicative of iron deficiency (79) and indicates that there is insufficient iron reaching the erythroid precursors for hemoglobin formation. A serum ferritin of less than 30 ng/ml indicates that iron stores are depleted since gastrointestinal iron absorption begins to increase at lower levels of serum ferritin (80). As long as the transferrin saturation remains above 16–20% there is sufficient iron for erythropoiesis regardless of the serum ferritin. However, knowledge of the serum ferritin is important because even though the percent transferrin saturation is adequate, iron stores could be so marginal that if an acute but mild blood loss occurred, there would be insufficient iron stores for maximal erythropoiesis despite epoetin therapy. Increasing the epoetin dose in this setting will only aggravate the iron deficiency, stimulating the need for more iron.

There are two forms of iron deficiency. Absolute iron deficiency occurs when the serum ferritin and percent transferrin saturation decrease below 30 ng/ml and 16–20%, respectively. However, the more common form of iron deficiency in epoetin-treated patients is a functional or relative iron deficiency (6). This is defined as a low transferrin saturation (less than 16–20%) but with a normal, or even elevated serum ferritin. Since these parameters can also be observed in inflammation because of the

acute phase reaction in which the serum ferritin suddenly increases to higher levels, it is necessary to document a serial reduction in serum ferritin levels in order to diagnose functional iron deficiency, hence the need to measure these iron parameters on a regular basis.

Unless iron overload is present (serum ferritin < 500 ng/ml), all patients treated with epoetin should receive oral iron, a minimum of 150–200 mg elemental iron a day. If absolute or functional iron deficiency develops despite compliant intake of oral iron, then intravenous iron is necessary to maintain optimal erythropoiesis with or without epoetin. Experience clearly indicates that a policy of maintaining adequate iron stores reduces the dose requirements of epoetin while maintaining a stable hematocrit.

Epoetin resistance

There are two forms of resistance to epoetin: primary and secondary unresponsiveness, the latter occurring after an initial response to epoetin.

The most common cause of a poor primary response to epoetin is an inadequate epoetin dose. The action of epoetin is dose dependent and not all respond to what has become the 'standard' dose of 50 U/kg, three times a week. There is a Gaussian distribution of dose requirements to maintain patients at a target hematocrit range, and those range of doses will vary depending upon the target hematocrit and whether the dose is given IV or SC. In the largest clinical trial with epoetin alfa, over 96% of iron replete patients responded (achieved a target hematocrit of 33–38 or increased the hematocrit by at least 6 points) with 150 U/kg, IV, three times a week. The median dose of epoetin to maintain the target hematocrit was 75 U/kg, IV, three times a week, with approximately 25% of the patients requiring 100 U/kg or more. If the target hematocrit is lower (i.e., 30–33), then the medium dose and range will be lower. The median dose will be even lower if the dose is given SC rather than IV.

The most common cause of resistance is inflammation or infection, which if present will blunt the action of epoetin (80). Examples include obvious infections, surgical inflammation and medical inflammatory disorders such as active systemic erythematosis and rheumatoid arthritis. This effect may be temporary lasting for a brief time after the inflammation has ceased and thus cause either a primary or secondary resistance. This cause of resistance can usually be suspected clinically, but is also associated with a decreased reticulocytosis and a decrease in serum iron and an increase in serum ferritin. When the serum iron and ferritin values revert to their prior values, then epoetin responsiveness should return. While the inflammatory effect of rheumatoid arthritis can be overcome with higher doses of epoetin (81, 82), and other inflammatory disorders can respond to larger doses of epoetin (83), to date this has not been documented to occur in dialysis patients. Therefore, one recommendation is to continue the same dose of epoetin while inflammation is present in order to maintain erythroid receptor-ligand interaction so that when the inflammatory response ceases, there will be no delay in the onset of subsequent erythropoiesis.

While inflammation and/or infection may be either primary or secondary causes of resistance to epoetin, secondary hyperparathyroidism with osteitis fibrosa and aluminum excess are usually causes of primary resistance. Such patients that require greater than 150 U/kg IV, or 100 U/kg SC, three times a week, assuming that iron stores are adequate, should be evaluated for osteitis fibrosa (84), aluminum excess (85, 86), and even thalessemia (87) and other rarer hematological entities such as folate deficiency and myelodysplasia. Osteitis fibrosa can be suspected by an increased alkaline phosphatase and intact parathyroid hormone level coupled with persistent hypercalcemia. Leukopenia and thrombocytopenia may also be present in severe osteitis fibrosa due to secondary hypersplenism. Hyperparathyroidism without osteitis fibrosa does not blunt the effect of epoetin. The definitive diagnosis of osteitis fibrosa requires a bone biopsy. The significance of erythropoietin levels increasing transiently after parathyroidectomy for secondary, but not primary hyperparathyroidism, is not clear (88). Occasionally this complication of severe secondary hyperparathyroidism can be reversed with intense medical therapy, but usually a surgical subtotal parathyroidectomy is necessary. Aluminum excess can be suspected in the iron replete patient by a low red cell mean corpuscular volume (MCV) and confirmed by an increased delta serum aluminum level after deferoxamine and/or positive staining for aluminum in a bone biopsy. After several months of weekly deferoxamine therapy the MCV reverts to normal and later anemia improves, with or without epoetin. Thalassemia, alpha and/or beta, may also blunt epoetin responsiveness. Alpha thalassemia, observed in an occasional patient of Chinese ancestry, is associated with a low MCV, and often requires more epoetin to obtain an erythropoietic response (89). A hemoglobin electrophoresis will establish the diagnosis. Hemoglobin H disease, common in South China, is associated with microcytosis and requires larger amounts of epoetin. Folate deficiency is associated with an elevated MCV, but the most common cause of an elevated MCV is due to epoetin itself. Epo releases larger marrow reticulocytes resulting in an increase in the MCV.

Adverse effects are uncommon

Contrary to early experiences in uncontrolled clinical trials, the adverse effects of epoetin therapy are infrequent and usually manageable. Iron deficiency is probably the most common 'adverse' development from epoetin therapy, but can be prevented if iron parameters are monitored and ample oral and/or IV iron is prescribed. Underdialysis and/or hyperkalemia is rare, although the dialysance of potassium and phosphorus does decrease with an increase in hematocrit (a reduction in plasma volume from which solutes diffuse during dialysis). An adjustment in the dialysis prescription occasionally may be necessary. Seizures were reported with increased frequency when epoetin was

first used (65, 91), and is usually, but not always, related to hypertensive encephalopathy, and occurs usually during the first 90 days of epoetin therapy when the target hematocrit is being attained (92). Subsequent experience has failed to record an increase in seizures above the known increased incidence associated with chronic renal failure and dialysis. Although epoetin alfa uses human albumin as a vehicle, allergic reactions, although reported, have not been serious enough to prevent successful retrial with the recombinant hormone (92).

The main adverse effects of most concern have to do with whether and how hypertension is induced or aggravated following epoetin therapy, and whether vascular access clotting is increased with epoetin or a rising red cell mass. Hypertension, defined as an increase in diastolic or mean arterial blood pressure of 10 mmHg or greater, was initially observed to develop in approximately 29% of 1,250 dialysis patients treated with epoetin in early clinical trials (5, 6, 65–70, 93–101). However, most of these studies were not controlled, and the incidence of hypertension is very high (80–90%) in chronic renal failure prior to the need for dialysis. Present experience with epoetin suggests that the incidence of a rise in diastolic pressure > 10 mmHg is closer to 20% when corrected for placebo effect (102). The pathogenesis of this hypertensive response in not clear, but has generated much discussion since some investigators think it is related to the effect of epoetin directly, while most suspect that hemodynamic changes related to the increasing red cell mass are responsible. The following observations have been claimed to support a direct pressor effect from epoetin: 1) blood pressure may increase prior to an increase in hematocrit (103); 2) infusion of epoetin into rat arteries results in vasoconstriction (104); 3) vascular endothelium has been found to contain a receptor for epoetin and epoetin stimulation, *in vitro*, results in endothelial proliferation (105) and 4) endothelin-1, a potent vasoconstrictor produced by the endothelial cell, increases following epoetin therapy (106). These findings, however, must be tempered by the following facts: 1) the pressor response following initiation of epoetin therapy occurs in only 20% of dialysis patients, and, if it does occur, usually develops after there has been a significant rise in hematocrit; 2) the amount of epoetin infused to cause renal artery vasoconstriction in the above quoted rodent models (104) was in supraphysiological amounts. Other studies using physiological amounts of epoetin have failed to document any direct vasoconstrictor activity in humans (107) or dogs (108); 3) there has been no confirmation that there is an endothelial cell erythropoietin receptor. Additionally, the plasma concentration of epoetin required to result in endothelial cell proliferation *in vitro* (> 2000 mU/ml) (105) is greater than what usually occurs after subcutaneous epoetin therapy. Although some investigators believe that hypertension does not develop after SC epoetin therapy (109), most studies have indicated a similarity in pressor response, regardless of the site of administration; 4) non-physiological amounts of epoetin were used to elicit the elevated *in vitro* endothelin-1 levels, and the clinical correlation was not consistent between hypertension and elevated endothelin-1 levels.

Vascular access clotting was thought to occur more frequently during the clinical trials with epoetin, but there were few placebo-controlled studies, and the nature of the vascular access was often not stated. Polytetrafluoroethylene (PTFE) arterio-venous grafts clot approximately three times as frequently as native arterio-venous fistulas (110). The only placebo-controlled study was for 6 months and suggested that epoetin increased access clotting (111). However, the type of vascular access was not mentioned. There continues to be disagreement about whether epoetin does (112) or does not (113) increase vascular access clotting. Because of the high frequency of PTFE graft clotting in the pre-epoetin era, it is very difficult to know whether epoetin, a rise in hematocrit, or neither, increases clotting in non-native vascular tissues. Most reports fail to substantiate an increase in clotting of PTFE or native arterio-venous fistulas in patients treated with epoetin (70, 98, 114, 115).

Ancillary measures to enhance erythropoiesis

Folic acid, multivitamin and amino acid supplements

Folic acid, multivitamins and occasionally amino acid supplements are given to dialysis patients to replace suspected deficiencies, either because of decreased dietary intake or dialysate-induced losses. Only folate deficiency can aggravate the hypoproliferative anemia by inducing a superimposed megaloblastic macrocytic anemia. A nonrestricted protein diet often compensates for dialysis-related folate losses. Histadine deficiency may aggravate the anemia of chronic renal failure (116), but replacement therapy has failed to improve the anemia (117). Dietary supplementation with essential amino acids (118) or multivitamins have proved ineffective in modifying the anemia of chronic renal failure.

Carnitine

L-carnitine, L-3hydroxy-4-N-triethylaminobutytric acid, is an intracellular compound that is the natural carrier of fatty acids from the cytoplasm to the mitochondria. It has been claimed to be necessary for red cell synthesis (119). Total and/or free plasma carnitine levels have been reported to be low in hemodialysis patients, and treatment with 2–4 mg/kg/dialysis, orally or intravenously, of L-carnitine, has resulted in a rise in hematocrit without (119) or with (120) epoetin, but results have been inconsistent. It is not clear whether total or free plasma carnitine levels reflect erythroid precursor carnitine levels or whether serum carnitine levels are related to the rate or degree of epoetin responsiveness. At the present time, there is insufficient data to recommend that all dialysis patients receive supplemental carnitine in order to optimize erythropoiesis. The presence of carnitine deficiency should be determined in patients who require unusually high doses of epoetin (i.e., > 300–450 U/kg, per week) assuming that other causes of epoetin 'resistance' have been excluded. If free plasma or total carnitine levels are low, then a 6 month trial of L-carnitine therapy might be warranted.

Androgens

Erythropoiesis can be increased in some dialysis patients with oral or intramuscular androgenic steroids. However, rarely can a normal red cell mass be attained, not everyone will have an erythropoietic response, and side effects have limited its long term usage, particularly in women. Nevertheless, because of the relative expense and rationing of epoetin in many countries, androgens have been used to try to amplify its erythropoietic effects. There is conflicting data as to whether androgens enhance the effectiveness of epoetin (121, 122). When a hormone is available to correct the anemia of chronic renal failure with relatively little side effects, adding another hormone with known adverse effects (123) in order to reduce overall costs, makes little scientific sense. But if epoetin is rationed (as it is in many countries), then it is a judgement decision as to whether the risks of adding androgen therapy is going to be cost-saving in the long run.

Improved dialysis clearance

There has long been the impression that 'better' dialysis (i.e., removal of more small and/or middle 'toxic' molecules) results in a higher hematocrit or hemoglobin. However, the data is not that convincing. In the early years of dialysis, switching from twice weekly to thrice weekly hemodialysis resulted in improved erythropoiesis (123), but the routine use of red cell transfusions, which suppress erythropoiesis, was discontinued at the same time. The National Cooperative Dialysis Study of over 10 years ago noted that better small molecule removal, with lower BUN levels, resulted in higher hematocrit levels (124). However, a prospective study of 6 months of reduced hemodialysis hours, three times a week, in which middle and small molecular clearances were decreased, disclosed no change in hematocrit levels (125). The European Dialysis & Transplant Association data of 1987, prior to the advent of epoetin, noted that over 6000 hemodialysis patients from Europe and the Middle East, who dialyzed longer than 15 hours per week, had a higher mean hemoglobin than those that dialyzed less than 11 hours per week (20). However, there was no evaluation of patient iron status nor statistical significance mentioned. Peritoneal dialysis has been claimed to result in higher hematocrit levels, due possibly to the removal of some toxic larger molecule not easily removed with hemodialyzer membranes. Another explanation for the higher red cell mass in peritoneally dialyzed patients is that they have better iron stores due to less blood loss (dialyzer and laboratory tests) which is common with in-center hemodialysis patients. For instance, although the percentage of

CAPD patients receiving epoetin is less than those on hemodialysis, the European-Middle Eastern study in the pre-epoetin era noted that the mean hemoglobin was not much different between home hemodialyis and CAPD patients (95.1 G/L, $n = 535$, *vs* 96.1 G/L, $n = 505$), respectively. A quantitative study of erythropoiesis, utilizing ferrokinetics, reticulocyte response, and transferrin receptor activity, noted that the erythropoietic response in hemodialysis subjects to 15, 50 or 150 U/kg of epoetin every other day for 4 doses, was similar to the responses in normal subjects given the same doses of epoetin (19). Therefore, for these hemodialysis patients, there was no blunting in the action of epoetin from the uremic solutes present in their circulation and suggests that 'better' dialysis is not necessarily going to improve erythropoiesis.

Exercise

Regular, fairly strenuous, exercise can improve erythropoiesis (126), although the mechanism for this is not clear. Since exercise is also good for the cardiovascular system, and may improve rehabilitation, a regular exercise program is recommended for all patients.

Red cell survival

Avoidance of drugs with hemolytic potential, such as penicillin, alpha methyldopa, and others, and proper preparation and monitoring of dialysate to avoid hemolysis from hyper-or hypotonicity (126), formaldehyde (128), copper contamination (129), chloramine (130), are necessary to prevent acute hemolysis. Chronic hemolysis may exist in any patient with splenomegaly or with severe osteitis fibrosa (131). Correction of the underlying cause(s) may improve the hematocrit, with or without epoetin. Although some studies suggest that improving red cell mass results in an improved red cell survival (132, 133), total correction of the anemia failed to improve red cell survival as determined by [51]Chromium red cell labelling (134). The chronic, mild shortening in red cell survival does not appear to be a major cause of the anemia of chronic renal failure and does not appear to affect the epoetin dose required to correct this anemia (11). All anemias of chronic disease are associated with a mild shortening in red cell survival (135), and most of these anemias can be corrected with epoetin (82, 83).

CLINICAL BENEFITS FROM EPOETIN THERAPY

Improvement in the anemia of chronic renal failure from epoetin therapy results in better tissue oxygenation. These clinical benefits of improved tissue oxygenation have been quantitated and include improved exercise capacity, cardiac, central nervous system function, endocrine, and skin circulation. In addition, the hematologic benefits of increased erythropoiesis include a reduction in iron overload, improved hemostasis and possibly improved immune responsiveness. The combined effect of these changes has led to an improved quality of life as quantitated by subjective questionnaire. The improvements in various organ systems that have occurred with partial correction in anemia indicate that uremia has not been the sole cause of the various clinical findings in chronic renal failure. The removal of the adverse effects of anemia should now allow investigators to have a better understanding of the role of uremia and perhaps other factors in the various end organ complications seen in chronic renal failure.

Exercise capacity

Partial correction of the anemia of hemodialysis patients has resulted in marked clinical improvement in exercise capacity as quantitated by measuring maximal oxygen uptake during progressive exercise on a cycle ergometer (136–138) and by isometric and isokinetics (139, 140). However, an increase in hematocrit from 22 to 30–35 results in an increase in maximal oxygen uptake from approximately 40% to only 50–60% of normal. After four months of maintaining a normal hematocrit, there is a further increase in oxygen consumption and duration of exercise, but not to normal (134). This dissociation between oxygen uptake and hemoglobin/hematocrit has recently been reviewed (141). There is lack of oxygen uptake by the 'uremic' myocyte despite adequate oxygen delivery, resulting in 'wasted' oxygen-more oxygen left over in the mixed venous blood than what was extracted. Muscle histomorphology is abnormal showing atrophy, and muscle fibers without adjacent capillaries (142). Of interest is that two dialysis patients were able to achieve normal oxygen utilization following aggressive exercise programs, one of whom had a hematocrit of 31 from epoetin therapy, and the other had a hematocrit of 34 without epoetin therapy (141). Whether they could have achieved even greater than normal oxygen utilizations, as occurs in well trained athletes with normal kidney function, remains to be determined. Exercise in dialysis patients has been shown to increase the ratio of capillaries to muscle fibers on biopsy. Therefore, a higher hematocrit/hemoglobin, with or without epoetin therapy unmasks muscle limitations in the ability to utilize oxygen. Efforts to increase exercise, prevent a sedentary lifestyle, and epoetin therapy prior to the onset of dialysis to prevent anemia should complement the positive effects of epoetin in improving exercise capacity. What direct effect uremia plays on this inability to optimize exercise capacity, is still unresolved.

Cardiac function

Anemia results in an increase in heart rate and cardiac contractility to optimize tissue oxygenation. This results in an increase in cardiac output, or cardiac index when adjusted to body size. The left ventricle dilates and initially there is a decrease in myocardial wall thickness, but the intracardiac wall stress increases by approximately 2.5 fold (143). To counteract this increased intracardiac pressure, left ventricular hypertrophy (LVH) develops initially as a compensatory process, but later evolves into a pathologic process leading to an increase in actual wall thickness. LVH results in diastolic dysfunction and non-atherosclerotic ischemia. LVH is a risk factor for survival. There is a definite inverse relationship between the degree of anemia and the extent of left ventricular end diastolic diameter (LVEDD) (144), the latter being a component of LVH (145). Partial correction of the anemia with epoetin has resulted in a decrease in LVEDD, sometimes to normal (146, 147), but not always (134, 145, 146, 148, 149). Cardiac output has also been reduced to near normal levels with improvement in the red cell mass (134, 146, 150, 151). Angina is reduced and ischemic changes on EKG may clear with improvement in the anemia (151–154). Angina seems best controlled with hematocrit levels greater than 33 (134, 154).

Since cardiovascular death is the greatest cause of demise of dialysis patients, and LVH is a significant risk factor for cardiovascular death, the reduction in heart rate and contractility reduces myocardial energy demand and should have a favorable influence in preventing or retarding the progression of heart disease in these patients (146).

Central nervous system function

Attention span, memory and cognitive function improve following partial correction of the anemia with epoetin therapy. This improvement has been quantitated with the Wechsler Adult Intelligence Scale (155, 156), and electroencephalography (157–159). Complete normalization of the abnormal EEG changes associated with anemia and renal failure, however, did not occur with partial correction of the anemia (hematocrit 30–35). Depression may also improve. Cerebral blood flow, which increases with anemia, returns to normal with improvement in the anemia (155, 160, 161) which is associated with improved neuropsychological performance. However, cerebral oxygen metabolism remains depressed even when the hematocrit is increased from 21 to 31%, as measured by positron emission tomography (161).

Endocrine changes

Sexual function improved in some men when their hematocrit increased with epoetin (162–168). The mechanisms for this improvement are not clear. Serum testosterone levels may initially be low and improve with improvement in the anemia (169). Serum follicle-stimulating hormone (FSH) levels may increase, suggesting a central mechanism for the improved sexual function. Other findings suggest a direct Leydig cell response since FSH and luteinizing hormone (LH) serum levels decreased as serum testosterone levels increased following epoetin therapy (170).

Others have found no relationship between serum testosterone levels and hematocrit in dialysis patients (164–166). There may be a modifying role of anemia, however, since testosterone levels, which fail to increase following administration of gonadal releasing hormone (GnRH) in anemic male patients with chronic renal failure, do increase to submaximal levels following GnRH therapy following months of epoetin therapy (171); FSH levels, which fail to increase following GnRH stimulation when patients are anemic, increase normally following partial correction of the anemia (171). This suggests that there are also anatomical reasons for decreased testosterone production in some male dialysis patients. Nevertheless, nocturnal penile tumescence has been documented to increase following improvement in the anemia, associated with an increase in the frequency of sexual intercourse (167, 168). Serum prolactin levels have decreased following epoetin therapy in some (166, 170), but not all (164, 165) male hemodialysis patients. Erythropoietin, per se, does not influence prolactin secretion in normal subjects (172).

Menstrual cycles are often abnormal and associated with amenorrhea in many women dialysis patients. Of those that are amenorrheic, many have had a resumption in menstruation following epoetin-induced improvement in their anemia (162, 173). Whether this improvement is related to a reduction in elevated serum prolactin levels as has been noted in some, but not all epoetin treated patients, is not clear. The incidence of pregnancy, which is decreased in patients with chronic renal failure, has not increased dramatically since the introduction of epoetin. Furthermore, the pregnancy outcome has not improved since the introduction of epoetin therapy (174), but the target hematocrit in this setting has usually not been to the normal range.

Other hormone levels have also been altered by epoetin therapy. Thyroid releasing hormone (TRH) increases the amount of thyroid stimulating hormone that is released from the hypothalamus. This effect is blunted in anemic patients with chronic renal failure, but is normalized after epoetin therapy (171). Growth hormone is increased following TRH administration in chronic renal failure, in contrast to normal subjects, but this abnormal response is normalized following epoetin therapy (171).

Immunological and other effects

There is some inconclusive evidence that immune reactivity is enhanced by epoetin therapy. Anti-HBs titers increased 5–8 fold in epoetin treated dialysis patients versus non-epoetin treated patients following hepatitis B vaccination (175). However, these results are difficult to interpret because the hematocrit remained unchanged despite epoetin, and red cell transfusions (which depress immunological responses) were greater in the non-epoetin treated group. The effects of epoetin on lymphocyte subsets is variable. Following epoetin therapy, there was a greater decrease in suppressor CD8 lymphocytes than CD4 helper cells, resulting in an increase in helper/suppressor cell ratio associated with an increase in hematocrit (176). However, in another study, CD4 cells, which are decreased in uremia, increased during 6 months of epoetin therapy associated with an increase in the hematocrit from 21.5 to 28 (177). Furthermore, delayed cutaneous hypersensitivity may improve after the hematocrit increases from 22 to 31 (176). The secretion of cytokines, such as IL-2, IFN and TNF may be blunted in uremia and contribute to the immune deficiency in uremia. Secretion of these cytokines, *in vitro*, from peripheral blood mononuclear cells, is enhanced following improvement in the anemia after epoetin therapy (178). Another mechanism suggested as to why immune responsiveness may improve following at least partial correction of the anemia, is that the expression of the erythrocyte complement receptor type 1 (CD35) increases following epoetin improvement in the hematocrit (178). E-CR1 appears to function by clearing immune complexes from the circulation and regulate antibody production . However, immature red cells, such as reticulocytes, express a greater amount of E-CD1, and it is not clear whether this response may have been solely due to the shift of younger and larger red cells into circulation as the result of epoetin. The same authors have noted that increasing the hematocrit from 32 to 42 with epoetin in patients with systemic lupus erythematosis (without renal failure) failed to modify their immune reactivity (180). Since infections are the second most common cause of death for dialysis patients, improvement in their immunological response is an important goal. Whether epoetin does have a significant impact upon immune reactivity in dialysis patients is still debatable. It is possible that any improvements are indirect as a result of overall improvement in health and activity following an increase in red cell mass.

Epoetin has also been claimed to decrease uremic pruritus by decreasing plasma histamine concentrations (181). However, pruritus continues to be a significant problem for many dialysis patients despite the use of epoetin. Epoetin therapy in hemodialysis patients to raise the hemoglobin from 7.7 to 9.9 g/dl has also been associated with a reduction in total cholesterol, apoprotein B levels and serum triglyceride levels (182). However, other studies have failed to detect any change in total cholesterol and triglyceride levels following epoetin therapy with hematocrit levels of 33-38 (65).

Hematological changes

The major effect of epoetin is to stimulate the proliferation and differentiation of erythrocyte progenitor cells, BFU-E and CFU-E, which leads to an increased release of premature reticulocytes and a subsequent increase in total circulating red cells. In almost all iron replete, stable patients with the hypoproliferative anemia of chronic renal failure, the hematocrit can be increased to any desired target if enough epoetin is given. Red cell transfusions, which were the only consistent way to treat this anemia in the past, were regularly used in up to 33% of dialysis patients prior to the availability of epoetin. According to the United States Renal Data System (USRDS), the outpatient transfusion rate has decreased from 16% to less than 4% of the in-center hemodialysis population since the onset of epoetin therapy (183). However, while this change seems impressive, total red cell transfusions may not have changed much, since transfusions during hospitalizations have increased, at least in the greater Seattle area (184). Nevertheless, iron overload, a serious metabolic complication due to repeated transfusions, is much less common, and theoretically, should no longer be a treat to patients with chronic renal failure. Also as a consequence of a reduction in transfusions, exposure to HLA antigens has decreased resulting in a decrease in panel reactive antibody (PRA) titers (185) allowing more such sensitized dialysis patients to have access to a kidney transplant. Presurgical autodonation of red cells is now possible for the dialysis patient, just as it is for any elective presurgical patient, except that the hematocrit must be increased to 38-40 to safely allow the removal of 2-4 units during the four weeks preceding the planned surgery (184).

There are other hematological changes that have also been noted. The MCV may increase as a result of a shift of larger reticulocytes into circulation, so that an elevated MCV does not necessarily indicate folate or vitamin B12 deficiency. The platelet count may increase transiently during initiation of epoetin therapy, but never to abnormally elevated levels. This slight, but statistically significant increase in platelets, is not necessarily related to iron deficiency (which can also increase platelet levels) and does not adversely effect thrombotic tendencies (186). Since the megakaryocyte has a receptor for Epo (186, 187), it is likely that there is some increase in thrombocytogenesis, but the effect appears to be transient and of no clinical significance. Megakaryopoiesis does not always occur following epoetin therapy, however (189). Platelet function and hemostasis are abnormal in renal failure, as noted by a prolonged bleeding time and abnormal *in vitro* platelet aggregation and adhesion studies. Increasing the hematocrit to above 27-30 by either red cell transfusion (190, 191), or by epoetin, has resulted in a reduction toward or to normal in the bleeding time (192-194) and improvement in platelet aggregation (194).

Quality of life

Initial clinical trials in 1986-1989 with epoetin indicated that most patients had a dramatic improvement in their quality of life as assessed by various subjective questionnaires (5, 6, 163, 195-198). However, more recent reports have indicated that quality of life has not improved as much as anticipated (199-201) There are several reasons for this discrepancy. The patients in the clinical trials were selected, and presumably they were more compliant; most of the early patients were iron overloaded and had brisk hematological responses; and the target hematocrit was higher in the early clinical trials than what has become standard in most countries with current therapy. The target hematocrit ranged from 35–40 (6), to 33–38 (65) in the early US trials, but the mean hematocrit of > 140,000 dialysis patients in the United States treated with epoetin as of December 1992 was less than 30 (183). Australia, Hong Kong, Japan, Europe, Canada also maintain target hematocrits levels of 28–33, yet quality of life evaluations usually suggest that patients are not doing as well as those treated in the earlier clinical trials, i.e., when hematocrit levels were higher. There are a number of reasons why the anemia is only being partially treated and not being corrected (184). Part of this is an exaggerated and inappropriate fear of serious complications expressed as '. . . a complete correction of renal anemia carries the risk of hypertension, encephalopathy, thrombosis, and hyperkalemia' (193), and 'disadvantages and risks of normal hematocrit dialysis' (202) (this latter reference was based on theoretical and not clinical experience). Such complications have not been associated with attaining a normal hematocrit with epoetin when the rate of rise in hematocrit is not rapid (134), nor have such complications been observed in increased frequency in those 3–5% of the dialysis population that maintain normal hematocrit levels without the need for exogenous Epo (203). Quality of life improved in 4 of 5 anemic patients with systemic lupus erythematosus not in renal failure whose hematocrit increased from 32 to 42 with epoetin therapy (180). Ideally, dialysis patients should have the opportunity to help determine what red cell mass is optimal for themselves, since there probably is a range (i.e., hematocrit 35–42) higher than present target levels, but costs, insurance and governmental regulations, and physician perceptions presently hamper the attainment of that goal.

Rehabilitation has not been improved with the use of epoetin in dialysis patients. One study suggested that earlier treatment of the anemia, that is prior to the need for dialysis, might result in keeping more patients working once dialysis is needed (7). Whether a more aggressive rehabilitation program with exercise conditioning and counseling, both prior to the need for dialysis, as well as in the early phase of dialysis, in addition to improving oxygen delivery to tissues with epoetin, will result in better rehabilitation remains to be determined, but clearly such programs are indicated.

Morbidity and mortality may also be positively impacted by epoetin therapy. Hospitalization rates have evidently decreased in Sweden, England, Canada (204) and Australia . Whether patient survival will improve has yet to be proved, although preliminary data suggests that hematocrit values of 33–38 attained with epoetin therapy have resulted in improved survival (205) and a higher hemoglobin (11.3 *vs* 9.9 g/dl) was the only factor that was associated with better survival of dialysis patients with

polycystic kidney disease vs those with glomerulonephritis in the pre-epoetin era (206).

SUMMARY

The anemia of chronic renal failure is primarily due to a relative deficiency in the renal hormone, erythropoietin. Epoetin can correct the anemia in the vast majority of dialysis patients. Since most patients are symptomatic when hematocrit levels decrease to or below 30, all such patients should be treated with epoetin assuming that iron stores are replete and blood pressure is controlled, and that other unusual causes of anemia have been excluded. Ideally, epoetin should be started when patients have progressive renal insufficiency prior to the need for dialysis, and given subcutaneously. The dose and frequency should be continued after dialysis is initiated; if epoetin is begun after dialysis is begun, it is best to be given SC three times a week until the target hematocrit is reached and then either the dose or frequency decreased in order to maintain a stable hematocrit. Although the FDA initially recommended a target hematocrit of 30–33, recently the target range has been increased to 30–36 (92). There is evidence that even a higher target (i.e., a normal hematocrit) would be more physiologic (134). Future studies should help establish what that target range should be. Iron parameters must be monitored frequently and iron repletion maintained in order to optimize epoetin therapy. Quality of life can be significantly improved by maintaining a near-normal to normal hematocrit, the morbidity of anemia can be decreased, and perhaps survival can be improved by not only ensuring adequate dialysis but also adequate hemoglobin levels to optimize tissue oxygenation. Future studies should reveal the extent of these improvements.

REFERENCES

1. Naets JP, Brauman H, Kraytman M: Etude de l'erythropoiese au cours de l'insuffisance renale aigue et chronique. *Acta Haematol* 24: 169, 1960
2. Emerson CP: The pathogenesis of anemia in acute glomerulonephritis. Estimations of blood production and blood destruction in a case receiving massive transfusions. *Blood* 3: 363, 1984
3. Eisenberg S: Blood volume in patients with acute glomerulonephritis as determined by radioactive chronium tagged red cells. *Am J Med* 27: 241, 1959
4. Eschbach JW, Adamson JW: Anemia of end-stage renal disease (ESRD). Editorial review. *Kidney Int* 28: 1, 1985
5. Winearls CG, Oliver DO, Pippard MJ, Reid C, Downing MR, Cotes PM: Effect of human erythropoietin derived from recombinant DNA on the anaemia of patients maintained by chronic haemodialysis. *Lancet* II: 1175, 1986
6. Eschbach JW, Egrie JC, Downing MR, Browne JK, Adamson JW: Correction of the anemia of end-stage renal disease with recombinant human erythropoietin: results

of a combined phase I and II clinical trail. *N Engl J Med* 316: 73, 1987

7. Eschbach JW, Kelly JR, Haley NR, Abels RI, Adamson JW: Treatment of the anemia of progressive renal failure with recombinant human erythropoietin. *N Engl J Med* 321: 158, 1989

8. Chaplin H, Mollison PL: Red cell life-span in nephritis and in hepatic cirrhosis. *Clinical Science* 12: 351, 1953

9. Stewart JW: Haemolytic anaemia in acute and chronic renal failure. *Q J Med* 36: 85, 1967

10. Eschbach JW: The anemia of chronic renal failure: pathophysiology and the effects of recombinant erythropoietin. *Kidney Int* 35: 134, 1989

11. Adamson JW, Egrie JC, Haley NR, Schneider GL, Sherrard DJ, Eschbach JW: Why do some hemodialysis patients need large doses of recombinant erythropoietin? *Kidney Int* 37: 235(A), 1990

12. Fisher JW: Mechanism of the anemia of chronic renal failure. Editorial review. *Nephron* 25: 106, 1980

13. McDermott FT, Galbraigh AJ, Corlett RJ: Inhibition of cell proliferation in renal failure and its significance to the uraemic syndrome: a review. *Scot Med J* 20: 317, 1975

14. Wallner SF, Vautrin RM: Evidence that inhibition of erythropoiesis is important in the anemia of chronic renal failure. *J Lab Clin Med* 97: 170, 1981

15. Delwiche F, Segal GM, Eschbach JW, Adamson JW: Hematopoietic inhibitors in chronic renal failure: lack of *in vitro* specificity. *Kidney Int* 29: 641, 1986

16. Segal GM, Eschbach JW, Egrie JC, Stueve T, Adamson JW: The anemia of end-stage renal disease: Hematopoietic progenitor cell response. *Kidney Int* 33: 983, 1988

17. Mladenovic J, Eschbach JW, Garcia JF, Adamson JW: The anaemia of chronic renal failure in sheep: Studies *in vitro*. *Br J Hematol* 58: 491, 1984

18. Eschbach JW, Mladenovic J, Garcia JF, Wahl PW, Adamson JW: The anemia of chronic renal failure in sheep: the response to erythropoietin-rich plasma *in vivo*. *J Clin Invest* 74: 434, 1984

19. Eschbach JW, Haley NR, Egrie JC, Adamson JW: A comparison of the responses to recombinant human erythropoietin in normal and uremic subjects. *Kidney Int* 43: 407, 1992

20. Geerling W, Morris RW, Brunner FP, Brynger H, Ehrich JHH, Fassbinder W, Rizzoni G, Selwood NH, Tufveson G, Wing AJ: Factors influencing anaemia in dialysis patients. A special survey by the EDTA-ERA registry. *Nephrol Dial Transplant* 8: 585, 1993

21. Egrie JC, Strickland TW, Lane J, Aoki K, Cohen AM, Smalling R, Trail G, Lin FK, Browne JK, Hines DK: Characterization and biological effects of recombinant human erythropoietin. *Immunobiology* 172: 213, 1986

22. Carnot P, Deflandre C: Sur l'activité hématopoietique de serum au cours de la regénération du sang. *C R Acad Sci (Paris)* 143: 384, 1906

23. Erslev AJ: Humoral regulation of red cell production. *Blood* 8: 349, 1953

24. Jacobson LO, Goldwasser E, Fried W, Plazk L: Role of the kidney in erythropoiesis. *Nature* 179: 633, 1957

25. Adamson JW: The erythropoietin/hematocrit relationship in normal and polycythemic man: Implications of marrow regulation. *Blood* 32: 597, 1968

26. Erslev AJ: *In vitro* production of erythropoietin by kidneys perfused with a serum-free solution. *Blood* 44: 77, 1974

27. Miyake T, Kung CKH, Goldwasser E: Purification of human erythropoietin. *J Biol Chem* 252: 5558, 1977

28. Lin F-K, Suggs S, Lin C-H, Browne JK, Smalling R, Egrie JC, Chen KK, Fox GM, Martin F, Stabinsky Z, Badrawi SM, Lai P-H, Goldwasser E: Cloning and expression of the human erythropoietin gene. *Proc Natl Acad Sci USA* 82: 7580, 1985

29. Jacobs K, Shoemaker C, Rudersdorf R, Neill SD, Kaufman RJ, Mufson A, Seehra J, Jones SS, Hewick R, Fritsch EF, Kawakita M, Shimizu T, Miyake T: Isolation and characterization of genomic and cDNA clones of human erythropoietin. *Nature Lond* 313: 806, 1985

30. Powell JS, Gerkner KL, Lebo RV, Adamson JW: Human erythropoietin gene: high level expresssion in stably transfected mammalian cells and chromosome localization. *Proc Natl Acad Sci USA* 83: 6465, 1986

31. Koury ST, Bondurant MC, Koury MJ: Localization of erythropoietin synthesizing cells in murine kidneys by *in situ* hybridization. *Blood* 71: 524, 1988

32. Lacombe C, DaSilva J-L, Bruneval P, Fournier J-G, Wendling F, Casadevall N, Camilleri J-P, Bariety J, Varet B, Tambourin P: Peritubular cells are the site of erythropoietin synthesis in the murine hypoxic kidney. *J Clin Invest* 81: 620, 1988

33. Bachmann S, LeHir M, Eckardt K-U: Co-localization of erythropoietin mRNA and ecto-5'-nucleotidase immunoreactivity in peritubular cells of rat renal cortex indicates that fibroblasts produce erythropoietin. *J Histochem Cytochem* 41: 335, 1993

34. Maxwell PH, Osmond MK, Pugh CW, Heryet A, Nicholls LG, Tan CC, Doe BG, Ferguson DJP, Johnson MH, Ratcliffe PJ: Identification of the renal erythropoietin-producing cells using transgenic mice. *Kidney Int* 44: 1149, 1993

35. Wang F, Fried W: Renal and extrarenal erythropoietin production in male and female rats of various ages. *J Lab Clin Med* 79: 181, 1972

36. Tan CC, Eckardt K-U, Firth JD, Ratcliffe PJ: Feedback modulation of renal and hepatic erythropoietin mRNA in response to graded anemia and hypoxia. *Am J Physiol* 263: F474, 1992

37. Koury ST, Bondurant MC, Koury MJ, Semenza GL: Localization of cells producing erythropoietin in murine liver by *in situ* hybridization. *Blood* 77: 2497, 1991

38. Meyrier A, Simon P, Boffa G, Brissot P: Uremia and the liver: the liver and erythropoiesis in chronic renal failure. *Nephron* 29: 3, 1981

39. Kolk-Vegter AJ, Bosch E, VanLeeuwen AM: Influence of serum hepatitis on haemoglobin level in patients on regular haemodialysis. *Lancet* I: 526, 1971

40. Brown S, Caro J, Erslev AJ, Murray TG: Spontaneous increase in erythropoietin and hematocrit value associated with transient liver enzyme abnormalities in an anephric patient undergoing hemodialysis. *Am J Med* 68: 280, 1980

41. Ratcliffe PJ: Molecular biology of erythropoietin. *Kidney Int* 44: 887, 1993

42. Schurek HJ, Jost U, Baumgartl H, Bertram H, Heckmann U: Evidence for a preglomerular oxygen diffusion shunt in rat renal cortex. *Am J Physiol* 259: F910, 1990

43. Echardt K-U, Kurtz A, Bauer C: Regulation of erythro-poietin production is related to proximal tubular functin. *Am J Physiol* 256: F942, 1989

44. Tan CC, Ratcliffe PJ: Oxygen sensing and erythropoi-etin mRNA production in isolated perfused rat kidneys. in *Pathophysiology and Pharmacology of Erythropoi-etin*, edited by Pagel H, Weiss C, Jelkmann W, Berlin, Springer-Verlag, 1992, p 57

45. Goldberg MA, Dunning SP, Bunn HF: Regulation of the erythropoieitn gene: evidence that the oxygen sensor is a heme protein. *Science* 242: 1412, 1988

46. Goldberg MA, Imagawa S, Dunning PS, Bunn HF: Oxy-gen sensing and erythropoietin gene regulation. in *Ery-thropoietin: From Molecular Structure to Clinical Appli-cation*, edited by Baldamus CA, Scigalla P, Wieczorek L, Koch KM, *Contrib Nephrol* 76: 39, 1989

47. Caro J, Schuster S, Raminez S: Regulating mechanisms involved in the expression of the erythropoietin gene. in *Erythropoietin: From Molecular Structure to Clinical Application*, edited by Baldamus CA, Scigalla P, Wiec-zorek L, Koch KM, *Contrib Nephrol* 76: 7, 1989

48. Koury MJ, Koury ST, Bondurant MC, Graber SE: Cor-relation of the molecular and anatomical aspects of renal erythropoietin production. in *Erythropoietin: From Mole-cular Structure to Clinical Application*, edited by Bal-damus CA, Scigalla P, Wieczorek L, Koch KM, *Contrib Nephrol* 76: 24, 1989

49. Erslev AJ, Caro J, Kansu E, Miller O, Cobbs E: Plasma erythropoietin in polycythemia. *Am J Med* 66: 243, 1979

50. Naets JP, Garcia JF, Tousaaint Ch, Buset M, Waks D: Radioimmunoassay of erythropoietin in chronic uraemia or anephric patients. *Scand J Haematol* 37: 390, 1986

51. Wide L, Bengtsson C, Birgegard G: Circadian rhythm of erythropoietin in human serum. *Br J Haematology* 72: 85, 1989

52. Coles GA, Liberek T, Davies ME, Robinson M, Jones J, Thomas G, Davies M, Macdougall IC, Williams JD: Estimation of erythropoietin secretion rate in normal and uremic subjects. *Am J Physiol* 263: F939, 1992

53. Jensen JD, Madsen JK, Jensen LW, Pedersen EB: Reduced production, absorption, and elimination of ery-thropoietin in uremia compared with healthy volunteers. *J Am Soc Nephrol* 5: 177, 1994

54. Wasley LC, Timony G, Murtha P, Stoudemire J, Dorner AJ, Caro J, Krieger M, Kaufman RJ: The importance of N and O-linked oligosaccharides for the biosynthesis and *in vitro* and *in vivo* biologic activities of erythropoietin. *Blood* 77: 2624, 1991

55. Salmonson T, Danielson BG, Wikstrom B: The phar-macokinetics of recombinant human erythropoietin after intravenous and subcutaneous administration to healthy subjects. *Br J Clin Pharmac* 29: 709, 1990

56. Brockmoller J, Kochling J, Weber W, Looby M, Roots I, Neumayer H-H: The pharmacokinetics and pharma-codynamics of recombinant human erythropoietin in haemodialysis patients. *Br J Clin Pharmac* 34: 499, 1992

57. McMahon FG, Vargas R, Ryan M, Jain AK, Abels RI, Perry B, Smith IL: Pharmacokinetics and effects of recombinant human erythropoietin after intravenous and subcutaneous injections in healthy volunteers. *Blood* 76: 1718, 1990

58. Piroso E, Erslev AJ, Flaharty KK, Caro J: Erythropoietin life span in rats with hypoplastic and hyperplastic bone marrows. *Am J Hematology* 36: 105, 1991

59. Dessypris EN, Graber SE, Krantz SB, Stone WJ: Effects of recombinant erythropoietin on the concentration and cycling status of human marrow hematopoietic progenitor cells *in vivo*. *Blood* 72: 2060, 1988

60. Sawada K, Krantz SB, Sawada ST, Civin CI: Quantitation of specific binding of erythropoietin to human erythroid colony-forming cells. *J Cell Physiol* 137: 337, 1988

61. D'Andrea AD, Zon LI: Erythropoietin receptor. Subunit structure and activation. *J Clin Invest* 86: 681, 1990

62. Mayeux P, Lacombe C, Casadevall N, Chretien S, Dusan-ter I, Gisselbrecht S: Structure of the murine erythropoi-etin receptor complex. Characterization of the erythro-poietin cross-linked proteins. *J Biol Chem* 266: 23380 1991

63. Koury MJ, Bondurant MC: Erythropoietin retards DNA breakdown and prevents programmed death in erythroid progenitor cells. *Science* 248: 378, 1990

64. Finch CA, Deubelbeiss K, Cook JD, Eschbach JW, Hark-er LA, Funk DD, Marsaglia G, Hillman RS, Slichter S, Adamson JW, Ganzoni A, Gilbert ER. Ferrokinetics in man. *Medicine* 49: 17, 1970

65. Eschbach JW, Abdulhadi MH, Browne JK, Delano BG, Downing MR, Egie JC, Evans RW, Friedman EA, Graber SE, Haley NR, Korbet S, Krantz SB, Lundin AP, Nis-senson AR, Odgen DA, Paganini EP, Rader B, Rutsky EA, Stivelman J, Stone WJ, Teschan P, Van Stone JC, Van Wyck DB, Zuckerman K, Adamson JW: Recombi-nant human erythropoietin in anemic patients with end-stage renal disease. *Ann Intern Med* 111: 992, 1989

66. Bommer J, Kugel M, Schoeppe W, Brunkhorst R, Samtleben W, Bramsiepe P, Scigalla P: Dose-related effects of recombinant human erythropoietin on erythro-poiesis. Results of a multicenter trial in patients with end-stage renal disease. *Contrib Nephrol* 66: 85, 1988

67. Urabe A, Takaku F, Mizoguchi H, Kubo K, Ota K, Shimizu N, Tanaka K, Mimura N, Nihei H, Koshikawa S, Akizawa T, Akiyama N, Otsubo O, Kawaguchi Y, Mae-da T: Effect of recombinant human erythropoietin on the anemia of chronic renal failure. *Intern J Cell Cloning* 6: 179, 1988

68. Canadian Erythropoietin Study Group: Association between recombinant human erythropoietin and qual-ity of life and exercise capacity of patients receiving haemodialysis. *Br Med J* 300: 573, 1990

69. Sundal E, Kaeser U: Correction of anaemia of chron-ic renal failure with recombinant human erythropoietin: safety and efficacy of one year's treatment in a Euro-pean multicentre study of 150 haemodialysis-dependent patients. *Nephrol Dial Transplant* 4: 979, 1989

70. Bennett WM: A multicenter clinical trial of epoetin beta for anemia of end-stage renal disease. *J Am Soc Nephrol* 1: 990, 1991

71. Ateshkadi A, Johnson CA, Oxton LL, Hammond TG, Bohenek WS, Zimmerman SW: Pharmacokinetics of intraperitoneal, intravenous, and subcutaneous recom-binant human erythropoietin in patients on continuous ambulatory peritoneal dialysis. *Am J Kidney Dis* 21: 635, 1993

72. Besarab A, Flaharty KK, Erslev AJ, McCrea JB, Vlasses PH, Medina F, Caro J, Morris E: Clinical pharmacology

and economics of recombinant human erythropoietin in end-stage renal disease: the case for subcutaneous administration. *J Am Soc Nephrol* 2: 1405, 1992

73. Boelaert JR, Schurgers ML, Mattysy EG, Belpaire FM, Daneel RF, De Cre MJ, Bogaert MG: Comparative pharmacokinetics of recombinant erythropoietin administered by the intravenous, subcutaneous, and intraperitoneal routes in countinuous ambulatory peritoneal dialysis (CAPD) patients. *Perit Dial Int* 9: 95, 1989

74. Kampf D, Kahl A, Passlick J, Pustelnik A, Echardt K-V, Ehmer B, Jacobs C, Baumelous A, Gransbensee B, Gahl HM: Single-dose kinetics of recombinant human erythropoietin after intravenous, subcutaneous and intraperitoneal adminsitration. *Contrib Nephrol* 76: 106, 1989

75. Granolleras C, Branger B, Beau MC, Deschodt G, Alsabadani B, Shaldon S: Experience with daily self-administered subcutaneous erythropoietin. *Contrib Nephrol* 76: 143, 1989

76. Eschbach JW, Haley NR, McCabe D, Egrie JC: Epoetin dosing: what route and frequency is best? *J Am Soc Nephrol* 2: 376(A), 1991

77. Eschbach JW, Haley NR, Adamson JW: The use of recombinant erythropoietin in the treatment of the anemia of chronic renal failure. in *Molecular and Cellular Controls of Hematopoiesis*, edited by Orlic D, New York Acad Sci, 554, 1989, p 225

78. Eschbach JW, Cook JD, Scribner BH, Finch CA: Iron balance in hemodialysis patients. *Ann Intern Med* 87: 710, 1977

79. Bainton DF, Finch CA: The diagnosis of iron deficiency anemia. *Am J Med* 37: 62, 1964

80. Adamson JW, Eschbach JW: The management of the anaemia of chronic renal failure with recombinant erythropoietin. *Quart J Med* 73: 1093, 1989

81. Means RT Jr, Olsen NJ, Krantz SB, Dessypris EN, Graber SE, Stone WJ, O'Neil VL, Pincus T: Treatment of the anemia of rheumatoid arthritis with recombinant human erythropoietin: clinical and *in vitro* studies. *Arth & Rheum* 32: 638, 1989

82. Gudbjornsson B, Hallgran R, Wide L, Birgegard G: Response of anaemia in rheumatoid arthritis to treatment with subcutaneous recombinant human erythropoietin. *Ann Rheum Dis* 51: 747, 1992

83. Horina JH, Petritsch W, Schmid CR, Reicht G, Wenzl H, Silly H, Krejs GJ: Treatment of anemia in inflammatory bowel disease with recombinant human erythropoietin: results in three patients. *Gastroent* 104: 1828, 1993

84. Sudhaker RD, Shih M-S, Mohini R: Effect of serum parathyroid hormone and bone marrow fibrosis on the response to erythropoietin in uremia. *N Engl J Med* 328: 171, 1993

85. Casati S, Passerini P, Campise MR, Graziani G, Cesana B, Perisic M, Ponticelli C: Benefits and risks of protracted treatment with human recombinant erythropoietin in patients having haemodialysis. *Br Med J* 295: 1017, 1987

86. Alfurayh O, Sobh M, Barri Y, Qunibi W, Taher S: Aluminum overload and response to recombinant human erythropoietin in patients under chronic haemodialysis. *Nephrol Dial Transplant* 7: 939, 1992

87. Cheng IKP, Lu H-B, Wei DCC, Cheng S-W, Chan C-Y, Lee FCP: Influence of thalassemia on the response to recombinant human erythropoietin in dialysis patients. *Am J Nephrol* 13: 142, 1993

88. Urena P, Echardt K-U, Sarfati E, Zingraff J, Zins B, Roullet JB, Roland E, Drueke T, Kurtz A: Serum erythropoietin and erythropoiesis in primary and secondary hyperparathroidism: effect of parathyroidectomy. *Nephron* 59: 384, 1991

89. Eschbach JW: (Panel discussion.) *Contrib Nephrol* 76: 216, 1989

90. Lazarus JM: Update on adverse reactions to erythropoietin therapy. *ASAIO J* 40: 70, 1994

91. Edmunds ME, Walls J: Pathogenesis of seizures during recombinant human erythropoietin therapy. *Sem Dial* 4: 163, 1991

92. Amgen Inc: Epogen (epoetin alfa) prescribing information. 29 June 1994

93. Samtleben W, Baldamus CA, Bommer J, Fassbinder W, Nonnast-Daniel B, Gurland HJ: Blood pressure changes during treatment with human erythropoietin. *Contrib Nephrol* 66: 114, 1988

94. Besarab A, Gaughan W, Medina F: Effect of erythropoietin on blood pressure in anemic hemodialysis patients. *Kidney Int* 35: 240(A), 1989

95. Schaefer R, Buerner B, Zech M, Denninger G, Borneff C, Heidland A: Treatment of the anemia of hemodialysis patients with recombinant human erythropoietin. *Int J Artif Organs* 11: 249, 1988

96. Dreis H, Zins B, Naret C, Casadevall N, Goureau Y, Peterlongo F, Varet B, Najean Y, Jacquot C, Drueke T: Recombinant erythropoietin: personal experience with a new treatment fo the anemia of chronic renal failure. *Transpl Proc* 21: 55, 1989

97. Nielsen OJ, Thaysen JH: Response to erythropoietin in anaemic haemodialysis patients. *J Int Med* 226: 89, 1989

98. Sundal E, Businger J, Kappeler A: Treatment of transfusion-dependent anaemia of chronic renal failure with recombinant human erythropoietin. *Nephrol Dial Transplant* 6: 955, 1991

99. Suzuki M, Hirasawa Y, Hirashima K, Arakawa M, Odaka M, Ogura Y, Yoshikawa Y, Sanaka T, Shinoda A, Morii H: Dose-finding, double-blind, clinical trial of recombinant human erythropoietin (Chugai) in Japanese patients with end-stage renal disease. *Contrib Nephrol* 76: 179, 1989

100. Duff MD, Golper TA, Sloan RS, Brier ME, Aronoff GR: Low-dose recombinant human erythropoietin therapy in chronic hemodialysis patients. *Am J Kidney Dis* 18: 60, 1991

101. Abraham PA, Macres MG: Blood pressure in hemodialysis patients during amelioration of anemia with erythropoietin. *J Am Soc Nephrol* 2: 927, 1991

102. Radermacher J, Koch KM: Erythropoietin and hypertension. in *Erythropoietin: Molecular Physiology and Clinical Applications*, edited by Bauer C, Koch KM, Scigalla P, Wieczorek L, New York, Marcel Dekker, 1993, p 129

103. Baskin S, Lasker N: Erythropoietin-associated hypertension. *N Engl J Med* 323: 999, 1990

104. Heidenrich S, Rahn K, Zidek W: Direct vasopressor effect of recombinant human erythropoietin on renal resistance vessel. *Kidney Int* 39: 259, 1991

105. Anagnostou A, Lee ES, Kessimian N, Levinson R, Steiner M. Erythropoietin has a mitogenic and positive chemotactic effect on endothelial cells. *Proc Natl Acad Sci* 87: 5978, 1990

106. Carlini RG, Dusso AS, Obialo CI, Alvarez UM, Rothstein M: Recombinant human erythropoietin (rHuEPO)

increases endothelin-1 release by endothelial cells. *Kidney Int* 43: 1010, 1993

107. Bund SJ, Heagerty A, Edmunds M, Walls J: Erythropoietin does not induce vasoconstriction directly in human subcutaneous resistance arterioles. *Nephron* 54: 173, 1989

108. Pagel H, Jelkmann W, Weiss Ch: Erythropoietin and blood pressure. *Horm Metabol Res* 21: 224, 1989

109. Carlini R, Obialo CI, Rothstein M: Intravenous erythropoietin (rHuEPO) administration increases plasma endothelin and blood pressure in hemodialysis patients. *Am J Hypertension* 6: 103, 1993

110. Churchill DN, Taylor DW, Cook RJ, LaPlante P, Barre P, Cartier P, Fay WP, Goldstein MB, Jindal K, Mandin H, Mckenzie JK, Muirhead N, Parfrey PS, Posen GA, Slaughter D, Ulan RA, Werb R: Canadian hemodialysis morbidity study. *Am J Kidney Dis* 19: 214, 1992

111. Muirhead N, Laupacis A, Wong C: Erythropoietin for anaemia in haemodialysis patients: results of a maintenance study (The Canadian Erythropoietin Study Group). *Nephrol Dial Transplant* 7: 811, 1992

112. Muirhead N: Erythropoietin is a cause of access thrombosis. *Sem Dial* 6: 184, 1993

113. Eschbach JW: Erythropoietin is not a cause of access thrombosis. *Sem Dial* 6: 180, 1993

114. Besarab A, Medina F, Musial E, Picarello N, Michael H: Recombinant human erythropoietin does not increase clotting in vascular accesses. *ASAIO Trans* 36: M749, 1990

115. Standage BA, Schuman EW, Ackerman D, Gross GF, Ragsdale JW: Does the use of erythropoietin in hemodialysis patients increase dialysis graft thrombosis rates? *Am J Surg* 165: 650, 1993

116. Kopple JD, Swendseid M: Evidence that histidine is an essential amino acid in normal and chronically uremic man. *J Clin Invest* 55: 881, 1975

117. Reeves RD, Barbour GL, Robertson CS, Crumb CK: Failure of histidine supplementation to improve anemia in chronic dialysis patients. *Am J Clin Nutr* 30: 579, 1977

118. Neuhauser M, Ulm A, Leber HW, Schutterle G: Influence of essential amino adids and keto acids on protein metabolism and the anaemia of patients on chronic intermittent haemodialysis. *Proc Eur Dial Transplant Assoc* 14: 557, 1978

119. Trovato GM, Ginardi V, Marco VD, Dell'aira AE, Corsi M: Long-term L-carnitine treatment of chronic anaemia of patients with end-stage renal failure. *Curr Ther Res* 31: 1042, 1982

120. Kooistra MP, Struyvenberg A, Van Es A: The response to recombinant human erythropoietin in patients with the anemia of end-stage renal disease is correlated with serum carnitine levels. *Nephron* 57: 127, 1991

121. Ballal SH, Domoto DT, Polack DC, Marciulonis P, Martin KJ: Androgens potentiate the effect of erythropoietin in the treatment of anemia of end stage renal disease. *Am J Kidney Dis* 17: 29, 1991

122. Berns JS, Rudnick MR, Cohen RM: A controlled trial of recombinant human erythropoietin and nandrolone decanoate in the treatment of anemia in patients on chronic hemodialysis. *Clin Nephrol* 37: 264, 1992

123. Eschbach JW, Adamson JW, Cook JD: Disorders of red blood cell production in uremia. *Arch Int Med* 126: 812, 1970

124. Santiago GC, Rao TKS, Laird NM: Effect of dialysis therapy on the hematopoietic system: The National Cooperative Dialysis Study. *Kidney Int* 23 (Suppl 13): 95S, 1983

125. Teschan PE, Ginn HE, Bourne JR, Ward JR, Schaffer JD: A prospective study of renal dialysis. *Trans Am Soc Artif Intern Organs J* 3: 108, 1983

126. Goldberg AP, Geltman EM, Hagberg JM, Gavin JR, Delmez JA, Carney RM, Naumowicz A, Oldfield MH, Harter HR: Therapeutic benefits of exercise training for hemodialysis patients. *Kidney Int* 24 (Suppl 16): 303S, 1983

127. Said R, Quintanilla A, Levin N, Ivanovich P: Acute hemolysis due to profound hypo-osmolality. A complication of hemodialysis. *J Dial* 1: 447, 1977

128. Pun KK, Yeung CK, Chan TK: Acute intravascular hemolysis due to accidental formalin intoxication during hemodialysis. *Clin Nephrol* 21: 188, 1984

129. Manzler AD, Schreiner AW: Copper-induced acute hemolytic anemia. A new complication of hemodialysis. *Ann Intern Med* 73: 409, 1970

130. Higgins MR, Gace M, Ulan RA: Anemia in hemodialysis patients. *Arch Intern Med* 137: 172, 1977

131. Weinberg SG, Lubin A, Wiener SN, Deoras MP, Ghose MK, Kopelman RC: Myelofibrosis and renal osteodystrophy. *Am J Med* 63: 755, 1977

132. Schwartz AB, Kahn SB, Kelch B, Kim KE, Pequignot E: RBC improved survival due to recombinant human erythropoietin explains effectiveness of less frequent, low dose subcutaneous therapy. *Clin Nephrol* 38: 283, 1992

133. Hughes RT, Cotes PM, Pippard MJ, Stevens JM, Oliver DO, Winearls CG, Royston JP: Subcutaneous adminstration of recombinant human erythropoietin to subjects on continuous ambulatory peritoneal dialysis: an erythrokinetic assessment. *Br J Haematol* 75: 268, 1990

134. Eschbach JW, Glenny R, Robertson T, Guthrie M, Rader B, Evans R, Chandler W, Davidson R, Easterling T, Denney J, Schneider G: Normalizing the hematocrit in hemodialysis patients with Epo improves quality of life and is safe. *J Am Soc Nephrol* 4: 425(A), 1993

135. Schilling RF: Anemia of chronic disease: a misnomer. *Ann Intern Med* 115: 572, 1991

136. Mayer G, Thum J, Cada E, Stummvoll HK, Graf H: Working capacity is increased following recombinant human erythropoietin treatment. *Kidney Int* 34: 525, 1988

137. Robertson HT, Haley NR, Gurthrie M, Cardenas D, Eschbach JW, Adamson JW: recombinant erythropoietin improves exercise capacity in anemic hemodialysis patients. *Am J Kidney Dis* 15: 325, 1990

138. Barany P, Freyschuss U, Pettersson E, Bergstrom J: Treatment of anaemia in haemodialysis patients with erythropoietin: long-term effects on exercsie capacity. *Clin Sci* 84: 441, 1993

139. Davenport A: The effect of treatment with recombinant human erythropoietin on skeletal muscle function in patients with end-stage renal failure treated with regular hospital hemodialysis. *Am J Kidney Dis* 22: 685, 1993

140. Guthrie M, Cardenas D, Eschbach JW, Haley NR, Robertson HT, Evans RW: Effects of erythropoietin on strength and functional status of patients on hemodialysis. *Clin Nephrol* 39: 97, 1993

141. Painter P, Moore GE: The impact of recombinant human erythropoietin on exercise capacity in hemodialysis patients. *Adv in Renal Repl Ther* 1: 55, 1994

142. Moore GE, Parsons DB, Stray-Gundersen J, Painter PL, Brinker KR, Mitchell JH: Uremic myopathy limits aerobic capacity in hemodialysis patients. *Am J Kidney Dis* 22: 277, 1993

143. Frenneaux M: Personal communication, 1994

144. London GM, Fabiani F, Marchais SJ, De Vernejoul M-Ch, Guerin AP, Safar ME, Metivier F, Llach F: Uremic cardiomyopathy: an inadequate left ventricular hyperthropy. *Kidney Int* 31: 973, 1987

145. Silberberg J, Racine N, Barre P, Sniderman AD: Regression of left ventricular hypertrophy in dialysis patients following correction of anemia with recombinant human erythropoietin. *Can J Cardiol* 6: 1, 1990

146. Low I, Grutzmacher P, Bergmann M, Schoeppe W: Echocardiographic findings in patients on maintenance hemodialysis substituted with recombinant human erythropoietin. *Clin Nephrol* 31: 26, 1989

147. Pascual J, Teruel JL, Moya JL, Liano F, Jimenez-Mena M, Ortunao J: Regression of left ventricular hypertrophy after partial correction of anemia with erythropoietin in patients on hemodialysis: a prospective study. *Clin Nephrol* 35: 280, 1991

148. Fellner SK, Lang RM, Neumann A, Lorcarz C, Borow KM: Cardiovascular consequences of correctin of the anemia of renal failure with erythropoietin. *Kidney Int* 44: 1309, 1993

149. London GM, Zins B, Pannier B, Naret C, Berthelot J-M, Jacquot C, Safar M, Drueke TB: Vascular changes in hemodialysis patients in response to recombinant human erythropoietin. *Kidney Int* 36: 878, 1989

150. Wizemann V, Schafer R, Kramer W: Follow-up of cardiac changes induced by anemia compensation in normotensive hemodialysis patients with left-ventricular hypertrophy. *Nephron* 62: 202, 1993

151. Morris KP, Skinner JR, Hunter S, Coulthard MG: Short term correction of anaemia with recombinant human erythropoietin and reduction of cardiac output in end stage renal failure. *Arch Dis Child* 68: 644, 1993

152. Macdougall IC, Lewis NP, Saunders MJ, Cochlin DL, Davies ME, Hutton RD, Fox KAA, Coles GA, Williams JD: Long-term cardiorespiratory effects of amelioration of renal anaemia by erythropoietin. *Lancet* 335: 489, 1990

153. Wizemann V, Kaufmann J, Kramer W: Effect of erythropoietin on ischemia tolerance in anemic hemodialysis patients with confirmed coronary artery disease. *Nephron* 62: 161, 1992

154. Steinman TI: Angina during hemodialysis: II. *Sem Dial* 6: 386, 1993

155. Horina JH, Fazekas F, Niederkorn K, Payer F, Valetitsch H, Winkler HM, Horner S, Freidl W, Pogglitsch H, Krejs GJ: Cerebral hemodynamic changes following treatment with erythropoietin. *Nephron* 58: 407, 1991

156. Temple RM, Langan SJ, Deary IJ, Winney RJ: Recombinant erythropoietin improves cognitive function in chronic haemodialysis patients. *Nephrol Dial Transplant* 7: 240, 1992

157. Grimm G, Stockenhuber F, Schneeweiss B, Madl C, Zeitlhofer J, Schneider B: Improvement of brain function in hemodialysis patients treated with erythropoietin. *Kidney Int* 38: 480, 1990

158. Marsh JT, Brown WS, Wolcott D, Carr CR, Harper R, Schweitzer SV, Nissenson AR: rHuEPO treatment improves brain and cognitive function of anemic dialysis patients. *Kidney Int* 39: 155, 1991

159. Sagales T, Gimeno V, Planella MJ, Raguer N, Bartolome J: Effects of rHuEPO on Q-EEG and event-related potentials in chronic renal failure. *Kidney Int* 44: 1109, 1993

160. Johnson WJ, McCarthy JT, Yanagihara T, Osmundson PJ, Ilstrup DM, Jenson BM, Bowie EJW: Effects of recombinant human erythropoietin on cerebral and cutaneous blood flow and on blood coagulability. *Kidney Int* 38: 919, 1990

161. Hirakata H, Yao H, Osato S, Ibayashi S, Onoyama K, Otsuka M, Ichiya Y, Kuwabara Y, Masuda Y, Fujishima M: CBF and oxygen metabolism in hemodialysis patients: effects of anemia correction with recombinant human EPO. *Am J Physiol* 262 (*Renal Fluid Electrolyte Physiol* 31): F737, 1992

162. Eschbach JW, Adamson JW: Recombinant human erythropoietin: implications for nephrology. *Am J Kidney Dis* 11: 203, 1988

163. Delano BG: Improvements in quality of life following treatment with rHuEpo in anemic hemodialysis patients. *Kidney Int* 14: 14, 1989

164. Bommer J, Kugel M, Schwobel B, Ritz E, Barth HP, Seelig R: Improved sexual function during erythropoietin therapy. *Nephrol Dial Transplant* 5: 204, 1990

165. Steffensen G, Au Aunsholt N: Does erythropoietin cause hormonal changes in haemodialysis patients? *Nephrol Dial Transplant* 8: 1215, 1993

166. Schaefer RM, Kokot F, Wernze H, Geiger H, Heidland A: Improved sexual function in hemodialysis patients on recombinant erythropoietin: a possible role for prolactin. *Clin Nephrol* 31: 1, 1989

167. Imagawa A, Kawanishi Y, Numata A: Is erythropoietin effective for impotence in dialysis patients? *Nephron* 54: 95, 1990

168. Sobh MA, Abd el Hamid I, Atta MG, Refaie AF: Effect of erythropoietin on sexual potency in chronic haemodialysis patients. *Scand J Urol Nephrol* 26; 181, 1992

169. Haley NR, Matsumoto AM, Eschbach JW, Adamson JW: Low testosterone levels increase in male hemodialysis patients treated with recombinant human erythropoietin. *Kidney Int* 35: 193(A), 1989

170. Kokot F, Wiecek A, Grzeszczak W, Klepacka J, Klin M, Lao M: Influence of erythropoietin treatment on endocrine abnormalities in haemodialyzed patients. *Contrib Nephrol* 76: 257, 1989

171. Ramirez G, Bittle PA, Sanders H, Bercu BB: Hypothalamo-hypophyseal thryoid and gonadal function before and after erythropoietin therapy in dialysis patients. *J Clin End & Metab* 74: 517, 1992

172. Bernini GP, Mariotti F, Brogi G, Cerri F, Santoni M, Ciardella F, Franchi F: Effects of erythropoietin adminstration on prolactin secretion in normal subjects. *Nephron* 65: 522, 1993

173. Schaefer RM, Kokot F, Heidland A: Impact of recombinant erythropoietin on sexual function in hemodialysis patients. *Contrib Nephrol* 76: 273, 1989

174. Hou SH: Frequency and outcome of pregnancy in women on dialysis. *Am J Kidney Dis* 23: 60, 1994

175. Sennesael JJ, Van der Niepen P, Verbeelen DL: Treatment with recombinant human erythropoietin increases antibody titers after hepatitis B vaccination in dialysis patients. *Kidney Int* 40: 121, 1991

176. Pfafft W, Gross H-J, Neumeier D, Nattermann U, Samtleben W, Gurland HJ: Lymphocyte subsets and delayed cutaneous hypersensitivity in hemodialysis patients receiving recombinant human erythropoietin. *Contrib Nephrol* 66: 195, 1988

177. Ueki Y, Nagata M, Miyake S, Tominaga Y: Lymphocyte subsets in hemodialysis patients treated with recombinant human erythropoietin. *J Clin Immunol* 13: 279, 1993

178. Gafter U, Kalechman Y, Orlin JB, Levi J, Sredni B: Anemia of uremia is associated with reduced *in vitro* cytokine secretion: immunopotentiating activity of red blood cells. *Kidney Int* 45: 224, 1994

179. Hebert LA, Birmingham DJ, Dillon JJ, Cosio FG, Shen X-P: Erythropoietin therapy in humans increases erythrocyte expression of complement receptor type 1 (CD35). *J Am Soc Nephrol* 4: 1786, 1994

180. Hebert LA, Birmingham DJ, Shen X-P, Brandt JT, Sedmak DD, Dillon JJ: Effect of recombinant erythropoietin therapy on autoimmunity in systemic lupus erythrematosus. *Am J Kidney Dis* 24: 25, 1994

181. Marchi SD, Cecchin E, Villalta D, Sepiacci G, Santini G, Bartoli E: Relief of pruritis and decreases in plasma histamine concentrations during erythropoietin therapy in patients with uremia. *N Engl J Med* 326: 969, 1992

182. Pollock CA, Wyndham R, Collett PV, Elder G, Field M, Kalowski S, Lawrence JR, Waugh DA, George CRP: Effects of erythropoietin therapy on the lipid profile in end-stage renal failure. *Kidney Int* 45: 897, 1994

183. Eschbach JW: Erythropoietin: the promise and the facts. *Kidney Int* 45 (Suppl 44): 70S, 1994

184. United States Renal Data System: USRDS 1994 Annual Data Report. The National Institute of Health, National Institute of Diabetes and Digestive and Kidney Diseases, Bethesda, MD, June 1994

185. Grimm PC, Sinai-Trieman L, Sekiya NM, Robertson LS, Robinson BJ, Fine RN, Ettenger RB: Effects of recombinant human erythropoietin on HLA sensitization and cell mediated immunity. *Kidney Int* 38: 12, 1990

186. Kaupke CJ, Butler GC, Vaziri ND: Effect of recombinant human erythropoietin on platelet production in dialysis patients. *J Am Soc Nephrol* 3: 1672, 1993

187. Horina JH, Schmid CR, Roob JM, Winkler HM, Samitz MA, Hammer HF, Pogglitsch H, Krejs GJ: Bone marrow changes following treatment of renal anemia with erythropoietin. *Kidney Int* 40: 917, 1991

188. Ishibashi T, Koziol JA, Burstein SA: Human recombinant erythropoietin promotes differentiation of murine megakaryocytes *in vitro*. *J Clin Invest* 79: 286, 1987

189. Dessypris EN, Gleaton JH, Armstrong OL: Effect of human recombinant erythropoietin on human marrow megakaryocyte colony formation *in vitro*. *Br J Haematol* 65: 265, 1987

190. Livio M, Marchesi D, Remuzzi G, Gotti E, Medda G, De Gaetano G: Uraemic bleeding: role of anaemia and beneficial effect of red cell transfusions. *Lancet* II: 1013, 1982

191. Fernandez F, Goudable C, Sie P, Ton-That H, Durand D, Suc JM, Boneu B: Low haematocrit and prolonged bleeding time in uraemic patients: effect of red cell transfusions. *Br J Haematol* 59: 139, 1985

192. Moia M, Mannucci PM, Vizzotto L, Casati S, Cattaneo M, Ponticelli C: Improvement in the haemostatic defect of uraemia after treatment with recombinant human erythropoietin. *Lancet* II: 1227, 1987

193. Vigano G, Benigni A, Mendogni D, Mingardi G, Mecca G, Remuzzi G: Recombinant human erythropoietin to correct uremic bleeding. *Am J Kidney Dis* 18: 44, 1991

194. Cases A, Escolar G, Reverter JC, Ordinas A, Lopez-Pedret J, Revert L, Castillo R: Recombinant human erythropoietin treatment improves platelet function in uremic patients. *Kidney Int* 42: 668, 1992

195. Evans RW, Rader B, Manninen DL: The quality of life of hemodialysis recipients treated with recombinant human erythropoietin. *JAMA* 262: 825, 1990

196. Auer J, Oliver DO, Winearls CG: The quality of life of dialysis patients treated with recombinant human erythropoietin. *Scand J Urol Nephrol* 131 (Suppl): 55, 1990

197. Keown PA: Quality of life in end-stage renal disease patients during recombinant human erythropoietin therapy. *Contrib Nephrol* 88: 81, 1991

198. Barany P, Pettersson E, Bergstrom J: Erythropoietin treatment improves quality of life in hemodialysis patients. *Scand J Urol Nephrol* 131: 55, 1990

199. Disney APS (ed): Fifteenth Report of the Australia and New Zealand Dialysis and Transplant Registry (Anzdata), Sponsored by the Australian Kidney Foundation, October 1992

200. Levin NW, Lazarus JM, Nissenson AR: National cooperative rHu erythropoietin study in patients with chronic renal failure – an interim report. *Am J Kidney Dis* 22 (Suppl 1): 3, 1993

201. Ifudu O, Paul H, Mayers JD, Cohen LS, Brezsnyak WF, Herman AI, Avram MM, Friedman EA: Pervasive failed rehabilitation in center-based maintenance hemodialysis patients. *Am J Kidney Dis* 23: 394, 1994

202. Shinaberger JH, Miller JH, Gardner PW: Disadvantages and risks of normal hematocrit hemodialysis. *Kidney Int* 35: 264(A), 1989

203. George C, Lundin AP, Delano BG, Brown C, Friedman EA: Absence of anemia in maintenance hemodialysis patients. *Int J Artif Org* 4: 277, 1981

204. Sheingold S, Churchill D, Muirhead N, Laupacis A, Labelle R, Goeree R: The impact of recombinant human erythropoietin on medical care costs for hemodialysis patients in Canada. *Soc Sci Med* 34: 983, 1992

205. Eschbach JW, Aquiling T, Haley NR, Fan MH, Blagg CR: The long term effects recombinant human erythropoietin on the cardiovascular system. *Clin Nephrol* 38 (Suppl 1): 98S, 1992

206. Ritz E, Zeier M, Schneider P, Jones E: Cardiovascular mortality of patients with polycystic kidney disease on dialysis: is there a lesson to learn? *Nephron* 66: 125, 1994

ORGAN AND METABOLIC COMPLICATIONS: BLEEDING DISORDERS IN RENAL FAILURE

VILMA E. QUIJADA, ROBERT M. LINDSAY and JAMES F. WINCHESTER

INTRODUCTION

Coagulation abnormalities associated with renal diseases, are seen in chronic and acute renal failure, but also in nephrotic syndrome, glomerulonephritis, urogenital neoplasms, and renal transplantation. In this chapter we will discuss, specifically, uremia and acute renal failure, including disseminated intravascular coagulation, since the latter two conditions are often inextricably linked. For causes of, and manifestations of, bleeding/thrombosis in nephrotic syndrome, nephritis, genito-urinary cancer and transplantation the reader is referred to a recent review (1). Normal hemostasis is outlined in Figure 1.

CHRONIC RENAL INSUFFICIENCY

Platelets

The first reference to a coagulation disorder in uremia was by Bright in 1827 (2). Since then, coagulation abnormalities in the uremic syndrome have been studied in detail. While severe thrombocytopenia is infrequent, a lesser decrease in platelet count may be found in chronic uremia, mainly as a result of impaired thrombopoiesis (3), or of increased platelet turnover (particularly in patients on hemodialysis), and in heparin-induced thrombocytopenia (4). Uremia produces abnormalities in platelet function, vessel-wall coagulation and plasma coagulation factors. The main physiological abnormality of platelet function is decreased aggregability in response to epinephrine, adenosine diphosphate (ADP) and collagen (5–7). In predialysis patients, there is a strong correlation between serum creatinine and severe bleeding, especially when serum creatinine is above 500 mmol/l (6 mg/dl) (8) whereas normal platelet function occurs below this concentration. Decreased platelet aggregation may be due to phenolic compounds (9), guanidinosuccinic acid (10), urea (11), or uremic 'middle molecules' (12).

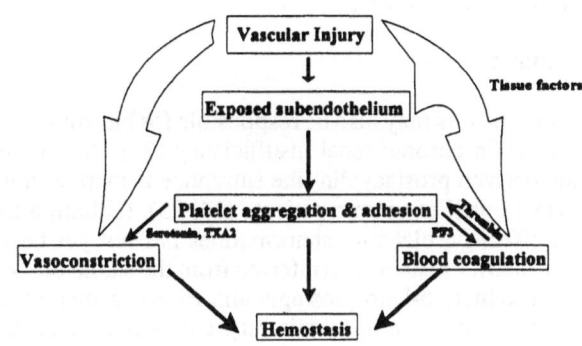

Figure 1. Normal hemostasis.

Thromboxane A_2 production in response to collagen, epinephrine or ADP induced platelet aggregation is decreased, while there is a normal response to administered exogenous arachidonic acid (13, 14), suggesting a defect in platelet formation (or release) of arachidonic acid from phospholipids. Elevation of plasma thromboglobulin and thrombospondin, two platelet-specific proteins released when platelets are disrupted or aggregated, is observed in severe renal failure, reflecting increased breakdown of platelets as seen in patients in hemodialysis (15, 16). Intracellular calcium concentration does not rise after a stimulus (ADP, and arachidonic acid) (17, 18), accounting for platelet aggregation abnormalities and the abnormal bleeding (19, 20). Improvement in bleeding time is seen with correction of the anemia (21) and prolonged hemodialysis time (8). Although a maximal improvement in platelet function was seen in one study of patients on continuous ambulatory peritoneal dialysis, (who have a different spectrum of uremic solutes removed through the peritoneal membrane compared to standard membranes for hemodialysis) (8), a further study has confirmed that platelet aggregation is corrected with hemodialysis, and that CAPD produces a platelet aggre-

Corrective action   **Abnormality**

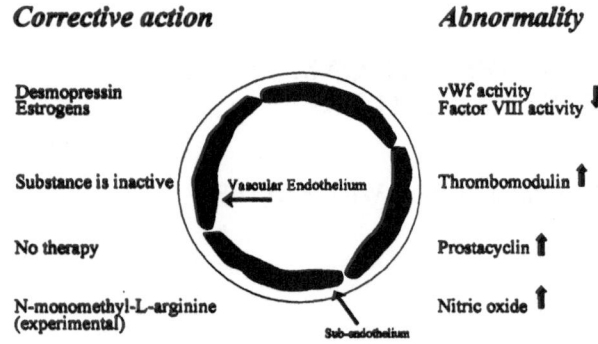

Figure 2. Vascular abnormalities and their potential correction in uremia.

gation profile intermediate between pre-hemodialysis and post-hemodialysis (22).

Vascular factors

Vascular factors may also be responsible for bleeding disturbances in chronic renal insufficiency (23). A venous tissue derived prostacyclin-like substance is increased in the vessel wall of uremic patients (24, 25), (although its exact effect on bleeding abnormalities has not yet been established). Prostacyclin (inferred from the stable breakdown product, 6-keto-prostaglandin-F_1 α) is increased in endothelial tissue in uremic rats, and while estrogens shorten bleeding time they had no effect on tissue prostacyclin concentrations (26). An endothelial derived protein, thrombomodulin, is increased in chronic renal failure; immunoblot analysis has shown that the substance is in the inactive degraded form which would be renally excreted if renal failure was not present (27). Nitric oxide (endothelial derived relaxing factor), may also be involved in the abnormal bleeding time of uremia; L-NMMA (N-monomethyl-L-arginine) an inhibitor of the formation of NO, shortens bleeding time in uremic animals, whereas the NO precursor, L-arginine, given simultaneously with L-NMMA, reverses the beneficial effect of L-NMMA (28). In hemodialysis patients, plasma L-arginine concentrations are higher than in controls, and uremic plasma is a potent inducer of NO synthesis in vascular endothelial cells (29). In addition, administration of L-arginine abolished the effect of estrogens on bleeding time (30). All of these factors lend credence to the importance of NO on bleeding and vascular reactivity in uremia.

Coagulation factors

Some coagulation factors and profibrinolytic plasma proteins have been found to be abnormal in uremic patients. The von Willebrand Factor (vWF) and Factor VIII, both of which are required for binding of platelets to subendothelial collagen, are elevated in uremic patients (31,

32), and have deficient biological activity, as measured by ristocetin cofactor activity. Ristocetin cofactor activity and Factor VIII coagulant activity increase with cryoprecipitate infusion (enriched with fibronectin, fibrinogen and Factor VIII (34), as well as desmopressin (deamino-D-arginine vasopressin (dDAVP)). The latter promotes von Willebrand factor release (35), and is associated with shortening of the bleeding time. Protein C activity, a vitamin K-dependent profibrinolytic activated plasma protein, is decreased in uremic patients (36, 37); this abnormality can be corrected by hemodialysis, suggesting the presence of a dialyzable inhibitor. Indeed, Faioni and colleagues have recently demonstrated the presence of a dialyzable factor in human uremic plasma which inhibits Protein C (38). Patients with end-stage renal disease, particularly on chronic hemodialysis, can also exhibit lupus-like anticoagulant activity, as has been found by some workers (39); this does not lead to increased bleeding and the incidence of hemorrhage is not higher compared to those with no lupus-like anticoagulant activity. A circulating lupus-like anticoagulant is demonstrable *in vitro* only, and is more likely associated with extrarenal and intrarenal thrombosis (40). Also described in uremia are the high plasma concentrations of fibrinogen and the decreased activity (16) of antithrombin III (AT-III) (41); these findings may be reflect a feed-back compensatory mechanism, since there is a correlation between depression of protein C activity and the severity of uremia (16, 37, 42).

These laboratory abnormalities explain high incidence of bruising, ecchymosis, purpura, prolonged bleeding from venipuncture sites, and gastrointestinal bleeding frequently seen in uremic patients (43). More severe complications have also been described, such as hemorrhagic pericarditis (with or without cardiac tamponade) (44), hemorrhagic pleural effusion, spontaneous subcapsular and retroperitoneal hematomata, and subdural hematomata, the latter of which carries a mortality rate as high as 90% (45–48).

Treatment

Treatment of chronic uremic patients with a bleeding diathesis is variable. Selection of a particular treatment regimen will depend on how rapid it is necessary to correct the abnormal bleeding, e.g., in the pre-surgical patient, or the patient with gastro-intestinal bleeding.

Whole blood or packed red-cell transfusion is known to decrease the bleeding time (49). Increased hematocrit is probably the cause for this finding, since the administration of erythropoietin has been shown to normalize the bleeding time in uremia (50). Erythropoietin, now a common therapy in dialysis patients, improves bleeding times, enhances platelet aggregation to ADP, etc, and elevates platelet counts, fibrinogen, factor VIII:C, vWF antigen, and vWF:ristocetin cofactor (20, 51). These coagulation changes were confirmed in another study, with the additional findings of transient elevations in pro-thrombotic

Table 1. Etiology and clinical consequences of coagulation disorders in renal failure

Disorder	Etiology
Prolonged bleeding time	Increased vascular prostacyclin, increased vascular nitric oxide, number and function of platelets, decreased circulating von Willebrand large multimers, decreased fibrinogen, anemia, uremic toxins.
Impaired platelet adhesion and aggregation	uremic toxins, decreased vascular thromboxane and vWf
Defective availability of platelet factor 3	uremic toxins
Poor clot retraction	defective coagulation
Increased plasma β-thromboglobulin	decreased renal clearance
Clinical consequences of the uremic bleeding disorder	
Minor:	Ecchymosis, purpura, epistaxis, gum bleeding, oozing from venepuncture sites
Major:	Gastrointestinal bleeding (peptic ulcer disease, angiodysplasia of stomach and duodenum, other arteriovenous malformations, etc), intracranial bleeds (subdural hematomata, etc), biopsy bleeding, subcapsular and retroperitoneal hematomata, etc

factors, thrombin-antithrombin III, protein C, and prostacyclin stimulating factor (52). The changes in platelet aggregation after erythropoietin therapy, as expected, are reversible with aspirin (53).

All dialysis modalities are associated with improvement in the bleeding time, particularly with prolonged hemodialysis and peritoneal dialysis (54). Infusion of cryoprecipitate, rich in Factor VIII, fibrinogen and fibronectin, will correct the bleeding tendency 1 hour after infusion, and the maximum effect may last for 4–12 hours, while improvement in bleeding time may last up to 24–36 hours after infusion (34, 55). Administration of dDAVP (0.3 μg/kg intravenously) will correct the bleeding time maximally 1–2 hours after the infusion, with no effect noticed if given over a prolonged period, due to temporary exhaustion of vWF and Factor VIII from the endothelium, since an effect occurs after time has elapsed between doses (35, 56). Subcutaneous injection of dDAVP has also been shown to be identical to intravenous dosing in correcting bleeding times in patients (57), and may be preferable for home use.

Conjugated estrogens have been used to correct the bleeding time, given intravenously (3 mg/kg for 5 days (58)), or orally (50 mg/day) (59). After IV treatment the effect is seen several hours later, but may last for up to 14 days; a significant decrease in the bleeding time is noticed from the second day. In a small placebo-controlled trial of Premarin® (a conjugated estrogen mixture of estrone, equilin, 17-α-dihydroequilin, 17-α-estradiol and others) in hemodialysis subjects with prolonged bleeding time, normalization of bleeding time, in the treatment but not in the placebo group, occurred after 7 days treatment (59). In rats 17-β-estradiol, of all the estrogens represented in the Premarin® mixture, was felt to be the key compound mediating the reduction in bleeding time, an effect blocked by the simultaneous administration of clomiphene and tamoxifen (60). Zearanolol, a beta-resorcyclic acid lactone (structurally very close to estrogens, but without their side-effects) has been tested in uremic rats, with significant and protracted shortening of the bleeding time (61). Clinical studies have not yet been performed in uremic patients to determine the efficacy of this product.

The dialysis patient also may be at risk of bleeding related to anticoagulation, whether systemic, or regional heparin, sodium citrate, or prostacyclin. Recently a glycosaminoglycan compound, dermatan sulfate, has undergone evaluation as an alternative to heparin (62). In addition uremic patients, in part because of pharmacokinetic disturbances, may be at greater risk of developing antibiotic induced coagulation disorders, with the induction of hypoprothrombinemia, such as seen with cephalosporins, etc (63).

Clinical and etiologic features of coagulation disturbances in uremia and acute renal failure are outlined in Table 1.

ACUTE RENAL FAILURE

Bleeding disorders are still extremely important determinants of morbidity and mortality in patients with acute renal failure. In acute renal failure of any etiology, the mortality rate associated with a hemorrhagic propensity ranges from 3 to 15% (64). Bleeding may be intracranial, gastrointestinal or from disseminated intravascular coagulopathy (DIC).

As in chronic renal failure, abnormalities in platelet adhesivity and aggregability *in vivo* and *in vitro* in response to potent stimuli are common. In the hemolytic uremic syndrome (HUS) (65), mediated by Escherichia coli verocytotoxin (66), and in thrombotic thrombocytopenic purpura (TTP) (67), abnormalities associated with the primary condition can be found. These are circulating high-molecular-weight polymers of vWF and Factor VIII:c, along with increased plasma concentrations of β-thromboglobulin, indicating activated clotting mechanisms and platelet disruption (68, 69). In acute renal failure due to snake bite (70), sepsis, and major obstetric catastrophes (71), DIC may be the main bleeding disorder. Up to 30% of patients present with overt DIC, mostly associated with obstetric complications, while DIC can occur in up to 50% of those without clinical signs (72). Correction of DIC is directed to correction of the primary condition.

Treatment

Treatment of bleeding in acute renal failure is directed to amelioration of the primary disorder. The often dramatic improvement in coagulation seen after dialysis in chronic renal failure patients, may not be seen in acute renal failure, since the primary stimulus for acute renal failure may also be primary instigator of the bleeding disorder. Thrombocytopenia may be due to sepsis, trauma and DIC. Cryoprecipitate infusion, dDAVP (73), and plasmapheresis have been reported to improve the hemorrhagic tendency in TTP and HUS; such measures are not likely to be effective in acute renal failure from sepsis, and surgical and obstetric complications, where attempts to correct the DIC should be concentrated on appropriate selection of antibiotics, dialysis and, if necessary, transfusion of fresh frozen plasma. When liver failure is present, such as in the hepatorenal syndrome, none of these measures is likely to be effective.

Hypercoagulability may also complicate acute renal failure, with extrarenal thrombosis occurring in up to 10% of cases (74, 75). Hyperfibrinogenemia, decreased fibrinolysis (76), and increased 'slow' antiplasmin activity (77), may also be observed.

REFERENCES

1. Quijada VE, Winchester JF: Renal Disease and Urology. in *Management of Bleeding Disorders in Surgical Practice*, edited by Forbes CD, Cuschieri A, Oxford, Blackwell Scientific Publications Ltd, 1993, p 149
2. Bright R: *Reports of Medical Cases Guy's Hospital of London*. Longman, Rees, Orme and Brown, London, 1827
3. Gafter U, Bessler H, Malachi T et al.: Platelet count and thrombopoietic activity in patients with chronic renal failure. *Nephron* 45: 207, 1987
4. Babcock RB, Dumper CW, Scharfman WB: Heparin induced immune thrombocytopenia. *N Engl J Med* 95: 237, 1976
5. George, JN and Shattil, SJ: The clinical importance of acquired abnormalities of platelet function. *N Engl J Med* 324: 27, 1991
6. Di Minno G, Martinez J, McKean ML et al.: Platelet dysfunction in uremia. Multifaceted defect corrected by dialysis. *Am J Med* 79: 552, 1985
7. Winchester JF, Forbes CD, Lang S et al.: Platelet function regulating agents – experimental data relevant to renal disease. in *Thromboembolism: A New Approach to Therapy*, edited by Mitchell JRA, Domenet JGI, London, Academic Press, 1977, p 84
8. Lindsay RM, Friesen M, Koens F et al.: Platelet function in patients on long term peritoneal dialysis. *Clin Nephrol* 6: 335, 1976
9. Rabiner SF, Molinas F: The role of phenol and phenolic acids on the thrombocytopathy and defective platelet aggregation of patients with renal failure. *Am J Med* 49: 346, 1970
10. Weiss, HJ: Acquired qualitative platelet disorders. in *Hematology*, edited by Williams WJ, Beutler E, Erslev, AJ et al., New York, McGraw-Hill, 1972, p 1171
11. Eknoyan G, Wacksman SJ, Gluek HI et al.: Platelet function in renal failure. *N Engl J Med* 280: 677, 1969
12. Bazilinski N, Shaykh M, Dunea G et al.: Inhibition of platelet function by uremic middle molecules. *Nephron* 40: 423, 1985
13. Remuzzi G, Benigni A, Dodesini P et al.: Reduced platelet thromboxane formation in uremia. Evidence for a functional cyclooxygenase defect. *J Clin Invest* 71: 762, 1983
14. Remuzzi G: Bleeding disorders in uraemia: pathophysiology and treatment. *Adv Nephrol* 18: 171, 1989
15. Gawaz MP, Ward RA: Effects of hemodialysis on platelet-derived thrombospondin (TSP). *Abstr Am Soc Nephrol* 398, 1990
16. Knudsen F, Dyerberg J: Platelets and antithrombin III in uraemia: the acute effect of haemodialysis. *Scand J Clin Lab Invest* 45: 341, 1985
17. Ware JA, Clark BA, Smith M et al.: Abnormalities in cytoplasmic Ca^{2+} in platelets from patients with uremia. *Blood* 73: 172, 1989
18. Steiner RW, Coggins C, Carvalho A: Bleeding time in uremia: a useful test to assess clinical bleeding. *Am J Hematol* 7: 107, 1979
19. Moosa A, Greaves M, Brown CB, MacNeil S: Elevated platelet-free calcium in uremia. *Br J Haematol* 74: 300, 1990
20. Cases A, Escolar G, Reverter JC et al.: Recombinant human erythropoietin treatment improves platelet function in uremic patients. *Kidney Int* 42: 668, 1992
21. Livio M, Gotti E, Marchesi D: Uraemic bleeding. Role of anaemia and beneficial effect of red cell transfusion. *Lancet* 2: 1013, 1982
22. Roger SD, Piper J, Tucker B, Raine AE, Baker LR, Kovacs IB: Comparison of haemostatic activity in haemodialysis and peritoneal dialysis patients with a novel technique, haemostatometry. *Nephron* 62: 422, 1992
23. Di Paolo N, Capotondo L, Rossi P et al.: Bleeding tendency of chronic uraemia improved by vascular factor. *Nephron* 52: 268, 1989
24. Remuzzi G, Cavenaghi AE, Mecca G et al.: Prostacyclin-like activity and bleeding in renal failure. *Lancet* 2: 1195, 1977
25. Slazus W: Increased platelet production of prostacyclin after injury to the microvasculature in uraemic platelets. *S Afr Med J* 81: 315, 1992
26. Zoja C, Vigano G, Bergamelli A, Benigni A, de Gaetano G, Remuzzi G: Prolonged bleeding time and increased vascular prostacyclin in rats with chronic renal failure:

effects of conjugated estrogens. *J Lab Clin Med* 112: 380, 1988

27. Takano S, Kimura S, Ohdama S, Aoki N: Plasma thrombomodulin in health and disease. *Blood* 76: 2024, 1990

28. Remuzzi G, Perico N, Zoja C, Corna D, Macconi D, Vigano G: Role of endothelium-derived nitric oxide in the bleeding tendency of uremia. *J Clin Invest* 86: 1768, 1990

29. Noris M, Begnini A, Boccardo P et al.: Enhanced nitric oxide synthesis in uremia: implications for platelet dysfunction and dialysis hypotension. *Kidney Int* 44: 445, 1993

30. Zoja C, Noris M, Corna D et al.: L-arginine the precursor of nitric oxide, abolishes the effect of estrogens on bleeding time in experimental uremia. *Lab Invest* 65: 479, 1991

31. Sakariassen KS, Bolhuis PA, Sixma JJ: Human blood platelet adhesion to artery subendothelium is mediated by Factor VIII-von Willebrand factor bound to the subendothelium. *Nature (London)* 279: 636, 1979

32. Kazatchkine N, Sultan V, Caen JP et al.: Bleeding in uremia: a possible cause. *Br Med J* 2: 612, 1976

33. Howard MA, Whitworth JA, Hendrix L et al.: Abnormal Factor VIII in chronic renal failure. *Med J Aust* 1: 148, 1979

34. Janson PA, Jubelirer ST, Weinstein MJ: Treatment of the bleeding tendency in uremia with cryoprecipitate. *N Engl J Med* 303: 1318, 1980

35. Mannuci PM, Remuzzi G, Pusineri F et al.: Deamino 8-D-arginine vasopressin shortens the bleeding time in uremia. *N Engl J Med* 308: 8, 1983

36. Sorensen PJ, Knudsen F, Nielsen A et al.: Protein C assays in uremia. *Thromb Res* 54: 301, 1989

37. Knudsen F, Sorensen PJ, Hoj A et al.: Inhibitors of coagulation in terminal renal failure and hemodialysis. *Nephron* 49: 335, 1988

38. Faioni EM, Franchi F, Krachmalnicoff A et al.: Low levels of the anticoagulant activity of protein c in patients with chronic renal insufficiency: an inhibitor of protein C is present in uremic plasma. *Thromb Haemost* 66: 420, 1991

39. Quereda C, Pardo A, Lamas S et al.: Lupus-like *in vitro* anticoagulant activity in end-stage renal disease. *Nephron* 49: 39, 1988

40. D'Agati V, Kunis Ch, Williams G: Anticardiolipin antibody and renal disease: a report of three cases. *J Am Soc Nephrol* 1: 777, 1990

41. Brand, TP, Jesperson, J, Sorensen, LH: Antithrombin III and platelets in hemodialysis patients. *Nephron* 28: 1, 1981

42. Allon M, Soffer O, Evatt B et al.: Protein S and C antigen levels in proteinuric patients. *Am J Hematol* 31: 96, 1989

43. Bronner M, Pati M, Cunningham C et al.: Estrogen-progesterone therapy for bleeding gastrointestinal telangiectasis in chronic renal failure. An uncontrolled trial. *Ann Intern Med* 105: 371, 1986

44. Suki WN: Pericarditis. *Kidney Int* 33(Suppl 24): 10S, 1988

45. Maher JF, Schreiner GE: Hazards and complications of dialysis. *N Engl J Med* 272: 370, 1966

46. Bechar M, Lakke JP et al.: Subdural hematoma during long term hemodialysis. *Arch Neurol* 26: 513, 1972

47. Tietjen DP, Moore J Jr, Gouge, SF: Hemodialysis associated acute subdural hematoma Interim management with peritoneal dialysis. *Am J Nephrol* 7: 478, 1987

48. Ingelberg R: Non-surgical treatment of subdural hematoma in hemodialysis patients. *Clin Neurol Neurosurg* 91: 85, 1989

49. Fernandez F, Goudable C, Su P et al.: Low hematocrit and prolonged bleeding time in uraemic patients: Effect of red cell transfusions. *Br J Haematol* 59: 139, 1985

50. Moia, M, Mannucci, PM, Vizzotto, I et al.: Improvement in the haemostatic defect of uraemia after treatment with recombinant human erythropoietin. *Lancet* 2: 1227, 1987

51. Huraib S, al-Momen AK, Gader AM, Mitwalli A, Sulimani F, Abu-Aisha H: The effects of recombinant human erythropoietin (sHuEpo) on the hemostatic system in chronic hemodialysis patients. *Clin Nephrol* 36: 252, 1991

52. Taylor JE, Belch JJ, McLaren M, Henderson IS, Stewart WK: Effect of erythropoietin therapy and withdrawal on blood coagulation and fibrinolysis in hemodialysis patients. *Kidney Int* 44: 182, 1993

53. Taylor JE, Henderson IS, Stewart WK, Belch JJ: Erythropoietin and spontaneous platelet aggregation in haemodialysis patients. *Lancet* 2: 1361, 1990

54. Rabiner, SF, Drake, RF: Platelet function as an indicator of adequate dialysis. *Kidney Int* 7 (Suppl 2): S144, 1975

55. Triulzi DJ, Blumberg N: Variability in response to cryoprecipitate treatment for hemostatic defects in uremia. *Yale J Biol Med* 63: 1, 1990

56. Ziegler ZR, Megaludis A, Fraley DS: Desmopressin (d-DAVP) effects on platelet rheology and von Willebrand factor activities in uremia. *Am J Hematol* 39: 90, 1992

57. Vigano GL, Mannucci PM, Lattuada A, Harris A, Remuzzi G: Subcutaneous desmopressin (DDAVP) shortens the bleeding time in uremia. *Am J Hematol* 31: 32, 1989

58. Liu Y, Kosfeld R, Marcum S: Treatment of uraemic bleeding with conjugated oestrogens. *Lancet* 2: 887, 1984

59. Shemin D, Elnour M, Amarantes B, Abuelo JG, Chazan JA: Oral estrogens decrease bleeding time and improve clinical bleeding in patients with renal failure. *Am J Med* 89: 436, 1990

60. Vigano G, Zoja C, Corna D et al.: 17 beta-estradiol is the most active component of the conjugated estrogen mixture active on uremic bleeding by a receptor mechanism. *J Pharmacol Exp Ther* 252: 344, 1990

61. Zoja C, Vigano, G, Corna, D et al.: Oral zeranol shortens the prolonged bleeding time of uremic rats. *Kidney Int* 38: 96, 1990

62. Ryan KE, Lane DA, Flynn A et al.: Antithrombotic effect of dermatan sulphate (MF 701) in haemodialysis for chronic renal failure. *Thromb Haemost* 68: 563, 1992

63. Manian FA, Stone WJ, Alford RH: Adverse antibiotic effects associated with renal insufficiency. *Rev Infect Dis* 12: 236, 1990

64. Steinman T, Lazarus JM: Organ system involvement in acute renal failure. in *Acute Renal Failure*, edited by Brenner BM, Lazarus JM, Philadelphia, Saunders, 1983, p 586

65. White DJ, Young F, McKendrick MW: Haemolytic uraemic syndrome in adults. *Br Med J* 296: 899, 1988

66. Kavi J, Wise R: Causes of the haemolytic uraemic syndrome. It might be verocytoxin produced by Escherichia coli. *Br Med J* 298: 65, 1989

67. Kelton JG, Moore JC, Murphy WG: Studies investigating platelet aggregation and releases initiated by sera from patients with thrombotic thrombocytopenic purpura. *Blood* 69: 924, 1987

68. Walters M, Levin M, Smith C et al.: Intravascular platelet activation in the hemolytic uremic syndrome. *Kidney Int* 33: 107, 1990

69. Monteagudo J, Pereira A, Roig S et al.: Investigation of plasma von Willebrand factor and circulating platelet aggregating activity in mitomycin C-related hemolytic uremic syndrome. *Am J Hematol* 33: 46, 1990

70. Chugh KS, Pal Y, Chakravarty RN et al.: Acute renal failure following poisonous snakebite. *Am J Kidney Dis* 4: 30, 1984

71. Stratta P, Canavese C, Goia L et al.: Clinical therapeutic correlations in consumption coagulopathy of obstetric acute renal failure. *Clin Exp Obstet Gynecol* 13: 43, 1986

72. Kanfer A: Coagulation and renal diseases. *Proc Eur Dial Transplant Assoc* 19: 703, 1982

73. Gotti E, Mecca G, Valentino C et al.: Renal biopsy in patients with acute renal failure and prolonged bleeding time. *Lancet* 2: 978, 1984

74. McMurray SD, Luft FC, Maxwell DR et al.: Prevailing patterns and predictor variables in patients with acute tubular necrosis. *Arch Intern Med* 138: 950, 1978

75. Kleinknecht D, Jungers P, Chanar, J et al.: Uremic and non-uremic complications in acute renal failure: Evaluation of early and frequent dialysis on prognosis. *Kidney Int* 1: 190, 1972

76. Larsson SO, Hedner U, Nilsson IM: On coagulation and fibrinolysis in acute renal insufficiency. *Acta Med Scand* 189: 443, 1971

77. Kanfer A, Vandewalle A, Beaufils M et al.: Enhanced antiplasmin activity in acute renal failure. *Br Med J* 4: 195, 1975

IMMUNOLOGICAL AND CHRONIC INFLAMMATORY ABNORMALITIES IN END STAGE RENAL DISEASE

BÉATRICE DESCAMPS-LATSCHA and PAUL JUNGERS

INTRODUCTION

In the late fifties, Dammin and coworkers (1) reported increased survival of skin homografts in patients with end stage renal disease (ESRD), suggesting for the first time that chronic uremia could be associated with a state of immune deficiency. The impaired immunity of ESRD patients has since been widely confirmed by numerous reports (reviewed in (2)) showing an enhanced susceptibility to certain infectious diseases, such as tuberculosis and listeriosis, an abnormally high incidence of tumors, anergy in cutaneous delayed-type hypersensitivity reactions and defective responses to vaccines against viral diseases such as influenza and hepatitis. A paradoxical observation is that maintenance dialysis does not improve but rather worsens this state of immune deficiency.

Several hypotheses have been put forward to elucidate the mechanisms of the immune system dysfunction observed in dialysis patients. A number of factors acting along both the humoral and the cellular axes of the immune system have been incriminated. Besides these factors, malnutrition, iron overload, zinc deficiency as well as circulating uremic toxins appear to be critical (3). One puzzling observation, emerging in particular from studies by our group (reviewed in (4)), is that the clinically and biologically immune deficiency paradoxically coexists with activation of most immunocompetent cells. This state of cellular activation is clinically expressed in one of the most serious complications linked to long-term dialysis, β2-microglobulin amyloidosis arthropathy (5).

This chapter will focus on the recent advances that have provided further insights into the complex pathophysiology of the immune deficiency associated with uremia and exacerbated by dialysis. After a brief survey of the clinical manifestations, the main disturbances in humoral and cellular factors of specific and non specific immunity will be reviewed with the aim of defining the respective role of chronic uremia and dialysis in this dysregulation of the immune system.

CLINICAL MANIFESTATIONS

We shall concentrate first on the increased susceptibility to infections, which clearly illustrates the underlying immune deficiency and is still a major problem in day-to-day management of dialysis patients, and second, on β2-microglobulin amyloid arthropathy which reflects the activation state of immunocompetent cells and is one of the main complications of long-term dialysis.

Bacterial infections

Despite improvements in dialysis and medical therapy, bacterial infections still represent a major cause of morbidity and mortality among dialysis patients (6–9). In a recent report on the main causes of death in North American dialysis centers over a 16-year period, bacterial infections accounted for 36% of deaths (9). Most studies have stressed the fact that infections in dialysis patients are not due to opportunistic organisms, but rather to common pathogens such as *Staphyloccocus aureus* and *Escherichia coli*. The high rate of chronic carriage and bacteremia is dictated by repetitive exposure to risk factors at their elective target sites, namely, vascular accesses for *S aureus* and the urinary tract for *E coli*. The abnormally high incidence of tuberculous (10) and non tuberculous intracellular pathogens such as *Legionella pneumophilia*, *Yersinia enterocolytica* and *Listeria monocytogenes* has suggested a defect in T cells that operate against such intracellular pathogens.

Besides the role of the vascular access as a portal of entry, comprehensive surveys of infectious complications in ESRD patients (7–9, 12, 13) have highlighted other factors involved in the pathogenesis of infections, including the direct immunosuppressive effects of uremic toxins; the indirect effects of metabolic abnormalities such as protein, trace-metal and vitamin deficiency; and the effects of dialysis membranes on complement and phagocytic cells. To some extent, the compounding effects of iron overload, zinc deficiency (8), protein malnutrition (14, 15), blood transfusions (16), and uremic toxins (17) contribute to the impairment of defenses against infections in ESRD patients on maintenance dialysis.

However, more recent reviews indicate that serious infections in ESRD patients on replacement therapy have become less common and are associated with a lower mortality rate than previously (12, 13), despite an increase in the proportion of elderly and diabetic patients accepted for hemodialysis. The advent of recombinant erythropoietin therapy may prove to have an indirect beneficial effect by reducing the frequency of blood transfusions in dialysis patients. This hypothesis is also supported by studies showing the disappearance of anti-HLA antibodies in highly sensitized patients treated with recombinant erythropoietin (18).

Viral infections

Unlike other immunocompromised patients who frequently develop varicella-zoster, patients on chronic dialysis seldom have overt clinical illnesses, but do show frequent reactivation of the virus. In contrast, the hemodialysis center has long been recognized as a high-risk environment for contamination by hepatitis B virus (HBV) and, more recently, hepatitis C virus (HCV) and human immunodeficiency virus (HIV).

Until 1981, when vaccination became available, HBV was a source of considerable morbidity and mortality among ESRD patients (19). Unlike healthy subjects, uremic patients infected with HBV had almost asymptomatic infection and, owing to their T cell defect, unless active-

ly immunized, such patients did not eradicate HBV and easily became chronic carriers (30% as compared to 5% in the normal population) (20, 21). The incidence of new cases of HBV among dialysis patients has also shown a decline because patients are exposed to a lower risk of infected blood products than in the past.

Active immunization with efficient vaccines against HBV has considerably lowered the incidence of HBV in dialysis units. However, as discussed below, nearly one third of patients do not respond to standard vaccination protocols (21, 22). Reinforced vaccination schedules with more frequent injections and/or higher antigen doses are necessary to induce and maintain protective antibody levels especially in elderly patients (22). Likewise various types of immunoadjuvant therapeutic protocols have been proposed (23, 24) with conflicting results. Without a doubt, the same problems that were encountered with HBV when vaccination was not yet available, will have to be faced with HCV infection (25). Since HCV transmission mainly originates from blood transfusions (26), both the development of more sensitive second generation tests for screening of blood donors (27, 28) and the reduced need for tranfusions in uremic patients with the advent of recombinant erythropoietin, have consistently reduced the incidence of HCV infection in dialysis centers. Finally, hepatitis Delta virus infection has been extremely rare in French ESRD patients relative to HBV reactivation or HCV infection (29).

Nephrologists dealing with HIV disease in ESRD patients have come up against a number of particular problems, including the influence of chronic uremia in asymptomatic HIV-seropositive patients, survival of HIV-infected patients on maintenance dialysis and the need for routine screening of patients and staff members (30–32). According to a recent report, HIV can be detected in the peritoneal fluid of HIV-positive patients treated by peritoneal dialysis (33), indicating that peritoneal fluid may be a source of viral transmission. HIV infection can also develop in patients who are already on maintenance dialysis, either through recognized risk factors or from infected blood products and donor organs. Lastly, nocosomial transmission of HIV, similar to that with HBV or HCV, may possibly occur in the dialysis environment.

β2-microglobulin amyloidosis

Osteoarticular amyloidosis deposits attributed to β2-microglobulin (34, 35) still represent a crucial problem of long-term dialysis (5).

β2-microglobulin is the 11 kD constant chain of HLA class I molecules, expressed at the surface of all nucleated cells. It is released in the plasma, essentially circulates as a monomeric form not bound to a transporter serum protein, and is filtered and metabolized by the kidney. Its level thus increases in parallel with the progression of renal failure. Increased synthesis and release of β2-microglobulin is seen in situations characterized by cell activation, in general including T cells, such as some inflammatory conditions and lymphoproliferative diseases.

Clinically two distinct forms of β2-microglobulin arthropathy have been described in dialysis patients: the carpal tunnel syndrome and a destructive arthropathy affecting medium-size and large joints. Based on clinical and radiologic criteria, the prevalence of osteoarticular lesions increases with the duration of hemodialysis, being present in almost all patients beyond 15 years of hemodialysis. Severe forms of arthropathy are less frequent in patients dialyzed with polyacrilonitrile than with cellulose membranes (36), and this is possibly related to the capacity of polyacrilonitrile to adsorb β2-microglobulin (37, 38).

The sequestration of β2-microglobulin depends on its plasma concentration (38) but one important question is whether synthesis and release of β2-microglobulin are increased in hemodialysis (5). A puzzling observation has been that β2-microglobulin arthropathy can be observed in non hemodialyzed patients (39). *In vitro* data suggest that peripheral blood cells from hemodialyzed patients exhibit increased levels of β2-microglobulin specific transcripts at the end of the session (5) and, if cultured, release high amounts of β2-microglobulin in the supernatant (40). *In vivo*, the presence of truncated β2-microglobulin fragments has recently been demonstrated in amyloid deposits (41) and it has been suggested that proteases and reactive oxygen species which are massively released by neutrophils activated by contact with cellulose membranes, participate in the fragmentation and secondary polymerization of β2-microglobulin (36, 42). Finally, the recent demonstrations that, on the one hand, a 9.5 kD β2-microglobulin fragment exerts a selective granulocyte inhibitory effect (8) and, on the other hand, that endothelial factors also contribute to the development of β2-microglobulin amyloidosis (43) reinforce the view of truncated β2-microglobulin as a cytokine in the cross-talk between neutrophils and other cells involved the dialysis-related systemic inflammatory process.

We shall now concentrate on the main abnormalities in the actors of specific and non specific immunity observed in chronic uremic and dialysis patients and schematically represented in Figure 1. In each section we will briefly review the recent knowledge in the normal host in referring to most recent overviews of immunological literature (44, 45).

SPECIFIC IMMUNITY

T and B cell cooperation

T lymphocytes, which are responsible for cell-mediated immunity, comprise three subpopulations defined on the basis of their function, i.e., helper T cells, cytotoxic T cells, and suppressor T cells (Figure 2). All three populations express CD2 and CD3 surface markers; helper T cells are CD4$^+$CD8$^-$, while cytotoxic T cells and suppressor T cells are CD4$^-$CD8$^+$. More precisely, CD4 and CD8 appear to be cell-interaction molecules which determine recognition by the T cell of major histocompatibility complex (MHC) determinants expressed by other cell types. The CD4 molecule interacts with a class II MHC determinant, and the CD8 molecule interacts with a class I MHC determinant (Figure 3).

B lymphocytes are endowed with humoral immunity. Their development is associated with expression of immunoglobulin (Ig) genes. Ig molecules are not only major products of B lymphocytes but also serve, in their membrane-associated form, as antigen-specific receptors. The specificity of all the surface Igs of a particular B cell is identical, and each B lymphocyte is committed to the antigen-binding specificity of its surface immunoglobulin molecule throughout its lifespan. Following stimulation with the antigenic determinant for which the Ig receptor is specific, the antibody molecules produced by the clonal progeny of a particular B lymphocyte will be the same as those of its surface Ig receptor for antigen. Besides endogenously produced surface Igs, B cells express cell membrane markers which are of central importance in the interaction with other elements of the immune system, e.g., MHC class II molecules and receptors for complement proteins C3b and C3d.

Antigen-specific T-cell responses require the presentation of processed peptides by antigen-presenting cells (APC), e.g. dendritic cells, monocyte-macrophages and B lymphocytes, and their recognition. These processes involve interaction between APC and the T cell receptor (TCR)/CD3 complex in conjunction with MHC class II glycoproteins, as well as accessory and co-stimulatory molecules including CD4 and adhesion molecules (e.g., ICAM-1/LFA-1). Antigen recognition by the TCR α/β is dependent upon a five-molecule complex known as CD3. Following occupancy of TCR/CD3 by antigen/MHC class II complexes, chains of the CD3 complex (γ) are phosphorylated (second messenger) and initiate several intracellular events. These processes also control and regulate T cell LFA-1 binding to monocyte ICAM-1 (strengthened adhesion), synthesis of IL-2 receptor (IL-2R), followed by IL-2 itself. The antigen signalling pathway depends on the number of receptors on the cell surface receptor.

Following cross-linkage by antigen binding to the B cell surface Ig complex, Ig molecules aggregate and form patches which travel to one pole of the B cell to form a cap. The antigen complex is then internalized by receptor-mediated endocytosis, and digested proteolytically into short peptide sequences that are then bound intracellularly by MHC class II molecules. These processed antigen-class II complexes are transported to and presented on the B-cell surface where they are accessible to helper T cells. Although B cells are not the only APC that can present antigens to helper T cells, B-cell antigen presentation appears to be very important in the secondary response.

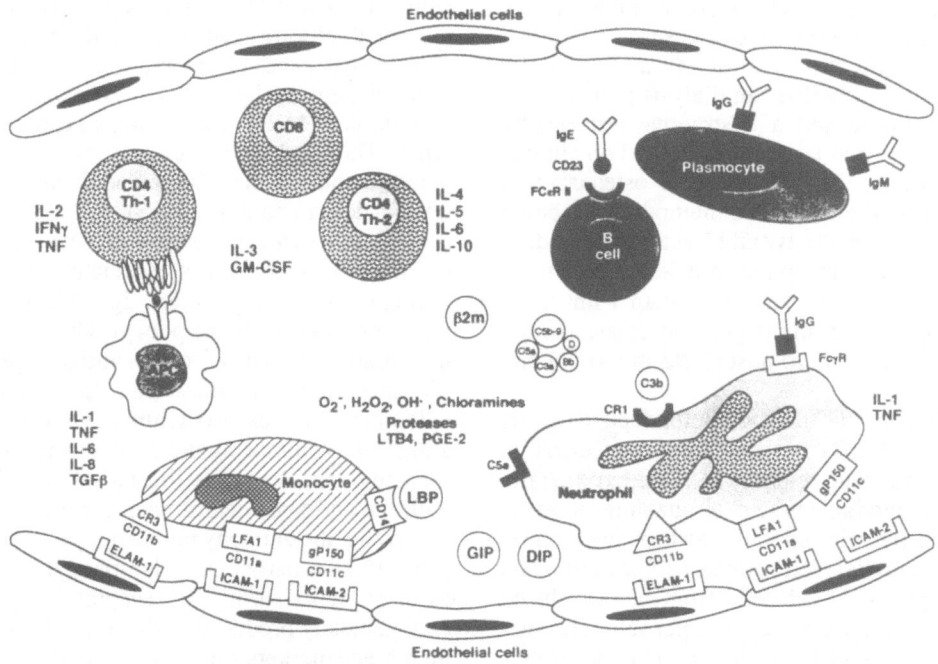

Figure 1. Schematic representation of the cellular actors and humoral factors of specific and non specific immunity possibly involved in immunological and chronic inflammatory abnormalities in ESRD.

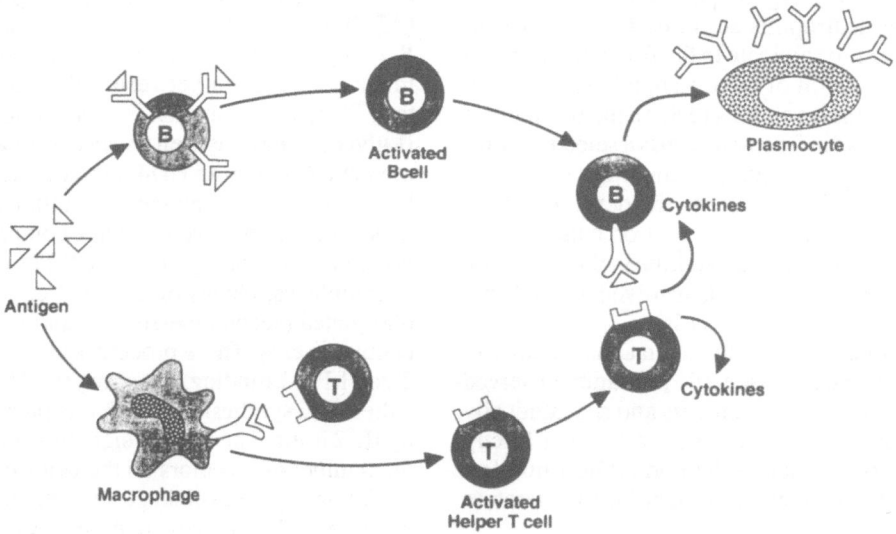

Figure 2. T and B cell cooperation. Following antigen presentation by macrophages, T cells are activated and produce cytokines which will help B cells to produce antibodies. B cells can also be activated by antigen and present antigen to helper T cells.

Following antigen recognition, the helper T cell undergoes blast transformation and clonal expansion. As a result of this activation, responding helper T cells produce a variety of lymphokines that influence the response of other cellular elements of the immune system. Among these, IL-2 binds to its receptor on the T cell, causing further T-cell proliferation, and gamma interferon (IFNγ) stimulates monocytes and macrophages to produce IL-1 which acts as a coactivator for T cells. Depending on the type of cytokine they produce, two types of helper T cell have been distinguished: *Th1 cells* which mainly produce IL-2 and IFNγ and are involved in hypersensitivity reactions,

NON SPECIFIC IMMUNITY   **HUMORAL AND CELLULAR SPECIFIC IMMUNITY**

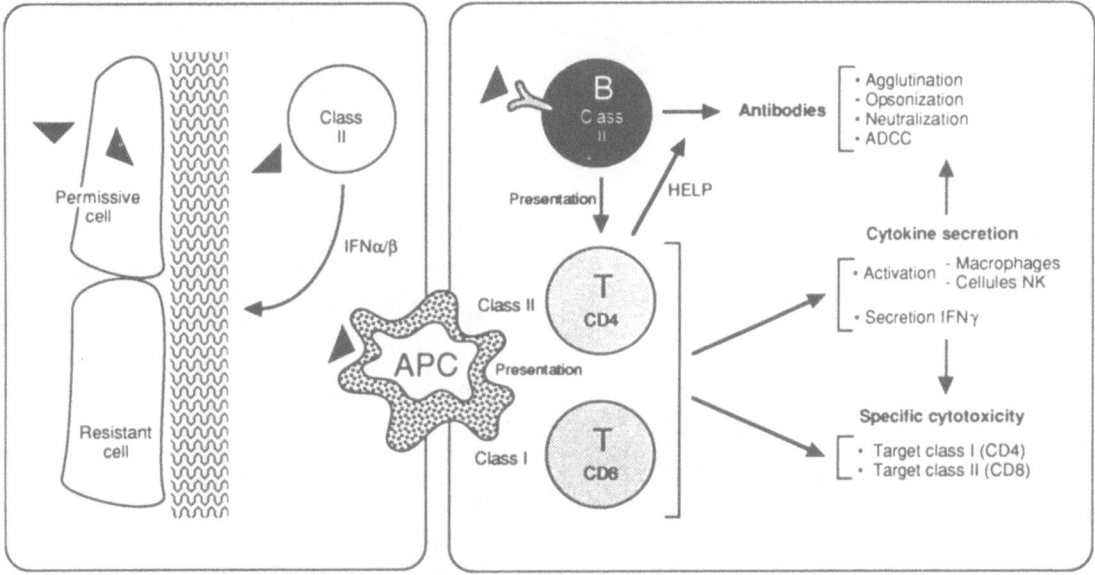

Figure 3. Cellular interactions in non specific and specific immunity. Macrophages or antigen presenting cells (APC) may recognize infectious agents either directly or, via permissive cells expressing class II antigens and producing IFNα and IFNβ. APC and B cells present antigens to CD4$^+$ T cells in association with HLA class II molecules while interaction between APC and CD8$^+$ T cells involves HLA class I molecules. CD4+ T cells help antibody production whereas CD8$^+$ T cells exert specific cytotoxicity. (Reproduced from JL Virelizier (44) with permission.)

and *Th2 cells* which mainly produce IL-4 and IL-6 which in turn act as B cell growth factors and differentiation factors, as well as IL-5 which acts on eosinophils and IL-10 which exerts suppressive effects on Th1 cells (Figure 4).

IL-2 is produced by T lymphocytes after antigenic or mitogenic stimulation. It has now been cloned and recombinant forms have been obtained. IL-2R is made up of at least two subunits, α and β. IL-2Rα (also known as the TAC antigen, CD25) is expressed *de novo* and is considered a marker of lymphocyte activation; IL-2Rβ is expressed constitutively on resting T cells but its increased expression is an index of T cell activation. Both subunits have low affinity for IL-2 but their combination gives rise to a receptor of high affinity which is involved in rapid internalization of IL-2 and mediates most of its biological activities. Production of IL-2 by T cells is regulated by monocytes and macrophages. Indeed, activated monocytes and macrophages produce IL-1, which is required for both IL-2 production and IL-2R expression; they also secrete PGE$_2$ which inhibits IL-2 production directly or indirectly by stimulating T cell suppressor activity. Antigen-activated B cells undergo blast transformation, clonal expansion and differentiation into plasma cells secreting antibody molecules of the IgM isotype. However, the lymphokines produced by antigen-activated helper T cells causes an isotype switch (from IgM to IgG, IgA or IgE).

It has become apparent in recent years that B cell-T cell interactions are two-way and that B cells can supply all the activation signals required for T cell proliferation. The B cell-T cell contact is additionally mediated by adhesion molecules which are present on both the B cell and the T cell and may bind ligands present on the other cell. Certain bacterial antigens, especially large polysaccharides with a repeating structure can elicit an immunoglobulin response without the action of helper T cells; these are called T-independent antigens.

Cytotoxic T lymphocytes (CTL) possess the potential to develop cytotoxic effector function following interaction with the antigenic determinant for which they possess the specific TCR. The TCR of CTL recognizes antigenic determinant in the context of class I MHC molecules, and in this way the CTL response is also 'restricted' by the MHC. A given CTL can kill multiple target cells that express the appropriate antigenic determinant. In performing its cytotoxic function the CTL first binds to the determinant on the target cell and then causes membrane damage and, lysis.

Less is known about the requirement for antigen recognition and activation in the case of *suppressor T cells*. Both antigen-specific and antigen-non-specific activation of suppressor T cells have been described, but the influence of the MHC in this activation process is not well defined. In appropriate conditions, helper T cells have been shown to act on helper T cells as well as on B cells,

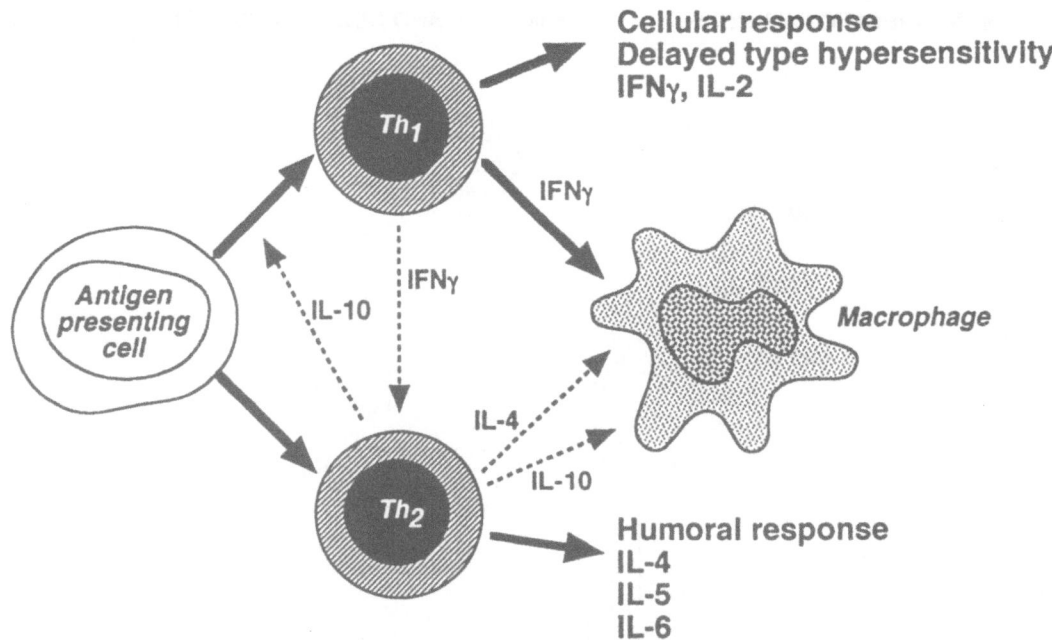

Figure 4. Dichotomy between helper CD4$^+$ T cells. Depending on the type of cytokines they produce, two types of helper T cell have been distinguished, namely Th1 cells which mainly produce IL-2 and IFNγ and are involved in hypersensitivity reactions, and Th2 cells which mainly produce IL-4, and IL-6 which in turn act as B cell growth factors and differentiation factors as well as IL-5 which acts on eosinophils and IL-10 which exerts suppressive effects on Th1 cells. (Reproduced from M Dy (44) with permission.)

and suppression appears to be mediated by soluble factors that are secreted by activated suppressor T cells.

T cells in chronic uremic and dialysis patients

T cell deficiency

Immunologists have long studied T cells to identify the origin of the immunodeficiency state associated with uremia. *In vivo*, no imbalance between CD4$^+$ and CD8$^+$ T cell subsets has been reported in ESRD patients (46), and the CD4/CD8 ratio does not appear to be influenced by the dialysis procedure (47, 48). However decreased delayed hypersensitivity reactions have been reported, and *ex vivo* uremic T lymphocytes exhibit impaired responses to mitogens and allogeneic lymphocytes (49).

The finding that T cell alterations are more marked in the presence of autologous serum, and that uremic plasma markedly reduces the proliferative response of normal T cells (51), suggested the involvement of circulating inhibitory substances. These include the guanidine derivatives, notably methylguanidine (52–54), non dialyzable protein factors (54, 55) and monocyte-derived suppressive factors such as prostaglandin E$_2$ (56, 57). More recent studies on the modulation of the TCR/CD3 complex in uremic patients suggest its down-regulation in the uremic environment (58, 59).

The hypothesis that monocytes are involved in these defective T cell responses was raised by the demonstration that T cell activation blockade is observed in monocyte-dependent stimulation (which is the case for all antigens, most mitogens and anti-CD3 antibody) but not in monocyte-independent stimulation (by anti-CD2 antibody) (60, 61). Whatever its underlying mechanisms, the defective proliferation of T cells is associated with abnormally low IL-2 and IFNγ production, a common finding which has recently been confirmed at the gene expression level (62).

Finally, an immunosuppressive effect of blood transfusions and subsequent iron overload (63–66) has been suggested and, interestingly, several reports have stressed the fact that recombinant erythropoietin partially corrects defective T cell responses (68, 69).

T cell activation

One puzzling observation is that despite their deficient responses to most pathogens and mitogens, T cells from dialysis patients show clear-cut signs of activation. This is manifested by increased numbers of cells expressing the Tac antigen or IL-2 receptor (IL-2R, CD25) (47, 49), higher density of IL-2R at the T cell surface (61) and increased levels of its soluble form in the circulation (70). The presence of such signs of activation in ESRD patients tested before the initiation of hemodialysis therapy suggested that uremia itself suffices to induce this cellular activation. This was further demonstrated in a more recent study by our group showing that both the number of T cells expressing CD25 and HLA-DR antigens and plasma levels of soluble CD25 were increased from the incipient stage of chronic renal failure, progressed with advancement of chronic renal failure and were even exacerbated in dialysis patients (data to be published). The prominent role of dialysis-membrane bioincompatibility in this accentuation of T cell activation has been elegantly illustrated by the group of Hakim (71) in a randomized crossover study involving a group of dialysis patients treated with complement-activating and non activating dialysis membranes.

The possibility of increased IL-2 consumption by its own receptor leading to decreased bioavailability for inducing the T cell response has been suggested (49) and at least partly verified by the observation that in uremic non responders to HBV vaccine, local injection of natural purified IL-2 together with a boost of the vaccine had a significant adjuvant effect (23). However, this was not confirmed in a recent randomized, placeco-controlled trial using recombinant IL-2 (2, 24). The dichotomy among helper T cells recently established on the basis of their cytokine profiles (see above), stresses the need for a more precise evaluation of the cytokine alterations related to uremia.

B cells in chronic uremic and dialysis patients

B cell deficiency

While plasma levels of IgG, IgM and IgA are usually in the normal range in ESRD patients, it is generally accepted that specific antibody responses of B cells, both *in vivo* and *in vitro* are abnormally depressed (reviewed in (72)). This is particularly well illustrated *in vivo* by the impaired antibody responses of ESRD patients (see below) to vaccines. However, since most of these vaccines involve T cell-dependent antigens, the possibility of an impaired cooperation between T and B cells should be reassessed, taking advantage of novel approaches for the evaluation of Th1 and Th2 cell types. Interestingly, administration of erythropoietin has been reported to improve B cell function (69, 73) as well as antibody titers after hepatitis B vaccination (74).

B cell activation

An increased incidence of autoantibodies has been reported in dialysis patients (75) and in patients on peritoneal dialysis (76). Likewise, the presence of IgE antibodies to the ethylene oxide used for sterilizing dialysis equipment (77) is also suggestive of abnormal sensitization in these patients, although this varies greatly among centers.

Finally, our finding of elevated plasma levels of the soluble form of the low-affinity Fc receptor of IgE (CD23), which is predominantly expressed on activated B cells is also suggestive of a B cell activation state (78). With regard to the biological significance of soluble CD23, its gradual accumulation during the progression of chronic renal failure along with the recent demonstration that it can be a cofactor in T cell activation (79), led us to propose this novel cytokine as 'the missing link' in the T cell activation associated with uremia (78).

Vaccination responses in chronic uremic and dialysis patients

Most studies of vaccination responses to T cell-independent vaccines, e.g., tetanus, diphtheria toxoid and varicella, have indicated that antibody titers in both uremic adults and children are lower than those achieved in the normal host and decline more quickly (80–85) with some exceptions (86, 87). This impaired response to vaccines is even more evident for vaccines against T cell-dependent antigens such as *Pneumococci* (84, 88, 89) and *Haemophilus influenzae* (90, 91) or, as mentioned above, HBV (20–22, 92, 93).

Several factors, such as age, renal failure, immunosuppression and type of administration are known to be associated with a decreased antibody responsiveness to vaccination. Genes within the MHC, which play a major role in the presentation of antigenic peptides to immunocompetent cells (see above), have also been shown to modulate immune responses to HBV in healthy subjects. An increased frequency of DR3 and DR7 alleles among non responders to HBs antigen has been reported (95–97). Special attention has also been focused on a recessive A1 B8 DR3 haplotype involved in a defective humoral response related to the absence of T cell help (97, 98). More recently, the HLA genetic heterogeneity of HBs vaccine response was reevaluated in a large series of hemodialyzed patients by using a DNA class II oligotyping technique (99). A significantly decreased DR2 frequency in non responders to hepatitis B was observed, while contrary to previous reports (97), the frequency of DR3 was not higher than in responders. These results argue in favor of the presence of HLA-linked immune response gene(s) controlling humoral response to HBs antigen rather than the presence of an immunosuppressive gene. Whether DR2 molecules are better presenters than other DR molecules remains to be investigated. Abnormalities in the expression of the TCR/CD3 antigen receptor complex (100, 101) together with disorders in accessory and adhesion molecule repertoires or selective blockade of monocyte-dependent T cell activation and IL-2 production (23, 60) have also been reported and attributed to the effect of the uremic environment and/or monocyte dysfunction. These observations have led to therapeutic trials combining cytokines such as IL-2, IFNγ and IFNα or thymopentin (23, 102, 103) with the HBV vaccine. Although promising results had been reported with natural IL-2 (23), these findings were not confirmed in a recent, randomized placebo-controlled trial using recombinant IL-2 (24).

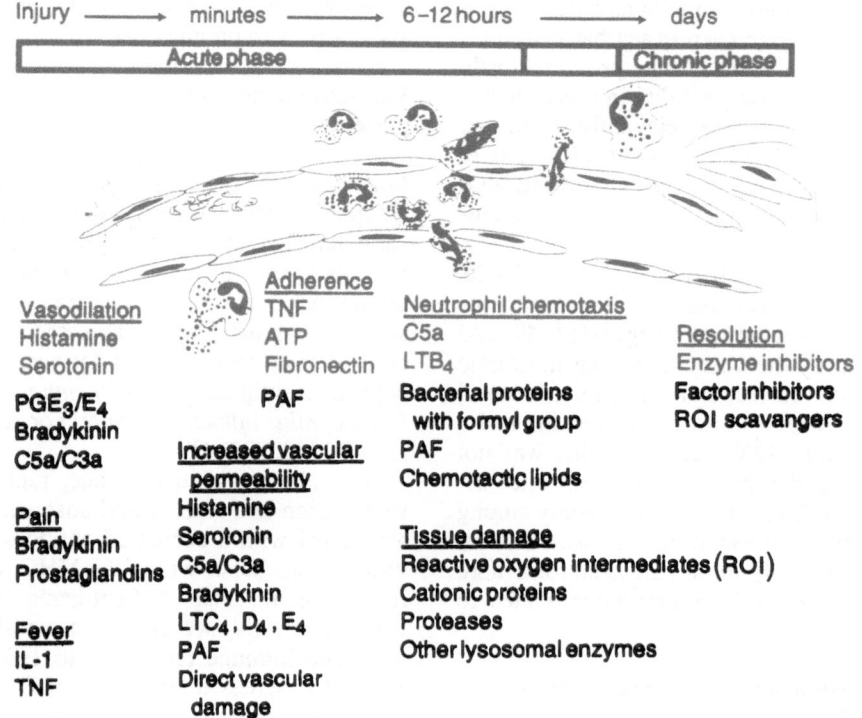

Figure 5. The acute and chronic phases of inflammatory response. (Reproduced from BAM Walker and JC Fantone (45) with permission.)

NON SPECIFIC IMMUNITY

Non specific immunity involves physical barriers, humoral factors (mainly derived from complement and coagulation systems), and cellular factors including polymorphonuclear and mononuclear phagocytes and natural killer (NK) cells. Changes in these factors result in acute and chronic phases of inflammation (Figure 5), which are a prerequisite for the development of the specific immune response (104).

Complement and coagulation systems

Complement activation schematically depicted in Figure 6 can result in direct plasma-mediated cytotoxicity. Generally, surface-bound immunoglobulins (IgG, IgM), aggregated antibodies, proteases, urate crystals and polynucleotides act through the classical pathway of the complement cascade by binding C1q to the plasma membrane. The alternative pathway is triggered by polysaccharides, fungi, bacteria, viruses or dialysis membranes through direct activation of C3. Activation of either pathway leads to the generation of C3a and C5a, as well as the formation of the membrane attack complex (MAC) (C6-C9).

Complement activation is one of the first responses to bacterial invasion via contact with surface polysaccharides, endotoxins, or surface-bound Igs. This pathway can

act as the first cytotoxic response to invasion while also initiating recruitment of leukocytes and vascular changes. Complement fragments C3a and C5a are referred to as anaphylatoxins. Both cause histamine release from mast cells and increase vascular permeability. C5a is also the most important chemotactic factor generated from plasma for neutrophils, monocytes, eosinophils and basophils. The best recognized function of the MAC is the formation of cytotoxic ion channels in both microbial pathogens and host cells upon which complement has been deposited. There is also experimental evidence indicating that the MAC or parts of it can aggregate platelets, prime leukocytes, and act as chemotactic factors.

The coating of particles with antibody or activated complement is referred to as opsonization. Opsonized particles, especially bacteria, are more readily recognized by neutrophils, monocytes and to a lesser extent eosinophils. These cells have specific receptors for C3b (CR1), C3bi (CR3) and the Fc portion of specific classes of Ig (FcRγ) which are used in recognition and phagocytosis of these particles. In addition, aggregate IgG is a stimulus for the production of toxic reactive oxygen intermediates and lysosomal enzyme release. Thus opsonization of pathogens provides an efficient system for recognition, uptake, and destruction by phagocytes.

The contact-activation system plays an important role in the inflammatory response, mainly through the gen-

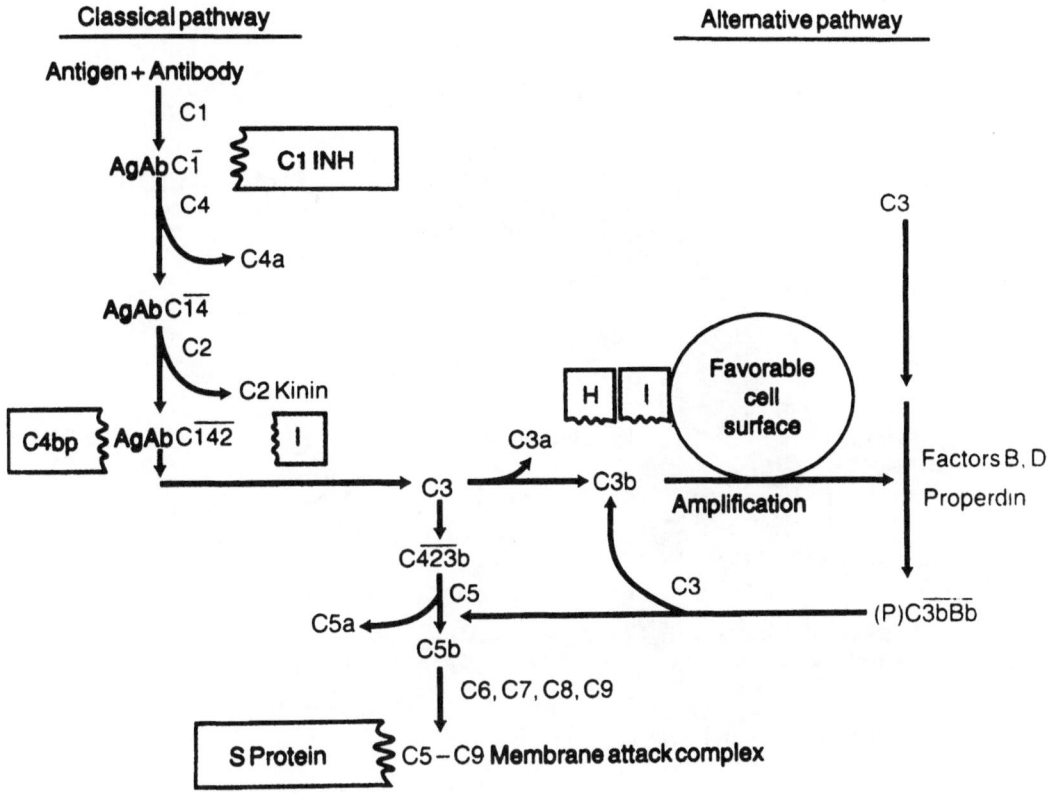

Figure 6. Sequence of activation of the complement components of the classical and alternative pathways. (Reproduced from F Eichenfield and RB Johnston (45) with permission.)

eration of bradykinine and activation of the coagulation system. To initiate this pathway, factor XII (Hageman factor) bound to a negatively charged surface is activated spontaneously or via proteolytic cleavage by kallikrein. Kallikrein is active in a number of reactions, including activation of factor XI, plasminogen, and C1q of the complement cascade. Its most important pro-inflammatory role is the cleavage of kininogen to bradykinin. Bradikinin increases vascular permeability, decreases arterial resistance, and causes smooth muscle contraction and, in combination with prostaglandins, is the major source of mediator-induced pain associated with the inflammatory response.

Complement and coagulation activation during dialysis

A great variety of intradialytic reactions have been ascribed to the activation of coagulation and complement factors which occurs following interaction between extracorporeal blood and dialysis membranes. According to a recent review (105), one may divide them into the more acute phenomena, such as activation of kallicrein, which is related to negative surface charges on membranes, causing hypotension particularly in dialysis patients treated with ACE inhibitors (106) or acute anaphylactoid reactions,

related in part to antibodies to ethylene oxide (ETO) (107), and in part to generation of complement-dependent anaphylatoxins C3a and C5a (108). These may be contrasted with more hypothetical adverse complement-related phenomena like Ba fragment-induced immunosuppression (109) and β2-microglobulin amyloid deposits.

Activation of the complement cascade received most attention in the early literature on the immune system in dialysis. It occurs in the early phase of the dialysis session, at the time of the nadir of leukopenia (110), mainly through the alternative pathway (108), and closely reflects dialysis membrane biocompatibility (111–114). The role of C5a and C3a, which was long restricted to their chemotactic activity, has been extended to several indices of neutrophil and/or monocyte activation such as a triggering of reactive oxygen intermediate production by neutrophils (115) and transcription (but not secretion) of interleukin-1 (IL-1) by monocytes (116). These new effects ascribed to activated complement components suggest a major contribution to dialysis-related complications and have opened the way to new approaches to the assessment of dialysis membrane biocompatibility.

It has also become evident that complement activation depends on a fine balance between various interactions which either favor or inhibit amplification of the alternative pathway (105). Among the inhibiting pathways, fac-

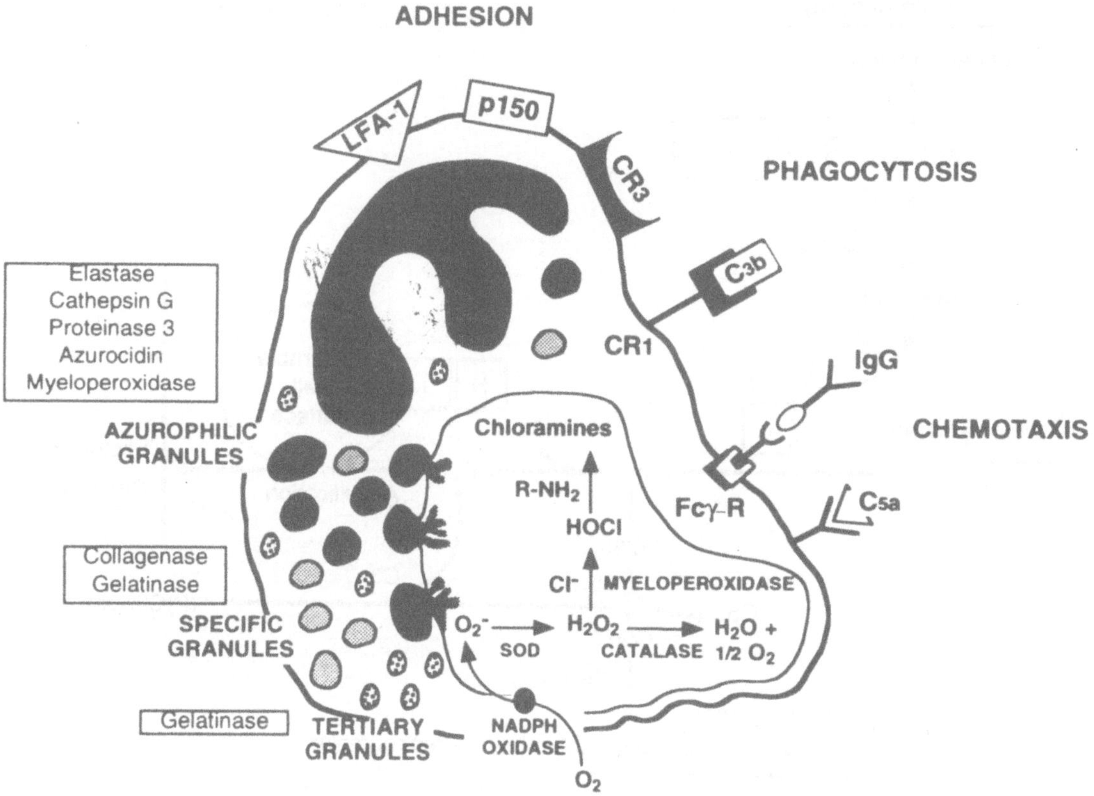

ADHESION

Figure 7. Scheme view of human polymorphonuclear cells. Phagocyte functions are under the control of membrane receptors, soluble mediators and a complex series of oxygen-dependent and independent lytic pathways. (Reproduced from V Witko-Sarsat and B Descamps-Latscha (121) with permission.)

tor H determines the rate of generation of active C3 convertase, mainly through competition between factor H and factor B for C3b (117). The local availability of factor H in proximity to C3b is now considered as the most important element determining whether a surface is activating or not. Among the biologically relevant amplifying pathways, factor D, a highly reactive serine protease generates C3 convertase by cleaving factor B bound to C3b (118). This low-molecular weight (24kD) compound is present at low concentration in plasma and accumulates in ESRD patients (119). Since it poises the complement system for strong activation and has no known endogenous inhibitor, factor D contributes to maintaining continuous low-grade turnover of the complement system and its accumulation might be relevant at sites of micro-inflammation such as amyloid deposits and atherosclerotic plaques. Interestingly, a recent report has shown that dialysis with poly-acrilonitrile membranes induces a significant drop (more than 80%) in plasma factor D concentrations and that this is also due to the adsorptive characteristics of the membrane (120).

Interest in complement activation products has been renewed following the observation of an increase in the terminal complement complex (C5b–9) closely reflecting membrane biocompatibility (105). In contrast to the transient release of C3a and C5a, C5-b9 is generated throughout the session. Among the potential consequences of such an ongoing generation, amplification of the non complement dependent cell activation signals through L-fucose-dependent steps as 'innocent bystander activation' was suggested by these authors.

Neutrophils and reactive oxygen intermediates

Neutrophils react to invading microorganisms and inflammatory mediators with a variety of coordinated responses including adherence to the vascular endothelium, transendothelial migration, cytoskeletal rearrangement in response to chemotactic agents, phagocytosis, and production of toxic mediators. Although critical to host defense, neutrophils can damage normal cells and dissolve connective tissues by the release of this complex assortment of deleterious agents including reactive oxygen species and proteases, leading to pathological process of inflammatory disorders. These functions are under the control of membrane receptors, soluble mediators and a complex series of oxygen-dependent and independent lytic pathways (Figure 7). Adherence to endothelium

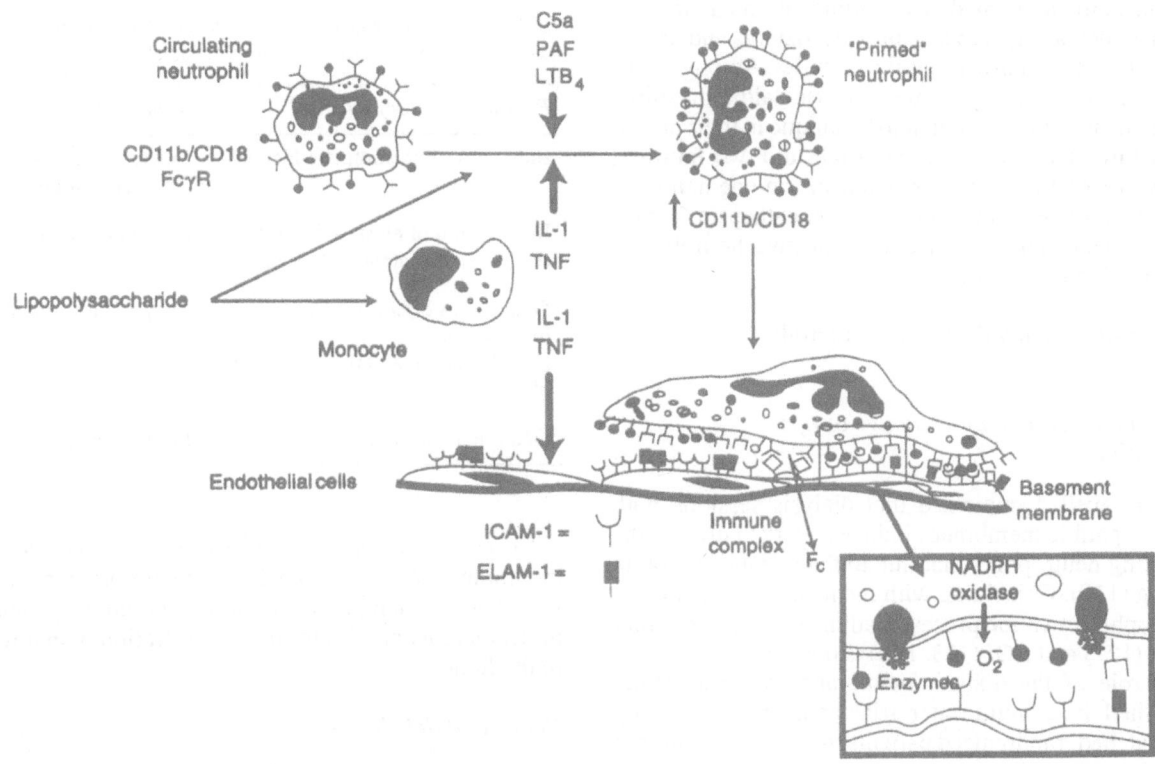

Figure 8. Adhesive interaction between neutrophils and endothelial cells induced by lipopolysaccharide. (Reproduced from BAM Walker and JC Fantone (45) with permission.)

is under the control of the β2 integrins CD11b/CD18 which can be activated by a wide variety of agonists, including chemoattractants (leukotriene B$_4$ (LTB$_4$), C5a, platelet activating factor (PAF) and pro-inflammatory cytokines such as tumor necrosis factor alpha (TNFα) (Figure 8). Some of these agonists also increase expression of endothelial cell ICAM-1, the counterreceptor for CD11b/CD18. Transendothelial migration appears to be regulated by the chemoatractant cytokine IL-8 which is released by the endothelial cells in response to agonists such as IL-1β, TNFα and LPS. IL-8 induces the neutrophil to shed selectin molecules, increases β2 integrin expression and provides a chemoattractant gradient across the endothelium. At the site of infection, neutrophils engulf the invading bacteria in a phagosome. This process involves the β2-integrin receptors and specific IgG Fc receptors which bind to complement fragment and immunoglobulins which coat the bacteria (opsonization process). Concerning bactericidal activity, it is still a convention to define two microbicidal pathways on the basis of their requirement for oxygen. The oxygen-dependent pathway depends on reactive oxygen intermediates (ROI) whose production follows the activation of NADPH oxidase, while the oxygen-independent pathway involves preformed enzymes and antimicrobial proteins stored in

neutrophil cytoplasmic granules and released upon activation (reviewed in (121)).

Oxidative metabolism activation, known as the respiratory burst, first involves NADPH-oxidase, which is an enzymatic complex composed of cytosolic and membrane proteins which ultimately translocate to the plasma membrane leading to the generation of superoxide anion (O2$^-$) and its dismutation product H$_2$O$_2$ at the inner surface of the phagososme. In the presence of chloride and H$_2$O$_2$, myeloperoxidase, an enzyme contained in azurophilic granules, can catalyse the formation of potent chlorinated oxidants such as hypochlorous acid (HOCl) and chloramines, the so-called long-lived oxidants. In distinction to ROI, which mainly act locally and have an extremely short life span, chloramines are long-lived oxidants which can be exported into the circulation and damage sites distant from their production. Several distinct mechanisms can be involved in the activation of the oxidase complex depending on the nature of the stimulus and its interaction pathway with the phagocyte membrane. Interestingly, the production of ROI can be triggered not only by bacteria, foreign particles and chemical substances, but also by physiological substances, e.g., antibodies, immune complexes, C5a, formylated peptides, PAF, LTB4, lipopolysaccharide (LPS) and cytokines such as TNFα and IFNγ.

Neutrophil non oxidative killing is mediated by enzymes such as myeloperoxidase, lysozyme, and antibiotic proteins stored in azurophilic granules. Among the 10 identified so far, lysozyme and bactericidal/permeability increasing protein are thought to be unique in their primary structure. The remaining eight fall into two families, each with four members: the defensins on one hand and the serine proteases including elastase, cathepsin G, proteinase 3 and their enzymatically inactive homologues azurocidin on the other hand.

Neutrophils in chronic uremic and dialysis patients

Neutrophil activation and reactive oxygen intermediates

It is now well documented that dialysis sessions with bioincompatible membranes induce a marked drop in the circulating neutrophil count due to their sequestration in the lung (110). Coinciding with the nadir of neutropenia, a neutrophil activation process leading to massive degranulation (122) and ROI (123, 124) is observed.

The role of the dialysis membrane has been firmly established in a multicenter trial comparing clinically well-matched, randomized patients treated with cellulose and polyacrilonitrile membranes (115). This study also showed a close correlation between the rise in C3a levels and the amount of reactive oxygen intermediates released by phagocytic cells in whole blood. Lastly, a study of the respective influence of uremia and dialysis showed that first dialysis sessions with cellulose membranes also induced ROI production, as measured by whole blood chemiluminescence level which was nonetheless significantly lower than that observed in chronic hemodialysis (125).

Increased malondialdehyde (MDA) serum levels (126), red blood cell membrane damage (127) and impaired deformability (128), and platelet dysfunction (129) reported in dialysis patients are also suggestive of oxidative stress (130).

Concerning the possible role of ROI in dialysis-related systemic inflammatory process (Table 1) one may speculate that these highly reactive molecules contribute to the dialysis-induced systemic inflammatory process by their capacity to induce the generation of chemotactic factors (131), to inactivate the elastase inhibitor (132) and to activate the latent collagenase of neutrophils (133). Likewise, their deleterious effects on cartilage (134) and β2-microglobulin (42) could contribute to amyloid arthropathy, and their DNA-denaturing effect to the premature aging of long-term dialysis patients (135). Lastly, since reactive oxygen intermediates may trigger T cell activation, they might contribute to the obscure mechanisms of T cell activation.

The activation state of neutrophils has recently been further documented by studies showing a significant modulation of their adhesion molecules during dialysis (136–

Table 1. Potential role of reactive oxygen species and long lived oxidants in inflammatory reactions associated with hemodialysis

Pro-inflammatory effects	Manifestations
Induction of chemotactic factors	Leukocyte pulmonary sequestration
Inactivation of elastase inhibitor. Activation of latent collagenase	Systemic inflammatory process
Deleterious effects on cartilage hyaluronate Fragmentation and polymerization of β2m	Amyloid arthropathy
DNA-denaturation	Premature aging

138). This effect which is selectively induced by cellulose membranes and correlates better than complement activation with changes in granulocyte counts, provides a molecular mechanism for the sequestration of neutrophils in the lung.

Neutrophil deficiency

An overall depression of the expected responses of neutrophils to pathogens, e.g., chemotactic, phagocytic and bactericidal activities, has been reported. Likewise their increased basal production of reactive oxygen intermediates contrasts with significantly decreased oxidative response capacity to both particulate and soluble stimuli (125, 139). A deactivation state, along with downregulation of C5a receptors (140) and opsonin receptors, could explain these defective responses of PMN, although uremic toxins, malnutrition and iron overload could also be involved (3, 8, 15). More recently, attention has been focused on a series of factors exerting such inhibitory effects on granulocyte functions. These include the 28 kD granulocyte-inhibiting protein (GIP), a 9.5-kD-β2-microglobulin fragment named GIP-2 (8) which also exerts a stimulatory effect on IgM production (141), and chemically distinguishable low molecular weight compounds (one hydrophilic and one lipophilic) which selectively inhibit neutrophil hexose monophosphate shunt activity (142).

Monocytes-macrophages and pro-inflammatory cytokines

As part of the first line of defence against invasion by infectious organisms, monocytes are attracted from the circulation to sites of infection, arriving much later than neutrophils. Like these latter, monocytes express receptors for IgG Fc fragment, complement components, and carbohydrate moities present on non encapsulated microorganisms and are likely to move to a site of infection. These receptors serve to enhance the capability of macrophages to bind and to phagocytize microorganisms and particulate antigens.

In addition to their phagocytic activity, monocytes and macrophages are involved in both the initiation and the effector phases of the immune response. Their expression of MHC class II determinants makes them effective as APCs (see above). Lymphokines such as IFNγ produced by antigen-stimulated T cells activate macrophages to become cytotoxic effector cells. Via their receptors for the Fc portion of IgG, macrophages act as effectors in ADCC (antibody dependent cellular cytotoxicity). This cytotoxic function of macrophages is important in defenses against tumors and virally infected cells.

To exert their effector function monocytes and macrophages secrete complement proteins a variety of enzymes, plasma proteins, prostaglandins, leukotrienes and cytokines including IFNα, and pro-inflammatory cytokines such as IL-1, tumor necrosis factor (TNFα) and IL-6. These cytokines are synthesized in response to infection, inflammation and immune challenge, and act on a variety of tissues by changing gene expression and cellular metabolism. They share with hormones the ability to act at picomolar or even fentomolar concentrations at sites distant from their production. They differ from hormones in that they are not required for the maintenance of homeostasis; their cell sources are not restricted to a given organ or tissue, and their genes are induced rather than constitutively expressed. Regardless of their mode of action, cytokines interact with their target cells via specific membrane receptors which may thus exert an inhibitory action. This can be induced by the shedding of soluble receptors, e.g., the soluble TNFα receptor, as well as through the action of receptor antagonists which compete for receptor occupancy despite a lack of demonstrable agonist activity, e.g., the IL-1 receptor antagonist (IL-1Ra).

Monocytes in chronic uremic and dialysis patients

Monocyte deficiency

As mentioned above, indirect evidence has been reported that monocytes could be involved in the T cell immunodeficiency observed in ESRD patients. Monocytes could effectively contribute to inhibiting T cell proliferative responses, as i) depletion of monocytes from T cell cultures improves T cell responses (143); ii) defective responses mainly involve monocyte-dependent stimulation (60, 61); and iii) inhibition of monocyte-derived immunosuppressive molecules such as prostaglandins with indomethacin at least partially restores lymphoproliferative responses (144).

More direct evidence has been provided by a study (145) showing that peripheral blood monocytes from ESRD patients with severe infections have defective FcRγ-mediated internalization of opsonized particles, suggesting defective antigen presentation.

Table 2. Potential role of pro-inflammatory cytokines in inflammatory reactions associated with hemodialysis

Sites of action	Manifestations
	Per dialytic clinical manifestations
Hypothalamus	Fever
Arteries	Hypotension
Central nervous system	Sleep anorexia
	Acute inflammatory reaction
Neutrophils	Degranulation,
	Reactive oxygen species production,
	Expression of adhesion molecules
Hepatocytes	Increased synthesis of
	fibrinogen
	serum amyloid A
	haptoglobin
	Chronic inflammatory reaction
Chondrocytes	Arthropathy
Endothelial cells	Atherosclerosis
Fibroblasts	Fibrosis
Articulations	β2-microglobulin amyloidosis

Monocyte activation and pro-inflammatory cytokines

The activation state of monocytes has been clearly illustrated by studies of their capacity to synthesize pro-inflammatory cytokines namely IL-1, TNFα and IL-6. IL-1, which is required for both IL-2 production and IL-2R expression, was first incriminated in acute and chronic inflammatory reactions associated with hemodialysis (146) based on observations that: i) both the clinical symptoms observed during dialysis sessions and the sites of complications in long-term hemodialyzed patients strikingly reflect the systemic effects and target organs of IL-1β (Figure 9 and Table 2); and ii) numerous HD-related factors can trigger the production of IL-1β by monocytes. This hypothesis was soon verified by several studies showing elevated levels of IL-1β in the plasma of dialysis patients (reviewed in reference (147)). It has been extended to the other major inflammatory cytokines, TNFα and IL-6, which share with IL-1β most of its biological activities and increased levels of TNFα (148, 149) and IL-6 (150, 151) have been reported in these patients. However, a lack of detectable IL-1β and TNFα in the circulation of dialysis patients has also been reported (152). It could be due to the concomitant presence of IL-1β and TNFα inhibitors capable of interfering in certain immunoassays (153).

At the cellular level, increased cell-associated IL-1 activity has also been reported (154), together with constitutively increased production of pro-inflammatory cytokines by cultured monocytes (155) from dialysis

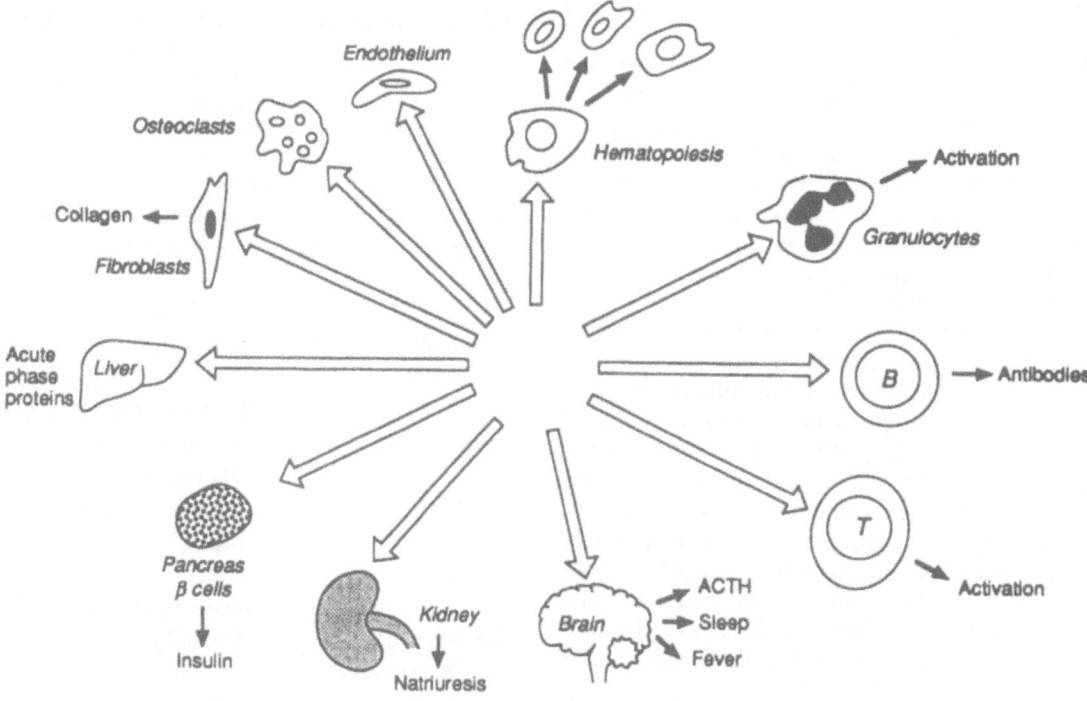

Figure 9. Main organ and cellular targets of interleukin-1. (Reproduced from M Dy (44) with permission.)

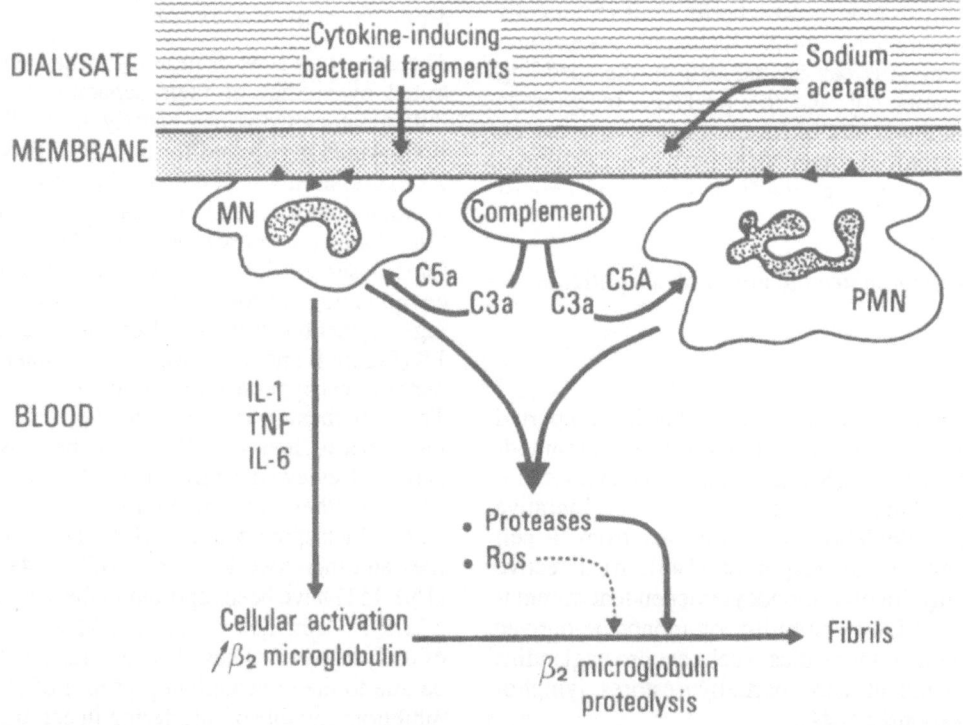

Figure 10. Dialysis-induced phagocyte activation in the generation of amyloid fibrils. Dialysate- and dialysis membrane-related factors contribute to activate polymorphonuclear neutrophils (PMN) and monocytes (MN) mainly via complement activated components leading to the generation of cytokines (IL-1, TNF and IL-6), proteases and reactive oxygen species (ROS) all of which might contribute to β2 microglobulin release, lysis and aggregation.

patients. Further evidence for a monocyte activation has been provided by several studies showing that dialysis induces the gene expression of IL-1β (156), TNFα (157) and IL-6 (158) in circulating monocytes. Lastly, our own studies showing that cell-associated levels of IL-1β (155) and plasma levels of both TNFα (149) and IL-6 (150) are elevated in nondialyzed ESRD patients, suggest that such monocyte activation is associated with uremia and not solely induced by dialysis.

Recent findings stress the fact that the potentially harmful effects of monocyte-derived pro-inflammatory cytokines are counteracted by specific inhibitors concomitantly synthesized in response to infectious or inflammatory challenge. TNF soluble receptors (TNF-sR55 and TNF-sR75) which bind to TNF and neutralize its effects and the IL-1Ra (IL-1 receptor antagonist) which competitively binds to the IL-1 receptor without triggering an activation signal, deserve special attention in dialysis patients (159). Increased plasma levels of TNF soluble receptors have already been reported in ESRD patients (160, 161) and in a recent study (162) we also found that both TNF-sR55 and TNF-sR75 were elevated at the incipient stage of chronic renal failure, increased in parallel with the progression of renal failure and further rose during the course of dialysis sessions; IL-1Ra levels were also elevated from the incipient stage of chronic uremia but were only moderately increased in the course of renal failure and contrary to TNF soluble receptors, tended to decrease during the dialysis session. Finally anti-cytokine autoantibodies (163) have also been reported in ESRD patients.

Another important issue in studies of pro-inflammatory cytokines in dialysis patients concerns the respective role of dialysis membrane biocompatibility and of endotoxins (lipopolysaccharide, LPS) which frequently contaminate the dialysate, in the induction of cytokine synthesis by monocytes. *In vitro* studies indicate that complement-activated components induce the transcription of IL-1β and TNFα in normal monocytes, but that LPS is required for subsequent protein synthesis (116). Most *in vivo* studies comparing complement-activating and non activating membranes concluded that the nature of the dialysis membrane had no major effect, at least with regard to predialysis cytokine production. Studies of the influence of dialysis membrane biocompatibility on perdialytic changes in cytokine levels have so far given controversial results.

The passage of cytokine-inducing substances by back-filtration from the dialysate into the blood compartment has been demonstrated (164–166). Among these, intact low-molecular-weight species of LPS that are unreactive with the *Limulus amoebocyte* assay have nonetheless been shown to have IL-1β inducing capacity (167). The permeability of dialysis membranes to TNFα-inducing substances has also been reported (164–168). Taken together these findings strongly suggest that monocyte activation may result from both complement activation with cellulose membranes and endotoxin transfer from the dialysate.

It can be assumed that with the increased popularity of high-flux dialysis membranes, there will be growing concern over potential transfer of cytokine-inducing substances across these more permeable membranes by back-filtration or back-diffusion. The use of high-flux membranes thus reinforces the need for ultrapure dialysate. As we have stated elsewhere (4), the search for biocompatible membranes has come up against a dilemma: dialysis membranes that are most compatible in terms of complement- and phagocyte oxidative burst-activating potential are those that may favor the transfer of cytokine-inducing substances.

Natural killer cells in chronic uremic and dialysis patients

Another important cell involved in nonspecific surveillance against malignant cells and virus-infected cells is the NK cell. The risk of malignancies in uremic patients is greater than in the general population, but evidence that NK cells could be altered in ESRD patients is still a matter of debate. In particular, it is unclear whether the NK cell deficiency noted by some groups measuring NK cell function is due to quantitative or qualitative abnormalities (169). Finally, flow cytometry analysis of NK cells in dialysis patients has recently shown that dialysis with bioincompatible membranes selectively alters NK cell number and activity, suggesting that a dysfunction in these cells could explain the impaired host resistance against tumors (170).

CONCLUSION

New insights into the humoral factors and cellular actors that could be involved in the immunodeficiency associated with uremia and exacerbated by dialysis suggest attractive hypotheses. Some of these such as the possible reduced bioavailability of IL-2, secondary to its overconsumption by activated T cells, or the defective antigen presenting capacity of monocytes to T cells prexist to the institution of dialysis therapy, whereas others like the reduced expression of phagocyte opsonin receptors and the impaired oxidative burst activity are more likely secondary to the recurrent perdialytic up-regulation of these receptors induced by bioincompatible dialysis membranes. The increased production of pro-inflammatory cytokines preexisiting to and exacerbated by dialysis has suggested that activated monocytes could play a significant role in the immune disorders observed in ESRD patients. Among dialysis-related factors, dialysate sterility has appeared more critical with the development of highly permeable dialysis membranes, thus reinforcing the need to develop ultrapure dialysis conditions. The recent challenges posed by the demonstration of the role of the progression of chronic renal failure itself in the induction of immune cell activation and dysfunction, and of the unique model of systemic inflammation represented by dialysis, is attracting the contribution of both basic scientists and clinical researchers. It is to be hoped that these efforts will lead not only to new knowledge but also to new immunointervention strategies of direct benefit to the patient.

ACKNOWLEDGEMENTS

We thank Dr Johanna Zingraff, Dr Christian Verger and Dr Anne Moynot for their participation to clinical investigation in dialysis patients. We are indebted to Dr Anh Thu Nguyen, Dr André Herbelin and Dr Lucienne Chatenoud for helpful contribution to laboratory studies and valuable discussions.

REFERENCES

1. Dammin GJ, Couch NP, Murray JE: Prolonged survival of skin homografts in uremic patients. *Ann NY Acad Sci* 64: 967, 1957
2. Descamps-Latscha B, Herbelin A, Nguyen AT, Zingraff J, Jungers P, Chatenoud L: Immune system dysregulation in uremia. *Seminars in Nephrology* 14: 253, 1994
3. Tolkoff-Rubin NE, Rubin RH: Uremia and host defenses. (Editorial Comment) *N Engl J Med* 322: 770, 1990
4. Descamps-Latscha B, Herbelin A: Long-term dialysis and cellular immunity. A critical survey. *Kidney Int* 43 (Suppl): 135S, 1993
5. Koch KM: Dialysis-related amyloidosis. *Kidney Int* 41: 1416, 1992
6. Keane WF, Maddy MF: Host defenses and infectious complications in maintenance hemodialysis patients. in *Replacement of Renal Function by Dialysis*, 3rd Edition, edited by JF Maher, Dordrecht/Boston, Kluwer Academic Publishers, 1989, p 865
7. Goldman M, Vanherweghem JL: Bacterial infections in chronic hemodialysis patients: epidemiologic and pathophysiologic aspects. *Adv Nephrol* 19: 315, 1990
8. Haag-Weber M, Horl WH: Uremia and infection: mechanisms of impaired cellular host defense. *Nephron* 63: 125, 1993
9. Mailloux LU, Bellucci AG, Wilkes BM et al.: Mortality in dialysis patients: analysis of the causes of death. *Am J Kidney Dis* 18: 326, 1991
10. Lundin AP, Adler AJ, Berlyne GM, Friedman EA: Tuberculosis in patients undergoing maintenance hemodialysis. *Am J Med* 67: 597, 1979
11. Garcia-Leoni ME, Martin-Scapa C, Rodeno P, Vaderrabamo F, Moreno S, Bouza E: High incidence of tuberculosis in renal patients. *Eur J Clin Microbiol Infect Dis* 9: 283, 1990
12. Kessler M, Hoen B, Mayeux D, Hestin D, Fontenaille C: Bacteremia in patients on chronic hemodialysis. *Nephron* 64: 95, 1993
13. Khan IH, Catto GRD: Long-term complications of dialysis. Infections. *Kidney Int* 43 (Suppl): 143S, 1993
14. Bergstrom J: Nutrition and adequacy of dialysis in hemodialysis patients. *Kidney Int* 43 (Suppl): 261S, 1993
15. Haag-Weber M, Horl WH: Altered cellular host defence in malnutrition and uremia. *Contrib Nephrol* 98: 105, 1992
16. Gafter U, Kalechman Y, Sredni B: Induction of a subpopulation of suppressor cells by a single blood transfusion. *Kidney Int* 41: 143, 1992
17. Vanholder R, Vanbiesen W, Ringoir S: Contributing factors to the inhibition of phagocytosis in hemodialyzed patients. *Kidney Int* 44: 208, 1993
18. Mourad G, Cristol JP, Chong G et al.: Disappearance of anti-HLA antibodies in highly sensitized patients treated with erythropoietin. *Transplant Proc* 24: 2512, 1992
19. Jungers P, Delagneau JF, Prunet P, Crosnier J: Vaccination against hepatitis B in hemodialysis centers. *Adv Nephrol* 11: 303, 1982
20. Crosnier J, Jungers P, Couroucé AM et al.: Randomized placebo-controlled trial of hepatitis B surface antigen vaccine in French haemodialysis units: II Haemodialysis patients. *Lancet* 1: 797, 1981
21. Mioli VA, La Greca G: A special issue on virus hepatitis and the kidney. *Nephron* 61: 251, 1992
22. Benhamou E, Courouce AM, Jungers P et al.: Hepatitis B vaccine: randomized trial of immunogenicity in hemodialysis patients. *Clin Nephrol* 21: 143, 1984
23. Meuer SC, Dumann H, Meyer Zum Buschenfelde KH, Kohler H: Low-dose interleukin-2 induces systemic immune responses against HBsAg in immunodeficient non-responders to hepatitis B vaccination. *Lancet* 1: 15, 1989
24. Jungers P, Devillier P, Salomon H, Cerisier JE, Courouce AM: Randomised placebo-controlled trial of recombinant interleukin-2 in chronic uraemic patients who are non-responders to hepatitis B vaccine. *Lancet* 344: 856, 1994
25. Jadoul M, Cornu C, van Ypersele de Strihou C, the UCL collaborative group: Incidence of risk factors for hepatitis C seroconversion in hemodialysis: a prospective study. *Kidney Int* 44: 1322, 1993
26. Knudsen F, Wantzin P, Rasmussen K et al.: Hepatitis C in dialysis patients: relationships to blood transfusions, dialysis and liver disease. *Kidney Int* 43: 1353, 1993
27. Chauveau P, Couroucé AM, Lemarec N et al.: Antibodies to hepatitis C virus by second generation test in hemodialyzed patients. *Kidney Int* 43 (Suppl): 149S, 1993
28. Vitale C, Tricerri A, Marangella M et al.: Epidemiology of hepatitis-C virus infection in dialysis units – 1st- versus 2nd-generation assays. *Nephron* 64: 315, 1993
29. Pol S, Dubois F, Mattlinger et al.: Absence of hepatitis Delta virus infection in chronic hemodialysis and kidney transplant patients in France. *Transplantation* 54: 1096, 1992
30. Glassock RJ, Cohen AH, Danovitch G, Parsa KP: Human immunodeficiency virus (HIV) infection and the kidney. *Ann Intern Med* 112: 35, 1990
31. Marcus R, Favero MS, Banerjee S et al.: Prevalence and incidence of human immunodeficiency virus among patients undergoing long-term hemodialysis. The Cooperative Dialysis Study Group. *Am J Med* 90: 614, 1991
32. Tebben JA, Rigsby MO, Selwyn PA, Brennan N, Kliger A, Finkelstein FO: Outcome of HIV infected patients on continuous ambulatory peritoneal dialysis. *Kidney Int* 44: 191, 1993

33. Breyer JA, Harbison MA: Isolation of human immuno-deficiency virus from peritoneal dialysis. *Am J Kidney Dis* 21: 23, 1993.

34. Gejyo F, Yamada T, Odani S et al.: A new form of amyloid protein associated with chronic hemodialysis was identi-fied as β2 microglobulin. *Biochem Biophys Res Commun* 129: 701, 1985

35. Gorevic PD, Munoz PC, Casey TT et al.: Polymerisation of intact β2 microglobulin in tissues causes amyloidosis in patients on chronic hemodialysis. *Proc Nat Acad Sci USA* 83: 7908, 1986

36. Van Ypersele C, Jadoul M, Malghem J, Maldague B, Jamart J: Effect of dialysis membrane and patient's age on signs of dialysis-related amyloidosis. *Kidney Int* 39: 1012, 1991

37. Zingraff J, Beyne P, Urena P et al.: Influence of haemodialysis membranes on β2-microglobulin kinetics: *in vivo* and *in vitro* studies. *Nephrol Dial Transplant* 3: 284, 1988

38. Chanard J, Vincent C, Caudwell V et al.: β2-microglobulin metabolism in uremic patients who are undergoing dialysis. *Kidney Int* 43 (Suppl): 83S, 1993

39. Zingraff J, Noël LH, Bardin T, Atienza C, Zins B, Drüeke T, Kuntz D: Beta 2 microglobulin amyloidosis in chronic renal failure. *N Engl J Med* 11 323, 1990

40. Zaoui PM, Stone WJ, Hakim RM: Effects of dialysis membranes on β2-microglobulin production and cellular expression. *Kidney Int* 38: 962, 1990

41. Linke RP, Keerling A, Rail A: Hemodialysis: demonstra-tion of truncated β2-microglobulin in AB amyloid *in situ*. *Kidney Int* 43 (Suppl): 100S, 1993

42. Capeillere-Blandin C, Delaveau T, Descamps-Latscha B: Structural modifications of human β2-microglobulin treated with oxygen-derived radicals. *Biochem J* 277: 175, 1991

43. Nakashima Y, Akizawa T, Nagai T, Koshikawa S: Role of uremic and endothelial factors in the development of β2-microglobulin amyloidosis. *Kidney Int* 41 (Suppl): 88S, 1993

44. Bach JF (ed): *Traité d'Immunologie*, Paris, Médecine Sciences Flammarion, 1993, 1205 pp

45. Sigal LH, Ron Y (eds): *Immunology and Inflamma-tion. Basic Mechanisms and Clinical Consequences*, New York, McGraw-Hill Inc, 1993, 805 pp

46. Raska K JR, Raskova J, Shea SM et al.: T cell subsets and cellular immunity in end-stage renal disease. *Am J Med* 75: 734, 1983

47. Chatenoud L, Dugas B, Beaurain G et al.: Presence of preactivated T cells in hemodialyzed patients: their pos-sible role in altered immunity. *Proc Natl Acad Sci USA* 83: 7457, 1986

48. Kurz P, Kohler H, Meuer S, Hutteroth T, Meyer Zum Buschenfelde KH: Impaired cellular immune responses in chronic renal failure: evidence for a T cell defect. *Kidney Int* 29: 1209, 1986

49. Beaurain G, Naret C, Marcon L et al.: *In vivo* T cell acti-vation in chronic uremic hemodialyzed patients. *Kidney Int* 36: 636, 1989

50. Newberry WM, Sanford JP: Defective cellular immunity in renal failure: depression of reactivity of lymphocytes to phytohemagglutinin by renal failure serum. *J Clin Invest* 50: 1262, 1971

51. Kamata K, Okubo M, Sada M: Immunosuppressive fac-tors in uraemic sera are composed of both dialysable and non-dialysable components. *Clin Exp Immunol* 54: 277, 1983

52. Barsotti G, Bevilacqua G, Morelli E et al.: Toxicity arising from guanidine compounds: role of methyl guanidine as uremic toxin. *Kidney Int* 7: S299, 1975

53. Hörl WH, Haag-Weber M, Georgopoulos A Block LH: Physicochemical charcterization of a polypeptide present in uremic serum that inhibits the biological activity of polymorphoniclear cells. *Proc Natl Acad Sci* 6353, 1990

54. Revillard JP: Immunologic alterations in chronic renal insufficiency. *Adv Nephrol* 8: 365, 1979

55. Nelson DS, Penrose JM: Effect of hemodialysis and trans-plantation on inhibition of lymphocyte transformation by sera from uremic patients. *Clin Immunol Immunopath* 4: 143, 1975

56. Chouaib S, Fradelizi D: The mechanism of inhibition of human IL-2 production. *J Immunol* 129: 2463, 1982

57. Chouaib S, Bertoglio JH: Prostaglandin E as modulators of the immune response. *Lymphokine Res* 7: 237, 1988

58. Sunder-Plassmann G, Heinz G, Wagner L, Prychzy B, Derfler K: T-cell selection and T-cell receptor variable beta-chain usage in chronic hemodialysis patients. *Clin Nephrol* 37: 252, 1992

59. Stachowski J, Pollok M, Burrichter H, Spithaler C, Bal-damus CA: Does uremic environment down-regulate T cell activation via TCR/CD3 antigen receptor complex? *J Clin Lab Immunol* 36: 15, 1991

60. Meuer SC, Hauer M, Kurz P, Meyer Zum Buschen-felde KH, Kohler H: Selective blockade of the antigen-receptor-mediated pathway of T cell activation in patients with impaired primary immune responses. *J Clin Invest* 80: 743, 1987

61. Stachowski J, Pollok M, Burrichter H, Baldamus CA: Immunodeficiency in ESRD-patients is linked to altered IL-2 receptor density on T cell subsets. *J Clin Lab Immunol* 34: 171, 1991

62. Gerez L, Madar L, Shkolnik T et al.: Regulation of interleukin-2 and interferon-gamma gene expression in renal failure. *Kidney Int* 40: 266, 1991

63. Keown P, Descamps-Latscha B: *In vitro* suppression of cell-mediated immunity by ferroproteins and ferric salts. *Cell Immunol* 80: 257, 1983

64. Smith MD, Hardy G, Williams JD, Coles GA: Suppressor cell numbers and activity in non-transfused renal dialysis patients. *Clin Nephrol* 20: 130, 1983

65. Bender BS, Curtis JL, Nagel JE et al.: Analysis of immune status of hemodialyzed adults: association with prior transfusions. *Kidney Int* 26: 436, 1984

66. De Sousa M: Immune functions in iron overload. *Clin Exp Immunol* 75: 1, 1989

67. Pfaffl W, Gross HJ, Neumeier D, Samtleben W, Gurland HJ: Lymphocyte subsets and delayed cutaneious hyper-sensitivity in hemodialysis patients receiving recombi-nant human erythropoietin. *Contrib Nephrol* 66: 195, 1988

68. Collart FE, Dratwa M, Wittek M, Wens R: Effects of recombinant human erythropoietin on T lymphocyte sub-sets in hemodialysis patients. *ASAIO Trans* 36: M219, 1990

69. Grimm PC, Sinai-Trieman L, Sekiya NM et al.: Effects of recombinant human erythropoietin on HLA sensitization and cell mediated immunity. *Kidney Int* 38: 12, 1990
70. Walz G, Kunzendorf U, Josimovic-Alasevic O et al.: Soluble interleukin 2 receptor and tissue polypeptide antigen serum concentrations in end-stage renal failure. *Nephron* 56: 157, 1990
71. Zaoui P, Green W, Hakim RM: Hemodialysis with cuprophane membrane modulates interleukin-2 receptor expression. *Kidney Int* 39: 1020, 1991
72. Descamps-Latscha B: The immune system in end stage renal disease. *Curr Opin Nephrol Hypert* 2: 883, 1993
73. Paczek L, Schaefer RM, Heidland A: Improved function of B lymphocytes in dialysis patients treated by recombinant human erythropoietin. *Contrib Nephrol* 87: 36, 1990
74. Sennesael JJ, Van Der Niepen P, Verbeelen DL: Treatment with recombinant human erythropoietin increases antibody titers after hepatitis B vaccination in dialysis patients. *Kidney Int* 40: 121, 1991
75. Nolph KD, Husted FC, Sharp GC, Siemsen AW: Antibodies to nuclear antigens in patients undergoing long-term hemodialysis. *Am J Med* 60: 673, 1976
76. Gagnon RF, Shuster J, Kaye M: Auto-immunity in patients with end-stage renal disease maintained on hemodialysis and continuous ambulatory peritoneal dialysis. *J Clin Lab Immunol* 11: 155, 1983
77. Rumpf KW, Seubert S, Seubert A et al.: Association of ethylene-oxide-induced IgE antibodies with symptoms in dialysis patients. *Lancet* 2: 1385, 1985
78. Descamps-Latscha B, Herbelin A, Nguyen AT et al.: Soluble CD23 as an effector of immune dysregulation in chronic uremia and dialysis. *Kidney Int* 43: 878, 1993
79. Mossalayi MD, Lecron JC, Dalloul AH et al.: Soluble CD23 (FcεRII) and interleukin-1 synergistically induce early human thymocyte maturation. *J Exp Med* 171: 959, 1990
80. Wilson WEC, Kirkpatrick CHH, Talmadge DW: Suppression of immunologic responsiveness in uremia. *Ann Intern Med* 62: 1, 1965
81. Boulton-Jones JM, Vick R, Cameron Js et al.: Immune responses in uremia. *Clin Nephrol* 1: 351, 1973
82. Byron PR, Mallick NP, Taylor G: Immune potential in human uraemia. 1. Relationship of glomerular filtration rate to depression of immune potential. *J Clin Pathol* 29: 765, 1976
83. Kleinknecht C, Margolis A, Bonnissol C, Gaiffe M, Sahyoun S, Broyer M: Serum antibodies before and after immunisation in haemodialysed children. *Proc Eur Dial Transpl Ass* 14: 209, 1977
84. Beaman M, Michael J, MacLennan IC, Adu D: T cell independent and T cell dependent antibody response in patients with chronic renal failure. *Nephrol Dial Transplant* 4: 216, 1989
85. Guérin A, Buisson Y, Nutini MT, Saliou P, London G, Marchais S: Response to vaccination against tetanus in chronic haemodialyzed patients. *Nephrol Dial Transplant* 7: 323, 1992
86. Stoloff IL, Stout R, Myerson RM, Havens WP: Production of antibody in patients with uremia. *N Engl J Med* 259: 320, 1958
87. Borradori L, Born B, Descoeudres C, Skvaril F, Morell A: Serum immunoglobulin levels and natural antibodies to haemophilus influenzae in hemodialysis patients: evidence for IgG subclass imbalances. *Nephron* 56: 35, 1990
88. Rytel MW, Dailey MP, Schiffman G, Hoffmann RG, Piering WF: Pneumococcal vaccine immunization of patients with renal impairment. *Proc Soc Exp Biol Med* 182: 468, 1986
89. Hibberd PL, Rubin RH: Approach to immunization in the immunosuppressed host. *Infect Dis Clin North Am* 4: 123, 1990
90. Abdulmassih Z, Duverlie G, Moriniere P et al.: Response to influenza vaccine in uremic patients: relation to erythrocyte magnesium and the value of a second injection. *Nephrologie* 8: 23, 1987
91. Rautenberg P, Teifke I, Schlegelberger T, Ullmann U: Influenza subtype-specific IgA, IgM and IgG responses in patients on hemodialysis after influenza vaccination. *Infection* 16: 323, 1988
92. Stevens CE, Alter HJ, Taylor PE, Zang EA, Harley EJ, Szuness W: Hepatitis B vaccine in patients receiving hemodialysis. *N Engl J Med* 311: 496, 1984
93. Kohler H, Arnold W, Renschin G, Dormeyer HH, Meyer Zum Buschenfelde KH: Active hepatitis B vaccination of dialysis patients and medical staff. *Kidney Int* 25: 124, 1984
94. Benhamou E, Courouce AM, Laplanche A, Jungers P, Tron JF, Crosnier J: Long-term results of hepatitis B vaccination in patients on dialysis. *N Engl J Med* 314: 1710, 1986
95. Weissman JY, Tsuchiyose MM, Tong MJ, Co R, Chin K, Ettenger RB: Lack of response to recombinant hepatitis B vaccine in non responders to the plasma vaccine. *JAMA* 260: 1734, 1988
96. Varla-Leftherioti M, Papanicolaou M, Spyropoulou M et al.: HLA-associated non-responsiveness to hepatitis B vaccine. *Tissue Antigens* 35: 60, 1990
97. Pol S, Legendre C, Mattlinger B, Berthelot P, Kreis H: Genetic basis of non-response to hepatitis B vaccine in hemodialyzed patients. *J Hepatol* 11: 385, 1990
98. Alper CA, Kruskall MS, Marcus-Bagley D et al.: Genetic pediction of nonresponse to hepatitis B vaccine. *N Engl J Med* 321: 708, 1989
99. Caillat-Zucman S, Giminez JJ, Albouze G et al.: HLA genetic heterogeneity of hepatitis B vaccine response in hemodialyzed patients. *Kidney Int* 43 (Suppl): 157S, 1993
100. Stachowski J, Pollock M, Burrichter H et al.: Relationships between TCR/CD3 receptor density on CD4 T cels and the anti-HBs antibody response to hepatitis B vaccination in ESRD patients. *Nephrol Dial Transplant* 7: 678, 1992
101. Stachowski J, Pollock M, Barth C, Maciejewski, Baldamus CA: Non-responsiveness to hepatitis B vaccination in haemodialysis patients: association with impaired TCR/CD3 antigen receptor expression regulating co-stimulatory processes in antigen presentation and recognition. *Nephrol Dial Transplant* 9: 144, 1994
102. Quiroga JA, Castillo I, Porres JC et al.: Recombinant gamma-interferon as adjuvant to hepatitis B vaccine in hemodialysis patients. *Hepatology* 12: 661, 1990
103. Dumann H, Meuer SC, Renschin G, Kohler H: Influence of thymopentin on antibody reponse, and monocyte and T cell function in hemodialysis patients who fail to respond to hepatitis B vaccination. *Nephron* 55: 136, 1990

104. Fauve RM: Inflammation and natural immunity. in *Progress in Immunology*, edited by Fougereau M, Dausset J, London, Academic Press, 1980, p 737

105. Deppish R, Ritz E, Hansch GM, Schols M, Rauterberg EW: Biocompatibility. Perspectives in 1993. *Kidney Int* 45 (Suppl): 77S, 1994

106. Tielemans CH, Madhoun P, Lenaers M, Schandene L, Goldman M, Vanherweghein JL: Anaphylactoid reactions on AN69 membranes in patients receiving ACE inhibitors. *Kidney Int* 38: 982, 1990

107. Bommer J, Ritz E: Ethylene oxide (ETO) as a major cause of anaphylactoid reactions in dialysis: a review. *Artif Organs* 11: 111, 1987

108. Hakim RM, Breillatt J, Lazarus JM, Port FK: Complement activation and hypersensitivity reactions to dialysis membranes. *N Engl J Med* 311: 878, 1984

109. Oppermann M, Kurts C, Zierz R, Quentin E, Weber Mh, Gotze O: Elevated plasma levels of the immunosuppressive complement fragment Ba in renal failure. *Kidney Int* 40: 939, 1991

110. Craddock PR, Fehr J, Dalmasso AP, Brighan KL, Jacob HS: Hemodialysis leukopenia. Pulmonary vascular leukostasis resulting from complement activation by dialyzer cellophane membranes. *J Clin Invest* 59: 879, 1977

111. Chenoveth DE, Cheung AK, Henderson LW: Anaphylatoxin formation during hemodialysis: effects of different dialyzer membranes. *Kidney Int* 24: 764, 1983

112. Kazatchkine MD, Carreno MP: Activation of the complement system at the interface between blood and artificial surfaces. *Biomaterials* 9: 30, 1988

113. Cheung AK, Parker CJ, Wilcox L, Janatova J: Activation of the alternative pathway of complement by cellulosic hemodialysis membranes. *Kidney Int* 36: 257, 1989

114. Cheung AK, Parker CJ, Wilcox LA, Janatova J: Activation of complement by hemodialysis mebranes: polyacrilonitrile binds more C3a than cuprophan. *Kidney Int* 37: 1055, 1990

115. Descamps-Latscha B, Goldfarb B, Nguyen AT et al.: Establishing the relationship between complement activation and stimulation of phagocyte oxidative metabolism in hemodialyzed patients: a randomized prospective study. *Nephron* 59: 279, 1991

116. Schindler R, Lonnemann G, Shaldon S, Koch KM, Dinarello CA: Transcription, not synthesis, of interleukin-1 and tumor necrosis factor by complement. *Kidney Int* 37: 85, 1990

117. Carreno MP, Labarre D, Maillet F, Josefowicz M, Kazatchkine MD: Regulation of the human alternative complement pathway: formation of a tertiary complex between factor H, surface bound C3b and chemical groups on non-activating surfaces. *Eur J Immunol* 19: 2145, 1989

118. Lesavre PH, Muller-Eberhard HJ: Mechanism of action of factor D of the alternative complement pathway. *J Exp Med* 148: 1498, 1978

119. Volanakis JE, Barnum SR, Giddens M, Galla JH: Renal filtration and catabolism of complement protein D. *N Engl J Med* 312: 395, 1985

120. Pascual M, Schifferli JA: Adsorption of complement factor D by polyacrilonitrile dialysis membranes. *Kidney Int* 43: 903, 1993

121. Witko-Sarsat V, Descamps-Latscha B: Neutrophil-derived oxidants and proteinases as immunomodulatory mediators in inflammation. *Mediat Inflamm* 3: 257, 1994

122. Horl WH, Riegel W, Steinhauer HB et al.: Granulocyte activation during hemodialysis. *Clin Nephrol* 26 (Suppl 1): 30, 1986

123. Ritchey EE, Wallin JD, Shah SV: Chemiluminescence and superoxide anion production by leukocytes from chronic hemodialysis patients. *Kidney Int* 19: 349, 1981

124. Nguyen AT, Lethias C, Zingraff J, Herbelin A, Naret C, Descamps-Latscha B: Hemodialysis membrane-induced activation of phagocyte oxidative metabolism detected *in vivo* and *in vitro* within microamounts of whole blood. *Kidney Int* 28: 158, 1985

125. Descamps-Latscha B, Herbelin A, Nguyen AT, Urena P: Respective influence of uremia and hemodialysis on whole blood phagocyte oxidative metabolism, and circulating interleukin-1 and tumor necrosis factor. *Adv Exp Med Biol* 297: 183, 1991

126. Richard MJ, Arnaud J, Jurkowitz C, Hachache T, Mefrahi H, Laporte F, Foret M, Favier A, Cordonnier D: Trace elements and lipid peroxidation abnormalities in patients with chronic renal failure. *Nephron* 57: 10, 1991

127. Giardini O, Taccone-Gallucci M, Lubrano R et al.: Evidence of red blood cell membrane lipid peroxidation in hemodialysis patients. *Nephron* 36: 235, 1984

128. Kikuchi Y, Koyama T, Koyama Y et al.: Red blood cell deformability in renal failure. *Nephron* 30: 8, 1982

129. Remuzzi G, Benigni A, Dodesini P et al.: Reduced platelet thromboxane formation in uremia: evidence for a cyclo-oxygenase defect. *J Clin Invest* 71: 762, 1983

130. Halliwell B: Oxidants and human disease: some new concepts. *FASEB J* 1: 358, 1987

131. Petrone WF, English DK, Wong K, McCord JM: Free radicals and inflammation: superoxide-dependent activation of a neutrophil chemotactic factor in plasma. *Proc Natl Acad Sci USA* 77: 1159, 1980

132. Carp H, Janoff A: *In vitro* suppression of serum elastase-inhibitory capacity by reactive oxygen species generated by phagocytosing polymorphonuclear leukocytes. *J Clin Invest* 63: 793, 1979

133. Weiss SJ, Peppin G, Ortiz X, Ragsdale C, Test ST: Oxidative autoactivation of latent collagenase by human neutrophils. *Science* 227: 747, 1985

134. Del Maestro RF: An approach to free radicals in medicine and biology. *Acta Physiol Scand Suppl* 492: 153, 1980

135. Memmos DE, Eastwood JB, Harris E, de Wardener HE: The 'shrinking man' syndrome. *Nephron* 30: 106, 1982

136. Himmerfarb J, Zaoui P, Hakim R: Modulation of granulocyte LAM-1 and MAC-1 during dialysis. A prospective, randomized controlled trial. *Kidney Int* 41: 388, 1992

137. Thylen P, Lundahl J, Fernvik E, Hed J, Svenson SB, Jacobson SH: Mobilization of an intracellular glycoprotein (Mac-1) on monocytes and granulocytes during hemodialysis. *Am J Nephrol* 12: 393, 1992

138. Tielemans CL, Delville JP, Husson CP et al.: Adhesion molecules and leukocyte common antigen on monocytes and granulocytes during hemodialysis. *Clin Nephrol* 39: 158, 1993

139. Vanholder R, Ringoir S, Dhondt A, Hakim R: Phagocytosis in uremic and hemodialysis: a prospective and cross sectional study. *Kidney Int* 39: 320, 1991

140. Lewis SL, Van Epps DE, Chenoweth DE: C5a receptor modulation on neutrophils and monocytes from chronic hemodialysis and peritoneal dialysis patients. *Clin Nephrol* 26: 37, 1986

141. Paczek L, Czarkowska B, Schaefer L, Schaefer RM, Heidland A: Effect of beta 2-microglobulin on immunoglobulin production. *Immunol Lett* 33: 87, 1992

142. Vanholder R, De Smet R, Hsu C, Vogeleere P, Ringoir S: Uremic toxicity. The middle molecule hypothesis revisited. *Seminars in Nephrol* 14: 205, 1994

143. Osaki K, Otsuka H, Uomizu K, Harada R, Otsuji Y, Hashimoto S: Monocyte-mediated suppression of mitogen responses of lymphocytes in uremic patients. *Nephron* 34: 87, 1983

144. Ruddy MC, Rubin AL, Novogrodsky A, Stenzel KH: Decreased macrophage-mediated suppression of lymphocyte activation in chronic renal failure. *Am J Med* 75: 571, 1983

145. Ruiz P, Gomez F, Schreiber AD: Impaired function of macrophage Fc receptors in end-stage renal disease. *N Engl J Med* 322: 717, 1990

146. Henderson LW, Koch KM, Dinarello CA, Shaldon S: Hemodialysis hypotension: the interleukin hypothesis. *Blood Purif* 1: 3, 1983

147. Dinarello CA: Cytokines: agents provocateurs in hemodialysis? *Kidney Int* 41: 683, 1992

148. Lonnemann G, Van Der Meer JW, Cannon JG et al.: Induction of tumor necrosis factor during extracorporeal blood purification letter. *N Engl J Med* 317: 963, 1987

149. Herbelin A, Nguyen AT, Zingraff J, Urena P, Descamps-Latscha B: Influence of uremia and hemodialysis on circulating interleukin-1 and tumor necrosis factor alpha. *Kidney Int* 37: 116, 1990

150. Herbelin A, Urena P, Nguyen AT, Zingraff J, Descamps-Latscha B: Elevated circulating levels of interleukin-6 in patients with chronic renal failure. *Kidney Int* 39: 954, 1991

151. Cavaillon JM, Poignet JL, Fitting C, Delons S: Serum interleukin-6 in long-term hemodialyzed patients. *Nephron* 60: 307, 1992

152. Powell AC, Bland LE, Oettinger CW et al.: Lack of plasma interleukin-1 beta or tumor necrosis factor-alpha elevation during unfavorable hemodialysis conditions. *J Am Soc Nephrol* 2: 1007, 1991

153. Haran N, Bar-Khayim Y, Frensdorff A, Barnard G: Tumor necrosis factor (TNF alpha) binding protein: interference in immunoassays of TNF alpha. *Kidney Int* 40: 1166, 1991

154. Haeffner-Cavaillon N, Cavaillon JM, Ciancioni C, Bacle F, Delons S, Kazatchkine MD: *In vivo* induction of interleukin-1 during hemodialysis. *Kidney Int* 35: 1212, 1989

155. Herbelin A, Urena P, Nguyen AT, Zingraff J, Descamps-Latscha B: Influence of first and long-term dialysis on uraemia-associated increased basal production of interleukin-1 and tumour necrosis factor alpha by circulating monocytes. *Nephrol Dial Transplant* 6: 349, 1991

156. Schindler R, Linnenweber S, Schulze M et al.: Gene expression of interleukin-1 beta during hemodialysis. *Kidney Int* 43: 712, 1993

157. Roccatello D, D'Alfonso S, Peruccio D et al.: Induction of mRNA for tumor necrosis factor alpha in hemodialysis. *Kidney Int* 39 (Suppl): 144S, 1993

158. Pertosa G, Gesualdo L, Tarantino EA, Ranieri E, Bottalico D, Schena FP: Influence of hemodialysis on interleukin-6 production and gene expression by peripheral blood mononuclear cells. *Kidney Int* 39 (Suppl): 149S, 1993

159. Dinarello CA: Interleukin-1 and tumor necrosis factor and their naturally occurring antagonists during hemodialysis. *Kidney Int* 38 (Suppl): 68S, 1992

160. Brockhaus M, Bar-Khayim Y, Gurwicz S, Frensdorff A, Haran N: Plasma tumor necrosis factor soluble receptors in chronic renal failure. *Kidney Int* 42: 663, 1992

161. Pereira BJG, Shapiro L, King AJ, Falagas ME, Strom JA, Dinarello CA. Plasma levels of IL-1 beta, TNF alpha and their specific inhibitors in undialyzed chronic renal failure, CAPD and hemodialysis patients. *Kidney Int* 45: 890, 1994

162. Descamps-Latscha B, Herbelin A, Nguyen AT et al.: Balance between IL-1β, TNFα, and their specific inhibitors in chronic renal failure and maintenance dialysis. *J Immunol* 154: 882, 1995

163. Sunder-Plassmann G, Sedlacek PL, Sunder-Plassmann R et al.: Anti-interleukin-1 alpha autoantibodies in hemodialysis patients. *Kidney Int* 40: 787, 1991

164. Lonnemann G, Behme TC, Lenzner B et al.: Permeability of dialyzer membranes to TNF alpha-inducing substances derived from water bacteria. *Kidney Int* 42: 61, 1992

165. Haeffner-Cavaillon N, Jahns G, Poignet JL, Kazatchkine MD: Induction of interleukin-1 during hemodialysis. *Kidney Int* 39 (Suppl): 139S, 1993

166. Kumano K, Yokota S, Nanbu M, Sakai T: Do cytokine-inducing substances penetrate through dialysis membranes and stimulate monocytes. *Kidney Int* 43 (Suppl): 205S, 1993

167. Urena P, Herbelin A, Zingraff J et al.: Permeability of cellulosic and non-cellulosic membranes to endotoxin subunits and cytokine production during *in-vitro* haemodialysis. *Nephrol Dial Transplant* 7: 16, 1992

168. Mege JL, Olmer M, Purgus R et al.: Haemodialysis membranes modulate chronically the production of TNF alpha, IL-1 beta and IL-6. *Nephrol Dial Transplant* 6: 868, 1991

169. Cala S, Maozuran R, Kordic D: Negative effect of uraemia and cuprophane haemodialysis on natural killer cells. *Nephrol Dial Transplant* 5: 437, 1990

170. Zaoui P, Hakim R: Natural killer cell function in hemodialysis patients: effect of the dialysis membrane. *Kidney Int* 43: 1298, 1993

HOST DEFENSES AND INFECTIOUS COMPLICATIONS IN MAINTENANCE HEMODIALYSIS PATIENTS

ANN RINEHART, ALLAN J. COLLINS and WILLIAM F. KEANE

INTRODUCTION

Prior to the advent of chronic hemodialysis, infection was a frequent terminal or pre-terminal event in patients with end-stage renal disease (ESRD). During the 1960s–1970s chronic hemodialysis therapy infectious complications resulted in significant morbidity and mortality, with up to one-third of deaths being attributable to infections (1–5). Despite improvement in dialysis and medical therapies, infection continues to account for a significant proportion (11 to 36%) of deaths in the chronic dialysis population (6–14). While this increased risk of infection is due to, in part, the necessity of blood access and/or complications of their underlying disease, there are abnormalities of the immune system in ESRD patients which may contribute to their predilection for infectious complications. In this chapter, we will review the incidence and types of infectious complications which occur in patients undergoing chronic hemodialysis, as well as outline our current understanding of the immune status of the dialysis patient. Quite importantly, the vast majority of infections are due to commonly occurring organisms, not opportunistic or unusual organisms, and repetitive exposure to infectious risk factors impacts on the types of infections observed.

UREMIA AS AN IMMUNOCOMPROMISED STATE

Several historic and more recent observations serve to outline the variety of immunologic perturbations of uremia. A delay in the rejection of both renal and skin allografts has been demonstrated in human as well as experimental uremic models (15–19). Clinically, an abnormal response to the hepatitis B virus, as evidenced by a milder but more prolonged infection and a higher incidence of chronic hepatitis, is well documented (20–23). A purported increase in the incidence of malignancy in ESRD patients has also been attributed to decreased immune system surveillance (24–27). Lastly, amelioration of the clinical manifestations of systemic lupus erythematosus in uremic and chronic hemodialysis patients suggests an alteration in immune system function (28). In addition to these clinical observations, numerous *in vivo* and *in vitro* tests have characterized the nature of the underlying mechanisms of these phenomena. Table 1 summarizes the results of the various studies used to define the alterations observed in the immunologic responsiveness of the uremic patient.

Humoral immunity

Serum levels of immunoglobulins A, G and M have generally been reported as normal (29–31), despite a consistently observed decrease in the B-lymphocyte cell population

Table 1. Immunology of uremia

	Result
Humoral immunity	
Immunoglobulin levels	N
Vaccination response	N, ↓
In vitro B cell response	↓
Lymphocyte function	
Lymphocyte number	↓
Blastogenic response	N, ↓
Cutaneous hypersensitivity	N, ↓
Cytokine production	↓
Helper/Suppressor ratios	N
Suppressor cell activity	N, ↑
Killer cell activity	N, ↓
Macrophage function	
Macrophage number	N, ↓
Phagocytosis	N, ↓
Mobility	N, ↓
Antigen presentation	↓
Suppressor activity	↑, ↓
Polymorphonuclear cell function	
PMN number	N
Chemotaxis	N, ↓
Adherence	↑
Phagocytosis	N, ↓
Intracellular killing	N, ↓

(29, 32, 33). This decline in B cell numbers may correct with initiation of dialysis (31, 32). An increased incidence of autoantibodies has been reported in dialysis patients, suggesting an intact humoral immune system (30, 34). In some cases, these autoantibodies are thought to be secondary to the hemodialysis procedure, such as anti-N-like antibodies from formaldehyde exposure or antinuclear antigen antibodies presumably secondary to repetitive exposure to nuclear material entrapped on the dialysis membrane (35–38). However, they are also present in the peritoneal dialysis population (34).

Although early studies of vaccination responses using tetanus or diphtheria toxoid suggested near normal antibody responses (39, 40), recent experience indicates that the uremic patient is less humorally responsive. Antibody levels after typhoid toxin or keyhole limpet hemocyanin are reduced (41–44). Antibody responses to influenza vaccine are generally comparable to controls (45–47), although one report showed a reduced response with severe uremia (48). After standard pneumococcal vaccination, antibody responses can be detected in the majority of ESRD patients, but in lower titers than observed in normals (49, 50). These titers are not as long-lasting in

ESRD patients receiving dialysis therapy, and antibody titers fall to unprotective levels more quickly (51, 52). In spite of recommendations to the contrary from the Center for Disease Control (53), some groups are recommending re-vaccination against pneumococci and have reported a low incidence of adverse reactions to re-vaccination (54). Hepatitis B vaccination has also resulted in an antibody response which is less than that seen in normal subjects (55–57). However, with the use of more potent vaccine, more frequent dosing schedules, or additional doses, higher rates of antibody response can be achieved (58–60), although antibody titers are not sustained (61, 62). Potentially underlying these abnormal responses, a decrease in IgG production by B lymphocytes from both uremic and hemodialyzed patients has been demonstrated *in vitro* (31, 32, 63–65).

One proposed mechanism for decreased humoral activity implicates elevated parathyroid hormone (PTH) levels generally found in chronic dialysis patients. PTH receptors have been found on B cells cultured from patients with Hodgkin's disease, acute leukemia, Burkitt's lymphoma and thymic hyperplasia. Gaciong et al. have demonstrated that IgG, IgA, and IgM production is suppressed in cultured B cells from dialysis patients versus controls. Both the intact molecule and N-terminal fragment of PTH inhibit B cell immunoglobulin production in normals and dialysis patients and only occurs with the hormone added at the initiation of the B cell culture, presumably affecting the initial stages of B cell proliferation and maturation. PTH may act through increased cAMP production, increasing cytosolic calcium in B cells (66).

In summary, humoral responses in dialysis patients are diminished compared to non-uremic subjects, both clinically and experimentally. Hyperparathyroidism is one potential etiology, but other factors are likely contributory.

Lymphocyte function

Delayed hypersensitivity as evaluated by skin testing is decreased to a variety of antigens in both dialyzed and uremic patients (30, 41, 43, 44, 67, 68). Patients with cutaneous anergy may have a normal cellular *in vitro* response to these antigens, indicating that the lack of reactivity is not due to an absence of antigen specificity (68).

A moderate decline in lymphocyte numbers involving both the B cell and T cell lines has generally been observed in ESRD patients (29–32, 68, 69). While the mechanism of this lymphopenia is unclear, with maintenance dialysis the lymphopenia may improve (33). The presence of lymphopenia has led to the suggestion that the defect in cell-mediated immunity is secondary to a decrease in cell numbers (41, 70). However, under conditions of equal cell numbers, the blastogenic response of uremic lymphocytes in autologous plasma to interleukin-2, mitogen stimulation (e.g., concanavalin-A or phytohemagglutinin), or to mixed lymphocyte culture has generally been observed to

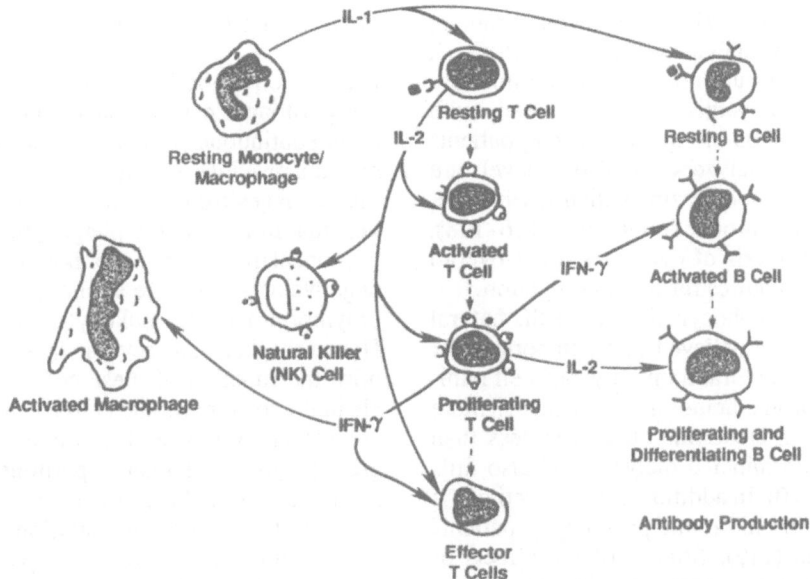

Figure 1. Cytokine pathways for immunomodulation. See text for detailed explanation. (IL= interleukin, IFN = interferon). From Fauci AS, Rosenberg SA, Sherwin SA, Dinarello CA, Longo DL, Lane HC: Immunomodulators in clinical medicine. *Ann Intern Med* 106: 421, 1987.

be decreased compared to non-uremic controls (67, 69, 71–74). In the majority of studies, uremic plasma suppresses normal T cell responses when tested *in vitro* (29, 73–78), and uremic cells function abnormally even when cultured in non-uremic plasma (29, 31, 58, 64, 71, 78, 79). Improvement of responses after dialysis or transplantation suggests that these changes are due to the uremic milieu (31, 44, 67, 69, 76). In this regard, middle molecules, such as guanidine derivatives, have been shown to suppress T cell function *in vivo* (80–83). Suppressive plasma factors, such as a very low density lipoprotein, have also been identified in experimental models of uremia (84–86). Thus, evidence supports both an inhibitory effect of uremic plasma and an intrinsic cellular defect as being responsible for the T cell dysfunction observed.

The presence of adherent cells in isolated lymphocyte preparations from rat models first suggested that abnormalities of immunologic cell/cell interaction may account for decreased lymphocyte responsiveness (87–89). Despite a decreased absolute number of helper cells in ESRD patients, the helper/suppressor T cell ratio, as determined by monoclonal antibodies, is unchanged (90–93). Suppressor T cells appear to be more active in these patients with their removal using OKT8 monoclonal antibodies improving lymphocyte mitogenic response (94, 95). Alternatively, depletion of monocyte/macrophage cells from cultures also improves lymphocyte responses (65, 96, 97). Arachidonic acid metabolites play a role in macrophage/lymphocyte immunomodulation, and inhibition of prostaglandin production with indomethacin alters lymphocyte blastogenic responses *in vitro* (96, 98). This supports the premise that the macrophage may be a

key factor in suppressing lymphocyte function in ESRD patients and is of even greater interest as the number of macrophages in end-stage renal disease patients is frequently increased (90, 91, 99).

Biochemical signaling between cells of the immune system is known to be important in their regulation (Figure 1). Production of these crucial cytokines appears to be altered in the uremic state. Interferon, necessary for optimal activation of macrophages, B lymphocytes and cytotoxic T cells, is produced in reduced amounts *in vitro* by lymphocytes from both uremic and hemodialyzed patients (100, 101). The production of interleukin-2, which serves to activate B cell antibody production, T cell differentiation, and natural killer cells, is also low in mitogen stimulated lymphocytes from hemodialyzed individuals (93). Interleukin 1 (IL-1), tumor necrosis factor α (TNFα) and interleukin-6 (IL-6) levels are all elevated in chronic hemodialysis patients. IL-1 production is stimulated during hemodialysis as detected by increased amounts of IL-1 β mRNA in peripheral blood monocytes(PBMC) leaving the dialyzer within five minutes of initiating hemodialysis. The increase in IL-1β mRNA has been significantly correlated with the increase in activated complement C5$_a$, with less complement-activating dialyzers, (polysulfone, hemophan, polyamide, or polyacrilonitrile) resulting in no detectable IL-1β mRNA production (102). Lipopolysaccharide (LPS) and acetate dialysate also stimulate IL-1 production, with the combination of LPS and C5$_a$ synergistic in its stimulation (103–110). TNFα secretion from PBMC rises in response to LPS *in vitro* in hemodialysis but not in CAPD patients, with the latter having the same response as controls (111). Higher basal TNFα levels which increase after dialysis are also found among patients using cuprophane dialyzers (112–114). Although their clinical relevance is currently unclear, plasma levels of TNF soluble receptors increase progressively with declining renal function and are highest among patients treated with cuprophane dialyzers (115). IL-6 levels are also elevated in uremic non-dialyzing patients, with LPS and $C5_a$ stimulating their production *in vitro* (116–118). Despite these elevated levels of cytokines, their overall biological significance requires further investigation.

The final arm of the lymphocyte network is the natural killer (NK) cell, which is believed to be important for tumor surveillance and antiviral immunity. NK cell number is decreased in chronic hemodialysis patients, more so than in patients with creatinine clearances less than 10 ml/min who had not initiated dialysis, and also falls during dialysis (119, 120). In addition, NK cell activity is also suppressed similarly in uremic pre-dialysis patients and in CAPD patients (119). Studies of the effects of dialyzer membrane type are conflicting. In two studies, cuprophane dialyzers decreased NK cell function (119, 121), while another study showed no effect of cuprophane versus an open membrane dialyzer (78). NK cell response to Il-2 is also depressed in chronic hemodialysis patients compared with healthy controls, and uremic sera also suppresses NK cell activity (78).

Thus, considerable evidence attests to functional abnormalities of lymphocytes and their decreased number in ESRD patients. These abnormalities appear to relate not only to intrinsic cellular defects due to the uremic milieu, but also to abnormal intercellular interactions and altered production of various cytokines.

Mononuclear phagocytic system function

The mononuclear phagocytic system, which includes circulating monocytes, activated macrophages, and resident macrophages of the reticuloendothelial system, has not been extensively studied in uremic or chronic hemodialysis patients. Responsible for antigen presentation to the lymphocyte, phagocytic activity, and immunomodulation, the mononuclear cell has a pivotal role in the immune system cascade. The phagocytic activity of macrophages from hemodialyzed patients is depressed as measured by the Rebuck window technique (122, 123), with ingestion of IgG coated red cells being decreased *in vitro* (124). Incubation of normal macrophages in uremic serum, specifically the high molecular weight fraction, also results in impaired phagocytic activity (125, 126). In experimental models and in hemodialyzed patients reportedly there is abnormal presentation of antigen to the T cell (127, 128). A decrease in C_{5a} binding by monocytes is demonstrated in both hemodialysis and peritoneal dialysis patients, suggesting that chronic complement activation (as evidenced by elevated plasma C_{3a}) may activate these cells and make them less responsive to infection (129).

Peritoneal macrophages

Elucidation of the pathogenetic mechanisms operative in the peritoneal cavity that could contribute to peritonitis in continuous ambulatory peritoneal dialysis (CAPD) patients provides a unique opportunity to evaluate tissue macrophages from uremic patients. *In vitro* studies suggest that in general the phagocytic capabilities of human peritoneal macrophages for both gram-positive and gram-negative organisms are similar to those of normal human polymorphonuclear leukocytes or monocytes (130–132). However, there are several factors that might compromise the function of these cells *in vivo*. Since IgG levels in the local peritoneal environment of CAPD patients are extremely low, and IgG is the principal opsonin for gram-positive organisms, peritoneal macrophages may not phagocytize these organisms. Likewise, due to low levels of C_3, opsonic recognition of gram-negative bacteria is impeded. (C_{3b}, the opsonic fragment of C_3, is a key opsonin for gram-negative bacteria). The low pH and high osmolality of dialysis solutions may also temporarily impair phagocytic cell function (133, 134). Low cytosolic calcium levels in peritoneal macrophages result in decreased macrophage superoxide production, leukotriene release, and bactericidal activity against *S epidermidis in vitro*. These abnormalities then reverse with incubation of the macrophages with high calcium levels and 1,25 dihydroxy Vitamin D (135, 136). Clinically, 1,25 mmol/l calcium dialysate is associated with an increased incidence of *S epidermidis* peritonitis compared with 1.75 mmol/l calcium dialysate (137). In addition to these deficits in opsonization, experimental data suggest that the ability of the peritoneal macrophage to kill certain strains of *S aureus, S epidermidis* as well as fungal organisms, such as *Candida albicans*, may be impaired (134, 138–142). Despite the presence of preopsonized organisms, effluent dialysate from infected patients also impairs neutrophil killing, suggesting the presence of an inhibitor. These combined deficits of opsonic molecules, as well as altered intracellular killing of these microorganisms, have been prospectively correlated with an increased incidence of clinical peritonitis in CAPD patients (143, 144). Intracellular bacterial sequestration without killing may offer bacteria protection from antibiotics and could explain peritonitis relapses (134, 142).

Polymorphonuclear cell function

Despite the demonstration of a granulopoietic inhibitor in the serum of uremic patients, neutrophil numbers in chronic renal failure and hemodialysis patients are generally reported to be normal to slightly elevated (145–147). This contrasts with the profound complement-mediated leukopenia demonstrated immediately after the initiation of hemodialysis (148). In addition, leukocyte response to acute infection may be blunted, and *in vivo* studies of neutrophil response are mixed, with a normal neutrophil inflammatory response being observed using the Rebuck window technique, but not with the intradermal or subcutaneous injection of urate crystals (123, 149–151). *In vitro*, polymorphonuclear cell functions are generally observed to be abnormal. Granulocyte adherence, the first step in neutrophil migration, is normal in undialyzed uremic patients but is abnormal in hemodialysis patients (152, 153). Decreased neutrophil chemotaxis is noted in untreated uremic patients, as well as in those treated by either peritoneal or hemodialysis, although the chemotactic response is more severely impaired in the hemodialyzed group (154–157). This defect is due to both an intrinsic cellular defect as well as to a circulating inhibitory factor. This serum factor has been further identified to be directed at C_{5a} mediated chemotaxis (158). Intrinsic cellular unresponsiveness to complement-mediated chemotaxis may be secondary to decreased C_{5a} receptor availability on polymorphonuclear leukocytes (129). This decrease in C_{5a} receptors is noted even in CAPD patients, suggesting that the apparent down-regulation of receptors is not just hemodialysis-associated but may be related to the uremic state as well. Levamisole has been shown to restore chemotaxis in uremic granulocytes to normal levels through unestablished mechanisms. Perhaps it may displace plasma factors bound to uremic granulocyte cell membrane receptors, permitting full expression of chemoattractant activity, or it may also restore the abnormally decreased intracellular cyclic GMP/cyclic AMP ratio (159).

Studies of the phagocytic capacity of neutrophils in uremia have been conflicting. Normal and depressed phagocytic activity has been seen in neutrophils from either uremic or hemodialyzed patients *in vitro* when studied either in uremic or in normal serum (29, 152, 154, 160–167). Decreased phagocytic activity, as manifested by reduced glucose uptake, oxygen consumption, and lactate production, has been correlated with several variables (167, 168). Elevated serum phosphorus levels have been implicated with the abnormality correcting after their normalization (161). In another study, a low-phosphorus, low-protein diet supplemented with ketoanalogues and essential amino acids resulted in marked improvement of phagocytosis (167). Vanholder et al. found that impaired phagocytosis *in vitro* was most highly correlated with time on dialysis and hematocrit. The PTH level was also a significant factor but was also highly correlated with time on dialysis, and may, therefore, not be an independent risk factor (169). In a different study, Vanholder et al. noted that phagocytic response was decreased to approximately half that of normal controls among pre-dialysis patients with serum creatinine levels > 6 mg/dl. In 15 patients prospectively followed from initiation of hemodialysis, the use of a cuprophane dialyzer further depressed the metabolic response to phagocytosis by 60%, while use of a synthetic membrane did not have any effect upon phagocytosis. After crossing over to the synthetic membranes, the phagocytic response then returned to baseline

pre-dialysis levels (170). Cuprophane dialyzers have been shown to induce a marked increase in C_{3a} antigen levels, which correlate with an elevated basal chemiluminescence response and a dramatic decrease in the chemiluminescence response to stimulating agents. Synthetic polyacrilonitrile membranes have evoked no such responses (171). Single hemodialysis sessions have also been shown to improve the phagocytic uptake of IgG coated particles to supranormal levels but this effect has not been correlated with any particular serum biochemical change (163). Iron overload also impairs phagocytosis that is not overcome by the provision of adequate opsonins, suggesting an effect directly on these phagocytic cells (164, 165). Following erythropoetin administration to hemodialysis patients with transfusional hemosiderosis, phagocytosis has improved as iron overload resolves (165).

The intracellular killing of PMNs, essential for combatting catalase-positive organisms, such as *S aureus*, *E Coli*, *Klebsiella aerogenes*, *Pseudomas aerguinosa*, *Proteus mirabilis*, and *Candida* species, is also impaired in hemodialysis patients (163–166). The production of hydrogen peroxide, a measure of respiratory burst activity and hence, intracellular killing ability, is reduced pre-dialysis but is improved, albeit to subnormal levels, immediately post-dialysis. After 2–3 days, the dysfunction recurs. CAPD and post-dialysis patients have similar degrees of PMN dysfunction, while there is little difference between uremic non-hemodialysis and control PMN hydrogen peroxide production. However, an inverse correlation is found between the hydrogen peroxide production and serum creatinine and BUN levels in pre-dialysis chronic renal failure patients (163). Iron overload also impairs neutrophilic killing and has specifically been studied in *Yersinia enterocolitica*. Killing is decreased in iron overloaded dialysis patients compared with normals and non-iron overloaded dialysis patients, but only in the presence of autologous serum (164, 165). Treatment with erythropoetin, with a reduction in iron overload, improves intracellular killing after 6 months (165). In this regard, recent studies suggest that higher hematocrits achieved with EPO are associated with a reduced infection-related mortality (see Mortality section).

Effects of nutrition

Protein calorie malnutrition, increased in prevalence in the dialysis population, has been demonstrated to produce lymphopenia, decreased lymphocyte function, and abnormal neutrophil function (168, 172–174). Amino acid losses during dialysis and decreased overall dietary intake have been implicated (175, 176). Indeed, the immune abnormalities of uremia bear a striking resemblance to those of malnutrition (176, 177). Clinically, malnutrition has been linked to increased infection-related hospitalization and death of dialysis patients and decreased lymphocyte function (178–181). The reversal of skin test anergy and lymphopenia have been demonstrated in two patients after three months of protein and calorie supplementation (182).

Other nutritional factors have also been studied. Vitamin B_6 deficiencies have been associated with an impairment of immune function, with low levels found in hemodialysis patients. Improvements in polymorphonuclear phagocytic activity and improved lymphocyte response to mitogens have been demonstrated with B_6 supplementation (183). Severe zinc deficiency can widely impair immune system function, and improvements in delayed hypersensitivity, mitogen-induced lymphocyte blastogenesis, and granulocyte mobility have been seen with zinc therapy in hemodialysis patients (184–186). Thus, nutritional abnormalities related to uremia and hemodialysis may contribute to abnormalities of immune function, but their relative contribution has not been clearly defined. However, recent studies have suggested that reduced albumin levels, an index of nutritional status, are associated with increased infection-related mortality (see Mortality section).

Effects of transfusion

Improved allograft survival has been reported in patients who have received multiple transfusions (187, 188). Improved graft survival in multiply transfused patients suggests a defect in cell mediated immunity secondary to transfusion. A comparison of previously transfused to non-transfused hemodialysis patients demonstrates a significant difference in the degree of lymphopenia, with the transfused patients showing the most marked lymphopenia (189). Lymphocytes from multiply transfused patients show a reduced mixed lymphocyte culture reactivity and a decreased phytohemagglutinin response. A decline in mixed lymphocyte culture response has been demonstrated immediately after transfusion in ESRD patients (190, 191). Individuals with greater than five transfusions compared to those with less than five blood transfusions demonstrated a significant difference in response to a battery of tests including spontaneous blastogenesis, mixed lymphocyte culture (MLC) and delayed cutaneous hypersensitivity (192). Importantly, this correlated significantly with graft survival.

The nature of this suppressive effect appears to be multifactorial. Anti-HLA antibodies produced by the non-specific stimulation of B cells in lymphocyte preparations could interfere with stimulated responses, and depletion of B cells from mixed lymphocyte cultures restores MLC reactivity to the normal range (190). This suggests that non-specific production of anti-HLA antibodies could have an immunosuppressive effect. Induction of suppressor cell activity has also been observed after blood transfusions in hemodialysis patients (192–195). Helper/suppressor ratios are also decreased in multiply transfused dialysis patients (189–192). Monocytes from patients with multiple transfusions demonstrate enhanced lymphocyte-suppressive activity, and treatment of cell preparations with indomethacin or radiation reduces transfusion induced suppression, further suggesting monocyte involvement in the induced suppression (192, 196, 197).

It is, therefore, intriguing to speculate whether many of the abnormalities of the ESRD patient's immune system are, in part, secondary to the tranfusions they receive. This, coupled with the interactions of nutrition factors, uremic toxins, differing dialysis techniques, and varying states of iron overload, may account for the tremendous heterogeneity observed in the immune responses of ESRD patients.

REVIEW OF INFECTIOUS COMPLICATIONS IN HEMODIALYSIS PATIENTS

Patient population

Only a few centers have attempted to longitudinally following chronic hemodialysis patients for the development of infectious complications. Four studies are noteworthy. The Canadian Hemodialysis Morbidity Study Group evaluated 496 patients for 18 months after initiation of hemodialysis who survived at least one month (181). Kessler et al. followed 1455 chronic hemodialysis patients in France from September 1989 to February 1990 (198). In Belgium, Goldman and Vanherweghem reported on two patient cohorts; 380 patients from 1965 to 1978, representing 6638 patient months, and 150 patients between 1979 to 1985, representing 5,280 patient-months (199). Keane et al. retrospectively analyzed 455 patients who survived one month on dialysis over a 42 month period between 1972 to 1975. They provided a total of 8,105 patient-months, 7,202 patient-months for non-diabetics and 903 patient-months for diabetics (200). Keane et al. reported a similar retrospective study for a 36 month period from 1982 to 1985. This study included 851 patients with a total of 15,486 patient-months; 569 non-diabetic and 282 diabetic hemodialysis patients with 10,729 and 4,757 patient-months, respectively (201). These four studies describe the types of infections experienced in the hemodialysis population worldwide, while the Minnesota/Belgium studies also attempt to identify time trends in infectious complications.

Mortality

Infection accounts for a significant proportion of deaths in hemodialysis patients. Early studies reported that between 12 to 38% of deaths were infection-related (1–8), and this frequency has remained relatively unchanged in recent reports (6, 9–14, 202–204). Two centers have attempted to analyze time trends in infectious death rates. Mailloux et al. reported on 532 patients from 1970 to 1985 and found that the infectious death rate fell from 44.4% from 1970–1973 to 21.6% from 1982–1985 (9). Keane et al.

reported that 19.8% of deaths were directly attributable to infection in the 1970s (200) and that 15.9% deaths seen from 1982–1985 were primarily caused by infection (201). Thus, a rate of 2.1 deaths/1,000 patient-months was observed in the Keane et al. 1980s series, lower, but not dramatically different than an incidence of 2.7/1,000 patient-months in their 1970s series.

Several risk factors for infectious deaths have been identified. Kjellstrand et al. have noted that proportionately more deaths are attributable to infectious diseases with greater time on dialysis, while the cardiovascular death rate decreases. In the same study, regardless of age, patients without any comorbid conditions at initiation were also more likely to experience an infectious death, while those with comorbidities more commonly died from cardiovascular causes (12). Mailloux et al. have reported that in their 16 year follow-up of 532 dialysis patients, the risk of infectious deaths increased with greater age at initiation of dialysis, but the impact of comorbidities on cause of death was not assessed (9). Keane et al. also identified advanced age at dialysis initiation to be a risk factor for infectious deaths (200, 201). Diabetes mellitus as the cause of ESRD was also a very important risk factor for infectious disease deaths (9, 200, 201). In Keane et al.'s 1970s and 1980s series, diabetic infection-related deaths were 4.4 and 2.7 deaths/1,000 patient-months, respectively. In comparison, non-diabetic infection-related deaths were 2.5 and 0.9 deaths/1,000 patient-months. Thus, infection-related deaths were two to three-fold more likely in diabetic patients.

More recently, low serum albumin concentration and hematocrit have been identified as risk factors for infectious deaths. Collins et al. have quantitated the relative risk for an infectious death among diabetics and non-diabetics with a serum albumin concentration $\leq$ 3.5 g/dl versus those with > 3.5 g/dl to be 3.24 and 4.23, respectively (205). Both were highly statistically significant. In the same study, Collins et al. also found that a serum hematocrit less than 29% was associated with a relative risk of infectious death of 2.51 in diabetics and 1.81 in non-diabetics (205).

Comparing the two series from Keane et al., the most common sources of infectious deaths have changed little over the last decade (Table 2). Access-related infection, pulmonary and intra-abdominal sepsis predominated in both series, with documented bacteremia being present in approximately half of the cases. The average length of time from the initiation of dialysis to infection-related death was 25 months in the earlier study, and 42 months in the later review (200, 201).

Bacteremia

Incidence

Bacteremia has been reported to occur with a prevalence of 3.8 to 20% in chronic hemodialysis patients (1, 181, 198–200, 206, 207). In the Keane et al. studies, bac-

teremia was defined as one or more positive blood cultures not felt to be a contaminant, based on clinical evidence of infection, such as fever, rigors, elevated white count or localizing symptoms. Using these criteria, their 1972 to 1975 study revealed 124 episodes of bacteremia in 91 patients over a 42 month period (200). This represents an incidence of 15.3 episodes of bacteremia per 1,000 patient-months and a prevalence of 20%. Incidences of 9.8–12.5 episodes/1,000 patient-months were reported by others during this same time period (199, 206). In comparison, the 36 month period in the 1980s demonstrated 97 episodes of bacteremia in 67 patients (201). This represents an incidence of 6.3/1,000 patient-months and a prevalence of 7.8%. These results suggest a reduction in the incidence of bacteremia in the Minnesota hemodialysis population over the course of the last 10 years. Other centers have reported incidences of 6.9–7.9 episodes/1,000 patient-months during this time (181, 198, 199).

Several risk factors for bacteremia have been noted in the Keane et al. 1970s experience. Diabetic patients developed bacteremia more often, with 32.1 episodes/1,000 patient-months versus only 13.2/1,000 patient-months in non-diabetic patients (200). In their follow-up period, minimal differences were found between diabetic and non-diabetic hemodialysis patients; indeed, diabetics had 4.6 episodes of bacteremia/1,000 patient-months while 6.0/1,000 patient-months were observed in non-diabetic patients (201). The Canadian Hemodialysis Study Group identified several risk factors for septicemia. For AV grafts compared to simple fistulae, the relative risk for sepsis was 5.85 (1.85 to 18.48). A serum albumin less than 3.0 g/dl carried a relative risk of 2.66 (1.31 to 5.39) compared with a serum albumin greater than 3.0 g/dl. The relative risk for septicemia for Native North American or Inuit persons was 3.83 (1.78 to 8.24) compared with non-aboriginals (181). Kessler et al. found that a surgical procedure within one month prior to sepsis was also a risk factor for bacteremia (198).

Infecting organisms

Gram-positive organisms have consistently been reported to be the most common infecting agent, accounting for 60–75% of isolates in the 1970s (199, 200, 206, 207). Few centers have published data on isolate distribution and time trends of infecting organisms. In all reported studies, gram-positive organisms predominate, although less dramatically in the two follow-up studies (Table 3). In the studies performed in the mid to late 1980s, gram-positive organisms account for 54 to 70% of the isolates.

Etiology of bacteremia

Access infection has been reported to account for 48–72% of all bacteremic episodes in hemodialysis patients in studies from the 1970s to early 1980s (200, 201, 206, 207). More recent studies would suggest that these findings have not changed (14, 198). In the ear-

Table 2. Association between primary site of infection and death

Source	(%) Blood access device	(%) Pulmonary	(%) Intra-abdominal	(%) Genitourinary	(%) Endocarditis[a]	(%) Meningitis	(%) Skin	(%) Other
1972–75 (n = 22) (201)	5	5	5	4	1	2	0	0
1982–85 (n = 32) (202)	8	7	7	2	2	0	2	4
Total (n = 54)	13 (24.1)[b]	12 (22.2)	12 (22.2)	6 (11.1)	3 (5.6)	2 (3.7)	2 (3.7)	4 (7.4)

[a]Does not include cases where endocarditis was felt to be secondary to another primary source such as access.
[b]Percent of all deaths.

Table 3. Isolates from bacteremic episodes

	Goldman (200)		Keane (201)	Keane (202)	Kessler (199)
	(1965–78)	(1979–85)	(1979–85)	(1972–75)	(1989–90)
Gram-positive organisms	–	–	95	53	44
S Aureus	53	11	40	24	39
S Epidermidis	0	9	30	7	3
Streptococcus sp	–	–	4	6	2
Listeria monocytogenes	1	1	2	1	–
Other gram-positive[a]	0	1	19	15	–
Gram-negative organisms	–	–	32	45	16
E Coli	15	17	16	18	12
Serratia sp	–	–	6	5	2
Pseudomonas sp	–	–	1	7	1
Other[b]	2	–	9	15	–
Anerobes Bacteroides fragilis	–	–	2	2	–
Miscellaneous	22	3	–	–	–

[a]Other gram-positive includes pneumococcus, enterococcus, bacillus sp and diphtheroids.
[b]Other gram-negative includes Klebsiella-Enterobacter, Proteus, Hemophilus, Eikenella corrodens, Achromobacter sp, and Citrobacter freundii.

ly 1970s, the access-related bacteremic rate was 8.5 episodes/1,000 patient-months, while in the 1980s, the rate fell to 3 episodes/1,000 patient-months. This change may be explained by the decreased use of the cannula as a blood access device, as these were responsible for 25% of access-related bacteremias (200, 201). Access-related bacteremic rates have again increased with the widespread usage of external silastic and polyethylene catheters, whose bacteremic rates have been reported to be 3.4–7.7/1,000 access-days (208–210).

S aureus is the predominant organism, accounting for 44–90% of all access-related bacteremias (198, 200, 201). In studies of external dialysis catheters, some series report *S aureus* to be the most common cause of bacteremia (210–214), while others note *S epidermidis* to be the most common isolate (208, 212, 215). Gram negative organisms account for approximately 10–34% of access septicemias (200, 201, 208, 210). Non-access related bac-

teremia appears to be responsible for 45% of total bacteremias in the 1970s (200). In subsequent series they contribute to 49–52% of all bacteremias, with the source unknown 32–44% of the time (198, 201). Non-access related sources were evenly dispersed among various sites in the Keane et al. series, but genitourinary sources predominated in the Kessler series (Table 4).

Mortality

Few centers have reported on bacteremic rates and associated mortality. The overall mortality from bacteremic episodes in Keane et al.'s 1970s series was 19 (15%) of 120 episodes (200). In comparison, in the 1980s study there were 14 deaths (14%) in 97 episodes (201). Kessler et al. have reported a bacteremia-related mortality of 6.3% (198). Mortality from access-related bacteremias also remains low; it was 10% in the Keane et al. 1970s

Table 4. Source of infection in access unrelated bacteremias

	Gastrointestinal tract (%)*	Genitourinary tract (%)*	Respiratory tract (%)*	Miscellaneous (skin, sinus, etc.) (%)*
1972–75 (n = 35) (201)†	12	7	7	9
1982–85 (n = 28) (202)†	6	10	7	5
Total (n = 63)	18 (29)*	17 (27)*	14 (22)*	14 (22)*
Kessler (199)*	3 (14)*	14 (67)*	0 (0)*	4 (19)*

*Percent of known sources. †Reference number.

study and 8.5% in the 1980s study, with other centers mortality rates being 0–7.7% (200, 201, 208, 209, 211).

Bacteriology

Gram-positive organisms, particularly S aureus, are the most common isolates (Table 3). One explanation for this finding is that 60% of hemodialysis patients have been shown to have S aureus colonization, a three-fold higher incidence than chronic renal failure patients not on dialysis (216). This appears to be specific to the hemodialysis patient, although the dialysis staff in the same unit have a colonization prevalence of 30%, which is several times higher than a normal healthy population. This high prevalence of staphylococcal carriage, not present at the initiation of dialysis, is acquired over the first several months (216). Cutaneous carrier states are significantly more likely to acquire staphylococcal access infections than non-carriers. With phage typing, the infecting organisms are identical to those present on the nose, throat, and skin, although it is unclear which site carries the highest risk of subsequent infection (213, 217–219). Methods aimed at decreasing this colonization, particularly the intermittent use of rifampin, have been shown to decrease shunt infections and bacteremia secondary to staphylococcal organisms (219). Nasal mupirocin ointment may also be of some benefit (220).

Numerous centers have identified dialysate fluid contamination to be a source of gram-negative bacteremia, with the most frequent culprits being Pseudomonas species. Xanthomonas maltophilia, Alcaligenes dentrificans, E casseliflavus (221–224). Despite dialysate bacterial counts substantially exceeding microbiologic standards in one center, bacteremia was a rare occurrence in 0.004% of hemodialysis runs, suggesting that dialysis membranes generally are effective barriers to bacteremia (221). However, colony counts less than microbiologic standards are not sufficient to prevent bacteremia. Incomplete mixing of the dialyzer sterilant appears to be a not infrequent cause of bacteremia (222, 224). Contamination of dialysis blood tubing with ultrafiltrate waste has also been implicated (223).

Complications of bacteremia

Several complications of bacteremia and access infection are well recognized in hemodialysis patients: bacterial endocarditis, osteomyelitis, septic arthritis and septic pulmonary emboli (200, 225–227). After a bacteremic episode, the incidence of a metastatic complication has been reported to be 10–27% (198, 200, 201). The potentially prolonged bacteremic state unique to access infections may contribute to the increased incidence of these otherwise unusual complications. In addition, the increased metabolic demands and catabolism of the septic state may have profound effects, especially if superimposed on a marginal nutritional status. Sepsis-related hypotension may further complicate the dialysis procedure itself at a time when dialysis requirements may be increased. The frequent onset of pericarditis after infection or surgery suggests that routine dialysis regimens may be inadequate during these hypermetabolic periods (228, 229).

Bacterial endocarditis

Only a few centers have compiled data on bacterial endocarditis in chronic dialysis patients. Early studies demonstrated a prevalence of 2.7 to 4.4% (230–233) with S aureus being the predominant organism and access infection the most common source of the organism. Overall mortality for this complication has been approximately 50% (234). In Keane et al.'s 1970s study, nine episodes of bacterial endocarditis were recorded, a rate of 1.2/1,000 patient-months and a prevalence of 2.0% (200). S aureus was the infecting organism in six of the cases, and the aortic valve was involved in eight of the nine. Six of the nine survived, with the other three dying as a consequence of acute cerebral embolic events. Successful valve replacement was accomplished in two of these patients.

In Keane et al.'s 1980s series, only four episodes of endocarditis were documented during the study period, an incidence of 0.26/1,000 patient-months and a prevalence of only 0.5% (201). However, three of the four patients died, two with S aureus infection, and one with E coli. The surviving patient had enterococcal mitral valve endocarditis which resolved with antibiotic therapy alone.

Osteomyelitis and septic arthritis

Metastatic infection of bones and joints is a well recognized complication in hemodialyzed patients, but scant published prevalence and incidence data are available (225, 227, 235–237). In Keane et al.'s 1970s study, 11 patients were found who had eight episodes of osteomyelitis and six episodes of septic arthritis with an overall incidence of 1.7 episodes/1,000 patient-months (200). Diabetic patients experienced an eight-fold higher incidence than non-diabetic counterparts (7.8 vs 1.0 episodes/1,000 patient-months). This predilection for the diabetic patient was also noted in the 1980s review with six cases of osteomyelitis being observed, five of them in diabetics (201). In the 1970s review, blood access devices were the origin of infection in eight cases (57%), and *S aureus* was isolated in 10 of the episodes (200). In some patients with osteomyelitis, more than one organism was isolated from the culture of the bony lesion.

The diagnosis of osteomyelitis still presents considerable difficulty. Non-specific symptoms such as a low grade fever, malaise and weight loss may dominate the clinical picture. The frequent lack of radiographic changes often delays diagnosis. In early studies, osteomyelitis was more common in vertebral bodies and in ribs (237), while in Keane et al.'s 1970s and 1980s experiences, the distal upper and lower extremities were the most frequent sites for infection (200, 201). Therapeutically, long-term antibiotics, combined with early debridement of the osteomyelitic lesion were usually successful. However, in diabetic patients, amputation of the affected limb was frequently necessary.

Septic arthritis most commonly involved the joints and wrist, and *S aureus* was the most frequent infecting organism (200). This experience is not dissimilar to that reported by others (235). In Keane et al.'s 1982 to 1985 bacteremia review, three patients were found to have metastatic joint infections, all of them with *S aureus*, including two in the shoulder joint and one in the acromioclavicular joint (201). In both series, all of the patients responded to systemic antimicrobial therapy without late sequela.

Septic pulmonary emboli

In dialysis patients with chronic or subcutaneous fistulas or external blood accesses subjected to repetitive venipuncture, the development of an infected thrombophlebitis or endarteritis associated with septic pulmonary emboli may occur (206, 207, 238–240). However, given the frequency of blood access device infections, this is clinically a rather uncommon complication. The incidence rate was 0.7 episodes/1,000 patient-months in Keane et al.'s 1972 to 1975 series, with no episodes recorded in the 1980s (200, 201). With the more frequent usage of the dual-lumen external catheter, whose known complication is subclavian vein thrombosis, septic pulmonary emboli may become more common in the future (210).

The diagnosis of septic pulmonary emboli should be considered if fever, cough and pleuritic chest pain devel-op during a dialysis treatment, especially in the setting of an underlying access infection or after thrombolytic therapy of a venous clot. While previous reports have emphasized that septic pulmonary emboli may develop in the absence of obvious access infection (238, 239), in Keane et al.'s series, evidence for an associated infection of blood access device was present in all episodes, five of them in cannulas, and two in bovine carotid fistulas. The infecting organisms in these cases were *S aureus* in three, *S epidermidis* in two, and one each of *S marcescens* and *E coli*. However, antibiotic therapy has been reported as successful treatment of septic pulmonary emboli, even without the removal of the blood access device (206, 207). All of the above cases were treated successfully with access removal and appropriate antimicrobial therapy.

Access infections

Infection of vascular access has always been a vexing problem and a cause of significant morbidity and mortality in the hemodialysis population. Access infections are consistently the leading cause of bacteremia in hemodialysis patients (14, 198, 200, 201, 206, 207), and one of the leading causes of access failure (181, 241–244). Blood access device infections, defined by the presence of a local inflammatory reaction and positive cultures obtained from the suppurative area, have rates varying with type of access. Internal fistulas carry a much lower risk of infection compared to external accesses, with simple AV fistulas having a rate of 8–20/1,000 access-days with an eventual infection occurrence of 1–5% (181, 200, 241, 243–248). Composed of either bovine carotid artery or polytetrafluorethylene (PTFE), prosthetic fistulas carry infection rates of 8–30/1,000 access-days, with 15–25% ultimately becoming infected (181, 200, 241, 243, 244, 247–252). With the acceptance of more elderly and diabetic patients with other medical comorbidities into the United States ESRD program, fewer simple AV fistulas are being placed in favor of prosthetic AV fistulas (181, 244). One could, therefore, anticipate accesses causing a greater proportion of infection in the future. Identified risk factors for infections in internal accesses include poor patient hygiene and the presence of diabetes mellitus (181, 244).

External accesses have evolved from the usage of cannulas with infection rates of 35–150/1,000 access-days, to dual-lumen catheters, providing temporary and sometimes permanent vascular access in selected patients (200, 245, 253). Comparison of infection rates between dual-lumen catheters and cannulas or internal accesses can be misleading, as the rate of infection in dual-lumen catheters increases with duration and number of dialyses usages, with infection eventually occurring if left in long enough (208, 210–212). Consequently, such catheters are often removed after a short period of time. The incidences of bacteremia and sepsis in subclavian polyurethane and polyethylene(Teflon) catheters have been reported to be

7.7/1,000 access-days, and 9.5/1,000 access-days, respectively (208). Others note that ultimately 7.2–37 percent of catheters develop local infections, and 6.8–20.3 percent cause bacteremia (209, 211, 212, 254). Silicone dual-lumen catheters with a Dacron cuff appear to have exit site infection rates of 5–5.3/1,000 access-days and a bacteremia rate of 0.29–3.4/1,000 access-days (209, 210, 255). Risk factors for infection with polyurethane and polyethylene catheters include the presence of diabetes mellitus and inexperienced hemodialysis nursing staff (209, 212). Carbon coated needle-free access devices such as Biocarbon® or Hemasite® were also associated with frequent infections occurring with a prevalence of approximately 25% and at a rate as high as 1.5 episodes/1,000 access-days (243, 251). Many of these devices were infected with gram-negative bacteria and resulted in a high incidence of bacteremia.

Bacteriology and treatment

Gram-positive organisms are responsible for 82–100% of all access-related infections. *S epidermidis* accounts for 11–86% of isolates with *S aureus* present 14–91% of the time. Gram-negative organisms, responsible for 0–18% of isolates, are fairly well dispersed among *E Coli*, Klebsiella, and Pseudomonas species (198, 200, 209, 210, 212, 213, 215). Most access infections in Keane et al.'s 1970 series were treated on an out-patient basis with systemic antibiotic therapy stressing good gram-positive coverage. However, 19.2% of these infections were severe enough to warrant hospitalization, with two-thirds of these patients demonstrating bacteremia. Among the hospitalized group, 60% required removal of the access device, most frequently external silastic catheters (200). Management of infected internal accesses is variable with some centers advocating ligation or removal of an access site felt to be the source of bacteremia. Others drain the abscess or resect the aneurysmal dilatation to avoid potential graft erosion (200, 243, 245, 247, 248, 250–252, 256, 257). Teflon catheters are, however, usually removed, while Dacron cuffed catheters may be treated and left in. However, sepsis often recurs (210, 255).

Methods to prevent vascular access infections have not been well developed. Sterile skin technique appears to have no benefit over clean technique. However, poor patient hygiene appears to be a risk factor for access infections, so that this may potentially be a remediable factor (213). Host nasal carriage of *S aureus* is an important risk factor for *S aureus* access infection. Boelaert et al. studied the thrice weekly nasal application of mupirocin ointment for culture positive patients and compared *S aureus* access infection rates six months prior to treatment and six months post-intervention. They demonstrated a trend in the fall of the *S aureus* bacteremia rate from 8.08/1,000 patient-months to 1.89/1,000 patient-months ($p = 0.08$). No bacterial resistance occurred in six months (220). Randomized controlled trials have yet to be performed. Intermittent prophylactic rifampin may also have potential benefit for reducing the incidence of staphylococcal access infections (219). Because a wide spectrum of organisms may be responsible for access infections, it is unlikely that a single antibiotic would be an effective prophylactic agent. The possibility of inducing resistant strains must also be considered. Prophylactic vancomycin was used in one uncontrolled study of 25 patients, where it was demonstrated that *S aureus* infections were reduced, but there was an increase in infections caused by organisms from the *Klebsiella enterobacter* group (258). Short term antibiotic prophylaxis, however, may be of value during procedures associated with transient bacteremias.

Systemic infections

Respiratory infection

A number of factors which may predispose hemodialysis patients to an increased risk of acquiring pulmonary infection have been identified. The permissive role of pathologic changes associated with uremic pulmonary edema, such as thick, tenacious mucous in the upper airways, the presence of hyaline-like membranes and alveolar fibrinous exudates could interfere with clearance of potential pathogens (259–262). A decreased pulmonary clearance for coagulase-positive staphylococci has been seen in experimental uremic models using mice (263). In addition, altered nasal-pharyngeal flora seen in chronically ill and hospitalized patients may predispose the hemodialysis patient to the development of pulmonary infections (264).

Keane et al. noted 40 episodes of pulmonary infections in 35 patients, an incidence of 5.7/1,000 patient-months (200). Others noted a similar rate of 6.9/1,000 patient-months (213). *Streptococcus pneumoniae* was isolated in 50% of the patients who were admitted with a primary diagnosis of pneumonia. In contrast, gram-negative organisms were frequently isolated in patients who developed pneumonias while in the hospital. There was no difference in the frequency of this infection between diabetic and non-diabetic patients. Death occurred in 12% of those patients who were admitted with a diagnosis of pneumonia, while 57% of those patients with hospital-acquired pneumonia eventually died. Chronic obstructive pulmonary disease and cardiac decompensation were commonly associated conditions in patients with respiratory infections. In comparison, an incidence of pulmonary infections as high as 51% has been reported by others with a mortality of approximately 50% (1). A baseline serum albumin level less than 3.0 mg/dl compared to greater than 3.0 mg/dl has been associated with a relative risk of 4.84 in acquiring pneumonia (181).

Urinary tract infections

With a decrease in urine output accompanying the development of renal failure, the subsequent stasis of urine flow might be expected to predispose the hemodialysis patient to an increased risk of urinary tract infection. Few studies have attempted to establish the prevalence of pyuria and bacteriuria and its clinical relevance. Bacteriuria has been reported in 28 to 58% of chronic hemodialysis patients (265–267). In a cross-sectional study of asymptomatic dialysis patients, 10 of 32 patients had greater than 10 WBC/HPF, and seven of these 10 grew out greater than 1×10^5 colonies/ml. Only urine with greater than 10 WBC/HPF demonstrated growth. Unlike normal hosts, *E Coli* was not the predominant organism. No predilection for cause of ESRD was noted. The long-term significance of bacteriuria and pyuria is unknown (267). Keane et al. previously documented 19 episodes of symptomatic urinary tract infections in 16 patients with an incidence of 2.3/1,000 patient-months (200). Polycystic kidney disease was the underlying diagnosis in 50%. In five of them, the clinical course was complicated by the development of a perinephric abscess refractory to systemic antibiotic therapy necessitating surgical nephrectomy, with three dying postoperatively. This experience is similar to that of others, whereby an incidence of symptomatic urinary tract infection of 11.6% has been shown, with four of the 11 patients having polycystic kidney disease as a cause of their renal failure (268). The treatment of urinary tract infections in hemodialysis patients may be difficult because in the absence of urinary flow, normal mechanisms for concentrating antibiotics at the site of infection may not be operative. This is particularly true for aminoglycosides. However, significant levels of antibiotics can be obtained in the urine using ampicillin or trimethoprim/sulfamethoxazole in patients with severe end-stage disease (269).

Unusual infections

The purported high incidence of mycobacterial infection may be presumptive evidence of the presence of defects in the immune system of hemodialysis patients. Rates of tuberculosis have been reported to be 10 to 15 times those found in the normal population, and they may account for approximately 1% of deaths of hemodialysis patients (270–276). Tuberculosis is particularly problematic in the Native American population, where incidence rates are 2–9 times those the general population, and ESRD has been shown to be a risk factor for active tuberculosis (277). Mortality from tubercular infection in hemodialysis patients ranges from 0 to 75%, and the diagnosis is frequently made at autopsy. Indeed, the non-specific symptoms of fever, anorexia and weight loss, plus the tendency for extrapulmonary disease, 80–90% in some series, make the diagnosis exceedingly difficult (273, 275). Routine cultures and skin tests are frequently negative, and the diagnosis is often delayed. The most reliable results for obtaining the diagnosis are culture of tissue biopsies from appropriate sources. Once the diagnosis is made, the response to therapy is usually good.

Another unusual pathogen is *Listeria monocytogenes*, which occasionally leads to clinical infections in renal transplant recipients, hemodialysis patients, or other immunosuppressed individuals. Reported as causing bacteremia and endocarditis in a number of hemodialysis patients, iron overload may be an etiologic factor in its development (230, 278–280).

Hemodialysis patients also appear predisposed to mucormycosis (*Rhizopus*) infections, with an international registry reporting 59 cases among dialysis patients. Presentations included dissemination in 44%, rhinocerebritis in 31%, and other sites in 25%. Unfortunately, the diagnosis was made predominantly at autopsy (61%). Without treatment, the case fatality rate was 86% and remained high at 72% despite amphotericin B. The major risk factor identified in this series was concurrent administration of deferoxamine, primarily indicated for aluminum overload. The deferoxamine-iron chelate, feroxamine, has been demonstrated to act as a siderophore to *Rhizopus* and to stimulate both growth and pathogenicity *in vitro* (281).

Dialysis patients may also be predisposed to *Clostridium difficile*-associated diarrhea. While they frequently are exposed to broad spectrum antibiotics, the major risk factor for this infection, impaired host defenses also have been implicated (282). Reviews of dialysis patients with *Clostridium difficile* diarrhea reveal that patients may be culture negative for *Clostridium difficile*, but all are either culture or toxin positive. Asymptomatic toxin positive patients were also noted. Clinical response to vancomycin is prompt, usually within 24–48 hours. The majority of patients previously received a cephalosporin or penicillinase-stable penicillin, although 27% received no prior antibiotics within 4 weeks of diarrhea onset (282–284). In comparing the colonic flora of 10 healthy dialysis patients to 10 healthy non-dialysis controls, the only statistically significant difference was a higher number of clostridia colonies in the uremic patient group. No *Clostridium difficile* strains were isolated from staff members or the ward environment. Treatment with lactobacillus acidophilus had no effect. The relapse rate was 25%.

SUMMARY

Infection in patients with ESRD receiving maintenance hemodialysis therapy remains a common cause of morbidity and mortality. The uremic state itself and contributing factors, such as nutritional deficiencies and presence of diabetes mellitus, create a population with an impaired immune response. The frequent and repetitive exposure of these patients to potential infectious agents during the normal course of their therapy represents a unique medical situation which enhances their susceptibility. One can only speculate that as older patients with more medical comorbidities who also preferentially use synthetic vascular access materials are accepted for chronic hemodialysis, infectious complications will pose even more challenging problems.

REFERENCES

1. Montgomerie JZ, Kalmanson GM, Guze LB: Renal failure and infection. *Medicine* 47: 1, 1968
2. Blagg CR, Hickman RO, Eschbach JW, Scribner BH: Home hemodialysis: six years' experience. *N Engl J Med* 283: 1126, 1970
3. Burton BT, Krueger KK, Bryan FA Jr: National registry of long-term dialysis patients. *JAMA* 218: 718, 1971
4. Gurland HJ, Brunner FP, Dehn Hv, Harlen H, Parsons FM, Schärer K: Combined report on regular dialysis and transplantation in Europe, III, 1972. *Proc Eur Dial Transplant Assoc* 10: XVII, 1973
5. Lowrie EG, Lazarus JM, Mocelin AJ, Bailey FL, Hampers CL, Wilson RE, Merrill JP: Survival of patients undergoing chronic hemodialysis and renal transplantation. *N Engl J Med* 288: 863, 1973
6. Johnson WJ, Kurtz SB, Anderson CF, Mitchell JC, III, Zincke H, O'Fallon WM: Results of treatment of renal failure by means of home hemodialysis. *Mayo Clin Proc* 59: 663, 1984
7. Johnson WJ, Kurtz SB, Mitchell JC, III, VanDenBerg CJ, Wochos DN, O'Fallon WM, Sterioff S: Results of treatment of center hemodialysis patients. *Mayo Clin Proc* 59: 669, 1984
8. Santiago A, Chazan JA: Factors associated with mortality among 405 chronic hemodialysis patients who died between 1973 and 1985. (Abstract) *Kidney Int* 31: 245, 1987
9. Mailloux LU, Bellucci AG, Wilkes BM, Napolitano B, Mossey RT, Lesser M, Bluestone PA: Mortality in dialysis patients: analysis of the causes of death. *Am J Kidney Dis* 18: 326, 1991
10. Morduchowicz G, Winkler J, Derzane E, Van Dyk DF, Wittenberg C, Zabludowski JR, Shohat J, Rosenfeld JB, Boner G: Causes of death in patients with end-stage renal disease treated by dialysis in a center in Israel. *Isr J Med Sci* 28: 776, 1992
11. Port FK: Mortality and causes of death in patients with end-stage renal failure. *Am J Kidney Dis* 15: 215, 1990
12. Kjellstrand CM, Fryd D, Najarian JS: Late deaths on dialysis and transplantation therapy. *Contrib Nephrol* 70: 64, 1989
13. Fernández JM, Carbonell ME, Mazzuchi N, Petruccelli D: Simultaneous analysis of morbidity and mortality factors in chronic hemodialysis patients. *Kidney Int* 41: 1029, 1992
14. Khan IH, Catto GRD: Long-term complications of dialysis: infection. *Kidney Int* 43 (Suppl 41): S143, 1993
15. Hume DM, Merrill JP, Miller BF, Thorn GW: Experiences with renal homotransplantation in humans. Report of nine cases. *J Clin Invest* 32: 327, 1955
16. Mannick JA, Powers JH, Mithoefer J, Ferrebee JW: Renal transplantation in azotemic dogs. *Surgery* 47: 340, 1960
17. Dammin GJ, Couch NP, Murray JE: Prolonged survival of skin homografts in uremia patients. *Ann N Y Acad Sci* 64: 967, 1957
18. Smiddy FG, Burwell RG, Parsons FM: The effect of acute uraemia upon the survival of skin homografts. The influence of uraemia upon certain aspects of lymph-node reactivity. *Br J Surg* 48: 328, 1960

19. Morrison AB, Maness K, Tawes R: Skin homograft survival in chronic renal insufficiency. *Arch Pathol* 75: 139, 1963
20. London WT, DiFiglia M, Sutnick AI, Blumberg BS: An epidemic of hepatitis in a chronic hemodialysis unit: Australia antigen and differences in host response. *N Engl J Med* 281: 571, 1969
21. London WT, Drew JS, Lustbader ED, Werner BG, Blumberg BS: Host responses to hepatitis B infection in patients in a chronic hemodialysis unit. *Kidney Int* 12: 51, 1977
22. Ribot S, Rothstein M, Goldblatt M, Grasso M: Duration of hepatitis B surface antigenemia (HBsAg) in hemodialysis patients. *Arch Intern Med* 139: 178, 1979
23. Szmuness W, Prince AM, Grady GF, Mann MK, Levine RW, Friedman EA, Jacobs MJ, Josephson A, Ribot S, Shapiro FL et al.: Hepatitis B infection. A point-prevalance study in 15 US hemodialysis centers. *JAMA* 227: 901, 1974
24. Matas AJ, Simmons RL, Kjellstrand CM, Buselmeier TJ, Najarian JS: Increased incidence of malignancy during chronic renal failure. *Lancet* 1: 883, 1975
25. Sutherland GA, Glass J, Gabriel R: Increased incidence of malignancy in chronic renal failure. *Nephron* 18: 182, 1977
26. Lindner A, Farewell YJ, Sherrard DJ: High incidence of neoplasia in uremic patients receiving long-term dialysis. *Nephron* 27: 292, 1981
27. Degoulet P, Reach I, Jacobs C: Cancer in patients on hemodialysis. *N Engl J Med* 300: 1279, 1979
28. Coplon NS, Diskin CJ, Peterson J, Sivenson RS: The long-term clinical course of systemic lupus erythematosus in end-stage renal disease. *N Engl J Med* 308: 186, 1983
29. Hosking CS, Atkins RC, Scott DF, Holdsworth SR, Fitzgerald MG, Shelton MJ: Immune and phagocytic function in patients on maintenance dialysis and post-transplantation. *Clin Nephrol* 6: 501, 1976
30. Casciani CU, DeSimone C, Bonini S, Gallucci MT, Matteucci G, Valesini G, Meli D, Masala C: Immunological aspects of chronic uremia. *Kidney Int* 13 (Suppl 8): S49, 1978
31. Raskova J, Ghobrial I, Czerwinski DK, Shea SM, Eisinger RP, Raska K Jr: B-cell activation and immunoregulation in end-stage renal disease patients receiving hemodialysis. *Arch Intern Med* 147: 89, 1987
32. Quadracci LJ, Ringdén O, Krzymanski M: The effect of uremia and transplantation on lymphocyte subpopulations. *Kidney Int* 10: 179, 1976
33. Hoy WE, Cestero RVM, Freeman RB: Deficiency of T and B lymphocytes in uremic subjects and partial improvement with maintenance hemodialysis. *Nephron* 20: 182, 1978
34. Gagnon RF, Shuster J, Kaye M: Auto-immunity in patients with end-stage renal disease maintained on hemodialysis and continuous ambulatory peritoneal dialysis. *J Clin Lab Immunol* 11: 155, 1983
35. Howell ED, Perkins HA: Anti-N-like antibodies in the sera of patients undergoing chronic hemodialysis. *Vox Sang* 23: 291, 1972
36. Crosson JT, Moulds J, Comty CM, Polesky HF: A clinical study of anti-N_{DP} in the sera of patients in a large repetitive hemodialysis program. *Kidney Int* 10: 463, 1976

37. Kaehny WD, Miller GE, White WL: Relationship between dialyzer reuse and the presence of anti-N-like antibodies in chronic hemodialysis patients. *Kidney Int* 12: 59, 1977

38. Nolph KD, Husted FC, Sharp GC, Siemsen AW: Antibodies to nuclear antigens in patients undergoing long-term hemodialysis. *Am J Med* 60: 673, 1976

39. Balch HH: The effect of severe battle injury and post-traumatic renal failure on resistance to infection. *Ann Surg* 142: 145, 1955

40. Stoloff IL, Stout R, Myerson RM, Havens WP Jr: Production of antibody in patients with uremia. *N Engl J Med* 259: 320, 1958

41. Wilson WEC, Kirkpatrick CH, Talmage DW: Suppression of immunologic responsiveness in uremia. *Ann Intern Med* 621: 1, 1965

42. Boulton-Jones JM, Vick R, Cameron JS, Block PH: Immune responses in uremia. *Clin Nephrol* 1: 351, 1973

43. Byron PR, Mallick NP, Taylor G: Immune potential in human uraemia. I. Relationship of glomerular filtration rate to depression of immune potential. *J Clin Path* 29: 765, 1976

44. Byron PR, Mallick NP, Taylor G: Immune potential in human uraemia. 2. Changes after regular haemodialysis therapy. *J Clin Path* 29: 770, 1976

45. Jordan MC, Rousseau WE, Tegtmeier GE, Noble GR, Muth RG, Chin TDY: Immunogenicity of inactivated influenza virus vaccine in chronic renal failure. *Ann Intern Med* 79: 790, 1973

46. Ortbals DW, Marks ES, Liebhaber H: Influenza immunization in patients with chronic renal disease. *JAMA* 239: 2562, 1978

47. Osanloo EO, Berlin BS, Popli S, Ing TS, Cummings JE, Ghandi VC, Geis WP, Hano JE: Antibody responses to influenza vaccination in patients with chronic renal failure. *Kidney Int* 14: 614, 1978

48. Pabico RC, Douglas RG, Betts RF, McKenna BA, Freeman RB: Influenza vaccination of patients with glomerular diseases. Effects on creatinine clearance, urinary protein excretion, and antibody response. *Ann Intern Med* 81: 171, 1974

49. Simberkoff MS, Schiffman G, Katz LA, Spicehandler JR, Moldover NH, Rahal J Jr: Pneumococcal capsular polysaccharide vaccination in adult chronic hemodialysis patients. *J Lab Clin Med* 96: 363, 1980

50. Linnemann CC Jr, First MR, Schiffman G: Response to pneumococcal vaccine in renal transplant and hemodialysis patients. *Arch Intern Med* 141: 1637, 1981

51. Nikoskelainen J, Koskela M, Forsström J, Kasanen A, Leinonen M: Persistence of antibodies to pneumococcal vaccine in patients with chronic renal failure. *Kidney Int* 28: 672, 1985

52. Rytel MW, Dailey MP, Schiffman G, Hoffman RG, Piering WF: Pneumococcal vaccine immunization of patients with renal impairment. *Proc Soc Exp Biol Med* 182: 468, 1986

53. Update: Pneumococcal polysaccharide vaccine usage – United States. Recommendations of the Immunization Practices Advisory Committee. *Ann Intern Med* 101: 348, 1984

54. Linnemann CC, First MR, Schiffman G: Revaccination of renal transplant and hemodialysis recipients with pneumococcal vaccine. *Arch Intern Med* 146: 1554, 1986

55. Stevens CE, Szmuness W, Goodman AI, Weseley SA, Fotino M: Hepatitis B vaccine: immune responses in haemodialysis patients. *Lancet* 2: 1211, 1980

56. Crosnier J, Jungers P, Courouce AM, Laplanche A, Benhamou E, Degos F, Lacour B, Prunet P, Cerisier Y, Guesry P: Randomised placebo-controlled trial of hepatitis B surface antigen vaccine in French haemodialysis units: II, haemodialysis patients. *Lancet* 1: 797, 1981

57. Stevens CE, Alter HJ, Taylor PE, Zang EA, Harley EJ, Szmuness W, and the dialysis vaccine trial study group: Hepatitis B vaccine in patients receiving hemodialysis. Immunogenicity and efficacy. *N Engl J Med* 311: 496, 1984

58. Desmyter J, Colaert J, DeGroote G, Reynders M, Reerink-Brongers EE, Lelie PN, Dees PJ, Reesink HW, and the Leuven renal transplantation collaborative group: Efficacy of heat-inactivated hepatitis B vaccine in haemodialysis patients and staff. *Lancet* 2: 1323, 1983

59. Benhamou E, Courouce AM, Jungers P, Laplanche A, Degos F, Brangier J, Crosnier J: Hepatitis B vaccine: randomized trial of immunogenicity in hemodialysis patients. *Clin Nephrol* 21: 143, 1984

60. Köhler H, Arnold W, Renschin G, Dormeyer HH, Zum Büschenfelde KHM: Active hepatitis B vaccination of dialysis patients and medical staff. *Kidney Int* 25: 124, 1984

61. de Graeff PA, Dankert J, de Zeeuw D, Gips CH, van der Hem GK: Immune response to two different hepatitis B vaccines in haemodialysis patients: a 2-year follow-up. *Nephron* 40: 155, 1985

62. Benhamou E, Courouce AM, Laplanche A, Jungers P, Tron JF, Crosnier J: Long-term results of hepatitis B vaccination in patients on dialysis. *N Engl J Med* 314: 1710, 1986

63. Kunori T, Fehrman I, Ringdén O, Möller E: *In vitro* characterization of immunological responsiveness of uremic patients. *Nephron* 26: 234, 1980

64. Kurz P, Köhler H, Meuer S, Hütteroth T, Zum Büschenfelde KHM: Impaired cellular immune responses in chronic renal failure: evidence for a T cell defect. *Kidney Int* 29: 1209, 1986

65. Osaki K, Otsuka H, Uomizu K, Harada R, Otsuji Y, Hashimoto S: Monocyte-mediated suppression of mitogen responses of lymphocytes in uremic patients. *Nephron* 34: 87, 1983

66. Gaciong Z, Alexiewicz JM, Linker-Israeli M, Shulman I, Pitts TO, Massry SG: Inhibition of immunoglobulin production by parathyroid hormone. Implications in chronic renal failure. *Kidney Int* 40: 96, 1991

67. Huber H, Pastner D, Dittrich P, Braunsteiner H: *In vitro* reactivity of human leukocytes in uraemia – a comparison with the impairment of delayed hypersensitivity. *Clin Exp Immunol* 5: 75, 1969

68. Selroos O, Pasternack A, Virolainen M: Skin test sensitivity and antigen-induced lymphocyte transformation in uraemia. *Clin Exp Immunol* 14: 365, 1973

69. Elves MW, Israëls MCG, Collinge M: An assessment of the mixed leucocyte reaction in renal failure. *Lancet* 1: 682, 1966

70. Sengar DPS, Hyslop DB, Rashid A, Harris JE: T-rosettes in hemodialysis patients and renal allograft recipients. *Cell Immunol* 20: 92, 1975

71. Kauffman CA, Manzler AD, Phair JP: Cell-mediated immunity in patients on long-term haemodialysis. *Clin Exp Immunol* 22: 54, 1975

72. Kamata K, Okubo M, Sada M: Immunosuppressive factors in uraemic sera are composed of both dialysable and non-dialysable components. *Clin Exp Immunol* 54: 277, 1983

73. Holdsworth SR, Fitzgerald MG, Hosking CS, Atkins RC: The effect of maintenance dialysis on lymphocyte function. I. Haemodialysis. *Clin Exp Immunol* 33: 95, 1978

74. Donati D, Degiannis D, Raskova J, Raska K: Uremic serum effects on peripheral blood mononuclear cell and purified T lymphocyte responses. *Kidney Int* 42: 681, 1992

75. Silk MR: The effect of uremic plasma on lymphocyte transformation. *Invest Urol* 5: 195, 1967

76. Newberry WM, Sanford JP: Defective cellular immunity in renal failure: depression of reactivity of lymphocytes to phytohemagglutinin by renal failure serum. *J Clin Invest* 50: 1262, 1971

77. Sengar DPS, Rashid A, Harris JE: *In vitro* reactivity of lymphocytes obtained from uraemic patients maintained on haemodialysis. *Clin Exp Immunol* 21: 298, 1975

78. Asaka M, Iida H, Izumino K, Sasayama S: Depressed natural killer cell activity in uremia. *Nephron* 49: 291, 1988

79. Nakhla LS, Goggin MJ: Lymphocyte transformation in chronic renal failure. *Immunology* 24: 229, 1973

80. Fehrman I, Ringdén O, Bergström J: MLC-blocking factors in uremic sera. *Clin Nephrol* 14: 183, 1980

81. Slavin RG, Fitch CD: Inhibition of lymphocyte transformation by guanidinosuccinic acid, a surplus metabolite in uremia. *Experientia* 27: 1340, 1971

82. Hanicki Z, Cichocki T, Sarnecka-Keller M, Klein A, Komorowska Z: Influence of middle-sized molecule aggregates from dialysate of uremic patients on lymphocyte transformation *in vitro*. *Nephron* 17: 73, 1976

83. Harris JE, Page D, Posen G, Stewart T. Suppression of *in vitro* lymphocyte function by uremic toxins. *J Urol* 108: 312, 1972

84. Raska K Jr, Morrison AB, Raskova J: Humoral inhibitors of the immune response in uremia. III. The immunosuppressive factor of uremic rat serum is a very low density lipoprotein. *Lab Invest* 42: 636, 1980

85. Stewart E, Miller TE: Host immune status in uraemia. II. Serum factors and lymphocyte transformation. *Clin Exp Immunol* 41: 123, 1980

86. Mezzano S, Pesce AJ, Pollak VE, Michael JG: Analysis of humoral and cellular factors that contribute to impaired immune responsiveness in experimental uremia. *Nephron* 36: 15, 1984

87. Raskova J, Morrison AB: A decrease in cell-mediated immunity in uremia associated with an increase in activity of suppressor cells. *Am J Pathol* 84: 1, 1976

88. Alevy YG, Slavin RG, Hutcheson P: Immune response in experimentally induced uremia. I. Suppression in mitogen responses by adherent cells in chronic uremia. *Clin Immunol Immunopathol* 19: 8, 1981

89. Raskova J, Raska K: Humoral inhibitors of the immune response in uremia. V. Induction of suppressor cells *in vitro* by uremic serum. *Am J Pathol* 111: 149, 1983

90. Lortran JE, Kiepiela P, Coovadia HM, Seedat YK: Suppressor cells assayed by numerical and functional tests in chronic renal failure. *Kidney Int* 22: 192, 1982

91. Raska Jr, Raskova J, Shea SM, Frankel RM, Wood RH, Lifter J, Ghobrial I, Eisinger RP, Homer L: T cell subsets and cellular immunity in end-stage renal disease. *Am J Med* 75: 734, 1983

92. Chida Y, Sakurai S, Yoshiyama N: The effect of hemodialysis on lymphocyte subsets during dialysis. *Clin Nephrol* 25: 159, 1986

93. Chatenoud L, Dugas B, Beaurain G, Touam M, Drüeke T, Vasquez A, Galanaud P, Bach JF, DelFraissy JF: Presence of preactivated T cells in hemodialyzed patients: their possible role in altered immunity. *Proc Natl Acad Sci USA* 83: 7457, 1986

94. Raskova J, Ghobrial I, Shea SM, Eisinger RP, Raska K: Suppressor cells in end-stage renal disease. Functional assays and monoclonal antibody analysis. *Am J Med* 76: 847, 1984

95. Guillon PJ, Woodhouse LF, Davison AM, Giles GR: Suppressor cell activity of peripheral mononuclear cells from patients undergoing chronic hemodialysis. *Biomedicine* 32: 11, 1980

96. Ruddy MC, Rubin AL, Novogrodsky A, Stenzel K: Decreased macrophage-mediated suppression of lymphocyte activation in chronic renal failure. *Am J Med* 75: 571, 1983

97. Tsakolos ND, Theoharides TC, Herdler ED, Guffinet J, Dwyer JM, Whisler HL, Askenase PW: Immune defects in chronic renal impairment: evidence for defective regulation of lymphocyte response by macrophages from patients with chronic renal impairment on haemodialysis. *Clin Exp Immunol* 63: 218, 1986

98. Kleiman KS, Zoschke DC: Suppression of human lymphocyte responses in chronic renal failure mediated by adherent cells: analysis in serum-free media. *J Lab Clin Med* 106: 262, 1985

99. Waltzer WC, Bachvaroff RJ, Raisbeck AP, Egelandsdal B, Pullis C, Shen L, Rapaport FT: Immunologic monitoring in patients with end-stage renal disease. *J Clin Immunol* 4: 364, 1984

100. Sanders Jr, Luby JP, Sanford JP, Hull AR: Suppression of interferon response in lymphocytes from patients with uremia. *J Lab Clin Med* 77: 768, 1971

101. Gál G, Toth M, Toth S: Interferon production by leukocytes of dialysed chronic uraemic patients. *Proc Eur Dial Transplant Assoc* 18: 188, 1981

102. Schindler R, Linnenweber S, Schulze M, Oppermann M, Dinarello CA, Shaldon S, Koch KM: Gene expression of interleukein-1β during hemodialysis. *Kidney Int* 43: 712, 1993

103. Dinarello CA: Interleukin-1 and tumor necrosis factor and their naturally occurring antagonists during hemodialysis. *Kidney Int* 42 (Suppl 38): S68, 1992

104. Ureña P, Herbelin A, Zingraff J, Lair M, Man NK, Descamps-Latscha B, Drueke T: Permeability of cellulosic and non-cellulosic membranes to endotoxin subunits and cytokine production during in-vitro haemodialysis. *Nephrol Dial Transplant* 7: 16, 1992

105. Luger A, Kovarik J, Stummvoll HK, Urbanska A, Luger TA: Blood-membrane interaction in hemodialysis leads to increased cytokine production. *Kidney Int* 32: 84, 1987

106. Herbelin A, Nguyen AT, Zingraff J, Urena P, Descamps-Latscha B: Influence of uremia and hemodialysis on circulating interleukin-1 and tumor necrosis factor α. *Kidney Int* 37: 116, 1990

107. Bingel M, Lonnemann G, Shaldon S, Koch KM, Dinarello CA: Human interleukin-1 production during hemodialysis. *Nephron* 43: 161, 1986

108. Lonnemann G, Koch KM, Shaldon S: Induction of interleukin-1 (IL-1) from human monocytes adhering to hemodialysis (HD) membranes. (Abstract) *Kidney Int* 31: 238, 1987

109. Shaldon S, Bingel M, Lonnemann G, Dinarello CA, Koch KM: Human interleukin-1 (IL-1) production is enhanced by sodium acetate. *Abstracts Am Soc Artif Intern Organs* 16: 33, 1987

110. Betz M, Haensch GM, Rauterberg EW, Bommer J, Ritz E: Cuprammonium membranes stimulate interleukin 1 release and arachidonic acid metabolism in monocytes in the absence of complement. *Kidney Int* 34: 67, 1988

111. Ryan JJ, Beynon HLC, Rees AJ, Cassidy MJD: *In vitro* production of tumor necrosis factor by monocytes cultured from dialysis patients. *Kidney Int* 43 (Suppl 41): S226, 1993

112. Roccatello D, D'Alfonso S, Peruccio D, Quattrocchio G, Cavalli G, Isidoro C, Piccoli G, Richiardi PM: Induction of mRNA for tumor necrosis factor α in hemodialysis. *Kidney Int* 43 (Suppl 39): S144, 1993

113. Descamps-Latscha B, Herbelin A, Nguyen AT, De Groote D, Chauveau P, Verger C, Jungers P, Zingraff J: Soluble CD23 as an effector of immune dysregulation in chronic uremia and dialysis. *Kidney Int* 43: 878, 1993

114. Pertosa G, Tarantino EA, Gesualdo L, Montinaro V, Schena FP: C5b–9 generation and cytokine production in hemodialyzed patients. *Kidney Int* 43 (Suppl 41): S221, 1993

115. Brockhaus M, Bar-Khayim Y, Gurwicz S, Frensdorff A, Haran N: Plasma tumor necrosis factor soluble receptors in chronic renal failure. *Kidney Int* 42: 663, 1992

116. Pertosa G, Gesualdo L, Tarantino EA, Ranieri E, Bottalico D, Schena FP: Influence of hemodialysis on interleukin-6 production and gene expression by peripheral blood mononuclear cells. *Kidney Int* 43 (Suppl 39): S149, 1993

117. Cavaillon JM, Poigner JL, Fitting C, Delons S: Serum interleukin-6 in long-term hemodialyzed patients. *Nephron* 60: 307, 1992

118. Herbelin A, Ureña P, Nguyen AT, Zingraff J, Descamps-Latscha B: Elevated circulating levels of interleukin-6 in patients with chronic renal failure. *Kidney Int* 39: 954, 1991

119. Cala S, Mazuran R, Kordic D: Negative effect of uraemia and cuprophane haemodialysis on natural killer cells. *Nephrol Dial Transplant* 5: 437, 1990

120. Pisa P, Jira M, Horky J, Strejcek J, Valek A: Depression in spontaneous cell-mediated cytotoxicity occurs during hemodialysis. *Clin Nephrol* 27: 289, 1987

121. Zaoui P, Hakim RM: Natural killer-cell function in hemodialysis patients: effect of the dialysis membrane. *Kidney Int* 43: 1298, 1993

122. Ringoir S, VanLooy L, Van de Heyning P, Leroux-Roels G: Impairment of phagocytic activity of macrophages as studied by the skin window test in patients on regular hemodialysis treatment. *Clin Nephrol* 4: 234, 1975

123. Hanicki Z, Cichocki T, Komorowska Z, Sulowicz W, Smolenski O: Some aspects of cellular immunity in untreated and maintenance hemodialysis patients. *Nephron* 23: 273, 1979

124. Urbanitz D, Sieberth HG: Impaired phagocytic activity of human monocytes in respect to reduced antibacterial resistance in uremia. *Clin Nephrol* 4: 13, 1975

125. Jorstad S, Viken KE: Inhibitory effects of plasma from uraemic patients on human mononuclear phagocytes cultured *in vitro*. *Acta Pathol Microbiol Scand (C)* 85: 169, 1977

126. Jorstad S, Kvernes S: Uraemic toxins of high molecular weight inhibiting human mononuclear phagocytes cultured *in vitro*. *Acta Pathol Microbiol Scand (C)* 86: 221, 1978

127. Alevy YG, Mueller KR, Slavin RG: Immune response in experimentally induced uremia. VI. Uremic macrophages are defective in their ability to present antigen to T cells. *Clin Immunol Immunopathol* 29: 433, 1983

128. Gibbons R, Martinez O, Lim V, Garovoy MR: Defective antigen presentation in uremia: a monocyte defect. *Kidney Int* 31: 232, 1987

129. Lewis SL, Van Epps DE, Chenoweth DE: C5a receptor modulation on neutrophils and monocytes from chronic hemodialysis and peritoneal dialysis patients. *Clin Nephrol* 26: 37, 1986

130. Keane WF, Comty CM, Verbrugh HA, Peterson PK: Opsonic deficiency of peritoneal dialysis effluent in continuous ambulatory peritoneal dialysis. *Kidney Int* 25: 539, 1984

131. Keane WF, Peterson PK: Host defense mechanisms of the peritoneal cavity and continuous ambulatory peritoneal dialysis. *Perit Dial Bull* 4: 122, 1984

132. Goldstein CS, Bomalaski JS, Zurier RB, Neilson EG, Douglas SD: Analysis of peritoneal macrophages in continuous peritoneal dialysis patients. *Kidney Int* 26: 733, 1984

133. Duwea K, Vas SI, Weatherhead JW: The effect of the composition of peritoneal dialysis fluid on chemiluminescence phagocytosis and bactericidal activity *in vitro*. *Infect Immun* 33: 130, 1981

134. Harvey DM, Sheppard KJ, Morgan AG, Fletcher J: Effect of dialysate fluids on phagocytosis and killing by normal neutrophils. *J Clin Microbiol* 25: 1424, 1987

135. Carozzi S, Nasini MG, Schelotto C, Caviglia PM, Barocci S, Cantaluppi A, Salit M: Peritoneal dialysis fluid (PDF) C++ and 1,25(OH)2D3 modulate peritoneal macrophage (PMO) antimicrobial activity in CAPD patients. *Adv Perit Dial* 6: 110, 1990

136. Carozzi S, Nasini MG, Cantaluppi A: Effects of long-term therapy with low Ca++ peritoneal dialysis solution (PDS) and I. P. 1,25(OH)2D3 (VD3) on peritoneal immune defense mechanisms in CAPD. (Abstract) *Perit Dial Int* 11 (Suppl 1): 42, 1991

137. Piraino B, Bernardini J, Holley JL, Perlmutter JA: Increased risk of staphylococcus epidermidis peritonitis in patients on dialysate containing 1.25 mmol/l calcium. *Am J Kidney Dis* 19: 371, 1992

138. Peterson PK, Gaziano E, Devalon M, Peterson LA, Keane WF: Antimicrobial activities of dialysate elicited and resident human peritoneal macrophages. *Infect Immun* 49: 212, 1985

139. Peterson PK, Lee D, Suh HJ, Devalon M, Nelson RD, Keane WF: Intracellular survival of Candida albicans in peritoneal macrophages from chronic peritoneal dialysis patients. *Am J Kidney Dis* 7: 146, 1986
140. Kleinman MF, Doehring RO, Furman KI et al.: Frontiers in peritoneal dialysis. in *Importance of Intracellular Organisms in CAPD,* edited by Maher JF, Winchester JF, New York, Field, Rich and Assoc, 1986, p 546
141. Verbrugh HA, Van Bronswizk H, Lien P: The fate of phagocytized Staphylococcus epidermidis: survival and growth in human mononuclear phagocytes as a potential pathogenic mechanism. in *Pathogenicity and Clinical Significance of Coagulase-negative Staphylococci,* edited by Pulverer G, Quie PG, Peters G, New York/Stuttgart, Gustav Fischer Verlag, 1987, p 55
142. Buggy BP, Schaberg DR, Swartz RD: Intraleukocyte sequestration as a cause of persistent Staphylococcus aureus peritonitis in continuous ambulatory peritoneal dialysis. *Am J Med* 76: 1035, 1984
143. Lamperi S, Carozzi S: Defective opsonic activity of peritoneal effluent during continuous ambulatory peritoneal dialysis (CAPD): importance and prevention. *Perit Dial Bull* 6: 87, 1986
144. Lamperi S, Carozzi S: Suppressor resident peritoneal macrophages and peritonitis incidence in continuous ambulatory peritoneal dialysis. *Nephron* 44: 219, 1986
145. Jensson O: Observations on the blood leukocytes in chronic renal insufficiency. *Br J Haematol* 4: 422, 1958
146. Riis P, Stougaard J: The peripheral blood leukocytes in chronic renal insufficiency. *Dan Med Bull* 6: 85, 1959
147. Vincent PC, Sutherland R, Morris TCM, Chapman GV: Inhibitor of *in vitro* granulopoiesis in plasma of patients with renal failure. *Lancet* 2: 864, 1978
148. Craddock PR, Fehr J, Dalmasso AP, Brigham KL, Jacob HS: Hemodialysis leukopenia. Pulmonary vascular leukostasis resulting from complement activation by dialyzer cellophane membranes. *J Clin Invest* 59: 879, 1977
149. Peresecenschi G, Blum M, Aviram A, Spirer ZH: Impaired neutrophil response to acute bacterial infection in dialyzed patients. *Arch Intern Med* 141: 1301, 1981
150. Brayton RG, Stokes PE, Schwartz MS, Louria DB: Effect of alcohol and various diseases on leukocyte mobilization, phagocytosis and intracellular bacterial killing. *N Engl J Med* 282: 123, 1970
151. Buchanan WW, Klinenberg JR, Seegmiller JE: The inflammatory response to injected microcrystalline monosodium urate in normal hyperuremic, gouty and uremic subjects. *Arthritis Rheum* 8: 361, 1968
152. Abrutyn E, Solomons NW, St Clair L, MacGregor RR, Root RK: Granulocyte function in patients with chronic renal failure: surface adherence, phagocytosis and bactericidal activity *in vitro. J Infect Dis* 135: 1, 1977
153. Lespier-Dexter LE, Guerra C, Ojeda W, Martinez-Maldonado M: Granulocyte adherence in uremia and hemodialysis. *Nephron* 24: 64, 1979
154. Salant DJ, Glover AM, Anderson R, Meyers AM, Rabkin R, Myburgh JA, Rabson AR: Depressed neutrophil chemotaxis in patients with chronic renal failure and after renal transplantation. *J Lab Clin Med* 88: 536, 1976
155. Siriwatratananonta P, Sinsakul V, Stern K, Slavin RG: Defective chemotaxis in uremia. *J Lab Clin Med* 92: 402, 1978

156. Greene WH, Ray C, Mauer SM, Quie PG: The effect of hemodialysis on neutrophil chemotactic responsiveness. *J Lab Clin Med* 88: 971, 1976
157. Björkstén B, Mauer SM, Mills EL, Quie PG: The effect of hemodialysis on neutrophil chemotactic responsiveness. *Acta Med Scand* 203: 67, 1978
158. Goldblum SE, Van Epps DE, Reed WP: Serum inhibitor of C5 fragment-mediated polymorphonuclear leukocyte chemotaxis associated with chronic hemodialysis. *J Clin Invest* 64: 255, 1979
159. Modai D, Weissgarten J, Zolf R, Peller S, Averbukh Z, Kaufman S, Shaked U, Cohen N, Golik A, Tieder M: Effect of levamisole on chemotaxis of granulocytes from uremic patients. *Nephron* 49: 237, 1988
160. Charpentier B, Lang P, Martin B, Noury J, Mathieu D, Fries D: Depressed polymorphonuclear leukocyte functions associated with normal cytotoxic functions of T and natural killer cells during chronic hemodialysis. *Clin Nephrol* 19: 288, 1983
161. Hällgren R, Fjellström KE, Håkansson L, Venge P: The serum-independent uptake of IgG-coated particles by polymorphonuclear leukocytes from uremic patients on regular dialysis treatment. *J Lab Clin Med* 94: 277, 1979
162. Montgomerie JZ, Kalmanson GM, Guze LB: Leukocyte phagocytosis and serum bactericidal activity in chronic renal failure. *Am J Med Sci* 264: 385, 1972
163. Hirabayashi Y, Kobayashi T, Nishikawa A, Okazaki H, Aoki T, Takaya J, Kobayashi Y: Oxidative metabolism and phagocytosis of polymorphonuclear leukocytes in patients with chronic renal failure. *Nephron* 49: 305, 1988
164. Cantinieaux B, Boelaert J, Hariga C, Fondu P: Impaired neutrophil defense against Yersinia enterocolitica in patients with iron overload who are undergoing dialysis. *J Lab Clin Med* 111: 524, 1988
165. Boelaert JR, Cantinieaux BF, Hariga CF, Fondu PG: Recombinant erythropoietin reverses polymorphonuclear granulocyte dysfunction in iron-overloaded dialysis patients. *Nephrol Dial Transplant* 5: 504, 1990
166. Haag-Weber M, Hable M, Schollmeyer P, Hörl WH: Metabolic response of neutrophils to uremia and dialysis. *Kidney Int* 36: S293, 1989
167. Aparicio M, Vincendeau P, Gin H, Potaux L, Boucher JL, Martin-Dupont P, Morel D, dePrecigout V, Bezian JH: Effect of a low-protein diet on chemiluminescence production by leukocytes from uremic patients. *Nephron* 48: 315, 1988
168. Chandra RK: Rosette-forming T lymphocytes and cell-mediated immunity in malnutrition. *Br Med J* 3: 608, 1974
169. Vanholder R, Van Biesen W, Ringoir S: Contributing factors to the inhibition of phagocytosis in hemodialyzed patients. *Kidney Int* 44: 208, 1993
170. Vanholder R, Ringoir S, Dhondt A, Hakim R, Waterloos MA, Van Lantschoot N, Gung A: Phagocytosis in uremic and hemodialysis patients: a prespective and cross sectional study. *Kidney Int* 39: 320, 1991
171. Descamps-Latscha B, Goldfarb B, Nguyen AT, Landais P, London G, Haeffner-Cavaillon N, Jacquot C, Herbelin A, Kazatchkine M: Establishing the relationship between complement activations and stimulation of phagocyte oxidative metabolism in hemodialized patients: a randomized prospective study. *Nephron* 59: 279, 1991

172. Schopfer K, Douglas SD: Neutrophil function in children with kwashiorkor. *J Lab Clin Med* 88: 450, 1976

173. Thunberg BJ, Swamy AP, Cestero RVM: Cross-sectional and longitudinal nutritional measurements in maintenance hemodialysis patients. *Am J Clin Nutr* 34: 2005, 1981

174. Guarnieri G, Ranieri F, Lipartiti T, Spangaro F, Giuntini D, Faccini L, Toigo G, Legnani F, Raimondi A, Campanacci L: Protein-calorie malnutrition in hemodialysis patients. *Int J Artif Organs* 3: 143, 1980

175. Comty CM, Wathen RL, Shapiro F: Protein metabolism in renal failure. *Urology* 1: 528, 1973

176. Mattern WD, Hak LJ, Lamanna RW, Teasley KM, Laffell MS: Malnutrition, altered immune function, and the risk of infection in maintenance hemodialysis patients. *Am J Kidney Dis* 1: 206, 1982

177. Glassock RJ: Nutrition, immunology, and renal disease. *Kidney Int* 74 (Suppl 16): S194, 1983

178. Acchiardo SR, Moore LW, Latour PA: Malnutrition as the main factor in morbidity and mortality of hemodialysis patients. *Kidney Int* 24 (Suppl 16): S199, 1983

179. Wolfson M, Strong CJ, Minturn D, Gray DK, Kopple JD: Nutritional status and lymphocyte function in maintenance hemodialysis patients. *Am J Clin Nutr* 39: 547, 1984

180. Collins A, Ma J, Umen A: Infectious and all-cause death rates in hemodialysis (HD) patients (PTS) are lower with a mean hematocrit (HCT) of 32% versus 26%. *Abstract XIIth International Congress of Nephrology*, Jerusalem, Israel, June 13–18, 1993

181. Churchill DN, Taylor W, Cook RJ, LaPlante P, Barre P, Cartier P, Fay WP, Goldstein MB, Jindal K, Mandin H et al.: Canadian hemodialysis morbidity study. *Am J Kidney Dis* 19: 214, 1992

182. Hak LJ, Leffell MS, Lamanna RW, Teasley KM, Bazzarre CH, Mattern WD: Reversal of skin test anergy during maintenance hemodialysis by protein and caloric supplementation. *Am J Clin Nutr* 36: 1089, 1982

183. Casciato DA, McAdam LP, Kopple JD, Bluestone R, Goldberg LS, Clements PJ, Knutson DW: Immunologic abnormalities in hemodialysis patients: improvement after pyridoxine therapy. *Nephron* 38: 9, 1984

184. Antoniou LD, Shalhoub RJ, Schechter GP: The effect of zinc on cellular immunity in chronic uremia. *Am J Clin Nutr* 34: 1912, 1981

185. Antoniou LD, Shalhoub RJ: Zinc-induced enhancement of lymphocyte function and viability in chronic uremia. *Nephron* 40: 13, 1985

186. Briggs WA, Pedersen MM, Mahajan SK, Sillix DH, Prasad AS, McDonald FD: Lymphocyte and granulocyte function in zinc-treated and zinc-deficient hemodialysis patients. *Kidney Int* 21: 827, 1982

187. Opelz G, Sengar DP, Mickey MR, Terasaki PI: Effect of blood transfusions on subsequent kidney transplant. *Transplant Proc* 5: 253, 1973

188. Opelz G, Terasaki PI: Improvement of kidney-graft survival with increased numbers of blood transfusions. *N Engl J Med* 299: 799, 1978

189. Bender BS, Curtis JL, Nagel JE, Chrest FJ, Kraus ES, Briefel GR, Adler WH: Analysis of immune status of hemodialyzed adults: association with prior transfusions. *Kidney Int* 26: 436, 1984

190. Fehrman I, Ringdén O, Möller E, Lundgren G, Goth CG: Is cell-mediated immunity in the uremic patient affected by blood transfusion? *Transplant Proc* 13: 164, 1981

191. Klatzmann D, Gluckman JC, Foucault C, Bensussan A, Assobga U, Duboust A: Suppression of lymphocyte reactivity by blood transfusions in uremic patients. I. Proliferative responses. *Transplantation* 35: 332, 1983

192. Kerman RH, Van Buren CT, Payne W, Flechner S, Agostino G, Conley S, Brewer E, Kahan BD: The influence of pretransplant blood transfusions from random donors on immune parameters affecting cadaveric allograft survival. *Transplantation* 36: 50, 1983

193. Smith MD, Hardy G, Williams JD, Coles GA: Suppressor cell numbers and activity in non-transfused renal dialysis patients. *Clin Nephrol* 20: 130, 1983

194. Smith MD, Williams JD, Coles GA, Salaman JR: The effect of blood transfusion on T-suppressor cells in renal dialysis patients. *Transplant Proc* 13: 181, 1981

195. Smith MD, Williams JD, Coles GA, Salaman JR: Blood transfusions, suppressor T cells, and renal transplant survival. *Transplantation* 36: 647, 1983

196. Klatzmann D, Bensussan A, Gluckman JC, Foucault C, Dausset J, Sasportes M: Blood transfusions suppress lymphocyte reactivity in uremic patients. II. Evidence for soluble suppressor factors. *Transplantation* 36: 337, 1983

197. Roy R, Lachance JG, Noel R, Grose JH, Beaudoin R: Improved renal allograft function and survival following nonspecific blood transfusions. I. Induction of soluble suppressor factors inhibiting the mitogenic response. *Transplantation* 41: 640, 1986

198. Kessler M, Hoen B, Mayeux D, Hestin D, Fontenaille C: Bacteremia in patients on chronic hemodialysis. *Nephron* 64: 95, 1993

199. Goldman M, Vanherweghem JL: Bacterial infections in chronic hemodialysis patients: epidemiologic and pathophysiologic aspects. *Adv Nephrol* 19: 315, 1990

200. Keane WF, Shapiro FL, Raij L: Incidence and type of infections occurring in 445 chronic hemodialysis patients. *Trans Am Soc Artif Intern Organs* 23: 41, 1977

201. Maddy M, Keane WF: Unpublished observations

202. Bradley JR, Evans DB, Calne RY: Long-term survival in haemodialysis patients. *Lancet* 1: 295, 1987

203. Charra B, Calemard E, Ruffet M, Chazot C, Terrat JC, Vanel T, Laurent G: Survival as an index of adequacy of dialysis. *Kidney Int* 41: 1286, 1992

204. Silins J, Fortier L, Mao Y, Posen G, Ugnat AM, Brancker A, Gaudette L, Wigle D: Mortality rates among patients with end-stage renal disease in Canada, 1981–86. *Can Med Assoc J* 141: 677, 1989

205. Keane WF, Collins AJ: Influence of comorbidity on mortality and morbidity in patients treated with hemodialysis. *Am J Kidney Dis* 24: 1010, 1994

206. Dobkin JF, Miller MH, Steigbigel NH: Septicemia in patients on chronic hemodialysis. *Ann Intern Med* 88: 28, 1978

207. Nsouli KA, Lazarus M, Schoenbaum SC, Gottlieb MN, Lowrie EG, Shocair M: Bacteremic infection in hemodialysis. *Arch Intern Med* 139: 1255, 1979

208. Cheesbrough JS, Finch RG, Burden RP: A prospective study of the mechanisms of infection associated with hemodialysis catheters. *J Infect Dis* 154: 579, 1986

209. Moss AH, McLaughlin MM, Lempert KD, Holley JL: Use of a silicone catheter with a dacron cuff for dialysis

short-term vascular access. *Am J Kidney Dis* 12: 492, 1988

210. Gibson SP, Mosquera D: Five years experience with the Quinton Permcath for vascular access. *Nephrol Dial Transplant* 6: 269, 1991

211. Vanholder R, Hoenich N, Ringoir S: Morbidity and mortality of central venous catheter hemodialysis: a review of 10 years' experience. *Nephron* 47: 274, 1987

212. Vanherweghem JL, Dhaene M, Goldman M, Stolear JC, Sabot JP, Waterlot Y, Serruys E, Thayse C: Infections associated with subclavian dialysis catheters: the key role of nurse training. *Nephron* 42: 116, 1986

213. Kaplowitz LG, Comstock JA, Landwehr DM, Dalton HP, Mayhall G: A prospective study of infections in hemodialysis patients: patient hygiene and other risk factors for infection. *Infect Control Hosp Epidemiol* 12: 534, 1988

214. Mulloy LL, Caruana RJ, Steele JCH, Wynn JJ: Polymicrobial bacteremia during long-term hemodialysis. *South Med J* 84: 594, 1991

215. Pezzarossi HE, Ponce de Leon S, Calva JJ, Lazo de la Vega SA, Ruiz-Palacios GM: High incidence of subclavian dialysis catheter-related bacteremias. *Infect Control Hosp Epidemiol* 7: 596, 1986

216. Kirmani N, Tuazon CU, Murray HW, Parrish AE, Sheagren JN: Staphylococcus aureus carriage rate of patients receiving long-term hemodialysis. *Arch Intern Med* 138: 1657, 1978

217. Goldblum SE, Ulrich JA, Goldman RS, Reed WP: Nasal and cutaneous flora among hemodialysis patients and personnel: quantitative and qualitative characterization and patterns of Staphylococcal carriage. *Am J Kidney Dis* 2: 281, 1982

218. Chow JW, Sorkin M, Goetz A, Yu VL: Staphylococcal infections in the hemodialysis unit: prevention using infection control principles. *Infect Control Hosp Epidemiol* 9: 531, 1988

219. Yu VL, Goetz A, Wagener M, Smith PB, Rihs JD, Hanchett J, Zuravleff JJ: Staphylococcus aureus nasal carriage and infection in patients on hemodialysis. Efficacy of antibiotic prophylaxis. *N Engl J Med* 315: 91, 1986

220. Boelaert JR, De Baere YA, Geernaert MA, Godard CA, Van Landuyt HW: The use of nasal mupirocin ointment to prevent Staphylococcus aureus bacteraemias in haemodialysis patients: an analysis of cost-effectiveness. *J Hosp Infect* 19: 41, 1991

221. Gordon SM, Oettinger CW, Bland LA, Oliver JC, Arduino MJ, Aguero SM, McAllister SK, Favero MS, Jarvis WR: Pyrogenic reactions in patients receiving conventional, high-efficiency, or high-flux hemodialysis treatments with bicarbonate dialysate containing high concentrations of bacteria and endotoxin. *J Am Soc Nephrol* 2: 1436, 1992

222. Beck-Sague CM, Jarvis WF, Bland LA, Arduino MJ, Aguero SM, Verosic G: Outbreak of gram-negative bacteremia and pyrogenic reactions in a hemodialysis center. *Am J Nephrol* 10: 397, 1990

223. Longfield RN, Wortham WG, Fletcher LL, Nauscheutz WF: Clustered bacteremias in a hemodialysis unit: cross-contamination of blood tubing from ultrafiltrate waste. *Infect Control Hosp Epidemiol* 13: 160, 1992

224. Vanholder R, Vanhaecke E, Ringoir S: Waterborne pseudomonas septicemia. *ASAIO Trans* 36: M215, 1992

225. Latos DL, Stone WJ, Alford RH: Staphylococcus aureus bacteremia in hemodialysis patients. *J Dial* 1: 399, 1977

226. Francioli P, Masur H: Complications of Staphylococcus aureus bacteremia. Occurrence in patients undergoing long-term hemodialysis. *Arch Intern Med* 142: 1655, 1982

227. Quarles LD, Rutsky EA, Rostand SG: Staphylococcus aureus bacteremia in patients on chronic hemodialysis. *Am J Kidney Dis* 6: 412, 1985

228. Comty CM, Cohen SL, Shapiro FL: Pericarditis in chronic uremia and its sequels. *Ann Intern Med* 75: 173, 1971

229. Bailey GI, Hampers CL, Hager EB, Merrill JP: Uremic pericarditis: clinical features and management. *Circulation* 38: 582, 1968

230. Leonard A, Raij L, Shapiro FL: Bacterial endocarditis in regularly dialyzed patients. *Kidney Int* 4: 407, 1973

231. Goodman JS, Crews HD, Ginn HE, Koenig MG: Bacterial endocarditis as a possible complication of chronic hemodialysis. *N Engl J Med* 280: 876, 1969

232. King LH Jr, Bradley KP, Shires DL Jr, Donohue JP, Glover JL: Bacterial endocarditis in chronic hemodialysis patients: a complication more common than previously suspected. *Surgery* 69: 554, 1971

233. Ribot S, Rothfeld D, Frankel HJ: Infectious endocarditis in maintenance hemodialysis patients. *Am J Med Sci* 264: 183, 1972

234. Keane WF, Raij LR: Host defenses and infectious complications in maintenance hemodialysis patients. in *Replacement of Renal Function by Dialysis*, 2nd Edition, edited by Drukker W, Parsons FM, Maher JF, The Hague, Martinus Nijhoff, 1983, p 646

235. Mathews M, Shen FH, Lindner A, Sherrard DJ: Septic arthritis in hemodialyzed patients. *Nephron* 25: 87, 1980

236. Parker MA, Tuazon CU. Cervical osteomyelitis. Infection due to Staphylococcus epidermidis in hemodialysis patients. *JAMA* 240: 50, 1978

237. Leonard A, Comty CM, Shapiro FL, Raij L: Osteomyelitis in hemodialysis patients. *Ann Intern Med* 78: 651, 1973

238. Goodwin NJ, Castronuovo JJ, Friedman EA: Recurrent septic pulmonary embolization complicating maintenance hemodialysis. *Ann Intern Med* 71: 29, 1969

239. Levi J, Robson M, Rosenfeld JB: Septicaemia and pulmonary embolism complicating use of arteriovenous fistula in maintenance haemodialysis. *Lancet* 2: 288, 1970

240. Shapiro FL, Messner RP, Smith HT: Satellite hemodialysis. *Ann Intern Med* 69: 673, 1968

241. Aman LC, Levin NW, Smith DW: Hemodialysis access site morbidity. *Proc Dial Transplant Forum* 10: 277, 1980

242. Porter JA, Sharp WV, Walsh EJ: Complications of vascular access in a dialysis population. *Curr Surg* 42: 298, 1985

243. Winsett OE, Wolma FJ: Complications of vascular access for hemodialysis. *South Med J* 78: 513, 1985

244. Windus DW, Jendrisak MD, Delmez JA: Prosthetic fistula survival and complication in hemodialysis patients: effects of diabetes and age. *Am J Kidney Dis* 19: 448, 1992

245. Ralston AJ, Harlow GR, Jones DM, Davis P: Infections of Scribner and Brescia arteriovenous shunts. *Br Med J* 3: 408, 1971

246. Kinnaert P, Vereerstraeten P, Toussaint C, Van Geertruyden J: Nine years' experience with internal arteriovenous fistulas for haemodialysis. *Br J Surg* 64: 242, 1977

247. Palder SB, Kirkman RL, Whittemore AD, Hakim RM, Lazarus JM, Tilney NL: Vascular access for hemodialysis. *Ann Surg* 202: 235, 1985

248. Zibari GB, Rohr MS, Landreneau MD, Bridges RM, DeVault GA, Petty FH, Costley KJ, Brown ST, McDonald JC: Complications from permanent hemodialysis vascular access. *Surgery* 104: 681, 1988

249. Vanderwerf BA, Rattazzi LC, Katzman KA, Schild AF: Three year experience with bovine graft arteriovenous (A-V) fistulas in 100 patients. *Trans Am Soc Artif Intern Organs* 21: 296, 1975

250. Yokoyama T, Bower R, Chinitz J, Schwartz A, Swartz C: Experience with 100 bovine arteriografts for maintenance hemodialysis. *Trans Am Soc Artif Intern Organs* 20: 328, 1974

251. Sabanayagam P, Schwartz AB, Soricelli RR, Lyons R, Chinitz J: A comparative study of 402 bovine heterografts and 225 reinforced expanded PTFE grafts as AVF in the ESRD patients. *Trans Am Soc Artif Intern Organs* 26: 88, 1980

252. Lilly L, Nghiem D, Mendez-Picon G, Lee HM: Comparison between bovine heterograft and expanded PTFE grafts for dialysis access. *Am Surg* 46: 694, 1980

253. Kaslow RA, Zellner SR: Infection in patients on maintenance hemodialysis. *Lancet* 2: 117, 1972

254. Dunea G, Domenico L, Gunnerson P, Winston-Willis F: A survey of permanent double lumen catheters in hemodialysis patients. *ASAIO Trans* 37: M276, 1991

255. Shusterman NH, Kloss K, Mullen JL: Successful use of double-lumen, silicone rubber catheters for permanent hemodialysis access. *Kidney Int* 35: 887, 1989

256. Bhat DJ, Tellis VA, Kohlberg WI, Driscoll B, Veith FJ: Management of sepsis involving expanded polytetrafluoroethylene grafts for hemodialysis access. *Surgery* 87: 445, 1980

257. Nghiem DD, Schulak JA, Corry RJ: Management of the infected hemodialysis access grafts. *Trans Am Soc Artif Intern Organs* 29: 362, 1983

258. Morris AJ, Bilinsky RT. Prevention of staphylococcal shunt infections by continuous vancomycin prophylaxis. *Am J Med Sci* 261: 88, 1971

259. Bass HE, Singer E: Pulmonary changes in uremia. *JAMA* 144: 819, 1950

260. Bass HE, Greenberg D, Singer E: Pulmonary changes in uremia. *JAMA* 148: 724, 1952

261. Hopps HC, Wissler RW: Uremic pneumonitis. *Am J Pathol* 31: 261, 1955

262. Rackow EC, Fein IA, Sprung C, Grodman RS: Uremic pulmonary edema. *Am J Med* 64: 1084, 1978

263. Goldstein E, Green GM: The effect of acute renal failure on the bacterial clearance mechanisms of the lung. *J Lab Clin Med* 68: 531, 1966

264. Johanson WG, Pierce AK, Sanford JP: Changing pharyngeal bacterial flora of hospitalized patients. Emergence of gram-negative bacilli. *N Engl J Med* 281: 1137, 1969

265. Jadav SK, Sant SM, Acharya VN: Bacteriology of urinary tract infection in patients of renal failure undergoing dialysis. *J Postgrad Med* 23: 10, 1977

266. Saitoh H, Nakamura K, Hida M, Satoh T: Urinary tract infection in oliguric patients with chronic renal failure. *J Urol* 133: 990, 1985

267. Chaudhry A, Stone WJ, Breyer JA: Occurrence of pyuria and bacteriuria in asymptomatic hemodialysis patients. *Am J Kidney Dis* 21: 180, 1993

268. Rault R: Symptomatic urinary tract infections in patients on maintenance hemodialysis. *Nephron* 37: 82, 1984

269. Bennett WM, Craven R: Urinary tract infections in patients with severe renal disease. *JAMA* 236: 946, 1976

270. Pradhan RP, Katz LA, Nidus BD, Matalon R, Eisinger RP: Tuberculosis in dialyzed patients. *JAMA* 229: 798, 1974

271. Papadimitriou M, Memmos D, Metaxas P: Tuberculosis in patients on regular hemodialysis. *Nephron* 24: 53, 1979

272. Andrew OT, Schoenfeld P, Hopewell PC, Humphreys M: Tuberculosis in patients with end-stage renal disease. *Am J Med* 68: 59, 1980

273. Lundin AP, Adler AJ, Berlyne GM, Friedman EA: Tuberculosis in patients undergoing maintenance hemodialysis. *Am J Med* 67: 597, 1979

274. Rutsky EA, Rostand SG: Mycobacteriosis in patients with chronic renal failure. *Arch Intern Med* 140: 57, 1980

275. Sasaki S, Akiba T, Suenaga M, Tomura S, Yoshiyama N, Nakagawa S, Shoji T, Sasaoka T, Takeuchi J: Ten years' survey of dialysis-associated tuberculosis. *Nephron* 24: 141, 1979

276. Belcon MC, Smith EKM, Kahana LM, Shimizu AG: Tuberculosis in dialysis patients. *Clin Nephrol* 17: 14, 1982

277. Mori MA, Leonardson G, Welty TK: The benefits of isoniazid chemoprophylaxis and risk factors for tuberculosis among Oglala Sioux Indians. *Arch Intern Med* 152: 547, 1992

278. Zeitlin J, Carvounis CP, Murphy RG, Tortora GT: Graft infection and bacteremia with Listeria monocytogenes in a patient receiving hemodialysis. *Arch Intern Med* 142: 2191, 1982

279. Woolridge TD, Cox JW: Graft infection and bacteremia. *Arch Intern Med* 143: 1070, 1983

280. Mossey RT, Sondheimer J: Listeriosis in patients with long-term hemodialysis and transfusional iron overload. *Am J Med* 79: 397, 1985

281. Van Cutsem J, Boelaert JR: Effects of deferoxamine, feroxamine and iron on experimental mucormycosis (zygomycosis). *Kidney Int* 36: 1061, 1989

282. Bárány P, Stenvinkel P, Nord CE, Bergström J: Clostridium difficile infection – a poor prognostic sign in uremic patients? *Contrib Nephrol* 38: 53, 1992

283. Leung ACT, Orange G, McLay A, Henderson S: Clostridium difficile-associated colitis in uremic patients. *Clin Nephrol* 24: 242, 1985

284. Aronsson B, Barany P, Nord CE, Nyström B, Stenvinkel P: Clostridium difficile-associated diarrhoea in uremic patients. *Eur J Clin Microbiol* 6: 352, 1987

VIRAL INFECTIONS IN DIALYSIS PATIENTS
PART A: HUMAN IMMUNODEFICIENCY VIRUS INFECTION IN DIALYSIS PATIENTS

T.K. SREEPADA RAO

VIRAL INFECTION IN DIALYSIS PATIENTS; HIV

Some of the important questions for nephrologists providing maintenance hemodialysis (MH) or peritoneal dialysis (PD) to patients with end stage renal disease (ESRD) who are also infected with various viral agents include:

a) What is the preferential mode of renal replacement therapy for ESRD patients, if the long-term prognosis is determined by the nature and severity of viral infection?

b) What are the different therapeutic strategies to treat these infected patients, such as the deployment of antiviral drugs, immunomodulators, and others, and their adverse effects in patients with compromised renal function?

c) What are the combined effects of superimposition of immunosuppression on chronic uremia, maintenance dialysis, renal transplantation, and immunosuppressive therapy, on the natural history of viral disease, especially in patients infected with the human immunodeficiency virus (HIV) which preferentially affects the T cell system?

d) What are the risks of nosocomial transmission of viral infections within a dialysis facility from patient to patient, patient to staff, and *vice versa*, and the precautions to be undertaken to prevent or minimize such a spread in dialysis units?

e) what are some of the legal issues surrounding patient and staff confidentiality, while providing patient care?

Many of the above issues which can lead to serious adverse consequences in dialysis patients and staff, are also valid in conjunction with many bacterial infections (staphylococcal, mycobacterium tuberculosis, etc). This chapter will be confined to a discussion of viral infections in ESRD patients, and in particular to HIV. Other viral diseases of concern in dialysis patients such as hepatitis B (HBV), hepatitis C (HCV), and cytomegalovirus (CMV), will not be discussed here.

In persons infected with HIV, a retro virus, clinical manifestations range from no obvious signs or symptoms (asymptomatic seropositive carriers), to a multisystem disease, namely, acquired immunodeficiency syndrome (AIDS). AIDS is characterized by severe constitutional symptoms, cachexia, life threatening conventional and opportunistic infections (OI), and development of unusual malignancies. The primary target of HIV is the CD4+ T lymphocyte, and a hallmark of the immunologic deficit in HIV disease is a progressive depletion of circulating CD4 cells, leading to immune deficiency, accompanied by the onset of clinical signs and symptoms at variable intervals. Clinical manifestations tend to occur in a temporal sequence, linked to the immune deficiency. For example, herpes zoster occurs earlier when immune function is relatively intact, oral thrush with moderate impairment of the immune system, and pneumocystis carinii pneumonia (PCP) and mycobacterium avium intracellularae (MAI) infection with advanced immunodeficiency. Prognosis depends on the stage of HIV infection, longer survival is seen in asymptomatic seropositive individuals, while patients with advanced clinical AIDS have the shortest survival. The factors which determine this variable (months to years), yet inexorable progression, from an intact immune status in the early stages, to onset of constitutional symptoms, multisystem disease, and functional disability leading to a very high mortality, are still poorly understood. Over the past decade, the Centers for Disease Control (CDC) has revised, several times, the classification system for HIV infection and guidelines for expanded surveillance case definition for the diagnosis of AIDS (1, 2). Under the recently modified guidelines, all patients with a CD4 count of $< 200/\mu l$ even without the presence of OI, and/or malignancies, are classified as having AIDS (2).

HIV ASSOCIATED RENAL DISORDERS

Infectious complications in the lungs, central nervous system, and gastrointestinal tract, malignancies such as Kaposi's sarcoma and lymphomas usually dominate the clinical features in most HIV patients. Renal manifestations which were first described in 1984 (3–5), are now recognized with increasing frequency both in the United States and elsewhere (6, 7). In the early 1980s, the diagnosis of AIDS was based on the clinical criteria of the presence of OI or unusual malignancy in persons with no known prior immunodeficiency. Consequently, initial descriptions of renal disease were referred to as AIDS associated nephropathy (AAN). The identification of HIV, and the introduction of serological markers to diagnose viral infection in its early stages, has resulted in the recognition of renal syndromes in many asymptomatic carriers of HIV. Hence, AAN is now changed to a comprehensive term HIV-associated nephropathy (HIVAN), to include renal manifestations in patients with all stages of HIV disease. From the studies published over the past decade, nephrologic problems associated with HIV infection can be broadly categorized into:

1. a spectrum of acute renal failure (ARF), the commonest being potentially reversible acute tubular necrosis,
2. HIV-associated nephropathy (HIVAN), manifested by nephrotic syndrome, focal and segmental glomerulosclerosis (FSGS), and rapid progression to ESRD,
3. ESRD from unrelated causes occurring in individuals with prior HIV infection,
4. patients undergoing maintenance hemodialysis (MH), peritoneal dialysis (PD), or renal transplantation (RT), acquiring HIV infection from blood transfusions, renal allografts, intravenous drug abuse (needle sharing), or through sexual contacts.

HIV infection, therefore, leads not only to the development of ESRD, but may also be a coincidental phenomenon in many subjects during the course of management of renal failure.

I. Acute Renal failure in HIV includes several heterogeneous disorders as listed in Table 1. For a detailed discussion of ARF in HIV disease, readers are referred to two current publications (8, 9). It is not surprising that ARF especially acute tubular necrosis (ATN), is a frequent occurrence in acutely ill hospitalized AIDS patients suffering from multiple infectious complications with hemodynamic compromise, and requiring the use of multiple nephrotoxic agents, such as radiocontrast agents, pentamidine, aminoglycoside antibiotics, etc, in their management. In many AIDS patients who are being treated in intensive care units, ATN may be a terminal event and dialysis support may be futile or not feasible. However in others, hemodialysis, peritoneal dialysis, or continuous arterio-venous hemofiltration (CAVH) for a brief duration, will result in the restoration of renal function, and patient survival. In other words, although the mortality from ARF is high in AIDS patients, with support-

Table 1. Acute renal disorders in HIV patients

Fluid, electrolyte, and acid-base derangements
1. Hypo and hypernatremia.
2. Inappropriate secretion of antidiuretic hormone (ADH).
3. Hypo and hyperkalemia.
4. Type IV renal tubular acidosis (hyporeninemic hypoaldosteronism).
5. Metabolic acidosis and alkalosis.
6. Hypo and hypercalcemia.
7. Hypomagnesemia.
8. Hypo and hyperphosphatemia.
9. Hypo and hyperuricemia.
10. Lactic acidosis.

Infections in the kidney
1. Renal micro abcesses from bacterial infections.
2. Tuberculosis of the kidney (Both typical and atypical mycobacterium).
3. Cytomegalovirus (other viral?) infections.
4. Candida, Cryptococcal, Aspergillous, mucormycosis, nocardial, and other fungal infections.

Infiltrative lesions of the kidney
1. Lymphoma of the kidney.
2. Kaposi's sarcoma.
3. Amyloidosis of the kidney.
4. Calcifications in the kidney.
5. Hypernephroma.
6. Other malignancies.

Acute renal failure (ARF)
1. Acute tubular necrosis from hypovolemic, anoxic, and toxic injuries.
2. Crystal induced renal failure (sulphadiazine and acyclovir).
3. Rhabdomyolysis and myoglobinuric renal failure.
4. Allergic interstitial nephritis from drugs such as trimethoprim sulphamethaxazole, phenytoin, and other agents.
5. Acute azotemia from non-steroidal anti-inflammatory drugs.
6. Plasmacytic Interstitial nephritis.
7. ARF from hemolytic uremic syndrome.
8. ARF from thrombotic thrombocytopenic purpura.
9. Post infectious immune complex glomerulonephritis.
10. Renal edema from massive proteinuria and severe hypoalbuminemia.
11. Multiple myeloma.
12. Urate deposits induced renal failure.
13. Obstructive nephropathy.
14. Retroperitoneal fibrosis.

ive care and dialysis, many will recover kidney function and survive for long periods to subsequently receive the benefits of anti-retroviral therapy. It is therefore essential that clinicians recognize reversible forms of ARF in HIV patients, and treat them aggressively with dialysis therapy. The choice between peritoneal or hemodialysis in the management of ARF in AIDS is dependent on the patient's hemodynamic status, and the availability of resources at the institution. We have generally employed repeated femoral vein cannulations, or indwelling subclavian or internal jugular vein catheters for vascular access for hemodialysis. While undergoing hemodialysis in intensive care units, hemodynamic parameters are monitored and pressor agents and fluid/colloids replacement are used as needed. We prefer the use of sorbent dialysis systems (such as the Redy system) to accomplish hemodialysis at the patient's bedside. On occasions, intermittent or continuous PD is employed in patients who cannot tolerate hemodialysis. Dialysis therapy is continued until recovery of renal function, or the patient's condition is considered terminal, and further treatment is unlikely to change the prognosis. In AIDS patients with ARF, withholding dialysis support must be individualized, taking into consideration a reasonable probability of salvagability, the wishes of patient and the family, in conjunction with the primary physicians. The precautions to be followed by staff while dialyzing HIV patients with ARF are similar to that during MD therapy in ESRD subjects (discussed later).

II. ESRD secondary to HIV infection: HIVAN, seen predominantly in young black men, and rare among caucasians, is characterized by nephrotic syndrome, FSGS, and a rapid fulminant progression to ESRD, in weeks to few months. HIVAN is not limited to patients with advanced clinical AIDS, but occurs in all stages of HIV infection. According to some workers, in about 30% of patients with HIVAN, nephrotic syndrome may be the initial presenting clinical feature, leading to the diagnosis of HIV infection in otherwise asymptomatic seropositive individuals (10). The unusual clinical aspect of HIVAN is the fulminant deterioration of renal function to irreversible uremia in the absence of contributing factors such as malignant hypertension, severe volume depletion, or exposure to nephrotoxic agents. Renal histology also fails to explain the rapid nature of renal functional loss. In most reports, progression to ESRD from the onset of massive proteinuria has ranged from a few weeks to few months (average about 4 months), although great variability exists. This observation contrasts strikingly with the clinical course of patients with idiopathic forms of FSGS, and that found in association with heroin addiction and other disorders. The typical renal histologic lesion consists of FSGS, glomerular collapse, marked epithelial cell changes, with intraglomerular deposition of IgM and C3. The most striking pathological features are seen in the renal tubules, and include severe tubular degenerative changes, tubular microectasia commonly referred to as 'microcystic dilatation', with the lumen filled with pale staining proteinaceous casts. Dilated tubules are present throughout the renal cortex and medulla. There is a notable absence of interstitial infiltrates, interstitial fibrosis, and arteriolar changes of hypertension. Under immunofluorescence microscopy, there is localization of IgM, C3, and C1q in the sclerosed segments, and in other mesangial regions. Characteristic ultrastructural lesions consist of multiple complex inclusions both in the nuclei and cytoplasm in a variety of cells, abundant tubuloreticular inclusions (TRI) in the vascular (glomerular, peritubular capillary, arterial and venular) endothelium, and interstitial cell cytoplasm (11, 12). Based on these findings, a viral etiology for HIVAN has been strongly suggested. The *in situ* hybridization studies demonstrating pro-viral HIV-DNA in renal tubular and glomerular epithelial cells offer strong support for the viral invasion theory in the causation of HIVAN (13). Recent studies strongly suggest a role for cytokines, such as transforming growth factor beta (TGF-β) in the pathogenesis of glomerulosclerosis in HIVAN (14–16).

In the early years of the AIDS epidemic, the survival of most patients with clinical AIDS and ESRD treated by MD was dismal. This outlook has changed significantly in recent years. As discussed later, survival in HIV disease patients with ESRD (irrespective of its cause) undergoing MD, is dependent on the clinical stage of viral infection.

III. ESRD secondary to other causes in HIV patients. It is estimated that there are more than a million HIV infected individuals in the US. It is therefore not surprising that diseases such as diabetes mellitus, hypertension, polycystic kidneys and others, leading causes of ESRD in population, can also occur in patients infected with HIV (7).

IV. HIV infection developing in patients prior to ESRD

1. ESRD subjects receiving renal replacement therapy may acquire HIV infection from blood transfusions, and renal allografts. With the introduction of mandatory screening of all transfused blood and organ donors, this mode of HIV transmission is likely to diminish and hopefully disappear.

2. Patients undergoing MD or RT can also acquire HIV infection through sexual contacts, and intravenous drug abuse.

Obviously, in this group of patients, since ESRD has preceded HIV infection, overall survival during renal replacement therapy can be expected to be much longer, than in those with a diagnosis of HIVAN in whom renal failure develops months to years after the onset of HIV infection.

HIV PROBLEMS IN DIALYSIS

The prevalence of HIV infection in the general population varies in different parts of the United States, with the highest incidence observed in some large metropolitan areas around the country. HIVAN is rare among caucasians, and hence ESRD secondary to HIVAN is a significant problem in certain large urban areas serving minorities. However, the disease is seen in all parts of the country. The USRDS 1993 annual data report, lists AIDS related nephropathy as a cause of ESRD in only 297 out of over 160,000 patients (< 0.2% overall) treated in the US between 1987 and 1990 (17), which obviously does not reflect the true prevalence. A recent annual report from the ESRD Network of NY, shows that there has been a progressive increase in the number of patients with HIV infection treated by MD in New York State from 18 in 1988 to 152 in 1992 (18). In the last ten years, the number of HIV patients with ESRD, in whom MH was initiated at Kings County Hospital Center in Brooklyn, NY, has varied between 15 to 35 each year (20 to 40% of all ESRD patients). However, in most dialysis centers in the US and elsewhere, the cause of ESRD in a majority of HIV seropositive patients is something other than HIVAN, and most would have acquired HIV infection through contaminated blood transfusions or via other known modes of transmission (sexual contact or needle sharing). While the number of patients with ESRD (from all causes) receiving renal replacement therapy in the US exceeded 180,000 in 1993, the latest CDC report indicates that 1.5% of 170,028 patients undergoing MD in 2170 dialysis centers in 1992 (approximately 2600), were infected with HIV (19). The incidence of HIV seropositivity in dialysis centers in the US has varied between 0% to 35% depending on the location of the facility, and the demographics of patients treated at the center (20). As summarized in Table 2, the incidence of HIV seropositivity in dialysis centers outside the US, is low and generally below 1% (20). In other words, the magnitude of HIV infection in an ESRD population receiving MD or PD is relatively small. Yet the issue is one of great significance in evoking many ethical and legal concerns among renal physicians.

PROGNOSIS IN HIV PATIENTS TREATED BY DIALYSIS

Prognosis of HIV infected ESRD patients treated by MD is dependent on the stage of HIV disease rather than the nature of the primary renal diagnosis. In the early years, before the introduction of serologic studies for HIV, the diagnosis of AIDS was established by clinical markers, and early asymptomatic patients could not be identified. Consequently, our initial observations in 1987, consisted of only those patients with advanced AIDS who were suffering from OI and or malignancies. The mean survival in 79 ESRD patients with AIDS who were treated by hemodialysis was only 3 months, with 2 patients surviving beyond 6 months, and none more than a year (21). These findings were substantiated by Ortiz et al. in 1988, who reported a mean survival of 93 ± 32 days (median 30

Table 2. HIV seropositivity in dialysis patients

Place[a]	No. tested/ no. positive	From transfusion
EDTA 1988	NR/277	72 of 127
Belgium	68/3 (4.4%)	3
Belgium	100/5 (5.0%)	3
Belgium	729/0	0
Italy	124/0	0
Italy	143/1 (0.7%)	1
Italy	87/0	0
Italy	320/0	0
Italy	645/2 (0.3%)	1
Frankfurt	1046/4 (0.4%)	NR
Berlin	434/0	0
Berlin	276/4 (1.4%)	4
Dusseldorf	02/4 (1.3%)	4
Vienna	110/1 (0.9%)	1
New Castle, UK	236/0	0
London, UK	137/0	0
Spain	308/2 (0.6%)	1
Brazil	132/19 (14.0%)	18
Cairo, Egypt	42/0	0
Paris	409/4 (1.0%)	3
Paris	49/1 (2.0%)	1
Japan	1066/0	0
Japan	248/0	0
Chicago, USA	83/0	0
Chicago, USA	520/4 (0.7%)	4
Virginia, USA	79/2 (2.5%)	2
Brooklyn, USA	67/5 (7.5%)	0
Brooklyn, USA	70/27 (39.0%)	2
Brooklyn, USA	155/16 (10.0%)	2
Miami, USA	129/22 (17.0%)	5
Miami, USA	80/9 (11.2%)	9
Jacksonville, USA	50/0	0
Pleasantville, USA	70/1 (1.4%)	0
Baltimore, USA	435/12 (2.8%)	12
Boston, USA	90/3 (3.3%)	3
Boston, USA	100/1 (1.0%)	1
Houston, USA	572/5 (0.9%)	5
Cleveland, USA	270/3 (1.1%)	NR
CDC 1988, USA	NR/1253	NR
CDC 1992, USA	NR/2600 (1.5%)	NR

NR: Not reported.
[a] See reference (20) for details.

days) in 17 AIDS patients (22). Furthermore, these workers also found a median survival of 420 days (mean 564 ± 191 days) in 5 patients with AIDS related complex (ARC). In a dialysis facility in Newark, NJ, 75% of AIDS patients with ESRD were dead in 6 months, and 88% in 12 months (23). In a short series of 5 AIDS subjects treated by Feinfeld *et al.* in 1989, a better mean survival of 13.2 ± 1.9 months was noted (24). In all these studies, death mainly resulted from opportunistic, and or intercurrent infections, and various malignancies. In addition, many AIDS patients exhibited a 'failure to thrive' syndrome manifested by severe cachexia unresponsive to nutritional supplementation. In many patients, death also resulted from suicide, and discontinuation of dialysis due to patient's and family preference. It was unclear whether such a poor prognosis noted in ESRD patients treated by maintenance dialysis was different from AIDS patients without renal failure. We have speculated that a persistent viremia, or other factors inherent to dialysis or chronic uremia *per se* (additional immunosuppression, severe anemia, malnutrition, cytokine disregulation such as excessive production of tumor necrosis factor, and other unknown factors), may be responsible for the poor survival in AIDS patients. On the other hand, prognosis in asymptomatic HIV carriers with ESRD undergoing MH was significantly better, with a mean survival of 488 ± 75 days in the studies by Ortiz *et al.* (22), and 15.7 ± 3.0 months in the experience of Feinfeld *et al.* (24). Chirgwin and co-workers, also reported a > 1 year survival in their HIV seropositive patients, with only one patient developing clinical AIDS during the 12 month observation period (25). During MD, some asymptomatic HIV carriers do progress to ARC and AIDS. In Miami, of the 28 asymptomatic HIV carriers beginning MD, 4 progressed to ARC and 3 to AIDS after 276 ± 81 days (median 180 days). Of the 17 ESRD patients with an initial diagnosis of ARC, 8 developed AIDS after 179 ± 35 days (median 210 days) of MH therapy (22). It is also unclear whether chronic uremia/maintenance dialysis *per se* can accelerate the progression from an HIV seropositive state to clinical AIDS. Limited data indicate that some HIV positive patients develop AIDS in about 7 months (22), while some continue to do well (25). However, the number of patients was small, and follow-up observation had been short.

Because of the gloomy results with MH in patients with AIDS, some nephrologists suggested the alternative deployment of continuous ambulatory peritoneal dialysis (CAPD). They felt that the glucose load from the dialysate may provide additional obligatory calories in improving the nutritional status in HIV patients, and prevent the inanition observed during MH. Another reason for this recommendation was also to minimize HIV transmission risks to staff members. Theoretically, exposure of staff to HIV infected patients is less during peritoneal dialysis than hemodialysis because: 1) peritoneal fluid may be less infectious than blood, 2) there is less likelihood of needle sticks, and 3) there is a different nature of staff to patient contact. Kimmel *et al.*, could not detremine any difference in the survival of patients treated by MH or CAPD. In their studies, a survival rate of 14.7 ± 8.5 months in 23 HIV patients treated by MH was similar to 17.9 ± 10.3 months in 8 receiving CAPD (26). All 31 patients in this study had either stage III or stage IV HIV disease. Another retrospective analysis of 39 HIV infected patients treated by CAPD, revealed one and two year survival rates of 58% and 54% respectively (27). Isolated observations from other centers also indicate similar rates of survival of HIV patients treated by MH or CAPD (28–30). A few case reports suggest an increased risk of peritonitis (fungal, tubercular, and unusual pathogens) in HIV patients undergoing CAPD therapy (31–34). However, other studies, with larger number of patients, do not support the fact that HIV patients treated by CAPD suffer from increased infection episodes (35). It is important to remember that the peritoneal dialysate is infectious and HIV has been isolated from the peritoneal fluid (36, 37). Therefore, the dialysate and all supplies used during CAPD must disposed of in the correct manner.

An essential point to keep in mind is that all of the above mentioned studies which have analyzed survival in HIV patients treated by MD, are retrospective observations. Most patients had not received anti-retroviral and other chemoprophylactic drugs employed in modern times. From the limited available information, it is unwise to draw firm conclusions regarding the prognosis of HIV infected ESRD patients undergoing renal replacement therapy.

Some recent observations indicate that the survival of ESRD patients with HIV disease is improving. A current analysis from our center showed that 41% of ESRD patients with advanced HIV disease were alive more than 15 months (38), many beyond 4 years. In the studies by Kimmel *et al.*, a mean survival of 15.5 ± 9.9 months in a group of 31 young HIV infected patients (mean age 37.5 ± 9.7 years) was seen which as expected, was significantly worse than the 44.0 ± 33.9 months survival in 361 non-HIV much older subjects (49.8 ± 15.7 years) (26). A report from the ESRD Network of New York, found a crude mortality rate in dialysis patients with HIV disease of 53.2% in 1989, which improved to 37.5% in 1992 (18). Unfortunately, overall survival data from US dialysis centers is not available.

The improvement in survival of HIV patients with or without renal disease in recent years, is related to better overall care, and may also in part be due to the widespread use of anti retroviral therapy, largely zidovudine (AZT). In the past, the recommended dose of AZT (usually 200 mg, five to six times daily), was associated even in non-renal patients with a high rate of side effects including gastrointestinal intolerance, insomnia, and myalgia. Other major side effects of AZT were bone marrow suppression leading to neutropenia, and severe anemia requiring blood transfusions, and discontinuation of the drug. In ESRD patients, AZT administration was especially difficult because of pre-existing anemia of chronic uremia. Until recently, there has been a great reluctance on the part of many physicians to use AZT in patients with uremia, primarily because of a lack of knowledge of the pharmacokinetics and side effect profile of AZT in the presence of renal insufficiency. At present, a reduction in dosage in all patients, and also a better understanding of the pharmacokinetics of AZT in patients with normal and severe renal failure, and in those undergoing MH or PD, has lead to wider use of AZT (39–42). The oral bioavailability of AZT is 60%, about 15–20% is excreted unchanged in the urine, with an elimination half life of one hour. AZT is metabolized in the liver to glucorinidated AZT (GAZT), whose half life is also about one hour. AZT is not nephrotoxic, and its renal clearance is 350 ml/min in a 70 kg man. In persons with normal GFR, with the administration of 200 mg every 4 hours, the peak plasma AZT concentration after 60 minutes is 0.62 μg/ml, and trough level of 0.16 μg/ml (both are virostatic concentrations). In dialysis subjects, peak plasma AZT concentration of 0.61 μg/ml after 40 minutes, and a trough level of 0.15 μg/ml is seen after a dose of 100 mg every 8 hours. The half life is not significantly altered compared to normals (although in one study both parameters were increased). GAZT, on the other hand, accumulates, and the plasma levels are greatly elevated in the presence of renal failure. During hemodialysis, the clearance of AZT has ranged between 63–102 ml/min (peritoneal clearance is negligible < 5 ml/min). Since this accounts for only about 5–8% of residual renal clearance, hemodialysis has no appreciable effect on AZT elimination, and supplemental doses are not needed. On the other hand, hemodialyzer clearance of GAZT is 71–91 ml/min in two studies which exceeds renal clearance. The biological effects of high levels of GAZT in renal failure patients are unknown. Although studies analyzing the toxicity in uremic patients are unavailable, limited experience by us and others indicate that anemia was a major limiting factor in the use of AZT. Anemia observed with AZT therapy in non-azotemic patients is associated with either low or high concentration of serum erythropoietin (EPO) (43). Those with low serum EPO levels respond well to exogenous recombinant human EPO (rHuEPO), with increase in hemoglobin and reduction in transfusion requirements (43). Recently we have also demonstrated that AZT induced anemia in HIV patients treated by MH is accompanied by low and high levels of serum EPO (44). The response to rHuEPO also correlates with low serum EPO levels in HIV patients receiving AZT and MH (44). In summary, 100 mg of AZT given three or four times a day may be appropriate in patients with renal failure, and the accompanying anemia can be effectively ameliorated with the use of rHuEPO.

Other therapeutic modalities in HIV patients include the use of newer anti-retroviral drugs such as 2',3'-dideoxyinosine (ddi), chemoprophylaxis (aerozolized pentamidine, and trimethoprim-sulfamethaxazole to prevent PCP, antitubercular drugs), and vaccination against pneumococci, influenza and others. For a detailed review of guidelines for usage of various drugs in HIV patients

with ESRD, readers are referred to a recent publication (45).

HIV disease, as well as chronic uremia irrespective of etiology, share a wide range of clinical and immune abnormalities (46–49). The hallmarks of both these syndromes are lymphocytopenia, defective cell mediated immunity, and decreased specific antibody production. Adoptive cell transfer experiments in animal models and *in vitro* studies have shown that a serum factor(s) is responsible for suppression of cell mediated immunity in uremia. In contrast, HIV induced immunosuppression involves intrinsic T-cell defects among a host of other abnormalities including decreased production of interferon-γ, and interleukin-2 (IL-2), but increased production of interleukin-6 (IL-6) and tumor necrosis factor (TNF) (50, 51). While uremia is characterized by decreased immunoglobulin levels, especially IgM, HIV disease typically manifests polyclonal hypergammaglobulinemia except during terminal AIDS. HIV infection is also associated with selective loss of CD4+, and CD29+ memory cells (48). This fact, coupled with the small number of reported cases of progression to AIDS in HIV seropositive dialysis patients has lead some to suggest that uremia may suppress the overt clinical expression of HIV in the absence of co-factors (52). HIV has tropism for T lymphocytes bearing the CD4 antigen, especially activated CD4 cells. In chronic uremia, the presence of qualitative and quantitative abnormalities of immune responses may limit (protect?) HIV replication. Patients undergoing MD, receive blood transfusions, and contract other viral infections (HBV, HBC, CMV and others), clinical events which will either stimulate or further depress the immune system. In urban centers such as Brooklyn, Miami, and Washington DC, many ESRD patients are narcotic addicts who continue to abuse drugs and share needles, risking repeated exposure to HIV and other infections, events which are likely to further exert a varying influence on the the immune status. In uremic patients treated by MD, the complicated interaction of these co-factors on the clinical progression of a latent HIV infection is not known. It might be argued that these co-factors act synergistically to stress a marginal immune system, thereby hastening the development of overt AIDS. The reported experience in dialysis patients does not support this argument, and prolonged survival of HIV seropositive individuals has been noted. In other words, it is unclear from the available data, whether chronic uremia/maintenance dialysis *per se* protects or adversely affects the natural history of HIV infection.

OTHER ISSUES IN HIV AND DIALYSIS

The other issues which need to be addressed by nephrologists in treating patients with HIV associated renal failure are:

1. Precautions during dialysis in patients with reversible ARF, and those with ESRD.
2. The need for routine screening for HIV antibody in patients and staff in dialysis units.
3. The risk to staff members and other patients of nosocomial transmission of HIV infection in dialysis units while providing care to HIV infected patients.
4. Renal transplantation in HIV disease patients.
5. Legal issues surrounding patient and staff confidentiality.

DIALYSIS GUIDELINES IN PATIENTS WITH HIV

Extensive epidemiologic studies led to the identification of patients at high risk for HIV infection in whom the mode of transmission of virus is similar to that of HBV. Dialysis units, very cognizant of the risk of hepatitis B to staff and patients, have followed infection control measures from the early 1970s, while caring for infected individuals. Those practices have been very effective in reducing the incidence of HBV infection by 93% (from 3% to 0.2%) among patients, and 96% (from 2.6% to 0.3%) among staff members (53). It was therefore logical, that even before HIV was identified, and serological markers of infection characterized, previously established HBV infection control precautions were used as a model to develop guidelines for health care and dialysis personnel to follow while treating AIDS patients. In the early days, misinformation and panic about the disease, created a great concern for administrative personnel about the safety of their dialysis staff regarding the risk of exposure to contaminated blood/peritoneal fluid, and needle stick injuries from infected patients during dialysis delivery. Extreme precautions which included strict isolation of patients, dedicated dialysis machines, caps, gowns, masks, goggles and booties for all medical, nursing and technical personnel were employed by us and others, in providing dialysis treatments for AIDS patients with acute and chronic uremia. With a better understanding of the low infectivity of HIV, the CDC proposed guidelines which does not currently advocate such ultra-conservative precautions during dialysis (54–56). The concentration of HIV in body fluids and blood is low, and the virus is easily inactivated by heating to 56°C for 8 minutes, or to 60°C for 6 minutes, or by exposure to 70% ethanol, 70% isopropanol or chlorine (50 mg/l) for 10–20 seconds (57, 58). CDC therefore recommends universal blood and body fluid precautions, and standard disinfection and sterilization strategies which are already employed in all dialysis units (55, 56). Isolation of patients with AIDS or asymptomatic carriers of HIV, the use of separate machines, the routine testing of staff and patients for HIV antibody for infection control purposes, are not recommended. The reuse of dialyzers in known HIV positive patients is also considered to be an acceptable procedure by the CDC.

We have successfully utilized the following more conservative guidelines in our unit in providing care for a large number of patients with AIDS or HIV seropositive individuals.

1. AIDS patients who are severely ill with renal failure and other complications such as diarrhea and respiratory symptoms are isolated from all other patients during dialysis. This is done primarily to prevent transmission of other communicable diseases.
2. Dialyzers or tubings are never reused.
3. The nursing, medical and technical staff wear protective gloves at all times and extreme care taken in the use and disposal of needles, and sharp objects. Immediately after use, all sharp objects and needles are deposited without capping or breaking, into nonpenetrable disposable containers.
4. After each use, the exterior of the dialysis machine is cleansed thoroughly with hypochlorite or other commonly used disinfectant solution, and the interior of the machine rinsed with formaldehyde solution.
5. For infection control purposes, routine screening of dialysis patients and staff for HIV antibody status is not conducted. However we feel strongly that there is a need for a systematic study to determine the risk of transmission among staff and patients in dialysis units who treat a large number of HIV infected patients.
6. An ongoing in service education program for staff and patients, and periodic monitoring of infection control procedures in dialysis units are very helpful in reinforcing policies, reducing unnecessary fear and panic among staff members, obtaining cooperation from all, and thus provide multidisciplinary and compassionate care to patients with AIDS.
7. It is important for all health care providers to realize that the infectivity of HIV is low, and that sterilization can be accomplished easily. Basic precautions followed diligently by dialysis personnel are sufficient to prevent transmission of the virus. Emotional over reactions from physicians and staff alike (especially the medical director of the unit, and the nursing supervisor) must be avoided.

To date, all workers who have performed serial HIV screening studies in dialysis patients and staff have failed to demonstrate nosocomial transmission of HIV from patient to patient, or patient to staff (59–63). One major observation which needs to be reemphasized is the fact that no maintenance dialysis patient lacking a known risk factor for HIV infection has developed seropositivity or AIDS either at Brooklyn or other dialysis facilities indicating a very low risk of nosocomial transmission of virus within a dialysis center. This may be related to the ease of disinfection of HIV in the environment, low transmittability of the virus during casual contact, and due to the universal precautions adopted by most dialysis units providing care. Nevertheless, it is imperative that dialysis staff treating HIV patients, observe infection control precautions adequately, and take extreme care in the disposal of contaminated materials. It is essential that dialysis administrators also periodically review the infection control procedures adopted and practiced by the medical, nursing and technical personnel in their respective units. Based on reported data, and from our large experience, we agree with the CDC recommendations that routine screening of dialysis patients for HIV infection is not necessary. We also feel that screening of dialysis patients is desirable, and should be encouraged because of the reasons outlined below:

a) Appropriate counseling to prevent transmission to sexual contacts.
b) Anti-retroviral (AZT, ddi) therapy, and vaccinations against pnemococcal pneumonia, influenza, and possibly against hepatitis B in seropositive patients.
c) Prophylaxis against PCP, candida, toxoplasma gondii, and herpes simplex infections.
d) Early diagnosis and treatment of tuberculosis (both typical, and atypical).
e) Surveillance for the onset of lymphomas, Kaposi's sarcoma, other opportunistic infections, and early intervention.
f) To secure social benefits for patients, obtain epidemiologic data, and accurate diagnosis of HIV infection.

RENAL TRANSPLANTATION IN HIV DISEASE

Few cases of transmission of HIV through the renal allograft have been reported both in Europe and the US. In each of these instances, the kidney donor either belonged to a group at high risk for HIV, or was the recipient of large quantities of blood prior to the harvesting of donor organs. Some recipients of an infected kidney have subsequently developed clinical AIDS, while others have continued to remain asymptomatic with good graft function despite immunosuppressive therapy. The current policy of routine testing of donors prior to transplantation, and exclusion of high risk individuals as organ and blood donors, should lead to a virtual disappearance of such HIV transmission in the future.

With regard to the feasibility of RT in asymptomatic HIV seropositive ESRD subjects, limited retrospective data available from many centers have been summarized in a recent review (64). In brief, the findings were as follows. In 11 patients (mean age 36.7 years, range 13–64 years), in whom HIV infection was present for an unknown duration prior to receiving the allograft, 3 developed AIDS after a mean duration of 17 months following RT, and 8 remained asymptomatic carriers of the virus with good graft function. In 48 patients (mean age 34.2 years, range 5–63 years) seronegative at the time of transplantation, the time to HIV seroconversion was 2 months post-transplant. HIV infection in these recipients were from a HIV positive donor in 8, blood transfusion in 13, high risk donor in 20 and unknown in the remaining 7

patients. Of the 48 recipients, 20 developed AIDS or ARC 3–60 months (mean 32 months) following RT, and 28 continue to be asymptomatic despite receiving corticosteroids and cyclosporine. Overall, 28 (76%) were alive with good graft function. The use of immunosuppressive drugs following transplantation has also led to an increased number of infectious complications accounting for patient mortality. In view of these uncertainties, and paucity of adequate information, at present most transplant centers are reluctant to undertake renal transplantation in asymptomatic HIV carriers.

LEGAL CONCERNS AND HIV

It is beyond the scope of this communication to discuss various legal ramifications surrounding HIV disease and patient and staff confidentiality. In brief, HIV screening of patients and staff should be performed after obtaining informed consent, respecting patient's desire for confidentiality, and with appropriate pre-test and post-test counseling. In our experience, a well informed patient rarely refuses HIV testing, requested by a concerned personal physician. Since many therapeutic approaches (mainly preventive) are available for the treatment of asymptomatic HIV seropositive individuals, it is very appropriate to encourage patients to undergo testing.

CONCLUSIONS

Renal physicians are faced with HIV related renal syndromes, some directly related to viral infection, and some coincidental to disease. Data is beginning to accumulate regarding the natural history of various HIV associated renal disorders. The ethical issue faced by nephrologists in caring for patients with AIDS and ESRD is a difficult one to deal with. In some patients, it is advisable to withhold maintenance dialysis therapy, while in others, provision of an opportunity for even a short period of anticipated survival may be desirable. We have always adopted the policy of individualizing the treatment options for each patient, taking into consideration the wishes of the patient, family, and companion in consultation with the primary physician(s). The next decade will be an era in which to judge whether or not we can prevent ESRD from HIVAN, and also improve survival and rehabilitation in HIV infected patients receiving renal replacement therapy.

REFERENCES

1. Revision of the CDC surveillance case definition for acquired immunodeficiency syndrome. *MMWR* 36 (No 1S): 3S, 1987

2. 1993 revised classification system for HIV infection and expanded case definition for AIDS among adolescents and adults. *MMWR* 41 (No RR-17): 1, 1992

3. Rao TKS, Filippone EJ, Nicastri AD, Landesman SH, Frank E, Chen CK, Friedman EA: Associated focal and segmental glomerulosclerosis in the acquired immunodeficiency syndrome. *N Engl J Med* 310: 669, 1984

4. Gardenswartz MH, Lerner CW, Seligson GR *et al.*: Renal disease in patients with AIDS: a clinicopathologic study. *Clin Nephrol* 21: 197, 1984

5. Pardo V, Aldana M, Colton RM *et al.*: Glomerular lesions in the acquired immunodeficiency syndrome. *Ann Intern Med* 101: 429, 1984

6. Rao TKS, Friedman EA, Nicastri AD: The types of renal disease in the acquired immunodeficiency syndrome. *N Engl J Med* 316: 1062, 1987

7. Rao TKS, Friedman EA: AIDS (HIV) associated nephropathy: does it exist? An in-depth review. *Am J Nephrol* 9: 441, 1989

8. Rao TKS, Friedman EA: Outcome of severe acute renal failure in patients with the acquired immunodeficiency syndrome. In press

9. Rao TKS, Berns JS: Acute renal failure in patients with HIV infection. in *Renal and urologic aspects of HIV infection*, edited by Kimmel PL, Berns JS, New York, Churchill Livingstone. In press

10. Bourgoignie JJ, Meneses R, Ortiz C, Jaffe D, Pardo V: The clinical spectrum of renal disease associated with human immunodeficiency virus. *Am J Kidney Dis* 12: 131, 1988

11. Chander P, Soni A, Suri A, Bhagwat R, Yoo J, Treser G: Renal ultrastructural markers in AIDS-associated nephropathy. *Am J Pathol* 126: 513, 1987

12. Chander P, Agarwal A, Soni A, Kim K, Treser G: Renal cytomembranous inclusions in idiopathic renal disease as predictive markers for the acquired immunodeficiency syndrome. *Hum Pathol* 19: 1060, 1988

13. Cohen AH, Sun NCJ, Shapshak P, Imagawa DT: Demonstration of human immunodeficiency virus in renal epithelium in HIV-associated nephropathy. *Modern Pathol* 2: 125, 1989

14. Kopp JB, Klotman ME, Adler SH *et al.*: Progressive glomerulosclerosis and enhanced renal accumulation of basement membrane components in mice transgenic for human immunodeficiency virus type 1 genes. *Proc Natl Acad Sci USA* 89: 1577, 1992

15. Kopp JB, Bruggeman LA, Klotman PE: Extracellular matrix gene expression in experimental glomerulonephritis. *Curr Opinions Nephrol Hypertension* 2: 609, 1993

16. Shukla RR, Kumar A, Kimmel PL: Transforming growth factor beta increases the expression of HIV-1 gene in transfected human mesangial cells. *Kidney Int* 44: 1022, 1993

17. United States Renal Data System: 1993 annual data report, p 24

18. ESRD Network of New York: 1992 annual report. July 1993

19. Tokras JI, Alter MJ, Favero MS, Moyer LA, Bland LA: National Surveillance of dialysis-associated diseases in the United States, 1992. *ASAIO J*. In press

20. Rao TKS: Acquired immunodeficiency syndrome human immunodeficiency virus and dialysis. in: *International Yearbook of Nephrology 1991*, edited by Andreucci VE, Fine LG, Boston, MA, Kluwer Academic publishers, 1990, p 199

21. Rao TKS: Maintenance dialysis in patients with human immunodeficiency virus infection. *Semin Dial* 1: 203, 1988

22. Ortiz C, Meneses R, Jaffe JA Fernandez JA, Perez G, Bourgoignie JJ: Outcome of patients with human immunodeficiency virus on maintenance hemodialysis. *Kidney Int* 34: 248, 1988

23. Ribot S, Dean D, Goldblat M, Saavedra M: Prognosis of HIV positive dialysis patients. *Kidney Int* 37: 315, 1990

24. Feinfeld DA, Kaplan R, Dressler R, Lynn I: Survival of human immunodeficiency virus-infected patients on maintenance dialysis. *Clin Nephrol* 32: 221, 1989

25. Chirgwin K, Rao TKS, Landesman SH: HIV infection in a high prevalence hemodialysis unit. *AIDS* 3: 731, 1989

26. Kimmel PL, Umana WO, Simmens SJ, Watson J, Bosch JP: Continuous ambulatory peritoneal dialysis and survival of HIV infected patients with end-stage renal disease. *Kidney Int* 44: 373, 1993

27. Tebben JA, Rigsby MO, Selwyn PA, Brennan N, Kliger A, Finkelstein FO: Outcome of HIV infected patients on continuous ambulatory peritoneal dialysis. *Kidney Int* 44: 191, 1993

28. Campbell J, Markowitz N, Fisher EJ, Cruz C: Continuous ambulatory peritoneal dialysis for the AIDS patient. in *Ambulatory Peritoneal dialysis*, edited by Avram MM, Giordano C, New York, Plenum Publishing Co, 1990, p 266

29. Diskin CJ: AIDS-related complex by continuous ambulatory peritoneal dialysis. *Nephron* 51: 548, 1989

30. Rubin J: Prevalence of HIV virus among patients undergoing continuous ambulatory peritoneal dialysis. *Trans Am Soc Artif Intern Organs* 35: 144, 1989

31. Baumgartner DD, Arterbery VE, Hale AJ, Gupta RK, Bradley SF: Peritoneal dialysis-associated tuberculous peritonitis in an intravenous drug user with acquired immunodeficiency syndrome. *Am J Kidney Dis* 14(2): 154, 1989

32. Dressler R, Peters AT, Lynn RI: Pseudomonal and candidal peritonitis as a complication of continuous ambulatory peritoneal dialysis in human immunodeficiency virus-infected patients. *Am J Med* 86: 787, 1989

33. Elsey RM, Carson RW, Dubose TD Jr: Pasteurella multocida peritonitis in an HIV-positive patient on continuous cycling peritoneal dialysis. *Am J Nephrol* 11: 61, 1991

34. Lewis M, Gorban-Brennan NL, Kliger A, Cooper K, Finkelstein FO: Incidence and spectrum of organisms causing peritonitis in HIV positive patients on CAPD. *Adv Perit Dial* 6: 136, 1990

35. Wasser WG, Boyle MJ, Brandon S, Gruber SJ, Winston RV, Feldman NS: HIV positivity does not predispose peritoneal dialysis patients to peritonitis. *J Am Soc Nephrol* 2: 369, 1991

36. Correa-Rotter R, Saldivar S, Soto LE, de Leon PS, Pena JC: Recovery of HIV antigen in peritoneal dialysis fluid. *Perit Dial Int* 10: 67, 1990

37. Breyer JA, Harbison MA: Isolation of human immunodeficiency virus from peritoneal dialysate. *Am J Kidney Dis* 21: 23, 1993

38. Shrivastava D, Delano BG, Lundin P, Rao TKS, Markell M, Friedman EA: Factors affecting survival of HIV+ patients undergoing maintenance hemodialysis. *J Am Soc Nephrol* 3: 320, 1992

39. Blum MR, Liao SHT, Good SS, Miranda PD: Pharmacokinetics and bioavailability of Zidovudine in humans. *Am J Med* 85 (Suppl 2A): 189, 1988

40. Gleason JR Jr, Brier ME: Zidovudine in renal failure. *Semin Dial* 3: 101, 1990

41. Paoli I, Dave M, Cohen BD: Pharmacodynamics of zidovudine in patients with end stage renal disease. *N Engl J Med* 326: 839, 1992

42. Kremer D, Munar MY, Kohlgepp SJ *et al.*: Zidovudine pharmacokinetics in five HIV seronegative patients undergoing continuous ambulatory peritoneal dialysis. *Pharmacotherapy* 12: 56, 1992

43. Spivak JL, Barnes DC, Fuchs E, Quinn TC: Serum immunoreactive erythropoietin in HIV-infected patients. *JAMA* 261: 3104, 1989

44. Shrivastava D, Rao TKS, Sinert R, Khurana E, Lundin AP, Friedman EA: The efficacy of erythropoietin in HIV infected end stage renal disease patients treated by maintenance hemodialysis. In press

45. Berns JS, Cohen RM, Rudnick MR, Bennett WM: Renal aspects of antimicrobial therapy for HIV infection. in *Renal and urologic aspects of HIV infection*, edited by Kimmel PL, Berns JS, New York, Churchill Livingstone. In press

46. Descamps-Latscha B, Herbelin A: Long-term dialysis and cellular immunity: a critical survey. *Kidney Int* 43 (Suppl 41): S135, 1993

47. Chatenoud L, Herbelin A, Beaurain G, Descamps-Latscha B: Immune deficiency of the uremic patient. *Adv Nephrol* 19: 259, 1990

48. Van Noesel: Functional and phenotypic evidence for selective loss of memory T cells in asymptomatic HIV infected men. *J Clin Invest* 86: 293, 1990

49. Pinching AJ: Antibody responses in HIV infection. *Clin Exp Immunol* 84: 181, 1989

50. Goldfeld AE, Birch-Limberger K, Schooley RT, Walker BD: HIV-1 infection does not induce tumor necrosis factor-alpha or interferon-beta gene transcription. *J Acquir Immune Defic Syndr* 4: 41, 1991

51. Munis JR, Richman DD, Kornbluth RS: Human immunodeficiency virus-1 infection of macrophages *in vitro* neither induces tumor necrosis factor (TNF)/cachectin gene expression nor alters TNF/cachectin induction by lipopolysaccharide. *J Clin Invest* 85: 591, 1990

52. Edelbaum DE: No AIDS among patients on dialysis? *N Engl J Med* 314: 187, 1986

53. Alter MJ, Favero MS, Moyer LA, Miller JK, Bland LA: National Surveillance of dialysis-associated diseases in the United States, 1988. *ASAIO Trans* 36: 107, 1990

54. Update: Universal precautions for prevention of transmission of human immunodeficiency virus, hepatitis B virus, and other bloodborne pathogens in health-care settings. *MMWR* 37: 377, 1988

55. Guidelines for for prevention of transmission of human immunodeficiency virus and hepatitis B virus to health-care and public safety workers. *MMWR* 38 (S-6): 1, 1989

56. Recommendations for preventing transmission of human immunodeficiency virus and hepatitis B virus to patients during exposure-prone invasive procedures. *MMWR* 40 (RR-8): 1, 1991

57. Martin LS, McDougal SJ, Loskoski SL: Disinfection and inactivation of Human T Lymphotropic virus type III/Lymphadenopathy-associated virus. *J Infect Dis* 152: 39, 1985

58. Shapshak P, McCoy CB, Rivers JE *et al.*: Inactivation of human immunodeficiency virus-1 at short time intervals using undiluted bleach. *J Acqd Immune Def Synd* 6: 218, 1993

59. Reiser I, Shapiro W, Porush J: The incidence and epidemiology of human immunodeficiency virus infection in 320 patients treated in an inner city hemodialysis center. *Am J Kidney Dis* 16: 26, 1990

60. Perez GO, Ortiz C, De Medina M, Schiff E, Bourgoignie JJ: Lack of transmission of human immunodeficiency virus in chronic hemodialysis patients. *Am J Nephrol* 8: 123,

61. Assogba U, Park A, Rey MA, Barthelemy A, Rottembourg J, Gluckman JC: Prospective study of HIV I seropositive patients in hemodialysis centers. *Clin Nephrol* 29: 312, 1988

62. Marcus R, Favero MS, Banerjee S *et al.*: Prevalence and incidence of human immunodeficiency virus among patients undergoing long-term hemodialysis. *Am J Med* 90: 614, 1991

63. Berlyne G, Kaczmarek RG, Hamburger S *et al.*: Seroprevalence of antibodies to the human immunodeficiency virus in dialysis workers: results of a multi-center study. *Nephron* 62: 441, 1992

64. Erice A, Rhame FS, Heussner RC, Dunn DL, Balfour HH Jr: Human immunodeficiency virus infection in patients with solid-organ transplants: report of five cases and review. *Rev Infect Dis* 13: 537, 1991

VIRAL INFECTIONS IN DIALYSIS PATIENTS
PART B: DIALYSIS ASSOCIATED HEPATITIS

FRANÇOISE DEGOS and PAUL JUNGERS

INTRODUCTION

Viral liver diseases, especially due to hepatitis B virus (HBV) and hepatitis C virus (HCV), were observed with a high frequency in hemodialysis units throughout the world. Due to the deficient immune response of uremic subjects, which renders them unable to eliminate viruses, hemodialysis patients act as reservoirs of the viruses and transmit infection to other patients, to the dialysis unit staff and eventually to their own family, in the case of infection with HBV.

Until 1982, important efforts were directed towards detection and isolation of infected patients, preventing first the spread of HBV and presently the spread of HCV which is a major problem in hemodialysis units in the early 1990s.

Only since the start of active immunization by hepatitis B vaccine in 1982 has a decline in the incidence of HBV infection been observed. At the present time, thanks to extensive vaccination (1), eradication of hepatitis B from dialysis units has been mostly obtained, and protection of health care workers is a fact. The epidemiology of HBV (2) and HCV (3) infection is now clearly identified due to the availability of tests detecting HBV and HCV infection. Clinical and epidemiological aspects of HBV and HCV infection are in fact quite different and will therefore be addressed separately.

HEPATITIS B VIRUS INFECTION

The clinical course of HBV infection in hemodialysis patients is remarkably asymptomatic, without jaundice and with a major risk of chronic progression. This tendency has been attributed to immunodepression due to chronic renal failure. A study of dialysis patients showed that both HBV chronic carriers and patients without evidence of past or present HBV infection had a significant decrease in both absolute number of lymphocytes and functional lymphocytes (4). There was no significant difference between the number of T lymphocytes in dialysis patients who normally cleared HBV infection as compared with healthy normal subjects, suggesting that the response to HBV may depend on the severity of immunodepression. However the importance of host factors is outlined by the higher frequency of chronic carriers in males as compared to females, and differences in the major histocompatibility system have been described (5).

Acute phase of HBV infection

Clinical symptoms of HBV infection can be marked by a preicteric phase with fever, arthalgias and skin rash. These symptoms usually resolve quickly with the onset of icterus and dark urine. With the onset of the icteric phase, symptoms of fatigue and abnormal anorexia typically worsen. Jaundice can last an average of 2 or 3 weeks. In many cases symptoms are lacking and HBV infection can be detected only by unusual asthenia, or by increase in serum transaminases.

The course of a typical case of acute hepatitis B infection is shown in Figure 1. The first serological marker detectable in the serum is HBsAg, which appears during the incubation period and persists in the serum throughout the symptomatic phase of the disease. Concurrently or shortly after the appearance of HBsAg in the serum, HBeAg and HBV DNA are detectable and rapidly increase, being thereafter undetectable within a few days to a few weeks. Indeed, disappearance of these serological markers indicates resolution of viral replication and thus predicts ultimate resolution of the hepatitis. In patients who develop chronic HBV infection, levels of HBV DNA and HBeAg remain high during the acute phase of the illness (6).

HBcAg is undetectable in the serum but detectable in the liver and is also a marker of viral replication. The first antibody to arise during the course of typical acute hepatitis B is antibody to HBc (anti-HBc). Initially, most of anti-HBc is of the IgM class. The IgM anti-HBc generally persists for only a few months after acute disease,

making detection of anti-HBc-IgM a valuable marker for the diagnosis of acute HBV infection. Anti-HBc antibody of the IgG type generally persists for life.

Antibody to HBsAg (anti-HBs) usually appears during convalescence, after clearance of HBsAg. It is considered as a marker of recovery and immunity to HBV. Patients who receive HBV vaccine will have anti-HBs and are protected against infection. Antibody to AgHBe commonly appears with clearance of AgHBe from the serum.

Consecutive to the acute phase of the disease, prospective studies have observed that 5 to 10% of adults can develop chronic liver disease, and the proportion of hemodialysis patients developing chronic HBV infection is approximately 30% (7). A small series of seven patients with acute HBV infection was reported in Spain. The occurrence of chronic liver disease was observed in 4/7 cases (8).

Chronic HBV infection and hepatocellular carcinoma

Most patients with chronic hepatitis B have no symptoms of liver disease. The most common symptom is fatigue, which tends to be intermittent. Myalgias, arthalgias and transient skin rashes are rare. Physical findings are rare, namely spider angiomata and tender hepatomegaly. Laboratory tests demonstrate increased ALT and AST, fluctuating over time and generally ranging from just above normal to 5–8-fold elevated. In hemodialysis patients the increase of transaminases activity is very mild, and may be absent, even though chronic liver disease can be demonstrated (6–8). The natural history of hepatitis B chronic infection leads to the occurrence of hepatocellular carcinoma. The role of HBV is multifactorial, and in most cases hepatocellular carcinoma is associated with cirrhosis (9–11).

Liver biopsy

Technique

The diagnosis must be assessed on histological examination of the liver, obtained by liver biopsy. The procedure of liver biopsy (12) in hemodialysis patients should be considered, as the risk involved in performing transparietal liver biopsy in these patients is certainly higher than in other patients; all teams have experienced severe complications such as hemoperitonitis or intrahepatic hematomas. Disorders of primary hemostasis, most of which are undetectable in usual tests, are probably responsible for such complications, and therefore the transvenous transjugular approach (13) should be recommended. This technique is safe and provides liver samples of sufficient size when performed in specialized centers. Due to the safety of the method, and to the important discrepancies between biochemical abnormalities and histological findings, liver biopsy should be performed to evaluate histological liver status of hemodialysis patients with HBV or HCV viral

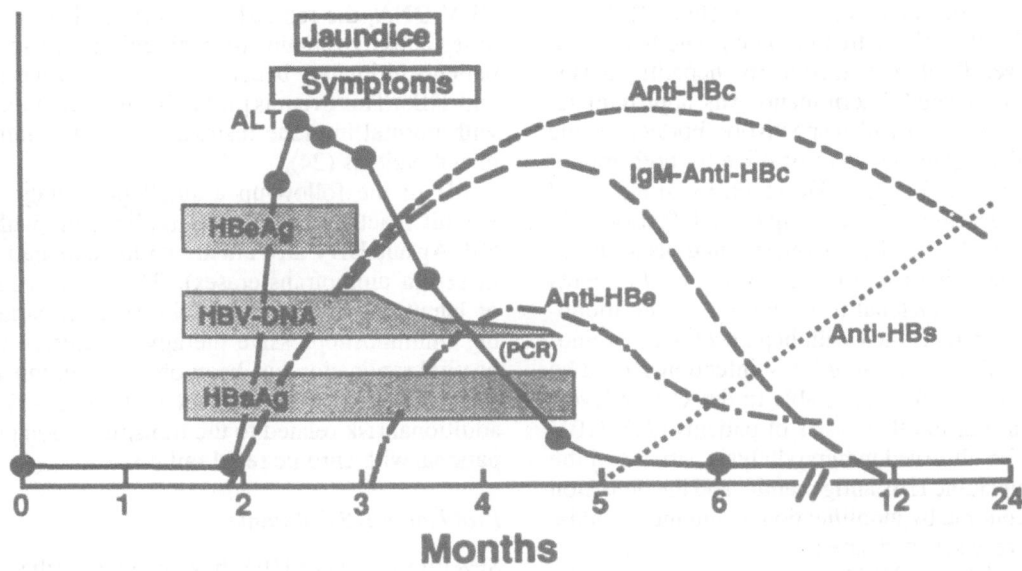

Figure 1. Serologic course of acute hepatities B. ALT = alanine aminotransferase, PCR = polymerase chain reaction.

markers in the serum, with or without biochemical abnormalities, prior to antiviral therapy or prior to the decision of renal transplantation.

Histological lesions

Liver lesions are those described in chronic hepatitis, namely necrosis, inflammatory infiltration and fibrosis (14), and the severity of liver lesions is usually evaluated according to the Knodell score (15); moreover, the presence of cirrhosis is associated with or without signs of activity of the disease (necrosis and inflammatory process). Lesions are especially mild in patients with immunodeficiency due to chronic renal failure, and fibrosis can be observed with a very mild inflammatory process (16). In immunocompromized patients, there is no correlation between the severity of liver lesions and the degree of biochemical abnormalities. The development of liver lesions from chronic hepatitis to cirrhosis can be observed without any clinical symptoms.

Specific aspects of HBV infection during hemodialysis

The histological status of 111 hemodialysis patients was studied in France when the prevalence of HBV infection in such patients was much higher than presently (7). However, this study was informative with regard to HBV related events in patients receiving regular hemodialysis treatment. Among the 111 patients studied, 51 were HBV carriers. Only 8 of the patients with HBV infection had normal liver, whereas this situation was noted in 50% of the patients without present HBV infection. Severe chronic hepatitis was observed in 21/51 patients with HBV infection. Among the 51 HBsAg carriers, viral

replication as evaluated by the detection of HBeAg in the serum (detection of HBV DNA was not available at the time of the study) was present in 30 patients. Replication was associated with severe histologic features, and was detectable in most (9/11) patients with active disease.

Histological follow-up

The progression of liver lesions during the hemodialysis period compared to the evolutive risk when renal failure is treated by transplantation remains the main question. Deterioration of the liver status has been observed in patients undergoing repeat liver biopsies (7), but clearance of HBsAg can be observed in some series. The clearance of the virus is usually associated with interruption of the histological activity of the disease. By contrast the clearance of viral replication (HBeAg, HBV DNA), and moreover of HBsAg, has been observed in very few patients treated by immunosuppressive therapy after renal transplantation (17).

Markers of HBV infection (18–19)

Serological tests for the detection of viral markers include HBsAg, HBeAg, anti-HBe, anti-HBc, anti-HBs and the direct approach of HBV replication by the detection of HBV DNA.

Tests

The detection of HBsAg by polyclonal radioimmunoassays (RIA) which was used in most centers in the past decade is now obsolete. In a recent large scale program, the use of monoclonal antibodies to HBsAg in hemodialysis patients gave informative data (20). This study was based on the use of polyclonal or monoclonal RIA in a population of 375 patients treated by chronic hemodialysis. The lower limit of detection for hepatitis B surface antigen-associated determinants was approximately 55 pg/ml and 125 pg/ml respectively. Forteen of the 375 hemodialysis patients were positive by both monoclonal and polyclonal assays. However, in addition, 17 patients were identified as harboring HBV infection only by the monoclonal assay. Moreover, serum transaminases activity was found increased in only 4 of the 17 patients detected by the monoclonal test, and one of the monoclonal positive patients died with hepatocellular carcinoma. Therefore, the detection of HBV infection should be performed with sensitive tests, able to detect low levels of HBsAg. Similar to other series of patients (21), HBV infection can be observed in hemodialysis patients in the absence of detectable HBs antigenemia, and the detection of the HBV genome by amplification technique could be of interest in very selected cases.

On a clinical basis, HBV DNA is measured by the hybridization technique (Genostix, Abbott, Chicago, Illinois), and this technique is able to detect levels of HBV DNA close to 10^5 genome equivalent per ml. This level of detection is well correlated with clinical symptoms and is very useful in clinical practice.

When the hybridization technique is unable to detect viral replication, HBV DNA can be detected by polymerase chain reaction (PCR). This technique is very sensitive and able to detect lower levels of HBV DNA (22). However, there is no correlation between results obtained by PCR and clinical symptoms. Therefore the hybridization technique should be preferred on a clinical basis.

Evolution of HBV markers

Serological markers in chronic hepatitis B are needed to determine the stage of infection and to predict outcome. The course of chronic HBV infection is shown in Figure 2 and can be divided into three phases (23):

(a) In the replicative phase, the onset is similar to that of acute hepatitis B: HBsAg, HBeAg, and HBV DNA are present in the serum. Aminotranferases remain elevated but do not reach the levels seen in typical, self limited acute hepatitis B (2–8 fold elevated).

(b) After several months or years of persistent HBV replication, spontaneous remission of the disease can occur. This remission is marked by the disappearance of HBV DNA from the serum followed by the loss of HBeAg, and then improvement of the serum aminotransferases activity. This phase is often marked by a transient worsening of disease activity, with a worsening of serum transaminases and symptoms including jaundice. This phase is called 'seroconversion' (conversion from HBeAg to anti-HBe) preceeds the third phase.

(c) The nonreplicative phase in which HBeAg is cleared and remission has occurred. Serum aminotransferases remain normal and symptoms have resolved. For most patients who enter remission with clearance of HBe and HBV DNA, the remission is sustained, serum transaminases activity remains normal and indeed some of these patients ultimately become HBsAg negative and develop anti-HBs. This event is probably more frequent in patients with normal immune response than in immunocompromized patients (24).

(d) In the follow-up a small percentage of patients exhibit reactivation of viral replication (with return of HBeAg and HBV DNA in the serum, and marked increase in serum aminotransferases). This event can be severe or latent and is frequently observed in patients receiving immunosuppressive therapy. Therefore reactivation of viral replication has been observed in most HBV carriers undergoing renal transplantation (25–27), and is an additional risk related to the transplantation procedure in patients with chronic renal failure.

Problem of HBV mutants

Several mutants of HBV have been described (28). From the clinical point of view, the most frequently observed is a mutant with a nucleotide substitution in the precore region (29, 30). This substitution prevents the production and secretion of HBeAg. Hepatocytes infected with precore defective mutants would not be able to produce HBeAg. Therefore the patients infected with this mutant have viral replication detected by HBV DNA in the absence of HBeAg, and with anti-HBe in the serum. It is not clear whether this substitution is observed with *de novo* infections or whether the mutation arises during infection, as a result of immune selection pressure.

The finding of HBV DNA in the serum of patients negative for all serological markers of HBV suggests that some genetic variants of HBV account for some cases of non-A, non-B hepatitis (31). The detection of HBV DNA is then possible with the PCR technique (32). The mutation is located in the 3′ end of the S genome (33). The situation of HBsAg negative/HBV DNA positive patients is probably relatively frequent in immunocompromised patients such as hemodialysis and transplant patients (25).

Delta virus

The delta virus, a defective RNA virus, occurs in the presence of HBsAg (34). Infection with delta virus may occur simultaneously with HBV infection (called co-infection) or as a superinfection in an HBV chronic carrier. Superinfection with delta virus has not been described in the literature in hemodialysis patients (35). It is a very rare event in renal transplant recipients, but two cases of fulminant hepatic failure due to superinfection with Delta virus were reported (36).

Value of screening for HBV markers in hemodialysis units

The screening of viral markers in hemodialysis units is now performed on a routine basis, and geographic variations are great, particularly concerning the epidemiology

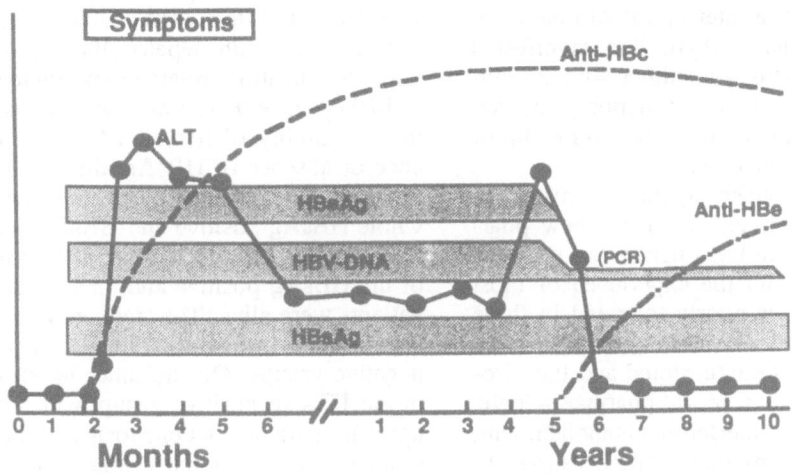

Figure 2. Serologic course of chronic hepatitis B. ALT = alanine aminotransferase, PCR = polymerase chain reaction.

of HBV. Ten years ago, in Dallas (Texas, USA) HBsAg was present in 2.7% of the patients entering the center. Contamination with HBV occurred in the center and was later documented in 10% of the cases, and evolution to chronic HBV infection was observed in approximately 30%. The possibility of the transient presence of anti-HBc or anti-HBs was also noted and interpreted as false positivity (37). This study also emphasized a minor variation of serum transaminases activity and the absence of correlation between biochemical and virological data. Such lack of relationship will become more obvious with concern to the detection of hepatitis C virus.

Treatment of chronic HBV infection

Alpha interferon

The most effective antiviral drug to inhibit viral replication is alpha interferon (38, 39). The aim of treatment is to reduce viral replication, and interferon should be given only during the replicative phase of the disease, when HBV DNA is present and stable in the serum (hybridization technique). Recommendations for therapy should be cautious, because the optimal dose and regimen remain unclear. Therapy is effective in 30 to 50% of non-immunocompromized patients, probably less in immunocompromized individuals, and side effects can be of concern.

Response to alpha interferon is defined by the loss of HBV DNA and HBeAg from serum, fall of serum transaminases activity into the normal range and subsequent improvement in liver histology. The serologic and biochemical pattern of a typical response to alpha interferon is marked by (38):

(a) Immediate decrease of serum HBV DNA, which is still detectable until 4 to 12 weeks of treatment, when it falls into undetectable range, assessed by the hybridization technique.

(b) Once HBV DNA has become undetectable, HBeAg is cleared, usually a few months later. The loss of HBeAg is usually followed by a fall of serum aminotransferases into the normal range and improvement of the histology. The clearance of HBeAg and HBV DNA during interferon therapy is usually accompanied by transient, subclinical exacerbation of the hepatitis as manifested by a 2 to 10 fold rise in serum transaminases levels. This pattern of response suggests that interferon acts by augmenting the immune response to HBV, triggering the inhibition of viral replication as well as having specific effects on cytotoxic T cells (39).

The optimal dose and duration of treatment is still uncertain. Most authors agree presently on a regimen of 4.5 to 5 million units daily or 9 to 10 million units three times a week for four months (38). Three formulations of alpha interferon are currently available: two recombinant interferon (Roferon A alpha 2a, Hoffmann LaRoche, and Intron A Alpha 2b, Schering-Plough), and the other is prepared from a lymphoblastoid cell line (Wellferon, Welcome).

Side effects are frequent and include both common early and late effects and unusual and severe side effects. A flu-like syndrome is generally observed during the first week of treatment, and can be managed by the use of acetaminophen within 3 hours preceding the injection. Malaise, muscle ache, headache, poor appetite, weight loss, increased need for sleep, irritability and hair loss are commonly observed. These side effects are highly individual and usually well tolerated. Fatigue is the most likely side effect. The most disturbing adverse effects of interferon therapy are psychological, including irritability and depression, and require interruption of treatment. Interferon can reveal or enhance thyroiditis, manifested as hyper- or hypothyroid status, sometimes with antithyroid antibodies, and checking thyroid function is mandatory before beginning treatment and in the follow up of patients receiving interferon therapy.

There are very few data concerning the administration of interferon to hemodialysis patients (40). Few pharmakokinetic studies (41) have been performed with the drugs presently available, and the experience of most clinicians is that interferon is poorly tolerated in these patients, and responsible for severe side effects. Therefore treatment has frequently to be interrupted and the virological effect is not obtained. A recent pharmakokinetic study demonstrated impaired interferon metabolism with increased bioavailability in hemodialysis patients (42). In any case, immunodeficiency is known to be a negative predictive factor of the antiviral effect of interferon therapy (40). Moreover, interferon acting as an immunostimulant has been responsible for rejection when prescribed to transplanted patients and should be administered under very careful care in this situation.

Vidarabine

Vidarabine is a nucleoside analogue, able to inhibit the DNA polymerase activity of the virus (43). This drug is effective, but severe neuromuscular side effects are considered very frequent. When such muscular pain occurs, definitive interruption of the drug is mandatory. Therefore this drug was not given on a large scale to hemodialysis patients. However, some experience is available concerning the administration of vidarabine to renal transplant recipients with satisfactory virological effect (clearance of HBV DNA and HBeAg in approximately 50% of the patients) (44), and tolerable side effects. Therefore there is probably a place for vidarabine in the treatment of HBV infection in renal transplant recipients.

Is hepatitis B a contraindication to renal transplantation in hemodialysis patients?

Whether related or not to HBV infection the morbidity and mortality of transplant recipients with liver diseases is a major problem, and few data are available on the subject (45–49). In a series of 82 renal transplant patients, hepatic dysfunction was reported in 31, as well as two deaths due to acute liver failure, but the report did not include any histopathological examination (47). Subsequently the incidence of liver dysfunction was evaluated as 10% in a series of 405 patients, with a mortality rate in this latter group of 45% as compared to 16% in the nonhepatitis group (48). Parfrey et al. reported a markedly decreased actuarial survival of patients with chronic liver disease compared to long surviving transplanted controls (49). Poor outcome due to HBV was observed in a group of 22

HBsAg positive renal transplant recipients whose serum transaminases were probably increased for at least one year. Eleven of them died of liver disease, five of hepatic failure, three with hepatocellular carcinoma, and three with complications related to portal hypertension.

In the Necker Hospital series, published in 1988 before the availability of hepatitis C virus markers, the presence or absence of HBsAg allowed distinction between two groups of patients (50). Patient survival curves of the whole HBsAg positive and HBsAg negative populations were similar (51). Ten years after transplantation, 81% of the HBsAg positive and 85% of the HBsAg negative patients were alive. The frequency of deaths from extrahepatic causes was similar in HBsAg positive and HBsAg negative groups. On the other hand, half of the deaths in the HBsAg positive group were related to liver failure; four patients had cirrhosis and died at a mean of 62 months (9 to 110 months) after transplantation. None of the HBsAg negative patients died from liver failure.

Considering histology as the most reliable means of patient classification (52, 53), liver changes could be compared to patient survival in the Necker Hospital series (44, 50, 51). Among 122 patients with liver biopsy obtained at the time of transplantation, 98 had chronic liver disease and 24 none. Cirrhosis was observed in 17% of the patients, the other 83% suffering from chronic hepatitis with or without histological activity. Serial biopsies were available from 70 patients and morphological deterioration of the liver status was noted in 56/70 (80%) of the cases. Death occurred in 22 HBsAg+ patients and was related to liver failure in four patients.

All these results question the indication of kidney transplantation in patients with liver disease (54). The selection criteria for kidney transplantation cannot be limited to serological data, but should also include histological findings. Immunosuppression, which is required for both prevention and treatment of graft rejection, potentiates replication of the virus. Such reactivation of viral replication was found in almost all the patients studied in the Necker Hospital series (25), whatever their HBe status, and was thereafter found by other studies (46). In addition, spontaneous disappearance of the viral replication is rare in immunocompromised patients. It is clear that the precise influence of transplantation on the prevalence and course of chronic liver disease is difficult to determine in the absence of randomized studies allowing comparison with patients treated by regular hemodialysis. Unfortunately, such studies were not performed when the prevalence of HBV infection in hemodialysis units was high.

Presently, due to the efforts to obtain HBV immunisation in patients with chronic renal failure (1), the prevalence of HBV infection has dropped dramatically and most of the patients with HBV chronic infection are not candidates for kidney transplantation due to extrahepatic contraindications. However, if the presence of chronic hepatitis *per se* can only be considered as an additive risk

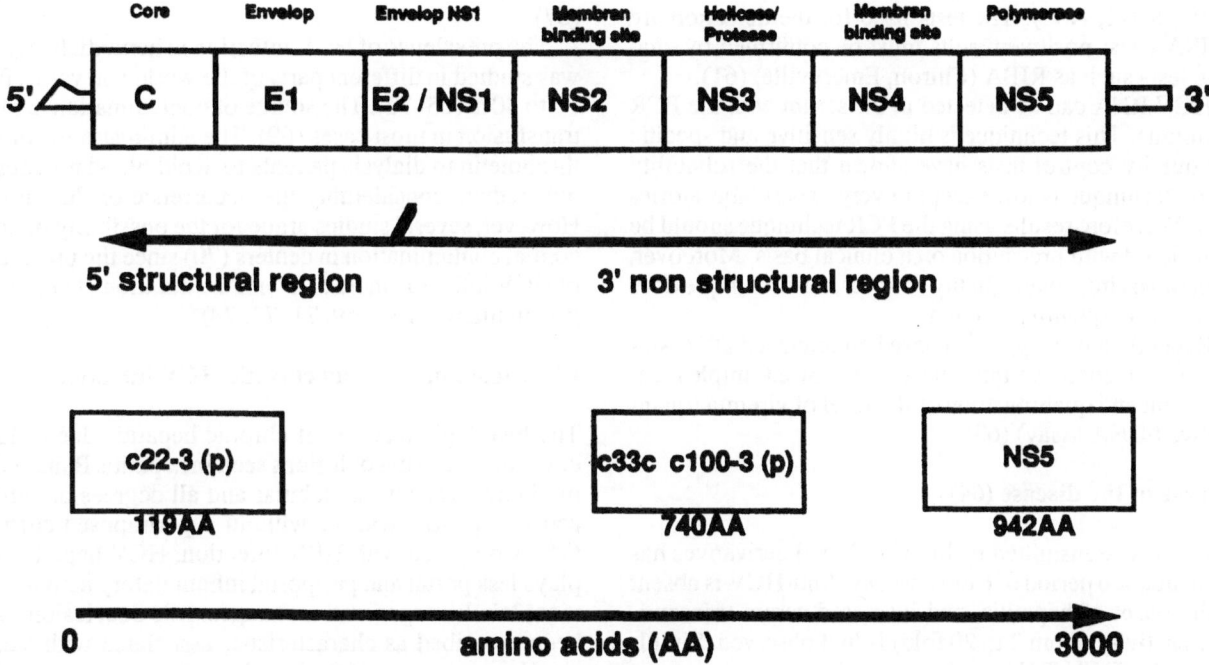

Figure 3. Genetic organization of hepatitis C virus genome.

for transplantation and requires very careful follow up after the transplantation procedure, a diagnosis of cirrhosis prior to transplantation is a contraindication to kidney transplantation since severe liver failure and death have been observed in nearly all patients with histologically documented cirrhosis prior to transplantation (50). The possibility of uncomplicated, inapparent cirrhosis justifies in our opinion liver biopsy (by the transvenous route) in all HBsAg positive patients who are candidates for kidney transplantation.

HEPATITIS C VIRUS INFECTION

The hepatitis C virus

Structure of HCV

The agent of parenterally transmitted non-A, non-B hepatitis has long been elusive. The breakthrough has been fostered by modern technology (3). Shotgun expression cloning of nucleic acid extracts from plasma containing the elusive non-A, non-B agent has led to the expression of a small protein fragment which bound IgG sera from patients convalescent from non-A, non-B hepatitis (55, 56). The cDNA clone expressing this protein fragment has allowed the cloning, sequencing and characterization of the whole genome. It is a single stranded RNA of 9400 kb. Its properties put HCV into the family of flaviviridiae. The virus has not been visualized in electron microscopy. The viral genome is made of three regions (Figure 3). The 5′ noncoding region is a very conserved region among the different subtypes of the virus. The structural region contains three genes, namely a capside gene (c) and two envelope genes (E1 and E2). The nonstructural region contains four domains, NS2, NS3, NS4 and NS5; these domains code for enzymes involved in HCV replication.

HCV genotypes

The determination of nucleotide sequences of HCV isolates showed a great variability of the genome and allowed the description of several genotypes (57). Presently several classifications are used. The main classifications are those of Okamoto (58) and of Simmonds (59). The high variability of the HCV genome might allow the virus to escape immune response and could explain the great number of chronic forms of the disease. The genotype is very probably involved in the outcome of the disease and response to treatment. Okamoto type II Simmonds 1b virus is obviously associated with severe outcome and the occurrence of cirrhosis.

Tests for the detection of HCV

The tests presently available are second and third generation tests, allowing a good sensitivity and specificity for the detection of antibodies to HCV (60). The tests use a capsid structural antigen (c22-3) and three nonstructural antigens coded by the NS3, NS4, and NS5 regions (c-200, c-100, 5-1-1, NS5). The tests used for the detection are ELISA tests; positive results must be confirmed by analytic tests such as RIBA (Chiron, Emeryville) (61).

HCV RNA can be detected in the serum with the PCR technique. This technique is highly sensitive and specific but quality control tests have shown that the reliability of the technique is low except in very expert laboratories (62). Therefore results using the PCR technique should be considered with precaution on a clinical basis. Moreover, even satisfying severe quality controls, this technique does not allow to quantify viremia.

Recently a new approach based on branched DNA signal amplification was introduced and allowed simple measurement and quantification of the level of viremia (quantitative bDNA assay) (63).

Course of the disease (64)

Hepatitis C transmitted by blood or blood derivatives has an incubation period of 6 to 12 weeks. Anti-HCV is absent at the onset of hepatitis, and increased serum transaminases activity (from 2 to 20 fold) is first observed. Simultaneously, HCV RNA is detectable in the serum. Antibodies to HCV are detectable in the serum after 2 to 4 weeks. This phase is asymptomatic in approximately 2/3 of the cases. Symptomatic cases present with dark urine or malaise, and abdominal discomfort. Several patterns of transaminases elevation can be observed: (a) polyphasic with fluctuations of enzyme levels, and sometimes periods with normal ALT between phases of biochemical abnormality; (b) a monophasic pattern with rapid increase to peak transaminases level followed by a rapid decline and eventual return to normal; (c) a plateau pattern with ALT persistently elevated without significant fluctuations. The acute phase often merges imperceptibly into a chronic outcome. This evolution is observed in at least 50% of the cases. Chronicity becomes probable when the elevation of transaminases persists for more than 6 months, but transition from acute to chronic hepatitis is mostly asymptomatic and silent. Chronic hepatitis is mostly diagnosed in the presence of ALT elevation lasting for more than 12 months.

In hemodialysis patients all available studies indicate that acute and chronic HCV infection are asymptomatic in most cases, even discovered on routine serologic tests in the absence of any biochemical abnormality. First generation tests gave a high rate of false positive and negative results in this situation, and detection of viremia by the PCR technique was positive in most cases (65). Moreover, the situation of positivity of the ELISA test, unconfirmed by analytic tests and with viremia confirmed by PCR, has been observed in the situation of immunodepression (66). Several studies report evidence of HCV infection with repeatedly normal transaminases activity (65, 67, 68), and severity of liver disease does not correlate with lev-

els of transaminases elevation or presence of HCV RNA (67).

The prevalence of HCV infection in hemodialysis units was studied in different parts of the world and varies from 10 to 40% (65–72). The source of contamination is blood transfusion in most cases (69). The administration of erythropoietin to dialysis patients to avoid blood transfusion will reduce considerably the occurrence of the disease. However, several studies argue for the possibility of nosocomial contamination in centers (70) since the prevalence of HCV infection increases with the duration of hemodialysis in many series (69, 71, 73, 74).

Liver histology during chronic HCV infection

The histologic features of chronic hepatitis due to HCV cover the spectrum of lesions seen in hepatitis B, including mild changes, chronic lobular and all degrees of chronic active hepatitis, with or without superimposed cirrhosis (75). Compared with HBV infection, HCV hepatitis displays less portal and periportal inflammatory activity, and more lobular degenerative changes. Bile duct lesions have been described as characteristic, associated with steatosis. However, none of the histologic features can be relied upon to establish a definitive diagnosis of chronic hepatitis due to HCV. In hemodialysis patients the signs of chronic hepatitis due to HCV are generally mild with minimal lobular infiltration and portal necrosis (75).

HCV-related autoimmune manifestations cirrhosis and hepatocellular carcinoma

Autoimmune associated diseases are frequent during HCV infection. In half of the cases, mixed cryoglobulinemia type II can be attributed to HCV infection (77). Conversely, asymptomatic cryoglobulinemia is frequent in patients with chronic HCV hepatitis. Membranoproliferative glomerulonephritis, which has to be distinguished from renal lesions due to cryoglobulinemia, has been related to HCV infection (78). Other autoimmune diseases, such as thyroiditis (79) Sjögren syndrome (80) and porphyria cutanea tarda (81) were recently described as associated with HCV chronic infection.

The evolution of chronic hepatitis to cirrhosis is the main concern with HCV infection. Very little data are available on the subject, and many authors agree that approximately 20% of HCV chronic carriers are at risk of cirrhosis (82). This risk is probably related to the genotype of the virus; however, some data suggest that transfusion-acquired hepatitis C is associated with more aggressive histological inflammatory activity than hepatitis resulting from intravenous drug abuse (83).

The occurrence of hepatocellular carcinoma in chronic HCV carriers concerns only patients with cirrhosis and is evaluated to approximately 20% of the patients suffering from cirrhosis (10, 84). In only very few cases of hepatocellular carcinoma in patients without cirrhosis, with

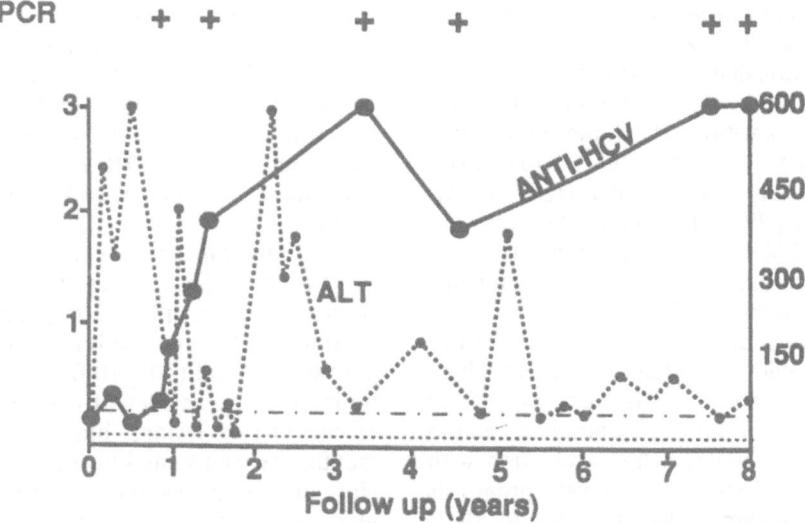

Figure 4. Serologic course of chronic hepatitis C. ALT = alanine aminotransferase, PCR = polymerase chain reaction.

HCV markers have been reported mostly with 1b geno-type (84b).

Treatment of HCV chronic infection

Even before HCV was identified, efforts began to pursue antiviral therapy for chronic non-A, non-B hepatitis. Early uncontrolled pilot trials of low dose interferon for chronic non-A, non-B hepatitis showed marked reduction of ALT levels and improvement in liver histology in 80% of treated patients (40). However responders often experienced a return of ALT levels to pretreatment values when interferon was stopped. Several controlled studies demonstrated that treatment with 1 to 5 million units of interferon given for 6 months induced a sustained response, with normal ALT several months after interruption of treatment in 20% of the cases (85). Molecular biology studies were able to show that the patients with sustained response had no detectable HCV replication demonstrated by the PCR technique in either the serum or the liver (86). Several ongoing studies suggest that higher doses and longer duration of treatment could increase the number of patients with sustained response to interferon. The level of viremia, assessed with the quantitative assay (bDNA) and the genotypes of the virus seem to be involved in the response to interferon.

In hemodialysis patients, treatment with interferon was used for chronic C hepatitis in Saudi Arabia on a small series of patients (87). The treatment induced a significant fall in ALT levels during the phase of therapy but the ALT level again reached pretreatment levels after interruption of interferon administration. Side effects were observed in 39% of the cases, but none of the patients required dosage reduction. By contrast, an Austrian series of 37 patients on hemodialysis receiving treatment by interfer-

on (88) provided results similar to those observed in other parts of Europe: treatment had to be stopped for severe side effects in 14/37 patients. However, when tolerated, the treatment was efficient and able to induce sustained suppression of viremia in 15/23 cases. This work suggested that interferon was effective in the treatment of HCV chronic hepatitis but the result was impaired by the degree of side effects. Therefore studies must be initiated to determine the acceptable dose of interferon to these patients.

Outcome of HCV infection after renal transplantation

The outcome of HCV infection in hemodialysis patients treated by renal transplantation is presently a major problem and the natural history of liver disease remains to be precisely determined. However, several series indicate that the presence of anti-HCV does not alter survival (73, 89–92) and actuarial curves (up to 210 months) did not show any difference in renal survival between HCV negative and positive recipients (91).

The overall prevalence in kidney recipients varies from 6 to 65% according to country (91–95). The presence of HCV is related in most series with the duration of dialysis, the number of blood transfusions prior to transplantation, the ethnic origin (higher prevalence in black kidney recipients) (96), and the possibility of drug addiction. However, the nosocomial route of contamination after renal transplantation cannot be excluded (91, 97). Due to this high prevalence in some series, HCV is the major cause of liver disease after kidney transplantation (92, 98, 99).

The outcome of HCV infection after renal transplantation is marked by several factors: 1) the frequency of asymptomatic infection and the lack of correlation between clinical symptoms, transaminases activity, and histological lesions (100, 101); 2) the possibility of community acquired infection demonstrated in several series by the increase of prevalence of anti-HCV in the first year following kidney transplantation (91); 3) the possible disappearance of anti-HCV in patients with obvious histologically documented liver disease, when HCV viremia can be demonstrated by PCR; in patients with or without circulating anti-HCV, semiquantitative evaluation of viremia showed the possibility of increasing viremia due to immunosuppressive therapy (65, 97, 98).

However, in all series, the presence of HCV, with or without viremia, and with or without histological liver lesions (except cirrhosis) does not affect patient survival and is therefore not considered as a contraindication to renal transplantation. By contrast, the association with HBV infection has obviously a more severe prognosis (89). The treatment of chronic hepatitis due to HCV with interferon has been proposed and considered as not suitable (101, 101b) after rénal transplantation (101b). Administration of interferon has two potential effects, 1) antiviral as it is able to reduce viremia with HCV RNA becoming undetectable after interferon administration, and 2) enhancer of immune response since kidney rejection was also observed in patients treated by interferon. Therefore such therapy should not be given except in very particular situations (40). The risks of administration of interferon after transplantation justifies the attempts to eradicate the virus during the hemodialysis period and, moreover, the preventive measures to avoid HCV infection in hemodialysis centers.

PREVENTION OF VIRAL HEPATITIS IN DIALYSIS UNITS

Sources and routes of HBV and HCV infection

Hepatitis B virus transmission

HBV infections mainly result from cross-infection of other patients and staff by patients with persistent HBV viremia, making them permanent virus reservoirs (102). Initially, blood transfusions were probably the main source of introduction of the virus into dialysis units (103). However, since 1970 only HBsAg-free blood has been used and blood transfusion is no longer a route of contamination. As a matter of fact, the subtypes of HBs Ag most frequently encountered in dialysis patients differ from those usually observed in blood donors in the same country (104). Since 1982, widespread vaccination of medical staff and patients together with confinement of HBsAg positive patients in separate units has rapidly led to a dramatic decrease in the incidence of HBV infections in both staff and uremic patients. As an example, at Necker hospital, whereas nearly half of dialysis patients at the time of kidney transplantation were HBsAg positive until 1980, this figure dropped to less than 5% after 1985 (105).

In parallel, the pool of chronic HBsAg carriers progressively decreased, thus reducing the risk of contamination. However, efforts directed toward systematic vaccination of medical staff should never be neglected because new patients, especially those arriving in emergency conditions, may introduce HBV in the unit with the risk of contamination of nurses and all other hospital personnel (106).

Transmission occurs via percutaneous or permucosal routes from blood spray during cannulation of arteriovenous fistulae, splashes or drops of blood (or serum) on skin, clothing or bedding, or from contact with used dialysis material (107–109). Members of the staff may be infected by accidental needle pricks, contamination of cuts or skin lesions, blood spraying into the eyes or mouth, or even by smoking or eating in the dialysis ward. Not only are nurses, physicians and technicians directly working in dialysis units at risk of HBV contamination, but also roentgenologists, surgeons, dentists and all other personnel involved in the care of infected patients, as well as laboratory personnel working in clinical or research laboratories and manipulating blood or serum specimens from infected subjects. Moreover, the presence of the virus has been demonstrated in saliva, vaginal secretions and semen (110). Thus, spouses or other intimate contacts of infected patients (or staff members) are also at high risk and need protection.

Hepatitis C virus transmission

The incidence of HCV infection in dialysis units has also strikingly decreased within the few past years, at least in countries of low endemicity, due to the combined influence of blood donor screening for HCV, and of the generalized use of recombinant erythropoietin which has sharply reduced transfusion requirements. Testing of blood for HCV serologic markers began in 1989 using first-generation ELISA tests, and since 1991 using the more sensitive second-generation ELISA-2 and RIBA-2 tests (111, 112). Concordant prospective studies involving serial determination of HCV serology in dialysis patients have reported a sharp decrease in the annual incidence of seroconversion in center-treated dialysis patients which, after the years 1990–1991 declined to 1 to 2% (111–115). Previously, a number of studies had shown a high prevalence of HCV positive subjects among dialysis patients, with a strong relationship between prevalence rate, length of time on dialysis and number of blood transfusions performed before blood testing was available, thus suggesting a prevalent role for blood transfusion as risk factor for transmission (111–119). As a matter of fact, a dramatic decrease in the incidence of post-transfusional hepatitis C was similarly reported in cardiac surgery patients following increasingly stringent screening of blood donors (120).

However, since HCV seroconversion has been observed in patients who had never received blood transfusion (111, 115, 116, 121–123), other factors than transfusion contribute to HCV transmission. Reports of outbreaks of hemodialysis-associated hepatitis C have implicated the contamination of hospital environmental surfaces and secondary patient-to-patient transmission due to poor aseptic techniques (125). In the report of Jadoul et al., clustering of three seroconverted patients in the same unit where they were dialyzed in the vicinity of HCV positive patients strongly supports the possibility of such nosocomial transmission (111). In this respect, the association between anti-HCV positivity and increasing duration on dialysis may reflect the cumulative risk of exposure to contamination in the dialysis environment (114, 119). However, by contrast to HBV infection, sexual transmission of HCV, especially from patient to spouse, is controversial and seems of limited consequence (114, 123), although injected drug abuse is an established risk factor for both viruses (121). Also, kidney transplants can transmit hepatitis C (126).

The prevalence of HCV infection in medical staff was reported to be low ($\leq$ 1%) even in the face of high prevalence among dialysis patients and before generalized blood screening for HCV was available (111, 112, 114, 121, 122). In recent prospective studies, annual incidence of HCV infection was reported to be nil in staff thus suggesting a much lower tendency for interindividual contamination with HCV than was observed with HBV (112, 114). However, the possible contamination from patient to patient through insufficiently protected manipulation, such as compression of fistula puncture site at the end of a dialysis session by the same nurse serving several patients in close vicinity, clearly stresses the importance of rigorous adherence to recommended precautions for preventing transmission of blood borne pathogens in health-care settings.

General prophylactic measures in dialysis units

Before passive and active immunization against HBV became available, the only means of preventing and controlling HBV infection in dialysis units was immediate detection and isolation of infected patients combined with strict cross-infection prophylaxis. Recommendations aimed at the prevention of spread of any type of hepatitis infection within dialysis centers were given in detail in the Public Health Laboratory Service (PHLS) report as early as 1968 (127). Their principles were: 1) immediate identification and exclusion from the HBV-free dialysis unit of any patient positive for HBsAg; 2) general hygienic precautions directed against spread of infective agents within the center; 3) prevention of spread of infection out of the dialysis unit, especially to the patient's family and to other hospital staff. Efficacy of such measures was clearly apparent in the United Kingdom where a nation-wide preventive program was started in 1968 (128, 129).

Measures aimed at preventing cross-contamination are detailed in the "Recommended precautions for patients undergoing hemodialysis who have AIDS or non-A non-

Table 1. Recommended precautions for patients undergoing hemodialysis

1. Scrupulous cleaning and disinfection of dialysis machines, other equipments, and environmental surfaces before and after each dialysis session.
2. Avoidance of sharing articles between patients.
3. Use of new disposable gloves before starting care of another patient, especially before compression of fistula puncture site at the end of dialysis sessions.
4. Regular screening for serum transaminase level.
5. Regular screening for HBV and HCV serologic markers.

B hepatitis" published in 1985 by the Centers for Disease Control (130) and updated in 1988 as "Universal precautions for prevention of transmission of blood borne pathogens in health-care settings" (131). They include cleaning and disinfection of instruments, machines and environmental surfaces that are routinely touched, avoidance of sharing articles between patients, frequent handwashing and use of disposable gloves. Specific measures recommended to dialysis units are summarized in Table 1.

These measures are exacting and time-consuming. They remain essential, however, because despite successful immunoprophylaxis against HB virus, they are still the only means of protection against the spread of other infective agents, especially hepatitis C virus (HCV) and human immunodeficiency virus (HIV). Whether or not HCV positive patients should be treated in separate facilities is still debated (132). Some authors suggest the need for such segregation in order to limit interindividual contamination (133). Recently the German Association of Clinical Nephrologists recommended isolating ELISA-2 positive patients with high ALT level (134). However, several arguments argue against such segregation (111). First, this measure would be ineffective because a substantial part of uremic patients with ELISA-2 positive serology or even with PCR-demonstrated HCV-RNA viremia exhibit no increase in ALT level (121, 133, 135), and viremia may be present in patients with negative serology due to the long time duration between contamination and detectable antibody by ELISA-2 test (136). Second, such segregation should be unfeasible, because isolation of patients with respect to HBV and HCV status would imply up to four separate facilities. Last, but not least, segregation of HCV positive patients may be hazardous because HCV exhibits a major genomic variability and cross-immunity between the various HCV strains has not been demonstrated, unlike for HBV. Sequential inoculation of chimpanzees with different HCV strains resulted in reappearance of viremia due to reinfection with the latest inoculated strain (137). Therefore, confining HCV positive patients in separate units should expose to the risk of acquiring multiple HCV strains, including those poorly responsive to antiviral therapy (111). In the present status of our knowledge, segregation of HCV positive patients is not yet warranted at least in countries of low HCV endemicity, but such separation may help to reduce the incidence of HCV contamination in countries of high endemicity.

Passive immunization against HBV

The protective efficacy of specific anti-hepatitis B human immunoglobulin preparations (HBIG) was first demonstrated in a study conducted on institutionalized mentally retarded children in whom HBV infection was endemic (138). This protective effect was confirmed subsequently in both medical personnel (139–141) and patients treated in dialysis units (142–144). Passive immunization with HBIG is presently used either for post-exposure protection after accidental inoculation in staff, or as regular preventive treatment in both health care personnel and dialysis patients when unresponsive to vaccination.

Post-exposure protection

Single injections of HBIG are still used for laboratory or hospital staff after accidental inoculation or transmucosal projection of HBsAg positive material. In 80 laboratory and dialysis staff members having received a single dose of HBIG within 7 days following accidental contamination, HBsAg-positive clinical hepatitis developed in only two, whereas eight developed active anti-HBs (140). Other trials of post-exposure passive immunization also showed high, although not absolute, protection (145). Iwarson questioned whether an accelerated vaccination protocol as tested by Wahl et al. (146) should afford better post-exposure protection than HBIG (147). Mitsui and coworkers evaluated the protective efficacy of combined HBIG and hepatitis B vaccine for postexposure prophylaxis after accidental hepatitis B virus inoculation, compared to HBIG injection alone (148). After combined injection of HB vaccine and HBIG within 48 hours of exposure (with vaccination repeated 1 and 3 months later), only 1 of 23 needlestick contaminated staff members contracted HBV infection, whereas 11 of 33 contaminated staff members who received only HBIG developed hepatitis B infection. Therefore, passive-active immunization with an accelerated vaccination protocol may be recommended in such situation as safer than simply passive protection, inasmuch as concomitant injection of HBIG has been proven not to inhibit the development of vaccine-induced antibody (149).

Long-term passive protection

HBIG are effective in preventing HBV infection provided the interval between two injections is not longer than 2 months in staff (139) and in dialysis patients as well (144). Passive-active immunization should be recommended in patients having to start dialysis treatment in emergency conditions, until a protective level of anti-HBs antibody has been elicited by repeated vaccine injections.

Long-term passive protection by means of regular HBIG injection in dialysis patients is now virtually confined to patients who do not respond to vaccination. However, the regular use of HBIG to prevent HBV infection in patients and staff of dialysis units, although effective, has several disadvantages. HBIG injections have to be repeated at short intervals (6 to 8 weeks) in order to maintain protective anti-HBs levels, and such repeated injections often become painful or even may lead to hypersensitivity, obliging termination (139). Moreover, HBIG preparations are expensive and a shortage of donors rich in anti-HBs antibody is to be anticipated, although anti-HBs titers in human donors may be increased by a booster injection of hepatitis B vaccine (150). Thus, clearly, only active immunization by vaccine can adequately solve the problem of large-scale, long-lasting prophylaxis in high-risk populations.

Active immunization

Principles of vaccine preparation

Active immunization against HBV is based on the production of anti-HBs antibodies in response to the injection of purified particles of the surface antigen of the virus.

First generation, plasma-derived vaccines

Because HB virus cannot be cultured in vitro, all first-generation vaccines were prepared from an unusual source of viral antigen, the plasma of chronic HBsAg carriers. Krugman and coworkers first demonstrated that a human plasma rich in HBsAg particles and containing complete virions, when heated for 1 mm at 98°C, lost infectivity but retained immunogenicity (151). Since that pioneer work, stringent procedures were developed to achieve purification and inactivation of human sera containing HBsAg particles in order to eliminate all proteins and viral contaminants, including human immunodeficiency virus (152–156). The Heptavax-B® vaccine produced by Merck, Sharp and Dohme is inactivated by pepsine digestion and urea denaturation and therefore devoid of pre-S2 determinant (153). The final antigen concentration is 20 mcg/dose for use in healthy subjects. The Hevac B® vaccine produced by Pasteur-Mérieux uses as starting material plasma from healthy donors devoid of HBeAg and of infective particles. Purification and inactivation are obtained by sequential zonal centrifugations without enzyme denaturation (156–158). This vaccine retains about 1% of pre-S2 determinant, and final antigen concentration is 5 mcg per dose. A heat-inactivated vaccine (CLB) had been developed in the Netherlands Red Cross blood center but is not licensed for worldwide utilization (159).

Second generation, DNA-recombinant vaccines

The basic principle for production of recombinant vaccines (160, 161) is to isolate the fraction of the HBV genome coding for selected envelope proteins and to transplant this fraction into a host cell, which can be a bacterium (such as E. coli), a yeast (such as Saccharomyces cerevisiae), or a mammalian cell (such as immortalized Chinese hamster ovary line). At the present time, three industrially manufactured recombinant vaccines have been licensed. Two are yeast-derived vaccines, containing only the S-region without any pre-S2 determinant of the HBV genome, one manufactured by Merck, Sharp and Dohme (Recombinax®), the other by Smith Kline Biologicals, Rixensart, Belgium (Engerix-B®). Another recombinant vaccine, using the Chinese hamster ovary cell line and containing both the S and the pre-S2 proteins is produced by Pasteur-Mérieux in France (Genhevac B®). The rationale for incorporating the pre-S2 region of the HBV genome (162) in the vaccine was based on the demonstration that the pre-S2 region is highly immunogenic and may enhance the production of anti-HBs antibody (163–166), and anti-pre-S2 antibody is important in the clearance of hepatitis B virus from infected hepatocytes (167).

Vaccination in healthy medical staff

Protective efficacy and immunogenicity of vaccines

The protective efficacy of the Merck vaccine had been initially tested in a placebo-controlled trial in male homosexuals in the New York area, a population at high risk of HBV infection (168, 169). This study first demonstrated that protection is in relation with the development of anti-HBs antibody at a minimum level which corresponds to what subsequently was estimated to be 10 mlU/ml (170). The protective efficacy of hepatitis B vaccines in healthy medical staff of dialysis units was demonstrated by placebo-controlled trials for the two licensed plasma-derived vaccines (171–173). The results of these controlled trials were confirmed by subsequent studies in hospital health care personnel (174–176). Taken together, they indicate that with any of the vaccines used, vaccination in healthy staff provides protective levels of anti-HBs (i.e., $\geq$ 10 mlU/ml) in at least 95% of subjects. Because a strong correlation was demonstrated between acquisition of an anti-HBs antibody level $\geq$ 10 mlU/ml and protection against HBV infection in the initial placebo-controlled trials using plasma-derived vaccines, only the immunogenic efficacy of recombinant vaccines had to be evaluated. All three licensed DNA-recombinant vaccines have been extensively tested and have been proven to be immunogenic in healthy subjects. Both yeast-derived vaccines at the usual dose of 20 mcg antigen exhibited a similar, or slightly lower potency to elicit production of anti-HBs antibody than the plasma-derived 20 mcg Merck vaccine, with seroconversion obtained in 95% or more of recipients (177–180). By contrast, the pre-S2 containing recombinant vaccine produced by Pasteur-Mérieux revealed more immunogenic than the corresponding plasma-derived vaccine (181).

Vaccination schedules and routes of injection

Vaccination protocols in healthy adults differ among countries. In the USA, a 0, 1, 6 month schedule is usually recommended, whereas in several European countries the usual schedule involves four injections at 0, 1, 2 and 12 months. The latter protocol induces comparable anti-HBs titers following primovaccination, but markedly higher titers following the booster injection at one year and may be more advantageous in terms of long-term protection (182).

The recommended route for all vaccines is intramuscular injection in the deltoid area (183) because intramuscular injections into the buttock, especially in obese subjects, as were previously performed, revealed often deceiving with no or poor response (184–186). In order to lower the cost of vaccination in large-scale vaccination campaigns, the intradermal route (with one-tenth of the dose used for intramuscular route for the corresponding vaccine) has been proposed to vaccine health care workers or medical students (187–191). However, the proportion of responders, antibody titers and duration of protection obtained using this technique appear to be lower than with protocols using intramuscular injections of usual antigen dose (192–194). Therefore, caution should be given when vaccinating health care workers exposed to a high risk of contamination, and control of acquired antibody titer should be advisable in such subjects.

Duration of protection

As expected, the duration of protection afforded by vaccination directly correlates with the peak concentration of anti-HBs antibody determined one month after booster injection, as demonstrated by longitudinal surveillance of healthy staff members in several studies (195–197). The time-course of decline in anti-HBs levels is similar in all vaccinees, with an initially rapid decrease of near 90% (i.e. about 1 log) within the first two years following the peak value, and thereafter a slower decline of about 50% during the subsequent two years. In our experience, an anti-HBs titer of 10 mlU/ml or more was present 5 years after booster in 93% of 143 healthy staff vaccinees (197, 198). The highest peak antibody levels following booster injection are observed when the 0, 1, 2, 12 month schedule is used or, at least, a 0, 1, 12 month schedule (199, 200). Based on the time-course of decline in antibody titer following the peak level, one can recommend that a second booster injection be done after 10 years in subjects with peak level $\geq$ 3000 mlU/ml, after 5 years with peak level between 1000 and 3000, and earlier when peak titer is under this value (201).

Low responses to the vaccine in healthy staff

Nevertheless, a small percentage (about 5%) of healthy subjects in all studies exhibit a lack of response or a very weak response (2 to 10 mlU/ml) to standard vaccination protocols. Some authors reported even lower seroconversion rates, of the order of 80% or less, in health-care workers (202). The reasons for such unresponsiveness in otherwise healthy adults are not fully understood. When excluding trivial factors such as inadequate storage temperature (204) or inappropriate site of injection (184–187), differences in individual genetic factors of immune responsiveness may be proposed as a possible explanation (205). The response to HBV surface antigen should depend on the presence of a dominant immune-response gene located in the major histocompatibility complex, the lack of such a gene being related to a low response. A greater-than-expected number of subjects homozygous for the extended haplotype HLA-B8, SC01, DR3 should be a marker of such a low response, as reported by Alper and coworkers (206). Fortunately, it has been shown that nearly half of healthy subjects who did not produce anti-HBs in response to the initial vaccine course may develop antibody following one or two additional doses (205). Repeated vaccine injections at short interval by the intradermal route were reported by Yasumura et al. to induce an immune response in health care workers who previously were non-responders (207). Also, an advanced age is a well-known factor of a weaker response to vaccine (208) and a higher antigen dosage may be preferred to overcome such weak response in subjects older than 40 years (209).

Observations of unpredictable low response suggest the need for serologic follow-up of highly exposed health care workers in order to ascertain whether or not they are effectively protected against HBV infection.

Vaccination in healthy subjects positive for HBV markers

An important issue is the safety of vaccinating healthy subjects positive for anti-HBc and/or anti-HBs, or for HBsAg. In all of the above-mentioned randomized efficacy trials, a number of HBV events, including seroconversion to HBsAg, occurred in vaccinees during the first months, at a time when antibody had not yet developed. In most cases, vaccination appeared to prevent persistent antigenemia and to limit viral replication (169–171). However, in chronic HBsAg carriers, vaccination was ineffective in suppressing antigenemia but appeared devoid of any adverse effect (210, 211).

Presence of isolated anti-HBs is found in a substantial proportion of hospital staff (212), especially in populations where a high prevalence of HBV markers exists (213), raising the question whether this represents previous unapparent HBV infection with immunity, or false positivity with non-protective antibody (211). Serologic response to vaccine may help discriminate between immune subjects, in whom vaccine should elicit a rapid,

frank "anamnestic" antibody response, whereas a slower, "primary-type" response, is expected in the other situation. Goudeau et al. (176) and Werner et al. (214) observed an anamnestic-type response following a single vaccine injection in only a few health care workers having isolated anti-HBs antibody.

The problem of healthy subjects with isolated high-titer ($\geq$ 70% inactivation) anti-HBc, although less frequent, is quite similar. An anamnestic response to a single dose of vaccine was very infrequently observed in such subjects in countries with low prevalence of natural HBV markers such as France (215) or the USA (216), whereas it was obtained in about half of the cases in countries with higher natural prevalence of HBV markers, such as Italy (217) or Greece (218). Thus, screening for anti-HBs and anti-HBc may be advisable prior to vaccine decision in health care workers in countries where a high prevalence of HBV markers exists (219), whereas in countries of low endemicity, screening for AgHBs, anti-HBs or anti-HBc in young adults is probably not cost-effective and vaccination of health care workers without screening prior to professional exposure is advisable because the vaccine causes no adverse effects in immune individuals (220).

Vaccination in uremic patients

Impaired immune responsiveness in dialysis patients

Whereas all of the available licensed vaccines provide active immunization to virtually all healthy subjects using standard vaccination protocols, effective immunization of dialysis patients still remains a problem. The development of anti-HBs antibody is inhibited in such patients by the immunodeficient state that characterizes uremia and which is not improved, or even worsened, by maintenance hemodialysis (221–225). The defects in immune response of uremics are both humoral and cellular (226). Evidence for a T-cell defect has been shown in dialysis patients as well as in predialysis patients (227–230). Similar impairment in immune responses is also observed in transplanted patients, even with a well functioning graft, due to the long-term use of immunosuppressive agents. Thus, impaired immune response to various vaccines is to be expected in uremic, dialyzed and transplanted patients. The mechanisms involved in uremia-associated defective immune response are discussed in detail in another chapter.

Immunogenicity and protective efficacy of vaccination in dialysis patients

The protective efficacy of vaccination against HBV infection in dialysis patients has been demonstrated by placebo-controlled trials using the plasma-derived Pasteur vaccine (231) and the Merck vaccine (232). However, both studies clearly showed a markedly lower rate of responders in dialysis patients than was previously observed in healthy subjects. Also, anti-HBs titers elicited in dialysis patients were considerably lower than in healthy staff members. A number of studies in all countries confirmed the poor immune response of dialyzed patients both in terms of responder rate and of antibody titers, when using the standard protocols recommended for healthy subjects, either with plasma-derived vaccines (233–244) or DNA-recombinant vaccines (245–248). Thus, the question arose whether reinforced protocols could overcome the deficient response of dialysis patients by increasing the dose of antigen, the number of injections, or both.

Reinforced vaccine protocols in dialysis patients
A comparative, randomized trial of immunogenicity was performed in 215 low-risk patients, treated either at home or in hepatitis-free centers in the Paris area (249, 250). Compared to the standard protocol (3 doses of 5 μg Hevac B vaccine at 0, 1, 2, months), two reinforced protocols (3 doses of 10 mg at 0, 1, 2 months or 4 single doses of 5 μg at 0, 1, 2 and 4 months) induced a significantly greater proportion of responders and significantly higher anti-HBs titers. As the results obtained by either of the two reinforced protocols did not differ statistically, the last schedule with 4 single injections of 5 μg, that had the best cost/efficacy ratio, was henceforth adopted as our recommended protocol for all dialyzed patients. In the experience of Goudeau et al. also using the Hevac B vaccine, the proportion of responders similarly rose from 56% following the third injection to 67% after a fourth injection given two months later (176). Another French group eventually obtained a responder rate of 90% in a population of aged dialysis patients by increasing the number of vaccine injections from 4 to 14 (251). Other reinforced protocols using increased doses of the plasma-derived Merck vaccine (40 μg/dose instead of 20 μg in healthy subjects) (234, 240), or of the heat-inactivated CLB vaccine (27 μg/dose instead of the 3 μg standard dose) (237, 239) were shown to improve the rate of responders up to 80% or more, together with an increase in anti-HBs titer.

Subsequently, DNA-recombinant vaccines have been extensively tested in dialysis patients. The SKF Engerix® vaccine has proven as immunogenic as the Merck plasma-derived vaccine in such patients, but use of a double-dose (40 μg instead of 20 μg) was proposed (246, 247). However, a 0, 1, 2, 6 or 0, 1, 2, 12 month vaccination schedule revealed more immunogenic that the standard 0, 1, 6 month schedule (252–255). The Merck Recombivax® vaccine even at double dose revealed to be less immunogenic than the plasma-derived vaccine in uremic patients (256) and is not recommended by the manufacturer in this indication. By contrast, the Pasteur-Mérieux pre-S2 containing DNA-recombinant vaccine revealed slightly more immunogenic than the plasma-derived vaccine (257).

Finally, chronic uremic patients act as "slow" responders who need more intense and/or more repeated antigenic stimulation to elicit antibody production than do healthy immunocompetent subjects. A consensus has emerged that the more efficient and cost-effective protocol is provided by repeated injections of standard doses of a highly immunogenic vaccine according to a 0, 1, 2, 4 (or 6) month schedule with a booster injection at the 12th month as standard protocol, with additional injections at 2–3 month intervals if no or poor response has been obtained following the fourth dose.

Duration of protection in dialysis patients
The duration of protection afforded by vaccination in dialysis patients has been studied by several groups. Protective anti-HBs levels lasted for at least 1 year in all patients who received a fourth injection in the study of Goudeau et al. (176). Benhamou et al. (258) longitudinally studied the time course of anti-HBs following the booster injection given at 1 year in patients participating in the above-mentioned efficacy trial (249). The rate of decline was parallel in all patients and the slope of the curves was similar to that observed in healthy staff, but the interval before anti-HBs titers fell below 10 mIU/ml was shorter than in healthy subjects because post-booster peak GMT values were, as a mean, 10 times lower. Projection of the curves showed that an anti-HBs level above 10 mIU/ml should be maintained for at least 2 years in patients having peak values of 1,000 mIU/ml or more. However, in patients exposed to a high risk of HBV infection, assessment of anti-HBs titer at regular intervals, especially in weak responders, should allow the best prediction of the optimal time for revaccination (248, 258).

Vaccination in chronic uremic patients prior to dialysis
As the impaired antibody production in dialysis patients is related to the uremic state, one could expect that vaccination started at an earlier stage of renal failure should obtain a better immune response. Therefore, several trials of vaccination prior to initiation of dialysis were performed in chronic uremic patients but all have shown that immune response to hepatitis B vaccine is impaired in uremic patients similar to those already on dialysis, even when vaccination is started at an early stage of chronic renal failure (234, 235, 259). However, reinforced protocols similar to those used in dialysis patients have been shown to improve immune response, either using plasma-derived vaccines (260, 261) or DNA-recombinant vaccines (256, 257).

Factors of impaired response in uremic patients
Although impaired response to hepatitis B vaccines is a universal finding in chronic uremic patients, either dialyzed or not, several factors may modulate the individual immune response in such patients (262).

A striking influence of age has been reported by several groups, with a markedly lower proportion of responders in dialysis patients over 50 or 60 than in younger patients (176, 231–233, 242, 243, 246, 248), at least in males (236) and, of note, the response rate in uremic children is especially high (263, 264). Others (240, 241, 262) did not observe an influence of age on the immune response, but they studied small series of dialyzed patients of whom most were aged 50 years or more. We observed a clear adverse influence of age in nondialyzed, chronic uremic patients, with a response rate of 81% in subjects under 40 compared to 42% in those over 60 using a plasma-derived vaccine (261), and the same tendency was observed when using the Pre-S2-containing recombinant vaccine (257). However, the mean antibody titer in responders did not differ whatever the age. Thus, the beneficial effect of multiple injections may be of special interest in older patients, who have the more delayed response, as shown in a population of aged dialysis patients (251).

By contrast, the influence of sex is much less apparent, although the response rate and antibody level have been reported to be slightly higher in female patients than in males (233, 249, 251, 261).

Immunogenetic factors were shown to influence the individual response to vaccine in uremics, as in healthy subjects. In dialysis patients, Pol et al. reported an increased frequency of the DR3 allele as well as of the extended HLA-A1, B8, DR3 haplotype in non-responders compared to responders (265). However, in a recent multicenter study bearing on 203 hemodialyzed patients, 45 non-responders exhibited a significantly lower frequency of the DR2 haplotype compared to responder patients or to 405 Caucasian controls (8.9% vs 21.5 and 26.2%, $p < 0.01$) whereas the DR3 haplotype frequency was not increased (266). This finding is now confirmed on an extended series of more than 400 dialysis patients.

The influence of recombinant erythropoietin therapy on immune response to vaccine is debated. Sennesael et al. reported a higher seroconversion rate and a five-fold greater mean antibody titer in 15 dialysis patients on erythropoietin therapy than in 22 patients who did not receive such treatment (267). However, others did not observe a different immune response whether or not patients received recombinant erythropoietin therapy (248, 268). Coexistent hepatitis C virus infection has been reported to be associated with a decrease in the antibody response of hemodialysis patients (268), but such a correlation was not observed by others (269). Response of renal allograft recipients to vaccine is very poor, whereas in patients vaccinated before transplantation, a booster injection is highly successful, and this is an additional argument to recommend hepatitis B vaccination prior to transplantation (270).

Combined immunostimulation and vaccination
Various attempts have been made to improve the defective immune response of uremic patients to hepatitis B vaccine by means of immunostimulation. Zinc supplementation was proposed as an adjuvant to hepatitis B vaccine in dialysis patients (271) but a beneficial influence of such supplementation was denied by others (272, 273). Subcutaneous injections of thymopentin combined to vaccine injections have been reported to improve the antibody response of dialysis patients previously unresponsive to a full vaccination course (274) but such beneficial effect

was not confirmed in two prospective controlled studies (275, 276). Gamma interferon was proposed by Quiroga et al. but a further prospective controlled study by the same authors failed to confirm a beneficial effect of IFγ associated to vaccine on response rate or antibody titer compared to recipients of vaccine alone (269).

In view of the defective bioavailability of Interleukin-2 (IL-2) in uremic patients (226, 227, 277), Meuer et al. tested the effects of local administration of an IL-2 preparation combined with hepatitis B vaccine in dialysis patients previously non-responders to the usual vaccination schedule (278). Seven of 10 patients developed antibody titers between 50 and 600 mIU/ml following vaccine reinjection together with IL-2. However, other authors using a recombinant IL-2 preparation failed to confirm such a beneficial effect (279). Similarly, in a prospective, placebo-controlled study in unresponsive uremic patients, we assessed the effects of concomitant administration of the pre-S2-containing recombinant vaccine together with 1 million units of recombinant IL-2 administered at the same site. We observed seroconversion in a substantial proportion of patients, but without significant difference in antibody response whether they received IL-2 or placebo (280). Similarly, IL-2 failed to improve primary antibody response to hepatitis B vaccine in healthy adults (281). Thus, at the present time, the search for effective immunoadjuvants is still an unsolved problem (282). However, several groups have reported seroconversion by repeated low-dose intradermal injections of recombinant hepatitis B vaccine at short time-intervals in dialysis patients (283, 284).

Results of vaccination and logistics of hepatitis prevention in dialysis units

Results of hepatitis B vaccination campaigns

In a few years since 1982, the generalized use of vaccination against HBV dramatically reduced the high morbidity and mortality due to HBV infection in nephrology units, at least in countries where extensive vaccination campaigns were actively pursued both in staff and patients.

The annual reports of the European Dialysis and Transplant Association from 1981 to 1991 clearly show a continuous reduction in the annual incidence of new cases of hepatitis B in staff and patients (285). As an example, the annual incidence of compensated virus B hepatitis cases in Belgium fell from 200 in 1980 to 40 in 1986, an 80% reduction (286). In the hospitals of the Paris area, which employ about 60,000 health care workers, vaccination was proposed in 1981 to highly exposed personnel, namely those working in nephrology units and blood centers, and was proposed in 1983 to all hospital health care workers. As a result, the mean annual incidence of recorded hepatitis B cases, which peaked at about 125 cases per year up to 1980, fell to 55 in 1984 and 16 in 1988, an 87% reduction from 1980 to 1988 (287).

Organizational aspects of hepatitis prevention in dialysis units

Logistic problems of vaccination differ between health care personnel and dialysis patients.

Vaccination against HBV in health care workers
As pointed out by Blumberg (288), health care institutions are morally and legally responsible for providing protection to their personnel. Thus, vaccination of all exposed health care personnel should be a legal requirement, or at least a strong recommendation. In healthy staff members, a consensus based on cost-effectiveness analysis, has emerged that in countries with low prevalence of natural HBV infection, generalized vaccination without pre screening for HBV markers should be recommended for large-scale programs at least in young medical personnel not yet exposed to the occupational risk of HBV contamination. However, in countries where there is a high prevalence of HBV markers in the general population and/or in hospital personnel, preliminary testing for HBV markers would be economically advisable, in order to exclude from vaccination subjects already positive for HBsAg or having a high anti-HBs titer, although there appears to be no disadvantage, other than cost, in vaccinating such patients (289).

Highly exposed hospital personnel who need priority vaccination include all those working in nephrology, dialysis and transplant units, blood banks, laboratories, operating and anesthetic wards, radiology, hepatology, hematology, infectious disease and intensive care units, this list being not limitative. In staff members exposed to a very high risk of infection, post-vaccination anti-HBs testing should be considered an important ethical issue, in view of the few, but unpredictable, subjects developing no or low response. Such subjects should be identified and offered an additional course of vaccination and, if still non-responsive, should be submitted to regular passive protection by HBIG or moved to less exposed work areas. Subjects having isolated anti-HBc and/or low-titer anti-HBs antibody should receive one vaccine dose and, if an "anamnestic" rise in anti-HBs titer is not developed, should complete a full vaccination course. A single anti-HBs determination one month following booster injection is usually sufficient for prediction of the optimal time for subsequent boostering.

Vaccination against HBV in uremic patients
The problem of dialyzed and of predialysis uremic patients is similar, due to their defective immune response which requires similarly reinforced protocols. However, when compared to the heavy cost of dialysis treatment and of transplantation, the cost of hepatitis B vaccination, even using larger or more frequent doses is not a limiting problem, as the cost of a full vaccination course is lower than that of a single dialysis session. Also, screening for HBV markers is part of routine surveillance of such patients and may result in significant savings. Therefore,

in view of the deleterious effects of HBV infection in dialyzed and in transplanted patients, effective immunization before starting dialysis treatment and kidney transplantation should be considered an important goal.

Reinforced protocols are needed in uremic patients, dialyzed or not, especially in older subjects. Based on extensive experience, the most efficient schedule comprises 4 doses at 0, 1, 2 and 4 months, followed by anti-HBs titration. Additional dose(s) should be given 2–3 months apart when no or poor (< 50 mIU/l) response has been elicited. In any case, a booster injection is to be given at month 12.

An important practical rule is to start the vaccination protocol early in the course of renal failure, ideally at least one year before the anticipated time of starting hemodialysis treatment. Thus, whenever possible, vaccination should be initiated in uremic patients when creatinine clearance has declined to 40–50 ml/mn or, more simply, when plasma creatinine concentration is in excess of 200 μmol/l. Such a policy should avoid the need for concomitant passive protection and allow the highest possible anti-HBs peak concentration to be achieved prior to start of dialysis.

Following booster injection, anti-HBs titer should be monitored at time-intervals adapted to the peak level, in order that subsequent booster injections may be given before anti-HBs has declined below the protective level, including after the start of dialysis treatment.

Prevention of HCV infection
At the present time, no vaccine against hepatitis C virus is available, nor predictable in a near future. The only means of preventing nosocomial transmission is scrupulous respect of the universal precautions for patients undergoing hemodialysis, which also apply to patients positive for the human immunodeficiency virus. Of note, no segregation for treatment in separate units is needed for patients positive for HCV or HIV, but careful cleaning and disinfection of dialysis equipment after each dialysis session and avoidance of dialyzer reutilization are of utmost importance.

CONCLUSION

In conclusion, the problem of viral hepatitis in dialysis units has been strikingly modified during the past decade. Due to sustained vaccination campaigns, hepatitis B virus infection has been virtually eradicated in staff, and nearly all uremic patients are now able to start dialysis and/or transplantation with a protective antibody level. The main persisting problem concerns dialyzed or transplanted patients who are chronic carriers of the HBV surface antigen and especially those with chronic active hepatitis. Further progress in antiviral therapy is needed to obtain eradication of viremia and stabilization of hepatic lesions.

The availability of routine serologic detection of hepatitis C virus infection has unmasked the high prevalence HCV infection in dialysis and transplant units. Both the generalized use of recombinant erythropoietin by reducing the need for blood transfusion, and universal screening of blood donors, strikingly lowered the incidence of new cases of HCV infection. However, as for hepatitis B virus the main present concern is for dialysis or transplant patients previously contaminated by hepatitis C virus who developed chronic non-A, non-B hepatitis. Again, further progress in antiviral therapy is needed to achieve suppression of viremia and healing of liver lesions. At the present time, vigilant vaccination policy against HBV and scrupulous respect of the universal precautions to prevent bloodborne and nosocomial infections are the best means of achieving eradication of HBV and HCV infection in dialysis units.

REFERENCES

1. Stevens CE, Taylor PE, Tong MJ, Toy PT, Vyas GN: Hepatitis B vaccine, an overview. in *Viral Hepatitis and Liver Disease*, edited by Vyas GN, Dienstag JL, Hoofnagle JH, Grune & Stratton, Orlando, 1984, p 275
2. Tiollais P, Pourcel C, Dejean A: The hepatitis B virus. *Nature* 317: 489, 1985
3. Houghton M, Richman K, Han J et al.: Hepatitis C virus (HCV): a relative of the pestiviruses and flaviviruses. in *Viral Hepatitis and Liver Disease*, edited by Hollinger FB, Lemon SM, Margolis H, Baltimore William & Wilkins, 1991, p 328
4. Degast GC, Houwen B, Van Der Hem JK, The JH: T lymphocyte number and function and the course of hepatitis B in hemodialysis patients. *Infect Immun* 14: 1138, 1976
5. Descamps B, Jungers P, Naret C, Zingraff J, Bach JF: HLA1 B8 phenotype association and HBs antigenemia evolution in 440 hemodialyzed patients. *Digestion* 15: 171, 1977
6. Hoofnagle JH, Di Bisceglie AM: Serodiagnosis of acute and chronic hepatitis. *Sem Liver Dis* 11: 73, 1991
7. Degott C, Degos F, Jungers P et al.: Relationship between liver histopathological changes and HBs Ag in 111 patients treated by long-term hemodialysis. *Liver* 3: 377, 1983
8. Bruguera M, Vidal L, Sanchez-Tapias JM, Casta J, Revert L, Rodes J: Incidence and features of liver disease in patients on chronic hemodialysis. *J Clin Gastroenterol* 12: 298, 1990
9. Paterlini P, Gerken G, Nakajima E et al.: Polymerase chain reaction to detect hepatitis B virus DNA and RNA sequences in primary liver cancers from patients negative for hepatitis B surface antigen. *N Engl J Med* 323: 80, 1990
10. Colombo M, De Franchis R, Del Ninno E et al.: Hepatocellular carcinoma in Italian patients with cirrhosis. *N Engl J Med* 325: 675, 1991
11. Schroeter GPJ, Weill R, Penn I et al.: Hepatocellular carcinoma associated with hepatitis B infection after kidney transplantation. *Lancet* 2: 381, 1982
12. Degos F, Degott C, Benhamou JP, Liver biopsy. in *Oxford Textbook of Clinical Hepatology*, edited by MacIntyre N, Benhamou JP, Bircher J, Rizzetto M, Rodes J, Oxford University Press 1991, p 320
13. Lebrec D, Goldfarb G, Degott C, Rueff B, Benhamou JP: Transvenous liver biopsy; an experience based on 1000 hepatic tissue samplings with this procedure. *Gastroenterology* 83: 338, 1982
14. Scheuer PJ: Classification of chronic viral hepatitis; need for reassessment *J Hepatol* 13: 372, 1991
15. Knodell RG, Ishak KG, Black WC et al.: Formulation and application of a numerical scoring system for assessing histological activity in asymptomatic chronic active hepatitis. *Hepatology* 1: 431, 1981
16. Gilli P, Cavazzini L, Stabellini N, Malacarne F, Soffritti S, Storari A: Histological features of non-A non-B hepatitis in hemodialysis patients. *Nephron* 61: 296, 1992
17. Parfrey PS, Forbes RDC, Hutchinson TA, Beaudoin JG, Dauphinee WD, Guttmann RD: The prevalence and progression of liver disease in renal transplant recipients: a histological study. *Transplant Proc* 16: 1103, 1984
18. Chu CM, Karayiannis P, Fowler MJF, Monjardino J, Liaw YF, Thomas HC: Natural history of chronic hepatitis B virus infection in Taiwan: studies of hepatitis B virus DNA in serum. *Hepatology* 5: 431, 1985
19. Lau JYN, Wright TL: Molecular virology and pathogenesis of hepatitis B. *Lancet* 342: 1335, 1993
20. Fujita YK, Kamata K, Kamena H, Isselbacher KJ, Wands JR: Detection of hepatitis B virus infection in hepatitis B surface antigen-negative hemodialysis patients by monoclonal radioimmunoassays. *Gastroenterology* 91: 1357, 1986
21. Brechot C, Degos F, Lugassy C et al.: Hepatitis B virus DNA in patients with chronic liver disease and negative tests for hepatitis B surface antigen. *N Engl J Med* 312: 270, 1985
22. Gerken G, Paterlini P, Manns M et al.: Assay of hepatitis B virus DNA by polymerase chain reaction and its relationship to pre-S and S-encoded viral surface antigens. *Hepatology* 13: 158, 1991
23. Nordenfeldt E, Lindholm T, Lofgren B, Moestrup T, Reinicke V: Different categories of chronic HBsAg carriers; a long term follow-up. in *Viral Hepatitis*, edited by Szmuness W, Alter HJ, Maynard JE, Philadelphia, Franklin Institute Press, 1981, p 237
24. Theilmann L, Gmelin K, Rambausek M et al.: HBV DNA and other hepatitis B virus markers in sera from long-term hemodialysis and kidney transplant patients. *Hepato-gastroenterol* 35: 147, 1988
25. Degos F, Lugassy C, Degott C et al.: HBV and HBV related viral infection in renal transplant recipients: a prospective study of 90 patients. *Gastroenterology* 94: 151, 1988
26. Hanson CA, Sutherland DE, Snover D: Fulminant hepatic failure in an HBsAg carrier renal transplant recipient following cessation of immunosuppressive therapy. *Transplantation* 39: 311, 1985
27. Marcellin P, Giostra E, Martinot Peignoux M et al.: Redevelopment of hepatitis B surface antigen after renal transplantation. *Gastroenterology* 100: 1432, 1991

28. Carman W, Thomas H, Domingo E: Viral genetic variation: hepatitis B virus as a clinical example. *Lancet* 341: 349, 1993

29. Bonino F, Brunetto MR, Rizzetto M, Will H: Hepatitis B virus unable to secrete e antigen. *Gastroenterology* 100: 1138, 1991

30. Carman WF, Jacyna MR, Hadziyannis S et al.: Mutation preventing formation of hepatitis B antigen in patients with chronic hepatitis B infection. *Lancet* 2: 588, 1989

31. Kremsdorf D, Thiers V, Garreau F et al.: Nucleotide sequence analysis of hepatitis B virus genomes isolated from serologically negative patients. in *Viral Hepatitis and Liver Disease*, edited by Hollinger FB, Lemon SM, Margolis, HS, Baltimore, William & Wilkins, 1991, p 222

32. Brechot C: Polymerase chain reaction for the diagnosis of hepatitis B and C viral hepatitis. *J Hepatol* 17: 35, 1993

33. Thiers V, Nakajima E, Kremsdorf D et al.: Transmission of hepatitis B from hepatitis-B-seronegative subjects. *Lancet* 2: 1273, 1988

34. Rizzetto M, Ponzetto A, Bonino F, Smedile A: Hepatitis Delta virus infection. Clinical and epidemiological aspects. in *Viral Hepatitis and Liver Disease*, edited by Zuckerman A, New York, Alan R Liss, 1988, p 389

35. Pol S, Dubois F, Mattlinger B et al.: Absence of hepatitis Delta virus infection in chronic hemodialysis and kidney transplant patients in France. *Transplantation* 54: 1096, 1992

36. Kharsha G, Degott C, Degos F, Carnot F, Potet F, Kreis H: Fulminant hepatitis in renal transplant recipients: the role of the Delta agent. *Transplantation* 44: 221, 1987

37. Ware AJ, Gorder NL, Gurian LE, Douglas C, Shorey JW, Parker T: Value of screening for markers of hepatitis in dialysis units. *Hepatology* 3: 513, 1983

38. Perillo RP: Treatment of chronic hepatitis B. in *Viral Hepatatis Liver Disease*, edited by Hollinger FB, Lemon SM, Margolis HS, Baltimore, William & Wilkins, 1991, p 616

39. Peters M: Mechanisms of action of interferons. *Semin Liv Dis* 9: 235, 1989

40. Davis G: Interferon treatment of viral hepatitis in immunocompromised patients. *Semin Liv Dis* 9: 267, 1989

41. Hirsch MS, Tolkoff-Rubin NE, Kelly AP, Rubin RH: Pharmakokinetics of human and recombinant leukocyte interferon in patients with chronic renal failure who are undergoing hemodialysis. *J Infect Dis* 148: 335, 1983

42. Buisson C, Degos F, Daniel F et al.: Pharmakokinetics of interferon Alpha 2b in hemodialysis. *Nephrol Dial Transpl* 9: 977, 1994

43. Marcellin P, Ouzan D, Degos F et al.: Randomized controlled trial of adenine arabinoside 5' monophosphate (ARA-AMP) in chronic active hepatitis: comparison of the efficacy in heterosexual and homosexual patients. *Hepatology* 10: 328, 1989

44. Pol S, Saltiel C, Legendre C et al.: Efficacy of Arabinoside 5' monophosphate in kidney recipients with chronic active hepatitis B: a pilot study. *Transplant Proc* 25: 1446, 1993

45. Degos F, Degott C: Hepatitis in renal transplant recipients. *J Hepatol* 9: 114, 1989

46. Dusheiko G, Song E, Bowyer S et al.: Natural history of hepatitis B virus infection in renal transplant recipients. A fifteen years follow-up. *Hepatology* 3: 330, 1983

47. Ware AJ, Luby JP, Eigenbrodt EH, Long DL, Hull AR: Spectrum of liver disease in renal transplant recipients. *Gastroenterology* 68: 755, 1975

48. LaQuaglia MP, Tolkoff-Rubin NE, Dienstag JL et al.: Impact of hepatitis on renal transplantation. *Transplantation* 32: 504, 1981

49. Parfrey PS, Forbes RDC, Hutchinson TA: The impact of renal transplantation on the course of hepatitis B liver disease. *Transplantation* 39: 610, 1985

50. Degos F, Debure A, Kreis H: Hepatitis in renal transplant recipients. *Transplantation Reviews* 1: 159, 1987

51. Pol S, Debure A, Degott C et al.: Chronic hepatitis in kidney allograft recipients. *Lancet* 335: 878, 1990

52. Rao JV, Kasiske BL, Anderson WR: Variability in the morphological spectrum and clinical outcome of chronic liver disease in hepatitis B-positive and B-negative renal transplant recipients. *Transplantation* 51: 391, 1991

53. Rao JV, Anderson WR, Kasiske BL, Dahl DC: Value of liver biopsy in the evaluation and management of chronic liver diseases in renal transplant recipients. *Am J Med* 94: 241, 1993

54. Fairley CK, Mijch A, Gust ID, Nichilson S, Dimitrakakis M, Lucas CR: The increased risk of fatal liver disease in renal transplant patients who are hepatitis Be antigen and/or HBV DNA positive. *Transplantation* 52: 497, 1991

55. Choo QL, Kuo G, Weiner AJ, Overby LR, Bradley DW, Houghton M: Isolation of a cDNA clone derived from a blood borne NANB viral hepatitis genome. *Science* 244: 359, 1989

56. Kuo G: An assay for circulating antibodies to a major etiologic virus of human NANB hepatitis. *Sciences* 244: 362, 1989

57. Brechot C, Kremsdorf D: Genetic variation of the hepatitis C virus (HCV) genome: random events or a clinically relevant issue? *J Hepatol* 17: 265, 1993

58. Okamoto H, Sugiyama Y, Okada S et al.: Typing hepatitis C virus by polymerase chain reaction with type-specific primers: application to clinical surveys and tracing infection sources. *J Gen Virol* 73: 673, 1992

59. Simmonds P, McOmis F, Yap PL et al.: Sequence variability in the 5' non coding region of hepatitis C virus: identification of a new virus type and restriction on sequence diversity. *J Gen Virol* 74: 661, 1993

60. Nakatsuji Y, Matsumoto A, Ogata H, Kiyosawa K: Detection of chronic hepatitis C virus infection by four diagnostic systems: first generation and second generation enzyme linked immunosorbent assay, second generation enzyme linked immunosorbent assay, second generation immunoblot assay, second generation recombinant immunoblot assay and nested polymerase chain reaction analysis. *Hepatology* 16: 300, 1992

61. Van der Poel CL, Cuypers HT, Reesink HW et al.: Confirmation of hepatitis C virus infection by new four antigen recombinant immunoblot assay. *Lancet* 337: 317, 1991

62. Zaaijer HL, Cuypers HTM, Reesink HW, Winkel IN, Gerken G, Lelie PN: Reliability of polymerase chain reaction for detection of hepatitis C virus. *Lancet* 341: 722, 1993

63. Lau JYN, Davis GL, Kniffen J et al.: Significance of serum hepatitis C virus RNA levels in chronic hepatitis C. *Lancet* 341: 1501, 1993

64. Tremolada F, Casarin C, Alberti A et al.: Long term follow-up of non-A, non-B (type C) post transfusion hepatitis. *Hepatology* 16: 273, 1992

65. Chan TM, Lok ASF, Cheng IKP, Chan RT: Prevalence of hepatitis C virus infection in hemodialysis patients: a longitudinal study comparing the results of RNA and antibody assays. *Hepatology* 17: 5, 1993

66. Almroth G, Ekermo B, Franzen L, Hed J: Antibodies responses to hepatitis C virus and its modes of transmission in dialysis patients. *Nephron* 59: 232, 1991

67. Camarelo C, Ortiz A, Aguilera B et al.: Liver disease patterns in hemodialysis patients with antibodies to hepatitis C virus. *Am J Kidney Dis* 22: 822, 1993

68. Mondelli MU, Smedile V, Piazza V et al.: Abnormal alanine aminotransferase activity reflects exposure to hepatitis C virus in haemodialysis patients. *Nephrol Dial Transplant* 6: 480, 1991

69. Stempel CA, Lake J, Kuo G, Vincenti F: Hepatitis C – its prevalence in end-stage renal failure patients and clinical course after kidney transplantation. *Transplantation* 55: 273, 1993

70. Vandelli L, Medici G, Savazzi AM et al.: Behavior of antibody profile against hepatitis C virus in patients on maintenance hemodialysis. *Nephron* 61: 260, 1992

71. Yamaguchi K, Nishimura Y, Fukioka N et al.: Hepatitis C virus antibodies in hemodialysis patients. *Lancet* 335: 1409, 1990

72. Kallinowski B, Theilmann L, Gmelin K et al.: Prevalence of antibodies to hepatitis C virus in hemod alysis patients. *Nephron* 59: 236, 1991

73. Elisaf M, Tsianos E, Mavridis A, Dardamanis M, Pappas M, Siamopoulos KC: Antibodies against hepatitis C virus (anti-HCV) in haemodialysis patients: association with hepatitis B serological markers. *Nephron Dial Transplant* 6: 476, 1991

74. Knudsen F, Wantzin P, Rasmussen K et al.: Hepatitis C in dialysis patients: relationship to blood transfusions, dialysis and liver disease. *Kidney Int* 43: 1353, 1993

75. Schauer PJ, Ashrafzadeh P, Sherlock S, Brown D, Dusheiko G: The pathology of hepatitis C. *Hepatology* 15: 567, 1992

76. Gilli P, Moretti M, Soffritti S, Menini C: Anti-HCV positive patients in dialysis units? *Lancet* 336: 243, 1990

77. Agnello V, Chung RT, Kaplan LM: A role for hepatitis C virus infection in type II cryoglobulinemia. *N Engl J Med* 327: 1490, 1992

78. Johnson RJ, Gretch DR, Yamabe H et al.: Membranoproliferative glomerulonephritis associated with hepatitis C virus infection. *N Engl J Med* 328: 1465, 1993

79. Tran A, Quaranta JF, Benzaken S et al.: High prevalence of thyroid autoantibodies in a prospective series of patients with chronic hepatitis before interferon therapy. *Hepatology* 18: 253, 1993

80. Haddad J, Deny P, Munz-Gotheil C et al.: Lymphocytic sialadenitis of Sjogren's syndrome associated with chronic hepatitis C virus liver disease. *Lancet* 339: 321, 1992

81. Fargion S, Piperno A, Capellini M et al.: Hepatitis C virus and porphyria cutanea tarda; evidence for a strong association. *Hepatology* 16: 1322, 1992

82. Seef LB, Buskell Bales Z, Wright EC et al.: Long term mortality after transfusion associated non-A, non-B hepatitis. *N Engl J Med* 327: 1906, 1992

83. Gordon SC, Elloway RS, Long JC, Dmuchowski CF: The pathology of hepatitis C as function of mode of transmission: blood transfusion vs. intravenous drug use. *Hepatology* 18: 1338, 1993

84. Caporaso N, Romano M, Marmo RS et al.: Hepatitis C virus infection is an additive risk factor for the development of hepatocellular carcinoma in patients with cirrhosis. *J Hepatol* 12: 367, 1991

84b. De Metri MS, Poussin K, Baccarini P et al.: HCV-associated liver cancer without cirrhosis. *Lancet* 345: 413, 1995

85. Tine F, Magrin S, Craxi A, Pagliaro L: Interferon for non-A, non-B chronic hepatitis. A meta-analysis of randomised clinical trials. *J Hepatol* 13: 192, 1991

86. Gil B, Qian C, Riezu JI, Civiera MP, Prieto J: Hepatic and extra-hepatic HCV RNA strands in chronic hepatitis C; different patterns of response to interferon treatment. *Hepatology* 18: 1050, 1993

87. Ellis ME, Alfurayh 0, Halim MA et al.: Chronic nonA nonB hepatitis complicated by end-stage renal failure treated with recombinant interferon alpha. *J Hepatol* 18: 210, 1993

88. Koenig P, Vogel W, Umlauft F et al.: Interferon treatment for chronic hepatitis C infection in uremic patients. *Kidney Int* 45: 1507, 1994

89. Huang CC, Liaw YF, Lai MK, Chu SH, Chuang CK, Huang JY: The clinical outcome of hepatitis C virus antibody-positive renal allograft recipients. *Transplantation* 53: 763, 1992

90. Roth D, Zucker K, Cirocco R et al.: The impact of hepatitis C virus infection on renal allograft recipients. *Kidney Int* 45: 238, 1994

91. Pol S, Legendre C, Saltiel CW et al.: Hepatitis C virus in kidney transplant recipients. Epidemiology and impact on renal transplantation. *J Hepatol* 15: 202, 1992

92. Ponz E, Campistol JM, Bruguera M et al.: Hepatitis C virus infection among kidney transplant recipients. *Kidney Int* 40: 748, 1991

93. Rohr MS, Lesniewski RR, Rubin CA et al.: Risk of liver disease in HCV-seropositive kidney transplant recipients. *Ann Surg* 217: 512, 1993

94. Roth D, Fernandez JA, Burke GW, Esquenazi V, Miller J: Detection of antibody to hepatitis C virus in renal transplant recipients. *Transplantation* 51: 396, 1991

95. Chan TM, Lok ASF, Cheng IKP, Ng IOL: Chronic hepatitis C after renal transplantation. *Transplantation* 56: 1095, 1993

96. Fritsche C, Brandes JC, Delaney SR et al.: Hepatitis C is a poor prognostic indicator in black kidney transplant recipients. *Transplantation* 55: 1283, 1993

97. Goffin E, Pirson Y, Cornu C et al.: Outcome of HCV infection after renal transplantation. *Kidney Int* 45: 551, 1994

98. Allison MC, Mowat A, McCruden EAB et al.: The spectrum of chronic liver disease in renal transplant recipients. *Quart J Med* 301: 355, 1992

99. Aroldi A, Tarantino A, Montagnino G et al.: Renal transplant recipients and chronic liver disease: statistical evaluation of predisposing factors. *Nephron* 61: 290, 1992

100. Lau JYN, Davis GL, Brunson ME et al.: Hepatitis C virus infection in kidney transplant recipients. *Hepatology* 18: 1027, 1993

101. Chan TM, Lok ASF, Cheng IKP, Chan RT: A prospective study of hepatitis C virus infection among renal transplant recipients. *Gastroenterology* 104: 862, 1993

101b. Rostaing L, Izopet J, Baron E et al.: Treatment of chronic hepatitis C with recombinant interferon alpha in kidney transplant recipients. *Transplantation* 59: 1426, 1995

102. Soulier JP, Jungers P, Zingraff J: Virus B hepatitis in hemodialysis centers. *Adv Nephrol* 6: 383, 1976

103. Reinicke V, Dybkjaer E, Poulsen H, Banke O, Lylloff K, Nordenfelt E: A study of Australia-antigen positive blood donors and their recipients with special reference to liver histology. *N Engl J Med* 286: 867, 1972

104. Couroucé-Pauty AM, Soulier JP: Further data on HBs antigen subtypes. Geographical distribution. *Vox Sang* 27: 533, 1974

105. Debure A, Degos F, Degott C et al.: Liver diseases and hepatic complications in renal transplant patients. *Adv Nephrol* 17: 375, 1988

106. Polakoff S, Cossart YE, Tillett HE: Hepatitis in dialysis units in the United Kingdom. *Br Med J* 3: 94, 1972

107. Pattison CP, Maynard JE, Berquist KR, Webster HM: Serological and epidemiological studies of hepatitis B in haemodialysis units. *Lancet* 2: 172, 1973

108. Dankert J, Uitentuis J, Houwen B, Tegzess AM, van der Hem GK: Hepatitis B surface antigen in environmental samples from hemodialysis units. *J Infect Dis* 134: 112, 1976

109. Maynard JE: Nosocomial viral hepatitis. *Am J Med* 70: 439, 1981

110. Heathcote H, Cameron CH, Dane DS: Hepatitis B antigen in saliva and semen. *Lancet* 1: 71, 1974

111. Jadoul M, Cornu C, Pais E: Second generation tests for hepatitis C virus in hemodialysis patients. *Ann Intern Med* 115: 747, 1991

112. Chauveau P, Couroucé AM, Lemarec C: Antibodies to hepatitis C virus by second generation test in hemodialyzed patients. *Kidney Int* 43 (Suppl 41): S149, 1993

113. Dentico P, Buongiorno R, Volpe A et al.: Prevalence and incidence of hepatitis C virus in hemodialysis patients: study of risk factors. *Clin Nephrol* 38: 49, 1992

114. Niu MT, Coleman PJ, Alter MJ: Multicenter study of hepatitis C virus infection in chronic hemodialysis patients and hemodialysis center staff members. *Am J Kidney Dis* 22: 568, 1993

115. Simon N, Couroucé AM, Le Marrec N, Ducamp S: A twelve year natural history of hepatitis C virus infection in hemodialyzed patients. *Kidney Int.* In press

116. Muller GY, Zabeleta ME, Arminio A et al.: Risk factors for dialysis-associated hepatitis C in Venezuela. *Kidney Int* 41: 1053, 1992

117. Dussol B, Chicheportiche C, Cantaloube C et al.: Detection of hepatitis C infection by polymerase chain reaction among hemodialysis patients. *Am J Kidney Dis* 22: 574, 1993

118. Bouchardeau F, Chauveau P, Le Marrec N, Girault A, Zins B, Couroucé AM: Detection of hepatitis C virus by polymerase chain reaction in hemodialyzed patients in relationship to anti-HCV status. *Res Virol* 144: 233, 1993

119. Conway M, Catterall AP, Brown EA et al.: Prevalence of antibodies to hepatitis C in dialysis patients and transplant recipients with possible routes of transmission. *Nephron Dial Transplant* 7: 1226, 1992

120. Donahue G, Munoz A, Ness PM et al.: The declining risk of post-transfusion hepatitis C virus infection. *N Engl J Med* 327: 369, 1992

121. Jeffers LJ, Perez GO, De Medina MD et al.: Hepatitis C infection in two urban hemodialysis units. *Kidney Int* 38: 320, 1990

122. Miyasaka M: Infection of hepatitis C virus in patients with chronic renal failure undergoing hemodialysis therapy and staff members. *Nippon Jinzo Gakkai Shi* 33: 989, 1991

123. Calabrese G, Vagelli G, Guaschino R, Gonella M: Transmission of anti-HCV within the household of haemodialysis patients. *Lancet* 338: 1466, 1991

124. Marchesi D, Arici C, Poletti E, Mingardi G, Minola E, Mecca G: Outbreak of non-A, non-B hepatitis in centre haemodialysis patients: a retrospective analysis. *Nephrol Dial Transplant* 3: 795, 1988

125. Niu MT, Alter MJ, Kristensen C, Margolis HS: Outbreak of hemodialysis-associated non-A, non-B hepatitis and correlation with antibody for hepatitis C virus. *Am J Kidney Dis* 19: 345, 1992

126. Pereira BJ, Milford EL, Kirkman RL, Levey AS: Transmission of hepatitis C virus by organ transplantation. *N Engl J Med* 325: 454, 1991

127. Public Health Laboratory Service: Infection risks of haemodialysis: some preventive aspects. *Br Med J* 3: 454, 1968

128. Public Health Laboratory Service Survey: Decrease in the incidence of hepatitis in dialysis units associated with prevention programme. *Br Med J* 4: 751, 1974

129. Public Health Laboratory Service: Hepatitis in retreat from dialysis units in United Kingdom in 1973. *Br Med J* 1: 1579, 1976

130. Favero MS: Recommended precautions for patients undergoing hemodialysis who have AIDS or non-A, non-B hepatitis. *Infect Control* 6: 301, 1985

131. Morbidity and mortality weekly report, Centers for Disease Control, Atlanta: Update: universal precautions for prevention of transmission of human immunodeficiency virus, hepatitis B virus, and other bloodborne pathogens in health-care settings. *JAMA* 260: 462, 1988

132. Vandelli L, Medici G, Savazzi AM, Lusvarghi E: Emergence of hepatitis C virus infection in haemodialysis units: must the patients be dialyzed in segregated sections? (abstract) *J Am Soc Nephrol* 10: 380A, 1990

133. Pol S, Romeo R, Zins B et al.: Hepatitis C virus RNA in anti-HCV positive hemodialyzed patients: significance and therapeutic implications. *Kidney Int* 44: 1097, 1993

134. Roggendorf M: Diagnosis and epidemiology of hepatitis C virus infection. *Mitteilungen der Deutschen Arbeitsgemeinschaft für Klinische Nephrologie* 21: 99, 1992

135. Willems M, DeJong G, Moshage H et al.: Surrogate markers are not useful for identification of HCV carriers in chronic hemodialysis patients. *J Med Virol* 35: 303, 1991

136. Wang JT, Wang TH, Lin JT, Shen JC, Lee CZ, Chen DS: Improved serodiagnosis of posttransfusion hepatitis C virus infection by a second-generation immunoassay based on multiple recombinant antigens. *Vox Sang* 62; 21, 1992

137. Farci P, Alter HJ, Govindarajan S et al.: Lack of protective immunity against reinfection with hepatitis C virus. *Science* 258: 135, 1992

138. Krugman S, Giles JP, Hammond J: Viral hepatitis, type B (MS-2 strain): prevention with specific hepatitis B immune serum globulin. *JAMA* 218: 1665, 1971

139. Courouce-Pauty AM, Delons S, Soulier JP: Attempt to prevent hepatitis by using specific anti-HBs immunoglobulin. *Am J Med* 270: 375, 1975

140. Iwarson S, Ahlmen J, Eriksson E et al.: Hepatitis B immune globulin in prevention of hepatitis B among hospital staff members. *J Infect Dis* 135: 473, 1977

141. Prince AM, Szmuness W, Mann MK et al.: Hepatitis B immune globulin: final report of a controlled multicentre trial of efficacy in prevention of dialysis-associated hepatitis. *J Infect Dis* 137: 131, 1978

142. Desmyter J, Bradburne AF, Vermylen C, Daneels R, Boelaert J: Hepatitis B immunoglobulin in prevention of HBs antigenaemia in haemodialysis patients. *Lancet* 2: 377, 1975

143. Surgenor DMacN, Chalmers TC, Conrad ME et al.: Clinical trials of hepatitis B immune globulin. *N Engl J Med* 293: 1060, 1975

144. Kleinknecht D, Courouce AM, Delons S et al.: Prevention of hepatitis B in hemodialysis patients using hepatitis B immunoglobulin. *Clin Nephrol* 8: 373, 1977

145. Grady GF, Lee VA, Prince AM et al. Hepatitis B immune globulin for accidental exposure among medical personnel: final report of a multicentre controlled trial. *J Infect Dis* 138: 625, 1978

146. Wahl M, Hermodsson S, Iwarson S: Hepatitis B vaccination with short dose intervals: a possible alternative for post-exposure prophylaxis? *Infection* 16: 229, 1988

147. Iwarson S: Post-exposure prophylaxis for hepatitis B: active or passive? *Lancet* ii: 146, 1989

148. Mitsui T, Iwano K, Suzuki S et al.: Combined hepatitis B immune/globulin and vaccine for postexposure prophylaxis of accidental hepatitis B virus infection in hemodialysis staff members: comparison with immune globulin without vaccine in historical controls. *Hepatology* 10: 324, 1989

149. Szmuness W, Stevens CE, Oleszko WR, Goodman A: Passive-active immunisation against hepatitis B: immunogenicity studies in adult American. *Lancet* i: 575, 1981

150. Courouce AM, Bouchardeau F, Le Marree N, Boulard G, Soulier JP: The use of hepatitis B vaccine as booster for donors immune to HBV for the production of hepatitis B immunoglobulin (HBIG). int *Second WHO IABS Symposium on Viral Hepatitis*, Basel, S. Karger, 1983, p 333

151. Krugman S, Giles JP, Hammond J: Viral hepatitis, type B (MS-2 strain): studies on active immunization. *JAMA* 217: 41, 1971

152. Jungers P, Delagneau JF, Prunet P, Crosnier J: Vaccination against hepatitis B in hemodialysis centers. *Adv Nephrol* 11: 303, 1982

153. Hilleman MR, Buynak EB, Roehm RR, Tytell AA, Bertland AV, Lampson GP: Purified and inactivated human hepatitis B vaccine: progress report. *Am J Med Sci* 270: 401, 1975

154. Jacobson IM, Dienstag JI: Viral hepatitis vaccines. *Ann Rev Med* 36: 241, 1985

155. Stevens CE, Taylor PE, Rubenstein P et al.: Safety of the hepatitis B vaccine. *N Engl J Med* 312: 375, 1985

156. Adamowicz P, Chabanier G, Hyafil F et al.: Elimination of serum proteins and potential virus contaminants during hepatitis B vaccine preparation. *Vaccine* 2: 209, 1984

157. Maupas P, Goudeau A, Coursaget P, Drucker J: Immunization against hepatitis B in man. *Lancet* 1: 1367, 1976

158. Adamowicz P, Gerfaux G, Platel A et al.: Large scale production of an hepatitis B vaccine. in *Hepatitis B Vaccine*, edited by Maupas P, Guesry P, Amsterdam, Elsevier-North Holland, 1981, p 37

159. Brummelhuis HGJ, Wilson-De Stüler LA, Raap AK: Preparation of hepatitis B vaccine by heat inactivation. in *Hepatitis B Vaccine*, edited by Maupas P, Guesry P, Amsterdam, Elsevier-North Holland, 1981, p 51

160. Zuckerman AJ: New hepatitis B vaccines. *Br Med J* 1: 492, 1985

161. Eddelston A: Modern vaccines: hepatitis. *Lancet* i: 1142, 1990

162. Neurath AR, Kent SBH, Strick NS, Taylor P, Stevens CE: Hepatitis B virus contains pre-S gene-encoded domains. *Nature* 315: 154, 1985

163. Coursaget P, Barrès JL, Chiron JP, Adamowicz P: Hepatitis B vaccines with and without polymerized albumin receptors. *Lancet* 1: 1152, 1985

164. Michel ML, Pontisso P, Sobczak E, Malpiece Y, Streek R, Tiollais P: Synthesis in animal cells of hepatitis B surface antigen particles carrying a receptor for polymerized human serum. *Proc Natl Acad Sci* 81: 7708, 1984

165. Milich D, Thornton G, Neurath R et al.: Enhanced immunogenicity of the pre-S region of hepatitis B surface antigen. *Science* 228: 1195, 1985

166. Itoh Y, Takai E, Ohnuma H et al.: A synthetic peptide vaccine involving the product of the PreS2 region of hepatitis B virus DNA: protective efficacy in chimpanzees. *Proc Natl Acad Sci USA* 89: 9174, 1986

167. Alberti A, Cavaletto D, Pontisso P, Chemello L, Tagariello G, Belussi F: Antibody response to pre-S2 and hepatitis virus induced liver damage. *Lancet* i: 1421, 1988

168. Szmuness W: Large-scale efficacy trials of hepatitis B vaccines in the USA: baseline date and protocols. *J Med Virol* 4: 327, 1979

169. Szmuness W, Stevens CE, Harley EJ et al.: Hepatitis B vaccine. Demonstration of efficacy in controlled clinical trial in a high-risk population in the United States. *N Engl J Med* 303: 833, 1980

170. Szmuness W, Stevens CE, Zang EA, Harley EJ, Kellner A: A controlled clinical trial of the efficacy of the hepatitis B vaccine (Heptavax B): a final report. *Hepatology* 1: 377, 1981

171. Crosnier J, Jungers P, Courouce AM et al.: Randomised placebo-controlled trial of hepatitis B surface antigen

vaccine in French haemodialysis units. I. Medical staff. *Lancet* 1: 455, 1981

172. Laplanche A, Couroucé AM, Benhamou E, Jungers P, Crosnier J: Response to hepatitis B vaccine. *Lancet* 1: 222, 1982

173. Szmuness W, Stevens CE, Harley EJ: Hepatitis B vaccine in medical staff of hemodialysis units: efficacy and subtype cross-protection. *N Engl J Med* 307: 1481, 1982

174. Desmyter J, Colaert J, De Groote G et al.: Efficacy of heat-inactivated hepatitis B vaccine in haemodialysis patients and staff. Double-blind placebo-controlled trial. *Lancet* 2: 1323, 1983

175. Dienstag JI, Werner BG, Polk BH et al.: Hepatitis B vaccine in health care personnel: safety immunogenicity and indicators of efficacy. *Ann Intern Med* 101: 34, 1984

176. Goudeau A, Dubois F, Barin F, Dubois MC, Coursaget P: Hepatitis B vaccines: clinical trials in high-risk setting in France (September 1975–September 1982). in *Second WHO/MBS Symposium on Viral Hepatitis*, Basel, Karger, 1983, p 267

177. Jilg W, Lobeer B, Schmidt M, Wilkse B, Zoulek G, Deinhardt F: Clinical evaluation of a recombinant hepatitis B vaccine. *Lancet* 2: 1174, 1985

178. Scolnick EM, McLean AA, West DJ, McAller WJ, Miller WJ, Buynack EB: Clinical evaluation in healthy adults of a hepatitis B vaccine made by recombinant DNA. *JAMA* 251: 2812, 1984

179. Brown SE, Stanley C, Howard CR, Zuckerman AJ, Steward MW: Antibody responses to recombinant and plasma derived hepatitis B vaccines. *Br Med J* 1: 159, 1986

180. Hollinger FB, Troisi CI, Pepe PE: Anti-HBs responses to vaccination with a human hepatitis B vaccine made by recombinant DNA technology in yeast. *J Infect Dis* 153: 156, 1986

181. Tron F, Degos F, Bréchot C et al.: Randomized dose range study of a recombinant hepatitis B vaccine produced in mammalian cells and containing the S and PreS2 sequences. *J Infect Dis* 160: 199, 1989

182. Scheiermann N, Gesemann M, Maurer C, Just M, Berger R: Persistence of antibodies after immunization with a recombinant yeast-derived hepatitis B vaccine following two different schedules. *Vaccine* 8: S44, 1980

183. Centers for Disease Control: Recommendations for protection against viral hepatitis. Recommendations of the immunization practices advisory committee. *Ann Intern Med* 103: 391, 1985

184. Ukena T, Esber H, Bessette R, Parks T, Crockers B, Shaw FE: Site of injection and response to hepatitis B vaccine. *N Engl J Med* 313: 579, 1985

185. Centers for Disease Control: Suboptimal response to hepatitis B vaccine given by injection into the buttock. *MMWR* 34: 105, 1985

186. Weber DJ, Rutala WA, Samsa GP, Santimaw JE, Lemon SM: Obesity as a predictor of poor antibody response to hepatitis B plasma vaccine. *JAMA* 254: 3187, 1985

187. Zuckerman AJ: Appraisal of intradermal immunisation against hepatitis B. *Lancet* i: 435, 1987

188. Gonzalez ML, Usandizaga M, Alomar P et al.: Intradermal and intramuscular route for vaccination against hepatitis B. *Vaccine* 8: 402, 1990

189. Bryan JP, Sjogren MH, Macarthy P, Cox E, Legters LJ, Perine PL: Persistence of antibody to hepatitis B surface antigen after low-dose, intradermal hepatitis B immunization and response to a booster dose. *Vaccine* 10: 33, 1992

190. Payton CD, Scarisbrick DA, Sikotra S, Flower AJ: Vaccination against hepatitis B: comparison of intradermal and intramuscular administration of plasma derived and recombinant vaccines. *Epidemiol Infect* 110: 177, 1993

191. Thompson SC, Darlington R, Tallent D, Robins-Browne R, Forsyth JR: Effectiveness of low-dose intradermal hepatitis B vaccination. Five years' experience of primary vaccination. *Med J Aust* 158: 372, 1993

192. Coleman PJ, Shaw FE, Serovich J, Hadler SC, Margolis HS: Intradermal hepatitis B vaccination in a large hospital employee population. *Vaccine* 9: 723, 1991

193. Centers for Disease Control: Inadequate immune response among public safety workers receiving intradermal vaccination against hepatitis B, United States 1990–1991. *J Am Med Assoc* 266: 1138, 1991

194. Struve J, Aronsson B, Frenning B, Granath F, von Sydow M, Weiland O: Intramuscular versus intradermal administration of a recombinant hepatitis B vaccine: a comparison of response rates and analysis of factors influencing the antibody response. *Scand J Infect Dis* 24: 423, 1992

195. Jilg W, Schmidt M, Deinhardt F, Zachoval R: Hepatitis B vaccination: how long does protection last? *Lancet* 2: 458, 1984

196. Grob PJ, Dufek A, Joller-Jemelka HI: Hepatitis B immunization – when is a booster injection necessary? *Schweiz Med Wschr* 115: 394, 1985

197. Jungers P, Couroucé AM, Laplanche A, Benhamou E: Hepatitis B vaccine. *N Engl J Med* 316: 47, 1987

198. Couroucé AM, Laplanche A, Benhamou E, Jungers P: Long-term efficacy of hepatitis B vaccination in healthy adults. in *Viral Hepatitis and Liver Disease*, edited by Dienstag J, Alan R. Liss, Inc, 1988, p 1002

199. Jilg W, Schmidt M, Deinhardt F: Prolonged immunity after late booster doses of hepatitis B vaccine. *J Infect Dis* 157: 1267, 1988

200. Bryan JP, Sjogren MH, Macarthy P, Cox B, Kao TC, Perine PL: Dosing schedule for recombinant hepatitis B vaccine. *J Infect Dis* 163: 1384, 1991

201. Laplanche A, Couroucé AM, Benhamou E, Jungers P: Timing of hepatitis B revaccination in healthy adults. *Lancet* i: 1206, 1987

202. Strickler AC, Kibsey PC, Vellend H: Seroconversion rates with hepatitis B vaccine. *Ann Intern Med* 101: 564, 1984

203. Schaaf DM, Lender M, Suedeker P, Graham LA: Hepatitis B vaccine in a hospital. *Ann Intern Med* 101: 720, 1984

204. Francis DP, Hadler SC, Thompson SE et al.: The prevention of hepatitis with vaccine: report of the Centers for Disease Control multi-center efficacy trial among homosexual men. *Ann Intern Med* 97: 362, 1982

205. Craven DE, Awdeh ZL, Kunches LM et al.: Non responsiveness to hepatitis B vaccine in health care workers: results of revaccination and genetic typings. *Ann Intern Med* 105: 356, 1986

206. Alper CA, Kruskall MS, Marcus-Bagley D et al.: Genetic prediction of non response to hepatitis B vaccine. *N Engl J Med* 321: 708, 1989

207. Yasumura S, Shimizu Y, Yasuyama T et al.: Intradermal hepatitis B virus vaccination for low- or non-responder health care workers. *Acta Med Okayama* 45: 457, 1991

208. Denis F, Mounier M, Hessel L et al.: Hepatitis B vaccination in the elderly. *J Infect Dis* 149: 1019, 1984

209. Treadwell TL, Keeffe EB, Lake J et al.: Immunogenicity of two recombinant hepatitis B vaccines in older individuals. *Am J Med* 95: 584, 1993

210. Dienstag JL, Stevens CE, Bhan AK, Szmuness W: Hepatitis B vaccine administered to chronic carriers of hepatitis B surface antigen. *Ann Intern Med* 96: 575, 1982

211. Dienstag JL, Ryan DM: Occupational exposure to hepatitis B virus in hospital personnel: infection or immunization? *Am J Epidemiol* 15: 26, 1982

212. Kessler HA, Haris AA, Payne JA, Hudson E, Potkin B, Levin S: Antibodies to hepatitis B surface antigen as the sole hepatitis B marker in hospital personnel. *Ann Intern Med* 103: 21, 1985

213. Kalish SB, Fisher B, Wallemark CB, Chniel JS, Phair JP: Prevalence of antibody to hepatitis B virus in foreign-born hospital employees. *Am J Med* 83: 824, 1987

214. Werner BG, Dienstag JL, Kuter BJ, Polk BF, Snydman DR, Craven DE, Crumpacker CS, Platt R, Grady GF: Isolated antibody to hepatitis B surface antigen and response to hepatitis B vaccination. *Ann Intern Med* 103: 201, 1985

215. Goudeau A, Dubois F: Immune status of anti-HBc positive individuals. *Lancet* 1: 396, 1984

216. Draelos M, Morgan T, Schifman RB, Sampliner RE: Significance of isolated antibody to hepatitis B core antigen determined by immune response to hepatitis vaccination. *JAMA* 258: 1193, 1987

217. Taliani G, Lece R, Furian C, Nuti M, Bernaschi P, de Bac C: Hepatitis vaccination for a wider diagnostic purpose? *Lancet* 2: 173, 1984

218. Hadziyannis SJ, Hatzakis A: Response to hepatitis B vaccine of anti-HBc positive subject. in *Hepatitis B Vaccine Symposium (Berne) New Findings and Perspectives*, edited by Tron F, Marnes-la-Coquette, Pasteur Vaccins, 1984, p 33.

219. Kane MA, Hadler SC, Maynard JE: Antibody to hepatitis B surface antigen and screening before hepatitis vaccination. *Ann Intern Med* 103: 791, 1985

220. Perrillo RP: Screening of health care workers before hepatitis B vaccination: more questions than answers. *Ann Intern Med* 103: 793, 1985

221. Goldblum SE, Reed WP: Host defenses and immunologic alterations associated with chronic hemodialysis. *Ann Intern Med* 93: 597, 1980

222. Revillard JP: Immunologic alterations in chronic renal insufficiency. *Adv Nephrol* 8: 365, 1979

223. Chatenoud L, Herbelin A, Beaurain G, Descamps-Latscha B: Immune deficiency of the uremic patients. *Adv Nephrol* 19: 259, 1990

224. Descamps-Latscha B: The immune system in end-stage renal disease. *Current Opinion in Nephrology and Hypertension* 2: 883, 1993

225. Chatenoud L, Jungers P, Descamps-Latscha B: Immunological considerations of the uremic and dialyzed patient. *Kidney Int* 45: S92, 1994

226. Kurz P, Köhler H, Meuer S, Hütteroth T, Meyer zum Büschenfelde KH: Impaired cellular immune responses in chronic renal failure: evidence for a T cell defect. *Kidney Int* 29: 1209, 1986

227. Meuer SC, Hauer M, Kurz P, Meyer zum Büschenfelde KH, Köhler H: Selective blockade of the antigen-receptor mediated pathway of T cell activation in patients with impaired primary immune responses. *J Clin Invest* 80: 743, 1987

228. Chatenoud L, Dugas B, Beaurain G et al.: Presence of preactivated T-cells in hemodialyzed patients: their possible role in altered immunity. *Proc Natl Acad Sci USA* 83: 7547, 1986

229. Beaurain G, Naret C, Marcon L et al.: *In vivo* T cell activation in chronic uremic hemodialyzed and non-hemodialyzed patients. *Kidney Int* 36: 636, 1989

230. Dumann H, Meuer S, Meyer zum Büschenfelde KH et al.: Hepatitis B vaccination and interleukin-2 receptor expression in chronic renal failure. *Kidney Int* 38: 1164, 1990

231. Crosnier J, Jungers P, Couroucé AM et al.: Randomised placebo-controlled trial of hepatitis B surface antigen vaccine in French haemodialysis units. II. Haemodialysis patients. *Lancet* 1: 797, 1981

232. Stevens CE, Alter HJ, Taylor PE, Zang EA, Harley EJ, Szmuness W: Hepatitis B vaccine in patients receiving hemodialysis. Immunogenicity and efficacy. *N Engl J Med* 311: 496, 1984

233. Stevens CE, Szmuness W, Goodman AI, Wesely SA, Fotino M: Hepatitis B vaccine: immune responses in haemodialysis patients. *Lancet* 2: 1211, 1980

234. Bommer J, Ritz E, Andrassy K et al.: Effect of vaccination schedule and dialysis on hepatitis B vaccination response in uraemic patients. *Proc Eur Dial Transplant Assoc Eur. Ren Assoc* 20: 161, 1983

235. Bommer J, Grussendorf M, Jilg W et al.: Vaccination against hepatitis B in patients with renal insufficiency. *Proc Eur Dial Transplant Assoc Eur Ren Assoc* 21: 300, 1984

236. Köhler H, Arnold W, Renschin G, Dormeyer HH, Meyer zum Büschenfelde KH: Active hepatitis B vaccination of dialysis patients and medical staff. *Kidney Int* 25: 124, 1984

237. De Graff PA, Dankert J, De Zeeuw D, Gips CH, van der Hem GK: Immune response to two different hepatitis B vaccines in haemodialysis patients: a 2-year follow-up. *Nephron* 40: 155, 1985

238. Carreno V, Mora I, Escuin F et al.: Vaccination against hepatitis B in renal dialysis units: short or normal vaccination schedule? *Clin Nephrol* 24: 215, 1985

239. Lelie PN, Reesink HW, De Jong-Van Manen S, Dees PJ, Rearink-Brongers EE: Immune response to heat-inactivated hepatitis B vaccine in patients undergoing hemodialysis. Enhancement of the response by increasing the dose of hepatitis B surface antigen from 3 to 27 μg. *Arch Intern Med* 145: 305, 1985

240. Van Geelen JA, Schalm SW, De Visser EM, Heigtink RA: Immune response to hepatitis B vaccine in hemodialysis patients. *Nephron* 45: 216, 1987

241. Pasko MT, Bartholomew WR, Beam TR, Jr, Amsterdam D, Cunningham EE: Long-term evaluation of the hepatitis B vaccine (Heptavax B) in hemodialysis patients. *Am J. Kidney Dis* 11: 316, 1988

242. Steketee RW, Ziarnik ME, Davis JP: Seroresponse to hepatitis B vaccine in patients and staff of renal dialysis centers, Wisconsin. *Am J Epidemiol* 127: 772, 1988

243. Smit-Leijs MBL, Kramer P, Heijtink RA, Hop WCJ, Schalm SW: Hepatitis B vaccination of haemodialysis patients: randomized controlled trial comparing plasma-derived vaccine with and without pre-S2 antigen. *Eur J Clin Invest* 20: 540, 1990

244. Albertoni F, Battilomo A, Di Nardo V et al.: Evaluation of a region-wide hepatitis B vaccination program in dialysis patients: experience in an Italian region. *Nephron* 58: 180, 1991

245. Jilg W, Schmidt M, Weinel B et al.: Immunogenicity of recombinant hepatitis B vaccine in dialysis patients. *J Hepatol* 3: 190, 1986

246. Bruguera M, Rodicio JL, Alcazar JM, Oliver A, Del Rio G, Esteban-Mur R: Effects of different dose levels and vaccination schedules on immune response to a recombinant DNA hepatitis B vaccine in haemodialysis patients. *Vaccine* 89 (Suppl): S47, 1990

247. Fleming SJ, Moran DM, Cooksley WGE, Faoagali JL: Poor response to a recombinant hepatitis B vaccine in dialysis patients. *J Infect* 22: 251, 1991

248. Buti M, Viladomiu L, Jardi R et al.: Long-term immunogenicity and efficacy of hepatitis B vaccine in hemodialysis patients. *Am J Nephrol* 12: 144, 1992

249. Benhamou E, Couroucé AM, Jungers P et al.: Hepatitis B vaccine: randomized trial of immunogenicity in hemodialysis patients. *Clin Nephrol* 21: 143, 1984

250. Couroucé AM, Jungers P, Benhamou E, Laplanche A, Crosnier J: Hepatitis B in dialysis patients. *N Engl J Med* 311: 1515, 1984

251. Michel P, Janin G, El Yafi S et al.: Improvement of immune response in dialysis patients to Hevac B vaccine after multiple injections of vaccine. *Proc Eur Dial Transplant Assoc Eur Ren Assoc* 22: 1077, 1985

252. Guan R, Tay HH, Choong HL, Yap I, Woo KT: Hepatitis B vaccination in chronic renal failure patients undergoing hemodialysis: the immunogenicity of an increased dose of a recombinant DNA hepatitis B vaccine. *Ann Acad Med Singapore* 19: 793, 1990

253. Dentico P, Buongiorno R, Volpe A et al.: Long-term immunogenicity and protective efficacy of recombinant DNA yeast-derived vaccine in hemodialysis patients. *J Nephrol* 6: 95, 1993

254. Bruguera M, Cremades M, Rodicio JL et al.: Immunogenicity of a yeast-derived hepatitis B vaccine in hemodialysis patients. *Am J Med* 87 (Suppl 3A): 30S, 1989

255. Joseph A, Rao TKS, Friedman EA: Long-term immunogenicity of two different four dose hepatitis B vaccination schedules in maintenance hemodialysis patients. *J Am Soc Nephrol* 4: 357A, 1993

256. Seaworth B, Drucker J, Starling J, Drucker R, Stevens C, Hamilton J: Hepatitis B vaccines in patients with chronic renal failure before dialysis. *J Infect Dis* 157: 332, 1988

257. Jungers P, Chauveau P, Couroucé AM et al.: Immunogenicity of the recombinant Genhevac B Pasteur Vaccine against hepatitis B in chronic uremic patients. *J Infect Dis* 169: 399, 1994

258. Benhamou E, Couroucé AM, Laplanche A, Jungers P, Tron F, Crosnier J: Long-term results of hepatitis B vaccination in patients on dialysis. *N Engl J Med* 314: 1710, 1986

259. Kurz P, Köhler H, Hütteroth T, Weber M, Meyer zum Büschenfelde KH: Immune defect in the early stage of chronic renal failure. *Proc Eur Dial Transplant Assoc Eur Ren Assoc* 22: 941, 1985

260. Jungers P, Chauveau P, Couroucé AM, Mattlinger B, Crosnier J: Hepatitis B vaccine in non-dialysed uraemic patients: preliminary results. *Proc Eur Dial Transplant Assoc Eur Ren Assoc* 22: 1073, 1985

261. Jungers P, Chauveau P, Loubaris T, Abbassi A, Couroucé AM: Immune response to hepatitis B vaccine in chronic uremic patients. in *Progress in Hepatitis B Immunization*, edited by Coursaget P, Tong MJ, John Libbey Eurotext Ltd, 1990, p 187

262. Walz G, Kunzendorf U, Haller H et al.: Factors influencing the response to hepatitis B vaccination of hemodialysis patients. *Nephron* 51: 457, 1989

263. Drachman R, Isacsohn M, Rudensky B, Drukker A: Vaccination against hepatitis B in children and adolescent patients on dialysis. *Nephrol Dial Transplant* 4: 372, 1989

264. Pillion G, Chiesa M, Maisin A, Schlegel N, Loirat C: Immunogenicity of hepatitis B vaccine (Hevac B) in children with advanced renal failure. *Pediatr Nephrol* 4: 627, 1990

265. Pol S, Legendre C, Mattlinger B, Berthelot P, Kreis H: Genetic basis of nonresponse to hepatitis B vaccine in hemodialized patients. *J Hepatol* 11: 385, 1990

266. Caillat-Zucman S, Gimenez JJ, Albouze G: HLA genetic heterogeneity of hepatitis B vaccine response in hemodialyzed patients. *Kidney Int* 41: S157, 1993

267. Sennesael JJ, Van der Niepen P, Verbeelen DL: Treatment with recombinant erythropoietin increases antibody titers after hepatitis B vaccination in dialysis patients. *Kidney Int* 40: 121, 1991

268. Navarro JF, Teruel JL, Mateos M, Ortuno J: Hepatitis C virus infection decreases the effective antibody response to hepatitis B vaccine in hemodialysis patients. *Clin Nephrol* 41: 113, 1994

269. Quiroga JA, Castillo I, Porres JC et al.: Recombinant gamma-interferon as adjuvant to hepatitis B vaccine in hemodialysis patients. *Hepatology* 12: 661, 1990

270. Lefebure AF, Verpooten GA, Gouttenye MM, De Broe ME: Immunogenicity of a recombinant DNA hepatitis B vaccine in renal transplant patients. *Vaccine* 11: 397, 1993

271. Rawer P, Willems WR, Breidenbach T, Guttman W, Pabst W, Schutterle G: Seroconversion rate, hepatitis B vaccination, hemodialysis, and zinc supplementation. *Kidney Int* 22: 149, 1987

272. Migneco G, Tripi S, Navetta A, La Ferla A, Vaccaro F: Serum zinc concentration and antibody response to hepatitis B vaccine in hemodialysis patients. *Minerva Ped* 81: 19, 1990

273. Kouw PM, Konings CH, De Vries PM, Van der Meulen J, Oe PL: Effects of zinc supplementation on zinc status and immunity in haemodialysis patients. *J Trace Elem Electrolytes Health Dis* 5: 115, 1991

274. Donati D, Gastaldi L: Controlled trial of thymopentin in hemodialysis patients who fail to respond to hepatitis B vaccination. *Nephron* 50: 133, 1988

275. Palestini M, Messina A, Ciaraffo S, De Sanctis GM, Errera G, Corradini SG: Brief treatment with thymopentin as adjuvant in vaccination for hepatitis B: controlled study in patients on periodic hemodialysis. *Riv Eur Sci Med Farmacol* 12: 135, 1990

276. Dumann H, Meuer SC, Renschin G, Köhler H: Influence of thymopentin on antibody response, and monocyte and T cell function in hemodialysis patients who fail to respond to hepatitis vaccination. *Nephron* 55: 136, 1990

277. Meuer SC, Hauer M, Kurz P, Meyer zum Büschenfelde KH, Köhler H: Monocyte defect in hemodialysis patients supports non-responsiveness in hepatitis B vaccination and development of HBsAg carrier state. in *Viral Hepatitis and Liver Disease*, edited by Zuckerman AI, New York, Alan Liss Inc, 1988, p 711

278. Meuer SC, Dumann H, Meyer zum BüschenfeWe KH, Köhler H: Low-dose interleukin-2 induces systemic immune responses against HBsAg in immunodeficient non-responders to hepatitis B vaccination. *Lancet* i: 15, 1989

279. Blankenstijn PJ, Van Hattum J, Boland GJ et al.: Hepatitis B vaccination of non-responder dialysis patients with recombinant hepatitis B vaccine in combination with interleukin-2. *J Am Soc Nephrol* 4: 334A, 1993

280. Jungers P, Devillier P, Salomon H, Cerisier JE, Couroucé AM: Randomised placebo-controlled trial of recombinant interleukin-2 in chronic uraemic patients who are non-responders to hepatitis B vaccine. *Lancet* 344: 856, 1994

281. Rose RM, Rey-Martinez J, Croteau C et al.: Failure of recombinant interleukin-2 to augment the primary humoral response to a recombinant hepatitis B vaccine in healthy adults. *J Infec Dis* 165: 775, 1992

282. Hibberd PL, Rubin RH: Immunization strategies for the immunocompromised host: the need for immunoadjuvants. *Ann Intern Med* 110: 955, 1989

283. Ono K, Kashiwagi S: Complete seroconversion by low-dose intradermal injection of recombinant hepatitis B vaccine in hemodialysis patients *Nephron* 58: 47, 1991

284. Waite N, Thomson L, Semple J, Goldstein M: Increase of hepatitis B antibody titre by repetitive administration of intradermal HB vaccine in chronic hemodialysis patients. *J Am Soc Nephrol* 3: 402A, 1992

285. Rodrigues I, Barros F, Guerra J, Cardoso C, Clemente J, Aguilar L: Intradermal vaccination against hepatitis B in hemodialysis patients. Influence of an immunomodulator. *Rev Port Nefrol Hipert* 8: 301, 1994

286. Poux JM, Ranger-Rogez S, Lagarde C, Benevent D, Denis F, Leroux-Robert C: Recombinant hepatitis B vaccine. Advantages of intradermal route in non-responsive dialysis patients. *Presse Med* 24: 803, 1995

287. Raine AEG, Margreiter R, Brunner FP et al.: Report on management of renal failure in Europe, XII, 1991. *Nephrol Dial Transplant* 7 (Suppl 2): 7, 1992

288. Lahaye D, Strauss P, Baleux C, Van Gause W: Cost-benefit analysis of hepatitis-B vaccination. *Lancet* ii: 441, 1987

289. Abiteboul D, Gouaille B: Bilan de la vaccination contre l'hépatite B à l'Assistance Publique – Hôpitaux de Paris. *Bulletin Epidémiologique Hebdomadaire* 41: 169, 1989

290. Blumberg BS: Feasibility of controlling or eradicating the hepatitis B virus. *Am J Med* 87 (Suppl 3A): 2S, 1989

291. Baker CH, Breunan JM: Legal aspects of hepatitis B immunization programs. *N Engl J Med* 331: 684, 1984

RENAL OSTEODYSTROPHY

FRANCISCO LLACH

INTRODUCTION

In this chapter, the term 'renal osteodystrophy' will be used in a generic sense to include all the clinical syndromes of skeletal disease and altered calcium (Ca) and phosphorus (P) homeostasis resulting from chronic renal failure (CRF). The skeletal pathology can include osteitis fibrosa and other features of secondary hyperparathyroidism, osteomalacia, aplastic or adynamic bone disease, osteoporosis, osteosclerosis, and in children, retardation of growth. Emphasis will be placed on the manifestations of these syndromes that occur in patients on maintenance dialysis with a consideration of pathogenesis, prevention and management.

Vitamin D

The term, vitamin D, is used to include vitamin D, or cholecalciferol, the naturally occurring sterol present in animals, and vitamin D, or ergocalciferol, a sterol generated through the ultraviolet irradiation of plant precursors. Vitamin D itself undergoes a two-step metabolism; first, in the liver, where it is converted to 25 hydroxyvitamin D (25(OH)D) and second in the kidney, where the biologically active form, (1,25(OH)$_2$D) is produced (Figure 1). Thus, the kidney plays an important endocrine role by producing 1,25(OH)$_2$D.

Vitamin D, itself is produced in the skin where ultraviolet irradiation converts 7 dihydrotachysterol to previtamin D, which in turn, is converted to vitamin D (1). The latter leaves the skin attached to a specific, high affinity carrier-protein in plasma, an alpha 2 globulin. Cholecalciferol is carried to the liver where it is converted to 25(OH)D. This conversion of vitamin D to 25(OH)D3 (or calcifediol) is not well regulated. The 25(OH)D which is carried bound to the same vitamin D-binding protein, has a very slow turnover rate, i.e. a half life of 20 to 25 days, and may represent a circulating, 'storage' form of vitamin D. The metabolic conversion of 25(OH)D3 to 1,25(OH)$_2$ D (or calcitriol) in the proximal tubular cells is highly regulated; this conversion is controlled by various factors that relate to the need of the organism for Ca and P(2). This conversion is stimulated by parathyroid hormone, hypophosphatemia (or low phosphate diet) and hypocalcemia (3). The metabolic conversion of calcitriol is also augmented during certain physiologic events such as pregnancy, lactation, and growth, which are associated with increased needs for calcium (4).

Calcitriol, or 1,25(OH)$_2$ D, is also bound to the vitamin D-binding protein but with less affinity than is 25(OH)D; it is carried to several target tissues, including the intestine, bone, kidney and parathyroid glands. Its best known action is on the intestine, where it enhances the active absorption of both Ca and P. It acts in the bone both to mobilize Ca, particularly in the presence of PTH, and to bring about the normal mineralization of osteoid. This may occur through elevation of serum Ca and P but also

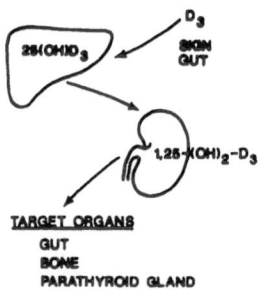

Figure 1. Schema showing the conversion of vitamin D$_3$ (D$_3$) to 25-hydroxyvitamin D$_3$ (25(OH)D$_3$ or calciferol) in the liver and subsequently to 1,25 dihydroxyvitamin D$_3$ (1,25(OH)$_2$D$_3$ or calcitriol) in the kidney.

through a specific action on collagen metabolism. There are also cellular receptors for calcitriol in the parathyroid glands, pancreas, kidneys, and salivary glands, although its action in these tissues are uncertain. Recently, calcitriol has been shown to play an important role in the regulation of the synthesis and secretion of PTH, which is independent of that occurring due to a rise in serum Ca (5) and may be related to the pathogenesis of hyperparathyroidism; this will be discussed in detail later. Calcitriol may also have an action on striated muscle, although receptors have not been identified. Most evidence indicates that calcitriol exerts its biological action in a manner similar to other steroid hormones (6). Thus, the sterol is bound to a specific cytosolic receptor and the receptor-hormone complex is transported from the cell cytosol to the nucleus where it induces the synthesis of messenger RNA, which in turn, may stimulate protein synthesis. The synthesis of one or more proteins, one of which may be Ca binding protein, facilitates the entry of Ca into the cell and induces its transepithelial transport.

In the absence of vitamin D, there is abnormally low intestinal absorption of Ca and to a lesser extent, of P. This results in hypocalcemia, which leads to secondary hyperparathyroidism and hypophosphatemia. There is impaired mineralization of osteoid (osteomalacia) and proximal myopathy a prominent feature of vitamin D deficiency, usually is present.

Another naturally occurring vitamin D sterol is 24,25 dihydroxivitamin D(24,25(OH)$_2$ D). This sterol is produced in the kidney but perhaps also in the intestine and bone. The absence or very low levels of serum 24,25(OH)$_2$ D in anephric animals and humans suggests that the kidney is primarily responsible for its generation. The biologic role of 24,25(OH)$_2$ D in man under natural circumstances and pathologic states is not clear.

Parathyroid hormone

Parathyroid hormone is a single chain polypeptide of 84 amino acids, which is secreted in response to a fall in blood Ca and to a lesser degree, by changes in the β adrenergic

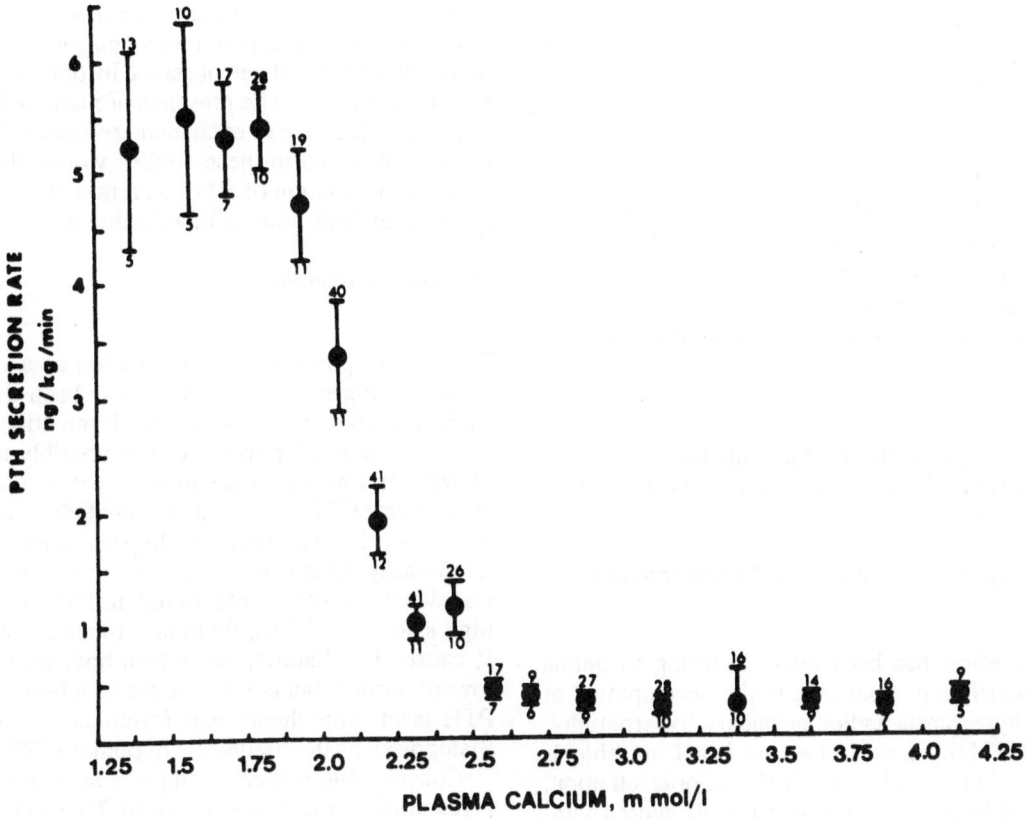

Figure 2. Secretory response of bovine parathyroid gland to changes in plasma Ca. The symbols and vertical bars indicate the secretory rate (mean ± SE). Note the sigmoidal nature of the relationship between secretory rate and plasma calcium concentration. (Modified after Mayer et al.)

(Ca: mmoles/l → mg/dl: multiply by 4

Ca: mmoles/l → mEq/l: multiply by 2)

system. Thus, there is a sigmoidal relationship between serum Ca and PTH, and small changes in blood Ca can influence hormonal secretion (7). Most changes in PTH occur as serum Ca varies from 7.5 to 10.5 mg/dl (1.88 to 2.63 mmol/1); changes in serum Ca above or below this range have minor effects on PTH secretion (Figure 2). A small but important fraction of PTH secretion is not affected by the blood Ca level, but some basal PTH secretion has been demonstrated in the presence of substantial hypercalcemia (8). The β-adrenergic system, epinephrine and norepinephrine, can augment PTH secretion, and acute hypermagnesemia can suppress PTH secretion, transiently at least (9, 10).

The intact PTH molecule, with a molecular mass of 9,500 Daltons, is secreted into the blood; it undergoes rapid cleavage in the liver and kidney with the release of several fragments (11). There are several biologically inactive carboxyterminal (C-terminal) fragments with molecular weights of approximately 7,000 which have circulating half-lives of 25 to 60 min; the small biologically active amino-terminal (N-terminal) fragment is metabolized primarily by the skeleton (12). The circulating

half-life of the C-terminal fragment is higher, and more often measured by available radioimmunoassay. Because the kidney is the only organ capable of degrading the C-terminal fragment, patients with renal insufficiency commonly have very high serum levels of PTH as measured by C-terminal assays.

Parathyroid hormone acts on the kidney and bone via activation of the adenylate cyclase system. In the kidney, PTH inhibits the reabsorption of Ca and stimulates the conversion of 25(OH)D to 1,25(OH)$_2$ D. With end stage renal failure, these biological actions become less important. In bone, PTH increases the conversion of mesenchymal cells to osteoclasts, increases bone resorption and activates osteoblasts. The effect of PTH is to increase bone resorption and formation with an increase in bone turnover.

PATHOGENESIS

The striking skeletal abnormalities observed in advanced CRF are believe to have their origin early in the course

Table 1. Factors contributing to the development of secondary hyperparathyroidism

---

Hypocalcemia
Phosphorus retention
Impaired calcemic response to PTH
    (skeletal resistance to PTH)
Altered vitamin D metabolism and resistance to calcitriol
Autonomous parathyroid cell proliferation
Altered degradation of PTH
Abnormal regulation of calcium-controlled PTH release

---

of renal disease. Since this chapter emphasizes features of advanced CRF, the early pathogenic events will be discussed briefly.

Secondary hyperparathyroidism. High turnover bone disease

Considerable effort has been made in trying to define the factors which may contribute to the development of parathyroid hyperplasia and/or secondary hyperparathyroidism (2°HPTH). These factors are listed in Table 1. They include: 1) hypocalcemia; 2) phosphorus retention; 3) impaired calcemic response to PTH; 4) altered vitamin D metabolism and resistance to calcitriol; 5) altered degradation of PTH by the kidney; 6) abnormal regulation of calcium-controlled PTH release (shift in the set point of calcium); and 7) autonomous proliferation. Importantly enough, these pathogenic factors are interrelated; thus, the problem often arises of isolating the importance of each factor. Furthermore, it is likely that one factor may exert a more prominent role than others at certain stages of CRF.

Hypocalcemia

Earlier, the main factor increasing PTH secretion and causing hyperplasia of the parathyroid glands in uremic patients was thought to be hypocalcemia. Thus, Bricker and Slatopolsky emphasized its importance in the genesis of 2°HPTH (13). Hypocalcemia has been shown to increase both synthesis and secretion of PTH (14, 15). Moreover, some of the factors mentioned above may lead to hypocalcemia and thus increase PTH production.

Observations in the last decade suggest that other factors may also be at work. First, studies in patients with early CRF have shown increases in serum PTH not associated with hypocalcemia (16, 17). Also, when oral physiologic doses of calcitriol are given to seemingly normocalcemic patients, a significant increase in serum calcium (Ca) is observed (18). Furthermore, Lopez-Hilker et al. have demonstrated that hypercalcemia did not prevent the development of 2°HPTH in azotemic dogs when calcitriol deficiency was present (19). Kaplan et al. also demonstrat-

ed increases in serum ionized Ca levels in uremic dogs with 2°HPTH as compared with control dogs (20). Similar results have also been observed by others after bilateral nephrectomy (21). The presence of increased PTH levels together with stable or even increased ionized Ca concentrations observed in these studies would also suggest a defective regulation of PTH secretion at the parathyroid gland level. This issue will be further discussed later.

Phosphorus retention

The role of phosphorus (P) retention as a major factor in the pathogenesis of 2°HPTH has been demonstrated by Slatopolsky et al. (22). As the P retention theory was initially proposed, a transient and possibly undetectable increase in serum P concentration was believed to occur in moderate CRF as a result of a small decrement in renal function (22). The transient hyperphosphatemia would temporarily reduce the concentration of blood ionized Ca, which in turn would stimulate PTH secretion. The high levels of PTH would reduce tubular reabsorption of P, cause phosphaturia, and return both serum P and Ca toward normal, but at the expense of a higher circulating PTH level. This theory was formulated by Bricker and Slatopolsky as the 'trade-off' hypothesis (23).

Considerable evidence supports an important role of P retention in the development of 2°HPTH. Reiss et al. demonstrated that a large oral P load led to an increase in serum P, a fall in ionized Ca, and an increase in serum PTH level in normal subjects (24). Others have shown that the long-term feeding of a high-P diet to animals caused parathyroid hyperplasia, high PTH, and mild hypocalcemia (25). Also, serum PTH levels correlated positively with the degree of hyperphosphatemia in dialysis patients (26). Furthermore, in experimentally induced CRF, the reduction of dietary P intake proportionally to the decrease in glomerular filtration rate (GFR) largely prevented the development of 2°HPTH in dogs with CRF (22). Nevertheless, when dietary P intake was reduced and an aluminum (Al) hydroxide gel was given to patients with CRF, serum PTH fell substantially but the values remained greater than normal. Also, only a mild reduction of PTH levels has been observed occasionally after P restriction in dialysis patients (27).

The available data suggest that though P retention is important in the development of 2°HPTH in advanced CRF, it may not be a factor in early CRF (28). Since we are focusing in ESRD and dialysis patients we will not discuss this issue in detail. As CRF progress P retention eventually will occur. Thus, in more advanced CRF there is impairment in P excretion following an oral P load (29). The fact that patients had a tendency to remain in P balance until the GFR is less than 20–25 ml/min was observed in 1954 (30). A decade later, it was noted that fractional excretion of P rises progressively in CRF as renal function worsens (31). and it is proportional to the level of PTH. Some of the factors that aggravate the

Table 2. Factors affecting serum phosphorus in dialysis patients

Residual renal function
Dietary phosphorus intake
Ingestion of phosphate-binding compounds
Intake of large amounts of supplemental calcium
Extent of vitamin D deficiency and treatment with active
    vitamin D compounds
Secretion of PTH; responsiveness of the skeleton to PTH
Rate of skeletal accretion (i.e., healing of osteomalacia or
    osteitis fibrosa)
Phosphate-containing enemas
Frequency, duration and efficiency of dialysis

degree of hyperphosphatemia in these patients are noted in Table 2.

Phosphorus retention can induce 2°HPTH through several mechanisms. As mentioned earlier, the reciprocal decrease in serum ionized Ca following an increase in serum P was considered the mechanism by which P retention induced 2°HPTH. Thus, in advanced CRF and during dialysis, hypocalcemia may be related to the marked elevation of serum P (44). However, an increase of P concentration *in vitro* within the usual range observed in dialysis patients did not reduce the ionized Ca concentration (32). In fact, in normal subjects, only a large increase in serum P (m) reduces total serum Ca by 0.18 mM (33). Phosphorus retention can also be at work through an indirect mechanism such as inhibiting the activity of the renal enzyme 1-a hydroxylase, which is responsible for the conversion of 25(OH) D to its active metabolite calcitriol (34). Phosphorus retention can also decrease the calcemic response to PTH (35).

A direct effect of P on the parathyroid gland has also been suggested. Lucas et al. (36) administered a low P diet to patients with advanced CRF for 3 months; while ionized Ca and calcitriol levels did not increase, an important decrease in serum PTH was observed. Similar results have been reported by others (37). These findings would suggest an effect of a low P diet in the control of PTH secretion. It has been recently shown in dogs that P restriction in advanced CRF improves 2°HPTH by a mechanism which may be independent of changes in serum Ca and calcitriol (35). Similarly, hemodialysis patients may have phosphorus-related changes in PTH without changes in serum Ca and calcitriol (37). Recently, we have also observed severe hyperphosphatemia worsening the 2°HPTH in dialysis patients receiving intravenous calcitriol (38). Finally, Yi et al. have shown, using Northern blot techniques, that moderate P restriction decreased the levels of PTH mRNA in rats with mild CRF independently of Ca and calcitriol (39).

Impaired calcemic response to PTH

A decreased calcemic response to the action of PTH is another cause of hypocalcemia in CRF. It was first described by Evanson in 1966; he noted that the calcemic response to an infusion of parathyroid extract was significantly lower in hypocalcemic patients with CRF than in normal subjects or in patients with primary hypoparathyroidism (40). Subsequently, Massry et al. observed that the calcemic response to a parathyroid extract in patients with moderate and advanced CRF was significantly lower than in normal individuals (41). This reduced calcemic response was unrelated to the initial levels of serum Ca, P or PTH. Llach et al. noted a delayed recovery from EDTA-induced hypocalcemia in patients with early CRF (creatinine clearances of 34 to 93 ml/min) as compared to normal subjects, despite higher PTH levels in the former (Figure 3) (35). Such observations indicate that the impaired calcemic response to PTH appears early in the course of CRF. Thus, a greater concentration of circulating PTH may be required to maintain a normal serum Ca level in patients with CRF.

Altered vitamin D metabolism and resistance to calcitriol

Abnormal conversion of vitamin D to its active form calcitriol probably plays a fundamental role in the development of 2°HPTH. The evidence that vitamin D metabolism is altered in advanced CRF is most convincing (42).

The kidney is the principal organ responsible for converting 25-(OH)D to calcitriol (43); this conversion is also the rate limiting step in the production of calcitriol. This discovery provided the framework for the hypothesis that vitamin D metabolism is altered in uremia. Anephric rats are unable to produce calcitriol from its precursor (44); an observation that led to speculation that impaired renal production of calcitriol accounts for impaired Ca absorption and osteomalacia in uremia. Several observations support this premise. Mawer et al. (45) and Schaefer et al. (46) have shown data providing indirect evidence for the failure of uremic patients to hydroxylase the 25-(OH)D at the C-1 position and thus produce calcitriol. Moreover, the serum levels of calcitriol have been uniformly noted to be decreased in patients with advanced CRF (42, 47).

The nature of the response to replacement with various vitamin D derivatives also supports the view that impaired conversion of 25-(OH)D to calcitriol is of importance in CRF. Thus, calcitriol in doses of 0.6 to 1.0 µg/day can increase [47]Ca absorption to normal in uremic patients (48), while the quantity of 25-(OH) D needed to augment Ca absorption in uremia is 100 to 500 µg (48); the amount of vitamin D needed, as stated before, is even greater (49). The relative effect of different vitamin D analogs on Ca absorption is shown in Figure 4. Though the levels of calcitriol have been found to be low in patients with advanced uremia, recent data indicate that abnormalities in calcitriol production may occur even in early CRF (50). Moreover,

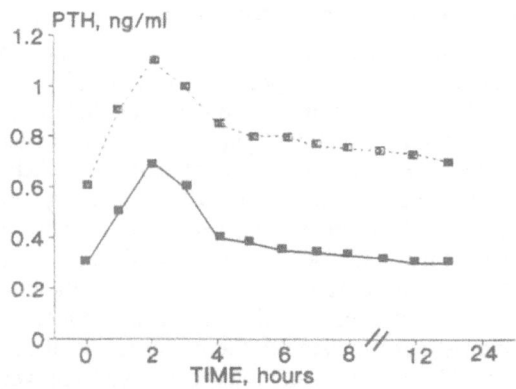

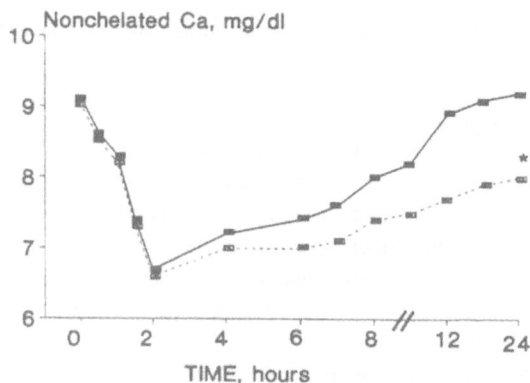

Figure 3. Mean values (± SE) of PTH and nonchelated calcium in relation to time during and after the infusion of EDTA, prior to calcitriol therapy. The shaded square-dotted line represent values from patients with early renal failure (ERF). The closed square-continuous line represent values from normal subjects. *p < 0.01. (From Llach et al. (28).)

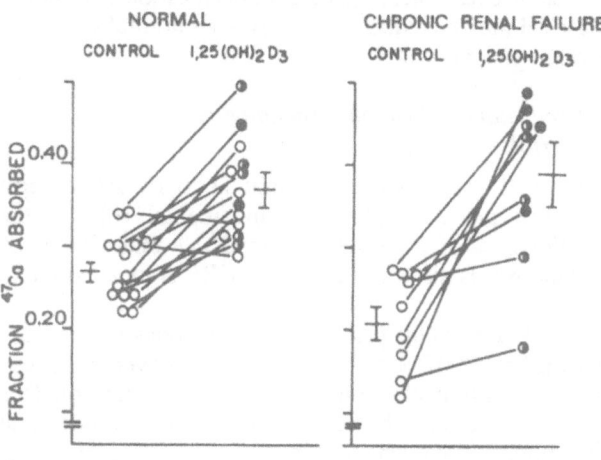

Figure 4. Changes in intestinal calcium absorption (^{47}Ca) in normal individuals and those with advanced chronic renal failure. Values were obtained before and after treatment with 1,25(OH)$_2$D$_3$, 0.6 to 2.7 μg/day, for 7 to 10 days. The horizontal bars and brackets indicate mean ± SEM (Reprinted from Brickman et al., with permission.)

since the 1α-hydroxylase is present in the mitochondria of proximal tubular cells, calcitriol synthesis may be more impaired in patients with tubulointerstitial renal disease. Thus, such patients have been described to have lower plasma levels of calcitriol even at early stages of CRF (51). Patients with chronic pyelonephritis developed a greater parathyroid gland mass than those with chronic glomerulonephritis. Vitamin D deficient osteomalacia also is observed more frequently in the former than in the latter (52). However, in other studies (53), the presence or absence of tubulointerstitial disease did not appear to affect calcitriol levels.

The pathophysiologic consequences of a reduced generation of calcitriol in renal insufficiency deserve further consideration. They include, as stated earlier, a decreased intestinal absorption of Ca (54) and a reduced calcemic response to PTH on the skeleton (35), thereby contributing to hypocalcemia. Moreover, it has been have shown that even despite the presence of hypercalcemia 2°HPTH develops when calcitriol deficiency is present (19). As will be discussed shortly, low serum calcitriol levels may lead to an increase in the synthesis and secretion of PTH (55).

Factors other than 2°HPTH may also play a role in the observed levels of calcitriol. Hsu et al. have shown that both the production rate and the metabolic clearance rate of calcitriol is decreased in uremic rats (56); also, they have observed in patients with moderate CRF (clearance of creatinine 34 ± 6 ml/min) that uremic plasma contains inhibitory factors that suppress not only the synthesis but also the degradation of calcitriol (57). They have also noted that uremic toxins suppress the genomic synthesis of the 24-hydroxylase, thereby reducing the metabolic clearance rate of calcitriol (58).

Interestingly, an increase in serum calcitriol levels following the administration of 25-(OH)D has also been observed in anephric patients undergoing hemodialysis (59). These results suggest extra-renal production of calcitriol in the presence of low calcitriol levels; moreover, they also suggest that physiological levels of calcitriol may regulate its own production (60). However, the source of calcitriol is not enough to correct the calcitriol deficit observed in CRF.

Regardless of the cause of decreased secretion of calcitriol, an important pathophysiologic consequence of this deficiency may be the absence of a modulating inhibitory action of this hormone on PTH synthesis and secretion, leading to 2°HPTH. A number of studies have shown that calcitriol exerts a negative feedback on the parathyroid glands. A significant suppression by calcitriol of mRNA coding for pre-pro-PTH (PTH mRNA) in bovine parathyroid cell cultures has been observed (61). This reduction in

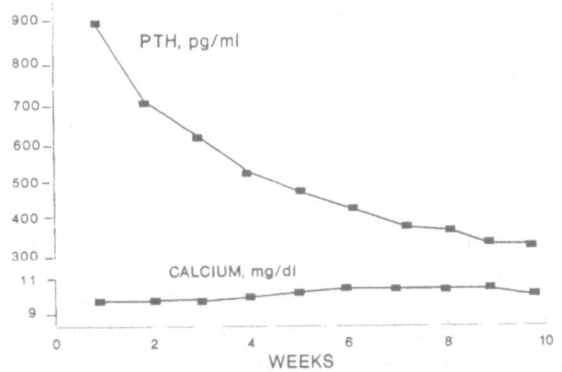

Figure 5. Baseline intact PTH and total serum calcium levels in patients with significant 2°HPTH during 10 weeks of intravenous calcitriol. Note the significant decrease in PTH (p < 0.01) in the absence of changes in serum calcium (Data from Dunlay et al. (66).)

PTH mRNA occurs primarily at the transcriptional level. Silver et al. have also shown that the administration of calcitriol to rats had a profound suppressive effect on *in vivo* PTH synthesis (62). Elevated PTH mRNA levels have also been demonstrated in experimental CRF and were attributed to reduced plasma levels of calcitriol (63). Thus, it seems that the major action of calcitriol on PTH secretion may occur by inhibiting transcription of DNA, thereby decreasing the synthesis of PTH available for secretion. Conversely, a decrease in the level of calcitriol would increase the synthesis and secretion of hormone by the parathyroid cell. These *in vitro* and experimental studies have been confirmed in hemodialysis patients (64). Thus, a direct suppressive effect of intravenously administered calcitriol on PTH secretion was observed in hemodialysis patients. In these patients, after the administration of intravenous calcitriol, serum PTH started to decrease before any change in blood ionized Ca level was detected. However, increased levels of serum Ca were observed later and were a contributory factor in the decrement of PTH. Delmez et al. also evaluated the inhibitory effect of intravenous calcitriol in dialysis patients with 2°HPTH (65). Serum ionized Ca and PTH (amino-terminal fragment) were determined before and after two weeks of intravenous calcitriol. Despite no significant changes in ionized Ca, PTH levels fell by 22%. Recently, we have also evaluated the direct inhibitory effect of calcitriol on parathyroid function in nine dialysis patients with severe hyperparathyroidism (66). They received intravenous calcitriol, 2 μg at the end of each dialysis for 10 weeks. In order to avoid hypercalcemia, the dialysate Ca concentration was reduced to 2.5 mEq/l. The basal PTH (intact molecule) fell from 902 ± 126 pg/ml to 466 ± 152 pg/ml after 10 weeks of therapy. This occurred in the absence of any significant changes in total serum Ca concentration (Figure 5).

Finally, like other steroid hormones, the biological actions of calcitriol appear to be mediated through a hormone cytoplasmatic receptor complex. The activated hormone-receptor complex then interacts with nuclear chromatin and binds a specific regulatory region of the 5'-flanking sequence of affected genes, altering DNA transcription of specific precursor-mRNA molecules (67). This vitamin D receptor (VDR) is wide spread in different tissues including intestine and parathyroid gland. A reduced density and binding of VDRs have been observed in parathyroid glands of both animals (68) and patients with CRF (69). Since the biological response to calcitriol is proportional to the density of VDR within the cell, a reduction in the number or inhibition of the VDR interaction with DNA may diminish the biological response to calcitriol. It is possible that reduced VDR number or function renders the parathyroid glands less responsive to the inhibitory action of calcitriol.

Autonomous proliferation

Secondary HPTH is characterized by marked enlargement of the parathyroid glands which, histologically, can be defined as diffuse and/or nodular hyperplasia; the latter being a more severe histological form (70). Earlier, the term 'tertiary hyperparathyroidism', describing the formation of an adenoma superimposed on diffuse hyperplasia was introduced (71). This term has been frequently applied to describe the condition when hypercalcemia develops in 2°HPTH (146–148). It is known that residual or transplanted parathyroid tissue containing nodular hyperplasia has a higher rate of recurrent hyperparathyroidism than that with diffuse hyperplasia (149–151). These areas of nodular hyperplasia may consist of cells with high secretory activity which are not suppressed normally by hypercalcemia. Furthermore, in parathyroid glands from hemodialysis patients, nodular hyperplasia is associated with a decrease in VDR density as compared with diffuse hyperplasia (74). Whether glands with nodular hyperplasia are less responsive to calcitriol treatment remains to be proven.

Altered degradation of PTH

An increased rate of secretion of PTH is the major mechanism responsible for high plasma levels of PTH in CRF. Considerable evidence demonstrates that the kidney plays an important role in the degradation of PTH and that the metabolic clearance of PTH is reduced in CRF (75); thus, reduced renal degradation of PTH may contribute to the hyperparathyroid state in uremia. Berson and Yalow reported immunochemical heterogeneity of PTH in the plasma of uremic patients; they suggested that the presence of more than one peptide fragment of PTH and altered metabolism of the hormone could account for the observed heterogeneity. This initial discovery was then followed by extensive research into the biochemistry and metabolism of PTH.

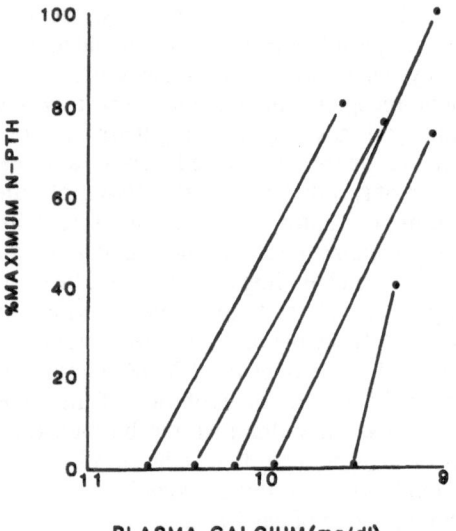

Figure 6. Response of PTH to changes in plasma calcium concentration induced by a low calcium dialysis in five patients with bone biopsy showing osteitis fibrosa. Note that despite a calcium concentration greater than 9 mg/dl (2.25 mmol/l), all patients responded with marked increase in PTH. Reproduced from Voigts et al., with permission of the publishers.

As discussed earlier, once intact PTH is secreted, the hormone is rapidly degraded, the amino-terminal portion is cleaved, and several inactive fragments from the carboxy-terminal fraction of the peptide appear in the serum. Because of the shorter half-life of both intact PTH and the amino-terminal fragment, the carboxy-terminal fragments become the predominant PTH peptide in the circulation. The intact parent peptide is rapidly degraded in the peripheral tissues, particularly in the kidney and the liver (76). The liver has a large capacity to degrade the peptide, but it may not play an important role in degradation of either the carboxy- or the amino-terminal fragments (75). By contrast, the kidney can extract and degrade the intact 84-residue molecule and both the carboxy- and amino-terminal fragments (77). Cathepsin D has been identified as one of the factors responsible for the intrarenal cleavage of intact PTH (78). In the presence of CRF, PTH metabolism is altered and the renal excretion of PTH and its fragments is decreased (79). Such altered PTH metabolism may additionally account for the elevated PTH levels observed in CRF; this was particularly relevant when PTH was measured with immunoassay which used an antiserum directed to the mid or, especially, the carboxy-terminal region. Also, different specificities of antisera probably accounted for the variability of PTH levels reported from various laboratories.

The advent of more advanced techniques such as the immunoradiometric (IRMA) or immunochemiluminescent (ICMA) assays has improved the diagnosis and management of patients with renal osteodystrophy (13, 80).

These new techniques use antibodies directed toward the intact PTH molecule and, thus, they avoid the measurement of various PTH fragments.

Abnormal regulation of calcium-controlled PTH secretion (set point of calcium)

Studies of the regulation of PTH secretion by Ca indicate a sigmoidal relationship between PTH secretion and ionized Ca over a narrow range of Ca concentration (7, 81). It has been shown recently that, in order to suppress the secretion of PTH, parathyroid cells from uremic patients require higher extracellular Ca concentrations than normal cells (83). Moreover, the adenylate cyclase of hyperplastic parathyroid glands is less susceptible to Ca-mediated inhibition (177). Thus, the 'set point' for Ca, the concentration of Ca required to inhibit 50% of maximal PTH secretion, is shifted toward the right. This abnormality may be an important factor in the abnormal secretion of PTH noted in uremia.

The earliest evidence suggesting an abnormal set point of Ca in CRF was presented by Voigts et al. in a report on dialysis patients with significant 2°HPTH (82). During acute hypocalcemia produced by a low-Ca dialysate (Figure 6), patients exhibited a marked increase in PTH levels as the serum Ca level decreased but was still within the normal range (greater than 9 mg/dl). Later, Delmez and associates demonstrated in dialysis patients that the administration of calcitriol for two weeks returned the abnormal set point for Ca toward normal (65). Thus, calcitriol appeared to have increased the sensitivity of the gland to changes in serum Ca concentration. However, the set point of Ca was estimated as a 50% decrease from basal levels of PTH, rather than from maximal PTH stimulation (65). Recently, we have assessed parathyroid gland function in nine patients with significant 2°HPTH (66). This was evaluated by inducing hypo- and hypercalcemia using a low- and a high-Ca dialysate during two separate dialyses performed 1 week apart. Parathyroid hormone values after dialysis-induced hypo- and hypercalcemia were plotted against ionized Ca for each patient, and the set point for Ca was determined. As can be appreciated in Figure 7, the PTH–Ca sigmoidal curve was shifted toward the right, After 10 weeks of intravenous calcitriol therapy ($2\ \mu g$ at the end of each dialysis), the curve was shifted to the left. Basal PTH levels fell from 902 ± 126 to 466 ± 152 pg/ml ($p < 0.01$) after calcitriol without any significant change in the serum total Ca concentration. The maximal PTH response during hypocalcemia decreased, after calcitriol therapy, from 1661 ± 485 to 1031 ± 280 pg/ml ($p < 0.05$). The PTH level at maximal inhibition during hypercalcemia decreased from 281 ± 76 to 192 ± 48 pg/ml. Although calcitriol reduced the PTH level at any Ca concentration, neither the set point of Ca nor the slope of the PTH–Ca curve was significantly different after 10 weeks of calcitriol. However, if a noncompliant patient who had persistent hyperphosphatemia is excluded, a significant change in the set point of Ca

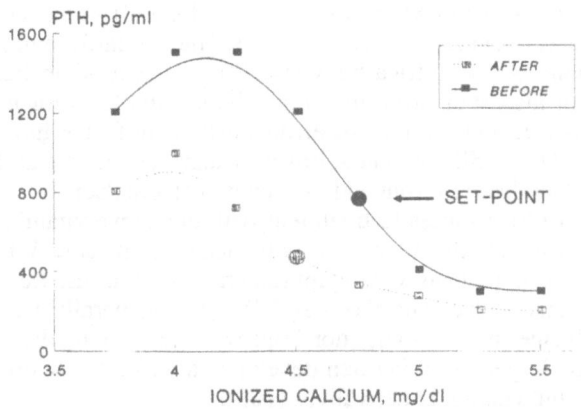

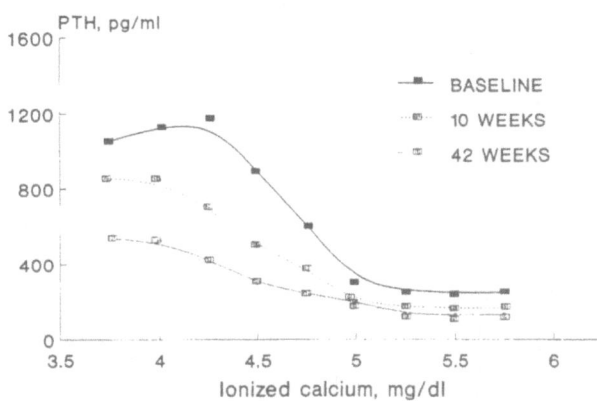

Figure 7. PTH–Ca curve in 9 patients with significant 2°HPTH before and after 10 weeks of intravenous calcitriol. One patient with hyperphosphatemia has been excluded. Then there is a significant shift of the set-point of calcium. (Data from Dunlay et al. (66).)

Figure 8. The effect of calcitriol treatment on the PTH–Ca curve is shown. The baseline (0 weeks) PTH–Ca curve is before calcitriol therapy, and the other two PTH–Ca curves are after 10 and 42 weeks of intravenous calcitriol. Between 0 weeks and both 10 and 42 weeks, significant differences were present in the hypocalcemic segment of the PTH–Ca curves. $^*p < 0.05$ *vs* 42 weeks. (From Rodriguez et al. (38).)

was observed (Figure 7). We have also evaluated the effect of long-term intravenous calcitriol administration in six patients which received calcitriol treatment during 42 weeks (38). At the end of the study, the slope of the PTH–Ca curve was decreased ($p < 0.05$) as compared with both 0 and 10 weeks (Figure 8). Malberti et al. have shown similar results in patients with 2°HPTH refractory to oral calcitriol (84). These patients received 2 μg of intravenous calcitriol three times a week for four months. They observed a shift in the set point of Ca and a decrease in the slope of the curve. These findings suggest that calcitriol: 1) reduced the functional mass of parathyroid cells (based on the significant decrease in maximal and minimal PTH) and 2) decreased the sensitivity of parathyroid cells.

Osteomalacia and adynamic bone disease. Low turnover bone diseases

Another skeletal lesion in patients with CRF is that represented by low bone-turnover states. The main bone features include a low bone formation rate and a defect in bone mineralization which, in severe cases, leads to osteomalacia. Recently, a new low bone-turnover entity has been identified: the aplastic or adynamic bone disease. There are few data on the pathogenesis of the low bone-turnover states. Earlier, it was thought that these states characterized by an impaired mineralization resulted from altered vitamin D metabolism; later, other pathogenic factors, including aluminum (Al) accumulation, were implicated.

The role of vitamin D

Despite the observations that plasma levels of calcitriol are low in most uremic patients and that intestinal Ca absorp-

tion is decreased in uremia (85), overt osteomalacia, or even histologic features suggestive of impaired mineralization, are noted rarely (86). Moreover, osteomalacia is often absent in anephric patients (86).

Defective skeletal mineralization may have been more common in the United Kingdom than in North America. Eastwood et al. noted that uremic osteomalacia correlated with decreased plasma levels of 25-(OH) D; the latter reflecting decreased vitamin D intake (87). Thus, relative vitamin D deficiency is more common in the United Kingdom and Scandinavian countries than in the United States because of less sunlight exposure and because the fortification of foods with vitamin D is not extensive in the former areas.

Since calcitriol production is impaired in CRF, it is not surprising that vitamin D deficiency leads to greater impairment of skeletal mineralization in patients with CRF. As patients with advanced CRF are often malnourished, low plasma levels of 25-(OH) D are also not infrequent (88). Plasma levels of 25-(OH) D have also been correlated with the protein content of the diet (88).

The mechanism whereby the absence of calcitriol impairs the mineralization of bone is not well understood. Whether vitamin D or calcitriol directly stimulates bone mineralization, or merely leads to bone mineralization by maintaining the appropriate milieu of Ca and P, remains controversial (89). Other vitamin D derivatives such as 25-(OH) D or 24,25-(OH)$_2$ D may also have an independent beneficial effect on bone mineralization (90, 91).

Aluminum accumulation

Convincing data indicate that accumulation of Al in patients with CRF can cause osteomalacia, hypercalcemia, encephalopathy, and hypochromic microcytic ane-

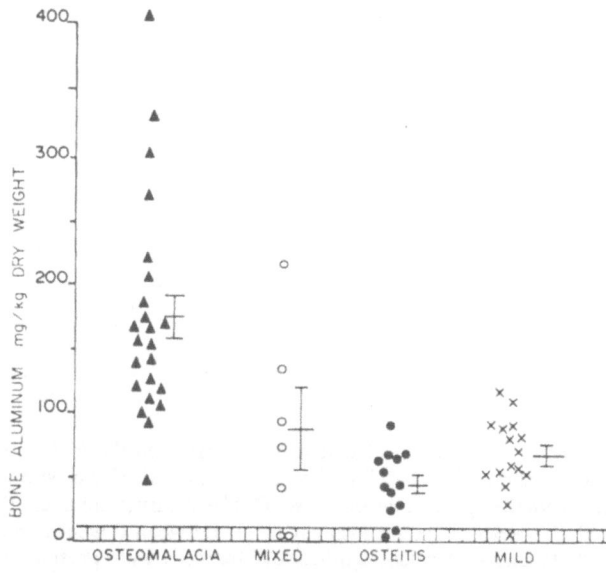

Figure 9. Bone Al content of patients with different types of renal bone disease. Some patients with mild and mixed disease probably had aplastic bone disease. Reproduced from Hodsman et al. (98) with permission of the publishers.

mia (92, 93). Outbreaks of fracturing 'dialysis osteomalacia' were first reported from dialysis centers in the United Kingdom; encephalopathy was also common in those patients (94). It was first postulated that this bone disease arose from fluoride accumulation or from P depletion (95), despite the rarity of hypophosphatemia in patients with advanced CRF. Then, Al levels were noted to be increased in the brain of patients dying with dialysis encephalopathy (96) and epidemiologic data showed a correlation between the incidence of osteomalacia, dialysis encephalopathy and high content of Al in water used for dialysis (97).

The Al content of bone was noted to be increased in most dialysis patients, whether measured by neutron activation, electron probe, atomic absorption spectroscopy, or a histochemical staining method (98, 99). Bone Al levels were observed to be markedly elevated in patients with refractory osteomalacia (Figure 9) and the Al content of bone correlated directly with the extent of osteomalacia in these patients (98). Moreover, Al deposits were noted along the mineralization front (99). Little or no tetracycline was incorporated along the surfaces with heavy Al staining indicating absent bone formation; the extent of surface Al staining correlated inversely with bone formation rate (99). In dialysis patients showing bone biopsy features of osteitis fibrosa, mixed features of osteomalacia plus osteitis fibrosa, or 'mild' disease (mild 2°HPTH), bone Al content has also been noted often above normal, but the values were generally less than those noted in patients with pure dialysis osteomalacia (99).

Rarely, other metals can also produce a low-turnover bone disease. Staining at the mineralization front for both

iron and Al (100) as well as iron alone (101) has been observed in some dialysis patients. The standard aluminon staining (auryl-tricarboxylic-acid) to detect Al in bone can also stain iron and, thus, bone samples with iron deposits in bone may be erroneously identified as having Al (102). Silicon and sulfur may also accumulate at the mineralization front and may cause osteomalacia.

Refractoriness to treatment with the active vitamin D sterol is another feature of Al-related osteomalacia. When dialysis patients with symptomatic Al bone disease are treated with calcitriol or $1\alpha(OH)$ D, they generally had no change in symptoms, nor improvement of bone disease and hypercalcemia often developed after only low doses of the vitamin D derivatives (103).

The clinical features of Al bone disease include progressive bone pain – affecting specially the axial skeleton – proximal muscle weakness, and fractures of the ribs, vertebrae, pelvis, and hips. Severe disability and skeletal deformities may occur (104). The biochemical findings of 131 hemodialysis patients comparing those with Al induced bone disease with those with osteitis fibrosa are displayed in Figure 10 (105). In patients with Al induced bone disease, serum Ca levels usually are normal or slightly increased; serum P concentration do not differ from other patients with advanced CRF but tend to be lower than in osteitis fibrosa; plasma Al levels are higher and PTH are inappropriately low. Some patients develop spontaneous hypercalcemia; in others hypercalcemia occurs during immobilization, while on vitamin D analogs, Ca-containing P binders, or with the use of high dialysate Ca concentration (103). Tumor-like calcification have been reported in association with severe Al intoxication (106) as well as improvement of a tumor-like calcification following appropriate therapy of Al intoxication and despite aggravation of 2°HPTH (73). In patients with Al intoxication, parathyroidectomy have been performed because these patients presented with hypercalcemia, fractures, bone pain and sometimes tumoral calcification; thus, they were erroneously diagnosed of having 2°HPTH (107). These patients may also have abnormal skeletal surveys suggestive of 2°HPTH which actually represent old erosions that were not mineralized as Al toxicity developed. Normal or elevated plasma alkaline phosphatase levels were noted (105). These differences may be in relation to the country of origin or the source of Al. Thus, plasma alkaline phosphatase levels are usually lower when the source of Al is parenteral intoxication and are usually high when the source is intestinal absorption of Al-containing phosphorus binders (108). Serum levels of calcitriol are low, as expected in end-stage renal disease. Serum levels of PTH often are lower than usual for dialysis patients (105) and fail to increase normally after the induction of hypocalcemia (Figure 11) (109). This most likely due to Al accumulation *per se* in the parathyroid gland, because of the increase in blood Ca concentration caused by Al effect either on bone or Ca-binding to serum proteins, or due to a combination of these effects.

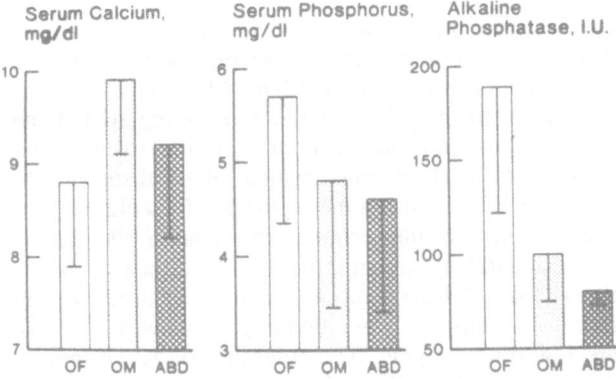

Figure 10a. Serum calcium and phosphorus concentration and alkaline phosphates activity in dialysis patients with osteitis fibrosa (OF), osteomalacia (OM), and aplastic bone disease (ABD); normal alkaline phosphatase, 30 to 100 IU/l. Reproduced from Llach et al. with permission of the publishers.

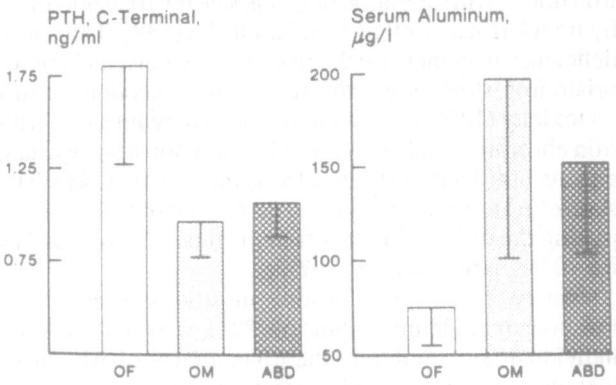

Figure 10b. Parathyroid hormone levels and aluminum concentrations in patients with osteitis fibrosa (OF), osteomalacia (OM), and aplastic bone disease (ABD). Normal range for PTH, 0.1 to 0.3 μg/ml; aluminium 2.3 to 6.4 μg/l. Reproduced from Llach et al. with permission of the publishers.

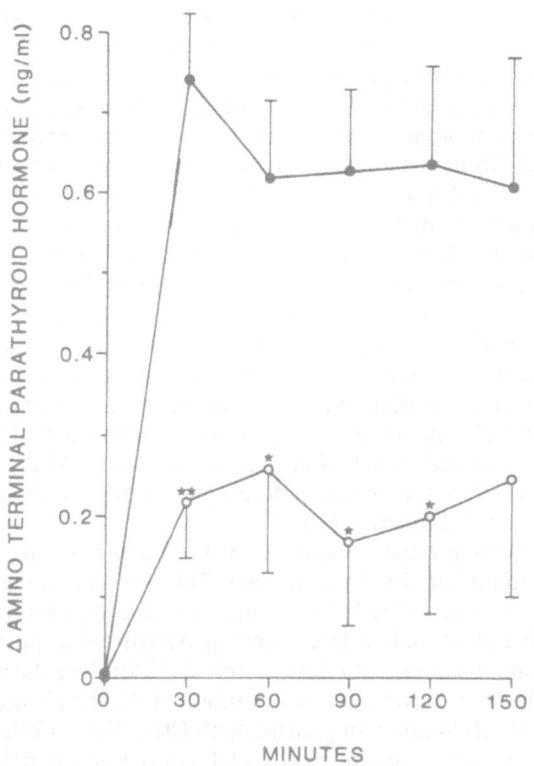

Figure 11. A comparison of PTH response to hypocalcemia in patients with biopsy proven osteomalacia (open circles) and osteitis fibrosa (closed circles). Observe the blunted PTH response in patients with osteomalacia. Reproduced from Andress et al. with permission of the publisher.

Aluminum-related bone disease may manifest following parathyroid surgery and after high PTH levels are reduced by treatment with vitamin D sterol (110). Bone surface Al deposits often increase after parathyroidectomy (110), and the decrease in PTH levels predispose to the appearance of osteomalacia. There is clinical and experimental evidence suggesting that high PTH may 'protect' from Al induced osteomalacia. Thus, in dialysis units with high dialysate Al content, those patients with severe osteitis fibrosa and high PTH levels rarely developed osteomalacia (111).

Also, the pattern of localization of Al in osteitis fibrosa may differ from that observed in osteomalacia. In the former, the Al is diffusely distributed in bone; in the latter, it is localized at the bone surface (112). However, Al-related bone disease may occasionally occur in patients with markedly elevated serum PTH levels (113). Also, the

clinical and histologic features of Al-related osteomalacia can improve substantially after the removal of only modest amounts of Al following infusions of deferoxamine and with only small increments in serum PTH levels (114). Removal of accumulated Al from dialysis patients leads to an increase in serum levels of both PTH and calcitriol (111). Thus, the mechanism whereby PTH modifies the features of Al-related bone disease remains unclear but it is likely that if bone turnover is reduced due to a decrease in PTH, Al may be redistributed in the bone predominantly in the mineralization front leading to an abnormal bone matrix synthesis and mineralization.

What are the sources of Al intoxication in patients with CRF? Although Al is ubiquitous in nature, the Al concentration is very low in biological systems since Al does not cross the skin and only small amounts are absorbed through the gastrointestinal tract. The first cases of Al-induced osteomalacia occurred in dialysis units using water with Al concentrations above 100 μg/l (94); however, a high incidence of bone disease has occurred in units using a dialysate Al near 50 μg/l (116). Since 80 to 95% of Al in plasma is protein-bound to transferrin and albumin (117), Al is transferred into the patient from the dialysate when the dialysate Al concentration exceeds the level of ultrafilterable Al in blood. Aluminum may also come from other sources: the cartridges used in the past for the regeneration of dialysate (sorbent system) released Al into dialysate (118); occasionally, preparations of peritoneal dialysate have had high concentrations of Al. Sorbent cartridges currently in use have proven to be safe and have not added Al to the dialysate, neither with acetate or bicarbonate(119). Similarly, samples of peritoneal dialysate recently evaluated have shown to be low in Al content ($< 7 \mu$g/l). On the basis of the available evidence, we recommend that dialysate Al levels be lower than 10 μg/l, and preferably below 5 μg/l. Significant amounts of Al have also been noted in albumin solutions (120) and in certain other constituents of parenteral solutions (121), including vesical irrigations with Alum (122). As mentioned earlier, if the parenteral load of Al is high enough, osteomalacia can develop even in patients with normal renal function (121).

Aluminum can accumulate in the body not only via parenteral but also the oral route. This was first noted by Berlyne et al. (123), but the evidence was largely ignored. Studies in normal subjects ingesting Al hydroxide indicate that small amounts of Al are absorbed (124); since the kidney is the sole route for the excretion of Al, the absorbed Al will accumulate in patients with CRF. The Al-related bone disease in uremic patients who have never had dialysis, but ingested only Al hydroxide, clearly indicates that Al toxicity can accumulate from an oral source (125). Moreover, close correlation has been noted between plasma Al concentration, which indicates recent Al loading (126), and the amount of ingested Al-containing P binders (127). Finally, after Al-containing P binders were discontinued in dialysis patients, plasma Al levels fell substantially, providing additional evidence for the contribution from an oral source (127). Aluminum toxicity and intestinal absorption can occur also with the ingestion of sucralfate (128). Evidence of brain accumulation of Al was noted in premature infants who had ingested a low-protein, low-phosphate formula that is often recommended for infants with CRF (129) although a subsequent prospective study failed to find any evidence of Al accumulation in 14 children who ingested this formula for up to 18 months (130).

The knowledge that oral absorption of Al is a major factor leading to Al accumulation in CRF has led to a consideration of the factors that augment its intestinal uptake. Many CRF patients can ingest Al gels for long periods with little accumulation, while others develop Al overload within a few months after they are given large doses of Al gels. The presence of uremia increases Al absorption (131), though the mechanism for this effect is uncertain. Both PTH and calcitriol have been implicated as increasing the intestinal absorption of Al (131); however, in other studies their effects were small or could not be detected (132). As mentioned earlier, patients with high PTH levels seem to be protected from the toxic effects of Al (111). The ingestion of Al compounds in conjunc-

tion with sodium citrate/citric acid – present in common drinks such as orange juice – may significantly enhance Al absorption (133). Severe and fatal Al toxicity has developed prior to dialysis in patients receiving Al gels and citric acid/sodium citrate (Shohl's solution) to correct acidosis (134). Marked enhancement of Al absorption has also been shown during the ingestion of Ca citrate (135), and certain over-the-counter compounds (Alka-Seltzer) which contain citrate and, thus, can augment Al absorption (136). All these compounds should be used with caution if not completely avoided in patients with CRF who are ingesting Al gels. The solubility of Al compounds increases substantially as the ph falls, indicating that gastric ph may modify Al absorption substantially. Thus, ranitidine, an H_2-receptor inhibitor, has been suggested to reduce Al toxicity in patients with CRF (137).

Iron stores may also modify Al kinetics since Al and iron share common pathways for intestinal absorption, serum transport and cellular uptake. Also, the degree of iron transferrin saturation may regulate the transport of Al by transferrin as well as cellular uptake (138). Thus, iron deficiency may increase the risk of Al toxicity, and appropriate iron stores seem to offer some protection against Al toxicity (139). Aluminum overload may interfere with iron absorption and be a causal factor in the iron-resistant anemia (140) and resistance to erythropoietin (141). The state of iron stores should also be considered when interpreting the deferoxamine test to diagnose Al overload as it will be discussed later (142).

Finally, certain host factors, mostly associated with low bone remodeling and/or low PTH, may make certain individuals susceptible to the toxic effects of Al. These include: prior parathyroidectomy (143); glucocorticoid treatment for a rejected renal transplantation (144); diabetes mellitus (145); decreasing PTH after calcitriol therapy (146); and bilateral nephrectomy (147).

Low serum PTH. 'Idiopathic' adynamic bone disease

Aplastic or adynamic bone-disease (ABD) has been recently described in uremic patients on chronic dialysis (148). This entity has been termed both 'aplastic' or 'adynamic' bone disease but, since the main diagnostic criterion is an abnormally low bone formation rate, the term 'adynamic' is preferred. Subsequently, it has been noted with increasing frequency in dialysis patients (149). Recently, 60% of patients undergoing peritoneal dialysis and 36% of hemodialysis patients were found to have ABD (149). Though this unusual high prevalence of the disease may be due to the inclusion of idiopathic and secondary forms of ABD and a greater awareness towards the disease, specific regional and local factors may also play a role. The afflicted patients have a low bone formation rate without osteoid accumulation (150). This latter finding is a major feature which distinguish this entity from osteomalacia. However, the diagnostic criteria of ABD may vary among different investigators and partially it could account for the observed differences in the prevalence of ABD. In addition to the osteoid surface, decreased osteoblast number and osteoblastic surfaces are also noted while osteoclast number and osteoclastic surfaces are usually normal or low (151).

In some patients, serial bone biopsies have shown the evolution from an aplastic state to osteomalacia, suggesting that the aplastic lesion may be a precursor of more typical osteomalacia. Conversion of the aplastic lesion to true osteomalacia suggests that the earliest abnormality may be inhibition of osteoid synthesis (a cellular insufficiency to form bone matrix), and that this is impaired to a greater extent than bone mineralization (151).

In previous observations, patients with histological features of ABD were noted to have significant Al deposits and were thought to have Al-related bone disease. For some investigators, the main etiological difference between Al-induced osteomalacia and ABD is the presence of a smaller Al burden in ABD as reflected by a lesser increase in plasma Al after a deferoxamine test. Thus, ABD has been described mainly in patients with relatively low Al overload; these patients were dialyzed with a dialysate not contaminated with Al and the main Al source was the ingestion of Al-containing P binders (105, 152). However, as it will be discussed later, Al is not the only cause of ABD.

An association between osteomalacia, ABD and the presence of low serum PTH was noted a decade ago. A smaller aluminum overload was observed in ABD by Andress et al. (152). However, we have shown important role of PTH in favoring osteomalacia rather than ABD (153). We noted in uremic parathyroidectomized rats that Al administration produced a bone lesion resembling ABD; the osteoid volume was higher when the parathyroid glands were present than when they were absent despite similar Al exposure. Thus, a potential contribution of low serum PTH to excessive reduction in bone turnover and the development of ABD has been raised (153).

A growing fraction of patients with ABD have been identified without Al deposits (148). Unlike aluminum bone disease, its incidence seems to be increasing and it is more frequently observed in the absence of Al accumulation (149). Furthermore, no difference in the incidence of ABD has been observed either in the presence or absence of Al deposits (148). Thus, factors other than Al have to be considered; they may include: age, hypothyroidism, corticosteroid treatment and Cushing syndrome, fluoride at toxic doses, iron, hypophosphatemia, and acidosis (see below) (150–152). Also, diabetic patients on chronic hemodialysis have been shown to have lower plasma PTH concentrations, lower bone formation and resorption than their matched nondiabetic controls (145), as well as diminished parathyroid gland responsiveness to an acute hypocalcemic challenge (154). In fact, diabetes has been associated with low PTH secretion and osteopenia even in the absence of CRF (155). Adynamic bone

disease has also been described without the presence of any of the above mentioned factors both in children (156) and in adults (150).

The real incidence of ABD is unknown; ranging from 10% to as high as 48% in those treated with continuous ambulatory peritoneal dialysis (CAPD); it has also been observed in 17% of hemodialysis patients (149). Thus, ABD seems to be more common in patients treated with CAPD. The continuous peritoneal exposure to a high dialysate Ca (3.5 mEq/l) increases serum Ca (157), which may suppress PTH secretion leading to a decrease in bone formation rate. This hypothesis though plausible is not proven, since older patients and a higher prevalence of diabetic patients are common among those treated with CAPD. However, a decrease in the peritoneal dialysate Ca to 2.0 mEq/l results in increased serum PTH, suggesting that the 'high' dialysate Ca contributes to the suppressed PTH levels (149).

The ingestion of large doses of Ca carbonate/acetate as P binders and an excessive parathyroid suppression with calcitriol also may be contributing factors in the development of ABD (151). Adynamic bone disease has also been associated to an overtreatment with vitamin D derivatives even in predialysis patients (146). Serum intact PTH levels have ranged from normal to 3 times the upper limit of normal in patients with ABD (149). It has been noted that normal bone formation rate in uremia corresponded to plasma intact PTH levels between 1.5–3 fold the upper limit of normal, suggesting that mild ° HPTH may be necessary to maintain normal bone formation rate. Until more is known about the natural history of ABD, it would seem prudent not to oversuppress intact PTH levels in dialysis patients to values lower than 2–3 fold the upper limit of normal.

Biochemically, ABD is characterized by normal or low alkaline phosphatase and osteocalcin. The measurement of bone alkaline phosphatase may be also useful since levels below 20 U/l have been shown to have a sensivity of 66% and a specificity of 86% for the diagnosis of ABD (153). Serum PTH levels are often above the normal range (149, 154) but lower than those observed in patients with osteitis fibrosa. More than 50% of the patients with biopsy-proven ABD may have normal intact PTH levels (155). Intact PTH levels greater than 200 pg/ml have a positive predictive value of 88% for the diagnosis of mild and severe 2°HPTH while a value below 65 pg/ml had a positive predictive value of 78% for ABD (156). Plasma Ca concentration tends to be high and/or increase rapidly when oral Ca, calcitriol or high dialysate Ca concentrations are used (148, 157).

While Al related ABD may be a symptomatic disease with patients having more frequent bone pain, fractures, and decreased bone density; patients with idiopathic ABD are often asymptomatic and without radiological abnormalities at the time of diagnosis. Thus, idiopathic ABD at present seems to be an histological finding rather than a disease. Moreover, no bone fracturing has been observed in conditions associated with low PTH levels such as primary or secondary hypoparathyroidism. Finally, in dialysis patients, ABD may reverse to a hyperparathyroid state, while persistence of this bone lesion is more likely after kidney transplantation due to the suppressive effect of corticosteroid on bone.

Hypophosphatemia

A low plasma P concentration may be the cause of low bone turnover (158). However, severe hypophosphatemia is rare in uremic patients. As early as 1966, Stanbury and Lumb observed an association between the presence of osteomalacia and a low plasma Ca×P product in patients with moderate to advanced CRF (159). In the United Kingdom, Kanis et al. noted an inverse relationship between the number of osteoid lamellae, an index of osteomalacia, and the predialysis plasma P levels in a large group of hemodialysis patients. Evidence for a mineralization defect was common in patients whose mean plasma P concentration was below the limit of normality. Since coexisting nutritional vitamin D deficiency could also be present, it is possible that the development of osteomalacia may require both a vitamin D deficiency and hypophosphatemia.

Altered synthesis and maturation of collagen

The formation of bone requires both synthesis and maturation of collagen. Without the maturation of collagen and the development of specific cross-linkages between collagen molecules, mineral deposition may not proceed normally. There is evidence of an abnormal collagen synthesis and maturation in uremia; rats with experimental uremia fail to develop mature, insoluble collagen and exhibit a preponderance of immature and soluble collagen that fails to mineralize normally. The underlying mechanism is unknown, but similarities exist between the abnormalities of collagen maturation observed in uremia and those noted in vitamin D deficiency (160). Russell and Avioli found that treatment of uremic animals with 25-(OH) D largely restored collagen maturation toward normal, providing additional evidence that altered vitamin D metabolism plays a role in defective collagen maturation (161). Whether these mechanisms are affected in uremic patients remain to be determined.

Maturation of bone crystals

The formation of mineralized bone involves the initial precipitation of amorphous Ca phosphate and its subsequent transformation into crystalline hydroxyapatite. This transformation and maturation of bone is required for the formation of bone of high structural quality. One characteristic of immature bone is the presence of large quantities of amorphous Ca phosphate and, thus, the evaluation of animals with CRF has revealed a correlation between the skeletal content of amorphous Ca phosphate and the quantity of immature, soluble collagen (162).

The reason for the delay in the maturation of bone mineral in uremia is uncertain; several factors may contribute. Thus, an increased bone magnesium content correlated with serum magnesium levels (162); an elevated pyrophosphate content (163) which may impair the normal conversion of amorphous Ca phosphate to crystalline apatite (164); and/or a diminished carbonate content, may be causative factors (162). It has been suggested that pyrophosphate may exist in the form of a magnesium salt and hence may be less susceptible to degradation by naturally occurring pyrophosphatases (163) or may slow the normal conversion of amorphous Ca phosphate to crystalline hydroxyapatite (164). In support of a role of magnesium is the observation that the rate of bone crystal maturation can be modified by altering the intake of magnesium (165). However, other authors observed that bone magnesium content positively correlated with bone calcium content and that bone magnesium did not reflect consistently serum magnesium levels (166).

The role of acidosis

The contribution of metabolic acidosis to the pathogenesis of mineral abnormalities in patients with CRF has yet to be clarified. A number of metabolic studies carried out in patients with uremia implicate acidosis in leading to negative Ca balance and thereby contributing to skeletal disease in CRF.

Pellegrino et al. (167) noted the reduction in carbonate and Ca content in uremic bone at autopsy to be proportional to the duration of uremia while Burnell et al. reported no correlation between the degree of acidosis and the quantity of bone carbonate in dialysis patients (168). They also observed an increase in P content of bone in patients treated with dialysis, (169) but Burnell et al. found no change in P content except a decrease in P in patients with marked osteitis fibrosa (168). Kaye et al. observed an increase in P content of bone in association with a decrease in carbonate (170). On the basis of the reciprocal relationship between changes in P and bicarbonate content, they suggested that a carbonate-deficient apatite is formed in uremia, where P is substituted by carbonate. The failure of Burnell et al. to detect an increase in P despite reduced carbonate content suggests that the loss of carbonate may not require P replacement; the data may also reflect a different degree of uremia and duration of dialysis treatment in the patients studied (168).

Certain observations suggest only a minor role of acidosis in leading to bone disease in uremia. Alkali therapy of patients suffering from overt renal osteodystrophy failed to produce healing of the bone lesion (171). Also, pharmacologic doses of vitamin D led to healing even in the presence of acidosis (172). Moreover, long-term acid feeding of animals produces skeletal lesions similar to osteoporosis or osteomalacia rather than producing osteitis fibrosa (173).

Lefebvre et al. in a prospective study done to evaluate the role of acidosis among dialysis patients, noted that lower doses of a vitamin D sterol were required to maintain normal serum Ca levels in the patients whose mild metabolic acidosis was corrected (174). In this study, a control group of dialysis patients with a dialysate bicarbonate of 33 mEq/l was followed and compared to an 'acidosis-corrected group', with dialysate bicarbonate increased by 7 to 15 mEq/l to maintain the predialysis plasma bicarbonate level at 24 mEq/l. In the control group, midregion PTH rose progressively, while the PTH values were stable in the 'corrected' group. Bone biopsies done prior to the study and after 18 months revealed a progressive increase of osteoid and osteoblast surface in the control patients while these alterations did not worsen in the 'acidosis-corrected' group. In patients who entered the study with an elevated bone formation rate, the basal high plasma osteocalcin levels increased further in the control group but were stable in the 'acidosis-corrected' group. Thus, there was evidence of progressive 2°HPTH in the group using a standard dialysate bicarbonate level, while the disease process was arrested with correction of metabolic acidosis. The investigators suggested that acidosis might enhance bone resorption and thereby release more P into extracellular fluid, with the latter being responsible for the worsening of 2°HPTH.

FEATURES OF RENAL OSTEODYSTROPHY

By the time symptoms appear, the patient usually has significant biochemical abnormalities and histologic evidence of bone disease. Thus, symptoms appear late in the course of renal osteodystrophy, they are rather nonspecific and usually subtle and insidious in onset. The severity of symptoms often does not correlate closely either with radiologic or histologic changes. Severely abnormal skeletal x-rays or bone biopsies may be observed in patients who are totally asymptomatic. So far, only the idiopathic form of adynamic bone disease has not been associated clearly with clinical signs or symptoms. Although beyond the scope of this chapter, the manifestations of the recently recognized 'Dialysis-related Amyloidosis' may be confused with other forms of renal osteodystrophy; therefore, we will include a brief mention of this disorder and refer the interested reader to published reviews (175, 176).

Signs and symptoms

Some signs and symptoms of renal osteodystrophy are noted in Table 3. Symptoms appear late in the course of renal osteodystrophy, they are rather nonspecific and usually are subtle and insidious in their onset.

Skeletal pain

Although not common, bone pain may develop and slowly progress to produce total disability (199). This can occur independently of skeletal pathology, whether primarily osteitis fibrosa, osteomalacia, or a mixture of both. How-

Table 3. Symptoms and signs of renal osteodystrophy

Bone pain and fractures
Acute periarthritis and pseudogout
Myopathy and muscular weakness
Spontaneous tendon rupture
Calciphylaxis
Corneal-conjunctival calcification: band keratopathy, red eye syndrome)
Pruritus
Skeletal deformities and retardation of growth
Anemia, pancytopenia, platelet dysfunction
Immunological abnormalities
Central nervous system disturbances and abnormal EEG
(?) Peripheral neuropathy
(?) Impotence
(?) Myocardial failure
Abnormal carbohydrate metabolism: Insulin resistance, hyperglycemia, hyperglucagonemia
(?) Hyperlipidemia and arteriosclerosis
Hypertension

ever, the most common cause of bone pain is osteomalacia and it is most often observed in Al-related bone disease. Pain is generally vague and deep-seated and may be diffuse or located in the low back, hips, knees, or legs. It often varies in intensity and is often aggravated by weight bearing or by sudden movement or pressure. Occasionally pain is localized around the knee, ankle, or heel, and it may be of such sudden appearance as to suggest acute arthritis. Pain in the low back may arise from collapse of a vertebral body; sharp chest pain may be the first indication of a rib fracture that has occurred during a cough, sneeze, or even during normal breathing. A change in position, such as sitting up from the supine position or spontaneous rolling over during sleep, may evoke generalized pain throughout the back, hips, and chest. Pain is not relieved by massage or local heat, and the patient usually perceives it as being more deeply seated than in the joints or muscles. Patients undergoing regular hemodialysis who are normally active and asymptomatic may develop, within several weeks to months, such severe pain as to make walking across a room difficult. Others experience such slow and gradual progression of symptoms that little notice is given until total debility has occurred.

Physical findings are frequently lacking; occasionally, localized tenderness may be apparent with pressure on the chest wall or lateral compression of the pelvis; tenderness may also be localized over the vertebral spinous processes or ribs. Spontaneous fractures can also be present. Commonly, the fractures involve the ribs, but any bone can be affected; the majority of fractures have been observed in low bone turnover Al-related bone disease. Bone pain can

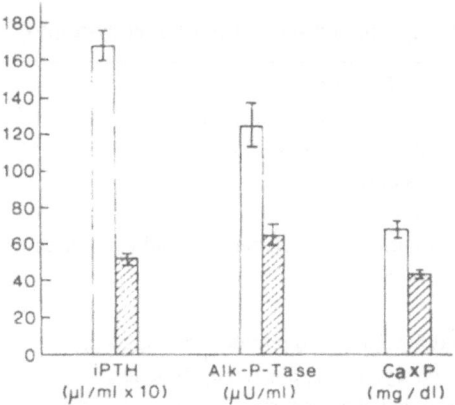

Figure 12. Values of iPTH, serum alkaline phosphatase and Ca×P observed in 12 patients with an acute monoarticular syndrome (open columns) compared to those of the other patients treated by dialysis (hatched columns). Reproduced from Llach et al. with permission.

also develop in association with dialysis-related amyloidosis.

Periarthritis-arthritis

This is manifested by acute pain, redness, stiffness and swelling around one or more joints. Rarely, pain may occur in the ankle or foot without local signs except for vague tenderness and can be associated with radiographic changes of subperiosteal resorption and/or periosteal new bone formation (178). Thus, this disorder may reflect overt 2°HPTH. The affected patients usually have higher levels of serum alkaline phosphatase activity, Ca×P product, and PTH levels than other dialysis patients (Figure 12) (179). Further evidence that such symptoms are related to 2°HPTH is provided by the observation that such discomfort can disappear completely within 1 to 2 weeks following subtotal parathyroidectomy. Occasionally, Ca deposits may be observed radiographically about the affected joints. Synovial biopsy may reveal crystals that, when studied by x-ray diffraction, are characteristic of hydroxyapatite. This syndrome must be differentiated from pseudogout or gouty arthritis; the last two are characterized by a true monarticular arthritis and can be differentiated by the identification of specific crystals of either Ca pyrophosphate or urate respectively, within the synovial fluid (180).

In general, periarthritis or arthritis responds well to treatment with anti-inflammatory agents such as indomethacin; medical treatment of 2°HPTH or parathyroidectomy, as mentioned above, may lead to marked improvement (178).

Erosive arthritis and joint effusions can be also skeletal manifestations of dialysis-related amyloidosis. Metacarpophalangeal or interphalangeal joints, shoulders, wrists and knees can be involved (180).

Pruritus

Itching is a common symptom in patients with advanced CRF, and it often improves and disappears following initiation of regular hemodialysis. However, pruritus may persist and can be of such intensity that it prevents sleep and interferes with patient's normal activities. Pruritus may reflect the presence of high PTH levels, hypercalcemia, high Ca×P product (> 70) or metastatic calcification. It may improve or, indeed, totally disappear within a few days after partial parathyroidectomy (181). Thus, the presence of refractory pruritus in a patient with CRF should alert the clinician to the possibility of 2°HPTH; if a patient with intractable itching has very high PTH levels parathyroidectomy should be considered, especially if refractoriness to appropriate medical treatment (i.e., intravenous calcitriol) is present.

The mechanism whereby 2°HPTH can lead to pruritus is uncertain. Elevated levels of Ca in the skin have been reported in such patients (181). However, the increased Ca content in the skin probably is not responsible for the itching, because the symptom improves within a few hours following surgery, while much more time is required before the skin Ca content decreases. Itching may develop in uremic patients with the administration of pharmacologic doses of vitamin D and during infusions of Ca; such observations suggest that an elevated concentration of ionic Ca in the extracellular fluid may be an important factor contributing to pruritus.

Observations that uremic pruritus may be relieved following the intravenous injection of lidocaine (181), irradiation with ultraviolet light (182), ingestion of activated charcoal (183), or erythropoietin therapy (184) point to the fact that uremic pruritus is multifactorial in nature. Thus, xerosis of the skin (185), peripheral neuropathy or the presence of increased histamine levels have been noted (186). In some cases severe pruritus did not improve after parathyroidectomy; thus, in the absence of specific evidence of 2°HPTH – i.e., very high levels of PTH, radiographic evidence of erosions, and/or bone biopsy features of osteitis fibrosa – parathyroid surgery should not be performed.

Red eye syndrome

This frequently occurs when the Ca×P product is high. The corneal calcification can even take a band-like configuration in the interpalpebral area, called band keratopathy (187). Usually asymptomatic, it can also result in ocular inflammation ('red eye syndrome') and decreased visual acuity (188). A rise in local pH due to the loss of CO_2 into the air has been suggested to predispose to ocular calcification.

Myopathy and muscular weakness

Muscular weakness is largely limited to the proximal musculature and can be a serious and debilitating problem even in patients without end-stage renal disease. This myopathy resembles in many ways the muscle weakness reported in vitamin D deficiency in patients without CRF or in patients with primary hyperparathyroidism (189). Plasma levels of muscle enzymes, such as creatine phosphokinase, are usually normal, and electromyographic abnormalities are either absent or nonspecific. The muscle weakness appears slowly, with the patient unable to climb stairs easily or to rise from a sitting position without help. The gait may become abnormal so that the patient waddles from side to side in a 'penguin' style. The afflicted patient may be confined to a wheelchair or may be unable to hold his or her arms above the head or to comb the hair because of shoulder-girdle weakness.

Proximal muscle weakness can be caused by P depletion (190), abnormal metabolism of vitamin D (191), Al loading (192), or 2°HPTH (193). Striking improvement in muscle weakness has been observed in some uremic children and adults following the administration of either calcitriol (1 to 5 μg/day) or 25(OH) D (10 to 100 μg/day) (193–195). Muscle biopsy, carried out in selected patients, has revealed mild, nonspecific myopathic alterations by light microscopy and severe degenerative changes by electron microscopy (196). Following treatment with 25(OH) D some findings have reverted to normal (196). Muscle weakness in uremic patients can promptly improve following treatment with calcitriol even before serum PTH levels fall, or with doses that are too low to reduce serum PTH (195); this suggests a role of vitamin D rather than 2°HPTH in certain patients. Muscle weakness may also be profound in patients with Al-related bone disease; furthermore, striking improvement has occurred after Al removal with deferoxamine, with little change in PTH status and without vitamin D therapy (196).

Other causes of muscular weakness can be noted in uremia such as peripheral neuropathy, electrolyte disturbances, iron overload and carnitine deficiency among others. Thus, not all muscle abnormalities present in uremia can be attributed to altered divalent ion metabolism. However, in patients with prominent symptoms of muscle pain and weakness, an empiric therapeutic trial of calcitriol or 25(OH) D is warranted and the presence of Al intoxication or severe 2°HPTH must be excluded.

Spontaneous tendon rupture

Spontaneous tendon rupture also occurs in patients with long-standing CRF and is usually associated with evidence of marked 2°HPTH (196). The syndrome has been reported in association with primary HPTH and other causes of 2°HPTH (197, 198). It had been suggested that an abnormality of collagen metabolism, which also affected the bone, may occur in tendons and cause weakening (199); an effect of systemic acidosis causing elastosis of tendons had also been proposed as a pathogenic mechanism (200). However, the histologic finding on biopsy specimens of excised quadriceps suggested that repeated minor fractures of the bone cortex had occurred at the site of tendon insertion and preceded the final total tendon rup-

ture. It was concluded that osteitis fibrosa was responsible for the minor fractures (201); the slow progressive rise in alkaline phosphatase over the preceding four to five years provided additional evidence for uncontrolled 2°HPTH as the most likely pathogenic factor in those ruptures.

Rupture occurs most commonly in the quadriceps or triceps tendons, or in extensor tendons of the fingers. Typically, the quadriceps tendon ruptures while the patient is walking, descending stairs, or after stumbling. Patients are usually unable to extend the affected leg and a palpable gap and ecchymoses above the tendon are characteristic. Surgical treatment with slow rehabilitation has shown satisfactory results (198). The presence of tendon ruptures should alert the clinician to inappropriate control of 2°HPTH although it has been also recently described in dialysis-related amyloidosis.

Calciphylaxis

Calciphylaxis is characterized by peripheral ischemic tissular necrosis, vascular calcification, and cutaneous ulcerations (202). Ischemic necrosis can affect also muscles and/or subcutaneous fat (203). This syndrome usually appears in patients with end-stage renal disease and is associated with a long-standing history of CRF, although patients have developed the syndrome following successful renal transplantation (204). The syndrome has been observed in association with renal diseases of varying causes and there is not predilection for a specific sex or age.

The skin lesions make their appearance as painful superficial violaceous discolorations in a mottled, circumscribed pattern involving the tips of the toes or fingers or occurring about the ankles, thighs, or buttocks. As these lesions progress, they become hemorrhagic with ischemic, 'dry' necrosis. Frequently, boring nonhealing ulcerations and eschares occur; lesions of the terminal phalanges are often clearly demarcated and toe or fingertips may even fall off (Figure 13). Such lesions resemble those that accompany vasculitis; however, biopsy specimens fail to show fibrinoid necrosis or granulomatous formation. All patients with calciphylaxis have demonstrated evidence of medial calcinosis of small and medium-sized arteries; skin biopsies generally reveal the presence of medial calcification and intimal thickening (203, 204). Ischemic myolysis, ischemic cardiac disease, and hemorrhagic panniculitis have been reported in individual cases.

The pathogenesis of this syndrome is uncertain. Extensive medial calcinosis of arteries can occur in patients with CRF and yet not lead to gangrene and ulceration; however, the possibility has been considered that Ca deposition may give rise to mechanical obstruction. The favorable response of some patients within several days of parathyroidectomy suggests that mechanical obstruction cannot totally explain the ischemia. Vascular spasms related to either hypercalcemia (205) or an effect of PTH itself may be implicated. The occurrence of such lesions after renal

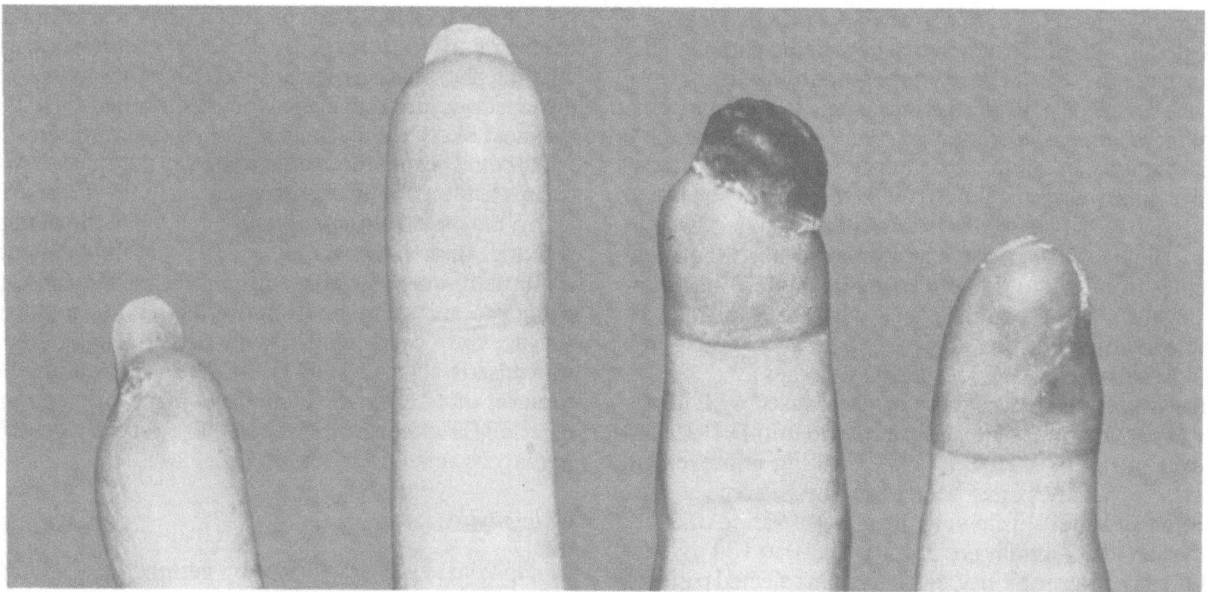

Figure 13. Ischemic necrosis involving the 2nd and 3rd digit of a uremic patient treated with maintenance hemodialysis. There was healing of the lesions following subtotal parathyroidectomy. (Case 3 from Gipstein et al.)

transplantation in patients receiving glucocorticoid raises the possibility that steroids may play a role (203, 204). Thus, Selye et al. showed in an animal model of this syndrome that calciphylaxis was more common in animals if they had been given large doses of glucocorticoid (206).

Most uremic patients presenting with this syndrome either previously had, or now have, evidence of overt 2°HPTH (203) and most have shown substantial improvement following partial parathyroidectomy (207). Nevertheless, calciphylaxis has been described after subtotal parathyroidectomy, suggesting other physiopathological pathways at work as well (208). Without treatment the lesions often progress with varying degrees of rapidity and a number of afflicted patients have died, usually from secondary uncontrollable sepsis (202, 207). Because of the poor prognosis, urgent partial parathyroidectomy is recommended when such lesions appear in conjunction with overt 2°HPTH (202, 207). In some patients serum PTH levels are not high; severe P restrictionmay reverse this syndrome (202). Patients with diabetes mellitus and CRF may also develop ischemic lesions, medial vascular calcification and a similar clinical picture. However, the lesions observed in diabetic patients rarely improve after parathyroidectomy.

Skeletal deformities

True deformities of bone are common in uremic children with long-standing CRF, in whom the bone undergoes rapid growth but skeletal deformities occasionally do occur in adults. Such deformities arise from abnormalities of skeletal remodeling and from recurrent fractures.

The deformities commonly observed in children include bowing of the long bones, especially tibia and femur, and defects arising from slipped epiphyses (208). Most commonly, slipped epiphyses become manifest in preadolescence. The hip is the most common site afflicted, followed by the radius and ulna; lower humeral, femoral, and tibial sites are more rarely involved (209). With hip involvement a limp is common and pain is often absent. When the radius and ulna are involved, local swelling and ulnar deviation of the hands appear. The histologic abnormalities associated with slipped epiphyses are those of 2°HPTH (210).

Since the pattern of bone deformity varies with age, in the patients younger than 3 to 4 years of age, changes of 2°HPTH often exhibit the typical radiographic findings of vitamin D deficiency (211). They include rachitic rosary, Harrison grooves and enlargement of the wrists and ankles due to a widening of the metaphysis beneath the growth plate in long bones (210). However, the radiographic features of a rickets-like lesion observed in uremic children has additional histologic features of 2°HPTH (208). Craniotabes and frontal bossing of the skull occur in children who develop CRF in the first two years of life (210). Uremia is a common cause of 'knock-knee,' or genu valgum at any age (212). This can appear within a few months; the presenting symptoms are difficulty in walking and pain in the knees.

In adults with CRF, particularly those with Al-related osteomalacia, skeletal deformities can be marked. They usually are confined to the axial skeleton. Lumbar scoliosis, thoracic kyphosis, and recurrent rib fracture may cause marked deformities to develop over 1 to 2 years in dialysis patients.

Retardation of growth

Growth retardation is an almost invariable finding in children with chronic renal insufficiency, both before and during management with maintenance hemodialysis or with CAPD (213). Growth can be impaired even without evidence of renal osteodystrophy. Before dialysis, one-third to one-half of children with a 'preterminal' stage of chronic CRF had heights below the third percentile (213); growth velocity was below normal limits for age in two-thirds of children under treatment with dialysis (214). Providing caloric supplements has been reported to improve growth (215), although this is not always successful (216). Studies showing that correction of acidosis can improve growth in children with renal tubular acidosis provide support to the idea that long-standing acidosis could have a deleterious effect on growth (217). Low levels of somatomedin have also been implicated in this complex problem (218). Improved or even catch-up growth has been observed in a few children after treatment with calcitriol (219). During treatment with calcitriol, catch-up growth did not occur during the early period of treatment when the serum PTH levels were still elevated and renal osteodystrophy was still evident; but it began after the apparent healing of the 2°HPTH. Nevertheless, the number of patients studied is small, and consistent increases in growth rate in subsequent reports in larger numbers of patients have not been observed in the majority of children undergoing maintenance dialysis during treatment with vitamin D, 1α(OH) D or calcitriol (214).

The more recent observations of strikingly improved growth velocity of children with CRF during therapy with *supraphysiologic* amounts of human growth hormone are of interest (220). The presence of resistance to the action of the growth hormone (221) as well as other hormones (PTH, insulin) (40, 222) has been described in CRF. The response to growth hormone is more pronounced when given before ages 8 to 10 years, and such treatment is associated with markedly increased plasma alkaline phosphatase, suggesting that there is increased osteoblastic activity (222, 223). The long-term results and potential side effects of such therapy are not known.

Anemia

Refractoriness to recombinant human erythropoietin treatment can be observed both in severe 2°HPTH and in Al-related bone disease. The former will be discussed later. The anemia of Al toxicity is usually mild and can be overcome by increasing the erythropoietin dose. At least two mechanisms seem to be involved: impaired iron uptake from transferrin into the erythrocyte precursor, and inhibition of iron incorporation into heme (224). Aluminum-induced resistance to erythropoietin therapy should be considered in patients with microcytic anemia and normal iron stores, and in those patients with refracto-

ry normochromic normocytic anemia with low-turnover bone disease. Therapy with deferoxamine may ameliorate the anemia but secondary iron deficiency should be avoided.

Central nervous system disturbances

Although central nervous system involvement is the most severe manifestation of Al intoxication (96), it is decreasing in frequency. Since symptoms and signs of brain and bone involvement may not occur together, the absence of findings in one does not preclude severe involvement in the other. Early symptoms are intermittent speech disturbances like stuttering and stammering; later, personality changes, apraxia, asterixis, seizures, and global dementia can appear. Signs and symptoms may be exacerbated by dialysis and by deferoxamine administration. The EEG may show characteristic multifocal bursts of delta and theta activity.

Central nervous system disturbances have also been related to 2°HPTH as it will be discussed shortly. A variety of symptoms may accompany even mild hypercalcemia in uremic patients, including mental confusion and lethargy (225).

Myocardial function abnormalities

Uremic patients often have cardiomyopathy. Uremia is associated with an increase in the Ca content of the myocardium; these changes may be due to excess PTH. Parathyroid hormone may also play an ancillary role in mitral annulus calcification (226). Bogin et al. examined the in vitro effects of PTH on cultured isolated heart cells (227). Both PTH fragments caused a significant increase in number of beats per minute, and the cells died earlier than control cells. In addition, sera from uremic parathyroidectomized rats did not affect heart rate, but sera from uremic rats had effects similar to those of PTH. Furthermore, London et al. noted, in dialysis patients studied by echocardiography, that left-ventricular hypertrophy was associated with the severity of 2°HPTH (228). Also, these patients had an increased heart rate, higher systolic pressure and end-systolic stress as well as increased velocity of fiber shortening and shorter left ventricular ejection time (229). These authors, as well as others, have observed a marked improvement in left ventricular function after parathyroidectomy (230, 231).

Aluminum may also affect myocardial function in patients with end-stage CRF. Thus, a high mortality from cardiac failure, often accompanied by cardiac arrhythmias has been noted in dialysis patients with evidence of Al overload, as determined by bone biopsy (233) or from the deferoxamine infusion test (153) Preferential accumulation of Al has been noted in the myocardium of uremic patients (92), and an association between left ventricular dysfunction or myocardial hypertrophy and the ultrastructural findings of myocardial Al accumulation has been observed (234). London et al., in hemodialysis patients, evaluated left ventricular function by echocardiography in relation to Al stores, as assessed by a bone biopsy and from the increment in plasma Al after deferoxamine (235). The patients without Al accumulation had significantly lower left ventricular mass and an increased velocity of myocardial fiber shortening compared to those with evidence of Al accumulation. Moreover, for the entire hemodialysis population Al stores correlated with increased left ventricular mass. Thus, these observations suggest that in uremic patients, left ventricular hypertrophy may be linked sometimes to increased Al stores.

Other uremic signs and symptoms related to 2°HPTH

A number of nonskeletal symptoms that commonly coexist in uremic patients with overt renal osteodystrophy may arise as a consequence of a common pathogenic mechanism leading to both the skeletal disease and the nonskeletal manifestations. Parathyroid hormone and the PTH-induced increase in intracellular Ca, may be uremic toxins (236, 237).

There is evidence that the 2°HPTH of experimental acute renal failure may lead to increased Ca content of the brain in association with an abnormal EEG (238). Probable relevance of these animal experiments to humans has been established by Cooper et al., who noted EEG abnormalities, increased levels of PTH, and increased brain Ca content occurred early in the course of acute renal failure (239). During the diuretic and recovery phases, serum PTH decreased to normal and the EEG became normal. A role for high PTH levels in altering central nervous system function in CRF and dialysis patients is less well established. The EEG abnormalities of uremia may revert toward normal with regular and adequate dialysis (240). Moreover, brain Ca levels were normal in most patients with CRF who were tested (239). Anecdotal experience has shown rather striking improvement in behavioral abnormalities following partial parathyroidectomy in some uremic patients with 2°HPTH, suggesting a neurotoxic role for PTH in some patients (241). Moreover, neural mechanisms of behavior and motor functions are affected by the cholinergic system, and CRF is associated with these abnormalities (242). Thus, it has been recently shown that uremia causes derangements in acetylcholine metabolism mainly due to reduced activity of choline kinase which mediated, at least partly, by 2°HPTH (243).

Although it has been suggested that peripheral neuropathy may occur with greater frequency in patients with 2°HPTH (244), this supposition has been challenged (245). Arieff and Schmidt noted that motor nerve conduction velocity was not associated with PTH levels (245). In acute uremia, increased nerve content of Ca and slowed motor nerve conduction velocity were related to increased parathyroid activity (246). Available information provides support for the view that PTH acts as a neurotoxin in the central nervous system abnormalities observed in acute CRF; whether it plays a role in peripheral neuropathy remains unclear (245).

The possibility that 2°HPTH contributes to impotence in patients with end-stage CRF has been suggested (236). In one prospective study, the administration of calcitriol was associated with an increase in potency in two of seven dialysis patients; a concomitant fall in plasma luteinizing hormone occurred in one of the two, and a rise in plasma testosterone in the other (247). However, another study showed no benefit following calcitriol administration (248). Thus, the impotence of chronic uremia is probably of multifactorial origin, but excess PTH may play a role in certain cases.

Extensive marrow fibrosis and sclerosis of bone can develop in uremic patients as a consequence of 2°HPTH; such alterations may contribute to the hematologic abnormalities present in uremia. An association between renal osteodystrophy, myelofibrosis, and abnormal hematopoiesis has been noted; (249) thus, patients with leukopenia, thrombocytopenia, and severe anemia are more likely to have overt bone disease than other dialysis patients. It has been suggested that splenomegaly may arise in certain uremic patients as a compensatory mechanism in response to the replacement of normal erythroid tissue by osteitis fibrosa. An increased incidence of anemia has been reported in patients with primary HPTH (250) and correlates with the extent of marrow fibrosis. In a recent report, refractoriness to recombinant erythropoietin treatment has also been related to the presence of bone marrow fibrosis (251). It has been also observed that the hematocrit may increase in uremic patients with severe 2°HPTH following partial parathyroidectomy (252). It appears that PTH may suppress erythropoietic function through local factors produced by marrow fibrosis. However, a direct effect of PTH on red blood cells is also possible. Meytes et al. examined the *in vitro* effects of intact PTH and some of its fragments on erythroid colony formation in human peripheral blood and mouse bone marrow (253). They observed that intact PTH and its carboxy-terminal fragment exert an inhibitory effect on erythropoiesis that might be overcome by increased erythropoietin levels. These observations are complemented by others, demonstrating inhibition of RNA and heme synthesis by PTH extracts (254). In addition, the amino-terminal PTH fragment has been shown to induce hemolysis of red blood cells (255). Thus, excess PTH could contribute to the shortened life span of red blood cells in uremia.

Inhibition of platelet function occurs in uremia and an inhibitory effect of PTH on platelet aggregation has also been noted (256). Thus, it is possible that excess PTH may be a contributing factor in the bleeding tendency of uremia.

Parathyroid hormone has also been implicated in the immunological abnormalities present in uremia (257).

Hypertriglyceridemia has been noted in a fraction of patients with uremia. Furthermore, parathyroidectomy partially inhibits the increase in lipids observed after bilateral nephrectomy, while the administration of parathy-

Table 4. Biochemical features of renal osteodystrophy

Hyperphosphatemia	Elevated plasma OH-proline
Hypocalcemia	Elevated plasma cyclic AMP
Elevated alkaline phospatase	Hypercalcemia
Hypermagnesemia	Hypophosphatemia
Elevated serum iPTH	Reduced calcitonin
Reduced plasma $1,25(OH)_2D$	Elevated bone aluminum
Reduced plasma $24,25(OH)_2D_3$	Elevated GLA protein
Increased Ca and Mg content of skin	

roid extract restores the hyperlipidemia in parathyroidectomized uremic rats (258). Such data provide support for the possibility that the hyperlipidemia of uremia may be related to an excess of PTH. Other observations suggest that the insulin secretion is impaired following chronic excess of PTH (259). PTH increases intracellular Ca of pancreatic islets due to both stimulation of camp generation and activation of protein kinase C (260). Thus, insulin resistance and hyperglycemia observed in uremia may be related to 2°HPTH.

BIOCHEMICAL FEATURES

The biochemical features of renal osteodystrophy are noted in Table 4.

Serum phosphorus

Serum P levels are usually slightly lower than normal (15, 97) or normal in early stages of CRF (30, 261). Hyperphosphatemia is generally absent until renal function falls to 20 to 30% of normal (30, 262). However, in patients with creatinine clearances below 20 ml/min, although hyperphosphatemia is common, serum P levels show wide variation, ranging from 2.5 to 15 mg/dl, and are mainly affected by dietary P intake. Some factors that can affect the serum P levels in patients with renal insufficiency are shown in Table 2. Of these the two most important are dietary P intake and the ingestion of P binding gels. Results from metabolic balance studies indicate that Al hydroxide gel, 75–200 ml/d increases fecal P by 30–44%. When dietary P intake is below 1 g/d and Al hydroxide is taken fecal P often exceeds dietary intake. However, when dietary P is increased to 2 g/d, fecal P is usually below dietary intake despite ingestion of the gels. Thus, a high P diet can offset the effect of Al hydroxide or carbonate, emphasizing the need for P restriction. A scheme showing quantitative relationship between dietary and fecal P and the influence of Al hydroxide is given in Figure 14.

The administration of vitamin D derivatives and the status of body stores of vitamin D (i.e., vitamin D deficiency), can also affect serum P levels. Vitamin D derivatives can directly change serum P by influencing P homeostasis or indirectly through PTH. Since a major action of calcitriol on P homeostasis is to enhance intestinal P absorption (263, 264), serum P may increase following the administration of calcitriol (Figure 15), specially in noncompliant patients with an unrestricted P diet (66). The administration of calcitriol often suppresses 2°HPTH in uremic patients; this may lead to reduced bone resorption with increased net deposition of Ca and P in bone. Thus, serum P levels sometimes decrease and a need for P binders are less during the first 2 to 3 months of treatment with calcitriol; later, once the period of rapid skeletal mineralization is complete, serum P may increase (265). However, increased serum P after calcitriol have also been reported; (266) differences in the dietary intake of P and calcitriol dosages could account for these differences.

Compliant patients, not taking vitamin D derivatives, can also have high P levels due to increased bone resorption secondary to severe 2°HPTH. Thus, serum P levels are often higher in patients with overt 2°HPTH (98, 267). Similarly, patients with severe 2°HPTH may be not only resistant to PTH inhibition by oral calcitriol but it may also further increase P absorption and aggravate the hyperphosphatemia, further aggravating 2°HPTH.

The ingestion of phosphate-binding compounds and the intake of large amounts of supplemental Ca can also lead to changes in serum P concentration. Serum P may also be influenced by the balance between synthesis and degradation of body proteins. Thus, marked hyperphosphatemia may appear during hypercatabolic states. Such an effect is magnified in a patient with markedly decreased renal function; thus, even a mild infection may be associated with disproportionate increases in serum urea nitrogen and P levels. Alternatively, periods of increased protein anabolism may be associated with the development of hypophosphatemia due to the intracellular shift of P. Hypophosphatemia may also occur with refeeding following starvation or protein depletion. Since dietary P is linked to the dietary protein content, the administration of diets markedly restricted in proteins and not supplemented with essential aminoacids may be associated with the appearance of marked hypophosphatemia (268). However, uremic patients ingesting a natural protein-restricted diet rarely develop hypophosphatemia, despite the limitation of P intake to 300 to 400 mg/day (269). Thus, the ingestion of essential amino acids may stimulate protein anabolism to a greater extent than that observed in patients receiving natural protein-restricted diets; this may usually result in a more significant hypophosphatemia. The infusion of amino acids and hypertonic glucose for total parenteral nutrition may also lead to substantial hypophosphatemia unless P is added to the parenteral solution.

Few uremic or dialysis patients exhibit normal or slightly low levels of plasma P concentration although they ingest a normal diet and are not taking P-binders (270). The reason for this is uncertain; some patients may have

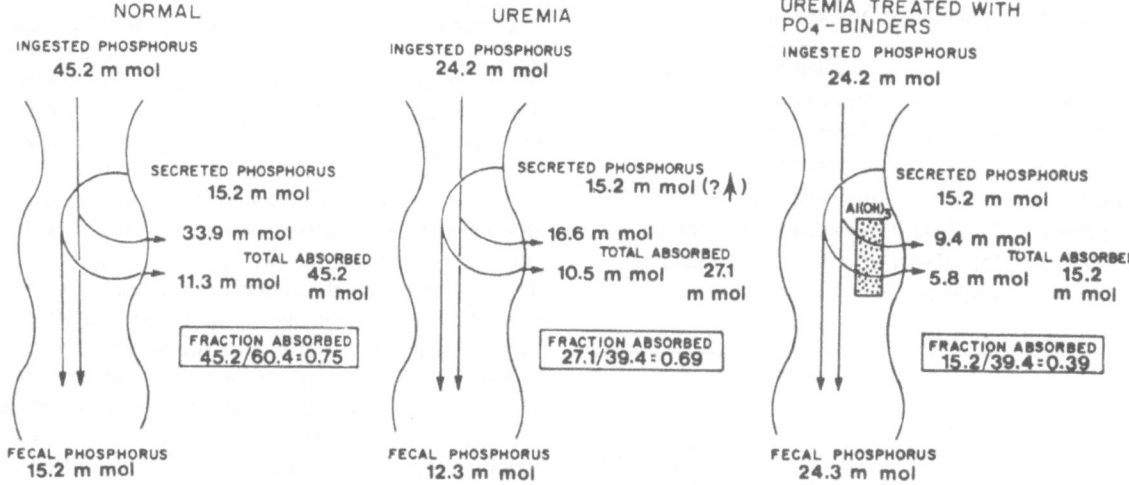

Figure 14. Schema showing approximate amount of phosphorus ingested, its fate in the intestine and the relative contribution of ingested and endogenously secreted phosphorus to total phosphorus lost in the feces. Representative values for a normal mean are shown on the left; in the middle are those for a typical uremic patient; the effect of a phosphate-binding gel on phosphorus absorption in uremic patients is shown on the right. (Modified from Coburn et al.)
(P [as phosphate] mmol → mg: multiply by 31)

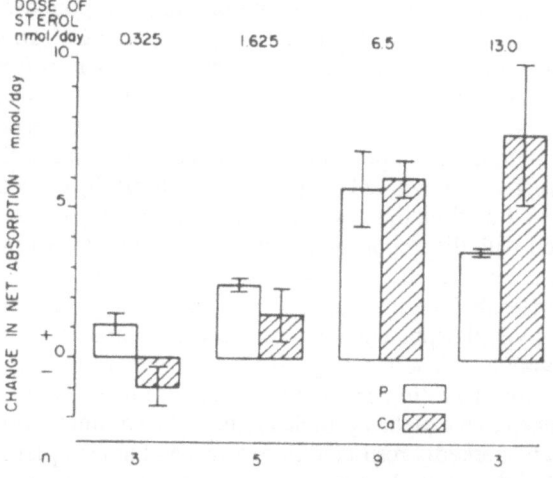

Figure 15. Changes in net absorption of calcium (Ca) and phosphorus (P) after varying daily doses of $1,25(OH)_2D_3$ or 1 alpha$(OH)D_3$. Data in normal subjects and patients with end-stage renal failure are combined (mean ± SEM). The doses of sterol correspond to 0.14, 0.68, 2.7 and 5 μg/day, respectively. (Modified after Coburn et al., with permission of the publisher.)
(Ca mmol → mg: multiply by 40.
P [as phosphate] mmol → mg: multiply by 31).

a greater degree of malabsorption of P than others. Since osteomalacia may be more common in uremic patients ingesting a low-P diet serum P levels must be monitored during P (or protein) restriction to avoid hypophosphatemia. Thus, the severity of features of osteomalacia

may correlate inversely with the predialysis P levels (Figure 12). Patients with stable CRF and those undergoing dialysis may be in a negative P balance and yet exhibit modest hyperphosphatemia (269). This negative balance does not correlate with the balance of either nitrogen or Ca, suggesting that excess P is deposited in soft tissues (269).

Serum calcium

Hypocalcemia

A detectable fall in total serum Ca concentration occurs, but not invariably, in patients with advanced CRF. The factors underlying such hypocalcemia have been previously discussed since they are of importance in the genesis of 2°HPTH. They may include a decreased intestinal Ca absorption, as a result of a reduced calcitriol synthesis or resistance to its action, hyperphosphatemia, and a decreased calcemic response to PTH.

Although both the mean total serum Ca level and the ionized Ca level are significantly lower in patients with advanced CRF (creatinine clearance 5 to 20 ml/min) than in normal subjects, total serum Ca levels were below the lower limits of normal in only 40% of uremic patients (271). Moreover, levels below 7.5 mg/dl are noted infrequently. The complexed Ca fraction is increased in advanced uremia because of increased binding of Ca to various anions (272). If the fraction of complexed Ca increases substantially, the level of ionized blood Ca may be low despite a normal total serum Ca level. A similar phenomenon may occur immediately after hemodialysis as hemoconcentration increases the protein-bound

Ca component (273). On the other hand, acidosis can decrease the degree of protein binding, and marked acidosis present in some uremic patients may induce this effect *in vivo*.

Low levels of total and ionized Ca are observed in uremic patients; however, the range of individual values is wide. The initiation of maintenance hemodialysis is often associated with an increase in total serum Ca concentration toward normal (268, 274). This increase in serum Ca has been observed despite persistent hyperphosphatemia and during the use of a dialysate Ca of 2.5 mEq/l (268). Such an observation, made several years ago when the control of hyperphosphatemia was poor, suggests the existence of some unknown factor, related to uremia and dialysis, that promotes correction of hypocalcemia. It may also be due to an improvement in the calcemic action of PTH since intestinal absorption of Ca is either unchanged or only slightly improved in regular hemodialysis (54, 275). When dialysis is carried out with more modern techniques and with the current therapeutic regimes to control renal osteodystrophy, the incidence of hypocalcemia is low and hypercalcemia becomes a more common problem.

Hypercalcemia

Hypercalcemia also occur in patients with CRF. Measurement of ionized Ca increases the sensitivity to recognize hypercalcemia, particularly in patients undergoing peritoneal dialysis (276), since their serum albumin levels are often below normal and lower than those observed in hemodialysis patients.

In general, it is known that the defect in intestinal Ca absorption can be surmounted with an increase in Ca intake or with calcitriol supplementation. The former will increase Ca absorption probably through simple ionic diffusion, a process not described to be affected by uremia; the latter will increase the carrier-mediated transport of Ca across the intestinal mucosa.

The recognized causes of hypercalcemia in patients with CRF are listed in Table 5. They must always be carefully delineated; in particular, Al toxicity and in general low bone-turnover states should be distinguished from overt 2°HPTH, since management is different. Thus, hypercalcemia in patients with overt 2°HPTH usually appear within months to years after hemodialysis has been initiated. Such hypercalcemia is usually related to a large mass of parathyroid tissue not inhibited by the presence of high serum Ca. As mentioned earlier, this condition has also been termed as 'tertiary hyperparathyroidism'. Hypercalcemia may also result from Al accumulation or, in general, a low bone-turnover state. Moreover, x-rays can show only 'osteopenia' though subperiosteal erosions may persist from earlier 2°HPTH that failed to mineralize when PTH synthesis was inhibited by Al accumulation (277). We have evaluated the mechanism for the hypercalcemia due to Al-related bone disease; thus, Al increases the protein-bound fraction of Ca and decreases ionized Ca. This, in turn, mobilizes Ca from bone and inter-

Table 5. Conditions associated with hypercalcemia in dialysis patients

Severe secondary hyperparathyroidism (tertiary hyperparathyroidism?)
Aluminum-related bone disease
High dietary calcium intake
Treatment with vitamin D metabolites
Use of high calcium dialysate (3.5 mEq/L or higher)
Phosphate restriction and hypophosphatemia
Immobilization*
Administration of thiazide diuretics
Use of calcium-exchange resins
Use of low-protein diets (usually low in phosphate)
Coexistence of other diseases causing hypercalcemia (multiple myeloma, sarcoidosis, tuberculosis, malignancy ...
After successful renal transplantation

stitium into the vascular space, leading to an increase in total Ca concentration (278). In addition, low bone formation rate and Al deposition along the mineralization front prevent the absorbed intestinal Ca to be incorporated into the bone.

Transient hypercalcemia can develop during therapy with large doses of oral Ca, especially in patients with advanced CRF (279), those treated with vitamin D derivatives, after the prolonged use of high dialysate Ca concentration (3.0 to 4.0 mEq/l) or the additional combined effect of these therapies. The hypercalcemia associated with low bone-turnover states may appear or become worse when any of these treatments, even in small doses, are used (105). Hypercalcemia may occur during treatment with Ca carbonate (279), Ca acetate, (280) or Ca-containing ion-exchange resins (281); in association with marked P restriction and hypophosphatemia (268), immobilization, and thiazide diuretics (282). Uremic patients may also develop hypercalcemia due to associated illnesses; e.g., multiple myeloma or malignancy. They may also develop hypercalcemia due to extrarenal synthesis of calcitriol, mostly in granulomatous diseases such as sarcoidosis or tuberculosis (283, 284). The hypercalcemia is usually prolonged and more marked in uremic patients because the loss of renal function eliminates the body's ability to excrete Ca mobilized from bone, absorbed through the intestine, or entering from the dialysate.

Serum magnesium levels

Serum magnesium (Mg) levels are commonly elevated in patients with advanced CRF. The homeostasis of Mg in CRF has received less attention than that of Ca or P. Normally the kidney is the main organ regulating body Mg; hence, the loss of renal excretory function leads to altered Mg homeostasis. Whether intestinal handling of Mg may be altered in uremia is controversial. Its net absorption is normal, and yet the jejunal and ileal transport of Mg has been reported to be reduced in uremic patients, as studied by perfusion of different intestinal segments. Treatment with calcitriol restores the Mg transport of a perfused intestine to normal (285), and yet there has been no detectable effect of either calcitriol or $1\alpha(OH)D$ on net intestinal absorption (286). The reasons for discrepancies between results from intestinal perfusion and those from metabolic balance studies have not been determined. It is possible that Mg transport is impaired in one portion of the intestine while it is normal or even increased in others, resulting in normal net Mg absorption through the entire gut. In general, in patients with advanced CRF, studies of Mg balance suggest that its net absorption is not markedly different from normal (286), although the intestinal absorption may be modestly decreased (287). With normal absorption and reduced renal excretion, a tendency to develop hypermagnesemia can be understood.

Serum Mg levels generally are normal until creatinine clearance rate is below 30 ml/min (262). With further impairment in renal function, there is a larger number of uremic patients exhibiting hypermagnesemia. A small increase in Mg intake in advanced CRF generally leads to an equal increase in urinary excretion of Mg, suggesting that Mg accumulates slowly (81). Approximately 20% of Mg is bound to albumin, a fraction that is unchanged in CRF despite an increase in total serum Mg level (162, 262). The increase in serum Mg levels is associated with an increase in skeletal Mg content (162, 262) and this may have an adverse effect on crystal bone formation (288) and the development of an osteomalacia-like picture (289). Other authors do not support this view (166).

In the patient with advanced CRF who is not on maintenance dialysis, the major factor that affects serum Mg levels is an increase in dietary Mg intake. With Mg-containing antacids, cathartics or enemas abrupt and marked hypermagnesemia may occur (290). In uremic patients undergoing dialysis, the Mg dialysate concentration is a major factor influencing serum Mg. Most dialysis centers have used 1.5 mEq/l, a level similar to the nonprotein-bound or diffusible Mg level in normal serum. With the use of this concentration, mildly elevated blood Mg levels of 2.5 to 4.0 mEq/l are common (262). The use of dialysate containing 0.5 to 0.8 mEq/l results in serum Mg concentrations in the upper range of normal or only slightly elevated in most dialysis patients (291). Centers using Mg-containing Ca salts as P binders should monitor serum Mg frequently and/or use a low or free Mg dialysate to avoid hypermagnesemia (282, 293).

The clinical consequences of hypermagnesemia and increased skeletal content of this cation in uremia are not known. Most uremic patients exhibit no known sequelae from the moderate hypermagnesemia, although the hypothermia of uremia has been attributed, in part, to Mg retention (294). When the serum Mg concentration is increased to levels above 3.5 to 5.0 mEq/l, flushing and burning of the skin may occur. Such symptoms have developed when the water purification system used for preparing dialysate fails (295). It has also been shown that an abrupt and marked elevation of serum Mg can suppress the secretion of PTH (296). However, no data are available to suggest that long-standing hypermagnesemia can reduce PTH secretion; Moreover, any suppressive effect of hypermagnesemia on PTH secretion would be offset by the stimulation of the parathyroid glands produced by the ensuing hypocalcemia.

On the other hand, hypomagnesemia may develop in uremic patients with an intestinal malabsorptive disease, poor nutritional intake or marked renal Mg wasting. Severe hypomagnesemia impairs the secretion and biological action of PTH as well as increases the metabolism of PTH resulting in marked hypocalcemia (297). Mg depletion may also cause a decrease in both osteoblast and osteoclast activity and lead to adynamic bone disease (289).

Biological markers of bone formation

Serum alkaline phosphatase

Serum alkaline phosphatase is made up of iso-enzymes produced by the intestine, liver, kidney, and bone. Despite the heterogeneity of this enzyme, the measurement of total alkaline phosphatase activity provides a rough indication of increased osteoblastic activity; Moreover, isoenzyme studies have shown that the increased alkaline phosphatase noted in uremia arises mainly from bone (290). Although high levels are observed in osteitis fibrosa, osteomalacia, or mixed lesions, markedly elevated levels are more characteristic of osteitis fibrosa (291). Moreover, serial measurements of plasma alkaline phosphatase activity usually identify the slow progression of skeletal disease in a uremic patient even if the rise is observed within the normal range (292). Serial measurements may also provide a useful clinical guide for monitoring the therapy of 2°HPTH with calcitriol. Thus, values that decrease over weeks or months usually indicate bone remineralization. However, uremic patients may have overt skeletal disease and normal plasma alkaline phosphatase level; thus, a normal alkaline phosphatase activity does not exclude significant skeletal disease in an individual patient.

Plasma alkaline phosphatase levels correlate with histologic features of 2°HPTH such as percentage of osteoblastic and active resorption surface (292, 293). Plasma alkaline phosphatase also frequently correlates with serum PTH levels (294). In low bone-turnover states (osteomalacia or aplastic bone disease) plasma alkaline phosphatase is usually not elevated (295). Normal alkaline phosphatase levels are more common in severe Al toxicity resulting from Al contaminated dialysate (291). It may reflect the toxic effect of Al on the osteoblast (296). Nevertheless, elevated alkaline phosphatase activity has been noted (297), especially if Al toxicity developed from the ingestion of Al containing P binders (105). Serum alkaline phosphatase levels may also increase early in the course of treatment with the chelating agent deferoxamine. In pediatric patients undergoing peritoneal dialysis, plasma alkaline phosphatase levels have been a poor predictor of histology (164). Thus, the alkaline phosphatase does not discriminate accurately between low and high-turnover bone disease.

Since hepatic abnormalities are common in dialysis patients, liver disease should be excluded as a cause of elevated alkaline phosphatase levels. Isoenzyme measurements often allow the identification of the source (290, 298). Also, recent preliminary observations have noted a low bone alkaline phosphatase activity in adynamic bone disease; low bone alkaline phosphatase had a sensitivity of 66% and a specificity of 86% when a value $\leq$ 20 U/l was used as a cut-off (153). However, these determinations are not widely available and further studies are still needed. A practical clinical approach is to measure the τ-glutamyl transpeptidase (GGT) or 5'-nucleotidase when the alkaline phosphatase is elevated. The finding of a normal value of these enzymes can largely exclude hepatic disturbances as the source of an elevated alkaline phosphatase.

Osteocalcin (bone GLA-protein)

Osteocalcin (bone GLA-protein, BGP or τ-carboxyglutamic acid-containing protein), is a recently discovered vitamin K dependent protein, produced by the osteoblast (299). It is the most abundant noncollagenous protein of bone and is delivered in the interstitial bone tissue from where it reaches the circulation fluids. Although osteocalcin levels reflect bone formation (300, 301), they are increased in CRF due to reduced renal clearance of the protein (447). Unlike total alkaline phosphatase, osteocalcin levels are normal in disorders not involving bone provided that renal function is normal (302).

Although absolute values are increased in patients with CRF, it has been suggested that osteocalcin can be helpful in separating patients with high-turnover from those with low-turnover bone lesions such as osteomalacia and adynamic bone disease (303). In a study of 30 patients undergoing maintenance dialysis, a correlation was observed between the plasma level of bone GLA-protein, histologic parameters of bone turnover and the degree of peritrabecular fibrosis (304). Osteocalcin averaged 8 times the normal value in the dialysis patients with low-turnover bone disease, but the values were greater than 40 times normal in patients with high bone turnover. The level of osteocalcin did provide a better separation of the two disorders than either alkaline phosphatase or amino-terminal PTH. In another study of 42 patients with mild to severe chronic CRF (serum creatinine 4.3 ± 2.0 mg/dl) the levels of osteocalcin were above normal in over 80% of the patients (305). There was a direct relationship between serum osteocalcin and serum creatinine levels, indicating the important role of renal function in determining the level of this peptide. In addition, there was a progressive rise in osteocalcin in patients not treated with calcitriol. In the treated group the osteocalcin levels either stabilized or fell. These observations indicate that the levels of osteocalcin may identify different conditions affecting bone in patients with CRF but, since the degree of CRF affects the osteocalcin level, it seems not yet possible to identify an individual renal patient as having a specific condition from the results of this measurement. In the same preliminary study mentioned before (153), low levels of osteocalcin had a sensitivity of 72% and a specificity of 77% in the diagnosis of adynamic bone disease in dialysis patients.

Preliminary data using an immunoradiometric assay (IRMA) or an enzyme immunoassay (306) which recognize the intact molecule of osteocalcin, have shown to be more discriminant than measurements by conventional RIA. This is probably because these new assays exclude fragment forms which are present in uremic sera. Since the residues of τ-carboxyglutamic acid are the responsible for the affinity of osteocalcin for bone mineral, the measurement of the biologically active carboxylated osteocalcin has been suggested to be more suitable to evaluate bone turnover in patients with end-stage renal disease (307).

Type I procollagen propeptide

Type I collagen is the major component (90%) of bone matrix and its circulating precursor levels may reflect type I collagen synthesis in tissues and has been developed as an index to investigate, among others, metabolic bone diseases, including renal osteodystrophy (308).

In the latter study, type I Procollagen did not correlate either with intact PTH, osteocalcin, alkaline phosphatase or with *static* histomorphometric parameters in the bone biopsy. However, and unlike osteocalcin, this marker correlated significantly with all *dynamic* parameters (308). The meaning of these observations are not clear.

Biological markers of bone resorption

Collagen breakdown products

Total and free hydroxyproline are released with the degradation of bone collagen and, normally, both are excreted in the urine (309). In patients with impaired urinary excretion due to CRF, the plasma levels of total and free hydroxyproline are increased. With an increase in bone resorption and collagen degradation plasma levels of hydroxyproline will increase even further (310). Thus, total plasma hydroxyproline may be a valuable index to assess the extent of bone resorption and the response to therapy (311). Plasma hydroxyproline usually decreases in association with improvement of skeletal disease following partial parathyroidectomy or treatment with calcitriol. Plasma concentration of free hydroxyproline correlates with bone histologic features suggestive of increased bone resorption (312). Despite the claims for its utility, the determination of hydroxyproline has not gained popularity. The recently developed measurement of collagen breakdown products such as *hydroxylysil pyridonoline* and *lysin pyridinoline* may prove more useful in the future (313).

Tartrate-resistant acid phosphatase

This is a bone resorption marker recently developed. Its isoenzyme b is synthesized by the osteoclast (314) and released into the circulation. Plasma tartrate-resistant acid phosphatase is increased in a variety of metabolic bone disorders with increased bone turnover (315). Preliminary studies seem to indicate that this marker, as the others, does not add further information and does not predict satisfactorily bone histology findings.

Other bone biological markers

Cyclic AMP

Cyclic AMP (Camp) is an important regulator of cell function acting as a 'second messenger' within the cell. Plasma levels of Camp are increased in uremic patients; normally, the plasma levels of Camp reflect PTH biological activity (316). However, no correlation has been noted between plasma Camp levels and the degree of 2°HPTH. Also, the levels can remain elevated for some time after parathyroidectomy (316). The reason for the presence of elevated levels of Camp in patients with CRF is unknown; it may be related to catecholamine or other peptide hormones for which Camp is also the second messenger.

Serum PTH

Serum PTH levels are elevated in most patients with CRF. A given PTH radioimmunoassay (RIA) can react with the amino-terminal region, the mid region, the carboxy-terminal region, or both the mid and carboxy-terminal region. Serum PTH levels are dramatically elevated when measured with an anti-serum directed primarily toward the mid or the carboxy-terminal region, while the degree of elevation is less when measured with an antiserum directed toward the amino-terminal region (75). Thus, the conventional RIA of PTH was limited by the measurement of biologically inactive mid-terminal and carboxy-terminal fragments generated by the metabolism of the hormone; this was even more important in patients with CRF, since these fragments are cleared by the kidney. With the advent of immunoradiometric assays (IRMA) which exclusively detect the intact PTH molecule, the evaluation of dialysis patients with 2°HPTH is more precise and in many instances the performance of bone biopsy may be avoided. Moreover, the IRMA assays have high specificity and sensitivity as well as excellent precision, allowing accurate measurements above, below and within the normal range. In addition to the diagnostic value, the IRMA assays have been instrumental in the dynamic evaluation of parathyroid gland function in dialysis patients, measuring acute changes in PTH levels (66, 317).

A large number of commercially available conventional radioimmunoassay for serum PTH provide no information about the predictive value of a given serum PTH level in regard to the severity of osteitis fibrosa. Thus, the discrimination between RIA-measured PTH levels in normal subjects from values in patients with primary hyperparathyroidism (154) provides little or no information about the meaning of a PTH level so measured in a patient with end-stage renal disease. Despite limitations, good correlations have been reported between the results of both midregion-carboxy-terminal and carboxy-terminal PTH assays (318, 319) and several histologic features of 2°HPTH in biopsies of hemodialysis patients; however these findings are not uniform. Furthermore, it has been often difficult to compare the results from different laboratories so that clinicians have had to use their experience in recognizing the clinical significance of a specific PTH level. Because the amino-terminal fragment of PTH is difficult to be detected in plasma, this assay may reflect 'intact' PTH. Thus, Voigts (82) and Andress (154) noted slightly better correlations with histologic features of 2°HPTH using the amino-terminal assay in comparison to results with the midregion or carboxy-terminal PTH.

Preliminary available data suggest that IRMA assays correlate with histologic features of bone disease in dialysis patients (7, 155). Moreover, these studies show a reasonably good separation of one type of bone disorder from another. Thus, in a recent study, Solal et al. compared intact, midregion and carboxy-terminal assays of PTH for the diagnosis of histological type of bone disease; they showed that the intact PTH measurement had the best correlation with the bone formation rate and was superior to the other assays for separating patients with 2°HPTH from those with adynamic lesions (155). The IRMA PTH assays also reveal remarkably similar ranges of normal values from one laboratory to another (320), thus allowing comparisons among different reports. Currently available evidence indicates that serum values 1.5–3 times above normal, using an intact PTH assay, correspond to a relatively normal bone formation rate on bone biopsies in patients with CRF (155). In summary, with the IRMA assay the diagnosis of 2°HPTH can be made accurately provided that Al toxicity is ruled out, and the therapeutic response to calcitriol therapy can be appropriately monitored (37).

Serum PTH levels are sometimes normal or undetectable in patients with CRF. Such a finding may occur in hypomagnesemia (297), low-turnover bone disease (155), excessive dosage of calcitriol (145), and obviously in parathyroidectomized patients.

Recently, a new immunochemiluminiscent assay also directed toward the intact PTH has become available (321) and its main advantage is that it avoids the radioisotopic hazard. A very good correlation (r = 0.93) was noted between an IRMA and an immunochemiluminiscent assay in 104 dialysis patients (322).

Plasma aluminum and the deferoxamine infusion test

Electrothermal atomic absorption spectroscopy provides an accurate means to measure plasma Al levels. The use of an international quality assessment program has improved the precision, accuracy and reproducibility of Al measurements (323). Tissue and plasma Al levels are substantially above normal in most patients with end-stage renal disease, particularly those who have taken Al-containing P binders or have been exposed Al contaminated dialysate (92). Plasma Al concentration largely reflects a recent 'load' of Al rather than Al toxicity (324) since plasma Al concentration does not correlate highly with tissue stores (126). However, most patients with Al-related bone disease have markedly elevated plasma Al concentrations (e.g., > 75 to 100 μg/l, compared to levels < 10 μg/l in normals. Also, patients with markedly elevated plasma Al levels (e.g., values above 150 to 200 μg/l) are very likely to develop Al-related bone disease and/or encephalopathy if the exposure to Al is maintained (126). In a large population study there were higher alkaline phosphatase levels and lower erythrocyte cell volume in dialysis patients with plasma Al levels above 100 μg/l compared to the group with levels below 100 μg/l (325). In yet another study, electroencephalographic features of encephalopathy were noted in 8 of 27 patients with plasma Al levels above 100 μg/l compared to none among 24 patients with plasma Al below 50 μg/l (326). It is of interest that only 5 of the 8 patients had any clinical manifestations of encephalopathy. In the former group, with plasma Al levels above 100 μg/l, the 8 patients with abnormal EEGs had higher plasma levels than the 19 patients with normal EEGs.

In patients who have been withdrawn from Al-containing P binders, plasma Al levels fall over the next 2–6 months, and thus, they are far less helpful in identifying those with clinically significant Al accumulation (e.g., greater than 25% surface stainable Al and subnormal bone formation rate). Plasma Al levels as low as 21 μg/l have been observed in a patient with biopsy evidence of Al-related bone disease when the ingestion of all Al-containing P binders was discontinued 18 months earlier (327).

It is important to monitor the Al content of dialysate. The maximum concentration permitted according to the American National Standard for HD Systems [Arlington, VA, AAMI, 1992 (RD-5-1992)] is 10 μg/l. Also, plasma Al concentrations should be measured at regular intervals in dialysis patients. We recommend measuring plasma Al every 4 months. Marked elevation of plasma Al levels in the majority of patients in a dialysis unit indicates that there has been exposure to unacceptably high concentrations of Al in the dialysate. This may indicate malfunctioning of the water treatment system or a dramatic increase in Al concentration in the water which may overwhelm the purification system. When only an isolated patient exhibits high concentrations of Al (e.g., >

40 μg/l), ingestion of excessive amounts of Al-containing P binders is usually present.

Bone, brain, heart and liver represent major sites of Al deposition within the body (92) but, as mentioned before, the degree of Al retention in these tissues does not correspond tightly with measurements in plasma. Measurement of the increment in plasma Al concentration following a standardized infusion of the chelating agent deferoxamine (DFO) has been proposed as a method to recognize dialysis patients with increased Al stores and a greater risk of Al-related bone disease (324). The relationship between the increment in plasma Al following DFO and the total Al content in bone is closer than that between the basal plasma Al and the bone Al content. However, it has been noted that the magnitude of the rise in plasma Al after DFO was not specific in all cases (328). Headsman et al. demonstrated that dialysis patients with 2°HPTH may have substantial increases in plasma Al following infusions of DFO despite little evidence of stainable Al in bone biopsy specimens (328). Such patients with 2°HPTH and a positive DFO infusion test may be, however, at increased risk for the development of Al-related bone disease after parathyroidectomy or if Al contamination is not avoided. Moreover, Al may not be distributed in tissues similarly in all patients, and a certain total quantity of Al in a tissue may not always be pathogenic. Once patients are protected from any Al exposure for several months (dialysate Al concentration below 10 μg/l and all Al-containing P binders avoided), both basal and the increment in plasma Al after DFO decrease substantially, even in the presence of Al staining at the bone mineralization front. Thus a certain pool of bone Al may be very resistant to removal, or is removed very slowly (121). The latter is particularly likely in a patient who has had prior parathyroidectomy.

Several factors may account for the variable results with the use of the DFO infusion test in the recognition of Al toxicity. The initial studies were done in patients with marked Al loading and severe symptomatic Al toxicity; Moreover, the patients continued either to be exposed to inappropriately elevated dialysate Al levels or to ingest Al-containing P binders. Studies in patients with mild Al toxicity indicate that the rise in plasma Al after DFO correlates well with bone Al content but it is not a good predictor of bone histology (329).

It appears that Al bone disease is decreasing in its frequency and severity (149). Thus, patients with Al bone disease are fewer but more difficult to diagnose. Some investigators have attempted to develop noninvasive strategies for the identification and serial monitoring of these patients. Thus, Al values < 30–40 μg/l makes Al-related bone disease unlikely but possible – especially if the patient has been totally withdrawn from Al exposure for 6–8 months or longer. As long as serum Al levels remain < 30 μg/l, it is also unlikely that such a patient could develop de novo Al toxicity. Between 40–100 μg/l the presence of this disease is likely, especially if associated with low PTH values, hypercalcemia or a positive DFO test; Al levels > 100 μg/l makes Al-related bone disease very probable, but it is not invariably present especially if serum PTH levels are high. In a recent report, using the combination of an intact PTH assay (IRMA) and the desferoxamine infusion test, the authors reported that an intact PTH level below 200 pg/ml and an increment of plasma Al, after DFO infusion ≥ 150 μg/l provided the best positive predictive value (≥ 95%) for Al bone disease in both peritoneal dialysis and hemodialysis patients; however, the sensitivity was only 35–45% (330). Moreover, this test cut-off would remain highly predictive even if the prevalence of the disorder decreases to as low as 5% for CAPD patients and 10% for the hemodialysis patients. The sensitivity of the combined PTH-DFO test evaluation was substantially lower in patients who had Al gels withdrawn for more than six months compared to those still ingesting Al-containing P binders. Other authors, using carboxy-terminal PTH, found that the combination of DFO test and PTH was helpful not to recognize but to exclude Al-related bone disease (331). 'Low-dose' DFO tests (0.5 g, 5 mg/kg) have been reported as useful in the diagnosis of Al-related bone disease (332). Thus, it is apparent that a bone biopsy may often be required for the diagnosis of Al toxicity in borderline and uncertain cases.

The state of iron stores may influence DFO test and, as such, status of iron stores should be considered in the interpretation of this test (102). Thus, patients with iron deficiency have higher increments of serum Al after DFO than those with iron overload. This may occur because DFO also mobilizes iron in addition to Al; thus, the more iron, the lesser the increment in serum Al after DFO. This may explain some of the frequent false negative responses observed in patients with obvious Al-induced bone disease.

Finally, the Al determination in the skin by inductively coupled plasma optical emission spectrometry has been suggested to be valuable for the evaluation of body Al content (333) although there is no uniform agreement (334).

Vitamin D levels

Under normal circumstances, serum calcitriol levels are either undetectable or below the normal range in patients with advanced CRF. Thus, the measurement of serum calcitriol is not usually helpful in the differential diagnosis of hypercalcemia in dialysis patients. However, if the cause of hypercalcemia is not identified and the patient is not receiving calcitriol treatment, an extrarenal production of calcitriol – such a granulomatous or a lymphoproliferative disorder (283, 284) should be suspected when calcitriol is in the normal range or higher.

DIALYSIS-RELATED AMYLOIDOSIS

This entity is observed in patients receiving long-standing maintenance dialysis and it is characterized by generalized arthralgia, bone cysts, scapulohumeral periarthritis, pathological fractures, carpal-tunnel syndrome and sometimes visceral involvement (335). The accumulation of a unique type of amyloid protein made up of β-2 microglobulin (an HLA Class I molecule, normally degraded by the kidney) is most likely responsible for this disorder (336). Although the pathophysiology of the process is not completely understood, these amyloid fibrils have a strong predilection to deposit in tendons, periarticular structures, at the end of long bones and within the intervertebral disks (175). The clinical manifestations of this entity almost never appear before 5 years of dialysis therapy and it is more common in patients who begin regular dialysis after the age of 50 years (180). The fraction of afflicted patients increases with the duration of dialysis therapy; thus, 70–80% of patients treated with hemodialysis for 10 years or more will accumulate β-2 amyloid in tissues (337).

Carpal tunnel syndrome (CATS) is the most prominent and usually first symptom of dialysis-related amyloidosis (338). Thus, CATS is not common in patients less than 5 years on dialysis and the incidence increases with the duration of maintenance dialysis. The reported incidence range from 30 to 100% in patients with more than 10 years on hemodialysis. Carpal tunnel syndrome results from entrapment of the median nerve by amyloid tissue deposits in the wrist, and the symptomatology of CATS is not different between uremic and nonuremic patients (180). It is usually bilateral and progressive, accompanied by numbness, paresthesia, hyperesthesia of the thumb, index, and middle fingers and the radial aspect of the fourth finger. As the CATS progresses, amyotrophy may develop. In contrast to osteitis fibrosa, pain often worsens at night and during dialysis. Amyloid fibril deposits have been noted in the transverse carpal ligament in 50% of patients affected by CATS. Surgical decompression is the treatment of choice since the response to local anesthetic agents and corticosteroid is only transient.

Severe arthralgia are also common in patients with dialysis-related amyloidosis. The affected joints are usually shoulders, knees, wrists, hip, ankle, elbow, small joints of the hand and occasionally the intervertebral discs. Scapulohumeral involvement with shoulder pain is a common clinical presentation. Joint effusion is reported to be as high as 50% of patients in hemodialysis for more than 10 years (339). Aspiration of the joint reveals a clear, sterile fluid, without inflammatory characteristics; the cell count ranges 50 to 5,000 cells/mm^3, and normal glucose levels and a low protein content are usually observed. Sometimes, centrifuged joint fluid stained with Congo red reveals the typical green birefringence of amyloid proteins. These findings strongly suggest dialysis-related amyloidosis, specially if they are associated to carpal tunnel syndrome, bone cysts, and pathological fractures. This arthropathy involves large and medium-sized joints. The lesion can start unilaterally, but usually the contralateral joint is affected. A pathological fracture may be the first manifestation of an affected joint (311). The spine can also be affected (340) destructive spondyloarthropathy, pseudotumor of the craniocervical junction causing serious spinal neurological complications (341). However, destructive spondyloarthropathy can also be due to 2°HPTH both with and without brown tumors, aluminum intoxication and apatite crystal deposition (341). The distinction between Dialysis-related Amyloidosis and the different forms of renal osteodystrophy can be difficult. Furthermore, β-2 amyloidosis may coexist with either high or low-turnover lesions of renal osteodystrophy.

Overall, the management of dialysis-related amyloidosis in patients with CRF is unsatisfactory. In the acute setting, treatment with nonsteroidal antiinflammatory drugs, corticosteroid and physical therapy are rarely useful. Shoulder arthroscopic synovectomy has shown to induce pain relief, and more radical open surgery may be of value in those patients who do not respond to conservative therapy (342). It has been shown that the use of highly permeable dialysis membranes can lower serum β-2 levels, but there is limited evidence that this has any effect on the progression of established disease; however, those patients treated with polyacrilonitrile dialysis membranes from the onset of the regular dialysis seem to have a lower incidence of the disease compared to patients treated with standard cellulosic membranes (337) The use of an specific adsorbent column has been also recently developed to be used in direct hemoperfusion, but experience is lacking regarding its effectiveness (343). Renal transplantation is the only alternative treatment, though the effectiveness of this modality to treat clinical manifestations of dialysis-related amyloidosis has been rarely reported (344). After successful renal transplantation, rapid normalization of β-2 microglobulin levels occur and the symptoms often disappear; (344) however, the histologic features of amyloid may persist (344).

RADIOGRAPHIC FEATURES OF RENAL OSTEODYSTROPHY

The radiographic features of renal osteodystrophy are listed in Table 6. Both the types of radiographic abnormality encountered and the incidence of specific bone radiographic alterations of dialysis patients vary considerably in reports from different centers (212). Such differences probably reflect some variation in the type of skeletal disease observed. Also, it is likely that differences both in the radiographic techniques employed, including type of film used, and knowledge of the radiologist are important. Thus, the apparent bone density in plain films is voltage-dependent; the higher the voltage, the more 'washed out' the bone appears (345). Also, the x-ray film and automatic film developing procedures currently in use result in

Table 6. Radiographic and other features of renal osteodystrophy

Osteopenia (reduced density)
Skeletal features of secondary hyperparathyroidism
   Subperiosteal resorption
   Cortical striations
   Cyst formation (brown tumor)
   Slipped epiphysis
   Mottled ('salt and pepper') skull
   Periosteal new bone formation
Abnormal enchondral ossification
   Rickets-like lesion
   Slipped epiphysis
Osteosclerosis
Pseudofractures (Looser's zones)
Genu valgum
Protrusio acetabuli
Endosteal bone resorption (metacarpal index)
Vertebral collapse (crush fracture)
Spontaneous rib fractures
Osteonecrosis (aseptic necrosis)
Soft tissue calcifications
   Periarticular calcification
   Tumoral calcifications
   Chondrocalcinosis
   Ocular calcification
Cutaneous calcification
   Visceral calcification
      Pulmonary (perfusion-ventilation abnormality)
      Cardiac (conduction, defect, congestive heart failure)
   Vascular calcification
      Medial
      Intimal
   Reduced mineral content
      Photon absorptiometry
      Neutron activation
   Abnormal scintiscan
      Increased uptake of ^{99m}Tc polyphosphate
      Symmetrical in osteitis fibrosa
      Identification of fractures (osteomalacia)

radiographs of much poorer quality than those available 30 to 40 years ago (346). Sensitive x-rays are particularly useful for radiographic views of the hands, and so should be done with fine-grain film; manual rather than automatic film developing should be used, and grid or screen techniques should be omitted. Magnification techniques can add further to the sensitivity. Meema et al. noted the phalanges to be normal in 67% of uremic patients using conventional techniques for x-ray films, and only 8% showed subperiosteal erosions (347). With the introduction of better films and use of magnification techniques, only 26%

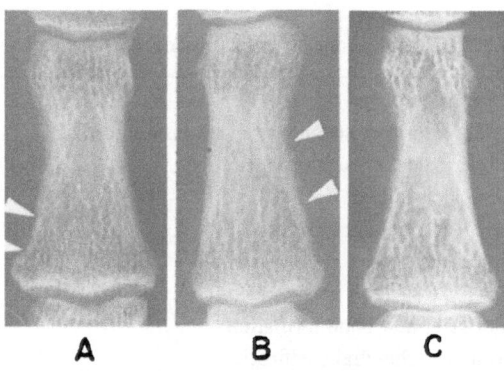

Figure 16. Appearance of subperiosteal erosions in 3 patients with renal osteodystrophy. A. There is an early saucer-shaped lesion with no overlying cortical bone on the lower radial shoulder (arrows). B. Moderately advanced erosion along the radial surface, but without an apparent break in the cortex (arrows). C. There is a cystic honeycomb appearance of the subperiosteal cortex (left). The erosions extend close to the distal interphalangeal joints. Reproduced from Parfitt with permission.

appeared normal, while 29% exhibited subperiosteal erosions. In our experience, there is a danger of over reading films when using these magnification techniques; familiarity with normal variation is required (348). It should also be mentioned that more than 50% of bone can be lost without any evidence in a radiograph since only the cortical bone is clearly noted and an important loss of cancellous bone can occur before it is appreciated (345).

Radiographic features of 2°HPTH

One of the principal radiographic features of 2°HPTH is the presence of *bone resorption* and *erosions*, which may occur on the subperiosteal, intracortical, and endosteal surface of cortical bone. Another radiographic feature is the presence of new bone formation at the periosteal surface, a process termed *periosteal neostosis* (349). Alterations of the trabecular volume of spongy bone may lead to both *osteosclerosis* or *osteopenia*.

Erosions occurring in conjunction with new bone formation may take the form of cysts or *osteoclastomas (brown tumors)*, although these occur less commonly in secondary than in primary HPTH (212). They may require the differential diagnosis with malignant tumors, metastasis or cysts related to dialysis amyloidosis. Occasionally, these brown tumors are accompanied by pain which does not increase during dialysis as it occurs in amyloidosis-related cysts. Although they can appear elsewhere, brown tumors develop most frequently in the maxillary region and may alter the configuration of the teeth. Subperiosteal erosions almost invariably accompany such lesions. With healing, the cystic areas may be replaced by areas of sclerosis.

Subperiosteal erosions of the phalanges identified with the use of fine-grain radiographs of the hands are the single most sensitive radiographic sign of 2°HPTH (350).

Abnormalities have been noted on radiographs in approximately 40 to 50% of the patients who show increased resorptive surfaces on bone biopsy (347); this frequency is increased with magnification of radiographs. The appearance of bone erosions has been shown to correlate well with serum PTH levels (348). The earliest lesions usually appear on the radial surface of the middle phalanges of the second or third digits of the dominant hand; they first appear as slight irregularities near either the proximal or distal shoulder formed by the metaphysis of the phalanx (212). As the lesions progress the erosions extend along a greater length of the radial surface of the phalanx (Figure 16) and involve other digits and adjacent proximal and distal phalanges; erosions eventually appear on the ulnar border. The evolution of such lesions has been described in detail by Parfitt (212). Although such erosions are generally asymptomatic, they occasionally produce erosive synovitis, which leads to soft tissue swelling, pain, and stiffness.

The tufts of the terminal phalanges of the second or third digit commonly show areas of resorption. Because of the natural occurrence of irregularities of the tuft, recognition of loss of the cortical margin may be difficult. Nonetheless, it has been possible quantify and grade the extent of such erosions (348). When the erosion of a terminal tuft is severe, marked loss of its structure may result, leading to collapse of the soft tissues; this can change the contour of the fingers to such an extent that they appear to show clubbing ('pseudo-clubbing') (351). Healing of erosions of the tuft and phalanges is believed to occur initially with replacement of poorly mineralized fibrous tissue and woven bone. Despite successful treatment and healing, the shape of the bone may not revert to normal (352). When Al overload occurs in conjunction with the presence of significant subperiosteal erosions, remineralization and normalization of radiographs may not occur when 2°HPTH is reversed by treatment with an active vitamin D sterol or by parathyroidectomy (277). Thus, some caution must be exercised in interpreting the presence of subperiosteal erosions as specific radiologic signs of osteitis fibrosa.

Other skeletal sites commonly showing subperiosteal erosions include the upper end of the tibia, the neck of the femur and humerus, the lower end of the radius and ulna, the ischium and pubis, the sacroiliac joints, the junction of the metaphysis and diaphysis of long bones and the distal end of the clavicles (212, 313). The predilection for subperiosteal erosions to occur near the junction of the metaphysis with the shaft is believed to occur because bone modeling during growth into a normal triangular shape with typical metaphyseal flaring requires that surplus bone on the outer cortex be removed. Consequently, the precursor cells of mesenchymal origin are more prone to differentiate into osteoclasts at this site. Such areas are often the first site of subperiosteal resorption in uremic children (209). Typical resorption of the phalanges may be uncommon in very young children, but it does

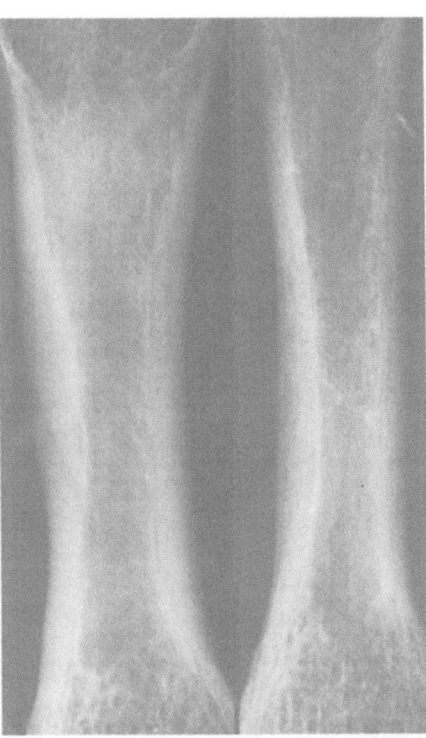

Figure 17. Left: cortical bone appears solid except for nutrients canal in the left cortex. Right: intracortical striations grade 3+ in a 30 year old female patient with end-stage renal failure.

occur in older adolescents and young adults; it is also less common in uremic patients over 40 years old (353). Resorption can be seen in the skull, leading to a mottled, lucent appearance; this is commonly associated with areas of osteosclerosis.

Erosions in the lamina dura are frequently noted in primary hyperparathyroidism, but are less commonly observed in uremic 2°HPTH (354). In the latter, increased resorption of bone also occurs in intracortical bone or in the Haversian canals and results in increased *intracortical striations* on radiographs (Figure 17). These cortical striations occur in a number of pathophysiologic processes associated with increased bone turnover: hyperthyroidism, acromegaly, and rapid growth spurt at adolescence. The striations are less specific for 2°HPTH than are subperiosteal erosions (355).

Periosteal neostosis, new woven bone arising within fibrous tissue overlying the periosteum, is separated from existing bone by a radiolucent area that represents the interposed area of fibrous tissue (349). As the process progresses, the fibrous tissue may calcify and the lucent zone disappear, and the existence of such new bone formation may be distinguished from an increased outer bone diameter.

Osteosclerosis arises because of an increase in the thickness and number of trabeculae in spongy bone. It is generally apparent only in skeletal areas composed large-ly of cancellous bone with little contribution of compact bone; these areas include the vertebrae, pelvis, skull, clavicle, proximal humerus, and proximal and distal femur and tibia. Patchy osteosclerosis may lead to a characteristic *'rugger jersey'* appearance on lateral views of the vertebrae and a *'salt and pepper'* appearance of the skull.

Radiographic alterations of the skull have been classified into four types (356): (1) a diffuse 'ground glass' appearance, with loss of sharp margins at the vascular grooves and diploic venous channels; (2) a diffuse mottled or granular appearance (the most frequent type), probably arising from a network of enlarged resorption spaces within the tables of the skull; (3) focal lucent defects, 1 to 3 cm in diameter, which may be present with or without a 'ground glass' or mottled appearance of surrounding areas; and (4) focal areas of sclerosis. The lesions may be confused with those of Paget's disease or multiple myeloma. These abnormalities of the skull may disappear after appropriate treatment (Figure 18).

Radiographic changes do not correlate well with histology (357). Such a lack of association may be related, in part, to the fact that radiographic abnormalities are most easily noted in cortical bone, while the bone biopsy primarily evaluates trabecular bone. Also, the presence of Al-related osteomalacia may prevent healing of erosions as 2°HPTH is reversed (277).

Radiographic features of osteomalacia

The radiographic features of osteomalacia are far less distinctive than those of 2°HPTH. Once the epiphyses have closed, the typical radiographic findings of rickets, i.e., widening and splaying of the epiphyseal growth plate, do not occur. The only pathognomonic finding of osteomalacia present in adults are *Looser zones* or *pseudofractures*. These are straight, wide bands of radiolucency that abuts the cortex and are usually perpendicular to the long axis of the bone; they may be bilateral and symmetrical and may or may not be accompanied by a narrow area of sclerosis or a small, poorly mineralized callus (212). Healing or callus formation is usually minimal unless specific treatment is given. The means for distinguishing a Looser zone from a stress fracture have been outlined by Parfitt (212). One important difference is that the initial hairline break of a stress fracture does not enlarge, but heals with minimal callus formation. In uremic patients spontaneous stress fractures commonly occur in the metatarsal or ribs with variable degrees of pain; these fractures tend to heal spontaneously but slowly with good callus formation. With mechanical stress or when vitamin D deficiency is very severe and prolonged, the Looser zone, like stress fractures, may extend across the full width of bone to produce a true fracture with displacement of the fragments (358). Looser zones have appeared remarkably infrequently in the authors' experience. Fewer than 2% of German dialysis patients exhibited Looser zones (359), although they were reported in 20% of uremic patients with symptomatic osteodystrophy in Australia (212). They can occur with

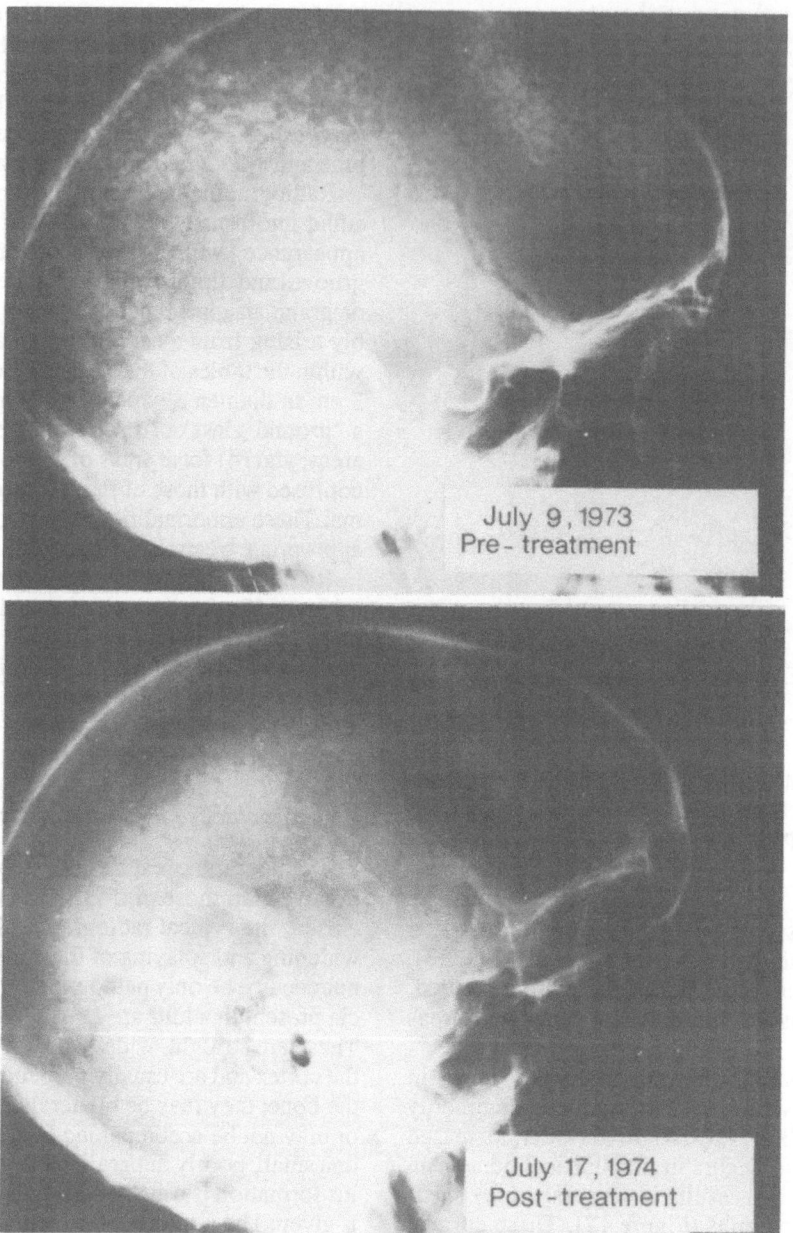

July 9, 1973
Pre-treatment

July 17, 1974
Post-treatment

Figure 18. Radiographs of the skull in a dialysis patient with overt renal osteodystrophy. The upper X-ray was taken before, and the lower after 10 months of treatment with $1,25(OH)_2D_3$.

osteomalacia due to Al accumulation, but are infrequent; true fractures may be seen more commonly. *True fractures* of the ribs and hips and compression fractures of the vertebral bodies are more common in dialyzed patients with osteomalacia than in those with osteitis fibrosa (233, 360).

Protusio acetabuli, identified as a convex bulging into the pelvis over the acetabulum, may be a specific feature of osteomalacia (361). Skeletal demineralization occurs with osteomalacia but is nonspecific. Features such as increased haziness or coarsening of the trabeculae, *biconcavity of the vertebral bodies* (particularly in association with normal bone density), and *bending deformities of long bones* are said to be typical of osteomalacia; however, few radiologists can make such distinctions (346). Uremic patients with osteomalacia may also have 2°HPTH; thus, bone erosions may coexist with osteomalacic features. In conclusion, since the features of osteomalacia are predominantly microscopic, this diagnosis can only be verified by bone histology.

Table 7. Frequency of periarticular calcification in dialysis patients

Author	Patients	Age	Calcification	
	n	(range or mean)	n	%
Rubin et al. (366)	59	54	7	12
Chou et al. (365)	68	51	5	7.5
Benhamou et al. (664)	72	56	32	44
Bardim et al. (367)	37	9	17	45
Kessler et al. (360)	171	59	33	19

Soft tissue calcification

Soft tissue calcification of several distinct types are common in patients with end-stage renal disease. The factors which predispose to their development include serum P levels greater than 8–9 mg/dl and/or an increase in the Ca×P product of plasma (greater than 70 mg), overt 2°HPTH, Al toxicity, high dialysate Ca concentration, the presence of alkalosis, and local tissue injury (362). Three major clinical varieties of extraskeletal calcification occur in uremia: (1) calcification of medium-sized arteries; (2) periarticular calcification; and (3) visceral calcification, which can involve the heart, lung, and kidney. Periarticular calcification have also been separated into three types (362): a) periarticular chondro-calcinosis, which can occur in both primary and 2°HPTH; b) calcific periarthritis, with associated calcification similar to those of typical dystrophic calcification; and c) tumoral calcinosis, which was common in early hemodialysis patients but still reported (73, 106). Periarticular calcification remain a problem in dialysis patients. Early reports from dialysis patients noted a prevalence as high as 52% (363). Though more effective control of hyperphosphatemia and 2°HPTH may have ameliorated this problem, it is still observed in 7 to 45% of hemodialysis patients (364, 365). Table 7 shows some observations in regard to the frequency of periarticular calcification. This is also a problem in CAPD patients, who have a frequency varying from 12 to 22% (366, 367). As mentioned before, tumoral or periarticular calcification may be occasionally associated with acute periarticular inflammation with pain, stiffness, and soft tissue swelling resembling acute arthritis.

The most frequent form of vascular calcification in patients with CRF is localized in the medial layer of small and medium-sized arteries (Monckeberg's type of arterial calcification); they are diffuse and continuous along the contour of the vessel wall. Involvement is most common in diabetic patients and the x-ray appearance contrasts with the dense, irregular, and discrete appearance of calcified plaques of the intimal layer of the vessel. Vascular calcification may be first detected as a 'ring' or 'tube' in the dorsalis pedis artery where it descends between the first and second metatarsal (353). Other common sites are

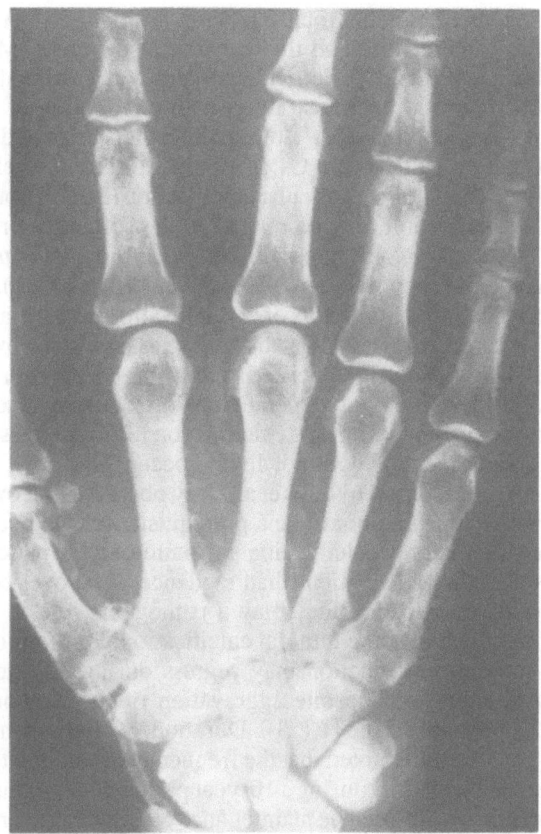

Figure 19. Radiograph showing marked calcification of the digital arteries; although intimal plaques may be present, the appearance is characteristic of extensive media calcification.

the ankles, feet, pelvis, hands, and wrists (Figure 19). Calcification of the medial layer often occur without any symptoms; however, the consequent rigidity and lack of compressibility of the vessel may make it difficult to palpate pulses or hear the Korotkov's sounds; also, vascular access for dialysis may be difficult to achieve. Vascular calcification are better detected by lateral views of the ankle or anterioposterior views of the hands or feet using magnification techniques (360). Occasionally, extensive vascular calcification are associated with ischemic lesions and calciphylaxis (202).

An evaluation of the incidence of vascular calcification suggests that they are age-related; vascular calcification were noted in 50% of dialysis patients aged 40 to 50, compared with 30% in the 15- to 30-year age group. Vascular calcification are quite uncommon but can occur in children with end-stage renal disease (369). Meema et al. documented the occurrence of calcification in 36% of uremic patients not treated with dialysis, 13% of patients who had received a renal transplant, and 8% of those undergoing hemodialysis (370).

The pathogenesis of these different types of extraskeletal calcification may vary; thus, visceral calcification can occur in patients totally lacking arterial and periarticular calcification, and the converse also occurs. Most authors agree that periarticular or tumoral calcification can be reversed by P restriction with a reduction of the Ca×P product in plasma. However, in other series of dialysis patients, the serum Ca×P product did not correlate with the extent of periarticular calcification (362). Though such calcification may be related to the solubility product of Ca and P, other possibilities exist; thus, PTH may enhance the accumulation of Ca in soft tissues (181), or poorly identified inhibitors of crystallization may be lacking. A direct role of PTH is difficult to assess, since overt 2°HPTH is usually associated with a high Ca×P product. Furthermore, though parathyroidectomy may lead to improvement of soft tissue calcification (371), regression of this calcification does not always occur (644).

In a recent report by Zins et al., they observed that overt 2°HPTH appeared not to be a prerequisite for the occurrence of tumoral calcification in hemodialysis patients (106). Eight of 10 patients had evidence of Al overload; thus, Al intoxication may play a pathogenic role in the development of some tumoral calcification. Furthermore, the tumoral calcification may regress during Al chelation therapy even despite aggravation of the concomitantly present 2°HPTH (73). Duration of dialysis may play a role; Tatler noted that the frequency of calcification increased with time during a 10-year period of hemodialysis treatment, despite the maintenance of an average serum P concentration and a Ca×P product below 70 (353). It is our strong impression that the dialysate Ca concentration may be also an important factor in the development of soft tissue calcification. During the last two decades, a dialysate Ca concentration of 3.5 mEq/l has been commonly used. The prevalence of soft tissue calcification has been shown decrease only from 68% in the period 1981–1983 to 57% (1991–1992) (372). As noted recently, the intradialytic Ca concentration dramatically increases in patients dialyzed with a 3.5 mEq/l dialysate Ca. Furthermore, the rate of Ca loss from the dialysate to the patient is very significant. The increment in serum Ca, totally disappears one hour after dialysis (Figure 20). Thus, it is quite possible that this decrement in serum Ca may represent rapid deposition of Ca into soft tissues.

Visceral calcification are rather infrequent and may differ from arterial and periarticular calcification on the basis of their chemical characteristics and pathogenesis (362); thus, visceral calcification are associated to factors such as tissue dystrophy (362). Visceral calcification exists as amorphous Ca phosphate. Usually, amorphous Ca phosphate is rapidly converted to apatite at a physiologic ph; the lack of such conversion led to the interference that increased pyrophosphate content of bone and serum might account for the occurrence of visceral calcification (163, 288). Contrary to the idea that soft tissue calcification may be associated with 2°HPTH, Contiguglia et al. noted that the degree of 2°HPTH, based on either parathyroid size at autopsy or serum Ca×P product, was not relat-

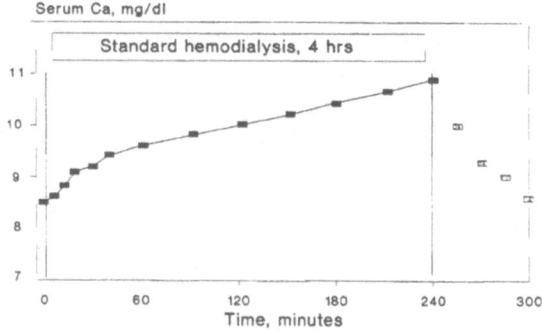

Figure 20. Intradialytic changes in serum calcium in 5 patients undergoing standard hemodialysis session of 4 hours (dialysate calcium 3.5 mEq/l). Note the increase in serum calcium and the fall to baseline values by one hour after dialysis. (From Llach et al., unpublished observations.)

ed to the extent of soft tissue calcification observed in uremic patients at autopsy (373). Kuzela et al. observed morphologic evidence of visceral calcification in 6 of 56 patients dying with CRF (374). Lungs, heart, kidneys, skeletal muscle and stomach are the mainly involved organs and visceral calcification may give rise to serious symptoms. Thus, atrioventricular block may occur on account of deposition of Ca in the cardiac conduction system; intractable cardiac failure has been related to the extensive replacement of myocardium with calcification (373). Extensive pulmonary calcification may lead to diffuse thickening of alveolar septa. Such calcification are only rarely extensive enough to be seen by radiography (375). Various alterations of pulmonary function, including reduced vital capacity, reduced carbon monoxide diffusion, and low pO_2 have been observed after death in patients subsequently shown to have severe pulmonary calcification. Such pulmonary calcification may be detected with the technetium pyrophosphate scan (376) but the disorder can often persist even after successful kidney transplantation and/or parathyroidectomy.

Finally, an increased Ca×P product may lead to increased Ca deposition in the kidney, and this may play a possible role in either accelerating or aggravating the progression of CRF (376–378). In the study of Lumlertgul et al. (378), P absorption was reduced by giving dihydroxyaluminum aminoacetate to the P-restricted rats, while the P-repleted group received glycine; the groups were pair-fed to ensure similar intakes of total calories, protein, carbohydrate, vitamins, and minerals. The tissue content of Ca in the heart, aorta, and kidneys was higher in the P-repleted than in the P-restricted group; there was more glomerular sclerosis, interstitial inflammation with fibrosis, and greater tubular atrophy in the P-repleted rats. Thus, phosphorus independent of protein restriction can retard the progression of renal insufficiency in rats following partial nephrectomy. Also, the use of a very low-P diet in partially nephrectomized rats was associated with little or no progression of renal insufficiency, whereas CRF progressed in animals receiving normal dietary levels of P (377). In clinical studies, Barsotti et al. (379) prospectively compared two groups of patients with moderate renal CRF who were placed on low-protein diets, one group receiving a low-P diet that provided P, 6.5 mg/kg/day, while the other group consumed a diet with 12 mg/kg/day of P. The rate of progression of CRF was greater in the group ingesting the higher protein intake. The provided data suggest that some benefit may be obtained in reducing P intake to decrease the rate of progression of CRF.

Osteopenia or osteoporosis

A common radiographic feature of patients with advanced CRF is decreased density of bone, which can arise from either 2°HPTH or osteomalacia and therefore is nonspecific. Parfitt et al. applied the term *dialysis osteopenia* to a syndrome characterized by a substantial reduction in bone density with an incidence of bone pain and fractures that is increased out of proportion to the radiographic and histologic evidence for either osteomalacia or osteitis fibrosa (380). The radiographic findings have been likened to those noted in the idiopathic osteoporosis of young adults. Features include loss of cortical bone from the endosteal surface, periarticular rarefaction, loss of trabecular bone with a honeycomb or fishnet pattern, and fractures that are somewhat intermediate in appearance between stress fractures and the typical Looser zones. Unfortunately, detailed biochemical and histologic studies with radiologic correlations in patients described two decades ago with this syndrome are not available; it is most likely that it represents the radiologic counterpart of Al-related bone disease with osteomalacia or adynamic bone disease.

Dialysis-related amyloidosis

Radiologic findings of dialysis-related amyloidosis are usually present before the onset of pain. A periarticular cystic bone lesion located in sites such as carpal and tarsal bones, femoral head, humeral head, distal radius, acetabula, pubic symphysis, and tibial plateau, strongly suggests dialysis-related amyloidosis (338, 381). Although these lesions can be characteristic, they are not pathognomonic and it is necessary to demonstrate the presence of β_2-amyloid deposit (382).

As mentioned before, brown-tumors should be distinguished from amyloid-related cysts; the former usually appear in the metaphysis and epiphysis of tubular bones and rarely are located in carpal bones. The amyloid-related cysts involve large joints and are restricted to the vicinity of synovial joints, without correlation with subperiosteal resorption. Thus, the occurrence of subchondral cysts appear to be specific of dialysis related amyloidosis (383). The presence of multiple rather than solitary cysts also suggests amyloid deposition. Fractures can develop in bones weakened by such cysts (180, 335). Also, bone cysts have been shown to persist even after successful kidney transplantation (384). Magnetic resonance imaging seems to be a well suited technique to show the extent and distribution of articular disease (395), including the upper cervical spine (386). Finally, ultrasonography has been shown to be helpful in the diagnosis of this disorder (see below) (387).

SCINTISCAN AND ULTRASONOGRAPHY

Skeletal scintigraphy using ^{99m}Tc pyrophosphate provides a sensitive method for the detection of skeletal alterations in patients with CRF. The technique allows for a noninvasive follow-up evaluation of the response to treatment. Although the mechanism responsible for the accumulation of pyrophosphate in bone has not been elucidated, evidence indicates that the pyrophosphate accumulates in areas of increased bone turnover (388). Rosenthal and Kaye suggested that pyrophosphate accumulates in skeletal areas with abnormal collagen metabolism, including either osteitis fibrosa or osteomalacia (389). From evaluation of the uptake of the isotopes over the distal femur, Lien et al. calculated the bone/soft tissue ratio of isotope uptake (390). Abnormal uptake was found in 78% of long-term dialysis patients and in a similar proportion of patients with chronic CRF who were not undergoing regular dialysis. On the basis of correlation between bone uptake of ^{99m}Tc pyrophosphate and urinary excretion of hydroxyproline, the authors concluded that increased skeletal uptake in uremia is related to the presence of immature collagen (390). Others have noted abnormal scintiscan in 13 of 14 patients undergoing dialysis (391). Symmetrically increased activity was noted over the skull, mandible, sternum, shoulders, vertebrae, and distal aspects of the femur and tibia. Uptake of the labeled pyrophosphate over certain areas, such as the mandible, was pronounced and appeared before radiographic abnormalities. Olgaard et al. noted that 90% of patients undergoing regular dialysis had pathologic pyrophosphate accumulation on scintigram, while radiographic abnormalities were present in only one-third (Figure 21) (392). The scintiscan can also be used to detect soft tissue calcification, particularly in the lungs (376). Finally, abnormal scintigram are more common in dialysis patients who previously received renal homograft; intensive glucocorticoid treatment may aggravate the abnormalities responsible for an abnormal scintiscan.

In the presence of low-turnover bone disease, bone scintiscan may reveal increased uptake at sites of either true fractures or pseudofractures, particularly the ribs, pelvis, and scapulae; these may be seen on scintiscan at a time when they cannot be detected by radiography (177). In general, however, pyrophosphate uptake is usually less in patients with Al-related osteomalacia than in those with osteitis fibrosa; the uptake may increase strikingly during chelation therapy. Thus, it is possible to differentiate between patients with osteitis fibrosa and osteomalacia from Al intoxication by the uptake of a bone scan (393).

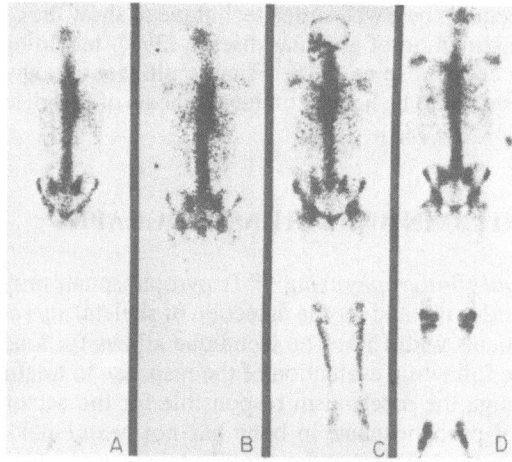

Figure 21. Skeletal scintigrams in a normal subject and patients with renal failure. A. Grade 0, normal scintigram; B. Grade 1, scintigram showing abnormal uptake in the femoral heads with an extension to the femoral neck and trochanteric region; C. Grade 2, scintigram showing abnormal uptake in the femoral head and neck and in the proximal half of the tibial shaft; D. Grade 3, scintigram showing extensive uptake in the femoral head and marked uptake in femoral and tibial condyles the tarsus and the proximal part of the metatarsus. Reproduced from Ølgaard et al. with permission of the publisher.)

However, patients with mixed lesions on biopsy specimens may be difficult to identify. Other authors noted that bone scans do not agree closely with the type or severity of renal osteodystrophy (394). Timing the hemodialysis sessions before scintigraphic imaging has been suggested to be helpful, since they seem to reduce unspecific high soft-tissue activity and thereby allowing bone uptake to be assessed more accurately (395). It appears that although bone scintiscan may help to establish the severity and/or type of bone disease in some patients, at present this technique is of limited value in the clinical evaluation of skeletal abnormalities in CRF.

Substraction ^{201}Tl-^{99m}Tc scintigraphy has been suggested as a valuable technique in the diagnosis of the localization of enlarged parathyroid glands. Thallium is a potassium analog and distributes in relationship to blood flow and state of the Na-K-atpase system (396). Both thyroid and parathyroid glands exhibit increased uptake of thallium relative to the surrounding tissue. By contrast, technetium is taken up only by the thyroid; thus, an image of the parathyroid gland can be obtained by subtracting the technetium from the thallium image. Substraction ^{201}Tl-^{99m}Tc scintigraphy is most useful prior to reoperation in patients with a failed initial surgery since the scan might aid in locating an ectopic gland or an abnormal gland in a patient with surgically altered anatomy (396). Scintigraphy with ^{201}Tl-^{131}I or ^{201}Tl-^{123}I can also be used to locate abnormal parathyroid glands with an efficacy at least similar than that with ^{201}Tl-^{99m}Tc (397).

Other scintigraphic techniques have been recently developed as noninvasive procedures to assess bone pathology in dialysis patients. Thus, it has been noted that serum PTH and the severity of subperiosteal resorption correlated with the ^{51}Cr-EDTA/^{99m}Tc-MAP ratio (398). EDTA and MAP are handled identically by the body except that the latter is taken up by osteoblasts; thus a low ratio indicates increased osteoblastic activity.

Finally, a radiodiagnostic test using serum amyloid P component labelled with ^{123}I has been shown to detect the amyloid fibrils ligand for this protein (399). Similarly, a ^{131}I-β_2-microglobulin has also been developed to assist the diagnosis of dialysis-related amyloidosis (400). The relative value of these techniques needs further evaluation (395).

Ultrasonography has been suggested as an useful non-invasive method in evaluating the size of the parathyroid glands in 2°HPTH. Patients with enlarged glands had a higher frequency of radiologic features of 2°HPTH as compared with those with undetected glands. Bone and joint pains and higher levels of serum alkaline phosphatase and intact PTH have also been noted in these patients (401). Ultrasonography has also been used to monitor the treatment of 2°HPTH with calcitriol; thus a decrease of the size of the glands has been reported after calcitriol therapy (402). Preliminary data also suggest that ultrasonography may be useful in the recognition and localization of graft-dependent recurrent 2°HPTH (403). However, there is not experience with this technique in the diagnosis 2°HPTH to reach a final conclusion. Ultrasonography has been also valuable in the diagnosis of Dialysis-related Amyloidosis; thus, it can detect and quantify the swelling of articular and periarticular soft tissue such as joint capsules, synovia and tendons usually seen in this disease (387, 404). In a recent study using high-resolution ultrasound of the shoulder, the presence of rotator cuffs greater than 8 mm in thickness and/or echogenic pads between muscle groups of the rotator cuff had a sensitivity of 72% and a specificity of 97% in the diagnosis of dialysis-related amyloidosis (387).

QUANTITATIVE MEASUREMENTS OF BONE MINERAL CONTENT

Metacarpal index

The metacarpal index can be obtained by measuring the dimensions of the cortex of a metacarpal bone on x-ray film using magnification and a special caliper (405). Normal data are available for the second left metacarpal, and the metacarpal index is the ratio of cortical to total bone width. On the basis of the assumption that this bone is a perfect cylinder, the ratio of cross-sectional cortical area to total cross section can be calculated (406). The metacarpal index has been validated by direct comparison to measurement of bone ash (407). Observations in patients with primary HPTH have suggested that total bone area is increased while the cortical area is reduced (408). In patients with CRF not treated with dialysis, the metacarpal index was found to be reduced in 20 to 40% (347, 355). One study suggested that the metacarpal index progressively decreases with duration of dialysis (409). Sugisaki et al., monitoring the metacarpal index, performed long-term observations over nine years in 44 hemodialysis patients in order to assess the combined effects of changes in therapeutic modality over this period of time (410). They observed that from 1980 to 1984, bone mineral content deteriorated significantly, but it improved from 1984 onwards. The combined effect of bicarbonate dialysate, the use of active derivatives of vitamin D and removal of aluminum are suggested explanations.

Photon absorptiometry

Another noninvasive method for the serial evaluation of the skeleton is *single photon absorptiometry* (411), in which the absorption of photons emitted from an isotopic source is used to assess the mineral content of bone. The isotopes employed, e.g., ^{125}I or ^{241}Am, emit photons of specific, narrow wave lengths and low energy (412). Such measurements are taken over the phalanges, the radius and ulna, and the femur. Hah et al. measured both the distal radius, which comprises primarily trabecular bone, and the midshaft of the radius, which represents compact bone; this has enabled them to evaluate the ratio of these two types of bone, which have different turnover rates (413). Griffith et al. noted the mineral content of the mid-radius and ulna to be lower in dialysis patients than in age-matched controls, they also observed a progressive loss of bone with increasing duration of dialysis treatment (414). In a subsequent study they reported that most women on dialysis maintained a stable bone mineral content, whereas 44% of males lost bone mass (415). No significant correlation was recently noted between single photon absortiometry scores and histomorphometric parameters (151).

Photon absorptiometry appears to be more accurate than the methods that measure bone density from radiographs; however, the measurements are limited to certain sites of the skeleton that primarily comprise cortical bone. It should be noted that bone mineral content can be reduced as a result of several causes: (1) primary reduction in volume of bone tissue, (2) increase in intracortical porosity as a consequence of enlarged Haversian canals, or (3) replacement of normally mineralized bone by unmineralized osteoid or poorly mineralized woven bone (212). The measurement of bone density by photon absorptiometry does not allow distinction between these causes; the technique is best used when serial measurements are obtained for quantifying bone mineral and the results are evaluated in conjunction with findings on fine-detail radiographs.

Dual-beam photon absorptiometry uses two separate isotopes or a dual photon source (gadolinium–153), permitting the subtraction of overlying soft tissue mass from that of bone. The technique can thus be used to measure the mineral content of sites of the skeleton lying deep within tissues; it is useful for assessing the mineral content of vertebral bodies and the femoral neck (416). With the advent of *dual energy x-ray bone absorptiometry*, a more precise and complete evaluation of bone mineral content can be obtained. Instead of a radioactive source of energy it uses x-rays at two energy levels. Preliminary observations with this more advanced technique suggest that it may be valuable in the follow-up of dialysis patients with bone disease rather than diagnosis (417). However, the presence of normal bone density by noninvasive techniques does not exclude the presence of bone disease (157).

Neutron activation

Neutron activation provides a more accurate method for measuring total Ca or bone mineral content either in the entire body or in isolated parts of the skeleton. This technique requires the availability of a neutron source in order to activate Ca and other elements in the skeleton, and an immediate access to a whole-body counter to measure the short-lived radionuclides. This technique has proved useful mainly in research studies of bone mineral content in uremic patients, and it may be particularly useful when serial measurements are used to evaluate the effects of a specific treatment modality (418).

Quantitative computed tomography

Computed tomography has been applied to measure the mineral content of the vertebral bodies (156, 419). Several computed tomography cuts of vertebra are compared with a standard. It is of value in conditions, such as osteoporosis, that primarily affect the trabecular bone and axial skeleton. It has also the theoretical advantage that is less affected by volume than dual photon absortiometry or the newest dual energy x-ray bone absorptiometry (420) but it gives a high radiation dose. It has not been applied widely to renal osteodystrophy but, recently, no significant correlation was noted between quantitative computed tomography and histomorphometric parameters (156).

HISTOLOGIC FEATURES OF BONE

Techniques for bone biopsy

The study of bone itself has evolved into a clinically useful tool for understanding the pathophysiologic processes involved and as a guide to the management of renal osteodystrophy. Under local anesthesia, a bone biopsy can easily and safely be obtained from the iliac crest. The sample, 5 × 20 mm, containing trabecular bone and both tables of cortices (421) is fixed in neutral formalin, then transferred to alcohol to prevent Ca loss, and embedded in a hard plastic, such as methacrylate. Thin sections of the undecalcified bone can be cut with a special micro-tome having a heavy steel blade. Uncalcified osteoid and calcified bone can be readily identified with such methods, unlike the specimen of bone prepared with the usual decalcification.

In addition to the qualitative interpretation of bone histology, quantification of various features and bone dynamics with tetracycline labeling can increase the sensitivity of the method and aid in comparison of biopsy samples. One method utilizes a grid eye-piece placed in the microscope (71); the surfaces of trabecular bone which intersect the grid markings are identified as forming (i.e., with osteoblasts and osteoid), resorbing (with osteoclasts and Howship's lacunae) or resting (bone surface without cellular activity). With another method, the microscopic image of bone is projected on a screen and each specific type of bone surface is traced with an electrical pencil attached to a computer and X-Y plotter (71). Quantitation of the surfaces occupied by active resorption, formation, or by inactive bone can provide static information but they may not provide data on the dynamics of bone formation, mineralization or resorption. Errors in static data may occur if the rate of metabolic activity varies (421); thus, the forming and resorbing surfaces could be twice normal, and yet skeletal dynamics can be normal if the activity of the osteoclasts and osteoblasts is reduced to half of normal. To obviate this problem, tetracycline, a fluorescent marker, which is rapidly incorporated into newly forming bone, is given on two separate occasions; this permits a measure of bone formation rate (72). In practice, the dynamics of trabecular bone are assessed after giving two separate doses of tetracycline, with the 'bone formation rate' quantitated as the distance between the two lines of fluorescence divided by the time between doses. The dynamics of trabecular bone turnover differ from those of cortical bone, which is organized into units called osteons, which surround a Haversian canal. Cortical bone turnover involves sequential osteoclastic resorption within the Haversian canal; this is followed by osteoblastic formation; also the numerous osteocytes, which are buried within the osteon, can participate in bone resorption through a 'osteocytic osteolysis'.

Osteitis fibrosa

Osteitis fibrosa, which presumably arises due to the high levels of PTH, is characterized by increased bone resorption and formation with a progressive increase in peritrabecular fibrosis (Figure 22A). A greater fraction of trabecular bone surface is occupied by resorption cavities filled with osteoclasts (Howship's lacunae); also, increased numbers of osteoblasts overlie the newly formed unmineralized matrix. As this process becomes severe, the narrow space is filled with fibrous tissue, creating typical 'osteitis fibrosa' (422). Double tetracycline labeling often reveals normal or increased bone turnover in patients with osteitis fibrosa (Figure 22B) (423).

Another feature of osteitis fibrosa is the alignment of collagen strands in an irregular, haphazard 'woven' pattern; this contrasts to the normal parallel alignment of strands of collagen in a lamellar manner. This disorganized structure of collagen in 'woven' bone may lead to defective physical properties of bone in response to stress, and a greater amount of inferior, 'woven bone' may be required to maintain mechanical stability (422). Also, increased mineralization of large quantities of 'woven bone' may contribute to the osteosclerosis seen in uremia.

Osteomalacia

Osteomalacia is characterized by an excess of unmineralized osteoid tissue; this arises from impaired mineralization of the protein matrix of bone. The major feature of osteomalacia is an increase in the width of unmineralized osteoid (Figure 22C). This is also found, to a certain extent, in osteitis fibrosa due to the delay of osteoid mineralization which is formed so rapidly. Therefore, the use of tetracycline labeling to identify impaired mineralization rate is useful in the identification of osteomalacia (Figure 22D). Nonetheless, the criteria employed in the recognition of osteomalacia include: 1) the measurement of the width of osteoid seams; 2) the specific number of osteoid lamellae in these seams; 3) the extent to which bone surface is covered with osteoid; 4) the volume of osteoid expressed as a fraction of total bone surface; and 5) a delayed rate of mineralization by tetracycline labeling (423).

The frequency of osteomalacia appears to have a marked geographic variation. Osteomalacia was initially noted in patients receiving maintenance dialysis (205, 206). Recently, osteomalacia has been observed in patients prior to the initiation of dialysis (52, 60). Epidemiologic evidence has implicated the presence of Al in the water since the incidence of osteomalacia is increased greatly in areas of high Al water content (97). Pretreatment oaf the water with reverse osmosis has decreased the incidence of osteomalacia (115). With the advent of the Maloney stain for Al, it has been shown that the great majority of osteomalacic dialysis patients have large deposits of Al in the bone (88). The characteristic pattern is a linear deposition of Al along the interface between trabecular bone and osteoid (99). The degree of osteomalacia has correlated closely with bone Al content, whether biochemically or histologically analyzed (98).

Aplastic (or adynamic) bone disease

Another type of bone lesion observed in dialysis patients is aplastic bone disease (148). This entity most likely is the result of Al toxicity. It is characterized by features similar to those of osteomalacia; the major difference is the absence of large osteoid seams. These patients also have a deficiency of cellular activity and absence of endosteal fibrosis; aluminum deposits are present both at the osteoid-bone interface and on the surface of trabecular bone. It seems that Al may be toxic to bone by simultaneously affecting bone formation and remodeling. While, aplastic bone disease may be a variant of osteomalacia; both are caused by Al accumulation. As mentioned previously, in the absence of PTH, Al toxicity may be more likely to result in aplastic bone disease rather than osteomalacia (153).

Mixed skeletal lesion

Another sub-group of patients exhibits wide osteoid seams combined with typical features of osteitis fibrosa. Such skeletal lesions are somewhat more common in young patients, in those with hypocalcemia, and in patients who have not undergone dialysis or treatment with vitamin D (424). These histologic features may be characteristic of vitamin D-deficiency itself, with components of both secondary hyperparathyroidism, which commonly occurs with vitamin D deficiency, and osteomalacia. Serum iPTH levels are significantly elevated in these patients (7).

There is disagreement as to whether dialysis treatment can lead to specific qualitative differences in skeletal disease or whether dialysis merely prolongs the lives of patients with end-stage uremia, thereby exposing them to the various pathogenic factors for a longer period of time. Certain incriminating factors unique to dialysis patients are administration of heparin, exposure to fluoridated water, exposure to high concentrations of acetate, periodic removal of bicarbonate, exposure to varying concentrations of Ca and Mg in dialysate, and the presence of Al, trace elements, and other substances in dialysate.

PREVENTION AND MANAGEMENT

The general objectives of management in dialysis patients are to suppress secondary hyperparathyroidism, produce normal mineralization, maintain normal concentration of Ca, Mg and P, prevent extaosseous calcification, and avoid aluminum toxicity. Therapeutic considerations will be classified as general management which apply to all dialysis patients and specific treatment from problems arising in certain patients.

General management

The management of altered divalent ion metabolism and osteodystrophy in patients with CRF is directed towards correcting the pathogenic factors already discussed. As such, important objectives in the clinical management of patients with renal osteodystrophy include: 1) maintenance of Ca and P as normal as possible; 2) to prevent the development of parathyroid hyperplasia or, if it has already occurred, to suppress parathyroid secretion and to reduce hyperplasia; 3) to avoid the exposure to toxic agents such as Al, iron or excess fluoride; 4) to restore the skeleton to near normal as possible; 5) to prevent and reverse extraskeletal calcification; and 6) to avoid the hazards inherent to the different treatment modalities.

The intensity of treatment and the specific treatment modality must vary depending on the stage of renal insufficiency, the presence or absence of overt bone disease, and whether regular dialysis has been initiated.

Control of hyperphosphatemia

Factors which contributes to hyperphosphatemia in dialysis patients are noted in Table 5. As already discussed, both phosphorus retention and hyperphosphatemia are major factors responsible for the development and maintenance of °HPTH in CRF. The high serum P is also an important factor in causing soft tissue calcification. Therefore, the goal of therapy must be to reduce serum P levels to normal or near normal as possible. In dialysis patients, predialysis serum P levels should be ideally maintained between 4.0 and 5.5 mg/dl.

The available options for reducing the P burden include: 1) reducing the intake of dietary P; 2) preventing the absorption of P with phosphate-binding agents; and 3) enhancing the removal of P from the body through more efficient dialysis in patients undergoing maintenance dialysis. Moreover, it is possible that with the improvement of 2°HPTH associated with P restriction, the control of hyperphosphatemia may become subsequently easier since the P efflux from bone decreases when PTH levels are lower. Conversely, compliant patients can show severe hyperphosphatemia which may be directly related to overt 2°HPTH.

$\longrightarrow$

Figure 22. A. A representative bone biopsy from a patient with osteitis fibrosa. Distinctive features include large multinucleated osteoclasts located in a resorption cavity; osteoid covered with multiple columnar osteoblasts (orange color) and marked endosteal fibrosis (Goldner stain × 200); B. Unstained section of a bone biopsy of a patient with osteitis fibrosa after double tetracycline label. Note the presence of active mineralization and bone formation as evidenced by the uptake of tetracycline and the presence of a double label (yellow bands). The lack of well demarcated label lines demonstrates a disorganized and abnormal mineralization (× 200); C. A representative bone biopsy from a patient with osteomalacia. Characteristic features include broad osteoid seams (red color), lack of cellular activity, irregular scalloped interface between osteoid and mineralized bone (green color) and the absence of marrow fibrosis (Goldner stain × 200); D. Unstained section of a patient with osteomalacia after double tetracycline label. Note the marked decrease in tetracycline uptake evidencing the lack of mineralization. The osteoid seams appear as a lighter shade of green than the mineralized bone (× 200).

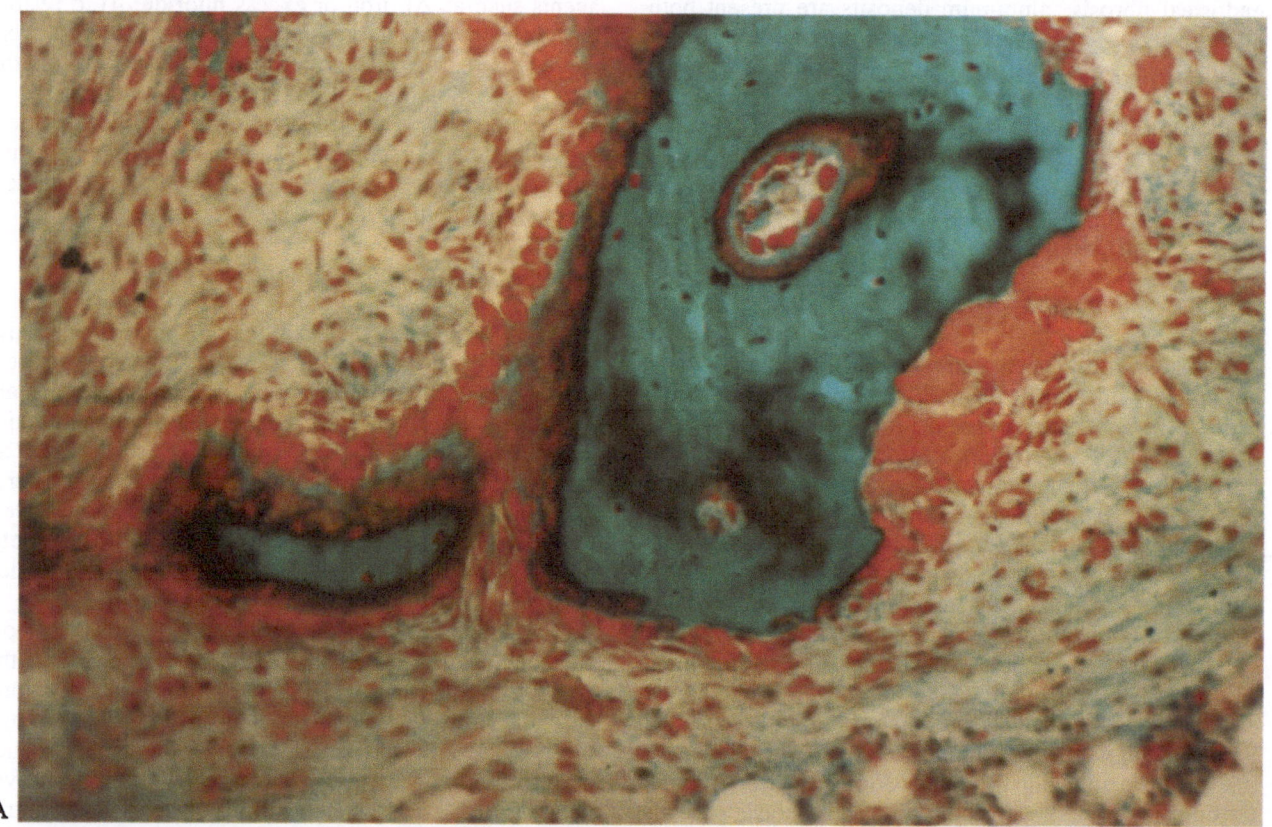

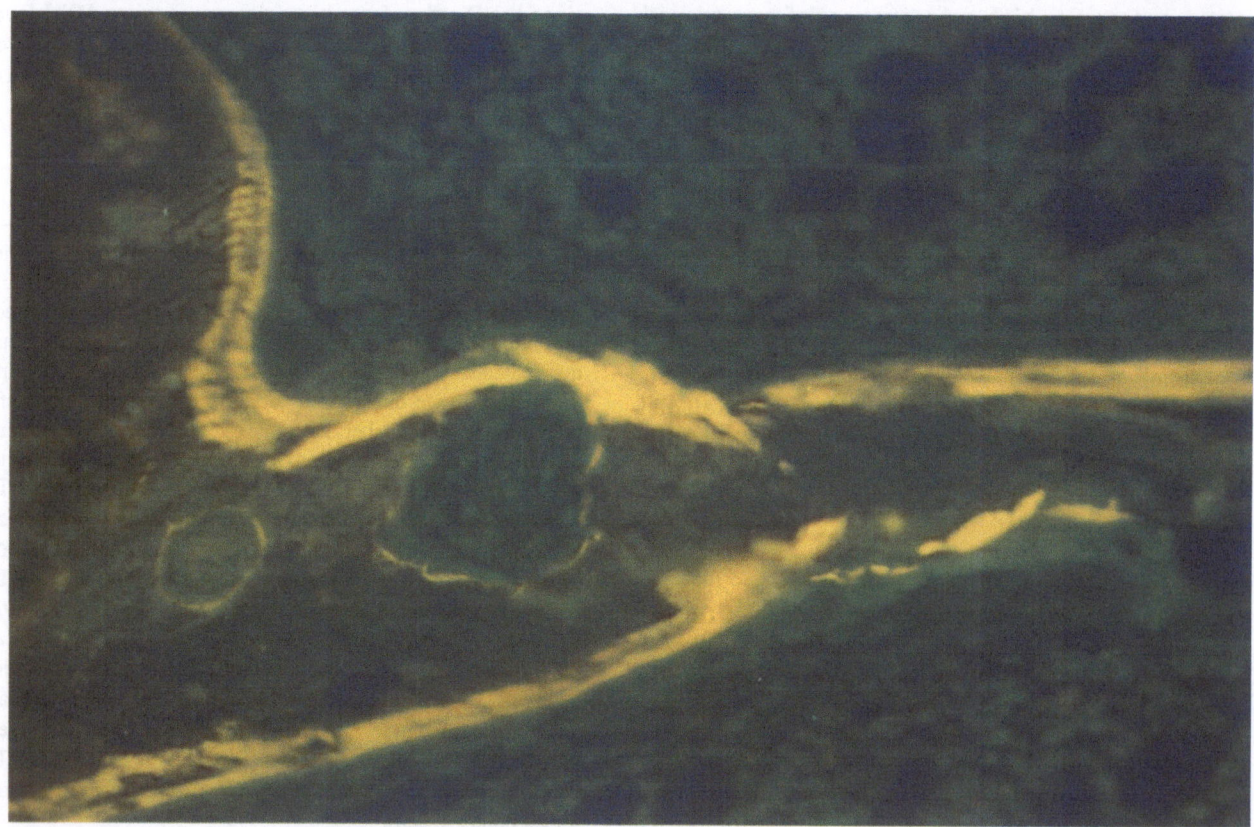

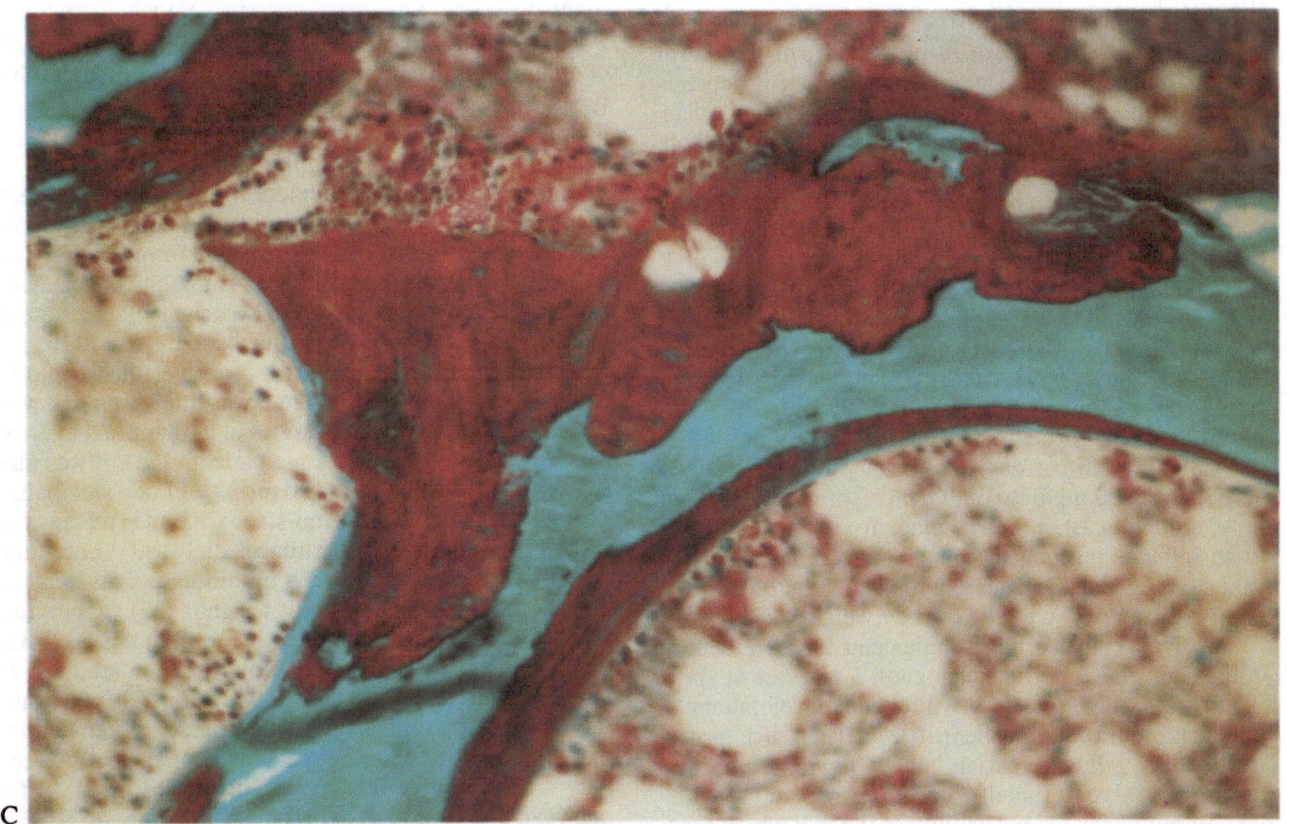

C

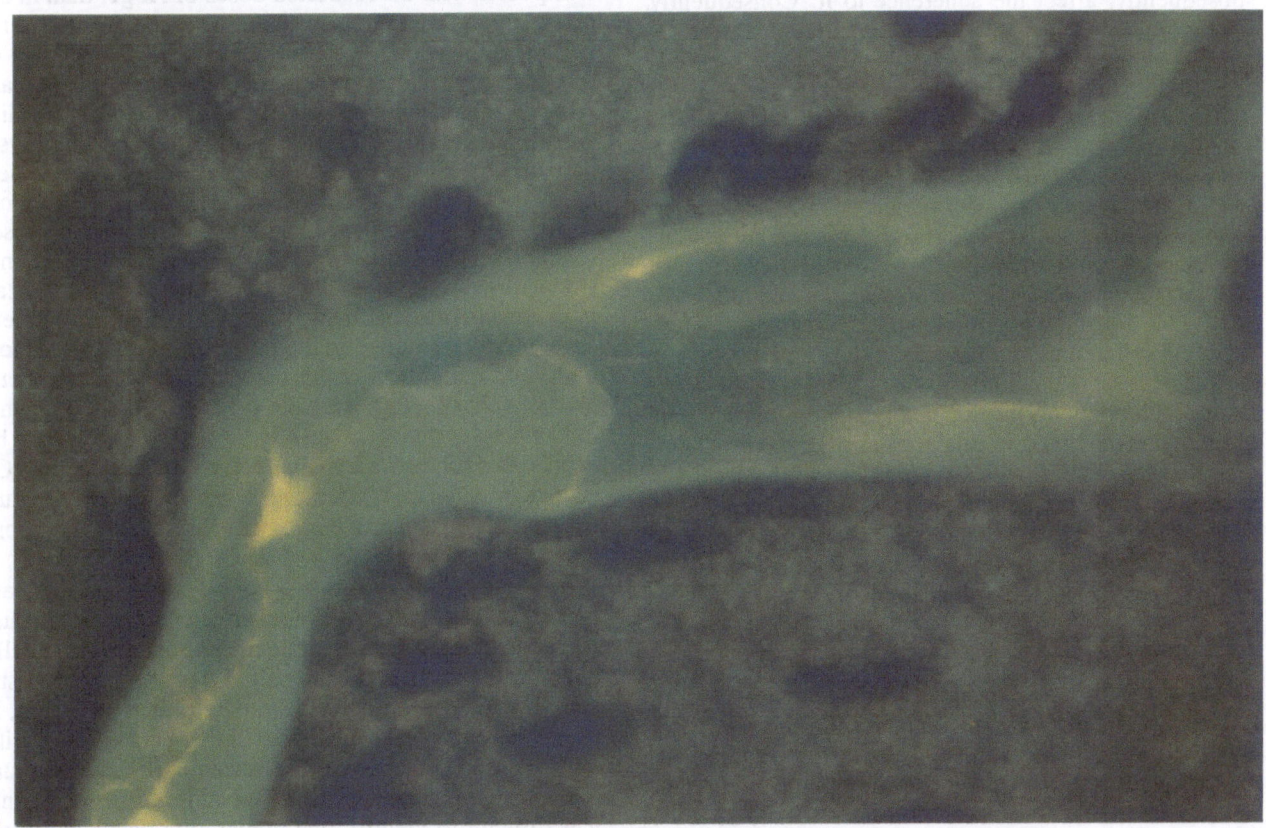

D

Dietary phosphorus restriction

Dietary P restriction is the main and first step in the control of hyperphosphatemia. The dietary intake of P depends primarily on consumption of meat and dairy products. Poultry, fish, most soft drinks (especially colas), whole grain breads and cereals, nuts and legumes are also foods especially high in P content. The usual intake of P by normal adults in the United States varies between 1 and 1.8 g/day (425). Theoretically, the dietary intake of P could be reduced in proportion to the decrease in GFR in patients with mild CRF. With elimination of dairy products and limitation to 40 g of protein per day, the dietary intake of P ranged from 650 to 1000 mg/day – a quantity that is approximately 60% of normal intake (426). With a more restricted protein diet (e.g., 20 g of high biological value protein per day), the dietary P intake ranged from 450 to 700 mg/day. With the preparation of special diets, utilizing pasta products made from starch and egg white and with prolonged boiling and washing of certain foods to remove P, Barsotti et al. lowered the P intake to 350 to 450 mg/day (6 mg/kg of body weight) (379). With a diet of vegetable origin supplemented with essential aminoacids and their ketoanalogues, Lafage et al. provided 3 to 5 mg/kg/day of P without the development of malnutrition in uremic patients (427). Thus, it is possible to reduce P intake substantially by modifying dietary intake, but this is difficult to achieve in practice without compromising the palatability of the diet which may, subsequently, affect the adherence to it. Consequently, restriction of dietary P intake in proportion to the decrease in GFR as the sole measure to avoid P retention is only feasible in patients with moderate CRF.

When patients enter onto maintenance dialysis and are prescribed diets with greater protein intake, the P intake also rises. The National Cooperative Dialysis Study (NCDS) suggested that with commencement of dialytic therapy, patients should ingest a diet containing at least 0.8 g/kg/day of protein (428). The average dietary intake of P in 162 hemodialysis patients who entered this study was 879 ± 248 mg/day. Although metabolic balance studies suggest that a minimum protein intake of 1 g/kg/day is necessary to maintain positive nitrogen balance, studies in CAPD patients noted a nearly neutral balance with a 1 g/kg/day of protein intake, and a positive balance was always achieved with 1.4 g/kg/day (429). Moreover, with a protein intake of 1 g/kg/day, the measured P intake ranged from 920 to 1200 mg/day, and when dietary protein was increased to 1.4 g/kg/day, the P intake was 1700 to 2400 mg/day.

Phosphorus-binding agents

Because it is difficult to achieve adequate dietary restriction of P, particularly in dialysis patients ingesting appropriate dietary protein, P-binding agents are required by most patients with end-stage CRF and by many patients with advanced CRF when the GFR decreases to 25–30% of normal (31) Phosphorus-binding agents lower intestinal P absorption by creating poorly soluble complexes of P in the intestinal tract. They can be mainly divided in Al-containing and Ca-containing P binders, although other types are also used.

Aluminum-containing phosphorus binders

Aluminum-containing P binders were the standard treatment prescribed for patients with end-stage CRF prior to 1985, then the risk of Al toxicity from oral Al was appreciated. As discussed earlier, Al toxicity is especially important in high risk conditions, such as diabetes, postparathyroidectomy and adynamic bone disease (430).

Are there any safe quantities of Al gels that could be used? It was suggested that there was little or no risk with the ingestion of up to six capsules or tablets of Al hydroxide per day in the adult uremic patient (126). It was also suggested that doses below 30 mg/kg of body weight had little risk in children with end-stage CRF (431). However, in children undergoing peritoneal dialysis, Al accumulation was noted even though the dosage of Al gels did not exceed 30 mg/kg of body weight (432). A progressive increase of mean plasma Al from 22 to 59 μg/l was observed in the children and young adults assigned to Al hydroxide, compared to a significant fall of plasma Al in the patients ingesting Ca carbonate. Moreover, one patient developed histologic evidence of skeletal Al toxicity after receiving this supposedly low dose of Al for one year. The control of hyperphosphatemia and 2°HPTH was poorer with the restricted doses of Al gel than in the group on Ca carbonate. Jenkins et al. noted, in adults limited to 6 tablets of Al hydroxide per day or 30 ml/day of a liquid suspension (maximum, 2.85 g/day), significant Al staining on bone biopsies in 2 of 16 adult hemodialyzed patients (433). Thus, a certain fraction of dialysis patients who ingest Al hydroxide, even in modest doses, may develop clinical evidence of Al toxicity. Larger doses are generally required in adult patients; thus the doses required to prevent serum P from rising in the National Cooperative Dialysis Study ranged from 3.5 to 4.9 g/day in the two major treatment groups with dialysis treatment schedules that resulted in the best survival and least morbidity (434). For the reasons noted above, we recommend that Al gels should not be the primary P-binding agents prescribed for patients with CRF. Aluminum gels may be needed in patients with side effects to Ca carbonate or Ca acetate or when a Ca salt alone is not effective. The latter patients often require a combination of either Ca carbonate or Ca acetate with an Al-based P binder (279).

When Al gels are needed, considerable data indicate that capsules or tablets are less effective than liquid suspensions (435); however, patient compliance is generally better with capsules than with the liquid forms. Constipation, which commonly accompanies their ingestion, is the most troublesome side effect limiting compliance with these agents. Because of wide variation in the individual patient's preference and 'taste' for different preparations, it is difficult to identify one preparation that satisfies all patients. Hence, efforts should be made to find a specific preparation that is suitable for each patient. Nevertheless, if Al-containing P binders need to be given, doses must be kept as low as possible, the duration of the treatment limited, the concurrent administration of citrate salts/citric acid discontinued and plasma Al levels monitored at regular intervals.

Calcium-containing phosphorus binders
It was known many years ago that large doses of Ca carbonate were effective in reducing the absorption of P from the gastrointestinal tract (436). A number of clinical studies have subsequently shown that Ca carbonate is an effective P-binding agent (437, 438). However, Ca carbonate had side effects such as hypercalcemia and gastrointestinal symptoms such as constipation, diarrhea (less common), changes in bowel habits, vague abdominal discomfort and dyspepsia. Occasionally these symptoms are so profound that patients have difficulty complying with the prescribed dosages. The long-term side effects of Ca-containing P binders are unknown; nevertheless, no difference in the incidence or extent of progression of extraskeletal calcification was noted in adult patients treated with Ca-containing P binders for as long as two or three years (439, 440).

Episodes of hypercalcemia have occurred in a substantial fraction of patients; (279) occasionally the hypercalcemia is severe enough to cause symptoms that require the withdrawal of the Ca salt. When ionized serum Ca was measured serially in dialysis patients started on Ca carbonate, the mean level increased significantly (441). In the United States many patients still undergo dialysis with a dialysate Ca of 3.0 to 3.5 mEq/l, and a positive balance for Ca is induced by dialysis with a dialysate Ca of 3.0 mEq/l or higher (442). Because of the development of hypercalcemia, the dialysate Ca has been reduced as Ca carbonate is widely used as a P binder (443, 444). Thus, dialysate Ca was lowered from 3.5 to 2.5 mEq/l (437) in a group of dialysis patients receiving 1.5 to 18 g/day of Ca carbonate; hyperphosphatemia was successfully managed, and the incidence of hypercalcemia was substantially reduced compared with an historical group receiving Ca carbonate and a dialysate Ca of 3.5 mEq/l. Sawyer et al. (443) utilized a stepwise reduction in dialysate Ca based on the serum ionized Ca when they initiated therapy with Ca carbonate; they lowered the dialysate Ca first to 2.7 mEq/l, and then, if necessary, to 2.1 mEq/l. In a large group of hemodialysis patients, they avoided hypercalcemia, achieved adequate P control, and noted a significant fall in intact PTH levels. In general, Ca carbonate has proven effective as the sole P-binder in 70–90% of adult and pediatric dialysis patients. However, others have observed only 50% of dialysis patients attaining adequate control of serum P levels when Ca carbonate was used as the sole P binder (445).

Calcium carbonate has been used together with severe dietary P restriction in the treatment of renal osteodystrophy. Thus, Lafage et al. (427) evaluated in patients with GFR $\leq$ 20 ml/min the efficacy of a very low-protein diet (0.3 g protein/kg body weight/day) supplemented with essential aminoacids, their ketoanalogues and 1 g of Ca carbonate – without pharmacological doses of vitamin D or physiological doses of 1α-hydroxylated derivatives – for a year. Despite the progression of CRF, they observed that P and PTH levels decreased significantly and low plasma bicarbonate returned to normal. Moreover, bone biopsies performed before and after one year showed an improvement of histodynamic parameters of osteitis fibrosa. In 5 of 9 patients histological changes were not different than normal and bone improved in the other 4 patients. Furthermore, in four patients with mixed osteodystrophy, the osteomalacic component was cured while the component of 2°HPTH was cured in two and improved in the remaining two. Only a noncompliant patient developed severe osteitis fibrosa during the follow-up.

Finally, it should be emphasized that although the ingestion of Ca salts can reduce the blood level of P, in patients with severe hyperphosphatemia the use of Ca-containing P binders must be avoided because the Ca×P product can increase above 70, predisposing to soft tissue calcification. In such patients, Al-containing P binders should be used first to lower the plasma P to a safer level (e.g., < 5.5–6 mg/dl) before Ca salts are initiated. The administration of large quantities of oral Ca should also be given cautiously when serum Ca is in the upper range of normal and vitamin D analogs are given. Under such circumstances, it is wise to use a dialysate Ca of 2.5 mEq/l to reduce the risk of hypercalcemia.

Quantitation and comparison of phosphorus-binders
Calcium carbonate contains 40% of elemental Ca, Ca acetate 25%, Ca lactate contains 12% and Ca gluconate 8%. Calcium chloride should be avoided in uremic patients because it causes metabolic acidosis.

Most observations with P-binders have been done in clinical trials with dosage adjustment to achieve adequate serum P levels; controls have been either patients receiving Al hydroxide, or a relatively brief control period with no binder ingested. Only a few studies have addressed the issue of the amount of a P binder required to bind the P in a diet. In metabolic balance studies, the administration of 100 ml/day of Al hydroxide gel caused a decrease in net absorption of P from 463 $\pm$ 108 mg/day to 128 $\pm$ 68 mg/day in five patients who ingested a diet containing 1135 $\pm$ 246 mg of P per day (446). In two other patients with dietary P intake below 700 mg/day, the dietary fecal losses of P exceeded the amount in the diet. In a few studies with the dosage of Al gel at 75 or 150 ml per day, the reduction of P absorption was similar to that with 100 ml per day (446).

Single meal studies have allowed to evaluate the effect of various P binders on intestinal P absorption (447, 448). In normal subjects the ingestion of 50 mEq of Al carbon-

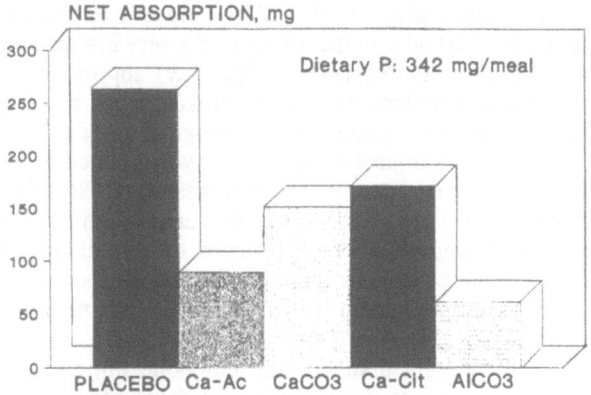

Figure 23. Effect of various phosphate binders on net intestinal absorption of phosphorus after a standardized meal containing 342 mg of phosphorus. (Modified from Sheikh et al. (448).)

ate, Ca carbonate, Ca citrate, and Ca acetate were compared, with the doses of Ca salts or Al containing preparations based on the dosage of Ca or Al provided. In normal subjects, the administration of Ca carbonate containing 1000 mg of Ca decreased the average net absorption from a meal with 342 mg of P from 263 mg to 151 mg, an average reduction in net absorption of 112 mg. The reduction of absorption with Ca acetate was 174 mg; with Al carbonate suspension, 202 mg; and with Ca citrate, 92 mg. The degrees of reduction with Ca acetate and Al carbonate were not different, but each was more effective than both Ca citrate and Ca carbonate (Figure 23) (448). In yet another study in normal subjects, the administration of 50 mEq of Ca acetate reduced the mean net absorption of P from a similar meal by 150 to 170 mg (449) when the agent was taken either immediately before or immediately after a meal. However, there was a significant reduction of the amount of P bound when the Ca acetate was taken 2 h after the meal.

In a recent report comparing patients receiving Ca acetate with those receiving Ca carbonate, serum P was controlled similarly by either binder (280). Although the daily amount of elemental Ca ingested by the patients taking Ca acetate was half of those ingesting Ca carbonate, the number of hypercalcemic episodes were small and comparable in both groups. Others in comparing the efficacy and side effects of Ca acetate and Ca carbonate in hemodialysis patients have not been able to identify a major advantage of Ca acetate over Ca carbonate (450). Thus, Ca carbonate still remains the most commonly used Ca-containing binder. Calcium acetate is more expensive, the size of tablets is rather large, it is less palatable and less tolerated. In addition, Ca acetate is not widely available.

It is important to 'titrate' the dose appropriately to the amount of P ingested in each meal. Large doses of binders may be required, particularly if there is an increase in dietary P. The average daily doses of Ca carbonate

employed in trials in dialysis patients have been 8.5 g/day (range 2.5 to 17 g) (279), 5.1 ± 2.5 g/day (130), and 5.8 ± 2.5g/day (451) in trials in the United States; reports in Europe described adequate control with use of 2.48 g (range 1 to 6 g) (443) and 2.57 g/day (range 1 to 6 g) (438); it is likely that such variations exist because of differences in dietary intake of P. In individual patients, the dose should be adjusted empirically according to the levels of serum P (445, 451). It must be emphasized that P binders, both Al or Ca based, are most effective when the dietary intake of P is below 1.0 g per day. With P intake > 2.0 g/day, their effectiveness is markedly reduced and hyperphosphatemia can persist despite their use. Finally, a variable efficacy of Ca carbonate tablets has been observed; preparations with inadequate solubility can render Ca carbonate ineffective (452).

Other phosphorus binders
Several other P-binding agents have been used in patients with CRF but they have certain disadvantages or have not been widely used. These include Ca citrate – 21% elemental Ca – (453), Mg carbonate or hydroxide (290, 293), and salts of polyuronic acid (413). Although Ca citrate is as effective a P binder as Ca carbonate, its use should be limited to certain specific situations, because Ca citrate, like other citrate salts, (133) markedly augments intestinal absorption of Al (135). Since some dialysis patients may need a small dose of Al gel with the Ca salt (279), there is a risk of acute Al toxicity – a condition with a high mortality (134). Magnesium carbonate in conjunction with Mg-free dialysate in patients undergoing regular hemodialysis was effective in controlling serum P (293); serum Mg levels did not change. However, other trials using Mg hydroxide have proven this salt ineffective or poorly tolerated (290, 454). When constipation accompanies the use of either Al-based P binders or Ca salts, the use of a free or lower-Mg dialysate combined with a modest ingestion of Mg salt, may be effective. Thus, Moriniere et al. have had success combining Ca carbonate with small doses of Mg hydroxide in long-term management of their patients (292). However, in more recent studies they were unsuccessful using Mg hydroxide as the sole P binder in the treatment of °HPTH with iv 1α(OH) D (455). The polyuronic acid derivatives have also been shown to be effective P binders (456). They are not available in the United States and have not been widely used in Europe. The use of these agents may be advisable in patients who are intolerant to Ca acetate, Ca carbonate or any of the P-binding Al gels.

Finally, it is important to consider that the fall in serum P level during dietary P restriction and therapy with P binders is often associated with a rise in serum Ca (267, 446). If the magnitude of the rise in serum Ca is adequate, the blood levels of PTH may further decrease (446). It is equally important to avoid lowering the concentration of serum P to levels lower than normal. A few patients require no P-binding agents; others require larger doses.

The overzealous use of P binders may result in hypophosphatemia, P depletion, and osteomalacia (190, 457).

Dialysance of phosphorus

Although removal of phosphorus by dialysis would seem appropriate to control hyperphosphatemia, the various dialytic techniques available cannot achieve this goal. The amount of P removed during hemodialysis varies mainly with the predialysis serum P level and also with the efficiency of the dialyzer being used. Kaye et al. (458) noted that the net P removal was 600 to 750 mg over 4 h of dialysis utilizing a 1.2 m^2 Cuprophan dialyzer when the predialysis serum P level varied from 5.0 to 7.0 mg/dl. Hou et al. (459) observed a high rate of P removal throughout the dialysis treatment (blood flow of 300 ml/min, dialysate flow of 500 ml/min, mean predialysis P levels 6.8mg/dl); however, the amount removed steadily declined during the 4 hours of treatment. Overall, 1 g of P was removed with each dialysis and this value was not affected by dialyzer membrane type, dialytic technique or dialysate Ca concentration in this particular study. Other studies observed that P removal was 587 ± 61 mg during 4 h of dialysis and 721 ± 53 mg with high flux hemodiafiltration carried out for 2 h with a blood flow of 500 ml/min (460, 461). With dialysis treatment targeted to achieve optimal urea removal, Shinaberger et al. (462) noted a 500 to 600 mg net removal of P during 4 h of conventional dialysis; removal of P increased only to 600 to 700 mg per dialysis during 3 h of high efficiency or high flux dialysis using cellulose acetate, polysulfone, and other highly permeable membranes. Interestingly, correction of anemia with erythropoietin resulted in a decreased P removal by 18%.

Several explanations account for the low mass transfer of P. First, the dialyzer clearances of P are somewhat lower than urea (40 to 50% of the rate for urea) although this difference is less with polysulfone dialyzers the differences become greater when blood flow is increased. Second, there is little or no removal of P from the erythrocyte and only plasma P is cleared by the dialyzer; and third, the excess of P which accumulates between two dialysis treatments has a volume of distribution well beyond the extracellular space so that the equilibration between the plasma P and extravascular compartment is delayed. Thus, serum P levels fall rapidly over the first 30 to 45 min of dialysis to values below 3.0 mg/100 ml (442, 460). This results in a low P gradient between plasma and dialysate, with less efficient mass transfer as the length of dialysis is extended. Moreover, the steady decrease in P removal efficiency during treatment is associated with an efflux of P from intracellular space and bone to the extracellular space as a result of the early decrease in serum P (459). In most patients, postdialysis serum P rapidly rebounds to predialysis values within two to three hours after completion of dialysis. In CAPD patients, the clearance of P is approximately 4.7 ml/min, and with each dialysate exchange 65 mg are removed, resulting in a daily removal of 307 mg (463). Thus, the net removal of P may be slightly higher in CAPD and this may explain some observations that serum P is easier to control during CAPD (464, 465).

With the widespread use of calcitriol, the control of hyperphosphatemia is of paramount importance. New dialyzer membranes have been used to improve P removal. The clearance ratios of plasma P to urea when a cellulose or a polycarbonate membrane is used are similar – that is, 64 and 78% respectively (466). High-flux hemodiafiltration improves the ratio to only 30% (460). However, the mass removal rates of P are similar regardless of the membrane used. For example, the total P removed during 4 h of hemodialysis using a Cuprophan membrane with a mean blood flow of 227 ml/min was 597 ± 61 mg per dialysis, while high-flux hemodiafiltration, at a blood flow rate of 504 ml/min, removed 721 ± 53 mg per dialysis. As mentioned before, the main factor in P removal is the predialysis serum P and the sharp decrease occurring during the first hour of dialysis (442) which precludes a higher P removal. It has been suggested that bicarbonate-based dialysate, compared to acetate, may increase the intracellular P pool and decrease serum P concentration; however, no differences in P transfer from the patient were noted in a preliminary comparison of dialysate solutions containing each of the two buffers (467). From all these observations and the mass balance calculations, it is apparent that although dialysis removes substantial amounts of P, additional efforts to control hyperphosphatemia are required in 80–90% of dialysis patients.

Failure to control hyperphosphatemia

The most common cause of hyperphosphatemia is poor compliance with both dietary P restriction and P-binders. Dietary training and support from the dietitian and nursing staff are of utmost importance. Reduced effectiveness of the P-binder may be another cause (452). Also, those patients with the most severe 2°HPTH present the most severe hyperphosphatemia; they may also have a more rapid rebound of serum P to higher levels during the interdialytic interval (468). The high serum P levels probably arise because bone resorption is markedly increased and P is released from bone into the blood. These patients may present a marked fall in serum P after parathyroidectomy or when PTH is decreased by intravenous calcitriol.

Nutritional calcium supplements

Calcium carbonate or Ca acetate are usually given, as described above, as P binders but they can also be used as a nutritional supplement. When either Ca carbonate or Ca acetate is given orally as a P binder, some Ca is inevitably absorbed. However, if Ca supplements are prescribed to reverse the negative Ca balance they should be administered between meals as opposed to its prescription as P-binders. Similarly, to maximize Ca absorption the amount prescribed should be ingested in several small doses throughout the day rather than one large dose.

The addition of Ca is important in patients with advanced CRF and those undergoing dialysis because, first, intestinal absorption of Ca is impaired in these patients; and second, the diets generally consumed by uremic patients contain reduced amounts of dairy products and, consequently, low quantities of Ca. The dietary Ca intake in patients with advanced CRF was noted to be 400 to 700 mg/day (469); a neutral or positive balance for Ca can be achieved in uremic patients by supplementation of the diet with Ca carbonate, Ca citrate, or Ca lactate (469), to increase the total intake of Ca to 1.5 g or more per day (269, 436). When, during the course of CRF, is the best time to add Ca supplements has not been resolved. Coburn et al. observed a normal intestinal Ca absorption in male patients with serum creatinine levels below 2.5 mg/dl (54), while Malluche et al. observed intestinal Ca absorption to be decreased in certain patients with GFR of 20 to 50 ml/min (470). Patients with more advanced CRF are more prone to develop hypercalcemia with oral Ca supplements, since they lack the renal route for Ca excretion.

Effects of long-term Ca supplementation for patients with advanced CRF have been reported. Makoff et al. gave 4 to 10 g of Ca carbonate per day to uremic patients not yet on dialysis. They observed a reduction of serum P, a slight rise in serum Ca, and a small increase in serum bicarbonate (471). Meyrier et al. gave 5 to 20 g of Ca carbonate per day to hemodialysis patients and compared them to other patients not receiving Ca carbonate (279). In the former group, bone biopsies showed less resorptive activity, radiographs showed less evidence of skeletal disease, and fewer fractures; less episodes of pseudo-gout and extraskeletal calcification were noted. Hypercalcemia, which was sometimes profound, resolved upon reduction of the Ca salt dosage. Plasma alkaline phosphatase and serum PTH concentration may decrease in uremic patients with overt 2°HPTH given supplements of either Ca carbonate or, in those with low serum P, Ca phosphate (429). Eastwood et al. compared bone biopsies from uremic patients with renal osteodystrophy treated with vitamin D with those from similar patients treated with Ca carbonate (351, 473). In patients receiving Ca carbonate, diffuse patchy deposition of Ca in osteoid was observed, and a distinct calcification front did not develop, while a calcification front was regularly observed in patients given vitamin D. This study provides evidence that vitamin D is more effective than Ca supplements in reversing overt uremic skeletal disease.

As mentioned before, treatment with oral Ca supplements is not free of risk. Large amounts of oral Ca compounds should be used cautiously in patients with marked hyperphosphatemia, because of the risk of elevating the Ca×P product and thereby predisposing to extraskeletal calcification. Hypercalcemia may develop in uremic patients, as in patients with normal renal function, during therapy with large quantities of oral Ca salts (279, 474). Hypercalcemia may be more common in patients with serum P concentrations below 3 mg/dl (268). Mild hypercalcemia (11 to 12 mg/dl) usually is not associated with symptoms; (127) but occasionally, uremic patients may exhibit symptoms despite only modestly elevated serum Ca levels. In addition to nausea, anorexia, vomiting, mental confusion, and lethargy, patients with advanced CRF may develop pruritus, 'red eye syndrome', band keratopathy and even a sharp elevation in blood pressure which can be clues for the suspicion of hypercalcemia.

Dialysate calcium concentration

Within a few months after initiation of regular hemodialysis, the basal concentration of serum Ca generally increases to between 9.0 and 10.0 mg/dl. This increase in serum Ca levels generally occurs in patients who were previously hypocalcemic, while little or no change occurs in patients with initial serum Ca levels near normal (274). Such increments in serum Ca may occur despite hyperphosphatemia or the use of a dialysate calcium lower than that in blood (268). The mechanism responsible for this increase in serum Ca is unknown; no improvement of the calcemic response to PTH has been detected with the initiation of dialysis (40) although uremic toxins have been shown to alter the calcemic response (475). Initiation of regular hemodialysis produces little or no change in intestinal Ca absorption (54), although a transient increase immediately after dialysis has been noted (476). With regular dialysis using the standard dialysate Ca content (3.5 mEq/l), there is a positive balance of Ca during the dialysis procedure; thus, it can explain the correction of hypocalcemia in some patients and the fact that predialysis serum Ca levels are sometimes normal. In a few patients, overt and persistent hypercalcemia appears some time after the initiation of hemodialysis (477).

The total serum Ca level almost invariably increases during the dialysis procedure. This may occur because of an increase in albumin level as a consequence of the ultrafiltration and hemoconcentration that accompanies hemodialysis; the affinity of plasma albumin for Ca may also be increased as a result of a rise in blood ph. Earlier studies carried out with Ca-specific electrodes indicate that the ionized blood Ca concentration can fall during hemodialysis with a dialysate Ca of 2.5 mEq/l even though total blood Ca level increases (273). However, more recent studies have failed to show a specific effect of hemoconcentration or change in ph on Ca binding to serum albumin (278). When the same evaluation is made during dialysis with a dialysate Ca level of 3.0 to 3.5 mEq/l, the ionized Ca level increases (442, 459).

It is likely that with a dialysate Ca concentration of either 3.0 or 3.5 mEq/l, patients receive too rapidly inappropriately large amounts of Ca with each dialysis. Recently, Argiles et al. have shown dramatic increments in intradialytic serum ionized Ca when a dialysate Ca

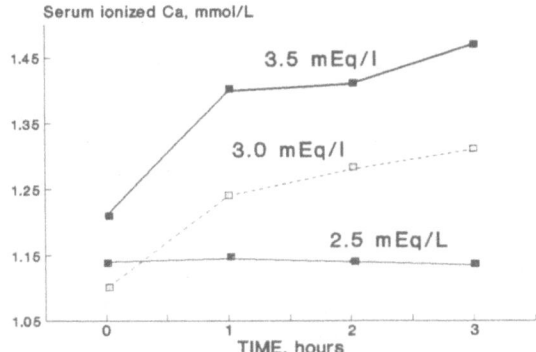
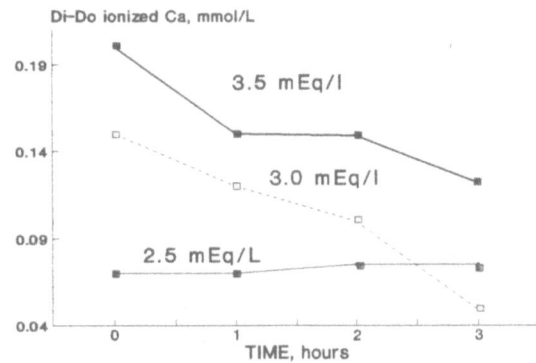

Figure 24. Shown on the left panel are the intradialytic calcium changes during regular hemodialysis with 3 different dialysate calcium concentrations (dCa) of 1.75, 1.5 and 1.25 mmol/l (3.5, 3 and 2.5 mEq/l). Shown on the right panel is the loss of calcium from dialysate ($D_i - D_o$) during hemodialysis using the same dCa concentrations. D_i = Dialysate inlet calcium. D_o = Dialysate outlet calcium. (Modified from Argiles et al. (442).)

concentration of 3.5 mEq/l was used; while no significant intradialytic changes in serum Ca were observed with a dialysate Ca of 2.5 mEq/l (Figure 24). Furthermore, significant intradialytic flux of ionized Ca from dialysate to patient was observed with both 3.5 and 3.0 mEq/l dialysate Ca and none with 2.5 mEq/l (442). These observations are similar to those of Hou et al. (459) who evaluated Ca fluxes across hemodialysis membrane in seven patients treated with 3.5, 2.5 and 1.5 mEq/l dialysate Ca. While dramatic positive Ca influx from dialysate to patients was observed in patients dialyzed against a 3.5 mEq/l dialysate Ca, only moderate Ca influxes were observed with a dialysate Ca of 2.5 mEq/l. Surprisingly, a dialysate Ca of 1.5 mEq/l resulted only in a moderate negative cumulative Ca efflux. Thus, these data strongly suggest that the standard 3.5 mEq/l dialysate Ca induces significant unwarranted intradialytic hypercalcemia. Our own observations support the above mentioned results. As we dialyzed patients with a standard dialysate Ca of 3.5 mEq/l for 4 hours, we measured serum Ca during dialysis at 1, 2, 3 and 4 hours, as well as 1, 2 and 3 hours postdialysis. There was the expected dramatic increase in serum calcium during dialysis; however, by the first hour postdialysis the high serum Ca returned to predialysis values (Figure 20). Thus, the question is: what is the fate of the acute and marked positive Ca balance induced during dialysis? It is likely that most of the intradialytic increment in serum Ca may rapidly deposit in soft tissues. In our view, the current use of a dialysate Ca of 3.5 mEq/l together with the use of Ca containing P binders and vitamin D analogs dialysate Ca may be an important factor in the development of soft tissue calcification.

The importance of a significant gradient of Ca between dialysate and patients's blood as a likely factor in soft tissue calcification is demonstrated by the recent observations of Fernandez and Montoliu (478). They evaluated a patient on dialysis with massive tumoral right shoulder calcification. Serum PTH (IRMA) was in the low-normal range, calcitriol was below normal and serum aluminum

was consistently less than 20 μg/l. As it can be noted in Figure 25, once the patient was placed on *daily* hemodialysis with a dialysate Ca concentration of 1 mEq/l, the predialysis serum Ca *increased* and it was maintained in the hypercalcemic range for six weeks. At the same time, the postdialysis serum Ca concentration steadily and significantly decreased with each dialysis; however, by the next dialysis the Ca values were back to the hypercalcemic range. Eight weeks later, because of the low postdialysis Ca, the patient was changed to 5 dialysis/week and dialysate Ca of 1.5 mEq/l. During the 12 month of frequent dialysis therapy, the tumoral calcification of the right shoulder progressively and dramatically disappeared and the patient's shoulder became functional. Moreover, during this period PTH levels remained below 20 pg/ml. In summary, this case exemplifies that a significant Ca gradient between dialyzer and patient resulted in the massive removal of Ca and P and disappearance of large soft tissue calcification. Thus, conversely, it is likely that a prolonged exposure to a positive Ca gradient may lead to soft tissue calcification.

Furthermore, a dialysate Ca of 2.5 mEq/l together with Ca carbonate may be effective in ameliorating 2°HPTH. Thus, recent studies evaluating the long-term effect of Ca carbonate and 2.5 mEq/l dialysate Ca in 21 hemodialysis patients noted not only that serum P was well controlled and serum Al fell significantly, but also that serum Ca increased and PTH decreased by 20% after 7 months of therapy (274); this suggests the presence of a positive Ca balance during this regimen. Moreover, the use of calcitriol promoted a more positive Ca balance. Thus, there is growing evidence that when Ca salts and/or calcitriol are used to treat 2°HPTH, the dialysate Ca should be reduced to 2.5 mEq/l (279, 437). In addition, such dialysate Ca concentration usually will allow patients to receive more appropriate doses of Ca salts and vitamin D derivatives which may result in a better control of the 2°HPTH (Figure 26). Fewer patients may develop hyper-

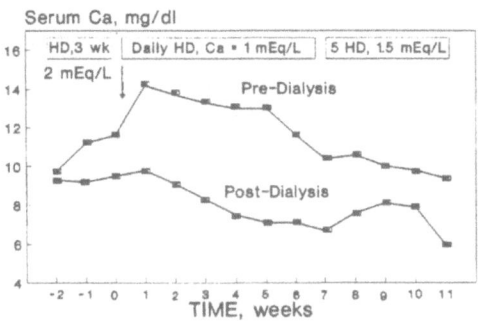
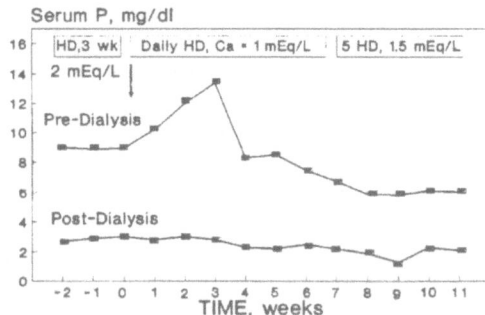

Figure 25. Shown on the left panel are pre- and postdialysis serum calcium changes in a patient with tumoral calcification of the shoulder. He was treated 3 times a week with a 2 mEq/l calcium dialysate, then switched to daily dialysis (for 8 weeks) using a 1 mEq/l dialysate calcium and finally, because of postdialysis hypocalcemia, the patient was treated 5 times a week with a dialysate calcium of 1.5 mEq/l. Shown on the right panel is the serum phosphorus during the above described treatment sequence. (Data from Fernandez and Montoliu (478).)

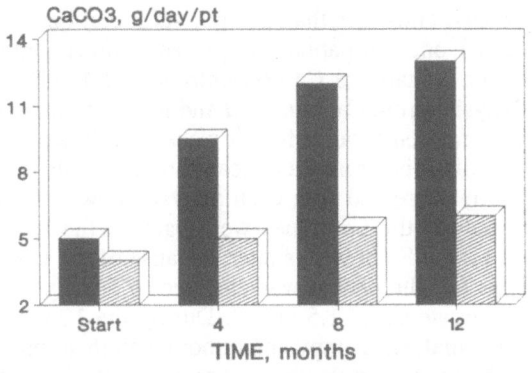
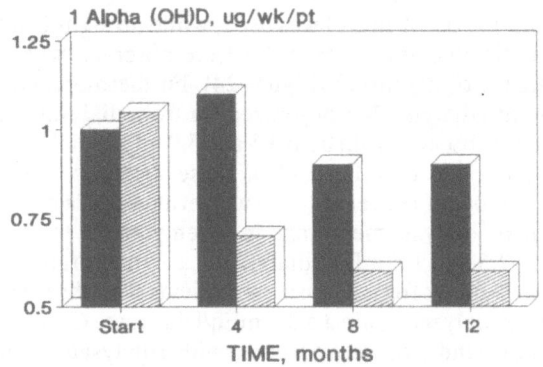

Figure 26. Calcium carbonate and oral 1α(OH)D treatments during one year follow-up. Open bars correspond to the control group maintained with dialysate Ca of 1.5 mmol/l (3 mEq/l) for 1 year, filled bars correspond to the study group (switched to a dialysate calcium of 1.25 mmol/l (2.5 mEq/l)). (Modified from Argiles et al. (442).)

calcemia with the dialysate Ca level of 2.5 mEq/l; in some patients with persistent hypercalcemia a dialysate Ca as low as 2.0 mEq/l may be used (443). Furthermore, a dialysate Ca of 2.5 mEq/l was only not associated with clinical intolerance but there was a postdialysis decrease in hypertension and blood pressure was easier to control (442). However, a greater reduction of the dialysate Ca may increase the risk of hypotension as a direct consequence of the lowered ionized Ca level (479).

In patients not taking Ca salts as a P binder or vitamin D, a number of earlier studies have evaluated the effect of various levels of Ca in dialysate (480). The use of dialysate Ca below 3.0 to 3.25 mEq/l was associated with more rapid loss of bone mineral than the use of dialysate Ca levels of 3.25 to 3.5 mEq/l (409, 412). Under these circumstances serum PTH levels have often slowly risen despite the increase in serum Ca concentration. Thus, there is little information to indicate that a dialysate Ca of 3.25 to 3.5 mEq/l per se may prevent the development of bone disease (353, 481). Earlier, the use of a lower concentra-

tion of 2.5 mEq/l was associated with progression of the bone disease; however, none of these patients received Ca salts or calcitriol (482). Recently, in 9 patients on hemodiafiltration, it was noted that intact PTH increased (from 94 ± 40 to 296 ± 99 pg/ml) after one year treatment with a dialysate Ca of 2.5 mEq/l while a dialysate Ca of 3.0 mEq/l showed no changes in PTH; this occurred despite the former group had an oral Ca intake almost double than the latter (442). However, when patients were treated for four months with intravenous 1α(OH) D a similar PTH reduction (72 and 75%) was noted in both groups. Thus, when a dialysate Ca of 2.5 mEq/l is used, efforts should be directed to ascertain that patients remain compliant with their prescribed Ca-containing P binders and a vitamin D metabolite is added in order to avoid a negative Ca balance. Regular measurements of intact PTH should also be performed.

It has also been recently reported that CAPD patients with the use of dialysate Ca of 3.5 mEq/l may have more sustained and higher Ca levels than patients on hemodialysis (157, 276); this may result in more effective PTH suppression than the intermittent Ca loading of hemodialysis. As mentioned before, the higher serum Ca may at least partly explain the high incidence of low-turnover bone lesions observed in peritoneal dialysis (148, 149). Peritoneal dialysate Ca of 2.5 mEq/l are now commercially available and there is growing evidence that, as it is already happening in hemodialysis patients, it may be desirable for patients treated with CAPD (483).

Use of vitamin D analogs

Despite dietary compliance with appropriate intake of Ca and restriction of P, the use of phosphate binders and an appropriate dialysate Ca, a significant number of patients develop 2°HPTH. Since a deficit in calcitriol is an important cause of 2°HPTH, the use of calcitriol and other analogs has become a widely accepted therapy. The widespread and appropriate use of vitamin D derivatives may be the most important single factor in the markedly decreased number of parathyroidectomies performed over the past decade (484, 485).

When uremic patients exhibit evidence of overt 2°HPTH with bone erosions, significant high levels of PTH and plasma alkaline phosphatase, treatment with vitamin D derivatives usually leads to clinical improvement. Pharmacologic doses of vitamin D (484, 485), dihydrotachysterol (486), 25(OH) D (487), 1α(OH) D (488), and 1,25(OH)$_2$D (485), have each led to improvement of symptoms and of x-rays toward normality, amelioration of bone pathology, and a fall in serum alkaline phosphatase and PTH concentration.

Although vitamin D and dihydrotachysterol have been available for a long time, there are only a few well documented reports on their efficacy. Vitamin D has been reported to induce more normal bone mineralization than Ca supplementation alone (3). Stanbury and Lumb as well as Dent et al. have shown that vitamin D at a dosage of 50,000 to 200,000 I/day improves overt skeletal disease in patients with advanced CRF (171, 489). However, the responsiveness of individual patients varied greatly. Similarly, Lumb et al. reported improvement of radiographic evidence of bone disease in children given 30,000 to 50,000 I/day of vitamin D for 5 to 13 months (486).

Several highly active, naturally occurring forms of vitamin D, 25(OH) D (calcifediol), 1,25(OH)$_2$ D (calcitriol), and 24,25(OH)$_2$ D have been evaluated in clinical trials (484, 485). Also, several synthetic vitamin D derivatives that bypass the need for renal 1α-hydroxylation have been introduced. These include 1α(OH) D; 5,6-trans-25(OH) D; and 5,6-trans D. Also, various synthetic analogues with some of the beneficial properties of vitamin D, such as inhibition of the synthesis of PTHmRNA but lacking inherent side effects, such as hypercalcemic activity – are being developed experimentally. Of all the above mentioned compounds, calcifediol, calcitriol, and 1α(OH) D have had the widest use (see below).

Calcifediol

Despite the availability of 25(OH) D (calcifediol) for research purposes since 1969, there are few reports of its use in patients with renal osteodystrophy (159). Intestinal absorption of Ca can be increased with 100 µg of calcifediol per day, while 20 µg/day is enough to augment Ca absorption in normal subjects (490). However, some data indicate that uremic patients may respond favorably to treatment with doses below 100 µg/day. Teitelbaum et al. treated five patients with 40 µg/day for 3 to 9 months; serum PTH and alkaline phosphatase decreased, and serial bone biopsies showed decreased numbers of osteoclasts, size of osteoid surface covered with active osteoblasts, and marrow fibrosis (491). Witmer et al. treated nine uremic children with calcifediol (487). Five had severe osteodystrophy that previously failed to respond to 13,000–27,000 I/day of vitamin D before calcifediol was given. Osteitis fibrosa improved, the number of osteoblasts and marrow fibrosis decreased in these five children receiving 25 to 200 µg/day of calcifediol. Other children with normal or near-normal skeletal x-rays at the initiation of hemodialysis, were given either 25 to 50 µg/day of calcifediol plus an oral Ca supplement or oral Ca alone. Bone lesions progressively worsened in the group receiving only oral Ca, but skeletal biopsies showed improved mineralization and decreased fibrosis in those given calcifediol. Fournier et al. noted a rise in plasma alkaline phosphatase activity and an increase in the active formation surface area of trabecular bone in three patients given 200 to 300 µg of calcifediol three times per week for 4 to 8 weeks (492). These effects differed from those observed in other patients given 1α(OH) D over the same period of time suggesting that calcifediol may have a specific effect on bone different from other vitamin D derivatives. Results from a five-center study have been summarized by Recker et al. (493). These hemodialysis patients received 200 µg of calcifediol three times weekly for 29 weeks, with the dose adjusted to avoid hypercalcemia; the final dose averaged 46 µg/day. As a group, the patients noted a significant improvement in musculoskeletal related symptoms and a better overall clinical status. Small increases in serum Ca and P concentrations were noted, and serum alkaline phosphatase activity fell. Plasma PTH concentration for the entire group did not change, although it decreased in individual patients. Bone biopsies showed an increased resorption surface area in conjunction with decreased fibrosis. Plasma levels of calcifediol rose to 200 to 300 µg/dl concurrently with the maximum elevation of serum Ca concentration. In each of the series reported, several patients developed hypercalcemia. The major disadvantages of calcifediol are that it is less potent than calcitriol and it has a greater half-life; thus, a greater number of days are also required for the episodes of hypercalcemia to resolve.

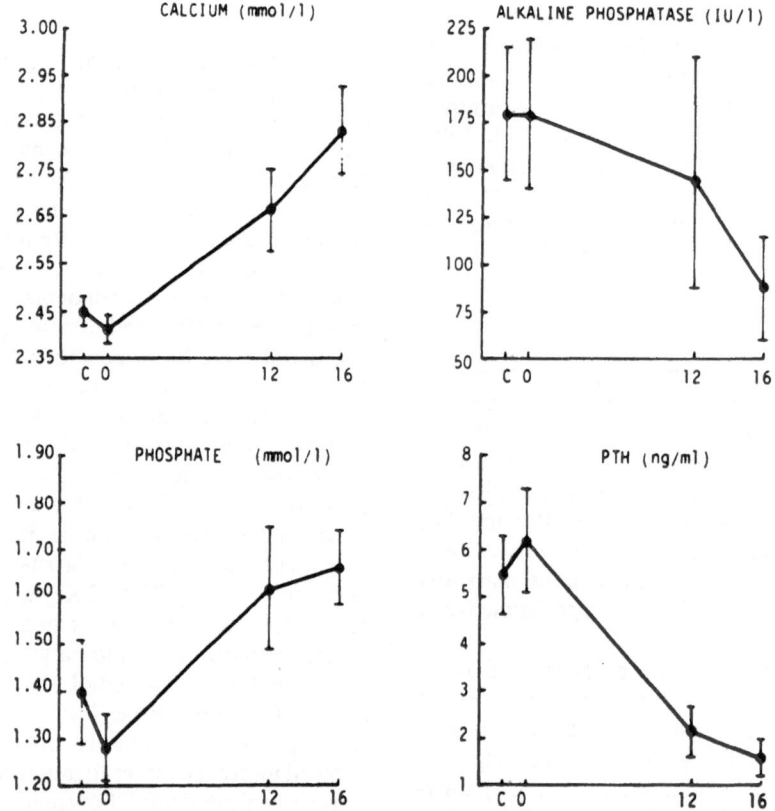

Figure 27. Mean values of plasma Ca, P, alkaline phosphatase, and serum immunoreactive PTH in 10 dialysis patients treated with 1-alpha-(OH)D₃ for 16 months. The initial dose was 1 µg/day, and the dose was adjusted in each patient during the trial. (Modified after Papapoulos et al.)
(Conversion factors: Ca mmol/l → mg/dl: × 4
P [as phosphate]: mmol/l → mg/dl: × 3.1)

Calcitriol

Oral calcitriol

In multiple clinical trials, calcitriol as well as 1α(OH)D has proven highly efficacious in the treatment of patients with renal osteodystrophy. They induced a marked decreased in alkaline phosphatase and PTH (Figure 27). In an early study, Brickman et al. reported observations in eight patients given 0.14 to 0.68 µg/day of oral calcitriol for 2 to 4 months. Patients with 2°HPTH and osteitis fibrosa showed decreases in serum PTH concentration, resorption surface area and marrow fibrosis (494). Those afflicted by muscle weakness improved their muscle strength. There was some improvement in the abnormal mineralization front in those with osteomalacia. Similar observations were reported by other authors (195). Eastwood et al. gave 0.54 to 1.35 µg/day of calcitriol to five patients for 4 weeks and noted an improvement in bone mineralization in three (495). Similarly, in a series of 40 patients treated with calcitriol at an average dose of 0.62 µg/day for 4 to 90 weeks (265), bone pain improved in 71% and muscle weakness in 85% of the patients. In patients with elevated serum PTH levels, these

levels often decreased and alkaline phosphatase activity declined toward normal. Bone biopsies improved and a close correlation was observed between improvement in the degree of osteitis fibrosa and reduction in serum PTH (496). A subgroup of patients with refractory osteomalacia developed hypercalcemia while receiving low doses of calcitriol; these patients were subsequently identified as having Al-related bone disease (452).

In many patients showing a favorable response, serum P concentration usually decreased within 1 to 3 months of treatment; subsequently, serum P often increased (Figure 28). Sherrard et al. evaluated pre- and post-treatment bone biopsies in uremic patients treated with calcitriol and two control groups of patients undergoing dialysis using a dialysate Ca of either 3.0 or 4.0 mEq/l (496). Pretreatment bone biopsies showed more extensive osteitis fibrosa in the calcitriol group. Nonetheless, there was a marked decrease in fibrosis in 10 of 11 patients with osteitis fibrosa, and increased mineralization in 16 of 17 patients treated with calcitriol. The patients treated with high dialysate Ca showed little or no improvement. Thus, the authors concluded that calcitriol was more effective

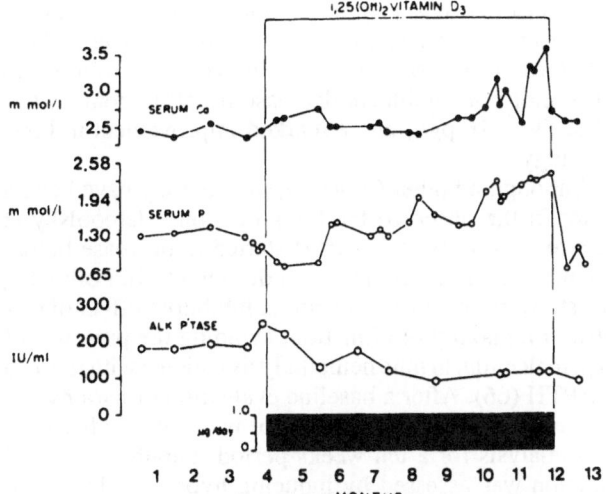

Figure 28. Treatment of renal osteodystrophy with 1,25(OH)₂D₃. Initially a decrease of serum P occurs suggesting remineralization of the skeleton. Later when mineralization slows and stimulation of calcium and phosphate absorption continues, hypercalcemia and hyperphosphatemia may develop. Both however, are rapidly reversed when the drug is discontinued or the dose is reduced. (Adapted from Coburn et al.)
(Conversion: Ca mmol/l → mg/dl: × 4
P [as Phosphate] mmol/l → mg/dl: × 3.1)

than Ca added to the dialysate in both improving mineralization and reversing °HPTH.

The studies reviewed above were carried out in patients with advanced CRF and overt °HPTH. Several controlled prospective studies have also been carried out in dialysis patients, including those who were asymptomatic. Thus, in a controlled double-blind study of 31 dialysis patients, Berl et al. gave either calcitriol, in an average dose of 0.82 µg/day, or vitamin D, in a dose of 400 I/day, for 12 weeks (494). They noted an increase in serum Ca from 9.05 ± 0.15 to 10.25 ± 0.20 mg/dl in those receiving calcitriol; serum Ca did not change in those receiving vitamin D. Serum PTH fell significantly in 11 of 13 patients receiving calcitriol; this response was not observed after vitamin D. Bone biopsies showed improvement of osteitis fibrosa in patients given calcitriol, but no change in those receiving vitamin D; osteomalacia failed to improve in patients receiving calcitriol. Maxwell et al. followed a similar protocol in a controlled study (497). They noted a significant decrease in plasma alkaline phosphatase activity in those receiving calcitriol, but no change in those receiving vitamin D. Hypercalcemia in patients taking calcitriol rapidly reversed after drug withdrawal.

In a double-blind trial Memmos et al. gave either 0.5 µg/day of calcitriol or a placebo to asymptomatic patients who had been on hemodialysis for at least one year; the trial lasted one or two years (498). At the end of one year 16 of the 30 patients receiving placebo, but only 1 of 27 patients receiving calcitriol, showed deterioration in

hand x-rays. Among the patients who entered the trial with abnormal skeletal x-rays, none receiving placebo showed improvement after two years, compared to 5 of 11 given calcitriol. Serum PTH, which were closely related to the severity of radiological °HPTH, and alkaline phosphatase levels showed a slight increase or no change, respectively, in the placebo group while both fell after calcitriol.

In a controlled study in asymptomatic dialysis patients with normal skeletal radiographs and good biochemical control of Ca and P levels, the frequency of new or worsened erosions was lower in patients given up to 1.0 µg/day of calcitriol, compared to placebo-treated patients (499). Serum PTH concentration was suppressed in a larger fraction of the patients treated with calcitriol, while PTH concentration more often increased in the control subjects. Analysis of the data in these patients disclosed considerable heterogeneity in the suppressibility of the parathyroid glands; a serum Ca of 10.0 to 10.8 mg/dl was needed in many patients to reduce serum PTH levels. Such observations are consistent with an increase in the set point of Ca; that is, in uremic patients a higher Ca concentration is required to suppress parathyroid gland activity.

In children with advanced CRF overt skeletal disease has a very high incidence compared with adults; those who received calcitriol have responded favorably. As mentioned before, improvement in growth or catch-up growth was initially reported in children receiving calcitriol (218), although subsequent observations have not confirmed such a beneficial effect (500). More recent observations in children undergoing treatment with CAPD suggest that the maintenance of normal serum Ca concentration during treatment with calcitriol may not invariably lead to reversal of the features of 2°HPTH (99). Indeed, it may be necessary to raise serum Ca concentration to levels slightly above normal to achieve a more consistent reversal of 2°HPTH (219).

In general, the trials with calcitriol and 1α(OH) D suggest that these sterol are the most effective in 2°HPTH, particularly when serum Ca concentration is normal or decreased; when osteomalacia and 2°HPTH coexist, a favorable response also occurs. Overall, oral calcitriol and 1α(OH) D appear to be similarly effective. Under some circumstances the bone can be restored largely to normal, but in other settings the elevated serum PTH levels persist and treatment with oral calcitriol is not successful in reversing the 2°HPTH. In this situation, as we will discuss later, intravenous calcitriol may be helpful.

The administration of calcitriol may help to predict the underlying bone disease. Thus, patients with low-turnover bone disease are prone to develop hypercalcemia with very low doses of calcitriol within the first several weeks of treatment as well as patients with severe 2°HPTH and marked parathyroid gland hyperplasia (22). When hypercalcemia develops after many weeks or months of treatment and phosphatase alkaline levels have returned to normal, it is very likely that osteitis fibrosa has substantially regressed.

As shown, the administration of oral calcitriol to dialysis patients – in many studies from 0.25 to 2 μg/day – is effective in reducing serum PTH levels and improving bone disease. In a recent study by Seidel et al. (501), a single oral dose of 2 μg of calcitriol induced a delayed (between 24 and 48 hours) but long-lasting (> 96 hours) decrease of intact PTH levels, even despite calcitriol levels returned to baseline levels earlier. Thus, new information on the kinetics of intact PTH after treatment with calcitriol may further provide new insights in the treatment schedules used, eventually improving results with less secondary effects.

Prophylactic treatment of dialysis patients with calcitriol may prevent the development of 2°HPTH. Preliminary data have suggested that the administration of calcitriol (or 1α(OH) D) in daily doses of 0.25–0.50 μg to patients with early to moderate CRF may reverse and/or prevent 2°HPTH and is rarely associated with hypercalcemia, hyperphosphatemia or impairment in renal function (502, 503). Moreover, careful monitoring is advised and if such complications arise, they are usually reversible. It should also be mentioned that there is evidence that calcitriol impairs creatinine secretion by the renal tubule; thus, serum creatinine levels may increase and the clearance of creatinine decrease without any change in true glomerular filtration rate (304). Thus, calcitriol therapy in early stages of CRF may prevent 2°HPTH. Moreover, patients such as children or those with very slow progression of CRF such in interstitial diseases may greatly benefit from early calcitriol therapy.

Intravenous calcitriol
The observation that calcitriol has a direct inhibitory effect on the parathyroid cell and that this effect is dose-related, makes the use of intravenous (iv) calcitriol an important alternative in the control of 2°HPTH. Thus, iv calcitriol administered three times weekly at the end of regular dialysis by inducing a higher peak in serum calcitriol concentration may result in a greater suppression of PTH and less undesirable hypercalcemic episodes (64–66). Earlier, the effects of oral versus intermittent iv calcitriol administration on the circulating plasma levels of calcitriol as well as on PTH secretion was compared (64). It was observed that oral administration of calcitriol in doses adequate to maintain serum Ca in the upper limits of normal did not alter PTH levels, whereas a marked suppression of PTH levels (70.1 ± 3.2%) was observed in 20 patients receiving iv calcitriol. Norris et al. also treated 10 patients with overt 2°HPTH with iv calcitriol (506). These patients received from 1 to 5 μg of calcitriol at the end of each dialysis for a period of 13 months. They observed a significant decrease in serum PTH (42 ± 4%) and alkaline phosphatase (62% ± 4); serum Ca increased from 10.1 to 11.2 mg/dl. Intravenous calcitriol has also been shown to improve histological features of 2°HPTH; thus, Andress et al. studied 12 hemodialysis patients with severe 2°HPTH refractory to oral calcitriol therapy (507). They were treated with

iv calcitriol, 1 to 2.5 μg three times a week given at the end of each dialysis, for 1 year or longer. The authors noted a mild increase in serum ionized Ca, from 2.5 to 2.6 mmol/l; a significant decrease in PTH, from 172 ± 34 to 69 ± 16 pg/l; and a marked improvement in bone histology.

Although a higher Ca levels, *per se*, may have been a factor in the observed PTH suppression, Slatopolsky et al. already observed that PTH started to decrease before any increment in serum Ca was detected (64). Following this study, we evaluated the direct inhibitory effect of calcitriol on parathyroid function, avoiding the presence of hypercalcemia, in nine hemodialysis patients with marked 2°HPTH (66). After a baseline evaluation of parathyroid function, we administered 2 μg of iv calcitriol after each hemodialysis for a ten weeks period. Parathyroid gland function was assessed by inducing hypo- and hypercalcemia using a low and a high Ca dialysate during two separate dialysis performed a week apart. In order to avoid the previously observed hypercalcemia during calcitriol administration, the dialysate Ca was reduced to 2.5 mEq/l. Parathyroid hormone values after dialysis induced hypo- and hypercalcemia were plotted against serum ionized Ca for each patient, and the sigmoidal relationship between PTH and Ca was evaluated. A sigmoidal relationship was established for each patient and the set point of Ca, as previously defined, was determined. The basal PTH levels fell from 902 ± 126 pg/ml to 466 ± 152 pg/ml (p < 0.01) after 10 weeks of calcitriol therapy. This occurred in the absence of any significant changes in serum Ca concentration (Figure 5). The PTH–Ca sigmoidal curve shifted to the left and downward after calcitriol therapy. Moreover, after calcitriol therapy, the maximum PTH response during hypocalcemia decreased from 1661 ± 485 pg/ml to 1031 ± 280 pg/ml (p < 0.05) and the minimal PTH level from 281 ± 76 to 192 ± 48 pg/ml (p < 0.05). However, neither the set point of Ca nor the slope of the PTH–Ca curve were significantly different after 10 weeks of calcitriol. If a noncompliant patient with persistent hyperphosphatemia was excluded, a significant shift of the set point of Ca to the left was noted (Figure 7).

Later, six patients continued to receive iv calcitriol and were re-evaluated after 42 weeks of treatment (37). The continued treatment with calcitriol resulted in a progressive decrease in serum PTH levels for a similar serum Ca concentration. In addition, the slope of the PTH–Ca curve was decreased at 42 weeks (p < 0.05) as compared with both 0 and 10 weeks (Figure 8). These findings suggest that calcitriol: 1) reduced the functional mass of parathyroid cells (based on the lower maximal PTH); and 2) decreased the sensitivity of parathyroid cells (difference in the slope of PTH–Ca curve with PTH as a percent of maximal PTH) as a result of long-term calcitriol treatment. Recently, Malberti et al. have reported similar results (84).

Hamdy et al. evaluated the effect of iv calcitriol in four patients with persistent hypercalcemia and marked

2°HPTH (508). These patients had been shown to be intolerant to oral administration of calcitriol. After each dialysis, calcitriol was administered iv in doses of 0.5–2.5 μg for 2 months. Calcitriol therapy continued for 7 and 8 months, respectively, in 2 of the 4 patients. After 4 weeks of therapy, a significant *decrease* in serum Ca was observed which was maintained throughout treatment as the dosage of iv calcitriol was increased. This was associated with a decrease in PTH levels. During the long-term administration of calcitriol, serum Ca values increased but lower concentrations of PTH were maintained. The authors concluded that the increment in serum Ca is not a prerequisite for the suppression of PTH secretion by calcitriol and that the presence of hypercalcemia does not preclude the use of iv calcitriol.

Finally, although the average dose has varied in different studies, most have used 0.5–1 μg/dialysis as a starting dose. Galena et al. used an average dose of 0.87 μg/dialysis in a large multicenter study which included 76 patients (266). Dressler et al. have recently evaluated 12 symptomatic hemodialysis patients with severe overt 2°HPTH (half of patients had PTH values ranging from 1500 to 3400 pg/ml) (509). Patients were selected for the presence of persistent or progressive 2°HPTH non responsive to oral calcitriol therapy; some patients were being considered for parathyroidectomy. They received iv calcitriol at the end of each dialysis for a mean period of 14 months. From an starting dose of 1 μg, calcitriol was dosed up to a maximum of 8 μg; the mean iv calcitriol dose administered was 4.4 μg. By the end of the study there was significant clinical improvement in all patients. In addition, PTH decreased from 1179 to 159 pg/ml. Serum Ca increased from 9.2 to 10.8 mg/dl. Hypercalcemic episodes were noted infrequently (mostly in 2 patients) while only 3 of them were placed on dialysate Ca of 2.5 mEq/l. No changes in serum P were observed except in a non compliant patient. These observations suggest that the severity of 2°HPTH may be an important factor in deciding what dose of iv calcitriol to use. Thus, the higher the levels of PTH, the higher the dose of calcitriol to be administered. In summary, the available data on iv calcitriol have shown to be a very effective therapy. In addition, it should be an alternative approach in patients who develop hypercalcemia or hyperphosphatemia after oral therapy; also, in those with overt 2°HPTH and in noncompliant patients.

Oral pulse therapy with calcitriol

Since the efficacy of the intermittent iv calcitriol most likely is related to the high peak of serum calcitriol achieved, the use of intermittent 'oral pulses' of calcitriol, ranging from 2 to 5 μg two or three times a week, has been evaluated (402, 510, 513). Thus, good results have been observed with such approach on the treatment of 2°HPTH (510, 513). Fukagawa et al. noted in patients with moderate 2°HPTH that a 4 μg of oral calcitriol twice weekly not only reduced the PTH levels but also the size of

the parathyroid glands by 41% as measured by ultrasound (402). This therapeutic regime has also proven effective in patients on CAPD with mild to moderate 2°HPTH (512). Recently, the efficacy of calcitriol on reduction of PTH mRNA and serum PTH levels was assessed when the calcitriol was administered as intermittent bolus or continuously by an osmotic minipump in an experimental model (514). The data showed that although the total increment (area under the curve) of serum calcitriol was smaller in the bolus group, the bolus administration resulted in a significant greater reduction of PTHmRNA than the continuous infusion of calcitriol (Figure 29). Thus, the more efficient suppression may be related to a higher peak calcitriol levels. Then, the response of parathyroid glands to calcitriol seems to be more influenced by short-term calcitriol peak levels than by long-term steady-state calcitriol levels. Similarly, a comparison of serum calcitriol levels after a single oral versus an iv dose revealed serum levels exceeding the normal range for a period up to 24 hours in both routes (472), but the overall area under the curve after iv calcitriol was 62% greater.

Other routes of administration

The intraperitoneal calcitriol administration has also proven effective in patients undergoing CAPD (515). More recently, the subcutaneous route has also been successfully tested in a few patients both in CAPD and hemodialysis (516, 517).

1α(OH) D

This synthetic form of calcitriol undergoes 25-hydroxylation in the liver to be converted to calcitriol before exerting its action. It is very active in patients with advanced uremia; the dose required to increase intestinal Ca absorption is only 1.5 to 2-fold of that needed for calcitriol (476). The improvement of hyperparathyroid bone disease and reversal of other features of 2°HPTH following its use are also similar to calcitriol although the required dosage is 50–75% higher (518). Both short-term and long-term clinical trials have shown 1α(OH) D to be effective in patients with CRF (488, 518). Not surprisingly, patients subsequently shown to have Al-related osteomalacia also failed to respond to 1α(OH) D (478), as did those treated with calcitriol (519).

The 1α(OH) D is widely used in Europe, Canada, and Japan, but only short-term trials have been carried out in the United States (518). The importance of concurrent use of P binders to control serum P concentration has been stressed by Davison et al. (520). Twenty patients receiving 1α(OH) D were compared with a group given Al hydroxide to reduce serum P to below 5.0 mg/dl before treatment with 1α(OH) D was initiated. In the former group the incidence of corneal calcification, pruritus, and radiographic evidence of soft extraskeletal calcification was higher. Bone erosions resolved in similar number of patients in both groups, but there was a higher incidence

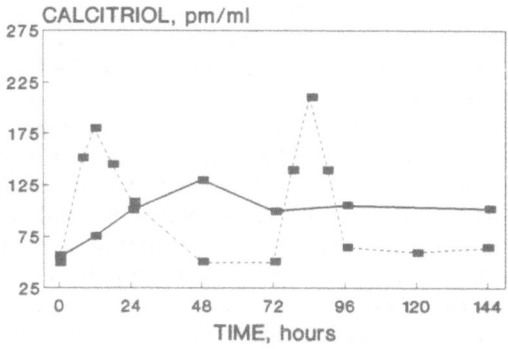

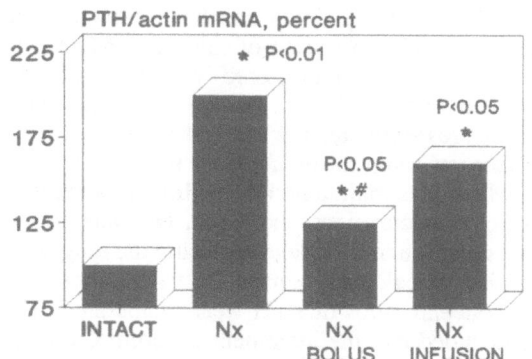

Figure 29. Comparison between intermittent bolus and continuous calcitriol administration in the rat with CRF and HPTH. On the left panel, blood levels of calcitriol during the continuous (solid line) as compared with bolus administration (dotted line). On the right panel, effect of bolus vs infusion on PTHmRNA. Nx = 5/6 nephrectomy (surgically induced CRF) (514).

of periosteal new bone formation in the group not given P binders.

Lind et al. and Brandi et al. have described the effect of iv administration of 1α(OH) D in patients on hemodialysis (521, 522). They observed a marked suppression of PTH and only a slight increase in serum ionized Ca. Thus, iv 1α(OH) D has an inhibitory effect on PTH secretion similar to that of calcitriol. More recently, Ljunghall et al. (523) studied normocalcemic patients treated for 12 weeks with an increasing dose of the sterol, but due to hypercalcemic episodes, the dose had to be reduced in most patients and withdrawn in three. At the end of the study, only six patients were receiving the maximal dose (4 μg/dialysis session) and in 17 patients the dose used was 1 μg per dialysis. Significant reductions of PTH were already observed after one week of treatment, and maximal suppression was obtained after 4 weeks. However, a mild increase in PTH levels was observed at the end of the study as a result of the dose adjustment done to avoid hypercalcemic episodes.

Long-term suppression of 2°HPTH by iv 1α(OH) D has also been evaluated. Thus, Brandi et al. also reported 13 patients who received intravenous 1α(OH) D; six of them up to 96 weeks (524). At the end of the study, PTH levels were still suppressed by 78 ± 4% after 300 days, 78 ± 9% after 550 days, and 85 ± 7% after 720 days.

Finally, in the choice of either 1α(OH) D or any D derivative lacking the 25-hydroxyl group it should be kept in mind that hepatic 25-hydroxylation is necessary before they become biologically active. Thus, simultaneous treatment with a drug such as phenobarbital, phenytoin, or glutethimide, as well as the presence of concomitant liver disease, may impair the hepatic 25-hydroxylation and may result in impaired action of the vitamin D sterol (525, 526).

Other vitamin D analogs

In addition to the sterol discussed above, several other synthetic vitamin D analogs have been used in short-term trials. Several of these sterol have the A ring of the steroid molecule rotated 180° about the 5,6 double bond; this converts the molecule from a *cis* to a *trans* configuration, with the normal 3-hydroxyl group assuming a geometric position equivalent to that of the 1a hydroxy moiety of calcitriol. This may be referred to as a 'pseudo 1a-hydroxyl' configuration. Several of such compounds can enhance Ca absorption in uremic patients (527); these include 5,6-*trans*-D and 5,6-*trans*-25-(OH)-D (527). These agents have been given to dialysis patients in Europe but it is not clear that these compounds have any advantage over calcitriol.

Another naturally occurring vitamin D sterol is 24,25(OH)$_2$ D. It would appear that there are qualitative differences between the effect of this sterol and that of calcitriol in patients with CRF (90, 91). Recently, favorable responses in a small number of patients whose osteomalacia was refractory to calcitriol alone responded to 24,25(OH)$_2$ D combined with calcitriol (528). Subsequently these patients were found to have Al-related osteomalacia (98), and their favorable responses have not been confirmed (529). Other studies have suggested that 24,25(OH)$_2$ D may have also a suppressive effect on the parathyroid glands (62, 530); however, other studies in patients with 2°HPTH and in dogs with experimental uremia failed to demonstrate this effect (521, 532). Nevertheless, recent observations strongly suggest that this sterol, unlike calcitriol, specifically inhibits bone resorption, and that this effect is independent of PTH (533). Thus, a study of 29 dialysis patients treated with either calcitriol or 24,25(OH)$_2$ D alone or both together showed that calcitriol inhibited PTH secretion and that 24,25(OH)$_2$ D decreased bone resorption and formation without any change in PTH levels. More important, the administration of both sterol together resulted in greater improvement in the abnormal bone resorption. Popovtzer et al. have evaluated the effect of $24,25(OH)_2$ D together with $1\alpha(OH)$ D in dialysis patients (90, 534). Osteoclastic parameters and bone mineralization improved significantly after 10–16 months only in the group receiving both sterol. Thus, these studies strongly suggest that combined treatment with $24,25-(OH)_2$ D and $1\alpha(OH)$ D or calcitriol may result in a greater improvement in bone histology.

Calcitriol analogues, mainly oxacalcitriol, are promising for the treatment of 2°HPTH. Thus, oxacalcitriol suppressed PTH synthesis and showed no hypercalcemic activity in experimental studies (535–537). However, a recent study has shown that such dissociative effect is not always present (538). The apparent discrepancy between these studies may be explained by the fact that in this recent study oxacalcitriol was administered in rats with more severe 2°HPTH. Thus, at present, it is not clear whether oxacalcitriol offers any advantage over calcitriol.

Treatment failures

The principal hazard in the use of vitamin D derivatives is hypercalcemia and when it occurs its resolution may require several weeks. The time required for the resolution of undesired hypercalcemia is related to the half-life of the vitamin D metabolite. Thus, one major feature of calcitriol and $1\alpha(OH)$ D is their rapid turnover compared to vitamin D itself. Kanis and Russell evaluated the rate of reversal of hypercalcemia or hypercalciuria induced by vitamin D, dihydrotachysterol, $1\alpha(OH)$ D, and calcitriol (539). The half-time for reversal of the effects was shorter after discontinuing calcitriol than was the case for $1\alpha(OH)$ D, vitamin D, or dihydrotachysterol; the differences were independent of the dose given or the length of treatment. Similar results were reported by Brickman et al. when comparing $1\alpha(OH)$ D and calcitriol (518). Thus, calcitriol shows the most rapid reversal of hypercalcemia, a useful feature should toxicity occur. Hypercalcemia has been suggested to be less frequent when oral calcitriol is given at night (540).

Likewise, intestinal absorption of P also augments after calcitriol therapy; (541) thus, hyperphosphatemia is not uncommon after oral calcitriol (Figure 25) (478). The magnitude of this increment seems to be lower with iv than with oral calcitriol. However, Galena et al. (266) have recently reported the effects of low-dose iv calcitriol (< 1 μg) in hemodialysis patients with significant 2°HPTH (mean intact PTH 767 ± 76 pg/ml); fifty-eight of 76 patients had a significant reduction on PTH levels. Although asymptomatic hypercalcemia was observed in 30% of the patients, hyperphosphatemia developed in 60%. In 12 of 22 patients who were taking Ca carbonate as the only P binder at the beginning of treatment, an Al-containing P binder had to be used to control their serum P levels.

Although vitamin D derivatives, either orally or intravenously, are effective decreasing synthesis and secretion of PTH (62), improving bone histology, suppressing parathyroid cell proliferation (542), decreasing the size of the hyperplastic parathyroid glands (402) and even triggering the apoptotic process (programmed cell death) of hyperplastic parathyroid cells (543), it should also be mentioned that a few patients do not experiment such improvement. Factors responsible for such therapeutic failures are not well known. Endogenous resistance to normal levels of calcitriol (544) and decreased vitamin D receptor density in nodular hyperplasia (74) could account for such failures. It has also been shown by in situ hybridization and cytometric DNA analysis that despite there were not differences in the amount of PTH mRNA in the cells from either diffuse or nodular hyperplastic glands, the recurrence of 2°HPTH may not be due to enhanced PTH synthetic activity but to the abnormal growth rate of the transplanted nodular graft (73, 545).

A known cause of failure to the treatment with calcitriol include an irregular administration of the sterol because of repeated episodes of hypercalcemia. Parathyroid size, in preliminary studies, has been noted to be critical for long-term prognosis of calcitriol therapy in dialysis patients (546). It is our impression that the larger the gland, the more severe the 2°HPTH and the more likely the presence of resistance to treatment. In this regard, the use of higher doses of intravenous calcitriol may correct the calcitriol resistance and avoid the need for parathyroidectomy even in patients with severe 2°HPTH (509).

Another emerging cause of failure to control 2°HPTH despite appropriate calcitriol therapy is the presence of significant hyperphosphatemia. Of particular interest is the observation in our previous study (38) in which in two patients, after the observed decreased in basal and maximal PTH levels following calcitriol treatment, they later developed severe hyperphosphatemia with a simultaneous worsening of the HPTH, despite continued calcitriol therapy (Figure 30). These findings suggest that P *per se* may lead to worsening of 2°HPTH and resistance to the inhibitory effect of calcitriol on PTH synthesis. Fernandez and Montoliu have recently evaluated parathyroid function and hyperphosphatemia in dialysis patients (478). As it is shown in Figure 31, severe hyperphosphatemia displaced the PTH–Ca curve toward the right in only 3 days. Figure 32 displays an schematic representation of the deleterious effects of hyperphosphatemia on PTH secretion and inhibitory action on calcitriol. Thus, hyperphosphatemia in the presence of calcitriol therapy may lead not only to an increase in the risk of soft tissue calcification through an increase in the Ca×P product (547), but it also may render calcitriol therapy ineffective and aggravate the 2°HPTH.

Finally, despite appropriate therapy with calcitriol, bone histology does not always return to normal in a substantial number of patients, clearly indicating the presence of factors other than calcitriol in the pathogenesis of 2°HPTH. It has also been observed in an experimental model that calcitriol failed to completely reverse hyper-

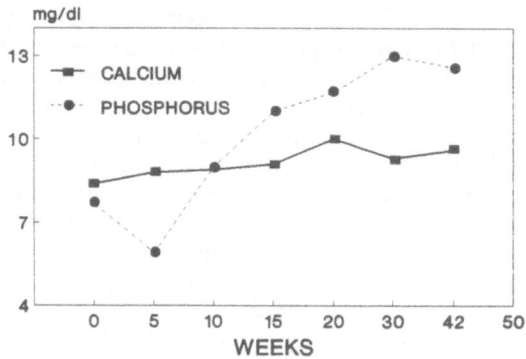
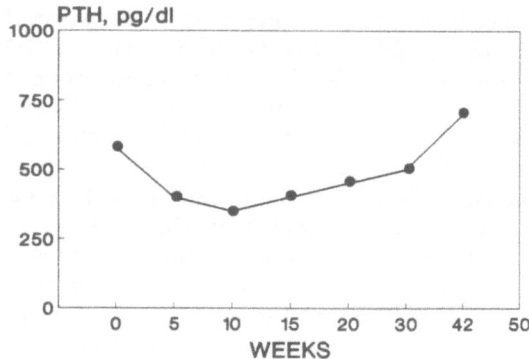

Figure 30.   A patient with 2°HPTH treated with intravenous calcitriol for 42 weeks. On the left panel serum calcium and phosphorus during this period are displayed. Shown on the right panel is the serum PTH. Note that while the patient developed severe hyperphosphatemia (dietary non compliance) and despite appropiate intravenous calcitriol treatment and serum calcium in the upper limit of normal, PTH progressively increased after the 5th week (38).

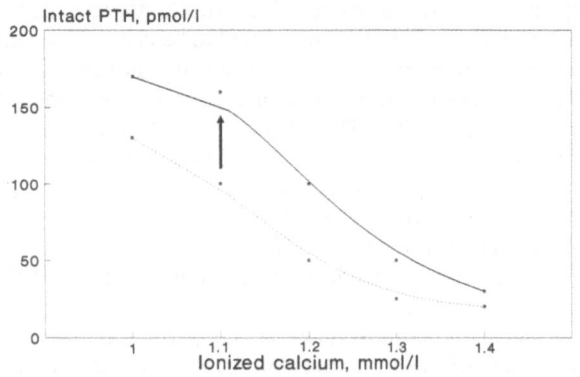

Figure 31.   Sigmoidal PTH–Ca relationship in a non compliant patient with severe hyperphosphatemia. The continuous line displays the PTH–Ca curve in the presence of severe hyperphosphatemia (10.5 mg/dl). The dotted line displays the PTH–Ca curve 3 days later after lowering serum phosphorus to 7.8 mg/dl. (Data from Fernandez and Montoliu (438).)

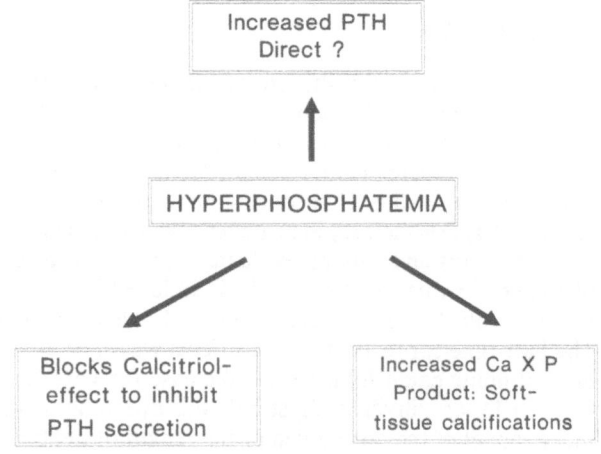

Figure 32.   Schematic representation of the deleterious effects of hyperphosphatemia.

plasia once the latter had been established (542). Also, parathyroid glands weights tend to be increased even after successful renal transplantation. We have observed that despite good clinical responses to calcitriol, a significant number of patients have a rebound in PTH to previous values once calcitriol is discontinued. Moreover, calcitriol did not have the same effect on the PTH–Ca sigmoidal curve than parathyroidectomy (84). Thus, medical parathyroidectomy with intravenous calcitriol is not equivalent to surgical parathyroidectomy. It is possible that with calcitriol the secretion of PTH decreases proportionally more than with a decrease in the mass of parathyroid cells (317).

Useful guidelines to therapy with calcitriol and other active vitamin D derivatives in patients on dialysis are the following: 1) In patients with intact PTH levels five-six fold greater than the upper limit of normality, calcitri-

ol should almost always be initiated; 2) In patients with intact PTH levels between 3–5 five fold normal, therapy at low doses might be considered, especially if serial determinations show a PTH increase; 3) In patients with intact PTH levels between 2–3 fold normal, calcitriol may not be advisable because of the risk of inducing low-turnover bone disease unless the cause is a rare severe malnutrition with nutritional vitamin D deficiency.

Patients who may benefit from intravenous calcitriol are: a) noncompliant patients; b) patients with overt 2°HPTH who cannot be treated with oral calcitriol therapy because of induced hypercalcemia; c) patients who develop hyperphosphatemia immediately after oral administration of calcitriol (they may respond to intravenous calcitriol with a lesser degree of hyperphosphatemia); and d) patients with marked 2°HPTH who are considered for parathyroidectomy (in some cases the administration of iv calcitriol may avoid surgery; the dosage of calcitriol may be increased as long as serum Ca and P are adequately controlled).

Parathyroidectomy

The medical management described above may not succeed, and the progression of overt 2°HPTH may necessitate parathyroidectomy (PTX). Thus, the clinical indications for parathyroid surgery include: *unequivocal evidence of 2°HPTH* (very high levels of serum PTH and the presence of osteitis fibrosa on bone biopsy), *exclusion of Al toxicity, and any of the following:* (1) persistent hypercalcemia not attributable to other causes, especially if hypercalcemia is symptomatic; (2) severe and intractable pruritus; (3) serum Ca×P product that consistently exceeds 70 to 80 together with progressive extraskeletal calcification; (4) progressive skeletal and articular pain, fractures or deformities; (5) symptomatic hypercalcemia after successful kidney transplantation; and (6) calciphylaxis. When a patient does not have a refractory hypercalcemia or hyperphosphatemia, a therapeutic trial with intravenous calcitriol should be tried prior to PTX.

Since Stanbury et al. carried out the first PTX in a patient with severe 2°HPTH (481), three surgical procedures for management of overt 2° HPTH have been developed. They are: 1) subtotal PTX; 2) total PTX with autotransplantation; and 3) total PTX without autotransplantation. Each procedure has its advocates (548–550); however, the most important factor is a surgeon who is highly skilled and experienced with parathyroid surgery and/or a particular technique. Some groups abrogate for the superiority of PTX with autotransplantation (551, 552), because of a re-operation in the forearm is technically simpler than in the neck. However, malignant degeneration of the autografted tissue has been reported (553) as well as muscle invasion by benign parathyroid hyperplasia (554). Recent observations surveying several hundred patients after PTX seems to indicate that similar results are obtained with subtotal PTX and total PTX with autotransplantation (549).

Substantial numbers of patients may have recurrence of 2°HPTH after PTX regardless of the procedure. Gagne et al. (421) noted that one third of the patients who underwent subtotal PTX or total PTX with autotransplantation had elevated intact levels of PTH. Because of the high rate of recurrence Kaye et al. favor total PTX without autotransplantation (550). In a recent long-term post-PTX follow-up (mean 3.8 years), 7 of 9 patients had measurable levels of intact PTH and one even mild 2°HPTH. All patients improved clinically and bone mineral density increased even in two-transplanted patients (550). Total PTX without autotransplantation remains controversial especially considering the propensity of these patients to develop Al-related bone disease and the unknown evolution of bone disease after an eventual kidney transplantation and corticosteroid treatment.

At surgery, it is imperative that *all* the parathyroid glands be identified. The number of glands normally varies from two to six (555); failure to recognize sites of normal fifth and sixth glands is a common cause of failure of parathyroid surgery (556). Good judgment and even more important, extensive experience of the parathyroid surgeon are clearly important for the identification and management of these atypical cases. When subtotal PTX is being performed, it is important that the most suitable gland be identified. Usually the gland that appears least hyperplastic but has an adequate blood supply is the best to partially resect; 40 to 60 mg of tissue should be left. After visually ascertaining that a satisfactory blood supply is preserved in the remaining parathyroid tissue, the surgeon can excise the other glands. The residual parathyroid tissue sometimes undergoes hyperplasia, necessitating a second surgical procedure; therefore, it is recommended that the remaining gland be marked by a metal clip and/or a long, black silk suture (557). When only two or three parathyroid glands in the neck or the upper anterior thorax are accessible at the time of neck exploration, the removal of all three glands is recommended under an assumption that the fourth gland is located elsewhere. Tissues should be maintained by cryopreservation in case that permanent hypoparathyroidism develops (558).

For parathyroid autotransplantation, parathyroid tissue, which has been identified by frozen section, is placed in chilled culture medium; then slices are implanted in multiple pockets in muscle on the lateral aspect of the flexor surface of the forearm of the nondominant arm (558). Nonabsorbable suture is used to secure the slices in the muscle pockets and to provide a marker for subsequent identification should surgical resection be required. Recently, the presternal subcutaneous implantation of the autograph has also been shown to be safe and effective (559). Finally, technical problems during the PTX should be few, and blood loss minimal. A dialysis patient should be treated with dialysis 1 day before the elective PTX and the hematocrit should be higher than 30% to assure the best possible coagulation. Usually the patient can leave the hospital within a week.

The most important problem in the postoperative period is hypocalcemia. Blood Ca levels almost invariably fall after removal of parathyroid tissue; the degree of hypocalcemia is related to the severity of histologic parameters of osteitis fibrosa (560). It is the so called 'hungry bone syndrome' since, in the absence of PTH, Ca influx to the bone dramatically increases and the resulting hypocalcemia is usually significant. The magnitude of Ca administration correlates closely with the severity of skeletal disease (561). Because of it, hypocalcemia is often more marked and prolonged than that observed in patients with primary HPTH after PTX. To minimize the postoperative hypocalcemia, 0.5 to 1.0 μg/day of oral calcitriol or 1.5–2 μg/dialysis of iv calcitriol, may be given for 4 to 6 days before PTX and immediately after it; also, oral Ca carbonate is given to provide 1 to 2 g of elemental Ca. Significant and often prolonged hypophosphatemia also develop after surgery due to the 'hungry bone'.

Tetany may occur during the postoperative period and usually occurs during the first hemodialysis sessions; this is most likely related to the ph increase induced by dialysis. The amount of oral Ca needed is often quite large; it can be increased 0.5 to 1.0 g/day at intervals of 3 to 7 days until serum Ca concentration begins to increase. If the concentration of serum Ca falls below 7.5 mg/dl, or if tetany appears, intravenous Ca should be given as well. Thus, after PTX careful monitoring of serum Ca is mandatory. Tetany occurring in a uremic patient with severe bone disease may be catastrophic; the simultaneous fracture of scapula, clavicle, and both femoral necks has been reported during an episode of tetany during dialysis (562). These major fractures have usually been observed 1 to 3 weeks after surgery. Interestingly, they often occurred late during the hemodialysis procedure. Seizures can also cause fractures and tendon avulsion. Such seizures may occur from 1–2 days up to 4 weeks after the surgery. In the postoperative management of patients with marked periarticular calcification, it may be wise to maintain a modest hypocalcemia – i.e., serum Ca concentration of 8.0 to 9.0 mg/dl – until the ectopic calcification have resolved. Similarly, the administration of Ca-containing P binders may be indicated to maintain serum P concentration in the range of 3.5 to 5.0 mg/dl.

In patients with marked skeletal disease, hypocalcemia may occasionally persist for 2 to 3 months after PTX. Large amounts of oral Ca supplements and appropriate doses of calcitriol usually are also successful in correcting hypocalcemia. Serum levels of P and Mg may also decrease during this time. If serum Mg falls below 1.5 mg/dl (1.2 mEq/l), oral supplemental Mg should be given. Administration of P salts aggravates hypocalcemia; thus patients should not receive P unless the serum P falls to very low levels (< 1.5–2 mg/dl). An increase in the calcitriol dosage may be needed. If the serum P concentration falls below 2.5 mg/dl, administration of P binders should be reduced or stopped, but no effort should be made to increase the P concentration above 3.5 to 4.0 mg/dl. Calcium carbonate or acetate are the agents of choice, and Al salts should be avoided (561).

During the period of hypocalcemia, remineralization of the skeleton is usually occurring; blood Ca concentration starts to rise and the requirement for Ca and calcitriol decrease markedly once bone remineralization is completed. If the doses of Ca and calcitriol are not reduced, hypercalcemia may ensue. The fall of a markedly elevated plasma alkaline phosphatase level to near normal may indicate that the bone is reaching a stage where healing is largely completed; when this occurs, the Ca supplements and vitamin D dosage should be reduced.

Failure of serum Ca concentration to decrease significantly after surgery may indicate either that too much residual parathyroid tissue was left behind or that missed, ectopic or supernumerary glands were present. Thus, several techniques such as ecography, CAT, ^{201}Tl-^{99m}Tc scintigraphy or a combination of these have been used for presurgical localization of parathyroid glands (396, 397, 563). Another cause of failure of serum Ca to decrease after PTX may be that severe osteitis fibrosa was not responsible for the hypercalcemia present prior to PTX. In this situation Al toxicity, a granulomatous or neoplastic disorder, among other causes, have to be excluded.

Hyperkalemia is another preventable complication after PTX (562). This is in agreement with recent information demonstrating an important role of PTH in regulating potassium homeostasis. When even modest hyperkalemia occurs in a dialysis patient during the immediate postoperative period, substantial electrocardiographic abnormalities may occur on account of the rise in potassium concentration and the concomitant hypocalcemia.

Another postoperative complication of PTX is the development of Al-related osteomalacia (143). The mechanism responsible for this is unclear; most likely, substantial accumulation of Al in bone had developed prior to the PTX, and the presence high PTH levels with an increased bone turnover rate may have protected the bone from the deleterious effect of Al. After PTX, bone turnover decreases markedly and Al is deposited on the mineralization front (143). The existence of symptomatic osteomalacia after PTX indicates that surgery may have not been indicated and hypercalcemia was due to preexisting Al-related bone disease. Furthermore, in the absence of PTH, removal of Al deposits from bone with DFO is more difficult.

Percutaneous ethanol injection

A new parathyroid ablative technique consisting of percutaneous fine-needle ethanol injection into enlarged parathyroid glands under ultrasonic guidance was developed by Giangrande et al. in 1982 (564). Their experience in fifty uremic patients already treated has been recently reviewed (499). Excellent results were also obtained in seven patients who had relapsed after subtotal PTX (565). The technique has also been proven effective by other groups (566, 567). Thus, this procedure may be an alternative to surgical treatment in selected cases. Side-effects have been reported to be rare, mild and transient.

TREATMENT OF ALUMINUM-RELATED BONE DISEASE

Patients with profound Al toxicity were initially difficult to manage. Hemodialysis employing Al-free water brought about the removal of only small quantities, because of substantial binding of Al to transferrin and other plasma proteins (566, 567); and some dialysis units continued to give Al gels. The management of Al toxicity with Al-free dialysate failed to produce clinical improvement if the patients continued to ingest Al-containing P binders (360). Prevention of this disease, which usually results from the use of Al contaminated water, is the most important single therapeutic first step. The finding of several patients with Al-related bone disease in a single dialysis unit should prompt reevaluation of the adequacy of the method used for water purification. Periodic sampling of plasma Al levels in a population of patients in a dialysis unit may provide the best indication of even intermittent contamination of water (126). Deionization and treatment with reverse osmosis are both effective methods for Al removal (570). However, reverse osmosis is inadequate as a sole purification method when the Al concentration of water exceeds 200 to 300 μg/l, as might arise when a municipal water treatment uses alum (aluminum sulfate) for the flocculation of water as part of the water treatment.

The second therapeutic step is the substitution of the Al-containing P binders for Ca carbonate or Ca acetate and the removal of other Al containing medications (such as albumin infusions, sucralfate or some hyperalimentation supplements). The implementation of these steps usually result in the healing of Al bone disease. Freemont et al. reported the improvement of bone biopsies 5 years after initiation of water purification combined with either withdrawal of Al hydroxide treatment or reduction of its dosage (571). Hercz et al. (125) reported substantial improvement of the histologic features of Al bone disease by 11 to 12 months after the afflicted patients had withdrawn Al-containing gels and underwent hemodialysis with low dialysate Al concentration (less than 10 μg/l).

Ackrill et al. first reported that the chelating agent deferoxamine (DFO) was effective for the removal of Al in a dialysis patient with encephalopathy; lifesaving improvement of both the neurologic features and the patients's musculoskeletal symptoms arising from osteomalacia was observed following treatment with DFO (572). Subsequently, this agent, which has a high affinity for Al as well as for iron, was also used in Al-related bone disease with dramatic favorable responses (114, 328).

Deferoxamine augments the removal of Al in two ways: it mobilizes Al from tissue stores, thereby increasing the plasma concentration of Al, and it increases the fraction of plasma Al that is ultrafilterable. Plasma Al is 80 to 90% protein bound, so that only 10–20% is ultrafilterable (569). This is the reason why Al is poorly removed during dialysis. After DFO, the absolute serum Al increases and most is in the form of aluminoxamine and feroxamine complexes, which are removable either by hemodialysis, peritoneal dialysis, using a charcoal hemoperfusion cartridge in combination with a dialysis membrane or hemofiltration (568, 573, 574).

Repeated infusion of DFO, 30–40 mg/kg/week during the last half hour of the preceding dialysis session, was associated with substantial clinical improvement in Al-related bone disease (114). A modest reduction of serum Ca was observed, and increments in plasma alkaline phosphatase levels occurred after 4 to 12 weeks of treatment; these observations are consistent with remineralization of bone. Moreover, bone biopsies have shown improvement with reduced Al staining and increased bone formation rate (114). Malluche et al. noted improved bone histology and an increase in the mineralization rate in three patients with mixed uremic bone disease that was characterized by Al deposits and yet normal bone formation (328). Ferritin levels usually decrease and, as mentioned above, PTH levels increase and signs of 2°HPTH may develop (especially in cases of mixed bone disease); indeed, some patients with low-turnover bone lesions may develop osteitis fibrosa (114). Erythrocyte mean corpuscular volume and hematocrit may also rise. Similarly, DFO has been noted to induce a greater response to erythropoietin therapy in patients who had minimal Al accumulation (575).

As these beneficial effects of therapy with DFO were being noted, a number of serious side effects were also recognized. Thus, retinal and auditory toxicity (576–578), hypotension, thrombocytopenia (579) and serious and even fatal cases of encephalopathy were noted (580). The risk of encephalopathy is lessened if the dose of DFO is decreased and adjusted periodically to limit the rise of serum Al 24–48 h after the DFO administration to values lower than 300 μg/l. Fatal infections with Yersinia species have been described (561–582). In addition, mucormycosis, a Rhizopus infection that is also commonly fatal, has also appeared among dialysis patients receiving long-term treatment with DFO (582, 583); the infection is most commonly disseminated; frequently following a rapidly fatal course; and commonly it is not suspected during life and recognized only at postmortem examination (582). Cultures of blood and other body fluids may not be positive even in cases of histologically proven infection. In regard to the probable mechanism of DFO-induced mucormycosis, it is likely that DFO, which is a microbial siderophore, stimulates the growth and pathogenicity of certain species of fungi by making environmental iron more available to the microorganism (584). This may occur as a result of receptors on the fungi for the DFO-iron complex (feroxamine), which then facilitates the uptake of iron by the microorganism (582). Iron and Al complexes of DFO are both cleared from the body largely by the kidneys; therefore, pharmacokinetics changes in uremia lead to a prolonged accumulation of feroxamine after DFO (585).

Because of the seriousness of these potential complications, and because they can appear after a short treatment with relatively low doses (582), DFO therapy should be limited to dialysis patients with proven Al encephalopathy or those with severe, symptomatic Al-related bone disease that has failed to respond to the withdrawal of Al-containing gels and the elimination of exposure to Al-contaminated dialysate. If DFO must be used, it should be given in the lowest possible doses (e.g., 5–15 mg/kg; every 7 to 10 days), and it is desirable that the dialysis performed after the treatment is done using a highly permeable dialysis membrane or the insertion of a charcoal cartridge that permits the rapid removal of DFO complexes of iron and Al (573, 574). Deferoxamine is increasingly being administered shortly before or at the beginning of the hemodialysis session (586). Serum Al levels should be measured repeatedly during treatment to minimize the risk of Al neurotoxicity and to titrate the DFO dosage (ideally serum aluminum should be between twice the basal value and always < 300 μg/l, when DFO is administered 24–48 hours before the measurement). With the recently available micromethod to determine DFO and its metallochelates aluminoxamine and feroxamine, it seems that DFO may be more appropriately dosaged (586) and in some patients weekly doses of 5 mg/kg of DFO may be sufficient (587).

The 1,2 dimethyl-3-hydroxipyrid-4-one (L1) is a new *oral* drug that has been safely used to treat thalassemic patients with iron overload. Preliminary data in the experimental animal noted the potential of the drug to increase ultrafilterable Al and mobilize Al from tissues (588). Further data is needed before its use is recommended in patients.

TREATMENT OF IDIOPATHIC ADYNAMIC BONE DISEASE

While the natural history of this entity is unknown, it seems advisable to prevent an excessive suppression of PTH (intact PTH lower than 1.5–3 fold the upper limit of normal) since mildly increased levels of PTH are associated with a normal bone formation rate in dialysis patients (146, 589). Dialysis patients with PTH levels in the normal range and without Al toxicity, may need to be treated with a dialysate Ca of 2.5 mEq/l or even lower to increase PTH and improve the low-turnover bone state. Recently, Hercz et al. have treated some of these patients with a 2.0 mEq/l dialysate Ca and noted an increase in PTH (149); an increase in the bone formation rate also occurred (590). While it is not known either the natural course or the morbidity of this disease, no general recommendations can be done.

OTHER TREATMENT CONSIDERATIONS

Calcitonin may be useful, in the future, in certain patients with inoperable 2°HPTH or patients that cannot be managed with calcitriol because of hypercalcemia (591). However, a report of its short-term administration in uremic patients showed little overall effect (592).

Biphosphonates are analogues of pyrophosphate with a potent inhibit effect on bone resorption (593). They inhibit osteoclast activity; recent reports also suggest that their effects could also be mediated by osteoblasts (594). There are only limited studies on the use of Biphospho-

nates in CRF and they are not conclusive. Indications for the use of these drugs in the future may be the hypercalcemic patients with increased bone turnover and those with extraosseous calcification due to high Ca×P product (595). Their side-effects, advantages and contraindications as well as details on dosage, administration and their use in combination therapy remain unknown.

Physicochemical properties of dialysis membranes other than permeability have a substantial effect decreasing intact PTH concentration during hemodialysis (596). However, PTH reverts to the previous level between hemodialysis sessions (596, 597). With the use of coated charcoal (150 g/cartridge) in combination with standard hemodialysis, a decrease in PTH levels – probably related to adsorption to the cartridge – has been observed (598). This decrease in PTH was associated with marked relief of pruritus and other symptoms. Thus, it was suggested that symptomatic patients with 2°HPTH prior to PTX, may be successfully treated with this therapeutic modality.

Patients undergoing regular dialysis receive periodic injections of heparin; clinical and experimental studies suggest that heparin, when given repeatedly, is associated with decreased skeletal mineralization and may predispose to fractures in patients without renal disease. In one study of bone mineral content in which hand radiographs were analyzed, a positive correlation was noted between the rate of decrease in bone mass and the regular dosage of heparin given to dialysis patients (599). Osteoporosis has been reported in patients receiving 15,000 to 30,000 U/day of heparin over long periods of time (535): multiple fractures and pseudoarthrosis have also been reported (600). Osteoporosis did not develop in patients receiving lower doses (i.e., 10,000 U/day), and dialysis patients may not receive quantities of heparin large enough to cause difficulties (601). However, a recent study using technetium-labeled heparin in 12 hemodialysis patients showed a greater accumulation of the tracer in knees and shoulders in hemodialyzed patients as compared with controls; this suggests that accumulation of heparin in bone tissue could play a role in causing osteopenia in hemodialysis patients (602). With the use of efficient dialyzers and shorter duration of dialysis, the quantity of heparin given is less, and the potential for any adverse effect of heparin on the skeleton are reduced.

Management of fractures

Rib fractures, probably the most frequent fractures in uremic patients, usually heal slowly over a period of several months. They are often asymptomatic and require little specific treatment. Traumatic fractures of the long bones and of the femoral neck may have a poor union even after several months. When fractures occur in patients with marked 2°HPTH it is mandatory to treat this patients with appropriate dose of calcitriol; often the fractures heal after calcitriol therapy. If the fracture does not heal, then the appropriate surgical repair should be considered, since prolonged immobilization can create even greater complications in such patients. In some patients with fractures due to Al-related osteomalacia, slow healing may occur even though Al accumulation has not been specifically treated. In such patients nonunion of the fracture occurs and the fracture may heal after DFO therapy. Successful use of femoral head prostheses has been noted in patients with end-stage CRF and in those on dialysis (537).

REFERENCES

1. Holick MF, McNeill SC, MacLaughlin JA et al.: The physiologic implications of the formation of previtamin D3 in skin. *Trans Assoc Am Phys* 92: 54, 1979
2. Gray, RW, Omdahl JL, Ghazarian JG, DeLuca HF: 25-hydroxycholecalciferol-1-hydroxylase. *J Biol Chem* 247: 7528, 1972
3. Hughes MR, Haussler MR, Wergedal J, Baylink DJ: Regulation of plasma 1 alpha,25-dihydroxyvitamin D3 by calcium and phosphate. *Clin Res* 23: 323A, 1975
4. Haussler MR, McCain TA: Basic and clinical concepts related to vitamin D metabolism and action. *N Eng J Med* 297: 974, 1041, 1977
5. Cantley LK, Russell J, Lettieri D, Sherwood LM: 1,25(OH)2 D-dihydroxyvitamin D3 suppresses parathyroid hormone secretion from bovine parathyroid cells in tissue culture. *Endocrinology* 117: 2114, 1985
6. DeLuca HF: Vitamin D endocrinology. *Ann Intern Med* 85: 367, 1976
7. Mayer GP, Hurst JG: Sigmoidal relationship between parathyroid hormone secretion rate and plasma calcium concentration in calves. *Endocrinology* 102: 1036, 1978
8. Mayer GP, Habener JF, Potts JF: Parathyroid hormone secretion *in vivo* demonstration of a calcium-independent nonsuppressible component of secretion. *J Clin Invest* 57: 678, 1976
9. Mayer GP, Hurst JG, Barto JA, Keaton JA, Moore MP: Effect of epinephrine on parathyroid hormone secretion in calves. *Endocrinology* 104: 1181, 1979
10. Habener JF, Potts JT Jr: Relative effectiveness of magnesium hormone *in vitro*. *Endocrinology* 98: 197, 1976
11. Habener JF, Mayer GP, Dee PC, Potts JT Jr: Metabolism of amino- and carboxyl-sequence immunoactive parathyroid hormone in the bovine: evidence for peripheral cleavage of hormone. *Metabolism* 25: 385, 1976
12. Martin KJ, Hruska K, Freitag JJ, Klahr S, Slatopolsky E: The peripheral metabolism of parathyroid hormone. *N Engl J Med* 301: 1092, 1979
13. Slatopolsky E, Caglar S, Pennell JP et al.: On the pathogenesis of hyperparathyroidism in chronic experimental insufficiency in the dog. *J Clin Invest* 50: 492, 1971
14. Russell J, Lettieri D, Sherwood LM: Direct regulation by calcium of cytoplasmatic messenger ribonucleic acid for preproparathyroid hormone in isolated bovine parathyroid cells. *J Clin Invest* 72: 1851, 1983
15. Yamamoto M, Igarashi T, Muramatsu M et al.: Hypocalcemia increases and hypercalcemia decreases the steady state level of parathyroid hormone messenger ribonucleic acid in the rat. *J Clin Invest* 83: 1053, 1989
16. Pitts TO, Piraino BH, Mitro R et al.: Hyperparathyroidism and 1,25-dihydroxyvitamin D deficiency in mild, moder-

ate, and severe renal failure. *J Clin Endocrinol Metab* 67: 876, 1988
17. Reichel H, Deibert B, Schmidt-Gayk H, Ritz E: Calcium metabolism in early chronic renal failure: Implications for the pathogenesis of hyperparathyroidism. *Nephrol Dial Transplant* 6: 162, 1991
18. Wilson L, Felsenfeld AJ, Drezner MK, Llach F: Altered divalent ion metabolism in early renal failure: Role of 1,25-(OH)2D. *Kidney Int* 27: 565, 1985
19. Lopez-Hilker S, Galceran T, Chan Y-L et al.: Hypocalcemia may not be essential for the development of secondary hyperparathyroidism in chronic renal failure. *J Clin Invest* 78: 1097, 1986
20. Kaplan MA, Canterbury JM, Jaffe D: Effect of dietary phosphorus (P) in the phosphaturic and calcemic response to parathyroid hormone (PTH) in the uremic dog. *Kidney Int* 18: 77, 1977
21. Tennant BJ, Lowe JE, Tasker JB: Hypercalcemia and hypophosphatemia in ponies following bilateral nephrectomy. *Proc Soc Exp Biol Med* 167: 365, 1981
22. Slatopolsky E, Caglar S, Gradowska L: On the prevention of secondary hyperparathyroidism in experimental chronic renal disease using 'proportional reduction' of dietary phosphorus intake. *Kidney Int* 2: 147, 1972
23. Bricker NS: trade off hypothesis. *N Engl J Med* 286: 1093, 1972
24. Reiss E, Canterbury JM, Bercovitz MA, Kaplan EL: The role of phosphate in the secretion of parathyroid hormone in man. *J Clin Invest* 49: 2146, 1970
25. Jowsey J, Reiss E, Canterbury JM: Long term effects of high phosphate intake on parathyroid hormone levels and bone metabolism. *Acta Orthop Scand* 45: 801, 1974
26. Fournier AE, Johnson WJ, Taves DR: Etiology of hyperparathyroidism and bone disease during chronic hemodialysis. I. Association of bone disease with potentially etiologic factors. *J Clin Invest* 50: 592, 1971
27. Fournier AE, Arnaud CD, Johnson WJ et al.: Etiology of hyperparathyroidism and bone disease during chronic hemodialysis. II. Factors affecting serum immunoreactive parathyroid hormone. *J Clin Invest* 50: 599, 1971
28. Llach F, Massry SG: On the mechanism of the prevention of secondary hyperparathyroidism in moderate renal insufficiency. *J Clin Endocrinol Metab* 61: 601, 1985
29. Maschio G et al.: Early dietary phosphorus restriction and calcium supplementation in the prevention of renal osteodystrophy. *Am J Clin Nutr* 33: 1546, 1980
30. Goldman R, Bassett SH: Phosphorus excretion in renal failure. *J Clin Invest* 33: 1623, 1954
31. Slatopolsky E, Gradowska L, Kashemsant C et al.: The control of phosphate excretion in uremia. *J Clin Invest* 45: 672, 1966
32. Adler AJ, Ferran N, Berlyne GM: Effect of inorganic phosphate on serum ionized calcium concentration *in vitro*: a reassessment of the 'trade-off hypothesis'. *Kidney Int* 28: 932, 1985
33. Hebert LA, Lemann J, Petersen JR, Lennon EJ: Studies of the mechanism by which phosphate infusion lowers serum calcium concentration. *J Clin Invest* 45: 1886, 1966
34. Portale AP, Halloran BP, Murphy MM, Morris RC Jr: Oral intake of phosphorus can determine the serum concentration of 1,25 D by determining its production rate in humans. *J Clin Invest* 77: 7, 1986

35. Rodriguez M, Martin-Malo A, Martinez ME et al.: Calcemic response to parathyroid hormone in renal failure: role of phosphorus and its effect on calcitriol. *Kidney Int* 40: 1055, 1991

36. Lucas PA, Brown RC, Woodhead JS, Coles G: 1,25 dihydroxycholecalciferol and parathyroid hormone in advanced renal failure: effect of simultaneous protein and phosphorus restriction. *Clin Nephrol* 25: 7, 1986

37. Tessitore N, Venturi A, Adami S et al.: Relationship between serum vitamin D metabolites and dietary intake of phosphate in patients with early renal failure. *Miner Electrolyte Metab* 13: 38, 1987

38. Rodriguez M, Felsenfeld AJ, Dunlay R et al.: The effect of long-term calcitriol administration on parathyroid function in hemodialysis patients. *J Am Soc Nephrol* 2: 1014, 1991

39. Yi H, Fukagawa M, Kurokawa K: Mild dietary phosphorus restriction directly prevents enhanced parathyroid hormone secretion and synthesis and proliferation of parathyroid cells in chronic renal failure in rats. *J Am Soc Nephrol* 3: 703, 1992

40. Evanson JM: The response to the infusion of parathyroid extract in hypocalcemic states. *Clin Sci* 31: 63, 1966

41. Massry SG, Coburn JW, Lee DBN et al.: Skeletal resistance to parathyroid hormone in renal failure: study in 105 human subjects. *Ann Intern Med* 78: 357, 1973

42. Christiansen C: Chronic renal failure and vitamin D metabolites: a status report. *J Steroid Biochem* 19: 517, 1983

43. Fraser DR, Kodicek E: Unique biosynthesis by kidney of a biologically active vitamin D metabolite. *Nature* 228: 764, 1970

44. Gray R, Boyle I, DeLuca HF: Vitamin D metabolism: The role of kidney tissue. *Science* 172: 1232, 1971

45. Mawer EB, Backhouse J, Taylor CM: Failure of formation of 1,25 dihydroxycholecalciferol in chronic renal insufficiency. *Lancet* 1: 626, 1973

46. Schaefer K et al.: Metabolism of 1,2 H3–4–C14-cholecalciferol in normal, uremic and anephric subjects. *Isr J Med Sci* 8: 80, 1972

47. Mason RS, Lissner d, Wilkinson M, Posen S: Vitamin D metabolites and their relationship to azotemic osteodystrophy. *Clin Endocrinol* 13: 375, 1980

48. Brickman AS, Coburn JW, Massry SG, Norman AW: 1,25 dihydroxyvitamin D3 in normal man and patients with renal failure. *Ann Intern Med* 80: 161, 1974

49. Brickman AS, Coburn JW, Norman AW: Action of 1,25 dihydroxycholecalciferol, a potent, kidney produced metabolite of vitamin D3 in uremic man. *N Engl J Med* 287: 891, 1972

50. Portale AP, Booth BE, Halloran BP, Morris RC Jr: Effect of dietary phosphorus on circulating concentrations of 1,25 dihydroxyvitamin D and immunoreactive parathyroid hormone in children with moderate renal insufficiency. *J Clin Invest* 73: 1580, 1984

51. Chesney RW, Hamstra AJ, Mazess RB: Circulating vitamin D metabolite concentrations in childhood renal diseases. *Kidney Int* 21: 65, 1982

52. Mora-Palma FJ, Lorenzo Sellares V, Ellis HL et al.: Osteomalacia in chronic renal failure before dialysis. *Proc Eur Dial Transplant Assoc* 19: 188, 1983

53. Cheung AK, Manolagas SC, Catherwood BC et al.: Determinants of serum 1,25 (OH)2D levels in renal disease. *Kidney Int* 24: 104, 1983

54. Coburn JW, Koppel MH, Brickman AS, Massry SG: Study of intestinal absorption of calcium in patients with renal failure. *Kidney Int* 3: 264, 1973

55. Chan YL, McKay C, Dye E, Slatopolsky E: The effect of 1,25-dihydroxycholecalciferol on parathyroid hormone secretion by monolayer cultures of bovine parathyroid cells. *Calcif Tissue Int* 3827: 2732, 1986

56. Hsu CH, Patel S, Young EW, Simpson RU: Production and degradation of calcitriol in renal failure rats. *Am J Physiol* 253: F1015, 1987

57. Hsu CH, Patel S, Buchsbaum BL: Calcitriol metabolism in patients with chronic renal failure. *Am J Kidney Dis* 17: 185, 1991

58. Hsu CH, Patel SR, Young EW: Mechanism of decreased calcitriol degradation in renal failure. *Am J Physiol* 262: F192, 1992

59. Dusso A, Lopez-Hilker S, Rapp N, Slatopolsky E: Extra-renal production of calcitriol. *Kidney Int* 34: 368, 1988

60. Dusso A, Finch J, Delmez J, Rapp N et al.: Extrarrenal production of calcitriol. *Kidney Int* 38: S36, 1990

61. Silver J, Russell J, Sherwood LM: Regulation by vitamin D metabolites of messenger ribonucleic acid for pre-proparathyroid hormone in isolated bovine parathyroid cells. *Proc Natl Acad Sci USA* 82: 4270, 1985

62. Silver J, Naveh-Many T, Mayer H: Regulation by vitamin D metabolites of parathyroid hormone gene *in vivo* by the rat. *J Clin Invest* 78: 1296, 1986

63. Shvil Y, Naveh-Many T, Barach P, Silver J: Regulation of parathyroid cell gene expression in experimental uremia. *J Am Soc Nephrol* 1: 99, 1990

64. Slatopolsky E, Weerts C, Thielan J et al.: Marked suppression of secondary hyperparathyroidism by intravenous administration of 1,25 dihydroxycholecalciferol in uremic patients. *J Clin Invest* 74: 2136, 1984

65. Delmez JA, Tindira C, Grooms P et al.: Parathyroid hormone suppression by intravenous 1,25 Dihydroxyvitamin D. A role for increased sensitivity to calcium. *J Clin Invest* 83: 1349, 1989

66. Dunlay R, Rodriguez M, Felsenfeld AJ, Llach F: Direct inhibitory effect of calcitriol on parathyroid function (sigmoidal curve) in dialysis patients. *Kidney Int* 36: 1093, 1989

67. Okazaki T, Igarashi T, Kronenberg KM: 5′ Flanking region of the parathyroid hormone gene mediates negative regulation by 1,25-(OH)2 vitamin D3. *J Biol Chem* 263: 2203, 1988

68. Merke J, Hugel U, Zlotkowski A et al.: Diminished parathyroid 1,25-(OH)2D3 receptors in experimental uremia. *Kidney Int* 32: 350, 1987

69. Korkor AB: Reduced binding of 3(H)1,25-dihydroxyvitamin D3 in the parathyroid glands of patients with renal failure. *N Engl J Med* 316: 1573, 1987

70. Malmaeus J, Grimelius L, Johansson H et al.: Parathyroid pathology in hyperparathyroidism secondary to chronic renal failure. *Scand J Urol Nephrol* 18: 157, 1984

71. St. Goar WT: Case records of the Massachusetts Genral Hospital. *N Engl J Med* 268: 943, 1963

72. McPhaul II, McIntosh DA, Hammond WS, Park OK: Autonomous secondary hyperparathyroidism. *N Engl J Med* 271: 1342, 1964

73. Tanaka Y, Seo H, Tominaga Y et al.: Factors related to the recurrent hyperfunction of autografts after total parathyroidectomy in patients with severe secondary hyperparathyroidism. *Surg Today* 23: 220, 1993

74. Fukuda N, Tanaka H, Tominaga Y et al.: Decreased 1,25-Dihydroxyvitamin D3 receptor density is associated with a more severe form of parathyroid hyperplasia in chronic uremic patients. *J Clin Invest* 92: 1436, 1993

75. Martin KJ, Hruska KA, Greenwalt A, Slatopolsky E: Selective uptake of intact parathyroid hormone by the liver. Differences between hepatic and renal uptake. *J Clin Invest* 58: 781, 1976

76. Catherwood BD et al.: Sites of clearance of endogenous parathyroid hormone in the vitamin D deficient dog. *Endocrinology* 98: 228, 1976

77. Hruska KA, Kopelman R, Rutherford WE: Metabolism of immunoreactive parathyroid hormone in the dog. The role of the kidney and the effects of chronic renal disease. *J Clin Invest* 56: 39, 1975

78. Zull JE, Chuang J: Characterization of parathyroid hormone fragments produced by cathepsin D. *J Biol Chem* 260: 1608, 1985

79. Freitag JJ, Martin KJ, Hruska KA et al.: Impaired parathyroid hormone metabolism in patients with chronic renal failure. *N Engl J Med* 298: 29, 1978

80. Segre GV, Sherrard DJ, Carlton EI: *Use of the PTH (IRMA) assay in patients with impaired renal function and renal osteodystrophy*, San Juan Capistrano, Nichols Institute, 1990, p 1

81. Mayer GP, Hurst JG: Sigmoidal relationship between parathyroid hormone secretion rate and plasma calcium concentration in calves. *Endocrinology* 102: 1036, 1978

82. Voigts A, Felsenfeld AJ, Andress DL, Llach F: Parathyroid hormone and bone histology: response to hypocalcemia in osteitis fibrosa. *Kidney Int* 25: 445, 1984

83. Brown EM, Wilson RE, Eastman R: Abnormal regulation of parathyroid hormone release by calcium in secondary hyperparathyroidism due to chronic renal failure. *J Clin Endocrinol Metab* 54: 172, 1982

84. Malberti F, Surian M, Cosci P: Effect of chronic intravenous calcitriol on parathyroid function and set point of calcium in dialysis patients with refractory secondary hyperparathyroidism. *Nephrol Dial Transplant* 7: 822, 1992

85. Coburn JW, Hartenbower DL, Massry SG: Intestinal absorption of calcium and the effect of renal insufficiency. *Kidney Int* 4: 96, 1973

86. Sherrard DJ, Baylink DJ, Wergedal JE, Maloney NA: Quantitative histological studies on the pathogenesis of uremic bone disease. *J Clin Endocrinol Metab* 39: 119, 1974

87. Eastwood JB, Harris E, Stamp TCB, De Wardener H: Vitamin D deficiency in the osteomalacia of chronic renal failure. *Lancet* 2: 1209, 1976

88. Offerman G, v.Herrath D, Schaefer K: Serum 25 hydroxycholecalciferol in uremia. *Nephron* 13: 269, 1974

89. Baylink DJ, Stauffer J, Wergedal JE, Rich C: Formation, mineralization and resorption of bone in vitamin D deficient rats. *J Clin Invest* 49: 112, 1970

90. Kanis JA, Cundy T, Bartlett M: Is 24,25 dihydroxycholecalciferol a calcium regulating hormone in man? *Br Med J* 1: 1382, 1978

91. Llach F, Brickman AS, Singer FR, Coburn JW: 24,25-Dihydroxycholecalciferol, a vitamin D sterol with qualitatively unique effects in uremic man. *Metab Bone Dis Rel Res* 2: 11, 1979

92. Alfrey AC, Hegg A, Craswell P: Metabolism and toxicity of aluminum in renal failure. *Am J Clin Nutr* 33: 1509, 1980

93. Wills MR, Savory J: Aluminum poisoning: dialysis encephalopathy, osteomalacia, and anaemia. *Lancet* 2: 29, 1983

94. Parkinson IS, Feest TG, Ward MK: Fracturing dialysis osteodystrophy and dialysis encephalopathy: an epidemiological survey. *Lancet* 1: 406, 1979

95. Siddiqui JY, Simpson W, Ellis HA, Kerr DNS: Fluoride and bone disease in patients on regular haemodialysis. *Proc Eur Dial Transplant Assoc* 8: 149, 1971

96. Alfrey AC, LeGendre GR, Kaehny WD: The dialysis encephalopathy syndrome. possible aluminum intoxication. *N Engl J Med* 294: 184, 1976

97. Ward MK, Feest TG, Ellis HA: Osteomalacic dialysis osteodystrophy: evidence for a waterborne etiological agent, probably aluminum. *Lancet* 1: 841, 1978

98. Hodsman AB, Sherrard DJ, Alfrey AC et al.: Bone aluminum and histomorphometric features of renal osteodystrophy. *J Clin Endocrinol Metab* 54: 539, 1982

99. Maloney NA, Ott SM, Alfrey AC et al.: Histologic quantitation of aluminum in iliac bone from patients with renal failure. *J Lab Clin Med* 99: 206, 1982

100. Pierce-Myli M, Pierides AM: Iron and aluminum osteomalacia during hemodialysis: a new syndrome. (Abstract) *Kidney Int* 25: 153, 1984

101. Phelps KR, Vigorita VJ, Bansal M, Einhorn T: Histological demonstration of iron but not aluminum in a case of dialysis associated osteomalacia. *Am J Med* 84: 775, 1988

102. Cannata JB, Diaz Lopez JB: Insights into the complex aluminium and iron relationship. *Nephrol Dial Transplant* 6: 605, 1991

103. Boyce BF, Fell GS, Elder H: Hypercalcemic osteomalacia due to aluminum toxicity. *Lancet* 2: 1009, 1982

104. Hodsman AB, Sherrard DJ, Wong EGC et al.: Vitamin D resistant osteomalacia in hemodialysis patients lacking secondary hyperparathyroidism. *Ann Intern Med* 94: 629, 1981

105. Llach F: Effects of renal failure and dialysis on divalent ion metabolism. in *Divalent Ion Homeostasis, Vol 11, Contemporary Issues in Nephrology*, edited by BM Brenner, JH Stein, New York, Churchill, Livingstone, Inc, 1983, p 291

106. Zins B, Zingraff J, Basile C et al.: Tumoral calcifications in hemodialysis patients: possible role of aluminum intoxication. *Nephron* 60: 260, 1992

107. Sherrard DJ, Ott SM, Andress DL: Pseudohyperparathyroidism: a syndrome associated with aluminum intoxication in chronic renal failure. *Am J Med* 79: 127, 1985

108. Norris KC, Crooks P, Nebeker HG et al.: Clinical and laboratory features of aluminum related bone disease: differences between sporadic and 'epidemic' forms of the syndrome. *Am J Kidney Dis* 6: 342, 1985

109. Andress DL, Felsenfeld AJ, Voigts A, Llach F: Parathyroid hormone response to hypocalcemia in hemodialysis patients with osteomalacia. *Kidney Int* 24: 364, 1983

110. Andress DL, Ott SM, Maloney NA, Sherrard DJ: Effect of parathyroidectomy on bone aluminum accumulation in chronic renal failure. *N Engl J Med* 312: 468, 1985

111. Ellis HA, Peart KM: Azotemic renal osteodystrophy; a quantitative study on iliac. *J Clin Pathol* 26: 83, 1973

112. Cournot-Witmer G, Zingraff J, Plachott JJ et al.: Aluminum localization in bone from hemodialyzed patients: relationship to matrix mineralization. *Kidney Int* 20: 375, 1981

113. Ellis HA: Aluminum and osteomalacia after parathyroidectomy. *Ann Intern Med* 96: 533, 1982

114. Ott SM, Andress DL, Nebeker HG et al.: Changes in bone histology after treatment with desferrioxamine. *Kidney Int* 29 (Suppl 18): S108, 1986

115. Fanti P, Faugere MC, Smith AJ, Malluche HH: Removal of aluminum is associated with increased production of 1, 25(OH)2 Vit. D in dialysis patients. (Abstract) *Kidney Int* 31: 346, 1987

116. Ricanati ES, Ott SM, Klein KL: Evaluation of bone in dialysis patients exposed to aluminum in dialysate. *Kidney Int* 21: 176, 1982

117. King SW, Savory J, Wills MR: Aluminum distribution in serum following hemodialysis. *Ann Clin Lab Sci* 12: 143, 1982

118. Mion C, Branger B, Issautier R: Dialysis fracturing osteomalacia without hyperparathyroidism in patients treated with HCO3 rinsed Redy cartridge. *Trans Amer Soc Artif Internal Organs* 27: 634, 1981

119. Llach F, Gardner PW, George CRP, Cairoli O: Aluminum kinetics using bicarbonate dialysate with the sorbent system. *Kidney Int* 43: 899, 1993

120. Milliner DS, Shinaberger JH, Shuman P, Coburn JW: Inadvertent aluminum administration during plasma exchange due to aluminum contamination of albumin-replacement solutions. *N Engl J Med* 312: 165, 1985

121. Klein GL, Ott SM, Alfrey AC et al.: Aluminum as a factor in the bone disease of long-term parenteral nutrition. *Trans Assoc Am Physicians* 95: 155, 1982

122. Moreno A, Dominguez P, Dominguez C, Ballabriga A: High serum aluminium levels and acute reversible encephalopathy in a 4-year-old boy with acute renal failure. *Eur J Ped* 150: 513, 1993

123. Berlyne GM, Ben-Ari J, Pest D: Hyperaluminaemia from aluminum resins in chronic renal failure. *Lancet* 2: 494, 1970

124. Kaehny WD, Hegg AP, Alfrey AC: Gastrointestinal absorption of aluminum from aluminum containing antacids. *N Engl J Med* 296: 1389, 1977

125. Hercz G, Andress DL, Nebeker HG et al.: Reversal of aluminum-related bone disease after substituting calcium carbonate for aluminum hydroxide. *Am J Kidney Dis* 11: 70, 1988

126. Winney RJ, Cowie JF, Robson JS: The role of plasma aluminum in the detection and prevention of aluminum toxicity. *Kidney Int* 29 (Suppl 18): S91, 1986

127. Salusky IB, Coburn JW, Foley J et al.: Effects of oral calcium carbonate on control of serum phosphorus and changes in plasma aluminum levels after discontinuation of aluminum-containing gels in children receiving dialysis. *J Pediatr* 108: 767, 1986

128. Robertson JA, Salusky IB, Goodman WG et al.: Sucralfate, intestinal aluminum absorption, and aluminum toxicity in a patient on dialysis. *Ann Intern Med* 111: 179, 1989

129. Freundlich M, Zilleruelo G, Abitbol C et al.: Infant formula as a cause of aluminum toxicity in neonatal uremia. *Lancet* 2: 527, 1985

130. Salusky IB, Coburn JW, Nelson P, Goodman WG: Prospective evaluation of aluminum loading from formula in infants with uremia. *J Pediatr* 116: 726, 1984

131. Ittel TH, Buddington B, Miller NL, Alfrey AC: Enhanced gastrointestinal absorption of aluminum in uremic rats. *Kidney Int* 32: 821, 1987

132. Nordal KP, Dahl E: Low dose calcitriol versus placebo in patients with predialysis chronic renal failure. *J Clin Endocrinol Metab* 67: 929, 1988

133. Slanina P, Frech W, Ekstrom L et al.: Dietary citric acid enhances absorption of aluminum in antacids. *Clin Chem* 32: 539, 1986

134. Bakir AA, Hryhorczuk DO, Berman E: Acute fatal hyperaluminemic encephalopathy in undialyzed and recently dialyzed patients. *Trans Am Soc Artif Intern Organs* 32: 171, 1986

135. Coburn JW, Mischel MG, Goodman WG, Salusky IB: Calcium citrate markedly enhances aluminum absorption from aluminum hydroxide. *Am J Kidney Dis* 17: 708, 1991

136. Sherrard DJ: Aluminum, Much ado about something. *N Engl J Med* 324: 558, 1991

137. Czapla K, Rodger RS, Halls DJ et al.: Ranitidine reduces aluminum toxicity in patients with renal failure. *Nephrol Dial Transplant* 7: 1246, 1992

138. Cannata JB, Fernandez-Soto I, Fernandez-Menendez MJ et al.: Role of iron metabolism in absorption and cellular uptake of aluminum. *Kidney Int* 39: 799, 1991

139. Cannata JB, Olaizola IR, Gomez-Alonso C et al.: Serum aluminum transport and aluminum uptake in chronic renal failure: role of iron and aluminum metabolism. *Nephron* 65: 141, 1993

140. Rosenlof K, Fyhrquist F, Tenhunen R: Erythropoietin, aluminium and anaemia in patients on haemodialysis. *Lancet* 335: 247, 1990

141. Casati S, Castelnovo C, Campise M, Ponticelli C: Aluminium interference in the treatment with human erythropoietin. *Nephrol Dial Transplant* 5: 441, 1990

142. D'Haese PC, De Broe ME: Aluminum toxicity. in *Handbook of Dialysis*, edited by Daugirdas JT, Ing TS, Boston/New York/Toronto/London, Little, Brown and Company, 1994, p 522

143. Felsenfeld AJ, Harrelson JM, Gutman RA: Osteomalacia after parathyroidectomy in patients with uremia. *Ann Intern Med* 96: 34, 1984

144. Alvarez-Ude F, Feest TG, Ward MK et al.: Hemodialysis bone disease: Correlation between clinical, histologic and other findings. *Kidney Int* 14: 68, 1978

145. Andress DL, Hercz G, Kopp JB et al.: Bone histomorphometry of renal osteodystrophy in diabetic patients. *J Bone Miner Res* 2: 525, 1987

146. Cohen-Solal ME, Sebert JL, Boudailliez B et al.: Non-aluminic adynamic bone disease in non-dialyzed uremic patients: a new type of osteopathy due to overtreatment? *Bone* 13: 1, 1992

147. Pei Y, Hercz G, Greenwood C et al.: Renal osteodystrophy in diabetic patients. *Kidney Int* 44: 159, 1993

148. Sherrard DJ, Ott S, Maloney N et al.: Renal osteodystrophy: clasification, cause and treatment. in *Clinical Disorders of Bone and Mineral Metabolism*, edited by Frame, B, Potts, JT Jr, Amsterdam, Excerpta Medica, 1983, p 254

149. Sherrard DJ, Hercz G, Pei Y et al.: The spectrum of bone disease in end-stage renal failure – an evolving disorder. *Kidney Int* 43: 436, 1993

150. Hercz G, Pei Y, Greenwood C et al.: Aplastic osteodystrophy without aluminum: the role of 'suppressed' parathyroid function. *Kidney Int* 44: 860, 1993

151. Malluche HH, Monier-Faugere MC: Risk of adynamic bone disease in dialyzed patients. *Kidney Int* (Suppl 38): S62, 1992

152. Andress DL, Maloney NA, Endres DB, Sherrard DJ: Aluminum-associated bone disease in chronic renal failure: high prevalence in a long-term dialysis population. *J Bone Miner Res* 1: 391, 1986

153. Rodriguez M, Lorenzo V, Felsenfeld AJ, Llach F: Effect of parathyroidectomy on aluminum toxicity and azotemic bone disease in the rat. *J Bone Miner Res* 5: 379, 1990

154. Heidbreder E, Gotz R, Schafferhans K, Heidland A: Diminished parathyroid gland responsiveness to hypocalcemia in diabetic patients with uremia. *Nephron* 42: 285, 1986

155. McNair P, Christensen MS, Madsbad S et al.: Hypoparathyroidism in diabetes mellitus. *Acta Endocrinol* 96: 81, 1981

156. Salusky IB, Coburn JW, Brill J: Bone disease in pediatric patients undergoing dialysis with CAPD or CCPD. *Kidney Int* 33: 975, 1988

157. Bender FH, Bernardini J, Piraino B: Calcium mass transfer with dialysate containing 1.25 and 1.75 mmol/L calcium in peritoneal dialysis patients. *Am J Kidney Dis* 20: 367, 1992

158. de Vernejoul MC, Marie P, Kuntz D et al.: Non-osteomalacic osteopathy associated with chronic hypophosphatemia. *Calcif Tissue Int* 34: 219, 1982

159. Stanbury SW, Lumb GA: Parathyroid function in chronic renal failure: a statistical survey of the plasma biochemistry in azotaemic renal osteodystrophy. *Q J Med* 35: 1, 1966

160. Mechanic GL et al.: Quantitative changes of bone collagen cross-links and precursors in vitamin D deficiency. *Biochem Biophys Res Comm* 47: 760, 1972

161. Russell JE, Avioli LV: 25 Hydroxycholecalciferol enhanced bone maturation in the parathyroprivic state. *J Clin Invest* 56: 792, 1975

162. Russell JE, Termine JD, Avioli LV: Abnormal bone mineral maturation in the chronic uremic state. *J Clin Invest* 52: 2848, 1973

163. Alfrey AC, Solomons CC: Bone pyrophosphate in uremia and its association with extraosseous calcification. *J Clin Invest* 57: 700, 1976

164. Termine JD, Posner AS: Amorphous/crystalline interrelationships in bone mineral. *Calcif Tissue Resch* 1: 8, 1967

165. Kaye M: Magnesium metabolism in the rat with chronic renal failure. *J Lab Clin Med* 84: 536, 1974

166. Giangrande A, Costantini S, Ballanti P et al.: Bone Mineral and Aluminum concentrations in patients undergoing CAPD. *Proc Eur Dialysis Transpl Assoc* 1991

167. Pellegrino ED, Biltz RM: The composition of human bone in uremia. *Medicine* 44: 397, 1965

168. Burnell JM, Teubner E, Wergedal JE, Sherrard DJ: Bone crystal maturation in renal osteodystrophy in humans. *J Clin Invest* 53: 52, 1974

169. Pellegrino ED, Biltz RM, Letteri JM: Interrelationships of carbonate, phosphate, monohydrogen phosphate, calcium, magnesium and sodium in uraemic bone: comparison of dialyzed and nondialyzed patients. *Clin Sci Molec Med* 53: 307, 1977

170. Kaye M, Fruch AJ, Silverman M: A study of vertebral bone powder from patients with chronic renal failure. *J Clin Invest* 49: 442, 1970

171. Stanbury SW, Lumb GA: Metabolic studies of renal osteodystrophy. I. Calcium, phosphorus and nitrogen metabolism in rickets, osteomalacia, and hyperparathyroidism complicating chronic uremia and in the osteomalacia of the adult Fanconi syndrome. *Q J Med* 35: 1, 1966

172. Barzel US, Jowsey J: The effects of chronic acid and alkali administration on bone turnover in adult rats. *Clin Sci* 36: 517, 1969

173. Cunningham J, Fraher LJ, Clemens TL et al.: Chronic acidosis with metabolic bone disease.Effect of alkali on bone morphology and vitamin D metabolism. *Am J Med* 73: 199, 1982

174. Lefebvre A, de Vernejoul MC, Gueris J et al.: Optimal correction of acidosis changes progression of dialysis osteodystrophy. *Kidney Int* 36: 1112, 198

175. Floege J, Schaffer J, Koch KM, Shaldon S: Dialysis related amyloidosis: a disease of chronic retention and inflammation? *Kidney Int* (Suppl 38): S78, 1992

176. Koch KM: Dialysis-related amyloidosis. *Kidney Int* 41: 1416, 1992

177. Wright RS, Mehls O, Ritz E, Coburn JW: Musculoskeletal manifestation of chronic renal failure, dialysis and transplantation. in *Renal Manifestations in Rheumatic Disease*, edited by Bacon P, Hadler N, London, Butterworth, 1982, p 352

178. Mirahmadi KS, Coburn JW, Bluestone R: Calcific periarthritis and hemodialysis. *JAMA* 229: 548, 1973

179. Hardouin P, Lecomte-Houcke M, Flipo RM et al.: Current aspects of osteoarticular pathology in patients undergoing hemodialysis: study of 80 patients. Part 2. Laboratory and pathologic analysis. Discussion of the pathogenic mechanism. *J Rheumatol* 14: 784, 1987

180. Massry SG et al.: Abnormalities of the musculoskeletal system in hemodialysis patients. *Semin Arthritis Rheum* 4: 321, 1975

181. Massry SG, Popovtzer MM, Coburn JW: Intractable pruritus as a manifestation of secondary hyperparathyroidism in uremia. Disappearance of itching following subtotal parathyroidectomy. *N Engl J Med* 279: 697, 1968

182. Gilchrest B et al.: Relief of uremic pruritus with ultraviolet phototherapy. *N Engl J Med* 297: 136, 1977

183. Pederson JA, Matter BJ, Czerwinski A, Llach F: Relief of idiopathic generalized pruritus in dialysis patients with activated oral charcoal. *Ann Intern Med* 93: 446, 1980

184. De Marchi S et al.: Relief of pruritus and decreases in plasma histamine concentrations during erythropoietin therapy in patients with uremia. *N Engl J Med* 326: 969, 1992

185. Nielsen T et al.: Pruritus and xerosis in patients with chronic renal failure. *Dan Med Bull* 27: 269, 1980

186. Stockenhuber F et al.: Increased plasma histamine levels in uraemic pruritus. *Clin Sci* 79: 477, 1990

187. Berlyne GM: Microcrystalline conjunctival calcification in renal failure: a useful clinical sign. *Lancet* 2: 366, 1968

188. Berlyne GM, Shaw AG: Red eyes in renal failure. *Lancet* 1: 4, 1967

189. Schott GD, Wills MR: Muscle weakness in osteomalacia. *Lancet* 1: 626, 1976

190. Baker LRI, Ackrill P, Cattell WR: Iatrogenic osteomalacia and myopathy due to phosphate depletion. *Br Med J* 3: 150, 1974

191. Smith R, Stern G: Myopathy, osteomalacia and hyperparathyroidism. *Brain* 90: 593, 1967

192. Coburn JW, Nebeker HG, Hercz G et al.: Role of aluminum accumulation in the pathogenesis of renal osteodystrophy, in *Nephrology, Vol II*, edited by Robinson RR, New York, Springer-Verlag, 1984, p 1383

193. Malette LE, Patten BM, Engel WK: Neuromuscular disease in secondary hyperparathyroidism. *Ann Intern Med* 82: 474, 1975

194. Brickman AS, Sherrard DJ, Jowsey J: 1,25 dihydroxycholecalciferol: effect on skeletal lesions and plasma parathyroid hormone in uremic osteodystrophy. *Arch Intern Med* 134: 883, 1974

195. Henderson RG, Russell RGG, Ledingham JG: Effects of 1,25 dihydroxycholecalciferol on calcium absorption, muscle weakness, and bone disease in chronic renal failure. *Lancet* 249: 83, 1974

196. Kanis JA, Cundy T, Earnshaw M et al.: Treatment of renal bone disease with 1α-hydroxylated derivitives of vitamin D₃: Clinical, biochemical, radiographic and histological responses. *Q J Med (New Series)* 48: 289, 1979

197. Cirincione R, Baker B: Tendon rupture with secondary hyperparathyroidism. *J Bone Joint Surg* 57: 852, 1975

198. Preston F, Adicoff A: Hyperparathyroidism with avulsion of three major tendons. *N Engl J Med* 266: 968, 1962

199. Avioli LV: Collagen metabolism, uremia and bone. *Kidney Int* 4: 105, 1973

200. Murphy KJ, McPhee I: Tears of major tendons in chronic acidosis with elastosis. *J Bone Joint Surg* 53: 510, 1971

201. Ryuzaki M, Konishi K, Kasuga A et al.: Spontaneous rupture of the quadriceps tendon in patients on maintenance hemodialysis-repor tof three cases with clinicopathological observations. *Clin Nephrol* 32: 144, 1989

202. Kurer MH, Baillod RA, Madgwick JC: Musculoskeletal manifestations of amyloidosis. A review of 83 patients on haemodialysis for at least 10 years. *J Bone Joint Surg* 73: 271, 1991

203. Gipstein R, Coburn JW, Adams D et al.: Calciphylaxis in man: A syndrome of tissue necrosis and vascular calcification in 11 patients with chronic renal disease. *Arch Intern Med* 136: 1273, 1976

204. Massry SG, Gordon A, Coburn JW: Vascular calcification and peripheral necrosis in a renal transplant recipient: Reversal of lesion following subtotal parathyroidectomy. *Am J Med* 49: 416, 1970

205. Weidmann P, Massry SG, Coburn JW: Effect of acute hypercalcemia on blood pressure in patients with chronic renal failure. *Ann Intern Med* 76: 741, 1972

206. Selye H: *Calciphylaxis*, Chicago, Univ of Chicago Press, 1982

207. Duh QY, Lim RC, Clark OH: Calciphylaxis in secondary hyperparathyroidism.Diagnosis and parathyroidectomy. *Arch Surg* 126: 1213, 1991

208. Poch E, Almirall J, Alsina M et al.: Calciphylaxis in a hemodialysis patient: Appearance after parathyroidectomy during a psoriatic flare. *Am J Kidney Dis* 19: 285, 1992

209. Mehls O, Ritz E, Krempien B: Roentgenological signs in the skeleton of uremic children. An analysis of the anatomical principles underlying the roentgenological changes. *Pediatr Radiol* 1: 183, 1973

210. Mehls O: Renal osteodystrophy in children: etiology and clinical aspects, in *Endstage Renal Disease in Children*, edited by Fine RN, Gruskin AB, Philadelphia, WB Saunders, 1984, p 227

211. Stanbury SW: The role of vitamin D in renal bone disease. *Clin Endocrinol* 7: 25S, 1977

212. Parfitt AM: Clinical and radiographic manifestations of renal osteodystrophy. in *Calcium Metabolism in Renal Failure and Nephrolithiasis*, edited by David DS, New York, John Wiley & Sons, 1977, p 150

213. Scharer K et al.: Growth in children with chronic renal failure. *Kidney Int* 13 (Suppl): S68, 1978

214. Chantler C, Donckerwolcke RA, Brunner FP et al.: Combined report on regular dialysis and transplantation of children in Europe. *Proc Eur Dial Transplant Assoc* 16: 74, 1979

215. Simmons JM, Wilson CJ, Potter DE, Holliday MA: Relation of caloric deficiency to growth failure in children on hemodialysis and the growth response to caloric supplementation. *N Engl J Med* 285: 653, 1971

216. Chantler C, Holliday M: Growth in children with renal disease, with special reference to the effects of caloric malnutrition: a review. *Clin Nephrol* 1: 230, 1973

217. McSherry E, Morris RC: Attainment and maintenance of normal growth status with alkali therapy in infants and children with classic renal tubular acidosis (RTA). *J Clin Invest* 61: 509, 1978

218. Saenger P, Wiedmann E, Schwartz E: Somatomedin and growth after renal transplantation. *Pediatr Res* 8: 163, 1974

219. Chesney RW, Moorthy A, Eisman JA et al.: Increased growth after long-term oral 1,25-vitamin D3 in childhood renal osteodystrophy. *N Engl J Med* 298: 238, 1978

220. Tonshoff B, Mehls O, Heinrich U et al.: Growth-stimulating effect of recombinant human growth hormone in children with end-stage renal disease. *J Pediatrics* 116: 561, 1990

221. Blum WF, Ranke MB, Kietzmann K et al.: Growth hormone resistance and inhibition of somatomedin activity by excess of insulin-like growth factor binding protein in uraemia. *Pediatr Nephrol* 5: 539, 1991

222. Eidemak I, Feldt-Rasmussen B, Strandgaard S et al.: Insulin resistance is present in moderate uraemia and correlated to the maximal aerobic work capacity. *J Am Soc Nephrol* 3: 281, 1992

223. Mehls O, Ritz E, Hunziker EB et al.: Improvement of growth and food utilization by human recombinant growth hormone in uremia. *Kidney Int* 33: 45, 1988

224. Stivelman JC: Refractoriness to recombinant human epoetin treatment. in *Dialysis Therapy*, edited by Nissenson AR, Fine RN, Philadelphia, Mosby-Year Book, 1993, p 236

225. Coburn JW, Massry SG, DePalma JS, Shinaberger JH: Rapid appearance of hypercalcemia with initiation of hemodialysis. *JAMA* 210: 2276, 1969

226. Mazzaferro S, Coen G, Bandini S et al.: Mitral annulus calcification in uremia. *Nephrol Dial Transplant* 8: 335, 1993

227. Bogin E, Massry SG, Harary I: Effect of parathyroid hormone on heart cells. *J Clin Invest* 67: 1215, 1981

228. London GM, Fabiani F, Marchais SJ et al.: Uremic cardiomyopathy: an inadequate left ventricular hypertrophy. *Kidney Int* 31: 973, 1987

229. London GM, de Vernejoul MC, Fabiani F et al.: Secondary hyperparathyroidism and cardiac hypertrophy in hemodialysis patients. *Kidney Int* 32: 900, 1987

230. Puschett JB, Moranz J, Kurnick WS: Evidence for a direct action of cholecalciferol and 25 hydroxycholecalciferol on the renal transport of phosphate, sodium and calcium. *J Clin Invest* 51: 373, 1972

231. Marchais SJ, Guerin AP, London AM et al.: Long-term effects of parathyroidectomy on left ventricular function in hemodialysis patients. *Blood Purif* 2: 155, 1992

232. Chazan J, Abuelo G, Blonsky S: Plasma aluminum levels (unstimulated and stimulated): clinical and biochemical findings in 185 patients undergoing chronic hemodialysis for 4 to 95 months. *Am J Kidney Dis* 13: 284, 1989

233. Llach F, Felsenfeld AJ, Coleman M et al.: The natural course of dialysis osteomalacia. *Kidney Int* 29: S74, 1986

234. Roth A, Nogues C, Galle P et al.: Multiorgan aluminum deposits in a chronic haemodialysis patient. Electron microscope and microprobe studies. *Virchows Arch (Pathol Anat)* 405: 131, 1984

235. London G, deVernejoul MC, Fabiani F et al.: Association between aluminum accumulation and cardiac hypertrophy in hemodialyzed patients. *Am J Kidney Dis* 13: 75, 1989

236. Massry SG, Goldstein D: Role of parathyroid hormone in uremic toxicity. *Kidney Int* 13 (Suppl): S39, 1978

237. Massry SG, Fadda GZ: Chronic renal failure is a state of cellular calcium toxicity. *Am J Kidney Dis* 21: 81, 1993

238. Arieff AI, Massry SG: Calcium metabolism of brain in acute renal failure. *J Clin Invest* 53: 387, 1974

239. Cooper JD, Lazarowitz V, Arieff AI: Neurodiagnostic abnormalities in patients with acute renal failure. Evidence for neurotoxicity of parathyroid hormone. *J Clin Invest* 61: 1448, 1978

240. Kiley JE et al.: Evaluation of encephalopathy by EEG frequency analysis in chronic dialysis patients. *Clin Nephrol* 5: 245, 1976

241. Ball JH et al.: The many facets of secondary hyperparathyroidism. *Arch Intern Med* 131: 746, 1973

242. Fraser CL, Arieff AI: Nervous system complications in uremia. *Ann Intern Med* 109: 143, 1988

243. Ni Z, Smogorzewski M, Massry SG: Derangements in acetylcholine metabolism in brain synaptosomes in chronic renal failure. *Kidney Int* 44: 630, 1993

244. Avram MM et al.: Search for the uremic toxin: Decreased motor nerve conduction velocity and elevated parathyroid hormone in uremia. *N Engl J Med* 298: 1000, 1978

245. Arieff AI, Schmidt R: Parathyroid hormone as a uremic neurotoxin. *N Engl J Med* 299: 362, 1978

246. Goldstein DA et al.: Effect of parathyroid hormone and uremia on peripheral nerve calcium and motor nerve conduction velocity. *J Clin Invest* 62: 88, 1978

247. Massry SG, Goldstein DA, Procci W, Kletsky OA: Impotence in patients with uremia: a possible role for parathyroid hormone. *Nephron* 19: 305, 1977

248. Blumberg A et al.: Influence of 1,25-dihydroxycholecalciferol on sexual dysfunction and related endocrine parameters in patients on maintenance hemodialysis. *Clin Nephrol* 13: 208, 1980

249. Weinberg SG et al.: Myelofibrosis and renal osteodystrophy. *Am J Med* 63: 755, 1977

250. Boxer M et al.: Anemia in primary hyperparathyroidism. *Arch Intern Med* 137: 588, 1977

251. Rao DS et al.: Effect of serum parathyroid hormone and bone marrow fibrosis on the response to erythropoietin in uremia. *N Engl J Med* 328: 171, 1993

252. Barbour GL: Effect of parathyroidectomy on anemia in chronic renal failure. *Arch Intern Med* 139: 889, 1979

253. Meytes D et al.: Effects of parathyroid hormone on erythrocytes. *J Clin Invest* 67: 1263, 1981

254. Zevin D et al.: Effect of parathyroid hormone and 1,25-dihydroxyvitamin D3 on RNA and heme synthesis by erythroid precursors. *Min Electrolyte Metab* 6: 125, 1981

255. Bogin E et al.: Effect of parathyroid hormone on osmotic fragility of human erythrocytes. *J Clin Invest* 69: 1017, 1982

256. Remuzzi G et al.: Parathyroid hormone inhibits human platelet function. *Lancet* 2: 1321, 1981

257. Alexiewicz JM, Gaciong Z, Klinger M et al.: Evidence of impaired T cell function in hemodialysis patients: potential role for secondary hyperparathyroidism. *Am J Nephrol* 10: 495, 1990

258. Cantin M: Kidney, parathyroid and lipemia. *Lab Invest* 14: 1691, 1965

259. Perna AF, Fadda GZ, Zhou XJ, Massry SG: Mechanisms of impaired insulin secretion following chronic excess of parathyroid hormone. *Am J Physiol* 259: F210, 1990

260. Fadda GZ, Thanakitcharu P, Smogorzewski M, Massry SG: Parathyroid hormone raises cytosolic calcium in pancreatic islets: study on mechanisms. *Kidney Int* 43: 554, 1993

261. Weeke E, Friis TH: Serum fractions of calcium and phosphorus in uremia. *Acta Med Scand* 189: 79, 1971

262. Walton J, Gray TK: Absorption of intestinal phosphate in the human intestine. *Clin Sci* 56: 407, 1979

263. Walling MW et al.: Jejunal phosphate (Pi) active transport: effects of phosphate depletion and vitamin D. *Fed Proc* 36: 1097, 1977

264. Walling MW: Intestinal Ca and phosphate transport: differential responses of vitamin D metabolites. *Am J Physiol* 133: 3488, 1977

265. Coburn JW, Brickman AS, Sherrard DJ: Clinical efficacy of 1,25 dihydroxyvitamin D3 in renal osteodystrophy. in *Vitamin D: Biochemical, Chemical and Clinical Aspects Related to Calcium Metabolism*, edited by Norman AW, Schaefer K, Coburn JW, Berlin, de Gruyter, 1977, p 657

266. Gallieni M, Brancaccio D, Padovese P et al., Italian Group for the Study of Intravenous Calcitriol: Low-dose intravenous calcitriol treatment of secondary hyperparathyroidism in hemodialysis patients. *Kidney Int* 42: 1191, 1992

267. Massry SG, Coburn JW, Popovtzer MM: Secondary hyperparathyroidism in chronic renal failure: the clinic

spectrum in uremia, during hemodialysis and after renal transplantation. *Arch Intern Med* 124: 431, 1969

268. Coburn JW, Brickman AS, Massry SG: Medical treatment in primary and secondary hyperparathyroidism. *Semin Drug Treat* 2: 117, 1972

269. Kopple JD, Coburn JW: Metabolic studies of low protein diets in uremia.II. Calcium, phosphorus and magnesium. *Medicine* 52: 597, 1973

270. Wiegmann TB, Kaye M: Malabsorption of calcium and phosphate in chronic renal failure: 32P and 45Ca studies in dialysis patients. *Clin Nephrol* 34: 35, 1990

271. Coburn JW, Popovtzer MM, Massry SG, Kleeman CR: The physiochemical state and renal handling of divalent ions in chronic renal failure. *Arch Intern Med* 124: 302, 1969

272. Walser M: The separate effects of hyperparathyroidism, hypercalcemia of malignancy, renal failure and acidosis on the state of calcium phosphate and other ions in plasma. *J Clin Invest* 41: 1454, 1962

273. Raman A, Chong YK, Sreenevasan G: Effects of varying dialysate calcium concentration on the plasma calcium fractions in patients on dialysis. *Nephron* 16: 181, 1976

274. Wing AJ, Curtis JR, Eastwood JB: Transient and persistent hypercalcaemia in patients treated by maintenance haemodialysis. *Br Med J* 4: 150, 1968

275. Messner RP et al.: The effect of hemodialysis, vitamin D, and renal homotransplantation on the calcium malabsorption of chronic renal failure. *J Lab Clin Med* 74: 472, 1969

276. Morton AR, Hercz G: Hypercalcemia in dialysis patients: comparison of diagnostic methods. *Dial Transplant* 20: 661, 1991

277. Shimada H, Makamura M, Marumo F: Influence of aluminum on the effect of 1 (OH)D3 on renal osteodystrophy. *Nephron* 35: 163, 1983

278. Rodriguez M, Felsenfeld AJ, Llach F: The role of aluminum in the development of hypercalcemia in the rat. *Kidney Int* 31: 766, 1987

279. Slatopolsky E, Weerts C, Lopez-Hilker S et al.: Calcium carbonate as a phosphate binder in patients with chronic renal failure undergoing dialysis. *N Engl J Med* 315: 157, 1986

280. Schaefer K, Scheer J, Asmus G et al.: The treatment of uraemic hyperphosphataemia with calcium acetate and calcium carbonate: a comparative study. *Nephrol Dial Transplant* 6: 171, 1991

281. Papadimitriou M, Gingell J, Chisholm G: Hypercalcemia from calcium ion exchange resins in patients on regular hemodialysis. *Lancet* 2: 948, 1968

282. Koppel MH, Massry SG, Shinaberger JH: Thiazide induced rise in serum calcium and magnesium in patients on maintenance hemodialysis. *Ann Intern Med* 72: 895, 1970

283. Barbour GL, Coburn JW, Slatopolsky E et al.: Hypercalcemia in an anephric patient with sarcoidosis, evidence for extrarenal generation of 1,25 dihydroxyvitamin D. *N Engl J Med* 305: 440, 1981

284. Felsenfeld AJ, Drezner MK, Llach F: Hypercalcemia and elevated calcitriol in a maintenance dialysis patient with tuberculosis. *Arch Intern Med* 146: 1941, 1986

285. Schmulen AC, Lerman M, Pak CYC et al.: Effect of 1,25-dihydroxyvitamin D3 therapy on jejunal absorption of magnesium in patients with chronic renal failure. *Am J Physiol* 238: 349G, 1980

286. Coburn JW, Hartenbower DL, Brickman AS: Intestinal absorption of calcium, magnesium, and phosphorus in chronic renal insufficiency. in *Calcium Metabolism in Renal Failure and Nephrolithiasis*, edited by David DS, New York, John Wiley & Sons, 1977, p 77

287. Brannan PG et al.: Magnesium absorption in the human small intestine: results in patients with absorptive hypercalciuria. *J Clin Invest* 57: 1412, 1976

288. Alfrey AC, Solomons CC, Ciricillo J, Miller NL: Extraosseous calcification. Evidence for abnormal pyrophosphate metabolism in uremia. *J Clin Invest* 57: 692, 1976

289. Wallach S: Relation of magnesium to osteoporosis and calcium urolithiasis. *Magnesium & Trace Elements* 10: 281, 1991

290. Guillot AP, Hood VL, Runge CF, Gennari FJ: The use of magnesium-containing phosphate binders in patients with end-stage renal disease on maintenance hemodialysis. *Nephron* 30: 114, 1982

291. Stewart WK, Fleming LW: The effects of dialysate magnesium on plasma and erythocyte magnesium and potassium concentrations during maintenance haemodialysis. *Nephron* 10: 221, 1973

292. Moriniere P, Fournier A, Westeel P et al.: Calcium carbonate and magnesium hydroxide in the prevention of renal osteodystrophy or the demise of aluminum toxicity in uremia. *Contrib Nephrol* 64: 58, 1988

293. O'Donovan R, Baldwin D, Hammer M, Moniz C: Substitution of aluminum salts by magnesium salts in control of dialysis hyperphosphataemia. *Lancet* i: 880, 1986

294. Freeman RM: The role of magnesium in the pathogenesis of azotemic hypothermia. *Proc Soc Exp Biol Med* 137: 1069, 1971

295. Freeman RM, Lawton RL, Chamberlain MA: Hard Water syndrome. *N Engl J Med* 276: 1113, 1967

296. Habener JF, Potts JT Jr: Relative effectiveness of magnesium and calcium on the secretion and biosynthesis of parathyroid hormone *in vitro*. *Endocrinology* 98: 197, 1976

297. Mennes P, Rosenbaum R, Martin KJ, Slatopolsky E: Hypomagnesemia and impaired parthyroid hormone secretion in chronic renal disease. *Ann Intern Med* 88: 206, 1978

298. Skillen AW, Pierides AM: Serum alkaline phosphatase isoenzyme patterns in patients with chronic renal failure. *Clin Chim Acta* 80: 339, 1977

299. Price PA et al.: New biochemical marker for bone metabolism. Measurement by radioimmunoassay of bone Gla protein in the plasma of normal subjects and patients with bone disease. *J Clin Invest* 66: 878, 1980

300. Delmas PD et al.: Assessment of bone turnover in postmenopausal osteoporosis by measurement of serum bone Gla-protein. *J Lab Clin Med* 102: 470, 1983

301. Slovid DM et al.: Clinical evaluation of bone turnover by serum osteocalcin measurements. *Calcif Tissue Int* 34: S15, 1982

302. Charhon SA, Delmas PD, Malaval L et al.: Serum bone Gla-protein in renal osteodystrophy: comparison with bone histomorphometry. *J Clin Endocrinol Metab* 63: 892, 1986

303. Epstein S, Traberg H, Raja R et al.: Serum and dialysate osteocalcin levels in hemodialysis and peritoneal dialysis patients and after renal transplantation. *J Clin Endocrinol Metab* 60: 1253, 1985

304. Malluche HH et al.: Plasma levels of bone Gla-protein reflect bone formation in patients on chronic maintenance dialysis. *Kidney Int* 26: 869, 1984

305. Coen G, Mazzaferro S, Bonucci E et al.: Bone GLA protein in predialysis chronic renal failure: Effects of 1,25(OH)2D3 administration in a long-term follow-up. *Kidney Int* 28: 783, 1985

306. Hosoda K, Eguchi H, Nakamoto T et al.: Sandwich immunoassay for intact human osteocalcin. *Clin Chem* 38: 2233, 1992

307. Saupe J, Konig M, Shearer MJ, Kohlmeier M: Carboxylated osteocalcin concentrations in plasma provide information about two independent bone modulating systems in end stage renal disease (ESRD). *J Am Soc Nephrol* 3: 676, 1992

308. Coen G, Mazzaferro S, Ballanti P et al.: Procollagen type I C-terminal extension peptide in predialysis chronic renal failure. *Am J Nephrol* 12: 246, 1992

309. Prockop D, Kivirikko K: Relationship of hydroxyproline excretion in urine to collagen metabolism. *Ann Intern Med* 66: 1243, 1967

310. Kowalewski J, Tomaszewski J, Hanzlik J: The elimination of free, peptide bound and protein bound hydroxyproline into dialysate during peritoneal dialysis in patients with renal failure. *Clin Chim Acta* 34: 123, 1971

311. Varghese Z et al.: Plasma hydroxyproline in renal osteodystrophy. *Proc Eur Dial Transplant Assoc* 10: 187, 1973

312. Hart W et al.: The hydroxyproline content of plasma of patients with impaired renal function. *Clin Nephrol* 4: 104, 1975

313. Eyre D: New biomarkers of bone resorption. *J Clin Endocrinol Metab* 74: 470A, 1992

314. Lam KW et al.: Tartrate-resistant (band 5) acid phosphatase activity measured by electrophoresis on acrylamide gel. *Clin Chem* 24: 309, 1978

315. Kraenzlin M, Lau KHW, Liang L: Development of an immunoassay for human serum osteoclastic tartrate-resistant acid phosphatase. *J Clin Endocrinol Metab* 71: 442, 1990

316. Hamet P et al.: Studies of the elevated extracellular concentration of cyclic AMP in uremic man. *J Clin Invest* 56: 339, 1975

317. Felsenfeld AJ, Llach F: Parathyroid gland function in chronic renal failure. *Kidney Int* 43: 771, 1993

318. Hruska KA, Teitelbaum SL, Kopelman R: The predictability of the histologic features of uremic bone disease by noninvasive techniques. *Metab Bone Dis Rel Res* 1: 39, 1978

319. Chan YL, Furlong TJ, Cornish CJ, Posen S: Dialysis osteodystrophy. A study involving 94 patients. *Medicine (Baltimore)* 64: 296, 1985

320. Nussbaum SR, Potts JT Jr: Immunoassays for parathyroid hormone 1–84 in the diagnosis of hyperparathyroidism. *J Bone Mineral Resch* 6 (Suppl 2): S43, 1991

321. Brown RC, Aston JP, Weeks I, Woodhead S: Circulating intact parathyroid hormone measured by a two-site immunochemiluminometric assay. *J Clin Endocrinol Metab* 65: 407, 1987

322. Morita A, Tabata T, Koyama H et al.: A two-site immunochemiluminometric assay for intact parathyroid hormone and its clinical utility in hemodialysis patients. *Clin Nephrol* 38: 154, 1992

323. Guillard O, Pineau A, Baruthlo F, Arnaud J: An international quality assessment program for measurement of aluminum in human plasma: a progress report. *Clin Chem* 34: 1603, 1988

324. Milliner DS, Ott SM, Nebeker HG: Deferoxamine infusion test for diagnosis of aluminum related osteomalacia. *Ann Intern Med* 101: 775, 1984

325. Piccoli A, Andriani M, Mattiello G et al.: Serum aluminium level in the Veneto chronic haemodialysis population: cross-sectional study on 1,026 patients. *Nephron* 51: 482, 1989

326. Rovelli E, Luciani L, Pagani C et al.: Correlation between serum aluminum concentration and signs of encephalopathy in a large population of patients dialyzed with aluminum free fluids. *Clin Nephrol* 29: 294, 1988

327. Norris KC, Sherrard DJ, Slatopolsky E, Coburn JW: Symptomatic renal bone disease: non-invasive parameters for diagnosis. (Abstract) *Abstract Book, XIth Internat Congr Nephrol* 405A, 1990

328. Malluche HH, Smith AJ, Abreo L, Faugere MC: The use of desferrioxamine in the management of renal patients with bone aluminum accumulation. *N Engl J Med* 311: 140, 1984

329. de Vernejoul MC, Marchais S, London G: Deferoxamine test and bone disease in dialysis patients with mild aluminum accumulation. *Am J Kidney Dis* 14: 124, 1989

330. Pei Y, Hercz G, Greenwood C et al.: Non-invasive prediction of aluminum bone disease in hemo- and peritoneal dialysis patients. *Kidney Int* 41: 1374, 1992

331. Mazzaferro S, Coen G, Ballanti P et al.: Deferoxamine test and PTHY serum levels are useful not to recognize but to exclude aluminum-related bone disease. *Nephron* 61: 151, 1992

332. Yaqoob M, Ahmad R, Roberts N, Helliwell T: Low-dose desferrioxamine test for the diagnosis of aluminum-related bone disease in patients on regular haemodialysis. *Nephrol Dial Transplant* 6: 484, 1991

333. Subra JF, Krari N, Tirot P et al.: Aluminium determination in the skin of patients with and without end-stage renal failure. *Nephron* 58: 170, 1991

334. Bindi P, Khayat R, Saiag P et al.: There is no aluminum accumulation in the skin of end-stage renal failure patients. *Nephron*, 1993

335. DiRaimondo CV, Casey T, Stone WJ: Pathologic fractures associated with idiopathic amyloidosis of bone in chronic hemodialysis patients. *Nephron* 43: 22, 1986

336. Gejyo F, Homma N, Suzuki M, Arakawa KM: Serum levels of β_2-microglobulin as a new form of amyloid protein in patients undergoing long-term hemodialysis. *N Engl J Med* 314: 585, 1986

337. van Ypersele de Strihou C, Jadoul M, Malghem J, Jamart J, the Working Party on Dialysis Amyloidosis: Effect of dialysis membrane and patient's age on signs of dialysis-related amyloidosis. *Kidney Int* 39: 1012, 1991

338. Fenves AZ, Emmett M, White MG et al.: Carpal tunnel syndrome with cystic bone lesions secondary to amyloidosis in chronic hemodialysis patients. *Am J Kidney Dis* 7: 130, 1986

339. Goldstein S, Winston E, Chung TJ et al.: Chronic arthropathy in long term hemodialysis. *Am J Med* 78: 82, 1985

340. Kuntz D, Naveau B, Bardin T et al.: Destructive spondylarthropathy in hemodialyzed patients. *Arthritis Rheum* 27: 369, 1984

341. Deforges-Lasseur C, Combe C, Cernier A et al.: Destructive spondyloarthropathy presenting with progressive paraplegia in a dialysis patient. Recovery after surgical spinal cord decompression and parathyroidectomy. *Nephrol Dial Transplant* 8: 180, 1993

342. Takenaka R, Fukatsu A, Matsuo S et al.: Surgical treatment of hemodialysis-related shoulder arthropathy. *Clin Nephrol* 38: 224, 1992

343. Gejyo F, Homma N, Hasegawa S, Arakawa M: A new therapeutic approach to dialysis amyloidosis: intensive removal of beta 2-microglobulin with adsorbent column. *Artif Organs* 17: 240, 1993

344. Nelson SR, Sharpstone P, Kingswoood JC: Does dialysis-associated amyloidosis resolve after transplantation? *Nephrol Dial Transplant* 8: 369, 1993

345. Poznanski AK: Radiologic Evaluation of Bone Mineral in Children. in *Primer on the Metabolic Bone Diseases and Disorders of Mineral Metabolism*, edited by Favus MJ, New York, Raven Press, 1993, p 115

346. Dent CE, Hodson C: Radiological changes associated with certain metabolic bone diseases. *Br J Radiol* 27: 605, 1954

347. Meema HE, Rabinovich S, Meema S et al.: Improved radiological diagnosis of azotemic osteodystrophy. *Radiology* 102: 1, 1972

348. Ritz E, Prager P, Krempien B: Skeletal x-ray findings and bone histology in patients on hemodialysis. *Kidney Int* 13: 316, 1978

349. Meema HE, Oreopoulos DG, Rabinovich S: Periosteal new bone formation (periosteal neostasis) in renal osteodystrophy. *Radiology* 110: 513, 1974

350. Doyle FH: Radiological patterns of bone disease associated with renal glomerular failure in adults. *Br Med Bull* 28: 220, 1972

351. Eastwood JB, Bordier PhJ, De Wardener H: Some biochemical, histological, radiological and clinical features of renal osteodystrophy. *Kidney Int* 4: 128, 1973

352. Glassford D, Remmers AR, Sarles H: Hyperparathyroidism in the maintenance dialysis patient. *Surg Gynecol Obstet* 142: 328, 1976

353. Tatler GL, Baillod RA, Varghese Z et al.: Evolution of bone disease over 10 years in 135 patients with terminal renal failure. *Br Med J* 4: 315, 1973

354. Prager P, Singer R, Ritz E, Krempien B: Diagnostischer Stellenwert der Lamina dura dentium beim sekundaren Hyperparathyreoidismus. *Fortschr Rontgenstrl* 129: 237, 1978

355. Meema HE, Meema S: Comparison of microradioscopic and morphometric findings in the hand bones with densitometric finding in the proximal radius in thyrotoxicosis and in renal osteodystrophy. *Invest Radiol* 7: 88, 1972

356. Ellis K, Hochstim RJ: The skull in hyperparathyroid bone disease. *Am J Roentgenol* 83: 732, 1960

357. Owen J, Parnell A, Keir M et al.: Critical analysis of the use of skeletal surveys in patients with chronic renal failure. *Clin Radiol* 39: 578, 1988

358. Chalmers J, Conacher WD, Gardner DL, Scott PJ: Osteomalacia – a common disease in elderly women. *J Bone Joint Surg* 49B: 403, 1967

359. Ritz E, Krempien B, Mehls O, Malluche HH: Skeletal abnormalities in chronic renal insufficiency before and during maintenance hemodialysis. *Kidney Int* 4: 116, 1973

360. Kessler M, Azoulay E, Netter P et al.: Arthropathie du dialyse: resultats d'une etude multicentrique realisee chez 171 malades hemodialyses depuis plus de 10 ans. in *Actualites en physiopathologie et pharmacologie acticulairs*, edited by Gaucher A, Pourel J, Netter P, Kessler M, Paris, Masson, 1989, p 272

361. Norfray J, Calenoff L, DelGreco F, Krumlovsky F: Renal osteodystrophy in patients on hemodialysis as reflected in the bony pelvis. *Am J Roentgenol* 125: 352, 1975

362. Parfitt AM: Soft tissue calcification in uremia. *Arch Intern Med* 124: 544, 1969

363. Jonhson C, Graham CB, Curtis FK: Roentgenographic manifestations of chronic renal disease treated by periodic hemodialysis. *Am J Radium Ther Nucl Med* 101: 915, 1967

364. Benhamou CL, Rouchon JP, Geslin N et al.: Arthropathies des membres chez les insuffisants renaux dialyses. *Presse med* 16: 119, 1987

365. Chou CT, Wassertein A, Schumacher HR, Fernandez P: Muskuloskeletal manifestations in hemodialysis patients. *J Rheumatology* 12: 1149, 1985

366. Rubin LA, Fam AG, Rubenstein J et al.: Erosive azotemic osteoarthropathy. *Arthritis Rheum* 27: 1086, 1984

367. Bardin T, Vasseur M, de Vernejoul MC et al.: Etude prospective de l'atteinte articulair des malades hemodialyses depuis plus de 10 ans. *Rev Rheum* 55: 131, 1988

368. Meema HE, Oreopoulos DG, Rapoport A: Serum magnesium level and arterial calcification in end stage renal disease. *Kidney Int* 32: 388, 1987

369. Ritz E, Mehls O, Bommer J: Vascular calcifications under maintenance hemodialysis. *Klin Wochenschr* 55: 375, 1977

370. Meema HE et al.: Arterial calcifications in severe chronic renal disease and their relationship to dialysis treatment, renal transplant, and parathyroidectomy. *Radiology* 121: 315, 1976

371. DeFrancisco AM, Ellis HA, Owen JP et al.: Parathyroidectomy in chronic renal failure. *Q J Med* 55: 289, 1985

372. Kainberger F, Traindl O, Baldt M et al.: Renale Osteodystrophie: Spektrum der Rontgensymptomatik bei modernen Formen der Nierentransplantation und Dauerdialysetherpie. *Rofo Fortschr geb Rontgenstr Neuen Bildgeb Verfahr* 157: 501, 1992

373. Contiguglia S, Alfrey AC, Miller NL: Nature of soft tissue calcification in uremia. *Kidney Int* 4: 229, 1973

374. Kuzela D, Huffer WE, Conger JD: Soft tissue calcification in chronic dialysis patients. *Am J Pathol* 86: 403, 1977

375. Conger JD, Hammond WS, Alfrey AC et al.: Pulmonary calcification in chronic dialysis patients. Clinical and pathologic studies. *Ann Intern Med* 83: 330, 1975

376. Davis B, Poulose K, Reba R: Scanning for uremic pulmonary calcifications. *Ann Intern Med* 85: 132, 1976

377. Ibels LS, Alfrey AC, Haut L, Huffer WE: Preservation of function in experimental renal disease by dietary restriction of phosphate. *N Engl J Med* 298: 122, 1991

378. Lumlertgul D, Burke TJ, Gillum D et al.: Phosphate depletion arrests progression of chronic renal failure independent of protein intake. *Kidney Int* 29: 658, 1986

379. Barsotti G, Giannoni A, Morelli E et al.: The decline of renal function slowed by very low phosphorus intake in chronic renal patients following a low nitrogen diet. *Clin Nephrol* 21: 54, 1984

380. Parfitt AM, Massry SG, Winfield A: Osteopenia and fractures occurring during maintenance hemodialysis. A 'new' form of renal osteodystrophy. *Clin Orthop* 87: 287, 1972

381. Homma N, Gejyo F, Kobayashi H et al.: Cystic radiolucencies of carpal bones, distal radius and ulna as a marker for dialysis-associated amyloid osteoarthropathy. *Nephron* 62: 6, 1992

382. Sole M et al.: Morphological and immunohistochemical findings in dialysis-related amyloidosis. *Appl Pathol* 7: 350, 1989

383. Zingraff J et al.: β2-microglobulin amyloidosis: esternoclavicualr joint biopsy study in hemodialysis patients. *Clin Nephrol* 33: 94, 1990

384. Zingraff J, Drueke T: Can the nephrologist prevent dialysis related amyloidosis? *Am J Kidney Dis* 18: 1, 1991

385. Cobby MJ, Adler RS, Swartz R, Martel W: Dialysis-related amyloid arthropathy: MR findings in four patients. *Am J Roentgenol* 157: 1023, 1991

386. Kroner G, Stabler A, Seiderer M et al.: Beta 2 microglobulin-related amyloidosis causing atlantoaxial spondyloarthropathy with spinal-cord compression in haemodialysis patients: detection by MRI. *Nephrol Dial Transplant* 6 (Suppl 2): 91, 1991

387. Kay J, Benson CB, Lester S et al.: Utility of high-resolution ultrasound for the diagnosis of dialysis-related amyloidosis. *Arthritis Rheum* 35: 926, 1992

388. Fleisch H, Russell RGG: Experimental clinical studies with pyrophosphate and diphosphonates. in *Calcium Metabolism in Renal Failure and Nephrolithiasis*, edited by David DS, New York, John Wiley & Sons, 1977, p 293

389. Rosenthal L, Kaye M: Observations on the mechanism of Tc labeled phosphate complex uptake in metabolic bone disease. *Nucl Med* 5: 59, 1976

390. Lien JW, Wiegmann TB, Rosenthall L, Kaye M: Abnormal Tc time pyrophosphate bone scans in chronic renal failure. *Clin Nephrol* 6: 509, 1976

391. Sy W, Mittal A: Bone scan in chronic dialysis patients with evidence of secondary hyperparathyroidism and renal osteodystrophy. *Br J Radiol* 48: 878, 1975

392. Olgaard K, Heerfordt J, Madsen S: Scintigraphic skeletal changes in uremic patients on regular hemodialysis. *Nephron* 17: 325, 1976

393. Karsenty G, Vigneron N, Jorgetti V: Value of the 99-mTc-methylene diphosphonate bone scan in renal osteodystrophy. *Kidney Int* 29: 1058, 1986

394. Hodson EM, Howman-Gilles RB, Evans RB et al.: The diagnosis of renal osteodystrophy: a comparison of technitium[99] pyrophosphate bone scintography with other techniques. *Clin Nephrol* 16: 24, 1981

395. de Jonge FA, Pauwels EK, Hamdy NA: Scintigraphy in the clinical evaluation of disorders of mineral and skeletal metabolism in renal failure. *Eur J Nuclear Med* 18: 839, 1991

396. Winzelberg GG: Parathyroid imaging. *Ann Intern Med* 107: 64, 1987

397. Suehiro M, Fukuchi M: Localization of hyperfunctioning parathyroid glands by means of thallium-201 and iodine-131 subtraction scintigraphy in patients with primary and secondary hyperparathyroidism. *Ann Nucl Med* 6: 185, 1992

398. Nisbet AP, Shaw P, Taube D et al.: 51Cr-EDTA/99mTc-MDP ratio: a simple non-invasive method for assessing renal osteodystrophy. *Br J Radiol* 62: 438, 1989

399. Hawkins PN et al.: Diagnostic radionuclide imaging of amiloid: biological targeting by circulating human serum amyloid P component. *Lancet* 1: 1413, 1988

400. Floege J et al.: Imaging of dialysis-related amyloid (AB-amyloid) deposits with 131I-β2-microglobulin. *Kidney Int* 38: 1169, 1990

401. Gladziwa U, Ittel TH, Dakshinamurty KV et al.: Secondary hyperparathyroidism and sonographic evaluation of parathyroid gland hyperplasia in dialysis patients. *Clin Nephrol* 38: 162, 1992

402. Fukagawa M, Okazaki R, Takano K et al.: Regression of parathyroid hyperplasia by calcitriol-pulse therapy in patients on long-term dialysis. *N Engl J Med* 323: 421, 1990

403. Winkelbauer F, Ammann ME, Langle F, Niederle B: Diagnosis of hyperparathyroidism with US after auto-transplantation: results of a prospective study. *Radiology* 186: 255, 1993

404. Jadoul M et al.: Ultrasonography detection of thickened joint capsules and tendons: an early marker of dialysis-related amyloidosis. (Abstract) *Nephrol Dial Transplant* 5: 727, 1990

405. Nordin BE, MacGregor J, Smith DA: The incidence of osteoporosis in normal women: Its relation to age and menopause. *Q J Med* 35: 25, 1966

406. Garn S, Poznanski A, Nagy M: Bone measurement in the differential diagnosis of osteopenia and osteoporosis. *Radiology* 100: 509, 1971

407. Gryfe CI et al.: Determination of the amount of bone in the metacarpal. *Age Ageing* 1: 213, 1972

408. Parfitt AM: The actions of parathyroid hormone on bone: relation to bone remodeling and turnover calcium homeostasis and metabolic bone disease. *Metabolism* 25: 909, 1976

409. Bone JM, Davison AM, Robson JS: Role of dialysate calcium concentration in osteoporosis in patients on hemodialysis. *Lancet* 1: 1047, 1972

410. Sugisaki H, Yamada K, Kataoka H, Kunitomo T: Long-term observation on renal osteodystrophy related parameters in dialysis patients. *Nephrol Dial Transplant* 6 (Suppl 2): 244, 1991

411. Rickers H, Christensen M, Podbro P: Bone mineral content in patients on prolonged maintenance hemodialysis: a three year follow-up study. *Clin Nephrol* 20: 302, 1983

412. Cameron JR, Mazess RB, Sorenson JA: Precision and accuracy of bone mineral determination by direct photon absorptiometry. *Invest Radiol* 3: 9, 1968

413. Hahn TJ, Hahn B: Osteopenia in patients with rheumatic diseases: principles of diagnosis and therapy. *Semin Arthritis Rheum* 6: 165, 1976

414. Griffiths HJ, Zimmerman RE, Bailey G, Snider R: The use of photon absorptiometry in the diagnosis of renal osteodystrophy. *Radiology* 109: 277, 1973

415. Griffiths HJ et al.: The long-term follow-up of 195 patients with renal failure: a preliminary report. *Radiology* 122: 643, 1977

416. Mazess RB, Peppler W, Chesnut C: Total body mineral and lead body mass by dual photon absorptiometry. *Calcif Tissue Int* 33: 361, 1981

417. Zanchetta J, Bogado: Bone mineral content in renal transplant patients. *Renal bone disease,parathyroid hormone and Vitamin D Singapore* 92, 1990

418. Denney JD, Sherrard DJ, Nelp WR: Total body calcium and long term calcium balance in chronic renal disease. *J Lab Clin Med* 82: 226, 1973

419. Cann CE, Genant HK, Ettinger B, Gordan G: Spinal mineral losses in oophorectomized women. *JAMA* 244: 2056, 1980

420. Funke M, Maurer J, Grabbe E, Scheler F: Vergleichende untersuchungen mit der quantitativen computertomographie und der Dual-Energy-X-Ray-Absortiometrie zur Knochendichte bei renaler osteopathie. *Rofo Fortschr geb Rontgenstr Neuen Bildgeb Verfahr* 157: 145, 1992

421. Gagne ER, Urena P, Leite-Silva S et al.: Short- and long-term efficacy of total parathyroidectomy with immediate autografting compared with subtotal parathyroidectomy in hemodialysis patients. *J Am Soc Nephrol* 3: 1008, 1992

422. Davies DR, Dent CE, Watson L: Tertiary hyperparathyroidism. *Br Med J* iii: 395, 1968

423. Black WC, Slatopolsky E, Elkan J, Hoffsten P: Parathyroid morphology in suppressible and non-suppressible renal hyperparathyroidism. *Lab Invest* 23: 497, 1970

424. Geffriaud C, Allinne E, Page B et al.: Decrease of tumor-like calcification in uremia despite aggravation of secondary hyperparathyroidism: a case report. *Clin Nephrol* 38: 158, 1992

425. Massry SG, Kopple JD: Requirements for calcium, phosphorus, and vitamin D. in *Nutrition and the Kidney*, edited by Mitch WE, Klahr S, Boston/New York/Toronto/London, Little Brown and Company, 1993, p 96

426. Coburn JW, Salusky IB: Control of serum phosphorus in uremia. *N Engl J Med* 320: 11402, 1989

427. Lafage M-H, Combe C, Fournier A, Aparicio M: Ketodiet, physiological calcium intake and native vitamin D improve renal osteodystrophy. *Kidney Int* 42: 1217, 1992

428. Schoenfeld P, Henry R, Laird N: Assessment of nutritional status of the National Cooperative Dialysis Study population. *Kidney Int* 23: 580, 1980

429. Blumenkrantz MJ, Kopple JD, Moran J, Coburn JW: Metabolic balance studies and dietary protein requirements in patients undergoing continuous peritoneal dialysis. *Kidney Int* 21: 849, 1982

430. Llach F, Nikakhtar B: Current advances in the therapy of secondary hyperparathyroidism and osteitis fibrosa. *Miner Electrolyte Metab* 17: 250, 1991

431. Sedman AB, Klein GL, Merritt RJ et al.: Evidence of aluminum loading in infants receiving intravenous therapy. *N Engl J Med* 312: 1337, 1985

432. Salusky IB, Foley J, Nelson P, Goodman WG: Aluminum accumulation from recommended doses of aluminum hydroxide in dialyzed children. *N Engl J Med* 324: 527, 1991

433. Jenkins DA, Gouldesbrough D, Smith GD et al.: Can low-dosage aluminum hydroxide control the plasma phosphate without bone toxicity? *Nephrol Dial Transplant* 4: 51, 1989

434. Harter HR, Laird NM, Teehan BP: Effects of dialysis prescription on bone and mineral metabolism: The National Cooperative Dialysis Study. *Kidney Int* 23 (Suppl 13): S73, 1983

435. Rutherford E, Mercado A, Hruska KA: An evaluation of a new and effective phosphous binding agent. *Trans Amer Soc Artif Internal Organs* 19: 446, 1973

436. Clarkson EM, Eastwood JB, Koutsaimanis K, De Wardener H: Net intestinal absorption of calcium in patients with chronic renal failure. *Kidney Int* 3: 258, 1973

437. Slatopolsky E, Weerts C, Norwood K et al.: Long term effects of calcium carbonate and 2.5 mEq/liter calcium dialysate on mineral metabolism. *Kidney Int* 36: 897, 1989

438. Malberti F, Surian M, Poggio F et al.: Efficacy and safety of long term treatment with calcium carbonate as a phosphate binder. *Am J Kidney Dis* 12: 487, 1988

439. Moriniere PG, Boudailliez B, Hocine C et al.: Prevention of osteitis fibrosa, aluminum bone disease and soft-tissue calcification in dialysis patients: a long term comparison of moderate doses of oral calcium ± Mg(OH)3 vs Al(OH)3 ± 1 alpha vitamin D3. *Nephrol Dial Transplant* 4: 1045, 1989

440. Renaud H, Atik A, Herve M et al.: Evaluation of vascular calcinosis risk factors in patients on chronic hemodialysis: Lack of influence of calcium carbonate. *Nephron* 48: 28, 1988

441. Sawyer N, Noonan K, Altmann P et al.: High dose calcium carbonate with stepwise reduction in dialysate calcium concentration: effective phosphate control and aluminum avoidance in haemodialysis patients. *Nephrol Dial Transplant* 4: 105, 1989

442. Argiles A, Kerr PG, Canaud B et al.: Calcium kinetics and the long-term effects of lowering dialysate calcium concentration. *Kidney Int* 43: 630, 1993

443. Sawyer N, Noonan K, Altmann P et al.: High dose calcium carbonate with stepwise reduction in dialysate calcium concentration: effective phosphate control and aluminum avoidance in haemodialysis patients. *Nephrol Dial Transplant* 3: 1, 1988

444. Cunningham J, Beer J, Coldwell RD et al.: Dialysate calcium reduction in CAPD patients treated with calcium carbonate and alphacalcidol. *Nephrol Dialysis Transplant* 7: 63, 1992

445. Fournier A, Moriniere P, Sebert JL et al.: Calcium carbonate, an aluminum free agent for control of hyperphosphatemia, hypocalcemia, and hyperparathyroidism. *Kidney Int* 29 (Suppl 18): S114, 1986

446. Clarkson EM, Luck VA, Hynson WV: The effect of aluminum hydroxide on calcium, phosphorus and aluminum balances, the serum parathyroid hormone concentration and the aluminum content of bone in patients with chronic renal failure. *Clin Sci* 43: 519, 1972

447. Mai M, Emmett M, Sheikh M et al.: Calcium acetate, an efective phosphorus binder in patients with renal failure. *Kidney Int* 36: 690, 1989

448. Sheikh M, Maguire J, Emmett M et al.: Reduction of Dietary Phosphorus Absorption by Phosphorus Binders. *J Clin Invest* 83: 66, 1989

449. Schiller L, Santa Ana CA, Sheikh M et al.: Effect of the time of administration of calcium acetate on phosphorus binding. *N Engl J Med* 320: 1110, 1989

450. Delmez JA, Tindira CA, Windus DW et al.: Calcium acetate as a phosphorus binder in hemodialysis patients. *J Am Soc Nephrol* 3: 96, 1992

451. Hercz G, Kraut JA, Andress DL: Use of calcium carbonate as a phosphate binder in dialysis patients. *Mineral Electrolyte Metab* 12: 314, 1986

452. Kobrin SM, Goldstein SJ, Shangraw RF, Raja RM: Variable efficacy of calcium carbonate tablets. *Am J Kidney Dis* 14: 461, 1989

453. Cushner HM, Copley J, Lindberg J, Foulks C: Calcium citrate, a non aluminum containing phosphate binding agent for treatment of CRF. *Kidney Int* 35: 95, 1988

454. Oe PL, Lips P, van der Muelen J et al.: Long-term use of magnesium hydroxide as a phosphate binder in patients on hemodialysis. *Clin Nephrol* 28: 180, 1987

455. Moriniere P, Maurouard C, Boudailliez B et al.: Prevention of hyperparathyroidism in patients on maintenance hemodialysis by intravenous 1 alpha hydroxyvitamin D3 in association with Mg(OH)2 as sole phosphate binder. A randomized comparative study with the association CaCO3±Mg(OH)2. *Nephron* 60: 154, 1992

456. Schneider HW, Kulbe KD, Weber H, Streicher E: *In vitro* and *in vivo* studies with a non-aluminum phosphate-binding compound. *Kidney Int* 29 (Suppl 18): S120, 1986

457. Mahoney J, Hayes J, Ingham J, Posen S: Hypophosphataemic osteomalacia in patients receiving hemodialysis. *Br Med J* 2: 142, 1976

458. Kaye M, Turner M, Ardila M et al.: Aluminum and phosphate. *Kidney Int* 33 (Suppl 24): S172, 1988

459. Hou SH, Zhao J, Ellman CF et al.: Calcium and phosphorus fluxes during hemodialysis with a low calcium dialysate. *Am J Kidney Dis* 18: 217, 1991

460. Albertini BV, Miller JH, Gardner PW, Shinaberger JH: High flux hemodiafiltration: under six hours/week treatment. *Trans Amer Soc Artif Internal Organs* 30: 227, 1984

461. Albertini BV, Miller JH, Gardner PW, Shinaberger JH: Performance characteristics of the hemoflow F60 in high-flux hemodiafiltration. *Contrib Nephrol* 46: 169, 1985

462. Shinaberger JH, Miller JH, Gardner PW: Characteristics of available dialyzers. edited by Nissenson AR, Fine RN, Genile D, Norwalk, Appleton Century Crofts, 1984

463. Delmez JA, Slatopolsky E, Martin KJ et al.: Minerals, vitamin D, and parathyroid hormone in continuous ambulatory peritoneal dialysis. *Kidney Int* 21: 862, 1982

464. Jaffe P, Podenphant J, Heaf JG: Bone histology in CAPD patients: a comparison with hemodialysis and conservatively treated chronic uremics. *Adv Perit Dial* 5: 171, 1989

465. Cannata JB, Briggs JD, Fell GS, Junor BJR: Comparison of control serum phosphate levels during continuous ambulatory peritoneal dialysis and during hemodialysis. *Perit Dial Bull* 3: 97, 1983

466. Fleming LW, Hudson SW, Stewart WK: Improved phosphate clearances with polycarbonate membranes. *Clin Exp Dialysis Apheresis* 6: 211, 1982

467. Miller JH, Gardner PW, Heinekin F et al.: Studies of inorganic phosphate removal during acetate and bicarbonate dialysis. *Proc Am Soc Artif Int Organs* 12: 57, 1983

468. Llach F, Nikakhtar B: Methods of controlling hyperphosphatemia in patients with chronic renal failure. *Current Opinion Nephrol Hypert* 2: 365, 1993

469. Clarkson EM, McDonald SJ, De Wardener H: The effect of a high intake of calcium carbonate in normal subjects and patients with chronic renal failure. *Clin Sci* 30: 425, 1966

470. Malluche HH, Werner E, Ritz E: Intestinal absorption of calcium and whole body calcium retention in incipient and advanced renal failure. *Mineral Electrolyte Metab* 1: 264, 1978

471. Makoff DL, Gordon A, Franklin SS et al.: Chronic calcium carbonate therapy in uremia. *Arch Intern Med* 123: 15, 1969

472. Curtis JR, De Wardener H, Gower P, Eastwood JB: The use of calcium carbonate and calcium phosphate without vitamin D in the management of renal osteodystrophy. *Proc Eur Dial Transplant Assoc* 7: 141, 1970

473. Eastwood JB, Bordier PhJ, De Wardener H: Comparison of the effect of vitamin D and calcium carbonate in renal osteomalacia. *Quart J Med* 40: 569, 1971

474. Ginsberg DS et al.: Hypercalcemia after oral calcium carbonate therapy in patients on chronic hemodialysis. *Lancet* 1: 1271, 1973

475. Somerville PJ, Kaye M: Resistance to parathyroid hormone in renal failure: role of vitamin D metabolites. *Kidney Int* 14: 245, 1978

476. Chanard J et al.: Rapid method for measurement of fractional intestinal absorption of calcium. *J Nucl Med* 15: 369, 1974

477. Katz A, Hampers CL, Merrill J: Secondary hyperparathyroidism and renal osteodystrophy in chronic renal failure. *Medicine* 48: 333, 1969

478. E Fernandez, J Montoliu: Succesful treatment of massive uraenic tumoral calcinosis with daily hemodialysis and very low calcium dialysate. *Nephrol Dial Transplant* 9: 1207, 1994

479. Lang RM, Fellner SK, Neumann A, Bushinsky DA: Left ventricular contractility varies directly with blood ionized calcium. *Ann Intern Med* 108: 424, 1988

480. Llach F, Coburn JW: Renal osteodystrophy and maintenance dialysis. in *Replacement of Renal Function by Dialysis*, edited by Maher JF, Dordrecht/Boston/Lancaster, Kluwer Academic Publishers, 1989, p 911

481. Regan RJ, Peacock M, Rosen SM: Effect of dialysate calcium concentration on bone disease in patients on hemodialysis. *Kidney Int* 10: 246, 1976

482. Catto GRD et al.: Haemodialysis therapy and changes in skeletal calcium. *Lancet* 1: 1150, 1973

483. Coburn JW: Mineral metabolism and renal bone disease: effects of CAPD versus hemodialysis. *Kidney Int* 43 (Suppl 40): S92, 1993

484. Voigts A, Felsenfeld AJ, Llach F: The effects of calciferol and its metabolites on patients with chronic renal failure. II. Calcitriol, hydroxyvitamin D and 24,25 dihydroxyvitamin D. *Arch Intern Med* 142: 1205, 1983

485. Voigts A et al.: The effects of calciferol and its metabolites on patients with chronic renal failure. I. Calciferol, dihydrotachysterol and calcifediol. *Arch Intern Med* 143: 960, 1983

486. Kaye M et al.: Arrest of hyperparathyroid bone disease with dihydrotachysterol in patients undergoing chronic hemodialysis. *Ann Intern Med* 73: 225, 1970

487. Witmer G, Margolis A, Fontaine O: Effects of 25 hydroxycholecalciferol on bone lesions of children with terminal renal failure. *Kidney Int* 10: 395, 1976

488. Peacock M: The clinical uses of 1α-hydroxyvitamin D₃. *Clin Endocrinol* 7 (Suppl): 1S, 1977

489. Dent CE, Harper CN, Philpot G: Treatment of renal glomerular osteodystrophy. *Q J Med* 30: 1, 1961

490. DeLuca HF, Avioli LV: Treatment of renal osteodystrophy with 25-hydroxycholecalciferol. *Arch Intern Med* 126: 896, 1970

491. Teitelbaum SL, Bone JM, Stein PM: Calcifedol in chronic renal insufficiency: skeletal response. *JAMA* 235: 164, 1976

492. Fournier A et al.: 1α-Hydroxycholecalciferol and 25-hydroxycholecalciferol in renal bone disease. *Proc Eur Dial Transplant Assoc* 12: 227, 1976

493. Recker R, Schoenfeld P, Letteri JM et al.: The efficacy of calcifediol in renal osteodystrophy. *Arch Intern Med* 138: 857, 1978

494. Berl T et al.: 1,25 Dihydroxycholecalciferol effects in chronic dialysis. A double-blind-controlled study. *Ann Intern Med* 88: 774, 1978

495. Eastwood JB, Phillips ME, De Wardener H: Biochemical and histological effects of 1,25-dihydroxycholecalciferol in the osteomalacia of chronic renal failure. in *Vitamin D and Problems Related to Uremic Bone Disease*, edited by Norman AW, Schaefer K, Grigoleit H-G, v Herrath D, Ritz E, Berlin, de Gruyter, 1975, p 595

496. Sherrard DJ, Brickman AS, Coburn JW: Skeletal response to treatment with 1,25 dihydroxyvitamin D in renal failure. *Contrib Nephrol* 18: 92, 1980

497. Maxwell D et al.: Calcitriol in dialysis patients. *Clin Pharmacol Therap* 23: 515, 1978

498. Memmos D et al.: Double-blind trial of oral 1,25-dihydroxy vitamin D3 versus placebo in asymptomatic hyperparathyroidism in patients receiving maintenance haemodialysis. *Br Med J* 282: 1919, 1981

499. Coburn JW et al.: Prospective, double blind trial with calcitriol in the prophylaxis of bone disease in asymptomatic dialysis patients. in *Vitamin D: Chemical, Biochemical and Clinical Endocrinology of Calcium Metabolism*, edited by Norman AW et al., Berlin, Walter de Gruyter, 1982, p 833

500. Chesney RW, Hamstra A, Jax DK: Influence of long term oral 1,25 dihydroxyvitamin D in childhood renal osteodystrophy. *Contrib Nephrol* 18: 55, 1980

501. Seidel A, Herrmann P, Klaus G et al.: Kinetics of serum 1,84 iPTH after high dose calcitriol in uremic patients. *Clin Nephrol* 39: 210, 1993

502. Massry SG et al.: Use of 1,25(OH)2D3 in the treatment of renal osteodystrophy in patients with moderate renal failure. in *Clinical Disorders of Bone and Mineral Metabolism*, edited by Frame B, Potts JT Jr, Amsterdam, Excerpta Medica, 1983, p 260

503. Goodman WG, Coburn JW: The use of 1,25-dihydroxyvitamin D₃ in early renal failure. *Annu Rev Med* 43: 227, 1992

504. Bertoli M, Luisetto G, Ruffatti A et al.: Renal function during calcitriol therapy in chronic renal failure. *Clin Nephrol* 33: 98, 1990

505. Oettinger CW, Oliver JC, Macon EJ: The effects of calcium carbonate as the sole phosphate binder in combination with low calcium dialysate and calcitriol therapy in chronic dialysis patients. *J Am Soc Nephrol* 3: 995, 1992

506. Norris KC, Kraut JA, Andress DL: Intravenous calcitriol for severe secondary hyperparathyroidism in dialysis patients. *Kidney Int* 27: 158, 1985

507. Andress DL, Norris KC, Coburn JW et al.: Intravenous calcitriol in the treatment of refractory osteitis fibrosa of chronic renal failure. *N Engl J Med* 321: 274, 1989

508. Hamdy NAT, Brown C, Kanis JA: Intravenous calcitriol lowers serum calcium concentrations in uraemic patients with severe hyperparathyroidism and hypercalcemia. *Nephrol Dial Transplant* 4: 545, 1989

509. Dressler R, Laut J, Lynn RI, Ginsberg N: Intravenous calcitriol for secondary hyperparathyroidism in patients with end-stage renal disease. *Clin Nephrol* 1995. In press

510. Klaus G, Mehls O, Hinderer J, Ritz E: Is intermittent oral calcitriol safe and effective in renal secondary hyperparathyroidism? *Lancet* 337: 800, 1991

511. Muramoto H, Haruki K, Yoshimura A et al.: Treatment of refractory hyperparathyroidism in patients on hemodialysis by intermittent oral administration of 1,25(OH)2VitaminD3. *Nephron* 58: 288, 1991

512. Martin KJ, Bullal HS, Domoto DT et al.: Pulse oral calcitriol for the treatment of hyperparathyroidism in patients on continuous ambulatory peritoneal dialysis: Preliminary observations. *Am J Kidney Dis* 19: 540, 1992

513. Tsukamoto Y, Nomura M, Takahashi Y et al.: The 'oral 1,25-dihydroxyvitamin D₃ pulse therapy' in hemodialysis patients with severe secondary hyperparathroidism. *Nephron* 57: 23, 1991

514. Reichel H, Szabo A, Uhl J et al.: Intermittent versus continuous administration of 1,25(OH)2D3 in experimental renal hyperparathyroidism. *Kidney Int* 44: 1259, 1993

515. Delmez JA, Dougan CS, Gearing BK et al.: The effects of intraperitoneal calcitriol on calcium and parathyroid hormone. *Kidney Int* 31: 795, 1987

516. Rolla D, Paoletti E, Marsano L et al.: Subcutaneous calcitriol in CAPD patients. *Perit Dial Int* 13: 118, 1993

517. Campistol JM, Torregrosa JV, Montesinos M et al.: Effectiveness of subcutaneous calcitriol (sCa) in the treatment of secondary hyperparathyroidism (HPT). *J Am Soc Nephrol* 4: 718, 1993

518. Brickman AS et al.: Comparison of effects of 1-α-hydroxyvitamin D3 and 1,25-dihydroxy-vitamin D3 in man. *J Clin Invest* 57: 1540, 1976

519. Coburn JW, Brickman AS, Sherrard DJ: Use of 1,25(OH)2vitamin D3 to separate 'types' of renal osteodystrophy. *Proc Eur Dial Transplant Assoc* 14: 442, 1977

520. Davison AM, Peacock M, Walker GS et al.: Phosphate and 1-alpha-hydroxyvitamin D3 therapy in haemodialysis patients. *Clin Endocrinol* 7 (Suppl): 91S, 1977

521. Brandi L, Daugaard H, Tvedegaard E et al.: Effects of intravenous 1α(OH)D3 on secondary hyperparathyroidism in chronic uremic patients on maintenance hemodialysis. *Nephron* 53: 294, 1989

522. Lind L, Wengle B, Wide L et al.: Suppression of serum parathyroid hormone levels by intravenous alphacalcidol in uremic patients on maintenance hemodialysis. *Nephron* 48: 296, 1988

523. Ljunghall S, Althoff P, Fellstrom B et al.: Effects on serum parathyroid hormone of intravenous treatment with alpha-

calcidol in patients on chronic hemodialysis. *Nephron* 53: 194, 1989

524. Brandi L, Daugaard H, Tvedegaard E et al.: Long-term suppression of secondary hyperparathyroidism by intravenous 1α-hydroxyvitamin D3 in patients on chronic hemodialysis. *Am J Nephrol* 12: 311, 1992

525. Pierides AM, Ellis HA, Ward MK: Barbiturate and anticonvulsant treatment in relation to osteomalacia with haemodialysis and renal transplantation. *Br Med J* 1: 190, 1976

526. Pierides AM, Kerr DNS, Ellis HA: 1α-hydroxycholecalciferol in hemodialysis renal osteodystrophy. Adverse effects of anticonvulsant therapy. *Clin Nephrol* 5: 189, 1976

527. Rutherford WE et al.: The effect of 5,6-trans vitamin D3 on calcium absorptin in chronic renal disease. *J Clin Endocrinol Metab* 40: 13, 1975

528. Hodsman J, Wong EG, Sherrard DJ: Preliminary trials with 24,25 dihydroxyvitamin D3 in dialysis osteomalacia. *Am J Med* 74: 407, 1983

529. Ott SM, Recker R, Coburn JW, Sherrard DJ: Vitamin D therapy in aluminum related osteomalacia. *Kidney Int* 32: 107, 1983

530. Canterbury JM et al.: Inhibition of parathyroid hormone secretion by 25-hydroxycholecalciferol and 24,25-dihydroxycholecalciferol in the dog. *J Clin Invest* 61: 1375, 1977

531. Friedlander MA, Horst RL, Hawker CC: Absence of effect of 24,25 dihydroxycholecalciferol on serum immunoreactive PTH in patients with persistent hyperparathyroidism after renal transplantation. *Clin Nephrol* 22: 206, 1984

532. Olgaard K, Finco D, Schwartz J: Effect of 24,25 dihydroxy-vitamin D3 on PTH levels and bone histology in dogs with chronic uremia. *Kidney Int* 25: 791, 1984

533. Dunstan CR et al.: Treatment of hemodialysis bone disease with 24,25(OH)2D3 and 1,25(OH)2D3 alone or in combination. *Mineral Electrolyte Metab* 11: 358, 1985

534. Popovtzer MM, Levi J, Bar-Khayim Y et al. Assessment of combined 24,25(OH)2D3 and 1 alpha (OH)D3 therapy for bone disease in dialysis patients. *Bone* 13: 369, 1992

535. Brown AJ, Ritter CR, Finch JL et al.: The noncalcemic analogue of vitamin D, 22 oxacalcitriol, suppresses parathyroid hormone synthesis and secretion. *J Clin Invest* 84: 279, 1989

536. Brown AJ, Finch JL, Lopez-Hilker S et al.: New active analogues of vitamin D with low calcemic activity. *Kidney Int* 29 (Suppl 29): S22, 1990

537. Slatopolsky E, Berkoben M, Kelber J et al.: Effects of calcitriol and non-calcemic vitamin D analogs on secondary hyperparathyroidism. *Kidney Int* Supplement 38: S43, 1992

538. Kubrusly M, Gagne E-R, Urena P et al.: Effect of 22-oxa-calcitriol on calcium metabolism in rats with severe secondary hyperparathyroidism. *Kidney Int* 44: 551, 1993

539. Kanis JA, Russell RGG: Rate of reversal of hypercalcemia and hypercalciuria induced by vitamin D and its 1ahydroxylated derivatives. *Br Med J* 1: 78, 1977

540. Schaefer K, Umlauf E, von Herrath D: Reduced risk of hypercalcemia for hemodialysis patients by administering calcitriol at night. *Am J Kidney Dis* 19: 460, 1992

541. Coburn JW et al.: Intestinal phosphate absorption in normal and uremic man: effects of 1,25(OH)2 vitamin D3 and 1(OH) vitamin D3. in *Phosphate metabolism*, edited by Massry SG, Ritz E, New York, Plenum Press, 1993

542. Szabo A, Merke J, Beier E et al.: 1,25(OH)2 vitamin D3 inhibits parathyroid cell proliferation in experimental uremia. *Kidney Int* 35: 1049, 1989

543. Fukagawa M, Wi H, Kurokawa K: Calcitriol induces apoptosis of hyperplastic parathyroid cells in uremia. *J Am Soc Nephrol* 2: 635, 1991

544. Fukagawa M, Kaname S, Igarashi T, Ogata E, Kurokawa K: Regulation of parathyroid hormone synthesis in chronic renal failure in rats. *Kidney Int* 39: 874, 1991

545. Tominaga Y, Tanaka Y, Sato K et al.: Recurrent renal hyperparathyroidism and DNA analysis of autografted parathyroid tissue. *W J Surg* 16: 595, 1992

546. Kitaoka M, Fukagawa M, Tanaka Y et al.: Parathyroid gland size is critical for longterm prognosis of calcitriol pulse therapy in chronic dialysis patients. (Abstract) *J Am Soc Nephrol* 2: 637, 1991

547. Mallick N, Berlyne G: Arterial calcification after vitamin D therapy in hyperphosphatemic renal failure. *Lancet* 2: 1316, 1968

548. Stanbury SW, Lumb GA, Nicholson WF: Elective subtotal parathyroidectomy for renal hyperparathyroidism. *Lancet* 1: 793, 1960

549. Llach F: Parathyroidectomy in chronic renal failure: indications, surgical approach and the use of calcitriol. *Kidney Int* 38: S62, 1990

550. Kaye M, Rosenthall L, Hill RO, Tabah RJ: Long-term outcome following total parathyroidectomy in patients with chronic renal disease. (Abstract) *Clin Nephrol* 39: 192, 1993

551. Baumann DS, Wells SA Jr: Parathyroid autotransplantation. *Surgery* 113: 130, 1993

552. Rothmund M, Wagner PK, Schark C: Subtotal parathyroidectomy versus total parathyroidectomy and autotransplantation in secondary hyperparathyroidism: a randomized trial. *W J Surg* 15: 745, 1991

553. White JV, LoGerfo P, Feind C, Weber C: Autologous parathyroid transplantation. *Lancet* 2: 461, 1983

554. Ellis HA: Fate of long term parathyroid autografts in patients with chronic renal failure treated by parathyroidectomy: a histopathological study of autografts, parathyroid glands and bone. *Histopathol* 13: 289, 1988

555. Gilmour JR: The gross anatomy of the parathyroid glands. *J Pathol Bacteriol* 46: 133, 1938

556. Wang C et al.: Hyperfunctioning supernumerary parathyroid glands. *Surg Gynecol Obstet* 148: 711, 1979

557. Gordon HE, Coburn JW, Passaro E: Surgical management of secondary hyperparathyroidism. *Arch Surg* 104: 520, 1972

558. Sicard GA, Wells SA Jr: Surgical treatment of secondary hyperparathyroidism. in *Surgery of the Thyroid and Parathyroid Glands*, edited by Kaplan EL, Edinburgh, Churchill Livingstone, 1983, p 243

559. Kinnaert P, Salmon I, Decoster-Gervy C et al.: Total parathyroidectomy and presternal subcutaneous implantation of parathyroid tissue for renal hyperparathyroidism. *Surg Ginec Obst* 176: 135, 1993

560. Felsenfeld AJ, Gutman RA, Llach F: Postparathyroidectomy hypocalcemia as an accurate indicator of

preparathyroidectomy bone histology in the uremic patient. *Mineral Electrolyte Metab* 10: 166, 1984

561. Litchman MB, Kinder BK, Johnson BM: Calcium requirements in ESRD patients after total parathyroidectomy with autotransplantation. *Dial Transplant* 16: 611, 1987

562. Shpitz B, Korzets Z, Dimbar A et al.: Immediate postoperative management of parathyroidectomy hemodialized patients. *Dial Transplant* 15: 507, 1986

563. Fine EJ: Parathyroid imaging: Its current status and future role. *Semin Nucl Med* 17: 350, 1987

564. Giangrande A, Cantu P, Solbiati L, Ravetto C: Ultrasonically guided fine-needle alcohol injection as an adjunct to medical treatment in secondary hyperparathyroidism. *Proc Eur Dial Transplant Assoc* 21: 895, 1984

565. Giangrande A, Castiglioni A, Solbiati L, Allaria P: Ultrasound-guided percutaneous fine-needle ethanol injection into parathyroid glands in secondary hyperparathyroidism. *Nephrol Dial Transplant* 7: 412, 1992

566. Page B, Zingraff J, Souberbielle JC et al.: Correction of severe hyperparathyroidism in two dialysis patients: surgical removal versus percutaneous ethanol injection. *Am J Kidney Dis* 19: 378, 1992

567. Takeda S, Michigishi T, Takazakura E: Successful ultrasonically guided percutaneous ethanol injection for secondary hyperparathyroidism. *Nephron* 62: 100, 1992

568. Milliner DS, Hercz G, Miller JH et al.: Clearance of aluminum by hemodialysis. Effect of desferrioxamine. *Kidney Int* 20 (Suppl 18): S100, 1986

569. Trapp G: Interactions of aluminum with cofactors, enzymes, and other proteins. *Kidney Int* 29 (Suppl 18): S12, 1986

570. De Broe ME, Drueke TB, Ritz E: Diagnosis and treatment of aluminium overload in end-stage renal failure patients. *Nephrol Dial Transplant* 8 (Suppl 1): 1, 1993

571. Freemont AJ et al.: Water treatment alone allows removal of aluminum from bone and reversal of the calcification defect in aluminum-related osteodystrophy. *Abstract Book, IXth International Congress Nephrology* 48A, 1984

572. Ackrill P, Ralston AJ, Day J, Hodge K: Successful removal of aluminum from patients with dialysis encephalopathy. *Lancet* 2: 692, 1980

573. Vasilakakis DM, D'Haese PC, Lamberts LV et al.: Removal of aluminoxamine and ferrioxamine by charcoal hemoperfusion and hemodialysis. *Kidney Int* 41: 1400, 1992

574. Molitoris BA, Alfrey AC, Alfrey PS: Rapid removal of DFO-chelated aluminum during hemodialysis using polysulfone dialyzers. *Kidney Int* 34: 98, 1988

575. Romero R, Novoa D, Otero S et al.: Direct effect of deferoxamine on hemoglobin synthesis in patients on hemodialysis treated with recombinant human erythropoietin. *Nephron* 63: 164, 1993

576. Gallant S, Boyden M, Gallant L et al.: Serial studies of auditory neurotoxicity in patients receiving deferoxamine therapy. *Am J Med* 83: 1085, 1987

577. Oliveri NF, Buncic R, Chew E: Visual and auditory neurotoxicity in patients receiving subcutaneous deferoxamine. *N Engl J Med* 314: 868, 1986

578. Cases A, Kelly J, Sabater J et al.: Acute visual and auditory neurotoxicity in patients with end-stage renal disease receiving desferrioxamine. *Clin Nephrol* 29: 176, 1988

579. Walker JA, Sherman RA, Eisinger RP: Thrombocytopenia associated with intravenous desferrioxamine. *Am J Kidney Dis* 6: 254, 1985

580. Sherrard DJ, Walker JA, Boykin J: Precipitation of dialysis dementia by deferoxamine treatment of aluminum related bone disease. *Am J Kidney Dis* 12: 126, 1988

581. Gallant T, Freedman MH, Vellend H, Francombe WH: Yersinia sepsis in patients with iron overload treated with deferoxamine. *N Engl J Med* 314: 1643, 1986

582. Boelaert JR, Fenves AZ, Coburn JW: Deferoxamine therapy and mucormycosis in dialysis patients: report of an international registry. *Am J Kidney Dis* 18: 660, 1991

583. Boelaert JR, van Roost G, Vergauwe PL et al.: The role of desferrioxamine in dialysis associated mucormycosisis. *Clin Nephrol* 29: 261, 1988

584. Van Cutsem J, Boelaert JR: Effects of deferoxamine, feroxamine and iron on experimental mucormyucosis (zygomycosis). *Kidney Int* 36: 10618, 1989

585. Boelaert JR, de Locht M, Van Cutsem J et al.: Mucormycosis during deferoxamine therapy is a siderophore-mediated infection: *in vitro* and *in vivo* animal studies. *J Clin Invest* 91: 19796, 1993

586. Cannata JB, Fernandez JL, Douthat W et al.: Aluminum (Al) transfer in dialysis: effect of different membranes, type of dialysis and forms of desferroxamine (DFO) administration. *J Am Soc Nephrol* 3: 671, 1992

587. Canavese C, Gurioli L, D'Amicone M et al.: Kinetics of aluminoxamine and feroxamine chelates in dialysis patients. *Nephron* 60: 411, 1992

588. Cannata JB, Elorriaga R, Menendez P et al.: A new orally active chelator in the treatment of aluminium (Al) overload. *J Am Soc Nephrol* 3: 671, 1992

589. Torres A, Hernandez D, Concepcion M et al.: Higher levels of intact parathyroid hormone (i-PTH) are necessary to maintain a normal bone remodelling in dialysis patients (DP). *J Am Soc Nephrol* 3: 677, 1992

590. Hercz G, Pei Y, Sherrard DJ, Chan W: Aplastic osteodystrophy: effect of lowering dialysate calcium. *J Am Soc Nephrol* 4: 697, 1993

591. Heynen G, Kanis JA, Oliver DO, Earnshaw M: Evidence that endogenous calcitonin protects against renal bone disease. *Lancet* 2: 1322, 1976

592. Delano BG et al.: A trial of calcitonin therapy in renal osteodystrophy. *Nephron* 11: 287, 1973

593. Fleisch H, Russell RGC, Francis MD: Diphosphonates inhibit hydroxiapatite dissolution *in vitro* and bone resorption in tissue culture and *in vivo*. *Science* 165: 1262, 1969

594. Sahni M, Guenther HL, Fleisch H et al.: Bisphosphonates act on rat bone resorption through the mediation of osteoblasts. *J Clin Invest*, 1993

595. Malluche HH: The possible use of bisphosphonates in the treatment of renal osteodystrophy. *Clin Nephrol* 38 (Suppl 1): S87, 1992

596. D'Amour P, Jobin J, Hamel L, L'Ecuyer N: iPTH values during hemodialysis: role of ionized Ca, dialysis membranes and iPTH assays. *Kidney Int* 38: 308, 1993

597. Gueris J, Fournier A, Sebert JL et al.: Comparative effects of dialysis with cuprophan versus polyacrilonitrile membranes on plasma immunoreactive parathyroid hormone levels in patients on chronic hemodialysis. *Calcif Tissue Res* 22: 34, 1977

598. Morachiello P, Landini S, Fracasso A et al.: Combined hemodialysis-hemoperfusion in the treatment of secondary hyperparathyroidism of uremic patients. *Blood Purif* 9: 148, 1991

599. Henderson RG, Russell RGG, Earnshaw M: Loss of metacarpal and iliac bone in chronic renal failure: influence of haemodialysis, parathyroid activity, type of renal disease, physical activity and heparin consumption. *Clin Sci* 56: 317, 1979

600. Jaffe MD, Wellis PW: Multiple fractures associated with long term sodium heparin therapy. *JAMA* 193: 152, 1965

601. Griffith GC, Nichols G, Asher JD, Flanagan B: Heparin osteoporosis. *JAMA* 195: 1089, 1966

602. Majdalani G, Chomant J, Kachko A et al.: Kinetics of technetium-labeled heparin in hemodialyzed patients. *Kidney Int* 43 (Suppl 41): S131, 1993

ORGAN AND METABOLIC COMPLICATIONS – ABNORMAL ENDOCRINE FUNCTION IN CHRONIC RENAL FAILURE

VICTORIA S. LIM and MICHAEL J. FLANIGAN

INTRODUCTION

Endocrine function is often abnormal in patients with chronic renal failure (CRF); these disturbances, though not life-threatening, diminish the quality of life and make interpretation of endocrine function tests difficult. The pathogenesis of these derangements are multi-factorial and complex in nature and can be classified as follows:

- Hormonal deficiency due to the absence of functioning renal mass – erythropoietin, 1,25 vitamin D_3, renin and osteogenic or bone morphogenic protein, a bone growth promoting factor (1).
- Hormonal deficiency due to uremia – Testosterone.
- Hormonal excess due to increased production – Parathyroid hormone (PTH), prolactin and growth hormone (GH).
- Hormonal excess due to decreased degradation – GH, prolactin, insulin and glucagon.
- Altered feedback regulation – gonadal dysfunction and excess GH and prolactin production.
- Altered hormone metabolism – impaired conversion of thyroxine to triiodothyronine.
- Altered end organ responsiveness – insulin and PTH resistance.

This chapter will attempt to address all the endocrine disturbances outlined above with the exception of erythropoietin and osteogenic protein deficiency and hyperparathyroidism.

GONADAL FUNCTION

Impotence, decreased libido, infertility, defective spermatogenesis and reduced testosterone production are common in men with CRF. The seminal fluid volume is small and the sperm count and percentage of motile sperms are reduced. Testicular histology varies from a mild maturation arrest to germinal cell aplasia. The most commonly observed characteristics are preservation of early spermatogenesis and depletion of more mature forms, notably, the spermatids. These are features typical of hormonal deficiency because the earlier stages of spermatogenesis are not hormone-dependent. By contrast, testicular damage induced by cytotoxic agents is characterized by disappearance of the earlier stages of spermatogenesis. In the circulation, testosterone binding globulin levels are normal, but total and free testosterone are reduced. Plasma luteinizing hormone (LH) is mildly elevated and plasma follicle-stimulating hormone (FSH) normal; the latter is only elevated in azoospermic patients (2).

In pre-menopausal women, amenorrhea, metromenorrhagia and infertility are common. Plasma levels of estradiol and progesterone are not different from those of normal subjects during the follicular phase of the menstrual cycle and plasma FSH and LH are normal as well. As illustrated in Figure 1, serial daily measurements of ovarian and pituitary hormones revealed that most women undergoing dialysis treatment have an anovulatory pattern characterized by oscillations of both LH and FSH without discernible peaks. Only a small fraction of uremic women have normal ovulatory hormonal profile (3).

In both male and female dialysis patients, clomiphene and GnRH administration resulted in a noticeable rise in plasma LH, and to a lesser extent, FSH. Clomiphene, a non-steroidal anti-estrogen competes with estrogen for hypothalamic receptors, instigates in an increased GnRH secretion and, secondarily, a rise in FSH and LH. This agent was used in CRF patients to test the integrity of the hypothalamic-pituitary axis. From these results, it appears that pituitary function is normal and the negative feedback loop between gonadal steroid and gonadotropin release is intact. This is further supported by the observation that post menopausal dialysis women have markedly elevated LH and FSH.

It has been suggested that uremic hypogonadism represents an end organ defect. The best evidence supporting this concept is derived from the work of Holdsworth

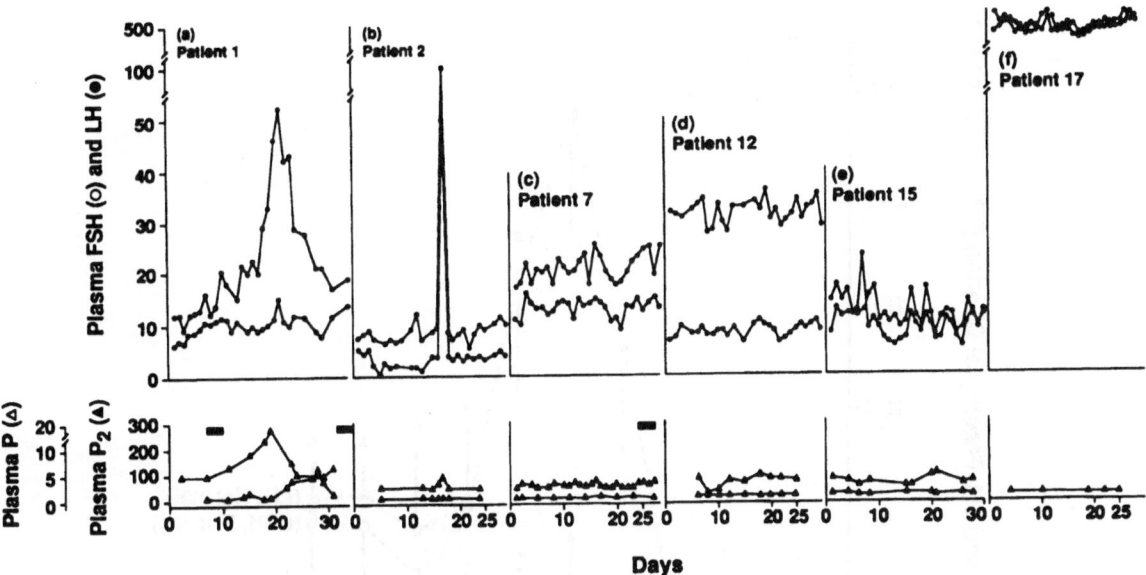

Figure 1. Plasma follicle-stimulating hormone (FSH), luteinizing hormone (LH), estradiol (E₂) and progesterone (P) levels during a 30-day period in six hemodialysis women; ▬ in the lower panels indicates menses. (a) Patient 1 had regular menses and normal ovulatory pattern. (b) Patient 2 had occassional scanty menses and her hormonal pattern was characterized by short LH and FSH surges, not preceeded by estradiol rise and was non-ovulatory as serum P did not increase. (c) Patient 7 had metromenorrhagia and galactorrhea, and her cycle was characterized by absence of estradiol peak, LH surge or a rise in progesterone. (d) Patient 12 had amenorrhea and galactorrhea, and she had an acyclic hormonal profile. (e) Patient 15 was a 20-year old woman with primary amenorrhea. She had acyclicity and her FSH and LH levels were low. (f) Patient 17 was post-menopausal; she had markedly elevated gonadotropins and her E₂ levels were non-detectable. (Reprinted with permission from the *Ann Int Med* 93: 21, 1980).

and colleagues who found a blunted testosterone response in CRF patients receiving human chorionic gonadotropin (hCG) injections (4).

We concur that there is end organ hypo-responsiveness with regard to steroidogenesis, but believe that there is a concomitant hypothalamic defect as evidenced by the following observations: (1) In a longitudinal study of male dialysis patients, a predictable rise of FSH was noted following successful transplantation. The FSH increment post transplant was marked and the elevation was sustained for many months; when sperm counts approached normal, FSH then declined. (2) The absence of cyclicity in female dialysis patients. (3) Estrogen supplementation with doses calculated to achieve estrogen peak during midcycle failed to induce a rise in serum LH in dialysis patients. In normal pre-menopausal women, similar estrogen doses resulted in a remarkable LH surge to levels greater than 200% above baseline (Figure 2). During the reproductive years, gonadotropin secretion in women is believed to consists of tonic and cyclic components. The former regulates basal gonadotropin secretion and is governed by a negative estrogen feedback. The latter depends upon the positive feedback of estrogen on the hypothalamus. In patients with renal failure, the negative feedback relation between estrogen and the tonic component of LH release is intact; the cyclic component of gonadotropin secretion, however, is impaired.

Recent studies centered on assessing hypothalamic function noted a reduction in the frequency of LH pulsatile secretion in both adult males and pubertal children with CRF (5). Furthermore, using a deconvolution analysis technique which takes into account simultaneous degradation and secretion, Veldhuis et al. showed a decrease in LH secretion rate and believe that the elevated serum LH concentration in CRF patients is due primarily to an increased circulating LH half-life (6).

In women, ovarian dysfunction does not appear to cause serious problems other than infertility, and perhaps decreased libido. The persistence of estrogen secretion and the lack of ovulation result in hormonal imbalance, metromenorrhagia and, less frequently, cystic ovaries. Dysfunctional uterine bleeding usually respond to progestational agents. Rupture of ovarian cysts may result in bloody peritoneal effluent. Since it is impractical to do serial daily sampling to determine the ovulatory pattern, contraception is advisable in female dialysis patients except for those with long standing amenorrhea.

In male patients, impotence may require medical attention. If nocturnal penile tumescence (NPT) is normal, patients merely need reassurance. Studies have shown a positive correlation between NPT and frequency of intercourse (7). If NPT is reduced, depot testosterone can be given to normalize the serum testosterone level. Generally, a replacement dose of 200 mg IM once every two weeks is

1238   *Victoria S. Lim and Michael J. Flanigan*

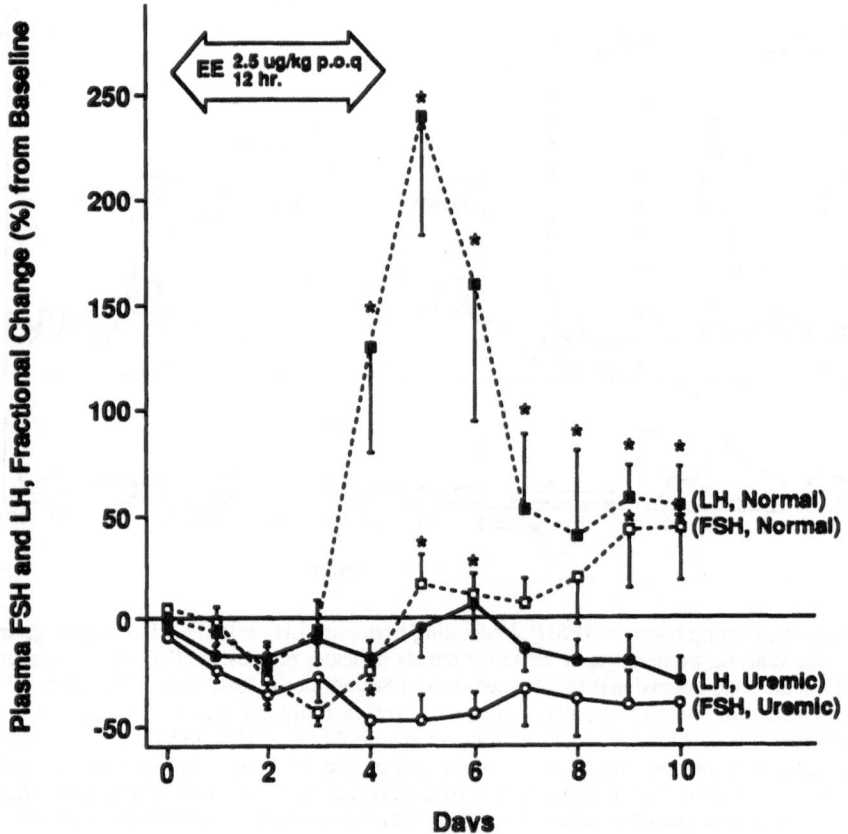

Figure 2. Plasma gonadotropin responses to ethinyl estradiol (EE) in 4 normal and 8 uremic pre-menopausal women. Both plasma LH (■, normal and ●, uremic) and FSH (□, normal and ○, uremic) levels are presented as % changes from baseline, i.e., before EE adminstration. Uremic patients showed a markedly blunted response to EE and * denotes *p* values ranged from < 0.05–< 0.001 by student's test. (Reprinted with permission from the *Ann Int Med* 93: 21, 1980).

sufficient. In the non-uremic hypogonadal state, androgen dosage and improvement in sexual function are generally well-correlated. In dialysis patients, such a correlation is lacking, making it difficult to attribute the sexual dysfunction soley to androgen deficiency. If zinc deficiency is documented, a trial of zinc therapy, administered orally as zinc acetate or in the dialysate as zinc chloride, is indicated with the goal of normalizing the serum zinc level (8). Short-term treatment with either hCG, clomiphen citrate or bromocriptine has been reported to improve sexual function in some patients (9). Bromocriptine is especially logical in patients with hyperprolactinemia. There are, however, no long-term studies on this matter. If hypothalamic dysfunction is the predominant defect in uremic hypogonadism, reproductive function could conceivably be improved by intermittent administration of rapidly metabolized GnRH or short-acting GnRH agonist to achieve pulsatile LH secretion. This type of treatment, though theoretically possible, has never been tried in dialysis patients because the need to restore fertility has not been an issue.

Since the introduction of erythropoietin, improved sexual function without a discernible rise in serum testosterone in men and resumption of regular menses in women, accompanied by a normalization of serum prolactin, have been reported (10).

HYPERPROLACTINEMIA

About 30% of dialysis patients exhibit hyperprolactinemia; the magnitude of the elevation is mild, about 3–6 times above normal. Hyperprolactinemia in these patients is due to a combination of decreased degradation and increased secretion (11). In contrast to other anterior pituitary hormones whose secretion is stimulated by hypothalamic releasing factors, prolactin secretion is tonically inhibited by dopaminergic mechanisms. Persistent prolactin elevation in CRF patients thus suggests disturbed dopaminergic regulation, either in the hypothalamus, or elsewhere in the central nervous system. The observation that neither oral L-dopa nor dopamine infused intravenously suppress plasma prolactin indicates that pituitary lactotrophs in these patients are resistant to dopamine (12). The presence of pituitary non-suppression made it difficult, it not impossible, to substantiate a concomitant central defect *in vivo*.

Because prolactin is known to inhibit gonadotropin secretion, the possibility that hyperprolactinemia may account for the hypogonadism commonly observed in dialysis patients remains an attractive hypothesis. Bromocriptine administration normalized serum prolactin and improved sexual function in a small number of patients (9).

THYROID FUNCTION

The most common thyroid abnormality observed in CRF patients is a reduction is serum total and free triiodothyronine (TT_3 and free T_3). Total thyroxine (TT_4), and less frequently, free T_4, are also reduced. The low T_3 is a result of impaired peripheral conversion of T_4 to T_3; the T_3 degradation rate remains normal (13).

Since thyroxine binding globulin (TBG) concentration is normal, reduced TT_4 is believed to be due to the presence of serum inhibitors which impair T_4 binding to TBG. Yet free T_4, measured indirectly as free T_4 index, is reduced as well. Moreover, several commercially available free T_4 assay kits also yield low free T_4 values in those patients whose TT_4 is reduced. These low free T_4 indices and low free T_4 values are explained on the basis that the binding inhibitors, which inhibit binding of T_4 to TBG, also inhibit the binding of T_4 to solid phase matrices, such as resin and activated charcoal, used in *in vitro* assay (14–16). Patients who are ingesting salicylates, non-steroidal anti-inflammatory agents and anti-convulsants can further aggravate this phenomenon of low TT_4 and low free T_4. Uremia decreases the binding of these drugs to serum proteins, leaving a higher free fraction of the drug which then secondarily displace T_4 from TBG and/or pre-albumin. Tracer equilibrium dialysis and direct equilibrium dialysis (non-tracer technique) have been touted to offer the most accurate free T_4 measurement. Unfortunately, even these techniques have yielded low free T_4 values in few CRF patients. The tracer equilibrium dialysis is also influenced by TBG and T_4 binding capacity. The low value from direct equilibrium dialysis is explained on the basis that the putative inhibitors may be dialyzable (17).

Serum total reverse T_3 (TrT_3), the inner ring 5-deiodination product of T_4, is invariably reduced in patients with hypothyroidism, increased in patients with a variety of non-renal non-thyroidal illnesses, but is normal in CRF patients. The normal TrT_3 in CRF is due to increased exit rate of rT_3 from the plasma to extravascular pool (18).

Serum TSH is normal and this is the single most important argument for euthyroidism. CRF patients who are truly hypothyroid can mount a definite TSH elevation. TSH response to thyrotropin-releasing hormone (TRH) is either normal or blunted. Hypothyroid subjects, even with CRF, have an exaggerated TSH response.

Low circulating thyroid hormones in CRF patients appear to have a protective effect on protein catabolism. Normalization of serum hormone profile following thyroid hormone supplementation results in increased nitrogen excretion and protein degradation as measured, respectively, by nitrogen balance and leucine flux (19, 20). Thus, thyroid hormone supplementation is indicated only when the diagnosis of hypothyroidism is unambiguous.

GROWTH HORMONE (GH) METABOLISM

CRF patients have elevated serum GH due to a combination of decreased degradation and increased secretion. Furthermore, hypoglycemia fails to stimulate GH secretion and hyperglycemia produces a paradoxical rise in serum GH. The rise in GH secretion following arginine infusion is also exaggerated (21).

GH affects skeletal growth indirectly by inducing hepatic synthesis of somatomedin (Sm) which in turn stimulates the growth of epiphyseal cartilage. Sm are now identified as insulin-like growth factors (IGF) I and II. In CRF patients, Sm is elevated when measured by radioimmunoassay, but is normal by bioassay. This discrepancy is thought to result from an Sm inhibitor in the uremic serum (22). Measurement of IGF I and II by radioimmunoassy showed variable levels.

Skeletal growth is impaired in children with CRF; height age is usually more retarded than bone age. Delayed bone age and delayed sexual maturation are actually beneficial in the sense that these delays prolong the opportunity for statural growth. Maneuvers useful to induce skeletal growth include adequate dialysis, increased nutritional intake, vitamin D administration, prevention of renal osteodystrophy, correction of metabolic acidosis, and recently, recombinant human growth hormone administration. With the latter treatment, CRF children exhibit a rise in growth velocity, an increase in body weight and mid-arm muscle circumference, all of which suggest a net anabolic effect (23). This salutary result has been obtained without glucose intolerance or accelerated decline in glomerular filtration rate. Moreover, this accelerated stutural growth did not hasten bone maturation, thus preserving further growth potential.

CARBOHYDRATE METABOLISM

In CRF patients, insulin clearance is reduced, its half-life prolonged, and the insulin effect on tissue glucose uptake is impaired. The prolonged half-life is due to a combination of diminished renal degradation and impaired hepatic clearance; the latter is improved by dialysis. Tissue insulin resistance is best characterized by euglycemic and hyperglycemic insulin clamps showing diminished body glucose uptake under the influence of insulin. Glucose uptake and utilization are also improved with dialysis treatment. In some patients, there may, additionally, be a component of reduced pancreatic β cell sensitivity (24, 25). Despite all these abnormalities, non-diabetic CRF patients have normal fasting blood glucose, basal insulin levels, however, are slightly higher than normal. In diabetic patients who develop renal failure, insulin dose may need adjustment. The direction of the dose adjustment will depend on which is the predominant disturbance, insulin resistance, impaired insulin clearance or reduced β cell secretion, at any one time.

Insulin resistance impairs lipoprotein lipase activity and hyperinsulinemia may stimulate very low density lipoprotein synthesis; both disturbances increase serum triglycerides, the most common lipid abnormality in end-stage renal disease (ESRD) patients. In peritoneal dialysis patients, the high glucose load and the increased insulin requirement may further aggravate the hypertriglyceridemia, and this defect is not improved by exogenous insulin administration.

Impaired glucagon and pro-glucagon degradation in CRF patients result in elevated serum glucagon levels. Feedback regulation of glucagon, however, is normal. Plasma glucagon is stimulated by arginine infusion and appropriately suppressed by glucose administration. Glucagon augments gluconeogenesis, and hyperglucagonemia may, in part, be responsible for the increased protein catabolism thought to be prevalent in ESRD patients (26, 27). Hypoglycemia has been reported both in diabetic and non-diabetic CRF patients. In the diabetics, the most common reason is failure to adjust the dose of insulin or oral hypoglycemic agent. Malnourished patients are more prone to hypoglycemia because of reduced hepatic glycogen storage. Symptomatic hypoglycemia in CRF patients has been attributed to β blockers resulting in inhibition of hepatic glucose production (28, 29).

ADRENAL FUNCTION

Glucocorticoid: Plasma cortisol half-life is prolonged and basal and integrated 24-hour plasma cortisol levels are frequently elevated in CRF patients. Plasma free cortisol is increased to a greater extent than total cortisol. This suggests a reduced cortisol binding by cortisol binding globulin. Plasma cortisol could be spuriously elevated secondary to cross-reactivity of some commercial antisera with steroid metabolites that accumulate in renal failure. This has been confirmed by the observation that a significant difference exists in the cortisol levels measured before and after chromatographic separation of plasma cortisol and cortisol metabolites. Because of this, an unexpectedly high level should be confirmed by an alternative assay procedure (30).

A diagnosis of hypoadrenocorticism is easily made because ACTH administration to CRF patients uniformly results in a rise in plasma cortisol levels. A diagnosis of hyperadrenocorticism, on the other hand, is difficult to establish because of the altered negative feedback control of the hypothalamo-pituitary-adrenocortical axis. A conventional 1 mg oral dexamethasone dose does not suppress cortisol secretion in the uremic patient. Although the 8 mg oral dose and the 1 mg intravenous dose suppress plasma cortisol to < 2 μg/dl, CRF patients generally escape the suppressive effect and resume cortisol secretion sooner than normal subjects. In non-uremic subjects with Cushing's syndrome, plasma cortisol levels remain > 10 μg/dl after 1 mg iv dexamethasone. Circadian cortisol rhythm, while lost in subjects with Cushing's sydrome, is maintained in CRF patients. Both normal and elevated plasma ACTH levels have been reported in CRF patients (31). Despite high circulating cortisol levels, CRF patients do not appear physically Cushingoid, and this has led investigators to hypothesize that CRF patients may have a tissue resistance to cortisol.

Adrenal Medullary Function: Resting plasma catecholamine levels are generally elevated in CRF patients (32). Since both tyrosine hydroxylase and dopamine hydroxylase, the catecholamine synthesizing enyzmes, are reduced, the increased levels are best attributed to decreased re-uptake or degradation. Reduced plasma catechol-O-methyl-transferase (COMT) activity found in CRF patients may result in decreased catecholamine degradation. Additionally, catecholamine depletion of the adrenergic nerve terminals in the salivary glands of uremic patients suggests reduces neuronal uptake or hightened degradation. Hemodialysis, by removing catecholamines, tends to reduce catecholamine levels.

Diagnosis of pheochromocytoma in CRF patients should utilize a combination of plasma catecholamine and appropriate imaging technique of the adrenal glands. The utility of clonidine suppression test has not been evaluated in this setting.

Renin-angiotensin-aldosterone system: Plasma renin activity (PRA) and plasma aldosterone are variable in dialysis patients, ranging from subnormal to elevated levels. The response of renin and aldosterone to volume contraction, assumption of upright posture and corticotropin stimulation is blunted. Angiotensin infusion also produced a blunted aldosterone response. Serum potassium appears to be the most important regulator of aldosterone secretion (33).

Because aldosterone not only increases urinary and fecal potassium excretion, but also enhances potassium transport into the cells, administration of fludrocortisone acetate (Florinef), a synthetic mineralo-corticoid, has been reported to reduce the severity of hyperkalemia in some patients.

Hypertension in dialysis patients is mostly treated by adequate ultrafiltration. In patients whose blood pressure is not volume-dependent, plasma renin may be elevated, and in such patients, ACE inhibitor may be useful.

HYPOTHALAMO-PITUITARY FUNCTION

Although hypothalamo-pituitary function has not been systematically assessed in CRF patients, aggregates of studies involving other endocrine systems suggest a definite derrangement of this central axis. Examples of these include hyperprolactinemia, hypothalamic amenorrhea, decreased frequency of pulsatile LH secretion, impaired cortisol suppression following dexamethasone administration, and paradoxical rise of growth hormone during glucose infusion. It is not clear whether these abnormalities are the result of dopaminergic deficiency or represent an imbalance between adrenergic, dopaminergic and serotoninergic input from the central nervous system.

CONCLUSIONS

Many of the endocrine disturbances described in this chapter including abnormal gonadal, thyroid and prolactin function are not unique to renal failure and reportedly accompany other chronic illnesses or malnutrition. In chronic renal failure, the severity of these disturbances vary with the general health status of the patients. Subjects who are well-dialyzed, well-nourished and with minimal concurrent diseases tend to have better preserved hormonal profile.

With few exceptions, all the endocrine abnormalities described here are corrected by successful renal transplantation. The exceptions are almost entirely due to the effects of glucocorticoids including inhibition of skeletal growth, carbohydrate intolerance and suppression of TSH response to TRH.

ACKNOWLEDGMENTS

We are grateful to our patients for their unquestionable trust and participation in our experiments, our colleagues at the University of Chicago and University of Iowa for their collaboration, the staff of the Dialysis Unit at the University of Iowa Hospitals for their continuing support, and Lisa Nelson and Bill Hufschmidt for secretarial help.

REFERENCES

1. Alper J: Boning Up: Newly isolated proteins heal bad breaks. *Science* 263: 324, 1994
2. Lim VS, Fang VS: Gonadal dysfunction in uremic men: a study of the hypothalamo-pituitary-testicular axis before and after renal transplantation. *Am J Medicine* 58: 655, 1975
3. Lim VS, Henriques C, Sievertson G, Frohman LA: Ovarian function in chronic renal failure: evidence suggesting hypothalamic anovulation. *Ann of Intern Med* 93: 21, 1980
4. Holdsworth S, Atkins RC, DeKrester DM: The pituitary-testicular axis in men with chronic renal failure. *N Engl J Med* 296: 1245, 1977
5. Talbot JA, Rodger RS, Robertson WR: Pulsatile bioactive luteinizing hormone secretion in men with chronic renal failure and following renal transplantation. *Nephron* 56: 66, 1990
6. Veldhuis JD, Wilkowski MJ, Zwart AD et al.: Evidence for attenuation of hypothalamic gonadotropin-releasing hormone (GnRH) impulse strength with preservation of GnRH pulse frequency in men with chronic renal failure. *J Clin Endocrinol Metab* 76: 648, 1993
7. Procci WR, Goldstein DA, Adelstein J et al.: Sexual dysfunction in the male patient with uremia: a reappraisal. *Kidney Int* 19: 317, 1981
8. Mahajan SK, Abasi AA, Prasad AS et al.: Effect of oral zinc therapy on gonadal function in hemodialysis patients. *Ann of Intern Med* 97: 357, 1982
9. Bommer J, del Pozo E, Ritz E, Bommer G: Improved sexual function in male hemodialysis patients on bromocriptine. *Lancet* 2: 496, 1979
10. Schaeffer RM, Kokot F, Wernze H et al.: Improved sexual funtion in hemodialysis patients on recombinant erythropoietin: a possible role for prolactin. *Clin Nephrol* 31: 1, 1989
11. Sievertson GD, Lim VS, Nakawatase C, Frohman LA: Metabolic clearance and secretion rates of human prolactin in normal subjects and in patients with chronic renal failure. *J Clin Endocrinol Metab* 50: 846, 1980
12. Lim VS, Kathpalia SC, Frohman LA: Hyperprolactinemia and impaired pituitary response to suppression and stimulation in chronic renal failure: reversal after transplantation. *J Clin Endocrinol Metab* 48: 101, 1979
13. Lim VS, Fang VS, Katz AI, Refetoff S: Thyroid dysfunction in chronic renal failure. *J Clin Invest* 60: 522, 1977
14. Oppenheimer JH, Schwartz HL, Mariash CN, Kaiser FE: Evidence for a factor in the sera of patients with nonthyroidal disease which inhibits iodothyronine binding in solid matrices, serum proteins, and hepatocytes. *J Clin Endocrinol Metab* 54: 757, 1982
15. Melmed S, Geola FL, Reed AW et al.: A comparison of methods for assessing thyroid function in nonthyroidal illness. *J Clin Endocrinol Metab* 54: 300, 1982
16. Kaptein EM, Macintyre SS, Weiner JM et al.: Free thyroxine estimates in nonthyroidal illness: comparison of eight methods. *J Clin Endocrinol Metab* 52: 1073, 1981
17. Nelson JC, Wilcox RB, Pandian MR: Dependence of free thyroxine estimates obtained with equilibrium tracer dialysis on the concentration of thyroxine-binding globulin. *Clin Chem* 38: 1294, 1992
18. Kaptein EM, Feinstein EI, Nicoloff JT, Massry SG: Serum reverse triiodothyronine and thyroxine kinetics in patients with chronic renal failure. *J Clin Endocrinol Metab* 57: 181, 1983
19. Lim VS, Flanigan MJ, Zavala DC, Freeman RM: Protective adaptation of low serum triiodothyronine in patients with chronic renal failure. *Kidney Int* 28: 541, 1985

20. Lim VS, Tsalikian E, Flanigan MJ: Augmentation of protein degradation by L-triiodothyronine in uremia. *Metabolism* 38: 1210, 1989

21. Ramirez G, O'Neill WM, Bloomer HA, Jubiz W: Abnormalities in the regulation of growth hormone in chronic renal failure. *Arch Intern Med* 138: 267, 1978

22. Phillips LS, Kopple JD: Circulating somatomedin activity and sulfate levels in adults with normal and impaired kidney function. *Metabolism* 30: 1091, 1981

23. Fine RN: Growth hormone and the kidney: the use of recombinant human growth hormone (rhGH) in growth-retarded children with chronic renal insufficiency. *J Am Soc Nephrol* 1: 1136, 1991

24. DeFronzo RA, Andres R, Edgar P, Walker WG: Carbohydrate metabolism in uremia: A review. *Medicine* 52: 469, 1973

25. DeFronzo RA: Pathogenesis of glucose intolerance in uremia. *Metabolism* 27 (Suppl 2): 1866, 1978

26. Kuku SF, Jaspan JB, Emmanouel DS et al.: Heterogeneity of plasma glucagon. Circulating components in normal subjects and patients with chronic renal failure. *J Clin Invest* 58: 742, 1976

27. Bilbrey GL, Faloona GR, White MG, Knochel JP: Hyperglucogonemia of renal failure. *J Clin Invest* 53: 841, 1974

28. Rabu M, Dor J, Adar R et al.: Spontaneous hypoglycemia in a diabetic patient with renal failure. *Isr J Med Sci* 9: 1036, 1973

29. Block MB, Rubenstein AH: Spontaneous hypoglycemia in diabetic paitents with renal insufficiency. *JAMA* 213: 1863, 1970

30. Nolan GE, Smith JB, Chavre VJ, Jubiz W: Spurious overestimation of plasma cortisol in patients with chronic renal failure. *J Clin Endocrinol Metab* 52: 1242, 1981

31. Rosman PM, Farag A, Peckham R et al.: Pituitary-adrenocortical function in chronic renal failure: blunted suppression and early escape of plasma cortisol levels after intravenous dexamethasone. *J Clin Endocrinol Metab* 54: 528, 1982

32. Campese VM, Romoff MS, Levitan D et al.: Mechanism of autonomic nervous system dysfunction in uremia. *Kidney Int* 20: 246, 1981

33. Weidmann P, Horton R, Maxwell MH et al.: Dynamic studies of aldosterone in anephric man. *Kidney Int* 4: 289, 1973

NEUROLOGICAL ASPECTS OF DIALYSIS PATIENTS

GÉRARD SAID

INTRODUCTION

This chapter is an update of the excellent one written by Jennekens and Jennekens-Schinkel in the previous edition of this textbook. Although there has been no breakthrough in the understanding of the neurological problems occurring in dialysis patients, the management of neurological patients has changed during the past few years, making it necessary to revise this chapter. Neurological complications in dialysis patients are common and diverse. Some relate to persistence of mild uraemia others complicate the dialysis procedure. A number of neurological disorders occur with relatively high frequency in patients requiring this form of therapy but do not relate to uraemia nor to the methods used for treatment.

CEREBRAL DISORDERS

Uraemic encephalopathy

The clinical syndrome of uraemic encephalopathy is presently observed only rarely on the hospital wards, owing to the efficiency of dialysis therapy. When dialysis treatment is not initiated early enough, the signs and symptoms of uraemic encephalopathy may remain subclinical for a long time provided that (a) renal function decreases gradually, (b) water and electrolyte imbalance is maintained, (c) blood pressure is kept within reasonable limits, (d) adequate food intake with protein restriction is observed, and (e) iatrogenic intoxication is avoided. In some patients, however, renal insufficiency progresses rapidly and the course of the disease is complicated by unexpected or unavoidable factors. Encephalopathy in these patients is not necessarily due to uraemic intoxication *per se* but to one or several other, often treatable conditions. It is often difficult to decide which manifestations result from uraemia and which from complicating disorders.

Clinical picture

The two main kinds of neurological changes to be distinguished in uraemic patients are those concerning complex mental functions and level of consciousness on the one hand and motor disturbances on the other hand. The initial neuropsychological changes involve decrease in alertness and attention span, inability to sustain attention and to concentrate on the tasks. Patients become irritable or apathic and incapable of performing their daily work. When the situation worsens, the sensorium becomes clouded and disoriented. Patients may be frightened and confused, and a delirious condition may develop. Often this can be attributed, however to concomitant disturbances of electrolyte and water homeostasis. In the final stage, patients hardly react and become comatose (1). The initial motor abnormality is *tremulousness*. This tremor is irregular in amplitude and has a frequency of 8 to 10/sec. It is only apparent during limb movements. The pathophysiology of this tremor is unknown. The second motor abnormality is called *asterixis* or flapping tremor. This phenomenon is not specific for uraemia but is also seen in other metabolic encephalopathies and occasionally in patients with focal brain lesions. Asterixis is caused by the inability to maintain a sustained position. When the hands are kept extended (or the feet dorsiflexed) a sudden interruption lasting only a few moments occurs, causing a downward flap. On electromyographic examination during this interruption there is electrical silence in the muscles involved which implies that the downward flap has to be attributed to a brief interruption of innervation (2). Malfunction of a hypothetical system concerned with maintenance of tonic postural contraction of muscle has been suggested as being responsible for the interruption (3). Bilateral and unilateral asterixis have been reported in patients with lesions in the pons, mesencephalon, thalamus and parietal lobe (4–8). *Myoclonus* is a third type of involuntary movement which develops in a late phase of uraemic encephalopathy. The term is used for twitching occurring irregularly and asymmetrically in the limbs, trunk and head. At rest the muscle contractions are slight (fascicular) and cause only fine movements or none at all. During passive or active movements or both and sometimes in response to sensory stimuli the contractions become stronger and are better described as jerks. In occasional patients the movements may even appear as ballistic. There are no concomitant specific EEG abnormalities. Patients in this condition have a clouded sensorium and are often stuporous. The jerks disappear after intravenous administration of clonazepam (0.75 to 1 mg in adults). Chadwick and French (9) called attention to the fact that uraemic myoclonus as described here resembles action (or intention) myoclonus and myoclonus in postanoxic encephalopathy. It has been suggested that this form of myoclonus is mediated by a spino-bulbarspinal reflex which is normally inhibited. The same authors point out that there is experimental evidence indicating that such myoclonus is caused by a functional disturbance of the reticular formation in the lower brainstem.

Generalized tonic and clonic convulsions are regularly seen in acute or advanced chronic renal failure. They are often indicative of non-uraemic complications as discussed later. In case of localized convulsions. focal brain lesions have to be considered. In the final stage patients are often mute and may be catatonic (10). The tendon reflexes may be brisk but in the terminal phase are often diminished.

Laboratory investigations and pathology

The cerebrospinal fluid (CSF) pressure is normal and the CSF protein content is often only slightly elevated. The CSF urea concentration is similar to that in serum. Pleocytosis has been reported previously but not in more recent publications (11–14). Electroencephalographic (EEG) changes develop concurrently with the clinical disorder and include disorganisation, slowing and loss of alpha frequency, diffuse slow wave bursts and specific paroxysmal discharges (15, 16). Visual and auditory evoked cortical responses are abnormal, that is response latencies are increased and peak amplitudes decreased (17–19). The classical study by Olsen (20) did not detect specific structural changes within the brain by light microscopy.

Effect of dialysis; pathophysiology and pathogenesis
Little is definitely established about the pathophysiology and pathogenesis of uraemic encephalopathy. Several hypotheses have been introduced and rejected; others are being evaluated. Whatever the pathogenesis, the lesion(s) is (are) obviously rapidly reversible and, therefore, to a large extent functional and not structural. In this respect, the reaction to dialysis treatment and renal transplantation is instructive. Even when the clinical manifestations are severe, the whole syndrome clears up within days or weeks after the onset of adequate dialysis treatment. An equally rapid improvement of EEG abnormalities occurs (21, 22). Increase of dialysis frequency from two to three times weekly is reflected in further improvement of the EEG frequencies. Mild slowing of EEG waves which has been present for many months during dialysis treatment may return to normal within 2 weeks following restoration of renal function by successful kidney transplantation (22).

Brain metabolism has been shown to be reduced in uraemia (23, 24) and oxygen utilisation is depressed. These changes may result from uraemic toxins, either by effects on neurotransmission (25) or by inhibition of enzyme activities. Activity of Na+-K+-ATPase in brain tissue of uraemic rats and activity of the Nat-K+-ATPase pump in brain synaptosomes of uraemic rats is decreased (26, 27). Inhibition of many other cerebral enzymes by constituents of uraemic dialysates has been demonstrated (28). The nature of the uraemic toxin(s) is still a matter of dispute. The available evidence points to effects of many toxic substances, i.e., calcium and perhaps sodium, some amino acids, other small molecules. Middle sized molecules and hormones produced in excess (29). A case has been made for parathyroid hormone (PTH) as one of the major uraemic toxins (see (30) for review). Plasma PTH levels have been reported to be raised even within 48 h of the onset of acute renal failure (31). PTH may affect cell processes in various ways. It increases calcium content of the brain and of other tissues. Intracellular calcium concentration affects regulation of many metabolic and enzymatic processes within the cell. Experimental investigations have demonstrated Ca++ accumulation in brain synaptosomes from uraemic rats and an effect of PTH on this accumulation has been reported (32). Increase of brain calcium content in acute experimental uraemia is associated with slowing of EEG waves. Increase in calcium content and changes in EEG frequencies are prevented by parathyroidectomy before the induction of uraemia (30). Changes closely resembling those associated with increase of brain calcium content in acute uraemia, are provoked in normal laboratory animals by administration of parathyroid extract. Patients with elevated plasma PTH have indeed a raised calcium concentration of brain tissue (31, 33).

Encephalopathy due to electrolyte disturbances and acidosis

Sodium imbalance
Experimental investigations have shown that the brain is protected to some extent against osmolar shifts; slow osmolar changes are tolerated better than rapid shifts (34). Acute hypo-osmolality or hyponatraemia may cause brain oedema because osmolality of brain tissue remains high in comparison to plasma osmolality attracting extracellular water (35). Subacute or chronic experimental hyponatraemia causes only a mild increase in brain water content, the osmolality of brain and plasma remaining equal. The critical factor for encephalopathy is probably the accumulation of water in the cells in the brain (36). A rapid fall in the plasma sodium level in patients to less than 130 mmol/l may cause neurological changes whilst a slow decrease need not become apparent neurologically until values of 120 mmol/l have been reached. There are many causes of hypo-osmolality and hyponatraemia in patients with renal failure, e.g., congestive heart failure, the nephrotic syndrome, impaired water excretion, excessive water ingestion or dialysis. The manifestations are non-specific and include headache, nausea. vomiting, drowsiness, muscle cramps, restless legs, asterixis, confusion, delirium, stupor and coma. Convulsions, either generalised or focal, are common. The CSF pressure is elevated and papilloedema may develop. The CSF protein is usually within normal limits. Hypernatraemia and hyperosmolality cause brain shrinkage and are rare in patients with renal failure. They may occur accidentally during haemodialysis with high sodium dialysis fluid. Clinical manifestations include drowsiness, delirium, stupor or coma. Generalised or focal seizures and stroke-like motor deficits may occur.

Potassium imbalance
Potassium imbalance, either with hypo- or hyperkalaemia causes neuromuscular and cardiac changes. Experimental investigations have elucidated that the mechanisms for potassium homeostasis in the CNS are highly efficient. This probably explains why potassium imbalance causes no clearly recognisable clinical manifestations of brain dysfunction (37).

Metabolic acidosis
Changes in pH profoundly affect cellular metabolism and function. The brain is protected by several mechanisms against arterial pH changes (38). The acid-base balance in the brain is reflected in the pH of the CSF. The blood-CSF barrier offers little resistance against diffusion of CO_2 but is relatively impermeable to bicarbonate. The decrease in the plasma bicarbonate level in metabolic acidosis is not followed by a similar decrease in the CSF. The compensatory fall in PCO_2 of the blood occurs rapidly; however the final effect of these two events results in a relatively stable CSF pH which initially even may show a temporary rise.

Correction of metabolic acidosis by intravenous administration of sodium bicarbonate solution is followed by a rise of PCO_2 in blood and CSF. The rise of CSF bicarbonate is much slower however, causing a decrease of CSF pH which induces deterioration of brain function.

Chronic metabolic acidosis in advanced chronic renal failure resulting from retention of non-volatile acids does not cause clinically manifest effects on the central nervous system functions. Rapidly developing severe metabolic acidosis, as occurs in acute renal failure, causes hyperventilation and substantial loss of CO_2 from the blood and the CSF. This is likely to be one of the factors causing confusion, stupor and eventually coma. Uraemic patients with convulsions are usually moderately or severely acidotic (39).

Calcium imbalance
Calcium ions play important roles in numerous cellular processes. It is therefore, not surprising that calcium imbalance results in functional disturbances of many organ systems including the nervous system. Experimental evidence shows that the CSF calcium concentration remains relatively constant during alterations in plasma calcium concentration (40, 41). The homeostatic mechanisms involved, however, do not offer absolute protection. Following experimental parathyroidectomy CSF calcium concentration decreases over a period of several weeks. It is therefore likely that brief changes in plasma calcium concentration induce only slight responses in CSF calcium concentration. An exchange between CSF and brain calcium has been demonstrated.

The total plasma calcium level in renal failure is characteristically depressed. Both the protein bound fraction and the ultrafiltrable portion decrease. Peripheral nervous system (CNS) manifestations of hypocalcaemia present as tetany. Due to the protective action of the blood-brain barrier the CNS is, in general, less sensitive to hypocalcaemia than the PNS. The main signs of the CNS dysfunction are generalised or focal seizures and mental changes: PNS manifestations include paraesthesiae, muscle cramps, carpopedal spasms and laryngeal stridor. Trousseau's sign (carpal spasm within 3 min following inflation of a blood pressure cuff around the upper arm to above the systolic pressure) and the Chvostek's sign (tapping on the facial nerve just in front of the ear elicits visible contractions in the facial musculature innervated by this nerve) may be positive. CNS manifestations of hypocalcaemia in uraemic patients are relatively small because the PTH levels are elevated and the calcium concentration in the brain is high (31, 33). Signs of peripheral nerve hyperexcitability are also observed only rarely, possibly because hypocalcaemia develops insidiously and peripheral nerve calcium concentrations remain relatively high.

Regardless of the cause, hypercalcaemic patients may present with evidence of encephalopathy such as impaired intellectual functioning, lethargy, confusion, hallucinations, delirium, stupor and coma (41, 42). Hypercalcaemia causes EEG changes strongly resembling those found in other metabolic encephalopathies. Inappropriately high dialysis fluid calcium concentrations have been reported to cause hypercalcaemia in patients on maintenance dialysis (43). In addition to the changes already mentioned, these patients also developed dysarthria, myoclonic jerks and seizures.

Magnesium imbalance

Plasma magnesium levels are raised in severe chronic renal failure, usually without inducing any neurological manifestations (39, 44), but when magnesium levels reach two or three times normal values drowsiness may develop. Levels of this magnitude may occur by excessive magnesium administration to patients with renal failure (44). Hypermagnesaemia affects the neuromuscular junction by inhibiting acetylcholine release (39).

Disequilibrium syndrome

Manifestations of neurological dysfunction may become apparent during the course of a dialysis treatment, usually during its last hour or shortly thereafter (34, 45). Mild symptoms such as headache, nausea and muscle cramps occur in many patients. More severe manifestations such as restlessness, confusion and generalised convulsions tend to develop during rapid dialysis, often in the early stages of the dialysis procedure. With the exception of the muscle cramps, the syndrome was originally attributed to a rapid decrease of plasma urea concentration, leaving the brain with a relatively high urea concentration. This osmotic gradient causes a shift of water into the brain inducing cerebral oedema and brain swelling. Results of animal investigations however, did not support the hypothesis that the osmotic gradient had to be attributed to urea or electrolytes (46, 47). Subsequently, the syndrome was considered to result from an osmotic gradient of unidentified, osmotically active agents and to lowering of the pH of the CSF and the brain cell water (48). It was shown that during rapid dialysis of uraemic dogs the arterial pH rose slightly, whereas a fall was registered in brain and CSF pH. It has been suggested that organic acids accumulating during dialysis cause the decline in pH. These substances might be sufficiently osmotically active to cause brain swelling. Prevention is possible by gradual correction of uraemia, particularly when initial blood urea concentrations are high. Intravenous use of osmotic agents such as glycerol can reduce the osmolar shift and may prevent neurological manifestations (49).

Intracranial neurological disorders tend to worsen during dialysis. When a presumed disequilibrium syndrome occurs in a patient fully adapted to a dialysis programme, a complicating intracranial disorder or errors in the composition of the dialysis fluid should be considered. La Greca et al. (50) measured the brain density on CT scans and found that uraemic individuals showed a consistent reduction in density during dialysis without change in brain volume.

Aluminium encephalopathy

Neurological manifestations associated with serum aluminium levels higher than 50 μg/l include speech disturbance, a mixture of dysarthria and non-fluent aphasia, wordfinding problems and dysgraphia. Behaviour and intellectual changes include apathy, depression, personality change, disorientation, apraxia and dyscalculia. The disorder may progress to a full picture of dementia associated with ataxia and myoclonus. Involuntary movements may be induced by sound, light or startle, or by movement (action myoclonus). Generalized seizures occur in about 60% of the patients, usually in the advanced phase of the disease (51).

EEG recording show paroxysmal bursts of irregular, generalised spike and wave activity (52). Evidence for an aluminium intoxication as a cause of this type of encephalopathy is provided by increased contents of aluminium in different organs, compared with uraemics controls. Also epidemics of encephalopathy occurred in regions with elevated aluminium concentration in the water supply and in dialysis units where there were failures in the dialysate purification systems (53). Although the role of aluminium is clear in many cases, there are some patients with similar patterns of dialysis encephalopathy without elevated serum aluminium level.

It is mandatory to routinely monitor aluminium levels in both haemodialysate and peritoneal dialysate. Values greater than 10 μg/l should prompt a full investigation of the purification system in the dialysis unit (51). The first step of treatment of established aluminium encephalopathy is to remove sources of aluminium such as oral phosphate binders containing aluminium such as aluminium hydroxide and to ensure that the dialysate is free of aluminium. Symptomatic treatment includes treatment of myoclonus with benzodiazepines, and of seizures by antiepileptic drugs.

Wernicke's encephalopathy and drug induced encephalopathy

A Wernicke's encephalopathy may develop after frequent vomiting in uraemic patients with restricted food intake (54). This syndrome is characterised by ataxia, changes in ocular motility and confusion. The ocular manifestations include nystagmus, abducens palsy or palsy of conjugate gaze. Ocular disturbances are almost a prerequisite for this diagnosis (55). Wernicke's encephalopathy is cured by early treatment with thiamine. If treatment with thiamine is not given early enough, Korsakoff's psychosis may remain as a permanent sequella, with characteristic defect in memorisation, resulting in disorientation with confabulation. Korsakoff's syndrome does not respond to thiamine.

Administration of drugs normally excreted by the kidneys, may cause neurotoxic effects in patients with renal failure. Penicillin is a well known example (56). In high doses it may cause myoclonus, hyperreflexia and coma. Cefazolin-induced encephalopathy in uraemia has been reported more recently (57).

Cerebrovascular disorders in dialysis patients

In the early 1970s reports of causes of death in patients treated with maintenance dialysis showed a high prevalence of vascular disorders. in particular ischaemic heart disease and cerebrovascular accidents (58, 59). It was suggested that the life span of dialysed patients was limited by accelerated atherosclerosis (58). Continued investigations raised doubt about this pessimistic view. It was argued that insufficient allowance had been made for pre-existing morbid conditions (60, 61). When patients known to have diabetes mellitus, atherosclerosis or a long history of hypertension prior to initiation of maintenance dialysis were excluded, and the age factor was sufficiently accounted for, the death rate due to atherosclerotic vascular diseases in dialysed patients was not significantly higher than in matched control populations. The accelerated atherosclerosis hypothesis remains unproved (62).

Cerebral lesions resulting from vascular disorders can be divided into two categories. The first category consists of diffuse or multifocal lesions or encephalopathies and the second comprises focal lesions. Among the diffuse lesions hypertensive encephalopathy is most frequent. Binswanger's encephalopathy may be present in an occasional patient.

Hypertensive encephalopathy

Hypertensive encephalopathy is related to a sudden rise in blood pressure to severely high levels. Hypertension may be of primary or secondary origin; renal lesions are commonly present. The association of hypertensive encephalopathy with other conditions is well documented. Eclampsia is a special form of hypertensive encephalopathy. Usually following an asymptomatic phase with moderate hypertension and proteinuria, patients develop an extremely high blood pressure (such as 250/150 mmHg) and neurological and ophthalmologic changes appear (63, 64) including severe headache with nausea and vomiting, drowsiness. confusion or agitation. Patients may have generalised or focal convulsions and an occasional patient

may display neck stiffness. Some patients present evidence of persistent focal neurological lesions but these do not belong to the basic manifestations of the syndrome. Such lesions result from vascular damage and are due to haemorrhage or thrombosis. Ophthalmologic investigation reveals papilloedema, retinal arteriolar abnormalities, 'cottonwool exudates' consisting of bundles of swollen axons (presumably resulting from ischaemia) and flame-shaped haemorrhages localised in the nerve fibre layer of the retina. The CSF pressure is raised and there may be a moderate rise in the CSF protein content. Lumbar puncture should however be avoided. Computed tomography (CT) scan of the brain, without contrast enhancement, often reveals brain swelling, with small ventricles and hyperlucency of the white matter. Magnetic resonance imaging of the brain can show periventricular areas of increased signals on T2 weighted images. If antihypertensive therapy is successful, the whole syndrome reverses rapidly with clearing of most manifestations, except for the focal changes. Anti-oedema therapy is often necessary in the acute phase.

The results of neuropathological investigations are of great interest. Apart from cerebral oedema and other changes present in brains from patients with and without malignant hypertension. three characteristic abnormalities are observed: (a) fibrinoid necrosis in the walls of intracerebral arterioles and small arteries. sometimes associated with fibrin thrombi, occluding the lumina and with extravascular deposits of fibrin, (b) focal or segmental changes in the walls of arterioles and small arteries consisting of fibrous thickening and hyalinisation and sometimes occlusion of the lumina. Because the clinical syndrome is entirely reversible, it is attributed by most authors to cerebral oedema, vasospasms and segmental dilatation of vessel walls. The latter are thought to be localised in parts of the vessels where muscular contractility of the wall has been surmounted by high intraluminar pressures (65). Changes in wall permeability of penetrating arterioles have been demonstrated rapidly after the onset of acute blood pressure elevation. For unknown reasons small arteries and arterioles penetrating into the brain seem particularly liable to permeability changes at the level of the second and third cortical cell layers (66).

The predilection for changes in small vessels may be explained by the role these vessels have in auto-regulation of cerebral blood flow. A rise in blood pressure is immediately followed by an increase in cerebrovascular resistance localised mainly in the intracerebral small arteries. A breakdown of this auto-regulatory system occurring during hypertensive episodes causes segmental dilatation of small vessels at sites where muscular contractility cannot withstand intra-arterial blood pressure.

Binswanger's encephalopathy (subcortical arteriosclerotic encephalopathy) SAE

Interest in this type of vascular encephalopathy has been recently revived by reports of diagnostically characteristic computerised tomographic (CT) scan appearances (67, 68).

The SAE syndrome may develop in patients with a long history of hypertension or other disorders predisposing to vascular damage, e.g., diabetes mellitus (69–74). At middle age or in early senescence a slowly progressive dementia develops. There is loss of spontaneity, with sluggishness and perseveration. Focal neurological manifestations including aphasia, unilateral neglect or visual defects are often associated with loss of memory. At the same time, neurological manifestations of motor and sensory dysfunctions become apparent, with difficulty in swallowing, walking and dysarthria. Some of these may be due to minor strokes but more often the neurological defects develop gradually over weeks or months. Periods of progression alternate with periods of stabilisation or improvement lasting for months or years.

CSF pressure remains normal: the protein content is slightly elevated in some patients. CT scans show diffuse low attenuation in the white matter. Neuropathological investigations reveal diffuse and focal loss of brain with gliosis in the subcortical areas. Lacunes are often present in the basal ganglia, thalamus and pons (74). The white matter loss has been attributed to ischaemia and oedema. The preferential localisation of the changes in the subcortical regions is unexplained. There is no essential difference between Bingswanger's encephalopathy and multi-infarct dementia.

Transient ischaemic attacks (TIA)

Transient ischaemic attacks (TIAs) are defined as temporary focal cerebral deficits, presumably related to ischaemia, lasting less than 24 h. TIAs are often associated with stenosis of extra- or intracranial arteries, they are predictors of cerebral infarcts and also of myocardial infarction (76–79). Thirty to 50% of patients with carotid territory TIAs have carotid occlusive disease. Carotid stroke from extracranial carotid occlusion is preceded in up to 50 to 70% by TIAs (80). TIAs may last a few seconds to several hours. Some patients have many attacks of exactly the same character, in others a stroke may follow the first TIA within days. Emboli consisting of fibrin platelet material from atherosclerotic sites are considered to be the cause for most TIAs. Diagnosis is not always easy as TIAs may be mimicked by many other disorders including focal epilepsy, syncope, Stokes Adams attacks, migraine and vertigo. The clinical manifestations of the attack depend on which artery is involved. Carotid territory produce contralateral weakness and paraesthesiae and ipsilateral visual disturbances. There may be aphasia when the hemisphere dominant for speech is involved. The visual disturbances are characterised by unilateral visual transient loss or blurring of the upper or lower half of one visual field (amaurosis fugax). Homonymous hemianopia may occur in TIAs of the vertebrobasilar system. Strongly indicative for the latter are also diplopia or dysarthria

and weakness or numbness on one or both sides of the body.

Cerebral infarcts

Although a thrombotic stroke may present as a single sudden attack, a gradual or a stuttering progressive course during several hours or days is not uncommon and this course is diagnostically helpful. The onset or progression occurs commonly during sleep or shortly after awakening.

The neurological picture is determined by the size and location of the infarct. When infarcts are large cerebral oedema may develop which may be life-threatening. Magnetic resonance imaging demonstrates the ischaemic zone within hours after stroke, CT scanning within days. Early CT scan shows slight hypodensity associated with increased blood brain barrier permeability and contrast enhancement. The main advantage of CT scan at that stage is to show absence of spontaneous hyperdensity characteristic of intracranial bleeding. Thus early scans must always be performed without contrast enhancement and, if necessary after iv injection of contrast medium.

In *cerebral embolism* the embolic material is derived commonly from a thrombus or an ulcerated atheromatous plaque in a carotid artery. The neurological defect appears suddenly, in a single attack. The brain region most commonly involved is the territory of the middle cerebral artery. A minority of the infarcts are haemorrhagic. The blood may reach the CSF but this is not usually the case. CT scans can demonstrate haemorrhagic infarcts. Cerebellar infarcts may justify surgical decompression because of the mass effect on the brainstem.

Treatment of TIAs and infarcts

The aim of treatment is to prevent infarct or further infarcts. Patients with TIAs or thrombotic infarcts are treated with drugs that prevent clotting and reduce the tendency of platelets to aggregate. The infarct preventing effect of aspirin in such patients has been demonstrated (79); the optimal daily dose has, however, not yet been established. Low doses, 100 mg per day or less, seem sufficient.

In patients with embolic infarcts the aim of treatment is to prevent further emboli. The heart is the main source of cerebral emboli and the most common cause is atrial fibrillation. Anticoagulants are effective in preventing embolism from heart disease (81), but anticoagulant therapy should be delayed for several days if the infarct is haemorrhagic. A CT must be performed before starting anticoagulation, to exclude intracerebral bleeding.

Intracerebral haemorrhage and subdural haematoma

The two main causes of non-traumatic intracranial haemorrhage are hypertension and anticoagulant therapy (82).

Many dialysis patients have a long history of hypertension and periods of hypertension are not uncommon during maintenance dialysis. Administration of heparin is necessary to carry out extracorporeal circulation and some patients are treated with warfarin or antiplatelet agents to maintain angio-access patency. Hence, cerebral haemorrhage is a risk in patients treated with regular dialysis.

Intracerebral hypertensive haemorrhages occur by ruptures of small penetrating arteries or arterioles with fibrinoid degeneration and microaneurysms. Extravasated blood forms an oval or roughly circular mass displacing and compressing adjacent brain tissue. Large haemorrhages may displace midline structures and vital centres may become compromised. Rupture or leakage through the cortical surface or into the ventricular system are common. The clinical picture is characterized by an abrupt onset and gradual or rapid evolution. CT scans accurately define and localise haemorrhages of 1.5 cm in diameter or larger, at least during the first 2 or 3 weeks after the onset (83). During these weeks the X-ray absorption coefficient of the haematoma decreases and a phase will be entered in which the density is equal to that of the surrounding brain substance. If CT scanning is not possible. examination of the CSF is necessary for diagnosis, but should be discouraged when signs of intracranial hypertension are present because of the increased risk of transtentorial herniation after CSF withdrawal. Usually the CSF will be bloody or xanthochromic. Apart from general medical care and antioedema treatment therapeutic possibilities are few. Surgical drainage of a large intracerebral supratentorial haematoma is usually considered futile in the acute phase. In acute or subacute cerebellar haemorrhages surgical drainage is the treatment of choice when the haematoma is large (more than 3 cm) and brainstem dysfunction is not yet severe and has lasted 12 h or less (84, 85). In general the prognosis is poor in patients with large haemorrhages. When the haematoma is small, restitution of function is often better than in patients with ischaemic infarcts, because the brain tissue is often more displaced than destroyed by the haematoma. Cerebellar infarcts can also induce intracranial hypertension requiring surgical drainage of the CSF.

Intracranial haemorrhages occurring during anticoagulant therapy are infrequent. They are usually localised in the subdural space (85–87). Subacute or chronic subdural haematoma may cause pseudodementia, drowsiness, confusion and mild hemiparesis. When the possibility of a haematoma in this location is considered, confirmation of the diagnosis is usually easy. The haematoma or hygroma may be visualised by CT scanning or arteriography. Exceptionally, an epidural haematoma causing spinal cord compression with bilateral weakness of the legs and loss of sensibility in the lower limbs may occur in patients on anticoagulant therapy.

Central nervous system infections

Infections are frequent complications in dialysis patients (see Chapter 41). Among these, intracranial infections are rare, but often life-threatening (88, 89). Intracranial infections may develop insidiously and patients may have few clinical symptoms. In patients with unusually severe headaches, meningitis should be considered. Signs of meningeal irritation (cervical rigidity and positive Kernig's sign) should be sought and the cerebrospinal fluid should be examined. CT scanning is of great value in the diagnosis of brain abscesses. The presence of sources for a direct spread of infection to the meninges, particularly mastoiditis and infection of nasal air sinuses should be ruled out. Uncommon types of infections such as cryptococcosis and cytomegalic virus infections have been reported in patients treated with immunosuppressive drugs.

Management of epilepsy

Renal failure may influence the response to anticonvulsants by altering the distribution, metabolism and clearance of the drugs. In patients with renal insufficiency the plasma protein binding of acidic drugs is decreased, whilst for basic drugs it is normal or decreased (87). The diminished protein binding is not, or only partly, due to decreased plasma protein concentrations. Several hypotheses have been put forward to explain this change in binding capacity of proteins. Either the binding capacity is inhibited competitively by uraemic toxins, or it is decreased by changes in properties of the proteins. The first hypothesis is the more likely since the impaired protein binding is reversible. It may be caused by organic acids known to be retained in renal insufficiency (90).

So far studies of anticonvulsants in uraemic patients have been limited mainly to phenytoin and valproic acid. It has been demonstrated that steady state total plasma concentrations of these drugs were lower in uraemic than in non-uraemic patients (92, 93). Due to decreased protein binding, however the free concentrations were relatively high. A further decrease in protein binding of valproic acid was observed during haemodialysis. This is possibly related to the administration of heparin which activates lipoprotein lipase (93). As a result the plasma level of non-esterified fatty acids increases and these compounds probably compete for binding sites with valproic acid.

Data presently available support the concept that no change in phenytoin and valproic acid dosages is required to treat epilepsy in uraemic patients. The lower steady state concentrations are compensated by higher free concentrations. Clinical experience conforms with this concept.

PERIPHERAL NEUROPATHIES

Uraemic polyneuropathy

Polyneuropathy is one of the principal and most frequent manifestations in chronic uraemia. At one time it was considered to be a potentially crippling disorder of patients on dialysis programmes, but it is now thought to be a calculable risk which can usually be prevented by early initiation of regular dialysis treatment. In a few patients, however, it may still cause serious problems.

Clinical features

The incidence of clinical polyneuropathy varies considerably from series to series, from 10 to 83% (51). This important range in the incidence of uraemic neuropathy is mainly due to the difficulty to agree on strict criteria for neuropathy. If minor electrophysiological abnormalities are taken into account, nearly all patients under dialysis treatment for chronic renal failure have some degree of alteration of nerve function, but the subtle abnormalities of nerve conduction velocity detected in nearly all patients under dialysis are not predictive of the occurrence of a symptomatic neuropathy, which affects approximately 10% of dialysis patients. In virtually every series males developed neuropathies several times more frequently than females.

Severity and progression of dialysis polyneuropathy are extremely variable. In most instances, both worsening and improvement evolve slowly over months, but on occasion neuropathy is fulminent in its course. Patients were reported in whom severe fulminant motor neuropathy occurred in the setting of sepsis and severe chronic renal failure, probably due to superimposed critical illness type of axonal polyneuropathy (95). Patients with rapidly evolving severe polyneuropathy but without sepsis are also reported (see review in (96, 97)).

Peripheral neuropathy is heralded by symptoms of dysfunction of lower motor neurones (LMN) or of primary sensory neurones. Whether or not muscle cramps in renal failure patients belong to this category is debated (94). Muscle cramps are recognised as early manifestations of LMN involvement in motor neurone disease (98) and many other neuropathies. They occur before the neurones have ceased to function, that is before muscle weakness occurs. Patients usually experience the cramps in the evening or late at night. The cramps are enhanced by preceding muscular exertion. Muscle cramps in chronic uraemia occur in a similar fashion. In favour of a relation with neuropathy is that the cramps occur predominantly in distal lower limb muscles. The nerve fibres innervating these muscles are the first to develop pathological changes.

The *restless legs syndrome* has been considered by some to be another symptom of peripheral neuronal dysfunction in uraemic patients (99). In the evening or when in bed, patients sense discomfort in the legs and feet and an urge to move the legs and to walk around. The syndrome has usually disappeared when clinical signs of neuropathy become apparent. The restless legs syndrome is, however. not a feature of lower motor diseases and is absent in most other peripheral neuropathies. It responds favourably to clonazepam (0.5 mg at bedtime) in a similar way as action or intention myoclonus does. It is considered by some to be of central origin (100).

When patients complain of paraesthesia (tingling or prickling) in the toes, feet or fingers, clinical signs of uraemic neuropathy are usually present and may even be severe (96). Burning feet occur only in a minority of patients (96). Pain is absent in the early stages of neuropathy but may be prominent in advanced and severe neuropathy (96, 101, 102). Depressed or abolished ankle reflexes and impaired vibration perception of the halluces are early and initially the only clinical signs of peripheral neuropathy (97). It is our experience that perception of light touch over distal lower limbs is affected first. In a minority of patients neuropathy progresses further. Atrophy and weakness of distal leg muscles may develop as well as disturbance of all sensory modalities in a stocking-like distribution. Clinical signs of neuropathy in the upper limbs occur only in severe cases, event though alterations of conduction velocity are present in all four limbs.

Although manifestations of *autonomic neuropathy* remain subclinical, laboratory investigations have shown that autonomic dysfunction is commonly present (96, 105–111). Some evidence indicates that reflexes involving thin unmyelinated nerve fibres are less impaired than those of myelinated nerve fibres in the parasympathetic vagal nerve. Whether the fall in blood pressure during haemodialysis can be ascribed to autonomic neuropathy is as yet undecided. The relation between somatic and autonomic neuropathy is weak.

In chronic uraemia increased susceptibility of peripheral nerves to pressure has not been demonstrated. Children with end-stage renal failure usually present no clinical evidence of peripheral neuropathy (112, 113).

Nerve conduction and quantitation of sensory loss

Electrophysiological investigations of patients with chronic uraemia have demonstrated slowing of conduction in all peripheral nerves studied (113, 114). Slowing occurs to almost the same degree in motor and sensory nerve fibres, in nerves of upper and lower limbs and in proximal and distal parts of limb nerves (115). In the most severe cases conduction may fall to 60 or 50% of the normal values. According to Nielsen (114) there is no critical degree of slowing of conduction indicating whether clinical signs of neuropathy will appear. Measurement of light touch and of vibratory perception thresholds is more suitable to evaluate progression or recovery of uraemic neuropathy than is measurement of nerve conduction velocity (97, 101). In a minority of the patients thermal sensitivity decreases before other sensory and motor functions are affected (116).

It important to consider the changes in the amplitude of the muscle response and of the sensory nerve action potentials because they reflect the number of functional axons in the nerve under study, while conduction velocity depends on the myelination of nerve fibres and on the density of larger myelinated fibres. It is thus not easy to interpret mild changes in nerve conduction velocity, especially when associated with loss of large myelinated fibres, which is the most constant morphological feature in uraemic neuropathy. It is our opinion that periodic electrophysiological studies are not necessary for monitoring dialysis. Indication of electrophysiological studies should be limited to patients who manifest symptoms of neuropathy, and include studies of nerve conduction velocity as well as of the amplitude of nerve action potentials. Important decrease of the sensory action potential means that the patient has lost a significant proportion of large myelinated fibres in the nerve studied.

The study of late responses, which are a sensitive measure of an electrodiagnostic abnormality, do not have a proven advantage as a serial measure (95).

Neuropathy and the degree of renal insufficiency

Manifestations of peripheral neuropathy are part of the terminal uraemic syndrome. In patients regularly controlled in outpatient departments, signs of neuropathy are generally lacking as long as the creatinine clearance exceeds 6 ml/min (94, 95). Exceptions to this rule occur, however. Septicaemia and catabolism may adversely affect the peripheral nerves and promote the development of neuropathy (117). In some patients the possibility of a preexisting or iatrogenic neuropathy should be considered. It is only in a minority of patients that a decrease of the creatinine clearance to less than 6 ml/min is accompanied by weakness of distal lower limb muscles and disturbance of sensation. In some this happens during a rapid exacerbation of chronic renal insufficiency. When it is possible to restore renal function to previous levels, the neuropathy persists and may now seem out of proportion to the degree of renal insufficiency (118).

Low protein, high calorie diet

Attempts have been made to prolong the non-dialysis period or the survival time of non-dialysable patients by prescribing low protein high calorie diets containing the minimal required amounts of essential amino acids. As far as neuropathy is concerned, a satisfactory result was claimed with a diet containing 15 to 20 g of protein and a supplement of essential amino acids and histidine (116, 117). Patients on these diets have a low plasma urea/creatinine ratio. It is conceivable that the toxin(s) inducing uraemic neuropathy accumulate(s) in the body fluids concomitantly with urea.

Effects of haemodialysis and continuous ambulatory peritoneal dialysis (CAPD)

In spite of variations in dialysis techniques and schedules there is general consensus as to the effect on peripheral neuropathy, adequate haemodialysis prevents deterioration of neuropathy and may even induce a slow improvement (96, 119, 120). Much less favourable is the effect on reduced nerve conduction velocities. Neuropathy usually creates no problem in patients on CAPD treatment. though worsening has been reported in individual cases (96, 120). On the basis of a careful study Tegner and Lindhohll (121) concluded that haemodialysis and CAPD did not result in differences in the 'clinical score' of their patients.

Of great interest are the changes in nerve function which are recorded after a single dialysis. Nerve conduction velocity is not influenced to a measurable extent (122) but the following occur: (a) a slight fall in the vibratory perception threshold (123), (b) an increase in the amplitude of nerve (and muscle) action potentials, (c) a change in resistance of the sensory action potential threshold to ischaemia (124), and (d) a decrease in the relative refractory period (125) which is lengthened in these patients. All these changes point to a reversal of functional membrane abnormalities. According to current opinion. serial measurements of nerve conduction velocity do not offer a reliable index for the adequacy of regular haemodialysis. If regular dialysis is obviously inadequate, as judged by the reappearance of uraemic symptoms, nerve conduction velocity does not necessarily worsen (126), because clinical manifestations are more closely related to loss of axons than to demyelination, and, as stated before, axon loss has much less influence on conduction velocity than loss of myelin. Serial determinations of clinical functions of large myelinated fibres, including study of vibratory perception thresholds and light touch sensation seem more suitable in detecting changes in nerve function than nerve conduction studies are.

The effect of transplantation

Successful kidney transplantation is followed by a two-phase course of recovery of neuropathy. The first phase is brief and begins within a few days after transplantation. Nerve conduction velocity increases and an amelioration of clinical signs rapidly becomes apparent (128–133). The second phase occurs slowly and lasts many months. Full clinical recovery is obtained in most patients and nerve conduction may attain normal levels, although persistence of some delay of conduction, particularly in lower limb nerves, is not unusual. Only in patients with very severe neuropathy do sequelae persist. There is no autonomic dysfunction in transplanted patients.

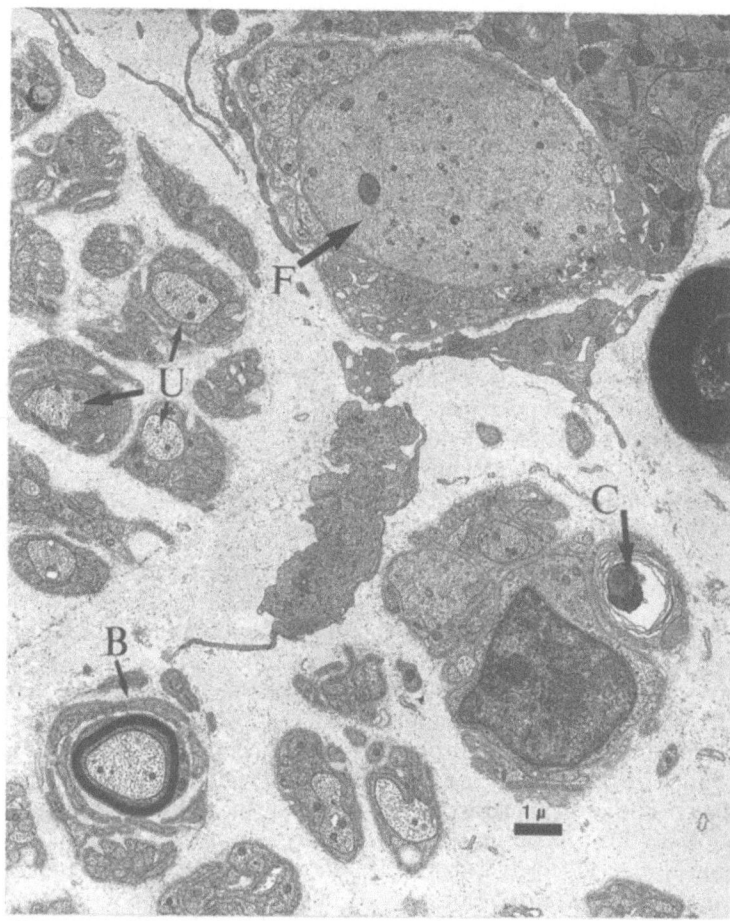

Figure 1. Electron micrograph of a nerve biopsy specimen from a patient with dialysis neuropathy. Note that the fibre F is a large, normally myelinated fibre, which is now demyelinated. B denotes a small myelinated fibre surrounded by a normal myelin sheath and several layers of Schwann cell processes forming onion bulb, often a sign of repeated demyelination and remyelination. In C there is a myelin and axonal debris of a fibre that has undergone axonal degeneration. Note that the unmyelinated fibres (U) are normal in aspect and density. Unmyelinated fibres convey pain sensation in peripheral nerves. Uranyl acetate and lead citrate.

Pathology and pathophysiology of uraemic polyneuropathy

Although much remains to be elucidated, studies of the pathology and pathophysiology of uraemic neuropathy have been informative and relevant to the whole of the uraemic syndrome and to disorders of the peripheral nervous system in general. Asbury et al. (134) and Forno and Alston (135) demonstrated that degeneration of nerve fibres in uraemic neuropathy was characterized by (a) structural impairment of axons and myelin sheaths and (b) demyelination of apparently unimpaired axons. These observations were confirmed by others (136, 137). It was accepted that demyelination was due to a metabolic disorder in the Schwann cells (138). It was also generally accepted that the slowing of nerve conduction could be explained by the demyelination (Figure 1). The classical concepts of the axon/Schwann cell relationships were questioned by Dyck and co-workers (139). However, they

suggested that demyelination in uraemic polyneuropathy should be considered as secondary to a primary axonal lesion. The main reason for this hypothesis was that demyelination did not occur at random but clustered in selected bundles of fibres which frequently showed evidence of axonal degeneration. They reported similar findings in another type of neuropathy (Friedreich's ataxia) which was generally accepted as a primary neuronal disease. Electrophysiological findings agreed with the concept according to which uraemic neuropathy in dialysis patients was a primary axonal disorder with little tendency to regeneration (140). Another major breakthrough was initiated by observations of the recovery process following renal transplantation.

The rapid, but usually mild, increase in nerve conduction velocity within a few days after successful transplantation (131) can be explained by remyelination and but not by regeneration which is a much slower process. Some functional disturbances may be caused by circulating toxins. The observations on changes in nerve function after a single dialysis confirmed the role of functional lesions. Although dialysis has a favourable effect it had to be assumed that regular dialysis treatment does not completely remove these toxins. Functional alterations together with morphological changes are held responsible for the slowing of nerve conduction.

Uraemic neuropathy in diabetic patients

In diabetic patients with renal insufficiency under dialysis treatment, the occurrence of severe axonal, length dependent, sensory and motor polyneuropathy is common. In such patients it is virtually impossible to ascribe with certainty specific signs or symptoms to one or to the other metabolic disturbance. However, severe symptomatic autonomic disturbances, pains, length dependent pattern of loss of temperature and pain sensation which point to predominant involvement of small myelinated and unmyelinated fibres are more characteristic of diabetic neuropathy (140). Conversely prominent motor deficit is in favour of a predominant role of uraemia. This discussion is not only academic because after renal transplantation, only the peripheral deficit which is related to uraemia is expected to improve.

Pathogenesis

The aetiology of uraemic polyneuropathy is complex. At least three pathogenetic mechanisms must be distinguished: deficiency, intoxication and hormonal imbalance. We shall briefly summarise the current views.

1. Uraemic polyneuropathy is due to vitamin B deficiency

Bl deficiency is the vitamin deficiency most likely implicated in view of the similarity of the neuropathies in uraemia and in conditions of Bl shortage (142). Vitamin B1 deficiency in uraemic patients with chronic renal failure has not been established, and there is no substantial loss of thiamine during dialysis probably because of its binding to plasma proteins. Administration of vitamin Bl neither cures nor prevents uraemic neuropathy

2. Inhibition of enzyme activity by uraemic toxins causes polyneuropathy

Babb et al. (143) suggested that a number of uraemic toxins had molecular masses in the 'middle' molecule range (300 to 2000 Daltons). Middle molecules would be less efficiently removed with haemodialysis than small molecules and accumulate in the body fluids. This hypothesis was supported by the observation that uraemic polyneuropathy was rarely seen in patients on long-term peritoneal dialysis perhaps because the peritoneal membrane is more permeable for middle molecules. Although this theory is attractive, the search for neurotoxic middle molecules has been disappointing (144, 145), and the occurrence of neuropathy is not correlated with middle molecule plasma

levels (97). Experimental investigations have demonstrated neurotoxic effects of several smaller substances, such as methylguanidine and myoinositol. The main argument against a pathogenetic role of these compounds is the lack of correlation between the plasma levels and the severity of polyneuropathy (146, 147).

The search for enzymes inhibited in uraemia has not been without success. Transketolase is a thiamine-dependent enzyme with a role in the pentose phosphate pathway. This enzyme is present in Schwann cells and in the CNS. Sterzel et al. (148) reported an increase of transketolase activity in post-dialysis erythrocytes compared to predialysis erythrocytes and postulated that this was secondary to the removal of an unknown inhibiting toxin. These findings however were not confirmed by others (149). Dobbelstein et al. (150) reported excessive stimulation of erythrocyte glutamic oxalacetic transaminase by exogenous pyridoxal phosphate, This was interpreted as indicative of endogenous pyridoxal phosphate deficiency and was thought to be caused by inhibition of pyridoxal phosphate kinase. Clinical manifestations associated with pyridoxal phosphate deficiency are epilepsy and polyneuropathy.

Dialysable substances have been shown to inhibit ouabain sensitive, sodium stimulated, potassium dependent ATPase and inhibition of this enzyme has been demonstrated *in vivo* in uraemic rats (26). Inhibition of sodium transport across cell membranes results in slowing of conduction along these membranes. Renal transplantation is followed by a rapid increase in activity of this enzyme. Its inhibition may underlie the rapidly reversible component of decreased nerve conduction velocity (151). An interesting observation concerns the decrease of the specific sodium permeability of the nodal membrane in acute uraemia (152). It was suggested that this decrease might relate to elevated intracellular calcium or intra-axonal accumulation of cationic metabolites.

3. Raised PTH blood levels in uraemic patients may cause neuropathy (possibly by increase of the peripheral nerve calcium concentration

This theory is supported by the following observations: (a) increased calcium concentrations in peripheral nerves and slowing of nerve conduction have been observed in uraemic dogs. Parathyroidectomy before the induction of uraemia prevented these changes (153). (b) In comparison with dialysis patients with normal or slightly elevated PTH levels, patients with high PTH blood levels show decreased motor nerve conduction velocities (154). Arguments against the role of PTH, however, are that (a) no correlation has been established in dialysis patients between four different immunochemically defined forms of PTH and nerve conduction velocity (155), (b) motor nerve conduction velocity in dialysis patients is not improved by parathyroidectomy (156), (c) polyneuropathy or slowing of nerve conduction is not a feature of hyperparathyroidism (157).

Mononeuropathy

A carpal tunnel syndrome (CTS) is a frequent complication of long-term haemodialysis. Twenty to 50% of the patients dialysed for 10 years or longer are reported to have CTS (158). The symptoms of tingling dysesthesias in median nerve distribution in the hand, particularly nocturnally, are the same for uraemic and non-uraemic patients, but in those on chronic haemodialysis the symptoms frequently are most noticeable during the procedure of dialysis itself. Though CTS has been stated to occur most frequently in limbs with arteriovenous shunts or fistulae (159–162), it is often bilateral. Its pathogenesis is likely to be multifactorial. All factors causing CTS in the normal population are also present in dialysed patients. Vascular access may he an additional factor. It leads to venous hypertension and in some cases to a certain degree of oedema in lower arm tissues which may narrow the carpal tunnel. Ischaemia due to a vascular steal mechanism may play a role in occasional patients. Aetiologically probably most important, however, are deposits of amyloid in the tissue surrounding the carpal tunnel. Amyloidosis is a complication of long term haemodialysis. The precursor protein of this form of amyloid is β_2 microglobulin (163). The plasma levels of β_2 microglobulin are persistently raised not only in patients on maintenance dialysis but also in patients on CAPD treatment (164). Ulnar nerve palsies develop in occasional dialysis patients (165, 166). A relation with raised venous pressure, predisposing to nerve compression in narrow tunnels was suggested (167) before the discovery of amyloidosis in long term dialysis. Severe nerve lesions obviously due to ischaemia have been reported in patients with bovine graft fistulae in the upper arm between the brachial artery and the cephalic vein (168).

Management of carpal tunnel syndrome in chronic renal failure depends on a judgment as to its basis. In most cases, the median nerve will be compressed by amyloid deposition or by the same factors that occur in non-uraemic individuals. In this situation, which is by far the most common, management is surgically carpal tunnel release. Care must be taken to obtain biopsy specimens of the flexor retinaculum for amyloid studies. Occasionally, the carpal tunnel syndrome may be related to the presence of an arteriovenous fistula in the forearm and be ischemic in origin. The management here, if the situation warrants, is closure of the fistula (96).

SKELETAL MUSCLE DISEASE

There are at least two causes for muscle weakness in patients with chronic renal failure.

1. Muscle weakness due to wasting and malnutrition is not rare in uraemic patients (169, 170). Such weakness is located predominantly in the proximal muscles and other anterior compartment muscles of the lower limbs. The histopathology of this condition is characterised by type II atrophy identical to that observed in cachexia (169). Biochemical investigations have disclosed a decrease in the energy rich phosphagens ATP and phosphocreatinine in muscle from uraemic patients (171).

2. Muscle weakness may be related to secondary hyperparathyroidism. A causal relation between primary hyperparathyroidism and proximal limb muscle weakness is well established (172). Secondary hyperparathyroidism commonly accompanies renal failure. Patients have bone pain and muscle atrophy. Microscopy reveals atrophy, predominantly of type II fibres. In transverse sections, the atrophic fibres are elongated in appearance as in neurogenic conditions. Serum creatine kinase activity is usually not raised.

Of interest is that carnitine levels in plasma and in muscle of dialysed patients may be decreased. Carnitine is a small molecule (165 Daltons) which is easily lost in the dialysate during dialysis. This decrease in plasma levels is, however, restored within 6 to 8 h after dialysis (174–177). Storage of lipid droplets in type I fibres is considered to be the hallmark of a myopathy, caused by carnitine deficiency (178). No lipid storage has been observed in skeletal muscle biopsies from dialysed patients (169).

Myasthenic syndrome in dialysis patients

Dialysis patients are sometimes given D,L carnitine to treat hypertriglyceridemia (179). In such patients a myasthenic syndrome with fluctuating diplopia, ptosis, dysphagia and proximal weakness, can develop. Weakness is dramatically improved by injection of pyridostigmine. Withdrawal of carnitine results in dramatic improvement (180, 181).

NEUROPSYCHOLOGICAL ASPECTS

A complete neuropsychological assessment is a prerequisite for accurate evaluation of the impairment of complex mental functioning. In most dialysis patients cognitive efficiency suffers. Using intelligence tests. such as Wechler's Adult Intelligence Scale. a deterioration of the total intelligence quotient (IQ) is found. This decline is partly due to slowness in performing the tests. In verbal tasks. requiring (over) learned knowledge, patients maintain their original level approximately. Performance IQ, as a measure of the ability to accomplish relatively new tasks with a visuo-spatial component under conditions of time pressure, deteriorates. Memory function is diminished particularly in registration, learning and reproduction of recently acquired data, the working memory being more vulnerable than retrieval from long term memory store. A mild disturbance of language function may become manifest in the rather non-specific symptom of word finding difficulty. Written language may suffer from control errors (e.g., anticipations and perseverations). A clear-cut dyscalculia is seldom present. Patients may sometimes, however, loose grip of number structure, as becomes apparent in errors when writing dictated numbers. Gnosis and praxis are usually intact, although minor deviations may occur, e.g., left-right mirroring and mild constructional disorders. Although patients are usually capable of sufficient mental tracking during examination many complain of problems in concentration which increase demonstrably during the intervals between dialysis treatments (182). Irritability and restlessness are prominent during the last hours of dialysis, and have to be considered as manifestations of the disequilibrium syndrome (183). The total neuropsychological picture is seen in encephalopathies of different aetiologies.

Few prospective studies comparing cognition before and during dialysis treatment have been published. Signs of a minor reduction in cognitive efficiency, possibly indicating cerebral dysfunction present before the start of dialysis treatment, have been found to regress during the treatment period and to have disappeared after 12 months of successful dialysis. Higher general intellectual level and fewer marked signs of pre-treatment cognitive dysfunction seem to result in a more rapid adjustment to the treatment. However, these factors were of no predictive value after 12 months of treatment (184).

According to Teschan and coworkers (185) the adequacy of the dialysis treatment may be monitored by repeated neuropsychological measurements. Cognition-dependent indices vary directly with the degree of uraemia, choice reaction time and continuous performance tests being sensitive indices.

REFERENCES

1. Raskin NH, Fishman RA: Neurological disorders in renal failure (first of two parts). *N Engl J Med* 294: 143, 1976
2. Leavitt S, Tyler HR: Studies in asterixis. *Arch Neurol* 10: 370, 1964
3. Shahani BT, Young RR: Asterixis – a disorder of the neural mechanisms underlying sustained muscle contraction. in *The Motor System: Neurophysiology and Muscle Mechanisms*, edited by Shahani M, Amsterdam, Elsevier Scientific Publishing Company, 1976, p 301
4. Young RR, Shahani BT: Unilateral asterixis produced by a discrete CNS lesion. *Trans Am Neurol Assoc* 101: 306, 1976
5. Ericson G, Warren SE, Gribik M: Unilateral asterixis in a dialysis patient. *JAMA* 240: 671, 1978
6. Degos JD, Verroust J, Bochareine A, Serdaru M, Barbizet J: Asterixis in focal brain lesions. *Arch Neurol* 36: 705, 1979
7. Donat JR: Unilateral asterixis due to thalamic haemorrhage. *Neurology* 30: 83, 1980
8. Kudo Y, Fukai M, Yamadori A: Asterixis due to pontine haemorrhage. *J Neurol Neurosurg Psychiatry* 48: 487, 1985
9. Chadwick D, French AT: Uraemic myoclonus: an example of reticular reflex myoclonus. *J Neurol Neurosurg Psychiatry* 12: 52, 1979
10. Steinman TI, Yager HM: Catatonia in uremia. *Ann Intern Med* 89: 74, 1978
11. Madonick MJ, Berke K, Schiffer I: Pleocytosis and meningeal signs in uremia: report on 62 cases. *Arch Neurol Psychiat* 64: 431, 1950
12. Schreiner GE, Maher JF: *Uremia. Biochemistry Pathogenesis and Treatment.* Springfield IL, Charles C Thomas, 1961, p 256
13. Tyler HR: Neurologic disorders in renal failure. *Am J Med* 44: 734, 1968
14. Jennekens FGI, Dorhout Mees EJ, Van der Most van Spijk D: Clinical aspects of uraemic polyneuropathy. *Nephron* 8: 414, 1971
15. Jacob JC, Gloor P, Elwan H: Electroencephalographic changes in chronic renal failure. *Neurology* 15: 419, 1965
16. Luyten JAFM, Storm van Leeuwen W, Jennekens FGI: EEG in uraemic patients with neuropathy. *Electroencephalogr Clin Neurophysiol* 28: 423, 190
17. Cohen SN, Syndulko K, Rever B, Krant J, Coburn I, Tourtelotte WW: Visual evoked potentials and long latency event-related potentials in chronic renal failure. *Neurology* 33: 1219, 1983
18. Komsuoglu SS, Mehta R, Jones LA, Harding GFA: Brainstem auditory evoked potentials in chronic renal failure and maintenance hemodialysis. *Neurology* 35: 419, 1985
19. Brown JJ, Sufit RL, Sollinger HW: Visual evoked potential changes following renal transplantation. *Electroencephalogr Clin Neurophysiol* 66: 101, 1987
20. Olsen S: The brain in uraemia. *Acta Psychiatr Scand* 36 (Suppl 156): 1, 1961
21. Kiley J, Hines O: Electroencephalographic evaluation of uremia, wave frequency evaluation on 40 uremic patients. *Arch Intern Med* 116: 67, 1965
22. Kiley JE, Woodruff MW, Pratt KL: Evaluation of encephalopathy by EEG frequency analysis in chronic dialysis patients. *Clin Nephrol* 5: 245, 1976
23. Heyman A, Patterson JL Jr, Jones RW Jr: Cerebral circulation and metabolism in uremia. *Circulation* 3: 558, 1951
24. Scheinberg P: Effects of uremia on cerebral blood flow and metabolism. *Neurology* 1: 101, 1954
25. Biasioli S, D'Andrea G, Feriani M, Chiarmante S, Fabris A, Ronco C, La Greca G: Uremic encephalopathy: an updating. *Clin Nephrol* 25: 57, 1986
26. Minkoff L, Gaertner G, Darab M, Levin ML: Inhibition of brain sodium-potassium ATPase in uremic rats. *J Lab Clin Med* 80: 71, 1972
27. Fraser CL, Sarnacki P, Arieff AI: Abnormal sodium transport in synaptosomes from brain of uremic rats. *J Clin Invest* 75: 2014, 1985
28. Hicks AM, Young DS, Wootton IDP: The effects of uraemic blood constituents on certain cerebral enzymes. *Clin Chim Acta* 9: 228, 1964
29. Bergström J: Uremia is an intoxication. *Kidney Int* 28 (Suppl 17): S2, 1985
30. Massry SG: Neurotoxicity of parathyroid hormone in uremia. *Kidney Int* 28 (Suppl 17): S5, 1985
31. Cooper JD, Lasarowitz VC, Arieff AI: Neurodiagnostic abnormalities in patients with acute renal failure. Evidence for neurotoxicity of parathyroid hormone. *J Clin Invest* 61: 1448, 1978

32. Fraser CL, Sarnacki P, Arieff A: Calcium transport abnormalities in uremic rat brain synaptosomes. *J Clin Invest* 76: 1789, 1985

33. Alfrey AC, Mishell JM, Burks J, Contiguglia SR, Rudolph H, Lewin E, Holmes JH: Syndrome of dyspraxia and multifocal seizures associated with chronic hemodialysis. *Trans Am Soc Artif Intern Organs* 18: 257, 1972

34. Plum F, Posner JB: *The Diagnosis of Stupor and Coma.* Third edition, Philadelphia, FA Davis Co, 1980, p 250

35. Arieff AI, Llach F, Massry SG: Neurological manifestations and morbidity of hyponatremia: correlation with brain water and electrolytes. *Medicine (Baltimore)* 55: 121, 1976

36. Fishman RA: Neurological manifestations of hyponatremia. in *Handbook of Clinical Nelarology*, Vol 28, edited by Vinken PJ and Bruyn GW, Amsterdam. North Holland Publishing Company, 1976, p 495

37. Reynolds EH: Neurological aspects of potassium imbalance. in *Handbook of Clinical Neurology*, Vol 28, edited by Vinken PJ and Bruyn GW, Amsterdam, North Holland Publishing Company, 1976, p 463

38. Lockman L: Neurological aspects of acid-base metabolism. in *Handbook of Clinical Neurology*, Vol 28, edited by Vinken PJ and Bruyn GW, Amsterdam, North Holland Publishing Company, 1976, p 507

39. Tyler HR: Neurological disorders in renal failure. in *Handbook of Clinical Neurology*, Vol 27, edited by Vinken PI and Bruyn GW, Amsterdam, North Holland Publishing Company, 1976, p 391

40. Bradbury M: *The Concept of a Blood Brain Barrier.* New York, John Wiley and Sons, 1979

41. Davis FA, Schauf CL: Neurological manifestations of calcium imbalance. in *Handbook of Clinical Neurology*, Vol 28, edited by Vinken PJ and Bruyn GW, Amsterdam, North Holland Publishing Company, 1976, p 527

42. Frame B: Neuromuscular manifestations of parathyroid disease. in *Handbook of Clinical Neurology*, Vol 27, edited by Vinken PJ and Bruyn GW, Amsterdam, North Holland Pubishing Company, 1976, p 283

43. Rivera-Vazques AB, Noriega-Sánchez A, Ramirez-Gonzalez R, Martinez-Maldonado M: Acute hypercalcemia in hemodialysis patients: distinction from 'dialysis dementia'. *Nephron* 25: 243, 1980

44. Durlach J: Neuromuscular manifestations of magnesium imbalance. in *Handbook of Clinical Neurology*, Vol 28, edited by Vinken PJ and Bruyn GW, Amsterdam, North Holland Publishing Company, 1976, p 545

45. Kennedy AC, Linton AL, Luke RG, Renfrew S, Dinwoodi A: The pathogenesis and prevention of cerebral dysfunction during dialysis. *Lancet* 1: 790, 1964

46. Arieff AI, Massry SG, Barientos A, Kleeman CR: Brain water and electrolyte metabolism in uremia: effects of slow and rapid hemodialysis. *Kidney Int* 4: 177, 1973

47. Mann H, Stiller S: Elimination of sodium chloride as the cause of dialysis disequilibrium syndrome. (Abstract) *Kidney Int* 17: 401, 1980

48. Arieff AI, Guisado R, Massry SG, Lazarowitz VC: Central nervous system pH in uremia and the effect of hemodialysis. *J Clin Invest* 58: 306, 1976

49. Arieff AI, Lazarowitz VC, Guisado R: Experimental dialysis disequilibrium syndrome: prevention with glycerol. *Kidney Int* 14: 270, 1978

50. La Greca G, Biasoli S, Chiaramonte S: Studies of brain density in hemodialysis and peritoneal dialysis. *Nephron* 21: 146, 1982

51. Bolton CF, Young GB: *Neurological Complications of Renal Disease.* Stoneham, MA, Butterworth-Heineman, 1990.

52. Hughes JR, Schreeder MT: EEG in dialysis encephalopathy. *Neurology (NY)* 30: 1148, 1980

53. Dunea G, Mahurkar SD, Mamdani B: Role of aluminum in dialysis dementia. *Ann Intern Med* 88: 502, 1978

54. Faris AA: Wernicke's encephalopathy a complication of chronic hemodialysis. *Arch Neurol* 18: 248, 1968

55. Victor M: The Wernicke Korsakoff syndrome. in *Handbook of Clinical Neurology*, Vol 28, edited by Vinken PJ and Bruyn GW, Amsterdam, North Holland Publishing Company, 1976, p 243

56. Dukes MNG: *Meyler's Side Effects of Drugs.* Ninth edition, Anmterdam, Excerpla Medica, 1980, p 416

57. Schwankhaus JD, Massucci EF, Kurtzke JF: Cefazolin-induced encephalopathy in a uremic patient. *Ann Neurol* 17: 211, 1985

58. Lindner A, Charra B, Sherrard DJ, Scribner BH: Accelerated atherosclerosis and prolonged maintenance hemodialysis. *N Engl J Med* 290: 679, 1974

59. Lazarus JM, Lowrie EG, Hampers CL, Merrill JP: Cardiovascular disease in uremic palients on hemodialysis. *Kidney Int* 7 (Suppl 2): S167, 1975

60. Burke JF Jr, Francos GC, Moore LL, Cho SY, Lasker N: Accelerated atherosclerosis in chronic dialysis: another look. *Nephron* 21: 181, 1978

61. Rostand SG, Greter JC, Kirk KA, Rutsky EA, Andreoli TE: Ischemic heart disease in patients with uremia undergoing maintenance hemodialysis. *Kidney Int* 16: 600, 1979

62. Lundin AP, Friedman EA: Vascular consequenees of maintenance hemodialysis. An unproven case. *Nephron* 21: 177, 1978

63. Dinsdale HB: Hypertension and the central nervous system. in *Current Neurology*, edited by Tyler HR, Dawson DM, Boston, Houghton Mifflin Publ, 1978, p 196

64. Dinsdale HB: Hypertensive encephalopathy. in *Stroke, Pathophysiology, Diagnosis and Management*, edited by Barnett HJM, Stein BM, Mohr JP, Yatsu FM, New York, Churchill Livingstone, 1986, p 896

65. Chester EM, Agamanolis DP, Banker BQ, Victor M: Hypertensive encephalopathy: a clinicopathologic study of 20 cases. *Neurology* 28: 928, 1978

66. Nag S, Robertson DM, Dinsdale HB: Cerebral cortical changes in acute experimental hypertension. An ultrastructural study. *Lab Invest* 36: 150, 1977

67. Rosenberg G, Kornfeld M, Stovring J, Bicknell JM: Subcortical arteriosclerotic encephalopathy (Bingswanger): computerized tomography. *Neurology* 29: 1102, 1979

68. Junck L, Herrick MK, Langston JW: CT-scan in subcortical arteriosclerotic encephalopathy. *Neurology* 30: 791, 1980

69. Olzewski J: Subcortical arteriosclerotic encephalopathy. *World Neurology* 3: 359, 1962

70. Biemond A: On Binswanger's subcortical arteriosclerotie encephalopathy and the possibility of its clinical recognition. *Psychiatr Neurol Neurosurg* 73: 413, 1970

71. Caplan LR, Schoene WC: Clinical features of subcortical arteriosclerotic encephalopathy. *Neurology* 28: 1206, 1978

72. Editorial (anonymous): Binswanger's encephalopathy. *Lancet* 1: 923, 1981

73. Nichols FT III, Mohr JP: Binswanger's subacute arteriosclerolic encephalopathy. in *Stroke, Pathophysiology, Diagnosis and Management*, edited by Barnett HJM, Mohr JP, Stein BM, Yatsu FM, New York, Churchill Livingstone, 1986, p 875

74. De Reuck J, Crevits L, De Coster W, Sieben G, van der Eecken H: Pathogenesis of Binswanger chronic progressive subconical encephalopathy. *Neurology* 30: 920, 1980

75. Reinmuth OM: Transient ischemic attacks. in *Current Neurology*, Vol 1, edited by Tyler HR, Dawson DM, Boston, Houghton Mifflin Publ, 1978, p 166

76. Mohr JP, Pessin MS: Extracranial carotid artery disease. in *Stroke, Pathophysiology, Diagnosis and Management*, edited by Barnett HJM, Mohr JP, Stein BM, Yatsu FM, New York, Churchill Livingstone, 1986, p 293

77. Toole JF, Yuson CP: Transient ischemic attacks with normal arteriograms. Serious or benign prognosis. *Ann Neurol* 1: 100, 1977

78. Pessin MS, Duncan GW, Mohr JP, Poskanzer DC: Clinical and angiographic features of carotid transient ischemic attacks. *N Engl J Med* 296: 358, 1977

79. Russo LS: Carotid system transient ischemic attacles: clinical, racial and angiographic correlations. *Stroke* 12: 470, 1982

80. Barnett HJM: Antithrombotic therapy in cerebral vascular disease; antispasmodics and fibrinolysins. in *Stroke, Pathohysiology, Diagnosis and Management*, edited by Barnett HJM, Mohr JP, Stein BM, Yatsu FM, New York, Churchill Livingstone, 1986, p 989

81. Gates PC, Barnett HJM, Silver MD: Cardiogenic stroke. in *Stroke, Pathophysiology, Diagnosis and Management*, edited by Barnett HJM, Mohr JP, Stein BM, Yatsu FM, New York, Churchill Livingstone, 1986, p 1085

82. Caplan LR: Intracranial hemorrhage. in *Current Neurology*, edited by Tyler HR, Dawson DM, Boston, Houghton Mifflin Publ, 1979, p 185

83. Little JR, Tubman DE, Ethier R: Cerebellar hemorrhage in adults: diagnosis by computerized tomography. *J Neurosurg* 48: 575, 1978

84. Crowell RM, Ojemann RG: Spontaneous brain hemorrhage, surgical considerations. in *Stroke, Pathophysiology, Diagnosis and Management*, edited by Barnett HJM, Mohr SP, Stein BM, Yatsu FM, New York, Churchill Livingstone, 1986, p 1191

85. Snyder M, Renaudin J: Intracranial hemorrhage associated with anticoagulation therapy. *Surg Neurol* 7: 31, 1977

86. Bechar M, Lakke JPW, Van der Hem GK, Beks JWF, Penning L: Subdural hematoma during long term hemodialysis. *Arch Neurol* 26: 513, 1972

87. Leonard A, Shapiro FL: Subdural hematoma in regularly hemodialyzed patients. *Ann Intern Med* 82: 650, 1975

88. Keane WF, Shapiro FL, Ray L: Incidence and type of infections occurring in 445 hemodialysis patients. *Trans Am Soc Artif Intern Organs* 23: 41, 1977

89. Nsouli KA, Lazarus JM, Schoenbaum SC, Gottlieb MN, Lowrie EG, Shocair M: Bacteremic infeclion in hemodialysis. *Arch Intern Med* 139: 1255, 1979

90. Reidenberg MM: The binding of drugs to plasma proteins and the interpretation of measurements of plasma concentration of drugs in patients with poor renal function. *Am J Med* 62: 466, 1977

91. Depner T, Gulyassy PF, Stanfel DA, Jarrard EA: Plasma protein binding in uremia: extraction and characterization of an inhibitor. *Kidney Int* 18: 86, 1980

92. Reynolds F, Jones NF, Zikoyanis PN, Smith SE: Salivary phenytoin concentrations in epilepsy and in chronic renal failure. *Lancet* 2: 384, 1976

93. Bruni J, Wang LH, Marbury TC, Lee CS, Wilder BJ: Protein binding of valproic acid in uremic patients. *Neurology* 30: 557, 1980

94. McGonigle RJS, Bewick M, Weston MJ, Parsons V: Progressive predominantly motor uraemic neuropathy. *Acta Neurol Scand* 71: 379, 1985

95. Bolton CF, Gilbert JJ, Hahn AF, Sibbald WJ: Polyneuropathy in critically ill patients. *J Neurol Neurosur Psychiatry* 47: 1223, 1984

96. Asbury AK: Neuropathies with renal failure, hepatic disorders, chronic respiratory insufficiency and critical illness. in *Peripheral Neuropathy*, edited by Dyck PJ, Thomas PK et al., Philadelphia, WB Saunders, 1993, p 1251

97. Said G, Boudier L, Selva J, Zingraff J, Drüecke T: Different patterns of uremic polyneuropathy: clinicopathologic study. *Neurology* 33: 567, 1983

98. Mulder DW: Motor neuron disease. in *Peripheral Neuropathy*, edited by Dyck PJ, Thomas PK, Lambert EH, Philadelphia, WB Saunders Co, 1975, p 759

99. Callaghan N: Restless legs syndrome in uremic neuropathy. *Neurology* 17: 359, 1966

100. Boghen D: Successful treatment of restless legs with clonazepam. *Ann Neurol* 6: 341, 1979

101. Jennekens FGI, Dorhout Mees EJ, Van der Most van Spijk D: Uraemic polyneuropathy. *Nephron* 8: 414, 1971

102. Nielsen VK: The peripheral nerve function in chronic renal failure. I Clinical symptoms and signs. *Acta Med Scand* 190: 105, 1971

103. Nielsen VK: The peripheral nerve function in chronic renal failure. VII Longitudinal course during terminal renal failure and regular dialysis. *Acta Med Scand* 195: 155, 1974

104. Nielsen VK: The peripheral nerve function in chronic renal failure. An analysis of the vibratory perception threshold. *Acta Med Scand* 191: 287, 1972

105. Hennessy WJ, Siemsen AW: Autonomic neuropathy in chronic renal failure. *Clin Res* 16: 385, 1968

106. Kersch ES, Krohnfield SJ, Unger A, Popper RW, Cantor S, Cohn K: Autonomic insufficiency in uremia as a cause of hemodialysis-induced hypotension. *N Engl J Med* 290: 650, 1974

107. Röckel A, Henneman H, Sternagel-Haase A, Heidhand A: Uraemic sympathetic neuropathy after haemodialysis and transplantation. *Eur J Clin Invest* 9: 23, 1979

108. Zuchelli P, Sturani A, Zuccala A, Santoro A, Degli Esposti E, Chiarini C: Dysfunction of the autonomic nervous system in patients with end-stage renal failure. *Contr Nephrol* 45: 69, 1985

109. Solders G, Persson A, Gutierrez A: Autonomic dysfunction in non-diabetic terminal uraemia. *Acta Neurol Scand* 71: 321, 1985

110. Mallamaci F, Zoccali C, Cicarelli M, Briggs JD: Autonomic function in uremic patients treated by hemodialysis or CAPD and in transplant patients. *Clin Nephrol* 25: 175, 1986

111. Solders G: Autonomic function tests in healthy controls and in terminal uraemia. *Acta Neurol Scand* 73: 638, 1986

112. Mentser MI, Clay S, Malekzadeh MH, Pennisi AJ, Ettenger RB, Uittenbogaart CH, Finc RN: Peripheral motor nerve conduction velocities in children undergoing chronic hemodialysis. *Nephron* 22: 337, 1978

113. Chan JC, Eng G: Long-term hemodialysis and nerve conduction in children. *Pediat Res* 13: 591, 1979

114. Nielsen VK: The peripheral nerve function in chronic renal failure. V Sensory and motor conduction velocity. *Acta Med Scand* 194: 445, 1973

115. Van der Most van Spijk D, Hoogland RA, Dijkstra S: Conduction velocities compared and related to degrees of renal insufficiency. in *New Developments in Electromyography and Clinical Neurophysiology*, Vol 2, edited by Desmedt JE, Basel, Karger, 1973, p 381

116. Dinn JJ, Crane DL: Schwann cell dysfunction in uraemia. *J Neurol Neurosurg Psychiatry* 33: 605, 1970

117. Bergström J, Lindblom U, Norée LO: Preservation of peripheral nerve function in severe uraemia during treatment with low protein, high calorie diet and surplus of essential amino-acids. *Acta Med Scand* 51: 99, 1975

118. Capelli P, Di Paolo B, Evangelista M, Di Marco T, Albertazzi A: Low protein diet supplemented with essential amino acids and keto analogues. Effects on uremic polyneuropathy and encephalopathy. *Contr Nephrol* 53: 58, 1986

119. Caccia MR, Mangili A, Mecca G, Ubiali E, Zanoni P: Effects of haemodialytic treatment on uremic polyneuropathy. *J Neurol* 217: 193, 1977

120. Cadilhac J, Mion C, Duday H, Dapres G, Georgesco M: Motor nerve conduction velocities as an index of the efficiency of maintenance dialysis in patients with end-stage renal failure. in *Peripheral Neuropathies*, edited by Canal N, Pozza G, Amsterdam, Elsevier, North Holland Biomedical Press, 1978, p 211

121. Kurts SB, Wong VH, Anderson CF, Vogel JP, McCarthy JT, Mitchell JC, Kumar R, Johnson WJ: Continuous ambulatory peritoneal dialysis. Three years' experience at the Mayo Clinic. *Mayo Clin Proc* 58: 633, 1983

122. Tegnér R, Lindholm B: Uremic polyneuropathy: different effects of hemodialysis and continuous ambulatory peritoneal dialysis. *Acta Med Scand* 218: 409, 1985

123. Stanley E, Brown JC, Pryor JS: Altered peripheral nerve function resulting from haemodialysis. *J Neurol Neurosurg Psychiatry* 40: 39, 1977

124. Edwards AE, Kopple JD, Kornfeld CM: Vibrotactile threshold in patients undergoing maintenance dialysis. *Arch Intern Med* 132: 706, 1973

125. Castaigne P, Cathala HP, Beaussart-Boulengé L, Petrover M: Effect of ischaemia on peripheral nerve function in patients with chronic renal failure undergoing dialysis treatment. *J Neurol Neurosurg Psychiatry* 35: 631, 1972

126. Lowitzsch K, Göhring U, Hecking E, Köhler H: Refractory period, sensory conduction velocity and visual evoked potentials before and after haemodialysis. *J Neurol Neurosurg Psychiatry* 44: 121, 1981

127. Dyck PJ, Johnson WJ, Lambert EH, O'Brien PC, Daube JR, Ovratt KF: Comparison of symptoms, chemistry and nerve function to assess adequacy of hemodialysis. *Neurology* 9: 1361, 1979

128. Nielsen VK: The peripheral nerve function in chronic renal failure. A survey. *Acta Med Scand* 573 (Suppl): 8, 1975

129. Ibraham MM, Crosland JM, Honigsberger L, Barnes AD, Dawson-Edwards P, Newman CE, Robinson BHB: Effect of renal transplantation on uraemic neuropathy. *Lancet* 2: 739, 1974

130. Nielsen VK: The peripheral nerve function in chronic renal failure. IX Recovery after transplantation. Electrophysiological aspects (sensory and motor nerve conduction). *Acta Med Scand* 195: 171, 1974

131. Oh SJ, Clements RS, Lee YW, Diethelm AG: Rapid improvement in nerve conduction velocity following renal transplantation. *Ann Neurol* 4: 369, 1978

132. Nielsen VK: The peripheral nerve function in chronic renal failure. VII Recovery after renal transplantation. Clinical aspects. *Acta Med Scand* 195: 163, 1974

133. Bolton CF: Electrophysiologic changes in uremic neuropathy after successful renal transplantation. *Neurology* 26: 152, 1976

134. Asbury AK, Victor M, Adams RD: Uremic polyneuropathy. *Arch Neurol* 8: 413, 1963

135. Forno L, Alston W: Uremic polyneuropathy. *Acta Neurol Scand* 43: 640, 1967

136. Jennekens FGI, Dorhout Mees EJ, van der Most van Spijk D: Nerve fibre degeneration in uraemic polyneuropathy. *Proc Eur Dial Transplant Assoc* 6: 191, 1969

137. Thomas PK, Hollinrake K, Lascelles RG, O'Sullivan DJ, Baillod RA, Moorhead JF, Mackenzie JC: The polyneuropathy of chronic renal failure. *Brain* 94: 761, 1971

138. Dayan AD, Gardner-Thorpe C, Down PF, Gleadle RI: Peripheral neuropathy in uremia. *Neurology* 20: 649, 1970

139. Dyck PJ, Johnson WJ, Lambert EH, O'Brien PC: Segmental demyelination secondary to axonal degeneration in uremic neuropathy. *Mayo Clin Proc* 46: 400, 1971

140. Hansen S, Ballantyne JP: A quantitative electrophysiological study of uraemic neuropathy. *J Neurol Neurosurg Psychiatry* 41: 128, 1978

141. Said G, Goulon-Goeau C, Slama G, Tchobroutsky G: Severe early-onset polyneuropathy in insulin-dependent diabetes mellitus. *N Engl J Med* 326: 1257, 1992

142. Pekelharing CA, Winkler C: Mitteilung über die Beriberi (Communication on beriberi). *Dtsch Med Wochenschr* 13: 845, 1887 (in German)

143. Babb AL, Popovich RP, Christopher TG, Scribner BH: The genesis of the square meter-hour hypothesis. *Trans Am Soc Artif Intern Organs* 17: 81, 1971

144. Tenckhoff H, Shilipetar G, Boen ST: One year's experience with home peritoneal dialysis. *Trans Am Soc Artif Intern Organs* 11: 11, 1968

145. Raskin NH, Fishman RA: Neurological disorders in renal failure (Second of two parts). *N Engl J Med* 294: 204, 1976

146. Merrill JP: The search for 'factor X'. *Clin Nephrol* 11: 56, 1979

147. Baker LRI, Marshall RD: A reinvestigation of methylguanidine concentration in sera from normal and uraemic subjects. *Clin Sci* 41: 563, 1971

148. Blumberg A, Esslen E, Bürgi W: Myoinositol – a uremic neurotoxin. *Nephron* 21: 186, 1971

149. Sterzel RB, Semar M, Lonergan ET, Treser G, Lange K: Relationship of nervous tissue transketolase to the neuropathy in chronic uremia. *J Clin Invest* 50: 2295, 1971

150. Kopple JD, Dirige OV, Jacob M, Wang M, Swenseid ME: Transketolase activity in red blood cells in chronic uremia. *Trans Am Soc Artif Intern Organs* 18: 250, 1972

151. Dobbelstein H, Körner WF, Mempel W, Grosse-Wilde H, Edel HH: Vitamin B6 deficiency in uremia and its implication for the depression of immune responses. *Kidney Int* 5: 233, 1974

152. Nielsen VK: Pathophysiological aspects of uraemic neuropathy. in *Peripheral Neuropathies*, edited by Canal N, Pozza G, Amsterdam, Elsevier/North Holland Biomedical Press, 1978, p 197

153. Brismar T, Tegnér R: Experimental uremic neuropathy. Part 2 (Sodium permeability decrease and inactivation in potential clamped nerve fibres). *J Neurol Sci* 65: 37, 1984

154. Goldstein DA, Chui LA, Massry SG: Effects of parathyroid hormone and uremia on peripheral nerve calcium and motor nerve conduction velocity. *J Clin Invest* 62: 88, 1978

155. Avram MM, Iancu M, Morrow P, Feinfeld D, Huatuco A: Uremic syndrome in man: new evidence for parathormone as a multisystem neurotoxin. *Clin Nephrol* 11: 59, 1979

156. Schaefer K, Offerman G, Von Herrath D, Schröter R, Stölzer R, Arntz HR: Failure to show a correlation between serum parathyroid hormone, nerve conduction velocity and serum lipids in hemodialysis patients. *Clin Nephrol* 14: 81, 1980

157. Drüeke T, Chkoff N, DiGiulo S, Zingraff J, Delons S, Man NK, Jungers P, Crosnier J: Absence of increased motor nerve conduction velocity after parathyroidectomy in dialysis patients. (Abstract) *Kidney Int* 15: 449, 1979

158. Layzer RB: *Neuromuscular Manifestations of Systemic Disease*, Philadelphia, FA Davis Co, 1985, p 112

159. Pagani, C, Zoerle, C, Guaita MC, Bazzi C, Sovgato G, Torgi G: Carpal tunnel syndrome in long-term dialyzed patients. *Contr Nephrol* 45: 72, 1985

160. Warren DJ, Otieno LS: Carpal tunnel syndrome in patients on intermittent haemodialysis. *Postgrad Med J* 51: 450, 1975

161. Bosanac PR, Bilder B, Grunberg RW, Banach SF, Kintzel JE, Stephens HW: Post-permanent access neuropathy. *Trans Am Soc Artif Intern Organs* 23: 162, 1977

162. Harding AE, LeFanu J: Carpal tunnel syndrome related to antebrachial Cimino–Brescia fistula. *J Neurol Neurosurg Psychiatry* 40: 511, 1977

163. Walts AE, Goodman MD, Matoru PA: Amyloid carpal tunnel syndrome and chronic hemodialysis. *Am J Nephrol* 5: 225, 1985

164. Chanard J, Lavaud S, Toupance O, Melin JP, Gillery P, Revillard JP: B2 microglobulin-associated amyloidosis in chronic haemodialysis patients. *Lancet* 1: 1212, 1986

165. Ballardie FW, Kerr DNS, Tennent G, Pepys MB: Haemodialysis versus CAPD: equal predisposition to amyloidosis. *Lancet* 1: 795, 1986

166. Hamilton DV, Evans DB, Henderson RG: Ulnar nerve lesion as complication of Cimino–Brescia arteriovenous fistula. *Lancet* 2: 1137, 1980

167. Ahmad R, Raichura N: Ulnar nerve lesion as complication of Cimino–Brescia arteriovenous fistula. *Lancet* 2: 1381, 1980

168. Bailey RR, Lynn KL: Arteriovenous shunts and nerve damage. *Lancet* 1: 211, 1981

169. Bolton CF, Driedger AA, Lindsay RM: Ischaemic neuropathy in uraemic patients caused by bovine arteriovenous shunt. *J Neurol Neurosurg Psychiatry* 42: 810, 1979

170. Ahonen RE: Light microscopic study of striated muscle in uremia. *Acta Neuropathol (Berl)* 49: 51, 1980

171. Kopple JD: Abnormal amino acid and protein metabolism in uremia. *Kidney Int* 14: 340, 1983

172. Alvestrand A, Fürst P, Bergström J: Intracellular amino acids in uremia. *Kidney Int* 24 (Suppl 16): 9, 1983

173. Jennekens FGI: Disuse, cachexia and ageing. in *Skeletal Muscle Pathology*, edited by Mastaglia FL, Walton JN, Edinburgh, London, New York, Churchill-Livingstone, 1981, p 605

174. DelCanale S, Fiaccadori E, Ronda N, Söderlund K, Antonucci C, Guariglia A: Muscle energy metabolism in uremia. *Metabolism* 35: 981, 1986

175. Bethlem J: *Myopathies*, Second edition, Amsterdam, Elsevier North Holland, 1980, p 269

176. Böhmer T, Bergrem H, Eiklid K: Carnitine deficiency induced during intermittent haemodialysis for renal failure. *Lancet* 1: 126, 1978

177. Mingardi G, Bizzi A, Cini M, Licini R, Mecca G, Garatini S: Carnitine balance in hemodialyzed patients. *Clin Nephrol* 13: 269, 1980

178. Bizzi A, Cini M, Garattini S, Mingardi G, Licini R, Mecca G: L-carnitine addition to haemodialysis liquid prevents plasma carnitine deficiency during dialysis. *Lancet* 1: 882, 1979

179. DiMauro S, Trevissan C, Hays A: Disorders of lipid metabolism in muscle. *Muscle Nerve* 3: 369, 1980

180. Lacour B, Chanard J, Haguet M, Basile D, Assan R, Di Giulio S, Ciancioni C, Lebkiri B, Drüeke T, Funck-Brentano JL: Carnitine improves lipid abnormalities in haemodialysis patients. *Lancet* 2: 763, 1980

181. Bazzato G, Coli U, Landini S, Mezzina C, Ciman M: Myasthenia-like syndrome after D,L- but not L-carnitine. *Lancet* 1: 1209, 1981

182. Clair F, Caillat S, Soufir JC, Lafforgue B, Drüeke T, Said G: Syndrome myasthénique induit par la D,L carnitine chez un hémodialysé chronique. *Press Méd* 13: 1154, 1984

183. West TPJ: A comparison of predialysis and postdialysis cognitive abilities. *Dial Transplant* 7: 809, 1978

184. Hagberg B: A prospective study of patients in chronic hemodialysis III. Predictive value of intelligence, cognitive deficit and ego defense structures in rehabilitation. *J Psychosom Res* 18: 151, 1974

185. Teschan PE, Ginn HE, Bourne JR, Ward JW: Neurobehavioral probes for adequacy of dialysis. *Trans Am Soc Artif Intern Organs* 23: 556, 1977

ORGAN AND METABOLIC COMPLICATIONS: TRACE ELEMENTS

ALLEN C. ALFREY

INTRODUCTION

A number of trace element disturbances have been recognized in uremic patients. This has been noted especially in patients receiving long term hemodialysis. There are a number of reasons that the patient with end-stage renal disease is at risk of developing trace element toxicity, as well as deficiency. As a direct result of loss of renal function, elements which are normally eliminated from the body through the kidney are retained. In proteinuric states metal binding proteins are also lost which can result in deficiencies of the elements being transported. With advanced renal failure the normal intestinal barriers, which exclude potentially toxic elements from being absorbed, are compromised. The artificial means by which patients are maintained following the development of end-stage renal disease can contribute further to elemental disturbances. Certain elements filtered, but normally retained by tubule function, may be lost across the dialyzing membrane. The body burden of other elements can be enriched from dialysis fluid contaminants, and transported to the patient during the procedure. Some of the elemental alteration from these various mechanisms have been associated with major clinical consequences.

TRACE ELEMENT DISTURBANCES

Blood is the tissue most widely used as in indicator of the status of body trace elements. However, it should be recognized that blood largely represents a transport system for most trace elements and alterations noted may not necessarily reflect the body burden of the element in question. The blood levels of a number of essential trace elements have usually been found to be decreased in both dialyzed and non-dialyzed uremic patients. Blood selenium has been found to be decreased in most but not all studies (1–8). Blood zinc levels have also been found to be decreased (9–11), as are serum manganese (12) and nickel (12–14). The level of copper in blood of uremic patients has usually been reported as normal (9, 15). Blood vanadium levels largely have been reported to be increased (16–20). Two other essential trace elements have also been found to be increased in the blood of uremic patients; chromium (15) and silicon (21–24). Of the non-essential elements blood levels of aluminum (12, 25) and lithium (26) have been found to be increased; whereas, blood rubidium and bromine have been found to be decreased (15, 27).

Multiple tissue trace element profiles have been characterized in both dialyzed and non-dialyzed uremic patients. As with blood a number of trace elements in other tissues have been found to be abnormal in uremic patients. These can be divided into three groups. The first group represents a similar disturbance in multiple tissues documenting an alteration in the total body burden of these elements. Six elements belong to this group. Total body aluminum, tin, zinc, and strontium are increased; whereas, total body rubidium is decreased in dialyzed and non-dialyzed uremic patients. Total body bromine is decreased only in dialyzed uremic patients (28, 29).

The second group of disturbances represents elements that may be increased or reduced in some tissues; whereas, they are either normal or actually affected in the opposite direction in other tissues. Examples of this alteration are the increased copper concentration in lungs associated with a reduced copper concentration in heart of both dialyzed and non-dialyzed uremic patients (28).

A third disturbance in trace elements would appear to be a translocation of an element from one organ to another. Two elements that fall into this group are cadmium and

Table 1. Mechanism of trace element disturbances with renal failure

1. Enhanced gastrointestinal absorption in the uremic state.
2. Inability to eliminate some elements because of reduced glomerular filtration rate.
3. Excess renal excretion, enhanced tubule secretion or loss of protein bound elements in proteinuric states.
4. Translocation of elements from a diseased system to other systems.
5. Enrichment from dialysis fluid contaminants.
6. Non-selective removal of elements by dialysis.

molybdenum, both of which are reduced in the diseased kidneys and increased in the liver (28).

Of the remaining essential trace elements tissue selenium levels have been found to be normal in uremic patients (28). Silicon has been found to be increased in spleen and liver in patients with chronic renal failure (30). Bone fluoride has been found to be increased in patients who have been exposed to dialysis fluid contaminated with fluoride (31). Vanadium has been reported to be increased in bones of uremic patients (32). With regard to non-essential elements tissue, stores of lead (28, 30, 32) and mercury (28) appear to be normal in most uremic patients. Uranium has been found to be increased in tissues from a limited number of dialysis patients.

MECHANISMS OF TRACE ELEMENT DISTURBANCES

It would appear, with few exceptions, that most trace element disturbances that occur in uremic patients are a result of uremia *per se* and not the dialysis procedure, since most elemental disturbances are shared by dialyzed and non-dialyzed uremic patients (28). However, the severity of the disturbances tend to be greater in dialyzed patients. For most elements, this presumably occurs because of the longer duration of uremia in the dialyzed patients. It is of interest that the four non-essential trace elements found consistently in all tissues in normal individuals (28, 33), strontium, aluminum, bromine, and rubidium, are altered in uremic patients.

Six mechanisms suggested for the altered tissue stores of trace elements found in uremic patients are listed in Table 1.

Enhanced gastrointestinal absorption in uremia

A number of animal studies (34, 35) and at least one human study (36) have shown that enhanced gastrointestinal absorption of aluminum occurs in the uremic state. Since aluminum absorption has been shown to occur passively through the paracellular pathway (37, 38) this would suggest the integrity of the paracellular pathway is compromised in uremia. In support of an anatomical alteration in the gastrointestinal tract is the finding of atrophic alterations of the intestinal mucosa in uremia (39). Similarly, enhanced aluminum absorption can be induced in animals by giving difluoromethylornithine, which causes atrophic lesions similar to those found in the uremic state (40). Other conditions, such as celiac disease and radiation enteropathy, accompanied by mucosal atrophy and leaky paracellular pathways, also have enhanced absorption of aluminum (36). At this time aluminum has been the only element documented to have increased absorption in the uremic state. However, it seems likely that other elements absorbed by similar mechanisms will also have enhanced absorption in the uremic state.

Inability to eliminate elements because of decreased glomerular filtration

For elements normally eliminated from the body by the kidney retention would be expected to result from loss of renal function. Two such elements whose elimination is largely if not entirely through the kidney are strontium and aluminum. The inability of the diseased kidney to eliminate adequately an increased systemic aluminum burden (resulting from both oral and parenteral sources) is well documented (41–43). Although not as well studied impaired renal function would be expected to retard the elimination of strontium as well.

Enhanced elimination of elements by renal mechanisms

One non-essential element, rubidium, is depleted in multiple tissues in both dialyzed and non-dialyzed uremic patients (28, 29). It has generally been assumed that rubidium and potassium are handled much alike in the body. However, tissue rubidium depletion (approximately 30%) far exceeds the 12.5% potassium depletion present in the same uremic population (28). This would suggest that in renal failure the renal clearance of rubidium exceeds the clearance of potassium.

Proteinuric states can represent another renal means of losing trace elements. A number of elements including iron, copper and zinc may be decreased as a result of urinary loss in association with their metal transporting proteins, respectively, ceruloplasmin, alpha globulin and transferrin (44–46).

Translocation from one organ to another

Two elements, molybdenum and cadmium appear to be translocated from the disease kidney to the liver (28). Cadmium is normally most concentrated in the kidneys, which contain about 30% of the total body cadmium. Probably because of decreased cadmium binding proteins in the diseased kidney, it is translocated to the liver. A similar mechanism might also account for the reduced levels of molybdenum in the diseased kidney.

EFFECT OF DIALYSIS ON TRACE ELEMENTS

The body burden of some elements has been enriched by the hemodialysis procedure as a result of being present in water supply used to prepare the dialysis fluid. A major example of this has been aluminum. The source of the aluminum was the water used for the preparation of the dialysis fluid (47–50). Fluoride represents another element commonly found in water supplies that also can be transported to the patient (31). In addition the dialysis fluid can act as an additional source of trace element enrichment. Numerous trace elements can contaminate the salts used in the preparation of hemodialysis fluid concentrate (51, 52) and peritoneal dialysis fluid (15, 51). As a result of differences in trace elements present in hemodialysis fluid because of contaminant in the salts or water used in its preparation, some elemental alterations found in hemodialysis patients are different from those found in peritoneal dialysis patients. As a consequence of being a contaminant in the preparative salts, chromium has been reported to be present in relatively high concentrations in dialysis solutions. Almost 50% of chromium in peritoneal dialysis solutions is transported to the patient during the dialysis procedure (15), in contrast to around 12.5% only, of chromium in hemodialysis solution transported to the patient during a procedure (51). It is felt that lactate in the peritoneal dialysis solution is at least partially responsible for the high transport of chromium in CAPD patients. As a result patients receiving CAPD have been found to have considerably higher blood chromium levels than other uremic patients (15).

Silicon and fluoride are rejected poorly by reverse osmosis treatment of water. In turn silicon and fluoride tend to be increased in some dialysis fluids. This has resulted in hemodialysis patients having higher blood fluoride and silicon levels than peritoneal dialysis patients (21, 53).

Elements can also be removed during the dialysis procedure. Bromine has been shown to be removed by both hemodialysis and peritoneal dialysis. Similarly, bromine tissue levels in hemodialysis patients (28) have been found to be reduced as well as blood bromine levels in both hemodialysis and peritoneal dialysis patients (15, 27). Another element significantly removed by the dialysis procedure is rubidium (15, 28). Although tissue rubidium levels are decreased in non-dialyzed uremic patients they are even further reduced in hemodialysis patients (28).

Table 2. Acute toxicity associated with the dialysis procedure

| Source | Acute Intoxication | |
	Element	Toxicity
Water supply		
Sewage and bacteria	NO_4	Methemoglobin
Water treatment facility		
Flocculation	Al	Neurological
Fluoridation	F	Cardiovascular
Water purification		
Exhausted anion column	H^+ (Cu leaching)	Hemolysis
	F	Cardiovascular
Dialysis fluid system		
Heater anodes	Al	Neurological
Regeneration system	Al	Neurological
Pumps	Al	Neurological
Copper tubing	Cu	Hemolysis
Galvanized holding tank	Zn	Gastrointestinal
Heater	Ni	Gastrointestinal

MECHANISM OF DIALYSIS INDUCED ACUTE TRACE ELEMENT TOXICITY

The dialysis procedure has been directly responsible for virtually all excess trace element exposure and toxicity described in uremic patients. To date no naturally occurring trace element in municipal water supplies has been shown to be responsible for any toxicity. Rather the use of unapproved water sources, the municipal water treatment facility or some component of the dialysis system has been responsible for causing the toxicity. The various trace elements responsible for toxic syndromes in dialysis patients are shown in Table 2.

Bacterial and sewage contamination in well water used to prepare dialysis fluid resulted in high nitrate levels. This caused methemoglobinemia in a dialysis patient manifested by nausea, vomiting, hypotension, lethargy and diaphoresis (54).

Acute aluminum and fluoride toxicity have resulted from the water treatment facility adding these two elements to the water supply (55, 56). Aluminum is added as a flocculating agent to remove turbidity from the water. There are no standards for aluminum in water so values vary greatly across the country (55). Using untreated municipal water for the preparation of the dialysis fluid has resulted in acute aluminum intoxication manifested primarily as seizures. Acute fluoride intoxication occurred in one group of dialysis patients as a consequence of a malfunction in a municipal water treatment facility which increased the fluoride content of the water 50 times normal

(56, 57). All patients developed gastrointestinal symptoms and one patient died after cardiac arrest (56, 57).

An additional source of trace element contamination has been the dialysis system hardware. Virtually all components of the system have been involved in producing toxicity. Aluminum has been dissolved from aluminum anodes (58) used in a water heating system, from an aluminum pump casing cover and impeller used to distribute acid dialysis fluid (59) and from cartridges used in a dialysis fluid regeneration system (60), causing aluminum neurotoxicity. Zinc has been leached from a galvanized tank used to store water for the preparation of dialysis fluid (61). This resulted in acute zinc intoxication manifested by repeated attacks of nausea, vomiting and fever during dialysis. Nickel has been leached from a stainless steel heating unit used to warm water after reverse osmosis treatment (62). During dialysis the patients experienced headache, dizziness, nausea and vomiting.

The improper use of water treatment equipment has also resulted in trace element contamination of the dialysis fluid. As a result of near exhaustion of the anion exchange resin fluoride has been displaced from the column by other anions with a higher affinity,thereby, enriching the dialysis fluid (63). Another consequence of exhaustion of the anion column is the lack of neutralizing the H^+ released from the cation exchange column. This caused acidification of the dialysis fluid, which in turn resulted in leaching of copper from copper tubing in the delivery system (64–67); acute copper intoxication manifested by fever, hemolysis, leukocytosis, metabolic acidosis and gastrointestinal symptoms, resulted.

All the acute trace element toxicity described above are easily preventible. This can be accomplished by treating adequately water used for the preparation of dialysis fluid, as well as maintaining the water treatment equipment as recommended by AAMI standards (68). In addition engineers or technicians responsible for creating and maintaining dialysis systems should be familiar with AAMI standards, and avoiding materials which contain potentially leachable elements, i.e., aluminum, nickel, zinc, and copper.

CHRONIC TOXICITY AND DEPLETION

Aluminum toxicity

The uremic patient is at risk of chronic aluminum loading and toxicity because of the potential for increased aluminum exposure, enhanced gastrointestinal absorption of aluminum and inability to eliminate any systemically administered aluminum because of compromised renal function. Approximately 85% of non-dialyzed patients with end-stage renal disease, who had no known history of ingesting aluminum containing compounds, were found to have elevated tissue stores of aluminum (42, 43). As stated above, in the uremic state, there is evidence that gastrointestinal aluminum absorption is enhanced, via derangements in paracellular pathway absorption. This augmented absorption of aluminum can even further be intensified by the concomitant administration of aluminum compounds and citrate (69–71).

The kidney's ability to excrete any absorbed or administered aluminum is critical in the prevention of an increased body burden of aluminum. Renal excretion has been shown to be the only means by which systemic aluminum burdens can be eliminated (41). The combination of reduction of renal function in association with parenteral loads of aluminum given during dialysis or enhanced gastrointestinal absorption (frequently in association with oral administration of aluminum compounds) can markedly increase the body burden of aluminum (42, 43).

Increased parenteral exposure to aluminum was first recognized in uremic patients chronically dialyzed with aluminum contaminated dialysis fluid (47–50). This resulted in the transfer of aluminum from the dialysis fluid to the blood during the dialysis procedure (25). As a result of plasma binding of the aluminum, largely to transferrin, the added aluminum was retained and the concentration gradient from dialysis fluid to blood maintained, further enhancing aluminum transport.

Clinical features of aluminum intoxication

It has been reasonably well established that aluminum can exert toxicity on the neurological (72), skeletal (73–76) and hematological (77, 78) systems in humans with advanced renal failure. It is less well established, if any toxicity, and under what circumstances, aluminum can be toxic in individuals with normal renal function.

In 1972 a new and distinct neurological disease was described in dialyzed uremic patients (79). This syndrome (dialysis encephalopathy or dialysis dementia) is characterized by an intermittent speech disturbance (stuttering or stammering), which is usually the first symptom noted. The speech disturbance is associated subsequently with personality changes, parietal lobe findings such as directional disorientation, seizures and auditory and visual hallucinations. As the disease progresses, the patient develops asterixis and myoclonus. All of the symptoms are markedly intensified by the dialysis procedure. Over a 7 to 9 month period following the onset of symptoms, the patient becomes totally mute and is unable to perform any purposeful movements. Death rapidly ensues (79, 80). Strikingly, the symptoms and course of this disease are similar among patients. The classical form of aluminum neurotoxicity has been confined largely to patients receiving dialysis in centers using dialysis fluid contaminated with aluminum over a long period of time. The aluminum contamination resulting from either municipal water supply (47–50, 81, 82), or materials (58–60) in the delivery system containing leachable aluminum.

An acute form of aluminum neurotoxicity has recently been described in uremic patients (69, 70). It occurs under three different conditions. These include dialysis

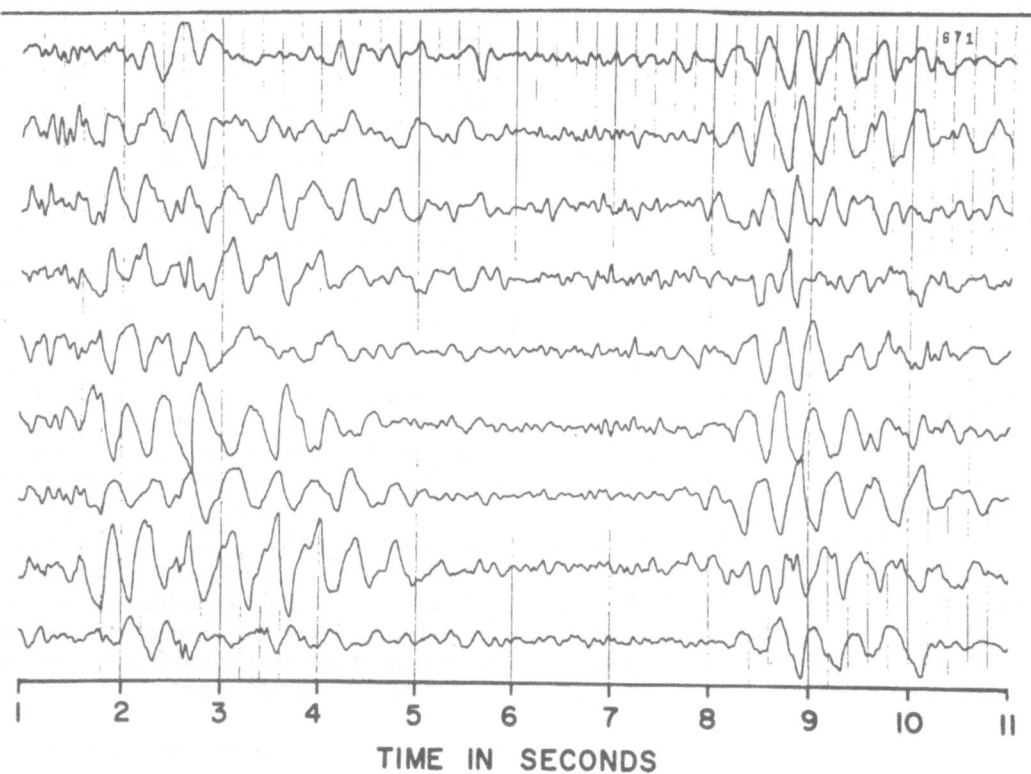

Figure 1. EEG alterations found in dialysis encephalopathy. Multifocal bursts of delta and occasional spike activity with relatively normal background rhythm.

performed with dialysis fluid highly contaminated with aluminum (59), the oral administration of citrate compounds in association with aluminum compounds (69, 70) and extreme elevation of plasma aluminum levels in association with deferoxamine therapy (83). It would appear that virtually all uremic children (84, 85) and non-dialyzed uremic adults (69, 70) who have developed acute aluminum neurotoxicity have done so from the ingestion of the combination of citrate and aluminum compounds. Although the patients may have some mild neurological findings of aluminum neurotoxicity, like the speech disturbance described above, more often there is an acute, explosive onset of symptoms. The major reported findings in adults include agitation, confusion, myoclonic jerks, grand mal seizures, obtundation, coma and death (69, 70). Aluminum neurotoxicity in children tends to be somewhat different in that it is manifested by regression of verbal and motor skills (84, 85), exemplified by the finding that children who have just started to walk and talk may lose these abilities.

If acute toxicity occurs as a consequence of high aluminum levels in the dialysis fluid it usually develops during the dialysis procedure. Symptoms related to deferoxamine therapy usually occur during or immediately following a dialysis where deferoxamine was administered (83). Although onset of symptoms of acute aluminum

intoxication may occur after months of ingestion of the combination of citrate and aluminum compounds, it is not uncommon for symptoms to develop in a matter of weeks following the combined ingestion of these two compounds (69, 70).

Diagnosis of aluminum neurointoxication is largely based on a history of either oral or parenteral exposure to aluminum in a uremic patient, demonstration of the classical clinical features and exclusion of other neurological conditions by appropriate studies. The most useful laboratory test supporting the diagnosis of aluminum neurotoxicity is the electroencephalogram (79, 80). Unlike most metabolic encephalopathies, including uremic encephalopathy, which exhibit a generalized slowing of the EEG, in aluminum intoxication the background rhythm is relatively normal with multifocal bursts of slow or delta waves frequently accompanied by spike activity (Figure 1). The CT scan may be normal or only show mild cortical atrophy. There are no cerebrospinal fluid abnormalities and aluminum levels in CSF are not increased. Histological changes that occur in the brains of patients dying of dialysis encephalopathy are non-specific and similar to changes seen in dialysis patients dying of other causes (80). Plasma aluminum levels in chronic intoxication are increased and frequently in the range of 100

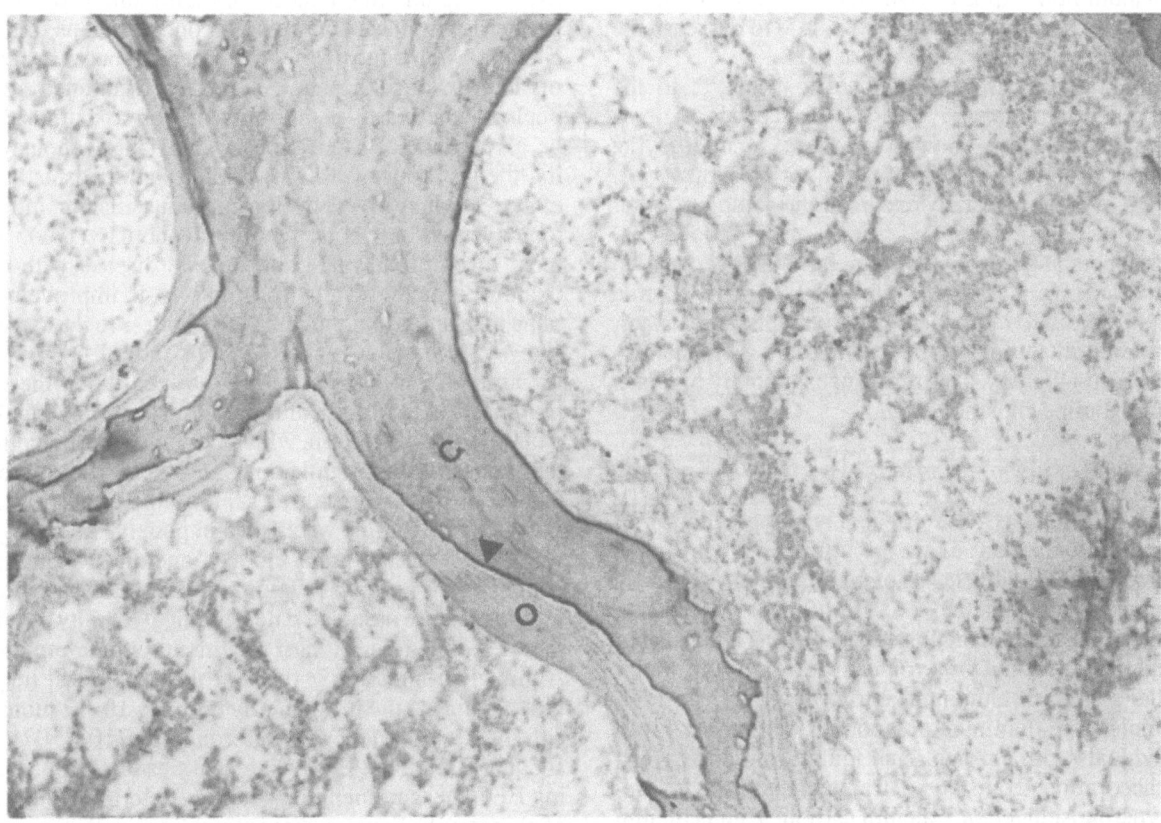

Figure 2. Bone histology present in aluminum associated bone disease. Classical features of osteomalacia with marked increase in non-calcified osteoid (O) tissue. Aluminum deposition is defined by the dark line (arrows) (Aluminon-stained) between calcified (C) and non-calcified bone (O).

to 200 μg/liter. With acute aluminum intoxication plasma aluminum levels are usually in excess of 500 μg/liter.

Aluminum skeletal toxicity is characterized by osteomalacia, bone pain, pathological fractures, proximal myopathy and failure to respond to any form of vitamin D therapy (73–76). Laboratory studies reveal relatively low, or normal, parathyroid hormone levels, usually normal alkaline phosphatase levels and mildly elevated serum calcium levels. Unlike virtually all other osteomalacic states serum phosphorus levels are either normal or more commonly slightly elevated. Evidence for the skeletal toxicity of aluminum is as convincing as it is for aluminum neurotoxicity. Aluminum associated fracturing osteomalacia was first recognized in association with dialysis encephalopathy in dialyzed uremic patients in areas with high aluminum levels in the water used to prepare the dialysis fluid (47, 48). As with encephalopathy, it was shown that fracturing osteomalacia could be largely prevented or would spontaneously heal by removing aluminum from the dialysis fluid (86). Besides parenteral exposure to aluminum, oral aluminum administration can also cause osteomalacia in uremic patients. Two studies in

which random bone biopsies were done in large dialysis populations showed that 25 to 30% of dialyzed uremic patient having no parenteral exposure to aluminum but routinely receiving oral aluminum containing phosphate binding gels, had aluminum-associated bone disease (87, 88). It has further been shown that virtually all osteomalacia which occurs in uremic patients is secondary to aluminum intoxication and that this form of bone disease does not result from uremia *per se* (89).

Diagnosis of aluminum associated bone disease is based on the clinical features of bone pain, pathological fractures, usually of the ribs and femoral neck, and proximal myopathy. Laboratory confirmation is made on bone biopsy showing classical osteomalacia with aluminum, as determined by aluminum staining, present between the junction of calcified and non-calcified bone (Figure 2). A marked increase in the quantity of bone aluminum is also observed (90). Initially it was felt that a second form of bone disease, adynamic bone disease, which is characterized by low turnover without hyperosteoidosis was also a result of aluminum intoxication. However, more recent studies do not support this contention, since avoidance of aluminum exposure (which has largely eliminated osteomalacic bone disease) has done little to decrease the incidence of adynamic bone disease (91).

Aluminum has also been shown to be toxic to the hematopoietic system (77, 78, 92). In uremic patients aluminum has been shown to cause a microcytic, hypochromic anemia in the setting of normal iron stores. This type of anemia usually occurs in the setting of other evidence of aluminum intoxication, such as bone disease or encephalopathy. Aluminum has also been shown to cause anemia in rats and rabbits (92). The anemia responds rapidly to aluminum chelation with deferoxamine. In addition aluminum induced anemia is resistant to erythropoietin therapy. This resistance is rapidly reversed by deferoxamine chelation (93).

Management of aluminum toxicity

A major impetus has been directed at the prevention of aluminum intoxication. There are now easily achievable standards for acceptable levels of aluminum in water used to prepare the dialysis fluid, ($< 10 \mu g$/liter). Materials in the dialysis system containing Al, as well as other leachable elements, should be avoided. Currently the major potential source of aluminum intoxication is from orally administered aluminum compounds commonly given to individuals with chronic renal failure to reduce phosphate absorption from the gastrointestinal tract to prevent hyperphosphatemia. Calcium carbonate and calcium acetate are being used increasingly as phosphate binders replacing aluminum containing phosphate binders (94, 95). Although the calcium salts are not as effective as aluminum in binding phosphate they are frequently adequate for controlling phosphate. Even when they are not adequate alone, when given in combination with aluminum containing phosphate binders they help reduce the amount of aluminum binders required to control serum phosphorus levels. To avoid toxicity patients with advanced renal failure receiving aluminum compounds should have plasma aluminum concentrations measured serially, and aluminum dosage modified if plasma aluminum levels exceed 20 to 25 μg/liter. Aluminum compounds should be avoided totally in uremic children.

Treatment of aluminum intoxication initially involves the removal of all parenteral and oral sources of aluminum. Following removal of parenteral exposure via dialysis fluid a number of patients with osteomalacia and far fewer with dialysis encephalopathy have recovered from aluminum intoxication without additional treatment (74, 75). Chelation therapy for aluminum intoxication has been widely used and adequately evaluated only in patients with dialysis dependent renal failure. (74, 75, 96–98). A number of different approaches to chelation have been recommended. Unlike iron, the amount of aluminum chelated appears to be determined by the size of the chelatable aluminum pool and not the dose of deferoxamine administered (97, 99, 100). It has been found that 1 or 2 grams of deferoxamine is equally as effec-

tive as 4 grams in chelation of aluminum as determined by the rise in plasma aluminum concentrations following chelation. The most effective spacing between dosage of deferoxamine has not been clearly defined so it is unclear whether 1 to 2 grams of deferoxamine should be given once or three times weekly intravenously during the last hour of dialysis. Deferoxamine is as equally effective when given by the intramuscular or intraperitoneal route, as when given intravenously (101). Treatment of aluminum associated bone disease with deferoxamine usually results in symptomatic improvement in bone pain and proximal muscle weakness in 2 to 3 months (94, 97, 98). However, treatment should be continued for around 6 months and discontinued when there is a minimal rise in plasma aluminum levels following deferoxamine administration, which demonstrates depletion of the chelatable aluminum pool. Symptomatic improvement has been found to occur as rapidly in patients given 0.5 grams deferoxamine weekly, as in patients given 6 grams weekly (97). Aluminum induced anemia responds in as similar a time period as symptomatic bone disease. In contrast aluminum associated neurological toxicity requires a more extended duration of treatment with deferoxamine. Although progression of the neurological disease may stabilize, improvement frequently requires 10–12 months of continuous treatment with deferoxamine (102, 107). With adequate treatment EEG abnormalities may resolve making EEG measurement important in determining duration of therapy. Following discontinuation of therapy, especially if too short, recurrence of aluminum neurotoxicity is not uncommon.

Therapy with deferoxamine is not without some risk. As described above patients with marked aluminum overload may develope acute neurological toxicity following deferoxamine therapy (83). Acute infections with Yersinia and mucormycosis have also been reported in patients receiving deferoxamine (104, 105). It is felt that feroxamine is an iron supplier promoting growth, of these non-siderophore producing organisms. Therefore, prior to treatment, the diagnosis of aluminum intoxication should be reasonably well established and evidence of aluminum overload demonstrated (either by a rise in plasma aluminum concentrations greater than 150 to 200 μg/liter following deferoxamine infusion or increased bone aluminum levels in association with classical histological findings of aluminum associated bone disease).

Cobalt intoxication

One well-documented case of cobalt-induced cardiomyopathy, characterized by extensive myocardial necrosis, has been reported in a dialysis patient receiving cobaltous chloride for treatment of anemia (106–108). High levels of cobalt were found in the myocardium of an additional four patients, but the histological features were much less distinctive.

Zinc deficiency

The second elemental alteration that has received considerable attention is zinc. Most studies have found decreased levels of zinc in serum, leukocytes and muscles of uremic patients (9–11). All other tissue stores of zinc have been found to be normal or increased in uremic patients (28). On the basis of low serum zinc levels, a number of investigators have suggested that certain symptoms and findings in renal failure such as hypogeusia, anorexia, impotence, and hormonal alterations (for example, low testosterone levels and increased LH, FSH and prolactin) are a result of zinc depletion. Zinc supplementation was reported to improve sexual function, increase testosterone levels and sperm counts, and decrease FSH, LH and prolactin levels in a group of dialysis patients (109–114). In a similar patient population however, zinc replacement had no effect on sexual function, testosterone levels nor gonadotrophin levels. Findings about zinc regarding smell, taste and appetite have also been conflicting (115–117).

CONCLUSIONS

The full importance of trace element disturbances in producing disease in dialyzed uremic patients has not been fully defined. At this time acute intoxication has been associated with aluminum, copper, zinc, nickel, fluoride and nitrates. Exposure to and toxicity from all of these elements has been a consequence of the delivery by dialysis fluid or from components of the dialysis system. No naturally occurring trace element constituent of municipal water supplies has yet been shown to produce toxicity. The only well documented chronic toxicity has resulted from aluminum. Exposure has resulted from either water contamination by aluminum or orally administered aluminum containing phosphate binding agents. No unequivocal essential trace element deficiency syndromes have been occured in either dialyzed or non-dialyzed uremic patients. Although a number of other trace element alterations have been documented in uremic patients their clinical significance, if any, awaits recognition.

REFERENCES

1. Dworkin B, Weseley S, Rosenthal WS, Schwartz EM, Weiss L: Diminished blood selenium levels in renal failure patients on dialysis: correlations with nutritional status. *Am J Med Sci* 293: 6, 1987
2. Turan B, Delilbasi E, Dalay N, Sert S, Afrasyap L, Sayal A: Serum selenium and glutathione-peroxidase activities and their interaction with toxic metals in dialysis and renal transplantation patients. *Biol Trace Elem Res* 33: 95, 1992
3. Foote JW, Hinks LJ, Lloyd B: Reduced plasma and white blood cell selenium levels in haemodialysis patients. *Clin Chim Acta* 164: 323, 1987
4. Girelli D, Olivieri O, Stanzial AM, Azzini M, Lupo A, Bernich P, Menini C, Gammaro L, Corrocher R: Low platelet glutathione peroxidase activity and serum selenium concentration in patients with chronic renal failure: relations to dialysis treatments, diet and cardiovascular complications. *Clin Sci* 84: 611, 1993
5. Kostakopoulos A, Kotsalos A, Alexopoulos J, Sofras F, Deliveliotis C, Dallistratos G: Serum selenium levels in healthy adults and its changes in chronic renal failure. *Int Urol Nephrol* 22: 397, 1990
6. Kallistratos G, Evangelou A, Seferiadis K, Vezyraki P, Barboutis K: Selenium and haemodialysis: serum selenium levels in healthy persons, non-cancer and cancer patients with chronic renal failure. *Nephron* 41: 217, 1985
7. Milly K, Wit L, Diskin C, Tulley R: Selenium in renal failure patients. *Nephron* 61: 139, 1992
8. Antos M, Jeren-Strujic B, Romic Z, Matanovic B, Gudel-Greguric J: Serum selenium levels in patients on hemodialysis. *Trace Elements in Medicine* 10: 173, 1993
9. Avasthi G, Singh HP, Katyal JC, Avasthi R, Aggarwal SP: Copper, zinc, calcium and magnesium in chronic renal failure. *J Assoc Phys India* 39: 531, 1991
10. Muirhead N, Kertesz A, Flanagan PR, Hodsman AV, Hollomby DJ, Valberg LS: Zinc metabolism in patients on maintenance Hemodialysis. *Am J Nephrol* 6: 422, 1986
11. Joven J, Villabona C, Rubies-Prat J, Espinel E, Galard R: Hormonal profile and serum zinc levels in uraemic men with gonadal dysfunction undergoing haemodialysis. *Clin Chim Acta* 148: 239, 1985
12. Hosokawa S, Oyamaguchi A, Yoshida O: Trace elements and complications in patients undergoing chronic hemodialysis. *Nephron* 55: 375, 1990
13. McNeely MD, Sunderman FW jr, Michay MW, Levine H: Abnormal concentrations of nickel in serum in case of myocardial infarction, stroke, burns, hepatic cirrhosis, and uremia. *Clin Chem* 17: 1123, 1971
14. Hosokawa S, Nishitani H, Umemura K, Tomoyoshi T, Sawanishi K, Osamu Y: Serum and corpuscular nickel and zinc in chronic hemodialysis patients. *Nephron* 45: 151, 1987
15. Wallaeys B, Cornelis R, Mees L, Lameire N: Trace elements in serum, packed cells and dialysis fluid of CAPD patients. *Kidney Int* 30: 599, 1986
16. Bello-Reuss EN, Grady TP, Mazumdar DC: Serum vanadium levels in chronic renal disease. *Ann Intern Med* 91: 743, 1979
17. Tsukamoto Y, Saka S, Kumano K, Iwanami S, Ishida O, Marumo F: Abnormal accumulation of vanadium in patients on chronic hemodialysis therapy. *Nephron* 56: 368, 1990
18. Hosokawa S, Yoshida O: Serum vanadium levels in chronic hemodialysis patients. *Nephron* 64: 388, 1993
19. Hosokawa S, Yoshida O: Vanadium in chronic hemodialysis patients. *Int J Artif Organs* 13: 197, 1990
20. Hosokawa S, Yamaguchi O, Yoshida O: Vanadium transfer during haemodialysis. *Int Urol Nephrol* 23: 407, 1991
21. Gitelman HJ, Alderman FR, Perry SJ: Silicon accumulation in dialysis patients. *Am J Kidney Dis* 19: 140, 1992

1268   *Allen C. Alfrey*

22. Berlyne G, Dudek E, Adler AJ, Rubin JE, Seidman M: Silicon metabolism: the basic facts in renal failure. *Kidney Int* 17 (Suppl) S175, 1985
23. Dobbie JW, Smith MJ: The silicon content of body fluids. *Scot Med J* 27: 17, 1982
24. Mauras Y, Riberi P, Cartier F, Allain P: Increase in blood silicon concentration in patients with renal failure. *Biomedicine* 33: 228, 1980
25. Kaehny WD, Alfrey AC, Holman RE, Shorr WJ: Aluminum transfer during hemodialysis. *Kidney Int* 12: 361, 1977
26. Durr JA, Miller NL, Alfrey AC: Lithium clearance derived from the natural trace blood and urine lithium levels. *Kidney Int* 28 (Suppl) S58, 1990
27. Rudolph H, Alfrey AC, Smythe WR: Muscle and serum trace element profile in uremia. *Trans Am Soc Artif Intern Organs* 19: 456, 1973
28. Smythe WR, Alfrey AC, Craswell PW, Crouch CA, Ibels LS, Kubo H, Nunnelley LL, Rudolph H: Trace element abnormalities in chronic uremia. *Ann Intern Med* 96: 302, 1982
29. Nunnelley LL, Smythe WR, Alfrey AC, Ibels LS: Uremic hyperstannum: elevated tissue tin levels associated with uremia. *J Lab Clin Med* 91: 72, 1978
30. Indraprasit S, Alexander GV, Gonick HC: Tissue composition of major and trace elements in uremia and hypertension. *J Chronic Dis* 27: 135, 1974
31. Cordy PE, Gagnon R, Taves DR, Kaye M: Bone disease in hemodialysis patients with particular reference to the effect of fluoride. *Can Med Assoc J* 110: 1349, 1974
32. Navarro JA, Granadillo VA, Salgado O, Rodriguez-Iturbe B, Garcia R, Delling G, Romero RA: Bone metal content in patients with chronic renal failure. *Clin Chem Acta* 211: 133, 1992
33. Tipton IH, Cook MJ: Trace elements in human tissue. Part II Adult subjects from the United States. *Health Physics* 9: 103, 1963
34. Ittel TH, Buddington B, Miller NL, Alfrey AC: Enhanced gastrointestinal absorption of aluminum in uremic rats. *Kidney Int* 32: 821, 1987
35. Ittel TH, Griessner A, Sieberth HG: Effect of lactate on the absorption and retention of aluminum in the remnant kidney rat model. *Nephron* 57: 332, 1991
36. Lindholm T, Thysell H, Ljunggren L, Divino JC, Schunnesson M, Stenstam M: Aluminum in patients with uremia and patients with enteropathy. *Nieren- und Hochdruckkrankheiten* 12: 192, 1983
37. Provan SD, Yokel RA: Aluminum uptake by the *in situ* rat gut preparation. *J Pharmacol Exp Ther* 245: 928, 1988
38. Froment DH, Molitoris BA, Buddington B, Miller NL, Alfrey AC: Site and mechanism of enhanced gastrointestinal absorption of aluminum by citrate. *Kidney Int* 36: 978, 1989
39. Goldstein DA, Horowitz RE, Petit S, Haldimann B, Massry SG: The duodenal mucosa in patients with renal failure: response to 1,25 (OH)$_2$D3. *Kidney Int* 19: 324, 1981
40. Ittel TH, Paulus CP, Handt S, Hofstadter F, Sieberth HG: Induction of intestinal mucosal atrophy by difluoromethylornithine: a nonuremic model of enhanced aluminum absorption. *Mineral Electrolyte Metab* 18: 15, 1992

41. Kovalchik MT, Kaehny WD, Hegg A, Jackson JT, Alfrey AC: Aluminum kinetics during hemodialysis. *J Lab Clin Med* 92: 712, 1978
42. Alfrey AC: Aluminum metabolism in uremia. *Neurotoxicology* 1: 43, 1980
43. Alfrey AC, Hegg A, Craswell P: Metabolism and toxicity of aluminum in renal failure. *Am J Clin Nutr* 33: 1509, 1980
44. Cartwright GE, Gubler CJ, Wintrobe MM: Studies on copper metabolism XI. Copper and iron metabolism in the nephrotic syndrome. *J Clin Invest* 33: 685, 1954
45. Ellis D: Anemia in the course of the nephrotic syndrome secondary to transferrin depletion. *J Pediatr* 90: 953, 1977
46. Brown EA, Sampson B, Muller BR, Curtis JR: Urinary iron loss in the nephrotic syndrome – an unusual cause of iron deficiency with a note on urinary copper losses. *Postgrad Med J* 160: 125, 1984
47. Parkinson IS, Ward MK, Feest TG, Fawcett RWP, Kerr DNS: Fracturing dialysis osteodystrophy and dialysis encephalopathy. An epidemiological survey. *Lancet* 1: 406, 1979
48. Platts MM, Goode GC, Hislop JS: Composition of the domestic water supply and the incidence of fractures and encephalopathy in patients on home dialysis. *Br Med J* 2: 657, 1977
49. Cartier F, Allain P, Garv J, Chatel M, Men Ault F, Pecker S: Encephalopathie myclonique progressive des dialyses. Role de l'eau utilisee pour l'hemodialyse. *Nouv Presse Med* 7: 97, 1978
50. McDermott JR, Smith AI, Ward MK, Faucett RWP, Kerr DNS: Brain-aluminum concentration in dialysis encephalopathy. *Lancet* 1: 901, 1978
51. Padovese P, Gallieni M, Brancaccio D, Pietra R, Fortaner S, Sabbioni E, Minoia C, Markakis K, Berlin A: Trace elements in dialysis fluids and assessment of the exposure of patients on regular hemodialysis, hemofiltration and continuous ambulatory peritoneal dialysis. *Nephron* 61: 442, 1992
52. Sabbioni E, Pietra R, Ubertalli L, Berlin A, Speziali M: Salts as a source of metals in dialysis fluids: an assessment study by means of neutron activation analysis. *Sci Total Environ* 84: 13, 1989
53. Bello VA, Gitelman HJ: High fluoride exposure in hemodialysis patients. *Am J Kidney Dis* 15: 320, 1990
54. Carlson DJ, Shapiro FL: Methemoglobinemia from well water nitrates: a complication of home dialysis. *Ann Intern Med* 73: 757, 1970
55. Miller RG, Kopfler FC, Kelty KC, Stober JA, Ulmer NS: The occurrence of aluminum in drinking water. *Am Water Works Assoc* 77: 84, 1984
56. Fatal fluoride intoxication in a dialysis unit. [News] *J Public Health Dent* 40: 360, 1980
57. McIvor M, Baltazar RF, Beltran J, Mower MM, Wenk R, Lustgarten J, Salomon J: Hyperkalemia and cardiac arrest from fluoride exposure during hemodialysis. *Am J Cardiol* 51: 901, 1983
58. Flendrig JA, Kruis H, Das HA: Aluminum intoxication: The cause of dialysis dementia? *Proc Eur Dial Transplant Assoc* 13: 355, 1976
59. Burwen DR, Olsen SM, Bland LA, Arduino MJ, Reid MH, Jarvis WR: Epidemic aluminium intoxication in

hemodialysis patients traced to use of an aluminum pump. *Kidney Int* 48: 469, 1995

60. Pierides AM, Frohnert PP: Aluminum related dialysis osteomalacia and dementia after prolonged use of the Redy cartridge. *Trans Am Soc Artif Intern Organs* 27: 629, 1981

61. Gallery ED, Blomfield J, Dixon SR: Acute zinc toxicity in haemodialysis. *Br Med J* 4: 331, 1972

62. Webster JD, Parker TF, Alfrey AC, Smythe WR, Kubo H, Neal G, Hull AR: Acute nickel intoxication by dialysis. *Ann Intern Med* 92: 631, 1980

63. Johnson WJ, Taves DR: Exposure to excessive fluoride during hemodialysis. *Kidney Int* 5: 451, 1974

64. Ivanovich P, Manzler A, Drake R: Acute hemolysis following hemodialysis. *Trans Am Soc Artif Intern Organs* 15: 316, 1969

65. Klein WJ Jr, Metz EN, Price AR: Acute copper intoxication. A hazard of hemodialysis. *Arch Intern Med* 129: 578, 1972

66. Lyle WH, Payton JE, Hui M: Haemodialysis and copper fever. *Lancet* 1: 1324, 1976

67. Lyle WH: Chronic dialysis and copper poisoning. *N Engl J Med* 276: 1209, 1967

68. AAMI: American National Standard for hemodialysis systems (ANSI/AAMI RD5-1981). Association for the Advancement of Medical Instrumentation, Arlington, VA, 1981

69. Kirschbaum BB, Schoolwerth AC: Acute aluminum toxicity associated with oral citrate and aluminum-containing antacids. *Am J Med Sci* 297: 9, 1989

70. Bakir AA, Hryhorczuk DO, Berman E, Dunea G: Acute fatal hyperaluminemic encephalopathy in undialyzed and recently dialyzed uremic patients. *Trans Am Soc Artif Intern Organs* 32: 171, 1986

71. Molitoris BA, Froment DH, Mackenzie TA, Huffer WH, Alfrey AC: Citrate: a major factor in the toxicity of orally administered aluminum compounds. *Kidney Int* 36: 949, 1989

72. Alfrey AC, LeGendre GR, Kaehny WD: The dialysis encephalopathy syndrome. Possible aluminum intoxication. *N Engl J Med* 294: 184, 1976

73. Ott SM, Maloney NA, Coburn JW, Alfrey AC, Sherrard DJ: The prevalence of bone aluminum deposition in renal osteodystrophy and its relation to the response to calcitriol therapy. *N Engl J Med* 307: 709, 1982

74. Pierides AM, Edwards WG Jr, Cullum UX Jr, McCall JT, Ellis HA: Hemodialysis encephalopathy with osteomalacic fractures and muscle weakness. *Kidney Int* 18: 115, 1980

75. Hodsman AB, Sherrard DJ, Alfrey AC, Ott S, Brickman AS, Miller NL, Maloney NA, Coburn JW: Bone aluminum and histomorphometric features of renal osteodystrophy. *Clin Endocrinol Metab* 54: 539, 1982

76. Hodsman AB, Sherrard D, Wong EGC, Brickman AS, Lee DBN, Alfrey AC, Singer SR, Norman AW, Coburn JW: Vitamin D-resistant osteomalacia in hemodialysis patients lacking secondary hyperparathyroidism. *Ann Intern Med* 94: 629, 1981

77. O'Hare JA, Murnaghan DJ: Reversal of aluminum-induced hemodialysis anemia by low-aluminum dialysis fluid. *N Engl J Med* 306: 654, 1982

78. Short ALK, Winney RJ, Robson JS: Reversible microcytic hypochromic anaemia in dialysis patients due to

aluminum intoxication. *Proc Eur Dial Transplant Assoc* 17: 226, 1980

79. Alfrey AC, Mishell MM, Burks J, Contiguglia SR, Rudolph H, Lewin E, Holmes JH: Syndrome of dyspraxia and multifocal seizures associated with chronic hemodialysis. *Trans Am Soc Artif Intern Organs* 18: 257, 1972

80. Burks JS, Alfrey AC, Huddlestone J, Norenberg MD, Lewin E: A fatal encephalopathy in chronic hemodialysis patients. *Lancet* 1: 764, 1976

81. Schreeder MT: Dialysis encephalopathy. *Arch Intern Med* 139: 510, 1979

82. Rozas VV, Port KF, Rutt WM: Progressive dialysis encephalopathy from dialysis fluid aluminum. *Arch Intern Med* 138: 1375, 1978

83. Sherrard DJ, Walker JV, Boykin JL: Precipitation of dialysis dementia by deferoxamine treatment of aluminum related bone disease. *Am J Kidney Dis* 12: 126, 1988

84. Sedman AB, Wilkening GN, Warady BA, Lum GM, Alfrey AC: Encephalopathy in childhood secondary to aluminum toxicity. *J Pediatr* 105: 836, 1984

85. Sedman AB, Miller NL, Warady BA, Lum GM, Alfrey AC: Aluminum loading in children with chronic renal failure. *Kidney Int* 26: 201, 1984

86. Milne FJ, Sharf B, Bell P, Meyer AM: The effect of low aluminum water and desferrioxamine on the outcome of dialysis encephalopathy. *Clin Nephrol* 20: 202, 1983

87. Llach F, Felsenfeld AJ, Coleman MD, Keveney JJ, Pederson JA, Medlock TR: The natural course of dialysis osteomalacia. *Kidney Int* 29 (Suppl 18): 74S, 1986

88. Chan Y-L, Furlong TJ, Cornish CJ, Posen S: Dialysis osteodystrophy – a study involving 94 patients. *Medicine* 64: 296, 1985

89. Dahl E, Nordal KP, Attramadal A, Halse J, Flatmark A: Renal osteodystrophy in predialysis patients without stainable bone aluminum. *Acta Med Scand* 224: 157, 1988

90. Maloney NA, Ott S, Alfrey AC, Coburn JW, Sherrard DJ: Histologic quanitation of aluminum in iliac bone from patients with renal failure. *J Lab Clin Med* 99: 206, 1981

91. Moriniere P, Cohen-Solal M, Belbrik S, Boudailliez B, Marie A, Westeel PF, Renaud H, Fievet P, Lalau JD, Sebert JL, Fournier A: Disappearance of aluminic bone disease in a long term asymptomatic dialysis population restricting Al(OH)$_3$ intake: emergence of an idiopathic adynamic bone disease not related to aluminum. *Nephron* 53: 93, 1989

92. Touam M, Martinez F, Lacour B, Zingraff J, DiGiulio S, Drueke T: Aluminum-induced, reversible microcytic anemia in chronic renal failure: clinical and experimental studies. *Clin Nephrol* 19: 295, 1983

93. Casati S, Castelnovo C, Campise M, Ponticelli C: Aluminum interference in the treatment of haemodialysis patients with recombinant erythropoietin. *Nephrol Dial Transplant* 5: 441, 1990

94. Fournier A, Moriniere P, Sebert J, Dkhiss H, Abssewe A, Leflow P, Renaud H, Gueris J, Gregoire I, Isrissi A, Garabedian M: Calcium carbonate, an aluminum-free agent for control of hyperphosphatemia, hypocalcemia and hyperparathyroidism in uremia. *Kidney Int* 29 (Suppl 18): 114S, 1986

95. Sheikh MS, Maquire JA, Emmett M, Santa Ana C, Nicar MK, Schiller LR, Fordtran JS: Reduction of dietary phos-

phorus absorption by phosphorus binders: a theoretical, *in vitro* and *in vivo* study. *J Clin Invest* 83: 66, 1989

96. Milne FJ, Hudson GA, Meyers AM, Baily P, Barmeir E, Dubowitz B, Reis P: Healing of fracturing bone disease occurring in patients on dialysis. *Afr Med J* 61: 955, 1982

97. Kurokawa K, Marumo F, Ogura Y, Ono T, Suzuki S: Aluminum associated bone disease: Considerations on the pathogenesis and the effects of deferoxamine treatment. *J Univ Occupational Environ Health* 9 (Suppl): 133, 1987

98. Nebeker HG, Milliner DS, Ott SM, Sherrard DJ, Alfrey AC, Abuelo JG, Wasserstein A, Coburn JW: Aluminum-related osteomalacia: clinical response to desferrioxamine. *Kidney Int* 25: 173, 1984

99. Ciancioni C, Poignet JL, Mauras Y, Panthier G, Delows S, Allain P: Plasma aluminum and iron kinetics in hemodialyzed patients after IV infusion of desferrioxamine. *Trans Am Soc Artif Intern Organs* 30: 479, 1984

100. Ciancioni C, Poignet JL, Naret C, Delows S, Mauras Y, Allain P, Man NK: Concomitant removal of aluminum and iron by haemodialysis and haemofiltration after desferrioxamine intravenous infusion. *Proc Eur Dial Transplant Assoc–Eur Renal Assoc* 21: 469, 1984

101. Molitoris BA, Alfrey PS, Miller NL, Hasbargen JA, Kaehny WD, Alfrey AC, Smith BJ: Efficacy of intramuscular and intraperitoneal deferoxamine for aluminum chelation. *Kidney Int* 31: 986, 1987

102. Ackrill P, Ralston A J, Day JP, Hodge KG: Successful removal of aluminum from patient with dialysis encephalopathy. *Lancet* 2: 692, 1980

103. Ackrill P, Ralston AJ, Day JP: The role of desferrioxamine in the treatment of dialysis encephalopathy. *Kidney Int* 29 (Suppl 18): S104, 1986

104. Veis JH, Contiguglia R, Klein M, Mishell J, Alfrey, AC, Shapiro JI: Mucormycosis in deferoxamine treated patients on dialysis. *Ann Intern Med* 107: 258, 1987

105. Brock JH: The effect of desferrioxamine on the growth of staphylococcus aureus, yersinia enterocolitica and streptococcus faecalis in human sera: uptake of deferoxamine-bound iron. *FEMS Microbiol Lett* 20: 439, 1983

106. Pehrsson K, Lins LE: Cobalt in uraemic cardiomyopathy. *Lancet* 2: 51, 1978

107. Lins LE, Pehrsson K: Cobalt intoxication in uraemic myocardiopathy? *Lancet* 1: 1191, 1976

108. Manifold IH, Platts MM, Kennedy A: Cobalt cardiomyopathy in a patient on maintenance haemodialysis. *Br Med J* 2: 1609, 1978

109. Atkin-Thor E, Goddard BW, O'Nion J, Stephen RL, Kolff WJ: Hypogeusia and zinc depletion in chronic dialysis patients. *Am J Clin Nutr* 31: 1948, 1978

110. Mahajan SK, Abbasi AA, Prasad AS, Briggs WA, McDonald FD: Effect of zinc therapy on uremic hypogonadism: a double blind study. *Proc Clin Dial Transplant Forum* 9: 260, 1979

111. Mahajan SK, Gardiner WH, Abbasi AA, Prasad AS, Briggs WA, McDonald FD: Hypogeusia in patients on hemodialysis. *Proc Clin Dial Transplant Forum* 8: 20, 1978

112. Mahajan SK, Prasad AS, Lambujon J, Abbasi AA, Briggs WA, McDonald FD: Improvement of uremic hypogeusia by zinc. *Trans Am Soc Artif Intern Organs* 25: 443, 1979

113. Mahajan SK, Abbasi AA, Prasad AS, Rabbani P, Briggs WA, McDonald FD: Effect of oral zinc therapy on gonadal function in hemodialysis patients. A double-blind study. *Ann Intern Med* 97: 357, 1982

114. Antoniou LD, Shalhoub RJ, Sudhakar T, Smith JC Jr: Reversal of uraemic impotence by zinc. *Lancet* 2: 895, 1977

115. Brook AC, Johnston DG, Ward MK, Watson MJ, Cook DB, Kerr DN: Absence of a therapeutic effect of zinc in the sexual dysfunction of haemodialysed patients. *Lancet* 2 (8195 pt 1): 618, 1980

116. Zetin M, Stone RA: Effects of zinc in chronic hemodialysis. *Clin Nephrol* 13: 20, 1980

117. Rodger RS, Brook AC, Muirhead N, Kerr DN: Zinc metabolism does not influence sexual function in chronic renal insufficiency. *Contrib Nephrol* 38: 112, 1984

MALNUTRITION AND DIALYSIS

DENIS FOUQUE and JOEL D. KOPPLE

NUTRITIONAL STATUS AS A RISK FACTOR FOR PATIENTS WITH END-STAGE RENAL DISEASE (ESRD)

Maintenance hemodialysis

Several studies indicate that in patients undergoing maintenance hemodialysis (MHD) or chronic peritoneal dialysis (CPD), a low dietary protein intake as well as biochemical markers of protein or calorie malnutrition are associated with increased morbidity and mortality. MHD patients with low serum urea nitrogen (SUN) levels or decreased protein nitrogen appearance (also referred to as PCR) have increased morbidity or mortality (1, 2). Since in MHD patients, low SUN is associated with low dietary protein intake, these data suggest that decreased dietary protein intake is a risk factor for mortality. In 98 non-diabetic MHD patients followed for 12 months, an inverse relationship has been observed between the protein nitrogen appearance and the frequency of hospitalizations and mortality rate (2). In 1990, Lowrie and Lew showed that, in over 12,000 MHD patients followed for

12 months, of various predialysis serum chemistries, the serum albumin exhibited the most striking odds ratio for survival (3). The odds ratio for mortality rose exponentially as serum albumin fell. Low serum cholesterol, urea, potassium, phosphorus and creatinine were also associated with increased mortality, but to a lesser extent. Since, in MHD patients these low values often reflect reduced dietary protein intake or muscle protein mass, these data provide further evidence that decreased nutritional intake is associated with increased mortality. These investigators later reported that most of the predictive power for the increased death risk associated with diabetes mellitus can be accounted for by the serum creatinine and albumin. The multicenter Canadian Hemodialysis Morbidity Study (4) reported a direct correlation between the serum albumin level and the morbidity and mortality risk in 486 MHD patients. A serum albumin level less than 3.0 g/dl was associated with a higher rate of arterio-venous shunt thrombosis, pulmonary edema, infections other than of vascular accesses, days of hospitalization and death. Two other recent studies also confirm that a low serum albumin

concentration is a strong predictor of high death rates (5, 6).

Chronic peritoneal dialysis

A study of 51 patients undergoing CAPD who were followed for five years showed that those patients who were not hospitalized had a higher normalized protein nitrogen appearance rate (nPNA or nPCR), a higher KT urea (the sum of the total dialysate and urinary urea clearances) and higher SUN (7). Patients who survived as compared to those who died had a greater serum albumin level (3.73 ± 37 *vs* 3.41 ± 0.34 g/dl, *p* < 0.01) and younger age. Also, a low serum albumin concentration was a strong predictor of death and number of hospitalization days. Neither Kt/V nor nPNA was correlated with these outcomes. Other workers reported that serum albumin was negatively correlated with the patients degree of fatigue as assessed by scoring on a scale of fatigue (8). In this latter study, serum albumin was also lower in diabetics than non-diabetics and in patients older than 65 years than in younger patients (8). Also, in 45 patients commencing CAPD who were followed for at least 12 months, serum albumin was the best predictor of mortality. Patients who were not hospitalized during the study had a significantly greater serum albumin level (9).

Furthermore, a recent large scale study involving 698 patients from 10 centers across the USA and Canada reported that serum albumin was the parameter most predictive of survival (10). Indeed, when serum albumin was greater than 3.5 g/dl, one and two year survival rates were 96 and 88% respectively, whereas the rates were only 89 and 68% when serum albumin was lower than 3.5 g/dl.

What is the clinical importance of these findings? About 25% of maintenance hemodialysis patients have a serum albumin lower than 3.7 g/dl and a serum cholesterol below 155 mg/dl (3). These values are associated with a higher mortality in MHD patients. It should be emphasized that these findings do not indicate that improving nutritional status by increasing nutritional intake or other maneuvers will reduce morbidity or mortality. Although, intuitively, this would seem to be a beneficial approach for improving outcome, it is also possible that the same illnesses that engender malnutrition will cause independently the high morbidity and mortality, and that the patient's protein-calorie malnutrition does not affect outcome. Although this latter explanation does not seem likely, further studies will be necessary to resolve this question.

The syndrome of protein and calorie malnutrition (Table 1)

Virtually every study of the nutritional status of chronically uremic patients and patients undergoing maintenance hemodialysis or chronic peritoneal dialysis indicates that such patients frequently manifest protein-calorie malnutrition (11–21). About one-third of patients have mild to

Table 1. Evidence for wasting or protein-calorie malnutrition in advanced chronic renal failure

Anthropometry, body composition	Biochemistry
Decrease in	*Decrease in*
Body weight	*Serum*
Height (children)	Total protein
Growth (children)	Albumin
Body fat	Transferrin
Fat-free solids	Prealbumin
Intra-cellular water	C1q
Muscle mass	C3
Total body potassium	Cholinesterase
(non-dialyzed patients)	Pseudocholinesterase
Total body nitrogen	
(CAPD patients)	*Plasma*
Total albumin mass,	Isoleucine
synthesis and catabolism	Leucine
Valine pools (non-dialyzed	Total tryptophan
patients)	Valine
	Tyrosine
	Valine/glycine ratio
	Essential/non-essential ratio
	Muscle
	3-Methyl histidine
	RNA/DNA ratio
	Valine
	Tyrosine
	Normal or increase in
	Plasma total non-essential amino acids
	Glycine

moderate malnutrition, and 6 to 8% have severe malnutrition. The evidence for malnutrition includes decreased relative body weight (RBW, the patient's body weight divided by the weight of normal people of the same age, height, gender and frame size), skinfold thickness (an estimation of body fat), arm muscle circumference and cross-sectional area (an indicator of total muscle or somatic protein mass), decreased serum albumin, transferrin, prealbumin, certain complement proteins and low growth rates in children. The pattern of plasma amino acids observed in chronic renal failure, although unique to this condition, shows many similarities to that observed in protein-calorie malnutrition. Total body nitrogen and bioelectrical impedance measurements also support the presence of a high incidence of protein-calorie malnutrition.

A high prevalence of protein-calorie malnutrition is present in patients commencing MHD or CPD (22). Those MHD patients who are malnourished at the onset of dialysis therapy are likely to be malnourished one to two years later. Conversely, those individuals who are well nourished at the onset of maintenance dialysis therapy are likely to remain well nourished. It is not uncommon for CPD patients to gain weight during the first six to 12 months of peritoneal dialysis treatment (23); however, this added weight appears to be at least largely fat and/or excess water (23). Recent evidence suggests that protein-calorie malnutrition often begins incipiently when the glomerular filtration rate (GFR) is about 28–35 ml/min/1.73 m^2 or even higher (24). However, patients usually do not become frankly malnourished until the GFR is 4–5 ml/min/1.73 m^2 or lower.

During CAPD, insufficient protein intake is potentially more serious because of the continuous nature of peritoneal protein losses, compared to minimal protein loss during hemodialysis treatment. It is also important to recognize that other types of nutritional deficits may exist in patients with chronic renal failure. This include deficiencies of 1,25 dihydroxycholecalciferol, vitamin B$_6$, folic acid, iron and possibly carnitine, zinc and selenium (25–32).

Causes of protein-calorie malnutrition in patients with chronic renal failure

There are many possible causes for protein-calorie malnutrition in patients with chronic renal failure or individuals receiving maintenance dialysis therapy. The most important cause is almost certainly inadequate nutrient intake due to anorexia. Anorexia may be caused by many factors including uremic toxins, gastrointestinal disorders such as peptic ulcers, gastritis or esophagitis (e.g., from gastroesophageal reflux), unpalatable medicines (e.g., phosphate binders or calcium supplements), superimposed acute or chronic illnesses (e.g., diabetes mellitus, vasculitides), and such emotional or psychosocial disorders like loneliness, depression and poverty (14–16, 18, 33–36). Before starting maintenance dialysis, routinely low protein and low phosphate diets are prescribed. These diets, even if carefully monitored, may be sometimes low in protein intake as well as hypocaloric (24, 37, 38) and therefore may be deleterious to the nutritional status before starting dialysis.

It is recognized commonly that maintenance dialysis patients spontaneously reduce their nutritional intake. This begins before the onset of end-stage renal disease. Indeed, spontaneous energy and protein intake are often reduced when the GFR falls below approximately 28 ml/min/1.73 m^2 (24). Dietary energy and protein intake gradually continue to fall as the GFR decreases below these values. When maintenance dialysis treatment is started, the spontaneous nutrient intake does not normalize. Jacob and colleagues (39) reported that 45% of 61 MHD patients had a protein intake less than 1.0 g/kg BW/d, whereas Bergström and associates found that 12% of 117 unselected MHD patients had a protein intake below 0.8 g/kg BW/d (36). A recent report of the pilot Mortality and Morbidity in Maintenance Hemodialysis (MMHD) study (40) showed a low energy intake (28 kcal/kg BW/d), that was further reduced in diabetic patients (25 kcal/kg BW/d). These energy intakes are substantially less than the 35 kcal/kg BW/d usually recommended for MHD patients or normal individuals, and may partly explain why long term hemodialysis patients are frequently malnourished.

The neuroregulation of appetite is far from understood in patients with chronic renal failure. Indeed, it has been suggested that, in addition to such factors as impaired gastrointestinal motility, poorly palatable diets and postdialysis malaise, some uremic toxins appear to directly affect appetite. Bergström and colleagues recently infused uremic ultrafiltrate into the peritoneal cavity of rats. Compared to rats infused with saline or plasma ultrafiltrate from healthy humans, the rats infused with uremic ultrafiltrate demonstrated a net reduction in their spontaneous food intake (41). Ultrafiltrate fractionation studies suggest that the molecular weight of the anorexia producing compound or compounds was about 1,000 to 5,000 Daltons (41).

These observations suggest that more intensive dialysis therapy might increase appetite by removing uremic toxins. Indeed, the dose of dialysis (Kt/V urea) is related to the UNA or PCR and, hence, dietary protein intake. Lindsay and associates increased the dose of dialysis in a group of MHD patients, and observed a spontaneous increase in PNA without evidence of catabolic events, suggesting that patients had increased their protein intake (42). Interestingly, for the same urea clearance, estimated protein intake was greater in CAPD patients with low Kt/V values and increased more rapidly when improving Kt/V compared to MHD patients (43). This fact suggests that the control of nutritional intake may be better achieved with CPD than MHD patients for comparable urea clearances. On the other hand, in many patients the PNA does not become normal when the Kt/V is increased. Although this might reflect the fact that Kt/V is not sufficiently high in these patients, it is possible that comorbid factors, poorly dialyzable compounds or other factors may contribute to the anorexia and that a high dose of dialysis, within a range that is attainable routinely may improve, but may not eradicate anorexia in many patients.

The dialysis procedure itself may promote wasting by removing nutrients and also, in the case of hemodialysis, by stimulating protein catabolism. Hemodialysis increases the urea nitrogen appearance (UNA or net urea generation), enhances net protein breakdown and promotes negative nitrogen balance (44, 45). During sham hemodialysis in normal volunteers, Guttierez et al. (45) reported an increased release of amino acids from the leg, indicating enhanced net muscle protein breakdown. Lim and coworkers were unable to confirm an effect of hemodialysis on protein catabolism, possibly because of the experimental methods employed (46). The bioincompatible nature of dialyzer membranes may stimulate the release of cytokines, such as interleukin-1, which may be the cause of the enhanced protein catabolism. Biocompatibility is discussed more fully elsewhere in this volume.

During a routine hemodialysis treatment using a low flux cuprophane membrane, 4–9 g of free amino acids may be lost through the dialyzer during fasting, and 8 to 10 g if patients are eating during the procedure (47, 48). Peptides are also removed at a magnitude of 2 to 3 g per dialysis (48), therefore leading to a net amino acid loss of 10 to 13 g per dialysis session (36). With high flux dialyzers in fasting patients about 8.0 ± 2.8 g (mean $\pm$ SD) of free amino acids are removed during a routine hemodialysis treatment (49). This is not different from the amount of free amino acids removed with low flux hemodialysis (12.6 ± 3.6 g) when patients receive intradialytic parenteral nutrition providing 42 g of amino acids and 200 g of dextrose monohydrate (50).

During hemodialysis with glucose-free dialysate, an average of 20 to 30 g of glucose is lost into the dialysate (51, 52). If dialysate containing 200 mg/dl (11 mmol/l) of glucose monohydrate (180 mg/dl of anhydrous glucose) is used, there is a net positive mass transfer to the patient of 10 to 30 g of glucose during each dialysis (51, 52).

Reuse of dialyzers has become a routine procedure in the United States (53). Although usually very small amounts of protein are lost during a single hemodialysis, Kaplan et al. (54) recently reported markedly increased protein losses when polysulfone membranes were reprocessed many times with bleach and formaldehyde. After 20 to 25 reuses, up to 17 g of protein were lost per hemodialysis (54). Protein losses do not seem to increase markedly until reprocessing exceed ten times. Interestingly, when the use of bleach for dialyzer reprocessing was discontinued, the patients underwent a significant increase in serum albumin, from 3.6 to 3.8 g/dl, which was considered to be due to reduced protein leakage through the dialyzers (54).

During CAPD, about 2 to 3.5 g of amino acids are lost to the dialysate (55, 56). Total daily protein losses are about 8.8 g; albumin accounts for about 6 g in the dialysate of healthy CAPD patients (57). However, protein losses may increase up to 15 to 20 g/d during mild bacterial peritonitis (57) and, in our experience, as high as 100 g/d before starting antibiotic therapy in patients with severe established peritonitis. With antibiotic treatment, protein losses fall rapidly but may remain elevated for days or weeks after the infection has come under control (57).

Deficiency of water soluble vitamins in maintenance dialysis patients results primarily from insufficient intake, losses in dialysate, or altered vitamin synthesis or metabolism or possibly the presence of inhibitors to the actions of the vitamins. Water-soluble vitamins and other bioactive compounds are removed both by hemodialysis and peritoneal dialysis (27, 58–60). These losses are offset to some extent by reduced urinary excretion and are to some extent replaced by the vitamins provided in a regular diet. If patients have low nutrient intakes, these losses may enhance malnutrition. In fact, the content of several vitamins in typical meals ingested by maintenance dialysis patients is less than the Recommended Dietary Allowances of the Food and Nutrition Board (27). However, the need for water-soluble vitamins may vary with the new types of dialyzers used. The more porous high flux dialyzers remove greater quantities of vitamins.

Patients with chronic renal failure often lose blood from occult gastrointestinal bleeding, frequent blood sampling for laboratory tests and from the sequestration of blood in the hemodialyzer (61, 62). Blood losses may contribute to protein wasting. For example, a patient with a hemoglobin of 120 g/l and a serum total protein of 70 g/l will lose approximately 16.5 g of protein per 100 ml of blood removed. Also, when performing nitrogen balance studies in these patients, blood volume drawn during the study should be taken into account when considering nitrogen output.

Endocrine and metabolic disorders are frequently observed during chronic renal failure. There is a state of resistance to many anabolic hormones including insulin, growth hormone and insulin-like growth factor-1 (IGF-1) (63, 64). In addition, increased plasma concentrations of glucagon are well established (65, 66) and hyperparathyroidism may promote catabolism in maintenance dialysis patients. Since 25-hydroxycholecalciferol has been reported to increase muscle protein synthesis *in vitro* (67), its deficiency might be associated with muscle protein wasting. It is possible that, among the plethora of metabolic derangements in patients with chronic renal failure, some may promote malnutrition. Acidemia, a condition frequently observed in renal failure patients, increases protein catabolism (68–70). Cytosolic calcium is increased in advanced renal failure (71). This disorder appears to promote a number of metabolic abnormalities (72, 73); it is not known whether any of those abnormalities cause malnutrition.

ASSESSMENT OF NUTRITIONAL STATUS

Assessment of dietary intake

Assessment of the patient's nutrient intake is one of the most important aspects of nutritional assessment. Unfortunately, there is no simple and easy method for estimating nutritional intake. Essentially two methods of dietary assessment are available. Dietary protein intake may be examined by UNA and PNA calculations. Intake of protein as well as all other nutrients may be assessed from dietary diaries with interviews and by food frequency assessment. The use of the UNA to estimate protein intake is convenient and inexpensive. Several techniques and equations have been developed specifically for hemodialysis and peritoneal dialysis (see below). It should be emphasized that the methods for estimating UNA from dialysis kinetic measurements are not very precise. In addition, although the UNA and PNA correlate well with dietary protein intake in patients who are not very catabolic or anabolic and who do not have large losses of body proteins, the correlation is not precise (74). Therefore, clinical judgement is necessary when utilizing the UNA to estimate dietary protein intake in MHD or CPD patients.

Three to five day dietary diaries monitored by the patient and followed by an interview with a dietician, if done carefully with an experienced dietitian may give information on dietary protein intake with an accuracy that is not much different from data observed from dialysis urea kinetics. In addition, the dietary diaries can provide information on a large array of nutrients including energy intake, which often may be a major contributor to malnutrition in renal failure patients. Since the analysis of food intake is performed by computer, it consumes virtually no additional time to obtain the intake of many nutrients as compared to protein alone. The content of some nutrients, particularly trace elements and vitamins, of various foods is often less well established and may vary substantially. Moreover, the use of three to five day diaries with interviews is laborious and time consuming for the dietitian.

It is important to conduct the dietary diary recall for a minimum of about three days to ascertain nutrient intake in MHD patients in both dialysis and non-dialysis days. Assessing intake during both weekdays and weekends is also helpful for obtaining an accurate estimate of the patient's usual intake during his weekly cycle. Food diaries are rarely obtained for more than five to seven consecutive days because the meticulous nature required for maintaining these records can lead patients to lose interest and become inaccurate.

Recently, a Finnish study examined the reliability of 2-day food diaries compared to tray composition in 121 healthy adults. The deviation between the patient-maintained diary intake and the observed intake was less than 15% for all nutrients and was not influenced by age or gender (75). Of special interest, the differences between the energy and protein intake determined from the diaries as compared to direct observation from the food consumed from the tray were +3% and −3%, respectively (75).

Urea nitrogen appearance (UNA)

In patients who are not very anabolic or catabolic, the dietary nitrogen intake is correlated directly with the measured total nitrogen output (TNO). TNO usually can be accurately estimated by the urea nitrogen appearance (UNA). UNA is the amount of urea nitrogen that appears or accumulates in body fluids and all outputs (e.g., urine,

dialysate, fistula drainage). UNA can be calculated as follows:

$$UNA \text{ (g/day)} = \text{urinary urea nitrogen (g/day)}$$
$$+ \text{ dialysate urea nitrogen (g/day)}$$
$$+ \text{ change in body urea-nitrogen (g/day)} \quad [1]$$

Change in body urea nitrogen (g/day)
$$= (SUN_f - SUN_i, \text{ g/l/day})$$
$$\times BW_i(kg) \times (0.60 \text{ l/kg}) + (BW_f - BW_i, \text{ kg/day})$$
$$\times SUN_f \text{ (g/l)} \times (1.0 \text{ l/kg}), \quad [2]$$

where $_i$ and $_f$ are the initial and final values for the period of measurement; SUN is serum urea nitrogen (g/l); BW is body weight (kg); 0.60 is an estimate of the fraction of body weight that is total body water; and 1.0 is the volume of distribution of urea in the weight that is gained or lost.

The estimated proportion of body weight that is water may be increased in patients who are edematous or lean, and decreased in individuals who are obese or very young. Changes in body weight during the 1- to 3-day period of measurement of UNA are assumed to be due entirely to changes in body water. In patients undergoing hemodialysis or intermittent peritoneal dialysis, the urea concentration in dialysate is low and difficult to measure accurately, and UNA is usually calculated during the interdialytic interval and then normalized to 24 hours.

The strong correlation between the UNA and nitrogen intake is useful for predicting the nitrogen intake in patients who are in neutral or slightly positive or negative nitrogen balance (74). However, in patients who are in very positive or negative balance such as in pregnancy or severe catabolic stress (infection, trauma), nitrogen output may not reflect intake. These latter situations are generally accompanied by obvious alterations of patients' clinical status and easy to identify.

In MHD patients, the use of dialysis kinetic techniques for determining UNA has been widely employed. Although generally useful, the dialysis kinetic approach is susceptible to several errors, including discrepancies between the published and actual clearance characteristics of individual hemodialyzers, unrecognized variations in blood and dialysate flow, and postdialysis disequilibrium between serum urea and other body urea pools (76). The recent development of an instrument that repetitively measures dialysate urea during hemodialysis treatment is very promising (77). In CPD patients, the relationship between dietary nitrogen intake, TNO and UNA is altered by the persistent peritoneal protein losses. Several equations have been developed, regarding the relationship between nitrogen intake and UNA, that adjust for these protein losses (78, 79).

Creatinine appearance

Since the quantity of creatinine in plasma or urine correlates with skeletal muscle mass, it has been proposed that creatinine appearance can be used to estimate skeletal muscle protein mass in CRF patients (80). Indeed, a correlation between lean body mass and creatinine appearance has been described in CPD patients (80). However, as of yet, healthy or desirable values for the creatinine appearance and the quantitative relation between skeletal muscle protein mass in maintenance dialysis patients have not been defined. Moreover, the relationship between skeletal muscle protein mass and creatinine appearance is complicated by the fact that dietary intake of skeletal muscle can substantially increase creatinine appearance, and that there is endogenous catabolism of creatinine which may be increased in uremic patients and which may be variable (81).

Chemical markers of nutritional status

Serum cholesterol

While serum cholesterol is often elevated in chronic renal failure patients, malnourished dialysis patients may have decreased cholesterol levels. A serum cholesterol lower than 150 mg/dl is often associated with severe malnutrition.

Serum albumin

The use of serum albumin to assess nutritional status has been reviewed in the previous section. It is important to note that the serum albumin varies according to the method of measurement (82). Blagg et al. repeatedly measured serum albumin in 235 unselected maintenance dialysis patients using different methods in the same specimens. These workers found a mean serum albumin value of 38 g/l with the bromcresol green technique and 33 g/l when serum was measured by the bromcresol purple or immuno-nephelometric procedures. Thus, the methods of measurement must be carefully noted when comparing serum albumin levels between different facilities (82), and specifically when reporting mortality and morbidity survival curves. These findings also raise the question as to whether the bromcresol green method is as accurate as bromcresol purple or immuno-nephelometry for measuring serum albumin in renal failure patients.

Serum transferrin

Serum transferrin has a shorter half-life (about 8 days) than albumin (about 19 days) and may be a more sensitive indicator of acute changes in protein metabolism. However, serum transferrin levels are influenced by iron metabolism, and also by infection and other acute inflammatory diseases. These factors must be taken into consideration when interpreting the serum transferrin. A serum transferrin level below 2000 mg/l may indicate malnutrition.

Serum prealbumin

Serum prealbumin, also called thyroxine-binding protein, has been reported to be elevated in chronic renal failure, even if malnutrition is present (83). This finding my be due to an increase in the prealbumin transporter, retinol binding protein (RBP). In CRF patients RBP may reduce the breakdown of free prealbumin and contribute to the increase in plasma total prealbumin concentrations. The increase in serum total prealbumin is directly correlated with the degree of renal failure. Thus interpretation of serum prealbumin is very difficult in patients who sustain acute changes in renal function. Several studies however, indicate that in MHD patients, other indicators of malnutrition appear to be strongly correlated with serum prealbumin levels less than 0.3 g/l (Figure 1) (84-87). A protein intake of 1.2 g/kg BW or more per day has been associated with a serum prealbumin value greater than 0.3 g/l (84). Also, in this same study, if the daily protein intake was greater than 1.4 g/kg BW, no further increment in serum prealbumin was observed (Figure 1) (84).

3-Methylhistidine (NT-methylhistidine)

In normal humans, 3-methylhistidine is a terminal degradation product amino acid from myofibrillar proteins and cannot be reused for protein synthesis. Therefore, its daily urinary excretion is highly correlated with total muscle mass and total fat-free mass in healthy adults (88). However, 3-methylhistidine directly reflects myofibrillar protein degradation and net muscle protein mass and in a number of clinical conditions, the muscle protein mass and balance may be discordant. In patients with balanced dietary intake of skeletal muscle, and muscle protein with unchanged GFR, a decrease in 3-methylhistidine may reflect reduction in the absolute rate of skeletal muscle protein degradation. It should be emphasized that urinary 3-methylhistidine excretion gives no information concerning the absolute rate of muscle protein synthesis.

Anthropometry and other body composition measurements

Every body compartment, including total body protein, lean body mass, adipose tissue, bone mass and total body water may vary in chronic renal failure patients. Weight, muscle mass and total body water also change over relatively short periods of time and therefore impair the accuracy of body composition measurements.

Weight

Monitoring the patient's body weight over time is one of the most useful anthropometric measurements. Because fluid is usually retained during the interdialytic period and edema is often present, the 'dry' weight is generally used. 'Dry' weight can be defined as the weight at which the patient is normotensive and edema is not present. One aim of dialysis is to remove sufficient fluid, to obtain the

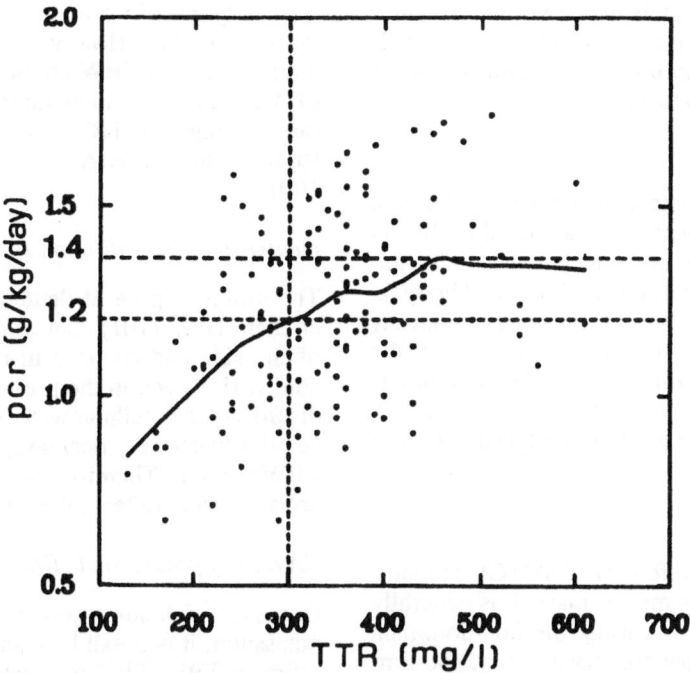

Figure 1. The relationship between serum prealbumin (transthyretin, TTR) and protein catabolic rate in 151 maintenance hemodialysis patients (Cleveland non-parametric smooting method) [from Cano et al., *Nephrol Dial Transplant* 7: 1069, 1992] (by permission of Oxford University Press).

patient's dry body weight by the end of the dialysis session without causing hypotension or cramps. Each weight must be measured in a standard fashion at each dialysis treatment using reliable scales, with the patient wearing similar types of clothes. Weight should be measured to the nearest 0.1 kg. Changes in dry body weight over time are usually reliable indices of alterations in nutritional status, and should be routinely monitored.

Body mass index (BMI)

BMI is calculated by dividing the patient's weight in kilograms by the square of the patient's height in meters. BMI is used to estimate total body fat. There are no tables for normal values for BMI. For men, a BMI greater than 30 kg/m^2 have approximately a 20% overweight (89) and an increased health risk. A BMI between 20 and 25 kg/m^2 is generally considered to indicate a healthy proportion of body fat (89). BMI calculated from the 1959 Metropolitan Life Insurances tables were between 21 and 22 kg/m^2. A BMI under 20 kg/m^2 may indicate protein-calorie malnutrition (89). For women, a BMI greater than 28 kg/m^2 indicates obesity; a BMI range of 19 to 24 kg/m^2 is considered desirable; a BMI below 15 kg/m^2 suggests protein-calorie malnutrition with and indicates 20% below ideal body weight (89). However, some heavy, muscular athletes may have a BMI in the obese range (90). Also, some highly conditioned athletes, such as long distance runners may have an abnormally low BMI. Quantitative predic-

tions of fat mass from BMI are rather inaccurate in the high range of BMI values. Smalley et al. recently reported that a BMI of 27 kg/m^2 can be associated with extreme values of total body fat content from 12 to 28% and 20 to 40% of body weight for males and females, respectively (91).

Weight standard

Weight standards refer either to normative standards derived from weights for different heights observed in the population or to functional standards such as those relating weight to morbidity or mortality. The United States National Health and Nutritional Evaluation Survey (NHANES) provides weights and other anthropometric measures in a large cohort of US residents classified according to their age, weight, gender and skeletal frame size (92). Data in these surveys are carefully collected by trained observers. These weights are often referred to as standard body weights. The ratio of a patient's weight ×100 to the weight of normal individuals of the same age, height gender and frame size is referred to as relative body weight (RBW). The Metropolitan Life Insurance actuarial tables published in 1959, and again in revised form, in 1983, indicate weight for age group, height, gender and frame size that are associated with the lowest mortality (93). These data in general are not obtained in such a precise manner. These weights tend to be about 8% less than standard weights. The weight of a patient ×100 divided by the weight of individuals of the same age range, height, gender, and frame size is referred to as desirable body weight (DBW). The normal or acceptable range for RBW and DBW is often 90 to 110%.

Skinfold thickness

Skinfold thicknesses correlate with total body fat, but accuracy of the measurements depends on the observer receiving careful training in the techniques. Quantitative relationships between skinfold thickness and body fat mass have been published (94). More accurate results may be obtained if at least three skinfolds are measured; the biceps, triceps, subscapular thickness and lateral thoracic skinfold are often measured (95). When edema is present, skinfold thickness may give a falsely high estimation of body fat.

Mid-arm muscle area

Mid-arm muscle area circumference (MAMC), or diameter, has been used to assess muscle mass. It is generally measured in the mid-arm area using the non-dominant arm, and in renal failure patients particularly, the arm that does not contain a vascular access. The following formula can be used to measure the mid-arm muscle circumference:

MAMC (cm) = mid-arm circumference (cm)

− 0.314 × triceps skinfold thickness (mm).   [3]

Lean body mass

Lean body mass is defined as the body weight minus total body fat. It includes the protein, carbohydrates, other non-fat organic compounds, and minerals in various organs and tissues, and also total body water (TBW). Lean body mass has been used extensively to describe body composition of obese individuals. However, in states such as renal failure, where the ability to regulate body water content is impaired and the percent body water is often abnormal, the use of lean body mass is misleading and theoretically could be harmful to the patient. For example, lean body mass may be increased, either because of increased protein mass, or increased body water. It is recommended that the term, lean body mass, should not be used to describe body composition of patients with renal disease or renal failure.

The following measurements of body composition, although less readily available in most centers, are being used or reported in the medical literature with sufficient frequency to justify comment.

Bioelectric impedance analysis (BIA)

The measurement of total body electrical resistance with surface electrodes gives a positive correlation between resistance and fat mass and a negative correlation between TBW and fat-free mass. Although BIA underestimates lean body mass by 5 to 6%, it is a reliable tool in healthy individuals (96). However, small or short-term (several day) changes in TBW are not reliably estimated by BIA (97). Furthermore, in maintenance hemodialysis patients, rapid changes in TBW affects the BIA results and few studies validating BIA in this condition are available (98–100).

Deuterated water dilution space

The dilution space of deuterated water is 3 to 4% larger than TBW (101), but allows an accurate estimation of the size and changes in total body water in healthy adults. However, in the presence of malnutrition or fluid disorders, extracellular water may increase whereas intracellular water may decrease, resulting in an unmodified TBW content. Therefore, in dialysis patients, TBW may not accurately reflect intracellular water or cell mass.

Total body potassium (TBK)

Because ^{40}K holds a constant relationship to total body potassium, it is possible, using a whole-body counter, to estimate TBK. TBK correlates with total body protein, and in individuals who can regulate total body water content normally, with body cell mass. However, in renal failure, the body cell mass may be altered due to changes in body water compartments. Furthermore, in renal failure patients, intracellular and extracellular potassium composition may be altered, and the relation between total body nitrogen (and hence body protein mass) and TBK may become altered.

Dual energy X-ray absorptiometry (DEXA)

Dual energy X-ray absorptiometry (DEXA) has been used for the measurement of bone-mineral density (102, 103). Regional measurements (hip, spine) can be performed with a minimum radiation dose. More recently, DEXA has been used for measuring the size and the proportion of fat in soft tissues, such as muscle, and in arms and legs. It is not yet accepted as a 'gold standard' for non-calcified tissue body composition (104). Studies in renal failure patients should become available in the near future (98). However, its use for the measurement of body composition in patients with renal failure has not yet been validated.

Other imaging procedures

Computed tomography (CT) and magnetic resonance imaging (MRI), both radiological techniques (105–107) can be used to measure total body fat and to identify the mass of different tissues (bone, muscle and fat) on cross-sectional areas or whole body sections. It is also possible to estimate visceral fat, which has been shown to correlate better than subcutaneous fat with some metabolic indices such as serum cholesterol, plasma lipoproteins or glucose tolerance (see review (107)). Precision and reproducibility of these methods are high in healthy adults (107). No data are yet available in renal failure patients.

Subjective global assessment (SGA)

SGA provides a rating of the protein-calorie nutritional status of individuals. Its advantages are: it combines disparate parameters of an individual's protein-calorie nutritional status into a single scope; it is easy to learn, convenient and quick to use; the scoring appears to be reproducible; it is inexpensive. The SGA is based on a medical history and physical examination (108, 109). The history is focused on recent weight loss and gastrointestinal disorders (anorexia, vomiting, diarrhea). The subcutaneous fat and muscle mass in the triceps and deltoid areas and lateral thoracic area are evaluated and the presence or absence of ankle edema is noted. The patient is characterized as having good nutritional status or moderate or severe malnutrition.

The use of SGA was originally reported in patients with gastrointestinal surgery. Recently, it has been applied to patients with renal failure. SGA has been reported in 36 MHD and 23 CAPD patients (110). In these patients using univariate analysis, SGA strongly correlated with serum albumin and the bioelectrical impedance analysis ($p < 0.001$), and acceptably with mid-arm muscle circumference (MAMC) ($p = 0.028$), percentage of total body fat ($p = 0.042$) and nPNA ($p = 0.027$). These data indicated that in these maintenance dialysis patients, the most important determinant of SGA was the estimations of the muscle mass and subcutaneous fat (110). Also, although a loss of body weight did not in itself indicate malnutrition, a constant body weight with development of ankle edema was clearly associated with malnutrition (110). At present, there are no published data of the prediction of morbidity or mortality by SGA in maintenance dialysis patients.

NUTRITIONAL REQUIREMENTS FOR MAINTENANCE DIALYSIS PATIENTS (TABLE 2)

Energy

Energy requirements do not appear to be different in patients undergoing maintenance dialysis therapy as compared to normal adults. Monteon et al. reported a similar rate of energy expenditure in normal adults, non-dialyzed CRF patients and MHD patients, both at rest and during physical activity (111). Also, Schneeweiss and colleagues recently reported that, in patients with predialysis CRF and in MHD patients, resting energy expenditure did not differ from normal adults, as long as sepsis was not present (112). Sufficient energy intake is necessary to maintain protein balance in MHD patients. Six sedentary MHD patients fed a constant protein intake of 1.1 g/kg

BW/day in a metabolic ward, were found to be in negative nitrogen balance when energy intake was approximately 25 kcal/kg BW/day, whereas they had neutral or positive nitrogen balance when energy intake was equal or greater than 35–38 kcal/kg BW/day (113). Thus, it MHD patients who do not engage in heavy physical activity should ingest about 35–38 kcal/kg BW/day. CPD patients probably should be given the same amount of energy, both from diet and dialysate as MHD patients. Patients over 60 years of age may be prescribed about 30 kcal/kg BW/day because normal individuals of this age seem to require less energy (114). Individuals who engage in more vigorous physical activity should receive higher energy intakes.

When dietary counseling is ineffective at increasing energy intake, the use of food supplements, intradialytic parenteral nutrition or tube feeding, including percutaneous gastric tube feeding, may be employed. Also, energy intake may be increased by adding glucose to the dialysate (115). When 10 mmol/l of glucose was added to dialysate, energy gain was about 100–120 kcal per session, whereas the use of glucose-free dialysis resulted in a net loss of 80–100 kcal. With a dialysate glucose concentration of 10 mM (180 mg/dl), no reduction in amino acid loss into hemodialysate was observed (115). With a dialysate glucose concentration of 25 mM (450 mg anhydrous glucose), amino acid losses into dialysate decreased substantially (48). This technique should be considered for malnourished MHD patients who have inadequate energy intake. For optimal sparing of protein, amino acids may also be added to the dialysate.

Protein

Most nitrogen balance studies suggest that maintenance hemodialysis patients require at least 1.0 g protein/kg/day (44, 113). Studies suggest that patients ingesting 1.0 to 1.2 g protein/kg/day are able to maintain nitrogen balance and tolerate this protein intake (14). To ensure sufficient protein intake, 1.2 g protein/kg/day is recommended. Intake should be composed of at least 50% of high value protein, i.e., from meat, fish and egg whites. It is possible, but not yet demonstrated, that as more porous dialyzer membranes are used, the dietary protein requirement may increase. These values may vary in the next years, because of modifications in dialysis membranes or techniques. For example, bleach reprocessing of polysulfone membranes has been shown to increase each dialysis protein loss from 1.2 to 17.5 g at the first, and until after the 23rd reuse (54).

Blumenkrantz et al. reported a curvilinear relationship (116) between dietary protein intake and nitrogen balance in CAPD patients. The data suggest that a protein intake of 1.2 to 1.3 g/kg/day may be necessary to ensure neutral to positive nitrogen balance in almost all clinically stable CAPD patients. There are virtually no studies of the dietary protein requirements in other forms of CPD (e.g., CCPD, NPD). A consideration of the probable pro-

Table 2. Recommended dietary nutrient intakes for patients undergoing maintenance hemodialysis or chronic peritoneal dialysis

	Maintenance hemodialysis (MHD)[a]	Chronic Peritoneal Dialysis (CPD)[a]
Protein	1.0–1.2 g/kg/day; $\geq$ 50% high biologic value protein	1.2–1.5 g/kg/day; $\geq$ 50% high biologic value protein
	1.2 g/kg/day is prescribed unless patient has normal protein status with intakes of 1.0–1.1 g protein/kg/day	1.2–1.3 g protein/kg/day is generally prescribed for malnourished patients, up to 1.5 g/kg/day may be given
Energy (kcal/kg/day)	$\geq$ 35 unless the patient's relative body weight is greater than 120% or the patient gains or is afraid of gaining unwanted weight	This refers to dietary intake. Energy intake from peritoneal dialysate is in addition to these values
Fat (percent of total energy intake)[b]	30–40	30–40
Polyunsaturated-saturated fatty acid ratio	1.0:1.0	1.0:1.0
Carbohydrate[c]	Rest of non-protein calories	
Total fiber intake (g/day)	20–25	20–25
Generals (range of intake)		
Sodium (mg/day)	1000 to 1500[d]	1000 to 2000[d]
Potassium (mEq/day)	40 to 70	40 to 70
Phosphorus (mg/kd/day)	8 to 17[e]	8 to 17[e]
Calcium (mg/day)	1400 to 1600[f]	800 to 1000[f]
Magnesium (mg/day)	200 to 300	200 to 300
Iron (mg/day)	$\geq$ 10 to 18	$\geq$ 10 to 18
Zinc (mg/day)	15	15
Water (ml/day)	Usually 750 to 1500[d]	Usually 1000 to 1500[d]
Vitamins	Diets to be supplemented with these quantities	
Thiamin (mg/day)	1.5	1.5
Riboflavin (mg/day)	1.8	1.8
Pantothenic acid (mg/day)	5	5
Niacin (mg/day)	20	20
Pyridoxine HCl (mg/day)	10	10
Vitamin B_{12} (μg/day)	3	3
Vitamin C (mg/day)	60	60
Folic acid (mg/day)	1	1
Vitamin A	No addition	No addition
Vitamin D	See text	See text
Vitamin E (IU/day)	15	15
Vitamin K	None[g]	None[g]

[a] When recommended intake is expressed per kilogram body weight, this refers to the standard weight as determined from NHANES data (92) or the adjusted body weight (ABW) for patients whose body weight differs by more than 15 to 20% from standard. ABW = standard weight + [(actual weight − standard weight) × 0.25].
[b] Refers to percent of total energy intake (diet plus dialysate).
[c] Should be primarily complex carbohydrates.
[d] Can be higher in CAPD patients or in hemodialysis patients who have greater urinary losses.
[e] Phosphate binders (aluminium carbonate or hydroxide, or calcium acetate, carbonate or citrate) often are also needed to maintain normal serum phosphorus levels.
[f] Dietary intake usually must be supplemented to provide these levels.
[g] Vitamin K supplements may be needed for patients who are not eating and who receive antibiotics.

tein and amino acid losses into peritoneal dialysate with these dialysis techniques suggests that the dietary protein requirements should be similar to that for CAPD.

Lipids and carnitine

There is a high incidence of elevated serum total triglycerides, low serum HDL cholesterol and high VLDL and IDL cholesterol in chronic renal failure. Serum LDL is often normal, possibly because of impaired conversion of VLDL and IDL to LDL. A number of abnormal serum apoprotein concentrations have been reported. Since there is a high prevalence of atherosclerosis during maintenance dialysis treatment, correction of these abnormalities should be considered.

An American Heart Association step 1 diet is recommended. This diet provides 30% of total calories from fat, in which saturated fat does not exceed 20% of total calories. Daily cholesterol intake is 300 mg or less. This diet usually lowers total serum cholesterol. If high triglycerides are present (100 mg/dl or more above the upper limit), a low intake of purified sugars is recommended. For patients with persistently increased serum LDL, VLDL, or IDL cholesterol, or very high serum triglycerides, more aggressive dietary therapy is proposed, including withdrawal of dietary alcohol and slowly digested complex, rather than purified, carbohydrates. Weight reduction diets for obese patients is routinely recommended. Medications that may reduce hypertriglyceridemia include, omega-3 fatty acids, up to 6 g/day, L-carnitine, 500 to 1000 mg/day if serum free carnitine levels are reduced. Fibric acid derivatives also may be employed to lower serum triglycerides. These latter compounds have altered pharmacokinetics in patients with chronic renal failure; the dosage must be reduced to avoid overdosage which may result in muscle cramps or rhabdomyolysis.

If high serum LDL cholesterol is not normalized by an appropriate diet (i.e., serum LDL cholesterol less than 160 mg/dl, and preferably less than 130 mg/dl) or if compliance to the diet prescription is not achieved, addition of hydroxymethylglutarate coenzyme A (HMG CoA) reductase inhibitor may be used.

Sodium and water

In patients with chronic renal failure, total body water is considered appropriate if blood pressure is normal or near-normal, edema is not present, and serum sodium is within the normal range. Thirst and ingestion of water play an important role in the regulation of water balance in these patients. Such factors as hyperglycemia (i.e., from poorly controlled diabetes mellitus), elevated dietary sodium intake, high dialysate sodium concentrations and certain psychogenic disorders are likely to increase thirst in MHD. Congestive heart failure, nephrotic syndrome, chronic portal hypertension may also increase sodium and water retention. In general, daily water intake should equal the urine output plus approximately 500 ml to replace insensible losses. Oliguric or anuric patients may be prescribed a sodium intake of 1000–1500 mg and a water intake of 750–1500 ml per day. In patients who are not anuric, high doses of loop diuretics (e.g., 500 to 1000 mg of furosemide daily) may increase sodium chloride and water excretion and, hence, the dietary allowance for these compounds.

Potassium

Maintenance dialysis patients usually do not become severely hyperkalemic because of increased fecal excretion of potassium, and the temporary transport of potassium into any the cells. The maintenance of a good urine output (e.g., 1000 ml/day or greater) also can cause substantial potassium excretion. Other conditions, in addition to oliguria or anuria, that predispose to hyperkalemia, include acidemia, insulinopenia, acute catabolic stresses, coronary angiography and such medications including non-steroidal antiinflammatory drugs, angiotensin converting enzyme inhibitors and B-receptor blockers. Also, insulin-dependent diabetic patients frequently may develop the hyporeninemic hypoaldosteronism syndrome with hyperkalemia (117). In general, maintenance dialysis patients are prescribed a dietary potassium intake of 70 mEq/day or less. Maintaining diuresis by loop diuretics may allow a sustained daily potassium excretion of 20 to 50 mEq. In addition, patients should receive detailed instructions on the potassium content of foods and should be advised to avoid high-potassium foods. When, despite these efforts, serum potassium is seriously elevated, ingestion of cation exchange resins (i.e., Kayexalate® may be added.

Magnesium

Magnesium is primarily excreted by the kidney. Since there is net gastrointestinal absorption of 40 to 50% of ingested magnesium (118), chronic renal failure patients are at risk for hypermagnesemia (119). There is often net bone accrual of magnesium in patients with chronic renal failure, which may contribute to renal osteodystrophy (120). In non-dialyzed CRF patients, magnesium balance may be attained with dietary magnesium intakes of 200 mg per day (118). Low-protein diets are also restricted in magnesium; the magnesium content of a 40 g protein diet is about 100 to 300 mg. Therefore, before dialysis, the serum magnesium levels in CRF patients are usually normal or slightly elevated, unless large amounts of magnesium-containing phosphate binders or laxatives are ingested. The optimal magnesium intake for maintenance dialysis patients is not well defined. Usually, hemodialysate containing 1.0 mEq per liter or peritoneal dialysate containing 0.50 to 0.75 mEq per liter of magnesium and a diet of a magnesium intake of 200 to 300 mg per day will maintain normal or slightly elevated serum magnesium concentrations.

Phosphorus and calcium

The dietary phosphorus requirement for MHD and CPD patients is about 8–10 mg/kg/day (114). Larger amounts of phosphorus are often allowed in order to increase the palatability of the diet. The dietary calcium content is about 1400 to 1600 mg/day in MHD patients and 800 to 1000 mg/day in CPD patients. The dietary calcium requirement will vary depending on calcium concentration of dialysate, particularly in CPD patients; if dialysate calcium is reduced below 3.5 mEq/l, the dietary calcium requirement will increase. Intake of 1,25 dihydroxycholecalciferol may decrease the dietary calcium need by facilitating intestinal calcium absorption.

The major challenge with regards to dietary phosphorus in maintenance dialysis patients is to reduce the phosphorus intake sufficiently to prevent hyperphosphatemia. Because phosphorus intake is directly correlated with the protein content of the diet, it is difficult to restrict phosphorus intake if large amounts of protein are ingested. Controlling high serum phosphorus is needed to avoid a high serum calcium-phosphorus product, and its deposition in soft tissues, and to better control serum parathormone levels. Two types of phosphorus binders may be used. Traditionally, aluminium carbonate and aluminium hydroxide phosphate binders were used, usually about six to twelve 500 mg capsules per day divided into three doses with meals. Due to the potential development of aluminium toxicity including bone disease, anemia and myopathy and also dialysis dementia, calcium-containing phosphate binders are generally preferred.

Three different calcium salts are commonly used. Calcium acetate has the greatest affinity for phosphorus and the lowest rate of intestinal calcium absorption. Hypercalcemia has been reported less frequently with the use of calcium acetate as compared to carbonate. Calcium carbonate is often the least expensive of the calcium binders. Calcium citrate should not be used together with aluminium salts because citrate enhances intestinal aluminium absorption. Indeed, due to the propensity of citrate to facilitate the intestinal absorption of other divalent or trivalent cations, including lead (121), calcium citrate is probably less preferable to calcium carbonate or calcium acetate as a phosphate binder. Usually, no more than 2000 mg/day of calcium (i.e., 5000 mg/day of calcium carbonate) is given as phosphate binders in order to prevent continued positive calcium balance and hypercalcemia. In a CRF patient commencing therapy with a very high serum phosphorus (e.g., above 6.5 mg/dl), aluminium phosphate binders rather than calcium salts may be used initially to decrease the serum phosphorus. This may reduce the risk of elevating the calcium-phosphorus product. When the serum phosphorus is reduced, calcium binders are then substituted for the aluminum salts. The calcium concentration

of peritoneal dialysate may need to be reduced (i.e., to 2.5 mEq/l) to prevent hypercalcemia in CPD patients who are taking calcium binders.

Vitamins and trace elements (Table 2)

Chronically uremic patients are reported to have a high incidence of vitamin deficiencies. 1,25-dihydrocholecalciferol production is impaired by the diseased kidney. Vitamin intake is often decreased in uremic patients because of anorexia and reduced food intake. Also, the diets prescribed for non-dialyzed chronic renal failure and maintenance dialysis patients frequently contain less than the recommended daily allowances for certain water-soluble vitamins (27). The metabolism of folate and pyridoxine is abnormal in renal failure (122), and many medicines have been reported to impair the pharmacology of vitamins (27). Water-soluble vitamins can also be removed by dialysis (58, 123).

Blood folate levels have been reported to be decreased in MHD patients not receiving supplements (124). When MHD patients were given folic acid supplements, their reticulocyte count and hematocrit rose (29). We have observed normal serum folate levels in virtually all MHD patients who receive 1.0 mg/day of folate supplement (unpublished observation).

Vitamin C losses into dialysate are substantial, and MHD patients often have low plasma and leukocyte ascorbic acid concentrations (60, 123, 125). Clinical signs suggesting mild scurvy have been described in MHD patients with a very low serum ascorbic acid level (125). A minimal oral daily amount of 60 mg of vitamin C is recommended. However, Descombes et al. reported that 27% of MHD patients receiving 400 to 600 mg of ascorbic acid weekly had plasma ascorbate values in the deficient range (126). After increasing vitamin C supplements to 1000–1500 mg/week, plasma ascorbate levels were above normal (up to 10 mg/l) in these patients. Also, in this latter study, MHD patients treated with polyacrylonitrile dialyzers had lower plasma ascorbate levels than those treated with cellulose acetate dialyzers (6.9 ± 3.6 vs 11.1 ± 4.9 mg/l, respectively, $p < 0.01$), possibly due to increased PAN dialyzer clearance of the vitamin (126). Large doses of vitamin C have been associated with high plasma oxalate levels in CRF patients, possibly increasing the risk of soft tissue deposition of oxalate.

Pyridoxine (vitamin B_6) has been reported to be low in plasma and red cells of MHD patients (29, 127, 128). Also, there may be an inhibitor of vitamin B_6 in uremic serum which is removed during hemodialysis (127). Pyridoxine supplements improve lymphocyte formation, and possibly immune function (127, 129). Indeed, a pyridoxine hydrochloride supplement of 10 mg/day completely restored erythrocyte glutamate-pyruvate transaminase activation index in stable MHD patients (128). A recent study confirmed the rapid improvement of these activities with 80–120 mg/week of pyridoxine hydrochloride in stable MHD patients (126).

Despite the water solubility of thiamine, riboflavin, pantothenic acid and biotin, these compounds are frequently found in the normal range in MHD patients. The losses of these vitamins into dialysate might be offset by the reduction in renal catabolism or urine loss in these patients. Therefore, the nutritional requirements for these vitamins are not well defined in MHD. However, since water-soluble supplements are safe, it would seem wise to prescribe them until these questions are more extensively studied.

Vitamin A is increased in serum of maintenance dialysis patients. Because bone toxicity has been reported with modest doses of vitamin A (i.e., 7500–15000 IU/day), it is not recommended for maintenance dialysis patients (130). Vitamin K deficiency is present infrequently in MHD patients. Patients receiving antibiotics that suppress intestinal bacteria for long periods of time may benefit from a supplement of vitamin K. Vitamin D administration has been extensively reviewed elsewhere in this volume.

Dietary requirements for trace elements have not been well defined in maintenance dialysis patients. Because of the pivotal role of the kidney in trace element excretion, it is not unexpected that, in maintenance dialysis patients, accumulation might occur. Also, because trace elements are avidly bound to serum proteins, small quantities of trace elements contained in dialysate (131) may be taken up against a concentration gradient.

Iron deficiency is common in CRF patients. Indeed, occult intestinal blood loss, repeated blood sampling, sequestration of blood into dialyzer and binding of iron to the dialyzer membrane frequently occur during MHD therapy (26, 28). Erythropoietin (EPO) may also rapidly deplete iron stores by enhancing erythropoiesis. Therefore, because of these potential iron deficiencies and before starting EPO therapy, body iron stores should be monitored and iron supplements might be administered. Ferrous sulfate, 300 mg, may be given three times a day one-half hour after meals to reduce gastric discomfort. Some patients may present nausea, constipation, anorexia or abdominal pain. These patients may better tolerate ferrous fumarate, gluconate or lactate. Intramuscular or intravenous iron supplements can also be used after a first test dose in order to detect allergic reactions.

Zinc deficiency may be present in chronic renal failure (30, 31, 132). In non-dialyzed CRF patients, total urinary excretion of zinc is reduced and fecal zinc excretion is increased (133). Some reports indicate that dysgeusia, and in males, impotency may be improved by giving patients zinc supplements (30, 31, 134). These findings have not been confirmed by Rodger et al. (135). Until this question is more extensively reviewed, maintenance dialysis patients should receive the Recommended Dietary Allowance for zinc, i.e., 15 mg/day (114).

In MHD patients, selenium levels have been reported to be low in serum (136, 137) and in the range of healthy adults when measured in plasma (138). Because selenium is a strong antioxidant compound, the question of selenium supplementation is of particular importance and deserves further studies.

DIALYSIS RELATED NUTRITIONAL SUPPORT

Some maintenance dialysis patients who have low nutrient intake and suffer from protein-calorie malnutrition may respond to dietary counseling or the use of oral food supplements. In some refractory patients, enteral tube feeding, sometimes through a percutaneous gastric feeding tube, or total parenteral nutrition are necessary. However, a number of malnourished maintenance dialysis patients ingest a daily diet which, although low, is not markedly deficient. These individuals might respond to supplemented parenteral nutrition either given intravenously during hemodialysis or added to peritoneal dialysate or hemodialysate. It should be emphasized that, although clinical research supports the benefits of these treatments in selected patients, definitive large scale clinical trials demonstrating the clinical value of these techniques are still lacking.

Intradialytic parenteral nutrition (IDPN) is a simple technique for increasing nutritional intake in malnourished MHD patients. There is no need for extra venous catheters or for hospitalization. Because of the elevated blood flow through the vascular access, high osmolar mixtures may be infused, composed either by lipids, or a so called three-in-one solution (dextrose, amino acids and lipids, also the assurance that prescribed nutritional treatment will be delivered to the patient. Some individual reports are encouraging (139). However, no methodologically adequate clinical trial has been carried out to examine benefits of treatment (140). Because these treatments are expensive, there is a need for cost-benefit studies. Furthermore, comparative studies between IDPN and food supplements or enteral feeding need to be performed (141).

Pharmacology of intradialytic parenteral nutrition

A commonly used solution for IDPN is composed of 15 to 20 kcal/kg body weight and 0.5 to 1 g protein/kg per dialysis session. A standard regimen (139) may provide 250 ml of 50% dextrose, 500 ml of 8.25% amino acids (1:1, essential to non-essential amino acid ratio) and 250 ml of a 20% lipid emulsion. If this supplement is added to the 25 to 27 kcal/kg and 0.8 to 1 g protein/kg, commonly reported to be ingested by malnourished MHD patients (40, 142), the accepted nutritional goals for such patients can be met (see Table 2). In general, such an IDPN solution should not be infused in less than four hours in order to allow to reduce the risk of hyperglycemia or hypertriglyceridemia.

Lipids

The inclusion of lipid infusion in IDPN infusates may be beneficial because: it will allow the glucose intake in the infusate to be reduced and, hence, the likelihood of developing hyperglycemia will be reduced; poly-non-saturated fatty acid deficiency is not uncommon in chronic renal failure (143); and the fact that lipid emulsions do not cross the dialyzer membrane and therefore will be retained by the patient. Lipid infusions have been reported to be well tolerated in MHD patients at a dose of 8 ml of a 20% emulsion/kg BW infused over four hours (144). However, if substantial hypertriglyceridemia is present, an uncommon occurrence in malnourished MHD patients, lipid administration is not recommended. Interestingly, lipid infusions may improve certain alterations of the lipoprotein profile of MHD patients (144). Indeed, after three months of administration of an IDPN solution containing lipids, essential and non-essential amino acids and glycyl-tyrosine, an increase in apo A1/apo B ratio has been observed, without a change in serum total cholesterol (142). More recently, these same workers reported that after one month of a lipid containing IDPN infusion given thrice weekly, serum lipoprotein (a) (Lpa) decreased, whereas the ratio apo C2/apo C3 increased. This suggests improved triglyceride transport and a reduction in atherogenic risk (144).

Amino acids

Losses of free amino acids during hemodialysis increase during IDPN by an amount equal to roughly 10% of the amino acids infused (50). Indeed, total amino acid losses into dialysate increased from 8.2 ± 0.1 to 12.6 ± 3.6 g during the procedure when patients received 39.5 g of an essential and non-essential amino acid solution and 200 g of dextrose (50). Compared to a saline infusion dialysis, plasma amino acids did not fall during IDPN (50). Recently, Chazot et al. (personal communication) have performed hemodialysis procedure with two different amino acid enriched hemodialysates in six MHD patients. The dialysate contained either 46.3 g (composition close to a normal plasma amino acid pattern) or 138.9 g (composition close to three times the normal plasma amino acid pattern) of amino acids for the entire HD procedure. Compared to regular bicarbonate dialysate (amino acid losses of 9.3 ± 2.7 g), there was no net loss of amino acids using the 46.3 g amino acid dialysate; with the high amino acid dialysate, there was a net gain of 39.1 ± 14.8 g per hemodialysis (Chazot et al., personal communication).

Infusion of amino acid into the peritoneal cavity may become a potential treatment for malnourished CPD patients. Indeed, a recent study reports the effects of

Table 3. Guidelines for IDPN

1. Low protein and/or energy intake associated with malnutrition diagnosed by standard procedures and measurements, including subjective global assessment.
2. Progressive weight loss.
3. Serum albumin equal or lower than 3.4 g/dl for two consecutive months.
4. Serum prealbumin below 300 mg/l.
5. Body weight below 90% of standard body weight from the NHANES data (92).
6. Failure of oral supplements to correct malnutrition.

an amino acid enriched peritoneal dialysate infusion in 19 malnourished CAD patients in a Clinical Research Center. After a 15 day control period, these patients received one to two daily exchanges containing 1.1% amino acid and no glucose instead of their usual dextrose solutions. The nitrogen balance increased from 0.5 ± 1.9 to 1.71 ± 2.4 g/day, $p < 0.001$. This indicates a clear anabolic response in these patients (145).

Clinical response to IDPN

Studies addressing the effects of intradialytic parenteral nutrition have been recently reviewed (140). Some studies have shown increases in serum albumin (142, 146, 147), creatinine and prealbumin (142). The fact that in some trials, patients' appetite improved shortly after starting IDPN has confounded interpretation of the effects of IDPN on nutritional status. IDPN therapy administered in a non-research setting to a large cohort of MHD patients was analyzed retrospectively (146). The patients that displayed reduced mortality in association with IDPN therapy, in comparison to retrospective controls, were those with a baseline serum albumin below 3.0 g/dl. A modest reduction in mortality was observed in patients with a serum albumin below 3.4 g/dl. However, increased mortality was observed in the IDPN treated patients having a baseline serum albumin greater than 3.5 g/dl, underscoring the potential hazards of this treatment (146).

In a recent retrospective study, Capelli et al. (147) reported by Cox analysis that IDPN treated patients had a better outcome than untreated patients. Serum albumin increased in both treated and untreated groups at six months of follow-up, but this effect was only sustained in the IDPN treated group. However, mortality rate was not different between groups at two years of treatment (147).

Several side-effects have been reported with the use of IDPN. Glucose infusion with concomitant endogenous insulin secretion may lead to reactive hypoglycemia when IDPN infusion is stopped. Hypophosphatemia may also occur after glucose infusion and insulin secretion; this may be enhanced by the loss of phosphate in the dialysis buffer. Liver function abnormalities have been reported, possibly from glucose overload or lipid metabolism abnormalities in these patients. Routine monitoring of serum electrolytes and liver enzymes should therefore be performed.

Guidelines proposed for IDPN therapy (148, 149) are given in Table 3.

IDPN support and growth factors

A recent study addressed the anabolic effects of combined recombinant human growth hormone and IDPN in seven malnourished MHD patients (150). The IDPN delivered 18 kcal and 0.69 g amino acid per kg BW and 50 g of fat thrice weekly. After six weeks of this IDPN, recombinant human growth hormone, 5 mg, was injected subcutaneously at the end of each dialysis, and the same IDPN regimen was maintained for another six weeks. Whereas energy and protein intake from patient reports did not vary before and during growth hormone treatment, serum insulin-like growth factor-1 (IGF-1) rose above baseline levels (115 vs 212 ng/ml, $p < 0.05$) and serum albumin increased significantly during the rhGH treatment period (3.5 vs 3.8 g/dl, $p < 0.04$) (150). However, it is difficult to clearly delineate the respective roles of IDPN and growth hormone in this study (150).

Preliminary results also suggest that administering recombinant insulin-like growth factor-1 (IGF-1) subcutaneously for 20 days results in a dramatically more positive nitrogen balance in six malnourished CPD patients (151).

REFERENCES

1. Shapiro JI, Argy WP, Rakowski TA, Chester A, Siemsen AS, Schreiner GE: The unsuitability of BUN as a criterion for prescription dialysis. *Trans Am Soc Artif Intern Organs* 29: 129, 1983
2. Acchiardo SR, Moore LW, Latour PA: Malnutrition as the main factor in morbidity and mortality of hemodialysis patients. *Kidney Int* 24: 199, 1983
3. Lowrie EG, Lew LN: Death risk in hemodialysis patients: the predictive value of commonly measured variables and an evaluation of death rate differences between facilities. *Am J Kidney Dis* 5: 458, 1990
4. Churchill DN, Taylor DW, Cook RJ et al.: Canadian hemodialysis morbidity study. *Am J Kidney Dis* 3: 214, 1992
5. Owen WF, Lew NL, Liu Y, Lowrie EG, Lazarus JM: The urea reduction ratio and serum albumin concentrations as predictors of mortality in patients undergoing hemodialysis. *N Engl J Med* 329: 1001, 1993
6. Collins AJ, Ma JZ, Umen A, Keshaviah P: Urea index (Kt/V) and other predictors of hemodialysis patient survival. *Am J Kidney Dis* 23: 272, 1994
7. Teehan BP, Schleifer CR, Brown JM, Sigler ME, Raimondo J: Urea kinetic analysis and clinical outcome on

8. Blake PG, Flowerdew G, Blake RM, Oreopoulos DG: Serum albumin in patients on continuous ambulatory peritoneal dialysis – predictors and correlations with outcomes. *J Am Soc Nephrol* 3: 1501, 1993
9. Rocco MV, Jordan JR, Burkart JM: The efficacy number as a predictor of morbidity and mortality in peritoneal dialysis patients. *J Am Soc Nephrol* 4: 1184, 1993
10. Keshaviah P, Churchill DN, Thorpe K, Taylor DW: Impact of nutrition on CAPD mortality. (Abstract) *J Am Soc Nephrol* 5: 494, 1994
11. Attman PO, Ewald J, Isaksson B: Body composition during long-term treatment of uremia with amino acid supplementation low-protein diet. *Am J Clin Nutr* 33: 801, 1980
12. Bianchi R, Mariani G, Toni MG, Carmassi F: The metabolism of human serum albumin in renal failure on conservative and dialysis therapy. *Am J Clin Nutr* 31: 1615, 1978
13. Heide B, Pierratos A, Khanna R et al.: Nutritional status of patients undergoing continuous ambulatory peritoneal dialysis (CAPD). *Perit Dial Bull* 3: 138, 1983
14. Kluthe R, Luttgren FM, Capetianu T, Heinze V, Katz N, Sudhoff A: Protein requirements in maintenance hemodialysis. *Am J Clin Nutr* 31: 1812, 1978
15. Kopple JD: Abnormal amino acid and protein metabolism in uremia. *Kidney Int* 14: 340, 1978
16. Salusky IB, Fine RN, Nelson P, Blumenkrantz MJ, Kopple JD: Nutritional status of children undergoing continuous ambulatory peritoneal dialysis. *Am J Clin Nutr* 38: 599, 1983
17. Thunberg BJ, Swamy AP, Cestero RV: Cross sectional and longitudinal nutritional measurements in maintenance hemodialysis patients. *Am J Clin Nutr* 34: 2005, 1981
18. Wolfson M, Strong CJ, Minturn D, Gray DR, Kopple JD: Nutritional status and lymphocyte function in maintenance hemodialysis patients. *Am J Clin Nutr* 39: 547, 1984
19. Young GA, Kopple JD, Lindholm B et al.: Nutritional assessment of continuous ambulatory peritoneal dialysis patients: an international study. *Am J Kidney Dis* 17: 462, 1991
20. Cano N, Fernandez JP, Lacombe P et al.: Statistical selection of nutritional parameters in hemodialysed patients. Proceedings of the fourth international congress on nutrition and metabolism in renal disease. *Kidney Int* 32 (Suppl 22): S178, 1987
21. Young GA, Swanepoel CR, Croft MR, Hobson SM, Parsons FM: Anthropometry and plasma valine, amino acids, and proteins in the nutritional assessment of hemodialysis patients. *Kidney Int* 21: 492, 1982
22. Blumenkrantz MJ, Kopple JD, Gutman YK: Methods for assessing nutritional status of patients with chronic renal failure. *Am J Clin Nutr* 33: 1567, 1980
23. Schilling H, Wu G, Pettit J et al.: Nutritional status of patients on long-term CAPD. *Perit Dial Bull* 5: 12, 1985
24. Kopple JD, Chumlea WC, Gassman JJ et al.: Relationship between GFR and nutritional status – results from the MDRD study. (Abstract) *J Am Soc Nephrol* 5: 335, 1994
25. Bellinghieri G, Savica V, Mallamace A et al.: Correlation between increased serum and tissue L-carnitine levels and

CAPD. A five year longitudinal study. *Adv Perit Dial* 6: 181, 1990 improved muscle symptoms in hemodialyzed patients. *Am J Clin Nutr* 38: 523, 1983

26. Delano BG, Manis JG, Manis T: Iron absorption in experimental uremia. *Nephron* 19: 26, 1977

27. Kopple JD, Swenseid ME: Vitamin nutrition in patients undergoing maintenance hemodialysis. *Kidney Int* 7 (Suppl 2): S79, 1975

28. Lawson DH, Boddy K, King PC, Linton AL, Will G: Iron metabolism in patients with chronic renal failure on regular dialysis treatment. *Clin Sci* 41: 345, 1971

29. Mackenzie JC, Ford JE, Waters AH, Harding N, Cattell WR, Anderson BB: Erythropoiesis in patients undergoing regular dialysis treatment (RDT) without transfusion. *Proc Eur Dialysis Transplant Assoc* 5: 172, 1968

30. Mahajan SK, Prasad AS, Lambujon J, Abbasi AA, Briggs WA, McDonald FO: Improvement of uremic hypogeusia by zinc. A double-blind study. *Am J Clin Nutr* 33: 1517, 1980

31. Sprenger KBG, Bundschu D, Lewis K, Spohn B, Schmitz J, Franz H: Improvement of uremic neuropathy and hypogeusia by dialysate zinc supplementation: a double-blind study. *Kidney Int* 24 (Suppl 16): S315, 1983

32. Consensus paper, chaired by Lasagna L and Schreiner G: Role of L-carnitine in treating renal dialysis patients. *Dial and Transplant* 23: 177, 1994

33. Carlson DM, Duncan DA, Naessens JM, Johnson WJ: Hospitalization in dialysis patients. *Mayo Clin Proc* 59: 769, 1984

34. Evans RW, Manninen DL, Garrison LP Jr et al.: The quality of life of patients with end-stage renal disease. *N Engl J Med* 312: 553, 1985

35. Grodstein GP, Blumenkrantz MJ, Kopple JD: Nutritional and metabolic response to catabolic stress in chronic uremia. *Am J Clin Nutr* 33: 1411, 1980

36. Bergström J: Nutrition and adequacy of dialysis in hemodialysis patients. *Kidney Int* 43 (Suppl 41): S261, 1993

37. Fouque D, Joly MO, Laville M et al.: Increase of serum Insulin-Like Growth Factor I (IGF 1) during chronic renal failure is reduced by low-protein diet. *Miner Electrolyte Metab* 18: 276, 1992

38. Ciancaruso B, Capuano A, D'amaro E et al.: Dietary compliance to a low protein and phosphate diet in patients with chronic renal failure. *Kidney Int* 36 (Suppl 27): S173, 1989

39. Jacob V, Le Carpentier JE, Salzano S et al.: IGF-1, a marker of undernutrition in hemodialysis patients. *Am J Clin Nutr* 52: 39, 1990

40. Eknoyan G, Beck GJ, Breyer JA et al.: Design and preliminary results of the mortality and morbidity of hemodialysis (MMHD) pilot study. (Abstract) *J Am Soc Nephrol* 5: 513, 1994

41. Bergström J, Mamoun H, Anderstam B, Södersten P: Middle molecules (MM) isolated from uremic ultrafiltrate (UF) and normal urine induce dose-dependent inhibition of appetite in the rat. (Abstract) *J Am Soc Nephrol* 5: 488, 1994

42. Lindsay RM, Spanner E: A hypothesis: the protein catabolic rate is dependent upon the type and amount of treatment in dialyzed uremic patients. *Am J Kidney Dis* 13: 382, 1989

43. Bergström J, Alvestrand A, Lindholm B, Tranaeus A: Relationship between Kt/V and protein catabolic rate

(PCR) is different in continuous peritoneal dialysis (CPD) and haemodialysis (HD) patients. (Abstract) *J Am Soc Nephrol* 2: 358, 1991

44. Borah M, Schoenfeld PY, Gotch FA, Sargent JA, Wolfson M, Humphreys MH: Nitrogen balance in intermittent hemodialysis therapy. *Kidney Int* 14: 497, 1978

45. Guttierez A, Alvestrand A, Wahren J, Bergström J: Effect of *in vivo* contact between blood and dialysis membranes on protein catabolism in humans. *Kidney Int* 38: 487, 1990

46. Lim VS, Bier DM, Flanigan MJ, Sum-Ping ST: The effect of hemodialysis on protein metabolism. A leucine kinetic study. *J Clin Invest* 91: 2429, 1993

47. Giordano C, DePascale C, De Cristofaro D et al.: Protein malnutrition in the treatment of chronic uremia. in *Nutrition in Renal Disease*, edited by Berlyne GM, Baltimore, Williams and Wilkins, 1968, p 23

48. Kopple JD, Swendseid ME, Shinaberger JH, Umezawa CY: The free and bound amino acids removed by hemodialysis. *Trans Am Soc Artif Intern Organs* 19: 309, 1973

49. Ikizler TA, Flakoll PJ, Parker RA, Hakim RM: Amino acid and albumin losses during hemodialysis. *Kidney Int* 46: 830, 1994

50. Wolfson M, Jones MR, Kopple JD: Amino acid losses during hemodialysis with infusion of amino acids and glucose. *Kidney Int* 21: 500, 1982

51. Wathen RL, Keshaviah P, Hommeyer P, Caldwell K, Comty CM: The metabolic effects of hemodialysis with and without glucose in the dialysate. *Am J Clin Nutr* 31: 1870, 1978

52. Gutierrez A, Bergström J, Alvestrand A: Hemodialysis-associated protein catabolism with and without glucose in the dialysis fluid. *Kidney Int* 46: 814, 1994

53. Levin NW: Dialyzer reuse. A currently acceptable practice. *Semin Dial* 6: 89, 1993

54. Kaplan AA, Halley SE, Lapkin RA, Graeber CW: Dialysate protein losses with bleach processed polysulphone dialyzers. *Kidney Int* 47: 573, 1995

55. Giordano C, DeSanto NG, Capodicasa G et al.: Amino acid losses during CAPD. *Clin Nephrol* 14: 230, 1980

56. Kopple JD, Blumenkrantz MJ, Jones MR, Moran JK, Coburn JW: Plasma amino acid levels and amino acid losses during continuous ambulatory peritoneal dialysis. *Am J Clin Nutr* 36: 395, 1982

57. Blumenkrantz MJ, Gahl GM, Kopple JD et al.: Protein losses during peritoneal dialysis. *Kidney Int* 19: 593, 1981

58. Andersen KEH: Folic acid status of patients with chronic renal failure maintained by dialysis. *Clin Nephrol* 8: 510, 1977

59. Rostand SG: Vitamin B12 levels and nerve conduction velocities in patients undergoing maintenance hemodialysis. *Am J Clin Nutr* 29: 691, 1976

60. Sullivan JF, Eisenstein AB, Mottola OM, Mittal AK: The effect of dialysis on plasma and tissue levels of vitamin C. *Trans Am Soc Artif Intern Organs* 18: 277, 1972

61. Linton AL, Clark WF, Dreidger AA, Werb R, Lindsay RM: Correctable factors contributing to the anemia of dialysis patients. *Nephron* 19: 95, 1977

62. Rosenblatt SG, Drake S, Fadem S, Welch R, Lifschitz MD: Gastrointestinal blood loss in patients with chronic renal failure. *Am J Kidney Dis* 1: 232, 1982

63. De Fronzo RA, Tobin JD, Rowe JW, Andres R: Glucose intolerance in uremia: quantification of pancreatic beta cell sensitivity to glucose and tissue sensitivity to insulin. *J Clin Invest* 62: 425, 1978

64. Fouque D: Insulin-like growth factor-1 (IGF-1) resistance in renal failure. *Miner Electrolyte Metab* 1995. In press

65. Kuku SF, Zeidler A, Emmanouel DS, Ratz AI, Rubenstein AH: Heterogeneity of plasma glucagon: patterns in patients with chronic renal failure and diabetes. *J Clin Endocrinol Metab* 42: 173, 1976

66. Fouque D, Peng S, Kopple JD: Impaired metabolic response to recombinant human insulin-like growth factor-1 in dialysis patients. *Kidney Int* 47: 876, 1995

67. Birge SJ, Haddad JG: 25-hydroxycholecalciferol stimulation of muscle metabolism. *J Clin Invest* 56: 1100, 1974

68. May RC, Kelly RA, Mitch WE: Mechanisms for defects in muscle protein metabolism in rats with chronic uremia. *J Clin Invest* 79: 1099, 1987

69. Mitch WE, May RC, Maroni BJ, Druml W: Protein and amino acid metabolism in uremia: influence of metabolic acidosis. *Kidney Int* 36 (Suppl 27): S205, 1989

70. Reaich D, Channon S, Scrisgeour CM, Daley SE, Wilkinson R, Goodship THJ: Correction of acidosis in humans with CRF decreases protein degradation and amino acid oxidation. *Am J Physiol* 265: E230, 1993

71. Raine AEG, Bedford L, Simpson AWM et al.: Hyperparathyroidism, platelet intracellular free calcium and hypertension in chronic renal failure. *Kidney Int* 43: 700, 1993

72. Akmal M, Massry SG, Goldstein DA, Fanti F, Weisz A, DeFronzo RA: Role of parathyroid hormone in the glucose intolerance of chronic renal failure. *J Clin Invest* 75: 1037, 1985

73. Akmal M, Barndt RR, Ansari AN, Mohler JG, Massry SG: Excess PTH in CRF induces pulmonary calcification, pulmonary hypertension and right ventricular hypertrophy. *Kidney Int* 47: 158, 1995

74. Gao XL, Kopple JD: Relationship between dietary protein, urea nitrogen appearance (UNA) and total nitrogen appearance (TNA) in patients with chronic renal failure. (Abstract) *J Am Soc Nephrol* 5: 491, 1994

75. Karvetti RL, Knuts LR: Validity of the estimated food diary: comparison of 2-day recorded and observed food and nutrient intakes. *J Am Diet Assoc* 92: 580, 1992

76. Daugirdas JT: Second generation logarithmic estimates of single-pool variable volume ST/V: an analysis of error. *J Am Soc Nephrol* 4: 1205, 1993

77. Poignet JL, Chauveau P, Desassis JF, Puget J: Adequacy of hemodialysis and nutrition: evaluation of an on-line urea monitor. (Abstract) *J Am Soc Nephrol* 5: 525, 1994

78. Blumenkrantz MJ, Kopple JD, Moran JK, Grodstein GP, Coburn JW: Nitrogen and urea metabolism during continuous ambulatory peritoneal dialysis. *Kidney Int* 20: 78, 1981

79. Bergström J, Furst P, Alvestrand A, Lindholm B: Protein and energy intake, nitrogen balance and nitrogen losses in patients treated with continuous ambulatory peritoneal dialysis. *Kidney Int* 44: 10481, 1993

80. Keshaviah PR, Nolph KD, Moore HL et al.: Lean body mass estimation by creatinine kinetics. *J Am Soc Nephrol* 4: 1475, 1994

81. Walser M: Creatinine excretion as a measure of protein nutrition in adults of varying age. *J Parenter Enteral Nutr* 11: 573, 1987

82. Blagg CR, Liedtke RL, Batjer JD et al.: Serum albumin concentration-related health care financing administration quality assurance criterion is method-dependent: revision is necessary. *Am J Kidney Dis* 21: 138, 1993

83. Cano N, DiCostanzo-Dufetel J, Calaf K et al.: Prealbumin-retinol-binding-protein-retinol complex in hemodialysis patients. *Am J Clin Nutr* 47: 664, 1988

84. Cano N, Stroumza P, Lacombe P, Labastie-Coeyrehourcq J, Durbec JP: Serum transthyretin and protein intake in haemodialysis patients. (Letter) *Nephrol Dial Transplant* 7: 1069, 1992

85. Cano N, Stroumza P, Lacombe P, Labastie-Coeyrehourcq J: Plasma prealbumin in hemodialysis patients. (Letter) *Am J Kidney Dis* 23: 621, 1994

86. Goldwasser P, Michel MA, Collier J et al.: Prealbumin and lipoprotein(a) in hemodialysis: relationships with patient and vascular access survival. *Am J Kidney Dis* 22: 215, 1993

87. Hakim RM, Levin N: Malnutrition in hemodialysis patients. *Am J Kidney Dis* 21: 125, 1993

88. Lukaski HC, Mendez J, Buskirk ER, Cohn SH: Relationship between endogenous 3-methylhistidine excretion and body composition. *Am J Physiol* 240: E302, 1981

89. Thomas AE, McKay DA, Cutlip MB: A nomograph method for assessing body weight. *Am J Clin Nutr* 29: 302, 1976

90. Heymsfield SB: Assessment of body composition. American Society for Parenteral and Enteral Nutrition annual meeting, San Diego, 1993, p 179

91. Smalley KJ, Knerr AK, Kendrick ZV, Colliver JA, Owen OE: Reassessment of body mass indices. *Am J Clin Nutr* 52: 405, 1990

92. Frisancho AR: New standards of weight and body composition by frame size and height for assessment of nutritional status of adults and the elderly. *Am J Clin Nutr* 40: 808, 1984

93. 1983 Metropolitan height and weight tables. Statistical Bull Metrop Insur Co 64: 3, 1983

94. Durnin JV, Womersley J: Body fat assessed from total body density and its estimation from skinfold thickness; measurements on 481 men and women aged from 16 to 72 years. *Br J Nutr* 32: 77, 1974

95. Blumenkrantz MJ, Kopple JD, Gutman RA et al.: Methods for assessing nutritional status of patients with renal failure. *Am J Clin Nutr* 33: 1567, 1980

96. Lukaski HC, Bolonchuk WW, Hall CB, Siders WA: Validation of tetrapolar bioelectrical impedance methods to assess human body composition. *J Appl Physiol* 60: 1327, 1986

97. Deurenberg P, Weststrate JA, Hautvast JGAJ: Changes in fat-free mass during weight loss measured by bioelectrical impedance and by densitometry. *Am J Clin Nutr* 49: 33, 1989

98. Charney DI, Leypoldt JK, Chan GM: Validity of dual-energy X-ray absorptiometry (DEXA) and single frequency bioelectrical impedance analysis (BIA) in chronic hemodialysis patients. (Abstract) *J Am Soc Nephrol* 4: 339, 1993

99. Dumler F, Schmidt R, Kilates C, Faber M, Lubkowski T, Frinak S: Use of bioelectrical impedance for the nutritional assessment of chronic hemodialysis patients. *Miner Electrolyte Metab* 18: 284, 1992

100. Spotti D, Librenti MC, Melandri M et al.: Bioelectrical impedance in the evaluation of the nutritional status of hemodialyzed diabetic patients. *Clin Nephrol* 39: 172, 1993

101. Wang J, Pierson RN, Kelly WG: A rapid method for the determination of deuterium oxide in man: application to the measurement of total body water. *J Lab Clin Med* 82: 170, 1983

102. Heymsfield SB, Wang J, Funfar J, Kehayias JJ, Pierson RN: Dual photon absorptiometry. Comparison of bone mineral and soft tissue mass measurement *in vivo* with established methods. *Am J Clin Nutr* 49: 1283, 1989

103. Going SB, Massett MP, Hall MC et al.: Detection of small changes in body composition by dual-energy X-ray absorptiometry. *Am J Clin Nutr* 57: 845, 1993

104. Roubenoff R, Kehayias JJ, Dawson-Hughes B, Heymsfield SB: Use of dual-energy x-ray absorptiometry in body-composition studies: not yet a 'gold standard'. *Am J Clin Nutr* 58: 589, 1993

105. Ross R, Leger L, Morris D, de Guise J, Guardo R: Quantification of adipose tissue by MRI: relationship with anthropometric variables. *J Appl Physiol* 72: 787, 1992

106. Brummer RJM, Rosen T, Bengtsson BA: Evaluation of different methods of determining body composition, with special reference to growth hormone-related disorders. *Acta Endocrinol* 128 (Suppl 2): 30, 1993

107. Sohlstrom A, Wahlund LO, Forsum E: Adipose tissue distribution as assessed by magnetic resonance imaging and total body fat by magnetic resonance imaging, underwater weighing, and body-water dilution in healthy women. *Am J Clin Nutr* 58: 830, 1993

108. Baker JP, Detsky AS, Wesson DE et al.: Nutritional assessment: a comparison of clinical judgement and objective measurements. *N Engl J Med* 306: 969, 1982

109. Detsky AS, McLaughlin JR, Baker JP et al.: What is subjective global assessment of nutritional status? *J Parenter Enteral Nutr* 11: 8, 1987

110. Enia G, Sicuso C, Alati G, Zoccali C: Subjective global assessment of nutritional in dialysis patients. *Nephrol Dial Transplant* 8: 1094, 1993

111. Monteon FJ, Laidlaw SA, Shaib JR, Kopple JD: Energy expenditure in patients with chronic renal failure. *Kidney Int* 30: 741, 1986

112. Schneeweiss B, Graninger W, Stockenhuber F et al.: Energy metabolism in acute and chronic renal failure. *Am J Clin Nutr* 52: 596, 1990

113. Slomowitz LA, Monteon FJ, Grosvenor M, Laidlaw SA, Kopple JD: Effect of energy intake on nutritional status in maintenance hemodialysis patients. *Kidney Int* 35: 704, 1989

114. Recommended Dietary Allowances. National Academy Press, 10th Edition, Washington DC, 1989

115. Guttierez A, Bergström J, Alvestrand A: Hemodialysis-associated protein catabolism with and without glucose in the dialysis fluid. *Kidney Int* 46: 814, 1994

116. Blumenkrantz MJ, Kopple JD, Moran JK, Coburn JW: Metabolic studies and dietary protein requirements in patients undergoing continuous ambulatory peritoneal dialysis. *Kidney Int* 21: 849, 1982

117. De Fronzo RA: Hyperkalemia and hyporeninemic hypoaldosteronism. *Kidney Int* 17: 118, 1980

118. Kopple JD, Coburn JW: Metabolic studies of low protein diets in uremia. II. Calcium, phosphorus and magnesium. *Medicine* 52: 597, 1973

119. Randall RE Jr, Cohen MD, Spray CC Jr et al.: Hypermagnesemia in renal failure: etiology and toxic manifestations. *Ann Intern Med* 61: 73, 1964

120. Wallach S: Effects of magnesium on skeletal metabolism. *Magnes Trace Elem* 9: 1, 1990

121. Rabinowitz MB, Kopple JD, Wetherill GW: Effect of food intake and fasting on gastrointestinal lead absorption in humans. *Am J Clin Nutr* 33: 1784, 1980

122. Toback FG: Amino acid treatment of acute renal failure. in *Acute Renal Failure*, edited by Brenner BM, Stein JH, London, Churchill Livingstone, 1980, p 202

123. Sullivan JF, Eisenstein AB: Ascorbic acid depletion during hemodialysis. *JAMA* 220: 1697, 1972

124. Whitehead VM, Comty CH, Posen GA, Kaye M: Homeostasis of folic acid in patients undergoing maintenance hemodialysis. *N Engl J Med* 279: 970, 1968

125. Sullivan JF, Eisenstein AB: Ascorbic acid depletion in patients undergoing chronic hemodialysis. *Am J Clin Nutr* 23: 1339, 1970

126. Descombes E, Hanck AB, Fellay G: Water soluble vitamins in chronic hemodialysis patients and need for supplementation. *Kidney Int* 43: 1319, 1993

127. Dobbelstein H, Korner WF, Mempel W, Grosse-Wilde H, Edel HH: Vitamin B6 deficiency in uremia and its implications for the depression of immune responses. *Kidney Int* 5: 233, 1974

128. Kopple JD, Mercurio K, Blumenkrantz MJ et al.: Daily requirement for pyridoxine supplements in chronic renal failure. *Kidney Int* 19: 694, 1981

129. Casciato DA, McAdam LP, Kopple JD et al.: Immunologic abnormalities in hemodialysis patients: improvement after pyridoxine therapy. *Nephron* 38: 9, 1984

130. Yatzidis H, Digenis P, Fountas P: Hypervitaminosis A accompanying advanced chronic renal failure. *Br Med J* 2: 352, 1975

131. Padovese P, Gallieni M, Brancaccio D et al.: Trace elements in dialysis fluids and assessment of the exposure of patients on regular hemodialysis, hemofiltration and continuous ambulatory peritoneal dialysis. *Nephron* 61: 442, 1992

132. Atkin-Thor E, Goddard BW, O'Nion J, Stephen RL, Kolff WJ: Hypogeusia and zinc depletion in chronic dialysis patients. *Am J Clin Nutr* 31: 1948, 1978

133. Mahajan SK, Bowersox EM, Rye DL et al.: Factors underlying abnormal zinc metabolism in uremia. *Kidney Int* 36 (Suppl 27): S269, 1989

134. Antoniou LD, Shalhoub RJ, Sudhakar T, Smith JC: Reversal of uremic impotence by zinc. *Lancet* ii: 895, 1977

135. Rodger RS, Sheldon WL, Watson MJ et al.: Zinc deficiency and hyperprolactinemia are not reversible causes of sexual dysfunction in uremia. *Nephrol Dial Transplant* 4: 888, 1989

136. Kallistratos G, Evangelou A, Seferiadis K, Vezyraki P, Barboutis K: Selenium and haemodialysis: serum selenium levels in healthy persons, noncancer and cancer patients with chronic renal failure. *Nephron* 41: 217, 1985

137. Cornelis R, Mees L, Ringoir S, Hoste J: Serum and red blood cell Zn, Se, Cs, and Rb in dialysis patients. *Miner Electrolyte Metab* 2: 88, 1979

138. Milly K, Wit L, Diskin C, Tulley R: Selenium in renal failure patients. *Nephron* 61: 139, 1992

139. Golper TA: Severe malnutrition II. *Semin Dial* 6: 362, 1993

140. Wolfson M: The cost and bother of intradialytic parenteral nutrition are not justified by available scientific studies. *ASAIO J* 39: 864, 1993

141. Wolfson M: Use of intradialytic parenteral nutrition in hemodialysis patients. *Am J Kidney Dis* 23: 856, 1994

142. Cano N, Labastie-Coeyrehourcq J, Lacombe P et al.: Perdialytic parenteral nutrition with lipids and amino acids in malnourished hemodialysis patients. *Am J Clin Nutr* 52: 726, 1990

143. Lacour B, Roullet JB, Drueke T: Les perturbations du métabolisme lipidique dans l'insuffisance rénale chronique. *Néphrologie* 4: 75, 1983

144. Cano N, Luc G, Stroumza P, Lacombe P, Durbec JP: Serum lipoprotein changes after prolonged intralipid infusion in malnourished haemodialysis patients. *Clin Nutr* 13: 111, 1994

145. Kopple JD, Bernard D, Messana J et al.: Treatment of malnourished CAPD patients with an amino acid based dialysate. *Kidney Int* 47: 1148, 1995

146. Chertow GM, Ling J, Lew NL, Lazarus JM, Lowrie EG: The association of intradialytic parenteral nutrition administration with survival in hemodialysis patients. *Am J Kidney Dis* 24: 912, 1994

147. Capelli JP, Kushner H, Camiscioli TC, Chen SM, Torres MA: Effect of intradialytic parenteral nutrition on mortality rates in end-stage renal disease care. *Am J Kidney Dis* 23: 808, 1994

148. Gupta BK, Plotner E, Spinowitz BS, Charytan C: Severe malnutrition IV. *Semin Dial* 6: 366, 1993

149. Cano N: Nutrition entérale et parentérale chez l'insuffisant rénal chronique hémodialysé. *Nutr Clin Métabol* 8: 205, 1994

150. Schulman G, Wingard RL, Hutchinson RL, Lawrence P, Hakim RM: The effects of recombinant human growth hormone and intradialytic parenteral nutrition in malnourished hemodialysis patients. *Am J Kidney Dis* 21: 527, 1993

151. Peng S, Fouque D, Kopple JD: Insulin-like growth factor 1 (IGF-1) causes anabolism in malnourished CAPD patients. (Abstract) *J Am Soc Nephrol* 3: 414, 1993

ORGAN AND METABOLIC COMPLICATIONS: β2-MICROGLOBULIN AMYLOIDOSIS

JUERGEN SCHAEFFER and KARL-MARTIN KOCH

HISTORY AND RECOGNITION OF THE SYNDROME

Five years after the initial publication on carpal tunnel syndrome in hemodialysis patients (1), Assenat et al. (2) were the first to point out an association of this syndrome with a local deposition of amyloid. In 1984, Charra et al. (3) reported a correlation of the shoulder pain syndrome in hemodialysis patients with amyloid-positive histology from carpal tunnel surgery, and described the presence of amyloid in synovial tissue. Bardin et al. (4) established amyloidosis as a prominent cause of carpal tunnel syndrome, finger flexor synovitis, and cystic bone radiolucencies, and coined the phrase 'dialysis amyloidosis'. The existence of a new form of amyloidosis peculiar to long-term hemodialysis patients underlying the amyloid arthropathy was suggested in 1985 (5), but the etiology and biochemical precursor were still unknown (6, 7).

Geyjo et al. (8, 9) were the first to identify, by size, amino acid composition and N-terminal sequencing, beta2-microglobulin (β2M) as the amyloid fibril protein. This was confirmed by Gorevic et al. (10) who in addition reported the presence of dimeric and polymeric aggregates of β2M in the amyloid. The characterization of 'dialysis-related amyloidosis' (11) was based on reports from the hemodialysis population; during the following years, a number of publications described the syndrome also in patients on peritoneal dialysis (12–16) and even single patients in the predialytic phase (17, 18). Systemic/visceral involvement of dialysis amyloidosis was recognized to have a low incidence, to occur late and to be generally of limited extent (19) although a few reports on excessive, clinically relevant visceral Aβ2M-deposits exist (20–22). A large amount of information has been accumulated on clinical and pathogenetic aspects of dialysis related or associated amyloidosis, or, as it is called now in accordance with WHO guidelines on the nomenclature of amyloidoses (23), Aβ2M-amyloidosis (24–27).

CLINCIAL FEATURES OF Aβ2M-AMYLOIDOSIS

The syndrome of Aβ2M-amyloidosis is characterized predominantly by the occurrence of a carpal tunnel syndrome and periarticular cystic bone lesions in combination with destructive arthropathy (11, 25, 26, 28); synovial tissue is the predominant site of amyloid deposition.

The symptomatology of carpal tunnel syndrome (CTS) in patients on long-term renal replacement therapy is identical to the idiopathic and other symtomatic carpal tunnel syndromes, with hypaesthesia, hypalgesia, nightly pains, thenar weakness and wasting, and an impairment of distal motor nerve conduction due to median nerve compression in the carpal tunnel bed (29–32). Surgical treatment of CTS consists of release of the transverse ligament and/or synovectomy of tendon sheaths (33). Postoperative recurrence of CTS after 2–3 years is observed in a significant proportion of patients (34). A clear predilection of CTS for the shunt arm does not exist (35). The incidence of CTS increases with time on dialysis, starting at about 6 to 8 years of treatment, rising to 50% at 15 years and 100% after 20 years of dialysis (35). Amyloid is usually found adjacent to collagen in carpal synovia, flexor tendon sheaths, transverse carpal ligament and perineural tissue (35). To which extent amyloid deposition in the carpal tunnel actually is responsible for development of the CTS remains unclear: the percentage of Aβ2M-positive biopsies, as well as the extent of amyloid deposition, vary widely between the published studies (3, 32). Although methodological differences and sampling errors may account for this, other pathogenetic mechanisms such as an increase in tissue fibrosis may also play a role, potentially reducing the importance of Aβ2M in some instances to an epiphenomenon. In extreme cases, on the other hand, Aβ2M-amyloidosis extends to tendons and tendon sheaths of the palm and fingers (4, 35), and a typical 'amyloid hand' with contraction of the hand and

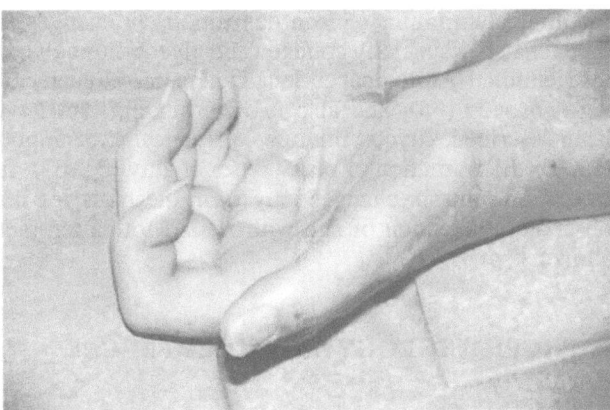

Figure 1. 'Amyloid hand'. Left hand in maximal extension: 44 year old patient after 20 years of hemodialysis.

Figure 2. Synovial deposition of Aβ2M-amyloid. Histology of hip synovia obtained at surgery: 42 year old patient after 18 years of hemodialysis. Staining with anti-β2M-antibody.

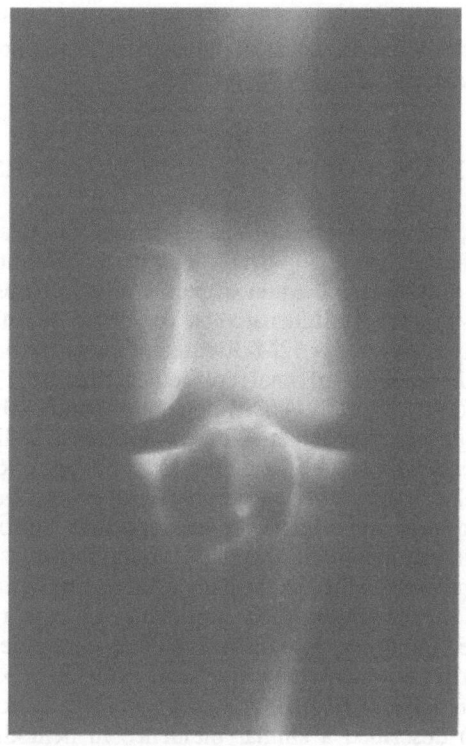

Figure 3. Radiotomography of knee with tibia cyst: 53 year old patient after 14 years of hemodialysis.

atrophy of digital muscles can develop in addition to CTS (Figure 1).

Joint manifestations of Aβ2M-amyloidosis (Figure 2) include a destructive arthropathy (5, 7, 36) with recurrent or persistent painful swelling and stiffening of large and medium sized joints, synovitis, joint effusions and erosions, as well as the occurrence of periarticular bone cysts (4). The cystic character of these lesions is derived from their X-ray appearance (radiolucency); histologically, Aβ2M-deposits have been shown in the cysts in addition to non-calcified collagenous matrix (37–39). Subchondral bone cysts are frequently seen – often bilaterally – in carpal bones, distal radius, humoral and femoral heads, acetabulum, and tibia plateau (Figure 3). Severe complications such as pathological fractures of the hips (37, 40) have occurred with increasing frequency in long-term dialysis patients.

Several forms of osteoarticular affections of the spine have been described in long-term dialysis patients. A dialysis-related spondylarthropathy has been attributed to hydroxylapatite crystal deposition in intervertebral discs, and is not necessarily related to amyloidosis (41). However, Aβ2M-amyloid does play a role in the pathogenesis of spondylarthropathy (42, 43), and Aβ2M-deposits were demonstrated at autopsy in preferentially cervical discs of renal failure patients (44). Cystic lesions, arthropathy with bone fragmentation and soft-tissue involvement may cause symptoms ranging from radiculopathy up to medullary compression or spinal fracture with resulting paraplegia (45, 46).

Swelling of articular and periarticular soft tissue (joint capsules, synovia, tendons) occurs and seems to be partly due to amyloid deposition; Aβ2M-amyloidosis may present as acute arthritis (47). Besides CTS symptoms, patients complain of articular and periarticular pain which can, especially in periarthritis humeroscapularis, be accentuated by the dialysis procedure.

Deposition of Aβ2M-amyloid in tissues other than the osteoarticular system has been observed in single instances, mostly localized in small blood vessels, and generally seems to be of a very limited amount and importance (19). Visceral symptoms have only rarely been observed, but occasionally severe complications of cardiac or intestinal Aβ2M-deposition were reported (20–22, 48, 49). Aβ2M-calculi have been described in the urinary tract of patients before and after start of dialysis (17, 50). Tumorlike subcutaneous deposits of Aβ2M were reported in a few cases (51–53), but random skin biopsies and abdominal fat aspirates usually tested negative for Aβ2M-amyloid (19, 48, 54, 55).

INCIDENCE AND PREDISPOSING FACTORS

Clearly, the appearance of Aβ2M-amyloid is related to a uremic state persisting over a long period of time (26). Aβ2M-amyloidosis has almost exclusively been observed in long-term renal failure patients. Very few cases of histologically confirmed Aβ2M-disease are known in patients *before* the initiation of renal replacement therapy (17, 18), and evidence for early Aβ2M-deposition (within the first year after initiation of hemodialysis) appears to be limited to patients who started treatment at an old age (56) (see also below). Most of the reported cases were patients on long-term treatment with conventional cuprophane hemodialysis membranes, but Aβ2M-amyloid does occur also in patients treated exclusively by high-flux hemodialysis or hemofiltration (57). A number of case reports indicated the occurrence of Aβ2M-disease in patients on long-term peritoneal dialysis who had not been exposed to hemodialysis (12–16), and more recently Maiorca et al. (58) described a similar incidence in hemodialysis and peritoneal dialysis populations, provided that time on treatment is comparable.

Maintenance of some residual renal function, with better preserved β2M-elimination, delays the appearance of Aβ2M-amyloidosis. Duration of renal replacement therapy, on the other hand, appears to have a strong impact on the development of Aβ2M-amyloidosis. This is clearly evident from clinical, radiological and scintigraphic data comparing the incidence of Aβ2M in relation to time on treatment (35, 57, 59–62). In these studies, the incidence range after 5 years of hemodialysis is 0–10%, after 10 years 15–65%, after 15 years 60–90%, and after 20 years 100%.

According to retrospective analysis of clinical (34, 56, 57) and scintigraphic data (63), age at the onset of dialysis treatment appears to be a very important predisposing factor in the genesis of Aβ2M-amyloidosis. Patients who started dialysis in their twenties may be free of clinically detectable Aβ2M-deposits even after 15 or more years of dialysis (64), while old patients can be affected already within the first few years (56). A role of secondary hyperparathyroidism or aluminium deposition in the pathogenesis of Aβ2M-disease has not been clearly established (64).

The unique distribution pattern of Aβ2M-amyloidosis in the synovia/osteoarticular system suggests that local predisposing factors may be important. Subjects of investigation and discussion have been: 1) cellular phenomena such as number and activity of macrophage-like synoviocytes, or migration of circulating inflammatory cells into the affected tissue sites, with a subsequent local cytokine action; 2) differences in local β2M concentration, pH,

calcium, aluminium, or iron deposition; 3) changes in tissue matrix, especially collagen and glycosaminoglycan distribution. Histological co-localization of β2M and collagen *in vivo* (65), and also *in vitro*-binding (66) have been described. Glycosaminoglycans appear to be important for the formation of many types of amyloid (67). In fact, tissue matrix changes may form the basis for the observed association of age with Aβ2M-formation (see above).

PATHOPHYSIOLOGY AND BIOCHEMICAL BASIS

On the basis of clinical, histological and biochemical data a variety of pathogenetic concepts and methodological approaches towards the problem of Aβ2M-amyloidosis have been established.

β2-microglobulin as the precursor protein

β2-microglobulin serum levels are increased 40–60 fold in patients with renal failure who lack the normal β2M excretory capacity by glomerular filtration and tubular breakdown (68). There is no doubt that β2M retention and accumulation form the physiological and biochemical basis for Aβ2M-formation; β2M is the characteristic circulating precursor protein incorporated into growing Aβ2M-amyloid fibrils (8–10). β2M monomers, dimeric and polymeric forms as well as different fragments of β2M (17, 69) were demonstrated biochemically in β2M amyloid material from various sites. Precipitation of amyloid-like fibrils from purified β2M *in vitro* has been described (70), but only under non-physiological conditions (evaporation of a salt-free β2M solution). Also, spontaneous β2M polymerization into amyloid fibrils was documented in mononuclear cell culture supernatants obtained from dialysis patients (71); however, the number of successful experiments was small, and the pathophysiological significance of this observation is not clear.

β2M levels, synthesis and removal rates

β2M serum levels show a wide overlap between patients with Aβ2M-amyloidosis and those without in cross-sectional studies (68, 72) and the incidence of Aβ2M appears to be related to the duration of β2M retention (3, 57) rather than serum concentrations. In fact, serum levels may even decline in the group of long-term patients with clinical evidence of Aβ2M (61). Nevertheless, possible alterations in β2M synthesis as well as efforts to enhance β2M removal by specific treatment techniques have received major attention, and the reported differences in the incidence of Aβ2M-amyloidosis between patient groups on different types of dialyzer membranes such as highly permeable, biocompatible polyacrilonitrile membranes versus less permeable, complement activating cellulosic membranes (38, 57) have stimulated interest in the underlying mechanisms.

In vivo, an increase in β2M synthesis by HLA-rich cells such as lymphocytes occurs in lymphoproliferative disorders. *In vitro*, increased synthesis and cellular release of β2M is induced in leucocytes by several proinflammatory agents and cytokines such as lipopolysaccharide, TNFalpha, IL-1, and others (73, 74). Cytokines are known to be induced during the dialysis procedure (75–77). The intensitiy of cytokine induction is related to the membrane type (75) and influenced by coexisting complement activation (78) as well as by the transmembrane passage of pyrogenic substances originating from bacterial contaminants of the dialysate (79–81). The extent of cytokine induction could well have an impact on β2M synthesis and thus on the kinetics of Aβ2M formation (see also section below on prevention and treatment).

Cell culture systems have been used to study the impact of chronic renal failure, dialysis treatment, and the type of dialysis membrane on β2M fibril production (82). However, the results of this and other studies on the effect of hemodialysis membranes on β2M synthesis and release by various blood-derived cells have been contradictory (83–86).

In vivo no significant intradialytic change in β2M serum concentration can be demonstrated once the effect of complex water shifts has been corrected for (87, 88). Kinetic studies in humans have demonstrated marginally increased whole-body β2M synthesis rates in dialysis patients treated with cellulosic or non-cellulosic membranes as compared to healthy controls (89–92); with the small number of patients studied, neither the differences between healthy controls and dialysis patients, nor between the patient groups on different membranes were statistically significant (91, 92). Larger studies with longitudinal follow-up in individual patients on different membranes would be needed to definitively answer this question (Figure 4).

Improving the β2M-removal capacity of renal replacement therapy, on the other side, has been a predominant objective of innovation in dialysis/treatment technology. Experimental and clinical evidence concerning this topic is discussed below in the section on treatment of Aβ2M-amyloidosis.

Altered processing of β2M

Similar to other forms of amyloidoses, an incomplete or atypical proteolysis has been proposed to enhance the amyloidogenicity of the β2M precursor protein. This idea is supported by the fact that biochemically altered β2M protein, typically fragments that have been cleaved by lysine-specific proteases (93), may occur in a significant proportion in various Aβ2M-deposits; such altered molecules could be more amyloidogenic due to changes in conformation or hydrophobicity. Theoretically, an atypical proteolysis can occur systemically, or locally at the

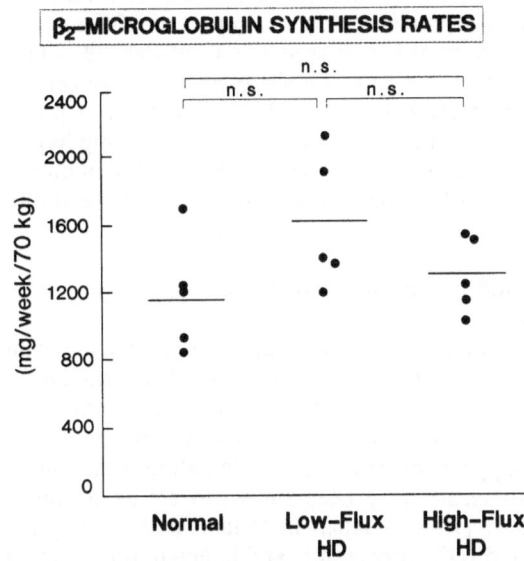

Figure 4. β2M-synthesis rates calculated from tracer kinetic study (^{131}I-β2M) in normal controls and patients on low-flux and high-flux hemodialysis.

synovial site of amyloid formation. Like β2M synthesis, β2M processing/proteolysis may be affected by a dialysis-related stimulation of inflammatory cells; an intradialytic release and/or activation of proteases has been described (94). An increased activity of antiprotease systems protecting β2M from proteolytic digestion has also been suggested to contribute to the incompleteness of β2M proteolysis and/or facilitate the persistence of Aβ2M-amyloid fibrils in tissue (95). This concept is based on the observation that various antiproteases such as alpha-2-macroglobulin can be detected in Aβ2M-deposits, but this is not a specific finding since they are also seen in amyloid-free tissue (96). The rise in plasma alpha-2-macroglobulin levels with dialysis which has been reported both on synthetic and cellulosic membranes (97) does not prove a causal relationship with Aβ2M development.

Biochemical and physiochemical alterations of β2M have been described that lead to a more acidic β2M molecule, and thereby may increase the tendency to aggregate and form amyloid fibrils. A single amino acid substitution in position 17 (aspartate for asparagin) has been described in β2M from plasma and amyloid fibrils of uremic patients (98, 99), but this observation has not been confirmed by others (100–102). More recently, Miyata et al. (103) demonstrated in Aβ2M-amyloid the presence of acidic β2M that is altered by the so-called Maillard reaction to contain advanced glycation endproducts (AGE). Advanced glycation endproducts appear to play a significant role in the pathogenesis of diabetic complications and in aging (104). AGE-modified β2M (brown in color, fluorescent and immunhistochemically stained by an anti-AGE antibody) was present not only in fibrils, but also (as a minor fraction) in serum and urine from long-term hemodialysis patients (103). An impact of AGE-modified proteins on cytokine systems has been described (105) and may be a link to macrophage and synovial cell participation in Aβ2M-genesis (106). However, at present there is only limited evidence for this intriguing hypothesis, and a higher incidence of Aβ2M-disease in diabetic patients with long-term renal failure has not been clinically described so far.

Role of inflammation: primary or secondary?

An inflammatory reaction as a primary event in the pathogenesis of β2M amyloid deposition could be triggered by complement activation and cytokine release from inflammatory cells after contact with the dialysis membrane (75–78); pyrogenic substances originating from contaminated dialysate have been shown to act as strong co-stimulators (78–81). Apart from increased β2M synthesis, altered β2M processing, and deficient proteolysis of β2M fibrils, such inflammatory mechanisms may also act through changes in local cellular activity and/or matrix composition. The role of underlying local inflammation is supported by one recent animal model approach, in which injection of β2M only together with the induction of an artificial joint inflammation in uremic rat knees led to local β2M-amyloid formation (107). However, an association of β2M amyloid deposits with inflammatory cells has not been consistently observed histologically, and the question whether inflammation or amyloidosis is first in the sequence of events remains controversial. In contrast to the concept that inflammatory cells facilitate pathological β2M processing and deposition in Aβ2M-amyloidosis, the morphological demonstration of moderate lymphocyte and macrophage infiltrates in advanced Aβ2M-amyloidosis may rather represent a secondary, foreign-body reaction of the body in the vicinity of Aβ2M-deposits (65, 108). On the other hand, recent autoradiographic data obtained after injection of radiolabelled β2M *in vivo* imply a significant participation of macrophages in the binding and incorporation of β2M into the amyloid (109). A participation of further local predisposing factors such as glycosaminoglycans (110) and collagen in the pathogenesis of Aβ2M-amyloidosis has been suggested, but their relative importance remains unknown. Collagen is known to bind β2M (66), filamentous or degenerative changes of collagen fibers in the skin have been described in cutaneous (not Aβ2M) amyloid (111) and may in analogous ways also contribute to Aβ2M-deposition. Various protein constituents other than β2M have been described in Aβ2M-amyloid (e.g., immunoglobulin light chains, amyloid P component, alpha2-macroglobulin, globin chains) (112, 113); however, their role in the pathogenesis of Aβ2M-amyloidosis remains speculative at present.

DIAGNOSIS OF Aβ2M-AMYLOIDOSIS

Early diagnosis is needed to relate various clinical symptoms to the presence of Aβ2M-amyloidosis, and to rule out alternative causes that could be treated. In later stages, the recognition of bone lesions at risk of fracture can lead to precautionary measures such as external (e.g., cervical spine cuff) or internal/surgical stabilization. The diagnosis of advanced Aβ2M-disease may be an indication to give a patient priority for urgent kidney transplantation (see section on treatment below). In addition, early diagnosis and adaequate follow-up of Aβ2M by preferably non-invasive, sensitive and specific diagnostic techniques is needed to evaluate prospectively the influence of different dialysis treatment strategies on the course of Aβ2M-amyloidosis.

Plasma levels of β2M are uniformly elevated about 30 to 60 fold in end-stage renal failure patients due to the absence of significant β2M excretion by the failing kidney. While retention of the β2M-molecule certainly forms a necessary basis for the build-up of Aβ2M-amyloid, a correlation between plasma levels and clinical or radiological evidence of Aβ2M has not been demonstrated (68, 114–116); thus, plasma concentrations cannot contribute to the diagnosis of Aβ2M-amyloidosis.

While clinical, sonographic and radiological evidence (as discussed below) serves to detect Aβ2M-amyloidosis, the definitive diagnosis can be made only from morphological study (65, 117–119). Representative tissue samples can be obtained at autopsy or during surgery. Alternatively, biopsy material can be gained from arthroscopic or blind puncture of joint synovia or by needle biopsy from joint cysts. Aspiration of joint effusion has been used to stain for tissue debris containing Aβ2M (118, 120), but is still invasive and not generally applicable for detection of Aβ2M. In analogy to other types of systemic amyloidoses, aspiration of abdominal fat, submucosal rectal biopsy and skin biopsy have been evaluated for diagnosis (19, 48, 54, 55, 118); however, due to the fact that Aβ2M is only occasionaly present in these tissues even in severe cases, these invasive methods are of limited value.

Appropriate histochemical investigation of possible Aβ2M-amyloidosis consists of alcaline congo-red staining according to Puchtler's method (121), demonstration of the typical apple-green bi-refringence under polarized light, and positive β2M-immunohistochemistry (65, 122). Further study by electron microscopy reveals characteristic parallel bundles of curvilinear, 8–10 nm thick fibrils which give an intense immunoreaction to anti-β2M antisera (65).

Obviously, the invasiveness of histological diagnosis of Aβ2M represents a major obstacle to morphological proof of suspected Aβ2M-disease, and even more for possible diagnostic screening purposes. Therefore, the mainstay of Aβ2M-diagnosis continues to be the typical constellation of clinical symptoms as outlined above, together with radiological signs suggestive of Aβ2M. A number of imaging techniques are used for diagnosis of Aβ2M-amyloidosis:

- Radiological examination shows destructive joint changes ranging from erosions and marginal defects (mainly at synovial insertion sites) to the characteristic periarticular bone cysts (39, 57). However, small cysts are commonly seen in healthy people especially in the carpal bones (123), and specific criteria have been suggested to classify a cyst as a correlate of Aβ2M-amyloidosis: size of at least 10 mm in shoulder and hip, 5 mm in the wrist; location outside areas that frequently show so-called synovial herniation pits; growth on follow-up examination of more than 30% per year; normal adjacent joint space to exclude cysts of osteoarthritic origin (57). Advanced radiological techniques such as tomography and computerized axial tomography may be helpful to further localize and describe the cystic abnormalities (124). In addition, nuclear magnetic resonance imaging is useful to investigate the extent of Aβ2M-lesions (26, 46, 125).

- Joint ultrasonography has increasingly been employed to detect and quantitatively evaluate thickened joint capsules and tendons in shoulder and hips (126–129). Increasing tendon diameter in correlation to increasing time on dialysis has been presumed to represent Aβ2M-deposition (130). However, sonography is susceptible to geometric errors due to non-standardized projections and techniques especially by inexperienced investigators. In addition, similar synovial changes occur in other, non-Aβ2M-related conditions including AL-amyloidosis (129), and so far no systematic studies on the specificity of joint sonography have been published. Echocardiography has been suggested to represent a valuable tool for search of visceral involvement of Aβ2M (48), but confirmation by other investigators is lacking so far.

Given the multilocular distribution of Aβ2M-amyloidosis throughout the osteoarticular system, scintigraphic imaging methods have been applied to achieve a whole-body oriented assessment. Since it was known that radionuclides used for bone scintigraphy were taken up by non-osseous amyloid tissue of the AL type (131), 99mTechnetium-Methyldiphosphonate (99mTc-MCP) was also evaluated for diagnostic imaging of dialysis related amyloidosis and arthropathy (132, 133), but has been largely abandoned due to the low diagnostic specificity.

In 1988 a new technique for in-vivo imaging of amyloid deposits was described in a mouse model of systemic amyloidosis (134), and subsequently applied in patients with different types of amyloidosis (135, 136). This method was based on the injection of radiolabelled serum amyloid P component (SAP), a nonfibrillar plasma glycoprotein synthetized by the liver, which undergoes non-covalent, calcium-dependent binding to amyloid fibrils and which has been shown to be a constituent of almost all types of amyloid. With ^{123}I-serum amyloid-P component scanning in chronic hemodialysis patients, focal tracer localization occurred at all sites where amyloid had been demonstrated histologically before, and at most sites of clinically diagnosed amyloid disease (137). As expected, the frequency of positive scans as well as the number of regions affected increased with duration of dialysis. Several results concerning the localization of tracer accumulation, however, were unexpected considering the known clinical and histological distribution pattern of Aβ2M: some commonly affected joints such as shoulders and hips had a surprisingly low frequency of tracer uptake (137); on the other hand, a high incidence of splenic tracer enrichment (30% of patients) was reported that is in contrast to autopsy data indicating that splenic Aβ2M-deposition is extremely rare, and even if so, amyloid is only present in minute amounts just like in other visceral organs (64, 138, 139). Short-term dialysis patients showed no evidence of local tracer uptake; likewise, no local tracer accumulation was noted in transplanted patients despite the fact that they had clinically and histologically proven Aβ2M before transplantation (137). It is unclear whether this latter observation indicates that previously existing amyloid deposits had disappeared, or whether it reflects a cessation of active amyloid deposition (including binding of SAP component) after transplantation (see below). Recently, another group has reproduced positive SAP-scintigraphy images in long-term dialysis patients with Aβ2M, but emphasized the limited specificity and sensitivity of this technique (140).

An alternative isotope method based on the administration of the radiolabelled immediate amyloid precursor molecule β2M, which could be assumed to be specific for Aβ2M-amyloidosis, was described in 1989 (141). β2-microglobulin was isolated and purified from hemofiltrate of a long-term dialysis patient who had over years consistently tested negative for hepatitis and human immunodeficiency viruses. After intravenous injection of radiolabelled ^{131}iodine-β2-microglobulin localized tracer enrichment could be detected and visualized by gamma-camera scintigraphy in sites of known or suspected Aβ2M-deposition.

The labelled β2M was taken up specifically into Aβ2M-amyloid as shown by autoradiography and confirmed also by numerous positive histologies from scan-positive sites, while it did not label sites of non-amyloid-related inflammation (62). On follow-up investigation in a small number of patients, the images obtained about one year after the initial study were highly reproducible. Evaluation of the scintigraphy results in the first 42 patients studied (62) showed that compared to clinical and radiological diagnosis of Aβ2M, β2M-scintigraphy was capable to detect more lesions, at an earlier time, and thus represents a more sensitive way to diagnose Aβ2M (Figure 5). Confirming data from a large retrospective clinical study (57) it was shown that the incidence and extent of Aβ2M diagnosed by ^{131}I-β2M scintigraphy increases

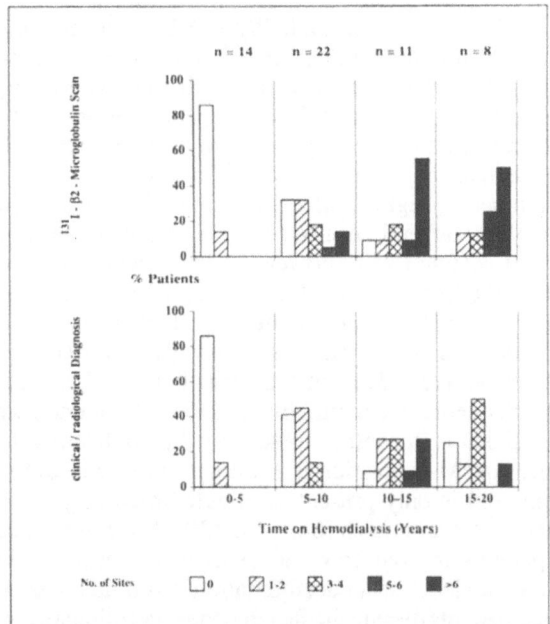

Figure 5. Presence of scintigraphic (^{131}I-β2M) versus clinical/radiological evidence of Aβ2M-amyloidosis (graded according to number of affected sites) depending on time on hemodialysis treatment.

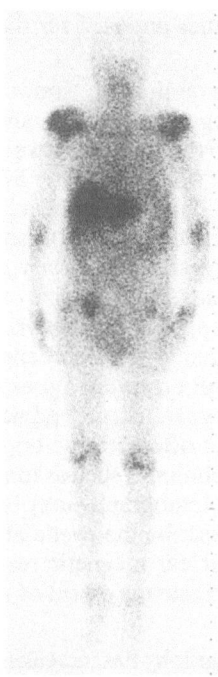

Figure 6. ^{111}In-β2M scintigraphy: ventral whole-body image of 59 year-old patient with severe Aβ2M-amyloidosis after 21 years of hemodialysis.

with time on hemodialysis, and in addition correlates positively with patient age at the onset of HD treatment (63). The usefulness ^{131}I-β2M scanning for the diagnosis of Aβ2M was also demonstrated in long-term chronic ambulatory peritoneal dialysis (CAPD) patients (142). In contrast, the technique does not work reliably in patients with significant residual renal function (e.g., pre-uremic or successfully transplanted patients), because, like endogenous β2M, labelled β2M is readily eliminated by functioning kidneys (91). ^{131}I-β2M scintigraphy has been reproduced with comparable results by groups in Spain (143) and Japan (144) using β2M obtained from urine or hemofiltrate.

The use of ^{131}Iodine for β2M scanning has been criticized because of the amount of radiation exposure due to the relatively long half-life and the significant contribution of β-emission (137). Recently, the labelling procedure was modified to employ the ^{111}indium isotope after covalent attachment of the chelator molecule diethyl-triamine-pentaacetic acid (DTPA) to β2M (145). Compared to ^{131}I-β2M scintigraphy, with the ^{111}In-DTPA-β2M technique better optical resolution is achieved at a significantly lower level of radiation exposure; the effective whole-body equivalent radiation dose in a completely anuric patient was calculated to be 5.3 mSv (Schaeffer et al., in preparation), close to the 4.5 mSv reported for the ^{123}I-SAP scan (136). The images obtained in by ^{111}In-β2M-scintigraphy so far confirmed the good agreement with the clinical and radiological distribution of Aβ2M as seen with the iodine method. Due to the enhanced optical resolution (Figure 6),

imaging of affected smaller joint areas (47, 56, 146) such as sternoclavicular and individual finger joints became possible.

Clinical and radiological signs will remain important clues for Aβ2M-diagnosis in long-term ESRD patients. Radiology and sonography will help to determine the extent of the disease and follow its course over time. β2M scintigraphy due to its non-invasiveness, sensitivity and specificity represents a valuable new approach towards earlier diagnosis of Aβ2M-amyloidosis. However, histomorphological demonstration of Aβ2M-amyloid by congo-red staining and immunohistochemical identification of Aβ2M-type amyloid will remain the diagnostic 'gold-standard'.

PREVENTION AND TREATMENT

One goal of better diagnostic techniques is to improve the therapeutic strategies for ESRD patients in order to avoid or at least delay the onset of Aβ2M-amyloidosis. Currently, kidney transplantation appears to be the only treatment of ESRD that is capable of preventing Aβ2M-formation, due to its capacity to reestablish renal β2M clearance (147, 148). As far as treatment of already existing Aβ2M-disease is concerned, transplantation leads to a rapid improvement in symptoms (possibly due to the administration of steroids), but not neccessarily to a disappearance of amyloid deposits (148–152).

The use of specific dialysis techniques may be related to the development of Aβ2M-amyloidosis (cf 153) on the basis of different mechanisms:

— Increased elimination of the precursor β2M by highly permeable membranes with higher transmembrane flux and possibly some additional adsorption of β2M (154, 155) may be advantageous, if reducing the precursor load (normal serum values cannot be achieved (156)) can slow down the progression of amyloid deposition (38, 157).

— On the other hand, membrane biocompatibility, e.g., the extent of complement stimulation and cytokine induction (75–78), might have an impact on overall β2M generation, or on local β2M processing by cells activated during the dialytic process. The experimental evidence regarding increased β2M generation is controversial: a stimulation of β2M production by mononuclear cells after contact with complement-activating dialysis membranes in-vitro was described in some reports (11, 85, 86); no difference in β2M generation was seen during incubation of whole blood with cellulosic versus polyacrylonitril membranes (83); kinetic studies *in-vivo* did not show a significant rise in β2M generation during the dialysis procedure (88–90, 92).

— Apart from biocompatibility of the membrane, pyrogens originating from bacterial contamination of the dialysate have been shown to permeate the dialyzer membrane (79, 80), and may strongly stimulate cytokine induction (78–81). The use of ultrapure, sterile and pyrogen-free dialysate has been reported to be associated with lower β2M serum concentrations (158), a reduced incidence of carpal tunnel syndrome (159), and a decreased degree of cytokine stimulation (160). Since all types of membrane may allow some pyrogen penetration, the employment of pyrogen-adsorbing ultrafilters in the dialysate circuit is advocated (81).

Clinically, a large retrospective study of dialysis patients treated with Cuprophane® and polyacrylonitril membranes did indeed show a difference in the incidence of cystic bone lesions ascribed to Aβ2M (57). These membranes differ not only in their β2M removal capacity, but also in respect to their biocompatibility, i.e., complement and cytokine induction. Concerning a definitive conclusion, the power of this comparison is somewhat limited due to its retrospective character and the fact that in both groups patients had also been treated (up to 10% of the dialysis duration) with the other type of membrane, and because the radiological diagnostic criteria employed – although well defined – still do not represent a specific diagnosis of Aβ2M-amyloidosis. With similar methodological limitations and smaller numbers, a significant difference between patients predominantly on polyacrilonitril- versus Cuprophane®-membranes was also observed by other authors in the incidence of CTS (161) and bone cysts (124).

Various studies failed to demonstrate a similar significant difference in manifestations of Aβ2M between patients on the different membrane types, but were criticized (162) for methodological reasons: in a study based on an EDTA questionnaire (163), bone cysts were used as the key indicator for Aβ2M-diagnosis, but no further qualification of these lesions was required; this report also indicates that many patients had been dialyzed with the other type of membrane for an extended period of time. Similarly, in another retrospective study (164) specific criteria for the classification of bone cysts were missing, and not β2M-specific forms of arthropathies such as spondylarthropathy were included for analysis. A third report (165), based on a small number of patients, used as an indicator of Aβ2M only the diagnosis of CTS which is not necessarily due to Aβ2M-deposition (as discussed above).

Attempts to reduce the β2M load by specific β2M-adsorbing devices (166) have been described, but their clinical usefulness remains to be established.

Because kidney transplantation is not an option for every patient on treatment for ESRD, and all other forms of renal replacement therapy can at best delay, but not prevent the development of Aβ2M-amyloidosis, symptomatic treatment remains a very important issue. In addition to physical therapy, non-steroidal antiinflammatory drugs and analgesics, corticosteroids are employed to reduce symptoms effectively in selected, severely affected patients (167). Besides carpal tunnel surgery, further operative interventions are removal of large synovial deposits, and preventive stabilizing bone surgery.

For the time being, preliminary guidelines for prevention of Aβ2M-amyloidosis (26, 27) are to aim for early transplantation, and to employ high-flux membranes (with high β2M-removal capacity and low levels of cytokine induction) in older patients with a life expectancy of < 10 years on treatment independent of potential transplantation, and young patients with a life expectancy < 10 years on treatment if transplantation is not possible.

OPEN QUESTIONS

Research on Aβ2M-amyloidosis is characterized by a gap between increasingly specific information and hypotheses on pathobiochemical aspects on one side, and the still increasing frequency and severity of clinical problems in the growing number of long-term ESRD patients on the other side. More knowledge about the underlying processes may help to find new ways to influence the course of the disease.

The question, whether or not the use of certain treatment modes does influence the long-term process of Aβ2M-development, cannot be answered unequivocally yet. Considering the retrospective clinical data, clean prospective multi-center studies will be needed. Well characterized patients, treated consistently with one type of membrane (cellulosic or synthetic) over a number of years, should be studied using well-defined, sensitive diagnostic criteria after certain time intervals for evidence of developing Aβ2M-deposits. Imaging of Aβ2M-amyloid deposits by β2M scintigraphy would serve as a useful tool for this purpose. Current efforts to employ recombinant human β2M as the protein source for β2M scintigraphy may further strengthen this technique.

Successful renal transplantation is the most effective treatment for Aβ2M-amyloidosis because it certainly stops its further progression, even though the question of regression of existing amyloid deposits (150) remains to be clarified.

REFERENCES

1. Warren DJ, Otieno LS: Carpal tunnel syndrome in patients on intermittent hemodialysis. *Postgrad Med J* 51: 450, 1975
2. Assenat H, Calemard E, Charra B, Laurent G, Terret JC, Vanel T: Hemodialyse syndrome du canal carpien et substance amyloide. *Nouv Presse Med* 9: 1715, 1980
3. Charra B, Calemard E, Uzan M, Terrat JC, Vanel T, Laurent G: Carpal tunnel syndrome, shoulder pain and amyloid deposits in long-term haemodialysis patients. *Proc EDTA–ERA* 21: 291, 1984
4. Bardin T, Kuntz D, Zingraff J, Voisin MC, Zelmar A, Lansaman J: Synovial amyloidosis in patients undergoing long-term hemodialysis. *Arthritis Rheum* 28: 1052, 1985
5. Munoz-Gómez J, Bergadá-Barado E, Gómez-Pérez R, Llopart-Buisán E, Subías-Sobrevía E, Rotés-Querol J, Solé-Arqués M: Amyloid arthropathy in patients undergoing periodical haemodialysis for chronic renal failure: a new complication. *Ann Rheum Dis* 44: 729, 1985
6. Morita T, Suzuki M, Kamimura A, Hirasawa Y: Amyloidosis of a possible new type in patients receiving long-term hemodialysis. *Arch Pathol Lab Med* 109: 1029, 1985
7. Rowe IF: Editorial: Amyloid arthropathy. *Ann Rheum Dis* 44: 727, 1985
8. Gejyo F, Yamada T, Odani S, Nakagawa Y, Arakawa M, Kunitomo T, Kataoka H, Suzuki M, Hirasawa Y, Shirahama T, Cohen AS, Schmid K: A new form of amyloid protein associated with chronic hemodialysis was identified as β_2-microglobulin. *Biochem Biophys Res Com* 129: 701, 1985
9. Gejyo F, Odani S, Yamada T, Homma N, Saito H, Suzuki Y, Nakagawa Y, Kobayashi H, Maruyama Y, Hirasawa Y, Suzuki M, Arakawa M: β_2-microglobulin: a new form of amyloid protein associated with chronic hemodialysis. *Kidney Int* 30: 385, 1986
10. Gorevic PD, Casey TT, Stone WJ, DiRaimondo CR, Prelli FC, Frangione B: Beta2-microglobulin is an amyloidogenic protein in man. *J Clin Invest* 76: 2425, 1985
11. Bardin T, Zingraff J, Kuntz D, Drüeke T: Dialysis-related amyloidosis. *Nephrol Dial Transplant* 1: 151, 1986
12. Benz RL, Siegfried JW, Teehan BP: Carpal tunnel syndrome in dialysis patients: comparison between continuous ambulatory peritoneal dialysis and hemodialysis populations. *Am J Kid Dis* 11: 473, 1988
13. Gagnon RF, Lough JO, Bourgouin PA: Carpal tunnel syndrome and amyloidosis associated with continuous ambulatory peritoneal dialysis. *Can Med Assoc J* 139: 753, 1988
14. Cornélis F, Bardin T, Faller B, Verger C, Allouache M, Raymond P, Rottembourg J, Tourlière, Benhamou C, Noel LH, Kuntz D: Rheumatic syndromes and β_2-microglobulin amyloidosis in patients receiving long-term peritoneal dialysis. *Arthritis Rheum* 32: 785, 1989
15. Brown E, Soldano L, Hendler E: Dialysis-related amyloidosis during peritoneal dialysis. *Trans Am Soc Artif Intern Organs* 36: 17, 1990
16. Jadoul M, Noel H, van Ypersele de Strihou C: β_2-microglobulin amyloidosis in a patient treated exclusively by continuous ambulatory peritoneal dialysis. *Am J Kid Dis* 15: 86, 1990
17. Linke RP, Bommer J, Ritz E, Waldherr R, Eulitz M: Amyloid kidney stones of uremic patients consist of beta$_2$-microglobulin fragments. *Biochem Biophys Res Comm* 136: 665, 1986
18. Morinière P, Marie A, El Esper N, Fardellone P, Deramond H, Remond A, Sebert JL, Fournier A: Destructive spondylarthropathy with β2-microglobulin amyloid deposits in a uremic patient before chronic hemodialysis. *Nephron* 59: 654, 1991
19. Noel LH, Zingraff J, Bardin T, Atienza C, Kuntz D, Drüeke T: Tissue distribution of dialysis amyloidosis. *Clin Nephrol* 27: 175, 1987
20. Maher ER, Hamilton Dutoit S, Baillod RA, Sweny P, Moorhead JF: Gastrointestinal complications of dialysis related amyloidosis. *Br Med J* 297: 265, 1988
21. Arakawa M, Geijo F, Oohara K, Homma N: Systemic deposition of beta-2 microglobulin amyloid. in *Dialysis Amyloidosis*, edited by Geijo F, Brancaccio D, Bardin T, Milan, Wichtig Editore, 1989, p 111
22. Shinoda T, Komatsu M, Aizawa T, Shirota T, Yamada T, Jhara T, Mizukami E: Intestinal pseudo-obstruction due to dialysis amyloidosis. *Clin Nephrol* 32: 284, 1989
23. WHO-IUS Nomenclature Sub-Committee: Nomenclature of amyloid and amyloidoses. *Bull World Health Org* 71: 105, 1993
24. Drüeke T, Zingraff J: Beta-2-microglobulin-related amyloidosis in long-term hemodialysis patients: possible pathogenetic mechanisms. *Contr Nephrol* 59: 99, 1987
25. Kleinman KS, Coburn JW: Amyloid syndromes associated with hemodialysis. *Kidney Int* 35: 567, 1989
26. Koch KM: Dialysis-related amyloidosis. *Kidney Int* 41: 1416, 1992
27. Floege J, Ehlerding G: Beta-2-microglobulin associated amyloidosis (Aβ2M-amyloidosis). *Nephron* 72: 9, 1996
28. Gravallese EM, Baker N, Lester S, Kay J, Owen WF: Musculoskeletal manifestations in β2-microglobulin amyloidosis. Case discussion. *Arthritis Rheum* 35: 592, 1992
29. Jain VK, Cestero RVM, Baum J: Carpal tunnel syndrome in patients undergoing hemodialysis. *J Am Med Assoc* 242: 2868, 1978
30. Halter SK, DeLisa JA, Stolov WC, Scardapane D, Sherrard DJ: Carpal tunnel syndrome in chronic renal dialysis patients. *Arch Phys Med Rehabil* 62: 197, 1981
31. Delmez JA, Holtmann B, Sicard GA, Goldberg AP, Harter HR: Peripheral nerve entrapment syndromes in chronic hemodialysis patients. *Nephron* 30: 118, 1982

32. Spertini F, Wauters JP, Poulenas I: Carpal tunnel syndrome: a frequent, invalidating, long-term complication of chronic hemodialysis. *Clin Nephrol* 21: 98, 1984

33. Corradi M, Paganelli E, Pavesi G: Internal neurolysis and flexor tenosynovectomy: adjuncts in the treatment of chronic median nerve compression at the wrist in hemodialysis patients. *Microsurgery* 10: 248, 1989

34. Kurer MH, Baillod RA, Madgwick JCA: Musculoskeletal manifestations of amyloidosis. *J Bone Joint Surg* 73-B: 271, 1991

35. Gejyo F, Homma N, Arakawa M: Carpal tunnel syndrome and β2-microglobulin-related amyloidosis in chronic hemodialysis patients. *Blood Purif* 6: 125, 1988

36. Rubin LA, Fam AG, Rubenstein J, Campbell J, Saiphoo C: Erosive azotemic osteoarthropathy. *Arthritis Rheum* 27: 1086, 1984

37. DiRaimondo CR, Casey TT, DiRaimondo CV, Stone WR: Pathologic fractures associated with idiopathic amyloidosis of bone in chronic hemodialysis patients. *Nephron* 43: 22, 1986

38. Vandenbroucke JM, Jadoul M, Maldague B, Huaux JP, Noel H, van Ypersele de Strihou C: Possible role of dialysis membrane characteristics in amyloid osteoarthropathy. *Lancet* i: 1210, 1986

39. Hurst NP, van den Berg R, Disney A, Alcock M, Albertyn L, Green M, Pascoe V: 'Dialysis related arthropathy': a survey of 95 patients receiving chronic haemodialysis with special reference to β2 microglobulin related amyloidosis. *Ann Rheum Dis* 48: 409, 1989

40. Onishi S, Andress DL, Maloney NA, Coburn JW, Sherrard DJ: Beta2-microglobulin deposition in bone in chronic renal failure. *Kidney Int* 39: 990, 1991

41. Kuntz D, Naveau B, Bardin T, Drüeke T, Treves R, Dryll A: Destructive spondylarthropathy in hemodialyzed patients. A new syndrome. *Arthritis Rheum* 27: 369, 1984

42. Sebert JL, Fardellone P, Marie A: Destructive spondylarthropathy in hemodialyzed patients: possible role of amyloidosis. *Arthritis Rheum* 29: 301, 1986

43. Bindi P, Chanard J: Destructive spondyloarthropathy in dialysis patients: an overview. *Nephron* 55: 104, 1990

44. Ohashi K, Hara M, Kawai R, Ogura Y, Honda K, Nihei H, Mimura N: Cervical discs are most susceptible to beta2-microglobulin amyloid deposition in the vertebral column. *Kidney Int* 41: 1646, 1992

45. Allain TJ, Stevens PE, Bridges LR, Phillips ME: Dialysis myelopathy: quadriparesis due to extradural amyloid of β2 microglobulin origin. *Br Med J* 296: 752, 1988

46. Kröner G, Stäbler A, Seiderer M, Moran JE, Gurland HJ: β2 Microglobulin-related spondylarthropathy with spinal-cord compression in haemodialysis patients: detection by MRI. *Nephrol Dial Transplant* 6 (Suppl 2): 91, 1991

47. Sethi D, Maher ER, Cary NRB: Dialysis amyloid presenting as acute arthritis. *Nephron* 30: 73, 1988

48. Campistol JM, Solé M, Munoz-Gómez J, Lopez-Pedret J, Revert L: Systemic involvement of dialysis amyloidosis. *Am J Nephrol* 10: 389, 1990

49. Takahashi S, Morita T, Koda Y, Murayama H, Hirasawa Y: Gastrointestinal involvement of dialysis-related amyloidosis. *Clin Nephrol* 30: 168, 1988

50. Watanabe K, Nakamura R, Kano S, Ohtake T, Hosoda Y, Saruta T: Amyloid urinary-tract calculi in patients on chronic dialysis. *Nephron* 52: 334, 1989

51. Brancaccio D, Gallieni M, Padovese P, Anelli A, Coggi G, Uslenghi C: Dialysis amyloidosis with massive popliteal deposition of beta2-microglobulin amyloid. *Lancet* ii: 802, 1988

52. Floege J, Brandis A, Nonnast-Daniel B, Westhoff-Bleck M, Tidow G, Linke RP, Koch KM: Subcutaneous amyloid-tumor of beta-2-microglobulin origin in a long-term hemodialysis patient. *Nephron* 53: 73, 1989

53. Athanasou NA, Ayers H, Rainey AJ, Oliver DO, Duthie RB: Joint and systemic distribution of dialysis amyloidosis. *Quart J Med* 78: 205, 1991

54. Campistol JM, Solé M, Ferrando J, Palou J, Munoz-Gómez J, López-Pedret J, Revert L: Negativeness of skin biopsy in dialysis amyloidosis. *Nephron* 48: 259, 1988

55. Varga J, Idelson BA, Felson D, Skinner M, Cohen AS: Lack of amyloid in abdominal fat aspirates from patients undergoing long-term hemodialysis. *Arch Int Med* 147: 1455, 1987

56. Stein G, Schneider A, Thoss K, Ritz E, Linke RP, Schaefer K, Sperschneider H, Abendroth K, Fünfstück R: Beta-2-microglobulin-derived amyloidosis: onset, distribution and clinical features in 13 hemodialysed patients. *Nephron* 60: 274, 1992

57. van Ypersele de Strihou C, Jadoul M, Malghem J, Maldague B, Jamart J, and the Working Party on Dialysis Amyloidosis: Effect of dialysis membrane and patient's age on signs of dialysis-related amyloidosis. *Kidney Int* 39: 1012, 1991

58. Maioraca R, Cancarini GC, Brunori G, Camerini C, Manili L: Morbidity and mortality of CAPD and hemodialysis. *Kidney Int* 43 (Suppl 40): S4, 1993

59. Schwarz A, Keller F, Seyfert S, Poll W, Molzahn M, Distler A: Carpal tunnel syndrome: a major complication in long-term hemodialysis patients. *Clin Nephrol* 22: 133, 1984

60. Haudoin P, Flipo RM, Foissac-Gegoux P, Thevenon A, Pouyol F, Duquesnoy B, Delcambre B: Current aspects of osteoarticular pathology in patients undergoing hemodialysis: study of 80 patients. Part 1. Clinical and radiological analysis. *J Rheumatol* 14: 780, 1987

61. Charra B, Calemard E, Laurent G: Chronic renal failure treatment duration and mode: their relevance to the late dialysis periarticular syndrome. *Blood Purif* 6: 117, 1988

62. Floege J, Burchert W, Brandis A, Gielow P, Nonnast-Daniel B, Spindler E, Hundeshagen H, Shaldon S, Koch KM: Imaging of dialysis-related amyloid (AB-amyloid) deposits with ^{131}I-β2-microglobulin. *Kidney Int* 38: 1169, 1990

63. Schaeffer J, Ehlerding G, Burchert W, Floege J, Shaldon S, Koch KM: Relationship of scintigraphically proven dialysis-related amyloidosis (DRA) to age and time on hemodialysis (HD). *J Am Soc Nephrol* 3: 392, 1992

64. Floege J, Schäffer J, Koch KM, Shaldon S: Dialysis related amyloidosis: a disease of chronic retention and inflammation? *Kidney Int* 42 (Suppl 38): S78, 1992

65. Coggi E, Maiorano E, Braidotti P, Dell'Orto P, Viale G: Beta-2 microglobulin amyloidosis in synovial membranes: histopathology, immunocytochemistry and electron microscopy. in *Dialysis Amyloidosis*, edited by

Gejyo F, Brancaccio D, Bardin T, Milan, Wichting Editore, 1989, p 57

66. Homma N, Geyjo F, Isemura M, Arakawa M: Collagen-binding affinity of β_2-microglobulin, a preprotein of hemodialysis-associated amyloidosis. *Nephron* 53: 37, 1989

67. Kisilevsky R, Snow AA: The potential significance of sulphated glycosaminoglycans as a common constituent of all amyloids: or, perhaps amyloid is not a misnomer. *Med Hypotheses* 26: 231, 1988

68. Gejyo F, Homma N, Suzuki Y, Arakawa M: Serum levels of β_2-microglobulin as a new form of amyloid protein in patients undergoing long-term hemodialysis. (Letter) *N Engl J Med* 314: 585, 1986

69. Linke RP, Hampl H, Barthel-Schwarze S, Eulitz M: β_2-microglobulin, different fragments and polymers therof in synovial amyloid in long-term hemodialysis. *Biol Chem Hoppe Seyler* 368: 137, 1987

70. Connors LH, Shirahama T, Skinner M,Fenves A, Cohen AS: *In vitro* formation of amyloid fibrils from intact β_2-microglobulin. *Biochem Biophys Res Comm* 131: 1063, 1985

71. Campistol JM, Sole M, Bombi JA, Rodriguez R, Mirapeix E, Munoz-Gomez J, Revert LI: *In vitro* spontaneous synthesis of beta-2-microglobulin amyloid fibrils in peripheral blood mononuclear cell culture. *Am J Pathol* 141: 241, 1992

72. Stein G, Schneider A, Thoss K, Ritz E, Schaefer K, Hüller M, Sperschneider H, Marzoll I: β_2-microglobulin serum concentration and associated amyloidosis in dialysis patients. *Nephrol Dial Transplant* 6 (Suppl 3): 57, 1991

73. Nachbaur K, Troppmair J, Bieling P, Kotlan B, König P, Huber CH: Cytokines in the control of β_2-microglobulin release. *In-vitro* studies on various hematopoietic cells. *Immunobiol* 177: 55, 1988

74. Nachbaur K, Troppmair J, Kotlan B, König P, Aulitzky W, Bieling P, Huber CH: Cytokines in the control of β_2-microglobulin release. *In vivo* studies with recombinant interferons and antigens. *Immunobiol* 177: 66, 1988

75. Lonnemann G, Koch KM, Shaldon S, Dinarello CA: Studies on the ability of hemodialysis membranes to induce, bind and clear human interleukin-1. *J Lab Clin Med* 112: 76, 1988

76. Haeffner-Cavaillon N, Cavaillon JM, Ciancioni C, Bacle F, Delons S, Katatchkine MD: *In vivo* induction of interleukin-1 during hemodialysis. *Kidney Int* 35: 1212, 1989

77. Schindler R, Linnenweber S, Schulze M, Oppermann M, Dinarello CA, Shaldon S, Koch KM: Gene expression of interleukin-1β during hemodialysis. *Kidney Int* 43: 712, 1993

78. Schindler R, Lonnemann G, Shaldon S, Koch KM, Dinarello CA: Transcription, not synthesis, of interleukin-1 and tumor necrosis factor by complement. *Kidney Int* 37: 85, 1990

79. Laude-Sharp M, Caroff M, Simard L, Pusineri C, Kazatchkine MD, Haeffner-Cavaillon N: Induction of IL-1 during hemodialysis: transmembrane passage of intact endotoxins (LPS). *Kidney Int* 38: 1089, 1990

80. Lonnemann G, Behme TC, Lenzner B, Floege J, Schulze M, Colton CK, Koch KM, Shaldon S: Permeability of dialyzer membranes to TNFalpha-inducing substances derived from water bacteria. *Kidney Int* 42: 61, 1992

81. Lonnemann G, Koch KM: Pyrogenic reactions. in *Replacement of Renal Function by Dialysis*, edited by Jacobs C, Kjellstrand C, Koch KM, Winchester JM, Dordrecht, Kluwer Academic Publishers, 1996, this volume

82. Campistol JM, Molin R, Bernard D, Rodriguez R, Mirapeix E, Munoz-Gomez J, Revert LI: *In vitro* synthesis of β_2-microglobulin: role of hemodialysis (HD), dialysis membranes, dialysis-amyloidosis (Aβ2M) and lymphokines. *Nephrol Dial Transplant* 7: 749, 1992

83. Zingraff J, Beyne P, Urena P, Uzan M, Nguyen Khoa Man, Descamps-Latscha B, Drüeke T: Influence of haemodialysis membranes on β_2-microglobulin kinetics: *in vivo* and *in vitro* studies. *Nephrol Dial Transplant* 3: 284, 1988

84. Paczek L, Schaefer RM, Heidland A: Dialysis membranes inhibit *in vitro* release of β_2-microglobulin from human lymphocytes. *Nephron* 56: 267, 1990

85. Zaoui PM, Stone WJ, Hakim RM: Effects of dialysis membranes on beta$_2$-microglobulin production and cellular expression. *Kidney Int* 38: 962, 1990

86. Jahn B, Betz M, Deppisch R, Janssen O, Hänsch GM, Ritz E: Stimulation of β_2-microglobulin synthesis in lymphocytes after exposure to Cuprophane dialyzer membranes. *Kidney Int* 40: 285, 1991

87. Hönig A, Marsden T, Schad S, Barth C, Pollok M, Baldamus CA: Correlation of β_2-microglobulin concentration changes to distribution volume. *Int J Artif Organs* 11: 459, 1988

88. Floege J, Granolleras C, Merscher S, Eisenbach GM, Deschodt G, Colton CK, Shaldon S, Koch KM: Is the rise in plasma beta-2-microglobulin seen during hemodialysis meaningful? *Nephron* 51: 6, 1989

89. Vincent C, Revillard JP, Galland M, Traeger J: Serum β_2-microglobulin in hemodialyzed patients. *Nephron* 21: 260, 1978

90. Odell RA, Slowiaczek P, Moran JE, Schindhelm K: Beta 2-microglobulin kinetics in end-stage renal failure. *Kidney Int* 39: 909, 1991

91. Floege J, Bartsch A, Schulze M, Shaldon S, Koch KM, Smeby LC: Clearance and synthesis rates of β_2-microglobulin in hemodialyzed patients and normals. *J Lab Clin Med* 118: 153, 1991

92. Vincent C, Chanard J, Caudwell V, Lavaud S, Wong T, Revillard JP: Kinetics of ^{123}I-β_2-microglobulin turnover in dialyzed patients. *Kidney Int* 42: 1434, 1992

93. Linke RP, Hampl H, Lobeck H, Rith E, Bommer J, Waldherr R, Eulitz M: Lysine-specific cleavage of β_2-microglobulin in amyloid deposits associated with hemodialysis. *Kidney Int* 36: 675, 1989

94. Hörl WH, Schaefer RM, Heidland A: Effect of different dialyzers on proteinases and proteinase inhibitors during hemodialysis. *Am J Nephrol* 5: 320, 1985

95. Argiles A, Mourad G, Atkins RC, Mion CM: New insights into the pathogenesis of hemodialysis-related amyloidosis. *Semin Dial* 3: 149, 1990

96. Campistol JM, Shirahama T, Abraham CR, Rodgers OG, Solé M, Cohen AS, Skinner M: Demonstration of plasma proteinase inhibitors in β_2-microglobulin amyloid deposits. *Kidney Int* 42: 915, 1992

97. Argiles A, Kerr PG, Mion C, Atkins RC: Serum alpha2-macroglobulin levels increase during dialysis indepen-

dent of the membrane used. *Nephrol Dial Transplant* 7: 748, 1992

98. Ogawa H, Saito A, Oda O, Nakajima M, Chung TG: Detection of novel beta2-microglobulin in the serum of hemodialysis patients and its amyloidogenic predisposition. *Clin Nephrol* 30: 158, 1988

99. Odani H, Oyama R, Titani K, Ogawa H, Saito A: Purification and complete amino acid sequence of novel beta2-microglobulin. *Biochem Biophys Res Commun* 168: 1223, 1990

100. Argiles A, Derancourt J, Jauregui-Adell J, Mion C, Demaille JG: Biochemical demonstration of serum and urinary beta 2-microglobulin in end-stage renal disease patients. *Nephrol Dial Transplant* 7: 1106, 1992

101. Vincent C, Dennoroy L, Revillard JP: Molecular variants of β2-microglobulin in renal insufficiency. *Biochem J* 298: 181, 1994

102. Linke RP: Altered β2-microglobulin in the genesis of AB-amyloidosis in uremic patients. *Rev Rhum* [Engl Ed] 61 (Suppl 9): 1, 1994

103. Miyata T, Oda O, Inagi R, Iida Y, Araki N, Yamada N, Horiuchi S, Taniguchi N, Maeda K, Kinoshita T: β2-microglobulin modified with advanced glycation end products is a major component of hemodialysis-associated amyloidosis. *J Clin Invest* 92: 1243, 1993

104. Kirstein M, Brett J, Radoff S, Ogawa S, Stern D, Vlassara H: Advanced protein glycasolation induces transendothelial human monocyte chemotaxis and secretion of platelet-derived growth factor: role in vascular disease of diabetes and aging. *Proc Natl Acad Sci USA* 87: 9010, 1990

105. Vlassara H, Brownlee M, Manogue KR, Dinarello CA, Pasagian A: Cachectin/TNF and IL-1 induced by glucose-modified protein: role in normal tissue remodeling. *Science* 240: 1546, 1988

106. Miyata T, Inagi R, Iida Y, Sato M, Yamada N, Oda O, Maeda K, Seo H: Involvement of β2-microglobulin modified with advanced glycation end products in the pathogenesis of hemodialysis-associated amyloidosis. *J Clin Invest* 93: 521, 1994

107. Ueda T: A histological study on the synovial tissue of rat knee joints in the experimental beta2-microglobulin derived amyloidosis. *Ryumachi (Japan)* 32: 308, 1992

108. Ehlerding G, Floege J, Schäffer J, Drommer W, Koch KM: No evidence for inflammatory or fibrotic synovial changes prior to deposition of dialysis related amyloid. *J Am Soc Nephrol* 4: 344, 1993

109. Gejyo F, Maruyama H, Teramura T, Kazama J, Ei I, Arahava N: Role of macrophages in β2-microglobulin-related dialysis amyloidosis. *Contr Nephrol* 112: 97, 1995

110. Ohishi H, Skinner M, Sato AN, Okuyama T, Geyjo F, Kimura A, Cohen AS, Schmid K: Glycosaminoglycans of the hemodialysis-associated carpal synovial amyloid and of amyloid-rich tissues and fibrils of heart, liver, and spleen. *Clin Chem* 36: 223, 1990

111. Ishii M, Kobayashi H, Chanoki M, Fukai K, Kono T, Hamada T, Muragaki Y, Ooshima A: Possible formation of cutaneous amyloid from degenerative collagen fibers. *Acta Derm Venerol* 70: 378, 1990

112. Brancaccio D, Garberi A, Ghiggeri GM, Zoni U, Braidotti P, Coggi G: B2M and Kii light chain are putative cofactors in the pathogenesis of dialysis amyloidosis. *J Am Soc Nephrol* 4: 335, 1993

113. Garcia-Garcia M, Garcia-Valero J, Mourad G, Argiles A: Protein constituents of amyloid deposits in beta2-microglobulin amyloidosis. *Rev Rhum* [Engl Ed] 61 (Suppl 9): 7S, 1994

114. Bommer J, Seelig P, Seelig R, Geerlings W, Bommer G, Ritz E: Determinants of plasma β2Microglobulin concentration: possible relation to membrane biocompatibility. *Nephrol Dial Transplant* 2: 22, 1987

115. Canaud B, Assounga A, Flavier JL, Slingeneyer A, Aznar R, Robinet-Levy M, Mion C: β-2 microglobulin serum levels in maintenance dialysis – what does is mean? *Trans Am Soc Artif Intern Organs* 34: 923, 1988

116. Sethi D, Gower PE: Dialysis arthropathy, β2-microglobulin and the effect of dialyser membrane. *Nephrol Dial Transplant* 3: 768, 1988

117. Hampl H, Lobeck H, Barthel-Schwarze S, Stein H, Eulitz M, Linke RP: Clinical, morphologic, biochemical, and immunohistochemical aspects of dialysis-associated amyloidosis. *Trans Am Soc Artif Intern Organs* 33: 250, 1987

118. Solé M, Cardesa A, Palacin A, Munoz-Gómez J, Campistol JM: Morphological and immunohistochemical findings in dialysis-related amyloidosis. *Appl Pathol* 7: 350, 1989

119. Nishi S, Gejyo F, Arakawa M: A histochemical study of hemodialysis related amyloidosis. *Acta Med Biol* 39 (Suppl): 75, 1991

120. Munoz-Gómez J, Gómez-Pérez R, Solé-Arques M, Llopart-Buisán E: Synovial fluid examination for the diagnosis of synovial amyloidosis in patients with chronic renal failure undergoing hemodialysis. *Ann Rheum Dis* 46: 324, 1987

121. Puchtler H, Sweat F, Levine M: On the binding of congo red by amyloid. *J Histochem Cytochem* 10: 335, 1962

122. Gejyo F, Homman N, Saito H, Arakawa M: Carpal tunnel sysdrome and beta-2 microglobulin amyloidosis: histological and biochemical aspects. in *Dialysis Amyloidosis*, edited by Geijo F, Brancaccio D, Bardin T, Milan, Wichtig Editore, 1989, p 35

123. Poznanski AK: *The Hand in Radiologic Diagnosis*, Ch. 8, Normal variation and congenital anomalies of the wrist, Philadelphia–London–Toronto, WB Saunders, 1974, p 128

124. Miura Y, Ishiyama T, Inomata A, Takeda T, Senma S, Okuyama K, Suzuki Y: Radiolucent bone cysts and the type of dialysis membrane used in patients undergoing long-term hemodialysis. *Nephron* 60: 268, 1992

125. Cobby MJ, Adler RS, Swartz R, Martel W: Dialysis-related amyloid arthropathy: MR findings in four patients. *Am Journal Roentgenol* 157: 1023, 1991

126. Jadoul M, Malghem J, Vandeberg B, van Ypersele de Strihou C: Ultrasonographic detection of thickened joint capsules and tendons: an early marker of dialysis-related amyloidosis. *Nephrol Dial Transplant* 5: 727, 1990

127. McMahon LP, Radford J, Dawborn JK: Shoulder ultrasound in dialysis related amyloidosis. *Clin Nephrol* 35: 227, 1991

128. Kay J, Benson CB, Lester S, Corson JM, Pinkus GS, Lazarus JM, Owen WF: Utility of high-resolution ultrasound for the diagnosis of dialysis-related amyloidosis. *Arthritis Rheum* 35: 926, 1992

129. Jadoul M, Malghem J, Vande Berg B, Van Ypersele de Strihou C: Ultrasonography of joint capsules and tendons

in dialysis-related amyloidosis. *Kidney Int* 43 (Suppl 41): 106, 1993

130. Calemard E, Charra B, Terrat JC, Vanei T, Chazot C, Laurent G, Pracros JP: Hip's synovial thickness and late dialysis arthropathy. *Nephrol Dial Transplant* 5: 725, 1990

131. Yood RA, Skinner M, Cohen AS, Lee VW: Soft tissue uptake of bone seeking radionuclide in amyloidosis. *J Rheumatol* 8: 760, 1981

132. Grateau G, Zingraff J, Fauchet M, Mundler O, Raymond P, Berthelot JM, Bardin T, Kuntz D, Drueke T: Radionuclide exploration of dialysis amyloidosis: preliminary experience. *Am J Kidney Dis* 9: 231, 1988

133. Sethi D, Naunton Morgan TC, Brown EA, Jewkes RF, Gower PE: Technetium-99-labelled methylene diphosphonate uptake scans in patients with dialysis arthropathy. *Nephron* 54: 202, 1990

134. Hawkins PN, Myers MJ, Epenetos AA, Caspi D, Pepys MB: Specific localization and imaging of mayloid deposits *in vivo* using ^{123}I-labelled serum amyloid P component. *J Exp Med* 167: 903, 1988

135. Hawkins PN, Myers MJ, Lavender JP, Pepys MB: Diagnostic radionuclide imaging of amyloid: biological targeting by circulating human serum amyloid P component. *Lancet* i: 1413, 1988

136. Hawkins PN, Lavender JP, Pepys MB: Evaluation of systemic amyloidosis by scintigraphy with ^{123}I-labelled serum amyloid P component. *N Engl J Med* 323: 508, 1990

137. Nelson SR, Hawkins PN, Richardson S, Lavender JP, Sethi D, Gower PE, Pugh CW, Winearls CG, Oliver DO, Pepys MB: Imaging of haemodialysis-associated amyloidosis with ^{123}I-serum amyloid P component. *Lancet* ii: 335, 1991

138. Zingraff J, Bardin T, Noel LH, Drüeke T: Lack of haemodialysis-associated amyloidosis. *Lancet* ii: 1089, 1991

139. Korzets A, Gafter U, Gal R, Schwartz A, Chagnac A, Weinstein T, Zevin D, Levi J: Hemodialysis associated amyloidosis (HAA) is a systemic disease. *J Am Soc Nephrol* 4: 362, 1993

140. Duquesnoy B, Flipo RM, Deveaux M, Foissac-Gegoux P, Marchandise X. Imaging of dialysis-related amyloid deposits with iodine-123-labeled serum amyloid P component. *Rev Rhum* [Engl Ed] 61 (Suppl 9): 33S, 1994

141. Floege J, Nonnast-Daniel B, Gielow P, Brandis A, Spindler E, Hundeshagen H, Koch KM, Shaldon S: Specific imaging of dialysis-related amyloid deposits using ^{131}I-β_2-microglobulin. *Nephron* 51: 444. 1989

142. Schaeffer J, Ehlerding G, Burchert W, Tsobanelis T, Jungheinrich C, Gruetzmacher P, Floege J: Imaging of dialysis-related amyloid (DRA) by ^{131}I β_2-microglobulin scan in CAPD. *Nephrol Dial Transplant* 7: 752, 1992

143. Ponz E, Piera C, Campistol JM, Lomena F, Deulofeu R, Munoz J, Revert L: Diagnostic imaging of dialysis amyloidosis (D-AM) with 131-β2 microglobulin (β2-M). Preliminary results. *Nephrol Dial Transplant* 5: 729, 1990

144. Kiyota A, Sugimura T, Yamagami S, Kishimoto T: Specific scintigraphy imaging of dialysis-related amyloid (DRA) deposits using ^{131}I-β_2-microglobulin (^{131}I-β_2-M). *J Am Soc Nephrol* 3: 374, 1992

145. Schäffer J, Burchert W, Floege J, Gielow P, Mahiout A, Nonnast-Daniel B, Shaldon S, Koch KM: Scan-

ning for dialysis related amyloidosis: improved resolution and reduced radiation exposure with ^{111}Indium-β_2-microglobulin. *J Am Soc Nephrol* 4: 382, 1993

146. Zingraff J, Noel LH, Bardin T, Kuntz D, Dubost C, Drueke T: β2-microglobulin amyloidosis: a sternoclavicular joint biopsy study in hemodialysis patients. *Clin Nephrol* 33: 94, 1990

147. Sethi D, Brown EA, Maini RN, Gower PE: Renal transplantation for dialysis arthropathy. *Lancet* ii: 448, 1988

148. Jadoul M, Malghem J, Prison Y, Maldague B, van Ypersele de Strihou C: Effect of renal transplantation on the radiological signs of dialysis amyloid osteoarthropathy. *Clin Nephrol* 32: 194, 1989

149. Sethi D, Brown EA, Cary NRB, Woodrow DF, Gower PE: Persistence of dialysis amyloid after renal transplantation. *Am J Nephrol* 9: 173, 1988

150. Nelson SR, Sharpstone P, Kingswood JC: Does dialysis-associated amyloid resolve after transplantation ? *Nephrol Dial Transplant* 8: 369, 1993

151. Kessler M, Netter P, Gaucher A: Outcome of dialysis-associated arthropathy and dialysis-related β2-microglobulin amyloidosis after renal transplantation. *Rev Rhum* [Engl Ed] 61 (Suppl 9:) 93S, 1994

152. Lebail-Darné JL, Bardin T, Zingraff J, Laredo JD, Voisin VC, Kreiss H, Kuntz D: The effect of renal transplantation on dialysis associated arthropathy. *Rev Rhum* [Engl Ed] 61 (Suppl 9): 89S, 1994

153. van Ypersele der Strihou C, Floege J, Jadoul M, Koch KM: Amyloidosis and its relationship to different dialysers. *Nephrol Dial Transplant* 9 (Suppl 2): 156, 1994

154. Floege J, Granolleras C, Deschodt G, Heck M, Baudin G, Branger B, Tournier O, Reinhard B, Eisenbach GM, Smeby LC, Shaldon S: High-flux synthetic versus cellulosic membranes for β2-microglobulin removal during hemodialysis, hemodiafiltration and hemofiltration. *Nephrol Dial Transplant* 4: 653, 1989

155. Floege J, Smeby L: Dialysis-related amyloidosis and high-flux membranes. *Contr Nephrol* 96: 124, 1992

156. Canaud B, Assounga A, Kerr P, Aznar R, Mion C: Failure of a daily haemofiltration programme using a highly permeable membrane to return β2-microglobulin concentrations to normal in haemodialysis patients. *Nephrol Dial Transplant* 7: 924, 1992

157. Drüeke T, Urena P, Man NK, Zingraff J: Membrane transfer, membrane adsorption and possible membrane-induced generation of beta-2-microglobulin. *Contr Nephrol* 74: 113, 1989

158. Quellhorst E, Schünemann B: Beta-2 amyloidosis and haemofiltration. in *Dialysis Amyloidosis*, edited by Gejyo F, Brancaccio D, Bardin T, Milan, Wichtig Editore, 1989, p 123

159. Baz M, Durand C, Ragon A, Jaber K, Andrieu D, Merzouk T, Purgus R, Olmer M, Reynier JP, Berland Y: Using ulatrpure water in hemodialysis delays carpal tunnel syndrome. *Int J Artif Organs* 14: 681, 1991

160. Schindler R, Lonnemann G, Schäffer J, Shaldon S, Koch KM, Krautzig S: The effect of ultrafiltered dialysate on the cellular content of interleukin-1 receptor antagonist in patients on chronic hemodialysis. *Nephron* 68: 229, 1994

161. Chanard J, Bindi P, Lavaud S, Toupance O, Maheut H, Lacour F: Carpal tunnel syndrome and type of dialysis membrane. *Br Med J* 298: 867, 1989

162. van Ypersele de Strihou C, Jadoul M, Jamart J: Highly permeable and biocompatible membranes. *Lancet* i: 1415, 1991

163. Brunner FP, Brynger H, Ehrich JHH, Fassbinder W, Geerlings W, Rizzoni G, Selwood NH, Tufveson G, Wing AJ: Case control study on dialysis arthropathy: the influence of two different dialysis membranes: data from the EDTA registry. *Nephrol Dial Transplant* 5: 432, 1990

164. Kessler M, Netter P, Maheut H, Wolf C, Prenat E, Huu TC, Gaucher A: Highly permeable and biocompatible membranes and prevalence of dialysis-associated arthropathy. (Letter) *Lancet* i: 1092, 1991

165. Simon P, Ang KS, Cavarle Y, Cam G, Catheline M, Genetet N: Does immunodeficiency in uremic patients promote dialysis-related amyloidosis? *Int J Artif Organs* 11: 102, 1988

166. Furuyoshi S, Matsumura T, Fujimoto T, Yasuda A, Takata S, Tani N, Nakazawa R, Honma N, Gejyo F, Arakawa M: Intensive removal of beta-2-microglobulin with adsorbent column. *Nephrol Dial Transplant* 7: 750, 1992

167. Bardin T: Low-dose prednisone in dialysis-related amyloid arthropathy. *Rev Rhum* [Engl Ed] 61 (Suppl 9): 97S, 1994

OPTIONS IN RENAL REPLACEMENT THERAPY

A.M. DAVISON

INTRODUCTION

Since the introduction over forty years ago of regular dialysis therapy for the management of end stage renal failure there have been dramatic changes in the way this treatment is provided. In pioneering days only a few highly selected patients were considered for treatment and only one treatment option was available (9). Generally, patients were treated twice weekly by haemodialysis for 14 hours with equipment which was, by present day standards, rather inefficient with little or no monitoring. Research and development has resulted in significant advances in dialyser design, membrane performance, and monitoring devices with the consequence that patients are now treated with expensive sophisticated equipment utilising computer assisted controls. Unlike the previous 'fixed' regimen patients now have the possibility of treatment 'tailored' to their individual requirement by using measurements of dialysis adequacy to determine the length of each dialysis session and currently patients' haemodialysis sessions vary from 2.5 to 6 hours twice or, more commonly, thrice weekly. This enables more patients to be treated as each dialysis machine may be used for two or three patients daily whereas previously with 14 hour sessions only one patient could be accommodated. In the late seventies continuous ambulatory peritoneal dialysis was introduced for the management of end stage renal failure (16). Previously peritoneal dialysis was virtually confined to the management of acute renal failure and was considered unsuitable for long-term management due to the lack of appropriate access to the peritoneal cavity and the almost invariable peritonitis due to poor technology relating to connecting and disconnecting the dialysis fluid. The development of soft permanent peritoneal catheters and improved design

of the lines and connections has however largely overcome the early difficulties with the consequence that peritoneal dialysis is now an effective and alternative additional therapeutic modality allowing for an increase in the numbers of patients receiving treatment. With these developments we have progressed to virtually unselected admissions to a programme which has multiple therapeutic options and as a consequence the physician managing a patient with terminal uraemia is required to make a series of decisions with respect to future management. These include:

1. Is dialysis appropriate treatment?
2. When is the most appropriate time to start dialysis support?
3. What is the most appropriate form of dialysis for the individual patient?
4. Where should dialysis be undertaken?
5. What is the potential for transplantation either before or after the commencement of dialysis?

Each of these questions has to be addressed separately and require full informed discussion with the patient and, where appropriate, relatives and/or carers. In the majority of instances the patient will be able to make an informed decision but in the case of young children, the elderly, and the mentally infirm it is necessary to consider the views of the family and other health care professionals such as the patient's general practitioner, involved nursing staff, and medical social workers. It is important to remember, however, that it is the responsibility of the attending physician to come to a decision and at all costs one must avoid management by committee whilst at the same time seeking a consensus view from all involved health care professionals. It is interesting to note how many people wish to take part in such discussions but thereafter leave the consequences to others. Patient confidentiality must be maintained at all times and equally important is to maintain the patient's confidence that his or her best interests will be sustained.

CAUSES FOR DIFFERENCES IN PRACTICE IN RENAL REPLACEMENT THERAPY

The answers which will evolve will depend on many factors not the least of which is the local availability of dialysis and transplantation facilities. It is interesting to note the diversity of practice which exists from country to country and between the industrialised and developing world. It would appear that each community has evolved its own particular practice and although it is tempting to compare, and as a consequence criticise, it is a fruitless exercise unless a very comprehensive evaluation is undertaken and all the factors influencing the evaluation of the particular service are known and understood.

There are indeed wide differences in renal replacement practice in different countries. It is not entirely clear why these differences have evolved, but it seems that almost every country has developed a unique response in providing a solution to coping medically with uraemia. Economic factors are of major importance in being able to provide an end stage renal failure programme including dialysis and transplantation. It has been estimated (23) that worldwide there are more than 500,000 cases of incident end stage renal disease annually and that more than 75% of these occur in the Third World. The provision of health care in any community is dependent on the wealth of the nation (15) and that, in Europe at least, there is a close correlation between the number of patients sustained on a renal replacement programme and the gross national product (24). Thus, whether dialysis therapy is an option for a patient will to some extent be dependent on the wealth of the community and the provision of service which has been developed. However, the economic state of a country is not the only factor to play an important role, because, even in industrialised nations there are marked differences in practice (7).

In Scandinavian countries for example there is considerable reliance placed on transplantation, particularly from related donors. On the other hand transplantation plays little part in the overall provision of treatment in countries such as Italy, while in Japan the contribution of transplantation is virtually zero. Dialysis regimens also vary from country to country with total treatment times being generally less in the United States of America when compared to Europe. The contribution of CAPD is greater in the United Kingdom than almost any other country. These wide divergencies and practice are not easy to explain and are clearly multifactorial. In considering options in renal replacement therapy the management plan for any particular patient will depend on available resources and local expertise. The over-riding principle must be to make the best use of the available resource to the maximum benefit of as many patients as possible. Choices have to be made because it is highly unlikely that any society will ever be able to finance, without some restrictions, the treatment of all patients with uraemia.

FOR WHOM IS RENAL REPLACEMENT THERAPY APPROPRIATE TREATMENT

Expansion of dialysis facilities in the developed world has reached the stage where every patient with chronic uraemia irrespective of age and presence of co-morbid factors should be considered for end stage renal failure treatment. This does not mean that all patients should receive dialysis and/or transplantation but that they should be assessed by a nephrologist so that an informed decision can be made based on current practice. Studies have indicated that referring physicians need to liaise with nephrologists otherwise the decisions they make regarding the suitability of an individual patient for dialysis are likely to be out of date (3). Improvements in technology and increasing experience has greatly widened the acceptance criteria as has the introduction of peritoneal dialysis.

Age, by itself, should be no bar to therapy being offered. In paediatric practice at one time it was difficult to treat patients whose weight was less than 15 kg due to difficulties with vascular access and lack of equipment using small extracorporeal blood volumes. In view of the growth suppression of uraemia this resulted in the majority of children less than 12–15 years old with long standing uraemia being unable to receive treatment. The introduction of CAPD and the miniaturisation of equipment has overcome these difficulties such that now even children of a few months old can benefit from treatment. At the other end of the age scale it was common that age was used as a means of controlling the numbers receiving dialysis although it is possible that elderly patients with the frequently associated cardiovascular disease would likely have had great difficulty with the equipment available at the time. In the elderly increasing experience has demonstrated that even patients in the ninth and tenth decade can benefit from dialysis providing there are no co-morbid factors preventing rehabilitation. Indeed, depending how survival is calculated, it might be proposed that elderly patients fare better than younger patients on dialysis particularly if the basis of success is measured by the prolongation of life compared to that which could be expected for a person of the same age and gender but without renal failure (17).

Extra-renal disease *per se* is no reason to deny a patient the opportunity of dialysis therapy providing that the quality of life which can be achieved is acceptable to the patient and family. Many patients with diabetes mellitus complicated by renal failure were not offered dialysis because of the known association of nephropathy with retinopathy, neuropathy, and vasculopathy. However, not all patients with diabetic nephropathy have widespread vascular disease to such an extent as to preclude satisfactory rehabilitation and so each patient should be considered individually and an appropriate decision made. It is the summative effect of diabetic complications which will determine whether a patient can be expected to achieve an acceptable quality of life. Similarly in other systemic diseases the extent and consequences of other organ involvement requires assessment and consideration before reaching any conclusion.

Usually malignant disease is considered an absolute contraindication to dialysis but this is inappropriate. Many malignancies are slowly progressive and a number, particularly lymphomas and leukaemias, are susceptible to chemotherapy. Myeloma and plasma cell dyscrasias may be controlled for many years and dialysis should be considered while therapeutic measures are introduced to induce remission (5). In general rapidly progressing malignancy, particularly if when recognised to be pre-terminal, should be a contraindication to dialysis. In other situations dialysis should be offered unless after informed discussion the patient declines.

If after careful consideration it is determined that dialysis is not a therapeutic option it is important to remember that much can be done to improve the clinical status of the patient. Blood pressure control should be achieved. Dietary measures such as reduction of protein intake frequently makes the patient feel better although not influencing renal function or progression. Control of plasma phosphate by a combination of dietary restriction and the use of binders such as aluminium hydroxide can significantly reduce pruritus and the irritating conjunctivitis which so frequently accompanies pre-terminal uraemia. Similarly achieving satisfactory salt and water balance can provide significant symptomatic improvement to the patient. Many patients with chronic illness do not fear death but rather they fear the mode of dying. In continuing to provide care during the terminal phase of uraemia the physician can do much to make remaining life more tolerable for the patient. To reject a patient just because they are unsuitable for dialysis treatment is unjustifiable.

In industrialised countries the criteria for admission to an end stage renal failure programme is thus the potential to achieve a satisfactory degree of rehabilitation when compared to a person of a similar age without renal failure. Although the term 'quality of life' is frequently used it is difficult to measure in spite of the fact that everyone will have a view as to what the term means. It should, however, assess physical function, social function, emotional and/or mental status, burden of symptoms, and perceived well-being (21). With increasing experience it is now recognised that many patients can lead a satisfactory, if restricted, life even in the presence of apparently severe disabilities and therefore all patients should have the benefit of careful assessment and where necessary a 'trial of therapy' should be undertaken as most clinicians are poor at being able to predict patient response to dialysis.

Dialysis treatment

In the early days of dialysis treatment, survival was an achievement in itself, but now there is an increasing requirement for treatment regimes to provide long term support. Now the physician is more interested in how well rather than how long the patient survives on dialysis. At one time dialysis was considered as a temporary treatment to be endured until a transplant became available. The strong emphasis on transplantation was due to the recognised inability of the artificial kidney to entirely replace the functions of a normal kidney. This in part remains true although the development of different dialysis membranes and the introduction of such medications as One Alpha Hydroxycholecalciferol and Human Recombinant Erythropoietin have had a major impact. Indeed the term 'artificial kidney' is inappropriate because the device we use only in part replaces the excretory function of the kidney and is incapable of mimicking the endocrine function. Furthermore the excretory function is not selective being based on molecular size, shape and charge rather than requirement for elimination.

Transplantation

Although transplantation remains the treatment of choice for many patients there is an increasing requirement to provide dialysis on a long term basis because of the increasing number of patients for whom transplantation is not a viable option. It is recognised that the results of transplantation in elderly patients is less satisfactory than that in younger patients (4) and, while it may be a useful therapeutic option, experience of transplantation in patients aged more than 70 years remains limited. Furthermore, a number of transplanted patients develop chronic rejection requiring a return to dialysis and in such patients further transplantation can be difficult due to the formation of cytotoxic antibodies and the greater difficulty in achieving a satisfactory match in a second as opposed to a first graft. The effect of this is that when accepting a patient for end stage renal failure management transplantation should be regarded as an option and one which may only be temporary. This then dictates a requirement for satisfactory long lasting vascular access, preservation of veins which may be required for vascular access, and careful patient management to avoid any complication which may make dialysis difficult or impossible should the transplant fail.

AIM OF THERAPY

The aim of renal replacement therapy is to provide for the maximum degree of patient rehabilitation that can be achieved. This does not solely relate to achieving certain biochemical targets, but relates to the physical, mental and social rehabilitation of the patient. This clearly varies with the age of the patient, but in general success can be considered when the patient achieves that which could be expected for their particular age. In addition to this, treatment should be also optimised to provide the patient with the least inconvenience. Dialysis will always impose certain limitations, but clearly, these should be reduced to an absolute minimum so as to interfere in the least possible way with the lifestyle of the patient.

A further aim of therapy is to avoid the development of complications which may arise during treatment. These can be attributed to the treatment itself, the continuing uraemia, or the late effects of treatment which was given during the phase of deteriorating renal function. In some circumstances, it is difficult to know which of these three possibilities is responsible. For instance patients on haemodialysis for longer than ten years are likely to develop an arthropathy which has been attributed to the deposition of β2-microglobulin associated amyloidosis (8) but whether this arises from minor repeated bioincompatibility reactions or from the continuing elevation of β2-microglobulin as a consequence of continuing uraemia is as yet uncertain. The increasing survival of patients receiving dialysis increases the importance of minimising potential therapy related complications.

WHEN SHOULD DIALYSIS BE STARTED

A decision as to the correct time to commence renal replacement therapy depends on the availability of facilities. If these are scarce, then strenuous attempts are made to delay the start of dialysis for as long as possible. This, however, has a cost to the patient in that prolonged dietary intervention may result in significant malnutrition and delay in starting treatment allows for the complications of uraemia such as osteodystrophy and neuropathy to further progress. It would seem prudent therefore, to commence dialysis at the earliest time that clinical benefit can be achieved.

It is not possible to separate the decision required with respect to commencing dialysis from the availability of facilities. At the time when dialysis was being introduced for the management of chronic renal failure few facilities were available and as a consequence few patients were accepted for treatment and every attempt was made to delay the start of dialysis for as long as possible by employing stringent dietary measures which included severe protein restriction, the 18 g Giovanetti diet, supplemented with increased carbohydrate and fat intake to make up for the 'lost' calories as a result of the protein restriction. In many parts of the world this is still practised due to inadequate availability of dialysis. Not surprisingly many patients entered a dialysis programme with considerable malnutrition and as a consequence rehabilitation was slow and frequently inadequately achieved. In addition, many patients had poorly controlled hypertension and it is now easy to see with hindsight that a considerable

amount of the atherosclerosis and peripheral vascular disease encountered in long-term dialysis patients must have been initiated or aggravated by their pre-dialysis dietary management. As dialysis facilities expanded there was less pressure to delay the start of treatment until the last possible moment and it is not surprising that the fitter the patient at the start of dialysis the shorter the time to achieve adequate rehabilitation.

The best outcome of treatment is achieved in patients referred to a specialist centre before dialysis is required (10). This allows for the gradual introduction of the patient to the concept of renal replacement therapy. Treatment options can be discussed and the patient given the opportunity of talking with dialysis patients and visiting the dialysis facility. In addition dietary measures can be introduced including protein restriction, sodium and potassium restriction, fluid control, and calorie control. Once the serum creatinine, in an adult patient of average size, is consistently in excess of 600 μmol/l it is advisable to establish vascular access – preferably a good arteriovenous fistula in the forearm. In patients who are identified at risk from progression to renal failure it is therefore vitally important to preserve all veins which may be required for vascular access. Thus intravenous infusions should be managed carefully to avoid thrombophlebitis – a useful habit is to resite peripheral intravenous lines daily. The majority of intravenous fluids are given over a 24 hour period but frequently this is not necessary and thought should be given to infusions being undertaken for only 12 hours daily. It is increasingly recognised that subclavian vascular access, if prolonged, can lead to stenosis and/or thrombosis (1) and should a fistula be subsequently inserted there is a risk of massive upper limb oedema. Finally when a patient is managed through a renal clinic prior to requiring dialysis some prediction can be made as to when dialysis will be required by plotting the reciprocal of the serum creatinine against time. There is no agreed level of renal function at which dialysis should be commenced but in general dialysis will be required when the serum creatinine is in the region of 1000 μmol/l although preferred practice would be to commence at any time the patient has symptoms which can be relieved by treatment. Using such projections it is frequently possible for the patient to make sensible forward planning with respect to holidays or important family events. In addition should there be a need for elective intercurrent surgical intervention this can be planned and thereby more safely undertaken. It is to be regretted that in spite of continued medical education approximately 50% patients requiring dialysis do not present until such treatment is urgently required.

Care is required in two circumstances. Firstly, in elderly patients the relationship between serum creatinine and renal function is altered due to the diminished muscle mass of elderly people and as a consequence the renal function is less for any given serum creatinine when compared to young adults (18). Secondly, in patients with failing transplant function it is advisable to return to dialysis at an early stage because of the adverse effects of continuing immunosuppression with or without corticosteroids, when it is obvious that progressive failure is inevitable. Thus in such circumstances once the serum creatinine is greater than 600 μmol/l it is prudent to withdraw immunosuppression, return to dialysis, and consider whether graft removal is required.

OPTIONS IN DIALYSIS THERAPIES

General considerations

Renal replacement therapy can be achieved by either dialysis or transplantation. The dialysis modalities include, haemodialysis and peritoneal dialysis. The haemodialysis modalities include haemofiltration and haemodiafiltration and may involve conventional membranes, and high flux membranes. Furthermore, current opinion dictates that the dialysis fluid employed should be bicarbonate based. The peritoneal dialysis techniques include continuous ambulatory peritoneal dialysis, continuous cyclical peritoneal dialysis, tidal dialysis, and intermittent dialysis.

Haemodialysis and peritoneal dialysis should not be seen as competing therapeutic options, rather, they are two methods of dealing with uraemia and each has certain advantages and disadvantages, and interestingly, in the short term at least, both appear to be equally effective in controlling the symptoms and signs of uraemia.

There are many patient factors which must be taken into account when determining the most appropriate therapeutic option. The expected duration of dialysis is clearly of prime importance. Those patients who can hope to obtain a cadaver or living related donor transplant within a short space of time are best suited to in-centre haemodialysis or CAPD. Improvements in the technology of CAPD has considerably reduced the incidence of peritonitis episodes and has the added advantage of avoiding the requirement for vascular access. Once treatment is initiated appropriate transplant work-up can be undertaken and a regular assessment of rehabilitation made to determine the most appropriate time to undertake transplantation. For patients who are unlikely to receive a transplant the therapeutic option will depend upon age, weight, co-morbidity, family support, and the requirement for nursing support during treatment. In general, children benefit from CAPD as this allows them to continue their school education. In elderly patients it has been suggested that CAPD is also the treatment of choice but unless there is good home support they may well feel isolated. Usually most patients will be suitable for either haemodialysis or CAPD and in such circumstances it becomes very much a matter of patient choice. For this to be properly exercised the patient has to be fully informed of the advantages and disadvantages of each technique so that an appropriate decision can be made. The use of suitably prepared videos and the oppor-tunity to meet with existing patients can be particularly helpful.

Haemodialysis

Haemodialysis was the first effective technique which was introduced for the long term management for patients with end stage renal failure and as a result most experience has been gained with this technique and it is considered as the gold standard. Many changes have taken place and the treatment has evolved from one which was administered for 14 hours twice weekly to one which is most commonly employed for 4 hours thrice weekly. Developments in dialyser design and membrane properties have significantly increased dialyser efficiency allowing for these very significant reductions in treatment times. In recent years high efficiency dialysis has been introduced using large surface area dialysers and increased flow rates of blood and dialysis fluid to achieve a greater rate of removal of solutes and fluid than in conventional haemodialysis with the objective being to further reduce treatment time. Generally high-efficiency dialysis has a treatment time of less than three hours, a blood flow rate of greater than 300 mls/min, and a dialysis fluid flow rate of greater than 500 mls/min.

Conventional membranes work predominantly in a diffusive mode where removal of solutes is determined by molecular size, shape, and charge, In an attempt to more accurately reproduce the functions of the glomerulus membranes have been developed which combine both diffusive and convective transport properties. This has allowed for the development of haemodiafiltration and high flux dialysis where there is a wider spectrum of molecular weights of substances removed. Whether this will result in a better control of uraemia is as yet undecided and we will have to await the results of long-term studies to determine whether either of these techniques is superior to conventional haemodialysis in the long term.

Haemodialysis is effective in controlling uraemia and prolonging life. Clearly however a dialyser only partially replaces some of the excretory functions of the kidney and does not replace the endocrine function. The introduction of one Alpha Hydroxycholecalciferol and Human Recombinant Erythropoietin has to a large extent overcome this problem. However, continuing uraemia remains with patients having a mean serum creatinine between 6 and 800 μmol/l and a mean serum urea of 15–20 mmols/l. Thus not only does haemodialysis only partially replace renal function it only partially corrects uraemia and this is probably the cause of many of the complications which arise in long-term therapy.

An essential requirement for good haemodialysis is satisfactory vascular access and in many patients this can prove difficult. Wherever possible the arterio-venous fistula should be inserted in the forearm of the non-dominant limb but where this is impracticable for any particular reason then the fistula can be fashioned in the antecubital fossa. In a small number of patients secondary vascular access procedures will be required employing the use of synthetic materials in either the upper limb or thigh. Care must be taken to preserve vascular access as haemodialysis may be required for many years.

Haemodialysis has many advantages, not the least of which is that treatment is usually required for 4 hours on two or three days each week. This leaves the remaining days of the week when the patient can pursue social or work activities. In comparison to CAPD there is less obesity, better nutrition and greater technique survival. Furthermore a major benefit is that, in general, patients on haemodialysis require less hospitalization than those maintained by CAPD.

The disadvantages of haemodialysis include the need for continual fluid and dietary restrictions. Between dialyses the weight gain should be restricted to less than 3% of body weight which depending on the residual renal function will restrict fluid allowance to about 1 litre daily. In addition sodium intake needs to be curtailed in view of its propensity to induce thirst and potassium intake has to be restricted otherwise dangerous hyperkalaemia may develop. Further disadvantages include the restrictions imposed on travel. In certain circumstances this can significantly affect employment prospects and the opportunity to undertake holidays. Travel limitations can be significantly eased with forward planning and the development of dialysis facilities in tourist resorts has allowed for holidays to be taken. Care has to be exercised however to avoid any potential for cross infection, particularly with Hepatitis B and HIV.

High efficiency and high flux dialysis have been introduced because of patient pressure to reduce treatment times. In addition the reduction in treatment time has the added advantage of reducing treatment costs as the major item in costings is staff salaries. Development became possible following the introduction of bicarbonate dialysis fluid and so overcoming the limitations of conventional haemodialysis imposed by the finite rate of acetate metabolism. It would appear that high efficiency and high flux dialysis is a treatment option for most patients. Haemofiltration should be considered for any patient who has disabling morbidity during haemodialysis and for whom CAPD is not an option. It is particularly useful for patients who develop profound hypotension during haemodialysis (6). It is, however, more expensive although for some may be the only form of symptom free treatment.

Psychological effects of long-term dialysis are not uncommon. Many patients after a period of time on dialysis become depressed as they come to realise the long-term nature of treatment. Many cope with this by anticipating successful transplantation at some undetermined time in the future.

Increasing attention is being paid to the issue of biocompatibility as repeated minor incompatibility reactions probably take place during each dialysis session. These

may have adverse cumulative effects resulting in the complications which are seen in long-term patients. These include β2-microglobulin related amyloidosis, peripheral vascular disease, and the increased incidence of myocardial disease.

In spite of all these potential disadvantages haemodialysis is a very satisfactory form of therapy for a terminal illness, an 80% survival at 5 years and a 50% survival at 10 years can be expected, although clearly survival depends on many factors such as age and the presence of co-morbid conditions. There are no absolute contraindications to selecting this option for patient management although good vascular access is an absolute requirement and cardiovascular stability an advantage.

Peritoneal dialysis

Peritoneal dialysis was used almost exclusively for the management of acute renal failure until the late seventies when the idea of a 'portable, wearable, equilibration peritoneal dialysis system' became reality with the development of permanent indwelling peritoneal catheters. The technique was rapidly accepted and introduced to clinical practice although it is now recognised that the major factor in this was financial rather than clinical. It was considered that peritoneal dialysis with its lack of a need for sophisticated expensive equipment would be much cheaper than haemodialysis as then practised. It is now recognised that this is a misconception although it has emerged that peritoneal dialysis is an effective and very satisfactory means of treating selected patients.

Continuous ambulatory peritoneal dialysis (CAPD) uses a relatively small volume of dialysis fluid with long equilibration times, most commonly 2 litres of fluid exchanged after intervals of 4–8 hours, i.e. four exchanges spaced throughout the day. The volume of exchange is adjusted for the patients' size and weight and ultrafiltration is achieved by alterations in tonicity by varying the concentration of dextrose. A steady state concentration of plasma creatinine, urea, electrolytes is achieved and thus the complications which arise as a result of disequilibrium are avoided.

CAPD is effective in the control of uraemia. An advantage of this technique is that residual renal function is better maintained than in patients managed by haemodialysis which may have implications in the control of β2-microglobulin with its associated amyloidosis. However symptomatic amyloidosis is uncommon before ten years of haemodialysis treatment and few CAPD patients have been maintained on treatment for this length of time and so it will be some time before this potential benefit can be ascertained.

CAPD appears to be as effective as haemodialysis in the control of hypertension and cardiac complications are probably as frequent in both groups. However CAPD may have an adverse effect on peripheral vascular disease due to its propensity for increasing atherosclerosis due to the effect of absorbed glucose from the dialysis fluid, on carbohydrate and lipid metabolism. Malnutrition may develop in about one third of patients and although the cause for this is uncertain many patients have an inadequate nutritional intake due to continuing anorexia and a sensation of abdominal fullness. Similar to other methods of treating renal failure CAPD has advantages and disadvantages.

Patients selected for CAPD require careful assessment if successful treatment is to be achieved. As the major cause of treatment failure is peritonitis it is important to assess the patients' ability to perform the procedure without introducing infection to the peritoneal cavity. The ability to satisfactorily undertake the required connection and disconnection of this dialysis fluid without risking the introduction of infection requires good vision although this is not absolute as devices are now available to aid the partially sighted or even patients totally blind. Manual dexterity is an obvious advantage although again aids are available to overcome difficulties.

Personal hygiene is clearly important as the majority of infections are with commensal organisms. Patient compliance is clearly very important but difficult to assess prior to starting treatment although those who have been unable to cope with simple drug regimens are unlikely to cope with the complexity of sterile 'no touch' techniques. Finally in the avoidance of infection the patient requires a clean environment in which to undertake bag exchanges. This can be achieved in the home or at work or even during travel although a degree of inventiveness may be required.

The advantages of CAPD compared to haemodialysis are considerable. There is no reduction in time spent each week on treatment. Most patients find that a bag exchange takes about 30 minutes which is equivalent to about 14 hours weekly (30 min × 4 daily) whereas haemodialysis is most commonly for 4 hours thrice weekly (12 hours). Of course as CAPD is undertaken at home the time taken to travel to and from the dialysis centre is avoided which could amount to a significant saving particularly for patients in rural areas. Vascular access is not required and this is obviously an advantage for those patients with obliterated forearm veins, hypoplastic vessels, and very small patients. Stable blood chemistry avoids the morbidity associated with disequilibrium e.g., headache, nausea, hypotension, and generally haemoglobin is greater when compared to patients on haemodialysis due to the avoidance of the small amount of red blood cells inevitably lost at each haemodialysis session. The greater freedom to travel without having to make careful and detailed forward planning to receive haemodialysis is much appreciated by many patients.

CAPD is not without its disadvantages which have to be carefully considered for each patient. There may be considerable psychological difficulties if patients present late in renal failure and thus have little time to come to terms with the consequences of their illness. The majority of patients commenced on CAPD will achieve a satis-

factory degree of training in 2–3 weeks after which they will undertake their treatment at home. This may result in isolation due to the lack of medical and nursing staff as well as the support gained from regular contact with similarly affected patients. The benefits of this peer support is often forgotten and this can be particularly important for the elderly if they are not well supported at home by family. In addition in time, many patients find that the requirement to undertake the dialysis procedure four times daily can be very demanding, tiring, and impossible to sustain. The term 'burn out' can be applied to this situation and requires transfer of the patient to an alternative form of therapy. Finally the change in body image from the catheter emerging through the abdominal wall and from the abdominal distention may be unacceptable. It is particularly distressing to the young slim female as friends and acquaintances may think that the distention is due to pregnancy and make inappropriate and distressing comments.

CAPD is a useful addition to the range of options available for the management of patients with end stage renal failure. It is the preferred method of treatment for patients with Hepatitis B or HIV carriers due to the reduced risk of transmission of infection to other patients and members of staff. It has also been suggested to be the treatment of choice for patients with diabetes mellitus due to the risk of intraocular haemorrhage during heparinisation and the commonly encountered difficulties with vascular access. Finally it is particularly useful for those patients with cardiovascular instability who develop profound hypotension during haemodialysis.

There are relatively few contraindications to CAPD but gross obesity, peritoneal adhesions, abdominal hernia and multiple abdominal surgical interventions all have the potential to make the treatment inadequate or impossible. In addition in patients who are frail, elderly, mentally infirm or demented are unsuitable unless there is adequate support from a family member or other carer. Thus in the selection of CAPD as a treatment option the physician has to consider medical, social and environmental factors before deciding that a satisfactory outcome is likely to be achieved.

Intermittent peritoneal dialysis is an alternative to patients in whom CAPD proves difficult to sustain. Intermittent peritoneal dialysis (IPD) is usually performed three or four times weekly during which there is manual exchange of dialysis fluid similar to CAPD but with considerably shortened dwell times, frequently 30 min to 1 hour. Nocturnal peritoneal dialysis has been used to describe the technique if it takes place overnight but it does not seem sensible to retain this term as it does nothing to explain the techniques other than the times at which it takes place. Continuous cyclic peritoneal dialysis (CCPD) is a technique involving a series of short exchanges, frequently at night, often undertaken with the assistance of an automated mechanical device relieving the patient of performing the exchanges. The various forms of intermittent peritoneal dialysis seem to be as efficient as CAPD providing that an adequate volume of dialysis fluid is employed.

IPD is most suitable for use in dialysis centres and is particularly of advantage to those patients for whom peritoneal dialysis in indicated but who have not been able to master the expertise needed to perform treatment safely and who do not have a partner who would be able to assist adequately to enable home treatment to succeed. CCPD is of most value for the management of patients who do not wish to undertake treatment during the day for social or employment reasons. It is of value in the management of children who need the assistance of a parent and for those children attending full time education for whom it avoids the constant reminder of their disability to their fellow pupils. In the elderly and mentally infirm it is also of value as it reduces the amount of time the carer has to spend assisting the patient. It does however have the disadvantage of additional cost due to the revenue expense of the lines and large fluid bags as well as the capital expense of the equipment.

SPECIFIC CIRCUMSTANCES

Children

Children present particular problems with respect to the provision of end stage renal failure management. The low incidence of end stage renal failure in children (approximately 5 pmp annually) presents logistical problems. There is a requirement for specialist centres employing paediatric trained staff and suitably adapted equipment. The multi-disciplinary team needs to include paediatric nephrologists, nursing staff, dietitians, medical social workers, and a teacher. As a significant number of the causes of end stage renal failure in children are due to developmental abnormalities a close liaison is required with a paediatric urologist.

The aim of treatment is not just the control of uraemia but avoidance of osteodystrophy, the maintenance of a good nutritional state, and maintenance of a normal growth pattern. These aims are difficult to achieve but the recent introduction of erythropoietin and human recombinant growth hormone has significantly improved the chances of achieving satisfactory growth.

The most appropriate time to commence therapy is earlier than that indicated for an adult. In the developing child the relationship between GFR and plasma creatinine changes with age; for instance in a six month old child a plasma creatine of 300 μmols/l probably represents renal function of less than 10% indicating that dialysis was required.

The choice of treatment should be discussed with the child and the parents. The threshold for achieving satisfactory haemodialysis is probably a weight of 15 kg. In children less than this weight it is unlikely that satisfacto-

ry vascular access will be achieved and therefore the only appropriate option would be CAPD or CCPD. In many circumstances for the very young child CCPD is the treatment of choice as treatment can be undertaken overnight reducing the time required by the parent to administer care.

A number of problems specifically arise in children maintained on dialysis. Many become dependent and strenuous efforts are often required to ensure that the child leads as normal a life as possible. There is clearly a need to maintain education and a close liaison with the child's school is essential. CCPD offers the child a greater chance of returning to full time education but should haemodialysis be the only option then there will be a need for a teacher to be specifically allocated to the paediatric unit. A further problem is the stress which parents feel in having to cope long-term with their child's illness. It is necessary to provide intermittent relief and some centres have given this by arranging to take the children away to a holiday camp, thereby giving the parents a welcome break from their responsibilities. It should also be remembered that siblings may feel neglected due to the amount of care and attention being devoted to the patient.

Growth failure and delayed puberty are common (19). This leads to particular problems with adolescence when serious psychological problems may arise. Although many children at the time of adolescence become somewhat rebellious this can be exaggerated in a child on dialysis and may become manifest by non-compliance particularly with respect to dietary restrictions, attendance at scheduled dialysis sessions, and missing bag exchanges for those on CAPD.

In summary, therefore, when determining the most appropriate therapeutic option for the paediatric patient CCPD would appear to be best for pre-school children and for school children in full time education. CAPD is a useful alternative if there are economic constraints on the provision of CCPD equipment. Peritoneal dialysis is particularly useful for those patients who live at a distance from a paediatric centre. Haemodialysis is an option once the child's weight is in excess of 15 kg but is dependent on suitable vascular access and close supervision may be required with respect to dietary non-compliance, particularly in the adolescent child. Home dialysis should be considered where peritoneal dialysis is not possible, e.g. in patients with the prune belly syndrome, and where transplantation is unlikely or has previously failed.

Elderly patients

In the developed countries there is an increasing number of elderly patients in the general population. This fact and increasing experience together with improvements in dialysis technology has resulted with an increasing acceptance of elderly patients for dialysis treatment. Such patients present a therapeutic challenge in view of the fact that they frequently have impaired cardiovascular responsiveness, impaired co-ordination, poor vision, poor mobility, and increased susceptibility to drug toxicity.

Cardiovascular instability and coronary insufficiency are two major problems which cause significant morbidity during haemodialysis. This can be lessened by using haemodiafiltration although in a number of patients troublesome symptoms will continue requiring a change to CAPD.

Haemodialysis in the elderly can offer a very satisfactory prolongation of life as well as achieving a very satisfactory quality of life. Although it is recognised that survival is less in elderly patients, 5 year survival 53% in those aged greater than 60 years of age compared with 68% in those aged less than 60 years (22), this is only to be expected. Elderly patients have also been shown to be capable of home haemodialysis with one centre reporting an impressive 80% survival at six years (13).

CAPD has been suggested as the most appropriate form of dialysis therapy for the elderly because of the increased incidence of cardiac disease and difficulties with vascular access due to peripheral vascular disease. Success with this technique however is dependent upon the degree of home support which is available for the patient. If such support is lacking then there is a tendency for the elderly patient to feel isolated and as a consequence is likely to become depressed and lack motivation. Many elderly patients prefer an hospital based treatment in view of the companionship which they gain by being treated with other patients in addition to their contact with nursing and other members of staff. Under such circumstances dialysis becomes an event to be enjoyed with the dialysis unit functioning in a way similar to that of day hospitals attached to geriatric departments.

Diabetes mellitus

The proportion of dialysis patients with an underlying diagnosis of end stage renal failure due to diabetic nephropathy is steadily increasing in all programmes. However, many such patients progressing to dialysis have other manifestations of diabetic angiopathy such as retinopathy, neuropathy, and peripheral vascular disease.

In general it would appear that CAPD is the treatment of choice for the diabetic patient and impressive survival figures can be obtained (11). Haemodialysis may be associated with a number of problems as in many vascular access may be difficult due to the associated peripheral vascular disease and fistula formation may precipitate distal ischaemia to such an extent that amputation is required. In addition the cardiovascular problems of the diabetic patient frequently lead to sudden and profound hypotension during haemodialysis. Finally retinopathy is common and intraocular bleeding may be precipitated by the heparinisation required during haemodialysis.

Although CAPD appears to be the treatment of choice it is not without complication in view of the increased susceptibility to infection, the visual impairment making bag exchanges difficult and the gastric atony with its accompanying nausea which may be aggravated by the intraperitoneal fluid.

WHERE SHOULD DIALYSIS BE UNDERTAKEN

The options available are dialysis within an hospital centre, satellite unit, minimal care unit, or at home. As with all aspects of dialysis each option has advantages and disadvantages which require to be taken into account when selecting the most appropriate treatment for an individual patient.

The hospital centre has an obvious advantage in that experienced nursing and medical staff are immediately available to deal with any problem which may arise. Furthermore other whole hospital services, such as a cardiac arrest team, are on site and can be called upon as required. Many patients feel 'secure' in such an environment and are reluctant to consider any alternative. Prior to commencing dialysis some patients may have experienced difficulties in their medical management because their renal failure was undiagnosed or ignored. Such patients come to view the dialysis centre as being the only place where they will receive appropriate treatment. Many patients have had little or no previous exposure to a clinical environment and few are conversant with the high technology of the dialysis unit and thus they find difficulty in believing that dialysis can be conducted in any area outside a major hospital and are therefore naturally reluctant to consider transfer to any other treatment area such as a satellite unit. For patients established on long-term treatment it is, however, not good management to dialyse them alongside patients commencing treatment and there is a need to split hospital units into high- and low-dependency areas so that the long-term patient receives treatment in a more tranquil surrounding where dialysis can be relegated to a routine matter rather than to a high drama status. Major hospital centres also have the disadvantage that they may be some distance from the patients' home requiring repetitive travel in all weathers.

The developments in dialysis facilities have often been driven by economic factors and this is certainly the case with respect to home haemodialysis. In the United Kingdom only few hospital centres were established and as a consequence they soon reached the limits of capacity with respect to patients. A solution was achieved by transferring the equipment to the patients home (20) and training the patients and an helper in the techniques of dialysis. The obvious advantage was that the patient did not have to travel and could undertake treatment at a time convenient to social and employment constraints. An added advantage was that it also placed the patient in charge of the treatment with an accompanying increase in self esteem which was reflected in increased physical and mental well-being. These advantages encouraged the expansion of home haemodialysis which was sustained to the late seventies after which there has been a steady decline in the number of patients managed in this way. The reasons for this decline have interestingly also been economic. The capital investment required to establish home haemodialysis is considerable and given the longevity of currently available dialysis machines it is unlikely that the equipment installed will ever be used to is maximum life. Home haemodialysis should therefore be reserved for patients who live in areas remote from a dialysis centre and for whom transplantation is not an option or following a failed transplant if there is little chance of retransplantation by virtue of the development of high titres of multispecific cytotoxic antibodies.

Home dialysis requires space either within the home or in a specially installed cabin. Many properties are unsuitable due to lack of space. Some favour an outside cabin because this removes from the home the 'hospital' environment due to the pervading odour of antiseptics. Home dialysis has a stressful effect on other members of the family and many find difficulty in coping with this stress. In almost all programmes there is a need to intermittently provide relief for the carer. The children of parents on home haemodialysis may develop emotional problems due to the regular required attention to the patient. Careful assessment of the family and environment is thus a mandatory pre-requisite before considering home haemodialysis as a therapeutic option.

Continuous ambulatory peritoneal dialysis is ideally suitable for home treatment and has the added advantage that the required capital investment is minimal. There is a need for storage space for the fluids and consumables and in certain homes this can produce almost insurmountable difficulties.

Minimal care units were established as a means of overcoming the economic problems of home haemodialysis. The conception was that an area could be provided in which a number of dialysis machines could be installed and used by a number of patients thus increasing cost effectiveness. The term minimal care was introduced as patients were trained and encouraged to undertake as much of their treatment as possible. They were trained to set up the machines – lining and priming – and also in the insertion of fistula needles, the management and control of the dialysis session, and with the cleaning up at termination. The minimum number of staff were present and in certain instances no staff were in attendance. The term minimal care is unfortunate in that the dialysis care received by the patient is identical to that in an hospital environment but it is the staffing which is minimal.

It soon became apparent that with the widening of the criteria for acceptance to a dialysis programme there was an increasing number of patients who were frail or who had co-morbid conditions which precluded their treatment in a minimally staffed unit. As a result the main centre had an increasing number of dependent patients. The solution was an increase in minimal care unit staffing to produce a satellite unit capable of accepting more dependent patients and those requiring assistance with their treatment.

Satellite haemodialysis units offer support to all patients except those with very particular nursing requirements. As with minimal care units the major advantage is close proximity to the patients' homes and the significant reduction in travelling time. An added advantage is that the presence of such a unit raises the profile of nephrology in the surrounding medical community with the frequent result that more patients are referred for consideration for treatment. Such units do not need medical staff to be present and while many are situated within an hospital this is not an absolute requirement. The development of major centres with surrounding satellite facilities is a most cost effective way of providing a renal failure service.

In conclusion haemodialysis can be undertaken in a major centre, a satellite unit, a minimal care unit, or the patient's home (CAPD has always been considered to be predominately a procedure to be carried out at home). It is the patient's need for support during dialysis and the local availability of facilities which will determine the appropriate option to be followed for any particular patient.

TRANSPLANTATION VERSUS DIALYSIS TREATMENTS

Transplantation is often considered by the patient to be the optimum therapeutic option in their end stage renal failure management. However, just as with haemodialysis and peritoneal dialysis, transplantation has advantages and disadvantages which must be carefully considered before a patient is entered to the transplant waiting list. An obvious advantage of transplantation is freedom from the tedium of routine haemodialysis or the bag exchanges of peritoneal dialysis. In essence the patient gains twelve to fourteen treatment free hours each week, as well as the obvious freedom of being able to travel without making forward planning arrangements for dialysis. The additional advantages are the return of endocrine and other metabolic functions which are not and never will be reproduced in an artificial kidney. For the health economist there are also important cost savings to be gained due to the very significantly less cost involved in post-transplant management compared to regular dialysis. It is important however to remember that dialysis and transplantation are not in competition but should rather be seen as alternatives in the management of end stage renal failure. Furthermore it would be wise to consider transplantation as a therapeutic option which may be temporary depending upon how well acute and chronic rejection processes are controlled by immunosuppressive therapy.

The disadvantages of transplantation is the requirement for the patient to remain on long term immunosuppressive therapy with the consequential risk of opportunistic infections and malignancy. Increasing experience has significantly altered immunosuppressive regimes such that currently patients are exposed to much lower doses of corticosteroids. As a consequence the adverse effects of steroid therapy have been significantly reduced and it is now less common for the post-transplant patient to develop steroid induced diabetes mellitus, a Cushingoid appearance, osteoporosis, avascular necrosis of the femoral head, and cataracts. The introduction of Cyclosporin as an immunosuppressive agent does not appear to have lessened the risk of malignancy and the tumours arising in transplant patients are most commonly skin but include lymphomas, solid tumours (stomach, colon, lung and breast) do not appear to be markedly increased by immunosuppressive therapy.

At one time it was considered that the results of transplantation were not as good in patients managed by CAPD but recent experience would suggest that patients transplanted from either modality appear to do equally well.

The results of transplantation in the pre-Cyclosporin era would appear to be less satisfactory in the elderly compared with younger patients (14). In the post-Cyclosporin era, however, it would appear that there is no significant difference in graft survival between younger and older patients although patient survival is significantly different with the elderly patients doing less well (12). It is likely that the differences in patients survival can be attributed to the increased morbidity of elderly patients particularly with respect to cardiovascular disease. If elderly patients are to be considered for transplantation then they require additional careful pre-transplant work up particularly with respect to cardiovascular status by echo and stress testing. A history of transient ischaemic attacks and cerebral vascular disease, particularly strokes, and the presence of peripheral vascular disease are relative contra-indications. All elderly male patients require examination to detect any prostatic hypertrophy which may produce obstructive uropathy after transplantation. Any patient known to have a malignancy should be excluded unless there has been a five year interval from successful treatment. As with younger patients the most common cause of mortality following transplantation is due to cardiovascular disease.

In the overall management of patients with end stage renal failure transplantation has a part to play and should be considered as a therapeutic option for all patients except those very young (i.e. less than 2 years old), those with malignant disease, HIV positive patients, and elderly patients in which there is evidence of cardiovascular disease. In patients with end stage renal failure due to diabetes mellitus consideration should be given to combined pancreas and kidney transplantation (2) in an attempt to relieve the patient of the limitations imposed by diabetic therapy and also to limit the recurrence of diabetic changes in the transplant.

DECISION TREE IN THE MANAGEMENT OF A PATIENT WITH END STAGE RENAL FAILURE

1. Suitable for a dialysis/transplant programme?
   - NO   Conventional management
     [Diet, fluid/electrolyte balance, bp control]
   - YES   Haemodialysis
     a. satellite centre
     b. home haemodialysis
     c. centre haemodialysis

     Peritoneal dialysis
     a. conventional CAPD
     b. CCPD
     c. IPD

2. Suitable for transplantation?
   - NO   continue dialysis regimen
   - YES   a. cadaver donor
     b. living related donor
     c. emotionally involved donor

3. Regular review
   Is most appropriate form of treatment being undertaken?
   - NO   change to that considered most appropriate
   - YES   continue

CONCLUSIONS

In the management of patients with end stage renal failure there is a requirement for the development of an integrated service involving both dialysis and transplantation. The dialysis options should include haemodialysis (hospital, satellite, home) and peritoneal dialysis. It may be that a unit is unable to provide the full range of services and in such a case it can be advantageous for a number of centres to combine together to ensure that their patients can receive the optimum therapy.

The most appropriate form of therapy can only be determined by careful consideration of the patient's clinical and social status together with a knowledge of the local availability of treatment options. It is important therefore to consider the various treatment options with the patient by explaining the various advantages and disadvantages of each form of treatment. Following this a treatment plan should be formulated taking account of all the various factors into consideration. Thereafter the physician should be prepared to regularly review the status of the patient to determine if their particular mode of therapy is appropriate so that changes can be made as required to ensure that the patient continues to receive the best therapeutic option.

REFERENCES

1. Barrett N, Spencer S, McIvor J, Brown E: Subclavian stenosis: a major complication of subclavian dialysis catheters. *Nephrol Dial Transplant* 3: 423, 1988
2. Brekke I, Drybekk D, Jakobsen, A et al.: Combined kidney and pancreas transplantation for diabetic nephropathy. *Transplant Proc* 18: 63, 1986
3. Challah S, Wing AJ, Bauer R et al.: Negative selection of patients for dialysis and transplantation in the United Kingdom. *Br Med J* 228: 1119, 1984
4. Cole EH: Renal transplantation in the elderly: the Toronto experience. in *Nephrology and Urology in the Aged Patient*, edited by Oreopoulos DG, Michelis MF, Herschorn S, Kluwer Academic Publishers, Dordrecht, 1993, p 349
5. Coward RA, Mallick NP, Delamore IW: Should patients with renal failure associated with myeloma be dialysed? *Br Med J* 287: 1575, 1983
6. Davison AM, Roberts TG, Mascie-Taylor BH, Lewins AM: Haemofiltration for profound dialysis induced hypotension: removal of salt and water without blood pressure change. *Br Med J* 285: 87, 1982
7. Fassbinder W, Brunner FP, Brynger H et al.: Combined report on regular dialysis and transplantation in Europe, XX, 1989. *Nephrol Dial Transplant* 6 (Suppl 1): 5, 1991
8. Gejyo F, Yamada T, Odani S et al.: A new form of amyloid protein associated with chronic haemodialysis was identified as β2-microglobulin. *Biochemical Biophysical Research Communications* 129: 701, 1985
9. Hegstrom RM, Murray JS, Pendras JP et al.: Hemodialysis in the treatment of chronic uraemia. *Trans Am Soc Artif Organs* 7: 136, 1966
10. Innes A, Rowe PA, Burden RP, Morgan AG: Early deaths on renal replacement therapy: the need for early nephrology referral. *Nephrol Dial Transplant* 7: 467, 1992
11. Maiorca R et al.: A six year comparison of patient and technique survivals in CAPD and HD. *Kidney Int* 34: 518, 1988
12. Morris GE, Jamieson NV, Small J, Evans DB, Calne R: Cadaveric renal transplantation in elderly patients: is it worthwhile? *Nephrol Dial Transplant* 6: 887, 1991
13. Ninon, C, Oules R, Canaud B et al.: Maintenance dialysis in the elderly: a review of 15 years' experience. *Proc EDTA-ERA* 21: 490, 1984
14. Ost L, Groth C-G, Lindholm B et al.: Cadaveric renal transplantation in patients of 60 years and above. *Transplant* 30: 339, 1980
15. Poikolainen K, Eskola J: Health services resources and their relation to mortality from causes amenable to health care intervention: a cross-national study. *Int J Epidemiol* 17: 86, 1988
16. Popovich RP, Moncrief JW, Dechard JF et al.: The definition of a novel portable/wearable equilibrium dialysis technique. *Trans Am Soc Artif Intern Organs* 5: 64, 1976
17. Rotellar E, Lubelza RA, Rotellar C et al.: Must patients over 65 be haemodialysed. *Nephron* 41: 152, 1985
18. Rowe JW, Andres R, Tobin JD et al.: The effect of age on creatinine clearance in man: a cross sectional and longitudinal survey. *J Gerentol* 31: 155, 1976
19. Schärer K et al.: Pubertal development in children with renal failure. *Pediatric and Adolescent Endocrinology* 20: 151, 1989
20. Shaldon S, Baillod RA, Compty C et al.: 18 months experience with a nurse-patient operated chronic dialysis unit. *Proc Eur Dial Transplant Assoc* 1: 233, 1964
21. Spitzer WO: State of science 1986: quality of life and functional status as target variables for research. *J Chron Dis* 40: 465, 1987
22. Tapsan JS, Rodger RSC, Mansy H et al.: Renal replacement therapy in patients aged over 60 years. *Postgrad Med J* 63: 1071, 1987
23. Woods HF: Perspectives on dialysis in the third world: a problem of economics. *Contrib Nephrol* 102: 237, 1993
24. Valek A, Wing AJ: Development of dialysis and transplant activity in the world in the seventies of the 20th century. *Z Exp Chir Transplant Künstliche Organe* 17: 69, 1984

PART A: HEMODIALYSIS-CLINICAL MANAGEMENT AND FOLLOW UP

BARBARA G. DELANO

INTRODUCTION

World wide, more than 500,000 patients are treated for End Stage Renal Disease. While transplantation and peritoneal dialysis are therapies to be considered, hemodialysis remains the mainstay of treatment. The tremendous and rapid growth of this therapy, which was first reported for the treatment of chronic renal failure in 1960 (1) has made it imperative for all health care providers to become familiar with the care of the dialysis patient. Most of the topics covered in this chapter are dealt with in greater detail in the rest of this book. The following will cover some practical aspects of how to initiate and monitor dialysis in routine and high risk patients.

INITIATION OF MAINTENANCE DIALYSIS

When?

The question as to what is the optimal time to start hemodialysis is not setteled. While there is no difficulty in deciding when to begin in a severely uremic patient, the asymptomatic patient, inexorably deteriorating in terms of measured renal function, creates a problem as when to abandon conservative therapy in favor of dialysis. Malangone and co-workers (2) examined clinical and laboratory data retrospectively in 402 patients at the start of dialysis. Initiation of therapy was decided on a clinical basis. They found a wide range of serum creatinine (3.5–35 mg/dl) and blood urea nitrogen levels (35–345 mg/dl), although the mean values were 11.7 ± 4.6 mg/dl and 122 ± 47 mg/dl respectively. In addition, 52% of the patients had hypoalbuminemia and 27% had hyponatremia. Male patients and diabetics had higher hematocrits at the onset of dialysis and significantly lower values of serum creatinine were found in women, diabetics and older patients.

Since 1975 Bonomini (3) has been advocating early initiation of maintenance hemodialysis (creatinine clearances of 15–21 ml/min). It is his belief that by doing so there will be fewer uremic complications, the effects of protein depletion will be eliminated and hormonal equilibrium will be better preserved (4). Indeed, Bonomini reported a 10 year survival of 88% in patients who initiated hemodialysis at a creatinine clearance of 10 ml/min or more, compared to a 55% ten year survival for patients started late, that is at a creatinine clearance of 2–4 ml/min (5). In addition, 'early' patients spent less time in the hospital (5 days/year/patient versus 14 days/year/patient) for late starters. There were also economic benefits revealing a 20% savings for a group of early starting patients if one considered the cost of dialysis sessions, hospitalizations and wages earned (6). Scribner points out that Bonomini's patients may be a selected group and not representative of the general dialysis population (7).

Ratcliffe et al. (8) compared two groups of patients initiating hemodialysis at creatinine clearances of either above or below 6 ml/min. Seventy percent of the late referral group had serious medical complications prolonging the initial hospitalization compared to 9% of the early starters.

Of interest is a study by Binik and coworkers (9) in which 204 patients with deteriorating renal function were identified before dialysis was required and randomly assigned to either an enhanced or standard educational program about renal disease. The enhanced program consisted of specially prepared slide lectures delivered by a trained research assistant. Among topics covered were basic kidney function, dietary management and renal replacement therapies. Surprisingly, patients in the enhanced education program started dialysis an average of 4.6 months latter that those in the standard program. The possible reasons for this were thought to be that by educating the patients they had induced dietary changes or that exposure may have allowed the patients to anticipate future health related changes and thus cope with them better.

At our institution we generally subscribe to about a 5 ml/min creatinine clearance as a starting point for maintenance hemodialysis. The patient's clinical condition however is much more important than laboratory measures.

We feel that maintenance of good nutrition is important and will pay particular attention to the patient's appetite and serum albumin level. It is not unusual to see someone with 'uremic symptoms' (i.e., nausea, vomiting, lassitude) at a serum creatinine of 5 mg/dl (442 umol/l), creatinine clearance approximately 10 ml/min or more, who subjectively feels much improved after initiation of hemodialysis. This is particularly true in patients with diabetes mellitus or other systemic diseases. In such patients early dialysis initiation seems indicated.

How? – Time to plan

Ideally, with the early recognition of the eventual need for renal replacement therapy, there can be a well thought out plan discussed before the patient becomes 'too uremic' to participate. We believe that the patient, family and other appropriate people should discuss the options available. The suitability of hemodialysis, peritoneal dialysis or transplant may vary according to the patient's age, diagnosis, location and preference. In our program we have a 'uremia nurse' who makes sure that the patient has an opportunity to meet with the transplant surgeon and nephrologist. Whenever possible, we have new patients meet with people who are leading fully active lives after many years of therapy.

If the decision is made for hemodialysis we like to have vascular access provided well in advance to allow the arteriovenous fistula to 'mature'. The Cimino-Brescia arteriovenous fistula (10) is the access of choice for most patients. If the surgeon does not think the patient's veins will support a good fistula a polytetraflouroethlene (PTFE) graft may be done (11). The patients are told to avoid blood drawing in their non-dominant arm to protect veins. We choose the non-dominant arm in the hope that the patient will opt for home or limited care hemodialysis with self puncture of the access. If a patients arrives in advanced uremia without an access, several different strategies may be tried. At our institution, most often permanent access is placed in the non-dominant arm and

either an internal jugular or less often, subclavian double lumen catheter (12) is placed or the patient has repeated percutaneous femoral venous catheterizations done until the fistula matures (13, 14). Another strategy is to place the permanent access in the non-dominant arm and maintain the patient by peritoneal dialysis through a Tenkoff catheter.

DIALYSIS PRESCRIPTION

When a patient is ready to start hemodialysis, a dialysis prescription must be written. Among the variables to be considered are the type of kidney to use, the hours of treatment, the dialysis bath and the blood flow. Patient characteristics include the size and age of the patient, residual renal function, dialysis access, fluid status and whether or not the patient has other non-renal conditions (see below).

DIALYZER SELECTION

In selecting a kidney for dialysis one may choose a 'conventional dialyzer', usually a cellulose kidney, or a 'high efficiency' dialyzer. The later is defined as a dialyzer that has an ultrafiltration coefficient of 10–19 ml/mmHg. These membranes have hydrophobic surfaces and high permeability to water and large molecular weight substances. Included in this category are membranes of the following materials: polysulfone (PS), polymethylmethacrylate (PMNA), polyacrylonitrile (PAN), polyamide (PA) and sulfonated polyacrylonitrile (AN69). These membranes clear small molecular weight substances in a manner similar to cellulose, but have a far greater permeability to water and increased permeability to high molecular weight solutes (15).

Because of the high ultrafiltration coefficient, they must be used in a delivery system that can control fluid removal. Systems currently available regulate ultrafiltration by withdrawing solution from a fixed volume circuit at a measured rate. Improved removal of small molecules can be obtained by increasing the blood flow rate to at least 400 ml/min (16, 17). However since small molecule transport can occur in both directions and as dialyzers become more efficient, there may be rapid entry of acetate into the circulation, most high efficiency therapy is performed using a bicarbonate bath.

Another potential advantage of the high efficiency membranes is the fact that they may be more 'biocompatible'. Dialysis with a cellulose type membrane may lead to complement activation, granulocytopenia, cytokine release and increased beta$_2$ microglobulin levels.

Beta$_2$ microglobulins have been associated with dialysis related amyloid in long term patients and it may be less prevalent in patients dialyzed with high flux membranes (18–20), although this is far from proven. The

Bergamo Collaborative Dialysis Study Group found no difference in acute intradialytic well-being, i.e., hypotension, headaches, nausea or pruritic in a double blind study that compared dialysis with a polysulfone and a cuprophan membrane (21). Among the disadvantages of high flux membranes are the potential for transport of contaminants from the dialysate to the blood, because of a hydrostatic pressure gradient from dialysate to blood or 'backfiltration'. Coupled with this is the fact that bicarbonate dialysate which is used with most high efficiency membranes is particularly vulnerable to bacterial contamination (22). Another disadvantage is the fact that these membranes are three to four times as expensive as cellulose kidneys. This means that those kidneys are frequently re-used.

At least in the United States at this time, the vast majority of dialyses are done using conventional cellulose type membranes. The physician should become familiar with several different models and prescribe from them. When using a conventional dialyzer for an adult patient, we use a hollow fiber kidney with a high *in vivo* small molecular clearance. The ultrafiltration coefficient chosen will vary according to the patients interdialytic weight gain. We believe patients should be dialyzed three times per week, usually for 4 h, although there is a move to shorten dialysis time with high efficiency kidneys (see below). A periodic measurement of the adequacy of dialysis should be done and appropriate adjustments made.

DIALYSIS SOLUTIONS

Several different concentrates are available. Attention must be paid to the following chemicals:

Sodium: Sodium is the major determinant of osmolality in the dialysate solution. The 'low sodium' bath that was originally used to control thirst and blood pressure led to excessive hypotension and cramping. For this reason, dialysis sodium is now in the range of 140–145 mg/l.

Potassium: For standard dialysis patients, a dialysis fluid potassium concentration of 2 mEq/l is routine. If the patient is catabolic or tends to have an excessive dietary intake of potassium, a zero or 1 mEg/l bath may be used. In a patient with heart disease or one receiving cardiac glycosides, the potassium concentration should be raised to 3 mEq/l.

Acetate vs bicarbonate: The choice of the appropriate buffer for a routine dialysis is not solved. With high-efficiency dialyzers most studies suggest that a bicarbonate bath should be used (23), although not everyone agrees with this (24). Because bicarbonate dialysate is prepared from concentrate that can support bacterial growth with endotoxin production, there is concern that the endotoxins or bacteria may cross or interact with the membranes and cause pyogenic reactions. Gordon, et al. (25) found a pyrogenic rate of 0.7/1000 treatments with no difference between conventional and high flux dialyzers. This rate

was reduced to 0.3/1000 treatments in a multicenter study that filtered the bicarbonate dialysate first with a polysulfone filter (26). This of course will increase the cost of a treatment. For a routine dialysis with a conventional dialyzer, it is still not clear if bicarbonate offers any major advantage compared to acetate as long as the sodium levels are equivalent. Comparative Doppler-echocardiographic studies of 12 patients in a cross-over manner found that while weight loss was equal, patients treated with acetate had a significant increase in heart rate and fractional shortening of the left ventricular diameter after acetate but those treated with bicarbonate did not (27). In another crossover study of patients on conventional dialysis, patients treated with acetate had equivalent weight loss, blood pressure and correction of acidosis as when they where treated with bicarbonate, however there were more symptoms like headache, malaise and vomiting (28). For all acute dialyses, in the elderly and in patients with significant heart disease the current standard of practice is to use a bicarbonate bath.

Calcium: The concentration of calcium in the dialysate has implications for the prevention and treatment of bone disease. The standard level is 1.25 to 1.5 mmol/l, however higher levels may result in a positive calcium balance in the patient. Saha, et al. (29) using a high calcium dialysate (1.75 mmol/l) were able to revert plasma parathyroid hormone (PTH) levels to normal in a group of ten patients. Another approach to treating hyperparathyroidism is to give large doses of IV cholecalciferol and use a low calcium dialysate to prevent hypercalcemia (30). A zero calcium bath is available and can be used as an acute treatment for dangerous levels of hypercalcemia from any cause.

Magnesium: Dialysate magnesium in standard solutions is absent or low (0.25–0.4 mm/l) because of the fear of producing hypermagnesemia in patients who cannot excrete magnesium through glomerular filtration (31). The serum magnesium that is frequently measured to be normal or high in dialysis patients is total magnesium. We measured ionized magnesium in 26 randomly selected hemodialysis patients using an ion-selective electrode and found that the ionized magnesium level was low, although the total magnesium was normal (32). Our patients also had an increased mean ionized calcium to ionized magnesium ratio which has been associated with atherogenesis in animal models (33). It may be that after further research the magnesium concentration of dialysate will be raised.

INITIATING DIALYSIS-FIRST TREATMENT

In 1962, a clinical syndrome of headaches, nausea, blurring of vision, tremors and seizures was described in patients which occurred most often after a rapid dialysis in people just beginning therapy. This has been called dialysis disequilibrium (34). The most consistent finding in patients with severe cases is an elevated cerebrospinal fluid pressure and cerebral edema. The exact mechanism by which this happens is not clear, although the possible causes for the increased brain H^+ ion concentration and brain osmolality that have been consistently found have recently been reviewed by Arieff (35).

With the advent of improving dialysis technology, widespread use of bicarbonate baths and earlier initiation of treatment, this condition is becoming rarer, however be aware that patients with pre-existing neurological conditions like head trauma, intracranial tumors and hematomas or malignant hypertension are at particular risk for the development of dialysis disequilibrium and subsequent brain damage (36). If a patient first comes to your attention with far advanced uremia you can attempt to minimize the syndrome by starting with short frequent treatment. Ideally, we dialyze for 2 h on day one, 2–4 h on day two, no dialysis on day three and then proceed with the usual thrice weekly schedule. Another possibility is to add osmotically active solutes (glucose, glycerol, albumin, urea, salt or mannitol) to the dialysate (37, 38). If the syndrome does occur, intravenous injection of 50 ml of 50% glucose or mannitol may improve the situation. These injections may be repeated two to three times over the next 2 h.

DURATION OF DIALYSIS-ADEQUACY OF TREATMENT

One of the most vociferous debates in Nephrology today has to do with the length of the individual dialysis treatment and what constitutes adequate dialysis. Since hemodialysis is time consuming and expensive, there is interest in shortening the hours of therapy and it is not unusual to have treatment times as disparate as 2 to 5 h (39). Hakim, Depner, and Parker (40) believe that there is good evidence that the dose of dialysis received by American patients is inadequate and plays a major role in the observed increasing mortality seen in the United States. Others agree with this. For instance, Held et al. (41), using a Cox proportion hazards model found that patients receiving an average dialysis treatment duration of less than 3.5 h had a relative mortality risk of 1.17 to 2.18 compared to those with treatment longer than 3.5 h (mortality risk 1.0). Perhaps the best dialysis survival data in the world comes from the Artificial Kidney Center in Tassin, France where cuprophan plate dialyzers are used and patients are treated for 8 h during each of three weekly sessions at a relatively low blood pump speed. In this center, 5 year survival of patients less than age 35 is 93%, and the same figure for patients greater than age 64 is an amazing 67% (42). To confuse the issue however are other studies that suggest that hours of treatment alone do not correlate with survival (43, 44). Adequate dialysis has still not been satisfactorily defined even after all these years (45). The trend recently is to have some objective quantitative measurement of adequacy. Statistical methods of assessing the adequacy of hemodialysis began with the dialysis index of Babb and Scribner (46, 47). Perhaps the most widely used is the Kt/V index popularized by Keshaviah and Collins (48). In this formula K = urea clearance (ml/min), t = treatment duration (min) and V = volume of distribution for urea. The National Association of Dialysis and Transplant patients have recently suggested that a Kt/V of 1.2 should be required for patients. Other numerical models include the percent reduction of urea (49) (using this formula a 65% reduction is considered desirable), or the DDQ (Direct Dialysis Quantification) (50).

Other workers continue to rely on such quantifiable tests as the EEG (51), vibration sensitivity threshold (52) and nerve conduction studies, although it is unclear whether the routine use of this is helpful in monitoring the adequacy of dialysis (53). The latest predictor of adequate dialysis, particularly as a function of patient survival, is the serum albumin. Owens, et al. (43) found that the serum albumin concentration was a more powerful predictor of death (21 times greater) than the urea reduction ratio. In their study of over 13,000 patients, 60% of the patients had serum albumin concentrations predictive of an increased risk of death, that is values below 4 g/dl. Indeed, it is felt that the excellent survival seen at the Tassen center is due to the fact that with long, slow dialysis, patients are seldom anorexic and consume adequate protein with a mean predialysis albumin level of 4.2 g/dl. In addition, the treatment leads to excellent blood pressure control with less than 5% of their patients on antihypertensives (42). The definition of adequate dialysis that DePalma suggested years ago (54), though imprecise, is still useful: 'Adequate dialysis is that which permits the patient to be rehabilitated, eat a reasonable diet, make blood, maintain a near normal blood pressure and prevent the development or progression of neuropathy'.

The biochemical changes that occur during a single dialysis depend on several factors: The concentration of the substance (e.g., urea), its rate of generation, the volume of distribution, the hemodialyzer clearance, and the elapsed dialysis time (55). The hemodialyzer clearance depends on the type of membrane, the surface area and the blood and dialysate flow rates. If one is not achieving the desired results, one can change the dialyzer to a more efficient type, increase the time of the treatment or increase the blood flow rate. Particularly with high flux dialyzers, blood flow rates of 400 ml/min are standard. Problems with blood delivery may be due to inadequate vascular access. A high venous pressure suggests there may be an access problem. Another question is whether or not blood recirculation is occurring? This can occur in the presence of a normal venous pressure and a good blood flow. To calculate recirculation, after dialysis has been occurring for a short period of time (1/2 hour) simultaneously draw a sample for BUN determination from the blood going to the dialyzer (Ca), from that returning from the dialyzer (Cv), and from the peripheral blood (Cp).

Then use the formula: $(Cp - Ca)/(Cp - Cv) \times 100 = \%$ recirculation. If more than 20% of the blood is recirculating, an angiogram with dilatation or corrective access surgery should be strongly considered. High blood flows used with the new dialyzers increase the percentage of blood that recirculates.

TERMINATION OF DIALYSIS

The issue of the voluntary withdrawal from long term dialysis was first addressed by Neu and Kjellstrand (56) when they reported that discontinuation of dialysis accounted for 22% of all deaths in a group of 1766 patients who started hemodialysis between 1966 and 1983. One half of the patients were competent when the decision was made, and although diabetes and other medical conditions were common in patients in whom dialysis was discontinued, 17% of patients had no associated conditions. Port and coworkers analyzing 5,208 patients in the Michigan registry initiating dialysis between 1980 and 1985 found that 9.4% of deaths were due to termination of dialysis. These patients were likely to be older (56% of patients greater than age 80, versus 0.1–3.4% for patents less than age 49), female, white and diabetic (57). Similarly, Mailloux, et al. (58) monitored 716 patients through 1989. Withdrawal from dialysis and cardiac events were the second leading cause of death, each accounting for 18.5% of deaths. Older age at initiation of dialysis, cancer, malnutrition, diabetes and dissatisfaction with life were important associations with the decision to withdraw.

Obviously there are opposing views on whether or not this decision should be suggested or supported in individual cases (59).

In the United States, congress has mandated that all facilities participating in the Medicare and Medicaid programs offer advanced directives to patients regarding their right to refuse medical treatment. The National Kidney Foundation has produced guidelines on how to implement this for dialysis units. In one report Holley and coworkers, found that after receiving written information on advanced directives, 48% of patients on chronic dialysis filled out forms and made their wishes known compared to 13% before (60).

A much easier problem is when to discontinue dialysis because of the return of significant renal function. In a study of 7,404 patients in the Michigan Kidney registry, this occurred in 2.8% of cases (61). Recovery of renal function has been reported in patients with malignant hypertension (62, 63), gout (64) scleroderma (65) systemic lupus erythematosus (66) and myeloma kidney (67).

Pichette and coworkers (68) noted the return of renal function in 342 of 14,318 registered dialysis patients (2.4%). This occurred after a mean of 8.9 ± 0.5 months of renal replacement therapy, with 52.3% of recoveries happening within the first 6 months. Using the Cox regression analysis, patients with myeloma, drug induced renal disease, vascular/hypertensive and systemic diseases were more likely to have return of renal function than others. Women were twice as likely to improve as men. In their study, 57% of patients were still off dialysis after 78 months. According to this data, it may be prudent to postpone transplantation for at least 1 year, particularly in young women with certain vascular renal diseases. A pre dialysis serum creatinine concentration equal to or lower than the previous post dialysis creatinine and an increase in the patient's urine volume are important clues suggesting the return of renal function.

MANAGEMENT OF THE ROUTINE DIALYSIS PATIENT

Monitoring of medical problems

Once the patient is stable and about to begin a maintenance program, the guidelines as in Tables 1–4 may be used for the routine management and follow up of common medical problems.

DIALYSIS IN HIGH RISK GROUPS

Diabetes Mellitus

Diabetes Mellitus accounts for approximately 25% of all people who are now on dialysis (95). Transplantation and peritoneal dialysis play a minor role in treating these patients. Early survival of diabetics on hemodialysis was dismal, but is improving (96). For 1990, The USRDS reported a 1 year survival of 74% and a 5 year of 19%. By comparison, the 1 and 5 yr survival for all ESRD patients was 78% and 40% respectively (95). Survival beyond the first decade has even been reported (97). Diabetics die from cardiovascular disease (20–50% of all deaths) (98). In one study (99), cardiovascular mortality was 4.8 times higher in type I patients and 3 times higher in type II patients than in controls.

Vascular access is a particular problem for diabetic patients and should be created early. Arterio-venous fistulae may mature poorly or not at all. In one study the synthetic PTFE graft survival was only slightly lower in diabetic patients than non-diabetic (100). For the best chance of maturation, access should be placed 3–6 months prior to anticipated use, and hemodialysis initiated early, i.e., a creatinine clearance of 10–20 ml/min (98).

The diabetic patient experiences many complications during treatment. Hypotension is common and sometimes occurs in the presence of clinical volume overload. The high prevalence of autonomic neuropathy makes it difficult for the patient's cardiovascular systems to compensate for rapid volume reduction during hemodialysis. A change of therapy to peritoneal dialysis is occasionally necessary.

Table 1. Routine tests at initial evaluation and at annual physical examination.

1. Bloods:
   Serum electrolytes, urea nitrogen (BUN), glucose, creatinine, Mg, lipid profile, Ca, PO_4, PTH, ferritin, uric acid, complete blood count, liver function tests, serological tests for syphilis and hepatitis B and C.
2. Electrocardiogram. Echocardiogram?
3. Chest X-ray, hand films.
4. Miscellaneous:
   Tine test, stool guaiac, mammogram for women over age 50. Offer hepatitis vaccination, HIV screening.
5. Assessment of vascular access:
   Physical exam, venous pressure, recirculation time and angiography if warranted (69).
6. Other: Discussion of consideration of home dialysis or transplantation.
7. Meeting with dietitian and social worker.

Monthly follow up
   Pre and post dialysis BUN, creatinine, electrolytes and glucose.
   Pre dialysis, liver profile, cholesterol, Ca, PO_4, hct.
   Some assessment of adequacy of dialysis (see above).

Fifty percent of diabetic dialysis patients require antihypertensive drugs compared to 28% of non-diabetics (101). In part this may be because there is a tendency toward higher interdialytic weight gains in diabetic patients (102). Antihypertensive medications must be chosen with care because of the tendency of Beta-blockers to mask hypoglycemia or to exaggerate lipid abnormalities. Calcium channel blockers are a good choice. In patients who develop angina during the dialysis treatment, 2% nitroglycerine ointment to the chest wall 30–60 minutes prior to therapy can be tried.

Ninety seven percent of newly evaluated uremic patients have significant retinopathy, and 25–30% are blind. While heparinization was once suspected of aggravating visual loss, this is no longer thought to be the case (103). Proliferative retinopathy is correlated with the duration of diabetes, female gender and the degree of blood pressure control. Aggressive treatment is needed to preserve vision and may be obtained by close association with an opthomologist and a regime of focal and panretinal laser photocoagulation or pars plane vitrectomy (104).

Adynamic bone disease is common in diabetic patients (105), and aluminum containing antacids should be particularly avoided in them because of the tendency for diabetics to have more aluminum accumulate in their bones (106).

Diabetic patients have more gastroparesis, more nausea and vomiting than other patients (107). These factors as well as diabetic diarrhea and possibly under dialysis because of poor vascular access results in a high degree

Table 2. Evaluation and treatment plan for anemia

It is now clear that the major cause of the anemia of uremia is erythropoietin deficiency (70, 71). A substantial clinical experience with the recombinant hormone has all but eliminated the role of shortened red cell survival or the presence of an inhibitor such as parathyroid hormone. Nonetheless, other factors may complicate the anemia of chronic renal failure and should be corrected. In addition, careful attention must be paid to iron balance when using erythropoietin. Conditions that cause resistance to this hormone must also be excluded (see table).

1. Diagnostic tests:
   a) Complete blood count, hemoglobin electrophoresis if indicated, serum folate and Vitamin B^{12} levels.
   b) Serum iron, iron binding capacity, ferritin, zinc and histidine levels. If iron low:
      Check stool for guaiac positive material.
      Check amount of blood lost through testing.
      Check for excess blood loss in dialyzer.
   c) Red cell indices:
      If evidence of hemolysis, eliminate possible causes such as copper, nitrate or chloramine toxicity, improperly mixed dialysate, drugs, hypophosphatemia or hemolysis due to antibodies from residual formaldehyde in reused dialyzers (72).
   d) Bone marrow in difficult cases.
2. Treatment:
   a) If serum folate low, give folic acid 1 mg/day.
   b) If Vitamin B^{12} low, give IM 1000 mg.
   c) If histidine low, give histidine 10 mg/day.
   d) Iron (will probably be needed for all patients treated with erythropoietin).
      Ferrous sulfate (oral 325 mg TID).
      Intravenous iron (Infed 100 mg times 10, or 500 mg times 2) (73).
   e) Erythropoietin 2,000–4,000 unit IV three times per week at the end of dialysis (74).
      1. If response inadequate give iron as above (75).
      2. Consider aluminum toxicity, infection, inflammation (76), folic acid deficiency or secondary hyperparathyroidism (77).
   f) If response inadequate, give 8–12,000 units.
   g) Consider subcutaneous erythropoietin which may have greater efficacy (78, 79).
   h) Daily moderate exercise (80).
   i) Transfuse only for:
      1. acute bleed,
      2. the elderly or patients with heart disease and Hct < 25 vols %.

---

of malnutrition. A diet of 25–30 Kcal/kg/d with 50% of calories from complex carbohydrates and 1.3–1.5 g/kg/d of protein is recommended.

Insulin requirements change with the initiation of hemodialysis and frequently increase. Careful blood glu-

Table 3. Uremic bone disease

Renal osteodystrophy continues to be a major problem for dialysis patients. In addition, it is an ever changing entity that now includes high-turnover bone disease (secondary hyperparathyroidism), low-turnover bone disease (osteomalacia and adynamic bone disease, with or without aluminum toxicity), a mixed bone picture and increasingly in long duration patients, amyloidosis (81). With the current understanding of the etiology of these syndromes, early management of patients with progressive renal insufficiency and attention to calcium and phosphorous balance it may be possible to prevent some of these conditions. If however the patient on dialysis has developed disease, the following table may be used as a guide for evaluation and treatment.

1. Initial evaluation:
   a) Biochemical
      1. Ca: If high, consider tertiary hyperparathyroidism, multiple myeloma, Vitamin D toxicity, solid tumors, sarcoidosis, immobilization, excess calcium ingestion or aluminum toxicity. If low, check serum albumin, consider liver disease, malabsorption, dietary lack, anticonvulsants or Vitamin D deficiency.
      2. Phosphorous: If high, reduce phosphate in diet to 400–800 mg/d or add phosphate binders (see below).
      3. Alkaline phosphatase: If high, fractionate to eliminate liver production.
      4. Serum parathormone level (Intact-PTH level best) (82).
   b) Radiology
      1. X-rays: Metabolic bone survey: Hand films best for subperiosteal reabsorption seen in hyperparathyroidism. Skull, pelvis, hands, chest, long bones helpful for determining the extent of disease and for finding other conditions such as demineralization and rarely, pseudofractures. Cystic changes, particularly multiple and in the metacarpal area and regions adjacent to large joints suggest amyloid.
      2. Bone scan-(technetium-labeled biphosphonates) cannot currently distinguish between high and low bone turnover states.
   c) Desferrioxamine infusion test (83) for aluminum intoxication.
   d) Bone biopsy in difficult cases with tetracycline labelling.
2. Management:
   a) Control phosphate to 4–5 mg/dl with binders. Calcium supplements: calcium carbonate 1–3 g/day with meals (watch for hypercalcemia), calcium acetate or aluminum hydroxide with meals for a short period of time (1–2 weeks).
   b) Use high calcium dialysate (3–4 mEq/l) to prevent hypocalcemia.
   c) 1, 25 vitamin D 0.25–1.5 ug/d orally (watch for hypercalcemia) (84).
   d) If PTH remains high, intravenous administration of cholecalciferol 1–3 ug/d (85). Consider using with low calcium dialysate if hypercalcemia develops.
   e) Parathyroidectomy with or without re-implantation of part of the gland (86).
   f) For aluminum bone disease, desferrioxamine infusion 1.5 g 1–2 times/week at end of dialysis.
   g) For amyloid bone disease consider high flux dialysis (not proven effective) or transplantation.

Table 4. 4-Hypertension: characterization and treatment

Hypertension is common in renal disease and multifactorial. In the majority of cases it is volume related and careful attention to salt and water balance can control the blood pressure in about 75% of patients on maintenance hemodialysis (87, 88). Recently however, Cheigh, et al. using 24 hour ambulatory blood pressure recordings found that only 51% of patients had significantly reduced blood pressure at the end of dialysis (89) and Sherman et al. found that weight gains commonly observed in patients undergoing dialysis had only a modest effect on predialyisis blood pressure (90). Other causes of hypertension include an increased activity of the renin-angiotensin-aldosterone system, the sympathetic nervous system and possibly reduced production of vasodilatory substances by the uremic kidney (91).

1. Mild (70–80% of patients):
   a) definition
      1. Pre dialysis diastolic blood pressure 100 mmHg or less.
      2. Plasma renin activity (PRA) usually normal.
   b) treatment
      1. Restrict dietary sodium to 80–100 mg/d.
      2. Ultrafiltration during dialysis.
2. Moderate (10–20% of patients):
   a) definition
      1. Pre dialysis diastolic blood pressure 100–120 mmHg.
      2. Blood pressure easily controlled with medications.
      3. PRA higher than group 1 but still normal.
   b) treatment
      1. As for group 1.
      2. Medications (first on non-dialysis days only).
      3. Alpha or Beta adrenoreceptor antagonists (Labetalol) 200 mg/d (theoretical advantage because of role of norepinephrine).
      4. Calcium channel blockers (Nifedipine or Verapamil) (92).
      5. Angiotensin Converting Enzyme (ACE) Inhibitors.
3. Severe (5–10% of patients):
   a) definition
      1. Diastolic blood pressure 120–140 mmHg or more.
      2. May be associated with cachexia, ascites and visual problems.
      3. PRA usually high.
   b) treatment
      1. As above.
      2. ACE Inhibitors (Enalapril, Captopril).
      3. Vasodilators (Minoxidil).
      4. Hemofiltration.
      5. Bilateral nephrectomy (rarely if ever needed with new drugs).
4. Others factors:
   a) Erythropoietin may increase blood pressure (93).
   b) Patients may have a delayed hypotensive response 1–5 h post dialysis (94).

cose monitoring, particularly in the early stages of therapy is important.

Pregnancy

Pregnancy is uncommon in woman undergoing hemodialysis because of a variety of hormonal and non-hormonal factors. Recently however, possibly because of erythropoietin and improved dialysis techniques, the number of dialysis patients who become pregnant is increasing. Hou (108) in a recent survey of American dialysis units found that over a 2 year period of time, 1.5% of women in the childbearing age became pregnant. Another report from Saudi Arabia (109) found an amazing 7.3% of married chronic dialysis patients under age 50 becoming pregnant.

These data suggest that birth control must be discussed with appropriate patients. Oral contraceptives may be contraindicated in women with hypertension and have been reported to increase vascular access clotting. Intrauterine devices can lead to heparin-associated bleeding. Barrier methods are the preferred choice (108).

If a patient becomes pregnant, there is high fetal wastage at all stages of pregnancy. The live birth outcome is at best 37% (110). Pregnancy is often diagnosed late. Missed periods are usual and urine pregnancy tests unreliable in dialysis patients. To increase the chances of a successful outcome a special dialysis strategy must be followed.

Dialysis time should be increased by 50% and if possible performed 5 times per week in an attempt to keep the predialysis BUN to less than 60–80mg/dl. Bicarbonate bath should be used.

Hypotension during dialysis should be avoided. Rapid fluctuations in intravascular volume may be controlled by limiting interdialytic weight gain to approximately 1 kg till late in pregnancy (111). Maternal hypertension occurs in approximately one-half of pregnant woman on dialysis and should be controlled. This can be accomplished by achieving euvolemia and medications if needed. Alphamethyldopa is the drug of choice, having the longest and most careful follow-up. Beta blockers, clonidine and labetalol may also be used (108). Angiotensin converting enzyme inhibitors are contra indicated as they are associated with increased fetal loss and bone deformities (112). The hematocrit should be maintained at a minimum of 30 vols %. This can probably be achieved safely with erthyropoietin as Hou and co-workers have shown, although the dose of the recombinant hormone may have to be increased (113). Iron saturation should be monitored closely and daily folate requirement increased to 1.8 mg. A diet prescription should include 1–1.5 g/kg of high biological protein and 30–35 cal/kg/d. In addition, 1500 mg of calcium, 80 mmol sodium, 50 mmol of potassium and water soluble vitamins should be included. Early and serial sonograms are needed for monitoring fetal growth. Polyhydramnios is common (114). The onset of labor has averaged 34 weeks and the birth weight of the infants is low (115).

Cardiac surgery in dialysys patients

Cardiac disease continues to be a major cause of mortality and morbidity in long term patients, so it is not surprising that the incidence of coronary artery bypass (CABP) and other heart surgery is rapidly increasing. Ko, Kreiger and Isom reviewed 25 patients who had cardiopulmonary bypass operations at their institution. Surgery was performed using standard bypass procedures with a Cobe membrane oxygenator and moderate hypothermia. As patients were given cardioplegic potassium, there was obvious concern for post operative potassium levels. Dialysis management consisted of having the patient dialyzed the day before the operation by their usual method. A peritoneal dialysis catheter was then placed and peritoneal dialysis started immediately on arrival of the patient to the Intensive Care Unit to relieve the extra fluid and potassium given during the procedure. This was continued for 7 days with prophylactic antibiotics added to the dialysis. The patients were then returned to hemodialysis. Intraoperatively, dialysis patients required more blood, platelets and fresh frozen plasma. Their operative mortality was 16% (116).

By contrast, Rostand et al. had an overall mortality of 42%. There were 4 deaths either intra or perioperatively for a hospital mortality of 20%. The usual hospital operative mortality for non-renal patients in their program is 1.2%. They managed the patients by having them dialyzed 24 h prior to surgery and within 24–48 h post operatively. They were also careful with fluid replacement (117). In another report of 39 patients, the operative mortality was 2.6% although 23% of the patients had pericarditis (118).

Pavie et al. also described their operative technique is 20 dialysis patients. During anesthesia and cardiopulmonary bypass, every effort was made to preserve the peripheral arterial and venous vessels for eventual dialysis access. This was done by using the jugular vein and dorsalis pedis arteries for monitoring. Arterial blood pressure was maintained above 60 mmHg and large doses of heparin were used to protect the arteriovenous shunts (119). Another group performed concurrent hemodialysis during the bypass procedure in one patient. They were thus able to delay further dialysis for 72 h (120).

Other strategies for operating on dialysis patients include:

1. Dialyze patient immediately after a diagnostic catheterization and cineangiogram. Limit the amount of dye used.

2. Maintain hematocrit at 30 vols %.

3. Pay careful attention to serum potassium.

4. Keep IV fluids to a minimum.

5. Protect the patient's fistula by padding. Do not perform blood pressure monitoring nor venipunctures in the access arm.

6. The timing of post operative hemodialysis can be dictated by the patient's status (121).

With erythropoietin it may be possible to increase a patient's hematocrit to 35 or 40 vols %, phlebotomize them and store their blood pre surgery.

The elderly

In 1989, 39% of dialysis patients were older than 65 years of age, and people over age 75 represented 13.3% (122). The remaining lifetime expectancy for elderly dialysis patients is considerably less than the general age matched US population and was reported in an excellent review of dialysis in the elderly by Ismail et al. (123). The vast majority of older patients are treated in center dialysis units. Experience with vascular access varies. Pourchez et al., were able to construct an arteriovenous fistulae in 41 of 47 patients aged 75 years or more, although others have successfully used this technique in only 25–30% of the elderly patients (124). Indeed, Hinsdale and coworkers reported that all fistulas placed in a group of patients over 65 years of age failed by 1 year. By contrast, the 1 year synthetic graft patency rate was 91% (125). Didlake reported on experience with PTFE grafts in 79 patients older that 65 years. There was no difference in the infection rate, aneurysms, flow problems or clotting when compared to a group of younger patients. One problem however for the older group was minor wound and skin changes. These authors thus recommend tunneling the graft slightly deeper than usual at each end to allow for a two-layer closure over the anastomoses. They also recommend absorbable subcuticular sutures to prevent erosion (126). The ability of older patients fistulae to delivery high blood flows for high-efficiency dialysis remains to be demonstrated.

Hypotension during dialysis is more frequent in the elderly and may lead to seizures, cerebral infarction, myocardial ischemia, aspiration pneumonia and vascular access thrombosis.

Chester and coworkers found twice as many medical problems in older patients, particularly more gastrointestinal bleeding and a higher transfusion requirement (127). This is not surprising since older people have a higher incidence of diverticular disease, angiodysplasia and gastritis particularly from the use of non-steroidal anti-inflammatory drugs.

Nutrition in dialysis patients is particularly important as malnutrition has a negative effect on survival (44). Hakim and Levine have pointed out that the elderly are particularly susceptible to malnutrition because of low income, social isolation, malabsorption, ill fitting dentures, depression, constipation and impaired taste acuity (128). Ifudu has recently pointed out the rehabilitation in the elderly is dismal (129).

A dialysis strategy for the elderly would be to maintain their hct at 30 vols %, make frequent reassessment of dry weight, avoid rapid ultrafiltration, hold antihypertensive drugs on the morning of dialysis and use a bicarbonate bath. If available, a volume controlled machine is helpful. Heparin should be minimal or bypassed if there is any evidence of gastrointestinal bleeding. Patients receiving digitalis may require a higher potassium concentrate. Frequent evaluations should be made of the vascular access to make sure it is not causing an excessive strain on the heart.

Special attention should be made to provide a palatable diet of at least 35 Kcal/kg/d with 1 g/kg/d of protein of which about 70% should be of high biological value. Pyridoxine 10 mg and folic acid 1 mg should be added.

Amyloidosis

Amyloidosis accounts for 1.3% of all patients admitted to dialysis centers in Europe (130). Although it is a serious systemic disease, survival of patients receiving renal replacement therapy is improving. For instance, Port and Nissenson reported on 321 such patients. Seventy five per cent received hemodialysis as their major form of therapy and 25% were treated by peritoneal dialysis. One and 3 year survival was 66% and 38% respectively (131). Moroni et al. reported very similar numbers, i.e., a 1 yr survival of 68% and 30% were alive at 5 yrs. In addition, they had 4 patients who were alive more than 10 yrs on dialysis (132). Patients who have a normal two-dimensional echocardiogram suggesting the absence of cardiac amyloidosis are most likely to derive long-term benefit from dialysis (133). The treatment of these patients is not without problems. Fistula failures are higher than controls and in 1 study occurred early with 31% of fistulas created lasting less than 2 days. A control group had 11% early occlusion (134). To prevent that, the authors suggest volume expansion post operatively. Hypotension and hemodynamic changes are major problems for amyloid patients. Martinez et al. reported permanent hypotension in 38% of their amyloid patients. Other problems that were more frequent than control patients were gastrointestinal hemorrhage, diarrhea, femoral neuropathy, ischemic colitis and early occlusion of access (135). Gastrointestinal involvement with amyloid can lead to malnutrition. Gertz stressed that these patients may die from intractable heart failure and arrhythmias if they have cardiac amyloid (133). Other causes of death included infection (136) and voluntary withdrawal from dialysis because of poor life quality.

Strategies for dealing with the profound hypotension have been to switch some patients to peritoneal dialysis. Others have infused large amounts of albumin (150–300 g/week) without benefit (137). Only bilateral surgical nephrectomy (138) or medical nephrectomy (destruction of residual renal function by nephrotoxic metallic salts)

(139) permitted the serum albumin to rise to a level to make dialysis feasible.

Multiple myeloma

When patients with multiple myeloma develop renal insufficiency it is regarded as a bad sign. While over 50% of patients develop some degree of renal impairment during the course of their illness, frequently it is secondary to dehydration, hypercalcemia, or the nephrotoxic effect of a drug and may be reversed (140). When the renal damage is irreversible is it worthwhile to use dialysis to prolong life? Brown et al. found a median duration of such patients on renal replacement therapy to be 7.5 months (141). Iggo and others reported on 23 patients who started chronic dialysis. While fifteen of their patients died, nine within the first six months, six patients survived more than 2 years. Actuarial survival was 45% at 12 months and 38% at 2 years (142). This is similar to the fairly optimistic 53% one year survival reported by Cosio and coworkers (143). Lazarus also had relatively long surviving patients, one who lived seven years (144). Some authors have suggested that myeloma patients be treated with peritoneal dialysis because of the potential to remove light chains from the patients organs (145), however the high incidence of infections in patients receiving chemotherapy makes the risk of peritonitis a factor to be considered. It may be prudent to begin chemotherapy while a patient is on hemodialysis and change to peritoneal treatment after two or more months (143). The use of erythropoietin in a report of four myeloma patients undergoing dialysis resulted in an increase in mean hematocrit from 23 ± 3 to 32 ± 4 vols %. Also those patients no longer needed blood transfusions and reported an improvement in well being (146). Another report of the use of this hormone in a very small group of patients questioned whether or not bone marrow proliferation from its use was responsible for the recurrence of myeloma in one patient. They also commented on the need for high doses of erythropoietin (320 U/kg/week) to achieve a response (147).

Liver disease

Performing hemodialysis in patients with severe liver disease, particularly with ascites is difficult. The treatment is frequently associated with hypotension requiring large volumes of salt-poor albumin, mannitol or saline (148). Hypotension may limit the amount of ultrafiltration possible thereby exaggerating the ascites. Marcus, Messana and Swartz switched nine patients with chronic renal and liver disease plus ascites to peritoneal dialysis. They found that this was a reasonable alternative in some patients (149). Excessive bleeding is another concern. Antithrombin III levels are low in hepatic failure and heparin kinetics are abnormal. Langley et al. thus performed a randomized trial of antithrombin III supplementation (3000 units before dialysis). This normalized antithrombin III lev-

els and reduced the total heparin required by the patients (150).

To optimize hemodialysis one should use bicarbonate as the buffer as it does not required hepatic metabolism. Liberal use of blood, albumin and fresh frozen plasma may be necessary. In patients with severe bleeding diathesis, a dialyzer that requires no heparin is appropriate.

Dialysis related ascites is an entity that develops in some patients once they are on hemodialysis. Etiologies are varied and include previous peritoneal dialysis, cirrhosis, tuberculosis, overhydration, infections, peritonitis, hemosiderosis, hepatitis, Hodgkins disease, portal hypertension (due to polycystic liver) and nephrotic syndrome (151, 152).

Dialysis ascites can occasionally be controlled by peritoneal-venous shunting or water immersion (153, 154). Another more novel approach recently reported by Okada and coworkers is to remove the ascitic fluid from the peritoneal cavity by a pump and then intravenously reinfuse it via the dialyzer along with the patients blood (155).

Intravenous drug abusers, HIV positive and AIDS patients

It is clear that in urban dialysis centers, HIV positive and AIDS patients are becoming increasingly frequent, particularly where there is widespread use of intravenous drugs with shared needles (156). The prognosis of patients with clinical AIDS is poor. Ribot et al. reported that only 12% of those with clinical AIDS were alive at 12 months, although patients who were just HIV positive fared better with a 54% five year survival (157). Zara and co-workers reported on a patient with clinical AIDS who survived 3.5 years on dialysis after the first episode of pneumocystis pneumonia (158).

Dialysis units should follow the CDC guidelines for hemodialysis in these patients which include universal precautions of blood and body fluids(159). Routine disinfection and sterilization strategies are felt to be adequate (160) and the use of separate machines not recommended. Although saliva has not been implicated in HIV transmission, resuscitation bags or other ventilation devices should be readily available to minimize the need for mouth to mouth resuscitation. In our dialysis unit, AIDS patients who are ill with complicating respiratory and diarrheal symptoms are isolated from other patients, to prevent the transmission of other communicable diseases. We use separate machines, dialyzers and tubing are not reused.

After each use, the exterior of the machines is thoroughly cleaned with hypochlorite and the interior rinsed with formaldehyde.

Problems encountered in dialyzing AIDS patients include difficulty in establishing vascular access in intravenous drug addicts who may have destroyed their veins from self-administered drugs, staphloccocal sepsis and bacterial endocarditis. Some patients are non-compliant with dialysis schedules and exhibit disruptive behavior in the unit. In HIV positive patients unexplained wasting which is unresponsive to hyperalimentation leads to several malnutrition which compromises survival (161).

Systemic lupus erythematosus

While once considered poor, the survival of patients with systemic lupus on hemodialysis has markedly improved. The Nissenson and Port study of 1029 patients had a 33 month survival of 73% (162) and others have found a 5 year survival of 89% (163). Cheigh and Stenzel note that 10–28% of patients with lupus nephritis severe enough to require dialysis will recover sufficient function to stop treatment (164). Extrarenal manifestation of lupus are diminished, but not abolished (163) and there is a case report of a patient who developed lupus after being on dialysis for two years (165). Vascular access complications are a continuing source of problems for these patients, and in some cases peritoneal dialysis may be appropriate (166). Patients with this disease frequently have high levels of antiphospholipid antibodies that are associated with venous thrombosis, however, no correlation was found between thrombotic events and raised anticardiolipin antibodies and lupus anticoagulant activity in a group of 45 dialysis patients (167). Early deaths are due to infectious complications of steroids, so that a prudent approach might be to initiate dialytic therapy early and markedly reduce steroid doses (168).

Sickle cell anemia

Patients with sickle cell anemia occasionally develop renal failure. In one study of 725 patients with this hemoglobinopathy, 4.2% developed renal failure at a median age of 23.1 years (169). Survival was not good with half of those patients dying an average of 4 years after exhibiting any degree of renal insufficiency. Deaths were primarily due to heart failure, pericardial and pleural effusions and hemorrhage. To optimize survival, careful attention should be given to fluid overload and dialysis instituted relatively early. In another study of 77 patients with sickle cell anemia on dialysis the 30 month survival was 59% (170). The dialysis course can be complicated by priapism (171) and ischemic intestinal necrosis (172). Among the strategies used to ensure a comfortable dialysis have been the use of frequent blood transfusions to maintain the sickle hemoglobin level less than 20%, and the use of 40% Oxygen so that the patients PO_2 is maintained at 95–125 mmHg, as hypoxia is a known stimulus to crises (173). The use of erythropoietin has not been very successful in these patients. Steinberg reported some improvement in anemia in two patients (174), however Rogers and coworkers found no improvement in one woman despite erythropoietin doses of 160 U/kg. Another patients had a slight response but the drug had to be stopped because he went onto sickle crises (175).

REFERENCES

1. Scribner BH, Buri R, Caner JEZ, Hegstrom R, Burnell JM: The treatment of chronic uremia by means of intermittent dialysis: a preliminary report. *Trans Am Soc Artif Intern Organs* 6: 114, 1960
2. Malangone JM, Abuelo JG, Pezzullo JC, Lund K, McGloin CA: Clinical and laboratory feature of patients with chronic renal disease at the start of dialysis. *Clin Nephrol* 31: 77, 1989
3. Bonomini V: On optimal dialysis. *Kidney Int* 7 (Suppl 3): 365S, 1976
4. Bonomini V: Long term early dialysis. (Abstract) *3rd Int Conf Uremia Capri* 7, 1980
5. Bonomini V: Early dialysis up-dated. *Int J Artif Organs* 4: 54, 1981
6. Bonomini V, Baldrati L, Stefoni S: Comparative cost/benefit analysis in early and late dialysis. *Nephron* 33: 1, 1983
7. Scribner BH: A critical comment. *Nephron* 16: 100, 1976
8. Ratcliffe PJ, Philips RE, Oliver, DV: Late referral for maintenance dialysis. *Br Med J* 288: 441, 1983
9. Binik YM, Devins GM, Barre PE et al.: Live and learn: patient education delays the need to initiate renal replacement therapy in end-stage renal disease. *J Nervous Mental Dis* 181: 371, 1993
10. Brescia MJ, Cimino JE, Appel K, Hurwich BJ: Chronic hemodialysis using venipuncture and a surgically created arterio-venous fistula. *N Engl J Med* 275: 1089, 1966
11. Kherlakian GM, Rodersheimer LR, King LR: Comparison of autogenous fistula versus expanded polytetrafluoroethyene graft fistula for angioaccess in hemodialysis. *Am J Surg* 152: 238, 1986
12. De Moor B, Vanholder R, Ringoir S: Subclavian vein hemodialysis catheters: advantages and disadvantages. *Artif Organs* 18: 293, 1994
13. Pascua LJ: Vascular access update. *Trans Am Soc Artif Intern Organs* 25: 526, 1979
14. Arana VA: Percutaneous femoral vein catheterization in patients requiring hemodialysis. *J Urol* 106: 492, 1971
15. Barth RH: High-Flux hemodialysis: overcoming the tyranny of time. *Contrib Nephrol* 102: 73, 1993
16. Barth RH, Rubin JE, Berlyne GM: Very high blood flow is safe and effective in hemodialysis. *ASAIO Abstr* 17: 58, 1988
17. Ronco C, Feriani M, La Greca G: Hemodynamic response to high blood flows and ultrafiltration modeling during short dialysis. *Kidney Int* 37: 317, 1990
18. Chanard J, Bindi P, Lavaud S, Toupance O, Malcut H, Lacour F: Carpal tunnel syndrome and type of dialysis membrane. *Br Med J* 298: 867, 1989
19. Miura Y, Ishiyama T, Inomata A et al.: Radiolucent bone cysts and the type of dialysis membrane used in patients undergoing long-term hemodialysis. *Nephron* 60: 268, 1992
20. Van Ypersele DO, Strichou C, Jadoul M, Malghem J, Maldague B, Jamart J: The working party on dialysis-related amyloidosis. *Kidney Int* 39: 1012, 1991
21. Bergamo Collaborative Dialysis Study Group: Acute intradialytic well-being: results of a clinical trail comparing polysulfone with cuprophan. *Kidney Int* 40: 714, 1991

22. Alter MJ, Favero MS, Moyer LA, Bland LA: National surveillance of dialysis-associated disease in the United States, 1989. *Trans Am Soc Artif Intern Organs* 37: 97, 1991

23. Collins AJ, Keshaviah P: High efficiency therapies for clinical dialysis. in *Clinical Dialysis*, 2nd Edition, edited by Nissenson AR, Fine RN, Gentile DE, Norwalk, Appleton & Lange, 1990, p 687

24. Civati G, Guastone C, Teatini U et al.: High flux acetate hemodialysis: a single-centre experience. *Nephrol Dial Transpl* 6 (Suppl 2): 75, 1991

25. Gordon SM, Oettinger CW, Bland LA et al.: Pyrogenic reactions in patients receiving conventional, high efficiency or high flux hemodialysis treatments with bicarbonate dialysate containing high concentration of bacteria and endotoxin. *J Am Soc Nephrol* 2: 1436, 1992

26. Pegus DA, Oettinger CW, Bland LA et al.: A prospective study of pyrogenic reaction in hemodialysis patients using bicarbonate dialysis fluids filtered to remove bacteria and endotoxin. *J Am Soc Nephrol* 3: 1002, 1992

27. Sztajzel J, Ruedin P, Stoermann C et al.: Effects of dialysate composition during hemodialysis on left ventricular function. *Kidney Int* 41: 60, 1993

28. Gurudev, KC, Pathak V, Prabhakar, KS, Bhaskar S, Prakash KC, Mani MK: Short term study of relative merits of acetate and bicarbonate dialysis. *J Assoc Physicians of India* 39: 921, 1991

29. Saha H, Pietila K, Mustonen J, Pasternack A, Morsky P: Acute effect of dialysate calcium concentration and intravenous Vitamin D3 on the secretion of parathyroid hormone in hemodialysis patients. *Clin Nephrol* 38: 145, 1992

30. Slatopolsky E, Weerts C, Norwood K: Long term effects of calcium carbonate and 0.5 mEq/l calcium dialysate on mineral metabolism. *Kidney Int* 36: 897, 1989

31. Valporean ML, Van Stone JC: Dialysate magnesium. *Semin Dial* 6: 46, 1993

32. Markell, MS, Altura BA, Sarn Y et al.: Deficiency of serum ionized magnesium in patients receiving hemodialysis or peritoneal dialysis. *ASAIO J* 39: 801, 1993

33. Altura BT, Brust M, Bloom S, Altura BM: Magnesium dietary intake modulates blood lipids and atherogenesis. *Proc Natl Acad Sci USA* 87: 1840, 1990

34. Kennedy AC, Linton AL, Eaton J: Urea levels in cerebrospinal fluid after hemodialysis. *Lancet* 1: 410, 1962

35. Arieff A: Dialysis Disequilibrium syndrome: current concepts on pathogenesis and prevention. *Kidney Int* 45: 629, 1994

36. Leonard A, Shapiro FL: Subdural hematoma in regularly hemodialylzed patients. *Ann Intern Med* 82: 650, 1975

37. Van Stone JC, Carey J, Meyer R Murrin C: Hemodialysis with glycerol containing dialysate. *Trans Amer Soc Artif Intern Organs* 2: 119, 1979

38. Rosa AA, Shideman J, McHugh R, Duncan D, Kjellstrand CM: The importance of osmolality fall and ultrafiltration rate on hemodialysis side effects. *Nephron* 27: 134, 1981

39. Goldwaser P, Mittman N, Antignani A et al.: Predictors of mortality in hemodialysis patients. *J Am Soc Nephrol* 3: 1613, 1993

40. Hakim RM, Depner TA, Parker TF: Adequacy of hemodialysis. *Am J Kidney Dis* 21: 567, 1993

41. Held PJ, Levin NW, Bovbjerg RR, Pauly MV, Diamond LH: Mortality and duration of hemodialysis treatment. *JAMA* 265: 871, 1991

42. Charra B: Does empirical long slow dialysis result in better survival? If so, how and why? *ASAIO J* 39: 819, 1993

43. Owens WF, Lew NL, Liu Y, Lowrie EG, Lazarus JM: The urea reduction ratio and serum albumin concentration as predictors of mortality in patients undergoing hemodialysis. *N Engl J Med* 329: 1001, 1993

44. Lowrie EG, Liu NL: Death risk of hemodialysis patients: the predictive value of commonly measured variables and evaluation of death rate differences between facilities. *Am J Kidney Dis* 15;458, 1990

45. Blagg CR: Adequacy of dialysis. *Am J Kidney Dis* 2: 218, 1984

46. Babb AL, Scribner BH: Quantitative description of dialysis treatment I. A dialysis index. *Kidney Int* 7 (Suppl 2): 23S, 1975

47. Ahmad S, Babb AL, Mulutinovic J, Scribner BH: Effect of residual renal function on minimal dialysis requirements. *Proc Euro Dial Tranpl Assoc* 16: 107, 1979

48. Keshaviah P, Collins A: Rapid high efficiency bicarbonate hemodialysis. *Trans Am Soc Artif Intern Organs* 32: 17, 1986

49. Basile C, Casino F, Lopez T: Percent reduction in blood urea concentration during dialysis estimates Kt/V in a simple and accurate way. *Am J Kidney Dis* 15: 40, 1990

50. Flanigan MJ, Fangman J, Lim VS: Quantitating hemodialysis: a comparison of three kinetic models. *Am J Kidney Dis* 17: 295, 1991

51. Teschan PE: Clinical estimates of treatment adequacy. *Artif Organs* 10: 201, 1986

52. Read DJ, Feest TG, Holmon RH: Vibratory sensory threshold: A guide to adequacy of dialysis. *Proc Eur Dial Transpl Assoc* 19: 253, 1983

53. Phillips LH, Williams FH: Are nerve conduction studies useful for monitoring the adequacy of renal dialysis? *Muscle and Nerve* 16: 970, 1993

54. DePalma JR: Adequate hemodialysis schedule. *N Engl J Med* 285: 353, 1972

55. Hakim RM, Lazarus JM: Medical aspects of hemodialysis. in *The Kidney*, edited by Brenner BM, Rector FC, Philadelphia, Saunders, 1986, p 1791

56. Neu S, Kjellstrand CM: Stopping long term dialysis. An empirical study of withdrawal of life supporting treatment. *N Engl J Med* 314: 14, 1986

57. Port FK, Wolfe RA, Hawthorne VM, Ferguson CW: Discontinuation of dialytic therapy as a cause of death. *Am J Nephrol* 9: 145, 1989

58. Mailloux LU, Bellucci AG, Napolitano B, Mossey RT, Wilkes BM, Bluestone PA: Death by withdrawal from dialysis: a 20 year clinical experience. *J Am Soc Nephrol* 3: 1631, 1993

59. Kjellstrand CM, Dolan JM, Rachels J, Epstein FH: Is one allowed to stop artificial organs allowing patients to die? *Trans Am Soc Artif Intern Organs* 32: 671, 1986

60. Holley JL, Nespor S, Rault R: The effects of providing chronic hemodialysis patients written material on advanced directives. *Am J Kidney Dis* 22: 413, 1993

61. Sekkarie MA, Port KF, Wolfe RA et al.: Recovery from end stage renal disease. *Am J Kidney Dis* 15: 61, 1990

62. Mitchell HC, Graham RM, Pettinger WA: Renal function during long treatment of hypertension with minoxidil. *Ann Intern Med* 93: 676, 1980

63. Bacon BR, Ricanati ES: Severe and prolonged renal insufficiency. Reversal in a patients with malignant hypertension. *JAMA* 239: 1159, 1978

64. Maxey RW, Rao TKS, Manis T, Delano BG, Friedman EA: Return of renal function after commencing maintenance hemodialysis. *Proc Clin Dial Transpl Forum* 5: 12, 1975

65. Steen VD, Constantino JP, Shapiro AP, Medsger TA: Outcome of renal crisis in systemic sclerosis: relation of availability of angiotensin converting enzyme inhibitors. *Ann Intern Med* 113: 352, 1990

66. Kimberly RP, Lockshin MD, Sherman RL, Mouradian J, Saal S: Reversible end-stage lupus nephritis. Analysis of patients able to discontinue dialysis. *Am J Med* 74: 361, 1983

67. Misani R, Tiraboschi G, Mingardi G, Mecca G: Management of myeloma kidney: an anti-light chain approach. *Am J Kidney Dis* 10: 28, 1987

68. Pichette V, Querin S, Desmeules M, Ethier J, Copleston P: Renal function recovery in end-stage renal disease. *Am J Kidney Dis* 22: 398, 1993

69. Richter M, Porile JL: Preservation of vascular access. *J Am Soc Nephrol* 4: 997, 1993

70. Esbach JW, Adamson JW: Recombinant human erythropoietin. *Implications for Nephrology* 9: 203, 1989

71. Eschbach JW: Erythropoietin: the promise and the facts. *Kidney Int* 45 (Suppl 4): 70S, 1994

72. Ng YY, Chow, MP, Lou JY et al.: Resistance to erythropoietin: immunohemolytic anemia induced by residual formaldehyde in dialyzers. *Am J Kidney Dis* 21: 213, 1993

73. Rault R, Nespor S, Holley J: Safety and efficacy of 500 mg of iron-dextran as a single IV infusion in patients on chronic dialysis. *Abs ASAIO* 23: 74, 1994

74. Amerling R, Levin NW: Erythropoietin update. *The Kidney* 26: 1, 1992

75. Van Wyck DB, Stivelman JC, Ruiz J, Kielin LF, Katz, MA, Ogden DA: Iron stores in patients receiving erythropoietin for dialysis associated anemia. *Kidney Int* 35: 712, 1989

76. Koury NJ: Investigating erythropoietin resistance. *N Engl J Med* 238: 205, 1993

77. Ra DS, Shah M, Muhinyo R: Effect of serum parathyroid hormone and bone marrow fibrosis on the response to erythropoietin in uremia. *N Engl J Med* 328: 171, 1993

78. Berersab A: Optimizing epoetin therapy in ESRD. The case for subcutaneous administration. *Am J Kidney Dis* 22: 23, 1993

79. Ashi NI, Paganini EP, Wilson JM: Erythropoietin: Intravenous versus subcutaneous administration. A review of the literature. *Am J Kidney Dis* 22 (Suppl 1): 23, 1993

80. Goldberg AP, Hagberg JM, Delmez, JA, Haynes ME: Metabolic effects of exercise training in hemodialysis patients. *Kidney Int* 18: 754, 1980

81. Goodman WG, Coburn JW, Ramirez JA, Slatopolsky E, Salusky IB: Renal osteodystrophy in adults and children. in *A Primer of Metabolic Bone Disease*, edited by Favus MJ, New York, Raven Press, 1993, p 304

82. Quarles DL, Davidal GA, Schwab SI, Bartholomey DW, Lobaugh B: Oral calcitriol and calcium: effective therapy for uremic hyperparathyroidism. *Kidney Int* 34: 840, 1988

83. McCarthy, JT, Milliner DS, Johnson WJ: Clinical experience with desferrioxamine in dialysis patients with aluminum toxicity. *Quart J Med* 74: 257, 1990

84. Quarles DL, Yohay Da, Carroll BA et al.: Prospective double blind placebo controlled trial of oral versus IV calcitriol in the treatment of hyperparathyroidism in ESRD. *J Am Soc Neprol* 4: 718, 1993

85. Andress DL, Norris KC, Coburn JW, Slatopolsky EA, Sherrard DJ: IV calcitriol in the treatment of refractory osteitis fibrosis of chronic renal failure. *N Engl J Med* 274: 274, 1989

86. Kaye M, D'Amons P, Henderson J: Elective total parathyroidectomy without autotransplant in ESRD. *Kidney Int* 35: 1390, 1989

87. Sulkova S, Valek A: The role of antihypertensive drugs in the therapy of patients on regular dialysis treatment. *Kidney Int* 34: S198, 1988

88. Acosta JH: Hypertension in chronic renal failure. *Kidney Int* 22: 702, 1982

89. Cheigh JS, Milite C, Sullivan J, Rubin AL, Stenzl KH: Hypertension is not adequately controlled in hemodialysis patients. *Am J Kidney Dis* 19: 453, 1992

90. Sherman RA, Daniel A, Cody RP: The effect of interdialytic weight gain on predialysis blood pressure. *Artif Organs* 17: 770, 1993

91. Ma, KW, Greene EL, Raij L: Cardiovascular risk factors in chronic renal failure and hemodialysis populations. *Am J Kidney Dis* 19: 505, 1992

92. Beyerlein C, Saszar G, Hollmann M, Schumacher A: Verapamil in antihypertensive treatment of patients on renal replacement therapy. *Eur J Clin Pharmac* 39: 35, 1991

93. Abraham PA, Opsahl JA, Kesaviah PR et al.: Body fluid spaces and blood pressure in hemodialysis patients during amelioration of anemia with erythropoietin. *Am J Kidney Dis* 16: 438, 1990

94. Battle, DC, Riotte AV, Land G: Delayed hypotensive response to dialysis in hypertensive patients with ESRD. *Am J Nephrol* 6: 14, 1986

95. United States Renal Data System: USRDS 1993 Annual Data Report. Bethesda, The National Institutes of Health, National Institute of Diabetes and Digestive and Kidney Diseases, Bethesda, MD, 1993

96. Ghavamian M, Gutch CF, Kopp KF, Kolff WJ: The sad truth about hemodialysis in diabetics. *JAMA* 222: 1386, 1972

97. Tzamaloukas, AH, Murphy G, Spalding CT: Diabetic nephropathy: eleven year survival with good quality of life. *Clin Nephrol* 38: 234, 1992

98. Miles AM, Friedman, EA: Dialytic therapy for diabetic patients with terminal renal failure. *Current Opinion in Nephrology and Hypertension* 2: 868, 1992

99. Ritz E, Strumpf C, Katz, F, Wing AJ, Quellhorst E: Hypertension and cardiovascular risk factors in hemodialyzyed diabetic patients. *Hypertension* 7 (Suppl 2): S118, 1985

100. Windus DW, Jendrisak MD, Delmez JA: Prosthetic fistula survival and complications in hemodialysis patients. Effects of Diabetes and age. *Am J Kidney Dis* 19: 448, 1992

101. Weinrauch LA, D'Eliz JA, Gleason RE et al.: Usefulness of left ventricular size and function in predicting survival in chronic hemodialysis patients with diabetes mellitus. *Am J Cardiol* 7: 300, 1992

102. Ifudu O, Dulin A, Lundin AP, Friedman EA: Diabetics manifest excess weight gain on maintenance hemodialysis. (Abstract) *ASAIO J* 21: 85, 1992

103. Diaz-Buxo JA, Burges NP, Greenman M, Chandeir JT, Farmer CP, Walker PJ. Comparison of peritoneal and hemodialysis. *Int J Artif Organs* 7: 257, 1984

104. Berman DH, Friedman EA, Lundin AP: Aggressive ophthalmological management in diabetic ESRD patients: a study of 31 consecutively referred patients. *Am J Nephrol* 12: 344, 1992

105. Vincenti F, Arnaud SB, Recker R et al.: Parathyroid and bone response of the diabetic patient to uremia. *Kidney Int* 25: 677, 1984

106. Andress DL, Kopp JB, Maloney NA, Coburn JW, Sherrard DJ: Early deposition of aluminum in bone in diabetic patients on hemodialysis. *N Engl J Med* 316: 292, 1987

107. Kjellstrand CM, Whitley K, Comty CM, Shapiro FL: Dialysis in patients with diabetes. *Diabetic Nephropathy* 2: 5, 1983

108. Hou S: Pregnancy and birth control in dialysis patients. *Dial Transpl* 23: 22, 1994

109. Souqiyyeh MZ, Huraib SO, Mohd-Saleh AG: Pregnancy in chronic hemodialysis patients in the kingdom of Saudi Arabia. *Am J Kidney Dis* 19: 235, 1992

110. Hou S: Frequency and outcome of pregnancy in women on dialysis. *Am J Kidney Dis* 23: 60, 1994

111. Davidson JM: Dialysis, Transplantation and Pregnancy. *Am J Kidney Dis* 17: 127, 1991

112. Anon: Are ACE Inhibitors safe in pregnancy? *Lancet* 2: 482, 1989

113. Hou S, Orlowski J, Pahl M: Pregnancy in women with end-stage renal disease: treatment of anemia and premature labor. *Am J Kidney Dis* 21: 16, 1993

114. Yasin SY, Beydown SW: Hemodialysis in pregnancy. *Obs Gyn Surg* 43: 655, 1988

115. Hou S: Pregnancy in women requiring dialysis for renal failure. *Am J Kidney Dis* 9: 368, 1987

116. Ko W, Kreiger KH, Isom OW: Cardiopulmonary bypass procedures in dialysis patients. *Ann Thorac Surg* 55: 677, 1993

117. Rostand SG, Kirk KA, Rutsky, EA, Pacifico AD: Results of cardiac bypass graft in ESRD. *Am J Kidney Dis* 12: 266, 1988

118. Opahl JA, Husebye DG, Helseth HK, Collins AJ: Cardiac bypass surgery in patients on maintenance dialysis: Long term survival. *Am J Kidney Dis* 12: 271, 1988

119. Pavie A, Mussat T, Valle D et al.: Open heart cardiac surgery in severe renal insufficiency and dialysis patients. *Arch Mal Coeur* 78: 242, 1985

120. Zawada ET Jr, Stinson JB, Done G: New perspective on coronary artery disease in hemodialysis patients. *South Med J* 75: 694, 1982

121. Laws KH, Merrill WH, Aammon JW Jr, Prager RL, Bender HW: Cardiac surgery in patients with chronic renal disease. *Ann Thorac Surg* 42: 152, 1986

122. Port FK: The end-stage renal disease program: trends over the past 18 years. *Am J Kidney Dis* 20: 3, 1992

123. Ismail NI, Hakim RM, Oreopoulos DG, Patrikarea A: Renal replacement therapies in the elderly. Part 1. Hemodialysis and chronic peritoneal dialysis. *Am J Kidney Dis* 22: 759, 1993

124. Pourchez T, Moriniere P, St Priest A: Outcome of vascular access for hemodialysis in the elderly (< 75 years). *Proc Eur Dial Transpl Assoc* 27: 160, 1990

125. Hinsdale JG, Lipcowitz GS, Hoover EL: Vascular access in the elderly. Results and perspectives in a geriatric population. *Dial Transpl* 14: 560, 1985

126. Didlake R, Raju S, Rhodes RS, Bower J: Dialysis access in patients older than 65 years. in *Vascular Access for Hemodialysis*, edited by Sommer BG, Henry ML, Boston, Precept Press, 1991, p 166

127. Chester AC, Rakowski, Argy WP Jr, Giacalone A, Sheiner GE: Hemodialysis in the eighth and ninth decade of life. *Arch Intern Med* 139: 1001, 1979

128. Hakim RM, Levin NL: Malnutrition in hemodialysis patients. *Am J Kidney Dis* 21: 125, 1993

129. Ifudu O, Mayers J, Matthew J, Tan CD, Cambridge A, Friedman EA: Dismal rehabilitation in geriatric inner-city hemodialysis patients. *JAMA* 5: 29, 1994

130. Banks RA, White HJO, MacKenzie JC, Tribe CR, Harrison PR: Replacement therapy in end stage renal amyloidosis. *J Royal Soc Med* 78: 593, 1985

131. Port FK, Nissenson AR: Outcome of ESRD in patients with rare causes of renal failure. II Renal or systemic neoplasm. *Quart J Med* 73: 1161, 1989

132. Moroni G, Banfi I: Chronic Dialysis in patients with systemic amyloidosis. The experience in Northern Italy. *Clin Nephrol* 38: 81, 1992

133. Gertz MA, Kyle RA, O'Falloon WM: Dialysis support of patients with primary systemic amyloidosis. A study of 211 patients. *Arch Intern Med* 152: 2245, 1992

134. Hashmoni M, Shapir Y, Chaimovitz C, Better OS, Schamek A: Blood access for hemodialysis in patients with end stage renal amyloid. *Dial Transpl* 11: 307, 1982

135. Martinez VA, Garcia C, Carreras M, Renert L, Olive JA: ESRD in systemic amyloidosis. Clinical course and outcome on dialysis. *Am J Nephrol* 10: 283, 1990

136. Ylinken K, Gronhagen C, Honkamen E, Ekstrand A, Metsarinne K, Kuhlback B: Outcome of patients with secondary amyloidosis in dialysis treatment. *Nephrol Dial Transpl* 7: 908, 1992

137. Rosansky SJ, Richards FW: Use of peritoneal dialysis in the treatment of patients with renal failure and paraproteinemia. *Am J Nephrol* 5: 361, 1985

138. Shapiro W, Chou SY, Porush JG: Nephrectomy for intractable proteinuria secondary to severe nephrotic syndrome. *Abs Am Soc Nephrol* 8: 824, 1975

139. Avram MM, Lapinid N, Lipner H: Medical nephrectomy. The use of metallic salts in uncontrollable massive nephrotic syndrome. *Trans Am Soc Artif Intern Organs* 22: 431, 1976

140. Mallick NP: Dialysis in the management of the renal failure of myeloma. *Quart J Med* 270: 871, 1989

141. Brown JH, Maxwell AP, Bruce I, Murphy BG, Doherty CC: Renal replacement therapy in multiple myeloma and systemic amyloidosis. *Irish J Med Sci* 162: 213, 1993

142. Iggo N, Palmer ABD, Severn A et al.: Chronic dialysis in patients with multiple myeloma and renal failure. A worthwhile treatment. *Quart J Med* 270: 903, 1989

143. Cosio FG, Pence TV, Shapiro FL, Kjellstrand CM: Severe renal failure in multiple myeloma. *Clin Nephrol* 15: 206, 1981

144. Lazarus HM, Adelstein DJ, Herzig RH, Smith MC: Long term survival of patients with multiple myeloma and acute renal failure at presentation. *Am J Kidney Dis* 2: 521, 1983

145. Randall RE, Williamson WC, Mullinax F, Tung MF, Still JS: Manifestations of systemic light chain deposition. *Am J Med* 60: 293, 1976

146. Ruedin P, Pechere Bertschi A, Chapuis B, Benedit P, Leski M: Safety and efficacy of recombinant human erythropoietin treatment of anemia associated with multiple myeloma in hemodialyzed patients. *Nephrol Dial Transpl* 8: 315, 1993

147. Caillette A, Barreto S, Gimenez E, Labeeuw M, Zech P: Is erythropoietin treatment safe and effective in myeloma patients receiving hemodialysis? *Clin Nephrol* 40: 176, 1993

148. Ellis D, Avner ED: Renal failure and dialysis therapy in children with hepatic failure in the perioperative period of orthotopic liver transplant. *Clin Nephrol* 25: 295, 1986

149. Marcus RG, Messana J, Swartz R: Peritoneal dialysis in end-stage renal disease patients with preexisting chronic liver disease and ascites. *Am J Med* 93: 35, 1992

150. Langley, PG, Keays R, Hughes Rd, Forbes A, Delvos U, Williams R: Antithrombin III supplementation reduces heparin requirement and platelet loss during hemodialysis of patients with fulminant hepatic failure. *Hepatology* 14: 251, 1991

151. Gotlieb L, Servadis C: Ascites in patients undergoing maintenance hemodialysis. *Am J Med* 101: 161, 1976

152. Arismendi GS, Izard MW, Hamptom WR, Maher JF: The clinical spectrum of ascites associated with maintenance dialysis. *Am J Med* 60: 46, 1976

153. Kearns PJ, Polhemus RJ, Oakes D, Rabkin R: Hepatorenal syndrome managed with hemodialysis, then reversed by peritoneovenous shunting. *J Clin Gastroenterol* 7: 341, 1985

154. Ponce P, Moreira P: Water immersion in an anuric cirrhotic patient. *Nephron* 43: 144, 1986

155. Okada K, Takahashi S, Higuch T, Maega H: Long term effect of intravenous reinfusion of unmodified autogenous peritoneal fluid combined with hemodialysis in a patient with dialysis related ascites. *Nephron* 65: 474, 1993

156. Reiser IA, Shapiro WB, Porush JG: The incidence and epidemiology of human immunodeficiency virus infection in 320 patients treated in an inner-city hemodialysis Unit. *Am J Kidney Dis* 16: 26, 1990

157. Ribot S, Dean D, Goldblat M, Saavedra M: Prognosis of HIV positive dialysis patients. *Kidney Int* 37: 325, 1990

158. Zara, AC, Berlyne GM, Barth RH: Prolonged survival in an AIDS patients with ESRD. *Kidney Int* 37: 325, 1990

159. Schoenfeld P, Feduska, NJ: Acquired immunodeficiency syndrome and renal disease: Report of the National Kidney Foundation-NIH Task Force in AIDS and kidney disease. *Am J Kidney Dis* 16: 14, 1990

160. Recommendation for prevention of HIV transmission in health care workers. *MMWR* 36 (Suppl 23): 1S, 1987

161. Rao TKS: Acquired immunodeficiency syndrome, HIV virus infection and dialysis. in *International Yearbook of Nephrology*, edited by Andreucci VE, Fein LG, Boston, Kluwer Academic Publishers, 1991, p 199

162. Nissenson AR, Port FK: Outcome of end-stage renal disease in patients with rare causes of renal failure III. Systemic vascular disorders. *Quart J Med* 74: 63, 1990

163. Nossent HC, Swaak TT, Berden JH: Systemic lupus erythematosus: Analysis of disease activity in 55 patients with end-stage renal failure treated with hemodialysis or CAPD. *Am J Med* 89: 169, 1990

164. Cheigh JS, Stenzel KH: End-stage renal disease in systemic lupus erythematosus. *Am J Kidney Dis* 21: 2, 1993

165. Hernandez, JJ, Bernis C, Paraiso V, Barril G, Alverez V, Traver JA: Development of systemic lupus erythematosus in a patients on hemodialysis. *Am J Nephrol* 112: 105, 1992

166. Stock GG, Krahe NK: Treatment of end-stage renal disease due to lupus nephritis: comparison of six patients treated with both peritoneal and hemodialysis. *Adv Perit Dial* 9: 147, 1993

167. Sitter T, Spannagl M, Schiffl H: Anticardiolipin antibodies and lupus anticoagulant in patients treated with different methods of renal replacement therapy in comparison to patients with systemic lupus erythematosus. *Ann Hematol* 65: 79, 1992

168. Coplon NS, Siegel R, Fries J: Hemodialysis in end stage lupus nephritis. *Trans Am Soc Artif Intern Organs* 19: 302, 1973

169. Prowars DR: Chronic renal failure in sickle cell anemia: Risk factors, clinical course and Mortality. *Ann Intern Med* 115: 614, 1991

170. Nissenson AR, Port FK: Outcome of ESRD in Patients with rare causes of renal failure. 1. Inherited and Metabolic Disorders. *Quart J Med* 73: 1055, 1989

171. Singhal PC, Lynn RI, Scharschmidt LA: Priapism and Dialysis. *Am J Nephrol* 6: 358, 1986

172. Tomson CRV: ESRD in sickle cell anemia. Future directions. *Postgraduate Med J* 68: 775, 1992

173. Gonzalez-Carrillo M, Rudge CJ, Parsons V, Bewick M, White JM: Renal transplantation in sickle cell disease. *Clin Nephrol* 18: 209, 1982

174. Steinberg MH: Erthryopoietin for anemia of renal failure in sickle cell anemia. *N Engl J Med* 324: 1369, 1991

175. Rogers SD, MacDougall JC, Thuraisinghen RC, Raine AEG: Erythropoietin in anemia of renal failure in sickle cell anemia. *N Engl J Med* 325: 1175, 1991

PART B: CLINICAL MANAGEMENT AND FOLLOW UP OF PD PATIENTS

C. VERGER

INTRODUCTION

The clinical management of patients treated by chronic peritoneal dialysis is basically the same as with other forms of dialysis. They are presented in other parts of this book, so we will focus on those aspects which are more specific to peritoneal dialysis. These specific aspects are related to the tolerance of the peritoneal membrane to a non physiological environment, to the permanent glucose load as well as protein losses and to the presence of the peritoneal catheter. Eventually the prevention of infection is the key factor of a successful peritoneal dialysis program. We must also underline that, due to the continuous treatment, variations in clinical status and blood chemistry on peritoneal dialysis are much slower than on haemodialysis: this often results in a non recognition of some complications that may therefore have a delayed diagnosis.

PARTICULARITIES OF NUTRITIONAL AND HYDRATION ASSESSMENT IN PERITONEAL DIALYSIS

Nutritional assessment

We wish to remind the reader that permanent assessment of nutritional status of the peritoneal dialysis patient is probably as important as the clinical detection of peritonitis. These patients have the particularity of being submitted to a permanent glucose load through the dialysate. This glucose load, associated with the feeling of abdominal plenitude, is source of anorexia. In addition dialysate exchanges induce a daily protein loss ranging from 4 to 10 g per day and even much more in case of peritonitis. Thus malnutrition may rapidly appear especially in elderly patients or even in younger ones during infectious episodes. However, as malnutrition is developed elsewhere in this book we will not go into further details in this chapter.

Hydration assessment

Control of dry weight on continuous peritoneal dialysis may be tricky. The continuous treatment prevents large variations in fluid shifts as usually observed on haemodialysis. Insidious over or under hydration may thus develop without clinical symptoms.

Overhydration

Overhydration seems more common that dehydration. This is due to the fact that physicians in charge of peritoneal dialysis patients are aware that the permanent glucose load, by peritoneal absorption, often provokes an increase of patients' body fat. So they have a tendency to neglect a progressive body weight increase that is supposed to be only 'dry weight' if the patient has no oedema, nor hypertension. However it is well known that CAPD patients who are transplanted have higher pulmonary arterial pressure than those on chronic haemodialysis (1). We recently observed a 22 year-old patient who had no oedema, whose blood pressure had been relatively well controlled for several years with hypotensive drugs and who was hospitalized for dyspnea and cardiac failure. A severe mitral insufficiency was diagnosed by echography and surgery was discussed for valvular replacement. However it was decided first to dehydrate the patient by using more hypertonic bags. He lost five kilograms, his cardiac volume decreased dramatically and his mitral insufficiency almost totally disappeared. This underlines the difficulty of defining the real dry weight in such patients. Oedema and hypertension are useful to detect overhydration but may appear late in young patients and be underestimated.

One way to detect these variations would be to use such techniques as impedancemetry, but they are not always reliable or even available (2). A cardiac ultrasonography per year and a chest X-ray every six months is advised to evaluate cardiac volume. Any increase must suggest overhydration and press the physician to a better control of his patients body weight.

Dehydration

Dehydration is as frequent as overhydration. It has the advantage to be more easily detected. First sign is often persistent orthostatic hypotension in the absence of hypotensive drugs, associated with muscle cramps. Blood chemistry usually confirms haemoconcentration with recent elevation of serum protein and haemoglobin. Dehydration is often observed in patients who are not able to adjust the glucose concentration of their dialysate and who continue to use hypertonic solutions without recognizing the cause of their troubles.

Management of patient hydration

Well trained patients can be taught to adjust themselves the ratio of their hypertonic to normotonic dialysis solutions according to their hydration status.

The treatment of hydration disturbances must always be directed at the minimal use of hypertonic solutions. So, in case of overhydration, we must first ask the patient to decrease his fluid intake. This can be obtained by decreasing beverages of course, but also in collaboration with a dietician, by analysing the patient's diet: soups, fruit, various vegetables in large quantity may be a hidden cause of water intake in amount larger than that eliminated by the peritoneum. If diet or fluid restriction is not sufficient, furosemide is precribed or increased if the patient has some residual function, otherwise he must be advised to increase the amount of hypertonic solutions. However this method should be used only for a short period of two or three days. The use of hypertonic solutions may induce hyperglycemia especially in diabetic patients if insulin is not adapted. In addition, hypertonic solutions are potentially agressive to the peritoneum. On a cycler, rapid exchanges with a normal sodium concentration may induce severe hypernatremia and, therefore, must be monitored (3). If the cause of hyperhydration is related to a temporary loss of ultrafiltration due to peritonitis, hypertonic exchanges should always be avoided as they can induce rapid submesothelial fibrosis (4).

The best way to control hypervolemia is probably to perform temporarily one or several haemodialysis sessions. In our experience we prefer to use temporary haemodialysis or haemofiltration rather than increasing hypertonic exchanges. However this means that a haemodialysis facility must be easily available as well as a close collaboration between teams in charge of haemodialysis and peritoneal dialysis patients; unfortunately this is not always possible in all centers. But we are convinced that the only way to perform peritoneal dialysis safely is to establish a close relationship between haemodialysis and peritoneal dialysis teams in the same department. In our experience one station for haemodialysis should always be reserved as a ratio for fifteen peritoneal dialysis patients treated at home.

The policy of using temporary haemodialysis each time when needed, means that peritoneal dialysis patients should have an arteriovenous fistula. This issue is controversial and will not be discussed extensively here. However there is no doubt that one is more reluctant to perform a haemodialysis session through a temporary central catheter than to punction a fistula. There is thus a trend in this case to use haemodialysis too late, whereas complications might have been rapidly solved by a single or two haemodialysis sessions. On the other hand, a fistula may sometimes induce cardiac failure in some patients, or may be never used and clot.

Our policy is the following: if the patient has no cardiac insufficiency and good peripheral vessels, we realize a fistula. If the first one is not successful, we do not try another one if there is no obvious need for it. We also realize a fistula if we have the feeling that the patient might present frequent hyperhydration episodes, otherwise we do not.

Dehydration is easily managed. The first step is to replace hypertonic solutions by 'isotonic' solutions. If this not efficient enough, the patient is advised to drink mineral water, preferably one which contains sodium bicarbonate, and/or to increase the salt content in his daily diet.

MECHANICAL COMPLICATIONS OF CAPD

Back pain

The permanent presence of two liters of dialysate in the abdomen may alter body posture as observed sometimes in pregnant women. This can be the cause of low back pain forcing sometimes to discontinuation of CAPD. Prevention and successful treatment may be obtained by regular exercises designed to strengthen the abdominal wall (5).

Hernias

There is a trend to an increased intra abdominal pressure on peritoneal dialysis that is even further increased with hypertonic solutions (6). This is often the cause of hernia in approximately 10% of CAPD patients, less frequently in patients on automated peritoneal dialysis, due to a probably lower intra abdominal pressure in recumbent position. In the series of Spinowitz (7) hernia developed in 28% of their population. The hernias were 30% incisional, 38% umbilical, 17% inguinal and 15% ventral. Most hernias developed within the first year with a higher incidence in patients with polycystic kidney disease, parous females and those with prior history of hernia surgery who deserve special vigilance.

CLINICAL MONITORING OF PERITONEAL STERILITY

Peritoneal infection has been long the main cause of CAPD drop out and it still appears as the Achilles' heel of peritoneal dialysis. Industry has designed numerous different systems to prevent peritoneal infection. Some of these systems may appear expensive sometimes but their efficacy in preventing extra cost due to increased morbidity must be considered. A retrospective study reports (8) that 40% of patients who had more than one peritonitis per year were transferred to in-center haemodialysis after 3 years, whereas only 18% of those with less than one episode every two years were transferred to haemodialysis during the same period. Thus, the increased cost of more expensive systems is balanced by the fact that

patients are maintained longer on home dialysis which is much cheaper than in center haemodialysis.

Efficient means were soon discovered to prevent peritonitis, among them the use of a filter on the infusion line (9, 10) and so called 'Y-line' based sytems that allow both to disconnect bags and lines and to flush away any organisms towards the drainage bag (11, 12). Filters have not been extensively used, due to esthetical concerns and because they were suspected to activate macrophages which increase production of interleukine-I that may cause sclerosing peritonitis (13). Almost ten years were necessary to convince the nephrological community that disconnect systems based on a Y-line with a 'Flush before fill' effect were very effective for preventing peritonitis (14–18). More recently other systems with UV irradiation (19), or heat sterelisation were also designed. The overall peritonitis rate in patients treated with modern systems ranges between one episode every two to four years.

Besides the design of systems, the quality of patient training by nurses is also of first importance. In the French Language Peritoneal Dialysis Registry it was demonstrated that patients trained carefully on standard systems averaged one episode every 30 months, whereas the peritonitis rate was one episode every 8 months when training was more casual or less sophisticated (20). So it appears that prevention of peritonitis is first dependent on the quality of training and clinical follow up.

The initial step of peritonitis diagnosis is almost always clinical (21). The key sign is an aspect of cloudy dialysate. Pain may be or not present. Usually ultrafiltration is decreased due to the inflammatory response which induces an hyperpermeability to glucose. However, decreased ultrafiltration may sometimes be observed before turbidity appears. In presence of such signs, a sample of dialysate must be collected for bacteriological examination. The diagnostic criteria for peritonitis are the presence of two of the three following conditions: 1) abdominal pain, 2) cloudy dialysate with more than 100 leucocytes per μl with 50% or more neutrophils, and 3) demonstration of bacteria in the peritoneal effluent by gram stain or culture.

In this chapter, we will not develop the treatment of bacterial peritonitis which is presented in details in other sections of this book. From a clinical point a view we must, however, underline some other modifications of the aspect of the effluent which are different from bacterial peritonitis.

Bloody effluent may sometimes be observed. In females it is usually associated with either ovulation or menstruation. It has no consequences and usually resolves with the one or two next exchanges. Temporary and slight peritoneal bleeding may also be observed after physical exercise as a long walk, running, biking or swimming. Much more of concern is the occurence of peritoneal bleeding in patients with polycystic kidney desease as it may be related to the developement of a carcinoma (22).

Chylous peritonitis: The clinical aspect is more a 'milky' than a cloudy aspect. Patients are not complaining about any pain, there is no loss or decrease in the ultrafiltration and cells count of effluent is low. This is due to the passage of lymph in the peritoneal cavity. It may be related to post operative trauma of lymphatic vessels (23–25) or to an increased lymphatic flow or to obstruction of lymphatic vessels by a tumor. Lymph flow in the thoracic duct may vary from 1 ml/kg/h to 200 ml/kg/h during a hyperlipemic meal (23, 26). This explains that the milky appearance of the dialysate may vary from one moment to another and is often dependent on the patient's diet. Main causes, besides surgical trauma during catheter implantation, are abdominal cancer (intestinal or gynecological), tuberculosis, cirrhosis, pancreatitis, cardiac failure. The treatment of these chylous ascites is the treatment of their etiology if possible. In addition an hyperprotidic diet has been proposed, associated with low fat and a high proportion of medium chain triglycerides (25).

CLINICAL MANAGEMENT OF THE PERITONEAL CATHETER AND ITS RELATED COMPLICATIONS

Care of peritoneal catheter

Different techniques are recommended during the first few days following the implantation. Every one agrees with the need of covering the catheter during the break-in period by non occlusive and air permeable gauze bandage. In addition every one agrees to immobilize the catheter against the skin. Some teams recommend to change the dressing daily or whenever they are noted to be discoloured by dialysate or blood. We have, with others, a different policy. We may admit that there is no more sterile atmosphere and environment than in the operating room. So during the first few days following implantation there is a high risk of contamination of the exit site wound if exposed to another less controlled atmosphere. This is why we never change the bandage before one week, even if it appears coloured with blood or dialysate leaks: with this technique we never observed a post operative infection and it appears very effective. After one week, until day 15, the dressings are changed by a nurse every other day and the patient is trained to do it him/herself during the next three weeks. After five weeks the catheter exit site may be left unprotected. Other prefer to keep a dressing and there is no consensus about that. The advantage of keeping a dressing is mainly to maintain the catheter immobilized. On the other hand some poorly compliant patients may keep the dressing for too long and provoke maceration; in addition allergy to dressing fixatives may occur and be source of bacterial colonization. Actually there is no consensus about a protocol for long term catheter care. Most teams agree to allow shower, even

bath, as far as the exit site is properly dried and desinfected after it has been wetted.

Late peritoneal leakage

Leakage of dialysis solution around chronic catheters usually occurs during the first weeks or months following implantation. Often such leaks are not apparent. In addition to overt fluid leakage at the skin exit site, leaks may manifest more insidiously by subcutaneous swelling and edema, weight gain without hypertension and diminished outflow volumes. Sometimes patients try to compensate a diminished drainage volume by increasing the number of hypertonic bags. This results in hypotension whereas body weight is rapidly increasing with appearance of subcutaneous abdominal edema. Early peritoneal leakage is usually related to a surgical problem. It should not be observed if a peritoneal leak is checked for before the patient leaves the operating room and if low initial volumes are used in the break-in period after catheter implantation.

Delayed leakage is often related to malnutrition or to previous history of steroïd therapy. In these patients, healing takes more time and normal volumes should be used no earlier than three weeks after catheter implantation. During this prolonged break-in period, it is advisable to perform, at least during the first week, a daily lavage, using small volumes (500 ml) in order to prevent catheter obstruction by fibrin.

Processus vaginalis, ombilical hernia

Other cause of leakage may be related to a patent processus vaginalis which may appear after several months or years. The main signs are groin or scrotal edema. Leakage related to a patent ombilical hernia may also be observed. These causes of leakage may be undetectable clinically and are only confirmed either with scintigraphy or tomodensitometry, using for the investigation a high volume with hypertonic bags in order to better visualize the source of leakage.

Pleural leak

Pleural effusion may be observed on CAPD rather than CCPD after several days or months of treatment. It is usually a massive right sided hydrothorax which is due to leakage of dialysate through a small, often congenital, diaphragmatic defect: usually high glucose and low protein concentrations reflects the origin of the fluid. It can also be diagnosed through injection of technetium-tagged macroaggregated albumin into the peritoneal space with subsequent testing of the pleural space for radioactivity in sampling the pleural fluid or by chest scanning using a gamma camera (27, 28). Management is to either stop peritoneal dialysis temporarily or change the patient to automated peritoneal dialysis on a cycler, using low volume-infusions.

In general, leakage is less frequent with automated peritoneal dialysis than with CAPD, because of diminished intraperitoneal pressure during recumbancy and the reduced volume present in the peritoneum during the day. Temporary transfer to CCPD may be used to stop leakage on CAPD. However the best way is to stop any form of peritoneal dialysis for 7 to 10 days, switching temporarily the patient to haemodialysis during this period. Most of the time peritoneal dialysis can be resumed without problem. However intraperitoneal pressure should be checked in these patients as described elsewhere in this Chapter to avoid too large infusion-volumes in patient with high intraabdominal pressure.

Outflow failure

Outflow failure may appear at any time in the course of peritoneal dialysis and be due to various causes.

Kinking

Kinking of the catheter within the subcutaneous tissue should not be observed with a good surgical technique as it is due usually to a subcutaneous curve with an acute angle or when deep and superficial cuffs have been implanted too close to each other. Obstruction due to kinking will usually become apparent soon after catheter placement; both inflow and outflow are slow and can be increased by pressing the subcutaneous tunnel. Replacement of the catheter is the only solution.

Catheter obstruction by fibrin

This may occur soon in the break-in period after implantation when the peritoneum is left empty for too long or sometimes after several months or years after a peritonitis. A mechanical method of desobstruction is often effective: Taking all aseptic precautions, fill a syringe with 20 ml of saline solution or dialysate, connect it to the catheter and press as hard and fast as possible. This method carries no risk and may be very effective. In contrast, one must NEVER try to aspirate, as it may suck fine particle of omentum and definitely obstruct the catheter. If desobstruction is not obtained, addition of heparin can be tempted but is usually ineffective. Urokinase (29) (better than streptokinase to avoid anaphylactic reaction (30)) may be used, but is seldom effective as well. Actually, when mechanical desobstruction, as described above, is not effective, one must suspect obstruction by omentum overlapping. In this case surgical replacement of the catheter is the only solution either by coelioscopy or laparatomy.

Catheter migration

When correctly implanted the extremity of the peritoneal catheter is situated in the lower abdominal pouch. The position of the catheter may be checked on an X-ray film. It is preferable to use a radiopaque-type peritoneal catheter in order to avoid the need for injecting a radiocontrast agent which may be a source of contamination.

Sometimes the intraperitoneal segment of the catheter migrates towards the upper left or right abdominal quadrant. If there is no consequence on drained volume and no pain, this complication may be totally unknown and only diagnosed on a abdominal X-ray film. However, most of time the first sign is a one way obstruction. The dialysate may be injected quite normally but drainage is very slow or quite impossible. If a straight catheter has been used, the catheter may be repositioned under fluoroscopy (31). After having premedicated the patient, a sterile, malleable metal rod, bent into a curve to facilitate passage through the catheter, is advanced to 4 cm of the catheter tip. Using the skin site as a fulcrum, the catheter is rotated gently so that the distal tip is moved to a better position. The function of the catheter may be tested immediately. However this is not posssible with a swan neck catheter. But most of time the displacement of the catheter is due to a colonization of holes by omentum and this procedure may be ineffective in 70% of cases. Peritoneoscopy may be more effective in about 50% (32–35). However catheter colonization is mostly due to the fact that the catheter lies on a large omentum, so if just attachments of the catheter to the omentum are disrupted, recurrence of obstruction and colonization may be observed and a definitive solution would be to use a surgical technique to replace the catheter and perform, at least a partial omentectomy.

Catheter exit site complications

External cuff erosion

Whereas most catheters are of the double cuff type, there is no consensus on the real need or not for using a single or double cuff. Most complications of double cuff catheters are related to the erosion of the subcutaneous track by too much superficial implantation of the external cuff. Poor vascularisation of subcutaneous tissue laying between the cuff and the epidermis, associated with the pressure of the catheter from deepness to surface is responsible for local ischemia and erosion. The next step is usually exsudation and colonization by microorganisms, mainly *staphylococcus aureus*. A primary cause of this complication is local skin ischemia. The use of local antibiotics is permanently ineffective per se and may result in a tunnel infection with resistant bacteria and eventually severe uncontrolled peritonitis. In our experience and those of others, incision of skin around the exit site, followed by careful 'cuff shaving' is often very effective. Il must be completed for ten days, twice a day, by local irrigation with polyvidone iodine the first day, then saline solution followed by local irrigation of adjusted antibiotics, mainly aminosides. Rifampicine with protamin may also be used, but rapidly associated with another antibiotic to prevent resistance. In our experience, this technique may be effective in 70% of cases. If three days after interruption of this treatment, infected exsudation is still present, or if a peritonitis occurs, the catheter must be removed immediately as there is a high probability of a deep cuff contamination. The first sign of this complication is the presence of redness around the exit site and the perception of the subcutaneous cuff when the finger is gently applied close to the exit site. There is no real effective technique to prevent evolution towards open erosion, besides avoiding traction on the catheter. This is why it must be immobilized as firmly as possible. There are some different types of immobilizers commercially available. However, tips and immobilizers can bring their own complications due to anergic local intolerance that may be sometimes difficult to solve.

Exit site infection without apparent risk of external cuff extrusion

The first sign is also redness, but palpation reveals a deep external cuff at least one centimeter away from the exit site. Exsudation and pus may be present at a later stage and cultures are positive. In this case local antibiotics may be tempted successfully but success depends on the causative organisms. Organisms other than *staphylococcus* or *pseudomonas* are the most responsive to treatment. Rifampicin may be very useful on *staphylococcus aureus* if rapidly associated with another synergistic antibiotic. However infections due to *pseudomonas aeruginosa* are usually resistant to all treatments, even if appropriate antibiotics are used and we advise to always remove the catheter when an exit site infection with this organism is observed. Local treatment consists in irrigation with the appropriate antibiotic, twice a day for ten days. Intraperitoneal antibiotherapy with the same or a synergistic antibiotic may also be initiated as well as oral antibiotherapy. If the exit site inflammation persists it may be necessary to remove the subcutaneous cuff following the same protocol as above, even if the external cuff is far from the exit site. After external cuff removal, irrigation of the subcutaneous tunnel must be continued for ten days.

Tunnel infection or deep cuff infection

Signs may be obvious, with pain along the tunnel, tenderness, redness and systemic signs with fever. Systemic antibiotherapy must be initiated either orally or intraperitoneally; at the same time, even without sign of exit site exsudation, the subcutaneous cuff must be extruded and 'shaved', the tunnel drained and tunnel instillations with antibiotics performed twice a day for ten days. If a peritonitis occurs, the catheter must be removed immediately. In other circumstances there are no clinical signs of exit site or tunnel infection, but the patient presents with relapsing peritonitis with the same organisms, mainly *staphylococcus epidermidis* or *aureus*, or *pseudomonas*. In such a case, there is a high suspicion of deeper cuff colonization and the catheter must be removed rapidly.

Pain during infusion

Pain during infusion occurs usually during the first week of treatment. It may be located in the pelvis or sometimes irradiating towards the shoulders. Temporary initial irritation of the peritoneum, as well initial high intraperitoneal pressure may be responsible. This pain may be reduced by increasing slowly the infusion volume during the first week following catheter implantation and by taking care of using prewarmed dialysate. Sometimes it is due to the attachement of part of the catheter by omentum colonization with traction during infusion: on the X-ray film the catheter is dislodged either towards the upper right or the upper left quadrant and it must be repositioned as described above. Another cause may be intolerance to low pH of the dialysis solution. Adding 4 to 5 mEq of sterile, pyrogen free sodium bicarbonate may be very effective (36). However any addition of a drug into the dialysate may potentially cause peritonitis and such a technique can only be used for a short period of time.

DIALYSIS ADEQUACY AND CLEARANCES

Adequacy

Adequacy has been described in detail elsewhere in this book. We must remind the reader that the main biological criteria admitted nowadays are a weekly KT/V index over 1.7 and a weekly total clearance (renal + peritoneal) over 50 liters (37). However Kt/V may not be reliable due to large variations of estimation of V and a 50 liter weekly clearance may not be enough in patients who have a high catabolic rate. So, other conventional biological or clinical criteria are still useful to appreciate the adequacy of dialysis: for example, anemia, not or unsatisfactorily corrected by erythropoietin in the absence of iron deficiency, is also a sign of underdialysis. Clinically, fatigue, breath amine odor, skin grey aspect, pruritus, anorexia, and insomnia are well known signs of underdialysis that may be observed on haemodialysis as well. Different clinical approaches have been tempted, among which the clinical subjective assessment (SGA) (38) and BRANDES index (39) are the most frequently used. These clinical index assess nutritional status as well as dialysis adequacy, due to the fact that both aspects are closely linked.

There are not many ways to increase the dose of dialysis on peritoneal dialysis. On CAPD the amount of fluid can be increased by using 2.5 or even 3 liter bags. However some patients may not tolerate such volumes and develop or increase respiratory insufficiency. In patients dialysed with only 3 exchanges, increasing the number of bags from 3 to four is usually well accepted. But from four to five, it may interfere excessively with social life and professional activity. In those patients who necessitate a large dose of dialysis, automated peritoneal dialysis appears as the best solution. Using large volumes, that is to say at least 20 to 25 liter per day, tidal peritoneal dialysis, and sometimes an extra bag during the day, it is possible to increase total mass transfer. However, patients with low peritoneal permeability may not benefit of increased peritoneal volume achieved by more rapid and numerous exchanges, since dialysate concentrations decrease with short dwell times. This is why it is important when a patient is switched from one modality of dialysis to another one to collect the total daily drainage and calculate the real mass transfer per day. When clinical or biological symptoms of underdialysis develop, or when the total time spent by the patient on peritoneal dialysis is interfering with social life and/or work, a transfer to haemodialysis is advisable.

Peritoneal dialysis clearance

Dwell time during CAPD ranges from 4 to 12 hours; as a result, dialysate to plasma equilibrium is usually obtained for small solutes (40) as urea or creatinine. Consequently it is more the total dialysate outflow than solute concentrations or peritoneal permeability which account for clearance evaluation when it is calculated after prolonged dwell time.

The best way to calculate peritoneal dialysis clearance delivered to the patient is to collect the 24 hour dialysate and pool the whole volume in the same container. One sample is collected to assay solute concentration. A blood sample is taken in the morning and clearance is calculated as $c = d.v24h/p$. More frequently clearance is expressed weekly, that is to say $Cw = C24.7$ days. It is usually admitted that in an anuric patient, Cw must be over 50 liters for $1.73\ m^2$ body surface.

Some teams have proposed to use a single exchange, during a four hour dwell to calculate clearance and extrapolate to the whole day. This method may be source of large under or over estimations as variations in dwell time, total volume drained, and convective transports depending on glucose concentration may interfere during a whole day when different dwell times are used with different glucose concentrations. This is why we recommend collecting the total 24 hour dialysate. For creatinine assay in the dialysate, it is better to use an enzymatic method in order to minimize interference with the glucose contained in dialysate (41).

It must be underlined that patients on peritoneal dialysis have often a residual renal function that can be maintained for a long time. This residual clearance must be taken into account when calculating the total clearance. So, in the follow up of peritoneal dialysis patients, both total renal clearance and weekly peritoneal clearances must be evaluated and the CAPD regimen adjusted in order to permanently obtain a total weekly clearance above 50 liters for creatinine.

CLINICAL MANAGEMENT OF PERITONEAL MEMBRANE PROPERTIES

As the peritoneal membrane is a living membrane, its permanent contact with a non physiological solution, as dialysate, may alter its properties in the long term. Besides modifications of quality of dialysis, more severe complications may appear as adhesions, sclerosis, calcifications (42). Morphological and structural alterations are most of the time detected at a severe stage when consequences on clearances and ultrafiltration are obvious or when digestive symptoms are present. Sometimes they are only detected at laparatomy, because the patient had no clinical symptom and because daily peritoneal clearances did not change. Indeed, due to the long dwell time, severe fibrosis and/or loss of peritoneal surface must be present before the dialysate appears non saturated after several hours.

Mass transfer area coefficient

Mathematical models have recently been designed to evaluate the quality of the peritoneal membrane, using more accurate methods than clearances after long dwell. Basically it is the mass transfer area coefficient (MTCA) that best characterizes the membrane. Initially described by Henderson and Nolph (43), it was improved by Popovich et al. (44, 45) and, more recently, by Krediet (46). It represents the peritoneal clearance at the very initial time. Whereas most techniques to measure MTCA need complicated computer programs and are not usable in current clinical practice, the model recently designed by Krediet appears more convenient. Its coefficient of variation is between 15 and 20% and is considered as sufficient for clinical purposes by the author (46).

Equilibration tests: different techniques and clinical significance

Currently, the methods most frequenlty used and recommended to follow up the peritoneal membrane properties are peritoneal equilibration tests.

Peritoneal structure background

The importance of the peritoneal permeability to glucose was pointed out by Tenchkoff in its 'Handbook on peritoneal dialysis' (47). In 1981 we described two groups of patients (48), one who had normal ultrafiltration with a relatively low absorption of glucose, and another group who presented with decreased ultrafiltration related to rapid glucose absorption. We demonstrated that this high permeability to glucose was initially mainly due to mesothelial desquamation and this was confirmed later in an animal model (49). It has been shown that the initial mesothelial desquamation may recover after temporary cessation of dialysis. However, if the mesothelial denudation is more extensive and lasts longer, fibrinolytic properties of the mesothelial layer disappear. This physiological modifications result in the progressive appearance of fibrin with subsequent development of intestinal loop adhesions. Sometimes a new fibrotic membrane covering the intestinal loop may develop and be responsible for an encapsulating peritonitis (50–57). Eventually the denuded mesothelium make the tissue underneath more susceptible to the aggression of high glucose concentrations (4). This is why it is recommended to avoid hypertonic solutions during peritonitis. When such a dramatic decrease of the surface of exchange is present, no exchange is possible anymore between the blood and the peritoneal compartment; in this case, the glucose concentration is permanently high in the dialysate, without transcapillary ultrafiltration. D/P urea and creatinine ratios are low.

Glucose and sodium equilibration curves

In order to detect peritoneal alterations by the means of peritoneal permeability profiles we designed a normogram using glucose absorption curves in CAPD patients (58, 59). The technique consisted in performing equilibration tests in patients who had been on CAPD for less than 6 months and had no history of peritonitis or previous abdominal surgery, using an hypertonic bag (40% dextrose, two liter infusion of a lactate buffered solution). With this protocol, normal ultrafiltration at 4 hours is 920 ± 415 ml (415 being the 90% interval of confidence), and, using the same interval of confidence, the average percentage of initial glucose concentrations at two hours is 30% to 70%; at 4 hours, 22% to 45%. In patients with normal transcapillary ultrafiltration a minimum of 5 mEq drop of the intraperitoneal sodium is observed, due to the fact that 50% of the transcapillary water removal is free water.

Thus by correlating glucose absorption, ultrafiltration and intraperitoneal sodium variations it is possible to detect peritoneal alterations. Table 1 shows the evolution of intraperitoneal glucose and sodium in three patients with different peritoneal permeabilities. Peritoneal permeability is dependent both on the integrity of the mesothelial layer and on the surface available for transperitoneal exchanges.

Loss of ultrafiltration

The frequency of decreased ultrafiltration varies from one publication to another between 10 to 20% and is dependent upon duration of dialysis, peritonitis rate and type of solutions used, but the understanding of its mechanisms is of first importance to detect peritoneal structure alterations. There are two main types of loss of ultrafiltration. *Type I* is due to hyperpermeability to glucose and appears to be linked to an enlargement of the peritoneal pores represented by the rupture of the mesothelial cells junctions or their desquamation. Most of the time this is reversible with temporary interruption of CAPD. On the other hand *type II loss* of ultrafiltration is associated with hypopermeability to glucose. Wu et al. (60) previously suggested that

this second type was the result of loss of surface, which was always confirmed in our experience by the discovery of either multiple adhesions or encapsulating peritonitis. It is extremely important to point out that none of our patients with loss of surface was clinically symptomatic and that usual examinations (echotomography, and small intestine transit radiography) were normal. Thus, analysis of equilibration tests during a loss of ultrafiltration appears to be the most precise way to early detect severe peritoneal injury and predict its anatomical aspect.

The measurement of sodium concentration during equilibration tests in presence of decreased ultrafiltration allows a more precise understanding. If a decreased ultrafiltration is observed whereas there is a normal glucose decrease and a normal drop of peritoneal sodium (that is to say more than 5 mEq, using the above protocol), it means that there is a normal transcapillary ultrafiltration; therefore, we must look for another explanation for the decreased drained volume. Usually such is due either to leakage around the catheter peritoneal entrance, a leakage through a non previously detected hernia (umbilical or unguinal) or possibly to exaggerated lymphatic absorption. In these cases hernia repair will allow to recover normal ultrafiltration. If the trouble is due to lymphatic absorption there is not any clinical possibility to interact; however Durand et al. suggested that high intraperitoneal pressure may sometimes be responsible for an increased lymphatic absorption; consequently, in this case, it is worthwhile to try and decrease the volume per exchange, provided total clearance is maintained by increasing the number of exchanges, or to switch the patient to another technique such as CCPD or TPD.

Temporary peritoneal rest

It has been demonstrated in rats that a peritoneum totally denuded of mesothelium may recover if dialysis is stopped. Both recovery of the mesothelial surface of ultrafiltration and permeability to solutes were observed. In rats remesothelialization takes no more than a few days (49). According to Dobbie (61) the remesotheliazation in humans may take two to four weeks, depending upon the severity and the extension of the initial peritoneal denudation. Miranda et al. (62) reported in seven patients with a type I loss of ultrafiltration a total recovery in 4 patients and a partial recovery of peritoneal permeability in the three others, after four weeks of temporary interruption of CAPD. During the interruption, patients were haemodialysed and 35 mg of heparin diluted in 100ml of dialysate were injected through the peritoneal catheter every 3 or 4 days. The lavage with heparin during the initial phase of interruption of CAPD is probably very important. We observed a patient (63) who stopped CAPD with a Type I loss of filtration which became a Type II loss of filtration after four weeks-interruption without lavage. At laparotomy she had developed an encapsulating peritonitis. This is probably due to the fact that type I losses of filtration are usually due to mesothelial denudation with consequent-

Table 1. Dialysate glucose and sodium concentrations during a 6 h dwell time in 3 CAPD patients with different types of peritoneal permeability (3.86% Dextrose solution – 2 l exchange)

Time (min)	Normal		Hyperpermeability		Loss of surface	
	Sodium (mmol/l)	Glucose (mmol/l)	Sodium (mmol/l)	Glucose (mmol/l)	Sodium (mmol/l)	Glucose (mmol/l)
0	134	201	133	196.1	133	203
30	125	153	131	94.7	133	175.5
60	120	134	132	90.2	132	163.2
90	118	116.7	132	73.7	132	151.6
120	117	102.1	133	59.0	132	135.6
150	116	90.9	134	48.5	132	133.0
180	117	84.8	135	41.0	132	122.9
210	117	78.12	135	32.8	132	115.6
240	118	73.26	136	27.8	132	108.1
270	118	69.48	136	22.8	133	100.1
300	119	65.52	136	21.0	133	83.0
330	120	62.16	136	18.2	133	88.2
360	121	58.8	137	16.08	133	81.8
Vol drained:	3000 ml		1900 ml		2030 ml	

ly a decreased fibrinolytic intraperitoneal activity associated with an increased production of fibrin in relation with the inflammatory state. In the other patients, when daily peritoneal lavages, even without heparin, were performed during the first two weeks, we never observed such an evolution and, often, at least a partial recovery of peritoneal permeability was achieved. It is possible that the variations in peritoneal permeability recovery from one patient to another, after temporay cessation of peritoneal dialysis, is dependent upon the severity of the initial lesion: the more extensive the lesion, the longer it takes to recover and the higher is the probability to develop sclerosis. This is why we recommend to temporarily interrupt peritoneal dialysis as soon as hyperpermeability appears. Again a close collaboration with a haemodialysis unit is therefore mandatory to achieve a safe peritoneal dialysis program.

If a progressive increase of peritoneal permeability with consequent low ultrafiltration may recover when recognized soon enough, severe hypopermeability is usually irreversible, since, it is due to either an important sclerosis or loss of surface of exchange in relation with multiple adhesions, mesenteric retraction or, seldom, an encapsulating peritonitis. The only logical attitude in this case is to stop CAPD definitely. Any sign of intestinal obstruction or digestive malabsorption should be investigated with tomodensitometry, barium meal, and sometime with laparatomy.

Peritoneal Equilibration Test

More recently Twardowski used these equilibrations curves in a different way from ours, to tailor peritoneal dialysis to patient's permeability profiles. Twardowski (64) gave a very successful name to these modified equilibration curves which he called PET test (for Peritoneal Equilibration Test). He used a different concentration of glucose, 2.50 instead of 3.86%), the volume injected being the same. Performing 103 PET test he separated his patients into different groups according to the ratio D/P (dialysate over plasma) for urea and creatinine concentrations and t/to (concentrations at time t divided by concentration at time to, immediately after the end of filling) of intraperitoneal glucose.

Moderately rapid transporters are those whose D/P urea and creatinine are less than one standard deviation below the average value, and whose t/to glucose are less than one standard deviation above the average. Very rapid transporters or very slow transporters are those whose difference with the mean is more than one standard deviation.

Various modifications of the PET test have been proposed to simplify the protocol or shorten the duration of dwell times. One approach is to collect 24 hour dialysate, mix the whole drained volume and calculate the D/P ratio for different solutes (65); in our opinion this is the best way to evaluate clearances but it may vary too much from day to day, depending on diffferences in dwell times, concentrations of glucose and patient's compliance, to detect small variations in peritoneal structure. In addition, prolonged dwell times for some exchanges may mask variations of peritoneal permeability for rapidly diffusive solutes, making this approach inaccurate to detect small alterations of peritoneal permeability; however, it may

Table 2. Classification of a patient's peritoneal transport using the Fast-PET (from Twardowski)

Transport classification	% of patients	Dialysate/plasma creatinine	Dialysate glucose	Ultrafiltration volume
Low	16	0.34–0.49	945–1214	2651–3326
Low average	34	0.50–0.64	724–944	2369–2650
Mean		0.65	723	2368
High average	34	0.66–0.81	502–722	2085–2367
High	16	0.82–1.03	230–501	1580–2084

be a simple approach to follow patients in clinical practice.

Another simplification proposed by Twardowski is what he called the Fast-PET (66). After an overnight dwell the patient is instructed to drain completely over for at least 20 minutes, then infuse two liters of 2.5% dextrose dialysis solution. The exact time at which infusion ends is noted. The patient must then arrange to be at the dialysis center to start drainage exactly four hours after the end of infusion. The volume drained is measured, an aliquot is taken for creatinine and glucose measurements, a blood sample is also obtained at the same time. Glucose has to be measured with hexokinase. Creatinine must be corrected for the interference with glucose or must be measured with an enzymatic method (41). The dialysate to plasma (D/P) creatinine ratio is then calculated. The results are compared in Table 2. The same protocol may be proposed to be done entirely by compliant patients at home; therefore, patients are just asked to bring their drained bag at the hospital. The problem is that some patients may not respect the exact protocol and it is thus estimated that at least 20% of them are unable to perform this investigation by themselves (67).

Whatever the fast PET test being performed entirely at home or in the hospital, it must be underlined that a single dosage at 4 hour may be source of large errors in non sufficiently trained teams and even in the laboratory. So a better accuracy is obtained by performing at least one extra dosage at 2 hour.

APEX

More recently we designed a new test that is easily performed during a two hour dwell (68, 69). Using the same protocol as for our initial equilibration tests (i.e., lactate solution, 2 liter bag, and 3.86% dextrose solution), we drew the equilibration curves of glucose and urea on the same graph. There is a time at which both curves cross each other (Figure 1). The higher the permeability, the shorter the time at which they cross, the lower the permeability, the longer the time. Unless a very severe hypopermeability is present, this time is less than two hours. That means that a two hour dwell is enough for a large majority of patients; this equilibration test thus needs only two

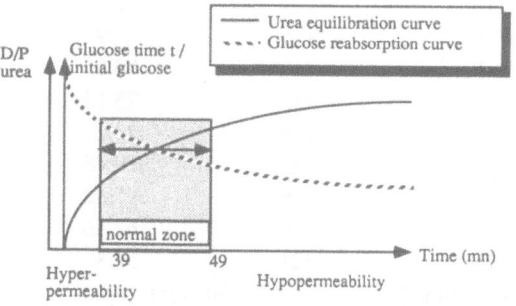

Figure 1. APEX: the time t represents the moment at which both urea equilibration curve and glucose reabsorption curve in percentages cross each other. Urea is expressed dialysate/plasma ratio, and intraperitoneal glucose as glucose time t divided by glucose immediately at the end of peritoneal filling.

hours and has been called Accelerated Peritoneal Equilibration Examination which is summarized by the acronym APEX, the crossing time being APEX-time. In a group of patients with normal permeability it was demonstrated in the range beween 39 minutes and 89 minutes. It is now extensively used in France both in children where the time is much shorter (70, 71) and in adults (68, 69). It has been recognized as reference and as a convenient and reliable test during a recent consensus conference in France (72). The advantages of this test are multiple: It summarizes permeability to both glucose and urea by a single number, facilitating comparison between patients or groups of patients; it is more precise and reliable than a single D/P, because it takes into account several measurements of solutes; and it is also at the same time more rapid to perform than a conventional four hour equilibration test and less expensive. Eventually it can be used the same way as a PET test to divide patients into low and rapid transporters by defining patients whose APEX-time is lower or higher than one standard deviation. We will discuss below the limitations for using these tests to tailor peritoneal dialysis.

Limits and reliability of equilibration tests

In order to check the reliability of peritoneal equilibration tests we performed in three different patients ten tests within less than 15 days, using a two hour dwell (73). All tests were performed using a 2 liter volume of a 3.86% dextrose concentration dialysis solution.Urea, glucose, creatinine were measured every 30 minutes and one blood sample was taken at the beginning of each test. Volumes drained were noted and ultrafiltration calculated by difference with the volume infused. At two hours the ratio final Glucose/initial glucose ranged from 37 to 52% in patient 1, it was 46 to 59% in patient 2 and 41 to 52% in the third patient. For urea D/P, ratios were respectively 66 to 75%, 63 to 70% and 85 to 89%. For APEX-times, variations were respectively 66 to 88 mn, 80 to 96 mn and 44 to 49 mn. The largest variations were observed in ultrafiltration, respectively 170 to 660 ml, 450 to 680 ml and 630 to 940 ml. Important variations can thus be observed in some patients from one day to another even when several equilibration tests are performed in the same conditions. However in our experience results always stayed in the normal range within which we never observed peritoneal damages. This means that all kinds of equilibration tests must be interpreted very carefully when used to prescribe dialysis modality, and probably three repeated tests should be done before taking a final decision. However these tests remain extremely useful to detect peritoneal membrane alteration, since we always observed some in cases of results beyond the normal range. Once again the APEX appeared the most convenient test as it had a coefficient of variation situated between those of glucose and urea, making a fair balance.

INFLUENCE OF INTRAPERITONEAL PRESSURE (IPP)

Net UF volume is strongly affected by IPP since a 1 cm H2O mean increase in IPP results in a 74 ml global UF in two hours. For Durand et al. (6, 76), intraperitoneal pressure may alter both lymphatic reabsorption and perhaps transcapillary UF. These authors also suggested that IPP modifies transperitoneal exchanges and may therefore interfere with evaluation of peritoneal permeability using equilibration tests and APEX. For these reasons IPP should be used when evaluating loss of ultrafiltration in correlation with equilibration tests. This influence of IPP has been confirmed by Abensur (75) who, in addition, demonstrated that the decreased ultrafiltration was positively correlated with lymphatic absorption. It is also possible that this variation of intra abdominal pressure explains the poor ultrafiltration sometimes observed during the post operative period after catheter implantation. Durand demonstrated that intraperitoneal pressure was higher during this period (76). This initial modifications are not explained but may be attributed to post operative pain and abdominal tension.

Importance of intraperitoneal pressure measurement to prescribe peritoneal dialysis

Patients with high intraperitoneal pressure on CAPD may benefit of automated peritoneal dialysis. In the latter case, both supine position and decreased intraperitoneal volumes may contribute to reduce intra abdominal pressure and consequently increase ultrafiltration (77). The follow up of intraperitoneal pressure may be useful to tailor peritoneal volumes immediately after catheter implantation.

Gotloib (78) demonstrated that IPP may influence cardiac ouput. In his experience the maximum IPP (with zero value at the level of umbilicus) was 14 cm of water and resulted in a 25% decrease of cardiac output. More recently, Durand et al. (79) used their technique of IPP measurement to determine the maximum intraperitoneal volume tolerable by correlating IPP and pulmonary vital capacity in the supine position. They showed that the maximum intraperitoneal volume corresponds to a mean intraperitoneal pressure of 18 cm and results in a 20% decrease of vital capacity. This upper limit tolerable volume is very variable from one patient to another, it ranged in their 20 patients between less than two liters up to 4.5 liters. It was positively correlated with patient's height. Therefore volumes used in automated peritoneal dialysis should always induce a supine intraperitoneal pressure less than 18 cm of water.This may be easily obtained by reducing the injection volume and increasing the number of exchanges. In other words, as well as the total peritoneal clearances must be individualized to each patient (taking in account D/P ratio, equilibration tests or APEX and total volumes), volume per exchange must also be monitored by intraperitoneal pressure measurement.

CONCLUSIONS

The main specific aspects of the clinical management of peritoneal dialysis patients are catheter related problems, peritoneal membrane permeability and nutrition status. The follow up of the peritoneal membrane may be scheduled as follows: An initial PET test or an APEX after 1 month and before 6 months of treatment should be systematically performed to act as a reference. Then daily ultrafiltration is estimated asking the patient to record the volume drained at each exchange by weighing his/her bags. If no modification is observed, one equilibration test per year, or every half year is enough.In case of peritonitis an extra equilibration test must be performed one month later if the volume drained per exchange has decreased. Nutritional assessment must be performed every six months and the amount of clearance delivered to the patient must take in account the evolution of his/her residual renal function. Renal and peritoneal clearances should be calculated every six months, as well as Kt/V and protein catabolic rate. Recurrent peritonitis, clinical signs of underdialysis, uncontrolled overhydration must press the physician to consider a transfer to haemodialysis, at least temporarily. When haemodialysis is used before the patient has been exhausted by the specific complications of peritoneal dialysis, he usually accepts easily to return to this method after recovery of a normal clinical status. Therefore both methods, haemodialysis and peritoneal dialysis, should never be considered as competitive, but as complementary. This approach and the availability of both treatments allow the physician to offer his patients the best suited treatment at the best moment during his/her life course on chronic replacement therapy.

APPENDIX 1. MEASUREMENT OF INTRAPERITONEAL PRESSURE (80)

The height of the dialysis fluid in the PD line is measured at atmospheric pressure before drainage. The maximal density of a dialysis fluid with a glucose concentrationof 3.86% being 1.017, the difference between the level of a dialysis fluid and a water column is less than 2%. Given the observed values and the range of normality, this difference may be neglected and the results may be expressed in centimeters of water (cmH20). Two measurements are made while the patient rests in a perfectly supine position on a strictly horizontal board. The first after deep inspiration (IPPinsp) and the second after deep expiration (IPPexp). Mean IPP is defined as (IPPinsp + IPPexp)/2. The level of the column is read with a scale graduated in cm after the height of the column has stabilized. The zero level of the column is set at the center of the abdominal cavity, on the medial axillary line. The peritoneal cavity is immediately emptied after taking the reading and the volume of the dialysis (IPV) fluid is measured. Mean intraperitoneal pressure with 2 liters of dialysate is approximately 11 cm of water. Using hypertonic solution with normal ultrafiltration, the final volume after a two hour dwell is 2820 ±319 ml with IPPinsp = 14 ±4 cm of water and IPPexp = 12 ±3 cm of water.

APPENDIX 2. EQUILIBRATION CURVES

Evaluation of equilibration tests

1. All studies are performed in the morning after a 30 min drainage.

2. Blood samples are taken at the beginning and end of dwell time for urea, sodium and glucose concentration measurements.

3. Only hypertonic bags buffered with lactate are used (2.25% in Twardowski's PET tests, 3.86% in Verger's Equilibration tests).

4. Bags are prewarmed before filling.

5. A 5 ml sample of dialysate is taken from the bag before filling to check the glucose measurement in the laboratory.

6. Immediately after filling of the peritoneal cavity, the bag is put down to a lower level to allow 100 cc of drainage. 5 cc are taken from the injection port and thrown away. Five more milliliters are taken and analyzed for glucose, sodium and urea. The remaining 90 cc are reintroduced into the peritoneal cavity. This is time t1. The same procedures are performed every 30 min until four hours (time t2, t3, ..., t9).

At the 4th hour the peritoneal cavity is totally drained. The ultrafiltration is the difference between the initial weight of the bag and final weight of the drainage bag.

APPENDIX 3. APEX

The technique is the same as in Appendix 2, but dextrose concentration is 3.86% and duration of dwell two hours. Urea and glucose equilibration curves are drawn on the same graph and time at which both curves cross is noted.

REFERENCES

1. Rottembourg J, Issad B, Benhmida M, Bitker MO et al.: CAPD renal transplantation: a successful strategy of treatment for patients with terminal uremia. in *Current Concepts in Peritoneal Dialysis*, edited by Ota K, Vth International Congres of Peritoneal Dialysis, 1990, p 747
2. Caillette A, Donia A, Labeeuw M, Zech P: Low values of total body water (TBW) in CAPD patients: results of 4 different estimations. *Perit Dial Int* 14 (Suppl 1): S52, 1994
3. Miller RB, Tassiro CR: Peritoneal dialysis. *N Engl J Med* 281: 945, 1969
4. Dobbie JW: Pathogenesis of peritoneal fibrosing syndromes (sclerosing peritonitis) in peritoneal dialysis. *Perit Dial Intern* 12: 14, 1992
5. Goodman CE, Husserl FE: Etiology, prevention and treatment of back pain inpatients undergoing continuous ambulatory peritoneal dialysis. *Perit Dial Bull* 1: 119, 1981
6. Durand PY, Chanliau J, Gambéroni J, Hestin D, Kessler M: Intraperitoneal hydrostatic pressure and ultrafiltration volume in CAPD. in *Advances in Peritoneal Dialysis*, edited by Khanna R, Nolph KD, Prowant BF, Twardowski ZJ, Oreoupoulos DG: 1993, Vol 9, p 46
7. Spinowitz B, Leggio A, Galler M, Golden R, Rascoff J, Charytan C: Prognostic indicators of hernia development in patients undergoing CAPD. in *Frontiers in Peritoneal Dialysis*, edited by Maher JF, Winchester JF, New York, Field, Rich and Associates Publishers, 1986, p 519
8. Faller B, Pierre D, Verger C, Gam G, Ryckelynck J-P, Bénévent D, Guiberteau R: French multicenter study on drop out and peritonitis rate in CAPD. in *Advances in Peritoneal Dialysis*, Proc 7th Ann CAPD Conference. *Perit Dial Bull* 179, 1987

9. Mion C, Slingeneyer A, Liendo-Liendo C, Perez C, Despaux E: Reduction in incidence of peritonitis associated with CAPD. *Proc Clin Dial Transplant Forum* 9: 63, 1979

10. Slingeneyer A, Liendo-Liendo C, Mion C: Continuous ambulatory peritoneal dialysis with a bacteriological filter on the dialysate infusion line. in *Proc of an International Symposium Paris*, editd by Legrain M, Amsterdam, Excerpta Medica Publishers, 1979, p 59

11. Bazzato G: CAPD by means of double bag, closed drainage infusio system. in *CAPD Proc Int Symp Paris 1979*, Amsterdam, Excerpta Medica, 1980, p 171

12. Bazzato G, Coli U, Landini S et al.: Six years' experience of CAPD with double bag system. *Perit Dial Bull* 4: S4, 1984

13. Shaldon S, Koch KM, Quelhorst E, Dinarello CA: Hazards of CAPD: interleukin-1 production. in *Frontiers in Peritoneal Dialysis*, edited by Maher JF, Winchester JF, New York Field, Rich and Associates Publishers, 1986, p 630

14. Maiorca E, Cantaluppi A, Cancarini GC et al.: 'Y' connector system for prevention of peritonitis in CAPD: a controlled study. *Proc EDTA* 20: 223, 1983

15. Ryckelynck J-Ph, Verger C, Cam, Faller B, Pierre D: Importance of the flush effect in disconnect systems. in *Advances in Peritoneal Dialysis*. Proc 8th Ann CAPD Conference. *Perit Dial Bull* 283, 1988

16. Verger C, Luzar M-A: *In vitro* study of CAPD Y-line systems. in *Advances in Peritoneal Dialysis*. Proc 6th Ann CAPD Conference. *Perit Dial Bull* 160, 1986

17. Buoncristiani U, Quintaliani G, Cozzari M, Carobi C: Current status of the Y-set. in *Advances in Peritoneal Dialysis*. Proc 6th Ann CAPD Conference. *Perit Dial Bull* 164, 1986

18. Verger C, Dumont M, Misrahi B et al.: CAPD without wearing bags: less peritonitis and more freedom. *EDTNA, London* 12: 38, 1983

19. Durand P-Y, Chanliau J, Gamberoni J, Mariot A, Kessler M: UV-flash: clinical evaluation in 97 patients; results of a french multicenter trial. *Perit Dial Int* 4: 219, 1994

20. Veniez G, Verger C, Ryckelynck J-P: Influence of the educational program on peritonitis rate on CAPD: analysis of data from the French Language peritoneal Dialysis Registry. *Perit Dial Int* 12: S1, 168, 1992

21. Rottembourg J, Jacq D, Singlas E, N'Guyen M: Medical management of peritonitis. *Proc Clin Dial Transplant Forum* 9: 248, 1979

22. Twardowski ZJ, Schreiber MJ, Burkhart JM: Peritoneal dialysis case forum: a 55 year old man with hematuria and blood tinged dialysate. *Perit Dial Int* 12: 61, 1992

23. Le Meur Y, Poux JM, Bénévent D, Leroux-Robert C: Ascite chyleuse chez quatre patientes traitées par dialyse péritonéale continue ambulatoire et revue de la littérature. *Bull Dial Perit* I: 23, 27, 1991

24. Humayun HM, Daugirdas JT, Ing TS, Leetey DJ, Gondhi VC, Popli S: Chylous ascitis in a patient treated with intermittent peritoneal dialysis. *Artif Organs* 8: 358, 1984

25. Pomeranz A, Reichenberg Y, Schuzz D, Drukker A: Chyloperitoneum: a rare complication of peritoneal dialysis. *Perit Dial Bull* 4: 35, 1984

26. Press OW, Press NO, Kaufman SD: Evaluation and management of chylous ascites. *Ann Intern Med* 96: 558, 1982

27. Spadaro JJ, Thakur V, Nolph KD: Technetium-99 m-labelled macroaggregated albumin in demonstration of

28. Walker F et al.: Intraperitoneal iopamidol, a new radiocontrast agent in the diagnosis of a pleuroperitoneal communication. *Perit Dial Bull* 6: 108, 1986

29. Parsoo I, McInstosh CG, Seedat YK: Urokinase infusion for obstructed catheter in CAPD. *Perit Dial Bull* 6: 105, 1986

30. Dykewicz MS et al.: Identification of patients at risk for anaphylaxis due to streptokinase. *Arch Intern Med* 146: 305, 1986

31. Degesys GE et al.: Tenckhoff peritoneal dialysis catheters: the use of fluoroscopy in management. *Radiology* 54: 819, 1985

32. Gaudry C, Nguyen Tan Lung R, Kourilsky O: Repositionnement d'un cathéter de dialyse péritonéale par coelioscopie. *Bull Dial Perit* 2: 143, 1992

33. Mutter D, Marichal JF, Petitjean P, Vix M, Evrard S, Marescaux J: Sauvegarde d'un cathéter de dialyse péritonéale chez l'insuffisant rénal chronique. Apport de la chirurgie laparascopique. *Press Medicale* 21: 1584, 1992

34. Schillinger F, Elhomsy G, Montagnac R, Matta W, Milcent T, Roussel G, Pelleger L: Implantation du cathéter de dialyse péritonéale par video-coelioscopie. *Bull Dial Périt* 3: 13, 1993

35. Ash SR, Handt AE, Bloch R: Peritoneoscopic placement of the Tenckhoff catheter: further clinical experience. *Perit Dial Bull* 3: 8, 1983

36. Henderson IS, Couper IA, Lumsden A: Potentially irritant glucose metabolites in unused CAPD fluid. in *Frontiers in Peritoneal Dialysis*, edited by Maher JF, Winchester JF, New York, Field, Rich and Associates Publishers, 1986, p 261

37. Nolph KD: Quantitating peritoneal dialysis delivery; a required standard of care. *Semin Dial* 4: 139, 1991

38. Young GA, Kopple JD, Lindholm B, Vonesh EF, De Vecchi A, Scalamogna A, Castelnova C, Oreopoulos DG, Anderson GH, Bergström J, Dichiro J, Gentile D, Nissenson A, Sakrani I, Brownjohn AM, Nolph KD, Prowant BF, Algrim CE, Martis L, Serkes KD: Nutritional assessement of Continuous Ambulatory Peritoneal Dialysis patients: an international study. *Am J Kidney Dis* 27: 462, 1991

39. Brandes JC, Piering WF, Beres JA: A method to assess efficacy of CAPD: a preliminary results. *Adv Perit Dial* 6: 192, 1990

40. Daugirdas JT, Ing TS, Gandhi VC, Hano JE, Chen WT, Yuan L: Kinetics of peritoneal fluid absorption in partients with chronic renal failure. *J Lab Clin Med* 95: 351, 1980

41. Larpent L, Verger C: The need for using an enzymatic colorimetric assay in creatinine determination for peritoneal dialysis solutions. *Perit Dial Bull* 10: 89, 1990

42. Failer B, Marichal JF, Brignon P, Benevent D, Pierre D, Ryckelynck J-P, Charra B, Verger C: Progressive calcifying peritonitis inperitoneal dialysis (two case histories). in *Advances in Continuous Ambulatory Peritoneal Dialysis*. Proc 7th Ann CAPD Conference. *Perit Dial Bull* 150, 1987

43. Henderson LW, Nolph KD: Altered permeability of peritoneal membrane after using hypertonic peritoneal dialysis fluid. *J Clin Invest* 38: 992, 1976

44. Popovich RP, Moncrief JW, Okutan M, Decherd JF: A model of the peritoneal dialysis system. *Proc 25th Ann Conf on Engr in Med and Biol* 14: 172, 1966

45. Popovich RP, Moncrief JW: Transport kinetics. in *Peritoneal Dialysis*, 2nd Edition, edited by Nolph KD, Boston, Martinus Nijhoff, 1985, p 115

46. Krediet RT, Boeschoten EW, Zuyderhoot FMJ, Arisz L: The relationship between peritoneal glucose absorption and body fluid loss by ultrafiltration during continuous ambulatory peritoneal dialysis. *Clin Nephrol* 27: 51, 1987

47. Tenckhoff H: *Chronic Peritoneal Dialysis: A Manual for Patients, Dialysis Personnel and Physicians*. Seattle, University of Washington School of Medicine Press, 1974

48. Verger C, Brunschvicg O, Le Charpentier Y, Lavergne A, Vantelon J: Structural and ultrastructural peritoneal membrane changes and permeabiliy alterations during continuous ambulatory peritoneal dialysis. *Proc Eur Dial Transplant Assoc* 18: 199, 1981

49. Verger C, Luger A, Moore HL, Nolph KD: Acute changes in peritoneal morphology and transport properties with infectious peritonitis and mechanical injury. *Kidney Int* 23: 823, 1983

50. Niaudet P, Berard E, Revillon Y, Lothon M, Broyer M: Sclerosing encapsulating peritonitis in children. *Control Nephrol* 57: 230, 1987

51. Lo WK, Chan KT, Leung ACT et al.: Sclerosing peritonitis complicating prolonged use of chlorhexidine in alcohol in the connection procedure for continuous ambulatory peritoneal dialysis. *Perit Dial Int* 2: 166, 1991

52. Rottembourg J, Gahl GM, Poignet JL, Mertani E, Strippoli P, Langlois P, Tranbaloc P, Legrain M: Severe abdominal complications in patients undergoing continuous ambulatory peritoneal dialysis. *Proc Eur Dial Transpl Assoc* 20: 236, 1983

53. Rottembourg J, Issad B, Langlois P, Cossette PY, Boudjemaa A, Mehamha H, Assogbau U, Gahl GM: Sclerosing peritonitis in patients treated by CAPD. in *CAPD Children*, edited by Fine RN et al., Berlin, Springer-Verlag, 1985, p 167

54. Slingeneyer A: Preliminary report on a cooperative international study on sclerosing encapsulating peritonitis. *Contr Nephrol* 57: 239, 1987

55. Slingeneyer A, Elie M: Cooperative international study on sclerosing encapsulating peritonitis. Preliminary report. in *Advances in Continuous Ambulatory Peritoneal Dialysis*, edited by Khanna R et al., Toronto, Perit Dial Bull Inc, 1985, Vol 1, p 118

56. Slingeneyer A, Mion C, Mourad G, Canaud B, Faller B, Beraud JJ: Progressive sclerosing peritonitis a late and severe complication of peritoneal dialysis. *Trans Am Soc Artif Intern Organs* 29: 633, 1983

57. Junor BJR, Briggs JD, Forwell MA et al.: Sclerosing peritonitis – the contribution of chlorhexidine in alcohol. *Perit Dial Bull* 5: 101, 1985

58. Verger C: Relationship between peritoneal membrane structure and its permeability: clinical implications. in *Advances in Continuous Ambulatory Peritoneal Dialysis*. Proc 5th Ann CAPD Conference. *Perit Dial Intern* 87, 1985

59. Verger C, Larpent L, Dumontet M: *Prognostic Value of Peritoneal Equilibration Curves in CAPD Patients: IIIrd International Symposium on Peritoneal Dialysis*, Washington DC, 1984

60. Wu G, Khanna R, Oreoupoulos DG, Vas SI: Incidence and pathogenesis of ultrafiltration failure among CAPD patients. *Kidney Int* 25: 262, 1984

61. Dobbie JW, Henderson I, Wilson LS: New evidence on the pathogenesis of sclerosing encapsulating peritonitis obtained from serial biopsies. in: *Advances in Continuous Ambulatory Peritoneal Dialysis*, edited by Khanna R et al., Toronto, Perit Dial Bull Inc, 1987, Vol 3, p 138

62. Miranda B, Selgas R, Celadilla O, Munoz J, SanchezSicilia L: Peritoneal resting and heparinization as an effective treatment for ultrafiltration failure in patients on CAPD. in *CAPD – A Decade of Experience*, edited by La Greca G et al., Basel, Karger, Contr Nephrol, Vol 89, 1991, p 199

63. Verger C, Celicout B: Peritoneal permeability and encapsulating peritonitis. *Lancet* April 27: 986, 1985

64. Twardowski ZJ, Nolph KD, Khanna R et al.: Peritoneal equilibration test. *Perit Dial Bull* 7: 138, 1987

65. Busch S, Schreiber M, Bodnar D, Buchler N, Fuchs J, Jackson-Bey D, Pearl J: The 24-hour D/P ratio is a convenient screen for identifying altered peritoneal transport rates. in *Advances in Peritoneal Dialysis*, Toronto, Peritoneal Dialysis Bulletin, 1993, Vol 9, p 119

66. Twardowski Z: The fast peritoneal equilibration test. *Semin Dial* 3: 141, 1990

67. Adcock A, Fox P, Walker P, Raymond K: Clinical experience and comparative analysis of the standard and fast peritoneal equilibration tests. in: *Advances in Peritoneal Dialysis*. Toronto, Peritoneal Dialysis Bulletin, 1992, Vol 8, p 59

68. Verger C, Larpent L, Veniez G: Mathematical determination of PET. (Abstract) *Perit Dial Intern* 10: S1, 1991

69. Verger C, Larpent L, Veniez G, Brunetot N, Corvaisier B: L'APEX ... description et utilisation. *Bull Dial Perit* 1: 36, 1991

70. Fischbach M, Mengus L, Birmelé B, Hamel G, Simeoni U, Geisert J: Point de croisement des courbes d'équilibration de l'urée et du glucose en dialyse péritonéale: description chez l'enfant. *Bull Dial Perit* 1: 127, 1991

71. Fischbach M, Mengus L, Birmelé B, Hamel G, Simeoni U, Geisert J: Solute equilibration curves, crossing time for urea and glucose during peritoneal dialysis: a function of age in children. *Adv Perit Dial* 7: 262, 1991

72. Conference de Consensus: La dialyse péritonéale, méthode de traitement de l'insuffisance rénale chronique. Conclusions. Eds: Pr JC Raphael Hôpital R Poincaré, 92380 Garches (France), and SANESCO, A Lam-Thanh, 47–49 ave E Vaillant, 92517 Boulogne Billancourt Cédex (France), 1993, p 10

73. Verger C, Larpent L, Corvaisier B, Stephan D, Veniez G: Repeatability of equilibration tests with special reference to the APEX technique. (Abstract) *Perit Dial Intern* 12: S1, 169, 1992

74. Twardowski ZJ, Prowant BF, Nolph KD et al.: High volume, low frequency continuous ambulatory peritoneal dialysis. *Kidney Int* 23: 64, 1983

75. Abensur H, Romao JE Jr, de Almeida Prado EB, Kakehashi E, Sabbaga E, Marcondes M: Influence of the hydrostatic intraperitoneal pressure and the cardiac function on the lymphatic absorption rate of the peritoneal cavity in CAPD. in *Advances in Peritoneal Dialysis*, edited by Khanna R, Nolph KD, Prowant BF, Twardowski ZJ, Oreoupoulos DG, 1993, Vol 9, p 41

76. Durand PY, Chanliau J, Gambéroni J, Hestin D, Kessler M: Evolution of intraperitoneal hydrostatic pressure following peritoneal catheter implantation. in *Advances in Peritoneal*

Dialysis, edited by Khanna R, Nolph KD, Prowant BF, Twardowski ZJ, Oreoupoulos DG, 1993, Vol 9, p 231

77. Twardowski ZJ, Khanna R, Nolph KD et al.: Intra-abdominal pressure during natural activities in patients treated with continuous ambulatory peritoneal dialysis. *Nephron* 44: 129, 1986

78. Gotloib L, Mines M, Garmozo L et al.: Hemodynamic effects of increasing intra-abdominal pressure in peritoneal dialysis. *Perit Dial Bull* 1: 41, 1981

79. Durand P-Y, Chanliau J, Gamberoni J, Hestin D, Kessler M: Comment mesurer le volume intrapéritonéal maximal admissible chez les patients en DPA? *Bull Dial Perit* 4: 219, 1994

80. Durand PY, Chanliau J, Gambéroni J, Hestin D, Kessler M: Intraperitoneal pressure, peritoneal permeability and volume of ultrafiltration in CAPD. in *Advances in Peritoneal Dialysis*, edited by Khanna R, Nolph KD, Prowant BF, Twardowski ZJ, Oreoupoulos DG, 1992, Vol 8, p 21

HOME HEMODIALYSIS AND SATELLITE HEMODIALYSIS

CHRISTOPHER BLAGG

INTRODUCTION

More than thirty years ago, hemodialysis was the first high-technology health care treatment to be transferred to the home and carried out by the patient with the help of a family member or other individual. Originally undertaken primarily for financial reasons, it soon became obvious that home hemodialysis increased the opportunity for patient independence and rehabilitation and provided an improved quality of life compared with patients dialyzing in a hospital or other outpatient dialysis facility. As financing improved for the treatment of end-stage renal disease (ESRD), the use of home hemodialysis declined and outpatient hemodialysis became the predominant treatment. Now, perhaps, the time is coming for home hemodialysis to come into its own again.

EARLY HISTORY OF HOME HEMODIALYSIS

Long term hemodialysis for ESRD first became practical in 1960 with development of the Teflon arteriovenous shunt (1). As a result, hemodialysis treatment programs began in some major teaching hospitals, and in 1962 the first free-standing (satellite) dialysis unit opened in Seattle (2). Probably the first use of home hemodialysis was in 1961 in Japan when Nosé used a coil dialyzer immersed in the tub of a commercial washing machine for this purpose (3). In 1963, Scribner visited India to train a physician to carry out hemodialysis in the home of a wealthy Madras businessman. Later that year, at least three nephrology programs were looking at using home hemodialysis as a less expensive alternative to outpatient hemodialysis in a hospital or a dialysis unit.

At this time, Scribner and Babb in Seattle were developing an automated dialysate production system. This used a central unit with proportioning pumps to mix dialysate concentrate and water to make dialysate for distribution to several dialysis stations at the University of Washington hospital (4). When the 15-year old daughter of one of Babb's friends developed chronic renal failure, the machine was miniaturized to make a single patient proportioning unit and several monitors were added to allow safe home hemodialysis (5). The patient and her mother used the device at home for several years without any major equipment-related problems. This machine, now in the Seattle Museum of History and Industry, was the prototype for all proportioning dialysis equipment.

About the same time, Merrill and co-workers in Boston began home hemodialysis using the twin-coil dialyzer, sending a nurse to the home to conduct each treatment (6). Concurrently, Shaldon in London began home hemodialysis using a system similar to that developed by Scribner and Babb (7), and it was Shaldon who first used overnight unattended home hemodialysis. The University of Washington team followed suit once a reliable arterial pressure monitor became available (8). Use of the low-resistance Kiil dialyzer allowed hemodialysis with cannulas without a blood pump, and required treatment for 8 to 10 hours three times weekly. Consequently it was logical to use overnight dialysis, with the patient sleeping at least some of the time.

It soon became apparent that home hemodialysis was as effective and much less expensive than outpatient hemodialysis in a hospital or free-standing dialysis unit because it did not require nursing staff. Consequently, Scribner and Shaldon pursued development of equipment to simplify the procedure and to ensure the equipment was as safe as possible. The fail-safe monitoring developed (9) is now a feature of almost all hemodialysis equipment.

Training in Seattle was conducted outside the dialysis unit from the beginning of the home dialysis program. The University of Washington team developed what became called the Coach House dialysis unit for this purpose. Several rooms in a local motel were modified for home hemodialysis training and to house the necessary patient support services. Over the next six years, more than 50 patients from the state of Washington and elsewhere in the US and abroad, were trained to do home hemodialysis at this unit (10). Experience with this program helped the staff of the Seattle Artificial Kidney Center as they developed their own home hemodialysis training program in response to a decision by the Center's Board of Trustees that all new patients were to do home hemodialysis. This was so the limited finds available at that time could be used to treat more patients. As a result, by 1970 more than 90% of dialysis patients in Washington State were being treated by home hemodialysis.

Because the number of patients continued to increase, the Center enlisted the aid of an educational consultant to examine and improve the patient training program. As a result, the Center was among the first programs to use video-tapes in dialysis training, and this shortened training time considerably (11).

Another home hemodialysis development pioneered in Seattle was the use of paid dialysis helpers. In the 1960s and early 1970s home hemodialysis was usually done by the patient with assistance from their spouse, other family member or a close friend. However, with increasing return of women to the work force and other changes in family structure and society, spouses or family members often were not available or willing to undertake the responsibility of helping with dialysis. The answer to this problem was to have the patient hire a home dialysis 'helper' to assist them. The helper was trained with the patient to do safe dialysis just as family members were, and no effort was made to have the helper become a trained dialysis technician. The helper worked for the patient as an independent contractor, and was reimbursed for their time through the patient. This proved to work extremely well and allowed many patients to do home hemodialysis who might not otherwise have been able to do so (12).

More recent history

Prior to establishment of the Medicare ESRD Program in 1973, funding was generally very limited in the US for treatment by dialysis and kidney transplantation, and so home hemodialysis became quite widely used to minimize cost to patients and institutions. As a result, the proportion of patients treated by home hemodialysis peaked in the early 1970s. In 1971, some 42% of the 10,000 or so dialysis patients were on home hemodialysis (13), but this then steadily declined to 12% by 1978 (14), 5.3% by 1984 (15), and less than 2% by 1991 (16).

In other westernized countries, home hemodialysis was also widely used for the same reasons. Thus, by 1977 more than 50% of Australian dialysis patients (17), and 25% of Canadian patients (18) were on home hemodialysis, and by 1980, 62% of British patients and some 20% of Danish, Swedish, Swiss, Irish, West German and French patients (19) were on home hemodialysis. In all these countries

there was unanimous agreement among those professionals experienced with home hemodialysis that this was the best treatment for many patients, provided appropriate training and support services were available.

However, in these countries too, the use of home hemodialysis began to decline, although somewhat later than in the US. For example, by 1985, only 31.8% of British patients and 8.2% of West German patients were on home hemodialysis (20), and by 1991 these figures had fallen to 11.9 and 3.0% respectively (21). Similarly, in 1992, the percentage of patients on home hemodialysis had declined to 10.9% in Canada (22), 18.1% in Australia and 28.8% in New Zealand (23).

Several factors contributed to this decline in the use of home hemodialysis, and although these differed to some degree from country to country, many related directly or indirectly to financing (24, 25). Financial concerns can affect dialysis facilities and physicians differently, or in some cases similarly, especially in the US where physicians may own one or more facilities.

In the US, for the first few years after its introduction in 1973, the Medicare ESRD Program provided much more generous funding for outpatient dialysis than for home dialysis. This led to a rapid proliferation of dialysis units across the country, vastly improving patient access to treatment, but at the same time leading to the decline in the use of home hemodialysis. Much of the increase in dialysis facilities over the years has been in proprietary or for-profit outpatient dialysis facilities, so that by 1993, there were 1,646 free-standing dialysis facilities in the US, of which 1,409 (85.6%) were for-profit facilities (26). For-profit dialysis facilities are less likely to treat patients by either home dialysis or transplantation (27). From the financial point of view, there is an incentive to keep facility dialysis stations in use so as to cover fixed costs and maximize profit. While physician reimbursement is by a monthly capitation fee and is the same, irrespective of the modality of dialysis, a number of nephrologists also have a direct financial interest in one or more facilities. In general, states with the highest proportion of patients treated by home dialysis are those in which the highest proportion of patients are treated by non-profit facilities (28, 29).

Economic factors have also impacted the use of home hemodialysis in other countries (25). For example, in Italy home hemodialysis is much less widely used in the south where regional reimbursement favors dialysis in centers, and there are many for-profit facilities which are prevented by law from overseeing home dialysis (30). In Japan, there has been almost no home hemodialysis because reimbursement is restricted to dialyses with a physician present, and self-administration of drugs in the home is illegal (31). Reimbursement to the facility and physician is also much less for continuous ambulatory peritoneal dialysis (CAPD) than for outpatient hemodialysis, and as 70% of Japanese dialysis patients are treated in private for-profit hospitals, this is a major financial disincentive. In the United Kingdom (32), home hemodialysis was widely used initially because of early experience with its advantages and because of cost constraints and limitations on facilities. More recently, CAPD has been increasingly used, primarily because originally the costs of this were applied to pharmacy budgets rather than the budgets of the dialysis programs.

Another major factor negatively affecting the use of home hemodialysis has been the relative lack of physicians and nurses with experience of this modality of treatment. In the US, during the years of rapid increase in the number of dialysis units, many nephrologists were trained in programs with little experience of dialysis, and very few were trained in programs which emphasized or had experience with home hemodialysis. Much the same happened in other countries.

One result of the decreased use of home hemodialysis was that when CAPD became available in the late 1970s, there was a pent up patient demand for some form of home dialysis. Thus, CAPD not only made home treatment available for the first time for many patients, it also resulted in a further reduction in the use of home hemodialysis. Two of the major advantages of CAPD are the brief time required for training, and the fact that patients can do this treatment themselves without assistance. As a result, the proportion of patients treated by home hemodialysis has continued to decline at the same time as a relatively rapid increase in patients treated by CAPD, continuous cycling peritoneal dialysis (CCPD), and other forms of peritoneal dialysis. In 1982, 1,793 patients were treated by home hemodialysis in the US. While this number was reported to almost triple over the next 4 years, much of this increase was probably spurious and due to earlier under-counting. In any case, the number declined again, and by 1991 was back down to 1,917, almost the same level as in 1982.

In contrast, over the same time period the number of patients treated by some form of peritoneal dialysis increased by some 350%, from 6,629 to 21,019 patients. As a percentage of all US dialysis patients, home hemodialysis patients declined from 6.89% in 1985 to 1.38% in 1991. During the same time period, the percentage of patients treated by peritoneal dialysis increased from 14.1 to 15.2% (33).

In theory, dialysis facility reimbursement in the US should favor home hemodialysis and CAPD because the costs of these are less than the cost of outpatient hemodialysis. Similarly, physician reimbursement is the same for all modalities of dialysis, while the amount of physician time required for support of home dialysis patients is usually less than for patients treated by outpatient dialysis. This was the rationale used by Medicare in the early 1980s in adopting reimbursement changes intended to provide an incentive for the use of home dialysis. Unfortunately, this had little effect on home hemodialysis, while making CAPD extremely profitable and so contributing to its increased use. Today, the use of CAPD in the US appears to be reaching a plateau, perhaps because even-

tually many such patients have to return to hemodialysis, either because of repeated peritonitis or because of concerns about the long term adequacy of this treatment.

At this time, home hemodialysis appears to be an endangered species in the US, used predominantly in the Northwest, and to a lesser extent elsewhere. In the years 1989 to 1991, in the Northwest Renal Network, covering Washington, Oregon, Alaska, Montana and Idaho, 8.97% of all ESRD patients were treated by home hemodialysis. The network serving Alabama, Mississippi and Tennessee had the next highest proportion of patients on home hemodialysis at 2.59% of all ESRD patients. The lowest rate was in the network serving Southern California where only 0.23% of patients were on home hemodialysis (33). In the Northwest Kidney Center's program, as of June 30th, 1994, there were 871 dialysis patients, of whom 224 (25.7%) were on home dialysis. Of these, 119 were on home hemodialysis (13.7% of all dialysis patients), and 105 (12.1%) were on some form of home peritoneal dialysis. Thus, it is still possible to maintain a relatively large population of patients on home hemodialysis in a program that is committed to this modality of treatment.

Selection of patients for home hemodialysis

Many factors are important in selection of patients for home hemodialysis (25). These include the medical condition of the patient, marital status, availability of suitable accommodation, the patient's learning ability, availability of either a family member as assistant or of a paid helper, and the patient and family's degree of anxiety and willingness to undertake this treatment at home. In Seattle, we have trained more than 2,500 patients to perform home hemodialysis over the last 30 years. Our experience has been that almost anyone physically capable of doing home hemodialysis can be successfully trained to do this, provided the patient is motivated and encouraged by the dialysis unit staff.

Various medical problems, such as severe cardiac disease resulting in arrhythmias or severe angina during dialysis may be contraindications to home hemodialysis. Nevertheless, other physical handicaps such as blindness, deafness, or relative immobility are not in themselves necessarily a contraindication to home hemodialysis (34, 35). Apart from severe cardiovascular problems, patient compliance with the dialysis regimen is perhaps the most important consideration in the decision to recommend home hemodialysis.

An essential requirement for successful home hemodialysis is good blood access that is easy for the patient to use. A native arteriovenous fistula is to be preferred over a vascular graft, and whenever possible surgery for this should be done some months before dialysis is started. This allows the fistula to mature, means the first dialyses by the unit staff will usually be free of access problems, and makes it easier for the patient to learn to stick their own fistula. It also means the patient can be taught to do this early on, so they have no qualms or difficulties with self-puncture by the time they start home hemodialysis training in earnest.

As far as age is concerned, home hemodialysis can be done by patients of all ages, with the possible exception of infants and very young children. For the latter, CAPD has proved particular useful while waiting for early renal transplantation. Early transplantation is also to be preferred for most older children and adolescents, but both home hemodialysis (36) and CAPD are very acceptable treatments for these patients. Home hemodialysis allows school attendance and adequate growth in pubertal, but not in prepubertal, children. While about 20% of children on home hemodialysis exhibit emotional disturbances, half the families of children exhibit stress symptoms. In adolescents treated by home hemodialysis, it may be necessary to provide the patient with a paid dialysis helper rather than use a family member, as this will help break dependency ties.

At the other extreme of age, there is a widespread belief among nephrologists that elderly patients are not good candidates for home hemodialysis. This has not been our experience. In Seattle, almost half the home hemodialysis patients are aged 60 years or older, and there have been many successful patients in their 70s and 80s. Apart from the greater likelihood of medical complications in older patients, the major problem for potential home hemodialysis patients is lack of a suitable family partner. In fact, this may be a problem for patients of all ages. In our experience, most patients now require the services of a paid dialysis helper (12), although unfortunately the Medicare ESRD Program does not cover the costs of this. If the spouse or other family member assists the patient we also pay them. It has not been our practice to encourage patients to undertake home hemodialysis on their own, although this has been done by others (37). Nevertheless, there is some increased risk in these circumstances.

For home hemodialysis, the patient must have suitable living accommodation with adequate plumbing and electricity and water supplies. This should be assessed by the unit's technical staff before training is started so any necessary changes can be carried out and inspected (38, 39). In addition, the patient can be given advice on how to make best use of the space available for dialysis and for storage of supplies.

A patient's ability to learn to do safe home hemodialysis does not appear to correlate with intelligence *per se*, but is closely related to motivation and desire for independence (40). Some years ago, we measured the intelligence quotient of 100 consecutive patients after successful completion of home hemodialysis training and found this to average 103, with a range from 78 to 147. This is very much what would be expected, as patients with serious intelligence deficits would not be considered candidates for home hemodialysis. Obviously, an illiterate patient or one who does not understand English will have more difficulties, but with the use of illustrations, videotapes, and translators we have been able to train a number of such patients.

Motivation and patient compliance are important, but another important psychological factor is the degree of anxiety shown by the patient or their family. The best way to alleviate this is to have the patient referred early to the training program, before the need to start dialysis. This allows them to learn about their disease and the dialysis procedure, and they and family members can meet with successful home hemodialysis patients. If possible, they should have the opportunity also to visit a patient during dialysis at home. For some patients who are anxious, CAPD may be a simple alternative which can be learned rapidly.

In Seattle, the Northwest Kidney Center also pioneered the use of a separate 'orientation unit' for the treatment of new patients. This allows new patients to dialyze in a single room where they can have social work, nutritional, financial, and vocational counselling, and exposure to exercise training, as well as close medical attention. During their dialysis in this unit new patients are able to review all modalities of treatment and to make an informed choice (41). This separate area and unbiased presentation of treatment options is important, because the initial mode of treatment and the attitudes of facility staff the patient meets are important factors influencing patient choice (42).

Patient selection for home hemodialysis is a topic that raises strong and varied opinions in nephrologists. Certainly, physician bias can have an important role in encouraging patients to consider home hemodialysis or CAPD rather than outpatient hemodialysis. One study compared opinions of nephrologists from North Carolina, Southern California, Australia and New Zealand. In general, if they had ESRD, physicians under the age of 50 would prefer home hemodialysis for themselves rather than a cadaveric transplant or CAPD (43). There was also a striking disparity between what physicians reported as their preferences for treating various patients and what they actually did in practice.

Other factors affecting selection of modality of dialysis include availability of resources, social issues and cultural habits (25). Thus, lack of available capital to establish new dialysis units or the presence of regulation to control the number of dialysis units, such as the Certificate of Need programs in some states in the US, can increase the utilization of home dialysis. Similarly, in the Canada and the US home dialysis is used more frequently in rural areas where there may be long distances to travel to a facility and where the population may be more independent and self-sufficient.

Other societal factors are also important. For example, in Australia, New Zealand and the South Pacific, ESRD in Polynesians and Aborigines is frequent and their social setting often precludes home dialysis. Similar problems affect much of the indigenous population of South America and Mexico. In the US, poor living conditions limit the use of home dialysis in some of the poor and the elderly. The small homes in Japan make home hemodialysis difficult, quite apart from the lack of reimbursement for this treatment. In Hong Kong, Chinese patients are averse to needle punctures, making home hemodialysis almost impossible, especially in light of the small living spaces in that country.

Home hemodialysis training

Several important general principles apply to training patients for home hemodialysis. Ideally, new patients should start their treatment in an area separate from that in which existing patients are treated by outpatient dialysis (41). Patient training, whether for home hemodialysis, CAPD or other forms of home peritoneal dialysis, should begin as soon as the patient is well enough to begin to absorb information. The first requirement is for the patient to learn to insert the needles for dialysis or other access procedure and care of the blood access. Fistula puncture is often a major obstacle for the patient to overcome, and so blood access, preferably a native fistula, should be established early whenever possible. This allows it time to mature prior to the patient starting hemodialysis.

At the same time as the patient is learning access procedures, they can begin to be exposed to information about the dietary regimen, their medical problems generally, and the various treatment options. If the patient was not seen before first starting on dialysis, this is also the time to begin social work intervention to support both patient and family, and to help with any financial or vocational issues. Where available, meetings with an exercise coach can also help ensure the patient realizes the importance of physical activity in maintaining and enhancing well being. Patients should be advised about use of their home for dialysis and need to learn details of the support services that will be available to them after they go home.

Once the patient is proficient in fistula puncture, the rest of the training is readily completed in three to six weeks. If training is also available on non-dialysis days this will speed up the process. However, it is important that whatever schedule is set up for dialysis and training, this should allow maximum opportunity for the patient to continue their employment or to have access to vocational and other rehabilitation services where appropriate. Home hemodialysis itself contributes to patient rehabilitation because patients learn new skills and develop self-confidence in their abilities to control their own treatment and eventually much of their life.

One of the most important characteristics of a successful home hemodialysis training program is commitment on the part of the staff to encourage independence and self-care. Training staff must be selected for their ability in teaching, and must be able to take a 'hands off' approach during dialysis, allowing patients to learn for themselves, even when they make mistakes. Training can be facilitated by the use of written materials, videotapes, films, posters, models and other educational aids (11, 44, 45).

Patients must be shown early on that hemodialysis is a relatively safe and simple procedure when carried out properly, and not an exotic, dangerous and complicated medical procedure. From the earliest dialysis, patients should learn that if a serious event such as a major blood leak occurs, dialysis can always be halted by clamping both arterial and venous blood lines, with no greater danger than loss of the blood in the dialyzer.

During training, the patient and their family member or paid helper should have their progress assessed at regular intervals to ensure they are acquiring the necessary knowledge. They have no need to learn the intricacies of the equipment, but rather must learn to carry out dialysis safely, learn the necessary emergency procedures for when medical or technical problems occur, and learn how and when to call for assistance or advice. This must always be available by telephone on a 24-hour basis, and ideally the nurse on call should be a member of the training staff so she is familiar with the patient's equipment, has access to their medical and dialysis records, and understands the needs of home hemodialysis patients.

In the US, training hemodialyses are reimbursed at a somewhat higher rate than routine outpatient dialysis. One study showed that home hemodialysis training cost about $8,300 more per patient than a comparable number of outpatient dialyses. However, because home hemodialysis costs less than outpatient dialysis (even though reimbursement is the same) these extra costs are recovered in 14 to 15 months (46).

Today, relatively few dialysis units have active home hemodialysis training programs. The average unit is relatively small and cannot be expected to train sufficient patients to attract and maintain good training staff. The solution to this is regional home hemodialysis training units. Patients who elect home hemodialysis can be referred to the unit for training while continuing to get medical care from their nephrologist. After going home, dialysis-related support can be provided through the training unit, but backup dialysis would be done at the original unit. An alterative approach is to send a training unit staff member into smaller units in the region to train patients. We have found this effective with units more than 100 miles away from Seattle. Again, after going home the patient's dialysis is monitored by the training staff, but medical care and backup dialysis are provided locally.

Support services for home hemodialysis

The home hemodialysis patient requires medical follow-up by a nephrologist, usually only on a monthly basis in the physicians office, unless there are problems. The patient should be taught to mail in a monthly blood sample to the laboratory for analysis, the reports on this going to the physician, the patient and the training program. The patient must also maintain records of each dialysis, and copies of the monthly dialysis log sheet must be returned to the training program and to the patient's physician.

Arrangements must be made to provide dialysis supplies to the patient's home on a regular basis and to provide technical support for maintenance and repair of the equipment. This can be done through a supplier or manufacturer, or, in the case of a large home hemodialysis program, these services can be provided directly by the training facility. The latter approach allows greater opportunities for contact with the patient and for visiting the home.

Besides availability of the patient's nephrologist for consultation, a home hemodialysis training nurse should be available by telephone at all times to answer patient questions and provide direction for any problem that may occur. In addition to talking the patient through problems, the nurse may refer the patient to their physician or for social work, financial, nutritional, or other consultation. Technical problems during dialysis may be dealt with directly by the nurse advising the patient on the actions to take, or by referring the patient for technical support next day. A training nurse should also visit the patient's home to observe a dialysis at least once a year, and preferably every six months. Following the visit, a detailed report should be sent to the training facility and to the patient's physician. In addition, there must be a system to keep patients aware of changes in techniques and procedures and of any other new information. When necessary, patient and assistant can return to the training unit for retraining on new procedures or for a refresher course.

In addition, there must be arrangements to provide back up outpatient hemodialysis for when the patient has medical, psychological, social or technical problems that preclude dialysis at home. These arrangements should also include opportunity for outpatient dialysis to provide relief or a vacation for the patient's assistant (47). Whenever possible, such backup dialyses should be provided either at the training unit itself, or at a nearby unit. This will enable training staff to check with the patient on problems, review dialysis procedures, and answer any questions.

Home hemodialysis patients are able to go on vacation or on business or other trips because arrangements can be made for them to dialyze in a center in many parts of the world. Alternatively, suitably trained patients can take with them portable dialysis equipment such as the sorbent-based Redy system (48). Patients of ours and of others have dialyzed in hotel rooms across the world, in camping trailers (49), in campsites and on mountain tops.

Patient survival with home hemodialysis

Survival with home hemodialysis has been reported to be at least as good, and probably better than survival with other dialysis modalities (50, 51). For example, in a large program in Mississippi the median survival in 150 home hemodialysis patients was 4,030 days. This compared with 3,600 days in patients treated by outpatient hemodialysis, and only 1,050 days in 230 patients treated by CAPD (52). Overall 15-year survival of the home hemodialysis patients was 40%. Similarly, an analysis of survival in 532 hemodialysis patients found a five and ten-year survival for home hemodialysis patients of 90%. Because this might reflect patient selection, a Cox proportional hazards regression model was used to correct for age and disease, and this still showed the best survival was in the home hemodialysis patients (53). Other studies have compared patient survival between home hemodialysis and CAPD, and have appeared to show this is better with home hemodialysis (54, 55). Again, this may in part reflect patient selection.

Recently, questions have also been raised about whether there may be an increased mortality with CAPD compared with hemodialysis (56). The largest series reported used data from a random sample of 4,136 patients starting dialysis in 1986 and 1987. Cox proportional hazards modelling was used to allow comparison of mortality while adjusting for patient characteristics, including comorbid conditions present at the onset of dialysis (57). No significant difference in mortality between the two treatments was found in non-diabetic patients. However, a higher adjusted mortality was found for CAPD patients with renal failure due to diabetes when compared with similar patients treated by hemodialysis (relative risk 1.26; $p = 0.03$). This difference was most marked in patients aged 58 years or older. There is need for further controlled studies addressing this comparison, and these, together with a study of survival with home hemodialysis are now being undertaken by the US Renal Data System (58).

Patient and technique survival

Some of the most impressive technique survival results come from the home hemodialysis program in Brooklyn run by the SUNY Health Science Center. This program, which has been in existence for more than 20 years, primarily treats an impoverished inner city population, some of whom might be regarded as highly unlikely candidates for home hemodialysis (59). Of 192 patients successfully trained for home hemodialysis, 36 (19%) were still on this treatment after 10 years (average duration 14 years), and 11 patients had been on home dialysis for more than 20 years (60). Long technique survival did not appear to correlate with age or sex, but appeared to be associated with white race and middle class origins, with white middle class males remaining on home hemodialysis the longest. In contrast, although CAPD has been used for some 17 years now, there are very few patients reported as still on this treatment even after only 10 years. This probably reflects the continuing problem of repeated peritonitis, the possibility of under-dialysis in at least some patients, and the effort required to do four exchanges a day, every day, for years on end.

A Scottish study has compared both patient and technique survival with home hemodialysis and with CAPD (55). Patient survival at 3 years was 93.8% with home hemodialysis and 86.2% with CAPD ($p < 0.05$); technique survival (excluding death and kidney transplantation) was 94.2 and 80.8% respectively ($p < 0.04$). Thus, the results with home hemodialysis appeared to be superior to those with CAPD, but this too may reflect patient selection. Again, it is to be hoped that analyses by the US Renal Data System using large numbers of patients will help give a better understanding of these issues.

Better nutrition may be important in the well being of home hemodialysis patients. Generally, they may be more compliant in terms of adherence to diet and fluid restriction than are patients on outpatient hemodialysis (61). However, our experience and that of others (62) is that many home hemodialysis patients do not practice significant dietary restrictions and yet are well rehabilitated and show little or no evidence of malnutrition.

Psychosocial aspects of home hemodialysis

Psychosocial adjustment is important in all dialysis patients and their immediate family members, but this differs somewhat for home hemodialysis patients. Generally, psychological distress is less in patients dialyzing at home rather than in a center. The spouses of home hemodialysis patients show scores for psychological distress that are similar to those of the spouses of patients on outpatient dialysis, although they report fewer social problems (63). Patient success with home hemodialysis appears to be positively correlated with denial (64) and to the presence of minimal psychiatric morbidity and physical symptoms, a coping spouse and continuing employment, house work or other activities (65). The probability of failure is said to be correlated with poorer compliance and increased anxiety and depression. Nevertheless, others have found that depressed patients starting home hemodialysis training usually have a remission of symptoms as training progresses and that depression does not affect outcome (66).

The prevalence of psychiatric morbidity is 31% in a population of home hemodialysis patients, and this is comparable to that of patients attending the office of a family doctor (67). In many ways there is as much or more stress on the spouse and family or the helper. Consequently, ongoing support and counselling should be available to all those involved in home hemodialysis, including the patient's family. There must also be provision for the person helping the patient to get relief or take a vacation, and this requires availability of outpatient dialysis for a short time (47).

In the case of children on home hemodialysis, there is a particular need for a comprehensive program of psychosocial support for parents as well as children. Parents suffer more stress than do the parents of children dialyzing as outpatients, while the children have more fears of complications and aggressive feelings. Nevertheless, the children are better than those treated as outpatients in terms of social contacts, school attendance, and education (36, 68). Parents and teachers need detailed instruction as to how to work with these children.

Patients on home hemodialysis are three times more likely ($p < 0.02$) to withdraw from dialysis without an obvious medical or technical reason than are patients on outpatient dialysis (69). It has been suggested that this difference may represent a response to the stress of home hemodialysis. However, it might also reflect the increased independence and control that home dialysis patients have over their life and treatment.

Quality of life with home hemodialysis

Several studies have compared quality of life and rehabilitation of patients treated by various modalities of dialysis and transplantation. These have generally confirmed the early impressions that home hemodialysis is the optimal treatment for patients who can do this. The two largest studies were done with 859 randomly selected patients from 11 dialysis and transplant units across the US (70), and with a similar number of patients from one geographic area in the Northeastern US (71). Both showed that quality of life and opportunity for rehabilitation were best in patients with a functioning renal transplant. Among patients treated by dialysis, home hemodialysis patients had a better quality of life and were more frequently judged to be rehabilitated than were patients treated by outpatient hemodialysis; CAPD patients fell between the two groups. These differences persisted after adjustment to allow for different medical and other demographic differences between the various patient groups. In general, home hemodialysis, CAPD and CCPD appear to offer the best opportunity for rehabilitation in patients who are not elderly or debilitated (72).

There are several possible reasons quality of life is better for home hemodialysis patients. The patient can select the day and time of dialysis and can dialyze longer or more frequently if he or she wishes to do so. This allows more adequate dialysis and avoids the time wasted in traveling to and from a center for treatment three times weekly, time that is generally longer than the time the patient takes in starting and ending their dialysis at home. The patient has a better opportunity to integrate dialysis into their life while continuing to work or carry out their usual daily activities. In this regard, home hemodialysis is generally better than CAPD, as patients on the latter treatment must take time out during every working day to exchange bags, and this may be very inconvenient.

By dialyzing at home, the patient is no longer in repeated contact with other dialysis patients, some of whom may have many medical problems. This avoids reinforcement of the 'sick' image that is all too easily fostered in patients with chronic disease, and especially in patients on outpatient hemodialysis. There is also less risk of exposure to hepatitis C and other infections that may be present in the environment of the health care facility.

Also important is the protection home hemodialysis offers from having the patient's blood access punctured by many different staff members of varying skill levels. No one can puncture their own fistula better than the confident well-trained home hemodialysis patient, and although no data have been published, it is our impression that home hemodialysis patients have fewer hospitalizations and other vascular access-related problems than do patients on outpatient hemodialysis.

SATELLITE HEMODIALYSIS

'Satellite dialysis' is one of the names used for outpatient dialysis done in a facility outside of a hospital setting and it also may imply that the unit is a satellite of a hospital or of a larger free standing dialysis program. Satellite dialysis is also called 'out-of-hospital dialysis' or 'limited care dialysis' and the facility in which it is done is variously called a 'free standing' or an 'independent' dialysis unit, or it may be a satellite unit of a hospital program that is situated outside the hospital. These names also generally imply dialysis done by nurses or technicians. However, another variant of facility dialysis outside a hospital is 'self-care dialysis' by a suitably trained patient, although, to increase the confusion, in some places this is also called 'limited care dialysis'. Of course, self-care dialysis in a facility must also be distinguished from home dialysis. Unfortunately, different countries and different authors use different nomenclature to describe outpatient dialysis.

Adding to the confusion, 'hospital dialysis' can mean inpatient dialysis for hospitalized patients who have acute renal failure or ESRD, but particularly in Europe this can also mean outpatient dialysis for patients with ESRD in a dialysis facility which is sited in a hospital. To complicate comparisons even further, such a hospital-based outpatient dialysis facility is likely to treat sicker and less medically stable patients than do many free standing dialysis facilities. Finally, particularly in the US, dialysis facilities may be proprietary or for-profit facilities owned by a chain organization or by individual entrepreneurs who are often physicians, or they may be not-for-profit facilities. In the US most free-standing facilities (85.6%) are for-profit, while only 4.1% of the hospital-based facilities are for-profit, and there are now many fewer hospital-based outpatient dialysis facilities than free-standing facilities.

For the sake of this discussion, the term satellite hemodialysis will mean hemodialysis in a free-standing or independent dialysis facility, outside the hospital setting. The term does not imply anything with regard to the ownership of the facility.

HISTORY OF SATELLITE HEMODIALYSIS

The first ever out-of-hospital dialysis facility was established in 1962 in Seattle as the Seattle Artificial Kidney Center. In 1960, working at the University of Washington's Clinical Research Center, Belding Scribner had shown that patients with ESRD could be kept alive with repeated hemodialysis (1). This new treatment changed a universally fatal disease to one that could be treated successfully. Research funds were not available to pay for the treatment of more than the original few patients, and insurance companies would not yet pay for dialysis for ESRD patients. As a result, Scribner turned to the community for support. He recognized that setting up a dialysis unit outside the hospital would reduce the fixed costs in comparison with hospital-based hemodialysis. However, this was not his only innovation. Up to then, hemodialysis had been seen as a complex and potentially dangerous procedure that could only be done with the direct supervision and participation of a physician or physicians. Scribner recognized that while this was true for most patients with acute renal failure, with appropriate training and organization, hemodialysis for ESRD patients could be done by nurses without direct involvement of a physician except when problems arose. This, too, resulted in significant cost saving.

With the support of Dr James Haviland, the King County Medical Society, and the Seattle Area Hospital Council, the Seattle Artificial Kidney Center began operations in January of 1962. Space for the unit was provided in the basement of the Swedish Hospital's nurses residence, and a three station outpatient hemodialysis unit was opened, supported by funds from the John A Hartford Foundation (73). This unit was the forerunner of the many out-of-hospital or satellite dialysis facilities around the world today.

In the US, as of the end of 1993, the Health Care Financing Administration reported there were total of 2,506 providers of services to ESRD patients and 35,267 approved dialysis stations. Providers included 64 transplant hospitals and 170 transplant/dialysis centers, 61 hospitals that provided inpatient care only, and 342 hospital outpatient dialysis units together with 223 'satellite' dialysis facilities. These latter were separate free-standing units belonging to hospital programs. There were also 1,646 independent (free-standing or satellite) dialysis units, of which 1,409 were proprietary for-profit dialysis units and 237 were non-profit units (26).

For-profit and not-for-profit hemodialysis

The preponderance of for-profit dialysis units is a phenomenon seen particularly in the US, although it occurs to a much lesser extent in some other western countries. For example, in 1987 there were 781 for-profit independent dialysis units in the US, and these accounted for 81.4% of all free standing dialysis units and 47.3% of all facilities (dialysis and transplant, hospital and free standing) serving ESRD patients. By the end of 1993, there were 1,409 for-profit independent dialysis units, almost a doubling in numbers over 6 years. These now accounted for 85.6% of all free standing dialysis units and 57.6% of all ESRD facilities (26). At the end of 1991 in the US, 96,228 dialysis patients were being treated in free-standing units, of whom 79,313 (82.4%) were in for-profit units, compared with 1982, when of the 34,081 patients, 26,278 (77.1%) were treated in for-profit units.

Many of the for-profit units in the US belong to so-called chain organizations, and these are in strong competition with each other to purchase dialysis units from non-profit organizations, hospitals and individual physician entrepreneurs. Popular wisdom has it that in 1994 the price of a dialysis facility on the open market was about $35,000 to $40,000 per dialysis patient.

What effect does the presence of so many for-profit dialysis units in the US have on the quality of care and other aspects of dialysis treatment? So far, this is a subject on which there is limited data. The Institute of Medicine report (74) noted that "The quality of care implications of the changing composition of the dialysis provider community need careful monitoring" and "The quality implications of the shift toward for-profit and physician ownership merit careful assessment. The committee is aware of no evidence that the shift from hospital-based to independent and from not-for-profit to for-profit dialysis facilities has resulted in problems of access or quality. The lack of systematic efforts to stress quality . . . preclude the development of such evidence at this time. *The committee recommends, however, that ownership changes be monitored closely over time and that means be developed to assess their implications for access and quality.*" (Their emphasis). This is yet to be done.

Only two recent papers have commented briefly on the question of quality of care and for-profit dialysis. In a paper relating use of short-time dialysis to the increased mortality with hemodialysis seen in the US compared with other developed countries, the comment was made ". . . patients treated with short-time dialysis were disproportionately treated in for-profit institutions . . ." (75). Similarly, in a review of hemodialysis prescription and actual delivery of treatment in dialysis units in the city of St. Louis, the adequacy of dialysis as measured by Kt/V was significantly lower in those patients treated in for-profit dialysis units (76).

Another aspect of quality is reflected by the rate of use of transplantation and home hemodialysis. As noted previously, studies have shown the greater opportunity for rehabilitation, independence and an optimal quality of life with these treatments (70, 71). In general, for-profit dialysis units have not given much encouragement for either treatment. A recent article examining data from the Health Care Financing Administration found this was consistent with the fact that "choices about type of treatment by proprietary facilities are influenced by financial incentives. For example, home dialysis was less likely to occur in areas where there was a higher proportion of for-profit facilities. These results are compelling because they are based on relatively small units of analysis (versus states), controlled for important contextual variables such as region and population growth, and adjusted for variables related to case mix" (27). This conclusion is also supported by data from the State of Washington where, in 1991, 27.6% of dialysis patients were on home hemodialysis and one kidney transplant was done for every 8 dialysis patients. This is a state with only 26 dialysis units and strong regulation of new dialysis units by Certificate of Need legislation. By comparison, two states without a Certificate of Need law, Louisiana and California, had 75 and 255 dialysis units respectively. In 1991, in Louisiana and in California, only 12.8% of dialysis patients were on home dialysis, and in Louisiana there was one transplant for every twenty dialysis patients (33). In Washington state at that time, only 2.4% of dialysis patients were treated in for-profit units, compared with 86.2% of patients in Louisiana and 71.1% in California (26).

The reasons for these differences almost certainly relate to reimbursement. General experience is that for-profit dialysis centers are more likely to use shortened dialysis times, fixed patient schedules, and different staffing levels in order to minimize cost and maximize profits. A recent study examined the effects of competition on dialysis facilities, service levels and patient selection (77). The most striking difference between for-profit and non-profit dialysis units was in staffing. Using 1990 data from the Health Care Financing Administration, the number of dialyses per staff hour was 0.34 in for-profit facilities and 0.27 in non-profit facilities. In other words, there was 26% more staff in non-profit facilities than in for-profit facilities. Corresponding ratios of technical staff to RNs were 2.67 and 0.91 respectively. Thus, there were less staff in for-profit units and a much higher ratio of technicians to nurses when compared with non-profit units. Such marked differences certainly have the potential to adversely affect quality of care.

THE FUTURE OF HOME HEMODIALYSIS AND SATELLITE DIALYSIS

There are some grounds now for optimism that the use of home hemodialysis will increase again in the future. There are several reasons for this.

One of the most important reasons is financial. In most countries in the developed world, the cost of health care is now a matter of great concern. With appropriate equipment, home hemodialysis would certainly be the most cost effective dialysis modality, provided the patient can do the this without assistance. This requires what Belding Scribner has called a 'one button machine'. At least two groups in the US are working on such a machine. This would not only be simple and safe for the patient to use for self care dialysis, but would also clean, reprocess and sterilize the dialyzer and tubing set, and be ready to use at the time for the next dialysis. Such a machine is already in use in the program of Professor Charles Mion in Montpellier in the south of France (78).

A most exciting new development is the report by Uldall and co-workers in Toronto of what they call 'simplified nocturnal home hemodialysis' (79). The approach being studied is the use of home hemodialysis for 8 hours while sleeping, 6 days weekly, using a 0.4 m^2 polysulphone dialyzer and a jugular venous catheter. This allows very adequate dialysis with a weekly Kt/V of 6.5. The equipment used performs *in situ* reuse of the dialyzer and blood lines, so minimizing patient work in starting and ending dialysis. Remote computerized monitoring of dialysis functions by modem is carried out by staff in the dialysis center. Such linkage should also allow transmission of dialysis data to the patient's physician. Another possible development is interactive visualization of the patient and staff member by each other using video, although this may raise privacy issues.

From the patient's point of view, this simplified home hemodialysis emphasizes again the advantages of home dialysis. First, there is the better quality of life and opportunity for independence and rehabilitation. Second, there is flexibility of scheduling dialysis, the possibility of dialyzing more than three times weekly, the saving in time otherwise spent in travelling to and from the dialysis unit three times weekly, and the opportunity to dialyze while sleeping. The increased adequacy of dialysis that can be achieved should result in improved patient survival, less morbidity, and reduced frequency of hospitalization, together with more opportunity to work or to spend time in other activities and with family and friends. All this will be achieved with only minimal if any involvement of family.

Another reason for believing the use of home hemodialysis will increase in the future is that patients are becoming better educated and more likely to realize that this treatment, among all dialysis modalities, has the most advantages to offer. Patients will also become aware that, while CAPD is a satisfactory and easily learnt form of home dialysis, it is not associated with such good quality of life, and there are concerns about long term adequacy and the possible increased mortality, particularly in older diabetic patients. There is also less risk of infection with home hemodialysis than with CAPD or CCPD because of the fewer connections required, and this will likely result in fewer episodes of hospitalization.

There will also be continuing pressure to move high technology medical care of all sorts into the home setting. Home care is being increasingly widely used in the US and elsewhere for purposes such as parenteral nutrition and other infusion treatments and for certain respiratory and cardiac treatments. A major reason for this is financial. Payment for these treatments is still relatively generous and primarily from private insurance, and so in recent years there has been rapid multiplication of for-profit companies providing these services. As the number of dialysis patients in the US is expected to more than double in the next ten years, the capital cost of providing facilities to treat these extra patients will increase correspondingly. As more user-friendly home hemodialysis equipment becomes available and patients demand this, facilities will soon become more willing to provide relatively profitable home hemodialysis.

Even so, because of the large increase in the number of dialysis patients in the future, the number of dialysis units and dialysis stations will also increase, there will be fewer hospital-based dialysis facilities, and for-profit dialysis corporations will become increasingly competitive with each other while providing both outpatient and home hemodialysis.

History repeats itself. Satellite dialysis began more than thirty years ago, and because of cost constraints home hemodialysis was developed. With financial constraints removed some twenty years ago, outpatient hemodialysis burgeoned, in part because it was easier to do. Fifteen years ago, CAPD began to meet the need for home dialysis for some patients, but now is beginning to be questioned as a long term treatment. Until the shortage of organs for transplantation is solved, the number of dialysis patients will continue to grow rapidly. As a result, the number of satellite units will also increase. Even so, with increasing cost constraints and the availability of suitable equipment, the time is ripe for home hemodialysis to begin flourishing once more.

REFERENCES

1. Quinton W, Dillard D, Scribner BH: Cannulation of blood vessels for prolonged hemodialysis. *Trans Am Soc Artif Intern Organs* 6: 104, 1960
2. Murray JS, Tu WH, Albers JB, Burnell JM, Scribner BH: A community hemodialysis center for the treatment of chronic uremia. *Trans Am Soc Artif Intern Organs* 8: 315, 1962
3. Nosé Y: Discussion. *Trans Am Soc Artif Intern Organs* 11: 15, 1965
4. Grimsrud L, Cole JJ, Lehman GA, Babb AL, Scribner BH: A central system for the continuous preparation and distribution of hemodialysis fluid. *Trans Am Soc Artif Intern Organs* 10: 107, 1964
5. Curtis FK, Cole JJ, Fellows BJ, Tyler LL, Scribner BH: Hemodialysis in the home. *Trans Am Soc Artif Intern Organs* 11: 7, 1965
6. Merrill JP, Schupak E, Cameron E, Hampers CL: Hemodialysis in the home. *JAMA* 190: 468, 1964
7. Baillod RA, Comty C, Ilahi M, Konotey-Ahulu FID, Sevitt L, Shaldon S: Overnight haemodialysis in the home. *Proc Eur Dial Transplant Assoc* 2: 99, 1965
8. Eschbach JW Jr, Wilson WE Jr, Peoples RW, Wakefield AW, Babb AL, Scribner BH: Unattended overnight home hemodialysis. *Trans Am Soc Artif Intern Organs* 12: 346, 1966

9. Grimsrud L, Cole JJ, Eschbach JW, Babb AL, Scribner BH: Safety aspects of hemodialysis. *Trans Am Soc Artif Intern Med* 13: 1, 1967

10. Blagg CR, Hickman RO, Eschbach JW, Scribner BH: Home hemodialysis: six years experience. *N Engl J Med* 283: 1126, 1970

11. Stinson JW, Clark MF, Sawyer TK, Blagg CR: Home hemodialysis training in three weeks. *Trans Am Soc Artif Intern Organs* 18: 66, 1972

12. Clark MF: Experience with paid dialysis helpers. *J Am Assoc Nephrol Nurses and Technicians* 4 (Suppl Edn): 39, 1977

13. Jenkins PG, Gutmann FD, Rieselbach RE: Self-hemodialysis. The optimal mode of dialytic therapy. *Archives of Internal Medicine* 136: 357, 1976

14. ESRD Facility Survey System, Dec 31, 1978. Washington, DC.: Department of Health, Education, and Welfare, 1978

15. Health Care Financing, Research Report, End-Stage Renal Disease, 1984: Baltimore, MD. US Department of Health and Human Services, Health Care Financing Administration, Bureau of Data Management and Strategy, Office of Research and Demonstrations, 1986

16. Health Care Financing, Research Report, End Stage Renal Disease, 1991: Baltimore, MD. Department of Health and Human Services, Health Care Financing Administration, Bureau of Data Management and Strategy, Office of Research and Demonstrations, 1993

17. Editorial: Dialysis and Transplantation. *Med J Aust* 1: 102, 1981

18. Shimizu A: Dialysis in Canada today. *Int J Artif Organs* 4: 41, 1981

19. Jacobs C, Broyer M, Brunner FP, Brynger H, Donckerwolcke RA, Kramer P, Selwood NH, Wing AJ, Blake PH: Combined report on regular dialysis and transplantation in Europe. *Proc Eur Dial Transplant Assoc* 18: 4, 1981

20. Broyer M, Brunner FP, Brynger H, Fassbinder W, Guillou PJ, Oules R, Rizzoni G, Selwood NH, Wing AJ, Challah S, Dykes SR: EDTA Registry Centre Survey, 1985: Report from the European Dialysis and Transplant Association Registry. *Nephrol Dial Transplant* 2: 475, 1987

21. Raine AEG, Margreiter R, Brunner FP, Ehrich JHH, Geerlings W, Landais P, Loirat C, Mallick NP, Selwood NH, Tufveson G, Valderrabano F: Report on management of renal failure in Europe. *Nephrol Dial Transplant* 7 (Suppl 2): 7, 1992

22. *Canadian Organ Replacement Register, 1992 Annual Report. Don Mills, Ontario, Canada*, Canadian Institute for Health Information, Don Mills, Ontario, March 1994

23. Disney APS ed: *Sixteenth Annual Report of the Australia and New Zealand Dialysis and Transplant Registry (ANZDATA), 1993*. Adelaide, South Australia. Australian Kidney Foundation, 1993

24. Rennie D, Rettig RA, Wing AJ: Limited resources and the treatment of end-stage renal failure in Britain and the United States. *Q J Med* 56: 321, 1985

25. Nissenson AR, Prichard SS, Cheng IKP, Gokal R, Kubota M, Maiorca R, Riella MC, Rottembourg J, Stewart JH: Non-medical factors that impact on ESRD modality selection. *Kidney Int* 43 (Suppl 40): S120, 1992

26. Health Care Financing Administration: End Stage Renal Disease Program Highlights 1993, 1994. Health Care Financing Administration, Bureau of Data Management and Strategy: Data from the Program Management and Medical Information System, 1987–1993

27. Cleary PD, Schlesinger M, Blumenthal D: Factors affecting the availability and use of hemodialysis facilities. *Health Care Financing Review* 13: 49, 1991

28. Schmidt RW, Blumenkrantz M, Wiegmann TB: The dilemmas of patient treatment for end-stage renal disease. *Am J Kidney Dis* 3: 37, 1983

29. Gardner K: Profit and the end-stage renal disease program. *N Engl J Med* 305: 461, 1981

30. D'Amico G: Treating end-stage renal-failure in Italy. in *Renal Failure. Who Cares?*, edited by Parsons FM, Ogg CS, Lancaster, England, MTP Press Ltd, 1983, p 89

31. Robin-Tani M: Worldwide renal care: Japanese methodology. *Contemp Dial* 11: 50, 1983

32. Wing AJ: A different view from different countries: United Kingdom. in *Ethical Problems in Dialysis and Transplantation*, edited by Kjellstrand CM, Dossetor JB, Dordrecht, The Netherlands, Kluwer Academic Publishers, 1993, p 207

33. US Renal Data System, USRDS 1994 Annual Data Report: Bethesda, MD. The National Institutes of Health, National Institute of Diabetes and Digestive and Kidney Diseases, 1994

34. Roberts CM: Home dialysis in the haemophiliac paraplegic patient. *Proc Eur Dial Transpl Nurses Assoc* 7: 62, 1979

35. Roberts CM, Davis B, Pavitt L: Home dialysis training in a blind patient and a deaf patient. *Proc Eur Dial Transpl Nurses Assoc* 1: 41, 1973

36. Wass VJ, Barratt TM, Howarth RV, Marshall WA, Chantler C, Ogg CS, Cameron JS, Baillod RA, Moorhead JP: Home haemodialysis in children. Report of the London Children's Home Dialysis Group. *Lancet* 1: 2426, 1977

37. Baillod RA, Moorhead JF: Review of ten years' home dialysis. *Proc Eur Dial Transplant Assoc* 11: 68, 1975

38. Baillod RA: Home dialysis. in *Replacement of Renal Function by Dialysis*, 2nd ed, edited by Drukker W, Parsons FM, Maher JF, Boston, Martinus Nijhoff, 1983, p 493

39. Sawyer TK, Blagg CR, Nissenson AR, Fine RN eds: *Dialysis Therapy*. 2nd ed. St Louis, The CV Mosby Co, 1992, Home preparation and installation for home dialysis. p 52

40. Snow W, Clark M: Understanding patient learning and performance capabilities for home dialysis training. *J Am Assoc Nephrology Nurses & Technicians* 3: 20, 1976

41. Eschbach JW, Seymour M, Potts A, Clark M, Blagg CR: A hemodialysis orientation unit. *Nephron* 33: 106, 1983

42. Smith MD, Hong BA, Michelman JE, Robson AM: Treatment bias in the management of end-stage renal disease. *Am J Kidney Dis* 3: 21, 1983

43. Mattern WD, McGaghie WC, Rigby RJ, Nissenson AR, Dunham CB, Khayrallah MA: Selection of ESRD treatment: an international study. *Am J Kidney Dis* 13: 457, 1989

44. Florkemeier V, Bayer H, Finke K, Schadlich HJ, Sieberth HG: An audio-visual teaching programme for training home dialysis patients. *Proc Eur Dial Transplant Assoc* 10: 538, 1973

45. Maiorca R, Castellani A, Cristinelli L, Migozzi G, Mileti M, Mombelloni S, Usberti M: A video box colour film for home dialysis training. *Proc Eur Dial Transplant Assoc* 10: 545, 1973

46. Delano BG, Feinroth MV, Feinroth M, Friedman EA: Home and medical center hemodialysis. Dollar comparison and payback period. *JAMA* 246: 230, 1981

47. Brown DJ, Craick CC, Davies SE, Johnson ML, Dawborn JK, Heale WF: Physical, emotional and social adjustments to home dialysis. *Medical Journal of Australia* 1: 245, 1978

48. Roberts M, Blumenkrantz MJ: Sorbent dialysis. in *Dialysis Therapy*, 1st ed, edited by Nissenson AR, Fine RN, Philadelphia, PA, Hanley and Belfus, Inc, 1986, p 222

49. Nikolay J, Gutmann A, Seybold D, Gessler U: Experiences with Redy-dialysis on a camper. *Life Support Systems* 1: 291, 1983

50. Roberts JL: Analysis and outcome of 1063 patients trained for home hemodialysis. *Kidney Int* 9: 363, 1976

51. Johnson WJ, Kurtz SB, Anderson CF, Mitchell JC, Zincke H, O'Fallon WM: Results of treatment of renal failure by means of home hemodialysis. *Mayo Clinic Proc* 59: 663, 1984

52. Rubin J, Hsu H, Bower J: Survival on dialysis therapy: one center's experience. *Am J Med Sci* 297: 80, 1989

53. Mailloux LU, Bellucci AG, Mossey RT, Napolitano B, Moore T, Wilkes BM, Bluestone PA: Predictors of survival in patients undergoing dialysis. *Am J Med* 84: 855, 1988

54. Gutman RA, Blumenkrantz MJ, Chan YK, Barbour GL, Gandhi VC, Shen FH, Tucker T, Murawski BJ, Coburn JW, Curtis FK: Controlled comparison of hemodialysis and peritoneal dialysis: Veterans Administration multicenter study. *Kidney Int* 26: 459, 1984

55. Gent AC, Rodger RS, Howie CA, Junor BJ, Briggs JD, Macdougall AI: Dialysis at home in the west of Scotland: a comparison of hemodialysis and continuous ambulatory peritoneal dialysis in age- and sex-matched controls. *Peritoneal Dialysis International* 12: 365, 1992

56. US Renal Data System, USRDS 1991 Annual Data Report. Bethesda, MD: National Institutes of Health, National Institute of Diabetes and Digestive and Kidney Diseases, 1991

57. Held PJ, Port FK, Turenne M, Gaylin DS, Hamburger RJ, Wolfe RA: Continuous ambulatory peritoneal dialysis and hemodialysis: comparison of patient mortality with adjustment for comorbid conditions. *Kidney Int* 45: 1163, 1994

58. Held, PJ: Personal communication, 1994

59. Delano BG, Lundin AP, Friedman EA: Successful home hemodialysis in purportedly unacceptable patients. *Nephron* 31: 191, 1982

60. Delano BG, Friedman EA: Correlates of decade-long technique survival on home hemodialysis. *ASAIO Transactions* 36: M337, 1990

61. Christensen AJ, Smith TW, Turner CW, Holman JM Jr, Gregory MC: Type of hemodialysis and preference for behavioral involvement: interactive effects on adherence in end-stage renal disease. *Health Psychology* 9: 225, 1990

62. Talemaitoga AS, Sanders BA, Hinton D, Lynn KL: Nutritional status of home hemodialysis patients. *Austral N Z J Med* 19: 303, 1989

63. Soskolne V, De-Nour AK: Psychosocial adjustment of home hemodialysis, continuous ambulatory peritoneal dialysis and hospital dialysis patients and their spouses. *Nephron* 47: 266, 1987

64. Richmond JM, Lindsay RM, Burton HJ, Conley J, Wai L: Psychological and physiological factors predicting the outcome on home hemodialysis. *Clin Nephrol* 17: 109, 1982

65. Farmer CJ, Bewick M, Parsons V, Snowden SA: Survival on home haemodialysis: its relationship with physical symptomatology, psychosocial background and psychiatric morbidity. *Psychological Medicine* 9: 515, 1979

66. Lowry MR, Atcherson E: A short-term follow-up of patients with depressive disorder on entry into home dialysis training. *Journal of Affective Disorders* 2: 219, 1980

67. Farmer CJ, Snowden SA, Parsons V: The prevalence of psychiatric illness among patients on home haemodialysis. *Psychological Medicine* 9: 509, 1979

68. Reichwald-Klugger E, Tieben-Heibert A, Korn R, Stein L, Weck K, Maiwald A, Mehls O, Diekmann L, Muller-Wiefel DE, Jochmus I et al.: Psychosocial adaptation of children and their parents to hospital and home hemodialysis. *International Journal of Pediatric Nephrology* 5: 45, 1984

69. Roberts JC, Kjellstrand CM: Choosing death. Withdrawal from chronic dialysis without medical reason. *Acta Medica Scandinavica* 223: 181, 1988

70. Evans RW, Manninen DL, Garrisson LPJ, Hart LG, Blagg CR, Gutman RA, Hull AR, Lowrie EG: The quality of life of patients with end-stage renal disease. *N Engl J Med* 312: 553, 1985

71. Bremer BA, McCauley CR, Wrona RM, Johnson JP: Quality of life in end-stage renal disease: a reexamination. *Am J Kidney Dis* 13: 200, 1989

72. Rubin J, Case G, Bower J: Comparison of rehabilitation in patients undergoing home dialysis. Continuous ambulatory or cyclic peritoneal dialysis vs home hemodialysis. *Arch Intern Med* 150: 1429, 1990

73. Haviland JW: Experiences in establishing a community artificial kidney center. *Trans Am Clin Clim Assoc* 77: 125, 1965

74. Rettig RA and Levinsky NG eds: *Kidney Failure and the Federal Government*. Washington DC, National Academy Press, 1991

75. Held PJ, Levin NW, Bovbjerg RR, Pauly MV, Diamond LH: Mortality and duration of hemodialysis treatment. *JAMA* 265: 871, 1991

76. Delmez JA, Windus DW and the St. Louis Nephrology Study Group: Hemodialysis prescription and delivery in a metropolitan community. *Kidney Int* 41: 1023, 1992

77. Farley DO: *Effects of Competition on Dialysis Facility Service Levels and Patient Selection*, Rand Graduate School, Santa Monica, CA, 1993

78. Mion C: Personal communication, 1994

79. Uldall R, Fraancoeur R, Ouwendyk M, Wallace L, Langos V, Ecclestone A, Vas S: Simplified nocturnal home hemodialysis (SNHHD). A new approach to renal replacement therapy. (Abstract) *JASN* 5(3): 428, 1994

LONG-TERM SURVIVAL IN DIALYSIS PATIENTS: A DEMOGRAPHIC OVERVIEW

C. JACOBS and N.H. SELWOOD

INTRODUCTION

Most of the data concerning survival of patients treated with maintenance dialysis therapies for end-stage renal disease (ESRD) published in the literature over the years are limited to up to 5–7 year survival after commencement of renal replacement therapy (RRT). This is true in particular for the data released on regular time-intervals through national or international renal data Registries such as the Registry of the European Dialysis and Transplant Association (EDTA-ERA) (1–3) or the United States Renal Data System (USRDS) (4), the Canadian Organ Transplant Register (5) or the Australia and New Zealand Dialysis and Transplant Registry (6). Comprehensive data relating to long-term survival for dialysis patients (10 or more years post start of treatment) are scarce (1) and usually display the experience of individual dialysis centres (7–11) or that of a small number of dialysis units operating within a limited geographical area (12). Overviews concerning experiences of very long survival on dialysis have also been reported on, or by, individual patients taken onto RRT during the early years of development of maintenance dialysis as a life-sustaining therapy for ESRD (13–16).

The EDTA-ERA Registry has been collecting data on patients submitted to various modes of RRT in the European countries and has published yearly a combined report on regular dialysis and transplantation in Europe for the past 23 years. As of December 1992, the Registry covered 36 countries located in Europe and in areas bordering the Mediterranean sea. 2762 Dialysis and Transplant Centres were known to the Registry with about 456,000 patients on file, among whom 168,214 were recorded as alive on RRT by December 1992 (2). This very comprehensive database which has been operating continuously for the past 25 years, thus provides an unique tool for a study on demographic and epidemiological aspects concerning the population of patients treated for up to 20–25 years by various modes of RRT.

METHODOLOGY

This study of long-term survivors is based on data collected on a yearly basis by the EDTA Registry through individual patient questionnaires which are completed and transmitted by the centres to the EDTA Registry Office in London (UK). The questionnaire records the patients' sex, date of birth, renal disease leading to ESRD, sequence of treatments according to time-course (hemodialysis (HD) peritoneal dialysis (PD), transplantation (TX) and also some technical features concerning dialysis therapy, transplantation management and the incidence and distribution of malignancies. The data processing and the resulting analyses are carried out on a VAX 3100 Computer System under the VMS operating system using applications software developed by Selwood (17).

The demographic and epidemiological analyses presented herein include patients reported as alive on 31 December 1992 and whose last known mode of therapy was hemodialysis (in-centre, satellite or home), whether or not HD had been preceded at some time by renal transplantation or peritoneal dialysis. Given the wide differences which have existed during the first two decades of implementation of RRT between many countries in Europe concerning the availability of dialysis or transplantation facilities as well as varying criteria for selection of patients for one or another (or not at all) technique of RRT, this survey of long survivors has been carried out according to a regional distribution of the European countries, a methodology which has been used in previous EDTA Registry reports (1).

The Western European Countries surveyed here were Austria, Belgium, France, West Germany, Luxembourg, the Netherlands, Switzerland and the United Kingdom. The average response rate to the patient-questionnaires in these 8 countries for the year 1992 was 71.3%, (ranging from 37% in the UK up to 100% in Luxembourg and the Netherlands).

Table 1. Patients alive on hemodialysis in December 1992

	Population (million)	Starting RRT 1974–1978		Starting RRT 1979–1983	
		N	pmp	N	pmp
East-Europ countries	90.1	138	1.5	5041	55.9
Mediter-countries	117.2	2110	18.0	4154	35.4
West-Europ countries	215.1	2752	12.8	5152	23.9
Nordic-countries	23	127	5.5	330	14.3
All four regions	445.4	5127	11.5	14677	32.9

The Mediterranean Countries included Greece, Italy, Portugal and Spain: the mean 1992 response-rate to the patient-questionnaires in these 4 countries was 62.7%, (ranging from 52% in Italy to 69% in Greece).

The Eastern European Countries comprised Bulgaria, (former) Czechoslovakia, Hungary and Poland. The mean 1992 patient-questionnaire response-rate for these 4 countries was 91.5% (72% for Czechoslovakia up to 100% in Bulgaria and Hungary).

The Nordic European Countries included Denmark, Finland, Norway and Sweden. The mean response-rate to the 1992 patient-questionnaires in these countries was 97.5%. The population figures of these countries used for calculating the prevalence data per million population (pmp) displayed hereunder are taken from the World Bank Atlas (1992 Edition).

RESULTS

In Table 1 are indicated the number and prevalence per million population (pmp) of patients alive on HD in December 1992 who were taken onto RRT in the years 1974 to 1978, that is 15 to 20 years ago. Almost no very long-term survivors are found in the Eastern European countries, most probably due to severe limitation of treatment facilities in these early times. The low prevalence of long survivors on HD in the Nordic countries may reflect the historically preferred strategy of renal transplantation as treatment for ESRD in these countries.

The picture changes notably for the patients who have started RRT in the 5 following years (1979–1983) that is 10 to 15 years ago. Here the highest stock of patients alive pmp on HD is now in the Eastern-European countries, most probably due to a delayed or very slow development of transplantation programmes in several of these countries. The same reason certainly applies to the Mediterranean countries, whereas the very active transplantation programmes developed in the Nordic countries may account for the rather small prevalence of long-term survivors currently maintained on HD therapy there.

Long-term survivors on RRT according to age at start of treatment

Figure 1 shows the distribution, according to age-groups at start of RRT, of patients alive on HD in December 1992 in the 4 above defined European regions and who had been taken on to RRT during the years 1974 to 1978, i.e., 15 to 20 years ago. Patients aged 15 to 34 years at start of RRT predominated in the East-European and Nordic countries and very likely being, at least in Nordic countries, the long-term survivors of previously transplanted patients having returned to HD after failure of one or more kidney grafts. There were 10% of patients who were aged 55 years or more when they started RRT between 15–20 years ago who were still alive on HD in the West European and Mediterranean Countries. By contrast, no such patients were recorded amongst the long survivors from East European countries.

The picture changes considerably for the population of patients taken onto RRT during the five following years (1979–1983), as shown in Figure 2. Here, 30% of the patients alive on HD in December 1992 in the East-European countries were aged 55 years or more at commencement of RRT more than 10 years earlier, a percentage similar to that recorded in the Western European countries. The high proportion of young patients (15–34 years at the start) on HD in the Nordic countries (33% *vs* about 20% in all the other three European areas) also probably reflects a more frequent than elsewhere temporary HD status prior to transplantation or after a failed transplant.

Long-time survivors according to primary renal disease (PRD)

The distribution of very long RRT survivors (starting treatment between 1974–1978) alive on HD in December 1992 according to their underlying renal disease is shown in Figure 3. Glomerulonephritis (GN) accounted for almost two thirds of the renal diseases identified in the few survivors recorded from the East-European countries, whilst patients with diabetic nephropathy or polycystic kidney disease (PCK: 5%) were 50 to 75% fewer than their coun-

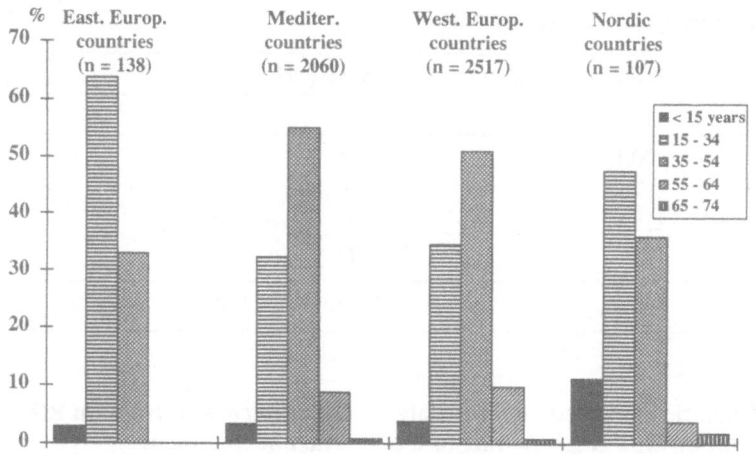

Figure 1. Patients alive on HD on 31st December 1992, who started RRT *between 1974–1978* according to age at initiation of RRT.

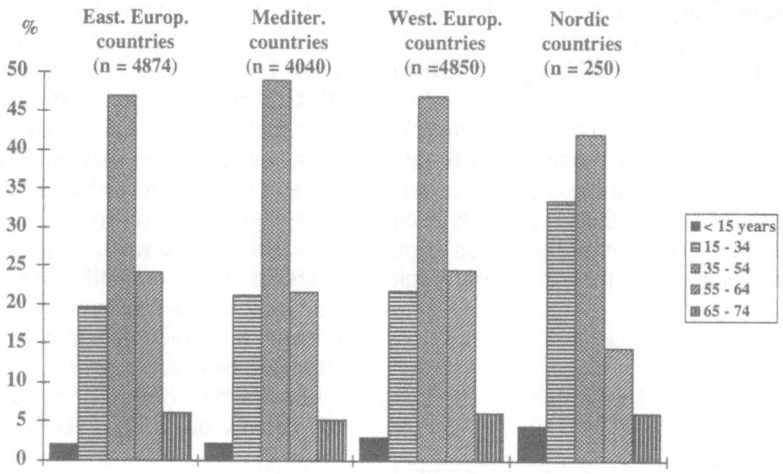

Figure 2. Patients alive on HD on 31st December 1992, who started RRT *between 1979–1983* according to age at initiation of RRT.

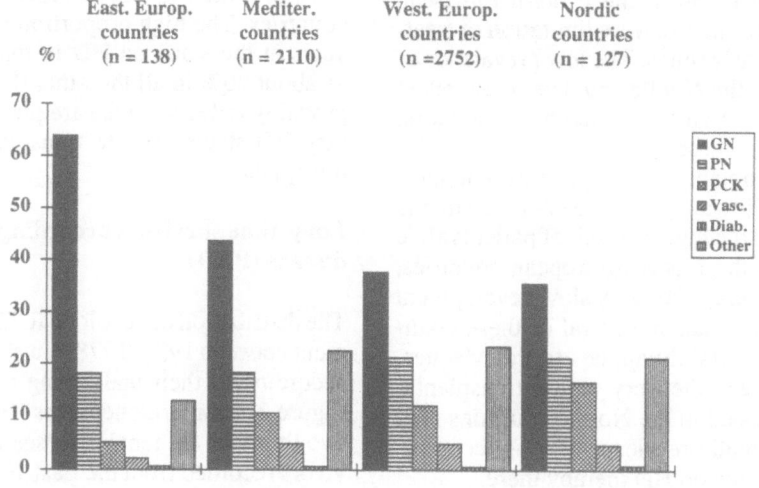

Figure 3. Patients alive on HD on 31st December 1992, who started RRT *between 1974–1978* according to underlying renal disease.

terparts recorded in the other European areas, very likely due to patient-selection according to age.

In the three other European areas, the proportions of long survivors with chronic pyelonephritis were similar at about 20%. Such was also the case for the very few patients with renal vascular diseases (less than 5%) whilst patients having diabetic nephropathy accounted for less than 1%, further indicating strong patient selection against this particular condition.

Among the patients who started RRT during the five following years (Figure 4), the proportions of those with primary GN ranges between 30% in the East, West and Mediterranean countries and 37% in the Nordic countries. Patients with PCK are now found in similar proportions in all the 4 investigated areas (around 14%), whereas diabetics now accounted for 1.2 to 2.6% of the survivors in three European Regions, the proportion being 3 to 5 times higher in the Nordic countries. This latter observation reflects the generally higher incidence of diabetes and its renal complications in some Nordic countries and a consequent stimulus to provide RRT in such patients (18–20).

Survival according to time on RRT

The differences evidenced according to time and geographical areas in Europe are confirmed by the results obtained in distributing the patient-populations more precisely into those submitted to RRT for less or more than 10 years and alive on HD by December 1992 (Table 2). Indeed, the number of patients pmp surviving for less than 10 years in the Eastern European Countries was 10 times higher than for those who had undergone RRT for more than 10 years. The higher prevalence of HD in patients treated for less than 10 years in the Mediterranean Countries similarly reflects the low contribution of transplantation in several of these countries (2), whereas it can be assumed that the relatively small number of patients remaining on HD in the Nordic countries may be composed mainly of those having returned to HD after a failed transplant.

The overall male to female ratio of patients submitted to RRT for more and less than 10 years having, or not, been temporarily transplanted and alive on HD in December 1992 is 1.15 and 1.31 respectively. The highest male predominance (1.47) is recorded in patients treated for less than 10 years and surviving on HD in the Nordic countries. An almost identical percentage of male and female long-term (> 10 years) survivors is found in the Western European countries, being 49.8 and 50.1% respectively (Table 3).

Tables 4 and 5 show the numbers, prevalence pmp and sex distribution of patients alive by December 1992 in the 4 defined European regions, according to whether the patients had or not received a kidney transplant at any time during their period on RRT.

Among the patients who had undergone RRT for more than 10 years (Table 4), the highest prevalence pmp of never grafted patients is found in the Mediterranean countries where no active transplantation programme was operative in the seventies or early eighties (21). In contrast, a very low prevalence pmp of long-term survivors on HD is recorded in the Eastern European and Nordic countries, for the already above indicated reasons, i.e., severe restrictions in patient uptake on RRT in the former countries and, on the other hand, as a result of a permanently active transplantation programme in the latter.

In the patients having received a kidney graft at some time, the male to female ratio is notably higher than in the group of non-grafted patients, with the exception of the Nordic countries where also the higher prevalence pmp of patients alive on HD at the end of 1992 may be the consequence of patients having returned to dialysis after a failed transplant.

Among the patients submitted to RRT for less than 10 years (Table 5), the prevalence pmp of never grafted patients alive on HD by December 1992 in the Eastern European countries has considerably increased (almost twentyfold) as compared to those having commenced RRT during the preceding decade (91 pmp vs 5.7). The high prevalence pmp of never grafted patients recorded in the Mediterranean Countries (216 pmp) results from a rapid development of dialysis facilities during the 1980s, mainly in Spain and Portugal, whilst transplantation either could not be offered or was considered as contra-indicated for an increasing number of patients taken onto RRT. As surmised above, the almost twofold difference in prevalence of previously grafted patients maintained on HD in the Nordic Countries vs the other European Regions may reflect the return to HD of patients with a failed kidney transplant.

Causes of death according to duration of renal replacement therapy

Causes of death have been analyzed for the patients who were taken onto RRT between 1974 and 1978 and who died while being treated with HD after less or more than 10 years after start of RRT (Figures 5 and 6).

In all the 4 European areas, cardiac causes of death were found in comparable proportions as well for patients submitted to RRT for more than 10 years (ranging between 36% and 40% in the Mediterranean and Nordic countries, respectively, (Figure 5) as in those who died after less than 10 years on RRT (Figure 6). Vascular causes of death were also found in similar proportions among the populations of patients in the 4 European areas, ranging between 13% and 19% of causes of death, culminating however at 22% in patients treated for less than 10 years in the Mediterranean countries.

Deaths from infectious causes were found to be highest in the East European and Nordic countries among patients who had been submitted to RRT for more than 10 years,

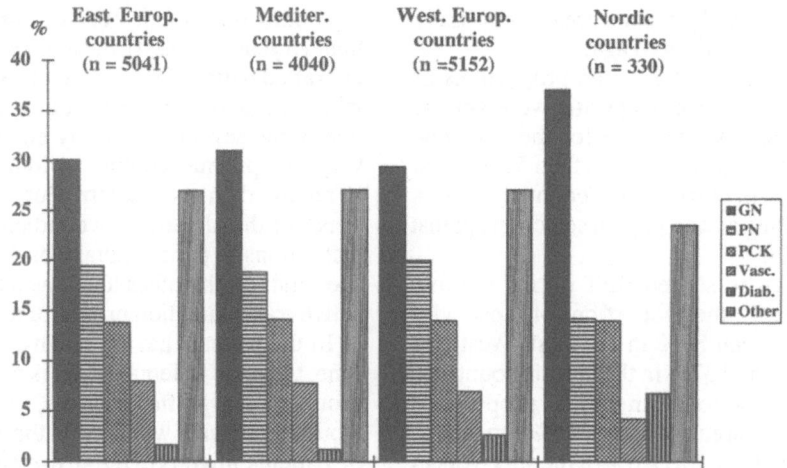

Figure 4. Patients alive on HD on 31st December 1992, who started RRT *between 1979–1983* according to underlying renal disease.

Table 2. Patients alive on hemodialysis in December 1992 on RRT for more or less than 10 years

	Population (million)	On RRT > 10 years		On RRT < 10 years	
		N	pmp	N	pmp
East-Europ countries	90.1	872	9.7	8779	97.4
Mediter-countries	117.2	7709	65.8	25973	221.6
West-Europ countries	215.1	6823	31.7	29151	135.5
Nordic-countries	23	507	22.0	3174	138
All four regions	445.4	15911	35.7	67077	15.6

Table 3. Distribution according to sex of patients alive on hemodialysis in December 1992, on RRT for more or less than 10 years, having on not been transplanted at some time

	On RRT > 10 years				On RRT < 10 years			
	N	Male %	Female %	M/F	N	Male %	Female %	M/F
East-Europ countries	872	58.7	41.3	1.42	8779	55.7	44.3	1.26
Mediter-countries	7709	56.3	43.7	1.29	25973	58.2	41.8	1.39
West-Europ countries	6823	49.9	50.1	0.99	29151	55.5	44.5	1.25
Nordic-countries	507	53.6	46.4	1.16	3174	59.5	40.5	1.47
All four regions	15911	54.6	45.4	1.15	67077	56.8	43.2	1.31

Table 4. Patients alive on hemodialysis in December 1992 never grafted or grafted at some time. Total RRT > 10 years

	Patients never grafted				Patients grafted at some time			
	All patients N	pmp	Male %	Female %	All patients N	pmp	Male %	Female %
East-Europ countries	515	5.7	56.1	43.9	357	4.0	62.5	37.5
Mediter-countries	6271	53.5	54.4	45.6	1438	12.3	64.4	35.6
West-Europ countries	4887	22.7	46.4	53.6	1936	9.0	58.5	41.5
Nordic-countries	153	6.6	44.4	55.6	354	15.4	57.6	42.4
All four regions	11826	26.5	51	49	4085	9.2	60.8	39.2

Table 5. Patients alive on hemodialysis in December 1992 never grafted or grafted at some time. Total RRT < 10 years

	Patients never grafted				Patients grafted at some time			
	All patients N	pmp	Male %	Female %	All patients N	pmp	Male %	Female %
East-Europ countries	8222	91	55.5	44.5	557	6.2	57.3	42.7
Mediter-countries	25324	216	58.1	41.9	649	5.5	62.4	37.6
West-Europ countries	28122	131	55.4	44.6	1029	4.8	59.9	40.1
Nordic-countries	2894	126	59.5	40.5	280	12.2	59.6	40.4
All four regions	64562	145	56.6	43.4	2515	5.6	59.9	40.1

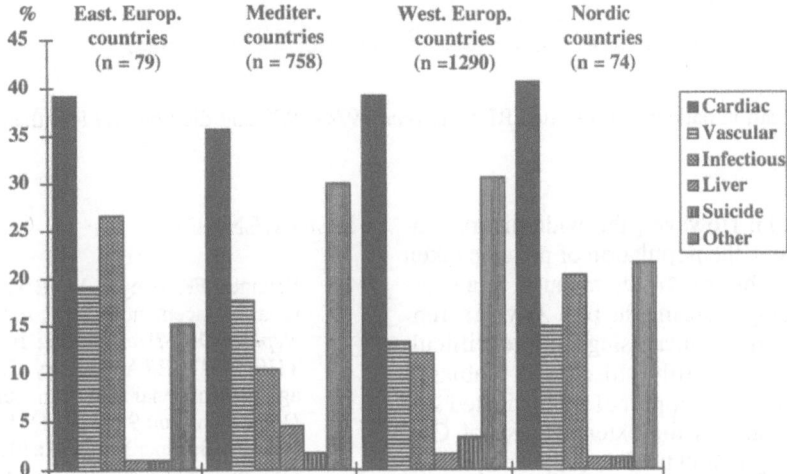

Figure 5. Causes of death in patients who started RRT *between 1974–1978* and died on HD more than 10 years after initiation of RRT.

being 27 and 20% respectively. A similar profile is found in patients submitted to RRT for less than 10 years (22 and 19% of all deaths). As suggested by the data presented above in this study, these lethal infections most probably occurred in long-term dialysis patients in the East-European countries and in previously transplanted patients in the Nordic countries. Less than 1% of deaths attributed to suicide or abandonment of treatment are reported for either group of patients in the East-European countries whereas these causes amounted to 3.2% of the deaths reported among the patients treated for less than 10 years who had died in the Nordic countries. This latter finding may reflect a higher suicide rate observed amongst the general population in some of the Scandinavian countries.

COMMENTS AND CONCLUSION

Less than 40 years ago terminal chronic renal failure was a 100% lethal disease. The mere fact that during the last two decades several thousands of patients in Europe did experience a 15–20 year survival on various modes of RRT, as documented in this study, clearly demonstrates the extraordinary performances that have been achieved with dialysis therapies and renal transplantation for sustaining life in patients otherwise doomed to an unavoidable death. These results, most certainly, exceed the most audacious expectations of the early pioneers in the field at a time when survival in uremic patients submitted to maintenance HD was registered in days or in months (22–24).

During the sixties and seventies the populations of patients having access to RRT increased rapidly in most of the economically developed countries and progressively included patients of increasing age and/or with more or less numerous serious co-morbid clinical conditions associated with renal insufficiency. Simultaneously, extensive knowledge on the pathophysiology of the uremic state was acquired while major technical advances improving the efficacy and safety of the dialysis techniques, as well as methods for assessing more objectively their performances and the results achieved, were made widely available to the medical community (25–27).

Amongst all the criteria that are taken into acount for assessing the 'adequacy' of dialysis treatments, patients'-

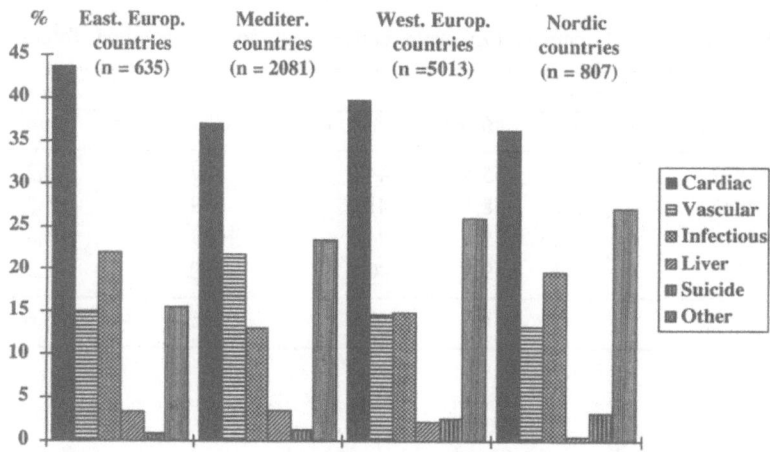

Figure 6. Causes of death in patients who started RRT *between 1974–1978* and died on HD less than 10 years after initiation of RRT.

survival ranks first (11). However, the wide diversification and heterogeneity in the population of patients taken onto RRT, as well as that of the therapeutic strategies which have been developed during the past 25 years, renders patient-survival studies increasingly more difficult to perform satisfactorily for truly objective or unbiased interpretations, even with the support of sophisticated statistical methods (28) such as the extensive use of Cox proportional hazards regression models (29). The present study did not attempt discussing the influence on patient-survival of on-going widely debated issues concerning various hemodialysis strategies (30–33), or the criteria used for assessing quantitative and qualitative results of RRT (34–36). Neither did we attempt comparing long-term survival between patients treated by HD or CAPD (37, 38) all the more so as, most probably, less than 100 patients worldwide have thus far been maintained exclusively on CAPD for 10 or more years (39).

The merely descriptive demographic data on a very large sample of patients having survived on RRT for as long as 20 years in four European geographical areas reflects well the impact on survival of modalities of patient-selection procedures and of the qualitative and quantitative availability of treatment methods in the different countries, depending on socio-economic factors, medical options and health-care policies.

In addition to purely medical and technical issues, these factors will certainly continue to play a key-role in the long-term results which will be achieved in the future for patients submitted to RRT, insofar as providing the most appropriate and safest mode of treatment for each individual patient at the lowest possible cost (36) still remains an unachieved goal for a large fraction of the population of terminally uremic patients worldwide.

REFERENCES

1. Brunner FP, Broyer M, Brynger H, et al.. Survival on renal replacement therapy: data from the EDTA Registry. *Nephrol Dial Transplant* 2: 109, 1988
2. THE EDTA-ERA Registry Committee: Report on management of renal failure in Europe XXIII, 1992. *Nephrol Dial Transplant* 9 (Suppl 1): 5, 1994
3. Held PJ, Brunner FP, Odaka M, Garcia JR, Port FK, Gaylin DS: Five-year survival for end stage renal disease patients in the United States, Europe and Japan 1982 to 1987. *Am J Kidney Dis* 15: 451, 1990
4. United States Renal Data System: USRDS 1989–1993 Annual Data Reports: The National Institutes of Health, National Institute of Diabetes and Digestive and Kidney Diseases, Bethesda, MD
5. Canadian Organ Replacement Register: Annual Report 1992. Canadian Institute of Information on Health. Don Mills (Ont) 195, 1994
6. Disney APS (ed): The 16th report of the Australia and New Zealand Dialysis and Transplant Registry (ANZDATA). Queen Elisabeth Hosp-Woodville, Adelaide, South Australia, 1994, p 60
7. Baillod RA, Vargheze Z, Fernando ON, Moorhead JF: Review of 71 patients receiving renal replacement for more than 10 years. in *Uremia: Pathobiology of Patients Treated for 10 Years or More*, edited by Giordano C, Friedman EA, Milan, Wichtig Editore, 1981, p 35
8. Zingraff J, Man NK, Drueke T, Jungers P, Crosnier J, Funck-Brentano JL: Long-term results in 40 uremic patients treated by hemodialysis for more than 10 years. in *Uremia: Pathobiology of Patients Treated for 10 Years or More*, edited by Giordano C, Friedman EA, Milan, Wichtig Editore, 1981, p 50
9. Laurent G, Calemard E, Charra B: Long dialysis: a review of 15 years experience in one centre 1968–1983. *Proc Eur Dial Transplant Ass* 20: 122, 1983
10. Raja R, Kramer M, Goldstein S, Caruana R, Lerner A: Short hemodialysis: 10 year follow-up. *Trans Am Soc Artif Int Org* 23: 374, 1986

11. Charra B, Calemard E, Ruffet M, Chazot Ch, Terrat JC, Vannel Th, Laurent G: Survival as index of adequacy of dialysis. *Kidney Int* 41: 1286, 1992
12. Iseki K, Kawasoe N, Osawa A, Fukiyama K: Survival analysis of dialysis patients in Okinawa, Japan (1971–1990). *Kidney Int* 43: 404, 1993
13. Eady RAJ: A patient's experience of over thousand hemodialyses. *Proc Eur Dial Transpl Assoc* 8: 50, 1971
14. Drukker W: Hemodialysis: a historical review. in *Replacement of Renal Function by Dialysis*, 3rd Edition, edited by Maher JF, Dordrecht, Kluwer Academic Publishers, 1989, p 21
15. Lundin, PA III: Prolonged survival on hemodialysis. in: *Replacement of Renal Function by Dialysis*, 3rd Edition, edited by Maher JF, Dordrecht, Kluwer Academic Publishers, 1989, p 1133
16. Scribner BH: A personalized history of chronic hemodialysis. *Am J Kidney Dis* 16: 511, 1990
17. Broyer M, Brunner FP, Brynger H, Donckerwolcke RA, Jacobs C, Kramer P, Selwood NH, Wing AJ: Combined report on regular dialysis and transplantation in Europe XIII. *Proc Eur Dial Transpl Assoc* 20: 13, 1983
18. Andersen AR, Christiansen JS, Andersen JT, Kreiner S, Deckert T: Diabetic nephropathy in type I (insulin-dependent) diabetes: an epidemiological study. *Diabetologia* 4: 97, 1985
19. Karvonen M, Tuomilehto J, Libmen I, Laporte R: A review of the recent epidemiological data on the worldwide incidence of type I (insulin-dependent) Diabetes Mellitus. *Diabetologia* 36: 883, 1993
20. Olivarius ND, Andreasen AH, Keiding N, Mögensen CE: Epidemiology of renal involment in newly diagnosed middle-aged and elderly diabetic patients. Cross sectional data from the population-based study diabetes care in general practice, Denmark. *Diabetologia* 36: 1007, 1993
21. Kramer P, Broyer M, Brunner FP, Brynger H, Doncker Wolke RA, Jacobs C, Selwood NH, Wing AJ: Combined report on regular dialysis and transplantation in Europe XII. *Proc Eur Dial Transpl Assoc* 19: 4, 1982
22. Scribner BH, Buri R, Caner JEZ, Hegstrom R, Burnell JM: The treatment of chronic uremia by means of intermittent dialysis: a preliminary report. *Trans Am Soc Artif Int Organs* 6: 114, 1960
23. Maher JF, Schreiner GE, Waters TJ. Successful intermittent hemodialysis: longest reported maintenance of life in true oliguria (181 days). *Trans Am Soc Artif Int Organs* 6: 123, 1960
24. Hegstrom RM, Murray JS, Pendras JR, Burnell JM, Scribner BH: Two-years experience with periodical hemodialysis in the treatment of chronic uremia. *Trans Am Soc Artif Int Organs* 8: 266, 1962
25. Van Holder RC, Ringoir SM: Adequacy of dialysis: a critical analysis. *Kidney Int* 42: 540, 1991
26. Hakim RM, Depner TA, Parker TF III: Adequacy of hemodialysis. *Am J Kidney Dis* 20: 107, 1992
27. Gotch T, Sargent JA: A mechanistic analysis of the National Cooperative dialysis study. *Kidney Int* 28: 526, 1985
28. United States Renal Data System: USRDS 1993 Annual Data Report, Section XIII: Analytical methods: technical notes. The National Institutes of Health, National Institute for Diabetes and Digestive and Kidney Diseases. Bethesda, MD, 1993, p 119
29. Cox DR: Regression models and life table. *JR Stat Soc (13)* 34: 187, 1972
30. Wizemann V, Kramer W: Short term dialysis, long-term complications: ten years experience with short duration renal replacement therapy. *Blood Purif* 5: 193, 1987
31. Held PJ, Levin NW, Bovbjerg RR, Pauly MV, Diamond LH: Mortality and duration of hemodialysis treatment. *JAMA* 265: 84, 1991
32. Charra B: Does empirical long slow dialysis result in better survival? If so, how and why? *ASAIO J* 39: 819, 1993
33. Parker TF III, Husni L, Huang W, Nancy L, Lowrie EG and Dallas Nephrology Associates: Survival of hemodialysis patients in the United States is improved with a greater quantity of dialysis. *Am J Kidney Dis* 23: 670, 1994
34. Gotch F, Sargent JA: A mechanistic analysis of the National Cooperative Dialysis Study (NCDS). *Kidney Int* 28: 528, 1985
35. Shaldon S: Unanswered questions pertaining to dialysis adequacy in 1992. *Kidney Int* 43 (Suppl 1): S274, 1993
36. National Institutes of Health Consensus Conference: Statement on morbidity and mortality of renal dialysis. *Ann Int Med* 121: 62, 1994
37. Maiorca R, Vonesh E, Cancarini GC et al.: A six-year comparison of patient and technique survivals in CAPD and HD. *Kidney Int* 34: 518, 1988
38. Wolfe RA, Port FK, Hawthorne VM, Guire KE: A comparison of survival among dialytic therapies of choice. *Am J Kidney Dis* 15: 443, 1990
39. Nolph KD: Update on peritoneal dialysis worldwide. *Perit Dial Intern* 13 (Suppl 2): 15, 1993

PART A: THE WORK OF THE REGISTRIES FOR RENAL DISEASE AND RENAL FAILURE: A CRITICAL REVIEW

N.P. MALLICK

Registries for renal disease have developed principally to track the way in which patients with end stage renal failure have been managed. The first such Registry was developed by the European Dialysis and Transplantation Association in the 1960's and then dealt principally with countries in the West of Europe where both dialysis and transplantation were being used as forms of renal replacement therapy.

In the earlier days it was exciting to watch the way in which more patients in ever more countries were treated and the way too in which the technology to treat them developed. Each meeting of the EDTA from its inception in 1964 for the next decade or so had its highlights in evidence of the tenacity of both patients and staff.

Today the management of patients by dialysis and transplantation is a much more established matter. As yet it is principally in Europe (now both 'East' and 'West'), in the United States, in Japan and in Australasia that attempts have been made comprehensively to provide services for all patients with end stage renal failure who require it from the earliest years of life to the eighth and ninth decades. Such explosive development has not been without its burdens both financial to the countries concerned and physical, mental and emotional to the staff, patients, and relatives involved. Nevertheless the frontiers have slowly been pushed back both by widening of age bands for patients for whom treatment can be achieved successfully and in another direction the widening of the range of conditions causing end stage renal failure (with associated co-morbidity) for which this form of therapy can be utilised.

While year on year change is barely perceptible both in the nature of patient population being treated and in the success or otherwise of the methods used to treat, overall the figures are impressive. The EDTA Registry covering as it does nearly 700,000,000 people in 36 countries treated in some 2,760 centres has records on 162,214 living patients and the end of 1992 on 456,055 who are or who have been managed by renal replacement therapy since the mid 1960s. Some details of the present database for other Registries are given in Table 1, together with the length of time for which they have collected data.

It can be recognised that Registries have charted the near explosive development of the stock of patients on

Table 1.

Country/ies	Data from	Population (m)	Total RRT 1992	PMP
Aust/NZ	1971	21.2	8788	414
Canada	1981	27.4	14211	518.5
Europe	1966	668.9	173404[a]	259[a]
United States	1988	255.4	188745[b]	739
Japan	1983	124.3	123926	996

[a] Data not complete.
[b] At end 1991.

renal replacement therapy. Also they have shown the increased longevity of these patients over the years (see succeeding chapters) and indicated the change in the percentage of patients with particular disease for whom treatment has been offered as confidence has increased in the effectiveness of renal replacement therapy (Figure 1). The ANZDATA has produced impressive data on their comprehensive analysis of these and associated matters.

Renal failure arises in individuals who otherwise are healthy, or in those with other illnesses. This is of importance for the future work of Registries in relation to the value of renal replacement therapy. Only recently has it been fully recognised that co-morbid illnesses – that is disease in organs other than the kidney, or disease which has arisen alongside the renal disease and is linked to the metabolic and other pathophysiological changes which accompany renal failure, is critically important in determining the benefit of RRT to individual patients. Thus, most of the data presently available subsumes the impact of *already established* disease on patients after RRT has commenced. As Port et al. point out in their chapter unaddressed these co-morbid factors significantly affect outcome.

The clear message from these studies to date both by Registries and others is that there is a need to look during the pre-end stage phase of renal disease (or even earlier than this) if such co-morbidity is to be minimised or treated and so the value of renal replacement therapy

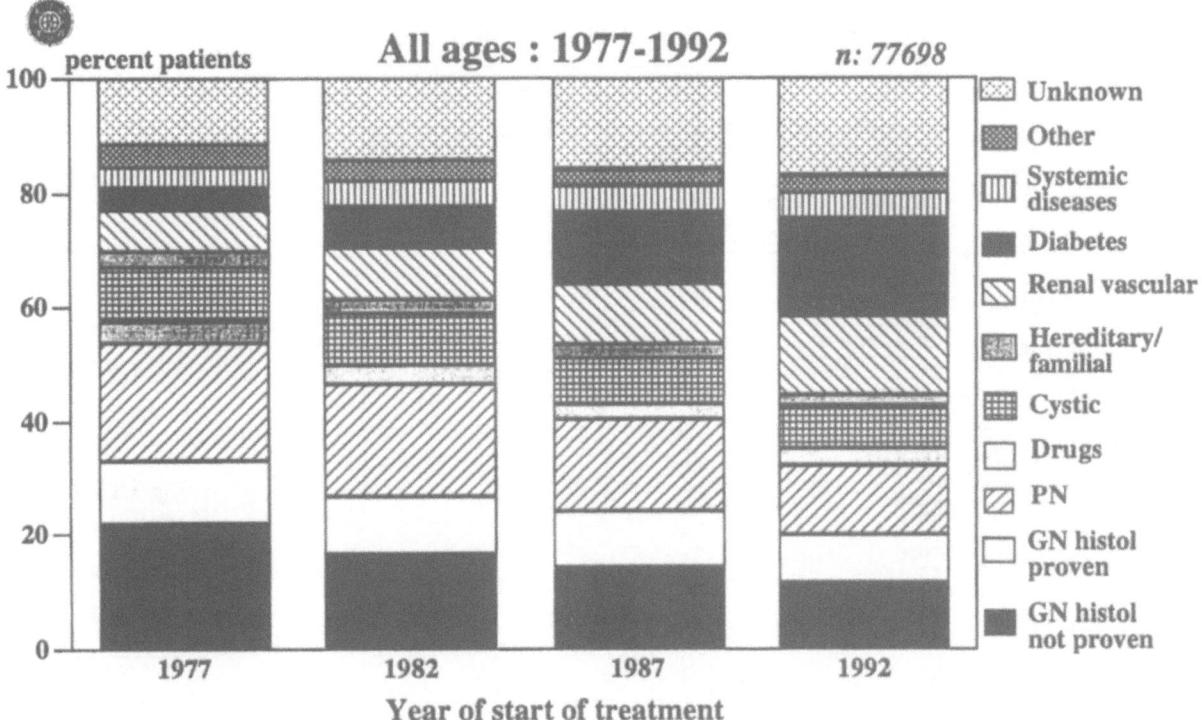

Figure 1.

enhanced. It must be recognised, too, that careful analysis of the influence of pre-existing comorbid conditions on the outcome of RRT may result in the conclusion, in some cases, that the cost-benefit of commencing RRT may be unacceptable, and that a patient is unlikely to have from RRT the gain in life and life quality that makes the therapy worthwhile.

The relatively simple database constructed for all patients in most Registries has been very valuable in pointing to the changing age pattern of new patients and of the stock of patients on therapy, to the changing pattern of primary renal disease from which they suffer and to the causes of death and to a lesser extent (because of data only just becoming available) on morbidity. The data on age are instructive. In some countries such as Italy the median age of entering renal replacement therapy is already 65. Thus one half of patients commencing therapy is already in the phase of formal retirement. However, whereas the median age for patients commencing RRT has risen by some 7 years across Europe as a whole (47 to nearly 60 years) in the last decade, the median age of the stock of patients has risen only by a year or so since 1977. This is because older patients die more quickly on dialysis and it is not yet clear whether this is inherently due to their naturally shorter life span (the figure suggests that death on renal replacement therapy is still significantly faster for any given age population than that of those without

such disease) or because of the impact of co-morbidity or other factors.

Furthermore, it must be remembered that well over 95% of all renal patients are managed in the home attending units for haemodialysis, or for assessment of CAPD, or for transplant follow-up. The majority of their time is in the community. This has a significant impact on their families and their work pattern. The, now many, retired and elderly patients treated by RRT provide a challenge to the social infrastructure and services available for the elderly, who are so often socially more isolated than their younger counterparts, even when in good health. Thus, the involvement of community services needs to be carefully charted by Registries across the world just as there is a need for a more careful examination of the impact of different morbid factors present before end stage has been reached on the quality of RRT.

Data have been instructive in a number of ways. For instance, it has been possible to chart the gradual decline of analgesic nephropathy as a cause of renal failure over the years, (Figure 2), to assess the potential neoplastic risk both of dialysis and transplantation, to investigate the cardiovascular risk in end stage renal failure at different ages and in different countries. However, the cross-sectional nature of much information and the difficulty in checking precisely the diagnostic criteria used both in the diagnosis of renal disease (for example, whether renal biopsy has been carried our or not or whether renovascular disease

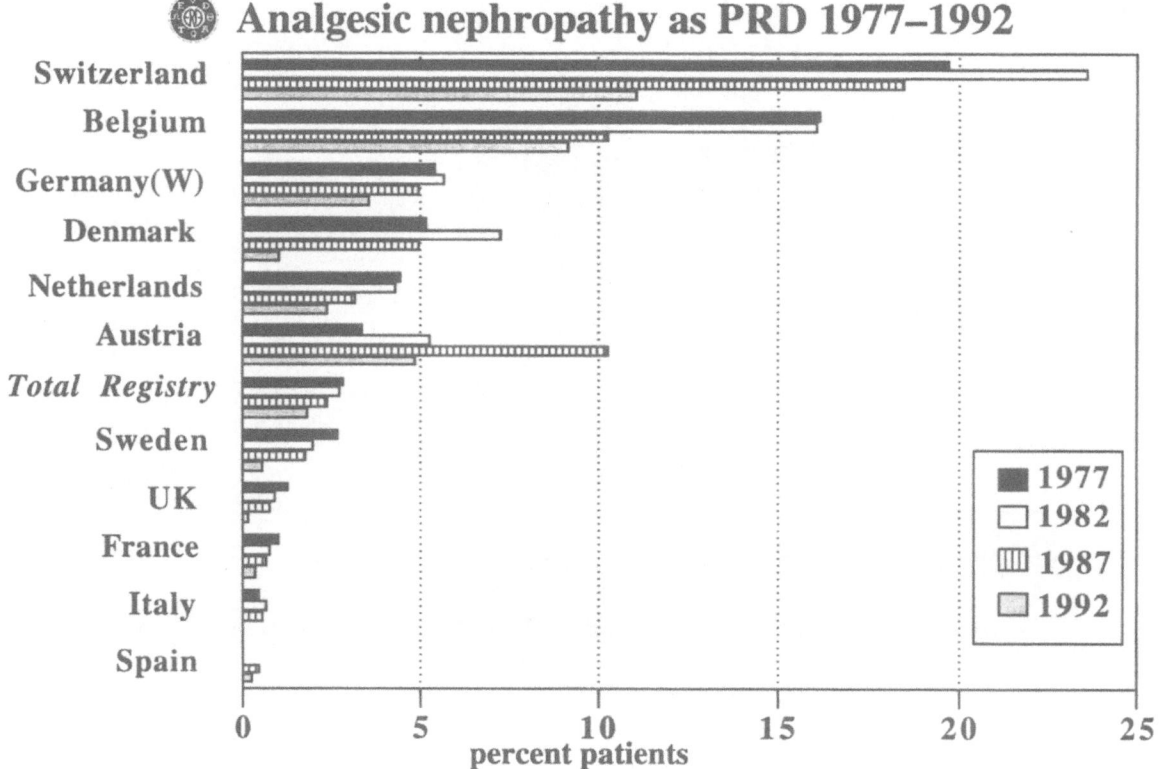

Figure 2.

has been diagnosed directly or inferred), or in charting complications (for example, on what criteria myocardial ischaemia or infarction have been diagnosed) make it difficult retrospectively to analyse the whole database.

It is clear that in order for this to be done large Registries such as the European one need to address their database on a more regional basis and this is more readily achieved if National Registries are developed and, if these National Registries have a sub-regional structure themselves. In this way the comprehensiveness of data returns can be checked locally and criteria on which particular categories are defined can be agreed. It then becomes possible to examine much more closely the way in which renal failure is managed and to assess the impact of various interventions (for example, the management of established cardiac disease before RRT commences, the careful control of blood pressure, the better control and support of patients with diabetic nephropathy, the assessment of the elderly in terms of their social as well as physical requirements once RRT is developed, exclusion criteria for transplantation). In this way it is possible to develop a sound base form which international comparisons can truly be established.

In some countries, notably the United States and Japan, quite precise figures are available for the cost of the renal replacement programme. These are not negligible. Thus, in the United States some \$30 per citizen, per year, is spent on the programme and in Japan this is over \$50. Put another way, 0.6–0.8% of the population might be consuming for renal services some 3% of the national health care budget.

Necessarily therefore as the stock of patients on renal replacement therapy rises, Governments are forced to take account of the costs this programme is entailing. It is incumbent on us to ensure that a cost effective service is maintained. There are a number of ways of addressing this. The first might be to determine the eventual stock of patients and the balance within that stock which is probable regarding patients surviving either with a functioning graft or on various forms of dialysis. At present these are difficult to assess individually. No consensus has emerged that CAPD or haemodialysis is the 'better' option overall and, indeed it is generally thought that either form of therapy can be effective in given patients and sometimes sequentially in the same patient, depending on clinical and other considerations.

While transplantation is generally accepted to be the optimal mode of therapy since it returns patients if successful to a near normal mode of life, the constraints on organ donation across the world makes it impracticable to consider transplantation for every patient who requires renal replacement therapy and, in any case, fac-

Table 2. Risk groups used in recent analysis of EDTA data

Standard	Age 15–54	No diabetes
Medium	Age 54–64	Diabetic 15–54
High	Age 65+	Diabetic 55+

tors such as co-morbidity, particularly cardiovascular disease or advanced age, in which the predicted life of the patient may be less than the predicted potential life of a graft, inevitably provide some modifying influences on who or who does not have a donor kidney offered.

Over and above these considerations it seems probable that the refined immunogenetic approaches now becoming available will increase confidence that proper typing and matching of donor and recipient is a better option that a mismatched graft with all the potential for possible enhanced rejection and of increased sensitisation of patients to previously unencountered HLA antigens. Despite many years of research the immunogenetic analysis of patient and graft has some way to go and remains a challenging field. Overall, therefore the lack of free access to donor organs will, for the foreseeable future, put a constraint on the cost effectiveness of renal replacement therapy, since inevitably some patients will be dialysed for whom transplantation would be a better option and there is the likelihood that a graft would be offered to those for whom there is the best chance of long term graft (as well as patient) survival. Registries have a pivotal role in focussing on the consequences both of 'good' tissue matching in ensuring optimal graft survival and on the consequences for an RRT programme of the restricted availability of organs for grafting.

In a number of European countries where transplantation has been practised actively some 50% of the renal replacement stock survives on a functioning graft. The proportion of patients on different dialysis modes differs widely. In Britain, for example, some 50% of the dialysis stock is on CAPD but this is much less in other European countries and somewhat less too in the United States There is also an age difference. Thus, in patients over 65 in Europe, only 2% of the stock of patients survive on a functioning transplant, the vast majority of the rest being on centre haemodialysis.

The complexity of the patient population and the choice of modality offered across the age and disease spectrum, varying in any case as it does form country to country, makes proper prediction of the likely eventual out-turn for the stock on renal replacement therapy very difficult. Nevertheless, this can be tackled. We and others (Wood, Roderick and Mallick unpublished) have recently revised our earlier modelling of stock at steady state (that is at which one patient entering the programme is balanced by one leaving it at death) and used EDTA and other data to establish survival rates and to estimate the steady state renal replacement therapy stock in risk groups

(see Table 2). It is possible then to produce an array of survival predictions which enable the pattern of eventual renal replacement stock to be determined according to the percentage of patients in each of the risk groups.

Taking recent evidence from the United Kingdom, that the percentage of patients being accepted in each group is standard risk 35%, medium risk 24%, high risk 41%, it is possible to predict that eventually if 30 kidneys per million population are available and at a take on rate of 80 per million population on average (an apparently realistic figure for a Caucasian population up to the age of 80), some 663 patients per million population might be on renal replacement therapy, of whom 273 would be transplanted, a ratio of dialysis to transplantation of 1.33 to 1. Figures can be adjusted according to take on rate and are robust to a 10% change in expected life as calculated on the whole EDTA database. Given such calculations it is possible to predict the likely cost of the programme but this only after fully accounting for the distribution of facilities to manage that programme and of the staff required for it too. Since take-on rates differ in ethnic groups a similar calculation can be applied to them too so that in any given country with a mixed ethnicity the overall take-on rate and predicted stock rates can be determined and the cost managing these programmes brought in to perspective.

The management of renal failure is an important but not the only aspect of renal disease for which Registries can be of service. The management of acute renal failure itself is posing increasing challenges in all countries particularly as the shift in the nature of the patients who develop this complication has changed. Many more patients now sustain acute renal failure when they are older and have complicating illnesses such as cardiovascular disease or other major trauma or surgery. On the other hand, it is less frequent in countries with well established obstetric services to see the earlier problems of septic abortion or of postpartum renal failure. From time to time, Registries have looked carefully at this problem across countries and in Europe, across the continent and the Mediterranean littoral which the EDTA Registry covers.

The nature of renal disease itself varies across the continent and across nations. It is well established now that some ethnic groups have a higher preponderance of renal failure than others and some of course have a higher preponderance of either type I (IDDM) or type II (NIDDM) diabetes mellitus. The diagnostic criteria for these groups needs particular assessment because of the influence of uraemia, and it is important to establish the way in which patients with diabetes mellitus are managed in different countries or regions. It is particularly relevant to see whether the involvement together of diabetologist and nephrologist, early in the course of diabetic nephropathy will result in decreased morbidity in this vulnerable group of patients as they approach end stage renal failure and require renal replacement therapy.

It is possible too through the use of both immunogenetic and clinical data to chart carefully the course of transplantation in different groups of patients selected either by disease, by age, by co-morbidity or by a combination of these factors.

For many of the purposes outlined above, prospective studies, in which a variety of factors must be charted carefully, are more likely to produce authoritative findings that retrospective or cross-sectional studies in which the full database required has not been obtained. Of course much depends here on the extent to which very detailed returns on each patient treated can be commanded by a Registry. If registration of patients in this way is not compulsory, only a basic data set for each patient may be obtainable. Then the collection of more detailed data requires prospective cohort studies. If however renal units are required to provide detailed data

on each of their patients on a regular basis, it is possible more readily to use the established database for the studies which are needed.

In either case the co-operation of experts both nephrologists and others in determining the sort of problems which should be addressed and in establishing the appropriate way in which these should be analysed is important. Integral to such groups of experts should be adequate statistical support to ensure that studies are properly structured. The Registries already established in the world are moving in this direction. They have the responsibility to show the way forward as other Registries develop in the very large portion of our world in which therapy for end stage renal failure remains yet unavailable.

PART B: OUTCOMES WITH ESRD THERAPY:
A CRITICAL OVERVIEW FROM THE UNITED STATES

FRIEDRICH K. PORT, MARC N. TURENNE and PHILIP J. HELD

INTRODUCTION

Patient survival is a very basic but important outcome of any therapeutic intervention. In the case of end stage renal disease (ESRD), outcome studies have included several other outcomes such as quality of life indicators, morbidity measures (e.g., hospitalizations), length of time on a treatment modality ('technique survival') and survival with a functioning kidney allograft (graft survival). The establishment of regional and national registries has markedly facilitated the evaluation of these outcomes in actual practice rather than in the referral practice or related multicenter environment. This chapter will focus primarily on population-based patient survival studies using information from the United States Renal Data System (USRDS) and the Michigan Kidney Registry.

METHODS FOR OUTCOMES RESEARCH

Survival probabilities can be estimated by an actuarial survival technique such as the Kaplan–Meier methodology (1). This approach describes the percent surviving at each point in time, while accounting for patients withdrawn from the analysis (censored), e.g., because of loss to follow-up, end of study, or, in the case of dialysis patient survival, renal transplantation. Such survival curves have frequently shown a steeper decline during the early months after initiation of ESRD therapy or early post transplantation, with a nearly constant death rate thereafter. When comparing survival curves on different modalities or for different patient groups (e.g., males versus females), it is important to consider differences in known predictors of survival such as differences in age between groups. This can be accomplished statistically by adjusting for the distribution of basic parameters such as age, sex, race, cause of ESRD and treatment modality. This approach is also useful for the assessment of time trends in actuarial survival by year of therapy, e.g.,

trends in first-year survival among patients starting ESRD therapy during different calendar years.

Adjusted analyses for comparative outcome studies can also be approached using a multifactorial analysis such as the Cox proportional hazards model (2). This methodology describes the relative mortality risk for one patient or treatment group relative to another group, labeled the reference group. A relative risk greater than 1.0 indicates a mortality risk greater than in the reference group. This approach provides for a more detailed analysis, allowing one simultaneously to examine the risk associated with such factors while adjusting for numerous other factors known to influence survival. This multivariate Cox analysis studies the days until death or until follow-up is censored, whichever occurs first. The method can be improved by considering interactions between some factors (e.g., age and treatment modality) or by allowing for a time dependent covariate, thereby removing the requirement of proportional hazards across time. Several of these approaches have been used in the analyses presented in this chapter.

For all outcome studies, the study design and methods of censoring require detailed attention. When outcome studies are to be used for advising patients regarding treatment choices, the intent-to-treat model is usually the best approach. For example, when assessing the survival benefits of CAPD versus hemodialysis for new ESRD patients, the model should keep the patient in the initially assigned group even when a change in dialytic modality occurs. A fraction of those patients choosing CAPD is expected to develop complications that require a switch to hemodialysis. On the other hand, a patient receiving a renal transplant would remain in the evaluation of all ESRD patient survival but not in the comparative dialysis patient survival, because transplantation is not considered a result of the dialytic choice but rather a desired change in therapy. The intent-to-treat model would keep the transplant recipient in the transplant group even after transplant failure and censor a patient only if lost to follow-up (e.g., moving out of the state or country) or if the patient was alive at the end

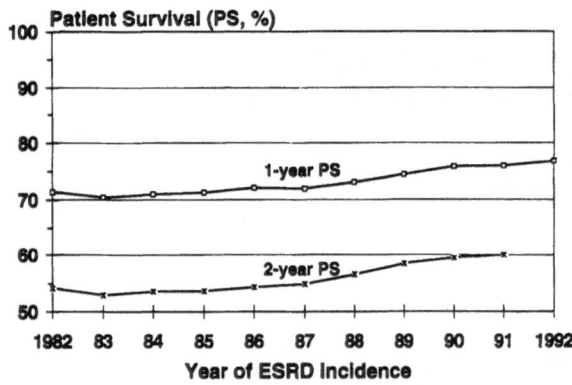

Figure 1. One and two-year dialysis patient survival by year of ESRD incidence, 1982–92, adjusted for age, sex, race and primary diagnosis. Medicare patients only. Estimates for the most recent year survival are preliminary. Sample size (n) ranges from 20,229 in 1982 to 51,078 in 1992. (Source: Reference 3)

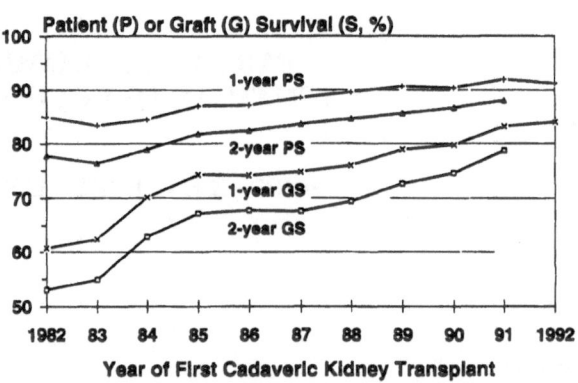

Figure 2. One and two-year patient and renal allograft survival probabilities for first cadaveric kidney transplant recipients, by year of transplantation, 1982–92, adjusted for age, sex, race and diagnosis. Medicare patients only. Estimates for the most recent year survival are preliminary. Sample size (n) ranges from 2,856 in 1982 to 6,067 in 1992. (Source: Reference 3)

of the follow-up period. A different analytical approach is used when the effectiveness of the treatment modality is assessed. In this case patients are removed from the study (censored) when a change in modality occurs, or more typically after a period of 30 or 60 days. This arbitrary carry-over period is used to consider a delayed mortality effect resulting from complications of the first modality. Thus, the study design varies greatly according to the specific question that is to be addressed.

SURVIVAL TRENDS

The USRDS has reported trends in one-year survival among patients new to ESRD (incident patients) and among patients alive on therapy (prevalent patients). Both analyses have shown an improvement over recent periods in adjusted actuarial Kaplan–Meier survival rate estimates when adjusting for the average mix of age, race, sex and cause of ESRD (3). This analysis censors dialysis patients at the time of transplantation. Figure 1 shows the one- and two-year survival probabilities for dialysis patients by year of initiation of ESRD therapy. Since data on new Medicare-insured patients may not be complete for the first 90 days of ESRD, this analysis starts on day 90 and considers the subsequent one or two years. There is a clear improving trend in dialysis patient survival in recent years while taking into account changes over time in the distribution of patients by age, race, sex and cause of ESRD. Changes in the presence of comorbid conditions at the start of therapy are not considered in this analysis but are not a plausible explanation for this observation, since comorbid conditions have likely increased rather than decreased over time. Reasons for these improvements in survival are unclear but may be, in part, related to documented increases in the prescribed and delivered dose (KT/V or

urea reduction ratio, URR) of dialysis (3, 4), increased use of bicarbonate dialysate, increased use of high flux or biocompatible dialyzers (5), and the introduction of human recombinant Erythropoietin.

For renal transplant recipients similar improvements have been shown according to adjusted actuarial one-year and two-year patient and graft survival rates (Figure 2). These analyses started on the day of transplantation and followed patients for the first one or two years by year of transplantation. Improvements in transplant outcomes are observed even after the introduction and wide-spread use of cyclosporine. The trends in one and two year actuarial patient survival estimates are depicted in Figure 2 and demonstrate continued improvements in recent years. Future research is needed to determine whether these recent improvements in short-term survival (e.g., at one and two years) continue and whether they are maintained over the longer term (e.g., five year graft and patient survival).

Comparison of these survival figures with those of other registries must consider the distribution of age, diabetes, transplantation rates and acceptance rates. Kjellstrand (6) has shown that higher acceptance rates are associated with higher percentages of diabetic and geriatric patients and are therefore suggestive of greater comorbidities. In international comparisons, where transplantation rates may differ widely by country, the overall ESRD patient survival rates, independent of the utilization of treatment modalities, may provide useful outcome comparisons (7, 8). However, completeness of death information may be critical for such comparisons. The USRDS captures deaths both through Social Security benefits and through reports from treatment centers. A recent analysis showed that the latter would report only approximately 90% of the deaths (3). Therefore, previous international comparisons showing a much lower survival in the United States

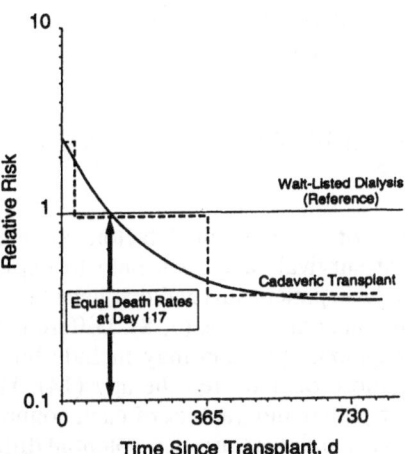

Figure 3. Relative risk (RR) of mortality over time for cadaveric transplant recipients versus wait-listed dialysis patients, 1984–89. A non-proportional Cox model was used to adjust survival for time since wait-listing, age, sex, race and primary diagnosis. RR is shown in both exponential form (continuous line) and at three distinct time intervals since date of transplantation (0–30, 31–365, and 365 + days, interrupted line). (Source: Reference 9)

(7, 8) may be explained in part by the virtually complete capturing of ESRD deaths in the United States compared to somewhat uncertain capture in other countries.

DIALYSIS VERSUS TRANSPLANT PATIENT OUTCOMES

Comparative outcomes studies for dialysis and transplant patients must be carefully designed, because of numerous potential biases: dialysis populations are not only older on average but also include patients who are not surgical candidates due to serious medical conditions. Furthermore, transplant recipients usually have to survive some time on dialysis, including the initial period of elevated mortality risk. There is also concern that the mortality risk after transplantation varies over time, since it is relatively high during the early postoperative period.

Analyses of data from the Michigan Kidney Registry dealt with these biases and limitations by only including patients who had passed medical evaluation and were placed on the waiting list for cadaveric renal transplantation (9). Starting the analyses with the date of wait-listing and using a time dependent (non-proportional) Cox model allowed a comparison of mortality risk among transplant recipients with dialysis patients who had been on the waiting list for the same length of time. The validity of the analysis was further improved by restricting the multivariate analysis to calendar years after the introduction of cyclosporine A and adjusting for the calendar year of transplantation. Figure 3 shows the main result from

this analysis of 1569 wait-listed dialysis patients and 799 transplant recipients. The mortality risk for transplant recipients was more than twice as high during the first month following transplantation and markedly reduced after the first year when compared to dialysis patients. Both the analysis by time interval and the continuous analysis provide a similar description of the relative mortality risk. Since this analysis was based on an intent-to-treat approach from date of listing for transplantation, it is most useful for discussing the benefits and risks of transplantation with potential transplant candidates. An analysis of the cumulative mortality risk comparison reveals that there is a net benefit from transplantation within 10 months of the date of transplant (9).

Patient survival is markedly superior for living-related donor transplantation compared to cadaveric transplantation. Thus, the described survival benefits of transplantation over dialysis are expected to be accentuated if one considers kidney transplants from a living related donor. Survival with a functioning renal allograft is also clearly superior for living donor compared to cadaveric donor transplants.

CAPD VERSUS HEMODIALYSIS PATIENT OUTCOMES

Several studies have compared survival among patients treated by the two major dialysis modalities, in-center hemodialysis and continuous ambulatory peritoneal dialysis (CAPD). In view of the observed large differences in the utilization of these dialytic modalities in international comparisons (3), such outcome studies may not be applicable across different health care systems.

A historical prospective study analyzed Michigan Kidney Registry data using both a treatment history and an intent-to-treat approach to compare outcomes for the two major dialytic treatment modalities (10). This study assigned patients to CAPD or center hemodialysis according to the treatment used on day 120 of ESRD and adjusted for age, sex, race and year of starting ESRD therapy. The main finding was that both patient groups had similar mortality risks for all cause of ESRD patient groups except for patients with diabetic ESRD. Although the mortality rates depended on whether intent-to-treat or treatment history was used for the analyses, the relative risks or comparative survivals did not differ appreciably by these analytical approaches. For diabetic patients this study showed a lower mortality risk for younger diabetic CAPD as compared to corresponding hemodialysis patients. This finding was statistically significant for ages 20–53 years. For ages 65–74, however, diabetic CAPD patients had a higher relative mortality risk than diabetic hemodialysis patients, while non-diabetic patients had similar results for the two treatment modalities (11).

This Michigan study was followed by a USRDS study of a national random sample of CAPD and center

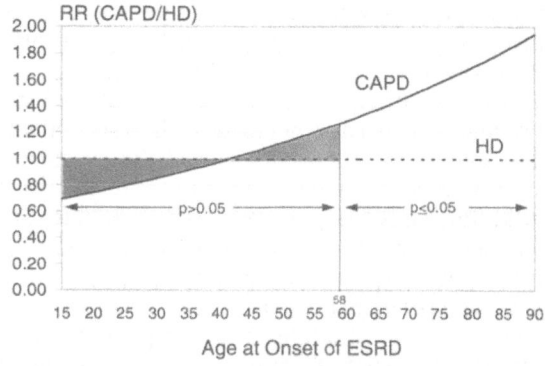

Figure 4. Relative risk (RR) of mortality for CAPD vs hemodialysis (HD), by age, 1986–87 incident diabetic patients. Adjusted in a Cox proportional hazards analysis for several demographic, comorbid and laboratory factors at onset of ESRD. (Source: derived from Reference 12)

hemodialysis patients, assigned according to their treatment modality on day 30 of ESRD (12). This study collected detailed information about comorbid risk conditions in addition to demographic variables at the start of ESRD. (These detailed factors were not available in the Michigan study.) The relative mortality risk with adjustment for these conditions also showed no differences by treatment modality among non-diabetic patients. However, among diabetic patients the mortality risk for CAPD patients was higher and statistically significant as compared with hemodialysis patients. The hypothesis of an age by treatment interaction that was developed in the Michigan study was tested in the USRDS study. As shown in Figure 4, this new USRDS analysis revealed that a statistically significant difference in mortality risk for CAPD versus hemodialysis was present only for ages above 58 years. Again, intent-to-treat and treatment history analyses gave similar comparative risks.

The strength of both studies is that they are based on defined populations (the state of Michigan and the Medicare population of the United States), rather than on data from selected collaborating centers. In contrast to the Michigan study, the USRDS study considered more adjustment factors, so that the latter would likely give a more reliable estimate. If younger diabetic CAPD patients had fewer comorbid conditions than corresponding hemodialysis patients, then the better outcomes for CAPD patients compared to hemodialysis patients in the Michigan study would be partly explained. The USRDS study actually confirmed such a difference by treatment modality for diabetic patients aged less than 65 years (12). Thus the two large population-based studies appear to be in excellent agreement. It remains unclear, however, whether unmeasured patient selection and differences in dialysis dose may have played a role in the findings among diabetic patients in both studies. Thus further research is

eeded, particularly since the dose of hemodialysis has been increasing in the US (4).

OTHER PREDICTORS OF PATIENT SURVIVAL IN THE US

Examination of the individual factors known to influence patient survival rates may help to explain differences in dialysis patient survival that have been observed in international comparisons (7, 8). Differences in treatment patterns exist (3), and may include both the type and quality/dose of delivered therapy (14). Differences in the underlying demographics of each country are also known to exist, and there are also potential differences in lifestyles and other factors that affect the overall health of each population.

Higher acceptance rates for ESRD have been documented in the US compared to other countries (3). Kjellstrand has suggested that higher acceptance rates for ESRD are related to ESRD treatment being extended to many patients who are sicker and require more complicated care (6). Factors of interest in international survival comparisons can be examined individually if one can adjust for possible confounding factors either by using a multivariate model or by normalizing certain characteristics of one population to the other population being compared (7, 8).

The Cox proportional hazards methodology has been used to conduct large-scale ESRD mortality analyses in the US with adjustment for extensive demographic and comorbid factors and other clinical indicators (9, 10, 12). Recent results from a national random sample of 1986–87 incident dialysis patients followed for up to four years (12) suggest statistically significant results ($p < 0.05$ unless otherwise noted) for many factors, including among diabetics and non-diabetics, respectively, age (RR ▬ 1.02 and 1.05 per year of age), race (RR ▬ 0.64 and 0.85 ($p = 0.10$) for blacks compared to whites) and sex (RR ▬ 0.88 ($p = 0.10$) and 0.76 for females compared to males). Many comorbid conditions and other factors were found to be predictive of mortality, including congestive heart failure (RR ▬ 1.31 and 1.23), peripheral vascular disease (RR ▬ 1.23 and 1.08 ($p = 0.46$)) and smoking (1.22 and 1.31). Higher mortality was also associated with lower serum albumin (RR ▬ 1.18 for 3.0–3.5 versus 3.6–4.0 g/dl) and lower serum creatinine (RR ▬ 0.96 per 1 mg/dl). Both measures suggest the importance of adequate patient nutrition.

The importance of the delivered dose of both hemodialysis and peritoneal dialysis is a topic that is beginning to receive widespread attention in the renal community in the US. At least one recent analysis has shown that the prescribed dose of hemodialysis is lower in the US than in the EDTA (14). The distribution of delivered Kt/V for a sample of 1990 prevalent US hemodialysis patients indicates that 38% of patients received a delivered Kt/V that was less than the minimum recommended by the National Cooperative Dialysis Study (4). The delivered dose of dialysis was associated with patient survival in a recent analysis by Owen et al. (15), providing evidence of a significant inverse correlation of dialysis dose (measured as URR) with mortality.

Mortality risks associated with many demographic, comorbid and other clinical factors have been documented in the United States. The proportional hazards methodology can be very useful in analyzing multiple factors predictive of mortality in ESRD patients, including those factors discussed in the present chapter and many other factors not considered. Documentation and analysis of risk factors in other countries may permit better comparison of mortality rates with adjustment for comorbid conditions.

ACKNOWLEDGEMENTS

The data reported in Figures 1 and 2 were published by the United States Renal Data System (USRDS, Reference 3). Figure 3 is reproduced from Reference 9. The data reported in Figure 4 are derived from Reference 12. The interpretation and reporting of these data are the responsibility of the authors and in no way should be seen as an official policy or interpretation of the US government.

References

1. Kaplan EL, Meier P: Nonparametric estimation from incomplete observations. *J Am Stat Assoc* 53: 457, 1972
2. Cox D: Regression models and life tables. *J R Stat Soc* 34: 187, 1972
3. United States Renal Data System: USRDS 1995 Annual Data Report. National Institutes of Health, National Institutes of Diabetes and Digestive and Kidney Diseases, Bethesda, MD, 1995, and *Am J Kidney Dis* 26 (Suppl 2): S1, 1995
4. Held PJ, Carroll CE, Liska DW, Turenne MN, Port FK: Hemodialysis therapy in the US: what is the dose and does it matter? *Am J Kidney Dis* 24: 974, 1994
5. Tokars JI, Alter MJ, Favero MS, Moyer LA, Bland LA: National surveillance of dialysis-associated diseases in the United States. *ASAIO Trans* 39: 71, 1993
6. Kjellstrand CM, Hylander B, Collins AC: Mortality on dialysis – on the influence of early start, patient characteristics, and transplantation and acceptance rates. *Am J Kidney Dis* 15: 483, 1990
7. Held PJ, Akiba T, Stearns NS et al.: Survival of middle aged dialysis patients in Japan and the US. in *Death on Dialysis; Preventable or Inevitable*, edited by Friedman EA, Dordrecht/Boston/London, Kluwer Academic Publishers, 1994, p 13
8. Held PJ, Brunner F, Odaka M, Garcia JR, Port FK, Gaylin DS: Five-year survival for end-stage renal disease patients in the United States, Europe, and Japan, 1982 to 1987. *Am J Kidney Dis* 15: 451, 1990
9. Port FK, Wolfe RA, Mauger EA, Berling DP, Jiang K: Comparison of survival probabilities for dialysis patients versus cadaveric renal transplant recipients. *JAMA* 270: 1339, 1993
10. Nelson CB, Port FK, Wolfe RA, Guire KE: Comparison of CAPD and hemodialysis patient survival with evaluation of trends during the 1980s. *J Am Soc Nephrol* 3: 1147, 1992
11. Port FK, Nelson CB, Wolfe RA: Mortality comparison for diabetic ESRD patients treated with CAPD versus hemodialysis. in *Death on Dialysis; Preventable or Inevitable*, edited by Friedman EA, Dordrecht/Boston/London, Kluwer Adademic Publishers, 1994, p 113
12. Held PJ, Port FK, Turenne MN, Gaylin DS, Hamburger RJ, Wolfe RA: Continuous ambulatory peritoneal dialysis and hemodialysis: comparison of patient mortality with adjustment for comorbid conditions. *Kidney Int* 45: 1163, 1994
13. United States Renal Data System: Patient selection to peritoneal dialysis versus hemodialysis according to comorbid conditions. *Am J Kidney Dis* 20: 20, 1992
14. Held PJ, Blagg CR, Liska DW, Port FK, Hakim R, Levin NW: The dose of hemodialysis according to dialysis prescription in Europe and in the United States. *Kidney Int* 42 (Suppl 38): S16, 1992
15. Owens WF, Lew NL, Yan Liu SM, Lowrie EG, Lazarus JM: The urea reduction ratio and serum albumin concentration as predictors of mortality in patients undergoing hemodialysis. *N Engl J Med* 329: 1101, 1993

PART C: REGISTRY REPORT OF DIALYSIS THERAPY IN JAPAN

SATOSHI TERAOKA, KENSHI MAEDA, HIROSHI TOMA, HIROSHI NIHEI, TETSUZO AGISHI, KAZUO OTA, ISAO ISHIKAWA, AKIRA SHINODA, TAKESHI SATO and SHOZO KOSHIKAWA

THE JAPANESE REGISTRY FOR DIALYSIS THERAPY AND ITS DATA BASE

The registry for dialysis therapy

An annual registry for dialysis therapies in Japan was started in 1983 following 15 years of preparation. The Japanese Society for Dialysis Therapy (JSDT) has a standing committee for statistics and investigation; its annual budget of $240,000 is funded by JSDT.

Inquiries and items for data base

JSDT questionnaires consist of four sheets. Sheet I was first used in 1968 and concerns facilities, such as the number of bedside monitors, medical staff members and dialysis patients, and the number of patients newly accepted and lost during the year. Individual registration and follow-up data of each patient were introduced in 1983 with sheets II–IV.

Sheets II and III are given to newly accepted patients to fill in name, gender, date of birth, date of the start of dialysis, coded original disease, prefecture residence, kind of dialysis modalities selected, and transfer or death. Since 1991 results of pre- and post-dialysis serum level, of urea nitrogen (SUN), creatinine (sCr) and phosphate, pre- and post-dialysis body weight, pre-dialysis serum albumin level, frequency of dialysis per week, and time of each dialysis session have been added. Sheet IV asks the same items as on sheets II and III of referred and unregistered patients.

Sheets I–IV are delivered to each dialysis center, and thereafter collected by the committee. In the 1992 registry, the recovery rate for sheet I was 99.45% (2520 dialysis centers out of 2534) and of sheets II–IV 95.46%. The collected data were analyzed by statistical methods including stepwise logistic regression analysis and have been published every year by JSDT as 'An overview of regular dialysis treatment in Japan' (1).

DEMOGRAPHIC FEATURES OF PATIENTS AND FACILITIES

Patients on regular dialysis treatment

Number of dialysis patients

The number of patients newly accepted to dialysis therapy in 1992 was 22,475 (yearly increment: 1598), while the number of dialysis patients who died in 1992 was 11,621 (yearly increment: 1899). Consequently, the net increase in dialysis patients in 1992 was 10,854 and the total number of dialysis patients was 123,926 (995.8 per million population) at the end of 1992 (Figure 1). Of these, 117,809 (95.1%) patients underwent hemodialysis (HD); 88,980 (71.8%) during the day time, 28,718 (23.2%) at night, and 111 (0.1%) at home; 6117 (4.9%) patients were maintained on peritoneal dialysis (PD), 6011 (4.9%) on

Number of patients

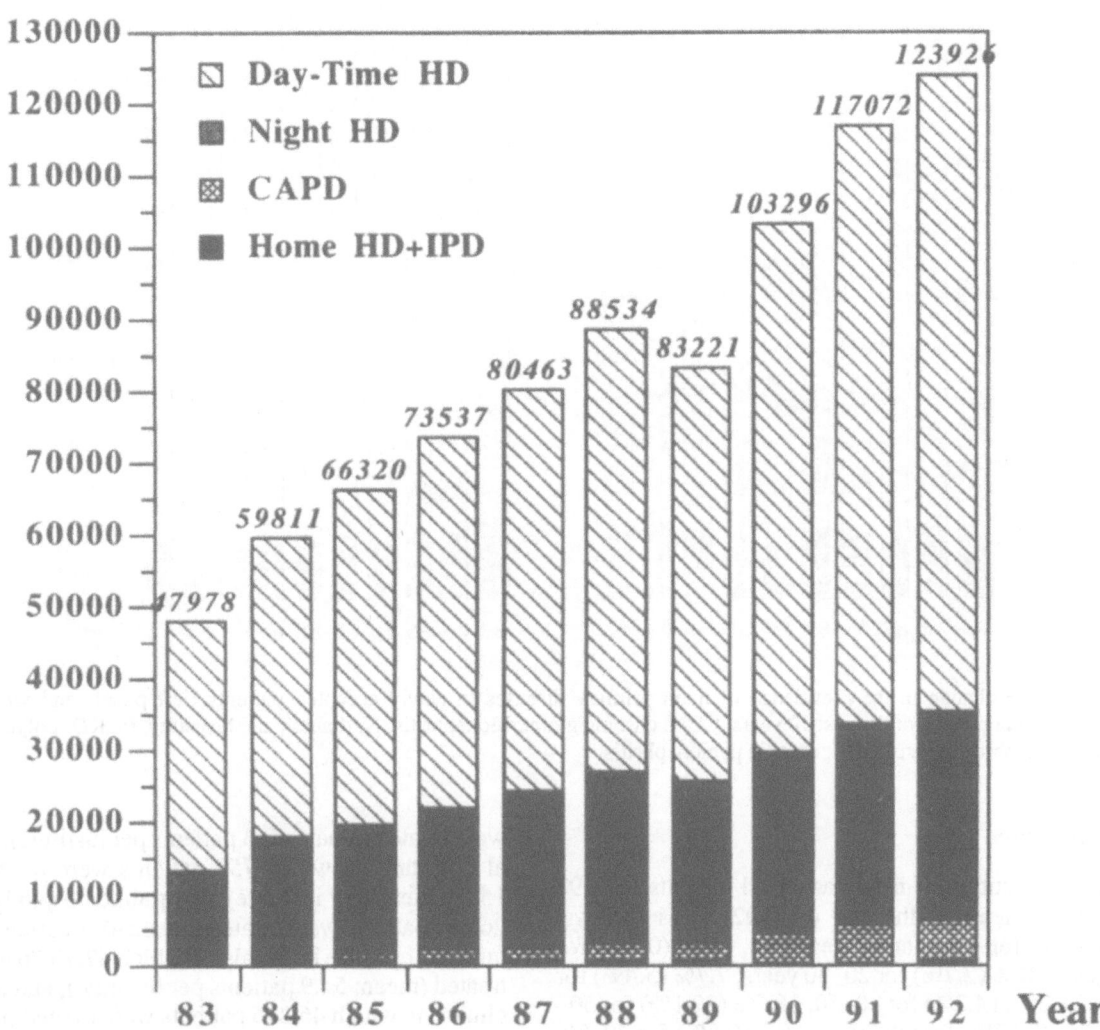

Figure 1. The number of patients on regular dialysis treatments by each therapeutic modality in the past 10 years.

continuous ambulatory PD (CAPD), and 106 (0.1%) on intermittent PD (IPD).

Primary diseases

The distribution of the primary diseases of newly accepted patients in 1992 is as follows: 42.2% for chronic glomerulonephritis (CGN), 28.4% for diabetic nephropathy, 5.9% for nephrosclerosis, 2.7% for polycystic kidney disease (PCKD), 1.6% for chronic pyelonephritis (CPN), 1.3% for systemic lupus erythematosus (SLE), 0.7% for rapidly progressive glomerulonephritis (RPGN), 0.7% for gout nephropathy, 0.7% for malignant hypertension, 0.6% for amyloid nephropathy, 0.5% for obstructive nephropathy, 0.5% for urological malignancy, 0.5% for unclassified glomerulonephritis, and others. The prevalence of main

primary diseases in the past 10 years is shown in Figure 2, with the progressive yearly increase in the percentage of diabetic nephropathy. The incidence of CGN as the primary disease for dialysis patients in Japan is much higher than in European countries, although it has been gradually decreasing. The incidence of biopsy-proven CGN was 68.8% in 1992, which is still high compared with European countries. However, the frequency of the biopsy-proven diagnosis was only 4.0% among the entire dialysis population. Furthermore, the biopsies were done to confirm the diagnosis in patients suspected of having CGN. The above-mentioned high incidence of biopsy-proven CGN, therefore, does not always mean a high incidence of CGN as the primary disease among the entire dialysis population.

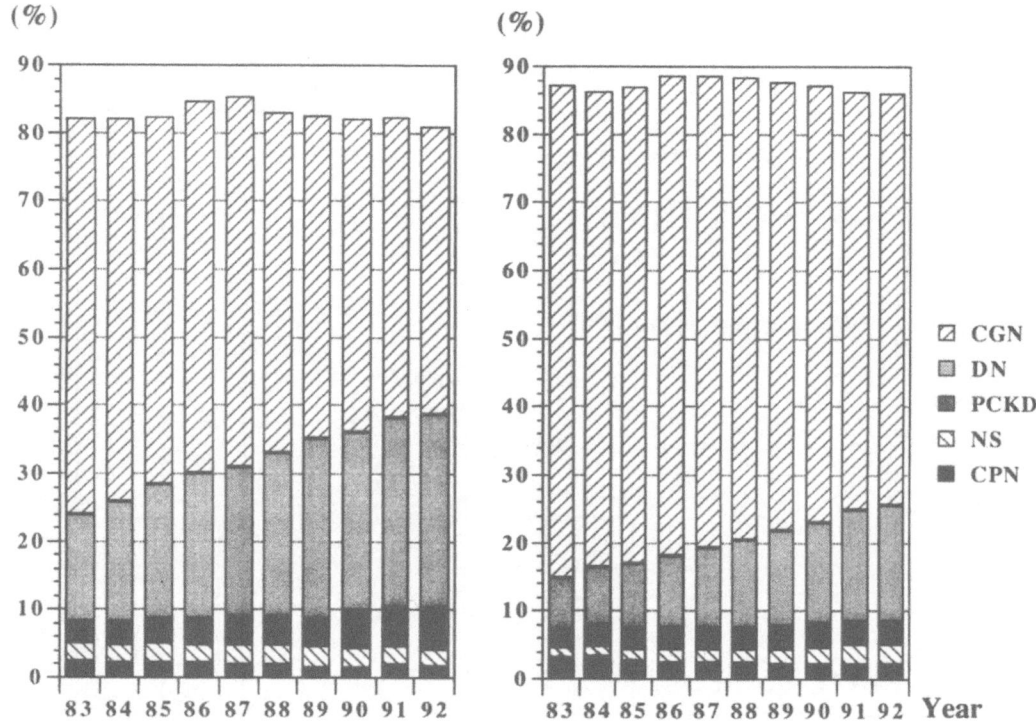

Figure 2. The change in the prevalence of main primary diseases in newly accepted patients (left panel) and whole dialysis populations (right panel) for the past 10 years. CGN: chronic glomerulonephritis, N: diabetic nephropathy, PCKD: polycystic kidney disease, NS: nephrosclerosis, CPN: chronic pyelonephritis.

Age distribution

The age distribution of newly accepted patients in 1992 (and total patients at the end of 1992) is as follows: 0.1% (0.1%) for less than 10 years old, 0.4% (0.7%) for teenages, 2.42% (2.7%) for 20–30 years, 7.7% (5.4%) for 30–40, 21.2% (14.3%) for 40–50, 26.6% (22.1%) for 50–60, 25.1% (27.2%) for 60–70, 13.1% (19.8%) for 70–80, 3.2% (5.9%) for 80–90, and 0.1% (0.3%) for 90+.

Time course of dialysis treatment

The number of patients maintained on regular dialysis therapy (RDT) for less than 5 years is 65,835 (54.1%), 29,775 (24.5%) for 5–10 years, 16,438 (13.5%) for 10–15 years, 8429 (6.9%) for 15–20 years, 1170 (1.0%) for 20–25 years, and 8 (0.0%) for more than 25 years.

Dialysis units

The total number of dialysis units in Japan was 2520 at the end of 1992, which possessed 49,650 bedside monitors. Compared to 1991, dialysis units and bedside monitors increased in number by 135 (5.7%) and 3968 (8.7%), respectively. The numbers of each type of dialysis unit and patients treated were as follows: 58 national universities, in which 660 patients were treated (mean: 11.4 patients per institute), 56 private universities, in which 2368 patients were treated (mean: 42.3 patients per institute), 49 national hospitals, in which 758 patients were treated (mean: 15.5 patients per institute), 604 public hospitals, in which 26,031 patients were treated (mean: 43.1 patients per institute), 861 private hospitals, in which 47,234 patients were treated (mean: 54.9 patients per institute), and 892 private clinics, in which 46,875 patients were treated (mean: 52.6 patients per institute; Figure 3).

SOCIOECONOMICAL BACKGROUND OF DIALYSIS TREATMENT PROGRAM IN JAPAN

Insurance system

All citizens and permanent foreign residents in Japan are supposed to join one of the medical care insurance systems, which are roughly divided into two categories: community insurance (National Health Insurance, NHI) and employees' insurance (Employees' Health Insurance, EHI) (2, 3). The latter is classified into society-managed health insurance for employees in giant companies and government-managed health insurance for employees in small-size enterprises, while the former is classified into the National Health Insurance Association and Municipalities Insurance for those not covered by employees' insur-

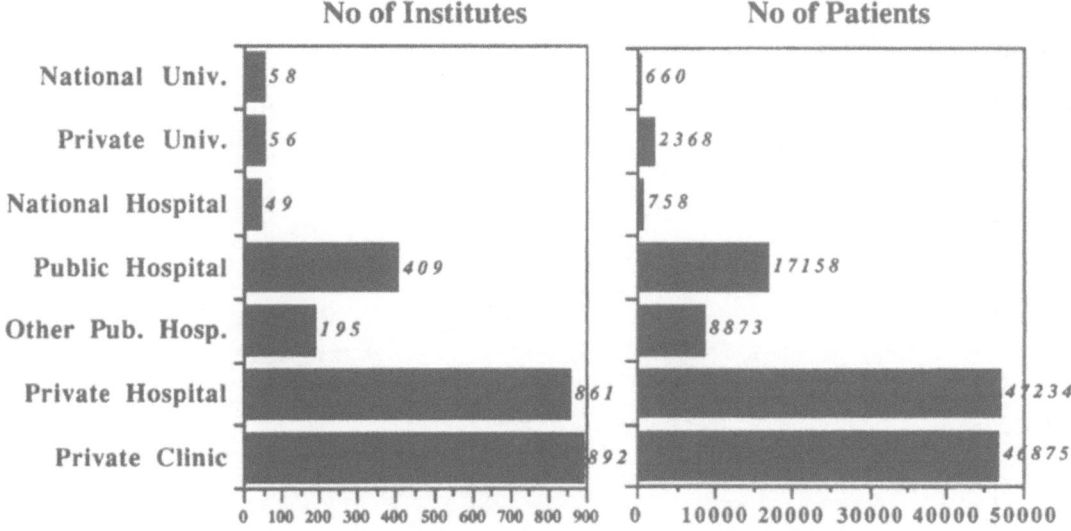

Figure 3. The number of each type of dialysis unit and patients treated in Japan.

ance schemes (2, 3). The insurance benefit is 90% of total medical costs for a person insured and 70% (outpatients) to 80% (inpatients) for dependents in case of employees' insurance, and 70% for both an insured person and his/her dependents in case of community insurance (2–4).

Payment system

The payment system for medical care in Japan is mainly based upon fee-for-service. One of the few exceptions is a fixed fee for RDT including management fee, technical fee and routine laboratory examinations for outpatients on RDT. Home and limited care dialysis are not officially approved. As the medical charge for RDT is set only for dialysis in hospitals and/or clinics, the number of patients on home-HD is quite limited in Japan.

Since 1972, Medical Care for Rehabilitation based on the Welfare Act for the Disabled enacted in 1942 has been applied to patients with end-stage renal disease (ESRD), now including both dialysis and kidney transplant patients (5). According to this system, individual charges vary with their income, but do not exceed $95 per month (5).

Patients pay 10% (insured persons in EHI) to 30% (dependents in EHI and all covered by NHI) of the medical fee to the hospital concerned, which is reimbursed later by the Medical Care for Rehabilitation in the case of patients on RDT. The hospital demands the remaining 70 to 90% from the Health Insurance Fund, which reimburses it after the assessment by the judging committee. The financial resources of the Health Insurance Fund consist of the citizens' contribution and governmental subsidy. Contribution rates range from 8.2 to 9.2% of income in EHI, and 1.07% of resident tax (3% of income) in addition to $150 per each family member in NHI (2–5).

Medical cost for dialysis therapy

The average monthly medical cost for a patient on RDT in Japan ranges from $4500 to $5000 for outpatients and from $8000 to $10,000 for inpatients. The estimated total annual medical expenses for patients on RDT in Japan amount to $700 billion. The government is aiming at cost control by cutting down the cost for HD and promoting kidney transplantation. There is, however, no law or restriction for or against a special modality of dialysis.

CLINICAL RESULTS OF REGULAR DIALYSIS TREATMENT PROGRAM

Survival rates

Overall actuarial survival rates of patients accepted for RDT after 1983 are shown in Figure 4. Overall, the 1, 5 and 9 year survivals are 83.95, 60.4 and 49.4%, respectively. Actuarial patient survival rates by age are shown in Figure 5. The survival rates of dialysis patients under 45 years old are superior, whereas those over 60 are poor, furthermore, those more than 75 years old are quite poor. Patient survival rates according to the main primary disease are shown in Figure 6, which presents a significantly lower survival rate for diabetic nephropathy and nephrosclerosis than that for CGN, PCKD and CPN. Survival rates for amyloid nephropathy, myeloma kidney and urological malignancies not shown here are extremely poor; however, this is attributed to the prognosis of the primary diseases.

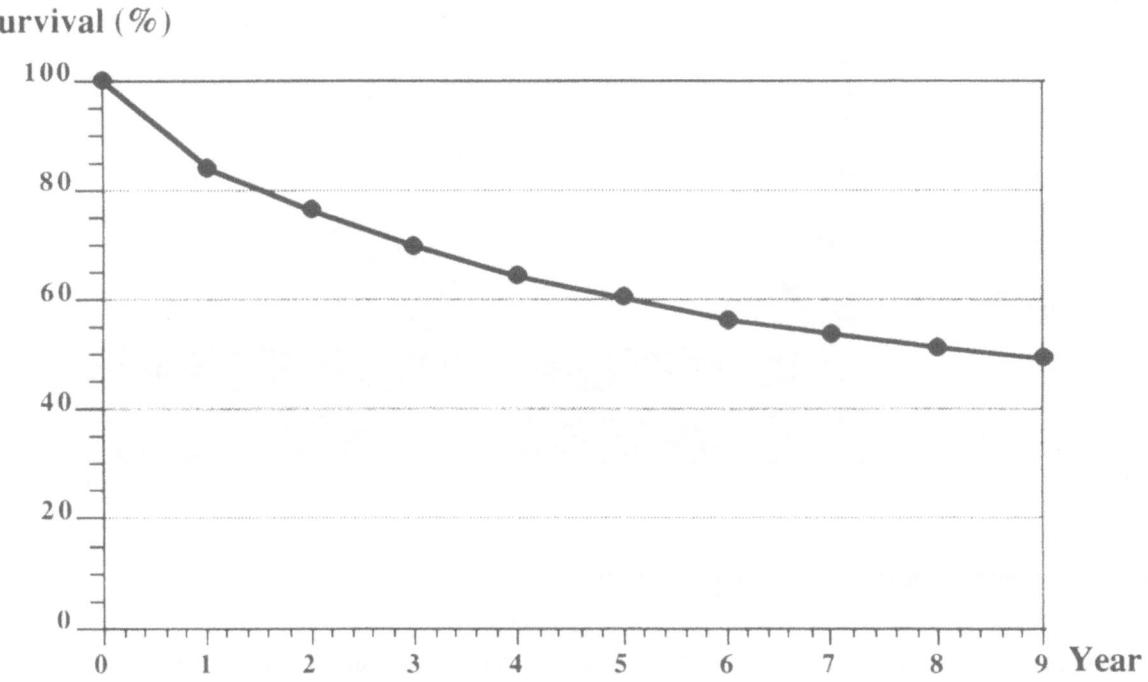

Figure 4. Overall actuarial survival rates of patients on regular dialysis treatment in Japan.

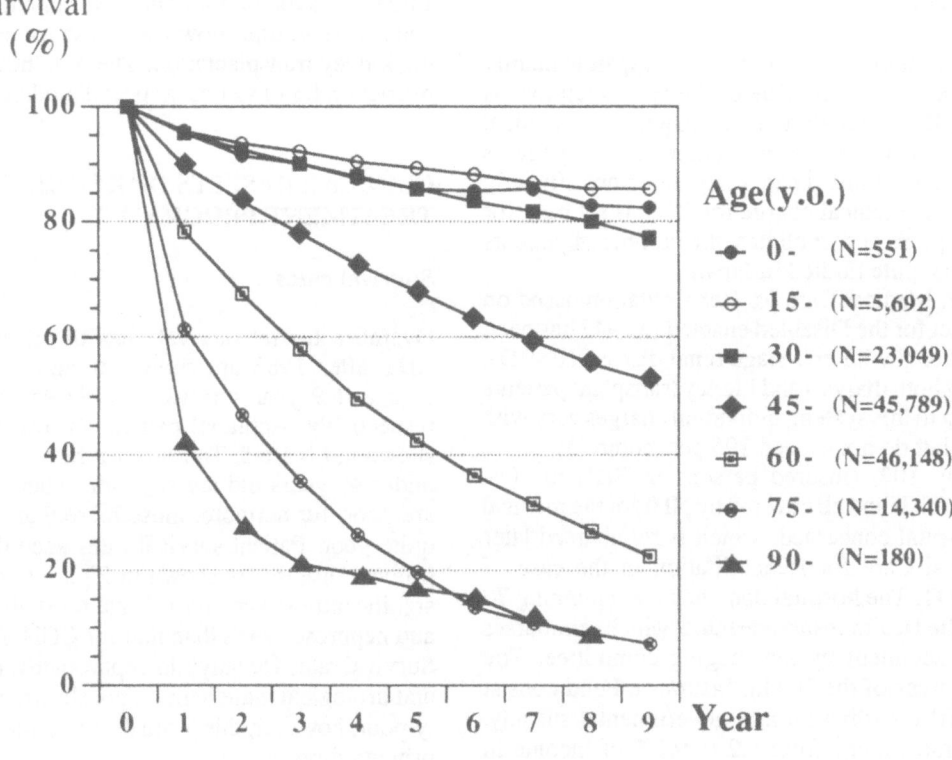

Figure 5. Actuarial survival rates of patients on regular dialysis treatment by age.

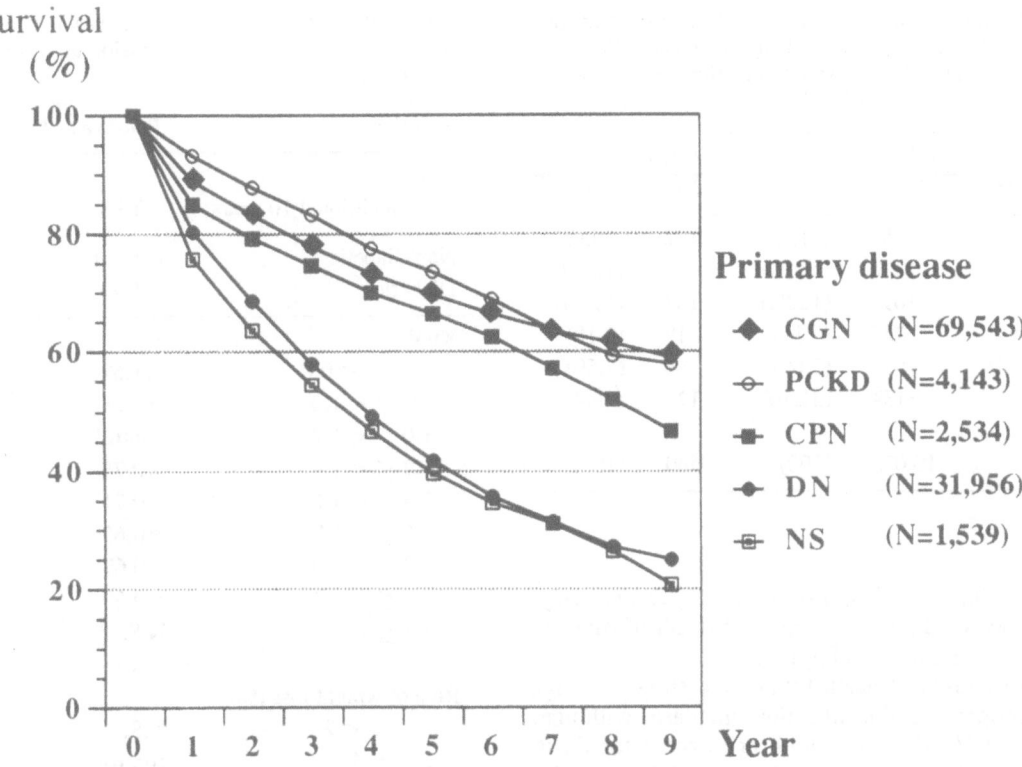

Figure 6. Actuarial survival rates of patients on regular dialysis treatment by main primary diseases.

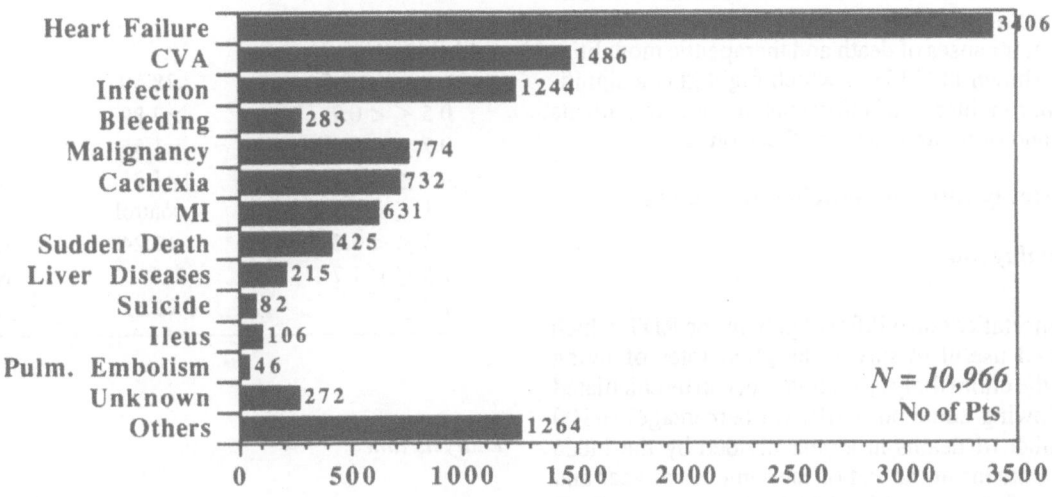

Figure 7. Causes of death among dialysis patients who died in 1992.

Causes of death

The causes of death of dialysis patients in 1992 are shown in Figure 7: 31.1% heart failure, 13.6% cerebrovascular accident (CVA), 11.3% infectious diseases, 7.1% malignancies, 6.7% cachexia/uremia, 5.8% myocardial infarc-tion, 3.9% hyperkalemia/sudden death, 2.6% hemorrhagic complications, 2.0% chronic liver diseases/liver cirrhosis, 1.0% ileus, 0.7% suicide, 0.4% pulmonary embolism, 8.7% unknown cause or undetermined, and 11.5% others. The overall percentage of causes of death among all patients since 1983 is 32.5, 12.5, 11.4, 7.2, 6.2, 5.5,

Table 1. The relationship of causes of death to therapeutic modalities in patients on regular dialysis treatment. CVA: cerebrovascular accident, MI: myocardial infarction, HD: hemodialysis, CAPD: continuous ambulatory peritoneal dialysis

Cause of death	HD		CAPD	
	No.	(%)	No.	(%)
Heart failure	3159	(31.35)	172	(29.66)
CVA	1380	(13.70)	73	(12.59)
Infection	1093	(10.85)	102	(17.59)
Malignancy	736	(7.31)	18	(3.10)
MI	573	(5.69)	44	(7.59)
Others	3134	(31.10)	171	(29.47)
Total	10,075	(100)	580	(100)

3.6, 4.3, 1.9, 0.6, 1.0, 0.6, 7.0 and 5.2%, respectively. The prevalence of the major causes of death of dialysis patients by year is shown in Figure 8.

The major causes of death by age are shown in Figure 9. The proportion of heart failure increases with age, while that of CVA decreases with age except for those 15–30 years old. The proportion of causes of death by the primary disease in dialysis patients is almost the same as that of the general dialysis population except for PCKD, in which the percentage of CVA is relatively increased while that of heart failure is lower (Figure 10). The relationship between major causes of death and therapeutic modalities of RDT is shown in Table 1, which highlights a significantly higher incidence of infectious diseases in patients on CAPD and of malignancies in those on HD.

Gross mortality rate and contributing factors

Gross mortality rate

The gross mortality rate (GMR) of patients on RDT, which is considered useful to survey the gross rates of living patients in the entire dialysis population, can be calculated by the following equation: GMR (in percentage) = 100 × the number of deaths in a year divided by the mean number of patients at the end of the same fiscal year and the previous fiscal year. The GMR of patients on RDT ranged from 7.4 to 9.0% from 1983, whereas it rose up to 9.7% in 1992, which was probably related to the change in the distribution of primary diseases and age among dialysis patients.

Age

The GMR of patients on RDT by age is shown in Figure 11, which demonstrates the increase in GMR with age.

Table 2. Risk factors and their relative risk in patients on regular dialysis treatment by logistic regression analysis. PCR: protein catabolic rate

Variables	Relative risk	P-value
Age every additional 10 years	×1.98	< 0.0001
Non-diabetic	control	control
Diabetic	×1.99	< 0.0001
Kt/V		
< 0.8	×1.62	< 0.0001
0.8 ≤ < 1.0	×1.28	< 0.002
1.0 ≤ < 1.2	control	control
1.2 ≤ < 1.4	×0.78	< 0.0001
1.4 ≤ < 1.6	×0.71	< 0.0001
1.6 ≤ < 1.8	×0.65	< 0.0001
1.8 ≤ < 2.0	×0.67	< 0.003
2.0 ≤ < 2.2	×0.50	< 0.004
2.2 ≤	N.S.	N.S.
Rate of weight loss (%)		
< 2	N.S.	N.S.
2 ≤ < 4	control	control
4 ≤ < 6	N.S.	N.S.
6 ≤ < 9	×1.33	< 0.0001
9 ≤	×2.17	< 0.0001
PCR (g/kg/day)		
< 0.5	×8.50	< 0.0001
0.5 ≤ < 0.7	×2.80	< 0.0001
0.7 ≤ < 0.9	×1.56	< 0.0001
0.9 ≤ < 1.1	×1.21	< 0.004
1.1 ≤ < 1.3	control	control
1.3 ≤ < 1.5	×1.24	< 0.05
1.5 ≤ < 1.7	N.S.	N.S.
1.7 ≤	×2.62	< 0.009

Dialysis time

The average time for each dialysis session in patients undergoing three sessions of HD, hemofiltration or hemodiafiltration every week was 4.30 ± 0.57 hours in 1991 and 4.17 ± 0.55 hours in 1992. The proportion of patients according to the average time of each dialysis session was 75.1% for 4–5 hours, 8.5% for less than 4 hours and 0.9% for more than 6 hours in 1992. The relationship of GMR to the average time of each dialysis session is shown in Figure 12, which demonstrates the increase in GMR with the decrease in average time of each dialysis session.

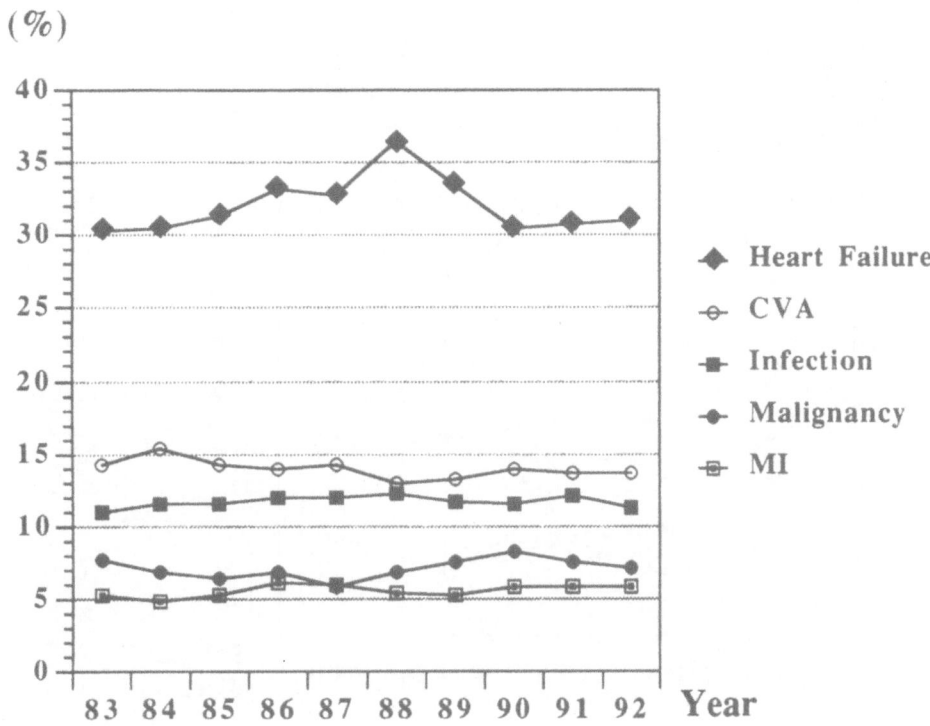

Figure 8. The prevalence of the major causes of death of dialysis patients by year.

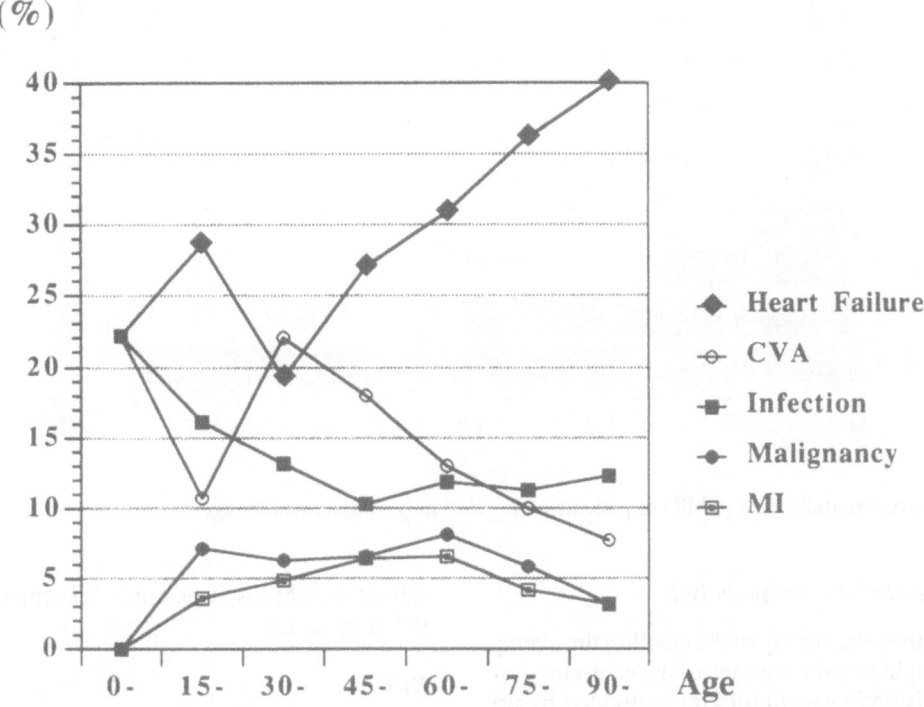

Figure 9. Major causes of death by age among dialysis patients who died in 1992.

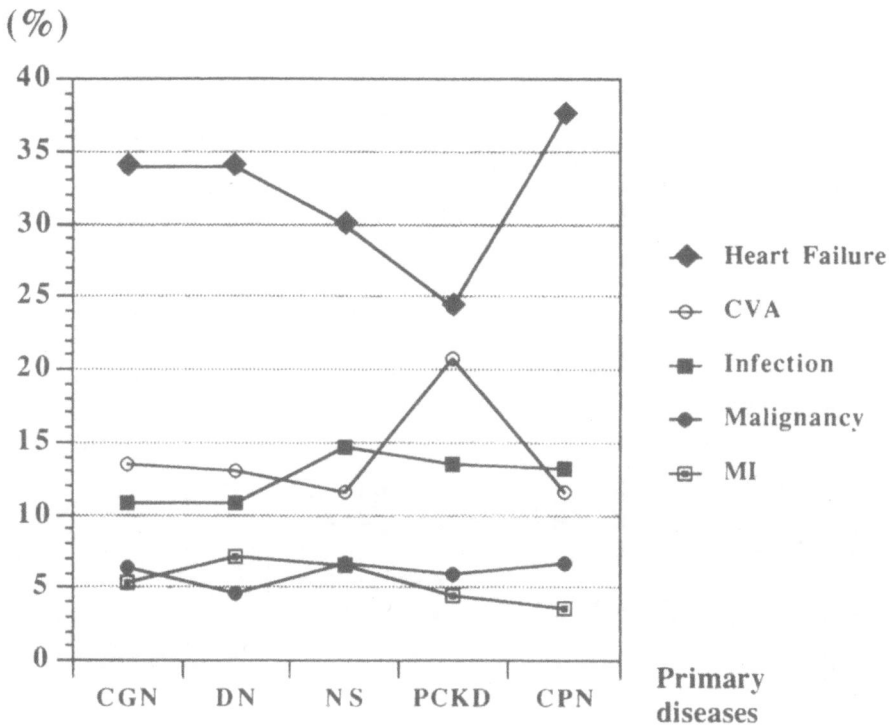

Figure 10. Major causes of death by the main primary diseases in dialysis patients.

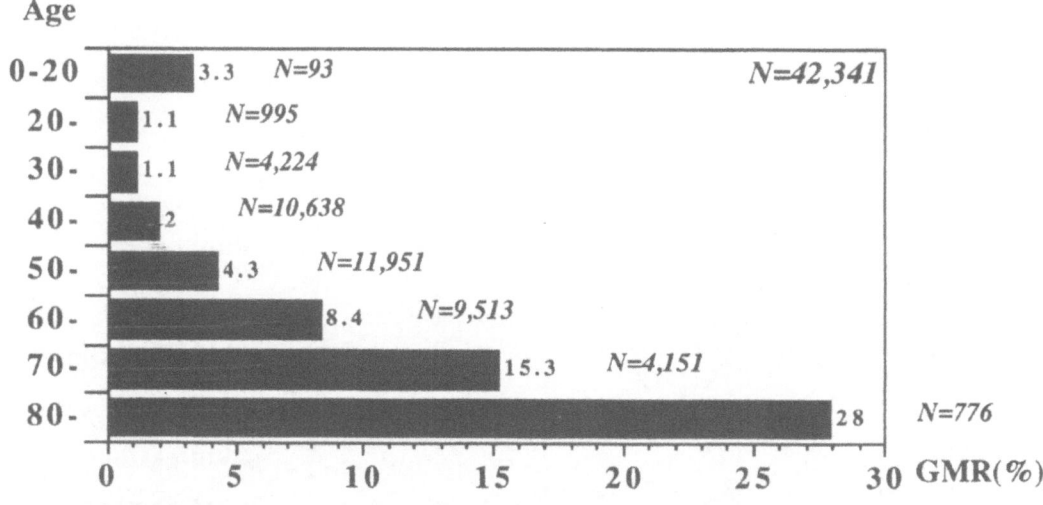

Figure 11. The gross mortality rate (GMR) of patients on regular dialysis treatment by age.

Rate of body weight loss during dialysis

With respect to the relationship of the GMR to the average rate of body weight loss during each dialysis session (pre- and post-dialysis body weight difference divided by pre-dialysis body weight), which roughly reflects the body weight change in the interval between two dialysis sessions, the gross mortality was increased when the average rate of weight loss was either less than 4% or more than 9% (Figure 13).

Kt/V

The average Kt/V in the collected data of dialysis patients was 1.32 ± 0.19 in 1991, and 1.32 ± 0.30 in 1992. As the value of Kt/V presented here was corrected by body

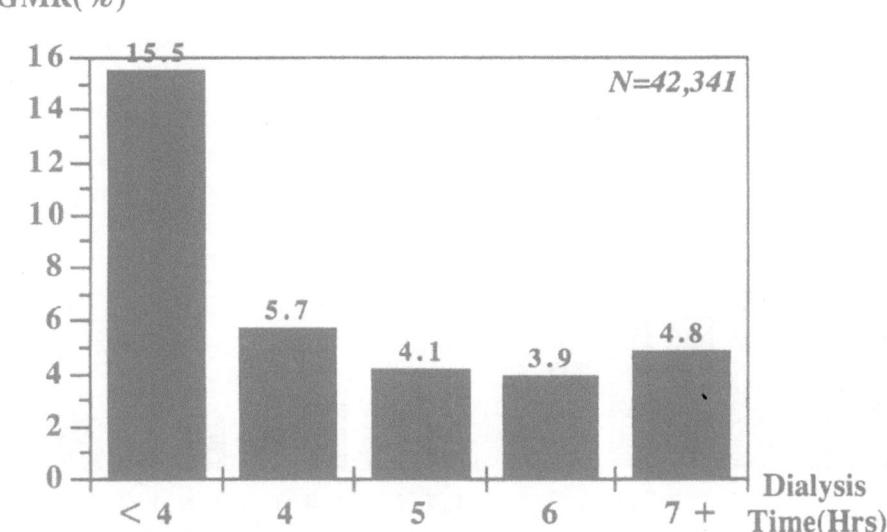

Figure 12. The relationship of the gross mortality rate (GMR) of patients on regular dialysis treatment to the average time of each dialysis session.

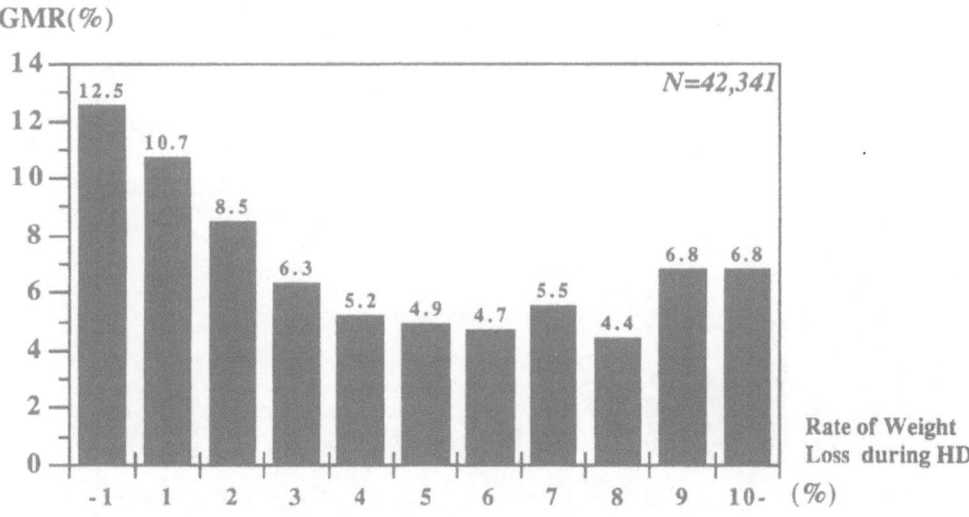

Figure 13. The relationship of the gross mortality rate (GMR) of patients on regular dialysis treatment to the average body weight loss during each dialysis session.

weight change, it is estimated to be 20% greater than that reported by Gotch et al. (6) in the National Cooperative Dialysis Study (NCDS). Thus, 1.0–1.1 can be regarded as the optimal value of the average Kt/V corrected by body weight change, corresponding to the value (0.9) which was proposed by Gotch based on non-collected data from NCDS (6). The average Kt/V was more than 1.0 in 88% of the total dialysis population in 1992. The relationship of the GMR to Kt/V is shown in Figure 14, in which the GMR increases as Kt/V decreases, especially when less than 1.0.

Protein catabolic rate

The average protein catabolic rate (PCR), which is regarded as equivalent to daily protein uptake, was 1.00 ± 0.20 g/kg/day in 1992. The PCR was more than 0.8 g/kg/day in 86.2% of the total dialysis population. The relationship of GMR to PCR is shown in Figure 15. GMR remains low if PCR is more than 1.0 g/kg/day, while it increases in geometric progression as PCR decreases. On the other hand, GMR is elevated as PCR exceeds 1.7 g/kg/day.

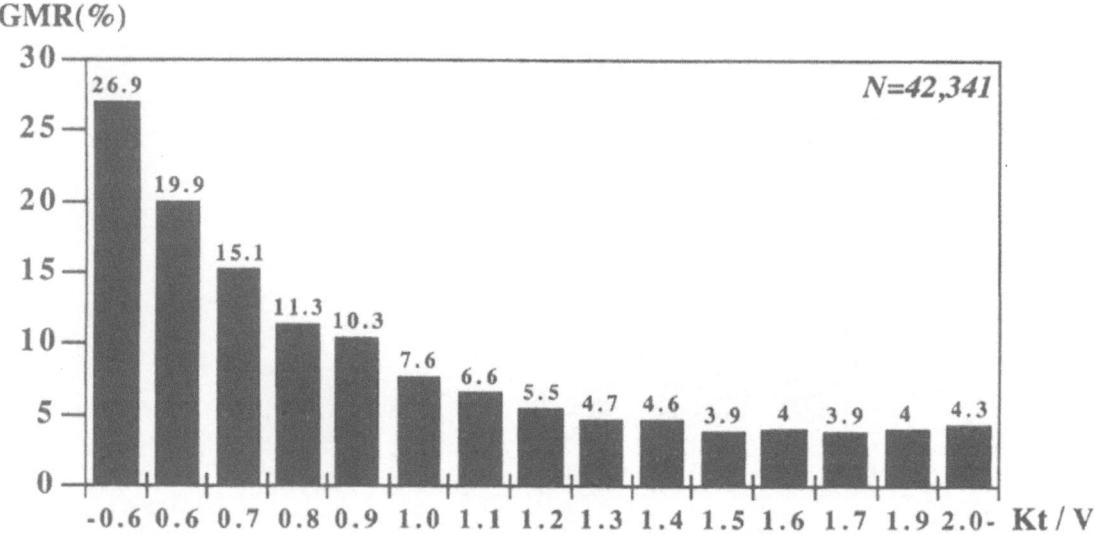

Figure 14. The relationship of the gross mortality rate (GMR) of patients on regular dialysis treatment to Kt/V.

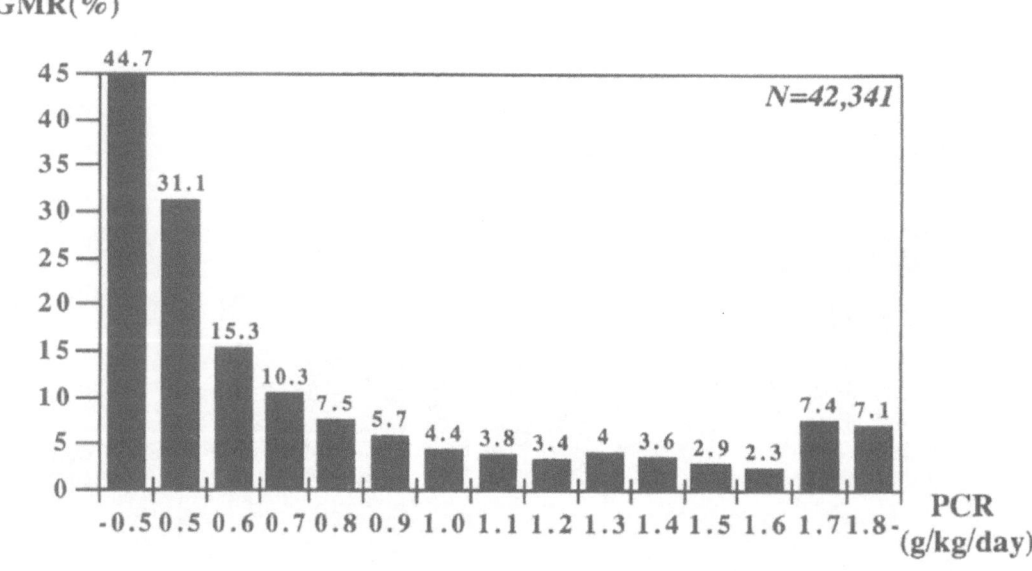

Figure 15. The relationship of the gross mortality rate (GMR) of patients on regular dialysis treatment to the protein catabolic rate (PCR).

Multivariate analysis by logistic regression model of risk factors in dialysis

Patients

The result of multivariate analysis by logistic regression model, in which age, primary disease (diabetic or non-diabetic), Kt/V, average rate of weight loss during each dialysis session and PCR were the independent variables, is shown in Table 2. Age (every additional 10 years), primary disease (diabetic), Kt/V (less than 1.0), weight loss during dialysis (more than 6%) and PCR (less than 1.1) had significant impacts on the survival rates. The relative risk of age was 1.98 times greater with every additional 10 years ($p < 0.0001$). The relative risk for diabetic patients was 1.99 times greater than that for non-diabetics ($p < 0.0001$). The relative risk was elevated significantly with increase in the rate of body weight loss during a dialysis session, when its rate was more than 6%. This result corresponds with that reported by Herd et al. (7). The relative risk was significantly lowered with the increase in Kt/V if Kt/V was less than 2.0–2.2, while it was not significantly different when Kt/V was greater than 2.2. The relative risk was significantly lowered with the increase in PCR if PCR was less than 1.5 g/kg/day, corresponding to the results reported by Gotch et al. (6) and Fernandez et al. (8), while it was elevated significantly for values greater than 1.7 g/kg/day ($p < 0.009$).

REFERENCES

1. Registration Committee of the Japanese Society for Dialysis Therapy: An overview of regular dialysis treatment in Japan (as of December 31, 1992). Japanese Society for Dialysis Therapy, Tokyo, 1993
2. Ministry of Health and Welfare: Medical care security. in *Health and Welfare in Japan*, edited by Ministry of Health and Welfare, Japan International Corporation of Welfare Services, Tokyo, 1989, p 14
3. Ministry of Health and Welfare: *Annual Report on Health and Welfare 1991–1992*, Japan International Corporation of Welfare Services, Tokyo, 1992, p 362
4. Health and Welfare Statistics Association: *Journal of Health and Welfare Statistics* 40(14): 7, 1993
5. Health and Welfare Statistics Association: *Journal of Health and Welfare Statistics* 40(9): 175, 1993
6. Gotch FA, Sargent JA: A mechanistic analysis of the National Cooperative Dialysis Study (NCDS). *Kidney Int* 28: 526, 1985
7. Herd PJ, Levin NW, Diamond LH et al.: Mortality and duration of hemodialysis treatment. *JAMA* 265(7): 871, 1991
8. Fernandez JM, Carbonell ME, Petrucelli D et al.: Simultaneous analysis of morbidity and mortality factors in chronic hemodialysis. *Kidney Int* 41: 1029, 1992

PART D: STRUCTURE AND OUTCOME MEASUREMENTS – EDTA-ERA REGISTRY

N.P. MALLICK

The European Renal Registry covers 36 countries of Europe and bordering the Mediterranean Sea. Countries vary widely in size from less than 5 to more than 80 million inhabitants. Overall nearly 700 million people are covered by the area of interest.

In such a diverse community it is difficult to be specific as to the health care systems to which renal data respond. Necessarily these vary as does the method of support for health care.

Data returns to our Registry are voluntary. Nevertheless, of the 2760 centres of which we are aware, some 70% return their centre data to us and between 50 and 65% (depending on the year at issue) return detailed analysis of individual patients to us. Where there is a National or Regional Registry there is virtually 100% return of patient data. This data is collected on the last day of the calendar year.

The different health care systems' methods of finance and the varied availability of computerised systems for data collection all work to make validation of our database a problem for us.

As, increasingly, national governments demand data so that individual units have to collect it and equally increasingly, as National Societies of Nephrology recognise the value of national or sub national regional registries and of patients on renal replacement therapy and for renal disease so does it become easier for us to have local sources of fully collected data on which to draw.

Table 1 indicates the range of dialysis centres as reported to the Registry on a country by country basis. Table 2 indicates the percentage of those centres which are reported to carry out transplantation.

The first report to an EDTA Congress was in 1964. Regular data collection began some four years later.

In Table 3 is shown the number of patients for whom records were available to us on 31 December 92. The actuarial survival for patients beginning treatment from 1986 is shown in Figure 1. This figure is refined for patients who have been solely on haemodialysis (up to the end of 1991) in Figure 2. While there is clearly a change in survival with age, it must be remembered that co-morbidity profoundly affects this.

Table 1.

	Population in millions)	Known dialysis centres
Nordic	23.247	118
Benelux	25.369	118
Spain	39.045	243
France	56.681	259
United Kingdom	57.536	89
Italy	57.718	566
Germany	78.028	501
Total Registry	668.868	

Table 2. Transplant centres as percentage of known RRT centres

Italy	2%
Germany	5%
Sweden	6%
Hungary	7%
Czechoslovakia	10%
Belgium	11%
Austria	12%
France	12%
Spain	12%
Netherlands	13%
Switzerland	13%
Denmark	23%
UK	37%

Table 3. Patient records on file 31 December 1992

Recorded alive on RRT	173403
Dead	180509
Status uncertain*	102143
Total	456055

Thus in recent data collected in the United Kingdom (as yet unpublished) it has been shown, using the EDTA database, that patients without other morbidity and aged 15 to 64 have the best survival unsurprisingly, but that for patients with diabetes mellitus and renal failure who are in the same age range, survival is virtually the same as that for patients without morbidity who are aged 65 to 74 (Wood IT, Roderick PR, Mallick NP unpublished).

These figures can be refined in a number of ways and this has been done increasingly in recent years both in Europe and in the United States. Apart from diabetes, cardiovascular disease is the principle other determinant of outcome. The fact that such co-morbid influences if present at the time when renal replacement therapy commences so profoundly influence the value of that therapy points decisively to the need to manage patients in the pre-end stage phase. This means that nephrologists must be early aware that such patients have been detected by other doctors and that sound nephrological opinion with an overall assessment of potential problems is made in good time.

The age distribution of patients beginning RRT in 1982, 1987 and 1992 is shown in Figure 3. When this is refined to look at the take-on rate in different age groups it is apparent that for major European countries patients up to the age of 64 are now receiving treatment probably in numbers close to the requirement. On the other hand the striking rise over these years in patients older than 65 is evident and has not appeared to have reached a plateau yet. Thus when examining the stock of patients on RRT (Figure 4) it is clear that this overall figure conceals a number of variables of age, co-morbidity and take-on rates at different ages together with the survival of patients defined by these parameters.

Furthermore these stock figures are influenced also by the factors mentioned above. As is shown in Figures 5 and 6, the proportion of patients in different age ranges who are treated by different forms of renal replacement therapy varies by country and also by underlying disease.

The stock figures depending as they do on such a complex series of variables can readily be misinterpreted.

Figures 7 to 9 show for three selective years and for last mode of therapy (haemodialysis, peritoneal dialysis or transplantation) the causes of death as recorded to us. These have changed in proportion little over time. Nevertheless some differences are clear in the significant increase in the number of patients who are now refusing to continue therapy (Figure 10). This is understandable and may reflect good medical practice in recognising that the value of therapy has changed for a given patient because of changes in their physical or other circumstances.

In Figure 11 is shown survival for two selected cohorts of patients after grafting. This takes in all patients by age or underlying illness. That there is an age related influence is shown in Figure 12. It is well known too that diabetic patients have poorer survival overall and this is shown in Figure 13 and this is represented by the Selwood analysis for standard PRD and diabetic patients in Figures 14 and 15.

Overall then survival in the European Registry has been calculated according to these broad parameters. Refinements are continually applied and analysis by country is also conducted. Varied approaches to renal replacement therapy across Europe are quite striking but analysis shows that even within a given country with an apparently homogeneous approach to care there are very wide differences also in the way patients are managed. It is the place for a Registry such as ours to gradually refine these differences and show which approaches are producing the best potential outcome.

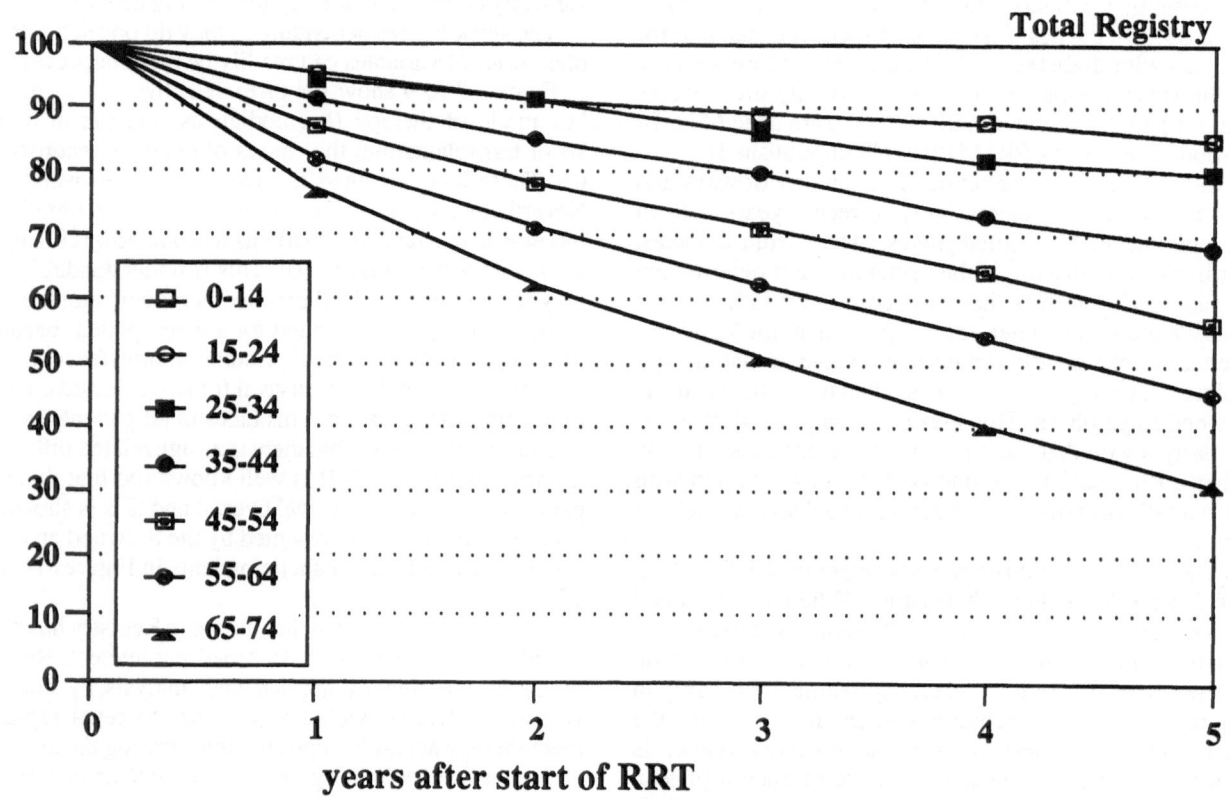

Figure 1. Actuarial survival for all patients beginning RRT in 1986–1991.

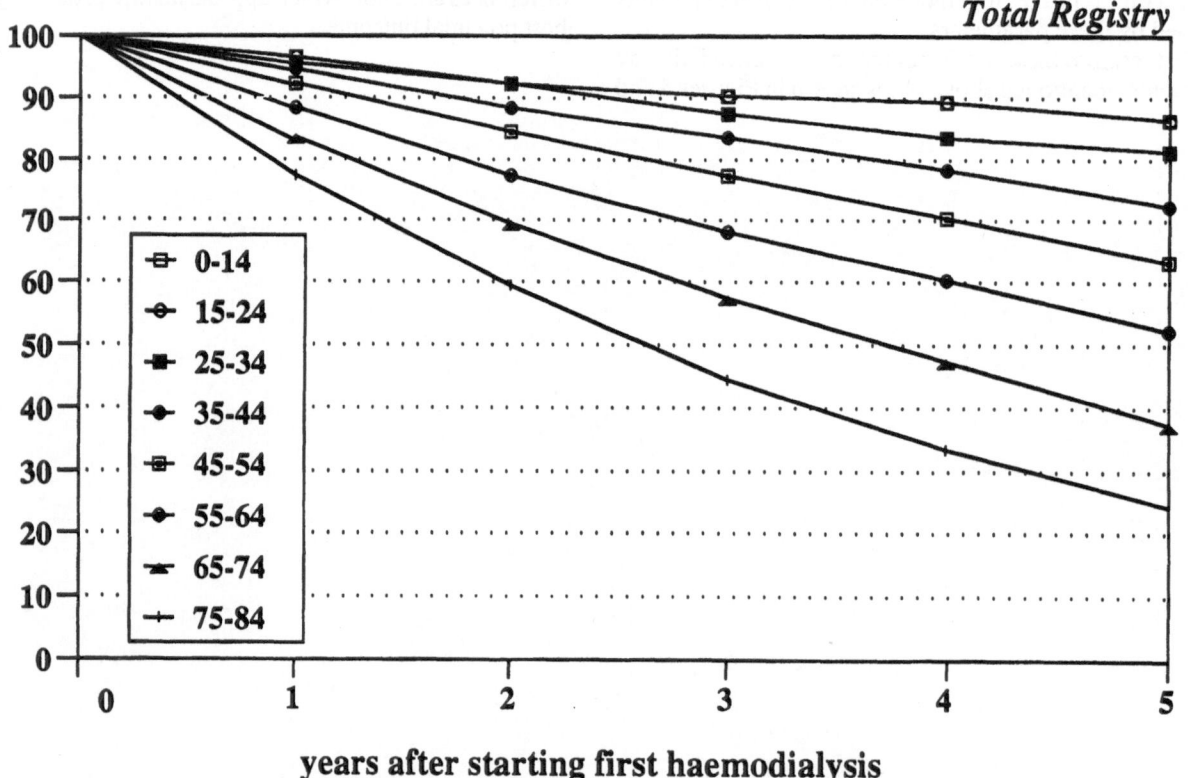

Figure 2. Survival on haemodialysis: all patients beginning RRT in 1986–1991.

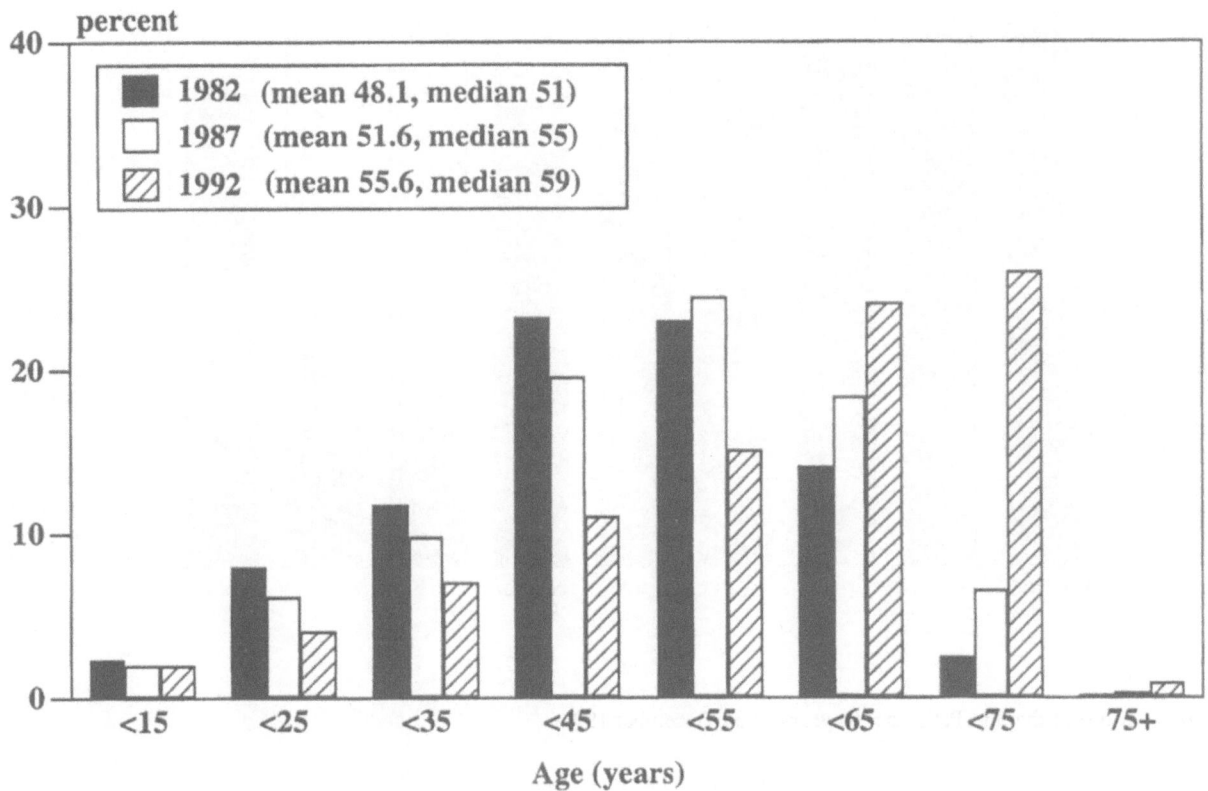

Figure 3. Age distribution of all patients beginning RRT in 1982, 1987 and 1992

	Transplant stock	Per million population	Dialysis stock	Per million population
Nordic	3843	165	2789	120
Benelux	5546	219	6421	253
Spain	8219	210	14000	359
France	11578	204	17062	301
United Kingdom	12011	209	10323	179
Italy	6721	116	22368	387
Germany	6973	89	20833	267
Total Registry	64296	96	118482	177

Figure 4. Number of patients on RRT at end of 1992.

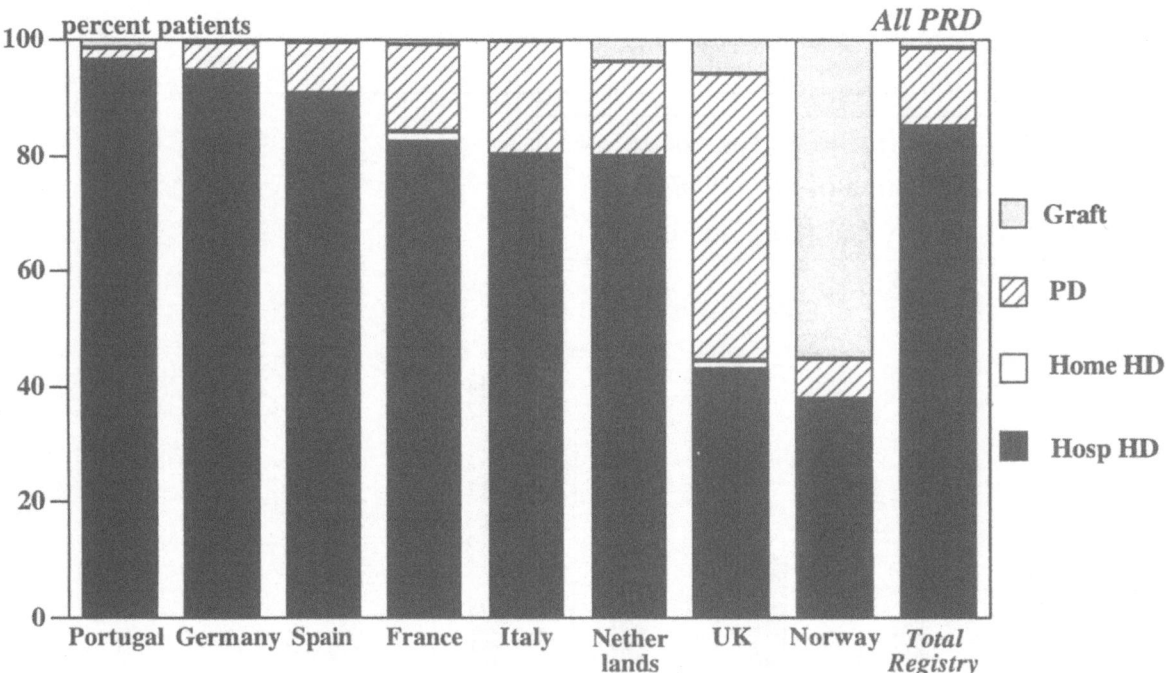

Figure 5. Mode of therapy. Patients > 65 years on 31 December 1992.

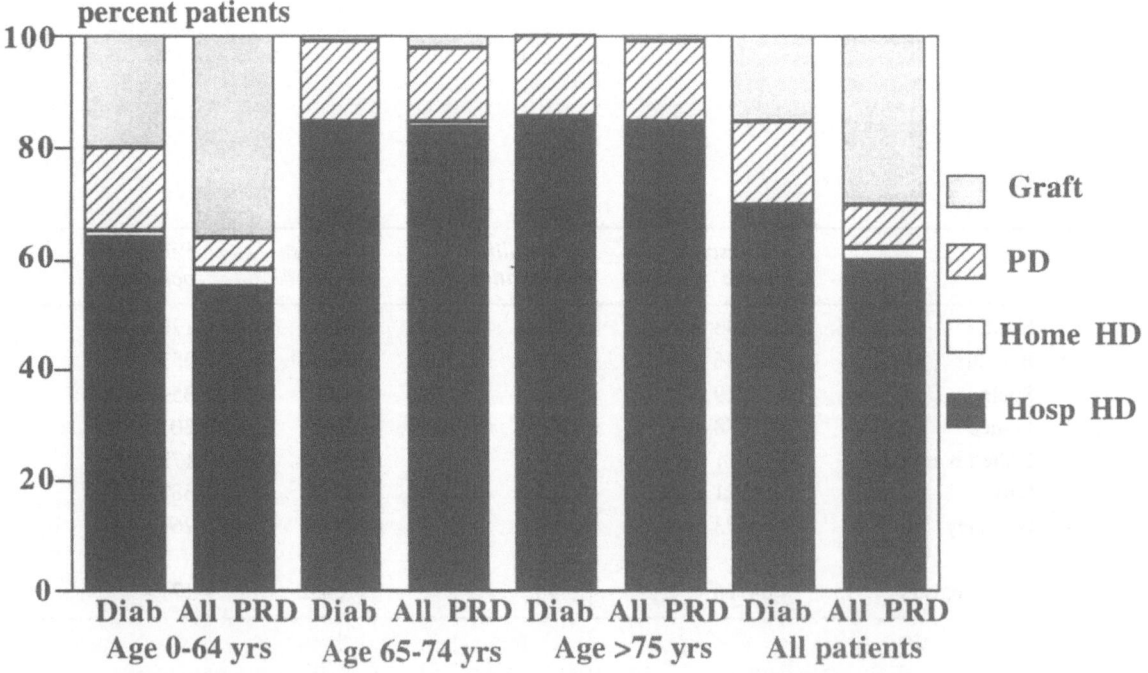

Figure 6. Diabetic patients vs all PRD on 31 December 1992.

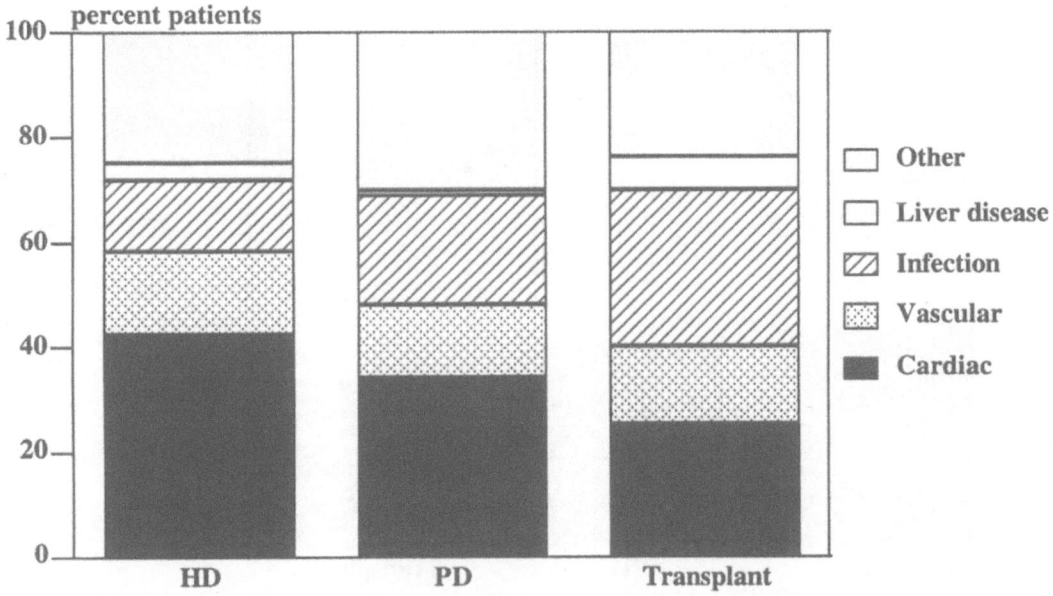

Figure 7. Causes of death in patients on RRT according to last mode of therapy 1982.

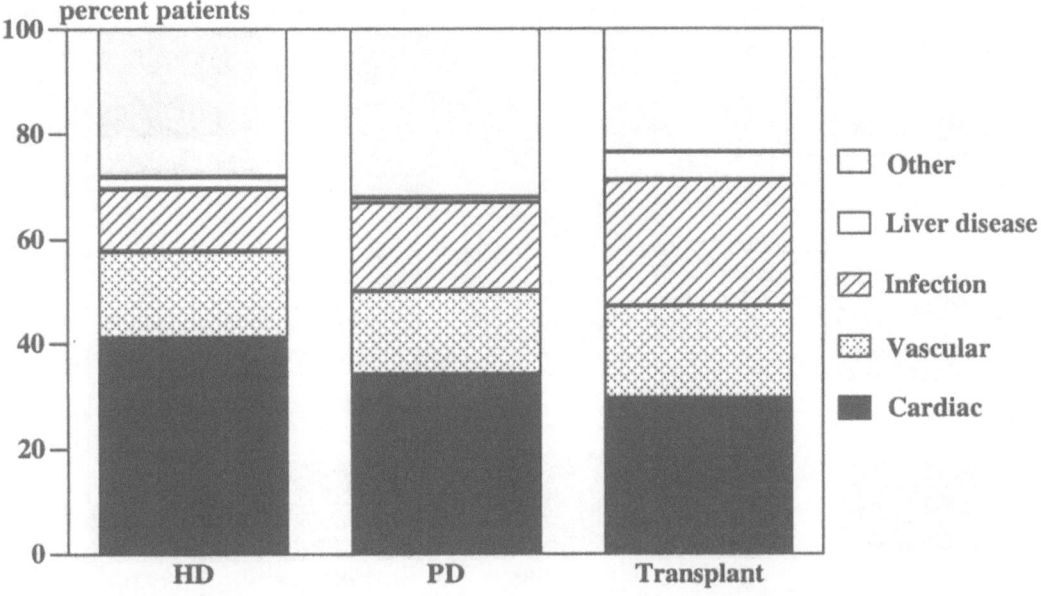

Figure 8. Causes of death in patients on RRT according to last mode of therapy 1986.

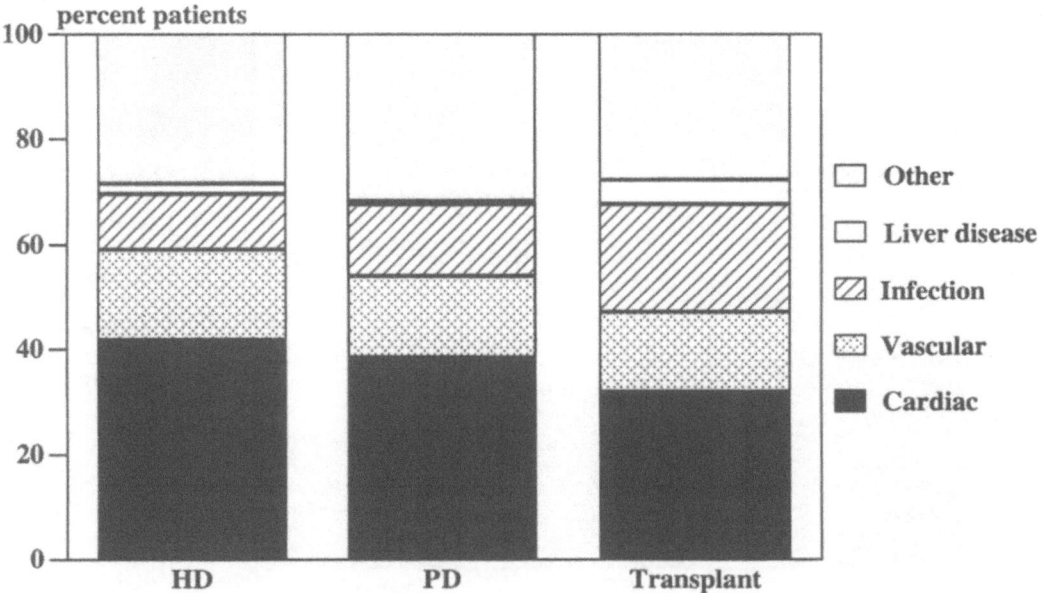

Figure 9. Causes of death in patients on RRT according to last mode of therapy 1991.

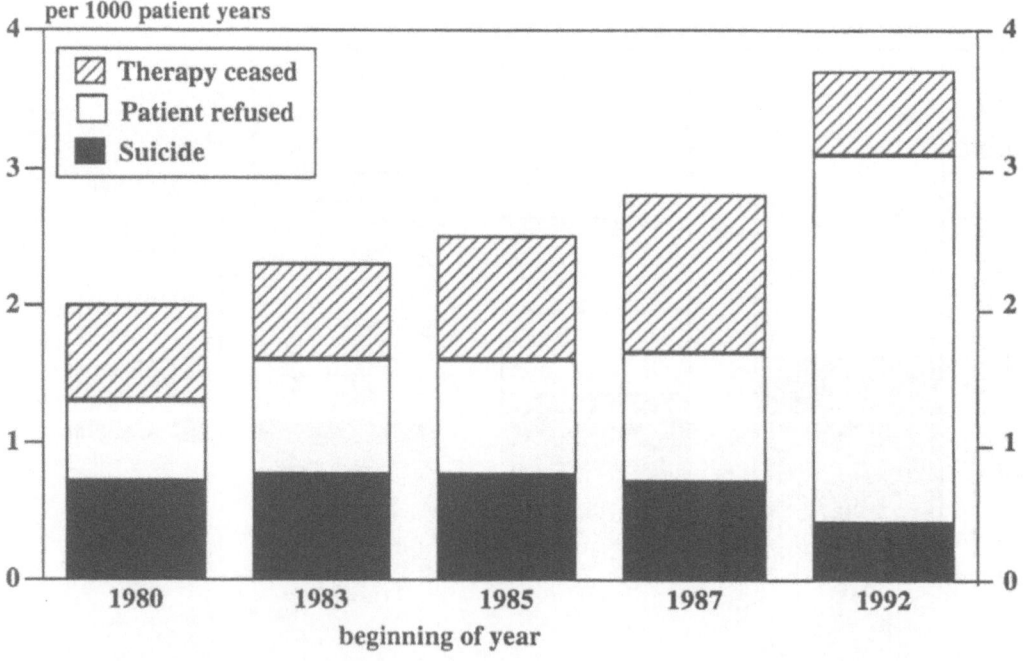

Figure 10. Death rate in all patients on HD.

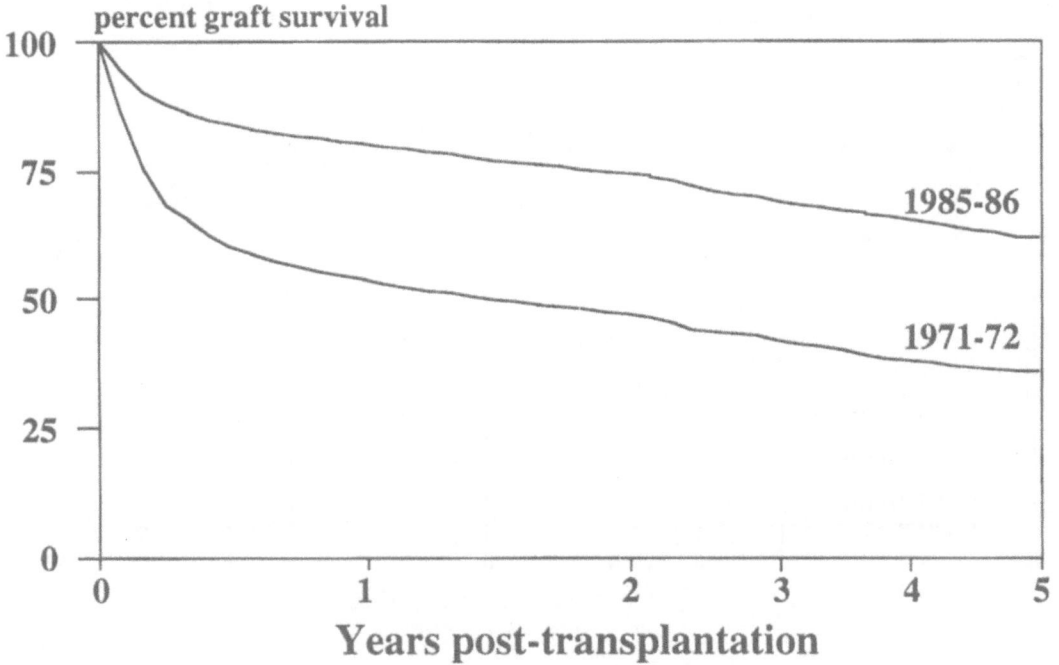

Figure 11. Graft survival of first CAD grafts performed in 1971–1972 and 1985–1986.

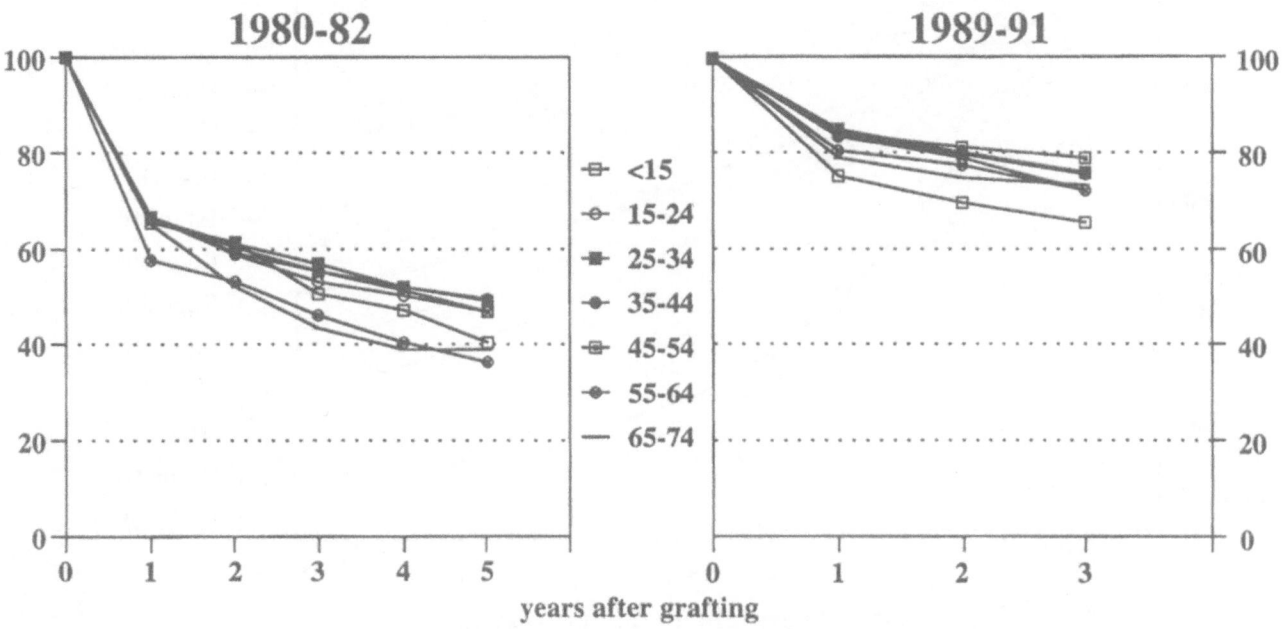

Figure 12. First CAD graft survival according to age of recipient – Total Registry.

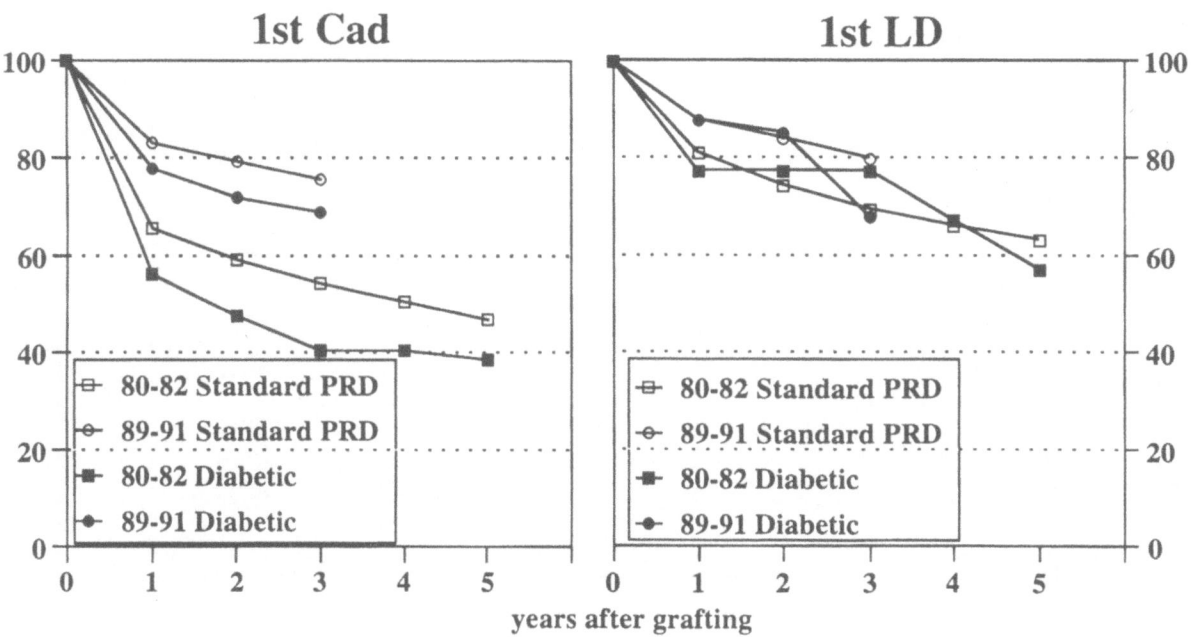

Figure 13. Graft survival according to PRD of recipient 1980–1982 and 1989–1991.

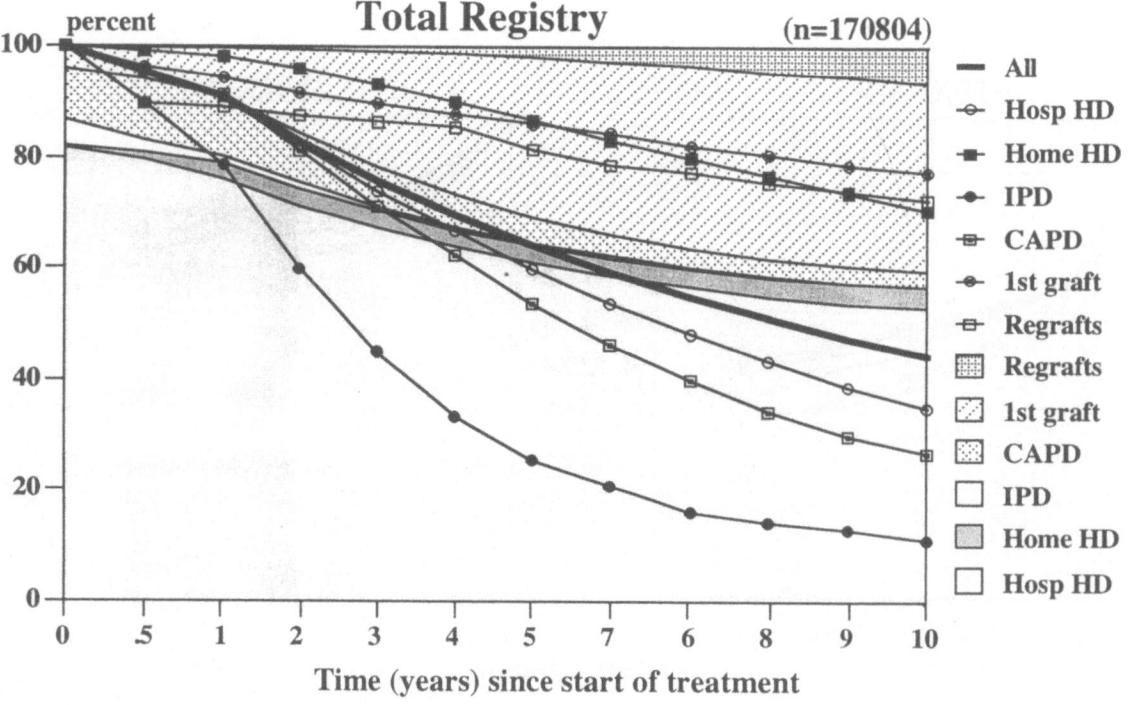

Figure 14. Patients starting treatment 1982–1991. Standard PRD, all ages.

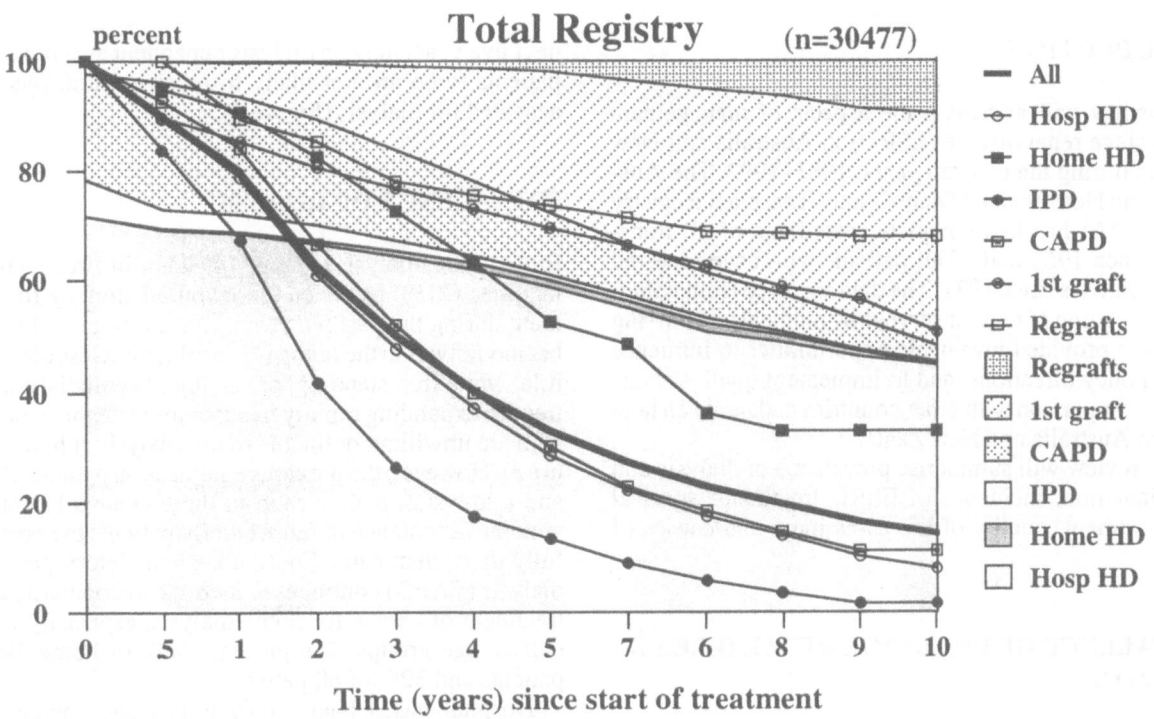

Figure 15. Patients starting treatment 1982–1991. Diabetics, all ages.

PART E: OUTCOMES – CRITICAL OVERVIEW: AUSTRALIAN REGISTRY

ALEX P.S. DISNEY

INTRODUCTION

This review will address some aspects of management of end stage renal disease (ESRD) in Australia and New Zealand during the past ten years, 1983–1992. The Australian and New Zealand Dialysis and Transplant Registry (ANZDATA) has had complete recordings of all transplants since 1965 and of all patients who have received regular dialysis since 1971. The data acquired from voluntary completion of regular surveys by medical and nursing staff have provided invaluable opportunities to influence health policy directions, and to implement quality assurance in comparison with other countries and between hospitals in Australia and New Zealand.

This review will summarise prevalence of dialysis and transplantation, incidence of ESRD treatment, survival with treatment, quality of life assessment and causes of death.

PREVALENCE OF END STAGE RENAL DISEASE PATIENTS

At 30 September 1993, there were 7388 patients (418 per million population (pmp)) in Australia and 1390 patients (397 pmp) in New Zealand either with a functioning renal transplant or dependent on dialysis; of these, 52% in Australia and 51% in New Zealand were transplant dependent. Only a small proportion of elderly patients had a functioning transplant: 23% of the 65–74 year group and 5% of the 75–84 year group. The comparative rates for the young and middle aged were 63% of those between 15–54 years, and 50% of those between 55–64 years (Figure 1). In the past ten years, improved graft survival rather than a higher transplantation rate has been responsible for increasing the proportion of patients kept alive by a functioning transplant. However, the majority of patients within the next five years may be dialysis dependent as more elderly patients (who are not likely to receive a transplant) are accepted for dialysis (Figure 2).

PREVALENCE OF DIALYSIS

In Australia, dialysis at home (49%) or in 'free-standing' facilities (21%) has been the favoured strategy for treatment during the past ten years. Current figures show that haemodialysis in the home is now playing a less prominent role, while free-standing, or satellite, haemodialysis centres are expanding rapidly to accommodate those patients who are unwilling or unable to use dialysis at home (Figure 3). However, the previous emphasis on patient self care and a low staff:patient ratio in these centres has shifted with the acceptance of more elderly patients to assisted or fully dependent care. Continuous ambulatory peritoneal dialysis (CAPD) continues to increase in popularity as the treatment of choice for home dialysis, especially for the elderly age groups. It represents 66% of home dialysis patients and 32% of all patients.

Hospital based haemodialysis has also increased in recent years, following a five-year lull in which satellite based haemodialysis and CAPD treatment expanded. The increasing age and hence frailty of dialysis patients, with concomitant vascular disease, may soon require the provision of free-standing units able to offer the intensity of nursing and medical services currently seen only in hospital based units. Alternatively, the costs of maintaining such a level of support at some distance from major hospitals may accelerate the relocation of these units closer too or even within the hospitals.

In New Zealand over the past ten years, home dialysis (either haemodialysis or CAPD) has increasingly predominated: in the past five years the prevalence of CAPD has also risen rapidly and now represents 56% of all patients and 68% of home dialysis patients.

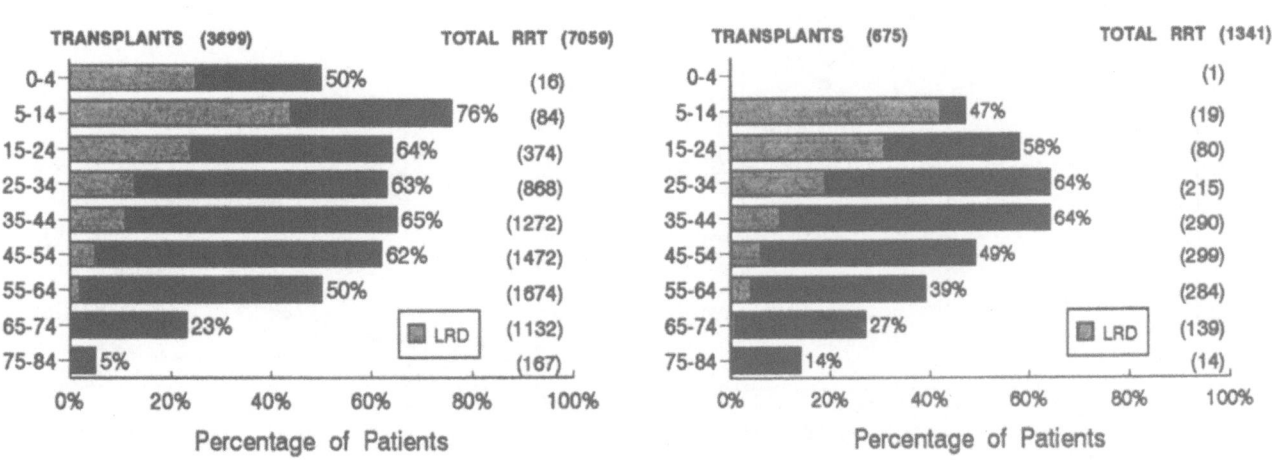

Figure 1. Proportion (%) of renal replacement treatment (RRT) patients (7059 in Australia, 1341 in New Zealand) dependent on a functioning transplant at 31 December 1992. The light coloured bars represent living donor kidneys, dark coloured bars represent cadaver donor kidneys. Age groups at 31 December 1992.

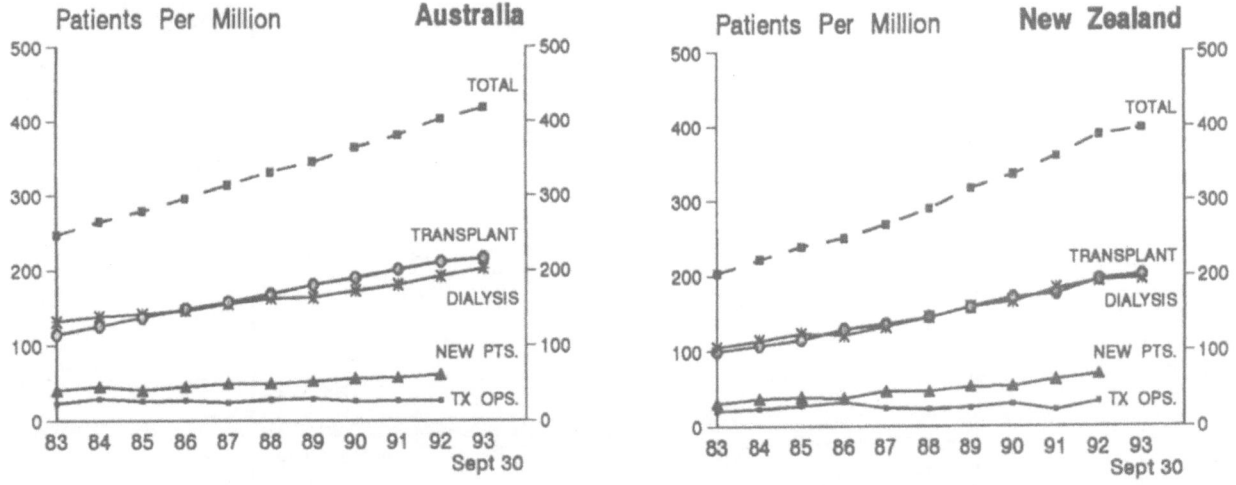

Figure 2. Population related number (pmp), 1) of all ESRD patients (total) with a functioning transplant or dependent on dialysis in Australia or New Zealand at 31 December each year, 1983–1992, and at 30 September 1993, 2) new patient incidence each year, 3) transplant operations each year.

PREVALENCE: TRANSPLANTS

Australia's annual transplantation rate of 27 pmp over the past five years has relied heavily on cadaver donor kidneys. Unfortunately, despite efforts to improve notification of transplant Coordinators about potential donors, the cadaver donor kidney rate in Australia remained only 22 pmp in the past year (Figure 2). Only 15% of transplanted kidneys have come from a living donor, and few of these operations have involved a living donor who was not related to the recipient. Living donor kidneys are now

being used more often because the waiting period for a cadaver donor organ is increasing, the median being eighteen months. Of those dialysis patients under 60 years old who were awaiting a transplant in 1992, just under 30% were transplanted during the year. The majority of donors have been young adults; however, the proportion in the middle-aged to elderly age group has been increasing. Similar transplant activity has been seen in New Zealand with the highest annual rate of 33 pmp being recorded in 1992.

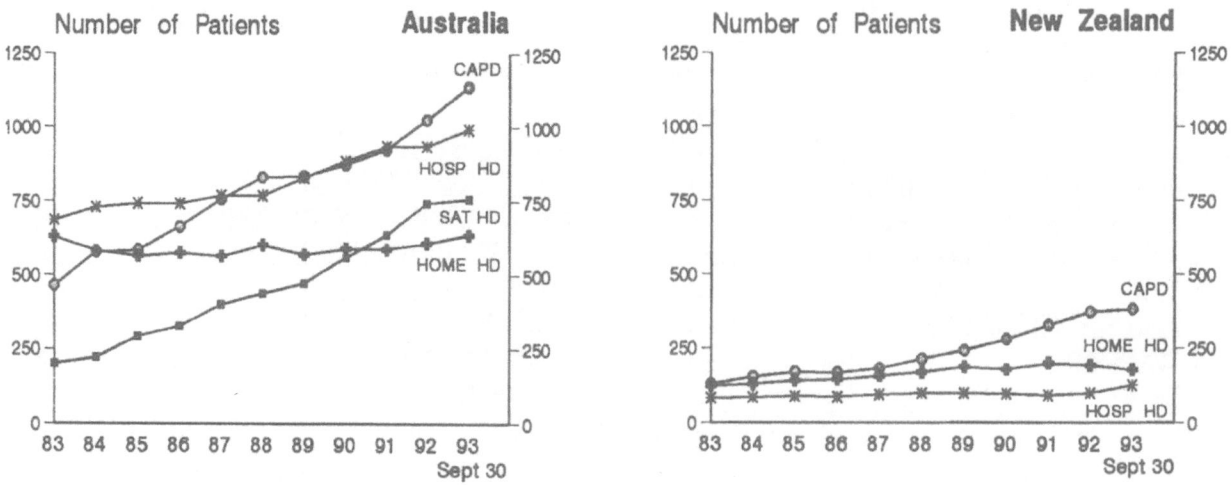

Figure 3. Prevalence of method and location of dialysis treatment for patients 1983–1992, and 30 September 1993, in Australia and New Zealand.

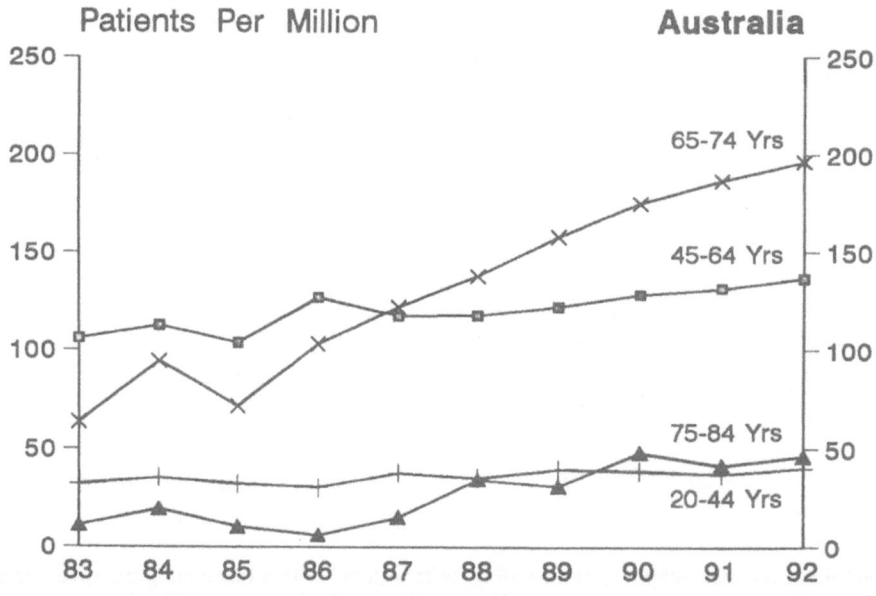

Figure 4. Age group specific annual incidence rate (pmp) of patients in Australia during the period 1983–1992 for age groups 20–44, 45–64, 65–74 and 75–84 years. Age at initial treatment.

INCIDENCE OF END STAGE RENAL DISEASE

Australia's annual incidence rate for end stage renal disease (ESRD) treatment rose markedly from 40 pmp in 1983 to 61 pmp in 1992; corresponding figures for New Zealand were 30 pmp to 69 pmp (Figure 2). Increasing acceptance of elderly patients for treatment in Australia was responsible for most of this change; the age group specific rate of new patients in the age group 65–74 years rose fourfold from 50 pmp in 1982 to 200 pmp by 1992. The rate in the older age group 75–84 years has risen from 5 to 50 pmp over the past five years (Figure 4). The steady rise in the age of new patients is reflected in the median age, this being 49 years in 1983 and 55 years (range 8 months to 87 years) in 1992. In 1992, 25% of new patients were aged over 65 years. (Figure 5).

Another significant factor in the rising incidence rate of new patients has been the increasing referral and acceptance of those with diabetic nephropathy, many of them from the indigenous racial groups. Indigenous races in both countries have a higher incidence of ESRD: in 1991 the Caucasoid group registered 48 pmp; Aboriginal, 196 pmp; Maori, 230 pmp; and Polynesian Pacific Islanders, 131 pmp.

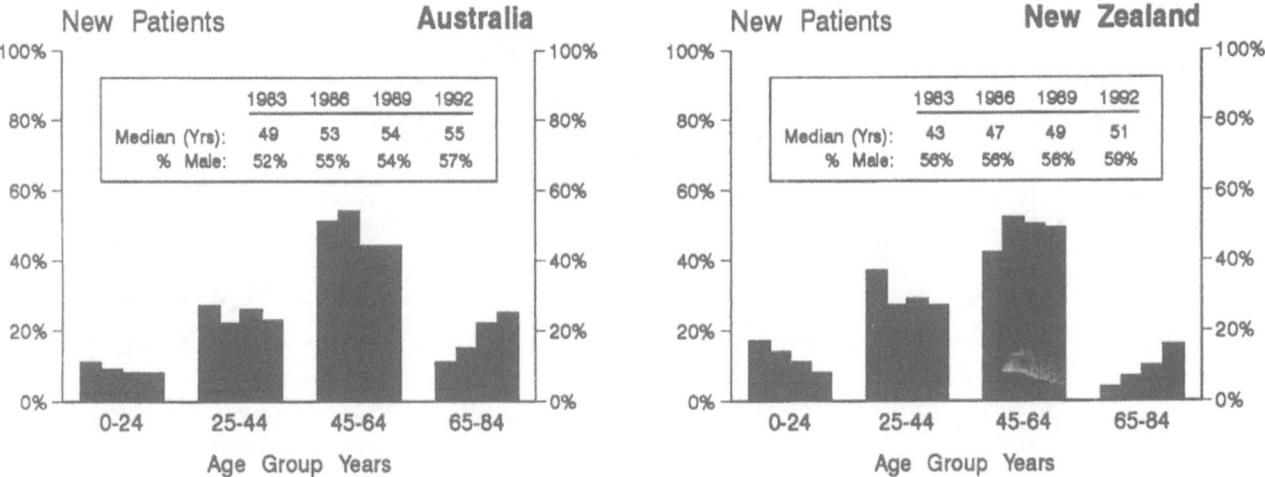

Figure 5. Proportion of new patients at 31st December for years 1983, 1986, 1989, 1992 in the age groups 0–24, 25–44, 45–64, 65–84 years, in Australia and New Zealand. Age at initial treatment. The median age (years) of new patients, and the proportion (%) of male patients are shown for the four selected years.

Co-morbid factors recorded for new patients during the past two years have shown 50% to be past or present smokers who had significantly greater risk of death within the first twelve months of treatment. As expected, coronary artery disease (33% of new cases) and peripheral vascular disease (21% of new cases) were associated with a greater risk of death in the same period: 3.5 and 4.5 times compared to patients without coronary or peripheral vascular disease respectively.

PRIMARY RENAL DISEASE

Glomerulonephritis remains the most common cause of renal failure in Australia; diabetes and renovascular disease/hypertension have increased as the age of patients has increased, and as more Aboriginals have received treatment. Most cases of diabetic nephropathy have been associated with Type II diabetes which is particularly common in the indigenous racial groups. There has been only a slight increase in the number of diabetics with Type I disease, which is believed to have resulted from improved management of blood glucose levels and blood pressure over the past 10–15 years. The higher incidence of diabetic nephropathy in New Zealand reflects the incidence of ESRD in Maori and Polynesian Pacific Islander patients of whom 45% have diabetic nephropathy compared to 11% of Caucasoid patients.

The fall in new cases of analgesic nephropathy from 18% in 1983 to 9% in 1992 has confirmed the success of a national education campaign and the legislation providing compound analgesics only by prescription.

INTEGRATED TREATMENT SURVIVAL
(Kaplan–Meier Method)

Although there has been a strong emphasis on transplantation, those unwilling or unsuitable for consideration for a graft have not been refused acceptance for dialysis. There have not been any financial incentives in Australia likely to promote dialysis at the expense of transplantation. Government has fully funded the renal failure treatment program since its inception nearly thirty years ago.

The longest surviving patient has had a functioning graft since 1965, and the longest dialysis survivor (without transplantation) started treatment in 1969. Recently, there were 189 patients surviving after 20 years, 73% with a functioning graft and 27% treated by dialysis (24% following a failed graft).

Age and primary renal disease have significantly influenced the outcome of treatment (Figure 6). The modal age group of new patients (45–64 years) have had a 66 month median survival with integrated dialysis and transplant treatment. The elderly and those with diseases associated with extensive vascular damage (diabetes, analgesic nephropathy, renovascular/hypertension) have had a meagre life expectancy. Such results have aroused debate about the quality and quantity of life related to the considerable expense.

DIALYSIS PRESCRIPTION

There has been only a mild trend towards short hours of dialysis with fast blood flow rates. The majority of patients undergo haemodialysis three times a week for a period of 12.5 hours per week (ranging from 4 to 24 hours) in Australia, and 14.5 hours (ranging from 4 to

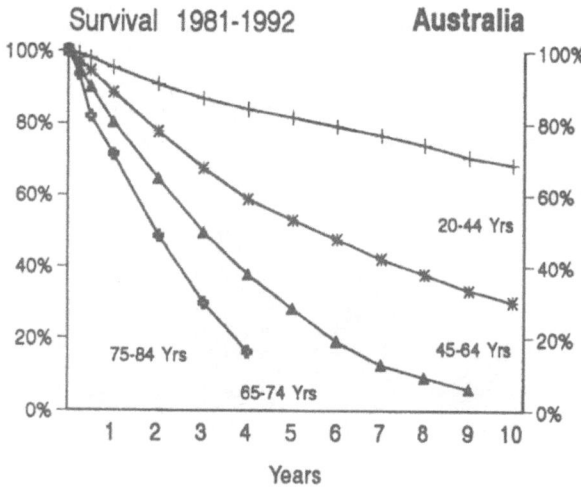
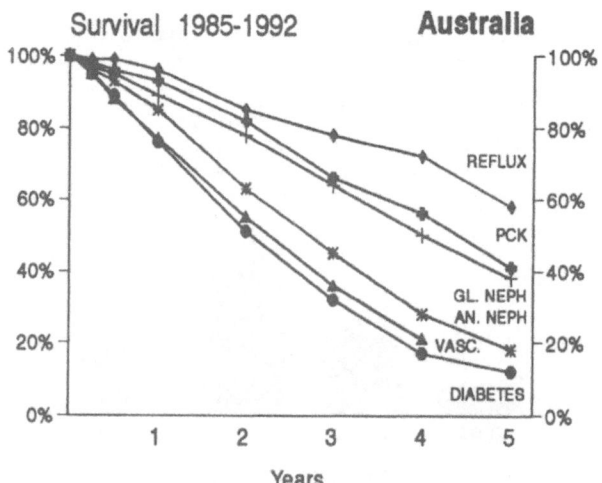

Figure 6. Patient survival (%) from initial treatment for ESRD patients in Australia, a) 1981–1992 related to age group (years) 20–44, 45–64, 65–74, 75–84 at initial treatment, b) 1985–1992 related to primary cause of renal disease; vesico-ureteric reflux (reflux), polycystic renal disease (PCK), glomerulonephritis (gl.neph), analgesic induced nephropathy (An.Neph), hypertension/renovascular disease (vasc.) and diabetic nephropathy (diabetes).

30 hours) in New Zealand. Individualised prescription of hours, blood flow rate, and membrane surface area based on urea clearance has influenced but not controlled dialysis treatment in most units: median treatment period 4 hours, blood flow rate 250 mls/min, surface area 1.1 m², with cuprophan or cellulose acetate based membranes. Use of bicarbonate based dialysate has extended to most patients in Australia (75%), but only a minority in New Zealand (25%).

Peritoneal dialysis prescription in Australia is almost exclusively CAPD, usually 56 litres per week, with a 'disconnect' system in most (82%) cases and a dialysate calcium concentration of 1.25 mmol/l in many cases (64%). In New Zealand, fewer (50%) use a disconnect system and the majority (88%) use a calcium concentration of 1.25 mmol/l.

SURVIVAL OF DIALYSED PATIENTS (TABLE 1)

There has been an integrated approach to the two main methods of dialysis – CAPD and haemodialysis – that does not encourage undue emphasis on comparison of their relative success. CAPD has been the preferred treatment for diabetics, the elderly and those with an unstable cardiovascular system, and has been the favoured option for units with insufficient haemodialysis facilities. The patient's perception of CAPD has been improved by the decreasing risk of peritonitis accompanying the more widespread use of disconnect systems. That many patients change electively from one form of dialysis to the other within the first three months is a measure of late referral, of

Table 1. Summary of Regular Dialysis Patient survival (%) at one and three years for Australia 1983–1992 (by Kaplan–Meier method) in relation to gender, method of dialysis, age at first dialysis treatment, race, primary renal disease and year of first treatments

Variable	1 yr	3 yr	Variable	1 yr	3 yr
Male	90	68			
Female	91	70	*Disease*		
			Glomerulonephritis	94	76
HD[a]	91	73	Analgesic	90	63
CAPD[b]	89	57	Vascular	84	54
			Polycystic	95	84
O–24 yr	98	94	Reflux	97	86
25–44 yr	96	85	Diabetic Neph	83	47
45–54 yr	93	77			
55–64 yr	88	62	*Year of Transplant*		
65–74 yr	83	54	1983	90	69
75–84 yr	73	34	1985	91	71
			1987	92	69
Caucasoid	91	69	1989	90	65
Aboriginal	86	66	1991	90	–
Maori	90	72			

[a] Haemodialysis.
[b] Continuous Ambulatory Peritoneal Dialysis.

unplanned initiation of treatment or of a preference for one form of dialysis in this initial phase of treatment.

The three-year survival rate of all dialysis patients treated during the past ten years is 69% in Australia and 65% in New Zealand, as shown in Table 1. Increasing age has had the strongest adverse influence on survival, with the range of three-year survival being 92% (0-24 years), 85% (25–44 years), 77% (45-54 years), 62% (55-64 years), 54% (65-74 years). The inclusion of age and primary renal disease in a Cox (2) model of proportional hazards indicates no adverse survival trend in patients who commenced dialysis in recent years. Significant variables have been age (risk 1.04 per year), female (risk 0.86), CAPD (risk 1.31), Aboriginal race (risk 1.66), primary renal disease diabetic nephropathy (risk 2.60), analgesic nephropathy (risk 1.51), hypertensive renal damage (risk 1.71) and polycystic renal disease (risk 0.68), with male Caucasoid, glomerulonephritis and haemodialysis treatment as the reference group.

While dependent on the chosen form of treatment, those using haemodialysis have had a lower risk of death than those using CAPD. Factors such as age and concomitant vascular conditions may have had some adverse influence, but most have been directly or indirectly included in the multifactorial analysis.

SURVIVAL OF TRANSPLANTED PATIENTS (TABLE 2)

As shown in Table 2, during the past ten years, successful graft survival has rapidly increased without change in patient survival. In 1991 the one-year patient and graft survivals for primary cadaver graft transplant operations in Australia were 93% and 84% respectively; in New Zealand 96% and 82% respectively. Primary cadaver donor graft survival has approached that of a living donor graft as shown in Table 2. The latest results for transplants performed in 1991 show regraft success has also reached encouraging levels. The patient and graft survival rates for all transplants performed in Australia during the period 1983–1992 were respectively 93 and 81% at one year, and 82 and 65% at five years; in New Zealand the survival rates were 92 and 73% at one year and 76 and 56% at five years. Most grafts have been functioning well at one year: serum creatinine < 200 μmol/l–84%, < 150 μmol/l– 52%.

The recipients' expectation of survival following transplantation decreased more rapidly as the age at transplantation increased; the median survival for the late middle-aged (55–64 years) has been half that of those twenty years younger (35-44 years) and only a third that of young adults (15–34 years): eight years, 17 years and 25 years respectively. Graft survival of those under 55 years has not been significantly influenced by age. The nature of the primary renal disease has had some influence on patient survival but considerably less on graft survival. Those with analgesic, diabetic or hypertensive/renovascular nephropathy have been more at risk of death or graft loss.

Unfortunately two of the indigenous racial groups, Aboriginal and Maori, have registered a significantly worse expectation of survival, both for the patient and the graft, than the Caucasoid (European descent) racial group. Many factors such as the high rate of diabetic nephropathy with concomitant vascular damage to other organs combined with lack of adherence to treatment have probably contributed to these disappointing results.

The cadaver donor kidney exchange program has allocated organs on the basis of HLA compatibility, with a bias towards the B locus and DR locus; few kidneys have been completely matched or mismatched for all three loci (A, B or DR). Grafts with one to three mismatches have had a significantly better survival rate than those with four or five mismatches. The one-year graft survival ranged from 92% (zero mismatch) to 87% (one to three mismatches) to 80% (four to five mismatches) during the past five years. Now that the graft survival of poorly matched grafts has improved, more highly mismatched organs have been allocated to those with blood group O or uncommon HLA antigens who are still awaiting a transplant after several years of dialysis treatment. Other risk factors for graft survival have been the age of the donor and rate of transplant activity in a unit. As the waiting lists for a transplant have lengthened, the acceptable age of a donor kidney has risen but has been accompanied by lower graft survival, caused in part by higher rates of vascular thrombosis in the early post-operative period. Greater attention is being directed to the assessment of the histological appearance or the functional capacity of the donor kidney before or after removal.

Kidneys from donors more than 54 years old registered shorter graft survival in association with higher rates of early post-operative vascular occlusions (3).

QUALITY OF LIFE (KARNOVSKY) (4)

The quality of life of patients has been recorded using the Karnovsky activity scale; there has been no widespread application of broader methods of assessing emotional and social interactive factors. Only a small proportion (12%) of dialysis patients were reportedly capable of entirely normal activity, but quite a large and increasing proportion were able to manage normal activity with minor effort (38%) or with moderate effort (25%). The remainder were capable of caring for daily needs, but many required considerable assistance; few were reported to be severely disabled or dependent on hospital care. As expected, activity decreased with age but the majority of elderly patients (65–84 years) who dialysed at home or in a satellite facility were still capable of normal activity with mild to moderate effort; those unable to do so were usually dependent on hospital based haemodialysis.

The new lease on life afforded by a transplant was evident from the capacity for normal activity reported by 95% of the patients (52% with no effort, 33% with minor effort and 10% with moderate effort).

Table 2. Summary of patient and graft survival (%) at one and five years following renal transplantation in Australia 1983–1992 (by the Kaplan–Meier method) in relation to source of donor kidney; age of recipient at transplantation; race; primary renal disease, and year of transplantation (primary cadaver graft only). Pacific Is = Pacific Islander (Polynesian). Maori is indigenous race (Polynesian) of New Zealander

Variable	Patient		Graft		Variable	Patient		Graft	
	1 yr	5 yr	1 yr	5 yr		1 yr	5 yr	1 yr	5 yr
Cad. donor (1)[a]	92	81	81	66	*Disease*				
Cad. donor (2)[a]	95	81	74	57	Glomerulonephritis	94	85	83	68
Living donor	96	87	90	75	Analgesic	85	71	75	62
0–14 yr	98	93	86	69	Vascular	90	77	82	62
15–34 yr	97	89	82	65	Polycystic	93	81	83	71
35–44 yr	94	86	83	69	Reflux	97	90	86	71
45–54 yr	92	79	80	65	Diabetic Neph	88	73	81	58
55–64 yr	87	67	78	59					
65–74 yr	82	–	72	–	*Year of Transplant*				
					1983	91	81	74	58
Caucasoid	93	83	83	68	1985	92	79	79	62
Aboriginal	91	63	81	45	1987	90	82	83	70
Maori[b]	87	66	67	48	1989	94	–	85	–
Pacific Is.[b]	92	81	76	61	1991	93	–	84	–

[a] Primary and Second Cadaver Donor.
[b] Australia and New Zealand.

REHABILITATION

The difficulties for dialysis patients, particularly the middle-aged, associated with retaining employment have increased during the recent period of economic recession. Patients under 65 years old were assessed for work (including home management) in the following categories: full time 33%, part time 20%, unable to get a job 15%, too sick 4%, retired 8%. As with the quality of life, those working were younger and dialysing at home or at a satellite haemodialysis facility; the elderly and infirm were dependent on hospital based haemodialysis. The likely long term social difficulties for the 18% of unemployed young adults emphasised the importance of early transplantation.

DEATH

In 1992, the death rate was 12% expressed in relation to the number of patients dialysed at any time during the year: 10 and 18% of those aged 45–64 years and 65–84 years old respectively. Cardiac events (myocardial ischaemia, sudden cardiac arrest, hyperkalaemia) have remained the major cause of death for dialysis dependent patients, particularly myocardial infarction which was recorded as the most common cardiac cause of death. The most at risk of a cardiac death were indigenous racial groups – Aboriginals (57% of deaths) and Maoris (59% of deaths) – and diabetic patients (53% of deaths).

Death caused by withdrawal from treatment has included those who have chosen to withdraw or those in terminal circumstances whose treatment has been discontinued following consultation with the patient and family. The frequency increased with age, reaching 11% of deaths of the 45–64 year age group and 16% of deaths of the 65–84 year age group. As a consequence, counselling, family support, 'permission to die' and hospice style facilities have assumed a more active and prominent role. While it was not as common amongst young patients, a few children and young adult diabetics withdrew from treatment.

Whereas only 2.4% of patients with a functioning graft died in 1992, the increasing prevalence of malignancy has been causing concern: 33% of deaths in that year. Common tumours occurred at a slightly higher rate than in the general population. Skin tumours, especially squamous cell carcinoma, occurred much more frequently, particularly in the tropical and sub-tropical regions. Lymphoma, Kaposi's Sarcoma and carcinoma of the cervix, female perineum or thyroid were far more common than in the general population. By 20 years, 20% of patients can expect to have a solid tumour or haemopoietic system malignancy. So far there has been no strong evidence to implicate particular immunosuppressive regimens in the development of malignancy. Use of anti T-cell antibodies for reversal of rejection decreased in recent years to 20% of primary grafts from a peak 25% of transplants performed in 1988.

CONCLUSION

As ESRD treatment is extended to those with high risk factors (elderly, vascular disease) there will be more assisted dialysis (probably in hospital based units), higher death rates, and increased expense for more intense assistance with dialysis involving use of bicarbonate based dialysate with volume controlled haemodialysis machines. There has been a dramatic improvement in the success of renal transplantation, which now must be directed to the sensitised patients with high cytoxic antibody reactivity. Finally, early prevention of renal failure and particularly the cardiovascular consequences must remain a top priority.

ACKNOWLEDGMENTS

The preparation of this report was dependent on the considerable efforts of all the health care professionals who complete the data survey forms from each contributing unit. Survival analysis was performed by Brian Livingston and Leigh Roeger. Lee Excell was invaluable with her untiring efforts to collate data, perform analyses and prepare tables and figures. Elisabeth Steinmetz typed and Karen Reid edited the manuscript with characteristic patience and attention to detail.

The ANZDATA Registry is funded by the Governments of Australia and New Zealand and the Australian Kidney Foundation.

REFERENCES

1. Kaplan EL, Meier P: Nonparametric estimation from incomplete observations. *J Am Statist Assoc* 53: 457, 1958
2. Peto R. Pike MC, Armitage P. Bresslow NE, Cox DR, Howard SV, Mantel N. McPherson K, Peto J, Smith PG: Design and analysis of randomised clinical trials requiring prolonged observation of each patient. II. Analysis and Examples. *Brit J Cancer* 35: 1, 1977
3. Penny MJ, Nankivell BJ, Disney APS, Blyth K, Chapman JR. Renal graft thrombosis: a survey of 134 consecutive cases. *Transplantation* 58: 565, 1994
4. Karnovsky DA, Burchenal JH: *Evaluation of Chemotherapeutic Agents* edited by MacLeod CM, New York, NY, Columbia University, 1949, p 191

PART F: RENAL REPLACEMENT THERAPY IN CANADA 1981–1992

STANLEY S.A.FENTON, PAULINE F. COPLESTON, MARIE DESMEULES,
GERALD S. ARBUS, DANIEL H. FROMENT, CARL M. KJELLSTRAND and JOHN J. JEFFERY

INTRODUCTION

The Canadian Organ Replacement Register (CORR) is a national information system on organ failure and transplantation with the mandate to provide the capability to record and analyze the level of activity and outcome of renal replacement therapy and vital organ transplantation.

CORR, operated by the Canadian Institute for Health Information, is administered by a Board of Directors consisting of individuals drawn from the various groups with an interest in CORR, including the Canadian Society of Nephrology, the Canadian Transplant Society, Canadian Association of Transplantation, consumer groups such as The Kidney Foundation, and the federal and provincial governments.

The day to day workings of CORR are overseen by its Management Committee, with representatives from each of the disciplines: kidney, heart, lung, liver, dialysis, and paediatrics. In turn, the Management Committee relies on two Data Advisory Committees, one for dialysis issues from the Canadian Society of Nephrology, and the other for transplantation issues from the Canadian Transplant Society.

A staff of 5 persons perform the data collection, maintenance, reporting, and system functions necessary to operate the Register.

The demography and the results of renal replacement therapy and renal transplantation in Canada, from 1981–1992, will be presented. These data have been collected by the Renal Failure Register (1), operated by Statistics Canada from 1981 to 1986, and by The Canadian Organ Replacement Register (2), operated by the Canadian Institute for Health Information (now incorporating the Hospital Medical Records Institute) from 1987 until the present.

METHODS

Data is collected from all dialysis and transplant centres, either using paper forms, or by transfer of electronic data files from local data bases. Centres using paper forms are encouraged to submit patient registrations at the time patients enter their programs. Two types of forms are used: the facility profile form, and patient specific forms. A facility profile form is completed by each dialysis and transplant program across the country, detailing the status of their program as of December 31st each year. Also, individual patient profile forms are completed for every new patient entering a renal replacement program, or receiving a transplant. Detailed information exists for all dialysis patients entering renal failure therapy since January 1, 1981, including basic transplant information. The current status of each patient is determined on December 31st of each year by the completion of an annual follow-up form which includes death, transplant, or change in modality information. For transplanted patients, the follow-up includes date and cause of graft failure and date and cause of death, as well as any return to dialysis information.

The Register either deals directly with the individual dialysis or transplant programs, or with provincial programs. Some provinces have, or are in the process of developing, provincial data collection systems, whereby the information will be collected at a provincial level and then forwarded to the national registry. Although participation in the registry is voluntary, on average, only one out of the 80 centres does not submit their data in time for inclusion in the annual report. Only 2% of patients are lost to follow up. Patient and kidney survival analyses have been carried out using the SAS Lifetest (3) method which incorporates the Kaplan Meier method (4). The Cox (5) proportional hazards model has been used to calculate the hazard ratios for the multiple regression analysis of factors influencing patient and kidney survival. The data is stored

Table 1. Incidence count of new patients entering renal replacement programs by age group, 1981–1992, Canada

	Total new pts.	Age 0–14	Age 15–44	Age 45–64	Age 65–74	Age 75+
CANADA						
1992	2,698	48	639	975	693	343
1991	2,629	54	632	905	701	337
1990	2,303	50	609	860	515	269
1989	2,128	46	578	782	503	219
1988	1,952	55	555	750	436	156
1987	1,831	55	493	665	464	154
1986	1,729	43	501	644	395	146
1985	1,567	36	490	609	317	115
1984	1,460	47	482	561	289	81
1983	1,314	27	481	503	233	70
1982	1,263	32	428	513	222	68
1981	1,215	40	394	497	216	68

Table 2. New case rate of patients entering renal replacement programs by age group, 1981–1992, Canada

	All ages	Age 0–14	Age 15–44	Age 45–64	Age 65–74	Age 75+
CANADA						
1992	98.4	8.4	49.3	178.0	361.9	261.6
1991	97.4	9.6	49.0	170.9	374.9	265.1
1990	86.6	9.0	47.6	165.8	282.5	219.1
1989	81.2	8.4	45.7	153.6	281.8	184.7
1988	75.3	10.1	44.1	149.8	249.7	137.7
1987	71.5	10.1	39.5	134.9	272.3	141.5
1986	68.2	8.0	40.5	132.0	239.2	139.3
1985	62.3	6.6	39.9	125.9	197.8	113.5
1984	58.5	8.6	39.6	116.8	185.6	82.7
1983	53.0	4.9	39.8	105.9	142.8	74.1
1982	51.4	5.9	35.7	109.1	147.2	74.5
1981	49.9	7.3	33.3	106.7	146.2	83.6

on a VAX 3100 model 80, with VMS operating system and Oracle relational data base management software.

RENAL REPLACEMENT FACILITIES

In 1992 there were 80 renal centres in Canada for a population of 27.4 million. Each centre serving, on average, a population base of 350,000. Twenty-four of these centres carry out renal transplants, with each transplant centre serving a population of about 1.4 million. Canada has 895 total care and 242 self care haemodialysis stations which represents 41.5 stations per million population.

Table 3. Incidence count of primary renal diagnoses for patients entering renal replacement programs, by age group, 1981–1992, Canada

	All ages	Age 0–14	Age 15–44	Age 45–64	Age 65+
Total	2,698	48	639	975	1,036
Unknown	384	5	64	105	210
Glomerulonephritis	516	7	187	165	157
Pyelonephritis	176	8	69	45	54
Drug induced	27	0	4	12	11
Polycystic kidney	143	1	29	86	27
Hypertension	275	1	28	84	162
Other renal vascular	187	0	8	53	126
Diabetes	657	0	150	323	184
Other	333	26	100	102	105

NEW CASE RATE

The Canadian population is mainly Caucasian (92%), with the largest visible minority being Asian (6%). Two percent of the population are Aboriginal North Americans and 1% are of African origin (6).

The number of new patients entering renal replacement programs has increased dramatically over the past 12 years, from 1,215 (49.9 pmp) in 1981, to 2,698 (98.4 pmp) in 1992 (Tables 1–2, Figure 1). In 1992, the age specific new case rate ranged from 8.4 per million for those aged 0–14 years to 361.9 per million for those aged 65–74 years. The largest increases have been seen in the 65–74 year and the over 75 year age groups (Figure 2).

PRIMARY RENAL DIAGNOSES

The leading causes of renal failure in Canadian patients in 1992 are diabetes (24.4%), glomerulonephritis (19.1%), and renal vascular disease including hypertension (17.1%). Diabetes has become the single most common cause, having increased from 15% in 1981 (Figure 3). Diabetes makes up 23% of the diagnoses in the 15–44 year age group, increasing to 33% in the 45–64 year age group. Glomerulonephritis declines from 29% in the 15–44 year age group to 15% in the over 65 year age group. Vascular diseases including hypertension augment with increasing age, from 5.6% in the 15–44 year age group to 30% in the over 65 year age group (Table 3, Figure 4).

PREVALENT CASE RATE

The prevalence of patients on renal replacement therapy has increased from 5,576 (229.1 per million population) in 1981 to 14,211 (518.5 per million population) by the

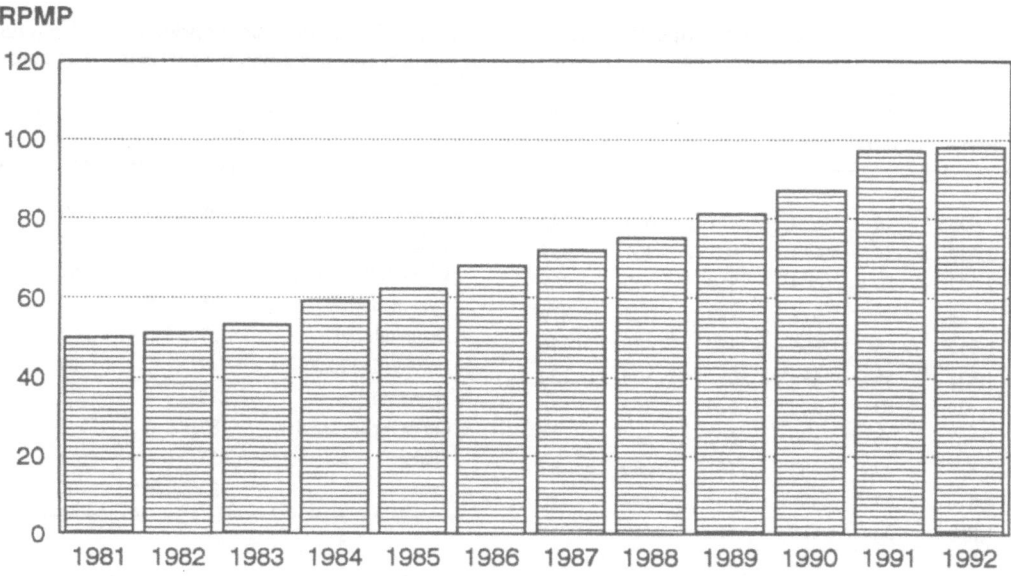

Figure 1. New case rate for patients entering renal replacement programs, 1981–1992, Canada

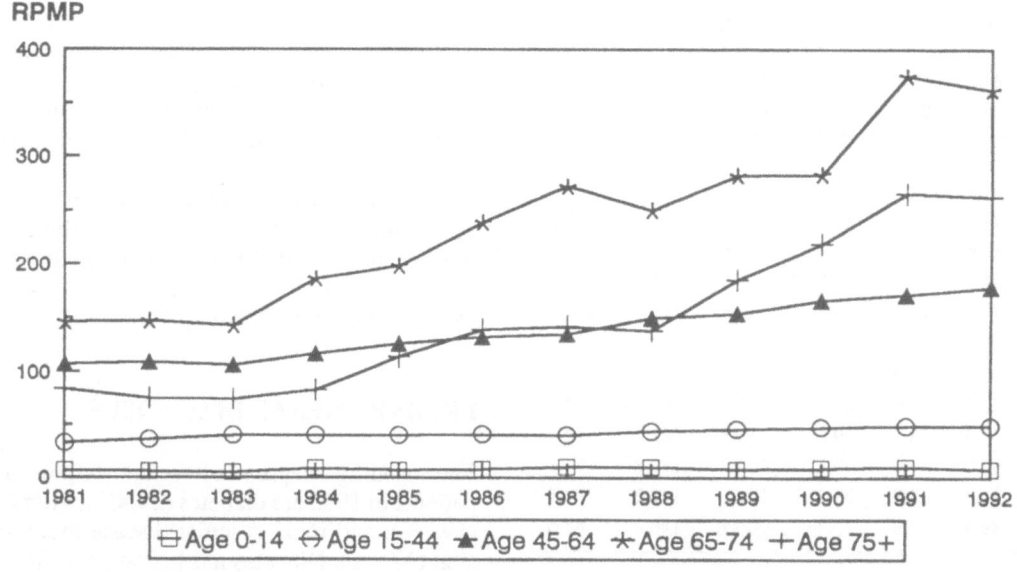

Figure 2. Age specific new case rate for patients entering renal replacement programs, 1981–1992, Canada.

end of 1992. Of these patients, 275.3 per million remain on dialysis and 243.1 per million remain alive with a functioning transplant at the end of 1992 (Tables 4–5, Figure 5).

MODALITY DISTRIBUTION

While the absolute number of patients has increased dramatically since 1981, the percent distribution by modality has remained relatively constant (Figure 6). Of the patients

on dialysis at the end of 1992, 62.6% (172.2 pmp) are on haemodialysis, and 37.4% (103.1 pmp) are on peritoneal dialysis.

The distribution between home/self care programs and centre based programs has also remained fairly stable, with 55.7% of patients receiving in centre dialysis and 44.3% receiving home/self care dialysis in 1992 (Figure 7). The home/self care dialysis population is comprised predominantly of patients on peritoneal dialysis, the peritoneal portion having increased from 55.7% in 1981 to 75.5% in 1992.

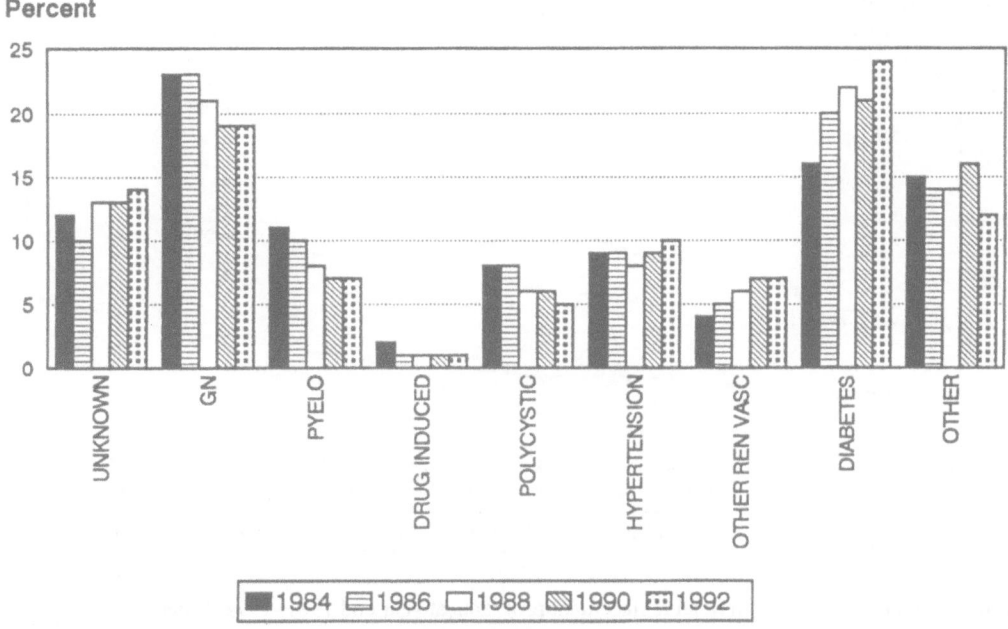

Figure 3. Distribution (%) of primary renal diagnoses for patients entering renal replacement programs in Canada in selected years. GN = glomerulonephritis, Pyelo = pyelonephritis, Ren Vasc = renal vascular.

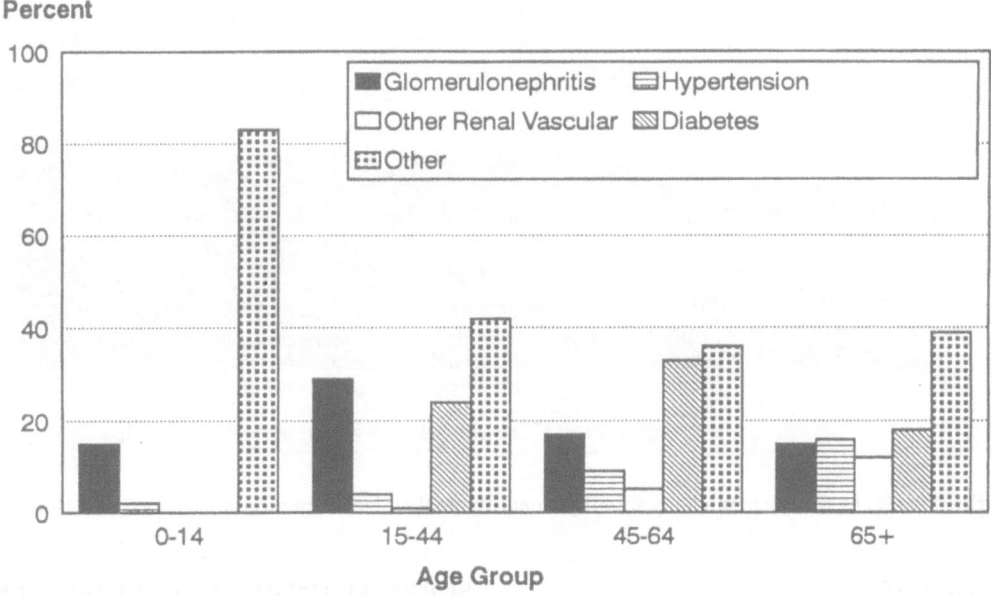

Figure 4. Distribution (%) of primary renal diagnoses by age group for new patients entering renal replacement programs, 1981–1992, Canada.

In 1992 54.4% of the new patients were trained for home dialysis, 94% of these for peritoneal dialysis, predominantly CAPD.

The technique failure rate for those beginning on peritoneal dialysis, mainly CAPD, remains high with 41% remaining on this treatment at 5 years, compared to 75% remaining on haemodialysis at 5 years (Figure 8).

RENAL TRANSPLANTATION

The number of kidney transplants increased from 487 (20 per million) in 1981 to 901 (34.8 per million) in 1988, but dropped to 755 (27.5 per million) in 1992 (Table 6, Figure 9). Approximately 80% of the transplants are from cadaveric donors and 20% from living donor sources.

Number of Patients

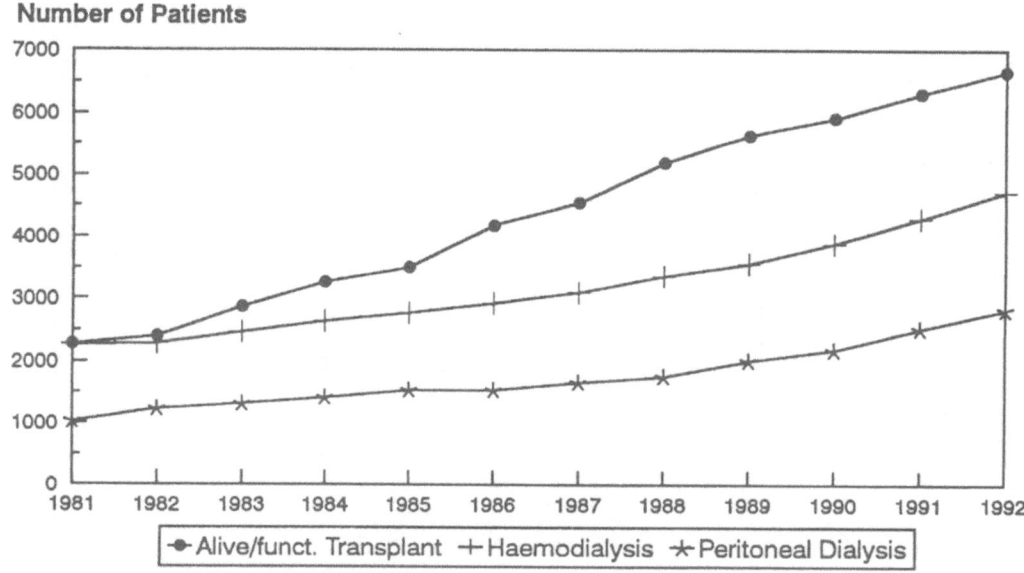

Figure 5. Prevalent count of all patients on renal replacement programs at year end 1981–1992, Canada.

Percent

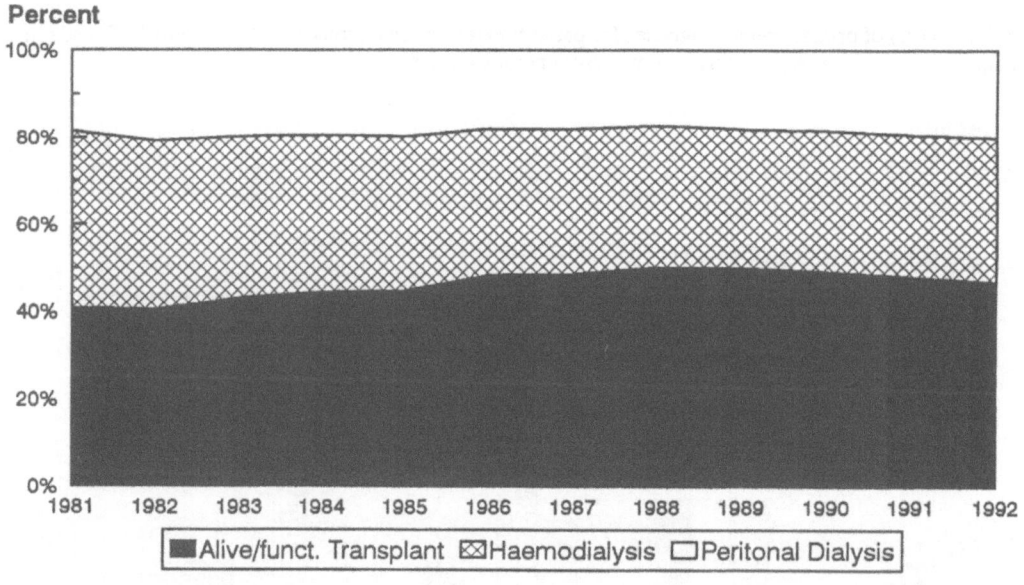

Figure 6. Distribution (%) by treatment modality for all patients on renal replacement programs at year end 1981–1992, Canada.

CAUSES OF DEATH

Cardiovascular disease is the most commonly reported cause of death at 42.8% of patients on all modalities who died in 1992. Uncertain causes make up the second largest group (15.9%), followed by social causes (mainly withdrawal from treatment), and infection (9.5%). The distribution of causes of death has remained relatively constant over the years (Figure 10).

SURVIVAL ON RENAL REPLACEMENT THERAPY

The two major risk factors affecting the survival of patients on renal replacement therapy are age and diabetes. Survival by age group of non-diabetic patients is shown in Figure 11, and that for diabetics is shown in Figure 12. The 15–44 year age group has the best survival in both groups, with 5 year survivals of 86 and 58% for non-diabetics and diabetics respectively. In the over 65 year age group, survival drops to 20 and 10% for non-diabetics and diabetics respectively.

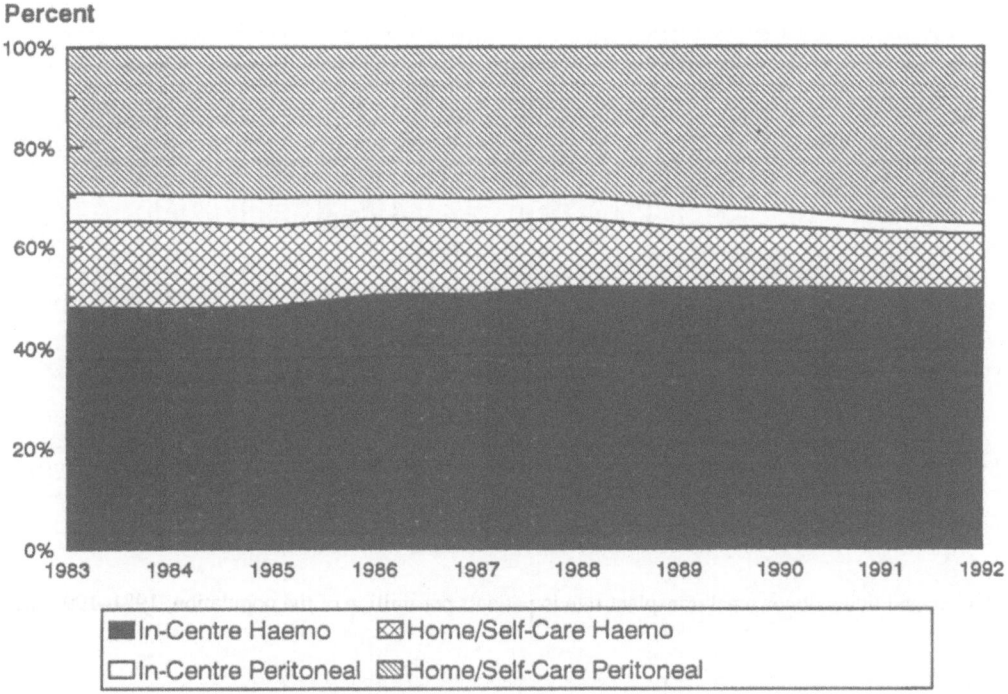

Figure 7. Distribution (%) by modality for all patients on dialysis at year end 1981–1992, Canada.

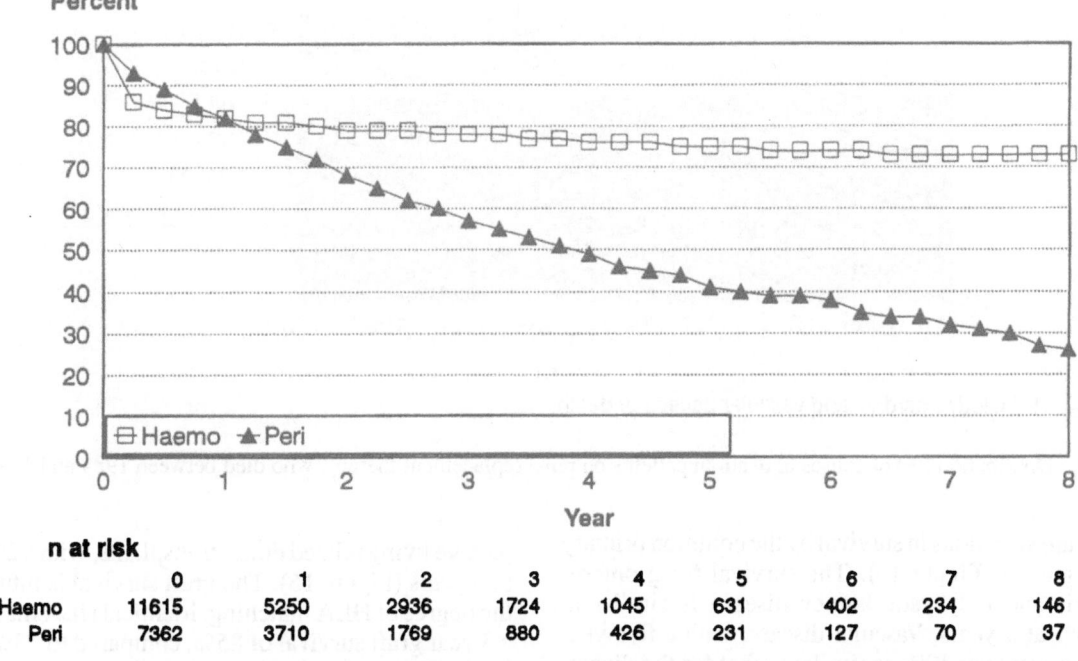

n at risk									
	0	1	2	3	4	5	6	7	8
Haemo	11615	5250	2936	1724	1045	631	402	234	146
Peri	7362	3710	1769	880	426	231	127	70	37

* Technique survival: calculated from the first treatment until a change to the alternate form of dialysis occurred. Transplant, recover function, and death were censored events.

Figure 8. Technique survival by type of first dialysis, all registered patients on renal replacement programs, 1981–1992, Canada.

RPMP

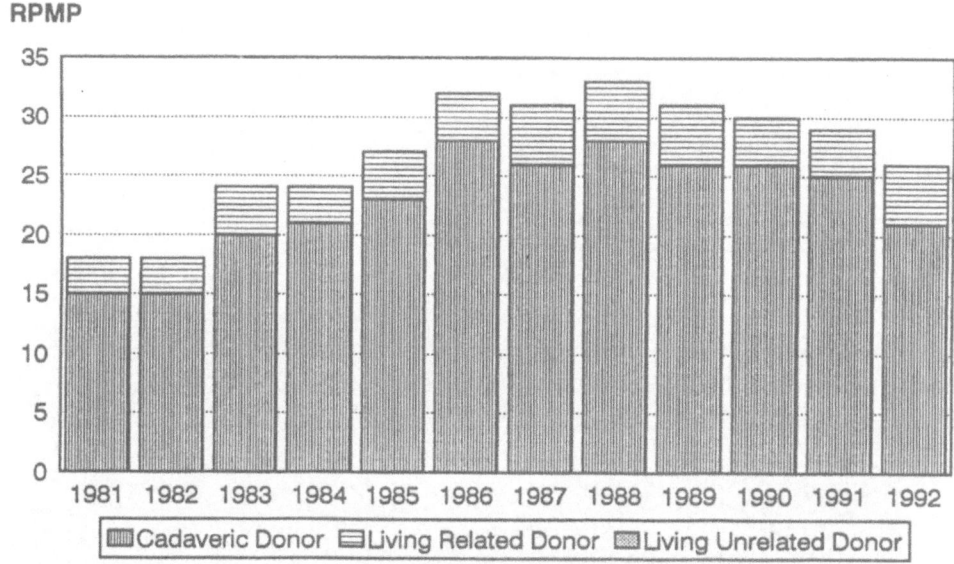

Figure 9. Cadaveric and living donor renal transplant rate in patients per million of the population, 1981–1992, Canada.

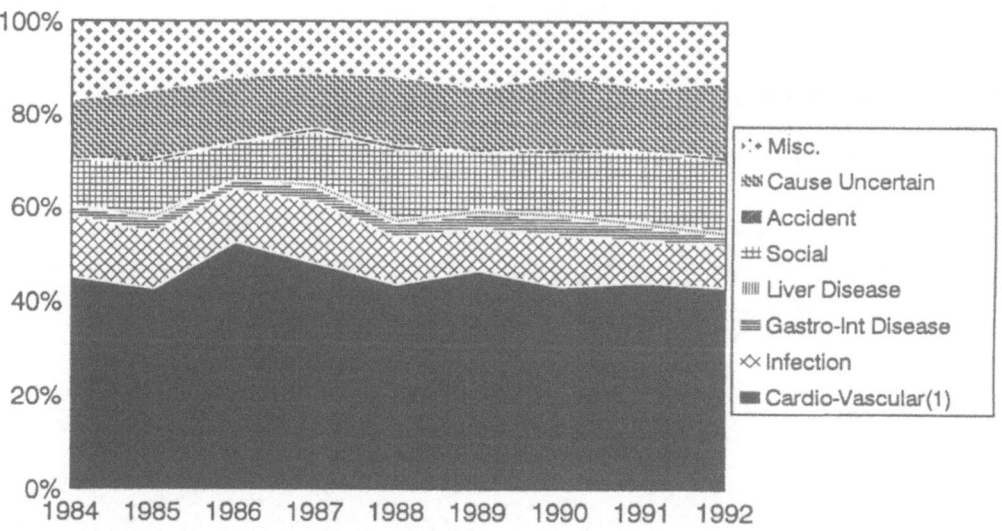

1. Includes cardiac and vascular causes of death

Figure 10. Distribution (%) of causes of death in patients on renal replacement therapy, who died between 1984 and 1992, Canada.

There are variations in survival by the common primary renal diagnoses (Figure 13). The survival for glomerulonephritis and polycystic kidney disease is similar at about 70% at 5 years. Vascular disease, with a five year survival of just over 30%, is similar to that for the diabetic. The survival of patients on renal replacement therapy with systemic diseases ranges from a five year survival of 60% for patients with systemic lupus erythematosus, to vasculitis (42%), scleroderma (35%), amyloid disease (22%) and myeloma (10%) (Figure 14).

The best long term patient survival is seen in those who receive living related donor transplants, with 92% survival at 5 years (Figure 15). The graft survival is influenced by the degree of HLA matching. Identical HLA matches have a 5 year graft survival of 85%, compared to 73% for the 1 haplo-identical matches (Figure 16).

The patient survival at 5 years for first cadaveric transplants is 82%, and falls to 75% for second cadaveric grafts (Figure 17). Similarly, the first cadaveric graft survival at 5 years is 65%, compared to 46% for second cadaveric grafts (Figure 18). Again, age has a strong influence on

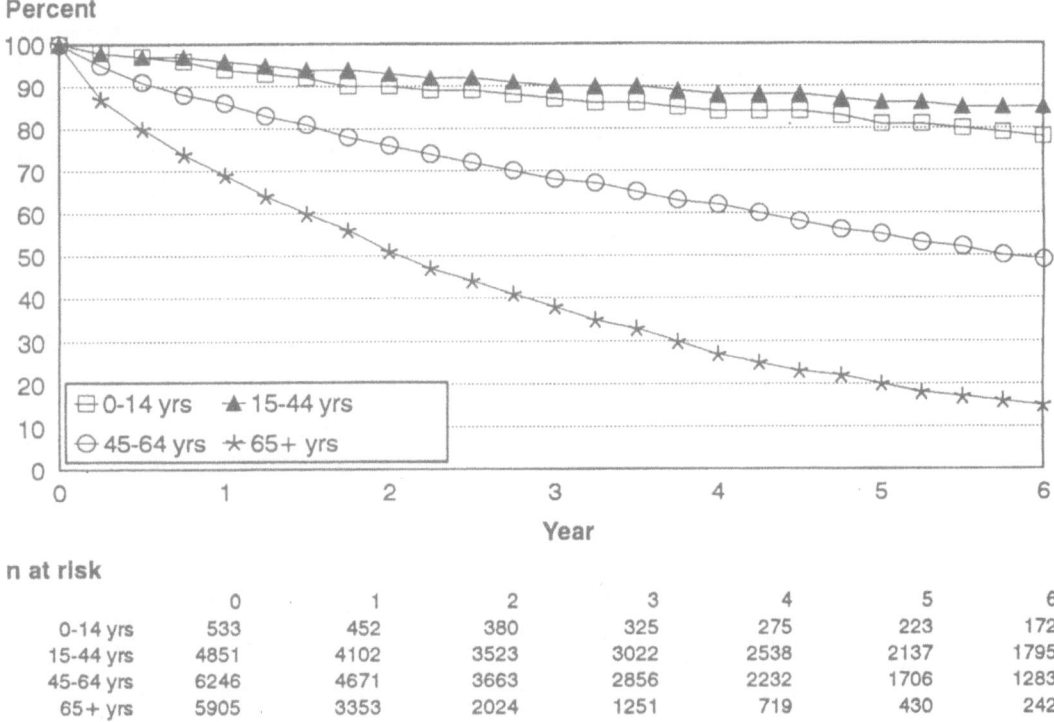

n at risk	0	1	2	3	4	5	6
0-14 yrs	533	452	380	325	275	223	172
15-44 yrs	4851	4102	3523	3022	2538	2137	1795
45-64 yrs	6246	4671	3663	2856	2232	1706	1283
65+ yrs	5905	3353	2024	1251	719	430	242

Figure 11. Survival of non-diabetic renal failure patients on all modalities of renal replacement therapy, by age group, 1981–1992, Canada.

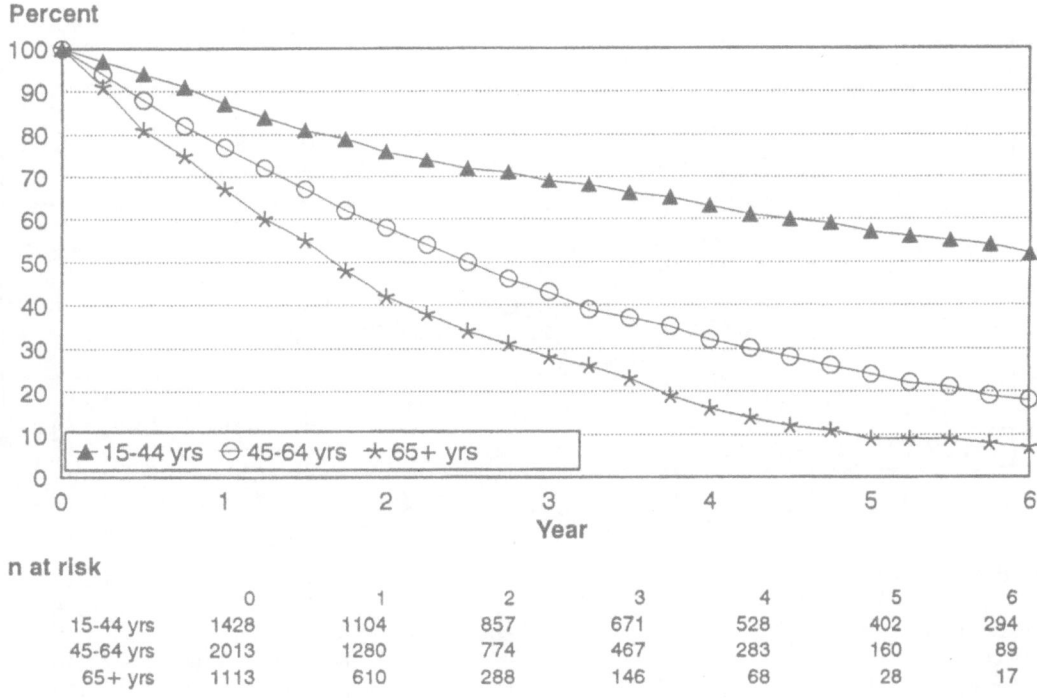

n at risk	0	1	2	3	4	5	6
15-44 yrs	1428	1104	857	671	528	402	294
45-64 yrs	2013	1280	774	467	283	160	89
65+ yrs	1113	610	288	146	68	28	17

Figure 12. Survival of diabetic renal failure patients on all modalities of renal replacement therapy, by age group, 1981–1992, Canada.

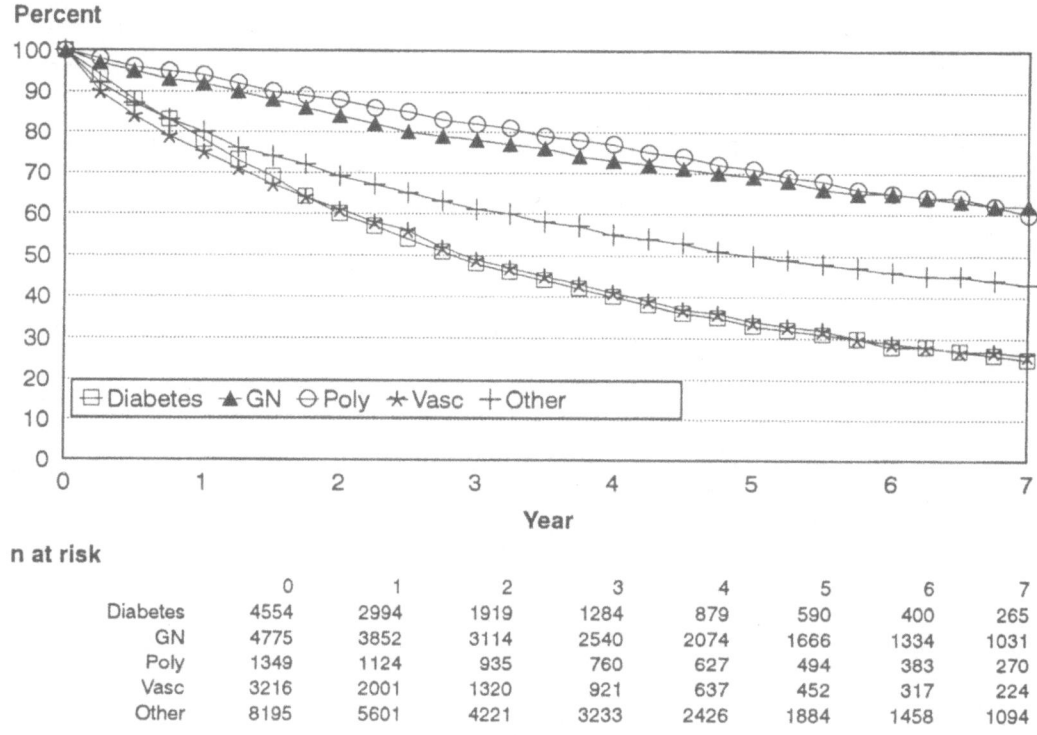

Figure 13. Survival of patients on all modalities of renal replacement therapy by primary diagnosis, 1981–1992, Canada. GN = glomerulonephritis, Poly = Polycystic disease, Vasc = Vascular diseases.

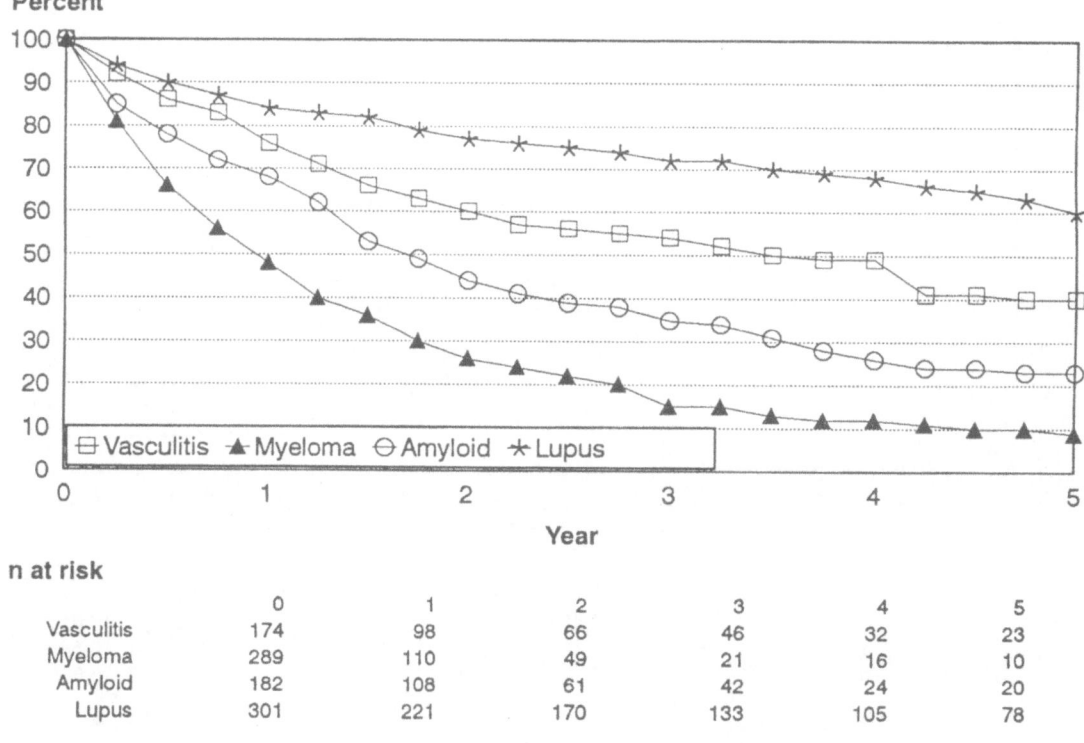

Figure 14. Survival of patients on all modalities of renal replacement therapy, by systemic disease type, 1981–1992, Canada.

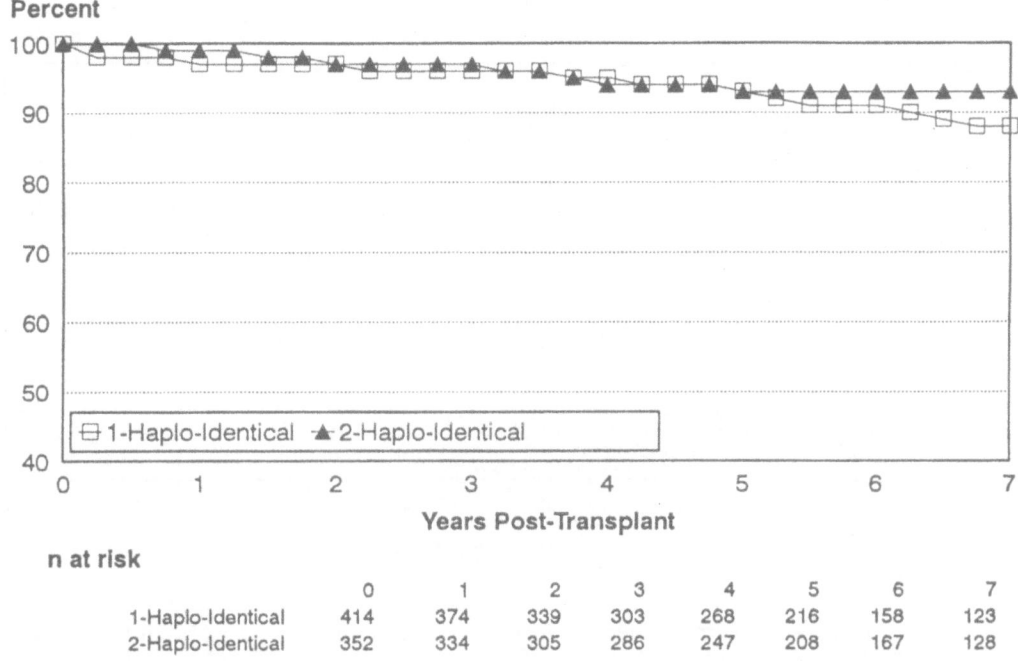

Figure 15. Patient survival for all patients receiving a living related donor transplant, by degree of HLA haplotype matching, 1981–1992, Canada.

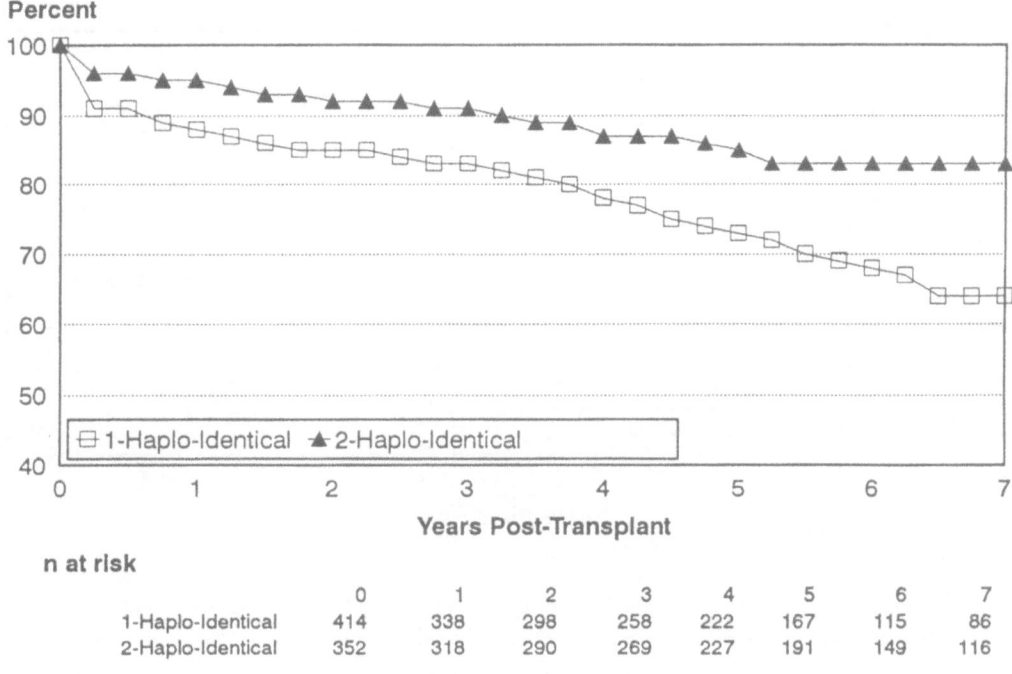

Figure 16. Graft survival for all patients receiving a living related donor transplant, by degree of HLA haplotype matching, 1981–1992, Canada.

survival. The 5 year survival for patients 0–14 years and 15–54 years is 85%, compared to only 70% for patients over 55 years (Figure 19). As far as graft survival by recipient age is concerned, the survival at 5 years is 54% for those 0–14 years, 67% for those aged 15–64 years, and 59% for those over 55 years (Figure 20). The prognosis for patients categorized as low risk (non-diabetic, Caucasian, 20–44 years at first treatment) is excellent, with

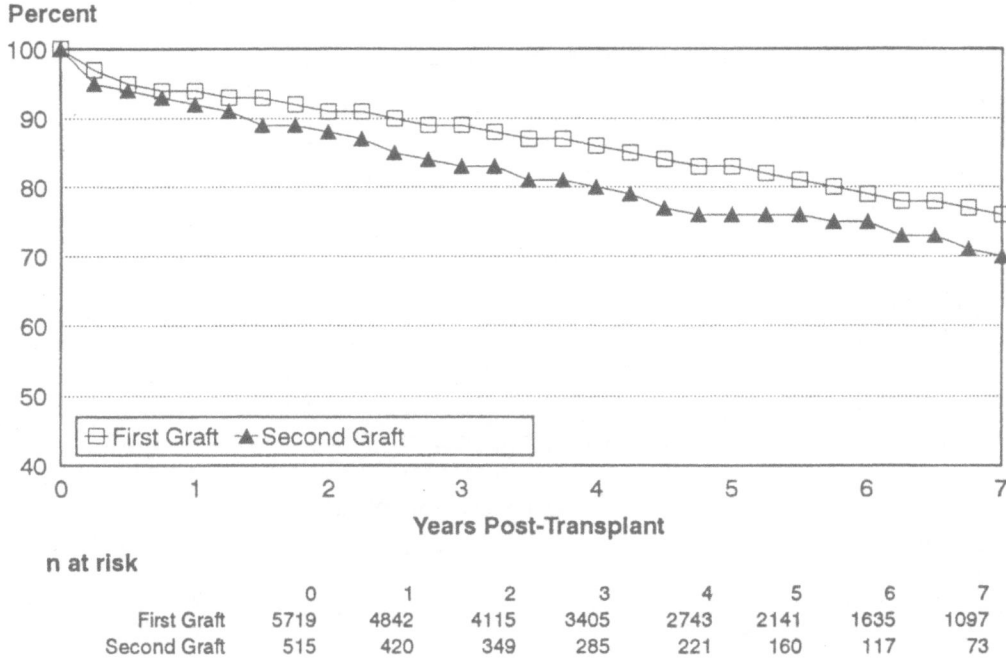

Figure 17. Patient survival for first cadaveric versus second cadaveric grafts, 1981–1992, Canada.

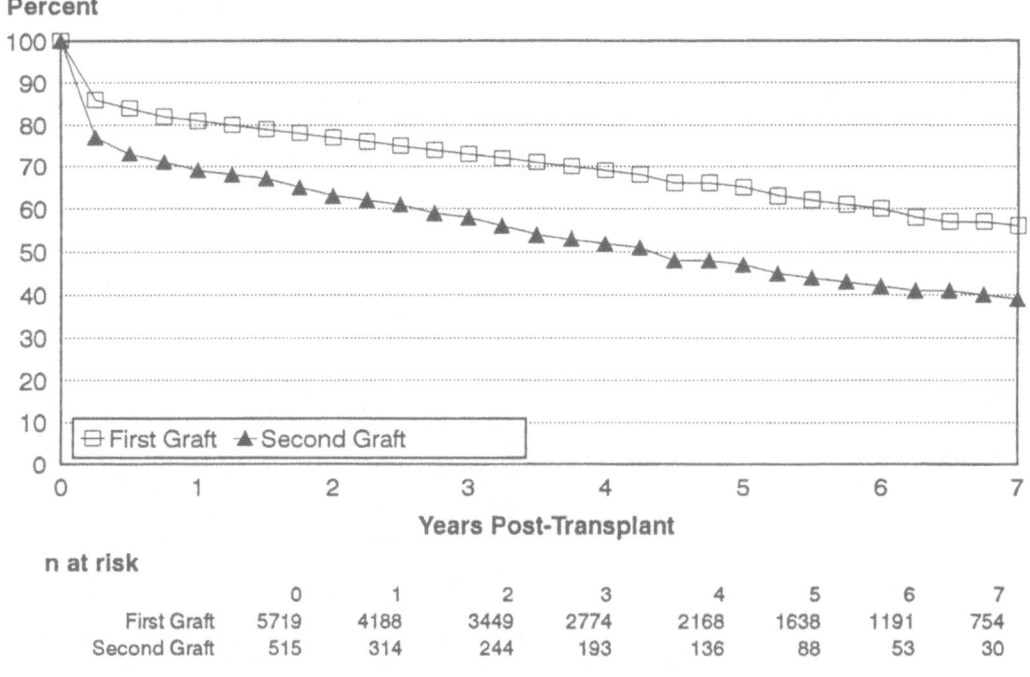

Figure 18. Graft survival for first cadaveric versus second cadaveric grafts, 1981–1992, Canada.

86% survival at 5 years compared to 50% survival at 5 years when all patients on renal replacement therapy are included (Figure 21).

COX REGRESSION ANALYSIS OF SURVIVAL

Cox proportional hazards model is a regression approach to survival analysis. As the survival of renal failure

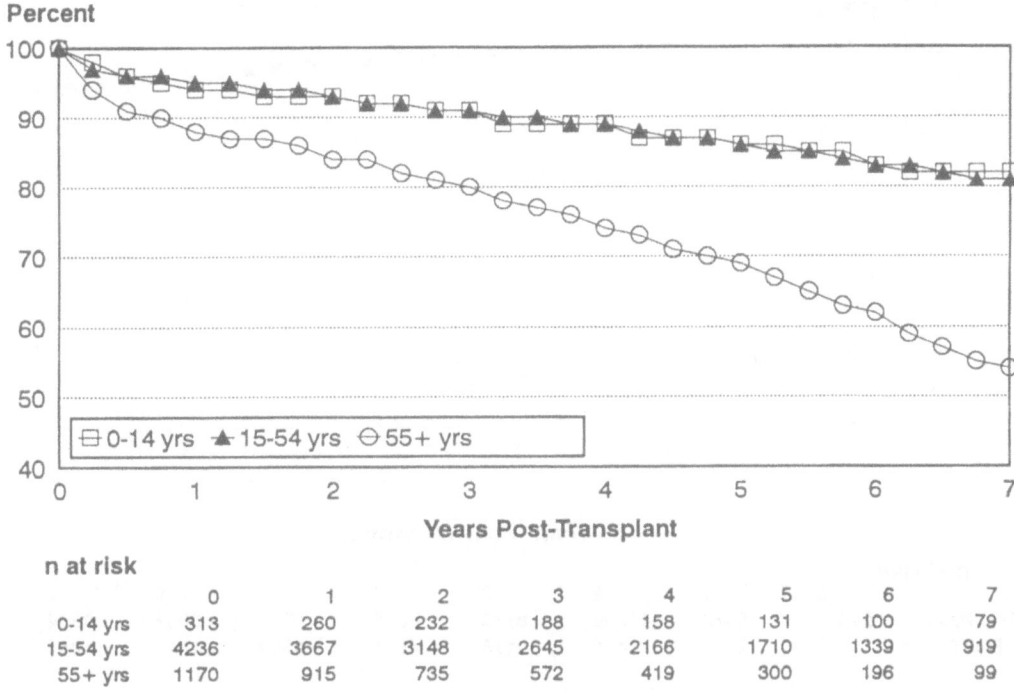

n at risk	0	1	2	3	4	5	6	7
0-14 yrs	313	260	232	188	158	131	100	79
15-54 yrs	4236	3667	3148	2645	2166	1710	1339	919
55+ yrs	1170	915	735	572	419	300	196	99

Figure 19. Patient survival of first cadaveric grafts by recipient age group, 1981–1992, Canada.

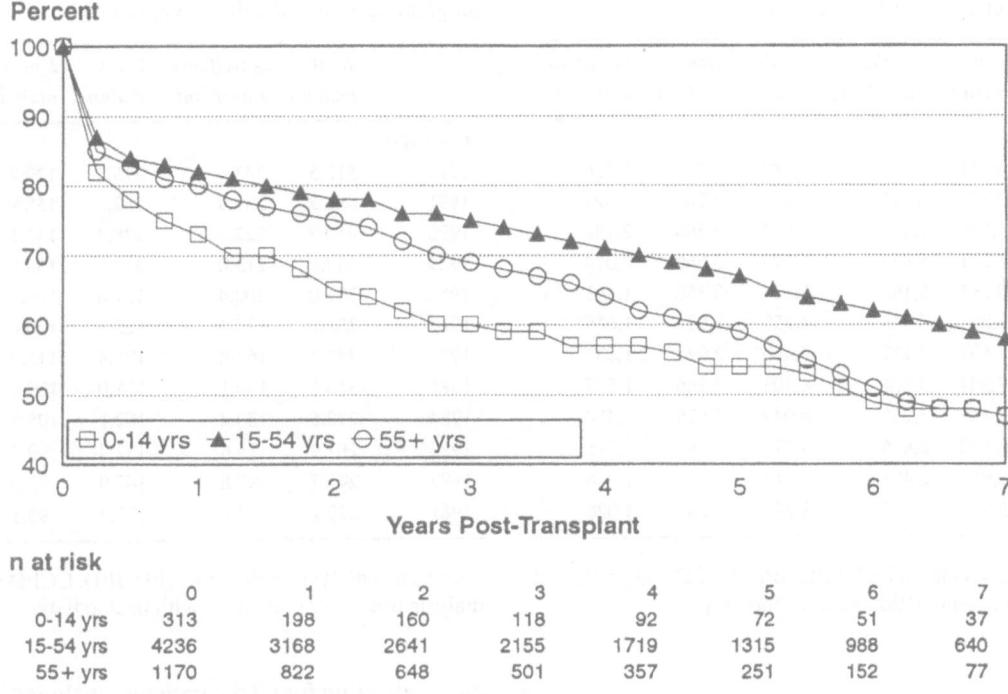

n at risk	0	1	2	3	4	5	6	7
0-14 yrs	313	198	160	118	92	72	51	37
15-54 yrs	4236	3168	2641	2155	1719	1315	988	640
55+ yrs	1170	822	648	501	357	251	152	77

Figure 20. Graft survival of first cadaveric grafts by recipient age group, 1981–1992, Canada.

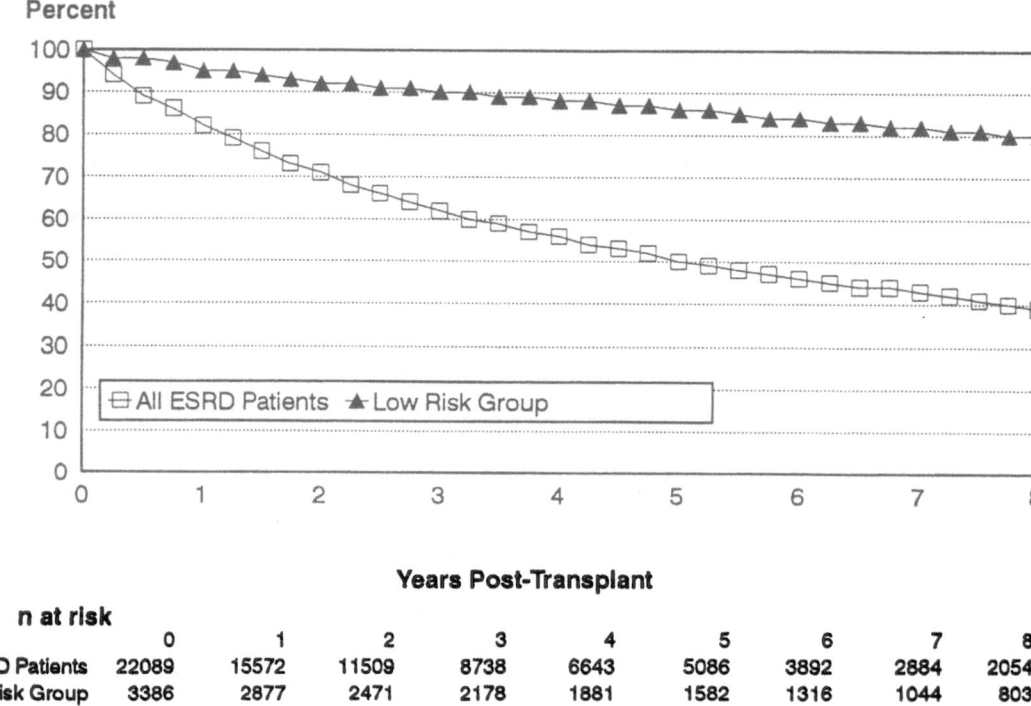

Years Post-Transplant

n at risk	0	1	2	3	4	5	6	7	8
All ESRD Patients	22089	15572	11509	8738	6643	5086	3892	2884	2054
Low Risk Group	3386	2877	2471	2178	1881	1582	1316	1044	803

Figure 21. Patient survival of all patients on renal replacement therapy compared to patients in the low risk group (non-diabetic, caucasian, 20–44 years at first treatment), 1981–1992, Canada. ESRD = end stage renal disease.

Table 4. Prevalent count of patients on renal replacement programs at year end 1981–1992, Canada

	Total patients	Alive/funct. transplant	Total dialysis	Haemo- dialysis	Peritoneal dialysis[a]
CANADA					
1992	14,211	6,664	7,547	4,721	2,826
1991	13,123	6,313	6,810	4,289	2,521
1990	11,986	5,914	6,072	3,884	2,188
1989	11,211	5,637	5,574	3,560	2,014
1988	10,313	5,192	5,121	3,358	1,763
1987	9,303	4,544	4,759	3,094	1,665
1986	8,637	4,177	4,460	2,923	1,537
1985	7,804	3,501	4,303	2,766	1,537
1984	7,305	3,256	4,049	2,635	1,414
1983	6,640	2,866	3,774	2,463	1,311
1982	5,916	2,403	3,513	2,287	1,226
1981	5,576	2,283	3,293	2,267	1,026

[a]Peritoneal dialysis includes CAPD, IPD, CCPD and peritoneal dialysis used in combination with haemodialysis.

Table 5. Prevalent case rate of all patients on renal replacement programs at year end 1981–1992, Canada

	Total patients	Alive/funct. transplant	Total dialysis	Haemo- dialysis	Peritoneal dialysis[a]
CANADA					
1992	518.5	243.1	275.3	172.2	103.1
1991	486.2	233.9	252.3	158.9	93.4
1990	450.9	222.5	228.4	146.1	82.3
1989	427.6	215.0	212.6	135.8	76.8
1988	398.0	200.4	197.6	129.6	68.0
1987	363.2	177.4	185.8	120.8	65.0
1986	340.7	164.8	175.9	115.3	60.6
1985	310.1	139.1	171.0	109.9	61.1
1984	292.5	130.4	162.1	105.5	56.6
1983	267.9	115.6	152.3	99.4	52.9
1982	240.7	97.8	142.9	93.0	49.9
1981	229.1	93.8	135.3	93.1	42.1

[a]Peritoneal dialysis includes CAPD, IPD, CCPD and peritoneal dialysis used in combination with haemodialysis.

patients is dependent on many factors, it is difficult to examine their effect by stratifying on all important variables because the sample sizes become too small. A regression approach solves this problem by simultane-

ously adjusting for all the variables included in the model. It is therefore possible, with Cox regression, to examine the effect of a certain factor on survival, while adjusting for the effect of all other variables.

Table 6. Renal transplant statistics, 1981–1992, Canada. Xplant = Transplants

	Transplant centres	Xplant number[b]	Xplant rpmp[a]	Cadaver organs	Total living donors	Living related donors	Living unrelated
CANADA							
1992	24	755	27.5	605	150	145	5
1991	24	843	31.2	711	132	126	6
1990	25	837	31.5	719	18	116	2
1989	25	858	32.7	720	138	131	7
1988	25	901	34.8	762	139	132	7
1987	25	826	32.2	701	125	124	1
1986	25	871	34.4	766	105	105	0
1985	24	738	29.3	635	103	103	0
1984	24	661	26.5	585	76	76	0
1983	24	642	25.9	537	105	105	0
1982	23	501	20.4	424	77	77	0
1981	23	487	20.0	413	74	74	0

[a]rpmp = rate per million population.
[b]Includes kidneys transplanted in combination with other organs.

Table 7. Cox regression analysis of patient survival, registered dialysis patients, age 0–64, 1981–1992, Canada

	Hazard ratio	95% Confidence interval
Dialysis		
Haemodialysis	1.00	
CAPD & CCPD	0.91*	(0.84, 0.98)
IPD	2.04*	(2.12, 2.73)
Primary Diagnosis		
Glomerulonephritis	1.00	
Polycystic	0.85	(0.72, 1.01)
Diabetes	2.11*	(1.90, 2.34)
Vascular	1.36*	(1.21, 1.54)
Other	1.34*	(1.21, 1.48)
Calendar Period		
1981–1984	1.00	
1985–1988	0.94	(0.88, 1.02)
1989–1992	0.59*	(0.54, 0.65)
Age		
0–14 years	2.17*	(1.71, 2.76)
15–44 years	1.00	
45–64 years	1.46*	(1.35, 1.59)

*Indicates a significant difference was found.

Table 8. Cox regression analysis of patient survival, registered dialysis patients, age 65+, 1981–1992, Canada

	Hazard ratio	95% Confidence interval
Dialysis		
Haemodialysis	1.00	
CAPD & CCPD	0.87*	(0.81, 0.94)
IPD	1.76*	(1.59, 1.94)
Primary diagnosis		
Glomerulonephritis	1.00	
Polycystic	0.65*	(0.52, 0.80)
Diabetes	1.53*	(1.37, 1.72)
Vascular	1.29*	(1.16, 1.43)
Other	1.24*	(1.13, 1.37)
Calendar period		
1981–1984	1.00	
1985–1988	0.95	(0.87, 1.02)
1989–1992	0.80*	(0.74, 0.87)
Age		
65–74 years	1.00	
75+ years	1.31*	(1.23, 1.40)

*Indicates a significant difference was found.

The hazard ratios corresponding to the different prognostic factors are obtained from the regression coefficients. They can be interpreted as a regular risk ratio:

Table 9. Cox regression analysis of patient survival, registered transplant patients, 1981–1992, Canada

	Hazard ratio	95% Confidence interval
Primary diagnosis		
Glomerulonephritis	1.00	
Polycystic	1.1	(0.85, 1.45)
Diabetes	3.41*	(2.81, 4.12)
Vascular	1.64*	(1.26, 2.12)
Other	1.13	(0.93, 1.36)
Calendar period		
1981–1984	1.00	
1985–1988	0.75*	(0.64, 0.88)
1989–1992	0.53*	(0.44, 0.64)
Donor source		
Cadaver	1.00	
Living	0.52*	(0.40, 0.68)
Age		
0–14 years	1.18	(0.78, 1.78)
15–44 years	1.00	
45–64 years	2.46*	(2.12, 2.86)
65+ years	5.27*	(3.96, 7.00)
Graft failure		
No	1.00	
Yes	4.59*	(3.99, 5.29)

*Indicates a significant difference was found.

Table 10. Cox regression analysis of graft survival, registered transplant patients, 1981–1982, Canada. Graft failure and death on the same day or the next day are censored observations

	Hazard ratio	95% Confidence interval
Primary diagnosis		
Glomerulonephritis	1.00	
Polycystic	0.88	(0.71, 1.08)
Diabetes	1.10	(0.94, 1.29)
Vascular	1.29*	(1.05, 1.59)
Other	1.06	(0.93, 1.19)
Calendar period		
1981–1984	1.00	
1985–1988	0.83*	(0.73, 0.94)
1989–1992	0.73	(0.64, 0.83)
Donor source		
Cadaver	1.00	
Living	0.54*	(0.46, 0.63)
Age		
0–14 years	1.26	(0.98, 1.62)
15-44 years	1.00	
45–64 years	0.86*	(0.77, 0.96)
65+ years	0.68*	(0.49, 0.94)

*Indicates a significant difference was found.

if they are below 1, the factor is protective, or increases survival; if they are above 1, the variable is a risk factor, or decreases survival. A hazard ratio is statistically significant if the 95% confidence limits do not encompass the value of 1.0. A hazard ratio of 1.12 would indicate that a patient's chance of dying within the analyzed time would be 1.12 times the reference. For example, if 20% of haemodialysis patients die at 1 year (reference ratio 1.0), the death rate for peritoneal dialysis patients would on average be 22.4% at 1 year (hazard ratio of 1.12).

Patients were categorized according to the following methodology. Follow-up was computed from initiation of treatment to death or the end of 1992. Patients were not censored if a change of treatment occurred, but were categorized according to the percentage of follow-up spent on each treatment. Patients who spent at least 90% of their follow-up time on haemodialysis were categorized into the haemodialysis group, those who spent at least 90% of their time on continuous ambulatory peritoneal dialysis (CAPD) or continuous cyclic peritoneal dialysis (CCPD) were categorized into the CAPD/CCPD group, and those who spent 90% of their follow-up time on intermittent peritoneal dialysis (IPD) were categorized into the IPD

group. The others, who received a mixture of dialysis modalities, were excluded from these analyses.

Cox regression models were fitted separately for dialysis and transplant patients. Different factors were examined; for dialysis patients, age at initiation of treatment, primary diagnosis and calendar period of registration were included in the model. For transplant patients survival, models also included donor source and graft failure status. Graft failure was a time-dependent variable in the regression model. Graft survival was also examined; graft failure was considered as an event, and deaths without failure (or deaths within one day of failure) were considered censored observations. On a subgroup of patients (approximately 10,300 patients), information on other comorbid conditions (angina, past myocardial infarction, pulmonary edema, cerebrovascular accident, peripheral vascular disease, lung disease) has been collected. The effect of these comorbid conditions on survival has been examined. The results of the Cox regression analyses are presented in Tables 7–11.

Among dialysis patients, separate analyses were performed for patients aged 0–64 years and 65+ to determine if prognostic factors had different effects in these two age groups. In both age groups, those who received CAPD seem to have higher survival than patients receiving only haemodialysis. Those on IPD dialysis have the lowest

Table 11. Cox regression analysis of patient survival, registered patients with information on comorbid conditions, 1988–1992, Canada

	Hazard ratio	95% Confidence interval
Treatment		
Tx within 6 months	1.00	
Haemo then Tx[b]	0.74	(0.51, 1.08)
Peri. then Tx[b]	0.72	(0.47, 1.10)
Haemodialysis	5.11[a]	(3.68, 7.09)
CAPD or CCPD	3.57[a]	(2.56, 4.98)
IPD	10.30*	(7.24, 14.65)
Primary diagnosis		
Glomerulonephritis	1.00	
Polycystic	0.78[a]	(0.61, 0.98)
Diabetes	1.93[a]	(1.69, 2.20)
Vascular	1.49[a]	(1.30, 1.71)
Other	1.47	(1.29, 1.67)
Age		
0–14 years	1.49	(0.96, 2.31)
15–44 years	1.00	
45–64 years	1.82[a]	(1.59, 2.08)
65+ years	2.68[a]	(2.34, 3.07)
Co-morbid conditions[c]		
(Diabetics excluded)		
None	1.00	
One	1.05	(0.93, 1.19)
More than one	1.72[a]	(1.53, 1.93)

[a]Indicates a significant difference was found.
[b]Period of dialysis was 6 months or greater.
[c]Comorbid conditions existing at time renal replacement therapy was started include: angina, past myocardial infarction, pulmonary edema, cerebrovascular accident, peripheral vascular disease and lung disease.

survival. Patients with primary diagnosis of glomerulonephritis and polycystic kidneys have better survival than others and diabetics have the poorest survival. A steady improvement in survival was noted by calendar period at registration. This improvement was more pronounced in the younger age group. The age group 15–44 years has the best survival (Tables 7–8).

Among transplant patients, a steady improvement in survival was also seen by calendar period of transplant. Age is an important determinant of patient survival; the 15–44 year age group demonstrates the highest survival. As expected, living donor recipients had better survival, and graft failure was a strong determinant of patient survival (Table 9).

Similar results were obtained for graft survival (Table 10). Graft survival improved dramatically between the calendar periods. Older patients were at a lower risk of graft failure than younger patients.

The separate analysis of patients with information on comorbid conditions indicated that, as expected, the presence of 2 or more of the following comorbid conditions (angina, past myocardial infarction, pulmonary edema, cerebrovascular accident, peripheral vascular disease, lung disease, excluding diabetes) decreases patient survival for all treatments combined. In this analysis, those patients not receiving a transplant have a much worse survival with relative risk of death ranging from 3.57 for CAPD/CCPD to 10.3 for those on IPD. There are many risk factors that are not collected by the Registry and therefore not included in this Cox model. These unknown modality selection factors mean that comparisons of outcome between modalities need to be interpreted with caution (Table 11).

ACKNOWLEDGEMENTS

The Canadian Organ Replacement Register is funded jointly by the federal and provincial governments, with 20% of funding from the federal government and 80% from the provincial/territorial ministries of health. Support is also obtained from The Kidney Foundation of Canada, and from the health care industry.

The collection of data and the maintenance of this Registry is made possible by the whole-hearted collaboration of the 80 individual renal programs across Canada.

The contribution of the current and past full time staff assigned to CORR at the Canadian Institute for Health Information (Formerly Hospital Medical Records Institute) has also been essential to the success of the Register.

The Canadian Society of Nephrology, The Canadian Transplant Society, The Canadian Association of Transplantation and the Canadian Association of Nephrology, Nurses and Technicians and their constituent members have also made an essential contribution to the Register since its inception in 1981.

REFERENCES

1. The Canadian Renal Failure Register: Annual Reports 1981 to 1986, Statistics Canada, Health and Welfare Canada, The Kidney Foundation of Canada, Suite 780, 5160, boulevard Décarie, Montreal, Canada, H3X 2H9
2. The Canadian Organ Replacement Register: Annual Reports 1987 to 1992, The Canadian Institute for Health Information, 250 Ferrand Drive, Don Mills, Ontario, Canada, M3C 2T9

3. SAS Technical Report: P-179, Release 6.03, SAS Institute Inc Cary, North Carolina, USA 1988, p 59

4. Kaplan EL, Meier P: Non parametric estimation from incomplete observations. *J Am Statist Assoc* 53: 457, 1958

5. Cox DR: Regression models and life tables. *J Royal Stat Soc* 34: 187, 1972

6. Statistics Canada, Census 1991, Ethnic Origins, Publication #93-315, 1993

ASSESSING THE PROGRESSION OF RENAL DISEASE

SAULO KLAHR

INTRODUCTION

Chronic renal insufficiency, once established, tends to progress to end-stage renal failure. The underlying mechanisms have been difficult to elucidate, because the glomerulus and the interstitium have a rather limited repertoire of responses to injury, and the kidney, therefore, responds to a variety of insults in a monotonous fashion. Diverse pathogenetic mechanisms, i.e., vascular, metabolic, or immunologic disorders, may lead to sclerosis, a process in which diverse renal structures are replaced by collagen, fibroblasts and mesenchymal matrix, resulting in disruption of normal renal function (1).

Glomerular injury may result from the deposition of compounds with biologic activity, i.e., immunoglobulins, components of complement, amyloid proteins, cryoglobulins, lipoproteins, toxins, and certain components of the cell wall of bacteria. Other factors may also initiate and sustain glomerular injury including intra or extracapillary coagulation, the accumulation of mesangial matrix, glomerular hypertrophy, and/or damage to epithelial cells. Glomerular injury may be initiated or facilitated by mechanical factors such as systemic hypertension and/or intraglomerular hypertension, or by metabolic abnormalities resulting from systemic diseases such as hyperlipidemia or diabetes. Various inflammatory and growth factors released from resident glomerular cells or from infiltrating cells, such as T cells, macrophages, neutrophils and platelets, may also contribute to renal injury.

Histologically, the end-result of progressive glomerular injury is frequently focal and segmental glomerulosclerosis accompanied by severe tubulointerstitial scarring. Diffuse fibrosis, the result of increased deposition of mesenchymal matrix, collagen and lipids, leads to progressive involvement both of segmental capillary loops within individual glomeruli and of additional, previously unaffected glomeruli.

Diseases affecting the kidney differ in their pathogenesis, histologic characteristics and rate of progression, but they all evoke similar alterations in renal function and a common constellation of chemical and physiologic abnormalities. The hallmark of chronic renal disease is a progressive decrease in glomerular filtration rate (GFR). Normal humans with approximately 2 million nephrons and a GFR of 120 ml/min can survive, albeit with difficulty, with less than 40,000 nephrons (2% of normal renal function). The challenge to survival posed by the loss of nephrons is met by a variety of adaptive mechanisms, most of which are not fully understood.

ASSESSING THE PROGRESSION OF RENAL DISEASE

Chronic renal failure is characterized by a progressive and usually irreversible decline in GFR. It is caused by numerous diseases. Three major mechanisms have been proposed to explain the progressive course of renal disease (1): a) persistent injury due to the initial pathogenic insult, b) secondary glomerular injury due either to adaptive changes in initially normal or minimally affected glomeruli or to intraglomerular coagulation, and c) secondary injury due to compensatory changes or to abnormalities in tubular and interstitial function. Distinguishing glomerular from tubular or interstitial abnormalities is sometimes difficult.

Measurements of GFR are used to estimate the mass of functional renal tissue or the number of functioning nephrons. The ideal markers of GFR are substances that are freely filtered across the glomerular capillaries, not secreted, reabsorbed, catabolized, or synthesized by the kidney. The substance should be harmless and easy to administer and measure accurately. Several exogenous compounds (inulin, ^{125}I-iothalamate, ^{99}Tc-DTPA, or ^{51}Cr-EDTA) fulfill these requirements. Although no endogenous substance is ideal for assessing GFR, clinically the clearance of endogenous creatinine is used for that purpose (2).

The concentrations of blood urea nitrogen (BUN) and serum creatinine have been used as indicators of the level of GFR. Urea is the final product of protein catabolism. It has a molecular weight of 60 and is freely filtered through the glomerulus. Subsequently about half of it diffuses back into the blood as the filtrate passes down the tubules. At low urine flow rates, tubular reabsorption of urea is enhanced, which leads to an increase in BUN. Increased protein intake and/or catabolism also increases BUN concentrations. Therefore, at any level of GFR, the BUN values may be affected by changes in urine flow and protein catabolism and/or protein intake.

Creatinine is produced from endogenous creatine and phosphocreatine in muscle (2). The quantity produced and excreted depends on muscle mass and, in a given individual, is relatively constant from day to day. Serum creatinine concentration is not affected by changes in protein catabolism but is affected by variations in dietary protein intake, particularly meat. Most of the creatinine excreted in the urine is filtered, but one component depends on tubular secretion. In general serum creatinine concentration rises when GFR falls. Changes in serum creatinine concentrations, particularly when GFR decreases to 60–90% of normal, may be relatively small, however, and values may remain within the accepted limits for serum creatinine levels in a normal population (2). Although creatinine clearance accurately measures GFR in individuals with normal renal function, with progressive renal disease the creatinine clearance does not parallel GFR. The ratio of creatinine clearance to true GFR increases progressively as GFR decreases because of an increasing contribution of creatinine secreted to the total amount of creatinine excreted in the urine (2).

Some investigators have proposed (3, 4) that in a particular patient, regardless of the etiology of the renal disease, a plot of the reciprocal of the serum creatinine concentration (l/serum creatinine) versus time is a linear function and that a change in the slope of this relationship indicates a change in the rate of progression of the renal disease. Another suggestion is that if a linear decline in l/serum creatinine is valid for all patients with a variety of renal diseases, then patients can serve as their own controls and there is no need to compare different patient groups (5). Although the l/serum creatinine versus time plots have been used to assess the progression of renal disease and the effect of therapeutic interventions, this approach has several drawbacks. In many of the published studies, failure to consider loss of muscle mass, changes in creatinine intake, spontaneous stabilization of renal function, and particularly the effects of frequent follow-up visits and blood pressure-control measures may account for the beneficial effects of protein restriction on the progression of renal disease as indicated by the reciprocal of serum creatinine concentration (6).

Table 1. Events that may decrease GFR transiently or permanently in patients with chronic renal disease

1. Extracellular fluid volume depletion
   Diarrhea, vomiting
2. Hypotension
   Due to volume depletion or drug-induced
3. Congestive heart failure
4. Infection
   Systemic, or of the urinary tract
5. Severe hypertension
6. Urinary tract obstruction
7. Nephrotoxic drugs
   Antibiotics, anesthetic agents, non-steroidal anti-inflammatory agents, cytotoxic agents, contrast material
8. Metabolic abnormalities
   Hypercalcemia, hyperuricemia

RISK FACTORS IN THE PROGRESSION OF RENAL DISEASE

Progression of chronic renal disease is mediated by several factors that operate either alone or in combination. These risk factors include systemic hypertension, proteinuria, hyperlipidemia, high protein or phosphorus intake or conditions that promote clotting or infiltration of the renal parenchyma by immune cells. Moreover, irrespective of the course of chronic renal failure several intercurrent events may accelerate the rate of loss of renal function. These events (see Table 1), which may cause a transient or permanent loss of renal function, are important, because their detection and correction may slow the progression of renal disease and delay the need for renal replacement therapy.

Systemic hypertension

Systemic hypertension, whether primary or secondary, may cause renal disease or may accelerate the loss of function in kidneys with established parenchymal disease (7).

Hypertension may damage the kidney by increasing arteriolar wall thickness, leading to ischemia and subsequent glomerulosclerosis, or it may damage the glomeruli directly through increased intraglomerular pressure (7). Although careful documentation of the effects of control of blood pressure on the progression of renal disease in humans is limited, most of the evidence suggests that ameliorating hypertension slows the progression of chronic renal failure.

The relationship between levels of blood pressure and rates of progression of renal disease has been studied extensively in experimental animal models. In sev-

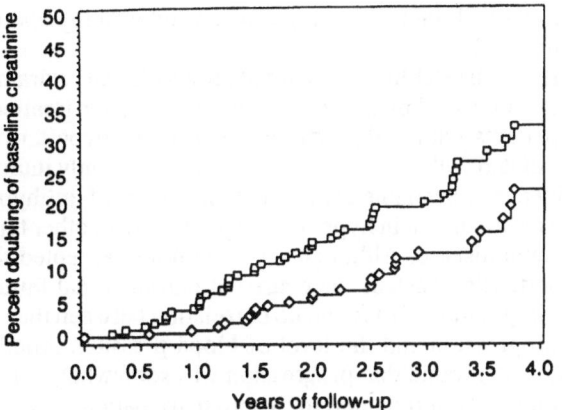

Figure 1. Time to doubling. For each treatment group (diamonds) the cumulative percentage of participants with doubling of serum creatinine to at least 177 μmol/l (2 mg/dl) over time is shown. (□), placebo; (◊), captopril. The percent risk reduction is 48.5 (16 to 69). P = 0.007. From (15), used with permission.

eral such models, hypertension accelerates proteinuria, mesangial expansion and glomerular sclerosis.

The Veterans Administration Cooperative Study established that control of hypertension reduces the frequency of progressive azotemia in patients with moderate and severe essential hypertension (8, 9). However, it is less clear that treatment of hypertension in patients with non-hypertensive renal disease has an effect on the rate of progression of renal insufficiency.

In specific diseases, particularly diabetic nephropathy, substantial evidence indicates that blood pressure reduction may prevent the progression of renal failure. Mogensen (10) reported initially in 1982 that treatment of hypertension in six patients with diabetic nephropathy led to a 60% reduction in their rate of loss of GFR. These observations were subsequently confirmed by Parving et al. (11) and Bjorck et al. (12). Each of these studies included only a small number of patients and in each case the investigator used the patients' rate of GFR loss prior to entry into the study as a control. A subsequent study (13) demonstrated in a randomized placebo-controlled trial that administration of enalapril significantly reduced blood pressure and proteinuria and increased GFR in normotensive patients with diabetic nephropathy. No such improvement was observed in the placebo-controlled patients. Although none of these patients had progressive renal insufficiency, the results of the study call into question the generally accepted blood pressure goal of 140/90 mmHg for patients with diabetic (or other forms of) nephropathy and suggest that there may be a special role for angiotensin-converting enzyme (ACE) inhibitors in the treatment of these patients.

Recently, the results of a randomized clinical trial of the effects of treatment with captopril, an angiotensin-converting enzyme inhibitor, in patients with insulin-dependent diabetes mellitus (IDDM) and diabet-

ic nephropathy have been published (14, 15). This study was designed to directly and prospectively test whether treatment of patients with IDDM and established diabetic nephropathy with an ACE inhibitor is associated with a reduction in the rate of progression of diabetic nephropathy. In contrast to previous studies, this trial was randomized, double-masked, and involved a large number – 409 – of relatively homogeneous patients with insulin-dependent diabetes, and incorporated a follow-up period sufficient for assessing the progression of renal insufficiency. Participants were randomized to receive either captopril, 25 mg orally three times a day, or placebo. In all participants, diastolic blood pressure was controlled at levels below 90 mmHg and systolic blood pressure at levels dependent on the patients' baseline blood pressures. Blood pressure control during the follow-up period in the placebo group was achieved using a variety of antihypertensives that excluded other ACE inhibitors or calcium channel blockers. The primary outcome of the study was the documentation of the time required for doubling of the baseline serum creatinine (Figure 1) to at least 177 μmol/l (2 mg/dl).

Secondary outcomes included a profile of urinary protein excretion and measurement of the duration of time preceding end-stage renal disease and death. During the scheduled follow-up visits there were no reported differences between the captopril-treated and placebo-treated groups in either blood sugar control as measured by glycosylated hemoglobin, or in protein intake as measured by 24-hour urinary urea excretion. As mentioned above, the primary outcome for this trial was documentation of the time required for doubling of the serum creatinine. During the period of follow-up, 25 of the participants receiving captopril reached the doubling of serum creatinine stop point, while 43 of those participants in the placebo-treated group reached that stop point. This difference between the captopril and placebo treated groups was significant. The time required for creatinine doubling in the captopril treated participants was longer than that in the placebo treated participants. The overall percent risk reduction conferred by captopril was 48.5% based on the proportion of hazard regression model (see Figure 2).

An important secondary outcome was the time interval before death, initiation of dialysis, or transplantation. In the captopril treated group there were 23 endpoints reached, representing single or combined endpoints (death, initiation of dialysis or transplantation), while in the placebo treated group there were 43 endpoints reached, with a percent risk reduction of 50.5% in those participants receiving captopril. Mean arterial blood pressure was approximately 4 mmHg lower during follow-up in the participants in the captopril treated group versus the placebo treated group. The lower blood pressure in the captopril treated group contributed only minimally to the more promising results in this group when data were analyzed by a proportional hazards regression model with blood pressure as a time-dependent covariate. Howev-

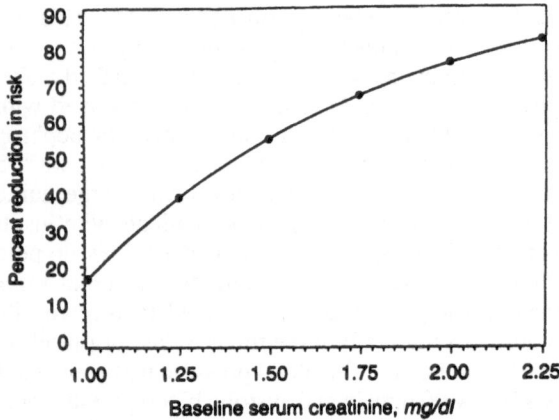

Figure 2. Percent reduction in risk with captopril as a function of baseline serum creatinine. From (15), used with permission.

er, it cannot be completely ruled out that blood pressure influenced the outcome of the study and had a role in the benefit provided. This study represents the largest cohort of patients with diabetic nephropathy in whom a beneficial effect of captopril on preserving renal function was demonstrated. These results suggest that ACE inhibitors have an effect beyond that of blood pressure reduction as compared to other antihypertensives. On the other hand, the difference of 4 mmHg in blood pressure may in itself be responsible for the differences in results obtained in the two groups. The authors also found that the medium protein excretion during follow-up decreased in the captopril treated participants compared to the placebo treated group. This is consistent with previous studies using meta regression analysis (16). The effect of captopril was influenced by the patients' serum creatinine level at entry into the study, since participants with worse renal insufficiency benefitted more from captopril. This in part reflects fewer doublings of serum creatinine in participants with lower serum creatinines at baseline and a longer time of observation required for doubling of serum creatinine in patients with higher GFRs. In summary, while angiotensin-converting enzyme inhibition with captopril significantly slowed the rate of decline of renal function in the patients with diabetic nephropathy, several questions remain unanswered by this study. The possible interaction between the use of ACE inhibitors and other interventions such as low protein diets, calcium channel blockers and tight blood sugar control were not addressed. This study was done using captopril as the ACE inhibitor and whether or not the results can be attributed to the ACE inhibitor effect of this agent or generalized to other ACE inhibitors is not known. It is possible that captopril could be exerting effects through mechanisms other than ACE inhibition. The free sulfhydryl group of captopril is a unique chemical feature of this ACE inhibitor. It has been reported to be responsible for scavenging free oxygen

radicals and attenuating reperfusion-induced myocardial injury (17).

It is well established that renal prognosis can be dramatically improved by aggressive antihypertensive treatment in patients with malignant hypertension or hypertension associated with scleroderma crisis. However, only indirect evidence is available for a beneficial effect of antihypertensive treatment in hypertensive patients with other types of renal disease. Although it is commonly accepted that hypertension hastens the course of chronic renal failure, one large study (18) found no correlation between the rate of progression and the level of blood pressure. Another study (19) found that progression was somewhat, but not significantly, more rapid in hypertensive patients. Several other large studies (20–22) reported a significant correlation between blood pressure and the rate of progression. Brazy et al. (21) found such a relationship only with diastolic but not with systolic pressure. None of these studies clarifies the central question of whether higher blood pressure levels accelerate the loss of renal function or, conversely, whether more rapidly progressing renal disease leads to higher blood pressures. It appears, however, that most of the evidence associates a reduction of blood pressure with a reduction in the rate of progression of renal disease. Alvestrand et al. (20) and Bergstrom et al. (23) attributed the reduced rate of progression of renal disease in their diet study patients, before any change of diet, to better control of blood pressure. These studies found a significant correlation between the degree of reduction in mean blood pressure after patients entered the study and the reduction of the rate of loss of renal function. Previously, Kajiwara (24) reported that propranolol use in glomerulonephritis patients led to a slower rate of progression of their renal disease. Similarly, Brazy et al. (21) found that patients successfully treated for hypertension demonstrate a slowing of the rate of progression. Yet none of these observations fully explain the association between hypertension and progressive loss of renal function. Since patients were not randomized in any of the above studies, it is possible that the patients with renal function declining more slowly for whatever reason had an associated reduction of blood pressure. That is, the blood pressure improvement might be the consequence of, and not the cause of, the improvement in the course of the underlying renal disease.

In the preliminary phase of the Modification of Diet in Renal Disease (MDRD) study, a significant correlation between the level of arterial pressure and the rate of progression was also noted in individuals who were normotensive by World Health Organization (WHO) criteria (22). This may imply that a graded renal risk exists even within the normotensive range (7). In the recently completed MDRD study (25) the effect of two levels of blood pressure control were also examined. In Study 1, 585 patients with GFR levels of 25–55 ml/min were randomly assigned to a usual or a low mean arterial pressure group (107 or 92 mmHg). In Study 2, 255 patients with GFR levels of 13–24 ml/min/1.73 m^2 were randomly assigned to a usual or low blood pressure group. In Study 1, patients assigned to the low blood pressure group as compared to the usual blood pressure group had a greater decline in GFR during the first four months after randomization. However, the decline in GFR from four months of follow-up to the end of the study was slower in the patients randomized to the low blood pressure group. The difference in mean blood pressure between the usual and low blood pressure groups during the follow-up period was 4.7 mmHg (p < 0.001) in both studies 1 and 2. The percent of patients taking antihypertensive (including diuretic) drugs for more than half of the follow-up period was 80% and 90%, respectively, in the usual and low blood pressure groups in Study 1 and 85% and 98%, respectively, in Study 2. The percent of patients taking ACE inhibitors alone or in combination for more than half of the follow-up period in Study 1 was 34% and 54% in the usual and low blood pressure groups, respectively, and 44% in both the usual and low protein diet groups. In Study 2, the percent of patients taking ACE inhibitors was, respectively, 27% and 43% in the usual and low blood pressure groups.

There was also in the MDRD study (25) a significant interaction between the prescribed blood pressure and the magnitude of proteinuria during the baseline period. This interaction affected the rate of decline in GFR beginning at four months of follow-up (p = 0.006) and the projected decline in GFR in three years of follow-up (p = 0.02). The beneficial effect of the low blood pressure intervention was greatest in the 54 patients in whom urinary protein excretion was greater than 3 g per day at baseline. The benefit was less vigorous in the 104 patients in Study 1 in whom proteinuria was 1–3 g/day and it was absent in the 420 patients in Study 1 in whom proteinuria was less than 1 g/day. We also found that 53 blacks in Study 1 had a more rapid projected decline in GFR (19 ml/min/3 years) than the 525 other patients (11 ml/min/3 years, p = 0.02). Blacks assigned to the low blood pressure group had a projected loss of GFR approximately half (14 ml/min/3 years) that of blacks in the usual blood pressure group (25 ml/min/3 years, p = 0.11). The lack of significance in this difference may be related to the small number of black patients enrolled in the MDRD study.

Proteinuria

The concept that proteinuria may be injurious to the glomerulus derives from the finding that the infusion of large amounts of heterologous albumin into normal animals produces an 'overflow' proteinuria that persists after the foreign protein has been excreted. There is vacuolization of glomerular epithelial cells and fusion of foot processes and focal sclerosis, the severity of which depends on the degree and chronicity of proteinuria (26). Progression to renal failure in the absence of proteinuria is extremely rare in glomerular disease. This may indicate

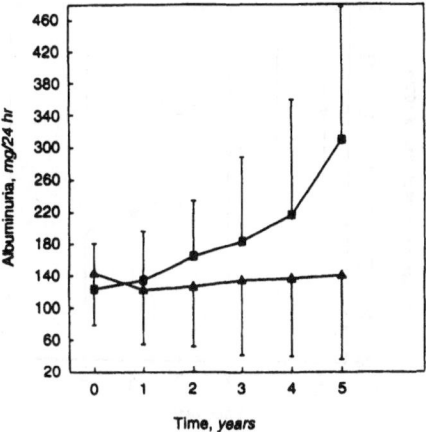

Figure 3. The evolution of mean albuminuria over five years in type II diabetics treated by enalapril (▲) versus placebo (■). From Ravid M, Savin H, Jutrin I, Bental T, Lang R, Lishner M: Long-term effect of ACE inhibition on development of nephropathy in diabetes mellitus type II. *Kidney Int* 45 (Suppl 45): S161, 1994. Used with permission.

that marked proteinuria is a sign of more severe and eventually progressive disease, or that profuse proteinuria is itself injurious and has a role in accelerating the original disease process or the development of glomerulosclerosis. Several retrospective studies indicate a greater likelihood for the development of end-stage renal failure in patients with severe glomerular disease and profuse continuing proteinuria (18). Prospective clinical studies examining this issue have not been conducted.

It would seem appropriate, however, to decrease the degree of proteinuria in chronic renal disease since many of the manifestations of the nephrotic syndrome (hypoalbuminemia, edema, hyperlipidemia) are related to protein losses in the urine. Depending on the etiology of the renal disease, proteinuria may be responsive to the administration of corticosteroids, immunosuppressive agents (cyclophosphamide, immuran, cyclosporine) or other drugs such as non-steroid anti-inflammatory agents (indomethacin). ACE inhibitors appear to be more effective than other antihypertensive agents in reducing proteinuria (27). Low-dose captopril reduced proteinuria in diabetics (13) and non-diabetic patients with nephropathy without affecting blood pressure. Thus, as suggested above, some of the effects of ACE inhibitors in the progression of renal failure may relate not only to control of blood pressure but also to diminished proteinuria (Figures 3 and 4). The long-term effects of ACE inhibition were evaluated in 22 mainly normotensive patients with non-diabetic renal disease and moderate to severe proteinuria (28). The patients with the greatest decrease in proteinuria initially showed less deterioration of renal function estimated from the slope of the reciprocal of serum creatinine versus time (see Figure 5).

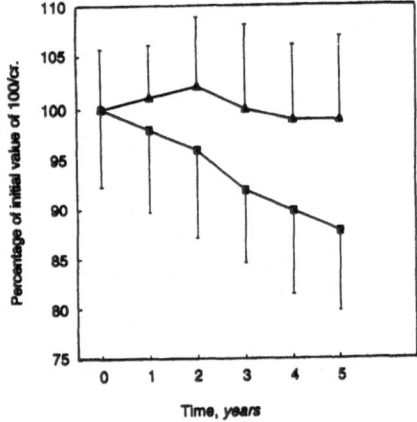

Figure 4. The decline in renal function expressed as percentage of initial value of reciprocal creatinine in type II diabetics treated by enalapril (▲) versus placebo (■). From Ravid M, Savin H, Jutrin I, Bental T, Lang R, and Lishner M. Long-term effect of ACE inhibition on development of nephropathy in diabetes mellitus type II: *Kidney Int* 45 (Suppl 45): S161, 1994. Used with permission.

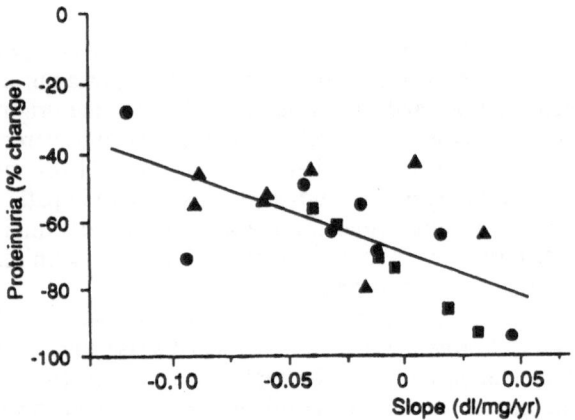

Figure 5. Correlation between the initial antiproteinuric response (percentage of change of proteinuria comparing the 2-month value with baseline) and the progression of renal function deterioration (r = 0.68; P < 0.001). The latter is expressed as the slope of the regression line plotted using the individual inverse serum creatinine levels at multiple study time points. Patients with membranous glomerulopathy (●), IgA nephropathy (■), and glomerulosclerosis (▲) are separately identified. From (28), used with permission.

It has been postulated that proteinuria results in the liberation of fatty acids during the reabsorption and catabolism of protein, particularly albumin, by proximal tubular cells. One or several of these fatty acids may act as chemoattractants for macrophages and lead to infiltration of the renal parenchyma by mononuclear cells. Macrophages, when activated, release a number of cytokines and growth factors that may influence the deposition of extracellular matrix and hence affect the progression of renal disease.

Williams et al. (18) reported that patients with diabetic nephropathy, chronic pyelonephritis, glomerulonephritis or polycystic kidney disease tend to have progressive renal failure, whereas the renal function of patients with hypertensive nephrosclerosis, analgesic nephropathy, and renal impairment following acute renal failure tends to be more stable despite comparable degrees of renal impairment. Similar results were obtained in the MDRD study (25), with polycystic disease patients and patients with glomerulonephritis demonstrating loss of renal function at a faster rate than those with other diagnostic entities. Patients with greater proteinuria also showed a more rapid progression of their renal disease. Aside from the importance of these observations in the design of clinical trials of dietary (or other) therapy for renal disease, the lack of progression of renal disease in certain patients challenges the hypothesis that it is the loss of renal tissue per se rather than the underlying renal disease that initiates the factors responsible for progressive renal insufficiency. In fact, if progression of renal disease is due to as many factors as there are different kinds of progressive renal disease, then it seems somewhat unlikely that a single therapeutic approach (such as diet) would be effective treatment in all cases. Indeed, some authors (29–31) who report an effect of dietary protein restriction on the progression of renal disease have found that this effect is more marked in patients with glomerulonephritis and tubulointerstitial nephritis than in patients with hypertensive nephropathy or polycystic kidney disease. Two groups of investigators (18, 29) found that larger degrees of proteinuria correlated with more rapid progression of renal disease and another group (30) reported that the dietary impact on the rate of progression could be predicted from the degree of reduction of proteinuria. Aside from identifying another factor to be controlled in future therapeutic trials, this observation is interesting because it suggests the possibility that dietary protein restriction has an effect on preservation of renal function through this mechanism which may or may not be due to changes in renal hemodynamics. In the MDRD study (25), it was also found that patients with proteinuria in excess of 3 g/day had a faster decline in GFR than those with proteinuria less than 1 g/day. Other baseline characteristics that correlated with progression of renal disease included gender (males progressed at a faster rate than females) and race (with blacks progressing at a faster rate than whites).

Hyperlipidemia

Numerous animal studies now exist to support a role of dietary induced hypercholesterolemia in the pathogenesis of progressive glomerular injury leading to focal glomerulosclerosis (FGS) (32–37). Hypercholesterolemia as a secondary consequence of glomerular proteinuria also appears to participate in progressive glomerular damage

(38–40). Thus, experimental data would seem to indicate that primary as well as secondary hyperlipidemia contributes to the pathogenesis of glomerular injury.

Various animal models of endogenous hyperlipidemia are known to develop progressive glomerular injury (38–40). Imai et al. described a strain of Sprague-Dawley rats with spontaneous hypercholesterolemia which developed moderate proteinuria and FGS by 9 months of age (38). Rats with the highest plasma cholesterol had the most significant reduction in renal function and the greatest degree of glomerular injury. Male rats had a significantly greater incidence of FGS than female rats. Not surprisingly, male rats had the higher serum cholesterol.

A number of studies have demonstrated that models of obesity and hyperlipidemia are associated with progressive glomerular injury (40–43). Zucker fatty rats have features of non-insulin-dependent diabetes mellitus (44), such as insulin resistance at the level of muscle and adipose tissue, mild glucose intolerance, pancreatic beta-cell hypertrophy, obesity, and hyperlipidemia (45, 46). Both proteinuria and progressive glomerular injury were noted to develop after hyperlipidemia occurred. There were no changes in single nephron GFR or intraglomerular pressure prior to the development of injury (41). Thus, in this model, hemodynamic factors did not appear necessary for the development of glomerular injury. Importantly, two structurally unrelated lipid-lowering drugs (lovastatin and clofibrate) significantly reduced proteinuria and glomerular injury without altering glomerular hemodynamics (47). These data suggested a pivotal role for lipid abnormalities in the pathogenesis of glomerular injury in the obese Zucker rat.

In studies of the nephrotic syndrome induced by the aminonucleoside of puromycin (PAN), reduction of circulating lipids by cholestyramine (48) or lovastatin (49) has been shown to reduce glomerular injury and preserve renal function. Thus, in models with hypercholesterolemia as a primary abnormality or in models with abnormalities of lipids occurring as a consequence of renal disease, pharmacologic modification of plasma lipids resulted in amelioration of glomerular injury. No comparable data on the role of hyperlipidemia in the progression of renal disease in humans are available, although several reports suggest a potential role of lipid abnormalities in this setting.

EFFECTS OF DIETARY PROTEIN RESTRICTION ON THE PROGRESSION OF RENAL DISEASE

During the last two decades clinical evidence has suggested a potentially important role for dietary protein restriction in slowing the progression of chronic renal failure (50). Many of the studies published have been criticized because of flaws in study design including the lack of randomization, the use of retrospective analysis, issues related to compliance, and the use of changes in the serum creatinine or creatinine clearance to assess progression.

Because of such considerations, clear guidelines proving the efficacy of dietary protein and phosphorus restriction on the progression of chronic renal failure in humans are at present tentative.

Several dietary regimens have been utilized to try to prevent the progression of chronic renal failure. These include: 1) a decrease in protein intake using a conventional protein diet containing 0.6 g of primarily high-quality protein per kilogram of body weight per day; 2) a more severely restricted diet of 0.3 g/kg body weight/day of predominantly vegetable proteins supplemented with a mixture of essential amino acids; or 3) 0.3 g protein/kg body weight/day supplemented with a mixture of keto acids. Since some of the diets utilized provide amounts of protein below the recommended standard for adequate nutrition, patients subjected to such diets should be closely monitored for early signs of protein depletion. They also need to be assessed for dietary compliance.

Dietary compliance is best assessed by determining the urea excretion in the urine. It is known that urea is the major component of urine nitrogen to vary with protein intake. Thus, it is important to measure the rate of urea production when evaluating protein intake. This is best done by collecting 24-hr urine specimens and measuring urea in such specimens. It is important at the same time to determine whether or not blood urea concentrations are relatively constant. If these levels are changing, urinary excretion of urea may be affected and consequently may not be an accurate reflection of protein intake. Urea balance can be calculated from changes in the urea pool, which can be obtained by multiplying the concentration of serum urea nitrogen in grams/liter by approximately 60% of body weight in kilograms, which is approximately the total body water. Once the size of the urea pool is calculated, the net production of urea, which is referred to as urea appearance rate, can be calculated as the sum of urinary urea nitrogen excretion plus accumulation (positive or negative) of urea nitrogen. If serum urea nitrogen and weight are stable, urea appearance rate equals the excretion rate.

Several authors have reported that decreasing protein intake with or without phosphorus restriction can slow the progression of chronic renal failure (50). As mentioned before, many of these studies utilized changes in serum creatinine or the reciprocal of serum creatinine to assess progression. However, protein intake may affect creatinine metabolism and concentrations without causing a commensurate effect on renal function. Hence, one may question the validity and conclusions reached in many of these studies. Williams et al. (18) reported a significantly slower rate of decline of the reciprocal of serum creatinine concentration in 41 of 47 patients with chronic renal disease eating a diet containing 0.6 g protein/kg body weight and approximately 320 mg of phosphorus during an average of 17 months. These patients had advanced chronic renal failure with serum creatinine values averaging 880 μmol/l (10 mg/dl). In a larger study, Rosman et al. (51) studied 149 patients with chronic renal disease for at least 18 months. These individuals had creatinine clearances less than 60 ml/min/1.73 m² and were stratified according to age, sex, and renal function, and then randomly assigned to a diet containing 0.4 to 0.6 g protein/kg body weight/day, or to an unrestricted diet. Compliance was monitored by measuring the 24-hr urea nitrogen excretion every three months. By analyzing changes in serum creatinine and the reciprocal, the investigators concluded that the diet reduced the average rate of progression by a factor of about 3. In contrast to previous results, it appeared that older patients and those with chronic glomerulonephritis had a better response than those with interstitial nephritis or polycystic kidney disease. Rosman and co-workers have also reported a 4-year follow-up of 153 of 248 patients initially entering the study (31). Although a significant benefit of dietary protein restriction was still noted, it was most apparent in those patients with more advanced renal insufficiency. Evidence for a beneficial response in women with chronic renal failure was minimal. From the data presented, slowing of progression was evident only in patients with glomerulonephritis. Progression in patients with polycystic kidney disease appeared to be related entirely to blood pressure control. A trial from Australia by Ihle et al. (52) examined in a randomized fashion the influence of a low protein diet on changes in the progression of renal disease. These patients ingested a diet containing 0.4 g protein/kg body weight/day, compared to an unrestricted protein intake in 64 subjects who were followed for 18 months. The groups were initially well matched for serum creatinine range 354–972 μmol/l (4–11 mg/dl), blood pressure, serum calcium and phosphorus concentration. Changes in GFR were assessed by chromium EDTA GFR determinations. End-stage renal failure developed in 9 (27%) of 33 patients who followed the unrestricted diet compared to only 2 (6%) of 31 who were believed to be compliant with the protein-restricted diet (p < 0.05). GFR decreased on average from about 15 to 6 ml/min in the former group but did not change significantly in the protein-restricted group (the average change was from about 14 to 12 ml/min). The outcome of patients who did not comply with the protein restriction was not detailed. As in the study of Rosman et al. (31), the estimated average protein intake was more than 0.7 g/kg body weight/day in the study of Ihle (52). Although serum albumin and anthropometric measurements did not change over the 18 months of follow up, weight, serum transferrin and total lymphocyte count decreased significantly. A study by Zeller et al. (53) examined the effect of decreases in protein content of the diet in patients with insulin-dependent diabetes. The investigators found a beneficial effect of protein restriction on the progression of renal disease. The MDRD study, a multicenter, prospective, randomized trial in 840 patients, examined the effects of protein restriction on the progression of chronic renal failure (25). In Study 1, 585 patients with GFRs of 25–55 ml/min were randomly assigned to a usual or a low protein diet (1.3 or 0.58 g/kg body weight/day). In Study 2, patients with GFRs of 13–24 ml/min were randomly assigned to the low or a very low (0.28 g/kg body weight/day) protein diet, supplemented with keto amino acids. The average follow-up of these patients was 2.2 years. Compared to the usual protein diet group, the low protein diet group had a greater decline in GFR during the first four months after randomization and a lesser decline thereafter. However, the total projected mean decline in GFR to 36 months did not differ between the diet groups. In Study 2, the very low protein diet had a marginal (p = 0.007) effect on GFR decline compared with the low protein diet. If one assumes that the initial decline in GFR in patients on a low protein diet in Study 1 is related to the hemodynamic effects of decreasing protein intake and one utilizes the subsequent slope in GFR from the follow-up visit at 4 months to the end of the study, one finds a 29% decrease in the rate of GFR loss in the patients ingesting the low protein diet as compared to those ingesting the usual protein diet. Compliance testing revealed that the patients on the usual diet ingested an average of 1.12 g protein/kg body weight as compared to approximately 0.7 g/kg body weight in those randomized to the low protein diet. It appears, therefore, that in most instances protein restrictions to 0.6 or to 0.4 g protein as a target have resulted in compliance rates that are closer to 0.7 g protein/kg body weight. In the MDRD study, no evidence emerged for the development of malnutrition or signs of protein depletion in the patients randomized to low protein diets. Overall, therefore, there is no clear definitive evidence that protein restriction ameliorates the progression of renal disease in humans. However, the overwhelming majority of data suggests a beneficial effect. Some degree of protein restriction may be recommended, but probably not to the extent that the eating patterns of patients are severely altered because of the dietary intervention.

EFFECTS OF PHOSPHORUS RESTRICTION ON THE PROGRESSION OF RENAL DISEASE

Several reports suggest an adverse effect of high phosphorus intake on renal function in both normal laboratory animals and those with reduced renal function, and it has been assumed that tissue injury in hyperphosphatemia results from calcium-phosphate deposition (54). A low-protein diet may affect progression of renal disease by decreasing the amount of phosphate in the diet. Whether the effects of dietary phosphate and protein are synergistic in slowing the progression of renal disease remains to be confirmed. Since phosphate restriction is required to prevent hyperparathyroidism and bone disease in patients with chronic renal failure, this maneuver is often recommended for patients with chronic renal disease, especially those with GFRs below 30 ml/min. Hyperphosphatemia is best treated by protein restriction and administration of phosphate-binding agents such as a calcium carbonate or calcium acetate.

ACKNOWLEDGEMENTS

Supported by Grant DK-09976, from the NIDDK, National Institutes of Health (USA). The author acknowledges with thanks the editorial assistance of Mr James Havranek.

REFERENCES

1. Klahr S, Schreiner G, Ichikawa I: The progression of renal disease. *N Engl J Med* 318: 1657, 1988
2. Levey AS, Perrone RD, Madias NE: Serum creatinine and renal function. *Ann Rev Med* 39: 465, 1988
3. Mitch WE, Walser M, Buffington GA, Lemann J: A simple method of estimating progression of chronic renal failure. *Lancet* 2: 1326, 1976
4. Rutherford WE, Blondin J, Miller JP, Greenwalt AS, Vavra JD: Chronic progressive renal disease: rate of change of serum creatinine concentration. *Kidney Int* 11: 62, 1977
5. Mitch WE: The influence of the diet on the progression of renal insufficiency. *Ann Rev Med* 35: 246, 1984
6. El Nahas AM, Coles GA: Dietary treatment of chronic renal failure: ten unanswered questions. *Lancet* 1: 597, 1986
7. Klahr S: The kidney in hypertension – villain and victim. *N Engl J Med* 320: 731, 1989
8. Veterans Administration Cooperative Study Group on Antihypertensive Agents: Effects of treatment on morbidity in hypertension: results in patients with diastolic blood pressures averaging 115 through 129 mmHg. *J Am Med Assoc* 202: 1028, 1967
9. Veterans Administration Cooperative Study Group on Antihypertensive Agents: Effects of treatment on morbidity in hypertension: II. Results in patients with diastolic blood pressure averaging 90 through 114 mmHg. *J Am Med Assoc* 213: 1143, 1970
10. Mogensen CE: Long-term antihypertensive treatment inhibiting progression of diabetic nephropathy. *Br Med J [Clin Res]* 285: 685, 1982
11. Parving H-H, Andersen AR, Smidt UM, Svendsen PA: Early aggressive antihypertensive treatment reduces rate of decline in kidney function in diabetic nephropathy. *Lancet* 1: 1175, 1983
12. Bjorck S, Nyberg G, Mulec H, Granerus G, Herlitz H, Aurell M: Beneficial effects of angiotensin converting enzyme inhibition on renal function in patients with diabetic nephropathy. *Br J Med [Clin Res]* 293: 471, 1986
13. Marre M, Leblanc H, Suarez L, Guyenne T-T, Menard J, Passa A: Converting enzyme inhibition and kidney function in normotensive diabetic patients with persistent microalbuminuria. *Br Med J [Clin Res]* 294: 1448, 1987
14. Lewis EJ, Hunsicker LG, Bain RP, Rohde RD, for the Collaborative Study Group: The effect of angiotensin-converting enzyme inhibition on diabetic nephropathy. *N Engl J Med* 329: 1456, 1993
15. Breyer JA, Hunsicker LG, Bain RP, Lewis EJ, the Collaborative Study Group: Angiotensin converting enzyme inhibition in diabetic nephropathy. *Kidney Int* 45 (Suppl 45): S156, 1994
16. Kasiske BL, Kalil RSN, Ma JZ, Liao M, Keane WF: Effect of antihypertensive therapy on the kidney in patients with diabetes: a meta-regression analysis. *Ann Intern Med* 118: 129, 1993
17. Westlin W, Mullane K: Does captopril attenuate reperfusion-induced myocardial dysfunction by scavenging free radicals? *Circulation* 77 (Suppl 1): 1–30, 1988
18. Williams PS, Fass G, Bone JM: Renal pathology and proteinuria determine progression in untreated mild/moderate chronic renal failure. *Q J Med* 67: 343, 1988
19. Maschio G, Oldrizzi L, Rugiu C: Role of hypertension on the progression of renal disease in man. *Blood Purif* 6: 250, 1988
20. Alvestrand A, Gutierrez A, Bucht H, Bergström J: Reduction of blood pressure retards the progression of chronic renal failure in man. *Nephrol Dial Transplant* 3: 624, 1988
21. Brazy PC, Stead WW, Fitzwilliam JF: Progression of renal insufficiency: role of blood pressure. *Kidney Int* 35: 670, 1989
22. Klahr S: The modification of diet in renal disease study. *N Engl J Med* 320: 864, 1989
23. Bergström J, Alvestrand A, Bucht H, Gutierrez A: Progression of chronic renal failure in man is retarded with more frequent clinical follow-ups and better blood pressure control. *Clin Nephrol* 25: 1, 1986
24. Kajiwara N: Therapy and prognosis of hypertension in chronic nephritis. *Jpn Circ J* 39: 779, 1975
25. Klahr S, Levey AS, Beck GJ, Caggiula AW, Hunsicker L, Kusek JW, Striker G, and the Modification of Diet in Renal Disease (MDRD) Study Group: The effects of dietary protein restriction and blood pressure control on the progression of chronic renal disease. *N Engl J Med* 330: 877, 1994
26. Oliver J, McDowell M, Lee YC: Cellular mechanisms of protein metabolism in the nephron I. The structural aspects of proteinuria; tubular absorption, droplet formation, and the disposal of proteins. *J Exp Med* 99: 589, 1954
27. Rosenberg ME, Hostetter TH: Comparative effects of antihypertensives on proteinuria: angiotensin-converting enzyme inhibitor *vs* α_1-antagonist. *Am J Kidney Dis* 18: 472, 1991
28. Gansevoort RT, de Zeeuw D, de Jong PE: Long-term benefits of the antiproteinuric effect of angiotensin-converting enzyme inhibition in nondiabetic renal disease. *Am J Kidney Dis* 22: 202, 1993
29. Oldrizzi L, Rugiu C, Valvo E, Lupo A, Loschiavo C, Gammaro L, Tessitore N, Fabris A, Panzetta G, Maschio G: Progression of renal failure in patients with renal disease of diverse etiology on protein-restricted diet. *Kidney Int* 27: 553, 1985
30. el Nahas AM, Masters-Thomas A, Brady SA, Farrington K, Wilkinson V, Hilson AJW, Varghese Z, Moorhead JF: Selective effect of low protein diets in chronic renal diseases. *Br Med J [Clin Res]* 289: 1337, 1984
31. Rosman JB, Donker AJ, Meijer S, Sluiter WJ, Piers-Becht TP, van der Hem GK: Two years' experience with protein restriction in chronic renal failure. *Contrib Nephrol* 53: 109, 1986

32. French JW, Yamanaka BS, Ostwald R: Dietary induced glomerulosclerosis in the guinea pig. *Arch Pathol* 83: 204, 1967

33. Wellman KF, Volk BW: Renal change in experimental hypercholesterolemia in normal and in subdiabetic rabbits. I. Short term studies. *Lab Invest* 22: 36, 1970

34. Peric-Golia L, Peric-Golia M: Aortic and renal lesions in hypercholesterolemic adult male, virgin Sprague-Dawley rats. *Atherosclerosis* 46: 57, 1983

35. Al-Shebeb T, Frohlich J, Magil AB: Glomerular disease in hypercholesterolemic guinea pigs: a pathogenetic study. *Kidney Int* 33: 498, 1988

36. Miyata J, Takebayashi S: Effect of hyperlipidemia on glomerular sclerosis in unilateral nephrectomized rats. *Acta Pathol Japn* 37: 1433, 1987

37. Diamond JR, Karnovsky MJ: Exacerbation of chronic aminonucleoside nephrosis by dietary cholesterol supplementation. *Kidney Int* 2: 671, 1987

38. Imai Y, Matsumura H, Miyajima H, Oka K: Serum and tissue lipids and glomerulonephritis in the spontaneously hypercholesterolemic (SHC) rat, with a note on the effects of gonadectomy. *Atherosclerosis* 27: 165, 1977

39. Kasiske BL, O'Donnell MP, Garvis WJ, Keane WF: Pharmacologic treatment of hyperlipidemia reduces glomerular injury in rat 5/6 nephrectomy model of chronic renal failure. *Circ Res* 62: 367, 1988

40. Kasiske BI, Cleary MP, O'Donnell MP, Keane WF: Effects of genetic obesity on renal structure and function in the Zucker rat. *J Lab Clin Med* 106: 598, 1985

41. O'Donnell MP, Kasiske BL, Cleary MP, Keane WF: Effects of genetic obesity on renal structure and function in the Zucker rat. II. Micropuncture studies. *J Lab Clin Med* 106: 605, 1985

42. Kolefsky S: Pathologic findings and laboratory data in a new strain of obese hypertensive rats. *Am J Pathol* 80: 129, 1975

43. Brobeck JR, Tepperman J, Long CNH: Experimental hypothalamic hyperphagia in albino rats. *Yale J Biol Med* 15: 831, 1943

44. Kasiske BL, O'Donnell MP, Keane WF: The obese Zucker rat model of glomerular injury in type II diabetes. *J Diabetic Compl* 1: 26, 1987

45. Bray GA: The Zucker fatty rat: a review. *Fed Proc* 36: 148, 1977

46. Schirandin H, Bach A, Schaeffer A, Bauer M, Weryha A: Biological parameters of the blood in the genetically obese Zucker rat. *Arch Int Physiol Biochim* 87: 275, 1979

47. Kasiske BL, O'Donnell MP, Cleary MP, Keane WF: Treatment of hyperlipidemia reduces glomerular injury in obese Zucker rats. *Kidney Int* 33: 667, 1988

48. Hanchak NA, Karnovsky MJ, Diamond JR: Cholestyramine resin lowers acute and recurrent proteinuria in chronic puromycin aminonucleoside nephrosis. (Abstract) *Kidney Int* 33: 376A, 1988

49. Harris KPG, Purkerson ML, Yates J, Klahr S: Lovastatin ameliorates the development of glomerulosclerosis and uremia in experimental nephrotic syndrome. *Am J Kidney Dis* 15: 16, 1990

50. Hunsicker LG: Studies of therapy of progressive renal failure in humans. *Semin Nephrol* 9: 380, 1989

51. Rosman JB, ter Wee PM, Meijer S, Piers-Becht TPM, Sluiter WJ, Donker AJM: Prospective randomised trial of early dietary protein restriction in chronic renal failure. *Lancet* 2: 1291, 1984

52. Ihle BU, Becker GJ, Whitworth JA, Charlwood RA, Kincaid-Smith PS: The effect of protein restriction on the progression of renal insufficiency. *N Engl J Med* 321: 1773, 1989

53. Zeller K, Whittaker E, Sullivan L, Raskin P, Jacobson H: Effect of restricting dietary protein on the progression of renal failure in patients with insulin-dependent diabetes mellitus. *N Engl J Med* 324: 78, 1991

54. Gimenez LF, Solez K, Walker WG: Relation between renal calcium content and renal impairment in 246 human renal biopsies. *Kidney Int* 31: 93, 1987

DIALYSIS IN DEVELOPING COUNTRIES

R.S. BARSOUM

INTRODUCTION

Of the hundreds of thousands of people with end-stage renal disease (ESRD), the majority are inhabitants of the Developing World. According to a recent World Bank's estimate (1), about 56% of the World's population live in countries with an annual gross national income (GNP) per capita less than 500 US dollars, indeed with an average of only 330 US\$. It is in those countries that renal disease is particularly common, and is notoriously associated with very high morbidity and mortality.

It is noteworthy that the term 'developing' is not restricted to economically compromised nations; it also includes those with indolent social, cultural or educational standards albeit reasonable financial standing. The problem of ESRD in these countries is less acute, but its management is often stunted by shortage of expertise and inadequacy of organization.

Dialysis services started in the Developing World by the early sixties, mainly for the management of acute renal failure. For almost two decades, only a few centers in the capital cities have been undergoing any regular dialysis for chronic renal failure (2). Yet over the past ten years or so, regular dialysis treatment became very widely, even wildly, spread all over the Developing World.

There is no doubt that acquisition of dialysis technology in that part of the world has saved many lives, paved the way for extensive renal transplant programs, and generated a lot of medical, nursing and technical skills which positively reflected, even beyond the scope of dialysis, on several other medical disciplines.

However, there is a growing concern among medical leaders in the Developing World about the issues of *optimization* and *side effects* of regular dialysis. For many reasons, the quality of service provided in a large proportion of units is sub-optimal leading to crippling and eventually fatal complications. Beyond individual limits, the most distressing side effects of dialysis in the Developing World extend to the community at-large, through a train of compound social, moral and economical impacts (3).

The background medical information needed for a dialysis-physician in this milieu should include a lot more than technique, Kt/V and a list of complications. He should be aware of local epidemiology, ecology, economy, politics, internal medicine and some nephrology! The target of this chapter is to provide the reader with a broad overview of the diverse dialysis experiences in this part of the world with brief emphasis on the particulars about certain regions.

EPIDEMIOLOGY

Renal failure profile in the Developing World

Acute renal failure

Acute renal failure remains fairly common (4–8). Its incidence, though not precisely defined in the vast majority of developing countries, seems to range between 100 and 150/million population per year. Among the leading causes are severe dehydration, obstetric accidents including hemorrhage and sepsis, ureteric obstruction usually by stones that often impact on schistosomal or tuberculous strictures, severe infections as *P. falciparum* malaria, and intoxication with drugs or 'traditional' medicines.

Chronic renal failure

The reported prevalence of ESRD ranges between 80 and 96/million population in South-East Asia (9, 10), 70–110/million in Arabia (11, 12), at least 120/million in

India (13) and 89 to 192/million in Africa (14–17) with a similar estimate in Latin America (18). Although the differences are, at least partly, related to local genetic and environmental factors (19, 20), a lot of bias is certainly incriminated. Many of the reported figures are crude estimates without definition of methodology. Slightly more reliable are those based on hospital admissions or analysis of death certificates (17, 21). Nevertheless, it is obvious that ESRD is highly prevalent in the Developing World as compared to Europe (around 40–80/million), though it matches with data on the United States (166/million) (22) particularly among the African- (376/million) (20) and Native- (269/million) Americans (23).

The reasons for this high prevalence differ according to regional ecological factors; infections, environmental pollution and inadequate health care being the most remarkable (19). Additional genetic influence may have an impact, which is difficult to assess.

Glomerulonephritis remains as the major cause of ESRD in the most compromised African countries as Ethiopia (58.4%) (6) and The Sudan (36%) (24). Its impact is much less prominent in other parts of the Developing World, varying between 18.2% (India) and 28.9% (Tunisia) (12, 15, 25–27). Proliferative glomerulonephritis constitutes the major bulk of primary etiology, in contrast to its remarkable decline in the developed world. This observation must be associated with the rich bio-ecological environment supervening in the South (19). Such glomerular lesions are commonly secondary to endemic infections including streptococcal skin lesions (Black Africa (8)), hepatosplenic schistosomiasis (North, East, West Africa, Arabia, South and Central America (28)), quartan malaria (British Guyana, Uganda, Kenya, Madagascar, Nigeria Ivory Coast, Sumatra and Yemen (29)), Hepatitis-B (South Africa (30), Zimbabwe (31)), and probably AIDS in Central Africa. IgA nephropathy, as a potential cause of proliferative glomerulonephritis, is quite rare in Africa (32–34) unless associated with hepatosplenic schistosomiasis (28). Yet the opposite seems to be the case in the South East Asia where a 30% incidence, close to that in the Pacific region, was reported in Hong Kong (27). It is difficult to assess its prevalence in many other parts of the Developing World, as appropriately explained in a recent report from India (25), owing to the lack of facilities for immunofluorescence examination of renal biopsy material.

With increasing industrialization, chronic interstitial nephritis emerges as a major cause of ESRD with a reported prevalence varying between 27.9 and 43.2% (Egypt, Kuwait, India) (25, 35, 36). While this is often attributed to the injudicious use of nephrotoxic medications (25), the role of environmental pollution remains questionable (37).

The reported contribution of diabetes is variable, ranging between 4.3 and 13.5% (6, 24, 26, 33, 38). However, there is an obvious trend of diabetic nephropathy to climb up the list in several Developing Countries reaching 20%

in Hong Kong (27), 21.2% in Kuwait (36) and as high as 26.8% in India (25).

The role of hypertensive nephrosclerosis is also variable, probably depending upon the definitions adopted, between 1.8 and 19.6%. Polycystic disease is rare (1.9–4.5%). Other causes of chronic renal failure are even less frequent (6, 24, 25, 32, 33).

Certain diseases have an unusually high frequency in particular countries, reflecting on the local epidemiological and clinical patterns of ESRD. In addition to those mentioned earlier as causes of glomerulonephritis, there is tuberculosis in India, Egypt and Saudi Arabia (19, 39–41) amyloidosis in East and North Africa and the adjacent Asian Mediterranean countries (6, 33, 42–44) and Ochratoxin-associated Balkan-type nephropathy in North Africa (45, 46) only to mention a few.

Availability of dialysis services in the Developing World

Acute dialysis

Hemodialysis is available for the management of acute renal failure in most of the major hospitals of the Capital cities all over the Developing World, Army and University hospitals usually taking the lead (6, 7, 15, 24, 47, 48). The efficiency of such setups depends on whether a chronic dialysis program is also running in the same hospital. Without this experience, the results of acute dialysis are often quite modest. Transportation of the critically ill patient with acute renal failure from a territorial hospital is a problem that often stunts the effectiveness of acute dialysis services even in the large medical centers.

For obvious reasons, acute peritoneal dialysis is more widely available. It is often implemented where limited or no specialized nephrological care is available, at least as a first line of therapy (2). Unfortunately, the prevailing hygienic conditions in such environment permits a high incidence of peritonitis.

Chronic dialysis

The numbers of patients treated by regular dialysis in the Developing World cannot be precisely defined, owing to the scarcity of reliable registries. Most of the currently available information is obtained from international registries, to which are linked only a few centers in the Developing World, that are neither representative nor regular in updating their data. A meta-analysis of a recent report of the EDTA Registry (49) suggests that, in the pooled experience of 7 participant developing countries, 31.8 patients/million population were alive on dialysis, and 7.8/million had functioning grafts by the end of 1991. The corresponding figures for Western Europe were 225.8 and 154.7 per million and for Eastern Europe 124.4 and 33.6 per million respectively.

This is undoubtedly an under-estimate. Contemporary data generated from sporadic publications (which are, unfortunately, mostly found in non-indexed local litera-

Table 1. Estimated numbers of patients currently receiving regular dialysis treatment in ten developing countries

| Country | Total population (millions) (1) | Dialysis population | | References |
		Total	Total/million	
Algeria	24.5	1,920	78.5	(50)
Brazil	147.0	18,200	123.6	(51)
Egypt	58.0	7,500	129.3	(50)
Hong Kong	5.7	1,400	245.6	(9)
Kuwait	2.0	196	98.0	(36, 53)
Saudi Arabia	13.6	2,085	153.3	(11)
Singapore	2.6	800	307.7	(10)
Sudan	24.4	120	4.9	(16)
Thailand	55.5	1,388	25.1	(54)
Tunisia	8.0	382	47.8	(55)

ture), national registries (by personal communication with colleagues in-charge) or supranational registries (as the African, Arabian and the Asian Pacific) suggest that the dialysis activity in the Developing World is much more extensive indeed (Table 1).

Availability of dialysis services in a certain country, particularly a *developing* one, does not reflect their *accessibility*. The customary expression of national dialysis activity as a 'Stock-and-Flow' pattern (Figure 1) provides a fairly accurate epidemiological evaluation and permits reasonable future projections. The 'stock', which includes the closely inter-related dialysis and transplant pools, reflects the *availability* of such treatments in a particular country; it is largely influenced by its wealth (2). On the other hand, 'flow' mirrors their *accessibility*; it generally indicates the adequacy of planning as well as the quality of technical and organizational performance.

There is a natural tendency for the 'stock' to keep expanding until the 'flow' is balanced by the equilibrium between total annual mortalities and new patient admissions. As *steady state* is achieved, the 'Stock-and-Flow' pattern provides an objective means for system evaluation, cost prediction and projection, and consideration of strategic amendments. A vast number of economically under-privileged countries are able to maintain *steady state* conditions with a relatively small 'stock' and a fast patient 'flow', at the expense of an exceptionally high mortality. This is a very frustrating situation, indeed, since improvement of the quality of service leading to a lower death rate either limits the rate of new patient acceptance or imposes an un-affordable 'stock' expansion.

In other countries, where the results of treatment are more comparable to international standards (56) (Figure 1), the proportional contribution of the principal treatment modalities significantly modifies the ultimate outcome of their ESRD programs. A fairly common pattern is that of countries where transplantation is not available at all. Under such circumstances, *steady state* cannot be achieved unless the 'stock' has more than tripled

the 'flow', while the clinical outcome is extremely modest, with a calculated median survival of only 2 years (Table 2).

The availability of transplantation significantly improves the outcome. When the main emphasis is laid on promoting such modality, as the case is for example in India, Iran and Latin America, median survival is considerably prolonged and the dialysis pool contracted. Although this approach provides significant financial advantages, it has its deleterious social implications (3).

This kind of strategy is not always possible, since local cultural factors often interfere with the establishment of extensive transplant activity. Given this constraint, as the situation is in the Far East, most of Africa and Arabia, and assuming that only one third of patients find their way for a transplant, *steady state* cannot be achieved unless the dialysis pool has doubled the size of annual 'flow' and the transplant has reached 5 folds such 'flow'. The anticipated median survival under such conditions would be 6.2 years.

THE DIALYSIS ENVIRONMENT

The patient

Young adults of the age range 20–50 constitute 70–80% of the Developing World dialysis population (13, 17, 21), which is attributed to the nature of prevailing primary diseases. There is a slight male preponderance, partly explained by the increased exposure to noxious environmental factors (*vide supra*). For similar reasons, the socio-economically underprivileged and the educationally compromised are the majority. This natural selection reflects on the outcome of dialysis treatment in two ways: *poor health conditions at the start* and *inadequate compliance*.

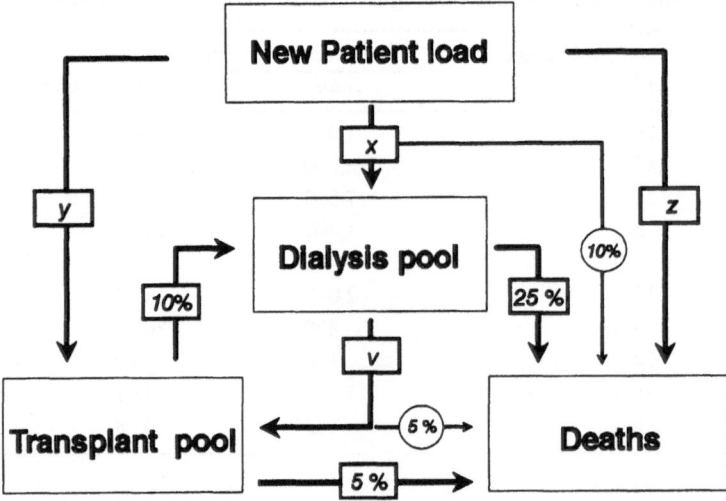

Figure 1. Typical 'Stock-and-Flow' pattern in a developing country. Figures in squares represent annual mortality rates, those in circles provide additional first year mortalities. Under *steady state* conditions, annual deaths should equal $x + y + z$. Explanation in text.

Table 2. Calculated steady-state 'Stock-and-Flow' patterns, median survivals and cost estimates for a program that accommodates 100 new patients per year, under four hypothetical treatment options

		Expected median survival on entry	*Option I* No transplants	*Option 2* Dialysis-restricted	*Option 3* Transplant-restricted	*Option 4* Both restricted
New patients		years				
Admitted for dialysis		2	100	33	67	33
Transplanted from dialysis pool[a]		9	0	100	68	43
Transplanted without prior dialysis		9	0	67	33	33
Total transplants			0	167	101	76
Untreated		0.25	0	0	0	34
		Annual cost per patient				
Steady state		US$				
Dialysis pool		13,433	330	131	205	129
Transplant pool	Initial	14,925	0	888	535	400
	Subsequent	4,478				
Option effectiveness						
Mean median survival[b]			2.0	7.8	6.2	5.3
Total median survival			200	1565	1040	758
Total annual cost[c]			4,410,376	8,217,834	6,636,738	4,653,483
Cost per patient year[d]			6,583	1,567	1,905	1,834

[a]Estimated according to the same restriction limits for those transplanted without prior dialysis.
[b]Computed according to the provisional survival rates given in Figure 1.
[c]Based on the average current costs in Egypt as shown in Figure 3.
[d]Based on the median survivals as shown in Figure 2.

Poor initial health: As mentioned earlier, terminal renal disease in the Developing World is often secondary to, or associated with other endemic disorders. Manifestations of such disorders (hepatosplenic schistosomiasis, tuberculosis, amyloidosis, protein-calorie malnutrition etc) are usually fully blown by the time the patient has reached renal failure, thereby imposing considerable modifications on the clinical patterns of ESRD and often influencing the choice of a particular dialysis modality.

Furthermore, delay in the detection of renal disease and institution of adequate initial management allows the establishment of irreversible uremic complications even before the first dialysis session. Most remarkable are anemia, cachexia, polyneuropathy, and sequelae of uncontrolled hypertension.

Hemodialysis access problems are fairly common, thanks to the imprudent use of the forearm veins for meaningless treatments such as the administration of concentrated glucose and certain herbal extracts.

Inadequate patient compliance: This problem is phenomenal in the Developing World dialysis experience. Compliance involves regularity of showing up for dialysis, sticking to proper dietary instructions, intake of medications and adequate rehabilitation. Poor compliance is often attributed to improper patient information, but the lack of motivation and financial shortcomings usually have a significant influence.

Medical staff

Shortage of adequately trained medical and paramedical local staff is the rule in the majority of developing countries. In the better-off nations, the teams often include expatriates in key positions. When this is un-affordable, unqualified teams simply take over. The author is aware of dialysis teams headed by General Practitioners, Gynecologists and even specialists in Chest Diseases, who never had any chance of proper training in dialysis and nephrology.

Several developing nations have developed their own training programs, which generate nephrologists and dialysis specialists, technicians and nurses. In-service training programs are already functional in a few countries, and successful regional conferences and post-graduate teaching courses have been conducted over the past decade. A lot of support in this area is provided by international and regional organizations.

Dialysis units

The reported number of dialysis units varies from less than one to 5 per million population (10, 13, 16, 51, 52, 55). When detailed figures are compared with the respective numbers of patients actually receiving regular dialysis, it can be appreciated that the units are not kept sufficiently busy. Reasons for non-functional equipment are many, including besides the lack of personnel,

such common developing world problems as shortage of running expenses, poor maintenance and inefficient organization.

State-sponsored, Insurance-sponsored and private units are available in most countries, in proportions that differ according to the political systems and GNPs. Excellent State-sponsored units are the majority in well-off countries (11, 36). In the majority, however, the standard of service in state-sponsored units is modest, which invites the active participation of the private sector. Political system permitting, as in Egypt, India, Brazil, Tunisia, and most of South-East Asia, private units tend to take the technical lead. Governments generally provide partial reimbursement for private dialysis in these countries. Insurance-sponsored units are also growing where health insurance systems are strong enough to substantiate the cost. The currently prevailing insurance policy is to reimburse subscribers for treatment in private units.

Most units are located in hospitals, with a few satellite units in the better developed countries. A few units accept the children and the old, but almost none is specialized in pediatric or geriatric dialysis.

Hard ware equipment is standard, mostly individual proportionating dialysis machines. An occasional unit would be equipped by central dialysate generation systems, of which some are locally manufactured (57), a distinct advantage when the maintenance problems are considered. The use of advanced technology depends on financing, but on the whole it remains very limited. For instance, the use of bicarbonate dialysis in the 7 Developing World centers reporting to the EDTA registry by 1991 was 7.3%, compared to 23.6% in Eastern European countries and 53.4% in Western Europe (49). The use of hemofiltration and hemodiafiltration is even more limited. Peritoneal dialysis Cyclers are barely used.

Adequate water treatment is compulsory for licensing a dialysis unit in a few developing countries. Even though, problems with optimal use, monitoring and maintenance often compromise the water quality. In a recent study, serum and bone aluminum concentrations were found to be extremely high in patients receiving their dialysis treatment in selected developing countries (58). The usual source of aluminum overload is water or concentrate (59) used for dialysate generation, but cooking pots and the intake of aluminum-based phosphate binders often contribute.

Cuprophane- or cellulose acetate-based hollow fibers are most commonly used and often re-used after manual washing and sterilization. High-flux dialyzers and biocompatible membranes are barely used. Little attention is usually paid to urea kinetics. Most patients are dialyzed with low-clearance dialyzers for an insufficient number of hours. Cost is only one explanation for that; negligence is certainly another.

Peritoneal dialysis fluid is frequently locally manufactured, though the better-off countries continue to import it particularly for CAPD. Problems with local manufacture

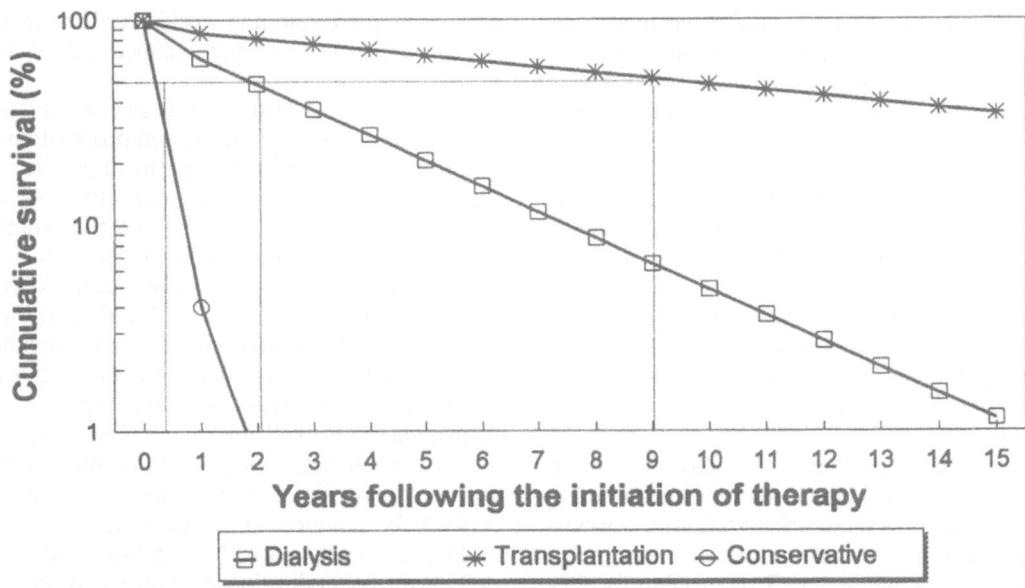

Figure 2. Calculated median survivals based on the rates shown in Figure 1. The *Median survival* is an expression of the time interval following initiation of therapy, at which 50% of a particular cohort of patients is expected to be still alive.

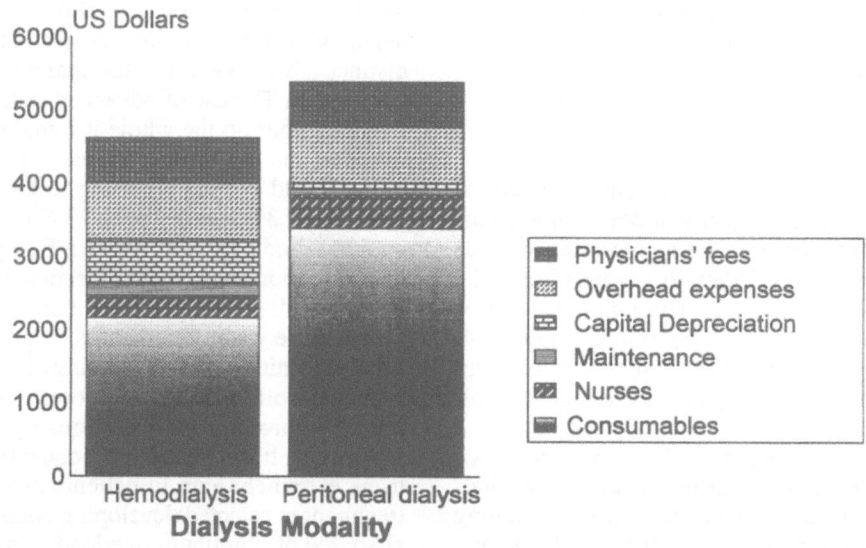

Figure 3. Items of dialysis cost in Egypt, 1993.

include certain technical details such as the water quality, pH control, purity of the chemicals and plastic connectors. Joint ventures between international and local firms are being established in quite a few developing countries, which should solve these problems.

Chronic dialysis modalities

Hemodialysis is the predominant dialysis modality in most developing countries, with a proportional contribu-

tion of 80 to 90% of the dialysis population (36, 49–51). In countries with the lowest GNPs, however, intermittent peritoneal dialysis is the inevitable alternative (6, 16, 47). The implementation of CAPD is widely variable, from sporadic center experiences (60, 61) to a national policy (Hong Kong – 70% (9), Thailand – 40% (54)). Most other countries refrain from CAPD because of the high cost (Figure 3), high incidence of infection, and poor patient compliance. Accordingly, CAPD is offered only as a second choice to selected patients of the higher social classes.

IPD is still carried out for high-risk patients as those with severe ischemic heart disease, complicated diabetes etc. On the whole, it accounts for at least 60.8% of all chronic peritoneal dialysis treatments in the Developing World, compared to 2.7% in Western Europe (49). Since adequate Kt/V can only be achieved by an impossible number of dialysis hours, IPD is associated with extremely poor median survival of the order of 1 year and modest quality of life (16, 47, 62). Although it is usually carried out in hospitals, the incidence of infection remains quite high.

Cost

The calculation of dialysis cost is a difficult and complex procedure. Besides the direct cost including the prices of consumable items, overhead expenses, salaries and fees, must include the cost of inter-dialytic therapy, transfusions, hospital admissions, transportation etc. In even broader terms, it should also consider the days off work and the reduced productivity of some patients.

The items of typical annual direct dialysis cost per capita in a developing country (52) are essentially the same; differences being mainly influenced by the proportion of imported versus locally manufactured material, and by the prevailing standards of salaries and professional fees which vary from 10 to 35% of the total cost (11, 62).

It is noteworthy, as shown in Figure 3, that peritoneal dialysis is the more expensive modality. The same conflicting fact is encountered in several other developing countries (e.g., India), but not in others (e.g., South East Asia). The major cost item in peritoneal dialysis is that of central preparation and sterilization of solutions and plastic bags which are manufactured on a small scale, with incredible overhead expenses. On the other hand, dialyzer re-use in certain centers is often responsible for effectively reducing the comparative cost of hemodialysis.

National kidney foundations

Very few developing countries have established independent national kidney foundations (21, 63) that take care of organization and funding of dialysis treatment, promote research and development, and support staff training. Unfortunately, this positive trend has a long way to go before it is publicized among other developing countries.

RESULTS OF TREATMENT

The reported annual mortality on all dialysis modalities, for all ages and irrespective of the primary renal disease in different Developing World countries varies from 15 to 35% (33, 38, 49). The first year mortality is about 10%

higher (i.e., 25–45%). The calculated average median survival, based on these figures is about 2 years (Figure 2). There is a considerable 'Center Effect', in favor of economically privileged units that can afford recruiting better equipment and staff (62).

Attention to the quality of life (30, 62) is proportionate to individual nations GNPs. In the poorer countries, which constitute the majority in the Developing World, this issue is not even raised. Patients are often contented by just being alive, even though disabled. The incidence of complications is quite high, mainly attributed to improper dialysis, aluminum intoxication, under-nutrition, dialysis-acquired infections and inadequate supplementary therapy.

Under-nutrition is predestined in certain countries, as a part of general starvation. Yet most physicians in the Developing World continue to recommend a protein-restricted diet to their patients on regular dialysis. Analysis of recent EDTA data (49) shows that 73.5% of uremic patients in developing countries are instructed to receive a daily protein intake less than 0.6 g/kg, as compared to 31.3% in Western Europe.

Dialysis-acquired infections are extremely common, mainly comprising the Hepatitis viri and Cytomegalovirus. The prevalence of HIV infection is also high in endemic areas; reports on its rate, epidemiological and clinical sequelae are awaited. Hepatitis-B infection, with a prevalence approaching 90% among dialysis patients in certain countries a couple of decades ago (2), has now regressed to 0–6.4% (49, 64). This decline is at least partly attributed to vaccination of the populations at risk. Unfortunately, HBV infection has been largely replaced by HCV, antibodies to which have been reported in 24.3 to about 70% from different developing countries, the latter figure is, indeed, the mode (64–66). Although the significance of HCV antibody detection remains unsettled, the available data from quite a few countries tend to support the presence of actual viraemia by positive PCR, and concomitant hepatocellular injury by remittent elevation of the hepatic transaminases. Nevertheless, clinically significant chronic liver disease is apparently not alarming.

Cytomegalovirus infection is often overlooked in the dialysis population, despite a prevalence amounting to 74% (67). This infection may lead to dialysis-associated rigors or pyrexia, yet its main importance lies in the potential risk that it imposes on the outcome of subsequent transplantation.

Similar implications seem to hold true for Salmonella infection, evidence of exposure to which having been detected in the pre-transplant assessment of a high percentage of patients (67).

Supplementary therapy: As a general rule, inter-dialytic medical care is extremely modest in the Developing World. Even such basic targets as blood pressure control, correction of anaemia, maintenance of the calcium and acid-base balance are often overlooked. Accessibility to active vitamin D and erythropoeitin is a matter of affordability. In 1991, 7.9% of patients on hemodialysis and 2.9% of those on peritoneal dialysis in the developing countries reporting to the EDTA Registry were treated with EPO, compared to 38.9% in Western Europe. The subsequent need for poly-transfusions certainly facilitates the spread of dialysis-associated viral infections.

SOCIO-ECONOMIC IMPACT

The scenario of dialysis treatment cannot be complete without emphasis on the social and economic dimensions. The meager social security services in the Developing World usually leave the patients, all by themselves, to face their physical disability, financial shortage and a shaken image within *family* and *community*. Their needs grow over the days, until they lose the dignity of personal *independence*. Disappointed in the outcome of treatment, they eventually become either hostile or submissive, yet almost always depressed, withdrawn, and reluctant. Towards this end, the deadly vicious circle of dialysis inadequacy, poor life quality and non-compliance is closed.

This raises the important philosophical question whether chronic dialysis under such circumstances is worthwhile. At least from the patient's point of view, it certainly is, otherwise he/she would not continue. Every dialysis patient has his/her own motive to do so; some form of rationalization for the commitment to *life*. Patients eventually learn to adapt, with a mixture of disability, dissatisfaction and a lot of *egocentrism*.

The medical profession is, unfortunately, the *scape goat* in this scenario. Renal physicians are often blamed, not only by the patients for the poor results of treatment, but also by the community at large for the modest cost-effectiveness of chronic dialysis therapy. It sometimes looks as though all parties had disregarded that *death* is the alternative! Physicians should realize, however, that in certain countries the cost of keeping one patient alive, but partially rehabilitated, on dialysis literally exceeds the average GNP generated by 10 citizens (2, 3). But what would be the meaning of 'community' if the healthy majority would not support a minority of the *sick*? How many folds as much would be willingly spent on importing cigarettes or buying weapons, as though the instinct of *death* supervenes on that for *life*?

Nationalization of the issue of renal failure management should be a pressing target of renal physicians in the Developing World. It cannot be over-emphasized that very little indeed can be achieved unless opinion leaders, politicians, fund-raising organizations and public information media are recruited into the same boat. Dialysis therapy is, after all, an undoubted blessing that every nation must learn how to enjoy.

ACKNOWLEDGMENT

The author acknowledges the willingness of leading colleagues in the Developing World to provide literature and data, without which this review would have been missing important information. Special thanks are due to Professor Kirpal Chug of India, Professor Aziz El-Matry of Tunisia, Professor Heonir Rocha of Brazil, Dr Faisal Shaheen of Saudi Arabia, and Professor Visith Sitprija of Thailand.

REFERENCES

1. The World Bank Atlas. International Bank for Reconstruction and Development/The World Bank. First Printing December 1990. ISBN 0 8213 1649 4
2. Barsoum R: Ethical and moral dilemmas arising from uremia therapy in the Third World – a 'KAP' review. *Prog Artif Organs* 85: 89, 1986
3. Barsoum R: Ethical problems in dialysis and transplantation: Africa. in *Ethical Problems in Dialysis and Transplantation*, edited by Kjellstrand C, Dossetor JB, Kluwer Academic Publishers, Dordrecht, Boston, London, 1991, p 169
4. Hadidy S, Asfari R, Shammaa M, Hanifi M: Acute renal failure among a Syrian population – incidence, etiology, treatment and outcome. *Int Urol Nephron* 21: 455, 1989
5. Mitwalli A, Al-Swailem A, Paul T, Aziz K, Aswad S, Wafa A: Acute renal failure in Al-Medina region, Kingdom of Saudi Arabia. *Saudi Kid Dis Transplant Bulletin* 3: 95, 1992
6. Habte B: Nephrology in Ethiopia. *Proc ISN-African Kid Electrolyte Conf, Cairo*, Cairo Univ Press, 1987, p 159
7. Sezi CL: Nephrology in Uganda. *Proc ISN-African Kid Electrolyte Conf, Cairo*, Cairo Univ Press, 1987, p 174
8. Akinkugbe O: The Nigerian scenario. *Proc ISN-African Kid Electrolyte Conf, Cairo*, Cairo Univ Press, 1987, p 189
9. Chan MK: Treatment of end stage renal failure in Hong Kong. in *Dialysis Therapy in the 1990's*, edited by Tanaka H, Contributions to Nephrology, Vol 82, Krager, Basel, Switzerland, 1990, p 25
10. Woo KT: *Renal Replacement Therapy in Singapore*. Contributions to Nephrology, Vol 82, Krager, Basel, Switzerland, 1990, p 30
11. Aldrees A, Paul T, Abu-Aisha H, Babiker M, Kurpad R, Aswad S: A cost evaluation of hemodialysis in Ministry of Health Hospitals, Saudi Arabia: an NKF study. *Saudi Kid Dis Transplant Bulletin* 2: 125, 1991
12. Aswad S: Causes of chronic renal failure in Saudi Arabia. *NKF Bulletin* 1: 8, 1986
13. Raj B, Jayaraman M: A global perspective. *Dial Transplant* 20: 470, 1991
14. Abdullah MS: Development of renal services in Kenya. *East African Med J* 58: 309, 1981
15. Mtabaji JP, Kitinya J: Diseases of the kidney and urinary tract in Tanzania: a case for more comprehensive renal services. *Proc ISN-African Kid Electrolyte Conf, Cairo*, Cairo Univ Press, 1987, p 167

16. Abboud O: Special problems and challenges with dialysis: Sudan. (Abstract) *Saudi Kid Dis Transplant Bulletin* 4 (Suppl 1): 35, 1993

17. Barsoum R, Rihan Z, Ibrahim A, Lebstein A: Long-term intermittent hemodialysis in Egypt. *Bull World Health Organ* 51: 674, 1974

18. Friedman EA, Delano BG: Can the World afford uremia therapy? *Proc VIII Int Congr Nephrol Athens*, 1981, p 57

19. Barsoum R: Nephrology and African ecology. An overview. *Artif Organs* 14: 235, 1991

20. Gordon D: Racial differences in ESRD. *Dial Transplant* 19: 114, 1990

21. Woods HF: A global perspective. *Dial Transplant* 20: 490, 1991

22. United States Renal Data System. Incidence and causes of treated ESRD. Annual data report. *Am J Kidney Dis* 18 (Suppl 2): 30, 1991

23. Newman JM, Marfin M, Eggers PW, Helgerson SD: End stage renal disease among Native Americans 1983–86. *Am J Public Health* 80: 318, 1990

24. Abboud O: Nephrology in the Sudan. *Proc ISN-African Kid Electrolyte Conf, Cairo*, Cairo Univ Press, 1987, p 157

25. Mani M: Chronic renal failure in India. *Nephrol Dial Transplant* 8: 684, 1993

26. Salah H: Nephrology in Algeria. *Proc ISN-African Kid Electrolyte Conf, Cairo*, Cairo Univ Press, 1987, p 176

27. Chan MK: Dialysis: a global perspective. *Dial Transplant* 20: 463, 1991

28. Barsoum R: Schistosomal glomerulopathies. *Kidney Int* 44: 1, 1993

29. Chug K, Sakhuja V: Tropical glomerulopathies. *Medicine Int* 86: 3548, 1991

30. Seedat YK: Glomerulonephritis in South Africa. *Nephron* 16: 257, 1992

31. Seggie J, Nathhoo K, Davies PG: Association of hepatitis-B (HBs) antigenemia and membranous glomerulonephritis in Zimbabwean children. *Nephron* 38: 115, 1984

32. Philibos M, Francis M, Barsoum R: The histopathologic pattern of glomerulonephritis in a single specialized center experience. (Abstract) *XI Egyptian Congress of Nephrology, Cairo* 1992, p 48

33. El-Matry A, Ben Abdullah T, Ben Maiz: Nephrology in Tunisia. *Proc ISN-African Kid Electrolyte Conf, Cairo*, Cairo Univ Press, 1987, p 178

34. Seedat Y, Nathoo B, Parag K, Naiker I, Ramsaroop R: IgA nephropathy in Blacks and Indians of Natal. *Nephron* 50: 137, 1988

35. El-Said W, Barakat S, Khedr E, Afifi A, El-Tayeb M: Complications of schistosomiasis among Egyptian dialysis patients. (Abstract) *II Int Congr Geographical Nephrol, Hurghada, Egypt* 1993, p 40

36. El-Reshaid K, Johny K, Sugathan T, Georgous M, Nampoory M: Epidemiological profile of end stage renal disease (ESRD) patients in Kuwait. (Abstract) *Saudi Kid Dis Transplant Bulletin* 4 (Suppl 1): 82, 1993

37. Barsoum R: Ecology and Egyptian nephrology. *Proc VIII Egypt Congr Nephron, Fayoum, Egypt*, 1989, p 4

38. Abdel-Samei M, Soliman A, Fayad T, Barsoum R, Kjellstrand C: Serious renal disease in Egypt. *Proc XIII Egypt Congr Nephron, Hurghada, Egypt*, 1993, p 32

39. Malhotra K, Parashar M, Sharma R et al.: Tuberculosis in maintenance hemodialysis patients. Study from an endemic area. *Post-graduate Med J* 57: 492, 1981

40. Pazianas M, Eastwood J, MacRae K, Phillips M: Racial origin and primary renal diagnosis in 771 patients with end-stage renal disease. *Nephrol Dial Transplant* 6: 931, 1991

41. Al-Khader A, Aswad S, Al-Suliman M, Babiker M: Prevalence of tuberculosis in the dialysis population of Saudi Arabia. *Saudi Kid Dis Transplant Bulletin* 1: 155, 1990

42. Barsoum R, Bassily S, Soliman M, Ramzy M, Milad M, Hassaballa A: Renal amyloidosis and schistosomiasis. *Trans R Soc Trop Med Hyg* 73: 367, 1979

43. Haddoum E, Rayane T, Mansouri R, Seba A, Benabadji M: Diseases associated with A-type renal amyloidosis in a Maghreb country. (Abstract) *Saudi Kid Dis Transplant Bulletin* 4 (Suppl 1): 118, 1993

44. Said R, Hamzeh Y, Said S, Tarawneh M, Al-Khateeb M: Spectrum of renal involvement in familial Mediterranean fever. (Abstract) *II Int Congr Geographical Nephrol, Hurghada, Egypt*, 1993, p 68

45. Achour A, Maaroufi K, Hammami M et al.: Chronic interstitial nephritis and Ochratoxin-A. (Abstract) *II Int Congr Geographical Nephron, Hurghada, Egypt*, 1993, p 52

46. Saadi MG, Abdulla E, Fadel F et al.: Prevalence of Ochratoxin-A (OT-A) among Egyptian children and adults with different renal diseases. (Abstract) *II Int Congr Geographical Nephron, Hurghada, Egypt*, 1993, p 22

47. Akinsola A, Adeiekun S: Renal replacement therapy in a Nigerian nephrological practice. (Abstract) *II Int Congr Geographical Nephron, Hurghada, Egypt*, 1993, p 67

48. Ankrah T: Nephrology in Ghana. *Proc ISN-African Kid Electrolyte Conf, Cairo*, Cairo Univ Press, 1987, p 186

49. Raine AEG, Margreiter R, Brunner F et al.: Report on the management of renal failure in Europe, XXII, 1991. *Nephrol Dial Transplant* 2 (Suppl): 7, 1992

50. Rayane T, Haddoum E: Chronic renal failure in Algeria. Renal replacement therapy strategies and progression. (Abstract) *Saudi Kid Dis Transplant Bulletin* 4 (Suppl 1): 118, 1993

51. Rocha H: Nefrologia no Brasil: alguns aspectos de sua evoluccao historica. *J Bras Neprologia* 15: 107, 1993

52. Barsoum R: Renal transplantation in a developing country. The Egyptian 17-year experience. *Afr J Health Sciences* 1: 30, 1994

53. El-Reshaid K, Johny K, Georgous M, Nampoory M, Al-Hilal N: The impact of Iraqi occupation on end-stage renal disease patients in Kuwait, 1990–1991. *Nephrol Dial Transplant* 8: 7, 1993

54. Sitprija V: Personal communication, 1994

55. El-Matry A, Kechrid R, Gafasi A, Ben Maiz H: La prise en charge du traitement de l'insuffisance renale chronique terminate en Tunisie. *La Tunisie Medicale* 72: 173, 1994

56. Gotch FA, Uehlinger DE: Mortality rate in US dialysis patients. *Dial Transpl* 20: 255, 1991

57. Barsoum R: A new locally constructed dialysis system. *Proc 1st Int Cong Biomed Engineering, Cairo*, 1976, C1

58. Haese PC, Couttenye M, Goodman W et al.: Value of the low-dose Desferrioxamine test (5–10 mg/kg) in the diagnosis of aluminum-related bone disease/aluminum overload. *Kidney Int.* Submitted for publication

59. Riad HS, Samuel H, Iskander I, De Broe M, Barsoum R: The dialysis concentrate as a source of aluminum intoxication in renal dialysis-treated patients. *Proc XII Egyptian Congress of Nephrology, Cairo*, 1992, p 84

60. Parsoo I, Seedat YK, Naiker S, Kallmeyer J: Continuous ambulatory peritoneal dialysis in South Africa – a 4-year experience. *Perit Dial Bull* 4: 78, 1984

61. Abu-Aisha H, Huraib S, Al-Wakeel J, Al-Gayyar F, Ali NZ: Attitudes towards CAPD and hemodialysis of patients who had the choice or experienced both modalities of therapy modules. (Abstract) *Saudi Kid Dis Transplant Bulletin* 4 (Suppl): 77, 1993

62. Barsoum R, Shahrezad S, Abdel-Azim O, Yassa H, Abdel-Samei M: Dialysis ward bio-ecology in a developing country. Effect on the results of treatment and impact of socio-economic factors. (Abstract) *VII World Congr Int Soc Artif Organs*, 1991, p 15

63. Aswad S, Paul T, Edrees A, Babiker M, Saleh A, Taha A, Al-Swailem A: The role of the National Kidney Foundation in cadaveric renal transplantation in Saudi Arabia. *Saudi Kid Dis Transplant Bulletin* 1: 145, 1990

64. Seedat YK, Macintosh C, Subban J: Quality of life for patients in an end-stage disease program. *South African Med J* 71: 500, 1987

65. El-Banawy S, Zaki A, Heghazi T, Mowafi N, Quiniti I, Renganathan E: Hepatitis C virus antibodies in hemodialysis patients. (Abstract) *II Int Congr Geographical Nephron, Hurghada, Egypt*, 1993, p 12

66. Tohamy M, Abdul-Naser M, Abdul Hafez Z, Kamel N, Sobh MA, Abdulla M: Hepatitis C infection in hemodialysis patients and staff in Assiut renal dialysis units. *Ain Shams Med J* 43: 625, 1992

67. Al-Arrayed A, Chandra S, Al-Arrayed A: Prevalence of hepatitis C antibodies in patients on chronic hemodialysis. (Abstract) *Saudi Kid Dis Transplant Bulletin* 4 (Suppl 1): 72, 1993

68. Barsoum R: The Egyptian transplant experience. *Transpl Proc* 24: 2417, 1992

PLANNING OF DIALYSIS FOR DISASTERS

KIM SOLEZ, IRAJ NADJAFI, ALI-REZE ATEF ZAFARMAND and ALLAN J. COLLINS

INTRODUCTION

Disasters requiring dialysis planning fall into two main categories: 1) disasters which interfere with treatment of pre-existing renal failure in developed countries by disrupting established dialysis services, and 2) disasters which cause substantial crush-injury-induced acute renal failure in underdeveloped countries which previously had limited or no dialysis facilities. The third potential category, crush-injury-induced acute renal failure in disasters in developed countries, is unusual owing to better standards of building construction in developed countries and better use of strategies which prevent acute renal failure (1). Even when it does occur the disruption of dialysis access for pre-existing renal failure patients is a greater problem. In the January 17, 1995 earthquake in Japan there were several hundred acute renal failure cases as a result of crush injury. However, well over 1,000 chronic renal failure patients had disruption of dialysis access (Dr Yoshihei Hirasawa, personal communication, 1995). The categories relating to domestic and foreign disasters are equally important, and the Public Education Committee of the US National Kidney Foundation has recently prepared a very instructive set of brochures dealing with planning for response to dialysis disruption in domestic disasters (2). However, in this chapter we will confine our attention to planning for dialysis needs for crush injury-induced acute renal failure in foreign disasters.

Acute renal failure as a consequence of a natural disaster was brought to the attention of the international medical community by the December 7th 1988 earthquake in the Armenian Federated Republic of the former Soviet Union (3–7). Because of the size and magnitude of the earthquake, centered near Spitak Armenia, a disaster search and rescue response unprecedented in scale was initiated (8, 9). Survivors were treated with conservative measures and appeared stable after extrication; however, many died suddenly from probable severe hyperkalemia in the field. The request for dialysis assistance catapulted the international community into an unparalleled disaster relief effort, teaching significant lessons to the world's response teams. It is now clear that search and rescue is only the first part of a multiphase response effort, especially if disaster-related acute renal failure is suspected. Secondary and tertiary phases of that response each need to be planned for and strengthened, including preventive measures to reduce the incidence of acute renal failure, as well as dialysis resources to be mobilized and made available to support teams.

This chapter will focus on the steps that search and rescue teams and advanced medical teams may use to reduce the potential for acute renal failure from crush injury in disasters, and to provide guidelines for the deployment of dialysis resources in the disaster setting.

EPIDEMIOLOGY OF ACUTE RENAL FAILURE IN DISASTERS

The occurrence of acute renal failure in disasters can be best understood by subdividing the types of disasters into major categories. The major source of acute renal failure in disasters is the massive damage caused by seismic events. In addition to seismic disasters (i.e., earthquakes), other events leading to acute renal failure include concussive or explosive-type disasters (i.e., building collapse from conventional or nuclear bombs; terrorist bombings like that in Lebanon, where a US army barracks was destroyed in 1982). These disasters are not the only types that may cause significant crush injury. Hurricanes and tornadoes also inflict major structural damage and victims may be caught under heavy debris, causing crush injury and the potential for acute renal failure.

The other major disaster category associated with acute renal failure centers on thermal injuries. These may be sustained during military explosions (such as on a naval vessel after a malfunctioned detonation of explosive charges), napalm bombings (Vietnam), and pipeline explosions like that occurring near Ufa, in the former Soviet Russian Federated Republic, in June of 1989. Such thermal injury may lead to severe volume loss, especially in children, and shock, with resultant acute renal failure if aggressive fluid therapy is not initiated. This was the case in the Ufa disaster, when 10 of 60 children with greater than 50% burns had acute renal failure (10).

The profound and rapid acute renal failure associated with crush injury has only recently been recognized as a major problem in disasters. The major earthquakes of recent years that have led to massive loss of life have been variably associated with acute renal failure. In the Mexico City earthquake of 1985, there were 3,000 to 4,000 deaths. Acute renal failure from crush injury was not, however, mentioned as a major epidemiologic or clinical concern during the relief effort (11–14). The next major earthquake associated with great loss of life was the Armenian quake of 1988 (8). Measuring approximately 6.9 on the Richter scale, this quake caused close to 25,000 deaths, with 100,000 injured, and between 400 and 600 victims suffering acute renal failure after extrication from the debris (4, 6). In the San Francisco earthquake of 1989, fewer than 60 people died, and only one case of acute renal failure from crush injury was identified. The 1990 earthquake in Iran caused at least 13,888 deaths. Reports of acute renal failure and requests for dialysis aid were made, and 156 patients were treated for acute renal failure (1, 15). In the 1990 quake in the Philippine Islands, close to 1,500 people died, but no cases of acute renal failure from crush injury were reported initially.

In reviewing the major earthquakes that have occurred in populated areas since 1985, some patterns do seem to emerge. Major loss of life appears to occur in areas where little of the sophistication of modern civil engineering and building techniques is available to create structures that can withstand seismic disturbances (11). Examples of this include the Armenian and Iranian earthquakes. Earthquakes that occur in modern cities, where modern construction materials and engineering techniques have led to more earthquake-resistant buildings, are associated with a considerably lower incidence of death, and the incidence of acute renal failure is almost nonexistent. Major disruptions of local services (hospitals, electrical power, communications, and transportation) were also considerably less in the Mexico, San Francisco, and Philippine earthquakes, allowing emergency teams to provide a more timely response to extricate victims. In Armenia and Iran, the major services and local support systems were almost entirely destroyed, severely inhibiting response time and causing delayed extrication of victims from the rubble (8). These delays contributed to the likelihood of prolonged crush injury and acute renal failure. Unfortunate-

ly, these recent disasters have only begun to set in motion an improved understanding of association between large-scale disasters and the development of acute renal failure. Changes in disaster responses need further study and testing to ensure that the most appropriate relief effort is mobilized.

CLINICAL PRESENTATION OF ACUTE RENAL FAILURE FROM CRUSH INJURY

The clinical presentation of acute renal failure in crush injuries has been described numerous times and has been well-reviewed by Better and Stein (16–19). Experience with crush injury victims in the bombings of London between 1940 and 1941, as first reported by Bywaters (20), provides a classic description of the hemoglobin, blood pressure, and urine output responses to acute renal failure from crush injury and rhabdomyolysis. Further clinical descriptions of hypocalcemia, myoglobinemia, myoglobinuria, severe hyperkalemia, and hyperphosphatemia, which define the syndrome, were reported, and the pathophysiologic mechanisms have been described (21, 22). The reader is referred to these listed references and more recent reviews for details of the pathophysiology and clinical consequences of rhabdomyolysis, myoglobinemia, and myoglobinuria (17, 18, 23–26).

The consequences of crush injury and rhabdomyolysis may vary considerably based on the speed with which the disaster team arrives at the site, extricates the victims, and initiates the aggressive management of the complications of acute renal failure. The experiences of several search and rescue teams providing care after the Armenian earthquake, particularly that of one of the authors, show that a considerable number of patients died of hyperkalemia postextrication from the rubble in Spitak, Leninakan, and Kirovakan (9). These deaths occurred after patients were stabilized with routine fluid management to return their blood pressures to normal. While patients were waiting for transportation to secondary and tertiary hospitals for subsequent care, unexpected sudden deaths occurred. Both the rapid demise of these patients and the association of the deaths with hyperkalemia led the Soviet Ministry of Health to request dialysis assistance from the international community. This sequence of extrication of victims with subsequent sudden death has led many to review the steps that may be taken in the field to prevent such a pattern and to develop algorithms to ensure consistent management of victims to reduce the need for large-scale high-technology relief efforts, if possible.

EARLY MANAGEMENT OF CRUSH INJURY

The prolonged compression of lower limbs, upper limbs, and trunk by fallen masonry provides the environment for the development of massive tissue injury. Such injury may result in rhabdomyolysis and the release of intracellular muscle constituents into the circulation, which then leads to metabolic acidosis, myoglobinemia, myoglobinuria, hyperkalemia, hyperphosphatemia, hyperuricemia, and coagulopathy. Deep muscle injury also leads to the sequestering of large amounts of fluid in the crushed tissues, with the rapid development of myoedema. The third spacing of fluids in the injured muscle beds can cause compartment compression syndrome, with further muscle injury as well as peripheral nerve damage (27–29). The considerable volume sequestered in the crushed tissues leads to intravascular volume depletion with resultant reduction in cardiac output, blood pressure, and renal blood flow (30). The consequent reduced renal perfusion leads to increased urinary concentration at a time when myoglobin and elevated levels of uric acid, also released from the injured muscles, are being excreted in the urine. All of these factors contribute to the precipitation of myoglobin in the renal tubules and tubular injury, resulting in acute renal failure (17, 18, 30).

The pathophysiologic changes in crush injury predispose the patient to severe hyperkalemia, hyperphosphatemia, and hypocalcemia during the resuscitation phase, which can lead to cardiac complications unless adequate measures are taken to alleviate the metabolic changes. Moderate amounts of resuscitation fluid may improve the intravascular volume deficit and increase blood pressure and perfusion pressure to the injured muscle bed. Once these muscle beds are reperfused, however, considerable amounts of formerly sequestered intracellular potassium will be released, as well as large amounts of organic acids. Both further exacerbate the release of potassium, resulting in severe hyperkalemia. This considerable acidosis also dramatically reduces renal blood flow and inhibits the kidney's ability to excrete this acid load, as well as interfering with adequate excretion of potassium. In the postresuscitative period and under conservative management, depending on the degree of muscle injury and delay in extrication of the victims, therefore, severe renal compromise and hyperkalemia of a life-threatening nature may develop, as noted in the resuscitated victims of the Armenian earthquake.

Alternative approaches to resuscitation of such patients have been developed that dramatically reduce the consequences of crush syndrome and the immediate postresuscitation risk of sudden death from hyperkalemia and acidosis in the setting of acute renal failure (30, 31). The early management of crush injury has been studied by Ron et al. (25), with victims from the 1982 building collapse in Lebanon. They prospectively studied a therapeutic approach aimed at the prevention of acute renal failure due to crush syndrome. Out of approximately 100 victims buried in the 1982 Lebanon incident, 20 survivors were located under the ruins. Medical crews were instructed to insert intravenous lines and infuse large quantities of crystalloid even before patients were extricated from beneath the rubble.

Seven patients identified as suffering from crush injury were evacuated by helicopter to the intensive care unit of the Rambam Medical Center in Haifa, Israel. The seven male patients had a mean age of 25 years, with all sustaining severe muscle injuries to the lower extremities and presenting with partial paralysis, absence of deep-tendon reflexes, and sensory deficits. Myoglobin was identified in the urine of all seven. Each man underwent surgical procedures such as external fixation, traction, and reduction of fractures. Laboratory evaluation on arrival at the medical center showed all patients had diminished platelet counts and no associated abnormal bleeding. The average anion gap was approximately 15 mEq/l. Three of the seven patients had potassium levels of 7 to 8.3 on admission to the hospital. Over a 60-hour period, potassium excretion averaged 387 mEq.

Aimed at avoiding acute renal failure, the objective of the study was defined as obtaining a diuresis of at least 300 ml/hour with a urine pH greater than 6.5. This was achieved by infusing, via central line, 300 ml/hour of half-normal saline with one ampule of sodium bicarbonate (44.5 mEq). If the central venous pressure rose more than 5 cm of water, the rate of intravenous infusion was decreased and 1 g/kg of mannitol was administered to the patient. Urine output and urine pH of the patient were checked hourly, and when urine pH was greater than 6.5 and plasma pH was greater than 7.45, acetazolamide was added intravenously to increase urinary alkalization. Further management of the patient was based on judgment to maintain central venous pressure within normal levels and to keep urine output at 300 ml/hour, as well as adjust the amount of sodium bicarbonate in the intravenous infusion and the urinary pH with additional doses of acetazolamide as necessary.

Initial volume assessment of the patients before starting the intensive fluid therapy showed central venous pressures varying between 0 and 2 cm of water. To reach a diuresis of more than 300 ml/hour, intravenous fluid therapy averaging 568 ml/hour over the first 60 hours was given. After approximately 60 hours, myoglobin was no longer evident in the urine and the kaliuresis decreased significantly, leading to the conclusion that cessation of active rhabdomyolysis and loss of muscle contents had occurred. The total fluid balance achieved in the first 60 hours was positive to approximately 12,000 mL of water and more than 1,200 mEq of sodium. The total amount of sodium bicarbonate used in those hours was over 685 mEq, to reach a urinary pH greater than 6.5. Intravenous bicarbonate therapy took an average of 4.2 hours to achieve the desired urinary pH level. The patients received significant volume expansion with large doses of sodium bicarbonate to correct acidosis, and alkalinization of urine with high urine output, which helped to reduce the precipitation of myoglobin in the tubules of the seven male patients with massive crush injury. None of the seven patients developed acute renal failure.

In contrast, a 36-year-old man injured at the same time, who was suspected of having a spinal cord injury and was treated at another ward, received only 2.5 l of fluid in the resuscitation period. By the time he was identified as suffering from crush injury, he had oliguria with a creatinine level of 4.8 mg/dl, and went into acute renal failure that required hemodialysis for 3 weeks. It appears from the experiences of Ron et al. that treatment of rhabdomyolysis with aggressive fluid and bicarbonate therapy prevented acute renal failure, in contrast to the alternative treatment given to the other patient.

The Lebanon incident illustrates one type of disaster and crush injury setting in which early intervention and rapid mobilization of search and rescue teams to the site resulted in early extrication of patients. In the earthquake disasters of Armenia and Iran, however, such significant delays occurred in the arrival of search and rescue teams at the disaster site that patients were pinned under large pieces of masonry and debris for over 48 to 72 hours. Such prolonged patient exposure, with its increasing levels of acidosis and hyperkalemia as well as volume depletion, may present a set of conditions different from those described by Ron et al.. Unfortunately, no clinical data are available to determine whether dialytic therapy could be significantly reduced by more rapid extrication in seismic disasters. Alternative and supportive plans need to be developed that not only incorporate early fluid management, but also address the monitoring of patients post-extrication to ensure early identification of hyperkalemia before victims are moved to secondary and tertiary hospital settings. Portable battery-powered electrocardiographic monitors provide an excellent method for diagnosing severe hyperkalemia in the field setting. The ISTAT point-of-care testing instrument which is capable of measuring plasma potassium, sodium, glucose, and urea nitrogen within 90 seconds also can be invaluable. Once identification of severe hyperkalemia has occurred, field medical teams can introduce appropriate management with sodium bicarbonate, calcium gluconate or calcium chloride, and sorbitol and sodium polystyrene sulfonate (Kayexalate). The use of 50% glucose in the field is advantageous; however, insulin therapy in the field is impractical because of the lack of refrigeration. As patients with severe hyperkalemia are identified, disaster response teams can triage patients based on the degree of hyperkalemia, the speed with which treatment is required, and the potential need for dialytic intervention.

DIALYSIS THERAPY FOR CRUSH INJURY IN SEISMIC DISASTERS

The introduction of dialysis into a disaster setting is difficult because of the requirements of equipment, supplies, and transport of skilled personnel. Because these resources are of a secondary and tertiary nature, adequate planning is needed to improve identification of the need as well as to provide rapid mobilization. Algorithms on mobilization of US dialysis teams have been developed at the Regional Kidney Disease Program in Minneapolis and coordinated with the US Office of Foreign Disaster Assistance in Washington, DC. Figure 1 (from Reference 3) depicts the sequence of mobilization of dialysis management teams to assess local needs for dialysis, as well as to determine area-wide needs for adequate distribution of the resources. A similar plan has been developed by Dr Norbert Lameire for Europe, under a plan utilizing resources of the Belgian Airforce, Doctors Without Borders, the European Union, and the Baxter Healthcare Corporation (1). The approaches allow teams of highly experienced technical engineers, nurses, and a physician executive manager to assess and deliver immediate dialysis. This team also can provide knowledgeable feedback to disaster organizations as the need arises for further dialysis teams, equipment, and supplies. Once a system for such mobilization is in place, the type of dialytic therapy being provided needs to be determined to ensure consistent rapid deployment.

Table 1 shows the advantages and disadvantages of different modes of dialytic therapy. The primary consideration in selecting a form of dialysis to be delivered in a disaster setting centers on a rapid but graded response. The severe weight restrictions in delivering medical supplies and the shortage of air freight space pose major problems in picking the type of dialytic therapy that will treat the greatest number of patients. Severe limitations in local airport unloading capabilities and ground transportation are equally important. Finally, local medical conditions relative to sanitation, electric power, water, and heating may also impact on the delivery of dialysis. With these limitations and local conditions in mind, a review of the types of dialysis and how they may be delivered is important.

Many types of dialytic techniques are available. The slow continuous forms of dialysis include slow continuous hemodialysis, slow continuous arteriovenous (AV) hemofiltration, and continuous ambulatory peritoneal dialysis (CAPD) (32, 33). Techniques that are intermittent in nature include intermittent hemodialysis, intermittent hemofiltration or diafiltration, and intermittent peritoneal dialysis. In the 1990s, intermittent peritoneal dialysis can only be performed with cyclers, with a resultant large fluid requirement to increase efficiency. The weight requirement would make intermittent peritoneal dialysis impractical in a disaster setting. The main focus, therefore, should be on the advantages and disadvantages of CAPD, slow continuous hemodialysis, AV hemofiltration, or intermittent hemodialysis.

Slow continuous AV hemodialysis and AV hemofiltration, as well as CAPD, have some obvious advantages. All of these therapies are technically simple to comprehend and the equipment is minimal. For CAPD, after placement of a peritoneal trochar or single-cuff Tenckhoff catheter, the only other requirements are the appropriate connection

Justification of Event by USGS, ISN Disaster Relief Task Force

Office of Foreign Disaster Assistance (OFDA) State Department

American and International Red Cross (ARC-IRC) (Develop emergency system contacts with IRC, WHO)

USGS and OFDA assess potential for crush injury

Contact made with advance dialysis management team to initiate official and unofficial contacts with host country

Advance dialysis team departs for site with primary rescue teams

Arrival of advance dialysis team:

1. Assess airport capacity
2. Assess local transportation
3. Deploy communication system
4. Survey primary sites for extent of crush injury
5. Survey hospitals for acute and chronic dialysis capabilities

Select number of US and European teams - Give details of site capability to receive teams to OFDA-IRC for mobilization

Implement triage system for dialysis
1. Aggressive fluid management
2. Develop dialysis sites
3. Transport patients to dialysis sites
4. Remove chronic dialysis patients from area if possible

Advance team to resurvey disaster sites and dialysis areas

Communicate to OFDA and IRC
US and European dialysis teams notified of mobilization

Dialysis team staff and equipment manufacturer notified

Team selected and proceeds to staging areas
1. Manufacturers provide transport of supplies to staging area
2. Teams given contacts in host country
3. Flight info relayed back to advance team to coordinate arrival of secondary teams
4. Teams depart to disaster site coordinate arrival of secondary teams

Teams' arrival in host country
1. Met by advance team
2. Secure visa entry
3. Secure cargo inventory unloading and clearance out of airport
4. Arrange transportation to dialysis sites

Dialysis team sites:
1. Dialysis locations and storage area
2. Unloading of supplies
3. Mechanical, electrical, and water system progress
4. Machine setup
5. Need for additional dialysis supplies
6. Coordinate dialysis requirement with conservative management

Figure 1. Mobilization chart for US Office and Disaster Assistance modified (from Reference 3).

Table 1. Techniques for dialysis (from Reference 3, used with permission)

Advantages and Disadvantages of Continuous Dialysis Techniques
    Types of Continuous Therapies:
        Slow continuous AV hemofiltration (CAVH)
        Continuous AV hemodialysis (CAVHD)
        Chronic ambulatory peritoneal dialysis (CAPD)
    Advantages of Hemo Continuous Therapies:
        Technically simple
        Management systems are easily maintained
        Less intense, easy training of local staff in techniques
        Continuous removal of solutes
        Continuous control of fluid balance
    Disadvantages of Hemo Continuous Therapies:
        CAVH and CAVHD, continuous heparinization
        One-on-one nursing management of patients in the field to ensure adequate fluid balance
        Infusion and ultrafiltration pumps requiring electrical supply and battery back-up
        Large fluid requirements with significant weight of supplies to be transported both by air and ground to field hospitals
        Slow removal of potassium and correction of acidosis related to limited clearance capability
        Minimal mobility of the patient
Advantages and Disadvantages of Chronic Ambulatory Peritoneal Dialysis
    Advantages:
        No blood access required
        Continuous control of fluid and solute removal
        Simple connection systems
        Provides additional glucose for nutrition
    Disadvantages:
        Sterile technique being required by local hospitals
        Further management of patients in secondary and tertiary centers after introduction of the catheter with an experienced staff
        Lack of availability of assistive devices for on and off techniques locally
        Large volume of fluid requirements, with significant weight for transportation
        Slow solute removal
Advantages and Disadvantages of Intermittent Hemodialysis
    Advantages:
        Blood access can be veno-venous by dual lumen catheters
        Avoids arterial access
        Efficient removal of solutes
        Lower weight requirements for supplies
        Rapid correction of hyperkalemia and acidosis
    Disadvantages:
        Requires sophisticated dialysis delivery systems and technical support
        Adequate water treatment to reduce machine problems and patient side effects
        Skilled, technical, and clinical staff
        Time delays in setting up equipment and water treatment
        Adequate spare parts to support technical equipment

---

systems for peritoneal fluid exchange and available skilled staff to ensure good sterile technique. In slow continuous AV hemofiltration, arteriovenous access is a necessary requirement. Short blood line sets, with the appropriate infusion pumps, are easy to comprehend, and fluid management can be easily monitored based on matching ultrafiltration and reinfusion. Slow continuous dialysis also has simplicity relative to short line sets and small dialyzers; in addition, dialysate infusion or dialysate outflow pumps are required for adequate ultrafiltration control.

The main advantages that have been outlined reflect the simplicity of these measures as applied in sophisticated medical settings by highly trained staff or in intensive care units used to caring for critically ill patients and having the necessary infusion pumps, wall suction, electric supplies, and sanitary techniques. All of these measures may not necessarily be available in the country of the disaster site or at local secondary and tertiary medical facilities. Therefore, although these methods of dialysis appear to have advantages in up-to-date medical facilities, they may not be practical in the setting of a seismic disaster.

There are potential additional drawbacks to slow therapies, which apply to both forms of dialysis. It is clear that continuous arteriovenous hemofiltration (CAVH) and continuous arteriovenous hemodialysis (CAVHD) require continuous heparinization of the patient, which can cause predisposition to gastrointestinal bleeding or at other injury site, as well as bleeding from the AV access. Techniques have been developed to perform regional protamine or even regional citrate therapy on CAVHD; these, however, increase the complexity and technical requirements for delivery of dialysis in the disaster setting and thus become disadvantages. Continuous arteriovenous hemofiltration and CAVHD also immobilize the patient, delaying movement through the disaster response system. Continuous monitoring of the infusion pumps and the particular requirements for electric supply or battery-powered equipment add increasing complexity to the management and movement of patients through the system – from field hospitals to secondary local hospitals to tertiary care areas for dialytic management. Another disadvantage is the requirement for large volumes of sterile fluid. The simplicity of the system in attaching either 2- or 5-l dialysate bags for patient management and the easy supply and transportation of such bags within Western countries may not necessarily be available in the local disaster setting. In fact, the weight requirements for managing a single patient in acute renal failure with slow continuous therapies may be four to six times that of intermittent hemodialysis that uses concentrates. The last and most significant disadvantage centers on the slow removal of potassium and correction of acidosis in the face of rapidly developing acute renal failure from rhabdomyolysis (33). The limitations of CAVH or CAVHD in the field setting therefore may very well outweigh the advantages of large-scale application of these therapies in a major disaster, in which crush injuries, severe hyperkalemia, and acidosis are not manageable by conservative measures and necessitate the use of dialytic techniques.

The advantages of CAPD have been outlined, but disadvantages of CAPD do exist, especially in the disaster setting. In Western medical centers good communication between patients and the medical staff allows teams to treat patients with peritoneal dialysis readily and safely. Similar suitable conditions may not be present in the host country. Patients' unfamiliarity with the placement of catheters in the abdominal cavity may prevent patient acceptance of the procedure. In addition, sterile technique and assist devices that are readily available in dialysis centers in the Western world may not necessarily be available in a disaster setting or in underdeveloped countries. The maintenance of these devices would be extremely difficult in the short-term disaster setting. Once again, the large volume of sterile fluid required to treat each patient creates weight and transportation difficulties within the disaster setting as well as difficulties in unloading at the host country. Local transportation out of airports and transportation over the ground may also be severely disrupted. Therefore the advantages and simplicity of CAPD may be outweighed by local logistic considerations in underdeveloped areas.

On balance intermittent hemodialysis seems to be the modality of choice in most post-disaster settings. Intermittent hemodialysis can be performed with venous-venous access via subclavian catheters or dual lumen femoral catheters. This central access is similar to the placement of other central fluid lines and is easily understood and practiced by medical personnel all over the world. Other advantages include extremely efficient treatment of a large number of patients with a limited amount of equipment in a fixed space. Patients who can be transported for dialysis treatment for severe hyperkalemia and acidosis can be treated with short high-efficiency treatments, eliminating the need for personnel to be involved in the ongoing fluid management is a situation in which skilled medical personnel may be extremely scarce. Another advantage of intermittent hemodialysis is the low volume of fluid and reduced transportation weight.

The disadvantages of intermittent therapy, however, are extremely important to consider. Intermittent hemodialysis requires a more sophisticated dialysis delivery system and technical support. To limit patient side effects from contaminated water, adequate water treatment is needed. This will also reduce machine problems. Time delays in setting up equipment and appropriate water treatment may contribute to patient morbidity. Finally, an adequate supply of spare parts is important to support the technical operation; without adequate backup equipment or spare parts, machine malfunctions would severely limit the dialysis team's ability to treat large numbers of patients.

It is clear that both slow continuous therapies and intermittent dialytic therapies have benefits and drawbacks that must be balanced when being applied to a specific disaster setting.

CLINICAL APPROACH TO DIALYTIC MANAGEMENT AFTER ESTABLISHED ACUTE RENAL FAILURE

In reviewing the advantages and disadvantages of the different techniques, CAPD and slow continuous therapies are seen to be problematic in the field setting when large numbers of patients need treatment and rapid transportation is needed. Intermittent dialytic therapies are extremely efficient and meet weight requirements, but also have disadvantages. The technical difficulties of intermittent hemodialysis can be overcome in such a way that a complete package of supplies and equipment with appropriate electric connectors and plumbing can be delivered, as was done in the Ufa disaster (6).

The experience gained in the Armenian earthquake disaster and subsequent work with the US Office of Foreign Disaster Assistance after the Ufa pipeline explosion have led to a rapid mobilization system for introduction of hemodialysis capability in a disaster setting (see Figure 1). This system first mobilizes a single dialysis team consisting of one physician, one dialysis nurse, and one dialysis technical engineer. All team members must be capable of dialyzing patients as well as contributing to set-up of water treatment and machine systems. The hemodialysis systems that have been proposed include basic water sediment cartridge filters, charcoal cartridge filters to remove chlorine, a small softener to remove calcium, and a reverse osmosis module to provide product water to the dialysis machines. All systems are configured to meet the local electric supply, and all plumbing is of a modular segment design, including tubing with quick connectors and a small water holding tank. The team brings the necessary electric wiring, outlet boxes, and plugs to ensure ability to tap local or emergency power. Hemodialysis machines of a mechanical-based nature are preferable to sophisticated electronic equipment. Heavily computerized equipment may experience difficulty in the face of electric instability and lack of computer parts in the field setting. If ultrafiltration control delivery systems are used, they must be able to operate in a manual mode.

Dialysate concentrate should be acetate-based to decrease the complexity of field application and to reduce shipping weight. Potassium content could be a standard zero or 3 mEq/l bath, with other concentrations being mixed if needed. Four dialysis machines would be capable of dialyzing 16 to 20 patients per 16-hour operation day. The maximum total patients managed could be 32 to 40 in the first week. Supplies needed the first week would be for 100 to 125 treatments; the total weight is approximately 8,000 pounds and can be transported by a small 8- to 10-passenger jet for quick response. This system effectively delivered dialysis capability to children in Ufa in June of 1989 within 18 to 24 hours. Finally, the dialysis supplies should contain dialyzers, bloodlines, and dialysis catheters for both adults and children. The team members need skill in both adult and pediatric dialysis techniques.

THE MOBILIZATION RESPONSE

Disaster response dialysis teams are best established on an international level to interface with major disaster international relief organizations. The Disaster Relief Task Force

of the International Society of Nephrology Commission on Acute Renal Failure has developed North American and European regional dialysis response coordinators who interface with their host countries (1). As the first dialysis management teams relay information back to relief organizations, additional teams already standing by can be mobilized. Additional supplies can be transported within 2 to 3 days to supply the primary teams as needed.

The initial dialysis teams, upon arrival, must acquire local information from the Minister of Health and assess immediate needs as well as determine whether any chronic dialysis capability exists in the area. One member of the team knowledgeable in dialysis systems and delivery should acquire the information and assist other members in securing movement of equipment and supplies from the airport to designated sites. After arrival at the sites established for dialysis, the team will split so the physician can review the number of patients needing dialysis with the local and foreign medical teams. Triaging of dialysis may be necessary initially if the demand is overwhelming, so patients with severe hyperkalemia, acidosis, or fluid overload receive priority. If chronic dialysis patients already exist in the host country, this may create additional difficulties if the previous dialysis capability was destroyed. Systems to move stable chronic patients to other areas may be needed to prevent overload of the acute dialysis capacity.

Overall, the keys to the teams' success are flexibility and sensitivity to the local community and conditions. Dialysis teams, like other disaster teams, are guests in the host country and should maintain a professional demeanor. Sensitivity to local customs and political environment is integral to the success not only of the search and rescue teams, but also dialytic management teams, which interface much more closely with the established medical community in the major secondary and tertiary hospitals. Conditions within the hospitals in the host country may be of varying quality, and considerable sensitivity in this area is necessary to ensure that the primary mission of the dialysis effort is not jeopardized. The experience gained in Armenia and Ufa also shows that the dialysis teams are consulted about numerous types of dialytic therapies that may be practiced in local hospitals. Team members have an advantage if they have knowledge in the practical delivery of all types of dialytic therapy to assist the host hospital if needed.

CONCLUSIONS AND RECOMMENDATIONS

The incidence of acute renal failure in seismic disaster is unknown and is highly dependent on the local area's builders' expertise in civil engineering. In Armenia in 1988, the number of patients dialyzed exceeded 150 and 400 to 600 patients were said to have acute renal failure. Early management of crush victims with administration of large amounts of intravenous fluid at the extrication site is critical to reduce the degree of acute renal failure and control the severe acidosis and hyperkalemia that can lead to postextrication cardiac arrhythmia and death. Portable electrocardiographic monitoring in the field can identify critical hyperkalemia requiring field treatment. Further aggressive fluid therapy with sodium bicarbonate and alkalinization of the urine can reduce the likelihood of acute renal failure development requiring dialysis. Field teams should be well versed in the recognition and conservative management of severe hyperkalemia.

Mobilization of dialysis teams may be needed if the host country fits the pattern of Armenia and Iran relative to stability of buildings. Demographic profiles of countries by disaster organizations are available and can assist in planning dialysis requirements. Dialytic therapies applied in a disaster setting must take into account not only the simplicity of bedside application, but also the volume and weight of supplies to be transported, the site of application, and the sophistication of the local medical system. All types of dialytic therapy were attempted in Armenia, with intermittent hemodialysis being the most successful in treating large numbers of patients.

The mobilization system should be an adjunct to a graded disaster response. Experienced dialysis teams with broad skills can meet immediate needs and have strong credibility in requesting additional teams through the host country and from relief organizations. Triaging of dialysis may be required so patients with severe hyperkalemia and acidosis receive priority, even over primary early treatment of those with uncomplicated uremia.

It is clear from the recent earthquake experience that graded disaster response systems are needed, not only to provide search and rescue teams and temporary housing for victims, but also to establish field intensive care units, specialized surgical and orthopedic teams, and dialysis capability at various levels. The US Office of Foreign Disaster Assistance and the International Society of Nephrology's Acute Renal Failure Task Forces have been in the forefront working with the experienced nephrology and critical care teams involved in the recent earthquakes, and will soon have in place the systems described in this article. Prevention of crush injury is clearly the cornerstone of management in these settings. Continued evaluation and epidemiologic data are needed to provide adequate planning.

Lastly, the introduction of dialysis into a host country with previously limited availability dramatically changes the local expectations for medical care. Dialysis teams cannot leave the local area without adequately training medical personnel to take over dialysis to treat patients who go on to chronic renal failure, and cannot fail to treat those patients with chronic renal failure discovered during the disaster response. These issues need to be considered as the primary and secondary phases of the disaster wind down and primary health care policy issues re-emerge for the host country. In the late 1990s, significant progress should be made in further improving disaster relief to the unfortunate victims of natural disasters, thereby improving survival rates through international cooperation.

EARLY LOW TECHNOLOGY INTERVENTION – LESSONS FROM THE 1990 EARTHQUAKE IN IRAN

(I Nadjafi and AR Atef Zafarmand)

An epidemiologic and prognostic evaluation of ARF in victims from the 1990 earthquake in Iran (15) may serve us as a model for future planning for such disasters.

Timing

Death in the victims of an earthquake occurs at two different times: 1) at the time of the disaster, from falling debris or collapsed masonry or while victims are trapped under the rubble, and 2) after the injured have been extricated. Although there has been no detailed studies showing cause of death in the first stage, it seems that the main causes are head trauma, spinal cord injury, suffocation and hemorrhage from various fractures and injuries.

In the 1990 Iran quake, 94% of the mortality occurred in the first stage (15). This figure was 97.8% in the 1985 earthquake in Mexico (34). Mortality in the second stage, after the victims have been extricated from the rubble, was due to three factors:

1. Surgical complications, fractures and visceral tears are the most important reasons for mortality and morbidity during this stage.
2. Rhabdomyolysis with hyperkalemic acute tubular necrosis (4, 19, 20, 35–39, 40). In the 1990 quake in Iran, in the evaluation of 495 patients at three university hospitals in Tehran, 32% of the 37 patients that died (12 patients) had ARF at the time of death (15). Among the patients transferred to these centres 10–15 hours after having been extricated from the rubble, three had been declard deceased as a result of hyperkalemia. (Similar cases have been reported in the Armenian earthquake (4, 6, 40).)
3. Other medical causes of death include: sepsis, myocardial infarction, adverse drug reactions, pancreatitis, etc.

From a medical standpoint we must concern ourselves more with reduction of the mortality rate in the second post-extrication stage of the disaster, which may start within a few hours of the onset of the catastrophe.

Incidence

It is important to know the exact incidence of kidney involvement in such disasters. This will help relief teams to prepare for renal complications and send sufficient dialysis personnel, equipment and supplies to the scene of the catastrophe. Such data is important to both civil defense planners, who have to deal with the aftermath of disaster, as well as health professionals who have to accept the responsibility for the care of the patients.

The reported incidence of ARF in major earthquakes varies greatly. In the Tangshen earthquake of 1976, 2–5% developed ARF (35). In the Armenian quake 400–600 patients required dialysis (4, 6). In contrast, in Nicaragua, El Salvador, Guatemala quake (42–44) ARF was rarely diagnosed. The 24.7% incidence of ARF reported by Villeo-Sahsyun (34) following the Mexico quake in 1985 is the highest so far reported in the literature. In Iran's earthquake the total number of patients receiving dialysis nationwide was very small, 154 (0.5%). This obviously represents the minimum number of patients with renal failure since many patients probably went unrecognized and died quickly from metabolic complications of ARF. Supporting this is the number of ARF cases in three teaching hospitals in Tehran, the capital of Iran, where 6% of admitted patients were dialyzed. We propose that underdiagnosis is the main reason explaining the very low incidence or even no ARF in some earthquakes.

The reported very high incidence of ARF in Mexico City is explained very easily by the fact that the earthquake damaged several major hospitals, resulting in loss of over 4000 beds (23%), as well as many health care workers. This loss resulted in a much higher threshold for admission to the hospitals. Only 9% of injured patients were hospitalized in Mexico City whereas in Iran 76% of the injured patients were hospitalized (33,615 of 43,390).

In general, the incidence of ARF is related to the severity of injuries in survivors which is a reflection of the severity of earthquake, population density, engineering characteristics of the buildings and many other variables, but we should expect that between 6–25% of admitted patients injured by the earthquake will need dialysis.

Early treatment with oral solutions

It is best to prevent ARF before it occurs. There is good evidence in the medical literature that prevention is possible (25, 31). It would be ideal to treat victims with 500 cc of normal saline, mannitol, bicarbonate and Lasix hourly for 60 hours (16, 47). But it is obvious that dealing with large numbers of victims in practice makes this impossible. Preparing this large number amount of ivs is completely impractical, even in a developed country.

In solving this problem we should pay attention to two factors: The first is proper decision-making regarding who should be treated and who is at risk to develop ARF. The second is the ability to use oral as well as iv fluids to rehydrate these patients.

In the Iranian experience, 25% of hospitalized patients had elevated muscle enzymes, of whom 20% developed ARF. The patients with ARF had at least 15 fold higher CPK, 10 fold higher SGOT and 3 fold higher LDH when compared with all other patients suffering rhabdomyolysis (15). In all patients with rhabdomyolysis urine Test-

Tape for blood was positive, but not all patients with Heme positive test had rhabdomyolysis. Ten percent of patients had true hematuria due to blunt trauma to the kidneys or pre-existing disease. In the next few days the specificity of this test decreases, because when ARF is stabilized, true hematuria frequently occurs. We observed that myoglobinuria often is observed even before physical examination shows limb swelling, stiffness and when swelling occured, it was too late to stop the process of ARF (unpublished data).

Paying attention to experimental models of rhabdomyolysis induced acute renal failure, it seems that oral rehydration therapy is also as good and sufficient as iv therapy (21, 54, 57–60). It is not only practical, cheap and feasible but also scientifically valid testing to prevent ARF in disaster victims by oral hydration of those at risk.

Based on physiologic and absorptive principles in the GI tract, we recommend the following solution: Na^+ 80 Meq/1\$Cl^-$ 50 Meq/1\$HCO^{3-}$ 30 Meq/1\Dextrose 100 Mosm/1. We can prepare this solution easily in the scene of catastrophe by adding 1 teaspoon of salt, 1 teaspoon sodium bicarbonate and 1 tablespoon of sugar to one litre of drinking water.

We propose to use 40 ml/kg/hour of oral solution for patients in shock and then 10 ml/kg/hour for the first few days after the signs of shock disappear. The reasons for choosing this formulation instead of for the Oral Rehydration Solution (ORS) powders available all over the world from WHO for treating diarrhea induced dehydration in children are:

1. We cannot treat these patients with potassium containing solutions, because virtually all are hyperkalemic and many die from this complication.
2. The solution must be iso-osmotic so that vomiting is not induced.
3. It should contain appropriate amounts of glucose to enhance sodium absorption through glucose dependent sodium absorption in the gut and to make the solution more palatable. The glucose will also counteract hyperkalemia.
4. It should contain bicarbonate for correcting acidosis and to induce an alkaline urine and counteract hyperkalemia.
5. It should have sodium as water-induced polyuria has little effect in preventing acute renal failure.

None of the iv solutions available on the market will fulfil these criteria. Therefore, they are not recommended to be used alone orally and also they are very expensive. The only limitation of oral rehydration is in those patients who are NPO It is logical that we start rehydration therapy as soon as possible, preferably less than six hours after the event, to be efficient (16–21, 47, 58). Better's protocol showed an incidence of ARF decreasing to 0% (47) with rapid intervation. In Iran even after a delay of 24 to 48 hours after the disaster, using a more conservative approach consisting of initial treatment of hypovolemia and followed by infusion of 3 1/24 hour of bicarbonate and diuretics, we were able to reduce the rate of ARF by 50%. (Perhaps by interfering with the consequences of second wave phenomenon of rhabdomyolysis starting 24 hours after the original insult (31–48).)

Summary of treatment

The best protocol we can propose is first to find patients at risk for developing ARF by checking urine for blood (myoglobin) with TestTape. If positive, this should be followed by checking muscle enzymes and potassium in blood, using small point-of-case testing machines which are available in the market. If these were high too, we must start iv hydration therapy or if it not available, oral hydration using the solution mentioned above. EKG should be checked regularly in hyperkalemic patients and treatment of hyperkalemia should be carried out on an emergent basis. For those developing ARF in spite of hydration protocols, dialysis has to be started. Peritoneal dialysis has no role in such a hypermetabolic and hyperkalemic patients as earthquake victims.

Approach to dialysis

The best hemodialysis apparatus which we suggest in these situations (paying attention to electricity and good water limitations) are Ready<reg> machines for hemodialysis, which need no more than a few litres of water and are battery operated also, no need for water treatment and can be operated in even the most rural location.

Calculation of the number of hemodialysis machines which are needed is very simple; for example, if we have 10,000 admissions and the average incidence of ARF is 10%, then 1,000 patients will need hemodialysis three times a week at least. It means 3,000 dialysis/weekly or 500 daily, now if a dialysis machine does four dialysis a day, it is obvious that 125 hemodialysis machines are needed (for at least one month). These machines are invaluable and useful tools for other events happening somewhere else in the future.

Finally, we strongly recommend that medical personnel responding to disasters make every effort to collect relevant medical data, to help provide a better approach in future disasters.

REFERENCES

1. Solez K, Bihari D, Collins AJ et al.: International dialysis aid in earthquakes and other disasters. *Kidney Int* 44: 479, 1993
2. National Kidney Foundation Public Education Committee: Planning for natural disasters: a guide for renal facilities; a guide for kidney patients. National Kidney Foundation, New York, 1994. In press
3. Collins AJ, Burzstein S: Renal failure in disasters. *Crit Care Clin* 7: 421, 1991
4. Collins AJ: Kidney dialysis treatment for victims of the Armenian earthquake. *N Engl J Med* 320: 1291, 1989
5. Mithias T, Sansom A: Successful haemodialysis of crush syndrome victims – the Armenian experience. Abstract presented at the 18th Annual Conference of the EDTNA–European Renal Care Association, 1989
6. Richards NT, Tattersall J, McCann M et al.: Dialysis for acute renal failure due to crush injuries after the Armenian earthquake. *Br Med J* 6671 (298): 443, 1989
7. Van Waeleghem JP, Verschoot M, Dewets JM et al.: Nephrology aid after seismic catastrophe in Armenia. Abstract presented at the 18th Annual Conference of the EDTNA–European Renal Care Association, 1989
8. Noji E: Medical and health care aspects of the Armenian Earthquake Reconnaissance Report. *Earthquake Spectra* 12 (Suppl): 161, 1989
9. Wyllie LA Jr, Filson JR: Armenian earthquake reconnaissance report. *Earthquake Spectra Professional Journal of the Earthquake Engineering Research Institute* 12: 161, 1989
10. Collins AJ: Report of dialysis assistance to victims of the Ufa team and pipeline explosion. Summary Report to the Office of Foreign Disaster Assistance, US State Department, Washington DC, 1989
11. Greg MB: Surveillance and Epidemiology. in *The Public Health Consequences of Disasters*, Washington DC, US Department of Health and Human Services, US Public Health Service Centers for Disease Control, 1989
12. Jones NP, Krimgold F, Noji EK et al.: Considerations in the epidemiology of earthquake injuries. in *International Workshop on Earthquake Injury Epidemiology for Mitigation and Response*, edited by Jones NP, Noji E, Baltimore, The Johns Hopkins University, July 10–12, 1989
13. Noji E: Evaluation of the efficacy of disaster response. *UNDRO News* Jun–Jul–Aug, 1987
14. Stratton JW: Earthquakes. in *The Public Health Consequences of Disasters*, Washington DC, US Department of Health and Human Services, US Public Health Service Centers for Disease Control, 1989
15. Atef Zafarmand MR, Nadjafi I, Broumand B, Rastegar A: Acute renal failure in earthquake victims in Iran: epidemiology and management. *Quart J Med* 87: 35, 1994
16. Better OS, Stein JH: Early management of shock and prophylaxis of acute renal failure in traumatic rhabdomyolysis. *N Engl J Med* 322 (Suppl 12): 825, 1990
17. Flamenbaum W, Gehr M, Gross M et al.: Acute renal failure associated with myoglobinuria and hemoglobinuria. in *Acute Renal Failure*, edited by Brenner BM, Lazarus JM, Philadelphia WB Saunders Company, 1983, p 269
18. Knochel JP: Rhabdomyolysis and myoglobinuria. in *The Kidney in Systemic Disease*, 2nd Edition, edited by Suki WN, Eknoyan G, New York, John Wiley, 1981, p 263
19. Ward MM: Factors predictive of acute renal failure in rhabdomyolysis. *Arch Intern Med* 148: 1553, 1988
20. Bywaters EGL, Beall D: Crush injuries with impairment of renal function. *Br Med J* 1: 427, 1941
21. Bywaters EGL, Popjak G: Experimental crushing injury: Peripheral circulatory collapse and other effects of muscle necrosis in the rabbit. *Surg Gynecol Obstet* 75: 612, 1942
22. Meroney WH, Arney GK, Segar WE et al.: The acute calcification of traumatized muscle with particular reference to acute post-traumatic renal insufficiency. *J Clin Invest* 36: 825, 1957

23. Honda N: Acute renal failure and rhabdomyolysis. *Kidney Int* 23: 888, 1983

24. Michaelson M, Taitelman U, Beshouty Z et al.: Crush syndrome: experience from the Lebanon war. *Isr J Med Sci* 20: 305, 1984

25. Ron D, Taitelman U, Michaelson M et al.: Prevention of acute renal failure in traumatic rhabdomyolysis. *Arch Intern Med* 144: 277, 1984

26. Santangelo ML, Usberti M, DiSalvo E: A study of the pathology of crush syndrome. *J Surg Gynecol Obstet* 154: 372, 1982

27. Matsen FA III: Compartmental syndrome: a unified concept. *Clin Orthop* 113: 8, 1975

28. Owen CA, Mubarak SJ, Hargens AR et al.: Intramuscular pressures with limb compression: Clarification of the pathogenesis of the drug-induced muscle-compartment syndrome. *N Engl J Med* 300: 1169, 1979

29. Whitesides TE, Haney TC, Morimoto K et al.: Tissue pressure measurements as a determinant for the need of fasciotomy. *Clin Orthop* 113: 43, 1975

30. Zager RA: Studies of mechanisms and protective maneuvers in myoglobinuric acute renal injury. *Lab Invest* 60: 619, 1989

31. Eneas JF, Schoenfeld PY, Humphreys MH: The effect of infusion of mannitol-sodium bicarbonate on the clinical course of myoglobinuria. *Arch Intern Med* 139: 801, 1979

32. Kaplan AA, Longnecker RE, Folkert VW: Continuous arteriovenous hemofiltration. *Ann Intern Med* 100: 358, 1984

33. Keshaviah P: Technical aspects of continuous and intermittent therapies. *ASAIO Trans* 34: 61, 1988

34. Villazon Sahagun A: Mexico City earthquake: Medical response. *J of World Association for Emergency & Disaster Medicine* 1: 35, 1986

35. Sheng CY: Medical support in the Tangshen earthquake: a review of the management of mass casualties and certain major injuries. *J Trauma* 27: 1130, 1987

36. Bywaters EGL, Stead JK: The production of renal failure following injection of solutions containing myohaemoglobin. *Quart J Exp Physiol* 33: 53, 1944

37. Kayem LJ: Myoglobinemia and myoglobinuria in patients with myositis. *Arth Rheum* 14: 457, 1971

38. Grossman RA: Nontraumatic rhabdomyolysis and acute renal failure. *N Engl J Med* 291: 807, 1974

39. Koffler A: Acute renal failure due to non-traumatic rhabdomyolysis. *Ann Intern Med* 85: 23, 1976

40. Tattersal JE, Richards NT, McCann M, Mathias T, Samson A, Jhonson A: Acute hemodialysis during the Armenian earthquake disaster. *Injury* 21: 25, 1990

41. Noji KN: Natural disasters. *Crit Care Med* 7: 271, 1991

42. Whittaker R, Fareed D: Earthquake disaster in Nicaragua: reflection on the initial management of massive casualties. *J Trauma* 14: 37, 1974

43. Durkin M: The San Salvador earthquake of October 19, 1986: casualties search and the health care system. *Earthquake Spectra* 3: 621, 1987

44. Deville de Goyeta C et al.: Earthquake in Guatemala; epidemiologic evaluation of the relief effort. *Bull Pan Health Org* 10: 95, 1976

45. Heppenstal RB, Sapega AA, Izank T, Fallon R, Shenton D, Park YS, Chance B: Compartment syndrome: a quantitative study of high-energy phosphorous compounds using 31P-magnetic resonance spectroscopy. *J Trauma* 29: 1113, 1989

46. Perry MO: Compartment syndromes and reperfusion injury. (Review) *Surg Clinics N Am* 68: 853, 1988

47. Better OS: The crush syndrome revisited. *Nephron* 55: 97, 1990

48. Knochel JP: Rhabdomyolysis and myoglobinuria. *Semin Nephrol* 1: 75, 1981

49. Odeh M: The role of reperfusion-induced injury in the pathogenesis of crush syndrome. *N Engl J Med* 324: 1417, 1991

50. Better OS, Abassi Z, Rubinstein I, Marom S, Winaver Y, Silberman M: The mechanism of muscle injury in crush syndrome: schemic versis pressure-stretch myopathy. *Mineral and Electrolyte Metabolism* 16: 181, 1990

51. Knochel JP: Serum calcium derangements in rhabdomyolysis. (Editorial) *N Engl J Med* 305: 61, 1991

52. Hostetter TH, Brenner BM: Renal circulatory and nephron function in experimental acute renal failure. in *Acute Renal Failure*, edited by Brenner BM, Lazarus JM, Philadelphia, WB Saunders Company, 1988, p 67

53. Corcoran AC, Page IH: Renal damage for ferroheme pigments, myoglobin, hematin. *Texas Report Biol Med* 3: 528, 1945

54. Zager RA: Studies of mechanisms and protective maneuvers in myoglobinuric acute renal injury. *Lab Invest* 60: 619, 1989

55. Knochel JP: Renal injury in muscle disease. in *The Kidney in Systemic Diseases*, edited by Suki WN, Eknoyan G, New York, Wiley Biomedical, 1976, p 129

56. Dubrow A and Flamenbaum W: Acute renal failure associated with myoglobinuria and hemoglobinuria. in *Acute Renal Failure*, edited by Brenner BM, Lazarus JM, Philadelphia, WB Saunders Company, 1988, p 279

57. Bauweiaa K, Hofbauer KG, Konrads A, Gross F: Effect of saralasin and serum in myohaemoglobinuric acute renal failure of rats. *Clin Sc Mel Med* 54: 555, 1987

58. Reineck HJ, O'Conno GJ, Lifschitz MD, Stein JH: Sequential studies on the pathophysiology of glycrol-induced acute renal failure. *J Lab Clin Med* 96: 356, 1980

59. Levinsky NG, Bernard D, Johnston PA: Mannitol and loop diuretics in acute renal failure. in *Acute Renal Failure*, edited by Brenner BM, Lazarus JM, Philadelphia, WB Saunders Company, 1988, p 712

60. Gacia G, Shider T, Feldman M et al.: Nephrotoxicity of myoglobin in the rat. (Abstract) *Kidney Int* 19: 1981, 200

PART A: PSYCHIATRIC ASPECTS OF THE DIALYSIS PATIENT

PETER G. WILSON

INTRODUCTION

Psychiatry and psychiatrists can help in the treatment of the dialysis patient, by being members of the caregiving team, and in diagnosing psychopathology in the patient, family and treatment team. Arrangements then can be made in setting up appropriate treatment for psychopathology, instituting treatment when indicated, and performing research in demographic, psychopathologic and outcome factors. This chapter will deal with adult problems and psychopathology, and not with the special problems of pediatric patients. Case reports are used in an illustrative fashion, to highlight symptoms and management of psychopathology.

The patient, as well as family, associates at work and dialysis staff, undergo many changes when he/she begins dialysis. The patient may begin these changes before the actual dialysis, because the disease has already had some impact on him or her. The family will certainly have already needed to look to the future and to prepare, associates at work may have to make changes in the job routine, and the dialysis staff must prepare to have another patient on the roster. The most difficult concept that a patient and family must face is that dialysis is not curative. Dialysis will keep the person alive, but cannot replace the native kidney functions, in the almost automatic way that we expect the kidneys to function. This is different from the way medicine and doctors are viewed by a patient coming for help. As Montagnac and colleagues (1) record, dialysis disorganizes the patient's world, through the need to see one's body differently, and see differently one's personal, professional and family roles. In the lay press, there are constant reminders of 'bleak US report on kidney-failure patients' (New York Times, November 4, 1993, p A17) and 'studies are grim on dialysis outlook' (New York Times, January 5, 1995, p A18). Galpin (2) has stressed that that the changes in body image, due to the invasiveness of the procedure, as well as the various nega-

tive reactions to the body, which has betrayed the person, and which over time begins to look quite different.

The variables that a patient brings to dialysis are significant, including patient disease, life style, personality and support (both family and other), family members and their reaction to the disease. Additional factors are personality, reaction of work mates to change in routine, and possible pressures on the dialysis staff when a new patient is added.

The type and longevity of the disease leading to end-stage renal disease (ESRD), may be of great importance. Patients who have a known family history of polycystic disease, may have prepared themselves for the eventuality and would be sensitive to the signs and symptoms of ESRD, while a patient with hypertension, may be confused by his/her decreased energy, nausea and other symptoms.

> Mrs W had a long family history of polycystic kidney disease, her mother and grandfather having died of this illness, during her lifetime. Because of her knowledge, she and her husband, decided to adopt children and prepared for the day when she would become symptomatic and need dialysis. They adopted when she was young. When symptoms showed, she was prepared, her children were mostly grown and she decreased her work load, to fit her dialysis schedule. It all worked as well as possible in this burdensome situation.

> Mrs N, a 24 year old woman, developed toxemia of pregnancy and immediately after delivery needed dialysis, without any time for preparation. She and her husband were presented with a new child and dialysis at the same time, leading to a chaotic family situation and ending in depression in the young mother.

The family may be well prepared for the eventuality of dialysis or it may hit them like a bolt of lightning.

Needless to say, advanced knowledge might make a large difference, because the strange symptoms and increasing disability can play havoc with family dynamics.

As dialysis delivery has become more competitive, dialysis staff has become more stressed with increasing patient load. This has meant that new patients are met with dismay and discouragement, hardly the greatest welcome to an already stressed individual.

> The week before Mrs A arrived at her dialysis center, there had been a 20% increase in the number of patients seen, at that center. Mrs A received a rather cool welcome and only months later, an explanation helped to clear the air.

Once dialysis has started, a honeymoon period may actually be at hand. Levy and colleagues (3) describe this interval beautifully, as many of the acute symptoms, i.e., nausea, low energy, disappear and the patient actually feels more comfortable and energized. The family may also feel better, since the chronic nature of dialysis has not sunk in, and there is a feeling that the need for dialysis will come to an end.

> Since he had not wanted to start dialysis Mr T had months of fatigue, inability to think straight, nausea and vomiting, which had made him unable to function. Brought into the Emergency Room, he started hemodialysis and a week later had fewer symptoms and was considering going back to his work as janitor. His wife and son, who had been exceedingly worried and hopeless about his situation, joined him in reveling in his newfound wellbeing and began to make plans to go on an extended vacation (forgetting that he needed thrice weekly dialysis).

The greatest difficulty occurs when there is little or no time to be made ready for dialysis. Where patient and family are thrust into the situation without preparation.

Age is an important variable in this early phase. Adolescents have great difficulty in acclimating to dialysis, fighting the process with non-compliance in coming to the sessions, not taking appropriate medication and not reporting symptoms. The older the patient, the more likely he/she accepts the situation of 'being tied' to dialysis. Gorynski and Knight (4) feel that a peer support group can be a valuable resource in the treatment of this complex younger age group.

> S, a 15 year old diabetic woman, had been grossly non-compliant with insulin therapy over the past 2 years. When dialysis became imperative, she missed numerous dialysis sessions, becoming cognitively impaired and impulsive, leading to further dangerous acts and life threatening situations. An adolescent group of dialysis patients made the situation more tolerable for both patients and dialysis staff.

FREQUENT PROBLEMS

Dialysis of all forms is invasive, confining the patient for hours, interrupting normal schedules with CAPD exchanges many times a day, etc. This engenders difficulties in acclimating to a new way of life. For people who are action oriented, lying down for 9–12 hours a week for hemodialysis is a real burden.

> Ms T was an important person in her industry, with many clients and very busy lifestyle. She rose at 6 AM and worked until 12 AM, with full energy. At 47 years of age, she needed dialysis for ESRD, but found that 12 hours/week was 'intolerable'. After numerous tries at center hemodialysis, she settled on IPD, with fair success. She had thought of 'taking my machine to restaurant meetings', she said laughingly, but sadly felt that 'nothing will ever really work and be the same'.

The dialysis patient becomes dependent on a whole battery of people, nephrologists, nurses, technicians, with a reliance on such people, which can lead to various scenarios, depending on one's personality.

> Mr F was a 61 year old CEO, who controlled the destiny of a large company. A man used 'to having my own way', he was horrified that he could not control the exact time of his dialysis and the schedule of the dialysis center workers. On the other hand, he felt safest in the center, because 'help is only a shout away'. This presented a quandary. He tried hiring someone to do his dialysis at home and then tried center dialysis, picking center dialysis in the end.

The patient may also develop the feeling of being 'hooked' forever to a machine that saves life, along with a sense of not having control over one's own being. Rittman and associates (5) outlined the pattern of control and the acclimation that a patient has to undergo.

> Ms E, a 56 year old housewife, mused about her experience of being on dialysis. 'I sit in the chair and look at the machine, with the blood coursing through it. It is my blood, and yet it is outside me. Horrors! Like a Dracula movie, but this thing is keeping me alive. Suppose something goes wrong? Suppose I feel worse? I feel all is out of control'.

As pointed out by Procci (6), both men and women develop sexual problems. Both have decreased libido and men become increasingly impotent. It was thought in the past that depression, anxiety and fatigue caused these problems, but we now know that the problem is in part due to zinc deficiency associated with dialysis. While depression, anxiety and fatigue may play a role and should be treated, the problem of decreased libido and male impotence is usually more physiologically based and certainly world wide (7).

> Ms F, a 45 year old married woman, had been on dialysis for 4 years, when she 'no longer desired my husband'. This was devastating to her, because

she feared 'that I no longer loved him'. Depression and anxiety were ruled out as primary causes and she was much relieved when she was told that her decrease libido seemed to be physiologically based. It was not her fault, and so she felt better.

When one does see anxiety and depression either primarily or secondarily, it should be treated, as described below.

Being on dialysis means living with a small or large level of physical pain. While it is true that people respond differently to the same stimulus of pain, the placing of the needles in HD, the fluid exchange in CAPD may cause pain. It is important to respectfully accept the vocalizations of the patient and do whatever possible to reduce the pain pharmacologically or through relaxation techniques. 'It is really nothing', 'It won't hurt much,' 'just grin and bear it', ' you are childish', are not helpful, frequently counterproductive and set up struggles that bode ill for future needed collaboration.

Yoshioka and associates (8) found that sleep disturbances were quite frequent in dialysis patients. Especially at risk, were patients on prolonged HD and those with advanced age. Interestingly, he also reported improvement with levodopa and carbamazepine. Sleep disturbance may be connected to depression and when this occurs, treatment of depression is the goal of choice.

WHAT HELPS

Preparation, and more preparation, are the prime considerations in making life easier for the patient and the family (9). This includes taking the patient on a tour of the dialysis facility, giving them literature to read, including the family in the preparatory process and giving the patients a sense of choice. When McKegney (10) offered patients the choice of dialysis or no dialysis (and dying), nearly all patients and their families chose dialysis. At our center, we frequently give the same choice, with the same results. It is most important that patients are involved in the choice of dialysis (when there is a real choice) and that they and the family feel part of the decision making process. Compliance is better when patient and family are involved. Some researchers have strong feelings about what is the most suitable type of dialysis (11), which may be true, but most researchers feel that patient participation is crucial for future compliance (12) and that health professionals, especially social workers and nurses (13) can be most influential in the decision. Of interest, Groome et al. (14) found that the number of times an item is mentioned in an interview, can determine the decision making process. Matching the patient to the type of dialysis (when possible), can pay large dividends in terms of compliance and psychopathology. Having an independent, active, working patient on CAPD, can give that person much needed leverage to live life as much as possible. A thorough evaluation

should include the concepts of dependence-independence, activity-passivity, control and mastery.

> Mr B, a 36 year old mechanic, worked with a close knit working group, people who covered for each other, but who were needed, every day on the job. He chose CAPD, so that he and his working group could schedule to cover work every day, including time for his dialysis exchanges.

To do home hemodialysis, one needs 'another' who is willing and able to take on a large and demanding responsibility. A mismatch here, can lead to great trouble, so that a thorough evaluation of 'another' must be done, with the understanding that they might opt out.

> Mr and Mrs D (he, on dialysis), decided on home hemodialysis. Actually, Mr D, who wanted the 'freedom' to work during the day, had chosen this modality. Mrs D, who also worked outside the home, acceded and they trained. After 2 months, Mrs D came to the nephrologist, saying that she could no longer go on with this routine, but was afraid to tell her husband. Their doctor, who had a good relationship with both people, saw them together and Mr D decided on IPD.

Patients are quite eloquent in what they think will help them. Bower (15), feels that the doctor-patient relationship needs much improvement, in that the doctors are not sensitive to patient needs, but frequently biologically and organically over involved. The doctors do not seem to listen to the patient's concerns, which are trivialized. Newmann (16) stresses education and patient empowerment (making choices) as the stimulus for what is needed and wanted by the patient.

PSYCHOPATHOLOGY AND ITS TREATMENTS

This section will include acute and chronic symptomatology, and previous psychopathology. Psychopathology in dialysis patients is world wide as reported by Kumar (17) who found that 52% of his dialysis patients in Pakistan had psychological problems, while Petrie (18), in New Zealand, found 43% with psychiatric morbidity.

DEPRESSION

Depression has been described as the most prevalent psychologic problem in patients on dialysis (19). Since depression is suffered by about 10% of the general population during their lifetime, many of the patients who come to dialysis will have suffered previous depression. Craven and others (20) found that about 8% of his sample had a current major depression, while Kimmel and others (21) concurring, stressed the importance of early treatment, because of the impact of depression on immunologic func-

Table 1. Criteria for major depressive episode

1. Depressed mood most of the day, nearly every day, as indicated by either subjective report (e.g., appears tearful)
    Note: In children and adolescents, depression can manifest as irritable mood.
2. Markedly diminished interest or pleasure in all, or almost all, activities most of the day, nearly every day (as indicated by either subjective account or observation made by others).
3. Significant weight loss when not dieting or weight gain (e.g., a change of more than 5% of body weight in a month), or decrease or increase in appetite nearly every day.
    Note: In children, consider failure to make expected weight gains.
4. Insomnia or hypersomnia nearly every day.
5. Psychomotor agitation or retardation nearly every day (observable by others, not merely subjective feelings of restlessness or being slowed down).
6. Fatigue or loss of energy nearly every day.
7. Feelings of worthlessness or excessive or inappropriate guilt (which may be delusional) nearly every day (not merely self-reproach or guilt about being sick).
8. Diminished ability to think or concentrate, or indecisiveness, nearly every day (either by subjective account or as observed by others).
9. Recurrent thoughts of death (not just fear of dying), recurrent suicidal ideation without a specific plan, or a suicide attempt or specific plan for committing suicide.

tion, nutrition and compliance, which in turn influence morbidity and mortality. Patterson and co-workers (22) in a prospective study, found that depression was an important variable in the two year mortality of ESRD patients. Driessen and Balk (23) found that the extent of depression was predictive of adjustment to kidney disease and compliance with treatment. If the patient had a history of a previous depression, they were more likely to have a recurrence, once on dialysis. This does not mean that dialysis causes depression, but that the patient's vulnerability to depression has increased. Other factors that make a patient more vulnerable to depression are: female sex, duration of dialysis, living alone, and unemployment (20). If there are symptoms of depression, depression should be treated. If the patient suffers from dysthymia, this also should be treated. If unsure, the patient can be given a general health questionnaire (24), scored and followed over time.

Definition of Depression as per DSM-4 is:

CRITERIA FOR MAJOR DEPRESSIVE EPISODE (25)

A. Five or more of the following symptoms have been present during the same 2-week period and represent a change from previous functioning; at least one of the symptoms is either (1) depressed mood or (2) loss of interest or pleasure (Table 1).
    Note Symptoms that are clearly due to a general medical condition, or mood-incongruent delusions or hallucinations, are not included.
B. The symptoms do not meet criteria for a mixed episode.

C. The symptoms cause clinically significant distress or impairment in social, occupational, or other important areas of functioning.
D. The symptoms are not due to the direct physiological effects of a substance (e.g., a drug of abuse, a medication) or a general medical condition (e.g., hypothyroidism).
E. The symptoms are not better accounted for by bereavement, i.e., after the loss of a loved one, the symptoms persist for longer than 2 months or are characterized by marked functional impairment, morbid preoccupation with worthlessness, suicidal ideation, psychotic symptoms, or psychomotor retardation.

DIAGNOSTIC CRITERIA FOR DYSTHYMIC DISORDER (25)

A. Depressed mood for most of the day, for more days than not, as indicated either by subjective account or observation by others, for at least 2 years.
    Note In children and adolescents, mood can be irritable and duration must be at least 1 year.
B. Presence, while depressed, of two (or more) of the criteria in Table 2.
C. During the 2-year period (1 year for children or adolescents) of the disturbance, the person has never been without the symptoms in criteria A and B for more than 2 months at a time.
D. No major depressive episode has been present during the first 2 years of the disturbance (1 year for children or adolescent); i.e., the disturbance is not better accounted for by chronic major depressive disorder, or major depressive disorder in partial remission.
    Note: There may have been a previous major depres-

Table 2. Diagnostic criteria for depression in dysthymic disorder

1. Poor appetite or overeating
2. Insomnia or hypersomnia
3. Low energy or fatigue
4. Low self-esteem
5. Poor concentration or difficulty making decisions
6. Feelings of hopelessness

sive episode provided there was a full remission (no significant signs or symptoms for 2 months), before development of the dysthymic disorder. In addition, after the initial 2 years (1 year in children or adolescents) of dysthymic disorder, there may be superimposed episodes of major depressive disorder, in which case both diagnoses may be given when the criteria are met for a major depressive episode.

E. There has never been a manic episode, a mixed episode or a hypomanic disorder and criteria have never been met for cyclothymic disorder.

F. The disturbance does not occur exclusively during the course of a chronic psychotic disorder, such as schizophrenia or delusional disorder.

G. The symptoms are not due to the direct physiological effects of a substance (e.g., a drug of abuse, a medication) or a general medical condition (e.g., hypothyroidism).

H. The symptoms cause clinically significant distress or impairment in social, occupational, or other important areas of functioning.

Specify if: early onset: if onset is before 21 years; late onset: if onset is 21 years or older, and (for most recent 2 years of dysthymic disorder): with atypical features.

Treatment of depression, as differentiated from mourning and the various adjustment reactions (26), should be a combination of psychotherapy and pharmacotherapy, which is successful in 85% of patients. Pharmacotherapy itself is successful in 65%, and psychotherapy in 50%, hence, the combination. Psychotherapy might be of short duration, and might also include, interpersonal therapy (27) or cognitive therapy (28). The selective serotonin reuptake inhibitors (SSRI) are the most used and safest of present anti-depressants and should be started in small doses and increased over time. Patients with ESRD should take one half to two thirds the usual dosage and have blood levels taken, when available (29).

> Mrs Q, a 56 year old woman, on dialysis for 5 years, began to complain of increasing pain and other somatic symptoms, transient thoughts of suicide, no joy in her grandchildren, friends and good deeds (previously a great pleasure). A 'good talking to', by her nephrologist produced no improvement and she was sent for psychiatric evaluation. Depression was diagnosed and she was started on sertraline hydrochloride 25 mg/day, which was gradually

increased to 75 mg, at which dose, after two weeks, there was considerable improvement in her mood and function.

A literature review reveals that 15–25% of the dialysis population seems to be depressed at any one time. This is higher than the national average. Since many depressive symptoms overlap with somatic symptoms in ESRD patients, depression is not an easy diagnosis to make. Most psychiatrists, however, feel that if there is a strong indication for depression or dysthymia it is better to treat than not, since depression adds to the debilitation of the ESRD, and to the already high suicidality in these patients. One should differentiate depression and dysthymia from adjustment disorders.

DIAGNOSTIC CRITERIA FOR ADJUSTMENT DISORDERS (25)

A. The development of emotional or behavioral symptoms in response to an identifiable stressor(s) occurring within 3 months of the onset of stressor(s).

B. Symptoms or behavior are clinically significant as evidenced either of the following:
   1. marked distress in excess of what would be expected from exposure to the stressor;
   2. significant impairment in social or occupational (academic) functioning.

C. The stress-related disturbance does not meet the criteria for another specific Axis I disorder and is not merely an exacerbation of a preexisting Axis I or Axis II disorder.

D. The symptoms do not represent bereavement.

E. Once the stressor (or its consequences) has terminated, the symptoms do not persist for more than an additional 6 months.

Specify if: acute: if the disturbance lasts less than 6 months; chronic: if the disturbance lasts for 6 months or longer treatment for adjustment reaction is usually psychotherapy.

DELIRIUM

Delirium is the great underdiagnosed psychopathology of ESRD. In DSM-4, delirium is defined as follows:

Diagnostic criteria for Delirium Due to . . . (indicating the general medical condition)

A. Disturbance of consciousness (i.e., reduced clarity of awareness of the environment) with reduced ability to focus, sustain, or shift attention.

B. A change in cognition (such as memory deficit, disorientation, language disturbance) or the development of a perceptual disturbance that is not better accounted for by a preexisting, established, or evolving dementia.

C. The disturbance develops over a short period of time (usually hours to days) and tends to fluctuate during the course of the day.

D. There is evidence from the history, physical examination, or laboratory findings that the disturbance is caused by the direct physiological consequences of a general medical condition.

If delirium is superimposed on a preexisting dementia of the Alzheimer's type, or vascular dementia, it is important to indicate the type of delirium by using the appropriate subtype of the dementia, e.g., dementia of the Alzheimer's type, with late onset, with delirium, and to indicate the name of the general medical condition on Axis I, e.g., delirium due to hepatic encephalopathy, and the general medical condition on Axis III.

Dialysis patients are exceptionally sensitive to this problem and are very disturbed by the symptoms.

> Mr W, a 48 year old man, on dialysis for four years, had been 'smiling a lot lately, talking more than usual'. On daily rounds, he was introduced to the staff psychiatrist, who asked about his well being. 'I feel great. Wouldn't you, lying here on the beach? 'When asked where he thought he was, he replied,'Miami'. On further examination, he was also disoriented to time and person, had poor recent memory, in addition to the obvious poor cognition.

Doctors and nurses are frequently annoyed by these patients, because of their extremely poor recent memory, since patients cannot do what we ask them to do, because of their poor recall. Family members are also angered, because of the episodes of disorientation (especially to time and place and sometimes to person). How can this person NOT recall meeting the physician or the family member? This frequently escalates into full fledged arguments and increasing agitation, as the delirium gets worse.

Treatment follows diagnosis of delirium, searching for and treating the etiology of the delirium. Agitation can be helped with small amounts of a phenothiazine, such as haloperidol 0.5 mg BID. Dosing must start low because of the ESRD, and a large bolus of drug will ensure a poor result, including worsening of delirium and Parkinson like symptoms. Some pharmacologists prefer quick acting benzodiazepines, such as lorazepam, which can calm, but has little antipsychotic potential. If either of these medications is given by mouth, it takes more than a few minutes to work, so that if there is little effect in 30 minutes, one should wait longer before giving another dose. Their duration of action is only a few hours, so that spaced doses, during the day, must be given.

> Ms V, a 39 year old woman, on dialysis for three years, began 'acting queer' according to her sister and her dialysis nurse. She became forgetful, argumentative, often became lost in her well known neighborhood, and came late for dialysis appointments. On further examination, she was found to have a slowly increasing creatinine and BUN, with increasing potassium, probably secondary to increasing dietary indiscretions, which she denied and probably did not recall. While investigating the etiology of these changes, she was offered haloperidol 0.5 mg, twice a day and became more compliant with dialysis and diet. When the physiologic parameters were improved, she was tapered from the haloperidol over a week's time.

Dialysis can be anxiety producing, especially at the initiation. If the patient is introduced to the machine slowly, helped by another dialysis patient, with explanation by the doctors and nurses, the anxiety usually decreases by the fourth to fifth week, although many patients do not settle down for eight to nine weeks. At this stage, informal psychotherapy, e.g. talking to the patient, having a relative along, etc, may prove more useful than using medication, but in some people it becomes necessary.

> Mr N, a 25 year old man with diabetes, had known for many years that he would need dialysis. He had never given himself the insulin injections, depending on his mother for this procedure. Even a gentle introduction, over time, to dialysis did not help in the terror that he felt, when dialysis was started. His mother being at the dialysis sessions helped a bit, but his outright crying and screaming made the dialysis team and other patients quite frightened. Lorazepam 0.5 mg given 30 minutes before the start of dialysis was quite helpful in getting him onto dialysis and another 0.5 mg, two hours into the dialysis was needed for the first three weeks. After two months on the machine, all medication could be discontinued, at first using lorazepam on alternating days, with the consent of the patient.

Medication also becomes necessary to alleviate the agitation in patients who must stay on the dialysis machine for prolonged therapy. If rapid anxiolysis is sought, lorazepam IV, is useful. If one wishes a longer anxiolytic effect, diazepam, is useful, again starting with small doses. Benzodiazepines lose their effectiveness after a few months (or sooner), so that the patient should be told that there is a finite time for this action and then the drug will be discontinued.

Relaxation techniques are often useful for these patients and can be given by any person trained in these techniques.

If the patient develops classic panic attacks, defined as:

CRITERIA FOR PANIC ATTACK (DSM-4) (25)

The specific diagnosis in which the panic attack occurs should be identified (e.g., panic disorder with agoraphobia. The diagnosis is made from the following; a discrete period of intense fear or discomfort, in which four (or more) of the symptoms in Table 3 developed abruptly and reached a peak within 10 minutes.

Table 3. Diagnostic criteria for panic attack

1. Palpitations, pounding heart, or accelerated heart
2. Sweating
3. Trembling or shaking
4. Sensations of shortness of breath or smothering
5. Feeling of choking
6. Chest pain or discomfort
7. Nausea or abdominal distress
8. Feeling dizzy, unsteady, lightheaded, or faint
9. Derealization (feelings of unreality) or depersonalization (being detached from oneself)
10. Fear of losing control or going crazy
11. Fear of dying
12. Paresthesias (numbness or tingling sensations)
13. Chills or hot flushes

Table 4. Criteria for adaptation to dialysis

1. Keeping distress within manageable limits
2. Maintaining sources of pleasure
3. Maintaining self-esteem
4. Continuing adequate relationships with others
5. Working out valued and socially acceptable roles
6. Sustaining some hope for the future
7. Effecting rehabilitation to patient's maximum physical capacity
8. Maintaining an effective and trusting relationship with the physician and staff

Here an SSRI can be very useful, as can cognitive restructuring training, by a trained professional.

With the increasing dialysis population, the number of patients with bipolar illness has also increased. Such patients require the constant use of lithium, valproic acid or carbamazepine.

> Mr U, a 25 year old man, on dialysis for one year, developed his third manic episode. He had stopped all medication six months before, and lithium had to be restarted at 300 mg/day. Blood levels, before dialysis and a few hours after dialysis were taken every time he came for dialysis. After ten days at a blood level of 0.5 mEq/L, his mania subsided.

If behavior is very disturbing, haloperidol in small doses might be used for the acute symptoms, in addition to the lithium, which usually takes one week after reaching therapeutic dose. Sometimes hospitalization might be necessary.

With the increasing number of people addicted to heroin, cocaine, and other illicit substances, as well as alcohol, it is imperative that we not pre-judge these individuals. Since these patients are frequently abusers of our health system and very difficult to deal with, they should be sent to centers that incorporate dialysis, detoxification and rehabilitation. Patients shoud be encouraged to join groups such as Alcoholics Anonymous.

Many patients with ESRD, also suffer from schizophrenia and must therefore be on phenothiazines, adjusting dosage for renal failure, frequently using half the usual therapeutic dose and starting with small doses.

> Ms O, a 36 year old woman, ill with schizophrenia for ten years and on dialysis for 6 months, became delusional and agitated and obviously needed a phenothiazine, which she had stopped taking just before starting dialysis. Her dose of haloperidol, needed to control her symptoms pre-dialysis had been 10 mg tid. She was now started with 2 mg tid and grad-

ually moved up to 6 mg tid, which controlled her symptoms.

ADAPTATION

Most dialysis patients really do well, most of the time. Stress is constant for them, in that they have lost control of a body function, are dependent on machine and staff for the dialysis, dependent on family for major support, etc. Despite more or less difficulty, they acclimate and adapt. Viederman (30) enumerated the criteria for good adaptation (Table 4).

Carbonell et al. (31), following over a hundred patients, found the following factors important in adaptation: marital status, religious beliefs, education level, occupation, means of transportation to get to the treatment center, self image before the illness, age and evaluation of the treatment, by the patient.

The family has a difficult time, when this chronic disease with dialysis, enters the family arena. The whole family system has to be rearranged in terms of responsibilities, work, family roles and stress management. At a time when the family in the Western world is already under the stress of many changes, add a serious, life threatening illness (ESRD). We know from the classic studies of Burton and colleagues (32), that support is crucial to morbidity, mortality, compliance, etc. To ask the family members to be maximally flexible to change, at a time when there are other gigantic changes producing stress, may jeopardise relationships. Couples, where a member has ESRD with dialysis are much more likely to separate than the average couple (where separation, already has been on the rise). Flaherty and O'Brien (33) make these points, but also looks at family styles, some of which will help (receptive family style)and some of which will hinder (remote family style) in the patient coping with dialysis. Naturally, it is the interface of family and patient, that makes for outcome. Reiss (34) also felt that family characteristics would influence medical outcome. In a very interesting study Rideout, Rodin and Littlefield (35), looked at depression in spouses of dialysis patients and found that 20% had symptoms of serious depression. When looking further at meaningful variables, social support from the ill partner was most significant, while social and financial stressors were important, but of less significance.

Since ESRD is a chronic illness, families should be seen and treated, over time. Paluszny et al. (36) summarize critical times: when the diagnosis is made, when symptoms present problems, when life crises occur, when developmental maladjustments interfere with compliance and when little else can be done. This last item, crucially important, is frequently missed, because we, the helpers, feel so helpless and hopeless. Yet, this is the time that patient and family need us most.

> Mrs B, an 83 year old woman, on dialysis for 15 years, with cardiac, hepatic, central nervous system and access problems, was clearly coming to the end of her life. As she came more infrequently for treatment, was more confused and more symptomatic, her family became more frantic about 'do something' and the staff indeed did more tests and procedures. In this setting, the patient became more agitated and frenzied and it was only with staff intervention with family, and helping them come to terms with the coming death of their mother, did the patient calm down.

The elderly may present different adaptational styles. Kutner and Brogan (37), point out that elderly patients frequently have lower expectations from dialysis and therefore may adapt better. Yet those elderly patients who were very active before dialysis and those who have to deal with many family relationship problems, have a more difficult time adapting to the dialysis.

COMPLIANCE

'How do we get patients to do what we believe is good for them?' asks one of our nephrologists. Usually we do know what would give the best results with our dialysis patients, 'but simply they will not do it'. Compliance does influence morbidity and mortality (38) and even as we tell them, it does not seem to make a difference. They remain 'difficult'. Our patients will only go along with a regimen, if they feel that it will directly benefit them, usually in the near future (39).

The usual definition of compliance might be, 'the extent to which patients take our prescriptions, as prescribed.' For many reasons, our recommendations are seen as impositions. There are factors that should alert us to possible non-compliance, especially as to taking medication (50.2%) and fluid restriction(49.5%) (40). Patient distress, decreasing satisfaction, poor attendance, severe untreatable illness, medically unexplained symptoms and co-existing social problems (41) were seen as crucial factors in compliance. Morduchowicz and others (42) isolated the following factors as crucial: serum potassium, serum phosphate, interdialysis weight gain, age, time on dialysis, place of birth, and whether patient comes accompanied to dialysis. One of the best parameters seems to be the percentage of time dialyzed compared with the total dialysis time prescribed (43). We use the Rogosin evaluation screen for compliance (Table 5).

The hardest realization for staff is that the ultimate responsibility for care rests with the patient and not with the staff. Early education by a team made up of health professionals and dialysis patients, has increased the compliance in our center. We try to build an alliance, in which we begin by educating the patient about their disorder and about dialysis. We listen respectfully to their symptoms and talk about possible treatments, or no treatment, when this is the fact. We try to engage a family member and feed back when the patient seems to be non-compliant, by physical parameters. Brock (44) found that 1) knowledge was negatively correlated to uncertainty, 2) level of education was positively correlated with coping effectiveness. Level of education can be enhanced through our educating the patient and family. Hegel et al. (45), have used a behavioral model consisting of positive reinforcement, shaping and self-monitoring, and found it quite useful.

Naturally, we must look for psychopathology, which frequently interferes with compliance. Depressed patients have a sense of 'doom and gloom' seeing no use in being compliant. 'It is too much trouble and it won't help anyway'. Treating the depression frequently helps.

Patients with delirium cannot recall our instructions and therefore cannot do what we suggest. In addition to trying to clear the delirium and using the proper pharmacotherapy, it is essential that a 'significant other' be recruited help with compliance.

Many patients quickly realize that if they eat forbidden food just before dialysis, or drink a great deal just before dialysis, they can 'get away with it'. Talking with some nephrologists, they agreed that frequently this type of 'getting away with it' might not be dangerous to the patient, but would be seen as 'being a bad patient'. This is not constructive to the doctor/patient relationship and it is important that we prioritize the non-compliant behavior and interfere only when necessary.

Studies on compliance show that age, number of side effects, number of procedures and medications, relationship with health care professionals and support systems are crucial. Children and adolescents are frequent non-compliers, while middle age people tend to be more compliant (46). People over 60 years, are more at risk for non-compliance, possibly due to impairment in recent memory. If medications can be combined or cut down, results are frequently better. In the classic studies of Burton et al. (32), the number and closeness of support persons, correlated closely with morbidity and mortality of patients on dialysis. The greater the number of support persons, the less morbidity and mortality.

The highest correlation is between compliance and relationship to the health care professionals. Those

Table 5. The Rogosin Institute Transplant Evaluation questionnaire

Patient Name _____

1.	Is the patient compliant with treatment?	YES	NO
	Does he/she do what staff ask him/her to do?	YES	NO
2	Does the patient miss more than 1 dialysis session per month (average)?	YES	NO
3.	a) Does the patient have potassium levels greater than 6.5%?	YES	NO
	b) How frequently (per month)?		
4.	Does the patient need extra dialysis sessions?	YES	NO
5.	a) Does the patient gain more than 3 kg between dialysis sessions?	YES	NO
	b) How frequently (per month)?		
6.	Does the patient show up for medical (non-dialysis) appointments? i.e., x-ray, EKG etc?	YES	NO
7.	Does the patient have disagreements with staff?	YES	NO
8.	a) Does the patient have BUN greater than 120?	YES	NO
	b) How frequently (per month)?		
9.	Does the patient take his/her medicine regularly?	YES	NO

patients who have a strong bond to us, will do more of what we want them to do, partly to please us, partly because they trust and understand what we try to do.

DYING AND DEATH

Patients frequently have thoughts that 'I have had enough', and I often get a call saying that 'the person is suicidal'. When I arrive, the patient may indeed 'have had enough', but seems calm and collected. As a psychiatrist I try to find out if the patient is depressed, has delirium, or an acute stressor that clouds the decision. The patient has the right to decide that he/she no longer wishes to dialyze, and thus die, if there is no psychopathology. This decision is not only explosive for the patient, but also for the family and for the dialysis staff. Family members are usually caught off guard, especially if they do not live with the patient. The significant other may not agree, but is usually aware of the decision. Children become panicky, when a parent 'has had enough', and for their own sake, wish to keep the person alive.

Staff has put in much time and effort, and see taking oneself off dialysis as a personal rejection of the staff and a hostile act. I am most useful when I can bring the various factions together, have the patient explain his/her

reasoning and concentrate on what is best for the patient. It is important that at this crucial junction, staff and a family NOT abandon the patient, even though they feel terribly sad and perhaps rejected and that plans be made for a 'good death'. This includes finding a place where the patient can have appropriate medication for sleep and anxiety, not be bothered with tests and have meaningful people around, who will hold and talk and make the person feel safe (47). Fukinishi (48) writes about the need for advanced directives, to make for a good death, and this is crucial to do, when the patient is still feeling well. Moss and others (49) have found that 92% of medical directors of nephrology units, felt that if the patient was competent, they would honor the patients wish to stop dialysis. This may be true for the nephrologist, but not for the nursing and social service staff.

USES OF PSYCHIATRISTS

Psychiatrists are most often called in consultation for patients that appear suicidal, have psychopathology such as depression, need treatment for psychopathology, are non-compliant with the dialysis regimen, or wish to terminate dialysis (and their lives). Psychiatrists are also consulted when dialysis patients' families develop psy-

Table 6. Obstacles to delivery of psychiatric care

---

1. Resistances of the patient
   a) fear of psychiatrists, who treat crazy people
   b) fear that anger and hostility will emerge, which will endanger the dialysis
   c) time is precious and consultations take time

2. Resistance created by the medical staff
   a) personal bias against psychiatry
   b) physicians general misunderstanding of how psychiatry works
   c) misunderstanding as to what depression and support really mean
   d) misuse of psychotropic drugs
   e) not understanding that the psychiatrists stance is essentially neutral, so that he is not there to 'convince the patient to do what you want', but to see why the patient will not do it, and through understanding, give the patient a conscious choice.

3. Resistances posed by psychiatrists
   a) use of psychoanalytic terms,not useful to the nephrologist
   b) not answering the question asked by the staff quickly and to the point i.e., looking at dynamics

---

chopathology, or when family friction leads to problems such as non-compliance.

In this chapter I have discussed psychopathology, non-compliance and termination of dialysis, and I would like to bring up areas where we and others have found that psychiatrists can be useful.

We have been involved with groups of nurses and social workers, in both in-patient and out-patient settings. These groups meet on a weekly basis and are patient problem orientated. Manley (50),describes the groups and mentions the types of problems, which have come up and been helpful: problems with compliance, problems between medical and non-medical staff, and emotional involvement with patients.

In these groups, it is important not to *therapize*, meaning doing treatment of the group or individual. Kaplan De-Nour and Czaczkes (51), specifically warns against doing group therapy. She feels that staff attitudes and reactions influence the patients adjustment and discussions of possible changes in attitude are frequently of help. Staff burnout has been a hot topic for many years. Kaplan De-Nour and Czaczkes (51) postulated that because of close and intense relationships over prolonged period of time would lead to problems of: guilt, possessiveness, overprotection, and withdrawal. Indeed much of our time in the group is spent on these topics.

Kalman (52) has postulated that there are obstacles to the delivery of psychiatric care, dividing the problems into three main areas as shown in Table 6.

CONCLUSION

If the above are taken into consideration, the psychiatric aspects of dialysis, in patient care, staff care and proper referral, can take place in a timely manner, so that we can take better care of our patients and ourselves.

REFERENCES

1. Montagnac R, Defert P, Schillinger F: Psychological impact periodic hemodialysis in the adult. (Editorial) *Nephrologie* 13: 145, 1992
2. Galpin C: Body image in end-stage renal failure. ıBr J Nursing 1: 21, 1992
3. Levy NB, Abram H, Kemph J et al.: Panel: living or dying. Adaption to haemodialysis. in *Living or Dying: Adaptation to Haemodialysis*, edited by Levy N, Springfield IL, CC Thomas, 1974
4. Gorynski L, Knight F: A peer support group for adolescent dialysis patients. *ANNA J* 19: 262, 1992
5. Rittman M, Northsea C, Hausauer N, Green C, Swanson L: Living with renal failure. *ANNA J* 20: 327, 1993
6. Procci WR: The study of sexual dysfunction in uremic males: problems for patients and investigators. *Clin Exp Dial Apheresis* 7: 289, 1983
7. Tabbane K, Ben-Rejeb R, Ghodhbane T, Douki S: *Annales-Medico-Psychologiques* 47: 325, 1989
8. Yoshioka M, Ishii T, Fukunishi I: Sleep disturbance of end-stage renal disease. *Japan J Psychiatr Neurol* 47: 847, 1993
9. Kopple JD, Hakim RM, Held PJ, Keane WF, King K, Lazarus JM, Parker III, TF, Teehan BP: Recommendations for reducing the high morbidity and mortality of United States maintenance dialysis patients. *Am J Kidney Dis* 24: 968, 1994
10. McKegney, FP: The patient's role in beginning and continuing maintenance haemodialysis. *Proc 4th Int Congr Nephrol* 3: 330, 1974
11. Nissenson AR: Measuring, managing, and improving quality in the end-stage renal disease treatment setting: peritoneal dialysis. *Am J Kidney Dis* 24: 368, 1994

12. Freeman RB: Passions in the arena. *Loss, Grief and Care* 5: 123, 1991

13. Holley JL, Barrington K, Kohn J, Hayes I: Patient factors and the influence of nephrologists, social workers and nurses on patient decisions to choose continuous peritoneal dialysis. *Adv Perit Dial* 7: 108, 1991

14. Groome PA, Hutchinson TA, Tousignant P: Content of a decision analysis for treatment choice in end-stage renal disease: who should be consulted. *Med Decision Making* 14: 91, 1994

15. Bower J: Doctor–patient relationship unique in dialysis, needs improvement. *Nephrol News Issues* 6: 47, 63, 1992

16. Newmann JM: Education and patient enpowerment will make rehabilitation work. *Nephrol News Issues* 8: 22, 26, 1994

17. Kumar H, Alam F, Naqvi SA: Experience of haemodialysis at the Kidney Centre. *J Pakistan Med Assoc* 42: 234, 1992

18. Petrie K: Psychological well-being and psychiatric disturbance in dialysis and renal transplant patients. *Br J Med Psych* 62: 91, 1989

19. Sno, H-N, Schoevers R-A, Wiltink, E-H, Molenaar D: Over spoelen en overspoeld raken. Psychiatrische complicaties bij dialyse patienten. On perfusion and confusion: Psychiatric complications in dialysis-patients. *Tijdschrift voor Psychiatrie* 34: 637, 1992

20. Craven JL, Rodin GM, Johnson L, Kennedy SH: The diagnosis of major depression in renal dialysis patients

21. Kimmel PL, Weihs K, Peterson RA: Survival in hemodialysis patients: the role of depression. *J Am Soc Nephrol* 4: 12, 1993

22. Peterson RA, Kimmel PL, Sacks CR, Mesquita ML, Simmens SJ, Reiss D: Depression, perception of illness and mortality in patients with end-stage renal disease. *Int J Psychiatr Med* 21: 343, 1991

23. Driessen M, Balk F: Chronic renal failure: predictors of good adjustment to disease and treatment (German); Original Title: Chronische Niereninsuffizienz: Pradiktoren fur eine gunstige Adaption an Krankheit und Behandlung. *Psychotherapie, Psychosomatik, Medizinische, Psychologie* 41: 363, 1991

24. Goldberg DP: *The Detection of Psychiatric Illness by Questionnaire: A Technique for the Identification and Assessment of Non-Psychotic Psychotic Psychiatric Illness*, Maudsley Monograph No 2, Oxford University Press, Oxford, 1972

25. DSM-IV: American Psychiatric Association Press, 1994

26. Streltzer J: Diagnostic and treatment considerations in depressed dialysis patients. *Clin Exp Dial Apheresis* 7: 257, 1983

27. Klerman GL, Weissman MM, Rounsaville BJ, Chevron ES: *Interpersonal Psychotherapy of Depression*, New York, Basic Books, 1984

28. Beck AT, Rush AJ, Shaw BF, Emery G: *Cognitive Therapy of Depression*, New York, Guilford Press, 1979

29. Levy NB: Psychopharmacology in patients with renal failure. *Int J Psychiatr Med* 20: 325, 1990

30. Viederman M: *Psychiatry*, Viederman & Rusk (Reference #1) cited in 37: 68, 1975

31. Carbonell Masia C, Hernandez Moreno L, Ramos Rieva J: Variables asociadas a la adaptacion psicosocial de los enfermos renales cronicos en tratamiento. *Actas Luso-*

Espanolas de Neurologia, Psiquiatria y Ciencias Afines 21: 1, 1993

32. Burton H, Kline S, Lindsay R, Heidenheim P: The sole of support in influencing outcome of end-stage renal disease. *Gen Hosp Psychiatr* 10: 260, 1988

33. Flaherty MJ, O'Brien ME: Family styles of coping in end stage renal disease. *ANNA J* 19: 345, 1992

34. Reiss D: Patient, family, and staff responses to end-stage renal disease. *Am J Kidney Dis* 15: 194, 1990

35. Rideout EM, Rodin GM, Littlefield CH: Stress, social support, and symptoms of deprssion in spouses of the medically ill. *Int J Psychiatr Med* 20: 37

36. Paluszny MJ, DeBeukelaer MM, Rowane WA: Families coping with the multiple crises of chronic illness. *Loss, Grief and Care* 5: 15, 1991

37. Kutner NG, Brogan D: Expectations and psychological needs of elderly dialysis patients. *Intl J Aging Human Dev* 31: 239, 1990

38. O'Brien ME: Compliance behavior and long-term maintenance dialysis. *Am J Kidney Dis* 15: 209, 1990

39. Schlenker BR, Britt TW, Pennington J, Murphy R, Doherty K: The triangle model of responsibility. *Psychol Rev* 101: 632, 1994

40. Bame SI, Petersen N, Wray NP: Variation in hemodialysis patient compliance according to demographic characteristics. *Soc Sci Med* 37: 1035, 1993

41. Sharpe M, Mayou R, Seagroatt V, Surawy C, Warwick H, Bulstrode C, Dawber R, Lane D: Why do doctors find some patients difficult to help? *Q J Med* 87: 187, 1994

42. Morduchowicz G, Sulkes J, Aizic S, Gabbay U, Winkler J, Boner G: Compliance in hemodialysis patients: a multivariate regression analysis. *Nephron* 64: 365, 1993

43. Kobrin SM, Kimmel PL, Simmens SJ, Reiss D: Behavioral and biochemical indices of compliance in hemodialysis patients. *ASAIO Trans* 37: M378, 1991

44. Brock J: Uncertainty, information needs, and coping effectiveness of renal families. *ANNA J* 17: 242, 1990

45. Hegel MT, Ayllon T, Thiel G, Oulton B: Improving adherence to fluid restrictions in male hemodialysis patients: a comparison of cognitive and behavioral approaches. *Health Psychology* 11: 324, 1992

46. Tebbi CK: Treatment compliance in childhood and adolescence. *Cancer* 71 (Suppl 10): 3441S, 1993

47. Wilson PG: Planning, dying and death in patients with end stage kidney disease. *Found Thanat* 2: 37, 1993

48. Fukunishi I: Anxiety associated with kidney transplantation. *Psychopathology* 26: 24, 1993

49. Moss AH, Stocking CB, Sachs GA, Siegler M: Variation in the attitudes of dialysis unit medical directors toward decisions to withhold and withdraw dialysis. *J Am Soc Nephrol* 4: 229, 1993

50. Manley M: The liaison psychiatrist and the outpatient hemodialysis unit, Part I: Reliability and validity of staff assessments of patient compliance on a hemodialysis unit. *Clin Exp Dial Apheresis* 7: 349, 1983

51. Kaplan De-Nour A, Czaczkes JW: in *Living or Dying: Adaptation to Haemodialysis*, edited by Levy N, Springfield IL, CC Thomas, 1974, p 102

52. Kalman, TP: Obstacles to the delivery of psychiatric care to transplant recipients and dialysis patients. *Clin Exper Dial Apheresis* 7: 335, 1983

PART B: QUALITY OF LIFE OF THE DIALYSIS PATIENT

J. AHLMÉN

QUALITY OF LIFE OF THE DIALYSIS PATIENT

Before 1972 the upper age limit for dialysis treatment in USA was 50 years. After this time the medical technology has contributed to an impressive long term patient survival on chronic dialysis. An increasing awareness of the need of the patient to live as close to normal life as possible has led to a concentration on problems concerned with the quality of life (QL). Initial studies to assess QL focused more on physical abilities than the studies with the more multi dimensional QL instruments used today.

To define the quality of life is very difficult if at all possible. It is, however, important to try to measure and quantify different aspects of QL. The wide variations in how to define QL may be divided into subjective and objective measures. Using only one research instrument may lead to a false QL interpretation if the result is depending on other not evaluated factors. Comprehensive correlations of different instruments indicated that they represented either function or feeling (1).

Research on different instruments has been persued for many years and is continuously going on to find reliable and valid instruments. The patient with chronic renal insufficiency who is offered the different modalities of active treatment of uremia is in a way fortunate to be able to prolong his life. The different limitations of transplantation, hemodialysis (HD) or peritoneal dialysis have a great impact on the patient's ordinary life. The mixing of different treatment modalities means a high and changing degree of adaptation for the individual patient. Survival of end stage renal disease (ESRD) as the most important quality of life measure is today quite good (2). The 20% annual mortality of chronic dialysis (USRDS 1992) will be discussed elsewhere.

Mortality is not only a result of the quality of medical treatment but also depending on social, economic and cultural factors. Patient survival in selected and matched materials of non-diabetic homehemodialysis

and continuous ambulatory peritoneal dialysis (CAPD) (3) patients showed significantly better survival for the homehemodialysis patients. Together with age, diabetes and comorbidity, psychosocial factors are important for patient survival.

The selection of patients to active treatment of uremia or not differs between countries mostly depending on resources for treatment. Comparisons of QL between patients with the different treatment modalities have been presented (4, 5) with the overall result that a patient with a successful renal transplantation have a higher QL than patients on homehemodialysis patients, on CAPD and patients on institutional hemodialysis respectively. Careful adjustments for case-mix influences of age and comorbid conditions decreased the differences between the different treatment modalities for ESRD in the pre-erythropoietin era. This was clearly demonstrated by Hart et al. (6) using the Sickness Impact Profile (SIP) for the evaluation mainly of the physical and psychosocial dimensions. The influence of selection criteria for the mode of treatment is great. In countries with a highly developed active treatment of uremia the choice of the patient after adequate information is very important. Wellinformed patients and their spouses prefer CAPD to HD (7) which ought to give a higher number of patients on peritoneal dialysis than is seen in most countries today. Some patients given the choice of having a kidney transplant may prefer to continue on chronic dialysis therapy (8). It can be expected that the motivation and the compliance to the treatment modality is higher when the patient's view has a great impact on the choice of therapy. Medical limitations and organ shortage decrease the number of patients suitable for kidney transplantation. Only about 28% of all patients on dialysis were suitable for kidney transplantation in Sweden 1990 (Ahlmén, Karlberg, Gäbel, unpublished), and this in a country with a high transplantation activity (2). The high number of elderly patients with about 1/3 of the dialysis patients above 70 years of age at the start of active treatment of uremia means that the majority of patients with chronic uremia will be chronically dialysed without the option of renal transplantation. Some patients above this age, however, want to receive a kidney transplant (9).

The historical development of the dialysis technique has made it possible to change the prospects of chronic dialysis from a fight for survival to a life with a high QL close to normal life. The understanding and introduction of therapy for renal osteodystrophy (10) together with the increasing routine use of Erythropoietin (Epo) (11) have meant important contributions to a higher QL for the dialysis patients. Quality of life is a multi dimensional concept and the optimal balance between subjective and objective QL assessments has not yet been settled. Many different methods have been suggested to set weights to the components included in the health status measures or in the QL measures. Aggregation of items or dimensions may be controversial. For ESRD patients as for other studied patients most methods of QL rely on responses to questionnaires sometimes combined with interviews and observations of personal status. The freedom of choice may be a very important factor in the evaluation of QL of a person. This evaluation may change for different reasons after a short or long time of dialysis treatment why the choice may be death. Kaye et al. (12) reported attitudes of both patients and staff regarding stopping treatment. The majority favoured discontinuation of therapy in patients definitely lacking decision making capacity but about 18% of both patients and staff wanted dialysis to continue. This problem is debated world-wide and constitutes one important QL aspect of chronic dialysis. This has lately been comprehensively reviewed by Rothemberg (13, 14). QL of the dialysis patient is the ultimate result of our quality efforts including quality improvement, quality assurance and quality management. A continuous and chronic treatment has implications not only on the patient's health status but on the psychological, social and economic well-being of the patient and on his closest net work of concerned persons. To perform comparisons of QL dimensions of dialysis patients with the general population and other disease categories are important to be able to evaluate where preventive QL-interventions can be expected to be most effective. Dialysis patients often score worse than other patient groups on QL-dimensions (15). Comparisons between patients (n = 60) and three other chronic disease groups (16) in the pre-Epo era did not show any significant differences in the Mental Health Index between the groups. All groups scored higher than a group of patients under treatment for depression. A consistent finding was an indication of a better Mental Health Index with advancing age in all of the investigated groups. This may mean that older people during life experiences have developed more effective skills to manage stressful life events. A truly randomized study when starting dialysis treatment may in some ways be helpful in describing the most important factors for a high QL on dialysis treat-

ment. The results of the different dialysis modalities today are similar enough to allow such a randomisation.

METHODS FOR MEASURING QUALITY OF LIFE

The number of used investigational instruments for QL is high. Many of the originally used methods were constructed for use in healthy adult people and not for ESRD patients. The choice of instruments for a clinial trial has to take into account the purpose of the study, the type of disease and treatment, if the material is to be used for comparisons with other disease groups and so on. The first appearing instruments as Karnofsky performance scale (KPS) (17), Campell's Index of Well-Being (18), Cantril's Self-Anchoring striving scale (19), Nottingham Health profile (NHP) (20, 21), Sickness Impact Profile (SIP) (22) have widely been used for QL aspects in ESRD patients often without a confirmation of their validity among these patient groups. Generic instruments are important for comparisons between different populations but may not be sensitive enough for measuring changes e.g. before and after Epo-therapy why there is a need also for validated, reliable specific instruments. The Kidney Disease Questionnaire (23) is one such developed instrument which limits the use of the instrument to patients with renal insufficiency. Self-Esteem Inventory (24, 25), Beck Depression Inventory (26), Spitzer's objective and subjective qualities of life instrument (27) are all examples of instruments involving satisfaction, happiness, depression and distress. The use of these instruments may give false impressions if the impact of comorbid non-renal diseases, age, sex and education are not accounted for which is known to influence subjective measurements of QL. The time trade off technique (28) is a generic instrument used to evaluate the utility of health state. It is not the purpose of these lines to include examples of all used questionnaires or structured interviews but only to bring about the necessity to use several validated investigational QL instruments simultaneously in combination with sociodemographic and medical investigations. Some researchers see QL as an entity and propose global measures for investigations while others propose the use of instruments made up of several different domains. These may be assessed with or without weighting.

The variability of the results between different QL methods ought to be as small as possible to reduce variations in e.g. cost-effectiveness analysis of patients' Quality-Adjusted life years, Value-Adjusted life years etc. of ESRD therapy (29). Multidisciplinary approach to QL evaluations of chronic dialysis is needed to include also cognitive functions and methods for determination of alexithymi (30).

Many instruments include different subscales to represent different dimensions of quality of life e.g. NHP, SIP. The use of multiple measures possibly also from multiple sources will increase the construct validity in defining the QL of dialysis patients. As there are no best measures for a given dimension several imperfect measures can be used. As they have different errors and biases the multiple measures together reflect desired QL dimensions better than a single instrument (31).

INFLUENCE OF MEDICAL FACTORS ON QL OF PATIENTS ON CHRONIC DIALYSIS

At present there is no evidence for differences in the mortality on HD compared to CAPD (32) especially after adjusting for different selection criteria (33). Comparisons are difficult as observed differences may entirely be due to differences in patient characteristics and case mix. The presence of comorbid factors and high age clearly show an increased risk of death for the dialysis patient (34). Failure to control blood pressure has a great impact on patient survival (35). Low serum albumin has also been reported to be an independent factor influencing dialysis mortality (36). It is difficult to positively change nutrient intake of dialysis patients resulting in increased serum albumin but education and increased nutrition knowledge may contribute to improved QL of hemodialysis patients (37).

Adequacy of dialysis with especially KT/V measurements has a great influence of both mortality (38, 39) and morbidity (40). It was not possible to detect a change from KT/V < 0.8 to >1.0 in QL in a small number of hemodialysis patients after a relatively short observation time with the Time Trade Off technique. (41). The Hemodialysis Quality of Life instrument as being a disease specific questionaire showed minor changes and was also considered non-responsive to detect this change of dialysis dose.

Morbidity seems to be higher for patients on CAPD compared to patients on intermittent HD. CAPD patients spent about twice as many days in hospital as HD patients (42). Hospital admissions were significantly higher for CAPD patients when 150 patients on homehemodialysis were retrospectively compared to 89 patients on CAPD (43). Comorbid conditions and patient selection influence the number of days spent in hospital. Meija et al. (44) reported that diabetics on hemodialysis spent significantly more days in hospital than diabetic patients on CAPD. The most important QL predictors for patient survival have been reported to be age and depression (45, 46). There are few reports concerned with depressive states that count for disease severity or underdialysis why the results may be debatable. An improvement of QL may be expected with longer observation time and more sensitive QL instruments as the number of hospitalizations has been shown to decrease with increasing KT/V (47). The results from long term therapy are scarce.

The influence on QL of medical factors seem to be small among patients above the age of 65 years (48) but of importance among younger patients. It is also important to note that in this study using the Cantril ladder scale (19) perceived overall life satisfaction did not show any signifant difference between the dialysis patients and a normal population. Age of the patient seem to have several important influences of QL of the dialysis patients. Children with chronic renal insufficiency are aimed for kidney transplantation as their ultimate active treatment of uremia. The literature is thus most comprehensive concerning QL in childen in conjunction with transplantation (49). The resilience of children with ESRD seemed to be good. Hemodialysis of adolescent patients in a small study had a worse functional outcome than patients on continuous peritoneal dialysis (50).

The QL of old patients on dialysis treatment have been studied for many years. Westlie et al. (51) investigated 1984 morbidity, mortality and life satisfaction of patients more than 70 years old. About 2/3 of these were able to carry out normal physical activity and enjoyed life. The cumulative survival of patients above the age of 70 years have been reported to be 25% after 5 years (52) and 17% after 7 years (51). McKevitt et al. (53) showed 1986 increased depressions and more physical limitations in patients above the age of 60 years compared to younger patients on dialysis. Medical complications are reported by Neu et al. 1986 (53) to be the most common reason (54) for stopping dialysis which appeared in one of six patients above the age of 60 years. Homehemodialysis treatment seemed in those days to be more common among patients who stopped dialysis (55) in contrast to the findings in a report by Wehle (56) from Sweden with a less developed homehemodialysis program. Dialysis was stopped in 9% of the patients. Among these 18% of the patients refused further treatment. Snach et al. found in 1988 (57) that the majority of hemodialysis patients above the age of 65 had a positive attitude towards the HD treatment but 15% of the patients showed depressive states. The principal reason was physical impairment by co morbid conditions but psycho-social factors were also important especially social isolation. The prevalence in a small study from Greece (58) of psychogeriatric morbidity did not seem to be depending on the treatment modality when HD was compared to CAPD. No significant relationship was found between age and an index of QL among patients in an outpatient hemodialysis centre (59). Kutner et al. (60) compared patients (1988) more than 60 years of age with control individuals without dialysis. The dialysis patients reported more functional disability, showed compromised psycho social function and lower levels of mastery over their lifes compared to age matched controls.

DIABETES

Diabetes mellitus is one of the most common causes of renal insufficiency. It is in itself a burden to the patients' QL because of the chronic development of degenerative complications. The patients choice of treatment for end-stage renal disease is thus even more difficult than for patients without diabetes. The diabetic patient on dialysis is therefore more dependent on their surrounding for their basic personal care needs than other patients on dialysis and also than a general population. Mortality for diabetic patients on hemodialysis and CAPD is higher than for organ replacement (61) but the selection of patients to the different treatment modalities is very strongly favoring a higher survival after kidney transplantation.

In the comprehensive study of Borgel et al. (62) with a mean age of the diabetic dialysis patients of 62 years the dependency was much higher compared to a general population above the age of 65. Among the 472 diabetic patients collected in a multicentre study 84% of the patients had chronic HD and the remaining patients chronic CAPD therapy. The Barthel Index (BI) used for evaluation of the dependency on activities of daily living showed significantly worse BI and thus more dependency for patients with diabetes type II compared to patients with diabetes type I. As the former patients were significantly older and had longer duration of the diabetes disease the BI differences became non-significant when age adjustment was performed. The QL investigations using visual analogue scales showed significantly worse scores for pain and fatigue for the dialysis patients compared to 121 non-dialysed diabetic patients (62, 63). No differences were found for the self-estimated QL or care burden between the dialysed and the non-dialysed patients. CAPD-patients showed a significantly lower BI than HD-patients. Both the pain, fatigue and the BI differences between diabetic patients on the different dialysis treatments might be quite different after the introduction of Epo and after another patient selection to the two dialysis modalities.

Diabetics are expected to have more dependency in their activities of daily living than other primary causes of uremia and chronic dialysis (64) because of the severe diabetic medical complications. Fukunishi reported that diabetic patients on dialysis have poor QL in the medical dimension, good QL in psychological and social dimensions but a high prevalence of alexithymia (65). In this study of 30 patients on HD and 28 patients on CAPD a small number of diabetic patients (8 and 7 patients respectively) were included. The diabetic patients were less depressive than the non-diabetic patients. The prevalence of alexithymia was 50% (75% of the diabetic and 41% of the non-diabetic patients) of the HD-patients. This was significantly higher than the prevalence of 18% of the CAPD-patients. The prevalence of alexithymia indicated a higher prevalence among the diabetic patients irrespective of the dialysis modality but this did not reach statistical significance in this small material.

The diabetic patient's acceptance of his situation rather than lack of knowledge may explain his optimistic view of his present health status. With the use of Cantril's self-anchoring striving scale Hoothay et al. (66) demonstrated that the 12 studied diabetic patients on chronic HD had high levels of their present subjective life satisfaction in spite of many diabetic complications. These patients also had an surprisingly optimistic view of their QL in the near future.

Psycho social problems within families are increasing as the diabetic patient on dialysis become less functional (67) but single exceptions with strong family support have been reported (68). In spite of a high degree of disability diabetic patients may return to the same degree of reabilitation and vocational status as before the start of dialysis therapy. Flynn (69) reported this for 23 out of 24 blind diabetic patients after starting CAPD. Sexual relations are reported to be poor but in most cases these problems often existed before the start of dialysis (70).

PSYCHOLOGICAL FACTORS AND ADJUSTMENT

When survivors (n – 204) and non-survivors (n – 37) on homedialysis were compared Wai et al. (71) were able to show the importance of depression, dialysis related stress score and age for patient survival. The majority of the patients had hemodialysis (62%). Medical factors as excessive interdialysis weight gain, hemoglobin levels and serum albumin levels discriminated significantly between survivors and non-survivors. The non-physiological factors, age, depression and stress score related to the dialysis process were, however, more powerful predictors for survival. Both functional status (Karnofsky scale) and quality of life (Spitzer QL index) among dialysis patients (n – 294, 84% HD, 16% CAPD) were independent risk factors correlated to the early mortality of dialysis patients (72). The subscale scores for activity, daily living, health and outlook were significantly higher for the survivors.

The non-compliance of dialysis patients concerning diet, medications and fluid restriction has several causes (73). It is also difficult without a comprehensive study to select the non-compliant dialysis patients from the compliant patients. Manley et al. (74) reported a poor relation between actual patient compliance and crude staff ratings of compliance. The problem of non-compliance arises already during the phase of renal insufficiency. Compliance may involve adaptive mechanisms of different kinds parallel to the changes of therapy for chronic renal disease (75).

Adjustment to a chronic disease may involve psychological well-being, good compliance and rehabilitation in connection with good medical status (76) or involve more specified factors (77). The interrelationship between the patient and his total environment includes the family, the dialysis and healthcare team, the social group and connections and the society at large. The majority of children living at home in a family with a dialysis patient in the pre-Epo era became more or less psychologically disturbed with anxiety, depression and behavioural problems (78).

In this study of 14 children there was no obvious differences between the reactions of the children in a family with a home hemodialysis patient or an incenter dialysis patient. The impact on family life is great and spouses have high rates of anxiety and depression (79). Even the sex of the dialysis patient may mean important differences in the adjustment and psychological distress of the family. Psychological distress may be associated with the cultural climate and the role expectations in the society. No significant differences in marital relations or psychologically well-being were found when patients and spouses were investigated in five different progression phases of chronic renal disease (80). These results were seen in spite of higher illness/treatment intrusiveness in the dialysis situation than in the non-diaysis situation. A significantly higher correlation between marital role strain and psychological distress was seen with increased illness/treatment intrusiveness. The dialysis partners rated themselves as less happy than the non-dialysis partners. The family adjustment seems to be more difficult if the dialysis patient is a woman (81). On the Psychosocial Adjustment to Physical Illness Scale the male patients had almost the same scores as their wives but more problems on the domestic environment domain. The female patients showed, however, more problems than the male patients. The female patients also showed significantly more problems when compared to their husbands in total scores, domestic environment and sexual relations. The psychological distress of both male and female patients and husbands were above the scores of a normal population.

The quality of care also influenzes the QL of the patients on chronic dialysis. This influence is continuous for a very long time. Long relationships between staff and patients are an important source of stress (82) of the dialysis staff and favour a certain working rotation. Burnout is a feared effect of emotional stress. Increased denial mechanisms of the staff may adversely affect patient care (79). In a wide in-unit adult hemodialysis population (n = 416) the overall satisfaction with care correlated moderately with QL with the used quality of life index (83). It was not clear wether the satisfaction with care was a cause or an effect. The strongest correlation was found between the overall satisfaction with care and the QL subscales of health and functioning. A weaker correlation was found between the psychological well-being and the tendency to be satisfied with care. Satisfaction with care was lower in patients who had more education and who had been on dialysis longer (84). A significant relationship exists between satisfaction with care and expectations (85) why these may increase with education and longer time on dialysis.

The psychological reactions of a patient on chronic HD have been described as three phases: honeymoon, disenchantment and discouragement and the long term adaption (86). The last two phases need interventions to preserve the QL of the patients.

Devins et al. (87) demonstrated that life satisfaction was significantly greater among CAPD-patients (n = 11) as compared to in centre hemodialysis patients (n = 39). Pessimism and hopelessness were significantly more prevalent among patients on centre hemodialysis treatment compared to transplant recipients. Two used depression-distress indices did not show any significant differences between HD, CAPD or kidney transplant patients. When homehemodialysis (n = 24), CAPD (n = 21) and in centre HD-patients (n = 24) were compared to transplant recipients (n = 69) total life satisfaction score was only significantly better for transplant recipients compared to patients on in centre dialysis (88).

A moderate prevalence of psychological distress was similar among transplant recipients (25%), patients on homehemodialysis (21%), patients on CAPD (33%) and on HD (33%) in a crossectional study based on questionnaires by Morris et al. (89). This was contradicted in study of Kock et al. (90) where transplant recipients (n = 76) estimated their posttransplant life to include significant reduction of sadness and depression. This was, however, the result of a retrospective evaluation using a visual analogue scale. HD-patients (n = 290) were more dissatisfied (30%) with their life in general compared to (n = 68) CAPD patients (17%) and transplant recipient (5%). The duration of the different dialysis treatments varied, however, with a twice as long mean time of renal failure for the HD patients compared to CAPD patients. This may be the main explanation for the difference in dissatisfaction between HD and CAPD. Patient selection is probably another.

When comparing matched CAPD (n = 33) and HD patients (n=33) (91) limited to ages 20–65 years on stable chronic dialysis they all demonstrated medium levels of self esteem. The majority of the patients showed high levels of control over their health outcome and moderate levels of psychological stress. There was no statistical difference concerning self esteem. However 56% of the CAPD patients and 42% of the hemodialysis patients had high self-esteem and low self-esteem was found in 19% and 31% respectively. Consequently perceptions of a distorted body image does not seem to have a greater influence on the self-esteem of CAPD patients compared to HD-patients. There was an indication in the Profile of Mood states of higher levels of emotional distress among HD-patients compared to CAPD- patients but statistical significance was only reached for anxiety. The CAPD-patients also rated their QL significantly higher than the HD-patients. The study also demonstrated the possibility of using global QL instruments for assessing the psychological state of the patients. High quality of life was correlated to high self-esteem and low levels of stress and mood disturbance. Self-rated global QL was quite high. This had been reported earlier (92) as a possible use of the mechanism of denial by the patient to his situation. Yanagida et al. (93) put forward that the higher the denial the lower the feelings of depression and dependency. When comparing different treatment modalities it is important to remember that individuals with ESRD have not been randomly assigned to a particular form of treatment.

In a comprehensive study by Theorell et al. (94) of 305 dialysis patients worse conditions in psychological health, self-reported depression, psychosomatic symptoms and sleep disturbances were more common among females younger than 44 years of age than among the other patients. Duration of dialysis treatment was not significantly correlated to these four QL indicators. Psychosomatic symptoms tended to be less frequent among peritoneal dialysis patients compared to HD-patients (p = 0.08). MANOVA testing revealed complicating diseases to be the most powerful explanatory factor in the analysis of depression.

The finding that young females showed worse adaption to dialysis is contradictory to the finding by Wolcott et al. (95) who found that men over 51 years of age had worse psychological adaptation than women and young dialysis patients. The reasons for the differences of these studies are unclear. Both studies were performed in the pre-Epo era and in both studies extensive investigational instruments were used. The differences might be explained by differences in cultural and health care systems. The distribution between the dialysis modalities also differed in the materials. In an early study by Livesley (96) a high incidence of anxiety and general distress was observed among hemodialysis patients (n = 85). About 1/3 of the studied patients thought that their problems started before the onset of the disease leading to dialysis treatment. Eight per cent indicated that their problems began before the start of dialysis but after the onset of renal disease. Fukunishi (30) demonstrated that anxiety and depressive symptoms were significantly more common among hemodialysis patients compared to CAPD-patients. Alexithymi was also demonstrated to be more common among HD-patients (15/30) than among CAPD-patients (5/28). This was confirmed in a study from Sweden where the prevalence of alexithymi among CAPD-patients peaked during the second half of the first year (Konarski, Westerlund, Ahlmén, Theorell, unpublished).

In a selected matched patient material (97) of successful non-diabetic transplant recipients (n = 31) and hospital dialysis patients (n = 31) the only significant differences were better psychosocial reactions in somatization of the former patients compared to HD-patients. Vocational rehabilitation in this selected material was high and psychological adjustment was similar in the two patient groups.

Parfrey et al. (98) could not demonstrate any significant differences in the subjective QL between hemodialysis patients and successfully transplanted kidney recipients. All were below the age of 50 years. Objective QL was significantly better for the transplant recipients. In a prospective study of 63 stable dialysis patients and 67 stable transplant patients who were interviewed one year apart the same main authors (99) showed small but significant improvements in the objective QL in the stable dialysis patients and small improvements in well-being and general affect in the stable transplant patients. Failed transplantation induced negative effects on well-being, life-satisfaction and subjective QL.

Fox et al. (100) using a Ql index showed that patients on homehemodialysis (n = 58) had a significantly higher Ql than both hospital HD-patients (n = 13) and CAPD-patients (n = 37). Periods of anxiety and depression were more common among CAPD-patients (49%) and hospital HD-patients (31%) than among homehemodialysis patients (19%). This variation may be questionned as, i.e., the number of hospital HD-patients were few compared to the number of patients in the other two groups. Tucker et al. (101) were not able to show any objective or subjective QL differences among in centre HD-patients and CAPD-patients.

PSYCHOSOCIAL FACTORS

Perceived illness intrusiveness investigated by Devins et al. (87) correlated significantly with, i.e., treatment time, uremic symptoms and intercurrent diseases. The overall levels of perceived intrusiveness did not differ between the three dialysis modalities: homehemodialysis, CAPD or institutional hemodialysis. The illness intrusiveness into the life domains of patients actively treated for uremia affected most physical well-being, work and to a lower extent social and family relations. Higher percieved intrusiveness of the dialysis regimen was associated with negative mood of the dialysis patients and lower perceived personal control over life activities. This is in accordance with the association of poor psychological adaptation and percieved health locus control described by Wolcott et al. 95). No significant difference was found in the family relationship domain (88) between transplant recipients and dialysis patients including sex life even if trends for higher life satisfaction scores were noted for transplanted patients. Among selected matched HD and CAPD-patients below 65 years of age (91) the CAPD-patients took significantly more part in community activities and showed a tendency for more active physical activities than HD-patients but both groups reported infrequent participation in most activities. This study also indicated that medical status, psychological status and social status variables are not as closely interrelated as might be expected. Dialysis patients who were able to work had a higher subjective QL (4). Only transplant (n = 144) patients and homehemodialysis patients (n = 287) showed subjective QL comparable to the general population. CAPD (n = 81) and in centre (n = 144) hemodialysis patients clearly showed a worse QL than GP. In spite of a few case mix calculations many questions remain unanswered in this comprehensive study.

The functional ability (Karnofsky index) of dialysis patients even after EPO-therapy (102) is lower than for transplant recipients. In this study (n = 329) a low number of dialysis patients returned to work. The ability to work was highest for homehemodialysis patients and lowest for CAPD-patients. 38% of the transplanted patients worked full-time or part-time compared to 27% of HD-patients and 23% of the CAPD-patients. These figures are in agreement with the studies of Lindsay et al. (43) after correction for age and sex.

When comparing HD-patients (n=15) and CAPD-patients (n = 15) with at least 6 months' treatment Schlebush found (92) that 34% of HD-patients and 20% of CAPD-patients worked part time or full time. Vocational adjustment was low in both patient groups and did not differ significantly between the different treatment modalities. Employment among Swedish both men and women below the age of 65 on dialysis was about 20% (94). Actively employed patients had significantly lower scores for depression. They reported lower psychological and intellectual demands than working men and women in the normal population younger than 65 years of age. Social support at work was experienced to be better in their work place for the dialysis patients than for the normal population. This pre-Epo study underlines active work as an indepent predictor of high QL of patients on chronic dialysis. It also indicated that active rehabilitation is a very important factor in dialysis care.

Many factors influence on the eventual return to an employment (103) among the dialysis patients. Procci et al. (104) showed that primarily treated stable patients on CAPD (n = 73) demonstrated a significantly higher degree of employment (27.4%) compared to in-center HD (n = 95) patients (9.6%) and patients who had failed CAPD (n = 46). Freeman et al. (105) demonstrated in 107 chronic dialysis patients (104 males and 3 females) that personality assessment was of predictive importance for vocational rehabilitation. Patients with normal profiles (Minnesota Multiphasic Personality Inventory) were more likely to return to full employment. Kock et al. (90) found that the increase in physical performance and leisure activities among transplant recipients did not improve the vocational situation. Work mobility and recreation were increased after Epo-therapy in an other study of in centre hemodialysis patients (106).

Case mix of therapies (5) have an impact on the vocational rehabilitation but significantly only for CAPD-patients (n = 510). Those who only had experience with CAPD-therapy showed the highest vocational rehabilitation of the non-diabetic dialysis patients in ages 19–56 years.

Sexual disturbancies among actively treated ESRD-patients were noted already in the early 1970s (107). Morris et al. (88) demonstrated several significant differences between transplanted patients and dialysis patients, but not in sex life or family relations.

Sexual dissatisfaction in the study of Simmons et al. (5) for male CAPD and HD-patients were similar (56 and 53% respectively) and significantly more problematic

than for transplant recipients (30%). Treatment modality had previously been reported to have no significant effect on the reduced sexual functioning (43) of dialysis patients (92). Stout et al. (108) investigated the patients' (n = 133) concerns and feeling of their sex life. There was no significant difference between CAPD-patients and HD-patients. About 40% of the patients reported no change in sexual relationships after the treatment start but 52% reported a significant deterioriation. 87% of 115 patients were very or moderately satisfied with their marriage but 63% of them had a very limited or non-existent sexual relationship on dialysis treatment.

ERYTHROPOIETIN

The introduction of Erythropoietin (Epo) in the clinical practice of patients on chronic dialysis (11, 109) started an impressive change in the life of patients on chronic dialysis treatment. The most striking effects have been a decrease in the need of blood transfusions and an increase in hemoglobin (Hb) values. Even a relatively moderate increase of hemoglobin had major effects on the QL of dialysis patients (106). The used instrument, sickness impact profile, showed significant improvements after Epo-therapy in the physical and psychosocial scores as in total scores. Most striking effects were found in the dimensions of ambulation, mobility, sleep disorders, social interaction, recreation and work. The improved work status did unfortunately not result in increased employment which just reflects the multi dimensional origin of vocational rehabilitation. Among important factors for vocational rehabilitation are comorbid conditions that limit the effect of Epo on the QL of dialysis patients. The effects of Epo seem to be significant after a relatively short time of therapy and further improvements on QL are less impressive with time (110). This may be a reflection of that further oxygen uptake after Epo-therapy after reaching Hb-values above 100 g/l are not significant (111). It seems, however, that the long term improvement of peripheral oxygen availability leads to a further increase of the anaerobic treshold in HD-patients without further increase of Hb-values. Hemodynamic changes and improvements in physical performance have also been demonstrated to appear after modest increments in hemoglobin (112) after Epo-therapy to 12 HD-patients. The reached test values were below matched non-uremic controls in spite of the increased Hb-values after Epo-therapy. Studies by Lewis et al. confirmed this (113).

Both children and adults with chronic renal failure suffer from impaired cognitive functions (114, 115). Hemodialysis alone seems to improve most of these functions (116, 117). In spite of these longterm improvements the hemodialysis procedure has been shown to impair the cognitive function of the patient compared to immediately before the start of the dialysis (118). Chronic anemia in itself is detrimental to the development of children even without renal failure. Epo has been shown to improve the cognitive functions in children on dialysis with e.g. increased ability to attend, concentrate and improved short term memory (119). Improved cognitive functions have also been registered in adults after Epo-treatment (117, 120–122). Cognitive functions may be investigated both as neuropsychologic and electrophysiologic tests. The former reflect motor and peripheral task performances. The latter reflect functions of the central nervous system. Stimulus related evoked potentials representing stable cortical sequences of EEG peaks improved significantly after Hb-increasing Epo-therapy (123). In the same study of 15 chronic HD-patients the psychometric trailmaking test showed a tendency to improvement. Both tests seem to confirm a positive effect of Epo on the brain dysfunction of anemic patients on chronic HD. Lundin (124) demonstrated with the use of cognitive event-related-potential that the amplitude of the so called component P3 latency improved after Epo-therapy. This P3 latency reflects the efficiency of information processing and is uneffected by mood. If the improvements after Epo-therapy only is an effect of increasing the Hb-value is still an open question. Some cognitive functional deficits have not been corrected until after a successful kidney transplantation.

In spite of the multitude of instruments used to measure QL all studies have shown an increased QL of the dialysis patients after a relatively short time after the start of regular use of Epo. Most apparent QL effects have been seen on physical symptoms. Wolcott et al. (121) demonstrated in a study of 15 relatively young patients on stable chronic hemodialysis, where a great number of QL investigational instruments was used, that Epo-therapy was associated with minimal improvements in social adaptation but marked improved energy levels and psychological improvements. Using an interviewer technique on complaints in a placebo controlled trial (125) significant improvements were found on the patient's fatigue, muscular weakness, palpitations, vertigo and dyspnoea. The comprehensive double blind randomised Canadian study including 118 patients on hemodialysis (23) verified these results including improved exercise results. This study, however, was more sensitive concerning changes in QL as three investigational instruments were used. After Epo-therapy for six months improvements were registered concerning relations and depression. The trade off technique did not demonstrate any improvement in overall quality of life. No improvement was detected in the aggregated psycho-social score investigated with the SIP instrument. Significant improvements were noted in the responses for the questions concerned with communication and, e.g., home maintenance. An improvement was also seen with the exercise test but not with a six minute walk test. This might reflect a difference between the patients' functional capacity and the physical symptoms reported by the patients in the kidney disease questionnaire (126). Delano (127) observed in 37 patients on hemodialysis after Epo-therapy an increased sense of well-being, less sleep distur-

bances, improvements in socializing and in sexual function. The impact of psychosocial factors and disturbed hormonal profiles in HD-patientes e.g. hyperprolactinemia (128) on sexual function is partly unclear. Improvement in sexual function has been confirmed by e.g. Bommer et al. in a small study of male HD-patients (129). In spite of the self reported improved sexual function after 10 months of Epo-therapy there was no significant changes in the profile of sexual hormones e.g. testosterone, estradiol, prolactin, luteinizing hormone or follicle stimulating hormone.

SIP and the Karnofsky performance scale (KPS) questionnaires were used by Valderrabano et al. (130) in 57 Epo-treated patients and 29 control patients on HD. The older patients showed indicators of worse QL before therapy than those below the age of 60 years. The improvements of QL after Epo-therapy seem to be of the same magnitude of patients above or below the age of 60 years. The KPS-score improved as well as the physical psychosocial and global score in SIP.

In a small number of patients responding to Epo an improvement in health satisfaction and well-being was found when investigated with a self report questionnaire (131). The latter was verified by Auer et al. (132). This study also indicated a decreased social isolation and better relationships including sex life. The used instrument (Nottingham Health Profile) made it possible to compare the QL of hemodialysis patients with scores of the general population (GP). The areas of energy, emotional well-being and pain were found to be equal to the general population. Social isolation, physical mobility and sleep disturbances remained to be worse among Epo-treated HD-patients in comparison with GP-norms. Comparisons with GP is important as there seems to be wide variations on the perspectives of QL among patients in active treatment of uremia. The subjective impression of QL increased after Epo-therapy to HD-patients to at least a level comparable to the GP and to patients with well functional kidney transplants (102). The overall life satisfaction results were also very high for the Epo-treated patients. The results were even higher than for the GP. This was also true for the subjective measure of happiness. Effective Epo-treatment of patients on CAPD have been reported to have a great impact on the QL of these patients (133). Significant improvements on energy and emotional well-being were seen. The above mentioned small changes in Epo-treated hemodialysis patients on psychosocial functions were more pronounced in CAPD patients. Both social adaptation and interests showed significant increases. It has also been reported that patients on CAPD show better scores on all neuropsychologic tests, show less mood disturbances and experience a higher QL than patients on HD (122). Again patient selection hampers adequate comparisons between patients on HD and CAPD.

The most constant adverse effect being an increase in diastolic blood pressure (23, 122, 126, 134) has not been

Table 1. Examples of the most often used quality of life instruments used among patients on chronic idalysis. (n) refers only to one example in the list of references. Some recent tests are included

Global instruments	
Sickness impact profile	(113)
Nottingham health profile	(134)
Spitzer quality of life index	(27)
Global adjustment to illness scale	(91)
Functional assessment instrument	
Karnofsky performance scale	(71)
Barthel index	(62)
Health assessment questionnaire	(139)
Activities of daily living index	(64)
ESRF activities of daily living scale	(142)
Disease specific instruments	
Kidney specific questionnaire	(140)
ESRD specific health questionnaire	(141)
Leicester uremic symptom scale	(142)
CAPD self-efficacy scale	(142)
Mental, psychological and emotional instruments	
General health questionnaire	(96)
Profile of mood states	(143)
Bradburn' affect balance scale	(144)
Campell' index of well-being	(18)
Cantril' life satisfaction scale	(66)
Psychological general well-being index	(145)
Beck' depression index	(26)
Hamilton depression scale	(58)
Wechsler adult intelligence scale	(117)
Self-esteem scale	(49)
Mental health index	(16)
Cognitive function tests	(122)
Perceived intrusiveness ratings scale	(87)

difficult to control. The registered increase in appetite results in an increase of ingested protein and an increased electrolyte imbalance which in turn may increase the need for dialysis. The risk of decreased compliance cannot be ignored. The increased blood viscosity (135) with Epo-treatment may lead to increased fistula clotting and an increased need of anticoagulants during dialysis. A careful clinical observation and monitoring of the Epo-dose minimizes these potentially adverse effects. A few cases of appearing anti Epo antibodies after Epo-therapy have been reported (136). The beneficial effects of Epo-therapy for the QL of patients on chronic dialysis are so great that manageable side effects should not preclude Epo-treatment in any patient on chronic dialysis therapy with low Hb-values.

COMMENTS

The technical and clinical development of all modes of dialysis has been rapid during the last decade why many early studies on QL of chronic dialysis patients have lost some relevance. The increased acceptance rate for dialysis of elderly patients, patients with serious comorbid diseases and the increased casemix increases the difficulties of measuring QL of patients on chronic dialysis. The impact on the social net work and on the renal staff has also increased parallell to the increased survival of the increased number of patients with non-renal complications. Harris et al. (137) demonstrated in 360 patients (60% of eligible patients) with moderate chronic renal insufficiency that these patients were significantly disabled compared to a general population even before reaching the state of uremia. The importance and association of sociodemographic factors, comorbid conditions and functional status was demonstrated with the sickness impact profile instrument, diagnoses, laboratory tests and sociodemographic data. Several factors were scewed in the material which decrease the total relevance of the study. The results are an important reminder of that QL investigations ought to start early in the course of chronic renal disease in order to alleviate or prevent the impact of active treatment of uremia on all aspects of QL of these patients.

CRUDE GUIDE LINES

It may be somewhat impertinent to try to present some rough guide lines in measuring the QL in the clinical setting of ESRD patients in chronic dialysis. Most QL instruments have been worked out and tested in university hospitals and similar environment by world experts in the different aspects of QL. It is of importance whether a nurse, social worker, physician or the patient himself should complete the appropriate questionnaire. Quality of life must be based on the patient's own opinions. This QL-picture may be completed by a spouse, close relative or other significant person in the patient's net work. Different medical disabilities may restrict the patient's own completing a questionnaire. In that situation one or two well informed and to the patient well known interviewers can be of help. An interaction between patient and interviewer is used in the kidney specific questionnaire (139). To measure QL is, however, very important wherever patients are treated with chronic dialysis. The individual variations in the valuation of quality of life are great why some estimation of each patient's concepts of his quality of life during the different treatment stages of ESRD are important to follow. When the patients are asked to define what they include in the term quality of life physical and social dimensions seem to be most important (145).

In the ideal situation medical decisions ought to be used together with different QL dimensions to make up the guide lines for interactive changes of the therapy for the individual patient. This makes great demands on the QL instruments.

As mentioned above cultural, social and comorbid conditions may differ and have such a great impact that one QL-instrument valuable in one geographical area is not sensitive enough in another area. It may be tempting to invent your own questionnaire or QL-instrument. The conditions for this procedure is a valuation to tested and accepted QL-instruments for a correct validation and reliability testing of the new test instrument. Reliability increases with the length of the instrument as the error of the measurements can be reduced. To use a single item is not acceptable as a measure of a latent QL dimension. An attractive way is to select a battery of subscales e.g. physical function from several different multi-item instruments to gain more depth in the QL dimension of special interest in the planned study. This battery approach has demonstrated good results in other medical situations (146).

Before starting investigations of QL you have to form the study design and intentions with the QL measurements. Secondly you have to try and define which aspects of medical and QL dimensions are needed for this goal. Thirdly you have to try and find one or probably a few QL-instruments that fulfil your intentional requirements. This has to be weighed against practical considerations as costs, time and mode of administration. All QL-instruments have drawbacks and limitations why probably two or three instruments will be needed for comprehensive QL valuations. If the planned investigation is to be performed at a single centre and be of cross-sectional character simpler instruments may be used than in studies of multicentric origin or in studies over long time. The sensitivity of the instrument to changes is then important (147). Special requirements have to be put to instruments intended to be used for comparisons with the general population. The relationship between health status and the quality of life measurements are complicated and may have to include the quality of environment and community life (148).

The question may arise if a disease specific instrument is to be used or a generic instrument (Table 1). Both kinds of instruments have their advantages. Disease specific instruments may indicate relatively little about the patient's overall well-being and health. Again a combination of instruments may be the best solution (149). Disease specific instruments are more responsive to changes e.g. in randomized trials than generic instruments. These may be advantageous in comparisons with the general population and may be of use as guide lines in resource allocations. Considerations of using a global index of quality of life is, however, in many ways not different from the process of making clinical decisions. The choice of psychometric scales are also important as the tests that rely very much on

somatic equivalents of depressions have demonstrated a higher prevalence of depressions among dialysis patients than tests that are not strongly relying on somatic symptoms (150). For measurements of changes over shorter periods of time visual analogue scales (151, 152) may be useful.

CONCLUSIVE REMARKS

The quality of life among patients on chronic dialysis is increasingly important when therapeutic interventions are planned e.g. the effect of growth hormone may be measured in controlled intervention trials. As the QL valuations differ among patients as a consequence of age, disease, education, mode of treatment etc. the need for longitudinal studies for the individual patient increases. QL instruments have to be reliable and have a high degree of validity. The ideal model for quality of life and health status outcome does not exist today. With increasing experience of which QL dimensions that are most important for the endstage renal disease patients a continuous change of QL-instruments can be expected. These have to be used together with clinical objective measurements for the benefit of the chonically dialyzed patient.

REFERENCES

1. Deniston L, Carpentier-Alting P, Kneisley J, Hawthorne V, Port F: Assessment of Quality of life in end-stage renal disease. *Health Services Research* 24: 555, 1989
2. Ehrlich J, Geerlings W, Jones E, Landais P, Loirat C, Mallick N, Margreiter R, Raine A, Saker L, Salmela K, Selwood N, Tufveson G, Valderrabano F: Report on management of renal failure in Europe. *XXIII* 9: 6, 1994
3. Grant A, Rodger S, Horwie C, Junor B, Briggs D, Macdougal A: Dialysis at home in the West of Scotland: a comparison of hemodialysis and continuous ambulatory peritoneal dialysis in age and sex-matched controls. *Perit Dial Int* 12: 365, 1992
4. Evans R, Manninen D, Garrison L, Hunt L, Blagg C, Gutman R, Hull A, Lowrie E: The quality of life of patients with end-stage renal disease. *N Eng J Med* 312: 553, 1985
5. Simmons R, Anderson C, Abress L: Quality of life and rehabilitation differences among four end-stage renal disease therapy groups. *Scand J Urol Nephrol* 24 (Suppl 131): 7, 1990
6. Hart G, Evans R: The functional status of ESRD patients as measured by the sickness impact profile. *J Chron Dis* 40 (Suppl 1): 117, 1987
7. Ahlmén J, Carlsson C, Schönborg C: Well-informed patients with end-stage renal disease prefer peritoneal dialysis to hemodialysis. *Perit Dial Int* 13 (Suppl 2): 196, 1993
8. Callender C, Jennings P, Bayton J, Flores J, Tagunicar H, Yeager C, Bond O: Psychologic factors related to dialysis in kidney transplant decisions. *Transplant Proc* 21: 1976, 1989

9. Kjellstrand CM: Age, sex and race inequality in renal transplantation. *Arch Intern Med* 148: 1305, 1988

10. Voigts A, Felsenfeld A, Llach F: The effects of calciferol and its metabolites on patients with renal failure. II. Calciferol, 1-alfha-hydroxy vitamin D3 and 24,25-dehydroxy vitamin D3. *Arch Intern Med* 143: 1205, 1983

11. Eschbach J, Egrie J, Downing M, Browne J, Adamson J: Correction of the anemia of end-stage renal disease with recombinant human erytropoietin, results of phase I and II clinical trial. *N Eng J Med* 316: 73, 1987

12. Kaye M, Lella J: Discontinuation of dialysis therapy in the demented patient. *Am J Nephrol* 6: 75, 1986

13. Rothenberg LS: Witholding and withdrawing dialysis from elderly ESRD patients. Part 1. A historical view of the clinical experience. *Geriatric Nephrology and Urology* 2: 109, 1992

14. Rothenberg L: Withholding and withdrawing dialysis from elderly ESRD patients: Part 2 – ethical and policy issues. *Geriatric Nephrology and Urology* 3: 23, 1993

15. Mandai T, Ohashi H, Ishii K, Ono M, Kishi K, Hashimoto Y, Minakata T, Tahagi J, Fujita A, Egoh Y, Tsuchiga K, Sacki H, Fakashima S, Asahi T, Mandai K, Adachi K, Maruyama S, Morimoto K: Quality of life in patients with hemodialysis, coronary artery by pass graft (CABG) surgery and mammary cancer. *Quality of Life Research* 3: 85, 1994

16. Casselith B, Lusk E, Strouse T, Miller D, Brown L, Cross P, Tenaglia A: Psychosocial status in chronic illness. A comparative analysis of six diagnostic groups. *N Eng J Med* 311: 506, 1984

17. Karnofsky D, Bucherval J: in *The Clinical Evaluation of Chemotherapeutic Agents in Cancer*, edited by Macleod CM, New York, Colombia University Press, 1949

18. Campell A, Converse P, Rodgers W: *The Quality of American Life*, New York, Russel Sage Foundation, 1976

19. Cantril H: *The Patterns of Human Concerns*, New Brunswick, Rutgers University press, 1965

20. Hunt S, McKenna S, McEwen J: The Nottingham Health Profile: subjective status and medical consultations. *Soc Sci Med* 15: 221, 1981

21. Hunt S, McKenna S, McEwen J, Buchett E, Williams J, Papp E: A quantitative approach to perceived health status: a validation study. *J Epidemiology and Community Health* 34: 281, 1980

22. Bergner M, Bobbitt R, Kressel S, Pollard W, Gibson B, Morris J: The Sickness Impact Profile: conceptual formulation and methology for the development of a health status measure. *Inf J Health Serv* 6: 393, 1978

23. Laupacis A, Canadian Erytropoietin Study Group: Association between recombinant human erytropoietin and quality of life and exercise capacity of patients receiving hemodialysis. *Br Med J* 300: 573, 1990

24. Wells L, Marwell G: *Self-Esteem: Its Conceptualization and Measurements*, Beverly Hills, California, Sage Publications Inc, 1976

25. Simmons RG, Klein SD, Simmons RL: *Gift of Life. The Effect of Organ Transplantation on Individual Family and Social Dynamics*, New Brunswick (USA) and Oxford (UK), Transaction Books, 1987

26. Beck AT, Ward C, Mendelsohn M, Mock J, Erbaugh J: An inventory for measuring depression. *Arch Gen Psychiatry* 4: 561, 1961

27. Spitzer W, Dobson A, Hall J, Cesterman E, Levi J, Shepherd R, Battista R, Catchlove B: Measuring the quality of life of cancer patients: a concise QL-index for use by physicians. *J Chron Dis* 34: 585, 1981

28. Churchill D, Torrance G, Taylor D, Barnes C, Ludwin D, Shimiza A, Smith E: Measurement of quality of life in end-stage renal disease: the time trade-off approach. *Clin Invest Med* 10: 14, 1987

29. Hornberger J, Redelmeier D, Petersen J: Variability among methods to assess patients' well-being and consequent effect on a cost-effectiveness analysis. *J Clin Epidemiol* 45: 505, 1992

30. Fukunishi J: Psychosomatic aspects of patients on hemodialysis. 3. Clinical usefulness of alexithymia. *Psychother Psychosom* 54: 214, 1990

31. Dew M, Simmons R: The advantage of multiple measures of quality of life. *Scand J Urol Nephrol* 24 (Suppl 131): 23, 1990

32. Wolfe R, Port F, Hawthorne W, Guire K: A comparison of survival among dialysis therapies of choice: in center hemodialysis versus continuous ambulatory peritoneal dialysis at home. *Am J Kidney Dis* 15: 433, 1990

33. Maiorca R, Vonesch EF, Cavalli P, de Vecchi A, Giangrande A, La Greca G, Scarpioni L, Bragantini L Castelnuovo C, Castiglioni A, Poisette P, Viglino G: A multicenter, selection adjusted comparison of patient and technique survival on CAPD and hemodialysis. *Perit Dial Int* 11: 118, 1991

34. Wright L: Survival in patients with end-stage renal disease. *Am J Kidney Dis* 17: 25, 1991

35. Lundin A, Adler A, Feinroth M: Maintenance hemodialysis. Survival beyond the first decade. *JAMA* 244: 38, 1983

36. Lowrie E, Lew N: Death risk in hemodialysis patients: the predictive value of commonly measured variables and an evaluation of death rate differences between facilities. *Am J Kidney Dis* 15: 458, 1990

37. Stewart J, Schvanefeldt N, Christensen N, Lauritzen G, Stein D: The effect of computerized dietary analysis, nutrition education on nutrition, knowledge, nutrition status, dietary compliance and quality of life of hemodialysis patients. *J Renal Nutrition* 3: 177, 1993

38. Gotch F, Yarian S, Keen M: A kinetic survey of US hemodialysis prescriptions. *Am J Kidney Dis* 15: 511, 1990

39. Acchiardo S, Runyan K, Hattem K, Ryson B, Faller J, Moore L, Jackson M: Impact of KT/V and protein catabolic rate (PCR) on hemodialysis (HD) mortality. (Abstract) *JASN* 3: 351, 1992

40. Ahmad S, Cole J: Lower morbidity associated with higher KT/V in stable hemodialysis patients. (Abstract) *JASN* 1: 346, 1990

41. Churchill D, Wallace J, Ludwin D, Beecroft M, Taylor W: A comparison of evaluative indices of quality of life and cognitive function in hemodialysis patients. *Controlled Clinical Trials* 12: 159, 1991

42. Kutner N, Brogan D, Kutner M: End-stage renal disease treatment modality and patients' quality of life. Longitudinal assessment. *Am J Nephrol* 6: 396, 1986

43. Lindsay R, Oreopoulus D, Burton H, Conley J, Wells G, Fenton S: Adaptation to home dialysis: a comparison of continuous ambulatory peritoneal dialysis and hemodialysis. in *Continuous Ambulatory Peritoneal Dialysis*, edit-

ed by Legrain M, Amsterdam, Excerpta Medica, 1980, p 120

44. Mejia G, Zimmerman S: Comparison of CAPD and hemodialysis for diabetics. *Perit Dial Bull* 5: 7, 1985
45. Burton H, Kline S, Lindsay R, Heidenheim A: The relationship of depression to survival in chronic renal failure. *Psychosomatic Medicine* 48: 261, 1986
46. Shulman R, Price J, Spinelli J: Bio psychosocial aspects of long term survival on endstage renal failure therapy. *Psychological Medicine* 19: 945, 1989
47. Gotch F, Sargent J: A mechnistic analysis of the National Cooperative Dialysis study (NCDS). *Kidney Int* 28: 526, 1985
48. Auer J, Gokal R, Stout J, Hillier V, Kincey J, Simon L, Oliver D: The Oxford-Manchester Study of dialysis patients. *Scand J Urol Nephrol* 24 (Suppl 131): 31, 1991
49. Klein S, Simmons R: The psychosocial impact of chronic kidney disease on children. in *Gift of Life*, edited by Simons RG, Klein SD, Simmons RL, New Brunswick (USA) and Oxford (UK), Transaction books, 1987, p 89
50. Roscoe J, Smith L, Williams A, Stein M, Morton R, Williamson Balfe J, Arbus G: Medical and social outcome in adolescents with endstage renal failure. *Kidney Int* 40: 948, 1991
51. Westlie L, Umen A, Nestrud S, Kjellstrand C: Mortality morbidity and life satisfaction in the very old dialysis patients. *Trans Am Soc Artif Intern Organs* 30: 21, 1984
52. Loew H: Die Dauerdialysebehandlung in hoheren Lebensalter. *Z Gerontol* 20: 52, 1987
53. McKevitt P, Jones J, Marion R: The elderly on dialysis: physical and psychosocial functioning. *Dialysis and Transplantation* 15: 130, 1986
54. Neu S, Kjellstrand C: Stopping long term dialysis: an empirical study of withdrawal of life supporting treatment. *N Eng J Med* 314: 14, 1986
55. Roberts J, Kjellstrand C: Choosing Death. *Acta Med Scand* 223: 181, 1988
56. Wehle B, Ahlmén J: Prudent withdrawal of chronic dialysis treatment. *Scand J Urol Nephrol* 24 (Suppl 131): 47, 1990
57. Schnack S, Eigler J, Schiffl H, Gurland H-J, Segerer W: Lebensqualität älterer Patienten unter den Bedingungen der Dauerdialyse. *Deutsch Med Wshr* 115: 1043, 1990
58. Iordanidis P, Alivanis P, Iakovidis A, Dombros N, Tsagalidis I, Balaskus E, Derveniotis V, Ierodiakonou C, Tourkantonis A: Psychiatric and psychosocial status of elderly patients undergoing dialysis. *Perit Dial Int* 13 (Suppl 2): 192, 1992
59. Morgan B: The relationship between chronological age and perceived quality of life of hemodialysis patients. *ANNA J* 17: 63, 1990
60. Kutner N, Brogan D: Assisted survival aging and rehabilitation needs: comparison of older dialysis patients and age-matched peers. *Arch Phys Med Rehabil* 73: 309, 1992
61. Jacobson S, Fryd D, Lins LE, Matson M, Sutherland D, Kjellstrand C: Transplantation, hemodialysis and continuous ambulatory peritoneal dialysis for end-stage renal disease in diabetic patients. *J Diabet Complications* 2: 150, 1988
62. Borgel F, Benhamou P, Zmirou D, Balducci F, Halimi S, Cordonnier D: Assessment of handicap in chronic dialysis diabetic patients (uremidiab § study). *Scand J Rehab Med* 24: 203, 1992

63. Borgel F, Pasqvier B, Benhamou P, Halimi S: Evaluation du handicap chez le patient diabetique. *Ann Readapt Med Phys* 33: 81, 1990
64. Julius M, Hawthorne V, Carpentier-Alting P, Kneisley J, Wolfe R, Port F: Independence in activities of daily living for end-stage renal disease patients: biomedical and demographic correlates. *Am J Kidney Dis* 13: 61, 1989
65. Fukunishi I: Psychosomatic aspects of patients on hemodialysis. Alexithymic trait of hemodialysis patients with diabetic nephropathy. *Psychother Psychosom* 52: 58, 1989
66. Hoothay F, De Stefano A, Leary E, Foley-Hartel T: Life Satisfaction and coping of diabetic hemodialysis patients. *ANNA J* 17: 361, 1990
67. Reiss D: Patient, family and staff responses to end-stage renal disease. *Am J Kidney Dis* 15: 194, 1990
68. Tzamaloukas A, Murphy G, Spalding T: Diabetic nephropathy eleven-year survival on hemodialysis. *Clin Nephrol* 38: 234, 1992
69. Flynn C: Why blind diabetics with renal failure should be offered treatment. *Br Med J* 287: 1177, 1983
70. Comty C, Leonard A, Shapiro F: Psychosocial problems in dialyzed diabetic patients. *Kidney Int* 6 (Suppl 1): 144, 1974
71. Wai L, Burton H, Richmond J, Lindsay R: Influence of psychosocial factors on survival of home-dialysis patients. *Lancet* ii: 155, 1981
72. McClellan W, Anson C, Birkeli K, Tuttle E: Functional status and quality of life: predictors of early mortality among patients entering treatment for end stage renal disease. *J Clin Epidemiol* 44: 83, 1991
73. King K: Noncompliance in the chronic dialysis population. *Dialysis & Transplantation* 20: 67, 1991
74. Manley M, Sweeney J: Assessment of compliance in hemodialysis adaptation. *J Psychosom Res* 30: 153, 1986
75. Kimmel P: Towards a developmental view of end-stage renal disease. *Am J Kidney Dis* 15: 191, 1990
76. Blodgett C: A selected review of the literature of adjustment to hemodialysis. *Int J Psychiatry Med* 11: 97, 1981
77. Kaplan De Nour A: Persönlichkeitsfaktorer und Adaptation. in *Psychonephrologie*, edited by Balch FB, Koch U, Speidel H, Berlin, Heidelberg, New York, Tokyo, Springer-Verlag, 1985, p 303
78. Friedlander R, Viedermann M: Children of dialysis patients. *Am J Psychiatry* 139: 100, 1982
79. Sensky T: Psychosomatic aspects of end-stage renal failure. *Psychother Psychosom* 59: 56, 1993
80. Chowance G, Binik Y: End stage renal disease and the marital dyad: an empirical investigation. *Soc Sci Med* 28: 971, 1989
81. Soskolne V, Kaplan De-Nour A: The psychosocial adjustment of patients and spouses to dialysis treatment. *Soc Sci Med* 29: 497, 1989
82. Kaplan De Nour A: Stresses and reactions of professional hemodialysis staff. *Dial Transplant* 13: 137, 1984
83. Ferrans C, Powers M: Quality of life index: development and psychometric properties. *Advances in Nursing Science* 8: 15, 1985
84. Ferrans C, Powers M, Kasch C: Satisfaction with health care of hemodialysis patients. *Research in Nursing & Health* 10: 367, 1987

85. Larsen D, Rootman I: Physician role performance and patient satisfaction. *Soc Sci Med* 10: 29, 1976
86. Levy N: Psychological reaction to machine dependency. *Psychiatry Clinics of North America* 13: 246, 1981
87. Devins G: Illness intrusiveness and quality of life in end-stage renal disease: comparison and stability across treatment modalities. *Health Psychology* 9: 117, 1990
88. Morris P, Jones B: Life satisfaction across treatment methods for patients with end-stage renal failure. *Med J Austr* 150: 428, 1989
89. Morris P, Jones B: Transplantation versus dialysis: a study of quality of life. *Transplant Proc* 20: 23, 1988
90. Koch V, Muthny F: Quality of life in patients with end-stage renal disease in relation to the method of treatment. *Psychother Psychosom* 54: 161, 1990
91. Wolcott D, Nissenson A: Quality of life in chronic dialysis patients: a critical comparison of continuous ambulatory peritoneal dialysis and hemodialysis. *Am J Kidney Dis* 9: 402, 1988
92. Schlebusch L, Botha G, Bosch B: Coping styles in hemodialysis and continuous peritoneal dialysis patients. *Dial Transplant* 13: 517, 1984
93. Yanagida E, Streltzer J, Siemsen A: Denial in dialysis patients: relationship to compliance and other variables. *Psychosomatic Medicine* 43: 271, 1981
94. Theorell T, Konarski-Svensson J, Ahlmén J, Perski A: The role of paid work in Swedish chronic dialysis patients nation – wide survey: paid work and dialysis. *J Int Med* 230: 501, 1991
95. Wolcott D, Nissenson A, Landswerk J: Quality of life in chronic dialysis patients. Factors unrelated to dialysis modality. *General Hospital Psychiatry* 10: 2647, 1988
96. Livesley J: Factors associated with psychiatric symptoms in patients undergoing chronic hemodialysis. *Can J Psychiatry* 26: 562, 1981
97. Sayag R, Kaplan De-Nour A, Shapira Z, Kahan E, Boner G: Comparison of psychosocial adjustment of male non diabetic kidney transplant and hospital hemodialysis patients. *Nephron* 54: 214, 1990
98. Parfrey P, Vavasour H, Bullock M, Harnett J, Gault M: Symptoms in end-stage renal disease: dialysis and transplantation. *Transplantation Proc* 19: 3407, 1987
99. Parfrey P, Vavasour H, Gault M: A prospective study of health status in dialysis and transplant patients. *Transplantation Proc* 20: 1231, 1988
100. Fox E, Peace K, Neale T, Morrison R, Hatfield P, Mellsop G: 'Quality of life for patients with end-stage renal failure. *Renal Failure* 13: 31, 1991
101. Tucker C, Ziller R, Smith W, Mars D, Coons M: Quality of life of patients on in-center hemodialysis versus continuous ambulatory peritoneal dialysis. *Perit Dial Int* 11: 341, 1991
102. Evans R: Recombinant human erythropoietin and the quality of life of end-stage renal disease patients: a comparative analysis. *Am J Kidney Dis* 18 (Suppl 1): 62, 1991
103. Julius M, Kneisley J, Carpentier-Alting P, Hawthorne V, Wolfe R, Port F: A comparison of employment rates of patients treated with continuous ambulatory peritoneal dialysis vs in center hemodialysis. *Arch Intern Med* 149: 839, 1989
104. Procci W: Male sexual functioning and maintenance hemodialysis: a prospective study. *Dial Transplant* 13: 100, 1984
105. Freeman C, Calsyn D, Sherrard D, Paige A: Psychological assessment of renal dialysis patients using standard psychomatric techniques. *J Consulting and Clinical Psychology* 48: 537, 1980
106. McMahon L, Dawborn J: Subjective quality of life assessment in hemodialysis patients at different levels of hemoglobin following use of recombinant human erytropoietin. *Am J Nephrol* 12: 162, 1992
107. Levy N: Sexual adjustment to maintenance hemodialysis and renal transplantation. National survey by questionnaire. Preliminary report. *Trans Am Soc Artif Intern Organs* 19: 138, 1973
108. Stout J, Auer J, Kincey J, Hillier U, Gokal R, Simon G, Oliver D: Sexual and marital relationships and dialysis – the patients's viewpoint. *Perit Dial Bull* 7: 97, 1987
109. Winearls C, Oliver D, Pippard M, Reid C, Downing M, Coles P: Effects of human erytropoietin derived from recombinant DNA on the anemia of patients maintained by chronic hemodialysis. *Lancet* ii: 1175, 1986
110. Wadhwa N, Friend R, Russo N, Cabralda T, Howell N, Suh H: Erytropoietin and quality of life in ESRD patients. (Abstract] *J Am Soc Nephrol* 2: 390, 1991
111. Mayer G, Thum J, Cada E, Stummvoll H, Graf H: Aerobic and anaerobic exercise capacity in patients on chronic hemodialysis and long-term recombinant human erytropoietin therapy. *Nephron* 51 (Suppl 1): 34, 1989
112. McMahon L, Johns J, McKenzie A, Austin M, Fowler R: Hemodynamic changes and physical performance at comparative levels of hemoglobin after long term treatment with recombinant erytopoietin. *Nephrol Dial Transplant* 7: 1199, 1992
113. Lewis N, Macdougall I, Coles G, Williams J, Fox K, Increased exercise capacity and reversal of exercise induced myocardial ischemia in hemodialysis patients treated with recombinant human erythropoietin. *Br Heart J* 61: 436, 1989
114. Osberg J, Meares G, McKee D, Burnett G: Intellectual functioning in renal failure and chronic dialysis. *J Chronic Dis* 35: 445, 1982
115. Fennell R, Rasbury W, Fennell E, Morris M: Effects of kidney transplantation on cognitive performance in a pediatric population. *Pediatrics* 74: 273, 1984
116. Corea A: Case management of the anemic patient: epoetin alfa-focus on cognitive function. *ANNA J* 20: 350, 1993
117. Nissenson A: Recombinant human erytropoietin: impact on brain and cognitive function, exercise tolerance, sexual potency and quality of life. *Semin Nephrol* 9 (Suppl 2): 25, 1989
118. Smith B, Winslow E, Cognitive changes in chronic renal patients during hemodialysis. *ANNA J* 17;283, 1990
119. Turner M, Ongkingco R, Hersch S, Moss H, El-Amin D, Ruley E: Effect of r-erythropoietin (Epo) on cognitive function of children with chronic failure. (Abstract) *J Am Soc Nephrol* 2: 390, 1991
120. Wolcott D, Schweitzer S, Marsh J, Nissenson A: Recombinant erythropoietin improves cognitive function and quality of life (QL) of chronic hemodialysis patients. (Abstract) *Kidney Int* 33: 242, 1988
121. Wolcott D, Marsch J, La Rue A, Carr C, Nissenson A: Recombinant human erythropoietin treatment may improve quality of life and cognitive function in chronic hemodialysis patients. *Am J Kidney Dis* 14: 478, 1989

122. Nissenson AR: Cognitive function in dialysis patients: impact of epoietin alfa. *New Directions in Anemia* 2: 1, 1991

123. Grimm G, Stockenhuber F, Schneweiss B, Madl C, Zeitlhofer J, Schneider B: Improvement of brain function in hemodialysis patients treated with erytropoietin. *Kidney Int* 38: 480, 1990

124. Lundin AP: Quality of life. subjective and objective improvements with recombinant human erythropoietin therapy. *Semin Nephrol* 9 (Suppl 1): 22, 1989

125. Lillevang S, Bangsgaard Pedersen F: The quality of life for hemodialysis patients before and after erythropoietin treatment. A double-blind, randomized placebo-controlled investigation. *Ugeskr Laeger* 152: 2999, 1990

126. Laupacis A, Wong C, Churchill D and the Canadian erythropoietin study group: The use of generic and specific Quality-of-life measures in hemodialysis patients treated with erythropoietin. *Controlled Clinical Trials* 12 (Suppl): 168S, 1991

127. Delano B: Improvements in quality of life following treatment with r-Hu Epo in anemic hemodialysis patients. *Am J Kidney Dis* 14 (Suppl 2): 14, 1989

128. Foulks C, Cushner H: Sexual dysfunction in the male dialysis patient: pathogenesis, evaluation and therapy. *Am J Kidney Dis* 8: 211, 1986

129. Bommer J, Kugel M, Schwobel B, Ritz E, Barth H, Seelig R: Improved sexual function during recombinant human erythropoietin therapy. *Nephrol Dial Transplant* 5: 204, 1990

130. Valderrabano F, Moreno F, Arucil FJ, Principe de Asturias H, Gregorio Maranon H: A controlled study of the effect of erythropoietin on the quality of life of elderly hemodialysis patients.(Abstract) *J Am Soc Nephrol* 3: 432, 1992

131. Barany P, Pettersson E, Bergström J: Erytropoietin treatment improves quality of life in hemodialysis patients. *Scand J Urol Nephrol* 24 (Suppl 131): 55, 1990

132. Auer J, Oliver D, Winearls C: The quality of life of dialysis patients treated with recombinant human erythropoietin. *Scand J Urol Nephrol* 131 (Suppl 1): 61, 1990

133. Auer J, Simon G, Stevens J, Griffiths P, Howarth D, Amastassiades E, Gokal R, Oliver D: Quality of life improvements in CAPD-patients treated with subcutaneosly administered erythropoietin for anemia. *Perit Dial Int* 12: 40, 1992

134. Lazarus M: Update on adverse reactions to erythropoietin therapy. *ASAIO J* 40: 70, 1994

135. Brown C, Kierman M, Zhao Z-H, Larsson R, Friedman E: Treatment of azotemic, anemic patients with recombinant human erythropoietin raises whole blood viscosity proportional to hematocrit. (Abstract) *Kidney Int* 33: 184, 1988

136. Bergrem H, Danielsson B, Eckhardt K-U, Kurtz A, Stridsberg M: A case of antierythropoietin antibodies following recombinant human erythropoietin treatment. in *Erythropoietin Molecular Physiology and Clinical Applications*, edited by Bauer C, Koch KM, Scigalla P, Wieczorelke L, New York, Marcel Dekker Inc, 1993, p 265

137. Harris L, Luft F, Rudy D, Tierny M: Clinical correlates of functional status in patients with chronic renal insufficiency. *Am J Kidney Dis* 21: 161, 1993

138. Fries J, Spitz P, Kraines R, Holman R: Measurement of patient outcome in arthritis. *Arthritis and Rheumatism* 23: 137, 1980

139. Laupacis A, Muirhead N, Keown P, Wong C: A disease-specific questionnaire for assessing quality of life in patients on hemodialysis. *Nephron* 60: 302, 1992

140. Parfrey P, Vavasour H, Bullock M, Henry S, Harnett J, Gault M: Development of a health questionaire specific for end-stage renal disease. *Nephron* 52: 20, 1989

141. Wright S, Stein A, Boyle H, Moorhouse J, Walls J: Health-related quality of life in end-stage renal failure. (Abstract) *Quality of Life Research* 3: 63, 1994

142. McNair D, Lorr M, Doppleman L: *Profile of Mood Status Manual*, San Diego, Education and Industrial Testing Service, 1971

143. Bradburn N: *The Structure of Psychological Well-Being*, Chicago, Aldine Publishing Company, 1969

144. Fazio A: A concurrent valuational study of the NHCS general well-being schedule. Vital and Health Statistics. DHEW publication no (HRA) 78-1347, National Center for Health Statistics, Hyattsville, MD, 1977

145. Ahlmén J: Quality of life: views among patients on active treatment of uremia. *Scand J Urol Nephrol* 131 (Suppl 1): 43, 1990

146. Croog S, Levine S, Testa M: The effects of antihypertensive therapy on the quality of life. *N Eng J Med* 314: 1657, 1986

147. Gayatt G, Deyo R, Charlson M: Responsiveness and validity in health status measurement: a clarification. *J Clin Epidem* 42: 403, 1989

148. Bergner M: Quality of life, health status and clinical research. *Medical Care* 27: 148, 1989

149. Mosteller F, Ware J, Levine S: Comments on the conference on Advances in Health Status Assessment. *Medical Care* 27: 282, 1989

150. Kutner N, Fair P, Kutner M: Assessing depression and anxiety in chronic dialysis patients. *J Psychosom Res* 29: 23, 1985

151. Lichert R: A technique for the measurements of attitudes. *Arch Psychol* 1: 140, 1932

152. Scott J, Huskisson E: Graphic representation of pain. *Pain* 2: 175, 1976

STOPPING DIALYSIS
PRACTICE AND CULTURAL, RELIGIOUS AND LEGAL ASPECTS

CARL M. KJELLSTRAND, RONALD CRANFORD and MICHAEL KAYE

INTRODUCTION

Stopping dialysis, as a cause of death is common, particularly in North America. In the USA it is now the third most common cause of death in dialysis patients, and in Canada the second most common cause, after vascular deaths, as illustrated in Figure 1.

When dialysis is stopped the patient who needs it will invariably die. In 155 dialysis patients, we studied the consequences of stopping dialysis. Death occurred after a mean of 8.1 days (range 1–28 days) (1). The number of days from the last dialysis to the death of each patient is shown in Figure 2. Port and co-workers doing a similar analysis in 282 patients concluded that it took somewhat longer, about 10 days (2). One reason for the difference may be that CAPD patients have better preserved renal function.

The general practical outline to stopping dialysis is presented in Table 1 (3).

Although the table presents the approach in logical stepwise fashion on three planes, in fact these considerations are simultaneously considered and intertwined.

ETHICAL ANALYSIS

The three ethical principles which bear on stopping life support are beneficence, non-maleficence and autonomy. Using these principles, three approaches to ethics analysis are suggested.

The first is Kantian deontology. There is an apparent inflexibility when staunch right-to-life arguments are applied in such a way that sanctity of life trumps all other duties, and prohibits all thought of termination of life-sustaining treatment. However, most physicians do not hold that beneficence is captured by absolute sanctity of life arguments. They also do not subscribe to a view that beneficence always takes priority over duties to avoid maleficence or promote patient autonomy. For them, the 'categorical imperative' (or unconditional principle that can be universally applied) becomes 'physician have obligations to promote patients' autonomy and their best interests, not 'physicians are always obliged to preserve life under all conceivable conditions.' Once this flexibility is introduced and understood, the objection that deontologic analysis can be too rigid, even cruel, in medical decision-making is negated.

The second analytic approach is existentialist. It is clear that only competent patients can quantitate burdens and benefits and then do the balancing that results in a decision, using whatever basis for judgement that seems right for them, as individuals. If the patient is incompetent, close relatives and friends must judge what the patient would have wished to be done. We have previously shown, that the decision made by competent patients is identical to that made by physicians and families on behalf of the incompetent patient (4). Thus. the argument that no-one can decide for someone else that it is better to be dead, is not correct. On the contrary, one can turn the tables and ask why one should force an incompetent patient to accept a treatment that a competent patient would not accept. After all, an incompetent patient no longer can appreciate the benefits and purpose of dialysis and thus suffers more than a competent patient who

Table 1. The analysis of *stopping dialysis*

PLANE I – ETHICAL ANALYSIS

1. *ETHICAL FRAMEWORK* – KANTIAN DEONTOLOGY

	BENEFICENCE	– ('Sanctity of Life')
	NON-MALEFICENCE	– Do Not Cause Suffering
	AUTONOMY	– Respect Dignity and Difference

2. *INTELLECTUAL/EMOTIONAL ANALYSIS* – EXISTENTIALISM

Weight Burden *vs* Benefit: Suffering *vs* Lifegain
Non-maleficence and Autonomy *vs* Beneficence

3. *PRACTICAL ANALYSIS* CONSEQUENCE – CLASSICAL UTILITARIANISM
What are the alternatives?

ACT	CONSEQUENCES
Do Everything	Analyze
Change Course	and
Do Less	Predict
Stop Everything	

PLANE II – PRACTICAL ANALYSIS

1. MEDICAL ASPECTS:	Disease Understood
	Prognosis Known
	Maximal Care Tried
	Do Experts Agree
2. WHY DO YOU WANT TO STOP	Patient's Best Interest
	Family Desperate
	Friends Squeamish
	Team Discouraged
	You Depressed and Tired
3. MAKING THE DECISION	Be Prepared
	DISCUSS-LISTEN-DOCUMENT
4. UNSOLVABLES:	Patient Undecided or Periodically Lucid
	Family Feuds
5. WHAT DO YOU PLAN TO DO:	DO NOT KILL
	Do Not Practice Medical
	Scrupulosity

PLANE III – AFTER DISCONTINUATION

1. AFTER STOPPING	– Visit Patient
	– Do No Bloodsamples
	– Watch and Prevent Pulmonary Edema
2. AFTER PATIENT IS DEAD	– Follow up with Family
	– Consequences for Family

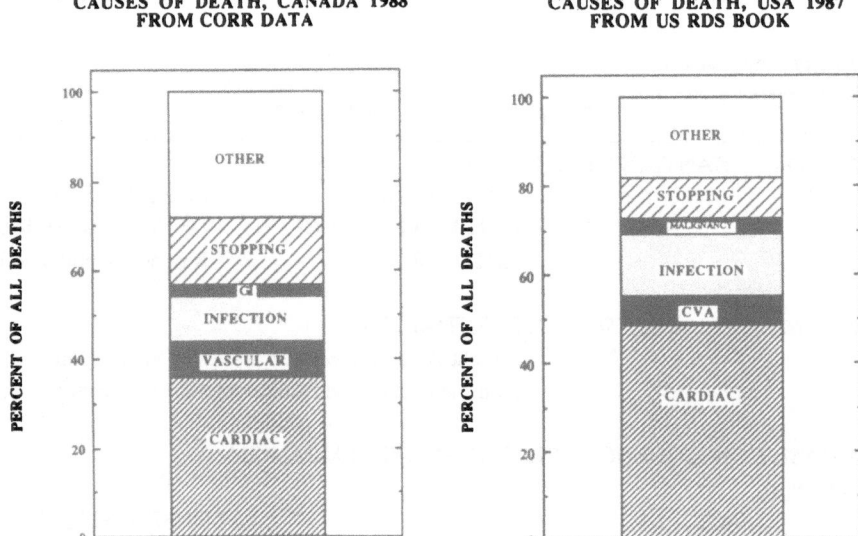

CAUSES OF DEATH, CANADA 1988
FROM CORR DATA

CAUSES OF DEATH, USA 1987
FROM US RDS BOOK

Figure 1. Causes of death in USA and Canada in the late 1980s. In Canada, stopping dialysis is the second most common cause of death, in the USA it is the third. CORR = Canadian Organ Replacement Registry, RDS = Renal Data System.

can still hopes for success or improvement. In such an analysis, one weighs non-maleficence and autonomy *versus* beneficence, here understood as sanctity of life. For the incompetent, the family and physician consider suffering and potential survival time and weigh these against each other to finally decide whether treatment should be continued or stopped. These family–physician considerations are similar to the Catholic church's consideration of extraordinary treatment where burdens against benefits are weighed (5). Obviously if patients are competent they do this weighing, using clear and accurate facts from their physicians, and emotional support from family, treatment team, physician and clergyman. An important duty here is for the physician to rule out underlying psychiatric abnormality which might induce the patient give up too early, and one must be sure that the patient has no treatable somatic complication which might tip the balance in favour of stopping treatment.

The third analytic approach is to perform an utilitarian analysis. One considers all possible treatment alternatives and tries to foresee positive and negative consequences and choose the course which maximizes benefit. Should one continue to do everything because there is a reasonable chance of improvement? Would shorter treatment times allow more freedom for the patient? Would dialysis away at a vacation facility be of help? Should one stop everything and let a patient die? Should one change course, is another dialysis method or dialysis place possible and would such a change help the patient? Would CAPD at home be more suitable for the in-centre patient, or would the reverse be true? Would it be better to stop treatment at home and transfer to in-centre to get the emotional support from the hospital team of caregivers?

In one article, it was more common for home dialysis patients than in-centre patients to stop treatment when there was no medical reason to do so (6). We speculated that at home, the patient was the only sick person with nobody but close family members on whom to vent anger and frustration, and was used to making important medical decisions alone. But the underlying equation was to maximize utility or most good for the patient – an exercise in act utilitarianism.

PRACTICAL ANALYSIS

Several medical aspects need consideration. Is the disease and its prognosis known and understood? The confusional dementia secondary to an acute illness such as septicemia in an old patient is different from the relentless downward course of dialysis dementia at the end-stage of aluminium intoxication or that secondary to many strokes. An endogenous depression may be treatable by antidepressants. Reactive depression secondary to a transient mishap in personal life is different from the truly miserable situation of the diabetic patient who progressively loses vision and then limbs through amputation. Kaye and associates have analyzed and defined the instances when one need not heed patients' wishes to stop treatment in order to allow time to overcome such transient setbacks (7).

Another important aspect is to be sure one has tried available therapy to the fullest extent. The Australian Anaesthesiology Association suggests employing maximal therapy for at least three weeks before one decides to withdraw it. In general, it appears unwise to discontinue chronic dialysis under the pressure of acute situations.

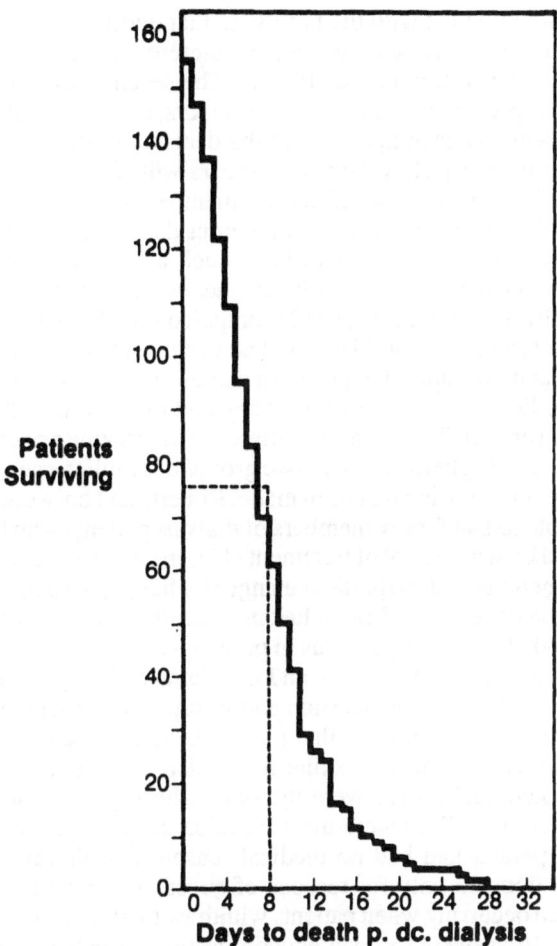

Figure 2. Time to death after last dialysis, in 155 patients who stopped dialysis.

Finally, it is important to make sure that necessary consultation has taken place, and that the consultants are in agreement that the situation is hopeless. Clearly, one should not stop therapy if a neurologist asks for a few more days to evaluate progress or to determine the irreversibility of dementia or cerebral damage caused by a stroke.

The second step in the common sense practical analysis is to reflect on why one is agreeing with a patient's wish to stop dialysis. Is it really in the patient's best interest? Is the situation truly hopeless? Is it really correct that conditions can only worsen. Are there other factors operating? Is the family desperate because things are going too slowly? Are the friends squeamish because of tubes, a respirator or temporary absence of control of bodily functions? Is the team of immediate care givers discouraged and demoralized? Have all relevant consultations been obtained?

In general, it appears that nurses tend to give up earlier than physicians. They are so much closer to the suffering, they see the patient continually. Physicians, on the

contrary, are more remote from the daily struggle and perhaps, therefore, tend to give up too late. Maybe these different points of view create a healthy tension in the team's view of the patient's situation and perhaps results in 'just enough care given.' Is the doctor recommending termination of treatment because he/she is depressed and tired of seeing the patient day after day? Is frustration at the dubious possibility of a solution in the foreseeable future unduly influencing judgement? When considering all these conflicting interests and wishes, it is obvious that the only valid decision is one which reflects the patient's wishes or, if the patient has lost capacity, the patient's best interests.

Several points need to be made concerning the actual decision to terminate treatment. First, one must be prepared to anticipate this possibility and discuss it frankly and openly, yet with sensitivity, with both patient and family earlier on in treatment, even before dialysis becomes necessary and again after completing several months of dialysis. This is the area of advance treatment directives. Questions of death, dying, and withdrawal of treatment are always difficult for physicians; they may judge them threatening and frightening to patients. Studies have shown that the opposite appears to be true. Bernard Lo, discussing the use of antibiotics, nasogastric feeding, feeding tubes and use of respirators with a group of gravely ill patients with heart conditions and cancer, found that 68% of these patients wished to have such discussions with physicians and that most of them wished the physician to originate the discussion (8). In actuality, only 6% had discussed life-sustaining treatment with a physician. When asked how the patients feel after this discussion, a questionnaire stated that 71% felt much better and that they had some control over these things, 53% felt relieved, and 53% felt cared for. Twenty-two percent said that they felt nervous about the discussion, 16% felt sad, and 6% felt like they wanted to give up. All in all, it appears clear that most patients want to have such discussion. Certainly, knowledge about the patient's wishes will considerably ease the decision-making later on, should the patient become incompetent. This is the objective sought by all forms of advance treatment directives.

When patients are making decisions to discontinue treatment three things are important for the caregivers:

1. Be open about details and discuss them.
2. Listen carefully to what different family members and other members of the team have to say. Ask them outright what they think about the situation, and understand that they often may have difficulty expressing an opposing view.
3. In case disagreements should arise in the future, the discussion must be carefully documented in the chart.

There are also instances where patient's decision to stop treatment must not be accepted – must be resisted. One is in the periodically undecided patient who may decide to stop treatment one day and continue treatment another. If so, one obviously proceeds until the patient had a prolonged period of lucidity and clarity and is capable of making a conclusive decision. The other outcome is when the patient becomes definitely incompetent. In that situation, the decision devolves onto family and caregivers, and if the family feuds over the decision, one has to continue treatment. When encountering such situations, the family should be told that their decision should be unanimous. If they are presently unable to reach a decision, they need to contemplate their positions, consider whether they need more medical information and whether they should confer with others, family friends or advisors or spiritual leaders for guidance. After a suitable period one can again bring up the question.

Consider carefully analgesics, fluid management and sedatives, but do not kill the patient. Only the Netherlands condones active killing of patients (9). Doing so in any other country would almost certainly lead to a murder charge. On the other hand, one must not practice what the Catholic church calls medical scrupulosity, that is, the using of technology simply because it is there; that is a sin. The moral and humane consequences of the technologies must be considered.

AWAITING DEATH

There are certain practical aspects in dealing with a patient who has decided to discontinue treatment and is waiting for death. The first is to warn the family that death may be a long time in coming, perhaps up to a month, so that they do not necessarily focus on the mean time of approximately one week. Secondly, they should be told that death in uremia is a comfortable death. The patient becomes increasingly lethargic and is usually found dead in bed, probably due to cardiac arrest secondary to hyperkalemia. However, progressive pulmonary edema leads to a horrible death, therefore fluid and sodium restriction needs to be maintained. Should fluid overload occur, oral or rectal Sorbitol can be used, or the patient can undergo ultrafiltration without dialysis. All other restrictions should be lifted.

One should not order any blood samples or absurd situations may arise, such as being called at night, or even worse having another on-call physician being asked to decide whether to treat hyperkalemia in the dying patient. Doing tests will indicate problems for which one would not contemplate doing anything. This is an unnecessary strain on everybody and a waste of resources. Do not do them!

However, patients awaiting death should be visited daily and contact should be maintained with their families. Listening to the chest, although it may appear an act of futility to the physician, is an act of kindness to the patient that tells him he has not been abandoned, and it eases the concern of the family that nobody cares any more.

Finally, there are two aspects to take care of, even after the patient has died. Some people have suggested a follow-up visit with the family, so that questions they are pondering may be answered, and therefore their grief and uncertainty diminished (10, 11). The second matter concerns preventing harms to the survivors, particularly if the patient was incompetent and the decision to discontinue was made by close family members with the caregivers. Deciding that the loved family member would be better off dead was obviously a momentous decision. Questions have been raised as to whether such a situation can do permanent harm to a family. Two teams have studied this. Walwork and associates (12) compared social functioning and grieving in families who had decided to stop respirator and life support of newborn babies to similar factors in families where the newborn baby had died while still on life support. There was no difference in grieving or social functioning between these two groups of families one year after the decision had been made. Roberts and co-workers wrote to 144 family members of dialysis patients who had died by withdrawal of treatment (13). In general, the family members felt no particular anger for having participated in the decision, and felt it had not disturbed their peace of mind. They were generous in praising nurses, physicians, residents, social workers and chaplains as being helpful both in making the decision and in supporting them after the decision. They felt that physician and residents were the most helpful in making the decision and that social workers and nurses were the ones who supported them afterwards. They were most troubled in the cases where the patient had had no medical reason to withdraw but had done so only for reasons of stress, a situation most often occurring when patients withdraw treatment at home (6). In answers to open ended questions, relatives were somewhat disappointed that physicians were so unwilling to talk to them about discontinuation of treatment, and suspected that physicians were overly optimistic and continued treatment for too long. They wished for more openness and truthfulness. No long term psychological harm seems to have come to relatives and family because of their involvement in the decision.

CULTURAL DIFFERENCES

There are great differences between different geographical regions in the incidence rates of suicide and stopping dialysis. Thus, stopping treatment or committing suicide in North America appears to be three times as common as in Europe and six times as common as in Japan.

Within the United States there are marked differences in the rate of stopping treatment, depending on race. Thus, in a review of the Michigan Dialysis Registry, Port et al. (2) found that stopping treatment was twice as common among whites as among blacks (Figure 3). One can only speculate about the reasons. Black patients seem to be more easer to get their older family members on dialysis. Kjellstrand and Logan found that the incidence of starting dialysis in blacks over the age of 64 years was twice that of

MICHIGAN DIALYSIS REGISTRY 1982 - 84

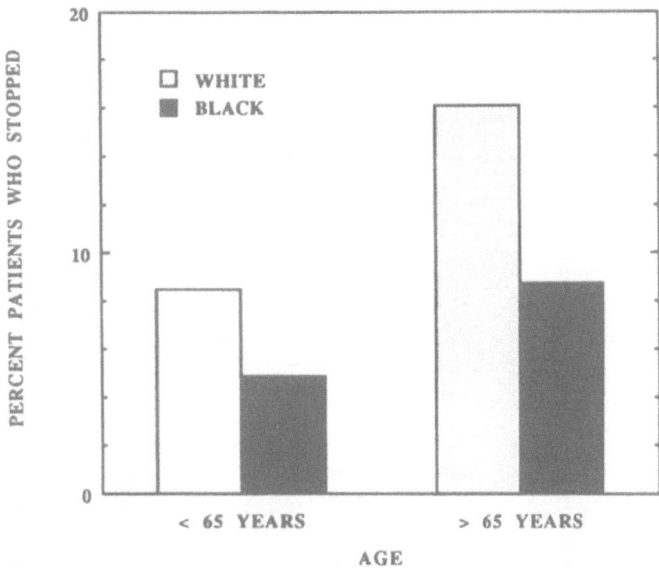

Figure 3. Stopping dialysis is twice as common among whites as among black patients (2).

whites when comparing those who choose to start dialysis to those who died of chronic kidney failure. The higher incidence of kidney failure in blacks thus does not explain this difference (14). Perhaps then this special care that black patients want to give their elderly is also reflected when the possibility of stopping treatment comes up. The other problem may be one of communication. Most physicians doing dialysis are white and perhaps communication problems exist more often between the white physicians and black patients (15). Dr Callender, a black transplant physician himself, has commented on the superstition, lack of education, and general distrust that black patients have of physicians (16, 17).

Superficially, even more profound differences can be found between Western Europe and North America. In Figure 4 are plotted data from Europe and Minnesota that are quite similar to that in USA and Canada (1, 18). While almost 9% of patients in Minnesota ultimately due because dialysis was stopped, this is true for only 3.1% of patients in Europe. However, when one examines age distribution, a startling difference is seen with older patients. In Europe these patients are not directly comparable because of different age limits. Perhaps the reason for the threefold difference in stopping treatment is that, in the United States, many more elderly patients are started on dialysis. This group have a particularly high rate of discontinuation of treatment, and in these elderly patients pre-existing disease is particularly common. It has been shown that pre-existing diseases are much more common among those patients who ultimately stop treatment (Figure 5).

Perhaps there is also a difference of attitude. In general, the European system appears more paternalistic than that in North America. Wehle and Ahlmén analyzing the pattern of stopping in Sweden, comment that 'the ultimate decision has to be made by the Head of the Department' (19). This indicates a more hierarchical type of decision-making than in North America where the decision is more a personal one, made between patient, physician and other caregivers, especially nurses, rather than by an official administrative physician, who may not know the patient well.

There are also some consequences of this difference in approach. In Europe, acute acts of deliberate suicide among dialysis patients are twice as common as in Minnesota (Figure 6). Perhaps desperate patients in Europe are more likely to end their lives in a violent fashion because bureaucratic physicians in Europe are less responsive to their needs than the more personal treatment team would be in North America.

In Japan the pattern of stopping dialysis is entirely different from that in Europe and North America (Figure 7). While stopping treatment and committing suicide shows a marked increase with age both in Europe and in North America (Figure 4), the reverse is true in Japan. Five percent of patients in Japan below the age of 30 end their lives by terminating therapy or committing suicide and this figure falls to less than 1% in patients over the age of 60 years. Thus, as a percentage of death, actually ending treatment or committing suicide is not more common in young patients in Europe and USA than in Japan, but in the patient above age 60 stopping therapy is 30 times

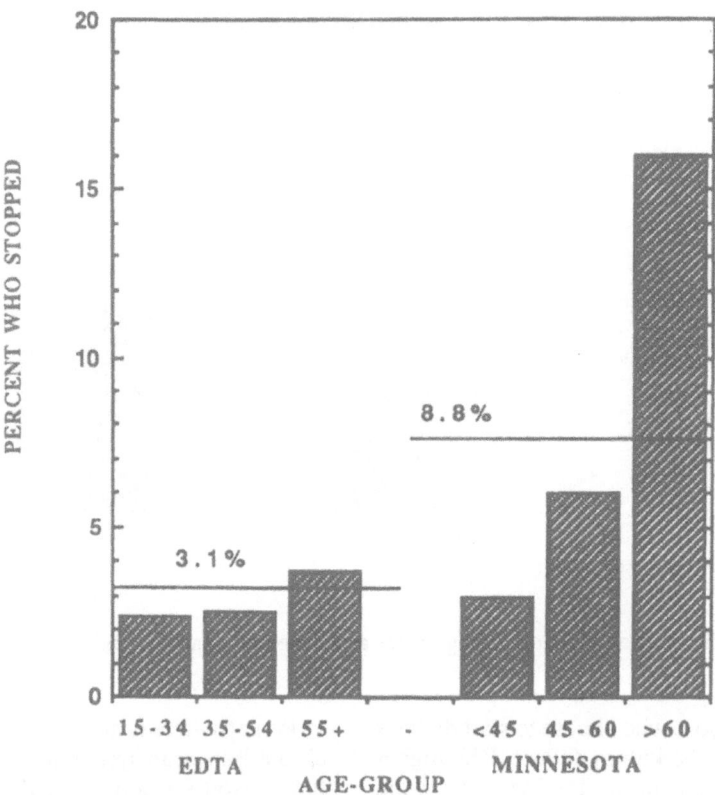

Figure 4. Stopping dialysis, a comparison of European and Minnesota Data. Overall stopping is three times as common in Minnesota, but part of this explanation may be that the US patients are older and more sick than European patients.

more common in USA than it is in Japan. Once can only speculate over the reasons. Perhaps the young patients in Japan feel particularly desperate as almost no transplants are done in this country, and it has been shown that it is the young who are particularly fervent about wishing to be transplanted, while this wish declines steeply with age (20). Patients in Europe or North America who are young can look forward almost with certainty to receiving a transplant. This is not the case in Japan. However, this does not explain the markedly low incidence of discontinuation of treatment and committing suicide in the old Japanese patients. Our understanding is that any prohibition against suicide cannot explain this difference as suicide as a solution to a difficult personal situation appears to be more acceptable to the Japanese than to almost any other culture. Perhaps it has to do with a general attitude to getting old. Clearly Western societies adulate the young and forget the old, but the reverse is true in Japan. To be old in Japan is to be considered not only wise, but to be a repository of knowledge, and to have the power of judgement that is admired and utilized and this may make the older Japanese patients feel a better sense of worth.

RELIGIOUS ASPECTS OF STOPPING TREATMENT

It is one of the paradoxes of history that believers in Judaism, Christianity or Islam have spent so much effort, time and blood in fighting among themselves and with each other yet there is so much that is common and jointly held by each of the three great monotheistic religions. All share the view of a single Deity who created the world and everything within it and at the centre of this creation is mankind, made in the image and likeness of the Creator. As each of these religious traditions developed, first Judaism, then Christianity and subsequently Islam, so each faith built on what had existed previously but added new insights and doctrines of its own. Without intending to trivialize the many differences between these three faiths, from a twentieth century secular viewpoint, their unity in a belief in a divine Being, in man's intimate relation to that Being and his purpose on earth to serve the Divine, provides far more apparent similarity than diversity.

It is against this framework, that the practicalities of ethical decision-making as it pertains to cessation of dialysis, require consideration. Excluded will be those whose

PRE-EXISTING DISEASES

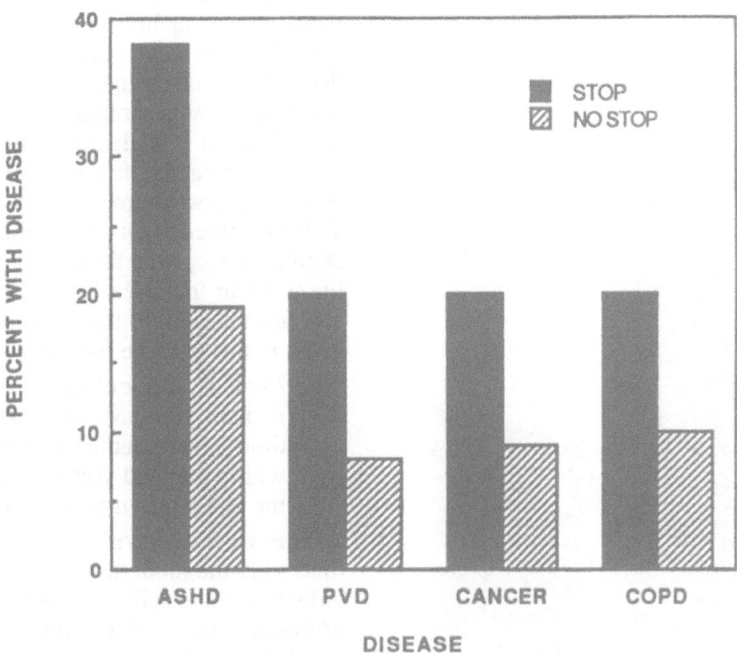

Figure 5. Stopping treatment as a cause of death, and pre-existing disease in Minnesota. Other serious diseases at start of dialysis are twice as common in patients who die from stopping dialysis as in the patients who do not stop therapy.

acceptance of their religious tradition is nominal only and who do not consider themselves as, in any way, bound by its precepts. The 'Christian' who is baptized, married and who will be buried by the Church but whose contact is limited to such rituals, is unlikely to seriously attempt to follow or be guided by the Church's moral and ethical teaching. While the individual, as part of a social group, may well follow certain practices and agree with certain views, this is more a form of group behaviour than a personal testimony arising from strong personal religious views. Such individuals – very many in the West – will not be the primary subjects of this chapter. Rather, the religious motivations of those for whom their beliefs form an important, often major place in their daily life, will be considered when the issue of discontinuation of dialysis arises.

Within the views of Judaism, Christianity and Islam, mankind is not alone, not a solitary agent, not an individual adrift in an ocean with only his own resources and responsibilities but instead is tied, related, serving something wholly other, outside of the person and bearing a special relation to him or her. As a result, life has a unique value and significance. It is not freely given or taken but instead carries a unique importance because the giver and supporter of that life is none other than the Divine Being. The earthly journey is not an enterprise undertaken without thought to any ultimate meaning or significance. On

the contrary, it is an event for which the individual is and will be held accountable. That person and group, with whom they associate, is compelled to consider standards for conduct and thought which have originated in the sacred words and books, are embedded in tradition and have survived through the centuries. From this basic rationale, the developments in biomedical ethics related to termination of life support must be viewed and will be arranged in order of increasing latitude of individual opinion and autonomy.

Islam

The Holy book, the Quran and the law, or Shari'a, form the basis for all behaviour. Man is the Divine viceregent (21) or deputy here and now, and the preservation conduct and enhancement of life on earth are paramount. Hence abortion is restricted and suicide and euthanasia are completely forbidden (22). The time of death is dependent on the will of Allah (23) and man has no right to terminate life except for judicial reasons (24).

Therefore, even with the most remote possibility of recovery, continuation of life support remains justified in Islamic thought. However, where any chance of recovery is absent, and life support is only prolonging the inevitability of death, there appears to be general agreement that it can be discontinued (25, 26). Death, if and when it occurs,

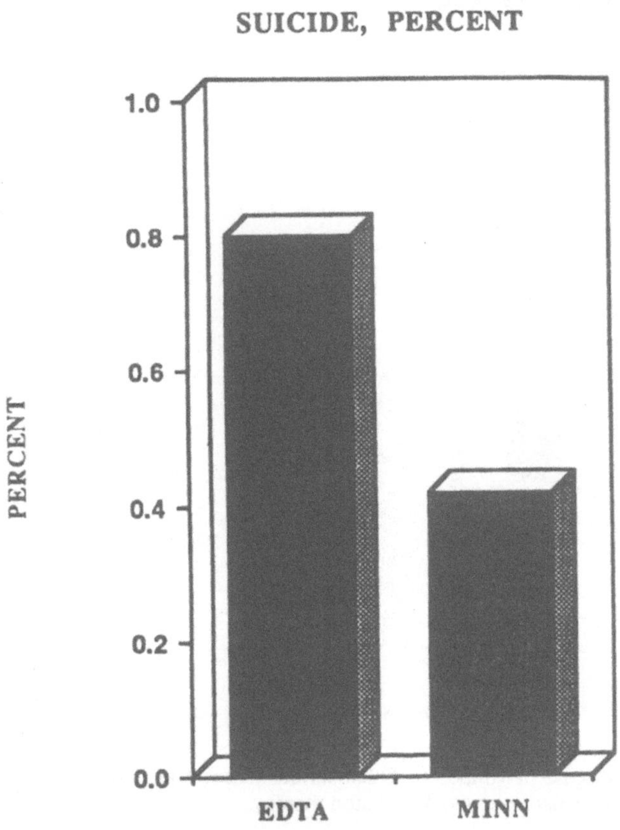

SUICIDE, PERCENT

Figure 6. Suicide is twice as common in dialysis patients in Europe as in Minnesota.

is then determined by Allah (27). Medical judgment is therefore necessary and differences of opinion may be present as to whether any possibility of recovery exists. In such circumstances, life support would be continued. As indicated, with the conscious, aware patient, the deliberate decision by the individual to stop dialysis would not be acceptable unless death was imminent from some condition other than renal failure. Suffering should be treated as competently as medically feasible but voluntary, premature death to escape suffering is impermissible.

Judaism

There is a wide range in ethical positions from the reform to that of classical orthodox Judaism. The latter is clear in its basic message although individual viewpoints vary. Because of man's unique relationship to, and creation by the Divine, life has special significance, both quantitatively and qualitatively. Suicide is forbidden and every effort has to be made to promote health and longevity. Even the addition of a short time period to the dying person is considered valuable unless suffering is of such magnitude that it eclipses any benefit. To promote health, save life or relieve suffering, numerous religious obser-

vations may be disregarded in favour of the greater good. The ill or dying person is obligated to receive treatment and every effort must be taken by the afflicted as well as those caring for him or her, to either restore the person to health or ameliorate their suffering. This singleminded, dedicated, even stringent approach to those who are sick, predicates that treatment cannot and must not be discontinued unless it is clearly futile (28, 29). Where dialysis or other forms of life support are merely prolonging the dying process, where recovery, even if limited, is impossible then there is agreement that these forms of treatment should be stopped, thereby allowing the termination of life to occur 'naturally' (30). The sense that only the Creator has the right to decide when this time has arrived is given in this passage from the Siddur.

> My God, the soul which you have placed within me is pure. you have created it; you have fashioned it; thou have breathed it into me and you preserve it within me, and you will, at some time, take it from me and return it to me in the time to come (31).

This view of Jewish law or Halakhah, therefore conflicts with the modern ethical stance inherent in the individual's right to self-determination and autonomy provided this does not conflict with societal rights. Halakhah, for the Orthodox, has a treasure trove of guidance for today's problems of ethical decision-making (32). The historical precedents and writings related to them, all based ultimately on the Torah, must not be disregarded. While at first no parallel or precedent may be seen, on closer scrutiny by those with the wisdom to understand, a way that is righteous and just will be found.

The principle whereby the individual has the right to forego life sustaning treatment represents an important distinction between Judaic and secular bioethics. As Shimon Glick has expressed it,

> beneficence takes precedence over autonomy (33).

In practical terms, there is the inherent uncertainty, in individual cases, as to whether the person has passed beyond the point of being helped by active treatment. In Halakhah, cessation of respiration signified death (34) but that was prior to the use of endotracheal tubes and respirators. In the setting of the intensive care unit, the absence of respiration calls for mechanical ventilation rather than pronouncement of death. As a result, treatment will be continued unless the medical view is that imminent (within a few days) death is inevitable and that treatment cannot influence this outcome. In most instances in practice, dialysis and other forms of life support are carried on until total collapse of bodily function takes place with the patient's demise a few minutes or hours later.

Movement from this traditional, orthodox viewpoint towards a looser, mature liberal Judaism allows a greater range of options and less consistency (35). Certainly, the importance and primacy attached to human life remains unchanged but there will be found a greater range of individual opinions which are acceptable to the community at large. The views of reform Judaism as they concern

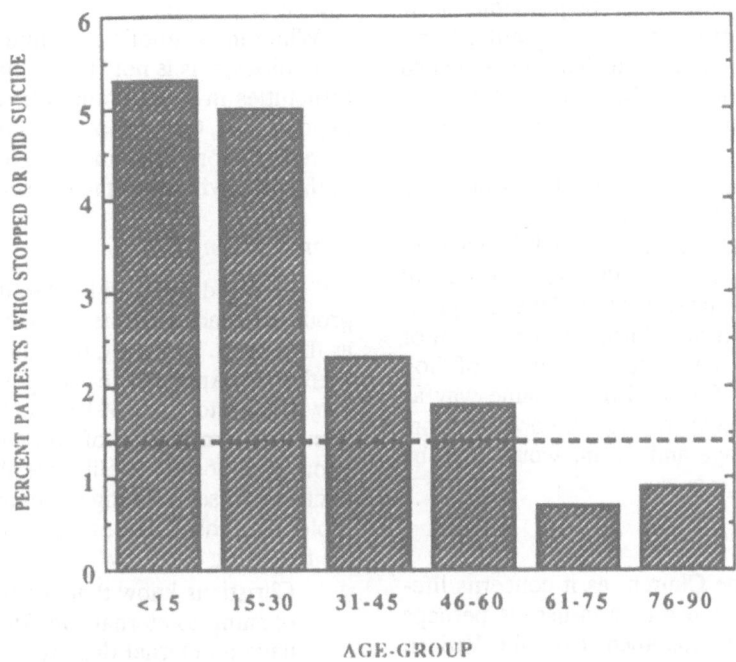

Figure 7. Stopping treatment and committing suicide as causes of death of dialysis patients in Japan. In Japan, contrary to USA and Europe, it is the young who stop treatment or commit suicide, not the old.

life support would overlap those of secular humanists. Mechanical and intrusive methods would be discarded once the chances of any recovery became increasingly unlikely, allowing death to occur, subsequent to this cessation, from whatever underlying physio-pathological processes are present. A viewpoint that humankind can, to some extent, control their own destinies and that the application of technology serving only to prolong existence is not consonant with man's unique sentient being and hence, its cessation should not cause disquiet. Censure, overt or implicit, by the religious authorities would not follow such a course, whereas, in both the conservative traditions of Islam and Orthodox Judaism such 'premature' hastening of death would be seen as a violation of the Divine prerogative which alone decides the beginning and end of man's time on earth and where an extra second of time may be worth as much or more than years of existence (36).

Christianity

For the most part, the major groupings within Christianity would have affinity toward the views discussed previously of reform Judaism and secular humanism as they apply to life support. In fact, one of the most renowned Protestant ethicists of this century. Reinhold Niebuhr has argued the

impossibility of deriving a social ethic (read biomedical ethic) from a pure religious ethic ...

(it) is not applicable to the problems of contemporary society nor yet to any conceivable society (37).

The uncertainty, the sense of continuing to understand and learn as we go along is very much a feature of Christian Protestant and, to an increasing extent, Roman Catholic biomedical ethics. This is expressed by Paul Ramsey in his influential writing 'The Patient as Person' when he states that

Medical ethics today must, indeed, be 'casuistry'; ... we can no longer be so confident that 'resolution' or 'solution' will be forthcoming (38).

The source for these views lies in epistemology. In particular, the importance placed on the foundation writings, the New Testament and, to a lesser extent, the Old Testament or Hebrew Bible. Unlike the Quran, which is considered to be as authoritative today as it was when written by the Prophet and to

represent the ultimate and permanent source of guidance (39)

the New Testament is viewed differently by most biblical scholars (40). The writings are not verbatim accounts of what Jesus said but rather they acquired their present form over many years with considerable selection and filtering in order to serve an expository function for whichever group the author was writing. The words of Jesus which have come down to us are applied to present day ethics only with varying degrees of license. The principles however, love, consideration, justice, concern, equality, dignity, stewardship and so on, remain valid. They have shaped the teaching of some of the most influential ethicists of our time (41). These attributes are now universally accepted, in theory at least if not always in practice; however, their applications in individual cases may be problematic because of conflicting claims and rights.

It should be noted that within most Christian subgroups, there are those who read the New Testament literally and would apply whatever is found there to problems of today with little, if any, further modification or adjustment (40). To them the Bible is the Word of God and therefore revered and followed in the same way as the Quran is for Islam. Ethical conduct for contraception, abortion, sexuality, marriage and so on, would then be dependent on biblical exegesis.

Roman Catholicism

The official teaching of the Church, as it concerns life-sustaining treatment and its use or non-use, is perhaps best expressed in a position statement from the Vatican in 1980 (42). The current position has not chanced. Life is seen as a gift of God with the use of that gift to be enjoyed in the service and love of God. Thus, the taking of life is prohibited, whether by 'mercy killing', suicide, abortion, or homicide. Suffering is seen as an inescapable aspect of our humanity. The use of technology to mitigate and relieve suffering is acceptable, even if to do so may indirectly shorten life. Here the intention is not to produce death but to give relief. Artificial methods of life support are permissible, indeed encouraged, but are not always mandatory and may be discarded if their use becomes unhelpful or if suffering is unrelieved and unremitting or when the burden of treatment is disproportionate to any benefit that may ensue.

The contrast between this view and the views of Orthodox Judaism and Islam is striking (43). Its origin lies in the Jesus of the New Testament who voluntarily followed a path to early death entailing much suffering but who overcame death to be with his Father. Thus, the Roman Catholic Church sees suffering and death as something to be avoided but, if unavoidable, then potentially the faithful may share in Christ's sufferings (44). Death, in itself, is not the end and therefore its inevitability does not have to be circumvented at all costs because beyond death lies paradise. The confluence of the Western democratic ideal –

over himself . . . the individual is sovereign (45)

with the ecclesiastical view that:

The time may come, therefore, when someone is reasonably convinced that life is coming to an end, and a prolongation of dying by additional complicated medical treatment is not the best investment the person can make of what remains (46).

highlights the importance of autonomy and self-determination in the dying process. Once it has progressed to a certain stage.

While the Catholic is willing to make use of modern technology, this is not always mandatory and there are no difficulties in abandoning treatment which fails to meet expectations. Cure is not to be pursued at all costs because there is a more fundamental good which, if not attained in this life, will await the believer in the next.

Protestantism

We are faced here with literally hundreds of different groupings, each with their own interpretation of the 'truth' as they see it. However, the mainline churches, Lutheran, Methodist, Anglican (Episcopal), and United hold views very similar to those of Roman Catholicism when it concerns the termination of life support. The majority are strongly opposed to deliberate abbreviation of life as distinct from discontinuing treatment that is futile or merely prolonging the dying process. This is well expressed in the following excerpts:

Christians know that death is not just an end but an opening to eternal life. Because we human beings have an eternal destiny, individuals have no right, even in the name of altruism, to cut short the earthly preparation of innocent human beings.

To prolong dying is not a doctor's duty . . .

Life supporting equipment such as respirators or dialysis machines, [should not] be withdrawn from patients who are not dying and who need them . . . This is not to be confused with the removal of a machine from a dying patient whose condition cannot be improved by it (47).

The significance of religious beliefs

The foregoing has looked briefly at a normative position of each of the three major world religions. It may be asked: To what extent do the faithful, in practice, actually follow and abide by these precepts?

There is little, if any, data on this subject in relation to life support. In a discussion on 'Exclusion from dialysis' in 1981, Fox at no point discusses religious constraints although the analysis focuses on sociological rather than medical and technical aspects (48). There are at least seven publications dealing with withdrawal of dialysis. They originate from Canada (49, 50), the United States' (1, 51), and Sweden (3, 52). In only one of these are religious factors mentioned by the authors (3). In a series of letters to the New England Journal of Medicine, in response to the Minneapolis paper, none of the correspondents refer to religion as a factor either for or against discontinuing treatment (53) and it is also not considered in an ethical forum on dialysis withdrawal (54). The reasons for this could be varied. The most obvious is that, faced with such an overwhelming, life threatening event as terminating dialysis, religious beliefs become unimportant. We would question this interpretation. All these studies have been retrospective and none have examined specifically the importance of religious values in the decision-making. As society is largely secular (although many nominally adhere to some religious group), the import of belief would be largely diluted. A recent prospective survey of hospitalized patients sought their attitude towards life support and the conditions determining refusal of such therapy (55). Again, religion was not discussed, suggesting either its lack of importance or possibly that religious views cannot be quantified. Perhaps they are too indefinite or that their consideration may actually be 'unscientific' and unfitting for a dispassionate, learned study!

Against these views is a remarkable paper showing that deaths of Jews were fewer than expected prior to the Passover in Los Angeles and higher after the holiday (56). This pattern was not present in Blacks, Orientals and Jewish infants. The indication is that death was in some way delayed to permit celebration of the religious event. We would interpret this as suggesting that religiosity is indeed very important but readily overlooked unless specifically looked for or studied in a homogeneous group of religious adherents. Thus, the 'official' statements by leading figures of the various religious groupings may well reflect, to some degree, the views of the 'people in the street' who are silent worshippers in the shrine, synagogue or church of their choice. If such indeed is the case, then care-giving professionals need to know more about the religious convictions of those they are trying to help. It would also be desirable for them to have at least a rudimentary understanding of some of the world's religions. Such an understanding could itself be beneficial in a world that is segmented and divided into multiple component parts. These divisions engender distrust and prejudice rather than tolerance and understanding. Patients' attitudes and coping mechanisms, in response to present day technology, will be influenced, not solely by their social and family ties, but also for many, by religious views and beliefs that originated millennia previously. Moving from Islam through Judaism, to Christianity the weight and significance of these views for the individual, and the society in which they live, become progressively diluted and secularized. However, their importance cannot be trivialized and we believe this to be particularly relevant for care-givers working in areas of life support.

Refusal of treatment

Differences of opinion may occur when patients wish to stop dialysis and their physicians believe they should continue. Frequently the wish to stop arises from a variety of social and/or medical concerns which are amenable to alteration. Given the appropriate modifications, these individuals may be content to continue treatment and some might eventually be transplanted. There are a few however-

er, in whom further improvement is apparently impossible, yet the physician's reluctance to stop treatment is at odds with the patient's wish to do so. The patients may have carefully considered the significance of their wishes as it affects their relationship with God and decided on this course, whereas the physician remains committed to a technological alternative. This dilemma is a particularly North American one and its resolution lies in the right of the individual to decide whether he or she does, or does not, want treatment. This is acknowledged for the competent individual, provided the person understands the significance and complications of stopping treatment. The rare instances where this right has been overridden has been described previously (7). These exceptions indicate the general rule that the competent individual, has the choice to either consent to, or refuse even life saving treatment for their own (religious or other) reasons.

LEGAL ASPECTS OF STOPPING DIALYSIS

We will here explore three major questions: in general, what is the current state of the law on termination of treatment decisions, what is the current law on stopping treatment in dialysis patients, and what are the unique features of stopping dialysis that make these decisions more, or less, legally problematic?

Current law

Legal and ethical dilemmas surrounding decisions to stop treatment are of relatively recent vintage. Legal decisions concerning the stopping of any form of medical treatment were essentially unheard of before the mid-1970s; emergence of the legal aspects of termination of treatment decisions can be traced to the *Quinlan* decision in 1975–1976 before the trial court and then the State Supreme Court of New Jersey. Since, then, the number of cases before the courts have increased almost exponentially. In *The Right to Die*, Alan Meisel cites 59 'significant reported' right-to-die legal cases in the United States from 1975 to 1990 (57). With regard to the withdrawal of artificial nutrition and hydration from critically ill patients, no significant cases came before the courts prior to 1983. During the period 1983 to the present, however, at least 50 court cases have focused on the withdrawal of this specific form of treatment (58). According to a report from the National Center of State Courts, there have been at least 7,000 court cases on termination of treatment in the United States (59).

In addition to court cases, there also has been a great deal of activity in the state legislatures (60, 61). Most states now have some form of advance directive legislation, e.g., living wills (41 states and the District of Columbia), or durable powers of attorney for health care (29 states and the District of Columbia). The courts and the legislatures have been somewhat divergent in their views, however. The courts, through a series of decisions, have tended to expand the rights of individual patients to discontinue treatment while the legislatures have in some ways restricted those same rights. Many living will statutes limit the termination of treatment to only those patients who are 'terminally ill'. Until recently, legislation in six states (Missouri, Connecticut, Wisconsin, Oklahoma, Maine, Georgia) forbids the withdrawal of artificial nutrition and hydration under nearly all circumstances (62). The Child and Abuse Amendment of 1984 also narrowly defines the circumstances in which nutrition and hydration may be stopped on critically ill newborns, though the language is unclear and the intent confusing (63).

Gradually, though, over the last fifteen years the legal system (in case law or statutes) has increasingly recognized the common law right of competent patients to refuse treatment. In 1990, the US Supreme Court in *Cruzan* recognized a federal constitutional right of patients to forego medical treatment. Some state courts have also recognized that patients have a state constitutional right to stop treatment.

A consensus is beginning to develop on some of the issues surrounding termination of treatment. A consensus is emerging, for example, that not only do competent patients have a constitutional and common-law right to discontinue treatment, but also that incompetent patients share in this same legal right. Further, a consensus is developing that not only respirators, but all tones of medical treatment may be discontinued.

However, at least two major issues remain legally problematic. The first issue concerns incompetent patients: what procedural mechanism should be established to protect their rights, and who is the appropriate surrogate decision-maker (64)? Some states have now erected stringent procedural safeguards for withdrawing treatment from incompetent patients. The New Jersey Supreme Court, acting partly from a lack of faith in the medical profession recommended in the *Conroy* decision a complicated system for protecting the rights of incompetent patients (65). However, this system, which included the involvement of the State Ombudsman's Office, turned out to be completely unworkable (66).

A second major issue that remains controversial is the withdrawal of artificial nutrition and hydration; however, here too a consensus seems to be emerging. All appellate court decisions (except for *Cruzan* in Missouri and *Grant* in Washington) have concluded that medical means of providing artificial nutrition and hydration are comparable to other life-sustaining medical treatments and can be discontinued according to the same principles and practices followed in the withdrawal of other forms of treatment (65, 67–75). Medical organizations and interdisciplinary authorities have articulated the same view (76–79). However, there continues to be some conflict between the parties moving toward consensus (i.e., medical organizations, interdisciplinary authorities and the courts) and

other deliberative bodies, such as some state legislatures and perhaps federal lawmakers.

Besides addressing the substantive questions of what constitutes medical treatment, and which medical conditions (terminally ill, imminently dying, permanently comatose, hopelessly ill) are appropriate for termination of treatment, the courts have tried to determine the best way to resolve who should make decisions for incompetents and how those decisions should be made (80). 'Substituted judgment' and 'best interests' are two common legal concepts. According to the standard of substituted judgment (which is considered subjective and highly individualistic), the decision to withdraw treatment is made after considering what the patient would have wanted. The more evidence there is of the patient's likely wishes (previous oral statements, written statements, and general life style), the more the standard of substituted judgment is satisfied. This standard does not specify who should decide, only that the surrogate decision-maker act in accordance with the patient's wishes. The 'best interests' standard is used when it is not known what the patient would have wanted. There is a great deal of confusion in both the legal and ethical literature on what constitutes 'best interests'. This standard is often followed by weighing the benefits and burdens of treatment against the benefits and burdens of continued existence for the patient.

Some states have adopted a more stringent evidentiary standard than others with regard to substituted judgment and have developed elaborate procedural standards to minimize abuse. That is, some states require more evidence than do other states as to the patient's likely wishes before they will accept that the substituted judgment standard has been satisfied. Most recently, State Supreme Court decisions in three states (Missouri, Maine, and New York) have articulated 'clear and convincing evidence standards (73, 81–84). Exactly how to apply these standards is a different matter. Individual trial court judges are free to decide whether the patient's previous views and life style meet a clear and convincing evidence standard. This standard then is highly individualistic, varying according to the particular trial court judge applying it. Other states have been less stringent in developing an evidentiary standard for incompetent patients. For example, the Minnesota State Supreme Court in *Torres* had little evidence of what Mr Torres would have wanted, and seemed to lean more toward a best interests standard (85).

Some states seem to place greater confidence in the family or friends to make decisions for incompetents, while other states have been reluctant to entrust family and health care providers with these decisions.

With this variety of judicial approaches to the termination of treatment, it should be remembered that in this country. decisions to limit treatment are made thousands of times each day – often in circumstances where the evidence of what the patient wants falls well short of a clear and convincing evidence standard, where the diagnosis and prognosis are less certain than the diagnosis of the persistent vegetative state, and where there is less unanimity among the immediate family members concerning the appropriate action. Recent studies have indicated that there may be at least one million deaths each year in the United States in which a conscious decision is made to limit treatment in some way (86). Very few of these cases reach the courts, nor could the courts, by whatever procedural mechanism they recommend, ever rule on even 1% of these cases in a strictly judicial setting.

What happens, then, when a ruling such as the *Saikewicz* decision by the Supreme Judicial Court in Massachusetts appears to require routine judicial review for all cases involving incompetent patients (87, 88)? In reality, what occurs is that these cases are not reviewed by the courts, and often treatment is continued far beyond the time when it should be discontinued (because of the fear of legal repercussions), or, the appropriate decisions are made, but more surreptitiously and quietly than they should be. Ultraconservative decisions advocating some form of routine judicial review in most termination of treatment decisions in incompetent patients will never work. There needs to be some compromise wherein the courts articulate policy, in conjunction with the legislatures, while ensuring their ability to resolve the more legally problematic cases. Since we are still basically in our infancy regarding the legal aspects of termination of treatment, how this area unfolds is still uncertain and will vary significantly in the individual states.

How does all of this relate to dialysis? What are the unique features of stopping dialysis that make this practice more or less legally problematic. Finally, how much have the courts been involved in dialysis cases?

Court cases

Of the major cases before the courts in this country on stopping treatment, only two have directly involved dialysis as the primary treatment to be discontinued. Earle N. Spring, 77, suffered from severe dementia ('advanced senility') and end-stage renal disease (89), and received 5-hour hemodialysis treatments three times a week. Heavy sedation was often used to overcome his resistance to treatment, and he often resisted transportation to dialysis treatment and pulled the dialysis needles out of his arm. Mr Spring experienced leg cramps, headaches and dizziness as side effects of the dialysis.

In January 1979, his wife of 55 years and his only son petitioned the probate court in Massachusetts for an order directing that dialysis be discontinued. The son had been appointed temporary guardian of his father, but in view of the request to discontinue treatment, the probate court also appointed a guardian *ad litem* to represent Mr Spring.

The probate court judge ruled in favour of discontinuing treatment but this decision was appealed by the guardian *ad litem* in December 1979 – almost one year after the court proceedings had begun. When the intermediate appellate court in Massachusetts affirmed the probate court's decision, the guardian *ad litem* appealed again. After 15 months of hearings, appeals, reversals, and stays the Massachusetts Supreme Judicial Court (SJC) finally issued its decision, one month after Mr Spring had died.

A major reason why the Massachusetts SJC decided to hear Mr Spring's case is that this case gave the court an opportunity to clarify what it had said in a previous decision in the matter of Joseph Saikewicz (90). In *Saikewicz*, the Massachusetts SJC appeared to say that all cases involving the discontinuation of treatment in incompetent patients should be a matter of routine judicial involvement (91, 100). In *Spring*, the court took the opportunity to say that this was not the intent of the *Saikewicz* decision. The justices clearly indicated that judicial approval was not always required before stopping treatment on incompetent patients. The court identified the following issues to be considered: the extent of impairment of the patient's mental faculties; whether the patient is in the custody of a state institution; the prognosis with or without proposed treatment; the complexity, risk, and novelty of such treatment; its possible side effects; the patient's level of understanding and probable reaction; the urgency of the decision; the consent of the patient's spouse or guardian; the good faith of those who participate in the decision; the clarity of professional opinion as to good medical practice; the interests of third persons; and the administrative requirements of any institution involved (92).

Unfortunately, the court did not prioritize these issues, nor did it indicate which ones needed to be reviewed by the probate courts in Massachusetts. Regarding criminal or civil liability for physicians in termination of treatment decisions, the Massachusetts SJC said, 'Little need be said about criminal liability: there is precious little precedent and what there is suggests that the doctor will be protected if he acts on a good faith judgment that is not grievously unreasonable by medical standards' (92).

Another case involving dialysis occurred in the State of New York in 1982 (93). Peter Cinque, a 41-year-old diabetic, was blind, had partial amputations of both legs, a bleeding gastrointestinal ulcer, and cardiovascular disease – all due to complications of diabetes. In addition to these complications, Mr Cinque was undergoing dialysis several days a week for end-stage renal disease. He was said to be receiving analgesic medications, including Demerol, for great pain, but was described as mentally alert and competent.

In early October, 1982, because of the pain and other complications Mr Cinque decided that he wished to discontinue dialysis and be allowed to die at home in the presence of his family. This decision was discussed with the entire family and a Catholic priest. Mr Cinque had several conversations with his nephrologist on October 12 and 14. The nephrologist and administrators at Lydia Hall Hospital told Mr Cinque he could stop his dialysis on October 15. Before this termination of treatment, he was removed from all sedative and analgestic medication so that he could be examined by two psychiatrists to determine his competency and ability to make his own decisions. After these examinations, he was found 'coherent and relevant' and unequivocal in his desire to stop dialysis and be allowed to die. On the same day he was examined, Mr Cinque signed two documents expressing his wishes (since he was blind, he signed with a mark).

Mark Cinque, one of Mr Cinque's brothers, commented that Peter Cinque 'was at last comforted and relieved' when the hospital appeared to agree with his wishes to discontinue dialysis. However, several hours later, the hospital had not only refused to discontinue treatment, but had gone to court. Mark Cinque described his brother as going through 'the most painful period of agony and suffering I had ever seen' (94).

Two days later, Mr Cinque sustained a respiratory arrest after which he lapsed into a coma and was maintained on a respirator. A trial court judge visited the bedside on October 19 and 21, 1982 and found him to be unconscious both times. The guardian *ad litem* appointed by the court agreed with the family that Mr Cinque had left unequivocal expressions of what he wanted prior to his present comatose state. The lower court found in favour of stopping treatment, but the case was immediately appealed to the highest court in New York, the Court of Appeals. The New York high court took the opportunity of Mr Cinque's dilemma to clarify its previous decisions in *Eichner* and *Storar* (81, 95) in which a clear and convincing evidence standard of the patient's wishes had been established before treatment could be stopped. The trial court judge felt that Mr Cinque's expressions before losing consciousness were so compelling that his statements satisfied a much more stringent standard than even 'clear and convincing,' that of 'beyond a reasonable doubt' and ordered the hospital to discontinue treatment on October 22. Unfortunately, in a bizarre and cruel turn of events, the hospital discontinued treatment immediately upon hearing of the court's decision without allowing his family to be present at Mr Cinque's bedside. Commenting on the Cinque case, Willard Gaylin, President of the Hastings Center, asked: 'How did we get into this 'Alice-in-Wonderland' world, where a man must beg for his legal rights, prove his sanity, endure court hearings and finally be reduced to a living cadaver to do what has generally been accepted as his privilege?' (96).

It is ironic that the day before Mr Cinque finally was allowed to die, the President's Commission for the Study of Ethical Problems in Medicine released a report on informed consent, pointing out that 4 of 5 Americans believe that the processes by which patients grant prior consent for hospital treatment are merely 'legal maneuvers to protect doctors from lawsuits' (97). The commission's Chairman, Morris B. Abrams, an attorney in New York City, called this finding dismal and startling (97). The commission said that in order for informed consent to be an effective process, it must be part of a larger process of shared decision-making and mutual respect between physician and patient. No case could more dramatically illustrate the failure of 'informed consent', 'shared decision-making,' and 'mutual respect between physician and patient' than the clash between Peter Cinque and medical and administrative personnel at Lydia Hall Hospital.

What general observations can we make from the Spring and Cinque cases, and how they were handled by the courts? First, quality of life was a major issue in both cases. It was obvious that quality of life was poor for both Mr Spring and Mr Cinque. Both situations are typical scenarios in which dialysis is often discontinued. In a study done by Neu and Kjellstrand of 66 patients who were incompetent at the time of stopping dialysis, 37 (56%) had 'advanced arteriosclerotic or dialysis dementia' and another 6 (9%) had severe memory/intellectual deficits that were secondary to strokes (1). In many of these cases, dialysis was stopped for the same reasons it was discontinued in Mr Spring.

Second, the courts seemed to view dialysis as a medical treatment with clear-cut benefits and side effects, and treated the termination of dialysis like the termination of other forms of medical treatment. The courts viewed stopping dialysis as being much less controversial than stopping artificial nutrition and hydration, or stopping life-saving medical treatment such as blood transfusions.

Third, these two cases reflect the early days of legal analysis. *Spring* was one of the earliest cases to reach the appellate court level in the United States (after *Quinlan*, *Saikewicz*, and *Dinnerstein*) (87, 98, 99). In Massachusetts, the higher courts were trying to clarify what they had said in *Saikewicz*, the second major right-to-die case in this country.

Fourth, the Cinque case illustrates how much easier it is for the courts to resolve issues when the patient is competent and his or her wishes concerning quality of life and medical treatment are clearly known. It also supports the movement towards advance directives. Thus, the courts focused on issues involving competent patients and the legal principle of substituted judgment rather than best interests. In the *Spring* case, however, the legal analysis focused more on the best interests standard. There was little offered at the probate-court level to identify what Mr Spring would have wanted, other than his wife's assertion, based on their long years of marriage, that 'he wouldn't want to live.' The higher court also took note of the fact that Mr Spring had led a vigorous active life, which he was no longer able to do.

Finally, Peter Cinque's dilemma exemplifies the extraordinary concerns about the liability of hospital and medical personnel. This concern about potential criminal and civil liability borders on hysteria; as in Mr Cinque's case, it compromises the ability of the medical profession to act in a humane, compassionate, common-sense way and brutalizes the patient and his family. It is hard to justify the actions of the hospital and physicians in his case, but three factors may partially explain what transpired. First, the case occurred at a time in the right-to-die movement when the law was much more unsettled than it is today. Second, the case was litigated in the State of New York, where the preoccupation with liability to the detriment of common sense and humane care is as great as it is anywhere in the country. Third, the highest court in New York had recently established an extremely high standard for knowing what incompetent patients would have wanted (erecting the clear and convincing evidence standard in the matters of *Eichner* and *Storar*); and physicians and hospital administrators may have been unclear on the full ramifications of these legal decisions.

Three other legal cases involving dialysis should be mentioned. In 1979, the Massachusetts SJC affirmed a trial-court order compelling an unconsenting, competent adult prisoner to submit to dialysis treatments that were considered life-saving (101). The higher court found that the prisoner's right to refuse life-saving treatment was outweighed by the state's interests in preserving life, in maintaining the ethical integrity of the medical profession and permitting hospitals to fully care for their patients, and in upholding orderly prison administration. This ruling, however, should not be considered a major legal decision on dialysis because it involved unique features of a termination of treatment decision not often seen. Essentially, the court felt that the prisoner was seeking to circumvent restrictions of the prison system by refusing dialysis.

A Minnesota case will help to dispel two commonly held myths in right-to-die cases, myths that have no solid foundation in theory or practice. The first is that there is a real possibility of civil or criminal liability in situations where the cases have been handled well by health care providers. The second myth, closely related to the first, is that family members, near or distant, who were not involved in the decision-making process leading to termination of treatment, may come forward at some later date and successfully sue physicians, even when the cases were handled well. A major problem, one that further perpetuates these fallacious views, is that many physicians seem to want complete immunity from civil or criminal liability for their actions, no matter how well or poorly they handle individual cases. To these physicians, any risk is too much risk. Their concerns about doing good for the individual patient are far outweighed by their concerns about liability. If individual cases are not handled well, either procedurally or substantively, then physicians should run a risk of sanction in some form, e.g., when a physician does not make a good faith effort to find family or friends or other appropriate surrogate decision-makers for an incompetent patient, or when a physician does not fully inform the patient of all the relevant benefits and risks of alternative forms of therapy. But, when the physicians handle cases appropriately, then the real risk of liability is small.

During the early 1970s a 62-year-old woman on chronic peritoneal dialysis in a large midwestern dialysis program became progressively demented and unable to care for herself at home. In the hospital, she would scream for no apparent reason, and her behaviour became increasingly disturbing to other patients. After numerous discussions with her husband which were extensively documented in the medical records, the attending nephrologist, with the consent of the husband, decided to discontinue dialysis, and the patient died shortly thereafter. Six months later, the patient's husband died.

Three years after the patient's death, shortly before the statute of limitations would have expired, two of the patient's children filed a civil law suit for abandonment against the nephrologist and the hospital. The plaintiffs argued that the nephrologist had abandoned the patient simply because he had discontinued dialysis. The decision was divided into two parts. First, the jury found that the defendants were not liable. The nephrologist had done nothing wrong legally by stopping dialysis on this patient with an extremely poor prognosis. Second, the jury found there would have been no monetary damages awarded to the plaintiffs, even if the physician had been found guilty of malpractice. Since the patient was totally disabled because of her illness, the jury reasoned no financial loss could result from her death.

Afterwards, one member of the jury asked the physician, 'Why did it take so long to make the decision (to discontinue dialysis)?' (102). Hopefully, this case will contribute to the view that doctors, acting in good faith and in accordance with reasonable standards of medical practice, need not fear frivolous law suits brought by disgruntled relatives.

Another court case involving dialysis occurred in New Mexico in 1983. The legal guardian for James R. Smith petitioned the lower court to authorize discontinuation of hemodialysis. This request was granted. However, the lower court's ruling was reversed on appeal to the Supreme Court of New Mexico who stated that there was no statute in New Mexico that would empower a guardian to discontinue hemodialysis on behalf of an incompetent patient. After this unfortunate ruling, the New Mexico legislature amended the state's right-to-die act by providing that, when an incompetent patient not executing a document under the right-to-die act is certified as terminally ill or in an irreversible coma, the physician may be allowed to remove medical treatment when all family members agree in good faith that the patient, if competent, would have chosen to forgo treatment. Thus, this case served as a stimulus for the New Mexico legislature to expand the rights of surrogates to discontinue treatment, and, indirectly, to expand the rights of patients to allow decisions to be made for them after they become incompetent (103).

Unique features of dialysis

What are the unique features of the withdrawal of dialysis that distinguishes it from the withdrawal of other forms of medical treatment? Why have there been so few dialysis cases before the courts? Will this trend of minimal legal involvement continue? What are the characteristics of cases involving cessation of dialysis that seem to make these decisions less legally troublesome?

Dialysis as 'high-tech' medical treatment

Where does dialysis lie on the continuum from highly technological, complicated, expensive, and burdensome medical treatments (e.g., respirators, cardiopulmonary resuscitation, heart-lung machines, extracorporeal membrane oxygenators) to simpler, less technological, less expensive and relatively non-burdensome medical treatments (e.g., antibiotics, artificial nutrition and hydration)? It seems clear that dialysis is perceived to be closer to the complex, technologic end of the continuum, thus decisions to stop dialysis are less legally problematic than decisions to forgo forms of treatment at the more basic end of the continuum.

Another reason why stopping dialysis may be less legally controversial is that in some cases it provides a stop-gap measure until transplantation can be done. When transplantation cannot be performed, or one or more transplants are unsuccessful, dialysis is still a treatment that is unquestionably life-prolonging. However, there often comes a time during the course of the progressive disease and its medical complications when the side effects of dialysis (which are rarely inconsequential, even in the early stages of renal failure) exceed the benefits. The long-term use of dialysis and subsequent determinations that its effectiveness has run its course and that it is now no longer beneficial, satisfies the medical-ethical (and legal) standard of a 'time-limited trial' of therapy (77).

Competent patients

Decisions to stop dialysis are often made by competent patients who have experienced the benefits and burdens of dialysis over a relatively long period of time, thus, there is no need to apply a substituted judgment or best interests standard, since the patient makes the decision as a direct expression of autonomy or self-determination. However, while many patients are clearly competent, others are comatose, severely demented, or their competency is unclear. These cases are more legally perplexing.

Quality of life

Decisions to discontinue dialysis are usually made after the treatment has been given an adequate trial, in order to see how much it helps the patient and to weigh the benefits and burdens of continued treatment in light of the progress of the underlying disease. In the Earle Spring case, for example the family became convinced that dialysis should be discontinued because Mr Spring had deteriorated mentally to the point where the family did not think dialysis was prolonging any meaningful existence. Similarly, Peter Cinque decided that the complications of diabetes were so devastating that he no longer wished to continue living with such severe disability and suffering.

Hence, some decisions are made after considering the advantages and disadvantages of both dialysis and other forms of treatment. The quality of life in cases resembling Earle Spring and Peter Cinque was so overwhelmingly poor that most people would not dispute decisions to discontinue dialysis. Unlike comparatively simple treatment such as antibiotics or artificial nutrition and hydration, the side effects, expense, and inconvenience of dialysis can be significant – especially when it sustains only marginal quality of life for the patient.

Dialysis is not curative; it does not cure the underlying disease process leading to kidney failure, nor is it life-saving in the same sense that surgery or blood transfusions sometimes are. It sustains life by replacing a basic biological function as do respirators and artificial nutrition and hydration. Dialysis is an 'artificial kidney,' just as a respirator is an 'artificial lung,' or artificial nutrition and hydration is an artificial gastrointestinal system.' Decisions to discontinue dialysis are no different from decisions to discontinue a respirator or to discontinue artificial nutrition and hydration. It is primarily the basic underlying condition of the patient that usually makes the treatment more or less advantageous or detrimental, and not the treatment itself. Decisions to discontinue dialysis, then, are often based not on the change in the benefit or burden accompanying the dialysis treatments themselves, but on the underlying quality of life of the patient. This is especially true when diabetes ravages the body and mind. If a patient has good health in all other respects, there should be little legal controversy surrounding a decision to continue dialysis. The improved quality of life would be such that most patients would accept the side effects of dialysis.

In many respects, then, dialysis decisions are less legally controversial than other non-treatment circumstances. However, three other features may make these cases more legally problematic.

Definition of terminal condition

The definition of 'terminal condition' has been significantly expanded and modified recently, and this has great bearing on the dialysis issue. In the 1985 version of the Uniform Rights of the Terminally Ill Act (URITA), a terminal condition was defined as a condition in which the patient would die within a relatively short period of time *with* continued medical treatment (104). According to the newer and much broader definition of terminal condition in the more recent URITA (1989), the patient will die within a relatively short period of time *without* medical treatment (105), thus, any patient who requires continuous life support systems to keep him or her alive and whose medical condition is 'incurable and irreversible' could be considered terminal. A patient in a persistent vegetative state, even though capable of living for an extended period of time (years, or decades) is terminal because he or she would die within a relatively short time (3–30 days, usually 7–14 days) after stopping artificial hydration. Recent court decisions (*Greenspan* in Illinois) have begun to reflect this newer definition (106). Renal failure by itself, as long as it is incurable and irreversible, could be considered a terminal condition: without continued dialysis the patient will die within a relatively short time, usually only a few weeks.

The newer definition of terminal condition gives patients greater control over their own lives. But this also means that the patient may elect to discontinue dialysis for reasons some would find questionable, such as temporary depression, marital strife, or other reasons that are more psychosociologic than medical.

Static versus progressive disease

In general, it is more legally controversial to discontinue treatment for a static disease process than for a progressive one. For example, withdrawal of the respirator seems to be more legally permissible in cases of a progressive neurologic disease such as amyotrophic lateral sclerosis, but more legally debatable when the patient's neurologic condition is static, as in a cervical cord injury. The courts and others have drawn distinctions between a progressive course and a static course because decisions to discontinue treatment in a static condition could have more negative impact on other categories of patients with a static condition, such as patients with cerebral palsy. This is why the *McAfee* case in Georgia (a man with a cervical cord injury who asked to have his respirator removed) was so controversial, why the disability groups were opposed to letting the courts allow Mr McAfee make the decision himself (107), and also why the *Bouvia* case in California was so controversial legally (108). Ms Bouvia had cerebral palsy her entire life. Her decision to withdraw artificial nutrition and hydration from herself was not, according to some, related to any progressive medical disease or increased suffering, but had more to do with psychological and social reasons.

In that the underlying renal failure is non-progressive, discontinuation of dialysis could be considered more controversial than discontinuations of other treatment. However, the basic disease process that led to the renal failure and other medical complications may be progressive, as in diabetes, and it is usually the underlying disease process and its effect on the person that is the primary reason for discontinuing dialysis.

Cost containment

A legally contentious situation could arise in the future should dialysis not be offered (or be withdrawn) based on social and economic considerations (109). Such a situation could easily arise as funds for dialysis become more limited than they have been since the enactment of the end-stage renal disease program in 1973. The British seem to encounter little legal difficulty regarding failure to offer dialysis, as opposed to deciding to withdraw it but find it more difficult to stop dialysis than to withhold it. However, the British medical and legal systems are

radically different from ours. A lack of litigation in Great Britain may be of little reassurance to those of us in the United States (110), where we seem to have more difficulty stopping treatment than starting it, although as Neu and Kjellstrand's study shows, and as others have now experienced, we have developed a much more humane, rational, common-sense basis for assessing the benefits and burdens of continued treatment and are more willing to discontinue dialysis for justifiable reasons than we have in the past.

Cruzan and constitutional law

What effect does the recent US Supreme Court ruling in the Nancy Cruzan case have on termination of treatment decisions in general, and dialysis decisions in particular? The *Cruzan* case is the first major termination of treatment case to be decided by the US Supreme Court (111). Its effects could be widespread or narrow, depending upon one's view of the decision (112).

Nancy Cruzan was 25 years old when she was involved in a single-car motor vehicle accident on a rural road in southwest Missouri on January 11, 1983. She was thrown 35 feet from the car and landed face down, causing obstruction of her airway. From the beginning, her prognosis for recovery of cognitive functions was felt to be extremely poor. She evolved into a persistent vegetative state over ensuing months and a gastrostomy tube was placed on February 7, 1983, approximately four weeks after the accident. In 1986, her parents, Joe and Joyce Cruzan, recognized that Nancy was in a persistent vegetative state and that her condition was hopeless. They further realized that Nancy would not want treatment under such circumstances. Nancy was described by her parents and friends as a proud, feisty, independent individual who took great pride in her physical appearance. The Cruzans began learning of similar cases in other states where feeding tubes had been removed from patients in a vegetative state, but they were told by the rehabilitation center where Nancy was staying that the feeding tube could not be removed without a court order.

In 1988, a trial court judge in Missouri ruled that it was permissible to discontinue Nancy's feeding tube in accordance with what the patient would have wanted and what the family wanted (113). The case was appealed to the Missouri State Supreme Court by the Attorney General of the State of Missouri and by the guardian *ad litem* appointed by the court to represent Nancy's interests. In a radical departure from nine previous appellate court decisions, the Missouri Supreme Court ruled in a 4-to-3 decision that Nancy's feeding tube could not be withdrawn (83). The family then appealed to the US Supreme Court which affirmed the ruling of the Missouri Supreme Court on June 25, 1990, and decreed that the Missouri courts were permitted (not required) constitutionally to erect a clear and convincing evidence standard for determining what an incompetent patient would have wanted concerning the stopping of artificial feeding.

There undoubtedly will be widespread misunderstanding concerning what the US Supreme Court did and did not say in *Cruzan*, so it is important to understand that the Court's decision was a very narrow one (114) which said in essence, that the states were free to develop procedural safeguards and evidentiary standards they feel appropriate. This is the only direct effect of the Court's ruling in *Cruzan*.

In addition to this narrow finding, however, the Court also made comments (*dicta*) on several other constitutional and legal aspects of stopping treatment which will have some indirect bearing on legal decisions in the individual states. For example, the Court ruled that a competent patient has a federal constitutional right to refuse treatment, but it did not rule on whether this right extends to incompetent patients. Most importantly, the Court, also by way of *dicta*, decided that there was no essential difference between the withdrawal of artificial nutrition and hydration and the withdrawal of other forms of medical treatment.

Further, five of the nine justices, including all of the dissenters, and Justice O'Connor in her concurring opinion, appeared to place great value on advance directives, especially durable power of attorney for health care and other means to designate surrogates for patients who are no longer competent. Justice O'Connor was fairly forceful in her opinion that there may be a constitutional right of liberty for incompetent patients to have treatment stopped when this decision is effectuated by an appropriately determined surrogate decision-maker. In Justice O'Connor's words, 'I also write separately to emphasize that the Court does not today decide the issue of whether a State must also give effect to the decisions of a surrogate decision-maker ... In my view, such a duty may well be *constitutionally required* to protect the patient's liberty interest in refusing medical treatment' (emphasis added) (111).

Conclusion

What conclusions can we draw from this review so that health care providers can be assured that dialysis decisions are correct (both substantively and procedural in the eyes of the law? As noted above, dialysis decisions will almost certainly be viewed as less controversial than other termination of treatment decisions such as artificial feeding or blood transfusions. Dialysis is viewed as a medical treatment located toward the technologically complex end of the treatment continuum; the quality of life for patients receiving such treatment is palpably poor. In perhaps half of the cases, the patient is competent and can make decisions consistent with his her values. In other cases, family members or friends are available to make decisions for the patient, in terms of either what the patient would have wanted (substituted judgment standard), or what the fam-

ily or friends perceive to be best for their loved one (best interests standard).

Some decisions to stop treatment may be more troubling and legally problematic as for example when there is a conflict among family members, or when there are no family members or appropriate surrogate decision-makers available at all. Decisions perceived as efforts to limit the use of resources will be considered more legally controversial.

As with other termination of treatment decisions, certain steps should be followed to ensure that decisions are legally acceptably from a procedural standpoint. A discussion of procedures that are both ethically and legally acceptable can be found in the Hastings Center Guidelines (77). Among the more important steps to follow, thorough documentation of all relevant circumstances is critical. The more complex and controversial the decision, the more documentation there should be. Also, formal written policies at the institutional level are of great value and the documentation in individual cases should note that practices in individual cases are in accordance with institutional policies.

Termination of treatment decisions are easier and less legally problematic when they are carried out in accordance with the patient's own wishes, expressed prior to incompetency. Patients should be encouraged to express what their wishes would be should this situation arise. Efforts to designate appropriate surrogate decision-makers should be commonplace, even when patients are relatively healthy, and the benefits of dialysis clearly outweigh any burdens. Health care providers, especially physicians, should become much more comfortable with discussing these decisions with patients and family far in advance of deteriorating health and impending incompetency and decisions to continue or discontinue dialysis should be part of an overall treatment plan reached through interdisciplinary care conferences and extensive discussions with all involved. Even though the patient is the central focus of these decisions, there should be an attempt to arrive at consensual decision-making. There also should be far greater emphasis (especially for dialysis) on the moral and legal legitimacy of stopping treatment rather than withholding treatment in the first place. Thus, the patient is given every opportunity to benefit from a dialysis program without fearing that he or she will become a prisoner of an unthinking, uncaring medical system that lacks the moral courage to stop treatment when it is no longer of value.

In the final analysis common sense and humane compassionate care consistent with current medical and ethical standards will almost always be legally acceptable. All discussions concerning what is legally acceptable should start with what makes the most sense and is most proper from an ethical standpoint. Good law follows good medicine and good ethics, not the reverse.

REFERENCES

1. Neu S, Kjellstrand CM: Stopping long-term dialysis. An empirical study of withdrawal of life-supporting treatment. *N. Engl J Med* 314: 14, 1986
2. Port FK, Wolfe RA, Hawthorne VM, Ferguson CW et al.: Discontinuation of dialysis therapy as a cause of death. *Am J Neph* 9: 145, 1989
3. Kjellstrand CM: Giving life – giving death. Ethical problems with high technology medicine. PhD Thesis. Karolinska Institute, Stockholm 1988 and *Acta Medica Scandinavica Supplementum* 1988, Suppl 725
4. Munoz JE, Kjellstrand CM: Withdrawing life support: do families and physicians decide as patients do? *Nephron* 48: 201, 1988
5. Sacred Congregation for the Doctrine of the Faith: Declaration on Euthanasia Ottawa, Ontario, Publication Service. Canadian Conference of Catholic Bishops 1980
6. Roberts J, Kjellstrand CM: Choosing death: withdrawal without medical reason from chronic dialysis. *Acta Med Scand* 223: 181, 1988
7. Kaye M, Bourgouin P, Low G: Physicians' noncompliance with patients' refusal of life-sustaining treatment. *Am J Nephrol* 7: 304, 1987
8. Lo B, McLeod GA, Saika G: Patient attitudes to discussing life-sustaining treatment. *Arch Intern Med* 146: 1613, 1986
9. Pence GE: Do not go slowly into that dark night: mercy killing in Holland. *Am J Med* 84: 139, 1988
10. Sandbert S, Holm L, Enger E: Veilednings – og omsorgsbehov hos etterlatte. *Tidskr Nor Lægeforen* 105: 1412, 1985
11. Tolle S, Bascom PB, Hickam DH et al.: Communication between physicians and surviving spouses following patient death. *J Gen Intern Med* 1: 309, 1986
12. Walwork E, Ellison PH: Follow up of families of neonates in whom life support was withdrawn. *Clin Ped* 24: 14, 1985
13. Roberts J, Snyder R, Kjellstrand CM: Withdrawal of life support – the survivors. *Acta Med Scand* 224: 141, 1988
14. Kjellstrand CM, Logan G: Racial, sexual and age inequalities in chronic dialysis. *Nephron* 45: 257, 1987
15. Kjellstrand CM: Racial, sexual and age inequalities in renal transplantation. *Arch Intern Med* 148: 1305, 1988
16. Callender CO: Organ donation in blacks: a community approach. *Transpl Proceed* 19: 1551, 1987
17. Callender CO: Organ donation in the black population: where do we go from here. *Transpl Proceed* 19 (Suppl 2): 36, 1987
18. Combined report on regular dialysis and transplantation in Europe 1979: in *Proceedings of the European Dialysis and Transplant Association*, edited by Robinson BHB, Hawkins JB, Vol 17. Pitman Medical Limited, London, 1980
19. Wehle B, Ahlmén J: Prudent withdrawal of chronic dialysis treatment. *Scand J Urol Nephrol Suppl* 131: 47, 1990
20. Kjellstrand CM, Lins LE, Ericson F et al.: On the wish for renal transplantation. *Transactions ASAIO* 35: 619, 1989
21. Quran: The meaning of the glorious Koran. *Mentor* 2: 30
22. Sahin AF: Islamic transplantation ethics. *Transpl Proc* 22: 939, 1990
23. Quran 39: 42
24. Darsh SM: *Islamic Health Rules*. Abul Qasim Publications, Jeddah, Saudi Arabia
25. Hathout H: Islamic basis for biomedical ethics. Fidia Research Foundation Symposium, Transcultural dimensions of medical ethics. National Academy of Sciences. Washington, DC, April 26–27, 1990
26. Darsh SM: *ibid*
27. Quran 40: 67, 68
28. Riemer J (ed): *Jewish Reflections on Death*. Schocken Books, New York, 1974
29. Glick S: A view from Sinai – a Jewish perspective on biomedical ethics. Fidia Symposium, *ibid*
30. Life-sustaining treatment: New York State task force on life and the law. July, 1987
31. Rosner F, Bleich JD (eds): Quoted by Bleich JD in *Jewish Bioethics*, Sanhedrin Press, New York, 1979, p 292
32. *ibid*
33. Glick S, *ibid*
34. Solovachik A: The Halakhic definition of death. in *Jewish Bioethics, ibid*
35. Life sustaining treatment. *ibid*
36. See comments by Bleich JD in *Jewish Bioethics*. The Quinlan case: a Jewish perspective. *ibid*
37. Niebuhr R: *An Interpretation of Christian Ethics*. Seaburg Press. New York, 1979, p 31
38. Ramsey P: *The Patient as Person*. Yale University Press, 1970, p 17
39. Bucaille M: *The Qur'an and Modern Science*. Abul Qasim Publications, Jeddah, Saudi Arabia
40. Kee HC, Young FW, Froehlich K: *Understanding the New Testament* 3rd Ed, Prentice-Hall, 1973
41. See: *J Med and Philosophy* 15: 1990
42. Declaration on Euthanasia, the Sacred Congregation for the Doctrine of the Faith. Vatican City, 1980. in *Deciding to forego life-sustaining treatment*. President's Commission for the Study of Ethical Problems in Medicine and Biomedical and Behavioural Research. US Government Printing Office, 1983
43. See: Life Support – Religious Considerations. in *Proc. 2nd International Congress on Ethics in Medicine*. New York, 1987
44. Philipp 3: 10. Common Bible. Revised Standard Version, Collins, 1970, p 186
45. Mill JS: *On Liberty*. Penguin Books, 1984, p 69
46. Ashley BM, O'Rourke KD: *Health Care Ethics. A Theological Analysis*. The Catholic Health Association of the United States, 1982, p 38
47. Grant S, Gentles I (ed): *Euthanasia in Care for the Dying and Bereaved*. Anglican Book Center, 1982
48. Fox RC: Exclusion from dialysis: a sociological and legal perspective. *Kidney Int* 19: 739, 1981
49. Rodin GM, Chmara BA, Ennis J et al.: Stopping life-sustaining medical treatment: psychiatric considerations in the termination of renal dialysis. *Can J Psychiatry* 26: 540, 1981
50. McKegney FP, Lange P: The decision to no longer live on chronic hemodialysis. *Amer J Psychiat* 128: 47, 1971
51. Silva JEM, Kjellstrand CM: Withdrawing life support. Do families and physicians decide as patients do? *Nephron* 48: 201, 1988
52. Dessner GH, Fisher SH, Curry E et al.: Stopping long-term dialysis. *N Engl J Med* 314: 1449, 1986

53. Lowance DC, Singer PA, Siegler M: Withdrawal from dialysis: an ethical perspective. *Kidney Int* 34: 124, 1988

54. Frankl D, Oye RK, Bellamy PE: Attitudes of hospitalized patients toward life support: a survey of 200 medical inpatients. *Amer J Med* 86: 645, 1989

55. Phillips DP, King EW: Death takes a holiday: mortality surrounding major social occasions. *Lancet* 2: 728, 1988

56. Meisel A: *The Right to Die*. 1990 Supplement. New York, Wiley Law Publications, 1990

57. Lynn J, Glover J: Ethical decision-making in enteral nutrition. in *Enteral and Tube Feeding*, edited by Rombeau P, Coldwell MD, 2nd edition, Philadelphia, WB Saunders, 1990, p 575

58. National Center for State Courts: Life-sustaining medical treatment: helping the courts decide. (Unpublished; final report to be released in 1991)

59. Society for the Right to Die: Legislation backgrounder, 1990

60. Right-to-die case and statutory citations: State-by-state listing. News from Society for the Right to Die 1990, August

61. Tube feeding laws in the United States. Society for the Right to Die Newsletter. New York: 15 October 1989

62. Child abuse and neglect prevention and treatment. 45 C.F.R. Sections 1340, 1-1340, 20: 1986

63. Weir RF, Gostin L: Decisions to abate life-sustaining treatment for nonautonomous patients. *JAMA* 264: 1846, 1990

64. In re Conroy, 98 N.J. 321, 486 A.2d 1209, 1985

65. Rhoden N: How should we view the incompetent? *Law, Medicine & Health Care* 17: 260, 1989

66. In re Hier, 18 Mass. App. 200, 464 N.E.2d 959, 1984, rev. denied, 392 Mass. 1102, 465 N.E.2d 261, 1984

67. In re Jobes, 108 H.J. 394, 529 A.2d 434, 1987

68. Corbett v D'Alessandro, 487 So.2d 368 (Fla. Dist. Ct. App.), review denied. 492 So.2d 1331: Fla., 1986

69. Brophy v New England Sinai Hosp., Inc. 398 Mass. 417, 497 N.E.2d 696; 1986

70. In re Peter, 108 N.J. 365, 529 A.2d 419, 1987

71. Delio v Westchester County Medical Center. 129 A.D.2d 1, 516 N.Y.S.2d 766, 1987

72. In re Gardner, 534 A.2d 947; Me. 1987

73. Gray v Romeo, 697 F. Supp. 580; D.R.I. 1988

74. McConnell v Beverly Enterprises-Connecticut, Inc., 209 Conn. 692, 553 A.2d 596, 1989

75. Deciding to forego life-sustaining treatment. Washington, DC: President's Commission for the Study of Ethical Problems in Medicine, 1983

76. Guidelines on the termination of life-sustaining treatment and the care of the dying. Briarcliff Manor, NY, The Hastings Center, 1987

77. Life-sustaining technologies and the elderly. Washington, DC, Office of Technology Assessment, 1987

78. See amicus curiae briefs filed to the US Supreme Court on behalf of petitioners in *Cruzan*: American Medical Association, American College of Surgeons, American Academy of Neurology, American Academy of Family Physicians, American Association of Neurological Surgeons, American Medical Women's Association, American Nurses Association, American Association of Nurse Attorneys, American College of Physicians, American Hospital Association, American Geriatrics Society, National Hospice Organization, Society for Critical Care Medicine

79. Rhoden NK: Litigating life and death. *Harvard Law Review* 102: 375, 1988

80. Eichner v Dillon, 52 N.Y.2d 363, 420 N.E.2d 64, 438 N.Y.S.2d 266, cert. denied, 454 U.S. 858, 1981

81. In re O'Connor 72, N.Y.2d 517, 531 N.E.2d 607, 534 N.Y.S.2d 866, 1988

82. Cruzan v Harmon, 760 S.W.2d 408 (Mo. 1988), cert. granted, 109 S. Ct. 3240, 1989

83. In re Chad Eric Swan, 569 A.2d 1202; Me, 1990

84. In re Torres, 357 N.W.2d 332; Minn. 1984

85. The American Hospital Association, in its amicus curiae brief to the US Supreme Court in *Cruzan*, stated that 70% of the 1.3 million patients who die in hospitals each year die after a decision to forgo life-sustaining treatment has been made. This number does not include patients who die at home or in nursing homes (1 Sept 1989, p 3)

86. Superintendent of Belchertown State School v Saikewicz, 373 Mass. 728, 370 N.E.2d 417, 1977

87. Relman AS: The Saikewicz decision: judges as physicians. *N Engl J Med* 289: 508, 1978

88. Weir RF: *Abating Treatment with Critically Ill Patients: Ethical and Legal Limits to the Medical Prolongation of Life*. New York, Oxford University Press, 1989, p 116

89. Liacos PJ: Dilemmas of dying. *Medicolegal News* 7: 4, 1979

90. Curran WJ: The Saikewicz decision. *N Engl J Med* 298: 499, 1978

91. In re Spring, 380 Mass. 629, 405 N.E.2d 115, 1980 – at 121

92. In re Lydia E. Hall Hosp., 116 Misc. 2d 477, 455 N.Y.S.2d 706 (Sup. Ct. 1982)

93. Barron JLI: Hospital tights patient's plea to end lifesaving treatment. *New York Times* 1982 Oct 21: 12

94. In re Storar, 52, N.Y.2d 363, 420 N.E.2d 64, 438 N.Y.S.2d 266, cert. denied, 454 U.S. 858, 1981

95. Gaylin W: A patient's rights must include power to refuse treatment. *Minneapolis Star and Tribune*, 1982 Oct 29, 16

96. Sullivan R: Panel criticizes procedures for patients' consent for treatments. *New York Times* 1982 Oct 22: 12

97. In re Quinlan, 70 N.J. 10, 355 A.2d 647, cert. denied, 429 U.S. 922, 1976

98. In re Dinnerstein, 6 Mass. App. 166, 380 N.E.2d 134, 1978

99. Relman A: The *Saikewicz* in decision: a medical viewpoint. *Am J of Law & Med* 4: 233, 1978

100. Commissioner of Correction v Myers, 399 N.E.2d 452: Mass., 1979

101. Shapiro F: Personal communication. 29 November 1990

102. New Mexico *ex rel* Smith v Fort, No 14, 768; N.M. 1983

103. Uniform Rights of the Terminally Ill Act [1985] 1–18, 9A U.L.A. 456; Supp. 1990

104. Uniform Rights of the Terminally Ill Act [1989], 1–18, 9A U.L.A. 456; Supp. 1990

105. In re Estate of Sidney Greenspan, No 67903; Ill. Sup Ct. July, 1990

106. State v McAfee, 385 S.E.2d 651; GA, 1989

107. Bouvia v Superior Court (Glenchur), 179 Cal. App. 3d 1127, 225 Cal. Rptr. 297, 1986

108. Hall MA: The malpractice standard under health care cost containment. *Law, Medicine & Health Care* 17: 347, 1989

109. Brahams D: When is discontinuation of dialysis justified? *Lancet* 1: 176, 1986

110. Cruzan *v* Director, Missouri Department of Health, 110 S. Ct. 2841, 1990

111. Annas GJ: Nancy Cruzan and the right to die. *N Eng J Med* 323: 670, 1990

112. In the estate of Nancy Beth Cruzan, Estate No CB384-9P, Probate Division, Circuit Court of Jasper County, Missouri, Judge Charles E. Teel, Jr., July 27, 1988

113. Annas GJ, Arnold B, Aroskar M et al.: Bioethicists' statement on the US Supreme Court's *Cruzan* decision. *N Engl J Med* 323: 686, 1990

COMBINED INDEX *

---

* Most important main entries are indicated in bold.